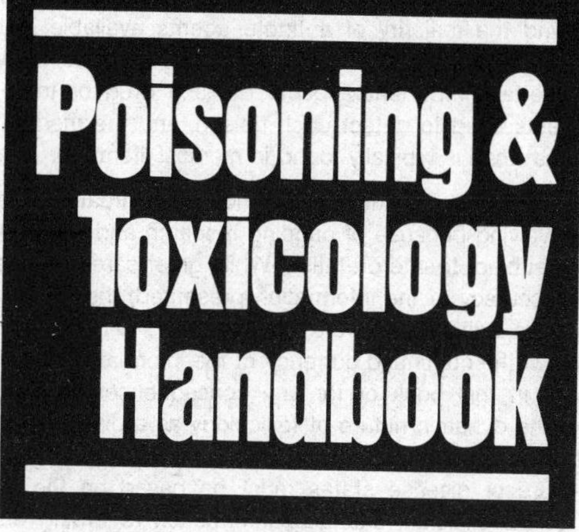

2nd Edition  **1996-97**

Jerrold B. Leikin, MD
Associate Director
Emergency Department
Rush Presbyterian-St Luke's Medical Center
Chicago, Illinois

Frank P. Paloucek, PharmD
Clinical Associate Professor
Pharmacy Practice
University of Illinois at Chicago
Chicago, Illinois

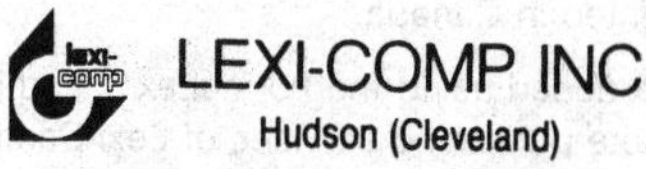

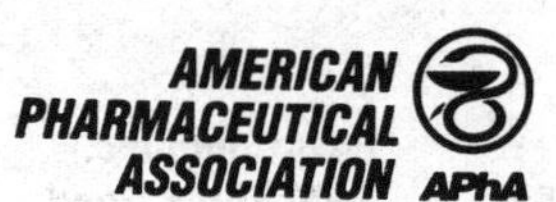

NOTICE

This handbook is intended to serve the user as a handy reference and not as a complete poisoning/toxicology resource. The publication covers adverse effects and overdoses of medicinal and nonmedicinal agents with empiric treatment recommendations, testing procedures necessary for diagnosis, and the majority of antidote agents available in the United States. The individual sections of this handbook are specifically designed to present certain important aspects of each drug or toxin exposure, laboratory tests used to detect each poison, and the therapy in a more concise format than is typically found in medical literature.

The nature of toxicology and the diagnosis and treatment is that it is constantly evolving because of ongoing research and clinical experience and is often subject to interpretation. While great care has been taken to ensure the accuracy of the information presented, the reader is advised that the authors, editors, reviewers, contributors, and publishers cannot be responsible for the continued currency of the information or for any errors or omissions in this book or for any consequences arising therefrom. Because of the dynamic nature of toxicology as a discipline, readers are advised that decisions regarding the diagnosis and treatment of specific toxin exposure or disease states must be based on the independent judgment of the clinician, changing information regarding drug therapy (eg, as reflected in the literature and drug manufacturer's most current product information), and changing medical practices. The editors are not responsible for any inaccuracy of quotation or for any false or misleading implication that may arise due to the text or formulas used or due to the quotation of revisions no longer official.

The editors, authors, and contributors have written this book in their private capacities. No official support or endorsement by any federal or state agency or pharmaceutical company is intended or inferred.

The publishers have made every effort to trace the copyright holders for borrowed material. If they have inadvertently overlooked any, they will be pleased to make the necessary arrangements at the first opportunity.

If you have any suggestions or questions
regarding any information presented in this handbook,
please contact our drug information pharmacist at

1-800-837-LEXI

This manual was produced using the FormuLex™ and Pathfinder™ programs — complete publishing services of Lexi-Comp Inc.

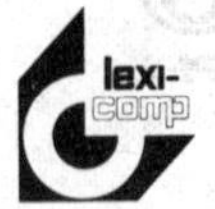

Lexi-Comp Inc.
1100 Terex Road
Hudson, Ohio 44236-3771
(216) 650-6506

ISBN 0-916589-30-7

Poisoning & Toxicology Handbook

2nd Edition 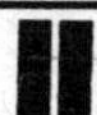 1996-97

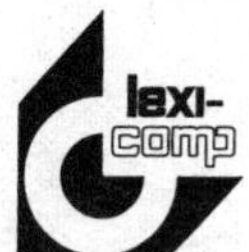

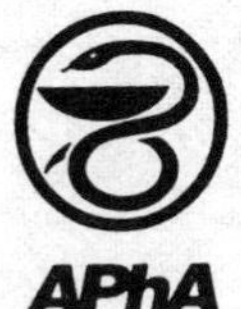

Dedications

To Robin Ellen, Scott Michael, and Eryn Nicole
for their inspiration, support, and unique contributions
to this book.

— Jerrold B. Leikin

To Sharon, Maggie, Robert, and Michael,
for your presence, inspiration, patience, and support,
and to all those responsible for
my being a pharmacist and clinical toxicologist today.

— Frank P. Paloucek

TABLE OF CONTENTS

TABLE OF CONTENTS

Comparison Charts

ABOUT THE AUTHORS

Jerrold Blair Leikin, MD, FACP, FACEP, DABMT

Dr Leikin received his Medical Doctorate degree from the Chicago Medical School in 1980. Following a combined residency in Internal Medicine and Emergency Medicine at Evanston Hospital and Northwestern Memorial Hospital, he then completed a fellowship in Medical Toxicology at Cook County Hospital in Chicago.

Dr Leikin was physician-in-charge of medicine at the University of Illinois Hospital Emergency Department and Section Chief of Emergency Medicine within the Department of Medicine. Upon transfer to Rush-Presbyterian-St Luke's Medical Center, Dr Leikin became Associate Director of the Emergency Department while also serving as the Medical Director of the Northeastern Illinois Regional Poison Control Center. He is also Medical Director of the United States Drug Testing Laboratory, Associate Director of the Toxicon Consortium, and holds an appointment as Associate Professor of Medicine at Rush Medical College.

Dr Leikin has presented over 100 abstracts at national meetings while publishing over 90 articles in peer-reviewed medical journals. He has written several chapters on the subject of toxicology in critical care medicine, internal medicine, and observational medicine textbooks. He is an active member of the American Academy of Clinical Toxicology, American College of Medical Toxicology, the American College of Emergency Physicians, and the American Medical Association. He is married and has two children.

Frank P. Paloucek, PharmD, ABAT

Dr Paloucek is currently a Clinical Associate Professor of Pharmacy Practice at the University of Illinois at Chicago. Dr Paloucek received his BS in Pharmacy from the University of Illinois in 1981 and his PharmD from the Philadelphia College of Pharmacy and Sciences in 1984. He completed a residency in pharmacy practice and a fellowship in clinical pharmacokinetics at the University of Illinois at Chicago.

His practice is in the Emergency Departments of the University of Illinois and at Michael Reese Hospital in Chicago and a pharmacy-based clinical toxicology at the latter. He is an Adjunct Assistant Professor in the Emergency Medicine Program and has been a faculty member of the American Academy of Clinical Toxicology since 1989 and a Diplomate of the American Board of Applied Toxicology since 1991. He has been a director of a postdoctoral clinical toxicology fellowship program since 1991 and is an original member of the Resident's Advisory Committee overseeing the education and training of postdoctoral trainees in pharmaceutical care at the University of Illinois Hospital. In addition to numerous scientific posters and clinical toxicology publications, Dr Paloucek is currently on the editorial board of *The Poison Review*. He has developed a reputation as an acknowledged expert on the pharmacist's role in emergency medicine and the interpretation of drug-toxin concentrations in poisoning patients.

Dr Paloucek is an active member of the American Society of Hospital Pharmacists, American Pharmaceutical Society, and the American College of Clinical Pharmacy. His research interests are toxicokinetics of medications in overdose, drug misadventures in the emergency department, and theophylline toxicity.

ABOUT THE CONTRIBUTORS

Anthony M. Burda, RPh, CSPI

Anthony Burda received his bachelor's degree in pharmacy in 1978 from the University of Illinois College of Pharmacy. Since February 1981, Mr Burda has been affiliated with the Chicago and Northeastern Illinois Regional Poison Control Center at Rush-Presbyterian-St Luke's Medical Center in Chicago. He has become certified as a specialist in poison information through the American Association of Poison Control Centers (AAPCC) in 1983, 1988, and 1993. His main responsibilities are providing immediate poison treatment information to healthcare professionals and the general public, while training and supervising fellows, residents, and students completing educational rotations in the poison center.

Mr Burda currently serves on the AAPCC Personnel Proficiency Committee which drafts criteria and examination questions for CSPI certification. He has lectured on and authored articles about management of intoxication and poison prevention.

Some of Mr Burda's other professional experiences include authoring several CE programs for pharmacists, lecturing in pharmacology/medications courses for nurses, and serving as a technical advisor to the executive director of a pharmacy association.

Andrew M. Davis, MD

Dr Davis is Acting Section Chief of Environmental and Occupational Medicine at Rush-Presbyterian-St Luke's Medical Center in Chicago. He is an associate professor, and holds joint appointments in Internal and Preventive Medicine.

Francine Dela Cruz, PharmD

Dr Dela Cruz has been a clinical pharmacist for 10 years in the areas of emergency medicine/clinical toxicology and neurology and is a board-certified pharmacotherapist. She currently works as a pharmacotherapist in the Emergency Departments at the University of Illinois and Michael Reese hospitals and holds a teaching position as a Clinical Assistant Professor in the College of Pharmacy at the University of Illinois at Chicago (UIC). Her practice and research areas of interest include the toxicology of antiepileptic agents and acetaminophen, acute treatment of ischemic stroke, and pharmacotherapy of epilepsy.

Dr Dela Cruz received a bachelor's degree from Oregon State University and her doctorate from the UIC. She is an active member of the American College of Clinical Pharmacy (ACCP), the Illinois College of Clinical Pharmacy (ICCP), the American Society of Hospital Pharmacists (ASHP), and the American Association of Clinical Toxicology (AACT).

John M. Eversole

Chief Eversole received his bachelor's degree in management at Lewis University. He joined the Chicago Fire Department in 1969. He is a certified Master Instructor through the Office of the Illinois State Fire Marshal. He teaches fire science programs for the Chicago City Wide Colleges and the University of Illinois. He is the Chairman of the Hazardous Materials Committee of the International Association of Fire Chiefs. He has been involved in a number of special programs such as the Deep Tunnel Project and the Hazardous Incident Team. At the present time, Chief Eversole is assigned as the Hazardous Materials Coordinator and is responsible for the Hazardous Materials HIT Team and coordinates all the Fire Department's units that make up the Hazardous Incident Task Force.

Teresa L. Hrones

Teresa Hrones received her bachelor's degree in journalism in 1989. She currently serves as spokesperson and media relations associate for Underwriters Laboratories Inc (UL) and serves on the Consumer Product Safety Commission Task Force concerning Professional and Consumer Education for Carbon Monoxide and Carbon Monoxide Detectors.

Brian E. Jahns, PharmD

Dr Jahns received his bachelor's degree in biology from the University of Western Ontario in 1988, and PharmD from Wayne State University in 1992. He completed a pharmacy practice residency at Detroit Receiving Hospital and University Health Clinics. He was a fellow in Emergency Medicine and Clinical Toxicology Pharmacotherapy at the University of Illinois College of Pharmacy, and University Hospital. He is now a clinical instructor and critical care pharmacist at St Michael's Hospital in Toronto.

Robert A. June, MD, PhD

Dr June received his master's and PhD degrees from Rush-Presbyterian-St Luke's Medical Center. He has worked at the Rush Poison Control Center for over 5 years. In addition to working at the Poison Control Center, Dr June is currently doing an emergency medicine residency and toxicology research at Cook County Hospital.

Jack W. Lipscomb, MM, RPh, ABAT

Jack Lipscomb received his bachelor's degree in pharmacy from the University of Illinois Medical Center in 1981, and his Master's of Management (MM) from Northwestern University in 1991. He received his board certification in clinical toxicology from the American Board of Applied Toxicology in 1992, and served as the Director of the Chicago and Northeastern Illinois Regional Poison Control Center at Rush-Presbyterian-St Luke's Medical Center in Chicago from 1982-1995.

Karen McAllister, RPh, CSPI

Karen McAllister received her bachelor's degree in pharmacy from the St Louis College of Pharmacy in 1991. She was certified as a Poison Information Specialist in 1993 through the American Association of Poison Control Centers (AAPCC). She currently practices at the Chicago and Northeastern Illinois Regional Poison Control Center at Rush-Presbyterian-St Luke's Hospital in Chicago.

Christine M. Moore, PhD

Dr Moore is currently the Associate Scientific Director of U.S. Drug Testing Laboratories, Chicago, a laboratory specializing in the detection of drugs in meconium, hair, and other less common sample matrices.

Following a PhD in Forensic Toxicology and postdoctoral work in Japan, Dr Moore served as a Research Associate at the University of Illinois and as Technical Services Manager of United Chemical Technologies, a manufacturer of solid-phases for use in clinical, drug testing, and pharmaceutical laboratories.

Paul E. Patty, PE

Paul Patty received his master's degree in business administration from Northern Illinois University, DeKalb in 1984 and a bachelor of science degree in engineering from Purdue University in 1973. He has worked for

Underwriters Laboratories Inc (UL) since 1973 and is responsible for the evaluation of life safety products including gas, smoke, and carbon monoxide detectors. Mr Patty has been a Registered Professional Engineer in Illinois since 1980.

Kevin O. Rynn, RPh, PharmD

Dr Rynn received his bachelor's degree from Rutgers University in 1990. He completed his PharmD degree at Duquesne University in 1992 and following a residency at Allegheny General Hospital, Dr Rynn completed an emergency medicine/toxicology fellowship at the University of Illinois in 1994. Currently, Dr Rynn is a pharmacotherapist at Michael Reese Hospital and Clinical Assistant Professor at the University of Illinois Hospital in Chicago.

Kim Sing, MD

Dr Sing graduated from the University of Illinois Emergency Medicine Residency Program in 1992. Dr Sing did a toxicology fellowship at Toxikon consortium at Cook County Hospital from 1992-1994. Currently, Dr Sing is at the University of Wisconsin Madison performing emergency medicine and toxicology duties.

Donald J. Tillman, PharmD

Donald Tillman received his PharmD degree from the University of Kansas in 1991. He then completed a pharmacy practice residency at the University of Illinois at Chicago Hospital in 1992. Dr Tillman subsequently completed a 2-year specialty residency and fellowship in emergency medicine and clinical toxicology at the University of Illinois at the Chicago College of Pharmacy. He is now employed as a clinical pharmacist in the Emergency Department for Kaiser Permanente in Denver, Colorado.

Elizabeth Young, PharmD

Dr Young received a bachelor's degree in zoology and master's degree in botany from Clemson University. Subsequent study in pharmacy was undertaken at the University of Illinois College of Pharmacy where she earned a PharmD degree and worked extensively in pharmacognosy research laboratories. After graduation, she completed a 1-year pharmacy practice residency at the University of Illinois. In 1995 she completed a 1-year specialized pharmacy residency in emergency medicine. She is now a clinical pharmacist in critical care and poison control at Memorial Mission Hospital, Asheville, North Carolina.

Michelle Zell-Kanter, PharmD

Michelle Zell-Kanter received her bachelor's degree in pharmacy from the University of Manitoba in 1978. In 1981, she received her PharmD degree from the Massachusetts College of Pharmacy and subsequently completed a clinical pharmacy residency at the University of Illinois Hospital in 1982. She was the clinical pharmacist for emergency services at the University of Illinois Hospital and a clinical assistant professor of pharmacy practice at the University of Illinois College of Pharmacy from 1982 until 1987. Since 1988, she has been the coordinator of the TOXIKON consortium at Cook County Hospital. She has also served on review panels for several journals. In 1991, she received diplomate status from the American Board of Applied Toxicology.

EDITORIAL ADVISORY PANEL

PREFACE FOR 2nd EDITION

While only about ten months have elapsed between editions of this handbook, a significant amount of information and refinement in practice has occurred. It has been our intent to incorporate this latest information in the ever-changing field of toxicology into this 2nd Edition of the Poisoning and Toxicology Handbook.

We have included, along with the updated information, and new to this edition, an additional 110 medicinal, 85 nonmedicinal, 10 biological, and 5 antidote monographs. The phone number index has been updated and the appendix has been expanded to contain over 179 pages of pertinent and valuable information including biological warfare agents, bioconcentration factors, and fat and salivary levels of toxin.

Our sincere thanks goes out to the staff of the Chicago and Northeastern Illinois Regional Poison Control Center, University of Illinois College of Pharmacy, Tom Quail, RN of Massachusetts Poison Control System, and the many reviewers across the country who gave us immeasurable assistance in helping develop and enhance this handbook.

ACKNOWLEDGMENTS

This handbook exists in its present form as a result of the concerted efforts of many individuals. The publisher and president of Lexi-Comp Inc, Robert D. Kerscher and the senior director of Programming and Publications, James P. Caro, American Pharmaceutical Association (APhA) deserve much of the credit for bringing the concept of such a book to fruition.

Other members of the Lexi-Comp staff whose contributions were invaluable and whose patience with the editors' enumerable drafts, revisions, deletions, additions, and enhancements was inexhaustible include: Lynn D. Coppinger, managing editor; Leonard L. Lance, BSPharm, pharmacy editor; John E. Janosik, PharmD; Diane Harbart, MT (ASCP), medical editor; Barbara F. Kerscher, production manager; Alexandra Hart, composition specialist; Jeanne Eads, Beth Daulbaugh, Julie Weekes, and Lisa Leukart, project managers; Jil Neuman, Jackie Mizer, Tracey J. Reinecke, and Jennifer Harbart, production assistants; Jeff J. Zaccagnini, Brian B. Vossler, and Jerry Reeves, sales managers; Edmund A. Harbart, vice-president, custom publishing division; and Jack L. Stones, vice-president, reference publishing division. The complex computer programming required for the typesetting of the book was provided by Jay L. Katzen, Dennis P. Smithers, David C. Marcus, Dale Jablonski, and Kenneth J. Hughes, system analysts, under the direction of Thury L. O'Connor, vice-president, and Alan R. Frasz, vice-president, information technologies.

Other APhA staff members whose contributions were important are Julian I. Graubart, Director Special Projects, Linda Sorin, Senior Director, Marketing, and James V. McGinnis, manager of art and production. A special thanks goes to Ronald Stewart, MS, for the use of his extensive library in the preparation of this handbook, and Chris Lomax, PharmD, director of pharmacy, Children's Hospital, Los Angeles, who played a significant role in bringing APhA and Lexi-Comp together.

Much of the material contained in the book was a result of pharmacy contributors throughout the United States and Canada. Lexi-Comp has assisted many medical institutions to develop hospital-specific formulary manuals that contain clinical drug information as well as dosing. Working with clinical pharmacists, hospital pharmacy and therapeutics committees, and hospital drug information centers, Lexi-Comp has developed an evolutionary drug database that reflects the practice of pharmacy in these major institutions.

In addition, the authors wish to thank their families, friends, and colleagues who supported them in their efforts to complete this handbook.

USE OF THE POISONING & TOXICOLOGY HANDBOOK

The *Poisoning & Toxicology Handbook* is organized into five major chapters, an appendix, numerical indices of Chemical Abstract Service (CAS) registry numbers (international system) and United Nations/United States Department of Transportation (DOT) numbers (used in the U.S.), a toxic symptoms index, and an alphabetical index.

Information is presented in a consistent format with extensive cross-referencing between chapters. Each chapter will provide the following fields of information.

MEDICINAL AGENTS

Generic Name	U.S. adopted name
Pronunciation Guide	
Related Information	Cross-reference to other pertinent drug information found in the Appendix
CAS Number	Chemical Abstract Service Registry Number, the international nomenclature system
UN Number	United Nations/Unites States Department of Transportation number. Identification nomenclature used for shipping in the United States; usually found on placard on side of vehicle.
Brand Names	Common trade names
Synonyms	Other names or accepted abbreviations for the generic drug
Use	Information pertaining to appropriate indications of the drug
Mechanism of Action	How the drug works in the body to elicit a response
Adverse Reactions	Side effects grouped by organ system affected
Signs & Symptoms of Acute Overdose	Primarily clinical effects of acute toxic exposure
Toxicodynamics/Kinetics	The magnitude of a drug's effect depends on the drug concentration at the site of action. The pharmacodynamics are expressed in terms of onset of action and duration of action. Pharmacokinetics are expressed in terms of absorption, distribution (including appearance in breast milk and crossing of the placenta), protein binding, metabolism, bioavailability, half-life, time to peak serum concentration, and elimination.
Usual Dosage	Information regarding the recommended final concentrations and rates for administration of the drug
Contraindications	Information pertaining to inappropriate use of the drug
Warnings	Hazardous conditions related to use of the drug and disease states or patient populations in which the drug should be cautiously used
Dosage Forms	Information with regard to form, strength, and availability of the drug
Stability	Storage, refrigeration, and compatibility information
Reference Range	Therapeutic and toxic serum concentrations listed when appropriate
Overdosage Treatment	Description of treatment modalities of adverse effects and overdosage, including decontamination, supportive therapy, and enhancement of elimination

Antidote	Cross references the reader to the drug and page where the antidote and its information can be located
Test Interactions	Listing of assay interferences when relevant; (B) = Blood; (S) = Serum; (U) = Urine
Diagnostic Tests Procedures	Directs the reader to the page in the handbook for information on the tests and/or procedures which should be considered in the treatment of the patient
Drug Interactions	Effects that may be potentially harmful or toxic when used with other medications
Pregnancy Risk Factor	Five categories established by the FDA to indicate the potential of a systemically absorbed drug for causing birth defects
Pregnancy Implications	Information which may be critical in the treatment of a pregnant patient
Administration	Specific instructions on proper procedure or information in relation to the administration of the drug
Monitoring Parameters	Laboratory tests and patient physical parameters that should be monitored for safety and efficacy of drug therapy are listed when appropriate
Patient Information Nursing Implications	Comments and/or considerations are offered when appropriate
Specific References	References used in the information of the monograph

NONMEDICINAL AGENTS

The same fields as in the Medicinal Agents section with the following additional field:

Commonly Includes

BIOLOGICAL AGENTS

The same fields as in the Medicinal Agents section with the following additional fields:

Scientific Name

Commonly Found In

LABORATORY TESTS

Synonyms	
Related Information	Cross-reference to other pertinent drug information found in the Appendix
Applies To	Other organisms included in the named genus
Test Includes or Procedure Commonly Includes	Laboratory tests or procedures that may occur when the named test is performed
Abstract	A brief description of the test and its use
Patient Preparation	Any special preparation that the patient must undergo prior to the procedure being performed
Aftercare	Special instructions or warnings for medical personnel for the care of the patient after the procedure is performed
Equipment	Equipment needed to perform the named procedure
Technique	Explanation of how procedure is performed
Specimen	Possible specimens that can be used for testing

Volume	Desirable amount of specimen needed for testing
Minimum Volume	Minimum amount of specimen required to perform testing
Container	Type of container required for acquiring and maintaining a usable specimen
Sampling Time	The time frame a specimen should be collected
Collection	General and specific collection instructions that should be followed to obtain a proper and usable specimen
Storage Instructions	The appropriate storage of the specimen after collection but prior to testing
Causes for Rejection	Possible reasons why a specimen may be rejected by the laboratory
Special Instructions	Specific instructions for the acquisition and handling of specimens
Reference Range	Therapeutic and toxic serum concentrations are listed when appropriate
Normal Range or Normal Findings	Serves as a general guideline. See specific testing facility for their ranges.
Critical Values Possible Panic Range	Values that alert the medical staff that the patient has reached a range or value that may be hazardous
Use	Common uses for the test/procedure
Limitations	Limits of the test/procedure
Contraindications	Reasons why this test should not be performed
Methodology	Testing methodologies available
Additional Information	Additional information about the test/procedure and its uses
Specific References	General references are provided

ANTIDOTES

The same fields as in the Medicinal Agents section.

FDA Pregnancy Categories

In many of the drug monographs throughout this book there is a field labeled Pregnancy Risk Factor (PRF) and the letter A, B, C, D, or X immediately following which signifies a category. The FDA has established these five categories to indicate the potential of a systemically absorbed drug for causing birth defects. The key differentiation among the categories rests upon the reliability of documentation and the risk:benefit ration. Pregnancy category X is particularly notable in that if any data exists that may implicate a drug as a teratogen and the risk:benefit ration is clearly negative, the drug is contraindicated during pregnancy.

These categories are summarized as follows.

A Controlled studies in pregnant women fail to demonstrate a risk to the fetus in the first trimester with no evidence of risk in later trimesters. The possibility of fetal harm appears remote.

B Either animal-reproductive studies have not demonstrated a fetal risk but there are no controlled studies in pregnant women, or animal-reproduction studies have shown an adverse effect (other than a decrease in fertility) that was not confirmed in controlled studies in women in the first trimester and there is no evidence of a risk in later trimesters.

C Either studies in animals have revealed adverse effects on the fetus (teratogenic or embryocidal effects or other) and there are no controlled studies in women, or studies in women and animals are not available. Drugs should be given only if the potential benefits justify the potential risk to the fetus.

D There is positive evidence of human fetal risk, but the benefits from use in pregnant women may be acceptable despite the risk (eg, if the drug is needed in a life-threatening situation or for a serious disease for which safer drugs cannot be used or are ineffective).

X Studies in animals or human beings have demonstrated fetal abnormalities or there is evidence of fetal risk based on human experience, or both, and the risk of the use of the drug in pregnant women clearly outweighs any possible benefit. The drug is contraindicated in women who are or may become pregnant.

SAFE WRITING

Health professionals and their support personnel frequently produce handwritten copies of information they see in print; therefore, such information is subjected to even greater possibilities for error or misinterpretation on the part of others. Thus, particular care must be given to how drug names and strengths are expressed when creating written healthcare documents.

The following are a few examples of safe writing rules suggested by the Institute for Safe Medication Practices, Inc.*

1. There should be a space between a number and its units as it is easier to read. There should be no periods after the abbreviations mg or mL.

Correct	**Incorrect**
10 mg	10mg
100 mg	100mg

2. Never place a decimal and a zero after a whole number (2 mg is correct and 2.0 mg is incorrect). If the decimal point is not seen because it falls on a line or because individuals are working from copies where the decimal point is not seen, this causes a tenfold overdose.

3. Just the opposite is true for numbers less than one. Always place a zero before a naked decimal (0.5 mL is correct, .5 mL is incorrect).

4. Never abbreviate the word unit. The handwritten U or u, looks like a 0 (zero) and may cause a tenfold overdose error to be made.

5. Q.D. is not a safe abbreviation for once daily, as when the Q is followed by a sloppy dot, it looks like QID which means 4 times daily.

6. O.D. is not a safe abbreviation for once daily, as it is properly interpreted as meaning "right eye" and has caused liquid medications such as saturated solution of potassium iodide and Lugol's solution to be administered incorrectly. There is no safe abbreviation for once daily. It must be written out in full.

7. Do not use chemical names such as 6-mercaptopurine or 6-thioguanine, as sixfold overdoses have been given when these were not recognized as chemical names. The proper names of these drugs are mercaptopurine or thioguanine.

8. Do not abbreviate drug names (5FC, 6MP, 5-ASA, MTX, HCTZ CPZ, PBZ, etc) as they are misinterpreted and cause error.

9. Do not use the apothecary system or symbols.

10. Do not abbreviate microgram as μg; instead use mcg as there is less likelihood of misinterpretation.

11. When writing an outpatient prescription, write a complete prescription. A complete prescription can prevent the prescriber, the pharmacist, and/or the patient from making a mistake and can eliminate the need for further clarification.

*From "Safe Writing" by Davis NM, PharmD and Cohen MR, MS, Lecturers and Consultants for Safe Medication Practices, 1143 Wright Drive, Huntingdon Valley, PA 19006. Phone: (215) 947-7566.

The legible prescriptions should contain:

a. patient's full name

b. for pediatric or geriatric patients: their age (or weight where applicable)

c. drug name, dosage form and strength; if a drug is new or rarely prescribed, print this information

d. number or amount to be dispensed

e. complete instructions for the patient, including the purpose of the medication

f. when there are recognized contraindications for a prescribed drug, indicate to the pharmacist that you are aware of this fact (ie, when prescribing a potassium salt for a patient receiving an ACE inhibitor, write "K serum leveling being monitored")

GENERAL REFERENCES

The following is a list of references utilized in the production of the individual monographs contained in this handbook.

1993 Emergency Response Guidebook, Washington DC: U.S. Department of Transportation (DOT), U.S. Government Printing Office, 1993.

Amdur MO, Doull J, and Klaasen CD, eds, *Casarett and Doull's Toxicology: The Basic Science of Poisons*, 4th ed, New York, NY: Pergamon Press, 1991.

Auerbach PS, ed, *Wilderness Medicine: Management of Wilderness and Environmental Emergencies*, 3rd ed, St Louis, MO: Mosby, 1995.

Auerbach PS, "A Medical Guide to Hazardous Marine Life," 2nd ed, St Louis, MO: Mosby, 1991.

Baselt RC and Cravey RH, eds, *Disposition of Toxic Drugs and Chemicals in Man*, 4th ed, Foster City, CA: Chemical Toxicology Institute 1995.

Billups NF, ed, *American Drug Index*, 38th ed, St Louis, MO: Facts and Comparisons, 1994.

Bleecker ML and Hansen JA, eds, *Occupational Neurology and Clinical Neurotoxicology*, Baltimore, MD: Williams and Wilkins, 1994.

Briggs GG, Freeman RK, and Yaffe Si, eds, *Drugs in Pregnancy and Lactation*, 4th ed, Baltimore, MD: Williams and Wilkins, 1994.

Bryson PD, ed, *Comprehensive Review in Toxicology*, 2nd ed, Rockville, MD: Aspen, 1989.

Cooney DO, *Activated Charcoal in Medical Applications*, New York, NY: Marcel Dekker, Inc, 1995.

Dorr RT and von Hoff DD, eds, *Cancer Chemotherapy Handbook*, 2nd ed, Norwalk, CT: Appleton and Lange, 1994.

Drugdex System: Gelman CR, Rumack BH, eds, Denver, CO: Drugdex Information System, Micromedex Inc, Vol 84.

Edmonds S, Stather R, *Reactions Weekly*, Langhorne, PA: Adis International Limited, 1995.

Ellenhorn MJ and Barceloux DG, eds, *Medical Toxicology; Diagnosis and Treatment of Human Poisoning*, New York, NY: Elsevier, 1988.

Ellis MD, ed, *Dangerous Plants, Snakes, Arthropods and Marine Life Toxicity and Treatment*, Hamilton, IL: Drug Intelligence Publications, Inc, 1978.

Gilman AG, Rall TW, Nies AS, et al, eds, *Goodman and Gilman's The Pharmacological Basis of Therapeutics*, 8th ed, New York, NY: Pergamon Press, 1990.

Goldfrank LR, Flomenbaum NE, Lewin NA, et al, eds, *Goldfrank's Toxicologic Emergencies*, 5th ed, Norwalk, CO: Appleton and Lange, 1994.

Grant WM, ed, *Toxicology of the Eye*, 3rd ed, Springfield, Charles C Thomas, 1986.

Haddad LM and Winchester JF, eds, *Clinical Management of Poisoning and Drug Overdose*, 2nd ed, Philadelphia, PA: WB Saunders Company, 1990.

Halstead BW and Halsted LG, eds, *Poisonous and Venomous Marine Animals of the World*, revised edition, Princeton, NY: Darwin Press, Inc, 1978.

Hayes WJ and Laws ER, eds, *Handbook of Pesticide Toxicology*, San Diego, CA: Academic Press, Inc, 1991.

Hodgson E and Levi PE, *A Textbook of Modern Toxicology*, New York, NY: Elsevier, 1987.

Isada CM, Kasten BL, Goldman, MP, et al, *Infectious Diseases Handbook*, Hudson, OH: Lexi-Comp Inc, 1994.

Jacobs DS, DeMott WR, Finley PR, et al, *Laboratory Test Handbook with Key Word Index*, 3rd ed, Hudson, OH: Lexi-Comp Inc, 1994.

Kingsbury JM, ed, *Poisonous Plants of the United States and Canada*, Englewood Cliffs, NJ: Prentice-Hall, 1964.

Knoben JE and Anderson PO, eds, *Handbook of Clinical Drug Data*, 7th ed, Hamilton, IL: Drug Intelligence Publications, Inc, 1993.

Koren G, ed, *Maternal-Fetal Toxicology: A Clinician's Guide*, 2nd ed, New York, NY: Marcel Dekker, Inc, 1994.

Lacy CF, Armstrong LL, Lipsy RJ, et al, *Drug Information Handbook*, 3rd ed, Hudson, OH: Lexi-Comp Inc, 1995.

Lampe KF and McCann MA, eds, *AMA Handbook of Poisonous and Injurious Plants*, Chicago, IL: American Medical Association, 1985.

Lance LL, Lacy C, and Goldman, MP, *Drug Information Handbook for the Allied Health Professional*, 2nd ed, Hudson, OH: Lexi-Comp Inc, 1995.

Lewis RJ, *Sax's Dangerous Properties of Industrial Materials*, 8th ed, New York, NY: Van Nostrand Reinhold, 1992.

Mandell GL, Bennett JE, and Dolin R, *Principles and Practice of Infectious Diseases*, 4th ed, New York, NY: Churchill Livingstone, 1995.

McEvoy GK, *AHFS 95 Drug Information American Hospital Formulary Service*, Bethesda, MD: American Society of Health-System Pharmacists, 1995.

Noji EK, Kelen GP, and Goessel TK, eds, *Manual of Toxicologic Emergencies*, Chicago, IL: Yearbook Medical Publisher, Inc, 1989.

Olin BR, ed, *Drug Facts and Comparisons*, St Louis, MO: Facts and Comparisons Inc, JB Lippincott Co, 1995.

Olin BR, ed, *Lawrence Review of Natural Products*, St Louis, MO: Facts and Comparisons, 1989 with updates to 1994.

Poisindex System: Rumack BH, Spoerke DG, eds, Denver, CO: Poisindex Information System, Micromedex Inc, Vol 85.

Reynolds JE, ed, *Martindale The Extra Pharmacopoeia*, 30th ed, London, England: The Pharmaceutical Press, 1993.

Russell RE, ed, *Snake Venom Poisoning*, Philadelphia, PA: JB Lippincott Co, 1980.

Schlesser JL, ed, *1991 Drugs Available Abroad*, Detroit, MI: Medec Books/Gale Research Inc, 1991.

Semla TP, Beizer JL, and Higbee MD, *Geriatric Dosage Handbook*, 2nd ed, Hudson, OH: Lexi-Comp Inc, 1995.

Shulman ST, Phair JP, and Sommers HM, eds, *The Biologic and Clinical Basis of Infectious Diseases*, 4th ed, Philadelphia, PA: WB Saunders Company, 1992.

Smith RP, *A Primer of Environmental Toxicology*, Philadelphia, PA: Lea and Febiger, 1992.

Spandorfer M, Curtiss D, and Snyder J, eds, *Making Art Safely*, New York, NY: Van Nostrand Reinhold, 1993.

Spoerke DG and Smolinske SC, eds, *Toxicity of Houseplants*, Boca Raton, FL: CRC Press, 1990.

Spoerke DG and Rumack BH, eds, *Handbook of Mushroom Poisoning, Diagnosis & Treatment*, Boca Raton, FL: CRC Press, 1994.

Sullivan JB and Krieger GR, eds, *Hazardous Material Toxicology: Clinical Principles of Environmental Health*, Baltimore, MD: Williams and Wilkins, 1992.

Taketomo CK, Hodding JH, and Kraus DM, *Pediatric Dosage Handbook*, 3rd ed, Hudson, OH: Lexi-Comp Inc, 1995.

Tarcher AB, ed, *Principles and Practice of Environmental Medicine*, New York, NY: Plenum Medical Book Company, 1992.

POISON INFORMATION CENTERS

Updated from "Poisoning Hotlines," *Emergency Medicine*, 1994, 26:96-102; and American Association of Poison Control Centers, *Vet Hum Toxicol*, 1994, 36:484-6.

*Denotes certified Regional Poison Control Centers by the American Association of Poison Control Centers (October, 1994).

Centers in each state are listed alphabetically by city.

ALABAMA

Regional Poison Control Center*
The Children's Hospital of Alabama
1600 7th Ave, S
Birmingham, AL 35233
(800) 292-6678 (Alabama only)
(205) 933-4050
939-9201
939-9202

The Alabama Poison Center*
408 A. Paul Bryant Dr, E
Tuscaloosa, AL 35401
(800) 462-0800 (Alabama only)
(205) 345-0600

ALASKA

Anchorage Poison Control Center
Providence Hospital Pharmacy
3200 Providence Dr
PO Box 6004
Anchorage, AK 99502
(800) 478-3193 (Alaska only)
(907) 261-3193

Fairbanks Poison Control Center
1650 Cowles St
Fairbanks, AK 99701
(907) 456-7182

ARIZONA

Samaritan Regional Poison Center*
Good Samaritan Regional Medical Center
1111 E McDowell Rd
Phoenix, AZ 85006
(602) 253-3334

Arizona Poison and Drug Information Center*
University of Arizona
Arizona Health Sciences Center
1501 N Campbell Ave, Rm 1156
Tucson, AZ 85724
(800) 362-0101 (Arizona only)
(602) 626-6016

ARKANSAS

Arkansas Poison and Drug Information Center
University of Arkansas for Medical Sciences
College of Pharmacy
Slot 522 (internal mailing)
4301 W Markham St
Little Rock, AR 72205
(800) 376-4766 (MDs and hospitals; Arkansas only)
(501) 661-6161
666-5532 (MDs and hospitals)

CALIFORNIA

Central California Regional Poison Control Center*
Valley Children's Hospital
3151 N Milbrook
Fresno, CA 93703
(209) 445-1222
(800) 346-5922

Los Angeles County Regional Drug and Poison Information Center
1200 N State St, Rm 1107A and B
Los Angeles, CA 90033
(800) 777-6476 (Los Angeles, Santa Barbara, and Ventura counties only)
(213) 222-3212
222-8086 (MDs and hospitals)

UC Davis Medical Center Regional Poison Control Center*
2315 Stockton Blvd, Rm HSF-124
Sacramento, CA 95817
(800) 342-9293 (northern California only)
(916) 734-3692

San Diego Regional Poison Center*
UCSD Medical Center
200 West Arbor Dr
San Diego, CA 92103
(800) 876-4766 (Imperial and San Diego counties only)
(619) 543-6000

San Francisco Bay Area Regional Poison Control Center*
San Francisco General Hospital
1001 Potrero Ave, Building 80, Rm 230
San Francisco, CA 94110
(800) 523-2222 (Del Norte, Humboldt, Mendocino, Sonoma, Napa, Marin, San Francisco, Contra Costa, Alameda, and San Mateo counties only)
(415) 476-6600

Santa Clara Valley Regional Poison Center*
Valley Health Center
750 S Bascom Ave, Suite 310
San Jose, CA 95128
(800) 662-9886 (Monterey, San Benito, San Luis Obispo, Santa Clara, and Santa Cruz counties only)
(408) 885-6000

COLORADO

Rocky Mountain Poison and Drug Center*
645 Bannock St
Denver, CO 80204
(800) 332-3073 (Colorado only)
525-5042 (Montana only)
446-6179 (Las Vegas only)
(303) 629-1123

Interstate Centers
The Poison Control Center
Omaha, NE
(800) 955-9119

CONNECTICUT

Connecticut Poison Control Center
University of Connecticut
Health Center
263 Farmington Ave
Farmington, CT 06030
(800) 343-2822 (Connecticut only)
(203) 679-3473 (Administration)
679-4346 (TDD)

DELAWARE

Interstate Centers
The Poison Control Center
Philadelphia, PA
(800) 722-7112

DISTRICT OF COLUMBIA

National Capital Poison Center*
George Washington University Medical Center
3201 New Mexico Ave, NW, Suite 310
Washington, DC 20016
(202) 625-3333 (Washington DC, suburban Maryland, and northern Virginia only)
362-8563 (TTY)

Interstate Centers
Blue Ridge Poison Center
Charlottesville, VA
(800) 451-1428

FLORIDA

Florida Poison Information Center at University Medical Center*
University of Florida Health Science Center
655 W 8th St
Jacksonville, FL 32209
(800) 282-3171 (Florida only)
(904) 549-4480 (Jacksonville)

Florida Poison Information Center and Toxicology Resource Center*
Tampa General Hospital
PO Box 1289
Tampa, FL 33601
(800) 282-3171 (Florida only)
(813) 253-4444 (Tampa)

Florida Poison Information Center/Miami
(800) 282-3171

GEORGIA

Georgia Poison Center*
Grady Memorial Hospital
80 Butler St, SE
Box 26066
Atlanta, GA 30335
(800) 282-5846 (Georgia only)
(404) 616-9000
525-3323 (TDD)

Medical Center of Central Georgia Regional Poison Control Center
777 Hemlock St
Macon, GA 31208
(912) 633-1427

HAWAII

Hawaii Poison Center
Kapiolani Women's and Children's Medical Center
1319 Punahou St
Honolulu, HI 96826
(800) 362-3585 (outer islands of Hawaii only)
362-3586
(808) 941-4411

IDAHO

Idaho Poison Center
3092 Elder St
Boise, ID 83705
(800) 632-8000 (Idaho only)
(208) 334-4580

ILLINOIS

Chicago & Northeastern Illinois Regional Poison Control Center
Rush-Presbyterian-St Luke's Medical Center
1653 W Congress Pkwy, Rm 432 Kellogg
Chicago, IL 60612
(800) 942-5969 (northern Illinois only)
(312) 942-5969

Swedish American Hospital
Rockford, IL
(800) 543-2022

Interstate Centers
Cardinal Glennon Children's Hospital Regional Poison Center
St Louis, MO
(800) 366-8888 (western Illinois only)

INDIANA

Indiana Poison Center*
Methodist Hospital of Indiana
I-65 at 21st St
PO Box 1367
Indianapolis, IN 46206
(800) 382-9097 (Indiana only)
(317) 929-2323
929-2336 (TTY)

Interstate Centers

Kentucky Regional Poison Center of Kosair Children's Hospital*
Louisville, KY
(502) 589-8222 (southern Indiana only)

IOWA

Mid-Iowa Club Poison and Drug Information Center
Iowa Methodist Medical Center
1200 Pleasant St
Des Moines, IA 50309
(800) 362-2327 (Iowa only)
(515) 241-6254

Poison Control Center
University of Iowa Hospitals and Clinics
200 Hawkins Dr
Iowa City, IA 52242
(800) 272-6477 (Iowa only)

St Luke's Poison Center
St Luke's Regional Medical Center
2720 Stone Park Blvd
Sioux City, IA 51104
(800) 352-2222 (western Iowa, northeastern Nebraska, and southern South Dakota only)
(712) 277-2222

Interstate Centers

McKennan Hospital Poison Center
Sioux Falls, SD
(800) 843-0505

KANSAS

Mid-America Poison Control Center
University of Kansas Medical Center
3901 Rainbow, Rm B-400
Kansas City, KS 66160
(800) 332-6633 (Kansas only)
(913) 588-6633 (Kansas and northern Missouri only)

HCA Wesley Poison Control Center Medical Center
550 N Hillside Ave
Wichita, KS 67214
(316) 688-2277

Interstate Centers

Cardinal Glennon Children's Hospital Regional Poison Control Center
St Louis, MO
(800) 366-8888 (Topeka only)

KENTUCKY

Kentucky Regional Poison Center of Kosair Children's Hospital*
PO Box 35070
Louisville, KY 40232
(800) 722-5725 (Kentucky only)
(502) 589-8222 (metropolitan Louisville and southern Indiana only)

LOUISIANA

Louisiana Drug and Poison Information Center
Northeast Louisiana University School of Pharmacy
Sugar Hall
Monroe, LA 71209
(800) 256-9822 (Louisiana only)
(318) 342-1710

MAINE

Maine Poison Control Center
Maine Medical Center
22 Bramhall St
Portland, ME 04102
(800) 442-6305 (Maine only)
(207) 871-2381 (ER)

MARYLAND

Maryland Poison Center*
University of Maryland School of Pharmacy
20 N Pine St
Baltimore, MD 21201
(800) 492-2414 (Maryland only)
(301) 528-7701

Interstate Centers
National Capital Poison Center*
3201 New Mexico Ave, NW, Suite 310
Washington, DC 20016
(202) 625-3333 (DC suburbs only)
362-8563 (TTY)

MASSACHUSETTS

Massachusetts Poison Control System*
300 Longwood Ave
Boston, MA 02115
(800) 682-9211
(617) 355-6609 (Administration)
355-6607 (Massachussetts)
232-2120 (Boston)

MICHIGAN

Poison Control Center*
Children's Hospital of Michigan
3901 Beaubien Blvd
Detroit, MI 48201
(313) 745-5711

Blodgett Regional Poison Center
Blodgett Memorial Medical Center
1840 Wealthy St, SE
Grand Rapids, MI 49506
(800) 632-2727 (616 area code only)
356-3232 (TTY)
(616) 774-7851 (Administration)

Bronson Poison Center
Bronson Methodist Hospital
252 E Lovell St
Kalamazoo, MI 49007
(800) 442-4112 (Michigan only)
(616) 341-6409

MINNESOTA

Hennepin Regional Poison Center*
Hennepin County Medical Center
701 Park Ave
Minneapolis, MN 55415
(612) 347-3141
337-7474 (TTY)
337-7387 (Petline)

Minnesota Regional Poison Center*
St Paul-Ramsey Medical Center
640 Jackson St
St Paul, MN 55101
(800) 222-1222 (Minnesota only)
(612) 221-2113

Interstate Centers
McKennan Hospital Poison Center
Sioux Falls, SD
(800) 843-0505

MISSISSIPPI

Forrest General Hospital Poison Center
400 S 28th Ave
PO Box 16389
Hattiesburg, MS 39401
(601) 288-4235

Mississippi Regional Poison Control Center
University Medical Center
2500 N State St
Jackson, MS 39216
(601) 354-7660

MISSOURI

Children's Mercy Hospital
2401 Gillham Rd
Kansas City, MO 64108
(816) 234-3430

Cardinal Glennon Children's Hospital Regional Poison Center*
1465 S Grand Blvd
St Louis, MO 63104
(800) 366-8888 (Missouri and western Illinois only)
(314) 772-5200
577-5336 (TTY)

MONTANA

Interstate Centers
Rocky Mountain Poison and Drug Center*
645 Bannock St
Denver, CO 80204
(303) 629-1123
(800) 525-5042

NEBRASKA

The Poison Center*
Childrens Memorial Hospital
8301 Dodge St
Omaha, NE 68114
(800) 955-9119 (Nebraska and Wyoming only)
(402) 390-5555 (Omaha)

Interstate Centers
McKennan Hospital Poison Center
Sioux Falls, SD
(800) 843-0505

St Luke's Medical Poison Center
2720 Stone Park Blvd
Sioux City, IA 51104
(800) 352-2222 (northeastern Nebraska only)

NEVADA

Interstate Centers
Rocky Mountain Poison and Drug Center
645 Bannock St
Denver, CO 80204
(800) 446-6179 (Las Vegas only)

Poison Center
Humana Hospital Sunrise
3186 Maryland Pkwy
Las Vegas, NV 89109
(800) 446-6179

Poison Center
Washoe Medical Center
77 Pringle Way
Reno, NV 89520
(702) 328-4144
328-4100

NEW HAMPSHIRE

New Hampshire Poison Information Center
Dartmouth Hitchcock Memorial Hospital
1 Medical Center Dr
Lebanon, NH 03756
(800) 562-8236 (New Hampshire only)
(603) 650-5000 (New Hampshire and bordering towns in Maine, Massachusetts, and Vermont only)

NEW JERSEY

New Jersey Poison Information and Education System*
Newark Beth Israel Medical Center
201 Lyons Ave
Newark, NJ 07112
(800) 962-1253 (New Jersey only)
(201) 926-8005
926-8008 (TTY)

Warren Hospital Poison Control Center
185 Roseberry St
Phillipsburg, NJ 08865
(800) 962-1253
(908) 859-6768

NEW MEXICO

New Mexico Poison and Drug Information Center*
University of New Mexico
Albuquerque, NM 87131
(800) 432-6866 (New Mexico only)
(505) 843-2551

NEW YORK

Western New York Regional Poison Control Center
Children's Hospital of Buffalo
219 Bryant St
Buffalo, NY 14222
(800) 888-7655 (New York only)
(716) 878-7654
878-7655

Long Island Regional Poison Control Center*
Winthrop-University Hospital
259 First St
Mineola, NY 11501
(516) 542-2323
542-2324
542-2325
542-3813

New York City Poison Control Center*
New York City Department of Health
455 First Ave, Rm 123
New York, NY 10016
(212) 340-4494
764-7667
689-9014 (TDD)

Hudson Valley Regional Poison Center*
Phelps Memorial Hospital Center
701 North Broadway
North Tarrytown, NY 10591
(800) 336-6997 (New York only)
(914) 366-3030

Finger Lakes Regional Poison Center/Life Line
University of Rochester Medical Center
Box 321
601 Elmwood Ave
Rochester, NY 14642
(800) 333-0542
(716) 275-5151
275-2700 (TTY)

Central New York Regional Poison Control Center
SUNY Health Science Center at University Hospital
750 E Adams St
Syracuse, NY 13210
(800) 252-5655 (New York only)
(315) 476-4766

NORTH CAROLINA

Western NC Poison Control Center
Memorial Mission Hospital
509 Biltmore Ave
Asheville, NC 28801
(800) 542-4225 (North Carolina only)
(704) 255-4490

Carolinas Poison Center*
Carolinas Medical Center
PO Box 32861
1000 Blythe Blvd
Charlotte, NC 28232
(800) 848-6946 (North Carolina and South Carolina only)
(704) 355-4000

Duke University Regional Poison Control Center
Duke University Medical Center
PO Box 3007
Durham, NC 27710
(800) 672-1697 (North Carolina only)
(919) 684-8111

Triad Poison Center at Moses H Cone Memorial Hospital
1200 N Elm St
Greensboro, NC 27401
(800) 953-4001 (Alamance, Forsyth, Guilford, Rockingham, and Randolph counties only)
(910) 574-8105

Catawba Memorial Hospital
Poison Control Center
810 Fairgrove Church Rd, SE
Hickory, NC 28602
(704) 322-6649

NORTH DAKOTA

North Dakota Poison Information Center
St Luke's Hospitals
720 Fourth St, N
Fargo, ND 58122
(800) 732-2200 (North Dakota, Minnesota only)
592-1889 (southeast North Dakota only)
(710) 234-5575 (local)

Interstate Centers
St Luke's Midland Regional Medical Center
Poison Control Center
Aberdeen, SD
(800) 592-1889

OHIO

Akron Regional Poison Center
1 Perkins Square
Akron, OH 44308
(800) 362-9922 (Ohio only)
(216) 379-8562
379-8446 (TTY)

Regional Poison Control System and Cincinnati Drug & Poison Information Center*
University of Cincinnati College of Medicine
231 Bethesda Ave, ML 144
Cincinnati, OH 45267
(800) 872-5111 (Cincinnati area)
762-0727 (southwest Ohio only)
(513) 558-5111

Greater Cleveland Poison Control Center
11100 Euclid Ave
Cleveland, OH 44106
(216) 231-4455

Central Ohio Poison Center*
Children's Hospital
700 Children's Dr
Columbus, OH 43205
(800) 682-7625 (Ohio only)
(614) 228-1323
228-2272 (TTY)
461-2012

Columbus Poison Center
700 Children's Dr
Columbus, OH 43205
(800) 762-0727 (Ohio only)
(513) 222-2227

Western Ohio Regional Poison and Drug Information Center
Children's Medical Center
1 Children's Plaza
Dayton, OH 45404
(800) 762-0727
(513) 222-2227

Firelands Community Hospital Poison Information Center
1101 Decatur St
Sandusky, OH 44870
(419) 626-7423

Poison and Drug Information Center of Northwest Ohio
Medical College of Ohio
3000 Arlington Ave
Toledo, OH 43614
(800) 589-3897 (northwestern Ohio and southeastern Michigan only)
(419) 381-3898

Mahoning Valley Poison Center
St Elizabeth Hospital Medical Center
1044 Belmont Ave
Youngstown, OH 44501
(800) 426-2348
(216) 746-2222
746-5510 (TDD)

Bethesda Poison Control Center
2951 Maple Ave
Zanesville, OH 43701
(614) 454-4221

Interstate Centers

Northwest Regional Poison Center
Erie, PA
(800) 822-3232 (northeastern Ohio only)

OKLAHOMA

Oklahoma Poison Control Center
Children's Hospital of Oklahoma
940 NE 13 St
Oklahoma City, OK 73104
(800) 522-4611 (Oklahoma only)
(405) 271-5454

OREGON

Oregon Poison Center*
Oregon Health Sciences University
3181 SW Sam Jackson Park Rd
Portland, OR 97201
(800) 452-7165 (Oregon only)
(503) 494-8968

PENNSYLVANIA

Poison Prevention Education Center
Geisinger Medical Center
100 N Academy Ave
Danville, PA 17821
(800) 352-7001 (Pennsylvania only)
(717) 275-6119

Central Pennsylvania Poison Center*
Milton S Hershey Medical Center
University Dr, PO Box 850
Hershey, PA 17033
(800) 521-6110
(717) 531-6111
531-6039

St Joseph Hospital and Health Care Center
250 College Ave
PO Box 3509
Lancaster, PA 17604
(717) 299-4546
291-8314
291-8425

The Poison Control Center*
Suite 220
3600 Market St
Philadelphia, PA 19104
(800) 722-7112 (Philadelphia, Montgomery, Delaware, Bucks, Chester, Berks, Lehigh, Northampton, Monroe, Carbon, and Schuylkill counties only)
(215) 386-2100

Pittsburgh Poison Center*
Children's Hospital of Pittsburgh
1 Children's Pl
3705 Fifth Ave at DeSoto St
Pittsburgh, PA 15213
(412) 681-6669

Interstate Centers
Mahoning Valley Poison Center
Youngstown, OH
(800) 426-2348 (Lawrence and Mercer counties only)

RHODE ISLAND

Rhode Island Poison Center*
Rhode Island Hospital
593 Eddy St
Providence, RI 02903
(401) 444-5727

SOUTH CAROLINA

Palmetto Poison Center
University of South Carolina
College of Pharmacy
Columbia, SC 29208
(800) 922-1117 (South Carolina and central Savannah River area of Georgia only)
(803) 777-1117 (Columbia area only)

SOUTH DAKOTA

Poison Control Center
St Luke's Midland Regional Medical Center
305 S State St
Aberdeen, SD 57401
(800) 592-1889 (South Dakota, North Dakota, Minnesota, and Wyoming only)
(605) 622-5678

Rapid City Regional Poison Control Center
353 Fairmont Blvd
Rapid City, SD 57709
(800) 232-2562
(605) 341-3333 (South Dakota only)

McKennan Poison Control Center
McKennan Hospital
800 E 21 St
PO Box 5045
Sioux Falls, SD 57117
(800) 952-0123 (South Dakota only)
843-0505 (Iowa, Minnesota, and Nebraska only)
(605) 336-3894

Interstate Centers
St Luke's Poison Center
Sioux City, IA
(800) 352-2222 (southeastern South Dakota only)

TENNESSEE

Southern Poison Center, Inc
847 Monroe Ave, Suite 230
Memphis, TN 38163
(901) 528-6048
448-6800
(800) 288-9999 (S Tennessee)

Middle Tennessee Regional Poison/Clinical Toxicology Center
1161 21st Ave S
501 Oxford House
Nashville, TN 37232
(800) 288-9999 (Tennessee only)
(615) 322-6435 (Nashville and adjacent counties only)
322-0157 (TDD)

TEXAS

Montgomery County Poison Control Center
Medical Center Hospital
504 Medical Center Blvd
Conroe, TX 77304
(409) 539-7700

North Texas Poison Center*
Parkland Hospital
5201 Harry Hines Blvd
PO Box 35926
Dallas, TX 75235
(800) 441-0040 (northern Texas only)
442-0410 (hospital and health-care providers only)
(214) 590-5000

El Paso Poison Control Center
RE Thomason General Hospital
4815 Alameda Ave
El Paso, TX 79905
(915) 533-1244

Southeast Texas Poison Center*
University of Texas Medical Branch
301 University Ave
Galveston, TX 77550-2780
(800) 392-8548 (MDs and ambulance personnel; Texas only)
(409) 765-1420 (Galveston only)
(713) 654-1701 (Houston only)

Central Texas Poison Center at Scott and White
2401 S 31st St
Temple, TX 76508
(817) 774-2005

UTAH

Poison Control Center
Columbia/HCA Davis Hospital and Medical Center
1600 W Antelope Dr
Layton, UT 84041
(801) 825-4357

Utah Regional Poison Control Center*
410 Chipeta Way, Suite 230
Salt Lake City, UT 84108
(800) 456-7707 (Utah only)
(801) 581-2151

VERMONT

Vermont Poison Center
Medical Center Hospital of Vermont
111 Colchester Ave
Burlington, VT 05401
(802) 658-3456 (Vermont and bordering New York towns only)

Interstate Centers
New Hampshire Poison Information Center
Lebanon, NH
(603) 650-5000

VIRGINIA

Blue Ridge Poison Center*
University of Virginia Health Sciences Center
Blue Ridge Hospital
Box 67
Charlottesville, VA 22901
(800) 451-1428 (Virginia, District of Columbia, Maryland, North Carolina, Tennessee, and West Virginia only)
(804) 924-5543

Virginia Poison Center
Virginia Commonwealth University
MCV Station, Box 522
Richmond, VA 23298
(800) 552-6337 (Virginia only)
(804) 828-9123 (local Richmond and TDD)

Interstate Centers
National Capital Poison Center*
3201 New Mexico Ave, NW, Suite 310
Washington, DC 20016
(202) 625-3333 (northern Virginia only)
362-8563 (TTY)

WASHINGTON

Washington Poison Center
PO Box L-5371
Seattle, WA 98105
(800) 732-6985 (Washington only)
572-0638
(206) 526-2121
517-2394 (TTD)
526-2223 (TTY)

WEST VIRGINIA

West Virginia Poison Center*
West Virginia University
Robert C. Byrd Health Sciences Center/Charleston Division
3110 MacCorkle Ave, SE
Charleston, WV 25304
(800) 642-3625 (West Virginia only)
(304) 348-4211

Poison Center
St Joseph's Hospital Center
19th St and Murdoch Ave
Parkersburg, WV 26101
(304) 424-4222

WISCONSIN

Green Bay Poison Center
St Vincent Hospital
PO Box 1997
Green Bay, WI 53201
(414) 433-8100

Regional Poison Control Center
University of Wisconsin Hospital and Clinics
600 Highland Ave
Madison, WI 53792
(608) 262-3702 (also TDD)

Milwaukee Poison Center
Children's Hospital of Wisconsin
9000 W Wisconsin Ave
PO Box 1997
Milwaukee, WI 53201
(414) 266-2222

WYOMING

Poison Control Center
St Lukes Midland Regional Medical Center
305 S State St
Aberdeen, WY 57401
(800) 592-1889 (Minnesota, North Dakota, South Dakota, and Wyoming only)
(605) 622-5678

Interstate Centers
The Poison Center*
8301 Dodge St
Omaha, NE 68114
(800) 955-9119 (NE & WY)
(402) 390-5555 (Omaha)

FOREIGN

†Denotes American Association of Poison Control Centers: Canadian Poison Center members.

CANADA

Alberta
PADIS (Poison and Drug Information Service)†
Foothills Provincial General Hospital
1403 29th St, NW
Calgary, Alberta T2N 2T9
(403) 670-1414 670-1059

British Columbia
BC Drug and Poison Information Centre†
St Paul's Hospital
1081 Burrard St
Vancouver, BC V6Z 1Y6
(604) 682-5050
682-2344

Manitoba
Poison Control Centre†
Children's Hospital
685 Bannatyne Ave
Winnipeg, Manitoba R3E OW1
(204) 787-2444

Nova Scotia
Izaak Walton Killan Children's Hospital
PO Box 3070
Halifax, Nova Scotia B3J 3G9
(800) 565-8161 (Prince Edward Island)
(902) 428-8161 (Nova Scotia)

Ontario
Provincial Regional Poison Control Centre
Children's Hospital
Eastern Ontario
401 Smyth Rd
Ottawa, Ontario K1H 8L1
(800) 267-1373
(613) 737-1100

Ontario Regional Poison Centre†
Hospital for Sick Children
555 University Ave
Toronto, Ontario M5G 1X8
(800) 263-9017
(416) 813-5823
813-5900

Quebec

Quebec Poison Control Center†
Centre Hospitalier de l'Universite Laval
2705 Boulevard Laurier; J-782
Sainte-Foy Quebec
Canada GIV 4G2
(418) 656-8090 654-2731

COSTA RICA

Centro Nacional de Control de Intoxicaciones
Hospital Nacional de Ninos
"Dr Carlos Saenz Herrera"
Apartado 1654
San Jose, Costa Rica
(506) 23-10-28

MEXICO

Centro Panamerico de Ecologia Humana y
Salud — Toxicologia
Rancho Guadalupe
Metepec, Edo de Mexico
Apartado 37-473
06696 Mexico, DF
52-(91-721)
6-44-04
6-43-44

PUERTO RICO

University of Puerto Rico
College of Pharmacy
GPO Box 5067
San Juan, Puerto Rico
(809) 758-2525 ext 1516
763-0196

GENERAL POISON INFORMATION SOURCES

Agency for Toxic Substances and Disease Registry
Atlanta, GA
(404) 639-6000

American Academy of Clinical Toxicology
Tampa, FL
(813) 251-6911 ext 14
254-2504 (Fax)

American Association of Poison Control Centers
3201 New Mexico Ave, NW
Suite 310
Washington, DC 20016
(202) 362-7217
362-8377 (Fax)

American College of Medical Toxicology
c/o Tanya Creaven
Pennsylvania Medical Society
777 E Park Dr
PO Box 8820
Harrisburg, PA 17105
(717) 558-7750 (ext 477)
558-7846
558-7841 (Fax)

American College of Occupational and Environmental Medicine
55 W Seegers Rd
Arlington Heights, IL 60005
(708) 228-6850

American Medical Association
Department of Drugs
(Identification of Foreign Drugs)
Chicago, IL 60610
(312) 464-4572

American Society of Addiction Medicine (ASAM)
4601 North Park Dr
Suite 101
Chevy Chase, MD 20815
(301) 656-3920

Association of Occupational and Environmental Clinics
1010 Vermont Ave, Suite 513
Washington, DC 20005
(202) 347-4976

Association of American Railroads
Bureau of Explosives
50 S Street, NW
Washington, DC
(202) 639-2222

Biological Effects of Low Level Exposures (BELLE)
Northeast Regional Environmental Public Health Center
University of Massachusetts
Amherst, MA
(413) 545-3164

Button Battery Hotline
Washington, DC
(202) 625-3333

Canadian Chemical Referral Center
Ottawa, Canada
(613) 237-6215

Canadian Transportation Emergency Center (CANVTEC)
Ottawa, Canada
(613) 996-6666

Cancer Information Service (National Cancer Institute) (ATSDR)
Office of Cancer Communication
NCI Building 31, Room 10A18
Bethesda, MD 20205
(800) 4-CANCER

CDC and Agency for Toxic Substances and Disease Registry (ATSDR)
Emergency Response Coordinators — 24 hours
(404) 639-0615
639-6300 (Division of Toxicology)

Center for Disease Control
Atlanta, GA
(404) 639-2888 (off hours)
639-3753 (days)

Center for Occupational Hazards (Art Hazards Information Center) — Center for Safety in the Arts
5 Beekman Street
New York, NY 10038
(212) 227-6220
Monday-Friday, 10 AM - 5 PM (EST)

Center for Substance Abuse Treatment (CSAT)
(800) 662-HELP

Chemical Spills Emergency Hotline
(800) 535-0202

Chemical Transportation Emergency Center (CHEMTREC)
2501 M Street, NW
Washington, DC 20037
(800) 424-9300
(202) 887-1258
463-1583 (Fax)
24 hours

Chevron/Ortho Emergency Information Center
(415) 233-3737 (collect)
(800) 454-2333
24 hours

Consumer Product Safety Commission
Washington, DC 20207
(800) 638-CPSC

Drug Abuse Warning Network (DAWN)
(Consumer Affairs)
Substance Abuse and Mental Health Services
Rockville, MD 20857
(301) 443-7934 (Administration Office of Applied Studies)
Room 16-105

Drugs and Crime Data Center and Clearinghouse
(800) 666-3332

Emergency Planning and Community Right-to-Know Hotline (EPA)
(800) 535-0202

Environmental Protection Agency (EPA)
Regional Offices
Region I: CT, ME, MA, NH, RI, VT
(617) 565-3420
Region II: NJ, NY, PR, VI
(212) 264-2657
Region III: DE, DC, MD, PA, VA, WV
(215) 597-9800
Region IV: AL, FL, GA, KY, MS, NC, SC, TN
(404) 347-4727
Region V: IL, IN, MI, MN, OH, WI
(312) 886-3000
Region VI: AR, LA, NM, OK, TX
(214) 655-6444
Region VII: IA, KS, MO, NE
(913) 551-7000
Region VIII: CO, MT, ND, SD, UT, WY
(303) 293-1603
Region IX: AM SAMOA, AZ, CA, GU, HI, NV,
Trust Territory of the Pacific Isl,
Marshall Isl, Palau, Ponape
(415) 744-1305
Region X: AK, ID, OR, WA
(206) 553-4973

EPA Safe Drinking Water Hotline
(800) 426-4791
Monday-Friday, 9 AM – 5:30 PM (EST)

EPA Hazardous Waste Hotline
(800) 535-0202

Food and Drug Administration
Office of Consumer Affairs (HFE-88)
5600 Fishers Lane
Rockville, MD 20857
(301) 443-3170
Monday-Friday, 8 AM – 5 PM (EST)

Food and Drug Administration
Surveillance and Data Processing Branch HFN-737
5600 Fishers Lane
Rockville, MD 20857
(301) 443-6260
Monday-Friday, 8 AM – 5 PM (EST)

Food and Safety Inspection Service
U.S. Department of Agriculture
Meat and Poultry Hotline
Room 1163S
Washington, DC 20250
(800) 535-4555
Monday-Friday, 10 AM – 4 PM (EDT)

Lungline/National Jewish Hospital
(800) 222-5864

Malignant Hyperthermia Association of the United States
PO Box 1069
Sherburne, NY 13460
(800) 644-9737
(800) 986-4287

Mead Data Center
9333 Springboro Pike
Dayton, OH 45401
(800) 227-4908
Medline/Gen Med

National Animal Poison Control Center
University of Illinois
College of Veterinary Medicine
2001 S Lincoln
Urbana, IL 61801
(900) 680-0000 $20 First 5 minutes/$2.95 each additional minute
(800) 548-2423 $30 Flat fee

National Center for Environmental Health (CDC)
(404) 488-7330

National DEET Registry (Pegus Research, Incorporated)
1425 South Seventh East
Salt Lake City, UT 84105
(800) 949-0089

National Inhalant Prevention Coalition
(Texas Prevention Partnership)
Austin, TX
(800) 269-4237

National Institute of Occupational Safety and Health (NIOSH)
4676 Columbia Pkwy
Cincinnati, OH 45226
(800) 356-4674
(513) 841-4491

National Lead Information Center
(800) LEAD-FYI

National Library of Medicine
MEDLARS Management Section
8600 Rockville Pike
Bethesda, MD 20209
(800) 638-8480
(301) 496-6193
Toxline (Toxicology Literature), Medline (Biomedical Literature), RTECS
Toxnet

National Pesticide Telecommunications Network
Department of Preventive Medicine, School of Medicine
Texas Technical University Health Sciences Center
Lubbock, TX 79430
(800) 858-7378 (toll-free in U.S.)
(806) 743-3091 (outside of U.S., non-toll-free)
743-3094 (Fax)
Monday-Friday, 8 AM – 6 PM (CST)

National Response Center (Oil and Chemical Spills)
U.S. Coast Guard Headquarters
2100 2nd St, SW, Rm 2611
Washington, DC 20593
(800) 424-8802
(202) 426-2675
24 hours

National Sexually Transmitted Disease Hotline
Atlanta, GA (CDC)
(800) 227-8922

North American Mycological Association
3556 Oakwood St
Ann Arbor, MI 48104
(313) 971-2552

NTIS (National Technical Information Service)
(703) 487-4600

Nuclear Regulatory Commission
Washington, DC
(202) 492-7000

Paraquat/Diquat Information
Zeneca, Inc, Agriculture Products
Wilmington, DE
(800) 327-8633

ICI Chipman
Stony Creek, Ontario
(800) 561-3636

Poisindex-Micromedex Inc
6200 S Syracuse Way, Suite 300
Englewood, CO 80111
(800) 525-9083
(303) 486-6400
486-6464 (Fax)

Rabies Immune Globulin (RIG) Producers
Connaught Laboratories
(800) 822-2463
Miles Pharmaceutical Division
(800) 288-8371
(203) 937-2242

Radiation Emergency Assistance Center/Training Site (REAC/TS)
Oak Ridge Institute for Science and Education
PO Box 117
Oak Ridge, TN 37831
(615) 576-3131 (days)
481-1000 (24-hour hotline)

Radon Hotline
(800) SOS-RADON

Seafood Safety Line
(Food and Drug Administration)
Rockville, MD
(800) 332-4010
Noon – 4 PM (EST)

Society of Forensic Toxicologists, Inc (SOFT)
PO Box 5543
Mesa, AZ 85211
(602) 839-9106

The Poison Review™
Box 775
3023 N Clark St
Chicago, IL 60657
(312) 563-1112

Teratogen Exposure Registry and Surveillance (TERAS)
Brigham and Women's Hospital
75 Francis St
Boston, MA 02115
(617) 732-6507

Therapeutic Antibodies, Inc
Nashville, TN
(615) 327-1027
320-1212 (Fax)

Toxic Chemical Release Inventory System (EPA)
(800) 535-0202

Toxic Substance Control Act
Assistance Office
Washington, DC
(202) 554-1404

Toxicology Information and Scientific Evaluation Group
National Toxicology Program
(919) 541-3391

Toxicology Information Response Center (TIRC)
Oak Ridge National Laboratory (ORHL)
(615) 576-1743

Information Centers
Chemicals (615) 574-7797
Environmental Mutagens (615) 574-7871
Environmental Teratology (615) 574-7871
Toxicology Data (615) 576-1746

"Turkey Talk" Line
(Butterball Turkey Company)
(800) 323-4848 (November-December only)

United States Drug Testing Laboratories
(Meconium/Hair Drug Analysis and Anabolic Steroid Testing)
Chicago, IL
(312) 421-7333

U.S. Drug Task Force
Investigation of Federal Drug Cases
Wheeling, WV
(800) 852-6946

Vaccine Adverse Event Reporting System
Rockville, MD
(800) 822-7967

Veterans Affairs Department
(800) 749-8387
7:30 AM – 8:30 PM CST weekdays

White House Office of National Drug Control Policy (ONDCP): Drugs and Crime Clearing House
Washington, DC
(800) 666-3332

TERATOGEN INFORMATION SERVICES

ARIZONA

Arizona Teratogen Information Program (ATIP)
University of Arizona, Department of Pediatrics
Section of Genetics/Dysmorphology
2504 East Elm St
Tucson, AZ 85716
(602) 795-5675; in Arizona, (800) 362-0101
626-4884 (Fax)
Dee Quinn, MS; H. Eugene Hoyme, MD; Lynn Hauck, MS

CALIFORNIA

California Teratogen Information Service & Clinical Research Program
University of California, San Diego
Department of Pediatrics
Division of Dysmorphology & Teratology
225 Dickinson St, #8446
San Diego, CA 92103-8446
(619) 294-6084; in California, (800) 532-3749
294-6217 (administrative only)
291-0946 (Fax)
Kenneth Lyons Jones, MD; Kathleen Johnson; Christina Chambers; Lyn Dick; Robert Felix

COLORADO

TIES
The Children's Hospital
B300 Genetics
1056 East 19th Ave
Denver, CO 80218
(800) 332-2082 (Colorado)
525-4871 (Wyoming)
(303) 861-6395
861-3992 (Fax)
Karen Prescott, MS; David Manchester, MD; Carol Walton, MS; Cathy Marquez

CONNECTICUT

Connecticut Pregnancy Exposure Information Service
Division of Human Generics, Room L-5072
University of Connecticut Health Center
263 Farmington Ave
Farmington, CT 06030
(203) 679-1502; in Connecticut, (800) 325-5391
679-1531 (Fax)
Glenda Lee Spivey, MS; Sally S. Rosengren, MD; Sharon Voyer, MS; Robert Pilarski, MS; Joanne Brochu

DISTRICT OF COLUMBIA

Reproductive Toxicology Center
2440 M St NW, Ste 217
Washington, DC 20037-1404
(202) 293-5137
293-7256 (Fax)
Anthony R. Scialli, MD; Armand Lione, PhD; G. Kay Padgett; Christine Colie, MD; Greta D. Ober

FLORIDA

Teratogen Information Services
Box 100296
University of Florida Health Science Center
Gainesville, FL 32610-0296
(904) 392-3050
392-3051 (Fax)
Donna H. Poynor, MM; Charles A. Williams, MD

Florida Teratogen Information Service
University of Miami School of Medicine
Mailman Center
PO Box 016820
Miami, FL 33101
(305) 547-6464
547-3919 (Fax)
Virginia H. Carver, PhD

Teratogen Information Service
University of South Florida
Department of Pediatrics, Box 15-G
12901 Bruce B. Downs Blvd
Tampa, FL 33613
(813) 974-2262
974-4985 (Fax)
Jaines K. Hartsfield, DMD; Boris G. Kousseff, MD; Suzanne R. Sage, RN, MS; Jamie L. Frias MD

GEORGIA

Centers for Disease Control
Division of Birth Defects and Genetic Diseases
Mail Stop F45
1600 Clifton Rd
Atlanta, GA 30333
(404) 488-4967
488-4643 (Fax)
Muin J. Khoury, MD, PhD; Jose F. Cordero MD, MPH

ILLINOIS

Illinois Teratogen Information Service
Northwestern University
333 E Superior, Ste 1543
Chicago, IL 60611
(312) 908-7441, (800) 252-4847
908-6643 (Fax)
Eugene Pergament MD, PhD

INDIANA

Indiana Teratogen Information Service
Department of Medical Genetics
Indiana University Medical Center
975 W Walnut St
Indianapolis, IN 46202
(317) 274-1071
274-2387 (Fax)
David D. Weaver, MD; Peg Davee, MS; Lola Cook, MS

IOWA

University of Iowa Prenatal Diagnostic Unit
Department of Obstetrics and Gynecology
University of Iowa
Iowa City, IA 52241
(319) 356-3561
355-6728 (Fax)
Roger Williamson, MD; Katherine Wenstrom, MD; Susan Sipes, MD; Stanley Grant, RN

University of Iowa Teratogen Information Service
Department of Pediatrics/Medical Genetics
University of Iowa Hospitals & Clinics
Iowa City, IA 52242
(319) 356-3347
James W. Hanson, MD; Ann Mullenburg, RN, MA

KANSAS

Prenatal Diagnostic & Genetic Clinic
HCA Wesley Medical Center
550 North Hillside
Wichita, KS 67214
(316) 688-2362
Sechin Cho, MD; Paula Floyd, RN, MN; Richard Lutz, MD; Nancy McMaster, RN, MEd

MASSACHUSETTS

Massachusetts Teratogen Information Service (MTIS)
National Birth Defects Center
30 Warren St
Boston, MA 02135
(617) 787-4957; in Massachusetts, (800) 322-5014
787-5834 (office)
787-6936 (Fax)
Susan Rosenwasser, MEd; Jane O'Brien, MD; Katryn Miller, MEd; Robin Maltz, MPH; Karen Treat, MS

Embryology Teratology Unit
Warren 801
Massachusetts General Hospital
Fruit St
Boston, MA 02114
(617) 726-1742
726-1866 (Fax)
Lewis B. Holmes, MD; Ailish M. Hayes, MD; Gerald V. Raymond, MD; Joan M. Stoler, MD

TERAS
c/o Dr Fred Bieber
Department of Pathology
Brigham & Women's Hospital
75 Francis St
Boston, MA 02115
(617) 732-6507
732-7513 (Fax)
Frederick R. Bieber, PhD; David Genest; George Mutter; Drucilla Roberts; Christopher Crum

MISSOURI

Columbia Teratogen Information Service
Department of Child Health
Medical Genetics Division
University of Missouri
1 Hospital Dr
Columbia, MO 65201
(314) 882-6991
882-2742 (Fax)
Virginia Proud, MD; Judith Miles, MD; Kathy Morris, MSSW

Genetics and Environmental Information Service (GENIS)
Washington University School of Medicine
Departments of Obstetrics & Gynecology and Genetics
216 South Kings Hwy
St Louis, MO 63110
(314) 454-8172
454-7358 (Fax)
Heidi Beaver, MPH; Sheri Babb; Laura Turlington, MS; Cindy Johnson, MS; James P. Crane, MD; Jeffrey M. Dicke; Jane E. Corteville; Diana L. Gray

NEBRASKA

Nebraska Teratogen Project
University of Nebraska Medical Center
600 S 42nd St
Omaha, NE 68198-5430
(402) 559-5071
559-5737 (Fax)
Beth Conover, RN, MS; Bruce Buehler, MD

NEW JERSEY

New Jersey Pregnancy Risk Information Service
University of Medicine and Dentistry of New Jersey-SOM
401 Haddon Ave
Camden, NJ 08103
(609) 757-7812; in New Jersey, (800) 441-0025
757-9792 (Fax)
Michael K. McCormack, PhD; Carol Zuber, MS; Charlotte Furey, BSN

NEW YORK

Perinatal Environmental and Drug Consultation Service (PEDECS)
Department of Obstetrics & Gynecology
PO Box 668
University of Rochester Medical Center
601 Elmwood Ave
Rochester, NY 14642
(716) 275-3638
244-2209 (Fax)
Richard K. Miller, PhD

Teratogen Information Service
1260 East and West Rd
Building 16
West Seneca, NY 14224
(716) 674-6300, x4812
Luther X. Robinson, MD; Sandra Gangell

NORTH DAKOTA

John T. Martsolf, MD
Division of Medical Genetics, Department of Pediatrics
University of North Dakota School of Medicine
501 Columbia Rd
Grand Forks, ND 58203
(701) 777-4277
777-3994 (Fax)
John T. Martsolf, MD; Mary Ebertowski, RN

PENNSYLVANIA

Pregnancy Healthline
Pennsylvania Hospital
Spruce Building, 7th Floor
8th and Spruce St
Philadelphia, PA 19107
(215) 829-3601
829-7423 (Fax)
Betsy Schick-Boschetto, MSN; Alan E. Donnenfeld, MD; Ronald J. Librizzi, DO

Pregnancy Safety Hotline
Department of Reproductive Genetics
School of Nursing, 2nd Floor
Western Pennsylvania Hospital
4800 Friendship Ave
Pittsburgh, PA 15224
(412) 687-SAFE
578-1125 (Fax)
Michael J. Kerr, MS; Kathy A. Bournikos, MS; Karen Filkins, MD; Christann Jackson, MD; Elizabeth Gettig, MS

Department of Reproductive Genetics
Magee-Women's Hospital
300 Halket St
Pittsburgh, PA 15213
(412) 647-4168
647-4343 (Fax)
Sandra G. Marchese, MS; Mona Penles Stadler, MS; Deanna P. Steele, MS; Luanne Fraer, MS; Amy Niklaus, MS; Faith Callif-Daley, MS; Dolores Pegram, MEd

SOUTH DAKOTA

Teratogen and Birth Defects Information Project
School of Medicine, University of South Dakota
414 E Clark
Vermillion, SD 57069
(800) 962-1642
(605) 677-5124 (Fax)
Virginia P. Johnson, MD; Patricia Skorey, MNS, BSN; Carol Strom, MS

TEXAS

Genetic Screening & Counseling Service
PO Box 2467
Denton, TX 76202-2467
(817) 383-3561
382-6235 (Fax)
Lori Wolfe, MS; Becky Althaus, MS; Donald W. Day, MD; Margaret Drummon-Borg, MD; Judith Martin, MD

UTAH

Pregnancy Riskline
44 Medical Dr
Salt Lake City, UT 84113
(801) 583-2229
584-8488 (Fax)
John Carey, MD; Marcia Feldkamp; Lynn Martinez; Marsha Leen - Mitchell

VERMONT

Vermont Pregnancy Risk Information Service
Vermont Regional Genetics Center
1 Mill St
Burlington, VT 05401
(802) 658-4310
Elizabeth F. Allen, PhD; Alan E. Guttmacher, MD

WASHINGTON

Central Laboratory for Human Embryology
Department of Pediatrics RD-20
School of Medicine
University of Washington
Seattle, WA 98195
(206) 543-3373
543-3184 (Fax)
Tom Shepard, MD; Alan Fantel, MD; Phil Mirkes

WISCONSIN

Teratogen Information Service
La Crosse Regional Genetic Services
PO Box 1326
La Crosse, WI 54602
(608) 791-6681; for Wisconsin, Iowa, and northern Illinois, (800) 362-9567
Janet Williams, MS

Great Lake Genetics
2323 N Mayfair Rd, Ste 410
Milwaukee, WI 53226
(414) 475-7400
475-7223
Loig Magnuson, RN; Jurgen Herrmann, MD; Bonnie-Jo Bates, MD

Eastern Wisconsin Teratogen Service
Medical Genetics Institute, SC
4555 W Schroeder Dr, Ste 180
Milwaukee, WI 53223
(414) 357-6555
357-9394 (Fax)
B. Rafael Elejalde, MD; Maria M. de Elejalde, MS, RN

CANADA

Safe Start Program
Chedoke-McMaster Medical Center
1200 Main St W, Rm 1E-1
Hamilton, Ontario L8N 3Z5
(416) 521-2100, x6788
521-5008 (Fax)
Elizabeth Chow Tung, PharmD

FRAME Program (Fetal Risk Assessment from Maternal Exposure)
800 Commissioners' Rd E
London, Ontario N6C 2V5
(519) 685-8293
685-8156 (Fax)
Michael J. Rieder, MD; Carlene Morrison

Motherisk Program
Division of Clinical Pharmacology and Toxicology
The Hospital for Sick Children
555 University Ave
Toronto, Ontario M5G 1X8
(416) 813-6780
813-7562 (Fax)
Gideon Koren, MD; Chris Eliopoulos; Natalie Horlatsh; Sheelagh Martin; Adrianne Einarson; Anne Pastuszak

Department of Medical Genetics
University of British Columbia
University Hospital-Shaughnessy Site
4500 Oak St
Vancouver, British Columbia V6H 3N1
(604) 875-2157
875-2376 (Fax)
J.M. Friedman, MD, PhD; Margot Van Allen, MD; Wendy Hird, MSc; Heidi Hogg, MSc

British Columbia Drug & Poison Information Centre
1081 Burrard St
Vancouver, British Columbia V6Z 1Y6
(604) 682-2344, x2126
631-5262 (Fax)
Janet Webb, MSc; Bev Louis, BSc (Pharm); Kathy McInnes, BSc (Pharm)

MEDICINAL AGENTS

APPROACH TO TOXICOLOGY

Peter Mere Latham (1789-1875) is credited with the statement, "Poisons and medicines are oftentimes the same substance given with different intents." While this remark was penned in a bygone era, it is probably more true today than it was then. For confirmation of this fact, one can open any clinical pharmacology textbook (or even the *Physician's Desk Reference*) and note therapeutic agents that can lead to specific toxic syndromes or toxidromes.[1] In this way, there are few fields in medicine that demand such immediate, decisive, and definitive treatment strategy with as small an information base as in the area of toxicologic emergencies. Despite the potential for the wide range of clinical presentations due to a virtually unlimited amount of toxins, <0.05% of all poison exposures called to a Poison Control Center result in death.[2] Although this statistic may be somewhat misleading because of a biased population sample, it is still evident that if one follows a consistent treatment algorithm of the poisoned patient, the outcome will be favorable in a vast majority of cases.[3-8]

PATTERNS OF MORTALITY RISK FROM DRUGS/SUBSTANCE OVERDOSE
A Theoretical Model

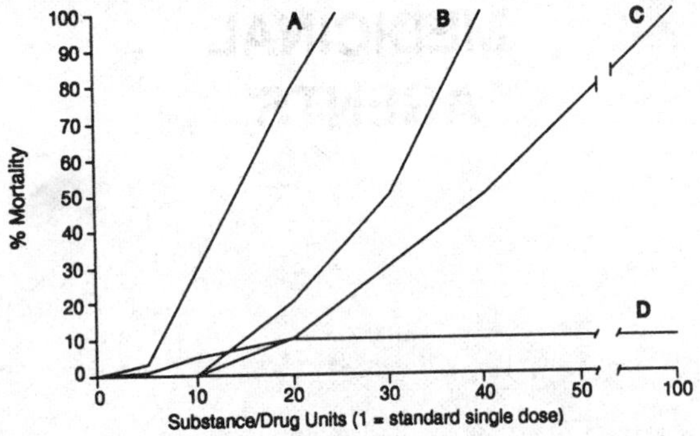

A - High toxicity: Digoxin, tricyclic antidepressant, theophylline, carbon monoxide, cyanide
B - Intermediate: Acetaminophen, salicylate, phenobarbital
C - Low: Propranolol
D - Threshold for overdose effect: Atropine, phenylpropanolamine

Theoretical model of patterns of mortality risk from drug or substance overdose. A = highly toxic substances that cause mortality with a dose-effect pattern (eg, digoxin, tricyclic antidepressants, theophylline, carbon monoxide, cyanide); B = other substances that react in a similar manner but require a larger dose or more time to reach 100% mortality (eg, acetaminophen, aspirin, iron); C = less toxic substances that act in a predictable dose-response relationship (eg, nonsteroidal anti-inflammatory drugs); D = substances that may cause mortality in a less predictable fashion where a clear dose-response relationship cannot be established (eg, atropine, phenylpropanolamine). (Courtesy of Yona Amitai, MD, Hadassah Medical Organization, Jerusalem, Israel)

Mortality from poisoning essentially follows two distinct patterns (see figure). Those toxins that cause mortality usually through cell necrosis by a dose-dependent mechanism are demonstrated in the figure by mortality curves A, B, and C. Highly toxic substances which can cause cellular damage and necrosis in a rapid dose-effect pattern are illustrated by mortality curve A. Moderately toxic agents, for which a higher dose is required to achieve 100% mortality, are illustrated by mortality curve B. Substances that are less toxic but whose dose-effect curve is more predictable (with a slope approaching 1) are illustrated by mortality curve C. Note that a definition of an antidote is any agent that moves a toxin mortality curve to the right. A second mechanism of toxin-induced mortality is demonstrated by curve D. This can be termed the "threshold effect", which is usually demonstrated by drugs that operate through a receptor mechanism (ie, atropine, beta-agonists, phenylpropanolamine). These drugs do not demonstrate a dose-dependent mortality curve but rather a plateau following a certain threshold dose whereupon maximal target organ response is achieved but no further mortality is expected to occur.

The recommended treatment plan for the poisoned patient is not unlike general treatment plans taught in advanced cardiac life support (ACLS) or advanced trauma life support (ATLS) courses. In this manner, the initial approach to the poisoned patient should be essentially similar in every case, irrespective of the toxin ingested, just as the initial approach to the trauma patient is the same irrespective of the mechanism of injury. This approach, which can be termed as routine poison management, essentially includes the following aspects.

- Stabilization: ABCs (airway, breathing, circulation); administration of glucose, thiamine, oxygen, and naloxone
- History, physical examination leading toward the identification of class of toxin (toxidrome recognition)
- Prevention of absorption (decontamination)
- Specific antidote, if available
- Removal of absorbed toxin (enhancing excretion)
- Support and monitoring for adverse effects

STABILIZATION OF THE PATIENT

In the initial evaluation of a toxic patient, the treating physician must remember that the most common cause of airway obstruction in the unconscious patient is passive obstruction by the tongue. In this way, the neck lift with jaw thrust may be the first maneuver performed by the physician on the unconscious poisoned patient followed by endotracheal intubation. Indications for endotracheal intubation in the poisoned patient include protection of the airway in the obtunded or comatose patient with a depressed or absent gag reflex to prevent aspiration during gastric lavage; controlled ventilation in patients who demonstrate respiratory depression or failure; removal of secretions in patients who develop pulmonary edema secondary to a toxic substance; and institution of positive end-expiratory pressure (PEEP) therapy for those patients who are at risk for developing adult respiratory distress syndrome (ARDS). A chest film should be obtained to note the position of the endotracheal tube.

Following evaluation of airway and breathing, the circulatory status needs to be assessed. Hypotension in the toxic patient must be addressed as quickly as possible in order to avoid the sequelae of shock. While hypotension in this group of patients may arise from a variety of mechanisms (ranging from decreased cardiac output due to myocardial depression; to venous pooling; to decreased peripheral resistance; or to hemorrhage), the initial treatment is essentially the same: intravenous fluid administration. A fluid challenge of 100-200 mL of a crystalloid solution (10-20 mL/kg in pediatrics) is often given at this time while urine output is monitored (0.5-1 mL/kg/hour). At this time, if the patient's mental status is altered or if hypotension exists, four essentially innocuous drugs (oxygen, naloxone, glucose, and thiamine) are administered for a combination of diagnostic and therapeutic reasons. See the following table.

Drugs to Be Utilized in the Toxic Patient With Altered Mental Status

Drug	Effect	Comment
25-50 g **dextrose** ($D_{50}W$) intravenously to reverse the effects of drug-induced hypoglycemia (adult) 1 mL/kg $D_{50}W$ diluted 1:1 (child).	This can be especially effective in patients with limited glycogen stores (ie, neonates and patients with cirrhosis).	Extravasation into the extremity of this hyperosmolar solution can cause Volkmann's contractures.
50-100 mg intravenous **thiamine**	Prevent Wernicke's encephalopathy	A water-soluble vitamin with low toxicity; rare anaphylactoid reactions have been reported.
Initial dosage of **naloxone** should be 2 mg in adult patients preferably by the intravenous route, although intramuscular, subcutaneous, intralingual, and endotracheal routes may also be utilized. Pediatric dose is 0.1 mg/kg from birth until 5 years of age. For potentially opioid-dependent patients with altered mental status, smaller doses (0.1-0.2 mg) could initially be used to increase arousal without producing withdrawal.	Specific opioid antagonist without any agonist properties.	It should be noted that some semisynthetic opiates (such as meperidine or propoxyphene) may require higher initial doses for reversal, so that a total dose of 6-10 mg is not unusual. If the patient responds to a bolus dose and then relapses to a lethargic or comatose state, a naloxone drip can be considered. This can be accomplished by administering two-thirds of the bolus dose that revives the patient per hour or injecting 4 mg naloxone in 1 L crystalloid solution and administering at a rate of 100 mL/hour (0.4 mg/hour).
Oxygen, utilized in 100% concentration	Useful for carbon monoxide, hydrogen, sulfide, and asphyxiants	While oxygen is antidotal for carbon monoxide intoxication, the only relative toxic contraindication is in paraquat intoxication (in that it can promote pulmonary fibrosis).

HISTORY AND PHYSICAL EXAMINATION

While the history and physical examination is the cornerstone of clinical patient management, it takes on special meaning with regard to the toxic patient. While taking a history may be a more direct method of the determination of the toxin, quite often it is not reliable. Information obtained may prove minimal in some cases and could be considered partial or inaccurate in suicide gestures and addicts. A quick physical examination often leads to important clues about the nature of the toxin. These clues can be specific symptom complexes associated with certain toxins and can be referred to as "toxidromes". See the following table.

Examples of Toxidromes

Toxidromes	Pattern	Example of Drugs	Treatment Approach
Anticholinergic	Fever, ileus, flushing, tachycardia, urinary retention, inability to sweat, visual blurring, and mydriasis. Central manifestations include myoclonus, choreoathetosis, toxic psychosis with lilliputian hallucinations, seizures, and coma.	Antihistamines Baclofen Benztropine Jimson weed Methylpyroline Phenothiazines Propantheline Tricyclic antidepressants	Physostigmine for life-threatening symptoms*
Cholinergic	Characterized by salivation, lacrimation, urination, defecation, gastrointestinal cramps, and emesis ("sludge"). Bradycardia and bronchoconstriction may also be seen.	Carbamate Organophosphates Pilocarpine	• Atropine* • Pralidoxime for organophosphate insecticides*
Extrapyramidal	Choreoathetosis, hyperreflexia, trismus, opisthotonos, rigidity, and tremor	Haloperidol Phenothiazines	• Diphenhydramine • Benztropine
Hallucinogenic	Perceptual distortions, synthesis, depersonalization, and derealization	Amphetamines Cannabinoids Cocaine Indole alkaloids Phencyclidine	Benzodiazepine
Narcotic	Altered mental status, unresponsiveness, shallow respirations, slow respiratory rate or periodic breathing, miosis, bradycardia, hypothermia.	Opiates Dextromethorphan Pentazocine Propoxyphene	Naloxone*

(continued)

Toxidromes	Pattern	Example of Drugs	Treatment Approach
Sedative/Hypnotic	Manifested by sedation with progressive deterioration of central nervous system function. Coma, stupor, confusion, apnea, delirium, or hallucinations may accompany this pattern.	Anticonvulsants Antipsychotics Barbiturates Benzodiazepines Ethanol Ethchlorvynol Fentanyl Glutethimide Meprobamate Methadone Methocarbamol Opiates Quinazolines Propoxyphene Tricyclic antidepressants	• Naloxone* • Flumazenil* • Urinary alkalinization (barbiturates)
Seizuregenic	May mimic stimulant pattern with hyperthermia, hyperreflexia, and tremors being prominent signs.	Anticholinergics Camphor Chlorinated hydrocarbons Cocaine Isoniazid Lidocaine Lindane Nicotine Phencyclidine Strychnine Xanthines	• Antiseizure medications • Pyridoxine for isoniazid* • Extracorporeal removal of drug (ie, lindane, camphor, xanthines) • Physostigmine for anticholinergic agents*

(continued)

Toxidromes	Pattern	Example of Drugs	Treatment Approach
Serotonin	Confusion, myoclonus, hyperreflexia, diaphoresis, tremor, facial flushing, diarrhea, fever, trismus	Clomipramine Fluoxetine Isoniazid L-tryptophan Moclobemide Paroxetine Phenelzine Sertraline Tranylcypromine Drug combinations include: MAO inhibitors with L-tryptophan Fluoxetine or meperidine Fluoxetine with carbamazepine or sertraline Clomipramine and meclobemide Trazadol and buspirone Paroxetine and dextromethorphan	Withdrawal of drug/benzodiazepine
Solvent	Lethargy, confusion, dizziness, headache, restlessness, incoordination, derealization, depersonalization	Acetone Chlorinated hydrocarbons Hydrocarbons Naphthalene Trichloroethane Toluene	Avoid catecholamines
Stimulant	Restlessness, excessive speech and motor activity, tachycardia, tremor, and insomnia — may progress to seizure. Other effects noted include euphoria, mydriasis, anorexia, and paranoia.	Amphetamines Caffeine (xanthines) Cocaine Ephedrine/pseudoephedrine Methylphenidate Nicotine Phencyclidine	Benzodiazepines
Uncoupling of oxidative phosphylation	Hyperthermia, tachypnea, diaphoresis, metabolic acidosis (usually)	Aluminum phosphide Aspirin/Salicylates 2,4-Dichlorophenol Di-n-Butyl Phthalate Dinitrophenols Dinitro cresols Hexachlorobutadiene Phosphorus Pentachlorophenol Tin (?) Zinc phosphide	• Sodium bicarbonate to treat metabolic acidosis • Patient cooling techniques • Avoidance of atropine or salicylate agents • Hemodialysis may be required for acidosis treatment

From Nice A, Leikin JB, Maturen A, et al, "Toxidrome Recognition to Improve Efficiency of Emergency Urine Drug Screens," *Ann Emerg Med*, 1988, 17:676-80. *See the Poison Control Center Antidote Chart.

The term toxidromes was originated by Mofensen in 1974 to assist the clinician in identifying the classification of toxins by toxin-specific symptom complexes. With the clinician focusing on the patient's vital signs, sensorium, motor signs, ocular findings, and other clinical abnormalities (eg, odor on breath, discoloration of urine), clinical toxin-pattern recognition can be achieved and an initial treatment plan formalized.

Sensorium: Determine whether the patient is comatose, stuporous, lethargic, confused, or alert.

Behavior and hallucinations: Often the hallucinatory pattern of the patient can be specific for certain drugs. For example, with atropine the patient experiences lilliputian hallucinations; with cocaine, there is a simple visual hallucinatory pattern with objects appearing in the periphery of vision; with phencyclidine, complex hallucinations are often indistinguishable clinically from a paranoid psychosis; and with LSD, the patient experiences a combination of illusions (seeing objects in altered forms), hallucination (experiencing sensations without external stimuli), and pseudohallucinations (knowing when one is hallucinating).[9]

Motor signs: Tremors, hyporeflexia and hyperreflexia, and even the nature of seizures can be useful diagnostic tools. Like hallucinations, seizures caused by specific toxins can exhibit certain specific properties. For example, strychnine is unique in that it can cause generalized seizures while the patient is alert. This can be referred to as a "spinal seizure." Other drug-induced seizures will respond only to specific antidotal therapies and not to conventional antiseizure medication. Examples of this property include anticholinergic-induced seizures, which may respond to physostigmine, and isoniazid-induced seizures, which respond to pyridoxine. Additionally, theophylline-induced seizures rarely respond to phenytoin alone and often only to multidrug therapy.

Vital signs: Sympathomimetics and anticholinergics essentially cause an increase in all of the vital signs parameters. This is particularly true for cocaine intoxication, where it has been noted that hyperthermia may be a particularly ominous sign for mortality. Conversely, organophosphates, opiates, barbiturates, beta-blockers, benzodiazepines, alcohol, and clonidine toxicities result in hypothermia, respiratory depression, and bradycardia.

Ocular findings: This can be divided into categories: pupillary size and reactivity, and demonstration of nystagmus.

Pupillary signs: Both anticholinergic and sympathomimetic substances can result in mydriasis, but in cocaine intoxication, the pupils will respond to light, whereas with anticholinergics the pupils will not. Agents that contribute to miosis include organophosphate insecticides, narcotics, bromide, acetone, clonidine, and nicotine. Phencyclidine has been known to cause either mydriasis or miosis.

Nystagmus: Alcohols are probably the most common etiology of horizontal nystagmus, although lithium, carbamazepine, solvents, meprobamate, quinine, and primidone can also result in horizontal nystagmus. Phencyclidine can cause a combination of vertical, horizontal, and even rotary nystagmus, as can phenytoin and sedative-hypnotics.

Other findings: In addition to these physical signs, odors emanating from the patient may also provide important directions in management. For example, a garlic odor is often caused by arsenicals, phosphorus compounds, or organophosphates. A rotten egg odor can be associated with decomposition of organic materials (hydrogen sulfide) or disulfiram.

Radiographs can be of some utility in toxic exposure analysis. Factors that influence radiodensity include molecular weight, atomic number, relative contrast to surrounding tissues, and compactness of the form of drug. Sustained-released medications can be more easily detected through digital enhancement of the radiograph.[10] It should be pointed out that this is not a reliable method for evaluating toxic exposure and should be utilized in only specific cases. These cases include evaluation of heavy metal exposure (including leaded paint chips), concretion formation of drugs (such as aspirin, meprobamate, glutethimide, barbiturates, iron, and sustained-release theophylline), and the body packing/stuffing phenomenon.

The clinical laboratory evaluation includes the assessment of the "three gaps of toxicology": anion gap (usually a type A lactic acidosis due to tissue hypoxia), osmolar gap, and oxygen saturation gap. What these "gaps" have in common is that the toxic substance accounts for a difference between calculated and measured determination. The following drugs are known to cause these gaps.

Toxins Affecting the Anion Gap

Drugs Causing Increased Anion Gap (>12 mEq/L)

Nonacidotic

Carbenicillin
Sodium salts

Metabolic Acidosis

Acetaminophen (ingestion >75-100 g)
Acetazolamide
Aluminum phosphate
Amiloride
Ammonium chloride
Ascorbic acid
Benzalkonium chloride
Bialaphos
2-Butanone
Carbon monoxide
Centrimonium bromide
Chloramphenicol
Cobalt
Colchicine
Cyanide
Dapsone
Dimethyl sulfate
Dinitrophenol
Endosulfan
Epinephrine (I.V. overdose)
Ethanol
Ethylene dibromide
Ethylene glycol
Fenoprofen
Fluoroacetate
Formaldehyde
Fructose (I.V.)
Glycol ethers
Hydrogen sulfide
Ibuprofen (ingestion >300 mg/kg)
Inorganic acid
Iodine
Iron
Isoniazid
Ketamine
Ketoprofen
Metaldehyde
Metformin
Methanol
Methenamine mandelate
Monochloracetic acid
Nalidixic acid
Naproxen
Niacin
Papaverine
Paraldehyde
Pennroyal oil
Pentachlorophenol
Phenelzine
Phenformin (off the market)
Phenol
Phenylbutazone
Phosphoric acid
Potassium chloroplatinite
Propofol
Propylene glycol
Salicylates
Sorbitol (I.V.)
Strychnine
Surfactant herbicide
Tetracycline (outdated)
Tienilic acid
Toluene
Tranylcypromine
Vacor
Verapamil
Zinc phosphide

Drugs Causing Decreased Anion Gap (<6 mEq/L)

Acidosis

- Acetazolamide
- Ammonium chloride
- Bromide
- Iodide
- Lithium
- Polymyxin B
- Spironolactone
- Sulindac
- Tromethamine

Drugs Causing Osmolar Gap

(by freezing-point depression, gap is >10 mOsm)

- Ethanol
- Ethylene glycol
- Glycerol
- Hypermagnesemia (>9.5 mEq/L)
- Isopropanol (acetone)
- Iodine (questionable)
- Mannitol
- Methanol
- Sorbitol

Toxins Associated With Oxygen Saturation Gap

(>5% difference between measured and calculated value)

- Carbon monoxide
- Cyanide (questionable)
- Hydrogen sulfide (possible)
- Methemoglobin

The Toxicology Laboratory is also very useful for determining levels of toxin in body fluids. Often these drug levels will guide therapy. For example, use of the Rumack-Matthew nomogram for acute acetaminophen poisoning can direct N-acetylcysteine therapy if the serum acetaminophen level falls above the treatment line.

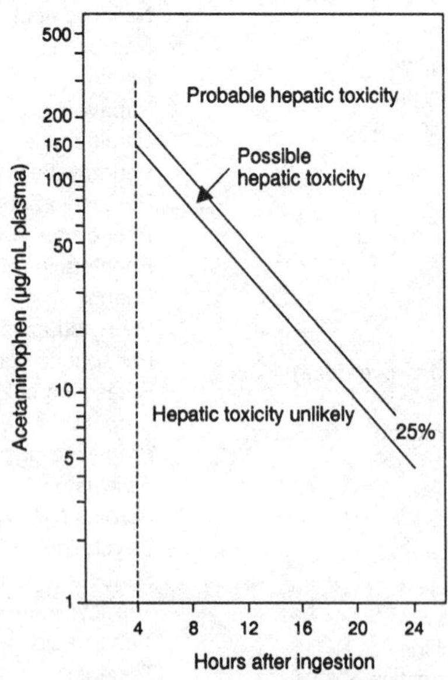

The Rumack-Matthew nomogram, relating expected severity of liver toxicity to serum acetaminophen concentrations. (From Smilkstein MJ et al, *Ann Emerg Med*, 1991, 10:1058.)

Similarly, the Done nomogram is somewhat useful in predicting salicylate toxicity in pediatric patients. Neither nomogram should be utilized with chronic ingestions. Recently, a nomogram has been devised for theophylline ingestion; see the following nomograms.

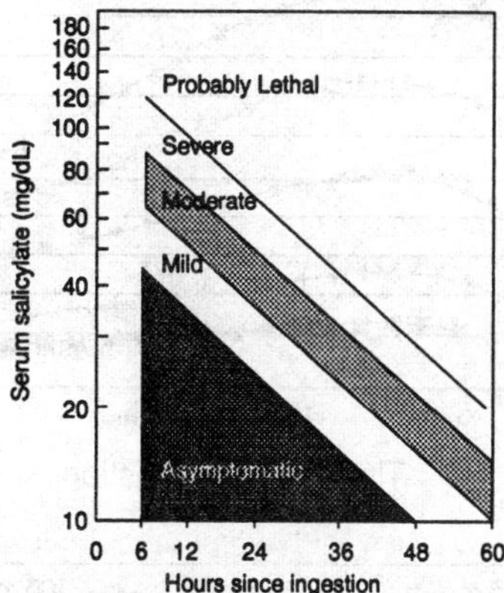

Done nomogram for salicylate poisoning. Note that this nomogram is not accurate for chronic ingestions. (From Done AK, "Salicylate Intoxication: Significance of Measurements of Salicylate in Blood in Cases of Acute Ingestions," *Pediatrics*, 1960, 26:800; copyright American Academy of Pediatrics, 1960.)

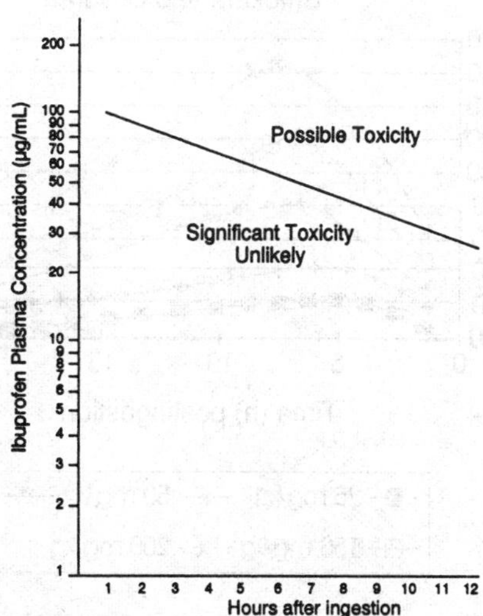

Ibuprofen nomogram, (From Hall AH, Smolinske SC, Stover B, et al, "Ibuprofen Overdose in Adults," *J Toxicol Clin Toxicol*, 1992, 30:34.)

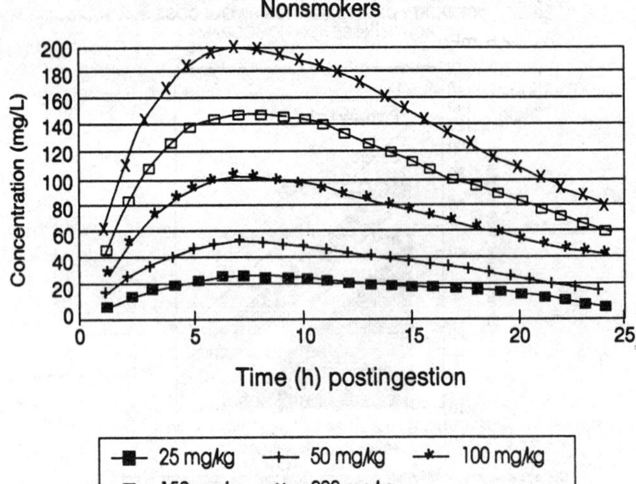

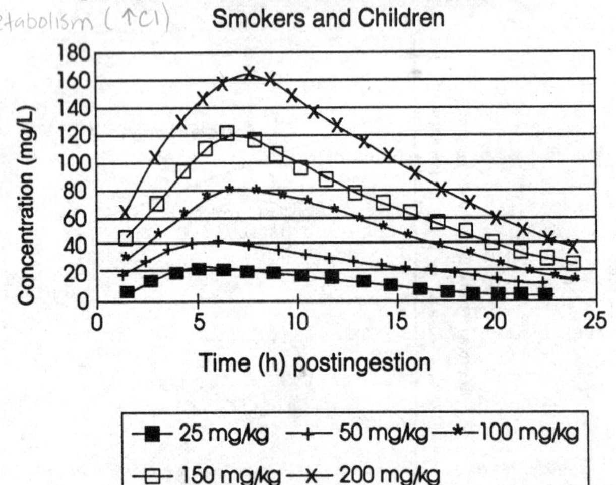

Nomogram for overdose of sustained-release theophylline in 1) nonsmoking adults, and 2) smokers and children. (Courtesy of Frank Paloucek, PharmD, College of Pharmacy, University of Illinois, Chicago.)

Additionally, certain serum levels demand immediate attention when they are obtained. For example, one should consider aggressive treatment in the setting of an acute exposure when one obtains a quantitative level of such toxins as a carboxyhemoglobin level >35% (hyperbaric oxygen), ethylene glycol >20 μg/dL (ethanol therapy with possible hemodialysis), methanol level >20 μg/dL (ethanol therapy with possible hemodialysis), lithium level >2.5 mEq/L (hemodialysis), iron level >350 μg/dL (deferoxamine), methemoglobin level >30% (methylene blue), salicylate level >100 mg/dL (hemodialysis), lead level >45 μg/dL (chelation), or mercury level >3 μg/dL (chelation).

PREVENTION OF ABSORPTION

Toxic substances can enter the body through the dermal, ocular, pulmonary, parenteral, and gastrointestinal routes. The basic principle of decontamination involves appropriate copious irrigation of the toxic substance relatable to the route of exposure. For example, with ocular exposure, this can be done with normal saline for 30-40 minutes through a Morgan therapeutic lens. With alkali exposures, the pH should be checked until the runoff of the solution is either neutral or slightly acidic. Skin decontamination involves removal of the toxin with nonabrasive soap. This should especially be considered for organophosphates, methylene chloride, dioxin, radiation, hydrocarbons, and herbicide exposure. Separate drainage areas should be obtained for the contaminated runoff.

Since >80% of incidents of accidental poisoning in children occur through the gastrointestinal tract, a thorough knowledge of gastric decontamination is essential. There are essentially four modes of gastric decontamination, of which three are physical removal (emesis, gastric lavage, and whole bowel irrigation). Activated charcoal associated with a cathartic is the fourth mode for preventing absorption.

Emesis: Emesis by means of syrup of ipecac (a derivative of the plant alkaloid emetine) has been one of the standards of gastric decontamination; utilized at a dose of 30 mL accompanied with 16 oz of fluid for adults (repeated in 20 minutes if no emesis). Dosage of 15 mL in children 1-12 years of age accompanied with 6-8 oz fluid, or 10 mL in infants 6-12 months of age with 4 oz fluid is virtually 100% effective in producing emesis. However, it is apparent that a 100% rate of emesis is not equatable to a 100% rate of removal of toxin. In the best of circumstances, only about a 30% to 40% removal rate can be achieved within 1-2 hours postingestion, although significantly higher removal rates can be achieved if emesis is obtained within 30 minutes postingestion. For this reason, while ipecac may be quite useful for home use (when administered in consultation with the appropriate healthcare professional), its use as a method of gastric decontamination in the hospital setting is decreasing.[11] The use of salt water, detergents, apomorphine, copper sulfate, and physical induction of emesis should be confined to the medical history books.

Gastric lavage: Gastric lavage through a 28- to 40-French Ewald tube is the second mode of physical removal of the ingested toxin. With the patient in the left lateral decubitus position, feet elevated 15°, approximately 200-300 mL saline is lavaged per run (10-15 mL/kg in children), with an additional 1-2 L used for irrigation after clearing. As with ipecac, an approximate 30% to 40% removal rate can be achieved. The contraindications are ingestion of caustic material, hydrocarbons, hemorrhagic diathesis, and seizures. Lavage should only be considered with an intubated airway with a cuffed endotracheal tube if the gag reflex is lost. Gastric lavage is not a routine procedure for all poisonings. Its use is reserved for life-threatening ingestions of selected agents within 1 hour of the ingestion.

Activated charcoal: The use of activated charcoal has had a resurgence over the past 10 years, with several studies comparing it favorably to the other forms of physical gastric decontamination. As an inert, nontoxic adsorbent with a surface area as high as 3000 m^2/g, it is quite effective in binding high molecular weight compounds due to intermolecular attractions (van der Waals forces). The dose of activated charcoal commonly used is 1 g/kg (can be instilled through an Ewald tube), although data (with theophylline and salicylate) suggest that the optimum dose is 10 g of activated charcoal for every gram of toxin ingested. While children may not want to drink activated charcoal because it is black and gritty, mixing it with juice may bring a higher acceptance rate. Tablets of activated charcoal should not be used for gastric contamination.

Activated charcoal is usually administered in conjunction with a cathartic to facilitate evacuation of the toxic substance. Cathartics most often administered are magnesium sulfate (15-20 g in a 10% solution), magnesium citrate (200-300 mL), sodium sulfate or sorbitol (100-150 mL in a 70% solution, or 0.5-3 mL/kg up to 50 g in pediatric patients). While cathartics may account for an additional 30% of more drug elimination, they should not be used in the presence of ileus. Additionally, recent reports of hypermagnesemia, in the setting of magnesium-containing cathartic administration with renal insufficiency and emesis associated with increasing amounts of sorbitol, indicate that cathartics are not a benign medication.

Whole bowel irrigation: Whole bowel irrigation with the use of GoLYTELY® has been advocated for certain intoxications, most particularly iron, lead, lithium, and the body packer phenomenon. At an adult infusion rate of 1-2 L/hour (250-500 mL/hour in children), it may take 4-6 hours (or 3 L) for complete bowel irrigation until the rectal effluent is clear. It should be considered as a first line decontamination procedure when one encounters a toxin that is not well adsorbed by activated charcoal within 2 hours of ingestion. Contraindications include adynamic ileus, hemorrhage, or bowel obstruction.

ANTIDOTES

One can use as a definition of an antidote any drug that increases the median lethal dose (LD_{50}) of a toxin. While certain drugs may modify symptoms produced by a toxin (ie, beta-blockers reducing heart rate in cocaine intoxication), only a relatively few toxins have specific antidotes (see Antidote chapter). The following table lists some of these antidotes that are commonly utilized.

Poison Control Center Antidote Chart

Antidote	Poison/Drug	Indications	Dosage	Comments
Acetylcysteine (Mucomyst®)	Acetaminophen	Unknown quantity ingested and <24 hours have elapsed since the time of ingestion or unable to obtain serum acetaminophen levels within 12 hours of ingestion. >7.5 g acetaminophen acutely ingested Serum acetaminophen level >150 μg/mL at 4 hours postingestion Acute ingested dose >200 mg/kg if no serum acetaminophen level is available. Evidence of hepatotoxicity or measurable acetaminophen levels more than 24 hours after an acute ingestion.	Dilute to 5% solutions with carbonated beverage, fruit juice, or water and administer orally. **Loading:** 140 mg/kg for 1 dose **Maintenance:** 70 mg/kg for 17 doses, starting 4 hours after the loading dose and given every 4 hours	SGOT, SGPT, bilirubin, prothrombin time, creatinine, BUN, blood sugar, and electrolytes should be obtained daily if a toxic serum acetaminophen level has been determined. **Note:** Activated charcoal has been shown to absorb acetylcysteine *in vitro* and may do so in patients. Serum acetaminophen levels may not peak until 4 hours postingestion, and therefore, serum levels should not be drawn earlier.
Amyl nitrate, sodium nitrate, sodium thiosulfate (cyanide antidote package)	Cyanide	Begin treatment at the first sign of toxicity if exposure is known or strongly expected.	Break ampul of amyl nitrate and allow patient to inhale for 15 seconds, then take away for 15 seconds. Use a fresh ampul every 3 minutes. Continue until injection of sodium nitrate (3% solution) 300 mg (0.15-0.33 mL/kg over 5 minutes in pediatric patients) can be injected at 2.5-5 mL/minute. Then immediately inject 12.5 g 25% sodium thiosulfate, slow I.V. (1.65 mL/kg in children).	If symptoms return, treatment may be repeated at half the normal dosages. For pediatric dosing see package insert. Do **not** use methylene blue to reduce elevated methemoglobin levels. Oxygen therapy may be useful when combined with sodium thiosulfate therapy.

(continued)

Antidote	Poison/Drug	Indications	Dosage	Comments
Antivenin (*Crotalidae*) polyvalent (equine origin)	Pit viper bites (rattlesnakes, cotton-mouths, copperheads)	Mild, moderate, or severe symptoms and history of envenomation by a pit viper **Mild:** Local swelling, (progressive) pain, no systemic systems **Moderate:** Ecchymosis and swelling beyond the bite site, some systemic symptoms and/or lab changes **Severe:** Profound edema involving entire extremity, cyanosis, serious systemic involvement, significant lab changes	**Mild:** 3-5 vials of antivenin in 250-500 mL NS **Moderate:** 6-10 vials of antivenin in 500 mL NS **Severe:** Minimum of 10 vials in 500-1000 mL NS Administer over 4-6 hours. Additional antivenin should be given on the basis of clinical response and continuing assessment of severity of the poisoning.	Draw blood for type and crossmatch, hematocrit, BUN, electrolytes, CBC, platelets, coagulation profile. Do **not** administer heparin for possible allergic reaction. A tetanus shot should also be given.
Atropine	Organophosphate and carbamate insecticides, mushrooms containing muscarine (inocybe or clitocybe)	Myoclonic seizures, severe hallucinations, weakness, arrhythmias, excessive salivation, involuntary urination, and defecation	**Children:** I.V.: 0.05 mg/kg **Adults:** I.V.: 1-2 mg Repeat dosage every 10 minutes until patient is atropinized (normal pulse, dilated pupils, absence of rales, dry mouth)	Caution should be used in patients with narrow-angle glaucoma, cardiovascular disease, or pregnancy. Plasma and/or erythrocyte cholinesterase levels will be depressed from normal. Atropine should only be used when indicated; otherwise, use may result in anticholinergic poisoning. For organophosphate poisoning, large doses of atropine may be required.
Calcium EDTA (calcium disodium versenate)	Lead	Symptomatic patients or asymptomatic children with blood levels >50 μg/dL	50-75 mg/kg/day deep I.M. or slow I.V. infusion in 3-6 divided doses for up to 5 days	If urine flow is not established, hemodialysis must accompany calcium EDTA dosing. In most cases, the I.M. route is preferred.

(continued)

Antidote	Poison/Drug	Indications	Dosage	Comments
Calcium gluconate	Hydrofluoric acid (HF), magnesium, fluoride	Calcium gluconate gel 2.5% for dermal exposures of HF <20% concentration S.C. injections of calcium gluconate for dermal exposures of HF in >20% concentration or failure to respond to calcium gluconate gel Intra-arterial use in a 10% to 20% solution can be utilized in distal extremity burns due to HF.	Massage 2.5% gel into exposed area for 15 minutes. Infiltrate each square centimeter of exposed area with 0.5 mL of 10% calcium gluconate S.C. using a 30-gauge needle. 1 mL/kg I.V. of a 10% solution for magnesium toxicity	Injections of calcium gluconate should not be used in digital area. With exposures to dilute concentrations of HF, symptoms may take several hours to develop. Calcium gluconate gel is not currently available. Contact your regional poison control center for compounding instructions.
Deferoxamine (Desferal®)	Iron	Peak serum iron: >350-500 μg/dL. Inability to obtain serum iron in a reasonable time and patient is symptomatic.	**Mild symptoms:** I.M.: 10 mg/kg up to 1 g every 8 hours **Severe symptoms:** I.V.: 10-15 mg/kg/hour not to exceed 6 g in 24 hours; rates up to 35 mg/kg have been given.	Passing of vin rose-colored urine indicates free iron was present. Therapy should be discontinued when urine returns to normal color. Monitor for hypotension, especially when giving deferoxamine I.V.
Digoxin immune Fab (ovine), (Digibind®)	Digoxin, digitoxin, oleander, foxglove, lily-of-the-valley (?), red squill (?)	Life-threatening cardiac arrhythmias, progressive bradyarrhythmias, second or third degree heart block unresponsive to atropine, serum digoxin level >10 ng/mL in an acute ingestion, potassium levels >5 mEq/L, or ingestion of >10 mg in adults (or 4 mg in children).	Multiply serum digoxin concentration at steady-state level by 5.6 and multiply the result by the patient's weight in kilograms, divide this by 1000 and divide the result by 0.6. This gives the dose in number of vials to use. For other dosing methods, see package insert.	Monitor potassium levels, continuous EKG. **Note:** Digibind® interferes with serum digoxin/digitoxin levels.

(continued)

Antidote	Poison/Drug	Indications	Dosage	Comments
Dimercaprol (BAL in oil)	Arsenic, lead, mercury, gold, trivalent antimony, methyl bromide, methyl iodide	Any symptoms due to arsenic exposure All patients with symptoms or asymptomatic children with blood levels >70 μg/dL Any symptoms due to mercury and patient unable to take D-penicillamine	3-5 mg/kg/dose deep I.M. every 4 hours until GI symptoms subside and patient switched to D-penicillamine 3-5 mg/kg/dose deep I.M. every 4 hours for 2 days then every 4-12 hours for up to 7 additional days 3-5 mg/kg/dose deep I.M. every 4 hours for 48 hours, then 3 mg/kg/dose every 6 hours, then 3 mg/kg/dose every 12 hours for 7 more days	Patients receiving dimercaprol should be monitored for hypertension, tachycardia, hyperpyrexia, and urticaria. Used in conjunction with calcium EDTA in lead poisoning. Cannot be given intravenously Rotate injection sites
Ethanol	Ethylene glycol or methanol	Ethylene glycol or methanol blood levels >20 mg/dL Blood levels not readily available and suspected ingestion of toxic amounts Any symptomatic patient with a history of ethylene glycol or methanol ingestion	**Loading dose:** I.V.: 7.5-10 mL/kg 10% ethanol in D_5W over 1 hour **Maintenance dose:** I.V.: 1.4 mL/kg/hour of 10% ethanol in D_5W. Maintain blood ethanol level of 100-200 mg/dL. Oral dosing: Loading dose: 600-700 mg/kg Maintenance: 125-150 mg/kg Diluted and administered orally as a 20% solution	Monitor blood glucose, especially in children, as ethanol may cause hypoglycemia. Do not use 5% ethanol in D_5W as excessive amounts of fluid would be required to maintain adequate ethanol blood levels. If dialysis is performed, adjustment of ethanol dosing is required.
Flumazenil (Romazicon®)	Benzodiazepine	As adjunct to conventional management of benzodiazepine overdose	I.V.: 0.2 mg over 30 seconds; wait another 30 seconds, and then give an additional 0.3 mg over 30 seconds. Additional doses of 0.5 mg over 30 seconds at 1-minute intervals up to a cumulative dose of 3 mg.	Onset of reversal usually within 1-2 minutes. Contraindicated in patients with epilepsy, increased intracranial pressure, or coingestion of seizuregenic agents (ie, cyclic antidepressant).

(continued)

Antidote	Poison/Drug	Indications	Dosage	Comments
Glucagon	Calcium channel blockers; beta-adrenergic blockers; hypoglycemic agents	Beta-adrenergic blocker or calcium channel blocker-induced cardiac dysfunction Treatment of hypoglycemia	S.C., I.M., or I.V.: 0.5-1 mg May repeat after 15 minutes	Requires liver glycogen stores for hyperglycemic response. Intravenous glucose must also be given in treatment of hypoglycemia.
Leucovorin (citrovorum factor, folinic acid)	Methotrexate, nitrous oxide (?), trimethoprim, pyrimethamine, methanol, trimetrexate	Methotrexate-induced bone marrow depression (methotrexate serum level $>1 \times 10^{-5}$ mmol/L); may also be useful in pyrimethamine-trimethoprim bone marrow depression	Dose should be equal to or greater than the dose of methotrexate ingested. Usually 10-100 mg/m^2 is given I.V. or orally every 6 hours for 72 hours.	Most effective if given within 1 hour after exposure. May not be effective to prevent liver toxicity. Monitor methotrexate levels. May enhance the toxicity of fluorouracil.
Methylene blue	Methemoglobin inducers (ie, nitrites, phenazopyridine)	Cyanosis Methemoglobin level >30% in an asymptomatic patient	I.V.: 1-2 mg/kg (0.1-0.2 mL/kg) per dose over 2-3 minutes. May repeat doses as needed clinically. Injection can be given as 1% solution or diluted in normal saline.	Treatment can result in falsely elevated methemoglobin levels when measured by a co-oximeter. Large doses (>15 mg/kg) may cause hemolysis.
Naloxone (Narcan®)	Opiates (eg, heroin, morphine, codeine)	Coma or respiratory depression from unknown cause or from opiate overdose	Give 0.4-2 mg I.V. bolus. Doses may be repeated if there is no response, up to 10 mg.	For prolonged intoxication, a continuous infusion may be used. See package insert for details or table previously presented in this text titled "Drugs to be Utilized in the Toxic Patient With Altered Mental Status."
D-penicillamine (Cuprimine®)	Arsenic, lead, mercury	Following BAL therapy in symptomatic acutely poisoned patients Asymptomatic patients with excess lead burden Patient symptomatic from mercury exposure or excessive levels	100 mg/kg/day up to 2 g in 4 divided doses for 5 days 1-2 g/day in 4 divided doses for 5 days **Children:** 100 mg/kg/day up to 1 g/day in 4 divided doses. Given for 3-10 days. **Adults:** P.O.: 250 mg 4 times/day	Possible contraindication for patients with penicillin allergy. Monitor heavy metal levels daily in severely poisoned patients. Monitor CBC and renal function in patients receiving chronic D-penicillamine therapy. Dosages given are for short-term acute therapy only.

(continued)

Antidote	Poison/Drug	Indications	Dosage	Comments
Physostigmine salicylate (Antilirium®)	Atropine and anticholinergic agents	Severe arrhythmias, anticholinergic delirium	**Children:** Slow I.V. push (over 3-5 minutes): 0.5 mg. Repeat as required for life-threatening symptoms **Adults:** Slow I.V. push (over 3-5 minutes): 0.5-2 mg	Dramatic reversal of anticholinergic symptoms after I.V. use. Should not be used just to keep patient awake. **Contraindications:** Asthma, gangrene; physostigmine use in cyclic antidepressant-induced cardiac toxicity it controversial. **Extreme caution** is advised — should be considered only in the presence of life-threatening anticholinergic symptoms.
	Intrathecal baclofen	Refractory seizures or arrhythmias unresponsive to conventional therapies	Same as above	
Pralidoxime (2-PAM, Protopam®)	Organophosphate, insecticides, tacrine	An adjunct to atropine therapy for treatment of profound muscle weakness, respiratory depression, muscle twitching	**Children:** 25-50 mg/kg in 250 mL saline over 30 minutes **Adults:** I.V.: 2 g at 0.5 g/minute or infused in 250 mL NS over 30 minutes	Most effective when used in initial 24-36 hours after the exposure. Dosage may be repeated in 1 hour followed by every 8 hours if indicated.
Phytonadione (vitamin K_1)	Coumarin derivatives, indandione derivatives	Large acute ingestion of warfarin rodenticides; chronic exposure or greater than normal prothrombin time	**Children:** I.M.: 1-5 mg. With severe toxicity, vitamin K_1 may be given I.V. **Adults:** I.M.: 10 mg	Vitamin K therapy is relatively contraindicated for patients with prosthetic heart valves unless toxicity is life-threatening.
Protamine sulfate	Heparin	Severe hemorrhage	Maximum rate of 5 mg/minute up to a total dose of 200 mg in 2 hours. 1 mg of protamine neutralizes 90 units of beef lung heparin or 115 units of pork intestinal heparin.	Monitor partial thromboplastin time or activated coagulation time. Effect may be immediate and can last for 2 hours. Monitor for hypotension.

(continued)

Antidote	Poison/Drug	Indications	Dosage	Comments
Pyridoxine (vitamin B_6)	Carbon disulfide (?), isoniazid monomethyl-hydrazine-containing mushrooms (Gyromitra); acrylamide, hydrazine	Unknown overdose or ingested isoniazid (INH) amount >80 mg/kg	I.V. pyridoxine in the amount of INH ingested or 5 g if amount is unknown given over 30-60 minutes.	Cumulative dose of pyridoxine is arbitrarily limited to 40 g in adults and 20 g in children.
Succimer (Chemet®)	Lead, arsenic, mercury	Asymptomatic children with venous blood lead 45-69 μg/dL. Not FDA approved for adult lead exposure or other metals.	P.O.: 10 mg/kg or 350 mg/m^2 every 8 hours for 5 days. Reduce to 10 mg/kg or 350 mg/m^2 every 12 hours for an additional 2 weeks.	Monitor liver function; emits "rotten egg" sulfur odor.

From Rush Poison Control Center, Rush-Presbyterian-St Luke's Medical Center, Chicago, IL 60612.

ENHANCEMENT OF ELIMINATION

Only recently has this aspect of poison management received more than cursory attention in practice and in the literature. The standard practice for enhancement of elimination consisted primarily of forced diuresis in order to excrete the toxin. However, the past 10 years experience has produced a radical change in the approach to this and therefore, a more focused methodology to eliminating absorbed toxins. Essentially, there are three methods by which absorbed toxins may be eliminated: recurrent adsorption with multiple dosings of activated charcoal, use of forced diuresis in combination with possible alkalinization of the urine, and use of dialysis or charcoal hemoperfusion.

Recently, multiple dosing of activated charcoal ("pulse dosing") has been advocated as a method for removal of absorbed drug. This procedure has been demonstrated to be efficacious in drugs that re-enter the gastrointestinal tract through enterohepatic circulation (ie, digitoxin, carbamazepine, glutethimide) and with drugs that diffuse from the systemic circulation into the gastrointestinal tract due to formation of a concentration gradient ("the infinite sink" hypothesis).

Toxins Eliminated by Multiple Dosing of Activated Charcoal

Baclofen (?)
Benzodiazepines (?)
Bupropion (?)
Carbamazepine
Chlordecone
Cyclosporine
Dapsone
Digitoxin
Digoxin (with renal impairment)
Glutethimide
Maprotiline
Meprobamate
Methotrexate
Methyprylon
Nadolol
Phencyclidine (?)
Phenobarbital
Phenylbutazone
Phenytoin (?)
Piroxicam
Propoxyphene
Salicylates (?)
Theophylline
Valproic acid

Essentially, this can be thought of as "intestinal dialysis". The toxins by which this method appears to be most efficacious are those with low volume of distribution (<1.0 L/kg), uncharged, low protein binding, long half-life, and that undergo enterohepatic circulation (although the latter property is not essential). Note that these are similar criteria required for a toxin to be removed by hemoperfusion.

Despite the above limitations, multiple dosing of activated charcoal is utilized quite often. The literature has demonstrated that only chlorpropamide clearance is not enhanced and the data on phenytoin and salicylates are somewhat equivocal due primarily to their high protein binding. The usual dosage of activated charcoal is 1 g/kg as the initial dose, followed by 0.5 g/kg every 2-4 hours. Usually at least three doses are required; cathartics should not be administered more than once daily. Multiple dosing of cholestyramine (4 g every 8 hours) resin may be useful in enhancing elimination of digitoxin, phenobarbital, warfarin, lorazepam, methotrexate, lindane, or chlordecone.

The practice of blindly overloading the toxic patient with intravenous fluids to promote diuresis is not been supported in the literature and is associated with an increased risk of pulmonary edema, hyponatremia, or increased intracranial pressure. Patients who exhibit the syndrome of inappropriate secretion of antidiuretic hormone (SIADH) should not undergo a diuresis. Ion trapping techniques are useful to increse renal excretion of polar drugs with a dissociable group that will carry a charge at a pH that is distant from their pKa. Thus, most of the drug will be ionic (either acidic or alkali) in the distal tubular lumen and in its ionic form will not undergo tubular reabsorption and thus enhance urinary excretion. The use of this modality (with or without ion trapping) should be limited to the following drugs.[12]

Toxins Eliminated by Forced Saline Diuresis

Barium
Bromides
Chromium
Cimetidine (?)
Cis-platinum
Cyclophosphamide
Hydrazine
Iodide
Iodine
Isoniazid (?)
Meprobamate
Methyl iodide
Mushrooms (Group I)
Nickel
Potassium chloroplatinite
Thallium

Toxins Eliminated by Alkaline Diuresis

2,4-D chlorophenoxyacetic acid
Barbital (serum levels >10 mg/dL)
Chlorpropamide
Fluoride
Isoniazid (?)
Mephobarbital
Methotrexate
Phenobarbital
Primidone
Quinolones antibiotic
Salicylates
Sulfisoxazole
Uranium

A urine flow of about 3 mL/kg/hour should be achieved with a combination of isotonic fluids or diuretics. Alkalinization can be achieved by administration of 44-88 mEq of sodium bicarbonate per liter to titrate a urine pH of 7.5; 20-40 mEq/L of potassium chloride may also be required (potassium should not be administered in patients with renal insufficiency). It should be noted that the efficacy of forced diuresis has only been studied for salicylates and phenobarbital. Although several drugs can exhibit enhanced elimination through an acidic urine (quinine, fenfluramine, strychnine, cathinone or khat, amphetamines, phencyclidine, nicotine, bismuth, ephedrine, flecainide), the practice of acidifying the urine should be discouraged in that it can produce metabolic acidosis and promote renal failure in the presence of rhabdomyolysis.

Hemodialysis can be used to increase clearance with the following drugs.

Drugs and Toxins Removed by Hemodialysis

Acetaminophen
Acyclovir
Aluminum
Amanita phalloides (?)
Amantadine (?)
Ammonium chloride
Amphetamine
Anilines
Antimony (Pentavalent) (?)
Atenolol
Boric acid
Bromides
Bromisoval
Calcium
Captopril (?)
Carbamazepine
Carbromal
Carisoprodol
Chloral hydrate
Chromium
Cimetidine (?)
Cyclophosphamide
Dapsone
Disopyramide
Enalapril (?)
Ethanol
Ethosuximide (?)
Ethylene glycol
Famotidine (?)
Fluoride
Folic acid
Formaldehyde
Foscarnet sodium
Gabapentin
Glycol ethers
Hydrazine (?)
Hydrochlorothiazide
Imipenem/Cilastatin
Iodides
Isoniazid
Isopropanol
Ketoprofen
Lithium
Magnesium
Meprobamate
Meropenem
Metal-chelate compounds
Metformin (?)
Methanol
Methaqualone
Methotrexate
Methyldopa
Methylprylone
Metronidazole
Monochloroacetic acid
Nadolol

- Oxalic acid
- Paraldehyde
- Phenelzine (?)
- Phenobarbital
- Phosphoric acid
- Potassium Chloride
- Procainamide
- Quinidine
- Ranitidine (?)
- Rifabutin
- Salicylates
- Sotalol
- Strychnine
- Succimer (?)
- Sulfamethoxazole
- Sulfisoxazole
- Thallium (?)
- Theophylline
- Thiocyanates
- Tranylcypromine sulfate (?)
- Valproic acid (?)
- Verapamil (?)

Hemodialysis is especially effective in correcting metabolic acidosis induced by certain toxins such as salicylates. Criteria utilized for hemodialysis include water solubility of the toxin, low volume of distribution (<1 L/kg), low protein binding (<70% to 80%), polarity, and low molecular weight (<500 daltons). Drugs in which hemodialysis is required at an early stage of intoxication include methanol, ethylene glycol, and boric acid. Hemodialysis also should be definitely used after heavy metal chelation in patients with renal failure.

A lipid-based dialysis (used by adding soy bean oil to an aqueous bath) may be useful in enhancing the elimination of such lipid soluble toxins as ethchlorvynol, glutethimide, camphor, or N,N-diethyltoluamide (DEET), although clinical studies with this modality are minimal. Complications of hemodialysis include hypotension, bleeding (due to systemic anticoagulation), nosocomial infection, or air embolism. Peritoneal dialysis should not be considered for the enhancement of elimination of drugs with the possible exception of vancomycin or boric acid.

Charcoal hemoperfusion can increase clearances of toxins that are absorbed by an adsorbent. Unlike hemodialysis, drug clearance through hemoperfusion is less dependent on water solubility, but on ability of the adsorbent to bind to the drug. Hemoperfusion is most efficacious for phenobarbital, glutethimide, theophylline, and paraquat. The complications of hemoperfusion are analogous to hemodialysis. Additionally, leukopenia, thrombocytopenia, or hypocalcemia may occur.

Drugs and Toxins Removed by Hemoperfusion (Charcoal)

- *Amanita phalloides* (?)
- Atenolol (?)
- Bromisoval
- Bromoethylbutyramide
- Caffeine
- Carbamazepine
- Carbon tetrachloride (?)
- Carbromal
- Chloral hydrate (trichloroethanol)
- Chloramphenicol
- Chlorpropamide
- Colchicine (?)
- Creosote (?)
- Dapsone
- Diltiazem (?)
- Disopyramide
- Ethchlorvynol
- Ethylene oxide
- Glutethimide
- Lindane
- Liotrix
- Meprobamate
- Methaqualone
- Methotrexate
- Methsuximide
- Methyprylon (?)
- Metoprolol (?)
- Nadolol (?)
- Oxalic acid (?)
- Paraquat
- Phenelzine (?)
- Phenobarbital
- Phenytoin
- Podophyllin (?)
- Procainamide (?)
- Quinidine (?)
- Rifabutin (?)
- Sotalol (?)
- Thallium (?)
- Thyroglobulin/Thyroid hormone
- Theophylline
- Verapamil (?)

Exchange transfusion is a useful modality to enhance drug elimination in neonatal or infant drug toxicity. Usually double or triple volume exchanges are performed. It has been utilized to treat barbiturate, iron, caffeine, sodium nitrite, or theophylline overdose.

SUPPORT AND MONITORING FOR ADVERSE EFFECTS

This aspect of poison management is the least studied. The usual disposition of the admitted poisoned patient is an intensive care unit bed or cardiac monitored bed to evaluate the late sequelae of the toxic agent. However, the practice of admitting the poisoned patient routinely to the intensive care unit is being questioned. A recent retrospective study identified eight clinical risk factors that predicted ICU interventions: (1) arterial carbon dioxide pressure ≥45 mm Hg, (2) need for emergency intubation, (3) seizures, (4) cardiac arrhythmia, (5) QRS duration ≥0.12 seconds, (6) systolic blood pressure <80 mm Hg, (7) second- or third-degree atrioventricular block, and (8) unresponsiveness to verbal stimuli.[13] If a toxic patient did not exhibit any of these characteristics, no ICU interventions (such as intubation, antiseizure therapy, intravenous vasopressors, antiarrhythmics, and dialysis or hemoperfusion) were performed.

Additionally, other risk factors that should be considered for ICU admission include the need for emergent hemodialysis or hemoperfusion, increasing metabolic acidosis, and any tricyclic or phenothiazine overdose manifesting anticholinergic signs of cardiac abnormalities.[14] While many drugs (such as ibuprofen) will manifest their toxicity within 4 hours after ingestion, tricyclic overdoses are renowned for their incidence of delayed complications.[15] It has been noted that most of these patients exhibited cardiac or neurologic abnormality prior to the delayed arrhythmia. The following are criteria for ICU admission.

Criteria for Admission of the Poisoned Patient to ICU

- Respiratory depression (pCO_2 >45 mm Hg)
- Emergency intubation
- Seizures
- Cardiac arrhythmia
- Hypotension (systolic blood pressure <80 mm Hg
- Unresponsiveness to verbal stimuli
- Second- or third-degree atrioventricular block
- Emergent dialysis or hemoperfusion
- Increasing metabolic acidosis
- Tricyclic or phenothiazine overdose manifesting anticholinergic signs, neurologic abnormality, QRS duration >0.12 second, or QT duration >0.5 seconds
- Administration of pralidoxime in organophosphate toxicity
- Pulmonary edema induced by drugs or toxic inhalation (ARDS)
- Drug-induced hypothermia or hyperthermia including neuroleptic malignant syndrome
- Hyperkalemia secondary to digitalis overdose
- Any use of digoxin-immune Fab fragments
- Body packers and stuffers
- Concretions secondary to drugs
- Emergent surgical intervention
- Antivenom administration in *Crotalidae*, coral snake, or arthropod envenomation
- Need for continuous infusion of naloxone

pCO_2 = carbon dioxide pressure
ARDS = adult respiratory distress syndrome

Adapted from Kulling P, Persson H, "Role of the Intensive Care Unit in the Management of the Poisoned Patient," *Med Toxicol*, 1986, 1:375-86 and Brett AS, Rothschild N, Gray R, et al, "Predicting the Clinical Course in Intentional Drug Overdose: Implication for Use of the Intensive Care Unit, *Arch Intern Med*, 1987, 147:133-7, and Callaham M, "Admission Criteria for Tricyclic Antidepressant Ingestion, *West J Med*, 1982, 137:425-9.

— This introductory text was written by
Jerrold B. Leikin, MD
Paul K. Hanashiro, MD
Rush-Presbyterian-St Luke's Medical Center

FOOTNOTES

1. Nice A, Leikin JB, Maturen A, et al, "Toxidrome Recognition to Improve Efficiency of Emergency Urine Drug Screens," *Ann Emerg Med*, 1988, 17(7):676-80.
2. Litovitz TL, Holm KC, Clancy C, et al, "Annual Report of the American Association of Poison Control Centers National Data Collection System," *Am J Emerg Med*, 1994, 12:546-84.
3. Noji EK and Kelen EK, eds, *Manual of Toxicologic Emergencies*, Chicago, IL: Year Book Medical Publishers, 1989.
4. Rumack BH and Spoerke DS, eds, *Poisondex* Information System, Denver: Micromedex, Inc, Vol 82, edition expires 11/30/94.
5. Goldfrank LR, ed, *Toxicologic Emergencies*, Norwalk, CT: Appleton-Century-Crofts, 5th ed, 1994.
6. Ellenhorn MJ and Barceloux DG, eds, *Medical Toxicology: Diagnosis and Treatment of Human Poisoning*, New York, NY, 1988.
7. Bryson PD, ed, *Comprehensive Review in Toxicology*, 2nd ed, Rockville, MD: Aspen Publications, 1989.
8. Kulig K, "Initial Management of Ingestions of Toxic Substances," *N Engl J Med*, 1992, 326(25):1677-81.
9. Leikin JB, Krantz A, Zell-Kanter M, et al, "Clinical Features and Management of Intoxication Due to Hallucinogenic Drugs," *Med Toxicol Adverse Drug Exp*, 1989, 4(5):324-53.
10. Tillman DJ, Ruggles DL, and Leikin JB, "Radiopacity Study of Extended-Release Formulations Using Digitalized Radiography," *Am J Emerg Med*, 1994, 12(3):310-4.
11. Merigian KS, Woodard M, Hedges JR, et al, "Prospective Evaluation of Gastric Emptying in the Self-Poisoned Patient," *Am J Emerg Med*, 1990, 8(6):479-83.
12. Garrettson LK and Geller RJ, "Acid and Alkaline Diuresis: When Are They of Value in the Treatment of Poisoning?" *Drug Saf*, 1990, 5(3):220-32.
13. Brett AS, Rothschild N, Gray R, et al, "Predicting the Clinical Course in Intentional Drug Overdose: Implications for Use of the Intensive Carte Unit," *Arch Intern Med*, 1987, 147(1):133-7.
14. Kulling P and Persson H, "Role of the Intensive Care Unit in the Management of the Poisoned Patient," *Med Toxicol*, 1986, 1(5):375-86.
15. Callaham M, "Admission Criteria for Tricyclic Antidepressant Ingestion," *West J Med*, 1982, 137(5):425-9.

REFERENCES

"Critical Care Toxicology," *Contemporary Management in Critical Care*, Vol 1, Hoffman RS and Goldfrank LR, eds, New York: Churchill Livingston, 1991.

Gentry CA, Paloucek FP, and Rodvold KA, "Prediction of Acetaminophen Concentrations in Overdose Patients Using a Bayesian Pharmacokinetic Model," *J Toxicol Clin Toxicol*, 1994, 32(1):17-30.

Hall AH, Smolinske SC, Stover B, et al, "Ibuprofen Overdose in Adults," *J Toxicol Clin Toxicol*, 1992, 30(1):23-37.

Hoffman RS and Goldfrank LR, "The Poisoned Patient With Altered Consciousness," *JAMA*, 1995, 274:562-9.

Newton EH, Shih RD, and Hoffman RS, "Cyclic Antidepressant Overdose: A Review of Current Management Strategies," *Am J Emerg Med*, 1994, 12(3):376-9.

Paloucek FP and Rodvold KA, "Evaluation of Theophylline Overdoses and Toxicities," *Ann Emerg Med*, 1988, 17(2):135-44.

Shannon M, "Hypokalemia, Hyperglycemia, and Plasma Catecholamine Activity After Severe Theophylline Intoxication," *J Toxicol Clin Toxicol*, 1994, 32(1):41-7.

248-2 *see* Tenidap *on page 725*

A-64077 *see* Zileuton *on page 811*

Abbokinase® Injection *see* Urokinase *on page 779*

Abciximab

Brand Names ReoPro®

Synonyms C7E3 FAB; C7EC

Use For patients undergoing coronary angioplasty or atherectomy to act as an antiplatelet agent; intended to use with aspirin and heparin with coronary ischemia

Mechanism of Action Fab antibody fragment of the chimeric human-murine monoclonal antibody 7E3; this agent binds to platelets resulting in steric hindrance, thus inhibiting platelet aggregation

Adverse Reactions

Cardiovascular: Hypotension, fibrillation (atrial) or flutter (3.5%), tachycardia (ventricular), complete A-V block

Central nervous system: Dizziness (2%), coma, insomnia, hyperesthesia, dysphonia

Dermatologic: Pruritus

Gastrointestinal: Diarrhea (1%), ileus

Genitourinary: Urinary retention, urinary tract infection

Neuromuscular & skeletal: Myopathy

Miscellaneous: Anaphylaxis, bleeding (~15%)

Signs & Symptoms of Acute Overdose Thrombocytopenia

Toxicodynamics/Kinetics Half-life: ~30 minutes

Usual Dosage I.V. bolus: 0.25 mg/kg given 10-60 minutes before the start of angioplasty followed by continuous I.V. infusion of 10 mcg/minute for 12 hours

Contraindications Acute internal bleeding, gastrointestinal or genitourinary bleeding within 6 weeks; history of stroke within 2 years or residual neurological deficit, bleeding diathesis, oral anticoagulants administration within 1 week (unless prothrombin time is <1.2 times control), major surgery or trauma within 6 weeks, intracranial neoplasm, arteriovenous malformation, aneurysm, uncontrolled high blood pressure, vasculitis, use of I.V. dextran, allergy to abciximab or murine proteins

Dosage Forms Injection, preservative free: 2 mg/mL (5 mL) (contains 10 ng of antibody Fab fragment)

Overdosage Treatment

Supportive therapy: Essentially no overdose experience; anaphylaxis may be treated with standard treatment; discontinue heparin; use pressure techniques if bleeding develops

Pregnancy Risk Factor C

Monitoring Parameters Bleeding time, prothrombin/coagulation parameters, CBC, platelet count

Additional Information Platelet aggregation returns to ≥50% baseline within 24 hours in 62% of patients and within 48 hours in 88% of patients; bleeding time falls <12 minutes within 12 hours in 75% of patients and within 24 hours in 90% of patients; may reduce restenosis rate. Risk factors for major bleeding episodes are female gender, increasing age, and lower body weight.

Specific References

Aguirre FV, Topol EJ, and Ferguson JJ, "EPIC Investigators: Bleeding Complications With the Chimeric Antibody to Platelet Glycoprotein IIb/IIIa Integrin in Patients Undergoing Percutaneous Coronary Intervention," *Circulation*, 1995, 91:2882-90.

Azrin MA, "The Use of Antibodies in Clinical Cardiology," *Am Heart J*, 1992, 124(3):753-68.

The EPIC Investigators, "Use of a Monoclonal Antibody Directed Against the Platelet Glycoprotein IIb/IIIa Receptor in High-Risk Coronary Angioplasty," *N Engl J Med*, 1994, 330(14):956-61.

Ward SR and Topol EJ, "New Strategies for the Prevention of Restenosis After Coronary Angioplasty," *Resident and Staff Physician*, 1995, 41(3):11-8.

Weitz J and Hirsh J, "New Anticoagulant Strategies," *J Lab Clin Med*, 1993, 122(4):364-73.

Abicol® *see* Reserpine *on page 678*

AC-4464 *see* Torsemide *on page 761*

Acalix® *see* Diltiazem *on page 287*

Accupril® *see* Quinapril Hydrochloride *on page 667*

Accuprin® *see* Quinapril Hydrochloride *on page 667*

Accupro® *see* Quinapril Hydrochloride *on page 667*

Accurbron® *see* Theophylline *on page 735*

Accutane® *see* Isotretinoin *on page 447*

Acebutolol Hydrochloride (a se byoo' toe lole)

Related Information

Beta-Blockers Comparison *on page 1644-1645*

CAS Number 37517-30-9; 34381-68-5

Brand Names Alol®; Prent®; Secadrex®; Sectral®; Wesfalin®

(Continued)

Acebutolol Hydrochloride *(Continued)*

Use Treatment of hypertension; ventricular arrhythmias; angina

Mechanism of Action Competitively blocks $beta_1$-adrenergic receptors with little or no effect on $beta_2$-receptors except at high doses; consider renal function. Exhibits membrane stabilizing and intrinsic sympathomimetic activity ("quinidine-like effect"); low lipid solubility, therefore, little crosses blood-brain barrier.

Adverse Reactions

Cardiovascular: Persistent bradycardia, hypotension, chest pain, edema, heart failure, cutaneous vasculitis, exacerbation of Raynaud's phenomenon

Central nervous system: CNS depression, confusion, dizziness, fatigue, drowsiness, night terrors, insomnia, headache, electroencephalogram abnormalities

Gastrointestinal: Constipation, diarrhea, nausea, vomiting

Genitourinary: Impotence

Hepatic: Elevated liver enzymes

Respiratory: Hypersensitivity pneumonitis, pleurisy, pulmonary granulomas

Miscellaneous: Hyperhidrosis, cold extremities, lupus syndrome

Signs & Symptoms of Acute Overdose Bradycardia, wheezing, dyspepsia, ataxia, flatulence, dyspnea, nocturia, insomnia, impotence, myalgia, hypoglycemia, depression, first degree A-V block, myasthenia gravis (exacerbation or precipitation of), hyperglycemia, heart failure, hypotension, QRS prolongation, cough, cardiovascular collapse, electromechanical dissociation, asystole

Toxicodynamics/Kinetics

Peak effect: 2.5-3.5 hours

Absorption: Oral: Well absorbed (70%)

Distribution: V_d: 1.2 L/kg; distributed into milk; low lipid solubility

Protein binding: 26%

Metabolism: Undergoes extensive first-pass metabolism; has active metabolite (diacetolol); undergoes extensive enterohepatic recirculation

Bioavailability: 40%

Half-life:

Acebutolol: 3-4 hours (in overdose it may be as long as 8 hours)

Diacetolol: 8-13 hours (in overdose 15 hours)

Time to reach peak serum concentration: Within 2-4 hours

Elimination: Primarily by bile and intestinal wall 50% to 60%; some hepatic occurs; renal excretion 30% to 40%; clearance: 615 mL/minute

Usual Dosage Adults: Oral: 400-800 mg/day in 2 divided doses

Dosing adjustment in renal impairment:

Cl_{cr} 10-50 mL/minute: Reduce dose by 50%

Cl_{cr} <10 mL/minute: Reduce dose by 75%

Not removed by hemodialysis or peritoneal dialysis

Dosing comments in hepatic impairment: Use with caution

Contraindications Uncompensated congestive heart failure; cardiogenic shock; bradycardia or heart block; hypersensitivity to acebutolol or related compounds

Warnings Abrupt withdrawal of beta-blockers may result in an exaggerated cardiac beta-adrenergic responsiveness. Symptomatology has included reports of tachycardia, hypertension, ischemia, angina, myocardial infarction, and sudden death. It is recommended that patients be tapered gradually off of beta-blockers over a 2-week period rather than via abrupt discontinuation. Use with caution in patients with diabetes, renal function decline, myasthenia gravis, and severe peripheral vascular disease.

Dosage Forms Capsule: 200 mg, 400 mg

Reference Range Fatalities associated with plasma levels >13,000 ng/mL (4 hours)

Overdosage Treatment

Decontamination: Lavage/activated charcoal with cathartic

Supportive therapy: Initiate support with fluids, epinephrine or dopamine may be useful; glucagon may be particularly effective for reversing cardiac manifestations; sympathomimetics (eg, epinephrine, dopamine, or amrinone), glucagon, or a pacemaker can be used to treat the toxic bradycardia, asystole, and/or hypotension

Enhancement of elimination: Multiple dose of activated charcoal may be effective

Test Interactions Increases triglycerides, potassium, uric acid, cholesterol (S), glucose; decreases HDL

Drug Interactions Nonsteroidal anti-inflammatory agents, salicylates, sympathomimetics, thyroid hormones, insulins, lidocaine, calcium channel blockers, nifedipine, catecholamine-depleting drugs, clonidine, disopyramide, prazosin, theophylline; enhanced effects with nicergoline (ergot alkaloid)

Pregnancy Risk Factor B (may induce fetal/neonatal bradycardia and tachypnea)

Monitoring Parameters Blood pressure, hypotension (orthostatic), heart rate, CNS effects

Patient Information Do not discontinue medication abruptly, sudden stopping of medication may precipitate or cause angina; consult pharmacist or physician before taking with other adrenergic drugs (eg, cold medications); notify physician if any of the following symptoms occur: difficult breathing, night cough, swelling of extremities, slow pulse, dizziness, lightheadedness, confusion, depression, skin rash, fever, sore throat, unusual bleeding or bruising; may produce drowsiness, dizziness, lightheadedness, blurred vision, confusion; use with caution while driving or performing tasks requiring alertness; may mask signs of hypoglycemia in diabetics; may be taken without regard to meals

Additional Information Since bioavailability increased in elderly about twofold, elderly patients may require lower maintenance doses; therefore, as serum and tissue concentrations increase, $beta_1$ selectivity diminishes

Specific References

Jean P, Arditti J, Jouglard J, et al, "Acute Acebutolol Poisoning," *Therapie*, 1984, 39(1):49-50.

Nicolas F, Villers D, Rozo L, et al, "Severe Self Poisoning With Acebutolol in Association With Alcohol," *Crit Care Med*, 1987, 15(2):173-4.

Sangster B, de Wildt D, and van Dijk A, "A Case of Acebutolol Intoxication," *Clin Toxicol*, 1983, 20(1):69-77.

Schmutz JL, Houet C, Trechot P, et al, "Sweating and Beta-Adrenoceptor Antagonists," *Dermatology*, 1995, 190(1):86.

Tanner LA, Bosco LA, and Zimmerman HJ, "Hepatic Toxicity After Acebutolol Therapy," *Ann Intern Med*, 1989, 111(6):533-4.

ACE Inhibitors Comparison *see page 1636*

Acephen® [OTC] *see* Acetaminophen *on this page*

Acepril® *see* Captopril *on page 181*

Acequin® *see* Quinapril Hydrochloride *on page 667*

Acetaminophen (a seet a min' oh fen)

Related Information

Oxycodone and Acetaminophen *on page 584*

Propoxyphene and Acetaminophen *on page 656*

CAS Number 103-90-2

Brand Names Acephen® [OTC]; Aceta® [OTC]; Anacin-3® [OTC]; Apacet® [OTC]; Banesin® [OTC]; Dapa® [OTC]; Datril® [OTC]; Dorcol® [OTC]; Feverall™ [OTC]; Genapap® [OTC]; Halenol® [OTC]; Liquiprin® Infant Drops [OTC]; Meda-Cap® [OTC]; Myapap® Drops [OTC]; Neopap® [OTC]; Panadol® [OTC]; Redutemp® [OTC]; Snaplets-FR® Granules [OTC]; Tempra® [OTC]; Tylenol® [OTC]; Ty-Pap [OTC]; Uni-Ace® [OTC]

Synonyms Paracetamol

Adverse Reactions

Cardiovascular: Rare cardiomyopathy, bradycardia

Central nervous system: Hypothermia

Dermatologic: Rash, toxic epidermal necrolysis

Endocrine & metabolic: Elevations of serum transaminases, hyponatremia, hypophosphatemia

Gastrointestinal: Vomiting, nausea, diarrhea, pancreatitis

Hepatic: Hepatic encephalopathy, fulminant hepatitis, jaundice, cirrhosis, liver transaminase rise may occur within 24 hours of ingestion

Ocular: Mydriasis, nystagmus, vision color changes (yellow tinge)

Renal: Renal injury with chronic use, acute tubular necrosis, renal failure (acute) is uncommon (0.4%) in overdose

Miscellaneous: Hypersensitivity reactions (rare)

Signs & Symptoms of Acute Overdose The acute symptomatic presentation of acetaminophen toxicity can be divided into 4 phases:

Phase I (up to 1 day): Gastrointestinal irritability predominates with nausea, vomiting, and sweating developing; large ingestions (>75 g in adults; >10 g in pediatric patients) can result in metabolic acidosis within 4 hours of ingestion; cardiac effects (arrhythmias, bradycardia) may develop

Phase II (1-3 days): Hepatic toxicity develops with elevation of hepatic enzymes, prothrombin time, and bilirubin; amylase elevation may peak at 2 days; patient may be otherwise asymptomatic. Oliguric renal failure may develop and may coincide with hepatic encephalopathy

Phase III (3-5 days): Hepatic necrosis continues with disseminated intravascular coagulation, hepatic encephalopathy, portal hypertension, and icterus developing; patient is at risk for hypoglycemia; renal insufficiency may also be present

Phase IV (5-14 days): Recovery with resolution of elevated hepatic enzymes usually occurring

Toxicodynamics/Kinetics

Distribution: V_d: 0.95 L/kg

Protein binding: <50%

Metabolism: Hepatic by glucuronidation (60%), sulfation (30%), and through N-acetyl-p-benzoquinoneimine (NAPQI-4%) which can cause hepatic necrosis in the setting of glutathione depletion

(Continued)

Acetaminophen *(Continued)*

Half-life: 2 hours

Usual Dosage Oral, rectal (if fever not controlled with acetaminophen alone, give with full doses of aspirin on an every 4- to 6-hour schedule):

Children <12 years: 10-15 mg/kg/dose every 4-6 hours as needed; do **not** exceed 5 doses (2.6 g) in 24 hours; alternatively, the following doses may be used; see table.

Acetaminophen Dosing

Age	Dosage (mg)	Age	Dosage (mg)
0-3 mo	40	4-5 y	240
4-11 mo	80	6-8 y	320
1-2 y	120	9-10 y	400
2-3 y	160	11 y	480

Adults: 325-650 mg every 4-6 hours or 1000 mg 3-4 times/day; do **not** exceed 4 g/day

Toxic dosage for hepatitis: 200 mg/kg

Dosing interval in renal impairment:

Cl_{cr} 10-50 mL/minute: Administer every 6 hours

Cl_{cr} <10 mL/minute: Administer every 8 hours (metabolites accumulate)

Dosing adjustment/comments in hepatic impairment: Appears to be well tolerated in cirrhosis; serum levels may need monitoring with long-term use

Nomogram: Plasma or Serum Acetaminophen Concentration vs Time Post Acetaminophen Ingestion*

Estimating potential for hepatotoxicity:
The following nomogram has been developed to estimate the probability that plasma levels in relation to intervals postingestion will result in hepatotoxicity.

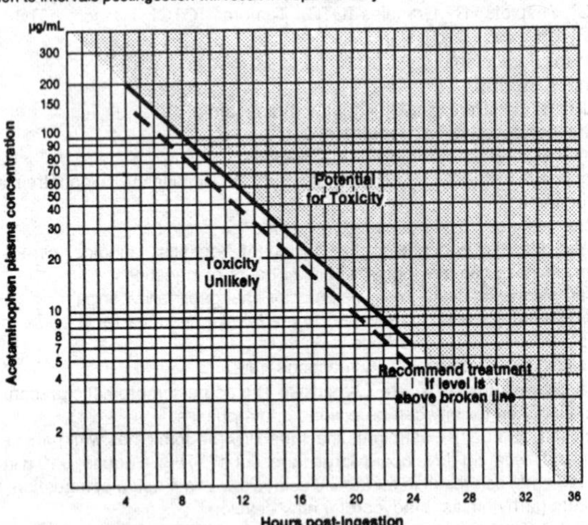

* Adapted from Rumack and Matthew, *Pediatrics*, 55:876, 1975.

If the acetaminophen level determined at least 4 hours following an overdose falls above the broken line, administer the entire course of acetylcysteine treatment.

If the acetaminophen level, determined at least 4 hours following an overdose, falls below the broken line, acetylcysteine treatment is not necessary or if already initiated may be discontinued. Serum levels drawn before 4 hours may not represent peak levels.

Cautions For Use of This Chart:

1. The time coordinates refer to time postingestion.
2. The graph relates only to plasma levels following a single acute overdose ingestion.
3. The broken line, which represents a 25% allowance below the solid line, is included to allow for possible errors in acetaminophen plasma assays and estimated time from ingestion of an overdose.

Dosage Forms

Caplet: 160 mg, 325 mg, 500 mg

Capsule: 325 mg, 500 mg
Drops: 100 mg/mL (15 mL); 120 mg/2.5 mL (35 mL)
Granules, premeasured packs: 80 mg (32s)
Elixir: 120 mg/5 mL (5 mL, 10 mL, 13.5 mL, 25 mL, 27 mL, 120 mL, 480 mL, 3780 mL); 130 mg/5 mL (12.5 mL, 25 mL); 160 mg/5 mL (5 mL, 10 mL, 20 mL, 120 mL, 240 mL, 500 mL, 3780 mL); 325 mg/5 mL (480 mL, 3780 mL)
Liquid, oral: 160 mg/5 mL (2.5 mL, 5 mL, 60 mL, 120 mL, 240 mL, 480 mL); 500 mg/15 mL (240 mL)
Powder, in capsules: 80 mg, 160 mg
Suppository, rectal: 120 mg, 125 mg, 300 mg, 325 mg, 650 mg
Suspension, oral: 48 mg/mL, 100 mg/mL, 160 mg/mL
Tablet: 120 mg, 325 mg, 500 mg, 650 mg
Tablet, chewable: 80 mg, 120 mg, 160 mg

Reference Range Patients with concentrations >150 mg/L before 4 hours can be empirically treated with acetylcysteine until repeat concentration after 4 hours has been obtained and interpreted; analgesic/antipyretic reference range: 10-30 mg/L (66-199 μmol/L)

Overdosage Treatment

Decontamination: Ipecac for ingestions >200 mg/kg if available at home or pre-hospital only; lavage within 1 hour of overdose, activated charcoal with cathartic if <4 hours following ingestion

Supportive therapy: Acetylcysteine (antidote) indicated for:

Any patient with a serum concentration above probable risk line on Rumack-Matthew nomogram

Any patient presenting ≥24 hours following an ingestion with evidence of hepatic toxicity

Empirically for any ingestion of ≥200 mg/kg where availability of serum concentration results exceeds 8 hours following ingestion; N-acetylcysteine is given 140 mg/kg followed by 70 mg/kg every 4 hours for 17 doses; although shorter 20-48 intravenous courses can be used also

STEPWISE MANAGEMENT
OF ACUTE ACETAMINOPHEN OVERDOSE

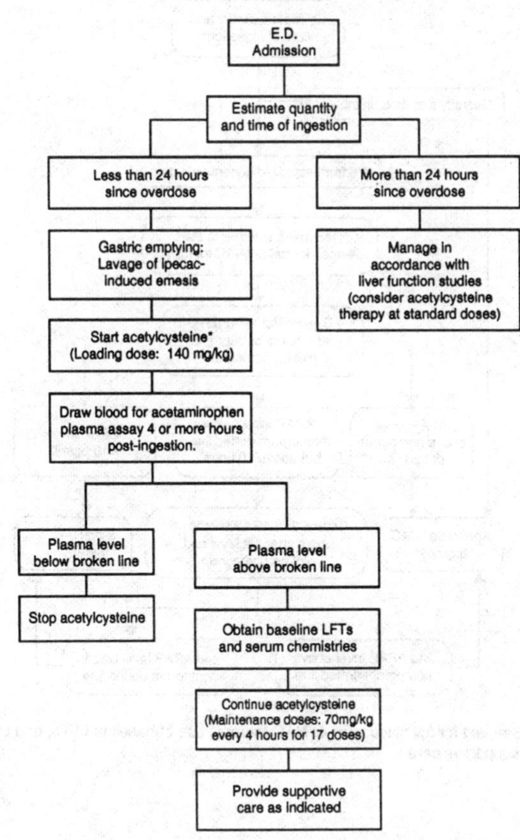

Enhancement of elimination: Multiple dosing of activated charcoal may be effective, but is usually not required if N-acetylcysteine therapy is given; forced diuresis is of no benefit; hemodialysis removes significant amounts of acetaminophen especially in patients with severe hepatic and renal dysfunction; usually not required if acetylcysteine given; moderately dialyzable (20% to 50%)

Antidote(s)

Acetylcysteine *on page 1388*

Test Interactions Can cause false elevation of urinary catecholamine levels

Diagnostic Tests/Procedures

Acetaminophen, Serum *on page 1180*

Drug Interactions Chronic ethanol abuse increases risk for acetaminophen hepatotoxicity; increased incidence of hepatotoxicity with concomitant administration of isoniazid

Pregnancy Risk Factor B

Pregnancy Implications Fetal liver toxicity can occur in overdose situations

Monitoring Parameters AST, ALT, PT, PTT, CBC, bilirubin, electrolytes, acetaminophen concentrations

Additional Information Cimetidine is not effective for hepatoprotection in acetaminophen overdose

MANAGEMENT OF ACUTE ACETAMINOPHEN (APAP) OVERDOSE TYLENOL® acetaminophen Extended Release

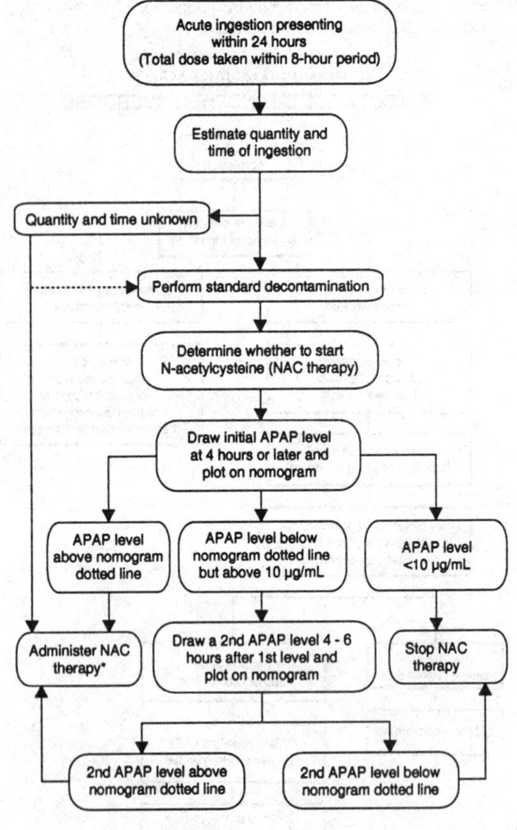

* See text for full discussion of NAC therapy, use of baseline LFTs, and other supportive care

The 4-hour serum concentration can be approximated by 0.59 x amount ingested as mg/kg; acetylcysteine is not useful for treatment of renal disease induced by acetaminophen. For extended relief product ingestions, draw an acetaminophen level at least 4 hours postingestion; a second and third acetaminophen level should be drawn every 4-6 hours after the initial level. These levels should be plotted on the Rumack/Matthew nomogram at the times each were drawn; if any of the plasma levels are above the hepatotoxic line on the Rumack/Matthew nomogram, the entire course of acetylcysteine treatment should be administered or if initiated, completed. Increased risk of liver toxicity in individuals ingesting 3 or more ethanol-containing beverages daily. See flow chart of "Management of Acute Acetaminophen Overdose for Tylenol® Extended Release."

Specific References

Burkhart KK, et al, "Cimetidine as Adjunctive Treatment for Acetaminophen Overdose," *Hum Exp Toxicol*, 1995, 14:299-304.

Douglas DR, Smilkstein MJ, and Sholar JB, "Overdose With Extended-Relief Acetaminophen: Is a New Approach Necessary?" *Acad Emerg Med*, 1995, 2:397.

Graudins A, Aaron CK, and Linden CH, "Overdose of Extended-Release Acetaminophen," *N Engl J Med*, 1995, 333:196.

Harrison PM, Keays R, Bray GP, et al, "Improved Outcome of Paracetamol-Induced Fulminant Hepatic Failure by Late Administration of Acetylcysteine," *Lancet*, 1990, 335(8705):1572-3.

Janes J and Routledge PA, "Recent Developments in the Management of Paracetamol (Acetaminophen) Poisoning," *Drug Saf*, 1992, 7(3):170-7.

Katzir Z, Baruch O, Hochman B, et al, "Spontaneous Remission of Paracetamol Induced Acute Renal Failure," *Clin Nephrol*, 1995, 43:346.

Knoop KJ, Snook CP, Stephan M, et al, "Failure of N-Acetylcysteine (NAC) to Prevent Acetaminophen-Induced Renal Failure," *Vet Hum Toxicol*, 1993, 35:336.

Lewis RK and Paloucek FP, "Assessment and Treatment of Acetaminophen Overdose," *Clin Pharm*, 1991, 10(10):765-74.

Singer AJ and Carracio TR, "Mofenson: The Temporal Profile of Increased Transaminase Levels in Patients With Acetaminophen-Induced Liver Dysfunction," *Ann Emerg Med*, 1995, 26:49-53.

Smilkstein MJ, Knapp GL, Kulig KW, et al, "Efficacy of Oral N-Acetylcysteine in the Treatment of Acetaminophen Overdose. Analysis of the National Multicenter Study (1976 to 1985)," *N Engl J Med*, 1988, 319(24):1557-62.

Whitcomb DC and Block GD, "Association of Acetaminophen Hepatotoxicity With Fasting and Ethanol Use," *JAMA*, 1994, 272:1845-50.

Acetaminophen and Aspirin

(a seet a min' oh fen, as' pir in, & kaf' een)

Brand Names Excedrin®, Extra Strength [OTC]

Use Relief of mild to moderate pain

Signs & Symptoms of Acute Overdose

Dermatologic: Rash

Gastrointestinal: Nausea, vomiting, gastrointestinal distress, bleeding,

Hematologic: Platelet inhibition, gastrointestinal bleeding

Hepatic: Hepatotoxicity

Renal: Renal injury with chronic use, tubular necrosis

Respiratory: Wheezing

Miscellaneous: Hypersensitivity reactions (rare)

Usual Dosage Adults: Oral: 1-2 tablets every 2-6 hours as needed for pain

Dosage Forms Tablet: Acetaminophen 125 mg and aspirin 240 mg with caffeine 32 mg; acetaminophen 250 mg and aspirin 250 mg with caffeine 65 mg

Overdosage Treatment See individual monographs for Acetaminophen and Aspirin

Pregnancy Risk Factor D

Acetaminophen and Oxycodone *see* Oxycodone and Acetaminophen *on page 584*

Aceta® [OTC] *see* Acetaminophen *on page 79*

Acetazolamide (a set a zole' a mide)

CAS Number 59-66-5

Brand Names AK-Zol®; Dazamide®; Diamox®

Use Lowers intraocular pressure to treat glaucoma, also as a diuretic, adjunct treatment of refractory seizures and acute altitude sickness; centrencephalic epilepsies (sustained release not recommended for anticonvulsant)

Mechanism of Action Reversible inhibition of the enzyme carbonic anhydrase resulting in reduction of hydrogen ion secretion at renal tubule and an increased renal excretion of sodium, potassium, bicarbonate, and water to decrease production of aqueous humor; also inhibits carbonic anhydrase in central nervous system to retard abnormal and excessive discharge from CNS neurons

Adverse Reactions

Cardiovascular: Cyanosis

(Continued)

Acetazolamide *(Continued)*

Central nervous system: Drowsiness, fatigue, dizziness, fever
Dermatologic: Melena, photosensitivity, rash, rosacea, rash
Endocrine & metabolic: Hypokalemia, hyperchloremic metabolic acidosis, loss of libido after 2 weeks of therapy, elevation of blood ammonia levels, hypocalcemia, impotence, hirsutism, hyperuricemia, hyperglycemia
Gastrointestinal: GI irritation, anorexia, nausea, vomiting, dry mouth
Hematologic: Bone marrow suppression, neutropenia, thrombocytopenia, aplastic anemia, porphyria
Hepatic: Hepatic insufficiency
Neuromuscular & skeletal: Muscle asthenia, paresthesia
Ocular: Myopia (transient), intraocular pressure (increased)
Renal: Dysuria, calculi (renal) (calcium phosphate/calcium oxalate), hematuria
Respiratory: Hyperpnea
Miscellaneous: Feces discoloration (black), porphyrinogenic

Toxicodynamics/Kinetics

Extended release capsule:
- Onset of action: 2 hours
- Peak effect: 3-6 hours
- Duration: 18-24 hours

Tablet:
- Peak effect: 1-4 hours
- Duration: 8-12 hours

I.V.:
- Onset of action: 2 minutes
- Peak effect: 15 minutes
- Duration: 4-5 hours

Distribution: Distributes into erythrocytes, kidneys; crosses blood-brain barrier; crosses placenta; distributes into milk to ~30% of plasma concentrations
Protein binding: 70% to 90%
Half-life: 2.4-5.8 hours
Elimination: 70% to 100% of I.V. or tablet dose is excreted unchanged in urine within 24 hours

Usual Dosage I.M. administration not recommended because of pain secondary to the alkaline pH

Children:
- Glaucoma:
  - Oral: 10-15 mg/kg/24 hours or 300-900 mg/m²/day in doses divided every 6-8 hours
  - I.V.: 5-10 mg/kg/dose every 6 hours not to exceed 1 g/day
- Edema: Oral, I.V.: 5 mg/kg or 150 mg/m² once every day or every other day in the morning
- Epilepsy: Oral: 8-30 mg/kg/day in 2-4 divided doses, not to exceed 1 g/day; sustained release capsule is not recommended for treatment of epilepsy
- Hydrocephalus in infancy: Oral, I.V.: Initial: 25 mg/kg/24 hours divided 3 times/day; increase by 25 mg/kg/24 hours to a maximum dosage of 100 mg/kg/24 hours in 3 divided doses
- Urine alkalinization: Oral: 5 mg/kg/dose repeated 2-3 times over 24 hours

Adults:
- Glaucoma:
  - Chronic simple (open-angle): Oral: 250 mg 1-4 times/day or 500 mg sustained release capsule twice daily
  - Secondary and acute (angle-closure): I.M., I.V.: 250-500 mg, may repeat in 2-4 hours to a maximum of 1 g/day
- Edema: Oral, I.V.: 250-375 mg once daily in the morning (alternate-day therapy may be more effective)
- Epilepsy: Oral: 8-30 mg/kg/day in 1-4 divided doses; sustained release capsule is not recommended for treatment of epilepsy
- Altitude sickness: Oral: 250 mg every 8-12 hours or 500 mg extended release every 12-24 hours (initiate 24-48 hours before ascent)

Dosing interval in renal impairment:
- Cl_{cr} 10-50 mL/minute: Administer every 12 hours
- Cl_{cr} <10 mL/minute: Avoid use → ineffective, may potentiate acidosis

In patients on hemodialysis, reduce dosage to 62.5 to 125 mg/day

Administration Reconstitute with at least 5 mL sterile water to provide an I.V. solution containing not more than 100 mg/mL; maximum concentration: 100 mg/mL; maximum rate of I.V. infusion: 500 mg/minute

Contraindications Hypersensitivity to acetazolamide or other sulfonamides; patients with hepatic insufficiency or significant renal insufficiency; decreased serum sodium and/or potassium levels; or patients with adrenocortical insufficiency; hyperchloremic acidosis

Warnings Use with caution in patients with respiratory acidosis and diabetes mellitus; impairment of mental alertness and/or physical coordination; I.M. administration is painful because of the alkaline pH of the drug

Dosage Forms

Capsule, sustained release: 500 mg

Injection: 500 mg/5 mL

Tablet: 125 mg, 250 mg

Stability Reconstituted solution may be stored under refrigeration (2°C to 8°C) for 24 hours (the product contains no preservative); discard unused solutions after 24 hours

Reference Range

Therapeutic range: 5-20 mg/L

Peak plasma level: 16 µg/mL after 250 mg of acetazolamide

Overdosage Treatment

Decontamination: Lavage/activated charcoal with cathartic

Enhancement of elimination: Hemodialysis may remove as much as 30% of dose if performed prior to significant distribution

Test Interactions May cause false-positive results for urinary protein with Albustix®, Labstix®, Albutest®, Bumintest®

Drug Interactions

Decreased effect: Increased lithium excretion (by 27% to 31%) and altered excretion; decreased hypoglycemia effect with gliclazide/glipizide of other drugs by alkalinization of urine (such as amphetamines, quinidine, procainamide, methenamine, phenobarbital, salicylates); primidone serum concentrations may be decreased

Increased toxicity: Cyclosporine trough concentrations may be increased resulting in possible nephrotoxicity and neurotoxicity

Enhanced diuresis with theophylline

Pregnancy Risk Factor C

Monitoring Parameters Intraocular pressure, potassium, serum bicarbonate; serum electrolytes, periodic CBC with differential

Patient Information Report numbness or tingling of extremities to physician; do not crush, chew, or swallow contents of long-acting capsule, but may be opened and sprinkled on soft food; ability to perform tasks requiring mental alertness and/or physical coordination may be impaired; take with food; may cause an alteration in taste, especially carbonated beverages

Nursing Implications Tablet may be crushed and suspended in cherry or chocolate syrup to disguise the bitter taste of the drug

Additional Information Sodium content of 500 mg injection: 47.2 mg (2.05 mEq)

Specific References

Corbett JT, "Acetazolamide and Purpura," *Br Med J*, 1985, 1:1122-3.

Vaziri ND, Saiki J, Barton CH, et al, "Hemodialyzability of Acetazolamide," *South Med J*, 1980, 73(4):422-3.

Schwenk MH, St. Peter WL, Meese MG, et al, "Acetazolamide Toxicity and Pharmacokinetics in Patients Receiving Hemodialysis," *Pharmacotherapy*, 1995, 15(4):522-7.

Wandstrat TL and Phillips J, "Pseudotumor Cerebri Responsive to Acetazolamide," *Ann Pharmacother*, 1995, 29:318.

Weiss IS, "Hirsutism After Chronic Administration of Acetazolamide," *Am J Ophthalmol*, 1974, 78(2):327-8.

Aceten® *see* Captopril *on page 181*

Acetic Acid (a see' tik)

CAS Number 64-19-7

Brand Names Aci-Jel®; Aquaear®; VōSol®

Synonyms Ethanoic Acid

Use Continuous or intermittent irrigation of the bladder; treatment of superficial bacterial infections of the external auditory canal and vagina; may be useful in jellyfish sting

Adverse Reactions

Dermatologic: Erythema/swelling may occur

Endocrine & metabolic: Systemic acidosis

Gastrointestinal (ingestion): Epigastric pain, pyloric stenosis, gastric perforation, achlorhydria

Ocular: Corneal irritation

Renal: Urologic pain, hematuria has occurred in patients receiving irrigation

Signs & Symptoms of Acute Overdose Tachypnea, coagulopathy, hematuria, cough, wheezing (all by inhalation); headache, nausea, vomiting (ingestion), hemolysis, disseminated intravascular coagulopathy

Usual Dosage

Irrigation: For continuous irrigation of the urinary bladder with 0.25% acetic acid irrigation, the rate of administration will approximate the rate of urine flow; usually 500-1500 mL/24 hours; for periodic irrigation of an indwelling urinary catheter to

(Continued)

Acetic Acid *(Continued)*

maintain patency, approximately 50 mL of 0.25% acetic acid irrigation is required. (Note: Dosage of an irrigating solution depends on the capacity or surface area of the structure being irrigated.)

Otic: Insert saturated wick, keep moist 24 hours; remove wick and instill 5 drops 3-4 times/day

Contraindications During transurethral procedures; hypersensitivity to drug or components

Warnings Use of irrigation in patients with mucosal lesions of urinary bladder may cause irritation from lesions and systemic acidosis may result from systemic absorption via lesions; not for internal intake or I.V. infusion; rectal administration is particularly hazardous and can cause bowel necrosis

Dosage Forms Solution:

Irrigation: 0.25% (1000 mL)

Otic: Acetic acid 2% in propylene glycol (15 mL, 30 mL, 60 mL)

Overdosage Treatment

Decontamination: Dilution of affected area; do not use ipecac or induce emesis

Supportive therapy: Inhalation 100% oxygen

Pregnancy Risk Factor C

Monitoring Parameters Obtain chest x-ray, respiratory status

Nursing Implications For continuous or intermittent irrigation of the urinary bladder, urine pH should be checked at least 4 times/day and the irrigation rate adjusted to maintain a pH of 4.5-5; topical use or irrigation use only

Additional Information Clear liquid with pungent odor; similar effects as hydrochloric acid but less corrosive

Specific References

Kawamata M, Fujita S, and Mayumi T, "Acetic Acid Intoxication by Rectal Administration," *J Toxicol Clin Toxicol*, 1994, 32(3):333-6.

Penner GE, "Acid Ingestion: Toxicology and Treatment," *Ann Emerg Med*, 1980, 9(7):374-9.

Acetohexamide (a set oh hex' a mide)

Related Information

Hypoglycemic Agents Comparison, Oral *on page 1650*

CAS Number 968-81-0

Brand Names Dimelor®; Dymelor®; Gamadiabet®

Use Adjunct to diet for the management of mild to moderately severe, stable, noninsulin-dependent (type II) diabetes mellitus

Mechanism of Action Causes hypoglycemia by stimulating pancreatic islet cells to release insulin; stimulates insulin release from the pancreatic beta cells; reduces glucose output from the liver; insulin sensitivity is increased at peripheral target sites; produces a mild diuretic effect and increases the urinary excretion of uric acid

Adverse Reactions

Central nervous system: Headache, ataxia, dizziness, fasciculations

Dermatologic: Skin rash, hives, photosensitivity

Endocrine & metabolic: Severe hypoglycemia, hyponatremia, syndrome of inappropriate antidiuretic hormone, hypoglycemia

Gastrointestinal: Nausea, vomiting, epigastric fullness, heartburn, diarrhea, anorexia, constipation

Hematologic: Aplastic anemia, hemolysis, bone marrow depression, thrombocytopenia, leukopenia, neutropenia, agranulocytosis, granulocytopenia

Hepatic: Cholestatic jaundice, cirrhosis

Ocular: Diplopia, photophobia

Toxicodynamics/Kinetics

Onset of effect: 1 hour

Peak hypoglycemic effects: 8-10 hours

Duration: 12-24 hours, prolonged with renal impairment

Distribution: Into breast milk

Protein binding: 85% to 88%

Metabolism: In the liver to hydroxyhexamide (active metabolite)

Half-life:

- Parent compound: 0.8-2.4 hours
- Metabolite: 5-6 hours

Elimination: Urinary excretion of <40% as unchanged drug; ~80% to 95% of dose excreted in urine within 24 hours; ~15% excreted in bile

Usual Dosage Adults: Oral (elderly patients may be more sensitive and should be started at a lower dosage initially): 250 mg to 1.5 g/day in 1-2 divided doses; doses >1.5 g/day are not recommended; if dose is ≤1 g, administer as a single daily dose

Dosing adjustment in renal impairment: Cl_{cr} <50 mL/minute: Avoid use; prolonged hypoglycemia occurs in azotemic patients

Dosing adjustment in hepatic impairment: Initiate therapy at lower than recommended doses

Contraindications Diabetes complicated by ketoacidosis, therapy of type I diabetes, hypersensitivity to sulfonylureas

Dosage Forms Tablet: 250 mg, 500 mg

Reference Range Glucose fasting: Adults: 80-140 mg/dL; Elderly: 100-180 mg/dL

Overdosage Treatment

Decontamination: Lavage/activated charcoal with cathartic

Supportive therapy: Glucose (25 g I.V.) is mainstay of therapy. Glucagon (1-5 mg I.V., I.M., or S.C.) (0.03-0.1 mg/kg in pediatrics) will have limited benefit; diazoxide is a third-line agent (3-8 mg/kg/24 hours)

Enhancement of elimination: Multiple dosing of activated charcoal may be effective. Peritoneal dialysis has been used with some success. Urine alkalinization is also useful.

Antidote(s)

Dextrose *on page 1409*

Glucagon *on page 1431*

Drug Interactions

Decreased effect: Decreases acetohexamide effect by oral anticoagulants, hydantoins, loop or thiazide diuretics, and phenylbutazone

Increased effect: Increases hypoglycemia when coadministered with salicylates or beta-adrenergic blockers; MAO inhibitors ↑ hypoglycemic response

Pregnancy Risk Factor D

Pregnancy Implications Can cause hypoglycemia in the fetus

Monitoring Parameters Monitor for signs and symptoms of hypoglycemia (fatigue, excessive hunger, profuse sweating, or numbness of extremities); fasting blood glucose, urine glucose, hemoglobin A_{1c} or fructosamine

Patient Information If nausea or stomach upset occurs, may be taken with food; take at the same time each day; avoid alcohol

Nursing Implications Advise patient to avoid alcohol or products containing alcohol; blood and urine glucose concentrations should be monitored when therapy is started; normally takes 7 days to determine therapeutic response

Specific References

Alexander RW, "Prolonged Hypoglycemia Following Acetohexamide Administration," *Diabetes*, 1966, 15(5):362-4.

Cowen DL, Burtis B, and Youmans J, "Prolonged Coma After Acetohexamide Ingestion," *JAMA*, 1967, 201(2):141-2.

Acetomorphine *see* Heroin Hydrochloride *on page 401*

Acetylsalicylic Acid *see* Aspirin *on page 133*

Acezide® *see* Captopril and Hydrochlorothiazide *on page 183*

Achromycin® *see* Tetracycline *on page 732*

Achromycin® V Oral *see* Tetracycline *on page 732*

Aciclovir *see* Acyclovir *on next page*

Acidulated Phosphate Fluoride *see* Fluoride *on page 355*

Acidum Etacrynicum *see* Ethacrynic Acid *on page 328*

Acidum Nicotinicum *see* Niacin *on page 554*

Aci-Jel® *see* Acetic Acid *on page 85*

Acrivastine (ak' ri vas teen & soo doe e fed' rin)

CAS Number 87848-99-5

Brand Names Duact®; Prolert®; Semprex-D®

Synonyms BW-825C

Use Allergic rhinitis, rash, atopic eczema, demographism

Mechanism of Action Analog of triprolidine, a potent antihistamine with sedative but no anticholinergic effects; histamine H_1-receptor antagonist

Adverse Reactions

Central nervous system: Lethargy, lightheadedness, headache, drowsiness, insomnia

Gastrointestinal: Dry mouth, nausea, diarrhea, dyspepsia

Toxicodynamics/Kinetics

Onset of action: Within 30 minutes

Absorption: Not affected by food

Protein binding: 50%

Metabolism: Hepatic to an active metabolite

Half-life: 1.4-2.5 hours

Elimination: Renal (65% eliminated unchanged)

Usual Dosage Oral: 8 mg every 4-6 hours

Contraindications Hypersensitivity to acrivastine or triprolidine

Warnings Use with caution in patients with renal insufficiency

Dosage Forms Capsule: Acrivastine 8 mg and pseudoephedrine hydrochloride 60 mg

(Continued)

Acrivastine *(Continued)*

Reference Range After a 12 mg oral dose, peak serum level is ~179 ng/mL within 1 hour of ingestion

Overdosage Treatment

Decontamination: Lavage/activated charcoal with cathartic

Supportive therapy: There is no specific treatment for an antihistamine overdose, however, most of its clinical toxicity is due to anticholinergic effects. Anticholinesterase inhibitors may be useful by reducing acetylcholinesterase. Anticholinesterase inhibitors include physostigmine, neostigmine, pyridostigmine and edrophonium. For anticholinergic overdose with severe life-threatening symptoms, physostigmine 1-2 mg (0.5 or 0.02 mg/kg for children) I.V., slowly may be given to reverse these effects.

Additional Information Often combined with pseudoephedrine (Duact®, Semprex-D®)

Specific References

Brogden RN and McTavish D, "Acrivastine: A Review of Its Pharmacological Properties and Therapeutic Efficacy in Allergic Rhinitis, Urticaria, and Related Disorders," *Drugs*, 1991, 41(6):927-40.

Levien TL and Baker DE, "Reviews of Acrivastine and Midotrine," *Hosp Pharmacy*, 1995, 30(3):229-35.

Actacode *see* Codeine *on page 238*

Actilyse® *see* Alteplase, Recombinant *on page 100*

Actimmune® *see* Interferon Gamma-1b *on page 436*

Actiplus® *see* Alteplase, Recombinant *on page 100*

Activase® Injection *see* Alteplase, Recombinant *on page 100*

Activated Ergosterol *see* Vitamin D *on page 797*

Actosolv® *see* Urokinase *on page 779*

Actrafan® HM *see* Insulin Preparations *on page 426*

Actrap® MC *see* Insulin Preparations *on page 426*

ACT® [OTC] *see* Fluoride *on page 355*

ACU-dyne® [OTC] *see* Povidone-Iodine *on page 635*

Acumen® *see* Deanol *on page 261*

Acupril® *see* Quinapril Hydrochloride *on page 667*

Acutrim® [OTC] *see* Phenylpropanolamine Hydrochloride *on page 622*

ACV *see* Acyclovir *on this page*

Acycloguanosine *see* Acyclovir *on this page*

Acyclovir (ay sye' kloe ver)

Related Information

Therapeutic Drugs Associated With Hallucinations *on page 1558-1559*

Valacyclovir Hydrochloride *on page 781*

CAS Number 59277-89-3; 69657-51-8

Brand Names Zovirax®

Synonyms Aciclovir; ACV; Acycloguanosine

Use Treatment of initial and prophylaxis of recurrent mucosal and cutaneous herpes simplex (HSV-1 and HSV-2) infections; herpes simplex encephalitis; herpes zoster; genital herpes infection; varicella-zoster infections

Mechanism of Action Inhibits DNA synthesis and viral replication by competing with deoxyguanosine triphosphate for viral DNA polymerase (thymidine kinase) and being incorporated into viral DNA

Adverse Reactions

Central nervous system: Headache, drowsiness, delirium, coma, dizziness, seizures, mania, psychosis, hyperacusis, pain, insomnia, visual and tactile hallucinations, confusion, agitation, encephalopathy, mental depression, fever, hyperthermia

Dermatologic: Skin rash

Gastrointestinal: Nausea, vomiting, anorexia, diarrhea, colitis

Hematologic: Bone marrow depression, thrombocytopenia, leukopenia

Hepatic: Elevation of liver enzymes

Local: Phlebitis at injection site, local pain and stinging with topical use

Neuromuscular & skeletal: Tremors, tremulousness, myoclonus

Renal: Can cause obstructive nephrotoxicity due to crystalluria at renal concentrations >2.5 mg/mL, impaired renal function (dose dependent)

Miscellaneous: Sore throat, sweating

Toxicodynamics/Kinetics

Absorption: Oral: 15% to 30%; food does not appear to affect absorption

Distribution: V_d: 0.7 L/kg; widely distributed throughout the body including brain, kidney, lungs, liver, spleen, muscle, uterus, vagina, and the CSF; lower in patients with renal failure

Protein binding: 15% to 30%

Metabolism: Small amount of hepatic metabolism

Half-life, terminal:

Neonates: 4 hours

Children 1-12 years: 2-3 hours

Adults: 3 hours

With renal failure: 20 hours

Time to peak serum concentration:

Oral: Within 1.5-2 hours

I.V.: Within 1 hour

Elimination: Primary route of elimination is the kidney; hemodialysis removes ~60% of the dose and to a much lesser extent by peritoneal dialysis

Usual Dosage

Dosing weight should be based on the smaller of lean body weight or total body weight

Adult determination of lean body weight (LBW) in kg:

LBW males: 50 kg + (2.3 kg x inches >5 feet)

LBW females: 45 kg + (2.3 kg x inches >5 feet)

Treatment of herpes simplex virus infections: I.V.:

Neonatal infection: 1500 mg/m^2/day divided every 8 hours or 30 mg/kg/day divided every 8 hours for 10-14 days

Children and Adults:

Mucocutaneous HSV infection: 750 mg/m^2/day divided every 8 hours or 5 mg/kg/dose every 8 hours for 5-10 days

HSV encephalitis: 1500 mg/m^2/day divided every 8 hours or 10 mg/kg/dose every 8 hours for 10 days

Adults:

Oral: Treatment: 200 mg every 4 hours while awake (5 times/day)

Prophylaxis: 200 mg 3-4 times/day or 400 mg twice daily

Topical: ½" ribbon of ointment every 3 hours (6 times/day)

Treatment of varicella-zoster virus infections:

Oral:

Children: 10-20 mg/kg/dose (up to 800 mg) 4 times/day

Adults: 600-800 mg/dose every 4 hours while awake (5 times/day) for 7-10 days or 1000 mg every 6 hours for 5 days

I.V.: Children and Adults: 1500 mg/m^2/day divided every 8 hours or 10 mg/kg/dose every 8 hours for 5-10 days

Prophylaxis in immunocompromised patients:

Varicella or herpes zoster in HIV-positive patients: Adults: Oral: 400 mg 5 times/day

Bone marrow transplant recipients: Children and Adults: I.V.:

Patients who are HSV seropositive: 5 mg/kg/dose divided every 8 hours

Patients who are CMV seropositive: 10 mg/kg/dose divided every 8 hours; for clinically significant CMV infections, ganciclovir should be used in place of acyclovir

Dosing interval in renal impairment:

Oral: HSV: Cl_{cr} <10 mL/minute: Administer every 12 hours

Oral: Varicella-zoster:

Cl_{cr} 10-25 mL/minute: Administer every 8 hours

Cl_{cr} <10 mL/minute: Administer every 12 hours

I.V.:

Cl_{cr} 25-50 mL/minute: 5-10 mg/kg/dose: Administer every 12 hours

Cl_{cr} 10-25 mL/minute: 5-10 mg/kg/dose: Administer every 24 hours

Cl_{cr} <10 mL/minute: 2.5 mg/kg/dose: Administer every 24 hours

Administration Reconstitute vial for injection with paraben-free sterile water; administer by slow I.V. infusion over at least 1 hour at a final concentration not to exceed 7 mg/mL; in patients who require fluid restriction, a concentration of up to 10 mg/mL has been infused; concentration >10 mg/mL increases the risk of phlebitis

Contraindications Hypersensitivity to acyclovir

Warnings Use with caution in patients with pre-existing renal disease or in those receiving other nephrotoxic drugs concurrently; maintain adequate urine output during the first 2 hours after I.V. infusion; use with caution in patients with underlying neurologic abnormalities, serious hepatic or electrolyte abnormalities, or substantial hypoxia; appears to reduce the length and severity of chickenpox, but should not be used unless patient is immunosuppressed

Dosage Forms

Capsule: 200 mg

Injection: 500 mg (10 mL); 1000 mg (20 mL)

Ointment, topical: 5% (3 g, 15 g)

(Continued)

Acyclovir *(Continued)*

Suspension, oral (banana flavor): 200 mg/5 mL (473 mL)
Tablet: 400 mg, 800 mg

Stability **Incompatible** with blood products and protein-containing solutions; reconstituted solutions remain stable for 24 hours at room temperature; do not refrigerate reconstituted solutions as they may precipitate

Reference Range Neurotoxicity associated with plasma levels of 470 μmol/mL

Overdosage Treatment

Decontamination: Ipecac or lavage/activated charcoal with cathartic

Supportive therapy: Renal toxicity and crystalluria can be managed with intravenous fluid hydration

Enhancement of elimination: Multiple dosing of activated charcoal may be effective; hemodialysis can remove about 60% of total body burden; exchange transfusion is not useful

Drug Interactions Increased effect with zidovudine (drowsiness, drowsiness), probenecid (CNS effects); probenecid increases plasma half-life

Pregnancy Risk Factor C

Pregnancy Implications Probably not harmful to fetus

Monitoring Parameters Urinalysis, BUN, serum creatinine, liver enzymes, CBC

Patient Information Patients are contagious only when viral shedding is occurring; recurrences tend to appear within 3 months of original infection; acyclovir is **not** a cure; avoid sexual intercourse when lesions are present

Nursing Implications Infuse over 1 hour; maintain adequate hydration of patient; check infusion site for phlebitis, rotate site to prevent phlebitis; wear gloves when applying ointment for self-protection

Additional Information Sodium content of 1 g: 4.2 mEq; not effective against cytomegalovirus

Specific References

Almond MK, Fan S, Dhillon S, et al, "Avoiding Acyclovir Neurotoxicity in Patients With Chronic Renal Failure Undergoing Haemodialysis," *Nephron*, 1995, 69:428-32.

Arndt KA, "Adverse Reactions to Acyclovir: Topical, Oral, and Intravenous," *J Am Acad Dermatol*, 1988, 18(1 Pt 2):188-90.

Eck P, Silver SM, and Clark EC, "Acute Renal Failure and Coma After a High Dose of Oral Acyclovir," *N Engl J Med*, 1991, 325(16):1178-9.

Feder HM, Goyal RK, and Krause PJ, "Acyclovir-Induced Neutropenia in an Infant With Herpes Simplex Encephalitis: Case Report," *Clin Infect Dis*, 1995, 20:1557-9.

Johnson GL, Limon L, Trikha G, et al, "Acute Renal Failure and Neurotoxicity Following Oral Acyclovir," *Ann Pharmacother*, 1994, 28(4):460-3.

Leikin JB, Shicker L, Orlowski J, et al, "Hemodialysis Removal of Acyclovir," *Vet Hum Toxicol*, 1995, 37(3):233-4.

McDonald LK, Tartaglione TA, Mendelman PM, et al, "Lack of Toxicity in Two Cases of Neonatal Acyclovir Overdose," *Pediatr Infect Dis J*, 1989, 8(8):529-32.

Adalat® *see* Nifedipine *on page 558*

Adamantanamine Hydrochloride *see* Amantadine Hydrochloride *on page 105*

Adapin® *see* Doxepin Hydrochloride *on page 301*

Adenocard® *see* Adenosine Triphosphate *on this page*

Adenosine Triphosphate

CAS Number 58-61-7; 56-56-5

Brand Names Adenocard®; Adenotriphos®; Atepodin®; Striadyne®; Trinosin®

Synonyms 6-Amino-9-Beta-D-Ribofuranosyl-9-H-Purine; 9-Beta-D-Ribofuranosyladenine

Use Treatment of paroxysmal tachycardia (ventricular) (PSVT); orphan drug for treatment of brain tumors in conjunction with BCNU

Mechanism of Action Endogenous nucleoside; produces transient atrioventricular block and coronary vasodilatation; slows conduction time through the A-V node, interrupting the re-entry pathways through the A-V node, restoring normal sinus rhythm

Adverse Reactions

Cardiovascular: Facial flushing, palpitations, chest pain, hypotension, fibrillation (atrial)

Central nervous system: Lightheadedness, dizziness, tingling in arms, numbness, fear, burning sensation, pain, headache, heaviness in arms, neck and back, migraine

Gastrointestinal: Nausea, metallic taste, tightness in throat, pressure in groin

Ocular: Blurred vision

Respiratory: Dyspnea, bronchospasm, chest pressure, hypoventilation

Miscellaneous: Sweating

Signs & Symptoms of Acute Overdose Bradycardia, wheezing, arrhythmias, lightheadedness, numbness, hypotension, urine discoloration (milky)

Toxicodynamics/Kinetics

Onset of action: Clinical effects occur rapidly

Duration: Very brief

Metabolism: In blood and tissue to inosine then to adenosine monophosphate (AMP) and hypoxanthine

Half-life: <10 seconds

Elimination: Excreted renally as uric acid

Usual Dosage Rapid I.V. push (over 1-2 seconds):

Children: Initial dose: 0.05 mg/kg; if not effective within 2 minutes, increase dose in 0.05 mg/kg increments every 2 minutes to a maximum dose of 0.25 mg/kg or until termination of PSVT; median dose required: 0.15 mg/kg; do not exceed 12 mg/dose; reduce dose if patient is taking dipyridamole

Alternatively: 0.1 mg/kg; if not effective, give 0.2 mg/kg; maximum: 12 mg/dose

Adults: 6 mg, if the dose is not effective within 1-2 minutes, a rapid I.V. dose of 12 mg may be given; may repeat 12 mg bolus if needed; doses >12 mg are not recommended

Note: Higher doses may be needed for administration via peripheral versus central vein

Contraindications Known hypersensitivity to adenosine, second and third degree A-V block or sick sinus syndrome unless pacemaker placed

Warnings Use with caution if wheezing is present; use with caution in patients with bronchospasm; use in patients with Wolff-Parkinson-White syndrome may be proarrhythmic

Dosage Forms Injection (prefilled disposable syringes): 6 mg, 12 mg

Reference Range 0.1-1.0 μmol/L

Overdosage Treatment

Supportive therapy: I.V. fluids for hypotensive effect; aminophylline may antagonize effects

Drug Interactions May not be as effective when used concurrently with methylxanthine; dipyridamole may enhance adenosine's effects; carbamazepine may increase degree of heart block

Pregnancy Implications Appears to be safe in pregnancy

Monitoring Parameters EKG, blood pressure

Additional Information No negative inotropic effect; may be effective against theophylline-induced seizures

Specific References

Brown SGA and Waterer GW, "Migraine Precipitated by Adenosine," *Med J Aust*, 1995, 162:389 & 391.

DeGroff CG and Silka MJ, "Bronchospasm After Intravenous Administration of Adenosine in a Patient With Asthma," *J Pediatr*, 1994, 125(5 Pt 1):822-3.

Exner DV, Muzyka T, and Gillis AM, "Proarrhythmia in Patients With Wolff-Parkinson-White Syndrome After Standard Doses of Intravenous Adenosine," *Ann Intern Med*, 1995, 122(5):351-2.

Furlong R, Gerhardt RT, Farber P, et al, "Intravenous Adenosine as First-Line Prehospital Management of Narrow-Complex Tachycardias by EMS Personnel Withhout Direct Physician Contact," *Am J Emerg Med*, 1995, 13:383-8.

Gausche M, Persse DE, and Sugarman T, "Adenosine for the Prehospital Treatment of Paroxysmal Supraventricular Tachycardia," *Ann Emerg Med*, 1994, 24(2):183-9.

Lee KL and Tai YT, "Adenosine in Wide Complex Tachycardia: Potential Pitfalls in Diagnostic Value," *Ann Emerg Med*, 1994, 24(4):741-7.

Madsen CD, Pointer JE, and Lynch TG, "A Comparison of Adenosine and Verapamil for the Treatment of Supraventricular Tachycardia in the Prehospital Setting," *Ann Emerg Med*, 1995, 25:649-55.

Nussbacher A, Arie S, Kalil R, et al, "Mechanism of Adenosine-Induced Elevation of Pulmonary Capillary Wedge Pressure in Humans," *Circulation*, 1995, 92:371-9.

Pelleg A and Porter RS, "The Pharmacology of Adenosine," *Pharmacotherapy*, 1990, 10(3):157-74.

Shannon M and Maher T, "Anticonvulsant Effects of Intracerebroventricular Adenocard in Theophylline-Induced Seizures," *Ann Emerg Med*, 1995, 26:6508.

Adenotriphos® *see* Adenosine Triphosphate *on previous page*

Adepril® *see* Amitriptyline Hydrochloride *on page 116*

Adepsine Oil *see* Mineral Oil *on page 534*

Adipex-P® *see* Phentermine Hydrochloride *on page 619*

ADR *see* Doxorubicin Hydrochloride *on page 303*

Adrenergic Agonists, Cardiovascular Comparison *see page 1638*

Adrenergic Agonists Drug Infusions Comparison *see page 1638*

Adriamycin PFS™ *see* Doxorubicin Hydrochloride *on page 303*

Adriamycin RDF™ *see* Doxorubicin Hydrochloride *on page 303*

Adrucil® Injection *see* Fluorouracil *on page 357*

Adsorbonac® [OTC] Ophthalmic *see* Sodium Chloride *on page 698*

Adumbran® *see* Oxazepam *on page 582*

Advil® [OTC] *see* Ibuprofen *on page 418*

Aeroaid® [OTC] *see* Thimerosal *on page 744*

Aerodine® [OTC] *see* Povidone-Iodine *on page 635*

Aerolate® *see* Theophylline *on page 735*

Aerolate III® *see* Theophylline *on page 735*

Aerolate JR® *see* Theophylline *on page 735*

Aerolate SR® S *see* Theophylline *on page 735*

Aeroseb-Dex® Topical Aerosol *see* Dexamethasone *on page 266*

Afrazine® *see* Oxymetazoline Hydrochloride *on page 586*

Afrinol® [OTC] *see* Pseudoephedrine *on page 661*

Afrin® Nasal Solution [OTC] *see* Oxymetazoline Hydrochloride *on page 586*

Afrodex® *see* Yohimbine Hydrochloride *on page 805*

Aftir Gel® *see* Malathion (Topical Lotion) *on page 489*

Agon® *see* Felodipine *on page 343*

Agoral® Plain [OTC] *see* Mineral Oil *on page 534*

AHD 2000® *see* Ethyl Alcohol *on page 336*

AK-Chlor® Ophthalmic *see* Chloramphenicol *on page 196*

AK-Dex® Ophthalmic *see* Dexamethasone *on page 266*

AK-Tracin® Ophthalmic *see* Bacitracin *on page 142*

AK-Zol® *see* Acetazolamide *on page 83*

Al *see* Aluminum *on page 104*

Ala-Tet® Oral *see* Tetracycline *on page 732*

Alaun *see* Aluminum *on page 104*

Albistat® *see* Miconazole *on page 530*

Albone *see* Hydrogen Peroxide *on page 408*

Albuterol (al byoo' ter ole)

CAS Number 18559-94-9

Brand Names Proventil®; Ventolin®

Synonyms Salbutamol

Use Bronchodilator in reversible airway obstruction due to asthma or COPD

Mechanism of Action Relaxes bronchial smooth muscle by action on beta$_2$-receptors with little effect on heart rate

Adverse Reactions

Cardiovascular: Tachycardia (slight), palpitations, hypertension, flushing, shortened P-R segment, lengthened Q-T segment, cardiac arrhythmias

Central nervous system: Dizziness, psychosis, headache, nervousness, CNS stimulation, hyperactivity, insomnia

Dermatologic: Maculopapular rash

Gastrointestinal: gastrointestinal upset

Neuromuscular & skeletal: Tremor

Signs & Symptoms of Acute Overdose Hypertension, thrombocytopenia, tachycardia, intraocular pressure (increased), seizures, diplopia, hypomagnesemia, angina, hypokalemia, hyperglycemia, agitation

Toxicodynamics/Kinetics

Onset of action: Peak bronchodilation: Within 30 minutes to 2 hours

Duration: 3-4 hours

Absorption:

Oral: Rapidly and well absorbed from gastrointestinal tract

Inhalation: Absorbed gradually from the bronchi with a portion of the swallowed fraction being absorbed from the gastrointestinal tract; system concentrations are low following inhalation of recommended doses because inhaled doses are only 5% of those required orally

Distribution: V_d: 2.2 L/kg; does not cross blood-brain barrier

Metabolism: By the liver to an inactive sulfate, with 28% appearing in the urine as unchanged drug

Half-life:

Oral: 3.7-5 hours

Inhalation: 3.8 hours

Elimination: ~76% excreted in urine over 3 days (most in first 24 hours); ~4% excreted in feces

Usual Dosage

Oral:

2-6 years: 0.1-0.2 mg/kg/dose 3 times/day; maximum dose not to exceed 12 mg/day (divided doses)

6-12 years: 2 mg/dose 3-4 times/day; maximum dose not to exceed 24 mg/day (divided doses)

>12 years: 2-4 mg/dose 3-4 times/day; maximum dose not to exceed 32 mg/day (divided doses)

Inhalation MDI: 90 mcg/spray:

<12 years: 1-2 inhalations 4 times/day using a tube spacer

≥12 years: 1-2 inhalations every 4-6 hours

Exercise-induced wheezing: 2 inhalations 15 minutes before exercising

Inhalation: Nebulization: 2.5 mg = 0.5 mL of the 0.5% inhalation solution to be diluted in 1-2.5 mL of NS

<5 years: 1.25-2.5 mg every 4-6 hours as needed

>5 years: 2.5-5 mg every 4-6 hours

Toxic dose requiring medical evaluation: 0.6 mg/kg

Contraindications Hypersensitivity to albuterol, adrenergic amines or any ingredients

Warnings Use with caution in patients with hyperthyroidism or diabetes mellitus; excessive use may result in tolerance; some adverse reactions may occur more frequently in children 2-5 years of age than in adults and older children; watch for excessive cardiovascular effects when combining inhaled albuterol with chronic oral sympathomimetic therapy

Dosage Forms

Aerosol, oral: 90 mcg/spray [200 inhalations] (17 g)

Capsule, microfine, for inhalation, as sulfate (Rotacaps®): 200 mcg

Solution, inhalation, as sulfate: 0.083% [0.83 mg/mL] (3 mL); 0.5% [5 mg/mL] (20 mL)

Syrup, as sulfate (strawberry flavor): 2 mg/5 mL (480 mL)

Tablet, as sulfate: 2 mg, 4 mg

Tablet, extended release: 4 mg

Reference Range Serum albuterol levels >25 ng/mL associated with increased cardiac toxicity

Overdosage Treatment In cases of overdose, supportive therapy should be instituted, and prudent use of a cardioselective beta-adrenergic blocker (eg, atenolol or metoprolol) should be considered, keeping in mind the potential for induction of bronchoconstriction in an asthmatic individual. Adenosine may be effective in the management of tachycardia (ventricular); dialysis has not been shown to be of value in the treatment of an overdose with this agent.

Diagnostic Tests/Procedures

Electrolytes, Blood *on page 1254*

Electrocardiography *on page 1253*

Drug Interactions Action of albuterol is antagonized by beta-adrenergic blocking agents such as propranolol; cardiovascular effects are potentiated in patients also receiving MAO inhibitors or tricyclic antidepressants

Pregnancy Risk Factor C

Monitoring Parameters Heart rate, CNS stimulation, asthma symptoms

Patient Information Do not exceed recommended dosage; rinse mouth with water following each inhalation to help with dry throat and mouth

Nursing Implications Before using, the inhaler must be shaken well; assess lung sounds, pulse, and blood pressure before administration and during peak of medication; observe patient for wheezing after administration, if this occurs, call physician

Additional Information Syrup is alcohol and sugar free

Specific References

Bartfield JM, Boenau IB, Lozon J, et al, "Comparison of Metered Dose Inhaler and Oral Administration of Albuterol in the Outpatient Treatment of Infants and Children," *Am J Emerg Med*, 1995, 13:375-8.

Cook P, Scarfone RJ, and Cook RT, "Adenosine in the Termination of Albuterol-Induced Supraventricular Tachycardia," *Ann Emerg Med*, 1994, 24(2):316-9.

Finnerty JP and Howarth PH, "Paradoxical Bronchoconstriction With Nebulized Albuterol But Not With Terbutaline," *Am Rev Respir Dis*, 1993, 148(2):512-3.

Hall MC, Schmidt G, et al, "Metered-Dose Inhaler Versus Nebulized Albuterol in Mechanically Ventilated Patients," *Am Rev Respir Dis*, 1993, 148:1567-70.

Leikin JB, Linowiecki KA, Soglin DF, et al, "Hypokalemia After Pediatric Albuterol Overdose: A Case Series," *Am J Emerg Med*, 1994, 12(1):64-6.

Lin R, Smith S, and Hergenroeder P, "High Serum Albuterol Levels and Tachycardia in Adult Asthmatics Treated With High-Dose continuously Aerosolized Albuterol," *Chest*, 1993, 103:221-5.

Mahajan M, Tucker J, and Dolgin J, "Protocol for Management of Accidental Pediatric Albuterol Ingestions," *Vet Hum Toxicol*, 1994, 36:361.

Spiller HA, Ramoska EA, Henretig FM, et al, "A Two-Year Retrospective Study of Accidental Pediatric Albuterol Ingestions," *Pediatr Emerg Care*, 1993, 9(6):338-40.

(Continued)

Albuterol *(Continued)*

Udezue E, D'Souza L, and Mahajan M, "Hypokalemia After Normal Doses of Neubulized Albuterol (Salbutamol)," *Am J Emerg Med*, 1995, 13(2):168-71.
Wiley JF 2nd, Spiller HA, Krenzelok EP, et al, "Unintentional Albuterol Ingestion in Children," *Pediatr Emerg Care*, 1994, 10(4):193-6.

Alcohol, Ethyl *see* Ethyl Alcohol *on page 336*
Aldace® *see* Spironolactone *on page 705*
Aldactone® *see* Spironolactone *on page 705*
Aldinamide® *see* Pyrazinamide *on page 663*
Aldocumar® *see* Warfarin Sodium *on page 800*
Aldomet® *see* Methyldopa *on page 519*
Aldopur® *see* Spironolactone *on page 705*

Alendronate

CAS Number 66376-36-1; 121268-17-5
Brand Names Fosamax®
Synonyms Alendronic Acid; Aminohydroxybutylidene Biphosphonate; Monosodium Alendronate
Use Investigational: Treat hypercalcemia, osteoporosis, and Paget's disease
Mechanism of Action Aminobiphosphonate which inhibits osteoclastic bone resorption by binding to hydroxyapatite

Adverse Reactions
Central nervous system: Fever
Endocrine & metabolic: Hypocalcemia (dose related)
Hematologic: Transient lymphopenia
Neuromuscular & skeletal: Arthralgia, myalgia

Toxicodynamics/Kinetics
Absorption: Oral: ~1% (reduced in presence of calcium and food)
Metabolism: None
Half-life: In bone: >10 years
Elimination: Renal: 50%

Usual Dosage
Hypercalcemia: I.V. 5-15 mg in 250 mL of normal saline given over a 2-hour period
Osteoporosis: Oral: 20-40 mg once daily (2 hours before or after meals)

Contraindications Hypersensitivity to alendronic acid or other biphosphonates
Warnings Renal insufficiency, congestive heart failure, hyperphosphatemia, hypocalcemia, liver disease, fever
Reference Range After a 10 mg I.V. dose, peak serum level of alendronic acid is ~309 ng/mL

Overdosage Treatment
Supportive therapy: Intravenous hydration; monitor urine flow and calcium and phosphorus level

Additional Information Better suited than etidronate for chronic therapy due to the fact that alendronic acid does not impair bone mineralization and thus does not increase the risk for osteomalacia; rapid injection can lead to renal failure due to calcium biphosphonate formation in renal tubules; alendronate is 200-1000 times more potent than etidronate

Specific References
Averbuch SD, "New Bisphosphonates in the Treatment of Bone Metastases," *Cancer*, 1993, 72(11 Suppl):3443-52.
Inzerillo MT, "Alendronate: An Investigational Agent for the Prevention and Treatment of Osteoporosis," *Pharm Therap*, 1994, 19:851-2.

Alendronic Acid *see* Alendronate *on this page*
Alergist® *see* Terfenadine *on page 728*
Aleve® [OTC] *see* Naproxen *on page 549*
Alfacalcidol *see* Vitamin D *on page 797*
Alfenta® Injection *see* Alfentanil Hydrochloride *on this page*

Alfentanil Hydrochloride (al fen' ta nill)

Related Information
Pharmacokinetics of Narcotic Agonist Analgesics *on page 1654*
CAS Number 71195-58-9; 64049-06-5; 70879-28-6
Brand Names Alfenta® Injection; Fanaxal®; Limifen®; Rapifen®
Use Analgesia; adjunct to anesthesia
Mechanism of Action Binds with stereospecific receptors at many sites within the CNS, increases pain threshold, alters pain perception, inhibits ascending pain pathways; is an ultra short-acting narcotic

Adverse Reactions

Cardiovascular: Bradycardia, hypotension, cardiac arrhythmias, hypotension (orthostatic), circulatory depression

Central nervous system: Drowsiness, confusion, CNS depression, seizures, mental depression, paradoxical CNS excitation or delirium, dizziness

Dermatologic: Skin rash, hives, itching

Gastrointestinal: Nausea, vomiting, biliary spasm

Genitourinary: Priapism

Neuromuscular & skeletal: Dysesthesia

Ocular: Blurred vision

Respiratory: Apnea, respiratory depression (at doses >1000 mcg), bronchospasm, sinus arrest, apnea, laryngospasm

Miscellaneous: Cold, clammy skin, physical and psychological dependence with prolonged use

Signs & Symptoms of Acute Overdose Miosis, respiratory depression, wheezing, hiccups, dysphagia, seizures, CNS depression, clammy skin

Toxicodynamics/Kinetics

Distribution: V_d:

Newborns, premature: 1 L/kg

Children: 0.163-0.48 L/kg

Adults: 0.46 L/kg

Protein binding: 92%

Metabolism: Hepatic to noralfentanil

Half-life, elimination:

Newborns, premature: 5.33-8.75 hours

Children: 40-60 minutes

Adults: 83-97 minutes

Obese patients: 172 minutes

Elderly: 137 minutes

Usual Dosage Doses should be titrated to appropriate effects; wide range of doses is dependent upon desired degree of analgesia/anesthesia

Children <12 years: Dose not established

Adults: Dose should be based on ideal body weight. See table.

Alfentanil

Indication	Approximate Duration of Anesthesia (min)	Induction Period (Initial Dose) (mcg/kg)	Maintenance Period (Increments/ Infusion)	Total Dose (mcg/kg)	Effects
Incremental injection	≤30	8-20	3-5 mcg/kg or 0.5-1 mcg/kg/min	8-40	Spontaneously breathing or assisted ventilation when required.
	30-60	20-50	5-15 mcg/kg	Up to 75	Assisted or controlled ventilation required. Attenuation of response to laryngoscopy and intubation.
Continuous infusion	>45	50-75	0.5-3.0 mcg/kg/min average infusion rate 1-1.5 mcg/kg/min	Dependent on duration of procedure	Assisted or controlled ventilation required. Some attenuation of response to intubation and incision, with intraoperative stability.
Anesthetic induction	>45	130-245	0.5-1.5 mcg/kg/min or general anesthetic	Dependent on duration of procedure	Assisted or controlled ventilation required. Administer slowly (over three minutes). Concentration of inhalation agents reduced by 30-50% for initial hour.

Administration Administer I.V. slowly over 3-5 minutes or by I.V. continuous infusion

Contraindications Hypersensitivity to alfentanil hydrochloride; increased intracranial pressure, severe respiratory depression

Warnings Rapid I.V. infusion may result in skeletal muscle and chest wall rigidity → impaired ventilation → respiratory distress/arrest; inject slowly over 3-5 minutes; nondepolarizing skeletal muscle relaxant may be required

Dosage Forms Injection, preservative free: 500 mcg/mL (2 mL, 5 mL, 10 mL, 20 mL)

Stability Dilute in D_5W, normal saline, or LR

(Continued)

Alfentanil Hydrochloride *(Continued)*

Reference Range 100-340 ng/mL (depending upon procedure); 310-340 ng/mL adequate anesthesia for intra-abdominal surgery; 190 ng/mL adequate for skin closure; 100-200 ng/mL adequate for superficial surgery

Overdosage Treatment

Decontamination: Lavage/activated charcoal with cathartic for oral ingestion

Supportive therapy: Naloxone in large doses and/or a continuous infusion may be necessary

Antidote(s)

Naloxone Hydrochloride *on page 1447*

Drug Interactions Increased toxicity: CNS depressants (eg, thiopental, benzodiazepines, barbiturates, phenothiazines, tricyclic antidepressants, centrally acting antihypertensives), erythromycin, cimetidine, MAO inhibitors

Pregnancy Risk Factor C

Pregnancy Implications Neonatal respiratory depression can occur

Monitoring Parameters Respiratory rate, blood pressure, heart rate

Additional Information Alfentanil may produce more hypotension compared to fentanyl, therefore, be sure to administer slowly and ensure patient has adequate hydration; half-life increased in burn patients; since this does not release histamine, it can be used safely in patients with pheochromocytoma

Specific References

Bodenham A and Park GR, "Alfentanil Infusions in Patients Requiring Intensive Care," *Clin Pharmacokinet*, 1988, 15(4):216-26.

Kirkham SR and Pugh R, "Opioid Analgesia in Uraemic Patients," *Lancet*, 1995, 345:1185.

Alferon® N *see* Interferon Alfa-N3 *on page 434*

Alglucerase (al glue' cir race)

CAS Number 143003-46-7

Brand Names Ceredase®

Use Orphan drug for treatment of Gaucher's disease

Mechanism of Action Glucocerebrosidase is an enzyme prepared from human placental tissue. Gaucher's disease is an inherited metabolic disorder caused by the defective activity of beta-glucosidase and the resultant accumulation of glucosyl ceramide laden macrophages in the liver, bone, and spleen. The disease affects an estimated 10,000-15,000 people in the United States, primarily of Eastern European Jewish descent, with up to 5,000 being symptomatic and requiring treatment; Ceredase® acts by replacing the missing enzyme associated with Gaucher's disease.

Adverse Reactions

Central nervous system: Slight fever, chills

Gastrointestinal: Abdominal discomfort, nausea, and vomiting

Local: Discomfort, burning, and swelling at the site of injection

Signs & Symptoms of Acute Overdose No obvious toxicity was detected after single doses of up to 234 units/kg

Usual Dosage Usually administered as a 20-60 units/kg I.V. infusion given with a frequency ranging from 3 times/week to once every 2 weeks

Warnings Prepared from pooled human placental tissue that may contain the causative agents of some viral diseases

Dosage Forms Injection: 10 units/mL (5 mL); 80 units/mL (5 mL)

Overdosage Treatment Supportive therapy: Acetaminophen for fever

Pregnancy Risk Factor C

Specific References

Whittington R and Goa KL, "Alglucerase: A Review of Its Therapeutic Use in Gaucher's Disease," *Drugs*, 1992, 44(1):72-93.

Algopent® *see* Pentazocine *on page 603*

Alimix® *see* Cisapride *on page 217*

Aliseum® *see* Diazepam *on page 271*

Alkaban-AQ® Injection *see* Vinblastine Sulfate *on page 790*

Alkeran® *see* Melphalan *on page 497*

Allegron® *see* Nortriptyline Hydrochloride *on page 571*

Aller-Chlor® [OTC] *see* Chlorpheniramine Maleate *on page 204*

Allerest® 12 Hours Nasal Solution [OTC] *see* Oxymetazoline Hydrochloride *on page 586*

Aller-eze® *see* Clemastine Fumarate *on page 223*

Allerplus® *see* Terfenadine *on page 728*

Allocaine *see* Procaine Hydrochloride *on page 644*

Allocar® *see* Digoxin *on page 284*

Allopurinol (al oh pure' i nole)

Related Information

Toxicities of Chemotherapeutic Agents *on page 1631-1633*

CAS Number 315-30-0

Brand Names Lopurin™; Zurinol®; Zyloprim®

Use Prevention of attack of gouty arthritis and nephropathy; also used to treat secondary hyperuricemia which may occur during treatment of tumors or leukemia; to prevent recurrent calcium oxalate calculi

Mechanism of Action Decreases the production of uric acid by inhibiting the action of xanthine oxidase, an enzyme that converts hypoxanthine to xanthine and xanthine to uric acid

Adverse Reactions

Central nervous system: Drowsiness, neuritis, fever

Dermatologic: Pruritic maculopapular rash, exfoliative dermatitis, erythema multiforme

Gastrointestinal: gastrointestinal irritation

Hematologic: Leukocytosis, leukopenia, thrombocytopenia, eosinophilia, bone marrow depression

Hepatic: Hepatitis

Ocular: Cataracts, diplopia

Renal: Renal impairment, proteinuria

Signs & Symptoms of Acute Overdose Most symptoms are from chronic use; nausea, vomiting, hepatitis, hypersensitivity, seizures, metallic taste, cerebral edema, myoglobinuria, leukopenia, toxic epidermal necrolysis, nephritis, Stevens-Johnson syndrome, pseudotumor cerebri, wheezing, hyperthermia, hematuria, dysosmia, neutropenia, agranulocytosis, granulocytopenia, alopecia, paresthesia

Toxicodynamics/Kinetics

Onset of action: Significant reduction of serum uric acid concentration usually occurs within 2 or 3 days

Duration: Serum uric acid concentration usually returns to the pretreatment value 1-2 weeks after discontinuation of therapy

Absorption:

Oral: ~80% from gastrointestinal tract

Rectal: <6%

Distribution: V_d: 2 L/kg; V_d oxypurinol: 1.6 L/kg; widely distributed to all extracellular fluid except brain

Protein binding: <1%

Metabolism: ~75% of the drug metabolized to active metabolites, chiefly oxypurinol

Half-life:

Parent: 1-3 hours

Oxypurinol: 18-30 hours in patients with normal renal function; 5-10 days in renal failure

Time to peak serum concentration: 0.5-2 hours for 300 mg dose

Elimination: Renal, up to 10% of dose excreted unchanged; remainder may be excreted by unidentified routes as other metabolites or in feces as unabsorbed allopurinol

Usual Dosage Oral:

Children: 10 mg/kg/day in 2-3 divided doses or 200-300 mg/m²/day in 2-4 divided doses, maximum: 600 mg/24 hours

Alternative dosing:

<6 years: 150 mg/day in 3 divided doses

6-10 years: 300 mg/day in 2-3 divided doses

Children >10 years and Adults: Daily doses >300 mg should be administered in divided doses

Myeloproliferative neoplastic disorders: 200-800 mg/day in 2-3 divided doses for prevention of acute uric acid nephropathy for 2-3 days starting 1-2 days before chemotherapy

Gout: 200-300 mg/day (mild); 400-600 mg/day (severe)

Maximum dose: 800 mg/day

Dosing interval in renal impairment: See table on next page.

Dosage supplement for hemodialysis: 50%

Contraindications Not to be used in pregnancy or lactation, or in patients with a previous severe allergy reaction

Warnings Do not use to treat asymptomatic hyperuricemia; reduce dosage in renal insufficiency, reinstate with caution in patients who have had a previous mild allergic reaction, use with caution in children; rash may be indicative of more serious hypersensitivity reaction, discontinue drug at first sign of rash

Dosage Forms Tablet: 100 mg, 300 mg

Stability Keep oral solution in refrigerator, remains stable for 56 days after preparation

(Continued)

Allopurinol *(Continued)*

Adult Maintenance Doses of Allopurinol*

Creatinine Clearance (mL/min)	Maintenance Dose of Allopurinol (mg)
140	400 qd
120	350 qd
100	300 qd
80	250 qd
60	200 qd
40	150 qd
20	100 qd
10	100 q2d
0	100 q3d

*This table is based on a standard maintenance dose of 300 mg of allopurinol per day for a patient with a creatinine clearance 100 mL/min.

Reference Range

Adults:

Males: 3.4-7.0 mg/dL (SI: 202-416 μmol/L) or slightly more

Females: 2.4-6.0 mg/dL (SI: 143-357 μmol/L) or slightly more

Uric acid, serum: An increase occurs during childhood. Values >7.0 mg/dL (SI: 416 μmol/L) are sometimes arbitrarily regarded as hyperuricemia, but there is no sharp line between normals on the one hand, and the serum uric acid of those with clinical gout. Normal ranges cannot be adjusted for purine ingestion, but high purine diet increases uric acid. Uric acid may be increased with body size, exercise, and stress. One fatal case was reported with levels of 230 μg/mL; death is rare.

Overdosage Treatment

Decontamination: Emesis in very early ingestions unless seizures present; lavage indicated in early ingestions

Supportive therapy: If significant amounts of allopurinol are thought to have been absorbed, it is a theoretical possibility that oxypurinol stones could be formed but no record of such occurrence in overdose exists. Alkalinization of the urine and forced diuresis can help prevent potential xanthine stone formation. Steroids and antihistamines are useful for hypersensitivity

Enhancement of elimination: Removed by hemodialysis, but of unknown value in overdose; renal clearance: 0.58 L/hour/kg; allopurinol and oxypurinol are dialyzable

Test Interactions Increases alkaline phosphatase, AST, ALT, decreases uric acid (S)

Drug Interactions Inhibits metabolism of azathioprine and mercaptopurine; use with ampicillin or amoxicillin may increase the incidence of skin rash; coadministration with thiazides may enhance hypersensitivity effects; may enhance hypoglycemia when given with chlorpropamide

Pregnancy Risk Factor C

Pregnancy Implications Distributes into breast milk

Monitoring Parameters CBC, serum uric acid levels, I & O, hepatic and renal function, especially at start of therapy

Patient Information Take after meals with plenty of fluid; discontinue drug and contact physician at first sign of rash, painful urination, blood in urine, irritation of eyes, or swelling of lips or mouth; may cause drowsiness

Additional Information Skin rash occurs most often in patients taking diuretics concurrently; may predispose patient to ampicillin-induced rash; alcohol decreases the effectiveness

Specific References

Elasy T, Kaminsky D, Tracy M, et al, "Allopurinol Hypersensitivity Syndrome Revisisted," *West J Med*, 1995, 162:360-1.

Ferner RE, Simmonds HA, and Bateman DN, "Allopurinol Kinetics After Massive Overdose," *Hum Toxicol*, 1988, 7(3):293-4.

McInnes GT, Lawson DH, and Jick H, "Acute Adverse Reactions Attributed to Allopurinol in Hospitalized Patients," *Ann Rheum Dis*, 1981, 40(3):245-9.

Parra E, Gota R, Gamen A, et al, "Granulomatous Interstitial Nephritis Secondary to Allopurinol Treatment," *Clin Nephrol*, 1995, 43:350.

Vinciullo C, "Allopurinol Hypersensitivity," *Med J Aust*, 1984, 141(7):449-50.

Almartyn® *see* Flecainide Acetate *on page 350*

Alodorm® *see* Nitrazepam *on page 562*

Alol® *see* Acebutolol Hydrochloride *on page 77*

Alomide® *see* Lodoxamide Tromethamine *on page 479*

Alophen Pills® [OTC] *see* Phenolphthalein *on page 617*

Alpha Alpha-Dimethyl Phenethylamine *see* Phentermine Hydrochloride *on page 619*

Alphakinase® *see* Urokinase *on page 779*

Alphamul® [OTC] *see* Castor Oil *on page 189*

Alprazolam (al pray' zoe lam)

Related Information

Benzodiazepines Comparison *on page 1643*

CAS Number 28981-97-7

Brand Names Tafil®; Trankimazin®; Valeans®; Xanax®; Xanor®

Replaces U-31889

Use Treatment of anxiety; adjunct in the treatment of depression; management of panic attacks; may be helpful in treating premenstrual syndrome (PMS)

Mechanism of Action Binds at stereospecific receptors at several sites within the central nervous system, including the limbic system, reticular formation; effects may be mediated through GABA. It is a triazolobenzodiazepine with some antidepressant activity.

Adverse Reactions

Cardiovascular: Hypotension

Central nervous system: Drowsiness, dizziness, confusion, sedation, slurred speech, headache, psychosis, ataxia

Gastrointestinal: Dry mouth, constipation, diarrhea, nausea, vomiting, absent bowel sounds

Hepatic: Acute hepatitis

Ocular: Blurred vision, diplopia, mydriasis

Miscellaneous: Physical and psychological dependence with prolonged use, combativeness

Signs & Symptoms of Acute Overdose Somnolence, delirium, depression, photosensitivity, dermatitis, insomnia, confusion, mania, coma, lightheadedness, leukocytosis, diminished reflexes, hypotension, respiratory depression, combativeness, hypothermia

Toxicodynamics/Kinetics

Onset of action:

- After single oral dose: Onset depends largely on absorption rate
- After multiple doses: Effects depend partly upon rate and extent of drug accumulation

Duration:

- After single dose: Depends upon rate and extent of drug distribution, as well as rate of elimination once distribution is completed
- After multiple doses: Depends on rate and extent of drug accumulation which in turn relates to elimination half-life and clearance

Absorption: Oral: Rapidly and well absorbed

Distribution: V_d: 0.9-1.6 L/kg

Protein binding: 80%

Metabolism: Extensive in the liver; major metabolite is inactive

Half-life:

- Parent compound: 12-15 hours
- Metabolite: 10-15 hours

Time to peak serum concentration: Within 1-2 hours

Elimination: Metabolites and parent compound in urine clearance: 1.4 mL/minute/kg

Usual Dosage Oral:

Children <18 years: Safety and dose have not been established

Adults: 0.25-0.5 mg 2-3 times/day, titrate dose upward; maximum: 4 mg/day

- Premenstrual syndrome: 1 mg/day in 4 divided doses from day 18 to first day of menses with a taper on first two menstrual days; may increase bedtime dosing to 0.5 mg after 3 days

Dosing adjustment in hepatic impairment: Reduce dose by 50% to 60% or avoid in cirrhosis

Note: Treatment >4 months should be re-evaluated to determine the patient's need for the drug

Contraindications Hypersensitivity to alprazolam or any component; possible cross-sensitivity with other benzodiazepines; severe uncontrolled pain, narrow-angle glaucoma, severe respiratory depression, pre-existing CNS depression; not to be used in pregnancy or lactation

(Continued)

Alprazolam *(Continued)*

Warnings Safety has not been established in children <18 years of age; withdrawal symptoms have occurred 18 hours to 3 days after abrupt discontinuation of alprazolam; when discontinuing therapy, decrease daily dose by no more than 0.5 mg every 3 days; reduce dose in patients with significant hepatic disease

Dosage Forms Tablet: 0.25 mg, 0.5 mg, 1 mg, 2 mg

Reference Range Toxic symptoms may occur at alprazolam plasma levels >350 mg/mL

Overdosage Treatment

Decontamination: Lavage/activated charcoal with cathartic

Supportive: Treatment for benzodiazepine overdose is supportive. Rarely is mechanical ventilation required. Flumazenil has been shown to selectively block the binding of benzodiazepines to CNS receptors, resulting in a reversal of benzodiazepine-induced CNS depression. Carbamazepine may be effective for withdrawal.

Enhancement of elimination: Multiple dosing of activated charcoal may be effective

Antidote(s)

Flumazenil *on page 1428*

Test Interactions Increases alkaline phosphatase; Visine®, Drano®, bleach may cause false-negative urine tests; oxazepam may interfere in giving falsely elevated glucose results

Drug Interactions Cimetidine may decrease and enzyme inducers may increase metabolism of alprazolam; CNS depressants may enhance CNS effects (ethanol, barbiturates); digoxin levels may triple when given with alprazolam; dextropropoxyphene may prolong its half-life; concomitant use of clomipramine with alprazolam can result in serotonin syndrome

Pregnancy Risk Factor D (may produce neonatal withdrawal)

Monitoring Parameters Respiratory and cardiovascular status

Patient Information May be taken with food; avoid alcohol ingestion; rise slowly to avoid fainting

Nursing Implications Assist with ambulation during beginning therapy

Additional Information Not intended for management of anxieties and minor distresses associated with everyday life; treatment longer than 4 months should be re-evaluated to determine the patient's need for the drug; 1 mg of alprazolam is equivalent approximately to 10 mg of diazepam in anxiolytic activity

Specific References

Cano-Munoz JL, Montejo-Iglesias ML, Yanez-Saez RM, et al, "Possible Serotonin Syndrome Following the Combined Administration of Clomipramine and Alprazolam," *J Clin Psychiatry*, 1995, 56:122.

Crome P and Ali C, "Clinical Features and Management of Self Poisoning With Newer Antidepressants," *Med Toxicol Adverse Drug Exp*, 1986, 1(6):411-20.

Fawcett JA and Kravitz HM, "Alprazolam: Pharmacokinetics, Clinical Efficacy, and Mechanism of Action," *Pharmacotherapy*, 1982, 2(5):243-54.

Freeman EW, Rickels K, Sondheimer SJ, et al, "A Double-Blind Trial of Oral Progesterone, Alprazolam, and Placebo in the Treatment of Severe Premenstrual Syndrome," *JAMA*, 1995, 274:51-7.

McCormick SR, Nielsen J, and Jatlow PI, "Alprazolam Overdose, Clinical Findings and Serum Concentrations in Two Cases," *J Clin Psychiatry*, 1985, 46(6):247-8.

Moulin CH, Rolachon A, Cohard M, et al, "Fulminant Hepatitis Secondary to Alprazolam," *Therapie*, 1994, 49(4):362-3.

Mumford GK, Evans SM, Fleishaker JC, et al, "Alprazolam Absorption Kinetics Affects Abuse Liability," *Clin Pharmacol Ther*, 1995, 57:356-65.

Prischl F, Donner A, Grimm G, et al, "Value of Flumazenil in Benzodiazepine Self-Poisoning," *Med Toxicol Adverse Drug Exp*, 1988, 3(4):334-9.

Alredase® *see* Tolrestat *on page 760*

AL-R® [OTC] *see* Chlorpheniramine Maleate *on page 204*

Altace™ Oral *see* Ramipril *on page 673*

Alteplase, Recombinant (al' te place)

CAS Number 105857-23-6

Brand Names Actilyse®; Actiplus®; Activase® Injection

Synonyms Tissue Plasminogen Activator, Recombinant; t-PA

Use Management of acute myocardial infarction for the lysis of thrombi in coronary arteries; management of acute massive pulmonary embolism (PE) in adults

Mechanism of Action Initiates local fibrinolysis by binding to fibrin in a thrombus (clot) and converts entrapped plasminogen to plasmin; does not initiate systemic fibrinolysis in absence of a thrombus

Adverse Reactions

Cardiovascular: Hypotension, reperfusion arrhythmia (bradycardia, premature ventricular contraction), pericardial effusion/pericarditis, chest pain

Central nervous system: Fever, seizures

Dermatologic: Ecchymosis

Gastrointestinal: Gastrointestinal hemorrhage, nausea, vomiting

Genitourinary: GU hemorrhage

Miscellaneous: Retroperitoneal hemorrhage, epistaxis, gingival hemorrhage, intracranial hemorrhage (0.6%); allergic reactions are rare (<0.02%)

Signs & Symptoms of Acute Overdose Increased incidence of intracranial bleeding or peripheral bleeding; coagulopathy, ocular hemorrhage, headache, hemoptysis, hematuria, gastrointestinal bleeding

Toxicodynamics/Kinetics

Duration of effect: 2 hours

Elimination: Cleared rapidly from circulating plasma at a rate of 550-650 mL/minute, primarily by the liver; >50% present in plasma is cleared within 5 minutes after the infusion has been terminated, and ~80% is cleared within 10 minutes

Usual Dosage

Acute myocardial infarction (administer as soon as possible after the onset of symptoms):

Accelerated infusion: Recommended total dose is based upon patient weight, not to exceed 100 mg

Patients weighing >67 kg: Recommended dose: 100 mg as a 15 mg I.V. bolus followed by 50 mg infused over the next 30 minutes, and then 35 mg infused over the next 60 minutes

Patients weighing ≤67 kg: Recommended dose: 15 mg I.V. bolus, followed by 0.75 mg/kg infused over the next 30 minutes not to exceed 50 mg, then 0.50 mg/kg over the next 60 minutes not to exceed 35 mg

The safety and efficacy of this accelerated infusion regimen has only been investigated with concomitant administration of heparin and aspirin; the bolus dose may be prepared in one of the following ways:

1. By removing 15 mL from the vial of reconstituted (1 mg/mL) Activase® using a syringe and needle (if this method is used with the 20 mg or 50 mg vials, the syringe should not be primed with air and the needle should be inserted into the vial stopper; if the 100 mg vial is used, the needle should be inserted away from the puncture mark made by the transfer device)
2. By removing 15 mL from a port (second injection site) on the infusion line after the infusion set is primed
3. By programming an infusion pump to deliver a 15 mL (1 mg/mL) bolus at the initiation of the infusion

The remainder of the dose may be administered as follows:

20 mg, 50 mg vials: Administer using either a polyvinyl chloride bag or glass vial and infusion set

100 mg vials: Insert the spike end of an infusion set through the same puncture site created by the transfer device in the stopper of the vial of reconstituted alteplase; hang vial from the plastic molded capping attached to the bottom of the vial

3-hour infusion: Recommended dose: 100 mg administered as 60 mg (34.8 million IU) in the first hour (of which 6-10 mg is administered as a bolus); 20 mg (11.6 million IU) over the second hour, and 20 mg (11.6 million IU) over the third hour; for smaller patients (<65 kg), a dose of 1.25 mg/kg administered over 3 hours, as described previously, may be used

Although the value of the use of anticoagulants during and following administration has not been fully studied, heparin has been administered concomitantly for 24 hours or longer in more than 90% of patients; aspirin and/or dipyridamole have been given to patients during and/or following heparin treatment

The bolus dose may be prepared in one of the following ways:

1. By removing 6-10 mL from the vial of reconstituted (1 mg/mL) alteplase using a syringe and needle (if this method is used with the 20 mg or 50 mg vials, the syringe should not be primed with air and the needle should be inserted into the vial stopper; if the 100 mg vial is used, the needle should be inserted away from the puncture mark made by the transfer device)
2. By removing 6-10 mL from a port (second injection site) on the infusion line after the infusion set is primed
3. By programming an infusion pump to deliver a 6-10 mL (1 mg/mL) bolus at the initiation of the infusion

The remainder of the dose may be administered as follows:

20 mg, 50 mg vials: Administer using either a polyvinyl chloride bag or glass vial and infusion set

100 mg vial: Insert the spike end of an infusion set through the same puncture site created by the transfer device in the stopper of the vial of reconstituted alteplase; hang the vial from the plastic molded capping attached to the bottom of the vial

Acute pulmonary embolism: 100 mg over 2 hours or 0.6 mg/kg over 2 minutes with heparin initiated immediately following infusion

Administration Do not use bacteriostatic water for reconstitution

Contraindications Active internal bleeding, history of cerebrovascular accident, intracranial neoplasm, aneurysm, or recent (within 2 months) intracranial or in-

(Continued)

Alteplase, Recombinant *(Continued)*

traspinal surgery or trauma; patients with known bleeding diathesis, arteriovenous malformation, or severe uncontrolled hypertension

Warnings Doses >150 mg have been associated with an increase of intracranial hemorrhage; use with caution in active menstrual bleeding

Dosage Forms Powder for injection, lyophilized: 20 mg [11.6 million units] (20 mL); 50 mg [29 million units] (50 mL); 100 mg [58 million units] (100 mL)

Stability Refrigerate; must be used within 8 hours of reconstitution; alteplase is **incompatible** with dobutamine, glyceryl trinitrate, dopamine, heparin, and nitroglycerin infusions; physically **compatible** with lidocaine, metoprolol, propranolol when administered via Y site

Reference Range Not routinely measured; literature supports therapeutic levels of 0.52-1.80 μg/mL

Overdosage Treatment

Supportive therapy: Treat bleeding complications with transfusions of red blood cells, fresh frozen plasma, and cryoprecipitate; do not administer dextran; although human overdose data is lacking, administration of aminocaproic acid (Amicar®) at a dose of 3-5 g I.V. followed by an infusion rate of 1-1.25 g/hour may be useful

Test Interactions Fibrinogen levels decrease 16% to 36%

Drug Interactions Increased therapeutic effect and toxicity: Oral anticoagulants, aspirin, dipyridamole, heparin

Pregnancy Risk Factor C

Monitoring Parameters Fibrinogen degradation products, blood pressure, PT, PTT, fibrinogen, platelet count, hematocrit

Nursing Implications Assess for hemorrhage during first hour of treatment

Additional Information Allergic reactions are unlikely; investigational for angina, deep vein thrombosis, catheter thrombosis, peripheral artery thrombosis, thrombotic stroke; has been used to treat acute myocardial infarction in a heart transplant recipient

Reimbursement Hotline: 1-800-879-4747

Professional Services (GENENTECH): 1-800-821-8590

Specific References

Astengo D, Badano L, and Bertoli D, "Recombinant Tissue Plasminogen Activator for Prosthetic Mitral-Valve Thrombosis," *N Engl J Med*, 1995, 333(4):259.

Bell WR, "Thrombolytic Therapy: Agents, Indications, and Laboratory Monitoring," *Med Clin North Am*, 1994, 78(3):745-64.

de Boer A and van Griensven JMT, "Drug Interactions With Thrombolytic Agents," *Clin Pharmacokinet*, 1995, 28:315-26.

Dehmer GJ, Gresalfi N, Daly D, et al, "Impairment of Fibrinolysis by Streptokinase, Urokinase, and Recombinant Tissue-Type Plasminogen Activator in the Presence of Radiographic Contrast Agents," *J Am Coll Cardiol*, 1995, 25(5):1069-75.

Geraets DR, Hoehns JD, Burke TG, et al, "Thrombolytic-Associated Cholesterol Emboli Syndrome: Case Report and Literature Review," *Pharmacotherapy*, 1995, 15(4):441-50.

Hagglund H, Ringden O, Ljungman P, et al, "No Beneficial Effects, But Severe Side-Effects by Recombinant Human Tissue Plasminogen Activator for Treatment of Hepatic Veno-Occlusive Disease After Allogensic Bone Marrow Transplantation," *Bone Marrow Transplant*, 1995, 15(Suppl 2):149.

Kalish SC, Gurwitz JH, Krumholz HM, et al, "A Cost-Effectiveness Model of Thrombolytic Therapy for Acute Myocardial Infarction," *J Gen Intern Med*, 1995, 10:321-30.

Krause J, "Catabolism of Tissue-Type Plasminogen Activator (t-PA), Its Variants, Mutants, and Hybrids," *Fibrinolysis*, 1988, 2:133-42.

Kurnick PB, "Circadian Variation in the Efficacy of Tissue-Type Plasminogen Activator," *Circulation*, 1995, 91(5):1341-6.

Lee TH, "Cost Effectiveness of Tissue Plasminogen Activator," *N Engl J Med*, 1995, 332:1443-4.

Mark DB, Hlatky MA, Califf RM, et al, "Cost Effectiveness of Thrombolytic Therapy With Tissue Plasminogen Activator as Compared With Streptokinase for Acute Myocardial Infarction," *N Engl J Med*, 1995, 332:1418-24.

Meyer BJ and Chesebro JH, "New Accelerated rt-PA Strategy Has Sufficient Advantage Over Older Streptokinase Strategies That it Should Be the Thrombolytic Strategy of Choice in Anterior and Large Infarctions," *Am J Ther*, 1995, 2:123-7.

Sloan MA, Price TR, Petito CK, et al, "Clinical Features and Pathogenesis of Intracerebral Hemorrhage After rt-PA and Heparin Therapy for Acute Myocardial Infarction: The Thrombolysis in Myocardial Infarction (TIMI) II Pilot and Randomized Clinical Trial Combined Experience," *Neurology*, 1995, 45:649-58.

The Gusto Angiographic Investigators, "The Effects of Tissue Plasminogen Activator, Streptokinase, or Both on Coronary-Artery Patency, Ventricular Function, and Survival After Acute Myocardial Infarction," *N Engl J Med*, 1993, 329(22):1615-22.

Thomas WO, Harris CN, D'Amore TF, et al, "Bilateral Forearm and Hand Compartment Syndrome Following Thrombolysis for Acute Myocardial Infarction: A Case Report," *J Emerg Med*, 1994, 12(4):467-72.

Virk AS, Antosia RE, and Partridge RA, "Use of Thrombolytic Therapy in a Heart Transplant Recipient With Acute Myocardial Infarction," *Ann Emerg Med*, 1995, 25:548-50.

White HD, "Comparative Safety of Thrombolytic Agents," *Am J Cardiol*, 1991, 68(16):30E-7E.

Woo KS and White HD, "Comparative Tolerability Profiles of Thrombolytic Agents," *Drug Saf*, 1993, 8(1):19-29.

ALternaGEL® [OTC] *see* Aluminum *on page 104*

Altretamine (al tret' a meen)

Related Information

Toxicities of Chemotherapeutic Agents *on page 1631-1633*

CAS Number 645-05-6

Brand Names Hexalen®; Hexastat®; Hexinawas®

Synonyms Hexamethylmelamine

Use Palliative treatment of persistent or recurrent ovarian cancer

Mechanism of Action Synthetic cytotoxic antineoplastic s-triazine derivative but the exact mechanism of action of the drug is unknown. Although altretamine clinical antitumor spectrum resembles that of alkylating agents, the drug has demonstrated activity in alkylator-resistant patients; probably requires hepatic microsomal mixed-function oxidase enzyme activation to become cytotoxic. The drug selectively inhibits the incorporation of radioactive thymidine and uridine into DNA and RNA, inhibiting DNA and RNA synthesis; metabolized to reactive intermediates which covalently bind to microsomal proteins and DNA. These reactive intermediates can spontaneously degrade to demethylated melamines and formaldehyde which are also cytotoxic.

Adverse Reactions

Central nervous system: Ataxia, agitation

Dermatologic: Alopecia, pruritus, eczema

Gastrointestinal: Nausea, vomiting, anorexia, diarrhea, abdominal cramps

Genitourinary: Cystitis

Hematologic: Thrombocytopenia and leukopenia occur during first week and reach a nadir at 3-4 weeks

Neuromuscular & skeletal: Paresthesia, hyporeflexia, muscle weakness, neuropathy (peripheral)

Toxicodynamics/Kinetics

Absorption: Oral: Well absorbed (75% to 89%)

Distribution: V_d: 460 L/m^2

Metabolism: Rapid and extensive demethylation in liver to nine metabolites; high concentrations in liver and kidney, but low concentrations in other organs

Half-life: 13 hours

Peak plasma levels: 0.3-3 hours

Elimination: In the urine (<1% unchanged); clearance: 0.7 L/minute/m^2

Usual Dosage

Adults: Oral (refer to protocol): 300 mg/m^2/day for 14-21 consecutive days in a 28-day cycle; in combination with other cytotoxic drugs, doses of 100-225 mg/m^2/day for 7-21 consecutive days in a 28-day cycle have been used

Maximum tolerated dose: 10-12 mg/kg/day for 21 consecutive days in 28-day cycle

Investigational parenteral administration: In 10% Intralipid® at an infusion rate of 2-8 mg/minute followed by 50 mL of saline

Contraindications Hypersensitivity to altretamine, pre-existing severe bone marrow depression or severe neurologic toxicity

Warnings Use with caution in patients with thrombocytopenia or leukopenia

Dosage Forms Capsule: 50 mg

Reference Range Peak plasma levels after a 200-300 mg/m^2 dose range from 0.3-20.8 mg/L

Overdosage Treatment

Decontamination: Lavage/activated charcoal with cathartic

Supportive therapy: Pyridoxine can be used to treat neuropathy (peripheral), although this mode of therapy is unproven

Antidote(s)

Pyridoxine Hydrochloride *on page 1465*

Drug Interactions

Decreased effect: Phenobarbital may increase metabolism

Increased toxicity: May cause severe hypotension (orthostatic) when administered with MAO inhibitors; concurrent use with MAO inhibitors and tricyclic antidepressants can result in syncope and dizziness within first week of treatment; increased toxicity with cimetidine (may decrease metabolism)

Pregnancy Risk Factor D

Monitoring Parameters WBC count, platelet count, CBC (monthly)

Additional Information Mucosal and dermal irritant

Specific References

Bruckner HW and Schleifer SJ, "Orthostatic Hypotension as a Complication of Hexamethylmelamine Antidepressant Interaction," *Cancer Treat Rep*, 1983, 67:516.

Damia G and D'Incalci M, "Clinical Pharmacokinetics of Altretamine," *Clin Pharmacokinet*, 1995, 28:439-48.

Hahn DA and Black C, "Hexamethylamine: A Review," *Drug Intell Clin Pharm*, 1980, 14:541-7.

Hansen LA and Hughes TE, "Altretamine," *DICP*, 1991, 25(2):146-52.

Manetta A, Mac Neill C, Lyter JA, et al, "Hexamethylmelamine as a Single Second-Line Agent in Ovarian Cancer," *Gynecol Oncol*, 1990, 36(1):93-6.

Alu-Cap® [OTC] *see* Aluminum *on this page*

Aluminum (a loo' mi num)

Related Information

Toxins Which Should be Lavaged With Solutions Other Than Water *on page 1635*

CAS Number 7429-90-5

UN Number 1309; 1396; 9260

Brand Names ALternaGEL® [OTC]; Alu-Cap® [OTC]; Alu-Tab® [OTC]; Amphojel® [OTC]; Dialume® [OTC]; Nephrox Suspension [OTC]

Synonyms Al; Alaun

Use Antacid; coloring agent in foods; antiperspirant; also found in sucralfate (207 mg aluminum per g dose)

Adverse Reactions

Central nervous system: Encephalopathy (dialysis dementia, drowsiness, hallucinations, coma), ataxia, parkinsonism, seizures
Dermatologic: Irritant dermatitis
Endocrine & metabolic: Hypercalcemia
Hematologic: Microcytic anemia
Neuromuscular & skeletal: Intention tremors, osteomalacia, osteodystrophy
Respiratory: Cough, pulmonary fibrosis, wheezing, cholestasis

Signs & Symptoms of Acute Overdose Toxicity is usually seen in the setting of water contamination used in hemodialysis, aluminum hydroxide toxicity in renal failure patients, contamination of total parenteral nutrition; solutions or human albumin solutions or industrial exposure inhibits brain glycolysis and microtubular polymerization; aluminum antacids may cause constipation, phosphate depletion, and bezoars or fecalith formation, feces discoloration (black), feces discoloration (white/speckling); in patients with renal failure, aluminum may accumulate to toxic levels; jaundice may also occur

Toxicodynamics/Kinetics

Absorption: 12% gastric, <1% oral
Protein binding: 50%
Half-life: 276 minutes
Elimination: Renal clearance 0.12 L/hour

Usual Dosage Oral:

Peptic ulcer disease:
- Children: 5-15 mL/dose every 3-6 hours or 1 and 3 hours after meals and at bedtime
- Adults: 15-45 mL every 3-6 hours or 1 and 3 hours after meals and at bedtime

Prophylaxis against gastrointestinal bleeding:
- Infants: 2-5 mL/dose every 1-2 hours
- Children: 5-15 mL/dose every 1-2 hours
- Adults: 30-60 mL/dose every hour
- Titrate to maintain the gastric pH >5

Hyperphosphatemia:
- Children: 50-150 mg/kg/24 hours in divided doses every 4-6 hours, titrate dosage to maintain serum phosphorus within normal range
- Adults: 500-1800 mg, 3-6 times/day, between meals and at bedtime

Antacid: Adults: 30 mL 1 and 3 hours postprandial and at bedtime

Dosage Forms

Capsule: 475 mg, 500 mg
Gel: 600 mg/5 mL (360 mL)
Suspension, oral: 320 mg/5 mL (500 mL)
Tablet: 300 mg, 500 mg, 600 mg

Reference Range Normal plasma aluminum levels are <10 μg/L; levels >100 μg/L are associated with toxicity; normal urinary aluminum level: 0.05-1 mg/L

Overdosage Treatment

Supportive therapy:
- Deferoxamine (15-20 mg/kg once weekly I.V.), traditionally used as an iron chelator, has been shown to increase urinary aluminum output
- Deferoxamine chelation of aluminum has resulted in improvements of clinical symptoms and bone histology
- Deferoxamine, however, remains an experimental treatment for aluminum poisoning and has a significant potential for adverse effects
- Deferoxamine infused 1-2 hours at the end of dialysis; monitor iron levels carefully along with platelet counts

Enhancement of elimination: Hemodialysis or charcoal hemoperfusion will also remove aluminum; aluminum-desferrioxamine complex can be efficiently removed with high flux dialysate membranes

Drug Interactions Aluminum hydroxide can decrease intestinal absorption of fluoride; aluminum phosphate gel can precipitate radioactive strontium in the gut

Pregnancy Risk Factor C

Additional Information Insoluble in water and alcohol; iron deficiency may increase aluminum absorption, possible association with dialysis, dementia, and renal osteodystrophy; aluminum comprises 8% of the earth's crust; bauxite is the main source of environmental aluminum

Aluminum only has one oxidation state (+3); background atmospheric aluminum levels range from 0.005-0.2 mg/m^3; baseline drinking water aluminum levels range from 0.003-1.6 mg/L; soil aluminum levels range from 700 mg/kg to over 100,000 mg/kg

Foods containing highest aluminum levels are ground coffee beans (52 mg/kg), salt (31-37 mg/kg), natural peanut butter (26-94 mg/kg), Oreo® chocolate cookie (12.7 mg/kg), pumpernickel bread (13.2 mg/kg), and lettuce (7.2 mg/kg)

Aluminum is not bioconcentrated in plants or terrestrial food chain; antacids/buffered aspirin can contain from 4-562 mg/kg of aluminum. Daily intake of aluminum is ~2-14 mg by food ingestion, 0.2 mg through drinking water, and 0.2 mg by inhalation; total body burden of aluminum is ~30-50 (50% in bone, 25% in lungs).

Specific References

Cumming RG and Klineberg RJ, "Aluminum in Antacids and Cooking Pots and the Risk of Hip Fractures in Elderly People," *Age Ageing*, 1994, 23:468-72.

Gupta S and Ahlaway SK, "Aluminum Phosphide POisoning - A Review," *Clin Toxicol*, 1995, 33:19-24.

Maher ER, Brown EA, Curtis JR, et al, "Accumulation of Aluminum in Chronic Renal Failure Due to Administration of Albumin Replacement Solutions," *Br Med J (Clin Res)*, 1986, 292(6516):306.

Monteagudo FS, Cassidy MJ, and Folb PI, "Recent Developments in Aluminum Toxicity," *Med Toxicol Adverse Drug Exp*, 1989, 4(1):1-16.

Robertson JA, Salusky IB, Goodman WG, et al, "Sucralfate, Intestinal Aluminum Absorption, and Aluminum Toxicity in a Patient on Dialysis," *Ann Intern Med*, 1989, 111(2):179-81.

U.S. Department of Health and Human Services, "Toxicological Profile for Aluminum TP-91/01," Agency for Toxic Substances and Diseases Registry, July 1992.

Aluminum Sucrose Sulfate *see* Sucralfate *on page 710*

Alupent® *see* Metaproterenol Sulfate *on page 506*

Alupram® *see* Diazepam *on page 271*

Alu-Tab® [OTC] *see* Aluminum *on previous page*

Aluzine® *see* Furosemide *on page 373*

Amantadine Hydrochloride (a man' ta deen)

Related Information

Therapeutic Drugs Associated With Hallucinations *on page 1558-1559*

CAS Number 665-66-7

Brand Names Symmetrel®

Synonyms Adamantanamine Hydrochloride

Use Symptomatic and adjunct treatment of parkinsonism; also used in prophylaxis and treatment of influenza A viral infection

Mechanism of Action As an antiviral, blocks the uncoating of influenza A virus preventing penetration of virus into host; antiparkinsonian activity may be due to its blocking the reuptake of dopamine into presynaptic neurons and causing direct stimulation of postsynaptic receptors

Adverse Reactions

Cardiovascular: Edema, hypotension (orthostatic), Q-T prolongation

Central nervous system: Dizziness, ataxia, confusion, insomnia, difficulty in concentrating, anxiety, restlessness, irritability, visual hallucinations, auditory hallucinations, headache, akathisia

Gastrointestinal: Nausea

Signs & Symptoms of Acute Overdose Nausea, vomiting, congestive heart failure, slurred speech, blurred vision, drowsiness, memory loss, mania, depression, coma, chorea (extrapyramidal), photosensitivity, night terrors, hyperthermia, myasthenia gravis (exacerbation or precipitation of), cardiac arrhythmias (including torsade de pointes), anticholinergic symptoms, CNS depression followed by stimulation, seizures, neuroleptic malignant syndrome, neutropenia, dystonic reactions, emesis, metabolic acidosis, psychosis, pulmonary edema, bradycardia, insomnia, fever, tachycardia

Toxicodynamics/Kinetics

Onset of action: Usually within 48 hours, antidyskinetic

Absorption: Well absorbed from gastrointestinal tract (55% to 90%)

Distribution: V_d: Normal: 4.4 ±0.2 L/kg; Renal failure: 5.1 ±0.2 L/kg; distributed to saliva, tear film, and nasal secretions; in animals, tissue (especially lung) concentrations higher than serum concentrations

Protein binding:

Normal renal function: ~67%

(Continued)

Amantadine Hydrochloride *(Continued)*

Hemodialysis patients: ~59%

Metabolism: Not appreciable, small amounts of an acetyl metabolite identified (5% to 15%)

Half-life:

Normal renal function: 10-28 hours

Elderly patients: 24-29 hours

Impaired renal function: 7-10 days

Hemodialysis patients: Usually within 48 hours

Time to peak serum concentration: 1-4 hours

Elimination: 80% to 90% unchanged in urine by glomerular filtration and tubular secretion

Usual Dosage

Children:

1-9 years: 4.4-8.8 mg/kg/day in 1-2 divided doses to a maximum of 150 mg/day

9-12 years: 100-200 mg/day in 1-2 divided doses

After first influenza A virus vaccine dose, amantadine prophylaxis may be administered for up to 6 weeks or until 2 weeks after the second dose of vaccine

Adults:

Parkinson's disease: 100 mg twice daily

Influenza A viral infection: 200 mg/day in 1-2 divided doses

Prophylaxis: Minimum 10-day course of therapy following exposure or continue for 2-3 weeks after influenza A virus vaccine is given

Elderly patients should take the drug in 2 daily doses rather than a single dose to avoid adverse neurologic reactions

Dosing interval in renal impairment:

Cl_{cr} 50-60 mL/minute: Administer 200 mg alternating with 100 mg/day

Cl_{cr} 30-50 mL/minute: Administer 100 mg/day

Cl_{cr} 20-30 mL/minute: Administer 200 mg twice weekly

Cl_{cr} 10-20 mL/minute: Administer 100 mg 3 times/week

Cl_{cr} <10 mL/minute: Administer 200 mg alternating with 100 mg every 7 days

Contraindications Hypersensitivity to amantadine hydrochloride or any component

Warnings Use with caution in patients with liver disease, a history of recurrent and eczematoid dermatitis, uncontrolled psychosis or severe psychoneurosis, epilepsy or other seizures and in those receiving CNS stimulant drugs

Dosage Forms

Capsule: 100 mg

Syrup: 50 mg/5 mL (480 mL)

Stability Protect from freezing

Reference Range Toxic and potentially fatal: 4-23 μg/mL

Overdosage Treatment

Decontamination: Emesis not recommended due to potential for seizures; lavage recommended in early ingestions after seizure control; activated charcoal with cathartic of value; multiple-dose activated charcoal not studied

Supportive therapy: If symptomatic, observe for 24-48 hours since cardiac symptoms are delayed; treatment should be directed at reducing the CNS stimulation and at maintaining cardiovascular function. Seizures can be treated with diazepam or lorazepam 5-10 mg I.V. every 15 minutes as needed; up to a total of 30 mg in adults (0.25-0.4 mg/kg/dose I.V. every 15 minutes as needed up to a total of 10 mg for children); lidocaine is drug of choice for arrhythmias followed by procainamide; bretylium, propranolol (if arrhythmias are due to beta-adrenergic excess); $MgSO_4$ for torsade de pointes; avoid class IA (other than procainamide) and class II agents; pulmonary edema may respond to steroids; norepinephrine may be effective for hypotension; physostigmine has been used and is recommended only in severe, life-threatening anticholinergic symptoms; ice baths, bromocriptine, and/or dantrolene may be effective for malignant hyperthermia, but clinical experience in this setting is limited.

Enhancement of elimination: Hemodialysis of minimal value, as is peritoneal dialysis; slightly dialyzable (5% to 20%)

Drug Interactions Additive anticholinergic effects in patients receiving drugs with anticholinergic activity; additive CNS stimulant effect with CNS stimulants

Pregnancy Risk Factor C

Pregnancy Implications Crosses placenta and blood-brain barrier; excreted in breast milk

Monitoring Parameters Renal function

Patient Information Do not abruptly discontinue therapy, it may precipitate a parkinsonian crisis; may impair ability to perform activities requiring mental alertness or coordination

Nursing Implications If insomnia occurs, the last daily dose should be taken several hours before retiring; assess parkinsonian symptoms prior to and throughout course of therapy

Specific References

Aoki FY and Sitar DS, "Clinical Pharmacokinetics of Amantadine Hydrochloride," *Clin Pharmacokinet*, 1988, 14(1):35-51.

Berkowitz CD, "Treatment of Acute Amantadine Toxicity With Physostigmine," *J Pediatr*, 1979, 95(1):144-5.

Miller KS and Miller JM, "Toxic Effects of Amantadine in Patients With Renal Failure," *Chest*, 1994, 105(5):1630.

Sartori M, Pratt CM, and Young JB, "Torsade de Pointe: Malignant Cardiac Arrhythmias Induced by Amantadine Poisoning," *Am J Med*, 1984, 77(2):388-91.

Amavil® *see* Amitriptyline Hydrochloride *on page 116*

Amaxin® *see* Chlorthalidone *on page 210*

Amazin® *see* Chlorpromazine Hydrochloride *on page 205*

Ambien™ *see* Zolpidem Tartrate *on page 814*

AmBisome® *see* Amphotericin B *on page 123*

Amboclorin® *see* Chlorambucil *on page 195*

Ambush Fog® *see* Permethrin *on page 608*

Americaine® [OTC] *see* Benzocaine *on page 149*

Amethocaine Hydrochloride *see* Tetracaine Hydrochloride *on page 731*

Amethopterin *see* Methotrexate *on page 515*

Amfebutamone *see* Bupropion *on page 170*

Amifostine

Related Information

Cisplatin *on page 218*

Cyclophosphamide *on page 249*

CAS Number 20537-88-6; 63717-27-1

Synonyms Ethiofos; Gammaphos

Use Investigational: In combination with cisplatin in treatment of metastatic melanoma and ovarian cancer

Mechanism of Action Organic thiophosphate compound which acts as a free radical scavenger agent; can be nephroprotective from alkylating agent effects; radioprotectant and can cause hypocalcemia through inhibition of bone resorption and parathyroid hormone secretion

Adverse Reactions

Cardiovascular: Hypotension (related to dose and infusion rates), flushing

Central nervous system: Drowsiness, sedation, fever

Endocrine & metabolic: Hypocalcemia, hypomagnesemia

Gastrointestinal: Nausea, vomiting

Respiratory: Sneezing

Toxicodynamics/Kinetics

Absorption: Oral: Poor

Distribution: V_d: 3.5 L

Metabolism: Hepatic dephosphorylation to two metabolites (WR-33278 and WR-1065)

Half-life: 9 minutes

Elimination: Renal; plasma clearance: 2.17 L/minute

Usual Dosage Given 15-20 minutes prior to cisplatin or cyclophosphamide therapy with adequate hydration and mannitol or furosemide

I.V.: 740-910 mg/m^2 over 15 minutes

Contraindications Amifostine hypersensitivity

Warnings Use with caution in patients with hypotension, cardiovascular disease, hypocalcemia, pregnancy, and breast feeding

Dosage Forms Amifostine 500 mg and mannitol 500 mg per 10 mL

Stability For 2 years in frozen conditions (-2°C to -10°C)

Reference Range Peak serum amifostine levels after an I.V. dose of 150 mg/m^2 ranges from 100-900 μmol/L

Overdosage Treatment Supportive therapy: Keep patient well hydrates; monitor renal status, calcium, and magnesium

Monitoring Parameters Calcium, magnesium, blood pressure

Additional Information Currently investigational and may be obtained through the National Cancer Institute Pharmaceutical Management Branch at (301) 496-5725 or 800-4-422-6237; use reconstituted solution within 8 hours; modulates hemotoxicity of ionizing radiation and cytotoxicity of cyclophosphamide, cisplatin; reduced mitomycin C induced thrombocytopenia; reduces toxicity in experimental animal models due to doxorubicin and carmustine; amifostine may be protective against cisplatin-induced neuropathy (peripheral), nephrotoxicity, and ototoxicity; may be protective against cyclophosphamide-related granulocytopenia, thrombocytopenia, and neurotoxicity

Specific References

Brown JM, "Sensitizers and Protectors in Radiotherapy," *Cancer*, 1985, 55(9 Suppl):2222-8.

(Continued)

Amifostine *(Continued)*

Glover D, Fox K, Weiler C, et al, "Clinical Trials of WR-2721 Prior to Alkylating Agent Chemotherapy and Radiotherapy," *Pharmacol Ther*, 1988, 39(1-3):3-7.

Shaw LM, Glover D, Turrisi A, et al, "Pharmacokinetics of WR-2721," *Pharmacol Ther*, 1988, 39(1-3):195-201.

Amikacin Sulfate (am i kay' sin)

Related Information

Aminoglycoside Dosing and Monitoring *on page 1490-1491*

CAS Number 39831-55-5

Brand Names Amikin® Injection

Use Treatment of documented gram-negative enteric infection resistant to gentamicin and tobramycin; documented infection of mycobacterial organisms susceptible to amikacin

Mechanism of Action Inhibits protein synthesis in susceptible bacteria by binding to ribosomal subunits

Adverse Reactions

Central nervous system: Myasthenia gravis (exacerbation or precipitation of)
Dermatologic: Rash
Neuromuscular & skeletal: Neuromuscular blockade
Otic: Ototoxicity, deafness, tinnitus
Renal: Nephrotoxicity

Signs & Symptoms of Acute Overdose Hypomagnesemia

Toxicodynamics/Kinetics

Distribution: Primarily distributes into extracellular fluid (highly hydrophilic); penetrates the blood-brain barrier when meninges are inflamed; crosses the placenta; however, CSF levels are inadequate

Half-life: 1.6-96 hours

Time to peak serum concentration:
- I.M.: Within 45-120 minutes
- I.V.: Within 30 minutes

Elimination: 94% to 98% excreted unchanged in urine via glomerular filtration within 24 hours; clearance dependent on renal function and patient age

Usual Dosage Individualization is critical because of the low therapeutic index. Use of ideal body weight (IBW) for determining the mg/kg/dose appears to be more accurate than dosing on the basis of total body weight (TBW). In morbid obesity, dosage requirement may best be estimated using a dosing weight of IBW + 0.4 (TBW - IBW). Initial and periodic peak and trough plasma drug levels should be determined, particularly in critically ill patients with serious infections or in disease states known to significantly alter aminoglycoside pharmacokinetics (eg, cystic fibrosis, burns, or major surgery).

Neonates: I.V.:
- <1200 g, 0-4 weeks: 7.5 mg/kg/dose every 12 hours
- Postnatal age <7 days:
  - 1200-2000 g: 7.5 mg/kg/dose every 12 hours
  - >2000 g: 10 mg/kg/dose every 12 hours
- Postnatal age >7 days:
  - 1200-2000 g: 7 mg/kg/dose every 8 hours
  - >2000 g: 7.5-10 mg/kg/dose every 8 hours

Infants, Children, and Adults: I.M., I.V.: 7.5 mg/kg/dose every 8 hours

Dosing interval in renal impairment: Loading dose: 5-7.5 mg/kg; subsequent dosages and frequency of administration are best determined by measurement of serum levels and assessment of renal insufficiency

Some patients may require larger or more frequent doses if serum levels document the need (ie, cystic fibrosis or febrile granulocytopenic patients)

Administration Administer by intermittent I.V. infusion over 30 minutes at a final concentration not to exceed 5 mg amikacin/mL

Contraindications Hypersensitivity to amikacin sulfate or any component; cross-sensitivity may exist with other aminoglycosides

Dosage Forms Injection: 50 mg/mL (2 mL); 250 mg/mL (2 mL, 4 mL)

Stability Stable for 24 hours at room temperature when mixed in D_5W, $D_5$1/4NS, $D_5$1/2NS, NS, LR

Reference Range

Therapeutic:
- Peak: 25-30 μg/mL
- Trough: 4-8 μg/mL

Toxic:
- Peak: >35 μg/mL
- Trough: >10 μg/mL

Overdosage Treatment Enhancement of elimination: Ticarcillin complexation or exchange transfusion does not appear to be of added benefit; saline diuresis may be of benefit; dialyzable (50% to 100%)

Drug Interactions

Increased/prolonged effect: Depolarizing and nondepolarizing neuromuscular blocking agents

Increased toxicity: Concurrent use of amphotericin may increase nephrotoxicity

Pregnancy Risk Factor C

Monitoring Parameters Urinalysis, BUN, serum creatinine, and be alert to ototoxicity

Patient Information Report loss of hearing, ringing or roaring in the ears, or feeling of fullness in head

Nursing Implications Aminoglycoside levels measured from blood taken from Silastic® central catheters can sometimes give falsely high readings; administer I.M. injection in large muscle mass; obtain culture for culture and sensitivity before first dose; weigh patient and obtain baseline renal function before therapy begins; monitor vital signs, serum levels are reportedly lower in patients with fever. Give around-the-clock rather than 3 times/day, to promote less variation in peak and trough serum levels; give other antibiotics at least 1 hour before or after amikacin.

Additional Information Sodium content of 1 g: 29.9 mg (1.3 mEq)

Specific References

Flandrois JP, Bouletreau P, Auboyer R, et al, "Accidental Amikacin Overdose in Man: Emergency Therapy by Extrarenal Dialysis," *Infection*, 1979, 7:190-1.

Green FJ, Lavelle KJ, and Arnoff GR, "Management of Amikacin Overdose," *Am J Kidney Dis*, 1981, 1:110-2.

Ho PW, Pien FD, and Kominami N, "Massive Amikacin Overdose," *Ann Intern Med*, 1979, 91:227-8.

Amikal® *see* Amiloride Hydrochloride *on this page*

Amikin® Injection *see* Amikacin Sulfate *on previous page*

Amilent® *see* Amitriptyline Hydrochloride *on page 116*

Amiloride Hydrochloride (a mill' oh ride)

CAS Number 2609-46-3; 2016-88-8; 17440-83-4

Brand Names Amikal®; Amilospare®; Kaluril®; Midamor®; Modamide®

Use Counteracts potassium loss induced by other diuretics in the treatment of hypertension or edematous conditions including CHF, hepatic cirrhosis, and hypoaldosteronism; usually used in conjunction with more potent diuretics such as thiazides or loop diuretics

Investigational: Cystic fibrosis

Mechanism of Action Interferes with potassium/sodium exchange in the distal renal tubule

Adverse Reactions

Cardiovascular: Orthostatic hypotension

Central nervous system: Headache, dizziness

Dermatologic: Pruritus, photosensitivity

Endocrine & metabolic: Hyperkalemia, hyponatremia

Gastrointestinal: Nausea, vomiting, abdominal pain, diarrhea, thirst

Neuromuscular & skeletal: Leg ischemia, muscle cramps, paresthesia

Respiratory: Cough, dyspnea

Signs & Symptoms of Acute Overdose Hypotension, encephalopathy, hyperuricemia, photosensitivity, impotence, numbness, cough, hyponatremia, constipation

Toxicodynamics/Kinetics

Onset of diuresis: 2-3 hours

Duration: 24 hours

Absorption: Oral: ~50%

Half-life: 6-9 hours

Elimination: Unchanged equally in urine and feces

Usual Dosage

Children: Although safety and efficacy have not been established by the FDA, a dosage of 0.625 mg/kg/day has been used in children weighing 6-20 kg

Adults: 5-10 mg/day (up to 20 mg)

Dosing adjustment in renal impairment:

Cl_{cr} 10-50 mL/minute: Administer 50% of normal dose

Cl_{cr} <10 mL/minute: Avoid use

Contraindications Hyperkalemia, potassium supplementation and impaired renal function, hypersensitivity to amiloride or any component

Warnings Use cautiously in patients with severe hepatic insufficiency; may cause hyperkalemia (serum levels >5.5 mEq/L) which, if uncorrected, is potentially fatal; medication should be discontinued if potassium level exceeds 6.5 mEq/L

Dosage Forms Tablet: 5 mg

Reference Range Peak serum amiloride level: 30-50 ng/mL after a 20 mg dose

(Continued)

Amiloride Hydrochloride *(Continued)*

Overdosage Treatment

Decontamination: Ipecac or lavage/activated charcoal with cathartic

Supportive therapy: Hyperkalemia can be treated with glucose/insulin and sodium bicarbonate (1 mEq/kg); sodium polystyrene sulfonate can also be given; I.V. fluids administration of 0.45% sodium chloride with furosemide (1 mg/kg, up to 40 mg) can be used to promote urine flow

Test Interactions ↑ potassium (S)

Drug Interactions

Amiloride reduces intestinal absorption of amoxicillin

Increased risk of hyperkalemia if given together with triamterene, spironolactone, angiotensin-converting enzyme (ACE) inhibitors

Increased toxicity of amantadine by decreasing its renal excretion; amiloride may enhance to proarrhythmic effects of quinidine on QRS duration

Pregnancy Risk Factor C

Monitoring Parameters Blood pressure, serum electrolytes, renal function

Additional Information Unlike triamterene, renal stone formation does not occur; diminishes the potassium excretion effects of thiazide diuretics

Specific References

Jaffey L and Martin A, "Malignant Hyperkalemia After Amiloride/Hydrochlorothiazide Treatment," *Lancet*, 1981, 1(8232):1272.

Kleyman TR and Cragoe EJ Jr, "The Mechanism of Action of Amiloride," *Semin Nephrol*, 1988, 8(3):242-8.

Wang L, Sheldon RS, Mitchell LB, et al, "Amiloride-Quinidine Interaction: Adverse Outcomes," *Clin Pharmacol Ther*, 1994, 56(6 Pt 1):659-67.

Westphal JF, Jehl F, Brogard JM, et al,"Amoxicillin Intestinal Absorption Reduction by Amiloride: Possible Role of the Na^+-H^+ Exchanger," *Clin Pharmacol Ther* 1995, 51:257-64.

Amilospare® *see* Amiloride Hydrochloride *on previous page*

2-Amino-6-Trifluoromethoxy-benzothiazole *see* Riluzole *on page 684*

6-Amino-9-Beta-D-Ribofuranosyl-9-H-Purine *see* Adenosine Triphosphate *on page 90*

Aminobenzylpenicillin *see* Ampicillin *on page 125*

Aminoglycoside Dosing and Monitoring *see page 1490*

Aminohydroxybutylidene Biphosphonate *see* Alendronate *on page 94*

Amino-Opti-E® Oral [OTC] *see* Vitamin E *on page 798*

Aminophylline (am in off' i lin)

CAS Number 317-34-0

Brand Names Phyllocontin®; Truphylline®

Synonyms Theophylline Ethylenediamine

Use Bronchodilator in reversible airway obstruction due to asthma or COPD as maintenance therapy only; for neonatal idiopathic apnea/bradycardia spells

Mechanism of Action Exact mechanism is unknown; probable mechanism involves increasing tissue concentrations of cAMP and/or occupying adenosine receptors as an antagonist and/or inhibition of phosphodiesterases, PDE III, PDE IV

Adverse Reactions Uncommon at serum theophylline concentrations ≤20 μg/mL

Cardiovascular: Palpitations, sinus tachycardia; fibrillation (atrial)

Central nervous system: Insomnia, agitation, irritability, seizures, nervousness, restlessness

Dermatologic: Skin rash

Gastrointestinal: Nausea, vomiting, epigastric pain

Neuromuscular & skeletal: Tremors

Miscellaneous: Allergic reactions

Signs & Symptoms of Acute Overdose Nausea, vomiting, diuresis, tachycardia (ventricular), insomnia, irritability, tachycardia, hyperglycemia, eczema, delirium, seizures, hypotension, hypokalemia, hypercalcemia, lactic acidosis, feces discoloration (black). Repetitive vomiting is an indication to hold theophylline therapy and rule out toxicity by serum concentrations.

Toxicodynamics/Kinetics

Absorption: Oral: Up to 100% of dose absorbed depending upon the formulation used

Distribution: V_d: 0.45 L/kg; rapid throughout extracellular fluid and tissues

Protein binding:

- Neonates: 36%
- Adults: 40% to 60%
- Patients with hepatic cirrhosis: 35%

Metabolism: In the liver by demethylation and oxidation

Half-life:
- Infants ≤6 months: >24 hours
- Children >6 months: 3.7±1.1 hours
- Adults:
  - Nonsmokers: 8.7±2.2 hours
  - Smokers (1-2 packs/day): 4-5 hours

Time to peak serum concentration:
- Oral: 1 hour
- Uncoated tablets: 2 hours
- Chewable tablets: 1-1.5 hours
- Enteric-coated tablets: 5 hours
- Extended-release capsules and tablets: 4-7 hours, in overdoses up to 27 hours
- Retention enema: 1-2 hours

Elimination: Excreted in urine; adults excrete 10% in urine as unchanged drug; neonates excrete a greater percentage of the dose unchanged in urine (up to 50%). See table.

Half-life (h)	Patient Population
7–9	Normal healthy
2–9	Children
15–58	Premature infants
18–24	Severe congestive heart failure
29	Cirrhosis

Usual Dosage

Neonates: Apnea of prematurity:
- Loading dose: 5 mg/kg for one dose
- Maintenance: I.V.:
  - 0-24 days: Begin at 2 mg/kg/day divided every 12 hours and titrate to desired levels and effects
  - >24 days: 3 mg/kg/day divided every 12 hours; increased dosages may be indicated as liver metabolism matures (usually >30 days of life); monitor serum levels to determine appropriate dosages
- Theophylline levels should be initially drawn after 3 days of therapy; repeat levels are indicated 3 days after each increase in dosage or weekly if on a stabilized dosage

Treatment of acute wheezing: Loading dose (in patients not currently receiving aminophylline or theophylline): 6 mg/kg (based on aminophylline) given I.V. over 20-30 minutes; administration rate should not exceed 25 mg/minute (aminophylline)

Approximate I.V. maintenance dosages are based upon **continuous infusions**; bolus dosing (often used in children <6 months of age) may be determined by multiplying the hourly infusion rate by 24 hours and dividing by the desired number of doses/day
- 6 weeks to 6 months: 0.5 mg/kg/hour
- 6 months to 1 year: 0.6-0.7 mg/kg/hour
- 1-9 years: 1-1.2 mg/kg/hour
- 12-16 years: 0.7 mg/kg/hour
- 9-12 years and young adult smokers: 0.9 mg/kg/hour
- Adults (healthy, nonsmoking): 0.7 mg/kg/hour
- Older patients and patients with cor pulmonale, patients with congestive heart failure or liver failure: 0.25 mg/kg/hour
- Dosage should be adjusted according to serum level measurements during the first 12- to 24-hour period; avoid using suppositories due to erratic, unreliable absorption. See table.

Guidelines for Drawing Theophylline Serum Levels

Dosage Form	Time to Draw Level
P.O. liquid, fast-release tab	Peak: 1 h post 4th dose Trough: just before 4th dose
P.O. slow-release product	Peak: 4 h post 3rd dose Trough: just before 3rd dose

Rectal: Adults: 500 mg 3 times/day

Administration Dilute with I.V. fluid to a concentration of 1 mg/mL and infuse over 20-30 minutes; maximum concentration: 25 mg/mL; maximum rate of infusion: 0.36 mg/kg/minute, and no greater than 25 mg/minute

(Continued)

Aminophylline *(Continued)*

Contraindications Uncontrolled tachyarrhythmias, hypersensitivity to ethylenediamine; use with caution in active peptic ulcer disease, seizure disorders

Dosage Forms Theophylline (anhydrous) equivalent listed in brackets
- Enema (Somophyllin®): 65.14 mg/mL [51.4 mg/mL]
- Injection, I.V. (Aminophyllin™): 25 mg/mL [19.7 mg/mL] (10 mL, 20 mL)
- Liquid, oral: 105 mg/5 mL [90 mg/5 mL] (240 mL)
- Suppository, rectal (Truphylline®): 250 mg [197.3 mg], 500 mg [394.5 mg]
- Tablet: 100 mg [85 mg], 200 mg [170 mg]
- Tablet (Aminophyllin™): 100 mg [79 mg], 200 mg [158 mg]
- Tablet, controlled release [12 hours] (Phyllocontin®): 225 mg [178 mg]
- Tablet, enteric coated: 100 mg [79 mg], 200 mg [158 mg]

Stability Store injection at room temperature, do not refrigerate; protect from heat and from freezing; use only clear solutions; stability of parenteral admixture at room temperature (25°C): 30 days

Reference Range
- Therapeutic (theophylline):
  - Neonatal apnea: 6-13 μg/mL
- Sample size: 0.5-1 mL serum (red top tube)
- Toxic: >20 μg/mL
- Timing of serum samples: If toxicity is suspected, draw a level at any time; if lack of therapeutic is effected, draw a trough immediately before the next oral dose

Overdosage Treatment
- Decontamination: Do not use ipecac; lavage should be performed if <1 hour after ingestion and >50 mg/kg was ingested/activated charcoal with cathartic; whole bowel irrigation should be considered for significant sustained release preparation ingestion
- Supportive therapy: Metoclopramide, ranitidine, or ondansetron can be used for vomiting; hypotension should be treated with intravenous normal saline hydration. Phenylephrine or levarterenol are preferred vasopressors that can be utilized for hypotension although an intravenous beta-adrenergic blocker (propranolol or esmolol) can be utilized in the patient without a history of bronchospastic disease. Seizures may require diazepam/lorazepam along with phenobarbital; phenytoin contraindicated; adenosine has had inconsistent effects in animal models. Lidocaine can be used for ventricular arrhythmias; must monitor for hypoglycemia.
- Enhancement of elimination: Multiple doses of activated charcoal can reduce the half-life of aminophylline/theophylline in half; do not use if an ileus is present. Charcoal hemoperfusion can increase the clearance of aminophylline/theophylline by approximately twofold to threefold over that of hemodialysis and is thus the extracorporeal modality of choice. Guidelines for charcoal hemoperfusion include a theophylline level >100 μg/mL in an acute overdose setting (or 50 μg/mL in a chronic setting), or the following signs if the level is >35 μg/mL: ventricular arrhythmias, metabolic acidosis, hypotension, refractory to vasopressors or fluid therapy, seizures, ileus. If a sustained release preparation is ingested or patient with charcoal ingestion is >60 years of age, the threshold for using charcoal hemoperfusion should be lower. If the patient is experiencing fluid overload due to congestive heart failure, hemodialysis can be performed to remove both theophylline/aminophylline and fluid.

Test Interactions Caffeine in high concentrations on selected procedures cross reacts as theophylline

Drug Interactions Changes in diet may affect the elimination of theophylline; theophylline may decrease the effects of phenytoin, adenosine, benzodiazepines, lithium, and neuromuscular blocking agents. Theophylline increases the excretion of lithium; theophylline may have synergistic toxicity with sympathomimetics, halothane. Cimetidine, allopurinol, propranolol, erythromycin, influenza virus vaccine, fluvoxamine, ciprofloxacin, clarithromycin, alcohol, enoxacin, interferon, propafenone, oral contraceptives, amiodarone, troleandomycin, clindamycin, and lincomycin may increase theophylline concentrations. Cigarette and marijuana smoking, rifampin, phenobarbital, phenytoin, and aminoglutethimide may decrease theophylline concentrations.

Pregnancy Risk Factor C

Pregnancy Implications Crosses the placenta and enters breast milk

Monitoring Parameters Monitor vital signs, I & O, mental status, EKG, serum theophylline concentration

Patient Information Oral preparations should be taken with a full glass of water; avoid drinking or eating large quantities of caffeine-containing beverages or food; take at regular intervals; take sustained release tablets whole; sustained release capsule forms may be opened and sprinkled on soft foods; do not chew beads

Nursing Implications Do not crush sustained release or enteric coated drug products
- Extravasation: Give hyaluronidase (1:10 dilution of a 1:150 unit vial in saline equivalent to 15 units/mL) S.C. in multiple (usually about 5) injections of 0.2 mL each to help increase absorption

Additional Information Elderly, acutely ill, and patients with severe respiratory problems, pulmonary edema, or liver dysfunction are at greater risk of toxicity because of reduced drug clearance; saliva levels are approximately equal to 60% of plasma levels; charcoal-broiled foods may increase elimination, reducing half-life by 50%; cigarette smoking may require an increase of dosage by 50% to 100%; aminophylline 100 mg is equivalent to theophylline 79 mg. Aminophylline (2.5 mg/kg) has been used to treat methotrexate-induced neurotoxicity in children.

Theophylline immediate release tablet/capsule: Bronkodyl®, Elixophyllin®, Quibron®-T, Slo-Phyllin®, Somophyllin®-T, Theolair™

Theophylline liquid: Accurbron®, Aerolate®, Aquaphyllin®, Asmalix®, Elixicon®, Elixophyllin®, Lixolin®, Theon®

Theophylline timed release capsule: Aerolate III®, Aerolate JR®, Aerolate SR®, Elixophyllin® SR, Lodrane®, Slo-bid™ Gyrocaps®, Slo-Phyllin® Gyrocaps®, Somophyllin®-CRT, Theobid®, Theoclear® L.A., Theophyl-SR®, Theospan®-SR, Theospan®-SR

Theophylline timed release tablet: Constant-T®, Duraphyl™, LaBID®, Quibron®-T/S, Respbid®, Sustaire®, Theochron®, Theo-Dur®, Theolair™-SR, Theo-Time®, Uniphyl®

Specific References

Bernini JC, Fort DW, Griener JC, et al, "Aminophylline for Methotrexate-Induced Neurotoxicity," *Lancet*, 1995, 345:544-7.

Henderson A, Wright DM, and Pond SM, "Management of Theophylline Overdose Patients in the Intensive Care Unit," *Anaesth Intensive Care*, 1992, 20(1):56-62.

Paloucek FP and Rodvold KA, "Evaluation of Theophylline Overdoses and Toxicities," *Ann Emerg Med*, 1988, 17(2):135-44.

Shannon M, "Predictors of Major Toxicity After Theophylline Overdose," *Ann Intern Med*, 1993, 119(12):1161-7.

Shannon MW and Maher TI, "Anticonvulsant Effects of Intracerebroventricular Adenosine in Theophylline-Induced Seizures," *Vet Hum Toxicol*, 1994, 36:350.

Strauss RE, Wertheim DL, Bonagura VR, et al, "Aminophylline Therapy Does Not Improve Outcome and Increases Adverse Effects in Children Hospitalized With Acute Asthmatic Exacerbations," *Pediatrics*, 1994, 93(2):205-10.

Wang RY, "Anticoagulant Effects of Adenosine in Aminophylline-Induced Seizures," *Vet Hum Toxicol*, 1994, 36:351.

Aminosalicylate Sodium *see* Para-Aminosalicylate Sodium *on page 592*

Amiodarone Hydrochloride (a mee' oh da rone)

CAS Number 1951-25-3; 19774-82-4

Brand Names Ancoron®; Atlansil®; Cordarone®; Maioda®; Miodaron®; Ortacrone®; Trangorex®

Replaces SKF-33-134-A

Use Management of resistant, life-threatening recurrent ventricular arrhythmias unresponsive to conventional therapy with less toxic agents; has also been used for treatment of supraventricular arrhythmias unresponsive to conventional therapy

Mechanism of Action Class III antiarrhythmic agent which inhibits adrenergic stimulation, prolongs the action potential and refractory period in myocardial tissue; decreases A-V conduction and sinus node function; structurally related to thyroxine

Adverse Reactions

Cardiovascular: Atropine-resistant bradycardia, heart block, sinus arrest, myocardial depression, chest pain, congestive heart failure, paroxysmal tachycardia (ventricular), hypotension, torsade de pointes with Q-T interval prolongation

Central nervous system: (20% to 40% incidence): Fatigue, malaise, abnormal gait, psychosis, dizziness, encephalopathy, insomnia, night terrors, extrapyramidal reaction, fever, headache, restlessness, abulia, ataxia parkinsonism

Dermatologic: Slate blue discoloration of skin, rash, alopecia, photosensitivity

Endocrine & metabolic: Hypothyroidism (or less commonly hyperthyroidism), hyperglycemia, increased triglycerides, gynecomastia

Gastrointestinal: Nausea, vomiting, anorexia, constipation, metallic taste

Genitourinary: Scrotal pain, epididymal pain and swelling

Hematologic: Coagulation abnormalities, thrombocytopenia

Hepatic: Increased liver enzymes, severe hepatic toxicity (potentially fatal), increased bilirubin, increased serum ammonia

Neuromuscular & skeletal: Tremors, proximal muscle asthenia, paresthesia

Ocular: Corneal microdeposits, diplopia; photophobia, optic neuropathy, cataract

Respiratory: (potentially fatal): Interstitial pneumonitis, hypersensitivity pneumonitis, pulmonary fibrosis; may present with cough, dyspnea

Miscellaneous: Sweating

Signs & Symptoms of Acute Overdose Extensions of pharmacologic effect, pseudotumor cerebri, hyperthyroidism, cirrhosis, syncope, A-V block, chest pain, myopathy, toxic epidermal necrolysis, thrombocytopenia, photosensitivity, sweating, sinus bradycardia and/or heart block, hypotension and Q-T prolongation; patients should be monitored for several days following ingestion; hemoptysis, night terrors, hypothyroidism, delirium insomnia

(Continued)

Amiodarone Hydrochloride *(Continued)*

Toxicodynamics/Kinetics

Onset of action: 3 days to 3 weeks after starting therapy

Peak effect: 1 week to 5 months

Duration: After discontinuation of therapy: 7-50 days; mean onset of effect and duration after discontinuation may be shorter in children vs adults

Absorption: Oral: Slow and variable, ~20% to 55%

Distribution: V_d: 66 L/kg (range: 18-148 L/kg)

Protein binding: 96%

Metabolism: In liver, major metabolite N-desethylamiodarone (active)

Bioavailability: ~50% (range: 20% to 80%)

Half-life: Parent compound (oral chronic therapy): 40-55 days (range: 26-107 days); half-life is shortened in children vs adults; metabolite: 60-92 days

Time to peak serum concentration: 3-7 hours

Elimination: Eliminated via biliary excretion; possible enterohepatic recirculation; <1% excreted unchanged in urine

Usual Dosage Oral (children <1 year should be dosed as calculated by body surface area):

Children: Loading dose: 10-15 mg/kg/day or 600-800 mg/1.73 m^2/day for 4-14 days or until adequate control of arrhythmia or prominent adverse effects occur (this loading dose may be given in 1-2 divided doses/day); dosage should then be reduced to 5 mg/kg/day or 200-400 mg/1.73 m^2/day given once daily for several weeks; if arrhythmia does not recur, reduce to lowest effective dosage possible; usual daily minimal dose: 2.5 mg/kg/day; maintenance doses may be given for 5 of 7 days/week

Adults: Ventricular arrhythmias: 800-1600 mg/day in 1-2 doses for 1-3 weeks, then 600-800 mg/day in 1-2 doses for 1 month; maintenance: 400 mg/day; lower doses are recommended for supraventricular arrhythmias

Dosing adjustment in hepatic impairment: Probably necessary in substantial impairment

Contraindications Hypersensitivity to amiodarone; severe sinus node dysfunction, marked sinus bradycardia; second and third degree A-V block; bradycardia-induced syncope, except if pacemaker is placed; thyroid disease

Warnings Not considered first-line antiarrhythmic due to high incidence of toxicity; 75% of patients experience adverse effects with large doses; discontinuation is required in 5% to 20% of patients; reserve for use in life-threatening arrhythmias refractory to other therapy; avoid during pregnancy and while breast-feeding

Dosage Forms Tablet: 200 mg

Stability May precipitate with heparin

Reference Range

Therapeutic: 1.5-2.5 mg/L (SI: 1-4 μmol/L) (parent); desethyl metabolite is active and is present in equal concentration to parent drug

Toxic effects can be observed at levels >2.5 mg/L for parent compound or 100 ng/dL for desethylamiodarone

Overdosage Treatment

Decontamination: Lavage/activated charcoal with cathartic

Supportive therapy: Intoxication with amiodarone necessitates EKG monitoring. When bradycardia occurs atropine may be given, however, atropine resistant bradycardia has been reported. In cases of difficult to treat amiodarone-induced bradycardia, injectable isoproterenol or a temporary pacemaker may be required.

Enhancement of elimination: Multiple dose of activated charcoal may be useful. Cholestyramine (4 g/hour for 4 hours) may be useful to decrease half-life. Dialysis is not useful.

Test Interactions Thyroid function tests: Amiodarone partially inhibits the peripheral conversion of thyroxine (T_4) to tri-iodothyronine (T_3); serum T_4 and reverse tri-iodothyronine (RT_3) concentrations may be increased and serum T_3 may be decreased; most patients remain clinically euthyroid, however, clinical hypothyroidism or hyperthyroidism may occur; hyperglycemia

Drug Interactions Amiodarone may increase plasma concentrations of digoxin and cardiac glycosides, flecainide, procainamide, quinidine, warfarin, and phenytoin resulting in toxicities; combined use with beta-blockers, digitalis or calcium channel blockers may result in bradycardia, sinus arrest; use with class I antiarrhythmics may cause ventricular arrhythmias; amiodarone + general anesthetics may result in bradycardia, hypotension, heart block; cholestyramine may possibly decrease amiodarone serum levels.

Pregnancy Risk Factor C (congenital hypothyroidism with goiter along with infant bradycardia can occur)

Pregnancy Implications Crosses placenta; distributes to breast milk in concentrations higher than maternal plasma concentrations

Monitoring Parameters Monitor heart rate and rhythm throughout therapy; EKG monitoring, baseline pulmonary function tests, thyroid function tests, and liver enzymes

Patient Information Take with food; use sunscreen or stay out of sun to prevent burns; skin discoloration is reversible; photophobia may make sunglasses necessary

Nursing Implications Assess patient for signs of thyroid dysfunction, drowsiness, edema of the hands, feet, weight loss, and pulmonary toxicity

Additional Information CNS symptoms normally develop within 7 days, muscle asthenia may present a great hazard for ambulation

Specific References

Ahmad S, "Amiodarone and Reversible Alopecia," *Arch Intern Med*, 1995, 155:1106.

Breithardt G, "Amiodarone in Patients With Heart Failure," *N Engl J Med*, 1995, 333:121-2.

Dotti MT and Federico A, "Amiodarone-Induced Parkinsonism: A Case Report and Pathogenetic Discussion," *Mov Disord*, 1995, 10:233-4.

Ector H, Rubens A, De Geest H, et al, "Amiodarone and Thyroid Function Tests," *Acta Cardiol*, 49:538-9.

Goddard CJ and Whorwell PJ, "Amiodarone Overdose and Its Management," *Br J Clin Pharmacol*, 1989, 43(5):184-6.

Magee LA, Downar E, Sarmer M, et al, "Pregnancy Outcome After Gestational Exposure to Amiodarone in Canada," *Am J Obstet Gynecol*, 1995, 172:1307-11.

Marchlinski FE, Gansler TS, Waxman HL, et al, "Amiodarone Pulmonary Toxicity," *Am J Med*, 1982, 97(6):839-45.

Nishimura H, Machida K, Shinozaki T, et al, "A Case of Depressive State Due to Amiodarone," *Seishin Igaku*, 1994, 26:1081-3.

Nitsch J and Luderitz B, "Acceleration of Amiodarone Elimination by Cholestyramine," *Dtsch Med Wochenschr*, 1986, 111(33):1241-4.

Podrid PJ, "Amiodarone: Reevaluation of an Old Drug," *Ann Intern Med*, 1995, 122:689-700.

Richer M and Robert S, "Fatal Hepatotoxicity Following Oral Administration of Amiodarone," *Ann Pharmacother*, 1995, 29:582-6.

Rigas B, Rosenfeld LE, and Barwick KW, "Amiodarone Hepatotoxicity," *Ann Intern Med*, 1986, 104(3):348-51.

Singh SN, Fletcher RD, Fisher SG, et al, "Aminodarone in Patients With Congestive Heart Failure and Asymptomatic Ventricular Arrhythmia," *N Engl J Med*, 1995, 333:77-82.

Snir Y, Pick N, Riesenberg K, et al, "Fatal Hepatic Failure Due to Prolonged Amiodarone Treatment," *J Clin Gastroenterol*, 1995, 20:265-6.

Tisdale JE, Follin SL, Ordelova A, et al, "Risk Factors for the Development of Specific Noncardiovascular Adverse Effects Associated With Amiodarone," *J Clin Pharmacol*, 1995, 35:351-6.

Valle JM, Alvarez D, Antinez J, et al, "Bronchiolitis Obliterans Organizing Pneumonia Secondary to Amiodarone: A Rare Etiology," *Eur Respir J*, 1995, 8:470-1.

Amitriptyline and Perphenazine

(a mee trip' ti leen & per fen' a zeen)

Brand Names Etrafon®; Perphenyline®; Triavil®; Triptazine®

Synonyms Perphenazine and Amitriptyline

Use Treatment of patients with moderate to severe anxiety and depression

Adverse Reactions

Cardiovascular: Postural hypotension, cardiac arrhythmias, tachycardia, sudden death

Central nervous system: Sedation, drowsiness, restlessness, anxiety, extrapyramidal reactions, pseudoparkinsonian signs and symptoms, seizures, altered central temperature regulation, neuroleptic malignant syndrome, neuroleptic malignant syndrome (NMS)

Dermatologic: Hyperpigmentation, pruritus, rash, photosensitivity

Endocrine & metabolic: Amenorrhea, galactorrhea, gynecomastia, syndrome of inappropriate antidiuretic hormone, weight gain

Gastrointestinal: Gastrointestinal upset, ileus, constipation dry mouth

Genitourinary: Urinary retention

Hematologic: Rarely neutropenia, granulocytopenia, eosinophilia, agranulocytosis (more often in women between fourth and tenth weeks of therapy), leukopenia (usually in patients with large doses for prolonged periods)

Hepatic: Jaundice

Ocular: Retinal pigmentation, blurred vision, intraocular pressure (increased)

Miscellaneous: Allergic reactions

Signs & Symptoms of Acute Overdose High prevalence of first degree A-V block, intraocular pressure (increased), stomatitis, neuroleptic malignant syndrome, myasthenia gravis (exacerbation or precipitation of), Q-T prolongation, impotence

Usual Dosage Oral: 1 tablet 2-4 times/day

Contraindications Hypersensitivity to amitriptyline, perphenazine or any component, cross-sensitivity with other phenothiazines may exist; avoid use in patients with narrow-angle glaucoma, bone marrow depression, severe liver or cardiac disease; avoid use during pregnancy and lactation

Warnings Safe use of tricyclic antidepressants in children <12 years of age has not been established; amitriptyline should not be abruptly discontinued in patients receiving high doses for prolonged periods

Dosage Forms Tablet:

2-10: Amitriptyline hydrochloride 10 mg and perphenazine 2 mg

(Continued)

Amitriptyline and Perphenazine *(Continued)*

4-10: Amitriptyline hydrochloride 10 mg and perphenazine 4 mg
2-25: Amitriptyline hydrochloride 25 mg and perphenazine 2 mg
4-25: Amitriptyline hydrochloride 25 mg and perphenazine 4 mg
4-50: Amitriptyline hydrochloride 50 mg and perphenazine 4 mg

Overdosage Treatment

Decontamination: Lavage/activated charcoal with cathartic; multiple dosing of activated charcoal is more effective

Supportive: Following initiation of essential overdose management, toxic symptoms should be treated. Ventricular arrhythmias often respond to phenytoin 15-20 mg/kg (adults) with concurrent systemic alkalinization (sodium bicarbonate 0.5-2 mEq/kg I.V.). Arrhythmias unresponsive to this therapy may respond to lidocaine 1 mg/kg I.V. followed by a titrated infusion. Physostigmine (1-2 mg I.V. slowly for adults or 0.5 mg I.V. slowly for children) may be indicated in seizures or movement disorders but should only be used **as a last resort**. Seizures usually respond to lorazepam or diazepam I.V. boluses (5-10 mg for adults up to 30 mg or 0.25-0.4 mg/kg/dose for children up to 10 mg/dose). If seizures are unresponsive or recur, phenytoin or phenobarbital may be required. Phenytoin is effective to decrease QRS complex interval. Do not use bretylium in hypotensive patients.

Antidote(s)

Sodium Bicarbonate *on page 1467*

Test Interactions See individual monographs for Amitriptyline and Perphenazine

Drug Interactions

Amitriptyline blocks the uptake of guanethidine and thus prevents the hypotensive effect of guanethidine; amitriptyline may be additive with or may potentiate the action of other CNS depressants such as sedatives or hypnotics; amitriptyline potentiates the pressor and cardiac effects of sympathomimetic agents such as isoproterenol, epinephrine, etc

With MAO inhibitors, fever, hypertension, tachycardia, confusion, seizures, and death have been reported

Additive anticholinergic effects seen with other anticholinergic agents

Cimetidine reduces the hepatiç metabolism of amitriptyline

Amitriptyline may increase the prothrombin time in patients stabilized on warfarin

Orthostatic hypotension increases when used with hexamethylmelamine; tremors increase with the addition of labetalol; amitriptyline may antagonize hypotensive effects of clonidine; lithium may promote seizures in patients taking amitriptyline; fenclonine reverses antidepressant effect; decreased gastrointestinal motility, seizures, respiratory depression, hypotension, tachycardia

Pregnancy Risk Factor D

Monitoring Parameters Monitor blood pressure and pulse rate prior to and during initial therapy; evaluate mental status; monitor weight, may increase appetite and possibly a craving for sweets; offer patient sugarless hard candy for dry mouth

Patient Information Do not drink alcoholic beverages

Specific References

Wilens TE, Stern TA, and O'Gara PT, "Adverse Cardiac Effects of Combined Neuroleptic Ingestion and Tricyclic Antidepressant Overdose," *J Clin Psychopharmacol*, 1990, 10(1):51-4.

Amitriptyline Hydrochloride (a mee trip' ti leen)

Related Information

Antidepressant Agents Comparison *on page 1639*

Therapeutic Drugs Associated With Hallucinations *on page 1558-1559*

CAS Number 549-18-8

Brand Names Adepril®; Amavil®; Amilent®; Anapsique®; Domical®; Elavil®; Endep®; Enovil®; Trepiline®; Tryptizol®

Use Treatment of various forms of depression, often in conjunction with psychotherapy; as an analgesic for certain chronic and neuropathic pain, migraine prophylaxis

Mechanism of Action Increases synaptic concentration of serotonin and/or norepinephrine in the central nervous system by inhibition of their reuptake by the presynaptic neuronal membrane

Adverse Reactions

Cardiovascular: Postural hypotension, cardiomyopathy, cardiac arrhythmias, tachycardia, sudden death, Q-T prolongation

Central nervous system: Sedation, asthenia, fatigue, anxiety, confusion, insomnia, psychosis, impaired cognitive function, seizures, extrapyramidal reaction are possible, restlessness, moderate to marked sedation can occur (tolerance to these effects usually occur), neuroleptic malignant syndrome, acute polyradiculopathy, visual hallucinations

Dermatologic: Photosensitivity

Endocrine & metabolic: Rarely syndrome of inappropriate antidiuretic hormone, weight gain

Gastrointestinal: Dry mouth, appetite (increased), constipation, adynamic ileus, lower esophageal sphincter tone may cause GE reflux
Genitourinary: Urinary retention
Hematologic: Rarely leukopenia, neutropenia, agranulocytosis, granulocytopenia, eosinophilia
Hepatic: Increased liver enzymes, cholestatic jaundice
Neuromuscular & skeletal: Tremors
Ocular: Blurred vision, photophobia, diplopia, increased intraocular pressure, mydriasis
Respiratory: Hyperventilation, adult respiratory distress syndrome
Miscellaneous: Allergic reactions

Signs & Symptoms of Acute Overdose Agitation, dental erosion, purpura, ejaculatory disturbances, photosensitivity, insomnia, lactation, hyperacusis, delirium, intraocular pressure (increased), paresthesia, hyponatremia, memory loss, mania, dementia, hyperthermia, myoglobinuria, confusion, periarteritis nodosa, hallucinations, extrapyramidal reaction, nystagmus, urinary retention, hypothermia, hypotension, neuroleptic malignant syndrome, tachycardia, QRS prolongation, respiratory depression, seizures, decreased gastrointestinal motility, bowel ischemia, fever, urine discoloration (blue-green)

Toxicodynamics/Kinetics
Onset of action: Therapeutic effects begin in 7-21 days
Absorption: Oral: Rapidly and well absorbed
Distribution: V_d: 8.3 L/kg
Protein binding: 90% or more in plasma and tissues
Metabolism: In the liver to nortriptyline (active), hydroxy derivatives and conjugated derivatives; impaired in elderly patients
Bioavailability: 30% to 60%
Half-life: Adults: 9-25 hours (15-hour average)
Time to peak serum concentration: Within 4 hours
Elimination: Renal excretion of 18% as unchanged drug; small amounts eliminated in feces by bile

Usual Dosage
Children: Pain management: Oral: Initial: 0.1 mg/kg at bedtime, may advance as tolerated over 2-3 weeks to 0.5-2 mg/day at bedtime

Adolescents: Oral: Initial: 25-50 mg/day; may give in divided doses; increase gradually to 100 mg/day in divided doses

Adults:
Oral: 30-100 mg/day single dose at bedtime or in divided doses; dose may be gradually increased up to 300 mg/day; once symptoms are controlled, decrease gradually to lowest effective dose
I.M.: 20-30 mg 4 times/day

Dosing interval in hepatic impairment: Use with caution and monitor plasma levels and patient response

Contraindications Hypersensitivity to amitriptyline (cross-sensitivity with other tricyclics may occur); narrow-angle glaucoma; patients receiving MAO inhibitors within past 14 days

Warnings To avoid cholinergic crisis, do not discontinue abruptly in patients receiving high doses chronically; use with caution in patients with cardiac conduction disturbances, history of hyperthyroidism, renal or hepatic impairment, bipolar illness; an EKG prior to initiation of therapy is advised

Dosage Forms
Injection: 10 mg/mL (10 mL)
Tablet: 10 mg, 25 mg, 50 mg, 75 mg, 100 mg, 150 mg

Stability Keep oral solution in refrigerator, remains stable for 7 days after preparation; protect injection and Elavil® 10 mg tablets from light

Reference Range
Therapeutic:
Amitriptyline and nortriptyline: 100-250 ng/mL (SI: 360-900 nmol/L)
Nortriptyline: 50-150 ng/mL (SI: 190-570 nmol/L)
Toxic: >500 ng/mL; seizures can occur at levels >1000 ng/mL (SI: >3605 nmol/L)

Overdosage Treatment
Decontamination: Lavage (within 2-3 hours)/activated charcoal with cathartic; do not induce emesis; multiple dosing of activated charcoal is more effective
Supportive therapy: Lavage within 6 hours of ingestion; following initiation of essential overdose management, toxic symptoms should be treated. Ventricular arrhythmias often respond to phenytoin 15-20 mg/kg (adults) with concurrent systemic alkalinization (sodium bicarbonate 0.5-2 mEq/kg I.V.). Arrhythmias unresponsive to this therapy may respond to lidocaine 1mg/kg I.V. followed by a titrated infusion. Physostigmine (1-2 mg I.V. slowly for adults or 0.5 mg I.V. slowly for children) may be indicated in seizures or movement disorders but should only be used as a last resort. Seizures usually respond to lorazepam or diazepam I.V. boluses (5-10 mg for adults up to 30 mg or 0.25-0.4 mg/kg/dose for chil-

(Continued)

Amitriptyline Hydrochloride *(Continued)*

dren up to 10 mg/dose). If seizures are unresponsive or recur, phenytoin or phenobarbital may be required. Phenytoin is effective to decrease QRS complex interval. Do not use bretylium in hypotensive patients. Norepinephrine is effective for hypotension. Avoid procainamide or other type Ia antiarrhythmics.

Antidote(s)

Sodium Bicarbonate *on page 1467*

Test Interactions Increases glucose, CPK, and LDH plasma catecholamine levels; cross reacts with phenothiazine levels

Drug Interactions Amitriptyline may decrease the effects of guanethidine and may increase the effects of other CNS depressants, adrenergic agents (epinephrine, isoproterenol), anticholinergic agents and warfarin. With MAO inhibitors, fever, tachycardia, hypertension, confusion, seizures, and death have been reported. Cimetidine and methylphenidate may decrease the metabolism and phenobarbital may increase the metabolism of amitriptyline; clonidine may cause hypertensive crisis and may accentuate toxicity.

Pregnancy Risk Factor D

Pregnancy Implications Crosses placenta; enters breast milk

Monitoring Parameters Monitor blood pressure and pulse rate prior to and during initial therapy, EKG for QRS widening or tachycardia; evaluate mental status; monitor weight, may increase appetite and possibly a craving for sweets

Patient Information Avoid alcohol ingestion; do not discontinue medication abruptly; may cause urine to turn blue-green; may cause drowsiness, dry mouth, constipation, blurred vision; rise slowly to prevent dizziness

Additional Information Plasma levels do not always correlate with clinical effectiveness; desired therapeutic effect (for depression) may take as long as 3-4 weeks, at that point dosage should be reduced to lowest effective level; when used for migraine headache prophylaxis, therapeutic effect may take as long as 6 weeks; a higher dosage may be required in a heavy smoker, because of increased metabolism

Specific References

Bosse GM, Barefoot JA, Pfeifer MP, et al, "Comparison of Three Methods of Gut Decontamination in Tricyclic Antidepressant Overdose," *J Emerg Med*, 1995, 13(2):203-4.

Ellison DW and Pentel PR, "Clinical Features and Consequences of Seizures Due to Cyclic Antidepressant Overdose," *Am J Emerg Med*, 1989, 7(1):5-10.

Foulke GE, "Identifying Toxicity Risk Early After Antidepressant Overdose," *Am J Emerg Med*, 1995, 13(2):123-6.

Guharoy SR, "Adult Respiratory Distress Syndrome Associated With Amitriptyline Overdose," *Vet Hum Toxicol*, 1994, 36(4):316-7.

Knudsen K and Abrahamsson K, "Effects of Epinephrine, Norepinephrine, Magnesium Sulfate, and Milrinone on Survival and the Occurrence of Arrhythmias in Amitriptyline Poisoning in the Rat," *Crit Care Med*, 1994, 22(11):1851-5.

Perrot LJ, "Amitriptyline Overdose Versus Sudden Infant Death Syndrome in a Two Month Old White Female," *J Forensic Sci*, 1988, 33(1):272-5.

Sasyniuk BI, Jhamandas V, Valois M, et al, "Experimental Amitriptyline Intoxication: Treatment of Cardiac Toxicity With Sodium Bicarbonate," *Ann Emerg Med*, 1986, 15(9):1052-9.

Stone CK, Kraemer CM, Carroll R, et al, "Does a Sodium-Free Buffer Affect QRS Width in Experimental Amitriptylline Overdose?" *Ann Emerg Med*, 1995, 26:58-64.

Tran P, Panacek EA, Rhee KJ, et al, "Is Norepinephrine More Efficacious Than Dopamine in Reversing Hypotension Caused by Cyclic Antidepressant Overdose?" *Ann Emerg Med*, 1995, 25(1):128-30.

Ammonium Chloride (a moe' nee um klor' ide)

CAS Number 12125-02-9

Brand Names Chlorammonia®; Darammon®; Dytuss®; Gen-Diur®; Hi-Amchol®; Pectomed®; Quelidrine®; Salmiac®

Synonyms Ammonium Muriate

Use Diuretic or systemic and urinary acidifying agent; treatment of hypochloremic states; industrial use: galvanizing procedures, fertilizer, electroplating, soldering, manufacture of dry batteries, deodorizer cleaners (Lysol®, Swish Toilet Bowl Cleaner®); may be useful in bromide toxicity

Mechanism of Action Increases acidity by increasing free hydrogen ion concentration; as an expectorant by irritating, the mucosa, causing reflex stimulation of the bronchial mucosal glands

Adverse Reactions

Cardiovascular: Bradycardia
Central nervous system: Mental confusion, coma, headache
Dermatologic: Rash
Endocrine & metabolic: Metabolic acidosis secondary to hyperchloremia
Gastrointestinal: gastrointestinal irritation
Local: Pain at site of injection
Respiratory: Hyperventilation

Signs & Symptoms of Acute Overdose Hyperchloremic, hypokalemic metabolic acidosis, hypomagnesemia, nausea, vomiting, headache, hyperventilation, diuresis, bradycardia, pulmonary edema, apnea

Toxicodynamics/Kinetics

Absorption: Rapid from gastrointestinal tract with absorption being complete in 3-6 hours

Distribution: Unknown

Metabolism: In the liver to urea

Elimination: In urine (1% to 3% in feces)

Usual Dosage Metabolic alkalosis: The following equations represent different methods of correction utilizing either the serum HCO_3^-, the serum chloride, or the base excess

Dosing of mEq NH_4Cl via the chloride-deficit method (hypochloremia):

Dose of mEq NH_4Cl = [0.2 L/kg x body weight (kg)] x [103 – observed serum chloride]; give 100% of dose over 12 hours, then re-evaluate

Note: 0.2 L/kg is the estimated chloride space and 103 is the average normal serum chloride concentration

Dosing of mEq NH_4Cl via the bicarbonate-excess method (refractory hypochloremic metabolic alkalosis):

Dose of NH_4Cl = [0.5 L/kg x body weight (kg) x (observed serum HCO_3^- - 24)]; give 50% of dose over 12 hours, then re-evaluate

Note: 0.5 L/kg is the estimated bicarbonate space and 24 is the average normal serum bicarbonate concentration

Dosing of mEq NH_4Cl via the base-excess method:

Dose of NH_4Cl = [0.3 L/kg x body weight (kg) x measured base excess (mEq/L)]; give 50% of dose over 12 hours, then re-evaluate

Note: 0.3 L/kg is the estimated extracellular bicarbonate and base excess is measured by the chemistry lab and reported with arterial blood gases

These equations will yield different requirements of ammonium chloride

Equation #1 is inappropriate to use if the patient has severe metabolic alkalosis without hypochloremia or if the patient has uremia

Equation #3 is the most useful for the first estimation of ammonium chloride dosage

Children: Urinary acidifying agents: Oral, I.V.: 75 mg/kg/day in 4 divided doses; maximum daily dose: 6 g

Adults: Urinary acidifying agent/diuretic:

Oral: 2-3 g every 6 hours

I.V.: 1.5 g/dose every 6 hours

Contraindications Severe hepatic and renal dysfunction; patients with primary respiratory acidosis

Warnings Safety and efficacy not established in children, use with caution in infants, or patients with impaired renal or hepatic function

Dosage Forms

Injection: 26.75% [5 mEq/mL] (20 mL)

Tablet: 500 mg

Tablet, enteric coated: 500 mg

Overdosage Treatment

Decontamination: Activated charcoal with cathartic

Supportive therapy: I.V. sodium bicarb for acidosis; replenish potassium

Test Interactions Increases ammonia (B), glucose (S); decreases potassium (S), sodium (S), urine pH

Drug Interactions Spironolactone and ammonium chloride may produce a profound acidosis

Pregnancy Risk Factor B

Monitoring Parameters Serum ammonia, potassium, serum pH

Patient Information Take oral dose after meals

Nursing Implications Rapid I.V. injection may increase the likelihood of ammonia toxicity; rate should not exceed 1 mEq/kg/hour; 26.75% solution must be diluted prior to administration

Additional Information Odorless, may produce explosive reaction (with potassium chlorate, nitrates, hydrogen cyanide)

TLV-TWA: 10 mg/m^3

PEL-TWA: 10 mg/m^3

Specific References

Bushinsky DA and Coe FL, "Hyperkalemia During Acute Ammonium Chloride Acidosis in Man," *Nephron*, 1985, 40(1):38-40.

Ammonium Muriate *see* Ammonium Chloride *on previous page*

Amoxapine (a mox' a peen)

Related Information

Antidepressant Agents Comparison *on page 1639*

Therapeutic Drugs Associated With Hallucinations *on page 1558-1559*

(Continued)

Amoxapine *(Continued)*

CAS Number 14028-44-5

Brand Names Asendin®; Demolox®; Moxadil®; Omnipres®

Use Treatment of neurotic and endogenous depression and mixed symptoms of anxiety and depression

Mechanism of Action Reduces the reuptake of serotonin and norepinephrine and blocks the response of dopamine receptors to dopamine; low effect on serotonin reuptake. Amoxapine is a metabolite of the antipsychotic agent loxapine.

Adverse Reactions

Anticholinergic: Extrapyramidal effects, tardive dyskinesia, blurred vision

Cardiovascular: Hypotension, sinus tachycardia; relatively low cardiac toxicity as compared to other tricyclic antidepressants

Central nervous system: Drowsiness, restlessness, dizziness, nervousness, insomnia, seizures, Parkinson's-like symptoms, chorea (extrapyramidal), tardive dyskinesia, fever, visual hallucinations, neuroleptic malignant syndrome, electroencephalogram abnormalities

Dermatologic: Rash, toxic epidermal necrolysis

Endocrine & metabolic: Amenorrhea, galactorrhea, syndrome of inappropriate antidiuretic hormone

Gastrointestinal: Constipation, dry mouth, pancreatitis

Hematologic: Leukopenia/neutropenia (agranulocytosis, granulocytopenia)

Ocular: Oculogyric crisis (extrapyramidal)

Signs & Symptoms of Acute Overdose Grand mal seizures, depression, photosensitivity, insomnia, hyperprolactinemia, mania, impotence, ejaculatory disturbances, extrapyramidal reaction, dementia, neuroleptic malignant syndrome, cognitive dysfunction, nystagmus, acidosis, coma, supraventricular arrhythmias, hematuria, incomplete right bundle-branch block, renal failure (acute), neurotoxic effects may be permanent, myoglobinuria, hematuria

Toxicodynamics/Kinetics

Onset of action: After 1-2 weeks

Absorption: Oral: Rapidly and well absorbed

Distribution: V_d: 60-70 L/kg

Protein binding: 90% or more

Metabolism: Extensive hydroxylation in the liver to active metabolites 8- and 7-hydroxyamoxapine which has dopamine-blocking effects

Half-life: 11-16 hours; 8-hydroxy metabolite is active, with a half-life (adults): 30 hours; half-life in overdoses may approach 40 hours

Time to peak serum concentration: Within 1-2 hours

Elimination: Metabolites and parent compound in urine, 7% to 18% excreted in feces

Usual Dosage Once symptoms are controlled, decrease gradually to lowest effective dose. Maintenance dose is usually given at bedtime to reduce daytime sedation. Oral:

Children <16 years: Not established

Adolescents: Initial: 25-50 mg/day; increase gradually to 100 mg/day; may give as divided doses or as a single dose at bedtime

Adults: Initial: 25 mg 2-3 times/day, if tolerated, dosage may be increased to 100 mg 2-3 times/day; may be given in a single bedtime dose when dosage <300 mg/day

Maximum daily dose:

Inpatient: 600 mg

Outpatient: 400 mg

Contraindications Hypersensitivity to amoxapine; cross-sensitivity with other tricyclics may occur; narrow-angle glaucoma; patients receiving MAO inhibitors within past 14 days

Warnings Do not discontinue abruptly in patients receiving high doses chronically; use with caution in patients with seizures, cardiac conduction disturbances, cardiovascular diseases, urinary retention, hyperthyroidism, or those receiving thyroid replacement

Dosage Forms Tablet: 25 mg, 50 mg, 100 mg, 150 mg

Reference Range

Therapeutic:

Amoxapine 20-100 ng/mL (SI: 64-319 nmol/L)

8-OH-amoxapine: 150-400 ng/mL (SI: 478-1275 nmol/L)

Both: 200-500 ng/mL (SI: 637-1594 nmol/L)

Fatal: 261 ng/mL

Overdosage Treatment

Decontamination: Lavage (up to 8 hours postingestion)/activated charcoal with cathartic; multiple dosing of activated charcoal may be effective; do not induce emesis

Supportive therapy: Following initiation of essential overdose management, toxic symptoms should be treated. Propofol (2.5 mg/kg bolus I.V. followed by infusion of 0.2 mg/kg/minute) has been effective in terminating amoxapine-induced seizures in a case report; ventricular arrhythmias often respond to phenytoin 15-20 mg/kg (adults) with concurrent systemic alkalinization (sodium bicarbonate 0.5-2 mEq/kg I.V.). Arrhythmias unresponsive to this therapy may respond to lidocaine 1 mg/kg I.V. followed by a titrated infusion. Seizures usually respond to lorazepam or diazepam I.V. boluses (5-10 mg for adults up to 30 mg or 0.25-0.4 mg/kg/dose for children up to 10 mg/dose). If seizures are unresponsive or recur, phenytoin or phenobarbital may be required. Use physostigmine only as **a last resort**.

Antidote(s)

Sodium Bicarbonate *on page 1467*

Test Interactions Increases glucose; may elevate prolactin level

Diagnostic Tests/Procedures

Amoxapine, Blood *on page 1190*

Drug Interactions May possibly decrease effects of clonidine and guanethidine; may increase effects of central nervous system depressants, adrenergic agents, anticholinergic agents; with monoamine oxidase inhibitors, fever, tachycardia, hypertension, seizures and death may occur; similar interactions as with other tricyclics may occur

Pregnancy Risk Factor C

Pregnancy Implications Distributes into breast milk

Monitoring Parameters Monitor blood pressure and pulse rate prior to and during initial therapy; evaluate mental status

Patient Information Dry mouth may be helped by sips of water, sugarless gum, or hard candy; avoid alcohol; very important to maintain established dosage regimen; photosensitivity to sunlight can occur; rise slowly to prevent dizziness

Nursing Implications May increase appetite and possibly a craving for sweets; recognize signs of neuroleptic malignant syndrome and tardive dyskinesia

Additional Information May take up to 2 weeks for full therapeutic effects to be apparent; maintenance dose is usually given at bedtime to reduce daytime sedation; tolerance develops in 1-3 months in some patients, close medical follow-up is essential

Specific References

Crome P and Ali C, "Clinical Features and Management of Self-Poisoning With Newer Antidepressants," *Med Toxicol Adverse Drug Exp*, 1986, 1(6):411-20.

Leonard BE, "Safety of Amoxapine," *Lancet*, 1989, 2(8666):808.

Litovitz TC and Troutman WG, "Amoxapine Overdose. Seizures and Fatalities," *JAMA*, 1983, 250(8):1069-71.

Mancias P, Kramer L, and Butler IJ, "Amoxapine Overdose in a Young Man: A Transient Mitochondrial Abnormality," *Pharmacotherapy*, 1995, 15(4):528-32.

Merigian KS, Browning RG, and Leeper KV, "Successful Treatment of Amoxapine-Induced Refractory Status Epilepticus With Propofol (Diprivan®)," *Acad Emerg Med*, 1995, 2:128-33.

Tasset JJ and Pesce AJ, "Amoxapine in Human Overdose," *J Anal Toxicol*, 1984, 8(3):124-8.

Amoxicillin (a mox i sill' in)

CAS Number 26787-78-0; 34642-77-8; 61336-70-7

Brand Names Amoxil®; Biomox®; Polymox®; Trimox®; Wymox®

Synonyms Amoxycillin; *p*-Hydroxyampicillin

Use Treatment of otitis media, sinusitis, and infections caused by susceptible organisms involving the respiratory tract, skin, and urinary tract; prophylaxis of bacterial endocarditis

Mechanism of Action Interferes with bacterial cell wall synthesis during active multiplication, causing cell wall death and resultant bactericidal activity against susceptible bacteria

Adverse Reactions

Central nervous system: Convulsions, fever

Dermatologic: rash (especially patients with mononucleosis), rash that appears after a few days of therapy may indicate hypersensitivity, erythema multiforme, Stevens-Johnson syndrome, bullous skin disease/pemphigoid

Gastrointestinal: Diarrhea (less than with ampicillin); esophageal ulcer

Hematologic: Hemolytic anemia, neutropenia, pancytopenia

Hepatic: Interstitial nephritis, hepatitis with cholestatic jaundice

Ocular: Diplopia

Miscellaneous: Superinfection

Signs & Symptoms of Acute Overdose Neuromuscular sensitivity, Stevens-Johnson syndrome, pemphigus, many beta-lactam containing antibiotics have the potential to cause neuromuscular hyperirritability or convulsive seizures

Toxicodynamics/Kinetics

Absorption: Oral: Rapid and nearly complete (89%); food does not interfere clinically

Distribution: V_d: 0.31 L/kg

Protein binding: 17% to 20%

Metabolism: Partial to penicilloic acid

Half-life:

Neonates, full-term: 3.7 hours

(Continued)

Amoxicillin *(Continued)*

Infants and Children: 1-2 hours
Patients with Cl_{cr} <10 mL/minute: 7-21 hours
Time to peak serum concentration:
Capsule: Within 2 hours
Suspension: 1 hour
Elimination: Renal excretion (80% as unchanged drug); lower in neonates

Usual Dosage Oral:
Children: 25-100 mg/kg/day in divided doses every 8 hours
Uncomplicated gonorrhea: ≥2 years: 50 mg/kg plus probenecid 25 mg/kg in a single dose; do not use this regimen in children <2 years of age, probenecid is contraindicated in this age group
Subacute bacterial endocarditis prophylaxis: 50 mg/kg 1 hour before procedure and 25 mg/kg 6 hours later
Adults: 250-500 mg every 8 hours; maximum dose: 2-3 g/day
Uncomplicated gonorrhea: 3 g plus probenecid 1 g in a single dose
Endocarditis prophylaxis: 3 g 1 hour before procedure and 1.5 g 6 hours later

Dosing interval in renal impairment:
Cl_{cr} 10-50 mL/minute: Administer every 12 hours
Cl_{cr} <10 mL/minute: Administer every 24 hours
Moderately dialyzable (20% to 50%)

Contraindications Hypersensitivity to amoxicillin, penicillin, or any component

Warnings In patients with renal impairment, doses and/or frequency of administration should be modified in response to the degree of renal impairment; high percentage of patients with infectious mononucleosis have developed rash during therapy with amoxicillin

Dosage Forms
Capsule: 250 mg, 500 mg
Powder for oral suspension: 125 mg/5 mL (5 mL, 80 mL, 100 mL, 150 mL, 200 mL); 250 mg/5 mL (5 mL, 80 mL, 100 mL, 150 mL, 200 mL)
Powder for oral suspension, drops: 50 mg/mL (15 mL, 30 mL)
Tablet, chewable: 125 mg, 250 mg

Stability Oral suspension and pediatric drops remain stable for 7 days at room temperature or 14 days if refrigerated

Reference Range After a 250 mg oral dose, peak plasma level of 5 µg/mL and urine level >300 µg/mL have been noted

Overdosage Treatment
Decontamination: Emesis or lavage rarely necessary/activated charcoal with cathartic can be used
Supportive therapy: Allergic reactions can be treated with epinephrine, diphenhydramine, and corticosteroids
Enhancement of elimination: Hemodialysis or charcoal hemoperfusion can be useful in removing penicillin; moderately dialyzable (20% to 50%)

Test Interactions ↑ AST, ALT, protein

Drug Interactions
Decreased effect of oral contraceptives; tetracyclines may decrease efficacy of penicillins; amiloride reduces intestinal absorption of amoxicillin
Increased levels with probenecid; allopurinol theoretically has an additive potential for amoxicillin rash; oral bioavailability increased by 16% when given with cimetidine

Pregnancy Risk Factor B

Monitoring Parameters With prolonged therapy, monitor renal, hepatic, and hematologic function periodically

Patient Information Report diarrhea promptly; entire course of medication (10-14 days) should be taken to ensure eradication of organism; should be taken in equal intervals around-the-clock to maintain adequate blood levels; may interfere with oral contraceptives, females should report symptoms of vaginitis; pediatric drops may be placed on child's tongue or added to formula, milk, etc

Nursing Implications Assess patient at beginning and throughout therapy for infection; give around-the-clock rather than 3 times/day to promote less variation in peak and trough serum levels.

Additional Information Food does not interfere with absorption; rash that appears after a few days of therapy may indicate hypersensitivity

Specific References

Dougall HT, et al, "The Effect of Amoxycillin on Salivary Nitrite Concentrations: An Important Mechanism of Adverse Reactions?" *Br J Clin Pharmacol*, 1995, 39:460-2.

Hautekeete ML, Brenard R, Horsmans Y, et al, "Liver Injury Related to Amoxycillin-Clavulanic Acid: Interlobular Bile-Duct Lesions and Extrahepatic Manifestations," *J Hepatol*, 1995, 22:71-7.

Jones KH and Hill SA, "The Toxicology Absorption and Pharmacokinetics of Amoxicillin," *Adv Clin Pharmacol*, 1974, 7:20.

Oe PL, et al, "Pharmacokinetics of the New Penicillins, Amoxicillin and Flucloxacillin in Patients With Terminal Renal Failure Undergoing Hemodialysis," *Chemotherapy*, 1973, 19:279.

Parry MF, "The Penicillins," *Med Clin North Am*, 1987, 71(6):1093-112.
Prignet JM, Galzin M, Duval JL, et al, "Amoxicillin-Induced Esophageal Ulcer With Intractable Hiccups as the Presenting Manifestation," *Semaine des Hopitaux*, 1995, 71:186-7.
Westphal JF, Jehl F, Brogard JM, et al,"Amoxicillin Intestinal Absorption Reduction by Amiloride: Possible Role of the Na^+-H^+ Exchanger," *Clin Pharmacol Ther*, 1995, 51:257-64.

Amoxil® *see* Amoxicillin *on page 121*

Amoxycillin *see* Amoxicillin *on page 121*

Amphojel® [OTC] *see* Aluminum *on page 104*

Ampho-Moronal® *see* Amphotericin B *on this page*

Amphotericin B (am foe ter' i sin)

Related Information

Antifungal Therapy *on page 1496-1497*

CAS Number 1397-89-3

Brand Names AmBisome®; Ampho-Moronal®; Funganiline®; Fungilin®; Fungizone®; Fungizone® Intravenous

Use Treatment of severe systemic infections and meningitis caused by susceptible fungi; fungal peritonitis; irrigant for bladder fungal infections; topically for cutaneous and mucocutaneous candidal infections

Mechanism of Action Binds to ergosterol altering cell membrane permeability in susceptible fungi and causing leakage of cell components with subsequent cell death

Adverse Reactions

Cardiovascular: Hypotension, hypertension, cardiac arrest, tachycardia, dilated cardiomyopathy, flushing

Central nervous system: Fever, chills, headache, malaise, delirium, seizures, psychosis, dysphoria, dizziness, Parkinsonian symptoms, hyperthermia, hemiparesis

Dermatologic: Maculopapular rash

Endocrine & metabolic: Hypokalemia, hypomagnesemia

Gastrointestinal: Anorexia, nausea, vomiting

Genitourinary: Urinary retention, anuria

Hematologic: Anemia, leukocytosis, coagulation defects, thrombocytopenia, agranulocytosis, leukopenia, bone marrow depression

Hepatic: Acute liver failure

Local: Thrombophlebitis

Neuromuscular & skeletal: Myalgia, paresthesia

Ocular: Vision changes, diplopia

Otic: Hearing loss

Renal: Renal tubular acidosis, renal failure, nephrotoxicity (cortical ischemia)

Respiratory: Dyspnea

Miscellaneous: Generalized pain, pain along lumbar nerves, arachnoiditis

Signs & Symptoms of Acute Overdose Renal dysfunction, deafness, hematuria, hypomagnesemia, hypokalemia, hyperthyroidism, encephalopathy, myoclonus, myalgia, meningitis, tubular necrosis, dysphoria, congestive heart failure, coagulopathy, delirium, feces discoloration (black), anemia, anorexia, thrombocytopenia, granulocytopenia, fever, nausea, and vomiting

Toxicodynamics/Kinetics

Absorption: Poor orally (9%) and by I.M. injection

Distribution: V_d: 3 L/kg; minimal amounts enter the aqueous humor, bile, CSF, amniotic fluid, pericardial fluid, pleural fluid, and synovial fluid

Plasma protein binding: 90%

Half-life, biphasic:

Initial: 15-48 hours

Terminal: 15 days

Time to peak serum concentration: I.V. infusion: During the first hour after a 4- to 6-hour infusion

Usual Dosage The minimum dilution for amphotericin B infusions is 0.1 mg/mL for peripheral lines and 1 mg/mL for central lines

Infants and Children:

Test dose: I.V.: 0.1 mg/kg/dose to a maximum of 1 mg; infuse over 30-60 minutes. If the test dose is tolerated, the initial therapeutic dose is 0.25 mg/kg. The daily dose can then be gradually increased, usually in 0.25 mg/kg increments on each subsequent day until the desired daily dose is reached.

Maintenance dose: 0.25-1 mg/kg/day given once daily; infuse over 2-6 hours. Once therapy has been established, amphotericin B can be administered on an every other day basis at 1-1.5 mg/kg/dose.

I.T.: 25-100 mcg every 48-72 hours; increase to 500 mcg as tolerated

Adults: I.V.:

Test dose: 1 mg infused over 20-30 minutes. Institute therapy with 0.25 mg/kg administered over 2-6 hours; the daily dose can be gradually increased on subsequent days to the desired level

(Continued)

Amphotericin B *(Continued)*

Maintenance dose: 0.25-1 mg/kg/day or 1.5 mg/kg every other day; do not exceed 1.5 mg/kg/day. If the test dose is tolerated, the initial therapeutic dose is 0.25 mg/kg. The daily dose can then be gradually increased, usually in 0.25 mg/kg increments on each subsequent day until the desired daily dose is reached.

Duration of therapy varies with nature of infection: Histoplasmosis, *Cryptococcus*, or blastomycosis may be treated with total dose of 2-4 g

I.T.: 25-300 mcg every 48-72 hours; increase to 500 mcg to 1 mg as tolerated

Children and Adults (doses up to 8 mg/kg in infants did not experience any permanent sequelae)

Bladder irrigation: 50 mg/day in 1 L of sterile water irrigation solution instilled over 24 hours for 2-7 days or until cultures are clear

Dialysate: 1-2 mg/L of peritoneal dialysis fluid either with or without low-dose I.V. amphotericin B (a total dose of 2-10 mg/kg given over 7-14 days)

Topical: Apply to affected areas 2-4 times/day for 1-4 weeks of therapy depending on nature and severity of infection

Dosing adjustment in renal impairment: If renal dysfunction is due to the drug, the daily total can be decreased by 50% or the dose can be given every other day; I.V. therapy may take several months

Administration Amphotericin is administered by I.V. infusion over 2-6 hours at a final concentration not to exceed 0.1 mg/mL. In patients unable to tolerate a large fluid volume, amphotericin B 0.25 mg/mL in D_5W given through a central venous catheter is the highest concentration reported to have been administered.

Contraindications Hypersensitivity to amphotericin or any component

Warnings Because of the nephrotoxic potential of amphotericin, other nephrotoxic drugs should be avoided; BUN and serum creatinine levels should be determined every other day while therapy is increased and at least weekly thereafter. I.V. amphotericin is used primarily for the treatment of patients with progressive and potentially fatal fungal infections; topical preparations may stain clothing

Dosage Forms

Cream: 3% (20 g)

Lotion: 3% (30 mL)

Ointment, topical: 3% (20 g)

Powder for injection, lyophilized: 50 mg

Stability Reconstitute only with sterile water without preservatives, not bacteriostatic water; benzyl alcohol, sodium chloride, or other electrolyte solutions may cause precipitation; for I.V. infusion, an in-line filter (>1 micron mean pore diameter) may be used; short-term exposure (<24 hours) to light during I.V. infusion does **not** appreciably affect potency

Reference Range Therapeutic: 1.0-2.0 μg/mL (SI: 1.0-2.2 μmol/L)

Overdosage Treatment

Supportive therapy: Premedication with hydrocortisone, diphenhydramine, or nonsteroidal anti-inflammatory agents can decrease chills; phosphate buffer or heparin can be added to amphotericin B infusions to decrease thrombophlebitis; simultaneous use of mannitol (1 g/kg) or sodium supplements may decrease renal failure incidence; meperidine (50-75 mg) may be used to prevent or treat chills; coadministration of amiloride (5 mg twice daily) can decrease incidence of hypokalemia

Enhancement of elimination: Exchange transfusion has been used with limited success in infants; no significant effect on amphotericin B plasma levels on double exchange transfusion and thus this modality is not recommended; poorly dialyzed

Test Interactions ↑ BUN (S); ↓ magnesium, potassium (S); decreased erythropoietin levels

Drug Interactions

Increased nephrotoxic effect of cyclosporine, aminoglycosides, foscarnet, pentamidine

Increased potassium depletion with corticosteroids; this may predispose patients receiving cardiac glycosides or skeletal muscle relaxants to toxicity secondary to hypokalemia

Enhanced antineoplastic effect with BCNU; synergistic antifungal effect with flucytosine; increased bone marrow toxicity when used with AZT

Pregnancy Risk Factor B

Monitoring Parameters Electrolytes, BUN, serum creatinine, hematocrit, liver function tests, CBC regularly; monitor input and output; monitor for signs of hypokalemia (muscle weakness, cramping, drowsiness, EKG changes, etc)

Patient Information Amphotericin cream may slightly discolor skin and stain clothing; personal hygiene is very important to help reduce the spread and recurrence of lesions; avoid covering topical applications with occlusive bandages; most skin lesions require 1-3 weeks of therapy; report any cramping, muscle weakness, or pain at or near injection site

Nursing Implications May premedicate patients with acetaminophen and diphenhydramine 30 minutes prior to the amphotericin infusion; meperidine (Demerol®) may help to reduce rigors

Additional Information Reversing sodium depletion may prevent amphotericin B-induced nephrotoxicity; dosage adjustments are not necessary with renal impairment; if decreased renal function is due to amphotericin, the daily dose can be decreased by 50% or the dose can be given every other day; due to increased pulmonary toxicity, granulocyte transfusion should be separated from amphotericin B administration as far as possible. Delivery of amphotericin B in a lipid diluent (20% fat emulsion) may decrease nephrotoxicity and rigors. Premedication is not effective in preventing fever or nausea.

Specific References

Anderson RP and Clark DA, "Amphotericin B Toxicity Reduced by Administration in Fat Emulsion," *Ann Pharmacother*, 1995, 29:496-500.

Arning M, Heer-Sonderhoff A, and Schneider W, "Cardiopulmonary Toxicity After Liposomal Amphotericin B (AmBisome®) in Neutropenic Patients With Acute Leukemia," *Onkologie*, 1994, 17:4.

Arsura EL, Ismail Y, Freedman S, et al, "Amphotericin B-Induced Dilated Cardiomyopathy," *Am J Med*, 1994, 97(6):560-2.

Benson JM and Nahata MC, "Clinical Use of Systemic Antifungal Agents," *Clin Pharm*, 1988, 7(6):424-38.

Brent J, Hunt M, Kulig K, et al, "Amphotericin B Overdoses in Infants: Is There a Role for Exchange Transfusion?," *Vet Hum Toxicol*, 1990, 32(2):124-5.

Devuyst O, Goffin E, and Van Ypersele de Strihou C, "Recurrant Hemiparesis Under Amphotericin B for *Candida albicans* Peritonitis," *Nephrol Dial Transplant*, 1995, 10:699-701.

Gales MA and Gales BJ, "Rapid Infusion of Amphotericin B in Dextrose," *Ann Pharmacother*, 1995, 29:523-9.

Goodwin SD, "Pretreatment Regimens for Adverse Events Related to Infusion of Amphotericin B," *Clin Infect Dis*, 1994, 20:755-61.

Jones RS, Barman A, Suh B, et al, "Successful Treatment of *Aspergillus vertebral* Osteomyelitis With Amphotericin B Lipid Complex," *Infect Dis Clin Prac*, 1995, 4:237-9.

Ampicillin (am pi sill' in)

CAS Number 69-53-4

Brand Names Marcillin®; Omnipen®; Omnipen®-N; Polycillin®; Polycillin-N®; Principen®; Totacillin®; Totacillin®-N

Synonyms Aminobenzylpenicillin

Use Treatment of susceptible bacterial infections; use for bacterial infections due to alkali burns

Mechanism of Action Interferes with bacterial cell wall synthesis during active multiplication, causing cell wall death and resultant bactericidal activity against susceptible bacteria

Adverse Reactions

Central nervous system: Convulsions

Dermatologic: Rash (more frequent in patients with Epstein-Barr virus infection), urticaria, bullous skin disease/pemphigoid

Gastrointestinal: Diarrhea, nausea, vomiting, glossitis, colitis

Hematologic: Eosinophilia, hemolytic anemia, thrombocytopenia, neutropenia

Ocular: Diplopia

Renal: Interstitial nephritis

Miscellaneous: Drug fever

Signs & Symptoms of Acute Overdose Cholestatic jaundice, erythema multiforme, toxic epidermal necrolysis, Stevens-Johnson syndrome, deafness, myocarditis, myalgia, hypoprothrombinemia, colitis, hypokalemia

Toxicodynamics/Kinetics

Absorption: Oral: 50%

Distribution: V_d: 0.17-0.31 L/kg; distributes into bile; penetration into CSF occurs with inflamed meninges only

Protein binding: 8% to 20%

Half-life:

- Neonates:
  - 2-7 days: 4 hours
  - 8-14 days: 2.8 hours
  - 15-30 days: 1.7 hours
- Children and Adults: 1-1.8 hours
- Anuric patients: 8-20 hours

Time to peak serum concentration: Oral: Within 1-2 hours

Elimination: ~90% of the drug excreted unchanged in urine within 24 hours

Usual Dosage

Neonates: I.M., I.V.:

- Postnatal age <7 days:
  - <2000 g: Meningitis: 50 mg/kg/dose every 12 hours; other infections: 25 mg/kg/dose every 12 hours
  - >2000 g: Meningitis: 50 mg/kg/dose every 8 hours; other infections: 25 mg/kg/dose every 8 hours

(Continued)

Ampicillin *(Continued)*

Postnatal age >7 days:

<2000 g: Meningitis: 50 mg/kg/dose every 8 hours; other infections: 25 mg/kg/dose every 8 hours

>2000 g: Meningitis: 50 mg/kg/dose every 6 hours; other infections: 25 mg/kg/dose every 6 hours

Infants and Children: I.M., I.V.: 100-200 mg/kg/day in 4-6 divided doses; meningitis: 200 mg/kg/day in 4-6 divided doses; maximum dose: 12 g/day

Children: Oral: 50-100 mg/kg/day divided every 6 hours; maximum dose: 2-3 g/day

Adults:

Oral: 250-500 mg every 6 hours

I.M.: 500 mg to 1.5 g every 4-6 hours

I.V.: 500 mg to 3 g every 4-6 hours; maximum dose: 12 g/day

Sepsis/meningitis: 150-250 mg/kg/24 hours divided every 3-4 hours

Dosing interval in renal impairment:

Cl_{cr} 10-30 mL/minute: Administer every 8-12 hours

Cl_{cr} <10 mL/minute: Administer every 12-24 hours

Administration Ampicillin can be administered IVP over 3-5 minutes at a rate not to exceed 100 mg/minute or I.V. intermittent infusion over 15-30 minutes; final concentration for I.V. administration should not exceed 100 mg/mL (IVP) or 30 mg/mL (I.V. intermittent infusion)

Contraindications Known hypersensitivity to ampicillin or other penicillins

Warnings Dosage adjustment may be necessary in patients with renal impairment; high percentage of patients with infectious mononucleosis have developed rash during therapy with ampicillin; use with caution in patients allergic to cephalosporins

Dosage Forms

Capsule, as anhydrous: 250 mg, 500 mg

Capsule, as trihydrate: 250 mg, 500 mg

Powder for injection, as sodium: 125 mg, 250 mg, 500 mg, 1 g, 2 g, 10 g

Powder for oral suspension, as trihydrate: 125 mg/5 mL (5 mL unit dose, 80 mL, 100 mL, 150 mL, 200 mL); 250 mg/5 mL (5 mL unit dose, 80 mL, 100 mL, 150 mL, 200 mL); 500 mg/5 mL (5 mL unit dose, 100 mL)

Powder for oral suspension, drops, as trihydrate: 100 mg/mL (20 mL)

Stability Oral suspension is stable for 7 days at room temperature or for 14 days under refrigeration; solutions for I.M. or direct I.V. should be used within 1 hour; solutions for I.V. infusion will be inactivated by dextrose at room temperature; if dextrose-containing solutions are to be used, the resultant solution will only be stable for 2 hours versus 8 hours in the 0.9% sodium chloride injection. D_5W has limited stability.

Minimum volume: Concentration should not exceed 30 mg/mL; manufacturer may supply as either the anhydrous or the trihydrate form

Overdosage Treatment

Decontamination: Emesis or lavage rarely necessary/activated charcoal with cathartic can be used; whole bowel irrigation is effective in decreasing bioavailability by 67%

Supportive therapy: Allergic reactions can be treated with epinephrine, diphenhydramine, and corticosteroids

Enhancement of elimination: Hemodialysis or charcoal hemoperfusion can be useful in removing penicillin; moderately dialyzable (20% to 50%)

Test Interactions ↑ protein; urinary glucose (Benedict's solution, Clinitest®); ↑ positive Coombs' [direct]

Drug Interactions

Decreased effect of oral contraceptives

Increased levels with probenecid; allopurinol theoretically has an additive potential for amoxicillin rash

Pregnancy Risk Factor B

Monitoring Parameters With prolonged therapy, monitor renal, hepatic, and hematologic function periodically

Patient Information Food decreases rate and extent of absorption, therefore, give on an empty stomach; report diarrhea promptly; entire course of medication (10-14 days) should be taken to ensure eradication of organism; should be taken in equal intervals around-the-clock to maintain adequate blood levels; females should report onset of symptoms of candidal vaginitis; may interfere with the effects of oral contraceptives

Nursing Implications Ampicillin and gentamicin should not be mixed in the same I.V. tubing or administered concurrently; give orally on an empty stomach (ie, 1 hour prior to, or 2 hours after meals) to increase total absorption. Give around-the-clock rather than 4 times/day to promote less variation in peak and trough serum levels.

Additional Information
Sodium content of 5 mL suspension (250 mg/5 mL): 10 mg (0.4 mEq)
Sodium content of 1 g: 66.7 mg (3 mEq)

Specific References

Tenenbein M, Cohen S, and Sitar DS, "Whole Bowel Irrigation as a Decontamination Procedure After Acute Drug Overdose," *Arch Intern Med*, 1987, 147(5):905-7.

Amrinone Lactate (am' ri none)

Related Information
Adrenergic Agonists, Cardiovascular Comparison *on page 1638*
Adrenergic Agonists Drug Infusions Comparison *on page 1638*

CAS Number 60719-84-8

Brand Names Inocor®; Wincoram®

Use Treatment of low cardiac output states (sepsis, congestive heart failure); adjunctive therapy of pulmonary hypertension; normally prescribed for patients who have not responded well to therapy with digitalis, diuretics, and vasodilators; effective for calcium channel blocker toxicity

Mechanism of Action Inhibits myocardial cyclic adenosine monophosphate (cAMP) phosphodiesterase activity and increases cellular levels of cAMP resulting in a positive inotropic effect; also possesses systemic and pulmonary vasodilator effects

Adverse Reactions
Cardiovascular: Hypotension, ventricular and supraventricular arrhythmias; may be related to infusion rate
Central nervous system: Headache, fever
Dermatologic: Yellow fingernail discoloration
Endocrine & metabolic: Nephrogenic diabetes insipidus
Gastrointestinal: Nausea, vomiting, abdominal pain, anorexia, hypogeusia, splenomegaly, stomatitis
Hematologic: Thrombocytopenia
Hepatic: Hepatotoxicity: Discontinue amrinone if significant increase in liver enzymes (serum lactic dehydrogenase or glutamic oxaloacetic transaminase) with symptoms of idiosyncratic hypersensitivity reaction (eg, eosinophilia) occurs
Neuromuscular & skeletal: Myalgia
Renal: Diuresis
Miscellaneous: Altered taste

Signs & Symptoms of Acute Overdose Hypotension, tachycardia, myalgia, lightheadedness, hyperthermia, diabetes insipidus, chest pain

Toxicodynamics/Kinetics
Onset of action: I.V.: Hemodynamic actions occur within 2-5 minutes
Peak effect: I.V.: Within 10 minutes
Duration: Dose dependent with low doses lasting approximately 30 minutes and higher doses lasting approximately 2 hours
Distribution: V_d:
- Neonates: 1.8 L/kg
- Infants: 1.6 L/kg
- Adults: 1.2 L/kg;

Protein binding: 10% to 49%
Metabolism: Liver
Half-life:
- Neonates 1-2 weeks: 22.2 hours
- Infants 6-38 weeks: 6.8 hours; negative correlation of age with half-life in infants 4-38 weeks of age
- Adults:
  - Normal volunteers: 3.6 hours
  - With CHF: 5.8 hours

Time to peak serum concentration: Within 10 minutes
Elimination: 60% to 90% as metabolites in urine within 24 hours; fecal elimination 18%

Usual Dosage Dosage is based on clinical response
Note: Dose should not exceed 10 mg/kg/24 hours

Neonates: 0.75 mg/kg I.V. bolus over 2-3 minutes followed by maintenance infusion 3-5 mcg/kg/minute; I.V. bolus may need to be repeated in 30 minutes

Children and Adults: 0.75 mg/kg I.V. bolus over 2-3 minutes followed by maintenance infusion 5-10 mcg/kg/minute; I.V. bolus may need to be repeated in 30 minutes

Dosing adjustment in renal failure: Cl_{cr} <10 mL/minute: Administer 50% to 75% of dose

Administration Should be administered solely via an I.V. pump

Contraindications Hypersensitivity to amrinone lactate or sulfites (contains sodium metabisulfite)

(Continued)

Amrinone Lactate *(Continued)*

Warnings Diuresis may result from improvement in cardiac output and may require dosage reduction of diuretics

Dosage Forms Injection: 5 mg/mL (20 mL)

Stability May be administered undiluted for I.V. bolus doses. For continuous infusion: Dilute with 0.45% or 0.9% sodium chloride to final concentration of 1-3 mg/mL; use within 24 hours; do not directly dilute with dextrose-containing solutions, chemical interaction occurs; may be administered I.V. into running dextrose infusions. Furosemide forms a precipitate when injected in I.V. lines containing amrinone.

Reference Range Plasma levels >2.5 μg/mL can be associated with toxicity

Overdosage Treatment Supportive therapy: There is no specific antidote for amrinone intoxication. Overdosage with amrinone has caused severe hypotension by vasodilation; if this occurs, general measures for circulatory support should be taken (isotonic saline, dopamine)

Test Interactions Lowers potassium

Drug Interactions When furosemide is admixed with amrinone, a precipitate immediately forms

Pregnancy Risk Factor C

Monitoring Parameters Monitor blood pressure and heart rate every 5 minutes during infusion; monitor cardiac index, stroke volume, systemic vascular resistance, and pulmonary vascular resistance (if Swan-Ganz catheter available); CVP, SBP, DBP, heart rate, platelet count, CBC, liver function and renal function tests. Monitor for hypotension, thrombocytopenia, hepatitis, and gastrointestinal effects; monitor fluids and electrolytes.

Patient Information Make position changes slowly because of hypotension (orthostatic)

Nursing Implications Patients should be carefully monitored for hemodynamic response (hypotension) and potential adverse effects (ie, thrombocytopenia, hepatitis, and gastrointestinal effects)

Additional Information Normally prescribed for patients who have not responded well to therapy with digitalis, diuretics, and vasodilators

Specific References

Lebovitz DJ, Lawless ST, and Weise KL, "Fatal Amrinone Overdose in a Pediatric Patient," *Crit Care Med*, 1995, 23:977-80.

Silverman BD, Merrill AJ, and Gerber L, "Clinical Effects and Side Effects of Amrinone," *Arch Intern Med*, 1989, 145(5):825-9.

Webster MW and Sharpe DN, "Adverse Effects Associated With the Newer Inotropic Agents," *Med Toxicol Adverse Drug Exp*, 1986, 1(5):335-42.

Anacin-3® [OTC] *see* Acetaminophen *on page 79*

Anacin® [OTC] *see* Aspirin *on page 133*

Anafranil® *see* Clomipramine Hydrochloride *on page 228*

Anaprox® *see* Naproxen *on page 549*

Anapsique® *see* Amitriptyline Hydrochloride *on page 116*

Anaspaz® *see* Hyoscyamine Sulfate *on page 415*

Anbesol® Maximum Strength [OTC] *see* Benzocaine *on page 149*

Ancoron® *see* Amiodarone Hydrochloride *on page 113*

Andriol® *see* Testosterone *on page 729*

Andro-Cyp® Injection *see* Testosterone *on page 729*

Andro® Injection *see* Testosterone *on page 729*

Andro-L.A.® Injection *see* Testosterone *on page 729*

Andronate® Injection *see* Testosterone *on page 729*

Andropository® Injection *see* Testosterone *on page 729*

Anemone Camphor *see* Camphor *on page 179*

Anergan® *see* Promethazine Hydrochloride *on page 650*

Anestacon® *see* Lidocaine Hydrochloride *on page 468*

Anethaine® *see* Tetracaine Hydrochloride *on page 731*

Aneurine Hydrochloride *see* Thiamine Hydrochloride *on page 741*

Angilol® *see* Propranolol Hydrochloride *on page 657*

Anginal® *see* Dipyridamole *on page 292*

Angioverin® *see* Papaverine *on page 591*

Anistal® *see* Ranitidine Hydrochloride *on page 675*

Anodyon *see* Ethyl Chloride *on page 337*

Ansaid® *see* Flurbiprofen Sodium *on page 364*

Ansamycin *see* Rifabutin *on page 681*

Anspor® *see* Cephradine *on page 191*

Antabuse® *see* Disulfiram *on page 296*

Antagosan® *see* Aprotinin *on next page*

Antaxone® *see* Naltrexone Hydrochloride *on page 548*

Antepsin® *see* Sucralfate *on page 710*

Anticode® *see* Edrophonium Chloride *on page 309*

Antidepressant Agents Comparison *see page 1639*

Antifungal Therapy *see page 1496*

Antihist-1® [OTC] *see* Clemastine Fumarate *on page 223*

Antihistamines

Commonly Found in Alkylamines, ethanolamines, ethylene diamines, phenothiazines, piperazines, piperidines by chemical structure; multiple other chemically unclassifiable, consider with OTC cough/cold, sinus, allergy, sleeping, antiemetic, and dizziness products

Use Rhinitis, rash, or allergic symptoms; antidote for scombroid fish poisoning and other natural toxins eliciting allergic manifestations

Mechanism of Action See individual monographs

Adverse Reactions Gastrointestinal, antimuscarinic, neurologic, psychosis, extrapyramidal, withdrawal syndromes; see individual monographs

Signs & Symptoms of Acute Overdose Nausea, ataxia, constipation, dry mouth, dry skin, vomiting, apnea, adynamic ileus; sedation, coma, seizures, hyperthermia, muscular rigidity, sinus tachycardia, hallucinations, urinary retention, mydriasis, CNS stimulation predominantly in children, CNS depression in adults; referral and treatment of ingestions >3 times usual dose suggested; sedation, coma, sinus tachycardia; excitation signs occur in children, CNS depression in adults

Warnings Many products containing antihistamines are sustained-release formulations

Overdosage Treatment Referral and treatment of ingestions >3 times usual dose suggested

Decontamination: Avoid ipecac (except prehospital), charcoal recommended; lavage indicated if obtunded or within 1 hour of ingestion or evidence of gastric hypomotility

Supportive therapy: There is no routine specific treatment; severe life-threatening symptoms may be treated with physostigmine; hypotension is best treated with norepinephrine or phenylephrine; seizures should be treated with benzodiazepines in absence of secondary complications (cardiac ischemia), sinus tachycardia does not require specific therapy; in presence of severe secondary complications, renal failure due to rhabdomyolysis, hemodialysis may be employed; sodium bicarbonate may be of some value in wide complex tachycardias

Diagnostic Tests/Procedures

Electrocardiography *on page 1253*

Blood Gases, Arterial *on page 1207*

Drug Interactions Erythromycin, ketoconazole, itraconazole can inhibit metabolism; antihistamines contribute to sedation with CNS depressants and add antimuscarinic activity to other antimuscarinics (monoamine oxidase inhibitors, atropine, tricyclic antidepressants); some agents have antiserotonin actions and may interact with other antiserotoninergic agents

Pregnancy Risk Factor B

Monitoring Parameters Vital signs, EKG

Additional Information Liquid preparations may also contain significant amounts of alcohol; topical administration on infants and small children has lead to severe systemic toxicity, particularly in presence of varicella infection

Specific References

Estelle F, Simons R, and Simons KJ, "Pharmacokinetic Optimisation of Histamine H_1-Receptor Antagonist Therapy," *Clin Pharmacokinet*, 1991, 21(5):372-93.

Feldman MD and Behar M, "A Case of Massive Diphenhydramine Abuse and Withdrawal From Use of the Drug," *JAMA*, 1986, 255(22):3119-20.

Maswosme JJ, et al, "Suspected Fatal Diphenhydramine Toxicity by Application to the Skin of an Infant With Varicella," *Hosp Pharm*, 1994, 29:26,28-30,53.

Uden DL, Huska DR, Kellenberger TA, et al, "Antihistamines: A Study of Pediatric Usage and Incidence of Toxicity," *Vet Hum Toxicol*, 1984, 26(6):469-72.

Antil® *see* Cimetidine *on page 212*

Antipsychotic Agents Comparison *see page 1642*

Antisacer® *see* Phenytoin *on page 623*

Antitirode G.W.® *see* Methimazole *on page 512*

Anti-Tuss® Expectorant [OTC] *see* Guaifenesin *on page 390*

Antituxil-Z® *see* Zipeprol Hydrochloride *on page 813*

Antivert® *see* Meclizine Hydrochloride *on page 494*

Antra® *see* Omeprazole *on page 576*

Antrizine® *see* Meclizine Hydrochloride *on page 494*

Anuject® *see* Procaine Hydrochloride *on page 644*

Anxanil® *see* Hydroxyzine *on page 414*

Apacet® [OTC] *see* Acetaminophen *on page 79*

APD: Aminohydroxypropylidene Disphosphonate *see* Pamidronate Disodium *on page 590*

Apekumarol® *see* Dicumarol *on page 277*

Aphilan R® *see* Buclizine Hydrochloride *on page 166*

Aphrodine Hydrochloride *see* Yohimbine Hydrochloride *on page 805*

Aphrodyne™ *see* Yohimbine Hydrochloride *on page 805*

Apo-dipyridamole® *see* Dipyridamole *on page 292*

Apodorm® *see* Nitrazepam *on page 562*

Apo-Nadol® *see* Nadolol *on page 545*

A-Poxide® *see* Chlordiazepoxide *on page 198*

Apresoline® *see* Hydralazine Hydrochloride *on page 405*

Aprotinin (ay proe ten' in)

CAS Number 9087-70-1

Brand Names Antagosan®; Fase®; Inibil®; Iniprol®; Kir Richter®; Midran®; Trasylol®

Synonyms Aprotininum

Use Treatment of life-threatening hemorrhage caused by increased plasmin concentration; prophylactic use to reduce perioperative blood loss in patients undergoing cardiopulmonary bypass in repeat coronary artery bypass graft surgery; may be effective against streptokinase-induced bleeding

Mechanism of Action Serine protease inhibitor; inhibits plasmin, kallikrein, and platelet activation; a weak inhibitor of plasma pseudocholinesterase

Adverse Reactions Increase in postoperative renal dysfunction compared to placebo; anaphylactic reactions have been reported in <0.5% of cases; such reactions are more likely to occur with repeated administration; bronchospasm

Signs & Symptoms of Acute Overdose Possible liver/tubular necrosis (acute) at a dose of 15 million KIU

Toxicodynamics/Kinetics Half-life: 150 minutes

Usual Dosage

Test dose: **All** patients should receive a 1 mL I.V. test dose at least 10 minutes prior to the loading dose to assess the potential for allergic reactions

Regimen A:
- 2 million units (280 mg) loading dose I.V. over 20-30 minutes
- 2 million units (280 mg) into pump prime volume
- 500,000 units/hour (70 mg/hour) I.V. during operation

Regimen B:
- 1 million units (140 mg) loading dose I.V. over 20-30 minutes
- 1 million units (140 mg) into pump prime volume
- 250,000 units/hour (35 mg/hour) I.V. during operation

Contraindications Hypersensitivity to aprotinin; thromboembolic disease requiring anticoagulation

Warnings Increased risk of hypersensitivity in patients previously exposed to aprotinin; use with caution in patients with renal insufficiency

Dosage Forms Injection: 1.4 mg/mL [10,000 units/mL] (100 mL, 200 mL)

Stability Incompatible with corticosteroids, heparin, tetracyclines

Reference Range Plasma concentration of 250 KIU/mL in patients after receiving 2 million KIU I.V. loading dose

Overdosage Treatment

Supportive therapy: Bronchospasm can be treated with beta agonist therapy; anaphylaxis can be treated with epinephrine, antihistamines, and corticosteroids

Drug Interactions Can potentiate tubocurarine chloride, succinylcholine when combined with heparin; whole blood activated clotting time may be further prolonged than when heparin is used alone

Pregnancy Risk Factor B

Specific References

Verstraete M, "Clinical Application of Inhibitors of Fibrinolysis," *Drugs*, 1985, 29(3):236-61.

Viby-Mogensen J, "Interaction of Other Drugs With Muscle Relaxants," *Semin Anesth*, 1985, 4:52-64.

Woodman RC and Harker LA, "Bleeding Complications Associated With Cardiopulmonary Bypass," *Blood*, 1990, 76(9):1680-97.

Aprotininum *see* Aprotinin *on previous page*

Apsolol® *see* Propranolol Hydrochloride *on page 657*

Aquachloral® Supprettes® *see* Chloral Hydrate *on page 193*

Aquaear® *see* Acetic Acid *on page 85*

Aquaphyllin® *see* Theophylline *on page 735*

Aquarid® *see* Furosemide *on page 373*

Aquasol A® *see* Vitamin A *on page 795*

Aquasol E® Oral [OTC] *see* Vitamin E *on page 798*

Aquazide-H® *see* Hydrochlorothiazide *on page 406*

Aqueous Testosterone *see* Testosterone *on page 729*

Aralen® Phosphate *see* Chloroquine Phosphate *on page 202*

Arcalion® *see* Thiamine Hydrochloride *on page 741*

Aredia™ *see* Pamidronate Disodium *on page 590*

Aredin® *see* Pamidronate Disodium *on page 590*

Arem® *see* Nitrazepam *on page 562*

Arfonad® *see* Trimethaphan Camsylate *on page 771*

Argesic®-SA *see* Salsalate *on page 689*

Arinol *see* Benzalkonium Chloride *on page 147*

Arlix® *see* Piretanide *on page 630*

Arm-a-Med® Metaproterenol *see* Metaproterenol Sulfate *on page 506*

Armil® *see* Benzalkonium Chloride *on page 147*

Armour® Thyroid *see* Thyroid *on page 749*

Arovit® *see* Vitamin A *on page 795*

Arrestin® *see* Trimethobenzamide Hydrochloride *on page 772*

Arret® *see* Loperamide Hydrochloride *on page 480*

Arteolol® *see* Carteolol Hydrochloride *on page 188*

Artha-G® *see* Salsalate *on page 689*

ASA *see* Aspirin *on page 133*

A.S.A. [OTC] *see* Aspirin *on page 133*

Asaurex® *see* Cimetidine *on page 212*

Ascorbic Acid (a skor' bik)

CAS Number 50-81-7

Brand Names Ascorbicap® [OTC]; C-Crystals® [OTC]; Cecon® [OTC]; Cetane® [OTC]; Cevalin® [OTC]; Ce-Vi-Sol® [OTC]; Dull-C® [OTC]; Flavorcee® [OTC]; Vita-C® [OTC]

Synonyms Cevitamic Acid; Vitamin C

Use Prevention and treatment of scurvy; urinary acidification; dietary supplementation; chromium nephrotoxicity/dermal burns due to chromium

Mechanism of Action Necessary for collagen formation and tissue repair in the body; involved in some oxidation-reduction reactions, as well as many other metabolisms

Adverse Reactions

Cardiovascular: Flushing, chest pain

Central nervous system: Faintness, dizziness, headache, fatigue

Gastrointestinal: Nausea, vomiting, heartburn, diarrhea, esophageal ulceration

Hematologic: Hemolysis (in patients with G-6-PD deficiency),

Renal: Hyperoxaluria

Signs & Symptoms of Acute Overdose Renal insufficiency, nephrotoxicity, esophageal ulceration, hematuria, nephropathy, dental erosion

Toxicodynamics/Kinetics

Absorption: Oral: Readily absorbed; absorption is an active process and is thought to be dose-dependent

Metabolism: In the liver by oxidation and hydrolyzed to 2-3 diketo-L-gluconic acid; eventually metabolized to L-threomic acid and oxalic acid

Elimination: Excreted in urine; there is an individual specific renal threshold for ascorbic acid; when blood levels are high, ascorbic acid is excreted in urine;

(Continued)

Ascorbic Acid *(Continued)*

whereas when the levels are subthreshold, very little if any ascorbic acid is cleared into urine

Usual Dosage Oral, I.M., I.V., S.C.:

Children:

Scurvy: 100-300 mg/day in divided doses for at least 2 weeks
Urinary acidification: 500 mg every 6-8 hours
Dietary supplement: 35-45 mg

Adults:

Scurvy: 100-250 mg 1-2 times/day
Urinary acidification: 4-12 g/day in 3-4 divided doses
Dietary supplement: 50-60 mg/day
Prevention and treatment of cold: 1-3 g/day
Recommended daily allowance: 60 mg

Chromium poisoning: I.V.: 1 g every 10-20 minutes, up to 3 g

Chromium dermal burns: 10% topical ascorbic acid along with 10 g of oral ascorbic acid

Contraindications Large doses during pregnancy

Warnings Diabetics and patients prone to recurrent calculi (renal) (eg, dialysis patients) should not take excessive doses for extended periods of time

Dosage Forms

Capsule, timed release: 500 mg
Crystals: 4 g/teaspoonful (1000 g)
Injection: 100 mg/mL; 250 mg/mL (2 mL, 30 mL); 500 mg/mL (1 mL, 2 mL, 50 mL)
Powder: 4 g/teaspoonful (1000 g)
Solution, oral: 35 mg/0.6 mL (50 mL); 100 mg/mL (50 mL)
Syrup: 500 mg/5 mL (5 mL, 10 mL, 120 mL, 480 mL)
Tablet: 25 mg, 50 mg, 100 mg, 250 mg, 500 mg, 1000 mg, 1500 mg
Tablet:

Chewable: 60 mg, 100 mg, 250 mg, 500 mg, 1000 mg
Effervescent: 1 g
Timed release: 500 mg, 1000 mg, 1500 mg

Stability Injectable form should be stored under refrigeration (2°C to 8°C); protect oral dosage forms from light; is rapidly oxidized when in solution in air and alkaline media

Reference Range Normal serum level: 10 μg/mL

Overdosage Treatment

Decontamination: Lavage/activated charcoal with cathartic; dilution with milk or water may minimize chances of esophageal injury

Test Interactions False-positive urinary glucose with cupric sulfate reagent, false-negative urinary glucose with glucose oxidase method; false-negative stool occult blood 48-72 hours after ascorbic acid ingestion; Hemoccult® and Gastroccult® tests can be unreliable in detecting gastrointestinal bleeding in iron overdoses treated with whole bowel irrigation (ferrous sulfate/ferrous gluconate: false-positive; ascorbic acid: false-negative)

Drug Interactions

Decreased effect of warfarin; decreased fluphenazine levels

Increased serum levels of estrogens; increased iron absorption; increased elimination of amphetamines, phencyclidine

Pregnancy Risk Factor A (C if used in doses above RDA recommendation)

Patient Information Do not take more than the recommended dose; take with plenty of water; report any pain on urination

Nursing Implications Avoid rapid I.V. injection

Additional Information Sodium content of 1 g: ~5 mEq

Specific References

Ballin A, Brown EJ, Koren G, et al, "Vitamin C-Induced Erythrocyte Damage in Premature Infants," *J Pediatr*, 1988, 113(1 Pt 1):114-20.

Giunta JL, "Dental Erosion Resulting From Chewable Vitamin C Tablets," *JAMA*, 1983, 107(2):253-6.

Korallus U, Harzdorf C, and Lewalter J, "Experimental Basis for Ascorbic Acid Therapy of Poisoning by Hexavalent Chromium Compounds," *Int Arch Occup Environ Health*, 1984, 53(3):247-56.

Lawton JM, Conway LT, Crosson JT, et al, "Acute Oxalate Nephropathy After Massive Ascorbic Acid Administration," *Arch Intern Med*, 1985, 145(5):950-1.

McAllister CJ, Scowden EB, Dewberry FL, et al, "Renal Failure Secondary to Massive Infusion of Vitamin C," *JAMA*, 1984, 252(13):1684.

Pru C, Eaton J, and Kjellstrand C, "Vitamin C Intoxication and Hyperoxalemia in Chronic Hemodialysis Patients," *Nephron*, 1985, 39(2):112-6.

Tunget CL, Clark RF, Manoguerra AS, et al, "Iron Overdose and Detection of Gastrointestinal Bleeding With the Hemoccult® and Gastroccult® Assays," *Ann Emerg Med*, 1995, 26:54-7.

Ascorbicap® [OTC] *see* Ascorbic Acid *on previous page*

Ascriptin® [OTC] *see* Aspirin *on next page*

ASE-136BS *see* Dirithromycin *on page 293*

Asendin® *see* Amoxapine *on page 119*

Asmalix® *see* Theophylline *on page 735*

Aspergum® [OTC] *see* Aspirin *on this page*

Aspirin (as' pir in)

CAS Number 50-78-2

Brand Names Anacin® [OTC]; A.S.A. [OTC]; Ascriptin® [OTC]; Aspergum® [OTC]; Bayer® Aspirin [OTC]; Bufferin® [OTC]; Easprin®; Ecotrin® [OTC]; Empirin® [OTC]; Measurin® [OTC]; Synalgos® [OTC]; ZORprin®

Synonyms Acetylsalicylic Acid; ASA

Use Treatment of mild to moderate pain, inflammation and fever; may be used as a prophylaxis of myocardial infarction and transient ischemic attacks (TIA)

Mechanism of Action Inhibits prostaglandin synthesis, acts on the hypothalamus heat-regulating center to reduce fever, blocks prostaglandin synthetase action which prevents formation of the platelet-aggregating substance thromboxane A_2; inhibits both vitamin K-dependent and independent clotting factors

Adverse Reactions

Cardiovascular: Fluid retention, circulatory collapse, pericardial effusion/pericarditis

Central nervous system: Headache, aseptic meningitis, psychosis, cognitive dysfunction, coma, seizures, electroencephalogram abnormalities

Dermatologic: Rash, pruritus, alopecia

Endocrine & metabolic: Hyperkalemia, anion gap metabolic acidosis, hypouricemia

Gastrointestinal: Abdominal pain, nausea, vomiting, bleeding, ulceration, constipation, diarrhea, dyspepsia

Hematologic: Leukopenia, neutropenia, agranulocytosis, granulocytopenia, aplastic anemia (rare), platelet inhibition, hypoprothrombinemia

Hepatic: Elevation of transaminases, fulminant hepatitis

Neuromuscular & skeletal: Rhabdomyolysis

Ocular: Diplopia

Otic: Ototoxicity, tinnitus

Renal: Renal failure (acute), albuminuria, nephrotic syndrome

Respiratory: Wheezing, adult respiratory distress syndrome, apnea, tachypnea, respiratory depression

Miscellaneous: Hypersensitivity, bezoars/concretions

Signs & Symptoms of Acute Overdose Nausea, colitis, wheezing, nephrotic syndrome, gout, delirium, deafness, vomiting, dry mouth, coagulopathy; Stevens-Johnson syndrome, stomatitis, cognitive dysfunction, chest pain, dementia, bezoars, gastrointestinal bleeding, hyperthermia, hematuria, hypoglycemia, nystagmus, ototoxicity, tinnitus, drowsiness; severe poisoning can manifest with coma, thirst, seizures, renal failure and or hepatic failure, hyponatremia, hypotension, respiratory depression, headache, dizziness, confusion, metabolic acidosis, fever, leukopenia, neutropenia, agranulocytosis, granulocytopenia, hyperglycemia, urine discoloration (pink), feces discoloration (black), feces discoloration (pink), feces discoloration (red), feces discoloration (tarry), pylorospasm, rhabdomyolysis

Phases of aspirin poisoning:

Phase I (up to 12 hours after ingestion): Tachypnea and hyperventilation predominate (respiratory alkalosis) with increased renal secretion of sodium, potassium, and bicarbonate resulting in both an alkaline urinary and serum pH

Phase II (12-24 hours after ingestion): Urine becomes more acidic as intracellular potassium decreases; while children <4 years of age may develop a pure metabolic acidosis, older patients will have significant respiratory compensation and thus serum pH can be alkalotic; coagulation abnormalities may occur

Phase III (over 24 hours after ingestion): Severe potassium and bicarbonate depletion occurs with hydrogen being excreted renally; serum pH becomes acidotic; infants may reach this phase within 6 hours

Toxicodynamics/Kinetics

Absorption: From the stomach and small intestine

Distribution: V_d: 0.2 L/kg (increases in overdose); distributes readily into most body fluids and tissues

Protein binding: 75% to 90%; salicylic acid: 80% at low serum concentrations; 50% at 70 mg/dL and 30% at 120 mg/dL

Metabolism: Hydrolyzed to salicylate (active) by esterases in the gastrointestinal mucosa, red blood cells, synovial fluid and blood; occurs primarily by hepatic microsomal enzymes; metabolic pathways are saturable

Half-life: 15-20 minutes; half-life is dose-dependent ranging from 3 hours at lower doses (300-600 mg), 5-6 hours (after 1 g) and 10 hours with higher doses

Time to peak serum concentration: About 1-2 hours

Elimination: Renal; primarily as free salicylic acid and conjugated metabolites

(Continued)

Aspirin *(Continued)*

Usual Dosage

Children:

Analgesic and antipyretic: Oral, rectal: 10-15 mg/kg/dose every 4-6 hours, up to a total of 60-80 mg/kg/24 hours

Anti-inflammatory: Oral: Initial: 60-90 mg/kg/day in divided doses; usual maintenance: 80-100 mg/kg/day divided every 6-8 hours, maximum dose: 3.6 g/day; monitor serum concentrations

Antirheumatic: Oral: 60-100 mg/kg/day in divided doses every 4 hours

Kawasaki disease: Oral: 80-100 mg/kg/day divided every 6 hours; after fever resolves: 8-10 mg/kg/day once daily; monitor serum concentrations

Adults:

Analgesic and antipyretic: Oral, rectal: 325-650 mg every 4-6 hours up to 4 g/day

Anti-inflammatory: Oral: Initial: 2.4-3.6 g/day in divided doses; usual maintenance: 3.6-5.4 g/day; monitor serum concentrations

TIA: Oral: 1.3 g/day in 2-4 divided doses

Toxic acute dose: 200 mg/kg

Lethal dose: 300 mg/kg

Myocardial infarction prophylaxis: 160-325 mg/day

Dosing adjustment in renal impairment: Cl_{cr} <10 mL/minute: Avoid use

Dosing adjustment in hepatic disease: Avoid use in severe liver disease

Contraindications Bleeding disorders, hypersensitivity to salicylates or other nonsteroidal anti-inflammatory drugs (NSAIDs)

Warnings Do not use aspirin in children <16 years of age for chickenpox or flu symptoms due to the association with Reye's syndrome; use with caution in patients with platelet and bleeding disorders, renal dysfunction

Dosage Forms

Suppository, rectal: 60 mg, 120 mg, 125 mg, 130 mg, 195 mg, 200 mg, 300 mg, 325 mg, 600 mg, 650 mg, 1200 mg

Tablet: 325 mg, 500 mg, 650 mg

Tablet:

Buffered:

325 mg with aluminum hydroxide 75 mg and magnesium hydroxide 75 mg

325 mg with aluminum hydroxide 150 mg and magnesium hydroxide 150 mg

500 mg with aluminum hydroxide 33 mg and magnesium hydroxide 150 mg

Chewable: 81 mg

Chewing gum: 227 mg

Controlled release: 800 mg

Enteric coated (delayed release): 80 mg, 165 mg, 325 mg, 500 mg, 650 mg, 975 mg

Timed release: 650 mg

Tablet, with caffeine: 400 mg and caffeine 32 mg; 500 mg and caffeine 32 mg

Stability Keep suppositories in refrigerator, do not freeze; hydrolysis of aspirin occurs upon exposure to water or moist air, resulting in salicylate and acetate, which possess a vinegar-like odor; do not use if a strong odor is present

Reference Range

Sample size: 1.5-2 mL blood (purple top tube)

Timing of serum samples: Peak levels usually occur 2 hours after ingestion; half-life increases with dosage (eg, the half-life after 300 mg is 3 hours, and after 1 g is 5-6 hours, and after 8-10 g is 10 hours)

Salicylate serum concentrations correlate with the pharmacological actions and adverse effects observed. See table.

Overdosage Treatment

Decontamination: Activated charcoal with cathartic is quite effective; each gram of activated charcoal can bind up to 550 mg of salicylic acid; whole bowel irrigation can also be used

Supportive therapy: Hypotension/dehydration can be managed with intravenous fluid therapy; acidosis should be treated with bicarbonates, seizures with benzodiazepines; blood products are indicated, as appropriate, for hemorrhage; antacids may promote gastric absorption

Enhancement of elimination: Forced alkaline diuresis with intravenous sodium bicarbonate to keep urine pH at 8 should be performed for salicylate levels >40 mg/dL; dialysis is indicated for secondary complications, acidosis, or renal failure and not toxin removal alone; consider hemodialysis for acute salicylate levels >100 mg/dL; multiple dosing of activated charcoal may not hasten elimination; dialyzable (50% to 100%)

Test Interactions False-negative results for glucose oxidase urinary glucose tests (Clinistix®); false-positives using the cupric sulfate method (Clinitest®); also, interferes with Gerhardt test, VMA determination; 5-HIAA, xylose tolerance test and T_3 and T_4

Drug Interactions Aspirin decreases serum concentrations probably by protein-binding displacement; there is an increased bleeding potential with concomitant warfarin therapy; may increase lithium and methotrexate concentrations by decreasing renal clearance; may decrease diuretic and hypotensive effects of thiazides, loop diuretics, ACE inhibitors, and beta-blockers; may increase nephrotoxicity of cyclosporine; salicylate absorption can be delayed with aluminum hydroxide, antihistamines, tricyclic antidepressants, isoniazid, opiates, neuroleptics, or sedative-hypnotics

Serum Salicylate: Clinical Correlations

Serum Salicylate Concentration (mg/dL)	Desired Effects	Adverse Effects/ Intoxication
~10	Antiplatelet Antipyresis Analgesia	GI intolerance and bleeding, hypersensitivity, hemostatic defects
15–30	Anti-inflammatory	Mild salicylism
25–40	Treatment of rheumatic fever	Nausea/vomiting, hyperventilation, salicylism, flushing, sweating, thirst, headache, diarrhea, and tachycardia
>40		Respiratory alkalosis, hemorrhage, excitement, confusion, asterixis, pulmonary edema, convulsions, tetany, metabolic acidosis, fever, coma, cardiovascular collapse, renal and respiratory failure

Aspirin Conversion Factor for NAS Compounds

Salicylate-Containing Product	ACF
Acetaminosalol	0.8290
Aloxipri	0.8333
Aluminum aspirin**	0.8956
Aminosalicylic acid	*
Ammonium salicylate	1.1611
Antipyrine salicylate	0.5520
Aspirin	1.0000
Benorylate	0.5750
Benzyl salicylate	0.9246
Bismuth subsalicylate	0.4975
Bromosalicylic acid acetate	0.6954
Calcium aminosalicylate	*
Calcium carbaspirin	0.3930
Carbamoylphenoxyacetic acid	0.9229
Choline salicylate	0.7466
Diethylamine salicylate	0.8526
Diflunisal	*
Ethyl salicylate	1.2244
Fendosal	0.4723
Glycol salicylate	0.9889
Homosalate	0.7154
Lithium salicylate	1.2512
Magnesium salicylate**	1.2068
Menthyl salicylate	0.6792
Methyl salicylate	1.3978
Octyl salicylate	0.7303
Phenazone salicylate	0.5519
Phenyl aminosalicylate	*
Phenyl salicylate	0.7469
Physostigmine salicylate	0.4360
Potassium aminosalicylate	*
Potassium salicylate	1.0224
Salicylamide	*
Salicylic acid	1.3043
Salsalate**	1.3953
Silver salicylate	0.7354
Sodium aminosalicylate	*
Sodium salicylate	1.1252
Sodium thiosalicylate	1.0226
Sulfasalazine	*
Thurfyl salicylate	0.8108
Triethanolamine Salicylate	0.6292

*Not converted to salicylate.

**Hydrolyzed to 2 molecules of salicylate.

Adapted from *Poisindex,* 1994, vol 81, Salicylates and Vandenberg S, *Vet Hum Toxicol,* 1989, 31:49–50.

Pregnancy Risk Factor C (D if full-dose aspirin in 3rd trimester)

Pregnancy Implications Late term fetus is more sensitive to adverse (acidotic) effects of aspirin; but with low dose aspirin, no evidence for increased frequency of abruptio placentae or perinatal mortality noted

Patient Information Watch for bleeding gums or any signs of gastrointestinal bleeding; take with food or milk to minimize gastrointestinal distress; notify physician if ringing in ears or persistent gastrointestinal pain occurs

Nursing Implications Administer with food or a full glass of water to minimize gastrointestinal distress; do not crush sustained release tablet; previous nonreaction does not guarantee future safe taking of medication

Additional Information To help evaluate the toxicity of nonaspirin salicylate agents, conversion to an aspirin equivalent dose (AED) may be necessary; by multiplying the dose ingested by the aspirin conversion factor (ACF) described in the table, the AED can be calculated. This calculation assumes that the nonaspirin salicylate is 100% absorbed and there is 100% conversion to salicylate and that the potency of the nonaspirin salicylate is equipotent with aspirin on a mole for mole basis.

Specific References

Abdel-Magid EH and el-Awad Ahmed FR, "Salicylate Intoxication in an Infant With Ichthyosis Transmitted Through Skin Ointment – A Case Report," *Pediatrics*, 1994, 94(6 Pt 1):939-40.

Bochner F and Lloyd JV, "Aspirin for Myocardial Infarction," *Clin Pharmacokinet*, 1995, 28:433-8.

Chapman BJ and Proudfoot AT, "Adult Salicylate Poisoning: Deaths and Outcome in Patients With High Plasma Salicylate Concentrations," *Q J Med*, 1989, 72(268):699-707.

Dugandric RM, Tierney MG, and Dickinson GE, "Evaluation of the Done Nomogram in the Management of Acute Salicylate Intoxication," *Ann Emerg Med*, 1989, 18(11):1186-90.

Fiske WD, Connell JM, and Benedek IH, "Lack of Pharmacokinetic Interaction Between Aspirin and Warfarin," *Am J Therap*, 1995, 2:407-13.

Govaert P, Staelens V, and Vanhaesebrouch P, "Perinatal Intracranial Hemorrhage Due to Maternal Salicylate Ingestion," *Clin Pediatr (Phila)*, 1995, 34:174-5.

Hauth JC, Goldenberg RL, Parker CR Jr, et al, "Low-Dose Aspirin: Lack of Association With an Increase in Abruptio Placentae or Perinatal Mortality," *Obstet Gynecol*, 1995, 85:1055-8.

Lee S, Johnson D, Klein J, et al, "Protein Binding of Acetylsalicylic Acid and Salicylic Acid in Porcine and Human Serum," *Vet Hum Toxicol*, 1995, 37(3):224-5.

Montgomery H, Porter JC, and Bradley RD, "Salicylate Intoxication Causing a Severe Systemic Inflammatory Response and Rhabdomyolysis," *Am J Emerg Med*, 1994, 12(5):531-2.

Palatnick W and Tenenbein M, "Increase Fetal Sensitivity in Aspirin Poisoning," *Vet Hum Toxicol*, 1994, 36:368.

Sibal BM, et al, "Low-Dose Aspirin in Nulliparous Women: Safety of Continuous Epidural Block and Correlation Between Bleeding Time and Maternal-Neonatal Bleeding Complications," *Am J Obstet Gynecol*, 1995, 172:1553-7.

Vandenberg SA, Smolinske SC, Spoerke DG, et al, "Nonaspirin Salicylates: Conversion Factors for Estimating Aspirin Equivalency," *Vet Hum Toxicol*, 1989, 31(1):49-50.

Verbeeck RK, "Pharmacokinetic Drug Interactions With Nonsteroidal Anti-inflammatory Drugs," *Clin Pharmacokinet*, 1990, 19(1):44-66.

Vertrees JE, McWilliams BC, and Kelly HW, "Repeated Oral Charcoal Administration for Treating Aspirin Overdose in Young Children," *Pediatrics*, 1990, 85(4):594-8.

Astemizole (a stem' mi zole)

Related Information

H1-Antihistamine Comparison *on page 1649*

CAS Number 68844-77-9

Brand Names Hismanal®

Use Perennial and seasonal allergic rhinitis and other allergic symptoms including rash

Mechanism of Action Peripheral H_1-receptor antagonist without anticholinergic or sedative effects; unrelated in structure to other nonsteroidals

Adverse Reactions

Cardiovascular: Palpitations, bradycardia, hypotension, torsade de pointes

Central nervous system: Headache, fatigue, nervousness, dizziness, depression, sedation, paradoxical excitement, insomnia, slight drowsiness, ataxia, EEG abnormalities

Dermatologic: Photosensitivity, alopecia, rash, angioedema

Gastrointestinal: Appetite increase, weight increase, nausea, diarrhea, abdominal pain, dry mouth

Genitourinary: Urinary retention

Hepatic: Hepatitis

Neuromuscular & skeletal: Arthralgia, myalgia, tremors, paresthesia

Ocular: Blurred vision, cycloplegia

Respiratory: Bronchospasm, thickening of bronchial secretions, pharyngitis

Miscellaneous: Edema, porphyrinogenic, epistaxis

Signs & Symptoms of Acute Overdose Nausea, flatulence, seizures, insomnia, depression, confusion, sedation, Q-T prolongation; myalgia, torsade de pointes, seizures, conjunctivitis

Toxicodynamics/Kinetics

Onset of action: Slow
Absorption: Rapid, reduced by food
Protein binding: 96% to 97%
Metabolism: Extensive
Half-life: 20-24 hours; elimination half-life: 7-11 days
Time to peak concentration: <1 hour
Elimination: 50% metabolites excreted in urine and feces

Usual Dosage Oral:

Children:
- <6 years: 0.2 mg/kg/day
- 6-12 years: 5 mg/day

Children >12 years and Adults: 10-30 mg/day; give 30 mg on first day, 20 mg on second day, then 10 mg/day in a single dose

Contraindications Hypersensitivity to astemizole or any component; hepatic dysfunction, pre-existing prolonged Q-T syndromes; concomitant erythromycin, itraconazole, or ketoconazole therapy

Warnings Doses >20 mg associated with severe cardiac manifestations

Dosage Forms Tablet: 10 mg

Overdosage Treatment

Decontamination: Lavage/activated charcoal
Supportive therapy: Lidocaine has been used successfully to treat cardiac arrhythmias; avoid type I antiarrhythmics, torsade may respond to I.V. magnesium

Drug Interactions Erythromycin, itraconazole, or ketoconazole inhibit astemizole metabolism predisposing to development of Q-T prolongation and ventricular arrhythmias

Pregnancy Risk Factor C

Monitoring Parameters EKG

Patient Information Take on an empty stomach at least 2 hours after a meal or 1 hour before a meal; may cause drowsiness; do not exceed recommended dose; notify physician or pharmacist if taking any heart medications

Nursing Implications Raise bed rails at night; may need assistance with ambulation

Additional Information Not likely to cause drowsiness; may be useful in treating granulocyte colony-stimulating bone pain

Specific References

Cunliffe NA, Barnes AJ, and Dunbar EM, "Stevens-Johnson Syndrome Following Astemizole Therapy," *Postgrad Med J*, 1995, 71:383.

Gudi R, Krishnomurthy M, and Pachter BR,"Astemizole in the Treatment of Granulocyte Colony Stimulating Factor-Induced Bone Pain," *Ann Intern Med*, 1995, 123(3):236-7.

Hoppu K, Tikanoja T, Tapanainen P, et al, "Accidental Astemizole Overdose in Young Children," *Lancet*, 1991, 338(8766):538-40.

Krstenansky PM and Cluxton RJ Jr, "Astemizole: A Long Acting Nonsedating Antihistamine," *Drug Intell Clin Pharm*, 1987, 21(12):947-53.

Simons FE, Kesselman MS, and Giddins NG, "Astemizole-Induced Torsade de Pointes," *Lancet*, 1988, 2(8611):624.

Snook J, Boothman-Burrell D, Watkins J, et al, "Torsade de Pointes Ventricular Tachycardia Associated With Astemizole Overdose," *Br J Clin Pract*, 1988, 42(6):257-9.

Wiley JF 2d and Gelber ML, "Cardiotoxic Effects of Astemizole Overdose in Children," *J Pediatr*, 1992, 120(5):799-802.

Astramorph™ PF *see* Morphine Sulfate *on page 539*

Atarax® *see* Hydroxyzine *on page 414*

Atazina® *see* Hydroxyzine *on page 414*

Atem® *see* Ipratropium Bromide *on page 438*

Atenol® *see* Atenolol *on this page*

Atenolol (a ten' oh lole)

Related Information

Beta-Blockers Comparison *on page 1644-1645*

CAS Number 29122-68-7; 60966-51-0

Brand Names Atenol®; Blokium®; Felobits®; Ibinolo®; Myocord®; Seles Beta®; Tenormin®; Vericordin®

Use Treatment of hypertension, alone or in combination with other agents; also used in management of angina pectoris; selective inhibitor of $beta_1$-adrenergic receptors; postmyocardial infarction patients; acute alcohol withdrawal

Mechanism of Action Competitively blocks response to beta-adrenergic stimulation; more hydrophilic than propranolol; not lipid soluble

(Continued)

Atenolol *(Continued)*

Adverse Reactions

Cardiovascular: Persistent bradycardia, hypotension, chest pain, edema, heart failure, A-V block, exacerbation of Raynaud's phenomenon

Central nervous system: Dizziness, fatigue, insomnia, drowsiness, confusion, psychosis, mental depression, depression, headache, night terrors

Dermatologic: Exacerbation of vitiligo

Gastrointestinal: Constipation, diarrhea, nausea, retroperitoneal fibrosis (rare)

Genitourinary: Impotence, sexual dysfunction

Hepatic: Cholestasis

Respiratory: Dyspnea has occurred when daily dosage exceeds 100 mg/day, wheezing

Miscellaneous: Cold extremities

Signs & Symptoms of Acute Overdose Bradycardia, dermatitis, depression, ataxia, night terrors, dry eyes, dry mouth, insomnia, impotence, A-V block, congestive heart failure, systemic lupus erythematosus (SLE), hypotension, wheezing, hypoglycemia, hypothermia

Toxicodynamics/Kinetics

Absorption: Incomplete from gastrointestinal tract; food reduces bioavailability

Distribution: V_d: 0.7 L/kg; does **not** cross the blood-brain barrier; low lipid solubility

Protein binding: 3% to 15%

Half-life: 6-9 hours (longest in patients with reduced renal function); 16 hours in neonates

Time to peak serum concentration: Oral: Within 2-4 hours

Elimination: 40% excreted as unchanged drug in urine, 50% in feces

Usual Dosage

Oral:

Children: 1-2 mg/kg/dose given daily

Adults:

Hypertension: 50 mg once daily, may increase to 100 mg/day; doses >100 mg are unlikely to produce any further benefit

Angina pectoris: 50 mg once daily, may increase to 100 mg/day; some patients may require 200 mg/day

Dosing interval in renal impairment:

Cl_{cr} 15-35 mL/minute: Administer 50 mg/day maximum

Cl_{cr} <15 mL/minute: Administer 50 mg every other day maximum

Postmyocardial infarction:

I.V.: Administer as soon as possible 5 mg over 5 minutes; follow with 5 mg I.V. 10 minutes later

Oral: Follow I.V. dose with 100 mg/day or 50 mg twice daily for 6-9 days postmyocardial infarction

Contraindications Pulmonary edema, cardiogenic shock, bradycardia, heart block, or uncompensated congestive heart failure, wheezing

Warnings Do not use in pregnant or nursing women; safety and efficacy in children have not been established; administer to CHF patients with caution; administer with caution to patients with bronchospastic disease, diabetes mellitus, hyperthyroidism. Abrupt withdrawal of the drug should be avoided, drug should be discontinued over 1-2 weeks. May potentiate hypoglycemia in a diabetic patient and mask signs and symptoms.

Dosage Forms

Injection: 0.5 mg/mL (10 mL)

Tablet: 25 mg, 50 mg, 100 mg

Reference Range Peak plasma level of 1-2 μg/mL 2-4 hours after 200 mg dose

Overdosage Treatment

Decontamination: Do not use ipecac; lavage/activated charcoal with cathartic is useful

Supportive therapy: Sympathomimetics (eg, epinephrine or dopamine), glucagon, atropine, or a pacemaker can be used to treat the toxic bradycardia, asystole, and/or hypotension. Initially, fluids may be the best treatment for toxic hypotension, with norepinephrine being used for refractory hypotension.

Enhancement of elimination: Multiple dosing of activated charcoal may be useful; hemodialysis may be of some benefit (moderately dialyzable 20% to 50%)

Test Interactions Increases triglycerides, potassium, uric acid, cholesterol (S), glucose; decreases HDL

Drug Interactions Additive effect with other hypotensive agents; bioavailability decreases when coadministered with ampicillin; complete heart block can occur with verapamil; indomethacin reduces hypotensive effects of atenolol; atenolol reduces disopyramide clearance by 20%; when used with thiazide diuretics, hypokalemia and increased serum triglycerides may occur

Pregnancy Risk Factor C

Pregnancy Implications May result in neonatal bradycardia, hypotension, or hypothermia if given near delivery; no apparent long-term effects

Monitoring Parameters Blood pressure, heart rate, fluid intake and output, daily weight, respiratory rate

Patient Information Adhere to dosage regimen; watch for hypotension (orthostatic); abrupt withdrawal of the drug should be avoided

Nursing Implications Patient's therapeutic response may be evaluated by looking at blood pressure, apical and radial pulses, fluid I & O, daily weight, respirations, and circulation in extremities before and during therapy; modify dosage in patients with renal insufficiency

Additional Information Most effective for treating hypertension in older, white patients

Specific References

Lewis RV and McDevitt DG, "Adverse Reactions and Interactions With Beta-Adrenoceptor Blocking Drugs," *Med Toxicol Adverse Drug Exp*, 1986, 1(5):343-61.

Schallreuter KU, "Beta-Adrenergic Blocking Drugs May Exacerbate Vitiligo," *Br J Dermatol*, 1995, 132:169.

Shanahan FL and Counihan TB, "Atenolol Self-Poisoning," *Br Med J*, 1978, 2(6139):773.

Stoschitzky K, Kahr S, Donnerer J, et al, "Stereoselective Increase of Plasma Concentrations of the Enantiomers of Propranolol and Atenolol During Exercise," *Clin Pharmacol Ther*, 1995, 57:543-51.

Yusof SW and Mishra RM, "Hepatic Dyspunction Associated With Atenolol," *Lancet*, 1995, 346:192.

Atenolol and Chlorthalidone (a ten' oh lole & klor thal' i done)

Brand Names Tenoret® 50; Tenoretic®

Use Treatment of hypertension with a cardioselective beta-blocker and a diuretic

Signs & Symptoms of Acute Overdose Hypokalemia (as per atenolol)

Usual Dosage Adults: Oral: Initial: One (50) tablet once daily, then individualize dose until optimal dose is achieved

Dosage Forms Tablet:

50: Atenolol 50 mg and chlorthalidone 25 mg

100: Atenolol 100 mg and chlorthalidone 25 mg

Overdosage Treatment

Decontamination: Do not use ipecac; lavage/activated charcoal with cathartic is useful

Supportive therapy: Sympathomimetics (eg, epinephrine or dopamine), glucagon, atropine, or a pacemaker can be used to treat the toxic bradycardia, asystole, and/or hypotension. Initially, fluids may be the best treatment for toxic hypotension, with norepinephrine being used for refractory hypotension.

Enhancement of elimination: Multiple dosing of activated charcoal may be useful; hemodialysis may be of some benefit (moderately dialyzable 20% to 50%)

Test Interactions Lowers magnesium and potassium more severely than either agent alone

Pregnancy Risk Factor D

Pregnancy Implications Do not use when breast-feeding

Additional Information May contain povidone as inactive ingredient

Specific References

Cocco G, Iselin HV, Strozzi C, et al, "Magnesium Depletion in Patients on Long-Term Chlorthalidone Therapy for Essential Hypertension," *Eur J Clin Pharmacol*, 1987, 32(4):335-8.

Atensine® *see* Diazepam *on page 271*

Atepodin® *see* Adenosine Triphosphate *on page 90*

Athymil® *see* Mianserin Hydrochloride *on page 529*

Ativan® *see* Lorazepam *on page 482*

Atlansil® *see* Amiodarone Hydrochloride *on page 113*

Atozine® *see* Hydroxyzine *on page 414*

Atrol® *see* Deanol *on page 261*

Atromid-S® *see* Clofibrate *on page 226*

Atropa belladonna *see* Belladonna *on page 144*

Atropine and Diphenoxylate *see* Diphenoxylate and Atropine *on page 291*

Atrovent® Aerosol Inhalation *see* Ipratropium Bromide *on page 438*

Audazol® *see* Omeprazole *on page 576*

Auranofin *see* Gold Compounds *on page 386*

Aurothioglucose *see* Gold Compounds *on page 386*

Auxina E® *see* Vitamin E *on page 798*

Aventyl® Hydrochloride *see* Nortriptyline Hydrochloride *on page 571*

Avermectin B_{1A} *see* Ivermectin *on page 449*

Avitina® *see* Vitamin A *on page 795*

Avlosulfon® *see* Dapsone *on page 260*

Axerophtholum *see* Vitamin A *on page 795*

Axid® *see* Nizatidine *on page 569*

Ayr® [OTC] *see* Sodium Chloride *on page 698*

Azantac® *see* Ranitidine Hydrochloride *on page 675*

Azatadine Maleate (a za' ta deen)

Related Information
H1-Antihistamine Comparison *on page 1649*

CAS Number 3978-86-7

Brand Names Optimine®

Use Treatment of perennial and seasonal allergic rhinitis and chronic rash

Mechanism of Action Azatadine is a piperidine-derivative antihistamine; has both anticholinergic and antiserotonin activity; has been demonstrated to inhibit mediator release from human mast cells *in vitro*; mechanism of this action is suggested to prevent calcium entry into the mast cell through voltage-dependent calcium channels

Adverse Reactions
Central nervous system: Slight to moderate drowsiness, dizziness, acute dystonic reactions (extrapyramidal reaction)
Gastrointestinal: Nausea, vomiting
Ocular: Blurred vision, diplopia
Respiratory: Thickening of bronchial secretions

Signs & Symptoms of Acute Overdose CNS depression or CNS stimulation, dry mouth, fixed pupils, mydriasis, apnea, flushing

Toxicodynamics/Kinetics
Absorption: Oral: Rapid and extensive
Half-life, elimination: ~8.7 hours
Peak concentration: 4 hours
Elimination: ~20% excreted unchanged in urine over 48 hours

Usual Dosage Children >12 years and Adults: Oral: 1-2 mg twice daily

Contraindications Hypersensitivity to azatadine or to other related antihistamines including cyproheptadine; patients taking monoamine oxidase inhibitors should not use azatadine

Dosage Forms Tablet: 1 mg

Overdosage Treatment
Decontamination: Activated charcoal with cathartic is recommended, gastric lavage is indicated with early presentations (≤1 hour) or evidence of slowed gastrointestinal motility or obtundation
Supportive therapy: There is no specific treatment for an antihistamine overdose, however, most of its clinical toxicity is due to anticholinergic effects. Anticholinesterase inhibitors may be useful by reducing acetylcholinesterase. Anticholinesterase inhibitors include physostigmine, neostigmine, pyridostigmine, and edrophonium. For anticholinergic overdose with severe life-threatening symptoms, physostigmine 1-2 mg (0.5 or 0.02 mg/kg for children) I.V., slowly may be given to reverse these effects.
Enhancement of elimination: Multiple dosing of activated charcoal may be effective

Pregnancy Risk Factor B

Patient Information May cause drowsiness; avoid alcohol; can impair coordination and judgment

Nursing Implications Assist with ambulation

Specific References
Joske DJ, "Dystonic Reaction to Azatadine," *Med J Aust*, 1984, 141(7):449.

3'-azido-2',3'-dideoxythymidine *see* Zidovudine *on page 807*

Azidothymidine *see* Zidovudine *on page 807*

Azithromycin (az ith roe mye' sin)

CAS Number 83905-01-5

Brand Names Zithromax™

Use Treatment of adult patients (>16 years of age) with mild to moderate infections of susceptible strains in upper and lower respiratory tract, skin and skin structure, and sexually transmitted diseases

Mechanism of Action Inhibits RNA-dependent protein synthesis at the chain elongation step; binds to the 50S ribosomal subunit resulting in blockage of transpeptidation

Adverse Reactions

Cardiovascular: Ventricular arrhythmias

Central nervous system: Headache, dizziness, fever

Dermatologic: Rash, angioedema

Gastrointestinal: Diarrhea (3.6%), nausea (2.6%), abdominal pain (2.5%), vomiting, cramping

Genitourinary: Nephritis

Hematologic: Eosinophilia

Hepatic: Elevation in hepatic enzymes, cholestatic jaundice

Local: Thrombophlebitis

Otic: Ototoxicity, tinnitus

Renal: Nephritis

Miscellaneous: Hypertrophic pyloric stenosis, myalgia, allergic reactions, feces discoloration (greenish gray), feces discoloration (white/speckling)

Toxicodynamics/Kinetics

Absorption: Oral: Rapid; food decreases absorption by 40% to 50%

Distribution: V_d: 23-31.1 L/kg; distributes well into skin, lungs, sputum, tonsils, and cervix; penetration into the CSF is poor

Protein binding: Variable, decreasing from 50% at 0.02 mcg/mL to 7% at 2 mg/mL

Bioavailability: 37%

Half-life: 68 hours

Time to peak: 2.5-3 hours; in elderly women, peak concentrations are increased to 30% to 50%; however no significant accumulation is seen

Elimination: Biliary excretion of unchanged drug is primary route of elimination with only 6% of unchanged drug in urine; renal clearance: 0.2-0.3 L/kg/hour

Usual Dosage Adults: Oral: 250 mg twice daily on day 1 and once daily on days 2-5

Chlamydia urogenital infections: 1 g as a single dose

Contraindications Hepatic impairment, known hypersensitivity to azithromycin, erythromycin, or any Zithromax™ components

Warnings Use with caution in patients with hepatic dysfunction; hepatic impairment with or without jaundice has occurred chiefly in older children and adults; it may be accompanied by malaise, nausea, vomiting, abdominal colic, and fever; discontinue use if these occur

Dosage Forms Capsule, as dihydrate: 250 mg

Reference Range Peak serum levels: 0.4-0.6 mg/L following a 500 mg dose

Overdosage Treatment

Decontamination: Lavage/activated charcoal with cathartic

Enhancement of elimination: Multiple dosing of activated charcoal may be effective

Drug Interactions

Decreased peak serum levels with aluminum- and magnesium-containing antacids by 24%

Increased effect/toxicity/levels of alfentanil, anticoagulants, astemizole, terfenadine, loratadine, bromocriptine, carbamazepine, cyclosporine, digoxin, ergots, disopyramide, theophylline, triazolam, and warfarin

Pregnancy Risk Factor C

Monitoring Parameters Liver function tests

Patient Information Take dose 1 hour prior to a meal or 2 hours after; do not take with aluminum- or magnesium-containing antacids

Additional Information Suggestion of improvement of cyclosporine-associated gingival hyperplasia with treatment of azithromycin

Specific References

Bahal N and Nahata MC, "The New Macrolide Antibiotics: Azithromycin, Clarithromycin, Dirithromycin, and Roxithromycin," *Ann Pharmacother*, 1992, 26(1):46-55.

Bendayan R, Georgis W, and Rafi-Tari S, "Interaction of 3'-Azido-d'-Deoxythymidine With the Oranic Base Transporter in a Cultured Renal Epithelium," *Pharmacotherapy*, 1995, 15(3):338-44.

Feldman RJ, Alcid DV, and Boruchoff SE, "Failure of Prolonged Azithromycin Therapy in Early Lyme Disease," *Infect Dis Clin Prac*, 1995, 4(3):230-2.

Guay DRP, "Pharmacokinetics of the New Macrolides," *Infect Med*, 1992, 9:9-13.

Ljuti D and Rumboldt Z, "Possible Interaction Between Azithromycin and Cyclosporin: A Case Report," *Nephron*, 1995, 70:130.

Neu HC, "New Macrolide Antibiotics: Azithromycin and Clarithromycin," *Ann Intern Med*, 1992, 116(6):517-9.

Wahlstrom E, Zamora JU, and Teichman S, "Improvement in Cyclosporin-Associated Gingival Hyperplasia With Azithromycin Therapy," *N Engl J Med*, 1995, 332(11):753-4.

Azolid® *see* Phenylbutazone *on page 620*

AZT *see* Zidovudine *on page 807*

Azubromaron® *see* Benzbromarone *on page 148*

Azulfidine® *see* Sulfasalazine *on page 712*

Azulfidine® EN-tabs® *see* Sulfasalazine *on page 712*

Azupamil® *see* Verapamil Hydrochloride *on page 787*

Azupentat® *see* Pentoxifylline *on page 607*

Babee® Teething Lotion [OTC] *see* Benzocaine *on page 149*

BAC *see* Benzalkonium Chloride *on page 147*

Baciguent® Topical [OTC] *see* Bacitracin *on this page*

Baci-IM® Injection *see* Bacitracin *on this page*

Bacitin® *see* Bacitracin *on this page*

Bacitracin (bass i tray' sin)

CAS Number 1405-87-4; 1405-89-6

Brand Names AK-Tracin® Ophthalmic; Baciguent® Topical [OTC]; Baci-IM® Injection; Bacitin®

Synonyms Bacitracinum

Use Treatment of susceptible bacterial infections (staphylococcal pneumonia and empyema); due to toxicity risks, systemic and irrigant uses of bacitracin should be limited to situations where less toxic alternatives would not be effective; oral administration has been successful in antibiotic-associated colitis; useful for gram-positive bacterial organisms

Mechanism of Action Inhibits bacterial cell wall synthesis by preventing transfer of mucopeptides into the growing cell wall

Adverse Reactions

Cardiovascular: Hypotension, tightness of chest

Dermatologic: Rash, itching, contact dermatitis, urticaria

Gastrointestinal: Anorexia, nausea, vomiting, diarrhea, rectal itching and burning

Hematologic: Blood dyscrasias

Ocular: Diplopia

Otic: Ototoxicity

Renal: Nephrotoxic when given parenterally (tubular or glomerular necrosis); hematuria, albuminuria (reversible)

Miscellaneous: Swelling of lips and face, pain, anaphylactic shock, sweating

Signs & Symptoms of Acute Overdose Tubular necrosis (acute), hypokalemia, myasthenia gravis (exacerbation or precipitation of)

Toxicodynamics/Kinetics

Duration of action: 6-8 hours

Absorption: Poor from mucous membranes and intact or denuded skin; rapidly absorbed following I.M. administration; not absorbed by bladder irrigation, but absorption can occur from peritoneal or mediastinal lavage

Protein binding: Minimally bound to plasma proteins

Half-life: 1.5 hours

Time to peak serum concentration: I.M.: Within 1-2 hours

Elimination: Slow elimination into urine with 10% to 40% of dose excreted within 24 hours; renal clearance: 154 mL/minute

Usual Dosage

Do not administer I.V.:

Infants:

$<$2.5 kg: 900 units/kg/day in 2-3 divided doses

$>$2.5 kg: 1000 units/kg/day in 2-3 divided doses

Children: 800-1200 units/kg/day divided every 8 hours

Adults: Not recommended

Antibiotic-associated colitis: Adults: Oral: 25,000 units 4 times/day for 7-10 days

Topical: Apply 1-4 times/day to infected area

Ophthalmic ointment: Instill $^1/_4$" to $^1/_2$" ribbon every 3-4 hours into conjunctival sac for acute infections or 2-3 times/day for mild to moderate infections for 7-10 days

Irrigation, solution: 50-100 units/mL in normal saline, lactated Ringer's, or sterile water for irrigation; soak sponges in solution for topical compresses 1-5 times/day or as needed during surgical procedures

Contraindications Hypersensitivity to bacitracin or any component; I.M. use is contraindicated in patients with renal impairment

Warnings Prolonged use may result in overgrowth of nonsusceptible organisms; I.M. use may cause renal failure due to tubular and glomerular necrosis; **do not** administer intravenously because severe thrombophlebitis occurs

Dosage Forms

Injection: 50,000 units

Ointment:

Ophthalmic: 500 units/g (1 g, 3.5 g, 454 g)

Topical: 500 units/g (1.5 g, 3.75 g, 15 g, 30 g, 120 g, 454 g)

Stability Sterile powder should be stored in the refrigerator; once reconstituted, bacitracin is stable for 1 week under refrigeration (2°C to 8°C); bacitracin sterile powder should be dissolved in 0.9% sodium chloride injection containing 2% procaine hydrochloride for I.M. use; do not use diluents containing parabens; bacitracin zinc is more stable than bacitracin

Reference Range Doses of 200-300 units/kg every 6 hours (I.M.) produce plasma levels of 2 units/mL

Overdosage Treatment Decontamination: Lavage/activated charcoal with cathartic with oral ingestion; irrigate dermal exposure with soap and water

Drug Interactions Increased toxicity: Nephrotoxic drugs; neuromuscular blocking agents and anesthetics (↑ neuromuscular blockade)

Pregnancy Risk Factor C

Monitoring Parameters I.M.: Urinalysis, renal function tests

Patient Information Ophthalmic ointment may cause blurred vision; topical bacitracin should not be used for longer than 1 week unless directed by a physician. Ophthalmic administration: Tilt head back, place medication in conjunctival sac and close eyes; apply light finger pressure on lacrimal sac for 1 minute following instillation. Do not share eye medications with others.

Nursing Implications For I.M. injection only, do **not** administer I.V.; confirm any orders for parenteral use; pH of urine should be kept >6 by using sodium bicarbonate

Additional Information 1 unit is equivalent to 0.026 mg

Specific References

Katz BE and Fisher AA, "Bacitracin: A Unique Topical Antibiotic Sensitizer," *J Am Acad Dermatol*, 1987, 17(6):1016-24.

Vale MA, Connolly A, Epstein AM, et al, "Bacitracin-Induced Anaphylaxis," *Arch Dermatol*, 1978, 114(5):800.

Westerman EL, "Toxicity of Mediastinal Irrigation With Bacitracin," *JAMA*, 1983, 250(7):899.

Bacitracinum *see* Bacitracin *on previous page*

Baclofen (bak' loe fen)

Related Information

Therapeutic Drugs Associated With Hallucinations *on page 1558-1559*

CAS Number 1134-47-0

Brand Names Lioresal®

Use Treatment of reversible spasticity associated with multiple sclerosis or spinal cord lesions

Mechanism of Action Inhibits transmission of both monosynaptic and polysynaptic reflexes at the spinal cord level, possibly by hyperpolarization of primary afferent fiber terminals, with resultant relief of muscle spasticity; a gamma aminobutyric acid ($GABA_B$) agonist

Adverse Reactions

Cardiovascular: Hypotension

Central nervous system: Drowsiness, fatigue, dizziness, psychiatric disturbances, psychosis, auditory and visual hallucinations, insomnia, slurred speech, headache, ataxia, hypotonia, electroencephalogram abnormalities

Dermatologic: Rash

Gastrointestinal: Nausea, constipation

Genitourinary: Urinary frequency

Ocular: Diplopia

Signs & Symptoms of Acute Overdose Vomiting, angina, euphoria, wheezing, insomnia, impotence, encephalopathy, dyspnea, mania, diarrhea, dementia, depression, hypothermia, muscle hypotonia, nystagmus, salivation, drowsiness, coma, seizures, respiratory depression, bradycardia, or tachycardia (ventricular) [flutter (atrial)], hypertension or hypotension

Toxicodynamics/Kinetics

Onset of action: Muscle relaxation effects require 3-4 days and maximal clinical effects are not seen for 5-10 days

Absorption: Oral: Rapid; absorption from the gastrointestinal tract is thought to be dose dependent

Distribution: V_d: 0.8 L/kg; distributed well in body; minimal amounts cross blood-brain barrier

Protein binding: 30%

Metabolism: Minimal in the liver

Bioavailability: 70% to 80%

Half-life: 3.5 hours

Time to peak serum concentration: Within 2-3 hours

Elimination: 85% of oral dose excreted in urine and feces as unchanged drug

Usual Dosage Oral:

Children:

2-7 years: Initial: 10-15 mg/24 hours divided every 8 hours; titrate dose every 3 days in increments of 5-15 mg/day to a maximum of 40 mg/day

≥8 years: Maximum: 60 mg/day in 3 divided doses

Adults: 5 mg 3 times/day, may increase 5 mg/dose every 3 days to a maximum of 80 mg/day

(Continued)

Baclofen *(Continued)*

Dosing adjustment in renal impairment: May be necessary to reduce dosage

Contraindications Hypersensitivity to baclofen or any component

Warnings Avoid abrupt withdrawal; use with caution in patients with seizure disorder, impaired renal function

Dosage Forms

Injection, intrathecal: 0.5 mg/mL (20 mL); 2 mg/mL (5 mL)

Tablet: 10 mg, 20 mg

Overdosage Treatment Supportive therapy: Following initiation of essential overdose management, symptomatic and supportive treatment should be instituted; physostigmine can alleviate drowsiness when intrathecal baclofen toxicity is present; atropine can be utilized for bradycardia; diazepam or lorazepam can be used for seizure management; dantrolene (10 mg/kg) has been used to treat hyperthermia due to baclofen withdrawal

Antidote(s)

Atropine Sulfate *on page 1395*

Physostigmine *on page 1457*

Test Interactions Increases alkaline phosphatase, AST, glucose, ammonia (B); decreases bilirubin (S)

Drug Interactions CNS depressants

Pregnancy Risk Factor C

Pregnancy Implications Crosses placenta

Patient Information Take with food or milk; abrupt withdrawal after prolonged use may cause anxiety, hallucinations, tachycardia or spasticity

Nursing Implications Epileptic patients should be closely monitored; supervise ambulation; avoid abrupt withdrawal of the drug

Additional Information Elderly are sensitive to this drug

Specific References

Cooke DE and Glasstone MA, "Baclofen Poisoning in Children," *Vet Hum Toxicol*, 1994, 36(5):448-50.

Khorasani A and Peruzzi WT, "Dantrolene Treatment for Abrupt Intrathecal Baclofen Withdrawal," *Anesth Analg*, 1995, 80:1054-6.

May CR, "Baclofen Overdose," *Ann Emerg Med*, 1983, 12:171-3.

Muller-Schwefe G and Penn RD, "Physostigmine in the Treatment of Intrathecal Baclofen Overdose. Report of Three Cases," *J Neurosurg*, 1989, 71(2):273-5.

Roberge RJ, Martin TG, Hodgman M, et al, "Supraventricular Tachyarrhythmia Associated With Baclofen Overdose," *J Toxicol Clin Toxicol*, 1994, 32(3):291-7.

BactoShield® Topical [OTC] *see* Chlorhexidine Gluconate *on page 200*

Bactrim™ *see* Co-trimoxazole *on page 242*

Bactrim™ DS *see* Co-trimoxazole *on page 242*

Baker's P&S [OTC] *see* Phenol *on page 616*

Balan® *see* Piperazine Citrate *on page 629*

Banesin® [OTC] *see* Acetaminophen *on page 79*

Barbita® *see* Phenobarbital *on page 614*

Barblac® *see* Pindolol *on page 627*

Base Ointment *see* Zinc Oxide *on page 813*

Bay Clor® *see* Chlorpromazine Hydrochloride *on page 205*

Bayer® Aspirin [OTC] *see* Aspirin *on page 133*

Baylocaine® *see* Lidocaine Hydrochloride *on page 468*

Bayotensin® *see* Nitrendipine *on page 562*

Baypresol® *see* Nitrendipine *on page 562*

Baypress® *see* Nitrendipine *on page 562*

Beaden® *see* Propranolol Hydrochloride *on page 657*

Beamat® *see* Cimetidine *on page 212*

Bechizolo® *see* Zipeprol Hydrochloride *on page 813*

Bedranol® *see* Propranolol Hydrochloride *on page 657*

Beef NPH Iletin® II *see* Insulin Preparations *on page 426*

Beef Regular Iletin® II *see* Insulin Preparations *on page 426*

Belladonna (bell a don' a)

Synonyms *Atropa belladonna*

Use Decrease gastrointestinal activity in functional bowel disorders and to delay gastric emptying as well as decrease gastric secretion

Mechanism of Action Belladonna is a mixture of the anticholinergic alkaloids atropine, hyoscyamine, and scopolamine (hyoscine). The belladonna alkaloids act primarily by competitive inhibition of the muscarinic actions of acetylcholine on structures innervated by postganglionic cholinergic neurons and on smooth muscle. The resulting effects include antisecretory activity on exocrine glands and intestinal mucosa and smooth muscle relaxation. The anticholinergic properties of scopolamine and atropine differ in that scopolamine has a more potent activity on the iris, ciliary body, and certain secretory glands; has more potent activity on the heart, intestine, and bronchial muscle, and a more prolonged duration of action; in contrast, hyoscyamine has actions similar to those of atropine, but is more potent in both its central and peripheral effects

Adverse Reactions

Cardiovascular: Orthostatic hypotension, fibrillation (ventricular), tachycardia, palpitations

Central nervous system: Confusion, lightheadedness, headache, loss of memory, hallucinations, drowsiness, tiredness, ataxia

Dermatologic: Skin rash

Gastrointestinal: Constipation, nausea, vomiting, bloated feeling

Genitourinary: Difficult urination

Neuromuscular & skeletal: Weakness

Ocular: Blurred vision, photophobia, vision color changes (red tinge), increased intraocular pain, intraocular pressure (increased)

Miscellaneous: Dry mouth, nose, throat, or skin; decreased flow of breast milk, difficulty in swallowing, enuresis, increased sensitivity to light, decreased sweating

Signs & Symptoms of Acute Overdose Anticholinergic toxicity may be caused by strong binding of a belladonna alkaloid to cholinergic receptors; anticholinesterase inhibitors reduce acetylcholinesterase, the enzyme that breaks down acetylcholine and thereby allows acetylcholine to accumulate and compete for receptor binding with the offending anticholinergic

Usual Dosage Tincture: Oral:

Children: 0.03 mL/kg 3 times/day

Adults: 0.6-1 mL 3-4 times/day

Contraindications Hypersensitivity to any components; glaucoma, elevated intraocular pressure, significant hepatic or renal disease, or pulmonary insufficiency

Dosage Forms Tincture: Belladonna alkaloids (principally hyoscyamine and atropine) 0.3 mg/mL with alcohol 65% to 70% (120 mL, 480 mL, 3780 mL)

Stability Store in tight, light-resistant container at 15°C to 30°C

Overdosage Treatment

Decontamination: With life-threatening symptoms, physostigmine 1-2 mg (0.5 or 0.02 mg/kg for children) S.C. or I.V. slowly may be given to reverse these effects

Pregnancy Risk Factor C

Monitoring Parameters CNS depression

Patient Information May cause drowsiness and blurred vision

Nursing Implications Assist patient with ambulation

Belladonna and Opium (bell a don' a & oh' pee um)

Brand Names B&O Supprettes®

Synonyms Opium and Belladonna

Use Relief of moderate to severe pain associated with rectal or bladder tenesmus that may occur in postoperative states and neoplastic situations; pain associated with ureteral spasm not responsive to non-narcotic analgesics and to space intervals between injections of opiates

Mechanism of Action Anticholinergic alkaloids act primarily by competitive inhibition of the muscarinic actions of acetylcholine on structures innervated by postganglionic cholinergic neurons and on smooth muscle; resulting effects include antisecretory activity on exocrine glands and intestinal mucosa and smooth muscle relaxation. Contains many narcotic alkaloids including morphine; its mechanism for gastric motility inhibition is primarily due to this morphine content; it results in a decrease in digestive secretions, an increase in gastrointestinal muscle tone, and therefore a reduction in gastrointestinal propulsion.

Adverse Reactions

Cardiovascular: Hypotension, bradycardia, peripheral vasodilation, intracranial pressure (increased), flushing, tachycardia, palpitations, fibrillation (ventricular), hypotension (orthostatic)

Central nervous system: CNS depression, drowsiness, sedation, dry mouth, nose, throat, or skin; loss of memory, asthenia, tiredness, headache, confusion, ataxia

Dermatologic: Skin rash

Endocrine & metabolic: Syndrome of inappropriate antidiuretic hormone (SIADH)

Gastrointestinal: Nausea, vomiting, constipation, bloated feeling, dysphagia

Genitourinary: Urinary retention

Local: Irritation at injection site

Ocular: Intraocular pain (increased), blurred vision

Renal: Dysuria

Respiratory: Apnea, respiratory depression, apnea

(Continued)

Belladonna and Opium *(Continued)*

Miscellaneous: Physical and psychological dependence, histamine release, decreased flow of breast milk, sensitivity to light (increased), decreased sweating, biliary or urinary tract spasm

Toxicodynamics/Kinetics

Onset of action:

Belladonna: 1-2 hours

Opium: Within 30 minutes

Metabolism: Opium metabolized in the liver with formation of glucuronide metabolites

Elimination: Belladonna excreted unchanged in urine

Usual Dosage Adults: Rectal: 1 suppository 1-2 times/day, up to 4 doses/day

Contraindications Glaucoma, severe renal or hepatic disease, bronchial asthma, respiratory depression, convulsive disorders, acute alcoholism, premature labor

Warnings Usual precautions of opiate agonist therapy should be observed; infants <3 months of age are more susceptible to respiratory depression, use with caution and generally in reduced doses in this age group

Dosage Forms Suppository, rectal:

#15A: Belladonna extract 15 mg and powdered opium 30 mg (12s)

#16A: Belladonna extract 15 mg and powdered opium 60 mg (12s)

Stability Store at 15°C to 30°C (avoid freezing)

Overdosage Treatment

Decontamination: Lavage and activated charcoal with cathartic

Supportive therapy: Naloxone should be given if patient has altered mental status; physostigmine should be given only for life-threatening anticholinergic symptoms

Antidote(s)

Naloxone Hydrochloride *on page 1447*

Physostigmine *on page 1457*

Test Interactions ↑ aminotransferase [ALT (SGPT)/AST (SGOT)] (S)

Drug Interactions

Decreased effect: Phenothiazines

Increased effect/toxicity: CNS depressants, tricyclic antidepressants

Pregnancy Risk Factor C

Patient Information May cause drowsiness and blurred vision

Nursing Implications Prior to rectal insertion, the finger and suppository should be moistened; assist with ambulation, monitor for CNS depression

Beloc® *see* Metoprolol Tartrate *on page 524*

Benazepril Hydrochloride (ben ay' ze prill)

Related Information

ACE Inhibitors Comparison *on page 1636-1637*

CAS Number 86541-75-5

Brand Names Lotensin®

Use Treatment of hypertension, either alone or in combination with other antihypertensive agents

Mechanism of Action Competitive inhibition of angiotensin I being converted to angiotensin II, a potent vasoconstrictor, through the angiotensin I-converting enzyme (ACE) activity, with resultant lower levels of angiotensin II which causes an increase in plasma renin activity and a reduction in aldosterone secretion

Adverse Reactions

Cardiovascular: Hypotension, tachycardia

Central nervous system: Fatigue, headache, dizziness, hypertonia

Dermatologic: Rash, photosensitivity

Endocrine & metabolic: Hyperkalemia, hypoglycemia

Gastrointestinal: Nausea

Hematologic: Leukopenia, eosinophilia

Renal: Proteinuria

Respiratory: Transient cough during early therapy

Miscellaneous: Hypersensitivity reaction

Signs & Symptoms of Acute Overdose Severe hypotension, dermatitis, hypertonia, drowsiness, renal insufficiency, leukopenia; myalgia, impotence, neutropenia; agranulocytosis; granulocytopenia

Toxicodynamics/Kinetics

Reduction in plasma angiotensin-converting enzyme activity:

Peak effect: Oral: 1-2 hours after administration of 2-20 mg dose

Duration: >90% inhibition for 24 hours has been observed after 5-20 mg oral dose

Reduction in blood pressure:

Single oral dose:

Peak effect: 2-6 hours
With continuous therapy:
Maximum response: 2 weeks
Duration: 2 years

Absorption: Rapid (37% of each oral dose); food does not alter significantly; metabolite (benazeprilat) itself unsuitable for oral administration due to poor absorption

Distribution: V_d: ~8.7 L

Metabolism: Rapid and extensive in the liver to its active metabolite, benazeprilat, via enzymatic hydrolysis; undergoes significant first-pass metabolism and is completely eliminated from plasma in 4 hours

Half-life:
Parent drug: 0.6 hours
Metabolite elimination: 22 hours (from 24 hours after dosing onward)

Time to peak serum concentration:
Unchanged parent: 30 minutes to 1 hour
Metabolite: 1½-2 hours after fasting or 2-4 hours after a meal

Elimination: Nonrenal clearance (ie, biliary, metabolic) appears to contribute to the elimination of benazeprilat (11% to 12%), particularly in patients with severe renal impairment; hepatic clearance is the main elimination route of unchanged benazepril

Usual Dosage Adults: Oral: 20-40 mg/day as a single dose or 2 divided doses

Dosing interval in renal impairment: Cl_{cr} <30 mL/minute: Administer 5 mg/day initially

Contraindications Renal impairment, collagen vascular disease, hypersensitivity to benazepril or any component

Warnings ACE inhibitors prevent potassium excretion, approximately as much as amiloride or spironolactone

Dosage Forms Tablet: 5 mg, 10 mg, 20 mg, 40 mg

Overdosage Treatment

Decontamination: Emesis or lavage/activated charcoal with cathartic

Supportive therapy: Following initiation of essential overdose management, toxic symptom treatment and supportive treatment should be initiated. Hypotension usually responds to I.V. fluids or Trendelenburg positioning. If unresponsive to these measures, the use of a parenteral inotrope may be required (eg, norepinephrine 0.1-0.2 mcg/kg/minute titrated to response). Seizures commonly respond to lorazepam or diazepam (I.V. 5-10 mg bolus in adults every 15 minutes if needed up to a total of 30 mg; I.V. 0.25-0.4 mg/kg/dose up to a total of 10 mg in children) or to phenytoin or phenobarbital.

Enhancement of elimination: Multiple dosing of activated charcoal may be effective; moderately dialyzable (20% to 50%); ~6% of metabolite was removed by 4 hours of dialysis following 10 mg of benazepril administered 2 hours prior to procedure; the parent compound was not found in the dialysate

Drug Interactions Probenecid increases benazepril levels, benazepril and diuretics have additive hypotensive effects; use potassium-sparing diuretics with care

Pregnancy Risk Factor D

Patient Information Administer 1 hour before meals

Nursing Implications Watch for hypotensive effect within 1-3 hours of first dose or new higher dose; many patients complain of transient cough during early therapy

Specific References

Herings RM, deBoer A, Stricker BH, et al, "Hypoglycemia Associated With Use of Inhibitors of Angiotensin Converting Enzyme," *Lancet*, 1995, 345:1195-8.

Waeber G, Fasanella d'Amore TF, Nussberger J, et al, "Effect on Blood Pressure and the Renin-Angiotensin System of Repeated Doses of the Converting Enzyme Inhibitor CGS 14824 A," *Eur J Clin Pharmacol*, 1987, 31(6):643-6.

Bencard® *see* Mianserin Hydrochloride *on page 529*

Benerva® *see* Thiamine Hydrochloride *on page 741*

Benicot *see* Niacinamide *on page 555*

Benirol *see* Benzalkonium Chloride *on this page*

Benozil® *see* Flurazepam Hydrochloride *on page 363*

Bensokain® *see* Benzocaine *on page 149*

Benylin® DM [OTC] *see* Dextromethorphan Hydrobromide *on page 270*

Benzalkonium Chloride (benz al koe' nee um)

CAS Number 8001-54-5

Brand Names Armil®; Benza® [OTC]; Capitol®; Germiphene®; Pameb®; Roccal®; Torbetol®; Zephiran® [OTC]

(Continued)

Benzalkonium Chloride *(Continued)*

Synonyms Arinol; BAC; Benirol; Bional; BTC 50; Zephirol

Use Surface antiseptic and germicidal preservative

Mechanism of Action Quaternary ammonium disinfectant (cationic)

Adverse Reactions

Cardiovascular: Hypotension

Central nervous system: Lethargy, seizures

Dermal: Bullous or pustular reactions, contact dermatitis

Gastrointestinal (ingestion): Emesis (hemetemesis), burning mouth/throat, pain, salivation, esophageal burns

Ocular: Corneal damage

Miscellaneous: Hypersensitivity; may be ototoxic, inhibits sperm motility; corrosive burn at concentrations >10%

Signs & Symptoms of Acute Overdose Elevated liver function tests, hypotension, metabolic acidosis, confusion, profuse diarrhea, muscle myoclonus/paralysis, seizures

Usual Dosage Thoroughly rinse anionic detergents and soaps from the skin or other areas prior to use of solutions because they reduce the antibacterial activity of BAC. To protect metal instruments stored in BAC solution, add crushed antirust tablets, 4 tablets/quart, to antiseptic solution, change solution at least once weekly. Not to be used for storage of aluminum or zinc instruments, instruments with lenses fastened by cement, lacquered catheters, or some synthetic rubber goods.

Contraindications Use in occlusive dressings, casts and anal or vaginal packs is inadvisable; irritation or chemical burns may result

Warnings Avoid contact with eyes; do not rely on antiseptic solutions to achieve complete sterilization

Dosage Forms

Concentrate, topical: 17% (500 mL, 4000 mL)

Solution, aqueous: 1:750 (60 mL, 120 mL, 240 mL)

Tincture: 1:750 (30 mL, 960 mL)

Tincture, spray: 1:750 (30 g, 180 g)

Tissue: 1:750 (packets)

Stability Foams when shaken; incompatible with iodine, soaps, anionic detergent, iodides, citrates, salicylates, silver nitrate, fluorescein, nitrates, peroxide, lanolin, potassium permanganate, aluminum, caramel, kaolin, pine oil, zinc sulfate, zinc oxide, and yellow mercuric oxide

Overdosage Treatment

Decontamination (ingestion): Activated charcoal with cathartic may be useful, dilute with milk or water; do not induce emesis

Supportive therapy: Treat hypotension with isotonic saline; endoscopy may be required to evaluated gastrointestinal burns

Enhancement of elimination: Hemodialysis or forced diuresis is not useful

Diagnostic Tests/Procedures

Complete Blood Count *on page 1236*

Electrocardiography *on page 1253*

Kidney Profile *on page 1279*

Monitoring Parameters EKG, complete blood count, and renal status

Specific References

van Berkel M and de Wolff FA, "Survival After Acute Benzalkonium Chloride Poisoning," *Hum Toxicol*, 1988, 7(2):191-3.

Wilson JT and Burr IM, "Benzalkonium Chloride Poisoning in Infant Twins," *Am J Dis Child*, 1975, 129(10):1208-9.

Benzamide Acetate *see* Flecainide Acetate *on page 350*

Benza® [OTC] *see* Benzalkonium Chloride *on previous page*

Benzatec® *see* Penicillin G, Parenteral, Aqueous *on page 600*

Benzbromaron *see* Benzbromarone *on this page*

Benzbromarone

CAS Number 3562-84-3

Brand Names Azubromaron®; De'suric®; Harolan®; Minuric®; Narcarcin®; Normurat®; Obarin®; Uricovac®; Urinorm®

Synonyms Benzbromaron

Use Uricosuric agent which lowers uric acid concentrations; used for hyperuricemia, gout, and Lesch-Nyhan syndrome

Mechanism of Action Blocks proximal tubular reabsorption of uric acid; also increases gastrointestinal elimination of uric acid

Adverse Reactions

Dermatologic: Petechiae

Gastrointestinal: Diarrhea, nausea

Genitourinary: Impotence

Hepatic: Elevated liver enzymes
Ocular: Allergic conjunctivitis
Miscellaneous: Gouty attacks, porphyrinogenic, elevated serum creatinine

Toxicodynamics/Kinetics
Onset of action: 3 hours
Peak effect: 8-12 hours
Duration: 15-21 hours
Absorption: Oral: 50%
Distribution: V_d: <0.3 L/kg
Protein binding: 99%
Metabolism: To benzarone and bromobenzarone
Half-life: 2.7 hours
Elimination: Feces (50%), renal

Usual Dosage 50-200 mg/day

Warnings Do not use during an acute gouty attack; reduce dosage in renal insufficiency; patient should have adequate urine output to prevent uric acid nephrolithiasis

Reference Range Peak serum level of 1.84 μg/mL after oral dose of 100 mg of benzbromarone

Overdosage Treatment
Decontamination: Ipecac or lavage/activated charcoal
Enhancement of elimination: Multiple dosage activated charcoal may be effective

Drug Interactions Additive uricosuric actions with allopurinol; reduced uricosuric effect with sulfinpyrazone, low doses of aspirin reduce the effectiveness of benzbromarone; may increase the anticoagulant activity of the warfarin-based oral anticoagulant effects

Additional Information Investigational (phase II trials) in the U.S.

Specific References

Babany G, Larrey D, Pessayre D, et al, "Chronic Active Hepatitis Caused by Benzarone," *J Hepatol*, 1987, 5(3):332-5.
Heel RC, Brogden RN, Speight TM, et al, "Benzbromarone: A Review of Its Pharmacological Properties and Therapeutic Use in Gout and Hyperuricemia," *Drugs*, 1977, 14:349-66.
Pevny I, "Benzaron Allergy," *Contact Dermatitis*, 1984, 11(2):122.

Benzene Hexachloride *see* Lindane *on page 470*

Benzocaine (ben' zoe kane)

CAS Number 94-09-7

Brand Names Americaine® [OTC]; Anbesol® Maximum Strength [OTC]; Babee® Teething Lotion [OTC]; Bensokain®; Benzocol®; BiCOZENE® [OTC]; Chiggertox® [OTC]; Dermoplast® [OTC]; Foille Plus® [OTC]; Hurricaine®; Merocaine®; Orabase®-B [OTC]; Orabase®-O [OTC]; Orajel® Brace-Aid Oral Anesthetic [OTC]; Orajel® Maximum Strength [OTC]; Orajel® Mouth-Aid [OTC]; Rhulicaine® [OTC]; Rid-A-Pain® [OTC]; Solarcaine® [OTC]; Spec-T®; Unguentine® [OTC]

Synonyms Ethoform; Ethyl Aminobenzoate; Orthocesin

Use Local anesthetic

Mechanism of Action Blocks both the initiation and conduction of nerve impulses by decreasing the neuronal membrane's permeability to sodium ions, which results in inhibition of depolarization with resultant blockade of conduction; a group I (ester) anesthetic; low water solubility

Adverse Reactions
Dermatologic: Eczema, urticaria
Gastrointestinal: Gastrointestinal irritation
Hematologic: Methemoglobinemia in infants
Local: Contact dermatitis, burning, stinging, tenderness, rash, edema

Signs & Symptoms of Acute Overdose Methemoglobinemia (within 1 hour), tachycardia, tachypnea, photosensitivity, eczema, drowsiness, cyanosis

Toxicodynamics/Kinetics
Onset of action: ~1 minute
Duration: 15-20 minutes
Absorption: Topical: Poor to intact skin, but well absorbed from mucous membranes and traumatized skin
Metabolism: Hydrolyzed in the plasma and to a lesser extent the liver by cholinesterase to aminobenzoic acid and ethanol
Elimination: Excretion of metabolites in urine

Usual Dosage
Mucous membranes: Dosage varies depending on area to be anesthetized and vascularity of tissues
Topical: Apply to affected area as needed

Contraindications Known hypersensitivity to benzocaine, other ester-type local anesthetics, or other components in the formulation

Warnings Not intended for use when infections are present

(Continued)

Benzocaine *(Continued)*

Dosage Forms Topical:

Aerosol: 5% (97.5 mL, 105 mL); 20% (20 g, 60 g, 120 g)
Cream: 5% (30 g, 454 g); 6% (28.4 g)
Liquid: With benzyl benzoate and soft soap (30 mL)
Lotion: 8% (90 mL)
Ointment: 5% (3.5 g, 30 g)

Overdosage Treatment

Decontamination: Lavage/activated charcoal with cathartic
Supportive therapy: Methylene blue for treatment of methemoglobinemia
Enhancement of elimination: Hyperbaric oxygen or exchange transfusion should be considered if patient does not respond to methylene blue; exchange transfusion should be considered if methemoglobin levels >70%

Diagnostic Tests/Procedures

Methemoglobin, Blood *on page 1296*

Drug Interactions May antagonize actions of sulfonamides

Pregnancy Risk Factor C

Monitoring Parameters Arterial blood gas

Methemoglobin levels:
15%: Chocolate colored blood is produced
20%: Symptomatic
40%: Tachycardia
50%: Stupor
70%: Lethal

Patient Information Do not eat for 1 hour after application to oral mucosa; chemical burns should be neutralized before application of benzocaine

Specific References

Anderson ST, Hajduczek J, and Barker SJ, "Benzocaine-Induced Methemoglobinemia in an Adult: Accuracy of Pulse Oximetry With Methemoglobinemia," *Anesth Analg*, 1988, 67(11):1099-101.

Bachmann P, Berthier JC, Storme B, et al, "Methemoglobinemia From Ingestion of Benzocaine. A Case of Pediatric Intoxication," *J Toxicol Clin Exp*, 1986, 6(2):123-8.

Guertler AT and Pearce WA, "A Prospective Evaluation of Benzocaine-Associated Methemoglobinemia in Human Beings," *Ann Emerg Med*, 1994, 24(4):628-30.

Shua-Haim JR and Gross JS, "Methemoglobinemia Toxicity From Topical Benzocaine Spray," *J Am Geriatr Soc*, 1995, 43:590.

Stein JM and Warfield CA, "Local Anesthetics: Principles of Safe Use," *Hosp Pract (Off Ed)*, 1983, 18(5):73-8.

Benzocaine, Butyl Aminobenzoate, Tetracaine, and Benzalkonium Chloride

(ben' zoe kane, byo' til a meen oh benz' oh ate, tet' ra kane, & (benz al koe' nee um klor' ide)

Brand Names Cetacaine®

Synonyms Tetracaine Hydrochloride, Benzocaine Butyl Aminobenzoate, and Benzalkonium Chloride

Use Topical anesthetic to control pain or gagging

Adverse Reactions

Hematologic: Methemoglobinemia in infants
Local: Contact dermatitis, burning, stinging, tenderness, rash, edema, aspiration

Usual Dosage Apply to affected area for approximately 1 second or less

Contraindications Hypersensitivity to benzocaine, tetracaine, benzalkonium chloride or any component; use in eyes and in secondary bacterial infection of the area; not for injection; do not use under dentures

Dosage Forms Aerosol: Benzocaine 14%, butyl aminobenzoate 2%, tetracaine 2%, and benzalkonium chloride 0.5% (56 g)

Overdosage Treatment

Decontamination: Lavage/activated charcoal with cathartic
Supportive therapy: Methylene blue for treatment of methemoglobinemia
Enhancement of elimination: Hyperbaric oxygen or exchange transfusion should be considered if patient does not respond to methylene blue; exchange transfusion should be considered if methemoglobin levels >70%

Pregnancy Risk Factor C

Patient Information Do not chew gum or eat within 1 hour after application to oral mucosa

Nursing Implications Topical anesthesia may impair swallowing, thus enhancing danger of aspiration; numbness of the tongue or buccal mucosa may increase the danger of biting trauma

Additional Information Only topical anesthetic which comes in an easy to spray bottle, however, sensitization may result from any one of the ingredients

Benzocol® *see* Benzocaine *on previous page*

Benzodiazepines Comparison *see page 1643*

Benzoylemethylecgonine Hydrochloride *see* Cocaine Hydrochloride *on page 236*

Benztropine Mesylate (benz' troe peen)

Related Information

Therapeutic Drugs Associated With Hallucinations *on page 1558-1559*

CAS Number 86-13-5

Brand Names Cogentin®

Use Adjunctive treatment of all forms of parkinsonism; also used in treatment of drug-induced extrapyramidal effects (except tardive dyskinesia) and acute dystonic reactions

Mechanism of Action Thought to partially block striatal cholinergic receptors to help balance cholinergic and dopaminergic activity

Adverse Reactions

Cardiovascular: Tachycardia

Central nervous system: Drowsiness, nervousness, visual hallucinations, restlessness, extrapyramidal reaction, hyperthermia, coma

Gastrointestinal: Nausea, vomiting, dry mouth, ileus

Genitourinary: Urinary retention

Ocular: Blurred vision, mydriasis

Signs & Symptoms of Acute Overdose CNS depression, seizures, chorea (extrapyramidal), impotence, confusion, nervousness, memory loss, dementia, hallucinations, dizziness, blurred vision, nausea, vomiting, hyperthermia, fever

Toxicodynamics/Kinetics

Onset of action:

Oral: Within 60 minutes

Parenteral: Within 15 minutes

Duration: 6-48 hours

Absorption: Well absorbed from gastrointestinal tract

Distribution: Largely unknown; however, drug crosses the blood-brain barrier

Metabolism: Unknown

Elimination: In urine as unchanged drug and metabolites; after oral therapy, small amounts are probably excreted in feces as unabsorbed drug

Usual Dosage

Extrapyramidal reaction, drug induced: Oral, I.M., I.V.:

Children >3 years: 0.02-0.05 mg/kg/dose 1-2 times/day

Adults: 1-4 mg/dose 1-2 times/day

Parkinsonism: Oral: 0.5-6 mg/day in 1-2 divided doses; if one dose is greater, give at bedtime

Titrate dose in 0.5 mg increments at 5- to 6-day intervals

Contraindications Children <3 years of age, use with caution in older children (dosage not established); patients with narrow-angle glaucoma, hypersensitivity to any component, pyloric or duodenal obstruction, stenosing peptic ulcers, bladder neck obstructions, achalasia, myasthenia gravis

Warnings Use with caution in hot weather or during exercise. Elderly patients frequently develop increased sensitivity and require strict dosage regulation – side effects may be more severe in elderly patients with atherosclerotic changes. Use with caution in patients with tachycardia, cardiac arrhythmias, hypertension, hypotension, prostatic hypertrophy (especially in the elderly) or any tendency toward urinary retention, liver or kidney disorders and obstructive disease of the gastrointestinal or GU tract. May exacerbate mental symptoms and precipitate a toxic psychosis when used to treat extrapyramidal reactions resulting from phenothiazines. When given in large doses or to susceptible patients, may cause asthenia and inability to move particular muscle groups. Tardive dyskinesia may occur with long-term therapy. Physostigmine can be used in treatment of overdose patients with extreme delirium; long-lasting seizures, life-threatening arrhythmias.

Dosage Forms

Injection: 1 mg/mL (2 mL)

Tablet: 0.5 mg, 1 mg, 2 mg

Overdosage Treatment Supportive therapy: Anticholinergic toxicity is caused by strong binding of the drug to cholinergic receptors. Anticholinesterase inhibitors reduce acetylcholinesterase, the enzyme that breaks down acetylcholine and thereby allows acetylcholine to accumulate and compete for receptor binding with the offending anticholinergic. For anticholinergic overdose with severe life-threatening symptoms, physostigmine 1-2 mg (0.5 or 0.02 mg/kg for children) S.C. or I.V., slowly may be given to reverse these effects.

Drug Interactions Central anticholinergic syndrome can occur when administered with narcotic analgesics; phenothiazines and other antipsychotics, tricyclic antidepressants, quinidine and some other antiarrhythmics, and antihistamines. May increase gastric degradation of levodopa and decrease the amount of levodopa absorbed by delaying gastric emptying – the opposite may be true for digoxin; delirium with fluoxetine or paroxetine

(Continued)

Benztropine Mesylate *(Continued)*

Pregnancy Risk Factor C

Pregnancy Implications May cross the placenta

Patient Information Take after meals; do not discontinue drug abruptly; notify physician if adverse gastrointestinal effects, fever, or heat intolerance occurs

Nursing Implications No significant difference in onset of I.M. or I.V. injection, therefore, there is usually no need to use the I.V. route. Improvement is sometimes noticeable a few minutes after injection. Titrate dose in 0.5 mg increments at 5- or 6-day intervals.

Specific References

Erwin WG and Turco TF, "Current Concepts in Clinical Therapeutics: Parkinson's Disease," *Clin Pharm*, 1986, 5(9):742-53.

Fahy P, Arnold P, Curry SC, et al, "Serial Serum Drug Concentrations and Prolonged Anticholinergic Toxicity After Benztropine (Cogentin®) Overdose," *Am J Emerg Med*, 1989, 7(2):199-202.

Harper G, Dawes M, Azlin C, et al, "Small Bowel Obstruction in a Child on an Antipsychotic," *J Child Adoles Psych Pharm*, 1995, 5:81-4.

Rosano TG, Meola JM, Wolf BC, et al, "Benztropine Identification and Quantitation in a Suicidal Overdose," *J Anal Toxicol*, 1994, 18(6):348-53.

Roth A, Akyol S, and Nelson JC, "Delirium Associated With the Combination of a Neuroleptic, an SSRI, and Benztropine," *J Clin Psychiatry*, 1994, 55(11):492-5.

Benzylpenicillin Potassium *see* Penicillin G, Parenteral, Aqueous *on page 600*

Benzylpenicillin Sodium *see* Penicillin G, Parenteral, Aqueous *on page 600*

Bepadil® *see* Bepridil Hydrochloride *on this page*

Bepridil Hydrochloride (be' pri dil)

CAS Number 49571-04-2; 64616-81-5; 64706-54-3; 74764-40-2

Brand Names Bepadil®; Cardiocal®; Cruor®; Vascor®

Use Treatment of chronic stable angina; only approved indication is hypertension, but may be used for congestive heart failure; doses should not be adjusted for at least 10 days after beginning therapy

Mechanism of Action Bepridil, a type 4 calcium antagonist, that possesses characteristics of the traditional calcium antagonist (nifedipine) but also possesses additional pharmacological properties. Similar to other calcium antagonists, bepridil relaxes vascular muscle, decreases pacemaker activity, and reduces cardiac muscle contractile force; however, a direct bradycardia effect of bepridil has been postulated, differing from calcium channel blockers. It is suggested that bradycardia effects arise out of direct action of bepridil on the S-A node; highly lipid soluble.

Adverse Reactions

Cardiovascular: Ventricular premature contractions, prolonged Q-T intervals, torsade de pointes, flattening or notched T waves

Central nervous system: Headache, dizziness

Dermatologic: Dermatitis, rash

Gastrointestinal: Anorexia, gastrointestinal upset, dyspepsia, nausea, diarrhea, constipation

Genitourinary: Sexual difficulties

Neuromuscular & skeletal: Tremors

Respiratory: Cough, nasal congestion, pharyngitis

Miscellaneous: Taste change, sweating, flu-like syndrome

Signs & Symptoms of Acute Overdose Nausea, asthenia, gingival hyperplasia, drowsiness, confusion, decreased cardiac output, second or third degree A-V block, ileus, hypotension, prolongation of Q-T interval, torsade de pointes, tachycardia (ventricular), bradycardia

Toxicodynamics/Kinetics

Distribution: V_d: 8.0 L/kg

Protein binding: 99%

Metabolism: Significant first-pass effect, metabolized to 4-hydroxyphenyl bepridil

Bioavailability: 59%

Half-life: 42 hours

Elimination: Renal: 66%; fecal: 22%

Usual Dosage Adults: Oral: Initial: 200 mg/day, then adjust dose at 10-day intervals until optimal response is achieved; maximum daily dose: 400 mg

Contraindications History of serious ventricular arrhythmias, sick sinus syndrome, or second or third degree A-V block (except in patients with a functioning ventricular pacemaker), hypotension, uncompensated cardiac insufficiency, congenital Q-T interval prolongation, and in patients taking other drugs that prolong the Q-T interval, or a history of hypersensitivity to bepridil

Warnings Reserve for patients in whom other antianginals have failed; use with caution in patients with hepatic or renal impairment and in patients with IHSS

Dosage Forms Tablet: 200 mg, 300 mg, 400 mg

Overdosage Treatment

Decontamination: Lavage/activated charcoal with cathartic

Supportive therapy: Fluids and vasopressors (dopamine, norepinephrine, or amrinone) are successful in treating hypotension and negative inotropic effects, calcium is often required to reverse chronotropic effects, ventricular arrhythmias should be treated with lidocaine or magnesium for torsade de pointes

Enhancement of elimination: Multiple dosing of activated charcoal may be effective

Antidote(s)

Calcium Gluconate *on page 1401*

Test Interactions Increases aminotransferases, CPK, LDH

Pregnancy Risk Factor C

Monitoring Parameters Frequent monitoring of EKG and serum electrolytes is required

Patient Information May cause cardiac arrhythmias if potassium is low; can be taken with food or meals, maintain potassium supplementation as directed, routine EKGs will be necessary during start of therapy or dosage changes; notify physician if the following occur: irregular heartbeat, dyspnea, pronounced dizziness, constipation, or hypotension

Specific References

Viallon A, Page Y, Lafond P, et al, "Bepridil and Torsade de Pointes: Are the Precautions of Use Respected?" *Therapie*, 1994, 49(5):431-4.

Zeller FP and Spinler SA, "Bepridil: A New Long-Acting Calcium Channel Blocking Agent," *Drug Intell Clin Pharm*, 1987, 21(6):487-92.

Beprolo® *see* Metoprolol Tartrate *on page 524*

Berkolol® *see* Propranolol Hydrochloride *on page 657*

Berkomine® *see* Imipramine *on page 422*

Berubigen® *see* Cyanocobalamin *on page 246*

Bespar® *see* Buspirone Hydrochloride *on page 171*

Betabion® *see* Thiamine Hydrochloride *on page 741*

Beta-Blockers Comparison *see page 1644*

Betadine® [OTC] *see* Povidone-Iodine *on page 635*

Betadren® *see* Pindolol *on page 627*

9-Beta-D-Ribofuranosyladenine *see* Adenosine Triphosphate *on page 90*

Betagan® [OTC] *see* Povidone-Iodine *on page 635*

Betalin® S *see* Thiamine Hydrochloride *on page 741*

Betaloc® *see* Metoprolol Tartrate *on page 524*

Betamin® *see* Thiamine Hydrochloride *on page 741*

Betapace® *see* Sotalol Hydrochloride *on page 703*

Betapressin® *see* Penbutolol Sulfate *on page 599*

Betaseron® *see* Interferon Beta-1b *on page 435*

Beta-Sol® *see* Thiamine Hydrochloride *on page 741*

Betatabs® *see* Thiamine Hydrochloride *on page 741*

Betaxin® *see* Thiamine Hydrochloride *on page 741*

Betaxina® *see* Nalidixic Acid *on page 547*

Betaxolol Hydrochloride (be tax' oh lol)

Related Information

Beta-Blockers Comparison *on page 1644-1645*

CAS Number 63659-18-7; 63659-19-8

Brand Names Betoptic®; Betoptic® S; Kerlone®

Use Treatment of chronic open-angle glaucoma, ocular hypertension; management of hypertension

Mechanism of Action Competitively blocks $beta_1$-receptors, with little or no effect on $beta_2$-receptors; lipophilic; no membrane stabilizing effect

Adverse Reactions

Cardiovascular: Bradycardia, palpitations, edema, congestive heart failure

Central nervous system: Dizziness, psychosis, fatigue, drowsiness, headache

Local: Mild ocular stinging and discomfort, tearing, erythema, itching

Ocular: Photophobia, decreased corneal sensitivity, keratitis

Miscellaneous: Cold extremities

Signs & Symptoms of Acute Overdose Bradycardia, photophobia, depression, ataxia, night terrors, hypotension

(Continued)

Betaxolol Hydrochloride *(Continued)*

Toxicodynamics/Kinetics

Onset of action:

Ophthalmic: Within 30-60 minutes with maximal effects occurring within 2 hours

Oral: Blood pressure significantly decreases within 3 hours

Duration: Oral: 25 hours

Absorption: May be systemically absorbed

Distribution: V_d: 4.9-13 L/kg

Protein binding: 50% to 60%

Metabolism: To multiple metabolites

Bioavailability: 75%

Half-life: 12-22 hours

Time to peak serum concentration: Ophthalmic solution or suspension: 2 hours

Elimination: Renal; clearance: 280 mL/kg/hour

Usual Dosage Adults:

Ophthalmic: Instill 1 drop twice daily

Oral: 10 mg/day; may increase dose to 20 mg/day after 7-14 days if desired response is not achieved; initial dose in elderly patients: 5 mg/day

Contraindications Bronchial asthma, sinus bradycardia, second and third degree A-V block, cardiac failure, cardiogenic shock, hypersensitivity to betaxolol or any component

Warnings Use with caution in patients with diabetes mellitus, asthma, cardiac failure

Dosage Forms

Solution, ophthalmic (Betoptic®): 0.5% (2.5 mL, 5 mL, 10 mL)

Suspension, ophthalmic (Betoptic® S): 0.25% (2.5 mL, 10 mL, 15 mL)

Tablet (Kerlone®): 10 mg, 20 mg

Stability Avoid freezing

Reference Range Oral dose of 20 mg produces a level of 42.6 ng/mL 4-6 hours after ingestion

Overdosage Treatment

Decontamination: Lavage/activated charcoal with cathartic for oral ingestion

Supportive therapy: Sympathomimetics (eg, epinephrine or dopamine), atropine, glucagon, or a pacemaker can be used to treat the toxic bradycardia, asystole, and/or hypotension; initially, fluids may be the best treatment for toxic hypotension

Enhancement of elimination: Multiple dosing of activated charcoal may be effective

Drug Interactions

Ophthalmic: Topical miotics, topical dipivefrin, topical epinephrine, systemic chronic anhydrous inhibitors, systemic beta-blockers, reserpine

Systemic: Other hypotensive agents, sympathomimetics, lidocaine, verapamil

Pregnancy Risk Factor C

Monitoring Parameters

Ophthalmic: Intraocular pressure <Pj[Systemic: Blood pressure, pulse

Patient Information Intended for twice daily dosing; keep eye open and do not blink for 30 seconds after instillation; wear sunglasses to avoid photophobic discomfort. Warn diabetic patients that betaxolol may mask the symptoms of hypoglycemia.

Additional Information Because of betaxolol's low lipid solubility, it is less likely to enter the CNS, decreasing the likelihood of CNS side effects

Specific References

Ball S, "Congestive Heart Failure From Betaxolol," *Arch Ophthalmol*, 1987, 105(3):320.

Bethanechol Chloride (be than' e kole)

CAS Number 590-63-6; 674-38-4

Brand Names Duvoid®; Myocholine®; Myo Hermes®; Myotonachol™; Myotonine®; Urecholine®; Urocarb®

Synonyms Carbamylmethycholine Chloride

Use Treatment of nonobstructive urinary retention and retention due to neurogenic bladder; treatment and prevention of bladder dysfunction caused by phenothiazines; diagnosis of flaccid or atonic neurogenic bladder

Mechanism of Action Stimulates cholinergic receptors in the smooth muscle of the urinary bladder and gastrointestinal tract resulting in increased peristalsis, increased gastrointestinal and pancreatic secretions, bladder muscle contraction, and increased ureteral peristaltic waves

Adverse Reactions

Cardiovascular: Hypotension, cardiac arrest, flushing (vasomotor response)

Central nervous system: Headache, extrapyramidal reaction, hypothermia

Gastrointestinal: Abdominal cramps, diarrhea, nausea, vomiting

Genitourinary: Urinary frequency

Ocular: Lacrimation

Respiratory: Bronchial constriction
Miscellaneous: Salivation, cholinergic toxicity, sweating

Signs & Symptoms of Acute Overdose Headache, drowsiness, A-V block, flushing, hypothermia, diarrhea, lacrimation, salivation, defecation, emesis, miosis, heart block

Toxicodynamics/Kinetics
Oral:
Onset of action: 0.5-1.5 hours
Duration: Up to 6 hours
S.C.: 5-15 minutes
Absorption: Oral: Variable

Usual Dosage
Children:
Oral:
Abdominal distention or urinary retention: 0.6 mg/kg/day divided 3-4 times/day
Gastroesophageal reflux: 0.1-0.2 mg/kg/dose given 30 minutes to 1 hour before each meal to a maximum of 4 times/day
S.C.: 0.15-0.2 mg/kg/day divided 3-4 times/day

Adults:
Oral: 10-50 mg 2-4 times/day
S.C.: 2.5-5 mg 3-4 times/day, up to 7.5-10 mg every 4 hours for neurogenic bladder

Contraindications Hypersensitivity to bethanechol; do not use in patients with mechanical obstruction of the gastrointestinal or GU tract or when the strength or integrity of the gastrointestinal or bladder wall is in question. It is also contraindicated in patients with hyperthyroidism, peptic ulcer disease, epilepsy, obstructive pulmonary disease, bradycardia, vasomotor instability, atrioventricular conduction defects, hypotension, or parkinsonism.

Warnings Potential for reflux infection if the sphincter fails to relax as bethanechol contracts the bladder; use with caution when administering to nursing women, as it is unknown if the drug is excreted in breast milk; safety and efficacy in children <5 years of age have not been established; syringe containing atropine should be readily available for treatment of serious side effects; for S.C. injection only; do not give I.M. or I.V. Cholinergic effects may occur with increased frequency in patients with diabetic neuropathy.

Dosage Forms
Injection: 5 mg/mL (1 mL)
Tablet: 5 mg, 10 mg, 25 mg, 50 mg

Overdosage Treatment
Decontamination: Lavage/activated charcoal with cathartic
Supportive therapy: Atropine (2-4 mg in adults or 0.04-0.08 mg/kg in children) should be given to control muscarinic symptoms; diazepam or lorazepam can be given for seizures

Antidote(s)
Atropine Sulfate *on page 1395*

Test Interactions ↑ lipase, amylase (S), bilirubin, aminotransferase [ALT (SGPT)/AST (SGOT)] (S)

Drug Interactions
Decreased effect: Procainamide, quinidine
Increased toxicity: Ganglionic blockers (critical decrease in blood pressure); adrenoblockers (hypothermia)

Pregnancy Risk Factor C

Patient Information Oral dose should be taken 1 hour before meals or 2 hours after meals to avoid nausea or vomiting; may cause abdominal discomfort, salivation, sweating, or flushing – notify physician if these symptoms become pronounced

Nursing Implications Contraindicated for I.M. or I.V. use due to a likely severe cholinergic reaction; for S.C. injection only – should never be give I.M. or I.V.; observe closely for side effects; have bedpan readily available if administered for urinary retention

Additional Information Cardiac effects less likely with bethanechol than acetylcholine chloride (Covochol®, Miochol®)

Specific References
Andersson KE, "Current Concepts in the Treatment of Disorders of Micturition," *Drugs*, 1988, 35(4):477-94.
Guerra MF and Ives TJ, "Bethanechol and Hypothermia," *Ann Intern Med*, 1983, 99(2):279-80.

Betim® *see* Timolol Maleate *on page 752*

Betoptic® *see* Betaxolol Hydrochloride *on page 153*

Betoptic® S *see* Betaxolol Hydrochloride *on page 153*

Bewon® *see* Thiamine Hydrochloride *on page 741*

Biamine® *see* Thiamine Hydrochloride *on page 741*

Biaxin™ Filmtabs® *see* Clarithromycin *on page 221*

BiCOZENE® [OTC] *see* Benzocaine *on page 149*

Bikalm® *see* Zolpidem Tartrate *on page 814*

Biocoryl® *see* Procainamide Hydrochloride *on page 642*

Bio E® *see* Vitamin E *on page 798*

Bio-Gan® *see* Trimethobenzamide Hydrochloride *on page 772*

Biomox® *see* Amoxicillin *on page 121*

Bional *see* Benzalkonium Chloride *on page 147*

Bionic *see* Niacin *on page 554*

Bio-Tab® Oral *see* Doxycycline *on page 305*

Biquin® *see* Quinidine *on page 668*

Bisacodyl (bis a koe' dill)

CAS Number 603-50-9; 1336-29-4

Brand Names Bisacodyl Uniserts®; Bisco-Lax® [OTC]; Carter's Little Pills® [OTC]; Clysodrast®; Dulcagen® [OTC]; Dulcolax® [OTC]; Fleet® Laxative [OTC]

Use Treatment of constipation; colonic evacuation prior to procedures or examination

Mechanism of Action Stimulates peristalsis by directly irritating the smooth muscle of the intestine, possibly the colonic intramural plexus; alters water and electrolyte secretion producing net intestinal fluid accumulation and laxation

Adverse Reactions

Endocrine & metabolic: Electrolyte and fluid imbalance (metabolic acidosis or alkalosis, hypocalcemia)

Gastrointestinal: Abdominal cramps, nausea, vomiting

Miscellaneous: Rectal burning

Signs & Symptoms of Acute Overdose Abdominal pain, proctitis, hypocalcemia, diarrhea, colonic atony

Toxicodynamics/Kinetics

Onset of action:
- Oral: 6-10 hours
- Rectal: 0.25-1 hour

Absorption: Oral, rectal: <5% absorbed systemically

Metabolism: In the liver to bis(parahydroxyphenyl) -pyridyl-2-methane (an active metabolite)

Elimination: Conjugated metabolites excreted in milk, bile, and urine

Usual Dosage

Children:
- Oral: >6 years: 5-10 mg (0.3 mg/kg) at bedtime or before breakfast
- Rectal suppository:
  - <2 years: 5 mg as a single dose
  - >2 years: 10 mg

Adults:
- Oral: 5-15 mg as single dose (up to 30 mg when complete evacuation of bowel is required)
- Rectal suppository: 10 mg as single dose
- Tannex:
  - Enema: 2.5 g in 1000 mL warm water
  - Barium enema: 2.5-5 g in 1000 mL barium suspension
  - Do not give >10 g within 72-hour period

Contraindications Do not use in patients with abdominal pain, obstruction, nausea or vomiting; do not administer bisacodyl tannex enema to children <10 years of age

Warnings Bisacodyl tannex should be used with caution in patients with ulceration of the colon and during pregnancy or lactation; safety of bisacodyl tannex usage in children <10 years of age has not been established; use with caution in patients with hemorrhoids

Dosage Forms

Enema: 10 mg/30 mL

Powder (Clysodrast®): 1.5 mg with tannic acid 2.5 g per packet (25s, 50s)

Suppository, rectal: 10 mg

Suppository, rectal, pediatric: 5 mg

Tablet, enteric coated: 5 mg

Overdosage Treatment

Decontamination: Lavage/activated charcoal (no cathartic)

Supportive therapy: Intravenous crystalloid hydration with potassium replacement

Drug Interactions Decreased effect with milk and antacids; decreased effect of warfarin

Pregnancy Risk Factor C

Patient Information Swallow tablets whole, do **not** crush or chew; do not take antacid or milk within 1 hour of taking drug

Nursing Implications Administer tablets 2 hours prior to, or 4 hours after antacids; increased pH may dissolve the enteric coating leading to gastrointestinal distress; do not crush enteric coated drug product

Specific References

Kjaergaard J, Christensen U, Stadil F, et al, "Colostomy Irrigation With Prostaglandin E2 and Bisacodyl: A Double-Blind Cross-Over Study," *Br J Surg*, 1984, 71(7):556-7.

Bisacodyl Uniserts® *see* Bisacodyl *on previous page*

Bisco-Lax® [OTC] *see* Bisacodyl *on previous page*

Bishydroxycoumarin *see* Dicumarol *on page 277*

Bismuth Subgallate (bis' muth sub gall' ate)

CAS Number 7440-69-9

Brand Names Devrom® [OTC]

Use Symptomatic treatment of mild, nonspecific diarrhea; skin protectant; antacid; in industry, used in boiler plugs, electrical fuses, solders, and dental techniques

Mechanism of Action Binds with thiol-containing enzyme in cerebrum; antimicrobial action against *Helicobacter pylori*

Adverse Reactions

Central nervous system: Headache, drowsiness, malaise, memory loss, seizures, ataxia, encephalopathy, tremors

Dermatologic: Oral lesions, bluish gum line, erythema, alopecia

Gastrointestinal: Stomatitis, nausea, vomiting, fecal impaction, anorexia

Hematologic: Methemoglobinemia

Neuromuscular & skeletal: Muscle myoclonus, osteoporosis

Miscellaneous: Bezoars, feces discoloration (black)

Signs & Symptoms of Acute Overdose Fever, methemoglobinemia, dementia, tongue discoloration, tubular necrosis, sweating, proteinuria, jaundice, memory loss, hyperthermia, confusion, stomatitis, hyperactivity, seizures

Toxicodynamics/Kinetics

Absorption: Poor through gastrointestinal tract and dermally (<1%)

Metabolism: Converted by bacteria in gastrointestinal tract to bismuth sulfide

Half-life: 5 days

Elimination: Urine

Usual Dosage Oral: 1-2 tablets 3 times/day with meals

Dosing adjustment in renal impairment: Should probably be avoided in patients with renal failure

Dosage Forms Tablet, chewable: 200 mg

Reference Range Plasma levels <5 μg/dL are not toxic

Overdosage Treatment

Decontamination: Emesis or lavage/activated charcoal with cathartic

Supportive therapy: D-penicillamine (15-40 mg/kg/day up to 250-500 mg 4 times/day in adults; 20-30 mg/kg/day orally in children before meals) has been tested in animal models; no human use experience. Methylene blue can be used for methemoglobinemia.

Antidote(s)

Methylene Blue *on page 1444*

Penicillamine *on page 1454*

Drug Interactions May reduce gastrointestinal absorption of tetracycline

Pregnancy Risk Factor C (D in 3rd trimester)

Additional Information Bismuth subsalicylate (Pepto-Bismol®) contains 58% bismuth and 42% salicylate; do not exceed 4.2 g/day dosage; bismuth is radiopaque

Specific References

Basinger MA, Jones MM, and McCroskey SA, "Antidotes for Acute Bismuth Intoxication," *J Toxicol Clin Toxicol*, 1983, 20(2):159-65.

Baxter GF, "Bismuth: From Alchemy to *Campylobacter*," *Pharm J*, 1989, 249:805-8.

Bradley B, Singleton M, and Po AL, "Bismuth Toxicity - A Reassessment," *J Clin Pharm Ther*, 1989, 14(6):423-41.

Gordon MF, Abrams RI, Rubin DB, et al, "Bismuth Subsalicylate Toxicity as a Cause of Prolonged Encephalopathy With Myoclonus," *Mov Disord*, 1995, 10:220-2.

Kruger G, Thomas DJ, Weinhardt F, et al, "Disturbed Oxidative Metabolism in Organic Brain Syndrome Caused by Bismuth in Skin Creams," *Lancet*, 1976, 2(7984):485-7.

Slikkerveer A and de Wolff FA, "Pharmacokinetics and Toxicity of Bismuth Compounds," *Med Toxicol Adverse Drug Exp*, 1989, 4(5):303-23.

Bisobloc® *see* Bisoprolol Fumarate *on this page*

Bisoprolol Fumarate (bis oh' proe lol)

CAS Number 66722-44-9; 66722-45-0; 104344-23-2

Brand Names Bisobloc®; Concor®; Detensiel®; Emconcor®; Emcor®; Euradal®; Monocor®; Soprol®; Zebeta®

(Continued)

Bisoprolol Fumarate *(Continued)*

Use Treatment of hypertension, alone or in combination with other agents

Mechanism of Action Selective inhibitor of $beta_1$-adrenergic receptors; competitively blocks $beta_1$-receptors, with little or no effect on $beta_2$-receptors at doses <10 mg

Adverse Reactions

Cardiovascular: Persistent bradycardia, hypotension, chest pain, edema, heart failure, exacerbation of Raynaud's phenomenon

Central nervous system: Fatigue, dizziness, insomnia, drowsiness, night terrors, CNS depression, confusion, headache

Gastrointestinal: Constipation, diarrhea, nausea

Genitourinary: Impotence

Miscellaneous: Cold extremities

Signs & Symptoms of Acute Overdose Bradycardia, hypotension, wheezing, ataxia, night terrors, cough, insomnia, impotence, hypoglycemia, cold extremities

Toxicodynamics/Kinetics

Absorption: Rapid and almost complete from gastrointestinal tract (90%)

Distribution: V_d: 2.9 L/kg; distributes widely to body tissues; highest concentrations in heart, liver, lungs, and saliva; crosses blood-brain barrier

Protein binding: 26% to 36%

Metabolism: Significant first-pass; extensively (50%) metabolized in the liver

Half-life: 9-13 hours; 21 hours in patients with liver disease

Time to peak serum concentration: 1.7-3 hours

Elimination: In urine (10% as unchanged drug) and feces (2% as unchanged drug)

Usual Dosage Adults: Oral: 5 mg once daily, may be increased to 10 mg, and then up to 20 mg once daily, if necessary; may be given without regard to meals

Contraindications Uncompensated congestive heart failure, cardiogenic shock, bradycardia, or heart block

Warnings Use with caution in patients with inadequate myocardial function; acute withdrawal may exacerbate symptoms; use with caution in patients undergoing anesthesia and in those with bronchospastic disease, hyperthyroidism, and impaired hepatic function

Dosage Forms Tablet: 5 mg, 10 mg

Reference Range Peak plasma level of 56 ng/mL after 10 mg dose and 445 ng/mL after 100 mg dose

Overdosage Treatment

Decontamination: Lavage/activated charcoal with cathartic; do not use ipecac

Supportive therapy: Glucagon (50-150 mcg/kg followed by continuous drip of 1-5 mg/hour) for positive chronotropic effect; atropine/isoproterenol can be utilized to increase heart rate; calcium chloride may also be effective; do **not** use epinephrine

Enhancement of elimination: Multiple dosing of activated charcoal is not likely to be of benefit; dialysis is not useful

Antidote(s)

Atropine Sulfate *on page 1395*

Glucagon *on page 1431*

Test Interactions ↑ thyroxine (S), glucose; no effect on lipid profile

Drug Interactions

Decreased effect/levels with barbiturates, rifampin, sulfinpyrazone

Increased effect/toxicity/levels of and with flecainide; increased effect of ritodrine; bradycardia with amiodarone

Pregnancy Risk Factor C

Pregnancy Implications Distributes into breast milk

Monitoring Parameters Blood pressure, EKG

Patient Information Do not discontinue abruptly; notify physician if CHF symptoms become worse; take at the same time each day; may mask diabetes symptoms, sweating will remain

Specific References

Lancaster SG and Sorkin EM, "Bisoprolol: A Preliminary Review of Its Pharmacodynamic and Pharmacokinetic Properties, and Therapeutic Efficacy in Hypertension and Angina Pectoris," *Drugs*, 1988, 36(3):256-85.

BL-191 *see* Pentoxifylline *on page 607*

Blanc de Zinc *see* Zinc Oxide *on page 813*

Blenoxane® *see* Bleomycin Sulfate *on this page*

Bleomycin Sulfate (blee oh mye' sin)

Related Information

Toxicities of Chemotherapeutic Agents *on page 1631-1633*

CAS Number 11056-06-7; 9041-93-4

Brand Names Blenoxane®; Bleo-S®; Oil Bleo®

Synonyms BLM

Use Treatment of squamous cell carcinomas, oral leukoplakia, melanomas, sarcomas, testicular carcinomas, Hodgkin's lymphoma, and non-Hodgkin's lymphoma; normalization of calcium in hypercalcemic patients

Unlabeled uses: Sclerosing agent for malignant pleural effusion

Mechanism of Action Inhibits synthesis of DNA; binds to DNA leading to single- and double-strand breaks

Adverse Reactions

Cardiovascular: Raynaud's phenomenon

Central nervous system: Chills, hypersomnia, personality changes, memory impairment, thermal dysfunction

Dermatologic: Alopecia, hyperpigmentation, nailbed changes, vesiculation

Gastrointestinal: Stomatitis, anorexia, nausea, vomiting, weight loss

Local: Mucocutaneous toxicity pain at tumor site, phlebitis

Pulmonary: Dose related when total dose is >400 units or with single doses >30 units; pathogenesis is poorly understood, but may be related to damage of pulmonary, vascular, or connective tissue. Manifested as an acute or chronic interstitial pneumonitis with interstitial fibrosis, hypoxia, and death. Symptoms include cough, dyspnea, and bilateral pulmonary infiltrates noted on CXR. It is controversial whether steroids improve symptoms of bleomycin pulmonary toxicity. Risk factors for development of pulmonary toxicity include cumulative dose >450 mg/m^2, age >70 years, pre-existing pulmonary disease, high oxygen therapy, concomitant chemotherapy, or thoracic irradiation.

Miscellaneous: Patients may become febrile after intracavitary administration

Signs & Symptoms of Acute Overdose Chills, fever, hyperthermia, thrombocytopenia, hypocalcemia, seizures, deafness, acrodynia, erythema, cystitis (hemorrhagic), pulmonary fibrosis, hyperpigmentation

Toxicodynamics/Kinetics

Absorption: I.M. and intrapleural administration produces serum concentrations of 30% of I.V. administration; intraperitoneal and S.C. routes produce serum concentrations equal to those of I.V.

Distribution: V_d: 0.3 L/kg; highest concentrations seen in skin, kidney, lung, heart tissues; low concentrations seen in testes and gastrointestinal tract; does not cross blood-brain barrier

Protein binding: 1%

Metabolism: By several tissue types, including the liver, gastrointestinal tract, skin, lungs, kidney, and serum

Half-life, biphasic: Dependent upon renal function:

- Normal renal function:
  - Initial: 1.3 hours
  - Terminal: 9 hours
- End-stage renal disease:
  - Initial: 2 hours
  - Terminal: 30 hours

Time to peak serum concentration: I.M.: Within 30 minutes

Elimination: 50% to 70% of dose excreted in urine as active drug; clearance: 0.07 L/kg/hour

Usual Dosage Refer to individual protocol; 1 unit = 1 mg

Children and Adults:

- Test dose for lymphoma patients: I.M., I.V., S.C.: 1-5 units of bleomycin before the first dose; monitor vital signs every 15 minutes; wait a minimum of 1 hour before administering remainder of dose
- I.M., I.V., S.C.: 10-20 units/m^2 (0.25-0.5 units/kg) 1-2 times/week in combination regimens; I.V. continuous infusion: 15-20 units/m^2/day for 4-5 days
- Maximum cumulative lifetime dose: 400 units

Dosing adjustment in renal impairment:

- Cl_{cr} 10-50 mL/minute: Administer 75% of normal dose
- Cl_{cr} <10 mL/minute: Administer 50% of normal dose

Not removed by hemodialysis

Adults: Intracavitary injection for pleural effusion: 60 units have been given in 50-100 mL SWI for malignant pleural effusion; intracavitary dose: 15-240 units

Administration Administer I.V. slowly over at least 10 minutes (no greater than 1 unit/minute) at a concentration not to exceed 3 units/mL; bleomycin for I.V. continuous infusion can be further diluted in normal saline (preferred) or D_5W

Contraindications Hypersensitivity to bleomycin sulfate or any component, severe pulmonary disease

Warnings Possible increased pulmonary toxicity to oxygen in scuba divers treated with bleomycin; the U.S. Food and Drug Administration (FDA) currently recommends that procedures for proper handling and disposal of antineoplastic agents be considered. Occurrence of pulmonary fibrosis is higher in elderly patients and in those receiving >400 units total and in smokers and patients with prior radiation therapy; a severe idiosyncratic reaction consisting of hypotension, mental confu-

(Continued)

Bleomycin Sulfate *(Continued)*

sion, fever, chills, and wheezing is possible; check lungs prior to each treatment for crackles.

Dosage Forms Powder for injection: 15 units

Stability Refrigerate powder, reconstituted at room temperature is stable for 28 days in refrigerator or for 14 days at room temperature; stability decreases in PVC bags; **incompatible** with carbenicillin, methotrexate, terbutaline, amino acid solutions, ascorbic acid, cefazolin, furosemide, diazepam, hydrocortisone, mitomycin, nafcillin, penicillin G, aminophylline; prolonged infusions in PVC containers should be avoided and glass bottles should be used; **compatible** with cyclophosphamide, doxorubicin, mesna, vinblastine, vincristine

Reference Range Steady-state levels for a dose of 20 units/day is from 50-200 milli-units/L

Overdosage Treatment
Supportive therapy: Use minimal amounts of oxygen; steroids are of uncertain benefit in preventing pulmonary fibrosis

Test Interactions Increases potassium (S)

Drug Interactions
CCNU: Increased severity of leukopenia
Cisplatin: Results in delayed bleomycin elimination due to decrease in creatinine clearance secondary to cisplatin; also increased incidence of Raynaud's phenomena noted
Digitalis glycosides: May decrease plasma levels and renal excretion of digoxin
Phenytoin: Results in decreased phenytoin levels, possibly due to decreased oral absorption
Vaccines: Impaired immune response to vaccines; possible infection after administration of live vaccines in patients receiving immunosuppressants

Pregnancy Risk Factor D

Monitoring Parameters Pulmonary function tests (total lung volume, forced vital capacity, carbon monoxide diffusion), renal function, chest x-ray, temperature initially, CBC with differential and platelet count; check body weight at regular intervals

Patient Information Hair should reappear after discontinuance of medication; maintain excellent oral hygiene habits; report any coughing, shortness of breath, or wheezing; skin rashes, shaking, chills, or transient high fever may occur following administration

Additional Information Myelosuppressive effects:
WBC: Rare
Platelets: Rare
Onset (days): 7
Nadir (days): 14
Recovery (days): 21

Specific References

Halsa T, Ueld K, and Yoshida S, "Toxic Effects of Bleomycin on the Hypothalamus Following Its Administration Into a Cystic Craniopharyngioma," *Br J Neurosurg*, 1994, 8(6):747-50.
Lamey PJ and Lewis MAO, "Oral Medicine in Practice: White Patches," *Br Dent J*, 1990, 168(4):147-52.
Nijjar T and Brandes LJ, "Bleomycin for Hypercalcemia Due to Cancer," *N Engl J Med*, 1983, 308:655.
Sostman HD, "Cytotoxic Drug-Induced Lung Disease," *Am J Med*, 1977, 62:608-15.
Toledo CH, Ross WE, Hood CI, et al, "Potentiation of Bleomycin Toxicity by Oxygen," *Cancer Treat Rep*, 1982, 66:359-62.
Zanetti CL, "Scuba Diving and Bleomycin Therapy," *JAMA*, 1990, 264(22):2869.

Bleo-S® *see* Bleomycin Sulfate *on page 158*

BLM *see* Bleomycin Sulfate *on page 158*

Blocadren® *see* Timolol Maleate *on page 752*

Blocotin® *see* Penbutolol Sulfate *on page 599*

Blokium® *see* Atenolol *on page 137*

Blox® *see* Loperamide Hydrochloride *on page 480*

BMY-27857 *see* Stavudine *on page 706*

Boestrol® *see* Diethylstilbestrol *on page 280*

Bolutol® *see* Gemfibrozil *on page 378*

Bolvidon® *see* Mianserin Hydrochloride *on page 529*

Bom-Bon® *see* Phenolphthalein *on page 617*

Bonine® [OTC] *see* Meclizine Hydrochloride *on page 494*

Boracic Acid *see* Boric Acid *on this page*

Boric Acid (bor' ik)

CAS Number 10043-35-3

Brand Names Borofax® [OTC]; Boroformol®; Borsyre®; Dri-Ear® [OTC]; Komex®; Sassolite®; Swim-Ear® [OTC]; Viskos®

Synonyms Boracic Acid; Orthoboric Acid

Use Food preservatives, emulsifiers, neutralizers, antifungal water softeners, contact lens cleaner, antiseptics, pesticides (for cockroaches)

Ophthalmic: Mild antiseptic used for inflamed eyelids

Topical ointment: Temporary relief of chapped, chafed, or dry skin, diaper rash, abrasions, minor burns, sunburn, insect bites, and other skin irritations

Mechanism of Action Disinfectant, astringent

Adverse Reactions

Central nervous system: CNS stimulation followed by CNS depression, fever

Dermatologic: Erythematous skin eruptions, pruritus, alopecia, erythrodermic desquamation (2-3 days after exposure) (boiled lobster appearance)

Gastrointestinal: gastrointestinal disturbance, vomiting, nausea, diarrhea

Hepatic: Elevated liver function tests

Miscellaneous: Feces discoloration (black), feces discoloration (blue), feces discoloration (blue-green)

Signs & Symptoms of Acute Overdose Elevated liver function tests, dry skin, dermatitis, desquamation, circulatory collapse, hyperthermia, toxic epidermal necrolysis, seizures, urine discoloration (blue-green), diarrhea, cardiovascular collapse, confusion

Toxicodynamics/Kinetics

Absorption: Not well absorbed through intact skin; absorbed well through inflamed skin

Half-life: 12 hours

Elimination: Renal, within 96 hours of ingestion

Usual Dosage Apply to lower eyelid 1-2 times/day

Contraindications Hypersensitivity to boric acid or any component; do not apply to inflamed skin

Dosage Forms

Ointment:

- Ophthalmic: 5% (3.5 g); 10% (3.5 g)
- Topical: 5% (52.5 g); 10% (28 g)
- Topical (Borofax®): 5% boric acid and lanolin (1¾ oz)

Solution, otic: 2.75% with isopropyl alcohol (30 mL)

Reference Range Normal boric acid levels: Children: 0.0-0.7 mg/dL; Adults: 0.0-0.2 mg/dL; levels of 2.0-15.0 mg/dL are associated with survival; levels >40.0 mg/dL are associated with lethality

Overdosage Treatment

Decontamination: Emesis or lavage for ingestions >200 mg/kg or 12 g total ingestion/activated charcoal with cathartic will not adsorb boric acid well; irrigate skin with soap and water for dermal exposure

Supportive therapy: Treat hypotension with isotonic saline, dopamine, or norepinephrine

Enhancement of elimination: Exchange transfusion or hemodialysis should be considered for serious toxic manifestations or if renal failure develops

Diagnostic Tests/Procedures

Liver Profile *on page 1286*

Drug Interactions Increases riboflavin excretion

Patient Information If irritation persists or increases, discontinue use

Nursing Implications Application to abraded skin or open wounds has caused fatal poisonings in infants

Additional Information Not a corrosive substance

Specific References

Baker MD and Bogema SC, "Ingestion of Boric Acid by Infants," *Am J Emerg Med*, 1986, 4(4):358-61.

Egfjord M, Jansen JA, Flachs H, et al, "Combined Boric Acid and Cinchocaine Chloride Poisoning in a 12-Month-Old Infant: Evaluation of Haemodialysis," *Hum Toxicol*, 1988, 7(2):175-8.

Linden CH, Hall AH, Kulig KW, et al, "Acute Ingestions of Boric Acid," *J Toxicol Clin Toxicol*, 1986, 24(4):269-79.

Litovitz TL, Klein-Schwartz W, Oderda GM, et al, "Clinical Manifestations of Toxicity in a Series of 784 Boric Acid Ingestions," *Am J Emerg Med*, 1992, 10:545-7.

Borofax® [OTC] *see* Boric Acid *on previous page*

Boroformol® *see* Boric Acid *on previous page*

Borsyre® *see* Boric Acid *on previous page*

B&O Supprettes® *see* Belladonna and Opium *on page 145*

Botulinum Toxin Type A (bot' yoo lin num)

Brand Names Oculinum®

Use Treatment of strabismus and blepharospasm; also used in spasmodic torticollis, occupational limb spasm

Investigational: Possibly indicated for achalasia; treatment improvement of oscillopsia due to acquired nystagmus

(Continued)

Botulinum Toxin Type A *(Continued)*

Mechanism of Action Botulinum A toxin is a neurotoxin produced by *Clostridium botulinum*, spore-forming anaerobic bacillus. Six distinct antigenic types of neurotoxins are generated by *Clostridium botulinum*, named from A to F, however, only the A toxin has been used clinically. Botulinum A toxin is a double-chain protein with a molecular weight of ~900,000; active portion of the molecule is the light chain and the heavy chain is inactive. The toxin appears to affect only one structure in humans, the presynaptic membrane of the neuromuscular junction, where it prevents calcium-dependent release of acetylcholine and produces a state of denervation. Following injection of the toxin into a muscle, the degree of resultant skeletal muscle asthenia or paralysis is dependent upon the dose administered. Muscle inactivation persists until new fibrils grow from the nerve and form junction plates on new areas of the muscle-cell walls. The antagonist muscle shortens simultaneously ("contracture"), taking up the slack created by agonist paralysis; following several weeks of paralysis, alignment of the eye is measurably changed, despite return of innervation to the injected muscle. In patients with sixth nerve palsy, the objective is to prevent contracture of the ipsilateral medial rectus muscle while the patient awaits recovery of the palsied lateral rectus muscle.

Adverse Reactions

Dermatologic: Diffuse skin rash

Local: Swelling of eyelid

Ocular: Blepharospasm, photophobia, diplopia, ptosis, vertical deviation, exacerbation of acute angle-closure glaucoma

Signs & Symptoms of Acute Overdose Neuromuscular paralysis, photophobia, dysphagia, dry eyes, dry mouth, dermatitis, mydriasis, lacrimation, cranial nerve palsies, corneal irritation, conjunctivitis, blurred vision

Usual Dosage The cumulative dose should not exceed 200 units in a 30-day period

Strabismus: 1.25-5 units (0.05-0.15 mL) injected into any one muscle

Blepharospasm: 1.25-5 units (0.05-0.15 mL) injected into the orbicularis oculi muscle

Achalasia: 80 units (20 units in each quadrant) injected directly into inferior esophageal sphincter through upper endoscopy

Acquired nystagmus: 25-30 units through retrobulbar injection

Warnings Use with caution in patients taking aminoglycosides or any other antibiotic or other drugs that interfere with neuromuscular transmission

Dosage Forms Powder for injection, lyophilized, preservative free: *Clostridium botulinum* Toxin type A 100 units

Stability Keep in undiluted vials in freezer; refrigerate reconstituted solution

Overdosage Treatment Supportive therapy: Treatment is entirely supportive; artificial ventilation may be required; antitoxins to botulism are of no benefit

Pregnancy Risk Factor C

Patient Information In strabismus, effect may take 2 days to occur and will last for 2-6 weeks; in blepharospasm, effect may take 3 days to occur and will last for 3 months; injections may be repeated indefinitely

Nursing Implications To alleviate spatial disorientation or double vision in strabismic patients, cover the affected eye; inject using a 27- to 30-gauge needle

Specific References

Borodic GE and Pearce LB, "New Concepts in Botulinum Toxin Therapy," *Drug Saf*, 1994, 11(3):145-52.

Bushara KO, Jones JW, and Park DM, "Localized Graying of Eyebrow Hair, A Side Effect of Botulinum Toxin Injections," *Mov Disord*, 1995, 10:382.

Cohen S and Parkman HP, "Treatment of Achalasia – Whalebone to Botulinum Toxin," *N Engl J Med*, 1995, 332(12):815-6.

Ferrari AP, Jr, Siqueira ES, and Brant CQ, "Treatment of Achalasia in Chagas' Disease With Botulinum Toxin," *N Engl J Med*, 1995, 332(12):824-5.

Jankovic J and Brin MF, "Therapeutic Uses of Botulinum Toxin," *N Engl J Med*, 1991, 324(17):1186-94.

Pasricha PJ, Ravich WJ, Hendrix TR, et al, "Intrasphincteric Botulinum Toxin for the Treatment of Achalasia," *N Engl J Med*, 1995, 322(12):774-8.

Pasricha PJ, Ravich WJ, Hendrix TR, et al, "Treatment of Achalasia With Intrasphincteric Injection of Botulinum Toxin," *Ann Intern Med*, 1994, 121(8):590-1.

Repka MX, Savino PJ, and Reinecke RD, "Treatment of Acquired Nystagmus With Botulinum Neurotoxin A," *Arch Ophthalmol*, 1994, 112(10):1320-4.

Sheean GL, Murray NM, and Marsden CD, "Pain and Remote Weakness in Limbs Injected With Botulinum Toxin A for Writer's Cramp," *Lancet*, 1995, 346:154-6.

Breezee® Mist Antifungal [OTC] *see* Miconazole *on page 530*

Brek® *see* Loperamide Hydrochloride *on page 480*

Breonesin® [OTC] *see* Guaifenesin *on page 390*

Brethaire® *see* Terbutaline Sulfate *on page 726*

Brethine® *see* Terbutaline Sulfate *on page 726*

Bretylate® *see* Bretylium Tosylate *on next page*

Bretylium Tosylate (bre til' ee um toss' a late)

CAS Number 59-41-6; 61-75-6

Brand Names Bretylate®; Bretylol®

Use Ventricular tachycardia and fibrillation; also used in the treatment of other serious ventricular arrhythmias resistant to lidocaine

Mechanism of Action Class II and class III antiarrhythmic properties; after an initial release of norepinephrine at the peripheral adrenergic nerve terminals, inhibits further release by postganglionic nerve endings in response to sympathetic nerve stimulation

Adverse Reactions

Cardiovascular: Hypotension (incidence 50% to 75%), transient initial hypertension, PVCs (increased), bradycardia, flushing

Central nervous system: Dizziness, syncope, confusion, fever, hyperthermia

Dermatologic: Rash

Gastrointestinal: Nausea, vomiting, rarely diarrhea, abdominal pain, parotid pain

Local: Muscle atrophy and necrosis with repeated I.M. injections at same site

Ocular: Conjunctivitis

Renal: Renal impairment

Respiratory: Nasal congestion

Miscellaneous: Hiccups

Signs & Symptoms of Acute Overdose Dyspnea, hypertension followed by hypotension, nausea, vomiting, renal dysfunction, ptosis, lightheadedness, paralysis, mydriasis

Toxicodynamics/Kinetics

Onset of action:

I.M.: May require 2 hours

I.V.: Antiarrhythmic effects seen within 6-20 minutes

Duration: 6-24 hours

Absorption: Well absorbed

Distribution: V_d: 5.9 L/kg; does not pass blood-brain barrier; widely distributed throughout body

Protein binding: 1% to 6%

Metabolism: Not metabolized

Half-life: 7-11 hours; average: 4-17 hours

Time to peak serum concentration: 1 hour

Elimination: Excreted unchanged in urine

Usual Dosage

Children:

I.M.: 2-5 mg/kg as a single dose

I.V.: Initial: 5 mg/kg, then attempt electrical defibrillation; repeat with 10 mg/kg if fibrillation (ventricular) persists at 15-minute intervals to maximum total of 30 mg/kg

Maintenance dose: I.M., I.V.: 5 mg/kg every 6-8 hours

Adults:

Immediate life-threatening ventricular arrhythmias; fibrillation (ventricular); unstable tachycardia (ventricular). **Note**: Patients should undergo defibrillation/cardioversion before and after bretylium doses as necessary:

Initial dose: I.V.: 5 mg/kg (undiluted) over 1 minute; if arrhythmias persist, give 10 mg/kg (undiluted) over 1 minute and repeat as necessary (usually at 15- to 30-minute intervals) up to a total dose of 30 mg/kg

Other life-threatening ventricular arrhythmias:

Initial dose: I.M., I.V.: 5-10 mg/kg, may repeat every 1-2 hours if arrhythmias persist; give I.V. dose (diluted) over 10-30 minutes

Maintenance dose: I.M.: 5-10 mg/kg every 6-8 hours; I.V. (diluted): 5-10 mg/kg every 6 hours; I.V. infusion (diluted): 1-2 mg/minute (little experience with doses >40 mg/kg/day)

Dosing adjustment in renal impairment:

Cl_{cr} 10-50 mL/minute: Administer 25% to 50% of dose

Cl_{cr} <10 mL/minute: Administer 25% of dose

Contraindications Digitalis intoxication-induced arrhythmias

Warnings Hypotension, patients with fixed cardiac output (severe pulmonary hypertension or aortic stenosis) may experience severe hypotension due to decrease in peripheral resistance without ability to increase cardiac output; reduce dose in renal failure patients; subtherapeutic doses may cause hypotension

Dosage Forms

Injection: 50 mg/mL (10 mL, 20 mL); 100 mg/mL

Injection, premixed in D_5W: 1 mg/mL (500 mL); 2 mg/mL (250 mL); 4 mg/mL (250 mL, 500 mL)

Stability Premixed infusion should be stored at room temperature and protected from freezing

(Continued)

Bretylium Tosylate *(Continued)*

Reference Range Fatal: 8.8 μg/mL

Overdosage Treatment

Supportive therapy: Administration of short-acting hypotensive agent (Nipride®) should be used for the hypertensive response; hypotension should be treated with fluid administration and dopamine; atropine is useful for bradycardia

Enhancement of elimination: Hemodialysis is of limited value; moderately dialyzable (20% to 50%)

Drug Interactions Other antiarrhythmic agents may potentiate or antagonize cardiac effects, toxic effects may be additive; the pressor effects of catecholamines may be enhanced by bretylium; may potentiate digitalis toxicity; quinidine or procainamide may cause hypotension when given with bretylium

Pregnancy Risk Factor C (may reduce uterine blood flow and cause fetal bradycardia)

Monitoring Parameters EKG, heart rate, blood pressure

Patient Information Anticipate vomiting

Nursing Implications I.M. injection should not exceed 5 mL volume in any one site

Additional Information Largest human overdose: 81 mg/kg of bretylium; patient expired 50 days later

Specific References

Bodnar T, Nowak R, Tomlanovich MC, et al, "Massive Intravenous Bolus Bretylium Tosylate," *Ann Emerg Med*, 1980, 9(12):630-3.

Gibson JS and Munter DW, "Intravenous Bretylium Overdose," *Am J Emerg Med*, 1995, 13(2):177-9.

Perlman PE, Adams WG Jr, and Ridgeway NA, "Extreme Pyrexia During Bretylium Administration," *Postgrad Med*, 1989, 85(1):111-2.

Thompson AE and Sussmane JB, "Bretylium Intoxication Resembling Clinical Brain Death," *Crit Care Med*, 1989, 17(2):14-9.

Bretylol® *see* Bretylium Tosylate *on previous page*

Brevibloc® Injection *see* Esmolol Hydrochloride *on page 323*

Brevital® Sodium *see* Methohexital Sodium *on page 514*

Bricanyl® *see* Terbutaline Sulfate *on page 726*

Britiazim® *see* Diltiazem *on page 287*

BRL 43694 *see* Granisetron *on page 388*

Bromarest® [OTC] *see* Brompheniramine Maleate *on next page*

Brombay® [OTC] *see* Brompheniramine Maleate *on next page*

Bromides

Commonly Found in Sodium, potassium, and ammonium bromide; also in multiple medications as salt form of drug; dextromethorphan hydrobromide, homatropine hydrobromide, neostigmine, potassium, propantheline, pyridostigmine, quinine hydrobromide, scopolamine hydrobromide; although this source of bromism has been rare in the U.S. since 1974.

Mechanism of Action Central nervous system depressant

Adverse Reactions

Central nervous system: Headache, slurred speech, hallucinations, retrograde amnesia

Dermatologic: Papules, erythematous pustular usually on legs, acneiform eruptions

Endocrine & metabolic: Hypochloremia

Gastrointestinal: Nausea, vomiting, anorexia

Neuromuscular & skeletal: Hypo- or areflexia, tremors, hyperesthesia, clonus

Miscellaneous: Hypothyroidism, feces discoloration (black)

Signs & Symptoms of Acute Overdose Vomiting, ataxia, pseudotumor cerebri, nausea, hypothyroidism, dementia, sedation, photophobia, hallucinations, nystagmus, dementia, slurred speech, tremors, ataxia, amnesia, mydriasis, erythema multiforme, decreased anion gap; chronic toxicity often causes acne-like rash, papilledema, gastric bezoar

Toxicodynamics/Kinetics

Absorption: ≥90%, can form bezoar

Distribution: V_d: 0.35-0.48 L/kg

Protein binding: 0%

Half-life: 9-15 days

Elimination: Via tubular secretion, renal clearance: 26 mL/kg/day

Reference Range >50 mg/dL generally toxic; normal blood bromide levels: 30-40 mg/dL

Overdosage Treatment

Decontamination: Emesis or lavage/activated charcoal with cathartic may be useful for organic bromide compounds (carbromal)

Supportive therapy: Intravenous administration of sodium chloride or, if salt loading is not desirable, ammonium chloride (2-3 g orally 3-4 times/day); monitor for acidosis

Enhancement of elimination: Forced saline diuresis to maintain a urine flow of 3-5 mL/kg/hour; hemodialysis can reduce half-life to 1-2 hours; furosemide (1 mg/kg up to 40 mg) can be added to ensure adequate urine output

Test Interactions Causes negative anion gap

Diagnostic Tests/Procedures

Anion Gap, Blood *on page 1193*

Bromide, Urine *on page 1212*

Pregnancy Implications Can cause fetal CNS depression; microcephaly, heart malformations, intrauterine growth retardation, club foot, hypotonia, polydactyly have been documented

Additional Information Transient rise in concentrations are often seen in initial days of treatment; radiopaque

Specific References

Battin D and Varkey T, "Neuropsychiatric Manifestations of Bromide Ingestion," *Postgrad Med J*, 1982, 58:523-4.

Carney MW, "Five Cases of Bromism," *Lancet*, 1971, 2(723):523-4.

Iberti TJ, Patterson BK, and Fisher CJ Jr, "Prolonged Bromide Intoxication Resulting From a Gastric Bezoar," *Arch Intern Med*, 1984, 144(2):402-3.

Brompheniramine Maleate (brome fen ir' a meen mal' ee ate)

Related Information

H1-Antihistamine Comparison *on page 1649*

CAS Number 980-71-2

Brand Names Bromarest® [OTC]; Brombay® [OTC]; Bromphen® [OTC]; Brotane® [OTC]; Chlorphed® [OTC]; Codimal-A®; Cophene-B®; Dehist®; Diamine T.D.® [OTC]; Dimetane® [OTC]; Dimetapp®; Histaject®; Nasahist B®; ND-Stat®; Oraminic® II; Sinusol-B®; Veltane®

Synonyms Parabromdylamine

Use Perennial and seasonal allergic rhinitis and other allergic symptoms including rash

Mechanism of Action Competes with histamine for H_1-receptor sites on effector cells in the gastrointestinal tract, blood vessels, and respiratory tract

Adverse Reactions

Central nervous system: Paradoxical excitation, drowsiness, dizziness, acute dystonic reactions

Dermatologic: Rash

Gastrointestinal: Nausea, anorexia, dry mouth

Hematologic: Blood dyscrasias (chronic)

Ocular: Diplopia

Signs & Symptoms of Acute Overdose Dry mouth, mydriasis, agranulocytosis, neutropenia, CNS depression, flushing

Toxicodynamics/Kinetics

Onset of action: Begins within 15-30 minutes; maximal clinical effects seen within 3-9 hours

Duration: Varies with formulation, up to 48 hours

Absorption: Well absorbed from gastrointestinal tract after administration

Distribution: Wide throughout body

Metabolism: Extensive by the liver

Half-life: 12-34 hours

Time to peak serum concentration: Within 2-5 hours

Elimination: In urine as inactive metabolites; 2% fecal elimination

Usual Dosage

Oral:

- Children:
  - <6 years: 0.125 mg/kg/dose given every 6 hours; maximum: 6-8 mg/day
  - 6-12 years: 2-4 mg every 6-8 hours; maximum: 12-16 mg/day
- Adults: 4 mg every 4-6 hours or 8 mg of sustained release form every 8-12 hours or 12 mg of sustained release every 12 hours; maximum: 24 mg/day

I.M., I.V., S.C.:

- Children <12 years: 0.5 mg/kg/24 hours divided every 6-8 hours
- Adults: 10 mg every 6-12 hours, maximum: 40 mg/24 hours

Contraindications Narrow-angle glaucoma, bladder neck obstruction, symptomatic prostate hypertrophy, asthmatic attacks, and stenosing peptic ulcer, hypersensitivity to brompheniramine or any component

Warnings Use with caution in patients with heart disease, hypertension, thyroid disease, and asthma

Dosage Forms

Elixir: 2 mg/5 mL with alcohol 3% (120 mL, 480 mL, 4000 mL)

Injection: 10 mg/mL (10 mL)

Tablet: 4 mg, 8 mg, 12 mg

Tablet, sustained release: 8 mg, 12 mg

(Continued)

Brompheniramine Maleate *(Continued)*

Stability Solutions may crystallize if stored below 0°C, crystals will dissolve when warmed

Reference Range Average steady-state concentrations: 18-22 ng/mL

Overdosage Treatment There is no specific treatment for an antihistamine overdose, however, most of its clinical toxicity is due to anticholinergic effects. Anticholinesterase inhibitors may be useful by reducing acetylcholinesterase. Anticholinesterase inhibitors include physostigmine, neostigmine, pyridostigmine and edrophonium. For anticholinergic overdose with severe life-threatening symptoms, physostigmine 1-2 mg (0.5 or 0.02 mg/kg for children) I.V., slowly may be given to reverse these effects.

Drug Interactions CNS depressants, MAO inhibitors

Pregnancy Risk Factor C

Patient Information Avoid alcohol; take with food or milk; swallow whole, do not crush or chew

Nursing Implications Raise bed rails, institute safety measures, aid patient with ambulation

Additional Information Causes less drowsiness than some antihistamines

Specific References

Lin CC, Kim HK, Lim J, et al, "Steady-State Bioavailability of Dexbrompheniramine and Pseudoephedrine From a Repeat-Action Combination Tablet," *J Pharm Sci*, 1985, 74(1):25-8.

Bromphen® [OTC] *see* Brompheniramine Maleate *on previous page*

Bronkodyl® *see* Theophylline *on page 735*

Bronocozina® *see* Zipeprol Hydrochloride *on page 813*

Bronx® *see* Zipeprol Hydrochloride *on page 813*

Brotane® [OTC] *see* Brompheniramine Maleate *on previous page*

Brumolin *see* Warfarin Sodium *on page 800*

BTC 50 *see* Benzalkonium Chloride *on page 147*

Bucladin®-S Softab® *see* Buclizine Hydrochloride *on this page*

Buclizine Hydrochloride (byoo' kli zeen)

CAS Number 129-74-8; 82-95-1

Brand Names Aphilan R®; Bucladin®-S Softab®

Use Prevention and treatment of motion sickness; symptomatic treatment of vertigo; adjunctive therapy for migraine headache

Mechanism of Action Buclizine acts centrally to suppress nausea and vomiting. It is a piperazine antihistamine closely related to cyclizine and meclizine. It also has CNS depressant, anticholinergic, antispasmodic, and local anesthetic effects, and suppresses labyrinthine activity and conduction in vestibular-cerebellar nerve pathways.

Adverse Reactions

Cardiovascular: Hypotension, palpitations

Central nervous system: Sedation, dizziness, paradoxical excitation, fatigue, insomnia

Gastrointestinal: Nausea, vomiting

Genitourinary: Urinary retention

Neuromuscular & skeletal: Tremors

Ocular: Blurred vision

Signs & Symptoms of Acute Overdose CNS stimulation or CNS depression; overdose may result in death in infants and children; facial flushing, insomnia, mydriasis

Usual Dosage Adults: Oral:

Motion sickness (prophylaxis): 50 mg 30 minutes prior to traveling; may repeat 50 mg after 4-6 hours

Vertigo: 50 mg twice daily, up to 150 mg/day

Contraindications Known hypersensitivity to buclizine

Dosage Forms Tablet, chewable: 50 mg

Overdosage Treatment There is no specific treatment for an antihistamine overdose, however, most of its clinical toxicity is due to anticholinergic effects. Anticholinesterase inhibitors may be useful by reducing acetylcholinesterase. Anticholinesterase inhibitors include physostigmine, neostigmine, pyridostigmine and edrophonium. For anticholinergic overdose with severe life-threatening symptoms, physostigmine 1-2 mg (0.5 or 0.02 mg/kg for children) I.V., slowly may be given to reverse these effects.

Pregnancy Risk Factor C

Patient Information May cause drowsiness

Nursing Implications Bucladin®-S Softab® may be chewed, swallowed whole, or allowed to dissolve in mouth

Specific References

Atkinson R and Appenzeller O, "Headache," *Postgrad Med J*, 1984, 60(710):841-6.

Bufferin® [OTC] *see* Aspirin *on page 133*

Bumetanide (byoo met' a nide)

CAS Number 28395-03-1

Brand Names Bumex®; Burinex®; Farmadiuril®; Fontego®; Fordiuran®

Use Management of edema secondary to congestive heart failure or hepatic or renal disease including nephrotic syndrome; may also be used alone or in combination with antihypertensives in the treatment of hypertension; can be used in furosemide-allergic patients; (1 mg is equivalent to 40 mg furosemide)

Mechanism of Action Inhibits reabsorption of sodium and chloride in the ascending loop of Henle and distal renal tubule, interfering with the chloride-binding cotransport system, thus causing increased excretion of water, sodium, chloride, magnesium, and calcium

Adverse Reactions

Cardiovascular: Hypotension
Central nervous system: Dizziness, asthenia, headache, encephalopathy
Endocrine & metabolic: Hyperglycemia, azotemia, hypokalemia, hypochloremia
Gastrointestinal: Cramps, nausea, vomiting
Genitourinary: Decreased uric acid excretion
Hepatic: Alteration of liver function test results
Renal: Serum creatinine (increased)

Signs & Symptoms of Acute Overdose Nausea, vomiting, Stevens-Johnson syndrome, diarrhea, hyponatremia, hypomagnesemia, hypokalemia, hyperuricemia, asterixis, dermatitis, xerostomia, chest pain, electrolyte depletion, volume depletion, hyperglycemia, leukopenia, neutropenia, agranulocytosis, granulocytopenia

Toxicodynamics/Kinetics

Onset of effect:
- Oral, I.M.: 30-60 minutes
- I.V.: Within a few minutes

Duration: 6 hours
Distribution: V_d: 13-25 L/kg
Protein binding: 95%
Metabolism: Partial, occurs in the liver
Bioavailability: Oral: 80% to 95%
Half-life:
- Infants <6 months: Possibly 2.5 hours
- Adults: 1-1.5 hours

Elimination: Majority of unchanged drug and metabolites excreted in urine

Usual Dosage

Children:
- <6 months: Dose not established
- >6 months:
  - Oral: Initial: 0.015 mg/kg/dose once daily or every other day; maximum dose: 0.1 mg/kg/day
  - I.M., I.V.: Dose not established

Adults:
- Oral: 0.5-2 mg/dose 1-2 times/day; maximum: 10 mg/day
- I.M., I.V.: 0.5-1 mg/dose; maximum: 10 mg/day
- Continuous I.V. infusions of 0.9-1 mg/hour may be more effective than bolus dosing

Administration Give I.V. slowly, over 1-2 minutes

Contraindications Hypersensitivity to bumetanide or any component, in anuria or increasing azotemia, severe fluid/electrolyte imbalance, hepatic failure, oliguria

Warnings Loop diuretics are potent diuretics; excess amounts can lead to profound diuresis with fluid and electrolyte loss; close medical supervision and dose evaluation is required

Dosage Forms

Injection: 0.25 mg/mL (2 mL, 4 mL, 10 mL)
Tablet: 0.5 mg, 1 mg, 2 mg

Stability I.V. infusion solutions should be used within 24 hours after preparation

Reference Range Effective plasma level: 40-80 ng/mL

Overdosage Treatment

Decontamination: Activated charcoal with cathartic
Supportive therapy: Hydration with 0.9% saline

Test Interactions Increased BUN, creatinine, ammonia (B), amylase (S), glucose, uric acid (S); decreased sodium, calcium, chloride, potassium

Drug Interactions Allergy to sulfonamides may result in cross-hypersensitivity to bumetanide; decreased blood pressure, when used with other antihypertensive

(Continued)

Bumetanide *(Continued)*

agents, may need to decrease dose of one or both agents; indomethacin may decrease bumetanide's effect; NSAIDs ↓ antihypertensive response

Pregnancy Risk Factor C

Monitoring Parameters Blood pressure, serum electrolytes, renal function, uric acid levels

Patient Information May be taken with food or milk; get up slowly from a lying or sitting position to minimize dizziness, lightheadedness, or fainting; also use extra care when exercising, standing for long periods of time, and during hot weather

Nursing Implications Be alert to complaints about hearing difficulty

Additional Information Patients with impaired hepatic function must be monitored carefully, often requiring reduced doses; larger doses may be necessary in patients with impaired renal function to obtain the same therapeutic response; can cause elevation of parathyroid hormone; patients allergic to sulfonamides may show allergy to bumetanide

Specific References

Ward A and Heel RC, "Bumetanide: A Review of Its Pharmacodynamic and Pharmacokinetic Properties and Therapeutic Use," *Drugs*, 1984, 28(5):426-64.

Bumex® *see* Bumetanide *on previous page*

Bupivacaine Hydrochloride (byoo piv' a kane)

CAS Number 2180-92-9; 14252-80-3; 18010-40-7

Brand Names Carbostesin®; Marcaine®; Sensorcaine®

Use Local anesthetic (injectable) for peripheral nerve block, infiltration, sympathetic block, caudal or epidural block, retrobulbar block

Mechanism of Action Blocks both the initiation and conduction of nerve impulses by decreasing the neuronal membrane's permeability to sodium ions, which results in inhibition of depolarization with resultant blockade of conduction; a group II (amide) anesthetic

Adverse Reactions

Cardiovascular: Cardiac arrest, hypotension, bradycardia, palpitation
Central nervous system: Convulsions, restlessness, anxiety, dizziness, asthenia
Gastrointestinal: Nausea, vomiting
Ocular: Blurred vision, diplopia
Otic: Ototoxicity, tinnitus
Respiratory: Apnea

Signs & Symptoms of Acute Overdose Cardiac depression, depression, nystagmus, ptosis, hypoglycemia, disorientation, myopathy, lightheadedness, seizures, cardiac arrest, cyanosis, ototoxicity; tinnitus, coma

Toxicodynamics/Kinetics

Onset of action: Dependent on route administered, but generally occurs within 4-10 minutes
Duration: 1.5-8.5 hours
Absorption: Complete systemic; rate influenced by site and route of administration, total dosage, administered, physical character of individual agent, and whether or not a vasoconstrictor is used concurrently
Distribution: V_d: 0.4-1 L/kg
Protein binding: 82% to 95% to alpha$_1$-acid glycoprotein
Metabolism: Liver metabolized to pipecolylxylidine
Half-life: Age-dependent
  Neonates: 8.1 hours
  Adults: 1.5-5.5 hours
Time to peak serum concentration: Usually 10-30 minutes; dependent upon factors affecting rate of absorption, may occur 1-2 minutes after intravascular or transtracheal injection
Elimination: Small amount (~6%) excreted in urine

Usual Dosage Dose varies with procedure, depth of anesthesia, vascularity of tissues, duration of anesthesia and condition of patient. Metabisulfites (in epinephrine-containing injection); do not use solutions containing preservatives for caudal or epidural block.

Caudal block (with or without epinephrine):
  Children: 1-3.7 mg/kg
  Adults: 15-30 mL of 0.25% or 0.5%

Epidural block (other than caudal block):
  Children: 1.25 mg/kg/dose
  Adults: 10-20 mL of 0.25% or 0.5%

Peripheral nerve block: 5 mL dose of 0.25% or 0.5% (12.5-25 mg); maximum: 2.5 mg/kg (plain); 3 mg/kg (with epinephrine); up to a maximum of 400 mg/day

Sympathetic nerve block: 20-50 mL of 0.25% (no epinephrine) solution

Contraindications Hypersensitivity to bupivacaine hydrochloride or any component, para-aminobenzoic acid or parabens; contraindicated in obstetrical paracervical block

Warnings Convulsions due to systemic toxicity leading to cardiac arrest have been reported, presumably following unintentional intravascular injection; use with caution in patients with liver disease. Some commercially available formulations contain sodium metabisulfite, which may cause allergic-type reactions. Pending further data, should not be used in children <12 years of age and the solution for spinal anesthesia should not be used in children <18 years of age. Do not use solutions containing preservatives for caudal or epidural block.

Dosage Forms Injection:

Bupivacaine:

Preservative free: 0.25% [2.5 mg/mL]; 0.5% [5 mg/mL]; 0.75% [7.5 mg/mL]

With preservative: 0.25% [2.5 mg/mL]; 0.5% [5 mg/mL]

Bupivacaine and epinephrine [1:200,000]:

Preservative free: 0.25% [2.5 mg/mL]; 0.5% [5 mg/mL]; 0.75% [7.5 mg/mL]

With preservative: 0.25% [2.5 mg/mL]; 0.5% [5 mg/mL]

Bupivacaine in dextrose [8.25%] (spinal): Preservative free: 0.75% [7.5 mg/mL]

Stability Solutions with epinephrine should be protected from light

Reference Range Therapeutic plasma levels: <3 μg/mL

Overdosage Treatment Supportive therapy: Treatment is primarily symptomatic and supportive. Termination of anesthesia by pneumatic tourniquet inflation should be attempted when the agent is administered by infiltration or regional injection. Seizures commonly respond to diazepam or lorazepam, while hypotension responds to I.V. fluids and Trendelenburg positioning. Bradyarrhythmias (when the heart rate is less than 60) can be treated with I.V., or S.C. atropine 15 mcg/kg. With the development of metabolic acidosis, I.V. sodium bicarbonate 0.5-2 mEq/kg and ventilatory assistance should be instituted.

Drug Interactions Vasopressors, ergot-type oxytocics, MAO inhibitors, TCAs, phenothiazines; ranitidine and cimetidine prolong bupivacaine's duration of action

Pregnancy Risk Factor C

Pregnancy Implications Can result in fetal bradycardia and fetal death

Monitoring Parameters Heart rate, blood pressure, respiratory rate; monitor fetal heart rate during paracervical anesthesia

Patient Information Do not chew food in anesthetized region to prevent traumatizing tongue, lip or buccal mucosa; single dose is usually sufficient in most applications

Additional Information Metabisulfites (in epinephrine-containing injection); do not use solutions containing preservatives for caudal or epidural block

Specific References

Lehmann LJ and Pallares VS, "Subdural Injection of a Local Anesthetic With Steroids: Complication of Epidural Anesthesia," *South Med J*, 1995, 88:467-9.

Long WB, Rosenblum S, and Grady IP, "Successful Resuscitation of Bupivacaine-Induced Cardiac Arrest Using Cardiopulmonary Bypass," *Anesth Analg*, 1989, 69(3):403-6.

Scott DB, Lee A, Fagan D, et al, "Acute Toxicity of Ropivacaine Compared With That of Bupivacaine," *Anesth Analg*, 1989, 69(5):563-9.

Tuominen MK, Pere P, and Rosenberg PH, "Unintentional Arterial Catheterization and Bupivacaine Toxicity Associated With Continuous Interscalene Brachial Plexus Block," *Anesthesiology*, 1991, 75(2):356-8.

Buprenex® *see* Buprenorphine Hydrochloride *on this page*

Buprenorphine Hydrochloride (byoo pre nor' feen)

CAS Number 52485-79-7; 53152-21-9

Brand Names Buprenex®

Use Management of moderate to severe pain

Mechanism of Action Opiate agonist/antagonist that produces analgesia by binding to kappa and mu opiate receptors in the CNS

Adverse Reactions

Cardiovascular: hypotension

Central nervous system: Drowsiness, psychosis, dizziness, headache, euphoria, slurred speech, malaise, dysphoria, hallucinations

Dermatologic: Allergic dermatitis

Gastrointestinal: Vomiting, nausea

Genitourinary: Urinary retention

Neuromuscular & skeletal: Paresthesia

Ocular: Blurred vision, miosis

Respiratory: Apnea, respiratory depression

Miscellaneous: Porphyrinogenic

Signs & Symptoms of Acute Overdose CNS depression, dysphoria, depression, pinpoint pupils, hypotension, bradycardia

Toxicodynamics/Kinetics

Onset of analgesia: I.M.: Within 10-30 minutes

(Continued)

Buprenorphine Hydrochloride *(Continued)*

Duration: Dose related; from 7 hours (1 mg total dose) to 24 hours (7 mg total dose)
Absorption:
I.M., S.C.: 90% to 100%
Sublingual: 31%
Distribution:
Children: V_d: 68.5 L
Adults: V_d: 97-187 L
Protein binding: 96%
Metabolism: Mainly in the liver; undergoes extensive first-pass metabolism to norbuprenorphine
Half-life: 2.2-3 hours
Elimination: 70% excreted in feces via bile and 20% in urine as unchanged drug

Usual Dosage I.M., slow I.V.:
Children ≥13 years and Adults: 0.3-0.6 mg every 6 hours as needed
Elderly: 0.15 mg every 6 hours; elderly patients are more likely to suffer from confusion and drowsiness compared to younger patients
Long-term use is not recommended
Maximum survivable dose: 16 mg

Contraindications Hypersensitivity to buprenorphine or any component

Warnings If used in narcotic dependent patients, may cause withdrawal effects; may increase cerebrospinal fluid pressure, use with caution in head injuries; can produce change in consciousness which hampers patient evaluation; naloxone may not be effective in reversing apnea; use with caution in the elderly, debilitated hypothyroidism, Addison's disease, prostatic hypertrophy; can increase intracholedochal pressure

Dosage Forms Injection: 0.3 mg/mL (1 mL)

Stability Protect from excessive heat or light

Reference Range I.V. dose of 0.3 mg results in a plasma buprenorphine level of 0.5 μg/L

Overdosage Treatment
Decontamination: Lavage/activated charcoal with cathartic for oral ingestion
Supportive therapy: Naloxone in large doses (5-10 mg) and/or a continuous infusion may be necessary to reverse respiratory depression

Antidote(s)
Naloxone Hydrochloride *on page 1447*

Test Interactions ↑ amylase, lipase

Drug Interactions Increased toxicity: Barbiturates, opiates, guanabenz, MAO inhibitors, biperiden, benzodiazepines (↑ CNS and respiratory depression); use with ketorolac (I.M.) with epidural buprenorphine can cause respiratory depression

Pregnancy Risk Factor C

Monitoring Parameters Pain relief, respiratory and mental status, blood pressure

Patient Information May cause drowsiness; avoid alcoholic beverages; may be habit forming

Nursing Implications Gradual withdrawal of drug is necessary to avoid withdrawal symptoms

Additional Information Buprenorphine 0.3 mg = morphine 10 mg = meperidine 75 mg; has longer duration of action than either agent

Specific References
Gal TJ, "Naloxone Reversal of Buprenorphine-Induced Respiratory Depression," *Clin Pharmacol Ther*, 1989, 45(1):66-71.
Jain PN and Shah SC, "Respiratory Depression Following Combination of Epidural Buprenorphine and Intramuscular Ketorolac," *Anaesthesia*, 1993, 48(10):898-9.
Mac Evilly M and O'Carroll C, "Hallucinations After Epidural Buprenorphine," *Br Med J*, 1989, 298(6678):928-9.

Bupropion (byoo proe' pee on)

Related Information
Antidepressant Agents Comparison *on page 1639*
Therapeutic Drugs Associated With Hallucinations *on page 1558-1559*

CAS Number 31677-93-7; 34911-55-2

Brand Names Wellbutrin®

Synonyms Amfebutamone

Use Treatment of depression

Mechanism of Action Bupropion is an antidepressant structurally different from all other previously marketed antidepressants; like other antidepressants the mechanism of bupropion's activity is not fully understood; the drug is a weak blocker of serotonin and norepinephrine re-uptake, inhibits neuronal dopamine re-uptake and is not a monoamine oxidase A or B inhibitor

Adverse Reactions
Cardiovascular: Hypertension

Central nervous system: Agitation, insomnia, seizures (0.5%), psychosis, fever, chills, headache, visual hallucinations, restlessness
Dermatologic: Pruritus
Endocrine & metabolic: Syndrome of inappropriate antidiuretic hormone
Gastrointestinal: Appetite (increased), nausea, vomiting, dry mouth
Genitourinary: Impotence
Neuromuscular & skeletal: Tremors
Ocular: Blurred vision
Otic: Ototoxicity, tinnitus

Signs & Symptoms of Acute Overdose Labored breathing, Parkinson's-like symptoms, delirium, insomnia, impotence, salivation, leukopenia, mania, arched back, ataxia, seizures (dose related), muscle rigidity, hypokalemia, confusion, vomiting, sinus tachycardia, slurred speech, fever

Toxicodynamics/Kinetics
Onset of action: 1-3 weeks
Absorption: Rapid from the gastrointestinal tract
Distribution: V_d: 27-63 L/kg; readily crosses blood-brain barrier
Protein binding: 75% to 88%
Metabolism: Extensive in the liver to multiple metabolites of which M-chlorohippuric acid is the major metabolite
Half-life: 14 hours (prolonged in cirrhotic patients)
Time to peak serum concentration: Oral: Within 3 hours
Elimination:
Renal: <1% excreted in urine unchanged; >60% excreted as metabolites within 24 hours; >80% within 96 hours
Hepatic: <10% (bupropion and metabolites) in feces

Usual Dosage Adults: Oral: 100 mg 3 times/day; begin at 100 mg twice daily; may increase to a maximum dose of 450 mg/day

Dosing adjustment/comments in renal or hepatic impairment: Patients with renal or hepatic failure should receive a reduced dosage initially and be closely monitored

Contraindications Seizure disorder, prior diagnosis of bulimia or anorexia nervosa, known hypersensitivity to bupropion

Warnings Estimated seizure potential is increased many fold in doses in the 450-600 mg/day dosage; giving a single dose of 150 mg or less will lessen the seizure potential; use in patients with renal or hepatic impairment increases the possibilities of possible toxic effects

Dosage Forms Tablet: 75 mg, 100 mg

Reference Range Blood levels >170 ng/mL associated with seizures

Overdosage Treatment
Decontamination: Lavage (within 12 hours)/activated charcoal with cathartic
Supportive therapy: I.V. diazepam or lorazepam is useful in treating seizures
Enhancement of elimination: Multiple dose of activated charcoal may be useful

Test Interactions May lower serum potassium; fluoxetine can interfere with bupropion quantitation by HPLC analysis in plasma or serum

Diagnostic Tests/Procedures
Potassium, Blood *on page 1328*

Drug Interactions Carbamazepine, phenytoin, cimetidine, phenobarbital, levodopa, MAO inhibitors

Pregnancy Risk Factor B

Pregnancy Implications Crosses the placenta; a study of one subject demonstrated that bupropion and its metabolites pass into breast milk

Monitoring Parameters Cardiac/neurological status

Patient Information Take in equally divided doses 3-4 times/day to minimize the risk of seizures; avoid alcohol

Nursing Implications Be aware that drug may cause seizures

Additional Information Does not have adverse anticholinergic effects; voluntarily withdrawn in 1986; reintroduced in 1989

Specific References
Davidson J, "Seizures and Bupropion: A Review," *J Clin Psychiatry*, 1989, 50(7):256-61.
Jennison TA, Brown P, Crossett J, et al, "A High-Performance Liquid Chromatographic Method for Quantitating Bupropion in Human Plasma or Serum," *J Anal Toxicol*, 1995, 19:69-72.
Van Wyck FJ, Manberg PJ, Miller LL, et al, "Overview of Clinically Significant Adverse Reactions to Bupropion," *J Clin Psychiatry*, 1983, 44(5 Pt 2):191-6.

Burinex® *see* Bumetanide *on page 167*
Buscapina® *see* Scopolamine *on page 691*
BuSpar® *see* Buspirone Hydrochloride *on this page*

Buspirone Hydrochloride (byoo spye' rone)

CAS Number 33386-08-2; 36505-84-7

Brand Names Bespar®; BuSpar®

Use Management of anxiety

(Continued)

Buspirone Hydrochloride *(Continued)*

Mechanism of Action Selectively antagonizes CNS serotonin 5-HT_1A receptors without affecting benzodiazepine-GABA receptors; an azaspirodecanedione derivative with lower potential for addition or sedation than other anxiolytics

Adverse Reactions

Cardiovascular: Bradycardia

Central nervous system: Sedation, disorientation, excitation, dizziness, dysphoria, extrapyramidal signs, lightheadedness, panic attacks, mania, fever, headache, ataxia

Dermatologic: Rash

Gastrointestinal: Nausea, vomiting, diarrhea, flatulence

Genitourinary: Urinary frequency

Hematologic: Leukopenia, eosinophilia

Hepatic: Elevated liver function tests

Neuromuscular & skeletal: Paresthesia

Ocular: Miosis

Respiratory: Nasal congestion

Signs & Symptoms of Acute Overdose Dizziness, drowsiness, depression, dysphoria, hyperprolactinemia, dry mouth, pinpoint pupils, memory loss, lightheadedness, extrapyramidal reaction, nausea, vomiting, bradycardia, seizures, leukopenia, neutropenia, agranulocytosis, granulocytopenia

Toxicodynamics/Kinetics

Onset of action: May require 1-2 weeks; because buspirone does not cause muscle relaxation or significant sedation, patient may not immediately notice effects of medication

Absorption: Rapid and complete from gastrointestinal tract

Distribution: V_d: 433 L/kg

Protein binding: 95%

Metabolism: In the liver by oxidation and undergoes extensive first-pass metabolism

Bioavailability: Extensive first-pass metabolism limits it

Half-life: 2-3 hours

Time to peak serum concentration: Within 40-60 minutes

Elimination:

Renal: 29% to 63% excreted in urine within 24 hours primarily as metabolites; clearance: 2.2 L/minute

Fecal: 18% to 38% excreted

Studies in the elderly found no significant changes in pharmacokinetic parameters

Usual Dosage Adults: Oral: 15 mg/day (5 mg 3 times/day); may increase in increments of 5 mg/day every 2-4 days to a maximum of 60 mg/day

Dosing adjustment in renal or hepatic impairment: Probably necessary

Contraindications Hypersensitivity to buspirone or any component

Warnings Safety and efficacy not established in children <18 years of age; avoid alcoholic beverages; causes less sedation than other anxiolytics, but patients should be cautioned about driving until they are certain buspirone does not affect them adversely; use in hepatic or renal impairment is not recommended

Dosage Forms Tablet: 5 mg, 10 mg

Reference Range Peak plasma levels ≤6 ng/mL noted up to 90 minutes after a 20 mg dose

Overdosage Treatment

Decontamination: Lavage/activated charcoal with cathartic

Supportive therapy: There is no known antidote for buspirone and most therapies are supportive and symptomatic in nature; diazepam or lorazepam may be used for seizures

Enhancement of elimination: Multiple dosing of activated charcoal would not be expected to be useful

Test Interactions Increases AST, ALT

Diagnostic Tests/Procedures

Liver Profile *on page 1286*

Drug Interactions MAO inhibitors, cimetidine, alcohol, highly protein bound drugs, haloperidol; metabolism is slowed with fluoxetine

Pregnancy Risk Factor B

Monitoring Parameters Mental status, neurologic status at least 6 hours, liver function tests

Patient Information May cause drowsiness or vertigo; take with food; report any change in senses (ie, smelling, hearing, vision); cautious use with alcohol is recommended; takes 2-3 weeks to see the full effect of this medication

Nursing Implications Monitor patient's mental status and for benzodiazepine withdrawal; food may increase the bioavailability of the drug

Additional Information Has shown little potential for abuse; related to ipsapirone; avoid when breast-feeding; unpleasant taste; buspirone (15-60 mg/day) may be useful in treatment of sexual dysfunction during treatment with a selective serotonin reuptake inhibitor

Specific References

Fanciullacci M, Sicuteri R, Alessandri M, et al, "Buspirone, But Not Sumatriptan, Induces Miosis in Humans: Relevance for a Serotoninergic Pupil Control," *Clin Pharmacol Ther*, 1995, 57:349-55.

Goetz CM, Krenzelok EP, Lopez G, et al, "Buspirone Toxicity: A Prospective Study," *Vet Hum Toxicol*, 1989, 31:371.

LeJoyeux M, et al, "Serotonin Syndrome: Incidence, Symptoms, and Treatment," *CNS Drugs*, 1994, 2:132-43.

McIvor RJ and Sinanan K, "Buspirone-Induced Mania," *Br J Psychiatry*, 1991, 158:136-7.

Norden MJ, "Buspirone Treatment of Sexual Dysfunction Associated With Selective Serotonin Re-Uptake Inhibitors," *Depression*, 1994, 2:109-12.

Preskorn SH, "Recent Pharmacologic Advances in Antidepressant Therapy for the Elderly," *Am J Med*, 1993, 94(5A):2S-12S.

Tiller JW, Burrows GD, and O'Sullivan BT, "Buspirone Overdose," *Med J Aust*, 1989, 150(1):54-5.

Busulfan (byoo sul' fan)

Related Information

Drugs and Chemicals Proven to be Teratogenic in Humans *on page 1572-1575*

Toxicities of Chemotherapeutic Agents *on page 1631-1633*

CAS Number 55-98-1

Brand Names Misulban®; Myleran®

Synonyms Buzulfan

Use Chronic myelogenous leukemia and bone marrow disorders, such as polycythemia vera and myeloid metaplasia, conditioning regimens for bone marrow transplantation

Mechanism of Action Reacts with N-7 position of guanosine and interferes with DNA replication and transcription of RNA (an alkylating agent). Busulfan has a more marked effect on myeloid cells (and is, therefore, useful in the treatment of CML) than on lymphoid cells. The drug is also very toxic to hematopoietic stem cells (thus its usefulness in high doses in BMT preparative regimens). Busulfan exhibits little immunosuppressive activity. Interferes with the normal function of DNA by alkylation and cross-linking the strands of DNA.

Adverse Reactions

Central nervous system: Dizziness, seizures, generalized or myoclonic seizures and loss of consciousness have been associated with high-dose busulfan (4 mg/kg/day)

Dermatologic: Hyperpigmentation, alopecia, dermal irritant, rash

Endocrine & metabolic: Addison-like syndrome, hyperuricemia

Fertility/carcinogenesis: Sterility, ovarian suppression, amenorrhea, azoospermia, and testicular atrophy; malignant tumors have been reported in patients on busulfan therapy

Gastrointestinal: Nausea, vomiting, diarrhea, mucositis

Hematologic: Porphyria; myelosuppression with nadirs of 14-21 days for leukopenia and thrombocytopenia; anemia, severe pancytopenia, bone marrow depression; since this is a delayed effect (busulfan affects the stem cells), the drug should be discontinued temporarily at the first sign of a large or rapid fall in any blood element. Some patients may develop bone marrow fibrosis or chronic aplasia which is probably due to the busulfan toxicity. In large doses, busulfan is myeloablative and is used for this reason in BMT.

Hepatic: Hepatic dysfunction, hepatic veno-occlusive disease, elevated liver function tests

Ocular: Blurred vision, cataract formation

Renal: Hemorrhagic cystitis

Respiratory: After long-term or high-dose therapy, a syndrome known as busulfan lung may occur; this syndrome is manifested by a diffuse interstitial pulmonary fibrosis and persistent cough, fever, rales, and dyspnea; may be relieved by corticosteroids

Miscellaneous: Pericardial fibrosis

Signs & Symptoms of Acute Overdose CNS depression, erythema multiforme, hyperuricemia, cholestatic jaundice, seizures, sexual dysfunction, periarteritis nodosa, myoclonus, hematuria, leukopenia, neutropenia, cataract, agranulocytosis, granulocytopenia

Toxicodynamics/Kinetics

Absorption: Oral: Rapidly and well absorbed

Distribution: V_d: ~1 L/kg; distributes into the CSF and saliva with levels similar to plasma

Protein binding: ~14%

Metabolism: Extensive in the liver (may induce own metabolism)

Half-life: 2-3 hours

Time to peak serum concentration:

- Oral: Within 4 hours
- I.V.: Within 5 minutes

(Continued)

Busulfan *(Continued)*

Elimination: 10% to 50% excreted in urine as metabolites within 24 hours; clearance rate of 4.5 mL/minute/kg

Usual Dosage Refer to individual protocols

Children: Oral: 0.06-0.12 mg/kg/day or 1.8-4.6 mg/m²/day; titrate dosage to maintain leukocyte count about 20,000/mm³ (dosages >4 mg/day are especially likely to reduce the leukocyte count)

Adults:

Bone marrow transplantation: 1 mg/kg ideal body weight 4 times/day for 4 days (total dose: 16 mg/kg) or as per protocol

Remission induction of CML: Oral: 4-8 mg/day (may be as high as 12 mg/day); Maintenance doses: Controversial, range from 1-4 mg/day to 2 mg/week; treatment continued until WBC reaches 10,000-20,000 cells/mm³ at which time drug is discontinued; when WBC reaches 50,000/mm³, maintenance dose is resumed

Unapproved uses:

Polycythemia vera: 2-6 mg/day

Thrombocytosis: 4-6 mg/day

Contraindications Hypersensitivity to busulfan or any component; failure to respond to previous courses; should not be used in pregnancy or lactation

Warnings The U.S. Food and Drug Administration (FDA) currently recommends that procedures for proper handling and disposal of antineoplastic agents be considered. May induce severe bone marrow hypoplasia; reduce or discontinue dosage at first sign, as reflected by an abnormal decrease in any of the formed elements of the blood; use with caution in patients recently given other myelosuppressive drugs or radiation treatment. If white blood count is high, hydration and allopurinol should be employed to prevent hyperuricemia.

Dosage Forms Tablet: 2 mg

Reference Range Mean peak serum level of a busulfan dose of 1 mg/kg is about 1080 ng/mL

Overdosage Treatment

Decontamination: Lavage/activated charcoal with cathartic

Enhancement of elimination: Multiple dosing of charcoal may be effective

Drug Interactions Thioguanine

Pregnancy Risk Factor D

Monitoring Parameters CBC with differential and platelet count, hemoglobin, liver function tests

Patient Information Watch for signs of bleeding; excellent oral hygiene is needed to minimize oral discomfort

Nursing Implications Avoid I.M. injection if platelet count falls <100,000/mm³

Additional Information Moderately radiopaque

Specific References

Buggia I, Locatelli F, Regazzi MB, et al, "Busulfan," *Ann Pharmacother*, 1994, 28(9):1055-62.

Marcus RE and Goldman JM, "Convulsions Due to High-Dose Busulphan," *Lancet*, 1984, 2(8417-18):1463.

Morris LE and Guthrie TH Jr, "Busulfan-Induced Hepatitis," *Am J Gastroenterol*, 1988, 83(6):682-3.

Butazolidin® *see* Phenylbutazone *on page 620*

Butorphanol Tartrate (byoo tor' fa nole)

CAS Number 42408-82-2; 58786-99-5

Brand Names Stadol®; Stadol® NS; Verstadol®

Use Management of moderate to severe pain

Mechanism of Action Mixed narcotic agonist-antagonist with central analgesic actions; binds to opiate receptors in the CNS (limbic system), causing inhibition of ascending pain pathways, altering the perception of and response to pain; produces generalized CNS depression

Adverse Reactions

Cardiovascular: Hypotension, flushing of the face, hypertension, bradycardia or tachycardia, hypotension

Central nervous system: CNS depression, anxiety, drowsiness, dizziness, lightheadedness, headache, malaise, restlessness, night terrors, asthenia, mental depression, confusion, hallucinations, false sense of well being, paradoxical CNS stimulation

Dermatologic: Skin rash, pruritus

Gastrointestinal: Anorexia, nausea, vomiting, stomach cramps, constipation, dry mouth

Genitourinary: Decreased urination, painful urination

Ocular: Blurred vision

Otic: Ototoxicity, tinnitus

Respiratory: Apnea, respiratory depression, dyspnea, troubled breathing

Miscellaneous: Dependence with prolonged use, increased sweating

Signs & Symptoms of Acute Overdose Coma, diplopia, lightheadedness, night terrors, euphoria, disorientation, pulmonary hypertension, biliary tract spasm, confusion

Toxicodynamics/Kinetics

Peak effect:

Oral: 1-1.5 hours

I.M.: Within 30-60 minutes

I.V.: Within 4-5 minutes

Absorption: Rapidly and well absorbed

Protein binding: 83%

Metabolism: In the liver with extensive first-pass effect

Half-life: 2.5-4 hours

Elimination: Excreted primarily in urine; 11% to 14% excreted in bile

Usual Dosage Adults:

I.M.: 1-4 mg every 3-4 hours as needed

I.V.: 0.5-2 mg every 3-4 hours as needed

Nasal spray: Headache: 1 spray in 1 nostril; if adequate pain relief is not achieved within 60-90 minutes, an additional 1 spray in 1 nostril may be given (each spray gives ~1 mg of butorphanol)

Dosing adjustment in renal impairment:

Cl_{cr} 10-50 mL/minute: Administer 75% of dose

Cl_{cr} <10 mL/minute: Administer 50% of dose

Contraindications Hypersensitivity to butorphanol or any component; avoid use in opiate-dependent patients who have not been detoxified, may precipitate opiate withdrawal

Warnings Use with caution in patients with hepatic/renal dysfunction

Dosage Forms

Injection: 1 mg/mL (1 mL); 2 mg/mL (1 mL, 2 mL, 10 mL)

Nasal spray: 10 mg/mL [14-15 doses] (2.5 mL)

Stability Store at room temperature, protect from freezing; **incompatible** when mixed in the same syringe with diazepam, dimenhydrinate, methohexital, pentobarbital, secobarbital, thiopental

Reference Range 0.7-1.5 ng/mL

Overdosage Treatment Supportive therapy: Naloxone hydrochloride (0.4-2 mg I.V., S.C., or through an endotracheal tube); a continuous infusion (at ⅔ the response dose/hour) may be required

Antidote(s)

Naloxone Hydrochloride *on page 1447*

Drug Interactions Increased toxicity: CNS depressants, phenothiazines, barbiturates, skeletal muscle relaxants, alfentanil, guanabenz, MAO inhibitors

Pregnancy Risk Factor B (D if used for prolonged periods or in high doses at term)

Pregnancy Implications Distributes into breast milk; crosses the placenta; sinusoidal fetal heart rate pattern described in two cases

Monitoring Parameters Pain relief, respiratory and mental status, blood pressure; monitor for CNS, respiratory depression

Patient Information May cause drowsiness; avoid alcohol

Nursing Implications Raise bed rails; aid with ambulation

Specific References

Gaver RC, Vasiljev M, Wong H, et al, "Disposition of Parenteral Butorphanol in Man," *Drug Metab Dispos Biol Fate Chem*, 1980, 8(4):230-5.

Pachter IJ and Evens RP, "Butorphanol," *Drug Alcohol Depend*, 1985, 14(3-4):325-38.

Srinivas NR, et al, "Lack of Pharmacokinetic Interaction Between Butorphanol Tartrate Nasal Spray and Sumatriptan Succinate," *J Clin Pharmacol*, 1995, 35:432-7.

Buzulfan *see* Busulfan *on page 173*

BW-430-C *see* Lamotrigine *on page 459*

BW-825C *see* Acrivastine *on page 87*

C7E3 FAB *see* Abciximab *on page 77*

C7EC *see* Abciximab *on page 77*

Cafatine® *see* Ergotamine *on page 317*

Cafatine-PB® *see* Ergotamine *on page 317*

Cafergot® *see* Ergotamine *on page 317*

Cafetrate® *see* Ergotamine *on page 317*

Caffeine (kaf' een)

CAS Number 58-08-2; 69-22-7; 5743-12-4

Brand Names Coffee Break®; Durvitan®; No-Doz® [OTC]; Percoffedrinol N®; Percutafeine®; Pro-Plus®; Vivarin® [OTC]

(Continued)

Caffeine *(Continued)*

Synonyms Guaranine; 7,Methyltheophylline; Theine; 1,3,7-Trimethylxanthine

Use Central nervous system stimulant; treatment of idiopathic apnea of prematurity; has several advantages over theophylline in the treatment of neonatal apnea, half-life is about 3 times as long, allowing once daily dosing, drug levels do not need to be drawn at peak and trough; has a wider therapeutic window, allowing more room between an effective concentration and toxicity

Mechanism of Action Increases levels of 3-5-AMP by inhibiting phosphodiesterase; methyl xanthine, CNS stimulant which increases medullary respiratory center sensitivity to carbon dioxide, stimulates central inspiratory drive, and improves skeletal muscle contraction (diaphragmatic contractility)

Adverse Reactions

Cardiovascular: Flushing

Central nervous system: Headache, dizziness, delirium, hallucinations, insomnia, fasciculations

Dermatologic: Urticaria

Gastrointestinal: Gastritis

Ocular: Miosis

Renal: Diuresis (<250 mg/day)

Signs & Symptoms of Acute Overdose Tachycardia, tachycardia (ventricular), tremors, hyperthermia, insomnia, nausea, vomiting, muscle twitching, diarrhea, premature ventricular contractions, tinnitus, delirium, seizures, myoglobinuria, hypokalemia, hyponatremia, hyperglycemia, hypercholesterolemia, hallucinations, leukocytosis, rhabdomyolysis

Toxicodynamics/Kinetics

Distribution: V_d:

Neonates: 0.8-0.9 L/kg

Adults: 0.5-0.7 L/kg

Protein binding: 17%

Metabolism: Hepatic

Half-life:

Neonates: 60-100 hours

Adults: 3-6 hours

Time to peak serum concentration: Oral: Within 1-1.5 hours

Usual Dosage Apnea of prematurity: Oral:

Loading dose: 10-20 mg/kg as caffeine citrate (5-10 mg/kg as caffeine base). If theophylline has been administered to the patient within the previous 5 days, a full or modified loading dose (50% to 75% of a loading dose) may be given at the discretion of the physician.

Maintenance dose: 5-10 mg/kg/day as caffeine citrate (2.5-5 mg/kg/day as caffeine base) once daily starting 24 hours after the loading dose. Maintenance dose is adjusted based on patient's response, (efficacy and adverse effects), and serum caffeine concentrations.

Contraindications Hypersensitivity to caffeine or any component

Warnings Use with caution in patients with a history of peptic ulcer; avoid in patients with symptomatic cardiac arrhythmias; parenteral caffeine is only available in the United States as a sodium benzoate salt. Due to reports of sodium benzoate inducing kernicterus by displacement of bilirubin and causing the gasping syndrome in newborns, use should be avoided in neonates.

Dosage Forms Tablet: 65 mg [anhydrous caffeine 32.5 mg]

Reference Range

Therapeutic: 8-14 μg/mL for neonatal apnea

Toxic: >30 μg/mL

Fatal: >80 μg/mL

Overdosage Treatment

Decontamination: Lavage/activated charcoal with cathartic

Supportive therapy: Seizures can be treated with diazepam or lorazepam or sodium pentobarbital; esmolol can be helpful for tachyarrhythmia; ventricular dysrhythmias and tachycardia (ventricular) with aberrancy have been successfully treated with procainamide in an adult (400 mg I.V. bolus followed by a 2 mg/minute infusion)

Enhancement of elimination: Multiple dosing of activated charcoal may be useful; exchange transfusion (in the neonate) or charcoal hemoperfusion for 4-5 hours can be useful

Test Interactions ↑ uric acid (S), slight increase in urine levels of VMA, catecholamines, can cause false elevations of serum theophylline levels

Diagnostic Tests/Procedures

Caffeine, Blood *on page 1214*

Drug Interactions Enhances the positive cardiac inotropic and chronotropic effects of beta-adrenergic agonists; increases absorption of ergotamines; caffeine elimination is increased (half-life reduced) with concomitant administration of phenytoin; caffeine elimination is reduced by mexiletine, ciprofloxacin, enoxacin, pipemidic acid, oral contraceptives, cimetidine, terbinafine, idrocilamide

Pregnancy Risk Factor B

Pregnancy Implications Teratogenic effects in animal studies at caffeine doses >40 mg/day; association with increased rate of spontaneous abortion, low birthweight, and premature delivery; data is conflicting and no definitive association shown

Additional Information Coffee beans contain 1% to 2% caffeine; 40% of the bronchodilatory activity of theophylline; lithium blood levels increase during caffeine withdrawal; analgesia from transcutaneous electrical nerve stimulation may be lessened with concomitant caffeine use

Lethal dose: Oral: 150-200 mg/kg

Caffeine content:
- Stimulants: 75-200 mg
- Coffee (5 oz): 100-150 mg
- Cola drinks (6 oz): 35-55 mg
- Cold preparations: 30-75 mg
- Tea: 30-50 mg
- Chocolate bar: 25 mg
- Guarana (800 mg): 24-40 mg
- Cocoa (5 oz): 2-20 mg
- Chocolate milk (8 oz): 2-7 mg

Specific References

Banner W Jr and Czajka PA, "Acute Caffeine Overdose in the Neonate," *Am J Dis Child*, 1980, 134(5):495-8.

Curatolo PW and Robertson D, "The Health Consequences of Caffeine," *Ann Intern Med*, 1983, 98(Pt 1):641-53.

Dalvi RR, "Acute and Chronic Toxicity of Caffeine: A Review," *Vet Hum Toxicol*, 1986, 28(2):144-50.

Dietrich AM and Mortensen ME, "Presentation and Management of an Acute Caffeine Overdose," *Pediatr Emerg Care*, 1990, 6(4):296-8.

Eisele JW and Reay DT, "Deaths Related to Coffee Enemas," *JAMA*, 1980, 244(14):1608-9.

Marchand S, Li J, and Charest J, "Effects of Caffeine on Analgesia From Transcutaneous Electrical Nerve Stimulation," *N Engl J Med*, 1995, 333(5):325-6.

Mester R, Toren P, Mizrachi I, et al, "Caffeine Withdrawal Increases Lithium Blood Levels," *Biol Psychiatry*, 1995, 37:348-50.

Calabren® *see* Glyburide *on page 384*

Calan® *see* Verapamil Hydrochloride *on page 787*

Calcifediol *see* Vitamin D *on page 797*

Calciferol™ *see* Vitamin D *on page 797*

Calcimar® *see* Calcitonin *on this page*

Calciparine® Injection *see* Heparin *on page 398*

Calcitonin (kal si toe' nin)

CAS Number 47931-85-1; 12321-44-7; 9007-12-9; 60731-46-6

Brand Names Calcimar®; Cibacalcin®; Miacalcin®

Synonyms Calcitonin (Human); Calcitonin (Pork); Calcitonin (Salmon); Elcatonin; Salcatonin

Use

Calcitonin (salmon): Treatment of Paget's disease of bone and as adjunctive therapy for hypercalcemia; also used in postmenopausal osteoporosis, cholecalciferol (vitamin D_3) induced hypercalcemia

Calcitonin (human): Treatment of Paget's disease of bone

Mechanism of Action Structurally similar to human calcitonin; regulates serum calcium concentration along with vitamin D and parathyroid hormone; acts on bone as well as kidneys and gastrointestinal tract; directly inhibits osteoclastic bone resorption; promotes the renal excretion of calcium, phosphate, sodium, magnesium, and potassium by decreasing tubular reabsorption; increases the jejunal secretion of water, sodium, potassium, and chloride

Adverse Reactions

Cardiovascular: Flushing of the face, swelling

Central nervous system: Dizziness, headache, tingling of palms and soles, chills

Dermatologic: Rash

Endocrine & metabolic: Hypocalcemia, hypophosphatemia

Gastrointestinal: Nausea, vomiting, diarrhea, anorexia

Neuromuscular & skeletal: Weakness

Renal: Diuresis, hypercalciuria

Respiratory: Dyspnea, nasal congestion

Toxicodynamics/Kinetics

Onset of action: Within 15 minutes

Duration:

I.M., S.C.: 8-24 hours

(Continued)

Calcitonin *(Continued)*

I.V.: 30 minutes to 12 hours
Distribution: Does not cross into the placenta
Metabolism: Rapidly metabolized by the kidneys but also in blood and peripheral tissues
Half-life: S.C.: 1.2 hours
Time to peak serum concentration: Hypercalcemia: 2 hours
Elimination: Excreted as inactive metabolites in the urine

Usual Dosage Dosage for calcitonin salmon is expressed in international units (IU); dosage of calcitonin human is expressed in mg; dosage for children not established

Hepatic osteodystrophy:
- Infants: 5-7 mcg/kg/day
- Children and Adults: 20-100 mcg/kg/day or every other day, titrate to obtain normal serum calcium/phosphate levels

Calcitonin salmon:
- Skin test: 1 unit/0.1 mL intracutaneously on the inner aspect of the forearm
  - The skin test is 0.1 mL of 10 IU dilution of calcitonin (must be prepared) injected intradermally; observe injection site for 15 minutes for wheal or significant erythema
- Paget's disease: S.C.: 100 units/day
- Postmenopause osteoporosis: I.M., S.C.: 100 units/day (concomitant therapy with supplemental calcium and vitamin D is recommended)
- Hypercalcemia: I.M., S.C.: 4 units/kg every 12 hours, may increase to maximum of 8 units/kg every 6 hours

Calcitonin human: I.M., S.C.: Paget's disease: 0.5 mg/day initially; some patients require as little as 0.25 mg or 0.5 mg 2-3 times/week; some patients require up to 0.5 mg twice daily

Contraindications Hypersensitivity to salmon protein or gelatin diluent with the salmon product

Warnings A skin test should be performed prior to initiating therapy of calcitonin salmon; have epinephrine immediately available for a possible hypersensitivity reaction

Dosage Forms Injection:
- Human (Cibacalcin®): 0.5 mg/vial
- Salmon:
  - Calcimar®: 200 units/mL (2 mL)
  - Miacalcin®: 100 units/mL (1 mL)

Stability Refrigeration is recommended for calcitonin salmon, is stable for up to 2 weeks at room temperature; NS has been recommended for the dilution to prepare a skin test; protect from light; calcitonin human may be stored at room temperature

Reference Range Therapeutic: <19 pg/mL (SI: 19 ng/L) basal, depending on the assay

Overdosage Treatment Supportive therapy: Intravenous hydration; monitor urine flow and calcium and phosphorus level

Test Interactions Decreases calcium (S)

Pregnancy Risk Factor B

Monitoring Parameters Serum calcium and electrolytes

Nursing Implications I.M. route is preferred; skin test should be performed prior to administration of salmon calcitonin; refrigerate when volume exceeds 2 mL

Specific References

Bergqvist E, Sjoberg HE, Hjern B, et al, "Calcitonin in the Treatment of Hypercalcaemic Crisis," *Acta Med Scand*, 1972, 192(5):385-9.

Stevenson JC, "Current Management of Malignant Hypercalcemia," *Drugs*, 1988, 36(2):229-30.

Calcitonin (Human) *see* Calcitonin *on previous page*

Calcitonin (Pork) *see* Calcitonin *on previous page*

Calcitonin (Salmon) *see* Calcitonin *on previous page*

Calcitriol *see* Vitamin D *on page 797*

Calcium Channel Blocking Agents Comparison *see page 1646*

Calmaxid® *see* Nizatidine *on page 569*

Calmazine® *see* Trifluoperazine Hydrochloride *on page 769*

Calmotal® *see* Promazine Hydrochloride *on page 649*

Calm-X® [OTC] *see* Dimenhydrinate *on page 289*

2-Camphanone *see* Camphor *on next page*

Campho-Phenique® *see* Camphor-Phenol *on page 180*

Camphor

CAS Number 76-22-2; 464-49-3; 464-48-2; 21368-68-3

UN Number 2717

Brand Names Mentholatum® Vapor Rub; Vicks® Vaporub®; Vicks® Vaposteam®

Synonyms Anemone Camphor; 2-Camphanone; Formosa Camphor; Gum Camphor; Huile de Camphre; Kampfer; Laurel Camphor; Matricaria Camphor

Use Plasticizer, moth repellent, preservative in pharmaceuticals and cosmetics, in lacquers and varnishes, explosives, and pyrotechnics; used as an antipruritic, topical rubefacient, aphrodisiac, abortifacient, contraceptive, cold remedy, suppressor of lactation, and antiseptic; camphorated liniment or oil usually contains 20% camphor; camphor spirits usually 10%

Mechanism of Action Stimulant of cerebral cortex

Adverse Reactions

Cardiovascular: Tachycardia

Central nervous system: Headache, dizziness, delirium, seizures, coma, fasciculations

Gastrointestinal: Nausea, vomiting

Genitourinary: Albuminuria

Hepatic: Elevated liver function tests

Neuromuscular & skeletal: Myoclonus

Ocular: Mydriasis, strabismus

Respiratory: Tachypnea

Signs & Symptoms of Acute Overdose Convulsions may occur suddenly without warning or may be preceded by fasciculations, dementia, hyperventilation, mental confusion, irritability, tremors, neuromuscular hyperactivity, and jerky movements of extremities; seizures may be followed by coma and apnea. Vomiting may occur shortly after ingestion (a gastrointestinal irritant); hepatic transaminase may be mildly and briefly elevated; chronic ingestion may cause granulomatous hepatitis; distinctive oral odor may be apparent; tachycardia, CNS depression, renal failure.

Toxicodynamics/Kinetics

Absorption: Readily through skin and mucous membranes

Distribution: V_d: 2-4 L/kg

Protein binding: 61%

Metabolism: Rapidly oxidized and conjugated in liver; metabolites may accumulate in fat stores

Half-life: 93-167 minutes

Peak effect: 90 minutes

Elimination: Odor of camphor may appear in urine; excreted primarily in urine; can also be excreted through the lungs

Usual Dosage Minimum lethal dose: 1 g (50 mg/kg)

Contraindications Do not use in infants

Dosage Forms Translucent crystalline mass, blocks, or powder

Reference Range Levels >14.5 mg/L associated with seizures

Overdosage Treatment

Decontamination: Lavage/activated charcoal with cathartic; do not use an oil base cathartic

Supportive therapy: Treat seizures with benzodiazepines, phenytoin, or phenobarbital; if seizures are refractory, pentobarbital should be initiated; ventilatory support may be required; do not give alcohols, oils, or fats because this will increase absorption

Enhancement of elimination: Lipid hemoperfusion and resin hemoperfusion has been reported to decrease levels in patients with refractory seizures; hemodialysis is ineffective; charcoal hemoperfusion may be helpful, although not as clear a benefit as resin hemoperfusion; all of these techniques are somewhat controversial

Pregnancy Risk Factor C

Pregnancy Implications Crosses placenta and has been associated with one fetal death; three other cases report healthy outcomes

Monitoring Parameters Liver/renal function; monitor neurologic status

Additional Information Odor is aromatic and pungent; aromatic taste produces sensation of cold; may mimic Reye's syndrome

TLV-TWA: 5 ppm

IDLH: 200 mg/m^3

Specific References

Antman E, Jacob G, Volpe B, et al, "Camphor Overdosage. Therapeutic Considerations," *N Y State J Med*, 1978, 78(6):896-7.

Kopelman R, Miller S, Kelly R, et al, "Camphor Intoxication Treated by Resin Hemoperfusion," *JAMA*, 1979, 241(7):727-8.

Koppel C, Martens F, Schirop T, et al, "Hemoperfusion in Acute Camphor Poisoning," *Intensive Care Med*, 1988, 14(4):431-3.

Mascie-Taylor BH, Widdop B, and Davison AM, "Camphor Intoxication Treated by Charcoal Haemoperfusion," *Postgrad Med J*, 1981, 57(673):725-6.

Siegel E and Wason S, "Camphor Toxicity," *Pediatr Clin North Am*, 1986, 33(2):375-9.

(Continued)

Camphor *(Continued)*

Winter ML, Rice BS, and Snodgrass WR, "Seizures and Serum Camphor Concentration in Man," *Vet Hum Toxicol*, 1991, 33:375.

Camphorated Tincture of Opium *see* Paregoric *on page 595*

Camphor-Phenol (kam' for-fee' nole)

Brand Names Campho-Phenique®

Use Relief of dry, itching skin, cold sores

Adverse Reactions

Cardiovascular: Hypotension
Gastrointestinal: Nausea, vomiting
Hepatic: Elevated liver enzymes
Ocular: Mydriasis
Miscellaneous: Sweating

Signs & Symptoms of Acute Overdose Convulsions, hypotension, tachypnea, coma

Usual Dosage Topical: Apply as needed for dry skin

Dosage Forms Lotion, topical: Camphor 0.5%, menthol 0.5%, and phenol 0.5% in emollient base (240 mL)

Overdosage Treatment

Decontamination: Do **not** use castor oil or ipecac; lavage (within 2 hours); activated charcoal with cathartic may be useful

Dermal: Polyethylene glycol can be used to irrigate if phenol concentrations are over 5%

Oral: Dilute with milk or water

Supportive therapy: Treat seizures with lorazepam, diazepam, barbiturates, or phenytoin

Enhancement of elimination: Charcoal or resin hemoperfusion may be useful as is lipid-based dialysis (Klung plate dialyzer) (see Camphor monograph)

Pregnancy Risk Factor C

Pregnancy Implications Camphor can cause fetal death

Monitoring Parameters Liver/renal function; monitor neurologic status

Additional Information Usually formulation involves about 4% to 10% camphor and 2% to 5% phenol

Specific References

Gibson DE, Moore GP, and Pfaff JA, "Camphor Ingestion," *Am J Emerg Med*, 1989, 7(1):41-3.

Mascie-Taylor BH, Widdop B, and Davison AM, "Camphor Intoxication Treated by Charcoal Hemoperfusion," *Postgrad Med J*, 1981, 57(673):725-6.

Capastat® Sulfate *see* Capreomycin Sulfate *on this page*

Capitol® *see* Benzalkonium Chloride *on page 147*

Capoten® *see* Captopril *on next page*

Capozide® *see* Captopril and Hydrochlorothiazide *on page 183*

Capreomycin Sulfate (kap ree oh mye' sin)

CAS Number 11003-38-6; 1405-37-4

Brand Names Capastat® Sulfate; Ogostal®

Use In conjunction with at least one other antituberculosis agent in the treatment of tuberculosis

Mechanism of Action Polypeptide antibiotic; bacteriostatic

Adverse Reactions

Central nervous system: Dizziness, fever
Dermatologic: Rash
Endocrine & metabolic: Hypokalemia, hypomagnesemia
Hematologic: Eosinophilia, neutropenia, leukocytosis, thrombocytopenia
Local: Pain induration, bleeding at injection site
Ocular: Vision color changes (white tinge)
Otic: Ototoxicity, deafness, tinnitus
Renal: Nephrotoxicity
Miscellaneous: Feces discoloration (greenish gray)

Toxicodynamics/Kinetics

Half-life: 2.5 hours
Elimination: Renal (50% to 60%)

Usual Dosage I.M.:

Infants and Children: 15-20 mg/kg/day, up to 1 g/day maximum

Adults: 15-30 mg/kg/day up to 1 g/day for 60-120 days, followed by 1 g 2-3 times/week

Dosing interval in renal impairment: Cl_{cr} <10 mL/minute: Decrease dose to ~33% of usual and administer every 48 hours; consult manufacturer's guidelines for specific dosing recommendations

Contraindications Known hypersensitivity to capreomycin sulfate

Warnings Use of capreomycin in patients with renal insufficiency or pre-existing auditory impairment must be undertaken with great caution, and the risk of additional eighth nerve impairment or renal injury should be weighed against the benefits to be derived from therapy. Since other parenteral antituberculous agents (eg, streptomycin) also have similar and sometimes irreversible toxic effects, particularly on eighth cranial nerve and renal function, simultaneous administration of these agents with capreomycin is not recommended. Use with nonantituberculous drugs (ie, aminoglycoside antibiotics) having ototoxic or nephrotoxic potential should be undertaken only with great caution. Care should be taken if administering with drugs with neuromuscular effects.

Dosage Forms Injection: 100 mg/mL (10 mL)

Reference Range 1 g administered I.M. gives a peak serum concentration of 30 μg/mL; desired serum steady-state level is 10 μg/mL

Overdosage Treatment

Enhancement of elimination: Hemodialysis if renal failure develops

Test Interactions Increases BUN, leukocytosis; decreases platelets, potassium

Pregnancy Risk Factor C

Patient Information Report any deafness to physician immediately; do not discontinue without notifying physician

Nursing Implications Solution for injection may acquire a pale straw color and darken with time; this is not associated with a loss of potency or development of toxicity

Captopril (kap' toe pril)

Related Information

ACE Inhibitors Comparison *on page 1636-1637*

CAS Number 62571-86-2

Brand Names Acepril®; Aceten®; Capoten®; Cor Tensobon®; Garranil®; Katopil®; Zorkaptil®

Use Management of hypertension and treatment of congestive heart failure; increase circulation in Raynaud's phenomenon; idiopathic edema

Mechanism of Action Competitive inhibitor of angiotensin-converting enzyme (ACE); prevents conversion of angiotensin I to angiotensin II, a potent vasoconstrictor; results in lower levels of angiotensin II which causes an increase in plasma renin activity and a reduction in aldosterone secretion

Adverse Reactions

Cardiovascular: Hypotension, chest pain, tachycardia, pericarditis
Central nervous system: Psychosis
Dermatologic: Rash, pruritus, exfoliative dermatitis, hyperpigmentation in children, pemphigus, lichenoid eruptions, angioedema
Endocrine & metabolic: Hyperkalemia, hyponatremia, hypoglycemia
Gastrointestinal: Tongue irritation; altered taste (2%)
Hematologic: Leukopenia/neutropenia (agranulocytosis, granulocytopenia)
Hepatic: Hepatitis
Neuromuscular & skeletal: Paresthesia
Renal: Proteinuria (1%), BUN (increased), serum creatinine (increased), reversible renal failure
Respiratory: Transient cough (10% to 25%), wheezing
Miscellaneous: Hyperhidrosis

Signs & Symptoms of Acute Overdose Severe hypotension, sweating, Stevens-Johnson syndrome, eosinophilia, pemphigus, dysosmia, bone marrow depression, hypoglycemia, diarrhea, coagulopathy, oliguria, lichenoid eruptions, hyperthermia, photosensitivity, cholestatic jaundice, night terrors, tubular necrosis, nephrotic syndrome, bullous skin disease/pemphigoid, pericarditis, hematuria, Parkinson's-like symptoms, hyperkalemia, hyponatremia, renal insufficiency, drowsiness, atrial ectopy, alopecia, fever, seizures, systemic lupus erythematosus (SLE), ototoxicity; tinnitus, wheezing

Toxicodynamics/Kinetics

Onset of action: Single dose: 15-60 minutes
Duration of hypotensive action: 5-10 hours
Absorption: Oral: 60% to 75% absorbed from gastrointestinal tract; reduced 30% to 40% in presence of food
Distribution: V_d: 0.7 L/kg; to all tissues except CNS
Protein binding: 25% to 30%
Metabolism: Hepatic, 50%
Half-life:
- Normal adult: Dependent upon renal and cardiac function: 1.9 hours
- Congestive heart failure: 2.06 hours
- Anuria: 20-40 hours

Time to peak serum concentration: Within 1-2 hours
Elimination: 95% excreted in urine in 24 hours

Usual Dosage Note: Dosage must be titrated according to patient's response; use lowest effective dose. Oral:

(Continued)

Captopril *(Continued)*

Neonates: Initial: 0.05-0.1 mg/kg/dose every 8-24 hours; titrate dose up to 0.5 mg/kg/dose given every 6-24 hours

Infants: Initial: 0.15-0.3 mg/kg/dose; titrate dose upward to maximum of 6 mg/kg/day in 1-4 divided doses; usual required dose: 2.5-6 mg/kg/day

Children: Initial: 0.5 mg/kg/dose; titrate upward to maximum of 6 mg/kg/day in 2-4 divided doses

Older Children: Initial: 6.25-12.5 mg/dose every 12-24 hours; titrate upward to maximum of 6 mg/kg/day

Adolescents and Adults: Initial: 12.5-25 mg/dose given every 8-12 hours; increase by 25 mg/dose to maximum of 450 mg/day

Note: Smaller dosages given every 8-12 hours are indicated in patients with renal dysfunction. Renal function and leukocyte count should be carefully monitored during therapy.

Dosing adjustment in renal impairment:

Cl_{cr} 10-50 mL/minute: Administer 75% of dose

Cl_{cr} <10 mL/minute: Administer 50% of dose

Contraindications Hypersensitivity to captopril or any component

Warnings Use with caution and modify dosage in patients with renal impairment; monitor BUN, serum creatinine, and renal function; use with caution in patients with collagen vascular disease

Dosage Forms Tablet: 12.5 mg, 25 mg, 50 mg, 100 mg

Stability Unstable in aqueous solutions; to prepare solution for oral administration, mix prior to administration and use within 10 minutes

Reference Range Plasma level of 6 μg/mL associated with hypotension while a level of 60 μg/mL associated with fatality

Overdosage Treatment

Decontamination: Ipecac or lavage/activated charcoal with cathartic

Supportive therapy: Following initiation of essential overdose management, toxic symptom treatment and supportive treatment should be initiated. Hypotension usually responds to I.V. fluids or Trendelenburg positioning. If unresponsive to these measures, the use of a parenteral inotrope may be required (eg, norepinephrine 0.1-0.2 mcg/kg/minute titrated to response). Seizures commonly respond to lorazepam or diazepam (I.V. 5-10 mg bolus in adults every 15 minutes if needed up to a total of 30 mg; I.V. 0.25-0.4 mg/kg/dose up to a total of 10 mg in children) or to phenytoin or phenobarbital. Naloxone (2 mg) may reverse hypotension. Sulindac may be useful for captopril-induced cough. Inhaled sodium cromoglycate (total dose: 40 mg/day) can decrease ACE-inhibitor cough by 50%.

Enhancement of elimination: Multiple dosing of activated charcoal or hemodialysis may be quite useful; moderately dialyzable (20% to 50%)

Antidote(s)

Naloxone Hydrochloride *on page 1447*

Test Interactions Increases BUN, creatinine, potassium, positive Coombs' [direct]; decreases cholesterol (S); May cause false-positive results in urine acetone determinations using sodium nitroprusside reagent

Diagnostic Tests/Procedures

Complete Blood Count *on page 1236*

Creatinine, Serum *on page 1243*

Protein, Semiquantitative, Urine *on page 1337*

Urea Nitrogen, Blood *on page 1370*

Drug Interactions Captopril + potassium-sparing diuretics cause an additive hyperkalemic effect; captopril + indomethacin or nonsteroidal anti-inflammatory agents cause a reduced antihypertensive response to captopril; leukopenia associated when given with azathioprine, can increase serum digoxin levels; use with cimetidine can cause paresthesia; allergic reactions including Stevens-Johnson syndrome associated with use of allopurinol

Pregnancy Risk Factor C (embryotoxicity at high doses in rabbits; thought to be involved with intrauterine growth retardation, and oliguria in neonatal exposed to captopril during gestation)

Pregnancy Implications Excreted in breast milk; neonatal renal failure can occur

Monitoring Parameters BUN, serum creatinine, urine dipstick for protein, complete leukocyte count, and blood pressure for up to 36 hours after ingestion

Patient Information Take 1 hour before meals; notify physician of persistent cough

Nursing Implications Watch for hypotensive effect within 1-3 hours of first dose or new higher dose; many patients complain of transient cough during early therapy

Additional Information Most effective for treating hypertension in young, white patients

Specific References

Augenstein WL, Kulig KW, and Rumack BH, "Captopril Overdose Resulting in Hypotension," *JAMA*, 1988, 259(22):3302-5.

Butt A and Burge SM, "Pemphigus Vulgaris Induced by Captopril," *Br J Dermatol*, 1995, 132(2):315-6.

Hargreaves MR and Benson MK, "Inhaled Sodium Cromoglycate in Angiotensin-Converting Enzyme Inhibitor Cough," *Lancet*, 1995, 345(8941):13-6.

Herings RM, deBoer A, Stricker BH, et al, "Hypoglycemia Associated With Use of Inhibitors of Angiotensin Converting Enzyme," *Lancet*, 1995, 345:1195-8.

Hirakata H, Onoyama K, Iseki K, et al, "Captopril (SQ 14225) Clearance During Hemodialysis Treatment," *Clin Nephrol*, 1981, 16(6):321-3.

Jeandidier N, Klewansky M, and Pinget M, "Captopril-Induced Acute Pancreatitis," *Diabetes Care*, 1995, 18:410-1.

Koutouby A and Habibullah J, "Reversible Neonatal Renal Failure Associated With Maternal Use of Captopril," *Saudi Med J*, 1995, 16:64-6.

Kuechle MK, Hutton KP, and Muller SA, "Angiotensin-Converting Enzyme Inhibitor-Induced Pemphigus: Three Case Reports and Literature Review," *Mayo Clin Proc*, 1994, 69(12):1166-71.

Lechleitner P, Dzien A, Haring C, et al, "Uneventful Self-Poisoning With a Very High Dose of Captopril," *Toxicology*, 1990, 64(3):325-9.

Varon J and Duncan SR, "Naloxone Reversal of Hypotension Due to Captopril Overdose," *Ann Emerg Med*, 1991, 20(10):1125-7.

Captopril and Hydrochlorothiazide

(kap' toe pril & hye droe klor oh thye' a zide)

Brand Names Acezide®; Capozide®

Use Management of hypertension and treatment of congestive heart failure

Adverse Reactions

Cardiovascular: Hypotension, tachycardia, pericarditis, hyperhidrosis

Dermatologic: Rash, exfoliative dermatitis, hyperpigmentation in children, pemphigus, lichenoid eruptions, angioedema

Endocrine & metabolic: Hyperkalemia, hyponatremia, syndrome of inappropriate antidiuretic hormone

Gastrointestinal: Tongue irritation, altered taste

Hematologic: Leukopenia/neutropenia (agranulocytosis, granulocytopenia)

Hepatic: Hepatitis

Neuromuscular & skeletal: Paresthesia

Renal: Increased BUN and serum creatinine, reversible renal failure, albuminuria

Respiratory: Transient cough, wheezing

Signs & Symptoms of Acute Overdose Severe hypotension, wheezing, sweating, pericarditis, pemphigus, hyperkalemia, hyponatremia, lichenoid eruptions, renal insufficiency, drowsiness, atrial ectopy

Usual Dosage Adults: Oral:

Hypertension: Initial: 25 mg 2-3 times/day; may increase at 1- to 2-week intervals up to 150 mg 3 times/day (captopril dosages)

Congestive heart failure: 6.25-25 mg 3 times/day (maximum: 450 mg/day) (captopril dosages)

Contraindications Hypersensitivity to captopril, hydrochlorothiazide, or any component

Warnings See individual monographs for Captopril and Hydrochlorothiazide

Dosage Forms Tablet:

25/15: Captopril 25 mg and hydrochlorothiazide 15 mg

25/25: Captopril 25 mg and hydrochlorothiazide 25 mg

50/15: Captopril 50 mg and hydrochlorothiazide 15 mg

50/25: Captopril 50 mg and hydrochlorothiazide 25 mg

Overdosage Treatment

Decontamination: Ipecac or lavage/activated charcoal with cathartic

Supportive therapy: Following initiation of essential overdose management, toxic symptom treatment and supportive treatment should be initiated. Hypotension usually responds to I.V. fluids or Trendelenburg positioning. If unresponsive to these measures, the use of a parenteral inotrope may be required (eg, norepinephrine 0.1-0.2 mcg/kg/minute titrated to response). Seizures commonly respond to lorazepam or diazepam (I.V. 5-10 mg bolus in adults every 15 minutes if needed up to a total of 30 mg; I.V. 0.25-0.4 mg/kg/dose up to a total of 10 mg in children) or to phenytoin or phenobarbital. Naloxone (2 mg) may reverse hypotension. Sulindac may be useful for captopril-induced cough.

Enhancement of elimination: Multiple dosing of activated charcoal or hemodialysis may be quite useful

Antidote(s)

Naloxone Hydrochloride *on page 1447*

Test Interactions Increases BUN, creatinine, potassium, positive Coombs' [direct]; decreases cholesterol (S); may cause false-positive results in urine acetone determinations using sodium nitroprusside reagent

(Continued)

Captopril and Hydrochlorothiazide *(Continued)*

Diagnostic Tests/Procedures
Complete Blood Count *on page 1236*
Creatinine, Serum *on page 1243*
Potassium, Blood *on page 1328*
Protein, Semiquantitative, Urine *on page 1337*
Urea Nitrogen, Blood *on page 1370*

Drug Interactions Captopril + potassium-sparing diuretics cause an additive hyperkalemic effect; captopril + indomethacin or nonsteroidal anti-inflammatory agents cause a reduced antihypertensive response to captopril; leukopenia associated when given with azathioprine can increase serum digoxin levels; use with cimetidine can cause paresthesia; allergic reactions including Stevens-Johnson syndrome associated with use of allopurinol

Pregnancy Risk Factor C

Monitoring Parameters See individual monographs for Captopril and Hydrochlorothiazide

Additional Information Contains 50 mg of captopril and 25 mg of hydrochlorothiazide

Carace C® *see* Lisinopril *on page 475*

Carafate® *see* Sucralfate *on page 710*

Carbamazepine (kar ba maz' e peen)

Related Information
Drugs and Chemicals Proven to be Teratogenic in Humans *on page 1572-1575*
Therapeutic Drugs Associated With Hallucinations *on page 1558-1559*

CAS Number 298-46-4

Brand Names Carbategretal®; Carbazep®; Epitrol®; Tegretol®

Synonyms Carbamazepinum; CBZ

Use Prophylaxis of generalized tonic-clonic, partial (especially complex partial), and mixed partial or generalized seizure disorder; may be used to relieve pain in trigeminal neuralgia or diabetic neuropathy; has been used to treat bipolar disorders

Mechanism of Action May depress activity in the nucleus ventralis of the thalamus or decrease synaptic transmission or to decrease summation of temporal stimulation leading to neural discharge by limiting influx of sodium ions across cell membrane or other unknown mechanisms; stimulates the release of ADH and potentiates its action in promoting reabsorption of water; chemically related to tricyclic antidepressants; in addition to anticonvulsant effects, carbamazepine has anticholinergic, antineuralgic, antidiuretic, muscle relaxant, and antiarrhythmic properties. May also decrease the turnover of γ-aminobutyric acid (GABA), an iminostilbene derivative.

Adverse Reactions
Cardiovascular: Edema, congestive heart failure, syncope, conduction disturbances (QRS prolongation, P-R interval prolongation)
Central nervous system: Sedation, dizziness, fatigue, headache, slurred speech, psychosis, dystonic reactions, seizures, visual hallucinations, ataxia
Dermatologic: Rash; but does not necessarily mean the drug should not be stopped; bullous eruption, erythema multiforme, toxic epidermal necrolysis, photosensitivity
Endocrine & metabolic: Hyponatremia
Gastrointestinal: Nausea, diarrhea, decrease in taste, anorexia
Genitourinary: Urinary retention
Hematologic: Neutropenia (can be transient), aplastic anemia (1 in 50,000 patients), thrombocytopenia, pseudolymphoma
Hepatic: Hepatitis
Neuromuscular & skeletal: Asterixis
Ocular: Nystagmus, diplopia, oculogyric crisis (extrapyramidal)
Miscellaneous: Can form bezoars, lupus erythematosus

Signs & Symptoms of Acute Overdose Dizziness, exfoliative dermatitis, Stevens-Johnson syndrome, hypothyroidism, hyponatremia, mania, chorea (extrapyramidal), toxic epidermal necrolysis, hyperreflexia, lichenoid eruptions, hyperthermia, dysosmia, extrapyramidal reaction, cognitive dysfunction, lymphoma, gingival hyperplasia, ileus, photosensitivity, bone marrow depression, leukemoid reaction, cholestatic jaundice, encephalopathy, jaundice, ataxia, A-V block, drowsiness, neuroleptic malignant syndrome, myoclonus, nausea, delirium, cough, vomiting, tremors, agitation, nystagmus, urinary retention, arrhythmias, coma, apnea, seizures, mydriasis, erythema multiforme, hypotension, drowsiness, hypothermia, leukocytosis, decrease gastrointestinal motility, oliguria, P-R prolongation, QRS prolongation, Q-T prolongation, alopecia, bradycardia, flushing, fever, systemic lupus erythematosus (SLE), leukopenia; neutropenia; agranulocytosis; granulocytopenia; bradycardia

Toxicodynamics/Kinetics

Onset of action: Anticonvulsant effect varies from hours to days, depending on individual patient; a stable therapeutic concentration may require a month to achieve due to to autoinduction of metabolism; relief of pain of trigeminal neuralgia occurs 8-72 hours; antimanic response, usually 7-10 days

Absorption: Slow from gastrointestinal tract

Distribution: Widely distributed in the body, especially in saliva, duodenal fluid, and bile; high concentrations in CSF

V_d:

- Neonates: 1.5 L/kg
- Children: 1.9 L/kg
- Adults: 0.59-2 L/kg
- Overdose: 3 L/kg

Protein binding: 75%; may be decreased in newborns

Metabolism: In the liver to active epoxide; induces liver enzymes to metabolite increase metabolism and shorten half-life over time

Bioavailability: Oral: 85% to 90%

Half-life:

- Initial: 18-55 hours
- Multiple dosing:
  - Children: 8-14 hours
  - Adults: 12-17 hours
  - Overdose: 24-26 hours

Time to peak serum concentration: Within 4-8 hours

Elimination: 1% to 3% excreted unchanged in urine; fecal excretion: 20% to 30%; first order elimination kinetics

Usual Dosage Oral (dosage must be adjusted according to patient's response and serum concentrations):

Children:

- <6 years: Initial: 5 mg/kg/day; dosage may be increased every 5-7 days to 10 mg/kg/day; then up to 20 mg/kg/day if necessary; administer in 2-4 divided doses/day
- 6-12 years: Initial: 100 mg twice daily or 10 mg/kg/day in 2 divided doses; increase by 100 mg/day at weekly intervals depending upon response; usual maintenance: 20-30 mg/kg/day in 2-4 divided doses/day; maximum dose: 1000 mg/day

Children >12 years and Adults: 200 mg twice daily to start, increase by 200 mg/day at weekly intervals until therapeutic levels achieved; usual dose: 800-1200 mg/day in 3-4 divided doses; some patients have required up to 1.6-2.4 g/day

Dosing adjustment in renal impairment: Cl_{cr} <10 mL/minute: Administer 75% of dose

Contraindications Hypersensitivity to carbamazepine or any component; may have cross-sensitivity with tricyclic antidepressants; should not be used in any patient with bone marrow depression, MAO inhibitor use

Warnings Potentially fatal blood cell abnormalities have been reported following treatment; early detection of hematologic change is important; advise patients of early signs and symptoms which are fever, sore throat, stomatitis, infections, easy bruising, petechial or purpuric hemorrhage; MAO inhibitors should be discontinued for a minimum of 14 days before carbamazepine is begun; administer with caution to patients with history of cardiac damage or hepatic disease

Dosage Forms

Suspension, oral (citrus-vanilla flavor): 100 mg/5 mL (450 mL)

Tablet: 200 mg

Tablet, chewable: 100 mg

Reference Range

Therapeutic: 4-12 μg/mL (SI: 17-51 μmol/L). Patients who require higher levels (8-12 μg/mL) (SI: 34-51 μmol/L) should be watched closely. Side effects including CNS effects occur commonly at higher dosage levels. If other anticonvulsants are given, therapeutic range is 4-8 μg/mL (SI: 17-34 μmol/L).

Ataxia and nystagmus is noted at levels >10 μg/mL (SI: >42 μmol/L); levels >30 μg/mL (SI: >127 μmol/L) associated with coma and respiratory depression

Fatal: Levels of 54 μg/L

Overdosage Treatment

Decontamination: Lavage/activated charcoal with cathartic is effective at binding certain chemicals and this is especially true for carbamazepine

Supportive therapy: Other treatment is supportive/symptomatic; flumazenil has been reported to reverse coma although its use is contraindicated in patients with seizure disorder; lithium, diltiazem, miconazole, and metoclopramide use with carbamazepine has been associated with neurotoxicity. Do not use physostigmine.

Enhancement of elimination: Multiple dose of activated charcoal is effective; charcoal hemoperfusion is also useful; forced diuresis is not effective

(Continued)

Carbamazepine *(Continued)*

Test Interactions Increases BUN, AST, ALT, ammonia, bilirubin, alkaline phosphatase (S); decreases calcium, T_3, T_4, sodium (S)

Diagnostic Tests/Procedures

Carbamazepine, Blood *on page 1219*

Carbamazepine-10,11-Epoxide *on page 1219*

Drug Interactions Erythromycin, isoniazid, propoxyphene, verapamil, diltiazem, and cimetidine may inhibit hepatic metabolism of carbamazepine with resultant increase of carbamazepine serum concentrations and toxicity; carbamazepine may induce the metabolism of imipramine, warfarin, haloperidol, doxycycline, oral contraceptives, phenytoin, theophylline, benzodiazepines, ethosuximide, valproic acid, corticosteroids and thyroid hormones; synergistic anticonvulsant effect with propranolol; metronidazole can increase carbamazepine plasma level; CNS disorders with concomitant erythromycin and clarithromycin

Pregnancy Risk Factor C

Pregnancy Implications Crosses the placenta; appears in breast milk in high concentrations; craniofacial defects, fingernail hypoplasia, and developmental delay correlated

Monitoring Parameters Neurologic/cardiac status, hematologic/liver function tests

Patient Information Take with food, may cause drowsiness, periodic blood test monitoring required

Nursing Implications Observe patient for excessive sedation

Additional Information Suspension dosage form must be given on a 3-4 times/day schedule versus tablets which can be given 2-4 times/day; EKG changes do **not** correlate with serum carbamazepine levels; it is hypothesized that hematological toxicity and immune system toxicity is due to 9-acridine carboxaldehyde metabolite

Specific References

Apfelbaum JD, Caravati EM, Kerns II WP, et al, "Cardiovascular Effects of Carbamazepine Toxicity," *Ann Emerg Med*, 1995, 25:631-5.

Cooney GF, Mochon M, Kaiser B, et al, "Effects of Carbamazepine on Cyclosporine Metabolism in Pediatric Renal Transplant Recipients," *Pharmacotherapy*, 1995, 15(3):353-6.

Furst SM and Uetrecht JP, "The Effect of Carbamazepine and Its Reactive Metabolite 9-Acridine Carboxaldehyde, on Immune Cell Function *In Vitro*," *Int J Immunopharmacol*, 1995, 17:445-52.

Gary N, Byra W, Eisinger R, "Carbamazepine Poisoning: Treatment by Hemoperfusion," *Nephron*, 1981, 27(4-5):202-3.

Iwahashi IS, Miyatake R, Suwaki H, et al, "The Durg-Drug Interaction Effects of Haloperidol on Plasma Carbamazepine Levels," *Clin Neuro Pharm*, 1995, 18:233-6.

Jones KL, Lacro RV, Johnson KA, et al, "Pattern of Malformation in the Children of Women Treated With Carbamazepine During Pregnancy," *N Engl J Med*, 1989, 320(25):1661-6.

Keating A and Blahunka P, "Carbamazepine-Induced Stevens-Johnson Syndrome in a Child," *Ann Pharmacother*, 1995, 29:538-9.

Montgomery VL, Richman BJ, Goldsmith LJ, et al, "Severity and Carbamazepine Level at Time of Initial Posion Center Contact Correlate With Outcome in Carbamazepine Poisoning," *J Toxicol Clin Toxicol*, 1995, 33(4):311-23.

Nilsson C, Sterner G, and Idvall J, "Charcoal Hemoperfusion for Treatment of Serious Carbamazepine Poisoning," *Acta Med Scand*, 1984, 216(1):137-40.

Ory JP, Bourscheld D, Lebrun C, et al, "Drug-Induced Pseudolymphoma in a Lupus Patient: One Case Due to Carbamazepine," *Clin Exp Rheumatol*, 1995, 12(Suppl 11):93.

Rispal P, Lasseur C, Labouyrie E, et al, "Carbamazepine-Induced Pseudolymphoma. Report of Two Cases," *Rev Med Interne*, 1995, 16:214-8.

Stafstrom CE, Nohria V, Loganbill H, et al, "Erythromycin-induced Carbamazepine Toxicity: A Continuing Problem," *Arch Pediatr Adolesc Med*, 1995, 149(1):99-101.

Stremski ES, Brady WB, Prasad K, et al, "Pediatric Carbamazepine Intoxication," *Ann Emerg Med*, 1995, 25:624-30.

Tohen M, Castillo J, Baldessarini RJ, et al, "Blood Dyscrasias With Carbamazepine and Valproate: A Pharmacoepidemiological Study of 2,228 Patients at Risk," *Am J Psychiatry*, 1995, 152(3):413-8.

Wason S, Baker RC, Carolan P, et al, "Carbamazepine Overdose – The Effects of Multiple Doses of Activated Charcoal," *J Toxicol Clin Toxicol*, 1992, 30(1):39-48.

Zuber M, Elsasser S, Ritz R, et al, "Flumazenil (Anexate®) in Severe Intoxication With Carbamazepine (Tegretol®)," *Eur Neurol*, 1988, 28(3):161-3.

Carbamazepinum *see* Carbamazepine *on page 184*

Carbamidine Hydrochloride *see* Guanidine Hydrochloride *on page 395*

Carbamylmethycholine Chloride *see* Bethanechol Chloride *on page 154*

Carbategretal® *see* Carbamazepine *on page 184*

Carbazep® *see* Carbamazepine *on page 184*

Carbocaine® *see* Mepivacaine Hydrochloride *on page 502*

Carbolic Acid *see* Phenol *on page 616*

Carbostesin® *see* Bupivacaine Hydrochloride *on page 168*

Cardem® *see* Celiprolol Hydrochloride *on page 191*

Cardiocal® *see* Bepridil Hydrochloride *on page 152*

Cardioquin® *see* Quinidine *on page 668*

Cardioreg® *see* Digoxin *on page 284*

Cardizem® *see* Diltiazem *on page 287*

Cardizem® CD *see* Diltiazem *on page 287*

Cardizem® SR *see* Diltiazem *on page 287*

Cardoxin® *see* Dipyridamole *on page 292*

Cardura® *see* Doxazosin *on page 300*

Carisoma® *see* Carisoprodol *on this page*

Carisoprodate *see* Carisoprodol *on this page*

Carisoprodol (kar eye soe proe' dole)

CAS Number 78-44-4

Brand Names Carisoma®; Flexartal®; Rela®; Sanoma®; Sodol®; Soma®; Soma® Compound; Somadril®; Soprodol®; Soridol®

Synonyms Carisoprodate; Isobamate; Isopropylmeprobamate

Use Skeletal muscle relaxant

Mechanism of Action Precise mechanism is not yet clear, but many effects have been ascribed to its central depressant actions

Adverse Reactions

Cardiovascular: Hypotension, tachycardia, tightness in chest, flushing of face

Central nervous system: Sedation, drowsiness, dizziness, fatigue, fainting, mental depression, lightheadedness, headache, clumsiness, insomnia, ataxia

Dermatologic: Skin rash, hives, erythema multiforme

Gastrointestinal: Nausea, vomiting, stomach cramps

Hematologic: Aplastic anemia, eosinophilia

Neuromuscular & skeletal: Trembling

Ocular: Diplopia, blurred vision, burning of eyes, nystagmus

Respiratory: Dyspnea

Miscellaneous: Hiccups, porphyrinogenic

Signs & Symptoms of Acute Overdose CNS depression, lightheadedness, insomnia, depression, erythema multiforme, stupor, coma, shock, respiratory depression

Toxicodynamics/Kinetics

Onset of action: Within 30 minutes

Duration: 4-6 hours

Distribution: Crosses the placenta; appears in high concentrations in breast milk

Metabolism: By the liver to meprobamate and hydroxymeprobamate

Half-life: 8 hours

Elimination: Excreted by kidneys

Usual Dosage Adults: Oral: 350 mg 3-4 times/day; take last dose at bedtime; compound: 1-2 tablets 4 times/day

Minimal lethal dose: 3.5 g (pediatrics)

Contraindications Acute intermittent porphyria, hypersensitivity to carisoprodol, meprobamate, tybamate, or any component

Warnings Use with caution in renal and hepatic dysfunction

Dosage Forms Tablet:

Rela®, Sodol®, Soma®, Soprodol®, Soridol®: 350 mg

Soma® Compound: Carisoprodol 200 mg and aspirin 325 mg

Reference Range 600 mg oral dose can produce peak carisoprodol plasma level between 9-20 mg/L; plasma levels >30 mg/L associated with stupor, coma, or death

Overdosage Treatment

Decontamination: Lavage/activated charcoal

Supportive therapy: Benzodiazepines for seizure control

Enhancement of elimination: Forced diuresis is not helpful; multiple dosing of activated charcoal may be helpful. Following attempts to enhance drug elimination; hypotension should be treated with I.V. fluids and/or Trendelenburg positioning.

Drug Interactions Potentiated with alcohol, guanabenz, meprobamate or other CNS depressants; enhance neuromuscular blockade when given with clindamycin; use with MAO inhibitors may cause hypotension and respiratory depression

Pregnancy Risk Factor C

Monitoring Parameters Look for relief of pain and/or muscle spasm and avoid excessive drowsiness

Patient Information May cause drowsiness or vertigo; avoid alcohol and other CNS depressants; may take with food if gastrointestinal upset occurs; if dizziness

(Continued)

Carisoprodol *(Continued)*

(hypotension (orthostatic)) occurs, avoid sudden changes in posture; use caution when climbing stairs etc

Nursing Implications Raise bed rails; institute safety measures; assist with ambulation

Specific References

Adams HR, Kerzee T, and Morehead CD, "Carisoprodol-Related Death in a Child," *J Forensic Sci*, 1975, 20:200-2.

Backer RC, Zumwalt R, McFeeley P, et al, "Carisoprodol Concentrations From Different Anatomical Sites: Three Overdose Cases," *J Anal Toxicol*, 1990, 14(5):332-4.

Goldberg D, "Carisoprodol Toxicity," *Milit Med*, 1969, 34:597-601.

Luehr JG, Meyerle KA, and Larson EW, "Mail-Order (Veterinary) Drug Dependence," *JAMA*, 1990, 263(5):657.

Carteolol Hydrochloride (kar' tee oh lole)

Related Information

Beta-Blockers Comparison *on page 1644-1645*

CAS Number 51781-06-7; 51781-21-6

Brand Names Arteolol®; Cartrol®; Endak®; Mikelan®; Ocupress®; Teoptic®

Use Management of hypertension; eye drops: open-angle glaucoma or intraocular hypertension

Mechanism of Action Blocks both $beta_1$- and $beta_2$-receptors and has mild intrinsic sympathomimetic activity; has negative inotropic and chronotropic effects and can significantly slow A-V nodal conduction

Adverse Reactions

Cardiovascular: Mesenteric arterial thrombosis, A-V block, persistent bradycardia, hypotension, chest pain, edema, heart failure, exacerbation of Raynaud's phenomenon

Central nervous system: Fatigue, dizziness, headache, insomnia, drowsiness, night terrors, CNS depression, confusion

Dermatologic: Purpura

Gastrointestinal: Ischemic colitis, constipation, nausea, diarrhea

Genitourinary: Impotence

Hematologic: Thrombocytopenia

Ocular: Corneal irritation, blurred vision with eye drop use

Respiratory: Wheezing

Miscellaneous: Cold extremities

Signs & Symptoms of Acute Overdose Severe hypotension, cough, ataxia, purpura, night terrors, insomnia, impotence, congestive heart failure, arrhythmias, colitis, sinus bradycardia, heart/respiratory failure and wheezing; pulmonary edema, mesenteric ischemia, cardiovascular collapse

Toxicodynamics/Kinetics

Protein binding: 23% to 30%

Metabolism: Hepatic (30% to 50%) to an active metabolite 8-hydroxycarteolol

Bioavailability: 85%

Half-life:

Parent compound: 6 hours

Metabolite: 8-12 hours

Time to peak plasma concentration: 1-3 hours

Elimination: Renal; clearance: 6.5 mL/minute/kg

Usual Dosage Adults:

Oral: 2.5 mg as a single daily dose, with a maintenance dose normally 2.5-5 mg once daily

Ophthalmic: Instill 1 drop in eye(s) twice daily

Contraindications Uncompensated congestive heart failure, cardiogenic shock, bradycardia or heart block

Dosage Forms

Solution, ophthalmic (Ocupress®): 1% (5 mL, 10 mL)

Tablet (Cartrol®): 2.5 mg, 5 mg

Overdosage Treatment

Decontamination: Lavage/activated charcoal with cathartic; do not use ipecac

Supportive therapy: Glucagon (50-150 mcg/kg followed by continuous drip of 1-5 mg/hour) for positive chronotropic effect; atropine/isoproterenol can be utilized to increase heart rate; calcium chloride may also be effective; do **not** use epinephrine

Enhancement of elimination: Multiple dosing of activated charcoal is not likely to be of benefit; dialysis is not useful

Pregnancy Risk Factor C

Monitoring Parameters Blood pressure, EKG, CVP

Additional Information Under investigation in phase II trials in the USA

Specific References

Ishizaki T, Ohnishi A, Sasaki T, et al, "Concentration-Effect and Time-Effect Relationships on Carteolol," *Eur J Clin Pharmacol*, 1983, 25(6):749-57.

Carter's Little Pills® [OTC] *see* Bisacodyl *on page 156*

Cartrol® *see* Carteolol Hydrochloride *on previous page*

Carvedilol

Related Information

Beta-Blockers Comparison *on page 1644-1645*

CAS Number 72956-09-3

Brand Names Kredex®

Use Investigational: Angina, hypertension, congestive heart failure

Mechanism of Action Noncardioselective beta-blocking agent with calcium channel blocking activity at higher dose (about 30 times the normal dose); similar to labetalol in that there is some $alpha_1$-adrenergic antagonist effect, thus acting as a vasodilator; less $alpha_1$ effect than labetalol or prazosin

Adverse Reactions

Cardiovascular: Bradycardia, hypotension (orthostatic) (especially in the elderly)
Central nervous system: Syncope, dizziness, headache
Dermatologic: Edema, pruritus
Gastrointestinal: Nausea, mild diarrhea
Respiratory: Wheezing

Toxicodynamics/Kinetics

Onset of action: 1 hour
Absorption: 22% to 24% (oral); not affected by food
Distribution: V_d: 1-2 L/kg
Protein binding: 90% to 95%
Metabolism: Hepatic with oxidation and glucuronide conjugation
Half-life: 4-8 hours
Elimination: Feces 60%; renal 16%

Usual Dosage

Angina: 25-50 mg twice daily (dose reduction in hepatic disease)
Hypertension: 25-50 mg twice daily

Contraindications Greater than a first degree heart block, hypersensitivity to beta-adrenergic blocking agents; cardiogenic shock and bradycardia

Warnings Use with caution in patients with bronchospasm, hepatic disease, intermittent claudication, elderly patients

Reference Range Peak serum levels of ~122 μg/L achieved after oral 50 mg dose

Overdosage Treatment

Decontamination: Gastric lavage with activated charcoal with cathartic is recommended; do not use ipecac

Supportive therapy: Sympathomimetics (eg, epinephrine or dopamine), atropine, glucagon or a pacemaker can be used to treat the toxic bradycardia, asystole, and/or hypotension; amrinone may also be effective for labetalol-induced hypotension; initially fluids may be the best treatment for toxic hypotension with norepinephrine being used for second-line therapy

Enhancement of elimination: Multiple dosing of activated charcoal may be useful; not dialyzable

Drug Interactions Increases absorption of digoxin

Additional Information High concentrations of carvedilol (>1 μmol/L) can cause calcium channel blocking effect; not useful for pheochromocytoma

Specific References

Cubeddu LX, Fuenmayor N, Varin F, et al, "Clinical Pharmacology of Carvedilol in Normal Volunteers," *Clin Pharmacol Ther*, 1987, 41(1):31-44.

Louis WJ, Krum H, and Conway EL, "A Risk-Benefit Assessment of Carvedilol in the Treatment of Cardiovascular Disorders," *Drug Saf*, 1994, 11(2):86-93.

McTavish D, Campoli-Richards D, and Sorkin EM, "Carvedilol: A Review of its Pharmacodynamic and Pharmacokinetic Properties and Therapeutic Efficacy," *Drugs*, 1993, 45(2):323-58.

Zhou HH and Wood AJ, "Stereoselective Disposition of Carvedilol Is Determined by CYP2D6," *Clin Pharmacol Ther*, 1995, 57:518-24.

Caryolysine® *see* Mechlorethamine Hydrochloride *on page 492*

Castor Oil (kas' tor)

CAS Number 8001-79-4

Brand Names Alphamul® [OTC]; Emulsoil® [OTC]; Fleet® Flavored Castor Oil [OTC]; Laxopol®; Neoloid® [OTC]; Palmil®; Purge® [OTC]; Ricifruit®; Unisol®

Synonyms Oleum Ricini; Ricinus Oil

Use Preparation for rectal or bowel examination or surgery; rarely used to relieve constipation; also applied to skin as emollient and protectant

Mechanism of Action Acts primarily in the small intestine; hydrolyzed to ricinoleic acid which reduces net absorption of fluid and electrolytes and stimulates peristalsis; oil is expressed from the seeds of *Ricinus communis*

Adverse Reactions

Central nervous system: Dizziness, hallucinations, syncope

(Continued)

Castor Oil *(Continued)*

Endocrine & metabolic: Electrolyte disturbance
Gastrointestinal: Abdominal cramps, nausea, diarrhea
Miscellaneous: Pelvic congestion

Toxicodynamics/Kinetics
Onset of action: Oral: 2-6 hours
Absorption: Orally
Metabolism: By pancreatic lipases to glycerol and ricinoleic acid

Usual Dosage Oral:
Liquid:
Infants <2 years: 1-5 mL or 15 mL/m²/dose as a single dose
Children 2-11 years: 5-15 mL as a single dose
Children ≥12 years and Adults: 15-60 mL as a single dose

Emulsified:
36.4%:
Infants: 2.5-7.5 mL/dose
Children <2 years: 5-15 mL/dose
Children 2-11 years: 7.5-30 mL/dose
Children ≥12 years and Adults: 30-60 mL/dose
60% to 67%:
Children <2 years: 1.25-5 mL
Children 2-12 years: 5-15 mL
Adults: 15-45 mL
95%, mix with ½ to 1 full glass liquid:
Children: 5-10 mL
Adults: 15-60 mL

Contraindications Known hypersensitivity to castor oil; nausea, vomiting, abdominal pain, fecal impaction, gastrointestinal bleeding, appendicitis, congestive heart failure, menstruation, dehydration

Warnings Use only when a prompt and thorough catharsis is desired; use with caution during menstruation

Dosage Forms
Emulsion, oral:
Alphamul®: 60% (90 mL, 3780 mL)
Emulsoil®: 95% (63 mL)
Fleet® Flavored Castor Oil: 67% (45 mL, 90 mL)
Neoloid®: 36.4% (118 mL)
Liquid, oral:
100% (60 mL, 120 mL, 480 mL)
Purge®: 95% (30 mL, 60 mL)

Stability Protect from heat (castor oil emulsion should be protected from freezing)

Overdosage Treatment
Decontamination: Lavage/activated charcoal without a cathartic
Supportive therapy: Intravenous fluid and electrolyte replacement; restrict solid food

Drug Interactions May decrease the effects of oral anticoagulants by decreasing absorption

Pregnancy Risk Factor X

Pregnancy Implications Can cause uterine contractures

Monitoring Parameters I & O, serum electrolytes, stool frequency

Patient Information Chill or take with juice or carbonated beverage to improve taste

Nursing Implications Do not administer at bedtime because of rapid onset of action

Additional Information Yellow liquid

Specific References
Brandle I, Bovjnah-Khovadja A, and Foussereau J, "Allergy to Castor Oil," *Contact Dermatitis*, 1983, 9:424-5.

Cataflam® *see* Diclofenac Sodium *on page 276*

Catapres® *see* Clonidine *on page 231*

Catapressan® *see* Clonidine *on page 231*

Catapres-TTS® *see* Clonidine *on page 231*

CBZ *see* Carbamazepine *on page 184*

CBZ *see* Cyclobenzaprine Hydrochloride *on page 248*

C-Crystals® [OTC] *see* Ascorbic Acid *on page 131*

2-CdA *see* Cladribine *on page 220*

CDDP *see* Cisplatin *on page 218*

Cebotid® *see* Flurbiprofen Sodium *on page 364*

Cecon® [OTC] *see* Ascorbic Acid *on page 131*

Cedilanid-D® *see* Deslanoside *on page 264*

Cedocard® *see* Isosorbide Dinitrate *on page 445*

Celectol® *see* Celiprolol Hydrochloride *on this page*

Celiprolol Hydrochloride

Related Information

Beta-Blockers Comparison *on page 1644-1645*

CAS Number 56980-93-9; 57470-78-7

Brand Names Cardem®; Celectol®; Corliprol®; Selecor®; Selectol®

Use Investigational: Hypertension, angina

Mechanism of Action Selective $beta_1$-adrenergic blocking agent with weak $alpha_2$ receptor blocking activity; no negative inotropic effect; may also stimulate $beta_2$ receptors resulting in vasodilitation

Adverse Reactions

Cardiovascular: Bradycardia, A-V block, Raynaud's syndrome, congestive heart failure

Central nervous system: Insomnia, dizziness, headache, vertigo, depression

Gastrointestinal: Nausea, diarrhea, dry mouth

Neuromuscular & skeletal: Tremors

Signs & Symptoms of Acute Overdose Hypoglycemia, A-V block, wheezing, insomnia

Toxicodynamics/Kinetics

Absorption: 30% to 74% (reduced by food)

Protein binding: 25%

Half-life: 4-10 hours

Peak plasma level: 2-4 hours

Elimination: Renal (50%)

Usual Dosage Oral: 200-600 mg once daily; no dosage alteration needed in elderly

Contraindications Hypersensitivity to celiprolol or other beta-blocking agents

Warnings Use with caution in patients with congestive heart failure, heart block, diabetics or oral hypoglycemic agents, patients with bronchospasm

Overdosage Treatment

Decontamination: Lavage/activated charcoal with cathartic; do not use ipecac

Supportive therapy: Glucagon (50-150 mcg/kg followed by continuous drip of 1-5 mg/hour) for positive chronotropic effect, amrinone may need to be added; atropine/isoproterenol can be utilized to increase heart rate; calcium chloride may also be effective but this approach has not thoroughly been investigated; do **not** use epinephrine in that unopposed alpha effects may occur; pacemaker or intra-aortic balloon counter pulsation may be required

Enhancement of elimination: Multiple dosing of activated charcoal is not likely to be of benefit; dialysis is not useful; not dialyzable (0% to 5%)

Antidote(s)

Glucagon *on page 1431*

Drug Interactions Decreased absorption with chlorthalidone, hydrochlorothiazide, and theophylline

Additional Information Can cause decrease in serum cholesterol; HDL increases noted; can cause increase in thyroid function tests; reduction in fibrinogen levels have been described

Specific References

Louis WJ, Krum H, and Conway EL, "A Risk-Benefit Assessment of Carvedilol in the Treatment of Cardiovascular Disorders," *Drug Saf*, 1994, 11(2):86-93.

Milne RJ and Buckley MMT, "Celiprolol: An Updated Review of Its Pharmacodynamic and Pharmacokinetic Properties and Therapeutic Efficacy in Cardiovascular Disease," *Drugs*, 1991, 41(6):941-69.

Pruss TP, Lamon KD, and Hagon NS, "Celiprolol – Overview of 6 Years of Clinical Trials Experience," *J Int Med Res*, 1988, 16(Suppl 1):17A-22A.

Celontin® *see* Methsuximide *on page 518*

Celupan® *see* Naltrexone Hydrochloride *on page 548*

Cenafed® [OTC] *see* Pseudoephedrine *on page 661*

Cena-K® *see* Potassium Chloride *on page 634*

Centralgine® *see* Meperidine Hydrochloride *on page 499*

Centrax® *see* Prazepam *on page 637*

Cepastat® [OTC] *see* Phenol *on page 616*

Cephradine (sef' ra deen)

CAS Number 38821-53-3; 31828-50-9; 58456-86-3

Brand Names Anspor®; Velosef®

Use Treatment of susceptible bacterial infections, including those caused by group A beta-hemolytic *Streptococcus*

(Continued)

Cephradine *(Continued)*

Mechanism of Action Bactericidal antibiotic with a mechanism similar to that of penicillins; after penetrating the bacterial cell wall, it stops cell synthesis and thereby kills the organism

Adverse Reactions

Dermatologic: Rash
Gastrointestinal: Nausea, vomiting, diarrhea, pseudomembranous colitis
Ocular: Nystagmus
Renal: Increased BUN and creatinine
Miscellaneous: Anaphylaxis, porphyrinogenic

Toxicodynamics/Kinetics

Absorption: Oral is faster than I.M., but well absorbed from all routes
Protein binding: 18% to 20%
Half-life: 1-2 hours
Time to peak serum concentration: Oral, I.M.: Within 1-2 hours
Elimination: ~80% to 90% unchanged drug is recovered in urine within 6 hours

Usual Dosage

Children ≥9 months:
Oral: 25-50 mg/kg/day in divided doses every 6 hours
I.M., I.V.: 50-100 mg/kg/day in equally divided doses every 6 hours up to 4 g/day

Adults:
Oral: 250-500 mg every 6-12 hours
I.M., I.V.: 1 g every 6 hours

Dosing adjustment in renal impairment:
Cl_{cr} 10-50 mL/minute: Administer 50% of dose
Cl_{cr} <10 mL/minute: Administer 25% of dose
or
Cl_{cr} 25-50 mL/minute: Administer every 12 hours
Cl_{cr} 10-25 mL/minute: Administer every 24 hours
Cl_{cr} <10 mL/minute: Administer every 36 hours

Contraindications Hypersensitivity to cephradine or any component or cephalosporins

Warnings Prolonged use may result in superinfection; use with caution in patients with a history of colitis or penicillin allergy; reduce dose in patients with renal dysfunction

Dosage Forms

Capsule: 250 mg, 500 mg
Powder for injection: 250 mg, 500 mg, 1 g, 2 g
Powder for oral suspension: 125 mg/5 mL (5 mL, 100 mL, 200 mL); 250 mg/5 mL (5 mL, 100 mL, 200 mL)

Stability Reconstituted solution is stable for 2 hours at room temperature and 24 hours when refrigerated; for I.V. infusion in NS or D_5W solution is stable for 10 hours at room temperature, 48 hours when refrigerated or 6 weeks when frozen; after freezing, thawed solution is stable for 10 hours at room temperature or 48 hours when refrigerated

Reference Range Oral doses of 1 g result in a peak plasma level of 24 μg/mL; intramuscular dose of 1 g results in a peak plasma level of 14 μg/mL

Overdosage Treatment

Decontamination: Emesis or lavage/activated charcoal with cathartic
Supportive therapy: Anaphylaxis can be treated with epinephrine, antihistamines, and corticosteroids
Enhancement of elimination: Multiple dosing of activated charcoal may be effective; hemodialysis or hemoperfusion can help enhance elimination

Test Interactions Positive Coombs' [direct]; ↑ glucose, protein; ↓ glucose

Drug Interactions Probenecid delays excretion

Pregnancy Risk Factor B

Pregnancy Implications Crosses the placenta; appears in breast milk

Patient Information Take until gone, do not miss doses; report diarrhea promptly; entire course of medication (10-14 days) should be taken to ensure eradication of organism; should be taken in equal intervals around-the-clock to maintain adequate blood levels; may interfere with oral contraceptives, females should report symptoms of vaginitis

Additional Information Sodium concentration: 6 mEq/g

Specific References

Wise R, "The Pharmacokinetics of the Oral Cephalosporins - A Review," *J Antimicrob Chemother*, 1990, 26(Suppl E):13-20.

Ceredase® *see* Alglucerase *on page 96*

Cerespan® *see* Papaverine *on page 591*

C.E.S. *see* Estrogens, Conjugated *on page 325*

Cesamet® *see* Nabilone *on page 542*

CES Congest® *see* Estrogens, Conjugated *on page 325*

Cetacaine® *see* Benzocaine, Butyl Aminobenzoate, Tetracaine, and Benzalkonium Chloride *on page 150*

Cetane® [OTC] *see* Ascorbic Acid *on page 131*

Cetobemidone *see* Ketobemidone Hydrochloride *on page 452*

Cevalin® [OTC] *see* Ascorbic Acid *on page 131*

Ce-Vi-Sol® [OTC] *see* Ascorbic Acid *on page 131*

Cevitamic Acid *see* Ascorbic Acid *on page 131*

Chiggertox® [OTC] *see* Benzocaine *on page 149*

Children's Hold® [OTC] *see* Dextromethorphan Hydrobromide *on page 270*

Chlo-Amine® [OTC] *see* Chlorpheniramine Maleate *on page 204*

Chloral *see* Chloral Hydrate *on this page*

Chloral Hydrate (klor al hye' drate)

CAS Number 302-17-0; 480-30-8

Brand Names Aquachloral® Supprettes®; Chloralix®; Kloral®; Noctec®; Rectules®; SK-Choral® Hydrate

Synonyms Chloral; Hydrated Chloral; Kloral Hydrat; Trichloroacetaldehyde Monohydrate

Replaces Knockout Drops

Use Short-term sedative and hypnotic (<2 weeks), sedative/hypnotic for dental and diagnostic procedures; sedative prior to EEG evaluations

Mechanism of Action Central nervous system depressant effects are due to its active metabolite trichloroethanol, mechanism unknown; highly lipid soluble

Adverse Reactions

Cardiovascular: Bigeminy, tachycardia (ventricular), hypotension; Q-T prolongation

Central nervous system: Disorientation, sedation, excitation (paradoxical), dizziness, fever, headache, ataxia

Gastrointestinal: Gastric irritation, nausea, vomiting, diarrhea, flatulence, gastric perforation

Hematologic: Leukopenia, eosinophilia

Hepatic: Hepatotoxicity

Local: Corrosive to skin

Ocular: Miosis

Respiratory: Laryngeal edema, aspiration

Miscellaneous: Physical and psychological dependence may occur with prolonged use of large doses, pear-like odor

Signs & Symptoms of Acute Overdose Hypotension, acne, tachycardia (ventricular), respiratory depression, hyporeflexia, laryngospasm, acetone breath, ileus, myoglobinuria, nystagmus, thirst, ptosis, jaundice, coma, hypothermia, cardiac arrhythmias, torsade de pointes, eczema, myocardial depression, ventricular ectopy, alopecia, cough, leukopenia, neutropenia, agranulocytosis, granulocytopenia, rhabdomyolysis

Toxicodynamics/Kinetics

Onset of action: Within 30-60 minutes

Duration: ~4-8 hours

Absorption: Oral, rectal: Well absorbed

Distribution: V_d: 0.75 L/kg; distributes well to all body fluids and tissues

Protein binding: 35% to 41%

Metabolism: Rapid to trichloroethanol; variable amounts metabolized in liver and kidney to trichloroacetic acid (inactive)

Half-life:

Trichloroethanol: 8-11 hours

Neonates: 3-5 hours

Elimination: Metabolites excreted in urine; small amounts excreted in feces via bile

Usual Dosage

Neonates: Oral, rectal: 25 mg/kg/dose for sedation prior to a procedure or 50 mg/kg as hypnotic

Children:

Sedation, anxiety: Oral, rectal: 5-15 mg/kg/dose every 8 hours, maximum: 500 mg/dose

Prior to EEG: Oral, rectal: 20-25 mg/kg/dose, 30-60 minutes prior to EEG; may repeat in 30 minutes to maximum of 100 mg/kg or 2 g total

Hypnotic: Oral, rectal: 20-40 mg/kg/dose up to a maximum of 50 mg/kg/24 hours or 1 g/dose or 2 g/24 hours

Sedation, nonpainful procedure: Oral: 50-75 mg/kg/dose 30-60 minutes prior to procedure; may repeat 30 minutes after initial dose if needed, to a total maximum dose of 120 mg/kg or 1 g total

(Continued)

Chloral Hydrate *(Continued)*

Adults: Oral, rectal:

Sedation, anxiety: 250 mg 3 times/day

Hypnotic: 500-1000 mg at bedtime or 30 minutes prior to procedure, not to exceed 2 g/24 hours

Dosing adjustment/comments in renal impairment: Cl_{cr} <50 mL/minute: Avoid use

Dosing adjustment/comments in hepatic impairment: Avoid use in patients with severe hepatic impairment

Contraindications Hypersensitivity to chloral hydrate or any component; hepatic or renal impairment; gastrointestinal upset or ulcers; severe cardiac disease

Warnings Trichloroethanol (TCE), a metabolite of chloral hydrate, is a carcinogen in mice; there is no data in humans; use with caution in patients with porphyria; use with caution in neonates, drug may accumulate with repeated use, prolonged use in neonates associated with hyperbilirubinemia

Dosage Forms

Capsule: 250 mg, 500 mg

Suppository, rectal: 324 mg, 500 mg, 648 mg

Syrup: 250 mg/5 mL (10 mL); 500 mg/5 mL (5 mL, 10 mL, 480 mL)

Stability Sensitive to light; exposure to air causes volatilization; store in light-resistant, airtight container; incompatible with alkali, soluble barbiturates

Reference Range Therapeutic: 2-12 μg/mL of trichloroethanol; 25 μg/mL of trichloroethanol correlated with fatalities

Overdosage Treatment

Decontamination: Lavage carefully due to risk of perforation/activated charcoal with cathartic

Supportive therapy: Treatment is supportive and symptomatic; lidocaine, metoprolol, or bretylium may be used for ventricular arrhythmias, while isoproterenol or atropine may be required for torsade de pointes; activated charcoal may prevent drug absorption; flumazenil may be effective

Enhancement of elimination: Multiple dosing of activated charcoal may be effective; hemodialysis and/or charcoal hemoperfusion is effective; exchange transfusion also may be useful for neonatal intoxication; dialyzable (50% to 100%)

Test Interactions False-positive urine glucose using Clinitest® method; may interfere with fluorometric urine catecholamine and urinary 17-hydroxycorticosteroid tests; causes proteinuria; well visualized on plain film x-ray; may interfere with BUN test

Diagnostic Tests/Procedures

Chloral Hydrate, Plasma *on page 1224*

Chloral Hydrate, Qualitative, Urine *on page 1224*

Drug Interactions May potentiate effects of warfarin, central nervous system depressants, alcohol; vasodilation reaction (flushing, tachycardia, etc) may occur with concurrent use of alcohol; concomitant use of furosemide (I.V.) may result in flushing, sweating, and blood pressure changes

Pregnancy Risk Factor C (may be a cause of neonatal withdrawal)

Pregnancy Implications Crosses the placenta; negligible amounts appear in breast milk

Monitoring Parameters Vital signs, O_2 saturation and blood pressure with doses used for conscious sedation

Patient Information Avoid alcohol and other CNS depressants; avoid activities needing good psychomotor coordination until CNS effects are known; drug may cause physical or psychological dependence; avoid abrupt discontinuation after prolonged use; if taking at home prior to a diagnostic procedure, have someone else transport

Nursing Implications Gastric irritation may be minimized by diluting dose in water or other oral liquid

Additional Information Tolerance to hypnotic effect develops, therefore, not recommended for use >2 weeks; taper dosage to avoid withdrawal with prolonged use; radiopaque; genotoxic; question of carcinogenesis is unanswered

Specific References

Buur T, Larsson R, and Norlander B, "Pharmacokinetics of Chloral Hydrate Poisoning Treated With Hemodialysis and Hemoperfusion," *Acta Med Scand*, 1988, 223(3):269-74.

Donovan KL and Fisher DJ, "Reversal of Chloral Hydrate Overdose With Flumazenil," *Br Med J (Clin Res)*, 1989, 298(6682):1253.

Meyer E, Van Bocxlaer JF, Lambert WE, et al, "Determination of Chloral Hydrate and Metabolites in a Fatal Intoxication," *J Anal Toxicol*, 1995, 19:124-6.

Mowry JB, Wilson GA, and Schreiner R, "Effect of Exchange Transfusion in Chloral Hydrate Overdose," *Vet Hum Toxicol*, 1983, 25:15-21.

Salmon AG, Kizer KW, Zeise L, et al, "Potential Carcinogenicity of Chloral Hydrate – A Review," *J Toxicol Clin Toxicol*, 1995, 33(2):115-21.

Seger D and Schwartz G, "Chloral Hydrate: A Dangerous Sedative for Overdose Patients?" *Pediatr Emerg Care*, 1994, 10(6):349-50.

Sing K, Erickson T, Amitai Y, et al, "Case Series of Chloral Hydrate Toxicity From Oral and Intravenous Administration," *Vet Hum Toxicol*, 1993, 35:339.

Chloralix® *see* Chloral Hydrate *on page 193*

Chlorambucil (klor am' byoo sil)

Related Information

Drugs and Chemicals Proven to be Teratogenic in Humans *on page 1572-1575*

Toxicities of Chemotherapeutic Agents *on page 1631-1633*

CAS Number 305-03-3

Brand Names Amboclorin®; Leukeran®; Linfolysin®

Use Management of chronic lymphocytic leukemia, Hodgkin's and non-Hodgkin's lymphoma; breast and ovarian carcinoma; Waldenström's macroglobulinemia, testicular carcinoma, thrombocythemia, choriocarcinoma

Mechanism of Action Interferes with DNA replication and RNA transcription by alkylation and cross-linking the strands of DNA; derived from mustine (a nitrogen mustard)

Adverse Reactions

Central nervous system: Confusion, agitation, hallucination; rarely generalized or focal seizures, drowsiness, psychosis, hallucinations, asthenia, ataxia

Dermatologic: Skin rashes, dermal irritant, toxic epidermal necrolysis

Endocrine & metabolic: Hyperuricemia

Gastrointestinal: Diarrhea, oral ulceration are infrequent

Genitourinary: Has caused chromosomal damage in man, oligospermia, both reversible and permanent sterility have occurred in both sexes; can produce amenorrhea in females; cystitis

Hematologic: Possible porphyria; use with caution when receiving radiation; bone marrow depression frequently occurs and occasionally bone marrow failure has occurred; blood counts should be monitored closely while undergoing treatment; leukopenia (at doses in excess of 6.5 mg/kg), lymphocytopenia, thrombocytopenia, anemia

Hepatic: Hepatotoxicity, hepatic necrosis

Neuromuscular & skeletal: Tremors, muscular myoclonus, paresthesia

Ocular: Transient blindness (at 1.5 mg/kg/day), keratitis

Miscellaneous: Pulmonary fibrosis at doses of 40 mg/kg, skin hypersensitivity, azoospermia, cardiotoxic, drug fever

Signs & Symptoms of Acute Overdose Convulsions, coma (at 5 mg/kg), hyperuricemia, ataxia, leukopenia, neutropenia, agranulocytosis, oligospermia, azoospermia, toxic epidermal necrolysis, granulocytopenia

Toxicodynamics/Kinetics

Absorption/Bioavailability: 70% to 80%; **food interferes with absorption** resulting in a 10% to 20% decrease in bioavailability

Distribution: V_d: 0.14-0.24 L/kg

Protein binding: ~99% bound to albumin; extensive binding to tissues and plasma proteins

Metabolism: In the liver to an active metabolite (phenylacetic acid mustard); parent compound: 1.5-2 hours

Half-life: 1.5-2 hours; active metabolite: 2.5 hours

Elimination: 60% excreted in urine within 24 hours, principally as metabolites

Usual Dosage Oral (refer to individual protocols):

Nephrotic syndrome: 0.1-0.2 mg/kg/day every day for 5-15 weeks with low-dose prednisone

Children: 0.1-0.2 mg/kg/day or 4-8 mg/m^2/day for 3-6 weeks for remission induction; maintenance therapy: 0.03-0.1 mg/kg/day

Adults: 0.1-0.2 mg/kg/day (4-8 mg/m^2/day) for 3-6 weeks, then adjust dose on basis of blood counts. Pulse dosing has been used in CLL as intermittent, biweekly, or monthly doses of 0.4 mg/kg and increased by 0.1 mg/kg until the disease is under control or toxicity ensues; an alternate regimen is 14 mg/m^2/day for 5 days, repeated every 21-28 days

Contraindications Previous resistance; hypersensitivity to chlorambucil or any component or other alkylating agents

Warnings The U.S. Food and Drug Administration (FDA) currently recommends that procedures for proper handling and disposal of antineoplastic agents be considered; disposal of urine must also be cautiously handled. Use with caution in patients with seizure disorder and bone marrow suppression; reduce initial dosage if patient has received radiation therapy, myelosuppressive drugs, or has a depressed baseline leukocyte or platelet count within the previous 4 weeks; can severely suppress bone marrow function; affects human fertility; carcinogenic in humans and probably mutagenic and teratogenic as well; chromosomal damage has been documented; secondary AML may be associated with chronic therapy.

Dosage Forms Tablet, sugar coated: 2 mg

Stability Protect from light

(Continued)

Chlorambucil *(Continued)*

Reference Range Peak plasma level after a dose of 0.6-1.2 mg/kg: 1 μg/mL

Overdosage Treatment

Decontamination: Lavage/activated charcoal with cathartic

Supportive therapy: Replace blood products/diazepam or lorazepam for seizures

Enhancement of elimination: Multiple dosing of activated charcoal may be effective; probably not dialyzable

Pregnancy Risk Factor D

Pregnancy Implications Urogenital malformation seen in rodent studies

Monitoring Parameters Liver function tests, CBC (for at least 3 weeks), leukocyte counts, platelets, serum uric acid

Patient Information Notify physician immediately if sore throat or bleeding occurs, contraceptive measures are recommended during therapy

Additional Information Myelosuppressive effects:

WBC: Moderate

Platelets: Moderate

Onset (days): 7

Nadir (days): 14-21

Specific References

Byrne TN Jr, Moseley TA III, and Finer MA, "Myoclonic Seizures Following Chlorambucil Overdose," *Ann Neurol*, 1981, 9(2):191-4.

Green AA and Naiman JL, "Chlorambucil Poisoning," *Am J Dis Child*, 1968, 116(2):190-1.

Harris J and Dodds LJ, "Handling Wastes From Patients Receiving Cytotoxic Drugs," *Pharm J*, 1985, 235:289-91.

Vandenberg SA, Kulig K, Spoerke DG, et al, "Chlorambucil Overdose: Accidental Ingestion of an Antineoplastic Drug," *J Emerg Med*, 1988, 6(6):495-8.

Chloramiphene *see* Clomiphene Citrate *on page 227*

Chlorammonia® *see* Ammonium Chloride *on page 118*

Chloramphenicol (klor am fen' i kole)

CAS Number 56-75-7; 530-43-8; 982-57-0

Brand Names AK-Chlor® Ophthalmic; Chloromycetin®; Chloroptic® Ophthalmic; Ophthochlor® Ophthalmic

Synonyms Cloranfenicol

Use Treatment of serious infections due to organisms resistant to other less toxic antibiotics or when its penetrability into the site of infection is clinically superior to other antibiotics to which the organism is sensitive; useful in infections caused by *Bacteroides*, *H. influenzae*, *Neisseria meningitidis*, *Salmonella*, and *Rickettsia*

Mechanism of Action Reversibly binds to 50S ribosomal subunits of susceptible organisms preventing amino acids from being transferred to growing peptide chains thus inhibiting protein synthesis

Adverse Reactions

Cardiovascular: Cardiotoxicity (left ventricular dysfunction); gray baby syndrome

Central nervous system: Nightmares, headache, depression

Dermatologic: Rash, epidermal necrolysis, rash, urticaria

Endocrine & metabolic: Metabolic acidosis (associated with serum levels >30 μg/mL),

Gastrointestinal: Diarrhea, stomatitis, enterocolitis, vomiting, glossitis, nausea, colitis

Hematologic: Bone marrow depression, aplastic anemia (prevalence 1/18,000 to 1/50,000), thrombocytopenia, hemolytic anemia in patients with G-6-PD deficiency, leukopenia, neutropenia, agranulocytosis, granulocytopenia, porphyria, coagulopathy

Hepatic: Hepatitis-pancytopenia syndrome

Neuromuscular & skeletal: Paresthesia

Ocular: Optic neuritis and papilledema especially noted in patients with cystic fibrosis; vision color changes (yellow tinge); nystagmus

Respiratory: Wheezing

Miscellaneous: Anaphylaxis, disulfiram-like reaction, feces discoloration (black), feces discoloration (blue), feces discoloration (blue-green), porphyrinogenic

Toxicodynamics/Kinetics

Absorption: Oral: 75% to 100%; in neonates, gastrointestinal absorption of chloramphenicol palmitate is slow and erratic

Distribution: V_d: 0.8-1.2 L/kg

Protein binding: 50%

Metabolism: Extensive in liver (90%) to inactive metabolites (monoglucuronide), principally by glucuronidation

Half-life: 1.6-3.3 hours (prolonged in neonates and with hepatic insufficiency); 3.5-3.9 hours in patients with renal failure

Neonates:

1-2 days postnatal: 24 hours

10-16 days postnatal: 10 hours

Time to peak serum concentration: Oral: Within 0.5-3 hours

Elimination: 5% to 15% excreted as unchanged drug in urine, 4% excreted in bile

Usual Dosage

Neonates: Initial loading dose: Oral, I.V. (I.M. is not recommended):

Postnatal age 0-4 weeks:

<2000 g: 25 mg/kg/day every 24 hours

<7 days, >2000 g: 25 mg/kg/day every 24 hours

7-28 days, >2000 g: 25 mg/kg/dose every 12 hours

Meningitis: Oral, I.V.: Infants >30 days and Children: 75-100 mg/kg/day divided every 6 hours

Other infections: Oral, I.V.:

Infants and Children: 50-75 mg/kg/day divided every 6 hours; maximum daily dose: 4 g/day

Adults: 50-100 mg/kg/day in divided doses every 6 hours; maximum daily dose: 4 g/day

Dosing adjustment/comments in hepatic impairment: Avoid use in severe liver impairment as increased toxicity may occur

Children and Adults:

Ophthalmic: Instill 1-2 drops or 1.25 cm (½") of ointment every 3-4 hours; increase interval between applications after 48 hours to 2-3 times/day

Otic solution: Instill 2-3 drops into ear 3 times/day

Topical: Gently rub into the affected area 1-4 times/day

Administration Can be administered IVP over 5 minutes at a maximum concentration of 100 mg/mL, or I.V. intermittent infusion over 15-30 minutes at a final concentration for administration of ≤20 mg/mL

Contraindications Hypersensitivity to chloramphenicol or any component

Warnings Use with caution in patients with impaired renal or hepatic function and in neonates; reduce dose with impaired liver function; use with care in patients with glucose 6-phosphate dehydrogenase deficiency. Serious and fatal blood dyscrasias have occurred after both short-term and prolonged therapy; should not be used when less potentially toxic agents are effective; prolonged use may result in superinfection.

Dosage Forms

Capsule: 250 mg

Cream (Chloromycetin®): 1% (30 g)

Ointment, ophthalmic (AK-Chlor®, Chloromycetin®, Chloroptic®): 1% [10 mg/g] (3.5 g)

Powder for injection, as sodium succinate: 1 g

Powder for ophthalmic solution (Chloromycetin®): 25 mg/vial

Solution:

Ophthalmic (AK-Chlor®, Chloroptic®, Ophthochlor®): 0.5% [5 mg/mL] (2.5 mL, 7.5 mL, 15 mL)

Otic (Chloromycetin®): 0.5% (15 mL)

Stability Refrigerate ophthalmic solution; constituted solutions remain stable for 30 days; use only clear solutions; frozen solutions remain stable for 6 months

Reference Range

Therapeutic: 10-25 μg/mL

Toxic: >25 μg/mL; Trough: 5-10 μg/mL

Timing of serum samples: Draw levels 1.5 hours and 3 hours after completion of I.V. or oral dose; trough levels may be preferred; should be drawn ≤1 hour prior to dose

Overdosage Treatment

Decontamination: Emesis or lavage (for doses >50 mg/kg)/activated charcoal with cathartic

Supportive therapy: For optic neuropathy or paresthesia, give pyridoxine (vitamin B_6 500 mg twice daily) and vitamin B_{12} (0.5 mg/day) orally

Enhancement of elimination: Multiple dosing of activated charcoal may be effective; hemodialysis may be effective and can reduce half-life to under 1 hour; hemoperfusion may also be effective; exchange transfusion may be helpful in neonates; slightly dialyzable (5% to 20%)

Antidote(s)

Pyridoxine Hydrochloride *on page 1465*

Test Interactions ↑ iron (B), prothrombin time (S); ↓ urea nitrogen (B); ↓ total iron binding capacity (S)

Diagnostic Tests/Procedures

Chloramphenicol, Serum *on page 1225*

Complete Blood Count *on page 1236*

Kidney Profile *on page 1279*

Liver Profile *on page 1286*

(Continued)

Chloramphenicol *(Continued)*

Iron and Total Iron Binding Capacity/Transferrin *on page 1275*

Drug Interactions

Decreased toxicity/levels with rifampin; decreased clearance of chloramphenicol with cimetidine

Increased effect/toxicity/levels of chlorpropamide, phenytoin, oral anticoagulants, and phenobarbital; disulfiram-like reaction with ethanol

Pregnancy Risk Factor C

Pregnancy Implications Readily crosses placenta; appears in breast milk; do not use chloramphenicol near term; avoid use of chloramphenicol during breast feeding

Monitoring Parameters CBC with reticulocyte and platelet counts, periodic liver and renal function tests, serum drug concentration

Patient Information Take on empty stomach; take with food if gastrointestinal upset, at evenly spaced intervals (every 6 hours around-the-clock); notify physician if persistent sore throat, tiredness, or unusual bleeding or bruising

Nursing Implications Give around-the-clock rather than 4 times/day to promote less variation in peak and trough serum levels

Additional Information Sodium content of 1 g (injection): 51.8 mg (2.25 mEq); gray baby syndrome occurs when neonates are given large doses of chloramphenicol and cardiovascular collapse occurs; it is associated with plasma levels of 50-100 μg/mL; blood dyscrasias can occur with ocular use

Specific References

Cocke JG Jr, "Chloramphenicol Optic Neuritis. Apparent Protective Effects of Very High Daily Doses of Pyridoxine and Cyanocobalamin," *Am J Dis Child*, 1967, 114(4):424-6.

Doona M and Walsh JB, "Use of Chloramphenicol as Topical Eye Medication: Time to Cry Halt? Bone Marrow Aplasia Also Occurs With Ocular Use," *Br Med J*, 1995, 319:1217-8.

Freundlich M, Cynamon H, Tamer A, et al, "Management of Chloramphenicol Intoxication in Infancy by Charcoal Hemoperfusion," *J Pediatr*, 1983, 103(3):485-7.

Kunin CM, Glazko AJ, and Finland M, "Persistence of Antibiotics in Blood of Patients With Acute Renal Failure. II. Chloramphenicol and Its Metabolic Products in the Blood of Patients With Severe Renal Failure Disease or Hepatic Cirrhosis," *J Clin Invest*, 1959, 38(9):1498-508.

Montoro A, Cao A, Ordoqui E, et al, "Contact Sensitivity to Chloramphenicol," *J Allergy Clin Immunol*, 1995, 95:291.

Ramilo O, Kinane BT, and McCracken GH Jr, "Chloramphenicol Neurotoxicity," *Pediatr Infect Dis J*, 1988, 7(5):358-9.

Yunis AA, "Chloramphenicol: Relation of Structure to Activity and Toxicity," *Annu Rev Pharmacol Toxicol*, 1988, 28:83-100.

Chloraseptic® [OTC] *see* Phenol *on page 616*

Chlorate® [OTC] *see* Chlorpheniramine Maleate *on page 204*

Chlordiazepoxide (klor dye az e pox' ide)

Related Information

Benzodiazepines Comparison *on page 1643*

Therapeutic Drugs Associated With Hallucinations *on page 1558-1559*

CAS Number 58-25-3; 438-41-5

Brand Names A-Poxide®; Equibral®; Libritabs®; Librium®; Mitran®; Resposan-10®; SK-Lygen®; Smail®; Solium®; Tropium®

Synonyms Methaminodiazepoxide Hydrochloride

Use Management of anxiety and as a preoperative sedative, symptoms of alcohol withdrawal

Mechanism of Action Benzodiazepine anxiolytic sedative that produces CNS depression at the subcortical level, except at high doses, whereby it works at the cortical level

Adverse Reactions

Cardiovascular: Hypotension, tachycardia, edema

Central nervous system: Drowsiness, confusion, mental impairment, visual hallucinations, ataxia

Dermatologic: Skin eruptions

Gastrointestinal: Nausea, constipation

Hematologic: Blood dyscrasias

Neuromuscular & skeletal: Reflex slowing

Ocular: Mydriasis, diplopia, nystagmus

Miscellaneous: Drug dependence, menstrual irregularities

Signs & Symptoms of Acute Overdose Hypotension, respiratory depression, coma, galactorrhea, myoglobinuria, hypothermia, lactation, ejaculatory disturbances, photosensitivity, cardiac arrhythmias, jaundice, hiccups, leukopenia, neutropenia, agranulocytosis, granulocytopenia, hyperglycemia, rhabdomyolysis

Toxicodynamics/Kinetics

Onset of action: 30-45 minutes; depends largely on absorption rate

Absorption: Well absorbed from gastrointestinal tract; may be slow and erratic depending upon the site of administration

Absorption rate:
I.M.: 15-30 minutes (erratic)
I.V.: 1-5 minutes
Distribution: V_d: 3.3 L/kg; widely distributed throughout body
Protein binding: 90% to 98%
Metabolism: Extensive in the liver to demoxepam (active), demethylchlordiazepoxide (active), and oxazepam (active)
Half-life:
Parent compound: 5-25 hours
Demoxepam: 24-96 hours
Time to peak serum concentration:
Oral: 1-4 hours
I.M.: 15-30 minutes
I.V.: 3-30 minutes
Elimination: Very little excretion in urine as unchanged drug; clearance: 0.4-0.5 mL/minute/kg

Usual Dosage I.M. route is not recommended
Children:
<6 years: Not recommended
>6 years: Anxiety: Oral, I.M.: 0.5 mg/kg/24 hours divided every 6-8 hours
Adults:
Anxiety:
Oral: 15-100 mg divided 3-4 times/day
I.M., I.V.: Initial: 50-100 mg followed by 25-50 mg 3-4 times/day as needed
Preoperative anxiety: I.M.: 50-100 mg prior to surgery
Alcohol withdrawal symptoms: Oral, I.V.: 50-100 mg to start, dose may be repeated in 2-4 hours as necessary to a maximum of 300 mg/24 hours

Dosing adjustment in renal impairment: Cl_{cr} <10 mL/minute: Administer 50% of dose

Dosing adjustment/comments in hepatic impairment: Avoid use

Contraindications Hypersensitivity to chlordiazepoxide or any component, preexisting CNS depression, severe uncontrolled pain

Warnings Mental impairment, reflex slowing, drug dependence; not considered a drug of choice in the elderly

Dosage Forms
Capsule, as hydrochloride: 5 mg, 10 mg, 25 mg
Powder for injection, as hydrochloride: 100 mg
Tablet: 5 mg, 10 mg, 25 mg

Stability Refrigerate injection; protect from light

Reference Range
Therapeutic: 0.1-3 μg/mL (SI: 0-10 μmol/L)
Toxic: >23 μg/mL (SI: >77 μmol/L); toxicity may be related to demoxepam levels >10 μg/mL
Urine drug screens can remain positive for 30 days

Overdosage Treatment
Decontamination: Lavage/activated charcoal with cathartic
Supportive therapy: Treatment for benzodiazepine overdose is supportive. Rarely is mechanical ventilation required. Flumazenil has been shown to selectively block the binding of benzodiazepines to CNS receptors, resulting in a reversal of benzodiazepine-induced CNS depression; do not use stimulants.
Enhancement of elimination: Multiple dosing of activated charcoal may be effective; not dialyzable (0% to 5%)

Antidote(s)
Flumazenil *on page 1428*

Test Interactions Visine®, Drano®, hand soap, or bleach can result in false-negative tests for benzodiazepines

Diagnostic Tests/Procedures
Chlordiazepoxide, Blood *on page 1225*

Drug Interactions Oral anticoagulants, alcohol, ketoconazole, tricyclic antidepressants, sedatives, hypnotics, and MAO inhibitors all increase CNS depression; oral contraceptives, cimetidine, and disulfiram inhibit chlordiazepoxide metabolism

Pregnancy Risk Factor D

Pregnancy Implications Crosses the placenta; appears in breast milk

Monitoring Parameters Respiratory and cardiovascular status

Patient Information Avoid alcohol and other CNS depressants; avoid activities needing good psychomotor coordination until CNS effects are known; drug may cause physical or psychological dependence; avoid abrupt discontinuation after prolonged use

Nursing Implications Up to 300 mg may be given I.M. or I.V. during a 6-hour period, but not more than this in any 24-hour period; do not use diluent provided with parenteral form for I.V. administration; dissolve with normal saline instead

(Continued)

Chlordiazepoxide *(Continued)*

Additional Information Often formulated with amitriptyline hydrochloride

Specific References

Bailey DN, "Blood Concentrations and Clinical Findings Following Overdose of Chlordiazepoxide Alone and Chlordiazepoxide Plus Ethanol," *Clin Toxicol*, 1984, 22(5):433-46.

Burkhart KK and Kulig KW, "The Diagnostic Utility of Flumazenil (A Benzodiazepine Antagonist) in Coma of Unknown Etiology," *Ann Emerg Med*, 1990, 19(3):319-21.

Minder EI, "Toxicity in a Case of Acute and Massive Overdose of Chlordiazepoxide and Its Correlation to Blood Concentration," *J Toxicol Clin Toxicol*, 1989, 27(1-2):117-27.

Chlorethyl *see* Ethyl Chloride *on page 337*

Chlorhexidine Digluconate *see* Chlorhexidine Gluconate *on this page*

Chlorhexidine Gluconate (klor hex' i deen)

CAS Number 55-56-1; 18472-51-0

Brand Names BactoShield® Topical [OTC]; Dyna-Hex® Topical [OTC]; Exidine® Scrub [OTC]; Hibiclens® Topical [OTC]; Hibistat® Topical [OTC]; Peridex® Oral Rinse

Synonyms Chlorhexidine Digluconate

Use Skin cleanser for surgical scrub, cleanser for skin wounds, germicidal hand rinse, and as antibacterial dental rinse. Chlorhexidine is active against gram-positive and gram-negative organisms, facultative anaerobes, aerobes, and yeast.

Mechanism of Action Chlorhexidine, a cationic polybiguanide, is an antiseptic and antimicrobial drug with bactericidal activity. At physiologic pH, chlorhexidine salts dissociate releasing a positively charged component. The bactericidal effect of chlorhexidine is a result of the binding of this cationic molecule to negatively charged bacterial cell walls and extramicrobial complexes. At low concentrations, this causes an alteration of bacterial cell osmotic equilibrium and leakage of potassium and phosphorous resulting in a bacteriostatic effect; at high concentrations of chlorhexidine, the cytoplasmic contents of the bacterial cell precipitate and result in cell death.

Adverse Reactions

Dermatologic: Facial edema, dermal hypersensitivity, urticaria

Local: Staining of oral surfaces (mucosa, teeth, dorsum of tongue), tartar on teeth (increased), altered taste, tongue irritation, oral irritation, contact dermatitis (8%)

Ocular: Corneal irritation

Respiratory: Dyspnea, nasal congestion

Miscellaneous: Desquamation/parotid gland swelling with mouthwash, methemoglobinemia caused by conversion to parachloraniline

Signs & Symptoms of Acute Overdose Hemolysis with systemic absorption, methemoglobinemia, bradycardia, gastritis, esophageal ulceration, deafness, tongue discoloration, fatty degeneration of liver, pulmonary edema

Usual Dosage

Oral rinse (Peridex®):

Precede use of solution by flossing and brushing teeth, completely rinse toothpaste from mouth; swish 15 mL undiluted oral rinse around in mouth for 30 seconds, then expectorate. Caution patient not to swallow the medicine; avoid eating for 2-3 hours after treatment. (The cap on bottle of oral rinse is a measure for 15 mL.)

When used as a treatment of gingivitis, the regimen begins with oral prophylaxis. Patient treats mouth with 15 mL chlorhexidine; swish for 30 seconds, then expectorate. This is repeated twice daily (morning and evening). Patient should have a re-evaluation followed by a dental prophylaxis every 6 months.

Cleanser:

Surgical scrub: Scrub 3 minutes and rinse thoroughly, wash for an additional 3 minutes

Hand wash: Wash for 15 seconds and rinse

Hand rinse: Rub 15 seconds and rinse

Contraindications Known hypersensitivity to chlorhexidine gluconate

Warnings Staining of oral surfaces, teeth, restorations, and dorsum of tongue may occur; keep out of eyes and ears; for topical use only; there have been several case reports of anaphylaxis following disinfection with chlorhexidine; rectal administration can result in ulcerative colitis

Dosage Forms

Foam, topical, with isopropyl alcohol 4% (BactoShield®): 4% (180 mL)

Liquid, topical, with isopropyl alcohol 4%:

Dyna-Hex® Skin Cleanser: 2% (120 mL, 240 mL, 480 mL, 960 mL, 4000 mL); 4% (120 mL, 240 mL, 480 mL, 4000 mL)

BactoShield® 2: 2% (960 mL)

BactoShield®, Exidine® Skin Cleanser, Hibiclens® Skin Cleanser: 4% (15 mL, 120 mL, 240 mL, 480 mL, 960 mL, 4000 mL)

Rinse:

Oral (mint flavor) (Peridex®): 0.12% with alcohol 11.6% (480 mL)

Topical (Hibistat® Hand Rinse): 0.5% with isopropyl alcohol 70% (120 mL, 240 mL)

Sponge/Brush (Hibiclens®): 4% with isopropyl alcohol 4% (22 mL)

Wipes (Hibistat®): 0.5% (50s)

Stability Incompatible with anionic soaps

Overdosage Treatment

Decontamination: Lavage/dilution with milk or water (4-8 oz or 15 mL/kg); activated charcoal with cathartic is not useful; irrigate skin/eyes

Supportive therapy: Methylene blue for methemoglobin toxicity

Test Interactions Elevates liver function tests

Pregnancy Risk Factor B

Pregnancy Implications No teratogenic effects reported

Patient Information Do not swallow, do not rinse after use; may cause reduced taste perception which is reversible; may cause discoloration of teeth

Specific References

Emerson D and Pierce C, "A Case of a Single Ingestion of 4% Hibiclens®," *Vet Hum Toxicol*, 1988, 30(6):583.

Massano G, Ciocatto E, Rosabianca C, et al, "Striking Aminotransferase Rise After Chlorhexidine Self-Poisoning," *Lancet*, 1982, 1(8266):289.

Quinn MW and Bini RM, "Bradycardia Associated With Chlorhexidine Spray," *Arch Dis Child*, 1989, 64(6):892-3.

Yong D, Parker FC, and Foran SM, "Severe Allergic Reactions and Intra-Urethral Chlorhexidine Gluconate," *Med J Aust*, 1995, 162(5):257-8.

1(2-(4-5-chloro-1-(4-fluorophenyl)-1H-indol-3-y1)-1-piperidinyl ethyl)-2-imidazoline *see* Sertindole *on page 695*

2-chlorodeoxyadenosine *see* Cladribine *on page 220*

Chloroethane *see* Ethyl Chloride *on page 337*

Chloromycetin® *see* Chloramphenicol *on page 196*

Chloroprocaine Hydrochloride (klor oh proe' kane)

CAS Number 133-16-4; 3858-89-7

Brand Names Nesacaine®

Use Infiltration anesthesia and peripheral and epidural anesthesia

Mechanism of Action Ester local anesthetic similar to procaine produces conduction block at nerve cell membrane

Adverse Reactions

Cardiovascular: Myocardial depression, hypotension, bradycardia, cardiovascular collapse, edema

Central nervous system: Anxiety, restlessness, disorientation, confusion, shivering, psychosis, seizures, drowsiness, unconsciousness, chills

Dermatologic: Urticaria

Gastrointestinal: Nausea, vomiting

Local: Transient stinging or burning at injection site

Neuromuscular & skeletal: Tremors

Ocular: Blurred vision, diplopia, nystagmus

Otic: Ototoxicity, tinnitus

Respiratory: Respiratory arrest

Miscellaneous: Anaphylactoid reactions

Signs & Symptoms of Acute Overdose Cardiac arrhythmias, seizures, coma, tachypnea progressing to apnea; tachycardia, hypertension, mydriasis

Toxicodynamics/Kinetics

Metabolism: Hydrolyzed by plasma cholinesterase

Half-life: 23 seconds

Usual Dosage Dosage varies with anesthetic procedure, the area to be anesthetized, the vascularity of the tissues, depth of anesthesia required, degree of muscle relaxation required, and duration of anesthesia

Infiltration and peripheral nerve block: 1% to 2%

Infiltration, peripheral and central nerve block, including caudal and epidural block: 2% to 3%, without preservatives

Contraindications Known hypersensitivity to chloroprocaine, or other ester type anesthetics; myasthenia gravis; concurrent use of bupivacaine; do not use for subarachnoid administration

Warnings Use with caution in patients with cardiac disease, hyperthyroidism, or with decreased pseudocholinesterase activity

Dosage Forms Injection:

Preservative free (Nesacaine®-MPF): 2% (30 mL); 3% (30 mL)

With preservative (Nesacaine®): 1% (30 mL); 2% (30 mL)

Stability May contain sodium bisulfite

(Continued)

Chloroprocaine Hydrochloride *(Continued)*

Overdosage Treatment

Decontamination: Lavage/activated charcoal with cathartic for oral ingestions

Supportive therapy: Treatment is primarily symptomatic and supportive. Termination of anesthesia by pneumatic tourniquet inflation should be attempted when the agent is administered by infiltration or regional injection. Seizures commonly respond to diazepam or lorazepam, while hypotension responds to I.V. fluids and Trendelenburg positioning. Bradyarrhythmias (when the heart rate is less than 60) can be treated with I.V., I.M. or S.C. atropine 15 mcg/kg. With the development of metabolic acidosis, I.V. sodium bicarbonate 0.5-2 mEq/kg and ventilatory assistance should be instituted. Chlorpromazine may be used to treat acute psychosis.

Enhancement of elimination: Multiple dosing of activated charcoal may be effective for oral ingestions

Drug Interactions Vasopressors, MAO inhibitors, TCA, phenothiazines, inhalation anesthetics, ergot-type oxytocics

Pregnancy Risk Factor C

Monitoring Parameters EKG, blood pressure, CBC with differential, platelet count

Nursing Implications Before injecting, withdraw syringe plunger to ensure injection is not into vein or artery

Specific References

Freeman DW and Arnold NI, "Paracervical Block With Low Doses of Chloroprocaine: Fetal and Maternal Effects," *JAMA*, 1975, 231(1):56-7.

Jankowsky EC, "Pharmacologic Aspects of Local Anesthetic Use," *Anesth Clin North Am*, 1990, 8:1-25.

Chloroptic® Ophthalmic *see* Chloramphenicol *on page 196*

Chloroquine Phosphate (klor' oh kwin)

CAS Number 50-63-5

Brand Names Aralen® Phosphate

Use Suppression or chemoprophylaxis of malaria; treatment of uncomplicated or mild-moderate malaria; extraintestinal amebiasis; rheumatoid arthritis; treatment of sideroblastic anemia and porphyria cutanea tarda

Mechanism of Action Binds to and inhibits DNA and RNA polymerase; interferes with metabolism and hemoglobin utilization by parasites; inhibits prostaglandin effects; additionally has quinidine-like cardiac effects

Adverse Reactions

Cardiovascular: Hypotension, extrapyramidal reaction, cardiomyopathy, Q-T prolongation, EKG changes (wide QRS tachycardia)

Central nervous system: Fatigue, psychosis, personality changes, headache, visual hallucinations

Dermatologic: Pruritus, hair bleaching, alopecia, erythema multiforme, photosensitivity

Gastrointestinal: Anorexia, nausea, vomiting, diarrhea, stomatitis

Hematologic: Blood dyscrasias such as dose-related leukopenia, neutropenia, agranulocytosis, granulocytopenia; and hemolytic anemia (especially in G-6-PD deficiency)

Ocular: Retinopathy (dose related, 5.1 mg/kg/day), blurred vision, cataract, diplopia, photophobia

Otic: Ototoxicity, deafness, tinnitus

Miscellaneous: Rust-yellow to brown color of urine

Signs & Symptoms of Acute Overdose Headache, methemoglobinemia, seizures, urine discoloration (brown), urine discoloration (milky), urine discoloration (rust), urine discoloration (yellow-brown), hypopigmented hair, myopathy, A-V block, Stevens-Johnson syndrome, arrhythmias, nystagmus, visual changes including blindness, corneal microdeposits, vision color changes (blue tinge), vision color changes (green tinge), vision color changes (yellow tinge); ptosis, myasthenia gravis (exacerbation or precipitation of), cardiovascular collapse, hypoglycemia, hypotension in a very rapid progression, hypokalemia; doses 20 mg/kg considered toxic

Toxicodynamics/Kinetics

Absorption: Oral: Rapid

Distribution: V_d (in plasma): 204 L/kg (range: 116-285 L/kg); may be as large as 800 L/kg; widely distributed in body tissues such as eyes, heart, kidneys, liver, and lungs where retention is prolonged

Protein binding: 50% to 65%

Metabolism: Partial hepatic metabolism occurs

Bioavailability: ~89%

Half-life: 3-5 days

Time to peak serum concentration: Within 1-2 hours

Elimination: ~70% excreted unchanged in urine; acidification of urine increases elimination of drug; small amounts of drug may be present in urine months following discontinuation of therapy

Usual Dosage Oral (dosage expressed in terms of mg of base):

Suppression or prophylaxis of malaria:

Children: Administer 5 mg base/kg/week on the same day each week (not to exceed 300 mg base/dose); begin 1-2 weeks prior to exposure; continue for 4-6 weeks after leaving endemic area; if suppressive therapy is not begun prior to exposure, double the initial loading dose to 10 mg base/kg and give in 2 divided doses 6 hours apart, followed by the usual dosage regimen

Adults: 300 mg/week (base) on the same day each week; begin 1-2 weeks prior to exposure; continue for 4-6 weeks after leaving endemic area; if suppressive therapy is not begun prior to exposure, double the initial loading dose to 600 mg base and give in 2 divided doses 6 hours apart, followed by the usual dosage regimen

Acute attack:

Children: 10 mg/kg on day 1, followed by 5 mg/kg 6 hours later and 5 mg/kg on days 2 and 3

Adults: 600 mg on day 1, followed by 300 mg 6 hours later, followed by 300 mg on days 2 and 3

Extraintestinal amebiasis:

Children: 10 mg/kg once daily for 2-3 weeks (up to 300 mg base/day)

Adults: 600 mg base/day for 2 days followed by 300 mg base/day for at least 2-3 weeks

Dosing adjustment in renal impairment: Cl_{cr} <10 mL/minute: Administer 50% of dose

To limit ocular effects, maximum daily dose should be 250 mg

Contraindications Retinal or visual field changes; patients with psoriasis; known hypersensitivity to chloroquine

Warnings Use with caution in patients with liver disease, G-6-PD deficiency, alcoholism or in conjunction with hepatotoxic drugs

Dosage Forms Tablet: 250 mg [150 mg base]; 500 mg [300 mg base]

Reference Range Average plasma concentrations 120-340 ng/L, toxicity associated with blood concentrations of 3-99 mg/L

Overdosage Treatment

Decontamination: Activated charcoal with cathartic, ipecac, if available, for prehospital use clearly indicated; lavage if patient is obtunded

Supportive therapy: Early administration of diazepam or lorazepam and epinephrine appears beneficial; avoid class I antiarrhythmics; 2 mg (I.V.) of clonazepam has terminated chloroquine-induced nonconvulsive status epilepticus

Enhancement of elimination: Minimally removed by hemodialysis; hemoperfusion useful early in course of ingestion, but toxicities often prevent use; multiple doses of activated charcoal may be effective

Antidote(s)

Epinephrine *on page 1422*

Diagnostic Tests/Procedures

Complete Blood Count *on page 1236*

Electrocardiography *on page 1253*

Electrolytes, Blood *on page 1254*

Urinalysis *on page 1373*

Drug Interactions Increased toxicity with cimetidine, kaolin, magnesium trisilicate, rabies vaccine (intradermally administered rabies vaccine)

Pregnancy Risk Factor B (C at high doses)

Pregnancy Implications Crosses the placenta; appears in breast milk; at high doses can cause spontaneous abortion, fetal retinal and vestibular effects noted at larger anti-inflammatory doses used for arthritis

Monitoring Parameters Periodic CBC, examination for muscular asthenia and ophthalmologic examination in patients receiving prolonged therapy

Patient Information Take with meals; report any visual disturbances or difficulty in hearing or ringing in the ears; tablets are bitter tasting

Specific References

August C, Holzhausen H-J, Schmoldt A, et al, "Histological and Ultrastructural Findings in Chloroquine-Induced Cardiomyopathy," *J Molecular Med*, 1995, 73:73-7.

Avina-Zubieta JA, Johnson ES, Suarez-Almazor ME, et al, "Incidence of Myopathy in Patients Treated With Antimalarials. A Report of Three Cases and a Review of the Literature," *Br J Rheumatol*, 1995, 34:166-70.

Curry S, Connor D, Holland D, et al, "Effect of I.V. $NaHCO_3$ on QRS Duration in Rats Poisoned With Chloroquine," *Vet Hum Toxicol*, 1994, 36:363.

Demaziere J, Fourcade JM, and Busseuil GT, "The Hazards of Chloroquine Self Prescription in West Africa," *J Toxicol Clin Toxicol*, 1995, 33(4):369-70.

Drenou B, Guyader D, Turlin B, et al, "Treatment of Sideroblastic Anemia With Chloroquine," *N Engl J Med*, 1995, 332(9):614

Jaeger A, Sauder P, Kopferschmitt J, et al, "Clinical Features and Management of Poisoning Due to Antimalarial Drugs," *Adverse Drug Exp Med Toxicol*, 1987, 2(4):242-73.

Mulhauser P, Allemann Y, and Regamey C, "Chloroquine and Nonconvulsive Status Epilepticus," *Ann Intern Med*, 1995, 123(1):77.

(Continued)

Chloroquine Phosphate *(Continued)*

Rajah A, "The Use of Diazepam in Chloroquine Poisoning," *Anaesthesia*, 1990, 45(11):955-7.
Riou B, Barriot P, Rimailho A, et al, "Treatment of Severe Chloroquine Poisoning," *N Engl J Med*, 1988, 318(1):1-6.
Schröder S, August C, Pompecki R, et al, "Fatal Vacuolar Cardiomyopathy in Chronic Chloroquine Drug Treatment," *Pathologe* 1995, 16(1):81-4.

Chlorphed®-LA Nasal Solution [OTC] *see* Oxymetazoline Hydrochloride *on page 586*

Chlorphed® [OTC] *see* Brompheniramine Maleate *on page 165*

Chlorpheniramine Maleate (klor fen ir' a meen mal' ee ate)

Related Information

H1-Antihistamine Comparison *on page 1649*
Therapeutic Drugs Associated With Hallucinations *on page 1558-1559*

CAS Number 113-92-8

Brand Names Aller-Chlor® [OTC]; AL-R® [OTC]; Chlo-Amine® [OTC]; Chlorate® [OTC]; Chlor-Pro® [OTC]; Chlor-Trimeton® [OTC]; Kloromin® [OTC]; Phenetron®; Telachlor®; Teldrin® [OTC]

Use Perennial and seasonal allergic rhinitis and other allergic symptoms including rash

Mechanism of Action Competes with histamine for H_1-receptor sites on effector cells in the gastrointestinal tract, blood vessels, and respiratory tract

Adverse Reactions

Central nervous system: Drowsiness, asthenia, headache, auditory and visual hallucinations, extrapyramidal reaction, electroencephalogram abnormalities
Dermatologic: Dermatitis
Gastrointestinal: Nausea, dry mouth
Genitourinary: Urinary retention
Hematologic: Blood dyscrasias
Ocular: Diplopia, blindness
Renal: Polyuria

Signs & Symptoms of Acute Overdose Dry mouth, mydriasis, CNS depression, extrapyramidal reaction, leukopenia, neutropenia, agranulocytosis, granulocytopenia, flushing

Toxicodynamics/Kinetics

Onset of action: 20-60 minutes
Duration: 8-12 hours
Absorption: Well from gastrointestinal tract; food in stomach delays absorption but does not affect bioavailability
Distribution: V_d:
- Children: 7 L/kg
- Adults: 3.2 L/kg

Protein binding: 69% to 72%
Metabolism: In the liver
Half-life:
- Children: 13 hours
- Adults: 20-24 hours
- Renal failure: 280-330 hours

Time to peak serum concentration: 2-6 hours
Elimination: Metabolites and parent drug (3% to 4%) excreted in urine; 35% of total within 48 hours

Usual Dosage

Children: Oral: 0.35 mg/kg/day in divided doses every 4-6 hours
- 2-6 years: 1 mg every 4-6 hours, not to exceed 6 mg in 24 hours
- 6-12 years: 2 mg every 4-6 hours, not to exceed 12 mg/day; sustained release: 8 mg at bedtime

Children >12 years and Adults: Oral: 4 mg every 4-6 hours, not to exceed 24 mg/day; sustained release: 8-12 mg every 8-12 hours, not to exceed 24 mg/day

Adults: Allergic reactions: I.M., I.V., S.C.: 10-20 mg as a single dose; maximum recommended dose: 40 mg/24 hours

Contraindications Hypersensitivity to chlorpheniramine maleate or any component; narrow-angle glaucoma, bladder neck obstruction, symptomatic prostate hypertrophy, asthmatic attacks, and stenosing peptic ulcer

Warnings Do not administer to premature or full-term neonates; young children may be more susceptible to side effects and CNS stimulation

Dosage Forms

Capsule: 12 mg
Capsule, timed release: 6 mg, 8 mg, 12 mg
Injection: 10 mg/mL (1 mL, 30 mL); 100 mg/mL (10 mL)
Syrup: 2 mg/5 mL (120 mL, 480 mL, 4000 mL)
Tablet: 4 mg, 8 mg, 12 mg

Tablet:
Chewable: 2 mg
Timed release: 8 mg, 12 mg

Overdosage Treatment There is no specific treatment for an antihistamine overdose, however, most of its clinical toxicity is due to anticholinergic effects. Anticholinesterase inhibitors may be useful by reducing acetylcholinesterase. Anticholinesterase inhibitors include physostigmine, neostigmine, pyridostigmine, and edrophonium. For anticholinergic overdose with severe life-threatening symptoms, physostigmine 1-2 mg (0.5 or 0.02 mg/kg for children) I.V., slowly may be given to reverse these effects.

Drug Interactions CNS depressants, monoamine oxidase inhibitors, epinephrine

Pregnancy Risk Factor B

Patient Information May cause drowsiness; swallow whole, do not crush or chew

Additional Information Not effective for nasal stuffiness

Specific References

Paton DM and Webster DR, "Clinical Pharmacokinetics of H_1-Receptor Antagonists (The Antihistamines)," *Clin Pharmacokinet*, 1985, 10(6):477-97.

Chlorpromazine Hydrochloride (klor proe' ma zeen)

Related Information

Antipsychotic Agents Comparison *on page 1642*
Doses and Administration of Several Frequently Used Antiemetic Agents *on page 1641*
Therapeutic Drugs Associated With Hallucinations *on page 1558-1559*

CAS Number 50-53-3; 69-09-0

Brand Names Amazin®; Bay Clor®; Dozine®; Hibanil®; Largactil®; Ormazine®; Prozil®; Repazine®; Thorazine®

Use Treatment of nausea and vomiting; psychoses; Tourette's syndrome; mania; intractable hiccups (adults); behavioral problems (children); tension and vascular headaches

Mechanism of Action Blocks postsynaptic mesolimbic dopaminergic receptors in the brain; exhibits a strong alpha-adrenergic blocking effect and depresses the release of hypothalamic and hypophyseal hormones; strongly anticholinergic

Adverse Reactions

Cardiovascular: Hypotension (especially with I.V. use), hypotension (orthostatic), tachycardia, cardiac arrhythmias
Central nervous system: Sedation, drowsiness, restlessness, anxiety, extrapyramidal reactions, pseudoparkinsonian signs and symptoms, tardive dyskinesia, neuroleptic malignant syndrome, seizures, altered central temperature regulation, auditory and visual hallucinations
Dermatologic: Hyperpigmentation, pruritus, rash, photosensitivity
Endocrine & metabolic: Amenorrhea, galactorrhea, gynecomastia, syndrome of inappropriate antidiuretic hormone, weight gain
Gastrointestinal: gastrointestinal upset, dry mouth, constipation
Genitourinary: Urinary retention, impotence, priapism
Hematologic: Leukopenia/neutropenia (agranulocytosis, granulocytopenia) (usually in patients with large doses for prolonged periods), thrombocytopenia, hemolysis, eosinophilia
Hepatic: Cholestatic jaundice (rare)
Ocular: Retinal pigmentation (>600 g total dosage), blurred vision, mydriasis, photophobia, nystagmus, diplopia, pigmentary deposits in the lens and cornea, epithelial keratopathy
Miscellaneous: Anaphylactoid reactions

Signs & Symptoms of Acute Overdose Deep sleep, hypoglycemia, coma, night terrors, Q-T prolongation, impotence, hypothermia, hyperprolactinemia, ejaculatory disturbances, toxic epidermal necrolysis, delirium, jaundice, neuroleptic malignant syndrome, photosensitivity, corneal microdeposits, extrapyramidal reaction, appetite (increased), Parkinson's-like symptoms, myasthenia gravis (exacerbation or precipitation of), hyperthermia, abnormal involuntary muscle movements, hypotension or hypertension, hirsutism, vision color changes (brown tinge), vision color changes (yellow tinge); systemic lupus erythematosus (SLE), urine discoloration (pink), urine discoloration (red), urine discoloration (red-brown)

Toxicodynamics/Kinetics

Onset of action:
Tablet: 30 minutes to 1 hour
Sustained released preparation: 30 minutes to 1 hour
Suppositories: 60 minutes

Duration: of action:
Tablet: 4-6 hours
Sustained release preparation: 10-12 hours
Suppositories: 3-4 hours

(Continued)

Chlorpromazine Hydrochloride *(Continued)*

Absorption:
- Oral: Erratic
- I.M.: Rapid

Distribution: V_d: 10-35 L/kg; widely distributed; accumulates in brain and other tissues with a rich blood supply

Protein binding: 92% to 98%

Metabolism: Extensive in the liver to active and inactive metabolites

Half-life:
- Biphasic: 30 hours
- Phase I: 2 hours

Time to peak serum concentration:
- Oral: 2-4 hours
- I.M.: 15-20 minutes

Elimination: <1% excreted as unchanged drug in urine within 24 hours

Usual Dosage

Children >6 months:

Psychosis:
- Oral: 0.5-1 mg/kg/dose every 4-6 hours; older children may require 200 mg/day or higher
- I.M., I.V.: 0.5-1 mg/kg/dose every 6-8 hours; maximum dose for <5 years (22.7 kg): 40 mg/day; maximum for 5-12 years (22.7-45.5 kg): 75 mg/day

Nausea and vomiting:
- Oral: 0.5-1 mg/kg/dose every 4-6 hours as needed
- I.M., I.V.: 0.5-1 mg/kg/dose every 6-8 hours; maximum dose for <5 years (22.7 kg): 40 mg/day; maximum for 5-12 years (22.7-45.5 kg): 75 mg/day
- Rectal: 1 mg/kg/dose every 6-8 hours as needed

Adults:

Psychosis:
- Oral: Range: 30-800 mg/day in 1-4 divided doses, initiate at lower doses and titrate as needed; usual dose: 200 mg/day; some patients may require 1-2 g/day
- I.M., I.V.: Initial: 25 mg, may repeat (25-50 mg) in 1-4 hours, gradually increase to a maximum of 2000 mg/day; usual dose: 300-800 mg/day

Nausea and vomiting:
- Oral: 10-25 mg every 4-6 hours
- I.M., I.V.: 25-50 mg every 4-6 hours
- Rectal: 50-100 mg every 6-8 hours

Dosing adjustment/comments in hepatic impairment: Avoid use in severe hepatic dysfunction

Contraindications Hypersensitivity to chlorpromazine hydrochloride or any component, cross-sensitivity with other phenothiazines may exist, avoid use in patients with narrow-angle glaucoma, bone marrow depression, severe liver or cardiac disease

Warnings Safety in children <6 months of age has not been established; use with caution in patients with cardiovascular disease or seizures; bone marrow depression, severe liver or cardiac disease; significant hypotension may occur, especially when the drug is administered parenterally; extended release capsules and injection contain benzyl alcohol; injection also contains sulfites which may cause allergic reaction

Dosage Forms

Capsule, sustained action: 30 mg, 75 mg, 150 mg, 200 mg, 300 mg
Concentrate, oral: 30 mg/mL (120 mL); 100 mg/mL (60 mL, 240 mL)
Injection: 25 mg/mL (1 mL, 2 mL, 10 mL)
Suppository, rectal, as base: 25 mg, 100 mg
Syrup: 10 mg/5 mL (120 mL)
Tablet: 10 mg, 25 mg, 50 mg, 100 mg, 200 mg

Stability Protect oral dosage forms from light; a slightly yellowed solution does not indicate potency loss, but a markedly discolored solution should be discarded; diluted injection (1 mg/mL) with NS and stored in 5 mL vials remain stable for 30 days; not soluble with alkali, aminophylline, ampicillin, chlorothiazide, methohexitone, phenobarbital, amphotericin, sulfadimidine

Reference Range

Therapeutic: 50-300 ng/mL (SI: 157-942 nmol/L)
Toxic: >750 ng/mL (SI: >2355 nmol/L)

Overdosage Treatment

Decontamination: Lavage/activated charcoal with cathartic

Supportive therapy: Following initiation of essential overdose management, toxic symptom treatment and supportive treatment should be initiated. Hypotension usually responds to I.V. fluids or Trendelenburg positioning. If unresponsive to these measures, the use of a parenteral inotrope may be required (eg, norepinephrine 0.1-0.2 mcg/kg/minute titrated to response). Seizures commonly respond to lorazepam or diazepam (I.V. 5-10 mg bolus in adults every 15 minutes if needed up to a total of 30 mg; I.V. 0.25-0.4 mg/kg/dose up to a total of 10 mg in children) or to phenytoin or phenobarbital. Also critical cardiac arrhythmias often respond to I.V. phenytoin (15 mg/kg up to 1 g), while other antiarrhythmics can be used. Neuroleptics often cause extrapyramidal reaction (eg, dystonic reactions) requiring management with diphenhydramine 1-2 mg/kg (adults) up to a maximum of 50 mg I.V. slow push followed by a maintenance dose for 48-72 hours. When these reactions are unresponsive to diphenhydramine, benztropine mesylate I.V. 1-2 mg (adults) may be effective. These agents are generally effective within 2-5 minutes.

Enhancement of elimination: Not dialyzable (0% to 5%); multiple dosing of activated charcoal would not be expected to be useful

Test Interactions False-positive for phenylketonuria, amylase, uroporphyrins, urobilinogen; possible false-negative pregnancy urinary test; may cause positive direct Coombs' test, thyroid function tests; may interfere with determinations of blood urea nitrogen, vitamin B_{12} tests

Drug Interactions Additive effects with other CNS-depressing agents; epinephrine may cause hypotension in patients receiving chlorpromazine due to phenothiazine-induced alpha-adrenergic blockade and unopposed epinephrine B_2 action; chlorpromazine may increase valproic acid serum concentrations; when given piperazine, seizures may occur; antacids, cimetidine may interfere with chlorpromazine absorption; nortriptyline or propranolol may increase chlorpromazine levels; salicylamide and acetanilide may displace chlorpromazine from its protein binding. H_2 antagonists decrease absorption of chlorpromazine.

Pregnancy Risk Factor C

Pregnancy Implications Crosses the placenta; appears in breast milk; may cause damage to fetal retina

Monitoring Parameters Periodic ophthalmologic exams, neurologic, cardiac status for 48 hours

Patient Information May cause drowsiness

Nursing Implications Dilute oral concentrate solution in juice before administration; avoid contact of oral solution or injection with skin (contact dermatitis); watch for hypotension when administering I.M. or I.V.

Additional Information Use decreased doses in elderly or debilitated patients; extrapyramidal reaction may be more common in patients with hypocalcemia; extrapyramidal reactions may be more common in pediatric patients, especially those with dehydration or acute illnesses (viral or CNS infections); avoid rectal administration in immunocompromised patients; may be useful in treating headaches due to meningitis

Specific References

Fernandes CM, "Parenteral Chlorpromazine and a Meningitis Headache," *J Emerg Med*, 1995, 13(4):577-9.

Knight ME and Roberts RJ, "Phenothiazine and Butyrophenone Intoxication in Children," *Pediatr Clin North Am*, 1986, 33(2):299-309.

Lipka LJ, Lathers CM, and Roberts J, "Does Chlorpromazine Produce Cardiac Arrhythmia Via the Central Nervous System," *J Clin Pharmacol*, 1988, 28(11):968-83.

Mitchell AC and Brown KW, "Chlorpromazine-Induced Retinopathy," *Br J Psychiatry*, 1995, 166:822-3.

Oshika T, "Ocular Adverse Effects of Neuropsychiatric Agents: Incidence and Management," *Drug Saf*, 1995, 12:256-63.

Rosenberg MR and Green M, "Neuroleptic Malignant Syndrome: Review of Response to Therapy," *Arch Intern Med*, 1989, 149(9):1927-31.

Chlorpropamide (klor proe' pa mide)

Related Information

Hypoglycemic Agents Comparison, Oral *on page 1650*

CAS Number 99-20-2

Brand Names Clordiabet®; Diabet®; Diabinese®; Gliconorm®; Glymese®; Hypomide®; Normoglic®

Use Controls blood sugar in adult onset, noninsulin-dependent diabetes (type II)

Mechanism of Action Stimulates insulin release from the pancreatic beta cells; reduces glucose output from the liver; insulin sensitivity is increased at peripheral target sites

Adverse Reactions

Cardiovascular: Edema

Central nervous system: Headache, dizziness, fasciculations

Dermatologic: Photosensitivity, rash, pruritus, hives

Endocrine & metabolic: Hypoglycemia, hyponatremia, syndrome of inappropriate antidiuretic hormone

Gastrointestinal: Anorexia, nausea, vomiting, diarrhea, abdominal cramps, constipation, heartburn, epigastric fullness

Hematologic: Blood dyscrasias: leukopenia, neutropenia, agranulocytosis, granulocytopenia, thrombocytopenia, aplastic anemia, hemolysis, bone marrow depression

(Continued)

Chlorpropamide *(Continued)*

Hepatic: Cholestatic jaundice
Ocular: Diplopia, photophobia
Miscellaneous: Feces discoloration (black), porphyrinogenic

Signs & Symptoms of Acute Overdose Hypoglycemia (may be prolonged), jaundice, leukopenia; photosensitivity, hyponatremia, lichenoid eruptions, ataxia, neutropenia; feces discoloration (black); erythema multiforme, agranulocytosis; Stevens-Johnson syndrome, granulocytopenia; colitis

Toxicodynamics/Kinetics
Peak effect: Oral: Within 6-8 hours
Distribution: V_d: 0.09-0.27 L/kg
Protein binding: 60% to 90%
Metabolism: Extensive in the liver, ~80%
Half-life: 30-42 hours; prolonged in elderly or with renal disease
Time to peak serum concentration: Within 3-4 hours
Elimination: 10% to 30% excreted in urine as unchanged drug

Usual Dosage The dosage of chlorpropamide is variable and should be individualized based upon the patient's response

Adults:
- Initial dose: 250 mg/day in mild to moderate diabetes in middle aged, stable diabetic; elderly patients: 100-125 mg/day
- Maintenance dose: 100-250 mg/day; severe diabetics may require 500 mg/day; avoid doses >500 mg/day

Dosing adjustment/comments in renal impairment: Cl_{cr} <50 mL/minute: Avoid use

Dosing adjustment in hepatic impairment: Dose reduction is recommended

Contraindications Cross-sensitivity may exist with other hypoglycemics or sulfonamides; do not use with type I diabetes, or with severe renal, hepatic, thyroid, or other endocrine disease

Warnings Patients should be properly instructed in the early detection and treatment of hypoglycemia; long half-life may complicate recovery from excess effects; because of chlorpropamide's long half-life, duration of action, and increased risk for hypoglycemia, not considered a hypoglycemic agent of choice in the elderly. May be porphyrinogenic; use with caution in patients with porphyria.

Dosage Forms Tablet: 100 mg, 250 mg

Reference Range
Glucose: Adults: 60-115 mg/dL
Elderly fasting glucose: 100-180 mg/dL
Chlorpropamide lethal level: >400 μg/mL in nondiabetic patients

Overdosage Treatment
Decontamination: Lavage/activated charcoal with cathartic
Supportive therapy: Glucose (25 g I.V.) is mainstay of therapy. Glucagon (1-5 mg I.V., I.M., or S.C.) will have limited benefit (0.03-0.1 mg/kg in pediatrics); diazoxide is a third-line agent
Enhancement of elimination: Multiple dosing of activated charcoal is not useful; alkalinization of urine is useful; charcoal hemoperfusion may remove as much as 80% of the body burden of chlorpropamide

Antidote(s)
Dextrose *on page 1409*

Drug Interactions
Decreased effect: Thiazides and hydantoins (eg, phenytoin), beta-adrenergic blockers, gemfibrozil, isoniazid, rifampin, chlorpromazine, oral contraceptives, thyroid hormone, diazoxide; ↓ chlorpropamide effectiveness → ↑ blood glucose
Increased toxicity: ↑ alcohol-associated disulfiram reactions; ↑ oral anticoagulant effect; salicylates → ↑ chlorpropamide effect → ↓ blood glucose; MAO inhibitors ↑ hypoglycemic response; sulfonamides → ↓ sulfonylureas clearance; indobufen, phenylbutazone, co-trimoxazole, chloramphenicol, monoamine oxidase inhibitors, fluconazole, methyldopa, ranitidine, enalapril, nortriptyline, sulfinpyrazone, miconazole

Pregnancy Risk Factor D

Pregnancy Implications Appears in breast milk

Monitoring Parameters Fasting blood glucose, normal Hgb A, C, or fructosamine levels; monitor for signs and symptoms of hypoglycemia, (fatigue, sweating, numbness of extremities); monitor urine for glucose and ketones

Patient Information Avoid alcohol; take at the same time each day

Specific References
Erickson T, Arora A, Lebby TI, et al, "Acute Oral Hypoglycemic Ingestions," *Vet Hum Toxicol*, 1991, 33(3):256-8.
Forrest JAH, "Chlorpropamide Overdosage: Delayed and Prolonged Hypoglycemia," *Clin Toxicol*, 1974, 7(1):19-24.
Gordon MR, Flockhart D, Zawadski JK, et al, "Hypoglycemia Due to Inadvertent Dispensing of Chlorpropamide," *Am J Med*, 1988, 85(2):271-2.

Graw RG and Clarke RR, "Chlorpropamide Intoxication - Treatment With Peritoneal Dialysis," *Pediatrics*, 1970, 45(1):106-8.

Seltzer HS, "Drug-Induced Hypoglycemia. A Review of 1418 Cases," *Endocrinol Metab Clin North Am*, 1989, 18(1):163-83.

Chlor-Pro® [OTC] *see* Chlorpheniramine Maleate *on page 204*

Chlorprothixene (klor proe thix' een)

CAS Number 113-59-7

Brand Names Taractan®; Tarasan®; Truxal®; Truxaletter®

Use Management of psychotic disorders, emotional disturbances

Mechanism of Action Low anticholinergic activity with similar properties as chlorpromazine

Adverse Reactions

Cardiovascular: Hypotension (especially with I.V. use), hypotension (orthostatic), tachycardia, cardiac arrhythmias, Q-T prolongation

Central nervous system: Sedation, drowsiness, restlessness, anxiety, extrapyramidal reactions, tardive dyskinesia, neuroleptic malignant syndrome, seizures, altered central temperature regulation, pseudoparkinsonian signs and symptoms

Dermatologic: Hyperpigmentation, pruritus, rash, photosensitivity

Endocrine & metabolic: Amenorrhea, galactorrhea, gynecomastia, weight gain

Gastrointestinal: gastrointestinal upset, dry mouth, constipation

Genitourinary: Urinary retention, impotence

Hematologic: Leukopenia/neutropenia (agranulocytosis, granulocytopenia) (usually in patients with large doses for prolonged periods), thrombocytopenia, hemolysis, eosinophilia

Hepatic: Cholestatic jaundice

Ocular: Retinal pigmentation, diplopia, blurred vision, mydriasis

Miscellaneous: Anaphylactoid reactions

Signs & Symptoms of Acute Overdose Deep sleep, coma, impotence, dry eyes, extrapyramidal reaction, Parkinson's-like symptoms, neuroleptic malignant syndrome, ejaculatory disturbances, neutropenia, jaundice, photosensitivity, abnormal involuntary muscle movements, hyperactivity, hypotension, oliguria with azotemia, systemic lupus erythematosus (SLE)

Toxicodynamics/Kinetics

Distribution: V_d: 11-23 L/kg

Protein binding: 99%

Metabolism: Hepatic to a sulfoxide metabolite

Half-life: 8-12 hours

Elimination: Renal: 29%, fecal: 41%

Usual Dosage

Children >6 years: Oral: 10-25 mg 3-4 times/day

Adults:

Oral: 25-50 mg 3-4 times/day, to be increased as needed; doses exceeding 600 mg/day are rarely required

I.M.: 25-50 mg up to 3-4 times/day

Contraindications Circulatory collapse, hypersensitivity to chlorprothixene or any component, comatose states due to central depressant drugs

Dosage Forms

Concentrate, oral, as lactate and hydrochloride (fruit flavor): 100 mg/5 mL (480 mL)

Injection, as hydrochloride: 12.5 mg/mL (2 mL)

Tablet: 10 mg, 25 mg, 50 mg, 100 mg

Reference Range

Therapeutic: 0.04-0.30 μg/mL

Fatal: 1.00-2.00 μg/mL

Overdosage Treatment

Decontamination: Lavage/activated charcoal with cathartic

Supportive therapy: Following initiation of essential overdose management, toxic symptom treatment and supportive treatment should be initiated. Hypotension usually responds to I.V. fluids or Trendelenburg positioning. If unresponsive to these measures, the use of a parenteral inotrope may be required. Seizures commonly respond to lorazepam or diazepam (I.V. 5-10 mg bolus in adults every 15 minutes if needed up to a total of 30 mg; I.V. 0.25-0.4 mg/kg/dose up to a total of 10 mg in children) or to phenytoin or phenobarbital. Also critical cardiac arrhythmias often respond to I.V. phenytoin (15 mg/kg up to 1 g), while other antiarrhythmics can be used. Neuroleptics often cause extrapyramidal reaction (eg, dystonic reactions) requiring management with benztropine mesylate I.V. 1-2 mg (adults) may be effective. These agents are generally effective within 2-5 minutes.

Enhancement of elimination: Multiple dosing of activated charcoal may be useful; combined hemodialysis/hemoperfusion over 4 hours may be beneficial; not dialyzable (0% to 5%)

(Continued)

Chlorprothixene *(Continued)*

Test Interactions Increases cholesterol (S), glucose; decreases uric acid (S)

Drug Interactions Ethanol has additive effects

Pregnancy Risk Factor C

Monitoring Parameters Renal and cardiac status for 48 hours

Patient Information May cause drowsiness; avoid alcohol

Additional Information Slight amine-like odor

Specific References

Koppel C, Schirop T, Ibe K, et al, "Hemoperfusion in Severe Chlorprothixene Overdose," *Intensive Care Med*, 1987, 13(5):358-60.

Scheithauer W, Ulrich W, Kovarik J, et al, "Acute Oliguria Associated With Chlorprothixene Overdosage," *Nephron*, 1988, 48(1):71-3.

Chlorthalidone (klor thal' i done)

CAS Number 77-36-1

Brand Names Amaxin®; Hydro-Long®; Hygroton®; Igrotin®; Thalitone®; Urolin®

Use Management of mild to moderate hypertension, used alone or in combination with other agents; treatment of edema associated with congestive heart failure, nephrotic syndrome, or pregnancy

Mechanism of Action Sulfonamide-derived diuretic that inhibits sodium and chloride reabsorption in the cortical-diluting segment of the ascending loop of Henle

Adverse Reactions

Cardiovascular: Hypotension

Dermatologic: Psoriasiform eruption, photosensitivity

Endocrine & metabolic: Hypokalemia, hypercalcemia, hypercholesterolemia, fluid and electrolyte imbalances (hypocalcemia, hypomagnesemia, hyponatremia), hyperuricemia, hyperglycemia

Gastrointestinal: Pancreatitis

Genitourinary: Impotence, prerenal azotemia

Hematologic: Rarely blood dyscrasias (ie, neutropenia, thrombocytopenia)

Miscellaneous: Periarteritis nodosa

Signs & Symptoms of Acute Overdose Hypermotility, hyperglycemia, photosensitivity, periarteritis nodosa, diuresis, impotence, LDL (increased), hyponatremia, hypomagnesemia, hypokalemia, hypocalcemia, nocturia, myopia, myasthenia gravis (exacerbation or precipitation of), vision color changes (yellow tinge), hyperuricemia, lethargy, confusion, muscle weakness

Toxicodynamics/Kinetics

Peak effect: 2-6 hours

Absorption: Oral: 65%

Distribution: V_d: 4 L/kg; crosses the placenta; appears in breast milk

Protein binding: 98% to red blood cells

Metabolism: In the liver

Half-life: 35-55 hours; may be prolonged with renal impairment, with anuria: 81 hours

Elimination: ~50% to 65% excreted unchanged in urine; clearance: 1.6 mL/kg/minute

Usual Dosage Oral:

Children: 2 mg/kg 3 times/week or 1-2 mg/kg/day

Adults: 25-100 mg/day or 100 mg 3 times/week

Dosing interval in renal impairment: Cl_{cr} <10 mL/minute: Avoid use or administer every 48 hours

Contraindications Hypersensitivity to chlorthalidone or any component, cross-sensitivity with other thiazides or sulfonamides; do not use in anuric patients

Warnings Hypokalemia, renal disease, hepatic disease, gout, lupus erythematosus, diabetes mellitus; use with caution in severe renal diseases

Dosage Forms Tablet:

Hygroton®: 25 mg, 50 mg, 100 mg

Thalitone®: 15 mg, 25 mg

Reference Range Peak serum chlorthalidone level of 6.3 mg/L after a single 200 mg dose

Overdosage Treatment

Decontamination: Lavage/activated charcoal

Supportive therapy: Intravenous fluid and electrolyte replacement

Test Interactions ↑ creatine phosphokinase [CPK] (S), ammonia (B), amylase (S), calcium (S), chloride (S), cholesterol (S), glucose, ↑ acid (S), ↓ chloride (S), magnesium, potassium (S), sodium (S)

Drug Interactions

Decreased effect of oral hypoglycemics; decreased absorption with cholestyramine and colestipol; decreased diuretic effect with naproxen

Increased effect with furosemide and other loop diuretics; increased toxicity/levels of lithium, diazide, pancuronium, calcium salts, vitamin D (increased calcium levels), antineoplastics (leukopenia), digoxin (arrhythmias with electrolyte imbalances); increased incidence of ventricular arrhythmias with ketaserin

Pregnancy Risk Factor D

Pregnancy Implications Decreased birth weight, neonatal hypoglycemia, or neonatal thrombocytopenia can occur

Monitoring Parameters Blood pressure, serum electrolytes, renal function

Patient Information May be taken with food or milk; take early in day to avoid nocturia; take the last dose of multiple doses no later than 6 PM unless instructed otherwise. A few people who take this medication become more sensitive to sunlight and may experience skin rash, redness, itching, or severe sunburn, especially if sun block SPF 15 or higher is not used on exposed skin areas.

Nursing Implications Assess weight, I & O reports daily to determine fluid loss; take blood pressure with patient lying down and standing

Additional Information Recent studies have found chlorthalidone effective in the treatment of isolated systolic hypertension in the elderly; avoid in breast-feeding mothers

Specific References

Freis ED, "The Efficacy and Safety of Diuretics in Treating Hypertension," *Ann Intern Med*, 1995, 122(3):223-6.

Mulley BA, Parr GD, Pau WK, et al, "Placental Transfer of Chlorthalidone and its Elimination in Maternal Milk," *Eur J Clin Pharmacol*, 1978, 13:129-31.

Chlor-Trimeton® [OTC] *see* Chlorpheniramine Maleate *on page 204*

Cholecalciferol *see* Vitamin D *on page 797*

Choline Magnesium Trisalicylate

(koe' leen mag nee' ze um sal iss' i late)

CAS Number 64425-90-7

Brand Names Tricosal®; Trilisate®

Use Management of osteoarthritis, rheumatoid arthritis, and other arthritides

Mechanism of Action Inhibits prostaglandin synthesis; acts on the hypothalamus heat-regulating center to reduce fever; blocks the generation of pain impulses

Adverse Reactions

Cardiovascular: Fluid retention, circulatory collapse

Central nervous system: Headache, aseptic meningitis, psychosis, cognitive dysfunction, coma, seizures

Dermatologic: Rash, pruritus

Endocrine & metabolic: Hyperkalemia, anion gap metabolic acidosis

Gastrointestinal: Abdominal pain, nausea, vomiting, bleeding, ulceration, constipation, diarrhea, dyspepsia

Hematologic: Leukopenia, neutropenia, agranulocytosis; granulocytopenia; aplastic anemia (rare), platelet inhibition

Hepatic: Elevation of transaminases, fulminant hepatitis

Otic: Ototoxicity, tinnitus

Renal: Renal failure (acute), albuminuria, nephrotic syndrome, chronic renal failure

Respiratory: Wheezing, respiratory depression

Miscellaneous: Hypersensitivity

Signs & Symptoms of Acute Overdose Nausea, hyponatremia, wheezing, nephrotic syndrome, cognitive dysfunction, gastrointestinal upset, gastrointestinal bleeding, bezoars, nystagmus, hypoglycemia, vomiting, ototoxicity, tinnitus, drowsiness; severe poisoning can manifest with coma, seizures, renal failure and or hepatic failure, hypotension, respiratory depression, tinnitus, hyperthermia, irritability, metabolic acidosis, hyperglycemia, urine discoloration (pink), feces discoloration (black), feces discoloration (pink), feces discoloration (red), feces discoloration (tarry)

Toxicodynamics/Kinetics

Absorption: From the stomach and small intestine within ~2 hours

Distribution: Readily into most body fluids and tissues

Protein binding: 75% to 90%

Metabolism: Hydrolyzed to salicylate in the liver

Half-life: Dose-dependent ranging from 2-3 hours at low doses to 30 hours at high doses

Time to peak serum concentration: 1-2 hours

Elimination: Excreted in urine

Usual Dosage Oral (based on total salicylate content):

Children <37 kg: 50 mg/kg/day given in 2 divided doses

Adults: 500 mg to 1.5 g 2-3 times/day; usual maintenance dose: 1-4.5 g/day

Dosing adjustment/comments in renal impairment: Avoid use in severe renal impairment

Contraindications Hypersensitivity to salicylates or any component or other nonacetylated salicylates

Warnings Use with extreme caution in patients with renal impairment, erosive gastritis, or peptic ulcer; avoid use in patients with suspected varicella or influenza

(Continued)

Choline Magnesium Trisalicylate *(Continued)*

(salicylates have been associated with Reye's syndrome in children <16 years of age when used to treat symptoms of chickenpox or the flu)

Dosage Forms

Liquid: 500 mg/5 mL [choline salicylate 293 mg and magnesium salicylate 362 mg per 5 mL] (237 mL)

Tablet:
- 500 mg: Choline salicylate 293 mg and magnesium salicylate 362 mg
- 750 mg: Choline salicylate 440 mg and magnesium salicylate 544 mg
- 1000 mg: Choline salicylate 587 mg and magnesium salicylate 725 mg

Reference Range

Salicylate blood levels for anti-inflammatory effect: 10-30 mg/dL

Analgesia and antipyretic effect: Up to 10 mg/dL

Overdosage Treatment

Decontamination: Lavage/activated charcoal with cathartic may be most efficacious

Supportive therapy: Hypotension/dehydration can be managed with intravenous fluid therapy; acidosis should be treated with bicarbonates, seizures with benzodiazepines; antacids, blood products are indicated, as appropriate, for hemorrhage

Enhancement of elimination: Dialysis is indicated for secondary complications, acidosis, or renal failure and not toxin removal alone; multiple dosing of activated charcoal may be effective

Test Interactions False-negative results for Clinistix® urine test; false-positive results with Clinitest®

Drug Interactions Aspirin decreases serum concentrations probably by protein-binding displacement; there is an increased bleeding potential with concomitant warfarin therapy; may increase lithium and methotrexate concentrations by decreasing renal clearance; may decrease diuretic and hypotensive effects of thiazides, loop diuretics, ACE inhibitors, and beta-blockers; may increase nephrotoxicity of cyclosporine

Pregnancy Risk Factor C

Pregnancy Implications Crosses the placenta; appears in breast milk

Monitoring Parameters Serum magnesium with high dose therapy or in patients with impaired renal function; serum salicylate levels

Patient Information Take with food; do not take with antacids

Nursing Implications Liquid may be mixed with fruit juice just before drinking

Additional Information Salicylate salts do not inhibit platelet aggregation and, therefore, should not be substituted for aspirin in the prophylaxis of thrombosis; total dose (mg) multiplied by 0.75 provides aspirin equivalent dose

Specific References

Chapman BJ and Proudfoot AT, "Adult Salicylate Poisoning: Deaths and Outcome in Patients With High Plasma Salicylate Concentrations," *Q J Med*, 1989, 72(268):699-707.

Dugandric RM, Tierney MG, and Dickinson GE, "Evaluation of the Done Nomogram in the Management of Acute Salicylate Intoxication," *Ann Emerg Med*, 1989, 18(11):1186-90.

Vandenberg SA, Smolinske SC, Spoerke DG, et al, "Nonaspirin Salicylates: Conversion Factors for Estimating Aspirin Equivalency," *Vet Hum Toxicol*, 1989, 31(1):49-50.

Verbeeck RK, "Pharmacokinetic Drug Interactions With Nonsteroidal Anti-inflammatory Drugs," *Clin Pharmacokinet*, 1990, 19(1):44-66.

Vertrees JE, McWilliams BC, and Kelly HW, "Repeated Oral Administration for Treating Aspirin Overdose in Young Children," *Pediatrics*, 1990, 85(4):594-8.

CI-719 *see* Gemfibrozil *on page 378*

CI-898 *see* Trimetrexate Glucuronate *on page 773*

CI-945 *see* Gabapentin *on page 374*

Cibacalcin® *see* Calcitonin *on page 177*

Cibalith-S® *see* Lithium *on page 476*

Ciclosporin *see* Cyclosporine *on page 252*

Cilipen® *see* Penicillin G, Parenteral, Aqueous *on page 600*

Ciloxan™ Ophthalmic *see* Ciprofloxacin Hydrochloride *on page 215*

Cimetidine (sye met' i deen)

Related Information

Therapeutic Drugs Associated With Hallucinations *on page 1558-1559*

CAS Number 51481-61-9

Brand Names Antil®; Asaurex®; Beamat®; Dyspamet®; Tagamet®; Zergamet®

Use Short-term treatment of active duodenal ulcers and benign gastric ulcers; long-term prophylaxis of duodenal ulcer; gastric hypersecretory states; gastroesophageal reflux; prevention of upper gastrointestinal bleeding in critically ill patients

Mechanism of Action Competitive inhibition of histamine at H_2-receptors of the gastric parietal cells resulting in reduced gastric acid secretion

Adverse Reactions

Cardiovascular: Bradycardia, hypotension, A-V block

Central nervous system: Dizziness, mental confusion, agitation, drowsiness, psychosis, delirium, fatigue, auditory and visual hallucination, fever, headache

Dermatologic: Rash, pruritus, alopecia, erythema annulare centrifugum, Stevens-Johnson syndrome, exfoliative dermatitis, rash, vasculitis

Endocrine & metabolic: Gynecomastia, reduces parathyroid hormone, diabetes insipidus, parotitis

Gastrointestinal: Mild diarrhea, pancreatitis

Genitourinary: Impotence, decreased libido

Hematologic: Neutropenia, thrombocytopenia, granulocytopenia, aplastic anemia

Hepatic: Elevated creatinine, elevated AST and ALT

Neuromuscular & skeletal: Myalgia

Ocular: Mydriasis, photophobia

Renal: Interstitial nephritis

Miscellaneous: Cutaneous lupus erythematosus

Signs & Symptoms of Acute Overdose Respiratory failure, Stevens-Johnson syndrome, depression, hyperthermia, impotence, extrapyramidal reaction, ileus, eosinophilia, hyperprolactinemia, galactorrhea, myopathy, myalgia, mania, leukocytosis, A-V block, delirium, disorientation, dementia, cholestatic jaundice, ataxia, bradycardia, mydriasis, coma, parotid pain, dry mouth, slurred speech, sweating, systemic lupus erythematosus (SLE), erythema multiforme, leukopenia; neutropenia; agranulocytosis; granulocytopenia

Toxicodynamics/Kinetics

Absorption: Oral: ~60% to 75%; may be affected by food

Distribution: V_d:

- Children: 1.2-2.1 L/kg
- Adults: 0.8 L/kg

Protein binding: 13% to 25%

Metabolism: In the liver to cimetidine sulfoxide, hydroxycimetidine, and guanyl urea cimetidine

Bioavailability: 60% to 70%

Half-life:

- Neonates: 3.6 hours
- Children: 1.4 hours
- Adults:
  - Normal renal function: 2 hours
  - Renal insufficiency: 3.7 hours
- Cimetidine sulfoxide: 2.6 hours
- Hydroxycimetidine: 4.7 hours

Time to peak serum concentration: Within 1 hour

Elimination: Principally as unchanged drug by the kidney; some excretion in bile and feces; renal clearance: 24-36 L/hour

Usual Dosage

Neonates: Oral, I.M., I.V.: 10-20 mg/kg/day divided every 4-6 hours

Children: Oral, I.M., I.V.: 20-40 mg/kg/day in divided doses every 4 hours

Adults: Short-term treatment of active ulcers:

- Oral: 300 mg 4 times/day or 800 mg at bedtime or 400 mg twice daily for up to 8 weeks
- I.M., I.V.: 300 mg every 6 hours or 37.5 mg/hour by continuous infusion; I.V. dosage should be adjusted to maintain an intragastric pH of ≥5

Patients with an active bleed: Give cimetidine as a continuous infusion (see above)

- Duodenal ulcer prophylaxis: Oral: 400-800 mg at bedtime
- Gastric hypersecretory conditions: Oral, I.M., I.V.: 300-600 mg every 6 hours; dosage not to exceed 2.4 g/day

Dosing adjustment/interval in renal impairment: Children and Adults:

- Cl_{cr} 20-40 mL/minute: Administer every 8 hours or 75% of normal dose
- Cl_{cr} 0-20 mL/minute: Administer every 12 hours or 50% of normal dose

Dosing adjustment/comments in hepatic impairment: Usual dose is safe in mild liver disease but use with caution and in reduced dosage in severe liver disease; increased risk of CNS toxicity in cirrhosis suggested by enhanced penetration of CNS

Contraindications Hypersensitivity to cimetidine or any component

Warnings Modify dosage in patients with renal and/or hepatic impairment

Dosage Forms

Infusion, as hydrochloride, in NS: 300 mg (50 mL)

Injection, as hydrochloride: 150 mg/mL (2 mL, 8 mL)

Liquid, oral, as hydrochloride (mint-peach flavor): 300 mg/5 mL with alcohol 2.8% (5 mL, 240 mL)

Tablet: 200 mg, 300 mg, 400 mg, 800 mg

Stability I.V. infusion solution with NS or D_5W solution is stable for 48 hours at room temperature; do not refrigerate injection since precipitation may occur

(Continued)

Cimetidine *(Continued)*

Reference Range Therapeutic: >1 µg/mL (SI: >4 µmol/L); confusion occurs in levels >2 µg/mL (SI: >8 µmol/L)

Overdosage Treatment

Decontamination: Emesis or lavage; activated charcoal with cathartic

Supportive therapy: Treatment is primarily symptomatic and supportive; routine use of physostigmine is not advised, although it can be used for life-threatening anticholinergic

Enhancement of elimination: Multiple dosing of activated charcoal may be beneficial; hemodialysis may be useful in reducing half-life; should be considered in patients experiencing severe toxicity or renal failure; slightly dialyzable (5% to 20%)

Test Interactions Increases AST, ALT, creatinine (S)

Drug Interactions Decreased elimination of lidocaine, theophylline, phenytoin, metronidazole, triamterene, procainamide, quinidine and propranolol; inhibition of warfarin metabolism, tricyclic antidepressant metabolism, diazepam elimination and cyclosporine elimination; metoclopramide and propantheline may reduce the absorption of cimetidine; ketoconazole

Pregnancy Risk Factor B

Pregnancy Implications Crosses the placenta; appears in breast milk

Monitoring Parameters Blood pressure with I.V. push ,administration; CBC

Patient Information Take with or immediately after meals

Nursing Implications Give with meals so that the drug's peak effect occurs at the proper time (peak inhibition of gastric acid secretion occurs at 1 and 3 hours after dosing in fasting subjects and approximately 2 hours in nonfasting subjects; this correlates well with the time food is no longer in the stomach offering a buffering effect); modify dosage in patients with renal impairment

Additional Information Cimetidine is not effective for hepatoprotection in acetaminophen overdose; may inhibit absorption of cobalamin; may increase HDL cholesterol concentrations; may cause phytobezoar formation; at doses >1 g/day of cimetidine, the risk of developing gynecomastia is 40 times that of nonusers; over-the-counter preparation marketed as Tagamet HB®

Specific References

Burkhart KK, et al, "Cimetidine as Adjunctive Treatment for Acetaminophen Overdose," *Hum Exp Toxicol*, 1995, 14:299-304.

Garcia Rodriguez LA and Jick H, "Risk of Gynaecomastia Associated With Cimetidine, Omeprazole, and Other Antiulcer Drugs," *BMJ*, 1994, 308(6927):503-6.

Inove A, Teramae H, Hisa T, et al, "Fixed Drug Eruption Due to Cimetidine," *Acta Derm Venereol*, 1995, 75:250.

Koren G and Zemlickis DM, "Outcome of Pregnancy After First Trimester Exposure to H_2-Receptor Antagonists," *Am J Perinatol*, 1991, 8(1):37-8.

Krenzelok EP, Litovitz T, Lippold KP, et al, "Cimetidine Toxicity: An Assessment of 881 Cases," *Ann Emerg Med*, 1987, 16(11):1217-21.

Mogelnicki SR, Waller JL, and Finlayson DC, "Physostigmine Reversal of Cimetidine-Induced Mental Confusion," *JAMA*, 1979, 241(8):826-7.

Penston J and Wormsley G, "Adverse Reactions and Interactions With H_2-Receptor Antagonists," *Med Toxicol Adverse Drug Exp*, 1986, 1(3):192-216.

Sawyer D, Conner CS, and Scalley, "Cimetidine: Adverse Reactions and Acute Toxicity," *Am J Hosp Pharm*, 1981, 38(2):188-97.

Cincain® *see* Dibucaine *on page 275*

Cinchocaine *see* Dibucaine *on page 275*

Cinetic *see* Thyroid *on page 749*

Cinobac® *see* Cinoxacin *on this page*

Cinobactin® *see* Cinoxacin *on this page*

Cinoxacin (sin ox' a sin)

CAS Number 28657-80-9

Brand Names Cinobac®; Cinobactin®; Nofrin®; Nossacin®; Noxigram®; Uronorm®; Uroxacin®

Use Urinary tract infections

Mechanism of Action Inhibits microbial synthesis of DNA with resultant problems in protein synthesis

Adverse Reactions

Central nervous system: Dizziness, insomnia, confusion, headache

Gastrointestinal: Nausea, vomiting, abdominal pain, diarrhea

Hematologic: Thrombocytopenia

Neuromuscular & skeletal: Tendon rupture

Ocular: Photophobia

Otic: Ototoxicity, tinnitus

Miscellaneous: Feces discoloration (greenish gray), feces discoloration (white/speckling)

Toxicodynamics/Kinetics

Absorption: Rapid and almost complete from gastrointestinal tract; delayed in presence of food

Distribution: V_d: 0.24-0.26 L/kg; concentrates in renal tissue

Protein binding: 60% to 80%

Metabolism: Probably hepatic; ~30% to 40% metabolizes to inactive metabolites

Half-life: 1.5 hours, prolonged in renal impairment

Time to peak serum concentration: Within 2-3 hours

Elimination: ~60% excreted as unchanged drug in urine

Usual Dosage Children >12 years and Adults: 1 g/day in 2-4 doses for 7-14 days

Dosing interval in renal impairment:

Cl_{cr} 20-50 mL/minute: 250 mg twice daily

Cl_{cr} <20 mL/minute: 250 mg/day

Contraindications History of convulsive disorders, hypersensitivity to cinoxacin or any component

Dosage Forms Capsule: 250 mg, 500 mg

Reference Range Mean urinary levels of ~300 μg/mL associated with an oral dose of 500 mg

Overdosage Treatment

Decontamination: Lavage/activated charcoal with cathartic

Drug Interactions Renal excretion is reduced with probenecid

Pregnancy Risk Factor B

Pregnancy Implications Crosses the placenta

Patient Information May be taken with food to minimize upset stomach; avoid antacid use; drink fluid liberally

Nursing Implications Hold antacids for 3-4 hours after giving

Specific References

Sisca TS, Heel RC, and Romankiewicz JA, "Cinoxacin: A Review of Its Pharmacological Properties and Therapeutic Efficacy in the Treatment of Urinary Tract Infections," *Drugs*, 1983, 25(6):544-69.

Stricker BH, Slagboom G, Demaeseneer R, et al, "Anaphylactic Reactions to Cinoxacin," *BMJ*, 1988, 297(6661):1434-5.

Szarfman A, Chen M, and Blum MD, "More on Fluoroquinolone Antibiotics and Tendon Rupture," *N Engl J Med*, 1995, 332(3):193.

Cin-Quin® *see* Quinidine *on page 668*

Cipro™ *see* Ciprofloxacin Hydrochloride *on this page*

Ciprofloxacin Hydrochloride (sip roe flox' a sin)

CAS Number 85721-33-1 (base); 86483-48-9 (hydrochloride)

Brand Names Ciloxan™ Ophthalmic; Cipro™

Use Treatment of documented or suspected pseudomonal infection in home care patients; documented multidrug resistant gram-negative organisms; documented infectious diarrhea due to *Campylobacter jejuni*, *Shigella*, or *Salmonella*; osteomyelitis caused by susceptible organisms in which parenteral therapy is not feasible; used ophthalmically for treatment of corneal ulcers and conjunctivitis due to strains of microorganisms susceptible to ciprofloxacin; typhoid fever (*Salmonella typhi*) and uncomplicated cervical/urethral gonorrhea (*Neisseria gonorrhoeae*)

Mechanism of Action Inhibits DNA-gyrase in susceptible organisms; inhibits relaxation of supercoiled DNA and promotes breakage of double-stranded DNA

Adverse Reactions

Cardiovascular: Hypertension

Central nervous system: Restlessness, night terrors, insomnia, dizziness, confusion, psychosis, mania, malaise, seizures, hemiplegia, depression, headache, dysphagia

Dermatologic: Rash, keratitis, photosensitivity, Henoch Schonlein *purpura*

Gastrointestinal: Nausea, vomiting

Hematologic: Anemia, eosinophilia, hemolytic anemia

Hepatic: Liver enzymes (increased), cholestatic jaundice, jaundice, hepatic necrosis

Neuromuscular & skeletal: Arthralgia, myalgia, tremors, tendon rupture

Ocular: Diplopia, photophobia

Renal: Renal failure (acute), nephritis, toxic epidermal necrolysis

Miscellaneous: Feces discoloration (greenish gray), feces discoloration (white/speckling), hematuria, serum sickness

Toxicodynamics/Kinetics

Absorption: Oral: Rapid from gastrointestinal tract following administration in a fasting state; absorption delayed in presence of food although overall absorption not substantially affected

Distribution: Distributes widely throughout body; tissue concentrations often exceed serum concentrations especially in the kidneys, gallbladder, liver, lungs, gynecological tissue, and prostatic tissue; distributes to saliva, nasal secretions,

(Continued)

Ciprofloxacin Hydrochloride *(Continued)*

aqueous humor, sputum, skin blister fluid, lymph, peritoneal fluid, bile, and prostatic secretions; also to skin, fat, muscle, bone, and cartilage; CSF concentrations reach 10% with noninflamed meninges and 14% to 37% with inflamed meninges

V_d:

Adults: 2-3 L/kg

Elderly: 1.0-1.6 L/kg

Protein binding: 16% to 43%

Metabolism: Partially in the liver to active metabolites

Bioavailability: Oral: 50% to 85%

Half-life:

Normal renal function: Parenteral: 5-6 hours

Impaired renal function: 6-8 hours

Elderly: ~6 hours

Time to peak serum concentration: Within 30 minutes to 2 hours

Elimination: 30% to 50% excreted as unchanged drug in urine; 20% to 40% excreted in feces primarily from biliary excretion

Usual Dosage Adults:

Oral: 250-750 mg every 12 hours, depending on severity of infection and susceptibility

I.V.: 200-400 mg every 12 hours depending on severity of infection

Ophthalmic:

Acute infections: Instill 1-2 drops every 15-30 minutes initially reducing the frequency of instillation gradually as the infection is controlled

Moderate infections: Instill 1-2 drops 4-6 times/day

Typhoid fever (*Salmonella typhi*): 500 mg twice daily for 10 days

Uncomplicated gonorrhea (*Neisseria gonorrhoeae*): 250 mg as a single dose

Dosing adjustment in renal impairment:

Cl_{cr} 10-50 mL/minute: Administer 50% of dose or administer every 18-24 hours

Cl_{cr} <10 mL/minute: Administer 33% of dose

Contraindications Hypersensitivity to ciprofloxacin, any component, or other quinolones

Warnings Prolonged use may result in superinfection; not recommended in children <18 years of age; ciprofloxacin causes arthropathy in immature animals; CNS stimulation may occur which may lead to tremor, restlessness, confusion and very rarely to hallucinations or convulsive seizures. Use with caution in patients with known or suspected CNS disorders. Discontinue use upon complaints of tendonitis.

Dosage Forms

Infusion, in D_5W: 400 mg (200 mL)

Infusion, in NS or D_5W: 200 mg (100 mL)

Injection: 200 mg (20 mL); 400 mg (40 mL)

Solution, ophthalmic: 3.5 mg/mL (2.5 mL, 5 mL)

Tablet: 250 mg, 500 mg, 750 mg

Stability Refrigeration and room temperature:

Prepared bags: 14 days

Premixed bags: Manufacturer expiration dating

Out of overwrap stability: 14 days

Reference Range

Peak plasma concentrations after a 750 mg oral dose: 3.0 μg/mL (9 μmol/g)

Therapeutic: 2.6-3.0 μg/mL

Toxic: >5.0 μg/mL

Overdosage Treatment

Decontamination: Lavage/activated charcoal with cathartic

Supportive therapy: Do **not** use flumazenil; diazepam, phenobarbital, or phenytoin can be used for seizures

Enhancement of elimination: Multiple dosing of activated charcoal may be effective; only small amounts of ciprofloxacin are removed by dialysis (<10%)

Drug Interactions Antacids may reduce absorption by up to 98%, if given at the same time; theophylline, probenecid, cyclosporine, warfarin, sucralfate

Pregnancy Risk Factor C

Pregnancy Implications Crosses the placenta; appears in breast milk

Monitoring Parameters Patients receiving concurrent ciprofloxacin and theophylline should have serum levels of theophylline monitored

Patient Information May be taken with food to minimize upset stomach; avoid antacid use; drink fluid liberally

Nursing Implications Hold antacids for 3-4 hours after giving

Additional Information 12 g ingestion resulted in mild symptoms in an adult; not effective in eliminating typhoid carrier state

Specific References

Cohen H and Francisco DH, "Twelve Gram Overdose of Ciprofloxacin With Mild Symptomatology," *Ann Pharmacother*, 1994, 28(6):805-6.

Gamboa F, Rivera JM, Mateos JMG, et al, "Ciprofloxacin-Induced Henoch-Schönlein Purpura," *Ann Pharmacother*, 1995, 29:84.

Guharoy SR, "Serum Sickness Secondary to Ciprofloxacin Use," *Vet Hum Toxicol*, 1994, 36(6):540-1.

Hooper DC and Wolfson JS, "Fluoroquinolone Antimicrobial Agents," *N Engl J Med*, 1991, 324(6):384-94.

Mackay AD and Mehta A, "Autoimmune Haemolytic Anemia Associated With Ciprofloxacin," *Clin Lab Haematol*, 1995, 17:97-8.

Rfidah EI, Findlay CA, and Beattie TJ, "Reversible Encephalopathy After Intravenous Ciprofloxacin Therapy," *Pediatr Nephrol*, 1995, 9:250-5.

Szarfman A, Chen M, and Blum MD, "More on Fluoroquinolone Antibiotics and Tendon Rupture," *N Engl J Med*, 1995, 332(3):193.

Villenueve JP, Davies C, and Cote J, "Suspected Ciprofloxacin-Induced Hepatotoxicity," *Ann Pharmacother*, 1995, 29:257-9.

Yew WW, Chau CH, Wong PC, et al, "Ciprofloxacin-Induced Renal Dysfunction in Patients With Mycobacterial Lung Infections," *Tubercle and Lung Lorazepam*, 1995, 76:173-5.

Cisapride (sis' a pride)

CAS Number 81098-60-4

Brand Names Alimix®; Prepulsid®; Propulsid®; Propulsin®

Synonyms R-51619

Use Treatment of nocturnal symptoms of gastroesophageal reflux disease (GERD), also demonstrated effectiveness for gastroparesis, refractory constipation, and nonulcer dyspepsia

Mechanism of Action Enhances the release of acetylcholine at the myenteric plexus. *In vitro* studies have shown cisapride to have serotonin-4 receptor agonistic properties (similar to metoclopramide) without dopamine-blocking activity.

Adverse Reactions

Central nervous system: Headache, insomnia, anxiety, nervousness, fever

Dermatological: Rash, pruritus

Gastrointestinal: Diarrhea, abdominal pain, nausea, constipation, flatulence, dyspepsia

Respiratory: Rhinitis, sinusitis, coughing, upper respiratory tract infection

Miscellaneous: Pain, increased incidence of viral infection; prolonged Q-T interval

Signs & Symptoms of Acute Overdose Diarrhea, abdominal cramping, seizures, insomnia

Toxicodynamics/Kinetics

Onset of effect: 0.5-1 hour

Distribution: V_d: 2.4 L/kg

Protein binding: 97.5% to 98%

Metabolism: Extensive to norcisapride, which is eliminated in urine and feces

Bioavailability: 35% to 40% (enhanced absorption by food)

Half-life: 7-10 hours

Elimination: <10% excreted into feces and urine

Usual Dosage Oral:

Children: Not recommended

Adults: Initial: 10 mg 4 times/day at least 15 minutes before meals and at bedtime; in some patients the dosage will need to be increased to 20 mg to obtain a satisfactory result

Contraindications Hypersensitivity to cisapride or any of its components; gastrointestinal hemorrhage, mechanical obstruction, gastrointestinal perforation, or other situations when gastrointestinal motility stimulation is dangerous

Warnings Pregnancy, lactation, may exacerbate tremor in Parkinson patients

Dosage Forms Tablet, scored: 10 mg, 20 mg

Reference Range Single oral dose of 10 mg results in plasma level of 41-65 mg/L

Overdosage Treatment

Decontamination: Lavage/activated charcoal with cathartic

Enhancement of elimination: Multiple dosing of activated charcoal may be effective

Drug Interactions

Decreased effect of digoxin (decreased absorption); decreased effect with atropine

Increased effect/toxicity of Coumadin® (warfarin), diazepam (increased levels), cimetidine, and ranitidine; increased effect with atropine; ventricular arrhythmias (torsade de pointes) can occur with combination of cisapride and ketoconazole, miconazole, or itraconazole

Pregnancy Risk Factor C

Pregnancy Implications Excreted in breast milk

Additional Information Rate of torsade de pointes associated with cisapride: 1:120,000 patients

Specific References

Barone JA, Huang YC, Bierman RH, et al, "Bioavailability of Three Oral Dosage Forms of Cisapride, a Gastrointestinal Stimulant Agent," *Clin Pharm*, 1987, 6(8):640-5.

Bran S, Murray WA, Hirsch IB, et al, "Long QT Syndrome During High-Dose Cisapride," *Arch Intern Med*, 1995, 155(7):765-8.

(Continued)

Cisapride *(Continued)*

Bucci KK, Haverstick DE, and Abercrombie SA, "Dystonic-like Reaction Following Cisapride Therapy," *J Fam Pract*, 1995, 40(1):86-8.

Koelz HR, "Treatment of Reflux Esophagitis With H_2-Blockers, Antacids, and Prokinetic Drugs," *Scand J Gastroenterol Suppl*, 1989, 156:25-36.

Olsson S and Edwards IR, "Tachycardia During Cisapride Treatment," *BMJ*, 1992, 305(6856):748-9.

Rizwanuddin S and Wolfe SM, "Cisapride and Torsade de Pointes," *Lancet*, 1995, 345:508.

Sempere AP, Duarte J, Cabezas C, et al, "Aggravation of Parkinsonian Tremor by Cisapride," *Clin Neuropharmacol*, 1995, 18:76-8.

Tack J, Coremans G, and Janssens J, "A Risk-Benefit Assessment of Cisapride in the Treatment of Gastrointestinal Disorders," *Drug Saf*, 1995, 12(6):384-92.

Cisplatin (sis' pla tin)

Related Information

Amifostine *on page 107*

Toxicities of Chemotherapeutic Agents *on page 1631-1633*

CAS Number 15663-27-1

Brand Names Platinol®; Platinol®-AQ

Synonyms CDDP

Use Head and neck, breast, testicular, and ovarian cancer; Hodgkin's and non-Hodgkin's lymphoma; sarcomas, bladder, gastric, lung, esophageal, cervical, and prostate cancer; myeloma, melanoma, mesothelioma, small cell lung cancer, and osteosarcoma

Mechanism of Action Inhibits DNA synthesis by the formation of DNA cross-links; denatures the double helix; covalently binds to DNA bases and disrupts DNA function; may also bind to proteins; the *cis*-isomer is 14 times more cytotoxic than the *trans*-isomer; both forms cross-link DNA but cis-platinum is less easily recognized by cell enzymes and, therefore, not repaired. Cisplatin can also bind two adjacent guanines on the same strand of DNA producing intrastrand cross-linking and breakage.

Adverse Reactions

Cardiovascular: Bradycardia, arrhythmias, tachycardia

Central nervous system: Convulsions, headache, visual hallucinations

Dermatologic: Mild alopecia

Endocrine & metabolic: Hypomagnesemia, hypocalcemia, hyponatremia, hypokalemia, hypophosphatemia, hyperuricemia

Gastrointestinal: Nausea, vomiting, diarrhea, thirst

Hematologic: Myelosuppression, leukopenia, thrombocytopenia, anemia

Hepatic: Elevation of liver enzymes (dose related)

Local: Phlebitis

Neuromuscular & skeletal: Paresthesia

Ocular: Papilledema, optic neuropathy, blurred vision, altered color vision, cortical blindness

Otic: Ototoxicity, tinnitus (especially pronounced in children and the elderly)

Renal: Nephrotoxicity (dose related proximal tubular defect usually seen in first month of treatment)

Miscellaneous: Anaphylactoid reactions

Signs & Symptoms of Acute Overdose Leukopenia or neutropenia (agranulocytosis, granulocytopenia), bone marrow depression; congestive heart failure, hypertension, Fanconi's syndrome; tubular necrosis, hypopigmented hair, hyperpigmented hair, thirst, hyperthermia, hypophosphatemia, hypomagnesemia, hyponatremia, migraine headache (exacerbation of), dermatitis, deafness, hypocalcemia, hyperuricemia, encephalopathy, cortical blindness, hypokalemia

Toxicodynamics/Kinetics

Distribution: I.V.: Rapidly distributes into tissue following administration; found in high concentrations in the kidneys, liver, ovaries, uterus, and lungs

Protein binding: >90%

Half-life:

- Initial: 20-30 minutes
- Beta: 1 hour
- Terminal: ~24 hours
- Secondary half-life: 44-73 hours

Metabolism: Undergoes nonenzymatic metabolism; the drug is inactivated (in both the cell and the bloodstream) by sulfhydryl groups; cisplatin covalently binds to glutathione and to thiosulfate

Elimination: >90% excreted in urine and 10% in bile; partially cleared by hemodialysis

Usual Dosage I.V. (**refer to individual protocols**):

An estimated Cl_{cr} should be on all cisplatin chemotherapy orders along with other patient parameters (ie, patient's height, weight, and body surface area).

It is recommended that a 24-hour urine creatinine clearance be checked prior to a patient's first dose of cisplatin and periodically thereafter (ie, after every 2-3 cycles of cisplatin).

Children: Various dosage schedules range from 30-100 mg/m^2 once every 2-3 weeks; may also dose similar to adult dosing

Adults:

Head and neck cancer: 100-150 mg/m^2 every 3-4 weeks

Testicular cancer: 10-20 mg/m^2/day for 5 days repeated every 3-4 weeks

Metastatic ovarian cancer: 50 mg/m^2 every 3 weeks

Rate of infusion varies from 30 minutes to 24-hour continuous infusion; cisplatin has been administered intraperitoneal with systemic sodium thiosulfate for ovarian cancer; doses up to 90-270 mg/m^2 have been administered and retained for 4 hours before draining

Dosing adjustment in renal impairment:

Cl_{cr} 10-50 mL/minute: Administer 50% to 75% of normal dose

Cl_{cr} <10 mL/minute: Administer 25% to 50% of normal dose

Administration I.V.: Rate of administration has varied from a 15- to 20-minute infusion, 1 mg/minute infusion, 6- to 8-hour infusion, 24-hour infusion, or per protocol

Contraindications Hypersensitivity to cisplatin or any other platinum-containing compounds or any component, anaphylactic-like reactions have been reported; pre-existing renal insufficiency, myelosuppression, hearing impairment

Warnings The U.S. Food and Drug Administration (FDA) currently recommends that procedures for proper handling and disposal of antineoplastic agents be considered. All patients should receive adequate hydration prior to and for 24 hours after cisplatin administration, with or without mannitol and/or furosemide, to ensure good urine output and decrease the chance of nephrotoxicity; reduce dosage in renal impairment. Cumulative renal toxicity may be severe; dose-related toxicities include myelosuppression, nausea, and vomiting; ototoxicity, especially pronounced in children, is manifested by tinnitus or loss of high frequency hearing and occasionally, deafness. **Serum magnesium, as well as other electrolytes, should be monitored both before and within 48 hours after cisplatin therapy.** Patients who are magnesium depleted should receive replacement therapy before the cisplatin is administered.

Dosage Forms

Injection, aqueous: 1 mg/mL (50 mL, 100 mL)

Powder for injection: 10 mg, 50 mg

Stability Incompatible with sodium bicarbonate; do not infuse in solutions containing <0.2% sodium chloride; do not refrigerate reconstituted solutions since precipitation may occur; protect from light; aluminum needles should not be used to administer the drug due to binding with the platinum

Reference Range Plasma levels for cytotoxicity: 50 mg/L at 1 hour or 5 mg/L at 8 hours

Overdosage Treatment

Supportive therapy: Erythropoietin can be given to prevent anemia; ondansetron, droperidol, metoclopramide, or corticosteroids can be given for emesis; sodium thiosulfate (7.5 g/m^2 I.V. followed by 2.13 g/m^2/hour over 12 hours) or mannitol (12.5 g) and/or furosemide can decrease nephrotoxicity. Tachycardia can be treated with intravenous verapamil; allopurinol (600-800 mg/day in divided doses) may be useful in managing hyperuricemia.

Enhancement of elimination: Hemodialysis is not effective

Antidote(s)

Mannitol *on page 1442*

Sodium Thiosulfate *on page 1470*

Diagnostic Tests/Procedures

Calcium, Serum *on page 1214*

Electrolytes, Blood *on page 1254*

Kidney Profile *on page 1279*

Magnesium, Serum *on page 1289*

Drug Interactions

Decreased toxicity: Sodium thiosulfate theoretically inactivates drug systemically; has been used clinically to reduce systemic toxicity with intraperitoneal administration of cisplatin

Increased toxicity: Delayed bleomycin elimination; ethacrynic acid has resulted in severe ototoxicity in animals

Pregnancy Risk Factor D

Pregnancy Implications May be toxic to fetal urogenital tract

Monitoring Parameters Renal function tests (serum creatinine, BUN, Cl_{cr}), electrolytes (particularly magnesium, calcium, potassium); hearing test, neurologic exam (with high dose), liver function tests periodically, CBC with differential and platelet count; urine output, urinalysis

Patient Information Drink plenty of fluids to maintain urine output, be prepared for severe nausea and vomiting following drug administration which can be delayed up to 48 hours; notify physician of numbness or tingling in extremities or deafness

(Continued)

Cisplatin *(Continued)*

Nursing Implications Needles, syringes, catheters, or I.V. administration sets that contain aluminum parts should not be used for administration of drug; perform pretreatment hydration with 1-2 liters of fluid infused for 8-12 hours prior to dose; monitor for possible anaphylactoid reaction

Additional Information Sodium content (10 mg): 35.4 mg (1.54 mEq)

Specific References

Bowman A, et al, "Effect of Adding Glutathione to Cisplatin in the Treatment of Stage I-IV Ovarian Cancer," *Br J Cancer*, 1995, 71(Suppl XXIV):14.

El Weshi A, Thieblemont C, Cottin V, et al, "Cisplatin-Induced Hyponatremia and Renal Sodium Wasting," *Acta Oncol*, 1995, 34:264-5.

Haupt R, Perin G, Dallorso S, et al, "Very High Dose Cis-Platinum (450 mg/sq m) in an Infant With Rhabdomyosarcoma," *Anticancer Rev*, 1989, 9(2):427-8.

Hebert ME, Bilvin JL, Kessler J, et al, "Anaphylactoid Reactions With Intraperitoneal Cisplatin," *Ann Pharmacother*, 1995, 29:260-3.

Higa GM, Wise TC, and Crowell EB, "Severe, Disabling Neurologic Toxicity Following Cisplatin Treatment," *Ann Pharmacother*, 1995, 29:134-7.

Howell SB, Pfeifle CL, Wung WE, et al, "Intraperitoneal Cisplatin With Systemic Thiosulfate Protection," *Ann Intern Med*, 1982, 97(6):845-51.

Rothmann SA and Weick JK, "Cisplatin Toxicity for Erythroid Precursors," *N Engl J Med*, 1981, 304(6):360.

Schilsky RL and Anderson T, "Hypomagnesemia and Renal Magnesium Wasting in Patients Receiving Cisplatin," *Ann Intern Med*, 1979, 90(6):929-31.

Shlebak AA, Clark PI, and Green JA, "Hypersensitivity and Cross-Reactivity to Cisplatin and Analogues," *Cancer Chemother Pharmacol*, 1995, 35(4):349-51.

13-*cis*-Retinoic Acid *see* Isotretinoin *on page 447*

Cistofuran® *see* Nitrofurantoin *on page 564*

***cis* Vitamin A Acid** *see* Isotretinoin *on page 447*

Cla *see* Clarithromycin *on next page*

Cladribine (kla' dri been)

CAS Number 4291-63-8

Brand Names Leustatin™

Synonyms 2-CdA; 2-chlorodeoxyadenosine; CldAdo

Use Hairy cell and chronic lymphocytic leukemias (HCL)

Mechanism of Action Purine nucleoside analogue; prodrug which is activated via phosphorylation by deoxycytidine kinase to a 5'-triphosphate derivative. This active form incorporates into susceptible cells and into DNA to result in the breakage of DNA strand and shutdown of DNA synthesis. This also results in a depletion of nicotinamide adenine dinucleotide and adenosine triphosphate (ATP). The induction of strand breaks results in a drop in the cofactor nicotinamide adenine dinucleotide and disruption of cell metabolism. ATP is depleted to deprive cells of an important source of energy. Cladribine is able to kill resting as well as dividing cells, unlike most other cytotoxic drugs.

Adverse Reactions

Bone marrow depression: Commonly observed in patients treated with cladribine, especially at high doses; at the initiation of treatment, however, most patients in clinical studies had hematologic impairment as a result of HCL. During the first 2 weeks after treatment initiation, mean platelet counts decline and subsequently increased with normalization of mean counts by day 12. Absolute neutrophil counts and hemoglobin declined and subsequently increased with normalization of mean counts by week 5 and week 6. Periodic assessment of peripheral blood counts, particularly during the first 4-8 weeks post-treatment, is recommended to detect the development of anemia, neutropenia, and thrombocytopenia and for early detection of any potential sequelae (ie, infection or bleeding).

Cardiovascular: Tachycardia

Central nervous system: Dizziness, insomnia, chills, malaise, fatigue, headache, asthenia

Dermatologic: Edema, pruritus, rash, erythema

Fever: Temperature ≥101°F has been associated with the use of cladribine in approximately 66% of patients in the first month of therapy. Although 69% of patients developed fevers, less than 33% of febrile events were associated with documented infection.

Gastrointestinal: Decreased appetite, constipation, abdominal pain, diarrhea; nausea and vomiting are not severe with cladribine at any dose level. Most cases of nausea were mild, not accompanied by vomiting and did not require treatment with antiemetics. In patients requiring antiemetics, nausea was easily controlled most often by chlorpromazine.

Local: Injection site reactions, pain

Neuromuscular & skeletal: Myalgia, arthralgia

Miscellaneous: Trunk pain, sweating

Signs & Symptoms of Acute Overdose Serum creatinine (increased), myalgia, bone marrow suppression, insomnia, quadriparesis, leukopenia; neutropenia; agranulocytosis; granulocytopenia

Toxicodynamics/Kinetics

Distribution: V_d: 4.52 ± 2.82 L/kg

Protein binding: 20% to plasma proteins

Bioavailability: Oral: 55%

Half-life: Biphasic:

Alpha: 25 minutes

Beta: 6.7 hours

Terminal, mean (normal renal function): 5.4 hours

Elimination: Mean: 978 ± 422 mL/hour/kg; estimated systemic clearance: 640 mL/hour/kg

Usual Dosage I.V.:

Children: Safety and effectiveness have not been established; in a phase I study involving patients 1-21 years of age with relapsed acute leukemia, cladribine was administered by continuous infusion at doses ranging from 3-10.7 mg/m²/day for 5 days (0.5-2 times the dose recommended in HCL). Investigators reported beneficial responses in this study; the dose-limiting toxicity was severe myelosuppression with profound neutropenia and thrombocytopenia.

Adults: 0.09-0.1 mg/kg/day continuous infusion for 7 consecutive days

Administration

Single daily infusion: Administer diluted in an infusion bag containing 500 mL of 0.9% sodium chloride and repeated for a total of 7 consecutive days

7-day infusion: Prepare with bacteriostatic 0.9% sodium chloride. Both cladribine and diluent should be passed through a sterile 0.22-micron hydrophilic filter as it is being introduced into the infusion reservoir. The calculated dose of cladribine (7 days x 0.09 mg/kg) should first be added to the infusion reservoir through a filter then the bacteriostatic 0.9% sodium chloride should be added to the reservoir to obtain a total volume of 100 mL.

Contraindications Patients with a prior history of hypersensitivity to cladribine

Warnings Because of its myelosuppressive properties, cladribine should be used with caution in patients with pre-existing hematologic or immunologic abnormalities; prophylactic administration of allopurinol should be considered in patients receiving cladribine because of the potential for hyperuricemia secondary to tumor lysis; appropriate antibiotic therapy should be administered promptly in patients exhibiting signs and symptoms of neutropenia and infection

Dosage Forms Injection, preservative free: 1 mg/mL (10 mL)

Stability Solutions should be administered immediately after the initial dilution or stored in the refrigerator (2°C to 8°C) for ≤8 hours. The use of dextrose 5% in water as a diluent is not recommended due to increased degradation of cladribine; should not be mixed with other intravenous drugs or additive or infused simultaneously via a common intravenous line. Admixtures for single daily infusion are stable for at least 24 hours at room temperature under normal room light in polyvinyl chloride infusion containers. Admixtures for 7-day infusion are stable (chemically and physically) for at least 7 days in the Pharmacia Deltec™ medication cassettes.

Reference Range Infusion of 8.9 mg/m²/day for 5 days results in a plasma concentration range of 20-54 nmol/L

Overdosage Treatment

Decontamination: Lavage/activated charcoal with cathartic

Enhancement of elimination: Multiple dosing of activated charcoal may be effective

Pregnancy Risk Factor D

Specific References

Baltz JK and Montello MJ, "Cladribine for the Treatment of Hematologic Malignancies," *Clin Pharm*, 1993, 12(11):805-13.

Beutler E, "Cladribine (2-Chlorodeoxyadenosine)," *Lancet*, 1992, 340(8825):952-6.

Piro LD, "2-Chlorodeoxyadenosine Treatment of Lymphoid Malignancies," *Blood*, 1992, 79(4):843-5.

Clarithromycin (kla rith' roe mye sin)

Related Information

Erythromycin *on page 319*

CAS Number 81103-11-9

Brand Names Biaxin™ Filmtabs®; Klacid®; Klaricid®

Synonyms Cla

Use Treatment against most respiratory pathogens (eg, *S. pyogenes*, *S. pneumoniae*, *S. agalactiae*, *S. viridans*, *M. catarrhalis*, *C. trachomatis*, *Legionella* spp., *Mycoplasma pneumoniae*[, *S. aureus*). Clarithromycin is highly active (MICs ≤0.25 mcg/mL) against *H. influenzae*, the combination of clarithromycin and its metabolite demonstrate an additive effect. Additionally, clarithromycin has shown activity against *C. pneumoniae* (including strain TWAR) and *M. avium* infection. Approved

(Continued)

Clarithromycin *(Continued)*

for pediatric use to treat *Mycobacterium avium* complex or otitis media. Clarithromycin may have some activity against *Cryptosporidia* and *Toxoplasma* encephalitis.

Mechanism of Action Exerts its antibacterial action by binding to 50S ribosomal subunit resulting in inhibition of protein synthesis. The 14-OH metabolite of clarithromycin is twice as active as the parent compound.

Adverse Reactions

Cardiovascular: Ventricular tachycardia, torsade de pointes

Central nervous system: Headache

Dermatologic: Urticaria

Gastrointestinal: Diarrhea, nausea, abnormal taste, dyspepsia, abdominal pain, pseudomembranous colitis

Hematologic: Decreased white blood count, elevated prothrombin time, eosinophilia, thrombocytopenia, thrombocytopenic purpura

Hepatic: Elevated AST, alkaline phosphatase, and bilirubin

Renal: Proteinuria, hematuria, elevated BUN and serum creatinine

Respiratory: Respiratory tract infection

Signs & Symptoms of Acute Overdose Nausea, vomiting, purpura, hematuria, diarrhea, eosinophilia, prostration, reversible pancreatitis, jaundice, tachycardia (ventricular), deafness with or without tinnitus or vertigo

Toxicodynamics/Kinetics

Absorption: Highly stable in the presence of gastric acid (unlike erythromycin)

Distribution: V_d: 243-266 L (metabolite: 304-309 L) Widely distributes into most body tissues with the exception of the CNS

Protein binding: 42% to 50%

Metabolism: Partially converted to the microbiologically active metabolite, 14-OH clarithromycin

Bioavailability: 50% (250 mg tablet)

Half-life, elimination: 3-4 hours with a 250 mg dose; 5-7 hours with a 500 mg dose; 14-hydroxyclarithromycin: 5-7 hours

Time to peak serum concentration: Oral: 2-4 hours

Elimination: Following 250 mg or 500 mg doses every 12 hours, ~20% to 30% of unchanged parent drug is excreted in urine

Usual Dosage Oral:

Children: 7.5 mg/kg twice daily (up to 1 g/day)

Adults: Usual dose: 250-500 mg every 12 hours for 7-14 days

- Upper respiratory tract: 250-500 mg every 12 hours for 10-14 days
  - Pharyngitis/tonsillitis: 250 mg every 12 hours for 10 days
  - Acute maxillary sinusitis: 500 mg every 12 hours for 14 days
- Lower respiratory tract: 250-500 mg every 12 hours for 7-14 days
  - Acute exacerbation of chronic bronchitis due to *M. catarrhalis* and *S. pneumoniae*: 250 mg every 12 hours for 7-14 days; *H. influenzae*: 500 mg every 12 hours for 7-14 days
  - Pneumonia due to *M. pneumoniae* and *S. pneumoniae*: 250 mg every 12 hours for 7-14 days
- Uncomplicated skin and skin structure: 250 mg every 12 hours for 7-14 days

Dosing adjustment in severe renal impairment: Decreased doses or prolonged dosing intervals are recommended

Contraindications Hypersensitivity to clarithromycin, erythromycin, or any macrolide antibiotic

Warnings In presence of severe renal impairment with or without coexisting hepatic impairment, decreased dosage or prolonged dosing interval may be appropriate; antibiotic associated colitis has been reported with use of clarithromycin; elderly patients experienced increased incidents of adverse effects due to known age-related decreases in renal function

Dosage Forms

Granules for oral suspension: 125 mg/5 mL (100 mL, 200 mL); 250 mg/5 mL (100 mL, 200 mL)

Tablet, film coated: 250 mg, 500 mg

Reference Range Steady-state levels of 250 mg/dose of clarithromycin: ~1 μg/mL

Overdosage Treatment

Decontamination: Lavage/activated charcoal with cathartic

Supportive therapy: Acute gastrointestinal irritation can be treated with milk or bismuth subsalicylate, lidocaine can be used for ventricular arrhythmias

Drug Interactions

Decreased serum levels of zidovudine can occur

Increased levels: Clarithromycin has been shown to increase serum **theophylline** levels by as much as 20%. **Carbamazepine** levels have been shown to increase after a single dose of clarithromycin; simultaneous use with erythromycin can result in elevated carbamazepine levels. While other drug interactions (digoxin, anticoagulants, ergotamine, triazolam) known to occur with erythromycin have not been reported in clinical trials with clarithromycin, concurrent use of these drugs should be monitored closely. Cyclosporine, terfenadine, astemizole levels may also be increased.

Increased toxicity: Concomitant use of clarithromycin with fluoxetine can result in fluoxetine intoxication manifesting as delirium

Pregnancy Risk Factor C

Monitoring Parameters Monitor patients receiving clarithromycin and drugs known to interact with erythromycin (ie, theophylline, digoxin, anticoagulants, triazolam) since there are still very few studies examining drug-drug interactions with clarithromycin; liver function tests

Patient Information May be taken with meals or without meals; may take with milk; finish all medication; do not skip doses

Nursing Implications Give every 12 hours rather than twice daily to avoid peak and trough variation

Additional Information In comparative trials, clarithromycin has been shown to be as effective treatment as penicillin for streptococcal pharyngitis, amoxicillin for acute maxillary sinusitis, ampicillin or erythromycin for acute bacterial exacerbations of chronic bronchitis, erythromycin for community acquired pneumonia, and erythromycin or cefadroxil for skin infections. In small studies, clarithromycin has also demonstrated efficacy in the treatment of *M. pneumoniae, C. pneumoniae*, and *Legionella pneumophila* respiratory tract infections. Additionally, the data from a short-term trial involving only small numbers of patients suggest that clarithromycin has clear activity against *M. avium* and may benefit patients with AIDS and disseminated *M. avium* infection.

Specific References

Guay DRP, "Pharmacokinetics of New Macrolides," *Infect Med*, 1992, 9(Suppl A):9-13.

Nightengale SD, Koster FT, Mertz GJ, et al, "Clarithromycin-Induced Mania in Two Patients With AIDS," *Clin Infect Dis*, 1995, 20:1563-4.

Oteo JA, Gomez-Cadinanos RA, Rosel L, et al, "Clarithromycin-Induced Thrombocytopenic Purpura," *Clin Infect Dis*, 1994, 19(6):1170-1.

Peters DH and Clissold SP, "Clarithromycin: A Review of its Antimicrobial Activity, Pharmacokinetic Properties, and Therapeutic Potential," *Drugs*, 1992, 44(1):117-64.

Pollak PT, Sketris IS, Mackenzie SL, et al, "Delirium Probably Induced by Clarithromycin in a Patient Receiving Fluoxetine," *Ann Pharmacother*, 1995, 29:486-8.

Stafstrom CE, Nohria V, Loganbill H, et al, "Erythromycin-induced Carbamazepine Toxicity: A Continuing Problem," *Arch Pediatr Adolesc Med*, 1995, 149(1):99-101.

Teare JP, Booth CL, Brown JL, et al, "Pseudomembranous Colitis Following Clarithromycin Therapy," *Eur J Gastroenterol Hepatol*, 1995, 7:275-7.

Claritin® *see* Loratadine *on page 481*

Claritine® *see* Loratadine *on page 481*

Clarityn® *see* Loratadine *on page 481*

Clarityne® *see* Loratadine *on page 481*

Clarmyl® *see* Clobazam *on next page*

Claudicat® *see* Pentoxifylline *on page 607*

CldAdo *see* Cladribine *on page 220*

Clemastine Fumarate (klem' as teen fume' a rate)

CAS Number 15686-51-8; 14976-57-9

Brand Names Aller-eze®; Antihist-1® [OTC]; Tavegil®; Tavist®; Tavist®-1 [OTC]

Synonyms Mecloprodin

Use Perennial and seasonal allergic rhinitis and other allergic symptoms including rash

Mechanism of Action Competes with histamine for H_1-receptor sites on effector cells in the gastrointestinal tract, blood vessels, and respiratory tract

Adverse Reactions

Cardiovascular: Palpitations, bradycardia

Central nervous system: Slight to moderate drowsiness, headache, fatigue, nervousness, dizziness, depression, ataxia

Dermatologic: Photosensitivity, rash, angioedema

Gastrointestinal: Appetite increase, weight increase, nausea, diarrhea, abdominal pain, dry mouth

Hepatic: Hepatitis

Neuromuscular & skeletal: Arthralgia, myalgia, paresthesia

Ocular: Diplopia, nystagmus

Respiratory: Pharyngitis, thickening of bronchial secretions, bronchospasm

Miscellaneous: Edema, epistaxis, porphyrinogenic

Toxicodynamics/Kinetics

Duration of effect: 10-12 hours

Peak therapeutic effect: Within 5-7 hours

Absorption: Almost 100% from gastrointestinal tract

(Continued)

Clemastine Fumarate *(Continued)*

Metabolism: In the liver (no enzyme induction)
Elimination: Excreted in urine

Usual Dosage Oral:

Children: <12 years: 0.4-1 mg twice daily

Children >12 years and Adults: 1.34 mg twice daily to 2.68 mg 3 times/day; do not exceed 8.04 mg/day; lower doses should be considered in patients >60 years; up to 6 mg/day given for angioedema

Contraindications Angle-closure glaucoma, hypersensitivity to clemastine or any component

Warnings Safety and efficacy have not been established in children <6 years of age; bladder neck obstruction, symptomatic prostate hypertrophy, asthmatic attacks, and stenosing peptic ulcer

Dosage Forms

Syrup (citrus flavor): 0.67 mg/5 mL with alcohol 5.5% (120 mL)
Tablet: 1.34 mg, 2.68 mg

Overdosage Treatment Supportive therapy: There is no specific treatment for an antihistamine overdose, however, most of its clinical toxicity is due to anticholinergic effects. Anticholinesterase inhibitors may be useful by reducing acetylcholinesterase. Anticholinesterase inhibitors include physostigmine, neostigmine, pyridostigmine and edrophonium. For anticholinergic overdose with severe life-threatening symptoms, physostigmine 1-2 mg (0.5 or 0.02 mg/kg for children) I.V., slowly may be given to reverse these effects.

Test Interactions May suppress wheal and flare response to antigen skin testing

Drug Interactions Increased toxicity (CNS depression): CNS depressants, MAO inhibitors, tricyclic antidepressants, phenothiazines, biperiden, guanabenz

Pregnancy Risk Factor C

Monitoring Parameters Look for a reduction of rhinitis, rash, eczema, pruritus, or other allergic symptoms

Patient Information Avoid alcohol; take with food; may cause drowsiness, may impair coordination or judgment

Nursing Implications Raise bed rails, institute safety measures, assist with ambulation

Additional Information Clemastine fumarate 1.34 mg = clemastine base 1 mg; offers no significant benefit over other antihistamines except that it may be dosed twice daily (in adults) as compared to other antihistamines with more frequent dosing

Specific References

Kok TH, Taitz LS, Bennett MJ, et al, "Drowsiness Due to Clemastine Transmitted in Breast Milk," *Lancet*, 1982, 1:914-5.

Clinoril® *see* Sulindac *on page 715*

Cliradon® *see* Ketobemidone Hydrochloride *on page 452*

Clobazam

CAS Number 22316-47-8

Brand Names Clarmyl®; Clopax®; Frisium®; Noiafren®; Sederlona®; Urbadan®; Urbanol®; Urbanyl®

Use Investigational: Antianxiety, anticonvulsant, and sedative agent

Mechanism of Action Facilitates gamma-aminobutyric acid neurotransmission; a 1,5 benzodiazepine derivative; weak hypnotic agent

Adverse Reactions

Cardiovascular: Orthostatic hypotension, syncope
Central nervous system: Sedation, dizziness, lightheadedness, headache, ataxia
Endocrine & metabolic: Weight gain
Gastrointestinal: Dry mouth

Signs & Symptoms of Acute Overdose Dizziness, confusion

Toxicodynamics/Kinetics

Distribution: V_d: 1 L/kg
Protein binding: 85% to 90%
Metabolism: Hepatic to active metabolite N-desmethyl clobazam
Half-life: 10-50 hours (parent drug); 77 hours (metabolite)
Peak plasma levels: Within 1.3 hours
Elimination: Renal

Usual Dosage

Adults: 20-30 mg/day in divided doses or at night; maximum daily dose: 60 mg
Elderly: 10-20 mg/day

Dosage Forms

Capsule: 10 mg
Tablet: 10 mg

Reference Range After a 40 mg oral dose, peak plasma levels are ~730 μg/L

Overdosage Treatment

Decontamination: Lavage/activated charcoal with cathartic

Supportive therapy: Rarely is mechanical ventilation required; flumazenil has been shown to selectively block the binding of benzodiazepines to CNS receptors, resulting in a reversal of benzodiazepine-induced CNS depression and respiratory depression

Enhancement of elimination: Multiple dose of activated charcoal is effective

Antidote(s)

Flumazenil *on page 1428*

Additional Information Used to relieve phantom limb pain; similar efficacy as with buspirone in treatment of anxiety/panic disorders; oral ingestion of 300 mg produced mental status changes; reduce dosage in elderly and cirrhosis

Specific References

Bohm C, Placchi M, Stallone F, et al, "A Double-Blind Comparison of Buspirone, Clobazam, and Placebo in Patients With Anxiety Treated in a General Practice Setting," *J Clin Psychopharmacol*, 1990, 10(3 Suppl):38S-42S.

Donlon PT and Singer JM, "Clobazam Versus Placebo for Anxiety and Tension in Psychoneurotic Outpatients: A Multicenter Collaborative Study," *J Clin Pharmacol*, 1979, 19:297-302.

Feely M, "Prescribing Anticonvulsant Drugs. 3. Clonazepam and Clobazam," *Prescribers J*, 1989, 29:111-5.

Rice-Oxley CP, "The Limited List: Clobazam for Phantom Limb Pain," *Br Med J*, 1986, 293(6557):1309.

Clofazimine Palmitate (kloe fa' zi meen)

CAS Number 2030-63-9

Brand Names Lamprene®

Use Treatment of dapsone-resistant leprosy; multibacillary dapsone-sensitive leprosy; erythema nodosum leprosum; *Mycobacterium avium* intracellular (MAI) infections

Mechanism of Action Binds preferentially to mycobacterial DNA to inhibit mycobacterial growth; also has some anti-inflammatory activity through an unknown mechanism

Adverse Reactions

Central nervous system: Dizziness, drowsiness

Dermatologic: Pink to brownish black discoloration of the skin and conjunctiva, dry skin, rash

Endocrine & metabolic: Hyperglycemia

Gastrointestinal: Constipation, abdominal pain, diarrhea, nausea, vomiting, ileus, gastrointestinal bleeding, red to brownish black feces discoloration

Ocular: Irritation of the eyes

Miscellaneous: Red to brownish black urine discoloration

Signs & Symptoms of Acute Overdose Nausea, hyperglycemia, photosensitivity, vomiting, diarrhea

Toxicodynamics/Kinetics

Absorption: Oral: Slow, 20% to 70%; bioavailability and rate of absorption increases with food

Distribution: Remains in tissues for prolonged periods; appears in breast milk; highly lipophilic; deposited primarily in fatty tissue and cells of the reticuloendothelial system; taken up by macrophages throughout the body; distributes into mesenteric lymph nodes, adrenal glands, subcutaneous fat, liver, bile, gallbladder, spleen, small intestine, muscles, bones, and skin; does not appear to cross blood-brain barrier

Metabolism: Partial in the liver to two metabolites

Half-life:

- Terminal: 8 days
- Tissue: 70 days

Time to peak serum concentration: 1-6 hours with chronic therapy

Elimination: Mainly in feces; negligible amounts excreted unchanged in urine; small amounts excreted in sputum, saliva, and sweat

Usual Dosage Oral:

Children: Leprosy: 1 mg/kg/day every 24 hours in combination with dapsone and rifampin

Adults:

- Dapsone-resistant leprosy: 100 mg/day in combination with one or more antileprosy drugs for 3 years; then alone 100 mg/day
- Dapsone-sensitive multibacillary leprosy: 100 mg/day in combination with two or more antileprosy drugs for at least 2 years and continue until negative skin smears are obtained, then institute single drug therapy with appropriate agent
- Erythema nodosum leprosum: 100-200 mg/day for up to 3 months or longer then taper dose to 100 mg/day when possible
- Pyoderma gangrenosum: 300-400 mg/day for up to 12 months

Dosing adjustment in hepatic impairment: Should be considered in severe hepatic dysfunction

(Continued)

Clofazimine Palmitate *(Continued)*

Warnings Use with caution in patients with gastrointestinal problems; well tolerated when administered in dosages ≤100 mg/day; dosages >100 mg/day should be used for as short a duration as possible

Dosage Forms Capsule: 50 mg, 100 mg

Reference Range Average plasma concentrations: 0.7-1.0 μg/mL

Overdosage Treatment

Decontamination: Lavage/activated charcoal with cathartic

Enhancement of elimination: Multiple dosing of activated charcoal may be effective

Drug Interactions Inhibits rifampin absorption

Pregnancy Risk Factor C

Pregnancy Implications Distributes into breast milk

Monitoring Parameters gastrointestinal complaints

Patient Information Drug may cause a pink to brownish-black discoloration of the skin, conjunctiva, tears, sweat, urine, feces, and nasal secretions

Nursing Implications Give with meals

Additional Information Crystal deposition in bowel can lead to ileus symptoms

Specific References

Freerksen E and Seydel JK, "Critical Comments on the Treatment of Leprosy and Other Mycobacterial Infections With Clofazimine," *Arzneimittelforschung*, 1992, 42(10):1243-5.

Holdiness MR, "Clinical Pharmacokinetics of Clofazimine: A Review," *Clin Pharmacokinet*, 1989, 16(2):74-85.

Moore VJ, "A Review of Side Effects Experienced by Patients Taking Clofazimine," *Lepr Rev*, 1983, 54(4):327-35.

Clofibrate (kloe fye' brate)

CAS Number 637-07-0; 882-09-7

Brand Names Atromid-S®

Use Adjunct to dietary therapy in the management of type III hyperlipidemias associated with high triglyceride levels

Mechanism of Action Mechanism is unclear but thought to reduce cholesterol synthesis and triglyceride hepatic-vascular transference (a fibric acid derivative)

Adverse Reactions

Cardiovascular: Angina, cardiac arrhythmias

Central nervous system: Headache, dizziness, fatigue, muscle cramping, aching, asthenia

Dermatologic: Skin rash, pruritus, dry brittle hair, alopecia, Stevens-Johnson syndrome

Endocrine & metabolic: Syndrome of inappropriate antidiuretic hormone

Gastrointestinal: Nausea which usually decreases with continued therapy or reduction in dosage, diarrhea, vomiting, dyspepsia, flatulence, abdominal distress, increased incidence of cholecystitis, gallstones

Genitourinary: Impotence

Hematologic: Anemia, eosinophilia, eosinophilic pneumonitis, leukopenia, neutropenia, agranulocytosis, granulocytopenia

Hepatic: Liver function test (increased)

Neuromuscular & skeletal: Myalgia

Ocular: Photophobia, myopathy (associated with hypoalbuminemia)

Renal: Rhabdomyolysis-induced renal failure, renal insufficiency, renal toxicity

Signs & Symptoms of Acute Overdose Lethargy, erythema multiforme, cholelithiasis, cardiomegaly, Stevens-Johnson syndrome, hyponatremia, hyperthermia, myalgia, photophobia, impotence, hematuria, fever, desquamation, dysuria, myoglobinuria, systemic lupus erythematosus (SLE)

Toxicodynamics/Kinetics

Absorption: Occurs completely; intestinal transformation is required to activate the drug

Distribution: V_d: 5.5 L/kg

Protein binding: 95% (75% in patients with nephrotic syndrome)

Metabolism: In the liver to an inactive glucuronide ester and an active metabolite (clofibric acid)

Half-life: 6-24 hours, increases significantly with reduced renal function; with anuria: 110 hours

Time to peak serum concentration: Within 3-6 hours

Elimination: 40% to 70% excreted in urine; clearance: 1.5-2.0 mL/minute

Usual Dosage Adults: Oral: 500 mg 4 times/day; some patients may respond to lower doses

Dosing interval in renal impairment:

Cl_{cr} 10-50 mL/minute: Administer every 12-18 hours

Cl_{cr} <10 mL/minute: Avoid use

Contraindications Hypersensitivity to clofibrate or any component, severe hepatic or renal impairment, primary biliary cirrhosis

Warnings Clofibrate has been shown to be tumorigenic in toxicity studies using rats; increased risk of cholelithiasis, cholecystitis; discontinue if lipid response is not obtained; no evidence substantiates a beneficial effect on cardiovascular mortality

Dosage Forms Capsule: 500 mg

Reference Range Therapeutic plasma level of parachlorophenoxyisobutyric acid: 80-150 μg/mL

Overdosage Treatment

Decontamination: Emesis or lavage/activated charcoal with cathartic

Enhancement of elimination: Multiple dosing of activated charcoal may be effective

Test Interactions Increased creatine phosphokinase [CPK], aldolase, serum glutamic-oxaloacetic acid level (S); decreased alkaline phosphatase (S), cholesterol (S), glucose, uric acid (S), fibrinogen, plasma thyroxine

Drug Interactions

Increased anticoagulant effect of warfarin; increased hypoglycemic effect with insulin/sulfonylureas

Increased toxicity/levels with probenecid; increased antidiuretic effect with desmopressin; increased diuretic effect with furosemide

Pregnancy Risk Factor C

Pregnancy Implications Crosses the placenta

Monitoring Parameters Serum lipids, LFTs, CBC

Patient Information If gastrointestinal upset occurs, may be taken with food, patient package insert available; notify physician of chest pain, dyspnea, irregular heartbeat, severe stomach pain with nausea and vomiting, persistent fever, sore throat, or unusual bleeding or bruising

Specific References

Cumming A, "Acute Renal Failure and Interstitial Nephritis After Clofibrate Treatment," *Br Med J*, 1980, 281(6254):1529-30.

Gugler R, "Clinical Pharmacokinetics of Hypolipidaemic Drugs," *Clin Pharmacokinet*, 1978, 3(6):425-39.

Wong SS, "Stevens-Johnson Syndrome Induced by Clofibrate," *Acta Dermato-Venereologica*, 1994, 74:475.

Clomid® *see* Clomiphene Citrate *on this page*

Clomiphene Citrate (kloe' mi feen)

CAS Number 911-45-5; 15690-57-0; 15690-55-8; 50-41-9; 7599-79-3; 7619-53-6

Brand Names Clomid®; Clomivid®; Milophene®; Omnifin®; Prolifen®; Serophene®

Synonyms Chloramiphene

Use Treatment of ovulatory failure in patients desiring pregnancy

Mechanism of Action Induces ovulation by stimulating the release of pituitary gonadotropins; triphenylethylene which binds to estrogen receptors; acts as an antagonist at low doses but is an estrogen agonist at doses >100 mg

Adverse Reactions

Central nervous system: Dizziness, psychosis, dementia, headache, ataxia

Dermatologic: Alopecia (reversible), rash

Endocrine & metabolic: Ovarian enlargement, ectopic pregnancy, gynecomastia, hot flashes, weight gain

Gastrointestinal: Distention, bloating, nausea, vomiting, stomatitis, abdominal/pelvic pain

Ocular: Blurring of vision (2% to 10%), photophobia, diplopia, cataract formation

Renal: Polyuria

Miscellaneous: Breast tenderness, anterior pituitary hemorrhage

Toxicodynamics/Kinetics

Metabolism: Hepatic

Half-life: 5-7 days

Elimination: Enterohepatically circulated; excreted primarily in feces with small amounts appearing in urine

Usual Dosage Adults: Female: Oral: 50 mg/day for 5 days (first course); start the regimen on or about the fifth day of cycle; if ovulation occurs, do not increase dosage; if ovulation does not occur, increase next course to 100 mg/day for 5 days. Three courses of therapy are an adequate therapeutic trial. Further treatment is not recommended in patients who do not exhibit ovulation.

Contraindications Pregnancy, liver disease, abnormal vaginal bleeding, endometrial cancer, ovarian cyst (other than polycystic ovary)

Dosage Forms Tablet: 50 mg

Overdosage Treatment

Decontamination: Lavage/activated charcoal with cathartic

Enhancement of elimination: Due to its enterohepatic recirculation, multiple dosing of activated charcoal may be effective

Test Interactions FSH/LH levels increase by ~150%

Drug Interactions Decreased response when used with danazol; decreased estradiol response when used with clomiphene

(Continued)

Clomiphene Citrate *(Continued)*

Pregnancy Risk Factor X

Pregnancy Implications Multiple births occur in ~10% of pregnancies with induced ovulation; increased frequency of delayed follicular rupture and ectopic pregnancy also noted

Additional Information Has been associated with testicular cancer, ectopic pregnancy, ovarian cancer

Specific References

Purvin VA, "Visual Disturbance Secondary to Clomiphene Citrate," *Arch Ophthalmol*, 1995, 113:482-4.

Sokol RZ, "Prevention and Management of Complications Occurring During Treatment With Clomifene," *Drug Saf*, 1990, 5(5):313-6.

Walker AB, Eldridge PR, and MacFarlane IA, "Clomiphene-Induced Pituitary Apoplexy in a Patient With Acromegaly," *J Endocrinol*, 1995, 144:29.

Clomipramine Hydrochloride (kloe mi' pra meen)

CAS Number 303-49-1; 17321-77-6

Brand Names Anafranil®

Use Treatment of obsessive-compulsive disorder (OCD)

Mechanism of Action Clomipramine appears to affect serotonin uptake while its active metabolite, desmethylclomipramine, affects norepinephrine uptake; a tricyclic tertiary amine antidepressant

Adverse Reactions

Cardiovascular: Orthostatic hypotension, tachycardia, flushing

Central nervous system: Convulsions, drowsiness, dizziness, neuroleptic malignant syndrome, psychosis, serotonin syndrome (confusion, restlessness, sweating, diarrhea)

Dermatologic: Photosensitivity

Endocrine & metabolic: Hyponatremia, syndrome of inappropriate antidiuretic hormone

Hepatic: Acute hepatitis

Neuromuscular & skeletal: Hyperreflexia

Signs & Symptoms of Acute Overdose Agitation, confusion, agranulocytosis, thrombocytopenia, photosensitivity, neuroleptic malignant syndrome, nystagmus, leukopenia, myoclonus, mania, memory loss, lactation, hallucinations, hyperprolactinemia, urinary retention, hyperthermia, hypotension, tachycardia, seizures, apnea

Toxicodynamics/Kinetics

Onset of action: 2-3 weeks

Absorption: Oral: Rapid

Distribution: V_d: 7-20 L/kg

Protein binding: Very highly protein bound in plasma and tissues (≥90%)

Metabolism: Extensive first-pass; metabolized to desmethylclomipramine (active) in the liver

Half-life: 20-30 hours; over 50 hours in an overdose setting

Usual Dosage Oral: Initial:

Children: 25 mg/day and gradually increase, as tolerated, to a maximum of 3 mg/kg/day or 200 mg/day, whichever is smaller

Adults: 25 mg/day and gradually increase, as tolerated, to 100 mg/day the first 2 weeks, may then be increased to a total of 250 mg/day maximum

Contraindications Patients in acute recovery stage of recent myocardial infarction; not to be used within 14 days of a MAO inhibitor

Warnings Seizures are likely and are dose related

Dosage Forms Capsule: 25 mg, 50 mg, 75 mg

Reference Range Level of 6560 ng/mL associated with fatality; serum levels may not peak until the fourth day

Overdosage Treatment

Decontamination: Lavage/activated charcoal with cathartic; multiple dosing of activated charcoal may be effective

Supportive therapy: Following initiation of essential overdose management, toxic symptoms should be treated. Ventricular arrhythmias often respond to phenytoin 15-20 mg/kg (adults) with concurrent systemic alkalinization (sodium bicarbonate 0.5-2 mEq/kg I.V.). Arrhythmias unresponsive to this therapy may respond to lidocaine 1 mg/kg I.V. followed by a titrated infusion. Physostigmine (1-2 mg I.V. slowly for adults or 0.5 mg I.V. slowly for children) may be indicated in reversing seizures or movement disorders, but **only as a last resort**. Seizures usually respond to lorazepam or diazepam I.V. boluses (5-10 mg for adults up to 30 mg or 0.25-0.4 mg/kg/dose for children up to 10 mg/dose). If seizures are unresponsive or recur, phenytoin or phenobarbital may be required. Clonidine is not effective.

Test Interactions Increases glucose, plasma catecholamine

Drug Interactions

Clomipramine blocks the uptake of guanethidine and clonidine and may prevent the hypotensive effects of these drugs; clomipramine and moclobemide may result in a fatal serotonin syndrome

CNS depressants: Clomipramine may be additive to the effects of CNS depressants
Sympathomimetic agents: Clomipramine potentiates the effects of sympathomimetic agents such as isoproterenol, epinephrine, etc
With MAO inhibitors: Fever, hypertension, tachycardia, seizures, agitation, delirium
Warfarin: Clomipramine may increase prothrombin time in patients stabilized on warfarin
Use with caution with oral contraceptives, may increase plasma concentrations; miconazole may inhibit metabolism of clomipramine; morphine increases availability of clomipramine; concomitant use of clomipramine with alprazolam can result in serotonin syndrome; seizures can result with concomitant clomipramine and fluoxetine therapy

Pregnancy Risk Factor D

Pregnancy Implications May cause neonatal hypotonia, hypoglycemia, and withdrawal at doses of 75 to 250 mg/day

Monitoring Parameters EKG/cardiac status

Patient Information May cause seizures, caution should be used in activities that require alertness like driving, operating machinery, or swimming; effect of drug may take several weeks to appear

Nursing Implications Monitor pulse rate and blood pressure prior to and during therapy, evaluate mental status

Additional Information May also relieve depression, panic attacks, and chronic pain; may be unsafe to use in patients with porphyria; not effective for sleep apnea

Specific References

Cano-Munoz JL, Montejo-Iglesias ML, Yanez-Saez RM, et al, "Possible Serotonin Syndrome Following the Combined Administration of Clomipramine and Alprazolam," *J Clin Psychiatry*, 1995, 56:122.
Dale O and Hole A, "Biphasic Time-Course of Serum Concentrations of Clomipramine and Desmethylclomipramine After a Near-Fatal Overdose," *Vet Hum Toxicol*, 1994, 36(4):309-10.
Hernandez AF, Montero MN, Pla A, et al, "Fatal Moclobemide Overdose or Death Caused by Serotonin Syndrome?" *J Forensic Sci*, 1995, 40(1):128-30.
Kuisma MJ, "Fatal Serotonin Syndrome With Trismus," *Ann Emerg Med*, 1995, 26:108.
Larrey D, Rueff B, Pessayre D, et al, "Cross Hepatotoxicity Between Tricyclic Antidepressants," *Gut*, 1986, 27(6):726-7.
LeJoyeux M, et al, "Serotonin Syndrome: Incidence, Symptoms, and Treatment," *CNS Drugs*, 1994, 2:132-43.
Ljungren B and Bojs G, "A Case of Photosensitivity and Contact Allergy to Systemic Tricyclic Drugs, With Unusual Features," *Contact Dermatitis*, 1991, 24(4):259-65.
Roberge RJ, Martin TG, Hodgman M, et al, "Acute Chemical Pancreatitis Associated With a Tricyclic Antidepressant (Clomipramine) Overdose," *J Toxicol Clin Toxicol*, 1994, 32(4):425-9.
Schimmell MS, Katz E, Shaag Y, et al, "Toxic Neonatal Effects Following Maternal Clomipramine Therapy," *J Toxicol Clin Toxicol*, 1991, 29(4):479-84.
Sternbach H, "Fluoxetine-Clomipramine Interaction," *J Clin Psychiatry*, 1995, 56:171-2.
Swanson-Biearman B, Goetz CM, Dean BS, et al, "Anafronil Overdose: A Fatal Outcome," *Vet Hum Toxicol*, 1989, 31:378.
Tueth MJ, "The Serotonin Syndrome in the Emergency Department," *Ann Emerg Med*, 1993, 22(8):1369.

Clomivid® *see* Clomiphene Citrate *on page 227*

Clonazepam (kloe na' ze pam)

Related Information

Benzodiazepines Comparison *on page 1643*
Flunitrazepam *on page 354*
Nitrazepam *on page 562*
Therapeutic Drugs Associated With Hallucinations *on page 1558-1559*

CAS Number 1622-61-3

Brand Names Iktorivil®; Klonopin™; Rivotril®

Use Prophylaxis of absence (petit mal), petit mal variant (Lennox-Gastaut), akinetic, and myoclonic seizures

Mechanism of Action Suppresses the spike-and-wave discharge in absence seizures by depressing nerve transmission in the motor cortex

Adverse Reactions

Cardiovascular: Hypotension
Central nervous system: Drowsiness, psychosis, changes in behavior or personality, dizziness, confusion; auditory, visual, and tactile hallucinations; CNS depression, disorientation, memory impairment, decreased concentration, headache, ataxia, hypotonia, choreiform movements
Dermatologic: Rash, alopecia
Gastrointestinal: Nausea, dry mouth, vomiting, diarrhea, constipation, anorexia
Hematologic: Thrombocytopenia, anemia, leukopenia, eosinophilia
Neuromuscular & skeletal: Staggering, falling, tremors
Ocular: Nystagmus, blurred vision
Respiratory: Hypersalivation and bronchial hypersecretion, respiratory depression, apnea

(Continued)

Clonazepam *(Continued)*

Miscellaneous: Physical and psychological dependence; precocious development in adolescents

Signs & Symptoms of Acute Overdose May produce somnolence, purpura, dysarthria, diplopia, confusion, ataxia, diminished reflexes, depression, hyperactivity, neuroleptic malignant syndrome, hirsutism, coma, hypotension, cyanosis, leukopenia; neutropenia; agranulocytosis; granulocytopenia

Toxicodynamics/Kinetics

Onset of action: 20-60 minutes

Duration:

Infants and young Children: Up to 6-8 hours

Adults: Up to 12 hours

Absorption: Oral: Well absorbed

Distribution: V_d: Adults: 1.5-4.4 L/kg; distributed widely throughout body; probably crosses blood-brain barrier and placenta

Protein binding: 50% to 85%

Metabolism: Extensive; undergoes nitro-reduction to inactive metabolites; principle metabolite: 7-aminoclonazepam

Half-life:

Children: 22-33 hours

Adults: 19-50 hours

Elimination: Metabolites excreted as glucuronide or sulfate conjugates; <2% excreted unchanged in urine

Usual Dosage Oral:

Children <10 years or 30 kg: Initial daily dose: 0.01-0.03 mg/kg/day (maximum: 0.05 mg/kg/day) given in 2-3 divided doses; increase by no more than 0.5 mg every third day until seizures are controlled or adverse effects seen; usual maintenance dose: 0.1-0.2 mg/kg/day divided 3 times/day; not to exceed 0.2 mg/kg/day

Adults: Initial daily dose not to exceed 1.5 mg given in 3 divided doses; may increase by 0.5-1 mg every third day until seizures are controlled or adverse effects seen; usual maintenance dose: 0.05-0.2 mg/kg; do not exceed 20 mg/day

Contraindications Hypersensitivity to clonazepam, any component, or other benzodiazepines; severe liver disease, acute narrow-angle glaucoma

Warnings Use with caution in patients with chronic respiratory disease or impaired renal function; abrupt discontinuance may precipitate withdrawal symptoms, status epilepticus or seizures

Dosage Forms Tablet: 0.5 mg, 1 mg, 2 mg

Reference Range

Sample size: 2 mL serum or plasma

Therapeutic: 10-50 ng/mL

Toxic: >80 ng/mL

Timing of serum samples: Peak serum levels occur 1-3 hours after oral ingestion

Overdosage Treatment

Decontamination: Lavage/activated charcoal with cathartic

Supportive therapy: Treatment for benzodiazepine overdose is supportive. Rarely is mechanical ventilation required. Flumazenil has been shown to selectively block the binding of benzodiazepines to CNS receptors, resulting in a reversal of benzodiazepine-induced CNS depression.

Enhancement of elimination: Multiple dose of activated charcoal may be effective

Antidote(s)

Flumazenil *on page 1428*

Drug Interactions CNS depressants, phenytoin, and barbiturates may enhance metabolism

Pregnancy Risk Factor C

Pregnancy Implications May cross the placenta

Patient Information May cause drowsiness

Nursing Implications Observe patient for excess sedation, respiratory depression

Additional Information Ethosuximide or valproic acid may be preferred for treatment of absence (petit mal) seizures; clonazepam-induced behavioral disturbances may be more frequent in mentally handicapped patients; may be effective therapy for tinnitus

Specific References

Barnett AM, "Treatment of Epilepsy With Clonazepam," *S Afr Med J*, 1973, 47(37):1683-6.

Bladin PF, "The Use of Clonazepam as an Anticonvulsant - Clinical Evaluation," *Med J Aust*, 1973, 1(14):683-8.

Brogden RN and Goa KL, "Flumazenil. A Preliminary Review of Its Benzodiazepine Antagonist Properties, Intrinsic Activity, and Therapeutic Use," *Drugs*, 1988, 35(4):448-67.

Clonidine (kloe' ni deen)

Related Information

Therapeutic Drugs Associated With Hallucinations *on page 1558-1559*

CAS Number 4205-90-7; 4205-91-8

Brand Names Catapres®; Catapressan®; Catapres-TTS®; Clonistada®; Dixart®; Hyposyn®; Ipotensium®; Isoglaucon®

Use Management of mild to moderate hypertension; either used alone or in combination with other antihypertensives; not recommended for first-line therapy for hypertension; also used for opiates withdrawal and in smoking cessation therapy; other uses may include prophylaxis of migraines, glaucoma, paralytic ileus, and diabetes-associated diarrhea

Mechanism of Action Stimulates alpha$_2$-adrenoreceptors in the brain stem, thus activating an inhibitory neuron, resulting in reduced sympathetic outflow, producing a decrease in vasomotor tone and heart rate

Adverse Reactions

Cardiovascular: Exacerbation of Raynaud's phenomenon, hypotension, bradycardia, palpitation, tachycardia, congestive heart failure, A-V block, transient paradoxical hypertension

Central nervous system: Drowsiness, dizziness, fatigue, insomnia, anxiety, auditory and visual hallucinations, headache

Dermatologic: Rash, pruritus

Endocrine & metabolic: Sodium and water retention

Gastrointestinal: Constipation, anorexia, dry mouth, nausea, vomiting, parotid pain

Genitourinary: Impotence

Hepatic: Hepatitis

Local: Skin reactions with patch

Ocular: Miosis, diplopia

Miscellaneous: Anogenital cicatricial pemphigoid

Signs & Symptoms of Acute Overdose Bradycardia, hypoglycemia, dry eyes, personality changes, insomnia, impotence, hyponatremia, syncope, A-V block, delirium, dementia, CNS depression, hypotension, ataxia, miosis, coma, dementia, hypotonia, hyporeflexia, hypothermia, nocturia, diarrhea, respiratory depression, apnea, irritability, seizures, paralytic ileus, heart block, hyperglycemia

Toxicodynamics/Kinetics

Onset of action: Oral: 30-60 minutes

Peak effect: Within 2-4 hours

Duration: 6-10 hours

Absorption:

Oral: Absorbed well

Transdermal: Absorbed mostly from chest and upper arm and least from thigh; absorbed through skin at a constant rate

Distribution: V_d: Adults: 2.1-4 L/kg; widely distributed throughout the body; crosses blood-brain barrier

Protein binding: 20% to 40%

Metabolism: Hepatic to inactive metabolites

Bioavailability: Oral: 75% to 95%

Half-life: Adults:

Normal renal function: 6-20 hours

Renal impairment: 18-41 hours

Time to peak serum concentration:

Oral: 3-5 hours

Transdermal: 2-3 days

Elimination: 65% excreted in urine (32% unchanged and 22% excreted in feces); clearance (renal): 3.1 mL/minute/kg

Usual Dosage

Children: Oral: Initial: 5-10 mcg/kg/day in divided doses every 8-12 hours; increase gradually at 5- to 7-day intervals to 25 mcg/kg/day in divided doses every 6 hours; maximum: 0.9 mg/day

Adults:

Oral: Initial dose: 0.1 mg twice daily, usual maintenance dose: 0.2-1.2 mg/day in 2-4 divided doses; maximum recommended dose: 2.4 mg/day

Transdermal: Apply once every 7 days; for initial therapy start with 0.1 mg and increase by 0.1 mg at 1- to 2-week intervals; dosages >2 x 0.3 mg do not improve efficacy

Dosing adjustment in renal impairment: Cl_{cr} <10 mL/minute: Administer 50% to 75% of normal dose

Contraindications Hypersensitivity to clonidine hydrochloride or any component

Warnings Do not abruptly discontinue; rapid increase in blood pressure, and symptoms of sympathetic overactivity (such as increased heart rate, tremor, agitation, anxiety, insomnia, sweating, palpitations) may occur; if need to discontinue, taper dose gradually over more than 1 week; dosage modification may be required in

(Continued)

Clonidine *(Continued)*

patients with renal impairment (reduce dose with decreased renal function); use with caution in cerebrovascular disease, coronary insufficiency, renal impairment, sinus node dysfunction; use with caution in patients unable to comply with the therapeutic regimen because of the risk of rebound hypertension

Dosage Forms

Patch, transdermal: 1, 2, and 3 (0.1 mg, 0.2 mg, 0.3 mg/day to 7-day duration)

Tablet, as hydrochloride: 0.1 mg, 0.2 mg, 0.3 mg

Reference Range Therapeutic: 1-2 ng/mL (SI: 4.4-8.7 nmol/L)

Overdosage Treatment

Decontamination: Lavage/activated charcoal with cathartic

Supportive therapy: Treatment is primarily supportive and symptomatic. Hypotension usually responds to I.V. fluids or Trendelenburg positioning. If unresponsive to these measures, the use of a parenteral vasoconstrictor may be required (eg, norepinephrine 0.1-0.2 mcg/kg/minute titrated to response). Naloxone may be utilized in treating the hypotension, CNS depression and/or apnea and should be given I.V. 0.01 mg/kg to 0.1 mg/kg, with repeats as needed. Atropine 15 mcg/kg I.V. or may be needed for symptomatic bradycardia. Tolazoline may be utilized to treat hypotension and bradycardia refractory to above therapy (initial dose of tolazoline is 10 mg I.V.).

Enhancement of elimination: Multiple dosing of activated charcoal may be effective; not dialyzable (0% to 5%)

Antidote(s)

Naloxone Hydrochloride *on page 1447*

Test Interactions Increases sodium (S); decreases catecholamines (U)

Drug Interactions Tricyclic antidepressants antagonize hypotensive effects of clonidine (no effect with maprotiline); beta-blockers may potentiate bradycardia in patients receiving clonidine and may increase the rebound hypertension seen with clonidine withdrawal; discontinue beta-blocker several days before clonidine is tapered off; nonsteroidal anti-inflammatory drugs may reduce clonidine's effect

Pregnancy Risk Factor C (not teratogenic in animals)

Monitoring Parameters Blood pressure, standing and sitting/supine, EKG for 48 hours

Patient Information Do not stop drug except on instruction of physician; check daily to be sure patch present

Nursing Implications Patches should be applied weekly at bedtime to a clean, hairless area of the upper outer arm or chest; rotate patch sites weekly

Additional Information Unsafe in patients with porphyria; rebound hypertension upon abrupt withdrawal usually occurs with doses >1.2 mg/day; appears to be the preferred "Mickey Finn" drug used by criminals in Moscow/Russia; addition of clonidine (75 µg to 150 µg) increased duration of analgesia produced by epidural morphine (2 mg) for cesarean delivery

Specific References

Capogna G, et al, "Addition of Clonidine to Epidural Morphine Enhances Postoperative Analgesia After Cesarean Delivery," *Reg Anaesth*, 1995, 20:57-61.

Corazza M, Mantovani L, Virgil A, et al, "Allergic Contact Dermatitis From a Clonidine Transdermal Delivery System," *Contact Dermatitis*, 1995, 32:246.

Fizer DH, Moss MN, and Walker W, "Critical Care for Clonidine Poisoning in Toddlers," *Crit Care Med*, 1990, 18(10):1124-8.

Klein MD, "An Unusual Cause of Clonidine Toxicity," *Am J Emerg Med*, 1991, 9(4):409-10.

Knapp JF, Fowler MA, Wheeler CA, et al, "A Two Year Old With Alteration of Consciousness," *Pediatr Emerg Care*, 1995, 11:62.

Kulig K, Duffy JP, Rumack BH, et al, "Naloxone for the Treatment of Clonidine Overdose," *JAMA*, 1982, 247(12):1697.

Clonistada® *see* Clonidine *on previous page*

Clopax® *see* Clobazam *on page 224*

Clopra® *see* Metoclopramide *on page 523*

Cloramin *see* Mechlorethamine Hydrochloride *on page 492*

Cloranfenicol *see* Chloramphenicol *on page 196*

ClorazeCaps® *see* Clorazepate Dipotassium *on this page*

Clorazepate Dipotassium (klor az' e pate)

Related Information

Benzodiazepines Comparison *on page 1643*

CAS Number 20432-69-3; 57109-90-7; 5991-71-9

Brand Names ClorazeCaps®; ClorazeTabs®; Gen-XENE®; Nansius®; Transene®; Tranxene®; Tranxilium®

Use Treatment of generalized anxiety and panic disorders; management of alcohol withdrawal; adjunct anticonvulsant in management of partial seizures

Mechanism of Action Facilitates gamma aminobutyric acid (GABA)-mediated transmission inhibitory neurotransmitter action, depresses subcortical levels of CNS

Adverse Reactions

Cardiovascular: Hypotension

Central nervous system: Drowsiness, psychosis, dizziness, confusion, amnesia, CNS depression, headache, ataxia

Dermatologic: Rash

Gastrointestinal: Nausea, dry mouth

Hepatic: Hepatic necrosis, jaundice

Ocular: Blurred vision, diplopia, nystagmus

Miscellaneous: Physical and psychological dependence with long-term use; long-term use may also be associated with renal or hepatic injury and reduced hematocrit

Signs & Symptoms of Acute Overdose Somnolence, confusion, ataxia, diminished reflexes, coma

Toxicodynamics/Kinetics Studies have shown that the elderly are more sensitive to the effects of benzodiazepines as compared to younger adults.

Onset of action: Depends largely upon absorption rate

Duration: 24 hours

Absorption: Rapidly decarboxylated to desmethyldiazepam (active) in acidic stomach prior to absorption

Distribution: V_d: 0.16-1.27 L/kg

Protein binding: 80% to 95%

Metabolism: In the liver to oxazepam (active) and desmethyldiazepam

Half-life: Adults:

Parent compound: >24 hours

Desmethyldiazepam: 48-96 hours

Oxazepam: 6-8 hours

Time to peak serum concentration: Oral: Within 1 hour

Elimination: Excreted primarily in urine; clearance: 1.8 mL/minute/kg

Usual Dosage Oral:

Children 9-12 years: Anticonvulsant: Initial: 3.75-7.5 mg/dose twice daily; increase dose by 3.75 mg at weekly intervals, not to exceed 60 mg/day in 2-3 divided doses

Children >12 years and Adults: Anticonvulsant: Initial: Up to 7.5 mg/dose 2-3 times/day; increase dose by 7.5 mg at weekly intervals; not to exceed 90 mg/day

Adults:

Anxiety: 7.5-15 mg 2-4 times/day, or given as single dose of 11.25 or 22.5 mg at bedtime

Alcohol withdrawal: Initial: 30 mg, then 15 mg 2-4 times/day on first day; maximum daily dose: 90 mg; gradually decrease dose over subsequent days

Contraindications Hypersensitivity to clorazepate dipotassium or any component; cross-sensitivity with other benzodiazepines may exist; avoid using in patients with pre-existing CNS depression, severe uncontrolled pain, or narrow-angle glaucoma

Warnings Not considered a drug of choice in the elderly; use with caution in patients with hepatic or renal disease; abrupt discontinuation may cause withdrawal symptoms or seizures

Dosage Forms

Capsule: 3.75 mg, 7.5 mg, 15 mg

Tablet: 3.75 mg, 7.5 mg, 15 mg

Tablet, single dose: 11.25 mg, 22.5 mg

Stability Unstable in water

Reference Range Therapeutic: 0.12-2.00 μg/mL (SI: 0.36-6.02 μmol/L)

Overdosage Treatment

Decontamination: Lavage/activated charcoal with cathartic

Supportive therapy: Treatment for benzodiazepine overdose is supportive; rarely is mechanical ventilation required. Flumazenil (Romazicon™) has been shown to selectively block the binding of benzodiazepines to CNS receptors, resulting in a reversal of benzodiazepine-induced CNS depression.

Antidote(s)

Flumazenil *on page 1428*

Drug Interactions Cimetidine may decrease hepatic clearance, CNS depressants; antacids may reduce bioavailability; oral contraceptives may inhibit hepatic metabolism

Pregnancy Risk Factor D

Pregnancy Implications Fetal malformations described with first trimester use; crosses the placenta; appears in breast milk

Monitoring Parameters Respiratory and cardiovascular status

Patient Information May cause drowsiness, use caution when driving; avoid alcohol and other CNS depressants

Nursing Implications Observe patient for excess sedation, apnea; raise bed rails, initiate safety measures, assist with ambulation

(Continued)

Clorazepate Dipotassium *(Continued)*

Additional Information Clorazepate offers no advantage over the other benzodiazepines; can cause fetal malformations

Specific References

Burkhart KK and Kulig KW, "The Diagnostic Utility of Flumazenil (A Benzodiazepine Antagonist) in Coma of Unknown Etiology," *Ann Emerg Med*, 1990, 19(3):319-21.

Patel DA and Patel AR, "Clorazepate and Congenital Malformations," *JAMA*, 1980, 244(2):135-6.

ClorazeTabs® *see* Clorazepate Dipotassium *on page 232*

Clordiabet® *see* Chlorpropamide *on page 207*

Cloretilo Chemirosa® *see* Ethyl Chloride *on page 337*

Cloretilo Vitulia® *see* Ethyl Chloride *on page 337*

Clotrimazole (kloe trim' a zole)

Related Information

Antifungal Therapy *on page 1496-1497*

CAS Number 23593-75-1

Brand Names Gyne-Lotrimin® [OTC]; Lotrimin®; Lotrimin AF® Cream [OTC]; Lotrimin AF® Lotion [OTC]; Lotrimin AF® Solution [OTC]; Mycelex®; Mycelex®-G

Use Treatment of susceptible fungal infections, including oropharyngeal candidiasis, dermatophytoses, superficial mycoses, and cutaneous candidiasis, as well as vulvovaginal candidiasis; clotrimazole troches are indicated for prophylaxis against oropharyngeal candidiasis in patients immunocompromised by therapy (including chemotherapy, radiation, or steroids) leukemia, solid tremors, or renal transplant (limited efficacy data for other etiologies of immunosuppressants)

Mechanism of Action An imidazole agent which binds to phospholipids in the fungal cell membrane altering cell wall permeability resulting in loss of essential intracellular elements

Adverse Reactions

Central nervous system: Drowsiness
Dermatologic: Contact dermatitis
Gastrointestinal: Nausea, vomiting, anorexia
Hepatic: Abnormal liver function tests
Miscellaneous: Mild burning, irritation, stinging to skin or vaginal area

Toxicodynamics/Kinetics

Absorption: Topical: Negligible through intact skin (0.5%)
Half-life: 3.5-5 hours
Time to peak serum concentration:
- Oral topical administration: Salivary levels occur within 3 hours following 30 minutes of dissolution time in the mouth
- Vaginal cream: High vaginal levels occur within 8-24 hours
- Vaginal tablet: High vaginal levels occur within 1-2 days

Elimination: Eliminated as metabolites via bile

Usual Dosage

Children >3 years and Adults:
- Oral: 10 mg troche dissolved slowly 5 times/day for 14 consecutive days
- Topical: Apply twice daily; if no improvement occurs after 4 weeks of therapy, reevaluate diagnosis

Children >12 years and Adults: Vaginal:
- Cream: Insert 5 g (= 1 applicatorful) of 1% vaginal cream daily for 7-14 days
- Tablets: Insert 100 mg/day for 7 days or 200 mg/day for 3 days or 500 mg single dose
- Patients treated for 14 days had a significantly higher cure rate

Contraindications Hypersensitivity to clotrimazole or any component

Warnings Clotrimazole should not be used for treatment of systemic fungal infection; safety and effectiveness of clotrimazole lozenges (troches) in children <3 years of age have not been established

Dosage Forms

Cream:
- Topical (Lotrimin®, Lotrimin® AF, Mycelex®, Mycelex® OTC) : 1% (15 g, 30 g, 45 g, 90 g)
- Vaginal (Gyne-Lotrimin®, Mycelex®-G): 1% (45 g, 90 g)

Lotion (Lotrimin®): 1% (30 mL)
Solution, topical (Lotrimin®, Lotrimin® AF, Mycelex®, Mycelex® OTC): 1% (10 mL, 30 mL)
Tablet, vaginal (Gyne-Lotrimin®, Mycelex®-G): 100 mg (7s); 500 mg (1s)
Troche (Mycelex®): 10 mg
Twin pack (Mycelex®): Tablet 500 mg (1's) and vaginal cream 1% (7 g)

Reference Range Peak serum levels after dermal cream application: <0.001 μg/mL; after vaginal tablet application, serum levels range from 0.02-0.05 μg/mL; peak serum levels after a 1.5 g oral dose ranges from 1-5 μg/mL

Overdosage Treatment
Decontamination: Ipecac or gastric lavage/activated charcoal
Enhancement of elimination: Multiple dosing of activated charcoal may be effective

Drug Interactions
Increased cyclosporine levels can occur
Enhanced hypoglycemic effects with sulfonylureas

Pregnancy Risk Factor B; C (oral)

Pregnancy Implications No congenital malformation association with topical use

Monitoring Parameters Periodic liver function tests during oral therapy with clotrimazole lozenges

Patient Information May cause irritation to the skin; lozenge (troche) must be dissolved slowly in the mouth

Nursing Implications Troche should be allowed to dissolve slowly in the mouth for maximum effect; when possible, obtain specimens for culture and sensitivity before the first dose; review allergy history

Additional Information Periodic assessment of hepatic function is advisable in patients with pre-existing hepatic impairment; re-evaluate topical therapy after one month

Specific References
Duhm B, Medenwalt H, Puetter J, et al, "The Pharmacokinetics of Clotrimazole," *Postgrad Med J*, 1974, 50(Suppl 1):13-7.
Hughes D and Kriedman T, "Treatment of Vulvovaginal Candidiasis With a 500 mg Vaginal Tablet of Clotrimazole," *Clin Ther*, 1984, 6(5):662-8.

Cloxazolam *see* Triazolam *on page 767*

Clozapine (kloe' za peen)

Related Information
Antipsychotic Agents Comparison *on page 1642*

CAS Number 5786-21-0

Brand Names Clozaril®; Leponex®

Use Management of schizophrenia

Mechanism of Action Tricyclic dibenzodiazepine structure; blocks dopamine receptors

Adverse Reactions
Cardiovascular: Orthostatic hypotension, tachycardia, myocarditis
Central nervous system: Hyperthermia, seizures, coma, dizziness, seizures, fatal neuroleptic malignant syndrome, electroencephalogram abnormalities
Endocrine & metabolic: Syndrome of inappropriate antidiuretic hormone
Gastrointestinal: Dry mouth, constipation, salivation
Genitourinary: Enuresis
Hematologic: Leukopenia/neutropenia (agranulocytosis, granulocytopenia)
Miscellaneous: Systemic lupus erythematosus-like reaction, hypertriglyceridaemia

Signs & Symptoms of Acute Overdose Coma, priapism, eosinophilia, seizures, neuroleptic malignant syndrome, salivation, impotence, enuresis, extrapyramidal reaction, delirium, cognitive dysfunction, nausea, hypoglycemia, hypertension, fasciculations, emesis, hypotension, agitation, disorientation, ataxia, nystagmus, torticollis, hypotonicity, Parkinson's-like symptoms, myoclonus, inability to urinate

Toxicodynamics/Kinetics
Distribution: V_d: 0.5-2.7 L/kg
Protein binding: 95%
Metabolism: Hepatic
Elimination: Feces (38%) and urine (54%)

Usual Dosage Adults: Oral: 25 mg once or twice daily initially and increased, as tolerated to a target dose of 300-450 mg/day after 2 weeks, but may require doses as high as 600-900 mg/day

Warnings Avoid in patients with closed-angle glaucoma, ileus, prostatic enlargement, or pre-existing bone marrow depression

Dosage Forms Tablet: 25 mg, 100 mg

Reference Range Therapeutic: 200-400 ng/mL; levels >500 ng/mL associated with change in mental status in children; levels >2000 ng/mL associated with CNS changes in adults; highest reported level with survival: 4400 ng/mL

Overdosage Treatment
Decontamination: Lavage/activated charcoal with cathartic
Supportive therapy: I.V. fluids for hypotension; lorazepam, diazepam, phenobarbital, or phenytoin for seizures; granulocyte colony-stimulating factor may be useful for agranulocytosis; clozapine-induced hypotension (orthostatic) can be treated with fludrocortisone 0.1 mg/day, with increasing doses to 0.3 mg/day over 2 weeks; desmopressin (intranasal: 10 mcg at bedtime) can be used to treat clozapine-induced enuresis
Enhancement of elimination: Multiple dose of activated charcoal may be useful

(Continued)

Clozapine *(Continued)*

Antidote(s)

Filgrastim *on page 1425*

Diagnostic Tests/Procedures

Liver Profile *on page 1286*

White Blood Count *on page 1380*

Drug Interactions Seizure has been reported with concomitant use of erythromycin; myoclonic seizures can result with concomitant fluoxetine and clozapine therapy

Pregnancy Risk Factor B

Monitoring Parameters White blood cell counts, EKG, liver function tests

Specific References

Anon, "Clozapine and Myocarditis," *Australian Adv Drug React Bull*, 1994, 13:14-15.

Aronowitz JS, Safferman AZ, Lieberman JA, "Management of Clozapine-Induced Enuresis," *Am J Psychiatry*, 1995, 152(3):472.

Campellone JV, McCluskey LF, and Greenspan D, "Fatal Outcome From Neuroleptic Malignant Syndrome Associated With Clozapine," *Neuropsychiatry, Neuropsychology, and Behavioral Neurology*, 1995, 8:70-3.

"Change in Clozapine Monitoring Requirements," *Pharm J*, 1995, 254:612.

Costello LE and Suppes T, "A Clinically Significant Interaction Between Clozapine and Valproate," *J Clin Psychopharmacol*, 1995, 15:139-41.

Funderberg LG, Vertrees JE, True JE, et al, "Seizure Following Addition of Erythromycin to Clozapine Treatment," *Am J Psychiatry*, 1994, 151(12):1840-1.

Gerson SL and Meltzer H, "Mechanisms of Clozapine-Induced Agranulocytosis," *Drug Saf*, 1992, 7(Suppl 1):17-25.

Ghaeli P and Dufresne RL, "Elevated Serum Triglycerides on Clozapine Resolve With Risperidone," *Pharmacotherapy*, 1995, 15:382.

Mady SP and Wax P, "Clozapine Intoxication in a Young Child," *Vet Hum Toxicol*, 1993, 35:338.

Pacia SV and Devinsky O, "Clozapine-Related Seizures: Experience With 5629 Patients," *Neurology*, 1994, 44(12):2247-9. <bp[Radford JM, Brown TM and Borison RL, "Unexpected Dysfonia While Changing From Clozapine to Risperidone," *J Clin Psychopharmacol*, 1995, 15:225-6.

Testani M Jr, "Clozapine-Induced Orthostatic Hypotension Treated With Fludrocortisone," *J Clin Psychiatry*, 1994, 55(11):497-8.

Welber MR and Nevins S, "Clozapine Overdose: A Case Report," *J Emerg Med*, 1995, 13(2):199-202.

Wickert WA, Campbell NR, and Martin L, "Acute Severe Adverse Clozapine Reaction Resembling Systemic Lupus/Erythematosus," *Postgrad Med J*, 1994, 70(830):940-1.

Wilson WH and Claussen AM, "Seizures Associated With Clozapine Treatment in a State Hospital," *J Clin Psychiatry*, 1994, 55(5): 184-8.

Wolf LR, and Otten EJ, "A Case Report of Clozapine Overdose," *Vet Hum Toxicol*, 1991, 33:370.

Clozaril® *see* Clozapine *on previous page*

Clysodrast® *see* Bisacodyl *on page 156*

Cobex® *see* Cyanocobalamin *on page 246*

Cocaine Hydrochloride (koe' kane)

Related Information

Principal Pharmacological Properties of Hallucinogenic Drugs *on page 1557*

CAS Number 53-21-4; 50-36-2

Synonyms Benzoylemethylecgonine Hydrochloride; Erythroxylon Coca

Use Topical anesthesia for mucous membranes

Mechanism of Action Blocks both the initiation and conduction of nerve impulses by decreasing the neuronal membrane's permeability to sodium ions, which results in inhibition of depolarization with resultant blockade of conduction; interferes with the uptake of norepinephrine by adrenergic nerve terminals producing vasoconstriction; a type I antiarrhythmic

Adverse Reactions

Cardiovascular: Decreased heart rate with low doses, tachycardia with moderate doses, hypertension, cardiomyopathy, cardiac arrhythmias, myocarditis

Central nervous system: Nervousness, restlessness, euphoria, excitation, headache, psychosis, hallucinations, agitation, seizures, slurred speech, hyperthermia, dystonic reactions, cerebral vascular accident, fasciculations

Dermatologic: Skin infarction, pruritus

Gastrointestinal: Nausea, anorexia

Genitourinary: Priapism

Hematologic: Thrombocytopenia, thrombosis

Neuromuscular & skeletal: Chorea (extrapyramidal), paresthesia

Ocular: Sloughing of the corneal epithelium, ulceration of the cornea, iritis, mydriasis, chemosis, tremors and clonic-tonic reactions

Renal: Myoglobinuria

Respiratory: Tachypnea, nasal mucosa damage (when snorting)

Miscellaneous: Madarosis, spontaneous bowel perforation

Signs & Symptoms of Acute Overdose Apnea, dental erosion, depression, sweating, photophobia, insomnia, hyperreflexia, nasal congestion, myocardial depression, mania, intracranial hemorrhage, ptosis, extrapyramidal reaction, dry mouth, euphoria, myalgia, lacrimation, coma, nystagmus, impotence, tachycardia (ventricular), epistaxis, dyspnea, migraine headache (exacerbation of), disorientation, paroxysmal tachycardia (ventricular), cardiomegaly, ataxia, corneal irritation, colitis, seizures, angina, blurred vision, respiratory depression, restlessness, respiratory alkalosis, hyperthermia, delirium, seizures, hallucinations, mydriasis, vomiting, muscular spasm, sensory aberrations, rhabdomyolysis, myoglobinuria, CNS hemorrhage, hypertension, chest pain

Toxicodynamics/Kinetics

Onset of action: Topical: Within 1 minute following administration to mucosa

Peak action: Within 5 minutes

Duration: ≥30 minutes, depending upon route and dosage administered

Absorption: Well absorbed through mucous membranes, limited by drug-induced vasoconstriction, and enhanced by inflammation

Distribution: V_d: 1.96-2.7 L/kg

Protein binding: ~90%

Metabolism: In the liver to benzoylecgonine, ecgonine methylester and norcocaine (active)

Bioavailability:

Oral: 30%

Nasal: 60%

Half-life: 75 minutes

Elimination: Excreted primarily in urine as metabolites (benzoylecgonine and ecgonine methylester) unchanged drug (<10%)

Usual Dosage Use lowest effective dose (contraindications of 1% to 4%); do not exceed 1 mg/kg; patient tolerance, anesthetic technique, vascularity of tissue, and area to be anesthetized will determine dose needed. For topical applications, solutions >4% are not advisable because of increased risk of systemic toxic reactions.

Contraindications Systemic use, hypersensitivity to cocaine or any component

Warnings Cocaine produces an addictive syndrome; use with caution in patients with hypertension, severe cardiovascular disease, or thyrotoxicosis and in infants; use with caution in patients with severely traumatized mucosa and sepsis in the region of intended application

Dosage Forms

Powder: 5 g, 25 g

Solution, topical: 4% [40 mg/mL] (2 mL, 4 mL, 10 mL); 10% [100 mg/mL] (4 mL, 10 mL)

Tablet, soluble, for topical solution: 135 mg

Stability Store in well closed, light-resistant containers

Reference Range

Therapeutic: 100-500 ng/mL (SI: 330 nmol/L)

Toxic: >1000 ng/mL (SI: >3300 nmol/L)

Overdosage Treatment

Decontamination: Activated charcoal with cathartic is useful for oral ingestion; whole bowel irrigation should be considered for body packers or body stuffers of cocaine packets; oral bicarbonate may decrease gastrointestinal cocaine absorption for body packers/stuffers in an *in vitro* model

Supportive therapy: Since no specific antidote for cocaine exists, serious toxic effects are treated symptomatically. Seizures are treated with lorazepam or diazepam. Benzodiazepines may be also useful for life-threatening arrhythmias, agitation, and/or hypertension; sodium bicarbonate may decrease QRS prolongation; phentolamine can be used of cocaine-induced vasoconstriction; do not use beta-blockers due to unopposed alpha-agonist effects; hypertension can be treated with nitroprusside (0.5-10 mcg/kg/minute), nitroglycerin (10 mcg/minute), phentolamine (5-10 mg I.V.), or enalaprilat (0.625-1.25 mg). Although lidocaine may promote cocaine-induced seizures, it is probably safe to use if used over 3 hours after cocaine use. The combination of esmolol and lorazepam has been advocated to treat hyperadrenergic crisis, but this combination has not been well studied.

Enhancement of elimination: Butyrylcholinesterase is strictly investigational; biscaodyl, psyllium, hydrophilic mucilloid, saline, or emollient laxative can be used to enhance fecal excretion of body packages.

Antidote(s)

Butyrylcholinesterase *on page 1399*

Strictly investigational

Phentolamine Mesylate *on page 1456*

Drug Interactions MAO inhibitors; epinephrine; use with ethanol may result in a toxic metabolite (cocaethylene) which may have active cardiac effects; use with naloxone; may have caused ventricular arrhythmias and fibrillation (atrial) in one case report; flumazenil has induced seizures in a cocaine rat model

(Continued)

Cocaine Hydrochloride *(Continued)*

Pregnancy Risk Factor C; (X if nonmedicinal use)

Pregnancy Implications Appears in breast milk; sustained arrhythmias may occur in the neonatal period; genitourinary abnormalities may occur

Monitoring Parameters Vital signs, cardiac/neurological status, CPK

Nursing Implications Use only on mucous membranes of the oral, laryngeal, and nasal cavities

Additional Information May cause cornea to become clouded or pitted, therefore, normal saline should be used to irrigate and protect cornea during surgery; not for injection; converted to cocaine sulfate as a drug of abuse; may precipitate porphyria; increased incidence of anticardiolipin antibody has been reported in cocaine abusers (especially with I.V. use); positive rheumatoid factor also has been noted in cocaine abusers. Incidence of acute myocardial infarction in patients with cocaine-associated chest pain is ~6%; initial EKG is only sensitive for 36% of acute myocardial infarction; ethanol plus cocaine use produces cocaethylene which has a longer half-life (~2 hours) than cocaine; while cocaethylene can produce tachycardia, myocardial depression, and is a competitive muscarinic antagonist, no direct effect on blood pressure is usually seen.

Specific References

Bailey DN, "Formation of Cocaisopropylene (Isopropylcocaine) by Human Liver *in vitro*," *J Anal Toxicol*, 1995, 19:205-8.

Beckman KJ, Parker RB, Hariman RJ, et al, "Hemodynamic and Electrophysiological Actions of Cocaine. Effects of Sodium Bicarbonate as an Antidote in Dogs," *Circulation*, 1991, 83(5):1799-807.

Brogan WC 3d, Lange RA, Glamann DB, et al, "Recurrent Coronary Vasoconstriction Caused by Intranasal Cocaine; Possible Role for Metabolites," *Ann Intern Med*, 1992, 116(7):556-61.

Frassica JJ, Orav EJ, Walsh EP, et al, "Arrhythmias in Children Prenatally Exposed to Cocaine," *Arch Pediatr Adolesc Med*, 1994, 148(11):1163-9.

Fritsma GA, Leikin JB, Maturen AJ, et al, "Detection of Anticardiolipin Antibody in Patients With Cocaine Abuse," *J Emerg Med*, 1991, 9(Suppl 1):37-43.

Haynes S, Stork CM, Hoffman RS, et al, "Letter to the Editor," *J Emerg Med*, 1995, 13(4):537-8.

Henning RJ, Wilson LD, and Glauser JM, "Cocaine Plus Ethanol Is More Cardiotoxic Than Cocaine or Ethanol Alone," *Crit Care Med*, 1994, 22(12):1896-906.

Hohm SP, "A 28-Year-Old Man With an Aortic Dissection and History of Cocaine Abuse," *J Emerg Nurs*, 1995, 21:199-201.

Hollander JE, Hoffman RS, Gennis P, et al, "Cocaine-Associated Chest Pain: One Year Follow-up," *Acad Emerg Med*, 1995, 2:179-84.

Hollander J, Hoffman RS, Shih RD, et al, "Coronary Artery Disease in Patients With Cocaine Associated Myocardial Infarction," *Acad Emerg Med*, 1995, 2:456.

Hollander JE, Burstein JL, Hoffman RS, et al, "Cocaine-Associated Myocardial Infarction," *Chest*, 1995, 107:5:1237.

Kain ZN, Kain TS, and Scarpelli EM, "Cocaine Exposure in Utero: Perinatal Development and Neonatal Manifestations - Review," *Clin Toxicol*, 1992, 30:607-36.

Kozlowski-Cepero K, "Cocaine-Induced Myocardial Infarction: Treatment With Thrombolytic Therapy," *J Emerg Nurs*, 1995, 21:109-11.

Merigian KS, "Cocaine-Induced Ventricular Arrhythmias and Rapid Atrial Fibrillation Temporally Related to Naloxone Administration," *Am J Emerg Med*, 1993, 11(1):96-7.

Merigian KS, Park LJ, and Leeper KV, et al, "Adrenergic Crisis From Crack Cocaine Ingestion: Report of Five Cases," *J Emerg Med*, 1994, 12(4):485-90.

Nicholson KE and Rogers JE, "Cocaine and Adrenaline Paste: A Fatal Combination?," *Br Med J*, 1995,311:250-1.

Pirwitz MJ, Willard JE, Landau C, et al, "Influence of Cocaine, Ethanol, or Their Combination on Epicardial Coronary Arterial Dimensions in Humans," *Arch Intern Med*, 1995, 155:1186-91.

Pugh CM, Mezghebe HM, and Leffall LS Jr, "Spontaneous Bowel Perforation in Drug Abusers," *Am J Emerg Med*, 1995, 13(1):113-4.

Richards CF, Clark RF, Holbrook T, et al, "The Effect of Cocaine and Amphetamines on Vital Signs in Trauma Patients," *J Emerg Med*, 1995, 13:59-63.

Riordan JP, Garvey JL, Schroeder JD, et al, "Effects of Cocaethylene and Cocaine in Isolated Rat Hearts," *Acad Emerg Med*, 1995, 2:395.

Rosenberg NM, Meert KL, Marino D, et al, "Occult Cocaine and Opiate Exposure in Children and Associated Physical Findings," *Pediatr Emerg Care*, 1995, 11(3):167.

Shannon RP, Manders WT, and Shen YT, "Role of Blood Doping in the Coronary Vasoconstrictor Response to Cocaine," *Circulation*, 1995, 92:96-105.

Todd K, Hollander JE, Heilpern K, et al, "Prevalence of the Use of Cocaine in Patients With Chest Pain," *Acad Emerg Med*, 1995, 2:344.

Uszenski RT, Gillis RA, and Schaer GL, "Additive Myocardial Depressant Effects of Cocaine and Ethanol," *Am Heart J*, 1992, 124(5):1276-83.

Wilson LD, Jeromin G, and Klein J, "Cocaine Causes Dose Dependent Cardiac Toxicity in an Animal Model of Cocaine Abuse," *Acad Emerg Med*, 1995, 2:344.

Codate *see* Codeine *on this page*

Co-Dax® *see* Doxepin Hydrochloride *on page 301*

Codeine (koe' deen)

Related Information

Pharmacokinetics of Narcotic Agonist Analgesics *on page 1654*

CAS Number 52-28-8; 76-57-3; 1420-53-7; 1422-07-7; 5913-76-8; 6854-40-6; 41444-62-6

Synonyms Actacode; Codate; Codeine Phosphate; Codeine Sulfate; Codlin; Methylmorphine; Paveral; Tricodein

Use Treatment of mild to moderate pain; antitussive in lower doses; dextromethorphan has equivalent antitussive activity but has much lower toxicity in accidental overdose

Mechanism of Action Binds to opiate receptors in the CNS, causing inhibition of ascending pain pathways, altering the perception of and response to pain; causes cough supression by direct central action in the medulla; produces generalized CNS depression; also has a dose-related histamine-releasing effect

Adverse Reactions

Cardiovascular: Palpitations, hypotension, bradycardia, peripheral vasodilation

Central nervous system: CNS depression, psychosis, intracranial pressure (increased), dizziness, drowsiness, sedation

Dermatologic: Pruritus

Endocrine & metabolic: Antidiuretic hormone release

Gastrointestinal: Nausea, vomiting, constipation, adynamic ileus

Ocular: Miosis

Respiratory: Apnea, respiratory depression, aspiration

Miscellaneous: Physical and psychological dependence, histamine release, biliary or urinary tract spasm

Signs & Symptoms of Acute Overdose Somnolence, constipation, miosis, hypocalcemia, vomiting, rhabdomyolysis, ataxia, syncope, erythema multiforme, syndrome of inappropriate antidiuretic hormone (SIADH), myasthenia gravis (exacerbation or precipitation of), respiratory failure, hallucinations, myoglobinuria, urine discoloration (milky)

Toxicodynamics/Kinetics

Onset of action:
- Oral: 30-60 minutes
- I.M.: 10-30 minutes

Peak action:
- Oral: 1-1.5 hours
- I.M.: 30-60 minutes

Duration: 4-6 hours

Absorption: Oral: Adequate

Distribution: V_d: 3.5 L/kg

Protein binding: 7%

Metabolism: Hepatic to morphine (active) and norcodeine along with other metabolites

Half-life: 3 hours

Elimination: 3% to 16% excreted in urine as unchanged drug, norcodeine, and free and conjugated morphine (to glucuronic acid)

Usual Dosage Doses should be titrated to appropriate analgesic effect; when changing routes of administration, note that oral dose is $^2/_3$ as effective as parenteral dose

Analgesic:
- Children: Oral, I.M., S.C.: 0.5-1 mg/kg/dose every 4-6 hours as needed; maximum: 60 mg/dose
- Adults: Oral, I.M., I.V., S.C.: 30 mg/dose; range: 15-60 mg every 4-6 hours as needed; maximum: 360 mg/24 hours

Antitussive: Oral (for nonproductive cough):
- Children: 1-1.5 mg/kg/day in divided doses every 4-6 hours as needed: Alternative dose according to age:
  - 2-6 years: 2.5-5 mg every 4-6 hours as needed; maximum: 30 mg/day
  - 6-12 years: 5-10 mg every 4-6 hours as needed; maximum: 60 mg/day
- Adults: 10-20 mg/dose every 4-6 hours as needed; maximum: 120 mg/day

Dosing adjustment in renal impairment:
- Cl_{cr} 10-50 mL/minute: Administer 75% of dose
- Cl_{cr} <10 mL/minute: Administer 50% of dose

Dosing adjustment in hepatic impairment: Probably necessary in hepatic insufficiency

Contraindications Hypersensitivity to codeine or any component

Warnings Use with caution in patients with hypersensitivity reactions to other phenanthrene-derivative opioid agonists (morphine, hydrocodone, hydromorphone, levorphanol, oxycodone, oxymorphone); respiratory diseases including asthma, emphysema, COPD, or severe liver or renal insufficiency; some preparations contain sulfites which may cause allergic reactions; may be habit-forming

Dosage Forms

Injection, as phosphate: 30 mg (1 mL, 2 mL); 60 mg (1 mL, 2 mL)

Solution, oral: 15 mg/5 mL

Tablet, as sulfate: 15 mg, 30 mg, 60 mg

(Continued)

Codeine *(Continued)*

Tablet, as phosphate, soluble: 30 mg, 60 mg
Tablet, as sulfate, soluble: 15 mg, 30 mg, 60 mg

Stability Store injection between 15°C to 30°C, avoid freezing; do not use if injection is discolored or contains a precipitate; protect injection from light

Reference Range
Therapeutic: Not established
Toxic: >1.1 μg/mL

Overdosage Treatment
Supportive therapy: Naloxone hydrochloride (0.4-2 mg I.V., S.C., or through an endotracheal tube); a continuous infusion (at ⅔ the response dose/hour) may be required
Enhancement of elimination: Multiple dosing of activated charcoal may be useful

Antidote(s)
Naloxone Hydrochloride *on page 1447*

Test Interactions ↑ aminotransferase [ALT (SGPT)/AST (SGOT)] (S)

Diagnostic Tests/Procedures
Codeine, Blood *on page 1235*

Drug Interactions
Decreased effect with cigarette smoking
Increased toxicity: CNS depressants, phenothiazines, TCAs, other narcotic analgesics, guanabenz, MAO inhibitors, neuromuscular blockers, quinidine

Pregnancy Risk Factor C (D if used for prolonged periods or in high doses at term)

Pregnancy Implications Crosses the placenta; appears in breast milk

Monitoring Parameters Pain relief, respiratory and mental status, blood pressure

Patient Information Avoid alcohol, may cause drowsiness, impaired judgment or coordination; may be addicting if used for prolonged periods

Nursing Implications Observe patient for excessive sedation, respiratory depression, implement safety measures, assist with ambulation

Specific References
Cardan E, "Fatal Case of Codeine Poisoning," *Lancet*, 1981, 1(8233):1313.
de Groot AC and Conemans J, "Allergic Urticarial Rash From Oral Codeine," *Contact Dermatitis*, 1986, 14(4):209-14.
Ivey HH and Kattwinkel J, "Danger of Actifed-C," *Pediatrics*, 1976, 57(1):164-5.

Codeine Phosphate *see* Codeine *on page 238*

Codeine Sulfate *see* Codeine *on page 238*

Codimal-A® *see* Brompheniramine Maleate *on page 165*

Codlin *see* Codeine *on page 238*

Coffee Break® *see* Caffeine *on page 175*

Cogentin® *see* Benztropine Mesylate *on page 151*

Cognex® *see* Tacrine Hydrochloride *on page 719*

Colace® [OTC] *see* Docusate *on page 297*

Colchicine (kol' chi seen)

CAS Number 64-86-8

Use Treat acute gouty arthritis attacks and to prevent recurrences of such attacks; management of familial Mediterranean fever; has been used to treat progressive systemic sclerosis (refractory)

Mechanism of Action Alkaloids from meadow saffron; mechanism of action is not completely understood; decreases leukocyte motility, decreases phagocytosis in joints, and lactic acid production, thereby reducing the deposition of urate crystals that perpetuates the inflammatory response; not an analgesic; antimitotic, may be responsible for toxicity

Adverse Reactions
Cardiovascular: Hypotension
Central nervous system: Dehydration, confusion, delirium, seizures
Dermatologic: Rash, alopecia
Gastrointestinal: Nausea, vomiting, diarrhea, abdominal pain
Genitourinary: Azoospermia
Hematologic: Leukopenia, neutropenia, agranulocytosis, thrombocytopenia, granulocytopenia, aplastic anemia
Hepatic: Hepatotoxicity
Neuromuscular & skeletal: Myopathy, peripheral neuritis, paralysis
Ocular: Diplopia
Renal: Hematuria
Respiratory: Apnea, respiratory depression, respiratory collapse
Miscellaneous: Feces discoloration (gray)

Signs & Symptoms of Acute Overdose Nausea, apnea, hypocalcemia, hematuria, purpura, ptosis, vomiting, hypothermia, rhabdomyolysis, oligospermia, leukocytosis, nephritis, hyperthermia, hypernatremia, sexual dysfunction, dysosmia, diarrhea, diabetes insipidus, bradycardia, myasthenia gravis (exacerbation or precipitation of), myoglobinuria, fever, feces discoloration (gray)

Toxicodynamics/Kinetics

Onset of action: Acute gouty arthritis (following first dose)
- Oral: 12 hours
- I.V.: 6-12 hours

Absorption: Rapid from gastrointestinal tract

Distribution: V_d: 2.2 L/kg; high concentrations appear in leukocytes, kidney, liver, spleen, and intestinal tract, but are absent in the heart, skeletal muscle, and brain

Protein binding: 10% to 31%

Metabolism: Partially deacetylated in the liver

Half-life: 12-30 minutes; prolonged in renal insufficiency

Time to peak serum concentration: Within 30-120 minutes then decline for 2 hours before increasing again due to enterohepatic recycling (important in toxicity)

Elimination: Primarily excreted in feces via bile; 10% to 20% excreted unchanged in urine

Usual Dosage

Prophylaxis of familial Mediterranean fever: Oral:
- Children:
  - ≤5 years: 0.5 mg/day
  - >5 years: 1-1.5 mg/day in 2-3 divided doses
- Adults: 1-2 mg/day in 2-3 divided doses

Adults:
- Oral: Acute attacks: Initial: 0.5-1.2 mg, then 0.5-0.6 mg every 1-2 hours or 1-1.2 mg every 2 hours until relief or gastrointestinal side effects (nausea, vomiting, or diarrhea) occur to a maximum total dose of 8 mg; wait 3 days before initiating another course of therapy
- I.V.: Initial: 2 mg, then 0.5 mg every 6 hours until response, not to exceed 4 mg/day; if pain recurs, it may be necessary to administer a daily dose of 1-2 mg for several days; however, do not give more colchicine by any route for at least 7 days after a full course of I.V. therapy (4 mg), transfer to oral colchicine in a dose similar to that being given I.V.
- Prophylaxis of recurrent attacks: Oral: 0.5-0.6 mg every other day
- Progressive systemic sclerosis: 1 mg twice daily (1 mg once daily in patients with renal failure)

Fatal dose: 0.8 mg/kg

Dosing adjustment in renal impairment:
- Cl_{cr} <50 mL/minute: Avoid chronic administration
- Cl_{cr} <10 mL/minute: Decrease dose by 50% for treatment of acute attacks

Contraindications Hypersensitivity to colchicine or any component; severe renal, gastrointestinal disease, or cardiac disorders

Warnings Use with caution in debilitated or elderly patients; severe local irritation can occur following S.C. or I.M. administration

Dosage Forms

Injection: 0.5 mg/mL (2 mL)

Tablet: 0.5 mg, 0.6 mg

Reference Range Plasma colchicine level of 12 ng/mL achieved after a 0.96 mg/kg overdose ingestion; patient was severely symptomatic

Overdosage Treatment

Decontamination: Emesis not recommended due to potential for seizures; lavage indicated if early in ingestion (control seizures with benzodiazepines prior to lavage); activated charcoal with sorbitol (first dose only) 1-2 g/kg at ½ first dose every 2-6 hours until toxic symptoms abate and patient is stable

Supportive therapy: Granulocyte colony-stimulating factor (300 mg/day S.C.) has been used to treat neutropenia; observe 2-12 hours due to latency of symptoms of toxicity; treat manifestations of toxicity accordingly; no specific antidote; supportive care is mainstay of treatment

Enhancement of elimination: Multiple dosing of activated charcoal may be useful; dialysis is not effective; not dialyzable (0% to 5%); colchicine specific antibodies are investigational

Antidote(s)

Filgrastim *on page 1425*

Test Interactions May cause false-positive results in urine tests for erythrocytes or hemoglobin; interferes with urine tests of hydrocorticoids

Drug Interactions Sympathomimetic agents, CNS depressants; vitamin B_{12} (malabsorption)

Pregnancy Risk Factor D

Monitoring Parameters CBC, electrolytes, fluid status, LFTS, BUN, creatinine

Nursing Implications Avoid I.M. and S.C. injection; injection should be made over 2-5 minutes into tubing of free-flowing I.V. with compatible fluid; **incompatible with dextrose**

(Continued)

Colchicine *(Continued)*

Additional Information Colchicine-specific Fab fragments are prepared from goat antiserum with an affinity constant of 2 x 10^{10} M_{-1}; total plasma colchicine level may rise 6- to 10-fold after infusion of antibody fragment; this treatment may not prevent bone marrow depression, but can improve hemodynamic status; may be useful in the treatment of Palmer fibromatosis

Specific References

Baud FJ, Sabouraud A, Vicaut E, et al, "Treatment of Severe Colchicine Overdose With Colchicine-Specific Fab Fragments," *N Engl J Med*, 1995, 332(10):642-5.

Burnakis TG, "Colchicine Treatment of Progressive Systemic Sclerosis," *Hospital Pharmacy*, 1995, 30:536-7.

Folpini A and Furfori P, "Colchicine Toxicity - Clinical Features and Treatment: Massive Overdose Case Report," *J Toxicol Clin Toxicol*, 1995, 33(1):71-7.

Heaney D, Derghazarian CB, Pineo GF, et al, "Massive Colchicine Overdose. A Report on the Toxicity," *Am J Med Sci*, 1976, 271(2):233-8.

Murray SS, Kramlinger KG, McMichan JC, et al, "Acute Toxicity After Excessive Ingestion of Colchicine," *Mayo Clin Proc*, 1983, 58(8):523-32.

Nagy LL, De Roos F, Hoffman RS, et al, "Colchicine-Induced Neutropenia, Treated With Granulocyte Colony Stimulating Factor," *Vet Hum Toxicol*, 1994, 36:366.

Pitts, Jr, FN, "Colchicine Therapy for Palmer Fibromatosis," *N Engl J Med*, 1995, 333(6):393.

Scherrmann JM, "Antibody Treatment of Toxin Poisoning - Recent Advances, " *J Toxicol Clin Toxicol*, 1994, 32(4):363-75.

Stapczynski JS, Rothstein RJ, Gaye WA, et al, "Colchicine Overdose: Report of Two Cases and Review of the Literature," *Ann Emerg Med*, 1981, 10(7):364-9.

Valenzuela P, Paris E, Oberpauer B, et al, "Overdose of Colchicine in a Three-Year-Old Child," *Vet Hum Toxicol*, 1995, 37(4):366-7.

Cologne Spirit *see* Ethyl Alcohol *on page 336*

Color-Pleon® *see* Sulfasalazine *on page 712*

Comizial® *see* Phenobarbital *on page 614*

Common Salt *see* Sodium Chloride *on page 698*

Compazine® *see* Prochlorperazine *on page 647*

Compound S *see* Zidovudine *on page 807*

Concor® *see* Bisoprolol Fumarate *on page 157*

Constant-T® *see* Theophylline *on page 735*

Contergan® *see* Thalidomide *on page 734*

Control® [OTC] *see* Phenylpropanolamine Hydrochloride *on page 622*

Converten® *see* Enalapril *on page 311*

Cophene-B® *see* Brompheniramine Maleate *on page 165*

Cordarone® *see* Amiodarone Hydrochloride *on page 113*

Cordil® *see* Isosorbide Dinitrate *on page 445*

Cordilox® *see* Verapamil Hydrochloride *on page 787*

Corgard® *see* Nadolol *on page 545*

Corliprol® *see* Celiprolol Hydrochloride *on page 191*

Corramedan® *see* Digitoxin *on page 283*

Correctol® Extra Gentle [OTC] *see* Docusate *on page 297*

Cortancyl® *see* Prednisone *on page 639*

Cor Tensobon® *see* Captopril *on page 181*

Corynathe Yohimbe *see* Yohimbine Hydrochloride *on page 805*

Corynine Hydrochloride *see* Yohimbine Hydrochloride *on page 805*

Cotrim® *see* Co-trimoxazole *on this page*

Cotrim® DS *see* Co-trimoxazole *on this page*

Co-trimoxazole (koe-trye mox' a zole)

CAS Number 8064-90-2

Brand Names Bactrim™; Bactrim™ DS; Cotrim®; Cotrim® DS; Septra®; Septra® DS; Sulfamethoprim®; Sulfatrim®; Sulfatrim® DS; Uroplus® DS; Uroplus® SS

Synonyms SMX-TMP; Sulfamethoxazole and Trimethoprim; TMP-SMX; Trimethoprim and Sulfamethoxazole

Use Treatment of urinary tract infections; acute otitis media in children; acute exacerbations of chronic bronchitis in adults; prophylaxis of *Pneumocystis carinii* pneumonitis (PCP); treatment of documented PCP, empiric treatment of highly suspected PCP in immunocompromised patients; treatment of documented or suspected shigellosis, typhoid fever, or *Nocardia asteroides* infection

Mechanism of Action Sulfamethoxazole interferes with bacterial folic acid synthesis and growth via inhibition of dihydrofolic acid formation from para-aminobenzoic acid; trimethoprim inhibits dihydrofolic acid reduction to tetrahydrofolate resulting in sequential inhibition of enzymes of the folic acid pathway

Adverse Reactions

Central nervous system: Confusion, dizziness, depression, hallucinations, seizures, fever, ataxia

Dermatologic: Rash (more common in patients taking large dosages or in patients with AIDS), erythema multiforme, epidermal necrolysis, Stevens-Johnson syndrome

Endocrine & metabolic: Hypoglycemia, hyponatremia, hyperkalemia

Gastrointestinal: Nausea, vomiting, glossitis, stomatitis, diarrhea, pseudomembranous colitis, pancreatitis, splenomegaly

Hematologic: Thrombocytopenia, anemia (megaloblastic), granulocytopenia, aplastic anemia, hemolysis (with G-6-PD deficiency), porphyria

Hepatic: Hepatitis, kernicterus in neonates

Local: Irritation, pain, phlebitis

Otic: Ototoxicity, tinnitus

Renal: Interstitial nephritis

Miscellaneous: Serum sickness, feces discoloration (black), urine discoloration (black), urine discoloration (brown), urine discoloration (rust), urine discoloration (yellow-brown)

Signs & Symptoms of Acute Overdose Leukopenia or neutropenia (agranulocytosis, granulocytopenia), blood dyscrasias, jaundice, cholestatic jaundice, coagulopathy, depression, toxic epidermal necrolysis, methemoglobinemia, meningitis, hyperkalemia, systemic lupus erythematosus (SLE), Stevens-Johnson syndrome, hypoglycemia, pseudotumor cerebri, erythema multiforme, colitis

Toxicodynamics/Kinetics

Absorption: Oral: 90% to 100%

Distribution: V_d:
- SMX: 0.21 L/kg
- TMP:1.2-2 L/kg

Protein binding:
- SMX: 68%
- TMP: 68%

Metabolism:
- SMX is N-acetylated and glucuronidated
- TMP is metabolized to oxide and hydroxylated metabolites

Half-life:
- SMX: 9 hours
- TMP: 6-17 hours, both are prolonged in renal failure

Time to peak serum concentration: Within 1-4 hours

Elimination: Excreted in urine as metabolites and unchanged drug

Usual Dosage Dosage recommendations are based on the trimethoprim component

Children >2 months:
- Mild to moderate infections: Oral, I.V.: 8 mg TMP/kg/day in divided doses every 12 hours
- Serious infection/*Pneumocystis*: I.V.: 20 mg TMP/kg/day in divided doses every 6 hours
- Urinary tract infection prophylaxis: Oral: 2 mg TMP/kg/dose daily
- Prophylaxis of *Pneumocystis*: Oral, I.V.: 10 mg TMP/kg/day or 150 mg TMP/m^2/day in divided doses every 12 hours for 3 days/week; dose should not exceed 320 mg trimethoprim and 1600 mg sulfamethoxazole 3 days/week

Adults:
- Urinary tract infection/chronic bronchitis: Oral: 1 double strength tablet every 12 hours for 10-14 days
- Sepsis: I.V.: 20 TMP/kg/day divided every 6 hours
- *Pneumocystis carinii*:
  - Prophylaxis: Oral, I.V.: 10 mg TMP/kg/day divided every 12 hours for 3 days/week
  - Treatment: I.V.: 20 mg TMP/kg/day divided every 6 hours

Dosing interval/adjustment in renal impairment:
- Cl_{cr} 30-50 mL/minute: Administer every 12-18 hours or reduce dose by 25%
- Cl_{cr} 15-30 mL/minute: Administer every 18-24 hours or reduce dose by 50%
- Cl_{cr} <15 mL/minute: Not recommended

Administration Infuse I.V. co-trimoxazole over 60-90 minutes; must be further diluted 1:25 (5 mL drug to 125 mL diluent, ie, D_5W); in patients who require fluid restriction, a 1:15 dilution (5 mL drug to 75 mL diluent, ie, D_5W) or a 1:10 dilution (5 mL drug to 50 mL diluent, ie, D_5W) can be administered

Contraindications Hypersensitivity to any sulfa drug or any component; porphyria; anemia (megaloblastic) due to folate deficiency; infants <2 months of age

Warnings Use with caution in patients with G-6-PD deficiency, impaired renal or hepatic function; adjust dosage in patients with renal impairment; injection vehicle

(Continued)

Co-trimoxazole *(Continued)*

contains benzyl alcohol and sodium metabisulfite; fatalities associated with sulfonamides, although rare, have occurred due to severe reactions including Stevens-Johnson syndrome, toxic epidermal necrolysis, hepatic necrosis, leukopenia; neutropenia; agranulocytosis; granulocytopenia; aplastic anemia and other blood dyscrasias; discontinue use at first sign of rash; elderly patients appear at greater risk for more severe adverse reactions

Dosage Forms The 5:1 ratio (SMX to TMP) remains constant in all dosage forms:

Injection: Sulfamethoxazole 80 mg and trimethoprim 16 mg per mL (5 mL, 10 mL, 20 mL, 30 mL, 50 mL)

Suspension, oral: Sulfamethoxazole 200 mg and trimethoprim 40 mg per 5 mL (20 mL, 100 mL, 150 mL, 200 mL, 480 mL)

Tablet: Sulfamethoxazole 400 mg and trimethoprim 80 mg

Tablet, double strength: Sulfamethoxazole 800 mg and trimethoprim 160 mg

Stability Do not refrigerate injection; is less soluble in more alkaline pH; protect from light; do not use NS as a diluent; injection vehicle contains benzyl alcohol and sodium metabisulfite

Stability of parenteral admixture at room temperature (25°C):

5 mL/125 mL D_5W = 6 hours
5 mL/100 mL D_5W = 4 hours
5 mL/75 mL D_5W = 2 hours

Reference Range Peak plasma concentrations of 20-50 mg/L (79-198 μmol/L) of SMZ and 0.9-1.9 mg/L (3.1-6.5 μmol/L) of TMP occur after oral ingestion of 800 mg of SMZ and 160 mg of TMP; plasma trimethoprim levels >5 mg/L (17 μmol/L) may be needed to treat *P. carinii* pneumonia

Overdosage Treatment

Decontamination: Lavage/activated charcoal with cathartic

Supportive therapy: Leucovorin (10 mg/m^2 every 6 hours for 72 hours) for trimethoprim bone marrow toxicity

Enhancement of elimination: Multiple dosing of activated charcoal may be effective

Test Interactions ↑ creatinine (Jaffé alkaline picrate reaction); increased serum methotrexate by dihydrofolate reductase method; does not interfere with RAI method

Drug Interactions

Decreased effect of cyclosporines

Increased effect of sulfonylureas and oral anticoagulants

Increased toxicity/levels of phenytoin; increased toxicity by displacing methotrexate from protein binding sites; increased nephrotoxicity of cyclosporines

Pregnancy Risk Factor C

Pregnancy Implications Crosses the placenta; distributes into breast milk

Monitoring Parameters CBC, renal function test, liver function test, urinalysis

Patient Information Take oral medication with 8 oz of water on an empty stomach (1 hour before or 2 hours after meals) for best absorption; report any skin rashes immediately; finish all medication, do not skip doses

Nursing Implications Infuse over 60-90 minutes, must dilute well before giving; may be given undiluted in a central line; not for I.M. injection; maintain adequate fluid intake to prevent crystalluria; give around-the-clock every 6-12 hours

Additional Information Injection vehicle contains benzyl alcohol and sodium metabisulfite; folinic acid should be given if bone marrow depression occurs; one double-strength tablet of trimethoprim-sulfamethoxazole 5 times/week has been demonstrated to aid in preventing spontaneous bacterial peritonitis in cirrhotic patients

Specific References

Bissuel F, Cotte L, Crapanne J-B, et al, "Trimethoprim-Sulphametohxazole Rechallene in 20 Previously Allergic HIV-Infected Patients After Homeopathic Desensitization," *AIDS*, 1995, 9:407-8.

Choo V, "UK Revises Indications for Co-Trimoxazole," *Lancet*, 1995, 346:175.

Dawkins B, Albury D, and Olsen TE, "Trimethoprim/Sulfamethoxazole-Induced Thrombocytopenia – A Case Report Supported by the Laboratory Diagnosis," *Aust N Z J Med*, 1995, 25:83.

Hennessy S, Strom BL, Berlin JA, et al, "Predicting Cutaneous Hypersensitivity Reactions to Co-Trimoxazole in HIV-Infected Individuals Receiving Primary *Pneumocystis carinii*, Pneumonia Prophylaxis," *J Gen Intern Med*, 1995, 10:380-6.

Jick H and Derbe LE, "A Large Population-Based Follow-Up Study of Trimethoprim-Sulfamethoxazole, Trimethoprim, and Cephalexin for Uncommon Serious Drug Toxicity," *Pharmacotherapy*, 1995, 15(4):428-32.

Jick H and Derbe LE, "Is Co-Trimoxazole Safe?" *Lancet*, 345:1118-9.

Masur H, "Prevention and Treatment of *Pneumocystis* Pneumonia," *N Engl J Med*, 1992, 327(26):1853-60.

Naguib MT, Lastrapes DL, Brandon FM, et al, "Trimethoprim-Sulfamethoxazole-Induced Renal Tubular Acidosis in a Patient With AIDS," *Clin Infect Dis*, 1995, 20:1435.

Noto H, Kaneko Y, Takano T, et al, "Severe Hyponatremia and Hyperkalemia Induced by Trimethoprim-Sulfamethoxazole in Patients With *Pneumocystis carinii* Pneumonia," *Intern Med*, 1995, 34:96-9.

Singh N, Gayowski T, Yu VL, et al, "Trimethoprim-Sulfamethoxazole for the Prevention of Spontaneous Bacterial Peritonitis in Cirrhosis: A Randomized Trial," *Ann Intern Med*, 1995, 122(8):595-8.

Coumadin® *see* Warfarin Sodium *on page 800*

Co-vidarabine *see* Pentostatin *on page 606*

Covostet® *see* Tetracaine Hydrochloride *on page 731*

Cozaar® *see* Losartan Potassium *on page 484*

CP-66 *see* Tenidap *on page 725*

CPA *see* Cyclophosphamide *on page 249*

CPM *see* Cyclophosphamide *on page 249*

CPT-II *see* Irinotecan *on page 439*

Crispin® *see* Tramadol Hydrochloride *on page 762*

Cromoglycic Acid *see* Cromolyn Sodium *on this page*

Cromolyn Sodium (kroe' moe lin)

CAS Number 16110-51-3; 15826-37-6

Brand Names Gastrocrom® Oral; Intal® Inhalation Capsule; Intal® Nebulizer Solution; Intal® Oral Inhaler; Nasalcrom® Nasal Solution; Opticrom®

Synonyms Cromoglycic Acid; Disodium Cromoglycate; DSCG

Use Adjunct in the prophylaxis of allergic disorders, including rhinitis, giant papillary conjunctivitis, and asthma; inhalation product may be used for prevention of exercise-induced bronchospasm; systemic mastocytosis, food allergy, and treatment of inflammatory bowel disease; **cromolyn is a prophylactic drug with no benefit for acute situations**; may be effective in decreasing ACE-inhibitor cough by 50%

Mechanism of Action Prevents the mast cell release of histamine, leukotrienes and slow-reacting substance of anaphylaxis by inhibiting degranulation after contact with antigens

Adverse Reactions

Cardiovascular: Pericarditis with pericardial tamponade

Central nervous system: Dizziness, headache

Dermatologic: Rash, eczema, angioedema

Gastrointestinal: unpleasant taste (inhalation aerosol), dry mouth, nausea, vomiting, diarrhea

Neuromuscular & skeletal: Joint pain, myositis

Ocular: Ocular stinging, lacrimation, chemosis

Renal: Dysuria

Respiratory: Coughing, hoarseness, sneezing, stuffy nose, wheezing

Miscellaneous: Eosinophilic pneumonia, anaphylactic reaction, nasal burning, throat irritation, pulmonary infiltrates

Signs & Symptoms of Acute Overdose Bronchospasm, dyspnea, pericarditis, wheezing, laryngeal edema, lacrimation, dysuria

Toxicodynamics/Kinetics Not effective for immediate relief of symptoms in acute asthmatic attacks; must be used at regular intervals for 2-4 weeks to be effective

Absorption:

- Inhalation: ~8% of dose reaches the lungs upon inhalation of the powder and is well absorbed
- Oral: 0.5% to 2% of dose
- Ophthalmologic: 0.03% of dose

Distribution: V_d: 0.2 L/kg

Protein binding: 57%

Half-life: 22 minutes

Time to peak serum concentration: Inhalation: Within 15 minutes

Elimination: Absorbed cromolyn is equally excreted unchanged in urine and feces (via bile); small amounts are exhaled; clearance: 0.35 L/kg/hour

Usual Dosage

Children and Adults:

- Inhalation (taper frequency to lowest effective dose):
  - >2 years: 20 mg 4 times/day by nebulization solution
  - >5 years: 2 inhalations 4 times/day by metered spray or 20 mg 4 times/day (Spinhaler®)
- For prevention of exercise-induced bronchospasm: Single dose of 2 inhalations (aerosol) or 20 mg (powder inhalation) just prior to exercise (no more than 1 hour)
- Nasal: >6 years: Instill 1 spray in each nostril 3-4 times/day

Mastocytosis: Oral:

- Children:
  - ≤2 years: 20 mg/kg/day 4 times/day up to 30 mg/kg/day
  - 2-12 years: 100 mg 4 times/day 15-20 minutes before meals, up to 40 mg/kg/day

(Continued)

Cromolyn Sodium *(Continued)*

Adults: 200 mg 30 minutes before meals and at bedtime

Administration For oral use, cromolyn powder is dissolved in hot water and taken at least 30 minutes before meals

Contraindications Hypersensitivity to cromolyn or any component; acute asthma attacks

Warnings Caution should be used when withdrawing the drug or tapering the dose as symptoms may reoccur; use with caution in patients with a history of cardiac arrhythmia; use with caution in patients with renal and hepatic impairment

Dosage Forms

Capsule:

Oral (Gastrocrom®): 100 mg

Oral inhalation (Intal®): 20 mg [to be used with Spinhaler® turbo-inhaler]

Inhalation, oral (Intal®): 800 mcg/spray (8.1 g)

Solution, for nebulization (Intal®): 10 mg/mL (2 mL)

Solution, nasal (Nasalcrom®): 40 mg/mL (13 mL)

Stability Nebulizer solution is **compatible** with metaproterenol sulfate, isoproterenol hydrochloride, 0.25% isoetharine hydrochloride, epinephrine hydrochloride, terbutaline sulfate, and 20% acetylcysteine solution for at least 1 hour after their admixture; store nebulizer solution protected from direct light

Reference Range Plasma levels not relatable to effect; peak plasma level after inhalation: ~15 ng/mL

Overdosage Treatment

Decontamination: Oral: Lavage/activated charcoal with cathartic

Supportive therapy: Treat inhalation exposure with 100% humidified oxygen; treat anaphylaxis with epinephrine and corticosteroids; albuterol can be given for bronchospasm

Drug Interactions Isoproterenol

Pregnancy Risk Factor B

Pregnancy Implications No known teratogenic effect

Monitoring Parameters Periodic pulmonary function tests

Patient Information Do not discontinue abruptly; not effective for acute relief of symptoms; must be taken on a regularly scheduled basis; do not mix oral capsule with fruit juice, milk, or foods

Nursing Implications Advise patient to clear as much mucus as possible before inhalation treatments

Additional Information Reserve systemic use in children <2 years of age for severe disease; avoid systemic use in premature infants

Specific References

Ahmad S, "Cromolyn Sodium and Anaphylaxis," *Ann Intern Med*, 1983, 99:882.

Hargreaves MR and Benson MK, "Inhaled Sodium Cromoglycate in Angiotensin-Converting Enzyme Inhibitor Cough," *Lancet*, 1995, 345(8941):13-6.

Slater EF, "Cardiac Tamponade and Peripheral Eosinophilia in a Patient Receiving Cromolyn Sodium," *Chest*, 1978, 73:838.

Walter SR, Evans ME, Richard AJ, et al, "The Fate of Disodium Cromoglycate in Man," *J Pharm Pharmacol*, 1972, 24:525-31.

Cruor® *see* Bepridil Hydrochloride *on page 152*

Crystalline Penicillin *see* Penicillin G, Parenteral, Aqueous *on page 600*

Crystamine® *see* Cyanocobalamin *on this page*

Crystapen® *see* Penicillin G, Parenteral, Aqueous *on page 600*

CS-045 *see* Troglitazone *on page 777*

CSA *see* Cyclosporine *on page 252*

CTX *see* Cyclophosphamide *on page 249*

Curling Factor *see* Griseofulvin *on page 389*

CV-205-502 *see* Quinagolide *on page 666*

CyA *see* Cyclosporine *on page 252*

Cyanocobalamin (sye an oh koe bal' a min)

CAS Number 68-19-9

Brand Names Berubigen®; Cobex®; Crystamine®; Cyanoject®; Cyomin®; Ener-B® [OTC]; Kaybovite-1000®; Redisol®; Rubramin-PC®; Sytobex®

Synonyms Vitamin B_{12}

Use Treatment of pernicious anemia; vitamin B_{12} deficiency; increased B_{12} requirements due to pregnancy, thyrotoxicosis, hemorrhage, malignancy, liver or kidney disease; water-soluble vitamin with a wide margin of safety

Mechanism of Action Coenzyme for various metabolic functions, including fat and carbohydrate metabolism and protein synthesis, used in cell replication and hematopoiesis

Adverse Reactions

Cardiovascular: Peripheral vascular thrombosis
Dermatologic: Itching, rash
Endocrine & metabolic: Hypokalemia
Gastrointestinal: Diarrhea
Miscellaneous: Allergic reactions, bezoar formation

Signs & Symptoms of Acute Overdose Hypokalemia

Toxicodynamics/Kinetics

Absorption: Absorbed from the terminal ileum in the presence of calcium; for absorption to occur gastric "intrinsic factor" must be present to transfer the compound across the intestinal mucosa
Distribution: Principally stored in the liver, also stored in the kidneys and adrenals
Protein binding: Bound to transcobalamin II
Metabolism: Converted in the tissues to active coenzymes methylcobalamin and deoxyadenosylcobalamin

Usual Dosage

Recommended daily allowance (RDA):
- Children 1-4 years: 3 mcg/day
- Adults: 6 mcg/day

Nutritional deficiency: 25-250 mcg/day

Children:
- Congenital pernicious anemia (if evidence of neurologic involvement): I.M.: 1000 mcg/day for at least 2 weeks; maintenance: 50 mcg/month
- Vitamin B_{12} deficiency: I.M., S.C.: 1-5 mg given in single or S.C. doses of 100 mcg/day over 2 or more weeks

Adults:
- Pernicious anemia: I.M., S.C.: 100 mcg/day for 6-7 days
- Vitamin B_{12} deficiency:
  - Oral: Usually not recommended, maximum absorbed from a single oral dose is 2-3 mcg
  - I.M., S.C.: 30 mcg/day for 5-10 days, followed by 100-200 mcg/month

Contraindications Hypersensitivity to cyanocobalamin or any component, cobalt; patients with hereditary optic nerve atrophy

Warnings Doses exceeding 10 mcg/day may produce hematologic response in patients with folate deficiency. Indiscriminate use may mask the true diagnosis of pernicious anemia. Single deficiency is rare (except multiple deficiencies). Monitor potassium concentrations during early therapy. Some products contain benzoyl alcohol.

Dosage Forms

Gel, nasal (Ener-B®): 400 mcg/0.1 mL
Injection: 30 mcg/mL (30 mL); 100 mcg/mL (1 mL, 10 mL, 30 mL); 1000 mcg/mL (1 mL, 10 mL, 30 mL)
Tablet [OTC]: 25 mcg, 50 mcg, 100 mcg, 250 mcg, 500 mcg, 1000 mcg

Stability Clear pink to red solutions are stable at room temperature; protect from light; **incompatible** with chlorpromazine, phytonadione, prochlorperazine, warfarin, ascorbic acid, dextrose, heavy metals, oxidizing or reducing agents

Reference Range The lower limit of normal (critical to the diagnosis of B_{12} deficiency/pernicious anemia) has not been firmly established; it is likely in the range of 100-250 pg/mL (SI: 74-185 pmol/L)

Overdosage Treatment

Supportive therapy: Allergic reactions can be treated with epinephrine, diphenhydramine, and corticosteroids

Test Interactions Methotrexate, pyrimethamine, and most antibiotics invalidate folic acid and vitamin B_{12} diagnostic microbiological blood assays

Drug Interactions Neomycin, colchicine, anticonvulsants → ↓ absorption, chloramphenicol → ↓ B_{12} effects

Pregnancy Risk Factor A (C if dose exceeds RDA recommendation)

Monitoring Parameters Serum potassium, erythrocyte and reticulocyte count, hemoglobin, hematocrit

Patient Information Pernicious anemia will require monthly injections for life

Nursing Implications I.M. or deep S.C. are preferred routes of administration; oral therapy is markedly inferior to parenteral therapy; monitor potassium concentrations during early therapy

Additional Information Radiopaque

Specific References

Schjonsby H, "Vitamin B_{12} Absorption and Malabsorption," *Gut*, 1989, 30(12):1986-91.
Silbergleit R and Lee DC, "Bowel Obstruction and Radiopaque Vitamin B_{12} "Pseudobezoar"," *Am J Emerg Med*, 1995, 13(1):112-3.

Cyanoject® *see* Cyanocobalamin *on previous page*

Cyater® *see* Terfenadine *on page 728*

Cyclizine (sye' kli zeen)

CAS Number 82-92-8 (base); 303-25-3 (hydrochloride); 5897-19-8 (lactate)

Brand Names Happy-Trip®; Marezine® [OTC]

Use Prevention and treatment of nausea, vomiting, and dizziness associated with motion sickness; control of postoperative nausea and vomiting

Adverse Reactions

Central nervous system: Drowsiness, dizziness, asthenia, headache, euphoria
Dermatologic: Dermatitis
Gastrointestinal: Nausea, dry mouth
Genitourinary: Polyuria, urinary retention
Hematologic: Blood dyscrasias, agranulocytosis
Hepatic: Hepatitis
Ocular: Diplopia

Signs & Symptoms of Acute Overdose Dry mouth, dry nose, euphoria, extrapyramidal reaction, insomnia, diarrhea, cholestatic jaundice, flushing, mydriasis, CNS depression

Toxicodynamics/Kinetics Duration of action: 4-6 hours

Usual Dosage

Children 6-12 years:
- Oral: 25 mg up to 3 times/day
- I.M.: Not recommended

Adults:
- Oral: 50 mg taken 30 minutes before departure, may repeat in 4-6 hours if needed, up to 200 mg/day
- I.M.: 50 mg every 4-6 hours as needed

Dosage Forms

Injection, as lactate: 50 mg/mL (1 mL)
Tablet, as hydrochloride: 50 mg

Reference Range Peak serum concentrations of 69 ng/mL after a 50 mg oral dose

Overdosage Treatment Decontamination: Lavage/activated charcoal with cathartic

Pregnancy Risk Factor B

Patient Information May cause drowsiness; avoid alcohol

Nursing Implications Raise bed rails, institute safety measures, assist with ambulation

Additional Information Commonly abused with opiates for euphoric effects

Specific References

Collier PM, "Agranulocytosis Associated With Oral Cyclizine," *Br Med J*, 1986, 292:174.
Gott PH, "Cyclizine Toxicity - Intentional Drug Abuse of a Proprietary Antihistamine," *N Engl J Med*, 1968, 279(11):596.
Kahn A and Harves GJ, "Increasing Misuse of Cyclizine," *Pharm J*, 1985, 235:773.

Cyclobenzaprine Hydrochloride (sye kloe ben' za preen)

CAS Number 303-53-7; 6202-23-9

Brand Names Flexeril®; Flexiban®; Lisseril®; Yurelax®

Synonyms CBZ; Propheptatriene

Use Treatment of muscle spasm associated with acute painful musculoskeletal conditions; supportive therapy in tetanus

Mechanism of Action Reduces tonic somatic motor activity influencing both alpha and gamma motor neurons; structurally related to amitriptyline

Adverse Reactions

Cardiovascular: Tachycardia, hypotension or hypertension, arrhythmias
Central nervous system: Drowsiness, headache, dizziness, fatigue, asthenia, nervousness, confusion, coma, visual hallucinations, seizures, manic psychosis
Dermatologic: Rash
Endocrine & metabolic: Syndrome of inappropriate antidiuretic hormone
Gastrointestinal: Dyspepsia, nausea, constipation, dry mouth, vomiting, urinary retention
Neuromuscular & skeletal: Myoclonus
Ocular: Blurred vision
Miscellaneous: Unpleasant taste, sweating

Signs & Symptoms of Acute Overdose Fever, diaphoresis, ataxia, mania, muscular rigidity, rhabdomyolysis, delirium, mydriasis, myalgia, hallucinations

Toxicodynamics/Kinetics

Onset of action: Commonly occurs within 1 hour
Absorption: Oral: Completely
Protein binding: 93%
Metabolism: Hepatic; may undergo enterohepatic recycling
Half-life: 1-3 days
Time to peak serum concentration: Within 3-8 hours
Elimination: Excreted renally (50%) as inactive metabolites and in feces (via bile) as unchanged drug

Usual Dosage Oral: **Note:** Do not use longer than 2-3 weeks

Children: Dosage has not been established

Adults: 20-40 mg/day in 2-4 divided doses; maximum dose: 60 mg/day

Toxic symptoms occur with ingestions >100 mg

Contraindications Hypersensitivity to cyclobenzaprine or any component; do not use concomitantly or within 14 days of MAO inhibitors

Warnings Hyperthyroidism, congestive heart failure, arrhythmias; cyclobenzaprine shares the toxic potentials of the tricyclic antidepressants; the usual precautions of tricyclic antidepressant therapy should be observed; use with caution in patients with urinary hesitancy or angle-closure glaucoma

Dosage Forms Tablet: 10 mg

Reference Range Therapeutic serum levels following a 40 mg dose: 10-40 ng/mL; a serum level of 260 ng/mL was associated with lethality

Overdosage Treatment

Decontamination: Lavage/activated charcoal with cathartic

Supportive therapy: Physostigmine can be utilized for severe life-threatening anticholinergic effects; hyperthermic states may require dantrolene and/or bromocriptine similar to the treatment of neuroleptic malignant syndrome

Enhancement of elimination: Multiple dosing of activated charcoal may be effective; dialysis is not useful

Antidote(s)

Physostigmine *on page 1457*

Drug Interactions Do not use concomitantly or within 14 days after MAO inhibitors; can cause fever and seizures

Increased effect/toxicity with alcohol, barbiturates, CNS depressants

Increased toxicity with MAO inhibitors, TCAs, anticholinergics

Can decrease the hypotensive effects of guanethidine

Pregnancy Risk Factor B

Patient Information Drug may impair ability to perform hazardous activities requiring mental alertness or physical coordination, such as operating machinery or driving a motor vehicle

Nursing Implications Raise bed rails, institute safety measures, assist with ambulation

Specific References

Ambre JJ, "Cyclobenzaprine Overdose," *Ann Intern Med*, 1985, 102(4):559-60.

Heckerling PS, Bartow TJ, "Paradoxical Diaphoresis in Cyclobenzaprine Poisoning," *Ann Intern Med*, 1984, 101(6):881.

Hucker HB, Stauffer SC, Albert KS, et al, "Plasma Levels and Bioavailability of Cyclobenzaprine in Human Subjects," *J Clin Pharmacol*, 1977, 17(11-12):719-27.

Linden CH, Mitchiner JC, Lindzon RD, et al, "Cyclobenzaprine Overdosage," *J Toxicol Clin Toxicol*, 1983, 20(3):281-8.

Spiller HA, Winter ML, Mann KV, et al, "Five Year Multicenter Retrospective Review of Cyclobenzaprine Toxicity," *Vet Hum Toxicol*, 1994, 36:370.

Theoharides TC, Harris RS, and Weckstein D, "Neuroleptic Malignant-Like Syndrome Due to Cyclobenzaprine," *J Clin Psychopharmacol*, 1995, 15:79-81.

Cyclomen® *see* Danazol *on page 257*

Cyclophosphamide (sye kloe foss' fa mide)

Related Information

Amifostine *on page 107*

Drugs and Chemicals Proven to be Teratogenic in Humans *on page 1572-1575*

Toxicities of Chemotherapeutic Agents *on page 1631-1633*

CAS Number 6055-19-2; 50-18-0

Brand Names Cytoxan®; Neosar® Injection

Synonyms CPA; CPM; CTX; CYT

Use Hodgkin's and non-Hodgkin's lymphoma, Burkitt's lymphoma, chronic lymphocytic leukemia, chronic granulocytic leukemia, AML, ALL, mycosis fungoides, breast cancer, multiple myeloma, neuroblastoma, retinoblastoma, rhabdomyosarcoma, Ewing's sarcoma; testicular, endometrium and ovarian, and lung cancer, and as a conditioning regimen for BMT; prophylaxis of rejection for kidney, heart, liver, and BMT transplants, severe rheumatoid disorders, nephrotic syndrome, Wegener's granulomatosis, idiopathic pulmonary hemosideroses, myasthenia gravis, multiple sclerosis, systemic lupus erythematosus, lupus nephritis, autoimmune hemolytic anemia, idiopathic thrombocytic purpura, macroglobulinemia, and antibody-induced pure red cell aplasia

Mechanism of Action Interferes with the normal function of DNA by alkylation and cross-linking the strands of DNA, and by possible protein modification; cyclophosphamide also possesses potent immunosuppressive activity; note that cyclophosphamide must be metabolized to its active form in the liver (an alkylating agent)

Adverse Reactions

Cardiovascular: High-dose therapy (>2.5 g/m²/day) may cause cardiac dysfunction manifested as congestive heart failure; cardiac necrosis or hemorrhagic

(Continued)

Cyclophosphamide *(Continued)*

myocarditis has occurred rarely, but is fatal; cyclophosphamide may also potentiate the cardiac toxicity of anthracyclines, tachycardia, facial flushing

Central nervous system: Headache, dizziness, fatigue

Dermatologic: Skin rash, skin hyperpigmentation (hyperpigmentation of palms and soles), transverse ridging of nails, hepatic toxicity, and dermatitis; allergic skin reactions (0.5%)

Alopecia: Frequent (occurs in 20% of patients), but hair will regrow although it may be of a different color or texture; hair loss usually occurs 3 weeks after therapy

Endocrine & metabolic: Hyperglycemia, hypokalemia

Gastrointestinal: Nausea and vomiting occur more frequently with larger doses, usually beginning 6-10 hours after administration; also seen are anorexia, diarrhea, stomatitis, pancreatitis, mucositis are seen occasionally; hemorrhagic colitis

Genitourinary: Oligospermia; acute cystitis (hemorrhagic) is believed to be a result of chemical irritation of the bladder by acrolein, a cyclophosphamide metabolite. Acute cystitis (hemorrhagic) occurs in 7% to 12% of patients and has been reported in up to 40% of patients. Hemorrhagic cystitis can be severe and even fatal. Patients should be encouraged to drink plenty of fluids (3-4 L/day) during therapy, void frequently, and avoid taking the drug at nighttime. If large I.V. doses are being administered, I.V. hydration should be given during therapy. The administration of mesna or continuous bladder irrigation may also be warranted.

Fertility: May cause sterility; interferes with oogenesis and spermatogenesis; may be irreversible in some patients; gonadal suppression (amenorrhea)

Hematologic: Porphyria, thrombocytopenia, anemia

Hepatic: Jaundice

Renal: Syndrome of inappropriate antidiuretic hormone has occurred with I.V. doses >50 mg/kg; tubular necrosis (acute) has also occurred, but usually resolves after the discontinuation of therapy; cystitis (hemorrhagic) may be severe

Respiratory: Interstitial pulmonary fibrosis with prolonged high dosage has occurred, rhinorrhea, sinus congestion, nasal stuffiness occurs when given in large I.V. doses

Miscellaneous: Patients experience runny eyes, sneezing during or immediately after the infusion, distortion, hyperuricemia, feces discoloration (black), sweating, anaphylaxis

Signs & Symptoms of Acute Overdose Hemorrhagic cystitis, hyponatremia, erythema multiforme, A-V block, hematuria, hypokalemia, hyperuricemia, Mees' lines, hyperpigmented hair, oligospermia, hypertension, hyperglycemia, tachycardia, leukopenia; neutropenia; agranulocytosis; granulocytopenia; azoospermia, colitis

Toxicodynamics/Kinetics

Absorption: Complete from gastrointestinal tract (>75%); can be absorbed dermally

Distribution: V_d: 0.48 L/kg (oral) to 0.71 L/kg (I.V.); well distributed; does cross into the CSF, but not in concentrations high enough to treat meningeal leukemia

Protein binding: 10% to 56%

Metabolism: In the liver to active metabolite (aldophosphamide); acrolein is also a metabolite which may result in bladder toxicity

Bioavailability: >75%

Half-life: 4-6.5 hours

Time to peak serum concentration: Oral: Within 1 hour

Elimination: In urine as unchanged drug (<30%) and as metabolites (85% to 90%)

Usual Dosage Refer to individual protocols

Children: Neuroblastomas/sarcomas: I.V.: 3 g/m^2/day for 2 days or 2 g/m^2/day for 3 days

Children and Adults:

Oral: 50-100 mg/m^2/day as continuous therapy or 400-1000 mg/m^2 in divided doses over 4-5 days as intermittent therapy

I.V.: 400-1500 mg/m^2 every 21-28 days

BMT-conditioning regimen: I.V.: 50 mg/kg/dose once daily for 3-4 days or 60 mg/kg/dose for 2 days

Nephrotic syndrome: Oral: 2-3 mg/kg/day every day for up to 12 weeks when corticosteroids are unsuccessful

Patients with compromised bone marrow function may require a 33% to 50% reduction in initial loading dose

Dosing adjustment in renal impairment:

Cl_{cr} 25-50 mL/minute: Administer 75% of normal dose

Cl_{cr} <25 mL/minute: Administer 50% of normal dose

Dosing adjustment in hepatic impairment:

Bilirubin 3.5-5 mg/dL or AST >180 IU: Administer 75% of normal dose
Bilirubin >5 mg/dL: Omit dose

Administration I.V. infusions may be administered over 1-2 hours; doses >500 mg to approximately 1 g may be administered over 20-30 minutes; may also be administered slow IVP in lower doses

Contraindications Hypersensitivity to cyclophosphamide or any component

Warnings The U.S. Food and Drug Administration (FDA) currently recommends that procedures for proper handling and disposal of antineoplastic agents be considered. Dosage adjustment needed for renal or hepatic necrosis; use with caution in patients with bone marrow depression; handle urine and feces from patients administered with cyclophosphamide with care.

Dosage Forms

Powder for injection: 100 mg, 200 mg, 500 mg, 1 g, 2 g
Powder for injection, lyophilized: 100 mg, 200 mg, 500 mg, 1 g, 2 g
Tablet: 25 mg, 50 mg

Stability I.V. solution is usually reconstituted in 20 mg/mL concentrations; solutions may be administered I.V., I.M., intraperitoneally, or intrapleurally; they may be infused I.V. in D_5W, 0.9% sodium chloride, D_5LR, lactated Ringer's, or 0.45% sodium chloride; prepared solutions should be used within 24 hours or may be stored up to 6 days under refrigeration; oral elixir may be prepared from the injectable preparation and is stable for 14 days if refrigerated

Overdosage Treatment

Decontamination: Emesis or lavage/activated charcoal with cathartic

Supportive therapy: Hyperuricemia can be treated with alkalinization of urine along with allopurinol; cystitis (hemorrhagic) can be controlled with bladder irrigation of 5% to 10% formalin glutathione, 2-mercaptoethane sulfonate (30 mg/kg/day for 4 doses) may be uroprotective; additionally, bladder irrigation with prostaglandin F_2-alpha (carboprost tromethamine) has been used; bladder spasm can be controlled with oxybutynin chloride 2.5-5 mg orally 3 times/day. For extravasation, hyaluronidase or chondroitin sulfatase injected S.C. can be utilized; do not use warm packs.

Enhancement of elimination: Multiple dosing of activated charcoal may be effective; hemodialysis may remove 36% of prodrug; moderately dialyzable (20% to 50%)

Test Interactions Hyponatremia can develop due to syndrome of inappropriate antidiuretic hormone, increases uric acid (S)

Drug Interactions

Decreased effect:

Digoxin: Cyclophosphamide may reduce digoxin serum levels

Phenobarbital and phenytoin induce hepatic enzymes and cause a more rapid production of cyclophosphamide metabolites with a concurrent decrease in the serum half-life of the parent compound

Increased toxicity:

Allopurinol may cause an increase in bone marrow depression and may result in significant elevations of cyclophosphamide cytotoxic metabolites

Anesthetic agents: Cyclophosphamide reduces serum pseudocholinesterase concentrations and may prolong the neuromuscular blocking activity of succinylcholine; use with caution with halothane, nitrous oxide, and succinylcholine

Chloramphenicol results in prolonged cyclophosphamide half-life to increase toxicity

Cimetidine inhibits hepatic metabolism of drugs and may reduce the activation of cyclophosphamide

Doxorubicin: Cyclophosphamide may enhance cardiac toxicity of anthracyclines

Indomethacin: Water intoxication may occur

Tetrahydrocannabinol results in enhanced immunosuppression in animal studies

Thiazide diuretics: Leukopenia may be prolonged

Pregnancy Risk Factor D

Pregnancy Implications Multiple anomalies (cleft palate, absent thumbs, dysmorphic facies, skeletal and CNS abnormalities noted); crosses the placenta; appears in breast milk

Monitoring Parameters CBC with differential and platelet count, ESR, BUN, UA, serum electrolytes, serum creatinine

Patient Information Drink plenty of fluids before and after doses; report any blood in urine

Nursing Implications Encourage adequate hydration and frequent voiding to help prevent cystitis (hemorrhagic)

Additional Information May be used in combination with a prophylactic agent for cystitis (hemorrhagic), such as mesna; transient myopia may occur in patients with systemic lupus erythematosus (SLE)

Amifostine may be protective against cyclophosphamide related granulocytopenia, thrombocytopenia, and neurotoxicity

(Continued)

Cyclophosphamide *(Continued)*

Myelosuppressive effects:
- WBC: Moderate
- Platelets: Moderate
- Onset (days): 7
- Nadir (days): 8-14
- Recovery (days): 21

Cardiac toxicity can occur at doses exceeding 2.4 g/m^2

Specific References

Arend SM, Hagen EC, Kroes AC, et al, "Activation of Chronic Hepatitis C Virus Infection by Cyclophosphamide in a Patient With cANCA-Positive Vasculitis," *Nephrol Dial Transplant*, 1995, 10(6):884-887.

Bressler RB and Huston DP, "Water Intoxication Following Moderate-Dose Intravenous Cyclophosphamide," *Arch Intern Med*, 1985, 145(3):548-9.

Bullock N and Whitaker RH, "Massive Bladder Haemorrhage," *Br Med J (Clin Res)*, 1985, 291(6508):1522-3.

Cognata CL, "Use of Prostaglandin F_2 Alpha for Cyclophosphamide-Induced Hemorrhagic Cystitis," *J Pharm Technol*, 1994, 10:204-6.

Garas G, Crawford GP, and Cain M, "Anaphylactic Reaction to Intravenous Cyclophosphamide," *Aust N Z J Med*, 1995, 25:59.

Garat JM, Martinez E, and Aragona F, "Open Instillation of Formalin for Cyclophosphamide-Induced Hemorrhagic Cystitis in a Child," *Eur Urol*, 1985, 11(3):192-4.

Kanwar VS, Albuquerque MLC, Ribeiro RC, et al, "Veno-occlusive Disease of the Liver After Chemotherapy for Rhabdomyosarcoma: Case Report With a Review of the Literature," *Med Pediatr Oncol*, 1995, 24:334-40.

Laufman LR, Jones JJ, Morrice B, et al, "Case Report of a Lethal Cardiac Toxic Effect Following High-Dose Cyclophosphamide," *J Natl Cancer Inst*, 1995, 87:539-40.

Mateu J, Alzamora M, Franco M, et al, "Ifosfamide Extravasation," *Ann Pharmacother*, 1994, 28(11):1243-4.

Moore MJ, "Clinical Pharmacokinetics of Cyclophosphamide," *Clin Pharmacokinet*, 1991, 20(3):194-208.

Vecchione A, "Boston Tragedy Underscores Need for System to Prevent Overdoses," *Hospital Pharmacist Report*, 1995, 9(4):15.

Wang LH, Lee CS, Majeske BL, et al, "Clearance and Recovery Calculations in Hemodialysis: Application to Plasma, Red Blood Cells, and Dialysate Measurements for Cyclophosphamide," *Clin Pharmacol Ther*, 1981, 29(3):365-72.

Cycloplegic Mydriatics Comparison *see page 1648*

Cyclosporin A *see* Cyclosporine *on this page*

Cyclosporine (sye' kloe spor een)

Related Information

Therapeutic Drugs Associated With Hallucinations *on page 1558-1559*

CAS Number 59865-13-3

Brand Names Sandimmune®

Synonyms Ciclosporin; CSA; CyA; Cyclosporin A

Use Immunosuppressant used with corticosteroids to prevent graft versus host disease in patients with kidney, liver, heart, and bone marrow transplants

Mechanism of Action Inhibition of production and release of interleukin II and inhibits interleukin II-induced activation of resting T lymphocytes

Adverse Reactions

Cardiovascular: Hypertension, hypotension, tachycardia, warmth, flushing, peripheral edema

Central nervous system: Convulsions, headache, psychosis, visual hallucinations, ataxia

Dermatologic: Hirsutism, gingival hyperplasia, acne, alopecia

Endocrine & metabolic: Hyperkalemia, hyperglycemia, hypomagnesemia, hyperuricemia, hyperlipidemia

Gastrointestinal: Abdominal discomfort, nausea, vomiting, colitis, pancreatitis

Genitourinary: Decreased urinary sodium/potassium excretion

Hematologic: Epithelial dysplasia, porphyria

Hepatic: Hepatotoxicity

Neuromuscular & skeletal: Tremors, myositis, leg cramps, paresthesia

Ocular: Cortical blindness, diplopia

Renal: Nephrotoxicity

Respiratory: Respiratory distress, sinusitis

Miscellaneous: Lymphoproliferative disorder, increased susceptibility to infection, sensitivity to temperature extremes, anaphylactic shock (may be due to polyoxyl 35 castor oil vehicle in the injectable solution), increased incidence of lymphoma, Kaposi's sarcoma

Signs & Symptoms of Acute Overdose Coma, dementia, colitis, cholestatic jaundice, hypomagnesemia, hyperuricemia, hypertriglyceridemia, hypertrichosis, deafness, hypertension, myoclonus, jaundice, eclampsia, leukopenia, dementia, [illegible]nia, myasthenia gravis (exacerbation or precipitation of), lymphoma, thrombo[illegible]enia, tubular necrosis, gingival hyperplasia, systemic lupus erythematosus

(SLE), gout, encephalopathy, dysphoria, delirium, seizures, cortical blindness, fibrillation (atrial), diarrhea, malaise, renal dysfunction, headache, metabolic acidosis, vomiting, facial flushing, dysgeusia, sweating, hypercalcemia, hyperglycemia

Toxicodynamics/Kinetics

Absorption: Oral: Incomplete and erratic

Distribution: V_d: 1.2 L/kg (1.5-7.5 L/kg in renal failure patients)

Protein binding: 90%

Metabolism: By mixed function oxidase enzymes in the liver to neurotoxic metabolite (M-17)

Bioavailability: 31% in pediatric renal transplant patients; gut dysfunction, commonly seen in BMT recipients, reduces oral bioavailability further

Half-life: Adults: 19-40 hours

Time to peak serum concentration: 3-4 hours

Elimination: Excreted primarily in bile; clearance is more rapid in pediatric patients than in adults. Clearance is decreased in patients with liver disease.

Usual Dosage Children and Adults: Oral dosage is ~3 times the I.V. dosage

Oral: Initial: 14-18 mg/kg/day, beginning 4-12 hours prior to organ transplantation; maintenance: 3-15 mg/kg/day divided every 12-24 hours

I.V.: Initial: 5-6 mg/kg/day beginning 4-12 hours prior to organ transplantation; patients should be switched to oral cyclosporine as soon as possible

Dosing adjustment in hepatic impairment: Probably necessary, monitor levels closely

Administration I.V. cyclosporine can be administered by I.V. intermittent infusion or continuous infusion; for intermittent infusion, administer over 2-6 hours at a final concentration not to exceed 2.5 mg/mL

Contraindications Hypersensitivity to cyclosporine or Cremophor EL™ (I.V. solution) or any component

Warnings Dosage needs to be adjusted in patients with hepatic and renal dysfunction; administer with adrenal corticosteroids; may increase the change of infection and possible development of lymphoma may result; make dose adjustments (to avoid toxicity or possible organ rejection) via cyclosporine blood levels because absorption is erratic; nephrotoxic, avoid concomitant use of other potentially nephrotoxic drugs (eg, acyclovir, aminoglycoside antibiotics, amphotericin B); deleterious in AIDS patients

Dosage Forms

Capsule: 25 mg, 100 mg

Injection: 50 mg/mL (5 mL)

Solution, oral: 100 mg/mL (50 mL)

Stability Do **not** store oral solution in the refrigerator; use contents of oral solution within 2 months after opening; I.V. cyclosporine prepared in normal saline or D_5W is stable 6 hours in PVC or 24 hours in a glass container or PAB container or Excel® container; do not freeze

Reference Range

Reference ranges are method-dependent and specimen-dependent. Trough levels should be obtained 12-18 hours after oral dose (chronic usage), 12 hours after I.V., dose, or immediately prior to next dose.

Therapeutic: Not well defined, dependent on organ transplanted, time after transplant, organ function and CSA toxicity

Toxic: Not well defined, nephrotoxicity usually occurs at whole blood trough levels above 150 ng/mL, but may occur at any level

Overdosage Treatment

Decontamination: Lavage/activated charcoal with cathartic

Supportive therapy: Diazepam, lorazepam, phenytoin, or phenobarbital for seizure control; calcium channel blockers are preferred agent for treatment of hypertension (nifedipine or verapamil)

Enhancement of elimination: Multiple dosing of activated charcoal can decrease half-life from 9 hours to under 3 hours (through enterohepatic recirculation of drug); hemodialysis is not useful

Test Interactions Specific whole blood, HPLC assay for cyclosporine may be falsely elevated if sample is drawn from the same line through which dose was administered (even if flush has been administered and/or dose was given hours before)

Diagnostic Tests/Procedures

Cyclosporine, Blood *on page 1247*

Drug Interactions

Decreased effect: Rifampin, phenytoin, barbiturates, intravenous sulfonamides/trimethoprim, carbamazepine, ethotoin, mephenytoin, and primidone ↓ plasma concentration of cyclosporine

Increased toxicity: Ketoconazole, androgens, diltiazem, methotrexate, methylprednisolone, erythromycin, oral contraceptives, verapamil, diltiazem and nicardipine ↑ plasma concentration of cyclosporine; melphalan, foscarnet, metolazone, ciprofloxacin, sulindac/diclofenac can increase nephrotoxicity; lovastatin

(Continued)

Cyclosporine *(Continued)*

with cyclosporine can result in myopathy; increased cyclosporine blood levels with concomitant use of danazol

Pregnancy Risk Factor C

Pregnancy Implications Distributes into breast milk; intrauterine growth retardation and osseous malformations can develop

Monitoring Parameters Cyclosporine levels, serum electrolytes (especially magnesium), renal function, hepatic function, blood pressure, pulse

Patient Information Use glass droppers or glass to hold dose; may mix with milk or juice for flavor; rinse container to get full dose

Nursing Implications Do not administer liquid from plastic or styrofoam cup; mixing with milk, chocolate milk, or orange juice preferably at room temperature, improves palatability; stir well and drink at once; do not allow to stand before drinking; rinse with more diluent to ensure that the total dose is taken; after use, dry outside of pipette; do not rinse with water or other cleaning agents; may cause inflamed gums

Additional Information Increases renin activity; grapefruit juice can inhibit cyclosporine metabolism in renal transplant patients; suggestion of improvement of cyclosporine-associated gingival hyperplasia with treatment of azithromycin

Specific References

Bachmann K, Sullivan TJ, Reese JH, et al, "The Influence of Dirithromycin on the Pharmacokinetics of Cyclosporine in Healthy Subjects and in Renal Transplant Patients," *Am J Therapeut*, 1995, 2:490-8.

Boni R and Dummer R, "Abscessed Inflammation as a Serious Complication of Low Dose Cyclosporin A in Atopic Dermatitis," *Eur J Dermatol*, 1995, 5:268-9.

Bulengo-Ransby SM, Sahn EE, Metcalf JS, et al, "Bowenoid Change in Association With Graft-Versus-Host Disease: A Cyclosporine Toxicity?" *J Am Acad Dermatol*, 1994, 31(6):1052-4.

Calonge MV, Glotz D, Bouscary D, et al, "Hemophagocytic Histiocytosis (HH) in Renal Transplant Recipients Under Ciclosporin Therapy: Report of the First Two Cases," *Clin Transpl*, 1995, 9:88-91.

Cooney GF, Mochon M, Kaiser B, et al, "Effects of Carbamazepine on Cyclosporine Metabolism in Pediatric Renal Transplant Recipients," *Pharmacotherapy*, 1995, 15(3):353-6.

Davies MG and Bowers PW, "Alopecia Areata Arising in Patients Receiving Cyclosporin Immunosuppression," *Br J Dermatol*, 1995, 132:835-6.

Ducharme MP, Warbasse LH, and Edwards DJ, "Disposition of Intravenous and Oral Cyclosporine After Administration With Grapefruit Juice," *Clin Pharmacol Ther*, 1995, 57:485-91.

Finieiz P, Mondon J-M, Chuet C, et al, "Drug Interactions Between Midecamycin and Cyclosporin," *Nephron*, 1995, 70:136.

Higgins EM, Hughes JR, Snowden S, et al, "Cyclosporin-Induced Periungual Granulation Tissue," *Br J Dermatol*, 1995, 132:829-30.

Hollander AA, Rooij J, Eef GWM, et al, "The Effect of Grapefruit Juice on Cyclosporine and Prednisone Metabolism in Transplant Patients," *Clin Pharmacol Ther*, 1995, 57:318-24.

Honcharik N and Anthone S, "Activated Charcoal in Acute Cyclosporine Overdose," *Lancet*, 1985, 1(8436):1051.

Hughes RL, "Cyclosporine-Related Central Nervous System Toxicity in Cardiac Transplantation," *N Engl J Med*, 1990, 323(6):420-1.

Kabeer MH, Filo RS, Milgrom ML, et al, "Central Pontine Myelinolysis Following Orthotopic Liver Transplant: Association With Cyclosporine Toxicity," *Postgrad Med J*, 1995, 71:239-41.

Kahan BD, "Cyclosporine," *N Engl J Med*, 1989, 321(25):1725-38.

Kino KJ and Wittkowsky AK, "Influence of Bile Acid Replacement on Cyclosporine Absorption in a Patient With Jejunoileal Bypass," *Pharmacotherapy*, 1995, 15(3):350-2.

Ljuti D and Rumboldt Z, "Possible Interaction Between Azithromycin and Cyclosporin: A Case Report," *Nephron*, 1995, 70:130.

McIntyre HD, Menzies B, Rigby R, et al, "Long-Term Bone Loss After Renal Transplantation: Comparison of Immunosuppressive Regimens," *Clin Transpl*, 1995, 9:20-4.

Morales JM, Muðz MA, Fernandez, et al, "Reversable Acute Renal Failure Caused by the Combined Use of Foscarnet and Cyclosporin in Organ Transplanted Patients," *Nephrol Dial Transplant*, 1995, 10(6):882-3.

Passfall J, Schuller I, and Keller F, "Pharmacokinetics of Cyclosporin During Administration of Danazol," *Nephrol Dial Transplant*, 1994, 9:1807-8.

Mernon M, deMagalhace-Silverman M, Bloom EJ, et al, "Reversible Cyclosporine-Induced Cortical Blindness in Allogeneic Bone Marrow Transplant Recipients," *Bone Marrow Transplant*, 1995, 15:283-6.

Scalzini A, Barni C, Stellini R, et al, "Fatal Invasive Aspergillosis During Cyclosporine and Steroids Treatment for Crohn's Disease," *Dig Dis Sci*, 1995, 40(3):528.

Tugwell P, Pincus T, Yocum D, et al, "Combined Therapy With Cyclosporine and Methotrexate in Severe Rheumatoid Arthritis," *N Engl J Med*, 1995, 333:137-41.

Wahlstrom E, Zamora JU, and Teichman S, "Improvement in Cyclosporin-Associated Gingival Hyperplasia With Azithromycin Therapy," *N Engl J Med*, 1995, 332(11):753-4.

Wallemacq PE and Lesne ML, "Accidental Massive I.V. Administration of Cyclosporine in Man," *Drug Intell Clin Pharm*, 1985, 19(1):29-30.

Yee GC and McGuire TR, "Pharmacokinetic Drug Interactions With Cyclosporine," *Clin Pharmacokinet*, 1990, 19(4):319-32 and 19(5):400-15.

Cylert® *see* Pemoline *on page 598*

Cymevene® *see* Ganciclovir *on page 377*

[illegible]t® *see* Moxonidine *on page 541*

[illegible]n® *see* Cyanocobalamin *on page 246*

Cyproheptadine Hydrochloride (si proe hep' ta deen)

Related Information

Antihistamines *on page 129*

CAS Number 129-03-3; 969-33-5; 41354-29-4

Brand Names Klarivitina®; Nuran®; Periactin®; Periactinol®

Use Angioedema, pruritus, urticaria (especially cold-induced urticaria), appetite stimulant, atopic dermatitis; useful in treating Cushing's syndrome, blepharospasm

Mechanism of Action Direct serotonin antagonist with anticholinergic and antihistamine effects

Adverse Reactions

Cardiovascular: Hypotension, palpitations, tachycardia

Central nervous system: Dizziness, fatigue, ataxia, euphoria, seizures, lethargy, hyperthermia

Endocrine & metabolic: Weight gain

Gastrointestinal: Nausea, vomiting, diarrhea

Genitourinary: Urinary retention, dysuria

Ocular: Diplopia, increased intraocular pressure, photosensitivity

Otic: Tinnitus

Respiratory: Bronchoconstriction

Toxicodynamics/Kinetics

Duration of action: 4-6 hours

Metabolism: Hepatic

Half-life: 16 hours

Elimination: Urine (57%) and feces (26%)

Usual Dosage

Children: 0.25 mg/kg/day or 8 mg/m^2/day in 2-3 doses

Adults: Therapeutic dosage range: 4-20 mg/day; usual adult therapeutic dosage range: 12-16 mg/day

Maximum daily adult dose: 0.5 mg/kg

Contraindications Lactation, hypersensitivity to cyproheptadine, narrow-angle glaucoma, symptomatic prostatic enlargement

Warnings Reduce dosage in patients with hepatic insufficiency; use with caution in patients with asthma, hyperthyroidism, stenosing peptic ulcer, bladder neck obstruction, gastrointestinal obstruction, hypertension; not to be used in combination with central nervous system depressants, MAO inhibitors, or ethanol

Dosage Forms

Syrup: 2 mg/5 mL with alcohol 5% (473 mL)

Tablet: 4 mg

Overdosage Treatment Referral and treatment of ingestions >3 times usual dose suggested

Decontamination: Avoid ipecac (except prehospital), charcoal recommended; lavage indicated if obtunded or within 1 hour of ingestion or evidence of gastric hypomotility

Supportive therapy: There is no routine specific treatment; severe life-threatening symptoms may be treated with physostigmine; hypotension is best treated with norepinephrine or phenylephrine; seizures should be treated with benzodiazepines in absence of secondary complications (cardiac ischemia), sinus tachycardia does not require specific therapy; in presence of severe secondary complications, renal failure due to rhabdomyolysis, hemodialysis may be employed; sodium bicarbonate may be of some value in wide complex tachycardias

Test Interactions Increases serum amylase; lowers serum prolactin; reduces hypoglycemia-induced growth hormone secretion; can cause false-positive serum tricyclic antidepressant screens

Drug Interactions

Decreased antidepressant effects of fluoxetine

Increased anticholinergic effect with use of MAO inhibitors

Pregnancy Risk Factor B

Additional Information Lowers serum prolactin levels; should not be administered during breast feeding; also has been used to treat serotonin syndrome induced by the combination of sertraline and isocarboxazid at a dose of 4 mg; can cause dependence

Specific References

Craven JL and Rodin GM, "Cyproheptadine Dependence Associated With an Atypical Somatoform Disorder," *Can J Psychiatry*, 1987, 32(2):143-5.

Herzog DB and Copeland PM, "Eating Disorders," *N Engl J Med*, 1985, 313(5):295-303.

Lappin RI and Auchincloss EL, "Treatment of the Serotonin Syndrome With Cyproheptadine," *N Engl J Med*, 1994, 331(15):1021-2.

Wians FH, Norton JT, and Wirebaugh, "False-Positive Serum Tricyclic Antidepressant Screen With Cyproheptadine," *Clin Chem*, 1993, 39(6):1355-6.

Cystit® *see* Nitrofurantoin *on page 564*

Cystodigin® *see* Digitoxin *on page 283*

Cystospaz® *see* Hyoscyamine Sulfate *on page 415*
Cystospaz-M® *see* Hyoscyamine Sulfate *on page 415*
CYT *see* Cyclophosphamide *on page 249*
Cytomel® *see* Liothyronine Sodium *on page 471*
Cytosafe® *see* Fluorouracil *on page 357*
Cytovene® *see* Ganciclovir *on page 377*
Cytoxan® *see* Cyclophosphamide *on page 249*
d4T *see* Stavudine *on page 706*
DADPS *see* Dapsone *on page 260*
Dagynil® *see* Estrogens, Conjugated *on page 325*
Daktar® *see* Miconazole *on page 530*
Daktarin® *see* Miconazole *on page 530*
Dalalone D.P.® Injection *see* Dexamethasone *on page 266*
Dalalone® Injection *see* Dexamethasone *on page 266*
Dalalone L.A.® Injection *see* Dexamethasone *on page 266*
Dalcaine® *see* Lidocaine Hydrochloride *on page 468*
Dal-E® *see* Vitamin E *on page 798*
Dalmane® *see* Flurazepam Hydrochloride *on page 363*
***d*-Alpha Tocopherol** *see* Vitamin E *on page 798*

Dalteparin (dal te' pa rin)

Brand Names Fragmin®; Fraxiparine®; Sandoparin®

Synonyms Tedelparin Sodium

Use Low molecular weight heparin indicated for deep vein thrombosis (DVT) prophylaxis and prophylaxis of surgical thromboembolic events

Mechanism of Action Low molecular weight heparin analog with a molecular weight of 4000-6000 daltons; the commercial product contains 3% to 15% heparin with a molecular weight <3000 daltons, 65% to 78% with a molecular weight of 3000-8000 daltons and 14% to 26% with a molecular weight >8000 daltons; while dalteparin has been shown to inhibit both factor Xa and factor IIa (thrombin), the antithrombotic effect of dalteparin is characterized by a higher ratio of antifactor Xa to antifactor IIa activity (ratio = 4)

Adverse Reactions
- Cardiovascular: Edema
- Central nervous system: Confusion, fever
- Dermatologic: Ecchymosis, pruritus
- Hematologic: Hemorrhage, thrombocytopenia, hematoma, erythema, hypochromic anemia, coagulopathy
- Gastrointestinal: Nausea
- Miscellaneous: Local irritation, pain

Toxicodynamics/Kinetics
- Distribution: V_d: 3-11 L
- Bioavailability: S.C.: 86%
- Peak serum concentrations: 4 hours
- Half-life, elimination: 2-5 hours (route dependent)
- Elimination: Renal

Usual Dosage S.C.: 2500 IU/day
- Acute venous thromboembolism:
  - I.V. bolus: 2500anti-Xa units
  - Continuous infusion: 15,000 anti-Xa units/24 hours for at least 5 days

Contraindications Active major bleeding or hemophilia; hypersensitivity to heparin or pork products; drug-induced thrombocytopenia

Warnings Heparin-induced thrombocytopenia, bacterial endocarditis, congenital or acquired bleeding disorders, active ulceration and angiodysplastic gastrointestinal disease, hemorrhagic stroke, status post brain, spinal, or ophthalmological surgery, uncontrolled arterial hypertension, recent CNS surgery, elderly, and lactation. Never give by intramuscular injection. Conventional heparin has possibly been associated with an increased risk of bleeding in females >60 years of age; it is unknown whether low molecular weight heparins pose the same risk; these agents should be used with caution in this population.

Dosage Forms Injection, preservative free: Anti-factor Xa 2500 units/0.2 mL (16 mL)

Reference Range Therapeutic plasma anti-Xa levels (antifactor Xa): 0.1-0.6 units/mL (antithrombotic activity); activated partial thromboplastin time (APTT) is not considered useful for dalteparin monitoring

Overdosage Treatment
- Supportive therapy: Protamine can be used for severe bleeding upon withdrawal of heparin (1 mg of protamine for every 1 mg of dalteparin [100 units] by slow I.V. push up to 50 mg)

Enhancement of elimination: While hemodialysis is not beneficial, exchange transfusion has been used successfully in a neonate and plasma exchange has been used successfully in four older patients for thrombocytopenia

Antidote(s)

Protamine Sulfate *on page 1463*

Drug Interactions Increased toxicity with oral anticoagulants, platelet inhibitors; increased risk of bleeding with aspirin use

Pregnancy Risk Factor B

Pregnancy Implications Does not cross the placenta

Monitoring Parameters Platelets, occult blood, PTT, and anti-Xa activity, if available

Nursing Implications Not intended for I.M. administration

Additional Information Molecular weight: 5000; sulfur content: 11%

Specific References

Harenberg J, "Pharmacology of Low Molecular Weight Heparins," *Semin Thromb Hemost*, 1990, 16(Suppl):12-8.

Thomas DP, "Bleeding After Low-Molecular Weight Heparin," *Lancet*, 1992, 339(8801):1119.

Verstraete M, "Pharmacotherapeutic Aspects of Unfractionated and Low Molecular Weight Heparins," *Drugs*, 1990, 40(4):498-530.

Danatrol® *see* Danazol *on this page*

Danazol (da' na zole)

CAS Number 17230-88-5

Brand Names Cyclomen®; Danatrol®; Danocrine®; Danol®; Ladazol®; Mastodanatrol®; Winobanin®

Use Treatment of endometriosis, fibrocystic breast disease, and hereditary angioedema; also used for refractory thrombocytopenic purpura in children

Unlabeled uses: Precocious puberty, gynecomastia, menorrhagia, idiopathic immune thrombocytopenia, lupus-associated thrombocytopenia, and autoimmune hemolytic anemia

Mechanism of Action Suppresses pituitary output of follicle-stimulating hormone and luteinizing hormone that causes regression and atrophy of normal and ectopic endometrial tissue; decreases rate of growth of abnormal breast tissue; reduces attacks associated with hereditary angioedema by increasing levels of C4 component of complement

Adverse Reactions

Cardiovascular: Hypertension, tachycardia

Central nervous system: Anxiety, depression

Dermatologic: Oily skin, acne, hirsutism, photosensitivity, cystic acne, seborrheic dermatitis, alopecia, erythema multiforme

Endocrine & metabolic: Amenorrhea, hyperglycemia, weight gain

Gastrointestinal: Pancreatitis

Genitourinary: Monilial vaginitis, testicular atrophy, enlarged clitoris, cystitis

Hematologic: Thrombocytopenia, thrombocytosis, hypercalcemia

Hepatic: Cholestatic jaundice

Neuromuscular & skeletal: Weakness

Otic: Hearing loss

Miscellaneous: Voice deepening, breakthrough bleeding, irregular menstrual periods, purpura, hematuria, hot flashes, decreased breast size, edema, virilization, clitoral hypertrophy, hypoestrogenism, bleeding gums, carpal tunnel syndrome, benign intracranial hypertension, hypogonadism, porphyrinogenic, peliosis of spleen and liver

Signs & Symptoms of Acute Overdose Systemic lupus erythematosus (SLE)

Toxicodynamics/Kinetics

Onset of therapeutic effect: Within 4 weeks following daily doses

Metabolism: Extensive hepatic metabolism, primarily to 2-hydroxymethylethisterone

Half-life: 4.5 hours (variable)

Time to peak serum concentration: Within 2 hours

Elimination: Excreted in urine

Usual Dosage

Children: Refractory thrombocytopenic purpura: 20-30 mg/kg/day in divided doses, up to 800 mg/day

Adults: Oral:

- Endometriosis: 100-400 mg twice daily for 3-6 months (may extend to 9 months)
- Fibrocystic breast disease: 50-200 mg twice daily for 2-6 months
- Hereditary angioedema: 400-600 mg/day in 2-3 divided doses

Contraindications Undiagnosed genital bleeding, hypersensitivity to danazol or any component, significant renal, hepatic, or cardiac impairment; pregnancy and lactation

Warnings Use with caution in patients with seizure disorders, migraine, impaired hepatic, renal, or cardiac disease; risk of bleeding increases in hemophilia

(Continued)

Danazol *(Continued)*

Dosage Forms Capsule: 50 mg, 100 mg, 200 mg

Reference Range Oral dose of 400 mg results in a peak plasma level of 0.08 ng/mL

Overdosage Treatment

Decontamination: Emesis with ipecac or lavage; activated charcoal with cathartic

Test Interactions Lowers FSH and LH; increased serum glucagon; decreased serum thyroxine levels

Drug Interactions

Decreased effect: Decreased insulin requirements

Increased toxicity: Warfarin may cause an anticoagulant effect; increased carbamazepine levels, cyclosporine (nephrotoxicity and hepatitis); possible increased tacrolimus levels

Inhibits carbamazepine metabolism; inhibition of clomiphene response

Increases cyclosporine levels; hypercalcemia when given with alfacalcidol

Pregnancy Risk Factor X

Pregnancy Implications Premature bone maturation, masculinization of urogenital sinus, clitoromegaly before 12th week of gestation in the female fetus; after the first trimester, clitoral hypertrophy would be primary effect in the female fetus

Monitoring Parameters Hepatic impairment

Patient Information Notify physician if masculinity effects occur

Nursing Implications Ensure patient is not pregnant before therapy

Specific References

Gately LE 3d and Andes WA, "Danazol and Erythema Multiforme," *Ann Intern Med*, 1988, 109(1):85.

Makdisi WJ, Cherian R, Vanveldhuizen PJ, et al, "Fatal Peliosis of the Liver and Spleen in a Patient With Agnogenic Myeloid Metaplasia Treated With Danazol," *Am J Gastroenterol*, 1995, 90(2):317-8.

Saenger P, "Abnormal Sex Differentiation," *J Pediatr*, 1984, 104(1):1-17.

Weinblatt ME, Kochen J, and Ortega J, "Danazol for Children With Immune Thrombocytopenic Purpura," *Am J Dis Child*, 1988, 142(12):1317-9.

Danlene® *see* Dantrolene Sodium *on this page*

Danocrine® *see* Danazol *on previous page*

Danol® *see* Danazol *on previous page*

Dantamacrin® *see* Dantrolene Sodium *on this page*

Dantralen® *see* Dantrolene Sodium *on this page*

Dantrium® *see* Dantrolene Sodium *on this page*

Dantrolene Sodium (dan' troe leen)

Related Information

Therapeutic Drugs Associated With Hallucinations *on page 1558-1559*

CAS Number 7261-97-4; 14663-23-1; 24868-20-0

Brand Names Danlene®; Dantamacrin®; Dantralen®; Dantrium®

Use Treatment of malignant hyperthermia, neuroleptic malignant syndrome, and serotonin syndrome; considered possibly beneficial for fever and rigidity due to carbon monoxide, cocaine poisoning, alcohol withdrawal "ecstasy"; hyperthermia due to baclofen withdrawal

Mechanism of Action Acts directly on skeletal muscle by interfering with release of calcium ion from the sarcoplasmic reticulum; prevents or reduces the increase in myoplasmic calcium ion concentration that activates the acute catabolic processes associated with malignant hyperthermia

Adverse Reactions

Cardiovascular/respiratory: Pleural effusion with pericarditis

Central nervous system: Convulsions, drowsiness, dizziness, lightheadedness, confusion, headache, fatigue, speech disturbances, tiredness, chills, fever, insomnia, nervousness, mental depression, auditory and visual hallucinations

Dermatologic: Rash

Gastrointestinal: Diarrhea, nausea, vomiting, severe constipation, anorexia, stomach cramps

Genitourinary: Urinary retention

Hepatic: Hepatitis, hepatitis

Neuromuscular & skeletal: Muscle asthenia

Ocular: Visual disturbances, diplopia

Otic: Ototoxicity, tinnitus

Renal: Hematuria

Respiratory: Apnea, respiratory depression

Miscellaneous: Slurred speech, lymphocytic lymphoma

Signs & Symptoms of Acute Overdose Lethargy, respiratory depression, pericarditis, nocturia, insomnia, hematuria, disorientation, neutropenia, jaundice, lightheadedness, crystalluria, seizures, hypotension

Toxicodynamics/Kinetics

Absorption: Slow and incomplete from gastrointestinal tract (70%)

Protein binding: Extensive

Metabolism: Slow in liver to weakly active metabolites
Half-life: 8.7 hours
Time to peak plasma concentration: 5 hours
Elimination: 25% excreted in urine as metabolites and unchanged drug, 45% to 50% excreted in feces via bile

Usual Dosage

Spasticity: Oral:

Children: Initial: 0.5 mg/kg/dose twice daily, increase frequency to 3-4 times/day at 4- to 7-day intervals, then increase dose by 0.5 mg/kg to a maximum of 3 mg/kg/dose 2-4 times/day up to 400 mg/day

Adults: 25 mg/day to start, increase frequency to 2-4 times/day, then increase dose by 25 mg every 4-7 days to a maximum of 100 mg 2-4 times/day or 400 mg/day

Malignant hyperthermia: Children and Adults:

Oral: 4-8 mg/kg/day in 4 divided doses

Preoperative prophylaxis: Begin 1-2 days prior to surgery with last dose 3-4 hours prior to surgery

I.V.: 1 mg/kg; may repeat dose up to cumulative dose of 10 mg/kg (mean effective dose is 2.5 mg/kg), then switch to oral dosage

Preoperative: 2.5 mg/kg ~$1\frac{1}{4}$ hours prior to anesthesia and infused over 1 hour with additional doses as needed and individualized

Contraindications Active hepatic disease; should not be used where spasticity is used to maintain posture or balance

Warnings Use with caution in patients with impaired cardiac function or impaired pulmonary function; has potential for hepatitis; overt hepatitis has been most frequently observed between the third and twelfth month of therapy; hepatic injury appears to be greater in females and in patients >35 years of age

Dosage Forms

Capsule: 25 mg, 50 mg, 100 mg
Powder for injection: 20 mg

Stability Reconstitute vial by adding 60 mL of sterile water for injection USP (**not bacteriostatic water for injection**); protect from light; use within 6 hours; avoid glass bottles for I.V. infusion

Overdosage Treatment

Decontamination: Lavage/activated charcoal with cathartic; do not use ipecac
Supportive therapy: Hypotension can be treated with isotonic I.V. fluids with the patient placed in the Trendelenburg position; dopamine or norepinephrine can be given if hypotension is refractory to above therapy

Antidote(s)

Dopamine Hydrochloride *on page 1418*
Norepinephrine Bitartrate *on page 1451*

Test Interactions Increases serum AST (SGOT), ALT (SGPT), alkaline phosphatase, LDH, BUN, and total serum bilirubin

Drug Interactions Increased toxicity with estrogens (hepatitis), CNS depressants (sedation), MAO inhibitors, phenothiazine, clindamycin (↑ neuromuscular blockade), verapamil (hyperkalemia and cardiac depression), theophylline (seizures)

Pregnancy Risk Factor C

Monitoring Parameters Motor performance should be monitored for therapeutic outcomes; nausea, vomiting, and liver function tests should be monitored for potential hepatitis

Patient Information Avoid unnecessary exposure to sunlight (or use sunscreen, protective clothing); avoid alcohol and other CNS depressants; patients should use caution while driving or performing other tasks requiring alertness

Nursing Implications 36 vials needed for adequate hyperthermia therapy; exercise caution at meals on the day of administration because difficulty swallowing and choking have been reported

Specific References

Britt BA, "Dantrolene," *Can J Anaesth*, 1984, 31(1):61-75.

Guerrero RM and Shifrar KA, "Diagnosis and Treatment of Neuroleptic Malignant Syndrome," *Clin Pharm*, 1988, 7(9):697-701.

May DC, Morris SW, Stewart RM, et al, "Neuroleptic Malignant Syndrome: Response to Dantrolene Sodium," *Ann Intern Med*, 1983, 98(2):183-4.

Paloucek FP, Erickson TE, Lundquist S, et al, "Oral Dantrolene Ingestion: A Case Series (Abstract)," *Vet Hum Toxicol*, 1991, 33:362.

Rosenberg MR and Green M, "Neuroleptic Malignant Syndrome. Review of Response to Therapy," *Arch Intern Med*, 1989, 149(9):1927-31.

Rubin AS and Zablocki AD, "Hyperkalemia, Verapamil, and Dantrolene," *Anesthesiology*, 1987, 66(2):248-9.

Tayeb OS, "A Serious Interaction of Dantrolene and Theophylline," *Vet Hum Toxicol*, 1990, 32(5):442-3.

Ward A, Chaffman MO, and Sorkin EM, "Dantrolene: A Review of Its Pharmacodynamic and Pharmacokinetic Properties and Therapeutic Use in Malignant Hyperthermia, the Neuroleptic Malignant Syndrome and an Update of Its Use in Muscle Spasticity," *Drugs*, 1986, 32(2):130-68.

Daonil® *see* Glyburide *on page 384*

Dapa® [OTC] *see* Acetaminophen *on page 79*

Dapsone (dap' sone)

Related Information

Therapeutic Drugs Associated With Hallucinations *on page 1558-1559*

CAS Number 80-08-0

Brand Names Avlosulfon®

Synonyms DADPS; DDS; Diaminodiphenylsulfone; Diaphenylsulfon; Diphenason; Sulphadine; Sulphon-mere

Use Treatment of leprosy, dermatitis herpetiformis, vasculitis, pemphigus, and generalized pustular psoriasis; has been given for treatment of brown recluse spider bites; prophylaxis and treatment of *Pneumocystis carinii*

Mechanism of Action Dapsone is a sulfone antimicrobial; mechanism of action of the sulfones is similar to that of the sulfonamides. Sulfonamides are competitive antagonists of para-aminobenzoic acid (PABA) and prevent normal bacterial utilization of PABA for the synthesis of folic acid.

Adverse Reactions

Central nervous system: Insomnia, psychosis, dizziness, headache, visual hallucinations

Dermatologic: Exfoliative dermatitis

Gastrointestinal: Nausea, vomiting

Hematologic: Hemolysis, methemoglobinemia, neutropenia, agranulocytosis, aplastic anemia, thrombocytosis

Hepatic: Hepatitis, cholestatic jaundice

Neuromuscular & skeletal: Paresthesia

Ocular: Blurred vision

Otic: Ototoxicity, tinnitus

Signs & Symptoms of Acute Overdose Can appear in a few minutes to within 24 hours following ingestion with methemoglobinemia and CNS stimulation being the most common; tachycardia, hypotension, dyspnea, hyperventilation, insomnia, aggressive behavior, hallucinations, oliguria, coma (with large overdose), paresthesia (distal motor axonopathy), toxic epidermal necrolysis, tubular necrosis, vomiting, nephrotic syndrome, elevated bilirubin, erythema multiforme, erythema, photosensitivity, cyanosis, elevated transaminases, hematuria have been reported in the overdose situation; methemoglobinemia is a common finding; sulfhemoglobinemia and aplastic anemia are rare; hemolysis with the appearance of Heinz bodies is common

Toxicodynamics/Kinetics

Absorption: Oral: 70% to 80%

Distribution: V_d: 1.5 L/kg; throughout total body water and present in all tissues, especially liver and kidney

Protein binding: Dapsone and its metabolites are highly protein bound (73%)

Metabolism: Acetylated to monoacetyl dapsone and can be deacetylated to dapsone; there are genetic determinators for a "fast" or "slow" acetylator within the population and may be limited to paresthesia. Dapsone is also hydroxylated to N-hydroxydapsone (NOH-dapsone) which may be responsible for the anemia

Half-life, elimination: 30 hours (range: 10-50 hours)

Time to peak serum concentration: Within 2-6 hours

Elimination: NOH-dapsone excreted in urine; 10% of dapsone is found in bile

Usual Dosage Oral:

Children: Leprosy: 1-2 mg/kg/24 hours; maximum: 100 mg/day

Adults:

Leprosy: 50-100 mg/day for 3-10 years

Dermatitis herpetiformis: Start at 50 mg/day, increase to 300 mg/day, or higher to achieve full control, reduce dosage to minimum level as soon as possible

PCP prophylaxis: 100 mg every other day or 50 mg/day

Brown recluse spider bites: 100 mg twice daily for 14 days

Dosing adjustment in renal impairment: Necessary, but no specific guidelines are available

Contraindications Hypersensitivity to dapsone or any component

Warnings Use with caution in patients with severe anemia, G-6-PD deficiency; hypersensitivity to other sulfonamides

Dosage Forms Tablet: 25 mg, 100 mg

Stability Protect from light

Reference Range Levels do not correlate with symptoms but may be used to confirm diagnosis; therapeutic concentrations: 0.5-5 µg/mL; toxic effects can occur at levels >10 µg/mL

Overdosage Treatment

Decontamination: Emesis, lavage/activated charcoal with cathartic

Supportive therapy: Monitor methemoglobin, CBC, blood smear, platelets, urinalysis, liver function tests, and ABGs; hemolysis may require transfusion; methylene blue 1-2 mg/kg (up to 4 mg/kg) may be required for symptomatic patients or those with a methemoglobin >30%; methylene blue may precipitate hemolytic anemia in large doses, in patients with G-6-PD deficiency and in one case of dapsone overdose; cimetidine may decrease the rate of toxic metabolite although has not been tried in the overdose situation

Enhanced elimination: Charcoal hemoperfusion may be useful (one case report) in patients who have clinical deterioration despite supportive care; hemodialysis has also been reported to decrease the half-life; plasma exchange has been utilized with varying degrees of success; multiple doses of activated charcoal enhance elimination and is considered treatment of choice and may be required for as long as 72 hours

Antidote(s)

Methylene Blue *on page 1444*

Drug Interactions

Decreased effect with para-aminobenzoic acid; decreased effect/levels with rifampin

Increased toxicity with folic acid antagonists

Pregnancy Risk Factor C

Pregnancy Implications Does cross placenta but there have been cases with normal pregnancy outcomes with mothers taking dapsone; however, because it has the capacity to induce methemoglobinemia and hemolytic anemia, it has been suggested to limit its use in pregnancy; overdose in pregnancy has not been reported; secreted in milk with a few reports of neonatal hemolytic anemia

Monitoring Parameters Monitor patient for signs of jaundice and hemolysis

Patient Information Frequent blood tests are required during early therapy; discontinue if rash develops and contact physician if persistent sore throat, fever, malaise, or fatigue occurs; may cause photosensitivity

Specific References

Hansen DG, Challoner KR, and Smith DE, "Dapsone Intoxication: Two Case Reports," *J Emerg Med*, 1994, 12(3):347-51.

McGoldrick MD and Bailie GR, "Severe Accidental Dapsone Overdose," *Am J Emerg Med*, 1995, 13:414-5.

Tracqui A, Gutbub AM, Kintz P, et al, "A Case of Acute Dapsone Poisoning. Toxicological Data and Review of the Literature," *J Anal Toxicol*, 1995, 19:229-35.

Wynn RF, Laing RB, and Leen CL, "Case Report of Dapsone-Related Thrombocytosis in an AIDS Patient," *Am J Med*, 1995, 98:602.

Darammon® *see* Ammonium Chloride *on page 118*

Daraprim® *see* Pyrimethamine *on page 664*

Darkene® *see* Flunitrazepam *on page 354*

Darvocet-N® *see* Propoxyphene and Acetaminophen *on page 656*

Darvocet-N® 100 *see* Propoxyphene and Acetaminophen *on page 656*

Darvon® *see* Propoxyphene *on page 655*

Darvon-N® *see* Propoxyphene *on page 655*

Datril® [OTC] *see* Acetaminophen *on page 79*

Dayto Himbin® *see* Yohimbine Hydrochloride *on page 805*

Dazamide® *see* Acetazolamide *on page 83*

DC 240® Softgel® [OTC] *see* Docusate *on page 297*

dCF *see* Pentostatin *on page 606*

ddC *see* Zalcitabine *on page 805*

ddCyd *see* Zalcitabine *on page 805*

DDI *see* Didanosine *on page 278*

DDS *see* Dapsone *on previous page*

Deaner® *see* Deanol *on this page*

Deanol

CAS Number 108-01-0; 3342-61-8; 968-46-7; 71-79-4

UN Number 2051

Brand Names Acumen®; Atrol®; Deaner®; Elevan®; Panclar®

Synonyms Demanol; 2-Dimethylaminoethanol

Use Psychostimulant, antispasmodic; not available in U.S. since 1983; has been used to reverse levodopa-induced dyskinesias; used for hyperkinetic children

Mechanism of Action Choline precursor which acts as a stimulant by enhancing central acetylcholine formation; dimethylaminoethanol salt of para-acetamidobenzoic acid

Adverse Reactions

Cardiovascular: Orthostatic hypotension (rare)

Central nervous system: Headache, insomnia, trismus

(Continued)

Deanol *(Continued)*

Dermatologic: Pruritus, rash
Gastrointestinal: Constipation

Usual Dosage

Reduce levodopa dyskinesias: Initial: 100 mg 3 times/day for 5 days; can increase dosage from 500-900 mg/day; improvement noted in 10-94 days

Hyperactivity syndrome: Children: Recommended daily dosage: 300 mg

Contraindications Seizures disorder

Dosage Forms

Injection: 1.5 g (15 mL), 3 g (15 mL)

Tablet:

- Deanol: 100 mg
- Deanol acetamidobenzoate: 100 mg
- Deanol benzilate: 0.3 mg

Overdosage Treatment

Decontamination: Lavage/activated charcoal

Supportive therapy: Although there is no data regarding its use, atropine may theoretically be useful to treat acetylcholine excess

Drug Interactions Avoid concomitant use of amphetamines

Additional Information Combined with various salts; often available in combination with PABA; if this combination is used in doses described above, must monitor for PABA toxicity, efficacy for uses described above is questionable

Specific References

Miller E, "Deanol in the Treatment of Levodopa-Induced Dyskinesias," *Neurology*, 1974, 24:116-9.

Decadron® *see* Dexamethasone *on page 266*

Decadron®-LA Injection *see* Dexamethasone *on page 266*

Decadron® Phosphate *see* Dexamethasone *on page 266*

Decadron® Phosphate Nasal Turbinaire® *see* Dexamethasone *on page 266*

Decadron® Phosphate Respihaler® Oral Inhaler *see* Dexamethasone *on page 266*

Decaject® Injection *see* Dexamethasone *on page 266*

Decaject-LA® Injection *see* Dexamethasone *on page 266*

Decaspray® Topical Aerosol *see* Dexamethasone *on page 266*

Decentan® *see* Perphenazine *on page 609*

Decofed® Syrup [OTC] *see* Pseudoephedrine *on page 661*

Decrelip® *see* Gemfibrozil *on page 378*

Dehist® *see* Brompheniramine Maleate *on page 165*

Dehydrobenzperidol *see* Droperidol *on page 307*

Deiten® *see* Nitrendipine *on page 562*

Dekasol® Injection *see* Dexamethasone *on page 266*

Dekasol-L.A.® Injection *see* Dexamethasone *on page 266*

Delatest® Injection *see* Testosterone *on page 729*

Delatestryl® *see* Testosterone *on page 729*

Delaxin® *see* Methocarbamol *on page 513*

Delix® *see* Ramipril *on page 673*

Delsym® [OTC] *see* Dextromethorphan Hydrobromide *on page 270*

Deltacortisone *see* Prednisone *on page 639*

Deltadehydrocortisone *see* Prednisone *on page 639*

Deltasone® *see* Prednisone *on page 639*

Demadex® *see* Torsemide *on page 761*

Demanol *see* Deanol *on previous page*

Demerol® *see* Meperidine Hydrochloride *on page 499*

Demetrin® *see* Prazepam *on page 637*

Demolox® *see* Amoxapine *on page 119*

Demorphan *see* Dextromethorphan Hydrobromide *on page 270*

Denan® *see* Simvastatin *on page 697*

Dendritis *see* Sodium Chloride *on page 698*

Deodorized Opium Tincture *see* Opium Tincture *on page 580*

Deoxycoformycin *see* Pentostatin *on page 606*

2'-deoxycoformycin *see* Pentostatin *on page 606*

Depakene® *see* Valproic Acid and Derivatives *on page 782*

Depakote® *see* Valproic Acid and Derivatives *on page 782*

Deponit® *see* Nitroglycerin *on page 566*

Depotest® Injection *see* Testosterone *on page 729*

Depo®-Testosterone Injection *see* Testosterone *on page 729*

Deprax® *see* Trazodone Hydrochloride *on page 765*

Deralin® *see* Propranolol Hydrochloride *on page 657*

Derbac-M® *see* Malathion (Topical Lotion) *on page 489*

Dermacaine® *see* Dibucaine *on page 275*

Dermoplast® [OTC] *see* Benzocaine *on page 149*

DES *see* Diethylstilbestrol *on page 280*

Desace® *see* Deslanoside *on next page*

Desacetyl-Lanatoside C *see* Deslanoside *on next page*

Desaci® *see* Deslanoside *on next page*

Desconex® *see* Loxapine *on page 486*

Desiccated Thyroid *see* Thyroid *on page 749*

Desipramine Hydrochloride (dess ip' ra meen)

Related Information

Antidepressant Agents Comparison *on page 1639*

CAS Number 50-47-5; 58-28-6

Brand Names Nebril®; Norpamin®; Nortimil®; Pertofrane®; Pertofrin®; Sertofren®

Synonyms Desmethylimipramine Hydrochloride

Use Treatment of various forms of depression, often in conjunction with psychotherapy; as an analgesic in chronic pain, peripheral neuropathies

Mechanism of Action Increases the synaptic concentration of serotonin and/or norepinephrine in the central nervous system by inhibition of their reuptake by the presynaptic neuronal membrane

Adverse Reactions

Cardiovascular: Cardiac arrhythmias

Central nervous system: Sedation, psychosis, confusion, dizziness, excitation, associated with falls, restlessness

Dermatologic: Photosensitivity

Endocrine & metabolic: Syndrome of inappropriate antidiuretic hormone, weight gain

Gastrointestinal: Constipation, nausea, vomiting, craving sweets, dry mouth, bowel ischemia

Genitourinary: Urinary retention

Hematologic: Blood dyscrasias

Hepatic: Hepatitis

Ocular: Blurred vision, diplopia, photophobia, intraocular pressure (increased), mydriasis

Otic: Ototoxicity, tinnitus

Miscellaneous: Hypersensitivity reactions

Signs & Symptoms of Acute Overdose Agitation, dental erosion, thrombocytopenia, photosensitivity, neuroleptic malignant syndrome, jaundice, hypertension, intraocular pressure (increased), dementia, coma, impotence, eosinophilia, dry mucous membranes, asystole, nystagmus, Q-T prolongation, confusion, hallucinations, hyperthermia, urinary retention, CNS depression, cyanosis, dry mucous membranes, leukopenia; neutropenia; agranulocytosis; granulocytopenia

Toxicodynamics/Kinetics

Onset of action: 2-3 weeks

Absorption: Well absorbed from gastrointestinal tract

Distribution: V_d: 33-42 L/kg; distributed widely into body including CNS

Protein binding: 92%

Metabolism: In the liver (hydroxylation and conjugation)

Half-life: Adults: 12-57 hours

Elimination: 70% excreted in urine; plasma clearance: 24 mL/hour/kg

Usual Dosage Oral (not recommended for use in children <12 years):

Adolescents: Initial: 25-50 mg/day; gradually increase to 100 mg/day in single or divided doses; maximum: 150 mg/day

Adults: Initial: 75 mg/day in divided doses; increase gradually to 150-200 mg/day in divided or single dose; maximum: 300 mg/day

(Continued)

Desipramine Hydrochloride *(Continued)*

Contraindications Hypersensitivity to desipramine (cross-sensitivity with other tricyclic antidepressants may occur); patients receiving MAO inhibitors within past 14 days; narrow-angle glaucoma

Warnings Some formulations contain tartrazine which may cause allergic reaction; do not discontinue abruptly in patients receiving long-term high-dose therapy; use with caution in patients with cardiovascular disease, conduction disturbances, urinary retention, seizure disorders, hyperthyroidism, or those receiving thyroid replacement

Dosage Forms

Capsule (Pertofrane®): 25 mg, 50 mg

Tablet (Norpramin®): 10 mg, 25 mg, 50 mg, 75 mg, 100 mg, 150 mg

Reference Range

Therapeutic: 150-300 ng/mL (SI: 560-1125 nmol/L)

Possible toxicity: >300 ng/mL (SI: >1070 nmol/L)

Toxic: >1000 ng/mL (SI: >3750 nmol/L)

Overdosage Treatment

Decontamination: Lavage/activated charcoal with cathartic; multiple dosing of activated charcoal is more effective

Supportive therapy: Lavage within 6 hours of ingestion; following initiation of essential overdose management, toxic symptoms should be treated. Ventricular arrhythmias often respond to phenytoin 15-20 mg/kg (adults) with concurrent systemic alkalinization (sodium bicarbonate 0.5-2 mEq/kg I.V.). Arrhythmias unresponsive to this therapy may respond to lidocaine 1 mg/kg I.V. followed by a titrated infusion. Seizures usually respond to lorazepam or diazepam I.V. boluses (5-10 mg for adults up to 30 mg or 0.25-0.4 mg/kg/dose for children up to 10 mg/dose). If seizures are unresponsive or recur, phenytoin or phenobarbital may be required. Phenytoin is effective to decrease QRS complex interval. Do not use bretylium in hypotensive patients. Extracorporeal membrane oxygenation for 60 hours has been used in an infant with some success for support of myocardial dysfunction

Antidote(s)

Sodium Bicarbonate *on page 1467*

Test Interactions Increases glucose

Drug Interactions May decrease effects of guanethidine and clonidine; may increase effects of CNS depressants, adrenergic agents, anticholinergic agents; with MAO inhibitors, fever, tachycardia, hypertension, seizures, and death may occur; interactions similar to other tricyclics may occur

Pregnancy Risk Factor C

Pregnancy Implications Distributes into breast milk

Monitoring Parameters Blood pressure, heart rate, mental status, weight, EKG for QRS widening

Patient Information Avoid alcohol ingestion; do not discontinue medication abruptly; may cause urine to turn blue-green; may cause drowsiness; avoid unnecessary exposure to sunlight

Nursing Implications Monitor blood pressure and pulse rate prior to and during initial therapy; may increase appetite

Additional Information May unmask pheochromocytoma

Specific References

Goodwin DA, Lally KP, and Null DM Jr, "Corporeal Membrane Oxygenation Support for Cardiac Dysfunction From Tricyclic Antidepressant Overdose," *Crit Care Med*, 1993, 21:625-7.

Riddle MA, Geller B, and Ryan N, "Another Sudden Death in a Child Treated With Desipramine," *J Am Acad Child Adolesc Psychiatry*, 1993, 32(4):792-7.

Tran P, Panacek EA, Rhee KJ, et al, "Is Norepinephrine More Efficacious Than Dopamine in Reversing Hypotension Caused by Cyclic Antidepressant Overdose?" *Ann Emerg Med*, 1995, 25(1):128-30.

Wallace DE, "Bowel Ischemia in Two Patients Following Tricyclic Antidepressant Overdose," *Vet Hum Toxicol*, 1989, 31:377.

Ware MR, "Tricyclic Antidepressant Overdose: Pharmacology and Treatment," *South Med J*, 1987, 80(11):1410-5.

Desitin® *see* Zinc Oxide *on page 813*

Deslanoside (des lan' oh side)

CAS Number 17598-65-1

Brand Names Cedilanid-D®; Desace®; Desaci®; Verdiana®

Synonyms Desacetyl-Lanatoside C

Use Rapid digitalizing effect in emergency treatment of congestive heart failure, paroxysmal atrial tachycardia, fibrillation (atrial) and flutter

Adverse Reactions

Cardiovascular: Sinus bradycardia, A-V block, S-A block, atrial or nodal ectopic beats, ventricular arrhythmias, bigeminy, trigeminy, atrial tachycardia with A-V block

Central nervous system: Drowsiness, fatigue, drowsiness, neuralgia, dizziness, disorientation, chorea (extrapyramidal), visual hallucinations, paranoia, headache

Endocrine & metabolic: Toxicity is enhanced by hypokalemia

Gastrointestinal: Vomiting, nausea, feeding intolerance, abdominal pain, diarrhea

Ocular: Blurred vision, halos, yellow or green vision, diplopia, photophobia, flashing lights

Signs & Symptoms of Acute Overdose Hyperkalemia, hypokalemia, neuropathy (peripheral), arrhythmias, tachycardia (ventricular), A-V block, fibrillation (ventricular) or asystole, vision color changes (blue tinge), vision color changes (green tinge), vision color changes (red tinge), vision color changes (yellow tinge); hypotension

Toxicodynamics/Kinetics Half-life: 33 hours

Usual Dosage I.M., I.V.:

Children:

Neonates, premature and full-term: 22 mcg divided into 2-3 doses every 3-4 hours

2 weeks to 3 years: 25 mcg/kg divided into 2-3 doses every 3-4 hours

>3 years: 22.5 mcg/kg divided into 2-3 doses every 3-4 hours

Children and Adults: Highly individualized

Adults: Loading dose: 1.2-1.6 mg in 2 divided doses over 24 hours

Contraindications Known hypersensitivity to deslanoside, patients who have received digitalis preparation with previous 2-3 weeks, tachycardia (ventricular) or fibrillation, severe pulmonary disease, idiopathic hypertrophic subaortic stenosis

Warnings Use with caution in patients with hypoxia, hypothyroidism, acute myocarditis, impaired renal function

Dosage Forms Injection: 0.2 mg/mL (2 mL)

Reference Range

Therapeutic: 0.5-2.0 ng/mL (SI: 0.6-2.6 nmol/L); Adults: <0.5 ng/mL (SI: <0.6 nmol/L) probably indicates underdigitalization unless there are special circumstances

Toxic: >2.0 ng/mL (SI: >2.6 nmol/L)

Fatal: >3.5 ng/mL (>4.8 nmol/L)

Overdosage Treatment

Decontamination: Lavage/activated charcoal with cathartic; whole bowel irrigation may be useful

Supportive therapy: Antidote: Life-threatening digoxin toxicity is treated with Digibind®; phenytoin, magnesium, and lidocaine are useful for arrhythmias; atropine is useful for bradycardia; avoid quinidine, bretylium, or cardioversion

Enhancement of elimination: Multiple dosing of activated charcoal may be useful; hemodialysis/hemoperfusion is ineffective

Test Interactions Digibind® will increase total serum digoxin level about 50-fold; digoxin-like immunoreactive substance (DLIS) which is an endogenous natriuretic substance may cause false elevation

Diagnostic Tests/Procedures

Digoxin, Blood *on page 1250*

Pregnancy Risk Factor C

Monitoring Parameters Routine serum level monitoring not recommended but is indicated to rule out toxicity, serum electrolytes (potassium, magnesium, calcium), heart rate; monitor blood pressure and EKG closely

Specific References

Bhatia SJS and Smith TW, "Digitalis Toxicity: Mechanisms, Diagnosis, and Management," *J Card Surg*, 1987, 2(4):453-65.

Woolf AD, Wenger TL, Smith TW, et al, "Results of Multicenter Studies of Digoxin-Specific Antibody Fragments in Managing Digitalis Intoxication in the Pediatric Population," *Am J Emerg Med*, 1991, 9(2 Suppl 1):16-20.

Desmethylimipramine Hydrochloride *see* Desipramine Hydrochloride *on page 263*

Desoxyephedrine Hydrochloride *see* Methamphetamine Hydrochloride *on page 510*

Desoxyn® *see* Methamphetamine Hydrochloride *on page 510*

Desoxyphenobarbital *see* Primidone *on page 641*

De'suric® *see* Benzbromarone *on page 148*

Desyrel® *see* Trazodone Hydrochloride *on page 765*

Detensiel® *see* Bisoprolol Fumarate *on page 157*

Devrom® [OTC] *see* Bismuth Subgallate *on page 157*

Dexacen® Injection *see* Dexamethasone *on next page*

Dexacen® LA Injection *see* Dexamethasone *on next page*

Dex-A-Diet® [OTC] *see* Phenylpropanolamine Hydrochloride *on page 622*

Dexametasone *see* Dexamethasone *on this page*

Dexamethasone (dex a meth' a sone)

Related Information

Doses and Administration of Several Frequently Used Antiemetic Agents *on page 1641*

CAS Number 50-02-2; 1177-87-3; 2265-64-7; 312-93-6; 3936-02-5; 2392-39-4

Brand Names Aeroseb-Dex® Topical Aerosol; AK-Dex® Ophthalmic; Dalalone D.P.® Injection; Dalalone® Injection; Dalalone L.A.® Injection; Decadron®; Decadron®-LA Injection; Decadron® Phosphate; Decadron® Phosphate Nasal Turbinaire®; Decadron® Phosphate Respihaler® Oral Inhaler; Decaject® Injection; Decaject-LA® Injection; Decaspray® Topical Aerosol; Dekasol® Injection; Dekasol-L.A.® Injection; Dexacen® Injection; Dexacen® LA Injection; Dexameth® Oral; Dexasone® Injection; Dexasone® L.A. Injection; Dexone® Injection; Dexone® LA Injection; Dexone® Tablet; Hexadrol® Phosphate Injection; Hexadrol® Tablet; Maxidex® Ophthalmic; Solurex® Injection; Solurex L.A.® Injection

Synonyms Dexametasone

Use Systemically and locally for chronic inflammation, allergic, hematologic, neoplastic, and autoimmune diseases; may be used in management of cerebral edema, as a diagnostic agent, antiemetic; to prevent neurologic sequelae in children with bacterial meningitis due to *Haemophilus influenzae* type b infections; no longer recommended for septic shock

Mechanism of Action Decreases inflammation by suppression of migration of polymorphonuclear leukocytes and reversal of increased capillary permeability; suppresses normal immune response

Adverse Reactions

Cardiovascular: Edema, hypertension, premature ventricular contraction

Central nervous system: Headache, mania, dizziness, seizures, psychosis, pseudotumor cerebri

Dermatologic: Acne, dermatitis, skin atrophy

Endocrine & metabolic: Pituitary-adrenal axis suppression, growth suppression, hyperthyroidism, glucose intolerance, hypokalemia, alkalosis, Cushing's syndrome, hyperglycemia

Gastrointestinal: Peptic ulcer, nausea, vomiting, pancreatitis

Hematologic: Eosinopenia, leukocytosis, leukemoid reaction, thrombocytopenia, porphyria

Neuromuscular & skeletal: Muscle asthenia, myalgia, osteoporosis, fractures

Ocular: Cataracts, ptosis, photophobia, diplopia, intraocular pressure (increased), glaucoma

Renal: Proteinuria

Miscellaneous: Feces discoloration (dark brown), hypertrichosis, porphyrinogenic, hiccups, blindness

Toxicodynamics/Kinetics

Time to peak serum concentration:

Oral: Within 1-2 hours

I.M.: Within 8 hours

Duration: Metabolic effect can last for 72 hours; acetate is a long-acting repository preparation with a prompt onset of action

Distribution: V_d: 0.8 L/kg

Protein binding: 68%

Metabolism: In the liver

Half-life: 2.4-3.5 hours

Elimination: Excreted in urine and bile; clearance: 0.2 L/hour/kg

Usual Dosage

Children:

Antiemetic (prior to chemotherapy): I.V.: 10 mg/m^2/dose (maximum: 20 mg) for first dose then 5 mg/m^2/dose every 6 hours as needed

Anti-inflammatory immunosuppressant: Oral, I.M., I.V.: 0.08-0.3 mg/kg/day or 2.5-10 mg/m^2/day in divided doses every 6-12 hours

Physiologic replacement: Oral, I.M., I.V.: 0.03-0.15 mg/kg/day or 0.6-0.75 mg/m^2/day in divided doses every 6-12 hours

Extubation or airway edema: Oral, I.M., I.V.: 0.5-2 mg/kg/day in divided doses every 6 hours beginning 24 hours prior to extubation and continuing for 4-6 doses afterwards

Cerebral edema: Loading dose: Oral, I.M., I.V.: 1-2 mg/kg/dose as a single dose; maintenance: 1-1.5 mg/kg/day (maximum: 16 mg/day) in divided doses every 4-6 hours for 5 days then taper for 5 days, then discontinue

Bacterial meningitis: 0.15 mg/kg within 4 hours of antibiotics and every 6 hours

Inhalation:

Oral: 2 inhalations 3-4 times/day to a maximum of 8 inhalations/day

Intranasal: 6-12 years: 1-2 sprays into each nostril twice daily to a maximum of 8 sprays/day

Adults:

Antiemetic (prior to chemotherapy): I.V.: 10 mg/m²/dose for first dose then 5 mg/m²/dose every 6 hours as needed

Anti-inflammatory: Oral, I.M., I.V. (I.M., I.V. should be sodium phosphate salt): 0.5-9 mg/day in divided doses every 6-12 hours

Cerebral edema: I.V. 10 mg stat, 4 mg I.M./I.V. every 6 hours until response is maximized, then switch to oral regimen, then taper off if appropriate. Dosage may be reduced after 2-4 days and gradually discontinued over 5-7 days

Unresponsive shock: I.V.: 1-6 mg/kg as a single I.V. dose, to 40 mg initially, followed by repeat doses every 2-6 hours while shock persists

Diagnosis for Cushing's syndrome: Oral: 1 mg at 11 PM, draw blood at 8 AM the following day for plasma cortisol determination

Acetate salt:

I.M.: 8-16 mg, may repeat in 1-3 weeks

Intralesional: 0.8-1.6 mg

Intra-articular/soft tissue: 4-16 mg, may repeat in 1-3 weeks

Phosphate salt: Intra-articular, intralesional, or soft tissue: 0.4-6 mg

Inhalation:

Oral: 3 inhalations 3-4 times/day to a maximum of 12 inhalations/day

Intranasal: 2 sprays into each nostril 2-3 times/day to a maximum of 12 sprays/day

Children and Adults:

Ophthalmic:

Ointment: Apply thin coating into conjunctival sac 3-4 times/day, gradually taper dose to discontinue

Suspension: Instill 2 drops into conjunctival sac every hour during the day and every other hour during the night; gradually reduce dose to every 3-4 hours, then to 3-4 times/day

Topical: Apply 1-4 times/day

Administration Administer undiluted solution IVP over 1-4 minutes if dose is <10 mg; high dose therapy must be administered by I.V. intermittent infusion over 15-30 minutes

Contraindications Active untreated infections; viral, fungal, or tuberculous diseases of the eye

Warnings Use with caution in patients with hypothyroidism, cirrhosis, hypertension, congestive heart failure, ulcerative colitis, thromboembolic disorders; fatalities have occurred due to adrenal cortical insufficiency in asthmatic patients during and after transfer from systemic corticosteroids to aerosol steroids; during this period, aerosol steroids do **not** provide the systemic steroid needed to treat patients having trauma, surgery, or infections; may retard bone growth

Dosage Forms

Dexamethasone **acetate**:

Injection: 8 mg/mL (5 mL)

Dalalone L.A.®, Decadron®-LA, Decaject-LA®, Dexasone® L.A., Dexone® LA, Solurex L.A.®: 8 mg/mL (1 mL, 5 mL)

Dalalone D.P.®: 16 mg/mL (1 mL, 5 mL)

Dexamethasone **base**:

Aerosol, topical:

Aeroseb-Dex®: 0.01% (58 g)

Decaspray®: 0.04% (25 g)

Elixir: 0.5 mg/5 mL (5 mL, 20 mL, 100 mL, 120 mL, 240 mL, 500 mL)

Decadron®, Hexadrol®: 0.5 mg/5 mL (100 mL, 120 mL, 237 mL)

Solution, oral: 0.5 mg/5 mL (5 mL, 20 mL, 500 mL)

Solution, oral concentrate: 0.5 mg/0.5 mL (30 mL)

Suspension, ophthalmic: 0.1% (5 mL)

Maxidex®: 0.1% (5 mL, 15 mL)

Tablet: 0.25 mg, 0.5 mg, 0.75 mg, 1 mg, 1.5 mg, 2 mg, 4 mg, 6 mg

Decadron®: 0.25 mg, 0.5 mg, 0.75 mg, 1.5 mg, 4 mg, 6 mg

Dexameth®: 0.5 mg, 0.75 mg, 1.5 mg, 4 mg

Dexone®: 0.5 mg, 0.75 mg, 1.5 mg, 4 mg

Hexadrol®: 1.5 mg, 4 mg

Therapeutic pack (Hexadrol®): Six 1.5 mg tablets and eight 0.75 mg tablets

Dexamethasone **sodium phosphate**:

Aerosol, nasal (Decadron® Phosphate Turbinaire®): 84 mcg/activation [170 metered doses] (12.6 g)

Aerosol, oral (Decadron® Phosphate Respihaler®): 84 mcg/activation [170 metered doses] (12.6 g)

Cream (Decadron® Phosphate): 0.1% (15 g, 30 g)

Injection: 4 mg/mL (1 mL, 2 mL, 5 mL, 10 mL, 30 mL); 10 mg/mL (1 mL, 10 mL)

Dalalone®, Decadron® Phosphate, Decaject®, Dexasone®, Hexadrol® Phosphate, Solurex®: 4 mg/mL (1 mL, 2 mL, 2.5 mL, 5 mL, 10 mL, 30 mL)

(Continued)

Dexamethasone *(Continued)*

Hexadrol® Phosphate: 10 mg/mL (1 mL, 10 mL); 20 mg/mL (5 mL)
Decadron® Phosphate: 24 mg/mL (5 mL, 10 mL)
Ointment, ophthalmic: 0.05% (3.5 g)
AK-Dex®, Baldex®, Decadron® Phosphate, Maxidex®: 0.05% (3.5 g)
Solution, ophthalmic: 0.1% (5 mL)
AK-Dex®, Baldex®, Decadron® Phosphate, I-Methasone®: 0.1% (5 mL)

Stability Injection of parenteral admixture:
Room temperature (25°C): 24 hours
Refrigeration (4°C): 2 days
Protect from light and freezing

Reference Range Dexamethasone suppression test, overnight: 8 AM cortisol <6 μg/100 mL (dexamethasone 1 mg)

Overdosage Treatment Decontamination: Emesis or lavage/activated charcoal with cathartic; acute overdose does not require tapering of dose

Test Interactions May result in false elevation of digoxin level (by radioimmunoassay)

Drug Interactions
Decreased effect with barbiturates, phenytoin, rifampin, aminoglutethimide
Decreased effect of salicylates, vaccines, toxoids, sulfonylureas

Pregnancy Risk Factor C

Monitoring Parameters Hemoglobin, occult blood loss, serum potassium, and glucose

Patient Information Notify physician of any signs of infection or injuries during therapy; inform physician or dentist before surgery if you are taking a corticosteroid; may cause gastritis; take with food; a thin film of cream or ointment is effective, do not overuse; do not use tight-fitting diapers or plastic pants on children being treated in the diaper area; use only as prescribed, and for no longer than the period prescribed; rub in lightly; avoid contact with eyes; notify physician if condition being treated persists or worsens

Nursing Implications Give oral formulation with meals to decrease gastritis; topical formation is for external use, do not use on open wounds; apply sparingly to occlusive dressings; should not be used in the presence of open or weeping lesions; **acetate injection is not for I.V. use**

Additional Information Not suitable for every other day dosing due to long duration of effect; intravenous dexamethasone (2 mg I.V.) can impair ethyl alcohol's ability to stimulate sympathetic nerve discharge and thus suppress alcohol-induced high blood pressure in the acute state

Specific References

Brophy TR, McCafferty J, Tyrer JH, et al, "Bioavailability of Oral Dexamethasone During High Dose Steroid Therapy in Neurological Patients," *Eur J Clin Pharmacol*, 1983, 24(1):103-8.
Duggan DE, Matalia N, Ditzler, CA, et al, "Bioavailability of Oral Dexamethasone," *Clin Pharmacol Ther*, 1975, 18(2):205-9.
Randin D, Vollenweider P, Tappy L, et al, "Suppression of Alcohol-Induced Hypertension by Dexamethasone," *N Engl J Med*, 1995, 332:1733-7.
Wald ER, Kaplan SL, and Mason, Jr EO, "Dexamethasone Therapy for Children With Bacterial meningitis," *Pediatrics*, 1994, 95(1):21-8.

Dexameth® Oral *see* Dexamethasone *on page 266*
Dexasone® Injection *see* Dexamethasone *on page 266*
Dexasone® L.A. Injection *see* Dexamethasone *on page 266*
Dexatrim® [OTC] *see* Phenylpropanolamine Hydrochloride *on page 622*
Dexedrina® *see* Dextroamphetamine Sulfate *on this page*
Dexedrine® *see* Dextroamphetamine Sulfate *on this page*
Dexnon® *see* Levothyroxine Sodium *on page 465*
Dexone® Injection *see* Dexamethasone *on page 266*
Dexone® LA Injection *see* Dexamethasone *on page 266*
Dexone® Tablet *see* Dexamethasone *on page 266*

Dextroamphetamine Sulfate (dex troe am fet' a meen)

Related Information
Principal Pharmacological Properties of Hallucinogenic Drugs *on page 1557*
Therapeutic Drugs Associated With Hallucinations *on page 1558-1559*

CAS Number 51-63-8; 51-64-9; 7528-00-9

Brand Names Dexedrina®; Dexedrine®; Ferndex®

Use Treatment of narcolepsy, abnormal behavioral syndrome in children, exogenous obesity

Mechanism of Action Blocks reuptake of dopamine and norepinephrine from the synapse, thus increases the amount of circulating dopamine and norepinephrine in cerebral cortex to reticular activating system; inhibits the action of monoamine oxidase and causes catecholamines to be released

Adverse Reactions

Cardiovascular: Hypertension, tachycardia (ventricular), tachycardia, palpitations, cardiac arrhythmias

Central nervous system: Insomnia, headache, nervousness, dizziness, seizures, mania, may precipitate Tourette's syndrome, depression, dysphonia, irritability, depression, agitation, fasciculations, euphoria, hallucination, extrapyramidal reaction, movement disorders

Endocrine & metabolic: Growth suppression, respiratory alkalosis, increased serum thyroxine (hyperthyroidism)

Gastrointestinal: Anorexia, nausea, vomiting, diarrhea, abdominal cramps, metallic taste, dry mouth

Genitourinary: Impotence

Hematologic: Porphyria

Neuromuscular & skeletal: Tremors, rhabdomyolysis

Renal: Myoglobinuria

Respiratory: Tachypnea

Miscellaneous: Porphyrinogenic

Toxicodynamics/Kinetics

Onset of action: 1-1.5 hours

Absorption: Food does not delay absorption

Distribution: V_d: 6.11 L/kg

Metabolism: In the liver

Half-life: Adults: 34 hours (pH dependent)

Time to peak serum concentration: Oral: Withih 3 hours

Elimination: Excreted in urine as unchanged drug and inactive metabolites after oral dose; excretion is enhanced in acidic urine

Usual Dosage Oral:

Children:

Narcolepsy: 6-12 years: Initial: 5 mg/day, may increase at 5 mg increments in weekly intervals until side effects appear; maximum dose: 60 mg/day

Attention deficit disorder:

3-5 years: Initial: 2.5 mg/day given every morning; increase by 2.5 mg/day in weekly intervals until optimal response is obtained, usual range: 0.1-0.5 mg/kg/dose every morning with maximum of 40 mg/day

≥6 years: 5 mg once or twice daily; increase in increments of 5 mg/day at weekly intervals until optimal response is reached, usual range: 0.1-0.5 mg/kg/dose every morning (5-20 mg/day) with maximum of 40 mg/day

Adults:

Narcolepsy: Initial: 10 mg/day, may increase at 10 mg increments in weekly intervals until side effects appear; maximum: 60 mg/day

Exogenous obesity: 5-30 mg/day in divided doses of 5-10 mg 30-60 minutes before meals

Contraindications Hypersensitivity to dextroamphetamine or any component; advanced arteriosclerosis, hypertension, hyperthyroidism, glaucoma, MAO inhibitors

Warnings Use with caution in patients with psychopathic personalities, cardiovascular disease, HTN, angina, and glaucoma; has high potential for abuse; use in weight reduction programs only when alternative therapy has been ineffective; prolonged administration may lead to drug dependence

Dosage Forms

Capsule, sustained release: 5 mg, 10 mg, 15 mg

Elixir (orange flavor): 5 mg/5 mL (480 mL)

Tablet: 5 mg, 10 mg

Stability Protect from light

Overdosage Treatment

Decontamination: Lavage/activated charcoal with cathartic

Supportive therapy: Seizures can be treated with lorazepam, diazepam, phenytoin, or phenobarbital; ventricular arrhythmias should be treated with lidocaine

Enhancement of elimination: Hemodialysis may be useful; do not acidify urine

Test Interactions False-positive amphetamine assays may occur from coadministration with ranitidine, phenylpropanolamine, brompheniramine, chlorpromazine, fluspiriline, or pipothiazine

Drug Interactions

Decreased effect of methyldopa, ethosuximide; decreased effect with acidifiers, psychotropics, lithium

Increased effect/toxicity of TCAs, phenytoin, MAO inhibitors, phenobarbital, general anesthetics, propoxyphene, norepinephrine, meperidine, acetazolamide, albuterol (cardiac effects)

Pregnancy Risk Factor C

Monitoring Parameters CNS activity

Patient Information Take during day to avoid insomnia; do not discontinue abruptly, may be addicting with prolonged use

(Continued)

Dextroamphetamine Sulfate *(Continued)*

Nursing Implications Last daily dose should be given 6 hours before retiring; do not crush sustained release drug product; dose should not be given in evening or at bedtime

Additional Information Illicit preparation may contain up to 24 g per spoon; 5 mg tablets contain tartrazine

Specific References

Grinstead GF, "Ranitidine and High Concentrations of Phenylpropanolamine Cross React in the EMIT Monoclonal Amphetamine/Methamphetamine Assay," *Clin Chem*, 1989, 35(9):1998-9.

Mattson RH and Calverley JR, "Dextroamphetamine-Sulfate-Induced Dyskinesias," *JAMA*, 1968, 204(5):400-2.

Richards CF, Clark RF, Holbrook T, et al, "The Effect of Cocaine and Amphetamines on Vital Signs in Trauma Patients," *J Emerg Med*, 1995, 13:59-63.

Segar DL, "Substances of Abuse: Topics," *Emerg Med*, 1985, 7:18-30.

Dextromethorphan Hydrobromide (dex troe meth or' fan)

Related Information

Therapeutic Drugs Associated With Hallucinations *on page 1558-1559*

CAS Number 125-69-9; 125-71-3; 6700-34-1

Brand Names Benylin® DM [OTC]; Children's Hold® [OTC]; Delsym® [OTC]; Hold® DM [OTC]; Pertussin® CS [OTC]; Pertussin® ES [OTC]; Robitussin® Cough Calmers [OTC]; Robitussin® Pediatric [OTC]; Scot-Tussin® DM Cough Chasers [OTC]; St. Joseph® Cough Suppressant [OTC]; Sucrets® Cough Calmers [OTC]; Suppress® [OTC]; Trocal® [OTC]; Vicks Formula 44® [OTC]; Vicks Formula 44® Pediatric Formula [OTC]

Synonyms Demorphan; d-Methorphan

Use Symptomatic relief of coughs caused by minor viral upper respiratory tract infections or inhaled irritants; most effective for a chronic nonproductive cough

Mechanism of Action Chemical relative of morphine lacking narcotic properties; controls cough by depressing the medullary cough center; has virtually no analgesic activity; acts through the sigma receptor with little dependence effect

Adverse Reactions

Central nervous system: Drowsiness, dizziness, coma, auditory and visual hallucinations, insomnia

Gastrointestinal: Nausea

Respiratory: Apnea, respiratory depression

Signs & Symptoms of Acute Overdose Excitation, respiratory depression, miosis, insomnia, tachycardia, coma, fever, hypertension, hyperthermia, hyperactivity, ataxia, tremors

Toxicodynamics/Kinetics

Onset of antitussive action: Within 15-30 minutes

Duration: Up to 6 hours

Metabolism: In the liver to an active metabolite (dextrophan)

Half-life: 2-4 hours

Time to peak: 2.5 hours

Elimination: Principally in urine

Usual Dosage Oral:

Children:

- 2-5 years: 2.5-7.5 mg every 4-8 hours; extended release is 15 mg twice daily (maximum: 30 mg/24 hours)
- 6-12 years: 5-10 mg every 4 hours or 15 mg every 6-8 hours; extended release is 30 mg twice daily (maximum: 60 mg/24 hours)

Children >12 years and Adults: 10-30 mg every 4-8 hours or 30 mg every 6-8 hours; extended release is 60 mg twice daily (maximum: 120 mg/24 hours)

Contraindications Hypersensitivity to dextromethorphan or any component

Warnings Use in children <2 years of age has not been proven safe and effective

Dosage Forms

Capsule (Drixoral® Cough Liquid Caps): 30 mg

Liquid:

- Pertussin® CS: 3.5 mg/5 mL (120 mL)
- Pertussin® ES, Vicks Formula 44®: 15 mg/5 mL (120 mL, 240 mL)
- Robitussin® Pediatric, St. Joseph® Cough Suppressant: 7.5 mg/5 mL (60 mL, 120 mL, 240 mL)

Liquid, sustained release, as polistirex (Delsym®): 30 mg/5 mL (89 mL)

Lozenges:

- Children's Hold®, Hold® DM, Robitussin® Cough Calmers, Sucrets® Cough Calmers: 5 mg
- Scot-Tussin® DM Cough Chasers: 2.5 mg
- Suppress®, Trocal®: 7.5 mg

Syrup:

- Benylin® DM: 10 mg/5 mL (120 mL, 3780 mL)
- Vicks Formula 44® Pediatric Formula: 15 mg/15 mL (120 mL)

Reference Range Serum level of 0.1 μg/mL associated with coma

Overdosage Treatment

Decontamination: Lavage is recommended for ingestions >10 mg/kg; activated charcoal with cathartic is useful

Supportive therapy: Naloxone hydrochloride (0.4-2 mg I.V., S.C., or through an endotracheal tube); a continuous infusion (at ⅔ the response dose/hour) may be required

Antidote(s)

Naloxone Hydrochloride *on page 1447*

Test Interactions Can give a false-positive on phencyclidine qualitative immunoassay screen

Drug Interactions Administration with monoamine oxidase inhibitors can cause hyperthermia

Pregnancy Risk Factor C

Patient Information Shake well; do not exceed recommended dosage; take with a large glass of water; if cough lasts more than 1 week or is accompanied by a rash, fever, or headache, notify physician

Nursing Implications Raise side rails, institute safety measures

Additional Information Monitor for bromide poisoning

Specific References

Bem JL and Peck R, "Dextromethorphan: An Overview of Safety Issues," *Drug Saf*, 1992, 7(3):190-9.

Katona B and Wason S, "Dextromethorphan Danger," *N Engl J Med*, 1986, 314(15):993.

LeJoyeux M, et al, "Serotonin Syndrome: Incidence, Symptoms, and Treatment," *CNS Drugs*, 1994, 2:132-43.

Pender ES and Parks BR, "Toxicity With Dextromethorphan-Containing Preparations: A Literature Review and Report of Two Additional Cases," *Pediatr Emerg Care*, 1991, 7(3):163-5.

Rammer L, Holmgren P and Sandler H, "Fatal Intoxication by Dextromethorphan: A Report on Two Cases" *Forensic Sci Int*, 1988, 37(4):233-6.

Taylor JA, Novack AH, Almquist JR, et al, "Efficacy of Cough Suppressants in Children," *J Pediatr*, 1993, 122(5 Pt 1):799-802.

Wolfe TR and Caravati EM, "Massive Dextromethorphan Ingestion and Abuse," *Am J Emerg Med*, 1995, 13(2):174-6.

Dextropropoxyphene *see* Propoxyphene *on page 655*

Dey-Dose® Metaproterenol *see* Metaproterenol Sulfate *on page 506*

DFMO *see* Eflornithine Hydrochloride *on page 310*

DHPG Sodium *see* Ganciclovir *on page 377*

Diabet® *see* Chlorpropamide *on page 207*

Diaβeta® *see* Glyburide *on page 384*

Diabetic Tussin EX® [OTC] *see* Guaifenesin *on page 390*

Diabewas® *see* Tolazamide *on page 756*

Diabinese® *see* Chlorpropamide *on page 207*

Diacetylmorphine *see* Heroin Hydrochloride *on page 401*

Dialose® [OTC] *see* Docusate *on page 297*

Dialume® [OTC] *see* Aluminum *on page 104*

Diamine T.D.® [OTC] *see* Brompheniramine Maleate *on page 165*

Diaminodiphenylsulfone *see* Dapsone *on page 260*

Diamorphine Hydrochloride *see* Heroin Hydrochloride *on page 401*

Diamox® *see* Acetazolamide *on page 83*

Diaphenylsulfon *see* Dapsone *on page 260*

Diaqua® *see* Hydrochlorothiazide *on page 406*

Diar-aid® [OTC] *see* Loperamide Hydrochloride *on page 480*

Diazemuls® *see* Diazepam *on this page*

Diazepam (dye az' e pam)

Related Information

Benzodiazepines Comparison *on page 1643*

Seizures, Neonatal Guidelines *on page 1604-1605*

Status Epilepticus Treatment Algorithm *on page 1608*

CAS Number 439-14-5

Brand Names Aliseum®; Alupram®; Atensine®; Diazemuls®; Lamra®; Solis®; Stesolid®; Tensium®; Valium®; Valrelease®; Vatran®; Vivol®; Zetran®

Use Management of general anxiety disorders, panic disorders, and to provide preoperative sedation, light anesthesia, and amnesia; treatment of status epilepticus, alcohol withdrawal symptoms; used as a skeletal muscle relaxant

(Continued)

Diazepam *(Continued)*

Mechanism of Action Depresses all levels of the CNS, including the limbic and reticular formation, probably through the increased action of gamma-aminobutyric acid (GABA), which is a major inhibitory neurotransmitter in the brain

Adverse Reactions

Cardiovascular: Cardiac arrest, hypotension, bradycardia, cardiovascular collapse

Central nervous system: Drowsiness, confusion, dizziness, amnesia, slurred speech, psychosis, hallucinations, paradoxical excitation or rage, ataxia

Endocrine & metabolic: Gynecomastia

Hematologic: Leukopenia, neutropenia, agranulocytosis, granulocytopenia

Local: Phlebitis, pain with injection

Neuromuscular & skeletal: Dysarthria

Ocular: Blurred vision, diplopia, mydriasis

Respiratory: Respiratory rate (decreased), apnea, laryngospasm

Miscellaneous: Physical and psychological dependence with prolonged use, dry mouth, hypersensitivity (type I) reactions

Signs & Symptoms of Acute Overdose Somnolence, hiccups, nystagmus, thrombocytopenia, eosinophilia, hypothermia, hyporeflexia, jaundice, memory loss, extrapyramidal reaction, gynecomastia, dysarthria, cognitive dysfunction, rhabdomyolysis, myoglobinuria, confusion, coma, hypoactive reflexes, renal failure, dyspnea, hypotension, slurred speech, ataxia, respiratory depression

Toxicodynamics/Kinetics

Onset of action:

- Oral: 30-60 minutes
- I.M.: 15-30 minutes
- I.V.: 1-5 minutes; onset almost immediate with short duration of action (20-30 minutes) when given I.V. for status epilepticus

Duration:

- Oral: ≤3 hours
- I.M. 15 minutes to 1 hour

Absorption: Oral: 83% to 100%

Distribution: V_d: 1.1 L/kg; widely distributed throughout body

Protein binding: 96%

Metabolism: In the liver; active major metabolite is desmethyldiazepam; other metabolites are methyl-lorazepam, oxazepam, and temazepam

Half-life:

- Increased in neonates, elderly, and those with severe hepatic disorders; desmethyldiazepam: 50-100 hours and can be prolonged in neonates
- Adults: 20-50 hours

Elimination: Excreted in urine with only small amounts in feces; renal clearance: 0.32-0.44 mL/minute/kg

Usual Dosage Oral absorption is more reliable than I.M.

Children:

- Sedation or muscle relaxation or anxiety:
  - Oral: 0.12-0.8 mg/kg/day in divided doses every 6-8 hours
  - I.M., I.V.: 0.04-0.3 mg/kg/dose every 2-4 hours to a maximum of 0.6 mg/kg within an 8-hour period if needed
- Status epilepticus: I.V.:
  - Neonates: 0.1-0.3 mg/kg/dose every 15-30 minutes given over 2-3 minutes, not to exceed 2 mg/24 hours
  - Infants 30 days to 5 years: 0.2-0.5 mg/dose given over 2-3 minutes, every 2-5 minutes to a maximum total dose of 5 mg
  - Children >5 years: 1 mg/dose given over 2-3 minutes, every 2-5 minutes to a maximum total dose of 10 mg

Adults:

- Anxiety/sedation/skeletal muscle relaxation:
  - Oral: 2-10 mg 2-4 times/day
  - I.M., I.V.: 2-10 mg, may repeat in 3-4 hours if needed
- Status epilepticus: I.V.: 5-10 mg every 10-20 minutes or 0.2-0.5 mg/kg/dose every 15-30 minutes, up to 30 mg; may repeat in 2-4 hours if necessary

Dosing adjustment in hepatic impairment: Reduce dose by 50% in cirrhosis and avoid in severe/acute liver disease

Contraindications Hypersensitivity to diazepam or any component; there may be a cross-sensitivity with other benzodiazepines; do not use in a comatose patient, in those with pre-existing CNS depression, respiratory depression, narrow-angle glaucoma, or severe uncontrolled pain

Warnings Do not use in pregnant women; because of its long half-life, not considered a drug of choice in the elderly; use with caution in patients receiving other CNS depressants, patients with low albumin, hepatic dysfunction, and in the elderly and young infants

Dosage Forms

Capsule, sustained release (Valrelease®): 15 mg

Injection: 5 mg/mL (1 mL, 2 mL, 5 mL, 10 mL)
Solution, oral (wintergreen-spice flavor): 5 mg/5 mL (5 mL, 10 mL, 500 mL)
Solution, oral concentrate: 5 mg/mL (30 mL)
Tablet: 2 mg, 5 mg, 10 mg

Stability Protect parenteral dosage form from light; potency is retained for up to 3 months when kept at room temperature; most stable at pH 4-8, hydrolysis occurs at pH <3; do not mix I.V. product with other medications

Reference Range Therapeutic:
Diazepam: 0.2-1.5 μg/mL (SI: 0.7-5.3 μmol/L)
N-desmethyldiazepam (nordiazepam): 0.1-0.5 μg/mL (SI: 0.35-1.8 μmol/L)
Urine drug screens can remain positive for 30 days

Overdosage Treatment
Decontamination: Lavage/activated charcoal with cathartic
Supportive therapy: Rarely is mechanical ventilation required; flumazenil has been shown to selectively block the binding of benzodiazepines to CNS receptors, resulting in a reversal of benzodiazepine-induced CNS depression and respiratory depression
Enhancement of elimination: Multiple dose of activated charcoal is effective

Antidote(s)
Flumazenil *on page 1428*

Test Interactions False-negative urinary glucose determinations when using Clinistix® or Diastix®; may inhibit thyroxine binding; may increase plasma testosterone

Diagnostic Tests/Procedures
Diazepam, Blood *on page 1249*

Drug Interactions CNS depressants (alcohol, barbiturates, opioids) may enhance sedation and respiratory depression of diazepam; enzyme inducers (nicotine, rifampin) may increase the hepatic metabolism of diazepam, propranolol, omeprazole, oral contraceptives; cimetidine may decrease the metabolism of diazepam; heparin, valproic acid may displace diazepam from binding sites which may result an increase in sedative effects; metoclopramide increases absorption as can antacids; diazepam levels increase with concomitant administration of fluvoxamine

Pregnancy Risk Factor D

Pregnancy Implications Possible fourfold increase in oral cleft lip in 1st trimester when given at time of delivery; hypotonia, hypothermia, and difficulties in sucking may occur

Monitoring Parameters Respiratory rate, heart rate, blood pressure

Patient Information Avoid alcohol and other CNS depressants; avoid activities needing good psychomotor coordination until CNS effects are known; drug may cause physical or psychological dependence; avoid abrupt discontinuation after prolonged use

Nursing Implications In children, do not exceed 1-2 mg/minute IVP; adults 5 mg/minute; provide safety measures (ie, side rails, night light, and call button); remove smoking materials from area; supervise ambulation; do not exceed 5 mg/minute IVP; provide safety measures (ie, side rails, night light, and call button); remove smoking materials from area; supervise ambulation

Additional Information Benzyl alcohol toxicity can develop after administration of high-dose intravenous diazepam (2.4 mg/kg/hour in 36 hours) in children; oral absorption more reliable than I.M.; intra-arterial injection may cause tissue necrosis

Specific References

Allikmets E, et al, "Long-term Use of Benzodiazepines: Abrupt Withdrawal Versus Withdrawal Under Nifedipine Cover," *Pharmacol Toxicol*, 1995, 76(Suppl 3):Abstr 8.
Traeger SM and Haug MT 3d, "Reduction of Diazepam Serum Half-Life and Reversal of Coma by Activated Charcoal in a Patient With Severe Liver Disease," *J Toxicol Clin Toxicol*, 1986, 24(4):329-37.
Votey SR, Bosse GM, Bayer MJ, et al, "Flumazenil: A New Benzodiazepine Antagonist," *Ann Emerg Med*, 1991, 20(2):181-8.

Diazoxide (dye az ox' ide)

CAS Number 364-98-7

Brand Names Eudemine®; Hyperstat® I.V.; Hypertonalum®; Proglycem® Oral

Synonyms Diazoxidum

Use
Oral: Hypoglycemia related to islet cell adenoma, carcinoma, hyperplasia, or adenomatosis, nesidioblastosis, leucine sensitivity, or extrapancreatic malignancy
I.V.: Emergency lowering of blood pressure

Mechanism of Action Inhibits insulin release from the pancreas; produces direct smooth muscle relaxation of the peripheral arterioles which results in decrease in blood pressure and reflex increase in heart rate and cardiac output

Adverse Reactions
Cardiovascular: Hypotension, cardiomyopathy, tachycardia, flushing, heart block, cardiomegaly

(Continued)

Diazoxide *(Continued)*

Central nervous system: Dizziness, asthenia, seizures, headache, extrapyramidal reaction (15%) and development of abnormal facies with chronic oral use,
Dermatologic: Rash, hirsutism (long-term treatment), edema,
Endocrine & metabolic: Hyperglycemia, ketoacidosis, labor (inhibition), hyperuricemia
Gastrointestinal: Nausea, vomiting, anorexia, constipation, pancreatitis
Hematologic: Leukopenia, thrombocytopenia, hemolysis
Local: Pain, burning, cellulitis/phlebitis upon extravasation
Ocular: Lacrimation, diplopia
Miscellaneous: Sodium and water retention

Signs & Symptoms of Acute Overdose Hyperglycemia, diplopia, hematuria, lacrimation, hyperuricemia, hypertrichosis, A-V block, hemiplegia, dysosmia, nephrotic syndrome, dermatitis, ketoacidosis, hypotension, lichenoid eruptions, hyperthermia, chest pain, bradycardia, leukopenia; galactorrhea, neutropenia; agranulocytosis; granulocytopenia; fever, congestive heart failure

Toxicodynamics/Kinetics

Hyperglycemic effects: Oral:
Onset of action: Within 1 hour
Duration: Normal renal function: 8 hours
Hypotensive effects: I.V.:
Peak effect: Occur within 5 minutes
Duration: Usually 3-12 hours
Distribution: V_d: 0.21 L/kg; crosses blood-brain barrier and placenta; distributed throughout the body; highest concentrations found in kidneys, liver, and adrenal glands
Protein binding: 90% (decreased in uremia)
Metabolism: Hepatic to 3-hydroxymethyl and 3-carboxy derivatives
Half-life:
Children: 9-24 hours
Adults: 20-45 hours
Elimination: 50% excreted unchanged in urine; clearance: 0.0036 L/hour/kg

Usual Dosage

Hyperinsulinemic hypoglycemia: Oral:
Newborns and Infants: 8-15 mg/kg/day in divided doses every 8-12 hours
Children and Adults: 3-8 mg/kg/day in divided doses every 8-12 hours

Hypertension: I.V.: Children and Adults: 1-3 mg/kg (maximum: 150 mg in a single injection); repeat dose in 5-15 minutes until blood pressure adequately reduced; repeat administration every 4-24 hours monitoring blood pressure closely; do not use longer than 10 days

Contraindications Hypersensitivity to diazoxide, thiazides, or other sulfonamide derivatives; aortic coarctation, arteriovenous shunts, dissecting aortic aneurysm; ineffective in hypertension due to pheochromocytoma

Warnings Use with caution in patients with diabetes mellitus, renal or liver disease, coronary artery disease, or cerebral vascular insufficiency

Dosage Forms

Capsule (Proglycem®): 50 mg
Injection (Hyperstat®): 15 mg/mL (1 mL, 20 mL)
Suspension, oral (chocolate-mint flavor) (Proglycem®): 50 mg/mL (30 mL)

Stability Protect from light, heat, and freezing; avoid using darkened solutions; virtually insoluble in water

Reference Range Plasma level of 35 mg/L (152 μmol/L) produces a 25% reduction of mean arterial pressure

Overdosage Treatment

Decontamination: Lavage/activated charcoal with cathartic
Supportive therapy: Insulin for hyperglycemia, fluid, and electrolyte restoration; place patient in Trendelenburg position if hypotensive; isotonic saline and/or dopamine or norepinephrine can be used
Enhancement of elimination: Low recovery with dialysis

Test Interactions Increases glucose, sodium (S), uric acid (S); false-negative insulin response to glucagon

Drug Interactions Diuretics and hypotensive agents may potentiate diazoxide adverse effects; diazoxide may increase phenytoin metabolism or free fraction; diazoxide may decrease warfarin protein binding; hyperglycemic effect may be exacerbated by chlorpromazine

Pregnancy Risk Factor C

Pregnancy Implications Can cause infantile alopecia along with neonatal hyperglycemia

Monitoring Parameters Blood pressure, serum uric acid; monitor blood glucose daily in patients receiving I.V. therapy

Patient Information Check blood glucose carefully

Nursing Implications I.V. diazoxide is given undiluted by rapid I.V. injection over a period of 30 seconds or less; shake suspension well before using; extravasation can be treated with warm compresses

Additional Information Patients may require a diuretic with repeated I.V. doses

Specific References

Lancaster-Smith M, Leigh NI, and Thompson HM, "Death Following Nonketotic Hyperglycemic Coma During Diazoxide Therapy and Peritoneal Dialysis," *Postgrad Med J*, 1974, 50:175-9.

Diazoxidum *see* Diazoxide *on page 273*

Dibucaine (dye' byoo kane)

CAS Number 61-12-1; 85-79-0

Brand Names Cincain®; Dermacaine®; Nupercainal® [OTC]; Nupercaine®; Percainal®

Synonyms Cinchocaine; Sovcainum

Use Fast, temporary relief of pain and itching due to hemorrhoids, minor burns, other minor skin conditions

Mechanism of Action Blocks both initiation and conduction of nerve impulses by decreasing the neuronal membrane's permeability to sodium ions, which results in inhibition of depolarization with resultant blockade of conduction; it is an amide anesthetic, one of the most potent and long-acting and more vasodilatory properties; quinolone derivative

Adverse Reactions

Cardiovascular: Edema

Dermatologic: Urticaria, cutaneous lesions

Gastrointestinal: Nausea, vomiting

Local: Burning, tenderness, irritation, inflammation, contact dermatitis, pruritus

Otic: Ototoxicity, tinnitus

Signs & Symptoms of Acute Overdose CNS/respiratory depression, ototoxicity; tinnitus, coma, ARDS, seizures, cough, vomiting

Toxicodynamics/Kinetics

Onset of action: Within 15 minutes

Duration: 2-4 hours

Absorption: Poor through intact skin, but well absorbed through mucous membranes and excoriated skin

Distribution: None

Metabolism: Hepatic

Elimination: None

Usual Dosage Children and Adults:

Rectal: Hemorrhoids: Insert ointment into rectum using a rectal applicator; administer each morning, evening, and after each bowel movement

Topical: Apply gently to the affected areas; no more than 30 g for adults or 7.5 g for children should be used in any 24-hour period

Contraindications Known hypersensitivity to amide-type anesthetics

Dosage Forms

Cream: 0.5% (45 g)

Ointment, topical: 1% (30 g, 60 g)

Stability Darkens on light exposure

Reference Range Plasma level of 71 ng/mL associated with seizures

Overdosage Treatment

Decontamination: Lavage/activated charcoal with cathartic

Supportive therapy: Treat seizures with lorazepam or diazepam; recurring seizures may require phenytoin or phenobarbital

Enhancement of elimination: Forced diuresis and hemodialysis may be beneficial

Pregnancy Risk Factor C

Monitoring Parameters Respiratory status

Patient Information If condition worsens, or if symptoms persist for >7 days, stop using the ointment and consult a physician; wash hands after use to avoid getting ointment in eyes

Nursing Implications Do not use near the eyes or over denuded surfaces or blistered areas

Additional Information Formerly marketed as Percaine; not available in the U.S. as an injectable

Specific References

Egfjord M, Jansen JA, Flachs H, et al, "Combined Boric Acid and Cinchocaine Chloride Poisoning in a 12-Month Old Infant: Evaluation of Haemodialysis," *Hum Toxicol*, 1988, 17(2):175-8.

Murphy JP and Anandaciva S, "Phantom Limb Pain and Spinal Anaesthesia," *Anaesthesia*, 1984, 39(2):188.

1-(2,6-Dichlorobenzylideneamine) Guanidine Acetate *see* Guanabenz Acetate *on page 391*

Diclofenac Sodium (dye kloe' fen ak)

Related Information

Nonsteroidal Anti-Inflammatory Comparison *on page 1655*

CAS Number 15307-79-6

Brand Names Cataflam®; Voltaren®

Use Acute and chronic treatment of rheumatoid arthritis, ankylosing spondylitis, and osteoarthritis; also used for juvenile rheumatoid arthritis, gout, dysmenorrhea, biliary and renal colic, fever, and pain relief; ophthalmic solution for postoperative inflammation after cataract extraction

Mechanism of Action Inhibits prostaglandin synthesis by decreasing the activity of the enzyme, cyclo-oxygenase, which results in decreased formation of prostaglandin precursors

Adverse Reactions

Cardiovascular: Fluid retention, circulatory collapse

Central nervous system: Headache, dizziness, aseptic meningitis, psychosis, cognitive dysfunction, coma, seizures

Dermatologic: Rash, pruritus

Endocrine & metabolic: Hyperkalemia, anion gap metabolic acidosis

Gastrointestinal: Abdominal pain, nausea, vomiting, bleeding, ulceration, constipation, diarrhea, dyspepsia

Hematologic: Leukopenia, neutropenia, agranulocytosis, granulocytopenia; aplastic anemia (rare), platelet inhibition, thrombocytopenia

Hepatic: Elevation of transaminases, fulminant hepatitis

Otic: Ototoxicity, tinnitus

Renal: Renal failure (acute), albuminuria, nephrotic syndrome, chronic renal failure

Respiratory: Wheezing, respiratory depression

Miscellaneous: Hypersensitivity

Signs & Symptoms of Acute Overdose Nausea, vomiting, wheezing, gastrointestinal upset, gastrointestinal bleeding, nephrotic syndrome, lichenoid eruptions, cognitive dysfunction, coagulopathy; ototoxicity, tinnitus, drowsiness; severe poisoning can manifest with coma, seizures, renal and or hepatic failure, hypotension, respiratory depression

Toxicodynamics/Kinetics

Absorption: Completely

Distribution: V_d: 0.55 L/kg

Protein binding: 99%

Metabolism: In the liver to inactive metabolites

Bioavailability: 50% to 60% secondary to first-pass metabolism

Half-life: 1-2 hours

Time to peak serum concentration: Within 2-3 hours

Elimination: Primarily in urine

Usual Dosage Adults:

Oral:

- Analgesia (Cataflam®): Starting dose: 50 mg 3 times/day
- Rheumatoid arthritis: 150-200 mg/day in 2-4 divided doses
- Osteoarthritis: 100-150 mg/day in 2-3 divided doses
- Ankylosing spondylitis: 100-125 mg/day in 4-5 divided doses

Ophthalmic: Instill 1 drop into affected eye 4 times/day beginning 24 hours after cataract surgery and continuing for 2 weeks

Contraindications Known hypersensitivity to diclofenac, any component, aspirin or other nonsteroidal anti-inflammatory drugs (NSAIDs); porphyria

Warnings Use with caution in patients with congestive heart failure, hypertension, decreased renal or hepatic function, history of gastrointestinal disease, or those receiving anticoagulants

Dosage Forms

Solution, ophthalmic, as sodium (Voltaren®): 0.1% (2.5 mL, 5 mL)

Tablet, enteric coated, as sodium (Voltaren®): 25 mg, 50 mg, 75 mg

Tablet, as potassium (Cataflam®): 50 mg

Overdosage Treatment

Decontamination: Ipecac or lavage/activated charcoal with cathartic

Supportive therapy: Hypotension/dehydration can be managed with intravenous fluid therapy; acidosis should be treated with bicarbonates, seizures with benzodiazepines; antacids, blood products are indicated, as appropriate, for hemorrhage

Enhancement of elimination: Dialysis or perfusion is indicated for secondary complications, acidosis, or renal failure and not toxin removal alone; multiple dosing of activated charcoal may be useful

Test Interactions Increases bleeding time

Drug Interactions Aspirin decreases serum concentrations probably by protein-binding displacement; there is an increased bleeding potential with concomitant warfarin therapy; may increase lithium, digoxin, and methotrexate concentrations by decreasing renal clearance; may decrease diuretic and hypotensive effects of thiazides, loop diuretics, ACE inhibitors, and beta-blockers; may increase nephrotoxicity of cyclosporine

Pregnancy Risk Factor B

Monitoring Parameters Monitor CBC, liver enzymes, occult blood loss; monitor urine output and BUN/serum creatinine in patients receiving diuretics

Specific References

Arnold MM and McKenna F, "A Double Blind Comparison of the Endoscopic and Clinical Effects of Tenoxicam and Diclofenac in Rheumatoid Arthritis," *Br J Rheumatol*, 1995, 34(Suppl 1):95.

Court H and Volans GN, "Poisoning After Overdose With Nonsteroidal Anti-inflammatory Drugs," *Adverse Drug React Acute Poisoning Rev*, 1984, 3(1):1-21.

George S and Rabi AH, "Thrombocytopenia Associated With Diclofenac Therapy," *Am J Health-System Pharmacy*, 1995, 52:420-1.

Helfgott SM, Sandberg-Cook J, Zakim D, et al, "Diclofenac-Associated Hepatotoxicity," *JAMA*, 1990, 264(20):2660-2.

Hoppmann RA, Peden JG, and Ober SK, "Central Nervous System Side Effects of Nonsteroidal Anti-inflammatory Drugs. Aseptic Meningitis, Psychosis, and Cognitive Dysfunction," *Arch Intern Med*, 1991, 151(7):1309-13.

Isdale A and Wright V, "Misoprostol/NSAID Fixed Combinations," *Drug Saf*, 1995, 12(5):291-8.

Kulling EJ, Beckman EA, and Skagius AS, "Renal Impairment After Acute Diclofenac, Naproxen, and Sulindac Overdoses," *J Toxicol Clin Toxicol*, 1995, 33(2):173-7.

Pillans PI and O'Connor N, "Tissue Necrosis and Necrotizing Fascitis After Intramuscular Administration of Diclofenac," *Ann Pharmacother*, 1995, 29:264-6.

Riad LE, Sawchuk RJ, McAlary MM, et al, "Effect of Food on the Multiple-Peak Behavior After a Single Oral Dose of Diclofenac Sodium Slow-Release Tablet in Humans," *Am J Ther*, 1995, 2:237-45.

Robinson MH, Wheatley T, and Leach IH, "Nonsteroidal Anti-inflammatory Drug-Induced Colonic Stricture; an Unusual Cause of Large Bowel Obstruction and Perforation," *Dig Dis Sci*, 1995, 40(2):315-9.

Robinson PM and Ahmed I, "Diclofenac and Post-Tonsillectomy Haemorrhage," *Clin Otolaryngol*, 1994, 19(4):344-5.

Smolinske SC, Hall AH, Vandenberg SA, et al, "Toxic Effects of Nonsteroid Anti-inflammatory Drugs in Overdose. An Overview of Recent Evidence on Clinical Effects and Dose-Response Relationships," *Drug Saf*, 1990, 5(4):252-74.

Vale JA and Meredith TJ, "Acute Poisoning Due to Nonsteroidal Anti-inflammatory Drugs," *Med Toxicol*, 1986, 1(1):12-31.

Verbeeck RK, "Pharmacokinetic Drug Interactions With Nonsteroidal Anti-inflammatory Drugs," *Clin Pharmacokinet*, 1990, 19(1):44-66.

Willkens RF, "Worldwide Clinical Safety Experience With Diclofenac," *Semin Arthritis Rheum*, 1985, 15(2 Suppl 1):105-10.

Dicorynan® *see* Disopyramide Phosphate *on page 294*

Dicoumarin *see* Dicumarol *on this page*

Dicoumarol *see* Dicumarol *on this page*

Dicumarol (dye koo' ma role)

Related Information

Warfarin Sodium *on page 800*

CAS Number 66-76-2

Brand Names Apekumarol®

Synonyms Bishydroxycoumarin; Dicoumarin; Dicoumarol; Dicumol

Use Prophylaxis and treatment of thromboembolic disorders

Mechanism of Action Depression of factors VII, IX, X, and II (sequential) - a hydroxycoumarin

Adverse Reactions More likely to have gastrointestinal side effects than warfarin

Cardiovascular: Circulatory collapse, pericardial effusion/pericarditis

Central nervous system: Fever

Dermatologic: Skin lesions, skin necrosis

Gastrointestinal: Anorexia, nausea, vomiting, diarrhea,

Hematologic: Hemorrhage, intracranial hemorrhage, ocular hemorrhage, bleeding gums, coagulopathy

Respiratory: Hemoptysis

Miscellaneous: Feces discoloration (black), feces discoloration (light brown), feces discoloration (pink), feces discoloration (red); priapism

Toxicodynamics/Kinetics

Duration of action: 5-6 days

Absorption: Oral: Well (but unpredictably) absorbed – affected by food

Distribution: V_d: 0.14 L/kg

Protein binding: 97%

Metabolism: In the liver

Half-life: Plasma: 1-2 days

Time to peak serum concentration: 1-9 hours

Elimination: In urine

Usual Dosage Adults: Oral: 25-200 mg/day based on prothrombin time (PT) determinations

Contraindications Severe liver or kidney disease, open wounds, uncontrolled bleeding, hypersensitivity to dicumarol or any component

(Continued)

Dicumarol *(Continued)*

Warnings Concomitant use with vitamin K may decrease anticoagulant effect; monitor carefully; concomitant use with ethacrynic acid, indomethacin, mefenamic acid, phenylbutazone, or aspirin increases warfarin's anticoagulant effect and may cause severe gastrointestinal bleeding; the duration of action is considerably longer than warfarin and prescribers should be aware of this difference; peak levels should be expected 1-2 weeks after dose adjustment

Dosage Forms Tablet: 25 mg, 50 mg, 100 mg

Stability Insoluble in water or alcohol

Reference Range

Normal: 20-30 μg/mL

Toxic: >70 μg/mL

Overdosage Treatment

Decontamination: Activated charcoal with cathartic should be given; lavage can be performed within 1 hour of ingestion

Supportive therapy: Vitamin K_1 should be given in doses as outlined in phytonadione; monitor PT and INR till normalization

Enhancement of elimination: Cholestyramine or multiple dosing of activated charcoal may be useful

Antidote(s)

Cholestyramine Resin *on page 1405*

Phytonadione *on page 1458*

Diagnostic Tests/Procedures

Bishydroxycoumarin, Blood *on page 1204*

Drug Interactions May accentuate toxicities of oral hypoglycemics and anticonvulsants. The following will decrease prothrombin time – antacids, antihistamines, phenobarbital, carbamazepine, cholestyramine, meprobamate, glutethimide, ethchlorvynol, oral contraceptives, ranitidine, chloral hydrate, diuretics. Increased prothrombin time due to allopurinol, amiodarone, cimetidine, clofibrate, dextran, diazoxide, diflunisal, diuretics, disulfiram, fenoprofen, ibuprofen, indomethacin, influenza virus vaccine, methyldopa, methylphenidate, MAO inhibitors, naproxen, nortriptyline, phenytoin, propylthiouracil, salicylates, quinidine, quinine, ranitidine, tolbutamide, thyroid drugs, sulindac, co-trimoxazole

Pregnancy Risk Factor D

Pregnancy Implications Safe in breast feeding

Additional Information

TLV-TWA: 0.1 mg/m^3

IDLH: 200 mg/m^3

Dicumol *see* Dicumarol *on previous page*

Didanosine (dye dan' oh seen)

CAS Number 69655-05-6

Brand Names Videx® Oral

Synonyms DDI

Use Treatment of advanced HIV infection in patients who are intolerant of zidovudine therapy or who have demonstrated significant clinical or immunologic deterioration during zidovudine therapy

Mechanism of Action Didanosine, a purine nucleoside analogue related to inosine and the deamination product of dideoxyadenosine (ddA), inhibits HIV replication *in vitro* in both T cells and monocytes. Didanosine is converted within the cell to the monophosphates, diphosphates, and triphosphates of ddA. These ddA-triphosphates act as substrate and inhibitor of HIV-reverse transcriptase substrate and inhibitor of HIV-reverse transcriptase thereby blocking viral DNA synthesis and suppressing HIV replication.

Adverse Reactions

Cardiovascular: Heart failure, thrombocytopenia, cardiomyopathy, Q-T prolongation, vasodilatation

Central nervous system: Headache (32% to 36%), asthenia, insomnia, malaise, CNS depression, cranial nerve palsies, fever, mania

Dermatologic: Rash, pruritus, erythema, eczema, alopecia

Endocrine & metabolic: Hypokalemia, hyperuricemia (dose related), hypomagnesemia, hypocalcemia

Gastrointestinal: Diarrhea (18%), nausea, dyspepsia, vomiting, anorexia, stomatitis, pancreatitis (9%), abdominal pain

Hepatic: Elevated liver enzymes, hepatic failure, fulminant hepatitis

Neuromuscular & skeletal: Paresthesia (34%)

Ocular: Retinal depigmentation, photophobia, diplopia, amblyopia, blindness

Respiratory: Cough, apnea, dyspnea

Signs & Symptoms of Acute Overdose Fanconi's syndrome, myalgia

Toxicodynamics/Kinetics

Absorption: 31% decrease if given with meals

Distribution: V_d: 1 L/kg; CSF levels equal 21% of serum levels
Protein binding: <5%
Bioavailability: 20% to 25% more bioavailable from the tablet than the powder form; absolute: 30% to 33%
Half-life:
Serum: 0.8-2.7 hours
Intracellular: Much longer (8-12 hours)
Time to peak plasma concentration: 30-60 minutes
Elimination: Renal (36% of dose with a clearance of 1 L/kg/hour)

Usual Dosage Oral (administer on an empty stomach):
Children: Dosing is based on body surface area (m^2):
<0.4: 25 mg tablets twice daily or 31 mg powder twice daily
0.5-0.7: 50 mg tablets twice daily or 62 mg powder twice daily
0.8-1: 75 mg tablets twice daily or 94 mg powder twice daily
1.1-1.4: 100 mg tablets twice daily or 125 mg powder twice daily

Adults: Dosing is based on patient weight:
35-49 kg: 125 mg tablets twice daily or 167 mg buffered powder twice daily
50-74 kg: 200 mg tablets twice daily or 250 mg buffered powder twice daily
≥75 kg: 300 mg tablets twice daily or 375 mg buffered powder twice daily

Note: Children >1 year and Adults should receive 2 tablets per dose and children <1 year should receive 1 tablet per dose for adequate buffering and absorption; tablets should be chewed

Dosing adjustment in renal impairment: Should be considered in patients with Cl_{cr} <60 mL/minute

Dosing adjustment in hepatic impairment: Should be considered

Contraindications Hypersensitivity to any component

Warnings Didanosine is indicated for treatment of HIV infection only in patients intolerant of zidovudine or who have failed zidovudine. Patients receiving didanosine may still develop opportunistic infections. Peripheral neuropathy occurs in ~35% of patients receiving the drug; pancreatitis, which in some cases can be fatal, occurs in ~17% of patients receiving didanosine; patients should undergo retinal examination every 6 months to 1 year. Use with caution in patients with decreased renal or hepatic function; in high concentrations, didanosine is mutagenic; use with caution in patients with edema or congestive heart failure; use with caution in patients with hyperuricemia.

Dosage Forms
Powder for oral solution:
Buffered (single dose packet): 100 mg, 167 mg, 250 mg, 375 mg
Pediatric: 2 g, 4 g
Tablet, buffered, chewable (mint flavor): 25 mg, 50 mg, 100 mg, 150 mg

Stability Pediatric oral solution is stable 30 days under refrigeration

Reference Range Peak plasma level of 1-29 μmol/L following oral dose of 0.8-33 mg/kg

Overdosage Treatment
Decontamination: Lavage/activated charcoal with cathartic
Enhancement of elimination: Multiple dosing of activated charcoal may be effective; hemodialysis may be effective in removing approximately 20% of dose

Test Interactions Lowers serum calcium, potassium, magnesium; increases serum triglycerides, uric acid

Diagnostic Tests/Procedures
Didanosine, Blood *on page 1249*

Drug Interactions Decreased absorption of tetracyclines, dapsone, itraconazole, ketoconazole, and quinolones if given together; can cause paresthesia when given with zalcitabine

Pregnancy Risk Factor B

Monitoring Parameters Serum potassium, uric acid, creatinine; hemoglobin, CBC with neutrophil, and platelet count, CD4 cells, liver function tests, amylase, weight gain, perform dilated retinal exam every 6 months

Patient Information Thoroughly chew tablets or manually crush or disperse 2 tablets in 1 oz of water prior to taking; for powder, open packet and pour contents into 4 oz of liquid; do not mix with fruit juice or other acid-containing liquid; stir until dissolved, drink immediately; do not take with meals

Nursing Implications Administer liquified powder immediately after dissolving; avoid creating dust if powder spilled, use wet mop or damp sponge

Additional Information
Contents of each tablet: 11.5 mEq of sodium, 15.7 mEq of magnesium, along with phenylalanine; tablets are buffered with dihydroxyaluminum sodium carbonate, magnesium hydroxide, and sodium citrate
Sodium content of each packet of buffered powder for oral solution: 60 mEq

Specific References

Bissuel F, Cotte L, Cruneel F, et al, "Didanosine-Induced Fulminant Hepatitis," 10th Internal Conference on AIDS, Abstract, 1994, 2:204.

(Continued)

Didanosine *(Continued)*

Bouvet E, Casalino E, Prevost MH, et al, "Fatal Case of 2',3'-Dideoxyinosine-Associated Pancreatitis," *Lancet*, 1990, 336(8729):1515.

Brouillette MJ, Chouinard G, and Lalonde R, "Didanosine-Induced Mania in HIV Infection," *Am J Psychiatry*, 1994, 151(12):1839-40.

Chidiac C, Alfandari S, Caron J, et al, "Diabetes Mellitus Following Treatment of AIDS With Didanosine," *AIDS*, 1995, 9:215-61.

Faulds D and Brogden RN, "Didanosine: A Review of Its Antiviral Activity, Pharmacokinetic Properties and Therapeutic Potential in Human Immunodeficiency Virus Infection," *Drugs*, 1992, 44(1):94-116.

May DB, Drew RH, Yedinak KC, et al, "Effect of Simultaneous Didanosine Administration on Itraconazole Absorption in Healthy Volunteers," *Pharmacotherapy*, 1994, 14(5):509-13.

Morse GD, Shelton MJ, and O'Donnell AM, "Comparative Pharmacokinetics of Antiviral Nucleoside Analogues," *Clin Pharmacokinet*, 1993, 24(2):101-23.

3',4'-Didehydro-4'-Deoxy-8'-Norvinca Leukoblastine Ditartrate *see* Vinorelbine Ditartrate *on page 794*

Dideoxycytidine *see* Zalcitabine *on page 805*

Didronate® *see* Etidronate Disodium *on page 338*

Didronel® *see* Etidronate Disodium *on page 338*

5,5-Diethyl-1-Methylbarbituric Acid *see* Mephobarbital *on page 501*

Diethylenediamine *see* Piperazine Citrate *on page 629*

Diethylstilbestrol (dye eth il stil bess' trole)

Related Information

Drugs and Chemicals Proven to be Teratogenic in Humans *on page 1572-1575*

CAS Number 56-53-1; 130-80-3

Brand Names Boestrol®; Distibene®; Stilphostrol® Injection; Stilphostrol® Oral

Synonyms DES; Stilbestrol; Stilboestrol

Use Palliative treatment of inopérable metastatic prostatic carcinoma and postmenopausal inoperable, progressing breast cancer

Mechanism of Action Competes with estrogenic and androgenic compounds for binding onto tumor cells and thereby inhibits their effects on tumor growth

Adverse Reactions

Cardiovascular: Hypertension, thromboembolism, myocardial infarction

Central nervous system: Headache, depression, dizziness, anxiety, stroke

Dermatologic: Rash, chloasma, melasma

Endocrine & metabolic: Gynecomastia, amenorrhea

Gastrointestinal: Nausea, anorexia, bloating, vomiting, diarrhea, gastrointestinal distress, pancreatitis

Genitourinary: Increased libido (female), decreased libido (male)

Hematologic: Thrombocytopenia, hemolytic anemia, pancytopenia, hypercalcemia

Hepatic: Cholestatic jaundice

Ocular: Intolerance to contact lenses

Miscellaneous: Peripheral edema, breast tenderness, breast tumors, alterations in frequency and flow of menses, edema, decreased glucose tolerance, increased triglycerides and LDL, increased susceptibility to *Candida* infection, increased risk of pre-eclampsia, porphyrinogenic

Signs & Symptoms of Acute Overdose Nausea, dysuria, depression, ectopic pregnancy, hirsutism, hypocalcemia, hyperprolactinemia, hyperactivity, gynecomastia, chest pain

Toxicodynamics/Kinetics

Absorption: Easily in gastrointestinal tract

Metabolism: In the liver

Elimination: Excreted in urine and feces

Usual Dosage Adults:

Male:

- Prostate carcinoma: Oral: 1-3 mg/day
- Diphosphate: Inoperable progressing prostate cancer:
  - Oral: 50 mg 3 times/day; increase up to 200 mg or more 3 times/day; maximum daily dose: 1 g
  - I.V.: Give 0.5 g, dissolved in 250 mL of saline or D_5W, administer slowly the first 10-15 minutes then adjust rate so that the entire amount is given in 1 hour; repeat for ≥5 days depending on patient response, then repeat 0.25-0.5 g 1-2 times for one week or change to oral therapy

Female: Postmenopausal inoperable, progressing breast carcinoma: Oral: 15 mg/day

Administration I.V. infusion: Dilute 0.5-1 g in 250-500 mL D_5W or NS; give 1-2 mL/minute for 10-15 minutes, then infuse remaining solution over 1 hour

Contraindications Undiagnosed vaginal bleeding, during pregnancy

Warnings Use with caution in patients with a history of thromboembolism, stroke, myocardial infarction (especially >40 of age who smoke), liver tumor, hypertension, cardiac, renal or hepatic insufficiency; estrogens have been reported to increase the risk of endometrial carcinoma; do not use estrogens during pregnancy

Dosage Forms

Injection, as diphosphate sodium (Stilphostrol®): 0.25 g (5 mL)

Tablet: 1 mg, 2.5 mg, 5 mg

Tablet (Stilphostrol®): 50 mg

Stability Intravenous solution should be stored at room temperature and away from direct light; solution is stable for 3 days as long as cloudiness or precipitation has not occurred

Overdosage Treatment

Decontamination: Emesis or lavage; activated charcoal with cathartic

Enhancement of elimination: Due to enterohepatic recirculation of drug, multiple dosing of activated charcoal may be effective

Test Interactions

Decreased antithrombin III; decreased serum folate concentration

Increased prothrombin and factors VII, VIII, IX, X; increased platelet aggregability; increased thyroid binding globulin; increased total thyroid hormone (T_4); increased serum triglycerides/phospholipids; increased prolactin level

Drug Interactions

Ascorbic acid can increase estrogen level; increased effect of corticosteroids, succinylcholine, TCAs

Decreased effect of oral anticoagulants; decreased DES levels: barbiturates, phenytoin, rifampin

Pregnancy Risk Factor X

Monitoring Parameters Mammography should be performed in all women prior to starting estrogen therapy and then annually; blood pressure, PAP smear annually

Patient Information Patients should inform their physicians if signs or symptoms of thromboembolic or thrombotic disorders including sudden severe headache or vomiting, disturbance of vision or speech, loss of vision, numbness or weakness in an extremity, sharp or crushing chest pain, calf pain, shortness of breath, severe abdominal pain or mass, mental depression or unusual bleeding.

Nursing Implications Note potency difference between DES base and DES diphosphonate

Additional Information Neoplasms associated with diethylstilbestrol use include renal, hepatic, angiosarcoma, breast, and clear-cell adenocarcinoma of the genital tract in women exposed to diethylstilbestrol *in utero*. The benefits of postmenopausal estrogen therapy may be substantial for some women. Diethylstilbestrol is not the drug of choice for vasomotor symptoms, to prevent bone loss, or to treat vaginal atrophy or urinary incontinence secondary to estrogen deficiency. Diethylstilbestrol does have a role in the treatment of inoperable, progressive prostatic carcinoma and inoperable, progressive breast cancer in select men and women. Risk of developing vaginal or cervical adenocarcinoma is 3 times greater with *in utero* exposure during first trimester as compared with fetal exposure after 13 weeks. *In utero* exposure to diethylstilbestrol does not appear to affect fertility or sexual function in males.

Specific References

Emens JM, "Continuing Problems With Diethylstilboestrol," *Br J Obstet Gynaecol*, 1994, 101(9):748-50.

Emens M, "Vaginal Adenosis and Diethylstilboestrol," *Br J Hosp Med*, 1984, 31(1):42-8.

Giusti RM, Iwamoto K, and Hatch EE, "Diethylstilbestrol Revisited: A Review of the Long-Term Health Effects," *Ann Intern Med*, 1995, 122(10):778-88.

Henriksson P, "Estrogen in Patients With Prostatic Cancer: An Assessment of the Risks and Benefits," *Drug Saf*, 1991, 6(1):47-53.

Hoch-Ligeti C, "Angiosarcoma of the Liver Associated With Diethylstilbestrol," *JAMA*, 1978, 240:1510-1.

Mittendorf R and Williams MA, "Stilboestrol Exposure *In Utero* and Risk of Pre-eclampsia," *Lancet*, 1995, 345(8944):265-6.

Wilcox AJ, Baird DD, Weinberg CR, et al, "Fertility in Men Prenatally to Diethylstilbestrol," *N Engl J Med*, 1995, 338:1411-6.

Diflucan® *see* Fluconazole *on page 353*

Diflunisal (dye floo' ni sal)

CAS Number 22494-42-4

Brand Names Dolobid®

Use Management of inflammatory disorders usually including rheumatoid arthritis and osteoarthritis; can be used as an analgesic for treatment of mild to moderate pain

Mechanism of Action Inhibits prostaglandin synthesis by decreasing the activity of the enzyme, cyclo-oxygenase, which results in decreased formation of prostaglandin precursors

(Continued)

Diflunisal *(Continued)*

Adverse Reactions

Cardiovascular: Tachycardia

Central nervous system: Dizziness, somnolence, insomnia, headache, sweating

Dermatologic: Rash, pruritus

Gastrointestinal: Nausea, dyspepsia, gastrointestinal pain, diarrhea, vomiting, constipation, flatulence, gastrointestinal bleeding/perforation

Genitourinary: Albuminuria

Otic: Tinnitus

Renal: Dysuria, interstitial nephritis, hematuria

Respiratory: Tachypnea

Miscellaneous: Hypersensitivity reactions

Signs & Symptoms of Acute Overdose Drowsiness, photosensitivity, dermatitis, Stevens-Johnson syndrome, gastrointestinal bleeding, malaise, depression, wheezing, thrombocytopenia, stomatitis, gastritis; lightheadedness, nephritis, insomnia, toxic epidermal necrolysis, neutropenia, myalgia, erythema multiforme, hyperthermia, nephrotic syndrome, eosinophilia, confusion, coagulopathy, cholestatic jaundice, hematuria, chills, nausea, vomiting, hyperventilation, tachycardia, ototoxicity, tinnitus, stupor, coma, fever

Toxicodynamics/Kinetics

Onset of analgesia: Within 60 minutes

Duration: 8-12 hours

Absorption: Well absorbed from gastrointestinal tract

Protein binding: 98% to 99%

Metabolism: Extensive in the liver

Half-life: 8-12 hours, prolonged with renal impairment

Time to peak serum concentration: Within 2-3 hours;

Elimination: Excreted in urine within 72-96 hours, ~3% as unchanged drug and 90% as glucuronide conjugates

Usual Dosage Adults: Oral:

Pain: Initial: 500-1000 mg followed by 250-500 mg every 8-12 hours; maximum daily dose: 1.5 g

Inflammatory condition: 500-1000 mg/day in 2 divided doses; maximum daily dose: 1.5 g

Dosing adjustment in renal impairment: Cl_{cr} <50 mL/minute: Administer 50% of normal dose

Contraindications Hypersensitivity to diflunisal or any component, may be a cross-sensitivity with other nonsteroidal anti-inflammatory agents including aspirin; should not be used in patients with active gastrointestinal bleeding

Warnings Peptic ulceration and gastrointestinal bleeding have been reported; platelet function and bleeding time are inhibited by diflunisal at higher doses; ophthalmologic effects; impaired renal function, use lower dosage; peripheral edema; possibility of Reye's syndrome; elevation in liver tests

Dosage Forms Tablet: 250 mg, 500 mg

Overdosage Treatment

Supportive therapy: Management of a nonsteroidal anti-inflammatory agent (NSAID) intoxication is primarily supportive and symptomatic. Fluid therapy is commonly effective in managing the hypotension that may occur following an acute NSAID overdose, except when this is due to an acute blood loss.

Enhancement of elimination: NSAID: Forced diuresis/hemodialysis are of no benefit

Test Interactions Increases chloride (S), glucose, ketone (U), uric acid (S), sodium (S); decreases uric acid (S), catecholamines (U), glucose, potassium (S), prothrombin time (S), uric acid (S); may cross-react with some salicylate assays

Drug Interactions Diflunisal - digoxin leads to increased digoxin plasma concentration; diflunisal - methotrexate may cause increased methotrexate plasma concentrations; diflunisal - anticoagulants leads to increased prothrombin time; hydantoins, sulfonamides, and sulfonylureas may be displayed may cause increase activity; lithium - diflunisal may cause increase lithium level; diflunisal - anticoagulants and thrombolytics increase bleeding without increased PT or PTT but with increased bleeding time

Pregnancy Risk Factor C

Pregnancy Implications Appears in breast milk

Patient Information May cause gastrointestinal upset, take with water, milk, or meals; do not take aspirin with diflunisal; swallow tablets whole, do not crush or chew

Specific References

Arias J, Fernandez-Rivas M, Moral A, et al, "Selective Adverse Reactions to Diflunisal," *Annals of Allergy, Asthma and Immunology*, 1995, 74:160-2.

Balali-Mood M and Prescott LF, "Failure of Alkaline Diuresis to Enhance Diflunisal Elimination," *Br J Clin Pharmacol*, 1980, 10(2):163-5.

Upadhyay HP and Gupta SK, "Diflunisal (Dolobid®) Overdosage," *Br Med J*, 1978, 2(6137):640.

Difosfen® *see* Etidronate Disodium *on page 338*

Digacin *see* Digoxin *on next page*

Digitoxin (di ji tox' in)

CAS Number 71-63-6

Brand Names Corramedan®; Cystodigin®; Digitoxine®; Digitrin®; Nativelle®; Purodigin®; Tardigal®

Use Congestive heart failure, fibrillation (atrial), flutter (atrial), paroxysmal atrial tachycardia, and cardiogenic shock

Mechanism of Action Indirect effect through vagal stimulation. Most clinically important actions of digitalis on the S-A and A-V nodes are mediated through the autonomic nervous system. Digitalis increases efferent vagal impulses, reflexly reduces sympathetic tone, and decreases the sinus rate. In a normal heart, the augmented vagal activity decreases the rate of generation of impulses in the S-A node. A decrease in sinus rate may not occur, but the maximum heart rate achieved during exercise is diminished. When the sinus rate is increased due to heart failure, digitalis has prominent negative chronotropic effects.

Adverse Reactions

Cardiovascular: Sinus bradycardia, A-V block, S-A block, atrial or nodal ectopic beats, ventricular arrhythmias, bigeminy, trigeminy, atrial tachycardia with A-V block

Central nervous system: Drowsiness, fatigue, drowsiness, neuralgia, disorientation, dizziness, visual hallucinations, headache

Endocrine & metabolic: Hyperkalemia with acute toxicity

Gastrointestinal: Vomiting, nausea, feeding intolerance, anorexia, abdominal pain, diarrhea

Hematologic: Thrombocytopenia

Ocular: Blurred vision, halos, yellow or green vision, diplopia, photophobia, flashing lights

Miscellaneous: Feces discoloration (black)

Signs & Symptoms of Acute Overdose Hyperkalemia, neuropathy (peripheral), Stevens-Johnson syndrome, photophobia, bowel ischemia, A-V block, depression, delirium, gynecomastia, arrhythmias, tachycardia (ventricular), fibrillation (ventricular), asystole, hypotension, ototoxicity; tinnitus, vision color changes (green tinge), vision color changes (blue tinge), vision color changes (red tinge), vision color changes (yellow tinge); tremors

Toxicodynamics/Kinetics

Onset of action: 1-2 hours

Peak effect: 4-12 hours

Distribution: V_d: 0.6 L/kg

Protein binding: 97%

Metabolism: Primarily hepatic to active metabolite digoxin

Bioavailability: 90% (gastrointestinal)

Half-life: 4-6 days

Usual Dosage Oral:

Children: Doses are very individualized; when recommended, digitalizing dose is as follows:

- <1 year: 0.045 mg/kg
- 1-2 years: 0.04 mg/kg
- 2 years: 0.03 mg/kg which is equivalent to 0.75 mg/mm^2
- Maintenance: Approximately $^1/_{10}$ of the digitalizing dose

Adults:

- Rapid loading dose: Initial: 0.6 mg followed by 0.4 mg and then 0.2 mg at intervals of 4-6 hours
- Slow loading dose: 0.2 mg twice daily for a period of 4 days followed by a maintenance dose
- Maintenance: 0.05-0.3 mg/day
- Most common dose: 0.15 mg/day

Dosing adjustment in renal impairment: Cl_{cr} <10 mL/minute: Administer 50% to 75% of normal dose

Dosing adjustment in hepatic impairment: Dosage reduction is necessary in severe liver disease

Contraindications Ventricular fibrillation, tachycardia (ventricular), hypersensitivity to digitoxin (rare)

Dosage Forms Tablet: 0.05 mg, 0.1 mg, 0.15 mg, 0.2 mg

Stability Insoluble in water

Reference Range

Therapeutic: 18-22 ng/mL (23-28 nmol/L)

Toxic: >25 ng/mL (>32 nmol/L)

Overdosage Treatment

Decontamination: Lavage/activated charcoal with cathartic

(Continued)

Digitoxin *(Continued)*

Supportive therapy: Antidote: Life-threatening digoxin toxicity is treated with Digibind®; ventricular pacing should be reserved for those patients not responding to Digibind®

Enhancement of elimination: Since enterohepatic recirculation accounts for a low percentage of digitoxin metabolism (6.6%/day), cholestyramine or multiple dosing of activated charcoal would have a minor effect on decreasing half-life; not dialyzable (0% to 5%)

Antidote(s)

Cholestyramine Resin *on page 1405*

Digoxin Immune Fab *on page 1411*

Test Interactions Digibind® will increase serum digitoxin level tenfold; digitoxin can interfere with urinary 17-hydroxycorticosteroid assay; digoxin-like immunoreactive substance (DLIS) which is an endogenous natriuretic substance may cause false elevation

Diagnostic Tests/Procedures

Digitoxin, Blood *on page 1249*

Drug Interactions Decreased gastrointestinal absorption: antacids, cholestyramine, colestipol; increased hepatic metabolism: phenytoin, phenobarbital, phenylbutazone, isoniazid, ethambutol, rifampin, spironolactone, aminoglycoside; decreased protein binding: phenylbutazone, sulfadimethoxine, phenobarbital, clofibrate, tolbutamide; increases levels: verapamil

Pregnancy Risk Factor C

Monitoring Parameters Monitor blood pressure and EKG closely

Patient Information Notify physician if loss of appetite or visual changes occur

Nursing Implications Check apical pulse before administering

Specific References

Baciewicz AM, Isaacson ML, and Lipscomb GL, "Cholestyramine Resin in the Treatment of Digitoxin Toxicity," *Drug Intell Clin Pharm*, 1983, 17(1):57-9.

Hess T, Riesen W, Scholtysik G, et al, "Digitoxin Intoxication With Severe Thrombocytopenia: Reversal by Digoxin-Specific Antibodies," *Eur J Clin Invest*, 1983, 13(2):159-63.

Park GD, Goldberg MJ, Spector R, et al, "The Effects of Activated Charcoal on Digoxin and Digitoxin Clearance," *Drug Intell Clin Pharm*, 1985, 19(12):937-41.

Taboulet P, Baud FJ, Bismuth C, et al, "Acute Digitalis Intoxication – Is Pacing Still Appropriate?" *Clin Toxicol*, 1993, 31:261-73.

Digitoxine® *see* Digitoxin *on previous page*

Digitrin® *see* Digitoxin *on previous page*

Digoxin (di jox' in)

Related Information

Therapeutic Drugs Associated With Hallucinations *on page 1558-1559*

CAS Number 20830-75-5

Brand Names Allocar®; Cardioreg®; Lanocor®; Lanoxicaps®; Lanoxin®; Lenoxin®; Purgoxin®

Synonyms Digacin

Use Treatment of congestive heart failure; slows the ventricular rate in tachyarrhythmias such as fibrillation (atrial), flutter (atrial), tachycardia (ventricular), paroxysmal atrial tachycardia, cardiogenic shock

Mechanism of Action Increases the influx of calcium ions, from extracellular to intracellular cytoplasm by inhibition of sodium and potassium ion movement across the myocardial membranes; this increase in calcium ions results in a potentiation of the activity of the contractile heart muscle fibers and an increase in the force of myocardial contraction (positive inotropic effect); inhibits adenosine triphosphatase (ATPase); decreases conduction through the S-A and A-V nodes

Adverse Reactions

Cardiovascular: Sinus bradycardia, A-V block, S-A block, atrial or nodal ectopic beats, tachycardia (ventricular), ventricular arrhythmias, bigeminy, trigeminy, atrial tachycardia with A-V block

Central nervous system: Drowsiness, fatigue, drowsiness, neuralgia, disorientation, dizziness, chorea (extrapyramidal), auditory and visual hallucinations, paranoia, headache

Endocrine & metabolic: Toxicity is enhanced by hypokalemia

Gastrointestinal: Vomiting, nausea, feeding intolerance, anorexia, abdominal pain, diarrhea

Hematologic: Thrombocytopenia

Ocular: Blurred vision, halos, yellow or green vision, diplopia, photophobia, flashing lights

Miscellaneous: Feces discoloration (black)

Signs & Symptoms of Acute Overdose Hyperkalemia, arrhythmias, Stevens-Johnson syndrome, photophobia, night terrors, heart block, A-V block, impotence, delirium, dementia, depression, hypokalemia, gynecomastia, dysphagia, seizures, neuropathy (peripheral), bowel ischemia, fibrillation (ventricular) or asystole, hypotension, ototoxicity; vision color changes (blue tinge), vision color changes (green tinge), vision color changes (red tinge); tinnitus, tremors

Toxicodynamics/Kinetics

Onset of action:
- Oral: 1-2 hours
- I.V.: 5-30 minutes

Peak effect:
- Oral: 2-8 hours
- I.V.: 1-4 hours

Duration: Adults: 3-4 days

Distribution: Minimal to body fat; high concentrations in myocardium, skeletal muscle, and kidney; crosses blood-brain barrier

V_d:
- Neonates, premature: 4.5 L/kg
- Neonates, full-term: 7.5-10 L/kg
- Children: 16 L/kg
- Adults: 7 L/kg; decreased V_d with renal disease

Protein binding: 23%

Metabolism: Small amount in the liver and gut by bacteria

Bioavailability: Dependent upon formulation, elixir: 70% to 85%, tablets: 60% to 80%, capsules: 90% to 100%

Half-life: Dependent upon age, renal and cardiac function
- Premature: 61-170 hours
- Neonates, full-term: 35-45 hours
- Infants: 18-25 hours
- Children: 35 hours
- Adults: 38-48 hours
  - Anephric: >4.5 days

Elimination: 50% to 70% excreted unchanged in urine

Usual Dosage When changing from oral (tablets or liquid) or I.M. to I.V. therapy, dosage should be reduced by 20% to 25%. See table.

Dosage Recommendations for Digoxin*

Age	Total Digitalizing Dose† (mcg/kg)		Daily Maintenance Dose‡ (mcg/kg)	
	P.O.	I.V. or I.M.	P.O.	I.V. or I.M.
Preterm infant	20–30	15–25	5–7.5	4–6
Full-term infant	25–35	20–30	6–10	5–8
1 mo–2 y	35–60	30–50	10–15	7.5–12
2–5 y	30–40	25–35	7.5–10	6–9
5–10 y	20–35	15–30	5–10	4–8
>10 y	10–15	8–12	2.5–5	2–3
Adults	0.75–1.5 mg	0.5–1 mg	0.125–0.5 mg	0.1–0.4 mg

*Based on lean body weight and normal renal function for age. Decrease dose in patients with ↓ renal function.

†Give one-half of the total digitalizing dose (TDD) in the initial dose, then give one-quarter of the TDD in each of two subsequent doses at 8–12 hour intervals. Obtain EKG 6 hours after each dose to assess potential toxicity.

‡Divided every 12 hours in infants and children <10 years of age. Given once daily to children >10 years and adults.

Dosing adjustment/interval in renal impairment:
- Cl_{cr} 10-50 mL/minute: Administer 25% to 75% of dose or every 36 hours
- Cl_{cr} <10 mL/minute: Administer 10% to 25% of dose or every 48 hours
- Reduce loading dose by 50% in ESRD

Contraindications Hypersensitivity to digoxin or any component; A-V block, idiopathic hypertrophic subaortic stenosis, or constrictive pericarditis, fibrillation (ventricular), tachycardia (ventricular)

Warnings Use with caution in patients with hypoxia, hypothyroidism, acute myocarditis, impaired renal function

Dosage Forms
- Capsule: 0.05 mg, 0.1 mg, 0.2 mg
- Elixir, pediatric (lime flavor): 0.05 mg/mL with alcohol 10% (60 mL)
- Injection: 0.25 mg/mL (1 mL, 2 mL)
- Injection, pediatric: 0.1/mL (1 mL)
- Tablet: 0.125 mg, 0.25 mg, 0.5 mg

(Continued)

Digoxin *(Continued)*

Stability Protect elixir and injection from light; solution compatibility: D_5W, $D_{10}W$, NS, sterile water for injection (when diluted fourfold or greater)

Reference Range

Therapeutic: 0.5-2.0 ng/mL (SI: 0.6-2.6 nmol/L); Adults: <0.5 ng/mL (SI: <0.6 nmol/L) probably indicates underdigitalization unless there are special circumstances

Toxic: >2.0 ng/mL (SI: >2.6 nmol/L); fatalities associated with levels >3.5 ng/mL (>4.8 nmol/L)

Overdosage Treatment

Decontamination: Lavage/activated charcoal with cathartic; whole bowel irrigation may be useful

Supportive therapy: Antidote: Life-threatening digoxin toxicity is treated with Digibind®; phenytoin, magnesium, and lidocaine are useful for cardiac arrhythmias; atropine is useful for bradycardia; avoid quinidine, bretylium, or cardioversion; ventricular pacing should be reserved for patients not responding to Digibind®l; delirium can respond to Digibind®

Enhancement of elimination: Multiple dosing of activated charcoal may be useful; exchange transfusion is of no benefit; hemodialysis/hemoperfusion is ineffective; not dialyzable (0% to 5%)

Antidote(s)

Cholestyramine Resin *on page 1405*

Digoxin Immune Fab *on page 1411*

Test Interactions Digibind® will increase total serum digoxin level about 50-fold; digoxin-like immunoreactive substance (DLIS) which is an endogenous natriuretic substance may cause false elevation

Diagnostic Tests/Procedures

Digoxin, Blood *on page 1250*

Drug Interactions Antacids, kaolin-pectin, cathartics, neomycin, colestipol, phenytoin, cholestyramine, and metoclopramide may decrease absorption of digoxin; quinidine, indomethacin, verapamil, amiodarone, diltiazem, erythromycin, tetracycline, and spironolactone may increase digoxin serum concentration; penicillamine may decrease digoxin's pharmacologic effects; propantheline and atropine may increase digoxin absorption

Pregnancy Risk Factor C

Pregnancy Implications Crosses the placenta; may appear in breast milk

Monitoring Parameters Routine serum level monitoring not recommended but is indicated to rule out toxicity, serum electrolytes (potassium, magnesium, calcium), heart rate; monitor blood pressure and EKG closely

Patient Information Instruct patients to notify physician if they suffer loss of appetite or visual changes

Nursing Implications Check apical pulse before administering

Additional Information

Toxic oral dose: 2 mg

Lethal dose:

- Children: 4 mg
- Adults: 10 mg

Death rate approaches 50% when serum digoxin levels are >6 ng/mL; digoxin-specific antibodies have reversed thrombocytopenia caused by digoxin

Specific References

Antman EM and Smith TW, "Digitalis Toxicity," *Annu Rev Med*, 1985, 36:357-67.

Chan T, Vilke GM, and Williams S, "Bidirectional Tachycardia Associated With Digoxin Toxicity," *J Emerg Med*, 1995, 13:89.

El-Mallakh RS, Hedges S, and Casey D, "Digoxin Encephalopathy Presenting as Mood Disturbance," *J Clin Psychopharmacol*, 1995, 15:82-3.

French JH, Thomas RG, Siskind AP, et al, "Magnesium Therapy in Massive Digoxin Intoxication," *Ann Emerg Med*, 1984, 13(7):562-6.

Gibson TP, "Hemoperfusion of Digoxin Intoxication," *Clin Toxicol*, 1980, 17(4):501-13.

Kaufman J, Leikin J, Kendzierski D, et al, "Use of Digoxin Fab Immune Fragments in a Seven-Day-Old Infant," *Pediatr Emerg Care*, 1990, 6(2):118-21.

Kinlay S and Buckley NA, "Magnesium Sulfate in the Treatment of Ventricular Arrhythmias Due to Digoxin Toxicity," *J Toxicol Clin Toxicol*, 1995, 33(1):55-9.

Moskovits N and Schweitzer P, "CVR and R Rounds: Digitalis-Induced Arrhythmias in a Patient With Normal Digoxin Blood Level," *Cardiovascular Reviews and Reports*, 1995, 16:49-52.

Steiner JF, Robbins LJ, Hammermeister KE, et al, "Incidence of Digoxin Toxicity in Outpatients," *West J Med*, 1994, 161(5):474-8.

Teague Ac, Garnett WR, Briggs GC, et al, "The Effect of Age and Everyday Exercise on Steady-State Plasma Digoxin Concentrations," *Pharmacotherapy*, 1995, 15(4)502-8.

Ujhelyi MR and Robert S, "Pharmacokinetic Aspects of Digoxin-Specific Fab Therapy in the Management of Digitalis Toxicity," *Clin Pharmacokinet*, 1995, 28:483-93.

Varriale P and Mossavi A, "Rapid Reversal of Digitalis Delirium Using Digoxin Immune Fab Therapy," *Clin Cardiol*, 1995, 18:351-2.

Woolf A, "Revising the Management of Digitalis Poisoning," *J Toxicol Clin Toxicol*, 1993, 31(2):275-6.

Dihydrohydroxycodeinone *see* Oxycodone Hydrochloride *on page 585*

Dihydromorphinone *see* Hydromorphone Hydrochloride *on page 409*

Dihydrotachysterol *see* Vitamin D *on page 797*

Dilacor™ XR *see* Diltiazem *on this page*

Diladel® *see* Diltiazem *on this page*

Dilantin® *see* Phenytoin *on page 623*

Dilart® *see* Papaverine *on page 591*

Dilaudid® *see* Hydromorphone Hydrochloride *on page 409*

Dilaudid-HP® *see* Hydromorphone Hydrochloride *on page 409*

Dilitrate®-SR *see* Isosorbide Dinitrate *on page 445*

Dilocaine® *see* Lidocaine Hydrochloride *on page 468*

Diltiazem (dil tye' a zem)

Related Information

Calcium Channel Blocking Agents Comparison *on page 1646-1647*

CAS Number 42399-41-7; 33286-22-5

Brand Names Acalix®; Britiazim®; Cardizem®; Cardizem® CD; Cardizem® SR; Dilacor™ XR; Diladel®; Dilzene®; Segontin®; Tildiem®; Zilden®

Synonyms Latiazem Hydrochloride

Use Management of angina pectoris due to coronary insufficiency, hypertension

Mechanism of Action A benzodiazepine calcium channel blocker which inhibits calcium ion from entering the "slow channels" or select voltage-sensitive areas of vascular smooth muscle and myocardium during depolarization, producing a relaxation of coronary vascular smooth muscle and coronary vasodilation; increases myocardial oxygen delivery in patients with vasospastic angina

Adverse Reactions

Cardiovascular: Arrhythmia, bradycardia, A-V block

Central nervous system: Dizziness, seizures, headache, restlessness, hypothermia

Dermatologic: Rash

Endocrine & metabolic: Hyperglycemia, gynecomastia

Gastrointestinal: Nausea, vomiting, ileus

Hepatic: Mild to marked elevations in liver function tests

Miscellaneous: Noncardiogenic pulmonary edema

Signs & Symptoms of Acute Overdose A-V block, toxic epidermal necrolysis, erythema multiforme, Stevens-Johnson syndrome, mania, myopathy, purpura, hyperglycemia, gynecomastia, gingival hyperplasia, hypotension, asystole, hypothermia, bradycardia, constipation, congestive heart failure

Toxicodynamics/Kinetics

Onset of action:

- Extended-release capsules: 2-3 hours
- Tablets: 30-60 minutes

Duration:

- Extended-release capsules: 12 hours
- Tablets: 4-8 hours

Absorption: ~40% (90% with long-term therapy)

Distribution: V_d:

- Oral: 3.1 L/kg
- I.V.: 11.1 L/kg

Protein binding: 77% to 85%

Metabolism: Extensive in the liver by deacetylation; undergoes extensive first-pass metabolism

Bioavailability: ~40% due to a significant first-pass effect following oral administration

Half-life: 4-6 hours (may increase with renal impairment); 36 hours in overdose setting

Time to peak serum concentration: Within 2-3 hours

Elimination: Excreted in urine and in bile mostly as metabolites

Usual Dosage Adults:

Oral:

- Capsule, sustained release:
  - Cardizem® CD: 180-300 mg once daily
  - Cardizem® SR: 60-120 mg twice daily
  - Dilacor™ XR: 180-240 mg once daily
- Tablet: 30-120 mg 3-4 times/day; dosage should be increased gradually, at 1- to 2-day intervals until optimum response is obtained; usual maintenance dose is usually 180-360 mg/day

(Continued)

Diltiazem *(Continued)*

I.V.: Initial: 0.25 mg/kg as a bolus over 2 minutes, if response is inadequate a second bolus dose may be administered after 15 minutes, then continuous infusion of 5-15 mg/hour for up to 24 hours; may also be utilized for continued heart rate reductions

Conversion from I.V. diltiazem to oral diltiazem: Start oral approximately 3 hours after bolus dose.

Oral dose (mg/day) is approximately equal to [rate (mg/hour) x 3 + 3] x 10

3 mg/hour = 120 mg/day
5 mg/hour = 180 mg/day
7 mg/hour = 240 mg/day
11 mg/hour = 360 mg/day (maximum recommended dose)

Toxic dose:
Children: 6 mg/kg
Adults: 2 g

Contraindications Severe hypotension or second and third degree heart block

Warnings Use with caution in titrating dosages for impaired renal or hepatic function patients; use with caution in patients with congestive heart failure; may be porphyrinogenic

Dosage Forms

Capsule, sustained release:
Cardizem® CD: 120 mg, 180 mg, 240 mg, 300 mg
Cardizem® SR: 60 mg, 90 mg, 120 mg
Dilacor™ XR: 180 mg, 240 mg
Injection (Cardizem®): 5 mg/mL (5 mL, 10 mL)
Tablet (Cardizem®): 30 mg, 60 mg, 90 mg, 120 mg

Reference Range Zero order kinetics are noted with massive ingestion relating to plasma levels >2000 ng/mL; therapeutic serum diltiazem levels: 50-200 ng/mL

Overdosage Treatment

Decontamination: Lavage/activated charcoal with cathartic is useful; ipecac-induced emesis can hypothetically worsen calcium antagonist toxicity, since it can produce vagal stimulation. The potential for seizures precipitously following acute ingestion of large doses of a calcium antagonist may also contraindicate the use of ipecac.

Supportive therapy: Supportive and symptomatic treatment, including I.V. fluids and Trendelenburg positioning, should be initiated as intoxication may cause hypotension. Intra-aortic balloon pump may be useful. Although calcium (calcium chloride I.V. 1-2 g in adults or 10-30 mg/kg in children over 5-10 minutes with repeats as needed) has been used as an "antidote" for acute intoxications, it should be reserved for those cases where definite signs of myocardial depression are evident. Diltiazem may be particularly unresponsive to calcium; heart block may respond to isoproterenol, glucagon, atropine and/or calcium, although a temporary pacemaker may be required. Refractory hypotension can be treated with norepinephrine, dopamine, or amrinone; use diazepam or lorazepam for seizures. Glucagon may increase myocardial contractility.

Enhancement of elimination: Multiple dosing of activated charcoal may not be effective; charcoal hemoperfusion may not be effective

Antidote(s)

Calcium Gluconate *on page 1401*
Glucagon *on page 1431*

Drug Interactions Diltiazem may increase beta-adrenergic blocking agents, cyclosporine, digoxin levels; cimetidine may increase diltiazem levels; diltiazem may increase carbamazepine toxicity; phenytoin decreases bioavailability of oral diltiazem; rifampin may markedly decrease diltiazem levels

Pregnancy Risk Factor C

Pregnancy Implications Appears in breast milk

Patient Information Do not discontinue abruptly; report any dizziness, dyspnea, palpitations, or edema

Nursing Implications Do not crush sustained release capsules

Additional Information Response to atropine may not be observed until after I.V. calcium administration; erythema may precede elevation of liver function tests by 3-5 days; most effective for treating hypertension in African-Americans

Specific References

Anthony T, Jastremski M, Elliott W, et al, "Charcoal Hemoperfusion for the Treatment of a Combined Diltiazem and Metoprolol Overdose," *Ann Emerg Med*, 1986, 15(11):1344-8.

Argenti D, Huang MY, Heald D, et al, "Comparative Pharmacokinetics and Bioavailability of Dilacor™ XR and Cardizem® CD in Healthy Volunteers," *Am J Ther*, 1995, 20-30.

Avila JR, Bejurano D, Gonzalez ML, et al, "Elevation of Hepatic Enzymes After Cutaneous Reaction Caused by Diltiazem," *Ann Pharmacother*, 1995, 29:317-8.

Baird MG, Juneau M, Nadeau C, et al, "Efficacy and Safety of Evening Administration of Controlled-Delivery Diltiazem Capsules in Chronic Stable Angina Patients," *Am J Therapeutics*, 1995, 2:401-6.

Ellenbogen KA, Dias VC, and Cardello FP, "Safety and Efficacy of Intravenous Diltiazem in Atrial Fibrillation or Atrial Flutter," *Am J Cardiol*, 1995, 75(1):45-9.

Fauville JP, Hantson P, Honore P, et al, "Severe Diltiazem Poisoning With Intestinal Pseudo-Obstruction: Case Report and Toxicological Data," *Clin Toxicol*, 1995, 33(3):273-7.

Ferner RE, Odemuyiwa O, Field AB, et al, "Pharmacokinetics and Toxic Effects of Diltiazem in Massive Overdose," *Hum Toxicol*, 1989, 8(6):497-9.

Howarth DM, Dawson AH, Smith AJ, et al, "Calcium Channel Blocking Drug Overdose: An Australian Series," *Hum Exp Toxicol*, 1994, 13(3):161-6.

Kalin JR, Wood KM, and Lee AJ, "A Possible Suicide by Diltiazem Overdose," *J Anal Toxicol*, 1994, 18(3):180-2.

Melanson P, Shih RD, DeRoos F, et al, "Intra-Aortic Balloon Counterpulsation in Calcium Channel Overdose," *Vet Hum Toxicol*, 1993, 35:345.

Proano L, Chiang WK, Wang RY, et al, "Calcium Channel Blocker Overdose," *Am J Emerg Med*, 1995, 13:444-50.

Roberts D, Honcharik N, Sitar DS, et al, "Diltiazem Overdose: Pharmacokinetics of Diltiazem and Its Metabolites and Effect of Multiple Dose Charcoal Therapy," *J Toxicol Clin Toxicol*, 1991, 29(1):45-52.

Snover SW and Bocchino V, "Massive Diltiazem Overdose," *Ann Emerg Med*, 1986, 15(10):1221-4.

Dilzene® *see* Diltiazem *on page 287*

Dimelor® *see* Acetohexamide *on page 86*

Dimenhydrinate (dye men hye' dri nate)

Related Information

Therapeutic Drugs Associated With Hallucinations *on page 1558-1559*

CAS Number 523-87-5

Brand Names Calm-X® [OTC]; Dimetabs®; Dinate®; Dramamine® [OTC]; Dramilin®; Hydrate®; Marmine® [OTC]; Nico-Vert®; Tega-Cert® [OTC]; TripTone® Caplets® [OTC]; Wehamine®

Use Treatment and prevention of nausea, dizziness, and vomiting associated with motion sickness

Mechanism of Action Competes with histamine for H_1-receptor sites on effector cells in the gastrointestinal tract, blood vessels, and respiratory tract; blocks chemoreceptor trigger zone, diminishes vestibular stimulation and depresses labyrinthine function through its central anticholinergic activity

Adverse Reactions

Cardiovascular: Hypotension

Central nervous system: Drowsiness, paradoxical CNS stimulation, dizziness, auditory and visual hallucinations, headache

Gastrointestinal: Anorexia

Genitourinary: Urinary frequency

Hematologic: Porphyria

Local: Pain at the injection site

Ocular: Blurred vision, affects color/night vision

Otic: Ototoxicity, tinnitus

Miscellaneous: Dry mucous membranes

Signs & Symptoms of Acute Overdose Toxicity may resemble atropine overdosage; CNS depression or CNS stimulation, mydriasis; dry mucous membranes

Toxicodynamics/Kinetics

Onset of action: Oral: Within 15-30 minutes

Duration: ~4-6 hours

Absorption: Well absorbed from gastrointestinal tract

Distribution: Wide throughout body

Metabolism: Extensive in the liver

Elimination: Renal

Usual Dosage

Children:

Oral:

2-5 years: 12.5-25 mg every 6-8 hours, maximum: 75 mg/day

6-12 years: 25-50 mg every 6-8 hours, maximum: 150 mg/day

I.M.: 1.25 mg/kg or 37.5 mg/m^2 4 times/day, not to exceed 300 mg/day

Adults: Oral, I.M., I.V.: 50-100 mg every 4-6 hours, not to exceed 400 mg/day

Contraindications Hypersensitivity to dimenhydrinate or any component, porphyria

Warnings Use with caution with prostatic hypertrophy, peptic ulcer, narrow-angle glaucoma, bronchial asthma, and cardiac arrhythmias

Dosage Forms

Capsule: 50 mg

Injection: 50 mg/mL (1 mL, 5 mL, 10 mL)

Liquid: 12.5 mg/4 mL

Tablet: 50 mg

Tablet, chewable: 50 mg

Overdosage Treatment

Supportive therapy: There is no specific treatment for an antihistamine overdose, however, most of its clinical toxicity is due to anticholinergic effects. Anticholin-

(Continued)

Dimenhydrinate *(Continued)*

esterase inhibitors may be useful by reducing acetylcholinesterase. Anticholinesterase inhibitors include physostigmine, neostigmine, pyridostigmine and edrophonium. For anticholinergic overdose with severe life-threatening symptoms, physostigmine 1-2 mg (0.5 or 0.02 mg/kg for children) I.V., slowly may be given to reverse these effects.

Drug Interactions CNS depressants, drugs with anticholinergic effects, ototoxic drugs

Pregnancy Risk Factor B

Pregnancy Implications Small amounts appear in breast milk; crosses placenta; possible oxytocic effect on the uterus at term

Patient Information May cause drowsiness

Nursing Implications I.V. injection must be diluted to 10 mL with NS and given at 25 mg/minute

Additional Information Dramamine® II contains meclizine

Specific References

Luria SM, Kinney JA, McKay CL, et al, "Effects of Aspirin and Dimenhydrinate (Dramamine®) on Visual Processes," *Br J Clin Pharmacol*, 1979, 7(6):585-93.

Dimethyl Sulfoxide

CAS Number 67-68-5

Brand Names Rimso®-50

Synonyms DMS0; Methyl Sulfoxide

Use Industrial solvent; only approved by FDA for treatment of interstitial cystitis; may be a vehicle for other agents; extravasation of chemotherapy agents

Investigational: I.V. use (dose 1 mg/kg) to reduce intracranial pressure in trauma patients

Signs & Symptoms of Acute Overdose Symptoms are rarely reported; facial flushing of face, photophobia, vasodilation, tachycardia, garlic-onion odor or breath, urine discoloration (red), headache, pruritus, dysosmia, agitation, and possible encephalopathy (rare), vomiting, diarrhea, mild elevation of liver function tests, possible hemolysis when given I.V., dizziness, hypernatremia, hemoglobinuria, altered taste

Toxicodynamics/Kinetics

Absorption: Well absorbed from all routes
Distribution: Rapid
Metabolism: Oxidized to dimethylsulfone and reduced to dimethylsulfide
Half-life: Parent drug: 11-14 hours; dimethylsulfone: 60-70 hours
Time to peak: Dermal: 4-8 hours
Elimination: Most DMS0 and metabolites excreted in urine

Usual Dosage Topical: 1.5 mL of a 90% solution every 6 hours for 2 weeks can be used to treat extravasation of anthracycline chemotherapeutic agents or mitomycin

Dosage Forms Solution: 50% [500 mg/mL] (50 mL)

Reference Range Dermal dose of 1 g/kg resulted in peak serum dimethylsulfoxide level of 504-506 mg/L and peak dimethylsulfone serum level of 333-514 mg/L; oral dose of 1 g/kg resulted in peak serum dimethylsulfoxide levels of 1029-3380 mg/L and peak dimethylsulfone level of 263-596 mg/L

Overdosage Treatment

Decontamination: Emesis, lavage/activated charcoal with sorbitol
Supportive therapy: Evaluate and monitor liver function, renal function, hemoglobin, and platelet count
Enhancement of elimination: No data; multiple dosing with activated charcoal may be effective; dialysis does not appear to be effective

Drug Interactions Increased toxicity with sulindac

Pregnancy Implications Unknown risk; appears to be teratogenic in animals

Monitoring Parameters May be analyzed but levels are not helpful

Additional Information Symptoms from DMS0 exposure may be due to other substances carried into the body; it may carry water soluble drugs and provide a dermal reservoir for sustained effect

Specific References

Bond GR, Curry SC, and Dahl DW, "Dimethylsulfoxide-Induced Encephalopathy," *Lancet*, 1989, 1(8647):1134-5.

Hucker HB, Miller JK, Hochberg A, et al, "Studies on the Absorption, Excretion, and Metabolism of Dimethylsulfoxide in Man," *J Pharmacol Exp Ther*, 1967, 155:309-17.
Muther RS and Bennett WM, "Effects of Dimethyl Sulfoxide on Renal Function in Man," *JAMA*, 1980, 244(18):2081-3.
Olver IN, Aisner J, Hament A, et al, "A Prospective Study of Topical Dimethyl Sulfoxide for Treating Anthracycline Extravasation," *J Clin Oncol*, 1988, 6(11):1732-5.

Dimipressin®, Iprogen® *see* Imipramine *on page 422*

Dinate® *see* Dimenhydrinate *on page 289*

Dintoina® *see* Phenytoin *on page 623*

Diocto-K® [OTC] *see* Docusate *on page 297*

Diocto® [OTC] *see* Docusate *on page 297*

Dioctyl Calcium Sulfosuccinate *see* Docusate *on page 297*

Dioctyl Potassium Sulfosuccinate *see* Docusate *on page 297*

Dioctyl Sodium Sulfosuccinate *see* Docusate *on page 297*

Dioeze® [OTC] *see* Docusate *on page 297*

Dipav® *see* Papaverine *on page 591*

Diphenason *see* Dapsone *on page 260*

Diphenoxylate and Atropine (dye fen ox' i late)

CAS Number 915-30-0; 3810-80-8

Brand Names Lofene®; Logen®; Lomanate®; Lomodix®; Lomotil®; Lonox®; Low-Quel®

Synonyms Atropine and Diphenoxylate

Use Treatment of diarrhea with nonbacterial causes

Mechanism of Action Diphenoxylate inhibits excessive gastrointestinal motility and gastrointestinal propulsion (an analogue of meperidine); commercial preparations contain a subtherapeutic amount of atropine to discourage abuse

Adverse Reactions Effects of atropine are noted first followed by diphenoxylate

Cardiovascular: Tachycardia, flushing

Central nervous system: Sedation, dizziness, asthenia, headache, hyperthermia, euphoria, drowsiness, irritability, seizures, coma, hallucination, hyperexcitability, ataxia

Dermatologic: Pruritus, rash

Gastrointestinal: Nausea, vomiting, abdominal discomfort, paralytic ileus, pancreatitis, dry mouth, anorexia, constipation

Genitourinary: Urinary retention

Ocular: Blurred vision

Respiratory: Apnea, respiratory depression (young children may be at greater risk)

Miscellaneous: Physical and psychological dependence with prolonged use

Signs & Symptoms of Acute Overdose Paralytic ileus

Toxicodynamics/Kinetics

Onset of action: Within 45-60 minutes

Peak effect: Within 2 hours

Duration: 3-4 hours

Absorption: Oral: Well absorbed

Distribution: V_d: 3.8 L/kg

Metabolism: Extensive in the liver to diphenoxylic acid (active)

Half-life: 2.5 hours; difenoxine: 4-7 hours

Time to peak serum concentration: 2 hours

Elimination: Primarily in feces (via bile); ~14% excreted in urine; <1% excreted unchanged in urine

Usual Dosage Use with caution in young children due to variable responses; if there is no response within 48 hours, the drug is unlikely to be effective and should be discontinued. Oral:

Children 2-12 years: 0.3-0.4 mg/kg/day of diphenoxylate in 2-4 divided doses

Adults: 15-20 mg/day of diphenoxylate in 3-4 divided doses

Contraindications Hypersensitivity to diphenoxylate, atropine or any component; severe liver disease, jaundice, dehydrated patient, and angle-closure glaucoma; it should not be used for children <2 years of age

Warnings High doses may cause addiction; use with caution in patients with ulcerative colitis, dehydration, and hepatic dysfunction; reduction of intestinal motility may be deleterious in diarrhea resulting from *Shigella*, *Salmonella*, toxigenic strains of *E. coli*, and from pseudomembranous enterocolitis associated with broad spectrum antibiotics; children may develop signs of atropinism (dryness of skin and mucous membranes, thirst, hyperthermia, tachycardia, urinary retention, flushing) even at the recommended dosages

Dosage Forms

Solution, oral: Diphenoxylate hydrochloride 2.5 mg and atropine sulfate 0.025 mg per 5 mL (4 mL, 10 mL, 60 mL)

(Continued)

Diphenoxylate and Atropine *(Continued)*

Tablet: Diphenoxylate hydrochloride 2.5 mg and atropine sulfate 0.025 mg

Reference Range Peak plasma level after 5 mg of diphenoxylate: 0.01 mg/L of diphenoxylate and 0.04 mg/L of difenoxine

Overdosage Treatment

Decontamination: Lavage/activated charcoal with cathartic

Supportive therapy: Naloxone for respiratory/central nervous system depression

Antidote(s)

Naloxone Hydrochloride *on page 1447*

Drug Interactions Increased toxicity: MAO inhibitors (hypertensive crisis), CNS depressants, antimuscarinics (paralytic ileus); may prolong half-life of drugs metabolized in liver

Pregnancy Risk Factor C

Pregnancy Implications Neonatal respiratory depression/withdrawal can occur

Monitoring Parameters Bowel frequency, symptoms of atropinism

Specific References

Cutler EA, Barrett GA, Craven PW, et al, "Delayed Cardiopulmonary Arrest After Lomotil® Ingestion," *Pediatrics*, 1980, 65(1):157-8.

Ginsburg GM, "Lomotil® (Diphenoxylate and Atropine) Intoxication," *Am J Dis Child*, 1973, 125(2):241-2.

Karim A, Ranney RE, Evernsen KL, et al, "Pharmacokinetics and Metabolism of Diphenoxylate in Man," *Clin Pharmacol Ther*, 1972, 13(3):407-19.

McCarron MM, Challoner KR, and Thompson GA, "Diphenoxylate-Atropine (Lomotil®) Overdose in Children: An Update (Report of Eight Cases and Review of the Literature)," *Pediatrics*, 1991, 87(5):694-700.

Diphenylan Sodium® *see* Phenytoin *on page 623*

Diphenylhydantoin *see* Phenytoin *on page 623*

Diphos® *see* Etidronate Disodium *on page 338*

Diprazinum *see* Promethazine Hydrochloride *on page 650*

Diprivan® Injection *see* Propofol *on page 653*

Dipropylacetic Acid *see* Valproic Acid and Derivatives *on page 782*

Dipyridamole (dye peer id' a mole)

CAS Number 58-32-2

Brand Names Anginal®; Apo-dipyridamole®; Cardoxin®; Natyl®; Persantine®; Plato®; Viscor®

Use Maintain patency after surgical grafting procedures including coronary artery bypass; with warfarin to decrease thrombosis in patients after artificial heart valve replacement; for chronic management of angina pectoris; with aspirin to prevent coronary artery thrombosis; in combination with aspirin or warfarin to prevent other thromboembolic disorders

Mechanism of Action Inhibits the activity of adenosine deaminase and phosphodiesterase, which causes an accumulation of adenosine, adenine nucleotides, and cyclic AMP; these mediators then inhibit platelet aggregation and may cause vasodilation; may also stimulate release of prostacyclin or PGD_2

Adverse Reactions

Cardiovascular: Vasodilatation, flushing, angina, pericardial effusion/pericarditis

Central nervous system: Dizziness, syncope, headache (dose related), asthenia

Dermatologic: Rash, pruritus

Gastrointestinal: Abdominal distress, nausea, vomiting

Respiratory: Asthma, pulmonary edema

Signs & Symptoms of Acute Overdose Hypotension, bradycardia, cholelithiasis, peripheral vasodilation, wheezing, coagulopathy, myalgia, metallic taste, chest pain

Toxicodynamics/Kinetics

Absorption: Readily from the gastrointestinal tract; variable and slow

Distribution: V_d: Adults: 2-3 L/kg; distributed widely in body tissues

Protein binding: 91% to 99%

Metabolism: Concentrated and metabolized in the liver; enterohepatic recirculation accounts for 16% of recycled dose

Bioavailability: 37% to 66%

Half-life, terminal: 10-12 hours; varies 1-12 hours

Time to peak serum concentration: Within 2-2.5 hours

Elimination: Excreted in feces via bile as glucuronide conjugates and unchanged drug

Usual Dosage

Oral:

Children: 4-10 mg/kg/day in 3 divided doses

Doses of 4-10 mg/kg/day have been used investigationally to treat albuminuria in pediatric renal disease

Adults: 75-400 mg/day in 3-4 divided doses

I.V.: 0.14 mg/kg/minute for 4 minutes; maximum dose: 60 mg

Contraindications Hypersensitivity to dipyridamole or any component

Warnings Safety and effectiveness in children <12 years of age have not been established; may further decrease blood pressure in patients with hypotension due to peripheral vasodilation

Dosage Forms

Injection: 10 mg/2 mL

Tablet: 25 mg, 50 mg, 75 mg

Stability Insoluble in water

Reference Range 300 mg oral dose associated with a serum dipyridamole level of 2.9 μg/mL

Overdosage Treatment

Decontamination: Ipecac or lavage/activated charcoal with cathartic

Supportive therapy: Fluids and vasopressors may be helpful although hypotension is often transient; coronary vasodilation may be reversed by aminophylline

Enhancement of elimination: Multiple dose of activated charcoal may be useful; dialysis unlikely to help because highly protein bound

Test Interactions May give falsely elevated lipoprotein level

Drug Interactions Heparin; can enhance the effect of adenosine

Pregnancy Risk Factor C

Pregnancy Implications Small amounts cross placenta

Monitoring Parameters Blood pressure, heart rate

Patient Information Notify physician or pharmacist if taking other medications that affect bleeding, such as NSAIDs or warfarin

Nursing Implications Dilute I.V. dipyridamole in at least a 1:2 ratio with D_5W

Additional Information Dipyridamole may also be given 2 days prior to open heart surgery to prevent platelet activation by extracorporeal bypass pump; doses of 4-10 mg/kg/day have been used investigationally to treat albuminuria in pediatric renal disease

Specific References

Blumenthal MS and McCauley CS, "Cardiac Arrest During Dipyridamole Imaging," *Chest*, 1988, 93(5):1103-4.

Nielsen-Kudsk F and Pedersen SK, "Pharmacokinetics of Dipyridamole," *Acta Pharmacol Toxicol (Copenh)*, 1979, 44(5):391-9.

Shannon M and Maher T, "Anticonvulsant Effects of Intracerebroventricular Adenocard in Theophylline-Induced Seizures," *Ann Emerg Med*, 1995, 26:6508.

Dirithromycin

CAS Number 62013-04-1

Brand Names Dynabac®

Synonyms ASE-136BS; LY-237216

Use Not yet FDA-approved for community-acquired pneumonia, pharyngitis/tonsilitis, bronchitis, skin and skin structure infections

Mechanism of Action Macrolide antibiotic similar to erythromycin, dirithromycin; inhibits RNA synthesis

Adverse Reactions

Central nervous system: Headache (5%), dizziness, asthenia

Dermatologic: Urticaria

Gastrointestinal: Abdominal pain (6%), diarrhea (5%), nausea (5%), dyspepsia

Toxicodynamics/Kinetics

Peak plasma level: 4-24 hours

Absorption: Food does not affect absorption

Protein binding: 15% to 32%

Metabolism: V_d: 800 L; hydrolysis to erythromycyclamine (active metabolite)

Half-life: 44 hours

Elimination: Fecal (81% to 97%), urine (1% to 3%)

Usual Dosage 500 mg/day

Contraindications Previous hypersensitivity to dirithromycin

Warnings Use with caution in patients with liver disease

Reference Range After a 500 mg oral dose, peak plasma level was 0.5 mg/L

Overdosage Treatment

Decontamination: Lavage/activated charcoal with cathartic

Supportive therapy: Acute gastrointestinal irritation can be treated with milk or bismuth subsalicylate; lidocaine can be used for ventricular arrhythmias

Elimination: Hemodialysis is not effective

Drug Interactions Fewer drug interaction effects than with erythromycin; antacids and H_2-blockers can increase absorption; concomitant therapy with theophylline can result in lower trough levels of theophylline (increased clearance)

Additional Information Effective against gram-positive organisms (*Legionella*, *Helicobacter pylori*, and *Chlamydia trachomatis*)

Specific References

Bachmann K, Sullivan TJ, Reese JH, et al, "The Influence of Dirithromycin on the Pharmacokine-

(Continued)

Dirithromycin *(Continued)*

tics of Cyclosporine in Healthy Subjects and in Renal Transplant Patients," *Am J Therapeut*, 1995, 2:490-8.

Brogden RN and Peters DH, "Dirithromycin: A Review of Its Antimicrobial Activity, Pharmacokinetic Properties, and Therapeutic Efficacy," *Drugs*, 1994, 48(4):599-616.

Disadine® *see* Povidone-Iodine *on page 635*

Disalcid® *see* Salsalate *on page 689*

Disalicylic Acid *see* Salsalate *on page 689*

Disne Asmol® *see* Ipratropium Bromide *on page 438*

Disodium Cromoglycate *see* Cromolyn Sodium *on page 245*

Disodium Difluoride *see* Fluoride *on page 355*

d-Isoephedrine Hydrochloride *see* Pseudoephedrine *on page 661*

Disonate® [OTC] *see* Docusate *on page 297*

Disoprivan® *see* Propofol *on page 653*

Disoprofol *see* Propofol *on page 653*

Disopyramide Phosphate (dye soe peer' a mide)

Related Information

Therapeutic Drugs Associated With Hallucinations *on page 1558-1559*

CAS Number 3737-09-5; 22059-60-5

Brand Names Dicorynan®; Napamide®; Norpace®; Rhythmodan®; Ritmilen®

Use Suppression and prevention of unifocal and multifocal premature, ventricular premature complexes, coupled tachycardia (ventricular); also effective in the conversion of fibrillation (atrial), flutter (atrial), and paroxysmal atrial tachycardia to normal sinus rhythm and prevention of the reoccurrence of these arrhythmias after conversion by other methods

Mechanism of Action Class IA antiarrhythmic: Decreases myocardial excitability and conduction velocity; reduces disparity in refractory between normal and infarcted myocardium; possesses anticholinergic, peripheral vasoconstrictive, and negative inotropic effects

Adverse Reactions

Cardiovascular: Congestive heart failure, edema, chest pain, syncope and hypotension; conduction disturbances including A-V block, QRS prolongation, Q-T prolongation

Central nervous system: Fatigue, malaise, nervousness, acute psychosis, depression, dizziness, asthenia, headache, auditory and visual hallucinations

Dermatologic: Generalized rashes

Endocrine & metabolic: Hypoglycemia, may initiate contractions of pregnant uterus, hyperkalemia may enhance toxicities, weight gain

Gastrointestinal: Constipation, nausea, vomiting, diarrhea, pain, gas, anorexia, dry mouth, decreased bowel sounds

Genitourinary: Urinary retention/hesitancy, impotence

Hematologic: Granulocytopenia

Hepatic: Hepatic cholestasis, elevated liver enzymes, increased cholesterol and triglycerides

Neuromuscular & skeletal: Paresthesia

Ocular: Blurred vision, photophobia, diplopia, mydriasis, acute angle-closure glaucoma

Respiratory: Dyspnea

Miscellaneous: Dry nose, eyes, and throat; anaphylactic shock

Signs & Symptoms of Acute Overdose Anticholinergic effects, hypotension, photosensitivity, impotence, hypoglycemia, A-V block, drowsiness, slurred speech, mydriasis, paroxysmal tachycardia (ventricular), jaundice, apnea, coma, heart block, loss of consciousness, respiratory arrest, intraocular pressure (increased), cardiac conduction disturbances, cardiac arrhythmias, QRS prolongation, Q-T prolongation, bradycardia, congestive heart failure, asystole, seizures, torsade de pointes, urine discoloration (milky), leukopenia; neutropenia; agranulocytosis; granulocytopenia

Toxicodynamics/Kinetics

Onset of action: 30-210 minutes

Duration of effect: 1.5-8.5 hours

Absorption: Rapid and nearly complete

Distribution: V_d: 0.5-1.3 L/kg; distributed well throughout extracellular fluid but is not extensively bound to tissues

Protein binding: 20% to 60%

Metabolism: In the liver to an active metabolite (mono-N-dealkylated pyramide)

Bioavailability: 60% to 83%

Half-life: Adults: 4-10 hours; increased half-life with hepatic or renal disease; sustained release: 11.7 hours

Time to peak serum concentration: 30 minutes to 3 hours

Elimination: Excreted 40% to 60% unchanged in urine and 10% to 15% in feces; clearance: 1.3 mL/minute/kg

Usual Dosage Oral:

Children:

- <1 year: 10-30 mg/kg/24 hours in 4 divided doses
- 1-4 years: 10-20 mg/kg/24 hours in 4 divided doses
- 4-12 years: 10-15 mg/kg/24 hours in 4 divided doses
- 12-18 years: 6-15 mg/kg/24 hours in 4 divided doses

Adults:

- <50 kg: 100 mg every 6 hours or 200 mg every 12 hours (controlled release)
- >50 kg: 150 mg every 6 hours or 300 mg every 12 hours (controlled release); if no response, may increase to 200 mg every 6 hours; maximum dose required for patients with severe refractory tachycardia (ventricular) is 400 mg every 6 hours

Dosing adjustment in renal impairment: 100 mg (nonsustained release) given at the following intervals: See table.

Creatinine Clearance (mL/min)	Dosage Interval
30–40	q8h
15–30	q12h
<15	q24h

Dosing interval in hepatic impairment: 100 mg every 6 hours or 200 mg every 12 hours (controlled release)

Contraindications Pre-existing second or third degree A-V block; cardiogenic shock or known hypersensitivity to the drug

Warnings May aggravate heart failure and cause hypotension; may be ineffective in hypokalemia and toxic effects enhanced in hyperkalemia; pre-existing urinary retention, family history or existing angle-closure glaucoma, myasthenia gravis, hypotension during initiation of therapy, congestive heart failure unless caused by an arrhythmia, widening of QRS complex during therapy or Q-T interval (>25% to 50% of baseline QRS complex or Q-T interval), sick sinus syndrome or WPW, renal or hepatic impairment require decrease in dosage

Dosage Forms

Capsule: 100 mg, 150 mg

Capsule, sustained action: 100 mg, 150 mg

Reference Range

Therapeutic:

- Atrial arrhythmias: 2.8-3.2 μg/mL (SI: 8.3-9.4 μmol/L)
- Ventricular arrhythmias: 3.3-7.5 μg/mL (SI: 9.7-22.0 μmol/L)

Toxic: >7.0 μg/mL (SI: >20.7 μmol/L)

Fatal: Levels >16.0 μg/mL

Overdosage Treatment

Decontamination: Lavage/activated charcoal with cathartic

Supportive therapy: Phenytoin and lidocaine are useful for ventricular arrhythmia; isoproterenol is useful to reverse cardiac depressant effects. Resuscitative effort may need to be prolonged. Calcium chloride may be useful for electromechanical disassociation.

Enhancement of elimination: Forced diuresis, charcoal hemoperfusion is effect; multiple dosing of activated charcoal may be effective; not dialyzable (0% to 5%)

Test Interactions Decreases glucose

Diagnostic Tests/Procedures

Disopyramide, Blood *on page 1251*

Drug Interactions Hepatic microsomal enzyme inducing agents (ie, phenytoin, phenobarbital, rifampin) may increase metabolism of disopyramide; erythromycin, quinidine, and atenolol may increase disopyramide serum concentrations; ethanol increases renal clearance

Pregnancy Risk Factor C (may cause uterine contractions)

Monitoring Parameters EKG, blood pressure, disopyramide drug level

Patient Information Notify physician if urinary retention or worsening CHF; do not break or chew sustained release capsules

Specific References

Accornero F, Pellanda A, Ruffini C, et al, "Prolonged Cardiopulmonary Resuscitation During Acute Disopyramide Poisoning," *Vet Hum Toxicol*, 1993, 35(3):231-2.

Hayler AM, Holt DW, and Volans GN, "Fatal Overdosage With Disopyramide," *Lancet*, 1978, 1(8071):468-9.

(Continued)

Disopyramide Phosphate *(Continued)*

Morady F, Scheinman MM, and Desai J, "Disopyramide," *Ann Intern Med*, 1982, 96(3):337-43.
Sathyavagiswaran L, "Fatal Disopyramide Intoxication From Suicidal/Accidental Overdose," *J Forensic Sci*, 1987, 32(6):1813-8.
Wayne K, Manolas E, and Sloman G, "Fatal Overdose With Disopyramide," *Med J Aust*, 1980, 1(5):231-2.

Dissenten® *see* Loperamide Hydrochloride *on page 480*

Distaval® *see* Thalidomide *on page 734*

Distibene® *see* Diethylstilbestrol *on page 280*

Disulfiram (dye sul' fi ram)

Related Information

Therapeutic Drugs Associated With Hallucinations *on page 1558-1559*

CAS Number 97-77-8

Brand Names Antabuse®

Use Management of chronic alcoholics; also used to treat allergic nickel dermatitis and can enhance the elimination of nickel

Mechanism of Action Disulfiram is a thiuram derivative which interferes with aldehyde dehydrogenase. When taken concomitantly with alcohol, there is an increase in serum acetaldehyde levels. High acetaldehyde causes uncomfortable symptoms, including flushing, nausea, thirst, palpitations, chest pain, dizziness, and hypotension. This reaction is the basis for disulfiram use in postwithdrawal long-term care of alcoholism. May also boost the immune function in HIV patients.

Adverse Reactions Alcohol-disulfiram reaction:

Cardiovascular: Flushing, cardiovascular collapse, myocardial infarction
Central nervous system: Dizziness, seizures, death, sweating, auditory and visual hallucinations, psychosis, headache
Gastrointestinal: Nausea, vomiting, metallic taste
Hepatic: Hepatitis
Ocular: Retrobulbar neuritis
Respiratory: Dyspnea, chest pain

Signs & Symptoms of Acute Overdose Nystagmus, paresthesia, ataxia, thrombocytopenia, facial flushing, numbness, impotence, syncope, ptosis, dysphoria, mania, memory loss, eczema, garlic-like breath, rotten egg breath, dementia, seizures, depression, metallic taste; blindness

Toxicodynamics/Kinetics

Peak effect: 8-12 hours
Absorption: 80% within 1 hour
Protein binding: 96%
Metabolism: To diethyldithiocarbamate (DDC) and methyl-DDC; DDC is then metabolized to diethylamine and carbon disulfide
Half-life:
- Disulfiram: 1-12 hours
- DDC: 15.5 hours
- Methyl-DDC: 22 hours
- Diethylamine: 14 hours
- Carbon disulfide: 9 hours

Elimination: Renal (<10%), fecal (20%), pulmonary (20% to 30%)

Usual Dosage Adults: Oral: Maximum daily dose: 500 mg/day in a single dose for 1-2 weeks; average maintenance dose: 250 mg/day; range: 125-500 mg; duration of therapy is to continue until the patient is fully recovered socially and a basis for permanent self control has been established; maintenance therapy may be required for months or even years

Contraindications Severe myocardial disease and coronary occlusion, hypersensitivity to disulfiram or any component, patient receiving alcohol, paraldehyde, alcohol-containing preparations like cough syrup or tonics

Warnings Should never be administered to a patient when he/she is in a state of alcohol intoxication, or without his/her knowledge; use with caution in patients with diabetes, hypothyroidism, seizure disorders, hepatic cirrhosis or insufficiency

Dosage Forms Tablet: 250 mg, 500 mg

Reference Range Peak blood disulfiram level after a 500 mg dose: 0.38 mg/L; peak DDC level is ~1.2 mg/L; peak carbon disulfide level is 14 mg/L; concomitant ethanol levels >0.12 g/dL associated with unconsciousness when ethanol is used with disulfiram

Overdosage Treatment Management of disulfiram reaction: Institute support measures to restore blood pressure (pressors and fluids); monitor for hypokalemia; metoclopramide or prochlorperazine can be used for vomiting; dopamine is not useful to treat disulfiram-ethanol induced hypotension; norepinephrine is the preferred agent; use of 4-methylpyrazole is investigational

Antidote(s)

Norepinephrine Bitartrate *on page 1451*

Test Interactions Decreases catecholamines (U); increases serum cholesterol acetone levels

Drug Interactions Increased toxicity of INH, metronidazole, phenytoin, alcohol, warfarin, diazepam, chlordiazepoxide; can cause elevation of theophylline

Pregnancy Risk Factor C

Pregnancy Implications Increased incidence of clubfoot, limb reduction, vertebral fusion have been reported

Monitoring Parameters Hypokalemia

Patient Information Do not drink any alcohol, including products containing alcohol (cough and cold syrups), or use alcohol-containing skin products for at least 3 days and preferably 14 days after stopping this medication or while taking this medication; not for treatment of alcohol intoxication; may cause drowsiness

Nursing Implications Administration of any medications containing alcohol including topicals is contraindicated

Specific References

Motte S, Vincent JL, and Gillet JB, "Refractory Hyperdynamic Shock Associated With Alcohol and Disulfiram," *Am J Emerg Med*, 1986, 4(4):323-5.

Pompidou A, Delsaux MC, Telvi L, et al, "Isoprinosine and Imuthiol, Two Potentially Active Compounds in Patients With AIDS-Related Complex Symptoms," *Cancer Res*, 1985, 45(9 Suppl):4671S-4673S.

Ditan® *see* Phenytoin *on page 623*

Diural® *see* Furosemide *on page 373*

Divalproex Sodium *see* Valproic Acid and Derivatives *on page 782*

Dixart® *see* Clonidine *on page 231*

Dizmiss® [OTC] *see* Meclizine Hydrochloride *on page 494*

***dl*-Alpha Tocopherol** *see* Vitamin E *on page 798*

***dl*-Norephedrine Hydrochloride** *see* Phenylpropanolamine Hydrochloride *on page 622*

d-Methorphan *see* Dextromethorphan Hydrobromide *on page 270*

DMSO *see* Dimethyl Sulfoxide *on page 290*

Docusate (dok' yoo sate)

CAS Number 128-49-4; 7491-09-0; 577-11-7

Brand Names Colace® [OTC]; Correctol® Extra Gentle [OTC]; DC 240® Softgel® [OTC]; Dialose® [OTC]; Diocto® [OTC]; Diocto-K® [OTC]; Dioeze® [OTC]; Disonate® [OTC]; DOK® [OTC]; DOS® Softgel® [OTC]; D-S-S® [OTC]; Kasof® [OTC]; Modane® Soft [OTC]; Pro-Cal-Sof® [OTC]; Regulax SS® [OTC]; Regutol® [OTC]; Silace® [OTC]; Sulfalax® [OTC]; Surfak® [OTC]

Synonyms Dioctyl Calcium Sulfosuccinate; Dioctyl Potassium Sulfosuccinate; Dioctyl Sodium Sulfosuccinate; DOSS; DSS

Use Stool softener in patients who should avoid straining during defecation and constipation associated with hard, dry stools

Mechanism of Action An emollient laxative which reduces surface tension of the oil-water interface of the stool resulting in enhanced incorporation of water and fat allowing for stool softening; also promotes intestinal secretion of potassium, water, sodium, and chloride

Adverse Reactions

Gastrointestinal: Intestinal obstruction, diarrhea, abdominal cramping

Miscellaneous: Throat irritation

Signs & Symptoms of Acute Overdose Abdominal cramps, diarrhea, fluid loss, hypokalemia, hypomagnesemia, nausea, vomiting

Toxicodynamics/Kinetics

Onset of action: 12-72 hours

Elimination: Biliary (primarily)

Usual Dosage Docusate salts are interchangeable; the amount of sodium, calcium, or potassium per dosage unit is clinically insignificant

Infants and Children <3 years: Oral: 10-40 mg/day in 1-4 divided doses

Children: Oral:

- 3-6 years: 20-60 mg/day in 1-4 divided doses
- 6-12 years: 40-150 mg/day in 1-4 divided doses

Adolescents and Adults: Oral: 50-500 mg/day in 1-4 divided doses

Older Children and Adults: Rectal: Add 50-100 mg of docusate liquid to enema fluid (saline or water); give as retention or flushing enema

Contraindications Concomitant use of mineral oil; intestinal obstruction, acute abdominal pain, nausea, vomiting; hypersensitivity to docusate or any component

Warnings Prolonged, frequent or excessive use may result in dependence or electrolyte imbalance

(Continued)

Docusate *(Continued)*

Dosage Forms

Capsule, as calcium:

DC 240® Softgel®, Pro-Cal-Sof®, Sulfalax®: 240 mg

Surfak®: 50 mg, 240 mg

Capsule, as potassium:

Diocto-K®: 100 mg

Kasof®: 240 mg

Capsule, as sodium:

Colace®: 50 mg, 100 mg

Correctol® Extra Gentle: 100 mg

Dioeze®: 250 mg

Disonate®: 100 mg, 240 mg

DOK®: 100 mg, 250 mg

DOS® Softgel®: 100 mg, 250 mg

D-S-S®: 100 mg

Modane® Soft: 100 mg

Regulax SS®: 100 mg, 250 mg

Liquid, as sodium (Diocto®, Colace®, Disonate®, DOK®): 150 mg/15 mL (30 mL, 60 mL, 480 mL)

Syrup, as sodium:

50 mg/15 mL (15 mL, 30 mL)

Colace®, Diocto®, Disonate®, DOK®, Silace®: 60 mg/15 mL (240 mL, 480 mL, 3780 mL)

Tablet, as sodium (Dialose®, Regutol®): 100 mg

Overdosage Treatment

Decontamination: Lavage/activated charcoal without a cathartic

Supportive therapy: Intravenous fluid and electrolyte replacement; restrict solid food

Test Interactions ↓ potassium (S), ↓ chloride (S); transaminases (elevated)

Drug Interactions Increased toxicity of mineral oil; leukopenia with liver enzyme elevation associated with concomitant use with danthron; hepatotoxic with oxyphenisatin or quinidine

Pregnancy Risk Factor C

Pregnancy Implications Can cause hypomagnesemia in the neonate; no evidence for congenital malformations

Patient Information Adults: Docusate should be taken with a full glass of water

Nursing Implications Docusate liquid should be given with milk, fruit juice, or infant formula to mask the bitter taste

Additional Information Docusate sodium 5-10 mg/mL liquid instilled in the ear as a ceruminolytic produces substantial ear wax disintegration within 15 minutes and complete disintegration after 24 hours. A safe agent to be used in elderly; some evidence that doses <200 mg are ineffective; stool softeners are unnecessary if stool is well hydrated or "mushy" and soft; shown to be ineffective used long-term.

Specific References

Pietrusko RG, "Use and Abuse of Laxatives," *Am J Hosp Pharm*, 1977, 34:291-300.

Schindler AM, "Isolated Neonatal Hypomagnesaemia Associated With Maternal Overuse of Stool Softener," *Lancet*, 1984, 2(8406):822.

Dofetilide

Synonyms UK-68-798

Use Prevention and treatment of fibrillation (atrial), flutter (atrial), paroxysmal tachycardia (ventricular), tachycardia (ventricular), fibrillation (ventricular); used in conjunction of implantable defibrillator

Mechanism of Action Selective class III antiarrhythmic agent (investigational agent undergoing phase III trials in U.S.); more potent than sotalol, it causes selective blockade of potassium channels in the myocardium that prolongs ventricular refractoriness

Adverse Reactions Cardiovascular: Prolongs Q-T intervals on EKG, bradycardia, possible increase in incidence of torsade de pointes

Toxicodynamics/Kinetics

Absorption: Oral: 100%; slightly delayed in presence of food

Distribution: V_d: 3.9 L/kg

Metabolism: Hepatic

Half-life:

I.V.: 7.5 hours

Oral: 7.1 hours

Peak plasma levels: 1-4 hours

Elimination: Renal

Usual Dosage

Oral: 0.25-1 mg twice daily in patients with sustained tachycardia (ventricular) (lower dose in patients with renal insufficiency)

I.V.:

Supraventricular tachycardia: 1-10 mcg/kg over 15 minutes followed by 0.12-0.5 mcg/kg maintenance infusion

Ventricular arrhythmia: 1.5-15 mcg/kg

Overdosage Treatment

Decontamination: Lavage/activated charcoal (for oral ingestion)

Supportive therapy: No human overdose experience since this agent inhibits intracellular potassium transport, agents such as glucose/insulin and hyperventilation may assist in creasing intracellular potassium concentrations; need to monitor for hypokalemia and torsade de pointes

Enhancement of elimination: Multiple dosing of activated charcoal may be effective

Drug Interactions Avoid agents that can induce torsade de pointes (such as cimetidine, haloperidol, erythromycin, terfenadine)

Additional Information Increases myocardial refractoriness

Specific References

Tran HT, Kuger J, and Chow MS, "Focus on Dofetilide: A Selective Class III Antiarrhythmic Agent," *Hosp Formul*, 1995, 30:23-7.

Dogmatil Forte® *see* Sulpiride *on page 717*

DOK® [OTC] *see* Docusate *on page 297*

Dolantin® *see* Meperidine Hydrochloride *on page 499*

Dolantina® *see* Meperidine Hydrochloride *on page 499*

Dolantine® *see* Meperidine Hydrochloride *on page 499*

Dolene® *see* Propoxyphene *on page 655*

Dolobid® *see* Diflunisal *on page 281*

Dolophine® *see* Methadone Hydrochloride *on page 508*

Dolosal® *see* Meperidine Hydrochloride *on page 499*

Domical® *see* Amitriptyline Hydrochloride *on page 116*

Domnamid® *see* Estazolam *on page 324*

Dopamet® *see* Methyldopa *on page 519*

Dopar® *see* Levodopa *on page 462*

Dopegyt® *see* Methyldopa *on page 519*

Doral® *see* Quazepam *on page 665*

Dorcol® [OTC] *see* Acetaminophen *on page 79*

Doriden® *see* Glutethimide *on page 383*

Dormalin® *see* Quazepam *on page 665*

Dormicum® *see* Midazolam Hydrochloride *on page 532*

Dormigen® *see* Nitrazepam *on page 562*

Dornase Alfa (door' nace al' fa)

Brand Names Pulmozyme®

Synonyms rDNase; Recombinant Human Deoxyribonuclease I

Use Management of cystic fibrosis patients to reduce the frequency of respiratory infections that require parenteral antibiotics, and to improve pulmonary function

Mechanism of Action The hallmark of cystic fibrosis lung disease is the presence of abundant, purulent airway secretions composed primarily of highly polymerized DNA. The principal source of this DNA is the nuclei of degenerating neutrophils, which is present in large concentrations in infected lung secretions. The presence of this DNA produces a viscous mucous that may contribute to the decreased mucociliary transport and persistent infections that are commonly seen in this population. Dornase alfa is a deoxyribonuclease (DNA) enzyme produced by recombinant gene technology. Dornase selectively cleaves DNA, thus reducing mucous viscosity and as a result, airflow in the lung is improved and the risk of bacterial infection may be decreased. Pulmonary function improves after 3 days of use.

Adverse Reactions

Cardiovascular: Chest pain

Dermatologic: Rash

Ocular: Conjunctivitis

Respiratory: Cough, dyspnea, pharyngitis, laryngitis, hoarse throat, wheezing, rhinitis, hemoptysis

Miscellaneous: Voice alteration (most noted in female patients)

Toxicodynamics/Kinetics Following nebulization, enzyme levels are measurable in the sputum within 15 minutes and decline rapidly thereafter

Usual Dosage Children >5 years and Adults: Inhalation: 2.5 mg once daily through selected nebulizers in conjunction with a Pulmo-Aide® or a Pari-Proneb® compressor

(Continued)

Dornase Alfa *(Continued)*

Contraindications Patients with known hypersensitivity to dornase alfa, Chinese hamster ovary cell products (eg, epoetin alfa), or any component

Warnings No clinical trials have been conducted to demonstrate safety and effectiveness of dornase in children <5 years of age, in patients with pulmonary function <40% of normal, or in patients for longer treatment periods of >12 months; no data exists regarding safety during lactation

Dosage Forms Solution, inhalation: 1 mg/mL (2.5 mL)

Stability Must be stored in the refrigerator at 2°C to 8°C (36°F to 46°F) and protected from strong light; should not be exposed to room temperature for a total of 24 hours

Overdosage Treatment Supportive therapy: 100% humidified oxygen; beta agonist bronchodilation for wheezing

Pregnancy Risk Factor B

Nursing Implications Should not be diluted or mixed with any other drugs in the nebulizer, this may inactivate the drug

Specific References

Fuchs HJ, Borowitz DS, Christiansen DH, et al, "Effect on Aerosolized Recombinant Human DNase on Exacerbations of Respiratory Symptoms and on Pulmonary Function in Patients With Cystic Fibrosis," *N Engl J Med*, 1994, 331(10):637-42.

Hubbard RC, McElvaney NG, Birrer P, et al, "A Preliminary Study of Aerosolized Recombinant Human Deoxyribonuclease I in the Treatment of Cystic Fibrosis," *N Engl J Med*, 1992, 326(12):812-5.

Doryx® Oral *see* Doxycycline *on page 305*

Doses and Administration of Several Frequently Used Antiemetic Agents *see page 1641*

DOS® Softgel® [OTC] *see* Docusate *on page 297*

DOSS *see* Docusate *on page 297*

Doxazosin (dox ay' zoe sin)

CAS Number 77883-43-3; 74191-85-8

Brand Names Cardura®

Use Alpha-blocking agent for treatment of hypertension; treatment of benign prostatic hyperplasia (BPH)

Mechanism of Action Doxazosin is a long-acting selective inhibitor of postjunctional alpha$_1$-adrenoceptors as demonstrated in isolated animal tissues and anesthetized healthy animals. Doxazosin is a water soluble quinazoline analogue of prazosin, and on a weight-for-weight basis is approximately half as potent as prazosin in postsynaptic alpha$_1$-adrenoceptor inhibition in animals and man. Inhibition of these alpha$_1$-adrenergic receptors in the peripheral vasculature prevents vasoconstriction from adrenergic stimulation; therefore, allowing vasodilation and a reduction in blood pressure. Because of doxazosin's and similar alpha$_1$-adrenergic blockers specificity, they preserve feedback control of transmitter norepinephrine release and, therefore, cause minimal reflex activation.

Adverse Reactions

Cardiovascular: Syncope, palpitation, edema, tachycardia
Central nervous system: Dizziness, lightheadedness, fatigue, drowsiness, asthenia, headache
Dermatologic: Rash
Gastrointestinal: Nausea, dry mouth
Genitourinary: Priapism
Respiratory: Nasal congestion

Signs & Symptoms of Acute Overdose Severe hypotension, lightheadedness, drowsiness, tachycardia

Toxicodynamics/Kinetics Increased age does not significantly affect the pharmacodynamics of doxazosin
Maximal effect: 2-6 hours after a dose
Duration of action: 24 hours
Distribution: V_d: 3.5 L/kg
Protein binding: 98%
Metabolism: Extensive in the liver
Half-life: 10-22 hours (no difference in renal failure); renal clearance: 2.2 mL/minute/kg
Time to peak serum concentration: 2.3 hours

Usual Dosage Adults: Oral: 1 mg once daily, may be increased to 2 mg once daily thereafter up to 4, 8, and 16 mg if needed

Contraindications Hypersensitivity to doxazosin or any component

Warnings Can cause marked hypotension and syncope with sudden loss of consciousness with the first few doses. Anticipate a similar effect if therapy is interrupted for a few days, if dosage is increased rapidly, or if another antihypertensive drug is introduced. Use with caution in patients with renal impairment, patients receiving first dose, or dosage increase of doxazosin.

Dosage Forms Tablet: 1 mg, 2 mg, 4 mg, 8 mg

Reference Range 8 mg dose is associated with a serum level of 60 ng/mL

Overdosage Treatment

Decontamination: Lavage/activated charcoal with cathartic

Supportive therapy: Treatment is supportive with fluids; use only pure alpha-adrenergic pressors for hypotension (norepinephrine, phenylephrine); dobutamine may also be helpful

Enhancement of elimination: Multiple dose of activated charcoal may be effective; not removed by dialysis

Antidote(s)

Dobutamine Hydrochloride *on page 1416*

Drug Interactions Other hypotensive agents

Pregnancy Risk Factor B

Monitoring Parameters Blood pressure, standing and sitting/supine

Patient Information Rise from sitting/lying carefully; may cause vertigo; take the first dose at bedtime

Nursing Implications Syncope may occur (usually within 90 minutes of the initial dose)

Specific References

Boston D and Collins C, "Safety, Efficacy, and Lipid Profile of Doxazosin at a VA Medical Center," *Hosp Formul*, 1995, 30:233-6.

Carlson RV, Bailey RR, Begg EJ, et al, "Pharmacokinetics and Effect on Blood Pressure of Doxazosin in Normal Subjects and Patients With Renal Failure," *Clin Pharmacol Ther*, 1986, 40(5):561-6.

Cubeddu LX, Fuenmayor N, Caplan N, et al, "Clinical Pharmacology of Doxazosin in Patients With Essential Hypertension," *Clin Pharmacol Ther*, 1987, 41(4):439-49.

Doxepin Hydrochloride (dox' e pin)

Related Information

Antidepressant Agents Comparison *on page 1639*

Therapeutic Drugs Associated With Hallucinations *on page 1558-1559*

CAS Number 1668-19-5; 1229-29-4

Brand Names Adapin®; Co-Dax®; Novoxapin®; Sinequan®; Triadapin®

Use Treatment of various forms of depression, usually in conjunction with psychotherapy; treatment of anxiety disorders; analgesic for certain chronic and neuropathic pain; topical preparation is used for pruritus

Mechanism of Action Increases the synaptic concentration of serotonin and/or norepinephrine in the central nervous system by inhibition of their reuptake by the presynaptic neuronal membrane; also an H_2-receptor antagonist

Adverse Reactions

Cardiovascular: Hypotension, cardiac arrhythmias

Central nervous system: Sedation, confusion, dizziness, visual hallucinations

Dermatologic: Photosensitivity

Endocrine & metabolic: Syndrome of inappropriate antidiuretic hormone

Gastrointestinal: Constipation, nausea, vomiting, dry mouth

Genitourinary: Urinary retention

Hematologic: Blood dyscrasias

Hepatic: Hepatitis

Ocular: Blurred vision, photophobia, mydriasis

Otic: Ototoxicity, tinnitus

Miscellaneous: Orthostasis, hypersensitivity reactions

Signs & Symptoms of Acute Overdose Confusion, dental erosion, priapism, photosensitivity, gynecomastia, hallucinations, ataxia, ejaculatory disturbances, extrapyramidal reaction, galactorrhea, seizures, rhabdomyolysis, myoglobinuria, nystagmus, urinary retention, hypoglycemia, hypothermia, hypotension, tachycardia, cyanosis, Q-T prolongation, respiratory depression

Toxicodynamics/Kinetics

Peak effect: Antidepressant effects usually occur after more than 2 weeks; anxiolytic effects may occur sooner

Absorption: Oral: Rapidly and well absorbed from gastrointestinal tract

Distribution: V_d: 20 L/kg; widely distributed into the body including CNS

Protein binding: 80% to 85%

Metabolism: Hepatically metabolized to metabolites, including desmethyldoxepin (active)

Half-life: Adults: 6-8 hours

Time to peak serum concentration: 2-4 hours

Elimination: Renal excretion, clearance: 14 mL/minute/kg

Usual Dosage

Oral (entire daily dose may be given at bedtime):

Adolescents: Initial: 25-50 mg/day in single or divided doses; gradually increase to 100 mg/day

(Continued)

Doxepin Hydrochloride *(Continued)*

Adults: Initial: 30-150 mg/day at bedtime or in 2-3 divided doses; may gradually increase up to 300 mg/day; single dose should not exceed 150 mg; select patients may respond to 25-50 mg/day

Dosing adjustment in hepatic impairment: Use a lower dose and adjust gradually

Topical: Adults: Apply in a thin film 4 times/day (with at least a 3- to 4-hour interval between applications); chronic use beyond 8 days may result in higher systemic levels

Contraindications Hypersensitivity to doxepin or any component (cross-sensitivity with other tricyclic antidepressants may occur); narrow-angle glaucoma

Warnings Do not discontinue abruptly in patients receiving chronic high-dose therapy; use with caution in patients with cardiovascular disease, conduction disturbances, seizure disorders, urinary retention, hyperthyroidism or those receiving thyroid replacement; avoid use during lactation; use with caution in pregnancy

Dosage Forms

Capsule: 10 mg, 25 mg, 50 mg, 75 mg, 100 mg, 150 mg

Concentrate, oral: 10 mg/mL (120 mL)

Cream: 5% (30 g)

Stability Protect from light

Reference Range

Therapeutic: 110-250 ng/mL

Toxic: >500 ng/mL

Overdosage Treatment

Decontamination: Lavage/activated charcoal with cathartic; multiple dosing of activated charcoal may be effective

Supportive therapy: Lavage within 6 hours of ingestion; following initiation of essential overdose management, toxic symptoms should be treated. Ventricular arrhythmias often respond to phenytoin 15-20 mg/kg (adults) with concurrent systemic alkalinization (sodium bicarbonate 0.5-2 mEq/kg I.V.). Arrhythmias unresponsive to this therapy may respond to lidocaine 1 mg/kg I.V. followed by a titrated infusion. Physostigmine (1-2 mg I.V. slowly for adults or 0.5 mg I.V. slowly for children) may be indicated in seizures or movement disorders but should only be used as **a last resort**. Seizures usually respond to lorazepam or diazepam I.V. boluses (5-10 mg for adults up to 30 mg or 0.25-0.4 mg/kg/dose for children up to 10 mg/dose). If seizures are unresponsive or recur, phenytoin or phenobarbital may be required. Quinidine, disopyramide, and procainamide are contraindicated.

Antidote(s)

Sodium Bicarbonate *on page 1467*

Test Interactions Increases glucose, catecholamine

Diagnostic Tests/Procedures

Doxepin, Blood *on page 1251*

Drug Interactions MAO inhibitors, guanethidine, clonidine, cimetidine inhibits elimination of doxepin; dextropropoxyphene inhibits metabolism of doxepin; tamoxifen may cause a decrease serum concentration of doxepin

Pregnancy Risk Factor C

Pregnancy Implications Do not give while breast-feeding, distributes into breast milk; crosses the placenta

Monitoring Parameters Blood pressure, heart rate, mental status, weight, EKG for QRS widening or tachycardia

Patient Information Avoid unnecessary exposure to sunlight; avoid alcohol ingestion; do not discontinue medication abruptly; may cause urine to turn blue-green; may cause drowsiness; may increase appetite

Additional Information Entire daily dose may be given at bedtime; avoid unnecessary exposure to sunlight; found in a 5% concentration in Zonalon® topical cream for pruritus

Specific References

Galynker II, Rosenthal RN, Perkel C, et al, "Doxepin Withdrawal Mania," *J Clin Psychiatry*, 1995, 56(3):122-3.

Jefferson JW, "Tamoxifen-Associated Reduction in Tricyclic Antidepressant Levels in Blood," *J Clin Psychopharmacol*, 1995, 15:223-4.

Tran P, Panacek EA, Rhee KJ, et al, "Is Norepinephrine More Efficacious Than Dopamine in Reversing Hypotension Caused by Cyclic Antidepressant Overdose?" *Ann Emerg Med*, 1995, 25(1):128-30.

Ware MR, "Tricyclic Antidepressant Overdose: Pharmacology and Treatment," *South Med J*, 1987, 80(11):1410-5.

Williams JO, "Respiratory Depression in Tricyclic Overdose," *Br Med J*, 1972, 1(800):631.

Doxoline® *see* Loxapine *on page 486*

Doxorubicin Hydrochloride (dox oh roo' bi sin)

Related Information

Toxicities of Chemotherapeutic Agents *on page 1631-1633*

CAS Number 25316-40-9; 23214-92-8

Brand Names Adriamycin PFS™; Adriamycin RDF™; Rubex®

Synonyms ADR; Hydroxydaunomycin Hydrochloride

Use Leukemias, lymphomas, multiple myeloma, osseous and nonosseous sarcomas, mesotheliomas, germ cell tumors of the ovary or testis, and carcinomas of the head and neck, thyroid, lung, breast, stomach, pancreas, liver, ovary, bladder, prostate, and uterus; neuroblastoma, osteosarcoma

Mechanism of Action Doxorubicin works through inhibition of topoisomerase-II at the point of DNA cleavage. A second mechanism of action is the production of free radicals (the hydroxy radical OH) by doxorubicin, which in turn can destroy DNA and cancerous cells. Doxorubicin is also a very powerful iron chelator, equal to deferoxamine. The iron-doxorubicin complex can bind DNA and cell membranes rapidly and produce free radicals that immediately cleave the DNA and cell membranes. Inhibits DNA and RNA synthesis by intercalating between DNA base pairs and by steric obstruction; active throughout entire cell cycle.

Adverse Reactions

Cardiovascular: Congestive heart failure, cardiotoxicity (transient type with abnormal EKG and arrhythmias, or a chronic, cumulative, dose-dependent type which progresses to congestive heart failure), cardiorespiratory decompensation, facial flushing, pericarditis

Dermatologic: Alopecia, hyperpigmentation of nail beds

Endocrine & metabolic: Hyperuricemia

Gastrointestinal: Stomatitis, esophagitis, nausea, vomiting, mucositis, diarrhea

Hematologic: Leukopenia (nadir: 10-14 days), thrombocytopenia, pancytopenia, hemolytic anemia

Local: Tissue necrosis upon extravasation, erythematous streaking along the vein if administered too rapidly

Ocular: Lacrimation (25%)

Miscellaneous: Urine discoloration (red)

Signs & Symptoms of Acute Overdose Leukopenia or neutropenia (agranulocytosis, granulocytopenia); hematuria, hyperuricemia, leukopenia, onycholysis, lacrimation, Mees' lines, myocardial depression, tongue discoloration, dysuria

Toxicodynamics/Kinetics

Absorption: Oral: Poor, <50%

Distribution: V_d: 25 L/kg; rapidly distributed into the liver, spleen, kidney, lung and heart

Protein binding: 70% bound to plasma proteins

Metabolism: In both the liver and in plasma to both active and inactive metabolites; doxorubicinol is active metabolite

Half-life, triphasic:

- Primary: 30 minutes
- Secondary: 3-3.5 hours for metabolites
- Terminal: 17-32 hours for doxorubicin and its metabolites

Elimination, triphasic: 80% eventually excreted in bile and feces

Usual Dosage Refer to individual protocols

I.V. (patient's ideal weight should be used to calculate body surface area):

Children: 35-75 mg/m^2 as a single dose, repeat every 21 days; or 20 mg/m^2 once weekly

Adults: 60-75 mg/m^2 as a single dose, repeat every 21 days or other dosage regimens like 20-30 mg/m^2/day for 2-3 days, repeat in 4 weeks or 20 mg/m^2 once weekly

The lower dose regimen should be given to patients with decreased bone marrow reserve, prior therapy or marrow infiltration with malignant cells

Currently the maximum cumulative dose is 550 mg/m^2; a baseline MUGA should be performed prior to initiating treatment. If the LVEF is <30% to 40%, therapy should not be instituted; LVEF should be monitored during therapy.

Doxorubicin has also been administered intraperitoneal (phase I in refractory ovarian cancer patients) and intra-arterially

Dosing adjustment in renal impairment: Cl_{cr} <10 mL/minute: Adjustments not required in mild to moderate renal failure

Reduce dose 75% in severe renal failure

Dosing adjustment in hepatic impairment:

Bilirubin 1.5-3 mg/dL or AST 60-180 IU: Administer 50% of dose

Bilirubin 3.1-5 mg/dL or AST >180 IU: Administer 25% of dose

Bilirubin >5 mg/dL: Avoid use

Administration May be further diluted in either NS of D_5W for I.V. administration

Contraindications Hypersensitivity to doxorubicin or any component, severe congestive heart failure, cardiomyopathy, pre-existing myelosuppression, patients with impaired cardiac function, patients who received previous treatment with complete cumulative doses of doxorubicin and/or daunorubicin

(Continued)

Doxorubicin Hydrochloride *(Continued)*

Warnings The U.S. Food and Drug Administration (FDA) currently recommends that procedures for proper handling and disposal of antineoplastic agents be considered. Reduce dose in patients with impaired hepatic function; severe myelosuppression is also possible. Total dose should not exceed 550 mg/m^2 or 400 mg/m^2 in patients with previous or concomitant treatment (with daunorubicin, cyclophosphamide, or irradiation of the cardiac region); irreversible myocardial toxicity may occur as total dosage approaches 550 mg/m^2. I.V. use only, severe local tissue necrosis will result if extravasation occurs.

Dosage Forms

Injection:
- Aqueous, with NS: 2 mg/mL (5 mL, 10 mL, 25 mL)
- Preservative free (Adriamycin PFS™): 2 mg/mL (5 mL, 10 mL, 25 mL, 100 mL)

Powder for injection, lyophilized: 10 mg, 20 mg, 50 mg
- Rubex®: 10 mg, 50 mg, 100 mg

Powder for injection, lyophilized, rapid dissolution formula (Adriamycin RDF™): 10 mg, 20 mg, 50 mg, 150 mg

Stability Protect from light, must be dispensed in an amber bag; store powder vials at room temperature, refrigerate liquid vials; reconstituted powder vials stable for 24 hours at room temperature and 48 hours if refrigerated; unstable in solutions with a pH <3 or >7. **Incompatible** with heparin, fluorouracil, aminophylline, cephalothin, methotrexate, dexamethasone, diazepam, hydrocortisone, furosemide. Y-site is **compatible** with doxorubicin, vincristine, cyclophosphamide, dacarbazine, bleomycin, vinblastine.

Reference Range No relationship between serum level and cytotoxicity; mean plasma doxorubicin level following 10-15 mg/m^2/day for 5 days of doxorubicin was 7.8-90 ng/mL

Overdosage Treatment

Supportive therapy: Prophylactically, dexrazoxane (Zinecard®) (1 g/m^2 I.V. prior to doxorubicin treatment) may reduce cardiotoxicity of doxorubicin; topical DMSO (1.5 mL of a 50% solution every 6 hours for 2 weeks) with cold compresses can be used to treat extravasation

Enhancement of elimination: While hemodialysis is not useful, Amberlite hemoperfusion may be effective if initiated within 1 hour of administration

Drug Interactions

Increased toxicity:
- Allopurinol may enhance the antitumor activity of doxorubicin (animal data only)
- Cyclophosphamide enhances the cardiac toxicity of doxorubicin by producing additional myocardial cell damage
- May decrease digoxin plasma levels and renal excretion
- Mercaptopurine ↑ toxicities
- Streptozocin greatly enhances leukopenia and thrombocytopenia
- Verapamil alters the cellular distribution of doxorubicin; may result in increased cell toxicity by inhibition of the P-glycoprotein pump
- On previously irradiated tissues

Pregnancy Risk Factor D

Pregnancy Implications Distributes into breast milk

Monitoring Parameters CBC with differential and platelet count, echocardiogram, liver function tests

Patient Information Discolors urine red/orange; immediately report any change in sensation (eg, stinging) at injection site during infusion (may be an early sign of infiltration)

Nursing Implications Local erythematous streaking along the vein and/or facial flushing may indicate too rapid a rate of administration; avoid extravasation, drug is a vesicant; if extravasation occurs, apply ice

Additional Information Cutaneous squamous-cell carcinoma (Marjolin's ulcer) has been associated at the site of doxorubicin extravasation 10 years after drug administration

Myelosuppressive effects:
- WBC: Moderate
- Platelets: Moderate
- Onset (days): 7
- Nadir (days): 10-14
- Recovery (days): 21-28

Specific References

Curran CF, "Acute Doxorubicin Overdoses," *Ann Intern Med*, 1991, 115(11):913-14.

Curran CF and Luce JK, "Accidental Acute Exposure to Doxorubicin," *Cancer Nurs*, 1989, 12(6):329-31.

Gordon KB, Tajuddin A, Guitart J, et al, "Hand-Foot Syndrome Associated With Liposome-Encapsulated Doxorubicin Therapy," *Cancer*, 1995, 75:2169-73.

Lauvin R, Miglianico L, and Hellegouarc'h R, "Skin Cancer Occurring 10 Years After the Extravasation of Doxorubicin," *N Engl J Med*, 1995, 332(11):754.

Seifert CF, Nesser ME, and Thompson DF, "Dexrazoxane in the Prevention of Doxorubicin-Induced Cardiotoxicity," *Ann Pharmacother*, 1994, 28(9):1063-72.

Speyer JL, Green MD, Kramer E, et al, "Protective Effect of the Bispiperazinedione ICRF-187 Against Doxorubicin-Induced Cardiac Toxicity in Women With Advanced Breast Cancer," *N Engl J Med*, 1988, 319(12):745-52.

Zimmerman S, Adkins D, Graham M, et al, "Case Report: Irreversible, Severe, Congestive Cardiomyopathy Occurring in Association With Interferon Alpha Therapy," *Cancer Biother*, 1994, 9(4):291-9.

Doxychel® *see* Doxycycline *on this page*

Doxycycline (dox i sye' kleen)

CAS Number 564-25-0; 17086-28-1; 83038-87-3; 10592-13-9; 24390-14-5

Brand Names Bio-Tab® Oral; Doryx® Oral; Doxychel®; Doxy® Oral; Monodox® Oral; Vibramycin®; Vibra-Tabs®

Synonyms Doxycycline Hyclate; Doxycycline Monohydrate

Use Principally in the treatment of infections caused by susceptible *Rickettsia*, *Chlamydia*, and *Mycoplasma* along with uncommon susceptible gram-negative and gram-positive organisms

Mechanism of Action Inhibits protein synthesis by binding with the 30S and possibly the 50S ribosomal subunit(s) of susceptible bacteria; may also cause alterations in the cytoplasmic membrane

Adverse Reactions

Central nervous system: Increased intracranial pressure, bulging fontanels in infants, headache

Dermatologic: Rash, photosensitivity, hyperpigmentation

Endocrine & metabolic: Fanconi-like reaction (polyuria, acidosis, albuminuria, hypokalemia, acidosis) with outdated drug

Gastrointestinal: Nausea, diarrhea, esophagitis and esophageal ulceration with the hyclate salt formulation, vomiting

Hematologic: Neutropenia, eosinophilia, porphyria

Hepatic: Hepatotoxicity

Local: Phlebitis (I.V. administration)

Miscellaneous: May cause discoloration of teeth in children, porphyrinogenic

Signs & Symptoms of Acute Overdose Leukopenia or neutropenia (agranulocytosis, granulocytopenia); photosensitivity, hypokalemia, flatulence

Toxicodynamics/Kinetics

Absorption: Almost completely from gastrointestinal tract; can be reduced with food or milk by 20%

Distribution: V_d: 0.75 L/kg

Protein binding: 88% to 90%

Metabolism: Not metabolized in the liver, instead is partially inactivated in the gastrointestinal tract by chelate formation

Half-life: 10-22 hours (usually increases to 22-24 hours with multiple dosing)

Time to peak serum concentration: Within 1.5-4 hours

Elimination: Excreted in urine (23%) and feces (30%); clearance: 0.032 L/hour/kg

Usual Dosage Oral, I.V. (do not administer S.C. or I.M.):

Children ≥8 years (<45 kg): 2-4 mg/kg/day in 1-2 divided doses, not to exceed 200 mg/day

Children >8 years (>45 kg) and Adults: 100-200 mg/day in 1-2 divided doses

Sclerosing agent for pleural effusion injection: 500 mg as a single dose in 30-50 mL of NS or SWI

Administration Slow I.V. intermittent infusion over a minimum of 1-2 hours at a concentration not to exceed 1 mg/mL (can be infused over 1-4 hours); concentrations <0.1 mg/mL are not recommended

Contraindications Hypersensitivity to doxycycline, tetracycline or any component; children <8 years of age; severe hepatic dysfunction

Warnings Use of tetracyclines during tooth development may cause permanent discoloration of the teeth and enamel hypoplasia; prolonged use may result in superinfection; photosensitivity reaction may occur with this drug; avoid prolonged exposure to sunlight or tanning equipment

Dosage Forms

Capsule, as hyclate: 50 mg, 100 mg

- Doxychel®, Monodox®, Vibramycin®: 50 mg
- Doxy®, Doxychel®, Monodox®, Vibramycin®: 100 mg

Capsule, coated pellets, as hyclate (Doryx®): 100 mg

Powder for injection, as hyclate: 100 mg, 200 mg

- Doxy®, Doxychel®, Vibramycin® IV: 100 mg, 200 mg

Powder for oral suspension, as monohydrate (raspberry flavor) (Vibramycin®): 25 mg/5 mL (60 mL)

Syrup, as calcium (raspberry-apple flavor) (Vibramycin®): 50 mg/5 mL (30 mL, 473 mL)

Tablet, as hyclate:

- Doxychel®: 50 mg

(Continued)

Doxycycline *(Continued)*

Bio-Tab®, Doxychel®, Vibra-Tabs®: 100 mg

Stability Tetracyclines form toxic products when outdated or when exposed to light, heat, or humidity; reconstituted solution is stable for 72 hours (refrigerated); for I.V. infusion in NS or D_5W solution, complete infusion should be completed within 12 hours; discard remaining solution

Reference Range Peak plasma level of 3 mg/L (6.5 μmol/L) following a 200 mg dose

Overdosage Treatment

Decontamination: Lavage/activated charcoal with cathartic; dilute with milk or water to avoid corrosive gastrointestinal effects

Supportive therapy: Antacids effective for gastrointestinal irritation

Enhancement of elimination: Multiple dosing of activated charcoal; can increase fecal elimination by binding to doxycycline after intestinal secretion; not dialyzable

Test Interactions False-negative urine glucose using Clinistix®, Tes-Tape®

Diagnostic Tests/Procedures

Complete Blood Count *on page 1236*

Liver Profile *on page 1286*

Drug Interactions

Decreased effect with antacids (aluminum, calcium, zinc, or magnesium), bismuth salts, sodium bicarbonate, barbiturates, carbamazepine, hydantoins; decreased effect of oral contraceptives

Increased effect of warfarin

Pregnancy Risk Factor D

Pregnancy Implications Appears in breast milk; can be taken for a short period of time during breast feeding

Monitoring Parameters Periodic monitoring of renal, hepatic, and hematologic function tests

Patient Information Avoid unnecessary exposure to sunlight; do not take with antacids, iron products, or dairy products; finish all medication; do not skip doses

Nursing Implications Infuse I.V. doxycycline over 1 hour

Additional Information Not as antianabolic as other tetracyclines

Specific References

Bryant SG, Fisher S, and Kluge RM, "Increased Frequency of Doxycycline Side Effects," *Pharmacotherapy*, 1987, 7(4):125-9.

Daunt N, Brodribb TR, and Dickey JD, "Oesophageal Ulceration Due to Doxycycline," *Br J Radiol*, 1985, 58(696):1209-11.

Francke EL and Neu HC, "Chloramphenicol and Tetracyclines," *Med Clin North Am*, 1987, 71(6):155-68.

Saivin S and Hovin G, "Clinical Pharmacokinetics of Doxycycline and Minocycline," *Clin Pharmacokinet*, 1985, 15:355-66.

Wilson WR and Cockerill FR 3d, "Tetracyclines, Chloramphenicol, Erythromycin, and Clindamycin," *Mayo Clin Proc*, 1987, 62(10):906-15.

Droperidol (droe per' i dole)

Related Information

Doses and Administration of Several Frequently Used Antiemetic Agents *on page 1641*

CAS Number 548-72-3

Brand Names Droleptan®; Inapsine®

Synonyms Dehydrobenzperidol

Use Tranquilizer and antiemetic in surgical and diagnostic procedures; antiemetic for cancer chemotherapy; preoperative medication

Mechanism of Action Alters the action of dopamine in the CNS, at subcortical levels, to produce sedation; it is a butyrophenone with phenothiazine-like properties

Adverse Reactions

Cardiovascular: Mild to moderate hypotension, tachycardia

Central nervous system: Drowsiness, restlessness, extrapyramidal reactions, restlessness, electroencephalogram abnormalities

Endocrine & metabolic: Syndrome of inappropriate antidiuretic hormone

Neuromuscular & skeletal: Tremors

Respiratory: Laryngospasm

Signs & Symptoms of Acute Overdose Hypotension, chills, wheezing, neuroleptic malignant syndrome, myasthenia gravis (exacerbation or precipitation of), tachycardia, Parkinson's-like symptoms, hallucinations, extrapyramidal reaction, coma

Toxicodynamics/Kinetics

Onset of action: 3-10 minutes

Peak effect: Within 30 minutes

Duration: 2-4 hours (may extend to 12 hours)

Absorption: I.M.: Absorbed well

Distribution: Crosses blood-brain barrier; goes into the CSF

Protein binding: Extensive

Metabolism: In the liver

Half-life: Adults: 2.3 hours

Elimination: Excreted in urine (75%) and feces (22%)

Usual Dosage Titrate carefully to desired effect

Children 2-12 years:

- Premedication: I.M.: 0.1-0.15 mg/kg; smaller doses may be sufficient for control of nausea or vomiting
- Adjunct to general anesthesia: I.V. induction: 0.088-0.165 mg/kg
- Nausea and vomiting: I.M., I.V.: 0.05-0.06 mg/kg/dose every 4-6 hours as needed

Adults:

- Premedication: I.M.: 2.5-10 mg 30 minutes to 1 hour preoperatively
- Adjunct to general anesthesia: I.V. induction: 0.22-0.275 mg/kg; maintenance: 1.25-2.5 mg/dose
- Alone in diagnostic procedures: I.M.: Initial: 2.5-10 mg 30 minutes to 1 hour before; then 1.25-2.5 mg if needed
- Nausea and vomiting: I.M., I.V.: 2.5-5 mg/dose every 3-4 hours as needed

Administration Administration recommendations for all doses: I.V.: Over 2-5 minutes

Contraindications Hypersensitivity to droperidol or any component

Warnings Use with caution in patients with myasthenia gravis or pheochromocytoma; may cause severe hypotension; use with caution in patients with hepatic or renal insufficiency; watch for hypotension when administering I.M. or I.V.; safety in children <6 months of age has not been established; use with caution in patients with cardiovascular disease or seizures; benefits of therapy must be weighed against risks of therapy

Dosage Forms Injection: 2.5 mg/mL (1 mL, 2 mL, 5 mL, 10 mL)

Stability Stability of parenteral admixture at room temperature (25°C): 24 hours

Overdosage Treatment

Decontamination: Lavage/activated charcoal with cathartic

Supportive therapy: Following initiation of essential overdose management, toxic symptom treatment and supportive treatment should be initiated. Hypotension usually responds to I.V. fluids or Trendelenburg positioning. If unresponsive to these measures, the use of a parenteral inotrope may be required (eg, norepinephrine 0.1-0.2 mcg/kg/minute titrated to response). Seizures commonly respond to lorazepam or diazepam (I.V. 5-10 mg bolus in adults every 15 minutes if needed up to a total of 30 mg; I.V. 0.25-0.4 mg/kg/dose up to a total of 10 mg in children) or to phenytoin or phenobarbital. Also critical cardiac arrhythmias often respond to I.V. phenytoin (15 mg/kg up to 1 g), while other antiarrhythmics can be used. Neuroleptics often cause extrapyramidal reaction (eg, dystonic reactions) requiring management with diphenhydramine 1-2 mg/kg (adults) up to a maximum of 50 mg I.M. or I.V. slow push followed by a maintenance dose for 48-72 hours. When these reactions are unresponsive to diphenhydramine, benztropine mesylate I.V. 1-2 mg (adults) may be effective. These agents are generally effective within 2-5 minutes.

(Continued)

Droperidol *(Continued)*

Drug Interactions Other CNS depressants (including ethanol and MAO inhibitors) may cause additive effects (CNS, respiratory depression, etc); droperidol plus fentanyl or other analgesics may cause an increase of blood pressure; conduction anesthesia may increase hypotension; droperidol plus epinephrine causes decreased blood pressure due to alpha-adrenergic blockade effects of droperidol. May enhance the effect of atropine on heart rate.

Pregnancy Risk Factor C

Pregnancy Implications Crosses the placenta

Monitoring Parameters Blood pressure, heart rate, respiratory rate

Patient Information Avoid alcoholic beverages

Additional Information Has good antiemetic effect as well as sedative and antianxiety effects

Specific References

Foster PN, Stickle BR, Dale M, et al, "Akathisia After Low-Dose Droperidol," *Br J Anaesth*, 1995, 74:477P.

Ghoneim MM and Korttila K, "Pharmacokinetics of Intravenous Anaesthetics: Implications for Clinical Use," *Clin Pharmacokinet*, 1977, 2(5):344-72.

Rosen C, Ratliff AF, Wolfe RW, et al, "The Efficacy of Droperidol in the Prehospital Setting," *Acad Emerg Med*, 1995, 2:446.

Drugs and Chemicals Proven to be Teratogenic in Humans *see page 1572*

Dry Thyroid *see* Thyroid *on page 749*

DSCG *see* Cromolyn Sodium *on page 245*

DSS *see* Docusate *on page 297*

D-S-S® [OTC] *see* Docusate *on page 297*

DTO *see* Opium Tincture *on page 580*

Duact® *see* Acrivastine *on page 87*

Duboisine *see* Hyoscyamine Sulfate *on page 415*

Dulcagen® [OTC] *see* Bisacodyl *on page 156*

Dulcolax® [OTC] *see* Bisacodyl *on page 156*

Dull-C® [OTC] *see* Ascorbic Acid *on page 131*

Duo-Trach® *see* Lidocaine Hydrochloride *on page 468*

DUP 753 *see* Losartan Potassium *on page 484*

Duradalat® *see* Nifedipine *on page 558*

Duragesic™ *see* Fentanyl Citrate *on page 347*

Duramorph® *see* Morphine Sulfate *on page 539*

Duranifin® *see* Nifedipine *on page 558*

Duraphyl™ *see* Theophylline *on page 735*

Durapindol® *see* Pindolol *on page 627*

Duratest® Injection *see* Testosterone *on page 729*

Durathate® Injection *see* Testosterone *on page 729*

Duration® Nasal Solution [OTC] *see* Oxymetazoline Hydrochloride *on page 586*

Durrax® *see* Hydroxyzine *on page 414*

Durvitan® *see* Caffeine *on page 175*

Duvoid® *see* Bethanechol Chloride *on page 154*

Dylate® *see* Papaverine *on page 591*

Dymelor® *see* Acetohexamide *on page 86*

Dynabac® *see* Dirithromycin *on page 293*

Dyna-Hex® Topical [OTC] *see* Chlorhexidine Gluconate *on page 200*

Dynalert® *see* Pemoline *on page 598*

Dynef® *see* Enalapril *on page 311*

Dyrenium® *see* Triamterene *on page 766*

Dyspamet® *see* Cimetidine *on page 212*

Dytac® *see* Triamterene *on page 766*

Dytuss® *see* Ammonium Chloride *on page 118*

Easprin® *see* Aspirin *on page 133*

Ebrantil® *see* Urapidil Hydrochloride *on page 778*

E-Caps® *see* Vitamin E *on page 798*

Economycin® *see* Tetracycline *on page 732*

Ecotrin® [OTC] *see* Aspirin *on page 133*

Ectasule® *see* Ephedrine Sulfate *on page 316*

Edecrin® *see* Ethacrynic Acid *on page 328*

Edecrina® *see* Ethacrynic Acid *on page 328*

Edrophonium Chloride (ed roe foe' nee um)

CAS Number 312-42-1; 116-38-1

Brand Names Anticode®; Enlon®; Reversol®; Tensilon®

Use Diagnosis and differentiation of myasthenia gravis; to reverse nondepolarizing neuromuscular blockers; treatment of paroxysmal atrial tachycardia; a curare antagonist, also used for curare overdose to treat respiratory depression, reverses neuromuscular block produced by curare

Mechanism of Action Inhibits destruction of acetylcholine by acetylcholinesterase which facilitates transmission of impulses across myoneural junction

Adverse Reactions

Cardiovascular: Arrhythmias, hypotension, bradyarrhythmias, ventricular asystole (after a dose of 10 mg)

Central nervous system: Convulsions, seizures

Gastrointestinal: Nausea, vomiting, diarrhea, excessive salivation

Genitourinary: Urinary frequency

Neuromuscular & skeletal: Weakness, muscle cramps

Ocular: Diplopia, photophobia, miosis, blurred vision

Respiratory: Laryngospasm, wheezing, respiratory paralysis, tachypnea, increased secretions

Miscellaneous: Sweating

Signs & Symptoms of Acute Overdose Muscle asthenia, nausea, vomiting, miosis, wheezing, respiratory paralysis, hypotension, fibrillation (atrial), seizures

Toxicodynamics/Kinetics

Onset of action:

I.M.: Within 2-10 minutes

I.V.: 30-60 seconds

Duration:

I.M.: 5-30 minutes

I.V.: 10 minutes

Distribution: V_d: 1.1 L/kg; crosses blood-brain barrier only at extremely high doses

Metabolism: Hydrolyzed by cholinesterase, metabolized by microsomal enzyme of liver

Half-life: 1.8 hours

Elimination: Renal

Usual Dosage I.V.:

Infants: Initial: 0.1 mg, followed by 0.4 mg if no response; total dose: 0.5 mg

Children:

Diagnosis: Initial: 0.04 mg/kg followed by 0.16 mg/kg if no response, to a maximum total dose of 5 mg for children ≤34 kg, or 10 mg for children >34 kg

Titration of oral anticholinesterase therapy: 0.04 mg/kg once; if strength improves, an increase in neostigmine or pyridostigmine dose is indicated

Adults:

Diagnosis: 2 mg test dose administered over 15-30 seconds; 8 mg given 45 seconds later if no response is seen; test dose may be repeated after 30 minutes

Titration of oral anticholinesterase therapy: 1-2 mg given 1 hour after oral dose of anticholinesterase; if strength improves, an increase in neostigmine or pyridostigmine dose is indicated

Differentiation of cholinergic from myasthenic crisis: 1 mg, may repeat after 1 minute (**Note:** Intubation and controlled ventilation may be required if patient has cholinergic crises.)

Reversal of nondepolarizing neuromuscular blocking agents (neostigmine with atropine usually preferred): 10 mg, may repeat every 5-10 minutes up to 40 mg

Termination of paroxysmal atrial tachycardia: I.V. rapid injection: 5-10 mg

Dosing adjustment in renal impairment: Dose may need to be reduced in patients with chronic renal failure

Contraindications Hypersensitivity to edrophonium or any component, gastrointestinal or GU mechanical obstruction

Warnings Atropine sulfate should always be readily available as an antagonist; use with caution in patients with bronchial asthma and those receiving a cardiac glycoside

(Continued)

Edrophonium Chloride *(Continued)*

Dosage Forms Injection: 10 mg/mL (1 mL, 10 mL, 15 mL)

Reference Range Dose of 0.5 μg/kg gives mean plasma concentration of 7.82 nmol/mL and will probably decrease cholinesterase levels by >80%

Overdosage Treatment Supportive therapy: Antidote is atropine for muscarinic symptoms; pralidoxime (2-PAM) may also be needed to reverse severe muscle asthenia or paralysis, although since edrophonium is such a short-acting drug, 2-PAM use is usually not necessary

Antidote(s)

Atropine Sulfate *on page 1395*

Pralidoxime Chloride *on page 1461*

Test Interactions Increases aminotransferase [ALT (SGPT)/AST (SGOT)] (S), amylase (S)

Drug Interactions Succinylcholine increases neuromuscular blockade; nondepolarizing muscle relaxants (eg, pancuronium, vecuronium) cause antagonized effects; digoxin increases cardiotoxic potential of edrophonium

Pregnancy Risk Factor C

Nursing Implications Atropine sulfate should be available at bedside

Additional Information Overdosage can cause cholinergic crisis which may be fatal; atropine should be readily available for treatment of cholinergic reactions; pralidoxime may reverse muscle asthenia

Specific References

Rossen RN, Krikorian J, and Hancock EW, "Ventricular Asystole After Edrophonium Chloride Administration," *JAMA*, 1976, 235(10):1041-2.

Youngberg JA, "Cardiac Arrest Following Treatment of Paroxysmal Atrial Tachycardia With Edrophonium," *Anesthesiology*, 1979, 50(3):234-5.

E.E.S.® Oral *see* Erythromycin *on page 319*

Efedron® *see* Ephedrine Sulfate *on page 316*

Eferox® *see* Levothyroxine Sodium *on page 465*

Effexor® *see* Venlafaxine *on page 786*

Eflornithine Hydrochloride (ee flor' ni theen)

CAS Number 96020-91-6

Brand Names Ornidyl®

Synonyms DFMO

Use Treatment of meningoencephalitic stage of *Trypanosoma brucei gambiense* infection (sleeping sickness), *P. carinii* infection, cryptosporidiosis infections in HIV-infected patients

Mechanism of Action Eflornithine exerts antitumor and antiprotozoal effects through specific, irreversible ("suicide") inhibition of the enzyme ornithine decarboxylase (ODC). ODC is the rate-limiting enzyme in the biosynthesis of putrescine, spermine, and spermidine, the major polyamines in nucleated cells. Polyamines are necessary for the synthesis of DNA, RNA, and proteins and are, therefore, necessary for cell growth and differentiation. Although many microorganisms and higher plants are able to produce polyamines from alternate biochemical pathways, all mammalian cells depend on ornithine decarboxylase to produce polyamines. Eflornithine inhibits ODC and rapidly depletes animal cells of putrescine and spermidine; the concentration of spermine remains the same or may even increase. Rapidly dividing cells appear to be most susceptible to the effects of eflornithine.

Adverse Reactions

Central nervous system: Convulsions

Dermatologic: Alopecia

Gastrointestinal: Diarrhea, vomiting

Hematologic: Anemia, leukopenia, thrombocytopenia

Otic: Hearing impairment, deafness

Signs & Symptoms of Acute Overdose In mice and rats, CNS depression, seizures, death have occurred human overdose cases are not published; leukopenia, neutropenia, agranulocytosis, granulocytopenia

Toxicodynamics/Kinetics

Absorption: Oral: ~60% readily absorbed

Half-life: 3-4 hours

Elimination: Unchanged primarily renally

Usual Dosage Adults: I.V. infusion: 100 mg/kg/dose given every 6 hours (over at least 45 minutes) for 14 days

Dosing adjustment in renal impairment: Dose should be adjusted although no specific guidelines are available

Dosage Forms Injection, concentrate: 200 mg/mL (100 mL)

Overdosage Treatment

Decontamination: Activated charcoal with cathartic

Supportive therapy: General poison management; no known antidote

Test Interactions Increases BUN; decreases RBC, WBC, platelets

Pregnancy Risk Factor C

Monitoring Parameters Complete blood count, mental status

Patient Information Report any persistent or unusual fever, sore throat, fatigue, bleeding, or bruising; frequent blood tests are needed during therapy

Nursing Implications Must be diluted before use and used within 24 hours of preparation

Specific References

Barbarash RA, Toll L, and Sahn SA, "Alpha-Difluoromethylornithine Infusion and Cardiac Arrest," *Ann Intern Med*, 1986, 105(1):141-2.

Haegele KD, Alken RG, Grove J, et al, "Kinetics of α-Difluoromethylornithine: An Irreversible Inhibitor of Ornithine Decarboxylase," *Clin Pharmacol Ther*, 1981, 30(2):210-7.

Efodine® [OTC] *see* Povidone-Iodine *on page 635*

Efudex® Topical *see* Fluorouracil *on page 357*

Egazil Duretter® *see* Hyoscyamine Sulfate *on page 415*

Elaldehyde *see* Paraldehyde *on page 593*

Elavil® *see* Amitriptyline Hydrochloride *on page 116*

Elcatonin *see* Calcitonin *on page 177*

Elevan® *see* Deanol *on page 261*

Elimite™ *see* Permethrin *on page 608*

Elixicon® *see* Theophylline *on page 735*

Elixomin® *see* Theophylline *on page 735*

Elixophyllin®-GG *see* Theophylline *on page 735*

Elixophyllin®-KI *see* Theophylline *on page 735*

Elixophyllin® SR *see* Theophylline *on page 735*

E-Lor® *see* Propoxyphene and Acetaminophen *on page 656*

Elorgan® *see* Pentoxifylline *on page 607*

Emconcor® *see* Bisoprolol Fumarate *on page 157*

Emcor® *see* Bisoprolol Fumarate *on page 157*

Emdopa® *see* Methyldopa *on page 519*

Emeside® *see* Ethosuximide *on page 333*

Empirin® [OTC] *see* Aspirin *on page 133*

Emulsoil® [OTC] *see* Castor Oil *on page 189*

E-Mycin® Oral *see* Erythromycin *on page 319*

Enable® *see* Tenidap *on page 725*

Enalapril (e nal' a pril)

Related Information

ACE Inhibitors Comparison *on page 1636-1637*

CAS Number 75847-73-3; 76095-16-4

Brand Names Converten®; Dynef®; Enapren®; Innovace®; Pres®; Reniten®; Vasotec®; Xanef®

Synonyms Enalaprilat; MK-421; N-(1-Ethoxycarbonyl-3-Phenylpropyl)-L-Anal-L-Proline Hydrogen Maleate

Use Management of mild to severe hypertension and congestive heart failure

Mechanism of Action Competitive inhibitor of angiotensin-converting enzyme (ACE); prevents conversion of angiotensin I to angiotensin II, a potent vasoconstrictor; results in lower levels of angiotensin II which causes an increase in plasma renin activity and a reduction in aldosterone secretion

Adverse Reactions

Cardiovascular: Hypotension, chest pain, syncope, diuresis, bradycardia

Central nervous system: Fatigue, psychosis, insomnia, dizziness, headache

Dermatologic: Rash, pemphigus, angioedema

Endocrine & metabolic: Hypoglycemia, gynecomastia, hyperkalemia

Gastrointestinal: Nausea, dyspepsia, diarrhea

Genitourinary: Impotence

Hematologic: Leukopenia/neutropenia (agranulocytosis, granulocytopenia), anemia

Neuromuscular & skeletal: Muscle cramps

Otic: Decreased hearing acuity

Renal: Deterioration in renal function, proteinuria

Respiratory: Cough

Miscellaneous: Loss of taste perception (less than with captopril), metallic taste

Signs & Symptoms of Acute Overdose Hypotension is usually not severe in

(Continued)

Enalapril *(Continued)*

overdose patients and manifests itself within 1 hour with a maximal effect at 4 hours; bradycardia, hypoglycemia, eosinophilia, azotemia, ototoxicity; tinnitus, pemphigus, thrombocytopenia, deafness, depression, insomnia, coagulopathy

Toxicodynamics/Kinetics

Onset of action: Oral: ~1 hour

Peak effect: Occurs in 4-8 hours

Duration: 12-24 hours

Absorption: Oral: 55% to 75% (enalapril) from gastrointestinal tract

Distribution: V_d: 1.7; full pattern unknown; does not appear to cross blood-brain barrier

Protein binding: 50% to 60%

Metabolism: Enalapril is a prodrug and undergoes biotransformation to enalaprilat in the liver (70% conversion of enalapril to enalaprilat)

Half-life:

- Enalapril:
  - Healthy adults: 1.3 hours
  - CHF adults: 3.4-5.8 hours
- Enalaprilat:
  - Infants 6 weeks to 8 months: 6-10 hours
  - Adults: 35-38 hours

Time to peak serum concentration: Within 30 minutes to 1.5 hours, while peak serum levels of enalaprilic acid (active) occur within 3-4.5 hours

Elimination: Principally in urine (60% to 80%) enalaprilic acid with some fecal excretion; renal clearance: 0.3 L/hour/kg

Usual Dosage Use lower listed initial dose in patients with hyponatremia, hypovolemia, severe congestive heart failure, decreased renal function, or in those receiving diuretics

Children:

- Investigational initial oral doses of **enalapril** of 0.1 mg/kg/day increasing over 2 weeks to 0.12-0.43 mg/kg/day have been used to treat severe congestive heart failure in infants (n=8)
- Investigational I.V. doses of **enalaprilat** of 5-10 mcg/kg/dose administered every 8-24 hours (as determined by blood pressure readings) have been used for the treatment of neonatal hypertension (n=10); monitor patients carefully; select patients may require higher doses

Adults:

- Oral: **Enalapril**: 2.5-5 mg/day then increase as required, usual therapeutic dose for hypertension: 10-40 mg/day in 1-2 divided doses; usual therapeutic dose for heart failure: 5-20 mg/day
- I.V.: **Enalaprilat**: 1.25 mg/dose, given over 5 minutes every 6 hours; doses as high as 5 mg/dose every 6 hours have been tolerated for up to 36 hours

Dosing adjustment in renal impairment:

- Oral: Enalapril:
  - Cl_{cr} 10-50 mL/minute: Administer 75% to 100% of usual dose
  - Cl_{cr} <10 mL/minute: Administer 50% of usual dose
- I.V.: Enalaprilat: Cl_{cr} <30 mL/minute: Start at 0.625 mg every 6 hours and increase dose based on response

Contraindications Hypersensitivity to enalapril, enalaprilat or any component

Warnings Use with caution and modify dosage in patients with renal impairment (especially renal artery stenosis), hyponatremia, hypovolemia, severe congestive heart failure or with coadministered diuretic therapy; experience in children is limited

Dosage Forms

Injection, as enalaprilat: 1.25 mg/mL (1 mL, 2 mL)

Tablet, as maleate: 2.5 mg, 5 mg, 10 mg, 20 mg

Stability Solutions for I.V. infusion mixed in NS or D_5W, are stable for 24 hours at room temperature

Reference Range Enalaprilat plasma level of 40 µg/L (104 mmol/L) can produce a mean blood pressure reduction of 12 mm Hg

Overdosage Treatment

Decontamination: Ipecac/lavage/activated charcoal with cathartic

Supportive therapy: Following initiation of essential overdose management, toxic symptom treatment and supportive treatment should be initiated. Hypotension usually responds to I.V. normal saline or Trendelenburg positioning. If unresponsive to these measures, the use of a parenteral inotrope may be required (eg, norepinephrine 0.1-0.2 mcg/kg/minute titrated to response). Seizures commonly respond to lorazepam or diazepam (I.V. 5-10 mg bolus in adults every 15 minutes if needed up to a total of 30 mg; I.V. 0.25-0.4 mg/kg/dose up to a total of 10 mg in children) or to phenytoin or phenobarbital. Naloxone may antagonize hypotensive effects. Inhaled sodium cromoglycate (total dose: 40 mg/day) can decrease ACE-inhibitor cough by 50%.

Enhanced elimination: Multiple dosing of activated charcoal may be effective

Test Interactions Increases BUN, creatinine, potassium, positive Coombs' [direct]; decreases cholesterol (S); may cause false-positive results in urine acetone determinations using sodium nitroprusside reagent

Drug Interactions Use with potassium-sparing diuretics may cause a additive hyperkalemic effect; hypotensive agent or diuretics leads to an increase of hypotensive effect; indomethacin may decrease hypotensive effect; may increase plasma concentrations of lithium

Pregnancy Risk Factor D

Monitoring Parameters Blood pressure, renal function, WBC, serum potassium

Patient Information Notify physician if vomiting, diarrhea, excessive sweating, or dehydration should occur; also if swelling of face, lips, tongue or difficulty in breathing occurs

Nursing Implications May cause depression in some patients; discontinue if angioedema of the face, extremities, lips, tongue, or glottis occurs

Additional Information Severe hypotension may occur in patients who are sodium and/or volume depleted, initiate lower doses and monitor closely when starting therapy in these patients; reduces albuminuria in sickle cell anemia by up to 70%

Specific References

Aoki RY and Saad ST, "Enalapril Reduces the Albuminuria of Patients With Sickle Cell Disease," *Am J Med*, 1995, 98:432-5.

Cleland JG, Dargie HI, McAlpine H, et al, "Severe Hypotension After First Dose of Enalapril in Heart Failure," *Br Med J (Clin Res)*, 1985, 291(6505):1309-12.

Gimenez JC, Diez JM, Solar MJ, et al, "Angioneurotic Edema Produced by Enalapril," *Ann Pharmacother*, 1995, 29:317.

Gonzalez-Fernandez RA, Altieri PI, Banchs HL, et al, "Effects of Enalaprilat on Regional Wall Stress in Patients With Angina Pectoris," *Am J Therap*, 1995, 2:395-400.

Hargreaves MR and Benson MK, "Inhaled Sodium Cromoglycate in Angiotensin-Converting Enzyme Inhibitor Cough," *Lancet*, 1995, 345(8941):13-6.

Herings RM, deBoer A, Stricker BH, et al, "Hypoglycemia Associated With Use of Inhibitors of Angiotensin Converting Enzyme," *Lancet*, 1995, 345:1195-8.

Lau CP, "Attempted Suicide With Enalapril," *N Engl J Med*, 1986, 315(3):197

Kuechle MK, Hutton KP, and Muller SA, "Angiotensin-Converting Enzyme Inhibitor-Induced Pemphigus: Three Case Reports and Literature Review," *Mayo Clin Proc*, 1994, 69(12):1166-71.

Poirier L, Bourgeois J, Lefebvre J, et al, "Ace Inhibitors as First-Line Treatment Agents: A Comparative Study of Trandolapril and Enalapril on Casual and Ambulatory Blood Pressures," *Am J Ther*, 1995, 2:159-64.

Spiller HA, Udicious TM, and Muir S, "Angiotensin-Converting Enzyme Inhibitor Ingestion in Children," *J Toxicol Clin Toxicol*, 1989, 27(6):345-53.

Todd PA and Heel PC, "Enalapril: A Review of Its Pharmacodynamic and Pharmacokinetic Properties and Therapeutic Use in Hypotension and Congestive Heart Failure," *Drugs*, 1986, 31(3):198-248.

Enalaprilat *see* Enalapril *on page 311*

Enapren® *see* Enalapril *on page 311*

Encainide Hydrochloride (en kay' nide)

CAS Number 66794-74-9; 37612-13-8; 66778-36-7

Brand Names Enkaid®

Use Ventricular arrhythmias; supraventricular arrhythmias; marketing discontinued in 1991

Mechanism of Action Encainide is a class IC agent that blocks the sodium channel of the Purkinje fibers; it slows conduction, reduces membrane responsiveness, increases the effective refractory period to the action potential and inhibits automaticity

Adverse Reactions

Cardiovascular: Arrhythmogenic effects range from an increased frequency of ventricular premature complexes (VPCs) to the development of new and/or more severe and potentially fatal ventricular tachyarrhythmias; bradycardia, first degree A-V block; negative inotropic effect; increased QRS, P-R, and Q-T_c intervals on EKG; congestive heart failure

Central nervous system: Dizziness, chills, headache, insomnia, seizures, ataxia

Endocrine & metabolic: Hyperglycemia, hypoproteinemia

Gastrointestinal: Dry mouth, metallic taste, nausea, constipation, diarrhea

Neuromuscular & skeletal: Tremors, myalgia

Ocular: Visual disturbances, diplopia, blurred vision (19%)

Toxicodynamics/Kinetics

Onset of action: 1-3 hours

Absorption: Well absorbed

Protein binding:

ODE: 75% to 85%

MODE: 92%

Metabolism: Extensively metabolized in the liver to two active metabolites, o-dimethyl encainide (ODE) and 3-methoxy-o-dimethyl encainide

(Continued)

Encainide Hydrochloride *(Continued)*

Bioavailability: Wide intrapatient differences
Half-life: 2.3-2.7 hours
Active metabolites:
ODE: 3-4 hours
MODE: 6-12 hours
Time to peak serum concentration: 0.5-1.5 hours
Elimination: Excreted in urine and bile

Usual Dosage Adults: Oral: 25 mg every 8 hours; may increase to 35 mg every 8 hours after 3-5 days if needed; increase to 50 mg every 8 hours in another 3-5 days if response is not achieved; maximum daily dosage: 200 mg

Administration Give around-the-clock rather than 4 times/day, 3 times/day, etc (ie, 12-6-12-6, not 9-1-5-9) to promote less variation in peak and trough serum levels

Contraindications Hypersensitivity to encainide or any component, second or third degree A-V block, premature ventricular complexes, nonsustained ventricular arrhythmias, cardiogenic shock

Warnings Can cause new or worsened arrhythmias; such proarrhythmic effects range from an increase in frequency of PVCs to the development of more severe tachycardia (ventricular) (ie, tachycardia that is more sustained or more resistant to conversion to sinus rhythm), with potentially fatal consequences; use with caution in patients with a history of congestive heart failure or myocardial dysfunction; use is recommended only in patients with life-threatening arrhythmias

Dosage Forms Capsule: 25 mg, 35 mg, 50 mg

Reference Range

Therapeutic: 50-85 μg/L (SI: 130-220 nmol/L)
ODE: 180-220 μg/L (SI: 460-565 nmol/L)
MODE: 140-185 μg/L (SI: 360-475 nmol/L) (normal phenotype)

Overdosage Treatment

Decontamination: Do not use ipecac; use lavage/activated charcoal with cathartic
Supportive therapy: Avoid type IA antiarrhythmic agents (quinidine, procainamide, disopyramide); intravenous sodium bicarbonate (1-2 mEq/kg) can be used for hypotension or ventricular arrhythmia; phenytoin (15 mg/kg up to 1 g I.V. slow administration of 50 mg/minute) is antiarrhythmic of choice; magnesium sulfate, lidocaine, bretylium, or propranolol can also be used for ventricular arrhythmias
Enhancement of elimination: Hemodialysis is not useful

Diagnostic Tests/Procedures

Electrocardiography *on page 1253*
Encainide, Blood *on page 1258*

Drug Interactions Beta-blockers (possible negative inotropic effects); quinidine reduced hepatic clearance in fast metabolizers

Pregnancy Risk Factor B

Pregnancy Implications Probably crosses the placenta; distributes into breast milk

Additional Information Based on adverse outcomes noted with encainide in the CAST trial, the FDA recommends that use of encainide be limited to patients with life-threatening ventricular arrhythmias

Specific References

Mortensen ME, Bolon CE, Kelley MT, et al, "Encainide Overdose in an Infant," *Ann Emerg Med*, 1992, 21(8):998-1001.
Pentel PR, Goldsmith SR, Salerno DM, et al, "Effect of Hypertonic Sodium Bicarbonate on Encainide Overdose," *Am J Cardiol*, 1986, 57(10):878-80.
Perry LL and Oszko MA, "Possible Encainide-Induced Hypoproteinemia," *J Fam Pract*, 1990, 31(1):90, 93.
Somberg JC, "New Directions in Antiarrhythmic Drug Therapy," *Am J Cardiol*, 1984, 54(4):8B-17B.
The Cardiac Arrhythmia Suppression Trial (CAST) Investigators, "Preliminary Report: Effect of Encainide and Flecainide on Mortality in a Randomized Trial of Arrhythmia Suppression After Myocardial Infarction," *N Engl J Med*, 1989, 321(6):406-12.
Turgeon J and Roden DM, "Pharmacokinetic Profile of Encainide," *Clin Pharmacol Ther*, 1989, 45(6):692-4.

Endak® *see* Carteolol Hydrochloride *on page 188*

Endep® *see* Amitriptyline Hydrochloride *on page 116*

Endone® *see* Oxycodone Hydrochloride *on page 585*

Ener-B® [OTC] *see* Cyanocobalamin *on page 246*

Enkaid® *see* Encainide Hydrochloride *on previous page*

Enlon® *see* Edrophonium Chloride *on page 309*

Enovil® *see* Amitriptyline Hydrochloride *on page 116*

Enoxacin (en ox' a sin)

Related Information

Therapeutic Drugs Associated With Hallucinations *on page 1558-1559*

CAS Number 74011-58-8

Brand Names Penetrex™

Use Complicated and uncomplicated urinary tract infections caused by susceptible gram-negative and gram-positive bacteria

Mechanism of Action Enoxacin exerts its antibacterial activity, as do other quinolone-azaquinolone antibiotics, by inhibition of bacterial DNA gyrase

Adverse Reactions

Central nervous system: Restlessness, dizziness, confusion, seizures, headache, depression, visual hallucinations
Dermatologic: Rash, photosensitivity
Gastrointestinal: Nausea, diarrhea, vomiting, gastrointestinal bleeding
Hematologic: Anemia
Hepatic: Liver enzymes (increased)
Neuromuscular & skeletal: Tremors, arthralgia, tendon rupture
Renal: Renal failure (acute), serum creatinine (increased) and BUN (increased)
Miscellaneous: Feces discoloration (white/speckling)

Toxicodynamics/Kinetics

Absorption: 98%
Distribution: Penetrates well into tissues and body secretions
Bioavailability: Essentially the bioavailability as I.V. administration; administration with food does not affect bioavailability
Half-life: 3-6 hours (average)
Elimination: Primarily excreted in urine, however, significant drug concentrations are achieved in feces

Usual Dosage Adults: Oral: 400 mg twice daily

Dosing adjustment in renal impairment: Cl_{cr} <50 mL/minute: Administer 50% of dose

Contraindications Hypersensitivity to enoxacin, any component, or other quinolones

Warnings Use with caution in patients with a history of seizures or epilepsy, renal dysfunction, psychosis, elevated intracranial pressure, prepubertal children, and pregnancy; nalidixic acid has been associated with erosions of the cartilage in weight-bearing joints and other signs of arthropathy in immature animals; similar precautions are advised for enoxacin although no data is available.

Dosage Forms Tablet: 200 mg, 400 mg

Reference Range Peak plasma level: 3 mg/L after a 750 mg oral dose

Overdosage Treatment

Decontamination: Lavage/activated charcoal with cathartic
Enhancement of elimination: Multiple dosing of activated charcoal may be effective

Pregnancy Risk Factor C

Specific References

Izu R, Gardeazabal J, Gonzalez M, et al, "Enoxacin-Induced Photosensitivity: Study of Two Cases," *Photodermatol Photoimmunol Photomed*, 1992, 9(2):86-8.
Szarfman A, Chen M, and Blum MD, "More on Fluoroquinolone Antibiotics and Tendon Rupture," *N Engl J Med*, 1995, 332(3):193.

Enoxaparine *see* Enoxaparin Sodium *on this page*

Enoxaparin Sodium (e nox ah pair' in)

CAS Number 74011-58-8

Brand Names Lovenox®

Synonyms Enoxaparine; LMWH; Low Molecular Weight Heparin; PK-10169

Use Prevention of deep vein thrombosis following hip replacement surgery

Mechanism of Action Inhibits thrombin

Adverse Reactions

Cardiovascular: Edema
Central nervous system: Confusion, fever
Dermatologic: Ecchymosis
Hematologic: Hemorrhage, thrombocytopenia, hematoma, rythema, hypochromic anemia, coagulopathy
Gastrointestinal: Nausea
Miscellaneous: Local irritation, pain

Toxicodynamics/Kinetics

Peak effect: 3 hours
Duration: 275 minutes
Bioavailability: S.C.: 91%
Half-life: 275 minutes
Elimination: In the kidney through glomerular filtration

(Continued)

Enoxaparin Sodium *(Continued)*

Usual Dosage S.C.: 30 mg within 24 hours of surgery, then twice daily for 7-10 days; 14 days maximum; a single daily dose of 40 mg has also been shown to be safe and effective in prevention of thromboembolism in patients undergoing orthopedic or gynecologic surgical procedures

Contraindications Active major bleeding or hemophilia; hypersensitivity to heparin or pork products; drug-induced thrombocytopenia

Warnings Heparin-induced thrombocytopenia, bacterial endocarditis, congenital or acquired bleeding disorders, active ulceration and angiodysplastic gastrointestinal disease, hemorrhagic stroke, status post brain, spinal, or ophthalmological surgery, uncontrolled arterial hypertension, recent CNS surgery, elderly, and lactation. Never give by intramuscular injection. Conventional heparin has possibly been associated with an increased risk of bleeding in females >60 years of age; it is unknown whether low molecular weight heparins pose the same risk; these agents should be used with caution in this population.

Dosage Forms Injection, preservative free: 30 mg/0.3 mL

Stability Incompatible with gentamicin

Reference Range Risk of bleeding increases when antifactor Xa levels exceed 0.4 unit/mL

Overdosage Treatment

Supportive therapy: Protamine can be used for severe bleeding upon withdrawal of heparin (1 mg of protamine for every 1 mg of enoxaparin by slow I.V. push)

Enhancement of elimination: While hemodialysis is not beneficial, exchange transfusion has been used successfully in a neonate and plasma exchange has been used successfully in four older patients for thrombocytopenia

Antidote(s)

Protamine Sulfate *on page 1463*

Drug Interactions Increased toxicity with oral anticoagulants, platelet inhibitors

Pregnancy Risk Factor B

Pregnancy Implications Does not cross the placenta

Monitoring Parameters Platelets, occult blood, PTT, and anti-Xa activity, if available

Additional Information About half the weight of heparin with 20% of the activity

Specific References

Buckley MM and Sorkin EM, "Enoxaparin: A Review of Its Pharmacology and Clinical Applications in the Prevention and Treatment of Thromboembolic Disorders," *Drugs*, 1992, 44(3):465-97.

Epanutin® *see* Phenytoin *on page 623*

Ephedrine Sulfate (e fed' rin)

Related Information

Therapeutic Drugs Associated With Hallucinations *on page 1558-1559*

CAS Number 134-72-5; 299-42-3; 50906-05-3

Brand Names Ectasule®; Efedron®; Ephedsol®; Fedrine®; Vicks Vatronol®

Use Bronchial asthma; nasal congestion; acute wheezing; acute hypotensive states

Mechanism of Action Releases tissue stores of epinephrine and thereby produces an alpha- and beta-adrenergic stimulation

Adverse Reactions

Cardiovascular: Hypertension, cardiomyopathy

Central nervous system: CNS-stimulating effects, nervousness, anxiety, fear, psychosis, tension, agitation, excitation, restlessness, asthenia, irritability, insomnia, auditory and visual hallucinations

Gastrointestinal: Nausea, anorexia

Neuromuscular & skeletal: Tremors

Signs & Symptoms of Acute Overdose Dysrhythmias, CNS depression, depression, insomnia, dry skin, respiratory depression, vomiting, respiratory alkalosis, seizures, mydriasis

Toxicodynamics/Kinetics

Onset of action: Oral: Bronchodilation within 15-60 minutes

Duration: 3-6 hours

Absorption: Rapid after administration

Distribution: Throughout body fluids; crosses the blood-brain barrier

Metabolism: Little hepatic metabolism

Half-life: 2.5-3.6 hours

Elimination: 60% to 77% excreted as unchanged drug in urine within 24 hours

Usual Dosage

Children: Oral, I.V., S.C.: 3 mg/kg/day or 100 mg/m^2/day in 4-6 divided doses

Adults:

Oral: 25-50 mg every 3-4 hours as needed

I.M., I.V., S.C.: 25-50 mg not to exceed 150 mg/24 hours

Contraindications Hypersensitivity to ephedrine or any component, cardiac arrhythmias, angle-closure glaucoma, patients on other sympathomimetic agents

Warnings Blood volume depletion should be corrected before ephedrine therapy is instituted; use with caution in patients with hypertension or hyperthyroidism; may cause hypertension

Dosage Forms

Capsule: 25 mg, 50 mg

Drops (Vicks Vatronol®): 0.5% (30 mL)

Injection: 25 mg/mL (1 mL); 50 mg/mL (1 mL, 10 mL)

Jelly (Kondon's Nasal®): 1% (20 g)

Spray (Pretz-D®): 0.25% (15 mL)

Stability Protect all dosage forms from light

Overdosage Treatment

Decontamination: Lavage/activated charcoal with cathartic

Supportive therapy: There is no specific antidote for ephedrine intoxication and the bulk of the treatment is supportive. Hyperactivity and agitation usually respond to reduced sensory input, however with extreme agitation haloperidol (2-5 mg I.M. for adults) may be required. Hyperthermia is best treated with external cooling measures, or when severe or unresponsive, muscle paralysis with pancuronium may be needed. Hypertension is usually transient and generally does not require treatment unless severe. For diastolic blood pressures >110 mm Hg, a nitroprusside infusion should be initiated. Seizures usually respond to diazepam or lorazepam I.V. and/or phenytoin maintenance regimens.

Drug Interactions Do not administer with other sympathomimetic agents; MAO inhibitors, general anesthetics, alpha- and beta-adrenergic blocking agents, cardiac glycosides, atropine, theophylline

Pregnancy Risk Factor C

Pregnancy Implications Crosses the placenta; appears in breast milk; fetal tachycardia can occur

Patient Information May cause wakefulness or nervousness

Nursing Implications Protect from light; do not administer unless solution is clear

Additional Information For I.V. administration, give undiluted injection slowly; additional I.V. doses may be given in 5-10 minutes if needed; do not exceed adult parenteral dose of 150 mg/24 hours; do not exceed pediatric dose of 3 mg/kg/24 hours; use the smallest effective dose; ephedrine is a precursor in the illicit manufacture of methamphetamine; ephedrine is extracted by dissolving ephedrine tablets in water or alcohol (50,000 tablets can result in 1 kg of ephedrine); conversion to methamphetamine occurs at a rate of 50% to 70% of the weight of ephedrine

Specific References

Pickup ME, May CS, Sendagire R, et al, "The Pharmacokinetics of Ephedrine After Oral Dosage in Asthmatics Receiving Acute and Chronic Treatment," *Br J Clin Pharmacol*, 1976, 3(1):123-34.

Ephedsol® *see* Ephedrine Sulfate *on previous page*

Epilim® *see* Valproic Acid and Derivatives *on page 782*

Epimorph Dolcontin® *see* Morphine Sulfate *on page 539*

Epinat® *see* Phenytoin *on page 623*

Epitrol® *see* Carbamazepine *on page 184*

EPO *see* Erythropoietin *on page 322*

Epoetin Alfa *see* Erythropoietin *on page 322*

Epogen® *see* Erythropoietin *on page 322*

Epoxitin® *see* Erythropoietin *on page 322*

Eprex® *see* Erythropoietin *on page 322*

Eptadone® *see* Methadone Hydrochloride *on page 508*

Equanil® *see* Meprobamate *on page 503*

Equibral® *see* Chlordiazepoxide *on page 198*

Ercaf® *see* Ergotamine *on this page*

Ergenyl® *see* Valproic Acid and Derivatives *on page 782*

Ergocalciferol *see* Vitamin D *on page 797*

Ergomar® *see* Ergotamine *on this page*

Ergostat® *see* Ergotamine *on this page*

Ergotamine (er got' a meen)

CAS Number 379-79-3

Brand Names Cafatine®; Cafatine-PB®; Cafergot®; Cafetrate®; Ercaf®; Ergomar®; Ergostat®; Lanatrate®; Medihaler Ergotamine™; Migergot®; Wigraine®

Use Vascular headache, such as migraine or cluster

Mechanism of Action Ergot alkaloid alpha-adrenergic blocker directly stimulates

(Continued)

Ergotamine *(Continued)*

vascular smooth muscle to vasoconstrict peripheral and cerebral vessels; may also have antagonist effects on serotonin

Adverse Reactions

Cardiovascular: Tachycardia, bradycardia, arterial spasm, portal hypertension, claudication and vasoconstriction, myocardial infarction

Central nervous system: Fasciculations, pallor

Gastrointestinal: Nausea, vomiting, diarrhea

Neuromuscular & skeletal: Weakness in the legs, myalgia, gangrene can develop, paresthesia, tremor

Miscellaneous: Rebound headache may occur with sudden withdrawal of the drug in patients on prolonged therapy, feces discoloration (tarry), renal tubule necrosis

Signs & Symptoms of Acute Overdose Symptoms include vasospastic effects, colitis, nausea, vomiting, drowsiness, impaired mental function, nystagmus, myalgia, asthenia, hypotension, chest pain, hypertension, bradycardia, vision color changes (red tinge), unconsciousness, seizures, shock and death

Toxicodynamics/Kinetics

Onset of action: Variable usually within 1-2 hours

Absorption: Oral, rectal: Erratic; absorption is enhanced by caffeine coadministration

Distribution: V_d: ~2 L/kg; crosses the blood-brain barrier; distributed widely throughout the body

Metabolism: Extensive in the liver

Bioavailability: <5%; rectal suppositories are ~20 times increased bioavailability than oral forms

Half-life: ~2 hours

Time to peak serum concentration: Within 30 minutes to 3 hours

Elimination: Excreted in bile as metabolites (90%)

Usual Dosage Adults:

Oral:

Cafergot®: 2 tablets at onset of attack; then 1 tablet every 30 minutes as needed; maximum: 6 tablets per attack; do not exceed 10 tablets/week

Ergostat®: 1 tablet under tongue at first sign, then 1 tablet every 30 minutes, 3 tablets/24 hours, 5 tablets/week

Rectal (Cafergot® suppositories, Wigraine® suppositories, Cafergot® P-B suppositories): 1 at first sign of an attack; follow with second dose after 1 hour, if needed; maximum dose: 2 per attack; do not exceed 5/week

Inhalation: Initial: 1 inhalation, followed by repeat inhalations 5 minutes apart to a maximum of 6 inhalations/24 hours or 15 inhalations/1 week

Contraindications Hypersensitivity to ergotamine, caffeine or any component; peripheral vascular disease, hepatic or renal disease, hypertension, peptic ulcer disease, sepsis, angina pectoris, anemia, phlebitis, sepsis, or thyrotoxicosis

Warnings Avoid during pregnancy; avoid prolonged administration or excessive dosage because of the danger of ergotism and gangrene

Dosage Forms

Aerosol, oral (Medihaler Ergotamine™): Ergotamine tartrate 360 mcg/metered spray [62.5 doses] (2.5 mL)

Suppository, rectal (Cafatine®, Cafergot®, Cafetrate®, Wigraine®): Ergotamine tartrate 2 mg and caffeine 100 mg (12s)

Tablet (Cafergot®, Ercaf®, Wigraine®): Ergotamine tartrate 1 mg and caffeine 100 mg

Tablet, sublingual (Ergostat®): Ergotamine tartrate 2 mg

Reference Range Serum levels >1.8 ng/mL are toxic

Overdosage Treatment

Decontamination: Gastric lavage, or induction of emesis or lavage, activated charcoal with cathartic, saline cathartic; keep extremities warm

Supportive therapy: Treatment is symptomatic with captopril, nifedipine, prazosin, vasodilators (nitroprusside) or nitroglycerin for hypertension; phentolamine can also be used; diazepam can be utilized for seizures; heparin, dextran, or corticosteroids can be used for hypercoagulable state; hyperbaric oxygen can be used as an adjunct to treat localized tissue hypoxia

Enhancement of elimination: Multiple dosing of activated charcoal may be effective

Drug Interactions

Propranolol: One case of severe vasoconstriction with pain and cyanosis has been reported

Erythromycin: Monitor for signs of ergot toxicity; troleandomycin

Pregnancy Risk Factor X

Pregnancy Implications Oxytocic effect

Patient Information Any symptoms such as nausea, vomiting, numbness or tingling, and chest, muscle, or abdominal pain should be reported to the physician. Initiate therapy at first sign of attack. Do **not** exceed recommended dosage.

Nursing Implications Do not crush sublingual drug product

Additional Information

Ergotamine tartrate: Ergostat®

Ergotamine tartrate and caffeine: Cafergot®

Ergotamine, caffeine, belladonna alkaloids and pentobarbital: Cafergot® P-B

Specific References

Edwards WM, "Accidental Poisoning of Newborn Infants With Ergonovine Maleate. A Lesson Application To All Delivery Rooms," *Clin Pediatr (Phila)*, 1971, 10(5):257-60.

Husum B, Metz P, and Rasmussen JP, "Nitroglycerin Infusion for Ergotism," *Lancet*, 1979, 2(8146):794-5.

McGuigan MA, "Ergot Alkaloids," *Clin Toxicol Rev*, 1984, 6:1-2.

Orton DA and Richardson RJ, "Ergotamine Absorption and Toxicity," *Postgrad Med J*, 1982, 58(675):6-11.

Eryc® Oral *see* Erythromycin *on this page*

EryPed® Oral *see* Erythromycin *on this page*

Ery-Tab® Oral *see* Erythromycin *on this page*

Erythrocin® Oral *see* Erythromycin *on this page*

Erythromycin (er ith roe mye' sin)

CAS Number 114-07-8; 134-36-1; 643-22-1; 96128-89-1; 3521-62-8; 41342-53-4; 304-63-2; 23067-13-2; 3847-29-8

Brand Names E.E.S.® Oral; E-Mycin® Oral; Eryc® Oral; EryPed® Oral; Ery-Tab® Oral; Erythrocin® Oral; Ilosone® Oral; PCE® Oral; Wyamycin® S Oral

Synonyms Erythromycin Base; Erythromycin Estolate; Erythromycin Ethylsuccinate; Erythromycin Gluceptate; Erythromycin Lactobionate; Erythromycin Stearate

Use Treatment of susceptible bacterial infections including *M. pneumoniae, Legionella* pneumonia, diphtheria, pertussis, chancroid, *Chlamydia*, and *Campylobacter* gastroenteritis; used in conjunction with neomycin for decontaminating the bowel

Unlabeled use: Gastroparesis

Mechanism of Action Inhibits RNA-dependent protein synthesis at the chain elongation step; binds to the 50S ribosomal subunit resulting in blockage of transpeptidation

Adverse Reactions

Cardiovascular: Ventricular arrhythmias, torsade de pointes and Q-T prolongation

Central nervous system: Fever, dizziness, hypothermia

Dermatologic: Skin rash

Gastrointestinal: Abdominal pain due to stimulation of gastrointestinal tract especially at doses exceeding 4 g/day; cramping, dyspepsia, nausea, vomiting, diarrhea, stomatitis, pancreatitis

Hematologic: Eosinophilia, porphyria

Hepatic: Cholestatic hepatitis, jaundice (more common in estolate salt)

Local: Thrombophlebitis (I.V. form)

Neuromuscular & skeletal: Myasthenia gravis (exacerbation or precipitation of with I.V. preparation)

Otic: Ototoxicity, deafness, tinnitus

Miscellaneous: Allergic reactions, anaphylactic shock, (in children), hypersensitivity reactions (0.5%), feces discoloration (greenish gray), feces discoloration (white/speckling)

Toxicodynamics/Kinetics

Absorption: Oral: 18% to 45%; variable but better with salt forms than with base form

Distribution: V_d: 0.72 L/kg

Protein binding: 75% to 80% (90% for estolate salt)

Metabolism: In the liver by demethylation

Half-life: 1.5-2 hours (peak), prolonged with reduced renal function (5-6 hours)

Time to peak serum concentration: 4 hours for the base, 3 hours for the stearate, 0.5-2.5 hours for the ethylsuccinate, 2-4 hours for the estolate; delayed in the presence of food except when using the estolate; due to differences in absorption, 200 mg erythromycin ethylsuccinate produces the same serum levels as erythromycin base or estolate

Elimination: Excretion of 2% to 15% unchanged drug in urine and major excretion in feces (via bile)

Usual Dosage

Neonates:

Postnatal age <7 days: Oral: 10 mg/kg/dose every 12 hours

Postnatal age >7 days: Oral:

<1200 g: 10 mg/kg/dose every 12 hours

≥1200 g: 10 mg/kg/dose every 8 hours

Ophthalmic: Prophylaxis of neonatal gonococcal or chlamydial conjunctivitis: 0.5-1 cm ribbon of ointment should be instilled into each conjunctival sac

(Continued)

Erythromycin *(Continued)*

Infants and Children:
- Oral: Do not exceed 2 g/day
  - Base and ethylsuccinate: 30-50 mg/kg/day divided every 6-8 hours
  - Estolate: 30-50 mg/kg/day divided every 8-12 hours
  - Stearate: 20-40 mg/kg/day divided every 6 hours
- Pre-op bowel preparation: 20 mg/kg erythromycin base at 1, 2, and 11 PM on the day before surgery combined with mechanical cleansing of the large intestine and oral neomycin
- I.V.: Lactobionate: 20-40 mg/kg/day divided every 6 hours, not to exceed 4 g/day

Children and Adults:
- Ophthalmic: Instill ½" (1.25 cm) 2-8 times/day depending on the severity of the infection
- Topical:
  - Gel/Solution: Apply twice daily to affected areas
  - Ointment: Apply every 3 hours 6 times/day for 1 week

Adults:
- Oral:
  - Base: 333 mg every 8 hours
  - Estolate, stearate or base: 250-500 mg every 6-12 hours
  - Ethylsuccinate: 400-800 mg every 6-12 hours
- Pre-op bowel preparation: 1 g erythromycin base at 1, 2, and 11 PM on the day before surgery combined with mechanical cleansing of the large intestine and oral neomycin
- I.V.: 15-20 mg/kg/day divided every 6 hours or given as a continuous infusion over 24 hours (maximum: 4 g/24 hours)

Administration Administer by I.V. intermittent or continuous infusion at a concentration of 1-2.5 mg/mL; maximum concentration: 5 mg/mL; I.V. intermittent infusions can be administered over 20-60 minutes

Contraindications Hepatic impairment, known hypersensitivity to erythromycin or its components

Warnings Should not be administered concurrently with astemizole, terfenadine; use with caution in patients with hepatic dysfunction; hepatic impairment with or without jaundice has occurred chiefly in older children and adults; it may be accompanied by malaise, nausea, vomiting, abdominal colic, and fever; discontinue use if these occur; avoid using erythromycin lactobionate in neonates since formulations may contain benzyl alcohol which is associated with toxicity in neonates

Dosage Forms

Erythromycin base:
- Capsule, delayed release: 250 mg
- Capsule, delayed release, enteric coated pellets (Eryc®): 250 mg
- Tablet:
  - Delayed release: 333 mg
  - Enteric coated (E-Mycin®, Ery-Tab®, E-Base®): 250 mg, 333 mg, 500 mg
  - Film coated: 250 mg, 500 mg
  - Polymer coated particles (PCE®): 333 mg, 500 mg

Erythromycin estolate:
- Capsule (Ilosone® Pulvules®): 250 mg
- Suspension, oral (Ilosone®): 125 mg/5 mL (480 mL); 250 mg/mL (480 mL)
- Tablet (Ilosone®): 500 mg

Erythromycin ethylsuccinate:
- Granules for oral suspension (EryPed®): 400 mg/5 mL (60 mL, 100 mL, 200 mL)
- Powder for oral suspension (E.E.S.®): 200 mg/5 mL (100 mL, 200 mL)
- Suspension, oral (E.E.S.®, EryPed®): 200 mg/5 mL (5 mL, 100 mL, 200 mL, 480 mL); 400 mg/5 mL (5 mL, 60 mL, 100 mL, 200 mL, 480 mL)
- Suspension, oral [drops] (EryPed®): 100 mg/2.5 mL (50 mL)
- Tablet (E.E.S.®): 400 mg
- Tablet, chewable (EryPed®): 200 mg

Erythromycin gluceptate: Injection: 1000 mg (30 mL)

Erythromycin lactobionate: Powder for injection, I.V.: 500 mg, 1000 mg

Erythromycin stearate: Tablet, film coated (Eramycin®, Erythrocin®, Wyamycin® S): 250 mg, 500 mg

Stability Erythromycin lactobionate should be reconstituted with sterile water for injection without preservatives to avoid gel formation; the reconstituted solution is stable for 2 weeks when refrigerated or 24 hours at room temperature. Erythromycin I.V. infusion solution is stable at pH 6-8. Do not use D_5W as a diluent unless sodium bicarbonate is added to solution.

Reference Range Peak plasma level after 500 mg dose is 0.3-1.9 μg/mL

Overdosage Treatment

Decontamination: Lavage/activated charcoal with cathartic

Supportive therapy: Acute gastrointestinal irritation can be treated with milk or bismuth subsalicylate; QT prolongation, hypotension, or ventricular arrhythmias can be treated with sodium bicarbonate; lidocaine can be useful for ventricular tachycardia; magnesium sulfate can be useful in treating torsade de pointes

Test Interactions False-positive urinary catecholamines and 17-hydroxycorticosteroids; estolate salt can result in false-positive elevation of serum aspartate aminotransferase when assayed colorimetrically

Diagnostic Tests/Procedures

Erythromycin, Blood *on page 1260*

Drug Interactions Increased effect/toxicity/levels of alfentanil, anticoagulants, astemizole, terfenadine, loratadine, bromocriptine, carbamazepine, cyclosporine, digoxin, disopyramide, theophylline, and triazolam; erythromycin coadministered with quinidine may reduce quinidine clearance; deafness reported with concomitant cimetidine; concomitant use of quinidine and erythromycin can result in increased quinidine levels; increased toxicity with ergots, methylprednisolone; odds ratio for QT_c prolongation with concomitant erythromycin and terfenadine use is 2.33; increased tacrolimus levels can occur with concomitant administration of erythromycin or rifampin; neutropenia and muscle pain can result if vinblastine and erythromycin are used together

Pregnancy Risk Factor B

Pregnancy Implications Crosses the placenta; appears in breast milk; avoid erythromycin estolate in that elevated serum aspartate aminotransferase can occur in 14% of patients (not a false-positive)

Monitoring Parameters Liver function tests

Patient Information Refrigerate after reconstitution, take until gone, do not skip doses; chewable tablets should not be swallowed whole; report to physician if persistent diarrhea occurs

Nursing Implications gastrointestinal upset, including diarrhea, is common; can give with food to decrease gastritis; some formulations may contain benzyl alcohol as a preservative; use with extreme care in neonates

Additional Information

Erythromycin base: E-Mycin®, Eryc®, Ery-Tab®, PCE®, Ilotycin®, Robimycin®

Erythromycin estolate: Ilosone®

Erythromycin ethylsuccinate: E.E.S.®, E-Mycin® E, EryPed®, Pediamycin®, Wyamycin® E

Erythromycin gluceptate: Ilotycin® Gluceptate

Erythromycin lactobionate: Erythrocin® Lactobionate-IV

Erythromycin stearate: Eramycin®, Erypar®, Erythrocin®, Ethril®, Wintrocin®, Wyamycin® S

Sodium content of oral suspension (ethylsuccinate) 200 mg/5 mL: 29 mg (1.3 mEq)

Sodium content of base Filmtab® 250 mg: 70 mg (3 mEq)

Specific References

Boyd I, "Erythromycin-Induced Hearing Loss," *Lancet*, 1991, 337(8733):113.

Catnach SM and Fairclough PD, "Erythromycin and the Gut," *Gut*, 1992, 33(3):397-401.

Furian V, Perello L, Jacquemin E, et al, "Interactions Between FK506 and Rifampicin or Erythromycin in Pediatric Liver Recipients," *Transplantation*, 1995, 59:1217-8.

Gholson CF and Warren GH, "Fulminant Hepatic Failure Associated With Intravenous Erythromycin Lactobionate," *Arch Intern Med*, 1990, 150(1):215-6.

Gumaste VV, "Erythromycin-Induced Pancreatitis," *Am J Med*, 1989, 86(6 Pt 1):725.

Hanrahan JP, Choo PW, Carlson W, et al, "Terfenadine-Associated Ventricular Arrhythmias and QT_c Interval Prolongation: A Retrospective Cohort Comparison With Other Antihistamines Among Members of a Health Maintenance Organization," *Ann Epidemiol*, 1995, 5:201-9.

Hassel B, "Hypothermia From Erythromycin," *Ann Intern Med*, 1991, 115(1):69-70.

Mogford N, Pallet A, and George C, "Erythromycin Deafness and Cimetidine Treatment," *BMJ*, 1994, 309(6969):1620.

Orban Z, MacDonald LL, Peters MA, et al, "Erythromycin-Induced Cardiac Toxicity," *Am J Cardiol*, 1995, 75:859-61.

Paris DG, Parente TF, Bruschetta HR, et al, "Torsade de Pointes Induced by Erythromycin and Terfenadine," *Am J Emerg Med*, 1994, 12(6):636-8.

Spinler SA, Cheng JWM, Kindwall KE, et al, "Possible Inhibition of Hepatic Metabolism of Quinidine by Erythromycin," *Clin Pharmacol Ther*, 1955, 57:89-94.

Stafstrom CE, Nohria V, Loganbill H, et al, "Erythromycin-induced Carbamazepine Toxicity: A Continuing Problem," *Arch Pediatr Adolesc Med*, 1995, 149(1):99-101.

Tobe SW, Siu LL, Jamal SA, et al, "Vinblastine and Erythromycin: An Unrecognized Serious Drug Interaction," *Cancer Chemother Pharmacol*, 1995, 35(3):188-90.

Erythromycin Base *see* Erythromycin *on page 319*

Erythromycin Estolate *see* Erythromycin *on page 319*

Erythromycin Ethylsuccinate *see* Erythromycin *on page 319*

Erythromycin Gluceptate *see* Erythromycin *on page 319*

Erythromycin Lactobionate *see* Erythromycin *on page 319*

Erythromycin Stearate *see* Erythromycin *on page 319*

Erythropoietin (e poe' e tin al fa)

Related Information

Therapeutic Drugs Associated With Hallucinations *on page 1558-1559*

CAS Number 113427-24-0; 122312-54-3

Brand Names Epogen®; Epoxitin®; Eprex®; Globuren®; Procrit®; Recormon®

Synonyms EPO; Epoetin Alfa; *r*HuEPO-α

Mechanism of Action Induces erythropoiesis by stimulating the division and differentiation of committed erythroid progenitor cells; induces the release of reticulocytes from the bone marrow into the blood stream, where they mature to erythrocytes. There is a dose response relationship with this effect. This results in an increase in reticulocyte counts followed by a rise in hematocrit and hemoglobin levels. Studies in lab animals suggest that epoetin may have an effect on megakaryoblast development, and increased platelet counts have been noted in dialysis patients receiving epoetin.

Adverse Reactions

Cardiovascular: Hypertension, edema, chest pain

Central nervous system: Fatigue, dizziness, headache, seizures, visual hallucinations

Dermatologic: Rash

Gastrointestinal: Nausea

Neuromuscular & skeletal: Arthralgias

Miscellaneous: Hypersensitivity reactions

Signs & Symptoms of Acute Overdose Hallucinations, polycythemia, coagulopathy, conjunctivitis

Toxicodynamics/Kinetics

Distribution: V_d: 0.3-0.6 L/kg

Bioavailability: 20% to 30% (S.C. injection)

Half-life: 9.3 hours (initial); 6.2 hours (multiple dose)

Elimination: 2.8 mL/kg/hour

Usual Dosage In patients on dialysis, epoetin alfa usually has been administered as an I.V. bolus 3 times/week. While the administration is independent of the dialysis procedure, it may be administered into the venous line at the end of the dialysis procedure to obviate the need for additional venous access; in patients with CRF not on dialysis, epoetin alfa may be given either as an I.V. or S.C. injection.

Dosing recommendations:

Dosing schedules need to be individualized and careful monitoring of patients receiving the drug is mandatory

*r*HuEPO-α may be ineffective if other factors such as iron or B_{12}/folate deficiency limit marrow response

Initial dose: I.V., S.C.: 50-150 units/kg 3 times/week

Dose should be reduced when the hematocrit reaches the target range of 30% to 33% (maximum: 36%) or a hematocrit increase of >4 points over any 2-week period

Dose should be held if the hematocrit exceeds 36% and until the hematocrit decreases to the target range (30% to 33%)

Dose should be increased by 25 units/kg 3 times/week if the hematocrit does not increase by 5-6 points after 8 weeks of therapy and hematocrit is below the target range; further increases of 25 units/kg 3 times/week may be made at 4- to 6-week intervals until the desired response is obtained. Doses exceeding 300 units/kg 3 times/week are not recommended because a greater biological response is not observed.

Maintenance dose: Should be individualized to maintain the hematocrit within the 30% to 33% target range

Anemia of prematurity: S.C.: 25-100 units/kg/dose 3 times/week

Zidovudine-treated HIV patients (available evidence indicates patients with endogenous serum erythropoietin levels >500 mU/mL are unlikely to respond); target hematocrit range: 36% to 40%

Cancer patients on chemotherapy (treatment of patients with endogenous serum erythropoietin levels >200 mU/mL is not recommended); target hematocrit range: 36% to 40%

Contraindications Known hypersensitivity to albumin human; uncontrolled hypertension

Warnings Use with caution in patients with history of epilepsy or seizures, thrombocytosis, chronic liver failure, malignancy, ischemic vascular disease, porphyria, hypertension; prior to and during therapy, iron stores must be evaluated

Pretherapy parameters:

Serum ferritin >100 ng/dL

Transferrin saturation (serum iron/iron binding capacity x 100) of >20%

Iron supplementation (usual oral dosing of 325 mg 2-3 times/day) should be given during therapy to provide for increased requirements during expansion of the red cell mass secondary to marrow stimulation by EPO.

For patients with endogenous serum EPO levels which are inappropriately low for hemoglobin level, documentation of the serum EPO level will help indicate which patients may benefit from EPO therapy.

Dosage Forms Injection, preservative free: 2000 units (1 mL); 3000 units (1 mL); 4000 units (1 mL); 10,000 units (1 mL)

Reference Range Transferrin soluble receptor (TSR) protein levels >3000 ng/mL in plasma associated with exogenous erythropoietin use (normal range: 1000-2000 ng/mL)

Overdosage Treatment Supportive therapy: Phlebotomy can be utilized for hypertension if standard antihypertensive treatment fails; I.V. hydration may also be required

Pregnancy Risk Factor C

Additional Information May require supplemental iron to keep ferritin levels >100 ng/dL; frequently used by athletes for "blood doping"; response to erythropoietin of metastatic renal cell carcinoma has been reported

Specific References

Brown KR, Carter W Jr, and Lombardi GE, "Recombinant Erythropoietin Overdose," *Am J Emerg Med*, 1993, 11(6):619-21.

Gareau R, Gagnon MG, Thellend C, et al, "Transferrin Soluble Receptor: A Possible Probe for Detection of Erythropoietin Abuse by Athletes," *Horm Metab Res*, 1994, 26(6):311-2.

MacDougall IC, "Adverse Reactions Profile: Erythropoietin in Chronic Renal Failure," *Prescribers J*, 1992, 32:40-4.

Rubins J, "Metastatic Renal Cell Carcinoma: Response to Treatment With Human Recombinant Erythropoietin," *Ann Intern Med*, 1995, 122:676-7.

Schwenk MH and Halstenson CE, "Recombinant Human Erythropoietin," *DICP*, 1989, 23(7-8):528-36.

Steinberg H, "Erythropoietin and Visual Hallucinations," *N Engl J Med*, 1991, 325(4):285.

Erythroxylon Coca *see* Cocaine Hydrochloride *on page 236*

Escopon® *see* Opium Alkaloids (Hydrochlorides) *on page 579*

Esidrix® *see* Hydrochlorothiazide *on page 406*

Esilgan® *see* Estazolam *on next page*

Eskalith® *see* Lithium *on page 476*

Eskalith CR® *see* Lithium *on page 476*

Eskazina® *see* Trifluoperazine Hydrochloride *on page 769*

Esmolol Hydrochloride (ess' moe lol)

Related Information

Beta-Blockers Comparison *on page 1644-1645*

CAS Number 84057-94-3; 81161-17-3; 103598-03-04

Brand Names Brevibloc® Injection

Use Treatment of tachycardia (ventricular), fibrillation (atrial)/flutter (primarily to control ventricular rate), and hypertension (especially perioperatively); may be effective for thyrotoxic crisis; has been used to treat tachycardia due to neonatal tetanus

Mechanism of Action Class II antiarrhythmic: Competitively blocks response to $beta_1$- and $beta_2$-adrenergic stimulation

Adverse Reactions

Cardiovascular: Hypotension (especially with doses >200 mcg/kg/minute), bradycardia, exacerbation of Raynaud's phenomenon

Central nervous system: Dizziness, somnolence, confusion, drowsiness, depression, headache, seizures

Gastrointestinal: Nausea, vomiting, dyspepsia, constipation

Local: Phlebitis (at concentrations >20 mg/mL), skin necrosis after extravasation

Otic: Ototoxicity, tinnitus

Respiratory: Bronchoconstriction (less than propranolol, but more likely with higher doses)

Miscellaneous: Other adverse reactions similar to other beta-blockers may occur, sweating

Signs & Symptoms of Acute Overdose Dose-related hypotension, lightheadedness, wheezing, dyspnea, hypoglycemia, dry mouth, ataxia, dizziness, A-V block, depression, headache, heart block

Toxicodynamics/Kinetics

Distribution: V_d: 3.5 L/kg

Protein binding: 55% (esmolol), 10% (ASL-8123)

Metabolism: Hydrolyzed by plasma esterases to ASL-8123 (acid metabolite) and methanol (which is not clinically significant)

Half-life: Adults: 9 minutes

Elimination: 17-20 L/kg/hour (285 mL/kg/min)

Usual Dosage I.V. (Must be adjusted to individual response and tolerance):

Children: An extremely limited amount of information regarding esmolol use in pediatric patients is currently available. Some centers have utilized doses of 100-

(Continued)

Esmolol Hydrochloride *(Continued)*

500 mcg/kg given over 1 minute for control of tachycardia (ventricular)s. Loading doses of 500 mcg/kg/minute over 1 minute with maximal doses of 50-250 mcg/kg/minute (mean 173) have been used in addition to nitroprusside in a small number of patients (7 patients, 7-19 years of age, median 13 years) to treat postoperative hypertension after coarctation of aorta repair.

Adults: Loading dose: 500 mcg/kg over 1 minute; follow with a 50 mcg/kg/minute infusion for 4 minutes; if response is inadequate, rebolus with another 500 mcg/kg loading dose over 1 minute, and increase the maintenance infusion to 100 mcg/kg/minute. Repeat this process until a therapeutic effect has been achieved or to a maximum recommended maintenance dose of 200 mcg/kg/minute. Usual dosage range: 50-200 mcg/kg/minute with average dose of 100 mcg/kg/minute.

Contraindications Sinus bradycardia, cardiac failure, or second or third degree heart block; uncompensated congestive heart failure; cardiogenic shock; hypersensitivity to esmolol, any component, or other beta-blockers

Warnings Use with extreme caution in patients with hyper-reactive airway disease; use lowest dose possible and discontinue infusion if wheezing occurs; use with caution in diabetes mellitus, hypoglycemia, renal failure; avoid extravasation; caution should be exercised when discontinuing esmolol infusions to avoid withdrawal effects

Dosage Forms Injection: 10 mg/mL (10 mL); 250 mg/mL (10 mL)

Reference Range Therapeutic: 1.0-1.5 mg/L (3.4-5.1 μmol/L); note that arterial esmolol levels are 7-fold higher than venous levels

Overdosage Treatment Supportive therapy: Usually discontinuation of the infusion will result in resolution of adverse effects within 30 minutes; hypotension can be treated with crystalloid infusion; beta agonist agents or aminophylline can be used for bronchoconstriction

Drug Interactions When given with succinylcholine (1 mg/kg I.V.) can cause attenuation of intubation-induced tachycardia; esmolol can cause a 9% to 19% increase in serum digoxin; warfarin may result in higher esmolol levels; morphine can cause a 46% increase in esmolol plasma levels

Pregnancy Risk Factor C

Specific References

Angaran DM, Schultz NJ, and Tschida VH, "Esmolol Hydrochloride: An Ultrashort-Acting, Beta-Adrenergic Blocking Agent," *Clin Pharm*, 1986, 5(4):288-303.

Brunette DD and Rothong C, "Emergency Department Management of Thyrotoxic Crisis With Esmolol," *Am J Emerg Med*, 1991, 9(3):232-4.

Gorczynski RJ, "Basic Pharmacology of Esmolol," *Am J Cardiol*, 1985, 56(11):3F-13F.

Gray RJ, "Managing Critically Ill Patients With Esmolol: An Ultra-Short Acting Beta-Adrenergic Blocker," *Chest*, 1988, 93(2):398-403.

Lowenthal DT, Porter RS, Saris SD, et al, "Clinical Pharmacology, Pharmacodynamics and Interactions With Esmolol," *Am J Cardiol*, 1985, 56(11):14F-18F.

Luyt D, Dance M, Litmanovich H, et al, "Esmolol in the Treatment of Severe Tachycardia in Neonatal Tetanus," *Anaesth Intensive Care*, 1994, 22(3):303-4.

Wiest DB, "Esmolol: A Review of Its Therapeutic Efficacy and Pharmacokinetic Characteristics," *Clin Pharmacokinet*, 1995, 28:190-202.

Wiest DB, Garner SS, and Childress LM, "Stability of Esmolol Hydrochloride in 5% Dextrose Injection," *Am J Health-Syst Pharm*, 1995, 52:716-8.

Espotabs® [OTC] *see* Phenolphthalein *on page 617*

Estazolam (ess ta' zoe lam)

CAS Number 29975-16-4

Brand Names Domnamid®; Esilgan®; Eurodin®; Nuctalon®; ProSom™

Use Short-term management of insomnia

Mechanism of Action Has not been fully elucidated in humans; the most promising hypothesis involves GABA transmission. GABA is a major inhibitory transmitter in the CNS. Benzodiazepines may exert their pharmacologic effect through potentiation of the inhibitory activity of GABA. Specific benzodiazepine receptors have been identified in the rat brain located in proximity to dense areas of GABA receptors, primarily in the frontal and occipital cortex. Benzodiazepines do not alter the synthesis, release, reuptake, or enzymatic degradation of GABA.

Adverse Reactions

Central nervous system: Drowsiness, amnesia, confusion, dizziness, headache, ataxia

Gastrointestinal: Nausea, vomiting, dry mouth

Hepatic: Cholestatic jaundice

Miscellaneous: Physical and psychological dependence may occur with prolonged use

Signs & Symptoms of Acute Overdose Somnolence, confusion, coma, diminished reflexes, mydriasis, respiratory depression

Toxicodynamics/Kinetics Studies have shown that the elderly are more sensitive to the effects of benzodiazepines as compared to younger adults

Metabolism: Rapid and extensive in the liver to inactive metabolites (1-oxo-estazolam)
Protein binding: 93%
Half-life: 8-31 hours (no significant changes in the elderly) (mean: 17 hours)
Time to peak serum concentration: Within 0.5-6 hours
Elimination: <5% excreted unchanged in urine, less than 4% excreted in feces

Usual Dosage Adults: Oral: 1 mg at bedtime, some patients may require 2 mg; start at doses of 0.5 mg in debilitated or small elderly patients

Dosing adjustment in hepatic impairment: May be necessary

Contraindications Hypersensitivity to estazolam, cross-sensitivity with other benzodiazepines may occur, severe uncontrolled pain, pre-existing CNS depression, narrow-angle glaucoma, sleep apnea

Warnings Abrupt discontinuance may precipitate withdrawal or rebound insomnia; has the potential for drug dependence and abuse

Dosage Forms Tablet: 1 mg, 2 mg

Overdosage Treatment

Decontamination: Lavage/activated charcoal with cathartic

Supportive therapy: Treatment for benzodiazepine overdose is supportive; rarely is mechanical ventilation required. Flumazenil (Romazicon™) has been shown to selectively block the binding of benzodiazepines to CNS receptors, resulting in a reversal of benzodiazepine-induced CNS depression. Do not use in concomitant tricyclic ingestion; treat hypotension with isotonic crystalloids, place in Trendelenburg position or give dopamine or norepinephrine.

Enhancement of elimination: Multiple dose of activated charcoal may enhance elimination

Antidote(s)

Flumazenil *on page 1428*

Test Interactions Visine®, Drano®, and bleach can cause false-negative urine tests

Drug Interactions CNS depressants may increase CNS adverse effects; cimetidine may decrease and enzyme inducers may increase the metabolism of estazolam

Pregnancy Risk Factor X (suggested to be teratogenic in animal and human data; can precipitate neonatal respiratory depression when given during delivery)

Monitoring Parameters Respiratory and cardiovascular status

Patient Information Avoid alcohol and other CNS depressants; avoid activities needing good psychomotor coordination until CNS effects are known; drug may cause physical or psychological dependence; avoid abrupt discontinuation after prolonged use

Nursing Implications Provide safety measures (ie, side rails, night light, and call button); remove smoking materials from area; supervise ambulation; avoid abrupt discontinuance in patients with prolonged therapy or seizure disorders

Specific References

Busto U, Bendayan R, and Sellers EM, "Clinical Pharmacokinetics of Nonopiate Abuse Drugs," *Clin Pharmacokinet*, 1989, 16(1):1-26.

Estigyn® *see* Ethinyl Estradiol *on page 331*

Estratab® *see* Estrogens, Esterified *on page 327*

Estrinyl® *see* Ethinyl Estradiol *on page 331*

Estrogenic Substances, Conjugated *see* Estrogens, Conjugated *on this page*

Estrogens, Conjugated (ess' troe jenz)

Brand Names CES Congest®; Dagynil®; Premarin® Injection; Premarin® Oral; Premarin® Vaginal; Presomen®; Progens®; Transannon®

Synonyms C.E.S.; Estrogenic Substances, Conjugated

Use Atrophic vaginitis; hypogonadism; primary ovarian failure; vasomotor symptoms of menopause; prostatic carcinoma; osteoporosis prophylactic

Mechanism of Action Increases the synthesis of DNA, RNA, and various proteins in target tissues; reduces the release of gonadotropin-releasing hormone from the hypothalamus; reduces FSH and LH release from the pituitary

Adverse Reactions

Cardiovascular: Hypertension, myocardial infarction, edema, thrombosis at doses >1.25 mg/day
Central nervous system: Headache, depression, dizziness, anxiety, stroke
Dermatologic: Chloasma, pruritus, melasma, rash
Gastrointestinal: Nausea, vomiting, diarrhea, bloating, anorexia, gastrointestinal distress, pancreatitis
Hepatic: Cholelithiasis, cholestatic jaundice
Local: Pain at injection

(Continued)

Estrogens, Conjugated *(Continued)*

Neuromuscular & skeletal: Chorea

Ocular: Intolerance to contact lenses

Miscellaneous: Peripheral edema, enlargement of breasts, breast tenderness, increased libido, site, breast tumors, amenorrhea, alterations in frequency and flow of menses, decreased glucose tolerance, increased triglycerides and LDL, increased susceptibility to *Candida* infection, thromboembolism, hypercalcemia with chronic use

Signs & Symptoms of Acute Overdose Fluid retention, jaundice, hypophosphatemia, impotence, gynecomastia, ectopic pregnancy, sexual dysfunction, depression, thrombophlebitis, dizziness

Toxicodynamics/Kinetics

Absorption: Readily absorbed from gastrointestinal tract and vaginal mucosa

Protein binding: 50% to 80%

Metabolism: To inactive compounds in the liver (estrone, estradiol)

Elimination: Bile and urine

Usual Dosage Adults:

Male: Prostate cancer: Oral: 1.25-2.5 mg 3 times/day

Female:

- Hypogonadism: Oral: 2.5-7.5 mg/day for 20 days, off 10 days and repeat until menses occur
- Abnormal uterine bleeding:
  - Oral: 2.5-5 mg/day for 7-10 days; then decrease to 1.25 mg/day for 2 weeks
  - I.M., I.V.: 25 mg every 6-12 hours until bleeding stops
- Moderate to severe vasomotor symptoms: Oral: 0.625-1.25 mg/day
- Postpartum breast engorgement: Oral: 3.75 mg every 4 hours for 5 doses, then 1.25 mg every 4 hours for 5 days
- Atrophic vaginitis, kraurosis vulvae: Vaginal: 2-4 g instilled/day 3 weeks on and 1 week off

Contraindications Undiagnosed vaginal bleeding; hypersensitivity to estrogens or any component; thrombophlebitis, liver disease, known or suspected pregnancy, carcinoma of the breast, estrogen dependent tumor

Warnings Use with caution in patients with asthma, epilepsy, migraine, diabetes, cardiac or renal dysfunction; estrogens may cause premature closure of the epiphyses in young individuals; safety and efficacy in children have not been established; estrogens have been reported to increase the risk of endometrial carcinoma

Dosage Forms

Cream, vaginal: 0.625 mg/g (42.5 g)

Injection: 25 mg (5 mL)

Tablet: 0.3 mg, 0.625 mg, 0.9 mg, 1.25 mg, 2.5 mg

Stability Refrigerate injection; reconstituted solution is stable for 60 days; injection is **compatible** with normal saline, dextrose, and invert sugar solutions; **incompatible** with proteins, ascorbic acid, or solutions with acidic pH

Reference Range

Children: <10 μg/24 hour (SI: <35 μmol/day) (values at Mayo Medical Laboratories)

Adults:

- Male: 15-40 μg/24 hours (SI: 52-139 μmol/day)
- Female:
  - Menstruating: 15-80 μg/24 hour (SI: 52-277 μmol/day)
  - Postmenopausal: <20 μg/24 hour (SI: <69 μmol/day)

Overdosage Treatment

Decontamination: Emesis or lavage; activated charcoal with cathartic

Enhancement of elimination: Due to enterohepatic recirculation of drug, multiple dosing of activated charcoal may be effective

Test Interactions

Decreased antithrombin III; decreased serum folate concentration

Increased prothrombin and factors VII, VIII, IX, X; increased platelet aggregability; increased thyroid binding globulin; increased total thyroid hormone (T_4); increased serum triglycerides/phospholipids

Drug Interactions

Decreased effect: Rifampin, barbiturates, phenytoin, carbamazepine decrease estrogen serum concentrations; estrogens may decrease effect of sulfonylureas, decreased oral hypoglycemic effect; decreased estrogen effect when used with phenytoin

Increased toxicity: Hydrocortisone increases corticosteroid toxic potential; increases potential for thromboembolic events with anticoagulants; increased toxicity with ascorbic acid; increased lethargy with tricyclic antidepressants; estrogens may increase metabolism of some benzodiazepines (lorazepam, oxazepam, temazepam), but decrease metabolism of others

Pregnancy Risk Factor X

Monitoring Parameters Dysfunctional uterine bleeding: Hematocrit, hemoglobin, PT

Patient Information Inform physician if signs or symptoms of any of the following occur: Thromboembolic or thrombotic disorders including sudden severe headache or vomiting, disturbance of vision or speech, loss of vision, numbness or weakness in an extremity, sharp or crushing chest pain, calf pain, shortness of breath, severe abdominal pain or mass, mental depression, or unusual bleeding; discontinue taking medication if you suspect you are pregnant or become pregnant. Patient package insert is available with product; insert vaginal product high into the vagina.

Nursing Implications May also be administered intramuscularly; give at bedtime to minimize occurrence of adverse effects; when administered I.V., drug should be administered slowly to avoid the occurrence of a flushing reaction

Specific References

Barrett-Connor E, Brown WV, Turner J, et al, "Heart Disease Risk Factors and Hormone Use in Postmenopausal Women," *JAMA*, 1979, 241:2167-9.

Christopherson WM, "Liver Tumours and the Pill," *Br Med J*, 1975, 4:756.

Cust MP, Ganagar KF, Hillard TC, et al, "A Risk-Benefit Assessment of Estrogen Therapy in Postmenopausal Women," *Drug Saf*, 1990, 5(5):345-58.

Estrogens, Esterified (ess' troe jens, es ter' i fied)

Brand Names Estratab®; Menest®; Neo-Estrone®

Use Atrophic vaginitis; hypogonadism; primary ovarian failure; vasomotor symptoms of menopause; prostatic carcinoma; osteoporosis prophylactic

Mechanism of Action All estrogens, including esterified estrogens, act in a similar manner. Estrogens exert their primary effects on the interphase DNA-protein complex (chromatin) by binding to a receptor (usually located in the cytoplasm of a target cell) and initiating translocation of the hormone-receptor complex to the nucleus. The specificity of estrogen action depends upon the presence and concentration of estrogen targets, which are defined as tissues containing a high concentration of estrogen receptors.

Adverse Reactions

Cardiovascular: Hypertension, myocardial infarction, edema, thromboembolism

Central nervous system: Headache, depression, dizziness, anxiety, stroke

Dermatologic: Chloasma, pruritus, melasma, rash,

Gastrointestinal: Nausea, anorexia, pancreatitis, bloating, vomiting, diarrhea, gastrointestinal distress

Hepatic: Cholestatic jaundice

Ocular: Intolerance to contact lenses

Miscellaneous: Peripheral edema, enlargement of breasts, breast tenderness, increased libido, breast tumors, amenorrhea, alterations in frequency and flow of menses, decreased glucose tolerance, increased triglycerides and LDL, increased susceptibility to *Candida* infection

Signs & Symptoms of Acute Overdose Fluid retention, jaundice, hypophosphatemia, sexual dysfunction, impotence, gynecomastia, migraine headache (exacerbation of); thrombophlebitis; toxicity is unlikely following single exposures of excessive doses

Toxicodynamics/Kinetics

Absorption: Readily absorbed from gastrointestinal tract

Protein binding: 50% to 80%

Metabolism: Rapid in the liver to less active metabolites

Elimination: Excreted in urine as unchanged compound and metabolites

Usual Dosage Adults: Oral:

Male: Prostate cancer (inoperable, progressing): 1.25-2.5 mg 3 times/day

Female:

Hypogonadism: 2.5-7.5 mg/day for 20 days, off 10 days and repeat until menses occur

Moderate to severe vasomotor symptoms: 0.3-1.25 mg/day

Breast cancer (inoperable, progressing): 10 mg 3 times/day for at least 3 months

Contraindications Known or suspected cancer of the breast, except in appropriately selected patients being treated for metastatic disease; known or suspected estrogen-dependent neoplasia; known or suspected pregnancy; undiagnosed abnormal genital bleeding; active thrombophlebitis or thromboembolic disorders; past history of thrombophlebitis, thrombosis, or thromboembolic disorders associated with previous estrogen use except when used in the treatment of breast or prostatic malignancy

Warnings Use with caution in patients with asthma, epilepsy, migraine, diabetes, cardiac or renal dysfunction; estrogens may cause premature closure of the epiphyses in young individuals; safety and efficacy in children have not been established; estrogens have been reported to increase the risk of endometrial carcinoma, do not use estrogens during pregnancy

Dosage Forms Tablet: 0.3 mg, 0.625 mg, 1.25 mg, 2.5 mg

Reference Range

Children: <10 μg/24 hour (SI: <35 μmol/day) (values at Mayo Medical Laboratories)

(Continued)

Estrogens, Esterified *(Continued)*

Adults:

Male: 15-40 μg/24 hours (SI: 52-139 μmol/day)

Female:

Menstruating: 15-80 μg/24 hour (SI: 52-277 μmol/day)

Postmenopausal: <20 μg/24 hour (SI: <69 μmol/day)

Overdosage Treatment

Decontamination: Emesis or lavage; activated charcoal with cathartic

Enhancement of elimination: Due to enterohepatic recirculation of drug, multiple dosing of activated charcoal may be effective

Test Interactions Endocrine function test may be altered

Decreased antithrombin III; decreased serum folate concentration

Increased prothrombin and factors VII, VIII, IX, X; increased platelet aggregability; increased thyroid binding globulin; increased total thyroid hormone (T_4); increased serum triglycerides/phospholipids

Drug Interactions

Decreased effect: Rifampin decreases estrogen serum concentrations

Increased toxicity: Hydrocortisone increases corticosteroid toxic potential; increases potential for thromboembolic events with anticoagulants

Pregnancy Risk Factor X

Patient Information Patients should inform their physicians if signs or symptoms of thromboembolic or thrombotic disorders occur including sudden severe headache or vomiting, disturbance of vision or speech, loss of vision, numbness or weakness in an extremity, sharp or crushing chest pain, calf pain, shortness of breath, severe abdominal pain or mass, mental depression or unusual bleeding; patients should discontinue taking the medication if they suspect they are pregnant or become pregnant.

Additional Information Esterified estrogens are a combination of the sodium salts of the sulfate esters of estrogenic substances; the principal component is estrone, with preparations containing 75% to 85% sodium estrone sulfate and 6% to 15% sodium equilin sulfate such that the total is not <90%

Specific References

Winship KA, "Unopposed Oestrogens," *Adverse Drug React Acute Poisoning Rev*, 1987, 6(1):37-66.

Estulic® *see* Guanfacine Hydrochloride *on page 394*

Etacrynate *see* Ethacrynic Acid *on this page*

Ethacrynic Acid (eth a krin' ik)

CAS Number 58-54-8

Brand Names Edecrin®; Edecrina®; Hydromedin®; Reomax®

Synonyms Acidum Etacrynicum; Etacrynate

Use Management of edema secondary to congestive heart failure; hepatic or renal disease, hypertension

Mechanism of Action Inhibits reabsorption of sodium and chloride in the ascending loop of Henle and distal renal tubule, interfering with the chloride-binding cotransport system, thus causing increased excretion of water, sodium, chloride, magnesium, and calcium

Adverse Reactions

Cardiovascular: Hypotension, diuresis

Dermatologic: Rash

Endocrine & metabolic: Fluid and electrolyte imbalances (fluid depletion, hypokalemia, hyponatremia, hyperglycemia), hyperuricemia

Gastrointestinal: gastrointestinal irritation, diarrhea, gastrointestinal bleeding (especially when used with warfarin)

Hematologic: Thrombocytopenia, leukopenia, neutropenia, agranulocytosis, granulocytopenia

Hepatic: Abnormal liver function tests

Otic: Ototoxicity, tinnitus, deafness

Renal: Renal injury

Miscellaneous: Feces discoloration (black)

Signs & Symptoms of Acute Overdose Hypoglycemia, hypotension, thrombocytopenia, hyponatremia, hypokalemia, hyperglycemia, nystagmus, myasthenia gravis (exacerbation or precipitation of), gout, dizziness, dysosmia, hypocalcemia, hyperuricemia, nocturia, hypomagnesemia, pancreatitis, leukopenia; neutropenia; agranulocytosis; granulocytopenia

Toxicodynamics/Kinetics

Oral:

Onset of diuretic effect: Within 30 minutes

Peak effect: 2 hours

Duration of action: 6-12 hours

I.V.:

Onset of diuresis: 5 minutes

Peak effect: 30 minutes

Duration of action: 2 hours

Protein binding: 90%

Bioavailability: Oral: ~100%

Half-life: 1-4 hours

Metabolism: In the liver to active cysteine conjugate

Elimination: Bile and urine

Usual Dosage

Children:

Oral: 25 mg/day to start, increase by 25 mg/day at intervals of 2-3 days as needed, to a maximum of 3 mg/kg/day

I.V.: 1 mg/kg/dose, (maximum: 50 mg/dose); repeat doses not recommended

Adults:

Oral: 50-100 mg/day in 1-2 divided doses; may increase in increments of 25-50 mg at intervals of several days to a maximum of 400 mg/24 hours

I.V.: 0.5-1 mg/kg/dose (maximum: 100 mg/dose); repeat doses not recommended

Dosing adjustment/comments in renal impairment: Cl_{cr} <10 mL/minute: Avoid use

Contraindications Hypersensitivity to ethacrynic acid or any component or other sulfonamides

Warnings Loop diuretics are potent diuretics, excess amounts can lead to profound diuresis with fluid and electrolyte loss; use with caution in patients with advanced hepatic cirrhosis, diabetes mellitus, hypotension, dehydration, history of water diarrhea from ethacrynic acid, hearing impairment; safety and efficacy in infants have not been established

Dosage Forms

Powder for injection, as ethacrynate sodium: 50 mg (50 mL)

Tablet: 25 mg, 50 mg

Overdosage Treatment

Decontamination: Activated charcoal with cathartic

Supportive therapy: Intravenous hydration with 0.9% saline; replace electrolyte deficiency

Drug Interactions

Decreased effect with indomethacin and other NSAIDs

Increased effect/toxicity/levels of warfarin, lithium; increased effect with thiazide diuretics

Pregnancy Risk Factor D

Monitoring Parameters Blood pressure, serum electrolytes, renal function, hearing, glucose

Additional Information Injection contains thimerosal

Specific References

Cowley AJ and Elkeles RS, "Diabetes and Therapy With Potent Diuretics," *Lancet*, 1978, 1(8056):154.

Gomolin IH and Garschick E, "Ethacrynic Acid-Induced Deafness Accompanied by Nystagmus," *N Engl J Med*, 1980, 303(12):702.

Lant A, "Diuretics: Clinical Pharmacology and Therapeutic Use," *Drugs*, 1985, 29(1):57-87.

Ethambutol Hydrochloride (e tham' byoo tole)

Related Information

Therapeutic Drugs Associated With Hallucinations *on page 1558-1559*

CAS Number 1070-11-7

Brand Names Myambutol®

Use Treatment of tuberculosis and other mycobacterial diseases in conjunction with other antituberculosis agents

Mechanism of Action Suppresses mycobacteria multiplication by interfering with RNA synthesis

Adverse Reactions

Central nervous system: Malaise, peripheral neuritis, mental confusion, fever, headache, visual hallucinations

Dermatologic: Rash, pruritus, angioedema

Endocrine & metabolic: Hyperuricemia

Gastrointestinal: Nausea, vomiting

Hepatic: Abnormal liver function tests

Ocular: Optic neuritis, photophobia

Miscellaneous: Anaphylactoid reactions, metallic taste

Signs & Symptoms of Acute Overdose Mental confusion, eosinophilia, disorientation, purpura, hyperuricemia, blindness, neutropenia, hallucinations, jaundice, nausea, vomiting, neuropathy (peripheral), optic neuropathy, fever, visual changes, anorexia, arthralgia, numbness of the extremities, toxic epidermal necrolysis, alopecia

(Continued)

Ethambutol Hydrochloride *(Continued)*

Toxicodynamics/Kinetics

Absorption: Oral: ~80%

Distribution: V_d: 1.6 L/kg; well distributed throughout the body with high concentrations in kidneys, lungs, saliva, and red blood cells

Protein binding: 10% to 30%

Metabolism: 20% by the liver to inactive metabolite

Half-life: 2.5-3.6 hours (up to 15 hours with renal impairment)

Time to peak serum concentration: Within 2-4 hours

Elimination: ~50% excreted in urine and 20% excreted in feces as unchanged drug

Usual Dosage Oral (not recommended in children <12 years of age):

Children >12 years: 15 mg/kg/day once daily

Adolescents and Adults: 15-25 mg/kg/day once daily, not to exceed 2.5 g/day

Dosing interval in renal impairment:

Cl_{cr} 10-50 mL/minute: Administer every 24-36 hours

Cl_{cr} <10 mL/minute: Administer every 48 hours and/or reduce daily dose

Contraindications Hypersensitivity to ethambutol or any component; optic neuropathy

Dosage Forms Tablet: 100 mg, 400 mg

Overdosage Treatment

Decontamination: Activated charcoal with cathartic/lavage

Supportive therapy: Replace potassium/sodium losses

Enhancement of elimination: Slightly dialyzable (5% to 20%) and possibly effective

Test Interactions Increases uric acid (S)

Drug Interactions Aluminum salts; aluminum hydroxide can decrease intestinal absorption of fluoride

Pregnancy Risk Factor B

Monitoring Parameters Periodic visual testing in patients receiving more than 15 mg/kg/day; periodic renal, hepatic, and hematopoietic tests

Additional Information Incidence of optic neuropathy increases significantly with dosages above 15 mg/kg/day but may be idiosyncratic

Specific References

Citron KM and Thomas GO, "Ocular Toxicity From Ethambutol," *Thorax*, 1986, 41(10):737-9.

Ducobu J, DuPont P, Laurent M, et al, "Acute Isoniazid/Ethambutol/Rifampicin Overdosage," *Lancet*, 1982, 1(8272):632.

Karnik AM, Al-Shamali MA, and Fenech FF, "A Case of Ocular Toxicity to Ethambutol - An Idiosyncratic Reaction?" *Postgrad Med J*, 1985, 61(719):811-3.

Ethanoic Acid *see* Acetic Acid *on page 85*

Ethanol *see* Ethyl Alcohol *on page 336*

Ethanol and Blood Alcohol Determination *see page 1176*

Ethatyl® *see* Ethionamide *on page 333*

Ethchlorvynol (eth klor vi' nole)

Related Information

Therapeutic Drugs Associated With Hallucinations *on page 1558-1559*

CAS Number 113-18-8

Brand Names Placidyl®

Use Short-term management of insomnia

Mechanism of Action A chlorinated acetylenic carbinol which causes nonspecific depression of the reticular activating system

Adverse Reactions

Cardiovascular: Bradycardia

Central nervous system: Facial numbness, residual sedation, headache, dizziness, psychosis, asthenia, nervousness, excitation, clumsiness, confusion, drowsiness (daytime), visual hallucinations

Dermatologic: Rash

Gastrointestinal: Nausea, vomiting, indigestion, stomach pain

Genitourinary: Urinary retention

Hematologic: Thrombocytopenia, porphyria, pancytopenia

Hepatic: Jaundice

Neuromuscular & skeletal: Trembling

Ocular: Blurred vision, diplopia, mydriasis, nystagmus

Renal: Myoglobinuria

Respiratory: Dyspnea

Miscellaneous: Slurred speech, retrograde amnesia, unpleasant aftertaste (mint-like)

Signs & Symptoms of Acute Overdose Hypotension, cough, pleural effusion, prolonged coma lasting over 100 hours, respiratory depression, ataxia, myopathy, numbness, pulmonary edema, rhabdomyolysis, hypothermia, bradycardia; bullous skin lesions

Toxicodynamics/Kinetics

Onset of action: 15-60 minutes

Duration: 5 hours

Absorption: Rapid from gastrointestinal tract

Distribution: V_d: 3-4 L/kg

Protein binding: 35% to 50%

Metabolism: In the liver

Half-life: 10-20 hours; over 100 hours in overdose

Time to peak serum concentration: 1.5 hours

Usual Dosage Adults: Oral: 500-1000 mg at bedtime

Dosing adjustment in renal impairment: Cl_{cr} <50 mL/minute: Avoid use

Contraindications Porphyria, hypersensitivity to ethchlorvynol or any component

Warnings Administer with caution to depressed or suicidal patients or to patients with a history of drug abuse; intoxication symptoms may appear with prolonged daily doses of as little as 1 g; withdrawal symptoms may be seen upon abrupt discontinuation; use with caution in the elderly and in patients with hepatic or renal dysfunction; use with caution in patients who have a history of paradoxical restlessness to barbiturates or alcohol; some products may contain tartrazine

Dosage Forms Capsule: 200 mg, 500 mg, 750 mg

Reference Range

Therapeutic: 2-8 μg/mL

Toxic: >13 μg/mL

Overdosage Treatment

Decontamination: Lavage/activated charcoal with cathartic

Supportive therapy: Hypotension can be treated with isotonic saline infusion (10-20 mL/kg), and or dopamine or norepinephrine

Enhancement of elimination: Multiple dosing of activated charcoal is effective for ingestions >10 g (or over 100 mg/kg); or for prolonged coma; hemodialysis (or preferably hemoperfusion) should be initiated; consider hemodialysis/hemoperfusion if ethchlorvynol serum levels are >10 μg/mL; monitor for rebound effect with redistribution of drug from fat storage; thus prolonged or repeated hemoperfusion may be needed

Antidote(s)

Dopamine Hydrochloride *on page 1418*

Norepinephrine Bitartrate *on page 1451*

Diagnostic Tests/Procedures

Ethchlorvynol, Blood *on page 1261*

Drug Interactions

Decreased effect of oral anticoagulants

Increased toxicity (CNS depression) with alcohol, CNS depressants, MAO inhibitors, TCAs (delirium)

Pregnancy Risk Factor C

Monitoring Parameters Cardiac and respiratory function and abuse potential

Patient Information May cause drowsiness, can impair judgment and coordination; avoid alcohol and other CNS depressants; ataxia can be reduced if taken with food; do not crush or refrigerate capsules

Nursing Implications Raise bed rails, institute safety measures, assist with ambulation

Specific References

Bertino JS Jr and Reed MD, "Barbiturate and Nonbarbiturate Sedative Hypnotic Intoxication in Children," *Pediatr Clin North Am*, 1986, 33(3):703-22.

Kathpalia SC, Haslitt JH, and Lim VS, "Charcoal Hemoperfusion for Treatment of Ethchlorvynol Overdose," *Artif Organs*, 1983, 7(2):246-8.

Kelner MJ and Bailey DN, "Ethchlorvynol Ingestion: Interpretation of Blood Concentrations and Clinical Findings," *J Toxicol Clin Toxicol*, 1983-84, 21(3):399-408.

Yell RP, "Ethchlorvynol Overdose," *Am J Emerg Med*, 1990, 8(3):246-50.

Ethinyl Estradiol (eth' in il ess tra dye' ole)

CAS Number 57-63-6

Brand Names Estigyn®; Estrinyl®; Feminone®; Primogyn C®; Progynon C®

Use Hypogonadism; primary ovarian failure; vasomotor symptoms of menopause; prostatic carcinoma; breast cancer

Mechanism of Action Increases the synthesis of DNA, RNA, and various proteins in target tissues; reduces the release of gonadotropin-releasing hormone from the hypothalamus; reduces FSH and LH release from the pituitary

Adverse Reactions

Cardiovascular: Hypertension, myocardial infarction, edema

Central nervous system: Headache, depression, dizziness, anxiety, stroke

Dermatologic: Chloasma, melasma, rash

Endocrine & metabolic: Hypercalcemia (in breast cancer patients), hyperglycemia, amenorrhea

Gastrointestinal: Nausea, vomiting, diarrhea, bloating, anorexia, gastrointestinal distress, pancreatitis

(Continued)

Ethinyl Estradiol *(Continued)*

Hepatic: Cholelithiasis, cholestatic jaundice
Neuromuscular & skeletal: Chorea
Ocular: Intolerance to contact lenses
Miscellaneous: Peripheral edema, enlargement of breasts, breast tenderness, increased libido, site, breast tumors, alterations in frequency and flow of menses, decreased glucose tolerance, increased triglycerides and LDL, increased susceptibility to *Candida* infection, thromboembolism, adrenal hyperplasia, porphyrinogenic

Signs & Symptoms of Acute Overdose Fluid retention, jaundice, hyperglycemia, thrombophlebitis, nausea; toxicity is unlikely following single exposures of excessive doses

Toxicodynamics/Kinetics

Absorption: Absorbed well from gastrointestinal tract (40% to 45%); unaffected with food
Protein binding: 97%
Peak plasma levels: 1.3 hours (delayed when given with mestranol)
Metabolism: Inactivated by liver
Half-life: 13-27 hours
Elimination: Eliminated by kidneys and bile

Usual Dosage Adults: Oral:

Male: Prostatic cancer (inoperable, progressing): 0.15-2 mg/day for palliation

Female:

- Hypogonadism: 0.05 mg 1-3 times/day for 2 weeks of a theoretical menstrual cycle followed by progesterone for 3-6 months
- Vasomotor symptoms: 0.02-0.05 mg for 21 days, off 7 days and repeat
- Breast cancer (inoperable, progressing): 1 mg 3 times/day for palliation
- Emergency contraception: 50 mcg taken within 72 hours will usually prevent pregnancy

Contraindications Thrombophlebitis, undiagnosed vaginal bleeding, hypersensitivity to ethinyl estradiol or any component, known or suspected pregnancy, carcinoma of the breast, estrogen-dependent tumor

Warnings Use with caution in patients with asthma, seizure disorders, migraine, cardiac, renal or hepatic impairment, cerebrovascular disorders or history of breast cancer, past or present thromboembolic disease, smokers >35 years of age

Dosage Forms Tablet: 0.02 mg, 0.05 mg, 0.5 mg

Reference Range Peak plasma level of ethinyl estradiol after a 0.05 mg dose: 100-200 pg/mL

Overdosage Treatment

Decontamination: Emesis or lavage; activated charcoal with cathartic
Enhancement of elimination: Due to enterohepatic recirculation of drug, multiple dosing of activated charcoal may be effective

Test Interactions

Decreased antithrombin III; decreased serum folate concentration; decreased zinc levels
Increased prothrombin and factors VII, VIII, IX, X; increased platelet aggregability; increased thyroid binding globulin; increased total thyroid hormone (T_4); increased serum triglycerides/phospholipids; increased serum cortisol level

Drug Interactions

Rifampin may decrease the effectiveness of oral contraceptives
Increased toxicity: Carbamazepine, tricyclic antidepressants, and corticosteroids; increased thromboembolic potential with oral anticoagulants; use with ascorbic acid may cause heavy vaginal bleeding

Pregnancy Risk Factor X

Monitoring Parameters Weight, blood pressure, glucose

Patient Information Inform your physician if signs or symptoms of any of the following occur: Thromboembolic or thrombotic disorders including sudden severe headache or vomiting, disturbance of vision or speech, loss of vision, numbness or weakness in an extremity, sharp or crushing chest pain, calf pain, shortness of breath, severe abdominal pain or mass, mental depression or unusual bleeding. Discontinue taking the medication if you suspect you are pregnant or become pregnant.

Nursing Implications Give at bedtime to minimize occurrence of adverse effects

Additional Information Estrinyl® contains tartrazine which can cause allergic reactions; 17-beta-estradiol modulates acetylcholine-induced coronary artery responses in postmenopausal women

Specific References

Collins P, Rosano GM, Sarrel PM, et al, "17 β-Estradiol Attenuates Acetylcholine-Induced Coronary Arterial Constriction in Women but Not Men With Coronary Heart Disease," *Circulation*, 1995, 92:24-30.

Goldzieher JW and Brody SA, "Pharmacokinetics of Ethinyl Estradiol and Mestranol," *Am J Obstet Gynecol*, 1990, 163(6 Pt 2):2114-9.

Ethiofos *see* Amifostine *on page 107*

Ethionamide (e thye on am' ide)

CAS Number 536-33-4

Brand Names Ethatyl®; Etiocidan®; Trecator®-SC

Use In conjunction with other antituberculosis agents in the treatment of tuberculosis and other mycobacterial diseases

Mechanism of Action Inhibits peptide synthesis

Adverse Reactions

Cardiovascular: Postural hypotension

Central nervous system: Drowsiness, psychosis, dizziness, seizures, headache, peripheral neuritis

Dermatologic: Rash, stomatitis

Endocrine & metabolic: Hypoglycemia, goiter, gynecomastia

Gastrointestinal: Nausea, vomiting, abdominal pain, diarrhea, anorexia, metallic taste

Hematologic: Thrombocytopenia, porphyria

Hepatic: Hepatitis

Ocular: Optic neuritis, photophobia, diplopia

Signs & Symptoms of Acute Overdose Paresthesias, neuropathy (peripheral), extensor plantar response, stomatitis, personality changes, vision color changes (increased color perception), hypoglycemia, anorexia, impotence, arthralgia

Toxicodynamics/Kinetics

Duration of action: 9 hours

Absorption: Rapid from gastrointestinal tract

Distribution: Distributed widely to most tissues and fluids including liver, kidneys, and spleen

Protein binding: 10%

Metabolism: Probably hepatic; metabolized to sulfoxide which is active to inactive metabolites

Bioavailability: 80%

Half-life: 2-3 hours

Time to peak serum concentration: Oral: Within 3 hours

Elimination: Excreted as metabolites (active and inactive) and parent drug in urine

Usual Dosage Oral:

Children: 15-20 mg/kg/day in 2 divided doses, not to exceed 1 g/day

Adults: 500-1000 mg/day in 1-3 divided doses

Dosing adjustment in renal impairment: Cl_{cr} <50 mL/minute: Administer 50% of dose

Contraindications Contraindicated in patients with severe hepatic impairment or in patients who are sensitive to the porphyria drug

Warnings Not used as a single agent; use with caution in patients receiving cycloserine or isoniazid

Dosage Forms Tablet, sugar coated: 250 mg

Reference Range Peak serum concentration: 2 µg/mL after an oral dose of 250 mg

Overdosage Treatment

Decontamination: Charcoal/lavage as indicated

Supportive therapy: Neurologic symptoms may resolve with pyridoxine or nicotinamide therapy

Test Interactions Decreases thyroxine (S)

Drug Interactions Cycloserine and isoniazid; increased hepatic damage with rifampin

Pregnancy Risk Factor C

Pregnancy Implications Crosses the placenta

Monitoring Parameters Initial and periodic serum AST and ALT

Patient Information Take with meals

Specific References

Pattyn SR, Janssens L, Bourland J, et al, "Hepatotoxicity of the Combination of Rifampin-Ethionamide in the Treatment of Multibacillary Leprosy," *Int J Lepr Other Mycobact Dis*, 1984, 52(1):1-6.

Ethocaine Hydrochloride *see* Procaine Hydrochloride *on page 644*

Ethoform *see* Benzocaine *on page 149*

Ethosuximide (eth oh sux' i mide)

Related Information

Therapeutic Drugs Associated With Hallucinations *on page 1558-1559*

CAS Number 77-67-8

Brand Names Emeside®; Zarontin®

Synonyms 2-ethyl-2-methylsuccinmide

Use Management of absence (petit mal) seizures, myoclonic seizures, and akinetic epilepsy

(Continued)

Ethosuximide *(Continued)*

Mechanism of Action Increases the seizure threshold and suppresses paroxysmal spike-and-wave pattern in absence seizures; depresses nerve transmission in the motor cortex

Adverse Reactions

Central nervous system: Sedation, dizziness, drowsiness, euphoria, visual hallucinations, insomnia, psychosis, agitation, behavioral changes, parkinsonism, headache

Dermatologic: Rashes, rash

Gastrointestinal: Nausea, vomiting, anorexia (dose related), abdominal pain (epigastric)

Hematologic: Leukopenia, aplastic anemia, thrombocytopenia

Hepatic: Liver enzyme elevation

Ocular: Photophobia, diplopia

Miscellaneous: Hiccups, lupus erythematosus

Signs & Symptoms of Acute Overdose Acute overdosage can cause CNS depression, ataxia, stupor, coma, hypotension; chronic overdose can cause skin rash, confusion, albuminuria, erythema multiforme, hepatic dysfunction, extrapyramidal reaction, dementia, hematuria, leukopenia; neutropenia; agranulocytosis; granulocytopenia; myasthenia gravis (exacerbation or precipitation of), insomnia, systemic lupus erythematosus (SLE), coma

Toxicodynamics/Kinetics

Absorption: Rapid and complete

Distribution: V_d: Adults: 0.62-0.72 L/kg; distributes to all body tissues except fat

Protein binding: 2% to 10%

Metabolism: ~80% in the liver to three inactive hydroxylated metabolites

Half-life:

- Children: 30 hours
- Adults: 50-60 hours

Time to peak serum concentration:

- Children: 3-7 hours
- Capsule: Within 2-4 hours
- Syrup: <2-4 hours

Elimination: Excreted slowly in urine as metabolites (50%) and as unchanged drug (10% to 20%); small amounts excreted in feces

Usual Dosage Oral:

Children 3-6 years: Initial: 250 mg/day (or 15 mg/kg/day) in 2 divided doses; increase every 4-7 days; usual maintenance dose: 15-40 mg/kg/day in 2 divided doses

Children >6 years and Adults: Initial: 250 mg twice daily; increase by 250 mg as needed every 4-7 days up to 1.5 g/day in 2 divided doses; usual maintenance dose: 20-40 mg/kg/day in 2 divided doses

Contraindications Known hypersensitivity to ethosuximide

Warnings When used alone in mixed seizures, ethosuximide may increase the frequency of tonic-clonic seizures. When patients with absence seizures also have tonic-clonic seizures, other anticonvulsants such as phenytoin or phenobarbital must be used in combination with ethosuximide. Avoid abrupt discontinuation of therapy; dosage should be reduced slowly to avoid precipitation of seizures. Use with caution in patients with hepatic or renal disease; may impair mental alertness and coordination.

Dosage Forms

Capsule: 250 mg

Syrup (raspberry flavor): 250 mg/5 mL (473 mL)

Reference Range

Therapeutic: 40-100 μg/mL (SI: 280-710 μmol/L)

Toxic: >150 μg/mL (SI: >1062 μmol/L); at steady-state, each 1 mg/kg will result in a serum rise of 2 μg/mL

Overdosage Treatment

Decontamination: Lavage/activated charcoal with cathartic

Supportive therapy: Treatment is supportive; benzodiazepine (diazepam or lorazepam) for seizures

Enhanced elimination: Hemoperfusion and hemodialysis may be useful; hemodialysis has an extraction efficiency of 61% to 100%; forced diuresis is not useful; multiple dosing of activated charcoal may be useful

Test Interactions Increases alkaline phosphatase (S); positive Coombs' [direct]; decreases calcium (S)

Diagnostic Tests/Procedures

Ethosuximide, Blood *on page 1261*

Drug Interactions Phenytoin, carbamazepine, primidone, phenobarbital may increase the hepatic metabolism of ethosuximide; isoniazid may inhibit hepatic metabolism with a resultant increase in ethosuximide serum concentrations

Pregnancy Risk Factor C (low teratogenicity in mice)

Pregnancy Implications Distributes into the fetus; breast milk-maternal serum ratio is 90%

Monitoring Parameters CBC, platelets, liver enzymes, trough ethosuximide serum concentration

Patient Information Take with food

Nursing Implications Observe patient for excess sedation

Additional Information Considered to be drug of choice for simple absence seizures

Specific References

Marbury TC, Lee CS, Perchalski RJ, et al, "Hemodialysis Clearance of Ethosuximide in Patients With Chronic Renal Disease," *Am J Hosp Pharm*, 1981, 38(11):1757-60.

Ethotoin (eth' o toin)

CAS Number 86-35-1

Brand Names Peganone®

Synonyms Ethylphenylhydantoin

Use Generalized tonic-clonic or complex-partial seizures

Mechanism of Action Exerts an anticonvulsant effect without causing general central nervous system depression. The mechanism of action is believed to be similar to that of phenytoin which appears to stabilize the normal seizure threshold and to prevent the spread of seizure activity rather than to abolish the primary focus of seizure discharges. Ethotoin is effective in protecting against electroshock seizures and, to a lesser extent, against pentylenetetrazol-induced seizures in laboratory animals.

Adverse Reactions

Cardiovascular: Hypotension, bradycardia, cardiac arrhythmias, cardiovascular collapse

Central nervous system: Drowsiness, drowsiness, slurred speech, dizziness, confusion, mood changes, fever, ataxia

Dermatologic: Rash

Gastrointestinal: Nausea, diarrhea, vomiting, gum tenderness, gingival hyperplasia

Hematologic: Blood dyscrasias

Local: Venous irritation and pain, thrombophlebitis

Neuromuscular & skeletal: Paresthesia

Ocular: Diplopia, photophobia,nystagmus, blurred vision

Miscellaneous: Lymphadenopathy, lupus erythematosus-like syndrome

Signs & Symptoms of Acute Overdose Ataxia, hypotension, numbness, gingival hyperplasia, insomnia, diplopia, bradycardia, anemia (megaloblastic), coma, systemic lupus erythematosus (SLE)

Toxicodynamics/Kinetics

Absorption: Rapidly although the extent of oral absorption is unknown

Metabolism: Exhibits saturable metabolism relative to the formation of n-diethyl and *p*-hydroxylethotoin which are the major metabolites

Half-life: 3-9 hours with low plasma levels (<8 μg/mL); average: ~5 hours; above this concentration, the half-life may be prolonged because of the nonlinear kinetics

Usual Dosage Oral:

Children: 30-60 mg/kg/day or 250 mg twice daily, may be increased up to 2-3 g/day

Adults: 250 mg 4 times/day after meals, may be increased up to 3 g/day in divided doses 4 times/day

Contraindications Hepatic abnormalities, hematologic disorders, known hypersensitivity to ethotoin

Dosage Forms Tablet: 250 mg, 500 mg

Reference Range Although the therapeutic range is poorly documented, most reports indicate that therapeutic plasma concentrations fall between 15-50 μg/mL

Overdosage Treatment

Decontamination: Lavage/activated charcoal with cathartic

Supportive: Bradycardia may be treated with atropine; benzodiazepine or phenobarbital for seizures

Enhancement of elimination: Multiple dosing of activated charcoal may be useful

Test Interactions Increases alkaline phosphatase (S); decreases calcium (S)

Drug Interactions Extreme paranoid symptoms have developed in patients receiving ethotoin and phenacemide concurrently

Pregnancy Risk Factor D

2-ethyl-2-methylsuccinmide *see* Ethosuximide *on page 333*

Ethyl Alcohol (al' koe hol, eth' il)

Related Information

Drugs and Chemicals Proven to be Teratogenic in Humans *on page 1572-1575*

CAS Number 64-17-5

UN Number 1170

Brand Names AHD 2000®; Lavacol® [OTC]

Synonyms Alcohol, Ethyl; Cologne Spirit; Ethanol; EtOH; Potato Alcohol; Spirits of Wine

Use Topical anti-infective; pharmaceutical aid; as an antidote for ethylene glycol overdose; as antidote for methanol overdose; may also be useful in propylene glycol

Mechanism of Action Central nervous system depressant

Adverse Reactions

Cardiovascular: Tachycardia, hypertension, atrial fibrillation
Central nervous system: Ataxia, dementia, Wenicke-Korsakoff syndrome
Gastrointestinal: Nausea, diarrhea, dyspepsia, vomiting, gastrointestinal hemorrhage, anorexia, pancreatitis
Hematologic: Porphyria
Hepatic: Hepatic cirrhosis, fatty degeneration of liver
Neuromuscular & skeletal: Dysarthria, peripheral neuropathy
Miscellaneous: Impaired judgment

Signs & Symptoms of Acute Overdose Atrial tachycardia, chorea (extrapyramidal), cardiomyopathy, tremors, thrombocytopenia, myocardial depression, impotence, acetone breath, dementia, depression, sedation, encephalopathy, leukocytosis, myopathy, hypocalcemia, hyporeflexia, hypophosphatemia, hyperuricemia, optic neuropathy, dysphagia, seizures, myoclonus, diplopia, apnea, lymphopenia, hyperventilation, numbness, respiratory depression, CNS depression, acidosis, hypokalemia, paresthesia, hypomagnesemia, hypothermia, hypoglycemia, gynecomastia, rhabdomyolysis, myoglobinuria, hyponatremia, fever, hypotension, methemoglobinemia, mydriasis, nystagmus, porphyria, ototoxicity; tinnitus

Toxicodynamics/Kinetics

Distribution: V_d: 0.6 L/kg
Metabolism: Hepatic to acetaldehyde by alcohol dehydrogenase at a rate of 10-30 mg/dL/hour

Usual Dosage I.V. doses of 100-125 mg/kg/hour to maintain blood levels of 100 mg/dL are recommended after a loading dose of 0.6 g/kg; maximum dose: 400 mL of a 5% solution within 1 hour

Administration Caution must be taken to avoid extravasation; administer only by slow I.V. infusion

Contraindications Patients with epilepsy

Warnings Administer only by slow I.V. infusion

Dosage Forms

Injection, absolute: 2 mL
Liquid, topical, denatured: 70% (473 mL)
Solution, inhalation: 20%, 40%

Reference Range Levels >100 mg/dL can cause nausea and vomiting; levels >300 mg/dL can be associated with coma and fatalities

Overdosage Treatment

Decontamination: Lavage within 2 hours/activated charcoal with cathartic
Supportive therapy: Flumazenil (2-5 mg) or naloxone may alleviate respiratory depression but not CNS depression; there is conflicting data regarding these two agents; crystalloid infusion for hypotension; monitor glucose; thiamine (50-100 mg) should also be given; monitor magnesium level; for rate control of atrial fibrillation, digoxin or intravenous diltiazem can be used
Enhancement of elimination: Hemodialysis removes 50% to 100%

Antidote(s)

Flumazenil *on page 1428*

Test Interactions Increases ammonia (B), creatine phosphokinase [CPK] (S); decreases glucose, magnesium; serum osmolarity gap increases an average of 20 for every 100 mg/dL of ethanol

Diagnostic Tests/Procedures

Alcohol, Blood
Alcohol, Semiquantitative, Urine *on page 1182*

Drug Interactions Chloral hydrate, disulfiram, guanethidine, methotrexate, metronidazole, nitroglycerin, phenytoin, CNS depressants enhance effect; may exacerbate acetaminophen toxicity; may increase nifedipine levels; probably no relevant clinical effect with H_2 blockers; disulfiram causes nausea/vomiting and hypotension; increases serum levels of phenytoin; shortens the half lives of tolbutamide, isoniazid, and warfarin; combination of methamphetamine with ethanol can increase heart rate and cardiac work

Pregnancy Risk Factor D (X if used for prolonged periods or in high doses at term)

Pregnancy Implications Causes fetal alcohol syndrome, facial dysmorphias, growth retardation

Additional Information Highest serum level recorded with full recovery: 1510 μg/dL (327.8 mmol/L) in an adult; in an adolescent it is 757 mg/dL; children who ingest a significant amount of alcohol should be monitored hourly for up to 6 hours; elevated serum lactate and lactate dehydrogenase levels may interfere with enzymatic ethanol assays; intravenous dexamethasone (2 mg I.V.) can impair ethyl alcohols ability to stimulate sympathetic nerve discharge and thus suppress alcohol-induced high blood pressure in the acute state

Odor threshold: 10 ppm

TLV-TWA: 1000 ppm

While the reduced risk for coronary heart disease by ethanol appears to be related to elevation of high density lipoprotein (HDL cholesterol) levels, the maximal benefit appears to be at the amount of one drink daily. Hepatic toxicity can occur at lower ethanol amounts in women as opposed to men.

Specific References

Brennan DF, Betzelos S, Reed R, et al, "Ethanol Elimination Rates in an ED Population," *Am J Emerg Med*, 1995, 13:276-80.

Cydulka RH, Eversman G, Sklar D, et al, "Alcoholic Patient: Recognition, Assessment, and Management of Urgent and Life Threatening Emergencies. Part I: Neurological, Cardiac, Pulmonary, and Renal Complications," *Emerg Med Rep*, 1995, 16(16):149-58.

Erstad BL and Cotugno CL, "Management of Alcohol Withdrawal," *Am J Health-Syst Pharm*, 1995, 52:697-709.

Gaziano JM, "Alcohol and Coronary Heart Disease," *BELLE Newsletter*, 1995, 4(1):1-5.

Guerin JM and Friedberg G, "Naloxone and Ethanol Intoxication," *Ann Intern Med*, 1982, 97(6):932.

Henning RJ, Wilson LD, and Glauser JM, "Cocaine Plus Ethanol Is More Cardiotoxic Than Cocaine or Ethanol Alone," *Crit Care Med*, 1994, 22(12):1896-906.

Holford NH, "Clinical Pharmacokinetics of Ethanol," *Clin Pharmacokinet*, 1987, 13(5):273-92.

Johnson RA, Noll EC, and Rodney WM, "Survival After a Serum Ethanol Concentration of 1.5%," *Lancet*, 1982, 2:1394.

Levitt MA, Staffeld Cook LA, Simon BC, et al, "Biochemical Markers of Cerebral Injury in Patients With Minor Head Trauma and Ethanol Intoxication," *Acad Emerg Med*, 1995, 2:675-80.

Linowiecki K, Paloucek F, Donnelly A, et al, "Reversal of Ethanol-Induced Respiratory Depression by Flumazenil," *Vet Hum Toxicol*, 1992, 34(5):417-9.

Maio RF, "Alcohol and Injury in the Emergency Department: Opportunities for Intervention," *Ann Emerg Med*, 1995, 26:221-3.

Mendelson J, Jones RT, Upton R, et al, "Methamphetamine and Ethanol Interactions in Humans," *Clin Pharmacol Ther*, 1995, 57:559-68.

Morgan DL, Durso MH, Rich BK, et al, "Severe Ethanol Intoxication in an Adolescent," *Am J Emerg Med*, 1995, 13:416-8.

Nine JS, Moraca M, Virji MA, et al, "Serum-Ethanol Determination: Comparison of Lactate and Lactate Dehydrogenase Interference in Three Enzymatic Assays," *J Anal Toxicol*, 1995, 19:192-6.

Pirwitz MJ, Willard JE, Landau C, et al, "Influence of Cocaine, Ethanol, or Their Combination on Epicardial Coronary Arterial Dimensions in Humans," *Arch Intern Med*, 1995, 155:1186-91.

Randin D, Vollenweider P, Tappy L, et al, "Suppression of Alcohol-Induced Hypertension by Dexamethasone," *N Engl J Med*, 1995, 332:1733-7.

Reily ME, Preedy VR, and Peters TJ, "Investigations Into the Toxic Effects of Alcohol on Skeletal Muscle," *Adverse Drug React Toxicol Rev*, 1995, 14(2):117-50.

Sucov A and Woolard RH, "Ethanol-Associated Hypoglycemia Is Uncommon," *Acad Emerg Med*, 1995, 2:185-9.

Vogel C, Caraccio T, Mofensen H, et al, "Alcohol Intoxication in Young Children," *J Toxicol Clin Toxicol*, 1995, 33(1):25-33.

Ethyl Aminobenzoate *see* Benzocaine *on page 149*

Ethyl Chloride (eth' il klor' ide)

CAS Number 75-00-3

UN Number 1037

Brand Names Cloretilo Chemirosa®; Cloretilo Vitulia®; WariActiv®

Synonyms Anodyon; Chlorethyl; Chloroethane; Kelene; Monochloroethane

Use Local anesthetic in minor operative procedures and to relieve pain caused by insect stings and burns and irritation caused by myofascial and visceral pain syndromes

Mechanism of Action Results in tissue hypothermia (-10°C) when used topically

Adverse Reactions Mucous membrane irritation

Signs & Symptoms of Acute Overdose Prolonged spraying may cause frostbite; laryngospasm, coma, respiratory, cardiac arrest when taken systemically

Toxicodynamics/Kinetics

Absorption: Readily through lungs

Half-life: 1-3 minutes (when taken systemically)

Elimination: Through lungs

Usual Dosage Dosage varies with use

Administration Spray for a few seconds to the point of frost formation when the tissue becomes white; avoid prolonged spraying of skin beyond this point; avoid broken skin or mucous membranes

(Continued)

Ethyl Chloride *(Continued)*

Contraindications Use near eyes or unbroken skin or mucous membranes, avoid repeated use over long periods

Warnings For external use only; ethyl chloride is highly flammable and explosive. Although it usually produces incomplete relaxation, it can induce laryngospasm, narcosis, cardiac depression, and even coma; because of its vapocoolant activity, excessive use may cause frostbite; inhalation of ethyl chloride should be avoided

Dosage Forms Spray: 100 mL, 120 mL

Stability Refrigerate; store in airtight containers preferably hermetically sealed at a temperature not exceeding 15°C; protect from light

Reference Range Serum ethyl chloride level of 200 mg/L associated with fatality following recreational use

Overdosage Treatment

Decontamination: Irrigate exposed areas with soap and water

Enhancement of elimination: Inhalation: 100% high humidity oxygen should be given

Pregnancy Risk Factor C

Additional Information Spray for a few seconds to the point of frost formation when the tissue becomes white; avoid prolonged spraying of skin beyond this point; highly flammable/air concentrations >5% may be explosive

TLV-TWA: 1000 ppm

IDLH: 20,000 ppm

PEL-TWA: 100 ppm

Specific References

Aberer W, "Local Anaesthesia With Ethyl Chloride Freezing: Problems Despite Proper Application," *Br J Dermatol*, 1991, 124(1):113-4.

Yacoub I, Robinson CA, Simmons GT, et al, "Death Attributed to Ethyl Chloride," *J Anal Toxicol*, 1993, 17(6):384-5.

Ethylphenylhydantoin *see* Ethotoin *on page 335*

Etidron® *see* Etidronate Disodium *on this page*

Etidronate Disodium (e ti droe' nate)

Related Information

Alendronate *on page 94*

CAS Number 7414-83-7; 2809-21-4

Brand Names Didronate®; Didronel®; Difosfen®; Diphos®; Etidron®; Osteum®

Use Symptomatic treatment of Paget's disease and heterotopic ossification due to spinal cord injury or after total hip replacement, hypercalcemia associated with malignancy

Mechanism of Action Decreases bone resorption by inhibiting osteocystic osteolysis; decreases mineral release and matrix or collagen breakdown in bone

Adverse Reactions

Endocrine & metabolic: Hyperphosphatemia, hypocalcemia

Gastrointestinal: Diarrhea, nausea, vomiting

Hematologic: Occult blood in stools

Neuromuscular & skeletal: Risk of fractures (increased), microfractures, increased bone pain, dose-related osteomalacia

Renal: Nephrotoxicity

Miscellaneous: Altered taste, hypersensitivity reactions

Signs & Symptoms of Acute Overdose Diarrhea, nausea, hypocalcemia

Toxicodynamics/Kinetics

Absorption: Is dependent upon dose administered; decreased oral absorption with calcium-rich foods

Distribution: ~½ absorbed dose is chemically absorbed to bone, presumably upon hydroxyapatite crystals, in areas of elevated osteogenesis

Metabolism: Not metabolized

Half-life: 5-7 hours in plasma; 90 days in bone

Elimination: Excreted as unchanged drug primarily in the urine with unabsorbed drug being eliminated in the feces

Onset of therapeutic effects: Within 1-3 months of therapy

Duration: 12 months without continuous therapy

Onset of action:

- Paget's disease: May be observed after 1 month of treatment; initially observed as a reduction in urinary hydroxyproline
- Hypercalcemia: Reductions in urinary calcium excretion which accompany reductions in bone resorption; may become apparent after 24 hours

Duration of action: Cleared from blood in 6 hours

Usual Dosage Adults:

Paget's disease: Oral: 5 mg/kg/day given every day for no more than 6 months; may give 10 mg/kg/day for up to 3 months; daily dose may be divided if adverse gastrointestinal effects occur

Heterotopic ossification with spinal cord injury: 20 mg/kg/day for 2 weeks, then 10 mg/kg/day for 10 weeks (This dosage has been used in children, however, treatment greater than 1 year has been associated with a rachitic syndrome)

Hypercalcemia associated with malignancy:

I.V. (Dilute dose in at least 250 mL NS): 7.5 mg/kg/day for 3 days; there should be at least 7 days between courses of treatment

Oral: Start 20 mg/kg/day on the last day of infusion and continue for 30-90 days

Dosing adjustment in renal impairment:

S_{cr} 2.5-5 mg/dL: Use with caution

S_{cr} >5 mg/dL: Do not use

Contraindications Patients with serum creatinine >5 mg/dL

Warnings I.V. form may be nephrotoxic and should be used with caution, if at all, and probably in reduced dosage in patients with impaired renal function (serum creatinine: 2.5-4.9 mg/dL); use with caution in patients with restricted calcium and vitamin D intake; dosage modification required in renal impairment

Dosage Forms

Injection: 50 mg/mL (6 mL)

Tablet: 200 mg, 400 mg

Stability Dilute I.V. dose in at least 250 mL NS; stable for 48 hours at room temperature or refrigerated

Reference Range Calcium (total): Adults: 9.0-11.0 mg/dL

Overdosage Treatment

Supportive therapy: Intravenous hydration; monitor urine flow and calcium and phosphorus level

Pregnancy Risk Factor B (oral)/C (parenteral)

Monitoring Parameters Serum calcium and phosphorous; serum creatinine and BUN

Patient Information Maintain adequate intake of calcium and vitamin D; take medicine on an empty stomach

Nursing Implications Dilute I.V. dose in at least 250 mL NS, ensure adequate hydration; dosage modification required in renal insufficiency

Specific References

Gray RE, "Severe Reaction to Diphosphonate," *BMJ*, 1988, 297(6655):1042.

Watts NB, Harris ST, Genant HK, et al, "Intermittent Cyclical Etidronate Treatment of Postmenopausal Osteoporosis," *N Engl J Med*, 1990, 323(2):73-9.

Etiocidan® *see* Ethionamide *on page 333*

Etodolac (ee toe doe' lak)

Related Information

Nonsteroidal Anti-Inflammatory Comparison *on page 1655*

CAS Number 41340-25-4

Brand Names Lodine®

Use Acute and long-term use in the management of signs and symptoms of osteoarthritis and management of pain

Mechanism of Action Inhibits prostaglandin synthesis by decreasing the activity of the enzyme, cyclo-oxygenase, which results in decreased formation of prostaglandin precursors

Adverse Reactions

Cardiovascular: Fluid retention, circulatory collapse

Central nervous system: Headache, aseptic meningitis, psychosis, cognitive dysfunction, coma, seizures

Dermatologic: Rash, pruritus

Endocrine & metabolic: Hyperkalemia, anion gap metabolic acidosis

Gastrointestinal: Abdominal pain, nausea, vomiting, bleeding, ulceration, constipation, diarrhea, dyspepsia

Genitourinary: Albuminuria

Hematologic: Leukopenia, neutropenia, agranulocytosis, granulocytopenia; aplastic anemia (rare), platelet inhibition

Hepatic: Elevation of transaminases, fulminant hepatitis

Otic: Ototoxicity; tinnitus, deafness

Renal: Renal failure (acute), nephrotic syndrome, chronic renal failure

Respiratory: Wheezing, respiratory depression

Miscellaneous: Hypersensitivity

Signs & Symptoms of Acute Overdose Nausea, flatulence, wheezing, vomiting, dysuria, hematuria, cognitive dysfunction, conjunctivitis, gastrointestinal bleeding, gastritis; nephrotic syndrome, ototoxicity, tinnitus, drowsiness; severe poisoning can manifest with coma, seizures, renal failure and or hepatic failure, hypotension, respiratory depression, leukocytes

Toxicodynamics/Kinetics

Absorption: Oral: Well absorbed

(Continued)

Etodolac *(Continued)*

Distribution: V_d: 0.4 L/kg
Protein binding: Highly protein bound
Half-life: 7 hours
Time to peak serum concentration: Within 1 hour

Usual Dosage Single dose of 76-100 mg is comparable to the analgesic effect of aspirin 650 mg; in patients ≥65 years, no substantial differences in the pharmacokinetics or side-effects profile were seen compared with the general population

Adults: Oral:
Acute pain: 200-400 mg every 6-8 hours, as needed, not to exceed total daily doses of 1200 mg; for patients weighing <60 kg, total daily dose should not exceed 20 mg/kg/day
Osteoarthritis: Initial: 800-1200 mg/day given in divided doses: 400 mg 2 or 3 times/day; 300 mg 2, 3 or 4 times/day; 200 mg 3 or 4 times/day; total daily dose should not exceed 1200 mg; for patients weighing <60 kg, total daily dose should not exceed 20 mg/kg/day

Contraindications Hypersensitivity to etodolac, aspirin or other NSAIDs

Warnings Risk of gastrointestinal ulceration, bleeding, and perforation with therapy

Dosage Forms Capsule: 200 mg, 300 mg

Reference Range After a 200 mg oral dose, peak plasma levels are ~12-16 mg/L; after a 400 mg oral dose, peak plasma level is ~21 mg/L

Overdosage Treatment

Decontamination: Ipecac or lavage/activated charcoal with cathartic
Supportive therapy: Hypotension/dehydration can be managed with intravenous fluid therapy; acidosis should be treated with bicarbonates, seizures with benzodiazepines; antacids, blood products are indicated, as appropriate, for hemorrhage
Enhancement of elimination: Dialysis or perfusion is indicated for secondary complications, acidosis, or renal failure and not toxin removal alone; multiple dosing of activated charcoal may be useful

Test Interactions False-positive for urinary bilirubin and ketone

Drug Interactions Aspirin decreases serum concentrations probably by protein-binding displacement; there is an increased bleeding potential with concomitant warfarin therapy; may increase lithium and methotrexate concentrations by decreasing renal clearance; may decrease diuretic and hypotensive effects of thiazides, loop diuretics, ACE inhibitors, and beta-blockers; may increase nephrotoxicity of cyclosporine

Pregnancy Risk Factor C

Monitoring Parameters Monitor CBC, liver enzymes, PT, PTT; monitor urine output and BUN/serum creatinine in patients receiving diuretics

Nursing Implications Do not crush tablets

Specific References

Boldy DA, Hale KA, and Vale JA, "Etodolac Overdose," *Hum Toxicol*, 1988, 7(2):203-4.
Court H and Volans GN, "Poisoning After Overdose With Nonsteroidal Anti-inflammatory Drugs," *Adverse Drug React Acute Poisoning Rev*, 1984, 3(1):1-21.
Hoppmann RA, Peden JG, and Ober SK, "Central Nervous System Side Effects of Nonsteroidal Anti-inflammatory Drugs. Aseptic Meningitis, Psychosis, and Cognitive Dysfunction," *Arch Intern Med*, 1991, 151(7):1309-13.
Mabee CL, Mabee SW, Baker PB, et al, "Fulminant Hepatic Failure Associated With Etodolac Use," *Am J Gastroenterol*, 1995, 90:659-61.
Smolinske SC, Hall AH, Vandenberg SA, et al, "Toxic Effects of Nonsteroid Anti-inflammatory Drugs in Overdose. An Overview of Recent Evidence on Clinical Effects and Dose-Response Relationships," *Drug Saf*, 1990, 5(4):252-74.
Vale JA and Meredith TJ, "Acute Poisoning Due to Nonsteroidal Anti-inflammatory Drugs," *Med Toxicol*, 1986, 1(1):12-31.
Verbeeck RK, "Pharmacokinetic Drug Interactions With Nonsteroidal Anti-inflammatory Drugs," *Clin Pharmacokinet*, 1990, 19(1):44-66.

EtOH *see* Ethyl Alcohol *on page 336*

Etrafon® *see* Amitriptyline and Perphenazine *on page 115*

Eudemine® *see* Diazoxide *on page 273*

Euflex® *see* Flutamide *on page 366*

Eukodal® *see* Oxycodone Hydrochloride *on page 585*

Eulexin® *see* Flutamide *on page 366*

Eulexine® *see* Flutamide *on page 366*

Eupasal® *see* Para-Aminosalicylate Sodium *on page 592*

Euphypnos® *see* Temazepam *on page 724*

Eupressyl® *see* Urapidil Hydrochloride *on page 778*

Euradal® *see* Bisoprolol Fumarate *on page 157*

Eurodin® *see* Estazolam *on page 324*

Euthroid® *see* Liotrix *on page 473*

Euthyrox® *see* Levothyroxine Sodium *on page 465*

Evac-U-Gen® [OTC] *see* Phenolphthalein *on page 617*

Evac-U-Lax® [OTC] *see* Phenolphthalein *on page 617*

Everone® Injection *see* Testosterone *on page 729*

E-Vimin® *see* Vitamin E *on page 798*

Evion® *see* Vitamin E *on page 798*

E-Vista® *see* Hydroxyzine *on page 414*

Excedrin®, Extra Strength [OTC] *see* Acetaminophen and Aspirin *on page 83*

Excedrin® IB [OTC] *see* Ibuprofen *on page 418*

Exhirud® *see* Hirudin *on page 404*

Exidine® Scrub [OTC] *see* Chlorhexidine Gluconate *on page 200*

Ex-Lax® [OTC] *see* Phenolphthalein *on page 617*

EXP-126 *see* Rimantadine Hydrochloride *on page 685*

Ezide® *see* Hydrochlorothiazide *on page 406*

Famciclovir (fam sye' kloe veer)

CAS Number 104227-87-4

Brand Names Famvir™

Use Management of acute herpes zoster (shingles)

Mechanism of Action Guanine derivative which inhibits viral DNA synthesis and replication through conversion to penciclovir in a similar manner as acyclovir

Adverse Reactions

Central nervous system: Headache, fatigue, fever, dizziness, somnolence

Gastrointestinal: Nausea, diarrhea, vomiting, constipation, anorexia, abdominal pain, pancreatitis

Neuromuscular & skeletal: Rigors, paresthesia

Toxicodynamics/Kinetics

Metabolism: Hepatic to penciclovir (active metabolite)

Bioavailability: 72% to 83%

Half-life: 2-3 hours

Elimination: Renal 73%, feces 27%

Usual Dosage Adult: Oral: 500 mg every 8 hours for 7 days

Contraindications Hypersensitivity to famciclovir

Dosage Forms Tablet: 500 mg

Overdosage Treatment

Decontamination: Ipecac or lavage/activated charcoal with cathartic

Supportive therapy: Renal toxicity and crystalluria can be managed with intravenous fluid hydration

Enhancement of elimination: Multiple dosing of activated charcoal may be effective; while no studies have been performed, hemodialysis would appear to be an effective modality for drug removal

Pregnancy Risk Factor B

Additional Information Most effective if therapy is initiated within 72 hours of initial lesion

Specific References

Boyd MR, Safrin S, and Kern ER, "Penciclovir: A Review of Its Spectrum of Activity, Selectivity, and Cross Resistance Pattern," *Antiviral Chem Chemother*, 1993, 4:3-11.

Daniels S and Schentagg JJ, "Drug Interaction Studies and Safety of Famciclovir in Healthy Volunteers: A Review." *Antiviral Chem Chemother*, 1993, 4:57-64.

De Clercq E, "Antivirals for the Treatment of Herpesvirus Infections," *J Antimicrob Chemother*, 1993, 32(Suppl A):121-32.

Goffin E, Horsmans Y, Pirson Y, et al, "Acute Necrotico-Hemorrhagic Pancreatitis After Famciclovir Prescription," *Transplantation*, 1995, 59:1218-9.

Hodge RA, "Famciclovir and Penciclovir: The Mode of Action of Famciclovir Including Its Conversion to Penciclovir," *Antiviral Chem Chemother*, 1993, 4:67-84.

Famodil® *see* Famotidine *on this page*

Famotidine (fa moe' ti deen)

CAS Number 76824-35-6

Brand Names Famodil®; Gaster®; Pepcid®; Pepcidine®; Pepdul®; Pepdulmite®

Use Therapy and treatment of duodenal ulcer, gastric ulcer, control gastric pH in critically ill patients, symptomatic relief in gastritis, gastroesophageal reflux, active benign ulcer, and pathological hypersecretory conditions

Mechanism of Action Competitive inhibition of histamine at H_2-receptors of the gastric parietal cells, which inhibits gastric acid secretion

(Continued)

Famotidine *(Continued)*

Adverse Reactions

Cardiovascular: Palpitations, hypertension, bradycardia, second degree A-V block
Central nervous system: Dizziness, asthenia, fatigue, seizures, insomnia, drowsiness, confusion, psychosis, headache (throbbing), fever
Dermatologic: Acne, pruritus, rash, dry skin
Gastrointestinal: Constipation, diarrhea, abdominal discomfort, flatulence, belching, anorexia
Hematologic: Thrombocytopenia
Hepatic: AST (increased), ALT (increased)
Neuromuscular & skeletal: Pain, paresthesia
Renal: Proteinuria, increased BUN and creatinine

Signs & Symptoms of Acute Overdose Hypotension, tachycardia, neutropenia, depression, dry skin, insomnia, impotence, seizures, A-V block, vomiting, CNS depression, confusion

Toxicodynamics/Kinetics

Onset of action: Gastrointestinal effects can be observed within 60 minutes following oral administration
Duration: 10-12 hours
Distribution: V_d: 1.1-1.4 L/kg; many body tissues
Protein binding: 15% to 20%
Metabolism: ~30% to 35% by the liver
Bioavailability: Oral: 40% to 50%
Half-life: 2.5-3.5 hours (increases with renal impairment; oliguric half-life: 20 hours)
Time to peak serum concentration: 1-3 hours
Elimination: Excreted as unchanged drug in urine

Usual Dosage

Children: Oral, I.V.: Doses of 1-2 mg/kg/day have been used; maximum dose: 40 mg

Adults:
- Oral:
  - Duodenal ulcer, gastric ulcer: 40 mg/day at bedtime for 4-8 weeks
  - Hypersecretory conditions: Initial: 20 mg every 6 hours, may increase up to 160 mg every 6 hours
  - GERD: 20 mg twice daily for 6 weeks
- I.V.: 20 mg every 12 hours

Dosing adjustment in renal impairment:

Cl_{cr} 30-50 mL/minute: Administer every 24 hours or 50% of dose
Cl_{cr} <30 mL/minute: Administer every 36-48 hours or 25% of dose

Contraindications Hypersensitivity to famotidine or other H_2 antagonist

Warnings Reduce dosage in decreased renal function

Dosage Forms

Infusion, premixed in NS: 20 mg (50 mL)
Injection: 10 mg/mL (2 mL, 4 mL)
Powder for oral suspension (cherry-banana-mint flavor): 40 mg/5 mL (50 mL)
Tablet, film coated: 20 mg, 40 mg

Stability Reconstituted I.V. solution is stable for 48 hours at room temperature; I.V. infusion in NS or D_5W solution is stable for 48 hours at room temperature; reconstituted oral solution is stable for 30 days at room temperature

Reference Range Serum level of 13 ng/mL will produce 50% inhibition of gastric acid secretion

Overdosage Treatment

Decontamination: Lavage/activated charcoal with cathartic
Supportive therapy: Treatment is primarily symptomatic and supportive
Enhancement of elimination: Hemodialysis may be useful, four- to sixfold increase in clearance

Drug Interactions Chlorpromazine absorption decreases

Pregnancy Risk Factor B

Pregnancy Implications Distributes into breast milk

Monitoring Parameters EKG, CBC, electrolytes

Nursing Implications Injection must be diluted prior to administration to a concentration of 20 mg/mL; reduce dosage in decreased renal function

Additional Information The expensive parenteral route should only be used when a patient is unable to take oral medication; less antiandrogenic than cimetidine; over-the-counter preparation marketed as Pepcid AC®

Specific References

Ahmad S, "Famotidine and Cardiac Arrhythmia," *DICP*, 1991, 25(3):315.

Gottlieb S, Decktor DL, Eckert JM, et al, "Efficacy and Tolerability of Famotidine in Preventing Heartburn and Related Symptoms of Upper Gastrointestinal Discomfort," *Am J Ther*, 1995, 2:314-9.

Inotsume N, Mishimura M, Nakano M, et al, "Removal of Famotidine by Haemodialysis in Elderly Anuric Patients," *Eur J Clin Pharmacol*, 1990, 38(3):313-4.

Simon TJ, Berlin RG, Gardner AH, et al, "Self-Directed Treatment of Intermittent Heartburn: A Randomized, Multicenter, Double-Blind, Placebo-Controlled Evaluation of Antacid and Low Doses of an H_2-Receptor Antagonist (Famotidine)," *Am J Ther*, 1995, 2:304-13.

Famvir™ *see* Famciclovir *on page 341*

Fanaxal® *see* Alfentanil Hydrochloride *on page 94*

Fargan *see* Promethazine Hydrochloride *on page 650*

Faril® *see* Nalidixic Acid *on page 547*

Farmadiuril® *see* Bumetanide *on page 167*

Fase® *see* Aprotinin *on page 130*

Fastin® *see* Phentermine Hydrochloride *on page 619*

Favistan® *see* Methimazole *on page 512*

Fedrine® *see* Ephedrine Sulfate *on page 316*

Feen-a-Mint® [OTC] *see* Phenolphthalein *on page 617*

Feldene® *see* Piroxicam *on page 631*

Felobits® *see* Atenolol *on page 137*

Felodipine (fe loe' di peen)

Related Information

Calcium Channel Blocking Agents Comparison *on page 1646-1647*

CAS Number 72509-76-3; 86189-69-7

Brand Names Agon®; Hydac®; Munobal®; Plendil®

Use Treatment of hypertension, also has been used in angina

Mechanism of Action Dihydropyridine calcium channel blocking agent similar to nifedipine; predominantly vasodilitary actions

Adverse Reactions

Cardiovascular: Peripheral edema, flushing, tachycardia

Central nervous system: Headache, dizziness, asthenia, insomnia, night terrors

Dermatologic: Urticaria, eczema

Gastrointestinal: Vomiting, dry mouth, flatulence, gingival hyperplasia, constipation

Respiratory: Cough

Signs & Symptoms of Acute Overdose Bradycardia, hypotension

Toxicodynamics/Kinetics

Distribution: V_d: 10 L/kg (normal patients); 5.6 L/kg (cirrhosis)

Protein binding: >99%

Metabolism: >99% in liver

Bioavailability: 15%

Half-life:

- Normal patients: 10-16 hours
- Renal failure: 2 hours

Elimination: Renal (70%), feces (30%)

Usual Dosage Oral: Initial: 5 mg once daily; may increase dose up to a maximum of 10 mg once daily; dosage range: 2.5-10 mg; starting dose recommended for elderly: 2.5 mg

Contraindications Hypersensitivity to felodipine, hypotension, and advanced aortic stenosis

Warnings Reduce dose in elderly, hepatic disease

Dosage Forms Tablet, extended release: 2.5 mg, 5 mg, 10 mg

Reference Range Therapeutic plasma level: 5-10 nmol/L; toxic: >30 nmol/L

Overdosage Treatment

Decontamination: Ipecac-induced emesis can hypothetically worsen calcium antagonist toxicity, since it can produce vagal stimulation. The potential for seizures precipitously following acute ingestion of large doses of a calcium antagonist may also contraindicate the use of ipecac. Lavage/activated charcoal with cathartic is useful. Whole bowel irrigation for sustained release preparations.

Supportive therapy: I.V. fluids and Trendelenburg positioning should be initiated as intoxication may cause hypotension. Calcium (calcium chloride I.V. 1-2 g in adults or 10-30 mg/kg in children over 5-10 minutes with repeats as needed) has been used as an "antidote" for acute intoxications, although its effectiveness is questionable in nifedipine overdose. Heart block may respond to isoproterenol, glucagon, atropine and/or calcium, although a temporary pacemaker may be required. Amrinone or dopamine may be required for hypotension. Glucagon may increase myocardial contractility.

Enhancement of elimination: Multiple dosing of activated charcoal is useful; ~9% of the parent drug can be removed by hemodialysis

Test Interactions May cause an increase in serum alkaline phosphatase, serum calcium, serum creatinine, serum gamma glutamyl transferase, serum norepinephrine, renin

(Continued)

Felodipine *(Continued)*

Drug Interactions May cause a transient increase in peak concentrations of digoxin; increased felodipine levels noted when given with cimetidine; lowered felodipine levels when administered with phenytoin, carbamazepine, or phenobarbital; increased felodipine toxicity with erythromycin

Pregnancy Risk Factor C

Additional Information Do not crush or chew pills; increased bioavailability when taken with grapefruit juice

Specific References

Buur T, Larsson R, Regardh CG, et al, "Pharmacokinetics of Felodipine in Chronic Hemodialysis Patients," *J Clin Pharmacol*, 1991, 31(8):709-13.

Todd PA and Faulds D, "Felodipine. A Review of the Pharmacology and Therapeutic Use of the Extended Release Formulation in Cardiovascular Disorders," *Drugs*, 1992, 44(2):251-77.

Wade JR and Sambol NC, "Felodipine Population Dose-Response and Concentration-Response Relationships in Patients With Essential Hypertension," *Clin Pharmacol Ther*, 1995, 57:569-81.

Feminone® *see* Ethinyl Estradiol *on page 331*

Femiron® *see* Iron *on page 439*

Femoxetine

CAS Number 59859-58-4

Use Investigational: Antidepressant, narcolepsy, tension headache

Mechanism of Action Selectively inhibits reuptake of serotonin

Adverse Reactions

Cardiovascular: Palpitations
Central nervous system: Nervousness, anxiety, insomnia, dizziness, headache
Dermatologic: Urticaria
Gastrointestinal: Nausea, dry mouth, constipation
Hepatic: Hepatitis
Neuromuscular & skeletal: Tremor
Renal: Dysuria
Respiratory: Nasal congestion
Miscellaneous: Diaphoresis

Toxicodynamics/Kinetics

Metabolism: Hepatic to inactive metabolites
Bioavailability: 5% to 10%
Half-life: ~20 hours
Elimination: Primarily renal

Usual Dosage

Depression: 300-600 mg in 3 divided doses; start at the lower dose
Narcolepsy: 300 mg twice daily
Tension headache: 100 mg 4 times/day

Dosing adjustment in hepatic impairment: Reduce initial dose to 100 mg/day

Contraindications Hypersensitivity to femoxetine

Warnings Use with caution in patients with previous hypersensitivity to this class of agents, patients with epilepsy, and in patients with hepatic disorders

Reference Range Peak serum levels following a 500-600 mg dose: 120 ng/mL

Overdosage Treatment

Decontamination: Lavage/activated charcoal with cathartic

Supportive therapy: Toxic symptoms should be treated. Ventricular arrhythmias often respond to phenytoin 15-20 mg/kg (adults) with concurrent systemic alkalinization (sodium bicarbonate 0.5-2 mEq/kg I.V.). Lidocaine may also be useful. Arrhythmias unresponsive to this therapy may respond to lidocaine 1 mg/kg I.V. followed by a titrated infusion. Physostigmine (1-2 mg I.V. slowly for adults or 0.5 mg I.V. slowly for children) may be indicated in reversing cardiac arrhythmias that are due to vagal blockade or for anticholinergic effects. Seizures usually respond to lorazepam or diazepam I.V. boluses (5-10 mg for adults up to 30 mg or 0.25-0.4 mg/kg/dose for children up to 10 mg/dose). If seizures are unresponsive or recur, phenytoin or phenobarbital may be required.

Enhancement of elimination: Multiple dosing of activated charcoal may not be useful; hemodialysis does not appear to be useful

Drug Interactions Concomitant administration with cimetidine can result in increased femoxetine levels

Additional Information Does not appear to be as effective as propranolol for migraine prophylaxis

Specific References

Aunsholt NA and Agnholt J, "Toxic Hepatitis Due to Femoxetine," *Acta Pharmacol Toxicol*, 1986, 58(4):253-4.

Schmidt J, Sorensen AS, Gjerris A, et al, "Femoxetine and Cimetidine: Interaction in Healthy Volunteers," *Eur J Clin Pharmacol*, 1986, 31(3):299-302.

Fenamon® *see* Nifedipine *on page 558*

Fenesin™ [OTC] *see* Guaifenesin *on page 390*

Fenfluramine (fen flure' a meen)

CAS Number 458-24-2

Brand Names Pondimin®

Use Anorectic agent

Signs & Symptoms of Acute Overdose Rapid onset of symptoms with relative short time between ingestion and death with a lack of response to normal supportive measures; tachycardia, mydriasis, seizures, occur within 30 minutes to 3½ hours postingestion; severe respiratory and/or cardiovascular complications occur within the first 4 hours; symptoms may last 2-3 days; arrhythmias reported are tachycardia, extrasystoles, asystole, and fibrillation (ventricular); facial flushing, sweating, night terrors, shivering, and hyperventilation have been reported; neurologic changes include tremors, nystagmus, seizures, ataxia, dementia, depression, diplopia, agitation, hypertension, impotence, hyperthermia, confusion, hyperreflexia, clonus, coma, hallucination, and psychosis

Toxicodynamics/Kinetics

Duration of action: 4-6 hours

Absorption: Rapid in gastrointestinal tract

Metabolism: Mainly in liver to N-triclyoromethylhippuric acid (66% to 92%); norfenfluramine (2% to 22%)

Time to peak: Within 1-2 hours

Elimination: Both parent and metabolite excreted in urine

Usual Dosage

Children: 1.5 mg/kg/day

Adults: 20 mg 3 times/day to a maximum of 40 mg 3 times/day

Minimum: <200 mg to 28.7 mg/kg

Maximum: <200 mg to 1600 mg

Symptoms usually at 4.6-6.2 mg/kg

Dosage Forms Tablet: 20 mg

Overdosage Treatment

Decontamination: No emesis, lavage/activated charcoal

Supportive therapy: Treatment of symptoms

Enhancement of elimination: Dialysis may help if renal function is impaired

Drug Interactions General anesthesia with halothane may have produced a fatal cardiac arrest in a patient taking fenfluramine; fenfluramine may potentiate effects of insulin causing hypoglycemia; this may be delayed in onset

Monitoring Parameters Fenfluramine in blood and urine within 1-2 hours postingestion

Specific References

Fleisher MR and Campbell DB, "Fenfluramine Overdosage," *Lancet*, 1969, 2(633):1306-7.

Melandri R, Re G, Morigi A, et al, "Whole Bowel Irrigation After Delayed Release Fenfluramine Overdose," *J Toxicol Clin Toxicol*, 1995, 33(2):161-3.

Veltri S and Temple AR, "Fenfluramine Poisoning," *J Pediatr*, 1975, 87(1):119-21.

Fenilcal® *see* Phenobarbital *on page 614*

Fenitoina *see* Phenytoin *on page 623*

Fenopraine *see* Propafenone Hydrochloride *on page 652*

Fenoprofen Calcium (fen oh proe' fen)

Related Information

Nonsteroidal Anti-Inflammatory Comparison *on page 1655*

CAS Number 53746-45-5

Brand Names Nalfon®

Use Symptomatic treatment of acute and chronic rheumatoid arthritis and osteoarthritis; relief of mild to moderate pain

Mechanism of Action Inhibits prostaglandin synthesis by decreasing the activity of the enzyme, cyclo-oxygenase, which results in decreased formation of prostaglandin precursors; proprionic acid derivative (like ibuprofen)

Adverse Reactions

Cardiovascular: Fluid retention, circulatory collapse

Central nervous system: Headache, aseptic meningitis, psychosis, cognitive dysfunction, coma, seizures

Dermatologic: Rash, pruritus

Endocrine & metabolic: Hyperkalemia, anion gap metabolic acidosis

Gastrointestinal: Abdominal pain, nausea, vomiting, bleeding, ulceration, constipation, diarrhea, dyspepsia

Genitourinary: Albuminuria

Hematologic: Leukopenia, neutropenia, agranulocytosis, granulocytopenia; aplastic anemia (rare), platelet inhibition

Hepatic: Elevation of transaminases, fulminant hepatitis

Ocular: Diplopia

(Continued)

Fenoprofen Calcium *(Continued)*

Otic: Ototoxicity, tinnitus
Renal: Renal failure (acute), nephrotic syndrome, chronic renal failure
Respiratory: Wheezing, respiratory depression
Miscellaneous: Hypersensitivity, feces discoloration (black)

Signs & Symptoms of Acute Overdose Nausea, vomiting, azotemia, wheezing, nephrotic syndrome, erythema multiforme, gastrointestinal bleeding, gastritis; cognitive dysfunction, coagulopathy, ototoxicity, tinnitus, drowsiness; severe poisoning can manifest with coma, seizures, renal failure and or hepatic failure, hypotension, respiratory depression, tachycardia, leukopenia, neutropenia, agranulocytosis, granulocytopenia, hypothermia

Toxicodynamics/Kinetics

Onset of action: Within 15-30 minutes
Duration: ~4-6 hours
Absorption: Rapid (to 80%) from upper gastrointestinal tract
Distribution: V_d: ~0.1 L/kg
Protein binding: 99%
Metabolism: Extensive in the liver
Half-life: 2.5-3 hours
Time to peak serum concentration: Within 2 hours
Elimination: Excretion in urine 2% to 5% as unchanged drug; small amounts appear in feces

Usual Dosage Adults: Oral:

Rheumatoid arthritis: 300-600 mg 3-4 times/day up to 3.2 g/day
Mild to moderate pain: 200 mg every 4-6 hours as needed

Contraindications Renal impairment, known hypersensitivity to fenoprofen or other NSAIDs

Warnings Use with caution in patients with congestive heart failure, hypertension, decreased renal or hepatic function, history of gastrointestinal disease, or those receiving anticoagulants

Dosage Forms

Capsule: 200 mg, 300 mg, 600 mg
Tablet: 600 mg

Reference Range Therapeutic: 20-65 μg/mL (SI: 82-268 μmol/L), not readily available

Overdosage Treatment

Decontamination: Ipecac or lavage/activated charcoal with cathartic
Supportive therapy: Hypotension/dehydration can be managed with intravenous fluid therapy; acidosis should be treated with bicarbonates, seizures with benzodiazepines; antacids, blood products are indicated, as appropriate, for hemorrhage
Enhancement of elimination: Dialysis or hemoperfusion is indicated for secondary complications, acidosis, or renal failure and not toxin removal alone; multiple dosing of activated charcoal may be useful

Test Interactions Increases chloride (S), sodium (S)

Diagnostic Tests/Procedures

Complete Blood Count *on page 1236*
Electrolytes, Blood *on page 1254*
Electrolytes, Urine *on page 1254*
Urinalysis *on page 1373*

Drug Interactions Aspirin decreases serum concentrations probably by protein-binding displacement of fenoprofen; there is an increased bleeding potential with concomitant warfarin therapy; may increase lithium and methotrexate concentrations by decreasing renal clearance; may decrease diuretic and hypotensive effects of thiazides, loop diuretics, ACE inhibitors, and beta-blockers; may increase nephrotoxicity of cyclosporine

Pregnancy Risk Factor B (D if used in the 3rd trimester or near delivery)

Pregnancy Implications Does not cross the placenta

Monitoring Parameters Monitor CBC, liver enzymes; monitor urine output and BUN/serum creatinine

Additional Information Generally nontoxic ingestions

Specific References

Appleby DH, "Fenoprofen (Nalfon®) Overdose," *Drug Intell Clin Pharm*, 1981, 15(2):129-30.
Court H and Volans GN, "Poisoning After Overdose With Nonsteroidal Anti-inflammatory Drugs," *Adverse Drug React Acute Poisoning Rev*, 1984, 3(1):1-21.
Hoppmann RA, Peden JG, and Ober SK, "Central Nervous System Side Effects of Nonsteroidal Anti-inflammatory Drugs. Aseptic Meningitis, Psychosis, and Cognitive Dysfunction," *Arch Intern Med*, 1991, 151(7):1309-13.
Kolodzik JM, Eilers MA, and Angelos MG, "Nonsteroidal Anti-inflammatory Drugs and Coma: A Case Report of Fenoprofen Overdose," *Ann Emerg Med*, 1990, 19(4):378-81.
Smolinske SC, Hall AH, Vandenberg SA, et al, "Toxic Effects of Nonsteroid Anti-inflammatory Drugs in Overdose. An Overview of Recent Evidence on Clinical Effects and Dose-Response Relationships," *Drug Saf*, 1990, 5(4):252-74.

Stotts JS, Fang ML, Dannaker CJ, et al, "Fenoprofen-Induced Toxic Epidermal Necrolysis," *J Am Acad Dermatol*, 1988, 18(4 Pt 1):755-7.

Vale JA and Meredith TJ, "Acute Poisoning Due to Nonsteroidal Anti-inflammatory Drugs," *Med Toxicol*, 1986, 1(1):12-31.

Verbeeck RK, "Pharmacokinetic Drug Interactions With Nonsteroidal Anti-inflammatory Drugs," *Clin Pharmacokinet*, 1990, 19(1):44-66.

Fentanest® *see* Fentanyl Citrate *on this page*

Fentanyl Citrate (fen' ta nil)

Related Information

Pharmacokinetics of Narcotic Agonist Analgesics *on page 1654*

CAS Number 437-38-7; 990-73-8

Brand Names Duragesic™; Fentanest®; Fentanyl Oralet®; Leptanal®; Sublimaze®; Tanyl®

Synonyms Phentanyl

Use Sedation, relief of pain, preoperative medication, adjunct to general or regional anesthesia, management of chronic pain (transdermal product)

Mechanism of Action Binds with stereospecific receptors at many sites within the CNS, increases pain threshold, alters pain reception, inhibits ascending pain pathways

Adverse Reactions

Cardiovascular: Hypotension, bradycardia

Central nervous system: CNS depression, drowsiness, dizziness, sedation, electroencephalogram abnormalities

Dermatologic: Erythema, pruritus

Endocrine & metabolic: ADH release

Gastrointestinal: Nausea, dyspepsia, vomiting, constipation

Local: Transdermal system: Edema, erythema, pruritus

Neuromuscular & skeletal: Skeletal and thoracic muscle rigidity especially following rapid I.V. administration

Ocular: Miosis

Respiratory: Apnea, respiratory depression, laryngospasm

Miscellaneous: Physical and psychological dependence with prolonged use, biliary or urinary tract spasm

Signs & Symptoms of Acute Overdose Apnea, flatulence, hypertension, pseudotumor cerebri, depression, confusion, hypertonia, laryngospasm, exfoliative dermatitis, coma, dyspnea, chest pain, respiratory depression (especially with doses >200 mcg), hiccups, hypotension, seizures

Toxicodynamics/Kinetics Respiratory depressant effect may last longer than analgesic effect

I.M.:

Onset of analgesia: 7-15 minutes

Duration: 1-2 hours

I.V.:

Onset of analgesia: Almost immediate

Duration: 0.5-1 hour

Transmucosal:

Onset of effect: 5-15 minutes with a maximum reduction in activity/fear

Peak analgesia: Within 20-30 minutes

Duration: Related to blood level of the drug

Absorption: Transmucosal: Rapid, ~25% from the buccal mucosa; 75% swallowed with saliva and slowly absorbed from gastrointestinal tract

Distribution: V_d: 4 L/kg; highly lipophilic, redistributes into muscle and fat

Protein binding: 80% to 86%

Metabolism: In the liver (N-dealkylation and hydroxylation); metabolites not active

Bioavailability: Transmucosal: ~50% (range: 36% to 71%)

Half-life: 2-4 hours

Transmucosal: 6.6 hours (range: 5-15 hours)

Elimination: Excreted in urine primarily as metabolites and 10% as unchanged drug

Usual Dosage Doses should be titrated to appropriate effects; wide range of doses, dependent upon desired degree of analgesia/anesthesia

Children 1-12 years:

Sedation for minor procedures/analgesia:

I.M., I.V.: 1-2 mcg/kg/dose; may repeat at 30- to 60-minute intervals. **Note:** Children 18-36 months of age may require 2-3 mcg/kg/dose

Transmucosal: 5 mcg/kg, if child is not fearful, fearful children and some younger children may require doses of 5-15 mcg/kg (which also carries an increased risk of hypoventilation); drug effect begins within 10 minutes, with sedation beginning shortly thereafter

Continuous sedation/analgesia: Initial I.V. bolus: 1-2 mcg/kg then 1 mcg/kg/hour; titrate upward; usual: 1-3 mcg/kg/hour

(Continued)

Fentanyl Citrate *(Continued)*

Pain control: Transdermal: Not recommended

Children >12 years and Adults:

Sedation for minor procedures/analgesia:

I.M., I.V.: 0.5-1 mcg/kg/dose; higher doses are used for major procedures

Transmucosal: 5 mcg/kg, suck on lozenge vigorously approximately 20-40 minutes before the start of procedure, drug effect begins within 10 minutes, with sedation beginning shortly thereafter

Preoperative sedation, adjunct to regional anesthesia, postoperative pain: I.M., I.V.: 50-100 mcg/dose

Adjunct to general anesthesia: I.M., I.V.: 2-50 mcg/kg

General anesthesia without additional anesthetic agents: I.V. 50-100 mcg/kg with O_2 and skeletal muscle relaxant

Pain control: Transdermal: Initial: 25 mcg/hour system; if currently receiving opiates, convert to fentanyl equivalent and administer equianalgesic dosage titrated to minimize the adverse effects and provide analgesia. To convert patients from oral or parenteral opioids to Duragesic™, the previous 24-hour analgesic requirement should be calculated. This analgesic requirement should be converted to the equianalgesic oral morphine dose. See tables.

Equianalgesic Doses of Opioid Agonists

Drug	Equianalgesic Dose (mg)	
	I.M.	P.O.
Codeine	130	200
Hydromorphone	1.5	7.5
Levorphanol	2	4
Meperidine	75	—
Methadone	10	20
Morphine	10	60
Oxycodone	15	30
Oxymorphone	1	10 (PR)

From *N Engl J Med,* 1985, 313:84–95.

Corresponding Doses of Oral/Intramuscular Morphine and Duragesic™

Oral 24-Hour Morphine (mg/d)	I.M. 24-Hour Morphine (mg/d)	Duragesic™ Dose (mcg/h)
45–134	8–22	25
135–224	28–37	50
225–314	38–52	75
315–404	53–67	100
405–494	68–82	125
495–584	83–97	150
585–674	98–112	175
675–764	113–127	200
765–854	128–142	225
855–944	143–157	250
945–1034	158–172	275
1035–1124	173–187	300

Product information, Duragesic™ — Janssen Pharmaceutica, January, 1991.

The dosage should not be titrated more frequently than every 3 days after the initial dose or every 6 days thereafter. The majority of patients are controlled on every 72-hour administration, however, a small number of patients require every 48-hour administration.

Elderly >65 years: Transmucosal: Dose should be reduced to 2.5-5 mcg/kg; elderly have been found to be twice as sensitive as younger patients to the effects of fentanyl

Dosing adjustment in renal impairment:

Cl_{cr} 10-50 mL/minute: Administer at 75% of normal dose

Cl_{cr} <10 mL/minute: Administer at 50% of normal dose

Administration Transmucosal product should begin 20-40 minutes prior to the anticipated start of surgery, diagnostic, or therapeutic procedure; foil overwrap should be removed just prior to administration; once removed, patient should place the unit in mouth and suck (not chew) it; unit should be removed after it is consumed or if patient has achieved an adequate sedation and anxiolytic level, and/or shows signs of respiratory depression

Contraindications Hypersensitivity to fentanyl or any component; increased intracranial pressure; severe apnea; severe liver or renal insufficiency;

Transmucosal is contraindicated in unmonitored settings where a risk of unrecognized hypoventilation exists or in treating acute or chronic pain

Warnings Fentanyl shares the toxic potentials of opiate agonists, and precautions of opiate agonist therapy should be observed; use with caution in patients with bradycardia; rapid I.V. infusion may result in skeletal muscle and chest wall rigidity → impaired ventilation → respiratory distress → apnea, bronchoconstriction, laryngospasm; inject slowly over 3-5 minutes; nondepolarizing skeletal muscle relaxant may be required; use transmucosal product with caution in patients with hepatic or renal disease, chronic obstructive pulmonary disease, patients with decreased respiratory reserve, and others with potentially compromised respiration; transmucosal product is not recommended for use in those who have received MAO inhibitors within 14 days; should be used with caution in patients with myasthenia gravis.

Dosage Forms

Injection, as citrate: 0.05 mg/mL (2 mL, 5 mL, 10 mL, 20 mL, 50 mL)

Lozenge, oral transmucosal (raspberry flavored): 200 mcg, 300 mcg, 400 mcg

Transdermal system: 25 mcg/hour [10 cm^2]; 50 mcg/hour [20 cm^2]; 75 mcg/hour [30 cm^2]; 100 mcg/hour [40 cm^2] (all available in 5s)

Stability Protect from light; incompatible when mixed in the same syringe with pentobarbital; incompatible with thiopental sodium and methohexital sodium

Transmucosal: Store at controlled room temperature of 15°C to 30°C (59°F to 86°F)

Reference Range

Therapeutic: 2-200 μg/L

Fatal: Serum level of 17.7 μg/L has been correlated with fatality

Overdosage Treatment

Decontamination: Lavage/activated charcoal with cathartic for oral ingestion

Supportive therapy: Naloxone in large doses and/or a continuous infusion may be necessary; laryngospasm and masseter muscle spasm also respond to naloxone

Antidote(s)

Naloxone Hydrochloride *on page 1447*

Diagnostic Tests/Procedures

Fentanyl, Blood or Urine *on page 1264*

Drug Interactions Increased toxicity with CNS depressants, cimetidine, thiopental, phenothiazine, TCAs, benzodiazepines; with midazolam, hypotension and respiratory depression have been noted. Decreased effect of epidural fentanyl when given with chloroprocaine.

Pregnancy Risk Factor B (D if used for prolonged periods or in high doses at term)

Pregnancy Implications Crosses the placenta

Monitoring Parameters Respiratory and cardiovascular status

Nursing Implications May cause rebound respiratory depression postoperatively; total dose of all narcotic analgesics administered, including transmucosal unit, should be considered before ordering narcotic analgesics during recovery from anesthesia; for patients who have received transmucosal product within 6-12 hours, it is recommended that if other narcotics are required, they should be used at starting doses $^1/_4$ to $^1/_3$ those usually recommended

Specific References

Baraka A, "Fentanyl-Induced Laryngospasm Following Tracheal Extubation in a Child," *Anaesthesia*, 1995, 50:375.

Bedforth NM and Lockey DJ, "Raynaud's Syndrome Following Intravenous Induction of Anaesthesia," *Anaesthesia*, 1995, 50:248-9.

Bennett MRD and Adams AP, "Postoperative Respiratory Complications of Opiates," *Clin Anaesthesiol*, 1983, 1:41-56.

Chaturvedi AK, Rao NG, and Baird JR, "A Death Due to Self-Administered Fentanyl," *J Anal Toxicol*, 1990, 14(6):385-7.

Furuya H and Okumura F, "Hemolysis After Administration of High Dose Fentanyl," *Anesth Analg*, 1986, 65(2):207-8.

Maurer PM and Bartkowski RR, "Drug Interactions of Clinical Significance With Opiad Analgesics," *Drug Saf*, 1993, 8(1):30-48.

Stoukides CA and Stegman M, "Diffuse Rash Associated With Transdermal Fentanyl," *Clin Pharm*, 1992, 11(3):222.

Fentanyl Oralet® *see* Fentanyl Citrate *on page 347*
Fentazin® *see* Perphenazine *on page 609*
Fenytoin® *see* Phenytoin *on page 623*
Feosol® *see* Iron *on page 439*
Feostat® *see* Iron *on page 439*
Feratab® *see* Iron *on page 439*
Fergon® *see* Iron *on page 439*
Fer-In-Sol® *see* Iron *on page 439*
Fer-Iron® *see* Iron *on page 439*
Ferndex® *see* Dextroamphetamine Sulfate *on page 268*
Fero-Gradumet® *see* Iron *on page 439*
Ferospace® *see* Iron *on page 439*
Ferralet® *see* Iron *on page 439*
Ferralyn® Lanacaps® *see* Iron *on page 439*
Ferra-TD® *see* Iron *on page 439*
Ferro-Sequels® *see* Iron *on page 439*
Ferrous Fumarate *see* Iron *on page 439*
Ferrous Gluconate *see* Iron *on page 439*
Ferrous Sulfate *see* Iron *on page 439*
Feverall™ [OTC] *see* Acetaminophen *on page 79*
Fibroblast Interferon *replaced by* Interferon Beta-1b *on page 435*
Fibrocit® *see* Gemfibrozil *on page 378*
FK506 *see* Tacrolimus *on page 720*
Flagyl® Oral *see* Metronidazole *on page 526*
Flavorcee® [OTC] *see* Ascorbic Acid *on page 131*

Flecainide Acetate (fle kay' nide)

Related Information
Lorcainide Hydrochloride *on page 484*

CAS Number 54143-55-4

Brand Names Almartyn®; Tambocor®

Synonyms Benzamide Acetate; R-818

Use Prevention and suppression of documented life-threatening ventricular arrhythmias (ie, sustained tachycardia (ventricular)); controlling symptomatic, disabling tachycardia (ventricular)s in patients without structural heart disease (class I agent)

Mechanism of Action Class IC antiarrhythmic; slows conduction in cardiac tissue by altering transport of ions across cell membranes; causes slight prolongation of refractory periods; decreases the rate of rise of the action potential without affecting its duration; increases electrical stimulation threshold of ventricle, HIS-Purkinje system; possesses local anesthetic and moderate negative inotropic effects

Adverse Reactions
Cardiovascular: Bradycardia, heart block, P-R prolongation, QRS prolongation, Q-T_c interval prolongation is minimal; worsening ventricular arrhythmias, congestive heart failure, palpitations, chest pain, edema, cardiac arrest, hypotension, syncope
Central nervous system: Dizziness, fatigue, nervousness, hypoesthesia, seizures, psychosis, visual hallucinations, headache
Dermatologic: Rashes, lupus-like syndrome
Gastrointestinal: Nausea, metallic taste, vomiting
Hematologic: Blood dyscrasias
Hepatic: Possible hepatic dysfunction
Neuromuscular & skeletal: Tremors, dysarthria, paresthesia
Ocular: Blurred vision, photophobia, diplopia
Respiratory: Dyspnea

Signs & Symptoms of Acute Overdose P-R prolongation, QRS prolongation, arthralgia, A-V block, Q-T prolongation increased amplitude of the T wave, impotence, heart block, reduced heart rate and myocardial contractility, syncope, conduction disturbances, congestive heart failure, neutropenia, blurred vision, tachycardia (ventricular), systemic lupus erythematosus (SLE), hypotension and death; primary arrhythmia noted: polymorphous or wide-complex tachycardia (ventricular), although wide-complex supraventricular arrhythmias can occur

Toxicodynamics/Kinetics
Absorption: Rapid from gastrointestinal tract
Distribution: V_d: Adults: 9 L/kg; distributes well throughout body

Protein binding: 40% to 50% (alpha$_1$ glycoprotein)
Metabolism: In the liver
Bioavailability: 5% to 90%
Half-life: Adults: 7-22 hours; increased half-life with congestive heart failure or renal dysfunction
Time to peak serum concentration: Within 1.5-3 hours
Elimination: 80% to 90% excreted in urine as unchanged drugs and metabolites (10% to 50%); 5% excreted in feces

Usual Dosage Oral:

Children: Initial: 3 mg/kg/day in 3 divided doses; usual 3-6 mg/kg/day in 3 divided doses; up to 11 mg/kg/day for uncontrolled patients with subtherapeutic levels

Adults: Initial: 100 mg every 12 hours, increase by 100 mg/day (given in 2 doses/day) every 4 days to maximum of 400 mg/day; for patients receiving 400 mg/day who are not controlled and have trough concentrations <0.6 μg/mL, dosage may be increased to 600 mg/day

Children and Adults:

Dosing adjustment in severe renal impairment: Cl_{cr} <10 mL/minute: Decrease usual dose by 25% to 50%

Dosing adjustment/comments in hepatic impairment: Monitoring of plasma levels is recommended because of significantly increased half-life

Contraindications Pre-existing second or third degree A-V block; right bundle-branch block associated with left hemiblock (bifascicular block) or trifascicular block; cardiogenic shock, myocardial depression; known hypersensitivity to the drug

Warnings The manufacturer and FDA recommend that this drug be reserved for life-threatening ventricular arrhythmias unresponsive to conventional therapy. Its use for symptomatic nonsustained tachycardia (ventricular), frequent premature ventricular complexes (PVCs), uniform and multiform PVCs and/or coupled PVCs is no longer recommended. Flecainide can worsen or cause arrhythmias with an associated risk of death. Proarrhythmic effects range from an increased number of PVCs to more severe tachycardia (ventricular)s (eg, tachycardias that are more sustained or more resistant to conversion to sinus rhythm). Use with caution in patients with pre-existing sinus node dysfunction, sick sinus syndrome, history of congestive heart failure or myocardial dysfunction; increases in P-R interval ≥300 MS, QRS ≥180 MS, Q-T_c interval increases and/or new bundle branch block; patients with pacemakers, renal impairment and/or hepatic impairment.

Dosage Forms Tablet: 50 mg, 100 mg, 150 mg

Reference Range

Therapeutic: 0.2-1.0 μg/mL (SI: 0.4-2.0 μmol/L)
Fatal: 21.3 μg/mL associated with fatality

Overdosage Treatment

Decontamination: Lavage/activated charcoal with cathartic
Supportive therapy: Monitoring; flecainide-induced tachycardia (ventricular) should be treated with ventricular pacing, antiarrhythmic drugs and/or cardioversion; however, it is commonly refractory to these measures; isoproterenol can be used for bradyarrhythmias; sodium bicarbonate (1-2 mg/kg) can be given for conduction delays
Enhancement of elimination: Multiple dosing of activated charcoal or charcoal hemoperfusion may be helpful; do not alkalinize the urine

Drug Interactions Increases plasma digoxin concentrations, possible additive negative inotropic effects with beta-blockers; alkalinizing agents (high-dose antacids, carbonic anhydrase inhibitors or sodium bicarbonate) may decrease flecainide's clearance

Pregnancy Risk Factor C

Pregnancy Implications Can cause transient neonatal conjugated hyperbilirubinaemia

Monitoring Parameters EKG and serum concentrations

Additional Information Based on adverse outcomes noted with flecainide in the CAST trial, the FDA recommends that use of flecainide be limited to patients with life-threatening ventricular arrhythmias

Specific References

Anderson IB and Olson KR, "Fatal Flecainide Poisoning in an Infant," *Vet Hum Toxicol*, 1994, 36:369.

Borgeat A, Biollaz J, Freymond B, et al, "Hemofiltration Clearance of Flecainide in a Patient With Acute Renal Failure," *Intensive Care Med*, 1988, 14(3):236-7.

Gotz D, Pohle S, and Barckow D, "Primary and Secondary Detoxification in Severe Flecainide Intoxication," *Intensive Care Med*, 1991, 17(3):181-4.

Muhiddin KA, Johnston A, and Turner P, "The Influence of Urinary pH on Flecainide Excretion and Its Serum Pharmacokinetics," *Br J Clin Pharmacol*, 1984, 17(4):447-51.

Salerno DM, Murakami MM, Johnston RB, et al, "Reversal of Flecainide-Induced Ventricular Arrhythmia by Hypertonic Sodium Bicarbonate in Dogs," *Am J Emerg Med*, 1995, 13:285-93.

Vanderhal AL, Cocjin J, Santulli Jr TV, et al, "Conjugated Hyperbilirubinemia in a Newborn Infant After Maternal (Transplacenta) Treatment With Flecainide Acetate For Fetal Tachycardia and Fetal Hydrops," *J Pediatr*, 1995, 126:988-90.

(Continued)

Flecainide Acetate *(Continued)*

Winkelmann BR and Leinberger H, "Life-Threatening Flecainide Toxicity. A Pharmacodynamic Approach," *Ann Intern Med*, 1987, 106(6):807-14.

Fleet® Relief *see* Pramoxine Hydrochloride *on page 636*

Fleet® Laxative [OTC] *see* Bisacodyl *on page 156*

Fleet® Flavored Castor Oil [OTC] *see* Castor Oil *on page 189*

Fleet® Mineral Oil Enema [OTC] *see* Mineral Oil *on page 534*

Fleroxacin

CAS Number 79660-72-3

Brand Names Megalone®; Quinodis®

Use Investigational: Urinary tract infections, sexually transmitted diseases, skin/soft tissue infections, bone and joint infections, respiratory tract infections, chancroid, bacterial diarrhea, typhoid fever, effective against *Enterobacteriacae, Acetobacter, Haemophilus, Neisseria, Moraxella*

Mechanism of Action Fluoroquinolone which inhibits bacterial DNA gyrase and thus has bactericidal activity

Adverse Reactions

Cardiovascular: Flushing

Central nervous system: Insomnia, headache, dizziness, night terrors, lethargy

Dermatologic: Photosensitivity (0.6%), pruritus

Gastrointestinal: Nausea (8%), vomiting, diarrhea, flatulence, dry mouth

Hematologic: Eosinophilia

Toxicodynamics/Kinetics

Distribution: V_d: 1.3-1.8 L/kg

Protein binding: 30%

Metabolism: Hepatic N-demethylation and N-oxidation to N-desmethylfleroxacin (active metabolite) and to fleroxacin-N-oxide (inactive)

Bioavailability: 96% to 100%

Half-life: 8.9-10.3 hours

Elimination: Urine

Usual Dosage

Oral:

- Uncomplicated urinary tract infection: 200 mg/day for 10 days
- Complicated urinary tract infection: 400 mg/day for 10 days
- Uncomplicated cervical or urethral gonorrhea: Single 400 mg dose
- Bronchitis: 400 mg once daily
- Skin/soft tissue infection: 400 mg/day
- Typhoid fever: 400 mg/day for 7 days

I.V.: Urinary tract infection: 400 mg

Contraindications Hypersensitivity to fleroxacin or other quinolones

Warnings Reduce dosage in renal insufficiency, elderly patients; use with caution in patients with central nervous system disorders, prepubertal children, psychiatric patients

Reference Range After an 800 mg oral dose, peak serum fleroxacin levels range from 7-15.6 μg/mL; therapeutic serum levels: 1-4 μg/mL

Overdosage Treatment

Decontamination: Lavage/activated charcoal with cathartic

Supportive therapy: Do **not** use flumazenil; diazepam, phenobarbital, or phenytoin for seizures

Enhancement of elimination: Multiple dosing of activated charcoal may be effective

Drug Interactions Antacids may decrease absorption as can sucralfate

Additional Information Less effective than other quinolones against *Streptococcus pneumoniae*, or *Pseudomonas aeruginosa*

Specific References

Bergeron MG, "The Pharmacokinetics and Tissue Penetration of the Fluoroquinolones," *Clin Invest Med*, 1989, 12(1):20-7.

Brouwers JR, "Drug Interactions With Quinolone Antibacterials," *Drug Saf*, 1992, 7(4):268-81.

Patel KB, Nicolau DP, Klepser ME, et al, "Focus on Fleroxacin: A New Once Daily Fluoroquinolone Antibiotic," *Formulary*, 1995, 30:261-7.

Stuck AE, Kim DK, and Frey FJ, "Fleroxacin Clinical Pharmacokinetics," *Clin Pharmacokinet*, 1992, 22(2):116-31.

Flexartal® *see* Carisoprodol *on page 187*

Flexeril® *see* Cyclobenzaprine Hydrochloride *on page 248*

Flexiban® *see* Cyclobenzaprine Hydrochloride *on page 248*

Flogotisol® *see* Thiamphenicol *on page 742*

Floxin® *see* Ofloxacin *on page 575*

Flucinome® *see* Flutamide *on page 366*

Fluconazole (floo koe' na zole)

Related Information

Antifungal Therapy *on page 1496-1497*

CAS Number 86386-73-4

Brand Names Diflucan®; Triflucan®

Use Treatment of susceptible fungal infections including oropharyngeal and esophageal candidiasis; treatment of systemic candidal infections including urinary tract infection, peritonitis, and pneumonia; treatment of cryptococcal meningitis; treatment of vaginal candidiasis

Mechanism of Action Interferes with cytochrome P-450 activity, decreasing ergosterol synthesis (principal sterol in fungal cell membrane) and inhibiting cell membrane formation

Adverse Reactions

Cardiovascular: Pallor
Central nervous system: Dizziness, seizures, headache
Dermatologic: Skin rash, exfoliative dermatitis
Endocrine & metabolic: Hypokalemia
Gastrointestinal: Nausea, abdominal pain, vomiting, diarrhea
Hematologic: Thrombocytopenia
Hepatic: Elevated AST, ALT, or alkaline phosphatase

Signs & Symptoms of Acute Overdose Convulsions, nausea, vomiting, hypokalemia, hepatic failure, hepatitis

Toxicodynamics/Kinetics

Absorption: Oral: Absorbed well
Distribution: V_d: 0.7-1.0 L/kg; widely distributed throughout body with good penetration into CSF, eye, and peritoneal fluid
Protein binding: 11% to 12%
Metabolism: Hepatic accounts for <10% of elimination
Bioavailability: oral: >90%
Half-life, normal renal function: 25-30 hours
Time to peak serum concentration: Within 2-4 hours
Oral: 1-2 hours
Intraperitoneal: ~7 hours
Elimination: 80% of dose excreted unchanged in urine

Usual Dosage The daily dose of fluconazole is the same for oral and I.V. administration

Indication	Day 1	Daily Therapy	Minimum Duration of Therapy
Oropharyngeal candidiasis	200 mg	100 mg	14 d
Esophageal candidiasis	200 mg	100 mg	21 d
Systemic candidiasis	400 mg	200 mg	28 d
Cryptococcal meningitis acute	400 mg	200 mg	10–12 wk after CSF culture becomes negative
relapse	200 mg	200 mg	

Efficacy of fluconazole has not been established in children; a small number of patients from 3-13 years of age have been treated with fluconazole using doses of 3-6 mg/kg/day once daily. Doses as high as 12 mg/kg/day once daily have been used to treat candidiasis in immunocompromised children.

Adults: Oral, I.V.: See table for once daily dosing
Vaginal candidiasis: Oral: 150 mg as a single dose

Dosing adjustment/interval in renal impairment:

Cl_{cr} 21-50 mL/minute: Administer 50% of recommended dose or administer every 48 hours

Cl_{cr} <20 mL/minute: Administer 25% of recommended dose or administer every 72 hours

Administration Parenteral fluconazole must be administered by I.V. infusion over approximately 1-2 hours; do not exceed 200 mg/hour when giving I.V. infusion

Contraindications Known hypersensitivity to fluconazole or other azoles

Warnings Patients who develop liver function tests (abnormal) during fluconazole therapy should be monitored closely for the development of more severe hepatic injury; if clinical signs and symptoms consistent with liver disease develop that may be attributable to fluconazole, fluconazole should be discontinued

(Continued)

Fluconazole *(Continued)*

Dosage Forms

Injection: 2 mg/mL (100 mL, 200 mL)

Tablet: 50 mg, 100 mg, 200 mg

Stability Parenteral admixture at room temperature (25°C): Manufacturer expiration dating; do not refrigerate

Overdosage Treatment Enhancement of elimination: 3-hour hemodialysis will remove 50% (unlikely to require this procedure)

Drug Interactions May increase cyclosporine levels when high doses used, may increase phenytoin serum concentration; may inhibit warfarins, terfenadine, astemizole, sulfonylureas metabolism; rifampin decreased concentrations of fluconazole

Pregnancy Risk Factor C

Monitoring Parameters Periodic liver function and renal function tests

Nursing Implications Monitor renal function as dosage adjustments are required with significant changes in renal function

Additional Information Expensive oral alternative to I.V. amphotericin B infusions; in some clinical studies it has been as effective as amphotericin B, but is less likely to cause serious adverse reactions; represents a significant advancement in the treatment of systemic cryptococcosis, including meningitis

Specific References

Force RW, "Fluconazole Concentrations in Breast Milk," *Pediatr Infect Dis J*, 1995, 14:235-6.

Grant SM and Clissold SP, "Fluconazole: A Review of Its Pharmacodynamic and Pharmacokinetic Properties and Therapeutic Potential in Superficial and Systemic Mycoses," *Drugs*, 1990, 39(6):877-916.

Mercurio MG and Elewski BE, "Thrombocytopenia Caused by Fluconazole Therapy," *J Am Acad Dermatol*, 1995, 32(3):525-6.

Fluimucil® *see* Thiamphenicol *on page 742*

Flumadine® *see* Rimantadine Hydrochloride *on page 685*

Flunitrazepam

Related Information

Clonazepam *on page 229*

Nitrazepam *on page 562*

CAS Number 1622-62-4

Brand Names Darkene®; Hypnoderm®; Hypnor®; Narcozep®; Noriel®; Roipnol®; Rophipnol®; Rophypnol®; Valsera®

Synonyms RO5-4200

Use Not marketed in United States, but is encountered in the U.S. as a drug of abuse; used for insomnia and sedation (short-term therapy) and anesthesia induction or supplementation in Europe

Mechanism of Action Intermediate to long-acting benzodiazepine, this agent facilitates the gamma-aminobuytric acid-mediated neuroreceptors

Adverse Reactions

Cardiovascular: Tachycardia, myocardial depression, hypotension

Central nervous system: Lethargy, dizziness, ataxia, headache, night terrors, porphyria

Gastrointestinal: Nausea, diarrhea

Neuromuscular & skeletal: Tremor

Respiratory: Cough, apnea

Miscellaneous: Hiccups

Signs & Symptoms of Acute Overdose Hypotension, apnea, coma, ataxia

Toxicodynamics/Kinetics

Absorption: Food can reduce absorption by 50%

Distribution: V_d: 3.4-5.5 L/kg

Protein binding: 80% to 90%

Metabolism: Hepatic to 7-aminoflunitrazepam and other metabolites

Bioavailability: 80% to 90%

Half-life: 19-22 hours

Elimination: Renal

Usual Dosage

Anesthesia induction: I.V.: 0.015-0.03 mg/kg slowly over 30-60 seconds

Premedication for anesthesia: I.M.: 0.015-0.03 mg/kg slowly over 30-60 seconds

Anesthesia maintenance: I.V.: 0.2-0.5 mg (0.005-0.01 mg/kg) 2-3 hours after anesthesia induction

Insomnia: Oral: 0.5-2 mg nightly; in elderly, 0.5 mg dose should be initiated

Contraindications Hypersensitivity to flunitrazepam, nitrazepam, or clonazepam

Warnings Use with caution in patients with porphyria, myasthenia gravis, cardiovascular disease, or hepatic/renal insufficiency; reduce dosage in elderly; dependence may occur

Dosage Forms

Injection: 2 mg/mL

Tablet: 0.5 mg, 1 mg, 2 mg

Reference Range Peak plasma levels after a 2 mg oral dose: 10-15 ng/mL

Overdosage Treatment

Decontamination: Lavage/activated charcoal with cathartic

Supportive therapy: Rarely is mechanical ventilation required; flumazenil has been shown to selectively block the binding of benzodiazepines to CNS receptors, resulting in a reversal of benzodiazepine-induced CNS depression and apnea; sedation also has been reversed with administration of aminophylline at a low dose of 2 mg/kg I.V.

Enhancement of elimination: Multiple dose of activated charcoal is effective

Antidote(s)

Flumazenil *on page 1428*

Drug Interactions Enhances sedative effects of ethanol and general anesthesias; with succinylcholine, increased intraovular pressure can occur; theophylline antagonizes sedative effects

Pregnancy Risk Factor D

Pregnancy Implications Can cross the placenta (no congenital malformations described) and accumulate in the fetus

Monitoring Parameters Blood pressure, heart rate, arterial blood gas

Additional Information About 10 times as potent as diazepam; insoluble in water; a growing drug of abuse in Europe and in the U.S. due to its euphoric producing qualities and low street price ($1-$3/tablet); usually several tablets are required for a euphoric effect; oral dose of 28 mg associated with fatality; psychomotor effects may last for 12 hours postdose; often abused in combination with heroin, ethanol, cocaine, or methamphetamine

Specific References

Gurel A, Elevli M, and Hamulu A, "Aminophylline Reversal of flunitrazepam Sedation," *Anesth Analg*, 1987, 66(4):333-6.

Heyndrickx B, "Fatal Intoxication With Flunitrazepam," *J Anal Toxicol*, 1987, 11(6):278.

Mattila MAK and Larni HM, "Flunitrazepam: A Review of Its Pharmacological Properties and Therapeutic Uses," *Drugs*, 1980, 20:353-74.

Fluopromazine *see* Triflupromazine Hydrochloride *on page 770*

Fluoride (flur' ide)

CAS Number 7681-49-4

UN Number 1690

Brand Names ACT® [OTC]; Fluorigard® [OTC]; Fluorinse®; Fluoritab®; Flura®; Flura-Drops®; Flura-Loz®; Gel Kam®; Gel-Tin® [OTC]; Karidium®; Karigel®; Karigel®-N; Listermint® With Fluoride [OTC]; Luride®; Luride® Lozi-Tab®; Luride®-SF Lozi-Tab®; Minute-Gel®; Pediaflor®; Pharmaflur®; Phos-Flur®; Point-Two®; Prevident®; Stop® [OTC]

Synonyms Acidulated Phosphate Fluoride; Disodium Difluoride; Sodium Fluoride; Sodium Hydrofluoride; Stannous Fluoride

Use Prevention of dental caries

Mechanism of Action Derived from hydrofluoric acid, reduces acid production by dental bacteria; increases tooth resistance to acid dissolution

Adverse Reactions

Central nervous system: Fasciculations

Dermatologic: Rash

Gastrointestinal: Gastrointestinal upset, nausea, feces discoloration (black), vomiting, stomach cramps

Neuromuscular & skeletal: Tremors, paresthesia

Miscellaneous: Products containing stannous fluoride may stain the teeth; ulceration of mucous membranes

Signs & Symptoms of Acute Overdose Gastrointestinal hemorrhage, delirium, apnea, slurred speech, tremors, tetany, seizures, hematuria, osteomalacia, hypothyroidism, hypotension, hypocalcemia, hypomagnesemia, hyperkalemia, fibrillation (ventricular), esophageal stricture, respiratory paralysis, mydriasis, urine discoloration (milky), nausea, vomiting, epigastric pain, diarrhea

Toxicodynamics/Kinetics

Absorption: Absorbed in gastrointestinal tract, lungs, and skin; calcium, iron, or magnesium may delay absorption

Distribution: V_d: 0.5-0.7 L/kg; 50% of fluoride is deposited in teeth and bone after ingestion; topical application works superficially on enamel and plaque

Half-life: 2-9 hours

Elimination: Urine and feces

Usual Dosage Oral:

Recommended daily fluoride supplement (2.2 mg of sodium fluoride is equivalent to 1 mg of fluoride ion): See table on next page.

Dental rinse or gel:

Children 6-12 years: 5-10 mL rinse or apply to teeth and spit daily after brushing

Adults: 10 mL rinse or apply to teeth and spit daily after brushing

Contraindications Hypersensitivity to fluoride or any component, or when fluoride content of drinking water exceeds 0.7 ppm

(Continued)

Fluoride *(Continued)*

Fluoride Ion

Fluoride Content of Drinking Water	Daily Dose, Oral (mg)
<0.3 ppm	
Birth – 2 y	0.25
2–3 y	0.5
3–12 y	1
0.3–0.7 ppm	
Birth – 2 y	0
2–3 y	0.25
3–12 y	0.5

Warnings Prolonged ingestion with excessive doses may result in dental fluorosis and osseous changes; do **not** exceed recommended dosage; some products contain tartrazine

Dosage Forms Fluoride ion content listed in brackets

Drops, oral, as sodium:
- Fluoritab®, Flura-Drops®: 0.55 mg/drop [0.25 mg/drop] (22.8 mL, 24 mL)
- Karidium®, Luride®: 0.275 mg/drop [0.125 mg/drop] (30 mL, 60 mL)
- Pediaflor®: 1.1 mg/mL [0.5 mg/mL] (50 mL)

Gel, topical:
- Acidulated phosphate fluoride (Minute-Gel®): 1.23% (480 mL)
- Sodium fluoride (Karigel®, Karigel®-N, PreviDent®): 1.1% [0.5%] (24 g, 30 g, 60 g, 120 g, 130 g, 250 g)
- Stannous fluoride (Gel Kam®, Gel-Tin®, Stop®): 0.4% [0.1%] (60 g, 65 g, 105 g, 120 g)

Lozenge, as sodium (Flura-Loz®) (raspberry flavor): 2.2 mg [1 mg]

Rinse, topical, as sodium:
- ACT®, Fluorigard®: 0.05% [0.02%] (90 mL, 180 mL, 300 mL, 360 mL, 480 mL)
- Fluorinse®, Point-Two®: 0.2% [0.09%] (240 mL, 480 mL, 3780 mL)
- Listermint® with Fluoride: 0.02% [0.01%] (180 mL, 300 mL, 360 mL, 480 mL, 540 mL, 720 mL, 960 mL, 1740 mL)

Solution, oral, as sodium (Phos-Flur®): 0.44 mg/mL [0.2 mg/mL] (250 mL, 500 mL, 3780 mL)

Tablet, as sodium: Chewable:
- Fluoritab®, Luride® Lozi-Tab®, Pharmaflur®: 1.1 mg [0.5 mg]
- Fluoritab®, Karidium®, Luride® Lozi-Tab®, Luride®-SF Lozi-Tab®, Pharmaflur®: 2.2 mg [1 mg]
- Flura®, Karidium®: 2.2 mg [1 mg]

Stability Store in tight plastic containers (not glass)

Reference Range Normal serum level of fluoride: 1.9-7.6 μg/dL (SI: 1-4 μmol/L); toxic urine fluoride level is >10 mg/L

Overdosage Treatment

Decontamination: Lavage with 10% calcium gluconate; if <8 mg/kg is ingested, dilute with milk; do not induce emesis; do not administer sodium bicarbonate; magnesium based cathartics are preferred; calcium binds to fluoride to decrease the absorption

Supportive therapy: Calcium gluconate to reduce tetanic contractures; quinidine may be particularly effective for treatment of ventricular arrhythmias; monitor magnesium

Enhancement of elimination: Hemodialysis can be utilized

Antidote(s)

Calcium Chloride *on page 1400*
Calcium Gluconate *on page 1401*

Test Interactions Low calcium, high potassium

Diagnostic Tests/Procedures

Fluoride, Serum *on page 1267*
Fluoride, Urine *on page 1267*

Drug Interactions Decreased effect/absorption with magnesium-, aluminum-, and calcium-containing products

Pregnancy Risk Factor C

Pregnancy Implications Crosses placenta; appears in breast milk

Patient Information Take with food (but not milk) to eliminate gastritis; with dental rinse or dental gel do **not** swallow, do **not** eat or drink for 30 minutes after use

Nursing Implications Avoid giving with milk or dairy products

Additional Information Odorless; not flammable; seafood can contain large amounts of fluoride (up to 28 mg/kg); tea can contain 0.5 mg/cup

PEL-TWA: 2.5 mg/m^3

IDLH: 500 mg/m^3

Total daily intake of fluoride: 2.1-2.4 mg (diet) and 2.8-5.9 mg (water)

In pediatrics, the therapeutic fluoride dosage is 0.05-0.07 mg/kg/day; fluorosis can develop at daily fluoride doses exceeding 0.1 mg/kg; fluoride supplementation should occur at age 6 months at a dose of 0.25 mg/day if their formulas or water contains <0.3 mg/L (0.3 ppm); this increases to daily supplementation of 0.5 mg at age 3 years and 1 mg at 6 years. Children >3 years of age require 0.25 mg/day of fluoride (0.5 mg/day at 6 years) if water fluoride ion level is 0.3-0.6 mg/L (0.3-0.6 ppm); fluoride levels in drinking water >0.6 mg/L (0.6 ppm) require no supplementation. Most fluoridated toothpastes contain ~1000 ppm of fluoride; thus, the daily dose of fluoride by brushing teeth is 0.134 mg from brushing once daily and 0.268 mg brushing twice daily. 53% of U.S. population drinks artificially fluoridated water at an optimal level of 1 mg/L (maximum allowable level 4 mg/L); carbonated beverages contain ~0.74 ppm of fluoride while tea contains ~2.6 ppm.

Specific References

Berman L, Taves D, Mitra S, et al, "Inorganic Fluoride Poisoning: Treatment by Hemodialysis," *N Engl J Med*, 1973, 289(17):922.

Cummings CC and McIvor ME, "Fluoride-Induced Hyperkalemia: The Role of Ca(2+)-Dependent K+ Channels," *Am J Emerg Med*, 1988, 6(1):1-3.

Fisher K, Picciotti M, Henretig F, et al, "Fluoride (F1) Toxicity From a Topical Dental Care Product (TDCP)," *Vet Hum Toxicol*, 1991, 33:365.

McIvor ME, "Acute Fluoride Toxicity. Pathophysiology and Management," *Drug Saf*, 1990, 5(2):79-85.

Pitt P and Berry H, "Fluoride Treatment in Osteoporosis," *Postgrad Med J*, 1991, 67(786):323-6.

Schuman AJ, "How Much Fluoride is Too Much?" *Contemporary Pediatrics*, 1995, 12(6):65-74.

U.S. Department of Health and Human Services, "Toxicological Profile for Fluorides, Hydrogen Fluoride, and Fluorine (F) TP-91/17," Agency for Toxic Substances and Diseases Registry, 1993.

Fluorigard® [OTC] *see* Fluoride *on page 355*

Fluorinse® *see* Fluoride *on page 355*

Fluoritab® *see* Fluoride *on page 355*

Fluoroplex® Topical *see* Fluorouracil *on this page*

Fluorouracil (flure oh yoor' a sill)

Related Information

Drugs and Chemicals Proven to be Teratogenic in Humans *on page 1572-1575*

Toxicities of Chemotherapeutic Agents *on page 1631-1633*

CAS Number 51-21-8

Brand Names Adrucil® Injection; Cytosafe®; Efudex® Topical; Fluoroplex® Topical; Fluroblastin®; Fluroblastine®

Synonyms 5-Fluorouracil; 5-FU

Use Treatment of carcinoma of stomach, colon, rectum, breast, and pancreas; also used topically for management of multiple actinic keratoses and superficial basal cell carcinomas

Mechanism of Action A pyrimidine antimetabolite that interferes with DNA synthesis by blocking the methylation of deoxyuricytic acid; 5-FU rapidly enters the cell and is activated to the nucleotide level; there it inhibits thymidylate synthetase (TS), or is incorporated into RNA (most evident during the gastrointestinal phase of the cell cycle). The reduced folate cofactor is required for tight binding to occur between the 5-FdUMP and TS.

Adverse Reactions

Cardiovascular: Cardiac arrhythmias, chest pain, heart failure, hypotension, coronary vasospasm, cardiomyopathy, tachycardia, heart failure

Central nervous system: Headache, gait and speech abnormalities, disorientation, dizziness, tingling of hands, cerebellar ataxia

Dermatologic: Alopecia, skin pigmentation, pruritic maculopapular rash, partial loss of nails or hyperpigmentation of nail bed, photosensitivity, dry skin

Gastrointestinal: Diarrhea, nausea, vomiting, anorexia, gastrointestinal hemorrhage, stomatitis, heartburn, gastrointestinal ulceration

Hematologic: Myelosuppression, bone marrow depression

Hepatic: Hepatotoxicity

Ocular: Visual disturbances, diplopia, nystagmus, lacrimation, optic neuropathy

Neuromuscular & skeletal: Rhabdomyolysis

Renal: Myoglobinuria

Respiratory: Dyspnea

Miscellaneous: Palmar-plantar erythrodysesthesia syndrome, feces discoloration (black)

Signs & Symptoms of Acute Overdose Alopecia, dermatitis, photosensitivity, hypotonia; pemphigus, lacrimation, coagulopathy, neutropenia, myocarditis, acro-

(Continued)

Fluorouracil *(Continued)*

dynia, hyperkeratosis, encephalopathy, coma, hypercalcemia, drowsiness, cardiogenic shock, bullous skin disease/pemphigoid

Toxicodynamics/Kinetics

Absorption: Oral: Erratic and rarely used

Distribution: V_d: 0.1-0.4 L/kg, ~22% of total body water; penetrates the extracellular fluid, CSF, and third space fluids (such as pleural effusions and ascitic fluid)

Protein binding: 8% to 12%

Metabolism: 5-FU must be metabolized to be active. 90% metabolized; accomplished by a dehydrogenase enzyme primarily found in the liver; dose may need to be omitted in patients with liver failure (bilirubin >5 mg/dL)

Bioavailability: <75%, erratic and undependable

Half-life (biphasic): Initial: 6-20 minutes; doses of 400-600 mg/m^2 produce drug concentrations above the threshold for cytotoxicity for normal tissue and remain there for 6 hours; two metabolites, FdUMP and FUTP, have prolonged half-lives depending on the type of tissue; the clinical effect of these metabolites has not been determined

Elimination: 5% of dose excreted as unchanged drug in the urine in 6 hours, and a large amount excreted as CO_2 from the lung

Usual Dosage Refer to individual protocols

Children and Adults:

I.V.: Initial: 12 mg/kg/day (maximum: 800 mg/day) for 4-5 days; maintenance: 6 mg/kg every other day for 4 doses

Single weekly bolus dose of 15 mg/kg can be administered depending on the patient's reaction to the previous course of treatment; maintenance dose of 5-15 mg/kg/week as a single dose not to exceed 1 g/week

I.V. infusion: 15 mg/kg/day (maximum daily dose: 1 g) has been given by I.V. infusion over 4 hours for 5 days repeated every 4-6 weeks

Alternatively:

I.V. infusion: 1000 mg/m^2 over 24 hours for 4-5 days, **or**

I.V. infusion: 3000 mg/m^2 over 24 hours once each week

Oral: 20 mg/kg/day for 5 days every 5 weeks for colorectal cancer

Dosing adjustment/comments in hepatic impairment: Bilirubin >5 mg/dL: Omit use

5-FU may also be administered intra-arterially or intrahepatically (refer to specific protocols)

Topical:

Actinic or solar keratosis: Apply twice daily for 2-6 weeks

Superficial basal cell carcinomas: Apply 5% twice daily for 3-12 weeks

Administration Administer by direct I.V. push injection (50 mg/mL solution needs no further dilution) or by I.V. infusion in D_5W or NS; toxicity may be reduced by giving the drug as a constant infusion; may be administered through a 25-gauge needle at any convenient rate

Contraindications Hypersensitivity to fluorouracil or any component; patients with poor nutritional status, bone marrow depression

Warnings The U.S. Food and Drug Administration (FDA) currently recommends that procedures for proper handling and disposal of antineoplastic agents be considered. Use with caution in patients who have had high-dose pelvic radiation or previous use of alkylating agents. Patient should be hospitalized during initial course of therapy. Impaired kidney or liver function. The drug should be discontinued if intractable vomiting or diarrhea, precipitous fall in leukocyte or platelet counts, or myocardial ischemia occurs.

Dosage Forms

Cream, topical:

Efudex®: 5% (25 g)

Fluoroplex®: 1% (30 g)

Injection (Adrucil®): 50 mg/mL (10 mL, 20 mL, 50 mL, 100 mL)

Solution, topical:

Efudex®: 2% (10 mL); 5% (10 mL)

Fluoroplex®: 1% (30 mL)

Stability Protect from light; slight discoloration of injection occurring during storage does not adversely affect potency or safety; but discard dark yellow solution; if precipitate forms, redissolve drug by heating to 140°F (60°C), shake well; allow to cool to body temperature before administration; **incompatible** with cytarabine, diazepam, doxorubicin, methotrexate. Concentrations of >25 mg/mL of fluorouracil and >2 mg/mL of leucovorin are **incompatible** (precipitation occurs). **Compatible** with vincristine, methotrexate, potassium chloride, magnesium sulfate.

Reference Range Plasma 5-FU level of 3.37 x $^{-6}$M with dose of 1.25 g/m^2/day

Overdosage Treatment

Decontamination: Emesis or lavage/activated charcoal with cathartic for oral ingestion

Supportive therapy: Allopurinol (300 mg 3 times/day) may be useful in decreasing toxicity

Enhancement of elimination: Forced diuresis or hemodialysis may enhance elimination

Test Interactions Fecal discoloration; may cause elevated total thyroxine level

Drug Interactions Methotrexate: This interaction is schedule dependent; **5-FU should be given following MTX, not prior to**

If MTX is given first: The cells exposed to MTX before 5-FU have a depleted reduced folate pool which inhibits the binding of the 5dUMP to TS. However, it does not interfere with FUTP incorporation into RNA. Polyglutamines, which accumulate in the presence of MTX, may be substituted for the folates and allow binding of FdUMP to TS. MTX given prior to 5-FU may activate 5-FU due to MTX inhibition of purine synthesis.

If 5-FU is given first: 5-FU inhibits the thymidine synthetase binding and thus the reduced folate pool is not depleted, thereby negating the effect of MTX.

Increased effect: Leucovorin: Increases the folate pool and in certain tumors, may promote TS inhibition and increase 5-FU activity. Must be given before or with the 5-FU to prime the cells; it is not used as a rescue agent in this case.

Decreased toxicity:

Allopurinol: Inhibits thymidine phosphorylase (an enzyme that activates 5-FU); antitumor effect of 5-FU appears to be unaltered, but the toxicity is decreased

Increased toxicity: Cimetidine, metronidazole

I.V. administration of fluorouracil and leucovorin are not compatible

Concomitant therapy with folic acid can cause bloody diarrhea

Pregnancy Risk Factor D

Monitoring Parameters CBC with differential and platelet count, renal function tests, liver function tests

Patient Information Avoid unnecessary exposure to sunlight; any signs of infection, easy bruising or bleeding, dyspnea, or painful or burning urination should be brought to physician's attention. Nausea, vomiting, or hair loss sometimes occur. Drug may cause permanent sterility and birth defects; may be excreted in breast milk, therefore, an alternative form of feeding your baby should be used.

Nursing Implications Cool to body temperature before using; after vial has been entered, any unused portion should be discarded within 1 hour; wash hands immediately after topical application of the 5% cream; I.V. formulation may be given orally mixed in water, grape juice, or carbonated beverage

Additional Information Myelosuppressive effects:

WBC: Mild

Platelets: Mild

Onset (days): 7-10

Nadir (days): 9-14

Recovery (days): 21

May be permeable to PVC gloves as opposed to latex gloves

Specific References

Curran CF and Luce JK, "Fluorouracil and Palmar-Plantar Erythrodysesthesia," *Ann Intern Med*, 1989, 111(10):858.

Diasio RB and Harris BE, "Clinical Pharmacology of 5-Fluorouracil," *Clin Pharmacokinet*, 1989, 16(4):215-37.

Kleiman NS, Lehane DE, Geyer CE Jr, et al, "Prinzmetal's Angina During 5-Fluorouracil Chemotherapy," *Am J Med*, 1987, 82(3):566-8.

Mainwaring P and Grygiel JJ, "Interaction of 5-Fluorouracil With Folates," *Aust N Z J Med*, 1995, 25:60.

Pottage A, Holt S, Ludgate S, et al, "Fluorouracil Cardiotoxicity," *Br Med J*, 1978, 1(6112):547.

Trissel LA, Martinez JF, and Xu QA, "Incompatibility of Fluorouracil With Leucovorin Calcium or Levoleucovorin Calcium," *Am J Health-Syst Pharm*, 1995, 52:710-5.

5-Fluorouracil *see* Fluorouracil *on page 357*

Fluoxetine Hydrochloride (floo ox' e teen)

Related Information

Antidepressant Agents Comparison *on page 1639*

CAS Number 54910-89-3

Brand Names Prozac®

Synonyms Fontex; LY-110140

Use Treatment of major depression, premenstrual dysphoria

Mechanism of Action Inhibits CNS neuron serotonin uptake; minimal or no effect on reuptake of norepinephrine or dopamine; does not significantly bind to alpha-adrenergic, histamine or cholinergic receptors; may therefore be useful in patients at risk from sedation, hypotension and anticholinergic effects of tricyclic antidepressants

Adverse Reactions

Cardiovascular: Tachycardia, tachycardia (ventricular) with Q-T interval prolongation, flutter (atrial), bradycardia

(Continued)

Fluoxetine Hydrochloride *(Continued)*

Central nervous system: Nervousness, insomnia, drowsiness, generalized seizures, anxiety, dizziness, fatigue, sedation, suicidal ideation, extrapyramidal reactions (rare), headache, ataxia

Dermatologic: Rash, pruritus, rash, alopecia

Endocrine & metabolic: Hypoglycemia, hyponatremia (elderly or volume-depleted patients), syndrome of inappropriate antidiuretic hormone

Gastrointestinal: Nausea, diarrhea, anorexia, dyspepsia, constipation, dry mouth

Neuromuscular & skeletal: Tremors

Ocular: Visual disturbances, blurred vision

Miscellaneous: Anaphylactoid reactions, excessive sweating, violent self injury

Signs & Symptoms of Acute Overdose Nausea, cystitis, hirsutism, tachycardia (ventricular), Q-T prolongation, insomnia, vasculitis, A-V block, myoclonus, eosinophilia, extrapyramidal reaction, cognitive dysfunction, lightheadedness, leukocytosis, depression, delirium, hallucinations, hyponatremia, hypokalemia, hypoglycemia, spontaneous vomiting, gout, rhabdomyolysis, myoglobinuria, agitation, hypomania, mania, generalized seizures, nystagmus, drowsiness, bradycardia

Toxicodynamics/Kinetics

Onset of action: 1-4 weeks

Peak effect: Antidepressant effects usually occur after more than 4 weeks; due to long half-life, resolution of adverse reactions after discontinuation may be slow

Absorption: Oral: Well absorbed

Distribution: V_d: 27 L/kg; readily crosses blood-brain barrier

Protein binding: 94.5%

Metabolism: To norfluoxetine (active)

Half-life:

Fluoxetine: 2-3 days (range: 1-9 days)

Norfluoxetine: 7-9 days (range: 3-15 days)

Time to peak serum concentration: Within 4-8 hours

Elimination: Excreted in urine as fluoxetine (2.5% to 5%) and norfluoxetine (10%); 15% excreted in feces; renal clearance: 0.6 L/hour/kg

Usual Dosage Oral:

Children <18 years: Dose not established

Adults: 20 mg/day in the morning; may increase after several weeks by 20 mg/day increments; maximum: 80 mg/day; doses >20 mg should be divided into morning and noon doses

Note: Lower doses of 5 mg/day have been used for initial treatment

Premenstrual dysphoria: 20 mg/day

Dosing adjustment in hepatic impairment:

Cirrhosis patients: Administer a lower dose or less frequent dosing interval

Compensated cirrhosis without ascites: Administer 50% of normal dose

Contraindications Hypersensitivity to fluoxetine; patients receiving MAO inhibitors currently or in past 2 weeks

Warnings Avoid alcoholic beverages; due to limited experience, use with caution in patients with renal or hepatic impairment, seizure disorders, cardiac dysfunction; diabetes mellitus; use with caution in patients at high risk for suicide

Dosage Forms

Capsule: 10 mg, 20 mg

Liquid (mint flavor): 20 mg/5 mL (120 mL)

Reference Range Therapeutic:

Fluoxetine: 100-800 ng/mL (SI: 289-2314 nmol/L); serum level of 1956 ng/mL (norfluoxetine level of 416 ng/mL) associated with seizure

Norfluoxetine: 100-600 ng/mL (SI: 289-1735 nmol/L)

Overdosage Treatment

Decontamination: Lavage/activated charcoal with cathartic

Supportive therapy: Toxic symptoms should be treated. Ventricular arrhythmias often respond to phenytoin 15-20 mg/kg (adults) with concurrent systemic alkalinization (sodium bicarbonate 0.5-2 mEq/kg I.V.). Lidocaine may also be useful. Arrhythmias unresponsive to this therapy may respond to lidocaine 1 mg/kg I.V. followed by a titrated infusion. Physostigmine (1-2 mg I.V. slowly for adults or 0.5 mg I.V. slowly for children) may be indicated in reversing cardiac arrhythmias that are due to vagal blockade or for life-threatening anticholinergic effects. Seizures usually respond to lorazepam or diazepam I.V. boluses (5-10 mg for adults up to 30 mg or 0.25-0.4 mg/kg/dose for children up to 10 mg/dose). If seizures are unresponsive or recur, phenytoin or phenobarbital may be required.

Enhancement of elimination: Multiple dosing of activated charcoal may not be useful; hemodialysis does not appear to be useful

Test Interactions Increases albumin in urine; fluoxetine can interfere with bupropion quantitation by HPLC analysis in plasma or serum

Diagnostic Tests/Procedures

Fluoxetine, Blood *on page 1267*

Drug Interactions With MAO inhibitors, fever, tremor, seizures, delirium, coma can occur; with tryptophan or selegiline may cause increased CNS and gastrointestinal toxic effects; fluoxetine may inhibit metabolism and increase effects of tricyclic antidepressants, trazodone, and possibly diazepam; may antagonize buspirone effects and may displace highly protein bound drugs; over 500 mg of fluoxetine combined with ethanol can lead to tachycardia, hypertension, and decrease in the level of consciousness; concomitant use of clarithromycin with fluoxetine can result in fluoxetine intoxication manifesting as delirium; seizures can result with concomitant clomipramine and fluoxetine therapy; myoclonic seizures can result with concomitant fluoxetine and clozapine therapy

Pregnancy Risk Factor B

Patient Information Avoid alcoholic beverages

Nursing Implications Offer patient sugarless hard candy for dry mouth

Additional Information EKG may reveal S-T segment depression; not shown to be teratogenic in rodents; plasma levels may be reliable in reflecting drug concentration in whole blood. Buspirone (15-60 mg/day) may be useful in treatment of sexual dysfunction during treatment with a selective serotonin reuptake inhibitor.

Specific References

Amitai Y, Kennedy E, De Sandre P, et al, "Red Cell and Plasma Concentrations of Fluoxetine and Norfluoxetine," *Vet Hum Toxicol*, 1993, 35(2):134-6.

Borys DJ, Setzer SC, Ling LJ, et al, "Acute Fluoxetine Overdose: A Report of 234 Cases," *Am J Emerg Med*, 1992, 10(2):115-20.

Borys DJ, Setzer SC, Ling LJ, et al, "The Effects of Fluoxetine in the Overdose Patient," *J Toxicol Clin Toxicol*, 1990, 28(3):331-40.

Braiberg G and Curry SC, "Seizure After Isolated Fluoxetine Overdose," *Ann Emerg Med*, 1995, 26:234-7.

Garcia-Monco JC, Padierna A, and Beldarrain MG, "Selegiline, Fluoxetine, and Depression in Parkinson's Disease," *Mov Disord*, 1995, 10:352.

Gardner SF, Rutherford WF, Munger MA, et al, "Drug-Induced Supraventricular Tachycardia: A Case Report of Fluoxetine," *Ann Emerg Med*, 1991, 20(2):194-7.

Gonzalez-Rothi RJ, Zander DS, and Ros PR, "Fluoxetine Hydrochloride (Prozac)-Induced Pulmonary Disease," *Chest*, 1995, 107:1763-5.

Grassi B, Gambini O, and Scarone S, "Severe Bradycardia Following Fluoxetine Administration: A Case Report in a Young HIV-1 Infected Woman," *Human Psychopharmacology: Clinical and Experimental*, 1995, 10:153-5.

Grounds D, Stocky A, Evans P, et al, "Antidepressants and Side Effects," *Aust N Z J Psychiatry*, 1995, 29:156-7.

Hofman M and Liu JK, "Conduction Abnormality and Ventricular Tachyarrhythmia Associated With Fluoxetine Overdose," *Vet Hum Toxicol*, 1994, 36:371.

Jackson C, Carson W, Markowitz J, et al, "SIADH Associated With Fluoxetine and Sertraline Therapy," *Am J Psychiatry*, 1995, 152:809-10.

Jennison TA, Brown P, Crossett J, et al, "A High-Performance Liquid Chromatographic Method for Quantitating Bupropion in Human Plasma or Serum," *J Anal Toxicol*, 1995, 19:69-72.

Kingsbury SJ and Puckett KM, "Effects of Fluoxetine on Serum Clozapine Levels," *Am J Psychiatry*, 1995, 152(3):473-4.

LeJoyeux M, et al, "Serotonin Syndrome: Incidence, Symptoms, and Treatment," *CNS Drugs*, 1994, 2:132-43.

McKenzie LJ and Risch SC, "Fibrocystic Breast Disease Following Treatment With Selective Serotonin Reuptake Inhibitors," *Am J Psychiatry*, 1995, 152(3):471.

Murthy R, Newton K, and Qureshi J, "The Association of Fluoxetine With Seizures," *J Psychopharmacology*, 1994, 8(3):187-8.

Norden MJ, "Buspirone Treatment of Sexual Dysfunction Associated With Selective Serotonin Re-Uptake Inhibitors," *Depression*, 1994, 2:109-12.

Pollak PT, Sketris IS, Mackenzie SL, et al, "Delirium Probably Induced by Clarithromycin in a Patient Receiving Fluoxetine," *Ann Pharmacother*, 1995, 29:486-8.

Spiller HA, Morse S, and Muir C, "Fluoxetine Ingestion: A One Year Retrospective Study," *Vet Hum Toxicol*, 1990, 32(2):153-5.

Steiner M, Steinberg S, Stewart D, et al, "Fluoxetine in the Treatment of Premenstrual Dysphoria,"*N Engl J Med*, 1995, 332:1529-34.

Sternbach H, "Fluoxetine-Clomipramine Interaction," *J Clin Psychiatry*, 1995, 56:171-2.

Fluphenazine (floo fen' a zeen)

Related Information

Antipsychotic Agents Comparison *on page 1642*

CAS Number 69-23-8; 2746-81-8; 146-56-5

Brand Names Moditen®; Permitil®; Prolixin®

Synonyms Fluphenazine Decanoate; Fluphenazine Enanthate; Fluphenazine Hydrochloride

Use Management of manifestations of psychotic disorders

Mechanism of Action Blocks postsynaptic mesolimbic dopaminergic receptors in the brain; exhibits a strong alpha-adrenergic blocking effect and depresses the release of hypothalamic and hypophyseal hormones

Adverse Reactions

Cardiovascular: Hypotension (especially orthostatic), tachycardia, cardiac arrhythmias, abnormal T waves with prolonged ventricular repolarization

Central nervous system: Sedation, drowsiness, restlessness, anxiety, extrapyramidal reactions, dystonic reactions, pseudoparkinsonian signs and symptoms, tardive dyskinesia, neuroleptic malignant syndrome, seizures, altered central temperature regulation

Dermatologic: Hyperpigmentation, pruritus, rash, contact dermatitis, photosensitivity (rare)

(Continued)

Fluphenazine *(Continued)*

Endocrine & metabolic: Amenorrhea, galactorrhea, gynecomastia, syndrome of inappropriate antidiuretic hormone, weight gain

Gastrointestinal: Constipation, adynamic ileus, gastrointestinal upset, dry mouth (problem for denture user), nausea, vomiting

Genitourinary: Urinary retention, overflow incontinence, priapism, sexual dysfunction

Hematologic: Leukopenia/neutropenia (agranulocytosis, granulocytopenia) (usually inpatients with large doses for prolonged periods)

Hepatic: Cholestatic jaundice

Ocular: Blurred vision, photophobia, diplopia, retinal pigmentation, pigmentary deposits in the lens and cornea, bilateral maculopathy

Signs & Symptoms of Acute Overdose Deep sleep, enuresis, hypotension or hypertension, photosensitivity, gynecomastia, lactation, neuroleptic malignant syndrome, ejaculatory disturbances, hyponatremia, depression, hypothermia, dystonic reactions, seizures, extrapyramidal reaction, respiratory failure, Parkinson's-like symptoms, hyperthermia, vision color changes (brown tinge), vision color changes (yellow tinge); Q-T (prolongation), systemic lupus erythematosus (SLE), urine discoloration (pink), urine discoloration (red), urine discoloration (red-brown)

Toxicodynamics/Kinetics

Onset of action: I.M. or S.C.: 24-72 hours

Peak neuroleptic effects: 48-96 hours; effects, onset, and duration are derivative dependent; the hydrochloride salt acts quickly and persist briefly, while the decanoate last the longest and requires more time for onset; following hydrochloride derivative administration, the onset of activity occurs within 1 hour yet persists for only 6-8 hours

Absorption: Varies with route of administration

Distribution: Widely distributed into body

Protein binding: ≥90%

Metabolism: In the liver

Half-life: Half-life is derivative dependent:

- Enanthate: 84-96 hours
- Hydrochloride: 33 hours
- Decanoate: 163-232 hours

Usual Dosage Adults:

Oral: 0.5-10 mg/day in divided doses at 6- to 8-hour intervals; some patients may require up to 40 mg/day

I.M.: 2.5-10 mg/day in divided doses at 6- to 8-hour intervals (parenteral dose is $\frac{1}{3}$ to $\frac{1}{2}$ the oral dose for the hydrochloride salts)

I.M., S.C. (decanoate): 12.5 mg every 3 weeks

Conversion from hydrochloride to decanoate I.M. 0.5 mL (12.5 mg) decanoate every 3 weeks is approximately equivalent to 10 mg hydrochloride/day

I.M., S.C. (enanthate): 12.5-25 mg every 3 weeks

Contraindications Hypersensitivity to fluphenazine or any component, cross-sensitivity with other phenothiazines may exist; avoid use in patients with narrow-angle glaucoma, bone marrow depression, severe liver or cardiac disease

Warnings Watch for hypotension when administering I.M. or I.V.; safety in children <6 months of age has not been established; use with caution in patients with cardiovascular disease or seizures; benefits of therapy must be weighed against risks of therapy; adverse effects may be of longer duration with depot form

Dosage Forms

Concentrate, as hydrochloride:

- Permitil®: 5 mg/mL with alcohol 1% (118 mL)
- Prolixin®: 5 mg/mL with alcohol 14% (120 mL)

Elixir, as hydrochloride (Prolixin®): 2.5 mg/5 mL with alcohol 14% (60 mL, 473 mL)

Injection, as decanoate (Prolixin Decanoate®): 25 mg/mL (1 mL, 5 mL)

Injection, as enanthate (Prolixin Enanthate®): 25 mg/mL (5 mL)

Injection, as hydrochloride (Prolixin®): 2.5 mg/mL (10 mL)

Tablet, as hydrochloride

- Permitil®: 2.5 mg, 5 mg, 10 mg
- Prolixin®: 1 mg, 2.5 mg, 5 mg, 10 mg

Reference Range Therapeutic: 5-20 ng/mL (SI: 10-40 nmol/L)

Overdosage Treatment

Decontamination: Lavage/activated charcoal with cathartic

Supportive therapy: Toxic symptom treatment and supportive treatment should be initiated. Hypotension usually responds to I.V. fluids or Trendelenburg positioning. If unresponsive to these measures, the use of a parenteral inotrope may be required (eg, norepinephrine 0.1-0.2 mcg/kg/minute titrated to response). Seizures commonly respond to lorazepam or diazepam (I.V. 5-10 mg bolus in adults every 15 minutes if needed up to a total of 30 mg; I.V. 0.25-0.4 mg/kg/dose up to a total of 10 mg in children) or to phenytoin or phenobarbital. Also critical cardiac arrhythmias often respond to I.V. phenytoin (15 mg/kg up to 1 g), while other antiarrhythmics can be used. Neuroleptics often cause extrapyramidal reaction (eg, dystonic reactions) requiring management with diphenhydramine 1-2 mg/kg (adults) up to a maximum of 50 mg I.M. or I.V. slow push followed by a maintenance dose for 48-72 hours. When these reactions are unresponsive to diphenhydramine, benztropine mesylate I.V. 1-2 mg (adults) may be effective. These agents are generally effective within 2-5 minutes. Ventricular arrhythmias often respond to quinidine or phenytoin; avoid quinidine or procainamide.

Enhancement of elimination: Multiple dosing of activated charcoal may be useful; not dialyzable (0% to 5%)

Test Interactions Increases cholesterol (S), glucose; decreases uric acid (S)

Diagnostic Tests/Procedures

Fluphenazine, Blood *on page 1268*

Drug Interactions Decreases barbiturate levels and decreases fluphenazine effectiveness when given together; with ethanol effects of both drugs may be increased; EPSEs and other CNS effects may be increased when coadministered with lithium; may potentiate the effects of narcotics including apnea; clonidine administration with fluphenazine may cause delirium

Pregnancy Risk Factor C (extrapyramidal reaction may develop in neonates from maternally administered drug)

Pregnancy Implications Crosses the placenta; appears in breast milk

Monitoring Parameters EKG monitoring for 48 hours

Patient Information Avoid alcoholic beverages

Nursing Implications Dilute oral concentrate solution in juice before administration; avoid contact of oral solution or injection with skin (contact dermatitis); watch for hypotension when administering I.M. or I.V.

Additional Information Oral liquid to be diluted in the following **only**: water, saline, 7-UP®, homogenized milk, carbonated orange beverages, pineapple, apricot, prune, orange, V8® juice, tomato, and grapefruit juices; benztropine can be used to treat nausea/vomiting

Specific References

Cheung HK and Yu EC, "Effect of 1050 mg Fluphenazine Decanoate Given Intramuscularly Over Six Days," *Br Med J (Clin Res)*, 1983, 286(6370):1016-7.

Fishbain DA, "Priapism Resulting From Fluphenazine Hydrochloride Treatment Reversed by Diphenhydramine," *Ann Emerg Med*, 1985, 14(6):600-2.

Oshika T, "Ocular Adverse Effects of Neuropsychiatric Agents: Incidence and Management," *Drug Saf*, 1995, 12:256-63.

Fluphenazine Decanoate *see* Fluphenazine *on page 361*

Fluphenazine Enanthate *see* Fluphenazine *on page 361*

Fluphenazine Hydrochloride *see* Fluphenazine *on page 361*

Flura® *see* Fluoride *on page 355*

Flura-Drops® *see* Fluoride *on page 355*

Flura-Loz® *see* Fluoride *on page 355*

Flurazepam Hydrochloride (flure az' e pam)

Related Information

Benzodiazepines Comparison *on page 1643*

CAS Number 17617-23-1; 1172-18-5

Brand Names Benozil®; Dalmane®; Staurodorm®

Use Short-term treatment of insomnia

Mechanism of Action Depresses all levels of the CNS, including the limbic and reticular formation, probably through the increased action of gamma-aminobutyric acid (GABA), which is a major inhibitory neurotransmitter in the brain

Adverse Reactions

Central nervous system: Drowsiness, dizziness, confusion, residual daytime sedation, paradoxical reactions, hyperactivity and excitation (rare), ataxia

Gastrointestinal: Dysgeusia

Hematologic: Porphyria

Miscellaneous: Physical and psychological dependence with prolonged use, porphyrinogenic

Ocular: Diplopia

Signs & Symptoms of Acute Overdose Apnea, respiratory depression, hyporeflexia, hypoactive reflexes, asterixis, unsteady gait, metallic taste, hypotension, coma, hyperactivity, drowsiness, ataxia, mydriasis, adult respiratory distress syndrome, nystagmus

Toxicodynamics/Kinetics

Onset of action: 15-20 minutes

Peak effect: 3-6 hours

Duration: 7-8 hours

(Continued)

Flurazepam Hydrochloride *(Continued)*

Absorption: Rapid through gastrointestinal tract
Distribution: V_d: 3.4 L/kg; widely distributed throughout the body
Protein binding: 97%
Metabolism: In the liver to N-desalkylflurazepam (active)
Half-life: Adults: 40-114 hours; N-desalkylflurazepam: 47-100 hours
Elimination: Prolonged in the elderly; accumulation of the parent drug and its metabolite occurs

Usual Dosage Oral:

Children:
- <15 years: Dose not established
- >15 years: 15 mg at bedtime

Adults: 15-30 mg at bedtime

Contraindications Hypersensitivity to flurazepam or any component (there may be cross-sensitivity with other benzodiazepines); pregnancy, pre-existing CNS depression, respiratory depression, narrow-angle glaucoma

Warnings Do not use in pregnant women; may cause drug dependency; safety and efficacy have not been established in children <15 years of age; use with caution in patients receiving other CNS depressants, patients with low albumin, hepatic dysfunction and in the elderly

Dosage Forms Capsule: 15 mg, 30 mg

Stability Store in light-resistant containers

Reference Range

Therapeutic: 0-4 ng/mL (SI: 0-9 nmol/L)
Metabolite N-desalkylflurazepam: 20-110 ng/mL (SI: 43-240 nmol/L)
Toxic: >0.12 μg/mL

Overdosage Treatment

Decontamination: Lavage/activated charcoal with cathartic

Supportive therapy: Treatment for benzodiazepine overdose is supportive. Rarely is mechanical ventilation required. Flumazenil has been shown to selectively block the binding of benzodiazepines to CNS receptors, resulting in a reversal of benzodiazepine-induced CNS depression. Hypotension can be treated with isotonic intravenous fluids with placement in Trendelenburg position; dopamine and norepinephrine can be used.

Enhancement of elimination: Forced diuresis or hemodialysis is not useful; multiple dosing of activated charcoal may be useful

Diagnostic Tests/Procedures

Flurazepam, Blood *on page 1268*

Drug Interactions Additive CNS depression with other CNS depressants, cimetidine may decrease and enzyme inducers may increase metabolism of flurazepam

Pregnancy Risk Factor X

Monitoring Parameters Respiratory and cardiovascular status

Patient Information Avoid alcohol and other CNS depressants; avoid activities needing good psychomotor coordination until CNS effects are known; drug may cause physical or psychological dependence; avoid abrupt discontinuation after prolonged use

Nursing Implications Provide safety measures (ie, side rails, night light, and call button); remove smoking materials from area; supervise ambulation; avoid abrupt discontinuance in patients with prolonged therapy or seizure disorders

Specific References

Ruff RL, Kutt H, and Hafler D, "Prolonged Benzodiazepine Coma," *N Y State J Med*, 1981, 81(5):776-7.

Stringer MD, "Adult Respiratory Distress Syndrome Associated With Flurazepam Overdose," *J R Soc Med*, 1985, 78(1)1:74-5.

Flurbiprofen Sodium (flure bi' proe fen)

Related Information

Ibuprofen *on page 418*
Nonsteroidal Anti-Inflammatory Comparison *on page 1655*

CAS Number 5104-49-4

Brand Names Ansaid®; Cebotid®; Froben®; Ocufen®; Ocuflur®

Use Inhibition of intraoperative miosis; acute or long-term treatment of signs of symptoms of rheumatoid arthritis and osteoarthritis; prevention and management of postoperative ocular inflammation and postoperative cystoid macular edema remains to be determined

Mechanism of Action Proprionic acid derivative (like ibuprofen); inhibits prostaglandin synthesis by decreasing the activity of the enzyme, cyclo-oxygenase, which results in decreased formation of prostaglandin precursors

Adverse Reactions

Cardiovascular: Fluid retention, circulatory collapse
Central nervous system: Headache, aseptic meningitis, psychosis, cognitive dysfunction, coma, seizures

Dermatologic: Rash, pruritus

Endocrine & metabolic: Hyperkalemia, anion gap metabolic acidosis

Gastrointestinal: Abdominal pain, nausea, vomiting, bleeding, ulceration, constipation, diarrhea, dyspepsia

Genitourinary: Albuminuria

Hematologic: Leukopenia, neutropenia, agranulocytosis, granulocytopenia; aplastic anemia (rare), platelet inhibition

Hepatic: Elevation of transaminases, fulminant hepatitis

Ocular: Diplopia

Otic: Ototoxicity, tinnitus

Respiratory: Wheezing, respiratory depression

Renal: Renal failure (acute), nephrotic syndrome, chronic renal failure

Miscellaneous: Hypersensitivity

Signs & Symptoms of Acute Overdose Nausea, vomiting, wheezing, gastrointestinal bleeding, gastritis; cognitive dysfunction, nephrotic syndrome, ototoxicity; tinnitus, drowsiness; severe poisoning can manifest with coma, seizures, renal and or hepatic failure, hypotension, respiratory depression

Toxicodynamics/Kinetics

Absorption: Rapid; penetrates cornea; significant systemic absorption may occur; peak concentrations at ~90 minutes

Distribution: V_d: 0.13 L/kg

Protein binding: 99%

Metabolism: Unknown

Half-life: 3.8 hours

Time to peak serum concentration: Within 1.5-2 hours

Elimination: Excreted by kidneys primarily as glucuronides and sulfates; clearance: 0.03-0.3 L/hour/kg

Usual Dosage

Oral: Rheumatoid arthritis and osteoarthritis: 200-300 mg/day in 2, 3, or 4 divided doses

Ophthalmic: Instill 1 drop every 30 minutes, 2 hours prior to surgery (total of 4 drops to each affected eye)

Dosage Forms

Solution, ophthalmic (Ocufen®): 0.03% (2.5 mL, 5 mL, 10 mL)

Tablet (Ansaid®): 50 mg, 100 mg

Reference Range

Mean steady-state levels: ~6 mg/mL (not age-dependent)

Peak serum flurbiprofen levels after a single 50 mg dose: ~8-9.4 mg/L

Overdosage Treatment

Decontamination: Ipecac or lavage/activated charcoal with cathartic

Supportive therapy: Hypotension/dehydration can be managed with intravenous fluid therapy; acidosis should be treated with bicarbonates, seizures with benzodiazepines; antacids, blood products are indicated, as appropriate, for hemorrhage

Enhancement of elimination: Dialysis or perfusion is indicated for secondary complications, acidosis, or renal failure and not toxin removal alone; multiple dosing of activated charcoal may be effective

Drug Interactions Aspirin decreases serum concentrations probably by protein-binding displacement; there is an increased bleeding potential with concomitant warfarin therapy; may increase lithium and methotrexate concentrations by decreasing renal clearance; may decrease diuretic and hypotensive effects of thiazides, loop diuretics, ACE inhibitors; may increase nephrotoxicity of cyclosporine; cimetidine (but not ranitidine) can increase flurbiprofen levels; flurbiprofen inhibits the metabolism of phenazone; actuates the hypotensive effect of propranolol (but not atenolol)

Pregnancy Risk Factor C

Pregnancy Implications Renal failure related to *in utero* exposure

Nursing Implications Care should be taken to avoid contamination of the solution container tip

Specific References

Albert KS, Gillespie WR, Raabe A, et al, "Determination of Flurbiprofen in Human Serum by Reverse-Phase High-Performance Liquid Chromatography With Fluorescence Detection," *J Pharm Sci*, 1984, 73(12):1823-5.

Brooks CD, Linet OI, Schellenberg D, et al, "Clinical Safety of Flurbiprofen," *J Clin Pharmacol*, 1990, 30(4):342-51.

Court H and Volans GN, "Poisoning After Overdose With Nonsteroidal Anti-inflammatory Drugs," *Adverse Drug React Acute Poisoning Rev*, 1984, 3(1):1-21.

Davis NM, "Clinical Pharmacokinetics of Flurbiprofen and its Enantiomers," *Clin Pharmacokinet*, 1995, 28(2):100-14.

Hoppmann RA, Peden JG, and Ober SK, "Central Nervous System Side Effects of Nonsteroidal Anti-inflammatory Drugs. Aseptic Meningitis, Psychosis, and Cognitive Dysfunction," *Arch Intern Med*, 1991, 151(7):1309-13.

Lesko SM and Mitchell AA, "An Assessment of the Safety of Pediatric Ibuprofen; A Practitioner-Based Randomized Clinical Trial," *JAMA*, 1995, 273(12):929-33.

(Continued)

Flurbiprofen Sodium *(Continued)*

Smolinske SC, Hall AH, Vandenberg SA, et al, "Toxic Effects of Nonsteroid Anti-inflammatory Drugs in Overdose. An Overview of Recent Evidence on Clinical Effects and Dose-Response Relationships," *Drug Saf*, 1990, 5(4):252-74.

Vale JA and Meredith TJ, "Acute Poisoning Due to Nonsteroidal Anti-inflammatory Drugs," *Med Toxicol*, 1986, 1(1):12-31.

Verbeeck RK, "Pharmacokinetic Drug Interactions With Nonsteroidal Anti-inflammatory Drugs," *Clin Pharmacokinet*, 1990, 19(1):44-66.

Fluroblastin® *see* Fluorouracil *on page 357*

Fluroblastine® *see* Fluorouracil *on page 357*

Flutamide (floo' ta mide)

CAS Number 13311-84-7

Brand Names Drogenil®; Euflex®; Eulexin®; Eulexine®; Flucinome®; Fugerel®; Niftolid®

Use Palliative treatment for prostatic carcinoma

Mechanism of Action Nonsteroidal antiandrogen with properties which block the action of dihydrotestosterone on the prostatic tissue and testes

Adverse Reactions

Cardiovascular: Hypertension

Dermatologic: Rash, photosensitivity

Endocrine & metabolic: Gynecomastia (10%), galactorrhea, hot flashes (60%), impotence (30%), sexual dysfunction

Gastrointestinal: Vomiting, nausea, diarrhea, anorexia (5%)

Hematologic: Anemia, leukopenia, thrombocytopenia

Hepatic: Hepatitis, jaundice

Signs & Symptoms of Acute Overdose Apnea, ataxia, hypoactivity, lacrimation, lethargy, vomiting, methemoglobinemia (up to 16.2% has been described)

Toxicodynamics/Kinetics

Protein binding: 92% to 96%

Metabolism: Primarily metabolite is 2-hydroxyflutamide (active); rapidly metabolized

Half-life: 2-hydroxyflutamide: 5-6 hours in healthy adults; 8 hours in elderly

Peak plasma level: 2-4 hours

Elimination: Renal (94%), feces (4%)

Usual Dosage Prostatic cancer: Oral: 250 mg every 8 hours (usually used in conjunction with leuprolide - a leuteinizing hormone-releasing hormone) to produce medical castration

Contraindications Hypersensitivity to flutamide

Dosage Forms Capsule: 125 mg

Reference Range At steady-state; plasma 2-hydroxyflutamide levels range from 1556-2284 ng/mL

Overdosage Treatment

Decontamination: Emesis or lavage/activated charcoal with cathartic

Supportive therapy: Treat symptomatic methemoglobinemia with methylene blue

Enhancement of elimination: Multiple dosing of activated charcoal may be beneficial; hemodialysis is not expect to be of benefit

Drug Interactions Increased prothrombin time and bleeding may occur with warfarin administration

Pregnancy Risk Factor D

Patient Information Male feminization is common

Additional Information Diarrhea may occur due to lactose intolerance; plasma testosterone and estradiol levels may be elevated

Specific References

Moller S, Iversen P, and Franzmann MB, "Flutamide-Induced Liver Failure," *J Hepatol*, 1990, 10(3):346-9.

Schott AM, Vial T, Gozzo I, et al, "Flutamide-Induced Methemoglobinemia," *DICP*, 1991, 25(4):600-1.

Yagoda A, "Flutamide-Induced Diarrhea Secondary to Lactose Intolerance," *J Natl Cancer Inst*, 1989, 81(23):1839-40.

Fluvoxamine

Brand Names Luvox®

Use Treatment of major depression and obsessive-compulsive disorder (OCD)

Mechanism of Action Serotonin reuptake inhibitor

Adverse Reactions

Central nervous system: Somnolence, headache, agitation, insomnia, dizziness, psychosis, syncope, tremors, hypokinesia, asthenia, akathisia, electroencephalogram abnormalities

Gastrointestinal: Dry mouth, nausea, vomiting, constipation

Hepatic: Elevated liver function tests

Signs & Symptoms of Acute Overdose No published reports; insomnia, coma, tachycardia, Stevens-Johnson syndrome, amenorrhea, mania, toxic epidermal necrolysis, depression, bradycardia, syndrome of inappropriate antidiuretic hormone (SIADH), hypotension, elevated liver function tests, seizures, death

Toxicodynamics/Kinetics

Absorption: Rapid and complete

Time to peak concentration: 5 hours

Distribution: V_d: 25 L/kg

Metabolism: Extensive to inactive metabolites

Half-life, elimination: 15 hours, increased in elderly

Usual Dosage Initiate at 50 mg/day; usual therapeutic dose: 100-300 mg/day in divided doses

Warnings Use with caution in patients with seizures

Dosage Forms Tablet: 50 mg, 100 mg

Overdosage Treatment

Decontamination: Lavage/activated charcoal with cathartic

Supportive therapy: Miaserin (15 mg at night) has been used to treat fluvoxamine-induced akathisia

Enhancement of elimination: Multiple dose activated charcoal may be useful

Drug Interactions Fluvoxamine inhibits cytochrome $P450IID_6$, $P450IIIA_4$ and may increase propranolol, warfarin, amitriptyline, clomipramine, imipramine, diazepam, alprazolam, terfenadine, astemizole; use with MAO inhibitors or other serotonin reuptake inhibitors, hyperpyrexia, tachycardia, seizures, death can occur

Pregnancy Risk Factor C

Pregnancy Implications No known data; excreted in breast milk at 30% serum concentrations

Specific References

Benfield P, and Ward A, "Fluvoxamine: A Review of Its Pharmacodynamic and Pharmacokinetic Properties, and Therapeutic Efficacy in Depressive Illness," *Drugs*, 1986, 32(4):313-34.

Grimsley SR, and Jann MW, "Paroxetine, Sertraline, and Fluvoxamine: New Selective Serotonin Reuptake Inhibitors," *Clin Pharm*, 1992, 11(11):930-57.

LeJoyeux M, et al, "Serotonin Syndrome: Incidence, Symptoms, and Treatment," *CNS Drugs*, 1994, 2:132-43.

Poyurovsky M, Meerovich I, and Weizman A, "Beneficial Effect of Low Dose Mianserin on Fluvoxamine-Induced Akathisia in an Obsessive-Compulsive Patient," *Clin Psychopharmaco*, 1995, 10:111-4.

Van Harten J, "Clinical Pharmacokinetics of Selective Serotonin Reuptake Inhibitors," *Clin Pharmacokinet*, 1993, 24(3):203-20.

Foille Plus® [OTC] *see* Benzocaine *on page 149*

Folex® *see* Methotrexate *on page 515*

Fontego® *see* Bumetanide *on page 167*

Fontex *see* Fluoxetine Hydrochloride *on page 359*

Fordiuran® *see* Bumetanide *on page 167*

Formosa Camphor *see* Camphor *on page 179*

Formula Q® [OTC] *see* Quinine Sulfate *on page 671*

Fortal® *see* Pentazocine *on page 603*

Fortral® *see* Pentazocine *on page 603*

Fortulgesic® *see* Pentazocine *on page 603*

Fortunan® *see* Haloperidol *on page 396*

Fortwin® *see* Pentazocine *on page 603*

Fosamax® *see* Alendronate *on page 94*

Foscarnet Sodium (fos kar' net)

CAS Number 63585-09-1; 34156-56-4

Brand Names Foscavir® Injection

Synonyms PFA; Phosphonoformate; Phosphonoformic Acid

Use Alternative to ganciclovir for treatment of CMV retinitis and other CMV infections; alternative to acyclovir for treatment of acyclovir-resistant HSV infections

Mechanism of Action Pyrophosphate analogue which acts as a noncompetitive inhibitor of many viral RNA and DNA polymerases as well as HIV reverse transcriptase. Inhibitory effects occur at concentrations which do not affect host cellular DNA polymerases; however, some human cell growth suppression has been observed with high *in vitro* concentrations. Similar to ganciclovir, foscarnet is a virostatic agent. Foscarnet does not require activation by thymidine kinase.

Adverse Reactions

Cardiovascular: Cardiomyopathy

Central nervous system: Fatigue, fever, headache, seizures (10%), hallucinations, electroencephalogram abnormalities

Endocrine & metabolic: Hypocalcemia, hypomagnesemia, hypokalemia, change in serum phosphorus, hypophosphatemia

(Continued)

Foscarnet Sodium *(Continued)*

Gastrointestinal: Nausea, diarrhea, dyspepsia, vomiting
Hematologic: Decreases in hemoglobin and hematocrit
Hepatic: Increases in liver enzymes
Local: Thrombophlebitis
Neuromuscular & skeletal: Paresthesia
Renal: Abnormal renal function including renal failure, albuminuria
Miscellaneous: Decreased creatinine clearance at continuous dosing of 130-230 mg/kg/day, penile ulceration (at 7-24 days), nephrogenic diabetes insipidus

Signs & Symptoms of Acute Overdose Seizures, wheezing, malaise, dementia, depression, hypercalcemia, thrombocytopenia, hypophosphatemia, lymphopenia, leukocytosis, dementia, hyponatremia, myalgia, meningitis, hypomagnesemia, nocturia, hypokalemia, leg cramps, dysuria, dysphagia, dry mouth, cough, renal dysfunction, perioral or limb paresthesias, hypocalcemia

Toxicodynamics/Kinetics

Absorption: Oral: Poor; I.V. therapy is needed for the treatment of viral infections in AIDS patients
Distribution: V_d: 0.3-0.6 L/kg; up to 28% of cumulative I.V. dose may be deposited in bone
Protein binding: 14% to 17%
Metabolism: Biotransformation does not occur
Half-life: ~3 hours
Elimination: Up to 28% excreted unchanged in urine

Usual Dosage See tables:

Dose Adjustment for Renal Impairment

The induction dose of foscarnet should be adjusted according to creatinine clearance as follows:

Creatinine Clearance (mL/min/kg)	Foscarnet Induction Dose (mg/kg q8h)
≥ 1.6	60
1.5	57
1.4	53
1.3	49
1.2	46
1.1	42
1	39
0.9	35
0.8	32
0.7	28
0.6	25
0.5	21
0.4	18

The maintenance dose of foscarnet should be adjusted according to creatinine clearance as follows:

Creatinine Clearance (mL/min/kg)	Foscarnet Maintenance Dose (mg/kg/day)
≥1.4	90–120
1.2–1.4	78–104
1–1.2	75–100
0.8–1	71–94
0.6–0.8	63–84
0.4–0.6	57–75

Induction treatment: 60 mg/kg 3 times/day for 14-21 days
Maintenance therapy: 90-120 mg/kg/day

Administration Administer diluted to 12 mg/mL through a peripheral line; may be administered undiluted through a central line; infuse over 1 hour

Contraindications Hypersensitivity to foscarnet, Cl_{cr} <0.4 mL/minute/kg during therapy

Warnings Renal insufficiency, concomitant administration of other potentially nephrotoxic drugs, patients should be adequately hydrated during therapy, frequent alterations in plasma electrolytes that have led to seizures; patients with history of seizures

Dosage Forms Injection: 24 mg/mL (250 mL, 500 mL)

Stability Do not admix or run with other drugs, multiple incompatibilities

Reference Range Therapeutic for CMV: 150 μg/mL

Overdosage Treatment

Supportive therapy: I.V. calcium salts for hypocalcemia; I.V. hydration is essential

Enhancement of elimination: Hemodialysis may be useful to aid in removal of the drug, although this has not been formally studied

Drug Interactions Concurrent use with pentamidine can cause severe hypocalcemia; additive effect on anemia when used in conjunction with zidovudine; concurrent use with cyclosporin can result in reversable renal failure

Pregnancy Risk Factor C

Monitoring Parameters Serum creatinine, calcium, phosphorus, potassium, magnesium; hemoglobin

Patient Information Foscarnet is not a cure; disease may progress; keep well hydrated; frequent ophthalmologic examinations and blood samples are needed

Nursing Implications Provide adequate hydration with I.V. normal saline prior to and during treatment to minimize nephrotoxicity

Specific References

Calligaro KD, Stern J, and DeLaurentis DA, "Foscarnet: A Possible Cause of Ulnar Artery Thrombosis in a Patient With AIDS," *J Vasc Surg*, 1994, 20(6):1007-8.

Jacobson MA, "Review of the Toxicities of Foscarnet," *J Acquir Immune Defic Syndr*, 1992, 5(Suppl 1):S11-7.

Morales JM, Munoz MA, Fernandez Zatarain G, et al, "Reversable Acute Renal Failure Caused by the Combined Use of Foscarnet and Cyclosporin in Organ Transplanted Patients," *Nephrol Dial Transplant*, 1995, 10:882-3.

Foscavir® Injection *see* Foscarnet Sodium *on page 367*

Fosinopril Sodium (foe sin' oh pril)

Related Information

ACE Inhibitors Comparison *on page 1636-1637*

CAS Number 97825-24-6; 88889-14-9

Brand Names Monopril®; Staril®

Use Treatment of hypertension, either alone or in combination with other antihypertensive agents; congestive heart failure

Mechanism of Action Competitive inhibition of angiotensin I being converted to angiotensin II, a potent vasoconstrictor, through the angiotensin I-converting enzyme (ACE) activity, with resultant lower levels of angiotensin II which causes an increase in plasma renin activity and a reduction in aldosterone secretion

Adverse Reactions

Cardiovascular: Orthostatic hypotension

Central nervous system: Headache, fatigue, dizziness, syncope, vertigo, insomnia

Dermatologic: Angioedema, rash

Endocrine & metabolic: Hypoglycemia, hyperkalemia

Gastrointestinal: Diarrhea, nausea, vomiting

Genitourinary: Sexual dysfunction, impotence

Hematologic: Neutropenia, agranulocytosis, anemia

Neuromuscular & skeletal: Muscle cramps

Renal: Deterioration in renal function, proteinuria

Respiratory: Cough (3%)

Miscellaneous: Loss of taste perception

Toxicodynamics/Kinetics

Protein binding: 95%

Metabolism: Fosinopril is a prodrug and is hydrolyzed to its active metabolite fosinoprilat via gut wall and hepatic esterases

Serum half-life: 3-4 hours; 12 hours for fosinoprilat

Bioavailability: 30% to 36%

Time to peak serum concentration: ~3 hours

Elimination: Eliminated in urine and bile as fosinoprilat, and it conjugates in roughly equal proportions; renal clearance: 17 mL/minute

Usual Dosage Adults: Oral: Initial: 10 mg/day and increase to a maximum dose of 80 mg/day; most patients are maintained on 20-40 mg/day

Contraindications Renal impairment, collagen vascular disease, hypersensitivity to fosinopril or any component

Warnings Use with caution and modify dosage in patients with renal impairment (decrease dosage) (especially renal artery stenosis), severe congestive heart failure or with coadministered diuretic therapy; experience in children is limited. Se-

(Continued)

Fosinopril Sodium *(Continued)*

vere hypotension may occur in patients who are sodium and/or volume depleted; initiate lower doses and monitor closely when starting therapy in these patients.

Dosage Forms Tablet: 10 mg, 20 mg

Reference Range Peak serum fosinoprilat level after a 40 mg dose: ~600 ng/mL

Overdosage Treatment

Decontamination: Lavage/activated charcoal

Supportive therapy: Following initiation of essential overdose management, toxic symptom treatment and supportive treatment should be initiated. Hypotension usually responds to I.V. fluids or Trendelenburg positioning. If unresponsive to these measures, the use of a parenteral inotrope may be required (eg, norepinephrine 0.1-0.2 mcg/kg/minute titrated to response). Seizures commonly respond to diazepam (I.V. 5-10 mg bolus in adults every 15 minutes if needed up to a total of 30 mg; I.V. 0.25-0.4 mg/kg/dose up to a total of 10 mg in children) or to phenytoin or phenobarbital. Naloxone has been shown to antagonize hypotensive effects of captopril, but routine use in an overdose situation due to this agent is uncertain.

Enhancement of elimination: Multiple dosing of activated charcoal may be effective; hemodialysis is not effective

Test Interactions Positive Coombs' [direct]; may cause false-positive results in urine acetone determinations using sodium nitroprusside reagent; may cause a falsely low serum digoxin level (with Digi-Tab® RIA kit)

Drug Interactions

Decreased effect: NSAIDs

Increased levels/toxicity: Lithium (3-fold level increase); hyperkalemia may occur with potassium-sparing diuretics

Pregnancy Risk Factor D

Monitoring Parameters Serum potassium

Patient Information Notify physician if vomiting, diarrhea, excessive perspiration, or dehydration should occur; also if swelling of face, lips, tongue or difficulty in breathing occurs or if persistent cough develops

Nursing Implications May cause depression in some patients; discontinue if angioedema of the face, extremities, lips, tongue, or glottis occurs; watch for hypotensive effects within 1-3 hours of first dose or new higher dose

Additional Information Some patients may have a decreased hypotensive effect between 12-16 hours; consider dividing total daily dose into 2 doses 12 hours apart; if patient is receiving a diuretic, a potential for first-dose hypotension is increased; to decrease this potential, stop diuretic for 2-3 days prior to initiating fosinopril if possible; continue diuretic if needed to control blood pressure

Due to frequent decreases in glomerular filtration (also creatinine clearance) with aging, elderly patients may have exaggerated responses to ACE inhibitors; differences in clinical response due to hepatic changes are not observed. ACE inhibitors may be preferred agents in elderly patients with congestive heart failure and diabetes mellitus. Diabetic proteinuria is reduced and insulin sensitivity is enhanced. In general, the side effect profile is favorable in elderly and causes little or no CNS confusion; use lowest dose recommendations initially.

Specific References

Anderson RJ, Duchin KL, Gore RD, et al, "Once-Daily Fosinopril in the Treatment of Hypertension," *Hypertension*, 1991, 17(5):636-42.

Binder SB, "ACE Inhibitors: Review of Four New Agents," *Am Fam Physician*, 1993, 48(5):851-7.

Guthrie R, "Fosinopril: An Overview," *Am J Cardiol*, 1993, 72(20):22H-4H.

Herings RM, deBoer A, Stricker BH, et al, "Hypoglycemia Associated With Use of Inhibitors of Angiotensin Converting Enzyme," *Lancet*, 1995, 345:1195-8.

Murdoch D and McTavish D, "Fosinopril: A Review of Its Pharmacodynamic and Pharmacokinetic Properties, and Therapeutic Potential in Essential Hypertension," *Drugs*, 1992, 43(1):123-40.

Fosphenytoin

Synonyms 3-Phosphoryloxymethyl Phenytoin Disodium

Use Investigational: Management of generalized tonic-clonic (grand mal), simple partial and complex partial seizures; prevention of seizures following head trauma/ neurosurgery; ventricular arrhythmias, including those associated with digitalis intoxication; beneficial effects in the treatment of migraine or trigeminal neuralgia in some patients; usually used in short-term seizure management

Mechanism of Action Diphosphate ester salt of phenytoin which acts as a water soluble pro-drug of phenytoin; after administration, plasma esterases convert to phenytoin as the active moiety

Adverse Reactions

Central nervous system: Slurred speech, dizziness, drowsiness, drowsiness, choreoathetosis, fever, visual hallucinations

Dermatologic: Rash, exfoliative dermatitis, erythema multiforme, facial edema, acne

Endocrine & metabolic: Folic acid depletion, osteomalacia, hyperglycemia, reduced plasma testosterone, gynecomastia

Gastrointestinal: Nausea, vomiting, gingival hyperplasia
Genitourinary: Priapism
Hematologic: Lymphadenopathy, neutropenia, thrombocytopenia, anemia (megaloblastic)
Local: Pain on injection
Neuromuscular & skeletal: Sensory paresthesia (long-term treatment)
Ocular: Nystagmus, blurred vision, diplopia
Renal: Nephrotic syndrome
Miscellaneous: Due to the fact that fosphenytoin is water soluble and has a lower pH (8.8) than phenytoin (12), necrosis or irritation at injection site is reduced

Signs & Symptoms of Acute Overdose Unsteady gait, tremors, hyperglycemia, chorea (extrapyramidal), gingival hyperplasia, gynecomastia, myoglobinuria, nephrotic syndrome, slurred speech, mydriasis, myoclonus, confusion, encephalopathy, hyperthermia, drowsiness, nausea, hypothermia, fever, hypotension, respiratory depression, leukopenia; neutropenia; agranulocytosis; granulocytopenia; hyperreflexia, coma, systemic lupus erythematosus (SLE), ophthalmoplegia

Toxicodynamics/Kinetics Pharmacokinetics appear to be similar to phenytoin
Onset of action: I.V.: 3-5 minutes
Absorption: Oral: Slow
Distribution: Into CSF, saliva, semen, gastrointestinal fluids, bile, and breast milk
V_d:
Premature Neonates: 1-1.2 L/kg
Full-term Neonates: 0.8-0.9 L/kg
Infants: 0.7-0.8 L/kg
Children: 0.7 L/kg
Adults: 0.6-0.7 L/kg
Protein binding: Adults: 90% to 95%, increased free fraction (decreased protein binding) in neonates (up to 20% free), infants (up to 15% free), and patients with hyperbilirubinemia, hypoalbuminemia, uremia
Metabolism: Broken down by phosphatases to phenytoin, formaldehyde, and phosphate; follows dose-dependent (Michaelis-Menten) pharmacokinetics with increased Vmax in infants >6 months and children vs adults; major metabolite (via oxidation) HPPA undergoes enterohepatic recycling
Bioavailability: I.M., I.V.: 100%
Half-life:
Fosphenytoin:
I.M.: 33 minutes
I.V.: 8 minutes
Phenytoin: 2-4 hours
Conversion to phenytoin:
I.M.: 32.7 minutes
I.V.: 7.6-8.9 minutes
Peak serum levels:
I.M.: 36-38.6 minutes
I.V.: 5.7-49 minutes
Elimination: Highly variable clearance, dependent upon intrinsic hepatic function and dose administered; elimination in urine as glucuronides; <5% excreted unchanged in urine; increased clearance and decreased serum concentrations with febrile illness

Usual Dosage
I.M.: Up to 450 mg has been used in adults
I.V.: 14-17 mg/kg (suggested); doses up to 3000 mg (38 mg/kg) have been used. Rates as high as 150-218 mg/minute have been administered. Usual infusion time: ~30 minutes

Contraindications Hypersensitivity to phenytoin or fosphenytoin; occurrence of any rash while on treatment; the drug should not be resumed if rash is exfoliative, purpuric, or bullous; not recommended for use in children <4 years of age

Warnings Use with caution in patients with severe cardiovascular, hepatic, renal disease or diabetes mellitus; avoid abrupt discontinuation; dosing should be slowly reduced to avoid precipitation of seizures; increased toxicity with nephrotic syndrome patient; may increase frequency of petit mal seizures; use with caution in patients with porphyria, fever, or hypothyroidism

Dosage Forms 150 mg (2 mL); 750 mg (10 mL)

Stability Refrigerated vials are stable for 2 years; at room temperature, stable for 3 months; I.V. solutions are stable for one day when refrigerated

Reference Range
Therapeutic: 10-20 μg/mL (SI: 40-79 μmol/L); toxicity is measured clinically, and some patients require levels outside the suggested therapeutic range
Toxic: 30-50 μg/mL (SI: 120-200 μmol/L)
Lethal: >100 μg/mL (SI: >400 μmol/L)

Manifestations of toxicity:
Nystagmus: 20 μg/mL (SI: 79 μmol/L)

(Continued)

Fosphenytoin *(Continued)*

Ataxia: 30 μg/mL (SI: 118.9 μmol/L)
Decreased mental status: 40 μg/mL (SI: 159 μmol/L)
Coma: 50 μg/mL (SI: 200 μmol/L)

Peak serum phenytoin level after a 375 mg I.M. fosphenytoin dose in healthy males: 5.7 μg/mL

Peak serum fosphenytoin levels and phenytoin levels after a 1.2 g infusion (I.V.) in healthy subjects over 30 minutes were 129 μg/mL and 17.2 μg/mL respectively

Overdosage Treatment

Supportive therapy: Treatment is supportive for hypotension; treat with I.V. fluids and place patient in Trendelenburg position; seizures may be controlled with lorazepam or diazepam 5-10 mg (0.25-0.4 mg/kg in children); intravenous albumin (25 g every 6 hours has been used to increase bound fraction of drug)

Enhancement of elimination: Multiple dosing of activated charcoal may be effective; peritoneal dialysis, diuresis, hemodialysis, hemoperfusion, and plasmapheresis is of little value

Test Interactions Increases glucose, alkaline phosphatase (S); decreases thyroxine (S), calcium (S); serum sodium increases in overdose setting

Diagnostic Tests/Procedures

Phenytoin, Blood *on page 1321*

Pregnancy Risk Factor D

Pregnancy Implications Distributes into breast milk; crosses placenta with fetal serum concentrations equal to those of mother; eye, cardiac, cleft palate, and skeletal malformations have been noted; fetal hydantoin syndrome associated with maternal ingestion of 100-800 mg/kg during 1st trimester

Monitoring Parameters Blood pressure, vital signs (with I.V. use), plasma level monitoring, CBC, liver function tests

Nursing Implications I.V. injections should be followed by normal saline flushes through the same needle or I.V. catheter to avoid local irritation of the vein; must be diluted to concentrations <6 mg/mL, in normal saline, for I.V. infusion

Additional Information 1.5 mg fosphenytoin is approximately equivalent to 1 mg phenytoin; equimolar fosphenytoin dose is 375 mg (75 mg/mL solution) to phenytoin 250 mg (50 mg/mL)

Water solubility: 142 mg/mL at pH of 9

Compatible with all diluents and does not require propylene glycol or ethanol for solubility; no drug interaction noted with diazepam; since there is no precipitation problem with fosphenytoin, no I.V. filter is required; antiarrhythmic effects may be similar to phenytoin; parenteral product contains no propylene sterol; this should allow for rapid intravenous bolus dosing without cardiovascular complications; formaldehyde production is not expected to be clinically consequential (about 200 mg) if used for one week

Specific References

Bebin M and Bleck TP, "New Anticonvulsant Drugs. Focus on Flunarizine, Fosphenytoin, Midazolam, and Stiripentol," *Drugs*, 1994, 48(2):153-71.

Jamerson BD, Dukes GE, and Brouwer KL, "Venous Irritation Related to Intravenous Administration of Phenytoin Versus Fosphenytoin," *Pharmacotherapy*, 1994, 14(1):47-52.

Leppik IE, Boucher R, Wilder BJ, et al, "Phenytoin Prodrug: Preclinical and Clinical Studies," *Epilepsia*, 1989, 30(Suppl 2):S22-6.

FPL-59002KP *see* Nedocromil Sodium *on page 551*

Fragmin® *see* Dalteparin *on page 256*

Fraxiparine® *see* Dalteparin *on page 256*

Freedox® *see* Tirilazad Mesylate *on page 754*

Frisium® *see* Clobazam *on page 224*

Fristamin® *see* Loratadine *on page 481*

Froben® *see* Flurbiprofen Sodium *on page 364*

Frusemide *see* Furosemide *on next page*

5-FU *see* Fluorouracil *on page 357*

Fugerel® *see* Flutamide *on page 366*

Fulvicin® P/G *see* Griseofulvin *on page 389*

Fulvicin-U/F® *see* Griseofulvin *on page 389*

Fumasorb® *see* Iron *on page 439*

Fumerin® *see* Iron *on page 439*

Funganiline® *see* Amphotericin B *on page 123*

Fungilin® *see* Amphotericin B *on page 123*

Fungizone® *see* Amphotericin B *on page 123*

Fungizone® Intravenous *see* Amphotericin B *on page 123*

Fungoid® Creme *see* Miconazole *on page 530*
Fungoid® HC Creme *see* Miconazole *on page 530*
Fungoid® Tincture *see* Miconazole *on page 530*
Furadantin® *see* Nitrofurantoin *on page 564*
Furalan® *see* Nitrofurantoin *on page 564*
Furan® *see* Nitrofurantoin *on page 564*
Furanite® *see* Nitrofurantoin *on page 564*
Furazosin *see* Prazosin Hydrochloride *on page 638*
Furil® *see* Nitrofurantoin *on page 564*

Furosemide (fur oh' se mide)

CAS Number 54-31-9

Brand Names Aluzine®; Aquarid®; Diural®; Impugan®; Lasilix®; Lasix®; Novosemide®; Puresis®; Urex®; Uritol®

Synonyms Frusemide

Use Management of edema associated with congestive heart failure and hepatic or renal disease; used alone or in combination with antihypertensives in treatment of hypertension; nebulized furosemide has been used to treat asthma

Mechanism of Action Inhibits reabsorption of sodium and chloride in the ascending loop of Henle and distal renal tubule, interfering with the chloride-binding cotransport system, thus causing increased excretion of water, sodium, chloride, magnesium, and calcium

Adverse Reactions

Cardiovascular: Diuresis

Central nervous system: Dizziness, myasthenia gravis (exacerbation or precipitation of), headache, fever

Dermatologic: Urticaria, Stevens-Johnson syndrome, exfoliative dermatitis, photosensitivity, lichenoid eruptions, erythema multiforme

Endocrine & metabolic: Hypokalemia, hypomagnesemia, hypercalcemia, hyponatremia, hypochloremia, alkalosis, hypocalcemia, hyperglycemia, dehydration, hyperuricemia

Gastrointestinal: Pancreatitis, nausea, oral solutions may cause diarrhea due to sorbitol content

Genitourinary: Prerenal azotemia, nocturia

Hematologic: Leukopenia/neutropenia (agranulocytosis, granulocytopenia), anemia, purpura, thrombocytopenia, eosinophilia

Otic: Potential ototoxicity, deafness, tinnitus

Renal: Nephrocalcinosis, proteinuria, interstitial nephritis, hypercalciuria

Signs & Symptoms of Acute Overdose Periarteritis nodosa, vision color changes (yellow tinge), photophobia

Toxicodynamics/Kinetics

Oral:

- Onset of diuresis: Within 0.5-1 hour
- Peak effect: Within 1-2 hours
- Duration: 6-8 hours

I.V.:

- Onset of diuresis: Within 5 minutes
- Duration: 2 hours

Absorption: Oral: 60% to 67%

Distribution: V_d: 0.1 L/kg

Protein binding: 91% to 99%

Half-life: 1.5 hours

Elimination: Renal (74%), 2 mL/minute/kg

Usual Dosage

Neonates, premature:

- Oral: Bioavailability is poor by this route; doses of 1-4 mg/kg/dose 1-2 times/day have been used
- I.M., I.V.: 1-2 mg/kg/dose given every 12-24 hours

Children and Infants:

- Oral: 2 mg/kg/dose increased in increments of 1 mg/kg/dose with each succeeding dose until a satisfactory effect is achieved to a maximum of 6 mg/kg/dose no more frequently than 6 hours
- I.M., I.V.: 1 mg/kg/dose, increasing by each succeeding dose at 1 mg/kg/dose at intervals of 6-12 hours until a satisfactory response up to 6 mg/kg/dose

Adults:

- Oral: 20-80 mg/dose initially increased in increments of 20-40 mg/dose at intervals of 6-8 hours; usual maintenance dose interval is twice daily or every day
- I.M., I.V.: 20-40 mg/dose, may be repeated in 1-2 hours as needed and increased by 20 mg/dose with each succeeding dose up to 1000 mg/day; usual dosing interval: 6-12 hours

(Continued)

Furosemide *(Continued)*

Dosing adjustment/comments in hepatic disease: Diminished natriuretic effect with increased sensitivity to hypokalemia and volume depletion in cirrhosis; monitor effects, particularly with high doses

Contraindications Hypersensitivity to furosemide or any component, anuria

Warnings Loop diuretics are potent diuretics, excess amounts can lead to profound diuresis with fluid and electrolyte loss; close medical supervision and dose evaluation is required

Dosage Forms

Injection: 10 mg/mL (2 mL, 4 mL, 5 mL, 6 mL, 8 mL, 10 mL, 12 mL)
Solution, oral: 10 mg/mL (60 mL, 120 mL); 40 mg/5 mL (5 mL, 10 mL, 500 mL)
Tablet: 20 mg, 40 mg, 80 mg

Reference Range

Therapeutic: 1-2 μg/mL (SI: 3-6 μmol/L)
Toxic: >50 μg/mL may be associated with toxicity

Overdosage Treatment

Decontamination: Activated charcoal with cathartic
Supportive therapy: Intravenous hydration with 0.9% saline

Test Interactions ↑ ammonia (B), ↑ amylase (S), ↑ glucose, ↑ uric acid (S); ↓ calcium (S), ↓ chloride (S), ↓ magnesium, ↓ sodium (S)

Drug Interactions Do not mix with highly acidic solutions of pH <5.5; a precipitate formed when mixed with gentamicin or netilmicin in 5% dextrose or 0.9% sodium chloride, but not with amikacin, kanamycin, or tobramycin; lithium → renal clearance decreased; furosemide interferes with hypoglycemic effect of antidiabetic agents; effects of antihypertensive agents may be enhanced; indomethacin may reduce natriuretic and hypotensive effects of furosemide; concomitant use of furosemide with aminoglycoside antibiotics or other ototoxic drugs should be avoided; NSAIDs ↓ antihypertensive response

Pregnancy Risk Factor C

Pregnancy Implications Neonatal hyponatremia/hyperuricemia can occur; possible increase in incidence of patent ductus arteriolysis

Additional Information Increased diuretic response in patients with cystic fibrosis; can cause elevation of parathyroid hormone; 40 mg furosemide is equivalent to 1 mg of bumetanide, 12 mg of piretanide, and 10-20 mg of torsemide; sodium content of 1 mL (injection): 0.162 mEq

Specific References

Bashey A and MacNee W, "Tetany Induced by Frusemide in Latent Hypoparathyroidism," *Br Med J (Clin Res)*, 1987, 295(6604):960-1.

Biano S, et al, "Protective Effect of Inhaled Furosemide on Allergen-Induced Early and Late Asthmatic Reactions," *N Engl J Med*, 1989, 321:1060-73.

Clegg HW, "Furosemide-Associated Fever," *J Pediatr*, 1995, 126:817-8.

Cutler RE, Forrey AW, Christopher TG, et al, "Pharmacokinetics of Furosemide in Normal Subjects and Functionally Anephric Patients," *Clin Pharmacol Ther*, 1974, 15(6):588-96.

Devito JM and Vance JR, "Furosemide-Induced Ototoxicity," *Clin Pharm*, 1983, 2(6):507-8.

Gifford RW Jr, "A Guide to Practical Use of Diuretics," *JAMA*, 1976, 235(17):1890-3.

Greger R and Wangemann P, "Loop Diuretics," *Renal Physiol*, 1987, 10(3-4):174-83.

Vargo DL, Kramer WG, Black PK, et al, "Bioavailability, Pharmacokinetics, and Pharmacodynamics of Torsemide and Furosemide in Patients With Congestive Heart Failure," *Clin Pharmacol Ther*, 1995, 57:601-9.

Gabapentin (ga' ba pen tin)

CAS Number 60142-96-3

Brand Names Neurontin®

Synonyms CI-945

Use Partial or secondary generalized seizures; possibly useful for pain relief due to reflex sympathetic dystrophy

Mechanism of Action Structural analog to gamma amino butyric acid (GABA). Binds to gabapentin receptors in hippocampus. No effect on GABA system.

Adverse Reactions

Central nervous system: Drowsiness, dizziness, impotence, ataxia
Dermatologic: Eczema
Endocrine & metabolic: Weight gain
Gastrointestinal: Nausea, vomiting, dry mouth
Neuromuscular & skeletal: Tremors
Ocular: Nystagmus
Respiratory: Cough

Toxicodynamics/Kinetics

Absorption: Oral: 50% to 60%
Distribution: V_d: 0.6-0.8 L/kg
Protein binding: 0%
Half-life: 5-6 hours
Elimination: Renal (56% to 80%)

Usual Dosage Children >12 years and Adults: Oral: 900-1800 mg/day administered in 3 divided doses; therapy is initiated with a rapid titration, beginning with 300 mg on day 1, 300 mg twice daily on day 2, and 300 mg 3 times/day on day 3

Dosing adjustment in renal impairment:

Cl_{cr} >60 mL/minute: Administer 1200 mg/day
Cl_{cr} 30-60 mL/minute: Administer 600 mg/day
Cl_{cr} 15-30 mL/minute: Administer 300 mg/day
Cl_{cr} <15 mL/minute: Administer 150 mg/day

Hemodialysis: 200-300 mg after each 4-hour dialysis following a loading dose of 300-400 mg

Dosage Forms Capsule: 100 mg, 300 mg, 400 mg

Reference Range Peak plasma level: 2 μg/mL 1.5-3 hours after a 200 mg dose

Overdosage Treatment

Decontamination: Lavage/activated charcoal with cathartic

Enhancement of elimination: Multiple dosing of activated charcoal may be useful; hemodialysis will be useful; see Usual Dosage

Drug Interactions Slight reduction in absorption with antacids

Pregnancy Risk Factor C

Pregnancy Implications No teratogenicity

Additional Information Not effective for absence seizures; benign pancreatic tumors noted in rodents administered high doses, ingestion of 48.9 g resulted in minimal symptoms

Specific References

Fischer JH, Barr AN, Rogers SL, et al, "Lack of Serious Toxicity Following Gabapentin Overdose," *Neurology*, 1994, 44(5):982-3.

Goa KL and Sorkin EM, "Gabapentin: A Review of Its Pharmacological Properties and Clinical Potential in Epilepsy," *Drugs*, 1993, 46(3):409-27.

Mellick LB and Mellick GA, "Successful Treatment of Reflex Sympathetic Dystrophy With Gabapentin," *Am J Emerg Med*, 1995, 13(1):96.

Short C and Cooke L, "Hypomania Induced by Gabapentin," *Br J Psychiatry*, 1995, 166:679-80.

Gallium Nitrate (gal' ee um)

CAS Number 13494-90-1; 135886-70-3

Brand Names Ganite™

Use Treatment of clearly symptomatic cancer-related hypercalcemia that has not responded to adequate hydration; Paget's disease

Mechanism of Action Gallium is a naturally occurring group IIIa heavy metal. It is the second metal, in addition to salts of platinum (group VIII metal), which has demonstrated significant clinical antitumor activity. The mechanism of hypocalcemia induced by gallium is primarily via inhibition of bone resorption with associated reduction in urinary calcium excretion. Gallium has increased the calcium content of newly mineralized bone following short-term treatment *in vitro*, and this effect combined with its ability to inhibit bone resorption has suggested the use of gallium for other disorders associated with increased bone loss. Gallium has produced significant decreases in urinary excretion of calcium and hydroxyproline in patients with solitary or multiple lytic bone metastases, and may be useful for preventing pathologic conditions in these patients.

Adverse Reactions

Endocrine & metabolic: Hypocalcemia, hypophosphatemia
Gastrointestinal: Nausea, vomiting
Hematologic: Anemia
Ocular: Optic neuritis
Otic: Hearing impairment
Renal: Renal toxicity

Toxicodynamics/Kinetics

Half-life, elimination (terminal): 25-111 hours
Elimination: Up to 70% of a dose is excreted by the kidneys

Usual Dosage Adults: I.V. infusion: 200 mg/m^2 for 5 consecutive days

Contraindications Should not be used in patients with a serum creatinine >2.5 mg/dL

Warnings Concurrent use of gallium nitrate with other potentially nephrotoxic drugs may increase the risk for developing severe renal insufficiency in patients with cancer-related hypercalcemia

Dosage Forms Injection: 25 mg/mL (20 mL)

Reference Range Steady-state gallium serum levels: Generally obtained within 2 days following initiation of continuous I.V. infusions of gallium nitrate

Overdosage Treatment Supportive therapy: Give calcium chloride for hypocalcemia

Drug Interactions Nephrotoxic drugs (eg, aminoglycosides, amphotericin B)

Pregnancy Risk Factor C

Pregnancy Implications Avoid breast feeding

Monitoring Parameters Urinary output, BUN, serum creatinine

Nursing Implications Patients should have adequate I.V. hydration, serum creatinine levels should be monitored during gallium nitrate therapy

Additional Information Has shown to be more effective in lowering serum calcium levels in patients with cancer-related hypercalcemia than calcitonin; due to the

(Continued)

Gallium Nitrate *(Continued)*

potential for drug-induced renal dysfunction, patients receiving gallium nitrate should be adequately hydrated to minimize risk

Specific References

"Hazards of Gallium for Treatment of Paget's Disease of Bone," *Lancet*, 1990, 335(8687):477.

Samson MK, Fraile RJ, Baker LH, et al, "Phase I-II Clinical Trial of Gallium Nitrate (NSC-15200)," *Cancer Clin Trials*, 1980, 3(2):131-6.

Warrell RP Jr, Coonley CJ, Straus DJ, et al, "Treatment of Patients With Advanced Malignant Lymphoma Using Gallium Nitrate Administered as a Seven-Day Continuous Infusion," *Cancer*, 1983, 51(11):1982-7.

Gamadiabet® *see* Acetohexamide *on page 86*

Gamma Benzene Hexachloride *see* Lindane *on page 470*

Gamma Hydroxybutyric Acid

CAS Number 502-85-2

Brand Names Gamma-OH®; Somatomax PM®; Somsanit®

Synonyms GHB; 4-Hydroxybutyrate; Sodium Oxybate

Use Narcolepsy; anesthetic agent

Mechanism of Action Central nervous system depressant which has anesthetic action; possible role as a neurotransmitter particularly in the substantia nigra influencing dopamine release

Adverse Reactions

Cardiovascular: Bradycardia, hypertension, hypotension

Central nervous system: Confusion, seizures, coma, dizziness, relaxation, euphoria, amnesia, hypotonia (dose related), ataxia, extrapyramidal reaction

Hematologic: Porphyria

Neuromuscular & skeletal: Tremors

Ocular: Nystagmus

Respiratory: Apnea, respiratory depression

Miscellaneous: Excessive salivation, urinary incontinence, fecal incontinence

Toxicodynamics/Kinetics

Onset of action:

- Oral: 15-30 minutes
- I.V.: 2-15 minutes

Duration of action: 3 hours

Distribution: V_d: 0.5 L/kg

Metabolism: Metabolized to succinic acid and carbon dioxide

Protein binding: 0%

Half-life: 0.3-1 hour

Usual Dosage Effects will occur at 3 g

Amnesia/hypotonia: 10 mg/kg

Lethargy, dizziness: 20-30 mg/kg

Coma, respiratory depression: 50-70 mg/kg

Usual illicit dose: Oral: 2.5 g (35 mg/kg)

Reference Range 4-butyrolactone plasma levels >2.5 mmol/L are associated with coma

Overdosage Treatment

Decontamination: Lavage/activated charcoal with cathartic

Supportive therapy: Atropine can be utilized for bradycardia; naloxone has been effective in reversing the effect in animals

Enhancement of elimination: Multiple dosing of charcoal may be effective

Antidote(s)

Naloxone Hydrochloride *on page 1447*

Test Interactions Elevates growth hormone and prolactin levels with a dose as little as 3 g; sodium salt can cause hypernatremia; hypokalemia has also been reported

Pregnancy Implications Has been used as an obstetric anesthetic agent; while GHB crosses the placenta, no fetal effects are known; can increase uterine contractions

Monitoring Parameters Respiratory status, EKG

Additional Information Recalled by the FDA in November 1990; found in certain ripe fruits such as guava; can be synthesized by titrating gamma butyrol lactone with sodium hydroxide to a pH of 6-7

Specific References

Dyer JE, "Gamma-Hydroxybutyrate: A Health-Food Product Producing Coma and Seizure-Like Activity," *Am J Emerg Med*, 1991, 9(4):321-4.

Dyer JE, Isaacs SM, and Keller KH, "Gamma Hydroxybutyrate (GHB)-Induced Coma With Serum and Urine Drug Levels," *Vet Hum Toxicol*, 1994, 36:348.

Gast JA and Frenia ML, "Gamma Hydroxybutyrate Toxicity," *Vet Hum Toxicol*, 1994, 36:348.

Helrich M, McAslan TC, Skolnick S, et al, "Correlation of Blood Levels of 4-Hydroxybutyrate With State of Consciousness," *Anesthesiology*, 1964, 25:771-5.

"Multistate Outbreak of Poisoning Associated With Illicit Use of Gamma Hydroxy Butyrate," *MMWR Morb Mortal Wkly Rep*, 1990, 39(47):861-3.

Snead OC 3d and Bearden LJ, "Naloxone Overcomes the Dopaminergic, EEG, and Behavioral Effects of Gamma Hydroxybutyrate," *Neurology*, 1980, 30(8):832-8.

Stephens BG and Baselt RC, "Driving Under the Influence of GHB?," *J Anal Toxicol*, 1994, 18(6):357-8.

Gamma-OH® *see* Gamma Hydroxybutyric Acid *on previous page*

Gammaphos *see* Amifostine *on page 107*

Ganciclovir (gan sye' kloe vir)

CAS Number 82410-32-0; 107910-75-8

Brand Names Cymevene®; Cytovene®

Synonyms DHPG Sodium; GCV Sodium; 2'NDG; Nordeoxyguanosine

Use CMV retinitis treatment of immunocompromised individuals, including patients with acquired immunodeficiency syndrome; treatment of CMV pneumonia in marrow transplant recipients, promising results have been achieved in AIDS patients and organ transplant recipients with CMV colitis, pneumonitis, and multiorgan involvement; attenuation of CMV infection in transplant patients

Mechanism of Action Ganciclovir is phosphorylated to a substrate which competitively inhibits the binding of deoxyguanosine triphosphate to DNA polymerase resulting in inhibition of viral DNA synthesis

Adverse Reactions

Cardiovascular: Edema, cardiac arrhythmias, hypertension, tachycardia (ventricular)

Central nervous system: Headache, seizures, confusion, nervousness, dizziness, psychosis, hallucinations, coma, fever, encephalopathy, malaise

Dermatologic: Rash

Endocrine & metabolic: Hypoglycemia

Gastrointestinal: Nausea, vomiting, diarrhea, anorexia

Hematologic: Reversible neutropenia (40%), thrombocytopenia (20%), leukopenia, anemia, eosinophilia

Hepatic: Elevation in liver function tests

Local: Phlebitis

Neuromuscular & skeletal: Myalgia

Ocular: Retinal detachment

Renal: Hematuria, increased BUN and serum creatinine

Respiratory: Dyspnea

Signs & Symptoms of Acute Overdose Leukopenia or neutropenia (agranulocytosis, granulocytopenia); hematuria, hypoglycemia, myalgia, tachycardia (ventricular), bone marrow depression

Toxicodynamics/Kinetics

Absorption: Oral: 4.6%

Distribution: 38% to 41% distributed into CSF; 99% distributed into lung

Protein binding: 1% to 2%

Half-life: 1.7-5.8 hours; increases to 29 hours with impaired renal function

Elimination: Majority (94% to 99%) is excreted as unchanged drug in urine

Usual Dosage Slow I.V. infusion (dosing is based on total body weight):

Children >3 months and Adults:

Induction therapy: 5 mg/kg/dose every 12 hours for 14-21 days followed by maintenance therapy

Maintenance therapy: 5 mg/kg/day as a single daily dose for 7 days/week or 6 mg/kg/day for 5 days/week

Dosing interval in renal impairment:

Cl_{cr} 50-79 mL/minute per 1.73 m^2: Administer 2.5 mg/kg/dose every 12 hours

Cl_{cr} 25-49 mL/minute per 1.73 m^2: Administer 2.5 mg/kg/dose every 24 hours

Cl_{cr} <25 mL/minute per 1.73 m^2: Administer 1.25 mg/kg/dose every 24 hours

Administration Administer by slow I.V. infusion over at least 1 hour at a final concentration for administration not to exceed 10 mg/mL

Contraindications Absolute neutrophil count <500/mm^3; platelet count <25,000/mm^3; known hypersensitivity to ganciclovir or acyclovir

Warnings Dosage adjustment or interruption of ganciclovir therapy may be necessary in patients with neutropenia and/or thrombocytopenia and patients with impaired renal function. Use with extreme caution in children since long-term safety has not been determined and due to ganciclovir's potential for long-term carcinogenic and adverse reproductive effects; ganciclovir may adversely affect spermatogenesis and fertility; due to its mutagenic potential, contraceptive precautions for female and male patients need to be followed during and for at least 90 days after therapy with the drug; take care to administer only into veins with good blood flow

Dosage Forms Powder for injection, lyophilized: 500 mg (10 mL)

Stability Reconstituted solution is stable for 12 hours at room temperature; **do not refrigerate**; reconstitute with sterile water **not** bacteriostatic water because parabens may cause precipitation

(Continued)

Ganciclovir *(Continued)*

Reference Range Peak steady state serum level of 5 mg/kg/dose: 15 μg/mL (44.5 μmol/L)

Overdosage Treatment

Decontamination: Emesis or lavage/activated charcoal with cathartic

Supportive therapy: Colony-stimulating factor may decrease hematologic toxicity

Enhancement of elimination: Multiple dosing may be effective; hemodialysis may be effective (40% to 50% removed by a 4-hour hemodialysis)

Test Interactions May increase serum alkaline phosphatase and serum bilirubin

Drug Interactions Increased effect/toxicity with probenecid, imipenem/cilastatin; increased toxicity in rapidly dividing cells with cytotoxic drugs; increased hematologic toxicity with zidovudine; increased nephrotoxicity when given with cyclosporine; seizures developed with imipenem and cilastatin

Pregnancy Risk Factor C

Pregnancy Implications Animal studies reveal growth retardation, cleft palate, microphthalmia, hydrocephaly

Monitoring Parameters CBC with differential and platelet count, serum creatinine, ophthalmologic exams

Patient Information Ganciclovir is not a cure for CMV retinitis; regular ophthalmologic examinations should be done; close monitoring of blood counts should be done while on therapy and dosage adjustments may need to be made

Nursing Implications Must be prepared in vertical flow hood; use chemotherapy precautions during administration; discard appropriately

Additional Information Sodium content of 500 mg vial: 46 mg

Questions about this drug can be directed to the Ganciclovir Study Center (301) 497-9888 or Syntex Laboratories (415) 496-3648

Specific References

Lake KD, Fletcher CV, Love KR, et al, "Ganciclovir Pharmacokinetics During Renal Impairment," *Antimicrob Agents Chemother*, 1988, 32(12):1899-900.

Morris DJ, "Adverse Effects and Drug Interactions of Clinical Importance With Antiviral Drugs," *Drug Saf*, 1994, 10(4):281-91.

Paul S and Dummer S, "Topics in Clinical Pharmacology, Ganciclovir," *Am J Med Sci*, 1992, 304(4):272-7.

Sommadossi JP, Bevan R, Ling T, et al, "Clinical Pharmacokinetics of Ganciclovir in Patients With Normal and Impaired Renal Function," *Rev Infect Dis*, 1988, 10(Suppl 3):S507-14.

Ganite™ *see* Gallium Nitrate *on page 375*

Gantrisin® Ophthalmic *see* Sulfisoxazole *on page 714*

Gantrisin® Oral *see* Sulfisoxazole *on page 714*

Garamycin® *see* Gentamicin Sulfate *on next page*

Gardenale® *see* Phenobarbital *on page 614*

Garranil® *see* Captopril *on page 181*

Gaster® *see* Famotidine *on page 341*

Gastrocrom® Oral *see* Cromolyn Sodium *on page 245*

Gastrolec® *see* Omeprazole *on page 576*

Gastrosed™ *see* Hyoscyamine Sulfate *on page 415*

GCV Sodium *see* Ganciclovir *on previous page*

Gee Gee® [OTC] *see* Guaifenesin *on page 390*

Gel Kam® *see* Fluoride *on page 355*

Gel-Tin® [OTC] *see* Fluoride *on page 355*

Gemfibrozil (jem fi' broe zil)

CAS Number 25812-30-0

Brand Names Bolutol®; Decrelip®; Fibrocit®; Gemlipid®; Lipozid®; Lipur®; Lopid®; Trialmin®

Synonyms CI-719

Use Treatment of hypertriglyceridemia in types III, IV, and V hyperlipidemia; type IIb dyslipidemia

Mechanism of Action Exact mechanism of action unknown, however, several theories exist regarding the VLDL effect; it can inhibit lipolysis and decrease subsequent hepatic fatty acid uptake as well as inhibit hepatic secretion of VLDL; together these actions decrease serum VLDL levels; increases HDL cholesterol; the mechanism behind HDL elevation is currently unknown

Adverse Reactions

Cardiovascular: Exacerbation of Raynaud's phenomenon

Central nervous system: Dizziness, drowsiness, somnolence, mental depression, frontal headache

Dermatologic: Exacerbation of psoriasis

Gastrointestinal: Abdominal pain, nausea, vomiting, diarrhea, constipation, flatulence, dry mouth

Genitourinary: Impotence
Hepatic: Cholelithiasis
Neuromuscular & skeletal: Paresthesia
Ocular: Blurred vision
Miscellaneous: Pulsatile

Toxicodynamics/Kinetics
Absorption: Well absorbed
Protein binding: 99%
Metabolism: In the liver by oxidation to two inactive metabolites
Half-life: 1.4 hours
Time to peak serum concentration: Within 1-2 hours
Elimination: A portion of the drug undergoes enterohepatic recycling; excreted in urine, primarily as unchanged drug (70%)

Usual Dosage Adults: Oral: 1200 mg/day in 2 divided doses, 30 minutes before breakfast and supper

Contraindications Renal or hepatic dysfunction, gallbladder disease, hypersensitivity to gemfibrozil or any component

Warnings Abnormal elevation of AST, ALT, LDH, bilirubin and alkaline phosphatase has occurred; if no appreciable triglyceride or cholesterol lowering effect occurs after 3 months, the drug should be discontinued; not useful for type I hyperlipidemia

Dosage Forms
Capsule: 300 mg
Tablet, film coated: 600 mg

Overdosage Treatment
Decontamination: Emesis or lavage/activated charcoal with cathartic
Enhancement of elimination: Multiple dosing of activated charcoal may increase clearance

Drug Interactions Increased effect of warfarin, glyburide; increased toxicity of lovastatin and other HMG-CoA reductase inhibitors

Pregnancy Risk Factor B

Monitoring Parameters Serum cholesterol

Patient Information May cause dizziness or blurred vision, abdominal or epigastric pain, diarrhea, nausea, or vomiting; notify physician if these become pronounced

Nursing Implications Monitor LFTs – abnormal elevation of AST, ALT, LDH, bilirubin and alkaline phosphatase have occurred; if no appreciable triglyceride or cholesterol, lowering effect occurs after 3 months, the drug should be discontinued

Specific References

Ahmad S, "Gemfibrozil Interaction With Warfarin Sodium," *Chest*, 1990, 98(4):1041-2.
Todd PA and Ward A, "Gemfibrozil: A Review of Its Pharmacodynamic and Pharmacokinetic Properties and Therapeutic Use in Dyslipidaemia," *Drugs*, 1988, 36(3):314-39.

Gemlipid® *see* Gemfibrozil *on previous page*
Gemonil® *see* Mephobarbital *on page 501*
Gemonil® *see* Metharbital *on page 512*
Genabid® *see* Papaverine *on page 591*
Genagesic® *see* Propoxyphene and Acetaminophen *on page 656*
Genapap® [OTC] *see* Acetaminophen *on page 79*
Genatuss® [OTC] *see* Guaifenesin *on page 390*
Gen-Diur® *see* Ammonium Chloride *on page 118*
Gen-K® *see* Potassium Chloride *on page 634*
Genoptic® Ophthalmic *see* Gentamicin Sulfate *on this page*
Genpril® [OTC] *see* Ibuprofen *on page 418*
Gentacidin® Ophthalmic *see* Gentamicin Sulfate *on this page*
Gent-AK® Ophthalmic *see* Gentamicin Sulfate *on this page*

Gentamicin Sulfate (jen ta mye' sin)

Related Information
Aminoglycoside Dosing and Monitoring *on page 1490-1491*
Therapeutic Drugs Associated With Hallucinations *on page 1558-1559*

CAS Number 1405-41-0

Brand Names Garamycin®; Genoptic® Ophthalmic; Gentacidin® Ophthalmic; Gent-AK® Ophthalmic; Gentrasul® Ophthalmic; G-myticin® Topical; Jenamicin® Injection

Use Treatment of susceptible bacterial infections, normally gram-negative organisms including *Pseudomonas*, *Proteus*, *Serratia*; treatment of bone infections, CNS infections, respiratory tract infections, skin and soft tissue infections, as well as abdominal and urinary tract infections, endocarditis, and septicemia

(Continued)

Gentamicin Sulfate *(Continued)*

Mechanism of Action Interferes with bacterial protein synthesis by binding to 30S and 50S ribosomal subunits resulting in a defective bacterial cell membrane

Adverse Reactions

Central nervous system: Gait instability, psychosis, dizziness, hallucinations, ataxia

Dermatologic: Rash

Endocrine & metabolic: Hypomagnesemia

Hematologic: Granulocytopenia

Hepatic: Elevated AST, ALT

Local: Thrombophlebitis

Neuromuscular & skeletal: Neuromuscular blockade

Ocular: Nystagmus

Otic: Ototoxicity, tinnitus (peak >12-15 μg/mL and high trough levels)

Renal: Nephrotoxicity (high trough levels) with albuminuria, reduction in glomerular filtration rate, increased serum creatinine, decrease in urine specific gravity, casts in urine and possible electrolyte wasting

Signs & Symptoms of Acute Overdose Leukopenia or neutropenia (agranulocytosis, granulocytopenia); hypokalemia, deafness, eczema, Fanconi's syndrome, thrombocytopenia, tubular necrosis, pseudotumor cerebri, myasthenia gravis (exacerbation or precipitation of), hypomagnesemia, seizures

Toxicodynamics/Kinetics

Absorption: Oral: <1%

Distribution: V_d: Increased by edema, ascites, fluid overload; decreased in patients with dehydration

- Neonates: 0.4-0.6 L/kg
- Children: 0.3-0.35 L/kg
- Adults: 0.2-0.3 L/kg

Protein binding: <30%

Half-life:

- Infants <1 week: 3-11.5 hours
- Infants 1 week to 6 months: 3-3.5 hours
- Adults: 1.5-3 hours; with anuria: 36-70 hours

Time to peak serum concentration: I.M.: Within 30-60 minutes

Elimination: Clearance is directly related to renal function, eliminated almost completely by glomerular filtration of unchanged drug with excretion in urine

Usual Dosage

Individualization is critical because of the low therapeutic index. Use of ideal body weight (IBW) for determining the mg/kg/dose appears to be more accurate than dosing on the basis of total body weight (TBW). In morbid obesity, dosage requirement may best be estimated using a dosing weight of IBW + 0.4 (TBW - IBW). Initial and periodic peak and trough plasma drug levels should be determined, particularly in critically ill patients with serious infections or in disease states known to significantly alter aminoglycoside pharmacokinetics (eg, cystic fibrosis, burns, or major surgery). Dose must be adjusted based on serum levels.

Neonates: I.M., I.V.:

- Postnatal age <7 days:
  - <1200 g, 0-4 weeks: 2.5 mg/kg/dose every 18-24 hours
  - >1200 g: 2.5 mg/kg/dose every 12-18 hours
- Postnatal age >7 days, >1200 g: 2.5 mg/kg/dose every 8-12 hours

Newborns: Intrathecal: 1 mg every day

Infants and Children:

- I.M., I.V.: 2.5 mg/kg/dose every 8 hours*
- Intrathecal: >3 months: 1-2 mg/day
- Ophthalmic:
  - Ointment: Instill ½" (1.25 cm) 2-3 times/day to every 3-4 hours
  - Solution: Instill 1-2 drops every 2-4 hours, up to 2 drops every hour for severe infections
- Topical: Apply 1-4 times/day to affected area

Adults:

- I.M., I.V.:
  - Severe life-threatening infections: 2-2.5 mg/kg/dose
  - Urinary tract infections: 1.5 mg/kg/dose
  - Synergy (for gram-positive infections): 1 mg/kg/dose
- Intrathecal: 4-8 mg/day

Dosing interval in renal impairment: Give an appropriate loading dose; subsequent doses and frequency of administration are best determined by measurement of serum levels and assessment of renal insufficiency**

* Some patients may require larger or more frequent doses (eg, every 6 hours) if serum levels document the need (ie, cystic fibrosis or febrile granulocytopenic patients)

** 2-3 serum level measurements should be obtained after the initial dose to measure the half-life in order to determine the frequency of subsequent doses

Ophthalmic:

Ointment: Instill ½" (1.25 cm) 2-3 times/day to every 3-4 hours

Solution: Instill 1-2 drops every 2-4 hours

Topical: Apply 1-4 times/day to affected area

Dosing adjustment/comments in hepatic disease: Monitor plasma concentrations

Administration Administer by I.V. slow intermittent infusion over 30 minutes; final concentration for administration should not exceed 10 mg/mL

Contraindications Hypersensitivity to gentamicin or other aminoglycosides

Warnings

Not intended for long-term therapy due to toxic hazards associated with extended administration; pre-existing renal insufficiency, vestibular or cochlear impairment, myasthenia gravis, hypocalcemia, conditions which depress neuromuscular transmission

Parenteral aminoglycosides are associated with significant nephrotoxicity or ototoxicity; the ototoxicity may be directly proportional to the amount of drug given and the duration of treatment; tinnitus or dizziness are indications of vestibular injury and impending deafness; renal damage is usually reversible

Dosage Forms

Cream, topical: 0.1% (15 g)

Injection: 40 mg/mL (1 mL, 2 mL, 10 mL, 20 mL)

Intrathecal: 2 mg/mL (2 mL)

Pediatric: 10 mg/mL (2 mL)

Ointment:

Ophthalmic: 0.3% (3.5 g)

Topical: 0.1% (15 g)

Solution, ophthalmic: 0.3% (1 mL, 5 mL, 15 mL)

Stability I.V. infusion solutions mixed in NS or D_5W solution are stable for 24 hours at room temperature; **incompatible** with penicillins

Reference Range

Therapeutic: Peak: 4-8 μg/mL (SI: 8-17 μmol/L); Trough: <2 μg/mL (SI: <4 μmol/L) (depends in part on the minimal inhibitory concentration of drug against organism being treated)

Toxic: Peak: >10 μg/mL (SI: >21 μmol/L); Trough: >2 μg/mL (SI: >8.4 μmol/L)

Overdosage Treatment Enhancement of elimination: While hemodialysis is of questionable benefit in those patients with normal renal function, it should be performed in patients with renal insufficiency; the addition of ticarcillin (2-5 g I.V. every 4-6 hours until gentamicin serum levels are <0.2 μg/mL) may complex with gentamicin and decrease the half-life of gentamicin by enhancing renal excretion

Test Interactions ↑ protein; ↓ magnesium; ↑ BUN, AST, GPT, alk phos, serum creatinine; ↓ potassium, sodium, calcium

Drug Interactions

Increased/prolonged effect: Depolarizing and nondepolarizing neuromuscular blocking agents can cause apnea

Increased toxicity: Concurrent use of amphotericin may increase nephrotoxicity; ototoxicity may be potentiated with administration of fludarabine

Pregnancy Risk Factor C

Pregnancy Implications Crosses the placenta

Monitoring Parameters Urinalysis, urine output, BUN, serum creatinine, peak and trough plasma gentamicin levels

Patient Information Report any dizziness or sensations of ringing or fullness in ears

Nursing Implications When injected into the muscles of paralyzed patients, the results are different than in normal patients; slower absorption and lower peak concentrations probably due to poor circulation in the atrophic muscles, suggest I.V. route; aminoglycoside levels measured in blood taken from Silastic® central catheters can sometime give falsely high readings. Monitor serum creatinine and urine output; obtain drug levels after the third dose. Peak levels are drawn 30 minutes after the end of a 30-minute infusion; trough levels are drawn within 30 minutes before the next dose; give other antibiotic drugs at least 1 hour before or after gentamicin. Hearing should be tested before, during, and after treatment.

Specific References

Ahkee S, Smith R, and Ritter GW, "Once-Daily Aminoglycoside Dosing in Lower Respiratory Tract Infections," *Pharm Therap*, 1995, 20:226-34.

Fuquay D, Koup J, and Smith AL, "Management of Neonatal Gentamicin Overdosage," *J Pediatr*, 1981, 99(3):473-6.

Lucena MI, Andrade RJ, Cabello MR, et al, "Aminoglycoside-Associated Nephrotoxicity in Extrahepatic Obstructive Jaundice," *J Hepatol*, 1995, 22:189-96.

Matz GJ, "Aminoglycoside Ototoxicity," *Am J Otolaryngol*, 1986, 7(2):117-9.

O'Brien RK and Sparling TG, "Gentamicin and Fludarabine Ototoxicity," *Ann Pharmacother*, 1995, 29:200.

(Continued)

Gentamicin Sulfate *(Continued)*

Schentag JJ, Simons GW, Schultz RW, et al, "Complexation Versus Hemodialysis to Reduce Elevated Aminoglycoside Serum Concentrations," *Pharmacotherapy*, 1984, 4(6):374-80.

Gentrasul® Ophthalmic *see* Gentamicin Sulfate *on page 379*

Gen-XENE® *see* Clorazepate Dipotassium *on page 232*

Gericin® *see* Nitrendipine *on page 562*

Germiphene® *see* Benzalkonium Chloride *on page 147*

GG *see* Guaifenesin *on page 390*

GG-Cen® [OTC] *see* Guaifenesin *on page 390*

GHB *see* Gamma Hydroxybutyric Acid *on page 376*

Gingicain® *see* Tetracaine Hydrochloride *on page 731*

Glibenclamide *see* Glyburide *on page 384*

Glibenese® *see* Glipizide *on this page*

Gliconorm® *see* Chlorpropamide *on page 207*

Glipizide (glip' i zide)

Related Information

Hypoglycemic Agents Comparison, Oral *on page 1650*

CAS Number 29094-61-9

Brand Names Glibenese®; Glucotrol®; Mindiab®; Minidiab®; Minodiab®

Synonyms Glydiazinamide

Use Management of noninsulin-dependent diabetes mellitus (type II)

Mechanism of Action Sulfonylurea which stimulates insulin release from the pancreatic beta cells; reduces glucose output from the liver; insulin sensitivity is increased at peripheral target sites

Adverse Reactions

Cardiovascular: Edema

Central nervous system: Headache, ataxia, dizziness, fasciculations

Dermatologic: Rash

Endocrine & metabolic: Hypoglycemia, syndrome of inappropriate antidiuretic hormone (SIADH), hyponatremia

Gastrointestinal: Anorexia, nausea, vomiting, diarrhea

Hematologic: Blood dyscrasias

Hepatic: Jaundice

Optic: Photosensitivity

Renal: Diuretic effect

Toxicodynamics/Kinetics

Duration of action: 12-24 hours

Peak blood glucose reductions: Within 1.5-2 hours

Absorption: Delayed when given with food; impaired in patients with hyperglycemia

Distribution: V_d: 0.2 L/kg

Protein binding: 92% to 99%

Metabolism: In the liver with metabolites (91% to 97%)

Half-life: 3-4 hours

Elimination: Metabolites (91% to 97%) excreted in urine (60% to 80%) and feces (11%)

Usual Dosage Oral (allow several days between dose titrations; administer 30 minutes before a meal for greatest reduction in postprandial hyperglycemia):

Adults: 2.5-40 mg/day; doses larger than 15-20 mg/day should be divided and given twice daily

Elderly: Initial: 2.5-5 mg/day; increase by 2.5-5 mg/day every 1-2 weeks

Dosing comment in renal impairment: Cl_{cr} <10 mL/minute: Some investigators recommend not using

Dosing adjustment in hepatic impairment: Initial dosages should be 2.5 mg/day; 5 mg has caused delayed hypoglycemia (11 hours) in a 13.2 kg child

Contraindications Hypersensitivity to glipizide or any component, other sulfonamides, type I diabetes mellitus

Warnings Use with caution in patients with severe hepatic disease; a useful agent since few drug to drug interactions and not dependent upon renal elimination of active drug

Dosage Forms Tablet: 5 mg, 10 mg

Reference Range Glucose: Adults: 80-140 mg/dL; Elderly: 100-180 mg/dL

Overdosage Treatment

Decontamination: Lavage/activated charcoal with cathartic

Supportive therapy: Glucose (25 g I.V.) is mainstay of therapy; glucagon (1-5 mg I.V., I.M., or S.C.) (0.03-0.1 mg/kg in pediatrics) will have limited benefit; diazoxide is a third-line agent (3-8 mg/kg/24 hours)

Enhancement of elimination: Multiple dosing of activated charcoal may be more effective for this agent than for other oral hypoglycemics due to enterohepatic recirculation of glipizide; peritoneal dialysis has been used with some success, but is not recommended as a routine procedure; urine alkalinization is also useful

Antidote(s)

Dextrose *on page 1409*

Glucagon *on page 1431*

Diagnostic Tests/Procedures

Electrolytes, Blood *on page 1254*

Glucose, Random *on page 1269*

Kidney Profile *on page 1279*

Drug Interactions

Increased effect: Histamine H_2 antagonists, anticoagulants, androgens, fluconazole, salicylates, gemfibrozil, sulfonamides, tricyclic antidepressants, probenecid, MAO inhibitors, methyldopa, digitalis glycosides, urinary acidifiers

Decreased effect: Beta-blockers, cholestyramines, hydantoins, rifampin, thiazide diuretics, urinary alkalines, charcoal

Pregnancy Risk Factor C

Monitoring Parameters Fasting blood glucose, hemoglobin A, C, fructosamine

Patient Information Patients must be counseled by someone experienced in diabetes education, signs and symptoms of hyper- and hypoglycemia, exercise and diet, blood glucose monitoring, and other related topics; eat regularly, do not skip meals; carry quick source of sugar; medical alert bracelet

Nursing Implications Monitor for signs and symptoms of hypoglycemia; patients who are anorexic or NPO, may need to have their dose held to avoid hypoglycemia

Additional Information Exhibits more of a diuretic action than chlorpropamide

Specific References

Berelowitz M, Fischette C, Cefalu W, et al, "Comparative Efficacy of a Once-Daily Controlled-Release Formulation of Glipizide and Immediate-Release Glipizide in Patients With NIDDM," *Diabetes Care*, 1994, 17(12):1460-4.

Frederick KA and Wang RY, "Delayed Hypoglycemia in a Child After Ingestion of a Single Glipizide Tablet," *Vet Hum Toxicol*, 1994, 35:365.

Goran B, Bo B, Martin F, et al, "Glipizide-Induced Severe Hypoglycemia," *Acta Endocrinol (Copenh)*, 1981, 98(Suppl 245):13.

Kilo C, Meenan A, and Bloomgarden Z, "Glyburide Versus Glipizide in the Treatment of Patients With Noninsulin Dependent Diabetes Mellitus," *Clin Ther*, 1992, 14(6):801-12.

Kradjan WA, Takeuchi KY, Opheim KE, et al, "Pharmacokinetics and Pharmacodynamics of Glipizide After Once-Daily and Divided Doses," *Pharmacotherapy*, 1995, 15(4):465-71.

Nadel HL, "Formulary Conversion From Glipizide to Glyburide: A Cost-Minimization Analysis," *Hosp Pharm*, 1995, 30:467-9, 472-4.

Globuren® *see* Erythropoietin *on page 322*

Glonoin *see* Nitroglycerin *on page 566*

Glucolon® *see* Glyburide *on next page*

Glucophage *see* Metformin *on page 507*

Glucophage® *see* Metformin *on page 507*

Glucotrol® *see* Glipizide *on previous page*

Glutethimide (gloo teth' i mide)

Related Information

Toxins Which Should be Lavaged With Solutions Other Than Water *on page 1635*

CAS Number 77-21-4

Brand Names Doriden®

Use Short-term treatment of insomnia; introduced in 1954

Mechanism of Action Central nervous system depressant with hypnotic action of phenobarbital and antimuscarinic effects

Adverse Reactions

Cardiovascular: Bradycardia, hypotension

Central nervous system: Convulsions, confusion, slurred speech, papilledema, dizziness, headache, prolonged coma, fever, ataxia, hypothermia

Dermatologic: Skin rash

Endocrine & metabolic: Hypocalcemia (with chronic use)

Gastrointestinal: Nausea, vomiting, ileus

Genitourinary: Urinary retention

Hematologic: Blood dyscrasias, methemoglobinemia, thrombocytopenia, leukopenia (with chronic use)

(Continued)

Glutethimide *(Continued)*

Neuromuscular & skeletal: Muscle spasm
Ocular: Nystagmus, mydriasis, diplopia
Respiratory: Apnea, respiratory depression, pulmonary edema
Miscellaneous: Porphyrinogenic

Signs & Symptoms of Acute Overdose Leukopenia or neutropenia (agranulocytosis, granulocytopenia); hypocalcemia, dry skin, bezoars, anemia (megaloblastic), methemoglobinemia, hyporeflexia, hypothermia, apnea

Toxicodynamics/Kinetics

Protein binding: 50%
Metabolism: Hepatic to an active metabolite (4-hydroxy-2-ethyl-2-phenylglutarimide); significant enterohepatic recirculation
Half-life: 5-22 hours

Usual Dosage Oral:

Adults: 250-500 mg at bedtime, dose may be repeated but not less than 4 hours before intended awakening; maximum: 1 g/day

Elderly/debilitated patients: Total daily dose should not exceed 500 mg
Overdose symptoms occur at 3 g ingestion

Lethal dose: 10 g

Contraindications Known hypersensitivity to glutethimide, porphyria

Dosage Forms Tablet: 250 mg, 500 mg

Reference Range

Therapeutic: 2-6 μg/mL
Toxic: >6 μg/mL

Overdosage Treatment

Decontamination: Aggressively lavage (with water or castor oil in a 1:1 mixture)/activated charcoal with cathartic (1 g for every 50 g of ingested drug)
Supportive therapy: Avoid overhydration, anticholinergic; treat methemoglobinemia with methylene blue agents
Enhancement of elimination: Multiple dosing of activated charcoal is effective; hemoperfusion is effective in removing metabolite and is preferred over hemodialysis (which is only about half as effective as charcoal hemoperfusion in removing glutethimide); considerations for extracorporeal removal of drug include ingestions >10 g (or a serum level >6 μg/mL), prolonged coma, flat line on EEG, or progressive systemic deterioration; do not alkalinize the urine

Antidote(s)

Methylene Blue *on page 1444*

Diagnostic Tests/Procedures

Electrocardiography *on page 1253*
Methemoglobin, Blood *on page 1296*

Drug Interactions Decreased effect of anticoagulants

Pregnancy Risk Factor C

Pregnancy Implications Neonatal respiratory depression/apnea have been noted as have neonatal withdrawal from chronic maternal use

Additional Information Often ingested with acetaminophen and codeine ("Fours and Doors")

Specific References

Baron JM and Tritch DL, "Castor Oil Catharsis in Acute Glutethimide Intoxication," *JAMA*, 1970, 211(6):1021-3.
Bender FH, Cooper JV, and Dreyfus R, "Fatalities Associated With Acute Overdose of Glutethimide (Doriden®) and Codeine," *Vet Hum Toxicol*, 1988, 30(4):332-3.
Raja RM, "Resin Hemoperfusion for Drug Intoxication - An Update," *Int J Artif Organs*, 1986, 9(5):319-22.
Sramek JJ and Khajawall A, "Loads," *N Engl J Med*, 1981, 305(4):231.

Glyate® [OTC] *see* Guaifenesin *on page 390*

Glyben® *see* Glyburide *on this page*

Glybenzcyclamide *see* Glyburide *on this page*

Glyburide (glye' byoor ide)

Related Information

Hypoglycemic Agents Comparison, Oral *on page 1650*

CAS Number 10238-21-8

Brand Names Calabren®; Daonil®; Diaβeta®; Glucolon®; Glyben®; Glynase™ PresTab™; Melix®; Micronase®

Synonyms Glibenclamide; Glybenzcyclamide

Use Management of noninsulin-dependent diabetes mellitus (type II)

Mechanism of Action A sulfonylurea which stimulates insulin release from the pancreatic beta cells; reduces glucose output from the liver; insulin sensitivity is increased at peripheral target sites

Adverse Reactions

Central nervous system: Headache, ataxia, dizziness

Dermatologic: Pruritus, rash, photosensitivity, skin rash, hives

Endocrine & metabolic: Hypoglycemia, syndrome of inappropriate antidiuretic hormone effect

Gastrointestinal: Nausea, epigastric fullness, heartburn, constipation, diarrhea, anorexia, epigastric fullness

Genitourinary: Nocturia

Hematologic: Thrombocytopenia, hemolysis, aplastic anemia, hypoglycemia (12-72 hours), leukopenia, neutropenia, agranulocytosis, granulocytopenia, bone marrow depression

Hepatic: Cholestatic jaundice

Neuromuscular & skeletal: Joint pain, paresthesia

Ocular: Myopia, optic atrophy (infant), diplopia

Signs & Symptoms of Acute Overdose Leukopenia or neutropenia (agranulocytosis, granulocytopenia); enuresis, eosinophilia, hyponatremia, photosensitivity, nocturia, exfoliative dermatitis, hypoglycemia, diuresis, coagulopathy

Toxicodynamics/Kinetics

Onset of action: Oral: Insulin levels in the serum begin to increase within 15-60 minutes after a single dose

Duration: Up to 24 hours

Distribution: V_d: 0.3 L/kg

Metabolism: To one moderately active and several inactive metabolites

Protein binding, plasma: High (97% to 99%)

Half-life: 3 hours; may be prolonged with renal insufficiency or hepatic insufficiency

Time to peak serum concentration: Adults: Within 2-4 hours

Elimination: 50% feces, 50% urine

Usual Dosage Oral:

Adults: 1.25-5 mg to start then increase at weekly intervals to 1.25-20 mg maintenance dose/day divided in 1-2 doses

Elderly: Initial: 1.25-2.5 mg/day, increase by 1.25-2.5 mg/day every 1-3 weeks

PresTab™: Initial: 0.75-3 mg/day, increase by 1.5 mg/day in weekly intervals, maximum: 12 mg/day

Dosing adjustment/comments in renal impairment:

Cl_{cr} 10-50 mL/minute: Use conservative initial and maintenance doses

Cl_{cr} <10 mL/minute: Avoid use

Dosing adjustment in hepatic impairment: Use conservative initial and maintenance doses and avoid use in severe disease

Contraindications Hypersensitivity to glyburide or any component, or other sulfonamides

Warnings Use with caution in patients with hepatic impairment. Elderly: Rapid and prolonged hypoglycemia (>12 hours) despite hypertonic glucose injections have been reported; age and hepatic and renal impairment are independent risk factors for hypoglycemia; dosage titration should be made at weekly intervals.

Dosage Forms

Tablet (Diaβeta®, Micronase®): 1.25 mg, 2.5 mg, 5 mg

Tablet, micronized (Glynase™ PresTab™): 1.5 mg, 3 mg

Reference Range

Normal fasting glucose:

Adults: 80-140 mg/dL

Elderly: 100-180 mg/dL

Therapeutic glyburide level: 40-50 ng/mL

Overdosage Treatment

Decontamination: Lavage/activated charcoal with cathartic

Supportive therapy: Glucose (25 g I.V.) is mainstay of therapy; glucagon (1-5 mg I.V., I.M., or S.C.) (0.03-0.1 mg/kg in pediatrics) will have limited benefit; diazoxide is a third-line agent (3-8 mg/kg/24 hours)

Enhancement of elimination: Multiple dosing of activated charcoal may be effective; peritoneal dialysis has been used with some success, but is not recommended as a routine procedure; urine alkalinization is also useful

Antidote(s)

Dextrose *on page 1409*

Glucagon *on page 1431*

Diagnostic Tests/Procedures

Electrolytes, Blood *on page 1254*

Glucose, Random *on page 1269*

Kidney Profile *on page 1279*

Drug Interactions

Decreased effect: Thiazides and beta-blockers may decrease effectiveness of glyburide

(Continued)

Glyburide *(Continued)*

Increased effect: Increased hypoglycemia with phenylbutazone, oral anticoagulants, hydantoins, salicylates, NSAIDs, MAO inhibitors

Increased toxicity: Increased disulfiram reactions with alcohol

Pregnancy Risk Factor D

Monitoring Parameters Fasting blood glucose, hemoglobin A_{2c}, fructosamine

Patient Information Patients must be counseled by someone experienced in diabetes education, signs and symptoms of hyper- and hypoglycemia, exercise and diet, blood glucose monitoring, and other related topics; eat regularly, do not skip meals; carry quick source of sugar; medical alert bracelet

Nursing Implications Monitor for signs and symptoms of hypoglycemia; patients who are anorexic or NPO, may need to have their dose held to avoid hypoglycemia

Additional Information More diuretic effect than chlorpropamide; glyburide-microsed dust may cause hypoglycemia by inhalation

Specific References

Gavin JR 3d, "Glyburide: New Insights Into Its Effects on the Beta Cell and Beyond," *Am J Med*, 1990, 89(Suppl 2A):1S-2S.

Nadel HL, "Formulary Conversion From Glipizide to Glyburide: A Cost-Minimization Analysis," *Hosp Pharm*, 1995, 30:472-74.

Nataas OB and Nesthus I, "Immune Haemolytic Anemia Induced by Glibenclamide in Selective IgA Deficiency," *Br Med J (Clin Res)*, 1987, 295(6594):366-7.

Schwinghammer TL, Antal ES, Kubacka RT, et al, "Pharmacokinetics and Pharmacodynamics of Glyburide in Young and Elderly Nondiabetic Adults," *Clin Pharm*, 1991, 10:532-8.

Sillence DO and Court JM, "Glibenclamide-Induced Hypoglycemia," *Br Med J*, 1975, 3(5981):490-1.

Glycerol Guaiacolate *see* Guaifenesin *on page 390*

Glyceryl Trinitrate *see* Nitroglycerin *on page 566*

Glycotuss® [OTC] *see* Guaifenesin *on page 390*

Glydiazinamide *see* Glipizide *on page 382*

Glymese® *see* Chlorpropamide *on page 207*

Glynase™ PresTab™ *see* Glyburide *on page 384*

Glytuss® [OTC] *see* Guaifenesin *on page 390*

G-myticin® Topical *see* Gentamicin Sulfate *on page 379*

Gold Compounds

Related Information

Radiation: Basics of Exposure *on page 1594-1600*

CAS Number 7440-57-5

Brand Names Myochrysine® Injection; Ridaura®; Solganal® Injection

Synonyms Auranofin; Aurothioglucose; Gold Sodium Thiomalate

Use Metallic use in dentistry; food coloring agent; auric drug used for treatment of progressive rheumatoid arthritis; adjunctive treatment in adult and juvenile active rheumatoid arthritis; alternative or adjunct in treatment of pemphigus; psoriatic patients who do not respond to NSAIDs

Mechanism of Action May inhibit phagocytosis and lysosomal enzyme

Adverse Reactions

Cardiovascular: Flushing

Dermatologic: Pruritus, hypersensitivity, alopecia, dermal eruption, rash, photosensitivity/phototoxicity, toxic epidermal necrolysis, exfoliative dermatitis, erythema

Endocrine & metabolic: Gynecomastia

Gastrointestinal: Nausea, vomiting, diarrhea

Hematologic: Thrombocytopenia, eosinophilia, leukopenia, anemia

Hepatic: Cholestatic jaundice, hepatitis, hepatic necrosis in overdose situation

Neuromuscular & skeletal: Paresthesia

Ocular: Corneal crystalline deposits that usually do not affect vision

Renal: Proteinuria, tubular necrosis (acute), interstitial nephritis (oral gold is less nephrotoxic than parenteral gold administration)

Respiratory: Wheezing, cough, interstitial lung disease

Miscellaneous: Drug-induced SLE, gingivitis

Signs & Symptoms of Acute Overdose Ventricular tachycardia, wheezing, photosensitivity, nephrotic syndrome, eosinophilia, hematuria, pancreatitis, metallic taste, lichenoid eruptions, dysosmia, dementia, crystalluria, toxic epidermal necrolysis, nystagmus, bleeding, feces discoloration (yellow-green); cataract, periarteritis nodosa, pemphigus, leukopenia; neutropenia; agranulocytosis; granulocytopenia, blood dyscrasias

Toxicodynamics/Kinetics

Distribution: V_d: 0.1 L/kg

Protein binding: 95%

Half-life: 5-16 days

Elimination: Normal urinary excretion is 0.1-1 mg/day; 10% to 40% excreted by feces

Usual Dosage

Auranofin: Oral:

Children: Initial: 0.1 mg/kg/day divided daily; usual maintenance: 0.15 mg/kg/day in 1-2 divided doses; maximum: 0.2 mg/kg/day in 1-2 divided doses

Adults: 6 mg/day in 1-2 divided doses; after 3 months may be increased to 9 mg/day in 3 divided doses; if still no response after 3 months at 9 mg/day, discontinue drug

Aurothioglucose: I.M.: Doses should initially be given at weekly intervals

Children 6-12 years: Initial: 0.25 mg/kg/dose first week; increment at 0.25 mg/kg/dose increasing with each weekly dose; maintenance: 0.75-1 mg/kg/dose weekly not to exceed 25 mg/dose to a total of 20 doses, then every 2-4 weeks

Adults: 10 mg first week; 25 mg second and third week; then 50 mg/week until 800 mg to 1 g cumulative dose has been given; if improvement occurs without adverse reactions, give 25-50 mg every 2-3 weeks, then every 3-4 weeks

Gold sodium thiomalate: I.M.:

Children: Initial: Test dose of 10 mg is recommended, followed by 1 mg/kg/week for 20 weeks; maintenance: 1 mg/kg/dose at 2- to 4-week intervals thereafter for as long as therapy is clinically beneficial and toxicity does not develop. Administration for 2-4 months is usually required before clinical improvement is observed.

Adults: 10 mg first week; 25 mg second week; then 25-50 mg/week until 1 g cumulative dose has been given; if improvement occurs without adverse reactions, give 25-50 mg every 2-3 weeks for 2-20 weeks, then every 3-4 weeks indefinitely

Dosage Forms

Capsule (Auranofin [Ridaura®]): 3 mg [gold 29%]

Injection (Gold Sodium Thiomalate [Myochrysine® Injection]): 25 mg/mL (1 mL); 50 mg/mL (1 mL, 10 mL)

Suspension, sterile (Aurothioglucose [Solganal®]): 50 mg/mL [gold 50%] (10 mL)

Reference Range

Gold:

Normal: 0-0.1 μg/mL (SI: 0-0.0064 μmol/L)

Therapeutic: 1-3 μg/mL (SI: 0.06-0.18 μmol/L)

Urine: <0.1 μg/24 hours

Peak serum gold levels after a 50 mg injection: 6-8 mg/L

Overdosage Treatment

Decontamination: Emesis or lavage/activated charcoal with cathartic

Supportive therapy: Lung toxicity can be treated with corticosteroids; for thrombocytopenia refractory to chelation therapy: cyclophosphamide (100 mg/day for 6 months or until platelet count was >100,000 with subsequent reduction of dose to 75 mg/day) can be utilized; high dose I.V. N-acetylcysteine may be useful to treat hematologic toxicity due to gold (2-9 g in 100 mL of D_5 ½NS over 2-6 hours, total dose: 13-153 g)

Enhancement of elimination: Chelation with BAL (dimercaprol) or D-penicillamine (250 mg 4 times/day for 11 days) can increase elimination; hemodialysis is not useful

Antidote(s)

Dimercaprol *on page 1414*

Penicillamine *on page 1454*

Diagnostic Tests/Procedures

Complete Blood Count *on page 1236*

Gold Level *on page 1270*

Protein, Quantitative, Urine *on page 1335*

Pregnancy Risk Factor C

Pregnancy Implications Teratogenic in animals; not proven to be teratogenic in humans; not compatible for breast feeding since it is excreted in breast milk

Monitoring Parameters CBC, liver function tests, renal function

Specific References

Bell RA and Dale IM, "Gold Secretion in Maternal Milk," *Arthritis Rheum*, 1976, 19(6):1374.

Bunch TW, "Gold Overdose Treated With BAL," *Arthritis Rheum*, 1974, 19(1):123-5.

Cook NJ, Owen ET, and Donlon JB, "A Further Possible Cause of Diarrhea Caused by Oral Gold," *Br J Rheumatol*, 1995, 34:395-6.

Davis CM, "D-Penicillamine for the Treatment of Gold Dermatitis," *Am J Med*, 1969, 46(3):472-6.

Fernandez-Herlihy L, "Requiem for Gold?" *Ann Intern Med*, 1991, 114(11):993-4.

Godfrey NF, Peter A, Simon TM, et al, "I.V. N-acetylcysteine Treatment of Hematologic Reactions to Chrysotherapy," *J Rheumatol*, 1982, 9(4):519-26.

Kozloff M, Votaw M, and Penner JA, "Gold-Induced Thrombocytopenia Responsive to Cyclophosphamide," *South Med J*, 1979, 72(11):1490-2.

Ulmeanu V, Toma M, Eugah B, et al, "Severe Thrombocytopenia Following Treatment With Gold Salts," *Clin Exp Rheumatol*, 12(Suppl 11):112.

Gold Sodium Thiomalate *see* Gold Compounds *on page 386*

Granisetron (gra ni' se tron)

CAS Number 109889-09-0

Brand Names Kytril®

Synonyms BRL 43694

Use Prophylaxis and treatment of chemotherapy-related emesis; may be prescribed for patients who are refractory to or have severe adverse reactions to standard antiemetic therapy. Granisetron may be prescribed for young patients (ie, <45 years of age who are more likely to develop extrapyramidal reactions to high-dose metoclopramide) who are to receive highly emetogenic chemotherapeutic agents as listed:

Agents with high emetogenic potential (>90%) (dose/m^2):
- Carmustine ≥200 mg
- Cisplatin ≥75 mg
- Cyclophosphamide ≥1000 mg
- Cytarabine ≥1000 mg
- Dacarbazine ≥500 mg
- Ifosfamide ≥1000 mg
- Lomustine ≥60 mg
- Mechlorethamine
- Pentostatin
- Streptozocin

or two agents classified as having high or moderately high emetogenic potential as listed:

Agents with moderately high emetogenic potential (60% to 90%) (dose/m^2):
- Carmustine <200 mg
- Cisplatin <75 mg
- Cyclophosphamide 1000 mg
- Cytarabine 250-1000 mg
- Dacarbazine <500 mg
- Doxorubicin ≥75 mg
- Ifosfamide
- Lomustine <60 mg
- Methotrexate ≥250 mg
- Mitomycin
- Mitoxantrone
- Procarbazine

Granisetron should not be prescribed for chemotherapeutic agents with a low emetogenic potential (eg, bleomycin, busulfan, cyclophosphamide <1000 mg, etoposide, 5-fluorouracil, vinblastine, vincristine)

Mechanism of Action Selective 5-HT$_3$ receptor antagonist, blocking serotonin, both peripherally on vagal nerve terminals and centrally in the chemoreceptor trigger zone

Adverse Reactions
- Cardiovascular: Transient blood pressure changes
- Central nervous system: Headache, somnolence, agitation, asthenia
- Endocrine & metabolic: Hot flashes
- Gastrointestinal: Constipation, diarrhea
- Hepatic: Liver enzyme elevations

Signs & Symptoms of Acute Overdose Somnolence, myalgia

Toxicodynamics/Kinetics
- Onset of action: Commonly controls emesis within 1-3 minutes of administration
- Duration: Effects generally last no more than 24 hours maximum
- Distribution: V_d: 2-3 L/kg; widely distributed throughout the body
- Metabolism: Hepatic
- Half-life:
  - Cancer patients: 10-12 hours
  - Healthy volunteers: 4-5 hours
- Elimination: Primarily nonrenal, 8% to 15% of dose excreted unchanged in urine; clearance: 0.2-0.5 L/hour/kg

Usual Dosage I.V.:

10-40 mcg/kg for 1-3 doses. Doses should be administered as a single IVPB over 5 minutes to 1 hour, given just prior to chemotherapy (15-60 minutes before).

As intervention therapy for breakthrough nausea and vomiting, during the first 24 hours following chemotherapy, 2 or 3 repeat infusions (same dose) have been administered, separated by at least 10 minutes

Dosing interval in renal impairment: Creatinine clearance values have no relationship to granisetron clearance

Contraindications Previous hypersensitivity to granisetron

Warnings Use with caution in patients with liver disease or in pregnant patients

Dosage Forms Injection: 1 mg/mL

Stability Stable when mixed in NS for at least 4 hours

Reference Range Peak serum levels: 11-124 ng/mL following a 40 mcg/kg dose

Overdosage Treatment

Decontamination: Lavage/activated charcoal with cathartic

Enhancement of elimination: Multiple dosing of activated charcoal may be effective

Diagnostic Tests/Procedures

Liver Profile *on page 1286*

Pregnancy Risk Factor B

Monitoring Parameters Liver function tests

Nursing Implications Doses should be given at least 15 minutes prior to initiation of chemotherapy

Specific References

Chung KC, Chin A, and Gill MA, "Stability of Granisetron Hydrochloride in a Disposable Elestomeric Infusion Device," *Am J Health-Syst Pharm*, 1995, 52:1541-3.

Joss RA and Dott CS, "Clinical Studies With Granisetron, a New 5-HT3 Receptor Antagonist for the Treatment of Cancer Chemotherapy-Induced Emesis," *Eur J Cancer*, 1993, 29A(Suppl 1):S22-9.

Plosker GL and Goa KL, "Granisetron: A Review of Its Pharmacological Properties and Therapeutic Use as an Antiemetic," *Drugs*, 1991, 42(5):805-24.

Grifulvin® V *see* Griseofulvin *on this page*

Grisactin® *see* Griseofulvin *on this page*

Grisactin® Ultra *see* Griseofulvin *on this page*

Griseofulvin (gri see oh ful' vin)

Related Information

Therapeutic Drugs Associated With Hallucinations *on page 1558-1559*

CAS Number 126-07-8

Brand Names Fulvicin® P/G; Fulvicin-U/F®; Grifulvin® V; Grisactin®; Grisactin® Ultra; Gris-PEG®

Synonyms Curling Factor; Griseofulvin Microsize; Griseofulvin Ultramicrosize

Use Treatment of susceptible tinea infections of the skin, hair, and nails (dermatophytes)

Mechanism of Action Inhibits fungal cell mitosis at metaphase; binds to human keratin making it resistant to fungal invasion

Adverse Reactions

Central nervous system: Fatigue, confusion, impaired judgment, insomnia, headache, dizziness, auditory hallucinations, ataxia

Dermatologic: Rash, photosensitivity reaction, erythema multiforme, angioedema, Stevens-Johnson syndrome, toxic epidermal necrolysis

Gastrointestinal: Nausea, vomiting, altered taste, diarrhea, dry mouth, stomatitis

Hematologic: Leukopenia, granulocytopenia

Hepatic: Hepatotoxicity

Neuromuscular & skeletal: Paresthesia

Renal: Proteinuria

Miscellaneous: Lupus-like syndrome, blurred vision, anaphylaxis, porphyrinogenic with chronic use

Signs & Symptoms of Acute Overdose Leukopenia or neutropenia (agranulocytosis, granulocytopenia); insomnia, porphyrinogenic, toxic epidermal necrolysis, depression, systemic lupus erythematosus (SLE), erythema multiforme, vision color changes (green tinge), photosensitivity, cholestatic jaundice

Toxicodynamics/Kinetics

Absorption: Absorption of ultramicrosize griseofulvin is almost complete; absorption of microsize griseofulvin is variable (25% to 70% of an oral dose); absorption is enhanced by ingestion of a fatty meal

Metabolism: Extensive in the liver

Half-life: 9-22 hours

Elimination: <1% excreted unchanged in urine; also excreted in feces and sweating

Usual Dosage Oral:

Children:

Microsize: 10-15 mg/kg/day in single or divided doses

Ultramicrosize: >2 months: 5.5-7.3 mg/kg/day in single or divided doses

Adults:

Microsize: 500-1000 mg/day in single or divided doses

Ultramicrosize: 330-375 mg/day in single or divided doses; doses up to 750 mg/day have been used for infections more difficult to eradicate such as tinea unguium and tinea pedis

Duration of therapy depends on the site of infection:

Tinea corporis: 2-4 weeks

Tinea capitis: 4-6 weeks or longer

(Continued)

Griseofulvin *(Continued)*

Tinea pedis: 4-8 weeks
Tinea unguium: 4-6 months

Contraindications Hypersensitivity to griseofulvin or any component; severe liver disease, porphyria (interferes with porphyrin metabolism)

Warnings Safe use in children <2 years of age has not been established; during long-term therapy, periodic assessment of hepatic, renal, and hematopoietic functions should be performed; may cause fetal harm when administered to pregnant women; avoid exposure to intense sunlight to prevent photosensitivity reactions; hypersensitivity cross reaction between penicillins and griseofulvin is possible

Dosage Forms

Microsize:

- Capsule (Grisactin®): 125 mg, 250 mg
- Suspension, oral (Grifulvin® V): 125 mg/5 mL with alcohol 0.2% (120 mL)
- Tablet:
  - Fulvicin-U/F®, Grifulvin® V: 250 mg
  - Fulvicin-U/F®, Grifulvin® V, Grisactin-500®: 500 mg

Ultramicrosize:

- Tablet:
  - Fulvicin® P/G: 165 mg, 330 mg
  - Fulvicin® P/G, Grisactin® Ultra, Gris-PEG®: 125 mg, 250 mg
  - Grisactin® Ultra: 330 mg

Reference Range Peak plasma griseofulvin level of 1 μg/mL after a 500 mg dose

Overdosage Treatment

Decontamination: Lavage/activated charcoal with cathartic

Enhancement of elimination: Multiple dosing of activated charcoal may be effective

Test Interactions False-positive urinary VMA levels

Diagnostic Tests/Procedures

Complete Blood Count *on page 1236*

Kidney Profile *on page 1279*

Liver Profile *on page 1286*

Drug Interactions

Decreased effect of anticoagulants, oral contraceptives; decreased effect/levels with barbiturates

Disulfiram-like reaction with alcohol

Pregnancy Risk Factor C

Pregnancy Implications Crosses the placenta; embryotoxic/teratogenic in cats and rodents; conjoined twins and mongolism noted in humans

Monitoring Parameters Periodic renal, hepatic, and hematopoietic function tests

Patient Information Avoid exposure to sunlight, take with fatty meal; if patient gets headache, it usually goes away with continued therapy; may cause dizziness, drowsiness, and impair judgment; do not take if pregnant; if you become pregnant, discontinue immediately

Additional Information

Microsize: Fulvicin-U/F®, Grifulvin® V, Grisactin®

Ultramicrosize: Fulvicin® P/G, Grisactin® Ultra, Gris-PEG®; gastrointestinal absorption of ultramicrosize is ~1.5 times that of microsize

Specific References

Kawabe Y, Mizuno N, Miwa N, et al, "Photosensitivity Induced by Griseofulvin," *Photodermatol*, 1988, 5(6):272-4.

Lecky BR, "Griseofulvin-Induced Neuropathy," *Lancet*, 1990, 335(8683):230-1.

Mion G, Verdon R, Le Gulluche Y, et al, "Fatal Toxic Epidermal Necrolysis After Griseofulvin," *Lancet*, 1989, 2(8675):1331.

Yang DJ and Rankin GO, "Nephrotoxicity of Antifungal Agents," *Adverse Drug React Acute Poisoning Rev*, 1985, 4(1):37-49.

Griseofulvin Microsize *see* Griseofulvin *on previous page*

Griseofulvin Ultramicrosize *see* Griseofulvin *on previous page*

Gris-PEG® *see* Griseofulvin *on previous page*

Guaifenesin (gwye fen' e sin)

CAS Number 93-14-1

Brand Names Anti-Tuss® Expectorant [OTC]; Breonesin® [OTC]; Diabetic Tussin EX® [OTC]; Fenesin™ [OTC]; Gee Gee® [OTC]; Genatuss® [OTC]; GG-Cen® [OTC]; Glyate® [OTC]; Glycotuss® [OTC]; Glytuss® [OTC]; GuiaCough® Expectorant [OTC]; Guiatuss® [OTC]; Halotussin® [OTC]; Humibid® L.A. [OTC]; Humibid® Sprinkle [OTC]; Hytuss® [OTC]; Hytuss-2X® [OTC]; Liquibid®; Malotuss® [OTC]; Medi-Tuss® [OTC]; Mytussin® [OTC]; Naldecon® Senior EX [OTC]; Pneumomist®; Respa-GF®; Robitussin® [OTC]; Scot-Tussin® [OTC]; Siltussin® [OTC]; Sinumist®-SR Capsulets® [OTC]; Touro Ex®; Uni-Tussin® [OTC]

Synonyms GG; Glycerol Guaiacolate

Use Temporary control of cough due to minor throat and bronchial irritation

Mechanism of Action Thought to act as an expectorant by irritating the gastric mucosa and stimulating respiratory tract secretions, thereby increasing respiratory fluid volumes and decreasing phlegm viscosity

Adverse Reactions

Central nervous system: Drowsiness, headache
Dermatologic: Rash
Gastrointestinal: Nausea, vomiting, stomach pain
Miscellaneous: Porphyrinogenic

Signs & Symptoms of Acute Overdose Vomiting, lethargy, coma, respiratory depression, nausea

Toxicodynamics/Kinetics

Absorption: Well absorbed from gastrointestinal tract
Distribution: V_d: 1 L/kg
Metabolism: Hepatic, 60%
Half-life: 1 hour
Elimination: Renal excretion of changed and unchanged drug

Usual Dosage Oral:

Children:

<2 years: 12 mg/kg/day in 6 divided doses
2-5 years: 50-100 mg (2.5-5 mL) every 4 hours, not to exceed 600 mg/day
6-11 years: 100-200 mg (5-10 mL) every 4 hours, not to exceed 1.2 g/day

Children >12 years and Adults: 200-400 mg (10-20 mL) every 4 hours to a maximum of 2.4 g/day (120 mL/day)

Contraindications Hypersensitivity to guaifenesin or any component

Warnings Not for persistent cough such as occurs with smoking, asthma, or emphysema or cough accompanied by excessive secretions

Dosage Forms

Caplet, sustained release (Touro Ex®): 600 mg
Capsule (Breonesin®, GG-Cen®, Hytuss-2X®): 200 mg
Capsule, sustained release (Humibid® Sprinkle): 300 mg
Liquid:

Diabetic Tussin EX®: 100 mg/5 mL (118 mL)
Naldecon® Senior EX: 200 mg/5 mL (118 mL, 480 mL)

Syrup (Anti-Tuss® Expectorant, Genatuss®, Glyate®, GuiaCough® Expectorant, Guiatuss®, Halotussin®, Malotuss®, Medi-Tuss®, Mytussin®, Robitussin®, Scot-Tussin®, Siltussin®, Uni-Tussin®): 100 mg/5 mL with alcohol 3.5% (30 mL, 120 mL, 240 mL, 473 mL, 946 mL)

Tablet:

Gee Gee®, Glytuss®: 200 mg
Glycotuss®, Hytuss®: 100 mg
Sustained release:

Fenesin™, Humibid® L.A., Liquibid®, Pneumomist®, Respa-GF®, Sinumist®-SR Capsulets®: 600 mg

Stability Protect from light

Reference Range 600 mg oral dose results in a peak guaifenesin blood level of 1.4 mg/L

Overdosage Treatment

Decontamination: Lavage/activated charcoal
Enhancement of elimination: Multiple dosing of activated charcoal may be effective

Test Interactions Possible color interference with determination of 5-HIAA and VMA; decreases serum uric acid (uricosuric)

Drug Interactions Disulfiram, MAO inhibitors, metronidazole, procarbazine

Pregnancy Risk Factor C

Monitoring Parameters Cough, sputum consistency and volume

Patient Information Take with a large quantity of fluid to ensure proper action; if cough persists for more than 1 week or is accompanied by fever, rash, or persistent headache, physician should be consulted

Specific References

Kuhn JJ, Hendley JO, Adams DF, et al, "Antitussive Effect of Guaifenesin in Young Adults With Natural Colds," *Chest*, 1982, 6:713-8.

Guanabenz Acetate (gwahn' a benz)

CAS Number 5051-62-7; 23256-50-0

Brand Names Rexitene®; Wytensin®

Synonyms 1-(2,6-Dichlorobenzylideneamine) Guanidine Acetate; WY-8678

Use Management of mild to moderate hypertension

Mechanism of Action Stimulates alpha$_2$-adrenoreceptors in the brain stem, thus activating an inhibitory neuron, resulting in reduced sympathetic outflow, producing a decrease in vasomotor tone and heart rate

Adverse Reactions

Cardiovascular: Bradycardia, chest pain

(Continued)

Guanabenz Acetate *(Continued)*

Central nervous system: Drowsiness, dizziness, asthenia, hypothermia, headache
Gastrointestinal: Nausea, dry mouth
Ocular: Miosis

Signs & Symptoms of Acute Overdose CNS depression, dyspnea, depression, impotence, gynecomastia, hypothermia, apnea, impotence, myalgia, bradycardia, drowsiness, diarrhea, hypotension, miosis, hyperglycemia and hypoglycemia

Toxicodynamics/Kinetics

Onset of action: Antihypertensive effects occur within 60 minutes
Duration: 12 hours
Absorption: Oral: ~75% from gastrointestinal tract
Distribution: V_d: 7.4-17 L/kg; widely distributed into body
Protein binding: 90%
Metabolism: Extensive
Bioavailability: Very low because of extensive first-pass metabolism
Half-life: 7-10 hours
Time to peak serum concentration: 2-5 hours
Elimination: <1% excreted as unchanged drug in urine

Usual Dosage Adults: Oral: Initial: 4 mg twice daily, increase in increments of 4-8 mg/day every 1-2 weeks to a maximum of 32 mg twice daily

Dosing adjustment in hepatic impairment: Probably necessary

Contraindications Hypersensitivity to guanabenz or any component

Warnings Not considered a drug of choice in the elderly; do not abruptly discontinue this medication

Dosage Forms Tablet: 4 mg, 8 mg

Stability Protect from light

Overdosage Treatment

Decontamination: Ipecac or lavage/activated charcoal with cathartic

Supportive therapy: Hypotension usually responds to I.V. fluids or Trendelenburg positioning. If unresponsive to these measures, the use of a parenteral vasoconstrictor may be required (eg, norepinephrine 0.1-0.2 mcg/kg/minute titrated to response). Naloxone may be utilized in treating the hypotension, CNS depression, and/or apnea and should be given I.V. 0.4-2 mg, with repeats as needed. Atropine 15 mcg/kg I.V. or I.M. may be needed for symptomatic bradycardia.

Enhancement of elimination: Multiple dosing of activated charcoal would not be useful; hemodialysis is not useful

Test Interactions Increases sodium (S)

Drug Interactions Other hypotensive agents

Pregnancy Risk Factor C

Monitoring Parameters Blood pressure, standing and sitting/supine

Patient Information May cause drowsiness; rise from sitting/lying position carefully, may cause dizziness

Additional Information Guanabenz is considered an alternate to clonidine; it causes less sodium retention than clonidine or methyldopa

Specific References

Hall AH, Smolinske SC, Kulig KW, et al, "Guanabenz Overdose," *Ann Intern Med*, 1985, 102(6):787-8.
Perrone J, Hoffman RS, Jones B, et al, "Guanabenz Induced Hypothermia in a Poisoned Elderly Female," *J Toxicol Clin Toxicol*, 1994, 32(4):445-9.
Rogers SJ, "Guanabenz Overdose," *Ann Intern Med*, 1986, 104(3):445.

Guanadrel Sulfate (gwahn' a drel)

CAS Number 22195-34-2; 40580-59-4

Brand Names Hylorel®

Use Step 2 agent in stepped-care treatment of hypertension, usually with a diuretic

Mechanism of Action Acts as a false neurotransmitter that blocks the adrenergic actions of norepinephrine; it displaces norepinephrine form its presynaptic storage granules and thus exposes it to degradation; it thereby produces a reduction in total peripheral resistance and therefore blood pressure

Adverse Reactions

Cardiovascular: Orthostatic hypotension, palpitations, chest pain
Central nervous system: Fatigue, dizziness, asthenia, headache, faintness, drowsiness
Gastrointestinal: Diarrhea, increased bowel movements
Genitourinary: Ejaculatory disturbances, nocturia
Ocular: Blurred vision
Respiratory: Dyspnea

Signs & Symptoms of Acute Overdose Hypotension, blurred vision, ejaculatory disturbances, dizziness, nocturia, nausea, vomiting

Toxicodynamics/Kinetics

Onset of action: 2 hours

Peak effect: Within 4-6 hours
Duration: 4-14 hours, average of 9 hours
Absorption: Oral: Rapid from gastrointestinal tract
Distribution: Hydrophilic and, therefore, does not cross the blood-brain barrier
Protein binding: 20%
Metabolism: Hepatic
Half-life: Initial: 1-4 hours, terminal: 5-45 hours
Time to peak serum concentration: Within 90-120 minutes
Elimination: Excreted in urine, 40% as unchanged drug; biphasic elimination

Usual Dosage Adults: Oral: Initial: 10 mg/day (5 mg twice daily); adjust dosage until blood pressure is controlled, usual dosage: 20-75 mg/day, given twice daily

Dosing in renal impairment:
Cl_{cr} 10-50 mL/minute: Administer every 12-24 hours
Cl_{cr} <10 mL/minute: Administer every 24-48 hours

Contraindications Known hypersensitivity to guanadrel, pheochromocytoma, congestive heart failure, patients taking MAO inhibitors

Warnings Not considered a drug of choice in the elderly

Dosage Forms Tablet: 10 mg, 25 mg

Overdosage Treatment
Decontamination: Ipecac or lavage/activated charcoal with cathartic
Supportive therapy: Hypotension usually responds to I.V. fluids or Trendelenburg positioning. If unresponsive to these measures, the use of a parenteral vasoconstrictor may be required (eg, dopamine 2-5 mcg/kg/minute titrated to 10 mcg/kg/minute). Naloxone may be utilized in treating the hypotension, CNS depression and/or apnea and should be given I.V. 0.4-2 mg, with repeats as needed. Atropine 15 mcg/kg I.V. or I.M. may be needed for symptomatic bradycardia.
Enhancement of elimination: Multiple dosing of activated charcoal may be effective

Test Interactions Increases sodium (S)

Drug Interactions Tricyclic antidepressants, sympathomimetics, vasodilators, alpha- or beta-blocking agents, reserpine, other hypotensive agents

Pregnancy Risk Factor B

Pregnancy Implications Crosses the placenta

Monitoring Parameters Blood pressure, standing and sitting/supine

Patient Information Change positions slowly; do not take any over-the-counter or prescription cold medications without consulting your physician

Nursing Implications Tablet may be crushed; assist patient with rising and ambulation

Additional Information Considered an alternative to guanethidine

Specific References

Finnerty FA Jr and Brogden RN, "Guanadrel: A Review of Its Pharmacodynamic and Pharmacokinetic Properties and Therapeutic Use in Hypertension," *Drugs*, 1985, 30(1):22-31.

Guanethidine Monosulfate *see* Guanethidine Sulfate *on this page*

Guanethidine Sulfate (gwahn eth' i deen)

CAS Number 55-65-2; 645-43-2

Brand Names Ismelin®

Synonyms Guanethidine Monosulfate; Guanetidine

Use Treatment of moderate to severe hypertension; also useful in treating vasopressin extravasation

Mechanism of Action Acts as a false neurotransmitter that blocks the adrenergic actions of norepinephrine; it displaces norepinephrine from its presynaptic storage granules and thus exposes it to degradation; it thereby produces a reduction in total peripheral resistance and therefore blood pressure

Adverse Reactions
Cardiovascular: Palpitations, chest pain, hypotension (orthostatic)
Central nervous system: Fatigue, hypoglycemia, dizziness, asthenia, drowsiness, faintness, headache
Gastrointestinal: Diarrhea, increased bowel movements
Genitourinary: Ejaculatory disturbances, nocturia
Ocular: Blurred vision, diplopia
Respiratory: Dyspnea
Miscellaneous: Hypertension in patients with pheochromocytoma

Signs & Symptoms of Acute Overdose Hypotension, ejaculatory disturbances, blurred vision, periarteritis nodosa, nocturia, ptosis, impotence, dizziness, syncope, nausea, vomiting

Toxicodynamics/Kinetics
Onset of action: 0.5-2 hours
Peak effect: 6-8 hours
Duration: 24-48 hours

(Continued)

Guanethidine Sulfate *(Continued)*

Absorption: Oral: Irregular (3% to 55%)

Distribution: Does not readily cross blood-brain barrier; distributed throughout body

Protein binding: None

Metabolism: Hepatic metabolism to inactive metabolites

Half-life: 5-10 days

Elimination: 25% to 60% of dose excreted unchanged in urine, small amounts also appear in feces

Usual Dosage Oral:

Children: Initial: 0.2 mg/kg/day, increase by 0.2 mg/kg/day at 7- to 10-day intervals to a maximum of 3 mg/kg/day

Adults:

Ambulatory patients: Initial: 10 mg/day, increase at 5- to 7-day intervals to a maximum of 25-50 mg/day

Hospitalized patients: Initial: 25-50 mg/day, increase by 25-50 mg/day or every other day to desired therapeutic response

Vasopressin extravasation: 10 mg in 0.9% saline (10 mL) with 1000 units of heparin either through offending I.V. cannulas or through multiple S.C. injections after removal of catheter; apply ice to affected area

Dosing interval in renal impairment: Cl_{cr} <10 mL/minute: Administer every 24-36 hours

Contraindications Pheochromocytoma, MAO inhibitors, hypersensitivity to guanethidine or any component

Warnings Orthostatic hypotension can occur frequently; avoid the use of guanethidine in the elderly

Dosage Forms Tablet: 10 mg, 25 mg

Reference Range Adrenergic blockade at plasma concentrations of 8 ng/mL

Overdosage Treatment Supportive therapy: Hypotension usually responds to I.V. fluids or Trendelenburg positioning. If unresponsive to these measures, the use of a parenteral vasoconstrictor may be required (eg, dopamine at 2-5 mcg/kg/minute titrated to 10 mcg/kg/minute). Treatment is primarily supportive and symptomatic; overdose symptoms usually last for 72 hours.

Test Interactions Increases sodium (S); decreases catecholamines (U)

Drug Interactions Tricyclic antidepressants, phenothiazines, anorexiants, haloperidol, maprotiline, methylphenidate and MAO inhibitors decrease antihypertensive efficacy, sympathomimetics (metaraminol, ephedrine)

Pregnancy Risk Factor C

Monitoring Parameters Blood pressure, standing and sitting/supine

Patient Information May cause drowsiness; rise from sitting/lying carefully, may cause dizziness

Nursing Implications Tablet may be crushed

Specific References

Kalmanovitch DV and Hardwick PB, "Hypotension After Guanethidine Block," *Anaesthesia*, 1988, 43(3):256.

MacCara ME, "Extravasation - A Hazard of Intravenous Therapy," *Drug Intell Clin Pharm*, 1983, 17:713.

Guanetidine *see* Guanethidine Sulfate *on previous page*

Guanfacine Hydrochloride (gwahn' fa seen)

CAS Number 29110-47-2

Brand Names Estulic®; Tenex®

Use Management of hypertension

Mechanism of Action False neurotransmitter ($alpha_2$-adrenoceptor agonist) that blocks the adrenergic actions of norepinephrine; displaces norepinephrine form its presynaptic storage granules and thus exposes it to degradation and, thereby, produces a reduction in total peripheral resistance and, therefore, blood pressure; structurally related to guanabenz, methyldopa, and clonidine

Adverse Reactions

Cardiovascular: Chest pain, bradycardia

Central nervous system: Drowsiness, dizziness, asthenia, headache

Gastrointestinal: Nausea, dyspepsia, dry mouth

Signs & Symptoms of Acute Overdose CNS depression, dermatitis, hypomagnesemia, insomnia, impotence, dysphagia, hypothermia, apnea, drowsiness, myalgia, leg cramps, diarrhea, hypotension (4-8 hours postingestion), bradycardia (within 2 hours of ingestion); paradoxical hypertension can occur

Toxicodynamics/Kinetics

Onset of action: Multiple doses within 1 week

Peak effect: Can be expected within 8-11 hours and can persist for 24 hours following a single dose

Absorption: Rapid and complete
Distribution: Widely to tissues
Protein binding: 70%
Metabolism: In the liver to glucuronide and sulfate metabolites
Bioavailability: 80% to 100%
Half-life: 17 hours
Time to peak serum concentration: Peak serum levels occur within 1-4 hours following oral administration
Elimination: Renal excretion of changed and unchanged drug (30%); 2% is recoverable in feces

Usual Dosage Adults: Oral: 1 mg usually at bedtime, may increase if needed at 3- to 4-week intervals to a maximum of 3 mg/day; 1 mg/day is most common dose

Contraindications Hypersensitivity to guanfacine or any component

Dosage Forms Tablet: 1 mg

Reference Range Adult therapeutic effect at serum levels of 1.5-2.0 ng/mL

Overdosage Treatment

Decontamination: Lavage/activated charcoal with cathartic
Supportive therapy: Hypotension usually responds to I.V. fluids or Trendelenburg positioning. If unresponsive to these measures, the use of a parenteral vasoconstrictor may be required (eg, norepinephrine 0.1-0.2 mcg/kg/minute titrated to response). Naloxone may be utilized in treating the hypotension, CNS depression and/or apnea and should be given I.V. 0.4-2 mg, with repeats as needed. Atropine 15 mcg/kg I.V. or I.M. may be needed for symptomatic bradycardia.
Enhancement of elimination: Hemodialysis is not useful due to its large volume of distribution.

Antidote(s)

Naloxone Hydrochloride *on page 1447*

Test Interactions Increases cholesterol, sodium (S), triglycerides, AST, GPT

Pregnancy Risk Factor B (no specific teratogenic effects noted in animals)

Monitoring Parameters Blood pressure, standing and sitting/supine, EKG

Patient Information May cause drowsiness, vertigo; do not discontinue this medication without consulting your physician; take at bedtime

Nursing Implications Tablet may be crushed; assist patient with rising and ambulation

Additional Information Usually given with a thiazide diuretic

Specific References

Cornish LA, "Guanfacine Hydrochloride: A Centrally Acting Hypertensive Agent," *Clin Pharm*, 1988, 7(3):187-97.

Granier P, Arsac P, and Debru JL, "Intoxication Par La Guanfacine," *Nouv Presse Med*, 1982, 11(21):1636-7.

Van Dyke MW, Bonace AL, and Ellenhorn MJ, "Guanfacine Overdose in a Pediatric Patient," *Vet Hum Toxicol*, 1990, 32(1):46-7.

Guanidine Hydrochloride (gwahn' i deen)

CAS Number 113-00-8; 50-01-1

Synonyms Carbamidine Hydrochloride; Iminourea Hydrochloride

Use Reduction of symptoms of muscle weakness associated with the myasthenic syndrome of Eaton-Lambert, not for myasthenia gravis; has been used in botulism (type B) to reverse neuromuscular blockade with disappointing results

Adverse Reactions

Cardiovascular: Bradycardia, A-V block
Central nervous system: Headache, seizures, dysphoria, drowsiness, ataxia
Endocrine & metabolic: Hypoglycemia
Gastrointestinal: Diarrhea, nausea, stomach cramps
Genitourinary: Urge to urinate
Local: Thrombophlebitis
Neuromuscular & skeletal: Muscle spasm, tremors, weakness
Ocular: Lacrimation, miosis, diplopia
Respiratory: Increased bronchial secretions, respiratory paralysis
Miscellaneous: Increased sweating and mouth watering, laryngospasm, hypersensitivity, hyper-reactive cholinergic responses, aplastic anemia

Usual Dosage Adults: Oral: Initial: 10-15 mg/kg/day in 3-4 divided doses, gradually increase to 40 mg/kg/day

Contraindications Hypersensitivity to drug

Dosage Forms Tablet: 125 mg

Overdosage Treatment

Decontamination: Lavage/activated charcoal
Supportive therapy: Treat bradycardia with atropine

Test Interactions Increase creatinine; hypoglycemia

Additional Information Primary effect on botulism is on improvement in ocular muscles; little effect on respiratory function

Specific References

Neal KR and Dunbar EM, "Improvement in Bulbar Weakness With Guanoxan in Type B Botulism," *Lancet*, 1990, 335(8700):1286-7.

(Continued)

Guanidine Hydrochloride *(Continued)*

Pugglari M and Cherington M, "Botulism and Guanidine," *JAMA*, 1978, 240:2276-7.

Guaranine *see* Caffeine *on page 175*

GuiaCough® Expectorant [OTC] *see* Guaifenesin *on page 390*

Guiatuss® [OTC] *see* Guaifenesin *on page 390*

Gum Camphor *see* Camphor *on page 179*

Gutron® *see* Midodrine Hydrochloride *on page 534*

GVG *see* Vigabatrin *on page 790*

G-well® *see* Lindane *on page 470*

Gyne-Lotrimin® [OTC] *see* Clotrimazole *on page 234*

H1-Antihistamine Comparison *see page 1649*

H_2O_2 *see* Hydrogen Peroxide *on page 408*

Habitrol™ Patch *see* Nicotine *on page 556*

Halcion® *see* Triazolam *on page 767*

Haldol® *see* Haloperidol *on this page*

Haldol® Decanoate *see* Haloperidol *on this page*

Halenol® [OTC] *see* Acetaminophen *on page 79*

Halite *see* Sodium Chloride *on page 698*

Haloneural® *see* Haloperidol *on this page*

Haloperidol (ha loe per' i dole)

Related Information

Antipsychotic Agents Comparison *on page 1642*

Doses and Administration of Several Frequently Used Antiemetic Agents *on page 1641*

CAS Number 52-86-8; 74050-97-8

Brand Names Dozic®; Fortunan®; Haldol®; Haldol® Decanoate; Haloneural®; Serenace®

Use Treatment of psychoses, Tourette's disorder, and severe behavioral problems in children; may be used for the emergency sedation of severely agitated or delirious patients

Mechanism of Action Competitive blockade of postsynaptic dopamine receptors in the mesolimbic dopaminergic system; depresses cerebral cortex and hypothalamus; exhibits a strong alpha-adrenergic and anticholinergic blocking activity

Adverse Reactions Sedation and anticholinergic effects are more pronounced than extrapyramidal effects; EKG changes, retinal pigmentation are more common than with chlorpromazine; concomitant therapy with perazine can cause agranulocytosis and hepatotoxicity

Cardiovascular: Hypotension (especially hypotension (orthostatic)), tachycardia, cardiac arrhythmias, abnormal T waves with prolonged ventricular repolarization

Central nervous system: Sedation, drowsiness, restlessness, anxiety, extrapyramidal reactions, dystonic reactions, pseudoparkinsonian signs and symptoms, tardive dyskinesia, neuroleptic malignant syndrome, seizures, altered central temperature regulation, electroencephalogram abnormalities

Dermatologic: Hyperpigmentation, pruritus, rash, contact dermatitis, photosensitivity (rare), alopecia

Endocrine & metabolic: Amenorrhea, galactorrhea, gynecomastia, syndrome of inappropriate antidiuretic hormone, weight gain

Gastrointestinal: Constipation, adynamic ileus, dyspepsia, gastrointestinal upset, dry mouth (problem for denture user)

Genitourinary: Urinary retention, overflow incontinence, priapism, sexual dysfunction

Hematologic: Leukopenia/neutropenia (agranulocytosis, granulocytopenia) (usually inpatients with large doses for prolonged periods)

Hepatic: Cholestatic jaundice

Ocular: Blurred vision, retinal pigmentation, ↓ visual acuity (may be irreversible)

Signs & Symptoms of Acute Overdose Deep sleep, hyperthermia, impotence, dementia, hyperreflexia, hyperprolactinemia, ejaculatory disturbances, chorea (extrapyramidal), hyperglycemia, ptosis, memory loss, lactation, hypopigmented hair, Parkinson's-like symptoms, confusion, dementia, gynecomastia, neuroleptic malignant syndrome, myasthenia gravis (exacerbation or precipitation of), hypoglycemia, hypothermia, disorientation, dysphagia, dystonic reactions, agitation, pulmonary edema, hypokalemia, arrhythmias, extrapyramidal reaction, Q-T prolongation, dry mouth, alopecia, bradycardia, fever, systemic lupus erythematosus (SLE), urine discoloration (pink), urine discoloration (red), urine discoloration (red-brown)

Toxicodynamics/Kinetics

Peak effect: Peak pharmacologic action and control of psychotic manifestation occurs within 30-40 minutes; decanoate form: Peak concentrations occur within about 6-7 days (range: 1-9 days)

Absorption: Well absorbed from the gastrointestinal tract

Distribution: V_d: 18-30 L/kg; widely distributed into the body

Protein binding: 90%

Metabolism: In the liver to inactive compounds

Bioavailability: Oral: 60%

Half-life: 20 hours; Decanoate: 3 weeks

Time to peak serum concentration:

- Oral: 3-6 hours
- I.M.: 10-20 minutes
- I.M. (long-acting): 3-9 days

Elimination: 33% to 40% excreted in urine within 5 days; an additional 15% excreted in feces

Usual Dosage

Children:

- 3-6 years (15-40 kg): Oral: Initial: 0.25-0.5 mg/day given in 2-3 divided doses; increase by 0.25-0.5 mg every 5-7 days; usual maintenance:
  - Agitation or hyperkinesia: 0.01-0.03 mg/kg/day once daily
  - Nonpsychotic disorders: 0.05-0.075 mg/kg/day in 2-3 divided doses
  - Psychotic disorders: 0.05-0.15 mg/kg/day in 2-3 divided doses
- 6-12 years:
  - Oral: Initial: 0.5-1.5 mg/day and increase gradually by 0.5 mg/24 hour increments to maintenance of 2-4 mg/24 hours
  - I.M. (as lactate): 1-3 mg/dose every 4-8 hours to a maximum of 0.1 mg/kg/day; change over to oral therapy as soon as able

Adults:

- Oral: 0.5-5 mg 2-3 times/day; maximum: 100 mg/day
- I.M. (as lactate): 2-5 mg every 4-8 hours as needed
- I.M. (as decanoate): Initial: 10-15 times the daily oral dose administered at 4-week intervals

Haloperidol lactate may also be administered intravenously

Contraindications Hypersensitivity to haloperidol or any component; narrow-angle glaucoma, bone marrow depression, CNS depression, severe liver or cardiac disease, parkinsonism

Warnings Safety and efficacy have not been established in children <3 years of age; watch for hypotension when administering I.M. or I.V.; use with caution in patients with cardiovascular disease or seizures; benefits of therapy must be weighed against risks of therapy; decanoate form should never be given I.V. Some tablets contain tartrazine which may cause allergic reactions; use caution in patients receiving anticonvulsant agents and in those with a history of seizures or EEG abnormalities

Dosage Forms

Concentrate, oral, as lactate: 2 mg/mL (5 mL, 10 mL, 15 mL, 120 mL, 240 mL)

Injection, as decanoate: 50 mg/mL (1 mL, 5 mL); 100 mg/mL (1 mL, 5 mL)

Injection, as lactate: 5 mg/mL (1 mL, 2 mL, 2.5 mL, 10 mL)

Tablet: 0.5 mg, 1 mg, 2 mg, 5 mg, 10 mg, 20 mg

Stability Protect oral dosage forms from light; insoluble in water

Reference Range

Therapeutic: 5-15 ng/mL (SI: 10-30 nmol/L) (psychotic disorders – less for Tourette's and mania)

Toxic: >42 ng/mL (SI: >84 nmol/L)

Overdosage Treatment

Decontamination: Lavage/activated charcoal with cathartic

Supportive therapy: Hypotension usually responds to I.V. fluids or Trendelenburg positioning. If unresponsive to these measures, the use of a parenteral inotrope may be required (eg, norepinephrine 0.1-0.2 mcg/kg/minute titrated to response). Seizures commonly respond to lorazepam or diazepam (I.V. 5-10 mg bolus in adults every 15 minutes if needed up to a total of 30 mg; I.V. 0.25-0.4 mg/kg/dose up to a total of 10 mg in children) or to phenytoin or phenobarbital. Also critical cardiac arrhythmias often respond to I.V. phenytoin (15 mg/kg up to 1 g), while other antiarrhythmics (ie, lidocaine) can be used. Neuroleptics often cause extrapyramidal reaction (eg, dystonic reactions) requiring management with diphenhydramine 1-2 mg/kg (adults) up to a maximum of 50 mg I.M. or I.V. slow push followed by a maintenance dose for 48-72 hours. When these reactions are unresponsive to diphenhydramine, benztropine mesylate I.V. 1-2 mg (adults) may be effective. These agents are generally effective within 2-5 minutes.

Enhancement of elimination: Multiple dosing of activated charcoal would not be expected to be useful

Test Interactions Decreases cholesterol (S)

(Continued)

Haloperidol *(Continued)*

Diagnostic Tests/Procedures
Haloperidol, Blood *on page 1271*

Drug Interactions CNS depressants may increase adverse effects; epinephrine may cause hypotension, carbamazepine and phenobarbital may increase metabolism and decreased effectiveness of haloperidol; haloperidol and anticholinergic agents may cause an increase in intraocular pressure; concurrent use with lithium has occasionally caused acute encephalopathy-like syndrome

Pregnancy Risk Factor C

Pregnancy Implications Crosses the placenta; appears in breast milk

Monitoring Parameters EKG, electrolytes

Patient Information May cause drowsiness

Nursing Implications Observe for extrapyramidal effects

Additional Information 5 mg of haloperidol (I.V.) followed by a bolus of 1 L of normal saline has been used to treat migraine headaches; may be used for the emergency sedation of severely agitated or delirious patients; call DIC for more information, ext 9125

Specific References

Aunsholt NA, "Prolonged Q-T Interval and Hypokalemia Caused by Haloperidol," *Acta Psychiatr Scand*, 1989, 79(4):411-2.

Bauer M, "Concurrent Agranulocytosis and Acute Hepatitis Resulting From Combination of Classic Neuroleptics and Subsequent Successful Clozapine Treatment," *Pharmacopsychiatry*, 1995, 28:29-31.

Di Salvo TG and O'Gara PT, "Torsade de Pointes Caused by High-Dose Intravenous Haloperidol in Cardiac Patients," *Clin Cardiol*, 1995, 18:285-90.

Doenecke AL and Heuermann RC, "Treatment of Haloperidol Abuse With Diphenhydramine," *Am J Psychiatry*, 1980, 137(4):487-8.

Fisher H, "A New Approach to Emergency Department Therapy of Migraine Headache With Intravenous Haloperidol: A Case Series," *J Emerg Med*, 1995, 13:119-22.

Harada H, Igarashi M, Sugae S, et al, "A Schizophrenic Patient Who Developed Extreme Hypothermia After an Increase in the Dose of Haloperidol: A Case Report," *Jpn J Psychiatry Neurol*, 1994, 48(3):595-8.

Kubota T, Ishikura T, and Jibiki I, "Alopecia Areata Associated With Haloperidol," *Jpn J Psychiatry Neurol*, 1994, 48(3):579-81.

Mahutte CK, Nakasato SK, and Light RW, "Haloperidol and Sudden Death Due to Pulmonary Edema," *Arch Intern Med*, 1982, 142(10):1951-2.

Schwartz M, Weller B, Erdreich M, et al, "Rabbit Syndrome and Tardive Dyskinesia: Two Complications of Chronic Neuroleptic Treatment," *J Clin Psychiatry*, 1995, 56:212.

Riker RR, Fraser GL, and Cox PM, "Continuous Infusion of Haloperidol Controls Agitation in Critically Ill Patients," *Crit Care Med*, 1994, 22(3):433-40.

Wilt JL, Minnema AM, Johnson RF, et al, "Torsade de Pointes Associated With the Use of Intravenous Haloperidol," *Ann Intern Med*, 1993, 119(5):391-4.

Halotussin® [OTC] *see* Guaifenesin *on page 390*

Haltran® [OTC] *see* Ibuprofen *on page 418*

Happy-Trip® *see* Cyclizine *on page 248*

Harolan® *see* Benzbromarone *on page 148*

HCTZ *see* Hydrochlorothiazide *on page 406*

Heavy Mineral Oil *see* Mineral Oil *on page 534*

Heitrin® *see* Terazosin *on page 725*

Hemocyte® *see* Iron *on page 439*

Hemovas® *see* Pentoxifylline *on page 607*

Heparin (hep' a rin)

CAS Number 9041-08-1; 9005-49-6; 37270-89-6

Brand Names Calciparine® Injection; Hep-Lock® Injection; Liquaemin® Injection

Synonyms Heparin Calcium; Heparin Lock Flush; Heparin Sodium

Use Prophylaxis and treatment of thromboembolic disorders

Mechanism of Action Potentiates the action of antithrombin III and thereby inactivates thrombin (as well as activated coagulation factors IX, X, XI, XII, and plasmin) and prevents the conversion of fibrinogen to fibrin; heparin also stimulates release of lipoprotein lipase (lipoprotein lipase hydrolyzes triglycerides to glycerol and free fatty acids)

Adverse Reactions
Cardiovascular: Cardiac tamponade
Central nervous system: Fever, headache, chills, hallucinations
Dermatologic: Urticaria, pruritus, eczema, alopecia, skin necrosis
Endocrine & metabolic: Hyperkalemia with prolonged therapy from hypoaldosteronism
Gastrointestinal: Nausea, vomiting
Genitourinary: Priapism

Hematologic: Hemorrhage (risk is threefold with APTT between 2-2.9 times control and eightfold when APTT is over 3 times control), thrombocytopenia (1.5%), incidence of thrombocytopenia is greater with bovine than porcine heparin preparations; intracranial hemorrhage, ocular hemorrhage, purpura, coagulopathy

Hepatic: Elevation of liver enzymes

Local: Irritation, ulceration, cutaneous necrosis have been rarely reported with deep S.C. injections

Neuromuscular & skeletal: Osteoporosis with doses >15,000 units/day or therapy of over 5 months

Miscellaneous: Urine discoloration (orange), urine discoloration (red), feces discoloration (black), feces discoloration (pink), feces discoloration (red); hematuria, conjunctivitis

Toxicodynamics/Kinetics

Onset of anticoagulation:
- I.V.: Immediate with use
- S.C.: Within 20-30 minutes

Absorption: Oral, I.M., rectal, sublingual: Erratic

Metabolism: Hepatic; believed to be partially metabolized in the reticuloendothelial system

Half-life:
- Mean: 1.5 hours
- Range: 1-2 hours; affected by obesity, renal function, hepatic function, malignancy, presence of pulmonary embolism, and infections

Elimination: Renal excretion, small amount excreted unchanged in urine

Usual Dosage

Line flushing: When using daily flushes of heparin to maintain patency of single and double lumen central catheters, 10 units/mL is commonly used for younger infants (eg, <10 kg) while 100 units/mL is used for older infants, children, and adults. Capped PVC catheters and peripheral heparin locks require flushing more frequently (eg, every 6-8 hours). Volume of heparin flush is usually similar to volume of catheter (or slightly greater). Additional flushes should be given when stagnant blood is observed in catheter, after catheter is used for drug or blood administration, and after blood withdrawal from catheter.

Addition of heparin (0.5-1 unit/mL) to peripheral and central TPN has been shown to increase duration of line patency. The final concentration of heparin used for TPN solutions may need to be decreased to 0.5 unit/mL in small infants receiving larger amounts of volume in order to avoid approaching therapeutic amounts. Arterial lines are heparinized with a final concentration of 1 unit/mL.

Children:
- Intermittent I.V.: Initial: 50-100 units/kg, then 50-100 units/kg every 4 hours
- I.V. infusion: Initial: 50 units/kg, then 15-25 units/kg/hour; increase dose by 2-4 units/kg/hour every 6-8 hours as required

Adults:
- Prophylaxis (low-dose heparin): S.C.: 5000 units every 8-12 hours
- I.V. infusion: Weight-based dosing:
  - Initial dose: 80 units/kg bolus then 18 units/kg/hour
    - APTT under 35 seconds (<1.2 x control): 80 units/kg bolus, then 4 units/kg/hour
    - APTT 35-45 seconds (1.2-1.5 x control): 40 units/kg bolus then 2 units/kg/hour
    - APTT 46-70 seconds (1.5-2.3 x control): No change
    - APTT 71-90 seconds (2.3-3 x control): Decrease infusion rate by 2 units/kg/hour
    - APTT over 90 seconds (over 3 x control): Hold infusion for one hour and then decrease infusion rate by 3 units/kg/hour

Contraindications Hypersensitivity to heparin or any component; severe thrombocytopenia, subacute bacterial endocarditis, suspected intracranial hemorrhage, uncontrollable bleeding (unless secondary to disseminated intravascular coagulation)

Warnings

Use with caution as hemorrhaging may occur; risk factors for hemorrhage include I.M. injections, peptic ulcer disease, increased capillary permeability, menstruation; severe renal, hepatic or biliary disease; use with caution in patients with shock, severe hypotension

Some preparations contain benzyl alcohol as a preservative. In neonates, large amounts of benzyl alcohol (>100 mg/kg/day) have been associated with fatal toxicity (gasping syndrome). The use of preservative-free heparin is, therefore, recommended in neonates. Some preparations contain sulfite which may cause allergic reactions.

Heparin does not possess fibrinolytic activity and, therefore, cannot lyse established thrombi; discontinue heparin if hemorrhage occurs; severe hemorrhage or overdosage may require protamine

Use caution with white clot syndrome (new thrombus associated with thrombocytopenia) and heparin resistance

(Continued)

Heparin *(Continued)*

Dosage Forms

Heparin sodium:

Lock flush injection:

Beef lung source: 10 units/mL (1 mL, 2 mL, 2.5 mL, 3 mL, 5 mL, 10 mL, 30 mL); 100 units/mL (1 mL, 2 mL, 2.5 mL, 3 mL, 5 mL, 10 mL, 30 mL)

Porcine intestinal mucosa source: 10 units/mL (1 mL, 2 mL, 10 mL, 30 mL); 100 units/mL (1 mL, 2 mL, 10 mL, 30 mL)

Porcine intestinal mucosa source, preservative free: 10 units/mL (1 mL); 100 units/mL (1 mL)

Multiple-dose vial injection:

Beef lung source, with preservative: 1000 units/mL (5 mL, 10 mL, 30 mL); 5000 units/mL (10 mL); 10,000 units/mL (4 mL, 5 mL, 10 mL); 20,000 units/mL (2 mL, 5 mL, 10 mL); 40,000 units/mL (5 mL)

Porcine intestinal mucosa source, with preservative: 1000 units/mL (10 mL, 30 mL); 5000 units/mL (10 mL); 10,000 units/mL (4 mL); 20,000 units/mL (2 mL, 5 mL)

Single-dose vial injection:

Beef lung source: 1000 units/mL (1 mL); 5000 units/mL (1 mL); 10,000 units/mL (1 mL); 20,000 units/mL (1 mL); 40,000 units/mL (1 mL)

Porcine intestinal mucosa: 1000 units/mL (1 mL); 5000 units/mL (1 mL); 10,000 units/mL (1 mL); 20,000 units/mL (1 mL); 40,000 units/mL (1 mL)

Unit dose injection:

Porcine intestinal mucosa source, with preservative: 1000 units/dose (1 mL, 2 mL); 2500 units/dose (1 mL); 5000 units/dose (0.5 mL, 1 mL); 7500 units/dose (1 mL); 10,000 units/dose (1 mL); 15,000 units/dose (1 mL); 20,000 units/dose (1 mL)

Heparin sodium infusion, porcine intestinal mucosa source:

D_5W: 40 units/mL (500 mL); 50 units/mL (250 mL, 500 mL); 100 units/mL (100 mL, 250 mL)

NaCl 0.45%: 2 units/mL (500 mL, 1000 mL); 50 units/mL (250 mL); 100 units/mL (250 mL)

NaCl 0.9%: 2 units/mL (500 mL, 1000 mL); 5 units/mL (1000 mL); 50 units/mL (250 mL, 500 mL, 1000 mL)

Heparin calcium:

Unit dose injection, porcine intestinal mucosa, preservative free (Calciparine®): 5000 units/dose (0.2 mL); 12,500 units/dose (0.5 mL); 20,000 units/dose (0.8 mL)

Stability Stable at room temperature; protect from freezing

Reference Range Therapeutic: 0.3-0.5 units/mL

Overdosage Treatment

Supportive therapy: Protamine can be used for severe bleeding upon withdrawal of heparin (1 mg of protamine for every 80-100 mg of heparin by slow I.V. push)

Enhancement of elimination: While hemodialysis is not beneficial, exchange transfusion has been used successfully in a neonate and plasma exchange has been used successfully in four older patients for thrombocytopenia

Antidote(s)

Protamine Sulfate *on page 1463*

Test Interactions Increased thyroxine (S) (competitive protein binding methods causing a false elevation); increased PT, increased PTT, increased bleeding time; interferes with calcium assay techniques leading to false depression of calcium. Note that serum electrolyte assay obtained through heparin-based cannulas can result in factitious hyperkalemia and/or hypernatremia.

Diagnostic Tests/Procedures

Complete Blood Count *on page 1236*

Drug Interactions

Decreased effect with digoxin, TCN, nicotine, antihistamine, I.V. NTG

Increased effect of sulfonylureas, angiotensin-converting enzymes; inhibitors can exacerbate heparin-induced hyperkalemia

Increased toxicity with NSAIDs, ASA, dipyridamole, dextran, hydroxychloroquine

Pregnancy Risk Factor C

Pregnancy Implications Does not cross placenta; does not appear in breast milk; while maternal thrombocytopenia and bleeding must be monitored, no congenital defects have been documented; heparin is probably safer than warfarin during pregnancy

Monitoring Parameters Platelet counts, PTT, hemoglobin, hematocrit, signs of bleeding

For intermittent I.V. injections, PTT is measured 3.5-4 hours after I.V. injection; for infusion, PTT can be performed 6 hours after a dosage change

Nursing Implications Do not administer I.M. due to pain, irritation, and hematoma formation

Additional Information Low molecular weight heparin agents carry a lower risk of thrombocytopenia; thrombocytopenia is more likely to occur with unfractionated heparin than low molecular weight heparin

Specific References

Aull L, Chao H, and Coy K, "Heparin-Induced Hyperkalemia," *DICP*, 1990, 24(3):244-6.

Becker PS and Miller VT, "Heparin-Induced Thrombocytopenia," *Stroke*, 1989, 20(11):1449-59.

Boon DMS, Kappers-Klunne MC, Michiels JJ, et al, "Heparin-Induced Thrombocytopenia and Thrombosis: A Potential Fatal Complication in a Routine Treatment," *Neth J Med*, 1995, 46:146-52.

Bouvier JL, Lefevre P, Villain P, et al, "Treatment of Serious Heparin-Induced Thrombocytopenia by Plasma Exchange: Report on 4 Cases," *Thromb Res*, 1988, 51(3):335-6.

Carter BL, "Therapy of Acute Thromboembolism With Heparin and Warfarin," *Clin Pharm*, 1991, 10(7):503-18.

Ginsberg JS and Hirsh J, "Optimum Use of Anticoagulants in Pregnancy," *Drugs*, 1988, 36(4):505-12.

Lee HN, Cook DJ, Sarabla A, et al, "Inadequacy of Intravenous Heparin Therapy in the Initial Management of Venous Thromboembolism," *J Gen Intern Med*, 1995, 10:342-5.

Raschke RA, Reilly BM, Guidry JR, et al, "The Weight-Based Heparin Dosing Nomogram Compared With a "Standard Care" Nomogram: A Randomized Controlled Trial," *Ann Intern Med*, 1993, 119(9):874-81.

Sawyer WT, "Management of Thromboembolic Disease," *US Pharm*, 1989, 14:H1-H29.

Scheffold N, Greinacher A, and Cyran J, "Atrial Thrombi in Heparin-Associated Type 11 Thrombocytopenia," *Dtsch Med Wochenschr*, 1995, 120:519-22.

Schreiner RL, Wynn RJ, and McNulty C, "Accidental Heparin Toxicity in the Newborn Intensive Care Unit," *J Pediatr*, 1978, 92(1):115-6.

Ulrick PJ and Manoharan A, "Heparin-Induced Skin Reaction," *Med J Aust*, 1984, 140(5):287-9.

Wagenknecht LE, Furberg CD, Hammon JW, et al, "Surgical Bleeding: Unexpected Effect of a Calcium Antagonist," *Br Med J*, 1995, 310:776-7.

Ward SR and Topol EJ, "How Best to Use Heparin in MI Patients Given Thrombolysis," *J Crit Illness*, 1995, 10(6):385-98.

Warkentin TE, Levine MN, Hirsch J, et al, "Heparin-Induced Thrombocytopenia in Patients Treated With Low-Molecular Weight Heparin or Unfractionated Heparin," *N Engl J Med*, 1995, 332:1330-5.

Wittkowsky AK and Kino KJ, "Heparin Monitoring Associated With Antiphospholipid Antibody Syndrome," *Pharmacotherapy*, 1995, 15(4):517-21.

Heparin Calcium *see* Heparin *on page 398*

Heparin Lock Flush *see* Heparin *on page 398*

Heparin Sodium *see* Heparin *on page 398*

Hep-Lock® Injection *see* Heparin *on page 398*

Herisan® *see* Zinc Oxide *on page 813*

Heroin Hydrochloride

Related Information

Principal Pharmacological Properties of Hallucinogenic Drugs *on page 1557*

CAS Number 561-27-3; 1502-95-0

Synonyms Acetomorphine; Diacetylmorphine; Diamorphine Hydrochloride

Use Most commonly a drug of abuse in the United States; used as an analgesic agent or cough suppressant in Britain

Mechanism of Action Acetylated morphine derivative with CNS depressant effects

Adverse Reactions

Cardiovascular: Hypotension

Central nervous system: Lethargy, coma, euphoria, hallucinations

Dermatologic: Pemphigus

Gastrointestinal: Constipation, dry mouth, nausea, vomiting

Genitourinary: Urinary retention

Hematologic: Thrombocytopenia

Neuromuscular & skeletal: Rhabdomyolysis, myoclonus

Ocular: Miosis, photophobia

Renal: Renal failure, proteinuria

Respiratory: Apnea, respiratory depression, bronchospasm (upon nasal insufflation), pulmonary edema, aspiration

Signs & Symptoms of Acute Overdose Amenorrhea, delirium, tongue discoloration, hypothermia, photophobia, pemphigus, nephrotic syndrome, myopathy, myocardial depression, impotence, extrapyramidal reaction, encephalopathy, dry mouth, dysphoria, disorientation, constipation

Toxicodynamics/Kinetics

Peak plasma level: 10 minutes after I.M. absorption

Distribution: V_d: 25 L/kg

Protein binding: 40%

Metabolism: Deacetylation to 6-acetylmorphine and then to morphine in the liver (both active metabolites)

(Continued)

Heroin Hydrochloride *(Continued)*

Half-life: 3-20 minutes

Elimination: Urine (as morphine glucuronides); total clearance: 31 mL/kg/minute

Usual Dosage

Analgesia (in Europe):

Oral: 5-10 mg

I.M., S.C.: 5 mg (usually I.V. dose)

As a drug of abuse:

Nasal insufflation, I.V., S.C.: Up to 200 mg; usual dose: ~2 mg

Contraindications Hypersensitivity to morphine or diamorphine, acute respiratory depression

Warnings May provoke hypertension and tachycardia in patients with pheochromocytoma; use with caution in renal/liver insufficiency, diarrhea associated with antibiotics; pulmonary disease, gallbladder disease, hypothyroidism, inflammatory bowel disease, prostatic hypertrophy, increased intracranial pressure

Reference Range Heroin doses of 150-200 mg can produce plasma morphine levels of 300 ng/mL; analgesic level: 20-65 ng/mL

Overdosage Treatment

Decontamination: Oral: Activated charcoal with cathartic; for asymptomatic body packers, whole bowel irrigation with polyethylene glycol (PEG) solution is recommended

Supportive therapy: Antidote of choice is naloxone (bolus: 0.4-2 mg I.V.); a continuous infusion may be required, especially in the management of a body stuffer/packer

Antidote(s)

Naloxone Hydrochloride *on page 1447*

Diagnostic Tests/Procedures

Morphine, Blood *on page 1300*

Morphine, Urine *on page 1300*

Drug Interactions Subcutaneous absorption may be delayed when coadministered with cocaine

Pregnancy Risk Factor B; D (if used for prolonged periods or near term)

Pregnancy Implications Associated with increased incidence of congenital abnomalies; higher rates of neonatal jaundice (due to accelerated liver maturity), lower birth rates, and perinatal mortality have been reported; narcotic withdrawal (incidence of 85% usually appearing within 48 hours) with associated elevated neonatal serum magnesium levels must be monitored; withdrawal is related to dose and length of exposure

Additional Information

Use and purity has been increasing; purity ranges from 3% to 30%; often combined with cocaine ("speedball") or phenobarbital/methaqualone ("karachi"); annual prevalence according to 1991 NIDA survey in U.S. population is ~0.3%

It appears that older users are more likely to inject while younger users are more likely to snort or smoke. Dark (Mexican) heroin is usually less potent than white (Asian) heroin. Urine drug screen will remain positive for about 40 hours; adulterants include talc, corn starch, quinine, lead, mannitol, sodium bicarbonate, and lidocaine.

Specific References

Cunningham EE, Zielezny MA, and Venuto RC, "Heroine-Associated Nephropathy," *JAMA*, 1983, 250:2935-6.

Inturrisi CE, Max BM, Foley KM, et al, "The Pharmacokinetics of Heroin in Patients With Chronic Pain," *N Engl J Med*, 1984, 310(19):1213-7.

Rothe M and Pragst F, "Solvent Optimization for the Direct Extraction of Opiates From Hair Samples," *J Anal Toxicol*, 1995, 19:236-40.

Sanders MN, Bernhisel-Broadbent J, and Staker LV, "Delayed Hypersensitivity Reaction to Heparin in a Pregnent Woman," *Int J Dermatol*, 1995, 34:443-4.

Sawynok J, "The Therapeutic Use of Heroin: A Review of the Pharmacological Literature," *Can J Physiol Pharmacol*, 1986, 64(1):1-6.

Sporer KA, Firestone J, and Isaacs SM, "The Prehospital Treatment of Heroin Overdoses," *Acad Emerg Med*, 1995, 2:448.

Utecht MJ, Stone AF, and McCarron MM, "Heroin Body Packers," *J Emerg Med*, 1993, 11(1):33-40.

Hexachlorocyclohexane *see* Lindane *on page 470*

Hexachlorophene (hex a klor' oh feen)

CAS Number 70-30-4

UN Number 2875

Brand Names Lotocreme®; pHisoHex®; Sapoderem®; Septisol®; Ster-Zac®

Use Surgical scrub and as a bacteriostatic skin cleanser; control an outbreak of gram-positive infection when other procedures have been unsuccessful

Mechanism of Action Bacteriostatic polychlorinated biphenyl which inhibits membrane-bound enzymes and disrupts the cell membrane

Adverse Reactions
Cardiovascular: Hypotension, bradycardia
Central nervous system: Convulsions, irritability, fever, pseudotumor cerebri, dementia, cerebral edema, confusion, drowsiness, coma
Dermatologic: Dermatitis, erythema, dry skin, photosensitivity
Gastrointestinal: Anorexia, nausea, vomiting, diarrhea
Ocular: Optic neuropathy, blindness, diplopia
Respiratory: Wheezing upon exposure to hexachlorophene powder; respiratory failure, respiratory arrest

Toxicodynamics/Kinetics
Absorption: Absorbed percutaneously through inflamed, excoriated, and intact skin
Metabolism: Hepatic
Half-life: 1 day; infants: 6.1-44.2 hours

Usual Dosage Children and Adults: Topical: Apply 5 mL cleanser and water to area to be cleansed; lather and rinse thoroughly under running water
Lethal oral dose: 2-10 g

Contraindications Known hypersensitivity to halogenated phenol derivatives or hexachlorophene; use in premature infants; use on burned or denuded skin; occlusive dressing; application to mucous membranes

Warnings Discontinue use if signs of cerebral irritability occur; exposure of preterm infants or patients with extensive burns has been associated with apnea, seizures, agitation and coma; do not use for bathing infants, premature infants are particularly susceptible to hexachlorophene topical absorption

Dosage Forms
Foam (Septisol®): 0.23% with alcohol 56% (180 mL, 600 mL)
Liquid, topical (pHisoHex®): 3% (8 mL, 150 mL, 500 mL, 3840 mL)

Stability Store in nonmetallic container (**incompatible** with many metals)

Reference Range Death in a child associated with a serum hexachlorophene level of 0.78 μg/mL

Overdosage Treatment
Decontamination:
Oral: Lavage/activated charcoal with cathartic for ingestions >0.5 mg/kg
Dermal: Vigorous irrigation with soap and water; olive oil or castor oil can dissolve hexachlorophene and also be utilized
Enhancement of elimination: Oral ingestion: Multiple dosing of activated charcoal may be effective

Pregnancy Risk Factor C

Pregnancy Implications Crosses the placenta; spongiform encephalopathy in low birth weight infants

Patient Information Do not leave on skin for prolonged contact; for external use only; discontinue product if condition persists or worsens and call physician; if suds enter eye, rinse out thoroughly with water

Additional Information In cosmetics, usually not at a concentration exceeding 0.1%

Specific References
Halling H, "Suspected Link Between Exposure to Hexachlorophene and Malformed Infants," *Ann N Y Acad Sci*, 1979, 320:426-35.
Lockhart JD, "How Toxic is Hexachlorophene?" *Pediatrics*, 1972, 50(2):229-35.
Marquardt ED, "Hexachlorophene Toxicity in a Pediatric Burn Patient," *Drug Intell Clin Pharm*, 1986, 20(7-8):624.
Nagy L and Orosz M, "Occupational Asthma Due to Hexachlorophene," *Thorax*, 1984, 39(8):630-1.

Hexacycline® *see* Tetracycline *on page 732*
Hexadrol® Phosphate Injection *see* Dexamethasone *on page 266*
Hexadrol® Tablet *see* Dexamethasone *on page 266*
Hexalen® *see* Altretamine *on page 103*
Hexamethylmelamine *see* Altretamine *on page 103*
Hexamidinum *see* Primidone *on page 641*
Hexastat® *see* Altretamine *on page 103*
Hexinawas® *see* Altretamine *on page 103*
h.g. Blending *see* Sodium Chloride *on page 698*
Hi-Amchol® *see* Ammonium Chloride *on page 118*
Hibanil® *see* Chlorpromazine Hydrochloride *on page 205*
Hibiclens® Topical [OTC] *see* Chlorhexidine Gluconate *on page 200*
Hibistat® Topical [OTC] *see* Chlorhexidine Gluconate *on page 200*

Hirucreme® *see* Hirudin *on this page*

Hirudin

Brand Names Exhirud®; Hirucreme®

Use Investigational: Thrombolysis in acute myocardial infarction to prevent reocclusion

Mechanism of Action Derived from the leech (*Hirudo medicinalis*), hirudin is a specific thrombin inhibitor; inhibits conversion of fibrinogen to fibrin

Adverse Reactions Hematologic: Bleeding, hemorrhage

Toxicodynamics/Kinetics

Absorption: S.C.: 36%

Half-life:

I.V.: 0.6-1.6 hours

S.C.: 0.6-3 hours

Elimination: Renal

Usual Dosage I.V.:

Bolus: 0.1-0.4 mg/kg

Infusion: 0.06-0.15 mg/kg/hour

Overdosage Treatment

Supportive therapy: Monitor aPTT; bleeding is dose related; treat hemorrhage with local therapy

Monitoring Parameters Activated PTT

Additional Information 1 mcg of hirudin inhibits ~10 units of human thrombin

Specific References

Adams SL, "The Medicinal Leech: A Page From the Annelids of Internal Medicine," *Ann Intern Med*, 1988, 109(5):399-405.

Nowak G, "Pharmacokinetics of Hirudin," *Semin Thromb Hemost*, 1991, 17(2):145-9.

Zeymer U and Neuhaus KL, "Hirudin and Excess Bleeding," *Drug Saf*, 1995, 12(4):234-9.

Hismanal® *see* Astemizole *on page 136*

Histaject® *see* Brompheniramine Maleate *on page 165*

Histerone® Injection *see* Testosterone *on page 729*

Histolyn-CYL® *see* Histoplasmin *on this page*

Histoplasmin (hiss toe plaz' min)

CAS Number 9008-05-3

Brand Names Histolyn-CYL®

Synonyms Histoplasmosis Skin Test Antigen

Use Diagnosing histoplasmosis; to assess cell-mediated immunity

Adverse Reactions Local: Vesiculation, ulceration, or necrosis at site of administration

Signs & Symptoms of Acute Overdose Excessive dosage may result in severe erythema and induration followed by necrosis and ulceration which may last for several weeks

Usual Dosage Adults: Intradermally: 0.1 mL of 1:100 dilution into volar surface of forearm; induration of ≥5 mm in diameter indicates a positive reaction

Contraindications Known hypersensitivity to phenol or polysorbate 80

Warnings Epinephrine should be available for immediate treatment of anaphylactic reaction; use with caution in patients with coccidioidal erythema nodosum; a dilution of 1:10,000 should be used for the initial skin test; resuscitative equipment should be available

Dosage Forms Injection: 1:100 (0.1 mL, 1.3 mL)

Stability Store in refrigerator (2°C to 8°C)

Overdosage Treatment Treatment is dilution of site of exposure

Drug Interactions Any live virus vaccine, corticosteroids, immunosuppressive agents may inhibit the immune response to the skin test

Pregnancy Risk Factor C

Nursing Implications Examine reaction site at 24-48 hours for cell-mediated immunity and 48-72 hours for histoplasmosis; use a $^3/_8$" to $^1/_2$" 26- or 27-gauge needle

Additional Information Some formulations may contain phenol

Specific References

Ahmed AR and Blose DA, "Delayed-Type Hypersensitivity Skin Testing," *Arch Dermatol*, 1983, 119(11):934-45.

Histoplasmosis Skin Test Antigen *see* Histoplasmin *on this page*

Hivid® *see* Zalcitabine *on page 805*

HN_2 *see* Mechlorethamine Hydrochloride *on page 492*

Hoe-118 *see* Piretanide *on page 630*

Hold® DM [OTC] *see* Dextromethorphan Hydrobromide *on page 270*

Homatropine and Hydrocodone *see* Hydrocodone and Homatropine *on page 407*

Hortetracin® *see* Tetracycline *on page 732*

Hostabloc® *see* Penbutolol Sulfate *on page 599*

Huile de Camphre *see* Camphor *on page 179*

Humibid® L.A. [OTC] *see* Guaifenesin *on page 390*

Humibid® Sprinkle [OTC] *see* Guaifenesin *on page 390*

HuMIST® [OTC] *see* Sodium Chloride *on page 698*

Humulin® *see* Insulin Preparations *on page 426*

Hurricaine® *see* Benzocaine *on page 149*

Hycodan® *see* Hydrocodone and Homatropine *on page 407*

Hydac® *see* Felodipine *on page 343*

Hydralazine Hydrochloride (hye dral' a zeen)

CAS Number 86-54-5; 304-20-1

Brand Names Apresoline®

Use Management of moderate to severe hypertension, congestive heart failure, hypertension secondary to pre-eclampsia/eclampsia; has been used to treat primary pulmonary hypertension

Mechanism of Action Direct vasodilation of arterioles (with little effect on veins) with decreased systemic resistance

Adverse Reactions

Cardiovascular: Palpitations, flushing, tachycardia, edema, myocardial ischemia
Central nervous system: Malaise, dizziness, dizziness, fever, headache, asthenia
Dermatologic: Rash, pruritus
Gastrointestinal: Anorexia, nausea, vomiting, diarrhea
Neuromuscular & skeletal: Arthralgia, peripheral neuritis, paresthesia
Ocular: Lacrimation, blurred vision, eyelid edema
Renal: Glomerulonephritis
Miscellaneous: Positive ANA, positive LE cells, feces discoloration (black)

Signs & Symptoms of Acute Overdose Hypotension, erythema multiforme, wheezing, lacrimation, impotence, cholestatic jaundice, tachycardia, thrombocytopenia, Stevens-Johnson syndrome, neuropathy (peripheral), hyperthermia, arrhythmias, shock, hypokalemia, lactic acidosis, leukopenia; neutropenia; agranulocytosis; granulocytopenia; systemic lupus erythematosus (SLE)

Toxicodynamics/Kinetics

Onset of action:
Oral: 20-30 minutes
I.V.: 5-20 minutes
Duration:
Oral: 2-4 hours
I.V.: 2-6 hours
Absorption: Well absorbed
Distribution: V_d: 1.6 L/kg
Protein binding: 85%
Metabolism: Large first-pass effect orally
Bioavailability: 30% to 50%
Half-life: 0.44-0.47 hours
Time to peak serum concentration: Oral: 60 minutes
Elimination:
Renal: 2% to 14% unchanged
Oral: 11% to 14% unchanged after I.V.
Feces: 3% to 12%

Usual Dosage Titrate dosage to patient's response

Children:
Oral: Initial: 0.75-1 mg/kg/day in 2-4 divided doses, not to exceed 25 mg/dose; increase over 3-4 weeks to maximum of 7.5 mg/kg/day in 2-4 divided doses; maximum daily dose: 200 mg/day
I.M., I.V.: 0.1-0.5 mg/kg/dose (initial dose not to exceed 20 mg) every 4-6 hours as needed

Adults:
Oral: Initial: 10 mg 4 times/day, increase by 10-25 mg/dose every 2-5 days to maximum of 300 mg/day
I.M., I.V.:
Hypertensive initial: 10-20 mg/dose every 4-6 hours as needed, may increase to 40 mg/dose; change to oral therapy as soon as possible
Pre-eclampsia/eclampsia: 5 mg/dose then 5-10 mg every 20-30 minutes as needed

(Continued)

Hydralazine Hydrochloride *(Continued)*

Dosing interval in renal impairment:

Cl_{cr} 10-50 mL/minute: Administer every 8 hours

Cl_{cr} <10 mL/minute: Administer every 8-16 hours in fast acetylators and every 12-24 hours in slow acetylators

Contraindications Hypersensitivity to hydralazine or any component, dissecting aortic aneurysm, mitral valve rheumatic heart disease, known or suspected coronary artery disease

Warnings Discontinue hydralazine in patients who develop SLE-like syndrome or positive ANA. Use with caution in patients with severe renal disease or cerebral vascular accidents. Some formulations may contain tartrazines or sulfites.

Dosage Forms

Injection: 20 mg/mL (1 mL)

Tablet: 10 mg, 25 mg, 50 mg, 100 mg

Stability Changes color after contact with a metal filter; do not store intact ampuls in refrigerator

Overdosage Treatment

Decontamination: Ipecac/lavage/activated charcoal with cathartic

Supportive therapy: Hypotension usually responds to I.V. fluids or Trendelenburg positioning. If unresponsive to these measures, the use of a parenteral vasoconstrictor may be required (eg, norepinephrine 0.1-0.2 mcg/kg/minute titrated to response). Treatment is primarily supportive and symptomatic. Verapamil, esmolol, or propranolol may be used to treat tachycardia.

Enhancement of elimination: Multiple dosing of activated charcoal may be useful

Test Interactions Increases calcium (S)

Drug Interactions MAO inhibitors may significantly decrease blood pressure; indomethacin may decrease hypotensive effects.

Pregnancy Risk Factor C (No reported adverse effects in pregnancy)

Pregnancy Implications Low levels in breast milk (safe for breast-feeding)

Monitoring Parameters Monitor blood pressure closely with I.V. use; monitor blood pressure standing and sitting/supine, renal function, urine output

Patient Information Report flu-like symptoms, check blood pressure, when rising from sitting/lying, do slowly

Nursing Implications Monitor blood pressure closely with I.V. use; dextrose solutions suggested

Additional Information Slow acetylators, patients with decreased renal function and patients receiving >200 mg/day (chronically) are at higher risk for systemic lupus erythematosus (SLE). Usually administered with diuretic and a beta-blocker to counteract side effects of sodium and water retention and reflex tachycardia although the beta-blocker may not be necessary in the elderly; odorless, bitter-tasting powder.

Specific References

Smith BA and Ferguson DB, "Acute Hydralazine Overdose: Marked ECG Abnormalities in a Young Adult," *Ann Emerg Med*, 1992, 21(3):326-30.

Hydrate® *see* Dimenhydrinate *on page 289*

Hydrated Chloral *see* Chloral Hydrate *on page 193*

Hydrea® *see* Hydroxyurea *on page 412*

Hydrochlorothiazide (hye droe klor oh thye' a zide)

CAS Number 58-93-5

Brand Names Aquazide-H®; Diaqua®; Esidrix®; Ezide®; HydroDIURIL®; Hydro-Par®; Hydro-T®; Mictrin®; Oretic®

Synonyms HCTZ

Use Management of mild to moderate hypertension; treatment of edema in congestive heart failure and nephrotic syndrome; diabetes insipidus, hypercalciuria

Mechanism of Action Inhibits sodium reabsorption in the distal tubules causing increased excretion of sodium and water as well as potassium and hydrogen ions; at high doses may inhibit carbonic anhydrase

Adverse Reactions

Central nervous system: Drowsiness, hyperthermia

Dermatologic: Photosensitivity

Endocrine & metabolic: Hypokalemia, hyperglycemia, hypochloremic metabolic alkalosis, hyperlipidemia, hyperuricemia, syndrome of inappropriate antidiuretic hormone

Gastrointestinal: Nausea, vomiting, anorexia

Genitourinary: Prerenal azotemia

Hematologic: Aplastic anemia, hemolysis, leukopenia, neutropenia, agranulocytosis, granulocytopenia, thrombocytopenia

Hepatic: Hepatitis, intrahepatic cholestasis

Neuromuscular & skeletal: Muscle asthenia, postural hypotension, paresthesia

Renal: Polyuria

Miscellaneous: Systemic lupus erythematosus (SLE)

Signs & Symptoms of Acute Overdose A-V block, cystitis, impotence, photosensitivity, hypokalemia, hyperuricemia, hyperglycemia, myocarditis, myalgia, diabetes insipidus, diuresis, nocturia, myasthenia gravis (exacerbation or precipitation of), systemic lupus erythematosus (SLE), vision color changes (yellow tinge), hyponatremia, pancreatitis, hyperperistalsis, hypercalcemia, leukopenia; neutropenia; agranulocytosis; granulocytopenia; fever

Toxicodynamics/Kinetics

Onset of diuretic action: Oral: Within 2 hours

Peak effect: 4 hours

Duration: 6-12 hours

Absorption: Oral: ~60% to 80%

Distribution: V_d: 1-4 L/kg

Protein binding: 40% to 64%

Half-life: 10-12 hours (may be up to 29 hours in patients with heart failure)

Elimination: Renal (95%), 4.9 mL/min/kg

Usual Dosage In pediatric patients, chlorothiazide may be preferred as there are more dosage forms (ie, suspension)

Oral (effect of drug may be decreased when used every day):

- Children (daily dosages should be decreased if used with other antihypertensives):
  - <6 months: 2-3 mg/kg/day in 2 divided doses
  - >6 months: 2 mg/kg/day in 2 divided doses
- Adults: 25-50 mg/day in 1-2 doses; maximum: 200 mg/day

Dosing adjustment/comments in renal impairment: Cl_{cr} <30 mL/minute: Not effective

Contraindications Pregnancy, anuria, renal decompensation, hypersensitivity to hydrochlorothiazide or any component, cross-sensitivity with other thiazides and sulfonamide derivatives

Warnings Use with caution in renal disease, hepatic disease, gout, lupus erythematosus, diabetes mellitus; some products may contain tartrazine

Dosage Forms

Solution, oral (mint flavor): 50 mg/5 mL (50 mL)

Tablet: 25 mg, 50 mg, 100 mg

Reference Range Serum level of 2 μg/mL associated with peak diuretic effect

Overdosage Treatment

Decontamination: Activated charcoal with cathartic

Supportive therapy: Intravenous hydration with 0.9% saline

Enhancement of elimination: Hemodialysis may be effective

Test Interactions ↑ creatine phosphokinase [CPK] (S), ammonia (B), amylase (S), calcium (S), chloride (S), cholesterol (S), glucose, ↑ acid (S), ↓ chloride (S), magnesium, potassium (S), sodium (S)

Drug Interactions

Decreased effect of oral hypoglycemics; decreased absorption with cholestyramine and colestipol

Increased effect with furosemide and other loop diuretics

Increased toxicity/levels of lithium; increases amantadine toxicity

Hyponatremia associated with trimethoprim or carbamazepine; calcium salt administration may result in milk-alkali syndrome; can produce elevation of plasma triglyceride concentrations when used with beta-blocking agents

Pregnancy Risk Factor D

Pregnancy Implications Neonatal side effects include decreased birth weight, hypoglycemia, thrombocytopenia, hyponatremia, hyperbilirubinemia

Monitoring Parameters Blood pressure, serum electrolytes, BUN, creatinine

Additional Information Inhibits insulin secretion/vitamin D synthesis

Specific References

Allen JH, McKenney JM, Stratton MA, et al, "Antihypertensive Effect of Hydrochlorothiazide Administered Once or Twice Daily," *Clin Pharm*, 1982, 1(3):239-43.

Materson BJ, "Diuretic-Associated Hypokalemia," *Arch Intern Med*, 1985, 145(11):1966-7.

Zahid M, Krumlovsky FA, Roxe D, et al, "Central Nervous System and Cardiac Manifestations of Hydrochlorothiazide Overdosage; Treatment With Hemodialysis," *Am J Kidney Dis*, 1988, 11(6):508-11.

Hydrocodone and Homatropine

(hye droe koe' done & hoe ma' toe peen)

Related Information

Pharmacokinetics of Narcotic Agonist Analgesics *on page 1654*

Brand Names Hycodan®; Hydromet®; Hydropane®; Hydrotropine®; Tussigon®

Synonyms Homatropine and Hydrocodone

Replaces Hydropane

Use Symptomatic relief of cough

(Continued)

Hydrocodone and Homatropine *(Continued)*

Adverse Reactions

Cardiovascular: Tachycardia

Central nervous system: Dizziness, sedation, lightheadedness, delirium, restlessness, headache

Dermatologic: Dry hot skin

Gastrointestinal: Impaired gastrointestinal motility (ileus)

Ocular: Mydriasis, blurred vision

Usual Dosage Oral (based on hydrocodone component):

Children: 0.6 mg/kg/day in 3-4 divided doses; do not administer more frequently than every 4 hours

A single dose should not exceed 1.25 mg in children <2 years of age, 5 mg in children 2-12 years, and 10 mg in children >12 years

Adults: 5-10 mg every 4-6 hours, a single dose should not exceed 15 mg; do not administer more frequently than every 4 hours

Contraindications Increased intracranial pressure, narrow-angle glaucoma, depressed ventilation, hypersensitivity to hydrocodone, homatropine, or any component

Warnings Use with caution in patients with hypersensitivity to other phenanthrene derivatives; use with caution in patients with respiratory diseases, or severe liver or renal failure; use with caution in children with spastic paralysis, in the elderly, and in patients with prostatic hypertrophy

Dosage Forms

Syrup (Hycodan®, Hydromet®, Hydropane®, Hydrotropine®): Hydrocodone bitartrate 5 mg and homatropine methylbromide 1.5 mg per 5 mL (120 mL, 480 mL, 4000 mL)

Tablet (Hycodan®, Tussigon®): Hydrocodone bitartrate 5 mg and homatropine methylbromide 1.5 mg

Reference Range 10 mg of hydrocodone given orally produces a serum level of 0.024 mg/L at 1.5 hours

Overdosage Treatment

Decontamination: Lavage/activated charcoal with cathartic

Supportive therapy: Naloxone should be given

Antidote(s)

Naloxone Hydrochloride *on page 1447*

Test Interactions ↑ ALT, AST (S)

Pregnancy Risk Factor C

Patient Information Avoid alcohol; may cause drowsiness and impair judgment or coordination; may be addicting if taken for prolonged periods; lack of saliva may enhance cavities; maintain good oral hygiene; use caution while driving; may cause blurred vision; notify physician if difficulty in urinating or constipation becomes severe

Nursing Implications Dispense in light-resistant container; observe patient for excessive sedation, respiratory depression, implement safety measures, assist with ambulation

HydroDIURIL® *see* Hydrochlorothiazide *on page 406*

Hydrogen Dioxide *see* Hydrogen Peroxide *on this page*

Hydrogen Peroxide (hye' droe jen per ox' ide)

CAS Number 7722-84-1

UN Number 2015

Brand Names Peroxyl®

Synonyms Albone; H_2O_2; Hydrogen Dioxide; Inhibine; Perhydrol; Peroxan; Peroxide

Commonly Found in Bleaching textiles, antiseptics, hair bleaching agents, loosens ear cerumen, recent intravenous use by AIDS patients to "cleanse blood." Household concentrations: 3%; industrial concentrations: 35%.

Use Cleanse wounds, suppurating ulcers, and local infections; used in the treatment of inflammatory conditions of the external auditory canal and as a mouthwash or gargle

Mechanism of Action Antiseptic oxidant that slowly releases oxygen and water upon contact with serum or tissue catalase; potent oxidizing agent

Adverse Reactions

Cardiovascular: Gas embolism

Gastrointestinal: Rupture of the colon, proctitis, ulcerative colitis, small bowel perforation

Hematologic: Hemolysis

Local: Irritation of the buccal mucous membrane, bleaching effect on hair

Neuromuscular & skeletal: Rhabdomyolysis

Respiratory: Interstitial lung disease

Renal: Myoglobinuria, renal failure

Signs & Symptoms of Acute Overdose Abdominal pain, colitis, coma, seizures

(35% hydrogen peroxide), dyspnea, chest pain, metabolic acidosis, gastric distention, gingival ulceration, vomiting, ocular exposure causes irritation, corneal ulceration, and lacrimation; oropharyngeal burns; systemic embolization can produce cardiac arrest; inhalation can cause cough and interstitial lung disease

Toxicodynamics/Kinetics Duration of action: Only while bubbling action occurs

Usual Dosage Children and Adults:

Mouthwash or gargle: Dilute the 3% solution with an equal volume of water; swish around in the mouth over the affected area for at least 1 minute and then expel; use up to 4 times/day (after meals and at bedtime)

Topical: 1.5% to 3% solution for cleansing wounds

Contraindications Should not be used in abscesses

Warnings Repeat use as a mouthwash or gargle may produce irritation of the buccal mucous membrane or "hairy tongue"; bandages should not be applied too quickly after its use

Dosage Forms

Gel, oral: 1.5% (15 g)

Solution:

Concentrate: 30.5% (480 mL)

Topical: 3% (120 mL, 480 mL)

Stability Keep tightly covered; decomposition is accelerated by metals and metallic salts; protect from heat and light

Overdosage Treatment

Decontamination: Dilute with water; use nasogastric tube for gastric decompression

Supportive therapy: Hyperbaric oxygen advocated for reducing size of gas emboli

Diagnostic Tests/Procedures

Blood Gases, Arterial *on page 1207*

Complete Blood Count *on page 1236*

Kidney Profile *on page 1279*

Potassium, Blood *on page 1328*

Monitoring Parameters CBC, renal status, x-rays

Patient Information Will bubble in mouth

Additional Information Clear, colorless fluid; bitter acid test; intravenous use associated with hemolytic anemia, and subsequent renal failure

TLV-TWA: 1 ppm

IDLH: 75 ppm

PEL-TWA: 1 ppm

Specific References

Dickson KF and Caravati EM, "Hydrogen Peroxide Exposure - 325 Exposures Reported to a Regional Poison Control Center," *J Toxicol Clin Toxicol*, 1994, 32(6):705-14.

Humberston CL, Dean BS, and Krenzelok EP, "Ingestion of 35% Hydrogen Peroxide," *J Toxicol Clin Toxicol*, 1990, 28(1):95-100.

Jordan KS, Mackey P, and Garvey E, "A 39 Year Old Man With Acute Hemolytic Crisis Secondary to Intravenous Injection of Hydrogen Peroxide," *J Emerg Nurs*, 1991, 17(1):8-10.

Luu TA, Kelley MT, Strauch JA, et al, "Portal Vein Gas Embolism From Hydrogen Peroxide Ingestion," *Ann Emerg Med*, 1992, 21(11):1391-3.

Sleigh JW and Linter SP, "Hazards of Hydrogen Peroxide," *Br Med J (Clin Res)*, 1985, 291(6510):1706.

Hydro-Long® *see* Chlorthalidone *on page 210*

Hydromedin® *see* Ethacrynic Acid *on page 328*

Hydromet® *see* Hydrocodone and Homatropine *on page 407*

Hydromorphone Hydrochloride (hye droe mor' fone)

Related Information

Pharmacokinetics of Narcotic Agonist Analgesics *on page 1654*

CAS Number 71-68-1; 466-99-9

Brand Names Dilaudid®; Dilaudid-HP®

Synonyms Dihydromorphinone

Use Management of moderate to severe pain; antitussive at lower doses

Mechanism of Action Binds to opiate receptors in the CNS, causing inhibition of ascending pain pathways, altering the perception of and response to pain; causes cough supression by direct central action in the medulla; produces generalized CNS depression

Adverse Reactions

Cardiovascular: Palpitations, hypotension, bradycardia, peripheral vasodilation

Central nervous system: CNS depression, intracranial pressure (increased), drowsiness, dizziness, sedation

Dermatologic: Pruritus

Endocrine & metabolic: Antidiuretic hormone release

Gastrointestinal: Nausea, vomiting, constipation

Ocular: Miosis

(Continued)

Hydromorphone Hydrochloride *(Continued)*

Respiratory: Apnea, respiratory depression

Miscellaneous: Physical and psychological dependence, histamine release, biliary or urinary tract spasm

Signs & Symptoms of Acute Overdose Apnea, respiratory depression, myasthenia gravis (exacerbation or precipitation of), coma, syndrome of inappropriate antidiuretic hormone (SIADH), flaccidity, hypotension, bradycardia, confusion

Toxicodynamics/Kinetics

Onset of analgesic effect: Within 15-30 minutes

Peak effect: Within 30-60 minutes

Duration: 4-5 hours

Distribution: V_d: 1.2 L/kg

Metabolism: Primarily in the liver

Bioavailability: 62%

Half-life: 2-3 hours

Elimination: Urine, principally as glucuronide conjugates

Usual Dosage

Doses should be titrated to appropriate analgesic effects; when changing routes of administration, note that oral doses are less than half as effective as parenteral doses (may be only one-fifth as effective)

Pain: Older Children and Adults:

Oral, I.M., I.V., S.C.: 1-4 mg/dose every 4-6 hours as needed; usual adult dose: 2 mg/dose

Rectal: 3 mg every 6-8 hours

Antitussive: Oral:

Children 6-12 years: 0.5 mg every 3-4 hours as needed

Children >12 years and Adults: 1 mg (5 mL) every 3-4 hours as needed

Dosing adjustment in hepatic impairment: Should be considered

Contraindications Hypersensitivity to hydromorphone or any component or other phenanthrene derivative

Warnings Tablet and cough syrup contain tartrazine which may cause allergic reactions; hydromorphone shares toxic potential of opiate agonists, and precaution of opiate agonist therapy should be observed; extreme caution should be taken to avoid confusing the highly concentrated injection with the less concentrated injectable product, injection contains benzyl alcohol; use with caution in patients with hypersensitivity to other phenanthrene opiates, in patients with respiratory disease, or severe liver or renal failure

Dosage Forms

Injection: 1 mg/mL (1 mL); 2 mg/mL (1 mL, 20 mL); 3 mg/mL (1 mL); 4 mg/mL (1 mL); 10 mg/mL (1 mL, 2 mL, 5 mL)

Suppository, rectal: 3 mg

Tablet: 1 mg, 2 mg, 3 mg, 4 mg

Stability Protect tablets from light; do not store intact ampuls in refrigerator; a slightly yellowish discoloration has not been associated with a loss of potency; I.V. is **incompatible** when mixed with minocycline, prochlorperazine, sodium bicarbonate, tetracycline, thiopental, dexamethasone

Reference Range 0.001-0.032 mg/L

Overdosage Treatment

Decontamination: Lavage/activated charcoal with cathartic

Supportive therapy: Naloxone hydrochloride (0.4-2 mg I.V., S.C., or through an endotracheal tube); a continuous infusion (at ⅔ the response dose/hour) may be required

Antidote(s)

Naloxone Hydrochloride *on page 1447*

Test Interactions ↑ aminotransferase [ALT (SGPT)/AST (SGOT)] (S)

Drug Interactions Increased toxicity with CNS depressants, phenothiazines, TCAs, MAO inhibitors, guanabenz, skeletal muscle relaxants (eg, tubocurarine)

Pregnancy Risk Factor B (D if used for prolonged periods or in high doses at term)

Pregnancy Implications Crosses the placenta

Monitoring Parameters Pain relief, respiratory and mental status, blood pressure

Patient Information May cause drowsiness; avoid alcohol; take with food or milk to minimize gastrointestinal distress

Nursing Implications Observe patient for oversedation, respiratory depression, implement safety measures

Additional Information Equianalgesic doses: Morphine 10 mg I.M. = hydromorphone 1.5 mg I.M.

Specific References

Honigberg IL, and Stewart JT, "Radioimmunoassay of Hydromorphone and Hydrocodone in Human Plasma," *J Pharm Sci*, 1980, 69(10):1171-3.

Inturrisi CE, "Narcotic Drugs," *Med Clin North Am*, 1982, 66(5):1061-71.

Hydropane® *see* Hydrocodone and Homatropine *on page 407*

Hydropane *replaced by* Hydrocodone and Homatropine *on page 407*

Hydro-Par® *see* Hydrochlorothiazide *on page 406*

Hydro-T® *see* Hydrochlorothiazide *on page 406*

Hydrotropine® *see* Hydrocodone and Homatropine *on page 407*

4-Hydroxybutyrate *see* Gamma Hydroxybutyric Acid *on page 376*

Hydroxycarbamide *see* Hydroxyurea *on next page*

Hydroxychloroquine Sulfate (hye drox ee klor' oh kwin)

CAS Number 747-36-4; 118-42-3

Brand Names Plaquenil®; Quensyl®

Synonyms Oxichlorochin

Use Suppresses and treats acute attacks of malaria; treatment of systemic lupus erythematosus and rheumatoid arthritis

Mechanism of Action Interferes with digestive vacuole function within sensitive malarial parasites by increasing the pH and interfering with lysosomal degradation of hemoglobin; inhibits locomotion of neutrophils and chemotaxis of eosinophils; impairs complement-dependent antigen-antibody reactions

Adverse Reactions

Cardiovascular: Hypotension, ventricular arrhythmia, torsade de pointes, bradycardia

Central nervous system: Insomnia, nervousness, night terrors, psychosis, headache, confusion, agitation, seizures, dizziness, ataxia

Dermatologic: Lichenoid dermatitis, exfoliative dermatitis, bleaching of the hair, hypopigmented hair, pruritus, phototoxicity

Endocrine & metabolic: Hypokalemia

Gastrointestinal: gastrointestinal irritation, anorexia, nausea, vomiting, diarrhea

Hematologic: Bone marrow depression, hemolysis, thrombocytopenia, leukopenia, neutropenia, agranulocytosis, granulocytopenia, aplastic anemia, porphyria

Neuromuscular & skeletal: Muscle asthenia

Ocular: Visual field defects, vision color changes (blue tinge); vision color changes (green tinge); vision color changes (yellow tinge); photophobia, blindness, diplopia, retinitis, retinopathy threshold dose is 7.8 mg/kg/day (less ocular toxicity than chloroquine)

Otic: Hearing loss

Miscellaneous: Porphyrinogenic

Signs & Symptoms of Acute Overdose Lymphocytosis

Toxicodynamics/Kinetics

Absorption: Oral: Complete

Protein binding: 55%

Metabolism: In the liver to desethylchloroquine and bisdesethylchloroquine

Half-life: 40 days

Elimination: Metabolites and unchanged drug slowly excreted in urine, may be enhanced by urinary acidification

Usual Dosage Oral:

Children:

- Chemoprophylaxis of malaria: 5 mg/kg (base) once weekly; should not exceed the recommended adult dose; begin 2 weeks before exposure; continue for 4-6 weeks after leaving endemic area
- Acute attack: 10 mg/kg (base) initial dose; followed by 5 mg/kg in 6 hours on day 1; 5 mg/kg in 1 dose on day 2 and on day 3
- JRA or SLE: 3-5 mg/kg/day divided 1-2 times/day to a maximum of 400 mg/day; not to exceed 7 mg/kg/day

Adults:

- Chemoprophylaxis of malaria: 2 tablets weekly on same day each week; begin 2 weeks before exposure; continue for 4-6 weeks after leaving endemic area
- Acute attack: 4 tablets first dose day 1; 2 tablets in 6 hours day 1; 2 tablets in 1 dose day 2; and 2 tablets in 1 dose on day 3
- Rheumatoid arthritis: 2-3 tablets/day to start taken with food or milk; increase dose until optimum response level is reached; usually after 4-12 weeks dose should be reduced by ½ and a maintenance dose of 1-2 tablets/day given
- Lupus erythematosus: 2 tablets every day or twice daily for several weeks depending on response; 1-2 tablets/day for prolonged maintenance therapy

To limit incidence of retinopathy, do not give more than 400 mg/day

Contraindications Retinal or visual field changes attributable to 4-aminoquinolines; hypersensitivity to hydroxychloroquine, 4-aminoquinoline derivatives, or any component

Warnings Use with caution in patients with hepatic disease, G-6-PD deficiency, psoriasis, and porphyria; long-term use in children is not recommended; perform

(Continued)

Hydroxychloroquine Sulfate *(Continued)*

baseline and periodic (6 months) ophthalmologic examinations; test periodically for muscle asthenia

Dosage Forms Tablet: 200 mg [base 155 mg]

Reference Range Peak serum level of hydroxychloroquine was 427 ng/mL after oral dose of 200 mg (155 mg base)

Overdosage Treatment

Decontamination: Emesis or lavage/activated charcoal with cathartic

Supportive therapy: Electrolyte balance should be monitored and treated, especially when refractory arrhythmias develop. Sodium bicarbonate 1-2 mEq/kg I.V. (or 0.5-1 mEq/kg in children) may decrease conduction defects. Phenytoin or lidocaine are often effective at controlling drug-induced arrhythmias, while phenytoin is preferred due to its beneficial effects on A-V conduction velocity. Torsade de pointes can be treated with magnesium sulfate or overdrive pacemaker.

Enhancement of elimination: Multiple dosing of activated charcoal is effective; exchange transfusion can be utilized to remove toxic metabolites; hemodialysis or charcoal hemoperfusion have little effect; slightly dialyzable (5% to 20%)

Drug Interactions Increased digoxin serum levels; blood dyscrasia with use with aurothioglucose

Pregnancy Risk Factor C

Pregnancy Implications No evidence of teratogenesis

Monitoring Parameters Ophthalmologic exam, CBC

Patient Information Take with food or milk; complete full course of therapy; wear sunglasses in bright sunlight; notify physician if blurring or other vision changes, ringing in the ears, or deafness occurs

Nursing Implications Periodic blood counts and eye examinations are recommended when patient is on chronic therapy; give with food or milk

Specific References

Bernstein HN, "Ocular Safety of Hydroxychloroquine," *Ann Ophthalmol*, 1991, 23(8):292-6.

Buchanan NM, Toubi E, Khamashta MA, et al, "The Safety of Hydroxychloroquine in Lupus Pregnancy: Experience in 27 Pregnancies," *Br J Rheumatol*, 1995, 34(Suppl 1):14.

Furst DE, "Rational Use of Disease-Modifying Antirheumatic Drugs," *Drugs*, 1990, 39(1):19-37.

Hart LE and Tugwell P, "The Use of Disease-Modifying Antirheumatic Drugs in the Management of Rheumatoid Arthritis," *Postgrad Med J*, 1989, 65(770):905-12.

Kutz DC and Bridges AJ, "Bullous Rash and Brown Urine in a Systemic Lupus Erythematosus Patient Treated With Hydroxychloroquine," *Arthritis Rheum*, 1995, 38(3):440-3.

Levy M, Buskila D, Gladman DD, et al, "Pregnancy Outcome Following First Trimester Exposure to Chloroquine," *Am J Perinatol*, 1991, 8(3):174-8.

Seguin P, Camus C, Leroy JP, et al, "Respiratory Failure Associated With Hydroxychloroquine Neuromyopathy," *Eur Neurol*, 1995, 35:236-7.

Hydroxydaunomycin Hydrochloride *see* Doxorubicin Hydrochloride *on page 303*

3-hydroxydiazepam *see* Temazepam *on page 724*

Hydroxyurea (hye drox ee yoor ee' a)

Related Information

Toxicities of Chemotherapeutic Agents *on page 1631-1633*

CAS Number 127-07-1

Brand Names Hydrea®; Litalir®; Onco-Carbide®

Synonyms Hydroxycarbamide

Use CML in chronic phase; preventing thrombosis in patients with essential thrombocythemia; radiosensitizing agent in the treatment of primary brain tumors; head and neck tumors; uterine cervix and nonsmall cell lung cancer; refractory psoriasis; sickle cell anemia and other hemoglobinopathies; hematologic conditions such as essential thrombocythemia, polycythemia vera, hypereosinophilia, and hyperleukocytosis due to acute leukemia. Has shown activity against renal cell cancer, malignant melanoma, ovarian cancer, head and neck cancer, and prostate cancer; may be useful in preventing sickle cell crisis.

Mechanism of Action Interferes with synthesis of DNA, during the S phase of cell division, without interfering with RNA synthesis; inhibits ribonucleoside diphosphate reductase, preventing conversion of ribonucleotides to deoxyribonucleotides; cell-cycle specific for the S phase and may hold other cells in the G_1 phase of the cell cycle.

Adverse Reactions

Central nervous system: Dizziness, disorientation, hallucinations, seizures, headache, drowsiness, fever, hyperthermia

Dermatologic: Maculopapular rash, dermatitis, facial erythema, hyperpigmentation, erythema of the hands and face, fingernail atrophy, dry skin, alopecia, ulcerated lichen planus of palms

Endocrine & metabolic: Hyperuricemia

Gastrointestinal: Nausea, vomiting, diarrhea, constipation, anorexia, stomatitis

Hematologic: Myelosuppression, thrombocytopenia, anemia (megaloblastic)
Hepatic: Elevation of hepatic enzymes
Renal: Dysuria, renal tubular function impairment
Miscellaneous: Carcinogenic potential, systemic lupus erythematosus (SLE), facial flushing, neurotoxicity

Toxicodynamics/Kinetics

Absorption: Readily absorbed from gastrointestinal tract (≥80%)
Distribution: Readily crosses the blood-brain barrier; well distributed into intestine, brain, lung, and kidney tissues
Metabolism: In the liver
Half-life: 3-4 hours
Time to peak serum concentration: Within 2 hours
Elimination: Renal excretion of urea (metabolite) and respiratory excretion of CO_2 (metabolic end product); 50% of the drug is excreted unchanged in urine

Usual Dosage Oral (**refer to individual protocols**):

Children: No dosage regimens have been established. Dosages of 1500-3000 mg/m^2 as a single dose in combination with other agents every 4-6 weeks have been used in the treatment of pediatric astrocytoma, medulloblastoma, and primitive neuroectodermal tumors

Adults: Dose should always be titrated to patient response and WBC counts. Usual oral doses range from 10-30 mg/kg/day or 500-3000 mg/day; if WBC count falls <2500 cells/mm^3, or the platelet count <100,000/mm^3, therapy should be stopped for at least 3 days and resumed when values rise toward normal
- Solid tumors: Intermittent therapy: 80 mg/kg as a single dose every third day; continuous therapy: 20-30 mg/kg/day given as a single dose/day
- Concomitant therapy with irradiation: 80 mg/kg as a single dose every third day starting at least 7 days before initiation of irradiation
- Resistant chronic myelocytic leukemia: 20-30 mg/kg/day as a single daily dose
- Essential thrombocythemia: 15 mg/kg/day (goal is platelet count of 600,000 mm^3)
- Prevention of sickle cell crisis: Initial dose: 15 mg/kg; increase dose 5 mg/kg/day every 12 weeks unless bone marrow depression occurs; if bone marrow depression occurs, stop treatment until marrow recovers and restart dose at 2.5 mg/kg lower than previous dose (folic acid at 1 mg/day can be given with hydroxyurea)

Dosing adjustment in renal impairment:
- Cl_{cr} 10-50 mL/minute: Administer 50% of normal dose
- Cl_{cr} <10 mL/minute: Administer 20% of normal dose

Contraindications Severe anemia, severe bone marrow depression; WBC <2500/mm^3 or platelet count <100,000/mm^3; hypersensitivity to hydroxyurea

Warnings The U.S. Food and Drug Administration (FDA) currently recommends that procedures for proper handling and disposal of antineoplastic agents be considered. Use with caution in patients with renal impairment, in patients who have received prior irradiation therapy, and in the elderly.

Dosage Forms Capsule: 500 mg

Stability Store capsules at room temperature; capsules may be opened and emptied into water (will not dissolve completely)

Overdosage Treatment

Decontamination: Lavage/activated charcoal with cathartic
Enhancement of elimination: Multiple dosing of activated charcoal may be useful

Test Interactions Elevation of serum uric acid, BUN, creatinine

Drug Interactions Increased toxicity: Fluorouracil: The potential for neurotoxicity may be increased with concomitant administration; exacerbates radiation-induced erythema

Pregnancy Risk Factor D

Pregnancy Implications Appears in breast milk

Monitoring Parameters CBC with differential, platelets, hemoglobin, renal function and liver function tests, serum uric acid

Patient Information Contents of capsule may be emptied into a glass of water if taken immediately; inform the physician if you develop fever, sore throat, bruising, or bleeding; may cause drowsiness, constipation, and loss of hair

Additional Information Handle urine from patients taking hydroxyurea with care

Myelosuppressive effects:
WBC: Moderate
Platelets: Moderate
Onset (days): 7
Nadir (days): 10
Recovery (days): 21

Specific References

Bauman JL, Shulruff S, Hasegawa GR, et al, "Fever Caused by Hydroxyurea," *Arch Intern Med*, 1981, 141(2):260-1.

Charache S, Terrin ML, Moore RD, et al, "Effect of Hydroxyurea on the Frequency of Painful Crises in Sickle Cell Anemia," *N Engl J Med*, 1995, 332:1317-22.

(Continued)

Hydroxyurea *(Continued)*

Cortelazzo S, Finazzi G, Ruggeri M, et al, "Hydroxyurea for Patients With Essential Thrombocythemia and a High Risk of Thrombosis," *N Engl J Med*, 1995, 332:1132-6.

Lossos IS and Matzner Y, "Hydroxyurea-Induced Fever: Case Report and Review of the Literature," *Ann Pharmacother*, 1995, 29:132-3.

Renfro L, Kamino H, Raphael B, et al, "Ulcerative Lichen Planus-Like Dermatitis Associated With Hydroxyurea," *J Am Acad Dermatol*, 1991, 24(1):143-5.

Rodgers GP, "Recent Approaches to the Treatment of Sickle Cell Anemia," *JAMA*, 1991, 265(16):2097-101.

Hydroxyzine (hye drox' i zeen)

CAS Number 68-88-2; 10246-75-0; 2192-20-3

Brand Names Anxanil®; Atarax®; Atazina®; Atozine®; Durrax®; E-Vista®; Hy-Pam®; Hyzine-50®; Masmoran®; Multipax®; Neucalm®; Quiess®; Rezine®; Ucerax®; Vamate®; Vistacon-50®; Vistaject-25®; Vistaject-50®; Vistaquel®; Vistaril®; Vistazine®

Synonyms Hydroxyzine Embonate; Hydroxyzine Hydrochloride; Hydroxyzine Pamoate

Use Treatment of anxiety, as a preoperative sedative, an antipruritic, an antiemetic, and in alcohol withdrawal symptoms

Mechanism of Action A piperazine compound which competes with histamine for H_1-receptor sites on effector cells in the gastrointestinal tract, blood vessels, and respiratory tract

Adverse Reactions

Cardiovascular: Palpitations, hypotension

Central nervous system: Slight to moderate drowsiness, headache, fatigue, nervousness, dizziness, depression, sedation, paradoxical excitement, insomnia, hyperthermia

Dermal: Photosensitivity, rash, angioedema

Gastrointestinal: Appetite increase, weight increase, nausea, diarrhea, abdominal pain, dry mouth

Genitourinary: Urinary retention

Hematologic: Hemolysis (I.V. administration)

Hepatic: Hepatitis

Neuromuscular & skeletal: Arthralgia, myalgia, tremors, paresthesia

Ocular: Blurred vision

Respiratory: Thickening of bronchial secretions, bronchospasm, pharyngitis

Miscellaneous: Epistaxis, porphyrinogenic

Signs & Symptoms of Acute Overdose Seizures, seizures, sedation, myalgia, depression, insomnia, impotence, hypotension

Toxicodynamics/Kinetics

Onset of effect: Within 15-30 minutes

Duration: 6-24 hours

Absorption: Oral: Rapid

Distribution: V_d:

- Children: 19 L/kg
- Adults: 16 L/kg
- Elderly: 23 L/kg

Metabolism: Exact metabolic fate is unknown

Half-life:

- Children: 7 hours
- Adults: 20 hours
- Elderly: 29 hours (25 hours citrizine)
- Biliary cirrhosis patients: 37 hours

Time to peak serum concentration: Within 2 hours

Usual Dosage

Children:

- Oral: 0.6 mg/kg/dose every 6 hours
- I.M.: 0.5-1 mg/kg/dose every 4-6 hours as needed

Adults:

- Antiemetic: I.M.: 25-100 mg/dose every 4-6 hours as needed
- Anxiety: Oral: 25-100 mg 4 times/day; maximum dose: 600 mg/day
- Preoperative sedation:
  - Oral: 50-100 mg
  - I.M.: 25-100 mg
- Management of pruritus: Oral: 25 mg 3-4 times/day

Dosing interval in hepatic impairment: Change dosing interval to every 24 hours in patients with primary biliary cirrhosis

Estimated lethal dose: 25-250 mg/kg

Administration For I.M. administration in children, injections should be made into the midlateral muscles of the thigh; hydroxyzine has been given slowly I.V. in diluted solution to oncology patients via central venous lines without problems; do **not** give subcutaneously or intra-arterially

Contraindications Hypersensitivity to hydroxyzine or any component

Warnings Should be used with caution in patients with angle-closure glaucoma, prostatic hypertrophy, and bladder neck obstruction; should also be used with caution in patients with asthma or COPD; subcutaneous, intra-arterial and I.V. administration **not** recommended since thrombosis and digital gangrene can occur; extravasation can result in sterile abscess and marked tissue induration

Dosage Forms

Hydrochloride:

Injection:

Vistaject-25®, Vistaril®: 25 mg/mL (1 mL, 2 mL, 10 mL)

E-Vista®, Hyzine-50®, Neucalm®, Quiess®, Vistacon-50®, Vistaject-50®, Vistaquel®, Vistaril®, Vistazine®: 50 mg/mL (1 mL, 2 mL, 10 mL)

Syrup (Atarax®): 10 mg/5 mL (120 mL, 480 mL, 4000 mL)

Tablet:

Anxanil®: 25 mg

Atarax®: 10 mg, 25 mg, 50 mg, 100 mg

Atozine®: 10 mg, 25 mg, 50 mg

Durrax®: 10 mg, 25 mg

Rezine®: 10 mg, 25 mg

Pamoate:

Capsule:

Hy-Pam®: 25 mg, 50 mg

Vamate®: 25 mg, 50 mg, 100 mg

Vistaril®: 25 mg, 50 mg, 100 mg

Suspension, oral (Vistaril®:) 25 mg/5 mL (120 mL, 480 mL)

Stability Protect from light; I.V. is **incompatible** when mixed with aminophylline, amobarbital, chloramphenicol, dimenhydrinate, heparin, penicillin G, pentobarbital, phenobarbital, phenytoin, ranitidine, sulfisoxazole, thioridazine, vitamin B complex with C

Reference Range Plasma hydroxyzine level of 5.6-41.8 μg/dL (13.2-102.0 nmol/L) therapeutic for pruritus in children; peak plasma level is 73 μg/L after 0.7 mg/kg dose in adults

Overdosage Treatment

Decontamination: Lavage/activated charcoal

Supportive therapy: Physostigmine should be utilized in severe life-threatening anticholinergic crisis

Enhancement of elimination: Multiple dosing of activated charcoal may be effective

Test Interactions Can suppress wheal and flare of antigen skin testing for 4 days

Drug Interactions Increased effect/toxicity: CNS depressants, anticholinergics

Pregnancy Risk Factor C

Pregnancy Implications Neonatal withdrawal syndrome may occur

Monitoring Parameters Relief of symptoms, mental status

Patient Information Will cause drowsiness, avoid alcohol and other CNS depressants, avoid driving and other hazardous tasks until the CNS effects are known

Nursing Implications Extravasation can result in sterile abscess and marked tissue induration; provide safety measures (ie, side rails, night light, and call button); remove smoking materials from area; supervise ambulation

Specific References

Hollister LE, "Hydroxyzine Hydrochloride: Possible Adverse Cardiac Interactions," *Psychopharmacol Comm*, 1971, 1:61-5.

Paton DM and Webster DR, "Clinical Pharmacokinetics of H_1-Receptor Antagonists (The Antihistamines)," *Clin Pharmacokinet*, 1985, 10(6):477-97.

Prenner BM, "Neonatal Withdrawal Syndrome Associated With Hydroxyzine Hydrochloride," *Am J Dis Child*, 1977, 131:529-30.

Simons FE, Simons KJ, and Frith EM, "The Pharmacokinetics and Antihistaminic of the H_1 Receptor Antagonist Hydroxyzine," *J Allergy Clin Immunol*, 1984, 73(1 Pt 1):69-75.

Hydroxyzine Embonate *see* Hydroxyzine *on previous page*

Hydroxyzine Hydrochloride *see* Hydroxyzine *on previous page*

Hydroxyzine Pamoate *see* Hydroxyzine *on previous page*

Hygroton® *see* Chlorthalidone *on page 210*

Hylorel® *see* Guanadrel Sulfate *on page 392*

Hyoscine *see* Scopolamine *on page 691*

Hyoscyamine Sulfate (hye oh sye' a meen)

CAS Number 101-31-5; 620-61-1; 6835-16-1

Brand Names Anaspaz®; Cystospaz®; Cystospaz-M®; Duboisine; Egazil Duretter®; Gastrosed™; Levsin®; Levsinex®; Neoquess®; Peptard®

Synonyms *l*-Hyoscyamine Sulfate

Use Treatment of gastrointestinal tract disorders caused by spasm, adjunctive therapy for peptic ulcers; also has been used in parkinsonism

(Continued)

Hyoscyamine Sulfate *(Continued)*

Mechanism of Action Blocks the action of acetylcholine at parasympathetic sites in smooth muscle, secretory glands and the CNS; increases cardiac output, dries secretions, antagonizes histamine and serotonin, antimuscarinic agent; found in the plant *Hyoscyamus niger*

Adverse Reactions

Cardiovascular: Tachycardia, palpitations, hypotension (orthostatic)

Central nervous system: Fatigue, delirium, restlessness, headache, lightheadedness, memory loss, ataxia

Dermatologic: Dry, hot skin; photosensitivity, skin rash

Gastrointestinal: Impaired gastrointestinal motility, constipation, dysphagia

Neuromuscular & skeletal: Tremors

Ocular: Mydriasis, blurred vision, intraocular pressure (increased)

Renal: Dysuria

Miscellaneous: Dry mouth, nose, or throat; irritation at injection site, decreased sweating

Signs & Symptoms of Acute Overdose Dilated unreactive pupils; impotence, blurred vision; facial flushing; dryness of mucous membranes; dysphagia, memory loss, foul breath, intraocular pressure (increased), diminished or absent bowel sounds, urinary retention, ileus, photophobia, tachycardia, lightheadedness, rhabdomyolysis, hyperthermia, hypertension, respiratory rate (increased), hallucinations (lilliputian), seizures, ataxia, coma, myoglobinuria

Toxicodynamics/Kinetics

Onset of effect: 2-3 minutes

Duration: 4-6 hours

Absorption: Oral: Absorbed well

Protein binding: 50%

Metabolism: In the liver

Half-life: 13% to 38%

Elimination: Excreted in urine

Usual Dosage

Children: Oral, S.L.: Dose as per table repeated every 4 hours as needed

Hyoscyamine

Weight (kg)	Dose (mcg)	Maximum 24-Hour Dose (mcg)
Children <2 y		
2.3	12.5	75
3.4	16.7	100
5	20.8	125
7	25	150
10	31.3–33.3	200
15	45.8	275
Children 2–10 y		
10	31.3–33.3	Do not exceed 0.75 mg
20	62.5	
40	93.8	
50	125	

Adults:

Oral or S.L.: 0.125-0.25 mg 3-4 times/day before meals or food and at bedtime

Oral: 0.375-0.75 mg (timed release) every 12 hours

I.M., I.V., S.C.: 0.25-0.5 mg every 6 hours

Contraindications Narrow-angle glaucoma, obstructive uropathy, obstructive gastrointestinal tract disease, myasthenia gravis, known hypersensitivity to belladonna alkaloids

Warnings Use with caution in children with spastic paralysis; use with caution in elderly patients. Low doses cause a paradoxical decrease in heart rates. Some commercial products contain sodium metabisulfite, which can cause allergic-type reactions. May accumulate with multiple inhalational administration, particularly in the elderly. Heat prostration may occur in hot weather. Use with caution in patients with autonomic neuropathy, prostatic hypertrophy, hyperthyroidism, congestive heart failure, cardiac arrhythmias, chronic lung disease, biliary tract disease

Dosage Forms

Capsule, timed release (Cystospaz-M®, Levsinex®): 0.375 mg
Elixir (Levsin®): 0.125 mg/5 mL with alcohol 20% (480 mL)
Injection (Levsin®): 0.5 mg/mL (1 mL, 10 mL)
Solution, oral (Gastrosed™, Levsin®): 0.125 mg/mL (15 mL)
Tablet:
Anaspaz®, Gastrosed™, Levsin®, Neoquess®: 0.125 mg
Cystospaz®: 0.15 mg

Stability Insoluble in ether; soluble in water

Overdosage Treatment

Decontamination: Lavage/activated charcoal with cathartic; do not induce emesis

Supportive therapy: Physostigmine should be used as a last resort for life-threatening seizures, arrhythmias, or hypertension that is refractory to standard supportive therapy; rhabdomyolysis can be treated with alkaline diuresis and mannitol; esmolol can be used for tachyarrhythmias; bethanechol (5-10 mg 3 times/day) can be given for peripheral anticholinergic signs

Enhancement of elimination: Multiple dosing of activated charcoal may be effective

Antidote(s)

Mannitol *on page 1442*
Physostigmine *on page 1457*

Drug Interactions

Decreased effect with antacids

Increased toxicity with amantadine, antimuscarinics, haloperidol, phenothiazines, TCAs, MAO inhibitors

Pregnancy Risk Factor C

Pregnancy Implications Crosses the placenta; small amounts appear in breast milk

Patient Information Maintain good oral hygiene habits, because lack of saliva may increase chance of cavities. Observe caution while driving or performing other tasks requiring alertness, as may cause drowsiness, dizziness, or blurred vision. Notify physician if skin rash, flushing or eye pain occurs; or if difficulty in urinating, constipation or sensitivity to light becomes severe or persists.

Nursing Implications Observe for tachycardia if patient has cardiac problems.

Specific References

Boyson SJ, "Bethanechol for Anticholinergic Side Effects," *Ann Neurol*, 1988, 23(4):422-3.
Rumack BH, "Anticholinergic Poisoning: Treatment With Physostigmine," *Pediatrics*, 1973, 52(3):449-51.
Shutt LE and Bowes JB, "Atropine and Hyoscine," *Anaesthesia*, 1979, 34(5):476-90.

Hy-Pam® *see* Hydroxyzine *on page 414*

Hypercal® *see* Rauwolfia Serpentina *on page 677*

Hyperstat® I.V. *see* Diazoxide *on page 273*

Hypertonalum® *see* Diazoxide *on page 273*

Hypnoderm® *see* Flunitrazepam *on page 354*

Hypnor® *see* Flunitrazepam *on page 354*

Hypnovel® *see* Midazolam Hydrochloride *on page 532*

Hypoglycemic Agents Comparison, Oral *see page 1650*

Hypolag® *see* Methyldopa *on page 519*

Hypomide® *see* Chlorpropamide *on page 207*

Hyposyn® *see* Clonidine *on page 231*

Hypoten® *see* Nitroprusside Sodium *on page 568*

Hypovase® *see* Prazosin Hydrochloride *on page 638*

Hytrin® *see* Terazosin *on page 725*

Hytrinex® *see* Terazosin *on page 725*

Hytuss-2X® [OTC] *see* Guaifenesin *on page 390*

Hytuss® [OTC] *see* Guaifenesin *on page 390*

Hyzine-50® *see* Hydroxyzine *on page 414*

Ibenzmethyzine *see* Procarbazine Hydrochloride *on page 645*

Ibidomide Hydrochloride *see* Labetalol Hydrochloride *on page 458*

Ibinolo® *see* Atenolol *on page 137*

Ibuprin® [OTC] *see* Ibuprofen *on next page*

Ibuprofen (eye byoo proe' fen)

Related Information

Flurbiprofen Sodium *on page 364*
Nonsteroidal Anti-Inflammatory Comparison *on page 1655*

CAS Number 15687-27-1

Brand Names Advil® [OTC]; Excedrin® IB [OTC]; Genpril® [OTC]; Haltran® [OTC]; Ibuprin® [OTC]; Ibuprohm® [OTC]; Ibu-Tab®; Medipren® [OTC]; Menadol® [OTC]; Midol® 200 [OTC]; Motrin®; Motrin® IB [OTC]; Nuprin® [OTC]; Pamprin IB® [OTC]; PediaProfen™; Rufen®; Saleto-200® [OTC]; Saleto-400®; Trendar® [OTC]; Uni-Pro® [OTC]

Synonyms *p*-Isobutylhydratropic Acid

Use Inflammatory diseases and rheumatoid disorders including juvenile rheumatoid arthritis; mild to moderate pain; fever; dysmenorrhea; gout

Mechanism of Action Inhibits prostaglandin synthesis by decreasing the activity of the enzyme, cyclo-oxygenase, which results in decreased formation of prostaglandin precursors

Adverse Reactions

Cardiovascular: Fluid retention, circulatory collapse

Central nervous system: Headache, aseptic meningitis, psychosis, cognitive dysfunction, dizziness, coma, seizures

Dermatologic: Rash, pruritus

Endocrine & metabolic: Hyperkalemia, anion gap metabolic acidosis

Gastrointestinal: Abdominal pain, nausea, vomiting, bleeding, ulceration, constipation, diarrhea, dyspepsia

Genitourinary: Albuminuria

Hematologic: Leukopenia, neutropenia, agranulocytosis, granulocytopenia; aplastic anemia (rare), platelet inhibition, hemolytic anemia (Coombs' positive)

Hepatic: Elevation of transaminases, fulminant hepatitis

Ocular: Diplopia

Otic: Ototoxicity, tinnitus

Renal: Renal failure (acute), nephrotic syndrome, chronic renal failure

Respiratory: Wheezing, respiratory depression, aspiration

Miscellaneous: Hypersensitivity, feces discoloration (black), amblyopia

Signs & Symptoms of Acute Overdose Nausea, vomiting, azotemia, wheezing, purpura, thrombocytopenia, nephrotic syndrome, hyperthermia, photosensitivity, depression, gastrointestinal bleeding, mental confusion, lightheadedness, hyponatremia, leukocytosis, hypoglycemia, gastritis; flatulence, Stevens-Johnson syndrome, erythema multiforme, cognitive dysfunction, systemic lupus erythematosus (SLE), coagulopathy, ototoxicity; tinnitus, drowsiness; severe poisoning can manifest with coma, seizures, renal and or hepatic failure, hypotension, hypothermia, respiratory depression, apnea, metabolic acidosis, nystagmus; more significant exposures associated with ingestions of >400 mg/kg, alopecia, fever, urine discoloration (red), urine discoloration (red-purple), feces discoloration (tarry)

Toxicodynamics/Kinetics

Onset of action: 30 minutes

Duration: 4-6 hours

Absorption: Oral: Rapid (85%) from gastrointestinal tract

Distribution: V_d: 0.11 L/kg; increased in patients with cystic fibrosis

Protein binding: 90% to 99%

Metabolism: In the liver by oxidation

Half-life: 2 hours

Time to peak serum concentration: Within 1-2 hours

Elimination: Urine (1% as free drug); some biliary excretion occurs; clearance: 0.045 L/hour/kg

Usual Dosage Oral:

Children:

- Antipyretic: 6 months to 12 years: Temperature <102.5°F (39°C): 5 mg/kg/dose; temperature >102.5°F: 10 mg/kg/dose given every 6-8 hours; maximum daily dose: 40 mg/kg/day
- Juvenile rheumatoid arthritis: 30-70 mg/kg/24 hours divided every 6-8 hours
  - <20 kg: Maximum: 400 mg/day
  - 20-30 kg: Maximum: 600 mg/day
  - 30-40 kg: Maximum: 800 mg/day
  - >40 kg: Adult dosage
- Start at lower end of dosing range and titrate upward; maximum: 2.4 g/day
- Analgesic: 4-10 mg/kg/dose every 6-8 hours

Adults:

- Inflammatory disease: 400-800 mg/dose 3-4 times/day; maximum dose: 3.2 g/day
- Analgesia/pain/fever/dysmenorrhea: 200-400 mg/dose every 4-6 hours; maximum daily dose: 3.4 g

Dosing adjustment/comments in severe hepatic impairment: Avoid use

Contraindications Hypersensitivity to ibuprofen, any component, aspirin or other nonsteroidal anti-inflammatory drugs (NSAIDs)

Dosage Forms

Suspension, oral: 100 mg/5 mL (120 mL, 480 mL)

Tablet: 200 mg [OTC], 300 mg, 400 mg, 600 mg, 800 mg

Reference Range Plasma concentrations >200 μg/mL (971 μmol/L) may be associated with severe toxicity; not readily available, thus not recommended; antipyretic effect can occur at plasma concentrations of 10 μg/mL (48 μmol/L)

Overdosage Treatment

Decontamination: Ipecac or lavage/activated charcoal with cathartic at ingestions >100 mg/kg; whole bowel irrigation is effective but usually not required

Supportive therapy: Hypotension/dehydration can be managed with intravenous fluid therapy; acidosis should be treated with bicarbonates, seizures with benzodiazepines; antacids, blood products are indicated, as appropriate, for hemorrhage

Enhancement of elimination: Dialysis or perfusion is indicated for secondary complications, acidosis, or renal failure and not toxin removal alone; multiple dosing of activated charcoal may be effective

Test Interactions Increases chloride (S), sodium (S)

Diagnostic Tests/Procedures

Anion Gap, Blood *on page 1193*

Blood Gases, Arterial *on page 1207*

Complete Blood Count *on page 1236*

Ibuprofen, Serum *on page 1273*

Stool Culture *on page 1356*

Urinalysis *on page 1373*

Drug Interactions Aspirin decreases serum concentrations probably by protein-binding displacement; there is an increased bleeding potential with concomitant warfarin therapy; may increase lithium and methotrexate concentrations by decreasing renal clearance; may decrease diuretic and hypotensive effects of thiazides, loop diuretics, ACE inhibitors, and beta-blockers; may increase nephrotoxicity of cyclosporine

Pregnancy Risk Factor B (D if used in the 3rd trimester)

Pregnancy Implications Renal failure related to *in utero* exposure

Monitoring Parameters CBC, liver enzymes; occult blood loss and periodic liver function test; monitor urine output, serum BUN and creatinine in patients with decreased renal function; with long-term therapy, periodic ophthalmic exams

Additional Information Each 5 mL of suspension contains 2.5 g of sucrose; nomogram available but relative lack of significant toxicity and inaccessibility of laboratory assay precludes use (see nomogram in the text preceding this chapter); high dose ibuprofen may be effective in treating lung disease in cystic fibrosis; largest ibuprofen ingested reported was 72 g in an adult; while hyperkalemia, metabolic acidosis, and rhabdomyolysis was noted, the patient did well with supportive therapy and did not require dialysis

Specific References

Castillo M, Lam, YWF, Dooley MA, et al, "Disposition and Covalent Binding of Ibuprofen and its Acyl Glucuronide in the Elderly," *Clin Pharmacol Ther*, 1995, 57:636-44.

Court H and Volans GN, "Poisoning After Overdose With Nonsteroidal Anti-inflammatory Drugs," *Adverse Drug React Acute Poisoning Rev*, 1984, 3(1):1-21.

Hall AH, Smolinske SC, Conrad FL, et al, "Ibuprofen Overdose: 126 Cases," *Ann Emerg Med*, 1986, 15(11):1308-13.

Hoppmann RA, Peden JG, and Ober SK, "Central Nervous System Side Effects of Nonsteroidal Anti-inflammatory Drugs. Aseptic Meningitis, Psychosis, and Cognitive Dysfunction," *Arch Intern Med*, 1991, 151(7):1309-13.

Kim J, Gazarian M, Verjee Z, et al, "Acute Renal Insufficiency in Ibuprofen Overdose," *Pediatr Emerg Care*, 1995, 11:107-8.

Konstan MW, Byard PJ, Hoppel CL, et al, "Effect of High-Dose Ibuprofen in Patients With Cystic Fibrosis," *N Engl J Med*, 1995, 332(13):848-54.

Lesko SM and Mitchell AA,"An Assessment of the Safety of Pediatric Ibuprofen. A Practitioner-Based Randomized Clinical Trial," *JAMA*, 1995, 273(12):929-33.

McElwee NE, Veltri JC, Bradford DC, et al, "A Prospective, Population-Based Study of Acute Ibuprofen Overdose: Complications are Rare and Routine Serum Levels are Not Warranted," *Ann Emerg Med*, 1990, 19(6):657-62.

Olsen KM, Gurley BJ, Davis GA, et al, "Comparison of Fluid Volumes With Whole Bowel Irrigation in a Simulated Overdose of Ibuprofen," *Ann Pharmacother*, 1995, 29:246-50.

Smolinske SC, Hall AH, Vandenberg SA, et al, "Toxic Effects of Nonsteroid Anti-inflammatory Drugs in Overdose. An Overview of Recent Evidence on Clinical Effects and Dose-Response Relationships," *Drug Saf*, 1990, 5(4):252-74.

Turturro MA, Paris PM, and Seaberg DC, "Intramuscular Ketorolac Versus Oral Ibuprofen in Acute Musculoskeletal Pain," *Acad Emerg Med*, 1995, 26:117-20.

Vale JA and Meredith TJ, "Acute Poisoning Due to Nonsteroidal Anti-inflammatory Drugs," *Med Toxicol*, 1986, 1(1):12-31.

Verbeeck RK, "Pharmacokinetic Drug Interactions With Nonsteroidal Anti-inflammatory Drugs," *Clin Pharmacokinet*, 1990, 19(1):44-66.

Wolfe TR, "Ibuprofen Overdose," *Am J Emerg Med*, 1995, 13:375.

Ibuprohm® [OTC] *see* Ibuprofen *on page 418*

Ibu-Tab® *see* Ibuprofen *on page 418*

ICI-194660 *see* Meropenem *on page 504*

Idasal® *see* Methoxamine Hydrochloride *on page 518*

Ido A50® *see* Vitamin A *on page 795*

Ido-E® *see* Vitamin E *on page 798*

IFLrA *see* Interferon Alfa-2a *on page 430*

IFN *see* Interferon Alfa-2a *on page 430*

IFN-alpha 2 *see* Interferon Alfa-2b *on page 432*

Igrotin® *see* Chlorthalidone *on page 210*

Ikacor® *see* Verapamil Hydrochloride *on page 787*

Iktorivil® *see* Clonazepam *on page 229*

Ilosone® Oral *see* Erythromycin *on page 319*

Imagotan® *see* Mesoridazine Besylate *on page 505*

Imex® *see* Tetracycline *on page 732*

Imidazole and Triazole Antifungal

Commonly Found in Fluconazole, itraconazole, ketoconazole, terconazole

Use Treatment of susceptible fungal infections, including candidiasis, oral thrush, blastomycosis, histoplasmosis, paracoccidioidomycosis, chronic mucocutaneous candidiasis, as well as certain recalcitrant cutaneous dermatophytoses; used topically for treatment of tinea corporis, tinea cruris, tinea versicolor and cutaneous candidiasis

Mechanism of Action Alters permeability of the cell wall; inhibits biosynthesis of triglycerides and phospholipids by fungi; inhibits several fungal enzymes that results in a build-up of toxic concentrations of hydrogen peroxide

Adverse Reactions See individual monographs for Fluconazole, Itraconazole, and Ketoconazole

Signs & Symptoms of Acute Overdose No published cases; generally an extension of known pharmacologic and toxicologic effects are seen; as a single agent it appears not to be significantly toxic; drug interactions can lead to serious sequelae and toxicity which must be recognized and considered

Toxicodynamics/Kinetics See individual monographs for Fluconazole and Ketoconazole

Overdosage Treatment

Decontamination: Ipecac or lavage/activated charcoal with cathartic

Enhancement of elimination: Multiple dosing of activated charcoal would not be expected to be helpful; not dialyzable (0% to 5%)

Diagnostic Tests/Procedures

Liver Profile *on page 1286*

Additional Information In some protocols, dosed at weekly intervals, still should be recognized as a contributor to toxicities

Imigran® *see* Sumatriptan Succinate *on page 717*

Iminourea Hydrochloride *see* Guanidine Hydrochloride *on page 395*

Imipem® *see* Imipenem/Cilastatin *on this page*

Imipemide *see* Imipenem/Cilastatin *on this page*

Imipenem/Cilastatin (i mi pen' em/sye la stat' in)

Related Information

Meropenem *on page 504*

CAS Number 64221-86-9; 74431-23-5; 82009-34-5; 81129-83-1

Brand Names Imipem®; Primaxin®; Tenacid®; Tienam®; Tracix®; Zienam®

Synonyms Imipemide

Use Treatment of documented multidrug-resistant gram-negative infection due to organisms proven or suspected to be susceptible to imipenem/cilastatin; treatment of multiple organism infection in which other agents have an insufficient spectrum of activity or are contraindicated due to toxic potential; imipenem is usually given with a dehydropeptidase I inhibitor cilastatin sodium which inhibits renal breakdown of imipenem

Mechanism of Action Inhibits bacterial cell wall synthesis by binding to one or more of the penicillin binding proteins (PBPs); which in turn inhibits the final transpeptidation step of peptidoglycan synthesis in bacterial cell walls, thus inhibiting cell wall biosynthesis. Bacteria eventually lyse due to ongoing activity of cell wall autolytic enzymes (autolysins and murein hydrolases) while cell wall assembly is arrested.

Adverse Reactions

Cardiovascular: Hypotension, palpitations, tachycardia
Central nervous system: Seizures, dizziness, vertigo, confusion
Dermatologic: Rash, pruritus, urticaria
Gastrointestinal: Nausea, diarrhea, vomiting, pseudomembranous colitis
Hematologic: Neutropenia, eosinophilia, thrombocytosis, aplastic anemia, leukopenia
Hepatic: Hepatotoxicity
Local: Phlebitis, pain at injection site
Neuromuscular & skeletal: Myasthenia gravis may worsen
Miscellaneous: Emergence of resistant strains of *P. aeruginosa*

Signs & Symptoms of Acute Overdose Seizures, tremors, myasthenia gravis (exacerbation or precipitation of)

Toxicodynamics/Kinetics

Distribution: V_d: 0.1-0.2 L/kg; neonates: 0.4 L/kg; imipenem appears in breast milk; crosses the placenta; distributed rapidly and widely to most tissues and fluids including sputum, pleural fluid, peritoneal fluid, interstitial fluid, bile, aqueous humor, reproductive organs, and bone; highest concentrations in pleural fluid, interstitial fluid, peritoneal fluid, and reproductive organs; low concentrations in cerebrospinal fluid
Protein binding: Imipenem: 20%; cilastatin: 40%
Metabolism: Imipenem is metabolized in the kidney by dehydropeptidase, this activity is blocked by cilastatin; cilastatin is partially metabolized in the kidneys
Half-life: Both: 60 minutes, extended with renal insufficiency
Elimination: Both: ~70% excreted unchanged in urine

Usual Dosage I.V. infusion (dosage recommendation based on imipenem component):

Children: 25 mg/kg every 6 hours
Adults: 1-4 g/day not to exceed 50 mg/kg/day; reduce dose in renal failure; usually given twice daily

Contraindications Hypersensitivity to imipenem/cilastatin or any component

Warnings Dosage adjustment required in patients with impaired renal function; safety and efficacy in children <12 years of age have not yet been established; prolonged use may result in superinfection; use with caution in patients with a history of seizures or allergy to any beta-lactams

Dosage Forms Powder for injection:

I.M.:
Imipenem 500 mg and cilastatin 500 mg
Imipenem 750 mg and cilastatin 750 mg
I.V.:
Imipenem 250 mg and cilastatin 250 mg (13 mL)
Imipenem 500 mg and cilastatin 500 mg (13 mL)

Stability Stable for 10 hours at room temperature following reconstitution with 100 mL of 0.9% sodium chloride injection; up to 48 hours when refrigerated at 5°C. If reconstituted with 5% or 10% dextrose injection, 5% dextrose and sodium bicarbonate, 5% dextrose and 0.9% sodium chloride, is stable for 4 hours at room temperature and 24 hours when refrigerated.

Reference Range Peak plasma imipenem concentration following a 500 mg I.V. dose of imipenem/cilastatin: ~40-50 μg/mL

Overdosage Treatment

Supportive therapy: Diazepam or phenytoin may be useful for treatment of seizures; fentanyl (100 mcg in adults) has been used with diazepam (5 mg) to treat tremors and seizures
Enhancement of elimination: Hemodialysis is particularly useful to increase clearance of imipenem and cilastatin; about 73% of imipenem and 82% of cilastatin are cleared by a 4-hour dialysis; peritoneal dialysis is not useful in enhancing elimination

Test Interactions Interferes with urinary glucose determination using Clinitest®; can cause false elevations of amylase and lipase

Drug Interactions Increased effect/toxicity with probenecid; theophylline and ganciclovir may potentiate seizures; aminoglycosides (synergy); can cause increase in cyclosporine levels

Pregnancy Risk Factor C

Monitoring Parameters Periodic renal, hepatic, and hematologic function tests

Nursing Implications Not for direct infusion; vial contents must be transferred to 100 mL of infusion solution; final concentration should not exceed 5 mg/mL; infuse over 30-60 minutes; watch for seizures; do not mix with or physically add to other antibiotics; however, may administer concomitantly

Additional Information

Seizure frequency is ~1.5% to 2% and usually occurs about 7 days after initiation of therapy; risk factors include brain lesions, epilepsy or previous seizure disorder, and renal insufficiency; the mechanism of action for seizures may be due to

(Continued)

Imipenem/Cilastatin *(Continued)*

binding of imipenem to gamma-aminobutyric acid (GABA) receptors in the central nervous system

Sodium content of 1 g injection:

I.M.: 64.4 mg (2.8 mEq)

I.V.: 73.6 mg (3.2 mEq)

Specific References

Barza M, "Imipenem: First of a New Class of Beta-Lactam Antibiotics," *Ann Intern Med*, 1985, 103(4):552-60.

Bomback T, Sesin GP, and Mucciardi N, "Possible Imipenem/Cilastatin-Induced Aplastic Anemia," *Pharmacy and Therapeutics*, 1995, 20(5):293-302.

Donowitz GR and Mandell GL, "Beta-Lactam Antibiotics," *N Engl J Med*, 1988, 318(7):419-26 and 318(8):490-500.

Hellinger WC and Brewer NS, "Imipenem," *Mayo Clin Proc*, 1991, 66(10):1074-81.

O'Riordan J, Jared M, Hutchinson M, et al, "Worsening of Myasthenia Gravis on Treatment With Imipenem/Cilastatin *J Neurol Neurosurg Psychiatry,*" , 1994, 57(3):383.

Leo RJ and Ballow CH, "Seizure Activity Associated With Imipenem Use: Clinical Case Reports and Review of the Literature," *DICP*, 1991, 25(4):351-4.

Norrby SR, "Carbapenems," *Med Clin North Am*, 1995, 79(4):745-60.

O'Donovan CA, White ML, Cheung A, et al, "Seizure Incidence With Imipenem Use at VA Hospital," *Hospital Formulary*, 1995, 30:172-5.

Park SY and Parker RH, "Review of Imipenem," *Infect Control*, 1986, 7(6):333-7.

Somani P, Freimer EH, Gross ML, et al, "Pharmacokinetics of Imipenem-Cilastatin in Patients With Renal Insufficiency Undergoing Continuous Ambulatory Peritoneal Dialysis," *Antimicrob Agents Chemother*, 1988, 32(4):530-4.

Imipramine (im ip' ra meen)

Related Information

Antidepressant Agents Comparison *on page 1639*

Therapeutic Drugs Associated With Hallucinations *on page 1558-1559*

CAS Number 50-49-7; 10075-24-8; 113-52-0

Brand Names Berkomine®; Dimipressin®, Iprogen®; Janimine®; Norpramin®; Presamine®; SK-Pramine®; Tofranil®; Tofranil-PM®

Synonyms Imipramine Hydrochloride; Imipramine Pamoate

Use Treatment of various forms of depression, often in conjunction with psychotherapy; enuresis in children; analgesic for certain chronic and neuropathic pain

Mechanism of Action Increases the synaptic concentration of serotonin, norepinephrine, and/or dopamine in the central nervous system by inhibition of their reuptake by the presynaptic neuronal membrane; peripheral alpha-receptor blockade may be the cause of hypotension (orthostatic).

Adverse Reactions

Cardiovascular: Cardiac arrhythmias, cardiomyopathy, hypotension, has been associated with falls (hypotension (orthostatic))

Central nervous system: Drowsiness, sedation, confusion, dizziness, asthenia, psychosis, restlessness, fatigue, anxiety, nervousness, sleep disorders, seizures, delirium, hyperthermia, visual hallucinations

Dermatologic: Rash, photosensitivity

Endocrine & metabolic: Syndrome of inappropriate antidiuretic hormone

Gastrointestinal: Nausea, vomiting, constipation, dry mouth

Genitourinary: Urinary retention

Hematologic: Blood dyscrasias

Hepatic: Hepatitis

Ocular: Blurred vision, photophobia, diplopia, intraocular pressure (increased), mydriasis

Miscellaneous: Hypersensitivity reactions

Signs & Symptoms of Acute Overdose Confusion, dental erosion, depression, impotence, eosinophilia, disorientation, colitis, jaundice, mania, lactation, ejaculatory disturbances, hypoglycemia, Q-T prolongation, ataxia, nystagmus, hallucinations, hyponatremia, hyperthyroidism, intraocular pressure (increased), seizures, (within 3 hours of ingestion), myasthenia gravis (exacerbation or precipitation of), hypotension, galactorrhea, cardiac arrhythmias, conduction defects; constipation, cyanosis, dementia, tachycardia (sinus); QRS prolongation, with rightward terminal 40 millisecond frontal plane of QRS vector, coma (mean duration: 6 hours); myoclonus, respiratory depression, pulmonary edema, leukopenia; neutropenia; agranulocytosis; granulocytopenia; alopecia, systemic lupus erythematosus (SLE), ototoxicity; tinnitus

Toxicodynamics/Kinetics

Maximum antidepressant effect: Usually after 2 weeks or more

Absorption: Oral: Well absorbed from gastrointestinal tract

Distribution: V_d: 15 L/kg; widely distributed into body including CNS

Protein binding: ≥85%

Metabolism: In the liver by microsomal enzymes to desipramine (active) and other metabolites; significant first-pass metabolism; undergoes enterohepatic recirculation

Half-life: 6-18 hours
Time to peak serum concentration:
Oral: 1-2 hours
I.M.: 30 minutes
Elimination: Almost all compounds following metabolism are excreted in urine

Usual Dosage Maximum antidepressant effect may not be seen for 2 or more weeks after initiation of therapy

Children: Oral:

Depression: 1.5 mg/kg/day with dosage increments of 1 mg/kg every 3-4 days to a maximum dose of 5 mg/kg/day in 1-4 divided doses; monitor carefully especially with doses ≥3.5 mg/kg/day

Enuresis: ≥6 years: Initial: 10-25 mg at bedtime, if inadequate response still seen after 1 week of therapy, increase by 25 mg/day; dose should not exceed 2.5 mg/kg/day or 50 mg at bedtime if 6-12 years of age or 75 mg at bedtime if ≥12 years of age

Adjunct in the treatment of cancer pain: Initial: 0.2-0.4 mg/kg at bedtime; dose may be increased by 50% every 2-3 days up to 1-3 mg/kg/dose at bedtime

Adolescents: Oral: Initial: 25-50 mg/day; increase gradually; maximum: 100 mg/day in single or divided doses

Adults:

Oral: Initial: 25 mg 3-4 times/day, increase dose gradually, total dose may be given at bedtime; maximum: 300 mg/day

I.M.: Initial: Up to 100 mg/day in divided doses; change to oral as soon as possible

Contraindications Hypersensitivity to imipramine (cross-sensitivity with other tricyclics may occur); patients receiving MAO inhibitors within past 14 days; narrow-angle glaucoma

Warnings Do not discontinue abruptly in patients receiving long-term high-dose therapy; some oral preparations contain tartrazine and injection contains sulfites both of which can cause allergic reactions; use with caution in patients with cardiovascular disease, conduction disturbances, seizure disorders, urinary retention, hyperthyroidism or those receiving thyroid replacement

Dosage Forms

Capsule, as pamoate (Tofranil-PM®): 75 mg, 100 mg, 125 mg, 150 mg
Injection, as hydrochloride (Tofranil®): 12.5 mg/mL (2 mL)
Tablet, as hydrochloride (Janimine®, Tofranil®): 10 mg, 25 mg, 50 mg

Stability Solutions stable at a pH of 4-5; turns yellowish or reddish on exposure to light. Slight discoloration does not affect potency; marked discoloration is associated with loss of potency. Capsules stable for 3 years following date of manufacture.

Reference Range

Therapeutic:

Imipramine and desipramine 150-250 ng/mL (SI: 530-890 nmol/L)
Desipramine 150-300 ng/mL (SI: 560-1125 nmol/L)

Metabolism may be impaired in elderly patients; toxic: >300 ng/mL (SI: >1070 nmol/L); serious symptoms are associated with levels >1000 ng/mL (SI: >3566 nmol/L)

Overdosage Treatment

Decontamination: Do not induce emesis; lavage is effective if performed within 90 minutes/activated charcoal with cathartic; multiple dosing of activated charcoal would be expected to be useful

Supportive therapy: Lavage within 6 hours of ingestion; following initiation of essential overdose management, toxic symptoms should be treated. Ventricular arrhythmias and ventricular conduction defects often respond to phenytoin 15-20 mg/kg (adults) with concurrent systemic alkalinization (sodium bicarbonate 0.5-2 mEq/kg I.V.). Titrate to a serum pH of 7.45-7.55. Arrhythmias unresponsive to this therapy may respond to lidocaine 1 mg/kg I.V. followed by a titrated infusion. Physostigmine (1-2 mg I.V. slowly for adults or 0.5 mg I.V. slowly for children) may be indicated for seizures or movement disorders but only as **a last resort**. Propranolol may also be utilized for supraventricular arrhythmias (rate: >160) at 1 mg/minute to a maximum of 5 mg in adults; pediatric dosage of 0.1 mg/kg/dose to 1 mg I.V.. Seizures usually respond to lorazepam or diazepam I.V. boluses (5-10 mg for adults up to 30 mg or 0.25-0.4 mg/kg/dose for children up to 10 mg/dose). If seizures are unresponsive or recur, phenytoin or phenobarbital may be required. Patients must be monitored for at least 24 hours if any signs or symptoms are exhibited. Dobutamine is preferred over dopamine for hypotension; glucagon (10 mg I.V.) can be given to treat hypotension. Flumazenil is contraindicated; magnesium has potentiated adverse cardiac effects (ie, asystole, decreased left ventricular pressure) in an animal model.

Antidote(s)

Sodium Bicarbonate *on page 1467*

Test Interactions Increases glucose; elevates plasma norepinephrine levels and plasma epinephrine levels threefold to fivefold; EMIT assays may give false-

(Continued)

Imipramine *(Continued)*

positive in presence of diphenhydramine, thioridazine, chlorpromazine, alimenazine, carbamazepine, cyclobenzaprine, or perphenazine

Diagnostic Tests/Procedures

Imipramine, Blood *on page 1274*

Drug Interactions May decrease or reverse effects of guanethidine and clonidine; may increase effects of CNS depressants, adrenergic agents, anticholinergic agents; with MAO inhibitors, fever, tachycardia, hypertension, seizures and death may occur; similar interactions as with other tricyclics may occur; carbamazepine enhances metabolism of imipramine

Pregnancy Risk Factor D (has been known to cause neonatal withdrawal consisting of tachypnea, restlessness, and insomnia)

Pregnancy Implications Crosses the placenta

Monitoring Parameters EKG for QRS widening or tachycardia, CBC, blood pressure, electrolytes, pH; monitor blood pressure and pulse rate prior to and during initial therapy; evaluate mental status; monitor weight

Patient Information May require 2-4 weeks to achieve desired effect; avoid alcohol ingestion; do not discontinue medication abruptly; may cause urine to turn blue-green; may cause drowsiness

Nursing Implications May increase appetite

Additional Information Imipramine hydrochloride: Tofranil®, Janimine® Imipramine Pamoate: Tofranil-PM®; monoclonal anti-imipramine antibodies are investigational

Specific References

Callaham M and Kassel D, "Epidemiology of Fatal Tricyclic Antidepressant Ingestion: Implications for Management," *Ann Emerg Med*, 1985, 14(1):1-9.

Cerva D, Graff J, and Flaherty JJ, "ARDS Associated With Massive Imipramine Overdose," *Am J Emerg Med*, 1986, 4(2):195-7.

Fouron JC and Chicoine R, "EKG Changes in Fatal Imipramine (Tofranil) Intoxication," *Pediatrics*, 1971, 48:777-81.

Frommer DA, Kulig KW, Marx JA, et al, "Tricyclic Antidepressant Overdose," *JAMA*, 1987, 257(4):521-6.

Hagerman GA and Hanashiro PK, "Reversal of Tricyclic Antidepressant-Induced Cardiac Conduction Abnormalities by Phenytoin," *Ann Emerg Med*, 1981, 10(2):82-6.

Kline JA, De Stefano AA, Schroeder JD, et al, "Magnesium Potentiates Imipramine Toxicity in the Isolated Rat Heart," *Ann Emerg Med*, 1994, 24(2):224-32.

Sener EK, Gabe S, and Henry JA, "Response to Glucagon in Imipramine Overdose," *J Toxicol Clin Toxicol*, 1995, 33(1):51-3.

Tran P, Panacek EA, Rhee KJ, et al, "Is Norepinephrine More Efficacious Than Dopamine in Reversing Hypotension Caused by Cyclic Antidepressant Overdose?" *Ann Emerg Med*, 1995, 25(1):128-30.

Tribble J, Weinhouse E, Garland J, et al, "Treatment of Severe Imipramine Poisoning Complicated by a Negative History of Drug Ingestion," *Pediatr Emerg Care*, 1989, 5(4):234-7.

Imipramine Hydrochloride *see* Imipramine *on page 422*

Imipramine Pamoate *see* Imipramine *on page 422*

Imitrex® *see* Sumatriptan Succinate *on page 717*

Immenoctal® *see* Secobarbital Sodium *on page 693*

Immune Interferon *replaced by* Interferon Gamma-1b *on page 436*

Imodium® *see* Loperamide Hydrochloride *on page 480*

Imodium® A-D [OTC] *see* Loperamide Hydrochloride *on page 480*

Imosec® *see* Loperamide Hydrochloride *on page 480*

Impugan® *see* Furosemide *on page 373*

Inapsine® *see* Droperidol *on page 307*

Inderal® *see* Propranolol Hydrochloride *on page 657*

Inderal® LA *see* Propranolol Hydrochloride *on page 657*

Indocin® *see* Indomethacin *on this page*

Indometacin *see* Indomethacin *on this page*

Indomethacin (in doe meth' a sin)

Related Information

Nonsteroidal Anti-Inflammatory Comparison *on page 1655*

Therapeutic Drugs Associated With Hallucinations *on page 1558-1559*

CAS Number 53-86-1 (Base); 74252-25-8 (Sodium)

Brand Names Indocin®

Synonyms Indometacin

Use Management of inflammatory diseases and rheumatoid disorders; moderate pain; acute gouty arthritis; I.V. form used as alternative to surgery for closure of patent ductus arteriosus in neonates

Mechanism of Action Inhibits prostaglandin synthesis by decreasing the activity of the enzyme, cyclo-oxygenase, which results in decreased formation of prostaglandin precursors

Adverse Reactions

Cardiovascular: Hypertension, edema

Central nervous system: Somnolence, fatigue, depression, confusion, dizziness, psychosis, frontal headache, visual and olfactory hallucinations

Dermatologic: Rash, alopecia, angioedema

Endocrine & metabolic: Hyperkalemia, dilutional hyponatremia (I.V.), hypoglycemia (I.V.)

Gastrointestinal: Nausea, vomiting, epigastric pain, abdominal pain, anorexia, gastrointestinal bleeding, ulcers, perforation, feces discoloration (black)

Hematologic: Hemolysis, bone marrow depression, leukopenia, neutropenia, agranulocytosis, granulocytopenia; platelet inhibition, aplastic anemia

Hepatic: Hepatitis

Ocular: Cataracts, diplopia

Otic: Ototoxicity, tinnitus

Renal: Renal failure, proteinuria, oliguria

Miscellaneous: Hypersensitivity reactions

Signs & Symptoms of Acute Overdose Nausea, colitis, wheezing, pseudotumor cerebri, gastrointestinal bleeding, photosensitivity, dementia, azotemia, impotence, hyponatremia, gastrointestinal hypoglycemia, esophageal ulceration; upset; syndrome of inappropriate antidiuretic hormone (SIADH), corneal microdeposits, hematuria, cholestatic jaundice, coagulopathy, vomiting, ototoxicity; tinnitus, drowsiness; severe poisoning can manifest with coma, seizures, blurred vision, renal and or hepatic failure, hypotension, respiratory depression, blindness, thrombocytopenia, hyperglycemia, urine discoloration (green), feces discoloration (green)

Toxicodynamics/Kinetics

Onset of action: Within 30 minutes

Duration: 4-6 hours

Absorption: Prompt and extensive from gastrointestinal tract

Distribution: V_d: 0.34-1.57 L/kg

Protein binding: 90%

Metabolism: In the liver with significant enterohepatic recycling

Half-life: $4\frac{1}{2}$ hours (longer in neonates)

Time to peak serum concentration: Within 3-4 hours

Elimination: Principally in urine as glucuronide conjugates; clearance: 0.12 L/hour/kg

Usual Dosage

Patent ductus arteriosus: Neonates: I.V.: Initial: 0.2 mg/kg; followed with: 2 doses of 0.1 mg/kg at 12- to 24-hour intervals if age <48 hours at time of first dose; 0.2 mg/kg 2 times if 2-7 days old at time of first dose; or 0.25 mg/kg 2 times if over 7 days at time of first dose; discontinue if significant adverse effects occur. Dose should be withheld if patient has anuria or oliguria.

Analgesia:

Children: Oral: Initial: 1-2 mg/kg/day in 2-4 divided doses; maximum: 4 mg/kg/day; not to exceed 150-200 mg/day

Adults: Oral, rectal: 25-50 mg/dose 2-3 times/day; maximum dose: 200 mg/day; extended release capsule should be given on a 1-2 times/day schedule

Contraindications Hypersensitivity to indomethacin, any component, aspirin, or other nonsteroidal anti-inflammatory drugs (NSAIDs); active gastrointestinal bleeding, ulcer disease; premature neonates with necrotizing enterocolitis, impaired renal function, IVH, active bleeding, platelet count <60,000/mm^3 or creatinine >1.6 mg/dL

Warnings Use with caution in patients with cardiac dysfunction, hypertension, renal or hepatic impairment, epilepsy, patients receiving anticoagulants and for treatment of JRA in children (fatal hepatitis has been reported)

Dosage Forms

Capsule: 25 mg, 50 mg

Capsule, sustained release: 75 mg

Powder for injection, as sodium trihydrate: 1 mg

Suppository, rectal: 50 mg

Suspension, oral: 25 mg/5 mL (237 mL, 500 mL)

Stability Protect from light; not stable in alkaline solution; reconstitute just prior to administration; discard any unused portion; do not use preservative containing diluents for reconstitution

Reference Range Therapeutic: 0.3-3.0 mg/L (0.8-8.0 μmol/L)

Overdosage Treatment

Decontamination: Ipecac or lavage/activated charcoal with cathartic

Supportive therapy: Hypotension/dehydration can be managed with intravenous fluid therapy; acidosis should be treated with bicarbonates, seizures with ben-

(Continued)

Indomethacin *(Continued)*

zodiazepines; antacids, blood products are indicated, as appropriate, for hemorrhage

Enhancement of elimination: Multiple doses of activated charcoal; dialysis or perfusion is indicated for secondary complications, acidosis, or renal failure and not toxin removal alone

Test Interactions Positive Coombs' [direct]

Drug Interactions Aspirin decreases serum concentrations probably by protein-binding displacement; there is an increased bleeding potential with concomitant warfarin therapy; may increase lithium and methotrexate concentrations by decreasing renal clearance; may decrease diuretic and hypotensive effects of thiazides, loop diuretics, ACE inhibitors, and beta-blockers; may increase nephrotoxicity of cyclosporine; cimetidine reduces absorption

Pregnancy Risk Factor B (D if used longer than 48 hours or after 34 weeks' gestation)

Pregnancy Implications May have adverse effects on fetus; crosses the placenta; appears in breast milk; renal failure related to *in utero* exposure

Monitoring Parameters BUN, serum creatinine, liver enzymes, CBC; ophthalmologic exams with chronic use

Nursing Implications Reconstitute just prior to administration; discard any unused portion; inject I.V. over 5-10 seconds; extended release capsules must be swallowed intact

Additional Information May affect platelet and renal function in neonates; misoprostol (200 μg) can reverse indomethacin-induced renal dysfunction in patients with stable alcoholic cirrhosis

Specific References

Bilimoria Y, Moy J, and Yu B, "Nephrotic Syndrome, Exfoliative Dermatitis, Eosinophilia, and Elevated IgE Associated With Indomethacin," *J Allergy Clin Immunol*, 1995, 95(2):287.

Court H and Volans GN, "Poisoning After Overdose With Nonsteroidal Anti-inflammatory Drugs," *Adverse Drug React Acute Poisoning Rev*, 1984, 3(1):1-21.

Hoppmann RA, Peden JG, and Ober SK, "Central Nervous System Side Effects of Nonsteroidal Anti-inflammatory Drugs. Aseptic Meningitis, Psychosis, and Cognitive Dysfunction," *Arch Intern Med*, 1991, 151(7):1309-13.

Sheehan TM, Boldy DA, and Vale JA, "Indomethacin Poisoning," *J Toxicol Clin Toxicol*, 1986, 24(2):151-8.

Smolinske SC, Hall AH, Vandenberg SA, et al, "Toxic Effects of Nonsteroid Anti-inflammatory Drugs in Overdose. An Overview of Recent Evidence on Clinical Effects and Dose-Response Relationships," *Drug Saf*, 1990, 5(4):252-74.

The International Agranulocytosis and Aplastic Anemia Study, "Risks of Agranulocytosis and Aplastic Anemia. A First Report of Their Relation to Drug Use With Special Reference to Analgesics," *JAMA*, 1986, 256(13):1749-57.

Vale JA and Meredith TJ, "Acute Poisoning Due to Nonsteroidal Anti-inflammatory Drugs," *Med Toxicol*, 1986, 1(1):12-31.

Verbeeck RK, "Pharmacokinetic Drug Interactions With Nonsteroidal Anti-inflammatory Drugs," *Clin Pharmacokinet*, 1990, 19(1):44-66.

Wong F, Massie D, and Hsu P, "The Effect of Misoprostol on Indomethacin-Induced Renal Dysfunction in Well-Compensated Cirrhosis," *J Hepatol*, 1995, 23:1-7.

InFed™ Injection *see* Iron *on page 439*

INH *see* Isoniazid *on page 443*

Inhibine *see* Hydrogen Peroxide *on page 408*

Inibil® *see* Aprotinin *on page 130*

Iniprol® *see* Aprotinin *on page 130*

Initard® *see* Insulin Preparations *on this page*

Innovace® *see* Enalapril *on page 311*

Inocor® *see* Amrinone Lactate *on page 127*

Insoma® *see* Nitrazepam *on page 562*

Insulatard® NPH *see* Insulin Preparations *on this page*

Insulin Preparations (in' su lin)

CAS Number 8049-62-5; 8063-29-4; 9004-10-8; 9004-12-0; 9004-21-1; 11061-68-0; 11070-73-8; 11091-62-6; 12584-58-6; 51798-72-2; 53027-39-7; 68859-20-1

Brand Names Actrafan® HM; Actrap® MC; Beef NPH Iletin® II; Beef Regular Iletin® II; Humulin®; Initard®; Insulatard® NPH; Lente® Iletin® I; Lente® Iletin® II; Lente® Purified Pork Insulin; Mixtard®; Neulente; Novolin®; NPH Iletin® I; Pork NPH Iletin® II; Pork Regular Iletin® II; Regular [Concentrated] Iletin® II U-500; Regular Iletin® I; Semilente® Iletin® I; Ultralente® Iletin® I; Ultratard; Velosulin®

Synonyms Insulinum; Lente; NPH; Semilente; Ultralente

Use Treatment of insulin-dependent diabetes mellitus, also noninsulin-dependent diabetes mellitus unresponsive to treatment with diet and/or oral hypoglycemics; to assure proper utilization of glucose and reduce glucosuria in nondiabetic patients receiving parenteral nutrition whose glucosuria cannot be adequately controlled with infusion rate adjustments or those who require assistance in achieving optimal caloric intakes; used to treat hyperkalemia

Mechanism of Action Replacement therapy for persons unable to produce the hormone naturally or in insufficient amounts to maintain glycemic control

Adverse Reactions Primarily symptoms of hypoglycemia

Cardiovascular: Palpitations, tachycardia, pallor

Central nervous system: Fatigue, tingling of fingers, mental confusion, loss of consciousness, headache, hypothermia, fasciculations

Dermatologic: Urticaria

Endocrine & metabolic: Hypoglycemia, hypokalemia

Gastrointestinal: Hunger, nausea, numbness of mouth

Local: Itching, redness, swelling, stinging, or warmth at injection site, atrophy or hypertrophy of S.C. fat tissue

Neuromuscular & skeletal: Muscle asthenia, tremors

Ocular: Transient presbyopia or blurred vision, nystagmus

Miscellaneous: Anaphylactoid reactions, sweating

Signs & Symptoms of Acute Overdose Hepatomegaly, seizures, dysarthria, numbness, parotid pain, ataxia, hypothermia, nystagmus, hyperglycemia, apnea, mydriasis, coma, periarteritis nodosa, noncardiogenic pulmonary edema, hypokalemia, hypoglycemia

Toxicodynamics/Kinetics

Onset and duration of hypoglycemic effects depend upon preparation administered; see table.

Insulin Preparations

Preparation	Onset of Action	Peak	Duration	pH
Regular	30 min	2.5-5 h	5-8 h	2.5-3.5
Semilente®	1-2 h	3-10 h	10-16 h	6.9-7.5
Lente®	2.5 h	7-15 h	18-23 h	6.9-7.5
NPH	90 min	10-20 h	24 h	6.9-7.5
PZI	4-8 h	14-24 h	<36 h	7.1-7.4
70/30	30 min	6-12 h	24 h	7.0-7.8
Isophane/Regular	6 h	4-8 h	24 h	6.9-7.5

Onset and duration: Biosynthetic NPH human insulin shows a more rapid onset and shorter duration of action than corresponding porcine insulins; human insulin and purified porcine regular insulin are similarly efficacious following S.C. administration. The duration of action of highly purified porcine insulins is shorter than that of conventional insulin equivalents. Duration depends on type of preparation and route of administration as well as patient related variables. In general, the larger the dose of insulin, the longer the duration of activity.

Absorption: Biosynthetic regular human insulin is absorbed from the S.C. injection site more rapidly than insulins of animal origin (60-90 minutes peak vs 120-150 minutes peak respectively) and lowers the initial blood glucose much faster.

Distribution: V_d: 0.37 L/kg

Protein binding: 5%

Metabolism: Hepatic

Bioavailability: Medium-acting S.C. Lente®-type human insulins did not differ from the corresponding porcine insulins

Elimination: Renal

Usual Dosage May administer I.V. (regular), I.M., S.C.

Diabetes mellitus:

Children and Adults: 0.5-1 unit/kg/day

Adolescents (growth spurts): 0.8-1.2 units/kg/day

Adjust dose to maintain premeal and bedtime blood glucose of 80-140 mg/dL (children <5 years: 100-200 mg/dL)

Hyperkalemia: Give calcium gluconate and $NaHCO_3$ first then 50% dextrose at 0.5-1 mL/kg and insulin 1 unit for every 4-5 g dextrose given

Diabetic ketoacidosis: Children and Adults: I.V. loading dose: 0.1 unit/kg, then maintenance continuous infusion: 0.1 unit/kg/hour (range: 0.05-0.2 units/kg/hour depending upon the rate of decrease of serum glucose – too rapid decrease of serum glucose may lead to cerebral edema).

Optimum rate of decrease (serum glucose): 80-100 mg/dL/hour

Note: Newly diagnosed patients with JODM presenting in DKA and patients with blood sugars <800 mg/dL may be relatively "sensitive" to insulin and should receive loading and initial maintenance doses approximately ½ of those indicated above.

(Continued)

Insulin Preparations *(Continued)*

Dosing adjustment in renal impairment (regular):

Cl_{cr} 10-50 mL/minute: Administer at 75% of normal dose

Cl_{cr} <10 mL/minute: Administer at 25% to 50% of normal dose; monitor blood glucose closely

Administration

I.V. infusions: To minimize adsorption problems to I.V. solution bag:

If new tubing is **not** needed: Wait a minimum of 30 minutes between the preparation of the solution and the initiation of the infusion

If new tubing is needed: After receiving the insulin drip solution, the administration set should be attached to the I.V. container and the line should be flushed with the insulin solution. The nurse should then wait 30 minutes, then flush the line again with the insulin solution prior to initiating the infusion.

If insulin is required prior to the availability of the insulin drip, regular insulin should be administered by I.V. push injection

Because of adsorption, the actual amount of insulin being administered could be substantially less than the apparent amount. Therefore, adjustment of the insulin drip rate should be based on effect and not solely on the apparent insulin dose. Furthermore, the apparent dose should not be used as the basis for determining the subsequent insulin dose upon discontinuing the insulin drip. Dose requires continuous medical supervision.

To be ordered as units/hour

Example: Standard diluent of regular insulin only: 100 units/100 mL NS (can be given as a more diluted solution, ie, 100 units/250 mL NS)

Insulin rate of infusion (100 units regular/100 mL NS)

1 unit/hour: 1 mL/hour
2 units/hour: 2 mL/hour
3 units/hour: 3 mL/hour
4 units/hour: 4 mL/hour
5 units/hour: 5 mL/hour, etc

Warnings Any change of insulin should be made cautiously; changing manufacturers, type and/or method of manufacture, may result in the need for a change of dosage; use with caution in patients with a previous hypersensitivity reaction; S.C. doses used in insulin-resistant patients must be reduced if given I.V., only regular insulin should be given I.V.

Dosage Forms All insulins are 100 units/mL (10 mL) except where indicated:

Rapid-acting:

- Regular beef and pork (Regular Iletin® I)
- Regular beef (purified) (Beef Regular Iletin® II)
- Regular human:
  - rDNA (Humulin® R)
  - rDNA, buffered (Humulin® BR)
  - Semisynthetic: Novolin® R, Novolin® R PenFil® (1.5 mL), Velosulin®
- Regular pork:
  - Purified (Pork Regular Iletin® II, Velosulin®)
  - Purified, concentrated (Regular [Concentrated] Iletin® II U-500): 500 units/mL (20 mL)
  - Regular Insulin
- Zinc suspension, prompt:
  - Beef (Semilente® Insulin)
  - Beef and pork (Semilente® Iletin® I)

Intermediate-acting:

- Isophane suspension:
  - Beef (NPH Insulin)
  - Beef and pork (NPH Iletin® I)
  - Beef (purified) (Beef NPH Iletin® II)
  - Human (rDNA) (Humulin® N)
  - Human (semisynthetic) (Novolin® N, Novolin® N PenFil®) (1.5 mL)
  - Pork (purified) (NPH Purified, Pork NPH Iletin® II, Insulatard® NPH)
- Zinc suspension:
  - Beef (Lente® Insulin)
  - Beef and pork (Lente® Iletin® I)
  - Beef (purified) (Lente® Iletin® II)
  - Human (rDNA) (Humulin® L)
  - Human (semisynthetic) (Novolin® L)
  - Pork (purified) (Lente® Iletin® II, Lente® Purified Pork Insulin)

Long-acting:

- Zinc suspension, extended:
  - Beef (Ultralente® Insulin)
  - Beef and pork (Ultralente® Iletin® I)
  - Human (rDNA) (Humulin® U)

Combinations:

Isophane insulin suspension (50%) and insulin injection (50%) human (rDNA) (Humulin® 50/50)

Isophane insulin suspension (70%) and insulin injection (30%) human (rDNA) (Humulin® 70/30)

Isophane insulin suspension (70%) and insulin injection (30%) human (semisynthetic) (Mixtard® Human 70/30, Novolin® 70/30)

Isophane insulin suspension (70%) and insulin injection (30%) human (semisynthetic) (Novolin® 70/30 PenFil®): 1.5 mL

Isophane insulin suspension (70%) and insulin injection (30%) pork (purified) (Mixtard®)

Stability Bottle in use is stable at room temperature up to 1 month; cold (freezing) causes more damage to insulin than room temperatures up to 100°F; avoid direct sunlight; cold injections should be avoided; do not carry in luggage hold of aircraft

Reference Range

Therapeutic, serum insulin (fasting): 5-20 μIU/mL (SI: 35-145 pmol/L)

Glucose:

Newborns: 20-80 mg/dL

Adults: 60-115 mg/dL

Elderly: 100-180 mg/dL

Peptide fragments are low (<0.5 ng/mL) in cases of exogenous insulin administration but high in insulinoma or sulfonylurea ingestion

Overdosage Treatment

Decontamination: Excision of tissue near insulin injection site can be performed

Supportive therapy: 50 mL $D_{50}W$ given intravenously; if no I.V. is available, glucagon 0.5-1 mg S.C. or I.M.; give 300 g of carbohydrates orally when patient awakens; insulin-induced peripheral and sacral edema has been successfully treated with oral ephedrine (15 mg every 8 hours)

Antidote(s)

Dextrose *on page 1409*

Glucagon *on page 1431*

Drug Interactions See table.

Environmental/Drug Interactions With Insulin Injection

Decrease Hypoglycemic Effect of Insulin	Increase Hypoglycemic Effect of Insulin	Unstable or Mixed Hypoglycemic Effect of Insulin
Chlorpromazine	Alcohol	Alcohol
Contraceptives, oral	Alpha-blockers	Beta-blockers
Corticosteroids	Anabolic steroids	Cyclophosphamide
Dextrothyroxine	Beta-blockers*	Isoniazid
Diltiazem	Captopril	Smoking
Dobutamine	Clofibrate	
Epinephrine	Enalapril	
Niacin	Fenfluramine	
Smoking	Guanethidine	
Thiazide diuretics	Hot baths	
Thyroid hormone	MAO inhibitors	
	Mebendazole	
	Pentamidine	
	Phenylbutazone	
	Salicylates	
	Sauna	
	Sulfinpyrazone	
	Tetracyclines	

*Nonselective beta-blockers may delay recovery from hypoglycemic episodes and mask signs/symptoms of hypoglycemia. Cardioselective agents may be alternatives.

Pregnancy Risk Factor B

Monitoring Parameters Urine sugar and acetone, serum glucose, electrolytes

Patient Information Do not change insulins without physician's approval; titrate vials to mix, do not shake; store in a cool place; when mixing insulins, draw up regular insulin into syringe first and use as soon as possible after mixing. Patients must be counseled by someone experienced in diabetes education, signs and symptoms of hyper- and hypoglycemia, exercise and diet, blood glucose monitoring, and other related topics.

Nursing Implications Patients using human insulin may be less likely to recognize hypoglycemia than if they use pork insulin; patients on pork insulin that have low blood sugar exhibit hunger and sweating; regular insulin is the only form for I.V. use; patients who are unable to accurately draw up their dose will need assistance such as prefilled syringes

(Continued)

Insulin Preparations *(Continued)*

Additional Information The term "purified" refers to insulin preparations containing no more than 10 ppm proinsulin (purified and human insulins are less immunogenic). Insulin abuse can be identified by presence of anti-insulin antibodies or decreased plasma C-peptide concentration; aspirin may be useful in alleviating hypersensitivity reactions

Specific References

Campbell IW and Ratcliffe JG, "Suicidal Insulin Overdosage Managed Exclusively by Excision of Insulin Injection Site," *Br Med J (Clin Res)*, 1982, 285(6339):408-9.

Hopkins DF, Cotton SJ, and Williams G, "Effective Treatment of Insulin-Induced Edema Using Ephedrine," *Diabetes Care*, 1993, 16(7):1026-8.

Levine DF and Bulstrode C, "Managing Suicidal Insulin Overdose," *Br Med J (Clin Res)*, 1982, 285(6346):974-5.

Mueller-Schoop J, "Accidental Intravenous Self-Injection With Insulin Pen," *Lancet*, 1993, 341(8849):894.

Pickup J, "Human Insulin: Problems With Hypoglycaemia in a Few Patients," *BMJ*, 1989, 299(6706):991-3.

Roberge RJ, Martin TG, and Delbridge TR, "Intentional Massive Insulin Overdose: Recognition and Management," *Ann Emerg Med*, 1993, 22(2):228-34.

Insulinum *see* Insulin Preparations *on page 426*

Intal® Inhalation Capsule *see* Cromolyn Sodium *on page 245*

Intal® Nebulizer Solution *see* Cromolyn Sodium *on page 245*

Intal® Oral Inhaler *see* Cromolyn Sodium *on page 245*

α-2-interferon *see* Interferon Alfa-2b *on page 432*

Interferon Alfa-2a (in ter feer' on)

Related Information

Toxicities of Chemotherapeutic Agents *on page 1631-1633*

CAS Number 76543-88-9

Brand Names Roferon-A®

Synonyms IFLrA; IFN; Recombinant Leukocyte A Interferon; rIFN-A

Use FDA approved: Patients >18 years of age: Hairy cell leukemia, AIDS-related Kaposi's sarcoma; multiple unlabeled uses; indications and dosage regimens are specific for a particular brand of interferon; used for treating adult patients with Philadelphia chromosome-positive chronic myelogenous leukemia

Mechanism of Action Inhibits cellular growth, alters the state of cellular differentiation, interferes with oncogene expression, alters cell surface antigen expression, increases phagocytic activity of macrophages and augments cytotoxicity of lymphocytes for target cells

Adverse Reactions Flu-like symptoms (fever, fatigue/malaise, myalgia, chills, headache, arthralgia, rigors) begin about 2-6 hours after the dose is given and may persist as long as 24 hours; usually patient can build up a tolerance to side effects

Cardiovascular: Tachycardia, cardiac arrhythmias, hypotension, edema

Central nervous system: Fatigue/malaise, dizziness, depression, confusion, sensory neuropathy, psychiatric effects, headache, EEG abnormalities, chills, abducent nerve paralysis

Dermatologic: Partial alopecia, rash, lichen planus

Endocrine & metabolic: Uric acid level (increased)

Gastrointestinal: Anorexia, dry mouth, nausea, vomiting, diarrhea, abdominal cramps, weight loss, change in taste

Genitourinary: Impotence

Hematologic: Leukopenia (mainly neutropenia), anemia, thrombocytopenia; decreased hemoglobin, hematocrit, platelets; neutralizing antibodies

Hepatic: ALT (increased) and AST (increased)

Neuromuscular & skeletal: Rigors

Ocular: Blurred vision

Renal: Proteinuria, creatinine (increased), BUN (increased)

Respiratory: Coughing, chest pain, nasal congestion

Miscellaneous: Thyroid dysfunction, sweating, subacute thyroiditis

Signs & Symptoms of Acute Overdose Hyperglycemia, leukopenia; neutropenia; agranulocytosis; granulocytopenia; impotence, Mees' lines, mania, A-V block, encephalopathy, coma

Toxicodynamics/Kinetics

Absorption: Filtered and absorbed at the renal tubule

Distribution: V_d: 31 L, but has been noted to be much greater (370-720 L) in leukemia patients receiving continuous infusion IFN; IFN does not penetrate the CSF

Metabolism: Majority of dose thought to be metabolized in the kidney

Bioavailability:

I.M.: 83%

S.C.: 90%

Half-life, elimination:

I.M., I.V.: 2 hours after administration

S.C.: 3 hours

Time to peak serum concentration: I.M., S.C.: ~6-8 hours
Elimination: Renal, 216 mL/minute

Usual Dosage Refer to individual protocols

Infants and Children: Hemangiomas of infancy, pulmonary hemangiomatosis: S.C.: 1-3 million units/m^2/day once daily

Adults >18 years: I.M., S.C.:

Hairy cell leukemia: Induction dose is 3 million units/day for 16-24 weeks; maintenance: 3 million units 3 times/week (may be treated for up to 20 consecutive weeks)

AIDS-related Kaposi's sarcoma: Induction dose is 36 million units/day for 10-12 weeks; maintenance: 36 million units 3 times/week (may begin with dose escalation from 3-9-18 million units each day over 3 consecutive days followed by 36 million units/day for the remainder of the 10-12 weeks of induction)

If severe adverse reactions occur, modify dosage (50% reduction) or temporarily discontinue therapy until adverse reactions abate

Contraindications Hypersensitivity to alfa-2a interferon or any component of the product

Warnings The U.S. Food and Drug Administration (FDA) currently recommends that procedures for proper handling and disposal of antineoplastic agents be considered. Use with caution in patients with seizure disorders, brain metastases, compromised CNS, multiple sclerosis, and patients with pre-existing cardiac disease, severe renal or hepatic impairment, or myelosuppression; safety and efficacy in children <18 years of age have not been established. Higher doses in the elderly or in malignancies other than hairy cell leukemia may result in severe obtundation.

Dosage Forms

Injection: 3 million units/mL (1 mL); 6 million units/mL (3 mL); 36 million units/mL (1 mL)

Powder for injection: 6 million units/mL when reconstituted

Stability Refrigerate; reconstituted solution is stable for 24 hours at room temperature and for 1 month when refrigerated

Reference Range Peak serum concentration following an I.V. dose of 36 million units: 10,400-17,470 pg/mL

Overdosage Treatment

Supportive therapy: Indomethacin or acetaminophen can be given for fever; avoid glucocorticoids

Enhancement of elimination: Hemodialysis is not useful

Test Interactions Increase in norepinephrine plasma levels

Drug Interactions

Increased effect:

Cimetidine: May augment the antitumor effects of interferon in melanoma

Theophylline: Clearance has been reported to be decreased in hepatitis patients receiving interferon

Increased toxicity: Vinblastine: Enhances interferon toxicity in several patients; increased incidence of paresthesia has also been noted

Pregnancy Risk Factor C

Monitoring Parameters Baseline chest x-ray, EKG, CBC with differential, liver function tests, electrolytes, platelets, weight; patients with pre-existing cardiac abnormalities, or in advanced stages of cancer should have EKGs taken before and during treatment

Patient Information Do not change brands as changes in dosage may result; possible mental status changes may occur while on therapy; report to physician any persistent or severe sore throat, fever, fatigue, unusual bleeding, or bruising; do not operate heavy machinery while on therapy since changes in mental status may occur

Nursing Implications Flu-like syndrome (fever, chills) occurs in the majority of patients 2-6 hours after a dose; use acetaminophen to prevent or partially alleviate headache and fever

Additional Information Indications and dosage regimens are specific for a particular brand of interferon; other brands of interferon (ie, Intron® A) have different indications and dosage guidelines; do not change brands of interferon as changes in dosage may result

Specific References

Barreca T, Corsini G, Franceschini R, et al, "Lichen Planus Introduced by Interferon-Alpha-2a Therapy for Chronic Active Hepatitis," *Eur J Gastroenterol Hepatol*, 1995, 7:367-8.

Fukumoto Y, Shigemitsu T, Kajii N, et al, "Abducent Nerve Paralysis During Interferon Alpha-2a Therapy in a Case of Chronic Active Hepatitis C," *Intern Med*, 1994, 33(10):637-40.

Gonzalez-Fernandez B, Arranz A, Penarrubia MJ, et al, "Subacute Thyroiditis Associated With Interferon-Alpha-2a Therapy," *Hormone & Metabolic Research*, 1995, 27:45-6.

Gori A, Caredda F, Franzetti F, et al, "Reversible Diabetes in a Patient With AIDS-Related Kaposi's Sarcoma Treated With Interferon Alpha-2a," *Lancet*, 1995, 345:1438-9.

Hirsch MS, Tolkoff-Rubin NE, Kelly AP, et al, "Pharmacokinetics of Human and Recombinant Leukocyte Interferon in Patients With Chronic Renal Failure Who Are Undergoing Hemodialysis," *J Infect Dis*, 1983, 148(2):335.

(Continued)

Interferon Alfa-2a *(Continued)*

Morris DJ, "Adverse Effects and Drug Interactions of Clinical Importance With Antiviral Drugs," *Drug Saf*, 1994, 10(4):281-91.

Read SJ, Crawford DHG, and Pender MP, "Trigeminal Sensory Neuropathy Induced by Interferon-Alpha Therapy," *Aust N Z J Med*, 1995, 25:54.

Soto Alvarez J, Sacristan JA, and Alsar MJ, "Interferon Alpha-2a-Induced Impotence," *DICP*, 1991, 25(12):1397.

Vial T and Descotes J, "Clinical Toxicity of the Interferons," *Drug Saf*, 1994, 10(2):115-50.

Wills RJ, "Clinical Pharmacokinetics of Interferons," *Clin Pharmacokinet*, 1990, 19(5):390-9.

Interferon Alfa-2b (in ter feer' on)

Related Information

Toxicities of Chemotherapeutic Agents *on page 1631-1633*

CAS Number 99210-65-8

Brand Names Intron® A

Synonyms IFN-alpha 2; α-2-interferon; rLFN-α2

Use FDA approved: Patients >18 years of age: Hairy cell leukemia, condylomata acuminata, AIDS-related Kaposi's sarcoma, chronic hepatitis non-A, non-B(C), chronic hepatitis B; indications and dosage regimens are specific for a particular brand of interferon

Mechanism of Action Alpha interferons are a family of proteins, produced by nucleated cells, that have antiviral, antiproliferative, and immune-regulating activity. There are 16 known subtypes of alpha interferons. Interferons interact with cells through high affinity cell surface receptors. Following activation, multiple effects can be detected including induction of gene transcription. Inhibits cellular growth, alters the state of cellular differentiation, interferes with oncogene expression, alters cell surface antigen expression, increases phagocytic activity of macrophages, and augments cytotoxicity of lymphocytes for target cells.

Adverse Reactions Flu-like symptoms (fever, fatigue/malaise, myalgia, chills, headache, arthralgia, rigors) begin about 2-6 hours after the dose is given and may persist as long as 24 hours; usually patient can build up a tolerance to side effects

Cardiovascular: Tachycardia, cardiac arrhythmias, hypotension, edema
Central nervous system: Fatigue/malaise, dizziness, depression, confusion, sensory neuropathy, psychiatric effects, fever, headache, EEG abnormalities, chills
Dermatologic: Partial alopecia, rash, purpura
Endocrine & metabolic: Uric acid level (increased)
Gastrointestinal: Anorexia, dry mouth, nausea, vomiting, diarrhea, abdominal cramps, weight loss, change in taste
Hematologic: Leukopenia (mainly neutropenia), anemia, thrombocytopenic thrombocytopenia, decreased hemoglobin, hematocrit, platelets; neutralizing antibodies
Hepatic: ALT (increased) and AST (increased)
Neuromuscular & skeletal: Myalgia, arthralgia, rigors, myasthenia gravis
Ocular: Blurred vision
Renal: Proteinuria, creatine and BUN (increased)
Respiratory: Coughing, chest pain, nasal congestion
Miscellaneous: Thyroid dysfunction, impaired spermatogenesis, sweating

Signs & Symptoms of Acute Overdose Hyperglycemia, encephalopathy, Mees' lines, leukopenia; neutropenia; agranulocytosis; A-V block, lymphopenia, granulocytopenia

Toxicodynamics/Kinetics

Absorption: Filtered and absorbed at the renal tubule
Distribution: V_d: is 31 L, but has been noted to be much greater (370-720 L) in leukemia patients receiving continuous infusion IFN; IFN does not penetrate the CSF
Metabolism: Majority of dose thought to be metabolized in the kidney
Bioavailability:
- I.M.: 83%
- S.C.: 90%

Half-life: Elimination:
- I.M., I.V.: 2 hours
- S.C.: 3 hours

Time to peak serum concentration: I.M., S.C.: ~6-8 hours
Elimination: Renal

Usual Dosage Adults (refer to individual protocols):

Hairy cell leukemia: I.M., S.C.: 2 million units/m^2 3 times/week for 2-≥6 months of therapy

AIDS-related Kaposi's sarcoma: I.M., S.C. (use 50 million units vial): 30 million units/m^2 3 times/week

Condylomata acuminata: Intralesionally (use 10 million units vial): 1 million units/lesion 3 times/week for 4-8 weeks; not to exceed 5 million units per treatment (maximum: 5 lesions at one time)

Chronic hepatitis C (non-A, non-B): I.M., S.C.: 3 million units 3 times/week for approximately a 6-month course

Chronic hepatitis B: I.M., S.C.: 5 million units/day or 10 million units 3 times/week for 16 weeks

If severe adverse reactions occur, reduce dosage 50% or temporarily discontinue therapy until adverse reactions abate

See table.

Decreased Granulocyte or Platelet Counts

Granulocyte Count	Platelet Count	Interferon 2b dose
<750/mm ^{3}	<50,000/mm ^{3}	Decrease by 50%
<500/mm ^{3}	<30,000/mm ^{3}	Interrupt

When platelet/granulocyte count returns to normal, reinstitute therapy

Contraindications Known hypersensitivity to interferon alfa-2b or any component

Warnings The U.S. Food and Drug Administration (FDA) currently recommends that procedures for proper handling and disposal of antineoplastic agents be considered. Use with caution in patients with seizure disorders, brain metastases, compromised CNS, multiple sclerosis, and patients with pre-existing cardiac disease, severe renal or hepatic impairment, or myelosuppression; safety and efficacy in children <18 years of age have not been established. Higher doses in the elderly or in malignancies other than hairy cell leukemia may result in severe obtundation.

Dosage Forms Powder for injection, lyophilized: 3 million units, 5 million units, 10 million units, 18 million units, 25 million units, 50 million units

Stability Refrigerate; reconstituted solution is stable for 1 month when refrigerated

Reference Range Peak serum level after I.V. infusion of 10 million units: 546 units/mL

Overdosage Treatment

Supportive therapy: Indomethacin or acetaminophen can be given for fever; avoid glucocorticoids

Enhancement of elimination: Hemodialysis is not useful

Drug Interactions

Increased effect: Cimetidine: May augment the antitumor effects of interferon in melanoma

Increased toxicity: Vinblastine: Enhances interferon toxicity in several patients; increased incidence of paresthesia has also been noted

Theophylline: Clearance has been reported to be decreased in hepatitis patients receiving interferon

Pregnancy Risk Factor C

Monitoring Parameters Baseline chest x-ray, EKG, CBC with differential, liver function tests, electrolytes, platelets, weight; patients with pre-existing cardiac abnormalities, or in advanced stages of cancer should have EKGs taken before and during treatment

Patient Information Do not change brands of interferon as changes in dosage may result; do not operate heavy machinery while on therapy since changes in mental status may occur; report to physician any persistent or severe sore throat, fever, fatigue, unusual bleeding, or bruising

Nursing Implications Use acetaminophen to prevent or partially alleviate headache and fever; do not use 3, 5, and 25 million unit strengths intralesionally, solutions are hypertonic; 50 million unit strength is not for use in condylomata

Additional Information Induction of insulin antibodies may result

Myelosuppressive effects:

- WBC: Mild
- Platelets: Mild
- Onset (days): 7-10
- Nadir (days): 14
- Recovery (days): 21

Specific References

Balmer CM, "The New Alpha Interferons," *Drug Intell Clin Pharm*, 1985, 19(12):887-93.

Batocchi AP, Evoli A, Servidei S, et al, "Myasthenia Gravis During Interferon Alfa Therapy," *Neurology*, 1995, 45(2):382-3.

Krug J, Fritzsch J, and Aust G, "Induction of Insulin Antibodies and Insulin Allergy Under Alpha-Interferon Treatment of Renal Cell Carcinoma in a Patient With Insulin-Treated Diabetes Mellitus – A Case Report," *Int Arch Allergy Immunol*, 1995, 106(2):169-72.

Murakami CS, Zeller K, Bodenheimer HC Jr, et al, "Idiopathic Thrombocytopenic Purpura During Interferon-Alpha2B Treatment for Chronic Hepatitis," *Am J Gastroenterol*, 1994, 89(12):2244-5.

(Continued)

Interferon Alfa-2b *(Continued)*

Poynard T, Bedossa P, Chevallier M, et al, "A Comparison of Three Interferon Alfa-2b Regimens for the Long-Term Treatment of Chronic Non-A, Non-B Hepatitis," *N Engl J Med*, 1995, 332:1457-62.

Sakano N, Yoshida T, Yoshioka K, et al, "Reversible Hypopituitarism After Interferon-Alfa Therapy," *Lancet*, 1995, 345:1305.

Spiegel RJ, "Intron® A (Interferon Alfa-2b) Clinical Overview and Future Directions," *Semin Oncol*, 1986, 13(3 Suppl 2):89-101.

Vial T and Descotes J, "Clinical Toxicity of the Interferons," *Drug Saf*, 1994, 10(2):115-50.

Zimmerman S, Adkins D, Graham M, et al, "Case Report: Irreversible, Severe, Congestive Cardiomyopathy Occurring in Association With Interferon Alpha Therapy," *Cancer Biother*, 1994, 9(4):291-9.

Interferon Alfa-N3 (in ter feer' on)

Related Information

Toxicities of Chemotherapeutic Agents *on page 1631-1633*

Brand Names Alferon® N

Use FDA approved: Condylomata acuminata, intralesional treatment of refractory or recurring genital or venereal warts; useful in patients who do not respond or are not candidates for usual treatments; indications and dosage regimens are specific for a particular brand of interferon

Mechanism of Action Alpha interferons are a family of proteins, produced by nucleated cells, that have antiviral, antiproliferative, and immune-regulating activity. There are 16 known subtypes of alpha interferons. Interferons interact with cells through high affinity cell surface receptors. Following activation, multiple effects can be detected including induction of gene transcription. Inhibits cellular growth, alters the state of cellular differentiation, interferes with oncogene expression, alters cell surface antigen expression, increases phagocytic activity of macrophages, and augments cytotoxicity of lymphocytes for target cells.

Adverse Reactions

Cardiac: Tachycardia, cardiac arrhythmias, chest pain, hypotension, SVT

Central nervous system: Dizziness, lightheadedness, tiredness, confusion, depression, sensory neuropathy, psychiatric effects, EEG abnormalities

Dermatologic: Skin rash, dry skin, alopecia

Endocrine & metabolic: Increased uric acid level

Gastrointestinal: Nausea, vomiting dry mouth, sweating, diarrhea, dizziness, abdominal cramps, weight loss, metallic tastes, stomatitis

Genitourinary: Albuminuria

Hematologic: Mildly myelosuppressive and well tolerated if used without adjunct antineoplastic agents; thrombocytosis has been reported, leukopenia (mainly neutropenia), anemia, thrombocytopenia, decreased hemoglobin, hematocrit, platelets

Hepatic: Hepatotoxicity, hepatic transaminase (increased), increased ALT and AST

Neuromuscular & skeletal: Leg cramps, paresthesia

Ocular: Blurred vision

Renal: Increased creatinine and BUN

Respiratory: Cough, nasal congestion, dyspnea

Miscellaneous: Neurotoxicity, flu-like syndrome, local sensitivity to injection, edema, neutralizing antibodies; usually patient can build up a tolerance to side effects, sweating

Signs & Symptoms of Acute Overdose Hyperglycemia, lightheadedness, encephalopathy, leukopenia; neutropenia; agranulocytosis; granulocytopenia; syndrome of inappropriate antidiuretic hormone (SIADH), coagulopathy

Toxicodynamics/Kinetics Elimination: Renal

Usual Dosage Adults: Inject 250,000 units (0.05 mL) in each wart twice weekly for a maximum of 8 weeks; therapy should not be repeated for at least 3 months after the initial 8-week course of therapy

Contraindications Patients with known hypersensitivity to alpha interferon, mouse immunoglobulin, or any component of the product

Warnings The U.S. Food and Drug Administration (FDA) currently recommends that procedures for proper handling and disposal of antineoplastic agents be considered. Use with caution in patients with seizure disorders, brain metastases, compromised CNS function, cardiac disease, severe renal or hepatic impairment, multiple sclerosis; safety and efficacy in children <18 years of age have not been established.

Dosage Forms Injection: 5 million units (1 mL)

Stability Store solution at 2°C to 8°C (36°F to 46°F); do not freeze or shake solution

Overdosage Treatment

Supportive therapy: Indomethacin or acetaminophen can be given for fever; avoid glucocorticoids

Enhancement of elimination: Hemodialysis is not useful

Drug Interactions

Increased effect: Cimetidine: May augment the antitumor effects of interferon in melanoma

Increased toxicity: Vinblastine: Enhances interferon toxicity in several patients; increased incidence of paresthesia has also been noted

Theophylline: Clearance has been reported to be decreased in hepatitis patients receiving interferon

Pregnancy Risk Factor C

Patient Information Warts are highly contagious until they completely disappear, abstain from sexual activity or use barrier protection; inform nurse or physician if allergy exists to eggs, neomycin, mouse immunoglobulin, or to human interferon alpha; acetaminophen can be used to treat flu-like symptoms

Nursing Implications Inject into base of wart with a small 30-gauge needle

Specific References

Vial T and Descotes J, "Clinical Toxicity of the Interferons," *Drug Saf*, 1994, 10(2):115-50.

Interferon Beta-1b (in ter feer' on)

Related Information

Toxicities of Chemotherapeutic Agents *on page 1631-1633*

CAS Number 9008-11-1

Brand Names Betaseron®

Synonyms rIFN-b

Replaces Fibroblast Interferon

Use Reduces the frequency of clinical exacerbations in ambulatory patients with relapsing-remitting multiple sclerosis (MS)

Mechanism of Action Interferon beta-1b differs from naturally occurring human protein by a single amino acid substitution and the lack of carbohydrate side chains; alters the expression and response to surface antigens and can enhance immune cell activities. Properties of interferon beta-1b that modify biologic responses are mediated by cell surface receptor interactions; mechanism in the treatment of MS is unknown.

Adverse Reactions Due to the pivotal position of interferon in the immune system, toxicities can affect nearly every organ system.

Cardiovascular: Palpitations, peripheral vascular disorders

Central nervous system: Depression (with suicidal ideations), somnolence

Dermatologic: Alopecia

Gastrointestinal: Gastrointestinal complaints, necrotizing ulcers

Hematologic: Blood dyscrasias

Local: Injection site reactions, injection site necrosis

Respiratory: Dyspnea

Miscellaneous: Flu-like symptoms, menstrual disorders, laryngitis, cystitis, albuminuria

Signs & Symptoms of Acute Overdose No human cases; probable response would be hypotension, fever, dry mouth, atrial tachycardia, personality changes, cough, pemphigus, disorientation, confusion, nausea, depression, vomiting, hypocalcemia, hyperkalemia

Toxicodynamics/Kinetics Bioavailability: Not bioavailable through oral route

Usual Dosage S.C.:

Children <18 years: Not recommended

Adults >18 years: 0.25 mg (8 million units) every other day

Contraindications Hypersensitivity to *E. coli* derived products

Warnings Lactation, depression, myelosuppression

Dosage Forms Powder for injection, lyophilized: 0.3 mg [9.6 million units]

Overdosage Treatment

Decontamination: Not necessary

Supportive therapy: Fever/chills can be treated with acetaminophen or nonsteroidal anti-inflammatory agent (indomethacin); hypotension can be treated with crystalloid infusion

Enhancement of elimination: Hemodialysis is not useful

Drug Interactions Decreases clearance of zidovudine thus increasing zidovudine toxicity

Pregnancy Risk Factor C

Monitoring Parameters Hemoglobin, liver function, and blood chemistries

Nursing Implications Patient should be informed of possible side effects, especially depression, suicidal ideations, and the risk of abortion; flu-like symptoms such as chills, fever, malaise, sweating, and myalgia are common

Additional Information May be available only in small supplies

Specific References

Nokta M, Loh JP, Douidar SM, et al, "Metabolic Interaction of Recombinant Interferon-Beta and Zidovudine in AIDS Patients," *J Interferon Res*, 1991, 11(3):159-64.

Quesada JR, Talpaz M, Rios A, et al, "Clinical Toxicity of Interferons in Cancer Patients: A Review," *J Clin Oncol*, 1986, 4(2):234-43.

Sheremata WA, Taylor JR, and Elgart GW, "Severe Necrotizing Cutaneous Lesions Complicating Treatment With Interferon Beta-1b," *N Engl J Med*, 1995, 332:1584.

Vial T and Descotes J, "Clinical Toxicity of the Interferons," *Drug Saf*, 1994, 10(2):115-50.

Interferon Gamma-1b (in ter feer' on)

Related Information

Toxicities of Chemotherapeutic Agents *on page 1631-1633*

CAS Number 98059-61-1

Brand Names Actimmune®

Replaces Immune Interferon; Interferon Gamma-2a

Use Reduce frequency and severity of serious infections associated with chronic granulomatous disease, Leishmanial infections

Investigational: Chronic lymphocytic leukemia, Hodgkin's disease, rheumatoid arthritis; may be useful in treatment for congenital osteopetrosis, toxoplasmosis, hyper-IgE states

Mechanism of Action Increases bone resorption in osteopetrosis

Adverse Reactions Similar neurotoxic effects (neurobehavioral changes) as with interferon alfa

Cardiovascular: Tachycardia, cardiac arrhythmias, hypotension, edema, syncope, cardiac ectopy

Central nervous system: Fatigue/malaise, dizziness, depression, confusion, sensory neuropathy, psychiatric effects, fever, headache, chills, seizures, in patients with brain metastasis, EEG abnormalities, parkinsonian syndrome

Dermatologic: Partial alopecia, rash, pruritus, erythema nodosum leprosum, exacerbation of psoriasis

Gastrointestinal: Anorexia, dry mouth, nausea, vomiting, diarrhea, abdominal cramps, stomatitis, sore throat, weight loss, flatulence

Hematologic: Leukopenia (mainly neutropenia), anemia, thrombocytopenia, decreased hemoglobin, hematocrit, platelets, flatulence

Hepatic: ALT (increased) and AST (increased)

Neuromuscular & skeletal: Myalgia, arthralgia, rigors

Ocular: Blurred vision

Renal: Proteinuria, uric acid level (increased), increased creatinine and BUN, oliguric or nonoliguric renal failure

Respiratory: Coughing, chest pain, nasal congestion

Miscellaneous: Change in taste, neutralizing antibodies, multiple sclerosis, sweating

Signs & Symptoms of Acute Overdose Leukopenia or neutropenia (agranulocytosis, granulocytopenia); hyperglycemia, hypertriglyceridemia, metallic taste, memory loss, wheezing, depression, systemic lupus erythematosus (SLE), hypocalcemia, A-V block

Toxicodynamics/Kinetics

Absorption: I.M., S.C.: 89%

Metabolism: Through liver

Half-life:

I.M.: 2.9 hours

I.V.: 30 minutes

S.C.: 5.9 hours

Usual Dosage Adults: S.C. (dosing is based on body surface (m^2)):

≤0.5: 1.5 mcg/kg/dose

>0.5: 50 mcg/m^2 (1.5 million units/m^2) 3 times/week

Osteopetrosis: 1.5 mcg/kg 3 times/week

Contraindications May exacerbate multiple sclerosis

Dosage Forms Injection: 100 mcg [3 million units]

Reference Range Peak serum level after an I.V. dose of 3000 mcg/m^2: 7.4-9.6 ng/mL; at 24 hours: 1 ng/mL

Overdosage Treatment

Supportive therapy: Indomethacin or acetaminophen can be given for fever; avoid glucocorticoids

Enhancement of elimination: Hemodialysis is not useful

Test Interactions Hypertriglyceridemia; rarely causes hyponatremia, hyperglycemia, hypocalcemia

Pregnancy Risk Factor C

Pregnancy Implications Contraindicated; causes decreased birth weight, increased rate of spontaneous abortion

Additional Information More heat- and acid-labile than alfa interferons

Specific References

Gallin JI, Farber JM, Holland SM, et al, "Interferon Gamma in the Management of Infectious Diseases," *Ann Intern Med*, 1995, 123:216-24.

Key, Jr LL, Rodriguiz RM, Willi SM, et al, "Long-Term Treatment of Osteopetrosis With Recombinant Human Interferon Gamma," *N Engl J Med* 1995, 332:1594-9.

Todd PA and Goa KL, "Interferon Gamma-1b: A Review of Its Pharmacology and Therapeutic Potential in Chronic Granulomatous Disease," *Drugs*, 1992, 43(1):111-22.

Unno N, Menconi MJ, Smith M, et al, "Nitric Oxide Mediates Interferon-γ-Induced Hyperpermeability in Cultured Human Intestinal Epithelial Monolayers," *Crit Care Med*, 1995, 23(7):1170-6.

Vassiliadis S and Athanassakis I, "Type II Interferon May be a Potential Hazardous Therapeutic Agent During Pregnancy," *Br J Haematol*, 1992, 82(4):782-3.

Vial T and Descotes J, "Clinical Toxicity of the Interferons," *Drug Saf*, 1994, 10(2):115-50.

Interferon Gamma-2a *replaced by* Interferon Gamma-1b *on previous page*

Intron® A *see* Interferon Alfa-2b *on page 432*

Inversine® *see* Mecamylamine Hydrochloride *on page 492*

Invite E® *see* Vitamin E *on page 798*

Iode *see* Iodine *on this page*

Iodex® Regular *see* Povidone-Iodine *on page 635*

Iodine (eye' oh din)

Related Information

Radiation: Basics of Exposure *on page 1594-1600*

Toxins Which Should be Lavaged With Solutions Other Than Water *on page 1635*

CAS Number 7553-56-2

Synonyms Iode; Iodine Crystals

Use Preoperatively to reduce vascularity of the thyroid gland prior to thyroidectomy; management of thyrotoxic crisis or recurrent hyperthyroidism; venous sclerosing agent; topical disinfectant; also found in marine life

Mechanism of Action Free iodine oxidizes microbial protoplasm making it effective against bacteria, fungi, yeasts, protozoa, and viruses; complexes with amino groups in tissue compounds to form iodophors from which the iodine is slowly released causing a sustained action

Adverse Reactions

Central nervous system: Fever, headache

Dermatologic: Skin rash, angioedema, rash, acne, contact dermatitis, erythema

Endocrine & metabolic: Hypothyroidism, hypercalcemia

Gastrointestinal: Mucosal hemorrhage, diarrhea, metallic taste

Hematologic: Eosinophilia

Hepatic: Elevated serum transaminases and bilirubin

Neuromuscular & skeletal: Arthralgia

Ocular: Swelling of eyelids

Respiratory: Pulmonary edema

Miscellaneous: Lymph node enlargement, feces discoloration (black), hypersalivation

Signs & Symptoms of Acute Overdose Hypothyroidism, dysphagia, fever, hypothyroidism, acneiform, rash, renal failure, sexual dysfunction, periarteritis nodosa, nausea, vomiting, hypercalcemia, gastroenteritis, circulation collapse, hypotension, swelling of glottis or larynx; renal failure (acute), metabolic acidosis with increased lactic acid, urine discoloration (blue-green); hypernatremia, elevated serum osmolarity, leukopenia; neutropenia; agranulocytosis; granulocytopenia; cough, tachycardia

Usual Dosage Adults: RDA: 150 mg; apply topically as necessary to affected areas of skin

Contraindications Hypersensitivity to iodide preparations; pregnancy, neonates, acute bronchitis

Warnings May be highly toxic if ingested, discontinue use if fever, skin rash, metallic taste, swelling/burning of mouth or throat, or other signs of iodine toxicity occur; use with caution in patients with tuberculosis

Dosage Forms

Solution: 2%

Tincture: 2%

Overdosage Treatment

Decontamination: Do not use ipecac; activated charcoal with cathartic is useful; gastric lavage with starch or 1% to 5% sodium thiosulfate will aid in removal (purple color of effluent)

Supportive therapy: Endoscopy may be required to evaluate gastrointestinal hemorrhage

Enhancement of elimination: Can be enhanced with osmotic diuresis or salt loading

Antidote(s)

Sodium Thiosulfate *on page 1470*

Test Interactions Interferes with thyroid function tests; falsely elevates chloride concentrations

Drug Interactions Lithium carbonate

Pregnancy Risk Factor D (can cause fetal goiter and hypothyroidism)

Monitoring Parameters Renal function, acid base status, electrolytes, CBC

Patient Information Take with food or milk; may stain skin and clothing

Nursing Implications Avoid tight bandages because iodine may cause burns on occluded skin

(Continued)

Iodine *(Continued)*

Additional Information IDLH - 10 ppm; iodophors/iodoform have low toxicity; acrid odor with sharp taste; vapor is violet when heated; lithium blood levels increase during caffeine withdrawal

Specific References

Dela Cruz F, Brown DH, Leikin JB, et al, "Iodine Absorption After Topical Administration," *West J Med*, 1987, 146(1):43-5.

Klein I and Levey GS, "Iodide Excess and Thyroid Function," *Ann Intern Med*, 1983, 98(3):406-7.

Iodine Crystals *see* Iodine *on previous page*

Ionamin® *see* Phentermine Hydrochloride *on page 619*

Ipersed® *see* Nitrazepam *on page 562*

Ipobar® *see* Penbutolol Sulfate *on page 599*

Ipotensium® *see* Clonidine *on page 231*

Ipratropium Bromide (i pra troe' pee um)

CAS Number 22254-24-6; 66985-17-9

Brand Names Atem®; Atrovent® Aerosol Inhalation; Disne Asmol®; Itrop®; Narilet®; Rinatec®

Use Anticholinergic for prevention of wheezing associated with COPD, bronchitis, and emphysema; good for cold-induced asthma and beta-blocking agent induced bronchospasm

Mechanism of Action Blocks the action of acetylcholine at parasympathetic sites in bronchial smooth muscle causing bronchodilation

Adverse Reactions

Cardiovascular: Palpitations
Central nervous system: Nervousness, dizziness, headache, fatigue
Dermatologic: Rash
Gastrointestinal: Nausea, dry mouth (25%), bitter taste (20% to 30%), buccal ulceration, paralytic ileus
Ocular: Blurred vision, exacerbation of closed-angle glaucoma, mydriasis
Respiratory: Cough, paradoxical wheezing

Toxicodynamics/Kinetics

Onset of bronchodilation: 1-3 minutes after administration
Peak effect: Within 1.5-2 hours
Duration: Up to 4-6 hours
Absorption: Not readily absorbed into the systemic circulation from the surface of the lung (0.03%) or from the gastrointestinal tract (2%)
Distribution: Inhalation: 15% of dose reaches the lower airways; does not penetrate CSF
Half-life: 3-4 hours
Elimination: Renal/feces

Usual Dosage Children >12 years and Adults: 2 inhalations 4 times/day up to 12 inhalations/24 hours

Contraindications Hypersensitivity to atropine or its derivatives

Warnings Use with caution in patients with angle-closure glaucoma, prostatic hypertrophy, or bladder neck obstruction

Dosage Forms Solution:

Inhalation: 18 mcg/actuation (14 g)
Nebulizing: 0.02% (2.5 mL)

Reference Range Inhalation of 555 μg of ipratropium results in peak plasma concentration of 0.06 ng/mL (0.03% of inhaled dose)

Overdosage Treatment Supportive therapy: Physostigmine should be administered for life-threatening anticholinergic poisoning; bethanechol (5-10 mg 3 times/day) can be given for peripheral anticholinergic side effects; esmolol can be used for tachyarrhythmia

Antidote(s)

Physostigmine *on page 1457*

Drug Interactions

Increased effect with albuterol
Increased toxicity with anticholinergics or drugs with anticholinergic properties (ie, nortriptyline), dronabinol

Pregnancy Risk Factor B

Patient Information Temporary blurred vision may occur if sprayed into eyes; shake canister well before each use of the inhaler

Specific References

Adlung J, Hohle KD, Zeren S, et al, "Studies of Pharmacokinetics and Biotransformation of Ipratropium Bromide in Man," *Arzneimittelforschung*, 1976, 26(5a):1005-10.

Connolly CK, "Adverse Reaction to Ipratropium Bromide," *Br Med J (Clin Res)*, 1982, 285(6346):934-5.

Cugell DW, "Clinical Pharmacology and Toxicology of Ipratropium Bromide," *Am J Med*, 1986, 81(5A):18-22.

Gross NJ, "Ipratropium Bromide," *N Engl J Med*, 1988, 319(8):486-94.

Osmond MH and Klassen TP, "Efficacy of Ipratropium Bromide in Acute Childhood Asthma: A Meta-Analysis," *Acad Emerg Med*, 1995, 2:651-6.

Roberts TE and Pearson DJ, "Wide-Eyed and Breathless," *Br Med J*, 1989, 299:1348.

Iproveratril Hydrochloride *see* Verapamil Hydrochloride *on page 787*

Ircon® *see* Iron *on this page*

Irinotecan

Synonyms CPT-II

Use Investigational: Antitumor agent utilized for treatment of small cell lung cancer, nonsmall cell lung cancer, ovarian, cervical and metastatic colon cancer

Mechanism of Action A derivative of camptothecin from the oriental tree *Camptotheca acuminata*; irinotecan inhibits the enzyme topoisomerase I which is involved in structural maintenance of DNA

Adverse Reactions

Cardiovascular: Flushing

Gastrointestinal: Diarrhea (may be severe), nausea, vomiting

Hematologic: Myelosuppression, anemia, thrombocytopenia, neutropenia

Ocular: Lacrimation

Miscellaneous: Sweating

Toxicodynamics/Kinetics

Metabolism: By intestinal flora, plasma, and liver to an active metabolite SN-38

Half-life:

- Parent drug: 8 hours
- Metabolite: 13 hours

Elimination: Primarily biliary

Usual Dosage Dosing regimens vary with usual dosage range of 40 mg/m^2/day to 250 mg/m^2/day up to a maximum of 750 mg/m^2/day; infusions are from 30-90 minutes and may vary from 3 times/week to weekly to every 3 weeks

Overdosage Treatment

Supportive therapy: Ondansetron (0.15 mg/kg I.V. or oral) with a corticosteroid is effective in preventing emesis; diphenhydramine can be used to decrease cholinergic reactions (lacrimation, sweating, flushing); loperamide (2 mg doses) is effective in treating diarrhea

Enhancement of elimination: Due to enterohepatic recirculation, multiple dosing of activated charcoal may be useful in enhancing clearance

Additional Information Diarrhea is dose related; high doses of loperamide can increase tolerated dose of irinotecan; used in combination with 5-FU and etoposide

Specific References

Fields SM and Burris HA, "Irinotecan: A New Topoisomerase I Inhibitor," *Highlights on Antineoplastic Drugs*, 1995, 12:68-71.

Iron

Related Information

Radiation: Basics of Exposure *on page 1594-1600*

CAS Number 1439-89-6

Brand Names Femiron®; Feosol®; Feostat®; Feratab®; Fergon®; Fer-In-Sol®; Fer-Iron®; Fero-Gradumet®; Ferospace®; Ferralet®; Ferralyn® Lanacaps®; Ferra-TD®; Ferro-Sequels®; Fumasorb®; Fumerin®; Hemocyte®; InFed™ Injection; Ircon®; Mol-Iron®; Nephro-Fer™; Simron®; Slow FE®; Span-FF®

Synonyms Ferrous Fumarate; Ferrous Gluconate; Ferrous Sulfate; Iron Dextran Complex

Commonly Found in Ferrous sulfate, ferrous gluconate, ferrous fumarate, ferrous chloride, ferrous carbonate, ferrous chloride

Use Prevention and/or treatment of iron deficiency anemias; prenatal supplementation

Mechanism of Action Essential component of hemoglobin, myoglobin, and multiple enzymes; supplementation is given to replenish lost iron stores

Adverse Reactions

Anaphylactoid reactions: Respiratory difficulties and cardiovascular collapse have been reported and occur most frequently within the first several minutes of administration

Cardiovascular: Hypotension, myocardial depression, flushing, tachycardia

Central nervous system: Dizziness, fever, headache, chills, sweating

Dermatologic: Urticaria

Gastrointestinal: Nausea, metallic taste, gastrointestinal irritation, epigastric pain, diarrhea, dark stools

Hematologic: Leukocytosis

Local: Pain, staining of skin at the site of I.M. injection, phlebitis

(Continued)

Iron *(Continued)*

Neuromuscular & skeletal: Arthralgia
Renal: Hematuria
Miscellaneous: Lymphadenopathy, aspiration, liquid preparations may temporarily stain the teeth
Note: Sweating, rash, arthralgia, fever, chills, dizziness, headache, and nausea may be delayed 24-48 hours after I.V. administration or 3-4 days after I.M. administration

Signs & Symptoms of Acute Overdose Fever, hypoglycemia, coagulopathy, hematuria, hyperventilation, bezoars, urine discoloration (black), hyperthermia, feces discoloration (black), feces discoloration (green); acute gastrointestinal irritation, esophageal ulceration; sweating, erosion of gastrointestinal mucosa, hepatic and renal impairment, sedation, coma, hematemesis, drowsiness, acidosis

There are essentially five stages of iron poisoning:
- Stage I (30 minutes to 6 hours): Predominately gastrointestinal irritation, due primarily to the corrosive effect of iron; nausea, vomiting, epigastric pain, gastrointestinal bleeding, drowsiness, and hypotension may occur; a metabolic acidosis, leukocytosis, or hyperglycemia may be present (due to vasodilatation)
- Stage II (6-24 hours): A latent period of symptom quiescence during which symptomatic improvement may be noted; in severe poisonings, there may be no latent period
- Stage III (6-48 hours): Metabolic and systemic derangement occur with cardiovascular collapse, coma, seizures, and coagulopathy (inhibition of thrombin and fibrinogen); pulmonary edema may occur due to cardiac failure
- Stage IV (2-7 days): Hepatotoxicity (jaundice) and coagulopathy occur; metabolic acidosis is present, and renal insufficiency may occur
- Stage V (1-8 weeks): Primarily delayed gastrointestinal complications, including gastric/duodenal fibrosis resulting in obstructive pattern; achlorhydria may develop

Toxicodynamics/Kinetics Total body stores are 3-4 g
Absorption: In ferrous state (Fe^{2+}) in duodenum and jejunum
Distribution: 70% as ferrous state in hemoglobin, 25% in ferric state as ferritin or hemosiderin, 0.1% in ferric state in plasma
Elimination: ~1 mg/day of iron is lost via urinary excretion, skin desquamation; this may increase to 2 mg/day when iron accumulates

Usual Dosage Oral **(dose expressed in terms of elemental iron):**
Recommended daily allowance:
- Male: 10 mg
- Female: 18 mg
- Pregnancy and lactation: 30-60 mg

Iron replacement:
- Infants: 10-25 mg/day in 3-4 divided doses
- Children:
  - 6 months to 2 years: Up to 6 mg/kg/day in 3-4 divided doses
  - 2-12 years: 3 mg/kg/day given 3-4 times/day
- Adults: 2-3 mg/kg/day given 3 times/day

Contraindications Hemosiderosis, hemochromatosis, hemolytic anemia, peptic ulcer disease, ulcerative colitis

Warnings Some products contain tartrazine which may cause allergic reactions

Dosage Forms Amount of elemental iron is listed in brackets
Ferrous fumarate:
- Capsule, controlled release (Span-FF®): 325 mg [106 mg]
- Drops (Feostat®): 45 mg/0.6 mL [15 mg/0.6 mL] (60 mL)
- Suspension, oral (Feostat®): 100 mg/5 mL [33 mg/5 mL] (240 mL)
- Tablet: 325 mg [106 mg]
  - Chewable (chocolate flavor) (Feostat®): 100 mg [33 mg]
  - Femiron®: 63 mg [20 mg]
  - Fumerin®: 195 mg [64 mg]
  - Fumasorb®, Ircon®: 200 mg [66 mg]
  - Hemocyte®: 324 mg [106 mg]
  - Nephro-Fer™: 350 mg [115 mg]
  - Timed release (Ferro-Sequels®): Ferrous fumarate 150 mg [50 mg] and docusate sodium 100 mg

Ferrous gluconate:
- Capsule, soft gelatin (Simron®): 86 mg [10 mg]
- Elixir (Fergon®): 300 mg/5 mL [34 mg/5 mL] with alcohol 7% (480 mL)
- Tablet: 300 mg [34 mg]; 325 mg [38 mg]
  - Fergon®, Ferralet®: 320 mg [37 mg]
  - Sustained release (Ferralet® Slow Release): 320 mg [37 mg]

Ferrous sulfate:
- Capsule:
  - Exsiccated (Fer-In-Sol®): 190 mg [60 mg]
  - Exsiccated, timed release (Feosol®): 159 mg [50 mg]
  - Exsiccated, timed release (Ferralyn® Lanacaps®, Ferra-TD®): 250 mg [50 mg]
  - Ferospace®: 250 mg [50 mg]
- Drops, oral:
  - Fer-In-Sol®: 75 mg/0.6 mL [15 mg/0.6 mL] (50 mL)
  - Fer-Iron®: 125 mg/mL [25 mg/mL] (50 mL)
- Elixir (Feosol®): 220 mg/5 mL [44 mg/5 mL] with alcohol 5% (473 mL, 4000 mL)
- Powder for injection: Deferoxamine: 500 mg vials
- Syrup (Fer-In-Sol®): 90 mg/5 mL [18 mg/5 mL] with alcohol 5% (480 mL)
- Tablet: 324 mg [65 mg]
  - Exsiccated (Feosol®) 200 mg [65 mg]
  - Exsiccated, timed release (Slow FE®): 160 mg [50 mg]
  - Feratab®: 300 mg [60 mg]
  - Mol-Iron®: 195 mg [39 mg]
  - Timed release (Fero-Gradumet®): 525 mg [105 mg]

Iron dextran complex: InFed™ injection: 50 mg/mL (2 mL, 10 mL)

Reference Range Levels >450-500 µg/dL associated with toxicity; consider treatment with levels ≥350 µg/dL; peak values are 2-4 hours after ingestion; standard measurement of total iron binding capacity (IBC) are unreliable and should not be used to assess the patient

Therapeutic:
- Male: 75-175 µg/dL (SI: 13.4-31.3 µmol/L)
- Female: 65-165 µg/dL (SI: 11.6-29.5 µmol/L); iron levels >300 µg/dL can be considered toxic and should be treated as an overdose

Overdosage Treatment

Determine amount of drug ingested based on mg/kg of elemental iron; doses <20 mg/kg are minimal to no toxicity; 20-60 mg/kg are mild to moderate; >60 mg/kg are potentially serious; see table.

Overdosage	Elemental Iron
Ferrous sulfate (hydrated)	20%
Ferrous fumarate	33%
Ferrous gluconate	12%
Ferrous chloride (hydrated)	28%
Ferric chloride (hydrated)	20%

Decontamination: Lavage with normal saline and/or whole bowel irrigation with polyethylene glycol electrolyte solution (GoLYTELY®); use WBI if radiopaque tablets present on KUB; charcoal is ineffective unless it is a multiple drug ingestion; oral deferoxamine is not effective

Supportive therapy: Shock can be treated with I.V. crystalloid fluids, blood products may be necessary; following treatment for fluid losses, metabolic acidosis, and shock, a severe iron overdose may be treated with deferoxamine. Deferoxamine may be administered I.V. (80 mg/kg over 24 hours) or I.M. (40-90 mg/kg every 8 hours). Lethal dose of elemental iron is 180-300 mg/kg.

Antidote: Deferoxamine is a chelating agent for iron; it binds free iron and some iron bound to ferritin and hemosiderin; the complex of iron and deferoxamine (ferrioxamine) is then excreted renally with a "vin rosé" color; color change is dependent on pH and concentrations with basic pH and higher concentrations being positively associated with the change in color.

Serum iron concentrations >500 µg/dL require treatment with deferoxamine; if severe ingestion is suspected, with while blood cell count >15,000/mm³, blood glucose >150 mg/dL, radiopaque tables on abdominal x-ray, spontaneous vomiting and diarrhea, and serum iron concentration delayed, consider treatment with deferoxamine.

Obtain baseline serum iron level and urine sample. Administration via I.V. route is preferred; give at 15 mg/kg/hour by continuous infusion. Doses up to 50 mg/kg/hour have been used for severe ingestion. Maximum recommended dose is 6 g/day; however, higher doses have been given. Continuous infusion of 15 mg/kg/hour should not be continued for longer than 24 hours without a "drug holiday." Monitor urine for "vin rosé" color change compared to baseline.

Endpoints of therapy include change in urine color back to baseline, serum concentrations of iron <100 mg/dL, and/or resolution of symptoms

Antidote(s)

Deferoxamine Mesylate *on page 1407*

Polyethylene Glycol *on page 1460*

Test Interactions Measured serum iron concentrations will be lowered in face of deferoxamine therapy; high serum iron may falsely increase total iron binding ca-

(Continued)

Iron *(Continued)*

pacity (TIBC) for most common assay; Hemoccult® and Gastroccult® tests can be unreliable in detecting gastrointestinal bleeding in iron overdoses treated with whole bowel irrigation (ferrous sulfate/ferrous gluconate: false-positive; ascorbic acid: false-negative)

Diagnostic Tests/Procedures

Complete Blood Count *on page 1236*

Iron and Total Iron Binding Capacity/Transferrin *on page 1275*

Drug Interactions Antacids decrease iron absorption; vitamin C increases gastrointestinal absorption; iron can inhibit tetracycline and penicillamine absorption

Pregnancy Risk Factor A; deferoxamine: C

Pregnancy Implications Although placental transport is poor and treatment of iron overdose in pregnancy should not be harmful, untreated patients may result in fetal and/or maternal morbidity and mortality

Nursing Implications Always obtain baseline urine before administration of deferoxamine; I.V. infusion may be prepared in saline or glucose

Additional Information Oral chelation with deferoxamine is not recommended; liver transplantation has been used for iron-induced hepatic failure 5 days after ingestion

Specific References

Bosse GM, "Conservative Management of Patients With Moderately Elevated Serum Iron Levels," *J Toxicol Clin Toxicol*, 1995, 33(2):135-40.

Cheney K, Gumbiner C, Benson B, et al, "Survival After a Severe Iron Poisoning Treated With Intermittent Infusions of Deferoxamine," *J Toxicol Clin Toxicol*, 1995, 33(1):61-6.

Engle JP, Polin KS, and Stile IL, "Acute Iron Intoxication: Treatment Controversies," *Drug Intell Clin Pharm*, 1987, 21(2):153-9.

Harju E, "Clinical Pharmacokinetics of Iron Preparation," *Clin Pharmacokinet*, 1989, 17(2):69-89.

Klein-Schwartz W, Oderda GM, Gorman RL, et al, "Assessment of Management Guidelines. Acute Iron Ingestion," *Clin Pediatr (Phila)*, 1990, 29(6):316-21.

Kozaki K, Egawa H, Garcia-Kennedy R, et al, "Hepatic Failure Due to Massive Iron Ingestion Successfully Treated With Liver Transplantation," *Clin Transpl*, 1995, 9:85-7.

Lacouture PG, Wason S, Temple AR, et al, "Emergency Assessment of Severity in Iron Overdose by Clinical and Laboratory Methods," *J Pediatr*, 1981, 99(1):89-91.

Tenenbein M and Yatscoff RW, "The Total Iron-Binding Capacity in Iron Poisoning, Is It Useful?" *Am J Dis Child*, 1991, 145(4):437-9.

Tunget CL, Clark RF, Manoguerra AS, et al, "Iron Overdose and Detection of Gastrointestinal Bleeding With the Hemoccult and Gastroccult Assays," *Ann Emerg Med*, 1995, 26:54-7.

Iron Dextran Complex *see* Iron *on page 439*

Ismelin® *see* Guanethidine Sulfate *on page 393*

Isobamate *see* Carisoprodol *on page 187*

Iso-Bid® *see* Isosorbide Dinitrate *on page 445*

Isocaine® HCl *see* Mepivacaine Hydrochloride *on page 502*

Isocainide Hydrochloride *see* Lorcainide Hydrochloride *on page 484*

Isocarboxazid (eye soe kar box' a zid)

CAS Number 59-63-2

Brand Names Marplan®

Use Symptomatic treatment of atypical, nonendogenous or neurotic depression

Mechanism of Action Thought to act by increasing endogenous concentrations of epinephrine, norepinephrine, dopamine, and serotonin through inhibition of the enzyme (monoamine oxidase) responsible for the breakdown of these neurotransmitters

Adverse Reactions

Cardiovascular: Hypotension, hypertension, edema, EKG changes (peaked T waves), palpitations

Central nervous system: Drowsiness, excitement, mania, coma, hallucinations, seizures, delirium, hyperthermia

Dermatologic: Skin rash

Endocrine & metabolic: Syndrome of inappropriate antidiuretic hormone, hyperhidrosis

Gastrointestinal: Dry mouth, constipation, nausea

Genitourinary: Urinary retention, ejaculatory disturbances

Ocular: Blurred vision, photophobia, ptosis, diplopia, mydriasis, "ping-pong" gaze, nystagmus

Neuromuscular & skeletal: Muscle rigidity, rhabdomyolysis, hyperreflexia

Renal: Myoglobinuria leading to renal failure

Respiratory: Tachypnea

Miscellaneous: Sweating

Usual Dosage Adults: Oral: 10 mg 3 times/day; reduce to 10-20 mg/day in divided doses when condition improves

Contraindications Uncontrolled hypertension, known hypersensitivity to isocarboxazid, pheochromocytoma, congestive heart failure, severe renal or hepatic impairment

Warnings Avoid tyramine-containing foods: red wine, cheese (except cottage, ricotta, and cream), smoked or pickled fish, beef or chicken liver, dried sausage, fava or broad bean pods, yeast vitamin supplements; avoid use with patients <16 or >60 years of age

Dosage Forms Tablet: 10 mg

Overdosage Treatment

Decontamination: Lavage/activated charcoal with cathartic

Supportive therapy: Diazepam or lorazepam can be used for agitation/seizures; dantrolene (2.5 mg/kg every 6 hours) can be used for muscle rigidity and hyperthermia; labetalol may be useful for hypertension, while norepinephrine is the preferred agent for treatment of hypotension; avoid bretylium for ventricular dysrhythmia, lidocaine or procainamide are preferred

Test Interactions ↓ glucose

Diagnostic Tests/Procedures

Creatine Kinase, Blood *on page 1242*

Electrocardiography *on page 1253*

Electrolytes, Blood *on page 1254*

Kidney Profile *on page 1279*

Drug Interactions

Decreased effect of antihypertensives

Increased toxicity with disulfiram (possible seizures), fluoxetine (and other serotonin active agents), TCAs (cardiovascular instability), meperidine (cardiovascular instability), phenothiazines (hyperpyretic crisis), levodopa, sympathomimetics (hyperpyretic crisis), barbiturates, rauwolfia alkaloids (eg, reserpine), dextroamphetamine (psychoses), foods containing tyramine (hypertension, headache, seizures); theophylline/caffeine (hyperthermia), cyclobenzaprine (fever/seizures)

Potentiation of hypoglycemia with oral hypoglycemic agents

Pregnancy Risk Factor C

Monitoring Parameters Blood pressure

Patient Information Avoid tyramine-containing foods and drinks

Nursing Implications Watch for hypotension (orthostatic); monitor blood pressure carefully, especially at therapy onset or if other CNS drugs or cardiovascular drugs are added; check for dietary and drug restriction

Specific References

Abrams JH, Schulman P, and White WB, "Successful Treatment of a Monoamine Oxidase Inhibitor-Tyramine Hypertensive Emergency With Intravenous Labetalol," *N Engl J Med*, 1985, 313(1):52.

Erich JL, Shih RD, and O'Connor R, "Ping-Pong Gaze Associated With Monoamine Oxidase Inhibitor Overdose," *Vet Hum Toxicol*, 1994, 36:371.

Vlahakis E, "Isocarboxazid Overdosage," *Med J Aust*, 1964, 506-8.

Isocardide® *see* Isosorbide Dinitrate *on page 445*

Isodine® [OTC] *see* Povidone-Iodine *on page 635*

Isoethadione *see* Paramethadione *on page 595*

Isoglaucon® *see* Clonidine *on page 231*

Isoket® *see* Isosorbide Dinitrate *on page 445*

Isonate® *see* Isosorbide Dinitrate *on page 445*

Isoniazid (eye soe nye' a zid)

Related Information

Therapeutic Drugs Associated With Hallucinations *on page 1558-1559*

CAS Number 54-85-3

Brand Names Laniazid®; Niconyl®; Nydrazid®; Triniad®; Uniad®

Synonyms INH; Isonicotinic Acid Hydrazide

Use Treatment of susceptible tuberculosis infections and prophylactically to those individuals exposed to tuberculosis

Mechanism of Action Inhibits myocolic acid synthesis resulting in disruption of the bacterial cell wall; inhibits pyridoxine use as a cofactor in production of gamma-aminobutyric acid (GABA), an inhibitory neurotransmitter

Adverse Reactions

Central nervous system: Peripheral neuritis, seizures, stupor, dizziness, psychosis, fever, auditory and visual hallucinations, ataxia

Dermatologic: Skin eruptions, angioedema

Endocrine & metabolic: Hyperglycemia

Gastrointestinal: Nausea, vomiting, epigastric pain, constipation, pancreatitis

Genitourinary: Urinary retention

Hematologic: Blood dyscrasias, hemolysis, eosinophilia, agranulocytosis

Hepatic: Hepatitis, elevated liver transaminase levels

Ocular: Optic neuritis, photophobia, diplopia

(Continued)

Isoniazid *(Continued)*

Otic: Ototoxicity (deafness), tinnitus

Signs & Symptoms of Acute Overdose Nausea, exfoliative dermatitis, Stevens-Johnson syndrome, eosinophilia, hyperreflexia, memory loss, hyperthermia, arthralgia, encephalopathy, deafness, vomiting, neuropathy (peripheral), myoglobinuria, nystagmus, systemic lupus erythematosus (SLE), myoclonus, hypoglycemia, slurred speech, dizziness, rhabdomyolysis, meningitis, metabolic acidosis, hyperglycemia, fever, blurred vision, hallucinations, paresthesia, hyperkalemia, stupor, coma, intractable seizures in acute; chronic overdosage has similar toxicities, though early signs of acute overdosage (nausea, vomiting) may not occur, leukopenia, neutropenia, agranulocytosis, granulocytopenia; tachycardia, hypotension, leukocytosis

Toxicodynamics/Kinetics

Absorption: Oral, I.M.: Rapid and complete; rate of absorption can be slowed when administered with food

Distribution: V_d: 0.57-0.76 L/kg; distributes into all body tissues and fluids including the CSF

Protein binding: 10% to 15%

Metabolism: By the liver with decay rate determined genetically by acetylation phenotype

Half-life:

- Fast acetylators: 30-90 minutes
- Slow acetylators: 2-5 hours
- Half-life may be prolonged in patients with impaired hepatic function or severe renal impairment

Time to peak serum concentration: Oral: Peak serum levels occur within 1-2 hours

Elimination: Excreted in urine (75% to 95%), feces, and saliva

Usual Dosage Oral, I.M. (recommendations often change due to resistant strains and newly developed information; consult MMWR for current CDC recommendations):

Children: 10-20 mg/kg/day in 1-2 divided doses (maximum: 300 mg total dose)

- Prophylaxis: 10 mg/kg/day given daily (up to 300 mg total dose) for 12 months

Adults: 5 mg/kg/day given daily (usual dose is 300 mg)

- Disseminated disease: 10 mg/kg/day in 1-2 divided doses
- Treatment should be continued for 9 months with rifampin or for 6 months with rifampin and pyrazinamide
- Prophylaxis: 300 mg/day given daily for 12 months

American Thoracic Society and CDC currently recommend twice weekly therapy as part of a short-course regimen which follows 1-2 months of daily treatment for uncomplicated pulmonary tuberculosis in compliant patients

- Children: 20-40 mg/kg/dose (up to 900 mg) twice weekly
- Adults: 15 mg/kg/dose (up to 900 mg) twice weekly

Toxic dose: 1.5 g

Lethal dose: 80-150 mg/kg

Dosing adjustment in hepatic impairment: Dose should be reduced in severe hepatic disease

Contraindications Acute liver disease; hypersensitivity to isoniazid or any component; previous history of hepatitis during isoniazid therapy

Warnings Severe and sometimes fatal hepatitis may occur or develop even after many months of treatment; patients must report any prodromal symptoms of hepatitis, such as fatigue, asthenia, malaise, anorexia, nausea, or vomiting; use with caution in patients with renal impairment and chronic liver disease

Dosage Forms

Injection: 100 mg/mL (10 mL)

Syrup (orange flavor): 50 mg/5 mL (473 mL)

Tablet: 50 mg, 100 mg, 300 mg

Stability Protect oral dosage forms from light

Reference Range

Therapeutic: 1-7 μg/mL (SI: 7-51 μmol/L)

Toxic: >10 μg/mL (SI: 73 μmol/L)

Overdosage Treatment

Decontamination: Do not use ipecac; gastric lavage (protect airway if gag reflex is negative) with activated charcoal with cathartic (lavage if obtunded)

Supportive therapy: Treat seizures with diazepam while awaiting pyridoxine; refractory seizures should be treated with thiopental or other short-acting barbiturates; acidosis should be appropriately treated with sodium bicarbonate; early consideration of intubation is recommended. Pyridoxine has been shown to be effective in the treatment of intoxication, especially when seizures occur. Pyridoxine I.V. is administered on a milligram to milligram dose. If the amount of isoniazid ingested is unknown, 5 g of pyridoxine should be given over 3-5 minutes and may be followed by an additional 5 g in 30 minutes; phenytoin is not useful;

pyridoxine can also be useful for coma or optic neuropathy. Because of the severe morbidity and high mortality rates with isoniazid overdose, patients who are asymptomatic after an overdose, should be monitored for 4-6 hours. Acute ingestions over 80 mg/kg should be given pyridoxine.

Enhancement of elimination: Dialysis may be useful (dialyzable 50% to 100%) as is hemoperfusion in refractory cases

Antidote(s)

Pyridoxine Hydrochloride *on page 1465*

Test Interactions False-positive urinary glucose with Clinitest®

Drug Interactions Phenytoin, carbamazepine, ketoconazole, fluconazole, diazepam, prednisone, disulfiram, aluminum salts, cycloserine, ethionamide

Pregnancy Risk Factor C

Pregnancy Implications Crosses the placenta; appears in breast milk

Monitoring Parameters Periodic liver function tests; monitoring for prodromal signs of hepatitis

Patient Information Report any prodromal symptoms of hepatitis (fatigue, asthenia, nausea, vomiting, dark urine, or yellowing of eyes) or any burning, tingling, or numbness in the extremities

Additional Information Children with low milk and low meat intake should receive concomitant pyridoxine therapy; most combination antituberculin products contain INH which generally should be regarded as the more significant toxin

Toxic dose: 1.5 g

Specific References

Askgaard DS, Wilcke T, and Dossing M, "Hepatotoxicity Caused by the Combined Action of Isoniazid and Rifampicin," *Thorax*, 1995, 50:213-4.

Bredemann JA, Krechel SW, and Eggers GW Jr, "Treatment of Refractory Seizures in Massive Isoniazid Overdose," *Anesth Analg*, 1990, 71(5):554-7.

Brent J, Vo N, Kulig K, et al, "Reversal of Prolonged Isoniazid-Induced Coma by Pyridoxine," *Arch Intern Med*, 1990, 150(8):1751-3.

Brown CV, "Acute Isoniazid Poisoning," *Am Rev Respir Dis*, 1972, 105(2):206-16.

Noble A, "Antituberculous Therapy and Acute Liver Failure," *Lancet*, 1995, 345(8953):867.

Rabassa AA, Trey G, Shukla U, et al, "Isoniazid-Induced Acute Pancreatitis," *Ann Intern Med*, 1994, 121(6):433-4.

Sharieff G and Shad JA, "Early Recognition of Isoniazid Overdose," *Hosp Physician*, 1995, 31(5):22-2.

Sievers ML and Herrier RN, "Treatment of Acute Isoniazid Toxicity," *Am J Hosp Pharm*, 1975, 32(2):202-6.

Wason S, LaCoutore PG, and Lovejoy FH Jr, "Single High-Dose Pyridoxine Treatment for Isoniazid Overdose," *JAMA*, 1981, 246(10):1102-4.

Isonicotinic Acid Hydrazide *see* Isoniazid *on page 443*

Isonipecaine Hydrochloride *see* Meperidine Hydrochloride *on page 499*

Isopropylmeprobamate *see* Carisoprodol *on page 187*

Isoptin® *see* Verapamil Hydrochloride *on page 787*

Isopto® Hyoscine *see* Scopolamine *on page 691*

Isorbil® *see* Isosorbide Dinitrate *on this page*

Isordil® *see* Isosorbide Dinitrate *on this page*

Isosorbide Dinitrate (eye soe sor' bide dye nye' trate)

Related Information

Therapeutic Drugs Associated With Hallucinations *on page 1558-1559*

CAS Number 87-33-2

Brand Names Cedocard®; Cordil®; Dilitrate®-SR; Iso-Bid®; Isocardide®; Isoket®; Isonate®; Isorbil®; Isordil®; Isotard®; Isotrate®; Soni-Slo®; Sorbid®; Sorbitrate®

Synonyms Sorbide Nitrate

Use Prevention and treatment of angina pectoris; for congestive heart failure; to relieve pain, dysphagia, and spasm in esophageal spasm with GE reflux

Mechanism of Action Reduces cardiac oxygen demand by decreasing left ventricular pressure and systemic vascular resistance by dilating coronary arteries and improving collateral flow to ischemic regions

Adverse Reactions

Cardiovascular: Postural hypotension, cutaneous flushing of head, neck, and clavicular area, tachycardia

Central nervous system: Dizziness, psychosis, visual hallucinations, seizures, headache

Dermatologic: Rash, facial flushing

Gastrointestinal: Nausea, gastrointestinal upset, diarrhea, vomiting

Hematologic: Hemolysis in G-6-PD deficient patients

Signs & Symptoms of Acute Overdose Hypotension, urinary frequency, cough, throbbing headache, dyspepsia, heart palpitations, ptosis, visual disturbances methemoglobin formation, cyanosis

(Continued)

Isosorbide Dinitrate *(Continued)*

Dosage Form	Onset of Action	Duration
Sublingual tablet	2–10 min	1–2 h
Chewable tablet	3 min	0.5–2 h
Oral tablet	45–60 min	4–6 h
Sustained release tablet	30 min	6–12 h

Toxicodynamics/Kinetics See table.

Onset of action:
- Sublingual: 3 minutes
- Tablet: 1 hour

Duration:
- Sublingual: 2 hours
- Tablet: 4-8 hours

Absorption: Well absorbed from the gastrointestinal tract

Distribution: V_d: 6.3-8.9 L/kg; widely distributed throughout the body

Metabolism: Extensive in the liver to conjugated metabolites, including isosorbide 5-mononitrate (active) and 2-mononitrate (active)

Bioavailability: 59% after sublingual administration, 22% after oral administration

Half-life:
- Parent: 1-4 hours
- 5-mononitrate: 4 hours

Elimination: Excreted in urine and feces

Usual Dosage Adults:

Oral: 5-40 mg every 6 hours or 40-80 mg every 8-12 hours in sustained release dosage form

Chewable: 5-10 mg every 2-3 hours

Sublingual: 2.5-10 mg every 4-6 hours

Contraindications Severe anemia, hypersensitivity to isosorbide dinitrate or any component

Warnings Do not crush or chew sublingual dosage form; do not crush chewable tablets before administration; increased intracranial pressure; do not use sustained-release products in patients with gastrointestinal hypermotility or malabsorption syndrome

Dosage Forms

Capsule, sustained release: 40 mg

Tablet:
- Chewable: 5 mg, 10 mg
- Oral: 5 mg, 10 mg, 20 mg, 30 mg, 40 mg
- Sublingual: 2.5 mg, 5 mg, 10 mg
- Sustained release: 40 mg

Reference Range Peak isosorbide plasma levels after a 5 mg oral and sublingual dose: 3.1 μg/L and 8.9 μg/L respectively

Overdosage Treatment

Decontamination: Ipecac or lavage/activated charcoal with cathartic

Supportive therapy: Formation of methemoglobinemia is dose related and unusual in normal doses; high levels can cause signs and symptoms of hypoxemia; treatment consists of placing patient in recumbent position and administering fluids; alpha-adrenergic vasopressors may be required; treat methemoglobinemia with oxygen and methylene blue at a dose of 1-2 mg/kg I.V. slowly; treat hypotension with isotonic fluid and Trendelenburg position; pressors rarely necessary unless ingestion is severe

Enhancement of elimination: Hemodialysis is not useful

Antidote(s)

Methylene Blue *on page 1444*

Test Interactions Decreases cholesterol (S)

Diagnostic Tests/Procedures

Methemoglobin, Blood *on page 1296*

Drug Interactions May antagonize the anticoagulant effect of heparin; ethanol potentiates toxicity

Pregnancy Risk Factor C

Monitoring Parameters Blood pressure, EKG

Patient Information Dispense drug in easy to open container; do not chew or crush sublingual or sustained-release dosage form

Nursing Implications Do not crush sustained release or sublingual drug product

Specific References

Aderka D, Garfinkel D, Bograd H, et al, "Isosorbide Dinitrate-Induced Hemolysis in G-6-PD-Deficient Subjects," *Acta Haematol*, 1983, 69(1):63-4.

Nakashima E, Rigod JF, Lin ET, et al, "Pharmacokinetics of Nitroglycerin and Its Dinitrate Metabolites Over a Thirty-Fold Range of Oral Doses," *Clin Pharmacol Ther*, 1990, 47(5):592-8.

Rosenthal R, "Visual Hallucinations and Suicidal Ideation Attributed to Isosorbide Dinitrate," *Psychosomatics*, 1987, 28(10):555-6.

Isotard® *see* Isosorbide Dinitrate *on page 445*

Isotrate® *see* Isosorbide Dinitrate *on page 445*

Isotretinoin (eye soe tret' i noyn)

Related Information

Drugs and Chemicals Proven to be Teratogenic in Humans *on page 1572-1575*

Vitamin A *on page 795*

CAS Number 4759-48-2

Brand Names Accutane®; Isotrex®; Roaccutan®; Roaccutane®; Roacutan®

Synonyms 13-*cis*-Retinoic Acid; *cis* Vitamin A Acid

Use Treatment of severe recalcitrant cystic and/or conglobate acne unresponsive to conventional therapy

Investigational: Treatment of children with metastatic neuroblastoma or leukemia that does not respond to conventional therapy; has been used in the treatment of juvenile chronic myelogenous leukemia

Mechanism of Action Reduces sebaceous gland size and reduces sebum production; regulates cell proliferation and differentiation

Adverse Reactions

Central nervous system: Mental depression, headache, tiredness, mood changes, psychosis, pseudotumor cerebri

Dermatologic: Dry skin, skin rash, skin peeling on hands or soles of feet, pruritus, alopecia, photosensitivity

Gastrointestinal: Stomach upset, inflammatory bowel disease, anorexia, nausea, vomiting, xerostomia

Hematologic: Hypertriglyceridemia, thrombocytopenia, agranulocytosis, hypercalcemia, hemolysis, decrease in hemoglobin and hematocrit

Hepatic: Hepatitis

Neuromuscular & skeletal: Myalgia, increased serum concentration of triglycerides, skeletal hyperostosis

Ocular: Burning, conjunctivitis, redness, itching of eye, dry eyes, photophobia, optic neuropathy, cataract, blepharo conjunctivitis (dose related)

Renal: Hypercalciuria

Miscellaneous: Cheilitis, dry mouth/nose, inflammation of lips, bleeding of gums, increase in erythrocyte sedimentation rate, thyrotoxicosis, epistaxis

Signs & Symptoms of Acute Overdose Headache, dermatitis, hyperuricemia, depression, photophobia, dry eyes, desquamation, vomiting, acrodynia, hyperthyroidism, eczema, ejaculatory disturbances, neutropenia, flushing, tachypnea, abdominal pain, hypercalcemia, hematuria, ataxia; all signs and symptoms have been transient

Toxicodynamics/Kinetics

Absorption: Oral: Demonstrates biphasic absorption; increased absorption with milk or food

Distribution: Crosses the placenta; appears in breast milk

Protein binding: 99% to 100%

Metabolism: In the liver; major metabolite: 4-oxo-isotretinoin (active)

Half-life, terminal:

- Parent drug: 10-20 hours
- Metabolite: 24-29 hours

Time to peak serum concentration: Within 3 hours

Elimination: Excreted equally in urine and feces

Usual Dosage Oral:

Children: Maintenance therapy for neuroblastoma: 100-250 mg/m^2/day in 2 divided doses has been used investigationally

Children and Adults: 0.5-2 mg/kg/day in 2 divided doses (dosages as low as 0.05 mg/kg/day have been reported to be beneficial) for 15-20 weeks or until the total cyst count decreases by 70%, whichever is sooner

Dosing adjustment in hepatic impairment: Dose reductions empirically are recommended in hepatitis disease

Contraindications Sensitivity to parabens, vitamin A, or other retinoids; patients who are pregnant or intend to become pregnant during treatment

Warnings Use with caution in patients with diabetes mellitus, hypertriglyceridemia; not to be used in women of childbearing potential unless woman is capable of

(Continued)

Isotretinoin *(Continued)*

complying with effective contraceptive measures; therapy is normally begun on the second or third day of next normal menstrual period; effective contraception must be used for at least 1 month before beginning therapy, during therapy, and for 1 month after discontinuation of therapy. Because of the high likelihood of teratogenic effects (~20%), do not prescribe isotretinoin for women who are or who are likely to become pregnant while using the drug.

Dosage Forms Capsule: 10 mg, 20 mg, 40 mg

Stability Store at room temperature and protect from light

Reference Range Therapeutic blood levels: 141-179 ng/mL

Overdosage Treatment

Decontamination: Emesis or lavage/activated charcoal

Supportive therapy: Hyperventilation, furosemide or mannitol (0.25-2 g/kg every 3-4 hours) for increased intracranial pressure

Enhancement of elimination: Due to enterohepatic recirculation, multiple dosing of activated charcoal may be effective

Drug Interactions

Decreased effect: Warfarin

Increased effect: Increased clearance of carbamazepine

Increased toxicity: Avoid other vitamin A products; may interfere with medications used to treat hypertriglyceridemia; increased hepatitis with methotrexate; increased risk of elevated intracranial pressure with tetracycline

Pregnancy Risk Factor X

Pregnancy Implications Associated with spontaneous abortion, cleft palate, microphthalmia, micrognatha, facial dysmorphia, mental retardation, limb reduction, CNS, heart, ear, thymus, and visual defects may occur; risk may be as high as 25%; usually associated with isotretinoin use during first month of gestation

Monitoring Parameters CBC with differential and platelet count, baseline sed rate, serum triglycerides, liver enzymes

Patient Information Avoid pregnancy during therapy; effective contraceptive measures must be used since this drug may harm the fetus; there is information from manufacturers about this product that you should receive; discontinue therapy if visual difficulties, abdominal pain, rectal bleeding, diarrhea; exacerbation of acne may occur during first weeks of therapy; avoid use of other vitamin A products; decreased tolerance to contact lenses may occur; do not donate blood for at least 1 month following stopping of the drug; loss of night vision may occur, avoid prolonged exposure to sunlight; do not double next dose if dose is skipped; avoid alcohol

Nursing Implications Capsules can be swallowed, or chewed and swallowed. The capsule may be opened with a large needle and the contents placed on apple sauce or ice cream for patients unable to swallow the capsule; administer with meals

Additional Information Not indicated for uncomplicated adolescent acne; because of the high likelihood of teratogenic effects, do not prescribe isotretinoin for women who are or who are likely to become pregnant while using the drug; patients should discontinue isotretinoin at least 30 days prior to attempting conception

Specific References

Boyd AS, "An Overview of the Retinoids," *Am J Med*, 1989, 86(5):568-74.

Castleberry RP, Emanuel PD, Zuckerman KS, et al, "A Pilot Study of Isotretinoin in the Treatment of Juvenile Chronic Myelogenous Leukemia," *N Engl J Med*, 1994, 331(25):1680-4.

Hepburn NC, "Deliberate Self-Poisoning With Isotretinoin," *Br J Dermatol*, 1990, 122(6):840-1.

LaFontaine N, Tousignant J, Rozenfarb E, et al, "Thyroglossal Cyst and Isotretinoin," *Eur J Dermatol*, 1995, 5:225-6.

Lammer EJ, Chen DT, Hoar RM, et al, "Retinoic Acid Embryopathy," *N Engl J Med*, 1985, 313(14):837-41.

Lee AG, "Pseudotumor Cerebri After Treatment With Tetracycline and Isotretinoin for Acne," *Cutis*, 1995, 55:165-8.

Lotan R, Xu XC, Lippman SM, et al, "Suppression of Retinoic Acid, Receptor-B in Premalignant Oral Lesions and Its Up-Regulation by Isotretinoin," *N Engl J Med*, 1995, 332:1405-10.

Mitchell AA, Van Bennekom CM, Louik C, et al, "A Pregnancy-Prevention Program in Women of Childbearing Age Receiving Isotretinoin," *N Engl J Med*, 1995, 333:101-6.

Rappaport EB and Knapp M, "Isotretinoin Embryopathy - A Continuing Problem," *J Clin Pharmacol*, 1989, 29(5):463-5.

Taillan B, Chichmanian RM, Vialla I, et al, "Paroxysmal Nocturnal Hemoglobinuria and Hemolysis Induced by Isotretinoin," *Therapie*, 1994, 49(5):468.

Isotrex® *see* Isotretinoin *on previous page*

Itraconazole (i tra koe' na zole)

Related Information

Antifungal Therapy *on page 1496-1497*

CAS Number 84625-61-6

Brand Names Sporanox® Oral

Use Treatment of susceptible fungal infections in immunocompromised and nonimmunocompromised patients including blastomycosis and histoplasmosis; treatment of AIDS-related disseminated histoplasmosis

Adverse Reactions

Cardiovascular: Hypertension, edema, bradycardia, arrhythmias

Central nervous system: Headache, euphoria, dizziness, insomnia

Dermatologic: Skin rash, exfoliative dermatitis

Endocrine & metabolic: Hypokalemia, hypertriglyceridemia, gynecomastia, adrenal cortical insufficiency

Gastrointestinal: Nausea, vomiting, dyspepsia, dry mouth, diarrhea, abdominal pain, anorexia, flatulence

Genitourinary: Impotence

Hepatic: Elevated AST, ALT, or alkaline phosphatase

Miscellaneous: Breast pain (male)

Toxicodynamics/Kinetics

Absorption: Rapid and complete

Protein binding: >99% protein bound

Metabolism: Hepatic, >97% to inactive metabolites

Elimination: 85% renally excreted, 40% as inactive metabolites

Usual Dosage Adults: Oral: 200 mg once daily, if no obvious improvement or there is evidence of progressive fungal disease, increase the dose in 100 mg increments to a maximum of 400 mg/day

Life-threatening: Loading dose: 200 mg 3 times/day (600 mg/day) should be given for the first 3 days

Contraindications Known hypersensitivity to itraconazole or other azoles; terfenadine

Warnings Coadministration with terfenadine is contraindicated; rare cases of serious cardiovascular adverse event, including death, tachycardia (ventricular) and torsade de pointes have been observed due to increased terfenadine concentrations induced by itraconazole; patients who develop liver function tests (abnormal) during itraconazole therapy should be monitored closely for the development of more severe hepatic injury; if clinical signs and symptoms consistent with liver disease develop that may be attributable to itraconazole, itraconazole should be discontinued

Dosage Forms Capsule: 100 mg

Overdosage Treatment

Decontamination: Ipecac or lavage/activated charcoal with cathartic

Enhancement of elimination: Multiple dosing of activated charcoal would not be expected to be helpful

Drug Interactions

Impaired absorption with antacids or H_2 blockers; decreases the metabolism of cyclosporine, digoxin, and terfenadine, while rifampin, phenytoin, and carbamazepine increases the elimination of itraconazole; both ketoconazole and itraconazole can increase peak concentration and elimination half-life of triazolam

Ventricular arrhythmias can occur with combination of cisapride and ketoconazole, miconazole, or itraconazole

Pregnancy Risk Factor C

Specific References

Kintzel PE, Rollins CJ, Yee CV, et al, "Low Itraconazole Serum Concentrations Following Administration of Itraconazole Suspension to Critically Ill Allogenic Bone Marrow Transplant Recipients," *Ann Pharmacother*, 1995, 29:140-3.

Tucker RM, Haq Y, Denning DW, et al, "Adverse Effects Associated With Itraconazole in 189 Patients on Chronic Therapy," *J Antimicrob Chemother*, 1990, 26(4):561-6.

Varhe A, Olkkola KT, and Neuvonen PJ, "Oral Triazolam is Potentially Hazardous to Patients Receiving Systemic Antimycotics Ketoconazole or Itraconazole," *Clin Pharmacol Ther*, 1994, 56(6 Pt 1):601-7.

Wheat J, Hafner R, Korzun AH, et al, "Itraconazole Treatment of Disseminated Histoplasmosis in Patients With the Acquired Immunodeficiency Syndrome," *Am J Med*, 1995, 98:336

Itrop® *see* Ipratropium Bromide *on page 438*

Ivermectin

CAS Number 70288-86-7; 70161-11-4; 70209-81-3

Brand Names Mectizan®

Synonyms Avermectin B_{1A}

Use Investigational: Onchocerciasis (*Onchocerca volvulus*), scabies, lymphatic filariasis (*Wucheria bancrofti*), and loiasis

Mechanism of Action Stimulates gamma aminobutyric acid (GABA) release and receptor binding; produced from streptomyces avermitilis

Adverse Reactions

Cardiovascular: Orthostatic hypotension

Central nervous system: Fever, headache, dizziness, hypothermia

Dermatologic: Rash, pruritus

(Continued)

Ivermectin *(Continued)*

Hematologic: Eosinophilia
Neuromuscular & skeletal: Arthralgia, myalgia, enlarged lymph nodes
Ocular: Mydriasis
Respiratory: Cough

Signs & Symptoms of Acute Overdose Tachycardia, hypotension, vomiting, abdominal pain, lethargy, pallor, pruritus, urticaria

Toxicodynamics/Kinetics
Half-life: 10-28 hours
Elimination: Feces

Usual Dosage
Onchocerciasis: Oral: 150-200 mcg/kg as a single dose
Scabies: Oral:
Uncomplicated: 200 mcg/kg as a single dose
With HIV infection: 200 mcg/kg as a single dose; may repeat as necessary in 2 weeks

Contraindications Hypersensitivity to ivermectin

Warnings May cause a mazzotti reaction (optic neuritis, pruritus, rash, edema, and proteinuria) due to killing of large numbers of microfilariae

Dosage Forms Tablet: 6 mg

Reference Range Doses of 50 mcg/kg can result in blood ivermectin levels of 9-13 ng/mL; adverse effects do not correlate with serum concentrations

Overdosage Treatment
Decontamination: Ipecac or lavage/activated charcoal with cathartic
Supportive therapy: Hypotension can be treated with intravenous fluids (ie, saline) and placement in Trendelenburg position; dopamine or norepinephrine can be used for refractory hypotension; antihistamines can be used for urticaria or pruritus

Additional Information Often used for prophylaxis against the heartworm (*Dirofilaria immitis*) in dogs; acceptable daily intake of ivermectin by World Health Organization is 0.2 mcg/kg; avoid use during breast feeding during first 3 months

Specific References

Aziz MA, "Chemotherapeutic Approach to Control of Onchocerciasis," *Rev Infect Dis*, 1986, 8(3):500-4.
"Ivermectin in Lymphatic Filariasis," *N Engl J Med*, 1990, 323(13):917-8.
Meinking TL, Taplin D, Hermida JL, et al, "The Treatment of Scabies With Ivermectin," *N Engl J Med*, 1995, 333:26-30.
Njoo FL, Beek WMS, Keukens HJ, et al, "Ivermectin Detection in Serum of Onchocerciasis Patients: Relationship to Adverse Reactions," *Am J Trop Med Hyg*, 1995, 52:94-7.
Taylor HR and Greene BM, "The Status of Ivermectin in the Treatment of Human Onchocerciasis," *Am J Trop Med Hyg*, 1989, 41(4):460-6.

Janimine® *see* Imipramine *on page 422*
Jatropur® *see* Triamterene *on page 766*
JB-11 *see* Trimetrexate Glucuronate *on page 773*
Jenamicin® Injection *see* Gentamicin Sulfate *on page 379*
Judolor® *see* Thiamine Hydrochloride *on page 741*
K+8® *see* Potassium Chloride *on page 634*
Kabikinase® *see* Streptokinase *on page 707*
Kaluril® *see* Amiloride Hydrochloride *on page 109*
Kampfer *see* Camphor *on page 179*
Kaochlor® S-F *see* Potassium Chloride *on page 634*
Kaon-CL® *see* Potassium Chloride *on page 634*
Kaopectate® II [OTC] *see* Loperamide Hydrochloride *on page 480*
Karidium® *see* Fluoride *on page 355*
Karigel® *see* Fluoride *on page 355*
Karigel®-N *see* Fluoride *on page 355*
Kasof® [OTC] *see* Docusate *on page 297*
Kato® *see* Potassium Chloride *on page 634*
Katopil® *see* Captopril *on page 181*
Kavrin® *see* Papaverine *on page 591*
Kaybovite-1000® *see* Cyanocobalamin *on page 246*
K-Dur® *see* Potassium Chloride *on page 634*
Keal® *see* Sucralfate *on page 710*
Kelene *see* Ethyl Chloride *on page 337*

Kendol® *see* Lorazepam *on page 482*

Kerlone® *see* Betaxolol Hydrochloride *on page 153*

Ketaject® *see* Ketamine Hydrochloride *on this page*

Ketalar® Injection *see* Ketamine Hydrochloride *on this page*

Ketamine Hydrochloride (keet' a meen)

Related Information

Therapeutic Drugs Associated With Hallucinations *on page 1558-1559*

CAS Number 6740-88-1; 1867-66-9

Brand Names Ketaject®; Ketalar® Injection; Ketanest®; Ketavet®

Use Induction of anesthesia; short surgical procedures; dressing changes

Mechanism of Action An N-methyl-D-aspartate (NMDA) neuroreceptor antagonist; some opiate agonist effect; while analgesic effect is rapid, laryngeal reflexes, muscle tone, and cardiopulmonary function is usually not affected; structurally related to phencyclidine

Adverse Reactions

Cardiovascular: Tachycardia, hypertension

Central nervous system: Visual hallucinations, delirium, dysphoric states, dystonic reactions, psychosis, dizziness, insomnia, ataxia, malignant hyperthermia, hypertonus, electroencephalogram abnormalities

Gastrointestinal: Increased salivation, nausea, vomiting

Ocular: Diplopia, lacrimation, increased intraocular pressure, nystagmus

Pulmonary: Edema, bronchodilitation, laryngospasm

Signs & Symptoms of Acute Overdose Seizures, apnea, delirium, fasciculations, extrapyramidal reaction, lacrimation, laryngospasm, insomnia, hyperglycemia, seizures, polyneuropathy, cardiac arrest

Toxicodynamics/Kinetics Duration of action (following a single dose):

Unconsciousness: 10-15 minutes

Analgesia: 30-40 minutes

Amnesia: May persist for 1-2 hours

Distribution: V_d: 3-5 L/kg

Protein binding: 30%

Metabolism: Hepatic to the active metabolite norketamine and dehydronorketamine

Half-life: 2.5 hours

Elimination: Renal

Usual Dosage

Anesthetic induction dose:

Oral: 4-5 mg/kg

I.M.: 5-10 mg/kg

I.V.: 1-2 mg/kg

Maintenance dose is ½, up to total induction dose as needed to maintain anesthesia

Duration of unconsciousness: 1 hour

Duration of amnesia: 2 hours

Contraindications Elevated intracranial pressure; patients with hypertension, aneurysms, thyrotoxicosis, congestive heart failure, angina, psychotic disorders; hypersensitivity to ketamine or any component

Warnings Should be used by or under the direct supervision of physicians experienced in administering general anesthetics and in maintenance of an airway, and in the control of respiration. Resuscitative equipment should be available for use.

Postanesthetic emergence reactions which can manifest as vivid dreams, hallucinations and/or frank delirium occur in 12% of patients; these reactions are less common in patients >65 years of age and when given I.M.; emergence reactions, confusion, or irrational behavior may occur up to 24 hours postoperatively and may be reduced by minimization of verbal, tactile, and visual patient stimulation during recovery or by pretreatment with a benzodiazepine.

Dosage Forms Injection: 10 mg/mL (20 mL, 25 mL, 50 mL); 50 mg/mL (10 mL); 100 mg/mL (5 mL)

Stability Do not mix with barbiturates or diazepam → precipitation may occur

Reference Range An I.V. dose of 2.5 mg/kg produces an average serum ketamine concentration of 1 mg/L at 12 minutes and 0.5 mg/L at 30 minutes, while doses of 4 mg/kg can produce a peak serum ketamine level of 6.3 mg/L

Overdosage Treatment

Decontamination: Lavage/activated charcoal

Supportive therapy: Benzodiazepines can be utilized for delirium, dysphoric reactions, or hallucinations; extrapyramidal reaction can be treated with diphenhydramine and/or benztropine. Benzodiazepines, alpha- and beta-adrenergic blockers, or verapamil can decrease cardiac stimulation; benzodiazepines are initial choice for seizure management. Atropine can be used to prevent excess salivation; positive end expiratory pressure can be used to treat laryngospasm.

(Continued)

Ketamine Hydrochloride *(Continued)*

Drug Interactions Elimination half-life and serum levels may be increased with concomitant administration of diazepam; thyroid therapy may enhance hypertensive effect; can enhance the effect of tubocurarine; naloxone can reverse the analgesia but not any other effect (ie, apnea); flumazenil can cause an increase in unpleasant emergence reactions when used with ketamine

Pregnancy Risk Factor D

Pregnancy Implications Crosses the placenta; fetal respiratory depression can occur

Additional Information Elevation of catecholamine levels occur

Specific References

Clements JA and Nimmo WS, "Pharmacokinetics and Analgesic Effect of Ketamine in Man," *Br J Anaesth*, 1981, 53:27-30.

Felser JM and Orban DJ, "Dystonic Reaction After Ketamine Abuse," *Ann Emerg Med*, 1982, 11:673-5.

Glickman A, "Ketamine: The Dissociative Anesthetic and the Development of a Policy for Its Safe Administration in the Pediatric Emergency Department," *J Emerg Nurs*, 1995, 21:116-24.

Moro-Sutherland DM and Shook JE, "Ketamine Use in a Pediatric Emergency Room," *Acad Emerg Med*, 1995, 2:428-9.

Winters WD, "Epilepsy or Anesthesia With Ketamine," *Anesthesiology*, 1972, 36:309-12.

Ketanest® *see* Ketamine Hydrochloride *on previous page*

Ketavet® *see* Ketamine Hydrochloride *on previous page*

Ketobemidone Hydrochloride

CAS Number 469-79-4

Brand Names Cliradon®; Ketogan®

Synonyms Cetobemidone

Use Pain relief in the postoperative period and during acute myocardial infarction; premedication for anesthesia

Mechanism of Action Opioid compound similar to meperidine structurally

Adverse Reactions

Central nervous system: Lethargy, headache, confusion, sedation (9%), dizziness, euphoria

Gastrointestinal: Ileus, nausea, vomiting, dry mouth, obstipation, constipation

Genitourinary: Urinary retention

Neuromuscular & skeletal: Smooth muscle spasm

Ocular: Blurred vision

Respiratory: Cough, apnea

Signs & Symptoms of Acute Overdose Apnea, coma

Toxicodynamics/Kinetics

Duration of effect: 4-5 hours

Distribution: V_d: 2-7.8 L/kg

Metabolism: Hepatic to norketobemidone and 4'-hydroxyketombemidone

Bioavailability: Oral (34%), rectal (44%)

Half-life: 2-2.4 hours

Elimination: Renal

Usual Dosage

I.M.: 5-7.5 mg every 6 hours

I.V.:

- Patient-controlled analgesia: 2-3 mg over one minute with each dose allowable per 15 minutes
- Postoperative pain: 3 mg/hour decreasing to 0.75 mg/hour after shivering cessation

Oral: 5-15 mg every 3-6 hours

Rectal: 10 mg every 3-4 hours

Contraindications Hypersensitivity to ketobemidone or acute respiratory depression

Warnings Use with caution in patients with renal, pulmonary, or hepatic disease, increased intracranial pressure, prostatic hypertrophy, gastrointestinal surgery

Dosage Forms

Injection: 5 mg/mL

Suppository: 10 mg

Tablet: 5 mg

Reference Range Following a 10 mg I.V. dose, peak serum levels are >500 ng/mL; following a 10 mg rectal dose, peak plasma levels range from 10-15 ng/mL; after a 10 mg oral dose, peak serum levels range from 10-30 ng/mL

Overdosage Treatment Supportive therapy: Naloxone hydrochloride (0.4-2 mg I.V., S.C., or through an endotracheal tube); a continuous infusion (at $^2/_3$ the response dose/hour) may be required

Antidote(s)

Naloxone Hydrochloride *on page 1447*

Additional Information Often combined with a spasmolytic agent W-N-dimethyl-3,3-diphenyl 1-methylallylamine (A-29) due to its effects on smooth muscle spasm

Specific References

Anderson P, Arner S, Bondesson U, et al, "Clinical Pharmacokinetics of Ketobemidone: Its Bioavailability After Rectal Administration," *Eur J Clin Pharmacol*, 1981, 19:217-23.

Holst-Larsen H, Aasen AO, and Rugstad HE, "Naloxone: A Potent Ketobemidone Antagonist in Man," *Acta Pharmacol Toxicol*, 1979, 45:91-5.

Ketoconazole (kee toe koe' na zole)

Related Information

Antifungal Therapy *on page 1496-1497*

CAS Number 65277-42-1

Brand Names Nizoral®

Use Treatment of susceptible fungal infections, including candidiasis, oral thrush, blastomycosis, histoplasmosis, paracoccidioidomycosis, chronic mucocutaneous candidiasis, as well as certain recalcitrant cutaneous dermatophytoses; used topically for treatment of tinea corporis, tinea cruris, tinea versicolor and cutaneous candidiasis

Mechanism of Action Alters permeability of the cell wall; inhibits biosynthesis of triglycerides and phospholipids by fungi; inhibits several fungal enzymes that results in a build-up of toxic concentrations of hydrogen peroxide

Adverse Reactions

Central nervous system: Psychosis

Dermatologic: Pruritus, rash

Endocrine & metabolic: Adrenal cortical insufficiency, gynecomastia

Gastrointestinal: Nausea, vomiting, abdominal discomfort, gastrointestinal bleeding, anorexia

Hematologic: Thrombocytopenia

Hepatic: Hepatotoxicity

Local: Irritation, stinging, phlebitis

Signs & Symptoms of Acute Overdose Dizziness, headache, nausea, photophobia, hypothyroidism, hyperuricemia, hypertriglyceridemia, sexual dysfunction, myalgia, vomiting, thrombocytopenia, diarrhea, paresthesias

Toxicodynamics/Kinetics

Absorption: Oral: Rapid (~75%)

Distribution: V_d: ~0.36 L/kg; well distributed to inflamed joint fluid, saliva, bile, urine, breast milk, sebum, cerumen, feces, tendons, skin and soft tissues, and testes; crosses blood-brain barrier poorly; only negligible amounts reach CSF; minimal distribution into the CNS

Protein binding: 93% to 96%

Metabolism: Partial in the liver by enzymes to inactive compounds

Bioavailability: Decreases as pH of the gastric contents increase

Half-life:

Biphasic, initial: 2 hours

Terminal: 8 hours

Time to peak serum concentration: Within 1-4 hours

Elimination: Primarily in feces (57%) with smaller amounts excreted in urine (13%)

Usual Dosage

Oral:

Children >2 years: 5-10 mg/kg/day divided every 12-24 hours for 2-4 weeks

Adults: 200-400 mg/day as a single daily dose

Shampoo: Apply twice weekly for 4 weeks with at least 3 days between each shampoo

Topical: Rub gently into the affected area once daily to twice daily

Dosing adjustment in hepatic impairment: Dose reductions should be considered in patients with severe liver disease

Contraindications Hypersensitivity to ketoconazole or any component; porphyria, CNS fungal infections (due to poor CNS penetration)

Warnings Has been associated with hepatitis, including some fatalities; perform periodic liver function tests; high doses of ketoconazole may depress adrenocortical function; life-threatening cardiac arrhythmias may occur in patients taking terfenadine concurrently with ketoconazole; gastric acidity is necessary for the dissolution and absorption of ketoconazole; avoid concomitant (within 2 hours) administration of antacids, H_2-blockers, anticholinergics; use with caution in patients with impaired hepatic function

Dosage Forms

Cream: 2% (15 g, 30 g, 60 g)

Shampoo: 2% (120 mL)

Suspension, oral: 100 mg/5 mL (120 mL)

Tablet: 200 mg

Reference Range Therapeutic: Peak: 1-4 mg/L; Trough: ≤1 mg/L

(Continued)

Ketoconazole *(Continued)*

Overdosage Treatment

Decontamination: Ipecac or lavage/activated charcoal with cathartic

Enhancement of elimination: Multiple dosing of activated charcoal would not be expected to be helpful; not dialyzable (0% to 5%)

Drug Interactions

Drugs that affect absorption (raise gastric pH) such as antacids, H_2-receptor blockers; drugs that decreases serum concentrations of ketoconazole (rifampin, isoniazid); drug concentrations that are increased by ketoconazole (phenytoin, cyclosporine, theophylline, terfenadine, warfarin); and drugs that cause hepatitis; terfenadine may cause life-threatening cardiac arrhythmias; both ketoconazole and itraconazole can increase peak concentration and elimination half-life of triazolam; ketoconazole can increase the plasma levels of triazolam; ketoconazole increases cisapride toxicity and can cause torsade de pointes

Ventricular arrhythmias can occur with combination of cisapride and ketoconazole, miconazole, or itraconazole

Pregnancy Risk Factor C

Pregnancy Implications Distributes into breast milk

Patient Information Cream is for topical application to the skin only; avoid contact with the eye; avoid taking antacids or H_2 antagonists at the same time as ketoconazole; take with food to alleviate gastric disturbance

Nursing Implications Administer 2 hours prior to antacids H_2-receptor antagonist to prevent decreased absorption due to the high pH of gastric contents

Specific References

Gorman SE, Dela Cruz F, and Paloucek F, "Ketoconazole and Zidovudine Overdose," *Am J Emerg Med*, 1995, 13(1):115-6.

Greenblatt DJ, von Moltke LL, Harmatz JS, et al, "Interaction of Triazolam and Ketoconazole," *Lancet*, 1995, 345(8943):191.

Hwang WL, Gau JP, Young JH, et al, "Ketoconazole and High-Dose Methylprednisolone Predisposing to Cyclosporine-Induced Seizures: A Report of Three Cases," *Acta Haematol*, 1992, 88(2-3):139-41.

Janssen PA and Symoens JE, "Hepatic Reactions During Ketoconazole Treatment," *Am J Med*, 1983, 74(1B):80-5.

Varhe A, Olkkola KT, and Neuvonen PJ, "Oral Triazolam is Potentially Hazardous to Patients Receiving Systemic Antimycotics Ketoconazole or Itraconazole," *Clin Pharmacol Ther*, 1994, 56(6 Pt 1):601-7.

Ketogan® *see* Ketobemidone Hydrochloride *on page 452*

Ketoprofen (kee toe proe' fen)

Related Information

Nonsteroidal Anti-Inflammatory Comparison *on page 1655*

CAS Number 22071-15-4 (Base); 57469-78-0 (Lysine); 57495-14-4 (Sodium)

Brand Names Orudis®

Use Acute or long-term treatment of rheumatoid arthritis and osteoarthritis; primary dysmenorrhea; mild to moderate pain

Mechanism of Action Inhibits prostaglandin synthesis by decreasing the activity of the enzyme, cyclo-oxygenase, which results in decreased formation of prostaglandin precursors

Adverse Reactions

Cardiovascular: Fluid retention, circulatory collapse

Central nervous system: Headache, aseptic meningitis, dizziness, psychosis, cognitive dysfunction, coma, seizures

Dermatologic: Rash, pruritus

Endocrine & metabolic: Hyperkalemia, anion gap metabolic acidosis

Gastrointestinal: Abdominal pain, nausea, vomiting, bleeding, ulceration, constipation, diarrhea, dyspepsia

Genitourinary: Albuminuria

Hematologic: Leukopenia, neutropenia, agranulocytosis, granulocytopenia; aplastic anemia (rare), platelet inhibition

Hepatic: Elevation of transaminases, fulminant hepatitis

Otic: Ototoxicity, tinnitus

Renal: Renal failure (acute), proteinuria, nephrotic syndrome, chronic renal failure

Respiratory: Wheezing, respiratory depression

Miscellaneous: Hypersensitivity

Signs & Symptoms of Acute Overdose Nausea, wheezing, insomnia, purpura, pseudotumor cerebri, photosensitivity, nephrotic syndrome, depression, conjunctivitis, gastrointestinal bleeding, impotence, myalgia, gastritis; exfoliative dermatitis, eczema, dyspnea, confusion, vomiting, cognitive dysfunction, ototoxicity; tinnitus, drowsiness; severe poisoning can manifest with coma, seizures, renal failure and or hepatic failure, hypotension, respiratory depression, apnea, metabolic acidosis, and nystagmus; leukocytosis

Toxicodynamics/Kinetics

Absorption: Almost completely from gastrointestinal tract

Distribution: V_d: 0.11 L/kg
Protein binding: High
Metabolism: In the liver, primarily as glucuronide conjugates
Half-life: 1-4 hours
Time to peak serum concentration: Within 30 minutes to 2 hours
Elimination: Renal excretion (60% to 75% of dose); remainder is biliary/fecal

Usual Dosage Oral:
Children 3 months to 14 years: Fever: 0.5-1 mg/kg every 6-8 hours
Children >12 years and Adults:
Rheumatoid arthritis or osteoarthritis: 50-75 mg 3-4 times/day up to a maximum of 300 mg/day
Mild to moderate pain: 25-50 mg every 6-8 hours up to a maximum of 300 mg/day

Contraindications Known hypersensitivity to ketoprofen or other NSAIDs/aspirin

Warnings Use with caution in patients with congestive heart failure, hypertension, decreased renal or hepatic function, history of gastrointestinal disease (bleeding or ulcers), or those receiving anticoagulants

Dosage Forms
Capsule (Orudis®): 25 mg, 50 mg, 75 mg
Capsule, extended release (Oruvail®): 100 mg, 150 mg, 200 mg

Overdosage Treatment
Decontamination: Ipecac or lavage/activated charcoal with cathartic
Supportive therapy: Hypotension/dehydration can be managed with intravenous fluid therapy; acidosis should be treated with bicarbonates, seizures with benzodiazepines; antacids, blood products are indicated, as appropriate, for hemorrhage
Enhancement of elimination: Dialysis or perfusion is indicated for secondary complications, acidosis, or renal failure and not toxin removal alone; multiple dosing of activated charcoal may be effective

Test Interactions Increases chloride (S), sodium (S)

Drug Interactions Aspirin decreases serum concentrations probably by protein-binding displacement; there is an increased bleeding potential with concomitant warfarin therapy; may increase lithium and methotrexate concentrations by decreasing renal clearance; may decrease diuretic and hypotensive effects of thiazides, loop diuretics, ACE inhibitors, and beta-blockers; may increase nephrotoxicity of cyclosporine

Pregnancy Risk Factor B

Nursing Implications Do not crush capsule

Specific References

Bond GR, Curry SC, et al, "Generalized Seizures and Metabolic Acidosis After Ketoprofen Overdose," *Vet Hum Toxicol*, 1989, 31:369.
Court H and Volans GN, "Poisoning After Overdose With Nonsteroidal Anti-inflammatory Drugs," *Adverse Drug React Acute Poisoning Rev*, 1984, 3(1):1-21.
Hoppmann RA, Peden JG, and Ober SK, "Central Nervous System Side Effects of Nonsteroidal Anti-inflammatory Drugs. Aseptic Meningitis, Psychosis, and Cognitive Dysfunction," *Arch Intern Med*, 1991, 151(7):1309-13.
Smolinske SC, Hall AH, Vandenberg SA, et al, "Toxic Effects of Nonsteroid Anti-inflammatory Drugs in Overdose. An Overview of Recent Evidence on Clinical Effects and Dose-Response Relationships," *Drug Saf*, 1990, 5(4):252-74.
Vale JA and Meredith TJ, "Acute Poisoning Due to Nonsteroidal Anti-inflammatory Drugs," *Med Toxicol*, 1986, 1(1):12-31.
Verbeeck RK, "Pharmacokinetic Drug Interactions With Nonsteroidal Anti-inflammatory Drugs," *Clin Pharmacokinet*, 1990, 19(1):44-66.

Ketorolac Tromethamine (kee' toe role ak trow meth' a meen)

Related Information
Nonsteroidal Anti-Inflammatory Comparison *on page 1655*

CAS Number 74103-06-3 (Base); 74103-07-4 (Tromethamine)

Brand Names Toradol®

Use Short-term management of pain; first parenteral NSAID for analgesia

Mechanism of Action Inhibits prostaglandin synthesis by decreasing the activity of the enzyme, cyclo-oxygenase, which results in decreased formation of prostaglandin precursors

Adverse Reactions
Cardiovascular: Fluid retention, circulatory collapse
Central nervous system: Headache, aseptic meningitis, psychosis, cognitive dysfunction, coma, seizures
Dermatologic: Rash, pruritus
Endocrine & metabolic: Hyperkalemia, anion gap metabolic acidosis
Gastrointestinal: Abdominal pain, nausea, vomiting, bleeding, ulceration, constipation, diarrhea, dyspepsia
Genitourinary: Albuminuria
Hematologic: Leukopenia, neutropenia, agranulocytosis, granulocytopenia; aplastic anemia (rare), platelet inhibition

(Continued)

Ketorolac Tromethamine *(Continued)*

Hepatic: Elevation of transaminases, fulminant hepatitis
Otic: Ototoxicity, tinnitus
Renal: Renal failure (acute), nephrotic syndrome, chronic renal failure
Respiratory: Wheezing, respiratory depression
Miscellaneous: Hypersensitivity

Signs & Symptoms of Acute Overdose Nausea, chills, wheezing, nephrotic syndrome, gastrointestinal bleeding, cognitive dysfunction, dry mouth, vomiting, coagulopathy, ototoxicity; tinnitus, drowsiness; severe poisoning can manifest with coma, seizures, renal and or hepatic failure, hypotension, respiratory depression

Toxicodynamics/Kinetics

Onset of action: I.M.: Within 10 minutes
Peak effect: Within 75-150 minutes
Duration: 6-8 hours
Absorption: Oral: Well absorbed
Protein binding: 99%
Metabolism: In the liver
Half-life: 5-6 hours, increased 30% to 50% in the elderly
Time to peak serum concentration: Within 30-40 minutes
Elimination: Renal excretion, 61% appearing in urine as unchanged drug

Usual Dosage

Adults (pain relief usually begins within 10 minutes):
- I.M., I.V.: Initial: 30-60 mg, then 15-30 mg every 6 hours as needed for up to 5 days maximum; maximum dose in the first 24 hours: 150 mg with 120 mg/24 hours for up to 5 days total
- Oral (use of oral ketorolac is only indicated as continuation therapy to parenteral ketorolac): 10 mg every 4-6 hours as needed for a maximum of 40 mg/day; on day of transition from I.M. to oral: maximum oral dose: 40 mg (or 120 mg combined oral and I.M.); maximum 5 days administration
- Ophthalmic: Instill 1 drop in eye(s) 4 times/day

Elderly >65 years: Renal insufficiency or weight <50 kg:
- I.M., I.V.: 15-30 mg, then 15 mg every 6 hours (parenteral) up to a maximum daily dose of 60 mg
- Oral dosage should not exceed daily amounts of 40 mg; maximum daily dose (including parenteral) should not exceed 120 mg

Administration When administering I.V., bolus should be administered no less than 15 seconds

Contraindications Patients who have developed nasal polyps, angioedema, or bronchospastic reactions to other NSAIDs; patients with active peptic ulcer disease, recent gastrointestinal bleeding, or in patients with a history of peptic ulcer disease or gastrointestinal bleeding, advanced renal impairment, hypovolemia; also contraindicated in patients with cerebrovascular bleeding, hemorrhagic diathesis, concomitant aspirin, other nonsteroidal or probenecid use, incomplete hemostasis, or those at high risk of bleeding. Due to platelet inhibition, do not use as a prophylactic analgesic before surgery or intraoperatively; due to its high alcohol content, it is not to be delivered through intrathecal or epidural routes; also contraindicated during labor and delivery due to its adverse effects on fetal circulation and its inhibition of uterine contractures; also contraindicated in nursing mothers.

Warnings Use of ketorolac at recommended doses for longer than 5 days is associated with an increased frequency and severity of adverse events; use extra caution and reduce dosages in the elderly because it is cleared renally somewhat slower and the elderly are also more sensitive to the renal effects of NSAIDs

Dosage Forms

Injection: 15 mg/mL (1 mL); 30 mg/mL (1 mL, 2 mL)
Solution, ophthalmic: 0.5% (5 mL)
Tablet: 10 mg

Stability Do not mix with morphine sulfate, meperidine hydrochloride, promethazine hydrochloride, or hydroxyzine hydrochloride in that precipitation may occur

Reference Range

Peak plasma level after a 60 mg dose (I.M.): 4-4.5 μg/mL
Serum concentration:
- Therapeutic: 0.3-5.0 μg/mL
- Toxic: >5.0 μg/mL

Overdosage Treatment

Decontamination: Ipecac or lavage/activated charcoal with cathartic
Supportive therapy: Hypotension/dehydration can be managed with intravenous fluid therapy; acidosis should be treated with bicarbonates, seizures with benzodiazepines; antacids, blood products are indicated, as appropriate, for hemorrhage
Enhancement of elimination: Dialysis or perfusion is indicated for secondary complications, acidosis, or renal failure and not toxin removal alone

Test Interactions Increases chloride (S), sodium (S), bleeding time

Drug Interactions Aspirin decreases serum concentrations probably by protein-binding displacement; there is an increased bleeding potential with concomitant warfarin therapy; may increase lithium and methotrexate concentrations by decreasing renal clearance; may decrease diuretic and hypotensive effects of thiazides, loop diuretics, ACE inhibitors, and beta-blockers; may increase nephrotoxicity of cyclosporine; concomitant administration of lithium and ketorolac can result in elevated lithium levels

Pregnancy Risk Factor B

Pregnancy Implications Distributes into breast milk

Monitoring Parameters BUN, serum creatinine, urinalysis, liver enzymes, occult blood loss; monitor for signs of pain relief, such as an increased appetite and activity

Additional Information 30 mg provides the analgesia comparable to 12 mg of morphine or 100 mg of meperidine; postmarketing surveillance of ketorolac indicated that the risk of clinically serious gastrointestinal bleeding was dose-dependent, particularly in elderly patients, who received doses exceeding 60 mg/day

Specific References

Buck ML, "Clinical Experience With Ketorolac in Children," *Ann Pharmacother*, 1994, 28(9):1009-13.

Court H and Volans GN, "Poisoning After Overdose With Nonsteroidal Anti-inflammatory Drugs," *Adverse Drug React Acute Poisoning Rev*, 1984, 3(1):1-21.

Gannon K, "Postmarketing Study Leads to Revamp of Toradol Labeling," *Hospital Pharmacist Report*, 1995, 9(4):98.

Hoppmann RA, Peden JG, and Ober SK, "Central Nervous System Side Effects of Nonsteroidal Anti-inflammatory Drugs. Aseptic Meningitis, Psychosis, and Cognitive Dysfunction," *Arch Intern Med*, 1991, 151(7):1309-13.

Jallad NS, Garg DC, Martinez JJ, et al, "Pharmacokinetics of Single-Dose Oral and Intramuscular Ketorolac Tromethamine in the Young and Elderly," *J Clin Pharmacol*, 1990, 30(1):76-81.

Langlois R and Paquette D, "Increased Serum Lithium Levels Due to Ketorolac therapy," *Can Med Assoc J*, 1994, 150(9):1455-6.

Logar BK, Friel PN, Peterson KL, et al, "Analysis of Ketorolac in Postmortem Blood," *J Anal Toxicol*, 1995, 19:61-4.

Pol Yanguas E, Blasco Segura P, and Costa LA, "A Case of Convulsive Crises Connected With the Use of Ketorolac," *Farmacia Clinica*, 1994, 11:687-90.

Quan DJ and Kayser SR, "Ketorolac Induced Acute Renal Failure Following a Single Dose," *J Toxicol Clin Toxicol*, 1994, 32(3):305-9.

Schaab KC, Dickinson ET, and Setzen G, "Acute Sensorineural Hearing Loss Following Intravenous Ketoralac Administration," *J Emerg Med*, 1995, 13(4):509-13.

Schoch PH, Ranno A, and North DS, "Acute Renal Failure in an Elderly Woman Following Intramuscular Ketorolac Administration," *Ann Pharmacother*, 1992, 26(10):1233-6.

Smolinske SC, Hall AH, Vandenberg SA, et al, "Toxic Effects of Nonsteroid Anti-inflammatory Drugs in Overdose. An Overview of Recent Evidence on Clinical Effects and Dose-Response Relationships," *Drug Saf*, 1990, 5(4):252-74.

Turturro MA, Paris PM, and Seaberg DC, "Intramuscular Ketorolac Versus Oral Ibuprofen in Acute Musculoskeletal Pain," *Acad Emerg Med*, 1995, 26:117-20.

Vale JA and Meredith TJ, "Acute Poisoning Due to Nonsteroidal Anti-inflammatory Drugs," *Med Toxicol*, 1986, 1(1):12-31.

Verbeeck RK, "Pharmacokinetic Drug Interactions With Nonsteroidal Anti-inflammatory Drugs," *Clin Pharmacokinet*, 1990, 19(1):44-66.

Kevadon® *see* Thalidomide *on page 734*

Kiditard® *see* Quinidine *on page 668*

Kinidin® *see* Quinidine *on page 668*

Kir Richter® *see* Aprotinin *on page 130*

Kisolu® *see* Urokinase *on page 779*

Klacid® *see* Clarithromycin *on page 221*

Klaricid® *see* Clarithromycin *on page 221*

Klarivitina® *see* Cyproheptadine Hydrochloride *on page 255*

Klonopin™ *see* Clonazepam *on page 229*

K-Lor™ *see* Potassium Chloride *on page 634*

Kloral® *see* Chloral Hydrate *on page 193*

Kloral Hydrat *see* Chloral Hydrate *on page 193*

Klor-con® *see* Potassium Chloride *on page 634*

Kloromin® [OTC] *see* Chlorpheniramine Maleate *on page 204*

Klorvess® *see* Potassium Chloride *on page 634*

Klotrix® *see* Potassium Chloride *on page 634*

K-Lyte/CL® *see* Potassium Chloride *on page 634*

Knockout Drops *replaced by* Chloral Hydrate *on page 193*

Komex® *see* Boric Acid *on page 160*

Kondremul® [OTC] *see* Mineral Oil *on page 534*

KP24® *see* Malathion (Topical Lotion) *on page 489*

Kredex® *see* Carvedilol *on page 189*

K-Tab® *see* Potassium Chloride *on page 634*

Kwell® *see* Lindane *on page 470*

Kwells® *see* Scopolamine *on page 691*

Kytril® *see* Granisetron *on page 388*

***L*-3-Hydroxytyrosine** *see* Levodopa *on page 462*

LAAM *see* Levomethadyl Acetate Hydrochloride *on page 463*

Labetalol Hydrochloride (la bet' a lole)

Related Information

Beta-Blockers Comparison *on page 1644-1645*

CAS Number 36894-69-6; 32780-64-6

Brand Names Labrocol®; Normodyne®; Trandate®

Synonyms Ibidomide Hydrochloride

Use Treatment of mild to severe hypertension; I.V. for hypertensive emergencies

Mechanism of Action Blocks alpha-, beta$_1$-, and beta$_2$-adrenergic receptor sites; elevated renins are reduced; roughly 80% beta-blocker and 20% alpha-blocker

Adverse Reactions

Cardiovascular: Orthostatic hypotension especially with I.V. administration, edema, congestive heart failure, A-V conduction disturbances, bradycardia

Central nervous system: Drowsiness, fatigue, dizziness, behavior disorders, headache

Dermatologic: Tingling in scalp or skin (transient with initiation of therapy), rash

Gastrointestinal: Nausea, dry mouth, vomiting, diarrhea

Genitourinary: Sexual dysfunction, urinary problems

Hematologic: Leukopenia

Neuromuscular & skeletal: Paresthesia, reversible myopathy

Ocular: Diplopia (dose-related)

Respiratory: Wheezing, nasal congestion

Miscellaneous: Systemic lupus erythematosus (SLE) syndrome

Signs & Symptoms of Acute Overdose Hypotension, claudication, priapism, cholestatic jaundice, night terrors, impotence, lightheadedness, ejaculatory disturbances, hypoglycemia, dyspepsia, depression, heart failure, wheezing, oliguric renal failure, bradycardia, systemic lupus erythematosus (SLE), leukopenia; neutropenia; agranulocytosis; granulocytopenia

Toxicodynamics/Kinetics

Onset of action:

- Oral: 20 minutes to 2 hours
- I.V.: 2-5 minutes

Peak effect:

- Oral: 1-4 hours
- I.V.: 5-15 minutes

Duration:

- Oral: 8-24 hours (dose-dependent)
- I.V.: 2-4 hours

Absorption: Oral: Rapid and complete

Distribution: V_d: Adults: 3-16 L/kg, mean: 9.4 L/kg; widely distributed throughout the body

Protein binding: 50%

Metabolism: Extensive first-pass effect; metabolized in liver primarily via glucuronide conjugation

Bioavailability: Oral: 25%; increased bioavailability with liver disease, elderly and concurrent cimetidine

Half-life: 5.5-8 hours

Elimination: Possible decreased clearance in neonates/infants; <5% excreted in urine unchanged; clearance rate: 1100 mL/minute

Usual Dosage Due to limited documentation of its use, labetalol should be initiated cautiously in pediatric patients with careful dosage adjustment and blood pressure monitoring

Children:

Oral: Limited information regarding labetalol use in pediatric patients is currently available in literature. Some centers recommend initial oral doses of 4 mg/kg/day in 2 divided doses. Reported oral doses have started at 3 mg/kg/day and 20 mg/kg/day and have increased up to 40 mg/kg/day.

I.V., intermittent bolus doses of 0.3-1 mg/kg/dose have been reported.

For treatment of pediatric hypertensive emergencies, initial continuous infusions of 0.4-1 mg/kg/hour with a maximum of 3 mg/kg/hour have been used.

Adults:

Oral: Initial: 100 mg twice daily, may increase as needed every 2-3 days by 100 mg until desired response is obtained; usual dose: 200-400 mg twice daily; not to exceed 2.4 g/day

I.V.: 20 mg or 1-2 mg/kg whichever is lower, IVP over 2 minutes, may give 40-80 mg at 10-minute intervals, up to 300 mg total dose

I.V. infusion: Initial: 2 mg/minute; titrate to response up to 300 mg total dose

Contraindications Asthma, cardiogenic shock, uncompensated congestive heart failure, bradycardia, pulmonary edema, or heart block

Warnings Orthostatic hypotension may occur with I.V. administration; patient should remain supine during and for up to 3 hours after I.V. administration; paradoxical increase in blood pressure has been reported with treatment of pheochromocytoma or clonidine withdrawal syndrome; use with extreme caution in patients with hyper-reactive airway disease, congestive heart failure, diabetes mellitus, hepatic dysfunction

Dosage Forms

Injection: 5 mg/mL (20 mL, 40 mL, 60 mL)

Tablet: 100 mg, 200 mg, 300 mg

Stability Stable in D_5W, saline for 24 hours; Incompatible with alkaline solutions, $NaHCO_3$; use only solutions that are clear or slightly yellow; may cause a precipitate if exposed to alkaline admixture; parenteral admixture at room temperature (25°C) or refrigeration (4°C): 24 hours

Reference Range Toxic: Serum levels >500 ng/mL

Overdosage Treatment

Decontamination: Gastric lavage with activated charcoal with cathartic is recommended; do not use ipecac

Supportive therapy: Sympathomimetics (eg, epinephrine or dopamine), atropine, glucagon, or a pacemaker can be used to treat the toxic bradycardia, asystole, and/or hypotension; amrinone may also be effective for labetalol-induced hypotension; initially fluids may be the best treatment for toxic hypotension with norepinephrine being used for second-line therapy

Enhancement of elimination: Multiple dosing of activated charcoal may be useful

Test Interactions False-positive urine catecholamines, VMA if measured by fluorometric or photometric methods; use HPLC or specific catecholamine radioenzymatic technique; can cause positive antinuclear antibody; a labetalol metabolite (3-amino-1-phenylbutane or APB) may cause a false-positive result with amphetamine/methamphetamine by thin-layer chromatography or immunoassay

Drug Interactions Cimetidine may potentiate labetalol action, additive hypotensive effects with other hypotensive drugs, halothane used concurrently may further decrease blood pressure, glutethimide may decrease labetalol concentrations. An increased incidence of tremor may be seen with concomitant tricyclic antidepressant use.

Pregnancy Risk Factor C

Pregnancy Implications Crosses the placenta; small amounts in breast milk

Monitoring Parameters Blood pressure, standing and sitting/supine, pulse; EKG for conduction defects

Patient Information Do not stop medication without consulting physician

Additional Information Not shown to be effective for cocaine-cardiovascular toxicity

Specific References

Cournat A, Merli I, Duchier J, et al, "Hemodynamic Effects of Dilevalol Following Acute and Long-Term Administration in Normal and Hypertensive Subjects," *Am J Ther*, 1995, 2:250-4.

Gibert RB, Peng PI, and Wong D, "A Labetalol Metabolite With Analytical Characteristics Resembling Amphetamines," *J Anal Toxicol*, 1995, 19:84-6.

Kollef MH, "Labetalol Overdose Successfully Treated With Amrinone and Alpha-Adrenergic Receptor Agonists," *Chest*, 1994, 105(2):626-7.

MacCarthy EP and Bloomfield SS, "Labetalol: A Review of Its Pharmacology, Pharmacokinetics, Clinical Uses, and Adverse Effects," *Pharmacotherapy*, 1983, 3(4):193-219.

Smit AJ, Mulder PO, de Jong PE, et al, "Acute Renal Failure After Overdose of Labetalol," *Br Med J (Clin Res)*, 1986, 293:1142-3.

Zell-Kanter M and Leikin JB, "Oral Labetalol in Hypertensive Urgencies," *Am J Emerg Med*, 1991, 9(2):136-8.

Labrocol® *see* Labetalol Hydrochloride *on previous page*

Ladazol® *see* Danazol *on page 257*

LAM *see* Levomethadyl Acetate Hydrochloride *on page 463*

Lamictal® *see* Lamotrigine *on this page*

Lamotrigine (la moe' tri jeen)

CAS Number 84057-84-1

Brand Names Lamictal®

Synonyms BW-430-C; LTG

(Continued)

Lamotrigine *(Continued)*

Use Partial/secondary generalized seizures, childhood epilepsy

Mechanism of Action Triazine derivative which inhibits release of glutamate (an excitatory amino acid)

Adverse Reactions

Cardiovascular: A-V block

Central nervous system: Dizziness, drowsiness, sedation, agitation, hyporeflexia, chills

Dermatologic: Hypersensitivity rash, Stevens-Johnson syndrome, angioedema

Endocrine & metabolic: Hypokalemia

Neuromuscular & skeletal: Ataxia

Ocular: Nystagmus, diplopia

Renal: Hematuria

Miscellaneous: Dry mouth, thick secretions

Toxicodynamics/Kinetics

Distribution: V_d: 1.1 L/kg

Protein binding: 55%

Metabolism: Hepatic and renal

Bioavailability: 97.6%

Half-life: 24 hours; increases to 59 hours with concomitant valproic acid therapy; decreases with concomitant phenytoin or carbamazepine therapy to 15 hours

Elimination: Hepatic and renal

Usual Dosage

Initial dose: 50-100 mg/day then titrate to daily maintenance dose of 100-400 mg/day in 1-2 divided daily doses

With concomitant valproic acid therapy: Start initial dose at 25 mg/day then titrate to maintenance dose of 50-200 mg/day in 1-2 divided daily doses

Reference Range Therapeutic: 2-4 μg/mL

Overdosage Treatment

Decontamination: Lavage/activated charcoal with cathartic

Enhancement of elimination: Multiple dosing of activated charcoal may be useful

Drug Interactions Decreased effectiveness when given with acetaminophen (increased renal clearance)

Pregnancy Implications Not teratogenic in animal studies

Additional Information Low water solubility

Specific References

Brodie MJ, "Lamotrigine," *Lancet*, 1992, 339(8806):1397-400.

Garnett WR and Pellock JM, "Focus on Lamotrigine: A New Antiepileptic Drug for Patients With Partial Seizures," *Hosp Formul*, 1994, 29:806-12.

Gilman JT, "Lamotrigine: An Antiepileptic Agent for the Treatment of Partial Seizures," *Ann Pharmacother*, 1995, 29:144-51.

Goa KL, Ross SR, and Chrisp P, "Lamotrigine: A Review of Its Pharmacological Properties and Clinical Efficacy in Epilepsy," *Drugs*, 1993, 46(1):152-76.

Harchelroad F, Lang D, and Valeriano J, "Lamotrigine Overdose," *Vet Hum Toxicol*, 1994, 36:372.

Schirop Th, Lufft H, Winkler M, et al, "Bronchial Mucosa Reaction in Lyell-Stevens-Johnson Syndrome Following Lamotrigine," *Intensivmedizin und Notfallmedizin*, 1994, 31:343.

Lamprene® *see* Clofazimine Palmitate *on page 225*

Lamra® *see* Diazepam *on page 271*

Lanatrate® *see* Ergotamine *on page 317*

Laniazid® *see* Isoniazid *on page 443*

Lannett® *see* Piperazine Citrate *on page 629*

Lanocor® *see* Digoxin *on page 284*

Lanophyllin® *see* Theophylline *on page 735*

Lanoxicaps® *see* Digoxin *on page 284*

Lanoxin® *see* Digoxin *on page 284*

Lansoprazole (lan soe' pra zole)

CAS Number 103577-45-3

Brand Names Lanzor®; Ogast®; Prevacid®

Use Peptic ulcer treatment, reflux esophagitis, Zollinger-Ellison syndrome

Mechanism of Action Similar to omeprazole; a proton pump inhibitor which decreases acid secretion in gastric parietal cells

Adverse Reactions

Central nervous system: Fatigue, dizziness, headache

Gastrointestinal: Diarrhea (21%), nausea, vomiting, thirst

Otic: Tinnitus

Toxicodynamics/Kinetics

Duration of effect: 1 day

Absorption: Food decreases absorption by 50%

Distribution: V_d: 0.5 L/kg

Protein binding: 97%

Metabolism: Hepatic oxidation to two metabolites (active)
Half-life:
Healthy patients: 1.5 hours
Elderly: 2.9 hours
Cirrhosis: 7 hours
Elimination: Renal

Usual Dosage Oral:
Peptic ulcer: 30 mg/day (once daily) for 4 weeks
Reflux esophagitis: 30 mg/day for 8 weeks
Zollinger-Ellison syndrome: 60-120 mg once daily or 60 mg twice daily

Contraindications Hypersensitivity to lansoprazole

Warnings Reduce dosage in patients with cirrhosis and elderly

Dosage Forms Capsule, enteric coated: 30 mg

Reference Range Peak serum level after a 60 mg oral dose: 2.2 μg/mL

Overdosage Treatment
Decontamination: Emesis or lavage/activated charcoal
Enhancement of elimination: Multiple dosing of activated charcoal may be effective
Not dialyzable

Test Interactions Increased plasma gastrin levels may occur

Additional Information May have activity against *Helicobacter pylori*

Specific References

Holt S, "Proton-Pump Inhibition for Acid-Related Disease," *South Med J*, 1991, 84(9):1078-87.
Landes BD, Petite JP, and Flouvat B, "Clinical Pharmacokinetics of Lansoprazole," *Clin Pharmacokinet*, 1995, 28:458-70.

Lantanon® *see* Mianserin Hydrochloride *on page 529*
Lanzor® *see* Lansoprazole *on previous page*
Laractone® *see* Spironolactone *on page 705*
Largactil® *see* Chlorpromazine Hydrochloride *on page 205*
Larodopa® *see* Levodopa *on next page*
Lasilix® *see* Furosemide *on page 373*
Lasipressin® *see* Penbutolol Sulfate *on page 599*
Lasix® *see* Furosemide *on page 373*
Lassar's Zinc Paste *see* Zinc Oxide *on page 813*
Latiazem Hydrochloride *see* Diltiazem *on page 287*
Latycin® *see* Tetracycline *on page 732*
Laudanum *see* Opium Tincture *on page 580*
Laurel Camphor *see* Camphor *on page 179*
Lavacol® [OTC] *see* Ethyl Alcohol *on page 336*
Laxopol® *see* Castor Oil *on page 189*
Lax-Pills® [OTC] *see* Phenolphthalein *on page 617*
LCR *see* Vincristine Sulfate *on page 792*
***L*-Dopa** *see* Levodopa *on next page*
Legatrin® [OTC] *see* Quinine Sulfate *on page 671*
Lemiserp® *see* Reserpine *on page 678*
Lenident® *see* Procaine Hydrochloride *on page 644*
Lenoxin® *see* Digoxin *on page 284*
Lente *see* Insulin Preparations *on page 426*
Lente® Iletin® I *see* Insulin Preparations *on page 426*
Lente® Iletin® II *see* Insulin Preparations *on page 426*
Lente® Purified Pork Insulin *see* Insulin Preparations *on page 426*
Leponex® *see* Clozapine *on page 235*
Leptanal® *see* Fentanyl Citrate *on page 347*
Leptilan® *see* Valproic Acid and Derivatives *on page 782*
Lesten® *see* Rauwolfia Serpentina *on page 677*
Lethobard® *see* Pentobarbital *on page 604*
Leukeran® *see* Chlorambucil *on page 195*
Leurocristine *see* Vincristine Sulfate *on page 792*
Leustatin™ *see* Cladribine *on page 220*

Leutrol® *see* Zileuton *on page 811*

Levanxol® *see* Temazepam *on page 724*

Levatol® *see* Penbutolol Sulfate *on page 599*

Levaxin® *see* Levothyroxine Sodium *on page 465*

Levodopa (lee voe doe' pa)

Related Information

Therapeutic Drugs Associated With Hallucinations *on page 1558-1559*

CAS Number 59-92-7

Brand Names Dopar®; Larodopa®

Synonyms *L*-3-Hydroxytyrosine; *L*-Dopa

Use Treatment of Parkinson's disease; diagnostic agent for growth hormone deficiency

Mechanism of Action Increases dopamine levels in the brain, then stimulates dopaminergic receptors in the basal ganglia to improve the balance between cholinergic and dopaminergic activity

Adverse Reactions

Cardiovascular: Palpitations, cardiac arrhythmias, hypotension (orthostatic)

Central nervous system: Memory loss, nervousness, anxiety, insomnia, fatigue, psychosis, auditory and visual hallucinations, dystonic reactions, ataxia, electroencephalogram abnormalities

Gastrointestinal: Nausea, vomiting, gastrointestinal bleeding, anorexia

Hematologic: Hemolytic anemia with positive direct and indirect Coombs' tests, leukopenia, neutropenia, agranulocytosis, granulocytopenia

Ocular: Blurred vision

Signs & Symptoms of Acute Overdose Palpitations, night terrors, hypokalemia, pseudotumor cerebri, Parkinson's-like symptoms, pemphigus, hyperpigmented hair, dysosmia, dementia, depression, chorea (extrapyramidal), memory loss, mania, leukocytosis, paroxysmal tachycardia (ventricular), confusion, delirium, euphoria, insomnia, thrombocytopenia, systemic lupus erythematosus (SLE), hyponatremia, hyperuricemia, congestive heart failure, gout, arrhythmias, fibrillation (atrial), eosinophilia, spasm, myoclonus, nausea, vomiting, restlessness, hypertension, respiratory dyskinesias, extrapyramidal reaction including chorioathetosis, malignant hyperthermia reported, leukopenia, neutropenia, agranulocytosis, granulocytopenia; alopecia, urine discoloration (black), urine discoloration (brown), urine discoloration (dark), feces discoloration (black)

Toxicodynamics/Kinetics

Onset of action: Significant improvement may occur in 2-3 weeks; some patients may require up to 6 months of continuous levodopa therapy to obtain optimal therapeutic benefit

Peak effect: Oral: Peak serum level occurs within 1-2 hours

Duration: Up to 5 hours/dose

Absorption: Rapid from small intestine by an active amino acid transport system

Distribution: V_d: 1.1 L/kg; widely distributed to most body tissues but not to CNS

Protein binding: Not significant

Metabolism: Majority of drug is peripherally decarboxylated in gastrointestinal wall to dopamine; small amounts of levodopa reach the brain where it is also decarboxylated to active dopamine

Half-life: 1-3 hours

Time to peak serum concentration: Within 1-2 hours

Elimination: Excreted primarily in urine (80%) as dopamine, norepinephrine, and homovanillic acid; clearance: 0.3 L/hour/kg

Usual Dosage Oral:

Children (given as a single dose to evaluate growth hormone deficiency): 0.5 g/m^2

or

<30 lbs: 125 mg

30-70 lbs: 250 mg

>70 lbs: 500 mg

Adults (administer with food): 500-1000 mg/day in divided doses every 6-12 hours; increase by 100-750 mg/day every 3-7 days until response or total dose of 8000 mg is reached

Significant therapeutic response may not be obtained for 6 months

Contraindications Hypersensitivity to levodopa or any component; narrow-angle glaucoma, MAO inhibitor therapy, melanomas or any undiagnosed skin lesions

Warnings Dosages >200 mg/kg/day have been shown to decrease fetal and postnatal growth and viability in animals; use with caution in patients with history of myocardial infarction, cardiac arrhythmias, asthma, wide-angle glaucoma, peptic ulcer disease; sudden discontinuation of levodopa may cause a worsening of Parkinson's disease. Safety for use during pregnancy has not been established. Use only where potential benefits outweigh potential hazards to fetus. Dosages >200 mg/kg/day have been shown to decrease fetal and postnatal growth and viability in animals.

Dosage Forms
Capsule: 100 mg, 250 mg, 500 mg
Tablet: 100 mg, 250 mg, 500 mg

Reference Range Peak serum level of 3.2 mg/L occurs after ingestion of 200 mg levodopa

Overdosage Treatment
Decontamination: Emesis may be of value in only very early ingestions; lavage preferred in early ingestions; activated charcoal with cathartic of use
Supportive therapy: Deanol and pyridoxine of questionable use for dyskinesias, but have been tried; dantrolene and/or bromocriptine has been used in malignant hyperthermia
Enhancement of elimination: Multiple dose activated charcoal has not been addressed

Test Interactions False-positive reaction for urinary glucose with Clinitest®; false-negative reaction using Clinistix®; false-positive urine ketones with Acetest®, Ketostix®, Labstix®; serum uric acid may be elevated

Drug Interactions Monoamine oxidase inhibitors can cause hypertension (protective if carbidopa used); decreased anti-Parkinson effect with papaverine, phenytoin, pyridoxine, or clonidine

Pregnancy Risk Factor C

Monitoring Parameters Serum growth hormone concentration, CBC, renal function, EKG, liver function tests, intraocular pressure

Patient Information Avoid vitamins with B_6 (pyridoxine); can take with food to prevent gastritis; do not stop taking this drug even if you do not think it is working; dizziness, lightheadedness, fainting may occur when you get up from a sitting or lying position

Additional Information Single dose is not usually associated with the above adverse reactions

Specific References

Hoehn MM and Rutledge CO, "Acute Overdose With Levodopa: Clinical and Biochemical Consequences," *Neurology*, 1975, 25(8):792-4.
Nutt JG and Fellman JH, "Pharmacokinetics of Levodopa," *Clin Neuropharmacol*, 1984, 7(1):35-49.
Sporer KA, "Carbidopa-Levodopa Overdose," *Am J Emerg Med*, 1991, 9(1):47-8.

Levo-Dromoran® *see* Levorphanol Tartrate *on next page*

Levomethadyl Acetate Hydrochloride (lee voe meth' a dil)

CAS Number 1477-40-3; 34433-66-4

Brand Names ORLAAM®

Synonyms LAAM; LAM; L-Methadyl Acetate

Use Management of opiate dependence

Mechanism of Action Derivative of methadone but with a longer half-life

Adverse Reactions
Cardiovascular: Bradycardia, peripheral vasodilation, hypotension, intracranial pressure (increased)
Central nervous system: Drowsiness, dizziness, sedation, CNS depression
Endocrine & metabolic: Antidiuretic hormone release
Gastrointestinal: Nausea, vomiting, constipation
Ocular: Miosis
Respiratory: Apnea, respiratory depression
Miscellaneous: Biliary or urinary tract spasm

Signs & Symptoms of Acute Overdose Bradycardia, hypotension, syndrome of inappropriate antidiuretic hormone (SIADH), coma

Toxicodynamics/Kinetics
Protein binding: 80%
Metabolism: Hepatic to L-alpha-noracetylmethadol and L-alpha-dinoracetylmethadol (active metabolites)
Half-life: 35-60 hours
Time to peak serum concentration: 1.5-6 hours
Elimination: Renal products as methadol and normethadol

Usual Dosage Adults: Oral: 20-40 mg 3 times/week, with ranges of 10 mg to as high as 140 mg 3 times/week; always dilute before administration and mix with diluent prior to dispensing

Warnings Not recommended for uses outside of the treatment of opiate addiction; shall be dispensed only by treatment programs approved by FDA, DEA, and the designated state authority. Approved treatment programs shall dispense and use levomethadyl in oral form only and according to the treatment requirements stipulated in federal regulations. Failure to abide by these requirements may result in injunction precluding operation of the program, seizure of the drug supply, revocation of the program approval, and possible criminal prosecution.

(Continued)

Levomethadyl Acetate Hydrochloride *(Continued)*

Dosage Forms Solution, oral: 10 mg/mL (474 mL)

Stability Store at room temperature

Reference Range A 60 mg dose can result in a peak serum level of 130 ng/mL; at 24 hours, it is 50 ng/mL

Overdosage Treatment

Decontamination: Lavage/activated charcoal with cathartic

Supportive therapy: If opiate withdrawal symptoms occur, small doses of methadone (5-15 mg) or clonidine (0.1 mg every 4-6 hours) or guanabenz may be given (4 mg every 4-6 hours); naloxone can be given for CNS depression

Antidote(s)

Naloxone Hydrochloride *on page 1447*

Test Interactions Can cause positive opiate urine screen

Drug Interactions Decreased effect/levels with phenobarbital

Pregnancy Risk Factor C

Monitoring Parameters Patient adherence with regimen and avoidance of illicit substances; random drug testing is recommended

Nursing Implications Drug administration and dispensing is to take place in an authorized clinic setting only; can potentially cause Q-T prolongation on EKG (not dose related)

Specific References

Blaine JD, Renault PR, Thomas DB, et al, "Clinical Status of Methadyl Acetate (LAAM)," *Ann N Y Acad Sci*, 1981, 362:101-15.

Kaiko RF and Inturrisi CE, "Disposition of Acetylmethadol in Relation to Pharmacologic Action," *Clin Pharmacol Ther*, 1975, 18(1):96-103.

Levorphanol Tartrate (lee vor' fa nole)

Related Information

Pharmacokinetics of Narcotic Agonist Analgesics *on page 1654*

CAS Number 77-07-6; 125-72-4; 5985-38-6

Brand Names Dromoran®; Levo-Dromoran®

Synonyms Levorphan Tartrate

Use Relief of moderate to severe pain; also used parenterally for preoperative sedation and an adjunct to nitrous oxide/oxygen anesthesia; 2 mg levorphanol produces analgesia comparable to that produced by 10 mg of morphine

Mechanism of Action Levorphanol tartrate is a synthetic opioid agonist that is classified as a morphinan derivative. Opioids interact with stereospecific opioid receptors in various parts of the central nervous system and other tissues. Analgesic potency parallels the affinity for these binding sites. These drugs do not alter the threshold or responsiveness to pain, but the perception of pain.

Adverse Reactions

Cardiovascular: Palpitations, hypotension, bradycardia, peripheral vasodilation

Central nervous system: CNS depression

Dermatologic: Pruritus

Endocrine & metabolic: Syndrome of inappropriate antidiuretic hormone (SIADH)

Gastrointestinal: Nausea, vomiting, constipation

Ocular: Miosis

Respiratory: Apnea, respiratory depression

Miscellaneous: Intracranial pressure (increased), physical and psychological dependence, histamine release, biliary or urinary tract spasm

Toxicodynamics/Kinetics

Onset of action: Analgesic effect: 10-30 minutes

Duration: 8 hours

Half-life: 12-16 hours

Usual Dosage Adults:

Oral: 2 mg every 6-24 hours as needed

S.C.: 2 mg, up to 3 mg if necessary, every 6-8 hours

Dosing adjustment in hepatic disease: Reduction is necessary in patients with liver disease

Contraindications Hypersensitivity to levorphanol or any component

Warnings Use with caution in patients with hypersensitivity reactions to other phenanthrene derivative opioid agonists (morphine, hydrocodone, hydromorphone, levorphanol, oxycodone, oxymorphone); respiratory diseases including asthma, emphysema, COPD or severe liver or renal insufficiency; some preparations contain sulfites which may cause allergic reactions; may be habit-forming; dextromethorphan has equivalent antitussive activity but has much lower toxicity in accidental overdose

Dosage Forms

Injection: 2 mg/mL (1 mL, 10 mL)

Tablet: 2 mg

Stability Store at room temperature, protect from freezing; I.V. is **incompatible** when mixed with aminophylline, barbiturates, heparin, methicillin, phenytoin, sodium bicarbonate

Overdosage Treatment Supportive therapy: Naloxone hydrochloride (0.4-2 mg I.V., S.C., or through an endotracheal tube); a continuous infusion (at ⅔ the response dose/hour) may be required

Antidote(s)

Naloxone Hydrochloride *on page 1447*

Drug Interactions

Increased effect with methylphenidate (↑ efficacy, ↓ respiratory depression)

Increased toxicity with CNS depressants (CNS depression); may potentiate toxicity (hyperthermia) of MAO inhibitors

Pregnancy Risk Factor B (D if used for prolonged periods or in high doses at term)

Monitoring Parameters Pain relief, respiratory and mental status, blood pressure

Patient Information Avoid alcohol, may cause drowsiness, impaired judgment or coordination; may be addicting if used for prolonged periods

Nursing Implications Observe patient for excessive sedation, respiratory depression, implement safety measures, assist with ambulation

Specific References

Sinclair JG and Lo GF, "The Blockade of Serotonin Uptake and the Meperidine-Monoamine Oxidase Inhibitor Interaction," *Proc West Pharmacol Soc*, 1977, 20:373-4.

Levorphan Tartrate *see* Levorphanol Tartrate *on previous page*

Levo-T™ *see* Levothyroxine Sodium *on this page*

Levothroid® *see* Levothyroxine Sodium *on this page*

Levothyroxine Sodium (lee voe thye rox' een)

Related Information

Liothyronine Sodium *on page 471*

Therapeutic Drugs Associated With Hallucinations *on page 1558-1559*

CAS Number 51-48-9; 55-03-8; 25416-65-3; 8065-29-0

Brand Names Dexnon®; Eferox®; Euthyrox®; Levaxin®; Levo-T™; Levothroid®; Levoxine®; Synthroid®; Thevier®; Thyrax®

Synonyms *L*-Thyroxine Sodium; T_4

Use Replacement or supplemental therapy in hypothyroidism; some clinicians suggest levothyroxine is the drug of choice for replacement therapy

Mechanism of Action Exact mechanism of action is unknown; however, it is believed the thyroid hormone exerts its many metabolic effects through control of DNA transcription and protein synthesis; involved in normal metabolism, growth, and development; promotes gluconeogenesis, increases utilization and mobilization of glycogen stores, and stimulates protein synthesis, increases basal metabolic rate

Adverse Reactions

Cardiovascular: Palpitations, tachycardia, cardiac arrhythmias

Central nervous system: Nervousness, insomnia, fever, headache, visual hallucinations

Dermatologic: Hair loss

Gastrointestinal: Diarrhea, abdominal cramps, weight loss, appetite (increased)

Neuromuscular & skeletal: Tremors

Miscellaneous: Sweating

Signs & Symptoms of Acute Overdose Tachycardia, hypertension, pseudotumor cerebri, agitation, insomnia, seizures (may occur up to 1 week postingestion), coma

Toxicodynamics/Kinetics

Oral: Onset of therapeutic effect: 3-5 days following administration

I.V.

- Onset of effect: Within 6-8 hours
- Peak effect: Within 24 hours

Absorption: Oral: Erratic (30% to 90%)

Metabolism: In the liver to tri-iodothyronine (active)

Half-life:

- T_3: 1 day; in overdose: 2.8 days
- T_4: 6 days; in overdose: 6 days

Time to peak serum concentration: 2-4 hours

Elimination: Excreted in feces (20%) and urine

Usual Dosage

Children:

Oral:

- 0-6 months: 8-10 mcg/kg/day or 25-50 mcg
- 6-12 months: 6-8 mcg/kg/day or 50-75 mcg
- 1-5 years: 5-6 mcg/kg/day or 75-100 mcg
- 6-12 years: 4-5 mcg/kg/day or 100-150 mcg
- >12 years: 2-3 mcg/kg/day or ≥150 mcg

(Continued)

Levothyroxine Sodium *(Continued)*

I.M., I.V.: 50% to 75% of oral dose

Adults:

Oral: 12.5-50 mcg/day to start, then increase by 25-50 mcg/day at intervals of 2-4 weeks; average adult dose: 100-200 mcg/day

I.M., I.V.: 50% of the oral dose

Myxedema coma or stupor: I.V.: 200-500 mcg one time, then 100-300 mcg the next day if necessary

Administration Dilute vial with 5 mL normal saline; use immediately after reconstitution; give by direct I.V. infusion over 2- to 3-minute period

Contraindications Recent myocardial infarction or thyrotoxicosis, uncorrected adrenal cortical insufficiency, hypersensitivity to active or extraneous constituents

Warnings Some preparations contain tartrazine; ineffective for weight reduction; high doses may produce serious or even life-threatening toxic effects particularly when used with some anorectic drugs; use cautiously in patients with pre-existing cardiovascular disease (angina, CHD), elderly since they may be more likely to have compromised cardiovascular functions; adrenal cortical insufficiency, myxedema, diabetes mellitus and insipidus may have symptoms exaggerated or aggravated; thyroid replacement requires periodic assessment of thyroid status. Chronic hypothyroidism predisposes patients to coronary artery disease. Elderly do not have a change in serum thyroxine associated with aging; however, plasma T_3 concentrations are decreased 25% to 40% in elderly. There is not a compensatory rise in thyrotropin suggesting that lower T_3 is not reacted upon as a deficiency by the pituitary. This indicates a slightly lower than normal dosage of thyroid hormone replacement is usually sufficient in older patients than in younger adult patients. TSH must be monitored since insufficient thyroid replacement (elevated TSH) is a risk for coronary artery disease and excessive replacement (low TSH) may cause signs of hyperthyroidism and excessive bone loss.

Dosage Forms

Powder for injection, lyophilized: 0.2 mg/vial (6 mL, 10 mL); 0.5 mg/vial (6 mL, 10 mL)

Tablet: 0.025 mg, 0.05 mg, 0.075 mg, 0.088 mg, 0.1 mg, 0.112 mg, 0.125 mg, 0.15 mg, 0.175 mg, 0.2 mg, 0.3 mg

Stability Protect tablets from light; do not mix I.V. solution with other I.V. infusion solutions; reconstituted solutions should be used immediately and any unused portions discarded

Reference Range Correlation is poor with symptomatology in acute overdose

Pediatrics: Cord T_4 and values in the first few weeks are much higher, falling over the first months and years

$\geq$10 years: ~5.8-11.0 μg/dL (SI: 75-142 nmol/L)

Borderline low: 4.5-5.7 μg/dL (SI: 58-73 nmol/L) or less

Low: $\leq$4.4 μg/dL (SI: $\leq$57 nmol/L); results <2.5 μg/dL (SI: <32 nmol/L) are strong evidence for hypothyroidism

Adults:

Approximate normal range: 4.0-12.0 μg/dL (SI: 51-154 nmol/L)

Borderline high: 11.1-13.0 μg/dL (SI: 143-167 nmol/L)

High: $\geq$13.1 μg/dL (SI: $\geq$169 nmol/L)

Normal range is increased in women on birth control pills (5.5-12.0 μg/dL)

Normal range in pregnancy: ~5.5-16.0 μg/dL (SI: ~71-206 nmol/L)

TSH: 0.4-10.0 (for those $\geq$80 years) mIU/L

T_4: 4.0-12.0 μg/dL (51-154 nmol/L)

T_3 (RIA) (total T_3): 80-230 ng/dL (1.2-3.5 nmol/L)

T_4, free: 0.7-1.8 ng/dL (9-23 pmol/L)

Overdosage Treatment

Decontamination: Gastric emptying indicated for ingestions >5 mg; ipecac or lavage with activated charcoal with cathartic

Supportive therapy: Propranolol may be used for hyperadrenergic signs (1 mg I.V. in adults, 0.01-0.1 mg/kg in pediatrics); sodium ipodate (3 g/1.7 m^2) has been used in acute ingestion to prevent T_4 to T_3 conversion

Enhancement of elimination: Plasmapheresis increases elimination 30-fold while charcoal hemoperfusion enhances T_4 elimination fivefold

Test Interactions Many drugs may have effects on thyroid function tests; para-aminosalicylic acid, aminoglutethimide, amiodarone, barbiturates, carbamazepine, chloral hydrate, clofibrate, colestipol, corticosteroids, danazol, diazepam, estrogens, ethionamide, fluorouracil, I.V. heparin, insulin, lithium, methadone, methimazole, mitotane, nitroprusside, oxyphenbutazone, phenylbutazone, PTU, perphenazine, phenytoin, propranolol, salicylates, sulfonylureas, and thiazides

Drug Interactions

Decreased effect: ↑ oral hypoglycemic requirements, phenytoin → ↓ levothyroxine levels, cholestyramine → ↓ absorption of levothyroxine

Increased effect: ↑ effect of oral anticoagulants

Increased toxicity: Tricyclic antidepressants → ↑ toxic potential of both drugs

Pregnancy Risk Factor A

Monitoring Parameters Thyroid function test (serum thyroxine, thyrotropin concentrations), resin tri-iodothyronine uptake (RT_3U), free thyroxine index (FTI), T_4, TSH, heart rate, blood pressure, clinical signs of hypo- and hyperthyroidism; TSH is the most reliable guide for evaluating adequacy of thyroid replacement dosage. TSH may be elevated during the first few months of thyroid replacement despite patients being clinically euthyroid. In cases where T_4 remains low and TSH is within normal limits, an evaluation of "free" (unbound) T_4 is needed to evaluate further increase in dosage

Patient Information Do not change brands without physician's knowledge; report immediately to physician any chest pain, increased pulse, palpitations, heat intolerances, excessive sweating; do not discontinue without notifying your physician

Nursing Implications I.V. form must be prepared immediately prior to administration; should not be admixed with other solutions

Additional Information Levothroid® tablets contain lactose; levothyroxine sodium is soluble in water

Specific References

Bauer LA, "Simulations of Levothyroxine Bioavailability Using a Single Dose Protocol," *Am J Therap*, 1995, 2:414-6.

Berkner PD, Starkman H, and Person N, "Acute L-Thyroxine Overdose: Therapy With Sodium Ipodate: Evaluation of Clinical and Physiologic Parameters," *J Emerg Med*, 1991, 9(3):129-31.

Binimelis J, Bassas L, Marruecos L, et al, "Massive Thyroxine Intoxication: Evaluation of Plasma Extraction," *Intens Care Med*, 1987, 13(1):33-8.

Escalante DA, Arem N, and Arem R, "Assessment of Interchangeability of Two Brands of Levothyroxine Preparations With a Third-Generation TSH Assay," *Am J Med*, 1995, 98:374.

Gorman RL, Chamberlain JM, Rose SR, et al, "Massive Levothyroxine Overdose: High Anxiety – Low Toxicity," *Pediatrics*, 1988, 82(4):666-9.

Kulig K, Golightly LK, and Rumack BH, "Levothyroxine Overdose Associated With Seizures in a Young Child," *JAMA*, 1985, 254(15):2109-10.

Mandel SH, Magnusson AR, Burton BT, et al, "Massive Levothyroxine Ingestion: Conservative Management," *Clin Pediatr (Phila)*, 1989, 28(8):374-6.

Mayor GH, Orlando T, and Kurtz N, "Limitations of Levothyroxine Bioequivalence Evaluation: Analysis of an Attempted Study," *Am J Therap*, 1995, 2:417-32.

Tunget CL, Clark RF, Turchen SG, et al, "Raising the Decontamination Level for Thyroid Hormone Ingestions," *Am J Emerg Med*, 1995, 13(1):9-13.

Levoxine® *see* Levothyroxine Sodium *on page 465*

Levsin® *see* Hyoscyamine Sulfate *on page 415*

Levsinex® *see* Hyoscyamine Sulfate *on page 415*

l-Hyoscyamine Sulfate *see* Hyoscyamine Sulfate *on page 415*

Libritabs® *see* Chlordiazepoxide *on page 198*

Librium® *see* Chlordiazepoxide *on page 198*

Lidocaine and Epinephrine (lye' doe kane & ep i nef' rin)

Brand Names Xylocaine® With Epinephrine

Use Local infiltration anesthesia

Mechanism of Action Lidocaine blocks both the initiation and conduction of nerve impulses via decreased permeability of sodium ions; epinephrine increases the duration of action of lidocaine by causing vasoconstriction (via alpha effects) which slows the vascular absorption of lidocaine

Adverse Reactions

Cardiovascular: Hypotension, bradycardia

Central nervous system: Lightheadedness, myasthenia gravis (exacerbation or precipitation of), nervousness, confusion, dizziness, drowsiness, seizures, confusion

Dermatologic: Urticaria

Neuromuscular & skeletal: Tremors

Ocular: Blurred vision

Otic: Ototoxicity, tinnitus

Respiratory: Wheezing

Toxicodynamics/Kinetics

Duration of action: 2-6 hours, dependent on dose and anesthetic procedure

Absorption: Completely systemic

Metabolism: Xylidine metabolites are actively toxic, but less so than the parent compound

Time to peak serum concentration: Usually 10-30 minutes; dependent upon factors affecting rate of absorption; may occur 1-3 minutes after intravascular or transtracheal injection

Elimination: Renal excretion primarily as metabolites, 10% unchanged

Usual Dosage Dosage varies with the anesthetic procedure

Children: Use lidocaine concentrations of 0.5% or 1% (or even more dilute) to decrease possibility of toxicity; lidocaine dose should not exceed 4.5 mg/kg/dose; do not repeat within 2 hours

Contraindications Hypersensitivity to local anesthetics of the amide type

Warnings Some products contain sulfites which may cause allergic reactions in

(Continued)

Lidocaine and Epinephrine *(Continued)*

sensitive individual; do not use solutions in distal portions of the body (digits, nose, ears, penis); do not use large doses in patients with conduction defects (eg, heart block)

Dosage Forms Injection with epinephrine:

1:200,000: Lidocaine hydrochloride 0.5% [5 mg/mL] (50 mL); 1% [10 mg/mL] (30 mL); 1.5% [15 mg/mL] (5 mL, 10 mL, 30 mL); 2% [20 mg/mL] (20 mL)

1:100,000: Lidocaine hydrochloride 1% [10 mg/mL] (20 mL, 50 mL); 2% [20 mg/mL] (1.8 mL, 20 mL, 50 mL)

1:50,000: Lidocaine hydrochloride 2% [20 mg/mL] (1.8 mL)

Stability Solutions with epinephrine should be protected from light; pH: 3.3-5.5

Overdosage Treatment Treatment is primarily symptomatic and supportive. Termination of anesthesia by pneumatic tourniquet inflation should be attempted when the agent is administered by infiltration or regional injection. Seizures commonly respond to diazepam or lorazepam, while hypotension responds to I.V. fluids and Trendelenburg positioning. Bradyarrhythmias (when the heart rate is less than 60) can be treated with I.V., or S.C. atropine 15 mcg/kg. With the development of metabolic acidosis, I.V. sodium bicarbonate 0.5-2 mEq/kg and ventilatory assistance should be instituted. Methemoglobinemia should be treated with methylene blue 1-2 mg/kg in a 1% sterile aqueous solution I.V. push over 4-6 minutes repeated up to a total dose of 7 mg/kg.

Antidote(s)

Methylene Blue *on page 1444*

Diagnostic Tests/Procedures

Methemoglobin, Blood *on page 1296*

Drug Interactions MAO inhibitors, tricyclic antidepressants

Pregnancy Risk Factor C

Nursing Implications Before injecting, withdraw syringe plunger to ensure injection is not into vein or artery

Additional Information Contains metabisulfites

Lidocaine Hydrochloride (lye' doe kane)

Related Information

Status Epilepticus Treatment Algorithm *on page 1608*

CAS Number 73-78-9; 6108-05-0

Brand Names Anestacon®; Baylocaine®; Dalcaine®; Dilocaine®; Duo-Trach®; LidoPen®; Nervocaine®; Norocaine®; Octocaine®; Xylocaine®

Synonyms Lignocaine Hydrochloride

Use Local anesthetic and acute treatment of ventricular arrhythmias from myocardial infarction, cardiac manipulation, digitalis intoxication

Mechanism of Action Class IB antiarrhythmic; suppresses automaticity of conduction tissue, by increasing electrical stimulation threshold of ventricle, HIS-Purkinje system, and spontaneous depolarization of the ventricles during diastole by a direct action on the tissues; blocks both the initiation and conduction of nerve impulses by decreasing the neuronal membrane's permeability to sodium ions, which results in inhibition of depolarization with resultant blockade of conduction

Adverse Reactions

Cardiovascular: Bradycardia, hypotension, heart block with sinus arrest, cardiac arrhythmias (tachycardia (ventricular)), cardiovascular collapse, torsade de pointes

Central nervous system: Lethargy, coma, agitation, slurred speech, seizures, psychosis, anxiety, euphoria, hallucinations, circumoral numbness

Gastrointestinal: Nausea, vomiting

Hematologic: Porphyria

Neuromuscular & skeletal: Paresthesia

Ocular: Blurred vision, diplopia, miosis

Otic: Ototoxicity, tinnitus

Respiratory: Depression or arrest

Miscellaneous: Porphyrinogenic

Signs & Symptoms of Acute Overdose Convulsions, asystole, methemoglobinemia, numbness, disorientation, respiratory failure, ptosis, mydriasis, A-V block, tachycardia (ventricular), diplopia, heart block, myoclonus, tremors, myasthenia gravis (exacerbation or precipitation of), delirium, slurred speech, agitation, coma, bradycardia, nystagmus, hypotension, cardiovascular collapse, euphoria, ototoxicity; tinnitus, methemoglobinemia may occur

Toxicodynamics/Kinetics

Onset of action: 45-90 seconds (single bolus dose)

Duration: 10-20 minutes

Absorption:

Oral: 30%

I.M.: Nearly complete

Distribution: V_d: Alterable by many patient factors; decreased V_d in CHF and liver disease; usually about 1.1 L/kg, although 2.2 L/kg has been described in a pediatric overdose; distributes rapidly into most body tissues; high affinity for adipose tissue

Protein binding: 60% to 80%; binds to alpha$_1$-acid glycoprotein

Metabolism: 95% in liver; active metabolites monoethylglycinexylidide (MEGX) and glycinexylidide (GX) can accumulate and may cause CNS toxicity

Half-life: Biphasic: Alpha: 7-30 minutes; Beta (terminal) adults: 1.5-2 hours; (terminal) premature infants: 3.2 hours; increased half-life with CHF, liver disease, shock, severe renal disease

Elimination: Renal excretion, 10% unchanged

Usual Dosage

Topical: Apply to affected area as needed; maximum: 3 mg/kg/dose; do not repeat within 2 hours

Injectable local anesthetic: Varies with procedure, degree of anesthesia needed, vascularity of tissue, duration of anesthesia required, and physical condition of patient; maximum: 4.5 mg/kg/dose; do not repeat within 2 hours

Children: E.T., I.V.: Loading dose: 1 mg/kg; may repeat in 10-15 minutes x 2 doses; after loading dose, start I.V. continuous infusion 20-50 mcg/kg/minute. Use 20 mcg/kg/minute in patients with shock, hepatic disease, mild congestive heart failure (CHF); moderate to severe CHF may require ½ loading dose and lower infusion rates to avoid toxicity. Dilute 150 mg x weight (kg) to 250 mL D_5W; then dose in mcg/kg/minute = 10 x infusion rate in mL/hour.

Endotracheal doses should be diluted to 1-2 mL with normal saline prior to endotracheal administration.

Adults: Antiarrhythmic:

I.M.: 300 mg may be repeated in 1-1.5 hours

E.T., I.V.: 50-100 mg bolus over 2-3 minutes; may repeat in 5-10 minutes up to 200-300 mg in a 1-hour period; continuous infusion of 20-50 mcg/kg/minute or 1-4 mg/minute; decrease the dose in patients with CHF, shock, or hepatic disease

Infusion pump should be used for I.V. infusion administration I.V. infusion rates (2 g/250 mL D_5W):

1 mg/minute: 7 mL/hour
2 mg/minute: 15 mL/hour
3 mg/minute: 21 mL/hour
4 mg/minute: 30 mL/hour

Contraindications Known hypersensitivity to amide-type local anesthetics; patients with Adams-Stokes syndrome, Wolff-Parkinson-White syndrome, or with severe degree of S-A, A-V, or intraventricular heart block (without a pacemaker)

Warnings Do not use preparations containing preservatives for spinal or epidural (including caudal) anesthesia; hepatic disease, heart failure, marked hypoxia, severe respiratory depression, hypovolemia or shock; incomplete heart block or bradycardia, fibrillation (atrial), renal dysfunction

Dosage Forms

Cream: 2% (56 g)

Injection: 0.5% [5 mg/mL] (50 mL); 1% [10 mg/mL] (2 mL, 5 mL, 10 mL, 20 mL, 30 mL, 50 mL); 1.5% [15 mg/mL] (20 mL); 2% [20 mg/mL] (2 mL, 5 mL, 10 mL, 20 mL, 30 mL, 50 mL); 4% [40 mg/mL] (5 mL); 10% [100 mg/mL] (10 mL); 20% [200 mg/mL] (10 mL, 20 mL)

Injection:

I.M. use: 10% [100 mg/mL] (3 mL, 5 mL)

Direct I.V.: 1% [10 mg/mL] (5 mL, 10 mL); 20 mg/mL (5 mL)

I.V. admixture, preservative free: 4% [40 mg/mL] (25 mL, 30 mL); 10% [100 mg/mL] (10 mL); 20% [200 mg/mL] (5 mL, 10 mL)

I.V. infusion, in D_5W: 0.2% [2 mg/mL] (500 mL); 0.4% [4 mg/mL] (250 mL, 500 mL, 1000 mL); 0.8% [8 mg/mL] (250 mL, 500 mL)

Jelly, topical: 2% (30 mL)

Liquid, viscous: 2% (20 mL, 100 mL)

Ointment, topical: 2.5% [OTC], 5% (35 g)

Solution, topical: 2% [20 mg/mL] (15 mL, 240 mL); 4% [40 mg/mL] (50 mL)

Stability I.V. infusion solutions admixed in D_5W is stable for a minimum of 24 hours; precipitates with amphotericin, methohexitone, or sulfadiazine

Reference Range

Therapeutic: 1.5-4.0 µg/mL (SI: 6.4-17.1 µmol/L), up to 6.0 µg/mL (SI: 25.6 µmol/L) if necessary

Toxic: >8.0 µg/mL (SI: >34.2 µmol/L)

Fatal: >15.0 µg/mL are associated with fatalities

Overdosage Treatment

Decontamination: Oral: Do not use ipecac due to possible development of seizures; lavage/activated charcoal with cathartic

Supportive therapy: Termination of anesthesia by pneumatic tourniquet inflation should be attempted when the agent is administered by infiltration or regional injection. Seizures commonly respond to diazepam or lorazepam, while hypo-

(Continued)

Lidocaine Hydrochloride *(Continued)*

tension responds to I.V. fluids and Trendelenburg positioning. Refractory hypotension can be treated with norepinephrine, dopamine, dobutamine, or intra-aortic balloons. Bradyarrhythmias (when the heart rate is less than 60) can be treated with I.V. atropine 15 mcg/kg, isoproterenol, or a pacemaker. With the development of metabolic acidosis, I.V. sodium bicarbonate 0.5-2 mEq/kg and ventilatory assistance should be instituted. Methemoglobinemia should be treated with methylene blue 1-2 mg/kg in a 1% sterile aqueous solution I.V. push over 4-6 minutes repeated up to a total dose of 7 mg/kg. Cardiopulmonary bypass and cardiac pacing has been utilized

Enhancement of elimination: Arteriovenous hemofiltration is also not useful; not dialyzable (0% to 5%)

Test Interactions Falsely lowered if blood makes contact with stopper of tube

Diagnostic Tests/Procedures

Lidocaine, Blood *on page 1284*

Drug Interactions Concomitant cimetidine or propranolol may result in increased serum concentrations of lidocaine with resultant toxicity; highly lipid soluble beta-blockers may impair lidocaine clearance

Pregnancy Risk Factor C (CNS and cardiac toxicity have been described in the setting of fetal acidosis)

Pregnancy Implications Crosses the placenta

Monitoring Parameters Monitor EKG continuously, serum lidocaine concentration, obtain methemoglobin level

Nursing Implications Local thrombophlebitis may occur in patients receiving prolonged I.V. infusions

Additional Information Odorless, bitter taste

Specific References

Amitai Y, Whitesell L, and Lovejoy FH Jr, "Death Following Accidental Lidocaine Overdose in a Child," *N Engl J Med*, 1986, 314(3):181-2.

Gonzalez del Rey J, Wason S, and Druckenbrod RW, "Lidocaine Overdose: Another Preventable Case," *Pediatr Emerg Care*, 1994, 10(6):344-6.

Krause RS, Filice M, Hughes D, et al, "Effect of Injection Speed on Pain of Lidocaine Infiltration," *Acad Emerg Med*, 1995, 2:463-4.

Noble J, Kennedy DJ, Latimer RD, et al, "Massive Lignocaine Overdose During Cardiopulmonary Bypass. Successful Treatment With Cardiac Pacing," *Br J Anaesth*, 1984, 56(12):1439-41.

Lidone® *see* Molindone Hydrochloride *on page 537*

LidoPen® *see* Lidocaine Hydrochloride *on page 468*

Lignocaine Hydrochloride *see* Lidocaine Hydrochloride *on page 468*

Limifen® *see* Alfentanil Hydrochloride *on page 94*

Lindane (lin' dane)

CAS Number 58-89-9

UN Number 2761

Brand Names G-well®; Kwell®; Scabene®

Synonyms Benzene Hexachloride; Gamma Benzene Hexachloride; Hexachlorocyclohexane

Use Treatment of scabies (*Sarcoptes scabiei*) and pediculosis (*Pediculus humanus capitis* – head lice, *Pediculus pubis* – crab lice)

Mechanism of Action Directly absorbed by parasites and ova through the exoskeleton; stimulates the nervous system resulting in seizures and death of parasitic arthropods; interferes with the gamma-aminobutyric acid A receptor chloride channel complex in the synapse

Adverse Reactions

Central nervous system: Dizziness, restlessness, seizures, headache, ataxia

Dermatologic: Eczema, contact dermatitis, urticaria

Gastrointestinal: Nausea, vomiting, diarrhea

Hematologic: Aplastic anemia

Hepatic: Hepatitis

Renal: Hematuria

Respiratory: Pulmonary edema, aspiration

Miscellaneous: Skin and adipose tissue may act as repositories

Signs & Symptoms of Acute Overdose Vomiting, restlessness, myoglobinuria, ataxia, seizures, blindness, nausea, rhabdomyolysis, neutropenia, arrhythmia, pulmonary edema, hematuria, hepatitis, respiratory depression, thrombocytopenia, agitation, lactic acidosis, disseminated intravascular coagulation, muscle necrosis

Toxicodynamics/Kinetics

Absorption: Systemic, up to 13% may occur; significantly absorbed through skin

Distribution: Stored in body fat

Metabolism: By the liver to 2,3,4,6-tetra chlorophenol

Half-life: Children: 17-22 hours

Time to peak serum concentration: Children: Topical: Within 6 hours after application

Elimination: Excreted in urine, feces, and breast milk

Usual Dosage Children and Adults: Topical:

Pediculosis/Scabies: Apply a thin layer of lotion or cream and massage it on skin from the neck to the toes (head to toe in infants). For adults, bathe and remove the drug after 8-12 hours; for children, wash off 6-8 hours after application (for infants, wash off 6 hours after application); repeat treatment in 7 days if lice or nits are still present.

Pediculosis, capitis and pubis: 15-30 mL of shampoo is applied and lathered for 4-5 minutes; rinse hair thoroughly and comb with a fine tooth comb to remove nits; repeat treatment in 7 days if lice or nits are still present

Contraindications Hypersensitivity to lindane or any component; premature neonates; acutely inflamed skin or raw, weeping surfaces; liver disease; patients with seizure disorder may be at increased risk for seizures

Warnings Use with caution in infants and small children; avoid contact with the face, eyes, mucous membranes, and urethral meatus

Dosage Forms

Cream: 1% (60 g, 454 g)

Lotion: 1% (60 mL, 473 mL, 4000 mL)

Shampoo: 1% (60 mL, 473 mL, 4000 mL)

Reference Range Lindane serum level of 0.13 μg/mL associated with seizures

Overdosage Treatment

Decontamination: Use soap and water to decontaminate the skin; cholestyramine may be effective in hastening elimination

Supportive therapy: Absorbed through skin and mucous membranes and gastrointestinal tract, has occasionally caused serious CNS, hepatic and renal toxicity when used excessively for prolonged periods, or when accidental ingestion has occurred; emesis should not be induced since seizures can occur within 15 minutes of ingestion; activated charcoal is effective. Do not give with milk, oil, or fatty food since it may enhance absorption. Diazepam and/or phenytoin can be used to treat seizures.

Enhancement of elimination: Hemoperfusion may be effective if performed early

Antidote(s)

Cholestyramine Resin *on page 1405*

Drug Interactions Oil-based hair dressing

Pregnancy Risk Factor B

Pregnancy Implications No fetal harm in animal studies receiving up to 10 times the normal dosage, do not use during breast feeding

Patient Information For topical use only; do not apply to face; avoid getting in eyes

Nursing Implications Drug should not be administered orally

Additional Information Consider alternative therapies (ie, crotamiton) for treatment of scabies in infants and children <10 years; drug has a bitter taste

Fatal oral dose: Adults: 28 g

TLV-TWA: 0.5 mg/m^3

IDLH: 1000 ppm

OSHA PEL-TWA: 0.5 mg/m^2

Specific References

Aks S, Krantz A, Hryhorczuk DO, et al, "Acute Accidental Oral Lindane Ingestions in Toddlers," *Vet Hum Toxicol*, 1994, 36:375.

Davies JE, Dedhia HV, Morgade C, et al, "Lindane Poisonings," *Arch Dermatol*, 1983, 119(2):142-4.

Kurt TL, Bost R, Gilliland M, et al, "Accidental Kwell® (Lindane) Ingestions," *Vet Hum Toxicol*, 1986, 28(6):569-71.

Solomon BA, Haut SR, Carr EM, et al, "Neurotoxic Reaction to Lindane in an HIV-Sero Positive Patient, An Old Medication's New Problem," *J Fam Pract*, 1995, 40(3):291-5-6.

Linfolysin® *see* Chlorambucil *on page 195*

Lioresal® *see* Baclofen *on page 143*

Liothyronine Sodium (lye oh thye' roe neen)

Related Information

Levothyroxine Sodium *on page 465*

CAS Number 55-06-1; 6893-03-3

Brand Names Cytomel®; Tertroxin®; Ti-Tre®; Triostat™

Synonyms Sodium *L*-Tri-iodothyronine; T_3 Sodium

Use Replacement or supplemental therapy in hypothyroidism, management of nontoxic goiter, chronic lymphocytic thyroiditis, as an adjunct in thyrotoxicosis and as a diagnostic aid; levothyroxine is recommended for chronic therapy. If rapid correction of thyroid is needed, T_3 is preferred but use cautiously and with lower recommended doses

(Continued)

Liothyronine Sodium *(Continued)*

Mechanism of Action Primary active compound is T_3 (tri-iodothyronine), which may be converted from T_4 (thyroxine) and then circulates throughout the body to influence growth and maturation of various tissues; exact mechanism of action is unknown; however, it is believed the thyroid hormone exerts its many metabolic effects through control of DNA transcription and protein synthesis; involved in normal metabolism, growth, and development; promotes gluconeogenesis, increases utilization and mobilization of glycogen stores, and stimulates protein synthesis, increases basal metabolic rate

Adverse Reactions

Cardiovascular: Palpitations, tachycardia, cardiac arrhythmias
Central nervous system: Nervousness, insomnia, fever, headache
Dermatologic: Hair loss
Gastrointestinal: Weight loss, appetite (increased), diarrhea, abdominal cramps
Neuromuscular & skeletal: Tremors
Miscellaneous: Sweating

Signs & Symptoms of Acute Overdose Tachycardia, hyperthyroidism, sweating, insomnia

Toxicodynamics/Kinetics

Onset of effect: Within 24-72 hours
Peak therapeutic effect: 72 hours
Duration: Up to 72 hours
Absorption: Oral: Well absorbed (~85% to 90%)
Metabolism: In the liver to inactive compounds
Half-life: 16-49 hours
Elimination: Urine

Usual Dosage

Congenital hypothyroidism: Children: Oral: 5 mcg/day increase by 5 mcg every 3 days to 20 mcg/day for infants, 50 mcg/day for children 1-3 years of age, and give adult dose for children >3.

Hypothyroidism: Oral:
Adults: 25 mcg/day increase by 12.5-25 mcg/day every 1-2 weeks to a maximum of 100 mcg/day
Elderly: Initial: 5 mcg/day, increase by 5 mcg/day every 1-2 weeks; usual maintenance dose: 25-75 mcg/day

T_3 suppression test: Oral: 75-100 mcg/day for 7 days; use lowest dose for elderly

Myxedema coma: I.V.: 25-50 mcg
Patients with known or suspected cardiovascular disease: 10-20 mcg
Note: Normally, at least 4 hours should be allowed between doses to adequately assess therapeutic response and no more than 12 hours should elapse between doses to avoid fluctuations in hormone levels. Oral therapy should be resumed as soon as the clinical situation has been stabilized and the patient is able to take oral medication. If levothyroxine rather than liothyronine sodium is used in initiating oral therapy, the physician should bear in mind that there is a delay of several days in the onset of levothyroxine activity and that I.V. therapy should be discontinued gradually.

Administration I.V. form must be prepared immediately prior to administration; dilute 200 mcg/mL vial with 2 mL of 0.9% sodium chloride injection and shake well until a clear solution is obtained; should not be admixed with other solutions

Contraindications Recent myocardial infarction or thyrotoxicosis, hypersensitivity to liothyronine sodium or any component, uncorrected adrenal cortical insufficiency

Warnings Use with extreme caution in patients with cardiovascular disease, adrenal cortical insufficiency, myxedema (including hypertension), or coronary artery disease; diabetes mellitus and insipidus may have symptoms exaggerated or aggravated; use with caution in elderly patients. Ineffective for weight reduction; high doses may produce serious or even life-threatening toxic effects particularly when used with some anorectic drugs; thyroid replacement requires periodic assessment or thyroid status. Chronic hypothyroidism predisposes patients to coronary artery disease. Short duration action permits fast dosage changes or diminishes toxicity rapidly; the rapid onset and dissipation of action make this a difficult agent to use in those likely to have adverse effects to thyroid such as elderly.

Elderly do not have a change in serum thyroxine associated with aging; however, plasma T_3 concentrations are decreased 25% to 40% in elderly. There is not a compensatory rise in thyrotropin suggesting that lower T_3 is not reacted upon as a deficiency by the pituitary. This indicates a slightly lower than normal dosage of thyroid hormone replacement is usually sufficient in older patients than in younger adult patients.

Dosage Forms

Injection: 10 mcg/mL (1 mL)
Tablet: 5 mcg, 25 mcg, 50 mcg

Stability Store between 2°C and 8°C (36°F to 46°F)

Reference Range Free T_3, serum: 250-390 pg/dL; TSH: 0.4 up to 10.0 (for those ≥80 years of age) mIU/L; remains normal in pregnancy

Overdosage Treatment

Decontamination: Gastric emptying indicated for ingestions >2 mg; ipecac or lavage with activated charcoal with cathartic

Supportive therapy: Propranolol may be used for hyperadrenergic signs (1 mg I.V. in adults, 0.01-0.1 mg/kg in pediatrics)

Enhancement of elimination: Plasmapheresis increases elimination 30-fold while charcoal hemoperfusion enhances T_4 elimination fivefold.

Test Interactions Many drugs may have effects on thyroid function tests; para-aminosalicylic acid, aminoglutethimide, amiodarone, barbiturates, carbamazepine, chloral hydrate, clofibrate, colestipol, corticosteroids, danazol, diazepam, estrogens, ethionamide, fluorouracil, I.V. heparin, insulin, lithium, methadone, methimazole, mitotane, nitroprusside, oxyphenbutazone, phenylbutazone, PTU, perphenazine, phenytoin, propranolol, salicylates, sulfonylureas, and thiazides

Drug Interactions

Decreased effect: Cholestyramine resin → ↓ absorption; antidiabetic drug requirements are ↑; estrogens → ↑ thyroid requirements

Increased effect: ↑ oral anticoagulant effect

Pregnancy Risk Factor A

Monitoring Parameters T_4, TSH, heart rate, blood pressure, clinical signs of hypo- and hyperthyroidism; TSH is the most reliable guide for evaluating adequacy of thyroid replacement dosage. TSH may be elevated during the first few months of thyroid replacement despite patients being clinically euthyroid. In cases where T_4 remains low and TSH is within normal limits, an evaluation of "free" (unbound) T_4 is needed to evaluate further increase in dosage.

Patient Information Do not change brands without physician's knowledge; report immediately to physician any chest pain, increased pulse palpitations, heat intolerances, excessive sweating; do not discontinue without notifying physician

Additional Information 15-37.5 mcg is equivalent to 0.05-0.06 mg levothyroxine; 60 mg thyroid USP; 45 mg Thyroid Strong®, and 60 mg thyroglobulin

Specific References

Dahlberg PA, Karlsson FA, and Wide L, "Triiodothyronine Intoxication," *Lancet*, 1979, 2(8144):700.

Liotrix (lye' oh trix)

CAS Number 8065-29-0

Brand Names Euthroid®; Thyrolar®

Synonyms T_3/T_4 Liotrix

Use Replacement or supplemental therapy in hypothyroidism (uniform mixture of T_4:T_3 in 4:1 ratio by weight); little advantage to this product exists and cost is not justified

Mechanism of Action The primary active compound is T_3 (tri-iodothyronine), which may be converted from T_4 (thyroxine) and then circulates throughout the body to influence growth and maturation of various tissues. Liotrix is uniform mixture of synthetic T_4 and T_3 in 4:1 ratio; exact mechanism of action is unknown; however, it is believed the thyroid hormone exerts its many metabolic effects through control of DNA transcription and protein synthesis; involved in normal metabolism, growth, and development; promotes gluconeogenesis, increases utilization and mobilization of glycogen stores and stimulates protein synthesis, increases basal metabolic rate.

Adverse Reactions

Cardiovascular: Palpitations, tachycardia, cardiac arrhythmias

Central nervous system: Nervousness, insomnia, fever, headache

Dermatologic: Hair loss

Gastrointestinal: Weight loss, appetite (increased), diarrhea, abdominal cramps

Neuromuscular & skeletal: Tremors

Miscellaneous: Sweating

Signs & Symptoms of Acute Overdose Tachycardia, hypertension, agitation, insomnia, seizures (may occur up to 1 week postingestion), coma

Toxicodynamics/Kinetics

Absorption: 50% to 95% from gastrointestinal tract

Time to peak serum concentration: 12-48 hours

Metabolism: Partially in the liver, kidneys, and intestines

Half-life: 6-7 days

Elimination: Partially excreted in feces and bile as conjugated metabolites

Usual Dosage Oral:

Congenital hypothyroidism:

- Children (dose/day):
  - 0-6 months: 8-10 mcg/kg
  - 6-12 months: 6-8 mcg/kg
  - 1-5 years: 5-6 mcg/kg

(Continued)

Liotrix *(Continued)*

6-12 years: 4-5 mcg/kg
>12 years: 2-3 mcg/kg

Hypothyroidism:

Adults: 30 mg/day, increasing by 15 mg/day at 2- to 3-week intervals to a maximum of 180 mg/day (usual maintenance dose: 60-120 mg/day)

Elderly: Initial: 15 mg, adjust dose at 2- to 4-week intervals by increments of 15 mg

Contraindications Hypersensitivity to liotrix or any component; recent myocardial infarction or thyrotoxicosis, uncomplicated by hypothyroidism; uncorrected adrenal cortical insufficiency, hypersensitivity to active or extraneous constituents

Warnings Ineffective for weight reduction; high doses may produce serious or even life-threatening toxic effects particularly when used with some anorectic drugs; use cautiously in patients with pre-existing cardiovascular disease (angina, CHD), elderly since they may be more likely to have compromised cardiovascular function. Patients with angina pectoris or other cardiovascular disease; adrenal cortical insufficiency, myxedema, diabetes mellitus and insipidus may have symptoms exaggerated or aggravated; thyroid replacement requires periodic assessment of thyroid status; TSH is the most reliable guide for evaluating adequacy of thyroid replacement dosage. Chronic hypothyroidism predisposes patients to coronary artery disease. Since T_3 is produced by monodeiodination of T_4 in peripheral tissues (80%) and since elderly have decreased T_3 (25% to 40%).

Elderly do not have a change in serum thyroxine associated with aging; however, plasma T_3 concentrations are decreased 25% to 40% in elderly. There is not a compensatory rise in thyrotropin suggesting that lower T_3 is not reacted upon as a deficiency by the pituitary. This indicates a slightly lower than normal dosage of thyroid hormone replacement is usually sufficient in older patients than in younger adult patients.

Dosage Forms Tablet: 30 mg, 60 mg, 120 mg, 180 mg [thyroid equivalent]

Reference Range

TSH: 0.4-10.0 (for those ≥80 years) mIU/L
T_4: 4.0-12.0 μg/dL (SI: 51-154 nmol/L)
T_3 (RIA) (total T_3): 80-230 ng/dL (SI: 1.2-3.5 nmol/L)
Free T_4: 0.7-1.8 ng/dL (SI: 9-23 pmol/L)

Overdosage Treatment

Decontamination: Gastric emptying indicated for ingestions >2 mg; ipecac or lavage with activated charcoal with cathartic

Supportive therapy: Propranolol may be used for hyperadrenergic signs (1 mg I.V. in adults, 0.01-0.1 mg/kg in pediatrics); sodium ipodate (3 g/1.7 m^2) has been used in acute ingestion to prevent T_4 to T_3 conversion.

Enhancement of elimination: Plasmapheresis increases elimination 30-fold while charcoal hemoperfusion enhances T_4 elimination fivefold

Test Interactions Many drugs may have effects on thyroid function tests; para-aminosalicylic acid, aminoglutethimide, amiodarone, barbiturates, carbamazepine, chloral hydrate, clofibrate, colestipol, corticosteroids, danazol, diazepam, estrogens, ethionamide, fluorouracil, I.V. heparin, insulin, lithium, methadone, methimazole, mitotane, nitroprusside, oxyphenbutazone, phenylbutazone, PTU, perphenazine, phenytoin, propranolol, salicylates, sulfonylureas, and thiazides

Drug Interactions

Decreased effect: ↑ hypoglycemic drug requirements, phenytoin → clinical lymphothyroidism; cholestyramine → ↓ drug absorption

Increased effect: ↑ oral anticoagulant effect

Increased toxicity: Tricyclic antidepressants → ↑ potential of both drugs

Pregnancy Risk Factor A

Monitoring Parameters T_4, TSH, heart rate, blood pressure, clinical signs of hypo- and hyperthyroidism; TSH is the most reliable guide for evaluating adequacy of thyroid replacement dosage. TSH may be elevated during the first few months of thyroid replacement despite patients being clinically euthyroid. In cases where T_4 remains low and TSH is within normal limits, an evaluation of "free" (unbound) T_4 is needed to evaluate further increase in dosage.

Patient Information Do not change brands without physician's knowledge; report immediately to physician any chest pain, increased pulse palpitations, heat intolerances, excessive sweating; do not discontinue without notifying your physician

Additional Information No advantage over synthetic levothyroxine sodium; 1 grain (60 mg) liotrix is equivalent to 0.05-0.06 mg levothyroxine; 60 mg thyroid USP and thyroglobulin; and 45 mg of Thyroid Strong®

Specific References

Berkner PD, Starkman H, and Person N, "Acute L-Thyroxine Overdose: Therapy With Sodium Ipodate: Evaluation of Clinical and Physiologic Parameters," *J Emerg Med*, 1991, 9(3):129-31.

Binimelis J, Bassas L, Marruecos L, et al, "Massive Thyroxine Intoxication: Evaluation of Plasma Extraction," *Intens Care Med*, 1987, 13(1):33-8.

Gorman RL, Chamberlain JM, Rose SR, et al, "Massive Levothyroxine Overdose: High Anxiety – Low Toxicity," *Pediatrics*, 1988, 82(4):666-9.

Kulig K, Golightly LK, and Rumack BH, "Levothyroxine Overdose Associated With Seizures in a Young Child," *JAMA*, 1985, 254(15):2109-10.

Mandel SH, Magnusson AR, Burton BT, et al, "Massive Levothyroxine Ingestion: Conservative Management," *Clin Pediatr (Phila)*, 1989, 28(8):374-6.

Liponorm® *see* Simvastatin *on page 697*

Lipozid® *see* Gemfibrozil *on page 378*

Lipur® *see* Gemfibrozil *on page 378*

Liquaemin® Injection *see* Heparin *on page 398*

Liquibid® *see* Guaifenesin *on page 390*

Liquid Paraffin *see* Mineral Oil *on page 534*

Liquid Pred® *see* Prednisone *on page 639*

Liquiprin® Infant Drops [OTC] *see* Acetaminophen *on page 79*

Lisino® *see* Loratadine *on page 481*

Lisinopril (lyse in' oh pril)

Related Information

ACE Inhibitors Comparison *on page 1636-1637*

CAS Number 76547-98-3; 83915-83-7

Brand Names Carace C®; Prinivil®; Zestril®

Use Treatment of hypertension, either alone or in combination with other antihypertensive agents

Mechanism of Action Competitive inhibition of angiotensin I being converted to angiotensin II, a potent vasoconstrictor, through the angiotensin I-converting enzyme (ACE) activity, with resultant lower levels of angiotensin II which causes an increase in plasma renin activity and a reduction in aldosterone secretion

Adverse Reactions

Cardiovascular: Hypotension (maximum hypotensive effect: 6 hours), syncope

Central nervous system: Fatigue, insomnia, dizziness, headache

Dermatologic: Rash, angioedema

Endocrine & metabolic: Hypoglycemia, hyperkalemia

Gastrointestinal: Nausea, diarrhea, altered taste

Genitourinary: Impotence, albuminuria

Hematologic: Leukopenia/neutropenia (agranulocytosis, granulocytopenia), anemia, aplastic anemia

Neuromuscular & skeletal: Muscle cramps

Renal: Deterioration in renal function

Respiratory: Cough (dry), wheezing

Signs & Symptoms of Acute Overdose Hypotension is usually not severe in overdose patients and manifests itself within 1 hour with a maximal effect at 4 hours; bradycardia, eosinophilia, hyperuricemia, azotemia, dyspepsia, thrombocytopenia, photophobia, insomnia, hypoglycemia, dyspnea, depression, dry mouth, gout, diplopia, confusion

Toxicodynamics/Kinetics

Absorption: Oral: Well absorbed, unaffected by food

Distribution: Widely in tissues

Protein binding: None

Metabolism: None

Half-life: 11-12 hours (in overdose patients: 34 hours)

Time to peak serum concentration: 7 hours

Elimination: Excreted almost entirely in urine as unchanged drug

Usual Dosage Adults: Oral: 10-40 mg/day in a single dose

Dosing adjustment in renal impairment:

Cl_{cr} 10-50 mL/minute: Administer 50% to 75% of normal dose

Cl_{cr} <10 mL/minute: Administer 25% to 50% of normal dose

Contraindications Hypersensitivity to lisinopril or any component

Warnings Use with caution and modify dosage in patients with renal impairment (decrease dosage) (especially renal artery stenosis), severe congestive heart failure or with coadministered diuretic therapy; experience in children is limited. Severe hypotension may occur in patients who are sodium and/or volume depleted, initiate lower doses and monitor closely when starting therapy in these patients.

Dosage Forms Tablet: 5 mg, 10 mg, 20 mg, 40 mg

Overdosage Treatment

Decontamination: Ipecac or lavage/activated charcoal with cathartic

Supportive therapy: Following initiation of essential overdose management, toxic symptom treatment and supportive treatment should be initiated. Hypotension usually responds to I.V. normal saline or Trendelenburg positioning. If unresponsive to these measures, the use of a parenteral inotrope may be required (eg, norepinephrine 0.1-0.2 mcg/kg/minute titrated to response). Seizures commonly

(Continued)

Lisinopril *(Continued)*

respond to lorazepam or diazepam (I.V. 5-10 mg bolus in adults every 15 minutes if needed up to a total of 30 mg; I.V. 0.25-0.4 mg/kg/dose up to a total of 10 mg in children) or to phenytoin or phenobarbital. Naloxone may antagonize hypotensive effects. Inhaled sodium cromoglycate (total dose: 40 mg/day) can decrease ACE-inhibitor cough by 50%.

Enhanced elimination: Multiple dosing of activated charcoal may be effective but not studied in an overdose setting; dialyzable (50%)

Antidote(s)

Naloxone Hydrochloride *on page 1447*

Test Interactions Increases BUN, creatinine, potassium, positive Coombs' [direct]; decreases cholesterol (S); may cause false-positive results in urine acetone determinations using sodium nitroprusside reagent

Pregnancy Risk Factor D (fetotoxicity in rabbits at doses ranging from 0.1-1 mg/kg/day)

Monitoring Parameters Blood pressure, renal function, WBC, serum potassium

Patient Information Notify physician if vomiting, diarrhea, excessive sweating, or dehydration should occur; also if swelling of face, lips, tongue or difficulty in breathing occurs or if persistent cough develops

Nursing Implications May cause depression in some patients; discontinue if angioedema of the face, extremities, lips, tongue, or glottis occurs; watch for hypotensive effects within 1-3 hours of first dose or new higher dose

Specific References

Dawson AH, Harvey D, Smith AJ, et al, "Lisinopril Overdose," *Lancet*, 1990, 335(8687):487-8.

Hargreaves MR and Benson MK, "Inhaled Sodium Cromoglycate in Angiotensin-Converting Enzyme Inhibitor Cough," *Lancet*, 1995, 345(8941):13-6.

Harrison BD, Laidlaw ST, and Reilly JT, "Fatal Aplastic Anaemia Associated With Lisinopril," *Lancet*, 1995, 346:247-8.

Herings RM, deBoer A, Stricker BH, et al, "Hypoglycemia Associated With Use of Inhibitors of Angiotensin Converting Enzyme," *Lancet*, 1995, 345:1195-8.

Kuo DC and Barish RA, "Isolated Uvular Angioedema Associated With ACE Inhibitor Use," *J Emerg Med*, 1995, 13(3):327-30.

Lisseril® *see* Cyclobenzaprine Hydrochloride *on page 248*

Listermint® With Fluoride [OTC] *see* Fluoride *on page 355*

Litalir® *see* Hydroxyurea *on page 412*

Lithane® *see* Lithium *on this page*

Lithium (lith' ee um)

Related Information

Drugs and Chemicals Proven to be Teratogenic in Humans *on page 1572-1575*

Therapeutic Drugs Associated With Hallucinations *on page 1558-1559*

CAS Number 554-13-2

Brand Names Cibalith-S®; Eskalith®; Eskalith CR®; Lithane®; Lithobid®; Lithonate®; Lithotabs®; PFI-Lith®; Phasal®

Synonyms Lithium Carbonate; Lithium Citrate

Use Management of acute manic episodes, bipolar disorders, and depression; industrial use: lubricants, alkaline storage batteries, nuclear reactors, alloys

Mechanism of Action Alters cation transport across cell membrane in nerve and muscle cells and influences reuptake of serotonin and/or norepinephrine

Adverse Reactions

Cardiovascular: T-wave flattening, conduction block, Q-T interval prolongation, chest pain, hypotension

Central nervous system: Lethargy, fatigue, fine hard dizziness, pseudotumor cerebri, cerebellar findings may be long term; visual hallucinations, hypothermia, fasciculations, electroencephalogram abnormalities

Dermatologic: Eruptions, atopic dermatitis, alopecia, folliculitis, pruritus, may exacerbate acne or psoriasis

Endocrine & metabolic: Hypothyroidism, goiter acneiform, hyperglycemia (diabetic ketoacidosis); increases parathyroid hormone secretion, hyperkalemia, polydipsia, hypermagnesemia, diabetes insipidus

Gastrointestinal: Nausea, anorexia, diarrhea, dry mouth, dysgeusia, mucosal ulcerations of mouth

Hematologic: Leukocytosis

Neuromuscular & skeletal: Muscle asthenia, cogwheel rigidity, chronic movements of the limbs, tremors

Ocular: Photophobia, exophthalmos, papilloedema, downbeat nystagmus

Renal: Nonspecific nephron atrophy, proteinuria, acidosis (renal tubular)

Miscellaneous: Excessive thirst, metallic taste

Signs & Symptoms of Acute Overdose Sedation, ataxia, cognitive dysfunction, impotence, hypothyroidism, hypothermia, hepatic failure, A-V block, encephalopathy, chorea (extrapyramidal), nystagmus, dementia, parotid pain, nocturia, hypokalemia, dysosmia, hypoglycemia, hyperthyroidism, hypertonia, hyperglycemia, neuroleptic malignant syndrome, mania, fever, photophobia, confusion, seizures, Graves' disease, thrombocytosis, rhabdomyolysis, myoglobinuria, hypercalcemia, ototoxicity, Parkinson's-like symptoms, tinnitus, heart block, tremors, arthralgia, systemic lupus erythematosus (SLE), leukopenia, neutropenia, agranulocytosis, granulocytopenia, visual changes, bradycardia, ventricular arrhythmia, myocardial infarction, hyperkalemia, polyuria, blurred vision, alopecia, hypotension; see table.

Lithium (acute ingestion)

Serum Level	Symptom
1.5–2.5 mEq/L	Polyuria, blurred vision, weakness, lethargy, dizziness, increased reflexes, fasiculations
2.5–3 mEq/L	Myoclonic twitching, incontinence, stupor, restlessness, coma
>3 mEq/L	Seizures, hypotension, cardiac arrhythmias

Toxicodynamics/Kinetics

Absorption: Rapid

Distribution: Crosses the blood-brain barrier; concentrates in thyroid gland, bone, and brain tissue

V_d: Initial, adults: 0.3-0.4 L/kg

V_{dss}: Adults: 0.7-1 L/kg

Protein binding: None

Metabolism: None

Half-life:

Adolescents: 18 hours

Adults: 24 hours

Terminal: 18-24 hours, can increase to more than 36 hours

Elderly or patients with renal impairment: Up to 36 hours

Time to peak serum concentration: Within 30 minutes to 2 hours

Time to peak CSF concentration: 24 hours

Elimination: 90% to 98% of dose excreted in urine as unchanged drug; other excretory routes include feces (1%) and sweat (4% to 5%)

Usual Dosage Oral: Monitor serum concentrations and clinical response (efficacy and toxicity) to determine proper dose

Children 6-12 years: 15-60 mg/kg/day in 3-4 divided doses; dose not to exceed usual adult dosage

Adults: 300-600 mg 3-4 times/day; usual maximum maintenance dose: 2.4 g/day or 450-900 mg of sustained release twice daily

Dosing adjustment in renal impairment:

Cl_{cr} 10-50 mL/minute: Administer 50% to 75% of normal dose

Cl_{cr} <10 mL/minute: Administer 25% to 50% of normal dose

Contraindications Hypersensitivity to lithium or any component; severe cardiovascular or renal disease

Warnings Lithium toxicity is closely related to serum levels and can occur at therapeutic doses; serum lithium determinations are required to monitor therapy; concomitant use of lithium with thiazide diuretics may decrease renal excretion and enhance lithium toxicity; diuretic dosage may need to be reduced by 30%; do not crush or chew, slow or extended release dosage form, swallow whole; use with caution in patients with cardiovascular or thyroid disease

Dosage Forms

Capsule, as carbonate: 150 mg, 300 mg, 600 mg

Syrup, as citrate: 300 mg/5 mL (5 mL, 10 mL, 480 mL)

Tablet, as carbonate: 300 mg

Tablet:

Controlled release, as carbonate: 450 mg

Slow release, as carbonate: 300 mg

Reference Range

Therapeutic: 0.6-1.2 mEq/L (SI: 0.6-1.2 mmol/L), for acute mania; 0.8-1.0 mEq/L (SI: 0.8-1.0 mmol/L) for protection against future episodes in most patients with bipolar disorder. A higher rate of relapse is described in subjects who are maintained below 0.4 mEq/L (SI: 0.4 mmol/L).

Toxic: >1.5 mEq/L (SI: >1.5 mmol/L); highest survival level: 14.6 mEq/L

Overdosage Treatment

Decontamination: 30-60 g of sodium polystyrene sulfonate may prevent absorption; whole bowel irritation with polyethylene glycol (2 L/hour for 5 hours in adults), may cause a 67% decrease in absorption; activated charcoal with cathartic may not be effective in adsorbing lithium but is not harmful if used.

(Continued)

Lithium *(Continued)*

Supportive therapy: There is no specific antidote for lithium poisoning. In the acute ingestion, following initiation of essential overdose management, correction of fluid and electrolyte imbalances should be commenced. Lithium-induced tachycardia (ventricular) may respond to I.V. magnesium sulfate.

Enhancement of elimination: Hemodialysis is the treatment of choice for severe intoxications; 50% to 100% dialyzable. Dialysis should be considered in a symptomatic patient with levels >2.5 mEq/L (acute ingestion) or >1.5 mEq/L in chronic toxicity setting. A level of 4 mEq/L is an absolute indication for dialysis; other indications for dialysis include neurologic toxicity, renal failure, or ingestions of sustained release preparations. Four hours of hemodialysis will reduce lithium concentrations by about 1 mEq/L, but due to a rebound effect, a usual dialysis time of 10-12 hours is recommended. Dialysis using a bicarbonate bath (35 millimole/L) may be more efficacious than an acetate bath in removing lithium.

Antidote(s)

Sodium Polystyrene Sulfonate *on page 1469*

Polyethylene Glycol *on page 1460*

Test Interactions Increases calcium (S), glucose, magnesium, potassium (S); decreases thyroxine (S); serum bicarbonate, urea levels elevated, serum bromide levels decreased; causes leukopenia, thrombocytopenia

Diagnostic Tests/Procedures

Lithium, Blood *on page 1285*

Lithium RBC/Plasma Ratio *on page 1286*

Drug Interactions Concomitant use of lithium with thiazide diuretics or nonsteroidal anti-inflammatory drugs (NSAIDs) may decrease renal excretion and enhance lithium toxicity; lithium and iodide salts (or iodine) may cause increased hypothyroid effects. Phenothiazines potentiate adverse neurologic effects as does verapamil and piroxicam; LSD and fluoxetine can cause seizures when taken with lithium. Theophylline, mannitol, and urea have all been shown to decrease serum lithium levels by enhancing its elimination. Carbamazepine can cause added neurotoxicity; lithium can interact with ACE inhibitors to decrease renal function. Captopril can cause an increase in lithium levels. Concomitant administration of lithium and ketorolac can result in elevated lithium levels.

Pregnancy Risk Factor D (use should be avoided in 1st trimester and just prior to delivery)

Pregnancy Implications Crosses the placenta; appears in breast milk at 35% to 50% the concentrations in serum; a transient syndrome of drowsiness, cyanosis, and hypotonia can occur in neonates whose mothers take lithium prior to delivery

Monitoring Parameters Lithium levels, fluid status, serum electrolytes, renal function, serum B_2 microglobulin may be indicator for renal disease

Patient Information Avoid tasks requiring psychomotor coordination until the CNS effects are known; blood level monitoring is required to determine the proper dose; maintain a steady salt and fluid intake especially during the summer months; do not crush or chew slow or extended release dosage form, swallow whole

Nursing Implications Give with meals to decrease gastrointestinal upset

Additional Information Lithium blood levels increase during caffeine withdrawal

Lithium citrate: Cibalith-S®

Lithium carbonate: Eskalith®, Lithane®, Lithobid®, Lithonate®, Lithotabs®

Specific References

Belanger DR, Tierney MG, and Dickinson G, "Effect of Sodium Polystyrene Sulfonate on Lithium Bioavailability," *Ann Emerg Med*, 1992, 21(11):1312-5.

Farag S, Watson RD, and Honeybourne D, "Symptomatic Junctional Bradycardia Due to Lithium Intoxication in Patient With Previously Normal Electrocardiogram," *Lancet*, 1994, 343(8909):1371.

Groleau G, "Lithium Toxicity," *Emerg Med Clin North Am*, 1994, 12(2):511-31.

Groleau G, Barish R, Tso E, et al, "Lithium Intoxication: Manifestations and Management," *Am J Emerg Med*, 1987, 5(6):527-32.

Hambrecht M, "Lithium and Pseudohallucinations: A Rare Side Effect," *Biol Psychiatry*, 1995, 37:120-1.

Joseph M and Vieweg V, "Electrocardiographic Changes of Sinus Bradycardia and Sinus Node Dysfunction Among Patients With Therapeutic Levels of Lithium," *Depression*, 1994-95, 2(4):226-31.

Langlois R and Paquette D, "Increased Serum Lithium Levels Due to Ketorolac Therapy," *Can Med Assoc J*, 1994, 150(9):1455-6.

Lehmann K and Ritz E, "Angiotensin-Converting Enzyme Inhibitors May Cause Renal Dysfunction in Patients on Long-Term Lithium Treatment," *Am J Kidney Dis*, 1995, 25(1):82-7.

Linakis JG, Hull KM, Lee CM, et al, "Effect of Delayed Tretment With Sodium Polystyrene Sulfonate on Serum Lithium Concentrations in Mice," *Acad Emerg Med*, 1995, 152:956-7.

Linakis JG, Savitt DL, Wu TY, et al, "Use of Sodium Polysytrene Sulfonate (SPS) for Reduction of Chronically Elevated Serum Lithium Concentrations in Mice," *Acad Emerg Med*, 1995, 2:395.

Moster R, Toren P, Mizrachi I, et al, "Caffeine Withdrawal Increases Lithium Blood Levels," *Biol Psychiatry*, 1995, 37:348-50.

Oshika T, "Ocular Adverse Effects of Neuropsychiatric Agents: Incidence and Management," *Drug Saf*, 1995, 12:256-63.

Palatnick W, Rowe B, Bell D, et al, "Diabetic Ketoacidosis Associated With Lithium Intoxication," *Vet Hum Toxicol*, 1993, 35:339.

Perrier A, Martin PY, Favre H, et al, "Very Severe Self-Poisoning Lithium Carbonate Intoxication Causing a Myocardial Infarction," *Chest*, 1991, 100(3):863-5.

Price LH and Heninger GR, "Lithium in the Treatment of Mood Disorders," *N Engl J Med*, 1994, 331(9):591-8.

Rampes H and Bhandari S, "Hypersalivation and Lithium Toxicity," *J Psychopharm*, 1994, 8(4):261.

Smith SW, Ling LJ, and Halstenson CE, "Whole Bowel Irrigation as a Treatment for Acute Lithium Overdose," *Ann Emerg Med*, 1991, 20(5):536-9.

Swanson Jr CL, Price WA, and McEvoy JP, "Effects of Concomitant Risperidone and Lithium Treatment," *Am J Psychiatry*, 1995, 152:1096.

Szerlip HM, Heeger P, and Feldman GM, "Comparison Between Acetate and Bicarbonate Dialysis for the Treatment of Lithium Intoxication," *Am J Nephrol*, 1992, 12:116-20.

Tomaszewski C, Musso C, and Pearson JR, "Lithium Absorption Prevented by Sodium Polystyrene Sulfonate in Volunteers," *Ann Emerg Med*, 1992, 21(11):1308-11.

Ward ME, Musa MN, Bailey L, "Clinical Pharmacokinetics of Lithium," *J Clin Pharmacol*, 1994, 34(4):280-5.

Watling SM, Gehrke JC, Gehrke CW, et al, "*In vitro* Binding of Lithium Using the Cation Exchange Resin Sodium Polystyrene Sulfonate," *Am J Emerg Med*, 1995, 13:294-6.

Worthley LT, "Lithium Toxicity and Refractory Cardiac Arrhythmia Treated With Intravenous Magnesium," *Anaesth Intensive Care*, 1974, 4:357-60.

Lithium Carbonate *see* Lithium *on page 476*

Lithium Citrate *see* Lithium *on page 476*

Lithobid® *see* Lithium *on page 476*

Lithonate® *see* Lithium *on page 476*

Lithotabs® *see* Lithium *on page 476*

Liticon® *see* Pentazocine *on page 603*

LM 427 *see* Rifabutin *on page 681*

L-Methadyl Acetate *see* Levomethadyl Acetate Hydrochloride *on page 463*

LMWH *see* Enoxaparin Sodium *on page 315*

Lodine® *see* Etodolac *on page 339*

Lodis® *see* Loperamide Hydrochloride *on next page*

Lodoxamide Tromethamine (loe dox' a mide tro meth' a meen)

CAS Number 53882-12-5; 53882-13-6; 63610-09-3

Brand Names Alomide®

Use Treatment of allergic keratoconjunctivitis, allergic conjunctivitis, and allergic keratitis

Mechanism of Action Mast cell stabilizer (similar to sodium cromoglycate) that inhibits the *in vivo* type I immediate hypersensitivity reaction to increase cutaneous vascular permeability associated with IgE and antigen-mediated reactions

Adverse Reactions

Central nervous system: Headache, dizziness, somnolence
Dermatologic: Rash
Gastrointestinal: Nausea, stomach discomfort
Local: Transient burning, stinging, discomfort
Ocular: Blurred vision, corneal erosion/ulcer, eye pain, corneal abrasion, blepharitis
Respiratory: Sneezing
Miscellaneous: Dry nose

Signs & Symptoms of Acute Overdose Feeling of warmth, headache, dizziness, fatigue, sweating, nausea, and loose stools following oral administration

Toxicodynamics/Kinetics Absorption: Topical: Very small and undetectable

Usual Dosage Children >2 years and Adults: Instill 1-2 drops in eye(s) 4 times/day for up to 3 months

Contraindications Hypersensitivity to any component of product

Warnings Safety and efficacy in children <2 years of age have not been established; not for injection; not for use in patients wearing soft contact lenses during treatment

Dosage Forms Solution, ophthalmic: 0.1% (10 mL)

Overdosage Treatment Decontamination: Lavage/activated charcoal with cathartic; for ocular exposure, irrigate with normal saline through a Morgans lens

Pregnancy Risk Factor B

Lofene® *see* Diphenoxylate and Atropine *on page 291*

Logen® *see* Diphenoxylate and Atropine *on page 291*

Lomanate® *see* Diphenoxylate and Atropine *on page 291*

Lomodix® *see* Diphenoxylate and Atropine *on page 291*

Lomotil® *see* Diphenoxylate and Atropine *on page 291*

Loniten® *see* Minoxidil *on page 536*

Lonox® *see* Diphenoxylate and Atropine *on page 291*

Lontanyl® *see* Testosterone *on page 729*

Lopemid® *see* Loperamide Hydrochloride *on this page*

Loperamide Hydrochloride (loe per' a mide)

CAS Number 53179-11-6; 34552-83-5

Brand Names Arret®; Blox®; Brek®; Diar-aid® [OTC]; Dissenten®; Imodium®; Imodium® A-D [OTC]; Imosec®; Kaopectate® II [OTC]; Lodis®; Lopemid®; Loperyl®; Orulop®; Pepto® Diarrhea Control [OTC]

Use Treatment of acute nonspecific diarrhea (including traveler's diarrhea) and chronic diarrhea associated with inflammatory bowel disease; decrease the volume of ileostomy discharge; also used as a prophylaxis for chemotherapy-induced diarrhea

Mechanism of Action Acts directly on intestinal muscles to inhibit peristalsis and prolong transit time

Adverse Reactions

Cardiovascular: Bradycardia

Central nervous system: Sedation, psychosis, restlessness, fatigue, dizziness, delirium

Dermatologic: Rash

Gastrointestinal: Nausea, vomiting, constipation, abdominal cramping, dry mouth

Genitourinary: Urinary retention, toxic megacolon

Signs & Symptoms of Acute Overdose CNS and respiratory depression, personality changes, dry mouth, dystonic reactions, gastrointestinal cramping, ileus, constipation, miosis

Toxicodynamics/Kinetics

Onset of action: Oral: Within 0.5-1 hour

Absorption: Oral: 40%; levels in breast milk expected to be very low

Protein binding: 97%

Metabolism: Hepatic (>50%) to inactive compounds

Half-life: 7-15 hours

Elimination: Fecal and urinary (1%) excretion of metabolites and unchanged drug (30% to 40%)

Usual Dosage Oral:

Children:

Acute diarrhea: 0.4-0.8 mg/kg/day divided every 6-12 hours, maximum: 2 mg/dose

Chronic diarrhea: 0.08-0.24 mg/kg/day divided 2-3 times/day, maximum: 2 mg/dose

Adults: Initial: 4 mg (2 capsules), followed by 2 mg after each loose stool, up to 16 mg/day (8 capsules)

Toxic dose: 2 mg/kg

Contraindications Hypersensitivity to loperamide or any component; patients who must avoid constipation; diarrhea resulting from some infections; patients with pseudomembranous colitis

Warnings Large first-pass metabolism, use with caution in hepatic dysfunction and ulcerative colitis; should not be used if diarrhea accompanied by high fever, blood in stool

Dosage Forms

Caplet: 2 mg

Capsule: 2 mg

Liquid, oral: 1 mg/5 mL (60 mL, 90 mL, 120 mL)

Tablet: 2 mg

Overdosage Treatment

Decontamination: Lavage/activated charcoal; do not use a cathartic if an ileus is present

Supportive therapy: Naloxone is useful to reverse CNS or apnea; dystonic reaction can be managed with benztropine (1-2 mg I.V.) or diphenhydramine (1 mg/kg up to 50 mg I.V.)

Antidote(s)

Naloxone Hydrochloride *on page 1447*

Test Interactions Increases glucose

Drug Interactions Increased toxicity with CNS depressants, phenothiazines, TCAs

Pregnancy Risk Factor B

Monitoring Parameters Stool frequency, fluid and electrolytes

Patient Information Do not take more than 8 capsules or 80 mL in 24 hours; if acute diarrhea persists for longer than 48 hours, etiology should be examined; drink plenty of fluids to help prevent dehydration

Additional Information If clinical improvement is not achieved after 16 mg/day for 10 days, control is unlikely with further use. Continue use if diet or other treatment does not control. Elderly are particularly sensitive to fluid and electrolyte loss. This generally results in lethargy, weakness, and confusion. Repletion and maintenance of electrolytes and water are essential in the treatment of diarrhea. Drug therapy must be limited in order to avoid toxicity with this agent.

Specific References

Bhutta TI and Tahir KI, "Loperamide Poisoning in Children," *Lancet*, 1990, 335(8685):363.

Ericsson CD and Johnson PC, "Safety and Efficacy of Loperamide," *Am J Med*, 1990, 88(6A):10S-14S.

Friedli G and Haenggeli CA, "Loperamide Overdose Managed by Naloxone," *Lancet*, 1980, 1:1413.

Schwartz RH and Rodriquez WJ, "Toxic Delirium Possibly Caused by Loperamide," *J Pediatr*, 1991, 118(4 Pt 1):656-7.

Loperyl® *see* Loperamide Hydrochloride *on previous page*

Lopid® *see* Gemfibrozil *on page 378*

Lopressor® *see* Metoprolol Tartrate *on page 524*

Lopurin™ *see* Allopurinol *on page 97*

Loram® *see* Lorazepam *on next page*

Loratadine (lor at' a deen)

Related Information

H1-Antihistamine Comparison *on page 1649*

CAS Number 79794-75-5

Brand Names Claritin®; Claritine®; Clarityn®; Clarityne®; Fristamin®; Lisino®

Synonyms SCH-29851

Use Relief of nasal and non-nasal symptoms of seasonal allergic rhinitis with little sedative properties

Mechanism of Action Long-acting tricyclic antihistamine with selective peripheral histamine H_1 receptor antagonistic properties; derived from azatadine

Adverse Reactions

Cardiovascular: Hypotension, hypertension, palpitations, tachycardia, fibrillation (atrial)

Central nervous system: Headache, somnolence, fatigue, anxiety, depression

Neuromuscular & skeletal: Hyperkinesia, arthralgias

Respiratory: Dyspnea, pharyngitis

Miscellaneous: Breast pain, nasal dryness, dry mouth, sweating

Signs & Symptoms of Acute Overdose Coma

Toxicodynamics/Kinetics

Onset of action: Within 1-3 hours

Peak effect: 8-12 hours

Duration: >24 hours

Absorption: Rapid

Protein binding: 98%; descarboethoxyloratadine: 73% to 77%

Metabolism: Extensive to an active metabolite (descarboethoxyloratadine)

Half-life: 12-15 hours; elderly: 18 hours; descarboethoxyloratadine: 18 hours

Elimination: Significant excretion into breast milk, feces, urine

Usual Dosage Children >12 years and Adults: Oral: 10 mg/day on an empty stomach

Dosing interval in liver impairment: 10 mg every other day to start

Contraindications Patients hypersensitive to loratadine or any of its components; use with caution in patients with asthma

Warnings Patients with liver impairment should start with a lower dose (10 mg every other day), since their ability to clear the drug will be reduced; use with caution in lactation, safety in children <12 years of age has not been established

Dosage Forms Tablet: 10 mg

Reference Range Peak serum level of 18 ng/mL 1 hour after a single 40 mg dose

Overdosage Treatment

Decontamination: Lavage/activated charcoal with cathartic

Enhancement of elimination: Hemodialysis is not useful; multiple dosing of activated charcoal may be useful

Drug Interactions Although there have not been any reports of interactions with triazole antifungals, cimetidine, ranitidine, theophylline, or macrolide antibiotics, extreme caution is still warranted when concurrently administered with these agents.

Increased toxicity: Procarbazine, other antihistamines, alcohol

Pregnancy Risk Factor B

(Continued)

Loratadine *(Continued)*

Patient Information Drink plenty of water; may cause dry mouth, sedation, drowsiness, and can impair judgment and coordination

Specific References

Clissold SP, Sorkin EM, and Goa KL, "Loratadine: A Preliminary Review of Its Pharmacodynamic Properties and Therapeutic Efficacy," *Drugs*, 1989, 37(1):42-57.

Lin CC, Radwanski E, Affrime M, et al, "Pharmacokinetics of Loratadine in Pediatric Subjects," *Am J Therap*, 1995, 2:504-8.

Luck JC and Evrard HM, "Atrial Fibrillation Associated With Loratadine Use," *J Allergy Clin Immunol*, 1995, 95(2):282.

Simons FE, "Loratadine, a Nonsedating H_1-Receptor Antagonist (Antihistamine)," *Ann Allergy*, 1989, 63(4):266-8.

Loraz® *see* Lorazepam *on this page*

Lorazepam (lor a' ze pam)

Related Information

Benzodiazepines Comparison *on page 1643*

Doses and Administration of Several Frequently Used Antiemetic Agents *on page 1641*

Seizures, Neonatal Guidelines *on page 1604-1605*

Therapeutic Drugs Associated With Hallucinations *on page 1558-1559*

CAS Number 846-49-1

Brand Names Ativan®; Kendol®; Loram®; Loraz®; Noxaben®; Punktyl®; Titus®

Use Management of anxiety, status epilepticus, delirium tremors, preoperative sedation, and amnesia, pain due to black widow spider bites

Mechanism of Action Depresses all levels of the CNS, including the limbic and reticular formation, probably through the increased action of gamma-aminobutyric acid (GABA), which is a major inhibitory neurotransmitter in the brain

Adverse Reactions

Cardiovascular: Cardiac arrest, hypotension, bradycardia, cardiovascular collapse

Central nervous system: Drowsiness, psychosis, confusion, dizziness, amnesia, slurred speech, paradoxical excitation or rage, orofacial dyskinesia, visual hallucinations, ataxia, delirium, persecutory delusions

Local: Phlebitis, pain with injection

Neuromuscular & skeletal: Myoclonus (in low birthweight neonates)

Ocular: Blurred vision, diplopia

Respiratory: Respiratory rate (decreased), apnea, laryngospasm

Miscellaneous: Physical and psychological dependence with prolonged use

Signs & Symptoms of Acute Overdose Symptoms of overdosage may be delayed for up to 7 hours; confusion, hypoactive reflexes, hyporeflexia, disorientation, rhabdomyolysis, nystagmus, myalgia, acute myoglobinuria, depression, visual and auditory hallucinations, dyspnea, labored breathing, "alpha" coma (alpha frequency rhythm on EEG), ataxia; onset of effects delayed as long as 7 hours in acute overdosage

Toxicodynamics/Kinetics Studies have shown that the elderly are more sensitive to the effects of benzodiazepines as compared to younger adults

Onset of action: I.M.: Hypnosis occurs in ~20-30 minutes; has been delayed in overdosage up to 7 hours

Duration: 6-8 hours

Absorption: Oral, I.M.: Prompt (83% to 100% orally)

Distribution: V_d: Neonates: 0.76 L/kg; adults: 1-1.3 L/kg; distributed widely throughout body

Protein binding: 88% to 92%, lower in elderly patients

Metabolism: In the liver to inactive compounds (piperazine N-oxide) with urinary excretion and minimal fecal clearance; metabolism is not significantly affected in the elderly

Half-life:

- Neonates: 40 hours
- Adults: 10-16 hours; one study found the half-life in the elderly to be 15.9 hours as compared to 14.1 hours in younger adults

Time to peak serum concentration:

- Oral: Within 5 hours
- I.M.: Within 2 hours

Elimination: In urine as glucuronide conjugates; 7% excreted in feces; clearance: 0.2 mL/kg/minute in neonates; 1.3 mL/kg/minute in adults

Usual Dosage

Antiemetic:

- Children 2-15 years: I.V.: 0.05 mg/kg (up to 2 mg/dose) prior to chemotherapy
- Adults: Oral, I.V.: 0.5-2 mg every 4-6 hours as needed

Anxiety and sedation:

- Infants and Children: Oral, I.V.: Usual: 0.05 mg/kg/dose (range: 0.02-0.09 mg/kg) every 4-8 hours

Adults: Oral: 1-10 mg/day in 2-3 divided doses; usual dose: 2-6 mg/day in divided doses

Insomnia: Adults: Oral: 2-4 mg at bedtime

Preoperative: Adults:

I.M.: 0.05 mg/kg administered 2 hours before surgery; maximum: 4 mg/dose

I.V.: 0.044 mg/kg 15-20 minutes before surgery; usual maximum: 2 mg/dose

Operative amnesia: Adults: I.V.: up to 0.05 mg/kg; maximum: 4 mg/dose

Status epilepticus: I.V.:

Neonates: 0.05 mg/kg over 2-5 minutes; may repeat in 10-15 minutes (see warning regarding benzyl alcohol)

Infants and Children: 0.1 mg/kg slow I.V. over 2-5 minutes, do not exceed 4 mg/single dose; may repeat second dose of 0.05 mg/kg slow I.V. in 10-15 minutes if needed

Adolescents: 0.07 mg/kg slow I.V. over 2-5 minutes; maximum: 4 mg/dose; may repeat in 10-15 minutes

Adults: 4 mg/dose given slowly over 2-5 minutes; may repeat in 10-15 minutes; usual maximum dose: 8 mg

Contraindications Hypersensitivity to lorazepam or any component; there may be a cross-sensitivity with other benzodiazepines; do not use in a comatose patient, those with pre-existing CNS depression, narrow-angle glaucoma, severe uncontrolled pain, severe hypotension

Warnings Dilute injection prior to I.V. use with equal volume of compatible diluent (D_5W, 0.9% sodium chloride, sterile water for injection); do **not** inject intra-arterially, arteriospasm and gangrene may occur; injection contains benzyl alcohol 2%, polyethylene glycol and propylene glycol; use caution in patients with renal or hepatic impairment, organic brain syndrome, myasthenia gravis or Parkinson's disease

Dosage Forms

Injection: 2 mg/mL (1 mL, 10 mL); 4 mg/mL (1 mL, 10 mL)

Solution, oral concentrated, alcohol and dye free: 2 mg/mL (30 mL)

Tablet: 0.5 mg, 1 mg, 2 mg

Stability Intact vials should be refrigerated, protect from light; may be stored at room temperature for up to 2 weeks; do not use discolored or precipitate containing solutions. Stability of parenteral admixture at room temperature (25°C): 4 hours. Insoluble in water.

Reference Range Therapeutic: 50-240 ng/mL (SI: 156-746 nmol/L)

Overdosage Treatment

Decontamination: Lavage/activated charcoal with cathartic

Supportive therapy: Treatment for benzodiazepine overdose is supportive; rarely is mechanical ventilation required. Flumazenil (Romazicon™) has been shown to selectively block the binding of benzodiazepines to CNS receptors, resulting in a reversal of benzodiazepine-induced CNS depression. Do not use in concomitant tricyclic antidepressant ingestion; treat hypotension with isotonic crystalloids, place in Trendelenburg position or give dopamine or norepinephrine.

Enhancement of elimination: Multiple dose of activated charcoal may enhance elimination

Antidote(s)

Flumazenil *on page 1428*

Test Interactions May increase the results of liver function tests; Visine®, Drano®, and bleach can cause false-negative urine tests

Drug Interactions Alcohol: Additive CNS depression, excessive or chronic alcohol ingestion should be avoided; probenecid inhibits clearance

Pregnancy Risk Factor X (suggested to be teratogenic in animal and human data; can precipitate neonatal respiratory depression when given during delivery)

Pregnancy Implications Crosses the placenta; enters breast milk

Monitoring Parameters Respiratory and cardiovascular status, creatine phosphokinase

Patient Information Potential for physical and psychological dependence with chronic use; advise patient of possible retrograde amnesia after I.V. or I.M. use; will cause drowsiness

Nursing Implications Keep injectable form in the refrigerator; inadvertent intra-arterial injection may produce arteriospasm resulting in gangrene which may require amputation; emergency resuscitative equipment should be available when administering by I.V.; prior to I.V. use, Ativan® injection must be diluted with an equal amount of compatible diluent; injection must be made slowly with repeated aspiration to make sure the injection is not intra-arterial and that perivascular extravasation has not occurred; provide safety measures (ie, side rails, night light, and call button); remove smoking materials from area; supervise ambulation

Additional Information Injectable form has a longer duration of action than diazepam; provides an amnestic effect, so is useful for preop and preadministration of chemotherapy

Specific References

Clark RF, Sage TA, Tunget C, et al, "Delayed Onset Lorazepam Poisoning Successfully Re-

(Continued)

Lorazepam *(Continued)*

versed by Flumazenil in a Child: Case Report and Review of the Literature," *Pediatr Emerg Care*, 1995, 11:32-4.

Guterman B, Sebastian P, and Sodha N, "Recovery From Alpha Coma After Lorazepam Overdose," *Clin Electroencephalogr*, 1981, 12(4):205-8.

Lapierre YD and Labelle A, "Manic-Like Reaction Induced by Lorazepam Withdrawal," *Can J Psychiatry*, 1987, 32(8):697-8.

Lee DSC, Wong HA, and Knoppert DC, "Myoclonus Associated With Lorazepam Therapy in Very-Low-Birth-Weight Infants," *Biol Neonate*, 1994, 66:311-5.

Lheureux P and Askenasi R, "Specific Treatment of Benzodiazepine Overdose," *Hum Toxicol*, 1988, 7(2):165-70.

McDermott CA, Kowalczyk AL, Schnitzler ER, et al, "Pharmacokinetics of Lorazepam in Critically Ill Neonates With Seizures," *J Pediatr*, 1992, 120(3):479-83.

Stanford GK and Pine RH, "Postburn Delirium Associated With Use of Intravenous Lorazepam," *J Burn Care Rehabil*, 1988, 9(2):160-1.

Lorcainide Hydrochloride

Related Information

Flecainide Acetate *on page 350*

CAS Number 59729-31-6; 58934-46-6

Brand Names Remivox®

Synonyms Isocainide Hydrochloride; Socainide Hydrochloride

Use Investigational: Management of ventricular/supraventricular arrhythmias

Mechanism of Action A class Ic antiarrhythmic agent with similar actions as flecainide acetate

Adverse Reactions

Cardiovascular: Bradycardia, heart block, P-R prolongation, QRS prolongation, Q-T_c interval prolongation is minimal; worsening ventricular arrhythmias, congestive heart failure, palpitations, chest pain, edema, cardiac arrest, hypotension, syncope

Central nervous system: Dizziness, headache, sleep disturbance

Miscellaneous: Hyponatremia, sweating

Signs & Symptoms of Acute Overdose Bradycardia, coma, A-V block, insomnia, hypotension, seizures, hyponatremia, widened ventricular complexes

Toxicodynamics/Kinetics

Absorption: Oral: Well absorbed

Protein binding: 83%

Distribution: V_d: 5-10 L/kg

Metabolism: Hepatic to norlorcainide (active metabolite)

Half-life: Lorcainide: 8 hours; norlorcainide: 27 hours

Elimination: Hepatic; clearance: 1500 mL/minute

Usual Dosage

Oral: 100 mg twice daily; maximum daily oral dose: 400 mg

I.V.: Initial: 2 mg/kg with an infusion rate of 10 mg/minute under EKG control

Contraindications Pre-existing second or third degree A-V block; right bundle-branch block associated with left hemiblock (bifascicular block) or trifascicular block; cardiogenic shock, myocardial depression; known hypersensitivity to the drug

Dosage Forms Tablet: 100 mg

Reference Range Serum therapeutic range: 150-400 ng/mL; serum lorcainide level of 1820 ng/mL and serum norlorcainide level of 450 ng/mL associated with fatality

Overdosage Treatment

Decontamination: Lavage/activated charcoal with cathartic

Supportive therapy: Benzodiazepines can be used for seizure control; bradycardia or hypotension can be managed with catecholamines; cardiac pacing will probably not be effective; multiple dosing of activated charcoal may be effective

Drug Interactions Rifampin can increase hepatic metabolism of lorcainide

Specific References

Evers J and Buttner-Belz U, "Fatal Lorcainide Poisoning," *J Toxicol Clin Toxicol*, 1995, 33(2):157-9.

Somani P and Temesy-Armos PN, "Efficacy and Hyponatremia With Lorcainide in Long-Term Treatment of Ventricular Arrhythmias," *J Clin Pharmacol*, 1990, 30:841.

Lorestat® *see* Tolrestat *on page 760*

Losartan Potassium

Brand Names Cozaar®

Synonyms DUP 753; MK 954

Use Investigational: Hypertension

Mechanism of Action Substituted imidazole which is an angiotensin II (AII) receptor antagonist; no increase in bradykinin noted

Adverse Reactions

Cardiovascular: Orthostatic hypotension

Central nervous system: Dizziness

Toxicodynamics/Kinetics

Duration of action: 24 hours

Absorption: Oral: 33% (not affected by food)

Protein binding:

Losartan: 98%

EXP 3174: 98%

Metabolism: Hepatic carboxylation to an active metabolite (EXP 3174)

Half-life:

Losartan: 2 hours

EXP 3174: 6 hours

Peak plasma level: 30 minutes

Usual Dosage Oral: 25-150 mg/day; although doses >80 mg/day do not exhibit any greater hypotensive effects

Dosage Forms Tablet: 25 mg, 50 mg

Overdosage Treatment

Decontamination: Ipecac/lavage/activated charcoal with cathartic

Supportive therapy: Following initiation of essential overdose management, toxic symptom treatment and supportive treatment should be initiated. Hypotension usually responds to I.V. normal saline or Trendelenburg positioning. If unresponsive to these measures, the use of a parenteral inotrope may be required (eg, norepinephrine 0.1-0.2 mcg/kg/minute titrated to response). Seizures commonly respond to lorazepam or diazepam (I.V. 5-10 mg bolus in adults every 15 minutes if needed up to a total of 30 mg; I.V. 0.25-0.4 mg/kg/dose up to a total of 10 mg in children) or to phenytoin or phenobarbital. Inhaled sodium cromoglycate (total dose: 40 mg/day) can decrease ACE-inhibitor cough by 50%.

Enhanced elimination: Multiple dosing of activated charcoal may be effective

Drug Interactions Increased hypotensive effects when used with diuretics

Additional Information Maximal antihypertensive effect seen in 3-6 weeks; lowers serum uric acid levels

Specific References

Caspi A, "Losartan, the First of a New Class of Antihypertensive Drugs," *P&T*, 1995, 20(6):341-52.

Krichbaum P and Abramowitz B, "Focus on Losartan: An Angiotensin II Receptor Antagonist for Treatment of Hypertension," *Hosp Formul*, 1994, 29:683-96.

Levien TL and Baker DE, "Losartan and Anagrelide," *Hosp Pharm*, 1995, 30(7):611-8.

Losec® *see* Omeprazole *on page 576*

Lotensin® *see* Benazepril Hydrochloride *on page 146*

Lotocreme® *see* Hexachlorophene *on page 402*

Lotrimin® *see* Clotrimazole *on page 234*

Lotrimin AF® Cream [OTC] *see* Clotrimazole *on page 234*

Lotrimin AF® Lotion [OTC] *see* Clotrimazole *on page 234*

Lotrimin AF® Solution [OTC] *see* Clotrimazole *on page 234*

Lotrimin® AF Powder [OTC] *see* Miconazole *on page 530*

Lotrimin® AF Spray Liquid [OTC] *see* Miconazole *on page 530*

Lotrimin® AF Spray Powder [OTC] *see* Miconazole *on page 530*

Lovastatin (loe' va sta tin)

CAS Number 75330-75-5

Brand Names Mevacor®; Mevinacor®

Synonyms Mevinolin; Mevlor; Monacolin K

Replaces MSD-803

Use Adjunct to dietary therapy to decrease elevated serum total and LDL cholesterol concentrations in primary hypercholesterolemia

Mechanism of Action Lovastatin acts by competitively inhibiting 3-hydroxyl-3-methylglutaryl-coenzyme A (HMG-CoA) reductase, the enzyme that catalyzes the rate-limiting step in cholesterol biosynthesis

Adverse Reactions

Central nervous system: Headache, psychosis

Dermatologic: Rash, pruritus

Endocrine & metabolic: Gynecomastia

Gastrointestinal: Flatulence, abdominal pain, cramps, diarrhea, pancreatitis, constipation, nausea

Ocular: Blurred vision, myositis

Signs & Symptoms of Acute Overdose Myoglobinuria, rhabdomyolysis, dyspepsia, myalgia, hyperthermia, gynecomastia, systemic lupus erythematosus (SLE), cholestatic jaundice

Toxicodynamics/Kinetics

Onset of effect: 3 days of therapy required for LDL cholesterol concentration reductions

(Continued)

Lovastatin *(Continued)*

Absorption: Oral: 30%
Protein binding: 95%
Half-life: 1.1-1.7 hours
Time to peak serum concentration: Oral: 2-4 hours
Elimination: ~80% to 85% of dose excreted in feces and 10% in urine following liver hydrolysis

Usual Dosage Adults: Oral: Initial: 20 mg with evening meal, then adjust at 4-week intervals; maximum dose: 80 mg/day

Contraindications Active liver disease, hypersensitivity to lovastatin or any component

Warnings May elevate aminotransferases; LFTs should be performed before and every 4- 6 weeks during the first 12-15 months of therapy and periodically thereafter; can cause myalgia and rhabdomyolysis; use with caution in patients who consume large quantities of alcohol or who have a history of liver disease

Dosage Forms Tablet: 10 mg, 20 mg, 40 mg

Overdosage Treatment Decontamination: Ipecac/lavage and activated charcoal with cathartic

Test Interactions ↑ liver transaminases (S), HDL cholesterol, CPK; ↓ VLDL and LDL levels

Drug Interactions
Increased effect/toxicity of levothyroxine (hyper-/hypothyroidism)
Increased toxicity with gemfibrozil (musculoskeletal effects such as myopathy, myalgia and/or muscle asthenia accompanied by markedly elevated CK concentrations, rash and/or pruritus); clofibrate, niacin (myopathy), erythromycin, cyclosporine, oral anticoagulants (increased PT)

Pregnancy Risk Factor X

Pregnancy Implications Interferes with fetal steroid synthesis. Congenital abnormalities (VATER) have been associated with 1st trimester use.

Monitoring Parameters Plasma triglycerides, cholesterol, and liver function tests

Patient Information Promptly report any unexplained myalgia, tenderness or asthenia, especially if accompanied by malaise or fever; do not interrupt, increase, or decrease dose without advice of physician

Nursing Implications Administer with meals, urge patient to adhere to cholesterol-lowering diet

Specific References
"HMG-CoA Reductase Inhibitors for Hypercholesterolemia," *N Engl J Med*, 1988, 319(18):1222-3.
Huchzermeyer H and Munzenmaier R, "Lovastatin-Induced Acute Cholestatic Hepatitis," *Dtsch Med Wochenschr*, 1995, 120(8):252-6.
Kogan AD and Orenstein S, "Lovastatin-Induced Acute Rhabdomyolysis," *Postgrad Med J*, 1990, 66(774):294-6.
The Lovastatin Study Group II, "Therapeutic Response to Lovastatin (Mevinolin) in Nonfamilial Hypercholesterolemia: A Multicenter Study," *JAMA*, 1986, 256(20):2829-34.

Lovenox® *see* Enoxaparin Sodium *on page 315*

Low Molecular Weight Heparin *see* Enoxaparin Sodium *on page 315*

Low-Quel® *see* Diphenoxylate and Atropine *on page 291*

Loxapac® *see* Loxapine *on this page*

Loxapine (lox' a peen)

Related Information
Antipsychotic Agents Comparison *on page 1642*

CAS Number 27833-64-3

Brand Names Desconex®; Doxoline®; Loxapac®; Loxitane®

Synonyms Loxapine Hydrochloride; Loxapine Succinate; Oxilapine Succinate

Use Management of psychotic disorders

Mechanism of Action Unclear mechanism of action; a dibenzoxazepine thought to be similar to chlorpromazine

Adverse Reactions
Cardiovascular: Hypotension, tachycardia, cardiac arrhythmias; abnormal T waves with prolonged ventricular repolarization, severe hypotension, arrhythmias, flutter (atrial)
Central nervous system: Sedation, drowsiness, restlessness, anxiety, extrapyramidal reactions, psychosis, dystonic reactions, pseudoparkinsonian signs and symptoms, seizures, altered central temperature regulation, tardive dyskinesia, neuroleptic malignant syndrome, CNS depression may occur
Dermatologic: Hyperpigmentation, pruritus, rash, photosensitivity
Endocrine & metabolic: Amenorrhea, galactorrhea, gynecomastia, syndrome of inappropriate antidiuretic hormone, weight gain
Gastrointestinal: Adynamic ileus, constipation, gastrointestinal upset, dry mouth (problem with denture users), nausea

Genitourinary: Urinary retention, overflow incontinence, priapism, sexual dysfunction

Hematologic: Agranulocytosis (more often in women between fourth and tenth weeks of therapy), leukopenia (usually in patients with large doses for prolonged periods)

Hepatic: Cholestatic jaundice

Ocular: Blurred vision, retinal pigmentation

Signs & Symptoms of Acute Overdose Deep sleep, Parkinson's-like symptoms, dysphagia, gynecomastia, dystonic reactions, syncope, neuroleptic malignant syndrome, rhabdomyolysis, agitation, CNS depression, ptosis, leukocytosis, sinus tachycardia, arrhythmias, extrapyramidal reaction, hypothermia, hypertension followed by hypotension, seizures, myoglobinuria, renal failure (acute), systemic lupus erythematosus (SLE), leukopenia; neutropenia; agranulocytosis; granulocytopenia

Toxicodynamics/Kinetics

Onset of action: Oral: Neuroleptic effects occur within 20-30 minutes

Peak effect: 90-180 minutes

Duration of effect: ~12 hours

Absorption: Completely from gastrointestinal tract

Distribution: Widely distributed in most tissues

Protein binding: 91% to 99%

Metabolism: Hepatic to amoxapine

Half-life:

Biphasic, initial: 5 hours

Terminal: 12-19 hours

Elimination: Urine, and to a smaller degree, in feces

Usual Dosage Adults:

Oral: 10 mg twice daily, increase dose until psychotic symptoms are controlled; usual dose range: 60-100 mg/day in divided doses 2-4 times/day; dosages >250 mg/day are not recommended

I.M.: 12.5-50 mg every 4-6 hours or longer as needed and change to oral therapy as soon as possible

Contraindications Hypersensitivity to chlorpromazine or any component, cross-sensitivity with other phenothiazines may exist; avoid use in patients with narrow-angle glaucoma, bone marrow depression, severe liver or cardiac disease; severe CNS depression, coma

Warnings Watch for hypotension when administering I.M. or I.V.; safety in children <6 months of age has not been established; use with caution in patients with cardiovascular disease or seizures; benefits of therapy must be weighed against risks of therapy

Dosage Forms

Capsule: 5 mg, 10 mg, 25 mg, 50 mg

Concentrate, oral: 25 mg/mL (120 mL dropper bottle)

Injection: 50 mg/mL (1 mL)

Overdosage Treatment

Decontamination: Lavage/activated charcoal with cathartic

Supportive therapy: Hypotension usually responds to I.V. fluids or Trendelenburg positioning. If unresponsive to these measures, the use of a parenteral inotrope may be required (eg, norepinephrine 0.1-0.2 mcg/kg/minute titrated to response). Seizures commonly respond to lorazepam or diazepam (I.V. 5-10 mg bolus in adults every 15 minutes if needed up to a total of 30 mg; I.V. 0.25-0.4 mg/kg/dose up to a total of 10 mg in children) or to phenytoin or phenobarbital. Also critical cardiac arrhythmias often respond to I.V. phenytoin (15 mg/kg up to 1 gram), while other antiarrhythmics can be used. Neuroleptics often cause extrapyramidal reaction (eg, dystonic reactions) requiring management with diphenhydramine 1-2 mg/kg (adults) up to a maximum of 50 mg I.M. or I.V. slow push followed by a maintenance dose for 48-72 hours. When these reactions are unresponsive to diphenhydramine, benztropine mesylate I.V. 1-2 mg (adults) may be effective. These agents are generally effective within 2-5 minutes.

Enhancement of elimination: Multiple dosing of activated charcoal would not be expected to be useful

Test Interactions False-positives for phenylketonuria, amylase, uroporphyrins, urobilinogen; increases glucose; elevates plasma norepinephrine levels and plasma epinephrine levels threefold to fivefold; EMIT assays may give false-positive in presence of diphenhydramine, thioridazine, chlorpromazine, alimenazine, carbamazepine, cyclobenzaprine, or perphenazine

Drug Interactions Other CNS depressants, anticonvulsants, lithium, metrizamide

Pregnancy Risk Factor C

Pregnancy Implications Crosses placenta; distributes into breast milk

Monitoring Parameters EKG, CBC, blood pressure, electrolytes, pH

Patient Information May cause drowsiness; avoid alcoholic beverages

Nursing Implications Injectable is for I.M. use only

(Continued)

Loxapine *(Continued)*

Additional Information

Loxapine hydrochloride: Loxitane® C oral concentrate, Loxitane® IM

Loxapine succinate: Loxitane® capsule

Specific References

Browne JL, Tsuang MT, and Perry PJ, "Amoxapine Neurotoxicity: A Case Report With Long-Term Follow-Up," *Drug Intell Clin Pharm*, 1982, 16(5):404-7.

Peterson CD, "Seizures Induced by Acute Loxapine Overdose," *Am J Psychiatry*, 1981, 138(8):1089-91.

Tam CW, Olin BR 3d, and Ruiz AE, "Loxapine-Associated Rhabdomyolysis and Acute Renal Failure," *Arch Intern Med*, 1980, 140(7):975-6.

Loxapine Hydrochloride *see* Loxapine *on page 486*

Loxapine Succinate *see* Loxapine *on page 486*

Loxitane® *see* Loxapine *on page 486*

L-PAM *see* Melphalan *on page 497*

L-Sarcolysin *see* Melphalan *on page 497*

LSD *see* Lysergic Acid Diethylamide *on this page*

LTG *see* Lamotrigine *on page 459*

***L*-Thyroxine Sodium** *see* Levothyroxine Sodium *on page 465*

Ludiomil® *see* Maprotiline Hydrochloride *on page 490*

Luminal® *see* Phenobarbital *on page 614*

Lumirelax® *see* Methocarbamol *on page 513*

Luride® *see* Fluoride *on page 355*

Luride® Lozi-Tab® *see* Fluoride *on page 355*

Luride®-SF Lozi-Tab® *see* Fluoride *on page 355*

Lusap® *see* Malathion (Topical Lotion) *on next page*

Lustral® *see* Sertraline Hydrochloride *on page 695*

Luvox® *see* Fluvoxamine *on page 366*

LY-110140 *see* Fluoxetine Hydrochloride *on page 359*

LY-139037 *replaced by* Nizatidine *on page 569*

LY-237216 *see* Dirithromycin *on page 293*

Lyphocin® Injection *see* Vancomycin Hydrochloride *on page 784*

Lysanxia® *see* Prazepam *on page 637*

Lysergic Acid Diethylamide

Related Information

Principal Pharmacological Properties of Hallucinogenic Drugs *on page 1557*

CAS Number 50-37-3

Synonyms LSD

Mechanism of Action Agonist at 5-hydroxtryptamine presynaptic receptor in midbrain

Signs & Symptoms of Acute Overdose Rhabdomyolysis, fear, tremors, delirium, hyperglycemia, leukocytosis, ataxia, psychosis, mydriasis, fever, sweating, flushing, tachycardia, hyper-reflexia, hallucinations (auditory and visual), vision color changes (increased color perception), euphoria, hypertonia, neuroleptic malignant syndrome, lacrimation, nausea, vomiting, diarrhea, hyperthermia, coma, seizures, tachypnea, respiratory arrest

Toxicodynamics/Kinetics

Onset of action: 20-90 minutes (10 minutes I.V.)

Duration: 6-8 hours

Distribution: V_d: 0.28 L/kg

Protein binding: 80%

Metabolism: To 2-oxy-lysergic acid diethylamide

Half-life: 3-5 hours

Usual Dosage

Hallucinogenic dose:

- Oral: 100-750 mcg
- I.V.: 50-500 mcg

Lethal dose: 0.2-1 mg/kg

Reference Range Dose of 500 mcg orally resulted in peak plasma levels of 4.2 ng/mL

Overdosage Treatment

Decontamination: Activated charcoal with cathartic with oral ingestion

Supportive therapy: Dantrolene (25 mg 3 times/day) should be given for neuroleptic malignant syndrome; diazepam or lorazepam can be used for agitation; haloperidol can be given for hallucinations

Diagnostic Tests/Procedures

Lysergic Acid Diethylamine Level *on page 1289*

Drug Interactions When combined with lithium and fluoxetine, can cause seizures; sertraline or paroxetine can incite occurrence of LSD flashback episodes (primarily visual)

Pregnancy Implications Can cause uterine contractions; effects on fetus is unknown, although increased incidence of limb defects and ocular abnormalities

Additional Information May be given as sugar cube, on filter or blotting paper, as a tablet or capsule; flashbacks may be induced by alcohol; urine may be positive for up to 120 hours by radioimmunoassay; odorless, colorless, tasteless

Specific References

Jackson TW and Hornfeldt CS, "Seizures Activity Following Recreational LSD Use in Patients Treated With Lithium and Fluoxetine," *Vet Hum Toxicol*, 1991, 33:387.

Kulig K, "LSD," *Emerg Med Clin North Am*, 1990, 8(3):551-8.

Leikin JB, Krantz AJ, Zell-Kanter M, et al, "Clinical Features and Management of Intoxication Due to Hallucinogenic Drugs," *Med Toxicol Adverse Drug Exp*, 1989, 4(5):324-50.

Long S, "Does LSD Induce Chromosomal Damage and Malformations? A Review of the Literature," *Teratology*, 1972, 6(1):75-90.

Markel H, Lee A, Holmes RD, et al, "LSD Flashback Syndrome Exacerbated by Selective Serotonin Reuptake Inhibitor Antidepressants in Adolescents," *J Pediatr*, 1994, 125(5 Pt 1):817-9.

Macrobid® *see* Nitrofurantoin *on page 564*

Macrodantin® *see* Nitrofurantoin *on page 564*

Maigret-50 *see* Phenylpropanolamine Hydrochloride *on page 622*

Maioda® *see* Amiodarone Hydrochloride *on page 113*

Malathion (Topical Lotion) (mal a thye' on)

CAS Number 121-75-5

UN Number 2783

Brand Names Aftir Gel®; Derbac-M®; KP24®; Lusap®; Malfesto®; Organoderm®; Ovide™ Topical; Prioderm®; Suleo-M®

Use Treatment of head lice and their ova (pediculosis)

Mechanism of Action A dimethoxy organophosphate insecticide with inherent toxicity

Adverse Reactions

Cardiovascular: Bradycardia

Central nervous system: Anxiety, clumsiness, confusion, dizziness, drowsiness, seizures

Dermatologic: Contact dermatitis, irritation of scalp

Gastrointestinal: Abdominal cramps, diarrhea

Ocular: Nystagmus

Signs & Symptoms of Acute Overdose Paresthesia

Usual Dosage Sprinkle Ovide™ lotion on dry hair and rub gently until the scalp is thoroughly moistened; pay special attention to the back of the head and neck. Allow to dry naturally – use no heat and leave uncovered. After 8-12 hours, the hair should be washed with a nonmedicated shampoo; rinse and use a fine-toothed comb to remove dead lice and eggs. If required, repeat with second application in 7-9 days. Further treatment is generally not necessary. Other family members should be evaluated to determine if infested and if so, receive treatment.

Contraindications Known hypersensitivity to malathion

Dosage Forms Lotion: 0.5% (59 mL)

Overdosage Treatment

Decontamination: Isolation, bagging, and disposal of all contaminated clothing and other articles; all emergency medical workers and hospital staff should follow appropriate precautions regarding exposure to hazardous material including the use of protective clothing, masks, goggles,and respiratory equipment

Dermal: Prompt thorough scrubbing of all affected areas with soap and water, including hair and nails

Gastric: Activated charcoal can be administered either orally or via a nasogastric tube; do not induce emesis because of danger of sudden respiratory compromise, alterations in mental status, seizures, coma, and possible aspiration of hydrocarbon vehicles

Ocular: Irrigation with copious tepid sterile water or saline

Supportive therapy: Including airway management, ventilatory assistance, humidified oxygen administration, and close monitoring for sudden respiratory failure

Enhancement of elimination: Dialysis and hemoperfusion is not indicated due to effectiveness of the prescribed treatment, large volume of distribution of organophosphates

Antidote:

Atropine: Administration should be guided by respiratory status, starting at 1-5 mg I.V. every 5-10 minutes as needed and should be titrated to the resolution

(Continued)

Malathion (Topical Lotion) *(Continued)*

of excess pulmonary secretions; frequent administration of large doses (cumulative doses >100 mg) may be necessary in massive exposures

Glycopyrrolate: May be administered if atropine is unavailable

2-PAM: For more significant exposures (ie, exposures requiring large doses of atropine, or with recurring symptoms, or exposures to more lipid soluble agents), administration should follow: 1-2 g I.V. over 5-10 minutes, repeated in 1 hour if asthenia reoccurs, then every 4-12 hours for recurring symptoms

Antidote(s)

Atropine Sulfate *on page 1395*

Pralidoxime Chloride *on page 1461*

Pregnancy Risk Factor B

Specific References

Burgess I, "Malathion Lotions for Head Lice - A Less Reliable Treatment Than Commonly Believed," *Pharm J*, 1991, 247:630-2.

Malfesto® *see* Malathion (Topical Lotion) *on previous page*

Mallisol® [OTC] *see* Povidone-Iodine *on page 635*

Mallorol® *see* Thioridazine Hydrochloride *on page 745*

Malogex® *see* Testosterone *on page 729*

Malotuss® [OTC] *see* Guaifenesin *on page 390*

Maprotiline Hydrochloride (ma proe' ti leen)

Related Information

Therapeutic Drugs Associated With Hallucinations *on page 1558-1559*

CAS Number 10347-81-6; 10262-69-8

Brand Names Ludiomil®

Use Treatment of depression and anxiety associated with depression

Mechanism of Action Increases the synaptic concentration of serotonin and/or norepinephrine in the central nervous system by inhibition of their reuptake by the presynaptic neuronal membrane

Adverse Reactions

Cardiovascular: Heart block, tachycardia

Central nervous system: Convulsions (dose-dependent), sedation, hand hypotonia, psychosis, dizziness, visual hallucinations

Endocrine & metabolic: Syndrome of inappropriate antidiuretic hormone, weight gain

Gastrointestinal: Constipation, increased appetite, extreme dry mouth

Genitourinary: Urinary retention

Hematologic: Leukocytosis, thrombocytopenia

Hepatic: Elevated liver function tests

Neuromuscular & skeletal: Tremor, myoclonus

Ocular: Blurred vision, intraocular pressure (increased)

Otic: Ototoxicity, tinnitus

Respiratory: Aspiration

Signs & Symptoms of Acute Overdose Agitation, confusion, Q-T prolongation, photosensitivity, A-V block, dental erosion, vasculitis, intraocular pressure (increased), bradycardia, eosinophilia, delirium, hypnopompic hallucinations, mania, urinary retention, hypothermia, hypotension, seizures, tachycardia, torsade de pointes, respiratory depression, leukopenia; neutropenia; agranulocytosis; granulocytopenia

Toxicodynamics/Kinetics

Onset of action: For desired therapeutic effect, up to 2-3 weeks, but sometimes within 7 days

Absorption: Slow

Distribution: V_d: 13-24 L/kg; chiefly distributed to brain, lungs, liver, and kidneys

Protein binding: 88%

Metabolism: In the liver to active and inactive compounds

Half-life: 51-58 hours

Time to peak serum concentration: Within 12 hours

Elimination: Urine (70%) and in feces (30%); also excreted in bile

Usual Dosage Oral:

Children 6-14 years: 10 mg/day, increase to a maximum daily dose of 75 mg

Adults: 75 mg/day to start, increase by 25 mg every 2 weeks up to 150-225 mg/day; given in 3 divided doses or in a single daily dose

Contraindications Narrow-angle glaucoma, hypersensitivity to maprotiline or any component

Warnings Maprotiline should not be abruptly discontinued in patients receiving high doses for prolonged periods; do not drink alcoholic beverages; use with caution in patients with cardiac conduction disturbances, history of hyperthyroid; safe use of tricyclic antidepressants in children <12 years of age has not been established

Dosage Forms Tablet: 25 mg, 50 mg, 75 mg

Reference Range Therapeutic: 100-150 ng/mL (SI: 361-540 nmol/L); levels >237 ng/mL can be associated with seizures

Overdosage Treatment

Decontamination: Emesis is contraindicated, lavage/activated charcoal with cathartic can be useful; multiple dosing of activated charcoal may be useful

Supportive therapy: Following initiation of essential overdose management, toxic symptoms should be treated. Ventricular arrhythmias often respond to phenytoin 15-20 mg/kg (adults) with concurrent systemic alkalinization (sodium bicarbonate 0.5-2 mEq/kg I.V.). Arrhythmias unresponsive to this therapy may respond to lidocaine 1 mg/kg I.V. followed by a titrated infusion. Physostigmine (1-2 mg I.V. slowly for adults or 0.5 mg I.V. slowly for children) may be used for seizures or movement disorders but only as **a last resort.** Seizures usually respond to lorazepam or diazepam I.V. boluses (5-10 mg for adults up to 30 mg or 0.25-0.4 mg/kg/dose for children up to 10 mg/dose). If seizures are unresponsive or recur, phenytoin or phenobarbital may be required. For hypotension, isotonic saline is effective; norepinephrine (adults: 8-12 mcg/minute or children 0.1-0.2 mcg/kg/minute) is most effective agent.

Antidote(s)

Sodium Bicarbonate *on page 1467*

Drug Interactions CNS depression synergism with ethanol use

Maprotiline blocks the uptake of guanethidine and thus prevents the hypotensive effect of guanethidine; maprotiline may be additive with or may potentiate the action of other CNS depressants such as sedatives or hypnotics; maprotiline potentiates the pressor and cardiac effects of sympathomimetic agents such as isoproterenol, epinephrine, etc

With MAO inhibitors, fever, hypertension, tachycardia, confusion, seizures, and death have been reported

Additive anticholinergic effects seen with other anticholinergic agents

Cimetidine reduces the hepatic metabolism of maprotiline

Maprotiline may increase the prothrombin time in patients stabilized on warfarin

Pregnancy Risk Factor B

Monitoring Parameters EKG (QRS widening)

Patient Information Avoid alcohol ingestion; do not discontinue medication abruptly; may cause drowsiness; full effect may not occur for 3-6 weeks; dry mouth may be helped by sips of water, sugarless gum, or hard candy

Nursing Implications Monitor blood pressure and pulse rate prior to and during initial therapy; evaluate mental status; monitor weight, may increase appetite and possibly a craving for sweets

Additional Information Odorless, bitter tasting; seizures rarely seen 5-30 hours postdrug ingestion

Specific References

Bergman RN and Watson WA, "Cardiac Toxicity Associated With Acute Maprotiline Self Poisoning," *Am J Emerg Med*, 1983, 2(2):144-6.

Wyss PA, Serena S, and Meier PJ, "Dose-Dependency of Seizures in Maprotiline (Ludiomil®) Intoxications," *Vet Hum Toxicol*, 1993, 35:341.

Marbaxin® *see* Methocarbamol *on page 513*

Marcaine® *see* Bupivacaine Hydrochloride *on page 168*

Marcillin® *see* Ampicillin *on page 125*

Marevan® *see* Warfarin Sodium *on page 800*

Marezine® [OTC] *see* Cyclizine *on page 248*

Marmine® [OTC] *see* Dimenhydrinate *on page 289*

Marplan® *see* Isocarboxazid *on page 442*

Masmoran® *see* Hydroxyzine *on page 414*

Mastodanatrol® *see* Danazol *on page 257*

Matricaria Camphor *see* Camphor *on page 179*

Matulane® *see* Procarbazine Hydrochloride *on page 645*

Maxeran® *see* Metoclopramide *on page 523*

Maxidex® Ophthalmic *see* Dexamethasone *on page 266*

Maximum Strength Desenex® Antifungal Cream [OTC] *see* Miconazole *on page 530*

Maxolon® *see* Metoclopramide *on page 523*

MDL-71754 *see* Vigabatrin *on page 790*

MDMA *see* Methamphetamine Hydrochloride *on page 510*

Measurin® [OTC] *see* Aspirin *on page 133*

Meballymal *see* Secobarbital Sodium *on page 693*

Mebaral® *see* Mephobarbital *on page 501*

Mecamylamine Hydrochloride (mek a mill' a meen)

CAS Number 60-40-2; 826-39-1

Brand Names Inversine®

Use Treatment of moderately severe to severe hypertension and in uncomplicated malignant hypertension

Mechanism of Action Mecamylamine is a ganglionic blocker. This agent inhibits acetylcholine at the autonomic ganglia, causing a decrease in blood pressure. Mecamylamine also blocks central nicotinic cholinergic receptors, which inhibits the effects of nicotine and may suppress the desire to smoke.

Adverse Reactions

Cardiopulmonary: Tachycardia

Central nervous system: Dizziness, syncope, asthenia, fatigue, hallucinations, confusion, sedation, psychosis, choreiform movements

Gastrointestinal: Loose stools, nausea, vomiting, anorexia, constipation

Genitourinary: Impotence, urinary retention

Neuromuscular & skeletal: Tremors

Ocular: Blurred vision, mydriasis

Miscellaneous: Dry mouth

Signs & Symptoms of Acute Overdose Hypotension, nausea, vomiting, impotence, urinary retention, constipation, seizures, diarrhea

Toxicodynamics/Kinetics

Absorption: Completely through gastrointestinal tract

Half-life, elimination: 6-8 hours

Time to peak plasma concentration: 1-2 hours

Elimination: 50% excreted renally within 1 day

Usual Dosage Adults: Oral: 2.5 mg twice daily after meals for 2 days; increased by increments of 2.5 mg at intervals of ≥2 days until desired blood pressure response is achieved; average daily dose: 25 mg

Dosing adjustment/comments in renal impairment: Use with caution, if at all, although no specific guidelines are available

Contraindications Coronary insufficiency, pyloric stenosis, glaucoma, uremia, recent myocardial infarction, unreliable, uncooperative patients

Warnings Use with caution in patients receiving sulfonamides or antibiotics that cause neuromuscular blockade; use with caution in patients with impaired renal function, previous CNS abnormalities, prostatic hypertrophy, bladder obstruction, or urethral strictive; do not abruptly discontinue

Dosage Forms Tablet: 2.5 mg

Overdosage Treatment

Decontamination: Lavage/activated charcoal with cathartic

Supportive therapy: Signs and symptoms are a direct result of ganglionic blockade; pressor amines may be used to correct hypotension; use caution as patients will be unusually sensitive to these agents. Physostigmine (0.5-1 mg I.V.) may be utilized to reverse adverse effects

Enhancement of elimination: Multiple dosing of activated charcoal may be useful

Antidote(s)

Physostigmine *on page 1457*

Pregnancy Risk Factor C

Patient Information Take after meals at the same time each day; notify physician immediately if frequent loose bowel movements occur; rise slowly from sitting or lying for prolonged periods; do not restrict salt intake

Nursing Implications Check frequently for hypotension (orthostatic); aid with ambulation

Specific References

Harington M and Kincaid-Smith P, "Psychosis and Tremor Due to Mecamylamine," *Lancet*, 1958, 1(7019):499-501.

Rokseth R and Storstein O, "Pulmonary Complications During Mecamylamine Therapy," *Acta Med Scand*, 1960, 167(1):23-7.

Mechlorethamine Hydrochloride (me klor eth' a meen)

Related Information

Drugs and Chemicals Proven to be Teratogenic in Humans *on page 1572-1575*

Toxicities of Chemotherapeutic Agents *on page 1631-1633*

CAS Number 51-75-2; 55-86-7

Brand Names Caryolysine®; Mustargen®

Synonyms Cloramin; HN_2; Mustine Hydrochloride; Nitrogen Mustard

Use Combination therapy for lymphomas and bronchogenic carcinoma; intracavitary use for malignant pleural effusions; topical application has been used for psoriasis, mycosis fungoides, skin lesions from chronic granulocytic leukemia and nonmalignant cutaneous Langerhans cell hystiocytosis

Mechanism of Action Bischloroethylamine which alkylates the N^7 position of quanine in DNA and RNA thus resulting in depurination of DNA-causing breakage

Adverse Reactions

Central nervous system: Headache, seizures
Gastrointestinal: Nausea, vomiting, dizziness, anorexia
Hematologic: Leukopenia (nadir: 6-8 days), thrombocytopenia (nadir: 10-16 days)
Hepatic: Jaundice
Neuromuscular & skeletal: Tremors
Otic: Tinnitus, deafness
Miscellaneous: Amenorrhea, hyperpigmentation

Signs & Symptoms of Acute Overdose Suppression of all formed elements of the blood, uric acid crystals, nausea, vomiting, deafness, diarrhea

Toxicodynamics/Kinetics

Absorption: Incomplete after intracavitary administration secondary to rapid deactivation by body fluids
Metabolism: I.V.: Drug undergoes rapid chemical transformation; unchanged drug is undetectable in the blood within a few minutes; rapidly metabolized to ethylene immonium ion
Half-life: <1 minute
Elimination: <0.01% of unchanged drug is recovered in urine

Usual Dosage As a single agent: 0.4 mg/kg/month (single dose) or 0.1 mg/kg on 4 successive days; up to 0.8 mg/kg may be given
Intracavitary: 0.2-0.4 mg/kg
Pericardial: 0.2 mg/kg
Topical: 10 mg/60 mL of water applied to affected area 1-2 times/day

Administration Administer I.V. push through a free flowing I.V. over 1-3 minutes at a concentration not to exceed 1 mg/mL

Contraindications Hypersensitivity to mechlorethamine or any component; preexisting profound myelosuppression or infection

Warnings The U.S. Food and Drug Administration (FDA) currently recommends that procedures for proper handling and disposal of antineoplastic agents be considered. Extravasation of the drug into subcutaneous tissues results in painful inflammation and induration; sloughing may occur. Patients with lymphomas should receive prophylactic allopurinol 2-3 days prior to therapy to prevent complications resulting from tumor lysis.

Dosage Forms Powder for injection: 10 mg

Stability Prepare solution immediately before each injection, since decomposition will occur upon standing; highly unstable in neutral or alkaline solutions; discard any unused drug after 15 minutes

Overdosage Treatment

Decontamination:
Dermal: Sodium thiosulfate $^1/_6$ molar solution: Mix 4 mL of 10% sodium thiosulfate with 6 mL of sterile water injected with fine hypodermic needle into area of extravasation; apply ice packs for 6-12 hours; a 1% lidocaine solution may also be infiltrated
Oral: Dilute with milk or water
Supportive therapy: Colony stimulating factor may be utilized to treat granulocytopenia

Test Interactions Increases potassium (S)

Drug Interactions Diethylmaleate, misonidazole, and buthionine sulfoximine (glutathione-depicting agents) can increase alkylating activity; narcotics and caffeine may potentiate toxicity

Pregnancy Risk Factor D

Pregnancy Implications Possibly teratogenic; oligodactyly and malformed kidneys have been described

Monitoring Parameters CBC with differential, hemoglobin and platelet count

Patient Information Protect skin from contact, will burn and irritate. Any signs of infection, easy bruising or bleeding, shortness of breath, or painful or burning urination should be brought to physician's attention. Nausea, vomiting, or hair loss sometimes occur. The drug may cause permanent sterility and may cause birth defects. The drug may be excreted in breast milk, therefore, an alternative form of feeding your baby should be used.

Nursing Implications Use within 1 hour of preparation

Additional Information Allopurinol may be given 2-3 days prior to treatment in lymphoma patients to prevent hyperuricemia; unused solutions can be neutralized by mixing with an equal volume of a solution containing 2.5% sodium bicarbonate and 2.5% sodium thiosulfate and letting stand for 45 minutes; equipment can be soaked (needles, gloves, etc) for 45 minutes in a 10% sodium thiosulfate bath before discarding; sodium thiosulfate has no effect on central nervous system effects

Specific References

Akintonwa A, "Potentiation of Nitrogen Mustard Toxicity by Narcotic Analgesics," *Clin Toxicol*, 1981, 18:451-8.

(Continued)

Mechlorethamine Hydrochloride *(Continued)*

Vonderheid EC, "Topical Mechlorethamine Chemotherapy: Considerations on its Use in Mycosis Fungoides," *Int J Dermatol*, 1984, 23(3):180-6.

Meclizine Hydrochloride (mek' li zeen)

CAS Number 1104-22-9 (anhydrous); 31884-77-2 (monohydrate); 569-65-3

Brand Names Antivert®; Antrizine®; Bonine® [OTC]; Dizmiss® [OTC]; Meni-D®; Ru-Vert-M®

Synonyms Meclozine Hydrochloride

Use Prevention and treatment of motion sickness; management of dizziness with diseases affecting the vestibular system

Mechanism of Action Has central anticholinergic action by blocking chemoreceptor trigger zone; decreases excitability of the middle ear labyrinth and blocks conduction in the middle ear vestibular-cerebellar pathways

Adverse Reactions

Central nervous system: Drowsiness, fatigue, sedation, dizziness, paranoia, extrapyramidal reaction

Gastrointestinal: Dry mouth, nausea, vomiting

Ocular: Blurred vision

Signs & Symptoms of Acute Overdose Excitation alternating with drowsiness, disorientation, confusion, respiratory depression, memory loss, hallucinations, flushing, mydriasis

Toxicodynamics/Kinetics

Onset of action: Within 1-2 hours

Duration: 8-24 hours

Distribution: Well distributed throughout the body

Metabolism: In the liver

Half-life: 6 hours

Elimination: Excreted as metabolites in urine and as unchanged drug in feces

Usual Dosage Children >12 years and Adults: Oral:

Motion sickness: 25-50 mg 1 hour before travel, repeat dose every 24 hours as needed

Vertigo: 25-100 mg/day in divided doses

Contraindications Hypersensitivity to meclizine or any component; pregnancy

Warnings Use with caution in patients with angle-closure glaucoma or prostatic hypertrophy

Dosage Forms

Capsule: 15 mg, 25 mg, 30 mg

Tablet: 12.5 mg, 25 mg, 50 mg

Tablet:

Chewable: 25 mg

Film coated: 25 mg

Reference Range Serum level of 10 ng/mL 12 hours after an oral dose of 75 mg

Overdosage Treatment

Decontamination: Lavage/activated charcoal with cathartic

Supportive therapy: There is no specific treatment for an antihistamine overdose, however, most of its clinical toxicity is due to anticholinergic effects. Anticholinesterase inhibitors may be useful by reducing acetylcholinesterase. Anticholinesterase inhibitors include physostigmine, neostigmine, pyridostigmine and edrophonium. For anticholinergic overdose with severe life-threatening symptoms, physostigmine 1-2 mg (0.5 or 0.02 mg/kg for children) I.V., slowly may be given to reverse these effects.

Drug Interactions CNS depressants, alcohol increases sedation

Pregnancy Risk Factor B

Pregnancy Implications Crosses the placenta

Patient Information Take after meals; do not discontinue drug abruptly; notify physician if adverse gastrointestinal effects, fever, or heat intolerance occurs; may cause drowsiness; avoid alcohol; adequate fluid intake or sugar free gum or hard candy may help dry mouth; adequate fluid and exercise may help constipation

Additional Information Moderately radiopaque

Specific References

Oosterveld WJ, "Vertigo: Current Concepts in Management," *Drugs*, 1985, 30(3):275-83.

Park J, Logan R, and Pottage A, "Drug-Induced Extrapyramidal Signs in Chronic Liver Disease - A Case Report," *Clin Toxicol*, 1977, 11(1):117-20.

Meclofenamate Sodium (me kloe fen am' ate)

Related Information

Nonsteroidal Anti-Inflammatory Comparison *on page 1655*

CAS Number 644-62-2 (Base); 6385-02-0 (Sodium)

Brand Names Meclomen®

Use Treatment of inflammatory disorders

Mechanism of Action Inhibits prostaglandin synthesis by decreasing the activity of the enzyme, cyclo-oxygenase, which results in decreased formation of prostaglandin precursors

Adverse Reactions

Cardiovascular: Fluid retention, circulatory collapse

Central nervous system: Headache, aseptic meningitis, psychosis, cognitive dysfunction, coma, seizures, dizziness

Dermatologic: Rash, pruritus

Endocrine & metabolic: Hyperkalemia, anion gap metabolic acidosis

Gastrointestinal: Abdominal pain, nausea, vomiting, bleeding, ulceration, constipation, diarrhea, dyspepsia

Genitourinary: Albuminuria

Hematologic: Leukopenia, neutropenia, agranulocytosis, granulocytopenia; aplastic anemia (rare), platelet inhibition, hemolytic anemia

Hepatic: Elevation of transaminases, fulminant hepatitis

Otic: Ototoxicity, tinnitus

Renal: Renal failure (acute), nephrotic syndrome, chronic renal failure

Respiratory: Wheezing, respiratory depression

Miscellaneous: Hypersensitivity

Signs & Symptoms of Acute Overdose Nausea, vomiting, wheezing, nephrotic syndrome, gastrointestinal bleeding, gastritis; cognitive dysfunction, ototoxicity; tinnitus, drowsiness; severe poisoning can manifest with coma, seizures, renal and or hepatic failure, hypotension, respiratory depression

Toxicodynamics/Kinetics

Duration of action: 2-4 hours

Absorption: Rapid and complete from gastrointestinal tract

Protein binding: 99%

Metabolism: In the liver

Half-life: 2-3.3 hours

Time to peak serum concentration: Within 30-90 minutes

Elimination: Principally in urine and feces (33%) as glucuronide conjugates

Usual Dosage Children >14 years and Adults: Oral:

Mild to moderate pain: 50 mg every 4-6 hours, not to exceed 400 mg/day

Rheumatoid arthritis/osteoarthritis: 200-400 mg/day in 3-4 equal doses

Contraindications Active gastrointestinal bleeding, ulcer disease, hypersensitivity to meclofenamate or other NSAIDs

Dosage Forms

Capsule: 50 mg, 100 mg

Tablet: 50 mg, 100 mg

Reference Range Steady-state meclofenamate plasma levels range from 10-20 μg/mL at a dose of 100 mg 3 times/day; one 100 mg dose results in a peak plasma level of 8-9 μg/mL

Overdosage Treatment

Decontamination: Ipecac or lavage/activated charcoal with cathartic

Supportive therapy: Hypotension/dehydration can be managed with intravenous fluid therapy; acidosis should be treated with bicarbonates, seizures with benzodiazepines; antacids, blood products are indicated, as appropriate, for hemorrhage

Enhancement of elimination: Dialysis is indicated for secondary complications, acidosis, or renal failure and not toxin removal alone; multiple dosing of activated charcoal may be effective

Test Interactions Increases chloride (S), sodium (S)

Drug Interactions Aspirin decreases serum concentrations probably by protein-binding displacement; there is an increased bleeding potential with concomitant warfarin therapy; may increase lithium and methotrexate concentrations by decreasing renal clearance; may decrease diuretic and hypotensive effects of thiazides, loop diuretics, ACE inhibitors, and beta-blockers; may increase nephrotoxicity of cyclosporine

Pregnancy Risk Factor B (D if used in the 3rd trimester)

Pregnancy Implications Crosses the placenta

Specific References

Court H and Volans GN, "Poisoning After Overdose With Nonsteroidal Anti-inflammatory Drugs," *Adverse Drug React Acute Poisoning Rev*, 1984, 3(1):1-21.

Glazko AJ, Chang T, Barondy PE, et al, "Metabolic Disposition of Meclofenamic Acid (Meclomen®) in Laboratory Animals and in Man," *Curr Ther Res*, 1978, 23:S22-41.

Hoppmann RA, Peden JG, and Ober SK, "Central Nervous System Side Effects of Nonsteroidal Anti-inflammatory Drugs. Aseptic Meningitis, Psychosis, and Cognitive Dysfunction," *Arch Intern Med*, 1991, 151(7):1309-13.

Preston SN, "Safety of Sodium Meclofenamate (Meclomen®)," *Curr Ther Res*, 1978, 23(Suppl 45):5107-12.

Smolinske SC, Hall AH, Vandenberg SA, et al, "Toxic Effects of Nonsteroid Anti-inflammatory Drugs in Overdose. An Overview of Recent Evidence on Clinical Effects and Dose-Response Relationships," *Drug Saf*, 1990, 5(4):252-74.

Vale JA and Meredith TJ, "Acute Poisoning Due to Nonsteroidal Anti-inflammatory Drugs," *Med Toxicol*, 1986, 1(1):12-31.

(Continued)

Meclofenamate Sodium *(Continued)*

Verbeeck RK, "Pharmacokinetic Drug Interactions With Nonsteroidal Anti-inflammatory Drugs," *Clin Pharmacokinet*, 1990, 19(1):44-66.

Meclomen® *see* Meclofenamate Sodium *on page 494*

Meclomid® *see* Metoclopramide *on page 523*

Mecloprodin *see* Clemastine Fumarate *on page 223*

Meclozine Hydrochloride *see* Meclizine Hydrochloride *on page 494*

Mectizan® *see* Ivermectin *on page 449*

Meda-Cap® [OTC] *see* Acetaminophen *on page 79*

Medihaler Ergotamine™ *see* Ergotamine *on page 317*

Medilax® [OTC] *see* Phenolphthalein *on page 617*

Medipren® [OTC] *see* Ibuprofen *on page 418*

Medi-Tuss® [OTC] *see* Guaifenesin *on page 390*

Medomet® *see* Methyldopa *on page 519*

Mefenamic Acid (me fe nam' ik)

Related Information

Nonsteroidal Anti-Inflammatory Comparison *on page 1655*

CAS Number 61-68-7

Brand Names Ponstel®

Use Short-term relief of mild to moderate pain including primary dysmenorrhea

Mechanism of Action Inhibits prostaglandin synthesis by decreasing the activity of the enzyme, cyclo-oxygenase, which results in decreased formation of prostaglandin precursors

Adverse Reactions

Cardiovascular: Fluid retention, circulatory collapse

Central nervous system: Headache, aseptic meningitis, psychosis, cognitive dysfunction, insomnia, coma, seizures, dizziness

Dermatologic: Rash, pruritus

Endocrine & metabolic: Hyperkalemia, anion gap metabolic acidosis

Gastrointestinal: Abdominal pain, nausea, vomiting, bleeding, ulceration, constipation, diarrhea, dyspepsia

Genitourinary: Albuminuria

Hematologic: Leukopenia, neutropenia, agranulocytosis, granulocytopenia; aplastic anemia (rare), platelet inhibition, hemolytic anemia

Hepatic: Elevation of transaminases, fulminant hepatitis

Otic: Ototoxicity, tinnitus

Renal: Renal failure (acute), nephrotic syndrome, chronic renal failure

Respiratory: Wheezing, respiratory depression

Miscellaneous: Hypersensitivity, feces discoloration (black)

Signs & Symptoms of Acute Overdose Nausea, vomiting, wheezing, nephrotic syndrome, thrombocytopenia, gastrointestinal bleeding, torticollis, insomnia, gastritis; cognitive dysfunction, colitis, bullous skin disease/pemphigoid, ototoxicity; tinnitus, drowsiness; severe poisoning can manifest with coma, seizures (38%), renal and or hepatic failure, hypotension, respiratory depression

Toxicodynamics/Kinetics

Onset of action: Within 2-4 hours

Duration: Up to 6 hours

Absorption: Slow from gastrointestinal tract

Protein binding: High

Metabolism: Conjugated in the liver

Half-life: 3.5 hours

Time to peak serum concentration:

- 250 mg dose: 2.5 hours
- 100 mg dose: 2-4 hours

Elimination: Urine (50%) and feces as unchanged drug and metabolites

Usual Dosage Children >14 years and Adults: Oral: 500 mg to start then 250 mg every 4 hours as needed; maximum therapy: 1 week

Seizuregenic dose:

- Children: 2 g
- Adults: 6 g

Dosing adjustment/comments in renal impairment: Not recommended for use

Contraindications Known hypersensitivity to mefenamic acid or other NSAIDs

Dosage Forms Capsule: 250 mg

Overdosage Treatment

Decontamination: Ipecac or lavage/activated charcoal with cathartic

Supportive therapy: Hypotension/dehydration can be managed with intravenous fluid therapy; acidosis should be treated with bicarbonates, seizures with benzodiazepines; antacids, blood products are indicated, as appropriate, for hemorrhage

Enhancement of elimination: Dialysis or perfusion is indicated for secondary complications, acidosis, or renal failure and not toxin removal alone; multiple dosing of activated charcoal may be effective

Test Interactions Increases chloride (S), sodium (S), positive Coombs' [direct]

Drug Interactions Aspirin decreases serum concentrations probably by protein-binding displacement; there is an increased bleeding potential with concomitant warfarin therapy; may increase lithium and methotrexate concentrations by decreasing renal clearance; may decrease diuretic and hypotensive effects of thiazides, loop diuretics, ACE inhibitors, and beta-blockers; may increase nephrotoxicity of cyclosporine

Pregnancy Risk Factor C

Specific References

Balali-Mood M, Critchley JA, Proudfoot AT, et al, "Mefenamic Acid Overdosage," *Lancet*, 1981, 2(8234):1354-6.

Court H and Volans GN, "Poisoning After Overdose With Nonsteroidal Anti-inflammatory Drugs," *Adverse Drug React Acute Poisoning Rev*, 1984, 3(1):1-21.

Gossinger H, Hruby K, Haubenstock A, et al, "Coma in Mefenamic Acid Poisoning," *Lancet*, 1982, 2(8294):384.

Hendrickse MT, "Mefenamic Acid Overdose Mimicking Brainstem Stroke," *Lancet*, 1988, 2(8618):1019.

Hoppmann RA, Peden JG, and Ober SK, "Central Nervous System Side Effects of Nonsteroidal Anti-inflammatory Drugs. Aseptic Meningitis, Psychosis, and Cognitive Dysfunction," *Arch Intern Med*, 1991, 151(7):1309-13.

Shipton EA and Muller FO, "Severe Mefenamic Acid Poisoning. A Case Report," *S Afr Med J*, 1985, 67(20):823-4.

Smolinske SC, Hall AH, Vandenberg SA, et al, "Toxic Effects of Nonsteroid Anti-inflammatory Drugs in Overdose. An Overview of Recent Evidence on Clinical Effects and Dose-Response Relationships," *Drug Saf*, 1990, 5(4):252-74.

Turnbull AJ, Campbell P, and Hughes JA, "Mefenamic Acid Nephropathy – Acute Renal Failure in Overdose," *Br Med J (Clin Res)*, 1988, 296(6622):646.

Vale JA and Meredith TJ, "Acute Poisoning Due to Nonsteroidal Anti-inflammatory Drugs," *Med Toxicol*, 1986, 1(1):12-31.

Verbeeck RK, "Pharmacokinetic Drug Interactions With Nonsteroidal Anti-inflammatory Drugs," *Clin Pharmacokinet*, 1990, 19(1):44-66.

Megalone® *see* Fleroxacin *on page 352*

Meleretten® *see* Thioridazine Hydrochloride *on page 745*

Melix® *see* Glyburide *on page 384*

Mellaril® *see* Thioridazine Hydrochloride *on page 745*

Mellaril-S® *see* Thioridazine Hydrochloride *on page 745*

Melphalan (mel' fa lan)

Related Information

Toxicities of Chemotherapeutic Agents *on page 1631-1633*

CAS Number 148-82-3

Brand Names Alkeran®

Synonyms L-PAM; L-Sarcolysin; Phenylalanine Mustard

Use Palliative treatment of multiple myeloma and nonresectable epithelial ovarian carcinoma; neuroblastoma, rhabdomyosarcoma, breast cancer, sarcoma; may be helpful in patients with primary amyloidosis

I.V. formulation: Use in patients in whom oral therapy is not appropriate

Mechanism of Action Alkylating agent which is a derivative of mechlorethamine that inhibits DNA and RNA synthesis via formation of carbonium ions; cross-links strands of DNA

Adverse Reactions

Cardiovascular: Vasculitis

Central nervous system: Fever

Dermatologic: Alopecia, rash, pruritus, vesiculation of skin

Endocrine & metabolic: Amenorrhea, hyponatremia, ovarian failure

Gastrointestinal: Nausea, vomiting, diarrhea, stomatitis, oral ulceration

Genitourinary: Bladder irritation,

Hematologic: Thrombocytopenia, anemia, leukopenia, neutropenia, agranulocytosis, granulocytopenia, hemolytic anemia

Local: Burning and discomfort at injection site

Renal: Hemorrhagic cystitis

Respiratory: Pulmonary fibrosis, cough, dyspnea

Miscellaneous: Hypersensitivity, feces discoloration (black)

Toxicodynamics/Kinetics

Absorption: Oral: Variable and incomplete (56%); food interferes with absorption

(Continued)

Melphalan *(Continued)*

Distribution: V_d: 0.5-0.6 L/kg throughout total body water
Protein binding: 55% initially; up to 90% after 12 hours of administration
Bioavailability: Unpredictable, decreasing from 85% to 58%
Half-life, terminal:
- Oral: 1.5 hours
- I.V.: 8 minutes

Time to peak serum concentration: Reportedly within 2 hours
Elimination: 10% to 15% excreted unchanged in urine; 20% to 50% excreted in stool after oral administration; clearance: 0.31 L/hour/kg

Usual Dosage Refer to individual protocols. Dose should always be adjusted to patient response and weekly blood counts.

Children:
- Oral: 4-20 mg/m²/day for 1-21 days
- Pediatric rhabdomyosarcoma: I.V.: 10-35 mg/m² bolus every 21-28 days
- Bone marrow transplant for neuroblastoma: 70-140 mg/m² on days 7 and 6 before BMT or 140-220 mg/m² as a single dose before BMT

Adults:
- Multiple myeloma:
  - Oral: 6 mg/day for 2-3 weeks or 10 mg/day for 7-10 days or 0.15 mg/kg/day for 7 days; labs should be carefully monitored during therapy and the drug may need to be discontinued after 2-3 weeks of treatment. Maintenance doses of 1-3 mg/day may be instituted after WBC recovery.
  - I.V.: 16 mg/m² over 15-20 minutes I.V. infusion and administered at 2-week intervals for 4 doses, then at 4-week intervals
- Bone marrow transplant: I.V.: 50-60 mg/m² (up to 140 mg/m²)
- Ovarian carcinoma: Oral: 0.2 mg/kg/day for 5 days, repeat every 4-5 weeks

Dosing adjustment in renal impairment:
- Cl_{cr} 10-50 mL/minute: Administer at 75% of normal dose
- Cl_{cr} <10 mL/minute: Administer at 50% of normal dose

Administration Reconstitute injection with special diluent 50 mg vial with special diluent to yield a 5 mg/mL solution; filter through a 0.45 μM Millex-HV filter; dilute the reconstituted solution with normal saline to a final concentration not to exceed 2 mg/mL; administer by I.V. infusion at a rate not to exceed 10 mg/minute, but total infusion should be given within 1 hour

Contraindications Hypersensitivity to melphalan or any component; severe bone marrow depression; patients whose disease was resistant to prior therapy

Warnings The U.S. Food and Drug Administration (FDA) currently recommends that procedures for proper handling and disposal for antineoplastic agents be considered. Is potentially mutagenic, carcinogenic, and teratogenic; produces amenorrhea. Reduce dosage or discontinue therapy if leukocyte count <3000/mm³ or platelet count <100,000/mm³; use with caution in patients with bone marrow suppression, impaired renal function, or who have received prior chemotherapy or irradiation. Toxicity to immunosuppressives is increased in elderly. Start with lowest recommended adult doses. Signs of infection, such as fever and WBC rise, may not occur. Lethargy and confusion may be more prominent signs of infection.

Dosage Forms
- Powder for injection: 50 mg, 100 mg
- Tablet: 2 mg

Stability Dilute I.V. formulation with diluent (to 5 mg/mL), then immediately further dilute to ≤0.45 mg/mL with 0.9% sodium chloride injection in a glass bottle and administer within 60 minutes; store at room temperature; protect from light; do not refrigerate reconstituted product; use within 1 hour of reconstitution

Reference Range At 0.6 mg/kg dose of melphalan, a peak plasma level of 280 ng/mL was obtained

Overdosage Treatment
- Decontamination: Lavage/activated charcoal with cathartic
- Supportive therapy: High-dose corticosteroids can be used for pulmonary fibrosis
- Enhancement of elimination: Multiple dosing of activated charcoal may be effective

Test Interactions False-positive Coombs' test [direct]

Diagnostic Tests/Procedures
- Complete Blood Count *on page 1236*

Drug Interactions
- Decreased effect: Cimetidine and other H_2 antagonists: The reduction in gastric pH has been reported to reduce the bioavailability of melphalan by 30%
- Increased toxicity:
  - Cyclosporine: Increased incidence of nephrotoxicity
  - Interferon alpha: Increased incidence of fever

Pregnancy Risk Factor D

Monitoring Parameters CBC with differential and platelet count, serum electrolytes, serum uric acid

Patient Information Any signs of infection, easy bruising or bleeding, dyspnea, or painful or burning urination should be brought to physician's attention. Nausea, vomiting, or hair loss sometimes occurs; drug may cause permanent sterility and birth defects. The drug may be excreted in breast milk, therefore, an alternative form of feeding your baby should be used.

Nursing Implications Protect from light; avoid skin contact with I.V. formulation

Additional Information Myelosuppressive effects:

WBC: moderate
Platelets: moderate
Onset (days): 7
Nadir (days): 10-18
Recovery (days): 42-50

Specific References

Alberts DS, Chang SY, Chen HS, et al, "Oral Melphalan Kinetics," *Clin Pharmacol Ther*, 1979, 26(6):737-45.
Coates TD, "Survival From Melphalan Overdose," *Lancet*, 1984, 2(8410):1048.
Kellie SJ and Kingston JE, "Ovarian Failure After High-Dose Melphalan in Adolescents," *Lancet*, 1987, 1(8547):1425.

Menadol® [OTC] *see* Ibuprofen *on page 418*

Menest® *see* Estrogens, Esterified *on page 327*

Meni-D® *see* Meclizine Hydrochloride *on page 494*

Mentholatum® Vapor Rub *see* Camphor *on page 179*

Meperidine Hydrochloride (me per' i deen)

Related Information

Pharmacokinetics of Narcotic Agonist Analgesics *on page 1654*

CAS Number 57-42-1; 50-13-5

Brand Names Centralgine®; Demerol®; Dolantin®; Dolantina®; Dolantine®; Dolosal®

Synonyms Isonipecaine Hydrochloride; Pethidine Hydrochloride

Use Management of moderate to severe pain; adjunct to anesthesia and preoperative sedation

Mechanism of Action Binds to opiate receptors in the CNS, causing inhibition of ascending pain pathways, altering the perception of and response to pain; produces generalized CNS depression; a cogenor of atropine

Adverse Reactions

Cardiovascular: Palpitations, hypotension, bradycardia, peripheral vasodilation, tachycardia (with I.V. injection), hypertension
Central nervous system: CNS depression, dizziness, drowsiness, sedation, seizures, psychosis, intracranial pressure (increased), parkinsonism especially associated with synthetic analogues (MPPP, MPTP, PEPAP), electroencephalogram abnormalities
Dermatologic: Pruritus
Endocrine & metabolic: Antidiuretic hormone release
Gastrointestinal: Nausea, vomiting, constipation (less likely than with morphine), licorice-like taste
Hematologic: Porphyria
Ocular: Miosis, mydriasis
Neuromuscular & skeletal: Myoclonus
Respiratory: Apnea, respiratory depression
Miscellaneous: Physical and psychological dependence, histamine release, biliary or urinary tract spasm

Signs & Symptoms of Acute Overdose Myoglobinuria, rhabdomyolysis, ejaculatory disturbances, syndrome of inappropriate antidiuretic hormone (SIADH), seizures

Toxicodynamics/Kinetics

Epidural: Onset of action: 5-30 minutes
Oral, I.M., S.C.:
  Onset of analgesic effect: Within 10-15 minutes
  Peak effect: Within 1 hour
  Duration: 2-4 hours
I.V.: Onset of effect: Within 5 minutes
Distribution: V_d: 3.1-5 L/kg
Protein binding: 55% to 75% in healthy patients; 32% in anuric patients
Metabolism: In the liver to normeperidine (demethylation)
Bioavailability: ~50% to 60%; increased with liver disease
Half-life:
  Parent drug: Terminal phase:
    Neonates: 23 hours; range: 12-39 hours
    Adults: 2.5-4 hours
    Adults with liver disease: 7-11 hours

(Continued)

Meperidine Hydrochloride *(Continued)*

Normeperidine (active metabolite):

Neonates: 20-80 hours

Adults: 15-30 hours; is dependent on renal function and can accumulate with high doses or in patients with decreased renal function

Usual Dosage Doses should be titrated to appropriate analgesic effect; when changing route of administration, note that oral doses are about half as effective as parenteral dose. Oral, I.M., I.V., S.C.:

Children: 1-1.5 mg/kg/dose every 3-4 hours as needed; 1-2 mg/kg as a single dose preoperative medication may be used; maximum: 100 mg/dose

Adults: 50-150 mg/dose every 3-4 hours as needed

Dosing adjustment in renal impairment:

Cl_{cr} 10-50 mL/minute: Administer at 75% of normal dose

Cl_{cr} <10 mL/minute: Administer at 50% of normal dose

Dosing adjustment/comments in hepatic disease: Increased narcotic effect in cirrhosis; reduction in dose more important for oral than I.V. route

Administration IVP meperidine should be given slowly

Contraindications Hypersensitivity to meperidine or any component; patients receiving MAO inhibitors presently or in the past 14 days

Warnings Use with caution in patients with pulmonary, hepatic, renal disorders, or increased intracranial pressure; use with caution in patients with renal failure or seizure disorders or those receiving high-dose meperidine; normeperidine (an active metabolite and CNS stimulant) may accumulate and precipitate twitches, tremors, or seizures; some preparations contain sulfites which may cause allergic reaction

Dosage Forms

Injection:

Multiple-dose vials: 50 mg/mL (30 mL); 100 mg/mL (20 mL)

Single dose: 10 mg/mL (5 mL, 10 mL, 30 mL); 25 mg/dose (0.5 mL, 1 mL); 50 mg/dose (1 mL); 75 mg/dose (1 mL, 1.5 mL); 100 mg/dose (1 mL)

Syrup: 50 mg/5 mL (500 mL)

Tablet: 50 mg, 100 mg

Stability Protect oral dosage forms from light; **incompatible** with aminophylline, heparin, phenobarbital, phenytoin, and sodium bicarbonate

Reference Range

Meperidine:

Therapeutic: 70-500 ng/mL (SI: 283-2020 nmol/L)

Toxic: >1000 ng/mL (SI: >4043 nmol/L)

Normeperidine: Toxic: >450 ng/mL

Overdosage Treatment Supportive therapy: Naloxone hydrochloride (0.4-2 mg I.V., S.C., or through an endotracheal tube); a continuous infusion (at ⅔ the response dose/hour) may be required

Antidote(s)

Naloxone Hydrochloride *on page 1447*

Test Interactions ↑ amylase (S), ↑ BSP retention, ↑ CPK (I.M. injections)

Drug Interactions

Decreased effect with phenytoin (↑ toxicity of meperidine and normeperidine concurrently)

Increased effect/toxicity of isoniazid (hypotension); increased effect/toxicity with MAO inhibitors (can be fatal), serotonin reuptake inhibitors (eg, fluoxetine), CNS depressants, TCAs, chlorpromazine, phenothiazines, barbiturates, amphetamines, cimetidine

Increased neurotoxicity with acyclovir

Pregnancy Risk Factor B (D if used for prolonged periods or in high doses at term)

Pregnancy Implications Crosses the placenta; appears in breast milk; fetal respiratory depression can occur

Monitoring Parameters Pain relief, respiratory and mental status, blood pressure

Patient Information Avoid alcohol, may cause drowsiness

Nursing Implications Observe patient for excessive sedation, CNS depression, seizures, respiratory depression

Additional Information Decrease the dose in patients with renal or hepatic impairment; equianalgesic doses: morphine 10 mg I.M. is equivalent to meperidine 75-100 mg I.M.

I.V. incompatible with barbiturates

Specific References

Armstrong PJ and Bersten A, "Normeperidine Toxicity," *Anesth Analg*, 1986, 65(5):536-8.

Buchanan JF and Brown CR, "Designer Drugs: A Problem in Clinical Toxicology," *Med Toxicol Adverse Drug Exp*, 1988, 3(1):1-17.

Kyff JV and Rice TL, "Meperidine-Associated Seizures in a Child," *Clin Pharm*, 1990, 9(5):337-8.

Miller RR and Jick H, "Clinical Effects of Meperidine in Hospitalized Medical Patients," *J Clin Pharmacol*, 1978, 18(4):180-9.

Stone PA, Macintyre PE, and Jarvis DA, "Norpethidine Toxicity and Patient Controlled Analgesia," *Br J Anaesth*, 1993, 71(5):738-40.

Mephobarbital (me foe bar' bi tal)

CAS Number 115-38-8

Brand Names Gemonil®; Mebaral®

Synonyms 5,5-Diethyl-1-Methylbarbituric Acid; Methylphenobarbital

Use Prophylactic management of tonic-clonic (grand mal) seizures and absence (petit mal) seizures

Mechanism of Action Increases seizure threshold in the motor cortex; depresses monosynaptic and polysynaptic transmission in the CNS

Adverse Reactions

Central nervous system: Drowsiness, drowsiness, paradoxical excitation (especially in children)

Dermatologic: Rash, including Stevens-Johnson syndrome or erythema multiforme

Gastrointestinal: Nausea, vomiting

Hematologic: Leukopenia/neutropenia (agranulocytosis, granulocytopenia), thrombocytopenic purpura

Miscellaneous: Psychological and physical dependence

Signs & Symptoms of Acute Overdose CNS depression, respiratory depression, nystagmus, hypothermia, tachycardia, hypotension, vision color changes (green tinge), vision color changes (yellow tinge); ptosis, renal failure, cyclic coma

Toxicodynamics/Kinetics

Onset of action: 20-60 minutes

Duration: 6-8 hours

Absorption: Oral: ~70%

Distribution: V_d: 2.6 L/kg; widely distributed throughout the body

Protein binding: 50%

Metabolism: Demethylated by the liver to phenobarbital (15%)

Half-life: 48-52 hours

Elimination: Excreted in urine

Usual Dosage Oral:

Epilepsy:

- Children: 6-12 mg/kg/day in 2-4 divided doses
- Adults: 200-600 mg/day in 2-4 divided doses

Sedation:

- Children:
  - <5 years: 16-32 mg 3-4 times/day
  - >5 years: 32-64 mg 3-4 times/day
- Adults: 32-100 mg 3-4 times/day

Dosing adjustment in renal or hepatic impairment: Use with caution and reduce dosages

Contraindications Hypersensitivity to mephobarbital or any component; preexisting CNS depression; apnea; severe uncontrolled pain; history of porphyria

Warnings Use with caution in patients with renal impairment and pulmonary insufficiency; avoid abrupt discontinuation of mephobarbital

Dosage Forms Tablet: 32 mg, 50 mg, 100 mg

Reference Range Phenobarbital level should be in the range of 15-40 μg/mL; levels of >80 μg/mL correlate with decreased mental status

Overdosage Treatment

Decontamination: Ipecac or lavage/activated charcoal with cathartic

Supportive therapy: Isotonic fluids for hypotension; dopamine or norepinephrine can be used

Enhancement of elimination: Repeated oral doses of activated charcoal significantly reduce the half-life of phenobarbital resulting from an enhancement of nonrenal elimination. The usual dose is 30-60 g every 4-6 hours for 3-4 days unless the patient has no bowel movement causing the charcoal to remain in the gastrointestinal tract. Assure adequate hydration and renal function. Urinary alkalinization with I.V. sodium bicarbonate also helps to enhance elimination. Hemodialysis or hemoperfusion is of uncertain value. Patients in stage four coma due to high serum barbiturate levels may require charcoal hemoperfusion.

Test Interactions Increases alkaline phosphatase (S), ammonia (B); decreases bilirubin (S), calcium (S)

Diagnostic Tests/Procedures

Mephobarbital, Blood *on page 1291*

Drug Interactions Mephobarbital is converted to phenobarbital in the liver; phenobarbital induces the liver enzyme involved with warfarin and doxycycline metabolism; ethanol and antihistamines may enhance adverse neurological effects

Pregnancy Risk Factor D

Monitoring Parameters Respiratory

(Continued)

Mephobarbital *(Continued)*

Patient Information May cause drowsiness, may impair coordination and judgment; do not discontinue abruptly; notify physician of dark urine, pale stools, jaundice, abdominal pain, persistent nausea, and vomiting; do not skip doses

Nursing Implications Observe patient for excessive sedation, apnea; raise bed rails, institute safety precautions, assist with ambulation

Additional Information Sometimes used in specific patients who have excessive sedation or hyperexcitability from phenobarbital; avoid abrupt discontinuation; phenobarbital is excreted in breast milk and may accumulate in the neonate

Specific References

Pond SM, Olson KR, Osterloh JD, et al, "Randomized Study of the Treatment of Phenobarbital Overdose With Repeated Doses of Activated Charcoal," *JAMA*, 1984, 251(23):3104-8.

Zawada ET, Nappi J, Done G, et al, "Advances in the Hemodialysis Management of Phenobarbital Overdose," *South Med J*, 1983, 76(1):6-8.

Mepivacaine Hydrochloride (me piv' a kane)

CAS Number 96-88-8; 1722-62-9

Brand Names Carbocaine®; Isocaine® HCl; Polocaine®; Scandicain®

Use Local anesthesia by nerve block; infiltration in dental procedures

Mechanism of Action Mepivacaine is an amino amide local anesthetic similar to lidocaine; like all local anesthetics, mepivacaine acts by preventing the generation and conduction of nerve impulses

Adverse Reactions

Cardiovascular: Bradycardia, myocardial depression, hypotension, cardiovascular collapse, edema

Central nervous system: Anxiety, restlessness, disorientation, confusion, shivering, seizures, drowsiness, unconsciousness, lightheadedness, headache, chills

Dermatologic: Urticaria

Gastrointestinal: Nausea, vomiting

Hematologic: Porphyria

Local: Transient stinging or burning at injection site

Neuromuscular & skeletal: Tremors

Ocular: Blurred vision

Otic: Ototoxicity, tinnitus

Respiratory: Respiratory arrest

Sensitivity reactions: Anaphylactoid reactions

Miscellaneous: Neonatal CNS depression following paracervical blocks from delivery, porphyrinogenic

Signs & Symptoms of Acute Overdose Dizziness, cyanosis, tremors, depression, bronchial spasm, seizures, nystagmus, muscle twitching, bradycardia, ototoxicity; tinnitus, apnea

Toxicodynamics/Kinetics

Onset of action: 7-15 minutes following epidural injection

Duration: 2-2.5 hours; similar onset and duration is seen following infiltration

Distribution: V_d: 1.2 L/kg

Protein binding: 70% to 85%

Metabolism: Chiefly in the liver by N-demethylation, hydroxylation, and glucuronidation; undergoes enterohepatic recirculation

Half-life:

- Neonates: 9 hours
- Adults: 2-3 hours

Elimination: Urinary excretion (95% as metabolites)

Usual Dosage Children and Adults: Injectable local anesthetic: Varies with procedure, degree of anesthesia needed, vascularity of tissue, duration of anesthesia required, and physical condition of patient

Contraindications A-V block, hypersensitivity to mepivacaine or any component, allergy to sodium bisulfate

Warnings Use with caution in patients with cardiac disease, renal disease, and hyperthyroidism; seizures due to systemic toxicity leading to cardiac arrest have been reported presumably due to intravascular injection

Dosage Forms Injection: 1% [10 mg/mL] (30 mL, 50 mL); 1.5% [15 mg/mL] (30 mL); 2% [20 mg/mL] (20 mL, 50 mL); 3% [30 mg/mL] (1.8 mL)

Reference Range

Therapeutic: Plasma levels are <5 μg/mL

Fatal: Fatalities are associated with levels >10 μg/mL

Overdosage Treatment

Decontamination: Lavage/activated charcoal with cathartic

Supportive therapy: Termination of anesthesia by pneumatic tourniquet inflation should be attempted when the agent is administered by infiltration or regional injection. Seizures commonly respond to diazepam or lorazepam, while hypotension responds to I.V. fluids and Trendelenburg positioning. Bradyarrhythmias (when the heart rate is less than 60) can be treated with I.V. atropine 15 mcg/kg.

With the development of metabolic acidosis, I.V. sodium bicarbonate 0.5-2 mEq/kg and ventilatory assistance should be instituted.

Enhancement of elimination: Exchange transfusion is of minimal benefit

Drug Interactions Beta-adrenergic blockers

Pregnancy Risk Factor C

Pregnancy Implications May cause neonatal depression or seizures

Monitoring Parameters EKG, respiratory status

Nursing Implications Before injecting, withdraw syringe plunger to ensure injection is not into vein or artery; solution is acidic

Additional Information Numbing, bitter taste

Specific References

Dodson WE, Hillman RE, and Hillman LS, "Brain Tissue Levels in a Fatal Case of Neonatal Mepivacaine (Carbocaine®) Poisoning," *J Pediatr*, 1975, 86(4):624-7.

Meprobam *see* Meprobamate *on this page*

Meprobamate (me proe ba' mate)

CAS Number 57-53-4

Brand Names Equanil®; Meprospan®; Miltown®; Neuramate®; Tenavoid®

Synonyms Meprobam

Use Management of anxiety disorders

Mechanism of Action Precise mechanisms are not yet clear, but many effects have been ascribed to its central depressant actions

Adverse Reactions

Cardiovascular: Syncope

Central nervous system: Drowsiness, cyanosis, slurred speech, headache, euphoria, dizziness, paradoxical excitation, ataxia

Ocular: Nystagmus, miosis, mydriasis

Hypersensitivity reactions:

- Mild: Rash, leukopenia, purpura, peripheral edema, angioedema, bullous dermatitis
- Severe: Fever, chills, wheezing, renal failure, dermatitis, stomatitis, Stevens-Johnson syndrome, agranulocytosis

Signs & Symptoms of Acute Overdose Drowsiness, bradycardia, drowsiness, wheezing, hyporeflexia, coma, respiratory depression, syncope, stupor, ataxia, areflexia, hypotension, tachycardia, bezoars, porphyria, leukopenia; neutropenia; agranulocytosis; granulocytopenia

Toxicodynamics/Kinetics

Onset of action: Oral: Within 60 minutes

Absorption: Oral: Well absorbed from gastrointestinal tract

Distribution: V_d: 0.75 L/kg; distributed throughout body

Protein binding: 20%

Metabolism: Promptly in the liver

Half-life: 10 hours; in overdose setting: >24 hours

Time to peak serum concentration: 1-3 hours

Elimination: Excreted in urine (8% to 20% as unchanged drug) and in feces (10% as metabolites)

Usual Dosage Oral:

Children 6-12 years: 100-200 mg 2-3 times/day

- Sustained release: 200 mg twice daily

Adults: 400 mg 3-4 times/day, up to 2400 mg/day

- Sustained release; 400-800 mg twice daily

Dosing interval in renal impairment:

- Cl_{cr} 10-50 mL/minute: Administer every 9-12 hours
- Cl_{cr} <10 mL/minute: Administer every 12-18 hours

Dosing adjustment in hepatic impairment: Probably necessary in patients with liver disease

Contraindications Hypersensitivity to meprobamate or any component, there may be a cross-sensitivity with other benzodiazepines; do not use in a comatose patient or in those with pre-existing CNS depression or narrow-angle glaucoma or severe uncontrolled pain

Warnings Physical and psychological dependence and abuse may occur; not recommended in children <6 years of age; allergic reaction may occur in patients with history of dermatological condition (usually by fourth dose)

Dosage Forms

Capsule, sustained release: 200 mg, 400 mg

Tablet: 200 mg, 400 mg, 600 mg

Reference Range

Therapeutic: 6-12 μg/mL (SI: 28-55 μmol/L)

Toxic: >60 μg/mL (SI: >275 μmol/L); coma is associated with levels >70 μg/mL

Fatal: Fatalities can occur with levels >142 μg/mL

(Continued)

Meprobamate *(Continued)*

Overdosage Treatment

Decontamination: Lavage/activated charcoal with cathartic

Supportive therapy: Following attempts to enhance drug elimination. Hypotension should be treated with I.V. fluids and/or Trendelenburg positioning.

Enhancement of elimination: Hemodialysis is recommended at plasma levels >20 mg/dL; charcoal hemoperfusion increases meprobamate clearance. Multiple dosing of activated charcoal may decrease half-life by 50%; forced diuresis with saline may be useful; moderately dialyzable (20% to 50%).

Drug Interactions CNS depressants, anticoagulants (not clinically significant), alcohol

Pregnancy Risk Factor D

Pregnancy Implications Crosses the placenta; appears in breast milk

Monitoring Parameters Mental status

Patient Information May cause drowsiness; avoid alcoholic beverages

Additional Information Can cause bezoars

Specific References

Hassan E, "Treatment of Meprobamate Overdose With Repeated Oral Doses of Activated Charcoal," *Ann Emerg Med*, 1986, 15(1):73-6.

Jacobsen D, Wiik-Larsen E, Saltvedt E, et al, "Meprobamate Kinetics During and After Terminated Hemoperfusion in Acute Intoxications," *J Toxicol Clin Toxicol*, 1987, 25(4):317-31.

Volturo GA, "Meprobamate and Bezoar Formation," *Ann Emerg Med*, 1987, 16(4):472-3.

Meprospan® *see* Meprobamate *on previous page*

Mercazolylum *see* Methimazole *on page 512*

Merocaine® *see* Benzocaine *on page 149*

Meropenem

Related Information

Imipenem/Cilastatin *on page 420*

CAS Number 96036-03-2

Synonyms ICI-194660; SM-7338

Use Carbapenem antibiotic useful against gram-positive and gram-negative (including *Pseudomonas aeruginosa*) organisms used in meningitis, skin, and soft tissue infections and in urinary tract infections

Mechanism of Action Interacts with proteins in bacterial cystoplasmic membrane; similar to imipenem

Adverse Reactions

Central nervous system: Headache

Gastrointestinal: Abdominal pain, vomiting, diarrhea, nausea

Hepatic: Elevation of liver function tests

Signs & Symptoms of Acute Overdose Convulsions

Toxicodynamics/Kinetics

Distribution: V_d: 13-21 L

Protein binding: Low

Metabolism: Extrarenal to a metabolite ICI-213689

Half-life: 1 hour (parent compound); 2 hours (metabolite)

Elimination: Renal (83%); clearance: 140-230 mL/minute

Usual Dosage I.V.:

Febrile neutropenia: 1 g every 8 hours

Meningitis: 2 g (38.5 mg/kg) every 8 hours

Skin/soft tissue infections: 0.5 g every 8 hours

Urinary tract infections: 0.5 g every 8 hours

Reduce dosage in elderly patients

Dosing interval in renal impairment: Prolong dose interval in patients with renal insufficiency

Cl_{cr} 30-50 mL/minute: Administer every 12 hours

Cl_{cr} <30 mL/minute: Administer every 24 hours

Contraindications Hypersensitivity to meropenem

Warnings Use with caution in patients with hypersensitivity to imipenem, penicillins, cephalosporin, history of asthma, renal insufficiency, epilepsy, elderly, liver dysfunction

Reference Range Peak serum meropenem levels after a 1 g dose: 55-62 μg/mL 30 minutes postinfusion

Overdosage Treatment

Supportive therapy: Benzodiazepines can be used for seizure control

Enhancement of elimination: Hemodialysis can effectively remove meropenem and its metabolite; dialysis clearance: 79-81 mL/minute

Drug Interactions Probenecid can increase half-life of meropenem to 1.3 hours

Specific References

Christensson BA, Nilsson-Ehle I, Hutchinson M, et al, "Pharmacokinetics of Meropenem in Sub-

jects With Various Degrees of Renal Impairment," *Antimicrob Agents Chemother*, 1992, 36(7):1532-7.
Mouton JW and van den Anker JN, "Meropenem Clinical Pharmacokinetics," *Clin Pharmacokinet*, 1995, 28:275-86.

Mersol® [OTC] *see* Thimerosal *on page 744*

Mesoridazine Besylate (mez oh rid' a zeen)

Related Information

Antipsychotic Agents Comparison *on page 1642*

CAS Number 5588-33-0; 32672-69-8

Brand Names Imagotan®; Serentil®

Replaces NC-123

Use Symptomatic management of psychotic disorders, including schizophrenia, behavioral problems, alcoholism as well as reducing anxiety and tension occurring in neurosis

Mechanism of Action Blockade of postsynaptic CNS dopamine receptors; a metabolite of thioridazine

Adverse Reactions

Cardiovascular: Hypotension (especially with I.V. use), hypotension (orthostatic), tachycardia, cardiac arrhythmias

Central nervous system: Sedation, drowsiness, restlessness, anxiety, extrapyramidal reactions, pseudoparkinsonian signs and symptoms, tardive dyskinesia, neuroleptic malignant syndrome, seizures, altered central temperature regulation

Dermatologic: Hyperpigmentation, pruritus, rash, photosensitivity

Endocrine & metabolic: Amenorrhea, galactorrhea, gynecomastia, syndrome of inappropriate antidiuretic hormone, weight gain

Gastrointestinal: gastrointestinal upset, dry mouth, constipation

Genitourinary: Urinary retention, impotence

Hematologic: Agranulocytosis, leukopenia (usually in patients with large doses for prolonged periods), thrombocytopenia, hemolysis, eosinophilia

Hepatic: Cholestatic jaundice

Ocular: Retinal pigmentation, nystagmus, blurred vision

Signs & Symptoms of Acute Overdose Deep sleep, coma, priapism, photophobia, impotence, enuresis, extrapyramidal reaction, neuroleptic malignant syndrome, ejaculatory disturbances, gynecomastia, Parkinson's-like symptoms, nystagmus, galactorrhea, abnormal involuntary muscle movements, hypotension, cardiac arrhythmias, QRS prolongation, vision color changes (brown tinge), vision color changes (yellow tinge); systemic lupus erythematosus (SLE), urine discoloration (pink), urine discoloration (red), urine discoloration (red-brown), leukopenia; neutropenia; agranulocytosis; granulocytopenia

Toxicodynamics/Kinetics

Onset of action: 30 minutes to 1 hour

Duration: 4-6 hours

Absorption: Very erratic, oral liquids are much more dependable

Distribution: V_d: 3-6 L/kg; widely distributed into body including breast milk

Protein binding: 91% to 99%

Metabolism: Hepatic

Half-life: 24-48 hours

Time to peak serum concentration: 2-4 hours; steady-state serum levels: 4-7 days

Elimination: Mostly excreted in urine

Usual Dosage Concentrate may be diluted just prior to administration with distilled water, acidified tap water, orange or grape juice; do not prepare and store bulk dilutions

Adults:

Oral: 25-50 mg 3 times/day; maximum: 100-400 mg/day

I.M.: 25 mg initially, repeat in 30-60 minutes as needed; optimal dosage range: 25-200 mg/day

Contraindications Hypersensitivity to mesoridazine or any component, cross-sensitivity with other phenothiazines may exist; avoid use in patients with narrow-angle glaucoma, bone marrow depression, severe liver or cardiac disease

Warnings Safety in children <6 months of age has not been established; use with caution in patients with cardiovascular disease or seizures; benefits of therapy must be weighed against risks of therapy

Dosage Forms

Injection: 25 mg/mL (1 mL)

Liquid, oral: 25 mg/mL (118 mL)

Tablet: 10 mg, 25 mg, 50 mg, 100 mg

Overdosage Treatment

Decontamination: Lavage/activated charcoal with cathartic

Supportive therapy: Following initiation of essential overdose management, toxic symptom treatment and supportive treatment should be initiated. Hypotension

(Continued)

Mesoridazine Besylate *(Continued)*

usually responds to I.V. fluids or Trendelenburg positioning. If unresponsive to these measures, the use of a parenteral inotrope may be required. Seizures commonly respond to lorazepam or diazepam (I.V. 5-10 mg bolus in adults every 15 minutes if needed up to a total of 30 mg; I.V. 0.25-0.4 mg/kg/dose up to a total of 10 mg in children) or to phenytoin or phenobarbital. Also critical cardiac arrhythmias and prolonged Q-T interval on EKG often respond to I.V. phenytoin (15 mg/kg up to 1 g), while other antiarrhythmics can be used. Neuroleptics often cause extrapyramidal reaction (eg, dystonic reactions) requiring management with benztropine mesylate I.V. 1-2 mg (adults) may be effective. These agents are generally effective within 2-5 minutes. Avoid use of quinidine, procainamide, or disopyramide

Enhancement of elimination: Multiple dosing of activated charcoal may be useful; not dialyzable (0% to 5%)

Test Interactions Increases cholesterol (S), glucose; decreases uric acid (S), calcium (S); may give false-positive when testing for tricyclic antidepressants through EMIT system

Drug Interactions

Other CNS depressants: Increased depression
Anticonvulsants: Decreased mesoridazine levels
Lithium: Oral solutions are incompatible when mixed
Metrizamide: Increases risk of seizures

Pregnancy Risk Factor C

Pregnancy Implications Distributes into breast milk

Monitoring Parameters EKG

Patient Information May cause drowsiness

Nursing Implications Watch for hypotension when administering I.M. or I.V.

Specific References

Marrs-Simon PA, Zell-Kanter M, Kendzierski DL, et al, "Cardiotoxic Manifestations of Mesoridazine Overdose," *Ann Emerg Med*, 1988, 17(10):1074-8.

Samet J and Surawicz B, "Cardiac Function in Patients Treated With Phenothiazines Comparison With Quinidine," *J Clin Pharmacol*, 1974, 14(11-12):588-96.

Metaprel® *see* Metaproterenol Sulfate *on this page*

Metaproterenol Sulfate (met a proe ter' e nol)

Related Information

Therapeutic Drugs Associated With Hallucinations *on page 1558-1559*

CAS Number 5874-97-5

Brand Names Alupent®; Arm-a-Med® Metaproterenol; Dey-Dose® Metaproterenol; Metaprel®; Prometa®

Synonyms Orciprenaline Sulfate

Use Bronchodilator in reversible airway obstruction due to asthma or COPD; because of its delayed onset of action (one hour) and prolonged effect (4 or more hours), this may not be the drug of choice for assessing response to a bronchodilator

Mechanism of Action Relaxes bronchial smooth muscle by action on $beta_2$-receptors with very little effect on heart rate

Adverse Reactions

Cardiovascular: Tachycardia (slight), palpitations, hypertension, flushing, shortened P-R segment, lengthened Q-T segment, cardiac arrhythmias
Central nervous system: Dizziness, headache, nervousness, CNS stimulation, hyperactivity, insomnia, visual and gustatory hallucinations
Dermatologic: Maculopapular rash
Gastrointestinal: gastrointestinal upset
Neuromuscular & skeletal: Tremors

Signs & Symptoms of Acute Overdose Angina, cardiac arrhythmias, tremors, dry mouth, insomnia

Toxicodynamics/Kinetics

Onset of action: Oral: Bronchodilation occurs within 15 minutes
Peak effect: Within 1 hour
Duration:
  Oral: Up to 4 hours
  Inhalation, aerosol: 1-5 hours
  Inhalation, handbulb nebulizer or IPPB: 2-6 hours
Absorption: Well from gastrointestinal tract
Distribution: Widely distributed throughout body
Metabolism: In the liver
Time to peak serum concentration:
  Inhalation, aerosol: ~1 hour
  Oral: Within 1 hour
Elimination: Primarily as glucuronic acid and conjugates in urine

Usual Dosage

Oral:

Children:

<6 years: 0.3-0.5 mg/kg/dose every 6-8 hours

6-9 years, <60 lbs: 10 mg 3-4 times/day

Children >9 years, >60 lbs and Adults: 20 mg 3-4 times/day

Inhalation: Children >12 years and Adults: 2-3 inhalations every 3-4 hours, up to 12 inhalations in 24 hours

Nebulizer:

Infants and Children: 0.01-0.02 mL/kg of 5% solution; minimum dose: 0.1 mL; maximum dose: 1 mL diluted in 2-3 mL normal saline every 4-6 hours (may be given more frequently according to need)

Adolescents and Adults: 5-20 breaths of full strength 5% metaproterenol **or** 0.2-0.3 mL of 5% metaproterenol in 2.5-3 mL normal saline until nebulized every 4-6 hours (can be given more frequently according to need)

Contraindications Hypersensitivity to metaproterenol or any component; pre-existing cardiac arrhythmias associated with tachycardia; use with a MAO inhibitor

Warnings Excessive or prolonged use may lead to tachyphylaxis; use with caution in patients with cardiovascular disorders, hyperthyroidism, seizure disorders, or diabetes mellitus; excessive use may result in cardiac arrest and death; do not use concurrently with other sympathomimetic bronchodilators

Dosage Forms

Aerosol, oral: 0.65 mg/dose (5 mL, 10 mL)

Solution for inhalation: 0.4% [4 mg/mL] (2.5 mL); 0.6% [6 mg/mL] (2.5 mL); 5% [50 mg/mL] (0.3 mL, 10 mL, 30 mL)

Syrup: 10 mg/5 mL (480 mL)

Tablet: 10 mg, 20 mg

Stability Store in tight, light-resistant container

Overdosage Treatment Beta-adrenergic stimulation can cause increased heart rate, decreased blood pressure, and CNS stimulation; heart rate can be treated with beta-blockers; decreased blood pressure can be treated with pure beta-adrenergic agents; diazepam 0.07 mg/kg or lorazepam can be used for excitation, seizures

Test Interactions Increases potassium (S)

Drug Interactions Other sympathomimetic agents exacerbate cardiac effects

Pregnancy Risk Factor C

Monitoring Parameters Heart rate, blood pressure, respiratory rate

Patient Information Do not exceed recommended dosage – excessive use may lead to adverse effects or loss of effectiveness. Shake canister well before use. Administer pressurized inhalation during the second half of inspiration, as the airways are open water and the aerosol distribution is more extensive. If more than one inhalation per dose is necessary, wait at least 1 full minute between inhalations – second inhalation is best delivered after 10 minutes for Alupent®. May cause nervousness, restlessness, insomnia – if these effects continue after dosage reduction, notify physician. Also notify physician if palpitations, tachycardia, chest pain, muscle tremors, dizziness, headache, flushing or if breathing difficulty persists.

Additional Information Because of its delayed onset of action (1 hour) and prolonged effect (4 or more hours), this may not be the drug of choice for assessing response to a bronchodilator

Specific References

Gilman MJ, Meyer L, Carter J, et al, "Comparison of Aerosolized Glycopyrrolate and Metaproterenol in Acute Asthma," *Chest*, 1990, 98(5):1095-8.

Jerrard DA, Olshaker J, Welebob E, et al, "Efficacy and Safety of a Rapid-Sequence Metaproterenol Protocol in the Treatment of Acute Adult Asthma," *Am J Emerg Med*, 1995, 13:392-5.

Metasedin® *see* Methadone Hydrochloride *on next page*

Metastron® *see* Strontium-89 Chloride *on page 709*

Metformin

Related Information

Hypoglycemic Agents Comparison, Oral *on page 1650*

CAS Number 657-24-9

Brand Names Glucophage®

Synonyms Glucophage

Use Noninsulin-dependent diabetes mellitus

Mechanism of Action Unclear, requires some endogenous insulin to act as antidiabetic

Adverse Reactions

Central nervous system: Fasciculations

(Continued)

Metformin *(Continued)*

Endocrine & metabolic: Lactic acidosis, hyponatremia, hypoglycemia, acidosis
Gastrointestinal: Diarrhea, metallic taste
Hematologic: Megaloblastic anemia, vitamin B_{12} deficiency
Miscellaneous: Vasculitis, sweating, hypersensitivity pneumonitis, porphyrinogenic

Toxicodynamics/Kinetics
Metabolism: No more than 20% metabolized
Distribution: V_d: 3.7 L/kg
Protein binding: 0%
Bioavailability: 30% to 60%
Half-life: 4-8 hours
Time to peak concentrations: 2-2.5 hours
Elimination: Renal, primarily unchanged

Usual Dosage Adults: Oral: 1500-1700 mg/day in divided doses

Warnings Use with caution in patients predisposed to developing lactic acidosis

Dosage Forms Tablet: 500 mg, 850 mg

Reference Range Peak plasma metformin level after a 1.5 g dose: ~3.1 mg/L; levels >45 mg/L associated with toxicity

Overdosage Treatment
Decontamination: Lavage/activated charcoal with cathartic
Supportive therapy: Glucose or glucagon for hypoglycemia; sodium bicarbonate for severe acidosis
Enhancement of elimination: Removed by hemodialysis; in presence of lactic acidosis, use nonlactate dialysate

Antidote(s)
Dextrose *on page 1409*
Glucagon *on page 1431*
Sodium Bicarbonate *on page 1467*

Drug Interactions Cimetidine inhibits metformin metabolism; steroids, alcohol increase risk of developing lactic acidosis

Additional Information Related to withdrawn phenformin; incidence of lactic acidosis approximately 6/10,000

Specific References

Callaghan TS, et al, "Megaloblastic Anemia Due to Vitamin B_{12} Malabsorption Associated With Long Term Metformin Treatment," *Br Med J*, 1980, 280:1214-5.
"Fatal Lactic Acidosis With Metformin," *Aust Adverse Drug Reactions Bulletin*, 1995, 14:6-7.
Gowardman JR and Havill J, "fatal Metformin Induced Lactic Acidosis: A Case Report," *N Z Med J*, 1995, 108:230-1.
Marchetti P and Navalesi R, "Pharmacokinetic-Pharmacodynamic Relationships of Oral Hypoglycemic Agents: An Update," *Clin Pharmacokinet*, 1989, 16(2):100-28.
Matthews SJ, "Focus on Metformin: A New Biguanide Antihyperglycemic Agent," *Formulary*, 1995, 30:383-7.
Paterson KR, Paice BJ, and Lawson DH, "Undesired Effects of Biguanide Therapy," *Adverse Drug React Acute Poisoning Rev*, 1984, 3(3):173-82.
Tymms DJ and Leatherdale BA, "Lactic Acidosis Due to Metformin Therapy in a Low Risk Patient," *Postgrad Med J*, 1988, 64(749):230-1.

Methadone Hydrochloride (meth' a done)

Related Information
Pharmacokinetics of Narcotic Agonist Analgesics *on page 1654*

CAS Number 76-99-3; 125-56-4; 297-88-1; 1095-90-5

Brand Names Dolophine®; Eptadone®; Metasedin®; Physeptone®; Symoron®

Use Management of severe pain, used in narcotic detoxification maintenance programs

Mechanism of Action Binds to opiate receptors in the CNS, causing inhibition of ascending pain pathways, altering the perception of and response to pain; produces generalized CNS depression

Adverse Reactions
Cardiovascular: Hypotension, bradycardia, peripheral vasodilation, palpitations
Central nervous system (toxicity may be delayed after 6 hours): CNS depression, intracranial pressure (increased), psychosis, drowsiness, dizziness, sedation (marked sedation seen after repeated administration), asthenia, tiredness, nervousness, headache, restlessness, malaise, confusion, mental depression, hallucinations, paradoxical CNS stimulation, choreic movements
Dermatologic: Skin rash, hives, pruritus
Endocrine & metabolic: Syndrome of inappropriate antidiuretic hormone (SIADH), hypoadrenalism
Gastrointestinal: Nausea, vomiting, constipation, dry mouth, anorexia, stomach cramps
Genitourinary: Decreased urination, ureteral spasm
Ocular: Miosis
Respiratory: Apnea, respiratory depression, troubled breathing, dyspnea
Miscellaneous: Histamine release, physical and psychological dependence with prolonged use, pain at injection site, paralytic ileus, biliary or urinary tract spasm

Signs & Symptoms of Acute Overdose Pulmonary edema, ejaculatory disturbances, respiratory depression, impotence, coma

Toxicodynamics/Kinetics

Oral:

Onset of action: Within 30-60 minutes

Duration: 6-8 hours; with repeated doses, increases to 22-48 hours

Parenteral:

Onset of action: Within 10-20 minutes

Peak effect: Within 1-2 hours

Enhanced analgesia has been seen in elderly patients on therapeutic doses of narcotics; duration of action may be increased.

Absorption: Absorbed well from gastrointestinal tract

Distribution: V_d: 3.8 L/kg; distributes widely to tissues

Protein binding: 80% to 89%

Metabolism: Liver metabolism (N-demethylation)

Bioavailability, oral: 92%

Half-life: 15-29 hours, half-life may be prolonged with alkaline pH

Elimination: Urine (<10% as unchanged drug); increased renal excretion with urine pH <6; clearance: 0.08 L/hour/kg

Usual Dosage Doses should be titrated to appropriate effects

Children: Analgesia:

Oral, I.M., S.C.: 0.7 mg/kg/24 hours divided every 4-6 hours as needed or 0.1-0.2 mg/kg every 4-12 hours as needed; maximum: 10 mg/dose

I.V.: 0.1 mg/kg every 4 hours initially for 2-3 doses, then every 6-12 hours as needed; maximum: 10 mg/dose

Adults:

Analgesia: Oral, I.M., I.V., S.C.: 2.5-10 mg every 3-8 hours as needed, up to 5-20 mg every 6-8 hours

Detoxification: Oral: 15-40 mg/day; should not exceed 21 days and may not be repeated earlier than 4 weeks after completion of preceding course

Maintenance of opiate dependence: Oral: 20-120 mg/day

Dosing adjustment in renal impairment: Cl_{cr} <10 mL/minute: Administer at 50% to 75% of normal dose

Dosing adjustment/comments in hepatic disease: Avoid in severe liver disease

Contraindications Hypersensitivity to methadone or any component

Warnings Tablets are to be used only for oral administration and **must not** be used for injection; use with caution in patients with respiratory diseases including: asthma, emphysema, or COPD and in patients with severe liver disease; because methadone's effects on respiration last much longer than its analgesic effects, the dose must be titrated slowly

Dosage Forms

Injection: 10 mg/mL (1 mL, 10 mL, 20 mL)

Solution:

Oral: 5 mg/5 mL (5 mL, 500 mL); 10 mg/5 mL (500 mL)

Oral, concentrate: 10 mg/mL (30 mL)

Tablet: 5 mg, 10 mg

Tablet, dispersible: 40 mg

Stability Highly **incompatible** with all other I.V. agents when mixed together

Reference Range

Therapeutic: 0.1-0.4 ng/mL (SI: 0.32-1.29 μmol/L)

Toxic: >2.0 μg/mL (SI: >6.46 μmol/L)

Overdosage Treatment

Decontamination: Lavage/activated charcoal with cathartic

Supportive therapy: Naloxone hydrochloride (0.4-2 mg I.V., S.C., or through an endotracheal tube); a continuous infusion (at ⅔ the response dose/hour) may be required

Antidote(s)

Naloxone Hydrochloride *on page 1447*

Test Interactions Increases thyroxine (S), aminotransferase [ALT (SGPT)/AST (SGOT)] (S)

Diagnostic Tests/Procedures

Methadone, Quantitative, Serum *on page 1293*

Methadone, Urine *on page 1293*

Drug Interactions

Decreased effect with phenytoin (↑ withdrawal), rifampin (→ withdrawal), pentazocine (→ withdrawal)

Increased effect/toxicity with CNS depressants, phenothiazines, TCAs, MAO inhibitors, cimetidine, diazepam

Pregnancy Risk Factor B (D if used for prolonged periods or in high doses at term)

Pregnancy Implications Crosses the placenta; appears in breast milk; neonatal respiratory depression

(Continued)

Methadone Hydrochloride *(Continued)*

Monitoring Parameters Pain relief, respiratory and mental status, blood pressure

Patient Information May cause drowsiness

Nursing Implications Observe patient for excessive sedation, respiratory depression, implement safety measures, assist with ambulation

Additional Information Not detected as an opioid in most urine immunoassays

Specific References

Gayle MO, Ryan CA, and Nazarali S, "Unusual Cause of Methadone Poisoning," *Acta Paediatr Scand*, 1991, 80(4):486-7.

Geller RJ and Garrettson LK, "Delayed Onset of Toxicity After Methadone Ingestion Due to Therapeutic Error," *Vet Hum Toxicol*, 1994, 36:367.

Molyneux E, Ahern R, and Baldwin B, "Accidental Ingestion of Methadone," *BMJ*, 1991, 303(6807):922-3.

Wasserman S and Yahr MD, "Choreic Movements Induced by the Use of Methadone," *Arch Neurol*, 1980, 37(11):727-8.

Wu CH and Henry JA, "Deaths of Heroin Addicts Starting on Methadone Maintenance," *Lancet*, 1990, 335(8686):424.

Methaminodiazepoxide Hydrochloride *see* Chlordiazepoxide *on page 198*

Methampex® *see* Methamphetamine Hydrochloride *on this page*

Methamphetamine Hydrochloride (meth am fet' a meen)

CAS Number 51-57-0; 537-46-2

Brand Names Desoxyn®; Methampex®

Synonyms Desoxyephedrine Hydrochloride; MDMA

Use Treatment of narcolepsy, exogenous obesity, abnormal behavioral syndrome in children (minimal brain dysfunction)

Adverse Reactions

Cardiovascular: Tachycardia, irregular heartbeat, hypertension, chest pain, dilated cardiomyopathy

Central nervous system: Irritability, insomnia, seizures, paranoia, false feeling of well being, agitation, nervousness, restlessness, insomnia, mood or mental changes, dizziness, lightheadedness, headache, visual hallucinations, delusional perceptions, CNS stimulation (severe), hyperthermia

Dermatologic: Skin rash, hives

Gastrointestinal: Diarrhea, nausea, vomiting, stomach cramps, constipation, anorexia, weight loss, dry mouth

Neuromuscular & skeletal: Tremors, choreoathetoid movements

Ocular: Blurred vision, mydriasis

Miscellaneous: Tolerance and withdrawal with prolonged use, changes in libido, Tourette's syndrome, increased sweating

Signs & Symptoms of Acute Overdose Pulmonary edema, respiratory alkalosis, gynecomastia, insomnia, hypertension, tachycardia or reflex bradycardia, periarteritis nodosa, tachypnea, delirium, rhabdomyolysis, confusion, mania, rigors, myoclonus, myoglobinuria, tremors, alopecia, feces discoloration (black)

Toxicodynamics/Kinetics

Duration of action: 8-24 hours

Metabolism: In liver to amphetamine (4% to 7%) and other metabolites

Half-life: 12-34 hours

Elimination: Renally

Usual Dosage

Attention deficit disorder: Children >6 years: 2.5-5 mg 1-2 times/day, may increase by 5 mg increments weekly until optimum response is achieved, usually 20-25 mg/day

Exogenous obesity: Children >12 years and Adults: 5 mg, 30 minutes before each meal; long-acting formulation: 10-15 mg in morning; treatment duration should not exceed a few weeks

Contraindications Known hypersensitivity to methamphetamine

Warnings Cardiovascular disease, nephritis, angina pectoris, hypertension, glaucoma, patients with a history of drug abuse

Dosage Forms

Tablet: 5 mg

Tablet, extended release (Gradumet®): 5 mg, 10 mg, 15 mg

Reference Range Therapeutic: 20-30 ng/mL

Overdosage Treatment

Decontamination: Lavage/activated charcoal with cathartic

Supportive therapy: Nitroprusside may be used for hypertension while diazepam or lorazepam can be used for agitation. Haloperidol can be used for hallucinatory behavior.

Enhancement of elimination: Multiple dosing of activated charcoal may be useful. While acid diuresis can increase excretion, it is not recommended due to renal effects.

Test Interactions A labetalol metabolite (3-amino-1-phenylbutane or APB) may cause a false-positive result with amphetamine/methamphetamine by thin-layer chromatography or immunoassay; false-positives by immunoassay can be seen with ranitidine, phenylpropanolamine, brompheniramine, chlorpromazine, fluspirilene or pipothiazine coingestion

Diagnostic Tests/Procedures

Methamphetamines, Serum *on page 1294*

Methamphetamines, Urine *on page 1294*

Drug Interactions Increased toxicity with MAO inhibitors (hypertensive crisis); combination of methamphetamine with ethanol can increase heart rate and cardiac work

Pregnancy Risk Factor C

Pregnancy Implications Crosses the placenta; can cause low birth weight/ premature birth; reportedly associated with increased obstetric complications and maternal death

Monitoring Parameters Heart rate, respiratory rate, blood pressure, and CNS activity

Patient Information Take during day to avoid insomnia; do not discontinue abruptly, may be addicting with prolonged use; do not crush or chew extended release tablet

Additional Information Illicit methamphetamine may contain lead; alkalinizing urine can result in longer methamphetamine half-life and elevated blood level; ephedrine is a precursor in the illicit manufacture of methamphetamine; ephedrine is extracted by dissolving ephedrine tablets in water or alcohol (50,000 tablets can result in 1 kg of ephedrine); conversion to methamphetamine occurs at a rate of 50% to 70% of the weight of ephedrine

Specific References

Catanzarite JA and Stein DA, "Crystal and Pregnancy: Methamphetamine-Associated Maternal Death," *West J Med*, 1995, 162:454-7.

Gibert RB, Peng PI,and Wong D, "A Labetalol Metabolite With Analytical Characterstics Resembling Amphetamines," *J Anal Toxicol*, 1995, 19:84-6.

McKinney PF, Tomaszewski C, Phillips S, et al, "Methamphetamine Toxicity Prevented by Activated Charcoal in a Mouse Model," *Ann Emerg Med*, 1994, 24(2):220-2.

Mendelson J, Jones RT, Upton R, et al, "Methamphetamine and Ethanol Interactions in Humans," *Clin Pharmacol Ther*, 1995, 57:559-68.

Nestor TA, Tamamoto WI, Kam TH, et al, "Acute Pulmonary Oedema Caused by Crystalline Methamphetamine," *Lancet*, 1989, 2(8674):1277-8.

Richards CF, Clark RF, Holbrook T, et al, "The Effect of Cocaine and Amphetamines on Vital Signs in Trauma Patients," *J Emerg Med*, 1995, 13:59-63.

Rothrock JF, Rubenstein R, and Lyden PD, "Ischemic Stroke Associated With Methamphetamine Inhalation," *Neurology*, 1988, 38(4):589-92.

Segar DL, "Substances of Abuse," *Topics Emerg Med*, 1985, 7:18-30.

Sperling LS and Horowitz JL, "Methamphetamine-Induced Choreoathetosis and Rhabdomyolysis," *Ann Intern Med*, 1994, 121(12):986.

Methaqualone Hydrochloride (meth a' kwa lone)

CAS Number 72-44-6; 340-56-7

Brand Names Normi-Nox®; Pallidan®; Somnomed®

Synonyms Quaalude®

Use Europeans use for insomnia; taken off the U.S. market in 1984

Mechanism of Action Nonbarbiturate hypnosedative

Adverse Reactions

Cardiovascular: Tachycardia

Central nervous system: Euphoria, slurred speech, salivation, ataxia, electroencephalogram abnormalities

Gastrointestinal: Emesis, necrotizing cystitis

Ocular: Nystagmus

Renal: Hematuria

Respiratory: Aspiration

Signs & Symptoms of Acute Overdose Hypotension, coma, hematuria, hyperreflexia, A-V block, erythema multiforme, dyspnea, hyperthermia, vision color changes (yellow tinge); respiratory depression, apnea, seizures, myoclonus

Toxicodynamics/Kinetics

Absorption: Complete within 2 hours

Distribution: V_d: 2.4-6.4 L/kg

Protein binding: 70% to 90%

Metabolism: Hepatic

Half-life: 33-40 hours

Usual Dosage

Insomnia: 150-300 mg at night

Lethal dose: 8 g

Reference Range A 600 mg dose will yield a peak plasma level of 7 mg/L; plasma level of methaqualone >20 mg/L is consistent with toxicity

Overdosage Treatment

Decontamination: Lavage (within 2 hours)/activated charcoal

Supportive therapy: Treat seizures with diazepam, phenobarbital, or phenytoin

(Continued)

Methaqualone Hydrochloride *(Continued)*

Enhancement of elimination: Hemodialysis or resin hemoperfusion can enhance elimination; do not use forced saline diuresis; multiple dosing of activated charcoal may be effective

Drug Interactions Enhances codeine analgesia

Additional Information Mandrax® also contains diphenhydramine

Specific References

Brown SS and Goenechea S, "Methaqualone: Metabolic, Kinetic, and Clinical Pharmacologic Observations," *Clin Pharmacol Ther*, 1973, 14(3):314-24.

Chang TMS, Coffey JF, Lister C, et al, "Methaqualone, Methyprylon, and Glutethimide Clearance by the ACAC Microcapsule Artificial Kidney: In Vitro and in Patients With Acute Intoxication," *Trans Am Soc Artif Intern Organs*, 1973, 19:87-91.

Kulberg A, "Substance Abuse: Clinical Identification and Management," *Pediatr Clin North Am*, 1986, 33(2):325-61.

Matthew H, Proudfoot AT, Brown SS, et al, "Mandrax Poisoning: Conservative Management in 116 Patients," *Br Med J*, 1968, 2(597):101-2.

Metharbital (meth ar' bi tal)

CAS Number 50-11-3

Brand Names Gemonil®

Synonyms Metharbitone

Use Control of grand mal, petit mal, myoclonic and mixed types of seizures

Adverse Reactions

Cardiovascular: Hypotension, circulatory collapse

Central nervous system: Drowsiness, paradoxical excitement, hyperkinetic activity, cognitive impairment, defects in general comprehension, short-term memory deficits, decreased attention span, ataxia

Dermatologic: Skin eruptions, skin rash, exfoliative dermatitis

Hematologic: Megaloblastic anemia

Hepatic: Hepatitis

Ocular: Vision color changes (yellow tinge)

Respiratory: Apnea, respiratory depression, apnea (especially with rapid I.V. use)

Miscellaneous: Psychological and physical dependence, ptosis

Toxicodynamics/Kinetics

Metabolism: Demethylated to barbital (active)

Elimination: Renal, 1% excreted unchanged; 9% excreted as barbital

Usual Dosage Oral:

Children: 5-15 mg/kg/day or 50 mg 1-3 times/day

Adults: 100 mg 1-3 times/day, adjust dosage to obtain optimal effect

Contraindications Suspected pregnancy, status asthmaticus, known hypersensitivity to metharbital (barbiturates)

Dosage Forms Tablet: 100 mg

Overdosage Treatment

Decontamination: Lavage/activated charcoal with cathartic

Enhancement of elimination: Multiple dosing of activated charcoal may be helpful

Test Interactions Increases alkaline phosphatase (S); decreases calcium (S)

Pregnancy Risk Factor D

Nursing Implications Solution is slightly acidic

Additional Information Faint, aromatic odor

Metharbitone *see* Metharbital *on this page*

Methimazole (meth im' a zole)

CAS Number 60-56-0

Brand Names Antitirode G.W.®; Favistan®; Strumazol®; Tapazole®; Thacupzol®; Thyrozol®; Tirodril®

Synonyms Mercazolylum; 1-Methylimidazole-2-thiol; Thiamazole; Tiamazol

Use Palliative treatment of hyperthyroidism, to return the hyperthyroid patient to a normal metabolic state prior to thyroidectomy, and to control thyrotoxic crisis that may accompany thyroidectomy

Mechanism of Action A thiourea which inhibits the synthesis of thyroid hormones by blocking the oxidation of iodine in the thyroid gland, blocking iodine's ability to combine with tyrosine to form thyroxine and tri-iodothyronine (T_3), does not inactivate circulating T_4 and T_3

Adverse Reactions

Cardiovascular: Edema

Central nervous system: Drowsiness, dizziness, headache

Dermatologic: Rash, pruritus, hair loss, skin pigmentation

Gastrointestinal: Loss of taste, nausea, vomiting

Hematologic: Leukopenia, neutropenia, agranulocytosis, granulocytopenia, hypoprothrombinemia

Hepatic: Cholestatic jaundice

Neuromuscular & skeletal: Arthralgia, paresthesia

Miscellaneous: Lupus-like syndrome, drug fever

Toxicodynamics/Kinetics

Bioavailability: 80% to 95%

Onset of antithyroid effect: Oral: Within 30-40 minutes

Duration: 2-4 hours

Protein binding: No plasma protein binding

Half-life: 4-13 hours

Elimination: Eliminated renally with ~12% excreted in urine within 24 hours

Usual Dosage Oral:

Children: Initial: 0.4 mg/kg/day in 3 divided doses; maintenance: 0.2 mg/kg/day in 3 divided doses up to 30 mg/24 hours maximum

Adults: Initial: 5 mg every 8 hours; maintenance dose: 5-15 mg/day up to 60 mg/day for severe hyperthyroidism

Adjust dosage as required to achieve and maintain serum T_3, T_4, and TSH levels in the normal range. An elevated T_3 may be the sole indicator of inadequate treatment. An elevated TSH indicates excessive antithyroid treatment.

Contraindications Hypersensitivity to methimazole or any component, nursing mothers

Warnings Use with extreme caution in patients receiving other drugs known to cause myelosuppression particularly agranulocytosis, patients >40 years of age; avoid doses >40 mg/day (↑ myelosuppression); may cause acneiform eruptions or worsen the condition of the thyroid

Dosage Forms Tablet: 5 mg, 10 mg

Stability Protect from light

Overdosage Treatment

Decontamination: Lavage/activated charcoal with cathartic

Enhancement of elimination: Multiple dosing of activated charcoal may be effective

Drug Interactions Increased toxicity: Iodinated glycerol, lithium, potassium iodide, anticoagulant activity increased

Pregnancy Risk Factor D

Pregnancy Implications Crosses the placenta; appears in breast milk (1:1)

Monitoring Parameters Monitor for signs of hypothyroidism, hyperthyroidism, T_4, T_3, CBC with differential, liver function (baseline and as needed), serum thyroxine, free thyroxine index

Patient Information Take with meals, take at regular intervals around-the-clock; notify physician if persistent fever, sore throat, fatigue, unusual bleeding or bruising occurs

Specific References

Hamor GH and Lafdjian A, "Dualistic Thiourea Moiety Taste Response of Methimazole," *J Pharm Sci*, 1967, 56(6):777-8.

Methioplequim *see* Trimethaphan Camsylate *on page 771*

Methocarbamol (meth oh kar' ba mole)

CAS Number 532-03-6

Brand Names Delaxin®; Lumirelax®; Marbaxin®; Relax Llano®; Robaxin®; Robomol®; Traumacut®; Tresortil®

Use Treatment of muscle spasm associated with acute painful musculoskeletal conditions; supportive therapy in tetanus, latrodectism

Mechanism of Action Causes skeletal muscle relaxation by reducing the transmission of impulses from the spinal cord to skeletal muscle

Adverse Reactions

Cardiovascular: Syncope, hypotension, bradycardia, flushing

Central nervous system: Lightheadedness, dizziness, drowsiness, seizures (rarely), headache

Gastrointestinal: Nausea

Ocular: Conjunctivitis, blurred vision, nystagmus (horizontal or vertical)

Renal: Renal impairment

Respiratory: Nasal congestion

Miscellaneous: Dry mouth, urine discoloration (brown/black), allergic manifestations

Signs & Symptoms of Acute Overdose Cardiac arrhythmias, nausea, vomiting, drowsiness, hypotension, apnea, coma, urine discoloration (black), urine discoloration (blue), urine discoloration (brown), urine discoloration (green)

Toxicodynamics/Kinetics

Onset of action:

Oral: Within 0.5 hours

I.V.: Immediately

Absorption: Rapid and complete

Distribution: Wide throughout the body

(Continued)

Methocarbamol *(Continued)*

Metabolism: In the liver
Half-life: 1-2 hours
Time to peak serum concentration: Within 1 hour
Elimination: Renally excreted over a 3-day period with a single dose

Usual Dosage

Children: Recommended **only** for use in tetanus I.V.: 15 mg/kg/dose or 500 mg/m^2/dose, may repeat every 6 hours if needed; maximum dose: 1.8 g/m^2/day for 3 days only

Adults: Muscle spasm:

Oral: 1.5 g 4 times/day for 2-3 days, then decrease to 4-4.5 g/day in 3-6 divided doses

I.M., I.V.: 1 g every 8 hours if oral not possible

Dosing adjustment/comments in renal impairment: Do not administer parenteral formulation to patients with renal dysfunction

Contraindications Renal impairment, hypersensitivity to methocarbamol or any component, comatose patients, myasthenia gravis, epilepsy

Dosage Forms

Injection: 100 mg/mL in polyethylene glycol 50% (10 mL)
Tablet: 500 mg, 750 mg

Reference Range Peak serum level after 2 g: 25.8 mg/L; peak serum levels after 4 g: 41 mg/L; blood levels >320 mg/L have been associated with fatalities

Overdosage Treatment

Decontamination: Lavage/activated charcoal with cathartic

Supportive therapy: Following attempts to enhance drug elimination, hypotension should be treated with I.V. fluids and/or Trendelenburg positioning

Enhancement of elimination: Dialysis and hemoperfusion might be useful in reducing serum drug concentrations; patient should be observed for possible relapses due to incomplete gastric emptying

Test Interactions May cause false elevation of urinary 5-hydroxyindoleacetic acid (5-HIAA)

Drug Interactions Potentiated with ethanol; will potentiate antimuscarinics and psychotropic agents

Pregnancy Risk Factor C

Monitoring Parameters Cardiac/respiratory

Patient Information May cause drowsiness

Nursing Implications Not recommended for S.C. administration; rate of injection should not exceed 3 mL/minute

Specific References

Lebby TI, Dugger K, Lipscomb JW, et al, "Skeletal Muscle Relaxant Ingestion," *Vet Hum Toxicol*, 1990, 32(2):133-5.

Preston KL, Guarino JJ, Kirk WT, et al, "Evaluation of the Abuse Potential of Methocarbamol," *J Pharmacol Exp Ther*, 1989, 248(3):1146-57.

Methohexital Sodium (meth oh hex' i tal)

CAS Number 309-36-4

Brand Names Brevital® Sodium

Use Induction and maintenance of general anesthesia for short procedures

Mechanism of Action Ultra short-acting I.V. barbiturate anesthetic

Adverse Reactions

Cardiovascular: Hypotension, peripheral vascular collapse
Central nervous system: Convulsions, CNS depression, headache
Gastrointestinal: Nausea, vomiting
Local: Pain on I.M. injection, thrombophlebitis
Neuromuscular & skeletal: Involuntary muscle movement, myoclonus, rigidity, tremors
Respiratory: Apnea, respiratory depression, laryngospasm, hiccups, coughing

Signs & Symptoms of Acute Overdose Apnea, tachycardia, ptosis, vision color changes (green tinge), vision color changes (yellow tinge); wheezing, hypotension

Toxicodynamics/Kinetics

Duration of action: 0.3 hours
Distribution: V_d: 1.1 L/kg
Half-life: 1-2 hours
Protein binding: 73%

Usual Dosage Doses must be titrated to effect

Children 3-12 years:

I.M.: Preop: 5-10 mg/kg/dose
I.V.: Induction: 1-2 mg/kg/dose
Rectal: Preop/induction: 20-35 mg/kg/dose; usual 25 mg/kg/dose; give as 10% aqueous solution

Adults: I.V.: Induction: 50-120 mg to start; 20-40 mg every 4-7 minutes

Lethal dose: 1-2 g

Dosing adjustment/comments in hepatic impairment: Lower dosage and monitor closely

Contraindications Porphyria, hypersensitivity to methohexital or any component

Warnings Use with extreme caution in patients with liver impairment, asthma, cardiovascular instability

Dosage Forms Injection: 500 mg, 2.5 g, 5 g

Stability Do not dilute with solutions containing bacteriostatic agents; solutions are alkaline (pH 9.5-11) and incompatible with acids (eg, atropine sulfate, succinylcholine), also incompatible with phenol-containing solutions and silicone

Overdosage Treatment

Decontamination: Lavage/activated charcoal with cathartic

Supportive therapy: Treatment is primarily supportive with mechanical ventilation if needed

Enhancement of elimination: Charcoal hemoperfusion may be of some benefit

Drug Interactions CNS depressants; seizures possible with concurrent use with paroxetine

Pregnancy Risk Factor C

Nursing Implications Avoid extravasation or intra-arterial administration

Specific References

Folkerts H, "Spontaneous Seizure After Concurrent Use of Methohexital Anesthesia For Electroconvulsive Therapy and Paroxetine: A Case Report," *J Nerv Ment Dis*, 1995, 183(2):115-6.

Forbes RB, Murray DJ, Dillman JB, et al, "Pharmacokinetics of Two Percent Rectal Methohexitone in Children," *Can J Anaesth*, 1989, 36(2):160-4.

Wells D, Davies G, and Wagner D, "Accidental Injection of Epidural Methohexital," *Anesthesiology*, 1987, 67(5):846-8.

Methotrexate (meth oh trex' ate)

Related Information

Drugs and Chemicals Proven to be Teratogenic in Humans *on page 1572-1575*

Toxicities of Chemotherapeutic Agents *on page 1631-1633*

Trimetrexate Glucuronate *on page 773*

CAS Number 59-05-2

Brand Names Folex®; Mexate®; Rheumatrex®

Synonyms Amethopterin; MTX

Use Treatment of trophoblastic neoplasms, leukemias, psoriasis, rheumatoid arthritis, osteosarcoma, non-Hodgkin's lymphoma

Mechanism of Action An antimetabolite that inhibits RNA and DNA synthesis and cell reproduction in cancerous cells; interferes with the conversion of folic acid to tetrahydrofolic acid by binding to the enzyme dihydrofolate reductase

Adverse Reactions

Cardiovascular: Vasculitis, pericarditis, pericardial effusion, pericardial effusion/pericarditis

Central nervous system: Malaise, fatigue, dizziness, encephalopathy, seizures, confusion, fever, chills, headache, hyperthermia

Dermatologic: Alopecia, rash, depigmentation or hyperpigmentation of skin, photosensitivity

Endocrine & metabolic: Hypoglycemia; diabetes

Gastrointestinal: Ulcerative stomatitis, nausea, abdominal distress, vomiting, diarrhea, anorexia, stomatitis, diarrhea, enteritis

Hematologic: Myelosuppression, leukopenia, hemorrhage

Hepatic: Cirrhosis (especially noted in diabetics and obese patients)

Neuromuscular & skeletal: Rarely arthralgia

Ocular: Blurred vision

Renal: Renal failure, cystitis

Respiratory: Interstitial pneumonitis, cough, dyspnea, crepitant rales

Miscellaneous: Decreased resistance to infection, mucositis, pancytopenia, feces discoloration (black), anaphylactic shock, metallic taste

Signs & Symptoms of Acute Overdose Bone marrow depression, tubular necrosis, cranial nerve palsies, pleural effusion, hemiplegia, dementia, coma, nausea, diarrhea, toxic epidermal necrolysis, sexual dysfunction, ataxia, oligospermia, myalgia, lymphoma, vomiting, alopecia, cirrhosis, azotemia, gynecomastia, melena, stomatitis, conjunctivitis, elevated AST, encephalopathy, leukopenia; neutropenia; agranulocytosis; granulocytopenia

Toxicodynamics/Kinetics

Absorption: Well absorbed orally at low doses (<30 mg/m^2); incomplete absorption after large doses; completely absorbed after I.M. injection

Distribution: V_d: 1.1 L/kg; distributed widely with highest concentrations in kidneys, gallbladder, spleen, liver, and skin; minimal passage across blood-brain barrier; does not achieve therapeutic concentrations in the CSF; sustained concentrations are retained in the kidney and liver

(Continued)

Methotrexate *(Continued)*

Protein binding: 50%

Metabolism: Hepatic; intracellular, enterohepatic

Half-life: 8-15 hours with high doses and 3-10 hours with low doses

Time to peak serum concentration:

Oral: Within 1-2 hours

Parenteral: Within 30-60 minutes

Elimination: Small amounts excreted in feces (10%); primarily excreted in urine (90%) via glomerular filtration and active transport; endogenous clearance: 1.5 mL/minute/kg

Usual Dosage Doses not requiring leucovorin rescue range from 30-40 mg/m^2 I.V. or I.M. repeated weekly, or oral regimens of 10 mg/m^2 twice weekly

High-dose MTX is considered to be >100 mg/m^2 and can be as high as 1500-7500 mg/m^2; these doses require leucovorin rescue, and patients receiving doses ≥1000 mg/m^2 should have their urine alkalinized with bicarbonate or Bicitra® prior to and following MTX therapy

Refer to individual protocols. MTX may be administered orally, I.M., I.V., S.C., intra-arterially, and intrathecally

Children:

Osteosarcoma:

I.V.: <12 years: 12 g/m^2 (12-18 g); >12 years: 8 g/m^2 (maximum dose: 18 g)

I.T.: 10-15 mg/m^2 (maximum dose: 15 mg) by protocol; ≤3 months: 3 mg; 4-11 months: 6 mg; <1 year: 6 mg; 1-2 years: 8 mg; 2-3 years: 10 mg; ≥3 years: 12 mg. I.T. doses are prepared with preservative-free MTX **only**. Hydrocortisone may be added to the I.T. preparation; total volume should range from 3-6 mL

Juvenile rheumatoid arthritis: Oral: 5-15 mg/m^2/week as a single dose or as 3 divided doses given 12 hours apart

Meningeal leukemia: I.V.: 6 g/m^2 loading dose over 1 hour, followed by I.V. continuous infusion: 1.2 g/m^2/hour for 23 hours

Acute lymphocytic leukemia (high-dose): I.V.: Loading dose: 200 mg/m^2 followed by 24-hour infusion of 1200 mg/m^2/day

ANLL: I.V.: 7.5 mg/m^2/day on days 1-5

Resistant ANLL: I.V.: 100 mg/m^2/dose on day 1

Non-Hodgkin's lymphoma: I.V.: 200-300 mg/m^2

Acute lymphoblastic leukemias: Oral, I.M., I.V.: Induction: 3.3 mg/m^2/day for 4-6 weeks; remission maintenance: 20-30 mg/m^2 twice weekly

Adults: I.V.: Range is wide from 30-40 mg/m^2/week to 100-7500 mg/m^2 with leucovorin rescue

Rheumatoid arthritis: Oral: 7.5 mg once weekly or 2.5 mg every 12 hours for 3 doses/week; not to exceed 20 mg/week

Elderly: Rheumatoid arthritis/psoriasis: 5 mg once weekly, if nausea occurs, split dose to 2.5 mg every 12 hours for day of administration; dose may be increased to 7.5 mg/week based on response (not >20 mg/week)

Dosing adjustment in renal impairment:

Cl_{cr} 10-50 mL/minute: Reduce dose to 50%

Cl_{cr} <10 mL/minute: Avoid use

Dosing adjustment in hepatic impairment:

Bilirubin 3.1-5 mg/dL or AST >180 units: Administer 75% of dose

Bilirubin >5 mg/dL: Do not use

Contraindications Hypersensitivity to methotrexate or any component; severe renal or hepatic impairment; pre-existing profound bone marrow depression in patients with psoriasis or rheumatoid arthritis

Warnings The U.S. Food and Drug Administration (FDA) currently recommends that procedures for proper handling and disposal of antineoplastic agents be considered. Because of the possibility of severe toxic reactions, fully inform patient of the risks involved; do not use in women of childbearing age unless benefit outweighs risks; may cause hepatitis, fibrosis and cirrhosis, along with marked bone marrow depression; death from intestinal perforation may occur; may cause photosensitivity type reaction; reduce dosage in patients with renal or hepatic impairment, ascites, and pleural effusion; use with caution in patients with peptic ulcer disease, ulcerative colitis, pre-existing bone marrow suppression.

Dosage Forms

Injection, as sodium: 2.5 mg/mL (2 mL); 25 mg/mL (2 mL, 4 mL, 8 mL, 10 mL)

Injection, as sodium, preservative free: 25 mg (2 mL, 4 mL, 8 mL, 10 mL)

Powder, for injection, as sodium: 20 mg, 25 mg, 50 mg, 100 mg, 250 mg, 1 g

Tablet: 2.5 mg

Tablet, dose pack: 2.5 mg (4 cards with 2, 3, 4, 5, or 6 tablets each)

Stability Store intact vials at room temperature; intrathecal solutions should be diluted immediately prior to use; reconstituted solutions remain stable for 4 weeks at room temperature and 3 months when refrigerated; protect from light

Reference Range Therapeutic range is dependent upon therapeutic approach. "High-dose" regimens produce drug levels between 10^{-6} M and 10^{-7} M 24-72 hours after drug infusion. Therapeutic range is dependent upon therapeutic approach. "High-dose" regimens produce drug levels between 10^{-6}M and 10^{-7}M 24-72 hours after drug infusion.

Toxic:
- Low-dose therapy: >9.1 ng/mL (SI: >20 nmol/L)
- High-dose therapy: >454 ng/mL (SI: >1000 nmol/L)

Overdosage Treatment

Decontamination: Ipecac or lavage/activated charcoal with cathartic

Supportive therapy: Severe bone marrow toxicity can result from overdose; leucovorin rescue can reduce the toxicity; administer as quickly as possible 10 mg/m^2 every 6 hours for 72 hours, follow serum methotrexate levels; aminophylline (2.5 mg/kg) has been used to treat methotrexate neurotoxicity in children

Enhancement of elimination: Multiple dosing of activated charcoal is effective; renal excretion is optimized at a urinary pH of 7.0. Charcoal hemoperfusion, hydration, and urinary alkalinization may enhance elimination and prevent precipitation in renal tubules; not dialyzable (0% to 5%)

Antidote(s)

Folic Acid *on page 1430*

Leucovorin Calcium *on page 1437*

Test Interactions Increases potassium (S)

Diagnostic Tests/Procedures

Methotrexate, Blood *on page 1297*

Drug Interactions Salicylates (may suppress MTX's clearance), sulfonamides, live virus vaccines, pyrimethamine, phenytoin, 5-FU, nonsteroidal anti-inflammatory drugs (NSAIDs); probenecid decreases renal elimination of MTX; tetracycline and phenytoin may displace methotrexate from albumin

Pregnancy Risk Factor D; X (psoriasis and rheumatoid arthritis); associated with birth defects

Pregnancy Implications Appears in small amounts into breast milk; crosses the placenta

Monitoring Parameters CBC with differential and platelet count, creatinine clearance, serum creatinine, BUN, and hepatic function tests; monitor for bleeding

Patient Information Any signs of infection, easy bruising or bleeding, dyspnea, or painful or burning urination should be brought to physician's attention. Nausea, vomiting or hair loss sometimes occur. The drug may cause permanent sterility and may cause birth defects. The drug may be excreted in breast milk, therefore, an alternative form of feeding your baby should be used.

Nursing Implications For intrathecal use, mix methotrexate without preservative with Elliott's B solution to concentration no greater than 2 mg/mL

Additional Information Low dose methotrexate (0.2 mg/kg/week) has been shown to be effective in treating idiopathic granulomatous hepatitis

Myelosuppressive effects:
- WBC: Mild
- Platelets: Moderate
- Onset (days): 7
- Nadir (days): 10
- Recovery (days): 21

Sodium content of 100 mg injection: 20 mg (0.86 mEq)

Sodium content of 100 mg (low sodium) injection: 15 mg (0.65 mEq)

Specific References

Bernini JC, Fort DW, Griener JC, et al, "Aminophylline for Methotrexate-Induced Neurotoxicity," *Lancet*, 1995, 345:544-7.

Berthelot JM, Planchon B, Barrier J, et al, "Pancytopenia and Methotrexate: 7 Cases (3 at the Very Beginning of Treatment)," *Revue du Rhumatisme*, 1994, 61:690.

Forbat LN, Hancock BW, and Gershlick AH, "Methotrexate-Induced Pericarditis and Pericardial Effusion: First Reported Case," *Postgrad Med J*, 1995, 71:244-5.

Grimes DJ, Bowles MR, Buttsworth JA, et al, "Survival After Unexpected High Serum Methotrexate Concentrations in a Patient With Osteogenic Sarcoma," *Drug Saf*, 1990, 5(6):447-54.

Henry MA and Gentry WL, "Single Injection of Methotrexate for Treatment of Ectopic Pregnancies," *Am J Obstet Gynecol*, 1994, 171(6):1584-7.

Knox TA, Kaplan MM, Gelfand JA, et al, "Methotrexate Treatment of Idiopathic Granulomatous Hepatitis," *Ann Intern Med*, 1995, 122(8):592-5.

LeGoff P, Chicault P, Guedes C, et al, "Reversible Lymphoma Occurring During Methotrexate Therapy for Rheumatoid Arthritis," *Clin Exp Rheumatol*, 1995, 1994, 12(Suppl 11):112.

Lobelle C, Lopez RM, Barreiro J, et al, "Anaphylactic Reaction to High-Dose Methotrexate," *Pediatric Hematology and Oncology*, 1995, 12:213-4.

Maillot F, Machet L, Mommeja-Marin H, et al, "Hyperthermia Due to Methotrexate in Still's Disease," *Therapie*, 1994, 49(6):520-1.

McIvor A, "Charcoal Hemoperfusion and Methotrexate Toxicity," *Nephron*, 1991, 58(3):378.

Minocha A, Dean HA, and Pittsley RA, "Liver Cirrhosis in Rheumatoid Arthritis Patients Treated With Long-Term Methotrexate," *Vet Hum Toxicol*, 1993, 35(1):45-8.

Shiroky JB, Neville C, Esdaile JM, et al, "Low-Dose Methotrexate With Leucovorin (Folinic Acid) in the Management of Rheumatoid Arthritis. Results of A Multicenter Randomized, Double-Blind, Placebo-Controlled Trial," *Arthritis Rheum*, 1993, 36(6):795-803.

(Continued)

Methotrexate *(Continued)*

Stephan M, Snook C, and Bausher J, "Pediatric Methotrexate (MTX) Ingestion: A Case Report," *Vet Hum Toxicol*, 1994, 36:366.

Tugwell P, Pincus T, Yocum D, et al, "Combination Therapy With Cyclosporine and Methotrexate in Severe Rheumatoid Arthritis," *N Engl J Med*, 1995, 333:137-41.

Methoxamedrine *see* Methoxamine Hydrochloride *on this page*

Methoxamine Hydrochloride (meth ox' a meen)

Related Information

Adrenergic Agonists, Cardiovascular Comparison *on page 1638*

CAS Number 61-16-5; 390-28-3

Brand Names Idasal®; Vasoxine®; Vasoxyl®

Synonyms Methoxamedrine

Use Treatment of hypotension occurring during general anesthesia; to terminate episodes of tachycardia (ventricular); treatment of shock

Mechanism of Action Direct-acting sympathomimetic amine with similar actions as phenylephrine; causes vasoconstriction primarily via alpha-adrenergic stimulation

Adverse Reactions

Cardiovascular: Ventricular ectopic beats, fetal bradycardia
Central nervous system: Headache, sweating
Gastrointestinal: Vomiting, nausea
Genitourinary: Urinary urgency
Ocular: Nystagmus

Signs & Symptoms of Acute Overdose Hypertension, bradycardia (reflex)

Toxicodynamics/Kinetics

Onset of action:
- I.M.: 15-20 minutes
- I.V.: Immediate

Duration:
- I.M.: 1.5 hours
- I.V.: 5-15 minutes

Distribution: Widely distributed in body fluids
Elimination: Not yet well defined

Usual Dosage Adults:

Emergencies: I.V.: 3-5 mg
Supraventricular tachycardia: I.V.: 10 mg
During spinal anesthesia: I.M.: 10-20 mg

Contraindications Hypersensitivity to methoxamine or any component

Dosage Forms Injection: 20 mg/mL (1 mL)

Overdosage Treatment Supportive therapy: Nitroprusside, labetalol, or phentolamine can be used for hypertension; atropine can be used for bradycardia

Pregnancy Risk Factor C

Specific References

Aviado DM Jr and Wnuck AL, "Mechanisms for Cardiac Slowing by Methoxamine," *J Pharmacol Exp Ther*, 1957, 119(1):99-106.

Methsuximide (meth sux' i mide)

CAS Number 77-41-8

Brand Names Celontin®

Use Control of absence (petit mal) seizures; useful adjunct in refractory, partial complex (psychomotor) seizures

Mechanism of Action Increases the seizure threshold and suppresses paroxysmal spike-and-wave pattern in absence seizures; depresses nerve transmission in the motor cortex

Adverse Reactions

Cardiovascular: Periorbital edema
Central nervous system: Sedation, dizziness, drowsiness, euphoria, nervousness, hallucinations, insomnia, agitation, behavioral changes, mental confusion, headache, Parkinson-like symptoms
Dermatologic: Rashes, rash, Stevens-Johnson syndrome
Gastrointestinal: Nausea, flatulence, vomiting, anorexia, abdominal pain
Hematologic: Leukopenia, aplastic anemia, thrombocytopenia, eosinophilia, pancytopenia, monocytosis
Ocular: Photophobia
Miscellaneous: Hiccups

Signs & Symptoms of Acute Overdose Dizziness, ataxia, hiccups, insomnia, dysarthria, stupor, relapsing coma, leukopenia; neutropenia; agranulocytosis; granulocytopenia

Toxicodynamics/Kinetics

Absorption: Rapidly and completely

Distribution: Widely throughout the body to all body tissues except fat
Protein binding: Not significant
Metabolism: Rapidly demethylated in the liver to N-desmethylmethsuximide (active metabolite)
Half-life: 2-4 hours; N-desmethylmethsuximide half-life may be 28-57 hours
Time to peak serum concentration: Within 1-4 hours
Elimination: <1% excreted in urine as unchanged drug

Usual Dosage Oral:
Children: Initial: 10-15 mg/kg/day in 3-4 divided doses; increase weekly up to maximum of 30 mg/kg/day

Adults: 300 mg/day for the first week; may increase by 300 mg/day at weekly intervals up to 1.2 g/day in 2-4 divided doses/day

Contraindications Known hypersensitivity to methsuximide

Warnings Use with caution in patients with hepatic or renal disease; avoid abrupt withdrawal of methsuximide

Dosage Forms Capsule: 150 mg, 300 mg

Stability Protect from high temperature

Reference Range
Therapeutic (normethsuximide): 10-40 μg/mL (SI: 53-212 μmol/L)
Toxic: >40 μg/mL (SI: >212 μmol/L); N-desmethylmethsuximide levels >150 μg/mL (SI: >738 μmol/L) associated with coma

Overdosage Treatment
Decontamination: Ipecac or lavage/activated charcoal with cathartic
Enhancement of elimination: Charcoal hemoperfusion (useful in removal of toxic metabolite) and hemodialysis may be useful

Test Interactions Increases alkaline phosphatase (S); decreases calcium (S)

Pregnancy Risk Factor C (may be teratogenic)

Monitoring Parameters CBC, hepatic function tests, urinalysis

Patient Information May cause drowsiness; periodic blood test monitoring required

Nursing Implications Observe patient for excess sedation

Specific References
Baehler RW, Work J, Smith W, et al, "Charcoal Hemoperfusion in the Therapy for Methsuximide and Phenytoin Overdose," *Arch Intern Med*, 1980, 140(11):1466-8.
Karch SB, "Methsuximide Overdose: Delayed Onset of Profound Coma," *JAMA*, 1973, 223(13):1463-5.
Miles MV, Tennison MB, and Greenwood RS, "Pharmacokinetics of N-desmethylsuximide in Pediatric Patients," *J Pediatr*, 1989, 114(4 Pt 1):647-50.

Methyldopa (meth ill doe' pa)

Related Information
Therapeutic Drugs Associated With Hallucinations *on page 1558-1559*

CAS Number 555-30-6; 41372-08-1

Brand Names Aldomet®; Dopamet®; Dopegyt®; Emdopa®; Hypolag®; Medomet®; Mopatil®; Novomedopa®

Synonyms Methyldopate Hydrochloride

Use Management of moderate to severe hypertension

Mechanism of Action Stimulation of alpha-adrenergic receptors by a false transmitter that results in a decreased sympathetic outflow to the heart, kidneys and peripheral vasculature (similar to clonidine)

Adverse Reactions
Cardiovascular: Orthostatic hypotension, bradycardia, edema
Central nervous system: Drowsiness, sedation, dizziness, headache, depression, psychosis, asthenia, memory lapse, seizures, fever, visual hallucinations
Dermatologic: Rash
Endocrine & metabolic: Sodium retention, syndrome of inappropriate antidiuretic hormone (SIADH), gynecomastia
Gastrointestinal: Nausea, vomiting, diarrhea, dry mouth, "black" tongue, pancreatitis
Genitourinary: Sexual dysfunction
Hematologic: Hemolysis, positive Coombs' test, leukopenia, thrombocytopenia
Hepatic: Hepatitis, liver enzymes (increased), jaundice, cirrhosis, hepatic necrosis
Respiratory: Nasal congestion

Signs & Symptoms of Acute Overdose Hypotension, hiccups, encephalopathy, photosensitivity, A-V block, hyperprolactinemia, gynecomastia, hyperthermia, ejaculatory disturbances, hypertension, dementia, depression, delirium, memory loss, lichenoid eruptions, galactorrhea, parotid pain, dementia, eczema, dermatitis, colitis, cognitive dysfunction, circulatory collapse, cholestatic jaundice, sedation, Parkinson's-like symptoms, bradycardia, dizziness, constipation or diarrhea, flatus, nausea, vomiting, hypothermia, CNS depression, leukopenia; neutropenia; agranulocytosis; granulocytopenia; alopecia, impotence, systemic lupus erythematosus (SLE), urine discoloration (black), urine discoloration (brown), urine discoloration (red), urine discoloration (red-brown)

(Continued)

Methyldopa *(Continued)*

Toxicodynamics/Kinetics

Onset of action: Oral, parenteral: Peak hypotensive effects occur within 3-6 hours

Duration: Variable:

Oral: 12-24 hours

I.V.: 10-16 hours

Absorption: From gastrointestinal tract is variable but averages ~50%

Distribution: V_d: 0.37 L/kg; distributed throughout the body

Protein binding: <15%

Metabolism: Intestinally and in the liver

Half-life: 75-80 minutes

Elimination: 85% metabolites excreted in urine

Usual Dosage

Children:

Oral: Initial: 10 mg/kg/day in 2-4 divided doses; increase every 2 days as needed to maximum dose of 65 mg/kg/day; do not exceed 3 g/day

I.V.: 5-10 mg/kg/dose every 6-8 hours up to a total dose of 65 mg/kg/24 hours or 3 g/24 hours

Adults:

Oral: Initial: 250 mg 2-3 times/day; increase every 2 days as needed; usual dose 1-1.5 g/day in 2-4 divided doses; maximum dose: 3 g/day

I.V.: 250-1000 mg every 6-8 hours; maximum dose: 1 g every 6 hours

Dosing interval in renal impairment:

Cl_{cr} >50 mL/minute: Administer every 8 hours

Cl_{cr} 10-50 mL/minute: Administer every 8-12 hours

Cl_{cr} <10 mL/minute: Administer every 12-24 hours

Contraindications Hypersensitivity to methyldopa or any component; (oral suspension contains benzoic acid and sodium bisulfite; injection contains sodium bisulfite); liver disease, pheochromocytoma

Warnings May rarely produce hemolytic anemia and liver disorders; positive Coombs' test occurs in 10% to 20% of patients; perform periodic CBCs; sedation usually transient may occur during initial therapy or whenever the dose is increased. Use with caution in patients with previous liver disease or dysfunction, the active metabolites of methyldopa accumulate in uremia. Patients with impaired renal function may respond to smaller doses. Elderly patients may experience syncope (avoid by giving smaller doses). Tolerance may occur usually between the second and third month of therapy. Adding a diuretic or increasing the dosage of methyldopa frequently restores blood pressure control.

Dosage Forms

Injection, as methyldopate hydrochloride: 50 mg/mL (5 mL, 10 mL)

Suspension, oral: 250 mg/5 mL (5 mL, 473 mL)

Tablet: 125 mg, 250 mg, 500 mg

Stability Injectable dosage form is most stable at acid to neutral pH; parenteral admixture at room temperature (25°C): 24 hours

Reference Range

Therapeutic: 1-5 µg/mL (SI: 4.7-23.7 µmol/L)

Toxic: >7 µg/mL (SI: >33.0 µmol/L)

Overdosage Treatment

Decontamination: Ipecac or lavage/activated charcoal with cathartic

Supportive therapy: Hypotension usually responds to I.V. fluids or Trendelenburg positioning. If unresponsive to these measures, the use of a parenteral vasoconstrictor may be required (eg, norepinephrine 0.1-0.2 mcg/kg/minute titrated to response). Treatment is primarily supportive and symptomatic. Use atropine to treat bradycardia.

Enhancement of elimination: Dialysis/hemoperfusion may be of some use; slightly dialyzable (5% to 20%)

Test Interactions Methyldopa interferes with the following laboratory tests: urinary uric acid, serum creatinine (alkaline picrate method), AST (colorimetric method), and urinary catecholamines (falsely high levels)

Drug Interactions Iron supplements can interact and cause a significant **increase** in blood pressure; methyldopa administration with lithium may cause increased lithium toxicity

Pregnancy Risk Factor C

Pregnancy Implications Crosses the placenta; appears in breast milk

Monitoring Parameters Blood pressure, standing and sitting/lying down

Patient Information May cause transient drowsiness; may cause urine discoloration; notify physician of unexplained prolonged general tiredness, fever or jaundice

Nursing Implications Transient sedation or depression may be common for first 72 hours of therapy; usually disappears over time; infuse over 30-60 minutes

Specific References

Brohee D and Cauchie P, "Lymphocyte Subsets in Immune Haemolytic Anaemia Induced by Alpha-Methyldopa," *Medical Science Research*, 1995, 23:67-8.

Johnston GD and Smith AM, "Management of Overdose Due to Antihypertensive Agents," *Adverse Drug React Acute Poisoning Rev*, 1990, 9(2):75-89.

Shnaps Y, Almog S. Halkin H, et al, "Methyldopa Poisoning," *J Toxicol Clin Toxicol*, 1982, 19(5):501-3.

Methyldopate Hydrochloride *see* Methyldopa *on page 519*

1-Methylimidazole-2-thiol *see* Methimazole *on page 512*

Methylmorphine *see* Codeine *on page 238*

Methylphenidate Hydrochloride (meth ill fen' i date)

Related Information

Therapeutic Drugs Associated With Hallucinations *on page 1558-1559*

CAS Number 113-45-1; 298-59-9

Brand Names Ritalin®; Ritalin-SR®; Rubifen

Use Treatment of attention deficit disorder and symptomatic management of narcolepsy; many unlabeled uses

Mechanism of Action Blocks the reuptake mechanism of dopaminergic neurons, appears to act at the cerebral cortex and subcortical structures

Adverse Reactions

Cardiovascular: Tachycardia, hypertension, hypotension, palpitations, cardiac arrhythmias

Central nervous system: Nervousness, insomnia, dizziness, drowsiness, movement disorders, precipitation of Tourette's syndrome, toxic psychosis (rare), fever, headache, visual hallucinations

Dermatologic: Rash

Endocrine & metabolic: Growth retardation, weight loss

Gastrointestinal: Anorexia, nausea, abdominal pain

Hematologic: Thrombocytopenia

Hepatic: Fulminant liver failure

Miscellaneous: Hypersensitivity reactions, talc retinopathy

Signs & Symptoms of Acute Overdose Tachypnea, seizures, agitation, insomnia, coma

Toxicodynamics/Kinetics

Immediate release tablet:

- Peak cerebral stimulation effect: Within 2 hours
- Duration: 3-6 hours

Sustained release tablet:

- Peak effect: Within 4-7 hours
- Duration: 8 hours

Absorption: Slow and incomplete from gastrointestinal tract

Distribution: V_d: 12-33 L/kg

Protein binding: 15%

Metabolism: In liver via hydroxylation to ritolinic acid

Half-life:

- Oral: 2-4 hours
- I.V.: 1-2 hours

Time to peak: 1-3 hours postingestion

Elimination: In urine as metabolites and unchanged drug with 45% to 50% excreted in feces via bile; urinary excretion is not pH dependent

Usual Dosage Oral:

Children ≥6 years: Attention deficit disorder: Initial: 0.3 mg/kg/dose or 2.5-5 mg/dose given before breakfast and lunch; increase by 0.1 mg/kg/dose or by 5-10 mg/day at weekly intervals; usual dose: 0.5-1 mg/kg/day; maximum dose: 2 mg/kg/day or 60 mg/day

Adults: Narcolepsy: 10 mg 2-3 times/day, up to 60 mg/day

Discontinue periodically to re-evaluate or if no improvement occurs within 1 month

Contraindications Hypersensitivity to methylphenidate or any component

Warnings Use with caution in patients with hypertension, seizures; has high potential for abuse; use with caution in patients with glaucoma, motor tics, Tourette's syndrome, patients with marked agitation, tension, and anxiety

Dosage Forms

Tablet: 5 mg, 10 mg, 20 mg

Tablet, sustained release: 20 mg

Reference Range Therapeutic: 5-40 ng/mL

Overdosage Treatment

Decontamination: Lavage/activated charcoal with cathartic

Supportive therapy: Nitroprusside may be used for hypertension while diazepam or lorazepam can be used for agitation. Haloperidol can be used for hallucinatory behavior.

Enhancement of elimination: Multiple dosing of activated charcoal may be useful; while acid diuresis can increase excretion, it is not recommended due to renal effects

(Continued)

Methylphenidate Hydrochloride *(Continued)*

Test Interactions False-positives by immunoassay can be seen with ranitidine, phenylpropanolamine, brompheniramine, chlorpromazine, fluspirilene or pipothiazine coingestion

Diagnostic Tests/Procedures

Methylphenidate, Blood *on page 1299*

Drug Interactions

Increased effect with MAO inhibitors; increased effect of guanethidine, bretylium

Increased serum concentrations of tricyclic antidepressants, warfarin, phenytoin, phenobarbital and primidone

Pregnancy Risk Factor C

Patient Information Last daily dose should be given several hours before retiring; do not abruptly discontinue; prolonged use may cause dependence

Nursing Implications Do not crush or allow patient to chew sustained release dosage form

Additional Information Chewing tablets instead of swallowing can lead to decreased efficacy and increase in side effects

Specific References

Berkovitch M, Pope E, Phillips J, et al, "Pemoline-Associated Fulminant Liver Failure: Testing the Evidence for Causation," *Clin Pharmacol Ther*, 1995, 57:696-8.

Friberg TR, Gragoudas ES, and Regan CD, "Talc Emboli and Macular Ischemia in Intravenous Drug Abuse," *Arch Ophthalmol*, 1979, 97(6):1089-91.

Parran TV Jr and Jasinski DR, "Intravenous Methylphenidate Abuse: Prototype for Prescription Drug Abuse," *Arch Intern Med*, 1991, 151(4):781-3.

Pleak RR, "Adverse Effects of Chewing Methylphenidate," *Am J Psychiatry*, 1995, 152:811.

Stecyk O, Loludice TA, Demeter S, et al, "Multiple Organ Failure Resulting From Intravenous Abuse of Methylphenidate Hydrochloride," *Ann Emerg Med*, 1985, 14(6):597-9.

Methylphenobarbital *see* Mephobarbital *on page 501*

Methyl Sulfoxide *see* Dimethyl Sulfoxide *on page 290*

7,Methyltheophylline *see* Caffeine *on page 175*

Methyprylon (meth i prye' lon)

CAS Number 125-64-4

Brand Names Noludar®

Mechanism of Action Similar to glutethimide; it is a piperidineclione which has sedative/hypnotic properties; water and lipid soluble

Adverse Reactions

Cardiovascular: Tachycardia, hypotension

Central nervous system: Headache, coma, dementia, seizures, hypothermia, hyperthermia

Gastrointestinal: Nausea, vomiting, diarrhea

Hematologic: Thrombocytopenia, neutropenia, porphyria

Hepatic: Jaundice, mild elevation of liver function tests

Ocular: Miosis, nystagmus

Neuromuscular & skeletal: Hyperreflexia

Respiratory: Respiratory failure, apnea, pulmonary edema

Miscellaneous: Porphyrinogenic

Signs & Symptoms of Acute Overdose Leukopenia or neutropenia (agranulocytosis, granulocytopenia); hypothermia

Toxicodynamics/Kinetics

Distribution: V_d: 1 L/kg

Protein binding: 60%; parent compound: 38% metabolites

Metabolism: Hepatic

Half-life: 4-16 hours (in overdose: 50 hours)

Elimination: Urine 60%, feces 20%

Usual Dosage

Usual daily dose: 200-400 mg at night

Minimum lethal dose: 6 g

Dosage Forms

Capsule: 300 mg

Tablet: 50 mg, 200 mg

Reference Range Therapeutic: 1 mg/dL; respiratory arrest can occur at plasma levels exceeding 6 mg/dL

Overdosage Treatment

Decontamination: Lavage/activated charcoal with cathartic

Supportive therapy: Hypotension can be treated with isotonic saline/Trendelenburg; dopamine or norepinephrine can then be used

Enhancement of elimination: Multiple dosing of activated charcoal probably is not effective; forced diuresis does not play any role; hemodialysis can remove ~20% of the dose; charcoal hemoperfusion is not effective in enhancing elimination

Diagnostic Tests/Procedures
Methyprylon, Blood *on page 1299*

Drug Interactions Ethanol potentiates sedative nature

Specific References

Mandelbaum JM and Simon NM, "Severe Methyprylon Intoxication Treated by Hemodialysis," *JAMA*, 1971, 216(1):139-40.

Meticorten® *see* Prednisone *on page 639*

Metoclopramide (met oh kloe pra' mide)

Related Information
Doses and Administration of Several Frequently Used Antiemetic Agents *on page 1641*

CAS Number 364-62-5; 7232-21-5; 54143-57-6

Brand Names Clopra®; Maxeran®; Maxolon®; Meclomid®; Metox®; Octamide®; Parmid®; Plasil®; Pramin®; Primperan®; Reclomide®; Reglan®

Use Symptomatic treatment of diabetic gastric paresis, gastroesophageal reflux; prevention of nausea associated with chemotherapy or postsurgery and facilitates intubation of the small intestine

Mechanism of Action Blocks dopamine receptors in chemoreceptor trigger zone of the CNS; enhances the response to acetylcholine of tissue in upper gastrointestinal tract causing enhanced motility and accelerated gastric emptying without stimulating secretions

Adverse Reactions
Cardiovascular: Bradycardia, hypotension/hypertension
Central nervous system: Extrapyramidal reactions, drowsiness, fatigue, restlessness, psychosis, anxiety, agitation, neuroleptic malignant syndrome
Dermatologic: Rash
Endocrine & metabolic: Gynecomastia
Gastrointestinal: Constipation, diarrhea
Genitourinary: Priapism
Hematologic: Methemoglobinemia (particularly in neonates); leukopenia, neutropenia, agranulocytosis, granulocytopenia, sulfhaemoglobinaemia
Neuromuscular & skeletal: Asterixis

Signs & Symptoms of Acute Overdose Drowsiness, ataxia, depression, chorea (extrapyramidal), gynecomastia, hyperprolactinemia, delirium, lactation, impotence, neuroleptic malignant syndrome, A-V block, galactorrhea, nystagmus, mania, Parkinson's-like symptoms, cognitive dysfunction, hyperthermia, wheezing, metallic taste, extrapyramidal reactions, seizures, hypertension, methemoglobinemia (in infants), muscle hypertonia, agitation, fever

Toxicodynamics/Kinetics
Onset of action:
- Oral: within 30-60 minutes
- I.V.: within 1-3 minutes

Duration: Therapeutic effects persist for 1-2 hours, regardless of route administered
Absorption: Rapid
Distribution: V_d: 3.5 L/kg; to most body tissues and fluids; crosses blood-brain barrier
Protein binding: 30%
Metabolism: Hepatic
Bioavailability: 30% to 100%
Half-life: 4-7 (half-life and clearance may be dose-dependent)
Time to peak serum concentration: 1-2 hours
Elimination: Primarily as unchanged drug in urine and feces

Usual Dosage
Children:
- Gastroesophageal reflux: Oral: 0.1 mg/kg/dose up to 4 times/day; efficacy of continuing metoclopramide beyond 12 weeks in reflux has not been determined; total daily dose should not exceed 0.5 mg/kg/day
- Gastrointestinal hypomotility: Oral, I.M., I.V.: 0.1 mg/kg/dose up to 4 times/day, not to exceed 0.5 mg/kg/day
- Antiemetic: I.V.: 1-2 mg/kg 30 minutes before chemotherapy and every 2-4 hours
- Facilitate intubation: I.V.: <6 years: 0.1 mg/kg; 6-14 years: 2.5-5 mg

Adults:
- Stasis/reflux: Oral: 10-15 mg/dose up to 4 times/day 30 minutes before meals or food and at bedtime; efficacy of continuing metoclopramide beyond 12 weeks in reflux has not been determined
- Gastrointestinal hypomotility: Oral, I.M., I.V.: 10 mg 30 minutes before each meal and at bedtime
- Antiemetic: I.V.: 1-2 mg/kg 30 minutes before chemotherapy and every 2-4 hours
- Facilitate intubation: I.V.: 10 mg

(Continued)

Metoclopramide *(Continued)*

Dosing adjustment in renal impairment:

Cl_{cr} 10-50 mL/minute: Administer at 75% of normal dose

Cl_{cr} <10 mL/minute: Administer at 50% of normal dose

Contraindications Hypersensitivity to metoclopramide or any component; gastrointestinal obstruction, pheochromocytoma, history of seizure disorder

Warnings Use with caution in patients with Parkinson's disease; dosage and/or frequency of administration should be modified in response to degree of renal impairment

Dosage Forms

Injection: 5 mg/mL (2 mL, 10 mL, 30 mL, 50 mL, 100 mL)

Solution, oral, concentrated: 10 mg/mL (10 mL, 30 mL)

Syrup, sugar free: 5 mg/5 mL (10 mL, 480 mL)

Tablet: 5 mg, 10 mg

Stability Protection of dilutions do not require light protection if used within 24 hours; stability of parenteral admixture at room temperature (25°C) and refrigeration (4°C): 2 days

Reference Range Dose of 10 mg results in a mean plasma level of 65 ng/mL

Overdosage Treatment

Decontamination: Ipecac or lavage/activated charcoal with cathartic

Supportive therapy: Metoclopramide often causes extrapyramidal reaction (eg, dystonic reactions) requiring management with diphenhydramine 1-2 mg/kg (adults) up to a maximum of 50 mg I.M. or I.V. slow push followed by a maintenance dose for 48-72 hours. When these reactions are unresponsive to diphenhydramine, benztropine mesylate I.V. 1-2 mg (adults) may be effective. These agents are generally effective within 2-5 minutes. Treat methemoglobin with methylene blue.

Enhancement of elimination: Multiple dosing of activated charcoal may be useful; hemodialysis is not useful; not dialyzable (0% to 5%)

Antidote(s)

Methylene Blue *on page 1444*

Test Interactions Increases aminotransferase [ALT (SGPT)/AST (SGOT)] (S), amylase (S)

Diagnostic Tests/Procedures

Methemoglobin, Blood *on page 1296*

Drug Interactions Anticholinergic agents, opiate analgesics

Pregnancy Risk Factor B (no adverse fetal effects have been observed)

Pregnancy Implications Crosses the placenta; appears in breast milk

Monitoring Parameters Periodic renal function test, methemoglobin in infants

Patient Information May impair mental alertness or physical coordination; avoid alcohol, barbiturates or other CNS depressants; take 30 minutes before meals; notify physician if involuntary movements occur

Nursing Implications Parenteral doses of up to 10 mg should be given I.V. push; higher doses to be given IVPB; infuse over at least 15 minutes

Additional Information Structurally similar to domperidone

Specific References

Hughes RL, "Hypotension and Dysrhythmia Following Intravenous Metoclopramide," *Anaesthesia*, 1984, 39(7):720.

Kearns GL and Fiser DH, "Metoclopramide-Induced Methemoglobinemia," *Pediatrics*, 1988, 82(3):364-6.

LeCouteur DG and Kay T, "Delayed Neuroleptic Malignant Syndrome Following Cessation of Prolonged Therapy With Metoclopramide," *Aust N Z J Med*, 1995, 25:261.

Low LC and Goel KM, "Metoclopramide Poisoning in Children," *Arch Dis Child*, 1980, 55(3):310-2.

Malkoff MD, Ponzillo JJ, Myles GL, et al, "Sinus Arrest After Administration of Intravenous Metoclopramide," *Ann Pharmacother*, 1995, 29:381-3.

Patterson JF, "Neuroleptic Malignant Syndrome Associated With Metoclopramide," *South Med J*, 1988, 81(5):674-5.

Scharman EJ, Lembersky R, and Krenzelok EP, "Efficiency of Whole Bowel Irrigation With and Without Metoclopramide Pretreatment," *Am J Emerg Med*, 1994, 12(3):302-5.

Van Veldhuizen PJ and Wyatt A, "Metoclopramide-Induced Sulfhemoglobinemia," *Am J Gastroenterol*, 1995, 90:1010-1.

Metoprolol Tartrate (me toe' proe lole)

Related Information

Beta-Blockers Comparison *on page 1644-1645*

CAS Number 54163-88-1; 37350-58-6; 56392-17-7

Brand Names Beloc®; Beprolo®; Betaloc®; Lopressor®; Metoros®; Prelis®; Selokeen®; Selo-Zok®; Toprol XL®

Use Treatment of hypertension and angina pectoris; prevention of myocardial infarction; selective inhibitor of $beta_1$-adrenergic receptors; migraine prophylaxis

Mechanism of Action Selective inhibitor of $beta_1$-adrenergic receptors; competitively blocks $beta_1$-receptors, with little or no effect on $beta_2$-receptors at doses <100 mg

Adverse Reactions

Cardiovascular: Persistent bradycardia, hypotension, chest pain, edema, heart failure, heart block, exacerbation of Raynaud's phenomenon

Central nervous system: Fatigue, dizziness, insomnia, drowsiness, night terrors, depression, confusion, headache, intermittent claudication

Dermatologic: Alopecia, psoriasiform eruptions, exacerbation of vitiligo

Gastrointestinal: Constipation, diarrhea, nausea, vomiting

Genitourinary: Impotence, penile fibrosis

Neuromuscular & skeletal: Arthralgia

Ocular: Diplopia

Otic: Loss of hearing

Respiratory: Wheezing

Miscellaneous: Cold extremities

Signs & Symptoms of Acute Overdose Bradycardia, hypotension, ataxia, seizures, insomnia, impotence, hyperreflexia, confusion, night terrors, heart failure, A-V block, asystole, cyanosis, wheezing, apnea, respiratory arrest, metabolic acidosis

Toxicodynamics/Kinetics

Onset of action: Oral: Peak antihypertensive effects occur within 1.5-4 hours

Duration: 10-20 hours

Absorption: Rapid and completely from gastrointestinal tract (90%)

Distribution: V_d: 4.2 L/kg; widely distributed to body tissues; highest concentrations in heart, liver, lungs, and saliva; crosses the blood-brain barrier; distributes into breast milk, lipid solubility is moderate

Protein binding: 8% to 12%

Metabolism: Significant first-pass metabolism; extensively metabolized in the liver

Half-life: 3-4 hours

Time to peak serum concentration: $1\frac{1}{2}$ to 4 hours

Elimination: Urine (3% to 10% as unchanged drug); clearance: 15 mL/minute/kg

Usual Dosage Safety and efficacy in children have not been established

Children: Oral: 1-5 mg/kg/24 hours divided twice daily; allow 3 days between dose adjustments

Adults:

Oral: 100-450 mg/day in 2-3 divided doses, begin with 50 mg twice daily and increase doses at weekly intervals to desired effect

Sustained release: 50-100 mg once daily; maximum: 400 mg/day

I.V.: 5 mg every 2 minutes for 3 doses in early treatment of myocardial infarction; thereafter give 50 mg orally every 6 hours 15 minutes after last I.V. dose and continue for 48 hours; then administer a maintenance dose of 100 mg twice daily

Dosing adjustment/comments in hepatic disease: Reduced dose probably necessary

Contraindications Uncompensated congestive heart failure, cardiogenic shock, bradycardia, or heart block

Warnings Use with caution in patients with inadequate myocardial function; acute withdrawal may exacerbate symptoms; use with caution in patients undergoing anesthesia, bronchospastic disease, hyperthyroidism, and impaired hepatic function

Dosage Forms

Injection: 1 mg/mL (5 mL)

Tablet: 50 mg, 100 mg

Tablet, sustained release: 50 mg, 100 mg, 200 mg

Reference Range Therapeutic: 20-340 ng/mL; survival has occurred with levels as high as 7,140 ng/mL

Overdosage Treatment

Decontamination: Ipecac or lavage/activated charcoal with cathartic

Supportive therapy: Sympathomimetics (eg, epinephrine or dopamine), atropine, glucagon, or a pacemaker can be used to treat the toxic bradycardia, asystole, and/or hypotension; initially fluids may be the best treatment for toxic hypotension

Enhancement of elimination: Charcoal hemoperfusion can be used to lower serum levels

Test Interactions Increases cholesterol (S), glucose

Drug Interactions Diuretics or other hypotensive drugs may increase the hypotensive effect of metoprolol; oral contraceptives may increase plasma metoprolol levels; cimetidine reduces clearance of metoprolol

Pregnancy Risk Factor B

Pregnancy Implications Pregnancy enhances the elimination of metoprolol

Monitoring Parameters Monitor hemodynamic status carefully after acute myocardial infarction; monitor cardiac status for at least 6 hours postingestion

Patient Information Do not stop taking drug abruptly

Nursing Implications Patient's therapeutic response may be evaluated by look-

(Continued)

Metoprolol Tartrate *(Continued)*

ing at blood pressure, apical and radial pulses, fluid I & O, daily weight, respirations, and circulation in extremities before and during therapy

Specific References

Anthony T, Jastremski J, Elliott W, et al, "Charcoal Hemoperfusion for the Treatment of a Combined Diltiazem and Metoprolol Overdose," *Ann Emerg Med*, 1986, 15(11):1344-8.

Love JN, "Beta-Blocker Toxicity: A Clinical Diagnosis," *Am J Emerg Med*, 1994, 12(3):356-7.

Moller BJ, "Massive Intoxication With Metoprolol," *Br Med J*, 1976, 1(6003):222.

Schallreuter KU, "Beta-Adrenergic Blocking Drugs May Exacerbate Vitiligo," *Br J Dermatol*, 1995, 132:169.

Shore ET, Cepin D, and Davidson MJ, "Metoprolol Overdose," *Ann Emerg Med*, 1981, 10(10):524-7.

Sire S, "Metoprolol Intoxication," *Lancet*, 1976, 2(7995):1137.

Wallin CJ and Hulting J, "Massive Metoprolol Poisoning Treated With Prenalterol," *Acta Med Scand*, 1983, 214(3):253-5.

Metoros® *see* Metoprolol Tartrate *on page 524*

Metox® *see* Metoclopramide *on page 523*

MetroGel® Topical *see* Metronidazole *on this page*

MetroGel®-Vaginal *see* Metronidazole *on this page*

Metro I.V.® Injection *see* Metronidazole *on this page*

Metronidaz *see* Metronidazole *on this page*

Metronidazole (me troe ni' da zole)

CAS Number 443-48-1; 13182-89-3; 69198-10-3

Brand Names Flagyl® Oral; MetroGel® Topical; MetroGel®-Vaginal; Metro I.V.® Injection; Protostat® Oral; Rosalox; Vagilen

Synonyms Metronidaz

Use Treat susceptible anaerobic bacterial and protozoal infections in the following conditions: amebiasis, symptomatic and asymptomatic trichomoniasis, bacterial vaginosis, skin and skin structure infections, CNS infections, intra-abdominal infections, systemic anaerobic infections; surgical prophylaxis; topically for the treatment of acne rosacea, and decubitus

Unlabeled uses: Crohn's disease, hepatic encephalopathy, as combination therapy for *Helicobacter pylori* in peptic ulcer; treat antibiotic-associated pseudomembranous colitis (AAPC)

Mechanism of Action Reduced to a product by a nitroreductase enzyme which interacts with DNA to cause a loss of helical DNA structure and strand breakage resulting in inhibition of protein synthesis and cell death in susceptible organisms

Adverse Reactions

Central nervous system: Headache, dizziness vomiting, seizures (dose related), psychosis, insomnia, ataxia, encephalopathy

Dermatologic: Pruritus

Gastrointestinal: Nausea, diarrhea, loss of appetite, change in taste sensation, dry mouth, metallic taste, pancreatitis, glossitis

Genitourinary: Vaginal candidiasis

Local: Thrombophlebitis

Neuromuscular & skeletal: Peripheral neuropathy (axonopathy), lethargy

Hematologic: Leukopenia, aplastic anemia

Ocular: Myopia, oculogyric crisis

Miscellaneous: Hypersensitivity, disulfiram-type reaction with alcohol, furry tongue, dark urine

Signs & Symptoms of Acute Overdose Hepatotoxicity (12.5 g ingestion), nausea, cystitis, vomiting, dysosmia, insomnia, neutropenia, gynecomastia, diplopia, dry skin, ataxia, seizures, neuropathy (peripheral)

Toxicodynamics/Kinetics

Absorption: Well absorbed, oral (100%), rectal (60% to 80%)

Distribution: V_d: 0.74 L/kg; excreted in breast milk

Protein binding: 10% to 20%

Metabolism: In the liver (30% to 60%) to an active hydroxy-metabolite

Half-life:

- Neonates: 25-75 hours
- Others: 6-8 hours, increases with hepatic impairment

Time to peak serum concentration: Within 1-2 hours

Elimination: Final excretion via urine (20% as unchanged drug) and feces (6% to 15%); clearance: 0.08 L/kg/hour

Usual Dosage

Neonates: Anaerobic infections: Oral, I.V.:

- 0-4 weeks: <1200 g: 7.5 mg/kg every 48 hours
- Postnatal age <7 days:
  - 1200-2000 g: 7.5 mg/kg/day given every 24 hours
  - >2000 g: 15 mg/kg/day in divided doses every 12 hours

Postnatal age >7 days:
1200-2000 g: 15 mg/kg/day in divided doses every 12 hours
>2000 g: 30 mg/kg/day in divided doses every 12 hours

Infants and Children:
Amebiasis: Oral: 35-50 mg/kg/day in divided doses every 8 hours
Other parasitic infections: Oral: 15-30 mg/kg/day in divided doses every 8 hours
Anaerobic infections: Oral, I.V.: 30 mg/kg/day in divided doses every 6 hours
Clostridium difficile (antibiotic-associated colitis): Oral: 20 mg/kg/day divided every 6 hours
Maximum dose: 2 g/day

Adults:
Amebiasis: Oral: 500-750 mg every 8 hours
Other parasitic infections: Oral: 250 mg every 8 hours or 2 g as a single dose
Anaerobic infections: Oral, I.V.: 30 mg/kg/day in divided doses every 8 hours; not to exceed 2 g/day
AAPC (*Clostridium difficile*): Oral: 250-500 mg 3-4 times/day for 10-14 days
Topical: Apply a thin film twice daily to affected areas
Vaginal: One applicatorful in vagina each morning and evening, as needed

Maximum tolerated exposure: 12 g

Administration Administer I.V. by slow intermittent infusion over 30-60 minutes at a final concentration for administration of 5-8 mg/mL

Contraindications Hypersensitivity to metronidazole or any component, 1st trimester of pregnancy

Warnings Use with caution in patients with liver impairment, blood dyscrasias, history of seizures; reduce dosage in patients with severe liver impairment, CNS disease

Dosage Forms
Gel:
Topical: 0.75% (30 g)
Vaginal: 0.75% (70 g)
Injection, ready to use, in normal saline: 5 mg/mL (100 mL)
Powder for injection, as hydrochloride: 500 mg
Tablet: 250 mg, 500 mg

Stability Reconstituted solution is stable for 96 hours when refrigerated; for I.V. infusion in normal saline or D_5W and neutralized (with sodium bicarbonate), solution is stable for 24 hours at room temperature; do not refrigerate neutralized solution because a precipitate will occur

Reference Range 500 mg oral dose results in a peak plasma level of 12 mg/L (70 μmol/L)

Overdosage Treatment
Decontamination: Lavage/activated charcoal; do not use a cathartic if an ileus is present
Supportive therapy: Benzodiazepines can be used for seizure control with phenobarbital in phenytoin used as second-line agent
Enhancement of elimination: Metronidazole and active metabolite are eliminated by hemodialysis; up to 45% of drug may be removed from 4 hours of hemodialysis; peritoneal dialysis can remove 10% of the dose (during a 7.5 hour period)

Test Interactions May cause falsely decreased AST and ALT levels

Drug Interactions
Decreased effect with barbiturates
Increased toxicity/levels of phenytoin, lithium, and warfarin; cimetidine may result in increased levels of metronidazole; disulfiram-like reaction with alcohol; coadministration of disulfiram and metronidazole may cause psychosis and confusion; metronidazole can increase carbamazepine plasma level

Pregnancy Risk Factor B

Pregnancy Implications Minimal teratogenic risk although midline facial defects during first trimester maternal usage have been noted

Monitoring Parameters WBC count

Patient Information Urine may be discolored to a dark or reddish-brown; do not take alcohol for at least 24 hours after the last dose; avoid beverage alcohol or any topical products containing alcohol during therapy; may cause metallic taste; may be taken with food to minimize stomach upset; notify physician if numbness or tingling in extremities occurs

Nursing Implications No Antabuse®-like reactions have been reported after **topical** application, although metronidazole can be detected in the blood; avoid contact between the drug and aluminum in the infusion set

Additional Information Sodium content of 500 mg (I.V.): 322 mg (14 mEq); D-lactic acidosis may develop in patients with short bowel syndrome due to overgrowth of D-lactate producing organisms (*Lactobacillus*, species, *Streptococcus bovis*, *Bifidobacterium* species or *Eubacterium*, species)

Specific References

Ahmed A, Loes DJ, and Bressler EL, "Reversible Magnetic Resonance Imaging Findings in Metronidazole-Induced Encephalopathy," *Neurology*, 1995, 45(3 Pt 1):588-9.

(Continued)

Metronidazole *(Continued)*

Belliveau PP, Nightingale CH, and Quintilani R, "Stability of Cefotaxime Sodium and Metronidazole in 0.9% Sodium Chloride Injection or in Ready-to-Use Metronidazole Bags," *Am J Health-Syst Pharm*, 1995, 52:1561-3.

Bradley WG, Karlsson IJ, and Russo ICG, "Metronidazole Neuropathy," *Br Med J*, 1977, 2:610-1.

Canto JM and Carcia-Cruz D, "Midline Facial Defect as a Teratogenic Effect of Metronidazole," *Birth Defects*, 1982, 18:85-8.

Cassey JG, Clark DA, Merrick P, et al, "Pharmacokinetics of Metronidazole in Patients Undergoing Peritoneal Dialysis," *Antimicrob Agents Chemother*, 1983, 24:950-1.

Coronado BE, Opal SM, and Yoburn DC, "Antibiotic-Induced D-Lactic Acidosis," *Ann Intern Med*, 1995, 122:839-42.

Falagas ME and Gorbach SL, "Clindamycin and Metronidazole," *Med Clin North Am*, 1995, 79(4):845-68.

Lam S and Bank S, "Hepatotoxiciy Caused by Metronidazole Overdose," *Ann Intern Med*, 1995, 122(10):803.

Lau AH, Chang CW, and Sabatini S, "Hemodialysis Clearance of Metronidazole and its Metabolites," *Antimicrob Agents Chemother*, 1986, 29(2):235-8.

Patterson BD, "Possible Interaction Between Metronidazole and Carbamazepine," *Ann Pharmacother*, 1994, 28(11):1303-4.

Ralph ED, "Clinical Pharmacokinetics of Metronidazole," *Clin Pharmacokinet*, 1983, 8:43-62.

Smogyi A, Kong C, Sabto J, et al, "Disposition and Removal of Metronidazole in Patients Undergoing Haemodialysis," *Eur J Clin Pharmacol*, 1983, 25:683-7.

Mevacor® *see* Lovastatin *on page 485*

Mevinacor® *see* Lovastatin *on page 485*

Mevinolin *see* Lovastatin *on page 485*

Mevlor *see* Lovastatin *on page 485*

Mexate® *see* Methotrexate *on page 515*

Mexiletine (mex' i le teen)

CAS Number 31828-71-4; 5370-10-4

Brand Names Mexitil®

Use Management of serious ventricular arrhythmias; suppression of PVCs

Mechanism of Action Class IB antiarrhythmic, structurally related to lidocaine, which may cause increase in systemic vascular resistance and decrease in cardiac output; no significant negative inotropic effect

Adverse Reactions

Excessive doses: 1.8-2.4 g: CNS depression

Cardiovascular: Palpitations, bradycardia, chest pain, syncope, hypotension, atrial or ventricular arrhythmias

Central nervous system: Dizziness, confusion, ataxia

Dermatologic: Rash

Gastrointestinal: Nausea, vomiting, diarrhea, hiccup, esophagitis associated with oral forms

Hematologic: Rarely thrombocytopenia

Hepatic: Hepatitis progressing to hepatic necrosis

Neuromuscular & skeletal: Tremors, paresthesia

Ocular: Diplopia

Otic: Ototoxicity, tinnitus

Respiratory: Dyspnea

Miscellaneous: Positive antinuclear antibody

Signs & Symptoms of Acute Overdose CNS depression, esophageal ulceration, dysphagia, impotence, bradycardia, dry mouth, malaise, memory loss, lightheadedness, left bundle-branch block, nausea, asystole, neutropenia, hypotension, QRS prolongation, congestive heart failure, paresthesia, seizures

Toxicodynamics/Kinetics

Onset of action: Oral: 30 minutes to 2 hours

Absorption: Well from upper intestinal section of gastrointestinal tract

Distribution: V_d: 5-7 L/kg

Protein binding: 50% to 70%

Metabolism: Extensive in the liver (some minor active metabolites)

Bioavailability: 88%

Half-life: Adults: 10-14 hours; Increase in half-life with hepatic or heart failure

Time to peak serum concentration: 2-3 hours

Elimination: 10% to 15% excreted unchanged in urine; urinary acidification increases excretion while alkalinization decreases elimination; clearance: 0.38 L/hour/kg

Usual Dosage Adults: Oral: 400 mg to start, then 200 mg in 8 hours, then 200-400 mg every 8 hours; adjust dose in 50-100 mg increments with a minimum of 2-3 days between doses; do not exceed 1200 mg/day

Dosing adjustment in renal impairment: Cl_{cr} <10 mL/minute: Administer at 50% to 75% of normal dose

Dosing adjustment/comments in hepatic disease: Reduce maintenance dose to 25% to 30% of normal dose; patients with severe liver disease may require lower dosages and must be monitored closely

Contraindications Cardiogenic shock, second or third degree heart block, hypersensitivity to mexiletine or any component

Warnings Exercise extreme caution in patients with pre-existing sinus node dysfunction; mexiletine can worsen bradycardias and other arrhythmias; A-V second or third degree block, sinus node dysfunction, intraventricular conduction abnormalities; follow closely in patients with liver disease, seizure disorder; avoid drugs or diets that greatly alter urinary pH; mexiletine can worsen arrhythmias; hepatic impairment prolongs half-life; elevations of AST; use with caution in patients with severe congestive heart failure, hypotension

Dosage Forms Capsule: 150 mg, 200 mg, 250 mg

Reference Range

Therapeutic: 0.75-2.00 μg/mL

Potentially toxic: >2.00 μg/mL; level of 20 μg/mL associated with seizures

Overdosage Treatment

Decontamination: Do not use ipecac; lavage/activated charcoal with cathartic is useful

Supportive therapy: Treatment includes supportive measures; atropine may be used for bradycardia; dopamine or norepinephrine can be used for hypotension

Enhancement of elimination: Forced diuresis with mannitol may be useful; do not alkalinize urine; hemodialysis may be useful, although there is no overdose experience of this modality

Test Interactions Abnormal liver function test, positive ANA, thrombocytopenia

Diagnostic Tests/Procedures

Mexiletine, Blood *on page 1299*

Drug Interactions Can increase serum theophylline levels; phenobarbital, phenytoin, rifampin, and other hepatic enzyme inducers may lower mexiletine plasma levels; cimetidine may increase mexiletine levels; antacids, narcotics, or anticholinergics may decrease rate of absorption; metoclopramide may increase rate of absorption; drugs or diets which affect urine pH can increase or decrease excretion of mexiletine; use with beta-blockers or calcium channel blockers may depress cardiac function; phenytoin or rifampin can enhance mexiletine metabolism

Pregnancy Risk Factor C

Pregnancy Implications Found in breast milk in similar concentrations as plasma

Patient Information Take with food; notify physician of side effects such as jaundice, fever, and sore throat

Additional Information I.V. form under investigation; bitter tasting

Specific References

Denaro CP and Benowitz NL, "Poisoning Due to Class 1B Antiarrhythmic Drugs. Lignocaine, Mexiletine, and Tocainide," *Med Toxicol Adverse Drug Exp*, 1989, 4(6):412-28.

Frank SE, Snyder JT, "Survival Following Severe Overdose With Mexiletine, Nifedipine, and Nitroglycerin," *Am J Emerg Med*, 1991, 9(1):43-6.

Kemptom J, Manoukian A, Levine B, et al, "A Mexiletine Intoxication," *J Anal Toxicol*, 1994, 18(6):346-7.

Nelson LS and Hoffman RS, "Mexiletine Overdose Producing Status Epilepticus Without Cardiovascular Abnormalities," *J Toxicol Clin Toxicol*, 1994, 32(6):731-6.

Mexitil® *see* Mexiletine *on previous page*

Miacalcin® *see* Calcitonin *on page 177*

Mianserin Hydrochloride (mee an' ser in)

CAS Number 24219-97-4; 21535-47-7

Brand Names Athymil®; Bencard®; Bolvidon®; Lantanon®; Norval®; Tetramide®; Tolvin®; Tovon®

Use Depression; has been used to treat fluvoxamine-induced akathisia

Mechanism of Action Tetracyclic piperazino-azepine antidepressant with few antimuscarinic effects; a central serotonin antagonist

Adverse Reactions

Cardiovascular: Bradycardia, hypotension (orthostatic)

Central nervous system: Drowsiness, seizures, restlessness

Dermatologic: Erythema multiforme, toxic epidermal necrolysis

Endocrine & metabolic: Hypokalemia, gynecomastia

Gastrointestinal: Glossitis

Hematologic: Leukopenia/neutropenia (agranulocytosis, granulocytopenia), aplastic anemia

Hepatic: Jaundice, elevation of liver function tests

Neuromuscular & skeletal: Polyarthralgia

Miscellaneous: Sweating

Signs & Symptoms of Acute Overdose Dizziness, hypotension, toxic epidermal necrolysis, heart block, hypokalemia, seizures, gynecomastia, prolonged sedation, tachycardia/bradycardia with conduction disturbances leading to complete A-V block, delirium

(Continued)

Mianserin Hydrochloride *(Continued)*

Toxicodynamics/Kinetics

Distribution: V_d: 16 L/kg

Protein binding: 90%

Metabolism: Hepatic to two active metabolites

Bioavailability: 70%

Half-life: 6-40 hours

Time to peak plasma levels: 1-3 hours

Elimination: Clearance: 0.5 L/hour/kg

Usual Dosage Initial dose: 30-40 mg/day; usual dose: 30-90 mg/day; maximum dose: 200 mg/day; for fluvoxamine-induced akathisia: 15 mg at night

Contraindications Severe liver disease, mania

Warnings Use with caution in patients with cardiac conduction abnormalities, diabetes mellitus, epilepsy, liver/renal disease; elderly at special risk for hematologic toxicity

Reference Range Peak serum level at a dose of 60 mg/day: 100-120 μg/L; a peak plasma level of 439 μg/L associated with heart block

Overdosage Treatment

Decontamination: Do not induce emesis; lavage/activated charcoal with cathartic

Supportive therapy: Treat seizures with diazepam or lorazepam; phenobarbital is second choice; atropine or isoproterenol can be used for bradycardia

Enhancement of elimination: Multiple dosing of activated charcoal or hemodialysis is not likely to be effective

Drug Interactions Phenytoin may reduce plasma levels of mianserin

Specific References

Carcone B, Vial T, Chaillet N, et al, "Symptomatic Bradycardia Caused by Mianserin at Therapeutic Doses," *Hum Exp Toxicol*, 1991, 10(5):383-4.

Green SD and Kendall-Taylor P, "Heart Block in Mianserin Hydrochloride Overdose," *Br Med J*, 1977, 2(6096):1190.

Haefeli WE, Schoenenberger RA, and Scholer A, "Recurrent Ventricular Fibrillation in Mianserin Intoxication," *BMJ*, 1991, 302(6773):415-6.

Marshall RJ, "The Pharmacology of Mianserin - An Update," *Br J Clin Pharmacol*, 1983, 15(Suppl 2):263S-8S.

Poyurovsky M, Meerovich I, and Weizman A, "beneficial Effect of Low Dose Mianserin on Fluvoxamine-Induced Akathisia in an Obsevvice Computsive Patient," *Int Clin Psychopharmacol*, 1995, 1011-4.

Micatin® Topical [OTC] *see* Miconazole *on this page*

Miconal® *see* Miconazole *on this page*

Miconazole (mi kon' a zole)

Related Information

Antifungal Therapy *on page 1496-1497*

CAS Number 22916-47-8; 22832-87-7

Brand Names Albistat®; Breezee® Mist Antifungal [OTC]; Daktar®; Daktarin®; Fungoid® Creme; Fungoid® HC Creme; Fungoid® Tincture; Lotrimin® AF Powder [OTC]; Lotrimin® AF Spray Liquid [OTC]; Lotrimin® AF Spray Powder [OTC]; Maximum Strength Desenex® Antifungal Cream [OTC]; Micatin® Topical [OTC]; Miconal®; Micotef®; Monistat-Derm™ Topical; Monistat i.v.™ Injection; Monistat™ Vaginal; Prilagin®; Zeasorb-AF® Powder [OTC]

Synonyms Miconazole Nitrate

Use

I.V.: Treatment of severe systemic fungal infections and fungal meningitis that are refractory to standard treatment (primarily amphotericin B)

Topical: Treatment of vulvovaginal candidiasis and a variety of skin and mucous membrane fungal infections

Mechanism of Action A synthetic l-phenethyl-imidazole antifungal agent which inhibits biosynthesis of ergosterol, damaging the fungal cell wall membrane, which increases permeability causing leaking of nutrients

Adverse Reactions I.V. adverse effect (ie, hyponatremia, dyspnea) may be due to injection vehicle (polyethoxylated castor oil)

Cardiovascular: Flushing of face or skin

Central nervous system: Dizziness, fever, chills, drowsiness

Dermatologic: Skin rash, itching

Endocrine & metabolic: Hyperlipidemia, syndrome of inappropriate antidiuretic hormone (SIADH)

Gastrointestinal: Anorexia, diarrhea, nausea, vomiting

Hematologic: Anemia, thrombocytosis

Local: Pain at injection site

Neuromuscular & skeletal: Tremors

Respiratory: Bronchospasm, dyspnea

Miscellaneous: Anaphylaxis, inappropriate secretion of antidiuretic hormone, porphyrinogenic

Signs & Symptoms of Acute Overdose Nausea, vomiting, wheezing, thrombocytosis, hyponatremia, drowsiness, dyspnea (I.V. dosage), tachycardia, seizures

Toxicodynamics/Kinetics

Absorption:

Oral: 25% to 30%

Dermal: 0.01% to 0.35%

Vaginal: 1% to 1.4%

Protein binding: 90% to 93%

Metabolism: In the liver

Half-life, multiphasic:

Initial: 40 minutes

Secondary: 126 minutes

Terminal phase: 24 hours

Elimination: ~50% excreted in feces and <1% in urine as unchanged drug

Usual Dosage

Children:

I.V.: 20-40 mg/kg/day divided every 8 hours

Topical: Apply twice daily for up to 1 month

Adults:

I.T.: 20 mg every 1-2 days

I.V.: Initial: 200 mg, then 1.2-3.6 g/day divided every 8 hours for up to 20 weeks

Topical: Apply twice daily for up to 1 month

Vaginal: Insert contents of 1 applicator of vaginal cream (100 mg) or 100 mg suppository at bedtime for 7 days, or 200 mg suppository at bedtime for 3 days

Not dialyzable (0% to 5%)

Administration Administer by slow I.V. intermittent infusion over 1-2 hours at a final concentration not to exceed 6 mg/mL

Contraindications Hypersensitivity to miconazole, fluconazole, ketoconazole, or polyoxyl 35 castor oil or any component

Warnings Administer I.V. with caution to patients with hepatic insufficiency; the safety of miconazole in patients <1 year of age has not been established; cardiorespiratory and anaphylaxis have occurred with excessively rapid administration

Dosage Forms

Cream:

Topical, as nitrate: 2% (15 g, 30 g, 56.7 g, 85 g)

Vaginal, as nitrate: 2% (45 g is equivalent to 7 doses)

Cream with hydrocortisone 1% (Fungoid® HC Creme): 2%

Injection: 1% [10 mg/mL] (20 mL)

Lotion, as nitrate: 2% (30 mL, 60 mL)

Powder, topical: 2% (45 g, 90 g, 113 g)

Solution, topical: 2% with alcohol (7.39 mL, 29.57 mL)

Spray, topical: 2% (105 mL)

Suppository, vaginal, as nitrate: 100 mg (7s); 200 mg (3s)

Stability Protect from heat; darkening of solution indicates deterioration; stability of parenteral admixture at room temperature (25°C): 2 days

Reference Range Peak plasma level after an I.V. dose of 1 g: 1 μg/mL

Overdosage Treatment

Decontamination: Dermal: Wash with soap and water

Supportive therapy: Seizures and anaphylaxis can be treated with standard therapy

Enhancement of elimination: Not dialyzable (0% to 5%)

Test Interactions Increased protein , hyponatremia

Drug Interactions

Increased effect of warfarin and sulfonylureas; increased levels of phenytoin

Increased toxicity (cardiac arrhythmia) with terfenadine, astemizole; increases trimetrexate toxicity

Decreased levels of cyclosporine; decreased levels of miconazole when given with rifampin; ventricular arrhythmias can occur with combination of cisapride and ketoconazole, miconazole, or itraconazole

Pregnancy Risk Factor B

Pregnancy Implications Increased fetal mortality in rabbit studies during first trimester, although no reported adverse effects reported in humans

Monitoring Parameters Hematocrit, hemoglobin, serum electrolytes and lipids

Patient Information Avoid contact with the eyes; for vaginal product, insert high into vagina and complete full course of therapy; notify physician if itching or burning occur; refrain from intercourse to prevent reinfection

Nursing Implications Administer I.V. dose over 2 hours; give around-the-clock to promote less variation in peak and trough serum levels

Additional Information Available without prescription

Miconazole: Monistat i.v.™

(Continued)

Miconazole *(Continued)*

Miconazole nitrate: Micatin®, Monistat™, Monistat-Derm™

No specific data for elderly; use does not require alteration in dose or dose intervals; assess patient's ability to self administer, may be difficult in patients with arthritis or limited range of motion

Specific References

Coulthard K, Martin J, and Matthews N, "Convulsions After Miconazole Overdose," *Med J Aust*, 1987, 146(1):57-8.

Fainstein V and Bodey GP, "Cardiorespiratory Toxicity Due to Miconazole," *Ann Intern Med*, 1980, 93:432-3.

Kanarek KS and Williams PR, "Toxicity of Intravenous Miconazole Overdosage in a Preterm Infant," *Pediatr Infect Dis*, 1986, 5(4):486-8.

Miconazole Nitrate *see* Miconazole *on page 530*

Micotef® *see* Miconazole *on page 530*

Micro-K® *see* Potassium Chloride *on page 634*

Micronase® *see* Glyburide *on page 384*

Mictrin® *see* Hydrochlorothiazide *on page 406*

Midamine® *see* Midodrine Hydrochloride *on page 534*

Midamor® *see* Amiloride Hydrochloride *on page 109*

Midaten® *see* Piretanide *on page 630*

Midazol *see* Midazolam Hydrochloride *on this page*

Midazolam Hydrochloride (mid' ay zoe lam)

Related Information

Benzodiazepines Comparison *on page 1643*

CAS Number 59467-70-8; 59467-96-8; 59467-94-6

Brand Names Dormicum®; Hypnovel®; Versed®

Synonyms Midazol

Use Preoperative sedation and provide conscious sedation prior to diagnostic or radiographic procedures

Mechanism of Action A short-acting triazolobenzodiazepine which depresses all levels of the CNS, including the limbic and reticular formation, probably through the increased action of gamma-aminobutyric acid (GABA), which is a major inhibitory neurotransmitter in the brain

Adverse Reactions

Cardiovascular: Cardiac arrest, hypotension, bradycardia, ventricular dysrhythmia

Central nervous system: Drowsiness, amnesia, dizziness, paradoxical excitation, psychosis, sedation, headache, delirium, ataxia, hypothermia

Gastrointestinal: Hiccups, nausea, vomiting

Local: Pain and local reactions at injection site (severity less than diazepam)

Neuromuscular & skeletal: Dysarthria

Ocular: Blurred vision, diplopia, mydriasis

Respiratory: Apnea, respiratory depression, apnea, laryngospasm, wheezing

Miscellaneous: Physical and psychological dependence with prolonged use

Signs & Symptoms of Acute Overdose Apnea, cough, chills, encephalopathy, hypothermia, hyperactivity, euphoria, dyspnea, respiratory depression, seizures, hypotension, coma, stupor, confusion, cardiovascular arrest

Toxicodynamics/Kinetics

Onset of action (sedation):

I.M.: Within 15 minutes

I.V.: Within 1-5 minutes

Peak effect: I.M.: 30-60 minutes

Duration: I.M.: Mean: 2 hours, up to 6 hours

Distribution: V_d: 0.8-2.5 L/kg; increased V_d with congestive heart failure (CHF) and chronic renal failure; widely distributed in body including CSF and brain

Protein binding: 95%

Metabolism: Extensive in the liver (microsomally) to alpha-hydroxymidazolam

Bioavailability: 35% to 44%

Half-life: 1-4 hours; increased half-life with cirrhosis, CHF, obesity, elderly

Time to peak serum concentration: I.M.: 15-60 minutes

Elimination: Excreted as glucuronide conjugated metabolites in urine, ~2% to 10% excreted in feces

Usual Dosage The dose of midazolam needs to be individualized based on the patient's age, underlying diseases, and concurrent medications. Personnel and equipment needed for standard respiratory resuscitation should be immediately available during midazolam administration.

Children:

Preoperative sedation:

I.M.: 0.07-0.08 mg/kg 30-60 minutes presurgery

I.V.: 0.035 mg/kg/dose, repeat over several minutes as required to achieve the desired sedative effect up to a total dose of 0.1-0.2 mg/kg

Rectal: 0.3 mg/kg diluted in 5 mL of saline

Adjunct use in anesthesia: Intranasal: 0.2-0.3 mg/kg

Conscious sedation during mechanical ventilation: I.V.: Loading dose: 0.05-0.2 mg/kg then follow with initial continuous infusion: 1-2 mcg/kg/minute; titrate to the desired effect; usual range: 0.4-6 mcg/kg/minute

Conscious sedation for procedures:

Oral, Intranasal: 0.2-0.4 mg/kg (maximum: 15 mg) 30-45 minutes before the procedure

I.V.: 0.05 mg/kg 3 minutes before procedure

Adolescents >12 years: I.V.: 0.5 mg every 3-4 minutes until effect achieved

Adults:

Preoperative sedation: I.M.: 0.07-0.08 mg/kg 30-60 minutes presurgery; usual dose: 5 mg

Conscious sedation: I.V.: Initial: 0.5-2 mg slow I.V. over at least 2 minutes; slowly titrate to effect by repeating doses every 2-3 minutes if needed; usual total dose: 2.5-5 mg; use decreased doses in elderly

Healthy Adults <60 years: Some patients respond to doses as low as 1 mg; no more than 2.5 mg should be administered over a period of 2 minutes. Additional doses of midazolam may be administered after a 2-minute waiting period and evaluation of sedation after each dose increment. A total dose >5 mg is generally not needed. If narcotics or other CNS depressants are administered concomitantly, the midazolam dose should be reduced by 30%.

Contraindications Hypersensitivity to midazolam or any component (cross-sensitivity with other benzodiazepines may occur); uncontrolled pain; existing CNS depression; narrow-angle glaucoma

Warnings Midazolam may cause respiratory depression/arrest; deaths and hypoxic encephalopathy have resulted when these were not promptly recognized and treated appropriately. The danger of apnea or underventilation is greater in the elderly; the peak effect may take longer; reduce dosage increments and slow the rate of injection. Impaired metabolism with cirrhosis. Use with caution in patients with congestive heart failure, renal impairment, pulmonary disease, hepatic dysfunction.

Dosage Forms Injection: 1 mg/mL (2 mL, 5 mL, 10 mL); 5 mg/mL (1 mL, 2 mL, 5 mL, 10 mL)

Stability Admixtures do not require protection from light for short-term storage

Overdosage Treatment

Supportive therapy: Rarely is mechanical ventilation required. Flumazenil (Romazicon™) has been shown to selectively block the binding of benzodiazepines to CNS receptors, resulting in a reversal of benzodiazepine-induced CNS depression. Acetaminophen can be used to mask the metallic bitter taste.

Enhancement of elimination: Hemodialysis is not useful; multiple dosing of activated charcoal may be useful

Antidote(s)

Flumazenil *on page 1428*

Test Interactions Visine®, Drano®, bleach, and soap may result in false-negative urine test

Drug Interactions CNS depressants, leads to increased sedation and apnea; doses of anesthetic agents should be reduced when used in conjunction with midazolam; cimetidine may increase midazolam serum concentrations; theophylline may antagonize the sedative effects of midazolam

Pregnancy Risk Factor D

Pregnancy Implications Avoid at 1st trimester and just prior to delivery; crosses placental barrier

Monitoring Parameters Respiratory and cardiovascular status

Nursing Implications Midazolam is a short-acting benzodiazepine. The onset of action of midazolam's sedation is 15 minutes with peak sedation at 30-60 minutes after intramuscular (I.M.) administration. Sedation occurs 3-5 minutes after intravenous (I.V.) administration. Recovery occurs within 2 hours in most patients, however, may require up to 6 hours in some cases; each mL contains 0.14 mEq of sodium.

Specific References

Allonen H, Ziegler, G, and Klotz U, "Midazolam Kinetics," *Clin Pharmacol Ther*, 1981, 30(5):653-61.

Arcos J, "Midazolam-Induced Ventricular Irritability," *Anesthesiology*, 1987, 67(4):612.

Davis P, Tome J, and McGowan F, "Preanesthetic Medication With Intranasal Midazolam for Brief Surgical Procedures," *Anesthesiology*, 1995, 82:2-5.

Doyle WL and Perrin L, "Emergence Delirium in a Child Given Oral Midazolam for Conscious Sedation," *Ann Emerg Med*, 1994, 24(6):1173-5.

Hughes J, Gill A, Leach HJ, et al, "A Prospective Study of the Adverse Effects of Midazolam on Withdrawal in Critically Ill Children," *Acta Paediatr*, 1994, 83(11):1194-9.

(Continued)

Midazolam Hydrochloride *(Continued)*

Votey SR, Bosse GM, Bayer MJ, et al, "Flumazenil: A New Benzodiazepine Antagonist," *Ann Emerg Med*, 1991, 20(2):181-8.

Midodrine Hydrochloride

CAS Number 42794-76-3; 3092-17-9

Brand Names Gutron®; Midamine®

Use Investigational: Hypotension (orthostatic), urinary incontinence, ejaculation disorders

Mechanism of Action Oral sympathomimetic agent which is an alpha$_1$-adrenergic agonist resulting in vasoconstriction; essentially a prodrug

Adverse Reactions

Cardiovascular: Tachycardia, bradycardia, supine hypertension, flushing

Central nervous system: Headache, insomnia, sleep disturbance, irritability

Dermatologic: Scalp pruritus

Gastrointestinal: Nausea, dry mouth

Miscellaneous: Piloerection, sweating

Toxicodynamics/Kinetics

Peak plasma concentration: 20-40 minutes

Absorption: Within 1 hour

Distribution: V_d: 4-4.6 L/kg

Metabolism: Hepatic to active metabolite (deglymidodrine)

Bioavailability: 93%

Half-life:

- Midodrine: 30 minutes
- Deglymidodrine: 2-3 hours

Elimination: Renal

Usual Dosage

Children: Oral: 0.06 mg/kg

Adults:

- Oral: 2.5-10 mg 3-4 times/day; maximum dose: 40 mg
- I.V.: 5-10 mg to treat hypotension

Contraindications Hypersensitivity to midodrine, hypertension

Warnings Use with caution in patients with congestive heart failure, cardiac disease, pheochromocytoma, nephritis, thyrotoxicosis, renal insufficiency

Reference Range After a 2.5 mg oral dose, peak serum level is ~11 μg/L at 0.5 hour; serum deglymidodrine level is 5 μg/L at 1-hour postingestion

Overdosage Treatment

Decontamination: Lavage/activated charcoal with cathartic

Supportive therapy: There is no specific antidote for midodrine intoxication and the bulk of the treatment is supportive. Hyperactivity and agitation usually respond to reduced sensory input, however with extreme agitation haloperidol (2-5 mg I.M. for adults) may be required. Hyperthermia is best treated with external cooling measures, or when severe or unresponsive, muscle paralysis with pancuronium may be needed. Hypertension is usually transient and generally does not require treatment unless severe. For diastolic blood pressures >110 mm Hg, a nitroprusside infusion should be initiated. Seizures usually respond to diazepam or lorazepam I.V. and/or phenytoin maintenance regimens.

Drug Interactions Avoid concomitant use of MAO inhibitors

Specific References

Levien TL and Baker DE, "Reviews of Acrivastine and Midodrine," *Hosp Pharmacy*, 1995, 30(3):229-35.

McTavish D and Goa KL, "Midodrine: A Review of Its Pharmacological Properties and Therapeutic Use in Orthostatic Hypotension and Secondary Hypotensive Disorders," *Drugs*, 1989, 38(5):757-77.

Midol® 200 [OTC] *see* Ibuprofen *on page 418*

Midran® *see* Aprotinin *on page 130*

Migergot® *see* Ergotamine *on page 317*

Miiolene® *see* Ritodrine Hydrochloride *on page 687*

Mikelan® *see* Carteolol Hydrochloride *on page 188*

Milkinol® [OTC] *see* Mineral Oil *on this page*

Milontin® *see* Phensuximide *on page 618*

Milophene® *see* Clomiphene Citrate *on page 227*

Miltown® *see* Meprobamate *on page 503*

Mindiab® *see* Glipizide *on page 382*

Mineral Oil (min' er al oyl)

CAS Number 8012-95-1

Brand Names Agoral® Plain [OTC]; Fleet® Mineral Oil Enema [OTC]; Kondremul® [OTC]; Milkinol® [OTC]; Neo-Cultol® [OTC]; Zymenol® [OTC]

Synonyms Adepsine Oil; Heavy Mineral Oil; Liquid Paraffin; Oil Mist; Petrolatum Oil; White Mineral Oil

Use Temporary relief of constipation, to relieve fecal impaction, preparation for bowel studies or surgery; baby oil can be used to remove tar/asphalt burns

Mechanism of Action An emollient laxative which eases passage of stool by decreasing water absorption and lubricating the intestine; low volatility; high viscosity

Adverse Reactions

Gastrointestinal: Nausea, vomiting, diarrhea, abdominal cramps, anal itching, intestinal obstruction from bezoar formation may result

Respiratory: Lipoid pneumonitis with aspiration

Signs & Symptoms of Acute Overdose Aspiration of oils may cause chemical pneumonitis with fever, leukocytosis, x-ray changes

Toxicodynamics/Kinetics

Onset of action: ~6-8 hours

Absorption: Limited from intestinal tract

Distribution: To mesenteric lymph nodes, intestinal mucosa, liver, and spleen

Metabolism: None

Elimination: Feces

Usual Dosage

Children:

Oral: 5-11 years: 5-20 mL once daily or in divided doses

Rectal: 2-11 years: 30-60 mL as a single dose

Children >12 years and Adults:

Oral: 15-45 mL/day once daily or in divided doses

Rectal: Retention enema, contents of one enema (range 60-150 mL)/day as a single dose

Contraindications Patients with colostomy or an ileostomy, appendicitis, ulcerative colitis, diverticulitis

Warnings Oral form should be avoided in children <6 years of age and bedtime doses should be avoided because of the risk of aspiration; do not administer in patients who have difficulty in swallowing

Dosage Forms

Emulsion, oral: 1.4 g/5 mL (480 mL); 2.5 mL/5 mL (420 mL); 2.75 mL/5 mL (480 mL); 4.75 mL/5 mL (240 mL)

Jelly, oral: 2.75 mL/5 mL (180 mL)

Liquid:

Oral: 30 mL, 180 mL, 500 mL, 1000 mL, 4000 mL

Rectal: 133 mL

Overdosage Treatment

Decontamination: Do not induce emesis; activated charcoal may be useful

Supportive therapy: Fluid/electrolyte replacement; pulmonary physiotherapy should be considered; corticosteroids are of unproven pulmonary benefit

Drug Interactions May impair absorption of fat-soluble vitamins (A,D,E,K), oral contraceptives, coumarin, sulfonamides; decreases absorption of beta-carotene and fat soluble vitamins

Pregnancy Risk Factor C

Monitoring Parameters Chest x-ray

Patient Information Do not take with food or meals; do not use if experiencing abdominal pain, nausea, or vomiting

Nursing Implications Administer on an empty stomach because of the risk of aspiration

Additional Information Associated with increased risk from bronchogenic carcinoma (from lipoid pneumonia), gastrointestinal tumors, and dermal tumors suppresses cough reflex; prolonged administration of mineral oil may decrease absorption of lipid-soluble vitamins A, D, E, and K. Light sterile mineral oils are not for injection. Gauze pads soaked with mineral oil compresses can be used to lyse eyelid adhesions due to cyanoacrylate adhesive; no ocular damage was reported over a 1½-day period.

Specific References

Ayvazian LF, Steward DS, Merkel CG, et al, "Diffuse Lipoid Pneumonitis Successfully Treated With Prednisone," *Am J Med*, 1967, 43:930-4.

Bock GW, "Skin Exposure to Cyanoacrylate Adhesive," *Ann Emerg Med*, 1984, 13(6):486.

Heckers H, Melcher FW, Dittmar K, et al, "Long-Term Course of Mineral Oil Pneumonia," *Lung*, 1978, 55:101-9.

Varkey B and Kutty AV, "Lipoid Pneumonia With Lipoid Granulomata in Scalene Node," *Ann Intern Med*, 1976, 84(2):176-7.

Minidiab® *see* Glipizide *on page 382*

Minims® *see* Tetracaine Hydrochloride *on page 731*

Minipress® *see* Prazosin Hydrochloride *on page 638*

Minitran® *see* Nitroglycerin *on page 566*

Minodiab® *see* Glipizide *on page 382*

Minodyl® *see* Minoxidil *on this page*

Minoxidil (mi nox' i dill)

CAS Number 38304-91-5

Brand Names Loniten®; Minodyl®; Regaine®; Rogaine®

Synonyms Minoxidilum

Use Management of severe hypertension; treatment of male pattern baldness (alopecia androgenetica)

Mechanism of Action Produces vasodilation by directly relaxing arteriolar smooth muscle, with little effect on veins, effects may be mediated by cyclic amp; stimulation of hair growth is secondary to vasodilation, increased cutaneous blood flow and stimulation of resting hair follicles

Adverse Reactions

Cardiovascular: Edema, chest pain, congestive heart failure, tachycardia, angina, pericardial effusion, pericardial effusion/pericarditis, EKG changes

Central nervous system: Dizziness, fatigue, headache

Dermatologic: Hypertrichosis (commonly occurs within 1-2 months of therapy), coarsening facial features, dermatologic reactions, rash, Stevens-Johnson syndrome, sunburn

Endocrine & metabolic: Sodium and water retention, weight gain, gynecomastia

Gastrointestinal: Vomiting

Local: Topical burning, itching

Ocular: Optic neuritis

Respiratory: Pulmonary hypertension/edema

Miscellaneous: Lupus erythematosus (SLE), hirsutism

Signs & Symptoms of Acute Overdose Hypotension, tachycardia, hyperglycemia, photosensitivity, pericardial effusion, pericarditis, hypertrichosis, thrombocytopenia, hair discoloration (red), erythema multiforme, coma, ototoxicity, tinnitus

Toxicodynamics/Kinetics

Absorption: 90% from gastrointestinal tract

Distribution: V_d: 2-3 L/kg; widely distributed throughout body

Protein binding: None

Metabolism: 88% primarily via glucuronidation

Bioavailability: Oral: 90%

Half-life: Adults: 3.5-4.2 hours

Time to peak serum concentration: 1 hour

Elimination: 12% excreted unchanged in urine; 3% excreted in feces

Usual Dosage

Children <12 years: Hypertension: Oral: Initial: 0.1-0.2 mg/kg once daily; maximum: 5 mg/day; increase gradually every 3 days; usual dosage: 0.25-1 mg/kg/day in 1-2 divided doses; maximum: 50 mg/day

Children >12 years and Adults:

- Hypertension: Oral: Initial: 5 mg once daily, increase gradually every 3 days; usual dose: 10-40 mg/day in 1-2 divided doses; maximum: 100 mg/day
- Alopecia: Topical: Apply twice daily; 4 months of therapy may be necessary for hair growth

Contraindications Pheochromocytoma, hypersensitivity to minoxidil or any component

Warnings Use with caution in patients with coronary artery disease or with recent myocardial infarction, pulmonary hypertension, significant renal dysfunction, congestive heart failure

Dosage Forms

Solution, topical: 2% = 20 mg/metered dose (60 mL)

Tablet: 2.5 mg, 10 mg

Reference Range Mean serum level (oral) for 5 mg: 59.2 ng/mL

Overdosage Treatment

Decontamination: Ipecac or lavage/activated charcoal with cathartic

Supportive therapy: Hypotension usually responds to I.V. fluids or Trendelenburg positioning. If unresponsive to these measures, the use of a parenteral vasoconstrictor may be required (eg, phenylephrine or dopamine). Treatment is primarily supportive and symptomatic.

Enhancement of elimination: Multiple dosing of activated charcoal is useful; hemodialysis may be useful; dialyzable (50% to 100%)

Test Interactions Increases alkaline phosphatase

Drug Interactions Concurrent administration with guanethidine may cause profound orthostatic hypotensive effects; additive hypotensive effects with other hypotensive agents or diuretics

Pregnancy Risk Factor C

Pregnancy Implications Distributes into breast milk

Monitoring Parameters Blood pressure, standing and sitting/supine, EKG

Patient Information Topical product must be used every day. Minoxidil is usually taken with at least two other antihypertensive medications. Take all medications as prescribed; do not discontinue any except on advice of physician. Notify the physician if any of the following occur: heart rate of ≥20 beats per minute over normal; rapid weight gain of >5 lb (2 kg); unusual swelling of extremities, face, or abdomen; breathing difficulty, especially when lying down; new or aggravated angina symptoms (chest, arm, or shoulder pain); severe indigestion, dizziness, lightheadedness, or fainting; nausea or vomiting may occur.

Nursing Implications May cause hirsutism

Additional Information Usually given in combination with a diuretic and beta-blocker

Specific References

Allon M, Hall D, and Macon EJ, "Prolonged Hypotension After Initial Minoxidil Dose," *Arch Intern Med*, 1986, 146(10):2075-6.

Isles C, Mackay A, Barton PJ, et al, "Accidental Overdosage of Minoxidil in a Child," *Lancet*, 1981, 1(8211):97.

Linas SL and Nies AS, "Minoxidil," *Ann Intern Med*, 1981, 94(1):61-5.

McCormick MA, Forman MH, and Manoguerra AS, "Severe Toxicity From Ingestion of a Topical Minoxidil Preparation," *Am J Emerg Med*, 1989, 7(4):419-21.

Poff SW and Rose SR, "Minoxidil Overdose With ECG Changes: Case Report and Review," *J Emerg Med*, 1992, 10(1):53-7.

Minoxidilum *see* Minoxidil *on previous page*

Minuric® *see* Benzbromarone *on page 148*

Minute-Gel® *see* Fluoride *on page 355*

Miodaron® *see* Amiodarone Hydrochloride *on page 113*

Mirsol® *see* Zipeprol Hydrochloride *on page 813*

Misulban® *see* Busulfan *on page 173*

Mitidin® *see* Nitrazepam *on page 562*

Mitran® *see* Chlordiazepoxide *on page 198*

Mixtard® *see* Insulin Preparations *on page 426*

MK-421 *see* Enalapril *on page 311*

MK 954 *see* Losartan Potassium *on page 484*

M-KYA® [OTC] *see* Quinine Sulfate *on page 671*

Moban® *see* Molindone Hydrochloride *on this page*

Modamide® *see* Amiloride Hydrochloride *on page 109*

Modane® Soft [OTC] *see* Docusate *on page 297*

Modane® [OTC] *see* Phenolphthalein *on page 617*

Moditen® *see* Fluphenazine *on page 361*

Mogadan® *see* Nitrazepam *on page 562*

Molindone Hydrochloride (moe lin' done)

Related Information

Antipsychotic Agents Comparison *on page 1642*

CAS Number 7416-34-4; 15622-65-8

Brand Names Lidone®; Moban®

Use Management of psychotic disorder

Mechanism of Action Mechanism of action mimics that of chlorpromazine; however, it produces more extrapyramidal effects and less sedation than chlorpromazine

Adverse Reactions

Cardiovascular: Hypotension, tachycardia, cardiac arrhythmias

Central nervous system: Sedation, drowsiness, restlessness, anxiety, extrapyramidal reactions, pseudoparkinsonian signs and symptoms, seizures, altered central temperature regulation, neuroleptic malignant syndrome (NMS), restlessness

Dermatologic: Hyperpigmentation, pruritus, rash, photosensitivity

Endocrine & metabolic: Amenorrhea, galactorrhea, gynecomastia, syndrome of inappropriate antidiuretic hormone, weight gain

Gastrointestinal: Dry mouth, constipation, gastrointestinal upset

Genitourinary: Urinary retention

Hematologic: Agranulocytosis (more often in women between fourth and tenth weeks of therapy), leukopenia (usually in patients with large doses for prolonged periods)

Hepatic: Elevated liver transaminases

Ocular: Blurred vision, retinal pigmentation

Signs & Symptoms of Acute Overdose Deep sleep, extrapyramidal reaction, priapism, gynecomastia, galactorrhea, Parkinson's-like symptoms, leukocytosis,

(Continued)

Molindone Hydrochloride *(Continued)*

neuroleptic malignant syndrome, rhabdomyolysis, cardiac arrhythmias, myoglobinuria with oliguria renal failure, systemic lupus erythematosus (SLE), leukopenia; neutropenia; agranulocytosis; granulocytopenia

Toxicodynamics/Kinetics

Duration of action: 24-36 hours

Absorption: Rapid from gastrointestinal tract

Distribution: V_d: 3-6 L/kg; widely distributed into body

Metabolism: In the liver

Half-life: 90 minutes

Time to peak serum concentration: Within 90 minutes

Elimination: Principally in urine and feces (90% within 24 hours)

Usual Dosage Oral:

Children:

3-5 years: 1-2.5 mg/day divided into 4 doses

5-12 years: 0.5-1 mg/kg/day in 4 divided doses

Adults: 50-75 mg/day increase at 3- to 4-day intervals up to 225 mg/day

Contraindications Narrow-angle glaucoma, bone marrow depression, CNS depression, liver or cardiac disease, hypersensitivity to molindone or any component

Warnings Avoid alcoholic beverages; use with caution in patients with cardiovascular disease or seizures

Dosage Forms

Concentrate, oral: 20 mg/mL (120 mL)

Tablet: 5 mg, 10 mg, 25 mg, 50 mg, 100 mg

Reference Range Antipsychotic range: 27-69 ng/mL; level of 152 ng/mL seen with rhabdomyolysis

Overdosage Treatment Following initiation of essential overdose management, toxic symptom treatment and supportive treatment should be initiated. Hypotension usually responds to I.V. fluids or Trendelenburg positioning. If unresponsive to these measures, the use of a parenteral inotrope may be required (eg, norepinephrine 0.1-0.2 mcg/kg/minute titrated to response). Seizures commonly respond to lorazepam or diazepam (I.V. 5-10 mg bolus in adults every 15 minutes if needed up to a total of 30 mg; I.V. 0.25-0.4 mg/kg/dose up to a total of 10 mg in children) or to phenytoin or phenobarbital. Also critical cardiac arrhythmias often respond to I.V. phenytoin (15 mg/kg up to 1 gram), while other antiarrhythmics can be used. Neuroleptics often cause extrapyramidal reaction (eg, dystonic reactions) requiring management with diphenhydramine 1-2 mg/kg (adults) up to a maximum of 50 mg I.M. or I.V. slow push followed by a maintenance dose for 48-72 hours. When these reactions are unresponsive to diphenhydramine, benztropine mesylate I.V. 1-2 mg (adults) may be effective. These agents are generally effective within 2-5 minutes.

Test Interactions May give false-positive result for the EMIT® system for tricyclics

Drug Interactions CNS depressants, antihypertensives, anticonvulsants; severe bradykinesia and tremor with paroxetine

Pregnancy Risk Factor C

Pregnancy Implications May appear in breast milk; not known if crosses the placenta

Monitoring Parameters Monitor blood pressure and pulse rate prior to and during initial therapy evaluate mental status; monitor weight; monitor WBC and liver transaminases along with CPK in overdoses; monitor EKG

Patient Information Avoid alcoholic beverages

Nursing Implications May increase appetite and possibly a craving for sweets; recognize signs of neuroleptic malignant syndrome and tardive dyskinesia

Specific References

Johnson SB, Alvarez WA, and Freinhar JP, "A Case of Massive Rhabdomyolysis Following Molindone Administration," *J Clin Psychiatry*, 1986, 47(12):607-8.

Katz SE, "Tardive Dyskinesia Associated With Molindone Treatment," *Am J Psychiatry*, 1990, 147(1):124-5, (letter).

Knight ME and Roberts RJ, "Phenothiazine and Butyrophenone Intoxication in Children," *Pediatr Clin North Am*, 1986, 33(2):299-309.

Malek-Ahmadi P and Allen SA, "Paroxetine-Molindone Interaction," *J Clin Psychiatry*, 1995, 56(2):82-3.

Molipaxin® *see* Trazodone Hydrochloride *on page 765*

Mol-Iron® *see* Iron *on page 439*

Monacolin K *see* Lovastatin *on page 485*

Monistat-Derm™ Topical *see* Miconazole *on page 530*

Monistat i.v.™ Injection *see* Miconazole *on page 530*

Monistat™ Vaginal *see* Miconazole *on page 530*

Monochloroethane *see* Ethyl Chloride *on page 337*

Monocor® *see* Bisoprolol Fumarate *on page 157*
Monodox® Oral *see* Doxycycline *on page 305*
Mono-Gesic® *see* Salsalate *on page 689*
Monohydroxybenzene *see* Phenol *on page 616*
Monopril® *see* Fosinopril Sodium *on page 369*
Monosodium Alendronate *see* Alendronate *on page 94*
Monoxidin *see* Moxonidine *on page 541*
Mopatil® *see* Methyldopa *on page 519*
Mopral® *see* Omeprazole *on page 576*

Morphine Sulfate (mor' feen)

Related Information

Pharmacokinetics of Narcotic Agonist Analgesics *on page 1654*
Principal Pharmacological Properties of Hallucinogenic Drugs *on page 1557*

CAS Number 57-27-2; 64-31-3; 6009-81-0; 6211-15-0

Brand Names Astramorph™ PF; Duramorph®; Epimorph Dolcontin®; MS Contin®; MSIR®; MST®; OMS®; Oramorph SR®; RMS®; Roxanol™; Roxanol SR™; Sevredol®; Statex®

Synonyms MS

Use Relief of moderate to severe acute and chronic pain; pain of myocardial infarction; relieves dyspnea of acute left ventricular failure and pulmonary edema; preanesthetic medication

Mechanism of Action Binds to opiate receptors in the CNS, causing inhibition of ascending pain pathways, altering the perception of and response to pain; produces generalized CNS depression

Adverse Reactions

Cardiovascular: Palpitations, hypotension, bradycardia, peripheral vasodilation
Central nervous system: CNS depression, psychosis, drowsiness, dizziness, sedation, intracranial pressure (increased)
Dermatologic: Pruritus (more common with epidural or intrathecal administration)
Endocrine & metabolic: Syndrome of inappropriate antidiuretic hormone (SIADH)
Gastrointestinal: Nausea, vomiting, constipation, adynamic ileus
Genitourinary: Urinary retention
Neuromuscular & skeletal: Myoclonus
Ocular: Miosis, nystagmus
Respiratory: Apnea, respiratory depression, aspiration
Miscellaneous: Physical and psychological dependence, histamine release, biliary or urinary tract spasm

Signs & Symptoms of Acute Overdose Apnea, encephalopathy, respiratory depression, hyponatremia, dry mouth, impotence, hypothermia, dysuria, constipation, myocardial depression, thirst, rhabdomyolysis, hypotension, seizures (in neonates), myoglobinuria, coma, miosis, pulmonary edema, hallucinations

Toxicodynamics/Kinetics

Absorption: Oral: Variable
Distribution: V_d: 3-4 L/kg; lower in elderly patients
Protein binding: 35%
Metabolism: In the liver via glucuronide conjugation
Half-life:
- Neonates: Prolonged 6% to 10%
- Adults: 1.5-2 hours

Elimination: Excreted unchanged in urine; renal clearance: 2 L/hour/kg
See table.

Dosage	Analgesia	
Form/Route	Peak	Duration
Tablets	1 h	4–5 h
Oral solution	1 h	4–5 h
Extended release tablets	1 h	8–12 h
Suppository	20–60 min	3–7 h
Subcutaneous injection	50–90 min	4–5 h
I.M. injection	30–60 min	4–5 h
I.V. injection	20 min	4–5 h

(Continued)

Morphine Sulfate *(Continued)*

Usual Dosage Doses should be titrated to appropriate effect; when changing routes of administration in chronically treated patients, please note that oral doses are approximately one-half as effective as parenteral dose

Infants and Children:

Oral: Tablet and solution (prompt release): 0.2-0.5 mg/kg/dose every 4-6 hours as needed; tablet (controlled release): 0.3-0.6 mg/kg/dose every 12 hours

I.M., I.V., S.C.: 0.1-0.2 mg/kg/dose every 2-4 hours as needed; usual maximum: 15 mg/dose; may initiate at 0.05 mg/kg/dose

I.V., S.C. continuous infusion: Sickle cell or cancer pain: 0.025-2 mg/kg/hour; postoperative pain: 0.01-0.04 mg/kg/hour

Sedation/analgesia for procedures: I.V.: 0.05-0.1 mg/kg 5 minutes before the procedure

Adolescents >12 years: Sedation/analgesia for procedures: I.V.: 3-4 mg and repeat in 5 minutes if necessary

Adults:

Oral: Prompt release: 10-30 mg every 4 hours as needed; controlled release: 15-30 mg every 8-12 hours

I.M., I.V., S.C.: 2.5-20 mg/dose every 2-6 hours as needed; usual: 10 mg/dose every 4 hours as needed

I.V., S.C. continuous infusion: 0.8-10 mg/hour; may increase depending on pain relief/adverse effects; usual range up to 80 mg/hour

Epidural: Initial: 5 mg in lumbar region; if inadequate pain relief within 1 hour, give 1-2 mg, maximum dose: 10 mg/24 hours

Intrathecal ($^1/_{10}$ of epidural dose): 0.2-1 mg/dose; repeat doses **not** recommended

Rectal: 10-20 mg every 4 hours

Dosing adjustment in renal impairment:

Cl_{cr} 10-50 mL/minute: Administer at 75% of normal dose

Cl_{cr} <10 mL/minute: Administer at 50% of normal dose

Dosing adjustment/comments in hepatic disease: Unchanged in mild liver disease; substantial extrahepatic metabolism may occur; excessive sedation may occur in cirrhosis

Administration When giving morphine I.V. push, it is best to first dilute in 4-5 mL of sterile water, and then to administer slowly (eg, 15 mg over 3-5 minutes)

Contraindications Known hypersensitivity to morphine sulfate; increased intracranial pressure; severe respiratory depression

Warnings Some preparations contain sulfites which may cause allergic reactions; infants <3 months of age are more susceptible to respiratory depression, use with caution and generally in reduced doses in this age group; use with caution in patients with impaired respiratory function or severe hepatic dysfunction and in patients with hypersensitivity reactions to other phenanthrene derivative opioid agonists (codeine, hydrocodone, hydromorphone, levorphanol, oxycodone, oxymorphone). Can cause hypertension in patients with pheochromocytoma. Use with caution in myasthenia gravis.

Dosage Forms

Injection: 0.5 mg/mL (10 mL); 1 mg/mL (10 mL, 30 mL, 60 mL); 2 mg/mL (1 mL, 2 mL, 60 mL); 3 mg/mL (50 mL); 4 mg/mL (1 mL, 2 mL); 5 mg/mL (1 mL, 30 mL); 8 mg/mL (1 mL, 2 mL); 10 mg/mL (1 mL, 2 mL, 10 mL); 15 mg/mL (1 mL, 2 mL, 20 mL)

Injection:

Preservative free: 0.5 mg/mL (2 mL, 10 mL); 1 mg/mL (2 mL, 10 mL)

I.V. via PCA pump: 1 mg/mL (10 mL, 30 mL, 60 mL); 5 mg/mL (30 mL)

I.V. infusion preparation: 25 mg/mL (4 mL, 10 mL, 20 mL)

Solution, oral: 10 mg/5 mL (5 mL, 10 mL, 100 mL, 120 mL, 500 mL); 20 mg/5 mL (5 mL, 100 mL, 120 mL, 500 mL); 20 mg/mL (30 mL)

Suppository, rectal: 5 mg, 10 mg, 20 mg, 30 mg

Tablet: 15 mg, 30 mg

Tablet:

Controlled release: 15 mg, 30 mg, 60 mg, 100 mg

Soluble: 10 mg, 15 mg, 30 mg

Sustained release: 30 mg, 60 mg, 100 mg

Stability Refrigerate suppositories; do not freeze; degradation depends on pH and presence of oxygen; relatively stable in pH 4 and below; darkening of solutions indicate degradation; usual concentration for continuous I.V. infusion = 0.1-1 mg/mL in D_5W; incompatible with acyclovir, furosemide, heparin, pethidine, prochlorperazine, promethazine

Reference Range

Therapeutic: Surgical anesthesia: 65-80 ng/mL (SI: 227-280 nmol/L)

Toxic: 200-5000 ng/mL (SI: 700-17,500 nmol/L)

Overdosage Treatment Supportive therapy: Naloxone hydrochloride (0.4-2 mg

I.V., S.C., or through an endotracheal tube); a continuous infusion (at $^2/_3$ the response dose/hour) may be required

Antidote(s)

Naloxone Hydrochloride *on page 1447*

Test Interactions ↑ aminotransferase [ALT (SGPT)/AST (SGOT)] (S), ↑ amylase

Diagnostic Tests/Procedures

Morphine, Blood *on page 1300*

Morphine, Urine *on page 1300*

Opiates, Qualitative, Urine *on page 1309*

Drug Interactions Increased toxicity with CNS depressants, cimetidine, MAO inhibitors, phenothiazines, tricyclic antidepressants, ethanol, thiopental, and hydroxyzine. Plasma morphine concentrations rise when co-administered with cisapride.

Pregnancy Risk Factor B (D if used for prolonged periods or in high doses at term)

Monitoring Parameters Pain relief, respiratory and mental status, blood pressure

Patient Information Avoid alcohol, may cause drowsiness, impaired judgment or coordination; may be addicting if used for prolonged periods

Nursing Implications Do not crush controlled release drug product, observe patient for excessive sedation, apnea; implement safety measures, assist with ambulation; use preservative-free solutions for intrathecal or epidural use

Additional Information Stimulates prolactin release; addition of clonidine (75-150 mcg) increased duration of analgesia produced by epidural morphine (2 mg) for cesarean delivery

Specific References

Brunk SF and Delle M, "Morphine Metabolism in Man," *Clin Pharmacol Ther*, 1974, 16(1):51-7.

Capogna G, et al, "Addition of Clonidine to Epidural Morphine Enhances Postoperative Analgesia After Cesarean Delivery," *Reg Anaesth*, 1995, 29:57-61.

Duthie DJ and Nimmo WS, "Adverse Effects of Opioid Analgesic Drugs," *Br J Anaesth*, 1987, 59(1):61-77.

Gerber N and Apseloff G, "Death From a Morphine Infusion During a Sickle Cell Crisis," *J Pediatr*, 1993, 123(2):322-5.

Groudine SB, Cresanti-Daknis C, and Lumb PD, "Successful Treatment of a Massive Intrathecal Morphine Overdose," *Anesthesiology*, 1995, 82(1):292-5.

Henry J and Volans G, "ABC of Poisoning. Analgesics: Opioids," *Br Med J (Clin Res)*, 1984, 289(6450):990-3.

Holdsworth MT, Adams VR, Chavez CM, et al, "Continuous Midazolam Infusion for the Management of Morphine-Induced Myoclonus," *Ann Pharmacother*, 1995, 29:25-9.

Inturrisi CE, "Narcotic Drugs," *Med Clin North Am*, 1982, 66(5):1061-71.

June HL, Stitzer ML, and Cone E, "Acute Physical Dependence: Time Course and Relation to Human Plasma Morphine Concentrations," *Clin Pharmacol Ther*, 1995, 57:270-80.

Schug SA, Zech D, and Grond S, "Adverse Effects of Systemic Opioid Analgesics," *Drug Saf*, 1992, 7(3):200-13.

Motrin® *see* Ibuprofen *on page 418*

Motrin® IB [OTC] *see* Ibuprofen *on page 418*

Moxadil® *see* Amoxapine *on page 119*

Moxonidine

CAS Number 75438-57-2

Brand Names Cynt®; Physiotens®

Synonyms Monoxidin

Use Investigational: Hypertension

Mechanism of Action Structurally similar to clonidine, moxonidine is a centrally active imidazoline and alpha$_2$-receptor antagonist; also promotes naturesis

Adverse Reactions

Cardiovascular: Orthostatic hypotension, edema, facial flushing

Central nervous system: Drowsiness, dizziness, headache, insomnia, vertigo

Gastrointestinal: Dry mouth (20%), thirst

Renal: Diuresis

Signs & Symptoms of Acute Overdose Hypotension

Toxicodynamics/Kinetics

Absorption: 80% to 90%

Distribution: V_d: 1.8-3 L/kg

Protein binding: 6% to 8% (not changed in renal failure)

Metabolism: To 4,5-dehydromoxonidine (10% to 20%)

Bioavailability: 89%

Half-life: 2.6 hours (increased in renal insufficiency)

Peak serum levels: 30-180 minutes

Elimination: Renal

Usual Dosage Starting dose: 0.2-0.4 mg/day; may increase after 3 weeks to 0.2-0.4 mg twice daily; maximum single dose: 0.4 mg

Contraindications Bradycardia, sick sinus syndrome, atrioventricular block, arrhythmias, severe congestive heart failure, severe coronary ischemia, unstable an-

(Continued)

Moxonidine *(Continued)*

gina pectoris, renal insufficiency (creatinine >1.8 mg/dL), angioedema, intermittent claudication, Raynaud's disease, Parkinson's disease, epilepsy, glaucoma, depression, pregnancy, lactation, children <16 years of age

Warnings Use with caution in patients with mild to moderate renal impairment (serum creatinine: 1.2-1.8 mg/dL)

Reference Range Peak serum moxonidine levels after 0.2 mg oral and intravenous administration were 1495 pg/mL and 3965 pg/mL respectively

Overdosage Treatment

Decontamination: Lavage/activated charcoal with cathartic

Supportive therapy: For hypotension, intravenous saline administration with placement of patient in Trendelenburg position; vasopressors may also be utilized

Enhancement of elimination: Multiple dosing of activated charcoal may be effective

Drug Interactions Concomitant use with beta-adrenergic blocking agents; abrupt withdrawal of moxonidine may lead to rebound hypertension

Specific References

Chrisp P and Faulds D, "Moxonidine: A Review of Its Pharmacology and Therapeutic Use in Essential Hypetension," *Drugs*, 1992, 44(6):993-1012.

Kirch W, Hutt HJ, and Plaenitz V, "The Influence of Renal Function on Clinical Pharmacokinetics of Moxonidine," *Clin Pharmacokinet*, 1988, 15(4):245-53.

MS *see* Morphine Sulfate *on page 539*

MS Contin® *see* Morphine Sulfate *on page 539*

MSD-803 *replaced by* Lovastatin *on page 485*

MSIR® *see* Morphine Sulfate *on page 539*

MST® *see* Morphine Sulfate *on page 539*

MTX *see* Methotrexate *on page 515*

Multipax® *see* Hydroxyzine *on page 414*

Munobal® *see* Felodipine *on page 343*

Muro 128® Ophthalmic [OTC] *see* Sodium Chloride *on page 698*

Muscatrol® *see* Permethrin *on page 608*

Mustargen® *see* Mechlorethamine Hydrochloride *on page 492*

Mustine Hydrochloride *see* Mechlorethamine Hydrochloride *on page 492*

Myambutol® *see* Ethambutol Hydrochloride *on page 329*

Myapap® Drops [OTC] *see* Acetaminophen *on page 79*

Mycelex® *see* Clotrimazole *on page 234*

Mycelex®-G *see* Clotrimazole *on page 234*

Mycobutin® *see* Rifabutin *on page 681*

Mycostatin® *see* Nystatin *on page 574*

Mykinac® *see* Nystatin *on page 574*

Myleran® *see* Busulfan *on page 173*

Myocholine® *see* Bethanechol Chloride *on page 154*

Myochrysine® Injection *see* Gold Compounds *on page 386*

Myocord® *see* Atenolol *on page 137*

Myo Hermes® *see* Bethanechol Chloride *on page 154*

Myotonachol™ *see* Bethanechol Chloride *on page 154*

Myotonine® *see* Bethanechol Chloride *on page 154*

Mysoline® *see* Primidone *on page 641*

Mytussin® [OTC] *see* Guaifenesin *on page 390*

N-(1-Ethoxycarbonyl-3-Phenylpropyl)-L-Anal-L-Proline Hydrogen Maleate *see* Enalapril *on page 311*

Nabilone (na' bi lone)

CAS Number 51022-71-0

Brand Names Cesamet®

Use Treatment of nausea and vomiting associated with cancer chemotherapy

Mechanism of Action Nabilone is a synthetic cannabinoid utilized as an antiemetic drug in the control of nausea and vomiting in patients receiving cancer chemotherapy; like delta-9-tetrahydrocannabinol (the active principal of marijuana), nabilone is a dibenzo(b,d)pyrans; has central CNS antiemetic action thorough the dopaminergic pathway

Adverse Reactions

Cardiovascular: Hypotension (5%), hypertension, tachycardia

Central nervous system: Changes of mood, confusion, hallucinations, depression, dizziness, drowsiness, headache

Gastrointestinal: Loss of appetite or appetite (increased), dry mouth

Ocular: Blurred vision

Respiratory: Difficulty in breathing

Toxicodynamics/Kinetics

Absorption: Oral: Rapid (96%)

Distribution: Rapid and extensive to body tissues

Metabolism: Undergoes rapid metabolism to one or more active metabolites

Bioavailability: 95.8%

Half-life: 35 hours (with metabolites); 2 hours (parent compound)

Elimination: Feces (65%) and urine (20%)

Usual Dosage Oral:

Children >4 years:

<18 kg: 0.5 mg twice daily

18-30 kg: 1 mg twice daily

>30 kg: 1 mg 3 times/day

Adults: 1-2 mg twice daily beginning 1-3 hours before chemotherapy is administered and continuing around-the-clock until 1 dose after chemotherapy is completed; maximum daily dose: 6 mg divided in 3 doses

Contraindications Nausea and vomiting not secondary to cancer chemotherapy

Warnings Use with caution in the elderly, those with pre-existing CNS depression, or a history of mental illness

Dosage Forms Capsule: 1 mg

Reference Range Peak serum levels after a 2 mg dose: 10 ng/mL

Overdosage Treatment

Decontamination: Ingestion: Lavage/activated charcoal

Supportive therapy: Benzodiazepines for agitation; hypotension can be treated with Trendelenburg/crystalloid infusion; tachycardia can be treated with beta-blockers

Drug Interactions CNS depression is potentiated with ethanol

Pregnancy Risk Factor C

Patient Information May cause drowsiness, impair judgment, coordination; avoid alcohol and other CNS depressants; can cause disorientation

Nursing Implications May cause drowsiness, euphoria; institute safety precautions

Specific References

Einhorn L, "Nabilone: An Effective Antiemetic Agent in Patients Receiving Cancer Chemotherapy," *Cancer Treat Rev*, 1982, 9(Suppl B):55-61.

Ward A and Holmes B, "Nabilone: A Preliminary Review of Its Pharmacological Properties and Therapeutic Use," *Drugs*, 1985, 30(2):127-44.

Nabumetone (na byoo' me tone)

Related Information

Nonsteroidal Anti-Inflammatory Comparison *on page 1655*

CAS Number 42924-53-8

Brand Names Relafen®

Use Management of osteoarthritis and rheumatoid arthritis

Mechanism of Action Nabumetone is a nonacidic, nonsteroidal anti-inflammatory drug that is rapidly metabolized after absorption to a major active metabolite, 6-methoxy-2-naphthylacetic acid. As found with previous nonsteroidal anti-inflammatory drugs, nabumetone's active metabolite inhibits the cyclo-oxygenase enzyme which is indirectly responsible for the production of inflammation and pain during arthritis by way of enhancing the production of endoperoxides and prostaglandins E_2 and I_2 (prostacyclin). The active metabolite of nabumetone is felt to be the compound primarily responsible for therapeutic effect. Comparatively, the parent drug is a poor inhibitor of prostaglandin synthesis.

Adverse Reactions

Cardiovascular: Fluid retention, circulatory collapse

Central nervous system: Headache, dizziness, aseptic meningitis, psychosis, cognitive dysfunction, coma, seizures

Dermatologic: Rash, pruritus

Endocrine & metabolic: Hyperkalemia, anion gap metabolic acidosis

Gastrointestinal: Abdominal pain, nausea, vomiting, bleeding, ulceration, constipation, diarrhea, dyspepsia

Genitourinary: Albuminuria

Hematologic: Leukopenia, neutropenia, agranulocytosis, granulocytopenia; aplastic anemia (rare), platelet inhibition

Hepatic: Elevation of transaminases, fulminant hepatitis

Otic: Ototoxicity, tinnitus

(Continued)

Nabumetone *(Continued)*

Renal: Renal failure (acute), nephrotic syndrome, chronic renal failure
Respiratory: Wheezing, respiratory depression
Miscellaneous: Hypersensitivity

Signs & Symptoms of Acute Overdose Nausea, vomiting, wheezing, photosensitivity, nephrotic syndrome, flatulence, gastritis; stomatitis, cognitive dysfunction, ototoxicity; tinnitus, drowsiness; severe poisoning can manifest with coma, seizures, renal and or hepatic failure, hypotension, respiratory depression

Toxicodynamics/Kinetics

Distribution: Diffusion occurs readily into synovial fluid with peak concentrations in 4-12 hours
Protein binding: >99%
Metabolism: Prodrug being rapidly metabolized to an active metabolite (6-methoxy-2-naphthylacetic acid); extensive first-pass hepatic metabolism
Half-life, elimination: Major metabolite: 24 hours
Time to peak serum concentration: Metabolite: Oral: Within 3-6 hours
Elimination: 80% recovered in urine and 10% in feces, with very little excreted as unchanged compound

Usual Dosage Adults: Oral: 1000 mg/day; an additional 500-1000 mg may be needed in some patients to obtain more symptomatic relief; may be administered once or twice daily

Dosing adjustment in renal impairment: None necessary; however, adverse effects due to accumulation of inactive metabolites of nabumetone that are renally excreted have not been studied and should be considered

Contraindications Hypersensitivity to nabumetone; should not be administered to patients with active peptic ulceration and those with severe hepatic impairment or in patients in whom nabumetone, aspirin, or other NSAIDs have induced asthma, rash, or other allergic-type reactions; fatal asthmatic reactions have occurred following NSAID administration

Warnings Elderly patients may sometimes require lower doses; patients with impaired renal function may need a dose reduction; use with caution in patients with severe hepatic impairment

Dosage Forms Tablet: 500 mg, 750 mg

Overdosage Treatment

Decontamination: Ipecac or lavage/activated charcoal with cathartic
Supportive therapy: Hypotension/dehydration can be managed with intravenous fluid therapy; acidosis should be treated with bicarbonates, seizures with benzodiazepines; antacids, blood products are indicated, as appropriate, for hemorrhage
Enhancement of elimination: Dialysis or perfusion is indicated for secondary complications, acidosis, or renal failure and not toxin removal alone; multiple dosing of activated charcoal may be effective

Drug Interactions Aspirin decreases serum concentrations probably by protein-binding displacement; there is an increased bleeding potential with concomitant warfarin therapy; may increase lithium and methotrexate concentrations by decreasing renal clearance; may decrease diuretic and hypotensive effects of thiazides, loop diuretics, ACE inhibitors, and beta-blockers; may increase nephrotoxicity of cyclosporine

Pregnancy Risk Factor C

Specific References

Bernhard GC, "Worldwide Safety Experience With Nabumetone," *J Rheumatol*, 1992, 19(Suppl 36):48-57.
Brier ME, Sloan RS, and Aronoff GR, "Population Pharmacokinetics of the Active Metabolite of Nabumetone in Renal Dysfunction," *Clin Pharmacol Ther*, 1995, 57:622-7.
Court H and Volans GN, "Poisoning After Overdose With Nonsteroidal Anti-inflammatory Drugs," *Adverse Drug React Acute Poisoning Rev*, 1984, 3(1):1-21.
Hoppmann RA, Peden JG, and Ober SK, "Central Nervous System Side Effects of Nonsteroidal Anti-inflammatory Drugs. Aseptic Meningitis, Psychosis, and Cognitive Dysfunction," *Arch Intern Med*, 1991, 151(7):1309-13.
Hyneck ML, "An Overview of the Clinical Pharmacokinetics of Nabumetone," *J Rheumatol*, 1992, 19(Suppl 36):20-4.
Jackson RE, Mitchell FN, and Brindley DA, "Safety Evaluation of Nabumetone in United States Clinical Trials," *Am J Med*, 1987, 83(4B):115-20.
Jenner PN, "A 12-Month Postmarketing Surveillance Study of Nabumetone: A Preliminary Report," *Drugs*, 1990, 40(Suppl 5):80-6.
Smolinske SC, Hall AH, Vandenberg SA, et al, "Toxic Effects of Nonsteroid Anti-inflammatory Drugs in Overdose. An Overview of Recent Evidence on Clinical Effects and Dose-Response Relationships," *Drug Saf*, 1990, 5(4):252-74.
Vale JA and Meredith TJ, "Acute Poisoning Due to Nonsteroidal Anti-inflammatory Drugs," *Med Toxicol*, 1986, 1(1):12-31.
Verbeeck RK, "Pharmacokinetic Drug Interactions With Nonsteroidal Anti-inflammatory Drugs," *Clin Pharmacokinet*, 1990, 19(1):44-66.

NaCl *see* Sodium Chloride *on page 698*

Nadolol (nay doe' lole)

Related Information

Beta-Blockers Comparison *on page 1644-1645*

CAS Number 42200-33-9

Brand Names Apo-Nadol®; Corgard®; Solgol®

Use Treatment of hypertension and angina pectoris; prevention of myocardial infarction; prophylaxis of migraine headaches

Mechanism of Action Competitively blocks response to beta-adrenergic stimulation; hydrophilic

Adverse Reactions

Cardiovascular: Persistent bradycardia, hypotension (orthostatic), Raynaud's syndrome, congestive heart failure, edema

Central nervous system: Fatigue, dizziness

Dermatological: Rash, alopecia

Gastrointestinal: Gastrointestinal discomfort, flatulence, nausea, diarrhea, pancreatitis

Genitourinary: Impotence

Respiratory: Wheezing, hypersensitivity, pneumonitis with elevated sedimentation rate, dyspnea, cough

Signs & Symptoms of Acute Overdose Hyperglycemia, ataxia, hyperkalemia, impotence

Toxicodynamics/Kinetics

Duration of effect: 24 hours

Absorption: Oral: 30% to 40%

Distribution: V_d: 2.1 L/kg; concentration in human breast milk is 4.6 times higher than serum

Protein binding: 25% to 28%

Half-life: Adults: 10-12 hours; increased half-life with decreased renal function

Time to peak serum concentration: Within 2-4 hours, persisting for 17-24 hours

Elimination: Renal 72%, feces 18%; clearance: 0.92 mL/min/kg

Usual Dosage Adults: Oral: Initial: 40 mg once daily; increase by 40-80 mg increments gradually at 3- to 7-day intervals; usual dosage: 40-80 mg/day; may need up to 240-320 mg/day; doses as high as 640 mg/day have been used

Dosing adjustment in renal impairment:

Cl_{cr} 10-50 mL/minute: Administer 50% of normal dose

Cl_{cr} <10 mL/minute: Administer 25% of normal dose

Contraindications Uncompensated congestive heart failure, cardiogenic shock, bradycardia or heart block

Warnings Increase dosing interval in patients with renal dysfunction; abrupt withdrawal of beta-blockers may result in an exaggerated cardiac beta-adrenergic responsiveness; symptomatology has included reports of tachycardia, hypertension, ischemia, angina, myocardial infarction, and sudden death; it is recommended that patients be tapered gradually off of beta-blockers over a period of 1-2 weeks rather than via abrupt discontinuation; use with caution in patients with bronchial asthma, wheezings, CHF, or diabetes mellitus

Dosage Forms Tablet: 20 mg, 40 mg, 80 mg, 120 mg, 160 mg

Reference Range Peak serum nadolol concentration of 5 ng/mL after a 2 mg dose; peak steady-state nadolol level after a 55 mg daily dose: 62 ng/mL

Overdosage Treatment

Decontamination: Lavage/activated charcoal with cathartic; do not use ipecac

Supportive therapy: Glucagon (50-150 mcg/kg followed by continuous drip of 1-5 mg/hour) for positive chronotropic effect; atropine/isoproterenol can be utilized to increase heart rate; calcium chloride may also be effective; do **not** use epinephrine

Enhancement of elimination: Hemodialysis may be useful; moderately dialyzable (20% to 50%)

Drug Interactions Increased effect with diuretics, other antihypertensives, verapamil

Pregnancy Risk Factor C

Monitoring Parameters Blood pressure, heart rate, fluid I&O, weight

Patient Information Adhere to dosage regimen; watch for hypotension (orthostatic); abrupt withdrawal of the drug should be avoided; take at the same time each day; may mask symptoms of diabetes; sweating will continue

Nursing Implications Patient's therapeutic response may be evaluated by looking at blood pressure, apical and radial pulses

Specific References

Hitzenberger G, "Initial Experience With a New Long-Acting Beta-Blocker, Nadolol, In Hypertensive Patients," *J Int Med Res*, 1979, 7(1):33-8.

Levy MB, Fink JN, and Guzzetta PA, "Nadolol and Hypersensitivity Pneumonitis," *Ann Intern Med*, 1986, 105(5):806-7.

Nalbuphine Hydrochloride (nal' byoo feen)

CAS Number 20594-83-6; 23277-43-2

Brand Names Nubain®

Use Relief of moderate to severe pain

Mechanism of Action Binds to opiate receptors in the CNS, causing inhibition of ascending pain pathways, altering the perception of and response to pain; produces generalized CNS depression. A 14-hydroxymorphine derivative. A kappa-receptor opioid agonist but a mu-receptor antagonist.

Adverse Reactions

Cardiovascular: Hypotension, flushing, hypertension, tachycardia

Central nervous system: CNS depression, dizziness, headache, asthenia, drowsiness, anxiety, mental depression, hallucinations, confusion, nervousness, restlessness, night terrors, insomnia, paradoxical CNS stimulation

Dermatologic: Urticaria, skin rash

Gastrointestinal: Nausea, vomiting, anorexia, dry mouth

Genitourinary: Ureteral spasm, decreased urination

Ocular: Blurred vision

Respiratory: Apnea, respiratory depression, dyspnea, pulmonary edema

Miscellaneous: Narcotic withdrawal, pain at injection site, histamine release, biliary spasm, toxic megacolon, sweating

Signs & Symptoms of Acute Overdose Coma, drowsiness, dysphoria, dyspepsia, depression, night terrors, insomnia, hypotension, miosis, clammy skin

Toxicodynamics/Kinetics

Peak effect:
- I.M.: 30 minutes
- I.V.: 1-3 minutes

Distribution: V_d: 2.9-14.4 L/kg

Metabolism: In the liver, no active metabolites

Bioavailability: Oral: 12%

Half-life:
- Children: 1 hour
- Adults: 2 hours
- Elderly: 2.3 hours

Time to peak serum concentration:
- I.M.: 30 minutes
- I.V.: 1-3 minutes

Elimination: Metabolites excreted primarily in feces (via bile) and in urine (~7%)

Usual Dosage I.M., I.V., S.C.:

Children 10 months to 14 years: Premedication: 0.2 mg/kg; maximum: 20 mg/dose

Adults: 10 mg/70 kg every 3-6 hours; maximum single dose: 20 mg; maximum daily dose: 160 mg

Dosing adjustment/comments in hepatic impairment: Use with caution and reduce dose

Contraindications Hypersensitivity to nalbuphine or any component

Warnings Use with caution in patients with recent myocardial infarction, biliary tract surgery, or sulfite sensitivity; may produce apnea; use with caution in women delivering premature infants; use with caution in patients with a history of drug dependence, head trauma or increased intracranial pressure, decreased hepatic or renal function, or pregnancy; some products may contain sulfites

Dosage Forms Injection: 10 mg/mL (1 mL, 10 mL); 20 mg/mL (1 mL, 10 mL)

Stability Incompatible with nafcillin, diazepam, or pentobarbital

Overdosage Treatment Supportive therapy: Naloxone hydrochloride (0.4-2 mg I.V., S.C., or through an endotracheal tube); a continuous infusion (at ⅔ the response dose/hour) may be required

Antidote(s)

Naloxone Hydrochloride *on page 1447*

Drug Interactions Increased toxicity: Barbiturate anesthetics causes increased CNS depression

Pregnancy Risk Factor B (D if used for prolonged periods or in high doses at term)

Pregnancy Implications May cause neonatal bradycardia or respiratory depression when used during labor.

Monitoring Parameters Relief of pain, respiratory and mental status, blood pressure

Patient Information Avoid alcohol, may cause drowsiness, impaired judgment or coordination; may be addicting if used for prolonged periods; will cause withdrawal in patients currently dependent on narcotics

Nursing Implications Observe patient for excessive sedation, apnea; implement safety measures, assist with ambulation; observe for narcotic withdrawal

Additional Information Little abuse potential

Specific References

Errick JK and Heel RC, "Nalbuphine: A Preliminary Review of Its Pharmacological Properties and Therapeutic Efficacy," *Drugs*, 1983, 26(3):191-211.

Leikin JB, Ehrenpreis ED, Barkin RL, et al, "Nalbuphine vs Meperidine in Sickle Cell Anemia," *DICP*, 1990, 24(7-8):781-2.

Yoo Y, Chung H, Kim I, et al, "Determination of Nalbuphine in Drug Abusers' Urine," *J Anal Toxicol*, 1995, 19:120-3.

Naldecon® Senior EX [OTC] *see* Guaifenesin *on page 390*

Nalfon® *see* Fenoprofen Calcium *on page 345*

Nalidixic Acid (nal i dix' ik)

Related Information

Therapeutic Drugs Associated With Hallucinations *on page 1558-1559*

CAS Number 389-08-2

Brand Names Betaxina®; Faril®; Nalissina®; NegGram®; Nogram®; Uriben®; Urogram®; Uropan®

Synonyms Nalidixinic Acid

Use Urinary tract infections

Mechanism of Action Inhibits DNA polymerization in late stages of chromosomal replication; direct antagonist of gabaergic neurotransmission

Adverse Reactions

Central nervous system: Fever, chills, malaise, drowsiness, dizziness, confusion, toxic psychosis, seizures, headache, visual hallucinations, intracranial pressure (increased)

Dermatologic: Rash, bullous eruptions, pruritus, photosensitivity reactions

Endocrine & metabolic: Metabolic acidosis

Gastrointestinal: Nausea, vomiting

Hematologic: Leukopenia, thrombocytopenia, hemolytic anemia

Hepatic: Hepatotoxicity (cholestatic)

Ocular: Visual disturbances, nystagmus

Miscellaneous: Feces discoloration (greenish gray), feces discoloration (white/speckling), porphyrinogenic

Signs & Symptoms of Acute Overdose Nausea, vomiting, pseudotumor cerebri, photosensitivity, erythema multiforme, eosinophilia, hyperthermia, dementia, thrombocytopenia, systemic lupus erythematosus (SLE), diplopia, dermatitis, coma, photophobia, toxic psychosis, seizures, intracranial pressure (increased), metabolic acidosis, leukopenia, neutropenia, agranulocytosis, granulocytopenia; vision color changes (blue tinge), vision color changes (violet tinge), vision color changes (yellow tinge); hyperglycemia

Toxicodynamics/Kinetics

Absorption: Rapid and almost completely from gastrointestinal tract

Distribution: Achieves significant antibacterial concentrations only in the urinary tract; small amounts appear in feces

Protein binding: 90%

Metabolism: Partly in the liver

Bioavailability: ~96%

Half-life: 6-7 hours (increases significantly with renal impairment)

Time to peak serum concentration: Oral: Within 1-2 hours

Elimination: Excreted in urine as unchanged drug and 80% as metabolites

Usual Dosage Oral:

Children 3 months to 12 years: 55 mg/kg/day divided every 6 hours; suppressive therapy is 33 mg/kg/day divided every 6 hours

Adults: 1 g 4 times/day for 2 weeks; then suppressive therapy of 500 mg 4 times/day

Dosing comments in renal impairment: Cl_{cr} <50 mL/minute: Avoid use

Contraindications History of convulsive disorders, hypersensitivity to nalidixic acid or any component; infants <3 months of age

Warnings Has been shown to cause cartilage degeneration in immature animals; usefulness may be limited by the emergence of bacterial resistance; use with caution in patients with impaired hepatic or renal function and prepubertal children; due to antagonism, do not use with nitrofurantoin

Dosage Forms

Suspension, oral (raspberry flavor): 250 mg/5 mL (473 mL)

Tablet: 250 mg, 500 mg, 1 g

Reference Range Peak plasma level of 20-50 μg/mL achieved 2 hours after oral dose of 1 g; urinary concentration after 1 g oral dose can range from 25-250 μg/mL

Overdosage Treatment

Decontamination: Lavage/activated charcoal with cathartic

Supportive therapy: Diazepam/lorazepam for seizures

Test Interactions False-positive urine glucose with Clinitest®, false increase in urinary VMA

Drug Interactions Warfarin (increased anticoagulant effect due to displacement from albumin-binding sites), antacids (decreases nalidixic acid absorption); re-

(Continued)

Nalidixic Acid *(Continued)*

duced urinary excretion by probenecid; gastrointestinal toxicity when used with melphalan

Pregnancy Risk Factor B

Pregnancy Implications Crosses the placenta; appears in breast milk with one case report of a neonate with G-6-PD deficiency developing hemolytic anemia

Patient Information Avoid undue exposure to direct sunlight; take 1 hour before meals

Specific References

Belton EM and Jones RV, "Haemolytic Anaemia Due to Nalidixic Acid," *Lancet*, 1965, 2(7414):691.

Leslie PJ, Cregeen RJ, and Proudfoot AT, et al, "Lactic Acidosis, Hyperglycaemia and Convulsions Following Nalidixic Acid Overdosage," *Hum Toxicol*, 1984, 3(3):249-53.

Nalidixinic Acid *see* Nalidixic Acid *on previous page*

Nalissina® *see* Nalidixic Acid *on previous page*

Nalorex® *see* Naltrexone Hydrochloride *on this page*

Naltrexone Hydrochloride (nal trex' one)

CAS Number 16590-41-3; 16676-29-2

Brand Names Antaxone®; Celupan®; Nalorex®; ReVia®; Trexan™

Use Adjunct to the maintenance of an opioid-free state in detoxified individual; approved for use in the treatment of ethanol abuse

Mechanism of Action Naltrexone is a cyclopropyl derivative of oxymorphone similar in structure to naloxone and nalorphine (a morphine derivative); it acts as a competitive antagonist at opioid receptor sites

Adverse Reactions

Cardiovascular: Hypertension, tachycardia

Central nervous system: Insomnia, irritability, anxiety, dysphoria, dizziness, headache

Dermatologic: Rash, acne, pruritus, alopecia, oily skin

Gastrointestinal: Nausea, vomiting, anorexia

Hematologic: Thrombocytopenia, agranulocytosis, hemolysis

Hepatic: Hepatitis

Neuromuscular & skeletal: Myalgia

Ocular: Blurred vision

Otic: Tinnitus

Miscellaneous: Narcotic withdrawal

Signs & Symptoms of Acute Overdose Hepatocellular damage, dysphoria, insomnia, leukopenia; neutropenia; agranulocytosis; granulocytopenia

Toxicodynamics/Kinetics

Duration of action:

- 50 mg: 24 hours
- 100 mg: 48 hours
- 150 mg: 72 hours

Absorption: Oral: Almost completely

Distribution: V_d: 3 L/kg; distributed widely throughout the body but considerable interindividual variation exists

Protein binding: 21%

Metabolism: Undergoes extensive first-pass metabolism to 6-β-naltrexol

Half-life: 4 hours; 6-β-naltrexol: 13 hours

Time to peak serum concentration: Within 60 minutes

Elimination: Principally in urine as metabolites and unchanged drug

Usual Dosage Do not give until patient is opioid-free for 7-10 days as required by urine analysis

Adults: Oral: 25 mg; if no withdrawal signs within 1 hour give another 25 mg; maintenance regimen is flexible, variable, and individualized (50 mg/day to 100-150 mg 3 times/week)

Alcoholism: 50 mg once day

Contraindications Acute hepatitis, liver failure, known hypersensitivity to naltrexone

Warnings Dose-related hepatocellular injury is possible; the margin of separation between the apparent safe and hepatotoxic doses appear to be only fivefold or less

Dosage Forms Tablet: 50 mg

Reference Range Peak plasma naltrexone level after a 100 mg oral dose: 44 μg/L

Overdosage Treatment

Decontamination: Ipecac or lavage/activated charcoal with cathartic

Supportive therapy: Dysmorphic/irritability can be treated by titrating with morphine

Test Interactions Elevates gonadotropin, serum cortisol

Diagnostic Tests/Procedures
Liver Profile *on page 1286*

Pregnancy Risk Factor C

Monitoring Parameters Liver function tests

Patient Information Will cause narcotic withdrawal; serious overdose can occur after attempts to overcome the blocking effect of naltrexone

Nursing Implications Monitor for narcotic withdrawal

Additional Information Up to 800 mg/day has been tolerated in adults without an adverse effect

Specific References

Kleber HD, "Naltrexone," *J Subst Abuse Treat*, 1985, 2(2):117-22.
Mitchell JE, "Naltrexone and Hepatotoxicity," *Lancet*, 1986, 1(8491):1215.

Nansius® *see* Clorazepate Dipotassium *on page 232*

Napamide® *see* Disopyramide Phosphate *on page 294*

Na-PAS® *see* Para-Aminosalicylate Sodium *on page 592*

Naprosyn® *see* Naproxen *on this page*

Naproxen (na prox' en)

Related Information
Nonsteroidal Anti-Inflammatory Comparison *on page 1655*

CAS Number 222-53-1; 26159-34-2

Brand Names Aleve® [OTC]; Anaprox®; Naprosyn®

Synonyms Naproxen Sodium

Use Management of inflammatory disease and rheumatoid disorders (including juvenile rheumatoid arthritis); acute gout; mild to moderate pain; dysmenorrhea; fever; menorrhagia

Mechanism of Action Inhibits prostaglandin synthesis by decreasing the activity of the enzyme, cyclo-oxygenase, which results in decreased formation of prostaglandin precursors

Adverse Reactions

Cardiovascular: Fluid retention, circulatory collapse
Central nervous system: Headache, aseptic meningitis, psychosis, cognitive dysfunction, dizziness, coma, seizures
Dermatologic: Rash, pruritus, increased incidence of shallow, facial scars (relative risk is 6) in children
Endocrine & metabolic: Hyperkalemia, anion gap metabolic acidosis
Gastrointestinal: Abdominal pain, nausea, vomiting, bleeding, ulceration, constipation, diarrhea, dyspepsia
Genitourinary: Albuminuria
Hematologic: Leukopenia, neutropenia, agranulocytosis, granulocytopenia; aplastic anemia (rare), platelet inhibition, eosinophilia
Hepatic: Elevation of transaminases, fulminant hepatitis
Otic: Ototoxicity, tinnitus
Renal: Renal failure (acute), nephrotic syndrome, chronic renal failure
Respiratory: Wheezing, pulmonary infiltrate, respiratory depression
Miscellaneous: Hypersensitivity

Signs & Symptoms of Acute Overdose Nausea, vomiting, wheezing, purpura, photosensitivity, nephrotic syndrome, night terrors, depression, impotence, gastrointestinal bleeding, stomatitis, intraocular pressure (increased), lightheadedness, gastritis; colitis, meningitis, cognitive dysfunction, gout, lichenoid eruptions, ejaculatory disturbances, ototoxicity; coagulopathy, systemic lupus erythematosus (SLE), tinnitus, drowsiness; severe poisoning can manifest with coma, seizures, renal and or hepatic failure, hypotension, respiratory depression, metabolic acidosis

Toxicodynamics/Kinetics

Onset of action: 1 hour
Duration: Up to 7 hours
Absorption: ~100% from gastrointestinal tract
Distribution: V_d: 0.1-0.3 L/kg
Protein binding: >99%; renal failure: 71%
Metabolism: Hepatic
Half-life: 9-20 hours
Time to peak serum concentration: Within 1-2 hours
Elimination: Renal, 95%

Usual Dosage Oral (as naproxen):

Children >2 years:
Fever: 2.5-10 mg/kg/dose; maximum: 10 mg/kg/day
Juvenile arthritis: 10 mg/kg/day in 2 divided doses

Adults:
Rheumatoid arthritis, osteoarthritis, and ankylosing spondylitis: 500-1000 mg/day in 2 divided doses; may increase to 1.5 g/day of naproxen base for limited time period

(Continued)

Naproxen *(Continued)*

Mild to moderate pain or dysmenorrhea: Initial: 500 mg, then 250 mg every 6-8 hours; maximum: 1250 mg/day naproxen base

Dosing adjustment in hepatic impairment: Reduce dose to 50%

Contraindications Hypersensitivity to naproxen, aspirin, or other nonsteroidal anti-inflammatory drugs (NSAIDs)

Warnings Use with caution in patients with gastrointestinal disease, cardiac disease, renal or hepatic impairment, and patients receiving anticoagulants

Dosage Forms

Suspension, oral (Naprosyn®): 125 mg/5 mL (480 mL)

Tablet, as sodium (Anaprox®): 275 mg (250 mg base); 550 mg (500 mg base)

Tablet:

Aleve® [OTC]: 200 mg

Naprosyn®: 250 mg, 375 mg, 500 mg

Reference Range Trough concentrations of >50 μg/L (217 μmol/L) are therapeutic in patients with rheumatoid arthritis; serum naproxen level of 414 mg/L associated with oral ingestion of 25 g and mild toxicity

Overdosage Treatment

Decontamination: Ipecac or lavage/activated charcoal with cathartic

Supportive therapy: Hypotension/dehydration can be managed with intravenous fluid therapy; acidosis should be treated with bicarbonates, seizures with benzodiazepines; antacids, blood products are indicated, as appropriate, for hemorrhage

Enhancement of elimination: Dialysis or perfusion is indicated for secondary complications, acidosis, or renal failure and not toxin removal alone; multiple dosing of activated charcoal may be effective

Test Interactions Increases chloride (S), sodium (S)

Drug Interactions Aspirin decreases serum concentrations probably by protein-binding displacement; there is an increased bleeding potential with concomitant warfarin therapy; may increase lithium and methotrexate concentrations by decreasing renal clearance; may decrease diuretic and hypotensive effects of thiazides, loop diuretics, ACE inhibitors, and beta-blockers; may increase nephrotoxicity of cyclosporine

Pregnancy Risk Factor B (D if used in the 3rd trimester or near delivery)

Pregnancy Implications Crosses the placenta; distributed into breast milk; maternal overdosage has lead to neonatal distress; drowsiness, hypotonia, edema

Monitoring Parameters Occult blood loss, periodic liver function test, hemoglobin, CBC, BUN, serum creatinine

Nursing Implications Administer with food, milk, or antacids to decrease gastrointestinal adverse effects

Additional Information Naproxen: Naprosyn® naproxen sodium: Anaprox®; 275 mg of Anaprox® equivalent to 250 mg of Naprosyn®; Aleve® [OTC] available in 1994

Specific References

Alun-Jones E and Williams J, "Hyponatremia and Fluid Retention in a Neonate Associated With Maternal Naproxen Overdosage," *J Toxicol Clin Toxicol*, 1986, 24(3):257-60.

Court H and Volans GN, "Poisoning After Overdose With Nonsteroidal Anti-inflammatory Drugs," *Adverse Drug React Acute Poisoning Rev*, 1984, 3(1):1-21.

Fredell EW and Strand LJ, "Naproxen Overdose," *JAMA*, 1977, 238(9):938.

Hoppmann RA, Peden JG, and Ober SK, "Central Nervous System Side Effects of Nonsteroidal Anti-inflammatory Drugs. Aseptic Meningitis, Psychosis, and Cognitive Dysfunction," *Arch Intern Med*, 1991, 151(7):1309-13.

Kulling EJ, Beckman EA, and Skagius AS, "Renal Impairment After Acute Diclofenac, Naproxen, and Sulindac Overdoses," *J Toxicol Clin Toxicol*, 1995, 33(2):173-7.

Martinez R, Smith DW, and Frankel LR, "Severe Metabolic Acidosis After Acute Naproxen Sodium Ingestion," *Ann Emerg Med*, 1989, 18(10):1102-4.

Nader DA and Schillaci RF, "Pulmonary Infiltrates With Eosinophilia Due to Naproxen," *Chest*, 1983, 83(2):280-2.

Smolinske SC, Hall AH, Vandenberg SA, et al, "Toxic Effects of Nonsteroid Anti-inflammatory Drugs in Overdose. An Overview of Recent Evidence on Clinical Effects and Dose-Response Relationships," *Drug Saf*, 1990, 5(4):252-74.

Vale JA and Meredith TJ, "Acute Poisoning Due to Nonsteroidal Anti-inflammatory Drugs," *Med Toxicol*, 1986, 1(1):12-31.

Verbeeck RK, "Pharmacokinetic Drug Interactions With Nonsteroidal Anti-inflammatory Drugs," *Clin Pharmacokinet*, 1990, 19(1):44-66.

Wallace CA, Farrow D, and Sherry DD, "Increased Risk of Facial Scars in Children Taking Nonsteroidal Anti-inflammatory Drugs," *J Pediatr*, 1994, 125(5 Pt 1):819-22.

Naproxen Sodium *see* Naproxen *on previous page*

Narcarcin® *see* Benzbromarone *on page 148*

Narcozep® *see* Flunitrazepam *on page 354*

Nardelzine® *see* Phenelzine Sulfate *on page 612*

Nardil® *see* Phenelzine Sulfate *on page 612*

Narilet® *see* Ipratropium Bromide *on page 438*

Nasahist B® *see* Brompheniramine Maleate *on page 165*

Nasalcrom® Nasal Solution *see* Cromolyn Sodium *on page 245*

Nasivin® *see* Oxymetazoline Hydrochloride *on page 586*

Natel® *see* Urokinase *on page 779*

Nativelle® *see* Digitoxin *on page 283*

Natulan® *see* Procarbazine Hydrochloride *on page 645*

Natulanar® *see* Procarbazine Hydrochloride *on page 645*

Natyl® *see* Dipyridamole *on page 292*

Navane® *see* Thiothixene *on page 747*

Navelbine® *see* Vinorelbine Ditartrate *on page 794*

NC-123 *replaced by* Mesoridazine Besylate *on page 505*

2'NDG *see* Ganciclovir *on page 377*

ND-Stat® *see* Brompheniramine Maleate *on page 165*

Nebivolol (ne biv' oh lole)

CAS Number 99200-09-6

Use Investigational; Hypertension

Mechanism of Action Selective $beta_1$-adrenoceptor antagonist which is mostly due to the d-isomer; L-isomer may improve left ventricular function

Adverse Reactions

Cardiovascular: Bradycardia, palpitations
Central nervous system: Headache, dizziness, somnolence
Gastrointestinal: Nausea
Genitourinary: Impotence
Neuromuscular & skeletal: Myalgia
Miscellaneous: Hypertriglycic eridemia (doses >30 mg)

Signs & Symptoms of Acute Overdose Hypotension, impotence

Toxicodynamics/Kinetics

Distribution: V_d: 10.1-39.4 L/kg
Protein binding: 98%
Metabolism: Hepatic (aromatic hydroxylation) to nebivolol glucuronide
Bioavailability: 12% (fast metabolizers); 96% (slow metabolizers)
Half-life: 8 hours (27 hours in slow metabolizers)

Usual Dosage Oral: 5 mg once daily

Contraindications Hypersensitivity to nebivolol, second or third degree heart block, bradycardia

Reference Range Peak plasma level of 1 μg/L in fast metabolizers and ~3 μg/L in slow metabolizers following a 5 mg oral dose; no change in plasma catecholamine levels (either at rest or during exercise)

Overdosage Treatment

Decontamination: Lavage/activated charcoal with cathartic; do not use ipecac
Supportive therapy: Glucagon (50-150 mcg/kg followed by continuous drip of 1-5 mg/hour) for positive chronotropic effect; atropine/isoproterenol can be utilized to increase heart rate; calcium chloride may also be effective
Enhancement of elimination: Multiple dosing of activated charcoal is not likely to be of benefit; dialysis is not useful; not dialyzable (0% to 5%)

Antidote(s)

Glucagon *on page 1431*

Specific References

Fitzgerald JD, "First International Nebivolol Investigators' Meeting," *Drug Investigation*, 1991, 3(Suppl 1):1-203.

Nebril® *see* Desipramine Hydrochloride *on page 263*

NebuPent™ *see* Pentamidine Isethionate *on page 601*

Nedocromil Sodium (ne doe kroe' mil)

CAS Number 69049-73-6; 69049-74-7; 101626-68-0

Brand Names Tilade® Inhalation Aerosol

Synonyms FPL-59002KP

Use Investigational: Adjunct in prophylaxis of asthma; seasonal allergic rhinitis; no benefit in acute asthmatic attacks

Mechanism of Action Disodium salt of a pyranoquinolone dicarboxylic acid which inhibits mediator release from inflammatory cells; can decrease bronchial hyper-reactivity; greater effect in inhibiting histamine release than cromolyn

Adverse Reactions

Cardiovascular: Chest pain

(Continued)

Nedocromil Sodium *(Continued)*

Central nervous system: Dizziness, headache, fatigue
Gastrointestinal: Nausea, vomiting, dry mouth, diarrhea, unpleasant taste
Respiratory: Coughing, pharyngitis, rhinitis, bronchitis, dyspnea, bronchospasm

Signs & Symptoms of Acute Overdose Bitter taste (13%), bronchospasm, headache, nausea, vomiting, dizziness

Toxicodynamics/Kinetics

Absorption:
- Oral: 2% to 3%
- Inhalation: 5% to 6%

Half-life: 2 hours
Elimination: Bile and urine

Usual Dosage Adults: Metered dose inhaler: 4 mg twice daily, up to 4 times/day

Contraindications Hypersensitivity to nedocromil or other ingredients in the preparation

Warnings Caution should be used when withdrawing the drug or tapering the dose as symptoms may reoccur; use with caution in patients with a history of cardiac arrhythmia; use with caution in patients with renal and hepatic impairment

Dosage Forms Aerosol: 1.75 mg/activation (16.2 g/canister)

Reference Range Peak plasma level after a 4 mg dose (inhalation): ~ 3.3 ng/mL in healthy patients and 2.8 ng/mL in asthmatic patients; levels not relatable to effect

Overdosage Treatment

Decontamination: Oral: Lavage/activated charcoal with cathartic
Supportive therapy: Treat inhalation exposure with 100% humidified oxygen; treat anaphylaxis with epinephrine and corticosteroids; albuterol can be given for bronchospasm

Pregnancy Risk Factor B

Monitoring Parameters Use of beta agonists (oral or inhaled), peak expiratory flow rates, frequency and severity of wheezing, coughing, chest tightness, shortness of breath or dyspnea

Additional Information Each canister provides about 112 inhalations; 1.75 g/actuation

Specific References

Gonzalez JP and Brogden RN, "Nedocromil Sodium. A Preliminary Review of its Pharmacodynamic and Pharmacokinetic Properties and Therapeutic Efficacy in the Treatment of Reversible Obstructive Airways Disease," *Drugs*, 1987, 34(5):560-77.

Nefazodone

Brand Names Serzone®

Use Antidepressant; treatment of major depression in adults

Mechanism of Action Chemically related to trazodone, 5-HT_2 receptor antagonist, also alpha$_1$-adrenergic antagonist; acts to inhibit neuronal uptake of serotonin and norepinephrine

Adverse Reactions

Cardiovascular: Postural hypotension, bradycardia
Central nervous system: Convulsions, lethargy, dizziness, confusion, asthenia, somnolence, lightheadedness, insomnia
Gastrointestinal: Dry mouth, nausea, constipation
Ocular: Visual changes, blurred vision, amblyopia

Signs & Symptoms of Acute Overdose Nausea, vomiting, lethargy

Toxicodynamics/Kinetics

Absorption: Rapid and complete
Protein binding: 99%
Distribution: V_d: 0.2-1 L/kg
Metabolism: Undergoes extensive first-pass metabolism; saturable and has active metabolite; metabolite also undergoes saturable metabolism; aliphatic hydroxylation in the liver to hydroxynefazodone (HO-NEF) and triazoledione; meta-chlorophenzyl piperazine is also produced
Bioavailability: 20%
Half-life:
- Nefazodone: 2-4 hours
- HO-NEF: 1.5-4 hours
- Triazoledione: 18 hours
- Meta-chlorohenylpiperazine: 4-8 hours

Peak plasma concentrations: Occur in 1 hour
Elimination: Renal (55%), feces (20% to 30%)

Usual Dosage Adults: 200 mg/day in 2 divided doses; can increase in increments of 100-200 mg/day at intervals no less than one week; usual effective daily dose: 300-600 mg; maximum daily dose: 600 mg; starting dose for elderly patients: 100 mg/day

Contraindications Hypersensitivity to nefazodone or other phenylpiperazine antidepressant or coadministration with terfenadine or astemizole

Warnings Coadministration with MAO inhibitors, alprazolam, triazolam (or other triazolobenzodiazepines); history of seizure disorders or cardiovascular disease

Dosage Forms Tablet: 100 mg, 150 mg, 200 mg, 250 mg

Reference Range After a 150 mg oral dose, peak plasma nefazodone, HO-NEF, and meta-chlorophenylpiperazine levels were 1200 ng/mL, 400 ng/mL, and 25 ng/mL respectively

TLC detection limit: 1 μg/mL

HPLC detection limit: 1-10 ng/mL

Overdosage Treatment

Decontamination (adults with ingestions >3 g): Lavage/activated charcoal with cathartic

Supportive therapy: Following initiation of essential overdose management, toxic symptoms should be treated. Ventricular arrhythmias often respond to phenytoin 15-20 mg/kg (adults) with concurrent systemic alkalinization (sodium bicarbonate 0.5-2 mEq/kg I.V.). Arrhythmias unresponsive to this therapy may respond to lidocaine 1 mg/kg I.V. followed by a titrated infusion. Treat bradycardia with atropine; benztropine may be useful to treat priapism. Seizures usually respond to lorazepam or diazepam I.V. boluses (5-10 mg for adults up to 30 mg or 0.25-0.4 mg/kg/dose for children up to 10 mg/dose). If seizures are unresponsive or recur, phenytoin or phenobarbital may be required. Priapism can be treated with alpha-adrenergic agonists.

Enhancement of elimination: Multiple dosing of activated charcoal may be effective; forced diuresis to remove active metabolite may not be beneficial

Drug Interactions Can result in serotonin syndrome with concomitant serotonin reuptake inhibitors, monoamine oxidase inhibitors; may inhibit metabolism of terfenadine or astemizole leading to Q-T prolongation and torsade de pointes; inhibits metabolism of benzodiazepines, especially alprazolam and triazolam

Pregnancy Risk Factor C

Additional Information May cause an increase in plasma prolactin levels; food delays absorption; inhibitor of cytochrome P-450 III4A and IID6; women and elderly receiving single doses attain significant higher peak concentrations than male volunteers

Specific References

Bristol-Myers Squibb Completing Comparisons of Serzone and SSRI Incidence of Sexual Dysfunction, Anxiety, and Sleep Disorders: Relapse Studies Ongoing, FDC Report - Pink Sheet, 1995, 11-2.

DeVane CL, "Nefazodone - Pharmacology and Efficacy of a New Antidepressant Agent: Formulary Considerations," *P & T*, 1995, 20(6):363-74.

Eison AS, Eison MS, Torrente JR, et al, "Nefazodone: Preclinical Pharmacology of a New Antidepressant," *Psychopharmacol Bull*, 1990, 26(3):311-5.

Fontaine R, "Novel Serotonergic Mechanisms and Clinical Experience With Nefazodone," *Clin Neuropharmacol*, 1993, 16(Suppl 3):S45-50.

Fontaine R, Ontiveros A, Elie R, et al, "A Double-Blind Comparison of Nefazodone, Imipramine, and Placebo in Major Depression," *J Clin Psychiatry*, 1994, 55(6):234-241.

Franc JE, Duncan GF, Farmen RH, et al, "High-Performance Liquid Chromatographic Method for the Determination of Nefazodone and Its Metabolites in Human Plasma Using Laboratory Robotics," *J Chromatogr*, 1991, 570(1):129-38.

Garside D and Goldberger, "Nefazodone," *Therapeutic Drug Monitoring and Toxicology In-Service Training and Continuing Education*, 1995, 16(5):109-10.

NegGram® *see* Nalidixic Acid *on page 547*

Nembutal® *see* Pentobarbital *on page 604*

Neo-Cultol® [OTC] *see* Mineral Oil *on page 534*

Neo-Estrone® *see* Estrogens, Esterified *on page 327*

Neofed® [OTC] *see* Pseudoephedrine *on page 661*

Neoloid® [OTC] *see* Castor Oil *on page 189*

Neopap® [OTC] *see* Acetaminophen *on page 79*

Neoquess® *see* Hyoscyamine Sulfate *on page 415*

Neosar® Injection *see* Cyclophosphamide *on page 249*

Neo-Synephrine® 12 Hour Nasal Solution [OTC] *see* Oxymetazoline Hydrochloride *on page 586*

Neovita® *see* Thiamine Hydrochloride *on page 741*

Nephro-Fer™ *see* Iron *on page 439*

Nephrox Suspension [OTC] *see* Aluminum *on page 104*

Nervocaine® *see* Lidocaine Hydrochloride *on page 468*

Nesacaine® *see* Chloroprocaine Hydrochloride *on page 201*

Neucalm® *see* Hydroxyzine *on page 414*

Neulente *see* Insulin Preparations *on page 426*

Neuramate® *see* Meprobamate *on page 503*

Neurontin® *see* Gabapentin *on page 374*

Neurostop® *see* Thiamine Hydrochloride *on page 741*

Neutrexin™ *see* Trimetrexate Glucuronate *on page 773*

Niacels™ [OTC] *see* Niacin *on this page*

Niacin (nye' a sin)

CAS Number 59-67-6

Brand Names Niac® [OTC]; Niacels™ [OTC]; Nicobid® [OTC]; Nicolar® [OTC]; Nicotinex [OTC]; Slo-Niacin® [OTC]

Synonyms Acidum Nicotinicum; Bionic; Nicotinic Acid; Vitamin B_3

Use Treatment of hyperlipidemias and hypercholesterolemia; treatment of pellagra; dietary supplement; treatment of hypoalphalipoproteinemia

Mechanism of Action Component of two coenzymes which is necessary for tissue respiration, lipid metabolism, and glycogenolysis; inhibits the synthesis of very low density lipoproteins while increasing high density cholesterol; water soluble vitamin B complex

Adverse Reactions

Cardiovascular: Hypotension, tachycardia, syncope, vasovagal attacks, flushing
Central nervous system: Dizziness, headache
Dermatologic: Pruritus, burning, tingling skin, increased sebaceous gland activity, hyperpigmentation
Endocrine & metabolic: Hyperuricemia, hyperglycemia
Gastrointestinal: gastrointestinal upset, nausea, vomiting, heartburn, diarrhea
Hematologic: Coagulopathy
Hepatic: Abnormal liver function tests, jaundice, and chronic liver damage
Ocular: Blurred vision, amblyopia
Neuromuscular & skeletal: Myopathy

Signs & Symptoms of Acute Overdose Delirium, nausea, thrombocytopenia, diarrhea, hepatitis, cholelithiasis, hyperuricemia, hyperglycemia, anorexia, arrhythmias, coagulopathy

Toxicodynamics/Kinetics

Peak serum concentrations: Oral: Within 45 minutes
Metabolism: Depending upon the dose, niacin converts to niacinamide; following this conversion, niacinamide is 30% metabolized in the liver
Half-life: 45 minutes
Elimination: Excreted in urine

Usual Dosage Give I.M., I.V., or S.C. only if oral route is unavailable and use only for vitamin deficiencies (not for hyperlipidemia)

Recommended daily allowances:
- 0-1 year: 6-8 mg/day
- 2-6 years: 9-11 mg/day
- 7-10 years: 16 mg/day
- >10 years: 15-18 mg/day

Children: Pellagra: Oral: 50-100 mg/dose 3 times/day

Adults: Oral:
- Hyperlipidemia: 1.5-6 g/day in 3 divided doses with or after meals
- Pellagra: 50-100 mg/dose 3-4 times/day; maximum: 500 mg/day
- Niacin deficiency: 10-20 mg/day, maximum: 100 mg/day

Contraindications Liver disease, peptic ulcer, known hypersensitivity to niacin

Warnings Monitor liver function tests, blood glucose; may elevate uric acid levels; use with caution in patients predisposed to gout; large doses should be administered with caution to patients with gallbladder disease, jaundice, liver disease, or diabetes; some products may contain tartrazine

Dosage Forms

Capsule, timed release: 125 mg, 250 mg, 300 mg, 400 mg, 500 mg
Elixir: 50 mg/5 mL (473 mL, 4000 mL)
Injection: 100 mg/mL (30 mL)
Tablet: 25 mg, 50 mg, 100 mg, 250 mg, 500 mg
Tablet, timed release: 150 mg, 250 mg, 500 mg, 750 mg

Stability Injection has a pH 4-6

Overdosage Treatment

Decontamination: Ipecac/lavage and activated charcoal with cathartic
Supportive therapy: Aspirin (160 mg or 325 mg) can reduce flushing due to niacin when given in a prophylactic manner; ibuprofen (200 mg) is also effective
Enhancement of elimination: Multiple dosing of activated charcoal may be effective

Test Interactions False elevations in some fluorometric determinations of urinary catecholamines; false-positive urine glucose (Benedict's reagent); increase in liver function test; glucose and uric acid

Diagnostic Tests/Procedures

Glucose, Random *on page 1269*
Liver Profile *on page 1286*
Uric Acid, Serum *on page 1371*

Drug Interactions

Decreased effect of oral hypoglycemics
Decreased toxicity (flush) with aspirin
Increased toxicity with lovastatin (myopathy) and possibly with other HMG-CoA reductase inhibitors

Pregnancy Risk Factor A (C if used in doses greater than RDA suggested doses)

Pregnancy Implications Excreted in breast milk

Monitoring Parameters Blood glucose, liver function tests, serum cholesterol

Patient Information May experience transient cutaneous flushing and sensation of warmth, especially of face and upper body; itching or tingling, and headache may occur, these adverse effects may be decreased by increasing the dose slowly or by taking aspirin or a NSAID 30 minutes to 1 hour prior to taking niacin; may cause gastrointestinal upset, take with food; if dizziness occurs, avoid sudden changes in posture; report any persistent nausea, vomiting, abdominal pain, dark urine, or pale stools to the physician; do not crush sustained release capsule

Nursing Implications Monitor closely for signs of hepatitis and myositis

Additional Information Pretreatment with 325 mg of aspirin prevents niacin-induced flushing

Specific References

Brown WV, "Niacin for Lipid Disorders," *Postgrad Med*, 1995, 98(2):185-93.
Dalton TA and Berry RS, "Hepatotoxicity Associated With Sustained-Release Niacin," *Am J Med*, 1992, 93(1):102-4.
Dunn Rt, Ford MA, Rindone JP, et al, "Low-Dose Aspirin and Ibuprofen Reduce the Cutaneous Reactions Follwoing Niacin Administration," *Am J Therap*, 1995, 2:478-80.
Lasagna L, "Over-the-Counter Niacin," *JAMA*, 1994, 271(9):709-10.
McKenney JM, Proctor JD, Harris S, et al, "A Comparison of the Efficacy and Toxic Effects of Sustained- vs Immediate-Release Niacin in Hypercholesterolemic Patients," *JAMA*, 1994, 271(9):672-7.
Schwab RA and Bachhuber BH, "Delirium and Lactic Acidosis Caused by Ethanol and Niacin Coingestion," *Am J Emerg Med*, 1991, 9(4):363-5.

Niacinamide (nye a sin' a mide)

CAS Number 98-92-0

Synonyms Benicot; Nicotinamide; Nicotinic Amide; Vitamin B_3

Use Prophylaxis and treatment of pellagra; treatment of N-d-pyridimethyl-N-P-nitrophenyl urea (PNU/Vacor®) toxicity

Mechanism of Action Used by the body as a source of niacin; water soluble vitamin B complex; less vasodilatory action than niacin

Adverse Reactions

Cardiovascular: Flushing, hypotension
Central nervous system: Headache
Dermatologic: Pruritus
Gastrointestinal: Vomiting
Ocular: Blurred vision

Toxicodynamics/Kinetics

Absorption: Rapid from gastrointestinal tract
Metabolism: In the liver
Half-life: 45 minutes
Time to peak serum concentration: 20-70 minutes
Elimination: Urine

Usual Dosage Oral:

Children: Pellagra: 100-300 mg/day in divided doses

Adults: 50 mg 3-10 times/day
Pellagra: 300-500 mg/day
Recommended daily allowance: 13-19 mg/day

Vacor® (PNU) toxicity: 500 mg I.M. or I.V. followed by 100-200 mg I.M. or I.V. every 4 hours up to 48 hours, then 100 mg orally 3-5 times/day for 2 weeks

Contraindications Liver disease, peptic ulcer, known hypersensitivity to niacin

Warnings Large doses should be administered with caution to patients with gallbladder disease or diabetes; monitor blood glucose; may elevate uric acid levels; use with caution in patients predisposed to gout; some products may contain tartrazine

Dosage Forms Tablet: 50 mg, 100 mg, 125 mg, 250 mg, 500 mg

Overdosage Treatment

Decontamination: Ipecac/lavage and activated charcoal with cathartic
Enhancement of elimination: Multiple dosing of activated charcoal may be effective

Test Interactions False elevations of urinary catecholamines in some fluorometric determinations

(Continued)

Niacinamide *(Continued)*

Diagnostic Tests/Procedures

Glucose, Random *on page 1269*
Liver Profile *on page 1286*
Uric Acid, Serum *on page 1371*

Drug Interactions

Decreased effect of oral hypoglycemics
Decreased toxicity (flush) with aspirin
Increased toxicity with lovastatin (myopathy) and possibly with other HMG-CoA reductase inhibitors

Pregnancy Risk Factor A (C if used in doses greater than RDA suggested doses)

Specific References

Gugler R, "Clinical Pharmacokinetics of Hypolipidaemic Drugs," *Clin Pharmacokinet*, 1978, 3(6):425-39.
LeWitt PA, "The Neurotoxicity of the Rat Poison Vacor. A Clinical Study of 12 Cases," *N Engl J Med*, 1980, 302(2):73-7.
Ovesen L, "Vitamin Therapy in the Absence of Obvious Deficiency: What Is the Evidence?" *Drugs*, 1984, 27(2):148-70.

Niac® [OTC] *see* Niacin *on page 554*
Nicobid® [OTC] *see* Niacin *on page 554*
Nicoderm® Patch *see* Nicotine *on this page*
Nicolar® [OTC] *see* Niacin *on page 554*
Niconyl® *see* Isoniazid *on page 443*
Nicorette® DS Gum *see* Nicotine *on this page*
Nicorette® Gum *see* Nicotine *on this page*
Nicotinamide *see* Niacinamide *on previous page*

Nicotine (nik oh teen')

Related Information

Toxins Which Should be Lavaged With Solutions Other Than Water *on page 1635*

CAS Number 54-11-5

UN Number 1654; 3144; 1655; 1656; 1657; 1658; 1659

Brand Names Habitrol™ Patch; Nicoderm® Patch; Nicorette® DS Gum; Nicorette® Gum; Nicotrol® Patch; ProStep® Patch

Commonly Found in Cigarettes (13-19 mg); nicotine gum (2-4 mg); cigars (15-40 mg); cigarette butt (5-7 mg); nicotine patch (8.3-114 mg); chewing tobacco (6-8 mg)

Use Insecticide, found in tobacco leaf (1% to 6% nicotine by weight) products

Mechanism of Action Direct stimulant to nicotinic acetylcholine receptor causing either sympathetic or parasympathetic effects

Adverse Reactions

Cardiovascular: Tachycardia, fibrillation (atrial)
Central nervous system: Salivation (increased), sweating, dizziness, headache, ataxia, fasciculations
Gastrointestinal: Nausea, emesis, altered taste
Neuromuscular & skeletal: Tremors
Ocular: Miosis
Miscellaneous: Oropharyngeal burning

Signs & Symptoms of Acute Overdose Nausea, cyanosis, hiccups, dry mouth, insomnia, dyspepsia, hyponatremia, blurred vision, hyperventilation, myalgia, hyperthermia, dementia, vomiting, nystagmus, hyperglycemia, lacrimation, A-V block, dysosmia, abdominal pain, mental confusion, diarrhea, apnea, salivation, lightheadedness, myoclonus, bronchial secretions (increased), muscle fasciculations/paralysis, paresthesia, respiratory depression, myasthenia gravis (exacerbation or precipitation of), mydriasis, tachycardia, hypertension then bradycardia, hypotension, diarrhea (may be delayed up to 24 hours in pediatric ingestion), seizures, methemoglobinemia, ototoxicity; tinnitus, hypotonia, hyperreflexia

Toxicodynamics/Kinetics

Absorption: Through skin and oral mucosa, gastrointestinal tract (except in stomach), respiratory tract; increased gastrointestinal, buccal, and dermal absorption in alkali medium
Distribution: V_d: 1-2 L/kg; higher in nonsmokers
Protein binding: 5% to 20%
Metabolism: Hepatic (cytochrome P-450) to cotinine and nicotine-N-oxide; large first-pass effect
Half-life:
Smokers: 0.8 hours

Nonsmokers: 1.3 hours
Cotinine: 15-20 hours
Gum/cigarette: 1-2 hours
Transdermal systems: 3-4 hours or higher

Elimination: 10% excreted unchanged, urine acidity with pH <5 may increase % excreted to 30%

Usual Dosage

Gum: Chew 1 piece of gum when urge to smoke, up to 30 pieces/day; most patients require 10-12 pieces of gum/day

Transdermal patches: Apply new patch every 24 hours to nonhairy, clean, dry skin on the upper body or upper outer arm; each patch should be applied to a different site; start with the 21 mg/day or 22 mg/day patch, except those patients with stable coronary artery disease should start with 14 mg/day; most patients the dosage can be reduced after 6-8 weeks; progressively lower doses are used every 2 weeks, with complete nicotine elimination achieved after 10 weeks

Contraindications Nonsmokers, severe angina pectoris, active temporomandibular joint disease

Warnings Nicotine is known to be one of the most toxic of all poisons; while the gum is being used to help the patient overcome a health hazard, it also must be considered a hazardous drug vehicle; use with caution in oropharyngeal inflammation and in patients with history of esophagitis or peptic ulcer

Dosage Forms

Patch, transdermal:
Habitrol™: 21 mg/day; 14 mg/day; 7 mg/day (30 systems/box)
Nicoderm®: 21 mg/day; 14 mg/day; 7 mg/day (14 systems/box)
ProStep®: 22 mg/day; 11 mg/day (7 systems/box)

Pieces, chewing gum, as polacrilex:
Nicorette®: 2 mg/square (96 pieces/box)
Nicorette® DS: 4 mg/square (96 pieces/box)

Reference Range A serum level of >50 ng/mL associated with toxicity; plasma nicotine level of 13,600 ng/mL associated with fatality; mean plasma level after smoking one cigarette: 5-30 ng//mL; plasma levels of cotinine averaged 0.001 mg/L in children from nonsmoking homes and 0.004 mg/L in children from homes with smoking cohabitants

Overdosage Treatment

Decontamination: Emesis not recommended due to potential for seizures; lavage with 1:10,000 potassium permanganate (100 mg/L) is recommended in ingestions after control of seizures; activated charcoal with cathartic use in acute ingestions not well established

For dermal exposures, wash area well with cool water and dry; soap (especially alkaline soaps) may increase absorption; remove any remaining transdermal systems; nicotine will continue to be absorbed several hours after removal due to depot in skin

Supportive therapy: Control seizures with benzodiazepines; if continuous, use phenytoin or phenobarbital; atropine can be utilized for cholinergic toxicity while phentolamine can be used for hypertension

Enhancement of elimination: Hemodialysis/hemoperfusion of unknown value; multiple doses probably necessary in ingestions of transdermal systems due to slow release of nicotine. While acidifying the urine may enhance elimination, this modality is not recommended due to inherent dangers; would proceed with forced diuresis.

Antidote(s)

Atropine Sulfate *on page 1395*

Diagnostic Tests/Procedures

Nicotine Level *on page 1308*

Pregnancy Risk Factor D (transdermal)/X (chewing gum)

Pregnancy Implications Pregnant smokers are almost twice as likely to have a spontaneous abortion or a low birth weight neonate (<2500 g); prematurity, placenta previa, and abruption rates are also increased in the smoker; nicotine is present in breast milk

Patient Information Wait 15 minutes after consuming acidic beverages or foods before using nicotine polacrilex

Nursing Implications Patients should be instructed to chew slowly to avoid jaw ache and to maximize benefit

Additional Information Symptoms usually do not occur in pediatric ingestions <1 mg/kg; not useful as maintenance therapy for ulcerative colitis

Lethal adult dose: 40 mg

Patients with deficiency of ability of C-oxidation of nicotine to cotinine will have decreased clearance and longer half-life of nicotine

Specific References

Benowitz NL, "Pharmacologic Aspects of Cigarette Smoking and Nicotine Addiction," *N Engl J Med*, 1988, 319(20):1318-30.

Benowitz NL, Jacob P III, and Sachs DPL, "Deficient C-oxidation of Nicotine," *Clin Pharmacol Ther*, 1995, 57:590-4.

(Continued)

Nicotine *(Continued)*

Blanchard J, "Nicotine," *Clin Toxicol Rev*, 1993, 15:11-2.

Harchelroad F, Potts K, Burdick J, et al, "Oral Absorption of Nicotine From Transdermal Therapeutic Systems," *Vet Hum Toxicol*, 1992, 34:332.

Luck W and Nau H, "Nicotine and Cotinine Concentrations in Serum and Urine of Infants Exposed Via Passive Smoking or Milk From Smoking Mothers," *J Pediatr*, 1985, 107(5):816-20.

McGee D, Brabson T, McCarthy J, et al, "Four-Year Review of Cigarette Ingestions in Children," *Pediatr Emerg Care*, 1995, 11(1):13-6.

Ottervanger JP, Festen JM, de Vries Ag, et al, "Acute Myocardial Infarction While Using The Nicotine," *Chest*, 1995, 107:1765-6.

Pattishall EN, Strope GL, Etzel RA, et al, "Serum Cotinine as a Measure of Tobacco Smoke Exposure in Children," *Am J Dis Child*, 1985, 139(11):1101-4.

Ross MP, Revolinski D, and Taurman L, "Green Tobacco Sickness Among Adults in Kentucky," *Vet Hum Toxicol*, 1994, 36:360.

Smolinske SC, Spoerke DG, Spiller SK, et al, "Cigarette and Nicotine Chewing Gum Toxicity in Children," *Hum Toxicol*, 1988, 7(1):27-31.

Svensson CK, "Clinical Pharmacokinetics of Nicotine," *Clin Pharmacokinet*, 1987, 12(1):30-40.

Thomas GA, Rhodes J, Mani V, et al, "Transdermal Nicotine as Maintenance Therapy for Ulcerative Colitis," *N Engl J Med*, 1995, 332(15):988-92.

Nicotinex [OTC] *see* Niacin *on page 554*

Nicotinic Acid *see* Niacin *on page 554*

Nicotinic Amide *see* Niacinamide *on page 555*

Nicotrol® Patch *see* Nicotine *on page 556*

Nico-Vert® *see* Dimenhydrinate *on page 289*

Nidrel® *see* Nitrendipine *on page 562*

Nifedipine (nye fed' i peen)

Related Information

Calcium Channel Blocking Agents Comparison *on page 1646-1647*

CAS Number 21829-25-4

Brand Names Adalat®; Duradalat®; Duranifin®; Fenamon®; Procardia®; Procardia XL®

Synonyms Nifedipinum

Use Angina, hypertrophic cardiomyopathy, hypertension (sustained release only)

Mechanism of Action Inhibits calcium ion from entering the "slow channels" or select voltage-sensitive areas of vascular smooth muscle and myocardium during depolarization, producing a relaxation of coronary vascular smooth muscle and coronary vasodilation; increases myocardial oxygen delivery in patients with vasospastic angina

Adverse Reactions

Cardiovascular: Flushing, hypotension, tachycardia, palpitation, syncope, peripheral edema

Central nervous system: Dizziness, giddiness, drowsiness, fever, chills, headache, psychosis

Dermatologic: Dermatitis, rash, photosensitivity reactions, flushing, purpura

Endocrine & metabolic: Gynecomastia

Gastrointestinal: Nausea, diarrhea, constipation, gingival hyperplasia, vomiting

Hematologic: Thrombocytopenia, leukopenia, anemia

Neuromuscular & skeletal: Joint stiffness, arthritis with elevated ANA

Ocular: Blurred vision, transient blindness

Respiratory: Dyspnea

Miscellaneous: Bezoars/concretions, sweating

Signs & Symptoms of Acute Overdose Hypotension, exfoliative dermatitis, wheezing, Q-T prolongation, gingival hyperplasia, memory loss, lightheadedness, depression, enuresis, bradycardia, gynecomastia, Raynaud's (exacerbation of), heart block, congestive heart failure, extrapyramidal reaction, peripheral vasodilation, nocturia, chest pain, reflex tachycardia, hyperthermia, constipation, pulmonary edema, hypokalemia, hyperglycemia, hyperkalemia, A-V block, leukopenia; neutropenia; agranulocytosis; granulocytopenia

Toxicodynamics/Kinetics

Onset of action:

- Oral: Within 20 minutes
- S.L.: Within 1-5 minutes

Duration: Capsules, tablets: 4-8 hours

Absorption: Rapid from gastrointestinal tract (60% to 75%)

Distribution: V_d: 0.8-1.4 L/kg

Protein binding: 92% to 98% (concentration-dependent)

Metabolism: In the liver to inactive metabolites capsules: 45% to 75%, sustained release: 65% to 86%

Bioavailability: 60% to 75%

Half-life:

- Normal adults: 2-5 hours

Cirrhosis: 7 hours
Overdose: 7.5 hours
Time to peak serum concentration:
Capsule: ~30-60 minutes
Tablet: 1-2 hours
Elimination: Excreted in urine (75% metabolites) and in feces (65% unchanged); renal clearance: 0.42 L/hour/kg

Usual Dosage
Children: Oral, S.L.:
Hypertensive emergencies: 0.25-0.5 mg/kg/dose
Hypertrophic cardiomyopathy: 0.6-0.9 mg/kg/24 hours in 3-4 divided doses

Adults: Oral: Initial: 10 mg 3 times/day as capsules or 30-60 mg once daily as sustained release tablet; maintenance: 10-30 mg 3-4 times/day (capsules); maximum: 180 mg/24 hours (capsules) or 120 mg/day (sustained release)

Dosing adjustment in hepatic impairment: Reduce oral dose by 50% to 60% in patients with cirrhosis

Contraindications Known hypersensitivity to nifedipine

Warnings Increased angina may be seen upon starting or increasing doses; may increase frequency, duration, and severity of angina during initiation of therapy; use with caution in patients with congestive heart failure or aortic stenosis (especially with concomitant beta-adrenergic blocker)

Dosage Forms
Capsule, liquid-filled (Adalat®, Procardia®): 10 mg, 20 mg
Tablet, extended release (Adalat® CC): 30 mg, 60 mg, 90 mg
Tablet, sustained release (Procardia XL®): 30 mg, 60 mg, 90 mg

Reference Range Therapeutic: 25-100 ng/mL; although levels >28 ng/mL correlate with negative inotropic effect after I.V. use

Overdosage Treatment
Decontamination: Ipecac-induced emesis can hypothetically worsen calcium antagonist toxicity, since it can produce vagal stimulation. The potential for seizures precipitously following acute ingestion of large doses of a calcium antagonist may also contraindicate the use of ipecac. Lavage/activated charcoal with cathartic is useful. Whole bowel irrigation for sustained release preparations.

Supportive therapy: I.V. fluids and Trendelenburg positioning should be initiated as intoxication may cause hypotension. Calcium (calcium chloride I.V. 1-2 g in adults or 10-30 mg/kg in children over 5-10 minutes with repeats as needed) has been used as an "antidote" for acute intoxications, although its effectiveness is questionable in nifedipine overdose. Heart block may respond to isoproterenol, glucagon, atropine and/or calcium, although a temporary pacemaker may be required. Amrinone or dopamine may be required for hypotension. Glucagon may increase myocardial contractility.
Enhancement of elimination: Multiple dosing of activated charcoal is useful

Antidote(s)
Calcium Chloride *on page 1400*
Calcium Gluconate *on page 1401*
Glucagon *on page 1431*

Drug Interactions Beta-blockers may increase cardiovascular adverse effects; anesthetic doses of fentanyl may causes hypotension; cimetidine may increase nifedipine serum concentration; nifedipine may increase phenytoin and possibly digoxin serum concentrations; nifedipine may increase quinidine levels and has an antiplatelet action that may increase bleeding time; rifampin may markedly decrease nifedipine levels

Pregnancy Risk Factor C

Pregnancy Implications Late decelerations of fetal heart rate can occur

Monitoring Parameters Blood pressure, EKG

Patient Information Do not chew or break sustained release capsules

Nursing Implications May cause some patients to urinate frequently at night; may cause inflamed gums; capsule may be punctured and drug solution administered sublingually or orally to reduce blood pressure in recumbent patient

Additional Information Capsule may be punctured and drug solution administered sublingually to reduce blood pressure in recumbent patient; tasteless; response to atropine may not be observed until after I.V. calcium administration

Specific References

Allikmets E, et al, "Long-term Use of Benzodiazepines: Abrupt Withdrawal Versus Withdrawal Under Nifedipine Cover," *Pharmacol Toxicol*, 1995, 76(Suppl 3):Abstr 8.

Clifton GD, Booth DC, Hobbs S, et al, "Negative Inotropic Effect of Intravenous Nifedipine in Coronary Artery Disease: Relation to Plasma Levels," *Am Heart J*, 1990, 119(2 Pt 1):283-90.

Ferner RE, Monkman S, Riley J, et al, "Pharmacokinetics and Toxic Effects of Nifedipine in Massive Overdose," *Hum Exp Toxicol*, 1990, 9(5):309-11.

Hata T, Manabe A, Hata K, et al, "Changes in Blood Velocities of Fetal Circulation in Association With Fetal Heart Rate Abnormalities: Effect of Sublingual Administration of Nifedipine," *Am J Perinatol*, 1995, 12:80-1.

(Continued)

Nifedipine *(Continued)*

Howarth DM, Dawson AH, Smith AJ, et al, "Calcium Channel Blocking Drug Overdose: An Australian Series," *Hum Exp Toxicol*, 1994, 13(3):161-6.
Kahn JK, "Nifedipine-Associated Acute Psychosis," *Am J Med*, 1986, 81(4):705-6.
Pearigen PD, "Death From Accidental Nifedipine Ingestion in a Toddler," *Vet Hum Toxicol*, 1993, 35:345.
Ramsdale DR, Morris JL, and Hardy P, "Gingival Hyperplasia With Nifedipine," *Br Heart J*, 1995, 73:115.
Whitebloom D and Fitzharris J, "Nifedipine Overdose," *Clin Cardiol*, 1988, 11(7):505-6.

Nifedipinum *see* Nifedipine *on page 558*

Niftolid® *see* Flutamide *on page 366*

Nilstat® *see* Nystatin *on page 574*

Nilvadipine

Related Information

Calcium Channel Blocking Agents Comparison *on page 1646-1647*

CAS Number 75530-68-6

Synonyms Nivadipine

Use Investigational: Hypertension; also may be useful in patients with cerebrovascular disease or stable exertional or variant angina pectoris

Mechanism of Action Dihydropyridine calcium channel blocking agent with properties similar to nifedipine

Adverse Reactions

Cardiovascular: Flushing, tachycardia, edema, hypotension, ventricular ectopy
Central nervous system: Headache, dizziness, sleep disturbances
Gastrointestinal: Nausea

Toxicodynamics/Kinetics

Protein binding: 98%
Distribution: V_d: 24-40 L/kg
Bioavailability: Oral: 14% to 19%
Half-life: 9.8-18.2 hours
Elimination: Renal; clearance: 1.08 L/kg/hour

Usual Dosage

Hypertension: 4-16 mg/day; reduce dosage to a maximum dose of 8 mg in patients with cirrhosis or with concomitant use with cimetidine
Cerebrovascular disease: 2-4 mg twice daily
Angina pectoris: 8-16 mg/day

Contraindications Acute apoplectic stroke, intracranial hemorrhage, raised intracranial pressure

Overdosage Treatment

Decontamination: Ipecac-induced emesis can hypothetically worsen calcium antagonist toxicity, since it can produce vagal stimulation. The potential for seizures precipitously following acute ingestion of large doses of a calcium antagonist may also contraindicate the use of ipecac. Lavage/activated charcoal with cathartic is useful. Whole bowel irrigation for sustained release preparations.

Supportive therapy: I.V. fluids and Trendelenburg positioning should be initiated as intoxication may cause hypotension. Calcium (calcium chloride I.V. 1-2 g in adults or 10-30 mg/kg in children over 5-10 minutes with repeats as needed) has been used as an "antidote" for acute intoxications, although its effectiveness is questionable in nifedipine overdose. Heart block may respond to isoproterenol, glucagon, atropine and/or calcium, although a temporary pacemaker may be required. Amrinone or dopamine may be required for hypotension. Glucagon may increase myocardial contractility.

Enhancement of elimination: Multiple dosing of activated charcoal is useful

Specific References

Kelly JG and O'Malley K, "Clinical Pharmacokinetics of Calcium Antagonists. An Update," *Clin Pharmacokinet*, 1992, 22(6):416-33.
"Nilvadipine: An Alternative Dihydropyridine for Treating Hypertension," *Drugs and Therapy Perspectives*, 1995, 5:(9)1-4.

Nimodipine (nye moe' di peen)

Related Information

Calcium Channel Blocking Agents Comparison *on page 1646-1647*

CAS Number 66085-59-4

Brand Names Nimotop®

Use Improvement of neurological deficits due to spasm following subarachnoid hemorrhage from ruptured congenital intracranial aneurysms who are in good neurological condition postictus

Mechanism of Action Nimodipine is a calcium channel blocker; animal studies indicate that nimodipine has a greater effect on cerebral arterials than other arterials; this increased specificity may be due to the drug's increased lipophilicity and cerebral distribution as compared to nifedipine indicated for patients with subarachnoid hemorrhage

Adverse Reactions

Cardiovascular: Reductions in systemic blood pressure, flushing, tachycardia, palpitations

Central nervous system: Dizziness

Dermatologic: Acne

Gastrointestinal: Nausea, constipation

Hematologic: Bleeding

Respiratory: Wheezing

Signs & Symptoms of Acute Overdose Hypotension, diarrhea, myalgia, lightheadedness, gingival hyperplasia, depression, hyponatremia, disorientation, peripheral vasodilation

Toxicodynamics/Kinetics

Absorption: Rapid

Distribution: V_d: 0.9 L/kg

Protein binding: >95%

Metabolism: Extensive in liver

Bioavailability: 13%

Half-life: 1-2 hours, increases with reduced renal function

Time to peak serum concentration: Within 1 hour

Elimination: Feces (32%) and urine (60% within 4 days)

Usual Dosage Adults: Oral: 60 mg every 4 hours for 21 days, start therapy within 96 hours after subarachnoid hemorrhage

Dosing adjustment in hepatic impairment: Reduce dosage to 30 mg every 4 hours in patients with liver failure

Contraindications Hypersensitivity to nimodipine or any component

Warnings Use with caution in impaired liver function; may increase frequency, duration, and severity of angina during initiation of therapy; use with caution in patients with congestive heart failure or aortic stenosis (especially with concomitant beta-adrenergic blocker)

Dosage Forms Capsule, liquid-filled: 30 mg

Overdosage Treatment

Decontamination: Ipecac-induced emesis can hypothetically worsen calcium antagonist toxicity, since it can produce vagal stimulation; lavage/activated charcoal with cathartic is useful. The potential for seizures precipitously following acute ingestion of large doses of a calcium antagonist may also contraindicate the use of ipecac.

Supportive therapy: Supportive and symptomatic treatment, including I.V. fluids and Trendelenburg positioning, should be initiated as intoxication may cause hypotension. Although calcium (calcium chloride I.V. 1-2 g in adults or 10-30 mg/kg in children over 5-10 minutes with repeats as needed) has been used as an "antidote" for acute intoxications, there is limited experience to support its routine use and should be reserved for those cases where definite signs of myocardial depression are evident. Heart block may respond to isoproterenol, glucagon, atropine and/or calcium, although a temporary pacemaker may be required; norepinephrine, dopamine, or amrinone for refractory hypotension.

Enhancement of elimination: Multiple dosing of activated charcoal may be useful

Antidote(s)

Calcium Chloride *on page 1400*

Calcium Gluconate *on page 1401*

Pregnancy Risk Factor C

Monitoring Parameters Blood pressure

Nursing Implications If the capsules cannot be swallowed, the liquid may be removed by making a hole in each end of the capsule with an 18-gauge needle and extracting the contents into a syringe; if given via NG tube, follow with a flush of 30 mL NS

Specific References

Ramoska EA, Spiller HA, and Myers A, "Calcium Channel Blocker Toxicity," *Ann Emerg Med*, 1990, 19(6):649-53.

Nimotop® *see* Nimodipine *on previous page*

Niotal® *see* Zolpidem Tartrate *on page 814*

Nipent™ Injection *see* Pentostatin *on page 606*

Nipride® *see* Nitroprusside Sodium *on page 568*

Niprina® *see* Nitrendipine *on next page*

Nipruss® *see* Nitroprusside Sodium *on page 568*

Nitrados® *see* Nitrazepam *on next page*

Nitrazepam

Related Information

Clonazepam *on page 229*
Flunitrazepam *on page 354*

CAS Number 146-22-5

Brand Names Alodorm®; Apodorm®; Arem®; Dormigen®; Insoma®; Ipersed®; Mitidin®; Mogadan®; Nitrados®; Nitrazepan®; Novanov®; Pelson®; Somnite®; Surem®; Tri®; Unisomnia®

Synonyms Nitrozepamum

Use Investigational: Short-term management of insomnia; treatment of infantile spasm and seizures

Mechanism of Action Facilitates gamma-aminobutyric acid neurotransmission; a 7-nitrobenzodiazepine derivative

Adverse Reactions

Central nervous system: Lethargy, disorientation, night terrors, opisthotonos, ataxia, headache, hypothermia
Endocrine & metabolic: Dysphagia, gout
Gastrointestinal: Salivation, dysphagia, anorexia
Hematologic: Porphyria
Ocular: Increased intraocular pressure

Signs & Symptoms of Acute Overdose Apnea, aspiration

Toxicodynamics/Kinetics

Peak serum levels: 1.4 hours
Duration of effect: 4-8 hours
Distribution: V_d: 2.4 L/kg (young patients); 4.8 L/kg (elderly)
Protein binding: 85% to 88%
Metabolism: Hepatic reduction
Bioavailability: 78%
Half-life: 24-29 hours
Elimination: Renal (80%), feces (20%)

Usual Dosage Oral:

Insomnia:
- Children:
  - 1-6 years: 2.5 mg
  - ≥7 years: 5 mg
- Adults: 5-10 mg at night

Epilepsy: Children and Adults: 1-6 mg/day; dosage should be decreased in elderly, hypothyroid patients, and cirrhosis
- Children maximum dose: 60 mg
- Adult maximum dose: 20 mg

Contraindications Hypersensitivity to nitrazepam, flunitrazepam, or clonazepam

Warnings Use with caution in patients with hypothyroidism, cirrhosis, elderly, pregnancy, and breast feeding

Reference Range Steady state plasma levels with a 5 mg/day oral dose: ~57 (±17) ng/mL; fatalities associated with postmortem blood levels of 1.2-9 mg/L

Overdosage Treatment

Decontamination: Lavage/activated charcoal with cathartic
Supportive therapy: Rarely is mechanical ventilation required; flumazenil has been shown to selectively block the binding of benzodiazepines to CNS receptors, resulting in a reversal of benzodiazepine-induced CNS depression and respiratory depression
Enhancement of elimination: Multiple dose of activated charcoal is effective

Antidote(s)

Flumazenil *on page 1428*

Drug Interactions Birth control pills, probenecid, and cimetidine can result in decreased nitrazepam clearance; rifampin can result in increased clearance of nitrazepam

Additional Information Hangover can occur at 20 mg oral doses; hallucinations from withdrawal can be treated with chlorpromazine

Specific References

Impallomeni M and Ezzat R, "Hypothermia Associated With Nitrazepam Administration," *Br Med J*, 1976, 1:223-4.
Murphy JV, Sawasky F, Marquardt KM, et al, "Deaths in Young Children Receiving Nitrazepam," *J Pediatr*, 1987, 111(1):145-7.
Nicholson AN, "Hypnotics: Their Place in Therapeutics," *Drugs*, 1986, 31(2):164-76.
Wyllie E, Wyllie R, Cruse RP, et al, "The Mechanism of Nitrazepam-Induced Drooling and Aspiration," *N Engl J Med*, 1986, 314(1):35-8.

Nitrazepan® *see* Nitrazepam *on this page*

Nitrendipine

Related Information

Calcium Channel Blocking Agents Comparison *on page 1646-1647*

CAS Number 39562-70-6

Brand Names Bayotensin®; Baypresol®; Baypress®; Deiten®; Gericin®; Nidrel®; Niprina®; Tensogradal®; Trendinol®

Use Investigational: Hypertension

Mechanism of Action Dihydropyridine calcium channel blocking agent with actions similar to nifedipine

Adverse Reactions

Cardiovascular: Flushing (4%), edema (6%), tachycardia
Central nervous system: Headache (10%), dizziness (6%), fatigue
Gastrointestinal: Nausea (7%)
Otic: Tinnitus

Toxicodynamics/Kinetics

Distribution: 6 L/kg
Protein binding: 98%
Metabolism: Hepatic to inactive metabolites
Bioavailability: 16% to 23%
Half-life: 8.6 hours
Elimination: Renal (80%), feces (8%)

Usual Dosage 20 mg/day (in patients with liver disease or in the elderly, an initial dose of 10 mg is recommended); maximum dose: 40 mg/day

Contraindications Hypersensitivity to other calcium channel blocking agents, hypotension, advanced aortic stenosis

Warnings Reduce dosage in elderly; use with caution in patients with liver insufficiency, digital ischemia, nonobstructive hypertrophic cardiomyopathy, Duchenne muscular dystrophy, or in combination with beta-blocking agents

Reference Range Peak plasma levels after a 20 mg oral dose: 5-40 μg/L

Overdosage Treatment

Decontamination: Ipecac-induced emesis can hypothetically worsen calcium antagonist toxicity, since it can produce vagal stimulation. The potential for seizures precipitously following acute ingestion of large doses of a calcium antagonist may also contraindicate the use of ipecac. Lavage/activated charcoal with cathartic is useful. Whole bowel irrigation for sustained release preparations.

Supportive therapy: I.V. fluids and Trendelenburg positioning should be initiated as intoxication may cause hypotension. Calcium (calcium chloride I.V. 1-2 g in adults or 10-30 mg/kg in children over 5-10 minutes with repeats as needed) has been used as an "antidote" for acute intoxications, although its effectiveness is questionable in nifedipine overdose. Heart block may respond to isoproterenol, glucagon, atropine and/or calcium, although a temporary pacemaker may be required. Amrinone or dopamine may be required for hypotension. Glucagon may increase myocardial contractility.

Enhancement of elimination: Multiple dosing of activated charcoal is useful

Drug Interactions Increased hypotensive effects with acebutolol, atenolol, carteolol, metoprolol

Additional Information Can cause an increase in plasma catecholamine, urinary aldosterone levels, and serum alkaline phosphatase levels; natriuresis and diuresis may also occur on a short-term basis

Specific References

Kelly JG and O'Malley K, "Clinical Pharmacokinetics of Calcium Antagonists. An Update," *Clin Pharmacokinet*, 1992, 22(6):416-33.

Moser M, "Nitrendipine in the Treatment of Mild to Moderate Hypertension," *Angiology*, 1988, 39(1 Pt 2):73-80.

Pedrinelli R, Fouad FM, Tarazi RC, et al, "Nitrendipine, A Calcium-Entry Blocker. Renal and Humoral Effects in Human Arterial Hypertension," *Arch Intern Med*, 1986, 146(1):62-5.

Santiago TM and Lopez LM, "Nitrendipine: A New Dihydropyridine Calcium-Channel Antagonist for the Treatment of Hypertension," *DICP*, 1990, 24(2):167-75.

Nitric Oxide

CAS Number 10102-43-9

UN Number 1660

Synonyms Nitrogen Monoxide; NO

Use Orphan drug status for treatment of primary pulmonary hypertension in the newborn; may be useful for septic shock, ARDS, or treatment of pulmonary effects of paraquat

Mechanism of Action Produces selective pulmonary vasodilatation without systemic vasodilatation through direct effect on smooth muscle of pulmonary vasculature

Adverse Reactions

Hematologic: Methemoglobinemia
Respiratory: Pulmonary fibrosis, rebound pulmonary hypertension from nitric oxide withdrawal

Toxicodynamics/Kinetics

Metabolism: Reacts with hemoglobin (at an affinity of 1400 times that of oxygen) to cause a nitrosyl-hemoglobin which is oxidized to methemoglobin and then into nitrate

(Continued)

Nitric Oxide *(Continued)*

Half-life: 5-50 seconds

Reference Range Normal plasma nitrate level: 24 μmol/L (range: 19-39 μmol/L); patients with congestive heart failure 56 μmol/L (range: 41-72 μmol/L)

Overdosage Treatment

Supportive therapy: Methylene blue for symptomatic methemoglobinemia

Antidote(s)

Methylene Blue *on page 1444*

Additional Information Flammable, can inactivate surfactant; colorless gas; paralysis (motor neuropathy) may develop in alcoholics

TLV-TWA: 25 ppm

IDLH: 100 ppm

Specific References

Collier J and Vallance P, "Physiological Importance of Nitric Oxide," *BMJ*, 1991, 302(6788):1289-90.

Fukuto JM and Chaudhuri G, "Inhibition of Constructive and Inducible Nitric Oxide Synthase," *Annu Rev Pharmacol Toxicol*, 1995, 35:165-94.

Groeneveld PH, Ringers J, van Dissel JT, et al, "Effect of Nitric Oxide on Renal Function in Septic Shock," *N Engl J Med*, 1994, 330(22):1620.

Koppel C, von Wissmann C, Barckow D, et al, "Inhaled Nitric Oxide in Advanced Paraquat Intoxication," *J Toxicol Clin Toxicol*, 1994, 32(2):205-14.

Miller OI, Tang SF, Keech A, et al, "Rebound Pulmonary Hypertension on Withdrawal From Inhaled Nitric Oxide," *Lancet*, 1995, 346:51-2.

Packer M, "Vasodilator Therapy for Primary Pulmonary Hypertension. Limitations and Hazards," *Ann Intern Med*, 1985, 103(2):258-70.

Petros AJ, Turner SC, and Nunn AJ, "Cost Implications of Using Inhaled Nitric Oxide Compared With Epoprostenol for Pulmonary Hypertension," *J Pharm Technol*, 1995, 11:163-6.

Roberts JD, Polaner DM, Lang P, et al, "Inhaled Nitric Oxide in Persistent Pulmonary Hypertension of the Newborn," *Lancet*, 1992, 340(8823):818-9.

Tsai GE and Gastfriend DR, "Nitric Oxide-Induced Motor Neuron Disease in a Patient With Alcoholism," *N Engl J Med*, 1995, 332(15):1036.

Winlaw DS, Smythe GA, Keogh AM, et al, "Increased Nitric Oxide Production in Heart Failure," *Lancet*, 1994, 344(8919):373-4.

Nitro-Bid® *see* Nitroglycerin *on page 566*

Nitrocap® TD *see* Nitroglycerin *on page 566*

Nitrocine® *see* Nitroglycerin *on page 566*

Nitrocontin® *see* Nitroglycerin *on page 566*

Nitroderm® *see* Nitroglycerin *on page 566*

Nitrodisc® *see* Nitroglycerin *on page 566*

Nitro-Dur® *see* Nitroglycerin *on page 566*

Nitrofurantoin (nye troe fyoor an' toyn)

CAS Number 67-20-9; 17140-81-7; 54-87-5

Brand Names Cistofuran®; Cystit®; Furadantin®; Furalan®; Furan®; Furanite®; Furil®; Macrobid®; Macrodantin®; Urodil®; Urolong®

Use Prevention and treatment of urinary tract infections caused by susceptible gram-negative and some gram-positive organisms; *Pseudomonas*, *Serratia*, and most species of *Proteus* are generally resistant to nitrofurantoin

Mechanism of Action Inhibits several bacterial enzyme systems including acetyl coenzyme A interfering with metabolism and possibly cell wall synthesis

Adverse Reactions

Central nervous system: Dizziness, headache, chills, fever, ataxia

Dermatologic: Rash, exfoliative dermatitis, rash, alopecia, toxic epidermal necrolysis

Gastrointestinal: Nausea, vomiting (dose-related), anorexia, pancreatitis, diarrhea

Hematologic: Hemolytic anemia, eosinophilia, leukopenia, thrombocytopenia, porphyria, methemoglobinemia

Hepatic: Hepatotoxicity (usually occurring in women after more than 1 year in use)

Neuromuscular & skeletal: Arthralgia, paresthesia

Ocular: Nystagmus, papilledema

Respiratory: Interstitial pneumonitis and/or fibrosis, dyspnea, cough, chest pain, pulmonary edema

Miscellaneous: Rust yellow to brown urine, lupus erythematosus-like reaction, porphyrinogenic

Signs & Symptoms of Acute Overdose Leukopenia or neutropenia (agranulocytosis, granulocytopenia); apnea; cholestatic jaundice, jaundice, hyperthermia, sexual dysfunction, pseudotumor cerebri, numbness, vision color changes (yellow tinge); methemoglobinemia, erythema multiforme, crystalluria

Toxicodynamics/Kinetics

Absorption: Well absorbed from gastrointestinal tract; the macrocrystalline form is absorbed more slowly due to slower dissolution, but causes less gastrointestinal distress; food may minimize adverse local gastrointestinal effects

Distribution: V_d: 0.8 L/kg
Protein binding: 60% to 90%
Metabolism: 60% of drug metabolized by body tissues throughout the body, with exception of plasma, to inactive metabolites
Bioavailability: Increased by presence of food
Half-life: 20-60 minutes; prolonged with renal impairment
Elimination: Excreted as metabolites and unchanged drug (40%) in urine and small amounts in bile; renal excretion via glomerular filtration and tubular secretion

Usual Dosage Oral:

Children >1 month: 5-7 mg/kg/day divided every 6 hours; maximum: 400 mg/day
Chronic therapy: 1-2 mg/kg/day in divided doses every 12-24 hours; maximum dose: 400 mg/day

Adults: 50-100 mg/dose every 6 hours (not to exceed 400 mg/24 hours); extended release: 100 mg every 12 hours with meals for 7 days
Prophylaxis: 50-100 mg/dose at bedtime

Dosing adjustment/comments in renal impairment: Cl_{cr} <50 mL/minute: Avoid use

Contraindications Hypersensitivity to nitrofurantoin or any component; renal impairment; infants <1 month (due to the possibility of hemolytic anemia)

Warnings Use with caution in patients with G-6-PD deficiency, patients with anemia, vitamin B deficiency, diabetes mellitus or electrolyte abnormalities; therapeutic concentrations of nitrofurantoin are not attained in urine of patients with Cl_{cr} <40 mL/minute; use with caution if prolonged therapy is anticipated due to possible pulmonary toxicity

Dosage Forms

Capsule: 50 mg, 100 mg
Capsule:
Extended release: 100 mg
Macrocrystal: 25 mg, 50 mg, 100 mg
Macrocrystal/monohydrate: 100 mg
Suspension, oral: 25 mg/5 mL (470 mL)
Tablet: 50 mg, 100 mg

Reference Range After an oral dose of 100 mg, urinary nitrofurantoin levels range from 50-100 μg/mL

Overdosage Treatment

Decontamination: Lavage/activated charcoal with cathartic
Supportive therapy: Treat symptomatic methemoglobinemia with methylene blue
Enhancement of elimination: Multiple dosing of activated charcoal may be effective

Antidote(s)

Methylene Blue *on page 1444*

Test Interactions Causes false-positive urine glucose with Clinitest®

Diagnostic Tests/Procedures

Complete Blood Count *on page 1236*
Methemoglobin, Blood *on page 1296*

Drug Interactions

Decreased effect with antacids (magnesium trisilicate), quinolone antibiotics, nalidixic acid
Increased effect/levels with probenecid, sulfinpyrazone

Pregnancy Risk Factor B

Pregnancy Implications Fetal hemolysis may occur; no congenital malformations documented; crosses the placenta; appears in breast milk

Monitoring Parameters Signs of pulmonary reaction, signs of numbness or tingling of the extremities, periodic liver function tests

Patient Information Take with food or milk; may discolor urine to a dark yellow or brown color; notify physician if fever, chest pain, persistent, nonproductive cough, or difficulty breathing occurs

Nursing Implications Higher peak serum levels may cause increased gastritis; give with meals to slow the rate of absorption and thus decrease adverse effects

Specific References

Burgert SJ, Burke JP, and Box TD, "Reversible Nitrofurantoin-Induced Chronic Active Hepatitis and Hepatic Cirrhosis in a Patient Awaiting Liver Transplantation," *Transplantation*, 1995, 59(3):448-9.

D'Arcy PF, "Nitrofurantoin," *Drug Intell Clin Pharm*, 1985, 19(7-8):540-7.

Penn RG and Griffin HP, "Adverse Reactions to Nitrofurantoin in the United Kingdom, Sweden, and Holland," *Br Med J (Clin Res)*, 1982, 284(6327):1440-2.

Nitrogard® *see* Nitroglycerin *on next page*

Nitrogen Monoxide *see* Nitric Oxide *on page 563*

Nitrogen Mustard *see* Mechlorethamine Hydrochloride *on page 492*

Nitroglicerina® *see* Nitroglycerin *on next page*

Nitroglycerin (nye troe gli' ser in)

CAS Number 55-63-0

Brand Names Deponit®; Minitran®; Nitro-Bid®; Nitrocap® TD; Nitrocine®; Nitrocontin®; Nitroderm®; Nitrodisc®; Nitro-Dur®; Nitrogard®; Nitroglicerina®; Nitroglyn®; Nitrol®; Nitrolan®; Nitrolingual®; Nitrong®; Nitrospan®; Nitrostat®; Sustachron®; Transdermal-NTG®; Transderm-Nitro®; Tridil®

Synonyms Glonoin; Glyceryl Trinitrate; Nitroglycerol; NTG; 1,2,3-Propanetriol Trinitrate; Trinitrin

Use Angina pectoris; I.V. for congestive heart failure (especially when associated with acute myocardial infarction); hypertension due to ergotism; pulmonary hypertension; hypertensive emergencies occurring perioperatively (especially during cardiovascular surgery); industrial uses: dynamite, cordite

Mechanism of Action Reduces cardiac oxygen demand by decreasing left ventricular pressure and systemic vascular resistance; dilates coronary arteries and improves collateral flow to ischemic regions

Adverse Reactions

Cardiovascular: Flushing, chest pain, hypotension, reflex tachycardia, severe hypotension, bradycardia, coronary vascular insufficiency, cardiac arrhythmias, palpitations

Central nervous system: Dizziness, restlessness, pallor, headache

Dermatologic: Allergic contact dermatitis, exfoliative dermatitis

Gastrointestinal: Nausea, vomiting, colic, diarrhea

Miscellaneous: Methemoglobinemia, alcohol intoxication, sweating and collapse

Signs & Symptoms of Acute Overdose Hypotension, throbbing headache, palpitations, bloody diarrhea, bradycardia, cyanosis, tissue hypoxia, metabolic acidosis, clonic seizures, circulatory collapse, methemoglobinemia

Toxicodynamics/Kinetics Onset and duration of action is dependent upon dosage form administered; see table.

Dosage Form	Onset of Effect	Peak Effect	Duration
Sublingual tablet	1–3 min	4–8 min	30–60 min
Lingual spray	2 min	4–10 min	30–60 min
Buccal tablet	2–5 min	4–10 min	2 h
Sustained release	20–45 min	45–120 min	4–8 h
Topical	15–60 min	30–120 min	2–12 h
Transdermal	40–60 min	60–180 min	8–24 h
I.V. drip	Immediate	Immediate	3–5 min

Absorption: Well from gastrointestinal tract

Distribution: V_d: 2.1-4.5 L/kg; distributed widely throughout the body

Protein binding: 60%

Metabolism: Extensive first-pass to inorganic nitrite

Half-life: S.L.: 1-4 minutes

Elimination: In urine; clearance: 140-320 mL/minute/kg

Usual Dosage Note: Hemodynamic and antianginal tolerance often develop within 24-48 hours of continuous nitrate administration

Children: Pulmonary hypertension: Continuous infusion: Start 0.25-0.5 mcg/kg/minute and titrate by 1 mcg/kg/minute at 20- to 60-minute intervals to desired effect; usual dose: 1-3 mcg/kg/minute; maximum: 5 mcg/kg/minute

Adults:

Buccal: Initial: 1 mg every 3-5 hours while awake (3 times/day); titrate dosage upward if angina occurs with tablet in place

Oral: 2.5-9 mg 2-4 times/day (up to 26 mg 4 times/day)

I.V.: 5 mcg/minute, increase by 5 mcg/minute every 3-5 minutes to 20 mcg/minute; if no response at 20 mcg/minute increase by 10 mcg/minute every 3-5 minutes, up to 200 mcg/minute

Ointment: 1" to 2" every 8 hours up to 4" to 5" every 4 hours

Patch, transdermal: Initial: 0.2-0.4 mg/hour, titrate to doses of 0.4-0.8 mg/hour; tolerance is minimized by using a patch-on period of 12-14 hours and patch-off period of 10-12 hours

Sublingual: 0.2-0.6 mg every 5 minutes for maximum of 3 doses in 15 minutes; may also use prophylactically 5-10 minutes prior to activities which may provoke an attack

Translingual: 1-2 sprays into mouth under tongue every 3-5 minutes for maximum of 3 doses in 15 minutes, may also be used 5-10 minutes prior to activities which may provoke an attack prophylactically

May need to use nitrate-free interval (10-12 hours/day) to avoid tolerance development; tolerance may possibly be reversed with acetylcysteine; gradually decrease dose in patients receiving NTG for prolonged period to avoid withdrawal reaction

Contraindications Hypersensitivity to nitroglycerin or any component; glaucoma; severe anemia

Warnings Do not chew or swallow sublingual dosage form; do not use extended release preparations in patients with gastrointestinal hypermotility or malabsorptive syndrome; use with caution in patients with hypovolemia, constrictive pericarditis, hypertension, and hypotension; use with caution in patients with increased intracranial pressure

Dosage Forms

Capsule, sustained release: 2.5 mg, 6.5 mg, 9 mg

Injection: 0.5 mg/mL (10 mL); 0.8 mg/mL (10 mL); 5 mg/mL (1 mL, 5 mL, 10 mL, 20 mL); 10 mg/mL (5 mL, 10 mL)

Ointment, topical (Nitrol®): 2% [20 mg/g] (30 g, 60 g)

Patch, transdermal, topical: Systems designed to deliver 2.5, 5, 7.5, 10, or 15 mg NTG over 24 hours

Spray, translingual: 0.4 mg/metered spray (13.8 g)

Tablet:

Buccal, controlled release: 1 mg, 2 mg, 3 mg

Sublingual (Nitrostat®): 0.15 mg, 0.3 mg, 0.4 mg, 0.6 mg

Sustained release: 2.6 mg, 6.5 mg, 9 mg

Stability I.V. infusion solution in NS or D_5W, is stable for 48 hours at room temperature, mixed and stored in glass containers; maximum concentration not to exceed 400 mcg/mL; do not mix with other drugs; store sublingual tablets and ointment in tightly closed container; store at 15°C to 30°C

Reference Range Concentrations of 1.2-11.0 ng/mL produce 25% decrease in capillary wedge pressure

Overdosage Treatment

Supportive therapy: Keep patient recumbent; elevate legs if needed; hypotension is treated with fluids and alpha-adrenergic pressors if needed; methylene blue treatment for methemoglobin

Enhancement of elimination: Forced diuresis may enhance elimination

Antidote(s)

Methylene Blue *on page 1444*

Test Interactions Increases catecholamines (U)

Diagnostic Tests/Procedures

Methemoglobin, Blood *on page 1296*

Drug Interactions I.V. nitroglycerin may antagonize the anticoagulant effect of heparin, monitor closely, may need to decrease heparin dosage when nitroglycerin is discontinued; alcohol, beta-blockers, calcium channel blockers may enhance nitroglycerin's hypotensive effect

Pregnancy Risk Factor C

Monitoring Parameters Blood pressure, heart rate

Patient Information Go to hospital if no relief after 3 sublingual doses; do not swallow or chew sublingual form

Nursing Implications I.V. must be prepared in glass bottles and use special sets intended for nitroglycerin; transdermal patches labeled as mg/hour

Additional Information I.V. preparations contain alcohol and/or propylene glycol; may need to use nitrate-free internal (10-12 hours/day) to avoid tolerance development; tolerance may possibly be reversed with acetylcysteine; gradually decrease dose in patients receiving NTG for prolonged period to avoid withdrawal reaction; monitor for ethanol toxicity due to diluent TLV-TWA 0.05 ppm; sweet, burning taste; tablets are not explosive. **Note**: Nitroglycerin tabs is a slang for heroin with intravenous nitroglycerin.

Specific References

Buckley R and Roberts R, "Symptomatic Bradycardia Following the Administration of Sublingual Nitroglycerin," *Am J Emerg Med*, 1993, 11(3):253-5.

Ehrenpreis ED, Young MA, and Leikin JB, "Symptomatic Nitroglycerin Toxicity From Erroneous Use of Topical Nitroglycerin," *Vet Hum Toxicol*, 1990, 32(2):138-9.

Khan AH and Carleton RA, "Nitroglycerin-Induced Hypotension and Bradycardia," *Arch Intern Med*, 1981, 141(8):984.

Marshall JB and Ecklund RE, "Methemoglobinemia From Overdose of Nitroglycerin," *JAMA*, 1980, 244(4):330.

Nitroglycerol *see* Nitroglycerin *on previous page*

Nitroglyn® *see* Nitroglycerin *on previous page*

Nitrol® *see* Nitroglycerin *on previous page*

Nitrolan® *see* Nitroglycerin *on previous page*

Nitrolingual® *see* Nitroglycerin *on previous page*

Nitrong® *see* Nitroglycerin *on previous page*

Nitropress® *see* Nitroprusside Sodium *on next page*

Nitroprussiat® *see* Nitroprusside Sodium *on this page*

Nitroprusside Sodium (nye troe pruss' ide)

CAS Number 13755-38-9; 14402-89-2

Brand Names Hypoten®; Nipride®; Nipruss®; Nitropress®; Nitroprussiat®

Synonyms Sodium Nitroferricyanide; Sodium Nitroprusside

Use Management of hypertensive crises especially due to ergotism; congestive heart failure; used for controlled hypotension to reduce bleeding during surgery

Mechanism of Action Causes peripheral vasodilation by direct action on venous and arteriolar smooth muscle, thus reducing peripheral resistance; will increase cardiac output by decreasing afterload; reduces aortal and left ventricular impedance

Adverse Reactions

- Cardiovascular: Excessive hypotensive response, palpitations, tachycardia followed by bradycardia
- Central nervous system: Restlessness, asthenia, disorientation, psychosis, increased intracranial hypertension, headache, delirium
- Endocrine & metabolic: Thyroid suppression, thiocyanate toxicity, hypothyroidism
- Gastrointestinal: Nausea, vomiting, adynamic ileus
- Hematologic: Thrombocytopenia
- Local: Transient phlebitis
- Neuromuscular & skeletal: Muscle spasm
- Otic: Ototoxicity, tinnitus
- Respiratory: Substernal distress, hypoxia, tachypnea
- Miscellaneous: Sweating

Signs & Symptoms of Acute Overdose Hypotension, vomiting, azotemia, methemoglobinemia, confusion, hypothyroidism, hyperventilation, bradycardia, muscular myoclonus, metabolic acidosis

Toxicodynamics/Kinetics

- Onset of action: Hypotensive effects occur in <2 minutes; following discontinuation of therapy, effects cease within 1-10 minutes
- Metabolism: Converted to cyanide by erythrocyte and tissue sulfhydryl group interactions; cyanide is converted in the liver by rhodanese to thiocyanate
- Half-life: <10 minutes; thiocyanate: 2.7-7 days (9 days in renal failure patients)
- Elimination: In urine

Usual Dosage I.V.:

- Children: Continuous infusion:
  - Initial: 1 mcg/kg/minute by continuous I.V. infusion; increase in increments of 1 mcg/kg/minute at intervals of 20-60 minutes; titrating to the desired response
  - Usual dose: 3 mcg/kg/minute; rarely need >4 mcg/kg/minute
  - Maximum (short term): 10 mcg/kg/minute. Dilute 15 mg x weight (kg) to 250 mL D_5W, then dose in mcg/kg/minute = infusion rate in mL/hour
- Adults: Begin at 2 mcg/kg/minute; increase in increments of 2-4 mcg/kg/minute (up to 20 mcg/kg/minute), then in increments of 10-20 mcg/kg/minute; titrating to the desired hemodynamic effect or the appearance of headache or nausea. When >500 mcg/kg is administered by prolonged infusion of faster than 2 mcg/kg/minute, cyanide is generated faster than an unaided patient can handle.
- Cyanide risk for for nitroprusside administration:
  - Low risk:
    - Short term (<8 hours) administration: 1.5 mg/kg total dose
    - Long term (>8 hours) administration: 2-4 mcg/kg/minute (at a dose of 5-10 mcg/kg/minute, cyanide toxicity can result in 5-10 hours)
  - Thiocyanide toxicity usually does **not** occur at total nitroprusside doses <70 mg/kg

Contraindications Hypersensitivity to nitroprusside or components; decreased cerebral perfusion; arteriovenous shunt or coarctation of the aorta (ie, compensatory hypertension)

Warnings Use only as an infusion with 5% dextrose in water; continuously monitor patient's blood pressure; excessive amounts of nitroprusside can cause cyanide toxicity (usually in patients with decreased liver function) or thiocyanate toxicity (usually in patients with decreased renal function, or in patients with normal renal function but prolonged nitroprusside use); use with caution in patients with increased intracranial pressure (head trauma, cerebral hemorrhage); severe renal impairment, hepatic failure, hypothyroidism, hyponatremia. Due to low endogenous thiosulfate production, postoperative patients receiving coronary artery bypass graft may be at risk for cyanide toxicity.

Dosage Forms Injection: 10 mg/mL (5 mL); 25 mg/mL (2 mL)

Stability Discard solution 24 hours after reconstitution and dilution in D_5W; promptly wrap in aluminum foil or other opaque material to protect from sunlight (incandescent light is safe); reconstituted solution should be very faint brown, discard if highly colored (blue, green or red); store powder in carton until use

Reference Range Cyanide levels

Whole blood levels: Smoker: ≤0.5 mg/L

Flushing and tachycardia seen at 0.5-1.0 mg/L; obtundation at 1.0-2.5 mg/L

Coma and death occur at >2.5 mg/L

Can also monitor thiocyanate levels if requiring prolonged infusion (>4 days) or ≥4 μg/kg/minute; therapeutic: 6-29 μg/mL (SI: 103-499 μmol/L)

Overdosage Treatment

Supportive therapy: Thiocyanate toxicity includes psychosis, tremor, delirium, hypothyroidism, hyperreflexia, confusion, asthenia, tinnitus, and coma; no metabolic acidosis is noted with thiocyanate toxicity; cyanide toxicity includes acidosis (decreased HCO_3, decreased pH, increased lactate), increase in mixed venous blood oxygen tension, tachycardia, altered consciousness, seizures, and almond smell on breath. Nitroprusside has been shown to release cyanide *in vivo* with hemoglobin. Cyanide toxicity does not usually occur because of the rapid uptake of cyanide by erythrocytes and its eventual incorporation into cyanocobalamin. However, prolonged administration of nitroprusside or its reduced elimination can lead to cyanide intoxication. In these situations, airway support with oxygen therapy is germane, followed closely with antidotal therapy of amyl nitrate perles, sodium nitrate 300 mg I.V. (10 mg/kg for children) and sodium thiosulfate 12.5 g I.V. (1.5 mL/kg for children). Sodium bicarbonate (1 mEq/kg) for treatment of acidosis; hydroxocobalamin or cobalt EDTA (Kelocyanor®) may also be effective against cyanide toxicity. Cyanide toxicity can be prevented by coadministration with hydroxocobalamin (2.4 g or 80 vials of hydroxocobalamin for every 100 mg of nitroprusside) or more practically with coadministration with sodium thiosulfate (1 g of sodium thiosulfate for every 100 mg of nitroprusside).

Enhancement of elimination: Hemodialysis may be effective when used in conjunction with above therapy

Antidote(s)

Cyanide Antidote Kit *on page 1406*

Hydroxocobalamin *on page 1433*

Diagnostic Tests/Procedures

Cyanide, Blood *on page 1246*

Drug Interactions May prolong the fibrinolytic activity of alteplase

Pregnancy Risk Factor C

Pregnancy Implications May decrease uterine blood flow by 25% to 35%

Monitoring Parameters Blood pressure, cardiac status, arterial blood gases, calculated and measured oxygen saturation, cyanide and thiocyanate levels

Nursing Implications I.V. infusion only, not for direct injection; protect from light; brownish solution is usable, discard if bluish in color

Additional Information Nitroprusside is converted to cyanide ions by the endothelium in the bloodstream; decomposes to prussic acid which in the presence of sulfur donor is converted to thiocyanate (liver and kidney rhodanase systems); thiocyanate is then renally eliminated

Specific References

Burke TG and Mutnick AH, "Treatment of Cyanide and Thiocyanate Toxicity Secondary to Sodium Nitroprusside," *J Pharm Technol*, 1994, 10:207-9.

Cohn JN and Burke LP, "Nitroprusside," *Ann Intern Med*, 1979, 91(5):752-7.

Harmon C and Wohlreich MM, "Sodium Nitroprusside-Induced Delirium," *Psychosomatics*, 1995, 36(1):83-5.

Palmer RF and Lasseter KC, "Drug Therapy: Sodium Nitroprusside," *N Engl J Med*, 1975, 292(6):294-7.

Schulz V, "Clinical Pharmacokinetics of Nitroprusside, Cyanide, Thiosulfate, and Thiocyanate," *Clin Pharmacokinet*, 1984, 9(3):239-51.

Vesey CJ and Cole PV, "Blood Cyanide and Thiocyanate Concentrations Produced by Long-Term Therapy With Sodium Nitroprusside," *Br J Anaesth*, 1985, 57(2):148-55.

Walters BN, "Urgent Treatment of Acute Hypertension," *Br J Hosp Med*, 1984, 31(1):49-52.

Wesson DE, Foley R, Sabatini S, et al, "Treatment of Acute Cyanide Intoxication With Hemodialysis," *Am J Nephrol*, 1985, 5(2):121-6.

Nitrospan® *see* Nitroglycerin *on page 566*

Nitrostat® *see* Nitroglycerin *on page 566*

Nitrozepamum *see* Nitrazepam *on page 562*

Nivadipine *see* Nilvadipine *on page 560*

Nix™ [OTC] *see* Permethrin *on page 608*

Nizatidine (ni za' ti deen)

CAS Number 76963-41-3

Brand Names Axid®; Calmaxid®; Nizax®

Replaces LY-139037

Use Treatment and maintenance of duodenal ulcer

Mechanism of Action Nizatidine is an H_2-receptor antagonist. In healthy volunteers, nizatidine has been effective in suppressing gastric acid secretion induced

(Continued)

Nizatidine *(Continued)*

by pentagastrin infusion or food. Nizatidine reduces gastric acid secretion by 29.4% to 78.4%. This compares with a 60.3% reduction by cimetidine. Nizatidine 100 mg is reported to provide equivalent acid suppression as cimetidine 300 mg. There has been a significant correlation between plasma nizatidine concentrations and gastric acid suppression, although not always reliable. Following a single oral nighttime dose of nizatidine 300 mg, acid suppression has been shown to last at least 10 hours. Although there does appear to be a correlation between acid suppression and ulcer healing, the relationship dose not always hold. The amount of nighttime acid secretion is believed to be an important factor in the development of ulcer disease. Thus, the inhibition of nocturnal acid secretion may be an important consideration in the therapy of duodenal ulcers. In comparison with placebo, nizatidine doses of 150 mg or 300 mg at bedtime reduce nighttime hydrogen ion concentration by 70% and 79% respectively. Cimetidine 800 mg at bedtime and ranitidine 300 mg at bedtime reduce nocturnal acid secretion by 76% and 95% respectively. These differences are not significant.

Adverse Reactions

Cardiovascular: Chest pain
Central nervous system: Somnolence, CNS depression, dizziness, headache
Dermatologic: Urticaria
Hematologic: Leukocytosis, eosinophilia, thrombocytopenia
Hepatic: Hepatic failure
Neuromuscular & skeletal: Myalgia
Renal: Renal failure
Miscellaneous: Sweating

Signs & Symptoms of Acute Overdose Muscular tremors, vomiting, impotence, dyspepsia, rapid respiration

Toxicodynamics/Kinetics

Distribution: V_d: 0.7-1.7 L/kg
Protein binding: 27% to 43%
Metabolism: In liver to N-demethylated metabolite (active)
Half-life, elimination: 1.3 hours
Elimination: Renal (50% unchanged)

Usual Dosage Adults: Active duodenal ulcer: Oral:

Treatment: 300 mg at bedtime or 150 mg twice daily
Maintenance: 150 mg/day

Dosing adjustment in renal impairment:

Cl_{cr} 50-80 mL/minute: Administer 75% of normal dose
Cl_{cr} 10-50 mL/minute: Administer 50% of normal dose or 150 mg/day for active treatment and 150 mg every other day for maintenance treatment
Cl_{cr} <10 mL/minute: Administer 25% of normal dose or 150 mg every other day for treatment and 150 mg every 3 days for maintenance treatment

Warnings Use with caution in children <12 years of age; use with caution in patients with liver and renal impairment; dosage modification required in patients with renal impairment

Dosage Forms Capsule: 150 mg, 300 mg

Overdosage Treatment

Decontamination: Ipecac or lavage/activated charcoal with cathartic
Supportive therapy: Treatment is primarily symptomatic and supportive
Enhancement of elimination: Multiple dosing of activated charcoal may be useful

Test Interactions False-positive urine protein using Multistix®, gastric acid secretion test, skin tests allergen extracts, serum creatinine and serum transaminase concentrations, urine protein test

Drug Interactions Decreased absorption of chlorpromazine

Pregnancy Risk Factor C

Pregnancy Implications No animal teratogenic effects at 1500 mg/kg/day

Patient Information It may take several days before this medicine begins to relieve stomach pain; antacids may be taken with ranitidine unless your physician has told you not to use them; wait 30-60 minutes between taking the antacid and ranitidine; avoid aspirin, cough and cold preparations; avoid use of black pepper, caffeine, alcohol, and harsh spices; may cause drowsiness or impair coordination and judgment

Nursing Implications Giving dose at 6 PM may better suppress nocturnal acid secretion than 10 PM

Additional Information LD_{50} ~80 mg/kg

Specific References

Callaghan JT, Bergstrom RF, Rubin A, et al, "A Pharmacokinetic Profile of Nizatidine in Man," *Scand J Gastroenterol Suppl*, 1987, 136:9-17.
Chey WD, Kochman ML, Traber PG, et al, "Possible Nizatidine-Induced Subfulminant Hepatic Failure," *J Clin Gastroenterol*, 1995, 20:164-7.
Knadler MP, Bergstrom RF, Callaghan JT, et al, "Nizatidine, An H_2-Blocker. Its Metabolism and Disposition in Man," *Drug Metab Dispos Biol Fate Chem*, 1986, 14(2):175-82.
Sullivan TJ, Reese JH, Buchmann KA, et al, "Bioavailability Study of Nizatidine When Administered in Food," *Am J Ther*, 1995, 2:275-8.

Vargas R, Ryan J, McMahon G, et al, "Pharmacokinetics and Pharmacodynamics of Oral Nizatidine," *J Clin Pharmacol*, 1988, 28(1):71-5.

Nizax® *see* Nizatidine *on page 569*
Nizoral® *see* Ketoconazole *on page 453*
Nostrilla® [OTC] *see* Oxymetazoline Hydrochloride *on page 586*
NaSal™ [OTC] *see* Sodium Chloride *on page 698*
N-methylhydrazine *see* Procarbazine Hydrochloride *on page 645*
NO *see* Nitric Oxide *on page 563*
Noctec® *see* Chloral Hydrate *on page 193*
No-Doz® [OTC] *see* Caffeine *on page 175*
Nofrin® *see* Cinoxacin *on page 214*
Nogram® *see* Nalidixic Acid *on page 547*
Noiafren® *see* Clobazam *on page 224*
Noludar® *see* Methyprylon *on page 522*
Nolvadex® Oral *see* Tamoxifen Citrate *on page 722*
Nonsteroidal Anti-Inflammatory Comparison *see page 1655*
Norcristine® *see* Vincristine Sulfate *on page 792*
Nordeoxyguanosine *see* Ganciclovir *on page 377*
Norflex® *see* Orphenadrine Citrate *on page 581*
Norglycin® *see* Tolazamide *on page 756*
Noriel® *see* Flunitrazepam *on page 354*
Normal Saline *see* Sodium Chloride *on page 698*
Normi-Nox® *see* Methaqualone Hydrochloride *on page 511*
Normison® *see* Temazepam *on page 724*
Normodyne® *see* Labetalol Hydrochloride *on page 458*
Normoglic® *see* Chlorpropamide *on page 207*
Normortmin® *see* Propafenone Hydrochloride *on page 652*
Normurat® *see* Benzbromarone *on page 148*
Norocaine® *see* Lidocaine Hydrochloride *on page 468*
Norpace® *see* Disopyramide Phosphate *on page 294*
Norpamin® *see* Desipramine Hydrochloride *on page 263*
Norpramin® *see* Imipramine *on page 422*
Nor-tet® Oral *see* Tetracycline *on page 732*
Nortimil® *see* Desipramine Hydrochloride *on page 263*
Nortrilen® *see* Nortriptyline Hydrochloride *on this page*

Nortriptyline Hydrochloride (nor trip' ti leen)

CAS Number 72-69-5; 894-71-3

Brand Names Allegron®; Aventyl® Hydrochloride; Nortrilen®; Norval®; Pamelor®

Use Treatment of various forms of depression, often in conjunction with psychotherapy

Mechanism of Action Increases the synaptic concentration of serotonin and/or norepinephrine in the central nervous system by inhibition of their reuptake by the presynaptic neuronal membrane

Adverse Reactions

- Cardiovascular: Postural hypotension, cardiac arrhythmias, tachycardia, sudden death
- Central nervous system: Sedation, restlessness, asthenia, fatigue, anxiety, psychosis, impaired cognitive function, and seizures have occurred occasionally
- Endocrine & metabolic: Syndrome of inappropriate antidiuretic hormone
- Gastrointestinal: Dry mouth, constipation, adynamic ileus
- Genitourinary: Urinary retention
- Hematologic: Rarely agranulocytosis, eosinophilia, porphyria
- Hepatic: Jaundice
- Neuromuscular & skeletal: Tremors
- Ocular: Blurred vision, photophobia, intraocular pressure (increased), mydriasis, nystagmus
- Respiratory: Hyperventilation
- Miscellaneous: Allergic reactions, porphyrinogenic

Signs & Symptoms of Acute Overdose Agitation, dental erosion, photosensitivity, insomnia, impotence, dysphagia, bone marrow depression, mania, intraocular

(Continued)

Nortriptyline Hydrochloride *(Continued)*

pressure (increased), ejaculatory disturbances, memory loss, A-V block, dementia, depression, delirium, thrombocytopenia, night terrors, hypoglycemia, confusion, heart block, hyponatremia, visual hallucinations, hyperthermia, respiratory depression, pulmonary edema, urinary retention, coma, hypothermia, hypotension, tachycardia, P-R prolongation, QRS prolongation, Q-T prolongation, measurement of QRS interval >0.10 seconds, may indicate significant toxicity; seizures within 3 hours of ingestion, leukopenia; neutropenia; agranulocytosis; granulocytopenia

Toxicodynamics/Kinetics

Peak effect: Maximal antidepressant effects may not occur for 2 weeks or more after therapy is begun

Absorption: Oral: Rapidly and well after administration

Distribution: V_d: 21 L/kg; widely distributed into body including CNS and breast milk

Protein binding: 93% to 95%

Metabolism: Undergoes significant first-pass metabolism; primarily detoxified in the liver

Half-life: 28-31 hours

Time to peak serum concentration: Within 7-8½ hours

Elimination: Excreted as metabolites and small amounts of unchanged drug in urine; small amounts of biliary elimination occurs

Usual Dosage Oral:

Nocturnal enuresis: Children:

- 6-7 years (20-25 kg): 10 mg/day
- 8-11 years (25-35 kg): 10-20 mg/day
- >11 years (35-54 kg): 25-35 mg/day

Depression: Adults: 25 mg 3-4 times/day up to 150 mg/day

Elderly and Adolescents: 30-50 mg/day in divided doses

Dosing adjustment in hepatic impairment: Lower doses and slower titration dependent on individualization of dosage is recommended

Contraindications Narrow-angle glaucoma, avoid use during pregnancy and lactation

Warnings Safe use of tricyclic antidepressants in children <12 years of age has not been established; nortriptyline should not be abruptly discontinued in patients receiving high doses for prolonged periods; do not drink alcoholic beverages; use with caution in patients with cardiac conduction disturbances, history of hyperthyroid; generic formulations may result in higher plasma levels

Dosage Forms

Capsule: 10 mg, 25 mg, 50 mg, 75 mg

Solution: 10 mg/5 mL (473 mL)

Stability Protect from light

Reference Range

Therapeutic: 50-150 ng/mL (SI: 190-570 nmol/L)

Toxic: >500 ng/mL (SI: >1900 nmol/L)

Overdosage Treatment

Decontamination: Lavage within 90 minutes/activated charcoal with cathartic; multiple dosing of activated charcoal would be expected to be useful

Supportive therapy: Following initiation of essential overdose management, toxic symptoms should be treated. Ventricular arrhythmias often respond to phenytoin 15-20 mg/kg (adults) with concurrent systemic alkalinization (sodium bicarbonate 0.5-2 mEq/kg I.V.). Titrate to a serum pH of 7.45-7.55. Arrhythmias unresponsive to this therapy may respond to lidocaine 1 mg/kg I.V. followed by a titrated infusion. Physostigmine (1-2 mg I.V. slowly for adults or 0.5 mg I.V. slowly for children) may be indicated for anticholinergic seizures or movement disorders, but only as **a last resort**. Propranolol may also be utilized for supraventricular arrhythmias (rate: >160) at 1 mg/minute to a maximum of 5 mg in adults; pediatric dosage of 0.1 mg/kg/dose to 1 mg I.V.. Seizures usually respond to lorazepam or diazepam I.V. boluses (5-10 mg for adults up to 30 mg or 0.25-0.4 mg/kg/dose for children up to 10 mg/dose). If seizures are unresponsive or recur, phenytoin or phenobarbital may be required. Patients must be monitored for at least 24 hours if any signs or symptoms are exhibited. Do not induce emesis; flumazenil is contraindicated.

Antidote(s)

Sodium Bicarbonate *on page 1467*

Test Interactions Increases glucose; elevates plasma norepinephrine levels and plasma epinephrine levels threefold to fivefold; EMIT assays may give false-positive in presence of diphenhydramine, thioridazine, chlorpromazine, alimenazine, carbamazepine, cyclobenzaprine, or perphenazine

Diagnostic Tests/Procedures

Nortriptyline, Blood *on page 1309*

Drug Interactions

Nortriptyline blocks the uptake of guanethidine and thus prevents the hypotensive effect of guanethidine; nortriptyline may be additive with or may potentiate the action of other CNS depressants such as sedatives or hypnotics; nortriptyline potentiates the pressor and cardiac effects of sympathomimetic agents such as isoproterenol, epinephrine, etc

With MAO inhibitors, fever, hypertension, tachycardia, confusion, seizures, and death have been reported

Additive anticholinergic effects seen with other anticholinergic agents

Cimetidine reduces hepatic metabolism of nortriptyline

Nortriptyline may increase the prothrombin time in patients stabilized on warfarin

Pregnancy Risk Factor D

Pregnancy Implications Distributes into breast milk

Monitoring Parameters EKG, cardiac monitoring

Patient Information Avoid alcohol ingestion; do not discontinue medication abruptly; may cause drowsiness

Nursing Implications Offer patient sugarless hard candy for dry mouth

Additional Information Maximum antidepressant effect may not be seen for 2 or more weeks after initiation of therapy

Specific References

Boehnert MT and Lovejoy FH Jr, "Value of the QRS Duration Versus the Serum Drug Level in Predicting Seizures and Ventricular Arrhythmias After an Acute Overdose of Tricyclic Antidepressants," *N Engl J Med*, 1985, 313(8):474-9.

Frommer DA, Kulig KW, Marx JA, et al, "Tricyclic Antidepressant Overdose," *JAMA*, 1987, 257(4):521-6.

Lipper B and Gaynor BD, "Value of Serum Tricyclic Antidepressant Levels With Massive Nortriptyline Overdose and Persistent Hypotension," *Am J Emerg Med*, 1995, 13(1):107.

Sunderrajan S, Brooks CS, and Sunderrajan EV, "Nortriptyline-Induced Severe Hyperventilation," *Arch Intern Med*, 1985, 145(4):746-7.

Tokarski GF and Young MJ, "Criteria for Admitting Patients With Tricyclic Antidepressant Overdose," *J Emerg Med*, 1988, 6(2):121-4.

Norval® *see* Mianserin Hydrochloride *on page 529*

Norval® *see* Nortriptyline Hydrochloride *on page 571*

Norzine® *see* Thiethylperazine Maleate *on page 743*

Nose-X® *see* Oxymetazoline Hydrochloride *on page 586*

Nossacin® *see* Cinoxacin *on page 214*

Novafed® *see* Pseudoephedrine *on page 661*

Novanov® *see* Nitrazepam *on page 562*

Novasoxazole® *see* Sulfisoxazole *on page 714*

Noveopen® *see* Penicillin G, Parenteral, Aqueous *on page 600*

Novocain® *see* Procaine Hydrochloride *on page 644*

Novocainamidum *see* Procainamide Hydrochloride *on page 642*

Novocamid® *see* Procainamide Hydrochloride *on page 642*

Novodorm® *see* Triazolam *on page 767*

Novoflurazine® *see* Trifluoperazine Hydrochloride *on page 769*

Novolin® *see* Insulin Preparations *on page 426*

Novomedopa® *see* Methyldopa *on page 519*

Novoridazine® *see* Thioridazine Hydrochloride *on page 745*

Novosemide® *see* Furosemide *on page 373*

Novoxapin® *see* Doxepin Hydrochloride *on page 301*

Novutox® *see* Procaine Hydrochloride *on page 644*

Noxaben® *see* Lorazepam *on page 482*

Noxigram® *see* Cinoxacin *on page 214*

NPH *see* Insulin Preparations *on page 426*

NPH Iletin® I *see* Insulin Preparations *on page 426*

NTG *see* Nitroglycerin *on page 566*

NTZ® Long Acting Nasal Solution [OTC] *see* Oxymetazoline Hydrochloride *on page 586*

Nubain® *see* Nalbuphine Hydrochloride *on page 546*

Nuctalon® *see* Estazolam *on page 324*

Numorphan® *see* Oxymorphone Hydrochloride *on page 587*

Nupercainal® [OTC] *see* Dibucaine *on page 275*

Nupercaine® *see* Dibucaine *on page 275*

Nuprin® [OTC] *see* Ibuprofen *on page 418*

Nuran® *see* Cyproheptadine Hydrochloride *on page 255*

Nydrazid® *see* Isoniazid *on page 443*

Nystatin (nye stat' in)

Related Information

Antifungal Therapy *on page 1496-1497*

CAS Number 1400-61-9

Brand Names Mycostatin®; Mykinac®; Nilstat®; Nystat-Rx®; Nystex®; O-V Staticin®

Use Treatment of susceptible cutaneous, mucocutaneous, and oral cavity fungal infections normally caused by the *Candida* species

Mechanism of Action Binds to sterols in fungal cell membrane, changing the cell wall permeability allowing for leakage of cellular contents

Adverse Reactions Dose of 10,000,000/day can produce mild nausea

Dermatologic: Contact dermatitis

Gastrointestinal: Nausea, vomiting, diarrhea

Local: Irritation

Respiratory: Cough, wheezing

Signs & Symptoms of Acute Overdose Nausea, vomiting, wheezing, Stevens-Johnson syndrome, diarrhea

Toxicodynamics/Kinetics

Absorption: Not absorbed through mucous membranes or intact skin; poorly absorbed from gastrointestinal tract; no detectable amount of drug is systemically available

Distribution: No detectable amount of drug is available for tissue distribution

Elimination: Excreted in feces as unchanged drug

Usual Dosage

Oral candidiasis: Suspension (swish and swallow orally):

- Neonates: 100,000 units 4 times/day or 50,000 units to each side of mouth 4 times/day
- Infants: 200,000 units 4 times/day or 100,000 units to each side of mouth 4 times/day
- Children and Adults: 400,000-600,000 units 4 times/day; troche: 200,000-400,000 units 4-5 times/day

Mucocutaneous infections: Children and Adults: Topical: Apply 2-3 times/day to affected areas; very moist topical lesions are treated best with powder

Intestinal infections: Adults: Oral tablets: 500,000-1,000,000 units every 8 hours

Vaginal infections: Adults: Vaginal tablets: Insert 1 tablet/day at bedtime for 2 weeks

Contraindications Hypersensitivity to nystatin or any component

Dosage Forms

Cream: 100,000 units/g (15 g, 30 g)

Ointment, topical: 100,000 units/g (15 g, 30 g)

Powder, for preparation of oral suspension: 50 million units, 1 billion units, 2 billion units, 5 billion units

Powder, topical: 100,000 units/g (15 g)

Suspension, oral: 100,000 units/mL (5 mL, 60 mL, 480 mL)

Tablet:

- Oral: 500,000 units
- Vaginal: 100,000 units (15 and 30/box with applicator)

Troche: 200,000 units

Stability Keep vaginal inserts in refrigerator; protect from temperature extremes, moisture and light

Reference Range A dose of 2,700,000 units/kg produces a plasma level of 9.8 units/mL; mean salivary levels were 1000 units/mL 2 hours after dissolution of 2 nystatin pastilles (400,000 units)

Overdosage Treatment

Decontamination: Activated charcoal with cathartic if emesis has not already occurred

Supportive therapy: General poison management

Pregnancy Risk Factor B

Patient Information Oral suspension should be swished about the mouth and retained in the mouth for as long as possible (several minutes) before swallowing. For neonates and infants, paint nystatin suspension into recesses of the mouth. Troches must be allowed to dissolve slowly and should not be chewed or swallowed whole.

Additional Information Very moist topical lesions are treated best with powder

Specific References

Wasilewski C Jr, "Allergic Contact Dermatitis From Nystatin," *Arch Dermatol*, 1971, 104(4):437.

Nystat-Rx® *see* Nystatin *on previous page*

Nystex® *see* Nystatin *on previous page*

Obarin® *see* Benzbromarone *on page 148*

Obermine® *see* Phentermine Hydrochloride *on page 619*

Ocean Nasal Mist [OTC] *see* Sodium Chloride *on page 698*

Octamide® *see* Metoclopramide *on page 523*

Octocaine® *see* Lidocaine Hydrochloride *on page 468*

OcuClear® [OTC] *see* Oxymetazoline Hydrochloride *on page 586*

Ocufen® *see* Flurbiprofen Sodium *on page 364*

Ocuflur® *see* Flurbiprofen Sodium *on page 364*

Oculinum® *see* Botulinum Toxin Type A *on page 161*

Ocupress® *see* Carteolol Hydrochloride *on page 188*

Ofloxacin (oh floks' a sin)

CAS Number 83380-47-6

Brand Names Floxin®

Use Quinolone antibiotic for skin and skin structure, lower respiratory and urinary tract infections, and sexually transmitted diseases

Mechanism of Action Ofloxacin, a fluorinated quinolone, is a pyridone carboxylic acid derivative which exerts a broad spectrum antimicrobial effect. Ofloxacin is related to the older quinolone derivatives, nalidixic acid, and oxolinic acid, and to the newer quinolone derivatives, norfloxacin and ciprofloxacin. Other "second generation" quinolones under investigation include pefloxacin, amifloxacin, enoxacin, and acrosoxacin. The primary target of the fluoroquinolones is DNA gyrase (topoisomerase II) an essential bacterial enzyme that maintains the superhelical structure of DNA. DNA gyrase is required for DNA replication and transcription, DNA repair, recombination, and transposition.

Adverse Reactions

Central nervous system: Sleep disorders, psychosis, nervousness

Dermatologic: Pruritus

Gastrointestinal: Decreased appetite

Genitourinary: Vaginal discharge

Neuromuscular & skeletal: Tendon rupture

Miscellaneous: Feces discoloration (greenish gray), feces discoloration (white/speckling)

Signs & Symptoms of Acute Overdose Nausea, vomiting, pseudotumor cerebri, photosensitivity, seizures

Toxicodynamics/Kinetics

Absorption: Well absorbed; administration with food causes only minor alterations in absorption

Distribution: V_d: 2.4-3.5 L/kg

Protein binding: 20%

Half-life, elimination: 5-7.5 hours

Elimination: Excreted primarily unchanged in urine

Usual Dosage

Children >1 year and Adults: Ophthalmic: Instill 1-2 drops in affected eye(s) every 2-4 hours for the first 2 days, then use 4 times/day for an additional 5 days

Adults: Oral, I.V.: 200-400 mg every 12 hours for 7-10 days for most infections or for 6 weeks for prostatitis

Dosing adjustment/interval in renal impairment:

Cl_{cr} 10-50 mL/minute: Administer 50% of normal dose or administer every 24 hours

Cl_{cr} <10 mL/minute: Administer 25% of normal dose or administer 50% of normal dose every 24 hours

Contraindications Hypersensitivity to ofloxacin or other members of the quinolone group such as nalidixic acid, oxolinic acid, cinoxacin, norfloxacin, and ciprofloxacin

Warnings Use with caution in patients with epilepsy or other CNS diseases which could predispose them to seizures; use with caution in patients with renal impairment

Dosage Forms

Injection: 200 mg (50 mL); 400 mg (10 mL, 20 mL, 100 mL)

Solution, ophthalmic: 0.3% (5 mL)

Tablet: 200 mg, 300 mg, 400 mg

Reference Range Overdose of 3 g ofloxacin (I.V.) yielded a peak plasma level of 39.3 μg/mL (patient had been administered 400 mg I.V. every 12 hours for 3 days previously)

(Continued)

Ofloxacin *(Continued)*

Overdosage Treatment

Decontamination: Emesis or lavage/activated charcoal with cathartic

Enhancement of elimination: Multiple dosing of activated charcoal may be effective; not removed by dialysis

Pregnancy Risk Factor C

Patient Information Report any skin rash or other allergic reactions; avoid excessive sunlight; do not take with food; do not take within 2 hours of any products including antacids which contain zinc, magnesium, or aluminum

Specific References

Kohler RB, Arkins N, and Tack KJ, "Accidental Overdose of Intravenous Ofloxacin With Benign Outcome," *Antimicrob Agents Chemother*, 1991, 35(6):1239-40.

Szarfman A, Chen M, and Blum MD, "More on Fluoroquinolone Antibiotics and Tendon Rupture," *N Engl J Med*, 1995, 332(3):193.

Ogast® *see* Lansoprazole *on page 460*

Ogostal® *see* Capreomycin Sulfate *on page 180*

Oil Bleo® *see* Bleomycin Sulfate *on page 158*

Oil Mist *see* Mineral Oil *on page 534*

Oleovitamin A *see* Vitamin A *on page 795*

Oleum Ricini *see* Castor Oil *on page 189*

Omapren® *see* Omeprazole *on this page*

Omeprazole (oh me' pray zol)

CAS Number 73590-58-6

Brand Names Antra®; Audazol®; Gastrolec®; Losec®; Mopral®; Omapren®; Parizal®; Prilosec™

Use Treatment of severe erosive esophagitis (grade 2 or above), diagnosed by endoscopy and treatment of symptomatic gastroesophageal reflux disease (GERD) poorly responsive to customary medical treatment; pathological hypersecretory conditions (Zollinger-Ellison syndrome); peptic ulcer disease

Mechanism of Action A benzimidazole compound prodrug which suppresses gastric acid secretion by inhibiting the parietal cell H+/K+ ATP pump

Adverse Reactions

Cardiovascular: Chest pain, tachycardia, bradycardia, hypertension

Central nervous system: Headache, dizziness, fever, fatigue, malaise, nervousness, asthenia

Dermatologic: Rash, dermatitis exfoliative

Endocrine & metabolic: Weight gain

Gastrointestinal: Diarrhea, nausea, abdominal pain, vomiting, constipation, abdominal swelling, anorexia, irritable colon, flatulence, dry mouth

Genitourinary: Urinary tract infection

Hematologic: Hypoglycemia, anemia, leukocytosis, pancytopenia, agranulocytosis, thrombocytopenia, neutropenia

Neuromuscular & skeletal: Back pain, myalgia, tremors, arthralgia

Respiratory: Cough

Miscellaneous: Lichen spinulosis, acute gout

Signs & Symptoms of Acute Overdose Hypothermia, sedation, depression, dry mouth, hypothermia, hypoglycemia, hyperhidrosis, urinary frequency, angioedema, nephritis, hyponatremia, gynecomastia, gout, dermatitis, confusion, blindness, seizures, hematuria, decreased respiratory rate demonstrated in animals only

Toxicodynamics/Kinetics

Onset of action: 1 hour

Duration of effect: 72 hours

Absorption: 40%

Distribution: V_d: 0.3-0.4 L/kg

Protein binding: 95%

Metabolism: Extensive in the liver

Half-life: 0.5-1.5 hours; 3 hours (liver disease); 5 hours (elderly)

Usual Dosage Oral:

Children: Dosage not established, but a starting dose of 0.7 mg/kg once daily in the morning is recommended; a second dose 12 hours later may be given if necessary; range of effective dosage: 0.7-3.3 mg/kg/day

Adults:

- Active duodenal ulcer: 20 mg/day for 4-8 weeks
- GERD or severe erosive esophagitis: 20 mg/day for 4-8 weeks
- Pathological hypersecretory conditions: 60 mg once daily to start; doses up to 120 mg 3 times/day have been administered; administer daily doses >80 mg in divided doses

Administration Administration via NG tube should be in an acidic juice

Contraindications Known hypersensitivity to omeprazole

Warnings In long-term (2-year) studies in rats, omeprazole produced a dose-related increase in gastric carcinoid tumors. While available endoscopic evaluations and histologic examinations of biopsy specimens from human stomachs have not detected a risk from short-term exposure to omeprazole, further human data on the effect of sustained hypochlorhydria and hypergastrinemia are needed to rule out the possibility of an increased risk for the development of tumors in humans receiving long-term therapy. Bioavailability may be increased in the elderly.

Dosage Forms Capsule: 20 mg

Stability Omeprazole stability is a function of pH; it is rapidly degraded in acidic media, but has acceptable stability under alkaline conditions. Prilosec™ is supplied as capsules for oral administration; each capsule contains 20 mg of omeprazole in the form of enteric coated granules to inhibit omeprazole degradation by gastric acidity; therefore, cannot recommend the extemporaneous preparation of an oral liquid form of Prilosec™ for administration into the stomach through an NG tube.

Overdosage Treatment

Decontamination: Emesis or lavage/activated charcoal

Enhancement of elimination: Multiple dosing of activated charcoal may be effective

Not dialyzable

Test Interactions Increase in gastric levels may result

Drug Interactions

Decreased effect of ketoconazole, itraconazole

Increased levels/toxicity of phenytoin, warfarin, benzodiazepines (oxidatively metabolized); dexamethasone may enhance antiemetic effect

Pregnancy Risk Factor C

Pregnancy Implications No fetotoxic effects known in either humans or animal models

Monitoring Parameters Improvement in gastrointestinal symptoms

Patient Information Take before eating

Nursing Implications Capsule should be swallowed whole; not chewed, crushed, or opened

Additional Information May be effective in preventing nonsteroidal anti-inflammatory drug-induced large gastric ulcers by inhibiting acid secretion; the incidence of side effects in elderly is not different than that of younger adults (≤65 years) despite slight decrease in elimination and increase in bioavailability. No dosage adjustments are necessary for elderly (≥65 years).

Specific References

Andersson T, "Omeprazole Drug Interaction Studies," *Clin Pharmacokinet*, 1991, 21(3):195-212.

Balian JD, Sukhova N, Harris JW, et al, "The Hydroxylation of Omeprazole Correlates With S-Mephenytoin Metabolism: A Population Study," *Clin Pharmacol Ther*, 1995, 57:662-9.

Berardi RR and Dunn-Kucharski VA, "Omeprazole: Defining Its Role in Gastroesophageal Reflux Disease," *Hosp Formul*: 1995, 30:216-25.

Beutler M, Hartmann K, Kuhn M, et al, "Arthralgias on Omeprazole," *BMJ*, 1994, 309(6969):1620.

Carulli MT, Epstein O, and Black CM, "Small Bowel Bacterial Overgrowth and Omeprazole in Patients With Sytemic Sclerosis," *Br J Rheumatol*, 1995, 34(Suppl 1):67.

Carvajal A and Arias LH, "Gynecomastia and Sexual Disorders After the Administration of Omeprazole," *Am J Gastroenterol*, 1995, 90:1028-9.

Coulter DM, "Monitoring of Omeprazole," *N Z Family Physician*, 1995, 22:76-7.

Friedman G, "Omeprazole," *Am J Gastroenterol*, 1987, 82(3):188-91.

Gonzalo FDE, Montagut LB, and Vecina ST, "Exfoliative Dermatitis Related to Omeprazole," *Ann Pharmacother*, 1995, 29:82-3.

Kraus A and Flores-Suarez LF, "Acute Gout Associated With Omeprazole," *Lancet*, 1995, 345(8947):461-2.

Larner AJ and Lendrum R, "Oesophageal Candidiasis After Omeprazole Therapy," *Gut*, 1992, 33(6):860-1.

Lindquist M and Edwards IR, "Endocrine Adverse Effects of Omeprazole," *Br Med J*, 1992, 305(6851):451-2.

Ottinger JP, Stricker BH, Kappelle JW, et al, "Omeprazole-Associated Agranulocytosis," *Eur J Haematol*, 1995, 54:279-80.

Soll AH, Weinstein WM, Kurata J, et al, "Nonsteroidal Anti-inflammatory Drugs and Peptic Ulcer Disease," *Ann Intern Med*, 1991, 114(4):307-19.

Teare JP, Spedding C, Whitehead MW, et al, "Omeprazole and Dry Mouth," *Scand J Gastroenterol*, 1995, 30:216-8.

Omnifin® *see* Clomiphene Citrate *on page 227*

Omnipen® *see* Ampicillin *on page 125*

Omnipen®-N *see* Ampicillin *on page 125*

Omnipres® *see* Amoxapine *on page 119*

Omnopon® *see* Opium Alkaloids (Hydrochlorides) *on page 579*

OMS® *see* Morphine Sulfate *on page 539*

Onco-Carbide® *see* Hydroxyurea *on page 412*

Oncovin® Injection *see* Vincristine Sulfate *on page 792*

Ondansetron (on dan' se tron)

Related Information

Doses and Administration of Several Frequently Used Antiemetic Agents *on page 1641*

CAS Number 99614-02-5; 116002-70-1; 103639-04-9

Brand Names Zofran® Injection; Zofran® Oral

Synonyms Ondansetron Hydrochloride Dihydrate

Use Prevention of postoperative nausea and vomiting; may be prescribed for patients who are refractory to or have severe adverse reactions to standard antiemetic therapy; utilized for prophylaxis of nausea and vomiting in postoperative patients. Ondansetron may be prescribed for young patients (ie, <45 years of age who are more likely to develop extrapyramidal reactions to high-dose metoclopramide) who are to receive highly emetogenic chemotherapeutic agents; see table in Appendix

Ondansetron should not be prescribed prophylactically for chemotherapeutic agents with a low emetogenic potential (eg, bleomycin, busulfan, cyclophosphamide <1000 mg, etoposide, 5-fluorouracil, vinblastine, vincristine)

Mechanism of Action Selective 5-HT_3 receptor antagonist, blocking serotonin, both peripherally on vagal nerve terminals and centrally in the chemoreceptor trigger zone

Adverse Reactions

Cardiovascular: Hypotension in overdose situation

Central nervous system: Sedation, seizures, extrapyramidal reactions, depression

Ocular: Blurred vision

Renal: Dysuria

Miscellaneous: Anaphylactoid reactions with I.V. reactions, pancreatitis

Signs & Symptoms of Acute Overdose Constipation, chest pain, dry mouth, diarrhea, headache, fever, abdominal cramps, jaundice, dizziness, dry mouth, skin rash, weakness, shortness of breath, wheezing, tachycardia, lightheadedness, seizures, rash, hypokalemia, transient elevations in serum levels of aminotransferases and bilirubin

Toxicodynamics/Kinetics

Absorption: Oral: 56%

Plasma protein binding: 70% to 76%

Metabolism: Extensively by hydroxylation, followed by glucuronide, sulfate conjugation, or demethylation

Half-life:

- Children <15 years: 2-3 hours
- Adults: 4 hours

Elimination: Excreted in urine and feces; <10% of parent drug recovered unchanged in urine

Usual Dosage

Oral:

- Children 4-11 years: 4 mg 30 minutes before chemotherapy; repeat 4 and 8 hours after initial dose
- Children >11 years and Adults: 8 mg 30 minutes before chemotherapy; repeat 4 and 8 hours after initial dose or every 8 hours for a maximum of 48 hours

I.V.: Administer either three 0.15 mg/kg doses or a single 32 mg dose; with the 3-dose regimen, the initial dose is given 30 minutes prior to chemotherapy with subsequent doses administered 4 and 8 hours after the first dose. With the single-dose regimen 32 mg is infused over 15 minutes beginning 30 minutes before the start of emetogenic chemotherapy. Dosage should be calculated based on weight:

- Children: Pediatric dosing should follow the manufacturer's guidelines for 0.15 mg/kg/dose administered 30 minutes prior to chemotherapy, 4 and 8 hours after the first dose. While not as yet FDA-approved, literature supports the day's total dose administered as a single dose 30 minutes prior to chemotherapy.
- Adults:
  - >80 kg: 12 mg IVPB
  - 45-80 kg: 8 mg IVPB
  - <45 kg: 0.15 mg/kg/dose IVPB

Dosing in hepatic impairment: Maximum daily dose: 8 mg in cirrhotic patients with severe liver disease

Administration Dilute in 50 mL I.V. fluid (maximum concentration: 0.64 mg/mL) and infuse over 15 minutes

Contraindications Hypersensitivity to ondansetron or any component

Warnings There is no information on dosage in children ≤3 years of age; ondansetron should be used on a scheduled basis, not as an "as needed" (PRN) basis, since data supports the use of this drug in the prevention of nausea and vomiting and not in the rescue of nausea and vomiting. Ondansetron is most effective in the first 24-48 hours of receiving chemotherapy.

Dosage Forms

Injection: 2 mg/mL (20 mL); 32 mg (single-dose vials)

Tablet: 4 mg, 8 mg

Stability The injection may be stored between 36°F and 86°F; stable when mixed in 5% dextrose or 0.9% sodium chloride for 48 hours at room temperature; does not need protection from light

Overdosage Treatment

Decontamination: Lavage/activated charcoal

Supportive therapy: Diphenhydramine can be used to manage pruritus, rashes, extrapyramidal signs (along with benztropine), and restlessness

Drug Interactions Metabolized by the hepatic cytochrome P-450 enzymes; therefore, the drug's clearance and half-life may be changed with concomitant use of cytochrome P-450 inducers (eg, barbiturates, carbamazepine, rifampin, phenytoin, and phenylbutazone) or inhibitors (eg, cimetidine, allopurinol, and disulfiram). Carmustine, etoposide, and cisplatin do not affect the pharmacokinetics of ondansetron in humans. Dexamethasone may enhance its antiemetic effects.

Pregnancy Risk Factor B

Monitoring Parameters Frequency of emesis

Patient Information May cause diarrhea and headache

Nursing Implications First dose should be given 30 minutes prior to beginning chemotherapy

Additional Information I.V. product has been successful when used orally; elderly have a slightly decreased hepatic clearance rate; this does not, however, require a dose adjustment. Not effective in preventing motion sickness; more effective than metoclopramide in preventing emesis in cisplatin treatment; may be useful in treating acetaminophen-induced or theophylline-induced vomiting.

Specific References

Alberti-Flor JJ, "Pancreatitis Associated With Ondansetron," *J Natl Cancer Inst*, 1995, 87:689-90.

Chaffee BJ and Tankanow RM, "Ondansetron – the First of a New Class of Antiemetic Agents," *Clin Pharm*, 1991, 10(6):430-6.

Chung KC, Moon YS, Chin A, et al, "Compatibility of Ondansetron Hydrochloride and Piperacillen Sodium-Tazobactam Sodium During Simulated Y-Site Administration," *Am J Health-Syst Pharm*, 1995, 52:1554-6.

Kirkham JC, Rutherford ET, Cunningham GN, et al, "Stability of Ondansetron Hydrochloride in a Tital Parental Nutrient Admixture," *Am J Health-Syst Pharm*, 1995, 52:1557-8.

Krstenansky PM, Petree J, and Long G, "Extrapyramidal Reaction Caused by Ondansetron," *Ann Pharmacother*, 1994, 28(2):280.

Milne RJ and Heel RC, "Ondansetron: Therapeutic Use as an Antiemetic," *Drugs*, 1991, 41(4):574-95.

Oren DA, "Dysphoria After Treatment With Ondansetron," *Am J Psychiatry*, 1995, 152:1101.

Sargent AI, Deppe SA, and Chan FA, "Seizure Associated With Ondansetron," *Clin Pharm*, 1993, 12(8):613-5.

Weissbach L, "Ondansetron," *Lancet*, 1991, 338:753.

Ondansetron Hydrochloride Dihydrate *see* Ondansetron *on previous page*

Operand® [OTC] *see* Povidone-Iodine *on page 635*

Ophthochlor® Ophthalmic *see* Chloramphenicol *on page 196*

Opialum *see* Opium Alkaloids (Hydrochlorides) *on this page*

Opiran® *see* Pimozide *on page 626*

Opium Alkaloids (Hydrochlorides) (oh' pee um)

Brand Names Escopon®; Omnopon®; Pantopon®

Synonyms Opialum; Papaveretum

Use Relief of severe pain

Adverse Reactions

Cardiovascular: Palpitation, hypotension, bradycardia, peripheral vasodilation

Central nervous system: CNS depression

Dermatologic: Pruritus

Endocrine & metabolic: Syndrome of inappropriate antidiuretic hormone (SIADH)

Gastrointestinal: Nausea, vomiting, constipation (more constipating than morphine)

Ocular: Miosis

Respiratory: Apnea, respiratory depression

Miscellaneous: Intracranial pressure (increased), physical and psychological dependence, histamine release, biliary or urinary tract spasm

Signs & Symptoms of Acute Overdose Apnea, delirium, dysphoria, respiratory depression, rhabdomyolysis, hypotension, ptosis, seizures (in neonates), myoglobinuria, coma, miosis, pulmonary edema

(Continued)

Opium Alkaloids (Hydrochlorides) *(Continued)*

Toxicodynamics/Kinetics

Absorption: Oral: Variable, more slowly absorbed than morphine

Distribution: V_d: 3-4 L/kg

Protein binding: 35%

Metabolism: In the liver via glucuronide conjugation

Half-life:

Neonates: Prolonged 6% to 10%

Adults: 2-4 hours

Elimination: Excreted unchanged in urine

Usual Dosage Adults: I.M., S.C.: 5-20 mg every 4-5 hours

Contraindications Known hypersensitivity to opium alkaloids

Dosage Forms Injection: 20 mg/mL (1 mL)

Overdosage Treatment Supportive therapy: Naloxone hydrochloride (0.4-2 mg I.V., S.C., or through an endotracheal tube); a continuous infusion (at ⅔ the response dose/hour) may be required

Antidote(s)

Naloxone Hydrochloride *on page 1447*

Pregnancy Risk Factor B (D if used for prolonged periods or in high doses at term)

Specific References

Robinson LQ and Stephenson TP, "Self Injection Treatment for Impotence," *BMJ*, 1989, 299(6715):1568.

Opium and Belladonna *see* Belladonna and Opium *on page 145*

Opium Tincture (oh' pee um)

Synonyms Deodorized Opium Tincture; DTO; Laudanum

Use Treatment of diarrhea or relief of pain

Mechanism of Action Contains many narcotic alkaloids including morphine; its mechanism for gastric motility inhibition is primarily due to this morphine content; it results in a decrease in digestive secretions, an increase in gastrointestinal muscle tone, and therefore a reduction in gastrointestinal propulsion

Adverse Reactions

Cardiovascular: Palpitations, hypotension, bradycardia, peripheral vasodilation

Central nervous system: CNS depression

Dermatologic: Pruritus

Endocrine & metabolic: Syndrome of inappropriate antidiuretic hormone (SIADH)

Gastrointestinal: Nausea, vomiting, constipation

Ocular: Miosis

Respiratory: Apnea, respiratory depression

Miscellaneous: Intracranial pressure (increased), physical and psychological dependence, histamine release, biliary or urinary tract spasm

Signs & Symptoms of Acute Overdose Apnea, respiratory depression, myasthenia gravis (exacerbation or precipitation of), ptosis, rhabdomyolysis, hypotension, seizures (in neonates), myoglobinuria, coma, miosis, pulmonary edema

Toxicodynamics/Kinetics

Duration of effect: 4-5 hours

Absorption: Variable from gastrointestinal tract

Metabolism: In the liver

Elimination: Eliminated in urine

Usual Dosage Oral:

Children:

Diarrhea: 0.005-0.01 mL/kg/dose every 3-4 hours for a maximum of 6 doses/24 hours

Analgesia: 0.01-0.02 mL/kg/dose every 3-4 hours

Adults:

Diarrhea: 0.3-1 mL/dose every 2-6 hours to maximum of 6 mL/24 hours

Analgesia: 0.6-1.5 mL/dose every 3-4 hours

Contraindications Increased intracranial pressure, severe respiratory depression, severe liver or renal insufficiency, known hypersensitivity to morphine sulfate

Warnings Opium shares the toxic potential of opiate agonists, and usual precautions of opiate agonist therapy should be observed; some preparations contain sulfites which may cause allergic reactions; infants <3 months of age are more susceptible to respiratory depression, use with caution and generally in reduced doses in this age group; this is **not** paregoric, dose accordingly

Dosage Forms Liquid: 10% [0.6 mL equivalent to morphine 6 mg]

Overdosage Treatment Supportive therapy: Naloxone hydrochloride (0.4-2 mg I.V., S.C., or through an endotracheal tube); a continuous infusion (at ⅔ the response dose/hour) may be required

Antidote(s)

Naloxone Hydrochloride *on page 1447*

Test Interactions ↑ aminotransferase [ALT (SGPT)/AST (SGOT)] (S)

Diagnostic Tests/Procedures
Morphine, Blood *on page 1300*
Morphine, Urine *on page 1300*
Opiates, Qualitative, Urine *on page 1309*

Drug Interactions
Increased effect with CNS depressants, cimetidine, MAO inhibitors, tricyclic antidepressants, ethanol, thiopental, and hydroxyzine
Phenothiazines may antagonize the analgesic effect of morphine and other opiate agonists
Dextroamphetamine may enhance the analgesic effect of morphine and other opiate agonists
Plasma morphine concentrations rise when co-administered with cisapride.

Pregnancy Risk Factor B (D if used for prolonged periods or in high doses at term)

Patient Information Avoid alcohol, may cause drowsiness, impair judgment, or coordination; may be addicting if used for prolonged periods

Nursing Implications Observe patient for excessive sedation, respiratory depression, implement safety measures, assist with ambulation

Opticrom® *see* Cromolyn Sodium *on page 245*

Optimine® *see* Azatadine Maleate *on page 140*

Orabase®-B [OTC] *see* Benzocaine *on page 149*

Orabase®-O [OTC] *see* Benzocaine *on page 149*

Orajel® Brace-Aid Oral Anesthetic [OTC] *see* Benzocaine *on page 149*

Orajel® Mouth-Aid [OTC] *see* Benzocaine *on page 149*

Orajel® Maximum Strength [OTC] *see* Benzocaine *on page 149*

Oramide® *see* Tolbutamide *on page 757*

Oraminic® II *see* Brompheniramine Maleate *on page 165*

Oramorph SR® *see* Morphine Sulfate *on page 539*

Orap™ *see* Pimozide *on page 626*

Orasone® *see* Prednisone *on page 639*

Orbinamon® *see* Thiothixene *on page 747*

Orciprenaline Sulfate *see* Metaproterenol Sulfate *on page 506*

Oretic® *see* Hydrochlorothiazide *on page 406*

Organoderm® *see* Malathion (Topical Lotion) *on page 489*

Orinase® *see* Tolbutamide *on page 757*

ORLAAM® *see* Levomethadyl Acetate Hydrochloride *on page 463*

Ormazine® *see* Chlorpromazine Hydrochloride *on page 205*

Ornidyl® *see* Eflornithine Hydrochloride *on page 310*

Orphenadrine Citrate (or fen' a dreen)

CAS Number 4682-36-4

Brand Names Norflex®

Use Treatment of muscle spasm associated with acute painful musculoskeletal conditions; supportive therapy in tetanus

Mechanism of Action Indirect skeletal muscle relaxant thought to work by central atropine-like effects; has some ephorogenic and analgesic properties

Adverse Reactions
Cardiovascular: Tachycardia
Central nervous system: Dizziness, asthenia, fatigue, drowsiness
Gastrointestinal: Dry mouth, nausea, constipation
Ocular: Blurred vision

Signs & Symptoms of Acute Overdose Blurred vision, tachycardia, rhabdomyolysis, confusion, seizures, respiratory arrest, arrhythmias, hypertension, vasodilation, anticholinergic symptoms, dystonic reactions, paralysis, psychosis, myoglobinuria

Toxicodynamics/Kinetics
Onset of action:
Oral: Within 1 hour
I.M.: 5 minutes
I.V.: Immediate
Duration: 12 hours
Peak effect: Within 2-4 hours
Absorption: Oral: Readily after administration from gastrointestinal tract; may be variable in overdose due to anticholinergic effects

(Continued)

Orphenadrine Citrate *(Continued)*

Distribution: Widely distributed throughout the body
Protein binding: 20%
Metabolism: Hepatic
Half-life: 14-16 hours
Time to peak serum concentration:
Oral: 6-8 hours
I.M.: 0.5 hours
I.V.: Immediate
Elimination: Primarily (60%) in urine (8% as unchanged drug)

Usual Dosage Adults:
Oral: 100 mg twice daily
I.M., I.V.: 60 mg every 12 hours

Contraindications Glaucoma, gastrointestinal obstruction, cardiospasm, myasthenia gravis, hypersensitivity to orphenadrine or any component

Dosage Forms
Injection: 30 mg/mL (2 mL, 10 mL)
Tablet: 100 mg
Tablet, sustained release: 100 mg

Reference Range
Toxic: 2-3 mg/mL
Fatal: 4-8 mg/L

Overdosage Treatment
Decontamination: Emesis not recommended due to potential for seizures; lavage in early ingestions after control of seizures; activated charcoal with cathartic of benefit
Supportive therapy: Treatment is predominantly symptomatic and supportive; physostigmine has been used for life-threatening anticholinergic symptoms; bethanechol has been used to control peripheral symptoms; alkaline diuresis/ mannitol has been used in rhabdomyolysis
Enhancement of elimination: Hemodialysis and peritoneal dialysis is ineffective; multiple-dose activated charcoal of unknown value, may be of benefit in ingestions of long-acting product

Pregnancy Risk Factor C

Patient Information May cause drowsiness; swallow whole, do not crush or chew sustained release product; avoid alcohol, may impair coordination and judgment

Nursing Implications Do not crush sustained release drug product; raise bed rails, institute safety measures, assist with ambulation

Additional Information Aplastic anemia has occurred rarely

Specific References

Beech M, Hell C, and Nightingale P, "Central Anticholinergic Syndrome," *Lancet*, 1987, 1(8541):1089.
Boyson SJ, "Bethanechol for Anticholinergic Side Effects," *Ann Neurol*, 1988, 23(4):422-3.
Clarke B, Mair J, and Rudolf M, "Acute Poisoning With Orphenadrine," *Lancet*, 1985, 1(8442):1386.
Danze LK and Langdorf MI, "Reversal of Orphenadrine-Induced Ventricular Tachycardia With Physostigmine," *J Emerg Med*, 1991, 9(6):453-7.

Ortacrone® *see* Amiodarone Hydrochloride *on page 113*
Orthoboric Acid *see* Boric Acid *on page 160*
Orthocesin *see* Benzocaine *on page 149*
Orudis® *see* Ketoprofen *on page 454*
Orulop® *see* Loperamide Hydrochloride *on page 480*
Ospronim® *see* Pentazocine *on page 603*
Osteum® *see* Etidronate Disodium *on page 338*
Ovide™ Topical *see* Malathion (Topical Lotion) *on page 489*
O-V Staticin® *see* Nystatin *on page 574*
Oxaminozoline *see* Rilmenidine *on page 684*

Oxazepam (ox a' ze pam)

Related Information
Benzodiazepines Comparison *on page 1643*

CAS Number 604-75-1

Brand Names Adumbran®; Serax®; Serenid® Forte

Replaces Wy-3498

Use Treatment of anxiety and management of alcohol withdrawal; may also be used as an anticonvulsant in management of simple partial seizures

Mechanism of Action Benzodiazepine anxiolytic sedative that produces CNS depression at the subcortical level, except at high doses, whereby it works at the cortical level

Adverse Reactions
Cardiovascular: Hypotension, bradycardia, cardiovascular collapse, cardiac arrest
Central nervous system: Drowsiness, confusion, dizziness, amnesia, slurred speech, paradoxical excitation or rage, ataxia
Dermatologic: Skin blisters
Hematologic: Porphyria
Local: Phlebitis
Ocular: Blurred vision, diplopia
Respiratory: Respiratory rate (decreased), apnea, laryngospasm
Miscellaneous: Physical and psychological dependence with prolonged use, porphyrinogenic

Signs & Symptoms of Acute Overdose Confusion, coma, hypoactive reflexes, hyporeflexia, dyspnea, nystagmus, slurred speech, unsteady gait, hyponatremia, hypochloremia, hyperglycemia (spurious)

Toxicodynamics/Kinetics Studies have shown that the elderly are more sensitive to the effects of benzodiazepine as compared to younger adults.
Absorption: Oral: Almost completely through gastrointestinal tract
Distribution: V_d: 0.6-2 L/kg; distributed widely throughout the body
Protein binding: 86% to 96%
Metabolism: In the liver to inactive compounds (primarily as glucuronides)
Half-life: 5-15 hours
Time to peak serum concentration: Within 2-3 hours
Elimination: Urinary excretion of unchanged drug (50%) and metabolites

Usual Dosage Oral:
Children: 1 mg/kg/day has been administered
Adults:
Anxiety: 10-30 mg 3-4 times/day
Alcohol withdrawal: 15-30 mg 3-4 times/day
Hypnotic: 15-30 mg

Contraindications Hypersensitivity to oxazepam or any component, cross-sensitivity with other benzodiazepines may exist; avoid using in patients with pre-existing CNS depression, severe uncontrolled pain, or narrow-angle glaucoma

Warnings Avoid using in patients with pre-existing CNS depression, severe uncontrolled pain, or narrow-angle glaucoma; use with caution in patients using other CNS depressants and in the elderly

Dosage Forms
Capsule: 10 mg, 15 mg, 30 mg
Tablet: 15 mg

Reference Range Therapeutic: 0.2-1.4 μg/mL (SI: 0.7-4.9 μmol/L)

Overdosage Treatment
Decontamination: Ipecac or lavage/activated charcoal with cathartic
Supportive therapy: Treatment for benzodiazepine overdose is supportive. Rarely is mechanical ventilation required. Flumazenil has been shown to selectively block the binding of benzodiazepines to CNS receptors, resulting in a reversal of benzodiazepine-induced CNS depression.
Enhancement of elimination: Multiple dosing of activated charcoal may be useful; not dialyzable (0% to 5%)

Antidote(s)
Flumazenil *on page 1428*

Test Interactions Visine®, Drano®, bleach may cause false-negative urine tests; oxazepam may interfere in giving falsely elevated glucose results

Diagnostic Tests/Procedures
Oxazepam, Serum *on page 1312*

Drug Interactions Ethanol delays absorption. Antiepileptics increase clearance.

Pregnancy Risk Factor D

Monitoring Parameters Respiratory and cardiovascular status

Patient Information May cause drowsiness, use caution when driving; avoid alcohol and drugs with CNS depressant effects

Nursing Implications Provide safety measures (ie, side rails, night light, and call button); remove smoking materials from area; supervise ambulation

Additional Information Excreted without need for liver metabolism

Specific References
Moshkowitz M, Pines A, Finkelstein A, et al, "Skin Blisters as a Manifestation of Oxazepam Toxicity," *J Toxicol Clin Toxicol*, 1990, 28(3):383-6.
Zileli MS, Teletar F, Deniz S, et al, "Oxazepam Intoxication Simulating Nonketo-Acidotic Diabetic Coma," *JAMA*, 1971, 215(12):1986.

Oxichlorochin *see* Hydroxychloroquine Sulfate *on page 411*

Oxilapine Succinate *see* Loxapine *on page 486*

Oxpentifylline *see* Pentoxifylline *on page 607*

Oxycodone and Acetaminophen

(ox i koe' done & a seet a min' oh fen)

Related Information

Acetaminophen *on page 79*
Oxycodone Hydrochloride *on next page*

Brand Names Percocet®; Roxicet®; Tylox®

Synonyms Acetaminophen and Oxycodone

Use Management of moderate to severe pain

Mechanism of Action Inhibits the synthesis of prostaglandins in the central nervous system and peripherally blocks pain impulse generation; produces antipyresis from inhibition of hypothalamic heat-regulating center; binds to opiate receptors in the CNS, causing inhibition of ascending pain pathways, altering the perception of and response to pain; produces generalized CNS depression

Adverse Reactions

Cardiovascular: Hypotension, bradycardia, peripheral vasodilation
Central nervous system: CNS depression, intracranial pressure (increased), drowsiness, sedation
Dermatologic: Pruritus
Endocrine & metabolic: Syndrome of inappropriate antidiuretic hormone (SIADH)
Gastrointestinal: Nausea, vomiting, constipation
Ocular: Miosis
Respiratory: Apnea, respiratory depression
Miscellaneous: Physical and psychological dependence, histamine release, biliary or urinary tract spasm

Signs & Symptoms of Acute Overdose Miosis, hypotension, respiratory depression, hepatic injury

Usual Dosage Oral (doses should be titrated to appropriate analgesic effects):

Children: Oxycodone: 0.05-0.15 mg/kg/dose to 5 mg/dose (maximum) every 4-6 hours as needed

Adults: 1-2 tablets every 4-6 hours as needed for pain
Maximum daily dose of acetaminophen: 8 g/day, in alcoholics: 4 g/day

Dosing adjustment in hepatic impairment: Dose should be reduced in patients with severe liver disease

Contraindications Hypersensitivity to oxycodone, acetaminophen or any component; severe respiratory depression

Warnings Use with caution in patients with hypersensitivity to other phenanthrene derivative opioid agonists (morphine, codeine, hydrocodone, hydromorphone, oxymorphone, levorphanol), asthma, COPD, severe liver or renal disease; some preparations may contain bisulfites which may cause allergies

Dosage Forms

Caplet: Oxycodone hydrochloride 5 mg and acetaminophen 500 mg
Capsule: Oxycodone hydrochloride 5 mg and acetaminophen 500 mg
Solution, oral: Oxycodone hydrochloride 5 mg and acetaminophen 325 mg per 5 mL (5 mL, 500 mL)
Tablet: Oxycodone hydrochloride 5 mg and acetaminophen 325 mg

Reference Range Acetaminophen: 20-110 ng/mL

Overdosage Treatment

Decontamination: Lavage/activated charcoal with cathartic
Supportive therapy: Naloxone hydrochloride (0.4-2 mg I.V., S.C., or through an endotracheal tube); a continuous infusion (at two-thirds the response dose/hour) may be required; N-acetylcysteine for acetaminophen toxicity

Antidote(s)

Acetylcysteine *on page 1388*
Naloxone Hydrochloride *on page 1447*

Test Interactions Serum digoxin-like immunoreactive substance found in acute acetaminophen overdose

Drug Interactions

Decreased effect with phenothiazines
Increased effect/toxicity with CNS depressants, TCAs, dextroamphetamine

Pregnancy Risk Factor C

Pregnancy Implications Appears in breast milk

Monitoring Parameters Pain relief, respiratory and mental status, blood pressure

Patient Information Avoid alcohol, may cause drowsiness, impaired judgment or coordination; may be addicting if used for prolonged periods

Nursing Implications Give with food, but high carbohydrate meal may retard absorption rate; observe patient for excessive sedation, apnea; implement safety measures, assist with ambulation

Additional Information Oxycodone and acetaminophen: Oxycet®, Percocet®, Roxicet®, Tylox®

Specific References

Sinatra RS and Harrison DM, "Oxymorphone in Patient-Controlled Analgesia," *Clin Pharm*, 1989, 8(8):541, 544.

Oxycodone Hydrochloride (ox i koe' done)

Related Information

Oxycodone and Acetaminophen *on previous page*

Pharmacokinetics of Narcotic Agonist Analgesics *on page 1654*

CAS Number 76-42-6; 124-90-3

Brand Names Endone®; Eukodal®; Roxicodone™; Supeudol®

Synonyms Dihydrohydroxycodeinone

Use Management of moderate to severe pain, normally used in combination with non-narcotic analgesics

Mechanism of Action Binds to opiate receptors in the CNS, causing inhibition of ascending pain pathways, altering the perception of and response to pain; produces generalized CNS depression

Adverse Reactions

Cardiovascular: Palpitations, hypotension, bradycardia, peripheral vasodilation

Central nervous system: CNS depression

Dermatologic: Pruritus

Endocrine & metabolic: Syndrome of inappropriate antidiuretic hormone (SIADH)

Gastrointestinal: Nausea, vomiting, constipation

Ocular: Miosis

Respiratory: Apnea, respiratory depression

Miscellaneous: Intracranial pressure (increased), physical and psychological dependence, histamine release, porphyrinogenic (possible), biliary or urinary tract spasm

Signs & Symptoms of Acute Overdose CNS depression, lightheadedness, respiratory depression, miosis, noncardiogenic pulmonary edema, coma

Toxicodynamics/Kinetics

Onset of pain relief: Oral: Within 15-30 minutes

Peak effect: 60 minutes

Duration: 3-6 hours

Metabolism: In the liver to noroxycodone by demethylation

Half-life: 2-5 hours

Elimination: Excreted in urine

Usual Dosage Oral:

Children:

6-12 years: 1.25 mg every 6 hours as needed

>12 years: 2.5 mg every 6 hours as needed

Adults: 5 mg every 6 hours as needed

Dosing adjustment in hepatic impairment: Reduce dosage in patients with severe liver disease

Contraindications Hypersensitivity to oxycodone or any component

Warnings Use with caution in patients with hypersensitivity reactions to other phenanthrene derivative opioid agonists (morphine, hydrocodone, hydromorphone, levorphanol, oxycodone, oxymorphone); respiratory diseases including asthma, emphysema, COPD, or severe liver or renal insufficiency; some preparations contain sulfites which may cause allergic reactions; may be habit-forming; dextromethorphan has equivalent antitussive activity but has much lower toxicity in accidental overdose

Dosage Forms

Liquid, oral: 5 mg/5 mL (500 mL)

Solution, oral concentrate: 20 mg/mL (30 mL)

Tablet: 5 mg

Reference Range Blood level of 5 mg/L associated with fatality

Overdosage Treatment Supportive therapy: Naloxone hydrochloride (0.4-2 mg I.V., S.C., or through an endotracheal tube); a continuous infusion (at ⅔ the response dose/hour) may be required

Antidote(s)

Naloxone Hydrochloride *on page 1447*

Diagnostic Tests/Procedures

Oxycodone, Blood or Urine *on page 1313*

Drug Interactions MAO inhibitors → ↑ adverse symptoms

Pregnancy Risk Factor B (D if used for prolonged periods or in high doses at term)

Monitoring Parameters Pain relief, respiratory and mental status, blood pressure

Patient Information Avoid alcohol; may cause drowsiness, impaired judgment or coordination; may be addicting if used for prolonged periods

Nursing Implications Observe patient for excessive sedation, respiratory depression, implement safety measures, assist with ambulation

Additional Information Oxycodone: Roxicodone™

Specific References

Kalso E and Vainio A, "Morphine and Oxycodone Hydrochloride in the Management of Cancer Pain," *Clin Pharmacol Ther*, 1990, 47(5):639-46.

Turturro MA and O'Toole KS, "Oxycodone-Induced Pulmonary Edema," *Am J Emerg Med*, 1991, 9(2):201-3.

Oxylin® *see* Oxymetazoline Hydrochloride *on this page*

Oxymetazoline Hydrochloride (ox i met az' oh leen)

CAS Number 1491-59-4;2315-02-8

Brand Names Afrazine®; Afrin® Nasal Solution [OTC]; Allerest® 12 Hours Nasal Solution [OTC]; Chlorphed®-LA Nasal Solution [OTC]; Dristan® Long Lasting Nasal Solution [OTC]; Drixine®; Drixoral®; Duration® Nasal Solution [OTC]; Nasivin®; Neo-Synephrine® 12 Hour Nasal Solution [OTC]; Nōstrilla® [OTC]; Nose-X®; NTZ® Long Acting Nasal Solution [OTC]; OcuClear® [OTC]; Oxylin®; Respir®; Sinarest® 12 Hour Nasal Solution; Sudafed® Nasal Spray; Tioclin®; Vicks Sinex® Long-Acting Nasal Solution [OTC]; Visine®; 4-Way® Long Acting Nasal Solution [OTC]; Zolin®

Use Symptomatic relief of nasal mucosal congestion and adjunctive therapy of middle ear infections, associated with acute or chronic rhinitis, the common cold, sinusitis, hay fever, or other allergies

Ophthalmic: Relief of redness of eye due to minor eye irritations, conjunctivitis

Mechanism of Action Sympathomimetic; stimulates alpha-adrenergic receptors in the arterioles of the nasal mucosa to produce vasoconstriction; imidazoline decongestant

Adverse Reactions Primarily local burning, hypothermia, dry mouth; may be porphyrinogenic; intra-arterial injection can cause localized gangrene due to ischemia; peripheral vasoconstriction due to nasal application is very rare

Cardiovascular: Bradycardia

Central nervous system: Headache, psychosis, mania, seizures (in children), insomnia

Toxicodynamics/Kinetics

Onset of effect: Intranasal: Within 5-10 minutes

Duration: 6-7 hours

Metabolism: Metabolic fate is unknown

Half-life: 5-8 hours

Elimination: Renal (30%) and feces (10%)

Usual Dosage Therapy should not exceed 3-5 days

Intranasal:

- Children 2-5 years: 0.025% solution: Instill 2-3 drops in each nostril twice daily
- Children ≥6 years and Adults: 0.05% solution: Instill 2-3 drops or 2-3 sprays into each nostril twice daily up to 3 days

Ophthalmic: Adults: 0.025% solution: Instill 1-2 drops into affected eye(s) every 6 hours up to 4 days

Contraindications Adrenergic agent hypersensitivity; narrow-angle glaucoma

Warnings Use with caution in patients with cardiac disease, thyroid disease, high blood pressure, diabetes mellitus, prostatic hypertrophy

Dosage Forms

Nasal solution:

- Drops:
  - Afrin® Children's Nose Drops: 0.025% (20 mL)
  - Afrin®, NTZ® Long Acting Nasal Solution: 0.05% (15 mL, 20 mL)
- Spray: Afrin®, Allerest® 12 Hours, Chlorphed®-LA, Dristan® Long Lasting, Duration®, 4-Way® Long Acting, Genasal®, Nasal Relief®, Neo-Synephrine® 12 Hour, Nōstrilla®, NTZ® Long Acting Nasal Solution, Sinex® Long-Acting, Twice-A-Day®: 0.05% (15 mL, 30 mL)

Ophthalmic solution (OcuClear®, Visine® L.R.): 0.025% (15 mL, 30 mL)

Stability Do not use if solution changes colors or becomes cloudy

Overdosage Treatment

Decontamination: Oral: Activated charcoal with cathartic

Supportive therapy: Seizures can be treated with benzodiazepines or phenytoin; nitroprusside can be used to treat hypertension

Drug Interactions Increased toxicity: MAO inhibitors

Pregnancy Risk Factor C

Patient Information Should not be used for self-medication for longer than 3 days, if symptoms persist, drug should be discontinued and a physician consulted; notify physician of insomnia, tremor, or irregular heartbeat; burning, stinging, or drying of the nasal mucosa may occur

Nursing Implications Spray/drops should not be used for >3 days without direct physician supervision

Additional Information Often best when used short-term in conjunction with long-term nasal corticosteroid

Specific References

Shukla PC, "Acute Ischemia of the Hand Following Intra-arterial Oxymetazoline Injection," *J Emerg Med*, 1995, 13:65-70.

Oxymorphone Hydrochloride (ox i mor' fone)

Related Information

Pharmacokinetics of Narcotic Agonist Analgesics *on page 1654*

CAS Number 76-41-5; 357-07-3

Brand Names Numorphan®

Use Management of moderate to severe pain and preoperatively as a sedative and a supplement to anesthesia

Mechanism of Action Oxymorphone hydrochloride (Numorphan®) is a potent narcotic analgesic with uses similar to those of morphine. The drug is a semisynthetic derivative of morphine (phenanthrene derivative) and is closely related to hydromorphone chemically (Dilaudid®).

Adverse Reactions

Cardiovascular: Palpitations, hypotension, bradycardia, peripheral vasodilation
Central nervous system: CNS depression
Dermatologic: Pruritus
Endocrine & metabolic: Syndrome of inappropriate antidiuretic hormone (SIADH)
Gastrointestinal: Nausea, vomiting, constipation
Ocular: Miosis
Respiratory: Apnea, respiratory depression
Miscellaneous: Intracranial pressure (increased), physical and psychological dependence, histamine release, biliary or urinary tract spasm

Toxicodynamics/Kinetics

Onset of analgesia:
- I.M., I.V., S.C.: Within 5-10 minutes
- Rectal: Within 15-30 minutes

Duration of analgesia: Parenteral, rectal: 3-6 hours
Metabolism: Conjugated with glucuronic acid
Peak effect: 30-60 minutes
Elimination: Excreted in urine

Usual Dosage Adults:

I.M., S.C.: 0.5 mg initially, 1-1.5 mg every 4-6 hours as needed
I.V.: 0.5 mg initially
Rectal: 5 mg every 4-6 hours

Contraindications Hypersensitivity to oxymorphone or any component, increased intracranial pressure; severe respiratory depression

Warnings Some preparations contain sulfites which may cause allergic reactions; infants <3 months of age are more susceptible to respiratory depression, use with caution and generally in reduced doses in this age group; use with caution in patients with impaired respiratory function or severe hepatic dysfunction and in patients with hypersensitivity reactions to other phenanthrene derivative opioid agonists (codeine, hydrocodone, hydromorphone, levorphanol, oxycodone, oxymorphone)

Dosage Forms

Injection: 1 mg (1 mL); 1.5 mg/mL (1 mL, 10 mL)
Suppository, rectal: 5 mg

Stability Refrigerate suppository

Overdosage Treatment Supportive therapy: Naloxone hydrochloride (0.4-2 mg I.V., S.C., or through an endotracheal tube); a continuous infusion (at ⅔ the response dose/hour) may be required

Antidote(s)

Naloxone Hydrochloride *on page 1447*

Drug Interactions

Decreased effect with phenothiazines
Increased effect/toxicity with CNS depressants, TCAs, dextroamphetamine

Pregnancy Risk Factor B (D if used for prolonged periods or in high doses at term)

Monitoring Parameters Respiratory rate, heart rate, blood pressure, CNS activity

Patient Information Avoid alcohol, may cause drowsiness, impaired judgment or coordination; may be addicting if used for prolonged periods

Nursing Implications Observe patient for excessive sedation, respiratory depression, implement safety measures, assist with ambulation

Specific References

Sinatra RS and Harrison DM, "Oxymorphone in Patient-Controlled Analgesia," *Clin Pharm*, 1989, 8(8):541, 544.

Oxyphenbutazone (ox i fen byoo' ta zone)

CAS Number 7081-38-1

Use Management of inflammatory disorders, as an analgesic in the treatment of mild to moderate pain and as an antipyretic; I.V. form used as an alternate to surgery in management of patent ductus arteriosus in premature neonates; acute gouty arthritis; removed from U.S. market

Mechanism of Action Anti-inflammatory effect is a prominent feature of the drug's pharmacology. Several hypotheses have been presented for the mode of

(Continued)

Oxyphenbutazone *(Continued)*

action. One of the main events in an inflammatory reaction is a leukocyte infiltration of the inflammatory site. An inhibition of leukocyte migration would restrict the entry of leukocytes and suppress, but not stop, the ensuing inflammation; has been observed to inhibit *in vitro* migration of total human leukocytes in a dose-dependent manner.

Adverse Reactions

Cardiovascular: Fluid retention, circulatory collapse

Central nervous system: Headache, aseptic meningitis, psychosis, cognitive dysfunction, coma, seizures

Dermatologic: Rash, pruritus

Endocrine & metabolic: Hyperkalemia, anion gap metabolic acidosis

Gastrointestinal: Abdominal pain, feces discoloration (black), nausea, vomiting, bleeding, ulceration, constipation, diarrhea, dyspepsia

Genitourinary: Albuminuria

Hematologic: Leukopenia, neutropenia, agranulocytosis, granulocytopenia; aplastic anemia (rare), platelet inhibition

Hepatic: Elevation of transaminases, fulminant hepatitis

Otic: Ototoxicity, tinnitus

Renal: Renal failure (acute), nephrotic syndrome, chronic renal failure

Respiratory: Wheezing, respiratory depression

Miscellaneous: Hypersensitivity

Signs & Symptoms of Acute Overdose Nausea, arthralgia, wheezing, nephrotic syndrome, gastrointestinal bleeding, gastritis; hypothyroidism, cognitive dysfunction, vomiting, ototoxicity; tinnitus, drowsiness; severe poisoning can manifest with coma, seizures, renal failure and or hepatic failure, hypotension, respiratory depression, apnea, feces discoloration (greenish gray), feces discoloration (pink), feces discoloration (pink), metabolic acidosis, nystagmus; leukocytosis

Usual Dosage Adults: Oral:

Rheumatoid arthritis: 100-200 mg 3-4 times/day until desired effect, then reduce dose to not exceeding 400 mg/day

Acute gouty arthritis: Initial: 400 mg then 100 mg every 4 hours until acute attack subsides, not longer than 1 week

Contraindications Active gastrointestinal bleeding, ulcer disease, hypersensitivity to oxyphenbutazone or any component

Warnings Use with caution in patients with congestive heart failure, hypertension, decreased renal or hepatic function, history of gastrointestinal disease (bleeding or ulcers), or those receiving anticoagulants; safety and efficacy in children <6 months of age have not yet been established; because of severe hematologic adverse effects, discontinue use if no favorable response is seen

Dosage Forms Tablet: 100 mg

Overdosage Treatment

Decontamination: Ipecac or lavage/charcoal

Supportive therapy: Hypotension/dehydration can be managed with intravenous fluid therapy; acidosis should be treated with bicarbonates, seizures with benzodiazepines; antacids, blood products are indicated, as appropriate, for hemorrhage

Enhancement of elimination: Dialysis or perfusion is indicated for secondary complications, acidosis, or renal failure and not toxin removal alone

Test Interactions Increases chloride (S), sodium (S), bleeding time

Drug Interactions Aspirin decreases serum concentrations probably by protein-binding displacement; there is an increased bleeding potential with concomitant warfarin therapy; may increase lithium and methotrexate concentrations by decreasing renal clearance; may decrease diuretic and hypotensive effects of thiazides, loop diuretics, ACE inhibitors, and beta-blockers; may increase nephrotoxicity of cyclosporine

Pregnancy Risk Factor D

Patient Information Take with food; may cause dizziness or drowsiness; notify physician and discontinue if persistent sore throat, fatigue, fever, or unusual bleeding or bruising occurs

Nursing Implications Do not crush tablet

Specific References

Court H and Volans GN, "Poisoning After Overdose With Nonsteroidal Anti-inflammatory Drugs," *Adverse Drug React Acute Poisoning Rev*, 1984, 3(1):1-21.

Hoppmann RA, Peden JG, and Ober SK, "Central Nervous System Side Effects of Nonsteroidal Anti-inflammatory Drugs. Aseptic Meningitis, Psychosis, and Cognitive Dysfunction," *Arch Intern Med*, 1991, 151(7):1309-13.

Smolinske SC, Hall AH, Vandenberg SA, et al, "Toxic Effects of Nonsteroid Anti-inflammatory Drugs in Overdose. An Overview of Recent Evidence on Clinical Effects and Dose-Response Relationships," *Drug Saf*, 1990, 5(4):252-74.

Vale JA and Meredith TJ, "Acute Poisoning Due to Nonsteroidal Anti-inflammatory Drugs," *Med Toxicol*, 1986, 1(1):12-31.

Verbeeck RK, "Pharmacokinetic Drug Interactions With Nonsteroidal Anti-inflammatory Drugs," *Clin Pharmacokinet*, 1990, 19(1):44-66.

Paclitaxel (pack li tax' el)

Related Information

Toxicities of Chemotherapeutic Agents *on page 1631-1633*

CAS Number 33069-62-4

Brand Names Taxol®

Synonyms Taxol A

Use Treatment of metastatic carcinoma of the ovary after failure of first-line or subsequent chemotherapy; treatment of metastatic breast cancer after failure of combination therapy for metastatic disease or relapse within 6 months of adjuvant chemotherapy

Mechanism of Action Derived from the Pacific yew tree (*Taxus brevifolia*), it induces microtubule formation while disrupting mitosis

Adverse Reactions

Cardiovascular: Hypotension, bradycardia, abnormal EKG, ventricular ectopy
Dermatologic: Alopecia, radiation recall dermatitis
Gastrointestinal: Nausea, vomiting, diarrhea
Hematologic: Neutropenia, leukopenia, thrombocytopenia, anemia
Hepatic: Abnormal liver function tests
Neuromuscular & skeletal: Myalgia, bone pain, neuropathy (peripheral) (at doses exceeding 250 mg/m^2), paresthesia
Respiratory: Pneumonitis
Miscellaneous: Hypersensitivity reactions

Signs & Symptoms of Acute Overdose Ventricular arrhythmias, erythema, congestive heart failure, dyspnea, neuropathy (peripheral), myopathy, dysphagia, diplopia, chest pain, stomatitis, wheezing, neuritis, leukopenia; neutropenia; agranulocytosis; granulocytopenia

Toxicodynamics/Kinetics Administered by I.V. infusion and exhibits a biphasic decline in plasma concentrations

Distribution: V_d: 67-182 L/m^2; initial rapid decline represents distribution to the peripheral compartment and significant elimination of the drug; later phase is due to a relatively slow efflux of paclitaxel from the peripheral compartment; mean steady state: 42-162 L/m^2, indicating extensive extravascular distribution and/or tissue binding

Protein binding: 89% to 98% bound to human serum proteins at concentrations of 0.1-50 mcg/mL

Metabolism: In the liver in animals and evidence suggests hepatic metabolism in humans

Half-life, mean, terminal: 5.3-17.4 hours after 1- and 6-hour infusions at dosing levels of 15-275 mg/m^2

Elimination: Urinary recovery of unchanged drug: 1.3% to 12.6% following 1-, 6-, and 24-hour infusions of 15-275 mg/m^2

Mean total body clearance range:
After 1- and 6-hour infusions: 5.8-16.3 L/hour/m^2
After 24-hour infusions: 14.2-17.2 L/hour/m^2

Usual Dosage Adults: I.V. infusion (refer to individual protocols):

Ovarian carcinoma: 135-175 mg/m^2 over 24 hours* administered every 3 weeks
Metastatic breast cancer: Treatment is still undergoing investigation; most protocols have used doses of 200-250 mg/m^2 over 24 hours*

*The results of an international study has demonstrated that a 3-hour infusion produces similar efficacy as a 24-hour infusion, but with less hematologic toxicity and less mucositis.

Contraindications History of hypersensitivity to any component or neutropenia <1500 cells/m^3

Warnings The FDA currently recommends that procedures for proper handling and disposal of antineoplastic agents be considered. Use with caution in patients with hepatic impairment, cardiovascular risk factors. All patients should be premedicated prior to Taxol® administration to prevent severe hypersensitivity reactions; premedication should consist of the following:

Dexamethasone 20 mg oral/I.V. administered 12 and 6 hours prior to Taxol®
Diphenhydramine (or equivalent) 50 mg I.V. 30-60 minutes prior to Taxol®
Cimetidine (300 mg) or ranitidine (50 mg) I.V. 30-60 minutes prior to Taxol®

Dosage Forms Injection: 6 mg/mL (5 mL)

Stability Vials must be stored under refrigeration 2°C to 8°C (36°F to 46°F) and protected from light. Dilute to a final concentration of 0.3-1.2 mg/mL in 0.9% sodium chloride injection, dextrose 5% in water, dextrose 5% in 0.9% sodium chloride, or dextrose 5% in Ringer's injection. These solutions are physically and chemically stable for up to 27 hours at ambient temperature (25°C) and room light; formulated in a vehicle known as Cremophor EL™ (polyoxyethylated castor oil). Cremophor EL™ has been found to leach the plasticizer DEHP from polyvinyl chloride infusion bags or administration sets. Taxol® solutions should be stored in glass bottles or polypropylene/polyolefin (Excel®) bags and administered through nonpolyvinyl chloride (ie, polyethylene-lined) administration sets; administer through I.V. tubing

(Continued)

Paclitaxel *(Continued)*

containing an in-line (0.22 micron) filter; administration through IVEX-2® filters (which incorporate short inlet and outlet polyvinyl chloride-coated tubing) has not resulted in significant leaching of DEHP; insoluble in water.

Reference Range Mean maximum serum concentrations: 435-802 ng/mL following 24-hour infusions of 200-275 mg/m^2 and were approximately 10% to 30% of those following 6-hour infusions of equivalent doses; not detected in cerebrospinal fluid

Overdosage Treatment Supportive therapy: Amitriptyline may be helpful for neuropathy; epinephrine, crystalloid fluids, diphenhydramine (25-50 mg in adults) and methylprednisolone (125 mg in adults) should be given for anaphylaxis; high-dose corticosteroids can be given to treat pneumonitis

Antidote(s)

Diphenhydramine Hydrochloride *on page 1415*

Test Interactions Elevates serum triglyceride levels/minor elevation of renal function or liver function test

Drug Interactions Increased toxicity: In phase I trials, myelosuppression was more profound when given after cisplatin than with alternative sequence; pharmacokinetic data demonstrates a decrease in clearance of ~33% when administered following cisplatin; possibility of an inhibition of metabolism in patients treated with ketoconazole

Pregnancy Risk Factor D

Monitoring Parameters Monitor for hypersensitivity reactions

Patient Information Alopecia occurs in almost all patients

Additional Information Skin necrosis can occur with subcutaneous extravasation

Specific References

Bitton RJ, Figg WD, and Reed E, "A Preliminary Risk-Benefit Assessment of Paclitaxel," *Drug Saf*, 1995, 12(3):196-208.

Del Priore G, Smith P, Warshal DP, et al, "Paclitaxel-Associated Hypersensitivity Reaction Despite High-Dose Steroids and Prolonged Infusions," *Gynecol Oncol*, 1995, 56(2):316-8.

Goldberg HL and Vannice SB, "Pneumonitis Related to Treatment With Paclitaxel," *J Clin Oncol*, 1995, 13(2):534-5.

Kingston DG, "The Chemistry of Taxol," *Pharmacol Ther*, 1991, 52(1):1-34.

Phillips KA, Urch M, and Bishop JF, "Radiation-Recall Dermatitis in a Patient Treated With Paclitaxel," *J Clin Oncol*, 1995, 13(1):305.

Rowinsky EK and Donehower RC, "Paclitaxel (Taxol®)," *N Engl J Med*, 1995, 332(15):1004-14.

Song JI and Dumais MR, "From Yew to Us: The Curious Development of Taxol," *JAMA*, 1991, 266(9):1281.

Weiss RB, Donehower RC, Wiernik PH, et al, "Hypersensitivity Reactions From Taxol," *J Clin Oncol*, 1990, 8(7):1263-8.

Pallidan® *see* Methaqualone Hydrochloride *on page 511*

Palmil® *see* Castor Oil *on page 189*

Pameb® *see* Benzalkonium Chloride *on page 147*

Pamelor® *see* Nortriptyline Hydrochloride *on page 571*

Pamidronate Disodium (pa mi droe' nate)

CAS Number 40391-99-9; 109552-15-0

Brand Names Aredia™; Aredin®

Synonyms APD: Aminohydroxypropylidene Disphosphonate

Use Hypercalcemia; primarily used in malignancy and Paget's disease

Mechanism of Action Inhibits osteoclastic bone resorption of calcium

Adverse Reactions

Central nervous system: Malaise, fever

Endocrine & metabolic: Hypocalcemia (20%), hypokalemia, hypomagnesemia, hypophosphatemia

Gastrointestinal: Vomiting, nausea, anorexia, constipation

Hematologic: Leukopenia (with oral therapy), thrombocytopenia, anemia

Local: Thrombophlebitis

Neuromuscular & skeletal: Bone pain

Ocular: Iritis, uveitis

Signs & Symptoms of Acute Overdose Hypotension, hypocalcemia, fever, hypophosphatemia, hypomagnesemia, hypokalemia, taste perversion

Toxicodynamics/Kinetics

Onset of action: 1-2 days

Absorption: Oral: 1% to 3%

Half-life: 27 hours

Elimination, biphasic: ~50% excreted unchanged in urine within 72 hours; clearance: 74 mL/minute

Usual Dosage

Oral: 300-600 mg/day in 2-3 divided doses prior to meals; maximum oral daily dose: 1.2 g (investigational in U.S.)

I.V.: 60-90 mg administered over 4-24 hours; may repeat after 7 days for moderate hypercalcemia

Paget's disease: Daily dose of 30 mg over 4-hour infusion period for 3 days has been utilized

Administration Administer in 0.5-1 L of normal saline or 5% dextrose; do not use Ringer's lactate

Contraindications Previous hypersensitivity to pamidronate or other biphosphonates

Warnings Use caution in patients with renal impairment as the potential nephrotoxic effects of pamidronate are not known; use caution in patients who are pregnant or in the breast-feeding period; leukopenia has been observed with oral pamidronate and monitoring of white blood cell counts is suggested; vein irritation and thrombophlebitis may occur with infusions; the position of the indwelling catheter should be changed at frequent intervals. Has not been studied exclusively in the elderly; monitor serum electrolytes periodically since elderly are often receiving diuretics which can result in decreases in serum calcium, potassium, and magnesium.

Dosage Forms Powder for injection, lyophilized: 30 mg, 60 mg, 90 mg

Reference Range Calcium (total): Adults: 9.0-11.0 mg/dL (SI: 2.05-2.54 mmol/L), may slightly decrease with aging; Phosphorus: 2.5-4.5 mg/dL (SI: 0.81-1.45 mmol/L)

Overdosage Treatment

Supportive therapy: Monitor for hypocalcemia; in one report (supplied by the drug company), fever and hypotension were corrected with use of steroids, but no formal studies could be found

Test Interactions Causes a decrease of serum calcium and phosphate

Drug Interactions Incompatible with calcium-containing I.V. fluids (ie, Ringer's solution); do not use concomitantly with foscarnet

Pregnancy Risk Factor C

Monitoring Parameters Serum calcium, phosphate, magnesium, potassium, serum creatinine, CBC with differential; pain, phlebitis at injection site

Specific References

Body JJ, Pot M, Borkowski A, et al, "Dose/Response Study of Aminohydroxypropylidene Biphosphonate in Tumor-Associated Hypercalcemia," *Am J Med*, 1987, 82(5):957-63.

De S, Meyer P, and Crisp AJ, "Pamidronate and Uveitis," *Br J Rheumatol*, 1995, 34:479.

Fitton A and McTavish D, "Pamidronate: A Review of Its Pharmacological Properties and Therapeutic Efficacy in Resorptive Bone Disease," *Drugs*, 1991, 41(2):289-318.

Ralston SH, Gallacher SJ, Patel U, et al, "Cancer-Associated Hypercalcemia: Morbidity and Mortality, Clinical Experience in 126 Treated Patients," *Ann Intern Med*, 1990, 112(7):499-504.

Pamine® *see* Scopolamine *on page 691*

Pamprin IB® [OTC] *see* Ibuprofen *on page 418*

Panadol® [OTC] *see* Acetaminophen *on page 79*

Panclar® *see* Deanol *on page 261*

Panmycin® Oral *see* Tetracycline *on page 732*

Pantopon® *see* Opium Alkaloids (Hydrochlorides) *on page 579*

Panwarfarin® *see* Warfarin Sodium *on page 800*

Papaveretum *see* Opium Alkaloids (Hydrochlorides) *on page 579*

Papaverine (pa pav' er een)

CAS Number 58-74-2; 61-25-6; 39024-96-9; 32808-09-6

Brand Names Angioverin®; Cerespan®; Dilart®; Dipav®; Dylate®; Genabid®; Kavrin®; Pavabid®; Pavagen®; Pavakey®; Pavaspan®; Pavasull®; Pavatab®; Pavatine® Pavased®; Pavatym®; Paverine Spancap®; Paverolan®; Therapav®; Vaso-Pav®

Synonyms 6,7-dimethoxy-1-vera trylisoquinoline

Use Relief of peripheral and cerebral ischemia associated with arterial spasm

Mechanism of Action Smooth muscle spasmolytic producing a generalized smooth muscle relaxation including vasodilatation, gastrointestinal sphincter relaxation, bronchiolar muscle relaxation and potentially a depressed myocardium; it is an inhibition of cellular respiration and phosphodiesterase along with being a calcium antagonist (inhibits uptake of adenosine)

Adverse Reactions

Cardiovascular: Flushing of the face, tachycardia, hypotension, cardiac arrhythmias with rapid I.V. use consisting of A-V block, premature ventricular contraction

Central nervous system: Depression, dizziness, drowsiness, sedation, drowsiness, headache

Dermatologic: Pruritus

Gastrointestinal: Dry mouth, nausea, constipation, vomiting, abdominal pain

(Continued)

Papaverine *(Continued)*

Genitourinary: Priapism with intracavernous injection,
Hematologic: Eosinophilia
Hepatic: Hepatic hypersensitivity, cirrhosis
Local: Thrombosis at the I.V. administration site
Respiratory: Apnea with rapid I.V. use
Miscellaneous: Sweating

Signs & Symptoms of Acute Overdose Constipation, coma, penile fibrosis, diplopia, asthenia, hypokalemia, coma, drowsiness, mydriasis, A-V block, liver damage, lactic acidosis, respiratory alkalosis, hyperglycemia

Toxicodynamics/Kinetics
Onset of action: Oral: Rapid
Absorption: Variable
Distribution: Tends to localize in adipose tissue and in liver; remainder distributes throughout the body
Protein binding: 90%
Metabolism: Rapid in the liver
Bioavailability: ~54%
Half-life: 30-120 minutes
Elimination: Primarily as phenolic metabolites in the urine

Usual Dosage
Children: I.M., I.V.: 1.5 mg/kg 4 times/day
Adults:
Oral: 100-300 mg 3-5 times/day
Oral, sustained release: 150-300 mg every 12 hours
I.M., I.V.: 30-120 mg every 3 hours as needed

Contraindications Complete atrioventricular block; Parkinson's disease

Warnings Use with caution in patients with glaucoma; administer I.V. cautiously since apnea and arrhythmias may result

Dosage Forms
Capsule, sustained release: 150 mg
Injection: 30 mg/mL (2 mL, 10 mL)
Tablet: 30 mg, 60 mg, 100 mg, 150 mg, 200 mg, 300 mg
Tablet, timed release: 200 mg

Stability Protect from heat or freezing; not do refrigerate injection; solutions should be clear to pale yellow; precipitates with lactated Ringer's; incompatible with bromides and iodides

Overdosage Treatment
Decontamination: Ipecac/activated charcoal with cathartic is useful
Supportive therapy: Lorazepam or diazepam 10-20 mg (0.25-0.4 mg/kg for children) is helpful for seizures; I.V. fluids and alpha-adrenergic pressors should be used for hypotension; sodium bicarbonate (1 mEq/kg) is useful to treat acidosis
Enhanced elimination: Multiple dosing of activated charcoal may be useful

Drug Interactions Additive effects with CNS depressants or morphine; papaverine decreases the effects of levodopa

Pregnancy Risk Factor C

Nursing Implications Rapid I.V. administration may result in arrhythmias and fatal apnea

Additional Information Therapeutic value is lacking

Specific References
Ilan Y and Gemer O, "Papaverine-Induced Coma," *Eur J Clin Pharmacol*, 1988, 33(6):651.
Jahr JS, Kan B, Paxtor CG, et al, "Hemodynamic Responses to Papaverine: Do Nitric Oxide, Cyclic GMP, or Calcium Mediate the Vasodilitation?" *Am J Ther*, 1995, 2:258-64.
Vaziri ND, Stokes J, and Treadwell TR, "Lactic Acidosis, A Complication of Papaverine Overdose," *Clin Toxicol*, 1981, 18(4):417-23.

Para-Aminosalicylate Sodium (a mee noe sal i' si late)

CAS Number 133-10-8; 6018-19-5

Brand Names Eupasal®; Na-PAS®; Salf-Pas®; Sodico®; Therapas®; Therazid®

Synonyms Aminosalicylate Sodium; PAS

Use Adjunctive treatment of tuberculosis

Adverse Reactions
Gastrointestinal: Nausea, vomiting, diarrhea
Endocrine & metabolic: Hypokalemia
Hepatic: Hepatitis, jaundice
Miscellaneous: Allergy, alopecia

Toxicodynamics/Kinetics
Absorption: Readily
Distribution: Widely distributed but appears in CSF only within inflamed meninges
Protein binding: 60% to 70%
Metabolism: Intestinal and liver
Half-life, elimination: ~1 hour

Peak concentrations: Within 1-4 hours
Elimination: Primarily in urine within 12 hours

Usual Dosage Oral:
Children: 240-360 mg/kg/day in 3-4 divided doses
Adults: 12-15 g/day in 3-4 divided doses

Contraindications Known hypersensitivity to para-aminosalicylate; G-6-PD deficiency

Warnings Avoid use in patients with hepatic or renal dysfunction, gastric bleeding disorders

Dosage Forms Tablet: 500 mg

Reference Range Inhibition of *Mycobacterium* tuberculosis at a level of 1 μg/mL

Overdosage Treatment
Decontamination: Lavage/activated charcoal with cathartic
Enhancement of elimination: Multiple dosing of activated charcoal may be effective

Test Interactions Urine glucose

Drug Interactions Interferes with rifampin absorption; displaces phenytoin from albumin thus raising free phenytoin levels; probenecid can increase serum concentration

Pregnancy Risk Factor C

Additional Information Capsules contain bentonite which may decrease absorption of concomitantly ingested drugs

Specific References

Rossouw JE and Saunders SJ, "Hepatic Complications of Antituberculous Therapy," *Q J Med*, 1975, 44(173):1-16.

Parabromdylamine *see* Brompheniramine Maleate *on page 165*

Paracetaldehyde *see* Paraldehyde *on this page*

Paracetamol *see* Acetaminophen *on page 79*

Paradione® *see* Paramethadione *on page 595*

Paral® *see* Paraldehyde *on this page*

Paraldehyde (par al' de hyde)

Related Information
Seizures, Neonatal Guidelines *on page 1604-1605*
Status Epilepticus Treatment Algorithm *on page 1608*

CAS Number 123-63-7

UN Number 1264

Brand Names Paral®

Synonyms Elaldehyde; Paracetaldehyde

Use Cyclic acetaldehyde trimer which is utilized as a treatment of status epilepticus and tetanus-induced seizures; has been used as a sedative/hypnotic, no longer used in the treatment of alcohol withdrawal symptoms

Mechanism of Action Unknown mechanism of action; causes depression of CNS, including the ascending reticular activating system to provide sedation/hypnosis and anticonvulsant activity

Adverse Reactions
Cardiovascular: Cardiovascular collapse, tachycardia
Central nervous system: Drowsiness, clumsiness, dizziness, "hangover effect"
Gastrointestinal: Strong and unpleasant breath, nausea, vomiting, stomach pain
Dermatologic: Skin rash, irritation of mucous membrane
Endocrine & metabolic: Metabolic acidosis
Hematologic: Leukocytosis
Hepatic: Hepatitis
Local: Thrombophlebitis
Renal: Renal tubular acidosis
Respiratory: Coughing, respiratory depression, pulmonary edema, laryngeal spasm
Miscellaneous: Psychological and physical dependence with prolonged use, albuminuria, porphyrinogenic

Signs & Symptoms of Acute Overdose Mild hypotension, dyspnea, confusion, hyperventilation, tachypnea, coma, respiratory depression, metabolic acidosis, pulmonary edema, pulmonary hemorrhage, mental confusion, acetone breath, stomatitis, myasthenia gravis (exacerbation or precipitation of), hemorrhagic gastritis, feces discoloration (black), renal failure; death has occurred with as little as 12-25 mL usually due to pulmonary edema

Toxicodynamics/Kinetics
Onset of hypnosis:
Oral: Within 10-15 minutes
I.M.: Within 2-3 minutes

(Continued)

Paraldehyde *(Continued)*

Duration: 6-8 hours
Absorption:
- Oral: 95%
- Rectal: 75%

Distribution: V_d: Neonates: 1.7 L/kg; adults: 0.9 L/kg; crosses the placenta
Metabolism: ~70% to 80% of a dose metabolized in the liver probably to acetaldehyde and then to acetic acid whereupon it is further metabolized via the Kreb's cycle to carbon dioxide and water
Half-life:
- Neonates: 10 hours
- Adults: 6-7.4 hours

Elimination: Renal (3%); lungs (28%)

Usual Dosage
Oral: Sedation:
- Children: 0.15-0.3 mL/kg
- Adults: 4-8 mL

I.M., I.V.: I.V. use is rare and should be diluted (4% to 5% solution): 0.1-0.3 mL/kg
Rectal:
- Children: 0.3 mL/kg to a maximum dose of 5 mL
- Adults: 4-8 mL diluted with sodium chloride

Minimal lethal dose:
- Oral: 25 mL
- I.V.: 35 mL
- Rectal: 12 mL

Administration
Oral: Dilute in milk or iced fruit juice
Rectal: Mix paraldehyde 2:1 with oil (cottonseed or olive)

Do **not** use any plastic equipment for administration, use glass syringes and rubber tubing

Contraindications Severe hepatic insufficiency, respiratory disease, gastrointestinal inflammation or ulceration, pregnancy, pulmonary disease

Warnings Use with caution in patients with asthma or other bronchopulmonary disease

Dosage Forms
Injection: 100% paraldehyde (5 mL ampul)
Liquid, oral or rectal: 1 g/mL (30 mL)

Stability Decomposes with exposure to air and light to acetaldehyde which then oxidizes to acetic acid; store in tightly closed containers; protect from light

Reference Range Antiseizure therapeutic blood level: 100-200 mg/L; blood levels approaching 1000 mg/L associated with fatality

Overdosage Treatment
Decontamination: Lavage (within 30 minutes)/activated charcoal; do not induce emesis
Supportive therapy: Treat acidosis with sodium bicarbonate; for hypotension, fluid challenge with isotonic saline or placement of patient in Trendelenburg position; vasopressors (dopamine or norepinephrine) can be used for refractory cases

Test Interactions Ketonuria may be present

Drug Interactions Barbiturates and alcohol may enhance CNS depression; "disulfiram reaction" with disulfiram

Pregnancy Risk Factor C

Patient Information Do not attempt tasks requiring psychomotor coordination until the CNS effects by the drug are known; do not drink alcohol; may cause physical and psychological dependence; do not use if solution has a brownish color

Nursing Implications Discard unused contents of any container which has been opened for more than 24 hours; do **not** use discolored solution; do **not** use any plastic equipment for administration; parenteral solution may be given orally; should be given in milk or iced fruit juice or dilute to 200 mL with saline

Additional Information Do not abruptly discontinue in patients receiving chronic therapy; decomposes to acetic aid in air; 4-8 mL of paraldehyde is equivalent to 30 mg of phenobarbital; was used for the treatment of delirium, tremors, but its use has been supplanted by benzodiazepines; odor of acetic acid indicates that decomposition has occurred; may be irritating to mucosa

Specific References

Bostrum B, "Paraldehyde Toxicity During Treatment of Status Epilepticus," *Am J Dis Child*, 1982, 136:414-5.

Ramsay RE, "Pharmacokinetics and Clinical Use of Parenteral Phenytoin, Phenobarbital, and Paraldehyde," *Epilepsia*, 1989, 20(Suppl 2):S1-3.

Paramethad *see* Paramethadione *on next page*

Paramethadione (par a meth a dye' one)

CAS Number 115-67-3

Brand Names Paradione®

Synonyms Isoethadione; Paramethad

Use Control absence (petit mal) seizures refractory to other drugs

Mechanism of Action Elevates the cortical and basal seizure thresholds, and reduces the synaptic response to low frequency impulses; similar properties to troxidone

Adverse Reactions

Central nervous system: Drowsiness, myasthenia gravis (exacerbation)

Dermatologic: Exfoliative dermatitis, rash, photosensitivity

Hematologic: Agranulocytosis, aplastic anemia, thrombocytopenia, exacerbation of porphyria

Hepatic: Hepatitis

Ocular: Blurred vision, nystagmus, photophobia

Renal: Nephrosis, proteinuria

Miscellaneous: Feces discoloration (black), systemic lupus erythematosus (SLE)

Signs & Symptoms of Acute Overdose Nausea, ataxia, visual disturbances, vision color changes (white tinge), systemic lupus erythematosus (SLE), leukopenia; neutropenia; agranulocytosis; granulocytopenia

Toxicodynamics/Kinetics

Absorption: Rapid from gastrointestinal tract

Distribution: Widely throughout the body

Protein binding: Insignificant

Metabolism: Hepatic metabolism via microsomal enzymes

Half-life: 12-24 hours

Elimination: Slow renal excretion (primarily as active metabolites)

Usual Dosage Oral:

Children: 300-900 mg/day in 3-4 equally divided doses

Adults: Initial: 900 mg/day in 3-4 equally divided doses, increase by 300 mg at weekly intervals to maximum of 2.4 g/day

Dosing adjustment in renal/hepatic impairment: Avoid use in patients with Cl_{cr} <10 mL/minute or with severe liver disease

Contraindications Blood dyscrasias, renal and hepatic impairment, known hypersensitivity to paramethadione, pregnancy

Warnings Because of the potential for fetal malformations, paramethadione should only be used when less toxic agents are ineffective; use with caution in patients with hepatic or renal impairment, systemic lupus erythematosus, retina or optic nerve disease, blood dyscrasias, or porphyria; some products may contain tartrazines

Dosage Forms Capsule: 150 mg, 300 mg

Overdosage Treatment

Decontamination: Lavage/activated charcoal with cathartic is useful

Enhanced elimination: Alkalinization of the urine increases elimination of the active metabolite; multiple dosing of activated charcoal may be useful

Test Interactions Increases alkaline phosphatase (S); decreases calcium (S), thyroxine (S)

Pregnancy Risk Factor D (associated with high incidence of congenital malformations, 4 times more hazardous than ethosuximide)

Patient Information Capsule must be swallowed whole; sunglasses may help in photophobic reaction; avoid excessive exposure to sunlight, use sunscreen or protective clothing; take with food or milk; do not abruptly discontinue or change dose, may cause drowsiness, impair coordination, or judgment; notify physician of persistent fever, sore throat, fatigue, skin rash, or unusual bleeding or bruising

Nursing Implications Raise side rails, institute safety measures, assist with ambulation

Additional Information Only supplied graduated dropper should be used to measure oral solution; clean, colorless liquid with aromatic odor

Specific References

Fabro S and Brown NA, "Teratogenic Potential of Anticonvulsants," *N Engl J Med*, 1979, 300(22):1280-1.

Paregoric (par e gor' ik)

CAS Number 8029-99-0

Synonyms Camphorated Tincture of Opium

Use Treatment of diarrhea or relief of pain; neonatal opiate withdrawal (heroin or methadone-induced withdrawal seizures)

Mechanism of Action Increases smooth muscle tone in gastrointestinal tract, decreases motility and peristalsis, diminishes digestive secretions

Adverse Reactions

Cardiovascular: Hypotension, bradycardia, vasodilation

(Continued)

Paregoric *(Continued)*

Central nervous system: CNS depression, intracranial pressure (increased), drowsiness, dizziness, sedation

Endocrine & metabolic: Syndrome of inappropriate antidiuretic hormone (SIADH)

Gastrointestinal: Nausea, vomiting, constipation

Genitourinary: Urinary retention, ADH release

Ocular: Miosis

Respiratory: Apnea, respiratory depression

Miscellaneous: Physical and psychological dependence, histamine release, urinary and biliary tract spasm

Toxicodynamics/Kinetics In terms of opium

Duration of action: 4-5 hours

Metabolism: In the liver

Elimination: Excreted in urine, primarily as morphine glucuronide conjugates and as parent compound (morphine, codeine, papaverine, etc)

Usual Dosage Oral:

Neonatal opiate withdrawal: 3-6 drops every 3-6 hours as needed, or initially 0.2 mL every 3 hours; increase dosage by approximately 0.05 mL every 3 hours until withdrawal symptoms are controlled; it is rare to exceed 0.7 mL/dose. Stabilize withdrawal symptoms for 3-5 days, then gradually decrease dosage over a 2- to 4-week period.

Children: 0.25-0.5 mL/kg 1-4 times/day

Adults: 5-10 mL 1-4 times/day

Contraindications Hypersensitivity to opium or any component; diarrhea caused by poisoning until the toxic material has been removed

Warnings Use with caution in patients with respiratory, hepatic or renal dysfunction, severe prostatic hypertrophy, or history of narcotic abuse; opium shares the toxic potential of opiate agonists, and usual precautions of opiate agonist therapy should be observed; some preparations contain sulfites which may cause allergic reactions; infants <3 months of age are more susceptible to respiratory depression, use with caution and generally in reduced doses in this age group

Dosage Forms Liquid: 2 mg morphine equivalent/5 mL [equivalent to 20 mg opium powder] (5 mL, 60 mL, 473 mL, 4000 mL)

Stability Store in light-resistant, tightly closed container

Overdosage Treatment Supportive therapy: Naloxone hydrochloride (0.4-2 mg I.V., S.C., or through an endotracheal tube); a continuous infusion (at ⅔ the response dose/hour) may be required

Antidote(s)

Naloxone Hydrochloride *on page 1447*

Test Interactions ↑ aminotransferase [ALT (SGPT)/AST (SGOT)] (S)

Drug Interactions Increased effect/toxicity with CNS depressants (eg, alcohol, narcotics, benzodiazepines, TCAs, MAO inhibitors, phenothiazine)

Pregnancy Risk Factor B (D when used long-term or in high doses)

Patient Information Avoid alcohol, may cause drowsiness, impaired judgment or coordination; may be addicting if used for prolonged periods

Nursing Implications Observe patient for excessive sedation, respiratory depression, implement safety measures, assist with ambulation

Additional Information Contains morphine 0.4 mg/mL and alcohol 45%

Specific References

Calabrese JR and Gulledge AD, "The Neonatal Narcotic Abstinence Syndrome: A Brief Review," *Can J Psychiatry*, 1985, 30(8):623-6.

Parizal® *see* Omeprazole *on page 576*

Parmid® *see* Metoclopramide *on page 523*

Parnate® *see* Tranylcypromine Sulfate *on page 763*

Paroxetine Hydrochloride (pa rox' e teen)

CAS Number 61869-08-7; 78246-49-8

Brand Names Paxil™; Seroxat®

Use Treatment of depression

Investigational: Obsessive-compulsive disorder

Mechanism of Action Paroxetine is a selective serotonin reuptake inhibitor (similar to fluvoxamine maleate), chemically unrelated to tricyclic, tetracyclic, or other antidepressants; presumably, the inhibition of serotonin reuptake from brain synapse stimulated serotonin activity in the brain; a phenylpiperidine derivative

Adverse Reactions

Cardiovascular: Bradycardia, hypotension, palpitation, vasodilation, hypotension (orthostatic)

Central nervous system: Headache, asthenia, nervousness, anxiety, somnolence, dizziness, insomnia, migraine, exacerbation of parkinsonism, extrapyramidal reaction, akathisia, electroencephalogram abnormalities

Dermatologic: Alopecia

Endocrine & metabolic: Amenorrhea, syndrome of inappropriate antidiuretic hormone, serotonin syndrome

Gastrointestinal: Constipation, diarrhea, nausea, dry mouth, anorexia, flatulence, vomiting, gastritis, thirst

Genitourinary: Ejaculatory disturbances, decreased libido, priapism

Hematologic: Granulocytopenia, anemia, leukopenia, neutropenia, agranulocytosis

Neuromuscular & skeletal: Arthritis, tremors, paresthesia

Ocular: Eye pain

Otic: Ear pain

Respiratory: Asthma

Miscellaneous: Bruxism, sweating

Signs & Symptoms of Acute Overdose Anxiety, confusion, dyspepsia, priapism, tachycardia, insomnia, hyponatremia, diarrhea, urinary frequency, fatigue, ejaculatory disturbances, extrapyramidal reaction, hypotension

Toxicodynamics/Kinetics

Distribution: V_d: 13 L/kg

Protein binding: 95%

Metabolism: Extensive by cytochrome P-450 enzymes to catechol and other inactive metabolites

Half-life: 21 hours; prolonged to 30-40 hours in elderly

Elimination: Metabolites are excreted in bile and urine

Usual Dosage Adults: Oral: 20 mg once daily (maximum: 50 mg/day), preferably in the morning; in elderly, debilitated, or patients with hepatic or renal impairment, start with 10 mg/day (maximum: 40 mg/day); adjust doses at 7-day intervals

Contraindications Do not use within 14 days of MAO inhibitors

Warnings Use cautiously in patients with a history of seizures, mania, renal disease, cardiac disease, suicidal patients, children, or during breast-feeding in lactating women; avoid ECT

Dosage Forms Tablet: 20 mg, 30 mg

Reference Range Oral doses of 40 mg produced a peak serum level of 26.6 ng/mL

Overdosage Treatment

Decontamination: Lavage/activated charcoal with cathartic

Supportive therapy: Crystalloid infusion for hypotension

Enhancement of elimination: Multiple dosing of activated charcoal may be effective

Test Interactions ↑ LFTs, hyponatremia (especially in elderly)

Drug Interactions

Decreased effect with phenobarbital, phenytoin

Increased effect/toxicity with alcohol, cimetidine, methohexital (seizures), MAO inhibitors (hyperpyrexic crisis); increased effect/toxicity of TCAs, fluoxetine, sertraline, phenothiazines, class 1C antiarrhythmics, warfarin (need to monitor for bleeding)

Increased toxicity (serotonin syndrome) when administered with over-the-counter cold medications (dextromethorphan); sertraline or paroxetine can incite occurrence of LSD flashback episodes (primarily visual); severe bradykinesia and tremor with molindone

Pregnancy Risk Factor B

Monitoring Parameters Hepatic and renal function tests, blood pressure, heart rate

Additional Information Similar properties to fluvoxamine maleate; buspirone (15-60 mg/day) may be useful in treatment of sexual dysfunction during treatment with a selective serotonin reuptake inhibitor

Specific References

Adler LA and Angrist BM, "Paroxetine and Akathisia," *Biol Psychiatry*, 1995, 37:336-7.

Ahmad S, "Paroxetine-Induced Priapism," *Arch Intern Med*, 1995, 155(6):645.

Bioch M, Stager SV, Braun AR, et al, "severe Psychiatric Symptoms Associated With Paroxetine Withdrawal," *Lancet*, 1995, 346:57.

Boyer WF and Blumhardt CL, "The Safety Profile of Paroxetine," *J Clin Psychiatry*, 1992, 53(Suppl):61-6.

Dechant KL and Clissold SP, "Paroxetine: A Review of Its Pharmacodynamic and Pharmacokinetic Properties and Therapeutic Potential in Depressive Illness," *Drugs*, 1991, 41(2):225-53.

Dunbar GC, "An Interim Overview of the Safety and Tolerability of Paroxetine," *Acta Psychiatr Scand*, 1989, 350:135-7.

Folkerts H, "Spontaneous Seizure After Concurrent Use of Methohexital Anesthesia for Electroconvulsive Therapy and Paroxetine: A Case Report," *J Nerv Ment Dis*, 1995, 183:115-6.

Gorman SE, Rice T, and Simmons HF, "Paroxetine Overdose," *Am J Emerg Med*, 1993, 11(6):682.

Greb WH, Buscher G, Dierdorf HD, et al, "Ability of Charcoal to Prevent Absorption of Paroxetine," *Acta Psychiatr Scand Suppl*, 1989, 350:156-7.

Jimenez-Jimenez FJ, Tejeiro J, Martinez-Junquera G, et al, "Parkinsonism Exacerbated by Paroxetine," *Neurology*, 1994, 44(12):2406.

Malek-Ahmadi P and Allen SA, "Paroxetine-Molindone Interaction," *J Clin Psychiatry*, 1995, 56(2):82-3.

(Continued)

Paroxetine Hydrochloride *(Continued)*

Markel H, Lee A, Holmes RD, et al, "LSD Flashback Syndrome Exacerbated by Selective Serotonin Reuptake Inhibitor Antidepressants in Adolescents," *J Pediatr*, 1994, 125(5 Pt 1):817-9.
McKenzie LJ and Risch SC, "Fibrocystic Breast Disease Following Treatment With Selective Serotonin Reuptake Inhibitors," *Am J Psychiatry*, 1995, 152(3):471.
Myers LB, Dean BS, and Krenzelok EP, "Paroxetine (Paxil®): Overdose Assessment of a New Selective Serotonin Reuptake Inhibitor," *Vet Hum Toxicol*, 1994, 36:370.
Nemeroff CB, "The Clinical Pharmacology and Use of Paroxetine, A New Selective Serotonin Reuptake Inhibitor," *Pharmacotherapy*, 1994, 14(2):127-38.
Norden MJ, "Buspirone Treatment of Sexual Dysfunction Associated With Selective Serotonin Re-Uptake Inhibitors," *Depression*, 1994, 2:109-12.
Reeves RR and Bullen JA, "Serotonin Syndrome Produced by Paroxetine and Low-Dose Trazodone," *Psychosomatics*, 1995, 36:159-60.
Skop BP, Finkelstein JA, Mareth TR, et al, "The Serotonin Syndrome Associated With Paroxetine, an Over-the-Counter Cold Remedy, and Vascular Disease," *Am J Emerg Med*, 1994, 12(6):642-4.

PAS *see* Para-Aminosalicylate Sodium *on page 592*
Pavabid® *see* Papaverine *on page 591*
Pavagen® *see* Papaverine *on page 591*
Pavakey® *see* Papaverine *on page 591*
Pavaspan® *see* Papaverine *on page 591*
Pavasull® *see* Papaverine *on page 591*
Pavatab® *see* Papaverine *on page 591*
Pavatine® Pavased® *see* Papaverine *on page 591*
Pavatym® *see* Papaverine *on page 591*
Paveral *see* Codeine *on page 238*
Paverine Spancap® *see* Papaverine *on page 591*
Paverolan® *see* Papaverine *on page 591*
Paxil™ *see* Paroxetine Hydrochloride *on page 596*
PBZ® *see* Tripelennamine *on page 776*
PBZ-SR® *see* Tripelennamine *on page 776*
PCE® Oral *see* Erythromycin *on page 319*
Pectomed® *see* Ammonium Chloride *on page 118*
PediaCare® Oral *see* Pseudoephedrine *on page 661*
Pediaflor® *see* Fluoride *on page 355*
PediaProfen™ *see* Ibuprofen *on page 418*
Peganone® *see* Ethotoin *on page 335*
Pelson® *see* Nitrazepam *on page 562*

Pemoline

Related Information

Therapeutic Drugs Associated With Hallucinations *on page 1558-1559*

CAS Number 2152-34-3; 68942-31-4; 18968-99-5

Brand Names Cylert®; Dynalert®; Tradon®; Volital®

Synonyms Phenoxazole; Phenylisohydantoin; Phenylpseudohydantoin

Use Controlling undirected hyperkinetic behavior; treat narcolepsy and antihistamine-induced drowsiness

Mechanism of Action Sympathetic amine similar in action to amphetamines; central nervous system stimulant

Adverse Reactions

Hepatic: Fulminant liver failure

Signs & Symptoms of Acute Overdose Choreoathetosis, rhabdomyolysis, hyperthermia, leukocytosis, mydriasis, vomiting, neutropenia, stuttering, dyskinesias, exacerbates Tourette's syndrome, anorexia, elevated liver function tests (1% to 2%), nystagmus, mania, insomnia, visual, tactile, and auditory hallucinations

Toxicodynamics/Kinetics

Protein binding: 50%
Distribution: V_d: 0.2-0.6 L/kg
Metabolism: Hepatic
Half-life:
 Children: 7 hours
 Adults: 12 hours
Elimination: Renal (50%)

Usual Dosage Oral: Initial: 37.5 mg increasing by 18.75 mg weekly; usual dose: 56.25-75 mg/day; maximum: 112.5 mg

Contraindications Hypersensitivity to pemoline; children with attention deficit disorder, concomitant Tourette's syndrome

Warnings Can produce dependence, can decrease seizure threshold; use with caution in patients with hepatic or renal dysfunction

Dosage Forms

Tablet: 18.75 mg, 37.5 mg, 75 mg

Tablet, chewable: 37.5 mg

Reference Range Therapeutic plasma range: 1-7 μg/mL

Overdosage Treatment

Decontamination: Lavage/activated charcoal with cathartic

Supportive therapy: Diazepam can be used to treat choreoathetosis and may be more effective than benztropine; alkaline diuresis with a diuretic (mannitol or furosemide) should be used to prevent renal failure due to rhabdomyolysis

Test Interactions May produce false elevations of acid phosphatase

Drug Interactions Do not use with MAO inhibitors in that hypertensive crisis can occur; magnesium hydroxide may increase absorption of pemoline

Pregnancy Risk Factor B

Additional Information Choreiform movements can occur in children at doses as low as 2 mg/kg; similar to dexamphetamine sulfate

Specific References

Bachman DS, "Pemoline-Induced Tourette's Disorder: A Case Report," *Am J Psychiatry*, 1981, 138:1116-7.

Berkovitch M, Pope E, Phillips J, et al, "Pemoline-Associated Fulminant Liver Failure: Testing the Evidence for Causation," *Clin Pharmacol Ther*, 1995, 57:696-8.

Briscoe JG, Curry SC, Gerkin RD, et al, "Pemoline-Induced Choreoathetosis and Rhabdomyolysis," *Med Toxicol*, 1988, 3(1):72-6.

Lindau W and de Girolami E, "Pemoline and the Prostate," *Lancet*, 1986, 1(8483):738.

Newlands WJ, "The Effect of Pemoline on Antihistamine-Induced Drowsiness," *Practitioner*, 1980, 224:1199-201.

Polchert SE and Morse RM, "Pemoline Abuse," *JAMA*, 1985, 254(7):946-7.

Sternbach H, "Pemoline-Induced Mania," *Biol Psychol*, 1981, 16:987-9.

Penbutolol Sulfate (pen byoo' toe lole)

Related Information

Beta-Blockers Comparison *on page 1644-1645*

CAS Number 38363-40-5; 38363-32-5

Brand Names Betapressin®; Blocotin®; Hostabloc®; Ipobar®; Lasipressin®; Levatol®

Use Treatment of mild to moderate arterial hypertension

Mechanism of Action Blocks both $beta_1$- and $beta_2$-receptors and has mild intrinsic sympathomimetic activity; has negative inotropic and chronotropic effects and can significantly slow A-V nodal conduction

Adverse Reactions

Cardiovascular: Exacerbation of Raynaud's phenomenon, persistent bradycardia, hypotension, congestive heart failure, A-V block, chest pain, edema, heart failure

Central nervous system: Nightmares, fatigue, insomnia, ataxia, drowsiness, depression, confusion, dizziness, headache

Gastrointestinal: Constipation, diarrhea, nausea, vomiting

Genitourinary: Impotence, nocturia, enuresis

Ocular: Diplopia

Respiratory: Chest pain

Miscellaneous: Cold extremities

Toxicodynamics/Kinetics

Absorption: Readily absorbed

Distribution: V_d: 0.5 L/kg

Protein binding: 80% to 98%

Metabolism: In liver (active metabolites)

Bioavailability: 100%

Half-life, plasma: 4.5 hours

Time to peak serum concentration: 1.5 hours

Elimination: 3% excreted as unchanged in 72 hours

Usual Dosage Adults: Oral: Initial: 20 mg once daily, full effect of a 20 or 40 mg dose is seen by the end of a 2-week period; doses of 40-80 mg have been tolerated but have shown little additional antihypertensive effects

Contraindications Uncompensated congestive heart failure, cardiogenic shock, bradycardia or heart block

Dosage Forms Tablet: 20 mg

Reference Range 50 mg dose results in peak serum concentration of 770 ng/mL after 1 hour

Overdosage Treatment

Decontamination: Lavage/activated charcoal with cathartic

Supportive therapy: Sympathomimetics (eg, epinephrine or dopamine), atropine, glucagon, or a pacemaker can be used to treat the toxic bradycardia, asystole,

(Continued)

Penbutolol Sulfate *(Continued)*

and/or hypotension; initially fluids may be the best treatment for toxic hypotension

Enhancement of elimination: Charcoal hemoperfusion can be used to lower serum levels

Pregnancy Risk Factor C

Specific References

Giudicelli JF, Richer C, and Chauvin M, "Comparative Beta-Adrenergic Receptor Block Effects and Pharmacokinetics of Penbutolol and Propranolol in Man," *Br J Clin Pharmacol*, 1977, 4(2):135-40.

Vallner JJ, Jun HW, and Needham TE, "Plasma Level Studies of Penbutolol After Oral Dose in Man," *J Clin Pharmacol*, 1977, 17(4):231-6.

Wilkinson J, "Beta Blocker Overdoses," *Ann Emerg Med*, 1986, 15(8):982.

Penetrex™ *see* Enoxacin *on page 315*

Penicillin G, Parenteral, Aqueous

(pen i sil' in gee, pa ren' ter al, aye' kwee us)

CAS Number 61-33-6; 69-57-8; 113-98-4

Brand Names Benzatec®; Cilipen®; Crystapen®; Noveopen®; Pentids®; Pfizerpen® Injection; Sodiopen®

Synonyms Benzylpenicillin Potassium; Benzylpenicillin Sodium; Crystalline Penicillin; Penicillin G Potassium; Penicillin G Sodium

Use Active against most gram-positive organisms except *Staphylococcus aureus*; some gram-negative such as *Neisseria gonorrhoeae* and some anaerobes and spirochetes; although ceftriaxone is now the drug of choice for Lyme disease and gonorrhea

Mechanism of Action Interferes with bacterial cell wall synthesis during active multiplication, causing cell wall death and resultant bactericidal activity against susceptible bacteria

Adverse Reactions

Central nervous system: Convulsions, anxiety, confusion, drowsiness, fever

Dermatologic: Rash, angioedema, urticaria

Endocrine & metabolic: Electrolyte imbalance, hypernatremia with sodium salt, hyperkalemia with potassium salt

Gastrointestinal: Nausea, diarrhea, pseudomembranous colitis

Hematologic: Hemolytic anemia, positive Coombs' reaction, neutropenia

Local: Thrombophlebitis

Neuromuscular & skeletal: Myoclonus

Renal: Acute interstitial nephritis (after large I.V. doses)

Miscellaneous: Jarisch-Herxheimer reaction, hypersensitivity reactions, anaphylaxis (0.05% frequency with injection); total allergic reactions (1% to 10%)

Signs & Symptoms of Acute Overdose Leukopenia or neutropenia (agranulocytosis, granulocytopenia); dyspnea, coagulopathy, tongue discoloration, pseudotumor cerebri, periarteritis nodosa, pemphigus, eosinophilia, colitis

Toxicodynamics/Kinetics

Absorption: Oral: 30%

Distribution: V_d: 0.2 L/kg; penetration across the blood-brain barrier is poor, despite inflamed meninges

Protein binding: 40% to 60%

Metabolism: In the liver (30%) to penicilloic acid

Half-life:

- Neonates:
  - <6 days: 3.2-3.4 hours
  - 7-13 days: 1.2-2.2 hours
  - >14 days: 0.9-1.9 hours
- Children and Adults with normal renal function: 20-50 minutes

Time to peak serum concentration:

- I.M.: Within 30 minutes
- I.V.: Within 1 hour

Elimination: Excreted in urine

Usual Dosage I.M., I.V. (do not give intrathecal):

Neonates:

- Postnatal age <7 days:
  - <2000 g: 25,000 units/kg/dose every 12 hours; meningitis: 50,000 units/kg/dose every 12 hours
  - >2000 g: 20,000 units/kg/dose every 8 hours; meningitis: 50,000 units/kg/dose every 8 hours
- Postnatal age >7 days:
  - <1200 g: 25,000 units/kg/dose every 12 hours; meningitis: 50,000 units/kg/dose every 12 hours
  - 1200-2000 g: 25,000 units/kg/dose every 8 hours; meningitis: 75,000 units/kg/dose every 8 hours

>2000 g: 25,000 units/kg/dose every 6 hours; meningitis: 50,000 units/kg/dose every 6 hours

Infants and Children (sodium salt is preferred in children): 100,000-250,000 units/kg/day in divided doses every 4 hours; maximum: 4.8 million units/24 hours
Severe infections: Up to 400,000 units/kg/day in divided doses every 4 hours; maximum dose: 24 million units/day

Adults: 2-24 million units/day in divided doses every 4 hours

Dosing interval in renal impairment:
Cl_{cr} 30-50 mL/minute: Administer every 6 hours
Cl_{cr} 10-30 mL/minute: Administer every 8 hours
Cl_{cr} <10 mL/minute: Administer every 12 hours

Toxic dose: 10,000,000 units (or 6 g)

Contraindications Known hypersensitivity to penicillin or any component

Warnings Avoid intravascular or intra-arterial administration or injection into or near major peripheral nerves or blood vessels since such injections may cause severe and/or permanent neurovascular damage; use with caution in patients with renal impairment, pre-existing seizure disorders, or with a history of hypersensitivity to cephalosporins

Dosage Forms
Injection, as sodium: 5 million units
Injection:
Frozen premixed, as potassium: 1 million units, 2 million units, 3 million units
Powder, as potassium: 1 million units, 5 million units, 10 million units, 20 million units

Stability Reconstituted parenteral solution is stable for 7 days when refrigerated; for I.V. infusion in NS or D_5W, solution is stable for 24 hours at room temperature; thawed solutions stable for 24 hours at room temperature or 14 days at refrigeration

Reference Range After 500 mg oral dose, peak plasma level is 1.5-2.7 mg/L

Overdosage Treatment
Decontamination: Emesis or lavage rarely necessary/activated charcoal with cathartic can be used
Supportive therapy: Allergic reactions can be treated with epinephrine, diphenhydramine, and corticosteroids
Enhancement of elimination: Hemodialysis or charcoal hemoperfusion can be useful in removing penicillin; moderately dialyzable (20% to 50%)

Antidote(s)
Epinephrine *on page 1422*

Test Interactions False-positive or negative urinary glucose determination using Clinitest®; positive Coombs' [direct]; false-positive urinary and/or serum proteins; interferes with the Guthrie test for phenylketonuria

Diagnostic Tests/Procedures
Electrolytes, Urine *on page 1254*

Drug Interactions Increased levels with probenecid

Pregnancy Risk Factor B

Pregnancy Implications Crosses the placenta; appears in breast milk

Patient Information Report any rash or dyspnea

Nursing Implications Administer I.M. by deep injection in the upper outer quadrant of the buttock; dosage modification required in patients with renal insufficiency; give around-the-clock to promote less variation in peak and trough levels

Additional Information
Penicillin G potassium: 1.7 mEq of potassium and 0.3 mEq of sodium per 1 million units of penicillin G
Penicillin G sodium: 2 mEq of sodium per 1 million units of penicillin G

Specific References
Wickerts CJ, Asaba H, Gunnarsson B, et al, "Combined Carbon Haemoperfusion and Haemodialysis in the Treatment of Penicillin Intoxication," *Br Med J*, 1980, 280(6226):1254-5.

Penicillin G Potassium *see* Penicillin G, Parenteral, Aqueous *on previous page*

Penicillin G Sodium *see* Penicillin G, Parenteral, Aqueous *on previous page*

Pentafen® *see* Pentazocine *on page 603*

Pentalgina® *see* Pentazocine *on page 603*

Pentam-300® *see* Pentamidine Isethionate *on this page*

Pentamidine Isethionate (pen tam' i deen eye se thi' o nate)

CAS Number 140-64-7

Brand Names NebuPent™; Pentam-300®

Use Treatment and prevention of pneumonia caused by *Pneumocystis carinii*; treatment of trypanosomiasis; leishmaniasis

(Continued)

Pentamidine Isethionate *(Continued)*

Mechanism of Action Interferes with RNA/DNA, phospholipids and protein synthesis, through inhibition of oxidative phosphorylation and/or interference with incorporation of nucleotides and nucleic acids into RNA and DNA, in protozoa

Adverse Reactions

Cardiovascular: Hypotension, tachycardia, hypotension (orthostatic), torsade de pointes

Central nervous system: Dizziness, fever

Dermatologic: Jarisch-Herxheimer-like reaction, rash

Endocrine & metabolic: Hypoglycemia, hyperglycemia, hypocalcemia

Gastrointestinal: Vomiting, metallic taste in mouth, pancreatitis

Hematologic: Megaloblastic anemia, granulocytopenia, leukopenia, thrombocytopenia, eosinophilia

Local: Pain at injection site

Renal/hepatic: Mild renal or hepatic injury

Respiratory: Irritation of the airway, cough, wheezing, bronchospasm

Signs & Symptoms of Acute Overdose Hypotension, azotemia, wheezing, anorexia, Q-T prolongation, Stevens-Johnson syndrome, cough, hypomagnesemia, toxic epidermal necrolysis, hypocalcemia, myoglobinuria, rhabdomyolysis, conjunctivitis, hypoglycemia, hyperglycemia, cardiac arrhythmias; no cases of acute oral overdose published, leukopenia, neutropenia, agranulocytosis, granulocytopenia

Toxicodynamics/Kinetics

Absorption: I.M.: Well absorbed

Distribution: V_d: Steady state: 3-32 L/kg; systemic accumulation of pentamidine does not appear to occur following inhalation therapy

Protein binding: 69%

Metabolism: Unknown

Half-life: Terminal: 6.4-9.4 hours; may be prolonged in patients with severe renal impairment

Elimination: 33% to 66% excreted in urine as unchanged drug

Usual Dosage

Children:

Treatment: I.M., I.V. (I.V. preferred): 4 mg/kg/day once daily for 14 days

Prevention:

I.M., I.V.: 4 mg/kg monthly or every 2 weeks

Inhalation (aerosolized pentamidine in children ≥5 years): 300 mg/dose given every 4 weeks via Respirgard® II inhaler (8 mg/kg dose has also been used)

Adults:

Treatment: I.M., I.V. (I.V. preferred): 4 mg/kg/day once daily for 14 days

Prevention: Inhalation: 300 mg every 4 weeks via Respirgard® II nebulizer

Dosing interval in renal impairment:

Cl_{cr} 10-50 mL/minute: Administer every 24-36 hours

Cl_{cr} <10 mL/minute: Administer every 48 hours

Contraindications Hypersensitivity to pentamidine isethionate or any component (inhalation and injection)

Warnings Patients receiving I.M. or I.V. pentamidine should be lying down and blood pressure should be monitored closely during administration of drug and several times thereafter until it is stable; use with caution in patients with diabetes mellitus, renal or hepatic dysfunction; hypertension or hypotension

Dosage Forms

Inhalation: 300 mg

Powder for injection, lyophilized: 300 mg

Stability Reconstituted solution is stable for 24 hours at room temperature; do not refrigerate due to the possibility of crystallization

Reference Range Peak plasma concentration after 2-hour I.V. infusion of 4 mg/kg pentamidine was 612 ng/mL

Overdosage Treatment

Supportive therapy: Bronchospasm can be treated with beta-agonist agents

Test Interactions Decreases glucose; elevates insulin levels

Diagnostic Tests/Procedures

Complete Blood Count *on page 1236*

Creatinine, Serum *on page 1243*

Liver Profile *on page 1286*

Drug Interactions Hypocalcemia with coadministration of foscarnet

Pregnancy Risk Factor C

Pregnancy Implications Based on animal data, the reference doses for embryolethality and for teratogenicity are estimated to be 0.08 mcg/kg/day and 4 mcg/kg/day, respectively. Aerosolized pentamidine can pass embryolethal doses to healthcare workers.

Monitoring Parameters Liver function tests, renal function tests, blood glucose, serum potassium and calcium, CBC with differential and platelet count, EKG, blood pressure

Patient Information PCP pneumonia may still occur despite pentamidine use; notify physician of fever, dyspnea, or coughing up blood

Nursing Implications Infuse I.V. slowly over a period of at least 60 minutes or administer deep I.M.

Additional Information Do not use NS as a diluent; NS is incompatible with pentamidine; infuse over at least 1 hour; hypotension associated with intravenous administration

Specific References

Comtois R, Pouliot J, Gervais S, et al, "High Pentamidine Levels Associated With Hypoglycemia and Azotemia in a Patient With *Pneumocystis carinii* Pneumonia," *Diagn Microbiol Infect Dis*, 1992, 15(6):523-6.

Conte JE Jr, "Pharmacokinetics of Intravenous Pentamidine in Patients With Normal Renal Function or Receiving Hemodialysis," *J Infect Dis*, 1991, 163(1):169-75.

Cortese LM, Gasser RA, Jr, Bjornson DC, et al, "Prolonged Recurrence of Pentamidine-Induced Torsade de Pointes," *Ann Pharmacother*, 1992, 26(11):1365-9.

Ito S and Koren G, "Estimation of Fetal Risk From Aerosolized Pentamidine in Pregnant Healthcare Workers," *Chest*, 1994, 106(5):1460-2.

Singh G, El-Gadi SM, and Sparks RA, "Pancreatitis Associated With Aerosolized Pentamidine," *Genitourin Med*, 1995, 71:130-1.

Pentazocine (pen taz' oh seen)

CAS Number 359-83-1; 2276-52-0; 17146-95-1; 64024-15-3

Brand Names Algopent®; Fortal®; Fortral®; Fortulgesic®; Fortwin®; Liticon®; Ospronim®; Pentafen®; Pentalgina®; Sosegon®; Sosenol®; Talwin®; Talwin® NX

Synonyms Pentazocine Hydrochloride; Pentazocine Lactate

Use Relief of moderate to severe pain; has also been used as a sedative prior to surgery and as a supplement to surgical anesthesia

Mechanism of Action Binds to opiate receptors in the CNS, causing inhibition of ascending pain pathways, altering the perception of and response to pain; produces generalized CNS depression; partial agonist-antagonist

Adverse Reactions

Cardiovascular: Palpitations, hypotension, tachycardia, peripheral vasodilation

Central nervous system: CNS depression, drowsiness, sedation, dizziness, euphoria, psychosis, lightheadedness (more frequently than morphine), hallucinations, confusion, disorientation, intracranial pressure (increased), seizures may occur in seizure-prone patients especially with large I.V. doses

Dermatologic: Pruritus, rash

Endocrine & metabolic: Syndrome of inappropriate antidiuretic hormone (SIADH)

Gastrointestinal: Nausea (more frequently than morphine), vomiting, constipation

Local: Tissue damage and irritation with I.M./S.C. use

Ocular: Miosis

Respiratory: Apnea, respiratory depression, laryngospasm

Miscellaneous: Physical and psychological dependence, histamine release, biliary or urinary tract spasm

Signs & Symptoms of Acute Overdose Hypertension, diarrhea, asterixis, toxic epidermal necrolysis, dry mouth, diplopia, nystagmus, myalgia, hyperthermia, erythema multiforme, tachycardia, seizures, respiratory depression, nephrotic syndrome, miosis, seizures

Toxicodynamics/Kinetics

Onset of action:

- Oral, I.M., S.C.: Within 15-30 minutes
- I.V.: Within 2-3 minutes

Duration:

- Oral: 4-5 hours
- Parenteral: 2-3 hours

Distribution: V_d: 4.4-7.8 L/kg

Protein binding: 61%

Metabolism: Large first-pass effect; metabolized in liver via oxidative and glucuronide conjugation pathways

Bioavailability, oral: ~20%; increased to 60% to 70% in patients with cirrhosis

Half-life: 2-3 hours; increased with decreased hepatic function

Elimination: Smaller amounts excreted unchanged in urine

Usual Dosage

Children: I.M., S.C.:

- 5-8 years: 15 mg
- 8-14 years: 30 mg

Children >12 years and Adults: Oral: 50 mg every 3-4 hours; may increase to 100 mg/dose if needed, but should not exceed 600 mg/day

Adults:

- I.M., S.C.: 30-60 mg every 3-4 hours, not to exceed total daily dose of 360 mg
- I.V.: 30 mg every 3-4 hours

(Continued)

Pentazocine *(Continued)*

Dosing adjustment in renal impairment:

Cl_{cr} 10-50 mL/minute: Administer 75% of normal dose

Cl_{cr} <10 mL/minute: Administer 50% of normal dose

Dosing adjustment in hepatic impairment: Reduce dose or avoid use in patients with liver disease

Contraindications Hypersensitivity to pentazocine or any component, increased intracranial pressure (unless the patient is mechanically ventilated)

Warnings Use with caution in seizure-prone patients, acute myocardial infarction, patients undergoing biliary tract surgery, patients with renal and hepatic dysfunction, head trauma, increased intracranial pressure, and patients with a history of prior opioid dependence or abuse; pentazocine may precipitate opiate withdrawal symptoms in patients who have been receiving opiates regularly; injection contains sulfites which may cause allergic reaction

Dosage Forms

Injection, as lactate: 30 mg/mL (1 mL, 1.5 mL, 2 mL, 10 mL)

Tablet: Pentazocine hydrochloride 50 mg and naloxone hydrochloride 0.5 mg

Stability Store at room temperature, protect from heat and from freezing; I.V. form is **incompatible** with aminophylline, amobarbital (and all other I.V. barbiturates), glycopyrrolate (same syringe), heparin (same syringe), nafcillin (Y-site)

Reference Range

Therapeutic: 0.05-0.2 mg/L

Fatal: >1.0 mg/L

Overdosage Treatment

Decontamination: Lavage/activated charcoal with cathartic; do not induce emesis

Supportive therapy: Naloxone hydrochloride (large doses may be required); seizures can be treated with diazepam, lorazepam, phenytoin, or phenobarbital

Antidote(s)

Naloxone Hydrochloride *on page 1447*

Diagnostic Tests/Procedures

Amylase, Serum *on page 1191*

Pentazocine, Urine *on page 1316*

Drug Interactions May potentiate or reduce analgesic effect of opiate agonist, (eg, morphine) depending on patients tolerance to opiates can precipitate withdrawal in narcotic addicts

Increased effect/toxicity with tripelennamine (can be lethal), CNS depressants (phenothiazines, tranquilizers, anxiolytics, sedatives, hypnotics, or alcohol)

Pregnancy Risk Factor B (D if used for prolonged periods or in high doses at term)

Pregnancy Implications Can cross the placenta

Monitoring Parameters Relief of pain, respiratory and mental status, blood pressure

Patient Information Avoid alcohol, may cause drowsiness, impaired judgment or coordination; may be addicting if used for prolonged periods; will cause withdrawal in patients currently dependent on narcotics

Nursing Implications Rotate injection site for I.M., S.C. use; avoid intra-arterial injection; observe patient for excessive sedation, respiratory depression, implement safety measures, assist with ambulation; observe for narcotic withdrawal

Additional Information Pentazocine hydrochloride: Talwin® NX tablet (with naloxone); naloxone is used to prevent abuse by dissolving tablets in water and using as injection; may be combined with tripelennamine (Ts and blues)

Specific References

Alexander JI and Spence AA, "Central Nervous Effects of Pentazocine," *Br Med J*, 1974, 2(912):224-5.

Challoner KR, McCarron MM, and Newton EJ, "Pentazocine (Talwin®) Intoxication: Report of 57 Cases," *J Emerg Med*, 1990, 8(1):67-74.

De Bard ML and Jagger JA, "T's and B's – Midwestern Heroin Substance," *Clin Toxicol*, 1981, 18(9):1117-23.

Martin WR, "Naloxone," *Ann Intern Med*, 1976, 85(6):765-8.

Reed DA and Schnoll SH, "Abuse of Pentazocine-Naloxone Combination," *JAMA*, 1986, 256(18):2562-4.

Pentazocine Hydrochloride *see* Pentazocine *on previous page*

Pentazocine Lactate *see* Pentazocine *on previous page*

Pentids® *see* Penicillin G, Parenteral, Aqueous *on page 600*

Pentobarbital (pen toe bar' bi tal)

CAS Number 76-74-4; 57-33-0

Brand Names Lethobard®; Nembutal®; Pentosol®; Repocal®; Sopental®

Use Short-term treatment of insomnia; preoperative sedation; high-dose barbiturate coma for treatment of increased intracranial pressure or status epilepticus unresponsive to other therapy

Mechanism of Action Short-acting barbiturate with sedative, hypnotic, and anticonvulsant properties

Adverse Reactions

Cardiovascular: Cardiac arrhythmias, hypotension

Central nervous system: Drowsiness, drowsiness, CNS stimulation or CNS depression, impaired judgment, decreased deep tendon reflexes, hypothermia

Dermatologic: Rash

Gastrointestinal: Nausea, vomiting

Renal: Oliguria

Respiratory: Laryngospasm, respiratory depression, apnea (especially with rapid I.V. use)

Miscellaneous: Physical and psychological dependency with chronic use

Signs & Symptoms of Acute Overdose Unsteady gait, slurred speech, rhabdomyolysis, confusion, bullous skin lesions, jaundice, ptosis, vision color changes (green tinge), vision color changes (yellow tinge); hypothermia, fever, hypotension, renal failure, myoglobinuria, hypoglycemia

Toxicodynamics/Kinetics

Onset of action:
- Oral or rectal: 15-60 minutes
- I.M.: Within 10-15 minutes
- I.V.: Within 1 minute

Duration:
- Oral or rectal: 1-4 hours
- I.V.: 15 minutes

Absorption: Oral, rectal: Rapid

Distribution: Widely throughout body
- V_d:
  - Children: 0.8 L/kg
  - Adults: 1 L/kg

Protein binding: 35% to 55%

Metabolism: Extensive in the liver via hydroxylation and oxidation pathways

Half-life: Terminal:
- Children: 25 hours
- Adults, normal: 22 hours
- Range: 35-50 hours

Elimination: <1% excreted unchanged renally

Usual Dosage

Children:
- Sedative: Oral: 2-6 mg/kg/day divided in 3 doses; maximum: 100 mg/day
- Hypnotic: I.M.: 2-6 mg/kg; maximum: 100 mg/dose
- Rectal:
  - 2 months to 1 year (10-20 lb): 30 mg
  - 1-4 years (20-40 lb): 30-60 mg
  - 5-12 years (40-80 lb): 60 mg
  - 12-14 years (80-110 lb): 60-120 mg **or**
  - <4 years: 3-6 mg/kg/dose
  - >4 years: 1.5-3 mg/kg/dose
- Preoperative/preprocedure sedation: ≥6 months:
  - Oral, I.M., rectal: 2-6 mg/kg; maximum: 100 mg/dose
  - I.V.: 1-3 mg/kg to a maximum of 100 mg until asleep
- Children 5-12 years: Conscious sedation prior to a procedure: I.V.: 2 mg/kg 5-10 minutes before procedures, may repeat one time

Adolescents: Conscious sedation: Oral, I.V.: 100 mg prior to a procedure

Adults:
- Hypnotic:
  - Oral: 100-200 mg at bedtime or 20 mg 3-4 times/day for daytime sedation
  - I.M.: 150-200 mg
  - I.V.: Initial: 100 mg, may repeat every 1-3 minutes up to 200-500 mg total dose
- Rectal: 120-200 mg at bedtime
- Preoperative sedation: I.M.: 150-200 mg

Children and Adults: Barbiturate coma in head injury patients: I.V.: Loading dose: 5-10 mg/kg given slowly over 1-2 hours; monitor blood pressure and respiratory rate; Maintenance infusion: Initial: 1 mg/kg/hour; may increase to 2-3 mg/kg/hour; maintain burst suppression on EEG

Dosing adjustment in hepatic impairment: Reduce dosage in patients with severe liver dysfunction

Contraindications Marked liver function impairment or latent porphyria; chronic or acute pain; hypersensitivity to barbiturates or any component

Warnings Use with caution in patients with hypovolemic shock, congestive heart failure, and hepatic impairment

Dosage Forms

Capsule, as sodium: 50 mg, 100 mg

Elixir: 18.2 mg/5 mL (473 mL, 4000 mL)

Injection, as sodium: 50 mg/mL (1 mL, 2 mL, 20 mL, 50 mL)

Suppository, rectal: 30 mg, 60 mg, 120 mg, 200 mg

(Continued)

Pentobarbital *(Continued)*

Stability Protect from light; aqueous solutions are not stable, commercially available vehicle (containing propylene glycol) is more stable; low pH may cause precipitate; use only clear solution; store in airtight container

Reference Range

Hypnotic: 1-5 μg/mL (SI: 4-22 μmol/L)
Drowsy: 6-10 μg/mL (SI: 44 μmol/L)
Stuporous: 11-17 μg/mL (SI: 46-76 μmol/L)
Coma: 20-50 μg/mL (SI: 88-221 μmol/L)

Overdosage Treatment

Decontamination: Lavage/activated charcoal with cathartic

Supportive therapy: If hypotension occurs, administer I.V. fluids and place the patient in the Trendelenburg position. If unresponsive, an I.V. vasopressor (eg, dopamine, epinephrine) may be required.

Enhancement of elimination: Forced alkaline diuresis is of no value in the treatment of intoxications with short-acting barbiturates. Charcoal hemoperfusion or hemodialysis may be useful in the harder to treat intoxications, especially in the presence of very high serum barbiturate levels with coma; multiple dosing of activated charcoal may be effective.

Test Interactions Increases ammonia (B); decreases bilirubin (S)

Drug Interactions Chloramphenicol, cimetidine, CNS depressants, doxycycline; can reduce effectiveness of beta-blockers

Pregnancy Risk Factor D (no correlation with development of congenital abnormalities demonstrated)

Pregnancy Implications Crosses placenta

Monitoring Parameters Respiratory status (for conscious sedation, includes pulse oximetry), cardiovascular status

Patient Information Avoid the use of alcohol and other CNS depressants; avoid driving and other hazardous tasks; avoid abrupt discontinuation; may cause physical and psychological dependence

Nursing Implications Parenteral solutions are highly alkaline; avoid extravasation; avoid rapid I.V. administration >50 mg/minute; institute safety measures to avoid injuries

Additional Information

Pentobarbital: Nembutal® elixir
Pentobarbital sodium: Nembutal® capsule, injection, and suppository

Specific References

McCarron MM, Schulze BW, Walberg CB, et al, "Short-Acting Barbiturate Overdosage. Correlation of Intoxication Score With Serum Barbiturate Concentration," *JAMA*, 1982, 248(1):55-61.
Wermeling D, Record K, Bell R, et al, "Hemodialysis Clearance of Pentobarbital During Continuous Infusion," *Ther Drug Monit*, 1985, 7(4):485-7.

Pentopuran® *see* Pentoxifylline *on next page*

Pentosol® *see* Pentobarbital *on page 604*

Pentostatin (pen' toe stat in)

CAS Number 53910-25-7

Brand Names Nipent™ Injection

Synonyms Co-vidarabine; dCF; Deoxycoformycin; 2'-deoxycoformycin

Use Orphan drug status in chronic lymphocytic leukemia and hairy cell leukemia; may be useful in *Mycosis fungoides*, refractory lymphomas

Mechanism of Action An irreversible inhibitor of adenosine deaminase (ADA) in the erythrocyte and lymphatic tissue which causes a build-up of deoxyadenosine thus inhibiting purine metabolism; also inhibits ribonucleotide reductase which blocks DNA synthesis

Adverse Reactions

Cardiovascular: Cardiomegaly, hypotension, flushing

Central nervous system: Lethargy, depression, coma, seizures, headache, fatigue, malaise, insomnia, dizziness, confusion, anxiety, ataxia, fever

Dermatologic: Dry skin, pruritus, eczema, alopecia, psoriasis

Endocrine & metabolic: Gynecomastia

Gastrointestinal: Anorexia, nausea, vomiting, constipation, diarrhea

Hematologic: Leukopenia (at doses >5 mg/m^2/day), lymphocytopenia, thrombocytopenia, anemia, eosinophilia, hemolysis, bone marrow depression, hemolytic anemia

Hepatic: Hepatotoxicity (which is reversible)

Neuromuscular & skeletal: Myalgia

Ocular: Keratoconjunctivitis, eye pain, photophobia

Renal: Renal failure at doses >5 mg/m^2/day, hematuria, dysuria

Respiratory: Bronchitis, dyspnea, cough

Miscellaneous: Hypersensitivity (11%), epistaxis

Toxicodynamics/Kinetics

Distribution: 20-23 L/m^2
Protein binding: 4%

Half-life: 4.9-6.2 hours
Elimination: Renal; clearance: 3.1 L/kg/hour

Usual Dosage Refractory hairy cell leukemia: Adults (refer to individual protocols): 4 mg/m^2 every other week; I.V. bolus over ≥3-5 minutes in D_5W or normal saline at concentrations ≥2 mg/mL; patients should receive previous I.V. hydration with 500-1000 mL of 0.45% saline; patient should also receive 500 mL of 0.45% saline with 5% dextrose after infusion; reassess after usually 6 months of treatment

Contraindications Prior hypersensitivity to pentostatin

Warnings Use with caution in myelosuppression, pregnancy, renal insufficiency, hepatic insufficiency; extensive pretreatment with chemotherapy or radiation therapy regimens

Dosage Forms Powder for injection: 10 mg/5 mL (50 mg mannitol per vial)

Reference Range Pentostatin plasma levels between 1-5 μM achieved after therapeutic dose

Overdosage Treatment Supportive therapy: Keep patient hydrated; erythrocyte transfusions may be indicated when the erythrocyte deoxyadenosine triphosphate to ATP ratio exceeds 1.0

Drug Interactions Increased cardiac toxicity (pulmonary edema, hypotension, ventricular arrhythmia) with associated use with cyclophosphamide; increased toxicity of pentostatin with allopurinol use may occur; intravenous formulations compatible with ondansetron and paclitaxel

Pregnancy Risk Factor D

Monitoring Parameters CBC, renal function tests

Additional Information Treatment with pentostatin should either be avoided or administered with great caution in patients with a history of fludarabine-associated hemolytic anemia; may contain sodium hydroxide or hydrochloric acid for pH adjustment (pH of solution 7-8.5); infections (particularly disseminated herpes zoster) may occur; withhold dose if serum creatinine increases; polyethylene gloves should be utilized when administering this agent; extravasation injuries not reported

Specific References

Byrd JC, Hertler AA, Weiss RB, et al, "Fatal Recurrence of Autoimmune Hemolytic Anemia Following Pentostatin Therapy in a Patient With a History of Fludarabine-Associated Hemolytic Anemia," *Ann Oncol*, 1995, 6:300-1.

Gryn J, Gordon R, Bapat A, et al, "Pentostatin Increases the Acute Toxicity of High Dose Cyclophosphamide," *Bone Marrow Transplant*, 1993, 12(3):217-20.

Spiers ASD, "Pentostatin (2'-Deoxycoformycin): Clinical Pharmacology, Role in Cancer Chemotherapy and Future Prospects," *Am J Ther*, 1995, 2:196-216.

Pentoxi® *see* Pentoxifylline *on this page*

Pentoxifylline (pen tox i' fi leen)

CAS Number 6493-05-6

Brand Names Azupentat®; Claudicat®; Elorgan®; Hemovas®; Pentopuran®; Pentoxi®; Torental®; Trental®

Synonyms BL-191; Oxpentifylline; Vasofirin

Use Symptomatic management of peripheral vascular disease, mainly intermittent claudication

Unapproved use: AIDS patients with increased TNF, CVA, cerebrovascular diseases, diabetic atherosclerosis, diabetic neuropathy, gangrene, hemodialysis shunt thrombosis, vascular impotence, cerebral malaria, septic shock, sickle cell syndromes, and vasculitis

Mechanism of Action Mechanism of action remains unclear; is thought to reduce blood viscosity and improve blood flow by altering the rheology of red blood cells

Adverse Reactions

Cardiovascular: Mild hypotension, angina
Central nervous system: Agitation, dizziness, headache
Gastrointestinal: Nausea, dyspepsia
Ocular: Blurred vision
Otic: Earache

Signs & Symptoms of Acute Overdose Fever, syncope, flushing, dyspepsia, thrombocytopenia, hypotension, seizures, laryngitis, atrioventricular block, agitation, tachycardia, mydriasis, hypokalemia, myoclonus, hyperglycemia, hypokalemia (lasts for 12 hours)

Toxicodynamics/Kinetics

Absorption: Oral: Well absorbed
Metabolism: Undergoes first-pass metabolism in the liver to active metabolites
Half-life:
Parent drug: 24-48 minutes
Metabolites: 60-96 minutes
Time to peak serum concentration: Within 2-3 hours after a 400 mg dose
Elimination: Mainly in urine (95%), feces (4%)

(Continued)

Pentoxifylline *(Continued)*

Usual Dosage Adults: Oral: 400 mg 3 times/day with meals; may reduce to 400 mg twice daily if gastrointestinal or CNS side effects occur

Contraindications Hypersensitivity to pentoxifylline or any component and other xanthine derivatives

Warnings Use with caution in patients with renal impairment or chronic occlusive arterial disease of the limbs

Dosage Forms Tablet, controlled release: 400 mg

Reference Range Therapeutic: 100-400 ng/mL; peak levels of 100 ng/mL obtained 2-3 hours after a 400 mg dose; serum level of 51,000 ng/mL associated with emesis, hypokalemia, and survival

Overdosage Treatment

Decontamination: Lavage/activated charcoal with cathartic; do not induce emesis

Supportive therapy: Seizures can be treated with diazepam, lorazepam, phenobarbital, or phenytoin. Hypotension can be treated with crystalloid infusion and Trendelenburg. Dopamine and norepinephrine can also be given for refractory hypotension.

Enhancement of elimination: Multiple dosing of activated charcoal may be effective; extracorporeal removal may also be effective although there is no experience with this modality

Test Interactions ↓ calcium (S), ↓ magnesium (S), false-positive theophylline levels are not likely

Drug Interactions Increased effect/toxic potential with cimetidine (↑ levels) and other H_2 antagonists, warfarin; increased effect of antihypertensives, insulin

Pregnancy Risk Factor C

Pregnancy Implications Distributes into breast milk

Patient Information Take with food or meals; if gastrointestinal or CNS side effects continue, contact physician; while effects may be seen in 2-4 weeks, continue treatment for at least 8 weeks

Specific References

Dolgin J, Abrams B, and Tucker J, "Survival With Massive Pentoxifylline Overdose and High Serum Levels," *Vet Hum Toxicol*, 1994, 36:369.

Garnier R, Riboulet-Delmas G, Chatenet T, et al, "Acute Pentoxifylline in Children," *Ann Pediatr Paris*, 1986, 33(1):62-3.

Sznajder IJ, Bentur Y, and Taitelman U, "First and Second Degree Atrioventricular Block in Oxpentifylline Overdose," *Br Med J (Clin Res)*, 1984, 288(6410):26.

Ward A and Clissold SP, "Pentoxifylline: A Review of Its Pharmacodynamic and Pharmacokinetic Properties and Its Therapeutic Efficacy," *Drugs*, 1987, 34(1):50-97.

Pepcid® *see* Famotidine *on page 341*

Pepcidine® *see* Famotidine *on page 341*

Pepdul® *see* Famotidine *on page 341*

Pepdulmite® *see* Famotidine *on page 341*

Peptard® *see* Hyoscyamine Sulfate *on page 415*

Pepto® Diarrhea Control [OTC] *see* Loperamide Hydrochloride *on page 480*

Perbilen® *see* Piretanide *on page 630*

Percainal® *see* Dibucaine *on page 275*

Percocet® *see* Oxycodone and Acetaminophen *on page 584*

Percoffedrinol N® *see* Caffeine *on page 175*

Percutafeine® *see* Caffeine *on page 175*

Perhydrol *see* Hydrogen Peroxide *on page 408*

Periactin® *see* Cyproheptadine Hydrochloride *on page 255*

Periactinol® *see* Cyproheptadine Hydrochloride *on page 255*

Periblastine® *see* Vinblastine Sulfate *on page 790*

Pericristine® *see* Vincristine Sulfate *on page 792*

Peridex® Oral Rinse *see* Chlorhexidine Gluconate *on page 200*

Permethrin (per meth' rin)

CAS Number 52645-53-1

Brand Names Ambush Fog®; Elimite™; Muscatrol®; Nix™ [OTC]; Permit®; Picket®

Use Single application treatment of infestation with *Pediculus humanus capitis* (head louse) and its nits, or *Sarcoptes scabiei* (scabies); also active against mosquitoes, blackflies, and tsetse flies

Mechanism of Action Inhibits sodium ion influx through nerve cell membrane channels in parasites resulting in delayed repolarization and thus paralysis of the pest (a pyrethroid)

Adverse Reactions
- Cardiovascular: Edema, tachycardia
- Central nervous system: Convulsions, headache
- Dermatologic: Pruritus, numbness or scalp discomfort, erythema, rash of the scalp
- Gastrointestinal: Vomiting, dizziness
- Local: Burning, stinging, tingling, cheek/perioral numbness
- Neuromuscular & skeletal: Paresthesia
- Respiratory: Sore throat, wheezing, dyspnea, sneezing

Signs & Symptoms of Acute Overdose Oral ingestion: Dizziness, anorexia, numbness, nausea, vomiting, headache, asthenia, coma, fasciculations, and seizures can occur at doses >200 mL

Toxicodynamics/Kinetics
- Duration of action: 14 days
- Absorption:
  - Oral: Readily absorbed
  - Topical: Minimal (<2%)
- Metabolism: In the liver, rapidly oxidized
- Elimination: Urine

Usual Dosage Topical:
- Head lice: Children >2 months and Adults: After hair has been washed with shampoo, rinsed with water, and towel dried, apply a sufficient volume of topical liquid to saturate the hair and scalp. Leave on hair for 10 minutes before rinsing off with water; remove remaining nits; may repeat in 1 week if lice or nits still present.
- Scabies: Apply cream from head to toe; leave on for 8-14 hours before washing off with water, a single application is usually adequate; may repeat in 1 week if lice or nits still present. For infants, also apply on the hairline, neck, scalp, temple, and forehead.

Contraindications Known hypersensitivity to pyrethyroid, pyrethrin or to chrysanthemums

Warnings Use during pregnancy only if clearly needed; do not use in infants; treatment with Nix™ may temporarily exacerbate the symptoms of itching, redness, swelling; for external use only

Dosage Forms
- Cream: 5% (60 g)
- Liquid, topical: 1% (60 mL)

Overdosage Treatment
- Decontamination: Emesis or lavage/activated charcoal with cathartic; wash exposed skin thoroughly with soap and water
- Supportive therapy: Epinephrine or diphenhydramine for allergic reactions; nebulized bronchodilators for wheezing; treat seizures with diazepam, lorazepam, phenytoin, or phenobarbital

Drug Interactions May result in progressive motor neurone disease when given with chlordane

Pregnancy Risk Factor B

Nursing Implications Avoid contact with eyes during administration; shake well before using

Additional Information Available in 1% formulation; suitable for aircraft disinfection

Specific References

Dorman DC and Beasley VR, "Neurotoxicology of Pyrethrin and the Pyrethroid Insecticides," *Vet Hum Toxicol*, 1991, 33(3):238-43.

He F, Wang S, Liu L, et al, "Clinical Manifestations and Diagnosis of Acute Pyrethroid Poisoning," *Arch Toxicol*, 1989, 63(1):54-8.

Permit® *see* Permethrin *on previous page*

Permitil® *see* Fluphenazine *on page 361*

Peroxan *see* Hydrogen Peroxide *on page 408*

Peroxide *see* Hydrogen Peroxide *on page 408*

Peroxyl® *see* Hydrogen Peroxide *on page 408*

Perphenazine (per fen' a zeen)

Related Information

Antipsychotic Agents Comparison *on page 1642*

CAS Number 58-39-9

Brand Names Decentan®; Fentazin®; Trilafon®

Use Symptomatic management of psychotic disorders, as well as severe nausea and vomiting

Mechanism of Action Blocks postsynaptic mesolimbic dopaminergic receptors in the brain; exhibits a strong alpha-adrenergic blocking effect and depresses the release of hypothalamic and hypophyseal hormones

(Continued)

Perphenazine *(Continued)*

Adverse Reactions

Cardiovascular: Hypotension, tachycardia, cardiac arrhythmias, bradycardia

Central nervous system: Sedation, drowsiness, restlessness, anxiety, extrapyramidal reactions, pseudoparkinsonian signs and symptoms, seizures, altered central temperature regulation

Dermatologic: Hyperpigmentation, pruritus, rash, photosensitivity reactions

Endocrine & metabolic: Amenorrhea, galactorrhea, gynecomastia, syndrome of inappropriate antidiuretic hormone, weight gain

Gastrointestinal: Dry mouth, constipation, gastrointestinal upset

Genitourinary: Urinary retention

Hematologic: Agranulocytosis (more often in women between fourth and tenth weeks of therapy), leukopenia (usually in patients with large doses for prolonged periods)

Neuromuscular & skeletal: Torticollis

Ocular: Blurred vision, nystagmus, photophobia, retinal pigmentation

Miscellaneous: Systemic lupus erythematosus (SLE)

Signs & Symptoms of Acute Overdose Deep sleep, dystonic reactions, galactorrhea, Parkinson's-like symptoms, agitation, coma, jaundice, Stevens-Johnson syndrome, neuroleptic malignant syndrome, gynecomastia, impotence, extrapyramidal reaction, thrombocytopenia, seizures, abnormal involuntary muscle movements, vision color changes (brown tinge), vision color changes (yellow tinge); urine discoloration (pink), urine discoloration (red), urine discoloration (red-brown), leukopenia; neutropenia; agranulocytosis; granulocytopenia

Toxicodynamics/Kinetics

Onset of action: 30 minutes to 1 hour

Absorption: Oral: Well absorbed

Distribution: To most body tissues and fluids with high levels in brain, lungs, liver, and spleen

Protein binding: 90% or more

Metabolism: In the liver; marked first-pass effect

Half-life: 9 hours

Time to peak serum concentration:
- Oral: Within 4-8 hours
- Decanoate injection: Within 7-8 days

Elimination: Urine and bile

Usual Dosage

Children:
- Psychoses: Oral:
  - 1-6 years: 4-6 mg/day in divided doses
  - 6-12 years: 6 mg/day in divided doses
  - >12 years: 4-16 mg 2-4 times/day
  - I.M.: 5 mg every 6 hours
- Nausea/vomiting: I.M.: 5 mg every 6 hours

Adults:
- Psychoses:
  - Oral: 4-16 mg 2-4 times/day not to exceed 64 mg/day
  - I.M.: 5 mg every 6 hours up to 15 mg/day in ambulatory patients and 30 mg/day in hospitalized patients
- Nausea/vomiting:
  - Oral: 8-16 mg/day in divided doses up to 24 mg/day
  - I.M.: 5-10 mg every 6 hours as necessary up to 15 mg/day in ambulatory patients and 30 mg/day in hospitalized patients
  - I.V. (severe): 1 mg at 1- to 2-minute intervals up to a total of 5 mg

Dosing adjustment in hepatic impairment: Dosage reductions should be considered in patients with liver disease although no specific guidelines are available

Contraindications Hypersensitivity to perphenazine or any component, cross-sensitivity with other phenothiazines may exist; avoid use in patients with narrow-angle glaucoma, bone marrow depression, severe liver or cardiac disease

Warnings Avoid alcoholic beverages; safety in children <12 years of age has not been established; use with caution in patients with cardiovascular disease or seizures; use with caution in patients with a history of seizures and in those receiving anticonvulsant agents

Dosage Forms

Concentrate, oral: 16 mg/5 mL (118 mL)

Injection: 5 mg/mL (1 mL)

Tablet: 2 mg, 4 mg, 8 mg, 16 mg

Reference Range 0.004-0.064 mg/L

Overdosage Treatment

Decontamination: Lavage/activated charcoal with cathartic

Supportive therapy: Following initiation of essential overdose management, toxic symptom treatment and supportive treatment should be initiated. Hypotension usually responds to I.V. fluids or Trendelenburg positioning. If unresponsive to these measures, the use of a parenteral inotrope may be required (eg, norepinephrine 0.1-0.2 mcg/kg/minute titrated to response). Seizures commonly respond to lorazepam or diazepam (I.V. 5-10 mg bolus in adults every 15 minutes if needed up to a total of 30 mg; I.V. 0.25-0.4 mg/kg/dose up to a total of 10 mg in children) or to phenytoin or phenobarbital. Also critical cardiac arrhythmias often respond to I.V. phenytoin (15 mg/kg up to 1 gram), while other antiarrhythmics can be used. Neuroleptics often cause extrapyramidal reaction (eg, dystonic reactions) requiring management with diphenhydramine 1-2 mg/kg (adults) up to a maximum of 50 mg I.M. or I.V. slow push followed by a maintenance dose for 48-72 hours. When these reactions are unresponsive to diphenhydramine, benztropine mesylate I.V. 1-2 mg (adults) may be effective. These agents are generally effective within 2-5 minutes.

Enhancement of elimination: Multiple dosing of activated charcoal may be useful; forced diuresis or hemodialysis is of no benefit; not dialyzable (0% to 5%)

Test Interactions Increases cholesterol (S), glucose; decreases uric acid (S)

Drug Interactions Other CNS depressants, anticonvulsants, disulfiram can enhance biotransformation of orally administered perphenazine, due to first-pass effect

Pregnancy Risk Factor C

Pregnancy Implications Crosses the placenta

Monitoring Parameters Cardiac, blood pressure, respiratory status

Patient Information May cause drowsiness

Nursing Implications Monitor for hypotension when administering I.M. or I.V.; dilute oral concentration to at least 2 oz with water, juice, or milk; for I.V. use, injection should be diluted to at least 0.5 mg/mL with NS and given at a rate of 1 mg/minute; can be combined with amitriptyline (Triavil®) which is moderately radiopaque

Specific References

Azaz-Livshits TL, Symmer LI, and Fraenkel YM, "Atypical Neuroleptic Malignant Syndrome Presenting as Rhabdomyolysis, Altered Consciousness, and Leukocytosis," *J Pharm Technol*, 1995, 11:173-5.

Hansen LB and Larsen NE, "Metabolic Interaction Between Perphenazine and Disulfiram," *Lancet*, 1982, 2(8313):1472.

Harper G, Dawes M, Azlin C, et al, "Small Bowel Obstruction in a Child on an Antipsychotic," *J Child Adoles Psychopharm*, 1995, 5:81-4.

Perphenazine and Amitriptyline *see* Amitriptyline and Perphenazine *on page 115*

Perphenyline® *see* Amitriptyline and Perphenazine *on page 115*

Persantine® *see* Dipyridamole *on page 292*

Persolu Richter® *see* Urokinase *on page 779*

Pertofrane® *see* Desipramine Hydrochloride *on page 263*

Pertofrin® *see* Desipramine Hydrochloride *on page 263*

Pertussin® CS [OTC] *see* Dextromethorphan Hydrobromide *on page 270*

Pertussin® ES [OTC] *see* Dextromethorphan Hydrobromide *on page 270*

Pethidine Hydrochloride *see* Meperidine Hydrochloride *on page 499*

Petrolatum Oil *see* Mineral Oil *on page 534*

PFA *see* Foscarnet Sodium *on page 367*

PFI-Lith® *see* Lithium *on page 476*

Pfizerpen® Injection *see* Penicillin G, Parenteral, Aqueous *on page 600*

Pharmacokinetics of Narcotic Agonist Analgesics *see page 1654*

Pharmaflur® *see* Fluoride *on page 355*

Phasal® *see* Lithium *on page 476*

Phenazine® *see* Promethazine Hydrochloride *on page 650*

Phencen® *see* Promethazine Hydrochloride *on page 650*

Phencyclidine Hydrochloride (fen sye' kli deen)

Related Information

Principal Pharmacological Properties of Hallucinogenic Drugs *on page 1557*

CAS Number 77-10-1; 956-90-1

Mechanism of Action Related to ketamine, PCP is an arylcyclohexylamine which stimulates alpha-adrenergic receptors

(Continued)

Phencyclidine Hydrochloride *(Continued)*

Adverse Reactions

Cardiovascular: Tachycardia

Central nervous system: Violent behavior, psychosis, paranoia, hallucinations, ataxia

Endocrine & metabolic: Hypoglycemia

Gastrointestinal: Vomiting

Ocular: Nystagmus, lacrimation, mydriasis (miosis in children)

Signs & Symptoms of Acute Overdose Myoglobinuria, fear, hyperuricemia, mania, delirium, hyperacusis, lacrimation, insomnia, ptosis, hypoglycemia, myopathy, impotence, fasciculations, depression, encephalopathy, hyperthermia, headache, rhabdomyolysis, fever, coma, sweating, respiratory depression, hypothermia, seizures, hypertension, tachycardia, myoclonus

Toxicodynamics/Kinetics

Distribution: V_d: 6.2 L/kg

Protein binding: 60% to 70%

Metabolism: Hepatic by oxidative hydroxylation

Half-life: 1 hour (in overdose: 17.6 hours)

Elimination: Renal (33 mL/minute)

Usual Dosage Joints are 100-400 mg PCP by weight; tablets are ~5 mg

Reference Range

Excitation: 20-30 ng/mL

Coma: 30-100 ng/mL

Seizures, fatalities: >100 ng/mL

Overdosage Treatment

Decontamination: Lavage/activated charcoal with cathartic for oral ingestions

Supportive therapy: Benzodiazepine for agitation; haloperidol (5 mg I.M.) improves psychotic symptoms; rhabdomyolysis can be treated with intravenous hydration, alkalinization, and mannitol; lorazepam or diazepam can be used to calm and sedate the patient

Enhanced elimination: Continuous gastric suction (due to gastric secretion of PCP) may increase elimination and should be considered in the comatose patient; multiple dosing of activated charcoal may be effective

Test Interactions Adulteration with bleach can cause false-negative urine immunoassays; doxylamine can cause a false-positive urine gas chromatographic result; dextromethorphan can give a false-positive on an immunoassay screen; ketamine is not expected to give a positive immunoassay

Pregnancy Implications Neonatal irritability, hypertonia, tremors

Specific References

McCarron MM, Schulze BW, Thompson GA, et al, "Acute Phencyclidine Intoxication: Clinical Patterns, Complications, and Treatment," *Ann Emerg Med*, 1981, 10(6):290-7.

McCarron MM, Schulze BW, Thompson GA, et al, "Acute Phencyclidine Intoxication: Incidence of Clinical Findings in 1000 Cases," *Ann Emerg Med*, 1981, 10(5):237-42.

Schaldenbrand JD, McClatchey KD, Patel JA, et al, "Doxylamine: A Cause for False-Positive Gas Chromatographic Assay for Phencyclidine," *Ther Drug Monit*, 1981, 3(2):181-3.

Tueth MJ, "Management of Behavioral Emergencies," *Am J Emerg Med*, 1995, 13:344-50.

Phenelzine Sulfate (fen' el zeen)

Related Information

Therapeutic Drugs Associated With Hallucinations *on page 1558-1559*

CAS Number 51-71-8; 156-51-4

Brand Names Nardelzine®; Nardil®

Synonyms Phenethylhydrazine Hydrogen Sulfate

Use Symptomatic treatment of atypical, nonendogenous or neurotic depression

Mechanism of Action Thought to act by increasing endogenous concentrations of epinephrine, norepinephrine, dopamine and serotonin through inhibition of the enzyme (monoamine oxidase) responsible for the breakdown of these neurotransmitters

Adverse Reactions

Cardiovascular: Hypotension, edema

Central nervous system: Drowsiness, psychosis, headache, auditory and visual hallucinations

Dermatologic: Skin rash

Endocrine & metabolic: Syndrome of inappropriate antidiuretic hormone

Gastrointestinal: Dry mouth, constipation, nausea

Genitourinary: Urinary retention

Hepatic: Jaundice

Neuromuscular & skeletal: Myoclonus

Ocular: Blurred vision, photophobia, mydriasis, nystagmus, amblyopia

Miscellaneous: Aplastic anemia, lupus-like reaction, serotonin syndrome (flushing, diarrhea)

Signs & Symptoms of Acute Overdose Sinus tachycardia, photosensitivity, exfoliative dermatitis, dry mouth, delirium, ejaculatory disturbances, rhabdomyolysis, myoglobinuria, palpitations, ptosis, mania, muscle myoclonus, impotence, extrapyramidal reaction, seizures, insomnia, neuroleptic malignant syndrome, restlessness, methemoglobinemia, transient hypertension, hypotension, drowsiness, fever, coma, muscle rigidity, hyperthermia, sweating, metabolic acidosis, flushing, tachypnea, mydriasis, hallucinations, nystagmus

Toxicodynamics/Kinetics

Onset of action: As early as 7-10 days in some patients but may take up to 4-8 weeks

Duration: At least 10 days for MAO activity to be recovered because of irreversible binding

Absorption: Oral: Well absorbed from gastrointestinal tract

Distribution: Not yet determined

Metabolism: Hepatic

Time to peak serum concentration: Oral: 2-4 hours

Elimination: Urine primarily as metabolites and unchanged drug

Usual Dosage Adults: Oral: 15 mg 3 times/day; may increase to 60-90 mg/day during early phase of treatment, then reduce to dose for maintenance therapy slowly after maximum benefit is obtained; takes 2-4 weeks for a significant response to occur

Contraindications Pheochromocytoma, hepatic or renal disease, cerebrovascular defect, cardiovascular disease, hypersensitivity to phenelzine or any component

Warnings Avoid tyramine-containing foods: red wine, cheese (except cottage, ricotta, and cream), smoked or pickled fish, beef or chicken liver, dried sausage, fava or broad bean pods, yeast vitamin supplements; safety in children <16 years of age has not been established; use with caution in patients with a history of seizures

Dosage Forms Tablet: 15 mg

Stability Protect from light

Overdosage Treatment

Decontamination: Do not induce emesis; lavage/activated charcoal with cathartic is useful

Supportive therapy: Competent supportive care is the most important treatment for an overdose with a monoamine oxidase (MAO) inhibitor. Both hypertension or hypotension can occur with intoxication. Hypotension may respond to I.V. fluids or vasopressors and hypertension usually responds to an alpha-adrenergic blocker. While treating the hypertension, care is warranted to avoid sudden drops in blood pressure, since this may worsen the MAO inhibitor toxicity. Muscle irritability and seizures often respond to diazepam or lorazepam, while hyperthermia is best treated antipyretics and cooling blankets. Cardiac arrhythmias are best treated with phenytoin or procainamide.

Enhancement of elimination: Charcoal hemoperfusion may be useful

Test Interactions Decreases glucose; peaked T waves noted on EKG

Drug Interactions Hypertensive crisis with foods containing tyramine (cheese, beer, wine); sympathomimetic drugs, meperidine, tricyclic antidepressants, phenothiazines, antihypertensives, disulfiram

Pregnancy Risk Factor C (no increase in congenital malformations noted when used in first trimester)

Monitoring Parameters Blood pressure, EKG, monitor glucose, electrolytes

Patient Information Avoid tyramine-containing foods: red wine, cheese (except cottage, ricotta, and cream), smoked or pickled fish, beef or chicken liver, dried sausage, fava or broad bean pods, yeast vitamin supplements

Nursing Implications Watch for hypotension (orthostatic); monitor blood pressure carefully, especially at therapy onset or if other CNS drugs or cardiovascular drugs are added; check for dietary and drug restriction

Specific References

Bass C and Kerwin R, "Rediscovering Monoamine Oxidase Inhibitors," *Br Med J (Clin Res)*, 1989, 298(6670):345-6.

Breheny FX, Dobb GJ, and Clarke GM, "Phenelzine Poisoning," *Anaesthesia*, 1986, 41(1):53-6.

Kaplan RF, Feinglass NG, Webster W, et al, "Phenelzine Overdose Treated With Dantrolene Sodium," *JAMA*, 1986, 255(5):642-4.

LeJoyeux M, et al, "Serotonin Syndrome: Incidence, Symptoms, and Treatment," *CNS Drugs*, 1994, 2:132-43.

Lichtenwalner MR, Tully Rg, Cohn RD, et al, "Two Fatalities Involving Phenelzine," *J Anal Toxicol*, 1995, 19:265-6.

Linden CH, Rumack BH, and Strehlke C, "Monoamine Oxidase Inhibitor Overdose," *Ann Emerg Med*, 1984, 13(12):1137-44.

Verrilli MR, Salanga VD, Kozachuk WE, et al, "Phenelzine Toxicity Responsive to Dantrolene," *Neurology*, 1987, 37(5):865-7.

Phenergan® *see* Promethazine Hydrochloride *on page 650*

Phenethylhydrazine Hydrogen Sulfate *see* Phenelzine Sulfate *on previous page*

Phenetron® *see* Chlorpheniramine Maleate *on page 204*

Phenobarbital (fee noe bar' bi tal)

Related Information

Seizures, Neonatal Guidelines *on page 1604-1605*
Status Epilepticus Treatment Algorithm *on page 1608*
Therapeutic Drugs Associated With Hallucinations *on page 1558-1559*

CAS Number 57-30-7; 50-06-6

Brand Names Barbita®; Comizial®; Fenilcal®; Gardenale®; Luminal®; Solfoton®

Synonyms Phenobarbital Sodium; Phenobarbitone; Phenylethylmalonylurea

Use Management of generalized tonic-clonic (grand mal) and partial seizures; prevention of febrile seizures in infants and young children; sedation; may also be used for prevention and treatment of neonatal hyperbilirubinemia and lowering of bilirubin in chronic cholestasis

Mechanism of Action Interferes with transmission of impulses from the thalamus to the cortex of the brain resulting in an imbalance in central inhibitory and facilitatory mechanisms

Adverse Reactions

Cardiovascular: Hypotension, cardiac arrhythmias, bradycardia, arterial spasm, and gangrene with inadvertent intra-arterial injection

Central nervous system: Drowsiness, drowsiness, CNS stimulation or CNS depression, impaired judgment, visual hallucinations, hypothermia, electroencephalogram abnormalities

Dermatologic: Rash

Gastrointestinal: Nausea, vomiting, ileus, hepatic dysfunction (idiosyncratic reaction), cholestasis

Local: Thrombophlebitis with I.V. use

Ocular: Nystagmus

Psychiatric: Depression

Renal: Oliguria, renal failure (secondary to hypotension)

Respiratory: Laryngospasm, respiratory depression, apnea (especially with rapid I.V. use)

Signs & Symptoms of Acute Overdose Unsteady gait, toxic epidermal necrolysis, asterixis, dysarthria, hyporeflexia, gingival hyperplasia, ataxia, myocardial depression, anemia (megaloblastic), hypothyroidism, ptosis, miosis, extrapyramidal reaction, cognitive dysfunction, pemphigus, rhabdomyolysis, hyperactivity, slurred speech, myoglobinuria, confusion, jaundice, hypothermia, fever, hypotension, bullous lesions, focal neurological signs, vision color changes (green tinge), pulmonary edema, methemoglobinemia, porphyria

Toxicodynamics/Kinetics

Onset of action:
- Oral: Within 20-60 minutes
- I.V.: Within 5 minutes with peak effect within 30 minutes

Duration:
- Oral: 6-10 hours
- I.V.: 4-10 hours

Absorption: Oral: 70% to 90%

Distribution: Widely in tissues and body fluids
- V_d:
  - Neonates: 0.8-1 L/kg
  - Infants: 0.7-0.8 L/kg
  - Children: 0.6-0.7 L/kg

Protein binding: 20% to 50%, decreased protein binding in neonates

Metabolism: In the liver via hydroxylation (60% to 75%) and glucuronide conjugation

Half-life:
- Neonates: 45-500 hours
- Infants: 20-133 hours
- Children: 37-73 hours
- Adults: 53-140 hours
- Overdose: 96-168 hours

Time to peak serum concentration: Within 1-6 hours

Elimination: 20% to 50% excreted unchanged in urine; clearance is 0.093 mL/minute/kg

Usual Dosage

Children:
- Sedation: Oral: 2 mg/kg 3 times/day
- Hypnotic: I.M., I.V., S.C.: 3-5 mg/kg at bedtime
- Preoperative sedation: Oral, I.M., I.V.: 1-3 mg/kg 1-1.5 hours before procedure

Anticonvulsant: Status epilepticus: **Loading dose:** I.V.:
- Neonates: 15-20 mg/kg in a single or divided dose
- Infants and Children: 10-20 mg/kg in a single or divided dose; in select patients may give additional 5 mg/kg/dose every 15-30 minutes until seizure is controlled or a total dose of 40 mg/kg is reached

Adults: 300-800 mg initially followed by 120-240 mg/dose at 20-minute intervals until seizures are controlled or a total dose of 1-2 g

Anticonvulsant maintenance dose: Oral, I.V.:

Neonates: 2-4 mg/kg/day in 1-2 divided doses; assess serum concentrations; increase to 5 mg/kg/day if needed (usually by second week of therapy)

Infants: 5-8 mg/kg/day in 1-2 divided doses

Children:

1-5 years: 6-8 mg/kg/day in 1-2 divided doses

5-12 years: 4-6 mg/kg/day in 1-2 divided doses

>12 years and Adults: 1-3 mg/kg/day in divided doses or 50-100 mg 2-3 times/day

Adults:

Sedation: Oral, I.M.: 30-120 mg/day in 2-3 divided doses

Hypnotic: Oral, I.M., I.V., S.C.: 100-320 mg at bedtime

Preoperative sedation: I.M.: 100-200 mg 1-1.5 hours before procedure

Dosing interval in renal impairment: Cl_{cr} <10 mL/minute: Administer every 12-16 hours

Dosing adjustment/comments in hepatic disease: Increased side effects may occur in severe liver disease; monitor plasma levels and adjust dose accordingly

Contraindications Hypersensitivity to phenobarbital or any component; preexisting CNS depression, severe uncontrolled pain, porphyria, severe respiratory disease with dyspnea or obstruction

Warnings Use with caution in patients with renal or hepatic impairment; abrupt withdrawal in patients with epilepsy may precipitate status epilepticus

Dosage Forms

Capsule: 16 mg

Elixir: 15 mg/5 mL (5 mL, 10 mL, 20 mL); 20 mg/5 mL (3.75 mL, 5 mL, 7.5 mL, 120 mL, 473 mL, 946 mL, 4000 mL)

Injection, as sodium: 30 mg/mL (1 mL); 60 mg/mL (1 mL); 65 mg/mL (1 mL); 130 mg/mL (1 mL)

Powder for injection: 120 mg

Tablet: 8 mg, 15 mg, 16 mg, 30 mg, 32 mg, 60 mg, 65 mg, 100 mg

Stability Protect elixir from light; not stable in aqueous solutions; use only clear solutions; do not add to acidic solutions, precipitation may occur

Reference Range

Therapeutic:

Infants and children: 15-30 μg/mL (SI: 65-129 μmol/L)

Adults: 20-40 μg/mL (SI: 86-172 μmol/L)

Toxic: >40 μg/mL (SI: >172 μmol/L); levels >80 μg/mL (SI: 344 μmol/L) are associated with coma

Fatal: 50-130 μg/mL (SI: 215-559 μmol/L)

Overdosage Treatment

Decontamination: Gastric lavage for life-threatening overdoses within 1 hour; activated charcoal with cathartic is effective

Supportive therapy: Hypotension: Isotonic intravenous fluid (10-20 mL/kg) is effective along with placement in Trendelenburg position; dopamine (2-5 mcg/kg progressing to 5-10 mcg/kg) or norepinephrine (0.1-0.2 mcg/kg/minute for children or 8-12 mcg/kg in adults to a maintenance dose of 2-4 mcg/minute) is effective.

Enhancement of elimination: Repeated oral doses of activated charcoal significantly reduce the half-life of phenobarbital resulting from an enhancement of nonrenal elimination. The usual dose is 30-60 g every 4-6 hours for 3-4 days unless the patient has no bowel movement causing the charcoal to remain in the gastrointestinal tract. Assure adequate hydration and renal function. Urinary alkalinization with I.V. sodium bicarbonate also helps to enhance elimination. Hemodialysis is of uncertain value. Patients in stage IV coma due to high serum barbiturate levels may require charcoal hemoperfusion; moderately dialyzable (20% to 50%).

Test Interactions Increases alkaline phosphatase (S), ammonia (B); decreases bilirubin (S), calcium (S)

Diagnostic Tests/Procedures

Phenobarbital, Blood *on page 1320*

Drug Interactions Phenobarbital may decrease the serum concentration or effect of ethosuximide, warfarin, oral contraceptives, phenylbutazone, chloramphenicol, griseofulvin, doxycycline, beta-blockers, theophylline, corticosteroids, tricyclic antidepressants, cyclosporine, quinidine, haloperidol, and phenothiazines; valproic acid, methylphenidate, chloramphenicol, propoxyphene, furosemide may inhibit the metabolism of phenobarbital with resultant increase in phenobarbital serum concentration; phenobarbital and benzodiazepines or other CNS depressants may cause an increase of CNS and respiratory depression (especially with I.V. loading doses of phenobarbital). Pyridoxine may reduce serum phenobarbital levels.

(Continued)

Phenobarbital *(Continued)*

Pregnancy Risk Factor D

Pregnancy Implications Crosses placenta, enters breast milk; no direct causal relationship established with congenital malformations; folate deficiency and hypoprothrombinemia has been noted in infants of mothers receiving phenobarbital

Monitoring Parameters Phenobarbital serum concentrations, mental status, CBC, LFTS, seizure activity

Patient Information Avoid the use of alcohol and other CNS depressants; avoid driving and other hazardous tasks; avoid abrupt discontinuation; may cause physical and psychological dependence; do not alter dose without notifying physician

Nursing Implications Parenteral solutions are highly alkaline; avoid extravasation; avoid rapid I.V. administration >50 mg/minute; avoid intra-arterial injection; institute safety measures to avoid injuries

Additional Information Sodium content of injection (65 mg, 1 mL): 6 mg (0.3 mEq); the elderly may be more sensitive to the sedative effects of phenobarbital

Specific References

Amitai Y and Degani Y, "Treatment of Phenobarbital Poisoning With Multiple Dose of Activated Charcoal in an Infant," *J Emerg Med*, 1990, 8(4):449-50.

Jacobsen D, Wiik-Larsen E, Dahl T, et al, "Pharmacokinetic Evaluation of Haemoperfusion in Phenobarbital Poisoning," *Eur J Clin Pharmacol*, 1984, 26(1):109-12.

Lin JL and Jeng LB, "Critical, Acutely Poisoned Patients Treated With Continuous Arteriovenous Hemoperfusion in the Emergency Department," *Ann Emerg Med*, 1995, 25:75-80.

Mockli G, Crowley M, Stern R, et al, "Massive Hepatic Necrosis in a Child After Administration of Phenobarbital," *Am J Gastroenterol*, 1989, 84(7):820-2.

Pond SM, Olson KR, Osterloh JD, et al, "Randomized Study of the Treatment of Phenobarbital Overdose With Repeated Doses of Activated Charcoal," *JAMA*, 1984, 251(23):3104-8.

Phenobarbital Sodium *see* Phenobarbital *on page 614*

Phenobarbitone *see* Phenobarbital *on page 614*

Phenol (fee' nole)

CAS Number 108-95-2

Brand Names Baker's P&S [OTC]; Cepastat® [OTC]; Chloraseptic® [OTC]

Synonyms Carbolic Acid; Monohydroxybenzene; Phenol Hydrate

Commonly Found in Production of resin; industrial coatings, adhesives, dyes, perfumes, textiles, lubricating oils, antiseptic agents

Use Relief of sore throat pain, mouth, gum, and throat irritations, neurologic pain, rectal prolapse, hemorrhoids, hydrocele

Adverse Reactions

Cardiovascular: Hypotension, cardiovascular collapse, tachycardia, atrial and ventricular arrhythmias

Central nervous system: CNS depression, slurred speech, coma, agitation, confusion, seizures

Dermatologic: Irritation, burns; white, red, or brown skin discoloration

Gastrointestinal: Nausea, vomiting, hemorrhage, ulceration, gastrointestinal bleeding

Renal: Nephritis

Respiratory: Pulmonary edema, wheezing, coughing, dyspnea, pneumonia

Miscellaneous: Green discoloration of urine, oral burns

Signs & Symptoms of Acute Overdose Urine discoloration (dark), urine discoloration (brown), urine discoloration (green), dermal burns, wheezing, hypothermia, nephritis, hematuria, cyanosis, seizures

Toxicodynamics/Kinetics

Absorption: Readily absorbed across mucous membranes, skin, or via inhalation

Distribution: Not known

Metabolism: In liver

Half-life:

- Conjugated phenol: 1 hour
- Elimination: 1-4.5 hours

Elimination: Renally with 52% unchanged

Usual Dosage Allow to dissolve slowly in mouth; may be repeated every 2 hours as needed

Lethal dose: 3 g

Contraindications Do not use in children <3 years of age

Dosage Forms

Liquid, topical (Baker's P&S): 1% with sodium chloride, liquid paraffin oil and water (120 mL, 240 mL)

Lozenge:

- Cēpastat®: 1.45% with menthol and eucalyptus oil
- Cēpastat® Cherry: 0.72% with menthol and eucalyptus oil
- Chloraseptic®: 32.5 mg total phenol, sugar, corn syrup

Mouthwash (Chloraseptic®): 1.4% with thymol, sodium borate, menthol, and glycerin (180 mL)

Solution (Liquified Phenol): 88% [880 mg/mL]

Reference Range

Normal total phenol level: 0.15-7.96 mg/100 mL

Lowest reported toxic serum level of phenol: 27 μg/mL

Toxic: >75 mg/L

Dinitrophenol or hydroquinone may produce methemoglobin BEI (urine) is 250 mg/g creatinine; serum levels <20 mg/L not associated with acute toxicity

Fatal: 1 g ingestion may be fatal

Overdosage Treatment

Decontamination:

Oral: Ipecac is contraindicated; lavage with water or polyethylene glycol/activated charcoal with cathartic

Dermal: Remove clothing, wash exposed skin with isopropyl alcohol, polyethylene glycol, or industrial methylated spirits; flush eyes with copious amounts of water (if exposed); methylene blue for symptomatic methemoglobinemia due to dinitrophenol or hydroquinol exposure

Inhalation: Remove from source and provide oxygen

Supportive therapy: Blood products for hemorrhage

Antidote(s)

Methylene Blue *on page 1444*

Diagnostic Tests/Procedures

Blood Gases, Arterial *on page 1207*

Complete Blood Count *on page 1236*

Electrolytes, Blood *on page 1254*

Liver Profile *on page 1286*

Methemoglobin, Blood

<sd[Phenol, Quantitative, Urine

Pregnancy Risk Factor C

Monitoring Parameters CBC, electrolytes, glucose, BUN

Additional Information Colorless or white crystals, acrid odor

Odor threshold of 0.05 ppm

TLV-TWA: 5 ppm

IDLH: 100 ppm

PEL-TWA: 5 ppm

Specific References

Bruce RM, Santodonato J, and Neal MW, "Summary Review of the Health Effects Associated With Phenol," *Toxicol Ind Health*, 1987, 3(4):535-68.

Hunter DM, Timerding BL, Leonard RB, et al, "Effects of Isopropyl Alcohol, Ethanol, and Polyethylene Glycol/Industrial Methylated Spirits in the Treatment of Acute Phenol Burns," *Ann Emerg Med*, 1992, 21(11):1303-7.

Liao JTF and Oehme FW, "Literature Reviews of Phenolic Compounds IV o-Phenylphenol," *Vet Hum Toxicol*, 1980, 22(6):406-8.

Nomoto Y, Fujita T, and Kitani Y, "Serum and Urine Levels of Phenol Following Phenol Blocks," *Can J Anaesth*, 1987, 34(3 Pt 1):307-10.

Soares ER and Tift JP, "Phenol Poisoning: Three Fatal Cases," *J Forensic Sci*, 1982, 27(3):729-31.

Phenolax® [OTC] *see* Phenolphthalein *on this page*

Phenol Hydrate *see* Phenol *on previous page*

Phenolphthalein (fee nole thay' leen)

CAS Number 77-09-8

Brand Names Alophen Pills® [OTC]; Bom-Bon®; Espotabs® [OTC]; Evac-U-Gen® [OTC]; Evac-U-Lax® [OTC]; Ex-Lax® [OTC]; Feen-a-Mint® [OTC]; Lax-Pills® [OTC]; Medilax® [OTC]; Modane® [OTC]; Phenolax® [OTC]; Prulet® [OTC]; Sure-Lax®

Synonyms Phenolphthalein, White; Phenolphthalein, Yellow

Use Stimulant laxative

Mechanism of Action A diphenylmethane compound which stimulates peristalsis by directly irritating the smooth muscle of the intestine, possibly the colonic intramural plexus

Adverse Reactions

Dermatologic: Rash, irritation and sensation of burning on rectal mucosa and proctitis, toxic epidermal necrolysis, erythema multiforme

Endocrine & metabolic: Electrolyte imbalance, hypoglycemia

Gastrointestinal: Abdominal cramps, nausea, vomiting

Signs & Symptoms of Acute Overdose Abdominal pain, toxic epidermal necrolysis, tongue discoloration, nephrotic syndrome, hypokalemia, feces discoloration (black); feces discoloration (red); diarrhea, hypoglycemia, pulmonary edema, hypotension, Stevens-Johnson syndrome, disseminated intravascular coagulation, seizures, pancreatitis

Toxicodynamics/Kinetics

Onset of action: Within 6-8 hours

(Continued)

Phenolphthalein *(Continued)*

Absorption: 5% to 15%

Elimination: Excreted in the feces and skin, with up to 15% excreted in the urine as the conjugate; enterohepatically recycled

Usual Dosage Oral:

Children: 15-60 mg

Adults: 60-200 mg preferably at bedtime

Toxic dose:

Children: 600 mg

Adults: 2 g

Contraindications Do not use in patients with abdominal pain, obstruction, nausea or vomiting; not to be used during pregnancy or lactation

Warnings Habit-forming and may result in laxative dependence and loss of normal bowel function with prolonged use, can cause skin hypersensitivity and fixed drug eruption

Dosage Forms

Gum: 97.2 mg

Tablet: 60 mg, 90 mg, 97.2 mg, 130 mg

Tablet, chewable: 65 mg, 90 mg, 97.2 mg, 120 mg

Wafer: 64.8 mg

Wafer, chewable: 80 mg

Reference Range Serum phenolphthalein level of 0.4 μg/L associated with fatality

Overdosage Treatment

Decontamination: Lavage/activated charcoal is useful (do not use a cathartic)

Supportive therapy: Intravenous fluid and electrolyte replacement

Enhancement of elimination: Multiple dosing of activated charcoal may be useful

Test Interactions ↓ calcium (S), ↓ potassium (S)

Pregnancy Risk Factor C

Monitoring Parameters Monitor stools daily or weekly; fluid/electrolyte status

Patient Information Do not exceed recommended doses; swallow tablet whole, do not crush or chew; do not take antacid or milk within 1 hour of taking tablet; if rectal bleeding or failure to respond occur, notify physician

Additional Information

Phenolphthalein, white: Alophen Pills® [OTC], Medilax® [OTC], Modane® [OTC], Modane® Mild [OTC], Phenolax® [OTC], Prulet® [OTC]

Phenolphthalein, yellow: Evac-U-Gen® [OTC], Evac-U-Lax® [OTC], Ex-Lax® [OTC], Feen-A-Mint® [OTC], Lax-Pills® [OTC] Yellow is 2-3 times more potent than white. Urine or stool may be red or pink; produces an alkaline stool; does not decrease food absorption.

The chronic use of stimulant cathartics is inappropriate and should be avoided although constipation is a common complaint from elderly, such complaints require evaluation; short term use of stimulants is best; if prophylaxis is desired, this can be accomplished with bulk agents (psyllium), stool softeners, and hyperosmotic agents (sorbitol 70%); stool softeners are unnecessary if stools are well hydrated, soft, or "mushy"

Specific References

Devore CD, Ulshen MH, and Cross RE, "Phenolphthalein Laxative and Factitious Diarrhea," *Clin Pediatr (Phila)*, 1982, 21:573-4.

Lambrianides AL and Rosin RD, "Acute Pancreatitis Complicating Excessive Intake of Phenolphthalein," *Postgrad Med J*, 1984, 60(705):491-2.

Sidhu PS, Wilkinson ML, Sladen GE, et al, "Fatal Phenolpthalein Poisoning With Fulminant Hepatic Failure and Disseminated Intravascular Coagulation," *Hum Toxicol*, 1989, 8(5):381-4.

Phenolphthalein, White *see* Phenolphthalein *on previous page*

Phenolphthalein, Yellow *see* Phenolphthalein *on previous page*

Phenoxazole *see* Pemoline *on page 598*

Phensuximide (fen sux' i mide)

CAS Number 86-34-0

Brand Names Milontin®

Use Control of absence (petit mal) seizures; ethosuximide must be used in combination with other anticonvulsants in patients with both absence and tonic-clonic seizures

Mechanism of Action Increases the seizure threshold and suppresses paroxysmal spike-and-wave pattern in absence seizures; depresses nerve transmission in the motor cortex

Adverse Reactions

Central nervous system: Dizziness, drowsiness, headache, aggressiveness, mental depression, night terrors, asthenia, tiredness, paranoid psychosis, ataxia

Dermatologic: Stevens-Johnson syndrome or SLE, rash, exfoliative dermatitis

Gastrointestinal: Anorexia, nausea, vomiting, weight loss

Hematologic: Agranulocytosis, leukopenia, aplastic anemia, thrombocytopenia, pancytopenia

Ocular: Photophobia

Miscellaneous: Hiccups, discolors urine to a pink-red to red-brown color

Signs & Symptoms of Acute Overdose Acute overdosage can cause CNS depression, blood dyscrasias, ataxia, stupor, coma, urinary frequency, photophobia, hypotension, night terrors, chronic overdose can cause skin rash, confusion, ataxia, albuminuria, hepatic dysfunction, hematuria

Toxicodynamics/Kinetics

Absorption: Oral: Well absorbed

Protein binding: 0%

Metabolism: In the liver to norphensuximide (30%)

Half-life: 5-12 hours (8 hours for metabolite)

Time to peak serum concentration: Within 1-4 hours

Elimination: In urine as active and inactive metabolites

Usual Dosage Children and Adults: Oral: 0.5-1 g 2-3 times/day

Contraindications Intermittent porphyria

Warnings Use with caution in patients with hepatic or renal disease; abrupt withdrawal of the drug may precipitate absence status

Dosage Forms Capsule: 500 mg

Reference Range Therapeutic: 10-20 μg/mL (SI: 57-114 μmol/L)

Overdosage Treatment

Decontamination: Do not induce emesis; lavage/activated charcoal

Enhancement of elimination: Forced diuresis is of no benefit; multiple dosing of activated charcoal may be useful; although data is lacking, hemodialysis or hemoperfusion may be effective

Test Interactions ↑ alkaline phosphatase (S); positive Coombs' [direct]; ↓ calcium (S)

Pregnancy Risk Factor D

Patient Information Take with food; do not discontinue abruptly; may cause drowsiness and impair judgment

Specific References

Porter RJ, Penry JK, Lacy JR, et al, "Plasma Concentrations of Phensuximide, Methsuximide, and Their Metabolites in Relation to Clinical Efficacy," *Neurology*, 1979, 29:1509-13.

Phentanyl *see* Fentanyl Citrate *on page 347*

Phentermine Hydrochloride (fen' ter meen)

CAS Number 122-09-8; 1197-21-3

Brand Names Adipex-P®; Fastin®; Ionamin®; Obermine®; Termine®; Zantryl®

Synonyms Alpha Alpha-Dimethyl Phenethylamine

Use Short-term adjunct in exogenous obesity

Mechanism of Action Phentermine is structurally similar to dextroamphetamine and is comparable to dextroamphetamine as an appetite suppressant, but is generally associated with a lower incidence and severity of CNS side effects. Phentermine, like other anorexiants, stimulates the hypothalamus to result in decreased appetite; anorexiant effects are most likely mediated via norepinephrine and dopamine metabolism. However, other CNS effects or metabolic effects may be involved.

Adverse Reactions

Cardiovascular: Hypertension, tachycardia, arrhythmias

Central nervous system: Euphoria, nervousness, insomnia, confusion, mental depression, restlessness, headache, paranoid psychosis

Dermatologic: Alopecia

Gastrointestinal: Nausea, vomiting, diarrhea, abdominal cramps, constipation

Genitourinary: Changes in libido

Hematologic: Blood dyscrasias

Neuromuscular & skeletal: Tremors, myalgia, rhabdomyolysis

Ocular: Blurred vision, mydriasis

Renal: Dysuria, polyuria

Respiratory: Dyspnea

Miscellaneous: Increased sweating

Signs & Symptoms of Acute Overdose Hyperactivity, agitation, hyperthermia, insomnia, hypertension, seizures

Toxicodynamics/Kinetics

Absorption: Well absorbed; resin absorbed slower and produces more prolonged clinical effects

Distribution: V_d: 3-4 L/kg

Half-life: 20 hours

Elimination: Primarily excreted unchanged in urine

Usual Dosage Oral:

Children 3-15 years: 5-15 mg/day for 4 weeks

Adults: 8 mg 3 times/day 30 minutes before meals or food or 15-37.5 mg/day before breakfast or 10-14 hours before retiring

(Continued)

Phentermine Hydrochloride *(Continued)*

Contraindications Known hypersensitivity to phentermine

Warnings Do not use in children <12 years of age; use with caution in patients with diabetes mellitus, cardiovascular disease, nephritis, angina pectoris, hypertension, glaucoma, patients with a history of drug abuse

Dosage Forms

Capsule: 15 mg, 18.75 mg, 30 mg, 37.5 mg

Capsule, resin complex: 15 mg, 30 mg

Tablet: 8 mg, 37.5 mg

Reference Range Therapeutic plasma level: 30-90 ng/mL

Overdosage Treatment

Decontamination: Do not induce emesis; lavage/activated charcoal

Supportive therapy: There is no specific antidote for phentermine intoxication and the bulk of the treatment is supportive. Hyperactivity and agitation usually respond to reduced sensory input, however with extreme agitation diazepam (10-20 mg orally in adults or 0.1 mg/kg in children) or I.V. droperidol (0.1 mg/kg) or haloperidol (0.1 mg/kg) may be required. Hyperthermia is best treated with external cooling measures, or when severe or unresponsive, muscle paralysis with pancuronium may be needed. Hypertension is usually transient and generally does not require treatment unless severe. For diastolic blood pressures >120 mm Hg, a nitroprusside infusion should be initiated. Seizures usually respond to diazepam IVP and/or phenytoin maintenance regimens. Alkaline diuresis with mannitol or furosemide may be required to treat rhabdomyolysis; do not acidify urine.

Enhancement of elimination: Multiple dosing of activated charcoal may be useful; extracorporeal removal has not been shown to be beneficial

Drug Interactions

Decreased effect of guanethidine; decreased effect with CNS depressants

Increased effect/toxicity with MAO inhibitors (hypertensive crisis), sympathomimetics, CNS stimulants

Pregnancy Risk Factor C

Monitoring Parameters CNS

Patient Information Take during day to avoid insomnia; do not discontinue abruptly, may be addicting with prolonged use

Nursing Implications Dose should not be given in evening or at bedtime

Specific References

Devan GS, "Phentermine and Psychosis," *Br J Psychiatry*, 1990, 156:442-3.

Hamer R and Phelps D, "Inadvertent Intra-arterial Injection of Phentermine: A Complication of Drug Abuse," *Ann Emerg Med*, 1981, 10:148-50.

Kokkinos J and Levine SR, "Possible Association of Ischemic Stroke With Phentermine," *Stroke*, 1993, 24(2):310-3.

Levine B, Caplan YH, and Dixon AM, "A Fatality Involving Phentermine," *J Forensic Sci*, 1984, 29(4):1242-5.

Phenylalanine Mustard *see* Melphalan *on page 497*

Phenylbutazone (fen ill byoo' ta zone)

CAS Number 50-33-9

Brand Names Azolid®; Butazolidin®

Use Management of inflammatory disorders, as an analgesic in the treatment of mild to moderate pain and as an antipyretic; I.V. form used as an alternate to surgery in management of patent ductus arteriosus in premature neonates; acute gouty arthritis

Mechanism of Action Phenylbutazone is an anti-inflammatory, antipyretic, uricosuric, and analgesic; mechanism of action is thought to be due primarily to prostaglandin inhibition, leukocyte migration inhibition, and lysosomal enzyme stabilization

Adverse Reactions

Cardiovascular: Tachycardia, hypotension

Central nervous system: Dizziness, drowsiness, headache, fatigue, seizures

Dermatologic: Rash, edema, erythema multiforme, toxic epidermal necrolysis

Gastrointestinal: Dyspepsia, heartburn, nausea, vomiting, abdominal pain, peptic ulcer, gastrointestinal bleeding, gastrointestinal perforation

Hematologic: Anemia, platelet inhibition, thrombocytopenia, coagulopathy, leukopenia, neutropenia, agranulocytosis, granulocytopenia

Hepatic: Hepatitis

Ocular: Vision changes

Otic: Ototoxicity, tinnitus

Renal: Renal failure (acute), myoglobinuria

Signs & Symptoms of Acute Overdose Drowsiness, exfoliative dermatitis, pericarditis, gastrointestinal bleeding, gastritis; toxic epidermal necrolysis, hematuria, periarteritis nodosa, coma, pemphigus, dysosmia, erythema multiforme, photosensitivity, stomatitis, hypothyroidism, lichenoid eruptions, dermatitis, colitis, ataxia, coagulopathy, cholestatic jaundice, jaundice, chest pain, abdominal pain, rhabdomyolysis, hypotension, agitation, diarrhea, hyperventilation, respiratory arrest, systemic lupus erythematosus (SLE), seizures, urine discoloration (red), urine discoloration (red-brown), feces discoloration (black), feces discoloration (greenish gray), feces discoloration (pink), feces discoloration (red), feces discoloration (red-brown)

Toxicodynamics/Kinetics

Onset of action: 30-60 minutes

Duration: 3-5 days

Absorption: Oral: Well absorbed from gastrointestinal tract

Distribution: Most body tissues and synovial spaces

Protein binding: 98%

Metabolism: To oxyphenbutazone and hydroxyphenbutazone in the liver

Half-life: 50-100 hours (increases with hepatic impairment)

Time to peak serum concentration: Within 30-60 minutes

Elimination: Urinary excretion primarily as metabolites (99%)

Usual Dosage Adults: Oral: Initial:

Rheumatoid arthritis: 100-200 mg 3-4 times/day until desired effect, then reduce dose to not exceeding 400 mg/day

Acute gouty arthritis: 400 mg, 100 mg every 4 hours until acute attack subsides, not to continue longer than 1 week

Dosing adjustment in hepatic impairment: Should not be administered to patients with liver dysfunction

Contraindications Active gastrointestinal bleeding, ulcer disease, hypersensitivity to phenylbutazone or any component

Warnings May cause agranulocytosis and aplastic anemia; is not just a simple analgesic; use only when other NSAIDs have failed; use with caution in patients with congestive heart failure, hypertension, decreased renal or hepatic function, history of gastrointestinal disease (bleeding or ulcers), or those receiving anticoagulants; safety and efficacy in children <6 months of age have not yet been established; because of severe hematologic adverse effects, discontinue use if no favorable response is seen

Dosage Forms

Capsule: 100 mg

Tablet: 100 mg

Reference Range

Therapeutic: 50-100 μg/mL (SI: 162-324 μmol/L)

Toxic: >100 μg/mL (SI: >324 μmol/L)

Overdosage Treatment

Supportive therapy: Management of a nonsteroidal anti-inflammatory agent (NSAID) intoxication is primarily supportive and symptomatic. Fluid therapy is commonly effective in managing the hypotension that may occur following an acute NSAID overdose, except when this is due to an acute blood loss. Seizures tend to be very short-lived and often do not require drug treatment; although, recurrent seizures should be treated with I.V. diazepam or lorazepam.

Enhancement of elimination: Since many of the NSAIDs undergo enterohepatic cycling, multiple doses of charcoal may be needed to reduce the potential for delayed toxicities; charcoal perfusion may remove 5% to 20% of drug

Test Interactions Decreases uric acid (S)

Drug Interactions May inhibit phenytoin or warfarin metabolism and methotrexate excretion

Pregnancy Risk Factor D

Pregnancy Implications Crosses the placenta; appears in breast milk

Patient Information Do not exceed recommended dosage; take with food; may cause dizziness or drowsiness; notify physician and discontinue if persistent sore throat, fatigue, fever, or unusual bleeding or bruising occurs

Specific References

Berlinger WG, Spector R, Flanigan MJ, et al, "Hemoperfusion for Phenylbutazone Poisoning," *Ann Intern Med*, 1982, 96(3):334-5.

Court H and Volans GN, "Poisoning After Overdose With Nonsteroidal Anti-inflammatory Drugs," *Adverse Drug React Acute Poisoning Rev*, 1984, 3(1):1-21.

Hoppmann RA, Peden JG, and Ober SK, "Central Nervous System Side Effects of Nonsteroidal Anti-inflammatory Drugs. Aseptic Meningitis, Psychosis, and Cognitive Dysfunction," *Arch Intern Med*, 1991, 151(7):1309-13.

"Phenylbutazone Ingestions Complicated by Coagulopathy and Suspected Rhabdomyolysis," *Vet Hum Toxicol*, 1994, 36:367.

Smolinske SC, Hall AH, Vandenberg SA, et al, "Toxic Effects of Nonsteroid Anti-inflammatory Drugs in Overdose. An Overview of Recent Evidence on Clinical Effects and Dose-Response Relationships," *Drug Saf*, 1990, 5(4):252-74.

Vale JA and Meredith TJ, "Acute Poisoning Due to Nonsteroidal Anti-inflammatory Drugs," *Med Toxicol*, 1986, 1(1):12-31.

Verbeeck RK, "Pharmacokinetic Drug Interactions With Nonsteroidal Anti-inflammatory Drugs," *Clin Pharmacokinet*, 1990, 19(1):44-66.

Phenylethylmalonylurea *see* Phenobarbital *on page 614*

Phenylisohydantoin *see* Pemoline *on page 598*

Phenylpropanolamine Hydrochloride

(fen ill proe pa nole' a meen)

CAS Number 154-41-6

Brand Names Acutrim® [OTC]; Control® [OTC]; Dex-A-Diet® [OTC]; Dexatrim® [OTC]; Maigret-50; Prolamine® [OTC]; Propadrine; Propagest® [OTC]; Rhindecon®; Stay Trim® Diet Gum [OTC]; Westrim® LA [OTC]

Synonyms *dl*-Norephedrine Hydrochloride; PPA

Use Anorexiant and nasal decongestant

Mechanism of Action Releases tissue stores of epinephrine and thereby produces an alpha- and beta-adrenergic stimulation; this causes vasoconstriction and nasal mucosa blanching; also appears to depress central appetite centers

Adverse Reactions

Cardiovascular: Palpitations, reflex bradycardia, cardiac arrhythmias, chest pain, hypertension, angina

Central nervous system: Anxiety, psychosis, nervousness, restlessness, headache

Genitourinary: Difficult urination

Ocular: Mydriasis

Signs & Symptoms of Acute Overdose Vomiting, hypertension, extrapyramidal reaction, seizures, cognitive dysfunction, hyperthermia, palpitations, paresthesia, tachycardia, anorexia, reflex bradycardia, renal failure

Toxicodynamics/Kinetics

Onset of action: Nasal decongestion: 15-30 minutes

Duration:

Tablet: 3 hours

Extended release: 12-16 hours

Absorption: Oral: Well absorbed

Distribution: V_d: 4.5 L/kg

Metabolism: In the liver to norephedrine

Bioavailability: ~100%

Half-life: 4.6-6.6 hours

Elimination: Primarily in urine as unchanged drug (80% to 90%)

Usual Dosage Oral:

Children: Decongestant:

2-6 years: 6.25 mg every 4 hours

6-12 years: 12.5 mg every 4 hours not to exceed 75 mg/day

Adults:

Decongestant: 25 mg every 4 hours or 50 mg every 8 hours, not to exceed 150 mg/day

Anorexic: 25 mg 3 times/day 30 minutes before meals or 75 mg (timed release) once daily in the morning

Precision release: 75 mg after breakfast

Contraindications Known hypersensitivity to drug

Warnings Use with caution in patients with high blood pressure, may cause excitement, acute narrow-angle glaucoma

Dosage Forms

Capsule: 37.5 mg

Capsule, timed release: 25 mg, 75 mg

Tablet: 25 mg

Tablet:

Precision release: 75 mg

Timed release: 75 mg

Reference Range Peak serum phenylpropanolamine: ~0.28 mg/L 6 hours after oral ingestion of 150 mg sustained release dose

Overdosage Treatment

Decontamination: Lavage/activated charcoal with cathartic

Supportive therapy: Lorazepam or diazepam 5-10 mg I.V. (0.25-0.4 mg/kg for children) or phenobarbital may be used for excitation and seizures; nitroprusside can be used for hypertension while labetalol or esmolol can be used for tachycardia; ventricular ectopy can be treated with lidocaine

Enhancement of elimination: Multiple dosing of activated charcoal should be performed for sustained release preparation

Pregnancy Risk Factor C

Patient Information Should not be used more than 3 consecutive weeks for weight loss; contact physician for insomnia, tremor, or irregular heartbeat

Nursing Implications Give dose early in day to prevent insomnia; observe for signs of nervousness, excitability

Specific References

Bernstein E and Diskant BM, "Phenylpropanolamine: A Potentially Hazardous Drug," *Ann Emerg Med*, 1982, 11(6):311-5.

Elkins B and Spoerke DG, "An Estimation of the Toxicity of Nonprescription Diet Aids From Seventy Exposure Cases," *Vet Hum Toxicol*, 1983, 25:81-5.

Forman HP, Levin S, Stewart B, et al, "Cerebral Vasculitis and Hemorrhage in an Adolescent Taking Diet Pills Containing Phenylpropanolamine: Case Report and Review of Literature," *Pediatrics*, 1989, 83(5):737-41.

Pentel P, "Toxicity of Over-the-Counter Stimulants," *JAMA*, 1984, 252(14):1898-903.

Puder KS and Morgan JP, "Persuading by Citation: An Analysis of the References of Fifty-Three Published Reports of Phenylpropanolamine's Clinical Toxicity," *Clin Pharmacol Ther*, 1987, 42(1):1-9.

3-Phenylpropiophenone *see* Propafenone Hydrochloride *on page 652*

Phenylpseudohydantoin *see* Pemoline *on page 598*

Phenytoin (fen' i toyn)

Related Information

Drugs and Chemicals Proven to be Teratogenic in Humans *on page 1572-1575*

Seizures, Neonatal Guidelines *on page 1604-1605*

Status Epilepticus Treatment Algorithm *on page 1608*

Therapeutic Drugs Associated With Hallucinations *on page 1558-1559*

CAS Number 57-41-0

Brand Names Antisacer®; Dilantin®; Dintoina®; Diphenylan Sodium®; Ditan®; Epanutin®; Epinat®; Fenytoin®

Synonyms Diphenylhydantoin; DPH; Fenitoina

Use Management of generalized tonic-clonic (grand mal), simple partial and complex partial seizures; prevention of seizures following head trauma/neurosurgery; ventricular arrhythmias, including those associated with digitalis intoxication; beneficial effects in the treatment of migraine or trigeminal neuralgia in some patients

Mechanism of Action Stabilizes neuronal membranes and decreases seizure activity by increasing efflux or decreasing influx of sodium ions across cell membranes in the motor cortex during generation of nerve impulses; prolongs effective refractory period and suppresses ventricular pacemaker automaticity, shortens action potential in the heart

Adverse Reactions

Dose related:

- Central nervous system: Slurred speech, dizziness, drowsiness, drowsiness, choreoathetosis, psychosis, fever, visual hallucinations
- Dermatologic: Rash, exfoliative dermatitis, erythema multiforme, facial edema, acne
- Endocrine & metabolic: Folic acid depletion, osteomalacia, hyperglycemia, reduced plasma testosterone, gynecomastia
- Gastrointestinal: Nausea, vomiting, gingival hyperplasia
- Genitourinary: Priapism
- Hematologic: Lymphadenopathy, neutropenia, thrombocytopenia, anemia (megaloblastic)
- Neuromuscular & skeletal: Sensory paresthesia (long-term treatment)
- Ocular: Nystagmus, blurred vision, diplopia
- Renal: Nephrotic syndrome
- Miscellaneous: Mutism

I.V.:

- Cardiovascular: Hypotension, bradycardia, cardiac arrhythmias, cardiovascular collapse (especially with rapid I.V. use)
- Central nervous system: Ataxia
- Dermatologic: Hirsutism, coarsening of facial features, Stevens-Johnson syndrome, pruritus
- Gastrointestinal: Gingival hyperplasia
- Hematologic: Blood dyscrasias, pseudolymphoma, lymphoma
- Hepatic: Hepatitis
- Local: Venous irritation and pain, thrombophlebitis
- Miscellaneous: Lymphadenopathy, urine discoloration (pink), urine discoloration (red), urine discoloration (red-brown), systemic lupus erythematosus-like syndrome

Signs & Symptoms of Acute Overdose Unsteady gait, toxic epidermal necrolysis, nephrotic syndrome, pseudotumor cerebri, acrodynia, hypocalcemia, enuresis, dementia, hypothyroidism, hyperprolactinemia, hyperglycemia, leukemoid reaction, gynecomastia, dysarthria, chorea (extrapyramidal), myasthenia gravis (exacerbation or precipitation of), extrapyramidal reaction, gingival hyperplasia, encephalopathy, delirium, vision color changes (white tinge, dysosmia, periarteritis nodosa, hirsutism, hypertrichosis, headache, cognitive dysfunction, tremors, Parkinson's-like symptoms, myoglobinuria, rhabdomyolysis, slurred speech, mydriasis, myoclonus, confusion, encephalopathy, hyperthermia, drowsiness, eosinophilia, nausea, hypothermia, fever, hypotension, respiratory depression, leuko-

(Continued)

Phenytoin *(Continued)*

penia); neutropenia; agranulocytosis; granulocytopenia; hyperreflexia, coma, systemic lupus erythematosus (SLE), erythema multiforme, ophthalmoplegia; see table. While toxicity from oral ingestion is relatively low, cardiac toxicity due to I.V. administration is primarily due to propylene glycol moiety.

Manifestations of Toxicity

Levels	Manifestation
20 mcg/mL (79 μmol/L)	Nystagmus
30 mcg/mL (118.9 μmol/L)	Ataxia
40 mcg/mL (159 μmol/L)	Decreased mental status
50 mcg/mL (200 μmol/L)	Coma

Toxicodynamics/Kinetics

Onset of action: I.V.: 3-5 minutes

Absorption: Oral: Slow

Distribution: Into CSF, saliva, semen, gastrointestinal fluids, bile, and breast milk

V_d:

Premature Neonates: 1-1.2 L/kg

Full-term Neonates: 0.8-0.9 L/kg

Infants: 0.7-0.8 L/kg

Children: 0.7 L/kg

Adults: 0.6-0.7 L/kg

Protein binding: Adults: 90% to 95%, increased free fraction (decreased protein binding) in neonates (up to 20% free), infants (up to 15% free), and patients with hyperbilirubinemia, hypoalbuminemia, uremia

Metabolism: Follows dose-dependent (Michaelis-Menten) pharmacokinetics with increased Vmax in infants >6 months and children vs adults; major metabolite (via oxidation) HPPA undergoes enterohepatic recycling

Bioavailability: Dependent upon formulation administered

Half-life: Changes with dose and serum concentrations; 8-60 hours after initiation of therapy with oral administration

Time to peak serum concentration: Dependent upon formulation administered; extended release capsule peak serum levels occur within 4-12 hours and within 2-3 hours after the immediate release preparation

Elimination: Highly variable clearance, dependent upon intrinsic hepatic function and dose administered; elimination in urine as glucuronides; <5% excreted unchanged in urine; increased clearance and decreased serum concentrations with febrile illness

Usual Dosage

Status epilepticus: I.V.:

Neonates: Loading dose: 15-20 mg/kg in a single or divided dose; maintenance dose: Initial: 5 mg/kg/day in 2 divided doses; usual: 5-8 mg/kg/day in 2 divided doses; some patients may require dosing every 8 hours

Infants and Children: Loading dose: 15-20 mg/kg in a single or divided dose; maintenance dose: Initial: 5 mg/kg/day in 2 divided doses, usual doses:

6 months to 3 years: 8-10 mg/kg/day

4-6 years: 7.5-9 mg/kg/day

7-9 years: 7-8 mg/kg/day

10-16 years: 6-7 mg/kg/day, some patients may require every 8 hours dosing

Adults: Loading dose: 15-20 mg/kg in a single or divided dose, followed by 100-150 mg/dose at 30-minute intervals up to a maximum of 1500 mg/24 hours; maintenance dose: 300 mg/day or 5-6 mg/kg/day in 3 divided doses

Anticonvulsant: Children and Adults: Oral:

Loading dose: 15-20 mg/kg; based on phenytoin serum concentrations and recent dosing history; administer oral loading dose in 3 divided doses given every 2-4 hours to decrease gastrointestinal adverse effects and to ensure complete oral absorption; maintenance dose: 300 mg/day or 5-6 mg/kg/day in 3 divided doses

Dosing adjustment/comments in renal impairment or hepatic disease: Safe in usual doses in mild liver disease; clearance may be substantially reduced in cirrhosis and plasma level monitoring with dose adjustment advisable. Free phenytoin levels should be monitored closely.

Contraindications Occurrence of any rash while on treatment; the drug should not be resumed if rash is exfoliative, purpuric, or bullous

Warnings Use with caution in patients with hepatic dysfunction; avoid abrupt discontinuation; dosing should be slowly reduced to avoid precipitation of seizures; increased toxicity with nephrotic syndrome patient; may increase frequency of petit mal seizures; I.V. form may cause hypotension, skin necrosis at I.V. site;

avoid I.V. administration in small veins; use with caution in patients with porphyria; discontinue if rash or lymphadenopathy occurs

Dosage Forms

Capsule, as sodium:
- Extended: 30 mg, 100 mg
- Prompt: 30 mg, 100 mg

Injection, as sodium: 50 mg/mL (2 mL, 5 mL)

Suspension, oral: 30 mg/5 mL (5 mL, 240 mL); 125 mg/5 mL (5 mL, 240 mL)

Tablet, chewable: 50 mg

Stability Parenteral solution may be used as long as there is no precipitate and it is not hazy; slightly yellowed solution may be used; refrigeration may cause precipitate, sometimes the precipitate is resolved by allowing the solution to reach room temperature again; drug may precipitate with pH ≤11.5; do not mix with other medications; may dilute with normal saline for I.V. infusion, but must be diluted to concentration <6 mg/mL

Reference Range

Therapeutic: 10-20 μg/mL (SI: 40-79 μmol/L); toxicity is measured clinically, and some patients require levels outside the suggested therapeutic range

Toxic: 30-50 μg/mL (SI: 120-200 μmol/L)

Lethal: >100 μg/mL (SI: >400 μmol/L)

Manifestations of toxicity:
- Nystagmus: 20 μg/mL (SI: 79 μmol/L)
- Ataxia: 30 μg/mL (SI: 118.9 μmol/L)
- Decreased mental status: 40 μg/mL (SI: 159 μmol/L)
- Coma: 50 μg/mL (SI: 200 μmol/L)

Overdosage Treatment

Decontamination: Emesis or lavage/activated charcoal with cathartic

Supportive therapy: Treatment is supportive for hypotension; treat with I.V. fluids and place patient in Trendelenburg position; seizures may be controlled with lorazepam or diazepam 5-10 mg (0.25-0.4 mg/kg in children); intravenous albumin (25 g every 6 hours has been used to increase bound fraction of drug)

Enhancement of elimination: Multiple dosing of activated charcoal may be effective; peritoneal dialysis, diuresis, hemodialysis, hemoperfusion, and plasmapheresis is of little value

Test Interactions Increases glucose, alkaline phosphatase (S); decreases thyroxine (S), calcium (S); serum sodium increases in overdose setting

Diagnostic Tests/Procedures

Phenytoin, Blood *on page 1321*

Drug Interactions Phenytoin may decrease the serum concentration or effectiveness of valproic acid, carbamazepine, ethosuximide, primidone, warfarin, oral contraceptives, corticosteroids, cyclosporine, theophylline, chloramphenicol, rifampin, doxycycline, quinidine, mexiletine, disopyramide, dopamine, or nondepolarizing skeletal muscle relaxants; protein binding of phenytoin can be affected by VPA or salicylates; serum phenytoin concentrations may be increased by cimetidine, disulfiram, trazodone, ethanol, halothane, phenylbutazone, azapropazone, ibuprofen, amiodarone, imipramine, miconazole, metronidazole, nifedipine, chloramphenicol, INH, trimethoprim, or sulfonamides and decreased by rifampin, cisplatin, vinblastine, bleomycin, folic acid, or continuous NG feeds, oxacillin, nitrofurantoin; phenytoin decreases the bioavailability of oral diltiazem; concomitant high-dose tamoxifen (200 mg/day) and phenytoin administration can result in increased serum phenytoin levels

Pregnancy Risk Factor D

Pregnancy Implications Distributes into breast milk; crosses placenta with fetal serum concentrations equal to those of mother; eye, cardiac, cleft palate, and skeletal malformations have been noted; fetal hydantoin syndrome associated with maternal ingestion of 100-800 mg/kg during 1st trimester

Monitoring Parameters Blood pressure, vital signs (with I.V. use), plasma level monitoring, CBC, liver function tests

Patient Information Shake oral suspension well prior to each dose; do not change brand or dosage form without consulting physician

Nursing Implications I.V. injections should be followed by normal saline flushes through the same needle or I.V. catheter to avoid local irritation of the vein; must be diluted to concentrations <6 mg/mL, in normal saline, for I.V. infusion

Additional Information Less than 5% of total body phenytoin is removed by plasmapheresis and rapid re-equilibration after plasmapheresis can occur resulting in increased free phenytoin levels; intravenous phenytoin salt has poor water solubility (0.02 mg/mL at a pH of 7) with a high PTT (12) and requires 40% propylene glycol and 10% ethanol

Phenytoin: Dilantin® chewable tablet and oral suspension

Phenytoin sodium, extended: Dilantin® Kapseal®

Phenytoin sodium, prompt: Diphenylan Sodium® capsule

Specific References

Berigan T and Watt TJ, "Dilantin Toxicity Presenting as Mutism Following Severe Head Injury: Case Report," *Milit Med*, 1994, 159:533-4.

(Continued)

Phenytoin *(Continued)*

Black J, Hannaman T, and Malone C, "The Relationship of Serum Albumin Level to Phenytoin Toxicity," *J Clin Pharmacol*, 1987, 27(3):249-50.

Dela Cruz FG, Kanter MZ, Fischer JH, et al, "Efficacy of Individualized Phenytoin Sodium Loading Doses Administered by Intravenous Infusion," *Clin Pharm*, 1988, 7(3):219-24.

Kerrick JM, Wolff DL, and Graves NM, "Predicting Unbound Phenytoin Concentrations in Patients Receiving Valproic Acid: A Comparison of Two Prediction Methods," *Ann Pharmacother*, 1995, 29:470-4.

Lombardi TP, Gailey RA, and Bryant BG, "Phenytoin Overdose in Neonate Attributable to Product Packaging Similarities," *Am J Hosp Pharm*, 1989, 46(10):1999-2000.

Mansur LI, Murrow RW, Garrelts JC, et al, "Rebound of Plasma Free Phenytoin Concentration Following Plasmapheresis in a Patient With Thrombotic Thrombocytopenic Purpura," *Ann Pharmacother*, 1995, 29:592-5.

Rabinowicz AL, Hinton DR, Dyck P, et al, "High-Dose Tamoxifen in treatment of Brain Tumors: interaction with Antiepileptic Drugs," *Epilepsia*, 1995, 36:513-5.

Rowden AM, Spoor JE, Bertino JS Jr, "The Effect of Activated Charcoal on Phenytoin Pharmacokinetics," *Ann Emerg Med*, 1990, 19(10):1144-7.

pHisoHex® *see* Hexachlorophene *on page 402*

Phos-Flur® *see* Fluoride *on page 355*

Phosphonoformate *see* Foscarnet Sodium *on page 367*

Phosphonoformic Acid *see* Foscarnet Sodium *on page 367*

3-Phosphoryloxymethyl Phenytoin Disodium *see* Fosphenytoin *on page 370*

***p*-Hydroxyampicillin** *see* Amoxicillin *on page 121*

Phyllocontin® *see* Aminophylline *on page 110*

Physeptone® *see* Methadone Hydrochloride *on page 508*

Physiotens® *see* Moxonidine *on page 541*

Picket® *see* Permethrin *on page 608*

Pimozide (pi' moe zide)

CAS Number 2062-78-4

Brand Names Opiran®; Orap™

Use Suppression of severe motor and phonic tics in patients with Tourette's disorder

Mechanism of Action A potent centrally-acting dopamine receptor antagonist resulting in its characteristic neuroleptic effects

Adverse Reactions

Cardiovascular: Ventricular arrhythmias, dose-related prolonged Q-T intervals

Central nervous system: Extrapyramidal effects, tardive dyskinesia, perioral numbness, fever

Endocrine & metabolic: Syndrome of inappropriate antidiuretic hormone, galactorrhea, hyponatremia

Gastrointestinal: Nausea, diarrhea, weight loss, anorexia, xerostomia

Genitourinary: Impotence, exacerbation of enuresis

Neuromuscular & skeletal: Tremors

Respiratory: Respiratory failure

Miscellaneous: Facial swelling

Signs & Symptoms of Acute Overdose Hypotension, enuresis, galactorrhea, impotence, respiratory depression, Parkinson's-like symptoms, EKG abnormalities, numbness, extrapyramidal reaction, drowsiness, seizures, QT interval prolongation, torsade de pointes

Toxicodynamics/Kinetics

Absorption: Oral: 50%; poor from gastrointestinal tract

Distribution: Widely into body

Protein binding: 99%

Metabolism: In the liver (with significant first-pass decay) to two inactive metabolites

Bioavailability: 50%

Half-life: 50 hours

Time to peak serum concentration: Within 6-8 hours

Elimination: 50% excreted in urine; 20%, fecal

Usual Dosage Children >12 years and Adults: Oral: Initial: 1-2 mg/day, then increase dosage as needed every other day; range is usually 7-16 mg/day, maximum dose: 20 mg/day or 0.3 mg/kg/day should not be exceeded

Dosing adjustment in hepatic impairment: Reduction of dose is necessary in patients with liver disease

Contraindications Simple tics other than Tourette's, history of cardiac arrhythmias, known hypersensitivity to pimozide

Dosage Forms Tablet: 2 mg

Reference Range 3 mg dose produces a plasma level of 3.3 ng/mL

Overdosage Treatment

Decontamination: Lavage/activated charcoal with cathartic

Supportive therapy: Following initiation of essential overdose management, toxic symptom treatment and supportive treatment should be initiated. Hypotension usually responds to I.V. fluids or Trendelenburg positioning. If unresponsive to these measures, the use of a parenteral inotrope may be required (eg, norepinephrine 0.1-0.2 mcg/kg/minute titrated to response). Seizures commonly respond to lorazepam or diazepam (I.V. 5-10 mg bolus in adults every 15 minutes if needed up to a total of 30 mg; I.V. 0.25-0.4 mg/kg/dose up to a total of 10 mg in children) or to phenytoin or phenobarbital. Also critical cardiac arrhythmias often respond to I.V. phenytoin (15 mg/kg up to 1 gram), while other antiarrhythmics can be used. Neuroleptics often cause extrapyramidal reaction (eg, dystonic reactions) requiring management with diphenhydramine 1-2 mg/kg (adults) up to a maximum of 50 mg I.M. or I.V. slow push followed by a maintenance dose for 48-72 hours. When these reactions are unresponsive to diphenhydramine, benztropine mesylate I.V. 1-2 mg (adults) may be effective. These agents are generally effective within 2-5 minutes.

Enhancement of elimination: Multiple dosing of activated charcoal may be useful; forced diuresis or hemodialysis is of no benefit

Pregnancy Risk Factor C

Additional Information Less sedation but more likely to cause extrapyramidal signs than chlorpromazine

Specific References

Bruun RD, "Subtle and Under-Recognized Side Effects of Neuroleptic Treatment in Children With Tourette's Disorder," *Am J Psychiatry*, 1988, 145(5):621-4.

Krähenbühl S, Sauter B, Kupferschmidt H, et al, "Case Report: Reversable QT Prolongation With Torsades de Pointes in a Patient With Pimozide Intoxication," *Am J Med sci*, 1995, 309:315-6.

Larkin C, "Epileptogenic Potential of Pimozide," *Am J Psychiatry*, 1983, 140(3):372-3.

Pinbetol® *see* Pindolol *on this page*

Pindolol (pin' doe lole)

Related Information

Beta-Blockers Comparison *on page 1644-1645*

Therapeutic Drugs Associated With Hallucinations *on page 1558-1559*

CAS Number 13523-86-9

Brand Names Barblac®; Betadren®; Durapindol®; Pinbetol®; Viskaldix®; Visken®

Use Management of hypertension

Mechanism of Action Blocks both $beta_1$- and $beta_2$-receptors and has mild intrinsic sympathomimetic activity; pindolol has negative inotropic and chronotropic effects and can significantly slow A-V nodal conduction

Adverse Reactions

Cardiovascular: Mesenteric arterial thrombosis, A-V block, chest tightness

Central nervous system: Auditory hallucinations, dizziness

Dermatologic: Purpura

Gastrointestinal: Ischemic colitis

Hematologic: Thrombocytopenia, leukopenia, neutropenia, agranulocytosis, granulocytopenia

Neuromuscular & skeletal: Fine tremors

Ocular: Diplopia

Respiratory: Wheezing

Miscellaneous: Lupus erythematous

Signs & Symptoms of Acute Overdose Severe hypotension, dry mouth, ataxia, insomnia, heart block, confusion, colitis, cold extremities, A-V block, myasthenia gravis (exacerbation or precipitation of), hypoglycemia, depression, bradycardia, impotence, heart failure and wheezing; hypertension and tachycardia also associated; coma, systemic lupus erythematosus (SLE)

Toxicodynamics/Kinetics

Onset of action: 3 hours

Duration: 24 hours; beta blockade lasted longer in elderly patients as compared to younger patients

Absorption: 50% to 95% of a dose is rapidly absorbed from gastrointestinal tract

Distribution: V_d: 1.2-2 L/kg; widely throughout body

Protein binding: 57%

Metabolism: In the liver (60% to 65%) to conjugates (no first-pass effect)

Bioavailability: 50% to 95%

Half-life: 2.5-4 hours (increased with renal insufficiency, age, and cirrhosis)

Time to peak serum concentration: Within 1-2 hours

Elimination: Urine (35% to 50% unchanged drug); clearance: 6.2 mL/minute/kg

Usual Dosage Adults: Oral: Initial: 5 mg twice daily, increase by 10 mg/day at 3- to 4-week intervals to a maximum of 60 mg/day

Dosing adjustment in renal and hepatic impairment: Reduction is necessary in severely impaired

(Continued)

Pindolol *(Continued)*

Contraindications Uncompensated congestive heart failure, cardiogenic shock, bradycardia or heart block, asthma, wheezing, COPD

Dosage Forms Tablet: 5 mg, 10 mg

Stability Protect from light

Reference Range Therapeutic: 0.02-0.04 μg/mL; 250 mg ingestion was associated with a serum level of 0.66 μg/mL; 500 mg ingestion produced a serum level of 1.5 μg/mL

Overdosage Treatment

Decontamination: Do not use ipecac; gastric lavage with activated charcoal with cathartic should be utilized

Supportive therapy: Sympathomimetics (eg, epinephrine or dopamine), glucagon or a pacemaker can be used to treat the toxic bradycardia, asystole, and/or hypotension; initially fluids may be the best treatment for toxic hypotension.

Enhancement of elimination: Multiple dosing of activated charcoal may be effective

Antidote(s)

Glucagon *on page 1431*

Test Interactions Increases cholesterol (S), glucose; decreases bilirubin (S)

Drug Interactions Nonsteroidal anti-inflammatory agents, salicylates, sympathomimetics, thyroid hormones, insulins, lidocaine, calcium channel blockers, nifedipine, catecholamine-depleting drugs, clonidine, disopyramide, prazosin, theophylline

Pregnancy Risk Factor B

Pregnancy Implications Excreted in breast milk

Monitoring Parameters Blood pressure, standing and sitting/supine, pulse

Patient Information Do not discontinue medication abruptly; consult pharmacist or physician before taking over-the-counter cold preparations

Additional Information May cause hypoglycemia during hemodialysis

Specific References

Meier J, "Pharmacokinetic Comparison of Pindolol With Other Beta-Adrenoceptor-Blocking Agents," *Am Heart J*, 1982, 104(2 Pt 2):364-73.

Offenstadt G, Hericord PH, and Amstrutz PH, "Voluntary Poisoning With Pindolol," *Nouv Presse Med*, 1976, 5(24):1539.

Thorpe P, "Prindolol in Hypertension," *Med J Aust*, 1971, 1(23):1242.

Weinstein RS, "Recognition and Management of Poisoning With Beta-Adrenergic Blocking Agents," *Ann Emerg Med*, 1984, 13(12):1123-31.

Piperacillin Sodium and Tazobactam Sodium

(pi per< a sill in so' dee um & ta zoe bak' tam so' dee um)

Brand Names Zosyn™

Use Treatment of infections of lower respiratory tract, urinary tract, skin and skin structures, gynecologic, bone and joint infections, and septicemia caused by susceptible organisms. Tazobactam expands activity of piperacillin to include beta-lactamase producing strains of *S. aureus*, *H. influenzae*, *Enterobacteriaceae*, *Pseudomonas*, *Klebsiella*, *Citrobacter*, *Serratia*, *Bacteroides*, and other gram-negative anaerobes.

Mechanism of Action Piperacillin interferes with bacterial cell wall synthesis during active multiplication, causing cell wall death and resultant bactericidal activity against susceptible bacteria; tazobactam prevents degradation of piperacillin by binding to the active side on beta-lactamase

Adverse Reactions

Cardiovascular: Hypertension, hypotension

Central nervous system: Convulsions, fever, headache, dizziness, confusion, drowsiness, agitation, insomnia

Dermatologic: Rash, exfoliative dermatitis

Endocrine & metabolic: Hypokalemia

Gastrointestinal: Diarrhea, nausea, vomiting, dyspepsia, *Pseudomonas* colitis

Hematologic: Hemolysis, eosinophilia, neutropenia, prolonged bleeding time, thrombocytopenia, positive Coombs' reaction, leukopenia

Hepatic: Elevated liver enzymes, cholestatic hepatitis

Local: Thrombophlebitis

Neuromuscular & skeletal: Myoclonus

Renal: Acute interstitial nephritis

Miscellaneous: Hypersensitivity reactions, anaphylactic shock, serum sickness-like reaction, wheezing, edema

Signs & Symptoms of Acute Overdose Leukopenia or neutropenia (agranulocytosis, granulocytopenia); eosinophilia, hypokalemia, insomnia, colitis

Toxicodynamics/Kinetics Both AUC and peak concentrations are dose proportional

Absorption: I.M.:

Piperacillin: 71%

Tazobactam: 84%

Distribution: V_d: Piperacillin: 0.3 L/kg; distributes well into lungs, intestinal mucosa, skin, muscle, uterus, ovary, prostate, gallbladder, and bile; penetration into CSF is low in subject with noninflamed meninges

Metabolism:
- Piperacillin: 6% to 9%
- Tazobactam: ~26%

Protein binding:
- Piperacillin: ~26% to 33%
- Tazobactam: 31% to 32%

Half-life:
- Piperacillin: 1 hour
- Metabolite: 1-1.5 hours
- Tazobactam: 0.7-0.9 hour

Elimination: Both piperacillin and tazobactam are directly proportional to renal function
- Piperacillin: 50% to 70% eliminated unchanged in urine, 10% to 20% excreted in bile
- Tazobactam: Found in urine at 24 hours, with 26% as the inactive metabolite

Hemodialysis removes 30% to 40% of piperacillin and tazobactam; peritoneal dialysis removes 11% to 21% of tazobactam and 6% of piperacillin; hepatic impairment does not affect the kinetics of piperacillin or tazobactam significantly

Usual Dosage Adults: I.V.: 3.375 g (3 g piperacillin/0.375 g tazobactam) every 6 hours

Dosing interval in renal impairment:
- Cl_{cr} <40 mL/minute: No change
- Cl_{cr} 20-40 mL/minute: Administer 2.25 g every 6 hours
- Cl_{cr} <20 mL/minute: Administer 2.25 g every 8 hours

Hemodialysis: Administer 2.25 g every 8 hours with an additional dose of 0.75 g after each dialysis

Contraindications Hypersensitivity to piperacillin, tazobactam, other penicillins, or any component

Warnings Use with caution in patients with known hypersensitivity to cephalosporins or other beta-lactamase inhibitors; not approved for use in patients <12 years of age; use with caution in patients with a history of seizures and in patients with renal function impairment

Dosage Forms Injection: Piperacillin sodium 2 g and tazobactam sodium 0.25 g; piperacillin sodium 3 g and tazobactam sodium 0.375 g; piperacillin sodium 4 g and tazobactam sodium 0.5 g (vials at an 8:1 ratio of piperacillin sodium to tazobactam sodium)

Stability Store at controlled room temperature; after reconstitution, stable for 24 hours at room temperature and 1 week when refrigerated; unused portions should be discarded after 24 hours at room temperature and 48 hours when refrigerated

Reference Range After a dose of 4 g piperacillin/500 mg tazobactam, mean serum piperacillin and tazobactam levels were 223.7 μg/mL and 27.2 μg/mL, respectively

Overdosage Treatment Enhancement of elimination: Combined charcoal hemoperfusion with hemodialysis may be useful, see Toxicodynamics

Test Interactions Positive Coombs' [direct] test 3.8%, ↑ ALT, ↑ AST

Drug Interactions
- Increased duration of neuromuscular blockers
- Increased/prolonged levels with probenecid

Pregnancy Risk Factor B

Nursing Implications Administer 1 hour apart from aminoglycosides; give around-the-clock (ie, 6-12-6-12)

Additional Information Total sodium content: 108 mg/vial

Specific References

Chung KC, Moon YS, Chin A, et al, "Compatibility of Ondansetron Hydrochloride and Piperacillin Sodium-Tazobactam Sodium During Simulated Y-Site Administration," *Am J Health-Syst Pharm*, 1995, 52:1554-6.

Jhee SS, Kern JW, Burm JP, et al, "Piperacillin-Tazobactam Pharmacokinetics in Patients With Intraabdominal Infections," *Pharmacotherapy*, 1995, 15(4):4f72-8.

Johnson CA, Halstenson CE, Kelloway JS, et al, "Single-Dose Pharmacokinetics of Piperacillin and Tazobactam in Patients With Renal Disease," *Clin Pharmacol Ther*, 1992, 51(1):32-41.

Sorgel F and Kinzig M, "The Chemistry, Pharmacokinetics and Tissue Distribution of Piperacillin/Tazobactam," *J Antimicrob Chemother*, 1993, 31(Suppl A):39-60.

Wickerts CJ, Asaba H, Gunnarsson B, et al, "Combined Carbon Hemoperfusion and Hemodialysis in Treatment of Penicillin Intoxication," *Br Med J*, 1980, 280(6226):1254-5.

Piperazidine *see* Piperazine Citrate *on this page*

Piperazine Citrate (pi' per a zeen)

CAS Number 110-85-0; 142-88-1; 144-29-6; 41372-10-5; 142-63-2; 14538-56-8; 18534-18-4

UN Number 2579

(Continued)

Piperazine Citrate *(Continued)*

Brand Names Balan®; Lannett®; Pipralen®; Richlyn®; Schein®; Uvilon®; Vermi®; Vermizine®; Wormex®

Synonyms Diethylenediamine; Piperazidine

Use Treatment of *Ascaris lumbricoides* (roundworm) and *Enterobius vermicularis*, (pinworm, threadworm); may be effective in treating tropical eosinophilia

Mechanism of Action Blocks acetylcholine response in smooth muscle causing flaccid paralysis; while the drug has its primary effect on the parasite in the gastrointestinal tract, there is no effect on larvae in tissues

Adverse Reactions

Central nervous system: Hypotonia, fever, dementia
Dermatologic: Urticaria, erythema multiforme
Gastrointestinal: Vomiting, diarrhea
Hematologic: Hemolytic anemia, thrombocytopenia
Hepatic: Hepatitis
Neuromuscular & skeletal: Arthralgia
Ocular: Nystagmus, eye irritant on direct contact, cataract, lacrimation
Respiratory: Bronchospasm, cough, rhinorrhea

Signs & Symptoms of Acute Overdose Nausea, ataxia, coma, seizures, lethargy, confusion, myoclonus, headache, vertigo, tremors, chorea hyporeflexia

Toxicodynamics/Kinetics

Bioavailability: 20% to 40%
Half-life: 2-6 hours
Elimination: Excreted in urine as metabolites and unchanged drug

Usual Dosage Oral (hexahydrate equivalent):

Ascaris lumbricoides:
Children: 75 mg/kg/day for 2 days (maximum daily dose: 3.5 g)
Adults: 3.5 g/day for 2 days

Enterobiasis:
Children: 65 mg/kg in one daily dose for 7 days (maximum daily dose: 2.5 g)
Adults: 65 mg/kg in one daily dose for 7 days (maximum daily dose: 2.5 g)

Tropical eosinophilia: Adults: 600 mg 3 times/day for 2 weeks

Contraindications Epilepsy, hepatic or renal insufficiency

Warnings Use with caution in patients with glucose-6-phosphate dehydrogenase deficiency, malnutrition, anemia, and pregnancy

Dosage Forms

Syrup: 500 mg/5 mL (473 mL, 4000 mL)
Tablet: 250 mg

Overdosage Treatment

Decontamination: Lavage/activated charcoal with cathartic
Supportive therapy: Seizures can be treated with a benzodiazepine, phenytoin, or phenobarbital

Drug Interactions Use with chlorpromazine may result in seizures; antihelmintic effect is decreased with pyrantel

Pregnancy Risk Factor B

Specific References

Conners GP, "Piperazine Neurotoxicity: Worm Wobble Revisited," *J Emerg Med*, 1995, 13(3):341-3.
Leach FN, "Management of Threadworm Infestation During Pregnancy," *Arch Dis Child*, 1990, 65(4):399-400.
Vaidya AB, et al, "Piperazine adipate in tropical eosinophilia," *Indian J Med Sci*, 1971, 25:684.

Pipralen® *see* Piperazine Citrate *on previous page*

Piretanide (peer et' a nide)

CAS Number 55837-27-9

Brand Names Arlix®; Midaten®; Perbilen®; Tauliz®

Synonyms Hoe-118

Use Investigational: Congestive heart failure, hypertension

Mechanism of Action Inhibits reabsorption of sodium and chloride in the ascending loop of Henle and distal renal tubule, interfering with the chloride-binding cotransport system, thus causing increased excretion of water, sodium, chloride, magnesium, and calcium

Adverse Reactions

Cardiovascular: Orthostatic hypotension
Central nervous system: Dizziness, headache
Dermatologic: Eczema, psoriasis, pruritus, exanthema
Endocrine & metabolic: Hyperglycemia, hypokalemia (less than with furosemide or hydrochlorothiazide), hypomagnesemia, hypercholesterolemia, hyperuricemia
Hepatic: Liver toxicity
Neuromuscular & skeletal: Joint pain

Signs & Symptoms of Acute Overdose Muscle cramps, hyperglycemia, hypomagnesemia, hypokalemia, hyperuricemia, hypotension

Toxicodynamics/Kinetics
Onset of diuresis: 30 minutes
Duration:
Oral: 3-4 hours
I.V.: 90 minutes
Distribution: V_d: 0.17-0.53 L/kg (uremic patients)
Protein binding: 94%
Bioavailability: Oral: 80%
Half-life: 1 hour
Elimination: Renal (45%)

Usual Dosage
Congestive heart failure:
Oral: 3-6 mg/day, up to 24 mg/day
I.V.: 6-12 mg every 12 hours
Hypertension: 6-12 mg/day
Renal failure: 6-96 mg/day

Contraindications Hypersensitivity to piretanide, hepatic coma, anuria, hypokalemia, hypovolemia, hyponatremia, hypotension

Warnings Use with caution in patients with diabetes mellitus, gout, liver disease, urinary retention

Reference Range Peak serum level after 12 mg oral dose: 775 ng/mL; peak serum level after 6 mg I.V. dose: 983 ng/mL

Overdosage Treatment
Decontamination: Activated charcoal with cathartic
Supportive therapy: Intravenous hydration with 0.9% saline

Drug Interactions Do not mix with highly acidic solutions of pH <5.5; a precipitate formed when mixed with gentamicin or netilmicin in 5% dextrose or 0.9% sodium chloride, but not with amikacin, kanamycin, or tobramycin; lithium → renal clearance decreased; furosemide interferes with hypoglycemic effect of antidiabetic agents; effects of antihypertensive agents may be enhanced; indomethacin may reduce natriuretic and hypotensive effects of furosemide; concomitant use of furosemide with aminoglycoside antibiotics or other ototoxic drugs should be avoided; NSAIDs ↓ antihypertensive response

Additional Information 6-12 mg of piretanide is equivalent to the antihypertensive effect of 100 mg of hydrochlorothiazide

Specific References
Beermann B and Grind M, "Clinical Pharmacokinetics of Some Newer Diuretics," *Clin Pharmacokinet*, 1987, 13(4):254-66.
Clissold SP and Brogden RN, "Piretanide: A Preliminary Review of Its Pharmacodynamic and Pharmacokinetic Properties and Therapeutic Efficacy," *Drugs*, 1985, 29(6):489-530.
Wells TG, "The Pharmacology and Therapeutics of Diuretics in the Pediatric Patient," *Pediatr Clin North Am*, 1990, 37(2):463-504.

Piroxicam (peer ox' i kam)

Related Information
Nonsteroidal Anti-Inflammatory Comparison *on page 1655*
Therapeutic Drugs Associated With Hallucinations *on page 1558-1559*

CAS Number 36322-90-4

Brand Names Feldene®

Use Management of inflammatory disorders; symptomatic treatment of acute and chronic rheumatoid arthritis, osteoarthritis, and ankylosing spondylitis

Mechanism of Action Inhibits prostaglandin synthesis by decreasing the activity of the enzyme, cyclo-oxygenase, which results in decreased formation of prostaglandin precursors

Adverse Reactions
Cardiovascular: Fluid retention, circulatory collapse
Central nervous system: Headache, aseptic meningitis, psychosis, cognitive dysfunction, dizziness, coma, seizures
Dermatologic: Rash, pruritus, photosensitivity/phototoxicity
Endocrine & metabolic: Hyperkalemia, anion gap metabolic acidosis
Gastrointestinal: Abdominal pain, nausea, vomiting, bleeding, ulceration, constipation, diarrhea, dyspepsia
Genitourinary: Albuminuria
Hematologic: Leukopenia, neutropenia, agranulocytosis, granulocytopenia; aplastic anemia (rare), platelet inhibition
Hepatic: Elevation of transaminases, fulminant hepatitis
Otic: Ototoxicity, tinnitus
Renal: Renal failure (acute), nephrotic syndrome, chronic renal failure
Respiratory: Wheezing, respiratory depression
Miscellaneous: Hypersensitivity

Signs & Symptoms of Acute Overdose Nausea, cognitive dysfunction, wheezing, toxic epidermal necrolysis, photosensitivity, pemphigus, nephrotic syndrome, hyponatremia, stomatitis, gastrointestinal bleeding, vomiting, gastritis; syndrome

(Continued)

Piroxicam *(Continued)*

of inappropriate antidiuretic hormone (SIADH), coagulopathy, ototoxicity; tinnitus, drowsiness; severe poisoning can manifest with coma, seizures, renal and or hepatic failure, hypotension, respiratory depression, blurred vision, tremors

Toxicodynamics/Kinetics

Onset of action: Within 1 hour

Duration: 24 hours

Absorption: Oral: Well absorbed from gastrointestinal tract; food delays absorption

Distribution: V_d: 0.12-0.14 L/kg

Protein binding: 98%

Metabolism: In the liver

Half-life: 30-86 hours

Time to peak serum concentration:
- Oral: 3-5 hours
- Rectal: 10 hours

Elimination: Excreted as unchanged drug (5%) and metabolites primarily in urine and in feces (33%)

Usual Dosage Oral:

Children: 0.2-0.3 mg/kg/day once daily; maximum dose: 15 mg/day

Adults: 10-20 mg/day once daily; although associated with increase in gastrointestinal adverse effects, doses >20 mg/day have been used (ie, 30-40 mg/day)

Dosing adjustment in hepatic impairment: Reduction of dosage is necessary

Contraindications Hypersensitivity to piroxicam, any component, aspirin or other nonsteroidal anti-inflammatory drugs (NSAIDs); active gastrointestinal bleeding

Warnings Use with caution in patients with impaired cardiac function, hypertension, impaired renal function, gastrointestinal disease and patients receiving anticoagulants, porphyria

Dosage Forms Capsule: 10 mg, 20 mg

Overdosage Treatment

Decontamination: Ipecac or lavage/activated charcoal with cathartic

Supportive therapy: Hypotension/dehydration can be managed with intravenous fluid therapy; acidosis should be treated with bicarbonates, seizures with benzodiazepines; antacids, blood products are indicated, as appropriate, for hemorrhage

Enhancement of elimination: Dialysis or perfusion is indicated for secondary complications, acidosis, or renal failure and not toxin removal alone; multiple dosing of activated charcoal may be effective

Test Interactions Increases chloride (S) sodium (S) bleeding time

Drug Interactions Aspirin decreases serum concentrations probably by protein-binding displacement; there is an increased bleeding potential with concomitant warfarin therapy; may increase lithium and methotrexate concentrations by decreasing renal clearance; may decrease diuretic and hypotensive effects of thiazides, loop diuretics, ACE inhibitors, and beta-blockers; may increase nephrotoxicity of cyclosporine

Pregnancy Risk Factor B (D if used in the 3rd trimester or near delivery)

Monitoring Parameters Occult blood loss, hemoglobin, hematocrit, and periodic renal and hepatic function tests; periodic ophthalmologic exams with chronic use

Nursing Implications Administer with food to decrease gastrointestinal adverse effect

Specific References

Chan TY, "Severe Asthma Attacks Precipitated by NSAIDs," *Ann Pharmacother*, 1995, 29:199.

Court H and Volans GN, "Poisoning After Overdose With Nonsteroidal Anti-inflammatory Drugs," *Adverse Drug React Acute Poisoning Rev*, 1984, 3(1):1-21.

Drouet A, Jean-Pastor MJ, and Valance J, "Visual Hallucinations Induced by Piroxicam," *Presse Med*, 1995, 24:504.

Gerber D, "Adverse Reactions of Piroxicam," *Drug Intell Clin Pharm*, 1987, 21(9):707-10.

Hoppmann RA, Peden JG, and Ober SK, "Central Nervous System Side Effects of Nonsteroidal Anti-inflammatory Drugs. Aseptic Meningitis, Psychosis, and Cognitive Dysfunction," *Arch Intern Med*, 1991, 151(7):1309-13.

Lo GC and Chan JY, "Piroxicam Poisoning," *Br Med J*, 1983, 287(6395):798.

MacDougall LG, Taylor-Smith A, Rothberg AD, et al, "Piroxicam Poisoning in a 2-Year Old Child. A Case Report," *S Afr Med J*, 1984, 66(1):31-3.

Mosvold J, Mellem H, Stave R, et al, "Overdosage of Piroxicam," *Acta Med Scand*, 1984, 216(3):335-6.

Smolinske SC, Hall AH, Vandenberg SA, et al, "Toxic Effects of Nonsteroid Anti-inflammatory Drugs in Overdose. An Overview of Recent Evidence on Clinical Effects and Dose-Response Relationships," *Drug Saf*, 1990, 5(4):252-74.

Vale JA and Meredith TJ, "Acute Poisoning Due to Nonsteroidal Anti-inflammatory Drugs," *Med Toxicol*, 1986, 1(1):12-31.

Verbeeck RK, "Pharmacokinetic Drug Interactions With Nonsteroidal Anti-inflammatory Drugs," *Clin Pharmacokinet*, 1990, 19(1):44-66.

p-Isobutylhydratropic Acid *see* Ibuprofen *on page 418*

PK-10169 *see* Enoxaparin Sodium *on page 315*

Placidyl® *see* Ethchlorvynol *on page 330*

Plaquenil® *see* Hydroxychloroquine Sulfate *on page 411*

Plasil® *see* Metoclopramide *on page 523*

Platinol® *see* Cisplatin *on page 218*

Platinol®-AQ *see* Cisplatin *on page 218*

Plato® *see* Dipyridamole *on page 292*

Plendil® *see* Felodipine *on page 343*

Pneumomist® *see* Guaifenesin *on page 390*

Pod-Ben-25® *see* Podophyllum *on this page*

Podocon-25® *see* Podophyllum *on this page*

Podofin® *see* Podophyllum *on this page*

Podophyllum (pode oh fil' um)

CAS Number 568-53-6; 518-29-6; 518-28-5; 8050-60-0

Brand Names Pod-Ben-25®; Podocon-25®; Podofin®

Use Topical treatment of condyloma acuminata (venereal warts); therapeutically dispersed as 25% podophyllum resin in tincture of benzoin or alcohol

Mechanism of Action Arrests cells in the metaphase of mitosis

Signs & Symptoms of Acute Overdose Develop 12-24 hours postexposure but may develop 4-8 hours after ingestion or topical application; hypotonia, nausea, vomiting, hallucinations, diarrhea, hypotension, tachycardia, psychosis, ataxia, fever, hallucinations, anuria may occur; within first week, pancytopenia and hepatic dysfunction may occur which resolves in 2-3 weeks, cardiotoxicity, memory loss, ileus, and coma may last 7-10 days; second week, polyneuropathy may appear and last for 2-3 months; hypotension (orthostatic) may last 6-9 months

Toxicodynamics/Kinetics Absorption: Absorbed well orally and cutaneously

Usual Dosage Apply topically to lesion twice daily for no more than 3 days

Maximum topical exposure: 0.5 mL/day or 10 cm^2

Maximum tolerated dose: 2.8 g

Minimum lethal exposure: Death occurred with 350 mg (topical) or 10 g (oral)

Dosage Forms Commercial preparations consist of 25% podophyllum in either tincture of benzoin or in 10% benzoin and 72% isopropyl alcohol; powdered form also available for compounding

Overdosage Treatment

Decontamination: Emesis or lavage/activated charcoal

Supportive therapy: Thrombocytopenia and leukopenia should be treated as needed; hypotension should be treated with isotonic intravenous fluids, Trendelenburg positioning, and dopamine or norepinephrine drips

Enhancement of elimination: Resin/charcoal hemoperfusion may facilitate neurologic recovery but should be reserved for those patients who deteriorate despite supportive care; hemodialysis may be helpful for those who develop anuria

Pregnancy Implications May be teratogenic when used orally during first trimester of pregnancy; use is discouraged in pregnancy

Additional Information Podophyllum is a mixture of 16 physiologic compounds: lignins (wood extracts) and flavonols; exists in rhizomes and roots of *Podophyllum peltatum* plant or "May apple" and contains at least 40% podophyllotoxin

Specific References

Campbell AN, "Accidental Poisoning With Podophyllin," *Lancet*, 1980, 1(8161):206-7.

Cassidy DE, Drewry J, and Fanning JP, "Podophyllum Toxicity: A Report of a Fatal Case and a Review of Literature," *J Toxicol Clin Toxicol*, 1982, 19(1):35-44.

Heath A, Mellstrand T, and Ahlmen J, "Treatment of Podophyllin Poisoning With Resin Hemoperfusion," *Hum Toxicol*, 1982, 1(4):373-8.

Holdright DR and Jahangiri M, "Accidental Poisoning With Podophyllin," *Hum Exp Toxicol*, 1990, 9(1):55-6.

Sundharam JA, "Is Podophyllin Safe for Use in Pregnancy?" *Arch Dermatol*, 1989, 125(7):1000-1.

Point-Two® *see* Fluoride *on page 355*

Polocaine® *see* Mepivacaine Hydrochloride *on page 502*

Polycillin® *see* Ampicillin *on page 125*

Polycillin-N® *see* Ampicillin *on page 125*

Polydine® [OTC] *see* Povidone-Iodine *on page 635*

Polymox® *see* Amoxicillin *on page 121*

Pondimin® *see* Fenfluramine *on page 345*

Ponstel® *see* Mefenamic Acid *on page 496*

Pontocaine® *see* Tetracaine Hydrochloride *on page 731*

Pork NPH Iletin® II *see* Insulin Preparations *on page 426*

Pork Regular Iletin® II *see* Insulin Preparations *on page 426*

Potasalan® *see* Potassium Chloride *on this page*

Potassium Chloride

CAS Number 7447-40-7

Brand Names Cena-K®; Gen-K®; K+8®; Kaochlor® S-F; Kaon-CL®; Kato®; K-Dur®; K-Lor™; Klor-con®; Klorvess®; Klotrix®; K-Lyte/CL®; K-Tab®; Micro-K®; Potasalan®; Rum-K®; Slow-K®

Use Replacement for potassium loss due to diuretics; treatment of hypokalemia and in metabolic acidosis; may be indicated in digitalis induced arrhythmias

Mechanism of Action As a principle intracellular ion, potassium serves as primary source for cellular electrical conduction

Signs & Symptoms of Acute Overdose Nausea, vomiting, diarrhea, weakness, paresthesia, muscle cramps, hypotension, peaked T waves, P-R prolongation, widened QRS, Q-T interval prolongation, bigeminy, ventricular arrhythmias, apnea, esophageal ulceration, GI bleeding, weakness, confusion, hyporeflexia

Toxicodynamics/Kinetics

Absorption: Well absorbed in small intestine

Half-life: 16 seconds

Elimination: Primarily renal (85%), feces (15%); daily losses: 10 mEq in feces, 7.5 mEq/L in sweat, 60-90 mEq in urine

Usual Dosage

Neonates: Oral, I.V.: 1-2 mEq/kg/day

Infants and older Children: 0.3 mEq/kg/hour

Adults:

I.V.: 10-15 mEq/hour, not to exceed 300 mEq/day if serum potassium is >2.5 mEq/L; at serum potassium levels <2.0 mEq/L, intravenous dose may be at a rate of 40 mEq/hour not to exceed 400 mEq/day

Oral: Replacement therapy due to diuretics: Usual: 60 mEq/day is sufficient, although doses up to 100 mEq/day may be required

Dosing adjustment in renal impairment: Reduce dose and use with caution

Contraindications Renal insufficiency, heat cramps, acute dehydration, Addison's disease

Warnings Use with caution in patients taking potassium-sparing diuretics, sickle cell disease

Dosage Forms

Capsule, controlled release, micro encapsulated (Micro-K®): 600 mg [8 mEq]; 750 mg [10 mEq]

Injection: 1.5 mEq/mL, 2 mEq/mL, 3 mEq/mL

Liquid, oral: 10 mEq/15 mL, 15 mEq/15 mL, 20 mEq/15 mL, 30 mEq/15 mL, 40 mEq/15 mL, 45 mEq/15 mL

Powder, oral: 15 mEq, 20 mEq, 25 mEq packet

Tablet:

Effervescent, as potassium chloride: 25 mEq

Effervescent, as potassium bicarbonate: 20 mEq, 25 mEq, 50 mEq

Sustained release, microcrystalloids (K-Dur®): 750 mg [10 mEq]; 1500 mg [20 mEq]

Wax matrix:

Kaon-Cl®: 500 mg [6.7 mEq]

K+8®: 600 mg [8 mEq]

Slow-K®: 600 mg [8 mEq]; 750 mg [10 mEq]

Reference Range Normal serum potassium: 3.5-5 mEq/L; symptoms can occur with serum levels >6.5 mEq/L; levels >8 mEq/L can be fatal

Overdosage Treatment

Decontamination: Ipecac or lavage; activated charcoal does not appear to be useful

Supportive therapy: Intravenous calcium antagonizes adverse cardiac effects, while sodium bicarbonate (1-2 mEq/kg), insulin, and glucose will enhance intracellular shift of potassium; sodium polystyrene sulfonate (adult dose: 15 g orally or 30-50 g as an enema, pediatric dose: 1 g/kg) will exchange potassium for sodium; hyaluronidase can be used for extravasation; inhalation beta-agonist agents (albuterol, salbutamol) can also result in rapid intravascular movement of potassium

Enhancement of elimination: Dialysis (hemodialysis or peritoneal dialysis) is useful in enhancing elimination

Antidote(s)

Hyaluronidase *on page 1432*

Sodium Bicarbonate *on page 1467*

Sodium Polystyrene Sulfonate *on page 1469*

Test Interactions Hyperkalemia may cause depression of serum sodium

Drug Interactions Use with potassium-sparing diuretics, ACE inhibitors, or indomethacin can result in hyperkalemia; may potentiate hypoglycemic effects of diazoxide; incompatible with intravenous solutions of amikacin, amphotericin B, diazepam, dobutamine, ergotamine, methylprednisolone, nitroprusside, penicillin G, phenytoin, promethazine

Pregnancy Risk Factor A

Pregnancy Implications High levels are detrimental to fetal cardiac function

Monitoring Parameters EKG, renal function, electrolytes

Additional Information Alkalosis decreases serum potassium levels, acidosis elevates serum potassium levels; do not chew or crush tablets; salt substitutes contain from 50-70 mEq potassium per teaspoon; safe for use during breast feeding; usually not irritating to the eye. Found in foods like cantaloupe, bananas, citrus fruits; potassium chloride is 13.3 mEq/g of salts (524 mg or 13.4 mmol); average daily intake of potassium by adults is 2.8-3.9 g (70-100 mEq); radiopaque; toxic oral dose with normal renal function: ~2 mEq/kg; lethal I.V. bolus dose: 0.75-0.9 mEq/kg; liquid preparations should be used as opposed to solid forms in patients with esophageal compression due to left atrial enlargement or bowel hypomotility; total body potassium content is ~3500 mEq in an adult male with 50 mEq being in extracellular fluid compartment.

Specific References

Chaturvedi AK, Rao NG, and Moon MD, "Poisoning Associated With Potassium," *Hum Toxicol*, 1986, 5(6):377-80.

Illingworth RN and Proudfoot AT, "Rapid Poisoning With Slow-Release Potassium," *Br Med J*, 1980, 281:485-6.

Saxena K, "Clinical Features and Management of Poisoning Due to Potassium Chloride," *Med Toxicol Adverse Drug Exp*, 1989, 4(6):429-43.

Potato Alcohol *see* Ethyl Alcohol *on page 336*

Potensan® *see* Yohimbine Hydrochloride *on page 805*

Povidone-Iodine (poe' vi done)

CAS Number 25655-41-8

Brand Names ACU-dyne® [OTC]; Aerodine® [OTC]; Betadine® [OTC]; Betagan® [OTC]; Disadine®; Efodine® [OTC]; Iodex® Regular; Isodine® [OTC]; Mallisol® [OTC]; Operand® [OTC]; Polydine® [OTC]; Videne®

Synonyms PVP-iodine

Use External antiseptic with broad microbicidal spectrum against bacteria, fungi, viruses, protozoa, and yeasts

Mechanism of Action Povidone-iodine is known to be a powerful broad spectrum germicidal agent effective against a wide range of bacteria, viruses, fungi, protozoa, and spores. It is an iodophor of which the polyvinylpyrrolidone is a solubilizing agent which liberates free iodine

Adverse Reactions

Central nervous system: Fever, headache

Dermatologic: Skin rash, angioedema, rash, acne, contact dermatitis, erythema

Endocrine & metabolic: Hypothyroidism

Gastrointestinal: Mucosal hemorrhage, diarrhea, metallic taste, elevated serum transaminases and bilirubin

Hematologic: Eosinophilia

Neuromuscular & skeletal: Arthralgia

Ocular: Swelling of eyelids

Respiratory: Pulmonary edema

Miscellaneous: Lymph node enlargement

Signs & Symptoms of Acute Overdose Gastroenteritis, circulation collapse, swelling of glottis or larynx; renal failure (acute), metabolic acidosis with increased lactic acid, hypernatremia, elevated serum osmolarity, hypothyroidism, leukopenia; neutropenia; agranulocytosis; granulocytopenia

Toxicodynamics/Kinetics Absorption: In normal individuals, topical application results in very little systemic absorption; with vaginal administration, however, absorption is rapid and serum concentrations of total iodine and inorganic iodide are increased significantly

Usual Dosage

Shampoo: Apply 2 tsp to hair and scalp, lather and rinse; repeat application 2 times/week until improvement is noted, then shampoo weekly

Topical: Apply as needed for treatment and prevention of susceptible microbicidal infections

Contraindications Hypersensitivity to iodine

Warnings Highly toxic if ingested; sodium thiosulfate is the most effective chemical antidote; avoid contact with eyes

Dosage Forms

Aerosol: 5% (90 mL)

Cleanser, topical: 7.5% (30 mL, 120 mL)

(Continued)

Povidone-Iodine *(Continued)*

Concentrate:
- Whirlpool: 10% (3840 mL)
- Perineal wash: 10% (240 mL)

Douche: 10% (0.5 oz/packet 240 mL)
Foam, topical: 10% (250 g)
Gel, vaginal: 10% (3 oz)
Mouthwash: 0.5% (180 mL)
Ointment, topical: 10% (0.9 g foil packet, 0.94 g, 28 g, 480 g)
Pads, antiseptic gauze: 10% (3" x 9", 5" x 9")
Scrub, surgical: 7.5% (480 mL, 946 mL)
Shampoo: 7.5% (120 mL)
Solution:
- Swab aid: 10% (100s)
- Swabsticks, 4": 10%
- Topical: 10% (240 mL, 480 mL, 946 mL)

Suppository, vaginal: 10%

Reference Range RDA in adults is 150 mg

Overdosage Treatment

Decontamination: Do not use ipecac; activated charcoal with cathartic is useful; gastric lavage with starch will aid in removal (purple color of effluent)

Enhancement of elimination: Can be enhanced with osmotic diuresis or salt loading

Test Interactions Interferes with thyroid function tests; falsely elevated chloride concentrations

Pregnancy Risk Factor D (can cause fetal goiter and hypothyroidism)

Monitoring Parameters Renal function, acid base status, electrolytes, CBC

Patient Information Do not swallow, avoid contact with eyes

Additional Information Antiseptic action is reduced by alkali solutions

Specific References

Apt L, Isenberg SJ, Yoshimori R, et al, "The Effect of Povidine-Iodine Solution at the Conclusion of Ophthalmic Surgery," *Am J Ophthalmol*, 1995, 119(6):701-5.

Dela Cruz F, Brown DH, Leikin JB, et al, "Iodine Absorption After Topical Administration," *West J Med*, 1987, 146(1):43-5.

Klein I and Levey GS, "Iodide Excess and Thyroid Function," *Ann Intern Med*, 1983, 98(3):406-7.

PPA *see* Phenylpropanolamine Hydrochloride *on page 622*

Prairie Gold® *see* Vitamin E *on page 798*

Pramace® *see* Ramipril *on page 673*

Pramin® *see* Metoclopramide *on page 523*

Pramocaine *see* Pramoxine Hydrochloride *on this page*

Pramoxine Hydrochloride (pra mox' een)

CAS Number 140-65-8; 637-58-1

Brand Names Fleet® Relief; Prax® [OTC]; Proctofoam® [OTC]; Tronolane® [OTC]; Tronothane® [OTC]

Synonyms Pramocaine

Use Temporary relief of pain and itching associated with anogenital pruritus or irritation; dermatosis, minor burns, or hemorrhoids

Mechanism of Action Pramoxine, like other anesthetics, decreases the neuronal membrane's permeability to sodium ions. Both initiation and conduction of nerve impulses are blocked, thus depolarization of the neuron is inhibited.

Adverse Reactions

Cardiovascular: Edema
Dermatologic: Urticaria, rash, contact eczema
Local: Burning, stinging

Signs & Symptoms of Acute Overdose Convulsions, respiratory failure, myoclonus, tremors, slurred speech, agitation, coma, bradycardia, hypotension, cardiovascular collapse, euphoria, ototoxicity; tinnitus, methemoglobinemia may occur

Toxicodynamics/Kinetics

Onset of action: Within 2-5 minutes
Duration: May last for several days

Usual Dosage Adults: Topical: Apply as directed, usually every 3-4 hours to affected area (maximum adult dose: 200 mg)

Contraindications Use in eyes or near nose, application over large areas, known hypersensitivity to pramoxine

Dosage Forms

Aerosol foam: 1% in an anesthetic mucoadhesive foam base (15 g)
Cream: 0.5% (60 g); 1% (28.4 g, 113.4 g, 454 g)
Gel: 1% (37.5 g)

Liquid: 1% (118 mL)
Lotion: 1% (15 mL, 120 mL, 240 mL)

Overdosage Treatment
Decontamination: Lavage/activated charcoal with cathartic
Supportive therapy: Seizures can be treated with diazepam, lorazepam, phenobarbital, or phenytoin; allergic reactions can be treated with epinephrine, diphenhydramine, and corticosteroids

Pregnancy Risk Factor C

Patient Information Discontinue if rash appears or if condition worsens or does not improve in 3-4 days

Nursing Implications Apply sparingly, use the minimal effective dose

Additional Information Less sensitization than benzocaine

Specific References

Fisher AA, "Allergic Reactions to Topical (Surface) Anesthetics With Reference to the Safety of Tronothane® (Pramoxine Hydrochloride)," *Cutis*, 1980, 25(6):584, 586, 589-91.
Van Ketel WG, "Allergy to Pramoxine (Pramocaine)," *Contact Dermatitis*, 1981, 7(1):49.

Prax® [OTC] *see* Pramoxine Hydrochloride *on previous page*

Prazepam (pra' ze pam)

CAS Number 2955-38-6

Brand Names Centrax®; Demetrin®; Lysanxia®; Trepidan®

Use Treatment of anxiety and management of alcohol withdrawal; may also be used as an anticonvulsant in management of simple partial seizures

Mechanism of Action Benzodiazepine anxiolytic sedative that produces CNS depression at the subcortical level, except at high doses, whereby it works at the cortical level

Adverse Reactions
Cardiovascular: Cardiac arrest, hypotension, bradycardia, cardiovascular collapse
Central nervous system: Drowsiness, confusion, dizziness, amnesia, slurred speech, paradoxical excitation or rage, delirium, persecutory delusions, ataxia
Local: Phlebitis, pain with injection
Neuromuscular & skeletal: Orofacial dyskinesia
Ocular: Blurred vision, nystagmus, diplopia
Respiratory: Respiratory rate (decreased), apnea, laryngospasm
Miscellaneous: Physical and psychological dependence with prolonged use

Signs & Symptoms of Acute Overdose Confusion, hypoactive reflexes, hyporeflexia, dry mouth, rhabdomyolysis, acute myoglobinuria, lightheadedness, visual and auditory hallucinations, dyspnea, labored breathing, "alpha" coma (alpha frequency rhythm on EEG), ataxia

Toxicodynamics/Kinetics Studies have shown that the elderly are more sensitive to the effects of benzodiazepines as compared to younger adults
Onset of action: Peak actions occur within 6 hours
Duration: 48 hours
Absorption: Readily from gastrointestinal tract
Distribution: V_d: 9.3-19.5 L/kg; distributed widely distributed throughout body
Protein binding: 85% to 97%
Metabolism: First-pass hepatic metabolism, primarily desmethyldiazepam (active)
Half-life:
- Parent: 78 minutes
- Desmethyldiazepam: 30-100 hours
- Half-life of desmethyldiazepam is significantly prolonged in elderly men (127.8 hours) as compared to young men (61.8 hours) and older women (75.4 hours); V_d is increased in the elderly

Time to peak serum concentration: Oral single dose: 2.5-6 hours
Elimination: Renal and feces (71%)

Usual Dosage Adults: Oral: 30 mg/day in divided doses, may increase gradually to a maximum of 60 mg/day

Contraindications Hypersensitivity to prazepam or any component, cross-sensitivity with other benzodiazepines may exist; avoid using in patients with pre-existing CNS depression, severe uncontrolled pain, or narrow-angle glaucoma

Warnings May cause drug dependency; avoid abrupt discontinuance in patients with prolonged therapy or seizure disorders; not considered a drug of choice in the elderly; safety and efficacy in children <18 years of age have not been established

Dosage Forms
Capsule: 5 mg, 10 mg, 20 mg
Tablet: 5 mg, 10 mg

Reference Range Therapeutic: 50-240 ng/mL (SI: 156-746 nmol/L)

Overdosage Treatment
Decontamination: Lavage/activated charcoal with cathartic
Supportive therapy: Treatment for benzodiazepine overdose is supportive; rarely is mechanical ventilation required. Flumazenil (Romazicon™) has been shown to

(Continued)

Prazepam *(Continued)*

selectively block the binding of benzodiazepines to CNS receptors, resulting in a reversal of benzodiazepine-induced CNS depression. Do not use in concomitant tricyclic ingestion; treat hypotension with isotonic crystalloids, place in Trendelenburg position or give dopamine or norepinephrine.

Enhancement of elimination: Multiple dose of activated charcoal may enhance elimination

Antidote(s)

Flumazenil *on page 1428*

Test Interactions May increase the results of liver function tests; Visine®, Drano®, and bleach can cause false-negative urine tests

Drug Interactions CNS depressants, disulfiram, cimetidine, levodopa, anticonvulsants, digoxin

Pregnancy Risk Factor X

Pregnancy Implications Suggested to be teratogenic in animal and human data; can precipitate neonatal respiratory depression when given during delivery; crosses placenta; appears in breast milk

Monitoring Parameters Respiratory and cardiovascular status

Patient Information May cause drowsiness, use caution when driving; avoid alcohol and drugs with CNS depressant effects

Nursing Implications Monitor for alertness

Additional Information Prazepam offers no significant advantage over other benzodiazepines

Specific References

Skielboe M, Anderson PM, Weber M, et al, "Reversal of Benzodiazepine Intoxication by Flumazenil," *Resuscitation*, 1991, 22:245-52.

Prazosin Hydrochloride (pra' zoe sin)

CAS Number 19216-56-9; 19237-84-4

Brand Names Hypovase®; Minipress®

Synonyms Furazosin

Use Hypertension, severe congestive heart failure (in conjunction with diuretics and cardiac glycosides)

Mechanism of Action Competitively inhibits postsynaptic alpha-adrenergic receptors which results in vasodilation of veins and arterioles and a decrease in total peripheral resistance and blood pressure; effective for ergotism-induced hypertension

Adverse Reactions

Cardiovascular: Orthostatic hypotension, syncope, palpitation, tachycardia, edema

Central nervous system: Dizziness, lightheadedness, night terrors, drowsiness, psychosis, asthenia, headache, hypothermia

Dermatologic: Rash, angioneurotic edema

Endocrine & metabolic: Fluid retention

Gastrointestinal: Nausea, dry mouth, fecal incontinence

Genitourinary: Urinary frequency, priapism, urinary incontinence, sexual dysfunction

Respiratory: Nasal congestion

Miscellaneous: Positive ANA

Signs & Symptoms of Acute Overdose Hypotension, drowsiness, bone marrow depression, enuresis, night terrors, impotence, syncope, ptosis, hypothermia, conjunctivitis, systemic lupus erythematosus (SLE), respiratory depression

Toxicodynamics/Kinetics

Onset of action: Hypotensive effect: Within 2 hours; Maximum decrease: 2-4 hours

Duration: 10-24 hours

Absorption: Well from gastrointestinal tract

Distribution: V_d: 0.5 L/kg (hypertensive adults); distributed widely to body tissues

Protein binding: 92% to 97%

Metabolism: Extensive in the liver

Bioavailability: Oral: 43% to 82%

Half-life: 2-4 hours; increased half-life with congestive heart failure

Time to peak serum concentration: 1-3 hours

Elimination: 6% to 10% excreted renally as unchanged drug; metabolites may be active; mainly in bile and feces

Usual Dosage Oral:

Children: Initial: 5 mcg/kg/dose (to assess hypotensive effects); usual dosing interval: every 6 hours; increase dosage gradually up to maximum of 25 mcg/kg/dose every 6 hours

Adults: Initial: 1 mg/dose 2-3 times/day; usual maintenance dose: 3-15 mg/day in divided doses 2-4 times/day; maximum daily dose: 20 mg

Contraindications Hypersensitivity to prazosin or any component

Warnings Can cause marked hypotension and syncope with sudden loss of consciousness with the first few doses. Anticipate a similar effect if therapy is interrupted for a few days, if dosage is increased rapidly, or if another antihypertensive drug is introduced.

Dosage Forms Capsule: 1 mg, 2 mg, 5 mg

Stability Store in airtight container; protect from light

Reference Range Plasma level of 47.6 ng/mL was noted in an overdose setting 11 hours after a 120 mg ingestion

Overdosage Treatment

Decontamination: Ipecac or lavage/activated charcoal with cathartic

Supportive therapy: Hypotension usually responds to I.V. fluids or Trendelenburg positioning. If unresponsive to these measures, the use of a parenteral vasoconstrictor may be required (eg, norepinephrine 0.1-0.2 mcg/kg/minute titrated to response). Treatment is primarily supportive and symptomatic.

Enhancement of elimination: Multiple dosing of activated charcoal may be effective

Antidote(s)

Norepinephrine Bitartrate *on page 1451*

Drug Interactions Diuretics and antihypertensive medications (especially beta-blockers) may increase prazosin's hypotensive effect

Pregnancy Risk Factor C

Monitoring Parameters Blood pressure, standing and sitting/supine

Patient Information Rise from sitting/lying carefully, may cause vertigo; take first dose at bedtime

Nursing Implications Syncope may occur usually within 90 minutes of the initial dose

Specific References

Lenz K, Druml W, Kleinberger G, et al, "Acute Intoxication With Prazosin: Case Report," *Hum Toxicol*, 1985, 4(1):53-6.

McClean WJ, "Prazosin Overdose," *Med J Aust*, 1976, 1(16):592.

Rygnestad TK and Dale O, "Self-Poisoning With Prazosin," *Acta Med Scand*, 1983, 213(2):157-8.

Vincent J, Meredith PA, Reid JL, et al, "Clinical Pharmacokinetics of Prazosin -- 1985," *Clin Pharmacokinet*, 1985, 10(2):144-54.

Prednicen-M® *see* Prednisone *on this page*

Prednisone (pred' ni sone)

CAS Number 53-03-1

Brand Names Cortancyl®; Deltasone®; Liquid Pred®; Meticorten®; Orasone®; Prednicen-M®; Sterapred®

Synonyms Deltacortisone; Deltadehydrocortisone

Use Treatment of a variety of diseases including adrenocortical insufficiency, hypercalcemia, rheumatic and collagen disorders; dermatologic, ocular, respiratory, gastrointestinal, and neoplastic diseases; organ transplantation and a variety of diseases including those of hematologic, allergic, inflammatory, and autoimmune in origin; not available in injectable form, prednisolone must be used

Mechanism of Action Decreases inflammation by suppression of migration of polymorphonuclear leukocytes and reversal of increased capillary permeability; suppresses the immune system by reducing activity and volume of the lymphatic system; suppresses adrenal function at high doses

Adverse Reactions

Cardiovascular: Edema, hypertension

Central nervous system: Dizziness, seizures, psychoses, pseudotumor cerebri, headache

Dermatologic: Acne, purpura, skin atrophy, angioedema

Endocrine & metabolic: Cushing's syndrome, pituitary-adrenal axis suppression, amenorrhea, growth suppression, glucose intolerance, hypokalemia, alkalosis

Gastrointestinal: Peptic ulcer, nausea, vomiting

Neuromuscular & skeletal: Muscle asthenia, osteoporosis, fractures

Ocular: Cataracts, glaucoma

Miscellaneous: Feces discoloration (black)

Signs & Symptoms of Acute Overdose Primarily neuropsychiatric, dementia, depression, hypokalemia, hyperuricemia, hyperglycemia, sexual dysfunction, lymphopenia, leukocytosis, intraocular pressure (increased), dementia, memory loss, thrombocytopenia, hirsutism, hypertrichosis, eosinopenia, gastrointestinal bleeding, mania, cognitive dysfunction

Toxicodynamics/Kinetics

Absorption: Oral: 78%

Distribution: V_d: 0.97 L/kg

Metabolism: Converted rapidly to prednisolone (active)

Elimination: Renal, 3.6 mL/min/kg

Usual Dosage Dose depends upon condition being treated and response of patient; dosage for infants and children should be based on severity of the disease and response of the patient rather than on strict adherence to dosage indicated

(Continued)

Prednisone *(Continued)*

by age, weight, or body surface area. Consider alternate day therapy for long-term therapy. Discontinuation of long-term therapy requires gradual withdrawal by tapering the dose.

Children: Oral:

- Anti-inflammatory or immunosuppressive dose: 0.05-2 mg/kg/day divided 1-4 times/day
- Acute asthma: 1-2 mg/kg/day in divided doses 1-2 times/day for 3-5 days
  - Alternatively (for 3- to 5-day "burst"):
  - <1 year: 10 mg every 12 hours
  - 1-4 years: 20 mg every 12 hours
  - 5-13 years: 30 mg every 12 hours
  - >13 years: 40 mg every 12 hours
- Asthma long-term therapy (alternative dosing by age):
  - <1 year: 10 mg every other day
  - 1-4 years: 20 mg every other day
  - 5-13 years: 30 mg every other day
  - >13 years: 40 mg every other day
- Severe refractory asthma: 5-10 mg/dose every day or 10-30 mg every other day
- Nephrotic syndrome: Initial: 2 mg/kg/day (maximum: 80 mg/day) in divided doses 3-4 times/day until urine is protein free for 5 days (maximum: 28 days); if albuminuria persists, use 4 mg/kg/dose every other day (maximum: 120 mg/day) for an additional 28 days; maintenance: 2 mg/kg/dose (maximum: 80 mg/dose) every other day for 28 days; then taper over 4-6 weeks

Children and Adults: Physiologic replacement: 4-5 mg/m^2/day

Adults: 5-60 mg/day in divided doses 1-4 times/day

Elderly: Use the lowest effective dose

Contraindications Serious infections, except septic shock or tuberculous meningitis; systemic fungal infections; hypersensitivity to prednisone or any component; varicella

Warnings Use with caution in patients with hypothyroidism, cirrhosis, hypertension, congestive heart failure, ulcerative colitis, thromboembolic disorders, and patients with an increased risk for peptic ulcer disease; gradually taper dose to withdraw therapy; may retard bone growth. Because of the risk of adverse effects, systemic corticosteroids should be used cautiously in the elderly, in the smallest possible dose, and for the shortest possible time.

Dosage Forms

Solution:

- Concentrate: 5 mg/mL (5 mL, 30 mL)
- Oral: 5 mg/5 mL (10 mL, 20 mL, 500 mL)

Syrup: 5 mg/5 mL (120 mL, 240 mL)

Tablet: 1 mg, 2.5 mg, 5 mg, 10 mg, 20 mg, 50 mg

Overdosage Treatment Decontamination: Emesis or lavage/activated charcoal with cathartic; acute overdose does not require tapering of dose

Test Interactions Skin tests

Drug Interactions Decreased effect: Barbiturates, phenytoin, rifampin ↓ corticosteroid effectiveness; ↓ salicylates, ↓ vaccines, ↓ toxoids effectiveness

Pregnancy Risk Factor B

Monitoring Parameters Blood pressure, blood glucose, electrolytes

Patient Information Notify surgeon or dentist before surgical repair; may cause gastritis; take with food; notify physician if any sign of infection occurs; avoid abrupt withdrawal when on long-term therapy

Nursing Implications Give with meals to decrease gastritis; withdraw therapy with gradual tapering of dose

Specific References

Boot Am, Nauta J, Hokken-Koelega AC, et al, "Renal Transplantation and Osteoporosis," *Arch Dis Child*, 1995, 72:502-6.

Frey BM and Frey FJ, "Clinical Pharmacokinetics of Prednisone and Prednisolone," *Clin Pharmacokinet*, 1990, 19(2):126-46.

Grotz WH, Mundinger FA, Gugel B, et al, "Bone Mineral Density After Kidney Transplantation: A Cross-Sectional Study in 190-Graft Recipients Up to 20 Years After Transplantation," *Transplantation*, 1995, 59:982-6.

Wolkowitz OM, "Long-Lasting Behavioral Changes Following Prednisone Withdrawal," *JAMA*, 1989, 261(12):1731-2.

Prelis® *see* Metoprolol Tartrate *on page 524*

Premarin® Injection *see* Estrogens, Conjugated *on page 325*

Premarin® Oral *see* Estrogens, Conjugated *on page 325*

Premarin® Vaginal *see* Estrogens, Conjugated *on page 325*

Prent® *see* Acebutolol Hydrochloride *on page 77*

Pre-Par® *see* Ritodrine Hydrochloride *on page 687*

Prepulsid® *see* Cisapride *on page 217*

Pres® *see* Enalapril *on page 311*

Presamine® *see* Imipramine *on page 422*

Presomen® *see* Estrogens, Conjugated *on page 325*

Pretz® [OTC] *see* Sodium Chloride *on page 698*

Prevacid® *see* Lansoprazole *on page 460*

Prevident® *see* Fluoride *on page 355*

Prilagin® *see* Miconazole *on page 530*

Prilosec™ *see* Omeprazole *on page 576*

Primaclone *see* Primidone *on this page*

Primavit® *see* Vitamin A *on page 795*

Primaxin® *see* Imipenem/Cilastatin *on page 420*

Primidone (pri' mi done)

Related Information

Seizures, Neonatal Guidelines *on page 1604-1605*

Therapeutic Drugs Associated With Hallucinations *on page 1558-1559*

CAS Number 125-33-7

Brand Names Mysoline®

Synonyms Desoxyphenobarbital; Hexamidinum; Primaclone

Use Prophylactic management of partial seizures with complex symptomatology (psychomotor seizures), generalized tonic-clonic, and akinetic seizure

Mechanism of Action Decreases neuron excitability, raises seizure threshold similar to phenobarbital

Adverse Reactions

Central nervous system: Drowsiness, dizziness, drowsiness, behavior change, psychosis, irritability, headache, asthenia, visual hallucinations, ataxia

Dermatologic: Rash

Gastrointestinal: Nausea, vomiting

Hematologic: Leukopenia, malignant lymphoma-like syndrome, anemia (megaloblastic), thrombocytopenia

Hepatic: Systemic lupus-like syndrome

Ocular: Diplopia, nystagmus, strabismus

Signs & Symptoms of Acute Overdose Unsteady gait, slurred speech, confusion, severe flapping tremors, loss of deep tendon reflexes, hypothyroidism, dementia, jaundice, hypothermia, fever, hypotension, ptosis, crystalluria (white, hexagonal crystals), ankle clonus, nystagmus, leukopenia; neutropenia; vision color changes (green tinge); agranulocytosis; granulocytopenia; systemic lupus erythematosus (SLE)

Toxicodynamics/Kinetics

Absorption: Rapid; usually complete with wide individual variation

Distribution: V_d: 0.6 L/kg; distributed widely throughout body

Protein binding: 0% to 19%

Metabolism: In the liver to phenobarbital (active) and phenylethylmalonamide (PEMA)

Bioavailability: 90% to 100%

Half-life:

Primidone: 3-24 hours

PEMA: 24-48 hours

Phenobarbital: 72-144 hours (age-dependent)

Time to peak serum concentration: Within 4 hours

Elimination: Urinary excretion of both active metabolites and unchanged primidone (15% to 25%); clearance: 0.78 mL/minute/kg

Usual Dosage Oral:

Neonates: Loading dose: 15-25 mg/kg/dose as a single dose; 12-20 mg/kg/day in divided doses 2-4 times/day; start with lower dosage and titrate upward

Children <8 years: Initial: 50-125 mg/day given at bedtime; increase by 50-125 mg/day increments every 3-7 days; usual dose: 10-25 mg/kg/day in divided doses 3-4 times/day

Children >8 years and Adults: Initial: 125-250 mg/day at bedtime; increase by 125-250 mg/day every 3-7 days; usual dose: 750-1500 mg/day in divided doses 3-4 times/day with maximum dosage of 2 g/day

Dosing interval in renal impairment:

Cl_{cr} 50-80 mL/minute: Administer every 8 hours

Cl_{cr} 10-50 mL/minute: Administer every 8-12 hours

Cl_{cr} <10 mL/minute: Administer every 12-24 hours

Contraindications Hypersensitivity to primidone or any component; porphyria

Warnings Avoid abrupt discontinuation; dosage should be slowly decreased to

(Continued)

Primidone *(Continued)*

avoid precipitation of seizures or status epilepticus; use with caution in patients with renal or hepatic impairment, pulmonary insufficiency

Dosage Forms

Suspension, oral: 250 mg/5 mL (240 mL)
Tablet: 50 mg, 250 mg

Stability Protect from light

Reference Range

Therapeutic:
- Children <5 years: 7-10 μg/mL (SI: 32-46 μmol/L)
- Adults: 5-12 μg/mL (SI: 23-55 μmol/L); toxic effects rarely present with levels <10 μg/mL (SI: <46 μmol/L) if phenobarbital concentrations are low

Dosage of primidone is adjusted with reference mostly to the phenobarbital level

Toxic: >15 μg/mL (SI: >69 μmol/L) associated with ataxia and/or drowsiness

Overdosage Treatment

Decontamination: Gastric lavage is effective even after 6 hours; activated charcoal with cathartic is effective

Supportive therapy: Hypotension: Isotonic intravenous fluid (10-20 mL/kg) is effective along with placement in Trendelenburg position; dopamine (2-5 mg/kg progressing to 5-10 mcg/kg) or norepinephrine (0.1-0.2 mcg/kg/minute for children or 8-12 mcg/kg in adults to a maintenance dose of 2-4 mcg/minute) is effective

Enhancement of elimination: Repeated oral doses of activated charcoal significantly reduce the half-life of primidone resulting from an enhancement of nonrenal elimination. The usual dose is 30-60 g every 4-6 hours for 3-4 days unless the patient has no bowel movement causing the charcoal to remain in the gastrointestinal tract. Assure adequate hydration and renal function. Urinary alkalinization with I.V. sodium bicarbonate also helps to enhance elimination. Hemodialysis is of uncertain value. Patients in stage IV coma due to high serum drug levels may require charcoal hemoperfusion; moderately dialyzable (20% to 50%)

Test Interactions Increases alkaline phosphatase (S); decreases calcium (S)

Diagnostic Tests/Procedures

Primidone, Blood *on page 1332*

Drug Interactions Phenytoin increases conversion of primidone to phenobarbital; valproic acid may increase phenobarbital concentrations derived from primidone; isoniazid may decrease metabolism of primidone; acetazolamide may reduce the absorption of primidone

Pregnancy Risk Factor D

Monitoring Parameters Serum primidone and phenobarbital concentration, CBC, SMA-12, urine analysis

Patient Information May cause drowsiness

Nursing Implications Observe patient for excessive sedation

Additional Information Hepatic metabolism to active products (phenylethylmalonamide and phenobarbital)

Specific References

Lane GP, Lewis CG, and Zail SC, "Macroscopic Crystalluria After Primidone Overdosage," *Med J Aust*, 1987, 147(11-12):624-5.

Schwankhaus JD, Kattah JC, Lux WE, et al, "Primidone/Phenobarbital-Induced Periodic Alternating Nystagmus," *Ann Ophthalmol*, 1989, 21(6):230-2.

Primogyn C® *see* Ethinyl Estradiol *on page 331*

Primperan® *see* Metoclopramide *on page 523*

Principal Pharmacological Properties of Hallucinogenic Drugs *see page 1557*

Principen® *see* Ampicillin *on page 125*

Prinivil® *see* Lisinopril *on page 475*

Prioderm® *see* Malathion (Topical Lotion) *on page 489*

Procainamide Hydrochloride (proe kane a' mide)

Related Information

Therapeutic Drugs Associated With Hallucinations *on page 1558-1559*

CAS Number 614-39-1; 51-06-9

Brand Names Biocoryl®; Novocamid®; Procan® SR; Pronestyl®; Pronestyl-SR®; Retard®; Rhythmin®

Synonyms Novocainamidum; Procaine Amide Hydrochloride

Use Ventricular tachycardia, premature ventricular contractions, paroxysmal atrial tachycardia, and fibrillation (atrial); to prevent recurrence of tachycardia (ventricular), paroxysmal tachycardia (ventricular), fibrillation (atrial) or flutter

Mechanism of Action Decreases myocardial excitability and conduction velocity and depresses myocardial contractility, by increasing the electrical stimulation threshold of ventricle, HIS-Purkinje system and through direct cardiac effects; classified as a Class IA antiarrhythmic agent

Adverse Reactions

Cardiovascular: Pericarditis, hypotension, tachycardia, cardiac arrhythmias, A-V block, Q-T prolongation, QRS prolongation

Central nervous system: Confusion, psychosis, disorientation, fever, visual hallucinations, ataxia

Dermatologic: Rash

Gastrointestinal: Nausea, vomiting, gastrointestinal complaints, diarrhea, dry mouth

Genitourinary: Urinary retention

Hematologic: Agranulocytosis, neutropenia, thrombocytopenia, hemolysis, positive Coombs' test

Hepatic: Granulomatous hepatitis

Neuromuscular & skeletal: Arthralgia, myalgia, myopathy

Ophthalmic: Blurred vision

Respiratory: Pleural effusion

Miscellaneous: Drug-induced systemic lupus erythematosus

Signs & Symptoms of Acute Overdose Hypotension, coagulopathy, QRS prolongation, torsade de pointes, hyperthermia, junctional tachycardia, hemoptysis, A-V block, intraventricular conduction delay, oliguria, myasthenia gravis (exacerbation or precipitation of), mania, drowsiness, confusion, renal failure, respiratory failure, anticholinergic toxidrome, systemic lupus erythematosus (SLE), leukopenia; neutropenia; agranulocytosis; granulocytopenia

Toxicodynamics/Kinetics

Onset of action: I.M.: 10-30 minutes

Absorption: Rapid; complete but may vary

Distribution: Widely in most body tissues, including CSF, liver, spleen, kidneys, lungs, muscles, brain, and heart

V_d:

Children: 2.2 L/kg, decreased V_d with renal failure, congestive heart failure, or shock; NAPA: 1.4 L/kg

Adults: 2 L/kg

Protein binding: 15% to 20%; NAPA: 10%

Metabolism: By acetylation in the liver to produce N-acetyl procainamide (NAPA) (active metabolite) which has been described as a Class III agent

Bioavailability: Oral: 75% to 95%

Half-life:

PCA:

Children: 1.7 hours; dependent upon hepatic acetylator

Adults with normal renal function: 2.5-4.7 hours; 10.4 hours in overdose setting

NAPA:

Children: 6 hours; dependent upon renal function

Adults with normal renal function: 6-8 hours; 35.9 hours in overdose setting

Time to peak serum concentration:

Capsule: Within 45 minutes to $2\frac{1}{2}$ hours

I.M.: 15-60 minutes

Elimination: Urinary excretion (25% as NAPA); renal clearance: 179-660 mL through glomerular filtration and active tubular secretion

Usual Dosage Must be titrated to patient's response

Children:

Oral: 15-50 mg/kg/24 hours divided every 3-6 hours; maximum: 4 g/24 hours

I.M.: 20-30 mg/kg/24 hours divided every 4-6 hours in divided doses; maximum: 4 g/24 hours

I.V.: Load: 3-6 mg/kg/dose over 5 minutes not to exceed 100 mg/dose; may repeat every 5-10 minutes to maximum of 15 mg/kg/load; maintenance as continuous I.V. infusion: 20-80 mcg/kg/minute; maximum: 2 g/24 hours

Adults:

Oral: 250-500 mg/dose every 3-6 hours or 500 mg to 1 g every 6 hours sustained release; usual dose: 50 mg/kg/24 hours; maximum: 4 g/24 hours

I.M.: 0.5-1 g every 4-8 hours until oral therapy is possible

I.V.: Loading dose: 1 g administered as slow infusion over 25-30 minutes or 100-200 mg/dose repeated every 5 minutes as needed to a total dose of 1 g; maintenance dose: 1-6 mg/minute by continuous infusion

Dosing interval in renal impairment:

Cl_{cr} 10-50 mL/minute: Administer every 6-12 hours

Cl_{cr} <10 mL/minute: Administer every 8-24 hours

Contraindications Complete heart block; second or third degree heart block without pacemaker; "torsade de pointes" (twisting of the points) an unusual tachycardia (ventricular); hypersensitivity to the drug or procaine, or related drugs; myasthenia gravis; systemic lupus erythematosus (SLE)

Warnings Long-term administration leads to the development of a positive antinuclear antibody test in 50% of patients which may lead to a lupus erythematosus-like syndrome (in 20% to 30% of patients); assess relative benefits and risks if ANA

(Continued)

Procainamide Hydrochloride *(Continued)*

titer becomes positive and consider alternative agent; discontinue procainamide with systemic lupus erythematosus (SLE) symptoms and change to alternative agent; do not chew or crush sustained-release dosage form, swallow whole; do not use sustained-release preparation for initial therapy; worsening of pre-existing myasthenia gravis; marked A-V conduction disturbances, bundle-branch block or severe cardiac glycoside intoxication, ventricular arrhythmias in patients with organic heart disease or coronary occlusion, supraventricular tachyarrhythmias unless digitalis levels adequate to prevent marked increases in ventricular rates; drug may accumulate in patients with renal or hepatic dysfunction; some tablets contain tartrazine; injection may contain bisulfite

Dosage Forms

Capsule: 250 mg, 375 mg, 500 mg
Injection: 100 mg/mL (10 mL); 500 mg/mL (2 mL)
Tablet: 250 mg, 375 mg, 500 mg
Tablet, sustained release: 250 mg, 500 mg, 750 mg, 1000 mg

Stability Use only clear or slightly yellow solutions; store in airtight containers
Stability of parenteral admixture at room temperature (25°C): 24 hours
Stability of parenteral admixture at refrigeration temperature (4°C): 24 hours

Reference Range Therapeutic: 4-10 μg/mL for procainamide, <16 μg/mL for sum of procainamide and N-acetyl procainamide; NAPA levels: 10-30 μg/mL. Optimal ranges must be ascertained for individual patients, with EKG monitoring.
Toxic (procainamide): >14 μg/mL (SI: >59.5 μmol/L)

Overdosage Treatment

Decontamination: Ipecac or lavage/activated charcoal with cathartic

Supportive therapy: Hypotension usually responds to I.V. fluids or Trendelenburg positioning. If unresponsive to these measures, the use of a parenteral inotrope may be required (eg, norepinephrine 0.1-0.2 mcg/kg/minute titrated to response). Concurrent sodium bicarbonate and sodium lactate infusions have been effective in reversing the drug-induced cardiac toxicity. Avoid quinidine, disopyramide, and beta-adrenergic blockers.

Enhancement of elimination: Multiple dosing of activated charcoal may be effective; hemodialysis or charcoal hemoperfusion are effective in decreasing half-life; NAPA is more effectively removed by hemoperfusion; forced diuresis in peritoneal dialysis is not effective; moderately dialyzable (20% to 50%)

Diagnostic Tests/Procedures

Procainamide, Blood *on page 1332*

Drug Interactions Cimetidine, ranitidine, and amiodarone may increase plasma PCA and NAPA concentrations, PCA dosage adjustment may be required; PCA may potentiate skeletal muscle relaxants and anticholinergic drugs may have enhanced effects

Pregnancy Risk Factor C

Monitoring Parameters EKG, blood pressure, CBC with differential, platelet count

Patient Information Do not discontinue therapy unless instructed by physician; notify physician or pharmacist if soreness of mouth, throat or gums, unexplained fever, symptoms of upper respiratory tract infection. Do not break or chew sustained release tablets. Sustained release tablets contain a wax core that slowly releases the drug. When this process is complete, the empty, nonabsorbable wax core is eliminated.

Nursing Implications Dilute I.V. with D_5W; maximum rate: 25-50 mg/minute

Specific References

Adams LE, Roberts SM, Donovan-Brand R, et al, "Study of Procainamide Hapten-Specific Antibodies in Rabbits and Humans," *Int J Immunopharmacol*, 1993, 15(8):887-97.

Braden GL, Fitzgibbons JP, Germain MJ, et al, "Hemoperfusion for Treatment of N-Acetylprocainamide Intoxication," *Ann Intern Med*, 1986, 105(1):64-5.

Prendergast MD and Nasca TJ, "Anticholinergic Syndrome With Procainamide Toxicity," *JAMA*, 1984, 251(22):2926-7.

Rosansky SJ and Brudy ME, "Procainamide Toxicity in a Patient With Acute Renal Failure," *Am J Kidney Dis*, 1986, 7(6):502-6.

Procaine Amide Hydrochloride *see* Procainamide Hydrochloride *on page 642*

Procaine Hydrochloride (proe' kane)

CAS Number 59-46-1; 51-05-8

Brand Names Anuject®; Lenident®; Novocain®; Novutox®; Venocaina®

Synonyms Allocaine; Ethocaine Hydrochloride

Use Produce spinal anesthesia and epidural and peripheral nerve block by injection and infiltration methods

Mechanism of Action Blocks both the initiation and conduction of nerve impulses by decreasing the neuronal membrane's permeability to sodium ions, which results in inhibition of depolarization with resultant blockade of conduction

Adverse Reactions

Central nervous system: Aseptic meningitis resulting in paralysis can occur, CNS stimulation followed by CNS depression, psychosis, paranoia, hallucinations, chills

Dermatologic: Skin discoloration

Gastrointestinal: Nausea, vomiting

Local: Burning sensation at site of injection, pain, tissue irritation

Ocular: Miosis, nystagmus, diplopia

Otic: Ototoxicity, tinnitus

Signs & Symptoms of Acute Overdose Cardiac arrhythmias, seizures, coma, tachypnea progressing to apnea; tachycardia, hypertension, mydriasis

Toxicodynamics/Kinetics

Onset of action: Within 2-5 minutes

Duration: 30-90 minutes (dependent upon patient, type of block, concentration, and method of anesthesia)

Absorption: Readily following parenteral administration

Distribution: V_d: 0.3-0.8 L/kg

Protein binding: Very low, 5% (primarily by alpha$_1$-acid glycoproteins)

Metabolism: Rapidly hydrolyzed by plasma enzymes to para-aminobenzoic acid and diethylaminoethanol (80% conjugated before elimination)

Half-life: 7.7 minutes

Elimination: In urine as metabolites and some unchanged drug (2%)

Usual Dosage Dose varies with procedure, desired depth, and duration of anesthesia, desired muscle relaxation, vascularity of tissues, physical condition, and age of patient

Contraindications PABA, parabens, cerebrospinal diseases, heart block, hypotension, hypertension, bowel pathology, gastrointestinal hemorrhage, known hypersensitivity to procaine

Warnings Patients with cardiac diseases, hyperthyroidism or other endocrine diseases may be more susceptible to toxic effects of local anesthetics

Dosage Forms Injection: 1% [10 mg/mL] (2 mL, 6 mL, 30 mL, 100 mL); 2% [20 mg/mL] (30 mL, 100 mL); 10% (2 mL)

Reference Range

Therapeutic: 3-11 μg/mL

Toxic: >20 μg/mL are associated with toxicity

Overdosage Treatment

Decontamination: Lavage/activated charcoal with cathartic for oral ingestions

Supportive therapy: Treatment is primarily symptomatic and supportive. Termination of anesthesia by pneumatic tourniquet inflation should be attempted when the agent is administered by infiltration or regional injection. Seizures commonly respond to diazepam or lorazepam, while hypotension responds to I.V. fluids and Trendelenburg positioning. Bradyarrhythmias (when the heart rate is less than 60) can be treated with I.V., I.M., or S.C. atropine 15 mcg/kg. With the development of metabolic acidosis, I.V. sodium bicarbonate 0.5-2 mEq/kg and ventilatory assistance should be instituted. Chlorpromazine may be used to treat acute psychosis.

Enhancement of elimination: Multiple dosing of activated charcoal may be effective

Drug Interactions Aminosalicylic acid, sulfonamides, digitalis, anticholinesterase, and succinylcholine

Pregnancy Risk Factor C

Specific References

Altman RS, Smith-Coggins R, and Ampel LL, "Local Anesthetics," *Ann Emerg Med*, 1985, 14(12):1209-17.

Hart D, "Psychotic Reaction to Procaine," *J Emerg Nurs*, 1984, 10(1):9-10.

Wikinski JA, Usubiaga JE, and Wikinski RW, "Cardiovascular and Neurological Effects of 4000 mg of Procaine," *JAMA*, 1970, 213(4):621-3.

Pro-Cal-Sof® [OTC] *see* Docusate *on page 297*

Procan® SR *see* Procainamide Hydrochloride *on page 642*

Procarbazine Hydrochloride (proe kar' ba zeen)

CAS Number 671-16-9; 366-70-1

Brand Names Matulane®; Natulan®; Natulanar®

Synonyms Ibenzmethyzine; N-methylhydrazine

Use Treatment of Hodgkin's disease, non-Hodgkin's lymphoma, brain tumor, bronchogenic carcinoma

Mechanism of Action Mechanism of action is not clear, methylating of nucleic acids; inhibits DNA, RNA, and protein synthesis; may damage DNA directly and suppress mitosis; metabolic activation required by host

Adverse Reactions

Cardiovascular: Orthostatic hypotension, hypertensive crisis

(Continued)

Procarbazine Hydrochloride *(Continued)*

Central nervous system: Mental depression, manic reactions, coma, hallucinations, psychosis, mania, dizziness, headache, nervousness, insomnia, night terrors, disorientation, foot drop, decreased reflexes, somnolence, confusion, and seizures, hyperpyrexia, irritability, ataxia

Dermatologic: Alopecia, pruritus, dermatitis, alopecia, hypersensitivity rash, hyperpigmentation

Gastrointestinal: Severe nausea and vomiting occur frequently and may be dose-limiting; anorexia, diarrhea, abdominal pain, stomatitis, dysphagia, diarrhea, and constipation; use a nonphenothiazine antiemetic, when possible

Hematologic: May be dose-limiting toxicity; procarbazine should be discontinued if leukocyte count is <4000 mL or platelet count <100,000 mL; leukopenia

Hepatic: Hepatotoxicity, jaundice

Neuromuscular & skeletal: Peripheral neuropathy, arthralgia, myalgia, tremors, paresthesia

Ocular: Nystagmus, diplopia, photophobia

Respiratory: Pleural effusion, cough, interstitial pneumonitis

Miscellaneous: Secondary malignancy, azoospermia, urinary frequency, nocturia, hematuria, hoarseness, flu-like syndrome, amenorrhea

Toxicodynamics/Kinetics

Absorption: Oral: Rapidly and well absorbed

Distribution: Crosses the blood-brain barrier and distributes into CSF

Metabolism: In the liver and kidney to N-isopropyl terephthalanic acid

Half-life: 10 minutes

Elimination: Urine and through respiratory tract (<5% as unchanged drug) and 70% as metabolites

Usual Dosage Oral (refer to individual protocols):

Children: 50-100 mg/m^2/day once daily; doses as high as 100-200 mg/m^2/day once daily have been used for neuroblastoma and medulloblastoma

BMT aplastic anemia conditioning regimen: 12.5 mg/kg/dose every other day for 4 doses

MOPP/C-MOPP regimens: 100 mg/m^2/day for 14 days and repeated every 4 weeks

Adults: Initial: 2-4 mg/kg/day in single or divided doses for 7 days then increase dose to 4-6 mg/kg/day until response is obtained or leukocyte count decreased <4000/mm^3 or the platelet count decreased <100,000/mm^3; maintenance: 1-2 mg/kg/day

Dose reductions are necessary in patients with reduced renal function, reduced hepatic function, and/or bone marrow disorders

Toxic dose: 1 g/m^2

Contraindications Hypersensitivity to procarbazine or any component, or pre-existing bone marrow aplasia, alcohol ingestion

Warnings The U.S. Food and Drug Administration (FDA) currently recommends that procedures for proper handling and disposal of antineoplastic agents be considered. Use with caution in patients with pre-existing renal or hepatic impairment; modify dosage in patients with renal or hepatic impairment or marrow disorders; reduce dosage with serum creatinine >2 mg/dL or total bilirubin >3 mg/dL; procarbazine possesses MAO inhibitor activity. Procarbazine is a carcinogen which may cause acute leukemia; procarbazine may cause infertility.

Dosage Forms Capsule: 50 mg

Stability Protect from light

Overdosage Treatment

Decontamination: Lavage/activated charcoal

Supportive therapy: Adverse effects, such as marrow toxicity may begin as late as 8 weeks after exposure

Test Interactions Increases potassium (S)

Drug Interactions Increased toxicity:

Procarbazine exhibits weak monoamine oxidase (MAO A and MAO B) inhibitor activity; foods containing high amounts of tyramine should, therefore, be avoided (ie, beer, yogurt, yeast, wine, cheese, pickled herring, chicken liver, and bananas). When a MAO inhibitor is given with food high in tyramine, a hypertensive crisis, intracranial bleeding, and headache have been reported. Meperidine, sympathomimetic amines (epinephrine and amphetamines) and antidepressants (tricyclics) should be used cautiously with procarbazine.

Barbiturates, narcotics, phenothiazines, and other CNS depressants can cause somnolence, ataxia, and other symptoms of CNS depression

Alcohol has caused a disulfiram-like reaction with procarbazine; may result in headache, respiratory difficulties, nausea, vomiting, sweating, thirst, hypotension, and flushing

Patients may experience impaired immune response to vaccines

Possible infection after administration of live vaccines in patients receiving immunosuppressants

Pregnancy Risk Factor D

Pregnancy Implications Teratogenic with genitourinary malformations, oligodactyly, ventricular septal defects, cerebral hemorrhage, growth retardation, and hemangiomas present

Monitoring Parameters CBC with differential, platelet and reticulocyte count, urinalysis, liver function test, renal function test.

Patient Information Avoid food with high tyramine content; obtain a list from your physician or pharmacist; do not take any new prescription or OTC drug without consulting your physician or pharmacist; avoid alcohol and alcohol containing products including topicals; notify physician of persistent fever, sore throat, bleeding, or bruising; may impair judgment and coordination; avoid prolonged exposure to sunlight

Nursing Implications Protect from light

Additional Information Myelosuppressive effects:

WBC: Moderate
Platelets: Moderate
Onset (days): 14
Nadir (days): 21
Recovery (days): 28

Specific References

Spivack SD, "Procarbazine," *Ann Intern Med*, 1974, 81:795-800.

Procardia® *see* Nifedipine *on page 558*

Procardia XL® *see* Nifedipine *on page 558*

Prochlorperazine (proe klor per' a zeen)

Related Information

Doses and Administration of Several Frequently Used Antiemetic Agents *on page 1641*

CAS Number 58-38-8

Brand Names Compazine®

Synonyms Prochlorperazine Edisylate; Prochlorperazine Maleate

Use Management of nausea and vomiting; acute and chronic psychosis

Mechanism of Action Blocks postsynaptic mesolimbic dopaminergic receptors in the brain, including the medullary chemoreceptor trigger zone; exhibits a strong alpha-adrenergic blocking effect and depresses the release of hypothalamic and hypophyseal hormones

Adverse Reactions

Cardiovascular: Hypotension (especially with I.V. use), hypotension (orthostatic), tachycardia, cardiac arrhythmias

Central nervous system: Sedation, drowsiness, restlessness, anxiety, extrapyramidal reactions, pseudoparkinsonian signs and symptoms, tardive dyskinesia, neuroleptic malignant syndrome, seizures, altered central temperature regulation

Dermatologic: Hyperpigmentation, pruritus, rash, photosensitivity

Endocrine & metabolic: Amenorrhea, galactorrhea, gynecomastia, syndrome of inappropriate antidiuretic hormone (SIADH), weight gain

Gastrointestinal: GI upset, dry mouth, constipation

Genitourinary: Urinary retention, impotence

Hematologic: Leukopenia, neutropenia, agranulocytosis, granulocytopenia; (usually in patients with large doses for prolonged periods), thrombocytopenia, hemolysis, eosinophilia

Hepatic: Cholestatic jaundice

Ocular: Retinal pigmentation, photophobia, blurred vision

Miscellaneous: Anaphylactoid reactions

Signs & Symptoms of Acute Overdose Deep sleep, coma, photosensitivity, extrapyramidal reaction, impotence, Parkinson's-like symptoms, systemic lupus erythematosus (SLE), neuroleptic malignant syndrome, vision color changes (brown tinge); nystagmus, urine discoloration (pink), urine discoloration (red), urine discoloration (red-brown), muscle spasm

Toxicodynamics/Kinetics

Onset of action:
- Oral: Within 30-40 minutes
- I.M.: Within 10-20 minutes
- Rectal: Within 60 minutes

Duration:
- Oral (immediate release), rectal doses: 3-4 hours
- Oral (extended release), I.M. doses: 12 hours

Distribution: Widely distributed into body

Protein binding: 90% or more

Metabolism: Primarily eliminated by hepatic metabolism

Half-life: 23 hours

(Continued)

Prochlorperazine *(Continued)*

Elimination: Primarily renal; some excreted in feces via biliary tract

Usual Dosage

Children >10 kg:

Oral, rectal: 0.4 mg/kg/24 hours in 3-4 divided doses; **or**

9-14 kg: 2.5 mg every 12-24 hours as needed; maximum: 7.5 mg/day

14-18 kg: 2.5 mg every 8-12 hours as needed; maximum: 10 mg/day

18-39 kg: 2.5 mg every 8 hours or 5 mg every 12 hours as needed; maximum: 15 mg/day

I.M.: 0.1-0.15 mg/kg/dose; usual: 0.13 mg/kg/dose; change to oral as soon as possible

I.V.: Not recommended in children <10 kg or <2 years

Adults:

Oral: 5-10 mg 3-4 times/day or sustained release twice daily; usual maximum: 40 mg/day; doses up to 150 mg/day may be required in some patients for treatment of severe psychotic disturbances

I.M.: 5-10 mg every 3-4 hours; usual maximum: 40 mg/day; doses up to 10-20 mg every 4-6 hours may be required in some patients for treatment of severe psychotic disturbances

I.V.: 2.5-10 mg; maximum 10 mg/dose or 40 mg/day; may repeat dose every 3-4 hours as needed

Rectal: 25 mg twice daily

Contraindications Children <2 years of age or weight <10 kg; not for use in pediatric surgery; hypersensitivity to prochlorperazine or any component; cross-sensitivity with other phenothiazines may exist; avoid use in patients with narrow-angle glaucoma; bone marrow depression; severe liver or cardiac disease

Warnings High incidence of extrapyramidal reactions occurs especially in children; hypotension with parenteral use; due to high incidence of extrapyramidal effects, injection contains sulfite which may cause allergic reactions in some patients; safety and efficacy have not been established in children <9 kg or <2 years of age; avoid in patients with Reye's syndrome

Dosage Forms

Capsule, sustained action, as maleate: 10 mg, 15 mg, 30 mg

Injection, as edisylate: 5 mg/mL (2 mL, 10 mL)

Suppository, rectal: 2.5 mg, 5 mg, 25 mg (12/box)

Syrup, as edisylate: 5 mg/5 mL (120 mL)

Tablet, as maleate: 5 mg, 10 mg, 25 mg

Stability Protect from light; clear or slightly yellow solutions may be used

Reference Range Blood level >1 μg/mL associated with toxicity

Overdosage Treatment

Decontamination: Lavage/activated charcoal; charcoal may need to be given in multiple doses for adequate decontamination

Supportive therapy: Initiate support with fluids, norepinephrine may be useful for hypotension; hypoperfusion states may respond to inotropic support with dobutamine. Bradyarrhythmia or ventricular dysrhythmia may respond to sodium bicarbonate or phenytoin; must avoid class 1A and 1C antiarrhythmics. Torsade de pointes may respond to magnesium; seizures should be managed with benzodiazepines or barbiturates; extrapyramidal reactions should be managed with diphenhydramine or benztropine.

Enhancement of elimination: Multiple dosing of charcoal may not be effective

Test Interactions False-positives for phenylketonuria, urinary amylase, uroporphyrins, urobilinogen

Diagnostic Tests/Procedures

Prochlorperazine, Blood *on page 1333*

Drug Interactions Additive effects with other CNS depressants; anticonvulsants; epinephrine may cause hypotension

Pregnancy Risk Factor C

Pregnancy Implications Crosses the placenta; appears in breast milk

Patient Information May cause drowsiness

Nursing Implications Avoid skin contact with oral solution or injection, contact dermatitis has occurred; observe for extrapyramidal reaction

Additional Information

Prochlorperazine: Compazine® suppository

Prochlorperazine edisylate: Compazine® oral solution and injection

Prochlorperazine maleate: Compazine® capsule and tablet

Specific References

Berk BZ, "Reaction to Prochlorperazine?" *Lancet*, 1969, 1(598):776.

Manser TJ and Warner JF, "Neuroleptic Malignant Syndrome Associated With Prochlorperazine," *South Med J*, 1990, 83(1):73-4.

Prochlorperazine Edisylate *see* Prochlorperazine *on previous page*

Prochlorperazine Maleate *see* Prochlorperazine *on previous page*

Procrit® *see* Erythropoietin *on page 322*

Proctofoam® [OTC] *see* Pramoxine Hydrochloride *on page 636*

Progan® *see* Promethazine Hydrochloride *on next page*

Progens® *see* Estrogens, Conjugated *on page 325*

Proglycem® Oral *see* Diazoxide *on page 273*

Prograf® *see* Tacrolimus *on page 720*

Progynon C® *see* Ethinyl Estradiol *on page 331*

Prolamine® [OTC] *see* Phenylpropanolamine Hydrochloride *on page 622*

Prolert® *see* Acrivastine *on page 87*

Prolifen® *see* Clomiphene Citrate *on page 227*

Prolixin® *see* Fluphenazine *on page 361*

Proloid® *see* Thyroglobulin *on page 748*

Proloide® *see* Thyroglobulin *on page 748*

Promahist® *see* Promethazine Hydrochloride *on next page*

Promazine Hydrochloride (proe' ma zeen)

Related Information

Antipsychotic Agents Comparison *on page 1642*

CAS Number 58-40-2; 53-60-1

Brand Names Calmotal®; Prozine-50®; Sparine®

Use Treatment of psychoses

Mechanism of Action Excess dopamine in the mesolimbic and mesocortical areas of the brain has been postulated to produce psychoses. Antipsychotics such as promazine act by blocking postsynaptic dopamine receptors, thus ameliorating psychotic symptoms. Promazine, an aliphatic phenothiazine, shares similar properties with chlorpromazine and thus produces a higher frequency of sedation and cardiovascular effects while producing only a moderate frequency of extrapyramidal reactions. Promazine has very weak antipsychotic activity.

Adverse Reactions

Cardiovascular: Hypotension (especially with I.V. use), hypotension (orthostatic), tachycardia, cardiac arrhythmias

Central nervous system: Sedation, drowsiness, restlessness, anxiety, extrapyramidal reactions, pseudoparkinsonian signs and symptoms, tardive dyskinesia, neuroleptic malignant syndrome, seizures, altered central temperature regulation

Dermatologic: Hyperpigmentation, pruritus, rash, photosensitivity

Endocrine & metabolic: Amenorrhea, galactorrhea, gynecomastia, syndrome of inappropriate antidiuretic hormone, weight gain

Gastrointestinal: gastrointestinal upset, dry mouth, constipation

Genitourinary: Urinary retention, impotence

Hematologic: Agranulocytosis, leukopenia (usually in patients with large doses for prolonged periods), thrombocytopenia, hemolysis, eosinophilia

Hepatic: Cholestatic jaundice, neonatal jaundice

Ocular: Retinal pigmentation, photophobia, blurred vision

Respiratory: Apnea, respiratory depression

Miscellaneous: Anaphylactoid reactions

Signs & Symptoms of Acute Overdose Deep sleep, coma, Parkinson's-like symptoms, impotence, hypoglycemia, galactorrhea, neuroleptic malignant syndrome, gynecomastia, dermatitis, extrapyramidal reaction, abnormal involuntary muscle movements, hypotension, seizures, respiratory depression, vision color changes (brown tinge); systemic lupus erythematosus (SLE), urine discoloration (pink), urine discoloration (red), urine discoloration (red-brown), leukopenia; neutropenia; agranulocytosis; granulocytopenia

Toxicodynamics/Kinetics Specific pharmacokinetics are poorly established but probably resemble those of other phenothiazines.

Absorption: Phenothiazines are only partially absorbed; great variability in plasma levels resulting from a given dose

Metabolism: Extensive in the liver

Half-life: Most phenothiazines have long half-lives in the range of 24 hours or more

Usual Dosage Oral, I.M.:

Children >12 years: Antipsychotic: 10-25 mg every 4-6 hours

Adults:

Psychosis: 10-200 mg every 4-6 hours not to exceed 1000 mg/day

Antiemetic: 25-50 mg every 4-6 hours as needed

Contraindications Narrow-angle glaucoma, bone marrow depression, hypersensitivity to promazine or any component

(Continued)

Promazine Hydrochloride *(Continued)*

Warnings Promazine shares the toxic potentials of other phenothiazines, and the usual precautions of phenothiazine therapy should be observed

Dosage Forms

Injection: 25 mg/mL (10 mL); 50 mg/mL (1 mL, 2 mL, 10 mL)

Tablet: 25 mg, 50 mg, 100 mg

Stability Protect from light; store in airtight container; not compatible with sodium bicarbonate, aminophylline, or phenobarbital

Overdosage Treatment

Decontamination: Lavage/activated charcoal with cathartic

Supportive therapy: Following initiation of essential overdose management, toxic symptom treatment and supportive treatment should be initiated. Hypotension usually responds to I.V. fluids or Trendelenburg positioning. If unresponsive to these measures, the use of a parenteral inotrope may be required (eg, norepinephrine 0.1-0.2 mcg/kg/minute titrated to response). Seizures commonly respond to lorazepam or diazepam (I.V. 5-10 mg bolus in adults every 15 minutes if needed up to a total of 30 mg; I.V. 0.25-0.4 mg/kg/dose up to a total of 10 mg in children) or to phenytoin or phenobarbital. Also critical cardiac arrhythmias often respond to I.V. phenytoin (15 mg/kg up to 1 gram), while other antiarrhythmics can be used. Neuroleptics often cause extrapyramidal reaction (eg, dystonic reactions) requiring management with diphenhydramine 1-2 mg/kg (adults) up to a maximum of 50 mg I.M. or I.V. slow push followed by a maintenance dose for 48-72 hours. When these reactions are unresponsive to diphenhydramine, benztropine mesylate I.V. 1-2 mg (adults) may be effective. These agents are generally effective within 2-5 minutes.

Enhancement of elimination: Multiple dosing of activated charcoal may be helpful; not dialyzable (0% to 5%)

Test Interactions Increases cholesterol (S), glucose; decreases uric acid (S)

Drug Interactions Antihypertensives, anticonvulsants, CNS depressants, MAO inhibitors, progesterone, oral contraceptives, and ethanol may accentuate toxicity

Pregnancy Risk Factor C (neonatal jaundice has been noted)

Patient Information May cause drowsiness, impair judgment and coordination; may cause photosensitivity; avoid excessive sunlight; notify physician of involuntary movements or feelings of restlessness

Nursing Implications I.M. injections should be deep injections; if giving I.V., dilute to at least 25 mg/mL and give slowly; watch for hypotension; protect injection from light

Additional Information More likely to cause seizures than other phenothiazines and has smaller amount protein bound than other phenothiazines

Specific References

Gold N, "Attempted Suicide With Chlorpromazine," *Med J Aust*, 1966, 1(12):492-4.

John E, "Promazine and Neonatal Hyperbilirubinemia," *Med J Aust*, 1975, 2(9):342-4.

Prometa® *see* Metaproterenol Sulfate *on page 506*

Prometh® *see* Promethazine Hydrochloride *on this page*

Promethazine Hydrochloride (proe meth' a zeen)

Related Information

H1-Antihistamine Comparison *on page 1649*

Therapeutic Drugs Associated With Hallucinations *on page 1558-1559*

CAS Number 58-33-3; 60-87-7

Brand Names Anergan®; Fargan; Phenazine®; Phencen®; Phenergan®; Progan®; Promahist®; Prometh®; Prorex®; V-Gan®

Synonyms Diprazinum

Use Symptomatic treatment of various allergic conditions, antiemetic, motion sickness, and as a sedative

Mechanism of Action Blocks postsynaptic mesolimbic dopaminergic receptors in the brain; exhibits a strong alpha-adrenergic blocking effect and depresses the release of hypothalamic and hypophyseal hormones; competes with histamine for the H_1-receptor; reduces stimuli to the brainstem reticular system; blocks acetylcholine

Adverse Reactions

Cardiovascular: Tachycardia, bradycardia, hypertension, hypotension

Central nervous system: Sedation (pronounced), confusion, fatigue, excitation, psychosis, extrapyramidal reactions, dystonic reactions, tardive dyskinesia, visual hallucinations

Dermatologic: Photosensitivity

Gastrointestinal: Dry mouth, gastrointestinal upset, constipation

Genitourinary: Urinary retention

Hematologic: Thrombocytopenia, leukopenia, agranulocytosis (rarely)

Hepatic: Cholestatic jaundice

Ocular: Blurred vision, nystagmus

Miscellaneous: Allergic reactions

Signs & Symptoms of Acute Overdose CNS depression, mydriasis, anticholinergic hallucinations, seizures, fever, tachycardia, leukemoid reaction, hyperthermia, eclampsia, coma, toxidrome, dry mouth, vision color changes (brown tinge); hyperreflexia myoclonus, impotence, flushing, urine discoloration (pink), urine discoloration (red), urine discoloration (red-brown), leukopenia, neutropenia, agranulocytosis, granulocytopenia

Toxicodynamics/Kinetics

Onset of effect: I.V.: Within 20 minutes (3-5 minutes with I.V. injection)

Duration: 4-6 hours

Distribution: V_d: 13.4 L/kg

Protein binding: 76% to 93%

Metabolism: In the liver

Time to peak plasma concentration: 3.4 hours

Elimination: Principally as inactive metabolites in urine and feces

Usual Dosage

Children:

- Antihistamine: Oral, rectal: 0.1 mg/kg/dose every 6 hours during the day and 0.5 mg/kg/dose at bedtime as needed
- Antiemetic: Oral, I.M., I.V., rectal: 0.25-1 mg/kg 4-6 times/day as needed
- Motion sickness: Oral, rectal: 0.5 mg/kg/dose 30 minutes to 1 hour before departure, then every 12 hours as needed
- Sedation: Oral, I.M., I.V., rectal: 0.5-1 mg/kg/dose every 6 hours as needed

Adults:

- Antihistamine (including allergic reactions to blood or plasma):
  - Oral, rectal: 12.5 mg 3 times/day and 25 mg at bedtime
  - I.M., I.V.: 25 mg, may repeat in 2 hours when necessary; switch to oral route as soon as feasible
- Antiemetic: Oral, I.M., I.V., rectal: 12.5-25 mg every 4 hours as needed
- Motion sickness: Oral, rectal: 25 mg 30-60 minutes before departure, then every 12 hours as needed
- Sedation: Oral, I.M., I.V., rectal: 25-50 mg/dose

Administration When administering IVP, do not give any faster than 25 mg/minute

Contraindications Hypersensitivity to promethazine or any component; narrow-angle glaucoma

Warnings Use with caution in patients with cardiovascular disease, impaired liver function, asthma, sleep apnea, seizures; do not give S.C. or intra-arterially, necrotic lesions may occur; injection may contain sulfites which may cause allergic reactions in some patients

Dosage Forms

Injection: 25 mg/mL (1 mL, 10 mL); 50 mg/mL (1 mL, 10 mL)

Suppository, rectal: 12.5 mg, 25 mg, 50 mg

Syrup: 6.25 mg/5 mL (5 mL, 120 mL, 240 mL, 480 mL, 4000 mL); 25 mg/5mL (120 mL, 480 mL, 4000 mL)

Tablet: 12.5 mg, 25 mg, 50 mg

Stability Protect from light and freezing; promethazine is **incompatible** when mixed with aminophylline, cefoperazone (Y-site), chloramphenicol, dimenhydrinate (same syringe), foscarnet (Y-site), furosemide, heparin, hydrocortisone, methohexital, penicillin G, pentobarbital, phenobarbital, thiopental

Reference Range

Therapeutic: 11-23 ng/mL

Toxic: >48 ng/mL

Fatal: 156 ng/mL (postmortem)

Overdosage Treatment

Decontamination: Lavage/activated charcoal with cathartic

Supportive therapy: Physostigmine should be used for acute life-threatening events; lorazepam, diazepam, phenytoin, or barbiturates for seizures

Enhancement of elimination: Multiple dosing of activated charcoal may be useful; not dialyzable (0% to 5%)

Antidote(s)

Physostigmine *on page 1457*

Test Interactions Alters the flare response in intradermal allergen tests

Drug Interactions Increased toxicity with epinephrine, CNS depressants; increased sedation when used with meperidine

Pregnancy Risk Factor C

Pregnancy Implications Can cause neonatal respiratory depression

Patient Information May cause drowsiness, impair judgment and coordination; may cause photosensitivity; avoid excessive sunlight; notify physician of involuntary movements or feelings of restlessness

Nursing Implications Rapid I.V. administration may produce a transient fall in blood pressure, rate of administration should not exceed 25 mg/minute; slow I.V. administration may produce a slightly elevated blood pressure; avoid extravasation since tissue necrosis has occurred with extravasation

(Continued)

Promethazine Hydrochloride *(Continued)*

Specific References

Buck ML and Blumer JL, "Phenothiazine-Associated Apnea in Two Siblings," *DICP*, 1991, 25(3):244-7.

Cleghorn C and Bourke G, "Physostigmine for Promethazine Poisoning," *Lancet*, 1980, 2(8190):368-9.

DeGrandi T and Simon JE, "Promethazine-Induced Dystonic Reaction," *Pediatr Emerg Care*, 1987, 3(2):91-2.

Shawn DH and McGuigan MA, "Poisoning From Dermal Absorption of Promethazine," *Can Med Assoc J*, 1984, 130(11):1460-1.

Pronestyl® *see* Procainamide Hydrochloride *on page 642*

Pronestyl-SR® *see* Procainamide Hydrochloride *on page 642*

Propacet® *see* Propoxyphene and Acetaminophen *on page 656*

Propadrine *see* Phenylpropanolamine Hydrochloride *on page 622*

Propafenone Hydrochloride (proe pa feen' one)

CAS Number 34183-22-7; 54063-53-5

Brand Names Normortmin®; Rhythmol®; Rytmonorm®

Synonyms Fenopraine; 3-Phenylpropiophenone

Replaces SA-79

Use Ventricular arrhythmia, fibrillation (atrial)/flutter supression

Mechanism of Action Type 1C antiarrhythmic agent with sodium channel and weak beta-blocking activity

Adverse Reactions

Cardiovascular: Sinus arrest, bradycardia, heart block, hypotension

Central nervous system: Convulsions, psychosis, dizziness, transient global amnesia

Gastrointestinal: Bitter taste, constipation

Genitourinary: Impotence

Hepatic: Elevated liver function tests, cholestatic jaundice

Neuromuscular & skeletal: Peripheral neuropathy

Respiratory: Wheezing

Signs & Symptoms of Acute Overdose Tachycardia, blood dyscrasias, impotence, granulocytopenia, seizures, third degree A-V block, myoclonus, QRS prolongation, metallic taste, hypotension, dizziness, Q-T prolongation

Toxicodynamics/Kinetics

Distribution: V_d: 0.7-3.6 L/kg

Protein binding: 77% to 95%

Metabolism: Hepatic to 5-hydroxypropafenone and N-depropylpropafenone

Bioavailability, oral: 12%

Half-life: In overdose, 12.3 hours

Elimination: Renal clearance: 0.2-0.09 L/hour/kg

Usual Dosage Adults: Oral: 150 mg every 8 hours, increase at 3- to 4-day intervals up to 300 mg every 8 hours; maximum daily dose: 1.2 g

Dosing adjustment in hepatic impairment: Reduction is necessary

Warnings May aggravate heart failure

Dosage Forms Tablet: 150 mg, 225 mg, 300 mg

Reference Range Therapeutic: 500-2000 ng/mL; serum propafenone level of 4839 ng/mL 5.5 hours postingestion is associated with severe toxicity

Overdosage Treatment

Decontamination: Ipecac/lavage, activated charcoal with cathartic

Supportive therapy: Avoid flecainide, encainide; pacemaker may be useful; sodium bicarbonate may be useful for A-V conduction disturbances or QRS prolongation along with reversing hypotension; atropine for bradycardia

Enhanced elimination: Hemodialysis is not useful

Test Interactions May cause elevated antinuclear antibody titer

Drug Interactions May enhance the effect of warfarin

Pregnancy Risk Factor C

Monitoring Parameters EKG

Additional Information Sudden death noted in young postoperative heart patients either on propafenone or withdrawn from it

Specific References

Burgess ED and Duff HJ, "Hemodialysis Removal of Propafenone," *Pharmacotherapy*, 1989, 9(5):331-3.

Galasso PJ, Stanton MS, and Vogel H, "Propafenone-Induced Peripheral Neuropathy," *Mayo Clin Proc*, 1995, 70:469-72.

Jancin B, "Propafenone Blamed for Deaths After Heart Surgery," *Internal News and Cardiology News*, 1993, 26:17.

Jones RJ, Brace SR, and Vander Tuin EL, "Probable Propafenone-Induced Transient Global Amnesia," *Ann Pharmacother*, 1995, 29:586-90.

McHugh TP and Perina DG, "Propafenone Ingestion," *Ann Emerg Med*, 1987, 16(4):437-40.

Perrone J, Blaustein B, Gindi M, et al, "Sodium Bicarbonate Reverses QRS Prolongation in Propafenone Overdose," *Vet Hum Toxicol*, 1994, 36:369.

Tyberg J, Macnaab J, Giesbrecht E, et al, "Toxicokinetics of Propafenone and its Metabolites in a Near Fatal Overdose," *Vet Hum Toxicol*, 1993, 35:344.

Propagest® [OTC] *see* Phenylpropanolamine Hydrochloride *on page 622*

1,2,3-Propanetriol Trinitrate *see* Nitroglycerin *on page 566*

Propheptatriene *see* Cyclobenzaprine Hydrochloride *on page 248*

Pro-Plus® *see* Caffeine *on page 175*

Propofol (proe' po fole)

CAS Number 2078-24-8

Brand Names Diprivan® Injection; Disoprivan®

Synonyms Disoprofol

Use Induction or maintenance of anesthesia for inpatient or outpatient surgery, sedation for the ICU patient; also has been used in tetanus, torticollis, and amoxapine-induced seizures

Mechanism of Action Propofol is a hindered phenolic (2,6-diisopropylphenol) compound with intravenous general anesthetic properties. The drug is unrelated to any of the currently used barbiturate, opioid, benzodiazepine, arylcyclohexylamine, or imidazole intravenous anesthetic agents. It is a gamma-aminobutyric acid ($GABA_A$) neurotransmitter complex agonist, possibly a glycine (neurotransmitter) antagonist.

Adverse Reactions

Cardiovascular: Hypotension, bradycardia, apnea, tachycardia, chest pain, flushing

Central nervous system: Fever, somnolence, agitation, confusion, syncope, electroencephalogram abnormalities

Dermatologic: Pruritus

Gastrointestinal: Nausea, vomiting, abdominal cramping, dry mouth, diarrhea

Neuromuscular & skeletal: Tremors, opisthotonos, myoclonus

Otic: Ear pain

Respiratory: Cough, bronchospasm, dyspnea, apnea

Miscellaneous: Causes green urinary discoloration on prolonged administration, porphyrinogenic

Signs & Symptoms of Acute Overdose Hypotension, bradycardia, myalgia, hiccups, A-V block, hair discoloration (green), seizures, cough, cardiovascular collapse, metabolic acidosis

Toxicodynamics/Kinetics

Onset of anesthesia: Within 30 seconds after bolus infusion

Duration: ~3-10 minutes depending on the dose and the rate of administration

Distribution: V_d: 2-6 mcg/mL during anesthesia; 1-2 mcg/mL upon awakening; large volume of distribution (2-15 L/kg - adults; 5-11 L/kg - children); highly lipophilic

Protein binding: 97% to 99%

Half-life, elimination (biphasic):

- Initial: ~40 minutes
- Terminal: ~200 minutes

Usual Dosage Dosage must be individualized based on total body weight and titrated to the desired clinical effect; however, as a general guideline:

No pediatric dose has been established; however, induction for children 1-12 years 2-2.8 mg/kg has been used

Induction: I.V.:

- Adults up to 55 years, and/or ASA I or II patients: 2-2.5 mg/kg of body weight (approximately 40 mg every 10 seconds until onset of induction)
- Elderly, debilitated, hypovolemic, and/or ASA III or IV patients: 1-1.5 mg/kg of body weight (approximately 20 mg every 10 seconds until onset of induction)

Maintenance: I.V. infusion:

- Adults up to 55 years, and/or ASA I or II patients: 0.1-0.2 mg/kg of body weight/minute (6-12 mg/kg of body weight/hour)
- Elderly, debilitated, hypovolemic, and/or ASA III or IV patients: 0.05-0.1 mg/kg of body weight/minute (3-6 mg/kg of body weight/hour)

I.V. intermittent: 25-50 mg increments, as needed

ICU sedation: Rapid bolus injection should be avoided. Bolus injection can result in hypotension, oxyhemoglobin desaturation, apnea, airway obstruction, and oxygen desaturation. The preferred route of administration is slow infusion. Doses are based on individual need and titrated to response.

Recommended starting dose: 1-3 mg/kg/hour

Adjustments in dose can occur at 3- to 5-minute intervals. An 80% reduction in dose should be considered in elderly, debilitated, and ASA II or IV patients. Once sedation is established, the dose should be decreased for the mainte-

(Continued)

Propofol *(Continued)*

nance infusion period and adjusted to response. The dose required for maintenance is 1.5-4.5 mg/kg/hour or 25-75 mcg/kg/minute. An alternative, but less preferred method of administration is intermittent slow I.V. bolus injection of 10-20 mg, administered over 3-5 minutes.

Amoxapine-induced seizures: I.V.: 2.5 mg/kg bolus followed by a 0.2 mg/kg/minute infusion

Contraindications When general anesthesia is contraindicated, hypersensitivity to propofol

Warnings Use slower rate of induction in the elderly; transient local pain may occur during I.V. injection; perioperative myoclonia has occurred; do not administer with blood or blood products through the same I.V. catheter; not for obstetrics, including cesarean section deliveries; not for use in neurosurgical anesthesia. Propofol administration should be avoided in patients with increased intracranial pressure or impaired cerebral circulation. Use in these patients may result in substantial decrease in mean arterial pressure and cerebral perfusion pressure. In addition, safety and effectiveness has not been established in children. Abrupt discontinuation prior to weaning or daily wake up assessments should be avoided. Abrupt discontinuation can result in rapid awakening, anxiety, agitation, and resistance to mechanical ventilation.

Dosage Forms Injection: 10 mg/mL (20 mL)

Stability Do not use if there is evidence of separation of phases of emulsion; discard any unused portions at end of the surgical procedure

Reference Range Propofol blood levels from 1.6-6.4 μg/mL associated with anesthetic action; levels from 1.0-2.2 μg/mL associated with regaining consciousness

Overdosage Treatment Supportive therapy: Hypotension usually responds to I.V. fluids and/or Trendelenburg positioning; parenteral inotropes may be needed

Test Interactions ↓ cholesterol (S)

Drug Interactions

Acts synergistically with midazolam

Decreased effect with theophylline (↓ sedative effects of propofol)

Increased effect/toxicity of alfentanil (↑ concentrations)

Increased toxicity with acetazolamide (cardiorespiratory instability), CNS depressants, atracurium (anaphylaxis), phenothiazines, fentanyl (↑ concentration of propofol), benzodiazepines, guanabenz, MAO inhibitors, narcotic analgesics, vecuronium (neuromuscular blockade), succinylcholine (severe bradycardia)

Pregnancy Risk Factor B

Monitoring Parameters Cardiorespiratory functions (eg, oxygen saturation, hypotension, apnea, airway obstruction, bradycardia) should be monitored in all patients. Patients receiving propofol by intermittent bolus injection should be closely monitored for respiratory depression, transient increase in sedation depth, and prolongation of recovery. Daily monitoring of serum lipids is recommended, especially in patients receiving high doses for long periods.

Patient Information Protect from light; shake well

Nursing Implications Changes urine color to green with prolonged use

Additional Information Not a cause of malignant hyperthermia; can reduce intracranial pressure

Specific References

Arndt GA, Reiss WG, and Bathke KA, "Computer-Assisted Continuous Infusion for the Delivery of Target-Controlled Infusions of Propofol During Outpatient Surgery," *Pharmacotherapy*, 1995, 15(4):512-6.

Bedforth NM and Lockey DJ, "Raynaud's Syndrome Following Intravenous Induction of Anaesthesia," *Anaesthesia*, 1995, 50:248-9.

Bennett Sn, McNeil MM, Bland LA, et al, "Postoperative Infections traced to Contamination of an Intravenous Anesthetic, Propofol," *N Engl J Med*, 1995, 333:147-54.

Borgeat A, "Efficiency of a Continuous Infusion of Propofol in a Patient with Tetanus," *Crit Care Med*, 1991, 19(2):295-7.

Borgeat A, "Usefulness of Propofol in Torticollis," *Br J Anaesth*, 1991, 66(4):530.

Brag RJ, "Fatal Myocardial Failure Associated With a Propofol Infusion in a Child," *Anaesthesia*, 1995, 50:94.

Cheong KF and Low TC, "Propofol and Postanaesthetic Shivering," *Anaesthesia*, 1995, 50:550-2.

Hullander RM, Leivers D, and Wingler K, "A Comparison of Propofol and Etomidate for Cardioversion," *Anesth Analg*, 1993, 77(4):690-4.

Langley MS and Heel RC, "Propofol: A Review of its Pharmacodynamic and Pharmacokinetic Properties and Use as an Intravenous Anaesthetic," *Drugs*, 1988, 35(4):334-72.

Merigian KS, Browning MD, and Leeper KV, "Successful Treatment of Amoxapine-Induced Refractory Status Epilepticus with Propofol (Diprivan®)," *Acad Emerg Med*, 1995, 21:128-33.

Mirenda J, "Proloonged Propofol Sedation in the Critical Care Unit," *Crit Care Med*, 1995, 23(7):1304.

Plummer D and Ross H, "Propofol in the E.D.," *Acad Emerg Med*, 1995, 2:462.

Strickland RA and Murray MJ, "Fatal Metabolic Acidosis in a Pediatric Patient Receiving an Infusion of Propofol in the Intensive Care Unit: Is There a Relationship?" *Crit Care Med*, 1995, 23(2):405-9.

Swanson ER, Seaberg DC, and Mathias S, "The Use of Propofol for Conscious Sedation in the Emergency Department," *Acad Emerg Med*, 1995, 2:462.

Swanson ER, Seaberg DC, Stypula RW, et al, "Propofol for Conscious Sedation: A Case Series," *Acad Emerg Med*, 1995, 2(7):661-2.

Propoxyphene (proe pox' i feen)

Related Information

Pharmacokinetics of Narcotic Agonist Analgesics *on page 1654*
Propoxyphene and Acetaminophen *on next page*
Therapeutic Drugs Associated With Hallucinations *on page 1558-1559*

CAS Number 469-62-5; 1639-60-7

Brand Names Darvon®; Darvon-N®; Dolene®

Synonyms Dextropropoxyphene; Propoxyphene Hydrochloride; Propoxyphene Napsylate

Use Management of mild to moderate pain

Mechanism of Action Binds to opiate receptors in the CNS, causing inhibition of ascending pain pathways, altering the perception of and response to pain; produces generalized CNS depression

Adverse Reactions

Cardiovascular: Hypotension
Central nervous system: Dizziness, lightheadedness, asthenia, sedation, paradoxical excitation and insomnia, headache, tiredness, psychosis, drowsiness, nervousness, restlessness, malaise, confusion, mental depression, auditory hallucinations
Dermatologic: Skin rash, hives
Gastrointestinal: gastrointestinal upset, nausea, vomiting, constipation, anorexia, stomach cramps, dry mouth, paralytic ileus
Genitourinary: Ureteral spasm, decreased urination
Hepatic: Liver enzymes (increased)
Neuromuscular & skeletal: Hyperreflexia
Respiratory: Troubled breathing, dyspnea, apnea
Miscellaneous: Psychologic and physical dependence, histamine release, pain at injection site, biliary spasm, intracranial pressure (increased)

Signs & Symptoms of Acute Overdose Vomiting, pulmonary edema, insomnia, impotence, hyperreflexia, disorientation, deafness, jaundice, hyperthermia, hypernatremia, dementia, thrombocytopenia, ptosis, neutropenia, nystagmus, seizures, rhabdomyolysis, diabetes insipidus, myoglobinuria, hypothermia, cyanosis, miosis, cardiac arrhythmia (ventricular), tremors, primary atrioventricular block, nodal tachycardia; dizziness, coma, death can occur within 1 hour

Toxicodynamics/Kinetics

Onset of effect: Oral: Within 30-60 minutes
Duration: 4-6 hours
Distribution: V_d: 12-26 L/kg
Protein binding: 78%
Metabolism: First-pass effect; metabolized in the liver to an active metabolite (norpropoxyphene) and inactive metabolites
Bioavailability: Oral: 30% to 70%
Half-life:
- Adults:
  - Parent drug: 8-24 hours (mean: ~15 hours)
  - Norpropoxyphene: 34 hours
- Elderly:
  - Parent drug: 37 hours
  - Norpropoxyphene: 42 hours

Elimination: 20% to 25% excreted in urine

Usual Dosage Adults: Oral:

Hydrochloride: 65 mg every 3-4 hours as needed for pain; maximum: 390 mg/day

Napsylate: 100 mg every 4 hours as needed for pain; maximum: 600 mg/day

Dosing comments in renal impairment: Cl_{cr} <10 mL/minute: Avoid use

Dosing adjustment in hepatic impairment: Reduced doses should be used

Contraindications Hypersensitivity to propoxyphene or any component

Warnings Give with caution in patients dependent on opiates, substitution may result in acute opiate withdrawal symptoms, use with caution in patients with severe renal or hepatic dysfunction; when given in excessive doses, either alone or in combination with other CNS depressants or propoxyphene products, propoxyphene is a major cause of drug-related deaths; do not exceed recommended dosage

Dosage Forms

Capsule, as hydrochloride: 32 mg, 65 mg
Suspension, oral, as napsylate: 50 mg/5 mL (480 mL)
Tablet, as napsylate: 100 mg

Reference Range

Therapeutic: 0.2 µg/mL, ranges published vary between laboratories and may not correlate with clinical effect

(Continued)

Propoxyphene *(Continued)*

Toxic: >0.5 μg/mL (SI: >1.5 μmol/L)

Overdosage Treatment

Decontamination: Lavage/activated charcoal with cathartic within 2 hours of ingestion

Supportive therapy: Naloxone hydrochloride for CNS depression, may also stop seizures and alleviate hypotension. Lidocaine or sodium bicarbonate can reverse QRS prolongation and ventricular arrhythmias.

Enhancement of elimination: Multiple dosing of activated charcoal is useful; not dialyzable (0% to 5%)

Antidote(s)

Naloxone Hydrochloride *on page 1447*

Test Interactions False-positive methadone test, ↓ glucose (S), ↑ LFTs, ↓ 17-OHCS (U)

Diagnostic Tests/Procedures

Propoxyphene, Blood or Urine *on page 1334*

Drug Interactions

Decreased effect with charcoal, cigarette smoking

Increased toxicity with CNS depressants; increased toxicity/effect of carbamazepine, phenobarbital, TCAs, warfarin, MAO inhibitors

Pregnancy Risk Factor C (D if used for prolonged periods)

Pregnancy Implications Possible human teratogen (cranial and facial abnormalities, prone peritoneum, absent limbs)

Monitoring Parameters Pain relief, respiratory and mental status, blood pressure

Patient Information May cause drowsiness, dizziness, or blurring of vision; avoid alcohol and other sedatives; may take with food; can impair judgment and coordination

Additional Information 100 mg of napsylate = 65 mg of hydrochloride

Propoxyphene hydrochloride: Darvon®

Propoxyphene napsylate: Darvon-N®

Specific References

Finkle BS, "Self-Poisoning With Dextropropoxyphene and Dextropropoxyphene Compounds: The USA Experience," *Hum Toxicol*, 1984, 3(Suppl):115S-134S.

Lawson AA and Northridge DB, "Dextropropoxyphene Overdose. Epidemiology, Clinical Presentation, and Management," *Adverse Drug Exp Med Toxicol*, 1987, 2(6):430-44.

Proudfoot AT, "Clinical Features and Management of Distalgesic Overdose," *Hum Toxicol*, 1984, 3(Suppl):85S-94S.

Stork CM, Redd JT, Fine K, et al, "Propoxyphene-Induced Wide QRS Complex Dysrhythmia Responsive to Sodium Bicarbonate – A Case Report," *J Toxicol Clin Toxicol*, 1995, 33(2):179-83.

Tennant FS Jr, "Complications of Propoxyphene Abuse," *Arch Intern Med*, 1973, 132(2):191-4.

Wetli CV and Bednarczyk LR, "Deaths Related to Propoxyphene Overdose: A Ten Year Assessment," *South Med J*, 1980, 73(9):1205-9.

Propoxyphene and Acetaminophen

(proe pox' i feen & a seet a min' oh fen)

Related Information

Acetaminophen *on page 79*

Pharmacokinetics of Narcotic Agonist Analgesics *on page 1654*

Propoxyphene *on previous page*

Brand Names Darvocet-N®; Darvocet-N® 100; E-Lor®; Genagesic®; Propacet®; Wygesic®

Synonyms Propoxyphene Hydrochloride and Acetaminophen; Propoxyphene Napsylate and Acetaminophen

Use Management of mild to moderate pain

Adverse Reactions

Central nervous system: Dizziness, lightheadedness, asthenia, sedation, paradoxical excitation, insomnia, headache

Dermatologic: Rashes

Gastrointestinal: gastrointestinal upset, nausea, vomiting, constipation

Hepatic: Liver enzymes (increased)

Respiratory: Troubled breathing, dyspnea, apnea

Miscellaneous: Psychologic and physical dependence

Signs & Symptoms of Acute Overdose Dizziness, coma, lightheadedness, death can occur within 1 hour

Usual Dosage Adults:

Darvocet-N®: 1-2 tablets every 4 hours as needed; maximum: 600 mg propoxyphene napsylate/day

Darvocet-N® 100: 1 tablet every 4 hours as needed; maximum: 600 mg propoxyphene napsylate/day

Contraindications Hypersensitivity to propoxyphene, acetaminophen or any component

Warnings When given in excessive doses, either alone or in combination with other CNS depressants, propoxyphene is a major cause of drug-related deaths; do not exceed recommended dosage; give with caution in patients dependent on opiates, substitution may result in acute opiate withdrawal symptoms

Dosage Forms Tablet:

Darvocet-N®: Propoxyphene napsylate 50 mg and acetaminophen 325 mg

Darvocet-N® 100: Propoxyphene napsylate 100 mg and acetaminophen 650 mg

E-Lor®, Genagesic®, Wygesic®: Propoxyphene hydrochloride 65 mg and acetaminophen 650 mg

Overdosage Treatment

Decontamination: Lavage/activated charcoal with cathartic within 2 hours of ingestion

Supportive therapy: Naloxone hydrochloride for CNS depression, may also stop seizures and alleviate hypotension. Lidocaine can reverse QRS prolongation and ventricular arrhythmias. Acetylcysteine should be used as per acetaminophen overdose protocol.

Enhancement of elimination: Multiple dosing of activated charcoal is useful; not dialyzable (0% to 5%)

Antidote(s)

Acetylcysteine *on page 1388*

Naloxone Hydrochloride *on page 1447*

Drug Interactions CNS depressants may potentiate pharmacologic effects; propoxyphene may inhibit the metabolism and increase the serum concentrations of carbamazepine, phenobarbital, tricyclic antidepressants and warfarin

Pregnancy Risk Factor C

Monitoring Parameters Pain relief, respiratory and mental status, blood pressure

Patient Information Do not exceed recommended dose; may cause drowsiness; avoid alcoholic beverages

Nursing Implications Monitor for excessive sedation

Additional Information

Propoxyphene hydrochloride and acetaminophen: Dolene® AP-65, Wygesic®, Genagesic®

Propoxyphene napsylate and acetaminophen: Darvocet-N®, Darvocet-N® 100; Propacet®

Propoxyphene napsylate 100 mg and propoxyphene hydrochloride contain same amount of propoxyphene; when using the acetaminophen nomograms, note that acetaminophen levels may rise after 4 hours when propoxyphene is coingested

Specific References

Bartle WR, Paradiso FL, Derry JE, et al, "Delayed Acetaminophen Toxicity Despite Acetylcysteine Use," *DICP*, 1989, 23(6):509.

Finkle BS, "Self-Poisoning With Dextropropoxyphene and Dextropropoxyphene Compounds: The USA Experience," *Hum Toxicol*, 1984, 3(Suppl):115S-134S.

Lawson AA and Northridge DB, "Dextropropoxyphene Overdose. Epidemiology, Clinical Presentation, and Management," *Adverse Drug Exp Med Toxicol*, 1987, 2(6):430-44.

Proudfoot AT, "Clinical Features and Management of Distalgesic Overdose," *Hum Toxicol*, 1984, 3(Suppl):85S-94S.

Tennant FS Jr, "Complications of Propoxyphene Abuse," *Arch Intern Med*, 1973, 132(2):191-4.

Tighe TV and Walter FG, "Delayed Toxic Acetaminophen Level After Initial Nontoxic Level," *Vet Hum Toxicol*, 1991, 33:356.

Wetli CV and Bednarczyk LR, "Deaths Related to Propoxyphene Overdose: A Ten Year Assessment," *South Med J*, 1980, 73(9):1205-9.

Propoxyphene Hydrochloride *see* Propoxyphene *on page 655*

Propoxyphene Hydrochloride and Acetaminophen *see* Propoxyphene and Acetaminophen *on previous page*

Propoxyphene Napsylate *see* Propoxyphene *on page 655*

Propoxyphene Napsylate and Acetaminophen *see* Propoxyphene and Acetaminophen *on previous page*

Propranolol Hydrochloride (proe pran' oh lole)

Related Information

Beta-Blockers Comparison *on page 1644-1645*

Therapeutic Drugs Associated With Hallucinations *on page 1558-1559*

CAS Number 525-66-6; 5051-22-9; 13013-17-7; 318-98-9; 13071-11-9; 4199-10-4; 3506-09-0

Brand Names Angilol®; Apsolol®; Beaden®; Bedranol®; Berkolol®; Deralin®; Inderal®; Inderal® LA

Use Management of hypertension, angina pectoris, pheochromocytoma, essential tremor, tetralogy of Fallot cyanotic spells, and arrhythmias (such as fibrillation (atrial) and flutter, A-V nodal re-entrant tachycardias, and catecholamine-induced arrhythmias); prevention of myocardial infarction, migraine headache; symptomatic treatment of hypertrophic subaortic stenosis; termination of thyrotoxic periodic paralysis

(Continued)

Propranolol Hydrochloride *(Continued)*

Mechanism of Action Competitively blocks response to beta$_1$- and beta$_2$-adrenergic stimulation; no intrinsic sympathomimetic or alpha-receptor antagonist activity; propranolol cardiotoxicity may be mediated through calcium dyshomeostasis

Adverse Reactions

Cardiovascular: Hypotension, impaired myocardial contractility, congestive heart failure, bradycardia, worsening of A-V conduction disturbances, abnormal T-wave inversion, claudication, syncope

Central nervous system: Lightheadedness, psychosis, insomnia, vivid dreams, asthenia, drowsiness, depression, auditory and visual hallucinations

Endocrine & metabolic: Hypoglycemia, hyperglycemia

Gastrointestinal: Nausea, vomiting, diarrhea, gastrointestinal distress

Genitourinary: Impotence, penile fibrosis

Hematologic: Agranulocytosis, thrombocytopenic purpura

Neuromuscular & skeletal: Myotonia, muscle asthenia, myasthenia gravis (exacerbation), arthralgia

Ocular: Diplopia

Respiratory: Wheezing

Miscellaneous: Cold extremities

Signs & Symptoms of Acute Overdose Severe hypotension, dyspnea, ataxia, impotence, hypoglycemia, hyperthyroidism, hyperreflexia, shock, retroperitoneal fibrosis, pemphigus, paranoia, hypothyroidism, urticaria, sexual dysfunction; A-V block, rhinorrhea, dementia, purpura, depression, hyperglycemia, cognitive dysfunction, sinus bradycardia, heart/respiratory failure and wheezing; myasthenia gravis (exacerbation or precipitation of), Graves' disease, pulmonary edema, mesenteric ischemia, cardiovascular collapse, alopecia, leukopenia; neutropenia; agranulocytosis; granulocytopenia

Toxicodynamics/Kinetics

Onset of action:
- Oral: Within 1-2 hours
- I.V.: 2 minutes

Duration:
- Oral: 6 hours
- I.V.: 3-6 hours

Absorption: Almost completely from gastrointestinal tract (90%)

Distribution: V_d: Adults: 3.9 L/kg; crosses blood-brain barrier; widely to body tissues; high lipid solubility

Protein binding:
- Newborns: 68%
- Adults: 93%

Metabolism: Extensive first-pass effect; metabolized in the liver to active and inactive compounds

Bioavailability: 30% to 40%; oral bioavailability may be increased in Down's syndrome children

Half-life:
- Children: 3.9-6.4 hours; possible increased half-life in neonates and infants, and overdose setting
- Adults: 4-6 hours

Time to peak serum concentration: 1-1.5 hours

Elimination: 1% excreted unchanged in urine; clearance: 12 mL/minute/kg

Usual Dosage

Tachyarrhythmias:
- Oral:
  - Children: Initial: 0.5-1 mg/kg/day in divided doses every 6-8 hours; titrate dosage upward every 3-7 days; usual dose: 2-4 mg/kg/day; higher doses may be needed; do not exceed 16 mg/kg/day or 60 mg/day
  - Adults: 10-80 mg/dose every 6-8 hours
- I.V.:
  - Children: 0.01-0.1 mg/kg slow IVP over 10 minutes; maximum dose: 1 mg
  - Adults: 1 mg/dose slow IVP; repeat every 5 minutes up to a total of 5 mg

Hypertension: Oral:
- Children: Initial: 0.5-1 mg/kg/day in divided doses every 6-12 hours; increase gradually every 3-7 days; maximum: 2 mg/kg/24 hours
- Adults: Initial: 40 mg twice daily or 60-80 mg once daily as sustained release capsules; increase dosage every 3-7 days; usual dose: ≤320 mg divided in 2-3 doses/day or once daily as sustained release; maximum daily dose: 640 mg

Migraine headache prophylaxis: Oral:
- Children: 0.6-1.5 mg/kg/day **or**
  - ≤35 kg: 10-20 mg 3 times/day
  - >35 kg: 20-40 mg 3 times/day
- Adults: Initial: 80 mg/day divided every 6-8 hours; increase by 20-40 mg/dose every 3-4 weeks to a maximum of 160-240 mg/day given in divided doses

every 6-8 hours; if satisfactory response not achieved within 6 weeks of starting therapy, drug should be withdrawn gradually over several weeks

Tetralogy spells: Children: Oral: 1-2 mg/kg/day every 6 hours as needed, may increase by 1 mg/kg/day to a maximum of 5 mg/kg/day, or if refractory may increase slowly to a maximum of 10-15 mg/kg/day

Thyrotoxicosis:

Neonates: Oral: 2 mg/kg/day in divided doses every 6-12 hours; occasionally higher doses may be required

Adolescents and Adults: Oral: 10-40 mg/dose every 6 hours

Adults: I.V.: 1-3 mg/dose slow IVP as a single dose

Adults: Oral:

Angina: 80-320 mg/day in doses divided 2-4 times/day or 80-160 mg of sustained release once daily

Pheochromocytoma: 30-60 mg/day in divided doses

Myocardial infarction prophylaxis: 180-240 mg/day in 3-4 divided doses

Hypertrophic subaortic stenosis: 20-40 mg 3-4 times/day

Essential tremor: 40 mg twice daily initially; maintenance doses: usually 120-320 mg/day

Dosing adjustment/comments in hepatic disease: Marked slowing of heart rate may occur in cirrhosis with conventional doses; low initial dose and regular heart rate monitoring

Contraindications Uncompensated congestive heart failure, cardiogenic shock, bradycardia or heart block, asthma, hyperactive airway disease, chronic obstructive lung disease, Raynaud's syndrome

Warnings In patients with angina pectoris, exacerbation of angina and, in some cases, myocardial infarction, occurred following abrupt discontinuance of therapy; use with caution in patients with renal or hepatic impairment

Dosage Forms

Capsule, sustained action: 60 mg, 80 mg, 120 mg, 160 mg

Injection: 1 mg/mL (1 mL)

Solution, oral (strawberry-mint flavor): 4 mg/mL (5 mL, 500 mL); 8 mg/mL (5 mL, 500 mL)

Solution, oral, concentrate: 80 mg/mL (30 mL)

Tablet: 10 mg, 20 mg, 40 mg, 60 mg, 80 mg, 90 mg

Stability Compatible in saline, incompatible with HCO_3^-; protect injection from light

Reference Range

Therapeutic: 50-100 ng/mL (SI: 190-390 nmol/L) at end of dose interval

Fatal: Levels >2000 ng/mL (SI: >7702 nmol/L)

Overdosage Treatment

Decontamination: Lavage/activated charcoal with cathartic; do not use ipecac

Supportive therapy: Glucagon (50-150 mcg/kg followed by continuous drip of 1-5 mg/hour) for positive chronotropic effect, amrinone may need to be added; atropine/isoproterenol can be utilized to increase heart rate; calcium chloride may also be effective but this approach has not thoroughly been investigated; do **not** use epinephrine in that unopposed alpha effects may occur; pacemaker or intra-aortic balloon counter pulsation may be required

Enhancement of elimination: Multiple dosing of activated charcoal is not likely to be of benefit; dialysis is not useful; not dialyzable (0% to 5%)

Antidote(s)

Glucagon *on page 1431*

Test Interactions Increases thyroxine (S), cholesterol (S), glucose

Drug Interactions Phenobarbital, rifampin may increase propranolol clearance and may decrease its activity; cimetidine may reduce propranolol clearance and may increase its effects; aluminum-containing antacid may reduce gastrointestinal absorption of propranolol; use of ipecac may precipitate cardiovascular collapse due to increased vagal tone; may enhance cardiac effects of digitalis; hypertension may occur with epinephrine

Pregnancy Risk Factor C (can cause intrauterine growth retardation)

Pregnancy Implications Crosses the placenta; small amounts appear in breast milk

Monitoring Parameters Blood pressure, EKG, CVP

Patient Information Do not discontinue abruptly; notify physician if CHF symptoms become worse; take at the same time each day; may mask diabetes symptoms

Nursing Implications I.V. dose much smaller than oral dose; I.V. administration should not exceed 1 mg/minute

Additional Information Healthy African-American individuals are more sensitive to beta-blockade effects of propranolol than healthy white individuals

Specific References

Elkharrat D and Bismuth C, "Acute Intoxication by Beta-Blocking Agents: No Mortality in Forty Cases," *Int J Clin Pharmacol Res*, 1982, 2:207-10.

Grandy W, "Severe Epinephrine-Propranolol Interaction," *Ann Emerg Med*, 1989, 18(1):98-9.

(Continued)

Propranolol Hydrochloride *(Continued)*

Jones JW, Clark MA, and Mullen BL, "Suicide by Ingestion of Propranolol," *J Forensic Sci*, 1982, 27(1):213-6.

Kerns W, Ransom M, Tomaszewski C, et al, "Mechanism of Propranolol Cardiotoxicity," *Vet Hum Toxicol*, 1994, 36:347.

Sato S, Tsuji MH, Okubo N, et al, "Combined Use of Glucagon and Milrinone may not be Preferable for Severe Propranolol Poisoning in the Canine Model," *J Toxicol Clin Toxicol*, 1995, 33:337-42.

Shayne P and Hart A, "Thyrotoxic Periodic Paralysis Terminated With Intravenous Propranolol," *Ann Emerg Med*, 1994, 24(4):736-40.

Sowinsky KM, Burlew BS, and Johnson JA, "Racial Differences in Sensitivity to the Negative Chronòtropic Effects of Propranolol in Healthy Men," *Clin Pharmacol Ther*, 1995, 57:678-83.

Stoschitzky K, Kahr S, Donnerer J, et al, "Stereoselective Increase of Plasma Concentrations of the Enantiomers of Propranolol and Atenolol During Exercise," *Clin Pharmacol Ther*, 1995, 57:543-51.

Propulsid® *see* Cisapride *on page 217*

Propulsin® *see* Cisapride *on page 217*

Propycil® *see* Propylthiouracil *on this page*

2-Propylpentanoic Acid *see* Valproic Acid and Derivatives *on page 782*

Propylthiouracil (proe pill thye oh yoor' a sill)

CAS Number 51-52-5

Brand Names Propycil®; Propyl-Thyracil®; Thyreustat II®; Tiotil®

Synonyms PTU

Use Palliative treatment of hyperthyroidism as an adjunct to ameliorate hyperthyroidism in preparation for surgical treatment or radioactive iodine therapy and in the management of thyrotoxic crisis

Mechanism of Action Inhibits the synthesis of thyroid hormones by blocking the oxidation of iodine in the thyroid gland; blocks synthesis of thyroxine and triiodothyronine

Adverse Reactions

Cardiovascular: Edema, cutaneous vasculitis, periarteritis

Central nervous system: Drowsiness, neuritis, dizziness, headache

Dermatologic: Rash, pruritus, exfoliative dermatitis, abnormal hair loss, skin pigmentation

Gastrointestinal: Nausea, vomiting, loss of taste

Hematologic: Agranulocytosis, thrombocytopenia, bleeding, hypoprothrombinemia

Hepatic: Jaundice, hepatitis

Neuromuscular & skeletal: Arthralgia

Renal: Nephritis

Respiratory: Interstitial pneumonitis

Miscellaneous: Drug fever

Signs & Symptoms of Acute Overdose Leukopenia or neutropenia (agranulocytosis, granulocytopenia); systemic lupus erythematosus (SLE), hyperthermia, deafness, myopathy, dysosmia, galactorrhea, enuresis

Toxicodynamics/Kinetics

For significant therapeutic effects, 24-36 hours are required and remissions of hyperthyroidism do not usually occur before 4 months of continued therapy

Distribution: V_d: 0.3-0.4 L/kg

Protein binding: 75% to 80%

Metabolism: Hepatic

Half-life: 1.5-5 hours

Time to peak serum concentration: Oral: Within 1 hour and persisting for 2-3 hours

Elimination: 35% excreted in urine, 1% in feces

Usual Dosage Oral: Administer in 3 equally divided doses at approximately 8-hour intervals; adjust dosage to maintain T_3, T_4, and TSH levels in normal range; elevated T_3 may be sole indicator of adequate treatment, elevated TSH indicates excessive antithyroid treatment

Neonates: 5-10 mg/kg/day in divided doses every 8 hours

Children: Initial: 5-7 mg/kg/day in divided doses every 8 hours **or**

6-10 years: 50-150 mg/day

>10 years: 150-300 mg/day

Maintenance: $\frac{1}{3}$ to $\frac{2}{3}$ of the initial dose in divided doses every 8-12 hours; this usually begins after 2 months on an effective initial dosage

Adults: Initial: 300-450 mg/day in divided doses every 8 hours (severe hyperthyroidism may require 600-1200 mg/day); maintenance: 100-150 mg/day in divided doses every 8-12 hours

Elderly: Use lower dose recommendations; initial dose: 150-300 mg/day

Dosing adjustment in renal impairment:

Cl_{cr} 10-50 mL/minute: Administer at 75% of normal dose

Cl_{cr} <10 mL/minute: Administer at 50% of normal dose

Contraindications Hypersensitivity to propylthiouracil or any component

Warnings Use with caution in patients >40 years of age because PTU may cause hypoprothrombinemia and bleeding, monitor prothrombin time during therapy; use with extreme caution in patients receiving other drugs known to cause decreased white blood cells; may cause agranulocytosis, thyroid hyperplasia, thyroid carcinoma (use >1 year).

Dosage Forms Tablet: 50 mg

Reference Range Peak serum level of 10 μg/mL following 400 mg ingestion; see table.

Laboratory Ranges

	Normal Values
Total T_4	5–11 mcg/dL
Serum T_3	85–185 ng/dL
TSH	0.4–4.8 μIU/mL

Overdosage Treatment Decontamination: Ipecac or lavage/activated charcoal with cathartic

Test Interactions Elevated alkaline phosphatase, decreased T_3, increased reverse T_3

Diagnostic Tests/Procedures

Thyroxine, Blood *on page 1361*

Drug Interactions Increased effect: ↑ anticoagulant activity

Pregnancy Risk Factor D

Monitoring Parameters CBC with differential, prothrombin time, liver function tests, thyroid function tests (T_4, T_3, TSH); periodic blood counts are recommended chronic therapy

Patient Information Do not exceed prescribed dosage; take at regular intervals around-the-clock; notify physician or pharmacist if fever, sore throat, unusual bleeding or bruising, headache or general malaise occurs

Additional Information The use of antithyroid thioamides is as effective in elderly as in younger adults; however, the expense, potential adverse effects, and inconvenience (compliance, monitoring) make them undesirable. The use of radioiodine, due to ease of administration and less concern for long-term side effects and reproduction problems, makes it a more appropriate therapy.

Specific References

Jackson GL, Flickinger FW, and Wells LW, "Massive Overdosage of Propylthiouracil," *Ann Intern Med*, 1979, 91(3):418-9.

Limaye A and Ruffolo R, "Propylthiouracil-Induced Fatal Hepatic Necrosis," *Am J Gastroenterol*, 1987, 82(2):152-4.

Propyl-Thyracil® *see* Propylthiouracil *on previous page*

2-Propylvaleric Acid *see* Valproic Acid and Derivatives *on page 782*

Prorex® *see* Promethazine Hydrochloride *on page 650*

ProSom™ *see* Estazolam *on page 324*

ProStep® Patch *see* Nicotine *on page 556*

Protostat® Oral *see* Metronidazole *on page 526*

Proventil® *see* Albuterol *on page 92*

Prozac® *see* Fluoxetine Hydrochloride *on page 359*

Prozil® *see* Chlorpromazine Hydrochloride *on page 205*

Prozine-50® *see* Promazine Hydrochloride *on page 649*

Prulet® [OTC] *see* Phenolphthalein *on page 617*

Pseudoephedrine (soo doe e fed' rin)

CAS Number 345-78-8

Brand Names Afrinol® [OTC]; Cenafed® [OTC]; Decofed® Syrup [OTC]; Neofed® [OTC]; Novafed®; PediaCare® Oral; Sudafed® [OTC]; Sudafed® 12 Hour [OTC]; Sufedrin® [OTC]

Synonyms *d*-Isoephedrine Hydrochloride; Pseudoephedrine Hydrochloride; Pseudoephedrine Sulfate

Use Temporary symptomatic relief of nasal congestion due to common cold, upper respiratory allergies, and sinusitis; also promotes nasal or sinus drainage

(Continued)

Pseudoephedrine *(Continued)*

Mechanism of Action Directly stimulates alpha-adrenergic receptors of respiratory mucosa causing vasoconstriction; directly stimulates beta-adrenergic receptors causing bronchial relaxation, increased heart rate and contractility

Adverse Reactions

Cardiovascular: Tachycardia, palpitation, cardiac arrhythmias, chest pain, myocardial ischemia

Central nervous system: Nervousness, excitation, dizziness, insomnia, drowsiness, psychosis, headache

Gastrointestinal: Nausea, vomiting

Genitourinary: Difficult urination

Neuromuscular & skeletal: Tremors

Signs & Symptoms of Acute Overdose Convulsions, nausea, depression, mydriasis, vomiting, insomnia, arrhythmias

Toxicodynamics/Kinetics

Onset of action: Within 15-30 minutes

Duration: 4-6 hours (up to 12 hours with extended release formulation administration)

Distribution: V_d: 2.74 L/kg; widely distributed throughout body

Metabolism: Partially in liver

Half-life: 9-16 hours

Elimination: 70% to 90% excreted in urine as unchanged drug and 1% to 6% as norpseudoephedrine (active)

Usual Dosage Oral:

Children (do not give sustained release tablets):

- <2 years: 4 mg/kg/day in divided doses every 6 hours
- 2-5 years: 15 mg every 6 hours; maximum: 60 mg/24 hours
- 6-12 years: 30 mg every 6 hours; maximum: 120 mg/24 hours

Adults: 30-60 mg every 4-6 hours, sustained release: 120 mg every 12 hours; maximum: 480 mg/24 hours

Dosing adjustment in renal impairment: Reduce dose

Contraindications Hypersensitivity to pseudoephedrine or any component; MAO inhibitor therapy, severe hypertension, severe coronary artery disease

Warnings Use with caution in patients with hyperthyroidism, diabetes mellitus, prostatic hypertrophy, ischemic, heart disease; use with caution in patients >60 years of age

Dosage Forms

Capsule: 60 mg

Capsule, timed release, as hydrochloride: 120 mg

Drops, oral, as hydrochloride: 7.5 mg/0.8 mL (15 mL)

Liquid, as hydrochloride: 15 mg/5 mL (120 mL); 30 mg/5 mL (120 mL, 240 mL, 473 mL)

Tablet, as hydrochloride: 30 mg, 60 mg

Tablet:

- Extended release, as sulfate: 120 mg
- Timed release, as hydrochloride: 120 mg

Overdosage Treatment There is no specific antidote for pseudoephedrine intoxication and the bulk of the treatment is supportive. Hyperactivity and agitation usually respond to reduced sensory input; however, with extreme agitation, haloperidol (2-5 mg I.M. for adults) may be required. Hyperthermia is best treated with external cooling measures, or when severe or unresponsive, muscle paralysis with pancuronium may be needed. Hypertension is usually transient and generally does not require treatment unless severe. For diastolic blood pressures >110 mm Hg, a nitroprusside infusion should be initiated. Seizures usually respond to lorazepam or diazepam I.V. and/or phenytoin maintenance regimens.

Drug Interactions MAO inhibitors, beta-adrenergic blocking agents; sympathomimetic agents

Pregnancy Risk Factor C

Pregnancy Implications Distributes into breast milk

Patient Information Do not exceed recommended dosage and do not use for longer than 3-5 days

Nursing Implications Do not crush extended release drug product

Additional Information

Pseudoephedrine hydrochloride: Cenafed® syrup [OTC], Decofed® syrup [OTC], Neofed® [OTC], Novafed®, Sudafed® [OTC], Sudafed® 12 Hour [OTC], Sudafed® Tablet [OTC], Sufedrin® [OTC]

Pseudoephedrine sulfate: Afrinol® [OTC]

Specific References

Pentel P, "Toxicity of Over-the-Counter Stimulants," *JAMA*, 1984, 252(14):1898-903.

Salmon J and Nicholson D, "DIC and Rhabdomyolysis Following Pseudoephedrine Overdose," *Am J Emerg Med*, 1988, 6(5):545-6.

Wright S and Tomassoni A, "Acute Myocardial Infarction Following Therapeutic Use of Pseudoephedrine," *Vet Hum Toxicol*, 1994, 36:366.

Pseudoephedrine Hydrochloride *see* Pseudoephedrine *on page 661*

Pseudoephedrine Sulfate *see* Pseudoephedrine *on page 661*

Psyquil® *see* Triflupromazine Hydrochloride *on page 770*

PTU *see* Propylthiouracil *on page 660*

Pulmozyme® *see* Dornase Alfa *on page 299*

Punktyl® *see* Lorazepam *on page 482*

Puresis® *see* Furosemide *on page 373*

Purex *see* Sodium Chloride *on page 698*

Purge® [OTC] *see* Castor Oil *on page 189*

Purgoxin® *see* Digoxin *on page 284*

Purochin® *see* Urokinase *on page 779*

Purodigin® *see* Digitoxin *on page 283*

PVP-iodine *see* Povidone-Iodine *on page 635*

Pyrazinamide (peer a zin' a mide)

CAS Number 98-96-4

Brand Names Aldinamide®; Zinamide®

Synonyms Pyrazinoic Acid Amide

Use Adjunctive treatment of tuberculosis when primary and secondary agents cannot be used or have failed

Mechanism of Action Converted to pyrazinoic acid in susceptible strains of *Mycobacterium* which lowers the pH of the environment

Adverse Reactions

Central nervous system: Malaise, seizures, fever

Dermatologic: Urticaria, rash, photosensitivity

Endocrine & metabolic: Gout, hyperuricemia

Gastrointestinal: Nausea, vomiting, anorexia

Hepatic: Hepatotoxicity, jaundice

Neuromuscular & skeletal: Arthralgia

Signs & Symptoms of Acute Overdose Gout, gastrointestinal upset, photophobia, hyperuricemia, hepatitis (>3 g/day dosage)

Toxicodynamics/Kinetics

Peak effect: Within 2 hours

Absorption: Oral: Well absorbed from gastrointestinal tract

Distribution: V_d: 0.57-0.74 L/kg; widely distributed into body tissues and fluids including the liver, lungs, and CSF

Protein binding: 10% to 20%

Metabolism: In the liver

Half-life: 9-10 hours, increased with reduced renal or hepatic function

Time to peak serum concentration: Within 2 hours

Elimination: Urine (4% as unchanged drug)

Usual Dosage Oral (calculate dose on ideal body weight rather than total body weight):

Children: 15-30 mg/kg/day in divided doses every 12-24 hours; daily dose not to exceed 2 g

Adults: 15-30 mg/kg/day in 3-4 divided doses; maximum daily dose: 3 g/day

Dosing adjustment in renal impairment: Cl_{cr} <50 mL/minute: Avoid use or reduce dose to 12-20 mg/kg/day

Dosing adjustment in hepatic impairment: Reduce dose

Contraindications Severe hepatitis, porphyria, hypersensitivity to pyrazinamide or any component

Warnings Administer with at least one other effective agent for tuberculosis; use with caution in patients with renal failure, gout, or diabetes mellitus

Dosage Forms Tablet: 500 mg

Overdosage Treatment

Decontamination: Ipecac or lavage/activated charcoal with cathartic

Enhancement of elimination: Multiple dosing of activated charcoal may be effective

Drug Interactions Isoniazid (decreased INH serum levels)

Pregnancy Risk Factor C

Monitoring Parameters Baseline liver function should be obtained prior to therapy then monitored during therapy; periodic liver function tests, serum uric acid

Patient Information Notify physician if fever, loss of appetite, malaise, nausea, vomiting, darkened urine occur

(Continued)

Pyrazinamide *(Continued)*

Specific References

Combs DL, O'Brien RJ, and Geiter LJ, "USPHS Tuberculosis Short-Course Chemotherapy Trial 21: Effectiveness, Toxicity, and Acceptability: The Report of Final Results," *Ann Intern Med*, 1990, 112(6):397-406.

Herlevsen P, Nielsen C, and Pedersen JT, "Convulsions After Treatment With Pyrazinamide," *Tubercle*, 1987, 68(2):145-6.

Lacroix C, Hoang TP, Nouveau J, et al, "Pharmacokinetics of Pyrazinamide and Its Metabolites in Healthy Subjects," *Eur J Clin Pharmacol*, 1989, 36(4):395-400.

Van Scoy RE and Wilkowske CJ, "Antituberculous Agents," *Mayo Clin Proc*, 1992, 67(2):179-87.

Pyrazinoic Acid Amide *see* Pyrazinamide *on previous page*

Pyribenzamine® *see* Tripelennamine *on page 776*

Pyrimethamine (peer i meth' a meen)

CAS Number 58-14-0

Brand Names Daraprim®

Use Prophylaxis of malaria due to susceptible strains of plasmodia; used in conjunction with quinine and sulfadiazine for the treatment of uncomplicated attacks of chloroquine-resistant *P. falciparum* malaria; used in conjunction with fast-acting schizonticide to initiate transmission control and suppression cure; synergistic combination with sulfonamide in treatment of toxoplasmosis

Mechanism of Action Inhibits parasitic dihydrofolate reductase, resulting in inhibition of tetrahydrofolic acid synthesis

Adverse Reactions

Central nervous system: Convulsions, ataxia

Gastrointestinal: Anorexia, abdominal cramps, vomiting, atrophic glossitis

Hematologic: Megaloblastic anemia, thrombocytopenia, leukopenia, neutropenia, agranulocytosis, granulocytopenia; pancytopenia

Neuromuscular & skeletal: Tremors

Respiratory: Respiratory failure

Signs & Symptoms of Acute Overdose Megaloblastic anemia, vomiting, seizures, fever, apnea, tachycardia

Toxicodynamics/Kinetics

Absorption: Oral: Well absorbed from intestinal tract

Distribution: V_d: Adults: 2.3-3.1 L/kg; widely distributed; mainly concentrated in blood cells, kidneys, lungs, liver, and spleen; crosses into CSF

Protein binding: 87%

Metabolism: Hepatic

Half-life: 80-95 hours

Time to peak serum concentration: Within 1.5-8 hours

Elimination: 20% to 30% excreted unchanged in urine

Usual Dosage Oral:

Malaria chemoprophylaxis:

- Children: 0.5 mg/kg once weekly; not to exceed 25 mg/dose **or**
- Children:
  - <4 years: 6.25 mg once weekly
  - 4-10 years: 12.5 mg once weekly
- Children >10 years and Adults: 25 mg once weekly
- Dosage should begin 1 day before entering endemic area and be continued for all age groups for at least 6-10 weeks after leaving endemic areas

Chloroquine-resistant *P. falciparum* malaria (when used in conjunction with quinine and sulfadiazine):

- Children 4-10 years: 25 mg/day once daily for 2 days
- Children >10 years and Adults: 25 mg twice daily for 2 days

Toxoplasmosis (with sulfadiazine or trisulfapyrimidines):

- Children: 1 mg/kg/day divided into 2 equal daily doses; decrease dose after 2-4 days by ½, continue for about 1 month; used with 100 mg sulfadiazine/kg/day divided every 6 hours; **or** 2 mg/kg/day divided every 12 hours for 3 days followed by 1 mg/kg/day (maximum: 25 mg/day) once daily for 4 weeks
- Adults: 50-75 mg/day together with 1-4 g of a sulfonamide for 1-3 weeks depending on patient's tolerance and response then reduce both drug dosages to ½ and continue for additional 4-5 weeks; leucovorin may be given to prevent hematologic problems due to folic acid deficiency

Contraindications Megaloblastic anemia; known hypersensitivity to pyrimethamine, chloroguanide; resistant malaria

Warnings When used for longer than 3-4 days, it is advisable to given leucovorin to prevent hematologic complications

Dosage Forms Tablet: 25 mg

Stability Pyrimethamine tablets may be crushed to prepare oral suspensions of the drug in water, cherry syrup or sucrose-containing solutions at a concentration of 1 mg/mL; stable at room temperature for 5-7 days

Overdosage Treatment

Decontamination: Activated charcoal with cathartic/lavage

Supportive therapy: Initiate with I.V. fluids; assure respiratory patency; treat seizures aggressively with benzodiazepines, follow with barbiturates, if necessary; other complications of seizures (acid base, etc), treat conventionally as necessary

Antidote: Leucovorin 10 mg/m^2 every 6 hours daily for 3 days followed by folic acid 10 mg/day if hematologic toxicity is present

Antidote(s)

Leucovorin Calcium *on page 1437*

Drug Interactions Para-aminobenzoic acid, sulfonamides

Pregnancy Risk Factor C

Pregnancy Implications Crosses placenta; appears in breast milk

Monitoring Parameters Monitor CBC and platelet counts every 2 weeks

Patient Information Take with meals to minimize vomiting; begin malaria prophylaxis at least 1 week prior to departure

Nursing Implications Monitor complete blood counts and platelet counts twice weekly

Additional Information Leucovorin may be given to prevent hematologic problems due to folic acid deficiency

Specific References

Akinyanju O, Goddell JC, and Ahmed I, "Pyrimethamine Poisoning," *Br Med J*, 1973, 4(885):147-8.

Chute JP, Decker CF, and Cotelingam J, "Severe Megaloblastic Anemia Complicating Pyrimethamine Therapy," *Ann Intern Med*, 1995, 122:884-5.

Phillips-Howard PA and West LJ, "Serious Adverse Drug Reactions to Pyrimethamine-Sulfadoxine, Pyrimethamine-Dapsone, and to Amodiaquine in Britain," *J R Soc Med*, 1990, 83(2):82-5.

White NJ, "Clinical Pharmacokinetics of Antimalarial Drugs," *Clin Pharmacokinet*, 1985, 10(3):187-215.

Quaalude® *see* Methaqualone Hydrochloride *on page 511*

Quazepam (kway' ze pam)

CAS Number 36735-22-5

Brand Names Doral®; Dormalin®; Temodal®

Use Short-term treatment of insomnia

Mechanism of Action Depresses all levels of the CNS, including the limbic and reticular formation, probably through the increased action of gamma-aminobutyric acid (GABA), which is a major inhibitory neurotransmitter in the brain

Adverse Reactions

Central nervous system: Daytime sedation, amnesia, confusion, dizziness, hallucinations, headache, ataxia

Gastrointestinal: Dry mouth, nausea, vomiting

Hepatic: Cholestatic jaundice

Miscellaneous: Physical and psychological dependence may occur with prolonged use

Signs & Symptoms of Acute Overdose Somnolence, confusion, coma, hyporeflexia, hypoactive reflexes, dyspnea, hypotension, slurred speech, ataxia

Toxicodynamics/Kinetics Studies have shown that the elderly are more sensitive to the effects of benzodiazepines as compared to younger adults

Absorption: Rapid through gastrointestinal tract

Distribution: V_d: 5-8.6 L/kg; distributed widely throughout body

Protein binding: 95%

Metabolism: In the liver to two active compounds (2-oxoquazepam and N-desalkyl-2-oxoquazepam)

Half-life:
- Parent: 25-41 hours
- Active metabolite: 40-114 hours
- In the elderly:
  - Parent: 53 hours
  - Active metabolite: 39-73 hours

Time to peak serum concentration: 2 hours

Elimination: Excreted in urine (31%) and feces (23%)

Usual Dosage Adults: Oral: Initial: 15 mg at bedtime, in some patients the dose may be reduced to 7.5 mg after a few nights

Dosing adjustment in hepatic impairment: Dose reduction may be necessary

Contraindications Narrow-angle glaucoma, known hypersensitivity to quazepam, cross-sensitivity with other benzodiazepines may occur; severe uncontrolled pain, sleep apnea

Warnings Abrupt discontinuance may precipitate withdrawal or rebound insomnia; has potential for drug dependence and abuse

(Continued)

Quazepam *(Continued)*

Dosage Forms Tablet: 7.5 mg, 15 mg

Reference Range Mean plasma level of 148 ng/mL 1.5 hours after ingestion of 25 mg

Overdosage Treatment

Decontamination: Ipecac or lavage/activated charcoal with cathartic

Supportive therapy: Treatment for benzodiazepine overdose is supportive. Rarely is mechanical ventilation required. Flumazenil has been shown to selectively block the binding of benzodiazepines to CNS receptors, resulting in a reversal of benzodiazepine-induced CNS depression.

Enhancement of elimination: Multiple dosing of activated charcoal may be useful

Antidote(s)

Flumazenil *on page 1428*

Drug Interactions CNS depressants may increase CNS adverse effects; cimetidine may decrease and enzyme inducers may increase the metabolism of quazepam

Pregnancy Risk Factor X

Pregnancy Implications Distributes into breast milk

Monitoring Parameters Respiratory and cardiovascular status

Patient Information Do not take any other CNS depressants, including alcohol; may cause daytime sedation

Nursing Implications Provide safety measures (ie, side rails, night light, call button); remove smoking materials from area; supervise ambulation

Additional Information More likely than triazolam to cause daytime sedation and fatigue; is classified as a long-acting benzodiazepine hypnotic (like flurazepam - Dalmane®), this long duration of action may prevent withdrawal symptoms when therapy is discontinued. There is little experience with this drug in the elderly; but because of its long duration of action, it is probably not a drug of choice.

Specific References

Chung M, Hilbert JM, Gural RP, et al, "Multiple Dose Quazepam Kinetics," *Clin Pharmacol Ther*, 1984, 35(4):520-4.

Hilbert JM, Gural RP, Symchowicz S, et al, "Excretion of Quazepam Into Human Breast Milk," *J Clin Pharmacol*, 1984, 24(10):457-62.

Quelidrine® *see* Ammonium Chloride *on page 118*

Quensyl® *see* Hydroxychloroquine Sulfate *on page 411*

Quibron®-T *see* Theophylline *on page 735*

Quibron®-T/SR *see* Theophylline *on page 735*

Quiess® *see* Hydroxyzine *on page 414*

Quinaglute® Dura-Tabs® *see* Quinidine *on page 668*

Quinagolide

CAS Number 87056-78-8; 94424-50-7

Synonyms CV-205-502

Use Treat hyperprolactinemia

Mechanism of Action Potent nonergot dopamine-D_2 receptor agonist; octahydrobenzoly (g) quinolone compound

Adverse Reactions

Cardiovascular: Hypotension (orthostatic), palpitations, pre-eclampsia

Central nervous system: Headache, dizziness, lethargy, psychosis, delusions

Endocrine & metabolic: Hot flashes

Gastrointestinal: Weight loss, nausea (60%), vomiting (35%), constipation, anorexia, dry mouth

Neuromuscular & skeletal: Muscle cramps

Respiratory: Nasal congestion

Toxicodynamics/Kinetics

Onset of action: 2 hours

Peak onset: 4 hours

Usual Dosage Hyperprolactinemia: 0.03-0.5 mg/day; usual dosage range: 0.05-0.1 mg/day at bedtime with food; maximum dose: 1.65 mg/day

Contraindications Hypersensitivity to quinagolide

Warnings Use with caution in patients with previous reactions to bromocriptine, pergolide, ergot derivatives, cardiovascular disease, pre-eclampsia, renal/hepatic insufficiency, psychiatric disorders, or abnormalities with normal menstruation

Overdosage Treatment

Decontamination: Lavage/activated charcoal with sorbitol

Enhancement of elimination: Multiple dosing of activated charcoal may be effective

Test Interactions Lowers serum prolactin level; may reduce serum thyroxine level; may increase serum estradiol levels

Additional Information Especially useful in patients resistant to bromocriptine; may be useful in the treatment of acromegaly, Parkinson's disease, or for use in lactation inhibition; promotes reduction in pituitary microadena size; decreases galactorrhea

Specific References

Barnett PS, Dawson JM, Butler J, et al, "CV205-502, A New Non-Ergot Dopamine Agonist, Reduces Prolactinoma Size in Man," *Clin Endocrinol (Oxf)*, 1990, 33(2):307-16.

Vance ML, Lipper M, Klibanski A, et al, "Treatment of Prolactin-Secreting Pituitary Macroadenomas With the Long-Acting Non-Ergot Dopamine Agonist CV 205-502," *Ann Intern Med*, 1990, 112(9):668-73.

Quinalan® *see* Quinidine *on next page*

Quinalbarbitone Sodium *see* Secobarbital Sodium *on page 693*

Quin-Amino® *see* Quinine Sulfate *on page 671*

Quinaminoph® *see* Quinine Sulfate *on page 671*

Quinamm® *see* Quinine Sulfate *on page 671*

Quinapril Hydrochloride (kwin' a pril)

Related Information

ACE Inhibitors Comparison *on page 1636-1637*

CAS Number 85441-61-8; 82586-55-8

Brand Names Accupril®; Accuprin®; Accupro®; Acequin®; Acupril®; Quinazil®

Use Treatment of hypertension either alone or in combination with other antihypertensive agents, congestive heart failure

Mechanism of Action Competitive inhibition of angiotensin I being converted to angiotensin II, a potent vasoconstrictor, through the angiotensin I-converting enzyme (ACE) activity, with resultant lower levels of angiotensin II which causes an increase in plasma renin activity and a reduction in aldosterone secretion

Adverse Reactions

Cardiovascular: Hypotension, myocardial infarction, angina pectoris, hypotension (orthostatic), rhythm disturbances, tachycardia, vasculitis, palpitations, syncope, flushing, peripheral edema

Central nervous system: Dizziness, headache, fatigue, malaise, depression, somnolence, insomnia, fever

Dermatologic: Urticaria, pruritus

Endocrine & metabolic: Hypoglycemia

Gastrointestinal: Diarrhea, abdominal pain, anorexia, constipation, flatulence, dry mouth, pancreatitis

Hematologic: Neutropenia, bone marrow depression

Hepatic: Hepatitis

Neuromuscular & skeletal: Gout, joint pain, shoulder pain

Ocular: Blurred vision

Renal: Increased BUN and serum creatinine

Respiratory: Upper respiratory symptoms, cough, bronchospasm, bronchitis, sinusitis

Miscellaneous: Chest discomfort, pharyngeal pain, sweating, diaphoresis

Toxicodynamics/Kinetics

Protein binding: 97%

Metabolism: Rapidly hydrolyzed to quinaprilat, the active metabolite

Half-life, elimination:

- Quinapril: 0.8 hours
- Quinaprilat: 2 hours

Time to peak serum concentration:

- Quinapril: 1 hour
- Quinaprilat: ~2 hours

Elimination: 50% to 60% of quinapril excreted in urine primarily as quinaprilat; renal clearance: 66 mL/minute

Usual Dosage Adults: Oral:

Hypertension: Initial: 10 mg once daily, adjust according to blood pressure response at peak and trough blood levels; in general, the normal dosage range is 20-80 mg/day

Congestive heart failure: Initial: 5 mg; normal dose: 5-30 mg/day

Dosing adjustment in renal impairment:

- Cl_{cr} >60 mL/minute: Administer 10 mg/day
- Cl_{cr} 30-60 mL/minute: 5 mg/day
- Cl_{cr} 10-30 mL/minute: 2.5 mg/day

Dosing comments in hepatic impairment: In patients with alcoholic cirrhosis, hydrolysis of quinapril to quinaprilat is impaired; however, the subsequent elimination of quinaprilat is unaltered

Contraindications Hypersensitivity to quinapril or history of angioedema induced by other ACE inhibitors

(Continued)

Quinapril Hydrochloride *(Continued)*

Warnings Use with caution in patients with renal insufficiency, autoimmune disease, renal artery stenosis; excessive hypotension may be more likely in volume-depleted patients; angioedema may occur during angiotensin-converting enzyme inhibitor therapy; quinapril should be discontinued if laryngeal stridor or angioedema of the face, tongue, or glottis is observed

Dosage Forms Tablet: 5 mg, 10 mg, 20 mg, 40 mg

Stability Store at room temperature

Reference Range Following a 10 mg dose, peak serum levels of quinapril and quinaprilat are 65 mg/mL and 223 ng/mL respectively

Overdosage Treatment

Decontamination: Lavage/activated charcoal

Supportive therapy: Following initiation of essential overdose management, toxic symptom treatment and supportive treatment should be initiated. Hypotension usually responds to I.V. fluids or Trendelenburg positioning. If unresponsive to these measures, the use of a parenteral inotrope may be required (eg, norepinephrine 0.1-0.2 mcg/kg/minute titrated to response). Seizures commonly respond to diazepam (I.V. 5-10 mg bolus in adults every 15 minutes if needed up to a total of 30 mg; I.V. 0.25-0.4 mg/kg/dose up to a total of 10 mg in children) or to phenytoin or phenobarbital. Naloxone has been shown to antagonize hypotensive effects of captopril, but routine use in an overdose situation due to this agent is uncertain.

Enhancement of elimination: Multiple dosing of activated charcoal may be effective; hemodialysis is not effective

Test Interactions ↑ potassium (S)

Drug Interactions

Decreased effect: NSAIDs

Increased levels/toxicity: Lithium, potassium or potassium-sparing diuretics (hyperkalemia), cyclosporine (nephrotoxicity)

Pregnancy Risk Factor D

Monitoring Parameters BUN, serum creatinine, renal function; nausea, headache, diarrhea, change in taste, cough

Patient Information Notify physician if vomiting, diarrhea, excessive perspiration, or dehydration should occur; also if swelling of face, lips, tongue, or difficulty in breathing occurs or if persistent cough develops

Nursing Implications May cause depression in some patients; discontinue if angioedema of the face, extremities, lips, tongue, or glottis occurs; watch for hypotensive effects within 1-3 hours of first dose or new higher dose

Additional Information

Patients taking diuretics are at risk for developing hypotension on initial dosing; to prevent this, discontinue diuretics 2-3 days prior to initiating quinapril; may restart diuretics if blood pressure is not controlled by quinapril alone

Due to frequent decreases in glomerular filtration (also creatinine clearance) with aging, elderly patients may have exaggerated responses to ACE inhibitors; differences in clinical response due to hepatic changes are not observed. ACE inhibitors may be preferred agents in elderly patients with CHF and diabetes mellitus. Diabetic proteinuria is reduced and insulin sensitivity is enhanced. In general, the side effect profile is favorable in elderly and causes little or no CNS confusion; use lowest dose recommendations initially.

Specific References

Alcocer L, Novoa G, and Sotres D, "Quinapril in the Treatment of Hypertension in Primary Care Centers," *Clin Ther*, 1993, 15(6):1021-30.

Hayaski H, Ohsugi S, Ishihara M, et al, "Effect of Quinapril on the Circadian Blood Pressure Pattern Evaluated by Periodic Analysis of Covariance," *Am J Ther*, 1995, 2:213-49.

Herings RM, deBoer A, Stricker BH, et al, "Hypoglycemia Associated With Use of Inhibitors of Angiotensin Converting Enzyme," *Lancet*, 1995, 345:1195-8.

Wadworth AN and Brogden RN, "Quinapril: A Review of Its Pharmacological Properties and Therapeutic Efficacy in Cardiovascular Disorders," *Drugs*, 1991, 41(3):378-99.

Quinazil® *see* Quinapril Hydrochloride *on previous page*

Quindan® *see* Quinine Sulfate *on page 671*

Quine® [OTC] *see* Quinine Sulfate *on page 671*

Quinidex® Extentabs® *see* Quinidine *on this page*

Quinidine (kwin' i deen)

Related Information

Therapeutic Drugs Associated With Hallucinations *on page 1558-1559*

CAS Number 27555-34-6; 50-54-4; 56-52-2; 6151-39-9; 63717-04-4; 65484-56-2; 6591-63-5; 7054-25-3; 72402-50-7; 747-45-4

Brand Names Biquin®; Cardioquin®; Cin-Quin®; Kiditard®; Kinidin®; Quinaglute® Dura-Tabs®; Quinalan®; Quinidex® Extentabs®; Quini® Durules®; Quinora®; Systodin®

Synonyms Quinidine Bisulfate; Quinidine Gluconate; Quinidine Hydrochloride; Quinidine Lactate; Quinidine Polygalacturonate; Quinidine Sulfate

Use Prophylaxis after cardioversion of fibrillation (atrial) and/or flutter to maintain normal sinus rhythm; also used to prevent reoccurrence of paroxysmal tachycardia (ventricular), paroxysmal A-V junctional rhythm, paroxysmal tachycardia (ventricular), paroxysmal fibrillation (atrial), and atrial or ventricular premature contractions; also has activity against *Plasmodium falciparum* malaria

Mechanism of Action Depresses phase O of the action potential; decreases myocardial excitability and conduction velocity, and myocardial contractility by decreasing sodium influx during depolarization and potassium efflux in repolarization; also reduces calcium transport across cell membrane; class I antiarrhythmic

Adverse Reactions

Cardiovascular: Syncope, hypotension, tachycardia, heart block, fibrillation (ventricular), vascular collapse, severe hypotension with rapid I.V. administration, torsade de pointes

Central nervous system: Dizziness, confusion, delirium, hallucinations, agitation, psychosis, headache

Dermatologic: Angioedema, pruritus, rash, may exacerbate psoriasis, eczematous dermatitis

Gastrointestinal: Nausea, vomiting, abdominal pain, cramps, diarrhea

Hematologic: Blood dyscrasias, thrombocytopenic purpura, hemolysis, agranulocytosis, aplastic anemia

Hepatic: Cholestatic jaundice

Ocular: Impaired vision, photophobia, diplopia

Otic: Ototoxicity, tinnitus

Respiratory: Apnea, respiratory depression

Miscellaneous: Fever with leukocytosis, can cause drug-induced systemic lupus erythematosus or SICCA syndrome or drug fever, cinchonism

Signs & Symptoms of Acute Overdose Ataxia, dementia, photosensitivity, drowsiness, rhabdomyolysis, respiratory distress with shallow respirations, thrombocytopenia, heart block, myoglobinuria, syncope, memory loss, lichenoid eruptions, hyperthermia, A-V block, dementia, coma, apnea, hypoglycemia, bradycardia, myasthenia gravis (exacerbation or precipitation of), mydriasis, depression, severe hypotension, anuria, absence of P waves, QRS prolongation, P-R prolongation, and Q-T prolongation, ventricular arrhythmias, hallucinations, and seizures, leukopenia; neutropenia; agranulocytosis; granulocytopenia

Toxicodynamics/Kinetics

Onset of action: I.M.: 15 minutes

Duration: Oral:

- Regular tablets or capsules: 6-8 hours
- Extended-release tablets: ~12 hours

Absorption: Well from gastrointestinal tract

Distribution: V_d: Adults: 2-3.5 L/kg, decreased V_d with congestive heart failure, malaria, increased V_d with cirrhosis; cirrhosis, or acute myocardial infarction; all tissues except brain; concentrates in heart, liver, kidneys, and skeletal muscle

Protein binding:

- Newborns: 60% to 70%
- Adults: 80% to 90%
- Decreased protein-binding with cyanotic congenital heart disease

Metabolism: Extensive in the liver

Bioavailability:

- Sulfate: 80%
- Gluconate: 70%

Half-life:

- Children: 2.5-6.7 hours
- Adults: 6-8 hours
- Increased half-life with elderly, cirrhosis and congestive heart failure

Time to peak plasma concentration: 1-3 hours

Elimination: Urine (15% to 25% as unchanged drug); clearance: 4.7 mL/minute/kg

Usual Dosage Note: Dosage expressed in terms of the salt: 267 mg of quinidine gluconate = 275 mg of quinidine polygalacturonate = 200 mg of quinidine sulfate

Children: Test dose for idiosyncratic reaction (sulfate, oral or gluconate, I.M.): 2 mg/kg or 60 mg/m^2

- Oral (quinidine sulfate): 15-60 mg/kg/day in 4-5 divided doses or 6 mg/kg every 4-6 hours; usual 30 mg/kg/day or 900 mg/m^2/day given in 5 daily doses
- I.V. **not** recommended (quinidine gluconate): 2-10 mg/kg/dose every 3-6 hours as needed

Adults: Test dose: Oral, I.M.: 200 mg administered several hours before full dosage (to determine possibility of idiosyncratic reaction)

- Oral (sulfate): 100-600 mg/dose every 4-6 hours; begin at 200 mg/dose and titrate to desired effect (maximum daily dose: 3-4 g); sustained release formulation: 300-600 mg every 8-12 hours

(Continued)

Quinidine *(Continued)*

Oral (gluconate): 324-972 mg every 8-12 hours
Oral (polygalacturonate): 275 mg every 8-12 hours
I.M.: 400 mg/dose every 4-6 hours
I.V.: 200-400 mg/dose diluted and given at a rate ≤10 mg/minute

Dosing adjustment in renal impairment: Cl_{cr} <10 mL/minute: Administer 75% of normal dose

Dosing adjustment/comments in hepatic impairment: Larger loading dose may be indicated, reduce maintenance doses by 50% and monitor serum levels closely

Contraindications Patients with complete A-V block with an A-V junctional or idioventricular pacemaker; patients with intraventricular conduction defects (marked widening of QRS complex); patients with cardiac glycoside-induced A-V conduction disorders; hypersensitivity to the drug or cinchona derivatives, myasthenia gravis

Warnings May cause syncope, most likely due to tachycardia (ventricular) or fibrillation, syncope may subside spontaneously, but occasionally may be fatal; discontinue quinidine if syncope occurs; myocardial depression, sick sinus syndrome, incomplete A-V block, cardiac glycoside intoxication, hepatic and/or renal insufficiency, myasthenia gravis; hemolysis may occur in patients with G-6-PD (glucose-6-phosphate dehydrogenase) deficiency; quinidine-induced hepatitis, including granulomatous hepatitis, increased serum AST and alkaline phosphatase concentrations, and jaundice may occur; use with caution in nursing women

Dosage Forms

Injection, as gluconate: 80 mg/mL (10 mL)
Tablet, as polygalacturonate: 275 mg
Tablet, as sulfate: 200 mg, 300 mg
Tablet:
Sustained action, as sulfate: 300 mg
Sustained release, as gluconate: 324 mg

Stability Do not use discolored parenteral solution

Reference Range Therapeutic: 2-5 μg/mL (SI: 6.2-15.4 μmol/L). Patient dependent therapeutic response occurs at levels of 3-6 μg/mL (SI: 9.2-18.5 μmol/L). Optimal therapeutic level is method dependent; >8 μg/mL (SI: >24 μmol/L) are associated with cinchonism while levels >14 ng/L are associated with cardiac toxicity

Overdosage Treatment

Decontamination: Emesis or lavage/activated charcoal with cathartic

Supportive therapy: Electrolyte balance should be monitored and treated, especially when refractory arrhythmias develop. Sodium bicarbonate 1-2 mEq/kg I.V. (or 0.5-1 mEq/kg in children) may decrease conduction defects. Phenytoin or lidocaine are often effective at controlling drug-induced arrhythmias, while phenytoin is preferred due to its beneficial effects on A-V conduction velocity. Torsade de pointes can be treated with magnesium sulfate or overdrive pacemaker.

Enhancement of elimination: Multiple dosing of activated charcoal is effective; hemodialysis or charcoal hemoperfusion have little effect; slightly dialyzable (5% to 20%)

Antidote(s)

Sodium Bicarbonate *on page 1467*

Test Interactions Increases prothrombin time (S) may interfere with urinary analysis of catecholamines; decreases glucose

Diagnostic Tests/Procedures

Quinidine, Serum *on page 1344*

Drug Interactions Quinidine potentiates nondepolarizing and depolarizing muscle relaxants; verapamil, amiodarone, alkalinizing agents, and cimetidine may increase quinidine serum concentrations; phenobarbital, phenytoin, and rifampin may decrease quinidine serum concentrations; quinidine may increase plasma concentration of digoxin, closely monitor digoxin concentrations, digoxin dosage may need to be reduced (by one-half) when quinidine is initiated, new steady-state digoxin plasma concentrations occur in 5-7 days; beta-blockers and quinidine may cause increased bradycardia; quinidine may enhance coumarin anticoagulants. Cimetidine impairs elimination of quinidine; quinidine and verapamil may result in severe hypotension; nifedipine may reduce serum quinidine levels. Amiloride may enhance to proarrhythmic effects of quinidine on QRS duration. Erythromycin coadministered with quinidine may reduce quinidine clearance; concomitant use of quinidine and erythromycin can result in increased quinidine levels.

Pregnancy Risk Factor C (no evidence for teratogenic effects)

Pregnancy Implications Crosses the placenta; excreted in breast milk

Monitoring Parameters Complete blood counts, liver and renal function tests, should be routinely performed during long-term administration

Patient Information Patients should notify their physician if rash, fever, unusual bleeding or bruising, ringing in the ears or visual disturbances occur

Nursing Implications When injecting I.M., aspirate carefully to avoid injection into a vessel; do not crush sustained-release drug product

Additional Information Sulfate form is the standard dosage preparation

Quinidine gluconate: Duraquin®, Quinaglute® Dura-Tabs®, Quinalan®, Quinatime®

Quinidine polygalacturonate: Cardioquin®

Quinidine sulfate: Cin-Quin®, Quinidex® Extentabs®, Quinora®

Specific References

Alloway JA and Salsta MP, "Quinidine-Induced Rheumatic Syndromes," *Semin Arthritis Rheum*, 1995, 24:315-22.

Bauman JL, Bauerfeind RA, Hoff JV, et al, "Torsade de Pointes Due to Quinidine: Observation in 31 Patients," *Am Heart J*, 1984, 107(3):425-30.

Daoud EG, Niebauer MJ, Man KC, et al, "Prospective Assessment of Quinidine-Induced Q-T Prolongation and Proarrhythmia in Hospitalized Patients," *J Am Coll Cardiol*, 1995, 220.

Haapanen EJ and Pellinen TJ, "Hemoperfusion in Quinidine Intoxication," *Acta Med Scand*, 1981, 210(6):515-6.

Lesne M, Devos M, and Reynaert M, "Enterogastric Cycle and Intoxication With Hydroquinidine: A Case Report," *Clin Toxicol*, 1981, 18(6):659-62.

Spinler SA, Cheng JW, Kindwall KE, et al, "Possible Inhibition of Hepatic Metabolism of Quinidine by Erythromycin," *Clin Pharmacol Ther*, 1955, 57:89-94.

Swiryn S and Kim SS, "Quinidine-Induced Syncope," *Arch Intern Med*, 1983, 143(2):314-6.

Wang L, Sheldon RS, Mitchell LB, et al, "Amiloride-Quinidine Interaction: Adverse Outcomes," *Clin Pharmacol Ther*, 1994, 56(6 Pt 1):659-67.

Quinidine Bisulfate *see* Quinidine *on page 668*

Quinidine Gluconate *see* Quinidine *on page 668*

Quinidine Hydrochloride *see* Quinidine *on page 668*

Quinidine Lactate *see* Quinidine *on page 668*

Quinidine Polygalacturonate *see* Quinidine *on page 668*

Quinidine Sulfate *see* Quinidine *on page 668*

Quini® Durules® *see* Quinidine *on page 668*

Quinine Sulfate (kwye' nine)

Related Information

Toxins Which Should be Lavaged With Solutions Other Than Water *on page 1635*

CAS Number 130-95-0

Brand Names Formula Q® [OTC]; Legatrin® [OTC]; M-KYA® [OTC]; Quin-Amino®; Quinaminoph®; Quinamm®; Quindan®; Quine® [OTC]; Quiphile®; Q-vel® [OTC]

Use Suppression or treatment of chloroquine-resistant *P. falciparum* malaria; treatment of *Babesia microti* infection; prevention and treatment of nocturnal recumbency leg muscle cramps

Mechanism of Action Not completely understood; depresses oxygen uptake and carbohydrate metabolism; intercalates into DNA, disrupting the parasite's replication and transcription; affects calcium distribution within muscle fibers and decreases the excitability of the motor end-plate region; interferes with function of plasmodial DNA; also, recent evidence suggests it may also do this through ↑ pH of plasmodial organelles; local anesthetic action and analgesic properties

Adverse Reactions

Cardiovascular: Flushing of the skin, angina, syncope, cardiac arrhythmias, hypotension

Central nervous system: CNS depression, seizures, fever, headache, fear, restlessness, psychosis, sweating, dizziness, ataxia, myasthenia gravis (exacerbation or precipitation of)

Dermatologic: Rash, pruritus, acne

Endocrine & metabolic: Hypoglycemia

Gastrointestinal: Nausea, vomiting, epigastric pain, altered taste

Hematologic: Hemolysis in G-6-PD deficiency, thrombocytopenia, leukopenia, neutropenia, agranulocytosis, granulocytopenia

Hepatic: Hepatitis, elevated liver function tests

Ocular: Nightblindness, diplopia, optic atrophy, blurred vision, photophobia

Otic: Ototoxicity, tinnitus

Respiratory: Apnea, respiratory depression

Miscellaneous: Symptoms of cinchonism, hypersensitivity reactions

Signs & Symptoms of Acute Overdose Cinchonism-ototoxicity; tinnitus, deafness, hypokalemia, headache, myoglobinuria, bradycardia, nausea, methemoglobinemia, abdominal pain, rhabdomyolysis, visual disturbance, A-V block, erythema multiforme, blood dyscrasias, mydriasis, photosensitivity, nephritis, toxic epidermal necrolysis, hypoglycemia, cardiac arrhythmias, nystagmus, hypotension, renal injury, coma, confusion, hemolysis, hypoprothrombinemia, vision color changes (green tinge), vision color changes (red tinge); urine discoloration (black), urine discoloration (brown), urine discoloration (dark), urine discoloration (red-brown)

(Continued)

Quinine Sulfate *(Continued)*

Toxicodynamics/Kinetics

Onset of action: 1-3 hours

Duration:

Regular: 6-8 hours

Extended: ~12 hours

Absorption: Oral: Readily absorbed, mainly from the upper small intestine even in diarrhea

Distribution: V_d: 1.2-1.7 L/kg; higher in convalescent malaria; distributed in all tissues except brain; concentrates in heart, liver, kidneys, and skeletal muscle

Protein binding: 70% to 95%

Metabolism: Primarily in the liver

Half-life: 6-12 hours; lower in active or convalescent malaria

Adults: 8-14 hours

Time to peak serum concentration:

Oral: 1-1.5 hours

I.M.: 1 hour

Elimination: Not effectively removed by peritoneal dialysis, removed by hemodialysis; excreted in bile and saliva with <5% excreted unchanged in urine; excretion in urine is twice as rapid if urine is acidic

Usual Dosage Parenteral dosage form may be obtained from Centers for Disease Control if needed. Oral:

Children: Chloroquine-resistant malaria and babesiosis: 25 mg/kg/day in divided doses every 8 hours for 7 days; maximum: 650 mg/dose

Adults:

Chloroquine-resistant malaria: 650 mg every 8 hours for 7 days in conjunction with another agent

Babesiosis: 650 mg every 6-8 hours for 7 days

Leg cramps: 200-300 mg at bedtime

Dosing interval/adjustment in renal impairment:

Cl_{cr} 10-50 mL/minute: Administer every 8-12 hours or 75% of normal dose

Cl_{cr} <10 mL/minute: Administer every 24 hours or 30% to 50% of normal dose

Contraindications Tinnitus, optic neuropathy, G-6-PD deficiency, hypersensitivity to quinine or any component, history of black water fever

Warnings Use with caution in patients with cardiac arrhythmias (quinine has quinidine-like activity) and in patients with myasthenia gravis, children <12 years of age, pregnancy

Dosage Forms

Capsule: 64.8 mg, 65 mg, 200 mg, 300 mg, 325 mg

Tablet: 162.5 mg, 260 mg

Reference Range

Therapeutic: 2.5-9.6 μg/mL

Toxic: >10.0 μg/mL

Fatal: >15.0 μg/mL

Overdosage Treatment

Decontamination: Emesis not recommended due to CNS depression and potential for seizures; control seizures with benzodiazepine prior to lavage; lavage with 1:10,000 potassium permanganate 100 mg in 1 L water, indicated if early in ingestion; forced diuresis is not recommended; charcoal hemoperfusion is not effective

Supportive therapy: Stellate ganglion block procedure has not been shown to be of clear benefit as blindness is usually reversible; effect of nitrates uncertain; treat acidosis, hypoglycemia accordingly; treat cardiac conduction defects with sodium bicarbonate (I.V. 1-3 mEq/kg), titrate to serum pH 7.45-7.50

Arrhythmias: Avoid disopyramide/procainamide (class IA and IC)

Ventricular tachycardia: Pacing, conversion, isoproterenol 2-10 mcg/minute (0.1-1 mcg/kg/minute (children))

Torsade de pointes: $MgSO_4$ 2 g, then drip at 3-20 mg/minute

Bradycardia: Pacing, standard therapy

Hypotension: Norepinephrine, isoproterenol effective

Enhancement of elimination: Despite relatively high volume of distribution and protein binding, as well as poor *in vitro* binding of quinine to charcoal, studies have demonstrated enhanced elimination with multiple dose charcoal; hemodialysis minimally effective (not recommended)

Antidote(s)

Norepinephrine Bitartrate *on page 1451*

Test Interactions Positive Coombs' [direct], Increases prothrombin time (S)

Drug Interactions Quinine potentiates nondepolarizing and depolarizing muscle relaxants; verapamil, amiodarone, alkalinizing agents, and cimetidine may increase quinine serum concentrations; phenobarbital, phenytoin, and rifampin may decrease quinine serum concentrations; quinine may increase plasma concentration of digoxin, closely monitor digoxin concentrations, digoxin dosage may need to be reduced (by one-half) when quinine is initiated, new steady-state digoxin plasma concentrations occur in 5-7 days; beta-blockers + quinine → ↑ bradycardia; quinine may enhance coumarin anticoagulants

Pregnancy Risk Factor X

Nursing Implications Administer by slow I.V. infusion

Additional Information Parenteral dosage form may be obtained from Centers for Disease Control if needed; common adulterant in street drugs

Specific References

Bateman DN, Blain PG, Woodhouse KW, et al, "Pharmacokinetics and Clinical Toxicity of Quinine Overdosage: Lack of Efficacy of Techniques Intended to Enhance Elimination," *Q J Med*, 1985, 54(214):125-31.

Boland ME, Roper SM, and Henry JA, "Complications of Quinine Poisoning," *Lancet*, 1985, 1(8425):384-5.

Dyson EH, Proudfoot AT, and Bateman DN, "Quinine Amblyopia: Is Current Management Appropriate?" *J Toxicol Clin Toxicol*, 1985-6, 23(7-8):571-8.

Jaeger A, Sauder P, Kopferschmitt J, et al, "Clinical Features and Management of Poisoning Due to Antimalarial Drugs," *Med Toxicol Adverse Drug Exp*, 1987, 2(4):242-73.

Lockey D and Bateman DN, "Effect of Oral Activated Charcoal on Quinine Elimination," *Br J Clin Pharmacol*, 1989, 27(1):92-4.

Quinodis® *see* Fleroxacin *on page 352*

Quinora® *see* Quinidine *on page 668*

Quiphile® *see* Quinine Sulfate *on page 671*

Q-vel® [OTC] *see* Quinine Sulfate *on page 671*

R-818 *see* Flecainide Acetate *on page 350*

R-51619 *see* Cisapride *on page 217*

R-64766 *see* Risperidone *on page 686*

Radiation: Basics of Exposure *see page 1594*

Ramace® *see* Ramipril *on this page*

Ramipril (ra mi' prill)

Related Information

ACE Inhibitors Comparison *on page 1636-1637*

CAS Number 87333-19-5

Brand Names Altace™ Oral; Delix®; Pramace®; Ramace®; Triatec®; Tritace®

Use Treatment of hypertension, alone or in combination with thiazide diuretics; congestive heart failure treatment postmyocardial infarction

Mechanism of Action Ramipril is a prodrug that is converted to ramiprilat in the serum (HOE 498); ramiprilat is an angiotensin-converting enzyme (ACE) inhibitor which prevents the formation of angiotensin II from angiotensin I and exhibits pharmacologic effects that are similar to captopril

Adverse Reactions

Cardiovascular: Tachycardia, chest pain, palpitations, hypotension
Central nervous system: Headache, dizziness, fatigue, malaise, insomnia
Dermatologic: Rash, pruritus, alopecia, psoriasiform eruption, angioedema
Endocrine & metabolic: Hyperkalemia, hyponatremia, hyperuricemia, hypoglycemia
Gastrointestinal: Abdominal pain, dyspepsia, vomiting, nausea, diarrhea, anorexia, constipation, dysgeusia
Genitourinary: Albuminuria
Hematologic: Neutropenia, agranulocytosis
Neuromuscular & skeletal: Paresthesia
Renal: Increased BUN, serum creatinine, oliguria
Respiratory: Transient cough (12%)

Signs & Symptoms of Acute Overdose Severe hypotension, hyponatremia, insomnia, hyperuricemia

Toxicodynamics/Kinetics

Onset of action: Reduction of blood pressure occurs in 2 hours
Peak: 6-8 hours
Duration: 24 hours
Absorption: Well absorbed from gastrointestinal tract
Protein binding:
- Ramipril: 1% to 73%
- Ramiprilat: 56%

Metabolism: Hepatically to the active form, ramiprilat (ramipril diacid)
Half-life:
- Ramipril: 5 hours; 1 hour (elderly); 2-5 hours (renal failure)
- Ramiprilat: 24-50 hours

Time to peak serum concentration: ~1 hour
Elimination: Ramipril and its metabolites are eliminated primarily through the kidneys (60%); fecal elimination accounts for 40%

(Continued)

Ramipril *(Continued)*

Usual Dosage Adults: Oral: 2.5-5 mg once daily, maximum: 20 mg/day

Dosing adjustment in renal impairment:

Cl_{cr} 10-50 mL/minute: Administer 50% to 75% of normal dose

Cl_{cr} <40 mL/minute: Patients should be started on 1.25 mg/day and titrated up to 5 mg/day maximum

Cl_{cr} <10 mL/minute: Administer 25% to 50% of normal dose

Contraindications Hypersensitivity to ramipril or ramiprilat

Warnings Use with caution and modify dosage in patients with renal impairment (decrease dosage) (especially renal artery stenosis), severe congestive heart failure, or with coadministered diuretic; severe hypotension may occur in patients who are sodium and/or volume depleted, initiate lower doses and monitor closely when starting therapy in these patients; should be discontinued if laryngeal stridor or angioedema of the face, tongue, or glottis is observed

Dosage Forms Capsule: 1.25 mg, 2.5 mg, 5 mg, 10 mg

Reference Range Serum ramipril blood level range: 4.7-8.8 ng/mL associated with a hypotensive effect (~20 mm Hg drop) in patients with severe hypertension; levels up to 357 ng/mL have been reported without adverse effects during long-term therapy

Overdosage Treatment

Decontamination: Ipecac or lavage/activated charcoal

Supportive therapy: Following initiation of essential overdose management, toxic symptom treatment and supportive treatment should be initiated. Hypotension usually responds to I.V. fluids or Trendelenburg positioning. If unresponsive to these measures, the use of a parenteral inotrope may be required (eg, norepinephrine 0.1-0.2 mcg/kg/minute titrated to response).

Enhancement of elimination: Multiple dosing of activated charcoal may be useful

Test Interactions Increases BUN, creatinine, potassium, positive Coombs' [direct]; decreases cholesterol (S); may cause false-positive results in urine acetone determinations using sodium nitroprusside reagent; increased erythrocyte sedimentation rate; reduces plasma aldosterone level by 50%

Drug Interactions

Decreased effect: Aspirin

Increased levels/toxicity: Lithium; chlorpromazine increases serum potassium when used with amiloride, spironolactone, triamterene; hypotension (orthostatic) with loop diuretics

Pregnancy Risk Factor D

Pregnancy Implications Malformations especially known in second or third trimester

Monitoring Parameters BUN, serum creatinine, renal function; nausea, headache, diarrhea, change in taste, cough

Patient Information Notify physician if vomiting, diarrhea, excessive perspiration, or dehydration should occur; also if swelling of face, lips, tongue, or difficulty in breathing occurs or if persistent cough develops

Nursing Implications May cause depression in some patients; discontinue if angioedema of the face, extremities, lips, tongue, or glottis occurs; watch for hypotensive effects within 1-3 hours of first dose or new higher dose

Additional Information Some patients may have a decreased hypotensive effect between 12 and 16 hours; consider dividing total daily dose into 2 doses 12 hours apart; if patient is receiving a diuretic, a potential for first-dose hypotension is increased; to decrease this potential, stop diuretic for 2-3 days prior to initiating ramipril; continue diuretic if needed to control blood pressure. Due to frequent decreases in glomerular filtration (also creatinine clearance) with aging, elderly patients may have exaggerated responses to ACE inhibitors; differences in clinical response due to hepatic changes are not observed. ACE inhibitors may be preferred agents in elderly patients with CHF and diabetes mellitus. Diabetic albuminuria is reduced and insulin sensitivity is enhanced. In general, the side effect profile is favorable in elderly and causes little or no CNS confusion; use lowest dose recommendations initially. Ramipril is effective and safe in reducing arterial pressure and reducing microalbuminuria in single-kidney patients without renovascular hypertension. Reduces mortality by 27% when given 3-10 days postmyocardial infarction.

Specific References

Aurell M, Delin K, Herlitz H, et al, "Pharmacokinetics and Pharmacodynamics of Ramipril in Renal Failure," *Am J Cardiol*, 1987, 59(10):65D-69D.

Becker RA and Scholkens B, "Ramipril: Review of Pharmacology," *Am J Cardiol*, 1987, 59(10):3D-11D.

Camaiti A, La Cava G, Del Rosso A, et al, "Efficacy and Safety of Ramipril in Hypertensive Single-Kidney Patients," *Am J Ther*, 1995, 2:328-32.

Herings RM, deBoer A, Stricker BH, et al, "Hypoglycemia Associated With Use of Inhibitors of Angiotensin Converting Enzyme," *Lancet*, 1995, 345:1195-8.

Todd PA and Benfield P, "Ramipril: A Review of its Pharmacological Properties and Therapeutic Efficacy in Cardiovascular Disorders," *Drugs*, 1990, 39(1):110-35.

Ranital® *see* Ranitidine Hydrochloride *on this page*

Ranitidine Hydrochloride (ra nye' te deen)

Related Information

Doses and Administration of Several Frequently Used Antiemetic Agents *on page 1641*

Therapeutic Drugs Associated With Hallucinations *on page 1558-1559*

CAS Number 66357-35-5

Brand Names Anistal®; Azantac®; Ranital®; Sostril®; Ulsal®; Zantac®; Zantan®

Use Short-term treatment of active duodenal ulcers and benign gastric ulcers; long-term prophylaxis of duodenal ulcer and gastric hypersecretory states, gastroesophageal reflux, recurrent postoperative ulcer, upper gastrointestinal bleeding, prevention of acid-aspiration pneumonitis during surgery, and prevention of stress-induced ulcers

Mechanism of Action Competitive inhibition of histamine at H_2-receptors of the gastric parietal cells, which inhibits gastric acid secretion

Adverse Reactions

Cardiovascular: Bradycardia

Central nervous system: Dizziness, sedation, malaise, mental confusion, auditory and visual hallucinations, psychosis, delirium, choreiform movements, dystonic reactions, headache, restlessness

Dermatologic: Contact dermatitis, rash, toxic epidermal necrolysis

Endocrine & metabolic: Gynecomastia (may be unilateral)

Gastrointestinal: Constipation, nausea, vomiting, hypergastrinemia

Genitourinary: Impotence

Hematologic: Thrombocytopenia, bone marrow hypoplasia (especially in renal failure)

Hepatic: Hepatitis, hepatitis (may be hypersensitivity reaction)

Neuromuscular & skeletal: Arthralgias

Renal: Allergic interstitial nephritis

Respiratory: Wheezing

Miscellaneous: Drug fever

Signs & Symptoms of Acute Overdose Muscular tremors, cognitive dysfunction, parotid pain, gynecomastia, insomnia, impotence, memory loss, leukemoid reaction, depression, extrapyramidal reaction, migraine headache (exacerbation of), hyperprolactinemia, mania, chest pain, disorientation, intraocular pressure (increased), cholestatic jaundice, diarrhea, vomiting, rapid respiration, bradycardia, leukopenia; neutropenia; agranulocytosis; granulocytopenia; chorea (extrapyramidal)

Toxicodynamics/Kinetics

Duration of action: 8-12 hours

Absorption: Oral: ~50%

Distribution: Minimally penetrates the blood-brain barrier; many body tissues

V_d:

Children: 1.6-2.4 L/kg

Adults: 1.2-1.9 L/kg

Protein binding: 15%

Metabolism: In the liver (30%)

Bioavailability: 50%

Half-life:

Children: 1.9-2.1 hours

Adults: 2-2.5 hours

Renal failure: 5.9-8.9 hours

Time to peak serum concentration: Within 2-3 hours

Elimination: Excreted primarily in urine (35% as unchanged drug) and in the feces; renal clearance: 24-32 L/hour

Usual Dosage Giving dose at 6 PM may be better than 10 PM bedtime, the highest acid production usually starts at approximately 7 PM, thus giving at 6 PM controls acid secretion better

Children:

Oral: 1.25-2.5 mg/kg/dose every 12 hours

I.M., I.V.: 0.75-1.5 mg/kg/dose every 6-8 hours, maximum daily dose: 400 mg

Continuous infusion: 0.1-0.25 mg/kg/hour (preferred for stress ulcer prophylaxis in patients with concurrent maintenance I.V.s or TPNs)

Adults:

Short-term treatment of ulceration: 150 mg/dose twice daily or 300 mg at bedtime

Prophylaxis of recurrent duodenal ulcer: 150 mg at bedtime

Gastric hypersecretory conditions: Oral: 150 mg twice daily, up to 6 g/day

I.M., I.V.: 50 mg/dose every 6-8 hours (dose not to exceed 400 mg/day)

Continuous I.V. infusion: 150 mg over 24 hours or 6.25 mg/hour titrated up to 2.5 mg/kg/hour or 220 mg/hour maximum

(Continued)

Ranitidine Hydrochloride *(Continued)*

Dosing adjustment in renal impairment:

Cl_{cr} 10-50 mL/minute: Administer at 75% of normal dose or administer every 18-24 hours

Cl_{cr} <10 mL/minute: Administer at 50% of normal dose or administer every 18-24 hours

Dosing adjustment/comments in hepatic disease: Unchanged

Contraindications Hypersensitivity to ranitidine or any component

Warnings Use with caution in children <12 years of age; use with caution in patients with liver and renal impairment; dosage modification required in patients with renal impairment

Dosage Forms

Capsule (GELdose™): 150 mg, 300 mg
Granules, effervescent (EFFERdose™): 150 mg
Infusion, preservative free, in NaCl 0.45%: 1 mg/mL (50 mL)
Injection: 25 mg/mL (2 mL, 10 mL, 40 mL)
Syrup (peppermint flavor): 15 mg/mL (473 mL)
Tablet: 150 mg, 300 mg
Tablet, effervescent (EFFERdose™): 150 mg

Stability Solution for I.V. infusion in NS or D_5W is stable for 48 hours at room temperature or 30 days when frozen; is stable for 24 hours in TPN solutions; is stable only for 12 hours in total nutrient admixtures (TPN) when lipids are added

Reference Range Plasma level of 100 ng/mL will cause 50% inhibition of gastric acid secretion

Overdosage Treatment

Decontamination: Ipecac or lavage/activated charcoal with cathartic

Supportive therapy: Treatment is primarily symptomatic and supportive

Enhancement of elimination: Multiple dosing of activated charcoal may be effective; slightly dialyzable (5% to 20%)

Test Interactions False-positive urine protein using Multistix®, gastric acid secretion test, skin tests allergen extracts, serum creatinine and serum transaminase concentrations, urine protein test

Drug Interactions Warfarin, procainamide (increased levels), ketoconazole, diltiazem

Pregnancy Risk Factor B (has been associated with eyelid hemangioma)

Pregnancy Implications Excreted in breast milk

Monitoring Parameters AST, ALT, serum creatinine; when used to prevent stress-related gastrointestinal bleeding, measure the intragastric pH and try to maintain pH >4

Patient Information It may take several days before this medicine begins to relieve stomach pain; antacids may be taken with ranitidine unless your physician has told you not to use them; wait 30-60 minutes between taking the antacid and ranitidine; avoid aspirin, cough and cold preparations; avoid the use of black pepper, caffeine, alcohol, and harsh spices

Nursing Implications I.M. solution does not need to be diluted before use; monitor creatinine clearance for renal impairment; giving dose at 6 PM be may better than 10 PM bedtime, the highest acid production usually starts at approximately 7 PM, thus giving at 6 PM controls acid secretion better; observe caution in patients with renal function impairment and hepatic function impairment

Additional Information Giving dose at 6 PM be may better than 10 PM bedtime, the highest acid production usually starts at approximately 7 PM, thus giving at 6 PM controls acid secretion better; give I.V. administration over a 30-minute period to avoid bradycardia; causes fewer adverse reactions and interactions than cimetidine; most patient's ulcers have healed within 4 weeks; long-term therapy may cause vitamin B_{12} deficiency; unlike cimetidine, there is no antiandrogen effect. Cimetidine (400 mg orally twice daily) has been used to treat ranitidine-induced hypergastrinemia.

Specific References

Balestrazzi P, Gregori G, Bernasconi S, et al, "Bradycardia and Neurologic Disorders Associated With Ranitidine in a Child," *Am J Dis Child*, 1985, 139(5):442.

Freeman HJ, "Ranitidine-Associated Interstitial Nephritis in a Patient With Celiac Sprue," *Can J Gastroenterol*, 1988, 2:35.

Lehmann AB, "Reversible Chorea Due to Ranitidine and Cimetidine," *Lancet*, 1988, 2(8603):158.

Maack DK and Spiller HA, "Rare Dystonic Reaction From Accidental Overdose of Ranitidine in a 3 Month Old," *Vet Hum Toxicol*, 1993, 35:343.

Miralles ES, Nunez M, del Olmo N, et al, "Ranitidine-related Toxic Epidermal Necrolysis in a Patient With Idiopathic Thrombocytopenic Purpura," *J Am Acad Dermatol*, 1995, 32(1):133-4.

Ohsawa T, Masuhara K, and Hirata W, "Reversal of Ranitidine-Induced Hypergastrinemia by Cimetidine," *Ann Pharmacother*, 1994, 28(11):1303.

Romaguera C, Grimalt F, and Vilaplana J, "Epidemic of Occupational Contact Dermatitis From Ranitidine," *Contact Dermatitis*, 1988, 18(3):177-8.

Souza Lima MA, "Hepatitis Associated With Ranitidine," *Ann Intern Med*, 1984, 101(2):207-8.

Rapidal® *see* Terfenadine *on page 728*

Rapifen® *see* Alfentanil Hydrochloride *on page 94*

Raudixin® *see* Rauwolfia Serpentina *on this page*

Rauverid® *see* Rauwolfia Serpentina *on this page*

Rauwolfia Serpentina (rah wool' fee a)

CAS Number 8063-17-0

Brand Names Hypercal®; Lesten®; Raudixin®; Rauverid®; Wolfina®

Synonyms Whole Root Rauwolfia

Use Mild essential hypertension; relief of agitated psychotic states

Adverse Reactions

Cardiovascular: Hypotension, tachycardia, flushing

Central nervous system: Drowsiness, fatigue, mental depression, coma, parkinsonism, hypothermia

Endocrine & metabolic: Sodium and water retention, gynecomastia, galactorrhea

Gastrointestinal: Abdominal cramps, nausea, vomiting, gastric acid secretion (increased), dry mouth, diarrhea

Ocular: Miosis, conjunctival flushing

Respiratory: Nasal congestion

Signs & Symptoms of Acute Overdose Hypotension, bradycardia, Parkinson's-like symptoms, galactorrhea, gynecomastia, CNS depression, hypothermia, vomiting, miosis, tremors, coma, extensor plantar response, facial flushing

Usual Dosage Adults: Oral: 200-400 mg/day in 2 divided doses

Contraindications Any ulcerative condition, gallstones, mental depression, electroshock therapy, hypersensitivity to reserpine or any component

Warnings Electroshock therapy: Discontinue reserpine 7 days before electroshock therapy; may increase gastrointestinal motility and secretions; acute hypersensitivity reactions may occur; tartrazine sensitivity; use cautiously in patients with renal insufficiency

Dosage Forms Tablet: 50 mg, 100 mg

Stability Protect from light

Overdosage Treatment

Decontamination: Emesis or lavage/activated charcoal with cathartic

Supportive therapy: Hypotension usually responds to I.V. fluids or Trendelenburg positioning. If unresponsive to these measures, the use of a parenteral inotrope may be required (eg, norepinephrine 0.1-0.2 mcg/kg/minute titrated to response). Anticholinergic agents may be useful in reducing the parkinsonian effects. Avoid the use of digoxin in these patients.

Enhancement of elimination: Multiple dosing of activated charcoal may be effective

Drug Interactions Use lower doses with diuretic treatment or other antihypertensive use

Pregnancy Risk Factor D (effects on neurobehavioral development in rodents)

Monitoring Parameters Blood pressure, standing and sitting/supine, EKG for 72 hours after ingestion

Patient Information Take with food or milk; impotency is reversible; notify physician if a weight gain of more than 5 pounds has taken place during therapy; may cause drowsiness

Specific References

McKown CH, Verhulst HL, and Crotty JJ, "Overdosage Effects and Dangers From Tranquilizing Drugs," *JAMA*, 1963, 185(6):425-30.

Walker WR and Mathis JL, "Rauwolfia Serpentia Revisited," *N C Med J*, 1981, 42(6):401-2.

rDNase *see* Dornase Alfa *on page 299*

Reclomide® *see* Metoclopramide *on page 523*

Recombinant Human Deoxyribonuclease I *see* Dornase Alfa *on page 299*

Recombinant Leukocyte A Interferon *see* Interferon Alfa-2a *on page 430*

Recormon® *see* Erythropoietin *on page 322*

Rectules® *see* Chloral Hydrate *on page 193*

Redisol® *see* Cyanocobalamin *on page 246*

Redutemp® [OTC] *see* Acetaminophen *on page 79*

Regaine® *see* Minoxidil *on page 536*

Reglan® *see* Metoclopramide *on page 523*

Regular Iletin® I *see* Insulin Preparations *on page 426*

Regular [Concentrated] Iletin® II U-500 *see* Insulin Preparations *on page 426*

Regulax SS® [OTC] *see* Docusate *on page 297*
Regutol® [OTC] *see* Docusate *on page 297*
Rela® *see* Carisoprodol *on page 187*
Relafen® *see* Nabumetone *on page 543*
Relax Llano® *see* Methocarbamol *on page 513*
Remivox® *see* Lorcainide Hydrochloride *on page 484*
Reniten® *see* Enalapril *on page 311*
Renormax® *see* Spirapril Hydrochloride *on page 704*
Reomax® *see* Ethacrynic Acid *on page 328*
ReoPro® *see* Abciximab *on page 77*
Repazine® *see* Chlorpromazine Hydrochloride *on page 205*
Repocal® *see* Pentobarbital *on page 604*

Reserpine (re ser' peen)

CAS Number 50-55-5

Brand Names Abicol®; Lemiserp®; Seominal®; Serpalin®; Serpasil®; SK-Reserpine®

Synonyms Reserpinum

Use Management of mild to moderate hypertension; possible use for tardive dyskinesia

Mechanism of Action Reduces blood pressure via depletion of sympathetic biogenic amines (norepinephrine and dopamine); this also commonly results in sedative effects

Adverse Reactions

Cardiovascular: Hypotension, tachycardia

Central nervous system: Drowsiness, fatigue, mental depression, coma, depression, psychosis, hallucinations, dizziness, parkinsonism, hypothermia

Dermatologic: Pruritus

Endocrine & metabolic: Sodium and water retention, gynecomastia, galactorrhea

Gastrointestinal: Abdominal cramps, nausea, vomiting, gastric acid secretion (increased), dry mouth, diarrhea

Ocular: Miosis, conjunctival flushing

Respiratory: Nasal congestion

Miscellaneous: Feces discoloration (black), systemic lupus erythematosus (SLE)

Signs & Symptoms of Acute Overdose Hypotension, galactorrhea, bradycardia, impotence, hyperglycemia, gynecomastia, Parkinson's-like symptoms, hypertension, depression, wheezing, CNS depression, hypothermia, syncope, sexual dysfunction, ptosis, vomiting, miosis, mydriasis, tremors, coma, extensor plantar response, flushing

Toxicodynamics/Kinetics

Onset of action: Within 3-6 days

Duration: 2-6 weeks

Absorption: Oral: ~40%

Distribution: Well distributed in body; crosses blood-brain barrier

Protein binding: 96%

Metabolism: Extensive in the liver (>90%)

Half-life: 50-100 hours

Time to peak plasma concentration: 1-3 hours

Elimination: Principal excretion in feces (30% to 60%) and small amounts in urine (10%)

Usual Dosage Oral (full antihypertensive effects may take as long as 3 weeks):

Children: 0.01-0.02 mg/kg/24 hours divided every 12 hours; maximum dose: 0.25 mg/day

Adults: 0.1-0.5 mg/day in 1-2 doses

Dosing adjustment in renal impairment: Cl_{cr} <10 mL/minute: Avoid use

Contraindications Any ulcerative condition, gallstones, mental depression, electroshock therapy, hypersensitivity to reserpine or any component

Warnings Electroshock therapy: Discontinue reserpine 7 days before electroshock therapy; may increase gastrointestinal motility and secretions; acute hypersensitivity reactions may occur; tartrazine sensitivity; use cautiously in patients with renal insufficiency

Dosage Forms Tablet: 0.1 mg, 0.25 mg, 1 mg

Stability Protect oral dosage forms from light; incompatible with ethacrynic acid

Overdosage Treatment

Decontamination: Emesis or lavage/activated charcoal with cathartic

Supportive therapy: Hypotension usually responds to I.V. fluids or Trendelenburg positioning. If unresponsive to these measures, the use of a parenteral inotrope may be required (eg, norepinephrine 0.1-0.2 mcg/kg/minute titrated to response). Anticholinergic agents may be useful in reducing the parkinsonian effects. Avoid the use of digoxin in these patients. Alprazolam can reverse reserpine-induced depression.

Enhancement of elimination: Multiple dosing of activated charcoal may be effective

Test Interactions Increases catecholamines (U) 1 or 2 days postingestion; elevates prolactin levels

Drug Interactions Monoamine oxidase inhibitors, other hypotensive agents, digoxin, quinidine, general anesthesia, sympathomimetics, tricyclic antidepressants; nonsteroidals, anti-inflammatory agents, may reduce reserpine's effectiveness

Pregnancy Risk Factor D (effects on neurobehavioral development in rodents)

Pregnancy Implications Crosses the placenta; appears in breast milk

Monitoring Parameters Blood pressure, standing and sitting/supine, EKG for 72 hours after ingestion

Patient Information Take with food or milk; impotency is reversible; notify physician if a weight gain of more than 5 pounds has taken place during therapy; may cause drowsiness

Nursing Implications Observe for mental depression and alert family members to report any symptoms

Additional Information Full antihypertensive effects may take as long as 3 weeks; at high doses, mental depression is possible and might lead to suicide

Specific References

Rogal PP, Rakitin VA, Boichak MP, et al, "Fatal Reserpine Poisoning," *Sud Med Ekspert*, 1989, 32(1):51-2.

Zsoter TT, Johnson GE, DeVeber GA, et al, "Excretion and Metabolism of Reserpine in Renal Failure," *Clin Pharmacol Ther*, 1973, 14(3):325-30.

Reserpinum *see* Reserpine *on previous page*

Respa-GF® *see* Guaifenesin *on page 390*

Respbid® *see* Theophylline *on page 735*

Respir® *see* Oxymetazoline Hydrochloride *on page 586*

Respirase® *see* Zipeprol Hydrochloride *on page 813*

Respirex® *see* Zipeprol Hydrochloride *on page 813*

Resposan-10® *see* Chlordiazepoxide *on page 198*

Restandol® *see* Testosterone *on page 729*

Restoril® *see* Temazepam *on page 724*

Retard® *see* Procainamide Hydrochloride *on page 642*

Retrovir® *see* Zidovudine *on page 807*

Reversol® *see* Edrophonium Chloride *on page 309*

ReVia® *see* Naltrexone Hydrochloride *on page 548*

Rexitene® *see* Guanabenz Acetate *on page 391*

Rezine® *see* Hydroxyzine *on page 414*

Rheumatrex® *see* Methotrexate *on page 515*

Rhindecon® *see* Phenylpropanolamine Hydrochloride *on page 622*

***r*HuEPO-α** *see* Erythropoietin *on page 322*

Rhulicaine® [OTC] *see* Benzocaine *on page 149*

Rhythmin® *see* Procainamide Hydrochloride *on page 642*

Rhythmodan® *see* Disopyramide Phosphate *on page 294*

Rhythmol® *see* Propafenone Hydrochloride *on page 652*

Ribavirin (rye ba vye' rin)

CAS Number 36791-04-5

Brand Names Viramid®; Virazid®; Virazide®; Virazole® Aerosol

Synonyms RTCA; Tribavirin

Use Treatment of patients with respiratory syncytial virus (RSV) infections; may also be used in other viral infections including influenza A and B and adenovirus; specially indicated for treatment of severe lower respiratory tract RSV infections in patients with an underlying compromising condition (prematurity, bronchopulmonary dysplasia, congenital heart disease, immunodeficiency, and immunosuppression); may be effective in treating Sabia virus infection (an arenavirus)

Mechanism of Action Inhibits replication of RNA and DNA viruses; inhibits influenza virus RNA polymerase activity and inhibits the initiation and elongation of RNA fragments resulting in inhibition of viral protein synthesis

(Continued)

Ribavirin *(Continued)*

Adverse Reactions

Cardiovascular: Hypotension, cardiac arrest
Central nervous system: Headache, fatigue, insomnia
Dermatologic: Rash, skin irritation
Gastrointestinal: Nausea, anorexia
Hepatic: Elevated bilirubin at doses exceeding 1 g/day
Ocular: Conjunctivitis
Respiratory: Mild wheezing, worsening of respiratory function
Miscellaneous: Reversible anemia with an increase in reticulocyte count

Toxicodynamics/Kinetics

Absorption: Absorbed systemically from the respiratory tract following nasal and oral inhalation; absorption is dependent upon respiratory factors and method of drug delivery; maximal absorption occurs with the use of the aerosol generator via an endotracheal tube; highest concentrations are found in the respiratory tract and erythrocytes
Protein binding: None
Metabolism: Occurs intracellularly to the inactive metabolite 1,2,4-triazole carboxamide and may be necessary for drug action
Bioavailability: Oral: 45%
Half-life, plasma:
Children: 6.5-11 hours
Adults: 24 hours, much longer in the erythrocyte (16-40 days), which can be used as a marker for intracellular metabolism
Time to peak serum concentration: Inhalation: Within 60-90 minutes
Elimination: Hepatic metabolism is major route of elimination with 40% of the drug cleared renally as unchanged drug and metabolites

Usual Dosage Infants, Children, and Adults:

Aerosol inhalation: Use with Viratek® small particle aerosol generator (SPAG-2) at a concentration of 20 mg/mL (6 g reconstituted with 300 mL of sterile water without preservatives)
Aerosol only: 12-18 hours/day for 3 days, up to 7 days in length
Arenavirus infection: Loading dose: 30 mg/kg, then 15 mg/kg every 6 hours for 4 days, then 7.5 mg/kg 3 times/day for 6 days

Toxicity associated with daily doses >2.4 g

Contraindications Females of childbearing age

Warnings Use with caution in patients requiring assisted ventilation because precipitation of the drug in the respiratory equipment may interfere with safe and effective patient ventilation; also monitor carefully in patients with COPD and asthma for deterioration of respiratory function. Ribavirin is potentially mutagenic, tumor-promoting, and gonadotoxic; there is evidence that ribavirin is teratogenic in small animals. Health care workers who are pregnant or may become pregnant should be advised of the potential risks of exposure and counseled about risk reduction strategies including alternate job responsibilities; virus resistance does not appear to develop; incubation period for RSV is 4-8 days.

Dosage Forms Powder for aerosol: 6 g (100 mL)

Stability Do not use any water containing an antimicrobial agent to reconstitute drug; reconstituted solution is stable for 24 hours at room temperature

Reference Range Cytotoxic at plasma levels >200 μg/mL; a 3 mg/kg dose produced a peak plasma level of 1-2 μg/mL

Overdosage Treatment

Decontamination: Emesis or lavage/activated charcoal with cathartic on oral ingestion
Enhancement of elimination: Hemodialysis is not useful

Test Interactions May cause transient elevation of serum iron level

Drug Interactions Decreased effect of zidovudine by inhibition of zidovudine phosphorylation; enhancement of antiviral activity with amantadine and interferon alfa

Pregnancy Risk Factor X

Pregnancy Implications Teratogenic in rodents (skeletal and gastrointestinal malformation)

Monitoring Parameters Respiratory function; hemoglobin and unconjugated bilirubin

Nursing Implications Keep accurate I & O record, discard solutions placed in the SPAG-2 unit at least every 24 hours and before adding additional fluid

Additional Information RSV season is usually December to April; viral shedding period for RSV is usually 3-8 days; surgical masks do not prevent inhalation

Specific References

Barry M, Russi M, Armstrong L, et al, "Breif Report: treatment of a Laboratory Acquired Saria Virus Virus Infection," *N Engl J Med*, 1995, 333(5):294-6.
Kramer TH, Gaar GG, Ray CG, et al, "Hemodialysis Clearance of Intravenously Administered Ribavirin," *Antimicrob Agents Chemother*, 1990, 34(3):489-90.

Morris DJ, "Adverse Effects and Drug Interactions of Clinical Importance With Antiviral Drugs," *Drug Saf*, 1994, 10(4):281-91.
Nicholson KG, "Properties of Antiviral Agents," *Lancet*, 1984, 2(8401):503-6 and 2(8402):562-4.
Van Bever HP, Desager KS, Van Hoeck K, et al, "Water Intoxication After Nebulised Tribavirin," *Lancet*, 1995, 345(8947):451.
Vogt MW, Hartshorn KL, Furman PA, et al, "Ribavirin Antagonizes the Effect of Azidothymidine on HIV Replication," *Science*, 1987, 235(4794):1376-9.

Richlyn® *see* Piperazine Citrate *on page 629*

Ricifruit® *see* Castor Oil *on page 189*

Ricinus Oil *see* Castor Oil *on page 189*

Rid-A-Pain® [OTC] *see* Benzocaine *on page 149*

Ridaura® *see* Gold Compounds *on page 386*

Ridazine® *see* Thioridazine Hydrochloride *on page 745*

Rifabutin (rif a bu' tin)

CAS Number 72559-06-09

Brand Names Mycobutin®

Synonyms Ansamycin; LM 427; Rifabutine

Use Prevention of disseminated *Mycobacterium avium* complex (MAC) in patients with advanced HIV infection

Mechanism of Action Inhibits DNA-dependent RNA polymerase at the beta subunit which prevents chain initiation

Adverse Reactions

Central nervous system: Fever, headache, seizures, confusion, insomnia
Dermatologic: Rash, skin erythema
Gastrointestinal: Abdominal pain, diarrhea, dyspepsia, nausea, vomiting, taste perversion, epigastric pain, anorexia, flatulence, eructation
Hematologic: Thrombocytopenia, anemia, leukopenia, neutropenia
Hepatic: Elevated liver enzymes, jaundice
Neuromuscular & skeletal: Arthralgia, myalgia
Ocular: Uveitis
Miscellaneous: Chest pain, taste perversion, discolored urine

Signs & Symptoms of Acute Overdose Polyarthralgia at doses >1 g/day; leukopenia; neutropenia; agranulocytosis; granulocytopenia

Toxicodynamics/Kinetics

Absorption: Oral: Readily absorbed 53%; delayed with high fat meal
Distribution: V_d: 9.32 L/kg; distributes to body tissues including the lungs, liver, spleen, eyes, and kidneys
Protein binding: 85%
Metabolism: To active (25-deacetylrifabutin) and inactive metabolites
Bioavailability: Absolute, 20% in HIV patients
Half life, terminal: 45 hours (range: 16-69 hours)
Peak serum level: Within 2-4 hours
Elimination: Renal and biliary clearance of unchanged drugs is 10%; 30% excreted in feces; 53% in urine unchanged; clearance: 0.14 L/kg/hour

Usual Dosage Oral:

Children: Efficacy and safety of rifabutin have not been established in children; a limited number of HIV-positive children with MAC (n=22) have been given rifabutin for MAC prophylaxis; doses of 5 mg/kg/day have been useful

Adults: 300 mg once daily; for patients who experience gastrointestinal upset, rifabutin can be administered 150 mg twice daily with food

Maximum dose: 1 g

Contraindications Hypersensitivity to rifabutin or any other rifamycins; rifabutin is contraindicated in patients with a WBC <1000/mm^3 or a platelet count <50,000 mm^3

Warnings Rifabutin as a single agent must not be administered to patients with active tuberculosis since its use may lead to the development of tuberculosis that is resistant to both rifabutin and rifampin; rifabutin should be discontinued in patients with AST >500 IU/L or if total bilirubin is >3 mg/dL. Use with caution in patients with liver impairment; modification of dosage should be considered in patients with renal impairment.

Dosage Forms Capsule: 150 mg

Reference Range Peak and trough plasma levels of a 600 mg dose twice daily is 900 ng/mL and 200 ng/mL respectively

Overdosage Treatment

Decontamination: Ipecac or lavage/activated charcoal with cathartic
Enhancement of elimination: Multiple dosing of activated charcoal may be effective; hemodialysis or charcoal hemoperfusion may be effective

Drug Interactions Decreased plasma concentration (because of induced liver enzymes) with coadministration of verapamil, methadone, digoxin, cyclosporine, cor-

(Continued)

Rifabutin *(Continued)*

ticosteroids, oral anticoagulants, theophylline, barbiturates, chloramphenicol, ketoconazole, oral contraceptives, quinidine, halothane; levels of zidovudine are decreased; may antagonize antimicrobial effect of ciprofloxacin on *Mycobacterium avium-intracellulare* complex (MAC); fluconazole and clarithromycin can increase rifabutin levels

Pregnancy Risk Factor B

Monitoring Parameters Periodic liver function tests, CBC with differential, platelet count, hemoglobin, hematocrit

Patient Information May discolor urine, tears, sweat, or other body fluids to a red-orange color; take 1 hour before or 2 hours after a meal on an empty stomach; soft contact lenses may be permanently stained; report to physician any severe or persistent flu-like symptoms, nausea, vomiting, dark urine or pale stools, or unusual bleeding or bruising; can be taken with meals or sprinkled on applesauce

Nursing Implications Administer with meals

Additional Information May discolor urine, saliva, and tears a brown-orange color; synergistic effects against *Mycobacterium avium* intracellulare complex (MAC) reported when combined with clarithromycin or clofazimine

Specific References

Dunn A-M, Tizer K, Cervia JS, et al, "Rifabutin-Associated Uveitis in a Pediatric Patient," *Pediatr Infect Dis J*, 1995, 14:246-7.

Havlir D, Torriani F, and Dube M, "Uveitis Associated With Rifabutin Prophylaxis," *Ann Intern Med*, 1994, 121(7):510-2.

Jacobs DS, Piliero PJ, Kuperwaser MG, et al, "Acute Uveitis Associated With Rifabutin Use in Patients With Human Immunodeficiency Virus Infection," *Am J Ophthalmol*, 1994, 118(6):716-22.

Karbassi M, and Nikou S, "Acute Uveitis in Patients With Acquired Immunodeficiency Syndrome Receiving Prophylactic Rifabutin," *Arch Ophthamol*, 1995, 113:699-701.

Kelleher P, Helbert M, Anderson J, et al, "Uveitis: Incidence Study," *AIDS*, 1994, 8(Suppl 4):18, abstract.

Levin RH and Bolinger AM, "Treatment of Nontuberculous Mycobacterial Infections in Pediatric Patients," *Clin Pharm*, 1988, 7(7):545-51.

Morris JT and Kelly JW, "Rifabutin-Induced Ageusia," *Ann Intern Med*, 1993, 119(2):171-2.

Rifai A, Peyman GA, Daun M, et al, "Rifabutin Associated Uveitis During Prophylaxis for Mycobacterium Avium Complex Infection," *Arch Ophthalmol*, 1995, 113:707.

Skinner MH and Blaschke TF, "Clinical Pharmacokinetics of Rifabutin," *Clin Pharmacokinet*, 1995, 28(2):115-25.

Rifabutine *see* Rifabutin *on previous page*

Rifadin® *see* Rifampin *on this page*

Rifampicin *see* Rifampin *on this page*

Rifampin (rif' am pin)

CAS Number 13292-46-1

Brand Names Rifadin®; Rimactane®

Synonyms Rifampicin

Use Management of active tuberculosis; eliminate meningococci from asymptomatic carriers; prophylaxis of *Haemophilus influenzae* type B infection

Mechanism of Action Inhibits bacterial RNA synthesis by binding to the beta subunit of DNA-dependent RNA polymerase, blocking RNA transcription

Adverse Reactions

Central nervous system: Drowsiness, fatigue, confusion, fever, headache, ataxia, electroencephalogram abnormalities

Dermatologic: Rash, pruritus

Gastrointestinal: Nausea, vomiting, diarrhea, stomatitis

Hematologic: Eosinophilia, blood dyscrasias (leukopenia, thrombocytopenia), agranulocytosis, granulocytopenia

Hepatic: Hepatitis

Local: Irritation at the I.V. site

Renal: Renal failure

Miscellaneous: Flu-like syndrome

Signs & Symptoms of Acute Overdose Nausea, vomiting, wheezing, dyspnea, pemphigus, colitis, hepatitis, Redman syndrome, myopathy, erythema multiforme, facial edema, toxic epidermal necrolysis, stomatitis, nephritis, scleral discoloration after 6-10 hours, pulmonary edema, abdominal pain, Stevens-Johnson syndrome, cholelithiasis, renal failure (acute), thrombocytopenia, skin discoloration, pruritus, hypersensitivity, hyperglycemia, urine discoloration (brown), urine discoloration (orange), urine discoloration (orange-red), urine discoloration (orange-yellow), urine discoloration (red), feces discoloration (orange-red), feces discoloration (red-brown), leukopenia, coma

Toxicodynamics/Kinetics

Absorption: Oral: Well absorbed from gastrointestinal tract (90%); food may delay or slightly reduce peak serum level

Distribution: V_d: 1.6 L/kg; distributed well to most body tissues and fluids including CSF, where concentrations are increased if meninges are inflamed; concentrations in liver, gallbladder, bile, and urine are higher than those found in blood; crosses the blood-brain barrier well; highly lipophilic

Protein binding: 80% to 90%

Metabolism: In the liver; undergoes enterohepatic recycling

Half-life: 3-4 hours, prolonged with hepatic impairment; increased in overdose

Time to peak serum concentration: Within 2-4 hours

Elimination: Principally in feces (60% to 65%) and urine (~30%); plasma rifampin concentrations are not significantly affected by hemodialysis or peritoneal dialysis; significant enterohepatic circulation and elimination in bile

Usual Dosage I.V. infusion dose is the same as for the oral route

Tuberculosis:

Children: 10-20 mg/kg/day in divided doses every 12-24 hours

Adults: 10 mg/kg/day; maximum: 600 mg/day

Treatment for 9 months with isoniazid or 6 months with isoniazid/pyrazinamide

American Thoracic Society and CDC recommendations should be consulted for current guidelines

Children: 10-20 mg/kg/dose (up to 600 mg) twice weekly under supervision to ensure compliance

Adults: 10 mg/kg (up to 600 mg) twice weekly

H. influenza prophylaxis:

Infants and Children: 20 mg/kg/day every 24 hours for 4 days

Adults: 600 mg every 24 hours for 4 days

Meningococcal prophylaxis:

<1 month: 10 mg/kg/day in divided doses every 12 hours

Infants and Children: 20 mg/kg/day in divided doses every 12 hours for 2 days

Adults: 600 mg every 12 hours for 2 days

Nasal carriers of *Staphylococcus aureus*: Adults: 600 mg/day for 5-10 days in combination with other antibiotics

Synergy for *Staphylococcus aureus* infections: Adults: 300-600 mg twice daily with other antibiotics

Dosing adjustment in hepatic impairment: Dose reductions are necessary to reduce hepatitis

Contraindications Hypersensitivity to rifampin or any component

Warnings Use with caution in patients with liver impairment; modification of dosage should be considered in patients with severe liver impairment

Dosage Forms

Capsule: 150 mg, 300 mg

Injection: 600 mg

Stability Reconstituted I.V. solution is stable for 24 hours at room temperature; rifampin oral suspension can be compounded with simple syrup or wild cherry syrup at a concentration of 10 mg/mL; the suspension is stable for 4 weeks at room temperature or in a refrigerator when stored in a glass amber prescription bottle

Overdosage Treatment

Decontamination: Immediate administration of activated charcoal inhibits absorption by 90%; emesis is not useful since vomiting is common in overdose; lavage useful in early ingestions; activated charcoal with cathartic of value, multiple-dose activated charcoal useful due to enterohepatic circulation

Supportive therapy: Mainly supportive and symptomatic treatment; overdose is rare and experience is limited; monitor hepatic and renal function

Enhancement of elimination: Multiple dosing of activated charcoal may be effective

Test Interactions Increases bilirubin (S), positive Coombs' [direct]; rifampicin can cause false-positive urine assay of opiates by kinetic interaction of microparticles in solution (KIMS) method up to a concentration of 0.9 μg/mL

Diagnostic Tests/Procedures

Complete Blood Count *on page 1236*

Drug Interactions Rifampin induces liver enzymes which may decrease the plasma concentration of the following drugs: verapamil, methadone, digoxin, cyclosporine, corticosteroids, oral anticoagulants, theophylline, barbiturates, chloramphenicol, ketoconazole, oral contraceptives, quinidine; halothane; ketoconazole; benzodiazepines; isoniazid; beta-adrenergic blockers

Rifampin may markedly decrease calcium channel blocker levels

Increased tacrolimus levels can occur with concomitant administration of erythromycin or rifampin

Pregnancy Risk Factor C

Pregnancy Implications Teratogenic in rodents

Monitoring Parameters Periodic monitoring of liver function (AST, ALT), CBC

Patient Information May discolor urine, tears, sweat, or other body fluids to a red-orange color; take 1 hour before or 2 hours after a meal on an empty stomach; soft contact lenses may be permanently stained

(Continued)

Rifampin *(Continued)*

Nursing Implications Evaluate hepatic status and mental status; give on an empty stomach (ie, 1 hour prior to, or 2 hours after meals) to increase total absorption

Additional Information Since resistant strains occur rapidly, normally used with other anti-TB drugs

Specific References

Acocella G, "Clinical Pharmacokinetics of Rifampicin," *Clin Pharmacokinet*, 1978, 3(2):108-27.

Askgaard DS, Wilcke T, and Dossing M, "Hepatotoxicity Caused by the Combined Action of Isoniazid and Rifampin," *Thorax*, 1995, 50:213-4.

Borcherding SM, Baciewicz AM, and Self TH, "Update on Rifampin Drug Interactions. II," *Arch Intern Med*, 1992, 152(4):711-6.

Furian V, Perello L, Jacquemin E, et al, "Interactions Between FK506 and Rifampicin or Erythromycin in Pediatric Liver Recipients," *Transplantation*, 1995, 59:1217-8.

Holdiness MR, "A Review of the Redman Syndrome and Rifampicin Overdose," *Med Toxicol Adverse Drug Exp*, 1989, 4(6):444-51.

Kindelan JM, Serrano I, Jurado R, et al, "Rifampin-Induced Severe Thrombocytopenia in a Patient With Pulmonary Tuberculosis," *Ann Pharmacother*, 1994, 28(11):1304-5.

Noble A, "Antituberculous Therapy and Acute Liver Failure," *Lancet*, 1995, 345(8953):867.

Orisakwe OE, Dioka CE, Orish CN, et al, "Charcoal and Rifampicin Pharmacokinetics," *Am J Ther*, 1995, 68-70.

Plomp TA, Battista HJ, Unterdorfer H, et al, "A Case of Fatal Poisoning by Rifampicin," *Arch Toxicol*, 1981, 48(4):245-52.

Trevilla PH, Jimenez EO, and Tena T, "Presence of Rifampicin in Urine Causes Cross-Reactivity With Opiates Using the KIMS Method," *J Anal Toxicol*, 1995, 19:200.

Walker-Renard P, "Pruritus Associated With Intravenous Rifampin," *Ann Pharmacother*, 1995, 29:267-8.

Wong P, Bottoroff MB, Heritage RW, et al, "Acute Rifampin Overdose: A Pharmacokinetic Study and Review of the Literature," *J Pediatr*, 1984, 104(5):781-3.

rIFN-A *see* Interferon Alfa-2a *on page 430*

Rilmenidine

CAS Number 54187-04-1

Synonyms Oxaminozoline

Use Investigational: Hypertension

Mechanism of Action Oxazoline derivative which has alpha$_2$-adrenergic receptor antagonist and an imidazoline receptor agonist with less sedation than clonidine

Adverse Reactions

Cardiovascular: Hypotension

Respiratory: Bronchospasm

Toxicodynamics/Kinetics

Distribution: V_d: 5 L/kg

Protein binding: <10%

Half-life: 8.31 hours

Time to peak plasma concentration: 2 hours

Elimination: Renal

Usual Dosage Oral: 1-2 mg/day in divided doses

Overdosage Treatment

Decontamination: Lavage/activated charcoal with cathartic

Supportive therapy: For hypotension, give intravenous saline; vasopressors may be necessary. Bronchospasm can be treated with beta-agonist agents

Enhancement of elimination: Multiple dosing of activated charcoal may be effective

Test Interactions May cause a decrease in plasma norepinephrine and epinephrine levels

Specific References

Fillastre JP and Vanhoutte PM, "Second International Symposium on Rilmenidine," *Am J Med*, 1989, 87(Suppl 3C): 15-74S.

Velasco M and Luchsinger A, "Central Acting Antihypertensive Drugs: Past, Present, and Future," *Am J Ther*, 1995, 2:255-7.

Velasco M, Soltero I, Sukerman M, et al, "Double-Blind, Randomized Study of the Efficacy, Tolerance, and Rebound Effects of the Antihypertensive Drug Rilmenidine: Comparative Evaluation With Clonidine," *Curr Ther Res*, 1993, 54:202-7.

Rilutek® *see* Riluzole *on this page*

Riluzole

Brand Names Rilutek®

Synonyms 2-Amino-6-Trifluoromethoxy-benzothiazole; RP54274

Use Investigational: May slow down progression of amyotrophic lateral sclerosis; may have some anticonvulsant properties

Mechanism of Action Glutamate neuroreceptor antagonist which promotes GABA activity

Adverse Reactions Hepatic: Elevated liver function tests, worsening of asthenia spasticity or stiffness

Usual Dosage Oral: 100 mg/day

Dosage Forms Tablet: 50 mg

Overdosage Treatment

Decontamination: Lavage/activated charcoal with cathartic

Additional Information May be obtained through Rhone-Poulenc Rorer Inc (Collegeville, PA) for compassionate use (through treatment IND process) by calling 800-727-6737 for treatment of amyotrophic lateral sclerosis; may be more effective for amyotrophic lateral sclerosis of bulbar onset; in animal models, riluzole was a potent inhibitor of seizures induced by ouabain

Specific References

Bensimon G, Lacomblez L, Meininger V, et al, "A Controlled Trial of Riluzole in Amyotrophic Lateral Sclerosis," *N Engl J Med*, 1994, 330(9):585-91.

Mantz J, Cheramy A, Thierry AM, et al, "Anesthetic Properties of Riluzole (54274 RP), A New Inhibitor of Glutamate neurotransmission," *Anesthesiology*, 1992, 76(5):844-8.

Mizoule J, Meldrum B, Mazadier M, et al, "2-Amino-6-Trifluoromethoxy-benzothiazole, A Possible Antagonist of Excitatory Amino Acid Neurotransmission--I. Anticonvulsant Properties," *Neuropharmacology*, 1985, 24(8):767-73.

Rowland LP, "Riluzole for the Treatment of Amyotrophic Lateral Sclerosis - Tco Soon to Tell?" *N Engl J Med*, 1994, 330(9):636-7.

Rimactane® *see* Rifampin *on page 682*

Rimantadine Hydrochloride (ri man' to deen)

CAS Number 1501-84-4; 13392-28-4

Brand Names Flumadine®; Roflual®

Synonyms EXP-126; Rimantadinum

Use Prophylaxis (adults and children) and treatment (adults) of influenza A viral infection

Mechanism of Action Similar to amantadine; inhibits viral RNA and protein synthesis

Adverse Reactions

Cardiovascular: Orthostatic hypotension, edema

Central nervous system: Dizziness, confusion, headache, insomnia, difficulty in concentrating, anxiety, restlessness, irritability, hallucinations

Gastrointestinal: Nausea, vomiting, dry mouth

Genitourinary: Urinary retention

Signs & Symptoms of Acute Overdose Convulsions (especially in the elderly), sedation

Toxicodynamics/Kinetics

Absorption: Oral: 92%

Metabolism: Liver

Half-life: 24-36 hours; renal failure: 48-72 hours

Elimination: Renal (75%)

Usual Dosage Oral:

Prophylaxis:

Children <10 years: 5 mg/kg give once daily

Children >10 years and Adults: 100 mg twice/day

Treatment: Adults: 100 mg twice/day

In patients with severe hepatic dysfunction or renal function, and in elderly nursing home patients, the dosage should be reduced to 100 mg/day

Contraindications Hypersensitivity to drugs of the adamantine class (rimantadine or amantadine)

Warnings Use with caution in patients with liver disease, a history of recurrent and eczematoid dermatitis, uncontrolled psychosis or severe psychoneurosis, seizures in those receiving CNS stimulant drugs

Dosage Forms

Syrup: 50 mg/5 mL (60 mL, 240 mL, 480 mL)

Tablet: 100 mg

Reference Range Peak serum levels: 240-320 ng/mL after a 200 mg dose

Overdosage Treatment

Decontamination: Lavage/activated charcoal with cathartic

Enhancement of elimination: Multiple dosing of activated charcoal may be useful

Pregnancy Risk Factor C

Specific References

Bentley DW, Karki SD, and Betts RF, "Rimantadine and Seizures," *Ann Intern Med*, 1989, 110(4):323-4.

Douglas RG Jr, "Prophylaxis and Treatment of Influenza," *N Engl J Med*, 1990, 322(7):443-50.

Wintermeyer SM and Nahata MC, "Rimantadine: A Clinical Perspective," *Ann Pharmacother*, 1995, 29:299-310.

Rimantadinum *see* Rimantadine Hydrochloride *on this page*

Rimso®-50 *see* Dimethyl Sulfoxide *on page 290*

Rinatec® *see* Ipratropium Bromide *on page 438*

Risperdal® *see* Risperidone *on this page*

Risperidone (ris per' i done)

CAS Number 106266-06-2

Brand Names Risperdal®

Synonyms R-64766

Use Management of psychotic disorders (eg, schizophrenia)

Mechanism of Action Risperidone is a benzisoxazole derivative, mixed serotonin-dopamine antagonist; binds to 5-HT_2 receptors in the CNS and in the periphery with a very high affinity; binds to dopamine-D_2 receptors with less affinity. The binding affinity to the dopamine-D_2 receptor is 20 times lower than the 5-HT_2 affinity. The addition of serotonin antagonism to dopamine antagonism (classic neuroleptic mechanism) is thought to improve negative symptoms of psychoses and reduce the incidence of extrapyramidal side effects.

Adverse Reactions

Cardiovascular: Palpitations, syncope, increases in blood pressure and heart rate

Central nervous system: Extrapyramidal reactions, headache, impaired concentration, dizziness, anxiety, sedation occurs at daily doses $\geq$20 mg/day, slurred speech, insomnia

Gastrointestinal: Nausea, anorexia

Genitourinary: Erection and ejaculatory disturbances, priapism

Neuromuscular & skeletal: Tremors

Ocular: Blurred vision

Miscellaneous: Dry mouth

Signs & Symptoms of Acute Overdose Hypotension, ejaculatory disturbances, neuroleptic malignant syndrome, mania, hallucinations, enuresis, palpitations

Toxicodynamics/Kinetics

Absorption: Oral: Rapid (not affected by food)

Metabolism: Extensive by cytochrome P-450 to 9-hydroxyrisperidone (active metabolite)

Protein binding: Plasma: 90%; 9-hydroxyrisperidone: 77%

Half-life: 24 hours (risperidone and its active metabolite)

Time to peak: Peak plasma concentrations within 1 hour

Usual Dosage

Recommended starting dose: 1 mg twice daily; slowly increase to the optimum range of 4-8 mg/day; daily dosages >10 mg do not appear to confer any additional benefit, and the incidence of extrapyramidal reactions is higher than with lower doses

Dosing adjustment in renal, hepatic impairment, and elderly: Starting dose of 0.5 mg twice daily is advisable

Contraindications Known hypersensitivity to any component of the product; use with caution in patients with breast cancer (can cause elevation of serum prolactin levels)

Dosage Forms Tablet: 1 mg, 2 mg, 3 mg, 4 mg

Reference Range Peak plasma level: 12 ng/mL within 2 hours of a 1 mg dose

Overdosage Treatment

Decontamination: Lavage/activated charcoal with cathartic

Supportive therapy: Lidocaine or phenytoin for ventricular arrhythmia

Enhancement of elimination: Multiple dosing of activated charcoal may be effective

Test Interactions Elevation of prolactin level

Drug Interactions Increased toxicity: Quinidine, warfarin

Pregnancy Risk Factor C

Nursing Implications Observe for extrapyramidal effects

Additional Information Temazepam (30 mg) can be used to treat insomnia

Specific References

Borison RL, Pathiraja AP, Diamond BI, et al, "Risperidone: Clinical Safety and Efficacy in Schizophrenia," *Psychopharmacol Bull*, 1992, 28(2):213-8.

Byerly MJ, Greer RA, and Evans DL "Behaviroal Stimulation Associated With Risperidone Initiation," *Am J Psychiatry*, 1995, 152:1096-7.

Cardoni AA, "Risperidone: Review and Assessment of Its Role in the Treatment of Schizophrenia," *Ann Pharmacother*, 1995, 29:610-8.

Gelders YG, "Thymosthenic Agents, a Novel Approach in the Treatment of Schizophrenia," *Br J Psychiatry Suppl*, 1989, 5:33-6.

Goss JB, "Concomitant Use of Thioridazine With Risperidone," *Am J Health-Syst Pharm*, 1995, 52:1012.

Heather GS and Vicas IM, "Risperidone Overdose: A Case Series," *Vet Hum Toxicol*, 1994, 36:371.

Meylan C, Bondolfi G, Aubert A-C, et al, "Reversible Neutropenia During a Cold: Possible Involvement of Risperidone? A Case Report," *Eur Neuropsychopharmacol*, 1995, 5:1-2.

Swanson Jr CL, Price WA, and McEvoy JP, "Effects of Concomitant Risperidone and Lithium Treatment," *Am J Psychiatry*, 1995, 152:1096.

Tekell JL, Smith EA, and Silva JA, "Prolonged Erection Associated With Risperidone Treatment," *Am J Psychiatry*, 1995, 152:1097.

Ritalin® *see* Methylphenidate Hydrochloride *on page 521*

Ritalin-SR® *see* Methylphenidate Hydrochloride *on page 521*

Ritmilen® *see* Disopyramide Phosphate *on page 294*

Ritodrine Hydrochloride (ri' toe dreen)

CAS Number 26652-09-5; 23239-51-2

Brand Names Miiolene®; Pre-Par®; Yutopar®

Use Inhibits uterine contraction in preterm labor

Mechanism of Action Tocolysis due to its uterine beta$_2$-adrenergic receptor stimulating effects; this agent's beta$_2$ effects can also cause bronchial relaxation and vascular smooth muscle stimulation

Adverse Reactions

Cardiovascular: Tachycardia, hypertension, palpitations, angina, chest pain

Central nervous system: Headache, migraine headache (exacerbation of)

Endocrine & metabolic: Hyperglycemia and insulin concentrations, galactorrhea, decreases serum potassium concentrations

Gastrointestinal: Vomiting

Hematologic: Leukocytosis, leukemoid reaction, neutropenia

Neuromuscular & skeletal: Tremors

Respiratory: Pulmonary edema

Signs & Symptoms of Acute Overdose Parotid pain

Toxicodynamics/Kinetics

Absorption: Oral: Rapid

Distribution: V_d: 0.7 L/kg

Protein binding: 32%

Metabolism: In the liver

Half-life: 15 hours

Bioavailability: 30%

Time to peak serum concentration: Within 0.5-1 hour

Elimination: In urine as unchanged drug and inactive conjugates; plasma clearance: 0.52 L/kg/hour

Usual Dosage Adults:

I.V.: 50-100 mcg/minute; increase by 50 mcg/minute every 10 minutes; continue for 12 hours after contractions have stopped

Oral: Start 30 minutes before stopping I.V. infusion; 10 mg every 2 hours for 24 hours, then 10-20 mg every 4-6 hours up to 120 mg/day

Contraindications Do not use before 20th week of pregnancy, cardiac arrhythmias, pheochromocytoma

Warnings Monitor hydration status and blood glucose concentrations; fatal maternal pulmonary edema has been reported, sometimes after delivery; fluid overload must be avoided, hydration levels should be monitored closely; if pulmonary edema occurs, the drug should be discontinued; use with caution in patients with moderate pre-eclampsia, diabetes, or migraine; some products may contain sulfites; maternal deaths have been reported in patients treated with ritodrine and concurrent corticosteroids (pulmonary edema)

Dosage Forms

Injection: 10 mg/mL (5 mL); 15 mg/mL (10 mL)

Tablet: 10 mg

Stability Stable for 48 hours at room temperature after dilution in 500 mL of NS, D_5W, or LR I.V. solutions

Reference Range After an oral 120 mg dose, maximum blood ritodrine level is 32 ng/mL

Overdosage Treatment

Decontamination: Lavage within 1 hour/activated charcoal with cathartic

Supportive therapy: Diazepam or lorazepam can be given for agitation; esmolol (50-100 mcg/kg I.V.) can be used for tachyarrhythmia

Enhancement of elimination: Multiple dosing of activated charcoal may be effective; hemodialysis may be effective

Diagnostic Tests/Procedures

Electrocardiography *on page 1253*

Drug Interactions

Decreased effect with beta-blockers

Increased effect/toxicity with meperidine, sympathomimetics, diazoxide, magnesium, betamethasone (pulmonary edema), potassium-depleting diuretics, general anesthetics

Pregnancy Risk Factor B

Pregnancy Implications Increased fetal heart rate; transient fetal hypoglycemia, hyperbilirubinemia in neonates have been noted; crosses the placenta

(Continued)

Ritodrine Hydrochloride *(Continued)*

Monitoring Parameters Hematocrit, serum potassium, glucose, colloidal osmotic pressure, heart rate, and uterine contractions

Patient Information Remain in bed during infusion

Nursing Implications Monitor amount of I.V. fluid administered to prevent fluid overload; place patient in left lateral recumbent position to reduce risk of hypotension; use microdrip chamber or I.V. pump to control infusion rate

Specific References

Bracero LA, Leikin E, Kirshenbaum N, et al, "Comparison of Nifedipine and Ritodrine for the Treatment of Preterm Labor," *Am J Perinatol*, 1991, 8(6):365-9.

Pisani RJ and Rosenow EC 3d, "Pulmonary Edema Associated With Tocolytic Therapy," *Ann Intern Med*, 1989, 110(9):714-8.

Rivotril® *see* Clonazepam *on page 229*

rLFN-α2 *see* Interferon Alfa-2b *on page 432*

rIFN-b *see* Interferon Beta-1b *on page 435*

RMS® *see* Morphine Sulfate *on page 539*

RO5-4200 *see* Flunitrazepam *on page 354*

Roaccutan® *see* Isotretinoin *on page 447*

Roaccutane® *see* Isotretinoin *on page 447*

Roacutan® *see* Isotretinoin *on page 447*

Ro-A-Vit® *see* Vitamin A *on page 795*

Robaxin® *see* Methocarbamol *on page 513*

Robitet® Oral *see* Tetracycline *on page 732*

Robitussin® Cough Calmers [OTC] *see* Dextromethorphan Hydrobromide *on page 270*

Robitussin® Pediatric [OTC] *see* Dextromethorphan Hydrobromide *on page 270*

Robitussin® [OTC] *see* Guaifenesin *on page 390*

Robomol® *see* Methocarbamol *on page 513*

Roccal® *see* Benzalkonium Chloride *on page 147*

Roferon-A® *see* Interferon Alfa-2a *on page 430*

Roflual® *see* Rimantadine Hydrochloride *on page 685*

Rogaine® *see* Minoxidil *on page 536*

Roipnol® *see* Flunitrazepam *on page 354*

Ronase® *see* Tolazamide *on page 756*

Rophipnol® *see* Flunitrazepam *on page 354*

Rophypnol® *see* Flunitrazepam *on page 354*

Rosalox *see* Metronidazole *on page 526*

Rotet® *see* Tetracycline *on page 732*

Roxanol™ *see* Morphine Sulfate *on page 539*

Roxanol SR™ *see* Morphine Sulfate *on page 539*

Roxicet® *see* Oxycodone and Acetaminophen *on page 584*

Roxicodone™ *see* Oxycodone Hydrochloride *on page 585*

RP54274 *see* Riluzole *on page 684*

RTCA *see* Ribavirin *on page 679*

Rubex® *see* Doxorubicin Hydrochloride *on page 303*

Rubifen *see* Methylphenidate Hydrochloride *on page 521*

Rubramin-PC® *see* Cyanocobalamin *on page 246*

Rufen® *see* Ibuprofen *on page 418*

Rum-K® *see* Potassium Chloride *on page 634*

Ru-Vert-M® *see* Meclizine Hydrochloride *on page 494*

Rytmonorm® *see* Propafenone Hydrochloride *on page 652*

SA-79 *replaced by* Propafenone Hydrochloride *on page 652*

Sabril® *see* Vigabatrin *on page 790*

Sabrilex® *see* Vigabatrin *on page 790*

Salazopyrin® *see* Sulfasalazine *on page 712*

Salbutamol *see* Albuterol *on page 92*

Salcatonin *see* Calcitonin *on page 177*

Saleto-200® [OTC] *see* Ibuprofen *on page 418*

Saleto-400® *see* Ibuprofen *on page 418*

Salflex® *see* Salsalate *on this page*

Salf-Pas® *see* Para-Aminosalicylate Sodium *on page 592*

Salgesic® *see* Salsalate *on this page*

Salicylazosulfapyridine *see* Sulfasalazine *on page 712*

Salicylsalicylic Acid *see* Salsalate *on this page*

Saline *see* Sodium Chloride *on page 698*

Saline® [OTC] *see* Sodium Chloride *on page 698*

Salmaterol *see* Salmeterol *on this page*

Salmeterol (sal me' te role)

CAS Number 89365-50-4; 94749-08-3

Brand Names Serevent®

Synonyms Salmaterol

Use Maintenance therapy for chronic asthma; prevention of exercise-induced asthma or nocturnal asthma

Mechanism of Action Relaxes bronchial smooth muscle by action on $beta_2$-receptors with little effect on heart rate; longer-acting than albuterol

Adverse Reactions

Cardiovascular: Tachycardia (slight), palpitations, hypertension, flushing, shortened P-R segment, lengthened Q-T segment, cardiac arrhythmias

Central nervous system: Dizziness, headache, nervousness, CNS stimulation, hyperactivity, insomnia

Dermatologic: Maculopapular rash, urticaria, pruritus

Gastrointestinal: gastrointestinal upset

Neuromuscular & skeletal: Tremor

Respiratory: Bronchospasm

Toxicodynamics/Kinetics

Onset of action: 30-60 minutes

Peak effect: 2 hours

Duration: 12 hours

Protein binding: 94% to 99%

Half-life: 3-4 hours

Elimination: Fecal

Usual Dosage Inhalation: Two inhalations (25 mcg) twice daily from a metered dose inhaler; maximum dose: 100 mcg twice daily

Contraindications Hypersensitivity to salmeterol, adrenergic amines, or any ingredients, children <12 years of age

Warnings Do not initiate in patients with significantly worsening or acutely deteriorating bronchospasm (acute asthmatic attacks); may cause paradoxical bronchospasm; use with caution in patients with cardiovascular disease, hypertension, hyperthyroidism, diabetes mellitus; avoid concomitant use of tricyclic antidepressants or MAO inhibitors

Dosage Forms Inhaler: 21 mcg/metered inhalation (60 & 120 doses)

Overdosage Treatment

Decontamination: Lavage/activated charcoal with cathartic for oral ingestion

Supportive therapy: Beta-blockers can be used for hyperadrenergic signs (use with caution in patients with wheezing)

Pregnancy Risk Factor C

Additional Information Tachyphylaxis usually does not occur

Specific References

Bone RC, "Another Word of Caution Regarding a new Long-Acting Bronchodilator," *JAMA*, 1995, 273(12):967-8.

Brogden RN and Faulds D, "Salmeterol Xinafoate: A Review of Its Pharmacological Properties and Therapeutic Potential in Reversible Obstructive Airways Disease," *Drugs*, 1991, 42(5):895-912.

Clark CE, Ferguson AD, and Siddorn JA, "Respiratory Arrests in Young Asthmatics on Salmeterol," *Respir Med*, 1993, 87(3):227-8.

Devoy MAB, Fuller RW, and Palmer JBD, "Are There any Detrimental Effects of the Use of Inhaled Long-Acting Beta-2-Agonists in the Treatment of Asthma?" *Chest*, 1995, 107:1116-24.

Hatton MQ, Allen MB, Mellor EJ, et al, "Salmeterol Rash," *Lancet*, 1991, 337(8750):1169-70.

Johnson M, "The Pharmacology of Salmeterol," *Lung*, 1990, 168(Suppl):115-9.

Salmiac® *see* Ammonium Chloride *on page 118*

Salsalate (sal' sa late)

CAS Number 552-94-3

Brand Names Argesic®-SA; Artha-G®; Disalcid®; Mono-Gesic®; Salflex®; Salgesic®; Salsitab®

(Continued)

Salsalate *(Continued)*

Synonyms Disalicylic Acid; Salicylsalicylic Acid

Use Treatment of minor pain or fever; rheumatoid arthritis, osteoarthritis, and related inflammatory conditions

Mechanism of Action Inhibits prostaglandin synthesis, acts on the hypothalamus heat-regulating center to reduce fever, blocks prostaglandin synthetase action which prevents formation of the platelet-aggregating substance thromboxane A_2

Adverse Reactions

Cardiovascular: Fluid retention, circulatory collapse

Central nervous system: Headache, aseptic meningitis, psychosis, cognitive dysfunction, dizziness, coma, seizures

Dermatologic: Rash, pruritus

Endocrine & metabolic: Hyperkalemia, anion gap metabolic acidosis

Gastrointestinal: Abdominal pain, nausea, vomiting, bleeding, ulceration, constipation, diarrhea, dyspepsia

Genitourinary: Albuminuria

Hematologic: Leukopenia, neutropenia, agranulocytosis, granulocytopenia; aplastic anemia (rare), platelet inhibition

Hepatic: Elevation of transaminases, fulminant hepatitis

Otic: Ototoxicity, tinnitus

Renal: Renal failure (acute), nephrotic syndrome, chronic renal failure

Respiratory: Wheezing, respiratory depression

Miscellaneous: Hypersensitivity

Signs & Symptoms of Acute Overdose Respiratory alkalosis, wheezing, gastrointestinal bleeding, gastritis; cognitive dysfunction, hyperthermia, nephrotic syndrome, bezoars, nystagmus, hyponatremia, hypoglycemia, tachypnea, tachypnea, nausea, vomiting, ototoxicity; tinnitus, drowsiness; severe poisoning can manifest with coma, seizures, renal failure and or hepatic failure, hypotension, respiratory depression, hyperglycemia, urine discoloration (pink), feces discoloration (black), feces discoloration (pink), feces discoloration (red), feces discoloration (tarry)

Toxicodynamics/Kinetics

Onset of action: Within 3-4 days of continuous dosing

Absorption: Oral: Completely from the small intestine

Distribution: Widely distributed to most body fluids and tissues

Protein binding: 75% to 90% (concentration dependent and decreases as serum concentrations increase)

Metabolism: Hydrolyzed in the liver to 2 moles of salicylic acid (active)

Half-life: 7-8 hours

Elimination: Almost totally excreted renally, about 1 hour

Usual Dosage Adults: Oral: 3 g/day in 2-3 divided doses

Dosing comments in renal impairment: In patients with end stage renal disease undergoing hemodialysis: 750 mg twice daily with an additional 500 mg after dialysis

Contraindications gastrointestinal ulcer or bleeding, known hypersensitivity to salsalate

Warnings Use with caution in patients with platelet and bleeding disorders, renal dysfunction, erosive gastritis, or peptic ulcer disease, previous nonreaction does not guarantee future safe taking of medication; do not use aspirin in children <16 years of age for chickenpox or flu symptoms due to the association with Reye's syndrome

Dosage Forms

Capsule: 500 mg

Tablet: 500 mg, 750 mg

Overdosage Treatment

Decontamination: Ipecac or lavage/activated charcoal with cathartic

Supportive therapy: Hypotension/dehydration can be managed with intravenous fluid therapy; acidosis should be treated with bicarbonates, seizures with benzodiazepines; antacids, blood products are indicated, as appropriate, for hemorrhage

Enhancement of elimination: Dialysis or perfusion is indicated for secondary complications, acidosis, or renal failure and not toxin removal alone; multiple dosing of activated charcoal may be effective; forced alkaline diuresis with intravenous bicarbonate to keep a urine pH >8 can hasten elimination

Test Interactions False-negative results for glucose oxidase urinary glucose tests (Clinistix®); false-positives using the cupric sulfate method (Clinitest®); also, interferes with Gerhardt test, VMA determination; 5-HIAA, xylose tolerance test and T_3 and T_4; a serum level of salicylate (by immunoassay) may underestimate salsalate levels; degradation of salsalate to salicylate can occur if specimens are allow to sit at room temperature

Drug Interactions Aspirin decreases serum concentrations probably by protein-binding displacement; there is an increased bleeding potential with concomitant warfarin therapy; may increase lithium and methotrexate concentrations by decreasing renal clearance; may decrease diuretic and hypotensive effects of thiazides, loop diuretics, ACE inhibitors, and beta-blockers; may increase nephrotoxicity of cyclosporine

Pregnancy Risk Factor C

Patient Information Avoid alcohol; do not self medicate with other drug products containing aspirin; use antacids to relieve upset stomach

Additional Information Does not appear to inhibit platelet aggregation; total dose (mg) multiplied by 1.4 gives aspirin equivalent dose

Specific References

Chapman BJ and Proudfoot AT, "Adult Salicylate Poisoning: Deaths and Outcome in Patients With High Plasma Salicylate Concentrations," *Q J Med*, 1989, 72(268):699-707.

Dugandric RM, Tierney MG, and Dickinson GE, "Evaluation of the Done Nomogram in the Management of Acute Salicylate Intoxication," *Ann Emerg Med*, 1989, 18(11):1186-90.

Spontak SF, Hassan FM, and Spadafora MP, "Salsalate Intoxication and Ramifications of Utilizing Nonspecific Analytical Methods in Estimating Quantitative Blood Concentrations," *J Anal Toxicol*, 1994, 18(4):229-31.

Vandenberg SA, Smolinske SC, Spoerke DG, et al, "Nonaspirin Salicylates: Conversion Factors for Estimating Aspirin Equivalency," *Vet Hum Toxicol*, 1989, 31(1):49-50.

Verbeeck RK, "Pharmacokinetic Drug Interactions With Nonsteroidal Anti-inflammatory Drugs," *Clin Pharmacokinet*, 1990, 19(1):44-66.

Vertrees JE, McWilliams BC, and Kelly HW, "Repeated Oral Administration for Treating Aspirin Overdose in Young Children," *Pediatrics*, 1990, 85(4):594-8.

Salsitab® *see* Salsalate *on page 689*

Salt *see* Sodium Chloride *on page 698*

Sandimmune® *see* Cyclosporine *on page 252*

Sandoparin® *see* Dalteparin *on page 256*

Sanoma® *see* Carisoprodol *on page 187*

Sapoderem® *see* Hexachlorophene *on page 402*

S.A.S.® *see* Sulfasalazine *on page 712*

Sassolite® *see* Boric Acid *on page 160*

Scabene® *see* Lindane *on page 470*

Scandicain® *see* Mepivacaine Hydrochloride *on page 502*

SCH-29851 *see* Loratadine *on page 481*

Sch-33844 *see* Spirapril Hydrochloride *on page 704*

Schein® *see* Piperazine Citrate *on page 629*

Scop *see* Scopolamine *on this page*

Scopex® *see* Scopolamine *on this page*

Scopine Tropate *see* Scopolamine *on this page*

Scopoderm® *see* Scopolamine *on this page*

Scopolamine (skoe pol' a meen)

Related Information

Cycloplegic Mydriatics Comparison *on page 1648*

Therapeutic Drugs Associated With Hallucinations *on page 1558-1559*

CAS Number 51-34-3; 114-49-8; 6533-68-2

Brand Names Buscapina®; Isopto® Hyoscine; Kwells®; Pamine®; Scopex®; Scopoderm®; Transderm Scop®; Vorigeno®

Synonyms Hyoscine; Scop; Scopine Tropate; Scopolamine Hydrobromide

Use Preoperative medication to produce amnesia and decrease salivation and respiratory secretions to produce cycloplegia and mydriasis; treatment of iridocyclitis, prevention of nausea and vomiting by motion; produces more CNS depression, mydriasis, and cycloplegia but less effective in preventing reflex bradycardia and effecting the intestines than atropine

Mechanism of Action Blocks the action of acetylcholine at parasympathetic sites in smooth muscle, secretory glands and the CNS; increases cardiac output, dries secretions, antagonizes histamine and serotonin; a tropane alkaloid

Adverse Reactions

Cardiovascular: Tachycardia, palpitations

Central nervous system: Disorientation, drowsiness, hallucinations, confusion, psychosis, delirium, electroencephalogram abnormalities

Gastrointestinal: Dry mouth, constipation

Genitourinary: Urinary retention

Ocular: Blurred vision, cycloplegia, mydriasis, photophobia, intraocular pressure (increased)

Miscellaneous: Anaphylactoid reactions, allergic reactions

Note: Systemic adverse effects have been reported with both the topical and ophthalmic preparations

(Continued)

Scopolamine *(Continued)*

Signs & Symptoms of Acute Overdose Mydriasis, confusion, bronchospasm, photophobia, dysuria, delirium, tachycardia, memory loss, intraocular pressure (increased), dementia, hypertension, seizures, coma, bradycardia, hyperthermia, visual hallucinations

Toxicodynamics/Kinetics

Absorption: Well absorbed by all routes of administration

Metabolism: Hepatic

Usual Dosage

Preoperatively:

Children: I.M., S.C.: 6 mcg/kg/dose (maximum: 0.3 mg/dose) or 0.2 mg/m^2 may be repeated every 6-8 hours **or** alternatively:

4-7 months: 0.1 mg

7 months to 3 years: 0.15 mg

3-8 years: 0.2 mg

8-12 years: 0.3 mg

Adults: I.M., I.V., S.C.: 0.3-0.65 mg; may be repeated every 4-6 hours

Motion sickness: Transdermal: Children >12 years and Adults: Apply 1 disc behind the ear at least 4 hours prior to exposure and every 3 days as needed; effective if applied as soon as 2-3 hours before anticipated need, best if 12 hours before

Ophthalmic:

Refraction:

Children: Instill 1 drop of 0.25% to eye(s) twice daily for 2 days before procedure

Adults: Instill 1-2 drops of 0.25% to eye(s) 1 hour before procedure

Iridocyclitis:

Children: Instill 1 drop of 0.25% to eye(s) up to 3 times/day

Adults: Instill 1-2 drops of 0.25% to eye(s) up to 4 times/day

Administration When giving I.V., must first be diluted with sterile water for injection

Contraindications Hypersensitivity to scopolamine or any component; narrow-angle glaucoma; acute hemorrhage

Warnings Use with caution with hepatic or renal impairment since adverse CNS effects occur more often in these patients; use with caution in infants and children since they may be more susceptible to adverse effects of scopolamine; use with caution in patients with gastrointestinal obstruction

Dosage Forms

Disc, transdermal: 1.5 mg/disc (4s)

Injection, as hydrobromide: 0.3 mg/mL (1 mL); 0.4 mg/mL (0.5 mL, 1 mL); 0.86 mg/mL (0.5 mL); 1 mg/mL (1 mL)

Solution, ophthalmic, as hydrobromide: 0.25% (5 mL, 15 mL)

Stability Avoid acid solutions, because hydrolysis occurs at pH <3

Reference Range Serum level of 890 pg/mL (SI: 7.93 nmol/L) correlated with psychosis

Overdosage Treatment

Decontamination: Lavage/activated charcoal with cathartic

Supportive therapy: Physostigmine can be utilized in life-threatening anticholinergic symptoms. Seizures can be treated with diazepam, lorazepam, phenobarbital, or phenytoin.

Enhancement of elimination: Multiple dosing of activated charcoal may be useful

Antidote(s)

Physostigmine *on page 1457*

Drug Interactions

Decreased effect of acetaminophen, levodopa, ketoconazole, digoxin, riboflavin, potassium chloride in wax matrix preparations

Increased effect/toxicity with anticholinergic agents

Pregnancy Risk Factor C

Pregnancy Implications Can cause neonatal drowsiness and tachycardia

Patient Information Report any changes of vision; wait 5 minutes after instilling ophthalmic preparation before using any other drops, do not blink excessively; put patch on day before traveling; once applied, do not remove the patch for 3 full days; may cause drowsiness, dizziness, and blurred vision; may impair coordination and judgment; report to physician any CNS effects; apply patch behind ear

Nursing Implications Topical disc is programmed to deliver *in vivo* 0.5 mg over 3 days; wash hands before and after applying the disc to avoid drug contact with eyes

Specific References

Bernstein S and Leff R, "Toxic Psychosis From Sleeping Medicines Containing Scopolamine," *N Engl J Med*, 1967, 277(12):638-9.

Hooper RG, Conner CS, and Rumack BH, "Acute Poisoning From Over-The-Counter Sleep Preparations," *JACEP*, 1979, 8(3):98-100.

Hughes SS and Zaloga GP, "Scopolamine Anisocaria," *Ann Emerg Med*, 1989, 18(4):423-4.
Osterholm RK and Camoriano JK, "Transdermal Scopolamine Psychosis," *JAMA*, 1982, 247(22):3081.

Scopolamine Hydrobromide *see* Scopolamine *on page 691*

Scot-Tussin® DM Cough Chasers [OTC] *see* Dextromethorphan Hydrobromide *on page 270*

Scot-Tussin® [OTC] *see* Guaifenesin *on page 390*

Secadrex® *see* Acebutolol Hydrochloride *on page 77*

Secobarbital Sodium (see koe bar' bi tal)

CAS Number 76-73-3

Brand Names Immenoctal®; Seconal™; Sedonal®; Seral®

Synonyms Meballymal; Quinalbarbitone Sodium

Use Short-term treatment of insomnia and as preanesthetic agent

Mechanism of Action Interferes with transmission of impulses from the thalamus to the cortex of the brain resulting in an imbalance in central inhibitory and facilitatory mechanisms

Adverse Reactions

Cardiovascular: Hypotension, cardiac arrhythmias, bradycardia

Central nervous system: Drowsiness, drowsiness, impaired judgment, CNS stimulation or CNS depression, hypothermia, electroencephalogram abnormalities

Dermatologic: Rash, mucosal ulcerations

Gastrointestinal: Nausea, vomiting

Local: Arterial spasm, and gangrene with inadvertent intra-arterial injection, thrombophlebitis with I.V. use

Renal: Oliguria

Respiratory: Laryngospasm, respiratory depression, apnea (especially with rapid I.V. use)

Signs & Symptoms of Acute Overdose Unsteady gait, slurred speech, myasthenia gravis (exacerbation or precipitation of), ptosis, vision color changes (green tinge); confusion, jaundice, hypothermia, nystagmus, fever, hypotension, CNS depression; can cause bezoars

Toxicodynamics/Kinetics

Onset of action: I.V.: Hypnosis occurs within 15-30 minutes

Duration: ~15 minutes

Absorption: Oral: Well absorbed (90%) from gastrointestinal tract; can also be absorbed through inhalation

Distribution: V_d: 1.5 L/kg; distributed rapidly throughout body tissues and fluids

Protein binding: 52% to 57%

Metabolism: In the liver

Half-life: 25 hours

Time to peak serum concentration: Within 2-4 hours

Elimination: Renally as inactive metabolites and small amounts as unchanged drug

Usual Dosage

Children:
- Hypnotic: I.M.: 3-5 mg/kg/dose; maximum: 100 mg/dose
- Preoperative sedation:
  - Oral: 50-100 mg 1-2 hours before procedure
  - Rectal: 5 mg/kg **or** <6 months: 30-60 mg; 6 months to 3 years: 60 mg; >3 years: 60-120 mg
- Sedation: Oral: 6 mg/kg/day divided every 8 hours

Adults:
- Hypnotic:
  - Oral, I.M.: 100-200 mg/dose
  - I.V.: 50-250 mg/dose
- Preoperative sedation: Oral: 100-300 mg 1-2 hours before procedure
- Sedation: Oral: 20-40 mg/dose 2-3 times/day

Fatal dose: 2-3 g

Contraindications CNS depression, uncontrolled pain, hypersensitivity to secobarbital or any component

Warnings Use with caution in patients with CHS, hepatic or renal insufficiency, marked liver impairment or latent porphyria; avoid alcoholic beverages; potential for drug dependency exists

Dosage Forms

Capsule: 100 mg

Injection: 50 mg/mL (2 mL)

Injection, rectal: 50 mg/mL (20 mL)

Tablet: 100 mg

Stability Do not shake vial during reconstitution, rotate ampul; aqueous solutions

(Continued)

Secobarbital Sodium *(Continued)*

are not stable reconstitute with aqueous polyethylene glycol; aqueous (sterile water) solutions should be used within 30 minutes; do not use bacteriostatic water for injection or lactated Ringer's; precipitates when used in solution with cimetidine

Reference Range

Therapeutic: 3-5 μg/mL (SI: 12.6-21.0 μmol/L)
Toxic: >5 μg/mL (SI: >21.0 μmol/L)

Overdosage Treatment

Decontamination: Lavage/activated charcoal with cathartic

Supportive therapy: If hypotension occurs, administer I.V. fluids and place the patient in the Trendelenburg position. If unresponsive, an I.V. vasopressor (eg, dopamine, epinephrine) may be required.

Enhancement of elimination: Forced alkaline diuresis is of no value in the treatment of intoxications with short-acting barbiturates. Charcoal hemoperfusion may be useful in the harder to treat intoxications, especially in the presence of very high serum barbiturate levels. Hemodialysis is less useful; slightly dialyzable (5% to 20%)

Diagnostic Tests/Procedures

Secobarbital, Blood *on page 1348*

Drug Interactions CNS depressants

Pregnancy Risk Factor D (fetal concentration is 70% of maternal)

Pregnancy Implications Crosses the placenta and appears in breast milk

Patient Information Food slows absorption

Nursing Implications I.V.: Give undiluted or diluted with sterile water for injection, normal saline, or Ringer's injection; maximum infusion rate: 50 mg/15 seconds

Specific References

Monteil RA, Raybaud H, Madinier I, et al, "Occurrence of Oral Mucosal Necrosis in a Patient With Barbiturate-Induced Coma," *Oral Surg Oral Med Oral Pathol*, 1991, 72(5):562-4.

Tracqui A, Kintz P, Mangin P, et al, "A Fatality Involving Secobarbital, Nitrazepam, and Codeine," *Am J Forensic Med Pathol*, 1989, 10(2):130-3.

Serpasil® *see* Reserpine *on page 678*

Sertindole

Synonyms 1(2-(4-5-chloro-1-(4-fluorophenyl)-1H-indol-3-y1)-1-piperidinyl ethyl)-2-imidazoline

Use Investigational: Antipsychotic agent

Mechanism of Action Antagonist of dopamine (d_2), serotonin, and norepinephrine (alpha$_1$-receptors); has limbic selectivity, somewhat similar to clozapine

Adverse Reactions

Cardiovascular: Orthostatic hypotension, syncope

Central nervous system: Lethargy, drowsiness, dizziness, headache (26%), dystonia

Genitourinary: Dry ejaculation

Neuromuscular & skeletal: Tremor, cogwheel rigidity

Respiratory: Nasal congestion

Toxicodynamics/Kinetics

Peak plasma level: 8-10 hours

Half-life: 60 hours (may exceed 100 hours in >10% of patients)

Protein binding: 99%

Metabolism: Hepatic to norsertindole and Lu28-092

Elimination: Fecal

Usual Dosage 4-32 mg/day; usual therapeutic dosage range: 16-20 mg/day

Overdosage Treatment

Decontamination: Lavage/activated charcoal with cathartic

Enhancement of elimination: Multiple dosing of activated charcoal may be effective

Additional Information Potent anxiolytic activity, low extrapyramidal reaction; no anticholinergic effects

Specific References

Hyttel J, Arnt J, Costall B, et al, "Pharmacological Profile of the Atypical Neuroleptic Sertindole," *Clin Neuropharmacol*, 1992, 15(Suppl 1 Pt A): 267A-8A.

Sertofren® *see* Desipramine Hydrochloride *on page 263*

Sertraline Hydrochloride (ser' tra leen)

Related Information

Antidepressant Agents Comparison *on page 1639*

CAS Number 79617-96-2; 79559-97-0

Brand Names Lustral®; Zoloft™

Use Treatment of major depression; also being studied for use in obesity and obsessive-compulsive disorder

Mechanism of Action Antidepressant with selective inhibitory effects on presynaptic serotonin (5-HT) reuptake; it is a naphthylamine derivative

Adverse Reactions

Cardiovascular: Palpitations, syncope, edema, either tachycardia or bradycardia

Central nervous system: Hypertonia, drowsiness, ataxia restlessness, dizziness, dystonic reactions

Dermatologic: Pruritus, hirsutism, acne, erythema multiforme

Endocrine & metabolic: Gynecomastia, serotonin syndrome (diarrhea, sweating, tremors), syndrome of inappropriate antidiuretic hormone

Gastrointestinal: Nausea, vomiting, diarrhea, dry mouth

Genitourinary: Ejaculatory disturbances (delay)

Neuromuscular & skeletal: Tremors, paresthesia

Ocular: Exophthalmos, photophobia, xerophthalmia, lacrimation, diplopia, mydriasis, anterior chamber hemorrhage

Psychiatric: Hypomania

Respiratory: Rhinitis, wheezing, cough, dyspnea, tachypnea

Miscellaneous: Sweating

Signs & Symptoms of Acute Overdose Tachycardia, conjunctivitis, dysuria, lacrimation, insomnia, hypoglycemia, hypertriglyceridemia, myoclonus, mania, myalgia, ejaculatory disturbances, fatigue, bone marrow depression, muscle twitching, purpura, hypertonia, hypertrichosis, dysphagia, gynecomastia, stomatitis, agitation, dermatitis, hirsutism, amenorrhea, drowsiness, hypertension, hypotension, chest pain

Toxicodynamics/Kinetics

Absorption: Slow

Distribution: V_d: 20 L/kg

Protein binding: 98%

Metabolism: Extensive to desmethylsertraline ($^1/_{10}$ the activity of parent compound)

Bioavailability, oral: 36%

Half-life, elimination: 24 hours

(Continued)

Sertraline Hydrochloride *(Continued)*

Time to peak plasma concentration: 8-12 hours

Elimination: Urine and feces

Usual Dosage Oral: Initial: 50 mg/day as a single dose, dosage may be increased at intervals of at least 1 week to a maximum recommended dosage of 200 mg/day

Warnings Do not use in combination with monoamine oxidase inhibitor or within 14 days of discontinuing treatment or initiating treatment with a monoamine oxidase inhibitor due to the risk of serotonin syndrome; use with caution in patients with pre-existing seizure disorders, patients in whom weight loss is undesirable, patients with recent myocardial infarction, unstable heart disease, hepatic or renal impairment, patients taking other psychotropic medications, agitated or hyperactive patients as drug may produce or activate mania or hypomania; because the risk of suicide is inherent in depression, patient should be closely monitored until depressive symptoms remit and prescriptions should be written for minimum quantities to reduce the risk of overdose

Dosage Forms Tablet: 50 mg, 100 mg

Reference Range 6 hours after doses of 400 mg and 200 mg, peak plasma levels were 253.2 ng/mL and 105.4 ng/mL respectively; plasma levels correlate poorly to clinical presentation; therapeutic clinical trials: 0.03-0.19 mg/L

Overdosage Treatment Overdose of <100 mg in children <5 years of age are tolerated well with decontamination and minimal supportive care

Decontamination: Lavage/activated charcoal with cathartic

Enhancement of elimination: Multiple dosing of activated charcoal may be effective

Test Interactions Elevates liver function tests, hypoglycemia, hypercholesterolemia, hypertriglyceridemia, decreases uric acid

Diagnostic Tests/Procedures

Sertraline, Blood *on page 1351*

Drug Interactions Decreases clearance of tolbutamide; increases free warfarin levels; use with ethanol may cause drowsiness; sertraline or paroxetine can incite occurrence of LSD flashback episodes (primarily visual)

Pregnancy Risk Factor B

Monitoring Parameters Uric acid, liver function, CBC

Patient Information If currently on another antidepressant drug, please notify physician. Although sertraline has not been shown to increase effects of alcohol, it is recommended that drinking be refrained from while on this medication. If pregnant or intent to become pregnant while on this drug, please alert physician to this fact; may experience some weight loss, but is usually minimal; if presently taking warfarin, digoxin, an oral hypoglycemic drug, or a drug having an effect on the central nervous system, such as a medication for insomnia or anxiety, please notify physician. There are no known interactions between sertraline and over-the-counter medications; however, they should be used with caution and the directions for their use should be followed carefully.

Additional Information Buspirone (15-60 mg/day) may be useful in treatment of sexual dysfunction during treatment with a selective serotonin reuptake inhibitor

Specific References

Brown DF and Kerr HD, "Sertraline Overdose," *Ann Pharmacother*, 1994, 28(11):1307.

Doogan DP and Caillard V, "Sertraline: A New Antidepressant," *J Clin Psychiatry*, 1988, 49(Suppl):46-51.

Hoaken PC, "An Alert to Extrapyramidal Side-Effects From SSRIs," *Can J Psychiatry*, 1995, 40(1):51.

Jackson C, Carson W, Markowitz J, et al, "SIADH Associated With Fluoxetine and Sertraline Therapy," *Am J Psychiatry*, 1995, 152:809-10.

Kassner J and Woolf A, "Sertraline HCl: A New Antidepressant," *Vet Hum Toxicol*, 1992, 34:343.

Kassner J and Woolf A, "Sertraline Hydrochloride: Correlation of Clinical Presentation With Plasma Concentration," *Vet Hum Toxicol*, 1993, 35:341.

Klein-Schwartz W and Anderson B, "Analysis of Sertraline Only Overdoses," *Vet Hum Toxicol*, 1994, 36:378.

Lau GT and Horwitz BZ, "Sertraline Overdose in 40 Patients," *Vet Hum Toxicol*, 1994, 36:370.

LeJoyeux M, et al, "Serotonin Syndrome: Incidence, Symptoms, and Treatment," *CNS Drugs*, 1994, 2:132-43.

Llorente MD, Gorelick M, and Silverman MA, "Sertraline as the Cause of Inappropriate Antidiuretic Hormone Secretion," *J Clin Psychiatry*, 1994, 55(12):543-4.

Markel H, Lee A, Holmes RD, et al, "LSD Flashback Syndrome Exacerbated by Selective Serotonin Reuptake Inhibitor Antidepressants in Adolescents," *J Pediatr*, 1994, 125(5 Pt 1):817-9.

Myers LB, Dean BS, and Krenzelok EP, "Sertraline (Zoloft™): Overdose Assessment of a New Antidepressant," *Vet Hum Toxicol*, 1993, 35:341.

Myers LB, Dean BS, and Krenzelok EP, "Sertraline (Zoloft™): A Pediatric Overdose Approach," *Vet Hum Toxicol*, 1994, 36:361.

Norden MJ, "Buspirone Treatment of Sexual Dysfunction Associated With Selective Serotonin Re-Uptake Inhibitors," *Depression*, 1994, 2:109-12.

Thornton SL and Resch DS, "SIADH Associated With Sertraline Therapy," *Am J Psychiatry*, 1995, 152:809.

Tueth MJ, "The Serotonin Syndrome in the Emergency Department," *Ann Emerg Med*, 1993, 22(8):1369.

Serzone® *see* Nefazodone *on page 552*

Sevredol® *see* Morphine Sulfate *on page 539*

Silace® [OTC] *see* Docusate *on page 297*

Siltussin® [OTC] *see* Guaifenesin *on page 390*

Simron® *see* Iron *on page 439*

Simvastatin (sim' va stat in)

CAS Number 79902-63-9

Brand Names Denan®; Liponorm®; Sinvacor®; Sivastin®; Zocor™; Zocord®

Use Adjunct to dietary therapy to decrease elevated serum total and LDL cholesterol concentrations in primary hypercholesterolemia

Mechanism of Action Simvastatin acts by competitively inhibiting 3-hydroxyl-3-methylglutaryl-coenzyme A (HMG-CoA) reductase, the enzyme that catalyzes the rate-limiting step in cholesterol biosynthesis

Adverse Reactions

Cardiovascular: Symptomatic hypotension

Central nervous system: Headache, psychosis

Gastrointestinal: Gastrointestinal symptoms

Hepatic: Persistent elevations in liver enzymes and CPK elevations (rarely) in the absence of clinical myopathy

Toxicodynamics/Kinetics Administered as a prodrug which is hydrolyzed in the liver to the hydroxy acid, its active form

Protein binding: 95%

Metabolism: First-pass extraction with hydrolysis to active metabolites

Time to peak serum concentration: 1-2 hours

Elimination: Primarily via the biliary tract (60%)

Usual Dosage Safety and efficacy in children and adolescents <20 years of age have not been established

Adults: Oral: Usual maintenance dose: 5-40 mg/day once daily in the evening

Dosing adjustment/comments in renal impairment: Recommended starting dose: 5 mg; patient should be closely monitored

Contraindications Previous hypersensitivity to simvastatin or lovastatin or other HMG-CoA reductase inhibitors; active liver disease or unexplained elevations of serum transaminases; pregnancy and lactation

Dosage Forms Tablet: 5 mg, 10 mg, 20 mg, 40 mg

Stability Tablets should be stored in well-closed containers at temperatures between 5°C to 30°C (41°F to 86°F)

Overdosage Treatment

Decontamination: Ipecac or lavage/activated charcoal with cathartic

Enhanced elimination: Multiple dosing of activated charcoal may be effective

Drug Interactions

Increased effect of warfarin

Increased toxicity of cyclosporin, gemfibrozil

Pregnancy Risk Factor X

Monitoring Parameters Creatine phosphokinase levels due to possibility of myopathy

Patient Information Report any unexplained myalgia, tenderness, or asthenia, especially if these symptoms are accompanied by malaise or fever

Nursing Implications Liver enzyme elevations may be observed during simvastatin therapy; combination therapy with other hypolipidemic agents may be required to achieve optimal reductions of LDL cholesterol; diet, weight reduction, and exercise should be attempted to control hypercholesterolemia before the institution of simvastatin therapy

Specific References

French J and White H, "Transient Symptomatic Hypotension in Patients on Simvastatin," *Lancet*, 1989, 2(8666):807-8.

Mauro VF and MacDonald JL, "Simvastatin: A Review of Its Pharmacology and Clinical Use," *DICP*, 1991, 25(3):257-64.

Mol MJ and Stalenhoef AF, "Adrenocortical Function in Patients on Simvastatin," *Lancet*, 1990, 335(8686):412-3.

Sinarest® 12 Hour Nasal Solution *see* Oxymetazoline Hydrochloride *on page 586*

Sinequan® *see* Doxepin Hydrochloride *on page 301*

Sinumist®-SR Capsulets® [OTC] *see* Guaifenesin *on page 390*

Sinusol-B® *see* Brompheniramine Maleate *on page 165*

Sinvacor® *see* Simvastatin *on this page*

Siquil® *see* Triflupromazine Hydrochloride *on page 770*

Sivastin® *see* Simvastatin *on previous page*

SK-Choral® Hydrate *see* Chloral Hydrate *on page 193*

SKF-33-134-A *replaced by* Amiodarone Hydrochloride *on page 113*

SK-Lygen® *see* Chlordiazepoxide *on page 198*

SK-Pramine® *see* Imipramine *on page 422*

SK-Reserpine® *see* Reserpine *on page 678*

Slo-bid™ *see* Theophylline *on page 735*

Slo-Niacin® [OTC] *see* Niacin *on page 554*

Slo-Phyllin® *see* Theophylline *on page 735*

Slo-Salt® [OTC] *see* Sodium Chloride *on this page*

Slow FE® *see* Iron *on page 439*

Slow-K® *see* Potassium Chloride *on page 634*

SM-7338 *see* Meropenem *on page 504*

Smail® *see* Chlordiazepoxide *on page 198*

SMX-TMP *see* Co-trimoxazole *on page 242*

Snaplets-FR® Granules [OTC] *see* Acetaminophen *on page 79*

Socainide Hydrochloride *see* Lorcainide Hydrochloride *on page 484*

Sodico® *see* Para-Aminosalicylate Sodium *on page 592*

Sodiopen® *see* Penicillin G, Parenteral, Aqueous *on page 600*

Sodium Benzoate (sow' dee um benz' oh ate)

CAS Number 532-32-1

Use Adjunctive therapy for the prevention and treatment of hyperammonemia due to suspected or proven urea cycle defects; used to treat urea cycle enzyme deficiency in combination with arginine

Adverse Reactions

Dermatologic: Urticaria

Gastrointestinal: Nausea, vomiting

Miscellaneous: Anaphylaxis

Toxicodynamics/Kinetics

Half-life: 0.75-7.4 hours

Elimination: Clearance is largely attributable to metabolism with urinary excretion of hippurate, the major metabolite

Usual Dosage Investigational use (not FDA approved): Children: Oral, I.V.: 0.25 g/kg bolus followed by 0.25-0.5 g/kg/day as continuous infusion or divided every 6-8 hours

Dosage Forms Powder: 454 g

Overdosage Treatment Supportive therapy: Treat rash with epinephrine, diphenhydramine and corticosteroids

Additional Information Not available commercially; oral solutions must be compounded using powder form; I.V. solutions must also be compounded and tested for sterility and pyrogenicity prior to use

Specific References

Michils A, Vandermoten G, Duchateau J, et al, "Anaphylaxis With Sodium Benzoate," *Lancet*, 1991, 337(8754):1424-5.

Sodium Chloride (sow' dee um klor' ide)

CAS Number 7647-14-5

Brand Names Adsorbonac® [OTC] Ophthalmic; Ayr® [OTC]; HuMIST® [OTC]; Muro 128® Ophthalmic [OTC]; NaSal™ [OTC]; Ocean Nasal Mist [OTC]; Pretz® [OTC]; Saline® [OTC]; Slo-Salt® [OTC]

Synonyms Common Salt; Dendritis; Halite; h.g. Blending; NaCl; Normal Saline; Purex; Saline; Salt

Use Prevention of muscle cramps and heat prostration; restoration of sodium ion in hyponatremia; induce abortion; restore moisture to nasal membranes; GU irrigant; reduction of corneal edema; source of electrolytes and water for expansion of the extracellular fluid compartment; intravenous sodium chloride use is essential in lithium or bromide toxicity

Mechanism of Action There is a fluid shift from intracellular to extracellular space centrally with acute salt poisoning resulting in dehydration of brain cells; principal extracellular cation; functions in fluid and electrolyte balance, osmotic pressure control, and water distribution

Adverse Reactions

Cardiovascular: Congestive conditions, thrombosis

Endocrine & metabolic: Hypernatremia, dilution of serum electrolytes, overhydration, hypokalemia
Hematologic: Hypervolemia
Local: Phlebitis, extravasation
Respiratory: Pulmonary edema

Signs & Symptoms of Acute Overdose Tachycardia, coma, congestive heart failure, thirst, fluid retention, hypokalemia, pulmonary edema, restlessness, irritability, dizziness, obtundation, seizures, nausea, vomiting, diarrhea, cramps; flat anterior fontanelle in infants

Toxicodynamics/Kinetics
Onset of action: Abortifacient: Labor usually starts within 12-24 hours
Absorption: Oral, I.V., dermal: Rapid
Distribution: V_d: 0.6 L/kg; widely distributed
Metabolism: Not significant
Elimination: Mainly in urine but also in sweat, tears, and saliva

Usual Dosage
Newborn electrolyte requirement:
Premature: 2-8 mEq/kg/24 hours
Term:
0-48 hours: 0-2 mEq/kg/24 hours
>48 hours: 1-4 mEq/kg/24 hours

Children: I.V.: Hypertonic solutions (>0.9%) should only be used for the initial treatment of acute serious symptomatic hyponatremia; maintenance: 3-4 mEq/kg/day; maximum: 100-150 mEq/day; dosage varies widely depending on clinical condition
Replacement: Determined by laboratory determinations mEq
Sodium deficiency (mEq/kg) = [% dehydration (L/kg)/100 x 70 (mEq/L) = [0.6 (L/kg) x (140 - serum sodium) (mEq/L)]
Nasal: Use as often as needed

Adults:
GU irrigant: 1-3 L/day by intermittent irrigation
Heat cramps: Oral: 0.5-1 g with full glass of water, up to 4.8 g/day
Replacement I.V.: Determined by laboratory determinations mEq
Sodium deficiency (mEq/kg) = [% dehydration (L/kg)/100 x 70 (mEq/L)] + [0.6 (L/kg) x (140 - serum sodium) (mEq/L)]

To correct acute, serious hyponatremia: mEq sodium = (desired sodium (mEq/L) - actual sodium (mEq/L) x 0.6 x wt (kg)); for acute correction use 125 mEq/L as the desired serum sodium; acutely correct serum sodium in 5 mEq/L/dose increments; more gradual correction in increments of 10 mEq/L/day is indicated in the asymptomatic patient
Chloride maintenance electrolyte requirement in parenteral nutrition: 2-4 mEq/kg/24 hours or 25-40 mEq/1000 kcals/24 hours; maximum: 100-150 mEq/24 hours
Sodium maintenance electrolyte requirement in parenteral nutrition: 3-4 mEq/kg/24 hours or 25-40 mEq/1000 kcals/24 hours; maximum: 100-150 mEq/24 hours. See table.

Approximate Deficits of Water and Electrolytes in Moderately Severe Dehydration

Condition	Water (mL/kg)	Na (mEq/kg)
Fasting and thirsting	100–200	5–7
Diarrhea		
isonatremic	100–120	8–10
hypernatremic	100–120	2–4
Hyponatremic	100–120	10–12
Pyloric stenosis	100–120	8–10
Diabetic acidosis		

*A **negative** deficit indicates total body **excess** prior to treatment.
Adapted from Vaughan VC III, McKay RJ Jr, and Behrman RE, eds, *Nelson Textbook of Pediatrics,* 11th ed, WB Saunders Co, 1979.

Nasal: Use as often as needed
Ophthalmic:
Ointment: Apply once daily or more often
Solution: Instill 1-2 drops into affected eye(s) every 3-4 hours
Abortifacient: 20% (250 mL) administered by transabdominal intra-amniotic instillation

(Continued)

Sodium Chloride *(Continued)*

Contraindications Hypersensitivity to sodium chloride or any component; hypertonic uterus, hypernatremia, fluid retention

Warnings Sodium toxicity is almost exclusively related to how fast a sodium deficit is corrected; both rate and magnitude are extremely important; use with caution in patients with congestive heart failure, renal insufficiency, liver cirrhosis, hypertension

Dosage Forms

- Drops, nasal: 0.9% with dropper
- Injection: 0.2% (3 mL); 0.45% (3 mL, 5 mL, 500 mL, 1000 mL); 0.9% (1 mL, 2 mL, 3 mL, 4 mL, 5 mL, 10 mL, 20 mL, 25 mL, 30 mL, 50 mL, 100 mL, 130 mL, 150 mL, 250 mL, 500 mL, 1000 mL); 3% (500 mL); 5% (500 mL); 20% (250 mL); 23.4% (30 mL, 100 mL)
- Injection:
  - Admixtures: 50 mEq (20 mL); 100 mEq (40 mL); 625 mEq (250 mL)
  - Bacteriostatic: 0.9% (30 mL)
  - Concentrated: 14.6% (20 mL, 40 mL, 200 mL); 23.4% (10 mL, 20 mL, 30 mL)
- Irrigation: 0.45% (500 mL, 1000 mL, 1500 mL); 0.9% (250 mL, 500 mL, 1000 mL, 1500 mL, 2000 mL, 3000 mL, 4000 mL)
- Ointment, ophthalmic (Muro 128®): 5% (3.5 g)
- Solution:
  - Irrigation: 0.9% (1000 mL, 2000 mL)
  - Nasal: 0.4% (15 mL, 50 mL); 0.6% (15 mL); 0.65% (20 mL, 45 mL, 50 mL)
  - Ophthalmic (Adsorbonac®): 2% (15 mL); 5% (15 mL, 30 mL)
- Tablet: 650 mg, 1 g, 2.25
- Tablet:
  - Enteric coated: 1 g
  - Slow release: 600 mg

Stability Store injection at room temperature; protect from heat and from freezing; use only clear solutions

Reference Range

- Serum/plasma levels:
  - Neonates:
    - Full-term: 133-142 mEq/L
    - Premature: 132-140 mEq/L
  - Children 2 months to Adults: 135-145 mEq/L

Neurologic symptoms occur when serum sodium reaches 150-160 mEq/L; serum sodium levels from 160-185 mEq/L will commonly cause seizures, especially if an attempt is made to rapidly lower serum sodium; >185 mEq/L, death will likely result

Overdosage Treatment

Supportive therapy: For hypernatremia, give 30-50 mEq/L of sodium (half chloride, half bicarbonate) by slow I.V. infusion; prepare solution by adding 15-25 mEq/L sodium chloride (2.5 mEq/mL) and 15-25 mEq sodium bicarbonate (1 mEq/mL) to 1 liter D_5W; administer at a rate of ⅔ maintenance with a goal of achieving normal serum sodium at 24-36 hours after initiating treatment; seizures may occur if serum sodium is lowered too quickly

Enhancement of elimination: Seizures can be treated with lorazepam or diazepam 0.1-0.25 mg/kg; hypernatremia is resolved through the use of diuretics and free water replacement. Peritoneal dialysis should be considered in infants who are salt poisoned; hemodialysis should be considered in patients who are refractory to other therapies on in patients with renal impairment.

Drug Interactions Corticosteroids, corticotropin

Pregnancy Risk Factor C

Pregnancy Implications Most of dose is concentrated in the decidua and fetal part of the placenta; some diffuses into maternal blood. When hypertonic sodium chloride is injected into the amniotic fluid, the following may result: Disseminated intravascular coagulation, renal necrosis, uterine and cervical lesions, pulmonary embolism, pneumonia, hemorrhage, death.

Monitoring Parameters Monitor I & O, weight, serum sodium, potassium, chloride, and bicarbonate levels

Patient Information Blurred vision is common with ophthalmic ointment; may sting eyes when first applied

Nursing Implications Bacteriostatic NS should not be used for diluting or reconstituting drugs for administration in neonates; I.V. infusion of 3% or 5% sodium chloride should not exceed 100 mL/hour and should be administered in a central line only; presence or worsening of rales and degree of peripheral edema with infusions

Additional Information Deaths have been reported in patients who have consumed salt water as an emetic; ingestion of 0.5-1 g/kg sodium chloride is likely to be toxic; tablets can be radiopaque; 1 tablespoon of tablet salt contains ~305 mEq of sodium and can cause an elevation of serum sodium by 30.5 mEq/L in a child 3 years of age

Lethal dose: 3 g/kg

Specific References

Barer J, Hill LL, Hill RM, et al, "Fatal Poisoning From Salt Used as an Emetic," *Am J Dis Child*, 1973, 125:889-90.

Gresham GS and Mashru MK, "Fatal Poisoning With Sodium Chloride," *Forensic Sci Int*, 1982, 20:87-8.

Meadow R, "Nonaccidental Salt Poisoning," *Arch Dis Child*, 1993, 68(4):448-52.

Moder KG and Hurley DL, "Fatal Hypernatremia From Exogenous Salt Intake: Report of a Case and Review of the Literature," *Mayo Clin Proc*, 1990, 65(12):1587-94.

Smith EJ, and Palevsky S, "Salt Poisoning in a Two-Year-Old Child," *Am J Emerg Med*, 1990, 8:571-2.

Sodium Fluoride *see* Fluoride *on page 355*

Sodium Hydrofluoride *see* Fluoride *on page 355*

Sodium *L*-Tri-iodothyronine *see* Liothyronine Sodium *on page 471*

Sodium Nitroferricyanide *see* Nitroprusside Sodium *on page 568*

Sodium Nitroprusside *see* Nitroprusside Sodium *on page 568*

Sodium Oxybate *see* Gamma Hydroxybutyric Acid *on page 376*

Sodium Salicylate (sow' dee um sal i' sil ate)

CAS Number 54-21-7

Brand Names Uracel®

Use Treatment of minor pain or fever; arthritis

Adverse Reactions

Dermatologic: Rash

Gastrointestinal: Nausea, vomiting, gastrointestinal distress, bleeding, ulcers

Hematologic: Platelet inhibition

Hepatic: Hepatotoxicity

Respiratory: Wheezing

Signs & Symptoms of Acute Overdose Nausea, vomiting, wheezing, bezoars, gastrointestinal bleeding, gastritis; hyperthermia, hypoglycemia, nystagmus, ototoxicity; tinnitus, drowsiness; severe poisoning can manifest with coma, seizures, renal failure and or hepatic failure, hyponatremia, hypotension, respiratory depression, headache, dizziness, confusion, metabolic acidosis, fever, leukopenia, neutropenia, agranulocytosis, granulocytopenia, hyperglycemia, urine discoloration (pink), feces discoloration (black), feces discoloration (pink), feces discoloration (red), feces discoloration (tarry), pylorospasm, rhabdomyolysis

Usual Dosage Adults: Oral: 325-650 mg every 4 hours

Dosage Forms Tablet, enteric coated: 325 mg, 650 mg

Reference Range

Sample size: 1.5-2 mL blood (purple top tube)

Timing of serum samples: Peak levels usually occur 2 hours after ingestion; half-life increases with dosage (eg, the half-life after 300 mg is 3 hours, and after 1 g is 5-6 hours, and after 8-10 g is 10 hours)

Salicylate serum concentrations correlate with the pharmacological actions and adverse effects observed; see table.

Serum Salicylate: Clinical Correlations

Serum Salicylate Concentration (mg/dL)	Desired Effects	Adverse Effects/ Intoxication
~10	Antiplatelet Antipyresis Analgesia	GI intolerance and bleeding, hypersensitivity, hemostatic defects
15–30	Anti–inflammatory	Mild salicylism
25–40	Treatment of rheumatic fever	Nausea/vomiting, hyperventilation, salicylism, flushing, sweating, thirst, headache, diarrhea, and tachycardia
>40		Respiratory alkalosis, hemorrhage, excitement, confusion, asterixis, pulmonary edema, convulsions, tetany, metabolic acidosis, fever, coma, cardiovascular collapse, renal and respiratory failure

Overdosage Treatment

Decontamination: Activated charcoal with cathartic is quite effective; each gram of activated charcoal can bind up to 550 mg of salicylic acid; whole bowel irrigation can also be used

(Continued)

Sodium Salicylate *(Continued)*

Supportive therapy: Hypotension/dehydration can be managed with intravenous fluid therapy; acidosis should be treated with bicarbonates, seizures with benzodiazepines; blood products are indicated, as appropriate, for hemorrhage; antacids may promote gastric absorption

Enhancement of elimination: Forced alkaline diuresis with intravenous sodium bicarbonate to keep urine pH at 8 should be performed for salicylate levels >40 mg/dL; dialysis is indicated for secondary complications, acidosis, or renal failure and not toxin removal alone; consider hemodialysis for acute salicylate levels >100 mg/dL; multiple dosing of activated charcoal may not hasten elimination; dialyzable (50% to 100%)

Additional Information Sodium content of 1 g: 6.25 mEq; less effective than an equal dose of aspirin in reducing pain or fever; patients hypersensitive to aspirin may be able to tolerate; total dose (mg) multiplied by 1.1 provides aspirin equivalent dose

Specific References

Chapman BJ and Proudfoot AT, "Adult Salicylate Poisoning: Deaths and Outcome in Patients With High Plasma Salicylate Concentrations," *Q J Med*, 1989, 72(268):699-707.

Dugandric RM, Tierney MG, and Dickinson GE, "Evaluation of the Done Nomogram in the Management of Acute Salicylate Intoxication," *Ann Emerg Med*, 1989, 18(11):1186-90.

Vandenberg SA, Smolinske SC, Spoerke DG, et al, "Nonaspirin Salicylates: Conversion Factors for Estimating Aspirin Equivalency," *Vet Hum Toxicol*, 1989, 31(1):49-50.

Verbeeck RK, "Pharmacokinetic Drug Interactions With Nonsteroidal Anti-inflammatory Drugs," *Clin Pharmacokinet*, 1990, 19(1):44-66.

Vertrees JE, McWilliams BC, and Kelly HW, "Repeated Oral Administration for Treating Aspirin Overdose in Young Children," *Pediatrics*, 1990, 85(4):594-8.

Sodium Valproate *see* Valproic Acid and Derivatives *on page 782*

Sodium Warfarin *see* Warfarin Sodium *on page 800*

Sodol® *see* Carisoprodol *on page 187*

Sofarin® *see* Warfarin Sodium *on page 800*

Solarcaine® [OTC] *see* Benzocaine *on page 149*

Solazine® *see* Trifluoperazine Hydrochloride *on page 769*

Solfoton® *see* Phenobarbital *on page 614*

Solganal® Injection *see* Gold Compounds *on page 386*

Solgol® *see* Nadolol *on page 545*

Solis® *see* Diazepam *on page 271*

Solium® *see* Chlordiazepoxide *on page 198*

Solurex® Injection *see* Dexamethasone *on page 266*

Solurex L.A.® Injection *see* Dexamethasone *on page 266*

Soma® *see* Carisoprodol *on page 187*

Soma® Compound *see* Carisoprodol *on page 187*

Somadril® *see* Carisoprodol *on page 187*

Somatomax PM® *see* Gamma Hydroxybutyric Acid *on page 376*

Somaz® *see* Temazepam *on page 724*

Somnite® *see* Nitrazepam *on page 562*

Somnomed® *see* Methaqualone Hydrochloride *on page 511*

Somsanit® *see* Gamma Hydroxybutyric Acid *on page 376*

Songar® *see* Triazolam *on page 767*

Soni-Slo® *see* Isosorbide Dinitrate *on page 445*

Sopental® *see* Pentobarbital *on page 604*

Soprodol® *see* Carisoprodol *on page 187*

Soprol® *see* Bisoprolol Fumarate *on page 157*

Sorbid® *see* Isosorbide Dinitrate *on page 445*

Sorbide Nitrate *see* Isosorbide Dinitrate *on page 445*

Sorbinil

CAS Number 68367-52-2

Use Investigational: Decrease the adverse effects of diabetes mellitus, specifically diabetic, nephropathy, retinopathy, neuropathy, and cataract formation

Mechanism of Action Aldose reductase inhibitor structurally related to hydantoin, decreased amounts of sorbitol and fructose are formed from glucose; thus, less water is drawn into the lens (through osmosis) and neurons, thus possibly leading to less diabetic complications

Adverse Reactions

Hematologic: Leukopenia, thrombocytopenia

Hepatic: Elevated liver function tests

Neuromuscular & skeletal: Myalgia

Miscellaneous: Hypersensitivity syndrome (maculopapular rash, toxic epidermal necrolysis, adult respiratory distress syndrome)

Toxicodynamics/Kinetics

Distribution: V_d: 0.7-1 L/kg

Half-life: 38-52 hours

Usual Dosage 200-250 mg once daily

Reference Range After a single 250 mg dose, peak plasma levels were 3.3 μg/mL in healthy young males, 5.4 μg/mL in elderly males, and 6.3 μg/mL in elderly females; after 5 days on above dose, plasma sorbinil levels can reach 10.6 μg/mL

Overdosage Treatment

Decontamination: Ipecac or lavage/activated charcoal with cathartic

Enhancement of elimination: Multiple dosing of activated charcoal may be effective

Specific References

Asbury AK, "Understanding Diabetic Neuropathy," *N Engl J Med*, 1988, 319(9):577-8.

Clark Jr CM and Lee DA, "Prevention and Treatment of the Complications of Diabetes Mellitus," *N Engl J Med*, 1995, 332:1210-7.

Marwick C, "NIH Testing Sorbinil to Prevent Diabetic Retinopathy," *JAMA*, 1984, 252(10):1263.

Raskin P and Rosenstock J, "Aldose Reductase Inhibitors and Diabetic Complications," *Am J Med*, 1987, 83(2):298-306.

Sorbitrate® *see* Isosorbide Dinitrate *on page 445*

Soridol® *see* Carisoprodol *on page 187*

Sosegon® *see* Pentazocine *on page 603*

Sosenol® *see* Pentazocine *on page 603*

Sostril® *see* Ranitidine Hydrochloride *on page 675*

Sotalol Hydrochloride (soe' ta lole)

Related Information

Beta-Blockers Comparison *on page 1644-1645*

CAS Number 959-24-0

Brand Names Betapace®

Use Treatment of ventricular arrhythmias, prevention of life-threatening arrhythmias, and sudden death postmyocardial infarction

Mechanism of Action Has both B- and B_2-receptor blocking activity; also passes some type III antiarrhythmic activity

Adverse Reactions

Cardiovascular: Hypotension (especially with higher doses), bradycardia, exacerbation of Raynaud's phenomenon, congestive heart failure, chest pain, tachycardia

Central nervous system: Dizziness, somnolence, confusion, drowsiness, mental depression, headache, drowsiness, insomnia, asthenia, tiredness, hallucinations, anxiety, diarrhea, night terrors

Dermatologic: Itching, skin rash; red, crusted skin

Gastrointestinal: Nausea, vomiting, stomach discomfort, constipation

Genitourinary: Decreased sexual ability, impotence

Hematologic: Leukopenia

Local: Skin necrosis after extravasation, phlebitis

Respiratory: Breathing difficulties, wheezing

Miscellaneous: Cold extremities, reduced peripheral circulation, sweating

Signs & Symptoms of Acute Overdose Leukopenia or neutropenia (agranulocytosis, granulocytopenia); Q-T prolongation; lightheadedness, depression, LDL (increased), eosinophilia, thrombocytopenia, myasthenia gravis (exacerbation or precipitation of), heart block, insomnia, impotence, hypoglycemia, bleeding

Toxicodynamics/Kinetics

Onset of action: Rapid, 1-2 hours

Peak effect: 3-4 hours

Absorption: ~70% which is decreased 20% to 30% by meals (especially milk products)

Distribution: V_d: 0.2-0.7 L/kg; low lipid solubility

Protein binding: Not protein bound (10%)

Bioavailability: 90% to 100%

Half-life: 7-15 hours

Elimination: Unchanged through kidney

Usual Dosage Adults: Oral: Initial: 80 mg twice daily; may be increased to 240-320 mg/day and up to 480-640 mg/day in patients with life-threatening refractory ventricular arrhythmias; adjust dose every 2-3 days

(Continued)

Sotalol Hydrochloride *(Continued)*

Dosing adjustment in renal impairment:

Cl_{cr} >60 mL/minute: Administer every 12 hours
Cl_{cr} 30-60 mL/minute: Administer every 24 hours
Cl_{cr} 10-30 mL/minute: Administer every 36-48 hours
Cl_{cr} <10 mL/minute: Individualize dose

Contraindications Uncompensated congestive heart failure, cardiogenic shock, bradycardia or heart block, pulmonary edema, asthma

Warnings Use with caution in patients with congestive heart failure, peripheral vascular disease, hypokalemia, hypomagnesemia, renal dysfunction, sick sinus syndrome; abrupt withdrawal may result in return of life-threatening arrhythmias; sotalol can provoke new or worsening ventricular arrhythmias

Dosage Forms Tablet: 80 mg, 160 mg, 240 mg

Reference Range Peak serum level: ~1.7 mg/L after 160 mg oral dose

Overdosage Treatment

Decontamination: Lavage/activated charcoal with cathartic; do not use ipecac

Supportive therapy: Glucagon (50-150 mcg/kg followed by continuous drip of 1-5 mg/hour) for positive chronotropic effect; glucagon can correct bradycardia and sinus arrest; atropine/isoproterenol can be utilized to increase heart rate; calcium chloride may also be effective

Enhancement of elimination: Multiple dosing of activated charcoal is likely to be of benefit; hemodialysis or hemoperfusion may be effective

Antidote(s)

Glucagon *on page 1431*

Drug Interactions Decreased effect/levels with coadministration of aluminum- and/or magnesium-containing antacids

Pregnancy Risk Factor B

Monitoring Parameters Serum magnesium, potassium, EKG

Patient Information Seek emergency help if palpitations occur; do not discontinue abruptly or change dose without notifying physician; take on an empty stomach

Nursing Implications Initiation of therapy and dose escalation should be done in a hospital with cardiac monitoring; lidocaine and other resuscitative measures should be available

Specific References

Blair AD, Burgess ED, Maxwell BM, et al, "Sotalol Kinetics in Renal Insufficiency," *Clin Pharmacol Ther*, 1981, 29:457-63.

Fernandes CMB and Daya MR, "Sotalol-Induced Bradycardia Reversed by Glucagon," *Can Fam Physician*, 1995, 41:659-65.

Pill MW and McCloskey WW, "Sotalol: What the Emergency Nurse Needs to Know," *J Emerg Nurs*, 1995, 21:229-31.

Sovcainum *see* Dibucaine *on page 275*

Span-FF® *see* Iron *on page 439*

Sparine® *see* Promazine Hydrochloride *on page 649*

Spec-T® *see* Benzocaine *on page 149*

Spirapril Hydrochloride (spye' ra pril)

Related Information

ACE Inhibitors Comparison *on page 1636-1637*

CAS Number 83647-97-6; 94841-17-5

Brand Names Renormax®

Synonyms Sch-33844

Use Treatment of hypertension, congestive heart failure

Mechanism of Action Angiotensin-converting enzyme inhibitor; inhibits renin-angiotensin system

Adverse Reactions

Central nervous system: Headache, dizziness, migraine headache (exacerbation of), hypoesthesia
Dermatologic: Skin rash
Gastrointestinal: Nausea, diarrhea, vomiting
Neuromuscular & skeletal: Back pain
Ocular: Conjunctivitis
Respiratory: Cough (1.5% to 4%)

Toxicodynamics/Kinetics

Absorption: Oral: 53% to 60% (delayed by high fat meals)
Distribution: V_d:
Oral: 270 L
I.V.: 28 L
Protein binding: 86% to 91%
Metabolism: Hepatic to active metabolite spiraprilat
Half-life: 1-2 hours
Elimination: Renal

Usual Dosage
Congestive heart failure: Oral: 1.5-6.25 mg
Hypertension: Starting dose: Oral: 12 mg/day in 1-2 divided doses; may increase dose in 2- to 4-week intervals

Contraindications Previous spirapril hypersensitivity

Warnings Use with caution in patients with previous hypersensitivity to other ACE inhibitors, pregnancy, renal/hepatic insufficiency, hyperkalemia, autoimmune disease

Dosage Forms Tablet: 3 mg, 6 mg, 12 mg, 24 mg

Reference Range After a 6 mg oral dose, peak plasma spirapril and spiraprilat level is ~20 ng/mL and 23 ng/mL respectively; after a 6 mg I.V. dose, peak serum spiraprilat level is ~45 ng/mL

Overdosage Treatment
Decontamination: Ipecac/lavage/activated charcoal with cathartic
Supportive therapy: Following initiation of essential overdose management, toxic symptom treatment and supportive treatment should be initiated. Hypotension usually responds to I.V. normal saline or Trendelenburg positioning. If unresponsive to these measures, the use of a parenteral inotrope may be required (eg, norepinephrine 0.1-0.2 mcg/kg/minute titrated to response). Seizures commonly respond to lorazepam or diazepam (I.V. 5-10 mg bolus in adults every 15 minutes if needed up to a total of 30 mg; I.V. 0.25-0.4 mg/kg/dose up to a total of 10 mg in children) or to phenytoin or phenobarbital. Naloxone may antagonize hypotensive effects. Inhaled sodium cromoglycate (total dose: 40 mg/day) can decrease ACE-inhibitor cough by 50%.
Enhanced elimination: Multiple dosing of activated charcoal may be effective

Specific References
Salvetti A, "Newer ACE Inhibitors: A Look at the Future," *Drugs*, 1990, 40(6):800-28.

Spirits of Wine *see* Ethyl Alcohol *on page 336*

Spirolone® *see* Spironolactone *on this page*

Spironolactone (speer on oh lak' tone)

CAS Number 52-01-7

Brand Names Aldace®; Aldactone®; Aldopur®; Laractone®; Spirolone®; Spironone®; Spirotone®; Tensin®; Uractone®

Use Management of edema associated with excessive aldosterone excretion; hypertension; primary hyperaldosteronism; treatment of hirsutism; acidosis

Investigational: Congestive heart failure

Mechanism of Action Competes with aldosterone for receptor sites in the distal renal tubules, increasing sodium chloride and water excretion while conserving potassium and hydrogen ions; may block the effect of aldosterone on arteriolar smooth muscle as well

Adverse Reactions
Central nervous system: Lethargy, headache, mental confusion, fever, ataxia
Dermatologic: Rash, alopecia
Endocrine & metabolic: Hyperkalemia (especially in patients with azotemia or receiving potassium supplements), dehydration, hyponatremia, hypokalemia, hyperchloremic metabolic acidosis, postmenopausal bleeding, amenorrhea, gynecomastia
Gastrointestinal: Anorexia, nausea, vomiting, diarrhea, gastritis
Hematologic: Eosinophilia
Hepatic: Hepatotoxicity
Ocular: Myopia
Renal: BUN (increased)
Miscellaneous: Development of systemic lupus erythematosus (SLE)

Toxicodynamics/Kinetics
Protein binding: 89%
Metabolism: In the liver to multiple metabolites, including canrenone (active)
Half-life: 1.4 hours (canrenone: 13-24 hours)
Time to peak serum concentration: Within 1-3 hours (primarily as the active metabolite)
Elimination: Urinary and biliary excretion

Usual Dosage Oral (to reduce delay in onset of effect, a loading dose of 2 or 3 times the daily dose may be administered on the first day of therapy):

Neonates: 0.5-1 mg/kg/dose every 8 hours

Children: 1-3.3 mg/kg/day in divided doses every 6-24 hours up to a maximum of 200 mg/day

Adults:
Edema, hypertension, hypokalemia: 25-200 mg/day in 1-2 divided doses
Diagnosis of primary aldosteronism: 100-400 mg/day in 1-2 divided doses

Dosing interval in renal impairment:
Cl_{cr} 10-50 mL/minute: Administer every 12-24 hours

(Continued)

Spironolactone *(Continued)*

Cl_{cr} <10 mL/minute: Avoid use

Contraindications Hypersensitivity to spironolactone or any component, hyperkalemia, anuria, renal failure, creatinine >2.5 mg/dL

Warnings Use with caution in patients with dehydration, hepatic disease, hyponatremia, renal sufficiency, patients receiving other potassium-sparing diuretics, ACE inhibitors, or potassium supplements; it is recommended the drug may be discontinued several days prior to adrenal vein catheterization

Dosage Forms Tablet: 25 mg, 50 mg, 100 mg

Reference Range Steady-state of canrenone levels (of spironolactone dosing 50 mg twice daily) are 50-70 ng/mL (trough) and 146-250 ng/mL (peak)

Overdosage Treatment

Decontamination: Ipecac or lavage/activated charcoal with cathartic

Supportive therapy: Hyperkalemia can be treated with glucose/insulin and sodium bicarbonate (1 mEq/kg); sodium polystyrene sulfonate can also be given; I.V. fluids administration of 0.45% sodium chloride with furosemide (1 mg/kg, up to 40 mg) can be used to promote urine flow

Test Interactions May cause false elevation in serum digoxin concentrations measured by RIA

Drug Interactions Increased serum potassium levels with potassium, potassium-sparing diuretics, indomethacin, angiotensin-converting enzymes inhibitors; reduces activity of warfarin; salicylates block spironolactone's diuretic effects; hyperkalemia can result with concomitant ACE inhibitor administration; cholestyramine and spironolactone can cause a hyperchloremic metabolic acidosis

Pregnancy Risk Factor D

Monitoring Parameters Blood pressure, serum electrolytes, renal function

Additional Information May be used in patients with hyperuricemia or gout

Specific References

Foukaridis GN, "Influence of Spironolactone and Its Metabolite Canrenone on Serum Digoxin Assays," *Ther Drug Monit*, 1990, 12(1):82-4.

Karim A, "Spironolactone: Disposition, Metabolism, Pharmacodynamics, and Bioavailability," *Drug Metab Rev*, 1978, 8(1):151-88.

Renkes P, Gaucher P, and Trechot P, "Spironolactone and Hepatic Toxicity," *JAMA*, 1995, 273(5):376-7.

Skluth HA and Gums JG, "Spironolactone: A Re-examination," *DICP*, 1990, 24(1):52-9.

Tweeddale MG and Ogilvie RI, "Antagonism of Spironolactone-Induced Natriuresis by Aspirin in Man," *N Engl J Med*, 1973, 289(4):198-200.

Zapater P and Alba D, "Acidosis and Extreme Hypokalemia Associated With Cholestyramine and Spironolactone," *Ann Pharmacother*, 1995, 29:199-200.

Spironone® *see* Spironolactone *on previous page*

Spirotone® *see* Spironolactone *on previous page*

Spondyvit® *see* Vitamin E *on page 798*

Sporanox® Oral *see* Itraconazole *on page 448*

S-P-T® *see* Thyroid *on page 749*

Stadol® *see* Butorphanol Tartrate *on page 174*

Stadol® NS *see* Butorphanol Tartrate *on page 174*

Stannous Fluoride *see* Fluoride *on page 355*

Staril® *see* Fosinopril Sodium *on page 369*

Statex® *see* Morphine Sulfate *on page 539*

Status Epilepticus Treatment Algorithm *see page 1608*

Staurodorm® *see* Flurazepam Hydrochloride *on page 363*

Stavudine (stav' yoo deen)

CAS Number 3056-17-5

Brand Names Zerit®

Synonyms BMY-27857; d4T

Use Treatment of adults with advanced HIV infection who are intolerant to approved therapies with proven clinical benefit or who have experienced significant clinical or immunologic deterioration while receiving these therapies, or for whom such therapies are contraindicated

Mechanism of Action Inhibits reverse transcriptase of the human immunodeficiency virus (HIV)

Adverse Reactions

Central nervous system: Excitability

Hematologic: Anemia

Hepatic: Elevated liver function tests

Neuromuscular & skeletal: Paresthesia (at doses >2 mg/kg/day)

Toxicodynamics/Kinetics

Distribution: V_d: 0.5 L/kg

Peak serum level: 1 hour after administration

Bioavailability: 82%
Half-life: 1-1.6 hours
Elimination: Renal (40%); clearance: 0.21 L/hour/kg

Usual Dosage Oral: Initial: 0.5-1 mg/kg/day in 3 divided doses; do not exceed a total dose of 2 mg/kg/day

Contraindications Hypersensitivity to stavudine

Warnings Use with caution in patients who demonstrate previous hypersensitivity to zidovudine, didanosine, zalcitabine, pre-existing bone marrow suppression, or renal insufficiency, paresthesia, folic acid or vitamin B_{12} deficiency

Dosage Forms Capsule: 15 mg, 20 mg, 30 mg, 40 mg

Reference Range Peak serum level after an oral dose of 4 mg/kg is 4.2 μg/mL

Overdosage Treatment

Decontamination: Ipecac or lavage/activated charcoal with cathartic
Enhancement of elimination: Multiple dosing of activated charcoal may be effective

Diagnostic Tests/Procedures

Complete Blood Count *on page 1236*

Specific References

Browne MJ, Mayer KH, Chafee SB, et al, "2',3'-Didehydro-3'-dexoxythymidine (d4T) in Patients With AIDS or AIDS-Related Complex - A Phase I Trial," *J Infect Dis*, 1993, 167(1):21-9.
Sandstrom E and Oberg B, "Antiviral Therapy in Human Immunodeficiency Virus Infections. Current Status," *Drugs*, 1993, 45(4):488-508.

Stay Trim® Diet Gum [OTC] *see* Phenylpropanolamine Hydrochloride *on page 622*
Steclin® *see* Tetracycline *on page 732*
Stelazine® *see* Trifluoperazine Hydrochloride *on page 769*
Stemetic® *see* Trimethobenzamide Hydrochloride *on page 772*
Sterapred® *see* Prednisone *on page 639*
Ster-Zac® *see* Hexachlorophene *on page 402*
Stesolid® *see* Diazepam *on page 271*
Stilbestrol *see* Diethylstilbestrol *on page 280*
Stilboestrol *see* Diethylstilbestrol *on page 280*
Stilnox® *see* Zolpidem Tartrate *on page 814*
Stilphostrol® Injection *see* Diethylstilbestrol *on page 280*
Stilphostrol® Oral *see* Diethylstilbestrol *on page 280*
St. Joseph® Cough Suppressant [OTC] *see* Dextromethorphan Hydrobromide *on page 270*
Stop® [OTC] *see* Fluoride *on page 355*
Streptase® *see* Streptokinase *on this page*

Streptokinase (strep toe kye' nase)

Related Information

Therapeutic Drugs Associated With Hallucinations *on page 1558-1559*

CAS Number 9002-01-1

Brand Names Kabikinase®; Streptase®

Use Thrombolytic agent used in treatment of recent severe or massive deep vein thrombosis (within 7 days), pulmonary emboli, peripheral arterial thrombosis, myocardial infarction, and occluded arteriovenous cannulas; can prevent venous valvular damage and development of venous hypertension; not effective for strokes

Mechanism of Action Activates the conversion of plasminogen to plasmin by forming a complex, exposing plasminogen-activating site, and clearing a peptide bond that converts plasminogen to plasmin; plasmin degrades fibrin, fibrinogen and other procoagulant proteins into soluble fragments; effective both outside and within the formed thrombus/embolus

Adverse Reactions

Cardiovascular: Hypotension, chest pain, arrhythmias, pericardial effusion/pericarditis
Central nervous system: Headache, chills, hallucinations
Dermatologic: Rash, angioneurotic edema
Gastrointestinal: Nausea, vomiting
Hematologic: Hemolytic anemia, anemia, eye hemorrhage, liver hemorrhage
Neuromuscular & skeletal: Guillain-Barré syndrome
Ocular: Ocular hemorrhage, periorbital edema
Respiratory: Bronchospasm
Miscellaneous: Periorbital swelling, anaphylaxis (2.5%), bleeding at sites of percutaneous trauma arrhythmias, sweating, epistaxis

(Continued)

Streptokinase *(Continued)*

Signs & Symptoms of Acute Overdose Epistaxis, confusion, wheezing, tubular necrosis, bleeding gums, hemoptysis, hematuria, ocular hemorrhage, leukocytosis, intracranial hemorrhage, jaundice, eczema, depression, coagulopathy, hematoma, spontaneous ecchymoses, oozing at catheter site

Toxicodynamics/Kinetics

Onset of action: Activation of plasminogen occurs almost immediately

Duration: Fibrinolytic effects last only a few hours, while anticoagulant effects can persist for 8-24 hours

Half-life: 83 minutes

Elimination: By circulating antibodies and via the reticuloendothelial system

Usual Dosage I.V.:

Children: Safety and efficacy not established; limited studies have used: 3500-4000 units/kg over 30 minutes followed by 1000-1500 units/kg/hour; clotted catheter: 25,000 units, clamp for 2 hours then aspirate contents and flush with normal saline

Adults (best results are realized if used within 5-6 hours of myocardial infarction; antibodies to streptokinase remain for 3-6 months after initial dose; use another thrombolytic enzyme (ie, urokinase), if thrombolytic therapy is indicated):

Guidelines for acute myocardial infarction (AMI):

1.5 million units infused over 60 minutes. Monitor for the first few hours for signs of anaphylaxis or allergic reaction. **Infusion should be slowed if blood pressure is lowered by 25 mm Hg or if asthmatic symptoms appear.** Begin heparin 5000-10,000 unit bolus followed by 1000 units/hour approximately 3-4 hours after completion of streptokinase infusion or when PTT is <100 seconds.

Guidelines for acute pulmonary embolism (APE):

3 million unit dose; administer 250,000 units over 30 minutes followed by 100,000 units/hour for 24 hours. Monitor for the first few hours for signs of anaphylaxis or allergic reaction. **Infusion should be slowed if blood pressure is lowered by 25 mm Hg or if asthmatic symptoms appear**. Begin heparin 1000 units/hour approximately 3-4 hours after completion of streptokinase infusion or when PTT is <100 seconds.

Thromboses: 250,000 units to start, then 100,000 units/hour for 24-72 hours depending on location

Cannula occlusion: 250,000 units into cannula, clamp for 2 hours, then aspirate contents and flush with normal saline

Administration I.V. infusion requires an infusion pump; streptokinase is administered by I.V., intra-arterial, or intracoronary infusion; may also be used to clear an occluded arteriovenous cannula

Contraindications Hypersensitivity to streptokinase or any component; recent strep infection; active internal bleeding, recent CVA (within 2 months), or intracranial or intraspinal surgery

Warnings Avoid I.M. injections; use with caution in patients with a history of cardiac arrhythmias, major surgery within last 10 days, gastrointestinal bleeding, recent trauma, severe hypertension, or in patients with recent exposure to streptokinase or anistreplase

Dosage Forms Powder for injection: 250,000 units (5 mL, 6.5 mL); 600,000 units (5 mL); 750,000 units (6 mL, 6.5 mL); 1,500,000 units (6.5 mL, 10 mL, 50 mL)

Stability Keep in refrigerator, use reconstituted solutions within 24 hours; store unopened vials at room temperature

Reference Range

Partial thromboplastin time (PTT) activated: 20.4-33.2 seconds

Prothrombin time (PT): 10.9-13.7 seconds (same as control)

Fibrinogen: 200-400 mg/dL

Drug Interactions

Decreased effect with antifibrinolytics (eg, aminocaproic acid)

Increased effect/toxicity with anticoagulants, antiplatelet drugs

Pregnancy Risk Factor C

Pregnancy Implications If streptokinase is used near term, delivery by Cesarean section should be considered

Monitoring Parameters Blood pressure, PT, APTT, fibrinogen, platelet count, hematocrit; bleeding, every 15 minutes for the first hour of therapy

Nursing Implications For I.V. or intracoronary use only; avoid I.M. injections; do not mix with other drugs

Additional Information Best results are realized if used within 5-6 hours of myocardial infarction; antibodies to streptokinase remain for 3-6 months after initial dose, use another thrombolytic enzyme (ie, urokinase) if repeat thrombolytic therapy is indicated; 6-month mortality rate in use for ischemic strokes is 44% higher in streptokinase group. Investigators applied analysis to data for patients ≥75 years of age from two large trials studying the impact of streptokinase on patient outcome after acute myocardial infarction; their conclusion was that age alone is not a contraindication to the use of streptokinase and that thrombolytic therapy is cost-effective and is beneficial toward the survival of elderly patients. Additional studies are needed to determine if a weight-adjusted dose will maintain efficacy but decrease adverse events such as stroke.

Specific References

Blum A and Shohat B, "CD-4 Lymphopenia Induced by Streptokinase," *Circulation*, 1995, 91(6):1899.

Cross DB and White HD, "Allergic Reactions to Streptokinase: Does Antibody Formation Prevent Reuse in a Second Myocardial Infarction?" *Clin Immunother*, 1994, 2:415-20.

de Boer A and van Griensven JMT, "Drug Interactions With Thrombolytic Agents," *Clin Pharmacokinet*, 1995, 28:315-26.

Dehmer GJ, Gresalfi N, Daly D, et al, "Impairment of Fibrinolysis by Streptokinase, Urokinase, and Recombinant Tissue-Type Plasminogen Activator in the Presence of Radiographic Contrast Agents," *J Am Coll Cardiol*, 1995, 25(5):1069-75.

Fears R, "Biochemical Pharmacology and Therapeutic Aspects of Thrombolytic Agents," *Pharmacol Rev*, 1990, 42(3):201-21.

Geraets DR, Hoehns JD, Burke TG, et al, "Thrombolytic-Associated Cholesterol Emboli Syndrome: Case Report and Literature Review," *Pharmacotherapy*, 1995, 15(4):441-8.

Hommel M, Boissel JP, Cornu C, et al, "Termination of Trial of Streptokinase in Severe Acute Ischaemic Stroke," *Lancet*, 1995, 345(8941):57.

Kalish SC, Gurwitz JH, Krumholz HM, et al, "A Cost-Effectiveness Model of Thrombolytic Therapy for Acute Myocardial Infarction," *J Gen Intern Med*, 1995, 10:321-30.

Krammer B, Steiner M, Burstein C, et al, "Spontaneous, Massive Liver Hemorrhage as a Complication of Thrombolysis With Ultra-high Dose Streptokinase in Deep Thrombophlebitis," *Vasa*, 1994, 23(4):373-6.

Lee TH, "Cost Effectiveness of Tissue Plasminogen Activator," *N Engl J Med*, 1995, 332:1443-4.

Marcus DM and Frederick AR, Jr, "Streptokinase-Induced Tenon's Hemorrhage After Retinal Detachment Surgery," *Am J Ophthalmol*, 1994, 118(6):815-7.

Mark DB, Hlatky MA, Califf RM, et al, "Cost Effectiveness of Thrombolytic Therapy With Tissue Plasminogen Activator as Compared With Streptokinase for Acute Myocardial Infarction," *N Engl J Med*, 1995, 332:1418-24.

Petch MC, "Dangers of Thrombolysis," *BMJ*, 1990, 300(6723):483-4.

Sleight P, "Streptokinase Is Still the Agent of Choice for Most Patients With Myocardial Infarction," *Am J Ther*, 1995, 2:128-35.

Taylor BV, Mastaglia FL, and Stell R, "Guillain-Barré Syndrome Complicating Treatment With Streptokinase," *Med J Aust*, 1995, 162(4):214-5.

Striadyne® *see* Adenosine Triphosphate *on page 90*

Strontium-89 Chloride (stron' shee um)

Related Information

Toxins Which Should be Lavaged With Solutions Other Than Water *on page 1635*

CAS Number 14158-27-1

Brand Names Metastron®

Use Relief of bone pain in patients with skeletal metastases

Mechanism of Action Similar to calcium; deposits in bone and teeth; stimulates bone formation while inhibiting bone resorption

Adverse Reactions Most severe reactions of marrow toxicity can be managed by conventional means; a flushing sensation has been observed in patients following rapid administration (usually over <30 seconds); thrombocytopenia

Signs & Symptoms of Acute Overdose Nausea, chills, vomiting, diarrhea, bone marrow suppression

Toxicodynamics/Kinetics Half-life: 50.5 days

Usual Dosage Adults: I.V.: 148 megabecquerel (4 millicurie) administered by slow I.V. injection over 1-2 minutes or 1.5-2.2 megabecquerel (40-60 microcurie)/kg; repeated doses are generally not recommended at intervals <90 days; measure the patient dose by a suitable radioactivity calibration system immediately prior to administration

Contraindications Pregnancy, lactation

Warnings Use caution in patients with bone marrow compromise; incontinent patients may require urinary catheterization. Body fluids may remain radioactive up to one week after injection. Not indicated for use in patients with cancer not involving bone and should be used with caution in patients whose platelet counts fall <60,000 or whose white blood cell counts fall <2400. A small number of patients have experienced a transient increase in bone pain at 36-72 hours postdose; this reaction is generally mild and self-limiting.

Dosage Forms Injection: 10.9-22.6 mg/mL [148 megabecquerel, 4 millicurrie] (10 mL)

Stability Store vial and its contents inside its transportation container at room temperature

Overdosage Treatment

Decontamination: Oral ingestion: Since absorption is rapid and water should not theoretically be used for gastric lavage, removal is probably not efficacious; give 1.5-10 g of sodium alginate (then 2-4 tablets every 2-4 hours for 24 hours) or 50-100 mL of aluminum phosphate gel (followed by 40 mL every 2 hours) or 65 mL of aluminum hydroxide orally (followed by 40 mL every 1-2 hours)

(Continued)

Strontium-89 Chloride *(Continued)*

Pregnancy Risk Factor D

Monitoring Parameters Complete blood count

Patient Information Eat and drink normally, there is no need to avoid alcohol or caffeine unless already advised to do so; may be advised to take analgesics until Metastron® begins to become effective; the effect lasts for several months, if pain returns before that, notify medical personnel

Nursing Implications During the first week after injection, strontium-89 will be present in the blood and urine, therefore, the following common sense precautions should be instituted:

1. Where a normal toilet is available, use in preference to a urinal, flush the toilet twice
2. Wipe away any spilled urine with a tissue and flush it away
3. Have patient wash hands after using the toilet
4. Immediately wash any linen or clothes that become stained with blood or urine
5. Wash away any spilled blood if a cut occurs

Additional Information Reacts with water (thermic reaction); does not emit gamma radiation

Specific References

Brandi ML, "New Treatment Strategies: Ipriflavone Strontium, Vitamin D Metabolites and Analogs," *Am J Med*, 1993, 95(Suppl 5A):5A-69S-5A-74S.

Lincoln TA, "Importance of Initial Management of Persons Internally Contaminated with Radionuclides," *Am Ind Hyg Assoc J*, 1976, 37(1):16-21.

Robinson RG, Preston DF, Schiefelbein M, et al, "Strontium 89 Therapy for the Palliation of Pain Due to Osseous Metastases," *JAMA*, 1995, 274:420-4.

Strumazol® *see* Methimazole *on page 512*

Sublimaze® *see* Fentanyl Citrate *on page 347*

Sucralfate (soo kral' fate)

CAS Number 54182-58-0

Brand Names Antepsin®; Carafate®; Keal®; Sugast®; Sulcrate®; Ulcogant®; U-One-S®

Synonyms Aluminum Sucrose Sulfate

Use Short-term management of duodenal ulcers; maintenance for duodenal ulcers; suspension may be used topically for treatment of stomatitis due to cancer chemotherapy and other causes of esophageal and gastric erosions

Mechanism of Action Forms a complex, a paste-like, cytoprotective substance, when combined with gastric acid that adheres to the damaged mucosal area. This selectively forms a protective coating that protects the lining against peptic acid, pepsin, and bile salts.

Adverse Reactions

Central nervous system: Dizziness, sleepiness

Dermatologic: Rash, pruritus

Gastrointestinal: Constipation, diarrhea, nausea, gastric discomfort, indigestion, dry mouth, intestinal obstruction may occur secondary to bezoars

Neuromuscular & skeletal: Back pain, dysarthria

Signs & Symptoms of Acute Overdose Toxicity is minimal, may cause constipation; encephalopathy, bezoars

Toxicodynamics/Kinetics

Onset of action: Paste formation and ulcer adhesion occur within 1-2 hours

Duration: Up to 6 hours; contains 207 mg of aluminum per dose which can dissociate at low pH

Absorption: Oral: <5% from gastrointestinal tract

Distribution: To many body tissues including liver and kidneys; acts locally at ulcer sites; unbound in gastrointestinal tract to aluminum and sucrose octasulfate

Metabolism: Not metabolized

Elimination: In urine as unchanged compounds; mostly fecal (90%)

Usual Dosage Oral:

Children: Dose not established; doses of 40-80 mg/kg/day divided every 6 hours have been used

Stomatitis: 2.5-5 mL (1 g/15 mL suspension), swish and spit or swish and swallow 4 times/day

Adults:

Duodenal ulcer treatment: 1 g 4 times/day, 1 hour before meals or food and at bedtime for 4-8 weeks, or alternatively 2 g twice daily

Duodenal ulcer maintenance therapy: 1 g twice daily

Stomatitis: 1 g/15 mL suspension, swish and spit or swish and swallow 4 times/day

Contraindications Hypersensitivity to sucralfate or any component

Warnings Use with caution in patients with chronic renal failure who have an impaired excretion of absorbed aluminum (small amounts of aluminum are absorbed from gastrointestinal tract); successful therapy with sucralfate should not be expected to alter the post-healing frequency of recurrence or the severity of duodenal ulceration

Dosage Forms

Suspension, oral: 1 g/10 mL (420 mL)
Tablet: 1 g

Stability Shake well and refrigerate suspension

Reference Range Normal serum aluminum levels are <15 μg/L (SI: <555 nmol/L); toxicity can occur at levels >100 μg/L (SI: >3706 nmol/L)

Overdosage Treatment Enhancement of elimination: Deferoxamine, traditionally used as an iron chelator, has been shown to increase urinary aluminum output. Deferoxamine chelation of aluminum has resulted in improvements of clinical symptoms and bone histology. Deferoxamine, however, remains an experimental treatment for aluminum poisoning and has a significant potential for adverse effects. Hemofiltration or hemodialysis can lower serum aluminum concentrations.

Drug Interactions Cimetidine, digoxin, phenytoin; because of the potential for sucralfate to alter the absorption of some drugs, separate administration (2 hours before or after) should be considered when alterations in bioavailability are believed to be critical; do not give antacids within 30 minutes of administration

Pregnancy Risk Factor B

Monitoring Parameters Aluminum

Patient Information Take before meals or on an empty stomach; may allow tablet to disintegrate in approximately 1 oz of room temperature water and drink the resulting suspension, if unable to swallow tablets whole; tablets may be disintegrated in water before taking

Nursing Implications Monitor for constipation; give 2 hours before or after administration of other oral drugs

Additional Information May decrease gastric emptying; little overdose experience; increased serum aluminum levels can occur after inadvertent I.V. administration

Specific References

Algozzine GJ, Hill G, Scoggins WG, et al, "Sucralfate Bezoar," *N Engl J Med*, 1983, 309(22):1387.
Domingo JL, Gomez M, Llobet JM, et al, "Comparative Effects of Several Chelating Agents on the Toxicity, Distribution, and Excretion of Aluminum," *Hum Toxicol*, 1988, 7(3):259-62.
Gonzalez Sanchez JM, Serna Juan SA, Galindo Sacristan E, et al, "Aluminum Intoxication After Parenteral Sucralfate Administration," *Farmacia Clinica*, 1994, 11:760-4.
Overdahl MC and Wewers MD, "Acute Occlusion of a Mainstem Bronchus by a Rapidly Expanding Foreign Body," *Chest*, 1994, 105(5):1600-2.
Robertson JA, Salusky IB, Goodman WG, et al, "Sucralfate, Intestinal Aluminum Absorption, and Aluminum Toxicity in a Patient on Dialysis," *Ann Intern Med*, 1989, 111(2):179-81.

Sucrets® Cough Calmers [OTC] *see* Dextromethorphan Hydrobromide *on page 270*

Sudafed® 12 Hour [OTC] *see* Pseudoephedrine *on page 661*

Sudafed® Nasal Spray *see* Oxymetazoline Hydrochloride *on page 586*

Sudafed® [OTC] *see* Pseudoephedrine *on page 661*

Sufedrin® [OTC] *see* Pseudoephedrine *on page 661*

Sufenta® *see* Sufentanil Citrate *on this page*

Sufentanil Citrate (soo fen' ta nil)

Related Information

Pharmacokinetics of Narcotic Agonist Analgesics *on page 1654*

CAS Number 56030-54-7; 60561-17-3

Brand Names Sufenta®

Use Analgesic supplement in maintenance of balanced general anesthesia

Mechanism of Action Binds with stereospecific receptors at many sites within the CNS, increases pain threshold, alters pain reception, inhibits ascending pain pathways; ultra short-acting narcotic; not a partial opiate antagonist

Adverse Reactions

Cardiovascular: Hypotension, hypertension, tachycardia, arrhythmia
Central nervous system: Electroencephalogram abnormalities
Dermatologic: Pruritus
Gastrointestinal: Nausea, vomiting
Neuromuscular & skeletal: Skeletal muscle rigidity
Respiratory: Apnea, respiratory depression, wheezing
Miscellaneous: Physical and psychological dependence with prolonged use; CNS depression

Signs & Symptoms of Acute Overdose Convulsions, myoclonus, biliary tract spasm, coma

Toxicodynamics/Kinetics

Onset of action: 1-3 minutes
Duration: Dose dependent; usually 30-60 minutes, may be up to 3.5 hours

(Continued)

Sufentanil Citrate *(Continued)*

Distribution: V_d: 2.9 L/kg
Protein binding: 92.5%
Metabolism: Primarily by the liver
Half-life: 158 minutes
Patients with cardiac surgery: 595 minutes
Patients with abdominal aortic surgery: 12 hours
Patients hyperventilating: 232 minutes
Obese patients: Increased half-life

Usual Dosage

Children <12 years: 10-25 mcg/kg with 100% O_2, maintenance: 25-50 mcg as needed

Adults: Dose should be based on body weight; **Note:** In obese patients (ie, >20% above ideal body weight), use lean body weight to determine dosage

1-2 mcg/kg with NO_2/O_2 for endotracheal intubation; maintenance: 10-25 mcg as needed

2-8 mcg/kg with NO_2/O_2 more complicated major surgical procedures; maintenance: 10-50 mcg as needed

8-30 mcg/kg with 100% O_2 and muscle relaxant produces sleep; at doses of $\geq$8 mcg/kg maintains a deep level of anesthesia; maintenance: 10-50 mcg as needed

Contraindications Hypersensitivity to sufentanil or any component

Warnings Sufentanil can cause severely compromised apnea; use with caution in patients with head injuries, hepatic or renal impairment or with pulmonary disease; sufentanil shares the toxic potential of opiate agonists, precaution of opiate agonist therapy should be observed; rapid I.V. infusion may result in skeletal muscle and chest wall rigidity → impaired ventilation → respiratory distress/arrest; inject slowly over 3-5 minutes; nondepolarizing skeletal muscle relaxant may be required

Dosage Forms Injection: 50 mcg/mL (1 mL, 2 mL, 5 mL)

Reference Range Peak serum sufentanil levels are about 11 μg/L ten minutes after I.V. administration of 1.5 μg/kg of the drug

Overdosage Treatment Supportive therapy: Naloxone hydrochloride (0.4-2 mg I.V., S.C., or through an endotracheal tube); a continuous infusion (at $\frac{2}{3}$ the response dose/hour) may be required

Antidote(s)

Naloxone Hydrochloride *on page 1447*

Drug Interactions Increased effect/toxicity with CNS depressants, beta-blockers; hypotension with midazolam

Pregnancy Risk Factor C

Nursing Implications Patient may develop rebound respiratory depression postoperatively

Specific References

Bovill JG, Sebel PS, Blackburn CL, et al, "The Pharmacokinetics of Sufentanil in Surgical Patients," *Anesthesiology*, 1984, 61(5):502-6.

Bowdle TA, "Myoclonus Following Sufentanil Without EEG Seizure Activity," *Anesthesiology*, 1987, 67(4):593-5.

Gust R and Böhrer H, "Stiff-Man Syndrome Associated With Continuous Sufentanil Administration," *Anaesthesia*, 1995, 50:575-6.

Rosow CE, "Sufentanil Citrate: A New Opioid Analgesic for Use in Anaesthesia," *Pharmacotherapy*, 1984, 4(1):11-9.

Sulfasalazine (sul fa sal' a zeen)

Related Information

Therapeutic Drugs Associated With Hallucinations *on page 1558-1559*

CAS Number 599-79-1

Brand Names Azulfidine®; Azulfidine® EN-tabs®; Color-Pleon®; Salazopyrin®; S.A.S.®; Sulazine®; Ulcol®

Synonyms Salicylazosulfapyridine

Use Management of ulcerative colitis, Crohn's disease; also may be effective in ankylosing spondylitis, scleroderma, rheumatoid arthritis, Behçet's disease and psoriasis; also may be useful in radiation, enteritis, and dermatitis herpetiformis

Mechanism of Action Acts locally in the colon to decrease the inflammatory response and systemically interferes with secretion by inhibiting prostaglandin synthesis

Adverse Reactions

Central nervous system: Fever, dizziness, encephalopathy, depression, headache, malaise, myopathy, visual hallucinations, confusion

Dermatologic: Itching, toxic epidermal necrolysis, skin rash, photosensitivity, Lyell's syndrome, Stevens-Johnson syndrome, alopecia

Gastrointestinal: Anorexia, nausea, vomiting, diarrhea, colitis

Genitourinary: Crystalluria

Hematologic: Granulocytopenia, leukopenia, thrombocytopenia, aplastic anemia, hemolytic anemia (Coombs' positive), lymphocytosis

Hepatic: Hepatitis, jaundice

Neuromuscular & skeletal: Chorea

Ocular: Vision color changes (red tinge)

Renal: Interstitial nephritis, acute nephrotoxicity, serum sickness-like reactions, urine discoloration (orange), urine discoloration (orange-yellow); hematuria, reversible oligospermia

Miscellaneous: Thyroid function disturbance, systemic lupus erythematosus (SLE), porphyrinogenic

Signs & Symptoms of Acute Overdose Headache, nausea, vomiting, diarrhea, confusion

Toxicodynamics/Kinetics

Absorption: 10% to 15% of dose is absorbed as unchanged drug from the small intestine

Distribution: Small amounts appear in feces and breast milk

Metabolism: Following absorption, both components are subject to polymorphic acetylation in the liver; split into sulfapyridine and 5-aminosalicylic acid (5-ASA) in the colon

Half-life: 5.7-10 hours; sulfasalazine: 0.6-1.4 hours (5-ASA)

Elimination: Primary excretion in urine (as unchanged drug, components, and acetylated metabolites)

Usual Dosage Oral:

Children >2 years: 40-60 mg/kg/day in 3-6 divided doses, not to exceed 6 g/day; maintenance dose: 20-30 mg/kg/day in 4 divided doses; not to exceed 2 g/day

Adults: 1 g 3-4 times/day, 2 g/day maintenance in divided doses; not to exceed 4 g/day

Dosing interval in renal impairment:

Cl_{cr} 10-30 mL/minute: Administer twice daily

Cl_{cr} <10 mL/minute: Administer once daily

Dosing adjustment in hepatic impairment: Avoid use

Toxic daily dose: 4 g

Contraindications Hypersensitivity to sulfasalazine, sulfa drugs, or any component; porphyria, gastrointestinal or GU obstruction; hypersensitivity to salicylates; children <2 years of age

Warnings Use with caution in patients with renal impairment; impaired hepatic function or urinary obstruction, blood dyscrasias, severe allergies or asthma, or G-6-PD deficiency

Dosage Forms

Suspension, oral: 250 mg/5 mL (473 mL)

Tablet: 500 mg

Tablet, enteric coated: 500 mg

Stability Protect from light; shake suspension well

Reference Range Toxic level of sulfapyridine: >50 mg/L (200 μmol/L)

Overdosage Treatment

Decontamination: Emesis or lavage/activated charcoal or cholestyramine can reduce sulfasalazine absorption

Supportive therapy: Anaphylaxis can be treated with standard therapy; acetylcysteine (24 g I.V. over 36 hours) has been used to treat sulfasalazine-induced hepatitis

Enhancement of elimination: Multiple dosing of activated charcoal may be effective

Drug Interactions Decreased effect with PABA or PABA metabolites of drugs (ie, procaine, proparacaine, tetracaine); decreases absorption of digoxin (by 25%) and folic acid; iron decreases sulfasalazine absorption; decreased effect of oral anticoagulants and oral hypoglycemic agents; decreased levels of digoxin or folic acid; decreased sulfasalazine levels with iron

Pregnancy Risk Factor B (D at term)

Monitoring Parameters Stool frequency, hematocrit, reticulocyte count, CBC, urinalysis, renal function tests, liver function tests

Patient Information Maintain adequate fluid intake; take after meals; may cause orange-yellow discoloration of urine and skin; take after meals or with food; do not

(Continued)

Sulfasalazine *(Continued)*

take with antacids; may permanently stain soft contact lenses yellow; avoid prolonged exposure to sunlight; shake well before using

Nursing Implications Gastrointestinal intolerance is common during the first few days of therapy; drug commonly imparts an orange-yellow discoloration to urine and skin. This drug should be administered after food to reduce gastrointestinal irritation; may cause orange-yellow discoloration of urine and skin.

Additional Information Since sulfasalazine impairs folate absorption, consider providing 1 mg/day folate supplement

Specific References

Gabay C, DeBandt M, and Palazzo E, "Sulphasalazine-Related Life-threatening Side Effects: Is N-acetylcysteine of Therapeutic Value?" *Clin Exp Rheumatol*, 1993, 11(4):417-20.

Haines JD, Jr, "Hepatotoxicity After Treatment With Sulfasalazine," *Postgrad Med*, 1986, 79(6):193-4, 197-8.

Jick H, Myers MW, and Dean AD, "The Risk of Sulfasalazine- and Mesalazine-Associated Blood Disorders," *Pharmacotherapy*, 1995, 15:176-81.

Peppercorn MA, "Sulfasalazine: Pharmacology, Clinical Use, Toxicity, and Related New Drug Development," *Ann Intern Med*, 1984, 101(3):377-86.

Tullien D, Wolkenstein P, Roupie E, et al, "Toxic Epidermal Necrolysis After Sulfasalazine Treatment of Mild Psoriatic Arthritis: Warning on the Use of Sulfasalazine for a New Indication," *Arthritis Rheum*, 1995, 38:573.

Veale DJ, Ho M, and Morley KD, "Sulphasalazine-Induced Lupus in Psoriatic Arthritis," *Br J Rheumatol*, 1995, 34:383-4.

Sulfatrim® *see* Co-trimoxazole *on page 242*

Sulfatrim® DS *see* Co-trimoxazole *on page 242*

Sulfisoxazole (sul fi sox' a zole)

CAS Number 80-74-0

Brand Names Gantrisin® Ophthalmic; Gantrisin® Oral; Novasoxazole®

Synonyms Sulfisoxazole Acetyl; Sulphafurazole

Use Treatment of lower, uncomplicated urinary tract infections, otitis media, *Chlamydia*; nocardiosis; treatment of acute pelvic inflammatory disease in prepubertal children

Mechanism of Action Interferes with bacterial growth by inhibiting bacterial folic acid synthesis through competitive antagonism of PABA

Adverse Reactions

- Central nervous system: Fever, dizziness, headache
- Dermatologic: Itching, skin rash, photosensitivity, Lyell's syndrome, Stevens-Johnson syndrome
- Gastrointestinal: Anorexia, nausea, vomiting, diarrhea
- Genitourinary: Crystalluria
- Hematologic: Granulocytopenia, leukopenia, thrombocytopenia, aplastic anemia, hemolytic anemia
- Hepatic: Hepatitis, jaundice
- Renal: Interstitial nephritis, acute nephropathy, hematuria
- Miscellaneous: Thyroid function disturbance, serum sickness-like reactions

Signs & Symptoms of Acute Overdose Drowsiness, dizziness, hematuria, nephrotoxicity, anorexia, abdominal pain, nausea, vomiting, hemolytic anemia, acidosis, jaundice, fever, agranulocytosis; doses of as little as 2-5 g/day may produce toxicity; the aniline radical is responsible for hematologic toxicity

Toxicodynamics/Kinetics

- Absorption: Sulfisoxazole acetyl is hydrolyzed in the gastrointestinal tract to sulfisoxazole which is readily absorbed (nearly 100%)
- Distribution: V_d: 0.16 L/kg; crosses the placenta; excreted into breast milk
- Protein binding: 85% to 88%
- Metabolized: In the liver by acetylation and glucuronide conjugation to inactive compounds
- Half-life: 4-7 hours, prolonged with renal impairment (to 11 hours)
- Time to peak serum concentration: Within 2-3 hours
- Elimination: Primarily in urine (95% within 24 hours), 40% to 60% as unchanged drug

Usual Dosage Not for use in patients <2 months of age

Children >2 months: Oral: 75 mg/kg stat, 120-150 mg/kg/day in divided doses every 4-6 hours; not to exceed 6 g/day

Adults: Oral: 2-4 g stat, 4-8 g/day in divided doses every 4-6 hours

Dosing interval in renal impairment:

Cl_{cr} 10-50 mL/minute: Administer every 8-12 hours

Cl_{cr} <10 mL/minute: Administer every 12-24 hours

>50% removed by hemodialysis

Children and Adults: Ophthalmic:

Ointment: Apply small amount to affected eye 1-3 times/day and at bedtime

Solution: Instill 1-2 drops to affected eye every 2-3 hours

Contraindications Hypersensitivity to any sulfa drug or any component, porphyria, pregnancy at term, infants <2 months of age (sulfas compete with bilirubin for protein binding sites), patients with urinary obstruction, sunscreens containing PABA

Warnings Use with caution in patients with G-6-PD deficiency (hemolysis may occur), hepatic or renal impairment; dosage modification required in patients with renal impairment; risk of crystalluria should be considered in patients with impaired renal function

Dosage Forms

Ointment, ophthalmic, as diolamine: 4% [40 mg/mL] (3.75 g)
Solution, ophthalmic, as diolamine: 4% [40 mg/mL] (15 mL)
Suspension, oral, pediatric, as acetyl (raspberry flavor): 500 mg/5 mL (480 mL)
Tablet: 500 mg

Stability Protect from light

Reference Range 2 g oral dose results in peak plasma level of 10-15 mg/L (37-56 μmol/L)

Overdosage Treatment

Decontamination: Ipecac or lavage/activated charcoal

Enhancement of elimination: Multiple dosing of activated charcoal may be effective; alkalinizing the urine decreases serum half-life by almost 30%; hemodialysis can enhance sulfisoxazole elimination

Test Interactions False-positive protein in urine; false-positive urine glucose with Clinitest®; can cause interference in serum calcium assays, thus giving the appearance of hypocalcemia

Drug Interactions

Decreased effect with PABA or PABA metabolites of drugs (ie, procaine, proparacaine, tetracaine, sunscreens with PABA)

Increased risk of bone marrow suppression with methotrexate; increased risk of nephrotoxicity with cyclosporine, but cyclosporine levels may decrease; increased effect of oral anticoagulants and oral hypoglycemic agents

Pregnancy Risk Factor B (D at term)

Pregnancy Implications Can cause kernicterus in neonates

Monitoring Parameters CBC, urinalysis, renal function tests

Patient Information Take with a glass of water on an empty stomach; avoid prolonged exposure to sunlight; report to physician any sore throat, mouth sores, rash, unusual bleeding, or fever

Nursing Implications Give around-the-clock to promote less variation in peak and trough serum levels; maintain adequate fluid intake

Specific References

Kaplan SA, Weinfold RE, Abruzzo CW, et al, "Pharmacokinetic Profile of Sulfisoxazole Following IM, IV, and PO Administration to Man," *J Pharm Sci*, 1972, 61:773.

Liston TE and Harbison R, "Sulfisoxazole Chemoprophylaxis for Frequent Otitis Media," *Pediatrics*, 1983, 71:524-30.

Sulfisoxazole Acetyl *see* Sulfisoxazole *on previous page*

Sulindac (sul in' dak)

Related Information

Nonsteroidal Anti-Inflammatory Comparison *on page 1655*

CAS Number 38194-50-2

Brand Names Clinoril®

Use Management of inflammatory disease, rheumatoid disorders; acute gouty arthritis; structurally similar to indomethacin but acts like aspirin; safest NSAID for use in mild renal impairment

Mechanism of Action Inhibits prostaglandin synthesis by decreasing the activity of the enzyme, cyclo-oxygenase, which results in decreased formation of prostaglandin precursors

Adverse Reactions

Cardiovascular: Fluid retention, circulatory collapse
Central nervous system: Headache, aseptic meningitis, psychosis, cognitive dysfunction, coma, seizures
Dermatologic: Rash, pruritus
Endocrine & metabolic: Hyperkalemia, anion gap metabolic acidosis
Gastrointestinal: Abdominal pain, nausea, vomiting, bleeding, ulceration, constipation, diarrhea, dyspepsia
Genitourinary: Albuminuria
Hematologic: Leukopenia, neutropenia, agranulocytosis, granulocytopenia; aplastic anemia (rare), platelet inhibition
Hepatic: Elevation of transaminases, fulminant hepatitis
Otic: Ototoxicity, tinnitus
Renal: Renal failure (acute), nephrotic syndrome, chronic renal failure
Respiratory: Wheezing, respiratory depression
Miscellaneous: Hypersensitivity

Signs & Symptoms of Acute Overdose Nausea, chills, azotemia, purpura,

(Continued)

Sulindac *(Continued)*

wheezing, Stevens-Johnson syndrome, nephrotic syndrome, nephritis, gastrointestinal bleeding, gastritis; leukemoid reaction, leukocytosis, photosensitivity, cognitive dysfunction, toxic epidermal necrolysis, thrombocytopenia, coagulopathy, vomiting, insomnia, hyperthermia, ototoxicity; tinnitus, drowsiness; severe poisoning can manifest with coma, seizures, renal and or hepatic failure, hypotension, respiratory depression, alopecia

Toxicodynamics/Kinetics

Absorption: Oral: 90% from gastrointestinal tract

Protein binding: 93%

Metabolism: Prodrug requiring metabolic activation; hepatic metabolism to sulfide metabolite (active) for therapeutic effects; also metabolized in the liver to sulfone metabolites (inactive)

Half-life:

Parent: 7 hours

Active metabolite: 18 hours

Time to peak serum concentration:

Fasting: Within 2 hours

With food: 3-4 hours

Elimination: Principally in urine (50%) with some biliary excretion (25%)

Usual Dosage Maximum therapeutic response may not be realized for up to 3 weeks. Oral:

Children: Dose not established

Adults: 150-200 mg twice daily or 300-400 mg once daily; not to exceed 400 mg/day

Dosing adjustment in hepatic impairment: Dose reduction is necessary

Contraindications Hypersensitivity to sulindac, any component, aspirin or other nonsteroidal anti-inflammatory drugs (NSAIDs)

Warnings Use with caution in patients with peptic ulcer disease, gastrointestinal bleeding, bleeding abnormalities, impaired renal or hepatic function, congestive heart failure, hypertension, and patients receiving anticoagulants

Dosage Forms Tablet: 150 mg, 200 mg

Reference Range Peak plasma levels after a 200 mg oral dose: ~4 mg/L (parent compound); 3 mg/L (sulfide metabolite); and 2 mg/L (sulfone metabolite)

Overdosage Treatment

Decontamination: Ipecac or lavage/activated charcoal with cathartic

Supportive therapy: Hypotension/dehydration can be managed with intravenous fluid therapy; acidosis should be treated with bicarbonates, seizures with benzodiazepines; antacids, blood products are indicated, as appropriate, for hemorrhage

Enhancement of elimination: Dialysis or perfusion is indicated for secondary complications, acidosis, or renal failure and not toxin removal alone; multiple dosing of activated charcoal may be effective

Test Interactions Increases chloride (S), sodium (S), bleeding time

Drug Interactions Aspirin decreases serum concentrations probably by protein-binding displacement; there is an increased bleeding potential with concomitant warfarin therapy; may increase lithium and methotrexate concentrations by decreasing renal clearance; may decrease diuretic and hypotensive effects of thiazides, loop diuretics, ACE inhibitors, and beta-blockers; may increase nephrotoxicity of cyclosporine

Pregnancy Risk Factor B (D during 3rd trimester or near delivery)

Monitoring Parameters Observe for edema and fluid retention; monitor blood pressure; liver enzymes, BUN, serum creatinine, CBC

Additional Information Structurally similar to indomethacin but acts like aspirin; associated with the highest incidence of upper gastrointestinal bleeds among NSAIDs; safest NSAID for use in mild renal impairment; maximum therapeutic response may not be realized for up to 3 weeks

Specific References

Court H and Volans GN, "Poisoning After Overdose With Nonsteroidal Anti-inflammatory Drugs," *Adverse Drug React Acute Poisoning Rev*, 1984, 3(1):1-21.

Harima Y, Maekawa T, Miyauchi Y, et al, "Intoxication With Sulindac, Tiaramide Hydrochloride and Diclofenac Sodium," *Intensive Care Med*, 1987, 13(5):361-2.

Hoppmann RA, Peden JG, and Ober SK, "Central Nervous System Side Effects of Nonsteroidal Anti-inflammatory Drugs. Aseptic Meningitis, Psychosis, and Cognitive Dysfunction," *Arch Intern Med*, 1991, 151(7):1309-13.

Kulling EJ, Beckman EA, and Skagius AS, "Renal Impairment After Acute Diclofenac, Naproxen, and Sulindac Overdoses," *J Toxicol Clin Toxicol*, 1995, 33(2):173-7.

Park GD, Spector R, Headstream T, et al, "Serious Adverse Reactions Associated With Sulindac," *Arch Intern Med*, 1982, 142(7):1292-4.

Smolinske SC, Hall AH, Vandenberg SA, et al, "Toxic Effects of Nonsteroid Anti-inflammatory Drugs in Overdose. An Overview of Recent Evidence on Clinical Effects and Dose-Response Relationships," *Drug Saf*, 1990, 5(4):252-74.

Vale JA and Meredith TJ, "Acute Poisoning Due to Nonsteroidal Anti-inflammatory Drugs," *Med Toxicol*, 1986, 1(1):12-31.

Verbeeck RK, "Pharmacokinetic Drug Interactions With Nonsteroidal Anti-inflammatory Drugs," *Clin Pharmacokinet*, 1990, 19(1):44-66.

Sulphadine *see* Dapsone *on page 260*

Sulphafurazole *see* Sulfisoxazole *on page 714*

Sulphon-mere *see* Dapsone *on page 260*

Sulpiride

CAS Number 15676-16-1; 23672-07-3

Brand Names Dogmatil Forte®; Sulpitil®; Tepavil®

Use Investigational: Antidepressive agent and antipsychotic agent

Mechanism of Action Substituted benzamide with selective dopamine receptor antagonism

Adverse Reactions

Cardiovascular: Palpitations, hypertension

Central nervous system: Dizziness, headache, neuroleptic malignant syndrome, neuroleptic malignant syndrome, sedation, Parkinson symptoms, extrapyramidal effects (30%)

Endocrine & metabolic: Galactorrhea

Gastrointestinal: Nausea, vomiting, dry mouth, constipation

Hepatic: Cholestatic jaundice

Ocular: Blurred vision

Miscellaneous: Anticholinergic effects, porphyrinogenic, sweating, diaphoresis

Toxicodynamics/Kinetics

Distribution: V_d: 1-2.7 L/kg

Protein binding: <40%

Bioavailability: Oral: 35% (food lowers absorption)

Half-life: 6-8 hours; 20-26 hours in renal failure

Elimination: Renal (clearance: 310 mL/minute)

Usual Dosage

Oral: 200-400 mg twice daily; may increase gradually to a maximum dose of 1.2 g/day

I.M.: 600-800 mg/day

Contraindications Hypersensitivity to sulpiride; pheochromocytoma; Parkinsonism

Warnings Reduce dosage in renal failure; use with caution in mania patients with epilepsy, urinary retention, hypertension

Reference Range After a 200 mg oral dose, peak plasma level ranges from 0.2-2 μg/mL

Overdosage Treatment

Decontamination: Emesis or lavage/activated charcoal with cathartic

Enhancement of elimination: Multiple dosing of activated charcoal may be effective

Drug Interactions Aluminum antacids or sucralfate will reduce sulpiride absorption

Additional Information Stimulates prolactin secretion; can exacerbate hypertension caused by pheochromocytoma, cross-hypersensitivity may exist with metoclopramide, tiapride, sultopride

Specific References

Caley CF and Weber SS, "Sulpiride: An Antipsychotic With Selective Dopaminergic Antagonist Properties," *Ann Pharmacother*, 1995, 29:152-60.

Sulpitil® *see* Sulpiride *on this page*

Sumatriptan Succinate (soo' ma trip tan)

CAS Number 103628-46-2; 103628-47-3; 103628-48-4

Brand Names Imigran®; Imitrex®

Use Acute treatment of migraine with or without aura

Unlabeled use: Cluster headaches

Mechanism of Action Selective agonist for serotonin (5HT, ID subtype receptor) in cranial arteries to cause vasoconstriction and reduces sterile inflammation associated with antidromic neuronal transmission correlating with relief of migraine

Adverse Reactions

Cardiovascular: Chest pain (7.9%), myocardial infarction, ventricular arrhythmia, tightness in chest, flushing (5.1%),

Central nervous system: Tingling lightheadedness, dizziness (8.1%), asthenia, drowsiness/sedation (7%), headache, numbness, neck pain, seizures, fatigue (4.6%)

Dermatologic: Skin rash

Endocrine & metabolic: Polydipsia, hot flashes, dysmenorrhea

Gastrointestinal: Nausea/vomiting (7.3%), abdominal discomfort, sore throat

Local: Injection site reaction, burning sensation

(Continued)

Sumatriptan Succinate *(Continued)*

Neuromuscular & skeletal: Myalgia, paresthesia (11.7%)
Renal: Dysuria, renal calculus
Respiratory: Dyspnea
Miscellaneous: Mouth discomfort, jaw discomfort, dehydration, feeling of heaviness (8%), sweating, hiccups

Signs & Symptoms of Acute Overdose Chest pain/angina, numbness, hypertension; fatalities due to myocardial infarction usually occur 3 or more hours after treatment

Toxicodynamics/Kinetics After S.C. administration:
Protein binding: 14% to 21%
Metabolism: Hepatic (80%)
Bioavailability: 97%
Half-life:
Distribution: 15 minutes
Terminal: 115 minutes
Time to peak serum concentration: 5-20 minutes
Elimination: In urine unchanged (22%), excreted as indole acetic acid metabolite (38%)

Usual Dosage Adults: S.C.: 6 mg; a second injection may be administered at least 1 hour after the initial dose, but not more than 2 injections in a 24-hour period

Contraindications I.V. use; use in patients with ischemic heart disease or Prinzmetal angina, patients with signs or symptoms of ischemic heart disease, uncontrolled HTN, use with ergotamine derivatives, hypersensitivity to any component, management of hemiplegic or basilar migraine

Warnings Use with caution in elderly, patients with hepatic or renal impairment; may cause mild, transient elevation of blood pressure; may cause coronary vasospasm

Dosage Forms Injection: 12 mg/mL (0.5 mL, 2 mL)

Stability Store at 2°C to 20°C (36°F to 86°F); protect from light

Reference Range Therapeutic range: 18-60 ng/mL

Overdosage Treatment
Decontamination for oral ingestion: Ipecac or lavage within 30 minutes/activated charcoal with cathartic
Supportive therapy: Nitroprusside, nifedipine, or hydralazine for hypertensive crisis; lidocaine or procainamide for ventricular ectopy; nitroglycerin can reverse sumatriptan-induced coronary artery vasoconstriction

Drug Interactions Increased toxicity: Ergot-containing drugs; avoid concomitant use with lithium and irreversible monoamine oxidase inhibitors; use with caution with concomitant serotonin reuptake inhibitor therapy

Pregnancy Risk Factor C (embryo lethal in rabbits)

Patient Information If pain or tightness in chest or throat occurs, notify physician; females should avoid pregnancy

Nursing Implications Do not administer I.V., may cause coronary vasospasm; pain at injection site lasts <1 hour

Additional Information May increase growth hormone level; oral dose of 100 mg is investigational; oral sumatriptan (100 mg) may prevent headache recurrence; may exacerbate depression

Specific References

Akpunonu BE, Mutgi AB, and Federman DJ, "Subcutaneous Sumatriptan for Treatment of Acute Migraine in Patients Admitted to the Emergency Department: A Multicenter Study," *Ann Emerg Med*, 1995, 25:464-9.

Blier P and Bergeron R, "The Safety of Concomitant Use of Sumatriptan and Antidepressant Treatment," *J Clin Psychopharmacol*, 1995, 15:106-9.

Boyd IW and Rohan AP, "Sumatriptan - Induced Chest Pain," *Lancet*, 1994, 344(8939):1704-5.

Curtin T, Brooks AP, and Roberts JA, "Cardiorespiratory Distress After Sumatriptan Given by Injection," *BMJ*, 1992, 305(6855):713-4.

La Porta LD, "Recurrent Depression After Sumatriptan Administration for Migraine," *J Clin Psychopharmacol*, 1995, 15:81-2.

Luman W and Gray RS, "Adverse Reactions Associated With Sumatriptan," *Lancet*, 1993, 341(8852):1091-2.

Stricker BH, "Coronary Vasospasm and Sumatriptan," *BMJ*, 1992, 305(6845):118.

Ottervanger JP, et al, "Characteristics of Sumatriptan-Induced Chest Pain," *Pharm World Sci*, 1995, 17:3.

Ottervanger JP, et al, "Determinants of Sumatriptan-Induced Chest Pain," *Pharm World Sci*, 1995, 17:7.

Ottervanger JP, van Witsen TB, Valkenburg HA, et al, "Adverse Reactions Attributed to Sumatriptan: A Postmarketing Study in General Practice," *Eur J Clin Pharmacol*, 1994, 47(4):305-9.

Palmer J, Feldman R, Mancini GB, et al, "Glyceryl Trinitrate Reversal of Post-Sumatriptan Coronary Artery Narrowing," *Lancet*, 1995, 345:1366.

Srinivas NR, et al, "Lack of Pharmacokinetic Interaction Between Butorphanol Tartrate Nasal Spray and Sumatriptan Succinate," *J Clin Pharmacol*, 1995, 35:432-7.

Walton-Shirley M, Flowers K, and Whiteside JH, "Unstable Angina Pectoris Associated With I Mitrex Therapy," *Cather Cardiovas*, 1995, 34:188.

Weidmann B, Jansen W, Bojko P, et al, "Sumatriptan-Induced Myocardial Infarction," *Intensivmedizin und Nofallmedizin*, 1994, 31:353.

Sumycin® Oral *see* Tetracycline *on page 732*

Super Blue *see* Tripelennamine *on page 776*

Supeudol® *see* Oxycodone Hydrochloride *on page 585*

Suppress® [OTC] *see* Dextromethorphan Hydrobromide *on page 270*

Sure-Lax® *see* Phenolphthalein *on page 617*

Surem® *see* Nitrazepam *on page 562*

Surfak® [OTC] *see* Docusate *on page 297*

Surmontil® *see* Trimipramine Maleate *on page 775*

Sustachron® *see* Nitroglycerin *on page 566*

Sustaire® *see* Theophylline *on page 735*

Swim-Ear® [OTC] *see* Boric Acid *on page 160*

Symmetrel® *see* Amantadine Hydrochloride *on page 105*

Symoron® *see* Methadone Hydrochloride *on page 508*

Synalgos® [OTC] *see* Aspirin *on page 133*

Synthroid® *see* Levothyroxine Sodium *on page 465*

Systodin® *see* Quinidine *on page 668*

Sytobex® *see* Cyanocobalamin *on page 246*

T_3 Sodium *see* Liothyronine Sodium *on page 471*

T_3/T_4 Liotrix *see* Liotrix *on page 473*

T_4 *see* Levothyroxine Sodium *on page 465*

Tacrine Hydrochloride (tak' reen)

CAS Number 321-64-2; 1684-40-8

Brand Names Cognex®

Synonyms Tacrinum; Tetrahydroaminoacrine; THA

Use Treatment of Alzheimer's disease

Mechanism of Action Inhibits cholinesterase activity similar to neostigmine

Adverse Reactions

Central nervous system: Agitation, dizziness

Dermatologic: Purpura

Gastrointestinal: Nausea, vomiting, diarrhea

Hepatic: Dose-related hepatitis

Signs & Symptoms of Acute Overdose Hypotension, bradycardia, depression, purpura, tachypnea, hallucination, confusion

Toxicodynamics/Kinetics

Absorption: Food decreases rate of absorption by 30% to 40%

Protein binding: 55%

Metabolism: Liver to velnacrine

Bioavailability: Oral: 17%

Half-life: 1.5-2 hours

Usual Dosage Adults: Initial: 10 mg 4 times/day; may increase by 40 mg/day adjusted every 6 weeks; maximum: 160 mg day; best administered separate from meal times; see table.

Dose Adjustment Based Upon Transaminase Elevations

ALT	Regimen
≤3 x ULN*	Continue titration
>3 to ≤5 x ULN	Decrease dose by 40 mg/day, resume when ALT returns to normal
>5 x ULN	Stop treatment, may rechallenge upon return of ALT to normal

*ULN = upper limit of normal.

Contraindications Patients previously treated with the drug who developed jaundice and in those who are hypersensitivity to acridine derivatives

Warnings Monitor liver enzymes weekly for at least the first 18 weeks, then once every 3 months; monitor weekly for 6 weeks after increasing dose. Patients with cardiovascular or liver disease, asthma, or peptic ulcer should use cautiously.

(Continued)

Tacrine Hydrochloride *(Continued)*

Dosage Forms Capsule: 10 mg, 20 mg, 30 mg, 40 mg

Reference Range

In clinical trials, serum concentrations >20 ng/mL were associated with a much higher risk of development of symptomatic adverse effects

Peak level: 6.5 ng/mL in 90 minutes after 50 mg dose

Overdosage Treatment Antidote is atropine for muscarinic symptoms; pralidoxime (2-PAM) may also be needed to reverse severe muscle asthenia or paralysis

Antidote(s)

Atropine Sulfate *on page 1395*

Pralidoxime Chloride *on page 1461*

Drug Interactions

Decreased effect of anticholinergics, cigarette smoking

Increased effect of theophylline, cimetidine, succinylcholine, cholinesterase inhibitors, or cholinergic agonists

Pregnancy Risk Factor C

Monitoring Parameters ALT (SGPT) levels and other liver enzymes weekly for at least the first 18 weeks, then monitor once every 3 months

Patient Information Effect of tacrine therapy is thought to depend upon its administration at regular intervals, as directed; possibility of adverse effects such as those occurring in close temporal association with the initiation of treatment or an increase in dose (ie, nausea, vomiting, loose stools, diarrhea) and those with a delayed onset (ie, rash, jaundice, changes in the color of stool); inform physician of the emergence of new events or any increase in the severity of existing adverse effects; abrupt discontinuation of the drug or a large reduction in total daily dose (80 mg/day or more) may cause a decline in cognitive function and behavioral disturbances; unsupervised increases in the dose may also have serious consequences; do not change dose without consulting physician

Specific References

Byrne J and Arie T, "Tetahydroaminoacridine (THA) in Alzheimer's Disease," *BMJ*, 1989, 298(6677):845-6.

Eagger SA, Levy R, Sahakian BJ, et al, "Tacrine in Alzheimer's Disease," *Lancet*, 1991, 338(8758):50-1.

Farlow M, Gracon SI, Hershey LA, et al, "A Controlled Trial of Tacrine in Alzheimer's Disease," *JAMA*, 1992, 268(18):2523-9.

Knapp MJ, Knopman DS, Solomon PR, et al, "A 30-Week Randomized Controlled Trial of High-Dose Tacrine in Patients With Alzheimer's Disease," *JAMA*, 1994, 271(13):985-91.

Madden S, Spaldin V, and Park BK, "Clinical Pharmacokinetics of Tacrine," *Clin Pharmacokinet*, 1995, 28:449-57.

Watkins PB, Zimmerman HJ, Knapp MJ, et al, "Hepatotoxic Effects of Tacrine Administration in Patients With Alzheimer's Disease," *JAMA*, 1994, 271(13):992-8.

Tacrinum *see* Tacrine Hydrochloride *on previous page*

Tacrolimus (ta kroe' li mus)

CAS Number 104987-11-3

Brand Names Prograf®

Synonyms FK506

Use Potent immunosuppressive drug used in liver, kidney, heart, lung, or small bowel transplant recipients

Mechanism of Action Suppressed humoral immunity (inhibits T-lymphocyte activation); produced by the fungus *Streptomyces* tsukubaensis

Adverse Reactions

Cardiovascular: Hypertension, cardiomyopathy

Central nervous system: Insomnia, headache, confusion, seizures, persistent coma, hyperesthesia

Endocrine & metabolic: Hyperglycemia

Gastrointestinal: Nausea, vomiting, and abdominal pain

Neuromuscular & skeletal: Mild tremors, dysarthria

Ocular: Photophobia

Renal: Elevated serum creatinine

Miscellaneous: Infections and malignant complications, including post transplant lymphoproliferative disorder, bacterial, viral, and fungal infections

Signs & Symptoms of Acute Overdose Coma, delirium, dyspnea, pleural effusion, night terrors, insomnia, hypomagnesemia, leukocytosis, thrombocytopenia, hypokalemia, hyperuricemia, hyperglycemia, hirsutism, encephalopathy, diarrhea, circumoral numbness

Toxicodynamics/Kinetics

Absorption: Better in small bowel patients with a closed stoma; unlike cyclosporine, clamping of the T-tube in liver transplant patients does not alter trough concentrations or area under the plasma concentration time curve; compared to fasting, the administration of tacrolimus 15 minutes after meals reduces the absorption an average of 27%; in blood, tacrolimus is primarily associated with RBCs such that the blood:plasma ratio ranges from 4-39; in plasma

Protein binding: 77% to 99%

Distribution: V_d: 0.9 L/kg; reaches concentrations 4 times greater than maternal plasma concentrations; concentrations in the breast are equivalent to the plasma

Metabolism: Hepatic, >99% metabolized, with at least 9 metabolites; liver dysfunction would be expected to increase the plasma concentration

Bioavailability: Oral: 5% to 67%, with an average of 30%

Half-life:

Health: 11.7

Liver transplant: 21.2 hours

Elimination: Pediatric patients clear the drug twice as rapidly as adults and require higher dose on a mg/kg basis to achieve similar concentrations in plasma; <1% of the dose is excreted in the urine as unchanged drug, 43 mL/minute/kg; elimination from the body is primarily via the bile

Usual Dosage

Initial: I.V. continuous infusion: 0.1 mg/kg/day until the tolerance of oral intake

Oral: Usually 3-4 times the I.V. dose, or 0.3 mg/kg/day in divided doses every 12 hours

Contraindications Hypersensitivity to tacrolimus, castor oils, or any component; do not use simultaneously with cyclosporine, discontinue cyclosporine for 24 hours before starting tacrolimus

Warnings Increased susceptibility to infection and the possible development of lymphoma may occur after administration of tacrolimus; it should not be administered simultaneously with cyclosporine; the pharmacokinetics of tacrolimus are highly variable between patients and within the same patient over time; monitoring of serum concentrations is essential to prevent organ rejection and reduce drug-related therapy

Dosage Forms

Capsule: 1 mg, 5 mg

Injection, with alcohol and surfactant: 5 mg/mL (1 mL)

Stability Twenty-four hours in dextrose 5% solutions or normal saline; tacrolimus is completely available from plastic syringes, glass or polyolefin containers; polyvinyl-containing sets (eg, Venoset®, Accuset®) adsorb significant amounts of the drug, and their use may lead to a lower dose being delivered to the patient

Reference Range Trough: 0.5-2 ng/mL (ELISA, plasma, extracted at 37 hours) for all transplant procedures (liver, heart, lung, kidney, small bowel)

Overdosage Treatment

Decontamination: Lavage/activated charcoal with cathartic

Enhancement of elimination: Multiple dosing of activated charcoal may be effective; dialysis/plasmapheresis not effective

Drug Interactions Separate administration of antacids from tacrolimus by at least 2 hours; erythromycin, clotrimazole, fluconazole, and methylprednisolone appear to increase plasma concentrations of tacrolimus in liver transplant recipients (in rats, ketoconazole, itraconazole, diltiazem, danazol, verapamil, and cimetidine also increase tacrolimus concentrations); cyclosporine is associated with synergistic immunosuppression and increased nephrotoxicity; nephrotoxic antibiotics and amphotericin B potentially increase nephrotoxicity; rifampin, phenytoin, and phenobarbital may decrease tacrolimus plasma concentrations

Pregnancy Risk Factor C

Pregnancy Implications Crosses the placenta; avoid breast feeding

Specific References

Atkison P, Joubert G, Barron A, et al, "Hypertrophic Cardiomyopathy Associated With Tacrolimus in Paediatric Transplant Patients," *Lancet*, 1995, 345:894-6.

Bronster DJ, Yonover P, Stein J, et al, "Demyelinating Sensorimotor Polyneuropathy After Administration of FK506," *Transplantation*, 1995, 59:1066-8.

Furian V, Perello L, Jacquemin E, et al, "Interactions Between FK506 and Rifampicin or Erythromycin in Pediatric Liver Recipients," *Transplantation*, 1995, 59:1217-8.

Kelly PA, Burckart GJ, and Venkataramanan R, "Tacrolimus: A New Immunosuppressive Agent," *Am J Health-Syst Pharm*, 1995, 52:1521-35.

Jusko WJ, Piekoszewski W, Kintmalm GB, et al, "Pharmacokinetics of Tacrolimus in Liver Transplant Patients," *Clin Pharmacol Ther*, 1995, 57:281-96.

MacDonald AS and Sketris IS, "Tacrolimus in Transplantation," *Am J Health-Syst Pharm*, 1995, 52:1569-71.

Natazuka T, Ogawa R, Kizaki T, et al, "Immunosuppressive Drugs and Hypertrophic Cardiomyopathy," *Lancet*, 1995, 345:1644.

Przepiorka D, Suzuki J, Ippoliti C, et al, "Blood Tacrolimus Concentration Unchanged by Plasmapheresis," *Am J Hosp Pharm*, 1994, 51(13):1708.

Starzl TE, Fung J, Jordan M, et al, "Kidney Transplantation Under FK506," *JAMA*, 1990, 264(1):63-7.

Winkler M and Christians U, "A Risk-Benefit Assessment of Tacrolimus in Transplantation," *Drug Saf*, 1995, 12(5):348-57.

Tafil® *see* Alprazolam *on page 99*

Tagamet® *see* Cimetidine *on page 212*

Talwin® *see* Pentazocine *on page 603*

Talwin® NX *see* Pentazocine *on page 603*

Tambocor® *see* Flecainide Acetate *on page 350*

Tamoxifen Citrate (ta mox' i fen)

Related Information

Toxicities of Chemotherapeutic Agents *on page 1631-1633*

CAS Number 10540-29-1; 54965-24-1

Brand Names Nolvadex® Oral

Use Palliative or adjunctive treatment of advanced breast cancer in men and women

Unlabeled use: Treatment of mastalgia, gynecomastia, and pancreatic carcinoma

Studies have shown tamoxifen to be effective in the treatment of primary breast cancer in elderly women. Comparative studies with other antineoplastic agents in elderly women with breast cancer had more favorable survival rates with tamoxifen. Initiation of hormone therapy rather than chemotherapy is justified for elderly patients with metastatic breast cancer who are responsive.

Mechanism of Action Competitively binds to estrogen receptors on tumors and other tissue targets, producing a nuclear complex that decreases DNA synthesis and inhibits estrogen effects; nonsteroidal agent with potent antiestrogenic properties which compete with estrogen for binding sites in breast and other tissues; cells accumulate in the G_0 and G_1 phases; therefore, tamoxifen is cytostatic rather than cytocidal

Adverse Reactions

Cardiovascular: Flushing

Central nervous system: Dizziness, psychosis, headache

Dermatologic: Rash, pruritus

Endocrine & metabolic: Vaginal bleeding or discharge, menstrual irregularities, hypercalcemia in patients with bony metastasis, (nocturnal), galactorrhea, hot flashes, ovarian cysts

Gastrointestinal: Nausea, vomiting is rare, cholestasis, steatohepatitis

Genitourinary: Priapism

Hematologic: Occasional leukopenia, thrombocytopenia, porphyria, agranulocytosis, thromboembolism (4.3%)

Ocular: Corneal opacification, reduced visual acuity, retinopathy at high doses (120 mg/day for 1 year)

Renal: Nephrotic syndrome

Miscellaneous: Porphyrinogenic

Signs & Symptoms of Acute Overdose Leukopenia or neutropenia (agranulocytosis, granulocytopenia); priapism, hypercalcemia, mental confusion, oligospermia, lactation, hirsutism, depression, sexual dysfunction, azoospermia, galactorrhea, cataract

Toxicodynamics/Kinetics

Absorption: Well absorbed from gastrointestinal tract

Time to peak serum concentration: Oral: Within 4-7 hours

Distribution: High concentrations found in uterus, endometrial and breast tissue

Metabolism: In the liver to N-desmethyltamoxifen (active)

Half-life: 4 days; N-desmethyltamoxifen: 9 days

Elimination: Undergoes enterohepatic recycling; excreted in feces, with only small amounts appearing in urine

Usual Dosage Adults: Oral: 10-20 mg twice daily in morning and evening; high-dose therapy is under investigation

Contraindications Hypersensitivity to tamoxifen

Warnings Use with caution in patients with leukopenia, thrombocytopenia, or hyperlipidemias; ovulation may be induced; "hot flashes" may be countered by Bellergal-S® tablets; decreased visual acuity, retinopathy and corneal changes have been reported with use for more than 1 year at doses above recommended; hypercalcemia in patients with bone metastasis; hepatocellular carcinomas have been reported in animal studies; endometrial hyperplasia and polyps have occurred

Dosage Forms Tablet: 10 mg

Reference Range Oral dose of 0.3 mg/kg yields a peak blood level of 0.06-0.14 μg/mL

Peak level of tamoxifen after a 20 mg dose: 42 μg/L

Peak level of N-desmethyltamoxifen after a 20 mg dose: 12 μg/L

Overdosage Treatment

Decontamination: Lavage/activated charcoal with cathartic

Enhancement of elimination: Multiple dosing of activated charcoal may be effective

Test Interactions T_4 elevations (no clinical evidence of hyperthyroidism)

Drug Interactions May cause 25% reduction of serum doxepin levels

Increased toxicity:

Allopurinol results in exacerbation of allopurinol-induced hepatitis

Cyclosporine may result in increased cyclosporine serum levels

Warfarin results in significant enhancement of the anticoagulant effect of warfarin; has been speculated that a decrease in antitumor effect of tamoxifen may also occur due to alterations in the percentage of active tamoxifen metabolites

Radiation recall (erythema) may occur

Concomitant high-dose tamoxifen (200 mg/day) and phenytoin administration can result in increased serum phenytoin levels

Pregnancy Risk Factor D

Monitoring Parameters Monitor WBC and platelet counts, tumor

Patient Information Report any vomiting that occurs after taking dose; patients should be advised to notify their physician of vaginal bleeding, asthenia, mental confusion; increased bone and tumor pain and local disease flare may occur with start of therapy

Nursing Implications Increase of bone pain usually indicates a good therapeutic response

Specific References

Cutuli B, Petit JC, Fricker JP et al, "Thromboembolic Accidents in Postmenopausal Patients Treated by Tamoxifen and Adjuvant Treatment: Frequency, Risk Factors, and Prevention," *Bull Cancer*, 1995, 82:51-6.

Cuzick J, Allen D, Baum M, et al, "Long Term Effects of Tamoxifen: Biological Effects of Tamoxifen Working Party," *Eur J Cancer*, 1992, 29A(1):15-21.

Dew JE and Eden JA, "Gynaecological Complications of Women Treated With Tamoxifen for Breast Cancer," *Aust N Z J Obstet Gynaecol*, 1995, 35:198-200.

Fernando IN and Tobias JS, "Priapism in Patient on Tamoxifen," *Lancet*, 1989, 1(8635):436.

Hochner-Celnikier D, Antaby E, and Yagel S, "Ovarian Cysts in Tamoxifen-Treated Premenopausal Women With Breast Cancer - A Management Dilemma," *Am J Obstet Gynecol*, 1995, 172:1323-4.

Jordan VC, "Tamoxifen: Toxicities and Drug Resistance During Treatment and Prevention of Breast Cancer," *Annu Rev Pharmacol Toxicol*, 1995, 35:195-212.

LiVolsi VA, Salhany KE, and Dowdy YG, "Endocervical Adenocarcinoma in Tamoxifen-Treated Patient," *Am J Obstet Gynecol*, 1995, 172:1065.

Parry BR, "Radiation Recall Induced by Tamoxifen," *Lancet*, 1992, 340(8810):49.

Pratt DS, Knox TA, and Erban J, "Tamoxifen-Induced Steatohepatitis," *Ann Intern Med*, 1995, 123(3):236.

Rabinowicz AL, Hinton DR, Dyck P, et al, "High-Dose Tamoxifen in Treatment of Brain Tumors: Interaction With Antiepileptic Drugs," *Epilepsia*, 1995, 36:513-5.

Ritchie LD and Grant SM, "Tamoxifen-Warfarin Interaction: The Aberdeen Hospitals Drug File," *BMJ*, 1989, 298(6682):1253.

Rutqvist LE, Johansson H, and Signomklao T, Stockholm Breast Cancer Study Group, "Adjuvant Tamoxifen Therapy for Early Stage Breast Cancer and Second Primary Malignancies," *J Natl Cancer Inst*, 1995, 87:645-51.

Spooner D and Evans BD, "Tamoxifen and Life-Threatening Hypercalcaemia," *Lancet*, 1979, 2(8139):413-4.

Tanyl® *see* Fentanyl Citrate *on page 347*

Tapazole® *see* Methimazole *on page 512*

Taractan® *see* Chlorprothixene *on page 209*

Tarasan® *see* Chlorprothixene *on page 209*

Tardigal® *see* Digitoxin *on page 283*

Tauliz® *see* Piretanide *on page 630*

Tavegil® *see* Clemastine Fumarate *on page 223*

Tavist® *see* Clemastine Fumarate *on page 223*

Tavist®-1 [OTC] *see* Clemastine Fumarate *on page 223*

Taxofit Vitamin E® *see* Vitamin E *on page 798*

Taxol® *see* Paclitaxel *on page 589*

Taxol A *see* Paclitaxel *on page 589*

TCN *see* Tetracycline *on page 732*

Tebamide® *see* Trimethobenzamide Hydrochloride *on page 772*

Tedelparin Sodium *see* Dalteparin *on page 256*

Tega-Cert® [OTC] *see* Dimenhydrinate *on page 289*

Tegretol® *see* Carbamazepine *on page 184*

Telachlor® *see* Chlorpheniramine Maleate *on page 204*

Teldane® *see* Terfenadine *on page 728*

Teldanex® *see* Terfenadine *on page 728*

Teldrin® [OTC] *see* Chlorpheniramine Maleate *on page 204*

Teline® Oral *see* Tetracycline *on page 732*

Tema³® *see* Temazepam *on next page*

Temaz® *see* Temazepam *on next page*

Temazepam (te maz' e pam)

Related Information

Benzodiazepines Comparison *on page 1643*

CAS Number 846-50-4

Brand Names Euphypnos®; Levanxol®; Normison®; Restoril®; Somaz®; Tema3®; Temaz®; Tenso®

Synonyms 3-hydroxydiazepam

Use Treatment of anxiety and as an adjunct in the treatment of depression; also may be used in the management of panic attacks; transient insomnia and sleep latency

Mechanism of Action Benzodiazepine anxiolytic sedative that produces CNS depression at the subcortical level, except at high doses, whereby it works at the cortical level

Adverse Reactions

Central nervous system: Drowsiness, confusion, dizziness, amnesia, night terrors, ataxia, electroencephalogram abnormalities

Dermatologic: Lichenoid drug eruption

Ocular: Mydriasis

Respiratory: Respiratory rate (decreased)

Signs & Symptoms of Acute Overdose Somnolence, diarrhea, confusion, night terrors, hyporeflexia, cognitive dysfunction, coma, hypoactive reflexes, dyspnea, hypotension, slurred speech, ataxia, hypothermia

Toxicodynamics/Kinetics

Onset of hypnotic effect: 30-60 minutes

Absorption: Nearly complete through gastrointestinal tract; slower through rectal route

Distribution: V_d: 1.4 L/kg; distributed widely throughout body

Protein binding: 96%

Metabolism: In the liver to oxazepam

Half-life: 10-15 hours

Time to peak serum concentration: Within 2-3 hours

Elimination: 80% to 90% excreted in urine as inactive metabolites; clearance: 0.69-1.05 mL/minute/kg

Usual Dosage Adults: Oral: 15-30 mg at bedtime; 15 mg in elderly or debilitated patients

Contraindications Hypersensitivity to temazepam or any component, severe uncontrolled pain, pre-existing CNS depression or narrow-angle glaucoma; not to be used in pregnancy or lactation

Warnings Use with caution in patients with mental impairment, reflex slowing, or the potential for drug dependence

Dosage Forms Capsule: 15 mg, 30 mg

Reference Range Therapeutic: 26 ng/mL after 24 hours; can be quantified by high performance liquid chromatography; postmortem levels >88.5 ng/mL have been correlated with fatalities

Overdosage Treatment

Decontamination: Lavage/activated charcoal with cathartic

Supportive therapy: Treatment for benzodiazepine overdose is supportive. Rarely is mechanical ventilation required. Flumazenil (Romazicon™) has been shown to selectively block the binding of benzodiazepines to CNS receptors, resulting in a reversal of benzodiazepine-induced CNS depression.

Enhancement of elimination: Multiple dosing of activated charcoal is effective; hemodialysis/forced diuresis is of no utility

Antidote(s)

Flumazenil *on page 1428*

Test Interactions Visine®, Drano®, bleach may cause false-negative urine tests; oxazepam may interfere in giving falsely elevated glucose results

Drug Interactions CNS depressants, alcohol, tricyclic antidepressants, unlike other benzodiazepines, there is minimal interaction with cimetidine, ranitidine, or oral contraceptives

Pregnancy Risk Factor X (when combined with diphenhydramine, may cause stillbirths)

Monitoring Parameters Respiratory and cardiovascular status

Patient Information Advise to avoid alcohol and other CNS depressants; avoid activities needing good psychomotor coordination until CNS effects are known; drug may cause physical or psychological dependence; avoid abrupt discontinuation after prolonged use

Nursing Implications Provide safety measures (ie, side rails, night light, and call button); remove smoking materials from area; supervise ambulation

Additional Information Causes minimal change in REM sleep patterns

Specific References

Grahame-Smith DG, "Misuse of Temazepam," *Br Med J (Clin Res)*, 1991, 302(6786):1210.

Ho PC, Triggs EJ, Heazlewood V, et al, "Determination of Nitrazepam and Temazepam in Plasma by High Performance Liquid Chromatography," *Ther Drug Monit*, 1983, 5(3):303-7.

Klotz U and Kanto J, "Pharmacokinetics and Clinical Use of Flumazenil (Ro 15-1788)," *Clin Pharmacokinet*, 1988, 14(1):1-12.

Temodal® *see* Quazepam *on page 665*

Tempra® [OTC] *see* Acetaminophen *on page 79*

Tenacid® *see* Imipenem/Cilastatin *on page 420*

Tenavoid® *see* Meprobamate *on page 503*

Tenex® *see* Guanfacine Hydrochloride *on page 394*

Tenidap

Brand Names Enable®

Synonyms 248-2; CP-66

Use Investigational: Rheumatoid arthritis, osteoarthritis

Mechanism of Action Inhibits cyclo-oxygenase and 5-lipoxygenase impairing prostaglandin and leukotriene production

Adverse Reactions

Central nervous system: Dizziness, headache

Gastrointestinal (noted in ~25% of patients): Nausea, constipation

Otic: Tinnitus

Renal: Reversible proteinuria

Toxicodynamics/Kinetics

Onset of action: Within 24 hours

Protein binding: 99%

Usual Dosage 120 mg/day (usually given in the morning)

Contraindications Hypersensitivity to any component, syndrome of nasal polyps, angioedema, and bronchospasm to aspirin

Warnings Use with caution in patients with peptic ulcer disease, renal/hepatic insufficiency, ulcerative colitis, hypertension, congestive heart failure, edema, anemia, allergy to nonsteroidal agents

Overdosage Treatment

Decontamination: Ipecac or lavage/activated charcoal with cathartic

Supportive therapy: Hypotension/dehydration can be managed with intravenous fluid therapy; acidosis should be treated with bicarbonates, seizures with benzodiazepines; antacids, blood products are indicated, as appropriate, for hemorrhage

Enhancement of elimination: Multiple doses of activated charcoal; dialysis or perfusion is indicated for secondary complications, acidosis, or renal failure and not toxin removal alone

Drug Interactions Tenidap decreases renal clearance of lithium, increases unbound phenytoin levels by 25%, and reduces antihypertensive effect of enalapril

Additional Information Oxindole-type nonsteroidal agent similar to indomethacin; may slow progressive joint erosion

Specific References

Blackburn WD Jr, Loose LD, Heck LW, et al, "Tenidap, in Contrast to Several Available Nonsteroidal Anti-inflammatory Drugs, Potently Inhibits the Release of Activated Neutrophil Collagenase," *Arthritis Rheum*, 1991, 34(2):211-6.

Brandt KD, "Toward Pharmacologic Modification of Joint Damage in Osteoarthritis," *Ann Intern Med*, 1995, 122:874-5.

Loose LD, Sipe JD, Kirby DS, et al, "Reduction of Acute-Phase Proteins With Tenidap Sodium, A Cytokine-Modulating Anti-Rheumatic Drug," *Br J Rheumatol*, 1993, 32(Suppl 3):19-25.

Matsushita I, Matsuno H, Kadowaki KM, et al, "Immunomodulating Effects of the New Antirheumatic Drug Tenidap on Collagen-Induced Arthritis," *Int J Immunopharmacol*, 1995, 17(3):213-20.

Tenoret® 50 *see* Atenolol and Chlorthalidone *on page 139*

Tenoretic® *see* Atenolol and Chlorthalidone *on page 139*

Tenormin® *see* Atenolol *on page 137*

Tensilon® *see* Edrophonium Chloride *on page 309*

Tensin® *see* Spironolactone *on page 705*

Tensium® *see* Diazepam *on page 271*

Tenso® *see* Temazepam *on previous page*

Tensogradal® *see* Nitrendipine *on page 562*

Teoptic® *see* Carteolol Hydrochloride *on page 188*

Tepavil® *see* Sulpiride *on page 717*

Terazosin (ter ay' zoe sin)

CAS Number 63590-64-7; 63074-08-8; 70024-40-7

Brand Names Heitrin®; Hytrin®; Hytrinex®; Vasocard®

Use Management of mild to moderate hypertension; benign prostate hypertrophy

(Continued)

Terazosin *(Continued)*

Mechanism of Action An $alpha_1$-specific blocking agent with minimal $alpha_2$ effects; this allows peripheral postsynaptic blockade, with the resultant decrease in arterial tone, while preserving the negative feedback loop which is mediated by the peripheral presynaptic $alpha_2$-receptors (similar in action to prazosin but longer duration of action)

Adverse Reactions

Cardiovascular: Orthostatic hypotension, syncope, palpitations, tachycardia, edema

Central nervous system: Dizziness, lightheadedness, night terrors, drowsiness, asthenia, headache, hypothermia

Dermatologic: Rash

Endocrine & metabolic: Fluid retention

Gastrointestinal: Nausea, dry mouth

Genitourinary: Urinary frequency, priapism, sexual dysfunction

Ocular: Blurred vision

Respiratory: Nasal congestion

Signs & Symptoms of Acute Overdose Hypotension, dyspnea, drowsiness, syncope, night terrors, impotence, hypothermia, shock

Toxicodynamics/Kinetics

Onset of action: 15 minutes

Duration: 24 hours

Absorption: Oral: Rapidly absorbed

Distribution: V_d: 17.7-30 L

Protein binding: 90% to 95%

Metabolism: Extensive in the liver to yield piperazine

Bioavailability: ~90%

Half-life: 9.2-12 hours

Time to peak serum concentration: Within 60 minutes

Elimination: Principally in feces (60%) and in urine (40%)

Usual Dosage Adults: Oral: 1 mg; slowly increase dose to achieve desired blood pressure or to desired urinary flow rates (BPH), up to 20 mg/day maximum

Contraindications Hypersensitivity to terazosin or any component

Warnings Syncope and hypotension (orthostatic) frequently occur with the first dose; use with caution in patients with confirmed or suspected coronary artery disease

Dosage Forms Tablet: 1 mg, 2 mg, 5 mg, 10 mg

Reference Range Single dose of 5 mg produces a peak concentration of 45 μg/L at 2 hours

Overdosage Treatment

Decontamination: Ipecac or lavage/activated charcoal with cathartic

Supportive therapy: Hypotension usually responds to I.V. fluids or Trendelenburg positioning. If unresponsive to these measures, the use of a parenteral vasoconstrictor may be required (eg, norepinephrine 0.1-0.2 mcg/kg/minute titrated to response). Treatment is primarily supportive and symptomatic.

Enhancement of elimination: Multiple dosing of activated charcoal would not be expected to be effective

Test Interactions No effect on lipid profile

Drug Interactions Ibuprofen

Pregnancy Risk Factor C

Monitoring Parameters Blood pressure, standing and sitting/supine; renal function

Patient Information Ambulation may be difficult because of hypotension (orthostatic); report any gain of body weight; fainting sometimes occurs after the first dose, take first dose at bedtime; rise from sitting/lying carefully, may cause dizziness

Additional Information Considered a step 2 drug in stepped approach to hypertension

Specific References

Kim J, Gazarian M, Verjee Z, et al, "Acute Renal Insufficiency in Ibuprofen Overdose," *Pediatr Emerg Care*, 1995, 11:107-8.

Luther RR, "Terazosin: A New Antihypertensive Agent With Favorable Effects on Lipids," *Int J Clin Pharmacol Ther Toxicol*, 1989, 27(7):313-9.

Sonders RC, "Pharmacokinetics of Terazosin," *Am J Med*, 1986, 80(Suppl 5B):20-4.

Titmarsh S and Monk JP, "Terazosin: A Review of Its Pharmacodynamic and Pharmacokinetic Properties, and Therapeutic Efficacy in Essential Hypertension," *Drugs*, 1987, 33(5):461-77.

Terbutaline Sulfate (ter byoo' ta leen)

CAS Number 23031-32-5

Brand Names Brethaire®; Brethine®; Bricanyl®

Use Bronchodilator in reversible airway obstruction and bronchial asthma; management of preterm labor

Mechanism of Action Relaxes bronchial smooth muscle by action on $beta_2$-receptors with less effect on heart rate

Adverse Reactions

Cardiovascular: Tachycardia (slight), palpitations, hypertension, flushing, shortened P-R segment, angina, lengthened Q-T segment, cardiac arrhythmias, fibrillation (atrial)

Central nervous system: Dizziness, headache, nervousness, CNS stimulation, hyperactivity, insomnia

Dermatologic: Maculopapular rash

Gastrointestinal: gastrointestinal upset

Neuromuscular & skeletal: Tremors

Signs & Symptoms of Acute Overdose Convulsions, nausea, hypokalemia, myoglobinuria, hepatitis, insomnia, hypocalcemia, rhabdomyolysis, vomiting, arrhythmias, hyperglycemia, chest pain

Toxicodynamics/Kinetics S.C. doses are more bioavailable and of quicker onset than oral doses

Onset of action:

- Inhalation: 5-30 minutes
- Oral: Within 60-120 minutes
- Parenteral: Within 15 minutes
- S.C.: 6-15 minutes

Duration:

- Inhalation: 3-6 hours
- Oral: 4-8 hours
- Parenteral: 1.5-4 hours

Absorption: 33% to 50% through gastrointestinal tract

Distribution: V_d: 1-2 L/kg; widely distributed throughout body

Protein binding: 25%

Metabolism: In the liver to inactive sulfate conjugates

Half-life: 11-16 hours

Elimination: Urine

Usual Dosage

Children <12 years:

- Oral: Initial: 0.05 mg/kg/dose 3 times/day, increased gradually as required; maximum: 0.15 mg/kg/dose 3-4 times/day or a total of 5 mg/24 hours
- S.C.: 0.005-0.01 mg/kg/dose to a maximum of 0.3 mg/dose every 15-20 minutes for 3 doses
- Nebulization: 0.1-0.3 mg/kg/dose up to a maximum of 10 mg/dose every 4-6 hours
- Inhalation: 1-2 inhalations every 4-6 hours

Children >12 years and Adults:

- Oral:
  - 12-15 years: 2.5 mg every 6 hours 3 times/day; not to exceed 7.5 mg in 24 hours
  - >15 years: 5 mg/dose every 6 hours 3 times/day; if side effects occur, reduce dose to 2.5 mg every 6 hours; not to exceed 15 mg in 24 hours
- S.C.: 0.25 mg/dose repeated in 15-30 minutes for one time only; a total dose of 0.5 mg should not be exceeded within a 4-hour period
- Nebulization: 0.1-0.3 mg/kg/dose every 4-6 hours
- Inhalation: 2 inhalations every 4-6 hours; wait 1 minute between inhalations

Dosing adjustment/comments in renal impairment:

Cl_{cr} 10-50 mL/minute: Administer at 50% of normal dose

Cl_{cr} <10 mL/minute: Avoid use

Contraindications Hypersensitivity to terbutaline or any component (may cause paradoxical bronchoconstriction, especially after repeated or excessive use)

Warnings Paradoxical bronchoconstriction may occur with excessive use, if it occurs, discontinue terbutaline immediately; use with caution in patients with diabetes mellitus, hypertension, hyperthyroidism, history of seizures, or cardiac disease

Dosage Forms

Aerosol, oral: 0.2 mg/actuation (10.5 g)

Injection: 1 mg/mL (1 mL)

Tablet: 2.5 mg, 5 mg

Stability Store injection at room temperature; protect from heat, light, and from freezing; use only clear solutions

Reference Range Peak plasma level after a 0.75 mg S.C. dose: ~10 μg/L 30 minutes after injection

Overdosage Treatment

Supportive therapy: In cases of overdose, prudent use of a cardioselective beta-adrenergic blocker (eg, atenolol or metoprolol) should be considered, keeping in mind the potential for induction of bronchoconstriction in an asthmatic individual; esmolol (150-300 mg/hour) can be safely used to treat tachycardia with hypotension even during pregnancy

Enhancement of elimination: Dialysis has not been shown to be of value in the treatment of an overdose with this agent.

(Continued)

Terbutaline Sulfate *(Continued)*

Drug Interactions MAO inhibitors, tricyclic antidepressants, beta-receptor blocking agents

Pregnancy Risk Factor B

Monitoring Parameters Serum potassium, heart rate, blood pressure, respiratory rate

Patient Information Separate administration of aerosol adrenocorticoid by 15 minutes; report any decreased effectiveness of drug

Nursing Implications Injection with S.C. use

Additional Information Used unofficially to delay delivery in preterm labor; has short-lived clinical effectiveness with development of tolerance with chronic use

Specific References

Kelly HW, McWilliams BC, Katz R, et al, "Safety of Frequent High Dose Nebulized Terbutaline in Children With Acute Severe Asthma," *Ann Allergy*, 1990, 64(2 Pt 2):229-33.

Lee DC, "Terbutaline Sulfate Overdose," *Ann Emerg Med*, 1995, 26:107-8.

Zehner WJ, Scott JM, Iannolo PM, et al, "Terbutaline vs Albuterol for Out-of-Hospital Respiratory Distress: Randomized Double-Blind Trial," *Acad Emerg Med*, 1995, 2:686-91.

Terfenadine (ter fen' a deen)

Related Information

H1-Antihistamine Comparison *on page 1649*

CAS Number 50679-08-8

Brand Names Alergist®; Allerplus®; Cyater®; Rapidal®; Seldane®; Teldane®; Teldanex®; Ternadin®; Triludan®

Use Perennial and seasonal allergic rhinitis and other allergic symptoms including rash; has drying effect in patients with asthma

Mechanism of Action Competes with histamine for H_1-receptor sites on effector cells in the gastrointestinal tract, blood vessels, and respiratory tract; binds to lung receptors significantly greater than it binds to cerebellar receptors, resulting in a reduced sedative potential; lacks anticholinergic activity

Adverse Reactions

Cardiovascular: Palpitations, bradycardia, hypotension, torsade de pointes

Central nervous system: Headache, fatigue, nervousness, dizziness, depression, sedation, dizziness, paradoxical excitement, insomnia, slight drowsiness, ataxia, electroencephalogram abnormalities

Dermatologic: Photosensitivity, rash, alopecia, angioedema

Gastrointestinal: Appetite increase, weight increase, nausea, diarrhea, abdominal pain, dry mouth

Genitourinary: Urinary retention

Hepatic: Hepatitis

Neuromuscular & skeletal: Arthralgia, myalgia, tremors, paresthesia

Ocular: Blurred vision, cycloplegia

Respiratory: Bronchospasm, thickening of bronchial secretions, pharyngitis

Miscellaneous: Edema, porphyrinogenic, epistaxis

Signs & Symptoms of Acute Overdose Nausea, confusion, sedation, insomnia, prolonged Q-T interval, torsade de pointes, seizures

Toxicodynamics/Kinetics

Duration of antihistaminic effect: Up to 12 hours

Protein binding: 97%

Metabolism: Extensive first-pass metabolism; metabolized in the liver to an active carboxylic acid metabolite and an inactive piperidine-carbinol metabolite

Half-life: 16-22 hours

Time to peak serum concentration: Within 1-2 hours

Elimination: Primarily excreted in feces (60%) and secondarily in urine (40%)

Usual Dosage Oral:

Children:

- 3-6 years: 15 mg twice daily
- 6-12 years: 30 mg twice daily

Children >12 years and Adults: 60 mg twice daily

Maximum daily dose: 120 mg, doses >1 g can produce arrhythmias

Contraindications Hypersensitivity to terfenadine or any component

Warnings Safety and efficacy in children <12 years of age have not been established; use with caution in patients with a history of cardiac conduction disturbances or cardiac arrhythmias, or those receiving antiarrhythmic medication

Dosage Forms Tablet: 60 mg

Stability Keep away from direct sunlight

Reference Range Terfenadine levels >10 ng/mL consistent with toxicity; carboxylic acid metabolite level between 250-300 ng/mL associated with steady-state dosing (60 mg twice daily)

Overdosage Treatment

Decontamination: Lavage/activated charcoal

Supportive therapy: Lidocaine has been used successfully to treat cardiac arrhythmias; avoid type I antiarrhythmics, torsade may respond to I.V. magnesium

Test Interactions Antigen skin testing procedures

Drug Interactions

Serious cardiac events have occurred with elevated terfenadine levels, which may occur with the use of ketoconazole, itraconazole, fluconazole, metronidazole, miconazole, erythromycin, troleandomycin, clarithromycin, fluoxetine, sotalol, troleandomycin, azithromycin, clarithromycin, cimetidine, fluoxetine, bepridil, sotalol; odds ratio for QT_c prolongation with concomitant erythromycin and terfenadine use is 2.33

Increased levels/toxicity of carbamazepine; increased toxicity of carbamazepine with displacement of carbamazepine from protein-binding sites by terfenadine

Pregnancy Risk Factor C

Monitoring Parameters Relief of symptoms

Patient Information Drink plenty of water; may cause dry mouth, sedation, drowsiness, can impair judgment and coordination

Nursing Implications Patient on medications that prolong the Q-T interval should be on a cardiac monitor when starting this drug

Additional Information Causes less drowsiness than other antihistamines; patients on medications that prolong the Q-T interval should be on a cardiac monitor when starting this drug

Specific References

Hanrahan JP, Choo PW, Carlson W, et al, "Terfenadine-Associated Ventricular Arrhythmias and QT_c Interval Prolongation: A Retrospective Cohort Comparison With Other Antihistamines Among Members of a Health Maintenance Organization," *Ann Epidemiol*, 1995, 5:201-9.

Jones SK and Morley WN, "Terfenadine Causing Hair Loss," *Br Med J*, 1985, 291:940.

Mathews DR, McNutt B, Okerholm R, et al "Torsades de Pointes Occurring in Association With Terfenadine Use," *JAMA*, 1991, 266(17):2375-6.

Woosley RL, Chen Y, Freiman JP, et al, "Mechanism of the Cardiotoxic Actions of Terfenadine," *JAMA*, 1993, 269(12):1532-6.

Terfluzin® *see* Trifluoperazine Hydrochloride *on page 769*

Teriam® *see* Triamterene *on page 766*

Termine® *see* Phentermine Hydrochloride *on page 619*

Ternadin® *see* Terfenadine *on previous page*

Tertroxin® *see* Liothyronine Sodium *on page 471*

Testo-Enant® *see* Testosterone *on this page*

Testosterone (tess toss' ter one)

CAS Number 5949-44-0; 2697-92-9; 15262-86-9; 58-22-0; 1045-69-8; 58-20-8; 5721-91-5; 315-37-7; 14191-92-5; 1255-49-8; 57-85-2

Brand Names Andriol®; Andro-Cyp® Injection; Andro® Injection; Andro-L.A.® Injection; Andronate® Injection; Andropository® Injection; Delatest® Injection; Delatestryl®; Depotest® Injection; Depo®-Testosterone Injection; Duratest® Injection; Durathate® Injection; Everone® Injection; Histerone® Injection; Lontanyl®; Malogex®; Restandol®; Testo-Enant®; Testoviron®; Testovis®; Testred®; Undestor®; Virilon®; Virormone®

Synonyms Aqueous Testosterone; Testosterone Cypionate; Testosterone Enanthate; Trans-Testosterone

Use Androgen replacement therapy in the treatment of delayed male puberty; postpartum breast pain and engorgement; inoperable breast cancer; male hypogonadism

Mechanism of Action Principal endogenous androgen responsible for promoting the growth and development of the male sex organs and maintaining secondary sex characteristics in androgen-deficient males

Adverse Reactions

Central nervous system: Euphoria, cerebrovascular accident

Dermatologic: Edema, acne, pruritus, exacerbation of psoriasis, hirsutism (increase in pubic hair growth)

Endocrine & metabolic: Gynecomastia, amenorrhea, hypercalcemia

Gastrointestinal: gastrointestinal irritation, nausea, vomiting

Genitourinary: Impotence, testicular atrophy, piloerection, clitoral enlargement, priapism, azoospermia, increased libido

Hematologic: Polycythemia, leukopenia

Hepatic: Hepatic dysfunction, hepatic necrosis (especially with water-based oral preparations), cholestatic hepatitis, hepatocellular carcinoma

Miscellaneous: Virilism, breast soreness, prostatic hypertrophy, prostatic carcinoma, hypersensitivity reactions

Signs & Symptoms of Acute Overdose Leukopenia or neutropenia (agranulocytosis, granulocytopenia); hirsutism, gynecomastia, hypertrichosis, oligospermia, jaundice, hypertension, depression, hypercalcemia, impotence, cholestatic jaundice

(Continued)

Testosterone *(Continued)*

Toxicodynamics/Kinetics

Absorption: From skin, gastrointestinal tract, oral mucosa

Duration of effect: Based upon the route of administration and which testosterone ester is used; the cypionate and enanthate esters have the longest duration, up to 2-4 weeks after I.M. administration

Protein binding: 98% (to transcortin and albumin)

Metabolism: In the liver to androsterone and etiocholanolone; methylation or alkylation at the 17-position of testosterone reduces hepatic metabolism

Half-life: 10-100 minutes

Elimination: Urine (90%) and feces via bile (6%)

Usual Dosage I.M.:

Delayed puberty: Children: 40-50 mg/m^2/dose (cypionate or enanthate) monthly for 6 months

Male hypogonadism: 50-400 mg every 2-4 weeks

Initiation of pubertal growth: 40-50 mg/m^2/dose (cypionate or enanthate) monthly until the growth rate falls to prepubertal levels (~5 cm/year)

During terminal growth phase: 100 mg/m^2/dose (cypionate or enanthate) monthly until growth ceases

Maintenance virilizing dose: 100 mg/m^2/dose (cypionate or enanthate) twice monthly or 50-400 mg/dose every 2-4 weeks

Inoperable breast cancer: Adults: 200-400 mg every 2-4 weeks

Hypogonadism: Adults:

Testosterone or testosterone propionate: 10-25 mg 2-3 times/week

Testosterone cypionate or enanthate: 50-400 mg every 2-4 weeks

Postpubertal cryptorchism: Testosterone or testosterone propionate: 10-25 mg 2-3 times/week

Dosing adjustment/comments in hepatic disease: Reduce dose

Contraindications Severe renal or cardiac disease, benign prostatic hypertrophy with obstruction, undiagnosed genital bleeding, males with carcinoma of the breast or prostate; hypersensitivity to testosterone or any component

Warnings Perform radiographic examination of the hand and wrist every 6 months to determine the rate of bone maturation; may accelerate bone maturation without producing compensating gain in linear growth; has both androgenic and anabolic activity, the anabolic action may enhance hypoglycemia

Dosage Forms Injection:

Aqueous suspension: 25 mg/mL (10 mL, 30 mL); 50 mg/mL (10 mL, 30 mL); 100 mg/mL (10 mL, 30 mL)

In oil, as cypionate: 100 mg/mL (1 mL, 10 mL); 200 mg/mL (1 mL, 10 mL)

In oil, as enanthate: 100 mg/mL (5 mL, 10 mL); 200 mg/mL (5 mL, 10 mL)

In oil, as propionate: 50 mg/mL (10 mL, 30 mL); 100 mg/mL (10 mL, 30 mL)

Reference Range

Testosterone, urine:

Male: 100-1500 ng/24 hours

Female: 100-500 ng/24 hours

Normal serum ranges (male): 12.1-35.7 nmol/L

Normal ratio of testosterone to epitestosterone: <6

Injected agents can be detectable in urine for 2 months while oral agents can be detectable for 2 weeks

Overdosage Treatment Decontamination: Oral: Ipecac or lavage/activated charcoal with cathartic

Test Interactions May cause a decrease in creatinine and creatine excretion and an increase in the excretion of 17-ketosteroids; decrease total T_4 serum level due to a decrease in thyroxine-binding globulin (free T_4 is unchanged)

Drug Interactions Increased toxicity: Oral anticoagulant and oral hypoglycemic agents effects may be enhanced, imipramine; also enhances toxicity of cyclosporine

Pregnancy Risk Factor X

Pregnancy Implications Crosses the placenta; appears in breast milk; fetal virilization

Monitoring Parameters Periodic liver function tests, radiologic examination of wrist and hand every 6 months (when using in prepubertal children)

Patient Information Virilization may occur in female patients; report menstrual irregularities; male patients report priapism; all patients should report persistent gastrointestinal distress, diarrhea, or jaundice

Nursing Implications Warming to room temperature and shaking vial will help redissolve crystals that have formed after storage; administer by deep I.M. injection into the upper outer quadrant of the gluteus maximus

Specific References

Borhan-Manesh F and Farnum JB, "Methyltestosterone-Induced Cholestasis. The Importance of Disproportionately Low Serum Alkaline Phosphatase Level," *Arch Intern Med*, 1989, 149(9):2127-9.

Cunningham GR, Cordero E, and Thornby JI, "Testosterone Replacement With Transdermal Therapeutic Systems. Physiological Serum Testosterone and Elevated Dihydrotestosterone Levels," *JAMA*, 1989, 261(17):2525-30.

Daigle RD, "Anabolic Steroids," *J Psychoactive Drugs*, 1990, 22(1):77-80.

Moller BB and Ekelund B, "Toxicity of Cyclosporine During Treatment With Androgens," *N Engl J Med*, 1985, 313(22):1416.

Ruch W and Jenny P, "Priapism Following Testosterone Administration for Delayed Male Puberty," *Am J Med*, 1989, 86(2):256.

Testosterone Cypionate *see* Testosterone *on page 729*

Testosterone Enanthate *see* Testosterone *on page 729*

Testoviron® *see* Testosterone *on page 729*

Testovis® *see* Testosterone *on page 729*

Testred® *see* Testosterone *on page 729*

Tetracaine Hydrochloride (tet' ra kane)

CAS Number 136-47-0; 94-24-6

Brand Names Anethaine®; Covostet®; Gingicain®; Minims®; Pontocaine®; Versola®

Synonyms Amethocaine Hydrochloride

Use Spinal anesthesia; local anesthesia in the eye for various diagnostic and examination purposes; topically applied to nose and throat for various diagnostic procedures

Mechanism of Action Blocks both the initiation and conduction of nerve impulses by decreasing the neuronal membrane's permeability to sodium ions, which results in inhibition of depolarization with resultant blockade of conduction

Adverse Reactions

Cardiovascular: Cardiac arrest, bradycardia
Central nervous system: CNS stimulation/depression
Dermatologic: Urticaria, contact dermatitis with topical form
Gastrointestinal: Nausea, vomiting
Local: Stinging
Ocular: Lacrimation, photophobia, corneal epithelial erosion, keratitis, corneal opacification
Respiratory: Respiratory arrest
Miscellaneous: Diabetes insipidus

Signs & Symptoms of Acute Overdose Apnea, respiratory depression, lacrimation, seizures, bradycardia, hypotension, ototoxicity; tinnitus, cataract

Toxicodynamics/Kinetics

Onset of action:
- Ophthalmic: Anesthetic effects occur within 60 seconds
- Topical: Within 3 minutes when applied to mucous membranes or when saddle block administered for spinal anesthesia

Duration: 1.5-3 hours
Absorption: Readily absorbed through mucous membranes into systemic circulation
Protein binding: 76%
Metabolism: By the liver and plasma to para-aminobenzoic acid
Elimination: Metabolites are renally excreted

Usual Dosage Maximum adult dose: 50 mg

Children: Safety and efficacy have not been established

Adults:
- Ophthalmic (not for prolonged use):
  - Ointment: Apply ½" to 1" to lower conjunctival fornix
  - Solution: Instill 1-2 drops
- Spinal anesthesia:
  - High, medium, low, and saddle blocks: 0.2% to 0.3% solution
  - Prolonged (2-3 hours): 1% solution
  - Subarachnoid injection: 5-20 mg
  - Saddle block: 2-5 mg; a 1% solution should be diluted with equal volume of CSF before administration
- Topical mucous membranes (2% solution): Apply as needed; dose should not exceed 20 mg
- Topical for skin: Ointment/cream: Apply to affected areas as needed

Contraindications Hypersensitivity to tetracaine or any component; ophthalmic secondary bacterial infection

Warnings No pediatric dosage recommendations; ophthalmic preparations may delay wound healing

Dosage Forms

Cream: 1% (28 g)
Injection: 1% [10 mg/mL] (2 mL)
Injection, with dextrose 6%: 0.2% [2 mg/mL] (2 mL); 0.3% [3 mg/mL] (5 mL)
Ointment:

(Continued)

Tetracaine Hydrochloride *(Continued)*

Ophthalmic: 0.5% [5 mg/mL] (3.75 g)
Topical: 0.5% [5 mg/mL] (28 g)
Solution:
Ophthalmic: 0.5% [5 mg/mL] (1 mL, 2 mL, 15 mL, 59 mL)
Topical: 2% [20 mg/mL] (30 mL, 118 mL)

Stability Store the solutions in the refrigerator; incompatible with alkalis

Overdosage Treatment

Decontamination: Lavage/irrigate/activated charcoal with cathartic

Supportive therapy: Treatment is primarily symptomatic and supportive. Termination of anesthesia by pneumatic tourniquet inflation should be attempted when the agent is administered by infiltration or regional injection. Seizures commonly respond to diazepam or lorazepam, while hypotension responds to I.V. fluids and Trendelenburg positioning. Bradyarrhythmias (when the heart rate is less than 60) can be treated with I.V., I.M., or S.C. atropine 15 mcg/kg. With the development of metabolic acidosis, I.V. sodium bicarbonate 0.5-2 mEq/kg and ventilatory assistance should be instituted.

Enhancement of elimination: Multiple dosing of activated charcoal may be effective

Drug Interactions Aminosalicylic acid, sulfonamides

Pregnancy Risk Factor C

Patient Information Report any rashes

Additional Information Approximately 10 times more potent than procaine

Specific References

Duffin RM and Olson RJ, "Tetracaine Toxicity," *Ann Ophthalmol*, 1984, 16(9):836, 838.

Garfield JM, Andriole GL, Vetto JL, et al, "Prolonged Diabetes Insipidus Subsequent to an Episode of Chemical Meningitis," *Anesthesiology*, 1986, 64(2):253-4.

Kintner JC, Grossniklaus HE, Lass JH, et al, "Infectious Crystalline Keratopathy Associated With Topical Anesthetic Abuse," *Cornea*, 1990, 9(1):77-80.

Tetracaine Hydrochloride, Benzocaine Butyl Aminobenzoate, and Benzalkonium Chloride *see* Benzocaine, Butyl Aminobenzoate, Tetracaine, and Benzalkonium Chloride *on page 150*

Tetracap® Oral *see* Tetracycline *on this page*

Tetracycline (tet ra sye' kleen)

Related Information

Drugs and Chemicals Proven to be Teratogenic in Humans *on page 1572-1575*

Therapeutic Drugs Associated With Hallucinations *on page 1558-1559*

CAS Number 60-54-8; 6416-04-2; 1336-20-5; 64-75-5

Brand Names Achromycin®; Achromycin® V Oral; Ala-Tet® Oral; Economycin®; Hexacycline®; Hortetracin®; Imex®; Latycin®; Nor-tet® Oral; Panmycin® Oral; Robitet® Oral; Rotet®; Steclin®; Sumycin® Oral; Teline® Oral; Tetracap® Oral; Tetralan® Oral; Tetralen®; Tetram® Oral; Topicycline® Topical; Triphacycline®

Synonyms TCN; Tetracycline Hydrochloride; Tetradecin; Tetraverine

Use Treatment of susceptible bacterial infections of both gram-positive and gram-negative organisms; also some unusual organisms including *Mycoplasma*, *Chlamydia*, and *Rickettsia*; may also be used for acne, exacerbations of chronic bronchitis, treatment of "seal finger", *Helicobacter pylori*, and treatment of gonorrhea and syphilis in patients that are allergic to penicillin

Mechanism of Action Inhibits bacterial protein synthesis by binding with the 30S and possibly the 50S ribosomal subunit(s) of susceptible bacteria; may also cause alterations in the cytoplasmic membrane

Adverse Reactions

Central nervous system: Pseudotumor cerebri, visual hallucinations

Dermatologic: Rash, exfoliative dermatitis, photosensitivity, toxic epidermal necrolysis, angioedema

Gastrointestinal: Nausea, vomiting, diarrhea, stomatitis, glossitis, antibiotic-associated pseudomembranous colitis, esophagitis, dry mouth, pancreatitis

Hematologic: Fanconi-like syndrome, neutropenia, hemolysis, hypoprothrombinemia, aplastic anemia

Hepatic: Hepatic steatosis (at doses >1 g/day I.V.); fatty degeneration of liver

Neuromuscular & skeletal: Injury to growing bones and teeth, myasthenia gravis (exacerbation)

Ocular: Myopia

Renal: Renal damage

Respiratory: Pulmonary infiltrates with eosinophilia

Miscellaneous: Hypersensitivity reactions, increased incidence of candidal superinfection, esophageal ulceration, exacerbation of systemic lupus erythematosus (SLE), intracranial hypertension, feces discoloration (black), feces discoloration (greenish gray), feces discoloration (red), feces discoloration (white/speckling), drug fever

Signs & Symptoms of Acute Overdose Nausea, diplopia; vomiting, tongue discoloration, coagulopathy, colitis, azotemia, metallic taste, lichenoid eruptions, toxic epidermal necrolysis, dysphagia, hypoglycemia, hypothermia, thrombocytopenia, Fanconi's syndrome, Stevens-Johnson syndrome, myasthenia gravis (exacerbation or precipitation of), systemic lupus erythematosus (SLE)

Toxicodynamics/Kinetics

Absorption: Oral: 75%

Distribution: V_d: 1-2 L/kg; small amount appears in bile

Protein binding: 20% to 60%

Half-life: Normal renal function: 8-11 hours

Time to peak serum concentration: Within 2-4 hours

Elimination: Primary route of elimination is the kidney, with 60% of a dose excreted as unchanged drug in urine

Usual Dosage

Children >8 years:

Oral: 25-50 mg/kg/day in divided doses every 6 hours; not to exceed 3 g/day

Ophthalmic:

Suspension: Instill 1-2 drops 2-4 times/day or more often as needed

Ointment: Instill every 2-12 hours

Adults:

Oral: 250-500 mg/dose every 6 hours

Ophthalmic:

Suspension: Instill 1-2 drops 2-4 times/day or more often as needed

Ointment: Instill every 2-12 hours

Topical: Apply to affected areas 1-4 times/day

Dosing interval in renal impairment:

Cl_{cr} 50-80 mL/minute: Administer every 8-12 hours

Cl_{cr} 10-50 mL/minute: Administer every 12-24 hours

Cl_{cr} <10 mL/minute: Administer every 24 hours

Dosing adjustment in hepatic impairment: Avoid use or maximum dose is 1 g/day

Contraindications Hypersensitivity to tetracycline or any component; do not administer to children ≤ 8 years of age

Warnings Use of tetracyclines during tooth development may cause permanent discoloration of the teeth and enamel, hypoplasia, and retardation of skeletal development and bone growth; use with caution in patients with renal or hepatic impairment and in pregnancy; pseudomotor cerebri has been reported with tetracycline use

Dosage Forms

Capsule: 100 mg, 250 mg, 500 mg

Ointment:

Ophthalmic: 1% [10 mg/mL] (3.5 g)

Topical: 3% [30 mg/mL] (14.2 g, 30 g)

Solution, topical: 2.2 mg/mL (70 mL)

Suspension:

Ophthalmic: 1% [10 mg/mL] (0.5 mL, 1 mL, 4 mL)

Oral: 125 mg/5 mL (60 mL, 480 mL)

Tablet: 250 mg, 500 mg

Stability Outdated tetracyclines have caused a Fanconi-like syndrome

Reference Range

Therapeutic: Not established

Toxic: >16 μg/mL

Overdosage Treatment

Decontamination: Emesis or lavage/activated charcoal with cathartic

Supportive therapy: Antacids can be given for epigastric pain; acetazolamide (500 mg twice daily) can be used to treat pseudotumor cerebri

Enhancement of elimination: Multiple dosing of activated charcoal may be effective; slightly dialyzable (5% to 20%)

Test Interactions False-negative urine glucose with Clinistix®

Drug Interactions

Decreased effect with antacids (aluminum, calcium, zinc, or magnesium), bismuth salts, sodium bicarbonate, barbiturates, carbamazepine, hydantoins; decreased effect of oral contraceptives

Increased effect of warfarin; increased nephrotoxicity with diuretics; increased benign intracranial hypertension with retinoids

Pregnancy Risk Factor D; B (topical)

Monitoring Parameters Renal, hepatic, and hematologic function test

Patient Information Take 1 hour before or 2 hours after meals with adequate amounts of fluid; avoid prolonged exposure to sunlight or sunlamps; avoid taking antacids, iron, or dairy products within 2 hours of taking tetracyclines; report persistent nausea, vomiting, yellow coloring of skin or eyes, dark urine, or pale stools;

(Continued)

Tetracycline *(Continued)*

ophthalmic may cause transient burning or pruritus; topical is for external use only and may stain skin yellow

Nursing Implications Give around-the-clock (ie, 6-12-6-12)

Additional Information May reduce serum vitamin B concentrations; D-lactic acidosis may develop in patients with short bowel syndrome due to overgrowth of D-lactate producing organisms (*Lactobacillus*, species, *Streptococcus bovis, Bifidobacterium* species or *Eubacterium*, species)

Tetracycline: Achromycin® V oral suspension, Sumycin® syrup, Tetralan® syrup

Tetracycline hydrochloride: Achromycin® injection, Achromycin® V capsule, Nortet® capsule, Panmycin® capsule, Robitet® capsule, Sumycin® capsule and tablet, Teline® capsule, Tetracyn® capsule, Tetralan® capsule

Specific References

Coronado BE, Opal SM, and Yoburn DC, "Antibiotic-Induced D-Lactic Acidosis," *Ann Intern Med*, 1995, 122:839-42.

Cuddihy J, "Case Report of Benign Intra-cranial Hypertension Secondary to Tetracycline," *Ir Med J*, 1994, 87(3):90.

Fox SA, Berenyi MR, and Straus B, "Tetracycline Toxicity Presenting as a Multisystem Disease," *Mt Sinai J Med*, 1976, 43(2):129-35.

Gardner K, Cox T, and Digre KB, "Idiopathic Intracranial Hypertension Associated With Tetracycline Use in Fraternal Twins: Case Reports and Review," *Neurology*, 1995, 45(1):6-10.

Lee AG, "Pseudotumor Cerebri After Treatment With Tetracycline and Isotretinoin for Acne," *Cutis*, 1995, 55:165-8.

Maroon JC and Mealy J Jr, "Benign Intracranial Hypertension. Sequel to Tetracycline Therapy in a Child," *JAMA*, 1979, 216(9):1479-80.

Sargent E, "Tetracycline for Seal Finger," *JAMA*, 1980, 244(5):437.

Walters BN and Gubbay SS, "Tetracycline and Benign Intracranial Hypertension: Report of Five Cases," *Br Med J (Clin Res)*, 1981, 282(6257):19-20.

Wandstrat TL and Phillips J, "Pseudotumor Cerebri Responsive to Acetazolamide," *Ann Pharmacother*, 1995, 29:318.

Tetracycline Hydrochloride *see* Tetracycline *on page 732*

Tetradecin *see* Tetracycline *on page 732*

Tetrahydroaminoacrine *see* Tacrine Hydrochloride *on page 719*

Tetralan® Oral *see* Tetracycline *on page 732*

Tetralen® *see* Tetracycline *on page 732*

Tetramide® *see* Mianserin Hydrochloride *on page 529*

Tetram® Oral *see* Tetracycline *on page 732*

Tetraverine *see* Tetracycline *on page 732*

T-Gen® *see* Trimethobenzamide Hydrochloride *on page 772*

THA *see* Tacrine Hydrochloride *on page 719*

Thacupzol® *see* Methimazole *on page 512*

Thalidomide

Related Information

Drugs and Chemicals Proven to be Teratogenic in Humans *on page 1572-1575*

CAS Number 50-35-1

Brand Names Contergan®; Distaval®; Kevadon®

Use Investigational: Treatment or prevention of graft-versus-host reactions after bone marrow transplantation; in aphthous ulceration in HIV-positive patients; reactional lepromatous or erythema nodosum leprosy; Langerhans cell histocytosis, Behçet's syndrome; hypnotic agent; also may be effective in rheumatoid arthritis, discoid lupus, and erythema multiforme; useful in type 2 lepra reactions, but not type 1

Mechanism of Action Mode of action for immunosuppression is unclear; inhibition of neutrophil chemotaxis and decreased monocyte phagocytosis may occur; may cause 50% to 80% reduction of tumor necrosis factor - alpha

Adverse Reactions

Cardiovascular: Tachycardia

Central nervous system: Dizziness, headache, irritability, lethargy, fever

Dermatologic: Edema, alopecia, pruritus

Endocrine & metabolic: Amenorrhea, sexual dysfunction

Gastrointestinal: Nausea, vomiting, dry mouth, constipation

Hematologic: Leukopenia

Neuromuscular & skeletal: Sensory neuropathy (peripheral) (after prolonged therapy due to neuronal degeneration), myoclonus

Toxicodynamics/Kinetics

Distribution: V_d: 120 L

Metabolism: Hepatic

Half-life: 8.7 hours

Peak plasma levels: 2-6 hours

Usual Dosage

Leprosy: Up to 400 mg/day; usual maintenance dose: 50-100 mg/day

Behçet's syndrome: 100-400 mg/day

Graft-vs-host reactions:

Children: 3 mg/kg 4 times/day

Adults: 100-1600 mg/day; usual initial dose: 200 mg 4 times/day for use up to 700 days

AIDS-related aphthous stomatitis: 200 mg twice daily for 5 days, then 200 mg/day for up to 8 weeks

Discoid lupus erythematosus: 100-400 mg/day; maintenance dose: 25-50 mg

Contraindications Pregnancy or women in childbearing years, neuropathy (peripheral), thalidomide hypersensitivity

Warnings Liver, hepatic, neurological disorders, constipation, congestive heart failure, hypertension

Reference Range Therapeutic plasma thalidomide levels in graft-vs-host reactions are 5-8 μg/mL, although it has been suggested that lower plasma levels (0.5-1.5 μg/mL) may be therapeutic; peak serum thalidomide level after a 200 mg dose: 1.2 μg/mL

Overdosage Treatment

Decontamination: Lavage/activated charcoal with sorbitol

Supportive therapy: Bisacodyl suppositories can be used for constipation

Pregnancy Risk Factor X

Pregnancy Implications Embryotoxic with limb defects noted from the 27th to 40th gestational day of exposure; fetal cardiac, gastrointestinal, and genitourinary tract abnormalities have also been described

Specific References

Beckman DA and Brent RL, "Mechanism of Known Environmental Teratogens: Drugs and Chemicals," *Clin Perinatol*, 1986, 13(3):649-87.

Gunzler V, "Thalidomide in Human Immunodeficiency Virus (HIV) Patients. A Review of Safety Considerations," *Drug Saf*, 1992, 7(2):116-34.

Schuler U and Ehninger G, "Thalidomide: Rationale for Renewed Use in Immunolgoical Disorders," *Drug Saf*, 1995, 12:364-9.

Thalitone® *see* Chlorthalidone *on page 210*

Theine *see* Caffeine *on page 175*

Theo-24® *see* Theophylline *on this page*

Theobid® *see* Theophylline *on this page*

Theochron® *see* Theophylline *on this page*

Theoclear® L.A. *see* Theophylline *on this page*

Theo-Dur® *see* Theophylline *on this page*

Theolair™ *see* Theophylline *on this page*

Theophylline (thee off' i lin)

Related Information

Therapeutic Drugs Associated With Hallucinations *on page 1558-1559*

CAS Number 58-55-9

Brand Names Accurbron®; Aerolate®; Aerolate III®; Aerolate JR®; Aerolate SR® S; Aquaphyllin®; Asmalix®; Bronkodyl®; Constant-T®; Duraphyl™; Elixicon®; Elixomin®; Elixophyllin®-GG; Elixophyllin®-KI; Elixophyllin® SR; Lanophyllin®; Quibron®-T; Quibron®-T/SR; Respbid®; Slo-bid™; Slo-Phyllin®; Sustaire®; Theo-24®; Theobid®; Theochron®; Theoclear® L.A.; Theo-Dur®; Theolair™; Theospan®-SR; Theovent®; Uniphyl®

Synonyms Theophylline Anhydrous

Use Bronchodilator in reversible airway obstruction due to asthma or COPD as maintenance therapy only; for neonatal apnea/bradycardia

Mechanism of Action Exact mechanism is unknown; probable mechanism involves increasing tissue concentrations of cAMP and/or occupying adenosine receptors as an antagonist and/or inhibition of phosphodiesterases, PDE III, PDE IV

Adverse Reactions Uncommon at serum theophylline concentrations ≤20 μg/mL

Cardiovascular: Palpitations, sinus tachycardia

Central nervous system: Insomnia, irritability, agitation, seizures, nervousness, psychosis, restlessness, visual hallucinations

Dermatologic: Skin rash

Gastrointestinal: Nausea, vomiting, epigastric pain

Neuromuscular & skeletal: Tremors

Miscellaneous: Allergic reactions, bezoars/concretions

Signs & Symptoms of Acute Overdose Nausea, esophageal ulceration, hypophosphatemia, hypomagnesemia, exfoliative dermatitis, leg cramps; paroxysmal tachycardia (ventricular), anorexia, diuresis, hyponatremia, bezoars, hypertension,

(Continued)

Theophylline *(Continued)*

fibrillation (atrial), vomiting, insomnia, irritability, tachycardia, seizures, delirium, hyperglycemia, hypotension, hypokalemia, hypercalcemia, lactic acidosis, feces discoloration (black). Repetitive vomiting is an indication to hold theophylline therapy and rule out toxicity by serum concentrations.

Toxicodynamics/Kinetics

Absorption: Oral: Up to 100% of dose absorbed, depending upon the formulation used

Distribution: V_d: 0.45 L/kg; rapid throughout extracellular fluid and tissues

Protein binding:
- Neonates: 36%
- Adults: 40% to 60%
- Patients with hepatic cirrhosis: 35%

Metabolism: In the liver by demethylation and oxidation

Half-life:
- Infants ≤6 months: >24 hours
- Children >6 months: 3.7±1.1 hours
- Nonsmokers: Adults: 8.7±2.2 hours
- Smokers (1-2 packs/day): 4-5 hours

Time to peak serum concentration:
- Oral: 1 hour
- Uncoated tablets: 2 hours
- Chewable tablets: 1-1.5 hours
- Enteric-coated tablets: 5 hours
- Extended-release capsules and tablets: 4-7 hours, in overdoses up to 27 hours
- Retention enema: 1-2 hours

Elimination: Urine; adults excrete 10% in urine as unchanged drug; neonates excrete a greater percentage of the dose unchanged in urine (up to 50%). See table.

Half-life (h)	Patient Population
7–9	Normal healthy
2–9	Children
15–58	Premature infants
18–24	Severe congestive heart failure
29	Cirrhosis

Usual Dosage Use ideal body weight for obese patients

Neonates:

Apnea of prematurity: Oral, I.V.: Loading dose: 4 mg/kg (theophylline); 5 mg/kg (aminophylline)

There appears to be a delay in theophylline elimination in infants <1 year of age, especially neonates; both the initial dose and maintenance dosage should be conservative

Approximate I.V. Theophylline Dosage for Treatment of Acute Bronchospasm

Group	Dosage for next 12 h*	Dosage after 12 h*
Infants 6 wk to 6 mo	0.5 mg/kg/h	
Children 6 mo to 1 y	0.6–0.7 mg/kg/h	
Children 1–9 y	0.95 mg/kg/h (1.2 mg/kg/h)	0.79 mg/kg/h (1 mg/kg/h)
Children 9–16 y and young adult smokers	0.79 mg/kg/h (1 mg/kg/h)	0.63 mg/kg/h (0.8 mg/kg/h)
Healthy, nonsmoking adults	0.55 mg/kg/h (0.7 mg/kg/h)	0.39 mg/kg/h (0.5 mg/kg/h)
Older patients and patients with cor pulmonale	0.47 mg/kg/h (0.6 mg/kg/h)	0.24 mg/kg/h (0.3 mg/kg/h)
Patients with congestive heart failure or liver failure	0.39 mg/kg/h (0.5 mg/kg/h)	0.08–0.16 mg/kg/h (0.1–0.2 mg/kg/h)

*Equivalent hydrous aminophylline dosage indicated in parentheses.

I.V.: Initial: Maintenance infusion rates:

Neonates:
- ≤24 days: 0.08 mg/kg/hour theophylline
- >24 days: 0.12 mg/kg/hour theophylline

Children >1 year and Adults:

Treatment of acute wheezing: I.V.: Loading dose (in patients not currently receiving aminophylline or theophylline): 6 mg/kg (based on aminophylline) given I.V. over 20-30 minutes; administration rate should not exceed 25 mg/minute (aminophylline). See table.

Approximate I.V. maintenance dosages are based upon **continuous infusions**; bolus dosing (often used in children <6 months of age) may be determined by multiplying the hourly infusion rate by 24 hours and dividing by the desired number of doses/day.

Dosage should be adjusted according to serum level measurements during the first 12- to 24-hour period.

Oral theophylline: Treatment of acute wheezing: Initial dosage recommendation: Loading dose (to achieve a serum level of about 10 μg/mL; loading doses should be given using a rapidly absorbed oral product **not** a sustained release product):

If no theophylline has been administered in the previous 24 hours: 4-6 mg/kg theophylline

If theophylline has been administered in the previous 24 hours, administer ½ the loading dose or 2-3 mg/kg theophylline can be given in emergencies when serum levels are not available.

On the average, for every 1 mg/kg theophylline given, blood levels will rise 2 μg/mL. Ideally, defer the loading dose if a serum theophylline concentration can be obtained rapidly. However, if this is not possible, exercise clinical judgment. If the patient is not experiencing theophylline toxicity, this is unlikely to result in dangerous adverse effects.

These recommendations, based on mean clearance rates for age or risk factors, were calculated to achieve a serum level of 10 μg/mL (5 μg/mL for newborns with apnea/bradycardia). In newborns and infants, a fast-release oral product can be used. The total daily dose can be divided every 12 hours in newborns and every 6-8 hours in infants. In children and healthy adults, a slow-release product can be used. The total daily dose can be divided every 8-12 hours.

Bronchial asthma: Oral theophylline: See table.

Age	Initial 3 Days	Second 3 Days	Steady-State Maintenance
<1 y	0.2 x (age in weeks) + 5		0.3 x (age in weeks) + 8
1-9 y	16 up to a maximum of 400 mg/24 h	20	22
9–12 y	16 up to a maximum of 400 mg/24 h	16 up to a maximum of 600 mg/24 h	20 up to a maximum of 800 mg/24 h
12–16 y	16 up to a maximum of 400 mg/24 h	16 up to a maximum of 600 mg/24 h	18 up to a maximum of 900 mg/24 h
Adults	400 mg/24 h	600 mg/24 h	900 mg/24 h

*Dose in mg/kg/24 hours of theophylline.

Increasing dose: The dosage may be increased in approximately 25% increments at 2- to 3-day intervals so long as the drug is tolerated or until the maximum dose is reached.

Maintenance dose (see table).

These recommendations, based on mean clearance rates for age or risk factors, were calculated to achieve a serum level of 10 μg/mL (5 μg/mL for newborns with apnea/bradycardia). In newborns and infants, a fast-release oral product can be used. The total daily dose can be divided every 12 hours in newborns and every 6-8 hours in infants. In children and healthy adults, a slow-release product can be used. The total daily dose can be divided every 8-12 hours.

Dose should be further adjusted based on serum levels; see table.

Guidelines for drawing theophylline serum levels are shown in the table.

Dosing adjustment/comments in hepatic disease: Higher incidence of toxic effects including seizures in cirrhosis; plasma levels should be monitored closely during long-term administration in cirrhosis and during acute hepatitis, with dose adjustment as necessary.

Rectal: Adults: 500 mg 3 times/day; avoid using suppositories due to erratic, unreliable absorption

Maintenance Dose for Acute Symptoms

Population Group	Oral Theophylline (mg/kg/day)	I.V. Aminophylline
Premature infant or newborn – 6 wk (for apnea/bradycardia)	4	5 mg/kg/day
6 wk – 6 mo	10	12 mg/kg/day or continuous I.V. infusion*
Infants 6 mo–1 y	12–18	15 mg/kg/day or continuous I.V. infusion*
Children 1–9 y	20–24	1 mg/kg/hour
Children 9–12 y, and adolescent daily smokers of cigarettes or marijuana, and otherwise healthy adult smokers younger than 50 y	16	0.9 mg/kg/hour
Adolescents 12–16 y (nonsmokers)	13	0.7 mg/kg/hour
Otherwise healthy nonsmoking adults (including elderly patients)	10 (not to exceed 900 mg/day)	0.5 mg/kg/hour
Cardiac decompensation, cor pulmonale and/or liver dysfunction	5 (not to exceed 400 mg/day)	0.25 mg/kg/hour

*For continuous I.V. infusion divide total daily dose by 24 = mg/kg/hour.

Dosage Adjustment After Serum Theophylline Measurement

Serum Theophylline		Guidelines
Within normal limits	10–20 mcg/mL	Maintain dosage if tolerated. Recheck serum theophylline concentration at 6–12 mo intervals.*
Too high	20–25 mcg/mL	Decrease doses by about 10%. Recheck serum theophylline concentration after 3 d and then at 6–12 mo intervals.*
	25–30 mcg/mL	Skip next dose and decrease subsequent doses by about 25%. Recheck serum theophylline.
	>30 mcg/mL	Skip next 2 doses and decrease subsequent doses by 50%. Recheck serum theophylline.
Too low	7.5–10 mcg/mL	Increase dose by about 25%.† Recheck serum theophylline concentration after 3 d and then at 6–12 mo intervals.*
	5–7.5 mcg/mL	Increase dose by about 25% to the nearest dose increment† and recheck serum theophylline for guidance in further dosage adjustment (another increase will probably be needed, but this provides a safety check).

From Weinberger M and Hendeles L, "Practical Guide to Using Theophylline," *J Resp Dis,* 1981, 2:12-27.

*Finer adjustments in dosage may be needed for some patients.
†Dividing the daily dose into 3 doses administered at 8-hour intervals may be indicated if symptoms occur repeatedly at the end of a dosing interval.

Guidelines for Drawing Theophylline Serum Levels

Dosage Form	Time to Draw Level
I.V. bolus	30 min after end of 30 min infusion
I.V. continuous infusion	12–24 h after initiation of infusion
P.O. liquid, fast-release tab	Peak: 1 h post a dose after at least 1 day of therapy Trough: Just before a dose after at least 1 day of therapy
P.O. slow-release product	Peak: 4 h post a dose after at least 1 day of therapy Trough: Just before a dose after at least 1 day of therapy

Contraindications Uncontrolled tachyarrhythmias, hyperthyroidism; use with caution in active peptic ulcer disease, seizure disorders

Dosage Forms

Capsule:

Immediate release (Bronkodyl®, Elixophyllin®): 100 mg, 200 mg

Timed release:

[8-12 hours] (Aerolate®): 65 mg [III]; 130 mg [JR], 260 mg [SR]
[8-12 hours] (Elixophyllin® SR): 125 mg, 250 mg
[8-12 hours] (Slo-bid™): 50 mg, 75 mg, 100 mg, 125 mg, 200 mg, 300 mg
[8-12 hours] (Slo-Phyllin® Gyrocaps®): 60 mg, 125 mg, 250 mg
[12 hours] (Theobid® Jr. Duracaps®): 130 mg
[12 hours] (Theobid® Duracaps®): 260 mg
[12 hours] (Theoclear® L.A.): 130 mg, 260 mg
[12 hours] (Theo-Dur® Sprinkle®): 50 mg, 75 mg, 125 mg, 200 mg
[12 hours] (Theospan®-SR): 130 mg, 260 mg
[12 hours] (Theovent®): 125 mg, 250 mg
[24 hours] (Theo-24®): 100 mg, 200 mg, 300 mg

Elixir (Asmalix®, Elixomin®, Elixophyllin®, Lanophyllin®): 80 mg/15 mL (15 mL, 30 mL, 480 mL, 4000 mL)

Infusion, in D_5W: 0.4 mg/mL (1000 mL); 0.8 mg/mL (500 mL, 1000 mL); 1.6 mg/mL (250 mL, 500 mL); 2 mg/mL (100 mL); 3.2 mg/mL (250 mL); 4 mg/mL (50 mL, 100 mL)

Solution, oral:

Theolair™: 80 mg/15 mL (15 mL, 18.75 mL, 30 mL, 480 mL)
Aerolate®: 150 mg/15 mL (480 mL)

Syrup:

Aquaphyllin®, Slo-Phyllin®, Theoclear-80®, Theostat-80®: 80 mg/15 mL (15 mL, 30 mL, 500 mL)
Accurbron®: 150 mg/15 mL (480 mL)

Tablet: Immediate release:

Slo-Phyllin®: 100 mg, 200 mg
Theolair™: 125 mg, 250 mg
Quibron®-T: 300 mg

Tablet:

Controlled release (Theox®): 100 mg, 200 mg, 300 mg

Timed release:

[12-24 hours]: 100 mg, 200 mg, 300 mg
[8-12 hours] (Constant-T®): 200 mg, 300 mg
[8-12 hours] (Quibron®-T/SR): 300 mg
[8-12 hours] (Respbid®): 250 mg, 500 mg
[8-12 hours] (Sustaire®): 100 mg, 300 mg
[8-12 hours] (T-Phyl®): 200 mg
[12-24 hours] (Theochron®): 100 mg, 200 mg, 300 mg
[8-24 hours] (Theo-Dur®): 100 mg, 200 mg, 300 mg, 450 mg
[8-24 hours] (Theo-Sav®): 100 mg, 200 mg, 300 mg
[8-24 hours] (Theolair-SR®): 200 mg, 250 mg, 300 mg, 500 mg
[24 hours] (Uniphyl®): 400 mg

Stability Store injection at room temperature, do not refrigerate; protect from heat and from freezing; use only clear solutions; stability of parenteral admixture at room temperature (25°C): 30 days

Reference Range Therapeutic (theophylline):

Neonatal apnea: 6-13 μg/mL
Therapeutic: 10-20 μg/mL
Toxic: 10-15 μg/mL

Timing of serum samples: If toxicity is suspected, draw a level at any time; if lack of therapeutic is effected, draw a trough immediately before the next oral dose

Overdosage Treatment

Decontamination: Do not use ipecac; lavage should be performed if <1 hour after ingestion and >50 mg/kg was ingested; activated charcoal with cathartic; whole bowel irrigation should be considered for significant sustained release preparation ingestion

(Continued)

Theophylline *(Continued)*

Supportive therapy: Metoclopramide, ranitidine, or ondansetron can be used for vomiting; hypotension should be treated with intravenous normal saline hydration. Phenylephrine or levarterenol are preferred vasopressors that can be utilized for hypotension although an intravenous beta-adrenergic blocker (propranolol or esmolol) can be utilized in the patient without a history of bronchospastic disease. Seizures may require diazepam/lorazepam along with phenobarbital; phenytoin contraindicated; adenosine has had inconsistent effects. Lidocaine can be used for ventricular arrhythmias; must monitor for hypoglycemia. Nitrazepam can be given if infantile spasm occur due to theophylline toxicity.

Enhancement of elimination: Multiple doses of activated charcoal can reduce the half-life of aminophylline/theophylline to 2-3 hours; do not use if an ileus is present. Charcoal hemoperfusion can increase the clearance of aminophylline/theophylline by approximately twofold to threefold over that of hemodialysis and is thus the extracorporeal modality of choice. Guidelines for charcoal hemoperfusion include a theophylline level >100 μg/mL in an acute overdose setting (or 50 μg/mL in a chronic setting), or the following signs if the level is >35 μg/mL: ventricular arrhythmias, metabolic acidosis, hypotension, refractory to vasopressors or fluid therapy, seizures, ileus. If a sustained release preparation is ingested or patient with chronic ingestion is >60 years of age, the threshold for using charcoal hemoperfusion should be lower. If the patient is experiencing fluid overload due to congestive heart failure, hemodialysis can be performed to remove both theophylline/aminophylline and fluid.

Test Interactions Caffeine in high concentrations on selected procedures cross reacts as theophylline

Diagnostic Tests/Procedures

Theophylline, Blood *on page 1359*

Drug Interactions Changes in diet may affect the elimination of theophylline; theophylline may decrease the effects of phenytoin, adenosine, benzodiazepines, lithium, and neuromuscular blocking agents. Theophylline increases the excretion of lithium; theophylline may have synergistic toxicity with sympathomimetics, halothane. Cimetidine, allopurinol, propranolol, erythromycin, influenza virus vaccine, oral contraceptives, amiodarone, fluvoxamine, ciprofloxacin, clarithromycin, alcohol, enoxacin, interferon, propafenone, troleandomycin, clindamycin, and lincomycin may increase theophylline concentrations. Cigarette and marijuana smoking, rifampin, phenytoin, carbamazepine, phenobarbital, and aminoglutethimide may decrease theophylline concentrations.

Pregnancy Risk Factor C

Pregnancy Implications Increased incidence of pre-eclampsia noted in patients taking theophylline; crosses placenta and enters breast milk

Patient Information Oral preparations should be taken with a full glass of water; avoid drinking or eating large quantities of caffeine-containing beverages or food; take at regular intervals; take sustained release tablets whole; sustained release capsule forms may be opened and sprinkled on soft foods; do not chew beads

Nursing Implications Do not crush sustained release or enteric coated drug products

Additional Information Elderly, acutely ill, and patients with severe respiratory problems, pulmonary edema, or liver dysfunction are at greater risk of toxicity because of reduced drug clearance; saliva levels are approximately equal to 60% of plasma levels; infantile spasm can occur; charcoal-broiled foods may increase elimination, reducing half-life by 50%; cigarette smoking may require an increase of dosage by 50% to 100%; aminophylline 100 mg is equivalent to theophylline 79 mg

Theophylline immediate release tablet/capsule: Bronkodyl®, Elixophyllin®, Quibron®-T, Slo-Phyllin®, Somophyllin®-T, Theolair™

Theophylline liquid: Accurbron®, Aerolate®, Aquaphyllin®, Asmalix®, Elixicon®, Elixophyllin®, Lixolin®, Theon®

Theophylline timed release capsule: Aerolate III®, Aerolate JR®, Aerolate SR®, Elixophyllin® SR, Lodrane®, Slo-bid™ Gyrocaps®, Slo-Phyllin® Gyrocaps®, Somophyllin®-CRT, Theobid®, Theoclear® L.A., Theophyl-SR®, Theospan®-SR, Theospan®-SR

Theophylline timed release tablet: Constant-T®, Duraphyl™, LaBID®, Quibron®-T/S, Respbid®, Sustaire®, Theochron®, Theo-Dur®, Theolair™-SR, Theo-Time®, Uniphyl®

Specific References

Hendeles L, Jenkins J, and Temple R, "revised FDA Labeling Guidelines for Theophylline Oral Dosage Forms," *Pharmacotherapy*, 1995, 15(4):409-27.

Henderson A, Wright DM, and Pond SM, "Management of Theophylline Overdose Patients in the Intensive Care Unit," *Anaesth Intensive Care*, 1992, 20(1):56-62.

Higgins RM, Hearing S, Goldsmith DJA, et al, "Severe Theophylline Poisoning: Charcoal Haemoperfusion or Haemodialysis?" *Postgrad Med J*, 1995, 71:224-6.

Lin JL and Jeng LB, "Critical, Acutely Poisoned Patients Treated With Continuous Arteriovenous Hemoperfusion in the Emergency Department," *Ann Emerg Med*, 1995, 25(1):75-80.

Matuschka PR and Vissing RS, "Clinafloxacin-Theophylline Drug Interaction," *Ann Pharmacother*, 1995, 29:378-80.

Minton NA and Henry JA, "Prevention of Drug Absorption in Simulated Theophylline Overdose," *J Toxicol Clin Toxicol*, 1995, 33(1):44-9.

Paloucek FP and Rodvold KA, "Evaluation of Theophylline Overdoses and Toxicities," *Ann Emerg Med*, 1988, 17(2):135-44.

Shannon M, "Predictors of Major Toxicity After Theophylline Overdose," *Ann Intern Med*, 1993, 119(12):1161-7.

Shannon M and Maher T, "Anticonvulsant Effects of Intracerebroventricular Adenocard in Theophylline-Induced Seizures," *Ann Emerg Med*, 1995, 26:6508.

Shields MD, Hicks EM, MacGregor DF, et al, "Infantile Spasms Associated With Theophylline Toxicity," *Acta Paediatr*, 1995, 84:215-7.

Stenius-Aarniala B, Riikonen S, and Teramo K, "Slow-Release Theophylline in Pregnant Asthmatics," *Chest*, 1995, 107(3):642-7.

Troger U and Meyer FP, "Influence of Endogenous and Exogenous Effectors on the Pharmacokinetics of Theophylline," *Clin Pharmacokinet*, 1995, 28:287-314.

Van den Brekel AM and Harrington L, "Toxic Effects of Theophylline Caused by Fluvoxamine," *Can Med Assoc J*, 1994, 151(9):1289-90.

Wang RY, "Anticoagulant Effects of Adenosine in Aminophylline-Induced Seizures," *Vet Hum Toxicol*, 1994, 36:351.

Theophylline Anhydrous *see* Theophylline *on page 735*

Theophylline Ethylenediamine *see* Aminophylline *on page 110*

Theospan®-SR *see* Theophylline *on page 735*

Theovent® *see* Theophylline *on page 735*

Therapas® *see* Para-Aminosalicylate Sodium *on page 592*

Therapav® *see* Papaverine *on page 591*

Therapeutic Drugs Associated With Hallucinations *see page 1558*

Therazid® *see* Para-Aminosalicylate Sodium *on page 592*

Thevier® *see* Levothyroxine Sodium *on page 465*

Thiamazole *see* Methimazole *on page 512*

Thiamine Hydrochloride (thye' a min)

CAS Number 59-43-8; 67-03-8

Brand Names Arcalion®; Benerva®; Betabion®; Betalin® S; Betamin®; Beta-Sol®; Betatabs®; Betaxin®; Bewon®; Biamine®; Judolor®; Neovita®; Neurostop®; Vitantial®

Synonyms Aneurine Hydrochloride; Thiaminium Chloride Hydrochloride; Vitamin B_1

Use Treatment of thiamine deficiency including beriberi, Wernicke's encephalopathy syndrome, and peripheral neuritis associated with pellagra, alcoholic patients with altered sensorium; various genetic metabolic disorders; dietary sources include legumes, pork, beef, whole grains, yeast, fresh vegetables; a deficiency state can occur in as little 3 weeks following total dietary absence

Mechanism of Action An essential coenzyme in carbohydrate metabolism by combining with adenosine triphosphate to form thiamine pyrophosphate

Adverse Reactions Hypersensitivity is rare

Cardiovascular: Warmth, tingling, cardiovascular collapse and death (primarily following repeated I.V. administration)

Dermatologic: Rash, pigmented purpura, angioedema, dermatitis

Toxicodynamics/Kinetics

Absorption:

Oral: Poor (5%)

I.M.: Rapid and complete

Elimination: Renally as unchanged drug (80% to 96%), and as pyrimidine after body storage sites become saturated

Usual Dosage Dietary supplement (depends on caloric or carbohydrate content of the diet):

Infants: 0.3-0.5 mg/day

Children: 0.5-1 mg/day

Adults: 1-2 mg/day

Note: The above doses can be found as a combination in multivitamin preparations

Children:

Noncritically ill thiamine deficiency: Oral: 10-50 mg/day in divided doses every day for 2 weeks followed by 5-10 mg/day for one month

Beriberi: I.M.: 10-25 mg/day for 2 weeks, then 5-10 mg orally every day for one month (oral as therapeutic multivitamin)

Adults:

Wernicke's encephalopathy: I.M., I.V.: 50 mg as a single dose, then 50 mg I.M. every day until normal diet resumed

Noncritically ill thiamine deficiency: Oral: 10-50 mg/day in divided doses

Beriberi: I.M., I.V.: 10-30 mg 3 times/day for 2 weeks, then switch to 5-10 mg orally every day for one month (oral as therapeutic multivitamin)

(Continued)

Thiamine Hydrochloride *(Continued)*

Administration Administer by slow I.V. injection

Contraindications Hypersensitivity to thiamine or any component

Warnings Use with caution for parenteral route (especially I.V.) of administration, see Adverse Reactions; large doses should be given in divided doses for better oral absorption; single vitamin B_1 deficiency is rare, check for other deficiencies

Dosage Forms

Injection: 100 mg/mL (1 mL, 2 mL, 10 mL, 30 mL); 200 mg/mL (30 mL)
Tablet: 50 mg, 100 mg, 250 mg, 500 mg
Tablet, enteric coated: 20 mg

Stability Protect oral dosage forms from light; **incompatible** with alkaline or neutral solutions and with oxidizing or reducing agents; exposure to heat may inactivate vitamin; incompatible with neutral or alkaline solutions; not compatible with barbiturates

Reference Range Therapeutic: 1.6-4 mg/dL

Overdosage Treatment

Decontamination: Oral: Emesis or lavage/activated charcoal with cathartic
Supportive therapy: For anaphylaxis, epinephrine, diphenhydramine, glucocorticoids should be given

Test Interactions False-positive for uric acid using the phosphotungstate method and for urobilinogen using the Ehrlich's reagent; large doses may interfere with the spectrophotometric determination of serum theophylline concentration

Drug Interactions Neuromuscular blocking agents; high carbohydrate diets or I.V. dextrose solutions increase thiamine requirement

Pregnancy Risk Factor A (C if dose exceeds RDA recommendation of 1.4-1.5 mg/day)

Patient Information Dietary sources include legumes, pork, beef, whole grains, yeast, fresh vegetables; a deficiency state can occur in as little 3 weeks following total dietary absence

Nursing Implications Parenteral form may be administered by I.M. or slow I.V. injection

Additional Information Found in green vegetables, pork, liver, fish, eggs; requires adequate magnesium for use as a coenzyme

Specific References

Doyon S and Roberts JR, "Reappraisal of the "Coma Cocktail": Dextrose, Flumazenil, Naloxone, and Thiamine," *Emerg Med Clin North Am*, 1994, 12(2):301-16.
Haecke PV, Ramaekers D, Vanderwegen L, et al, "Thiamine-Induced Anaphylactic Shock," *Am J Emerg Med*, 1995, 13:371.
Petrie WM and Ban TA, "Vitamins in Psychiatry. Do They Have a Role?" *Drugs*, 1985, 30(1):58-65.
Reuler JB, Girard DE, and Cooney TG, "Current Concepts: Wernicke's Encephalopathy," *N Engl J Med*, 1985, 312(16):1035-39.
Stephen JM, Grant R, and Veh CS, "Anaphylaxis From Administration of Intravenous Thiamine," *Am J Emerg Med*, 1992, 10(1):61-3.
Wrenn KD, Murphy F, and Slovis CM, "A Toxicity Study of Parenteral Thiamine Hydrochloride," *Ann Emerg Med*, 1989, 18(8):867-70.

Thiaminium Chloride Hydrochloride *see* Thiamine Hydrochloride *on previous page*

Thiamphenicol (thye am fen' i kole)

CAS Number 15318-45-3; 847-25-6; 2393-92-2; 2611-61-2

Brand Names Flogotisol®; Fluimucil®; Urfamycin®

Synonyms Thiophenicol; Vicemycetin

Use Gonorrhea, chancroid, *Gardnerella vaginalis*, vaginitis

Mechanism of Action Reversibly binds to 50S ribosomal subunits of susceptible organisms preventing amino acids from being transferred to growing peptide chains thus inhibiting protein synthesis

Adverse Reactions Dose-dependent reversible myelosuppression is more frequent than with chloramphenicol; not seen after single-dose use

Central nervous system: Headache, drowsiness, dizziness
Dermatologic: Pruritus
Gastrointestinal: Epigastric pain, nausea, vomiting
Neuromuscular & skeletal: Peripheral neuropathy with long-term use
Ocular: Optic neuritis

Toxicodynamics/Kinetics

Absorption:
- Oral: 75% to 91%
- I.M.: 100%

Distribution: V_d: ~0.5 L/kg
Protein binding: 10% to 20%
Half-life: 2.6-7 hours
Elimination: Renal

Usual Dosage

Oral: Single dose of 2.5 g (for uncomplicated gonorrhea) or 500 mg 3 times/day for 6 days

I.M.:

Children: 25-30 mg/kg/day

Adults: 1-3 g/day

I.V.: 750 mg to 1 g 3 times/day

Contraindications Hypersensitivity to thiamphenicol, bone marrow depression, pregnancy

Warnings Use with caution if other myelosuppressive drugs are given; reduce dose if multiple doses are required for renal failure and in elderly

Reference Range Serum levels after an I.V. dose of 10 mg/kg: ~13-14 μg/mL; after an oral dose of 2.5 g, peak serum thiamphenicol levels range from 16-18 μg/mL

Overdosage Treatment

Decontamination: Oral: Emesis or lavage/activated charcoal

Enhancement of elimination: Multiple dosing of activated charcoal may be effective; although there is no human overdose experience, hemodialysis or hemoperfusion may be effective

Pregnancy Implications Crosses the placenta, avoid during pregnancy

Additional Information Less likely than chloramphenicol to cause "gray syndrome" in neonates

Specific References

Fuglesang J and Bergan T, "Chloramphenicol and Thiamphenicol," *Antibiot Chemother*, 1982, 31:1-21.

Plomp TA, Moes RAA, and Thiery M, "Placental Transfer of Thiamphenicol in Term Pregnancy," *Eur J Obstet Gynecol Reprod Biol*, 1977, 7:383-8.

Thiethylperazine Maleate (thye eth il per' a zeen)

CAS Number 1179-69-7

Brand Names Norzine®; Torecan®

Use Relief of nausea and vomiting

Mechanism of Action Blocks postsynaptic mesolimbic dopaminergic receptors in the brain; exhibits a strong alpha-adrenergic blocking effect and depresses the release of hypothalamic and hypophyseal hormones; acts directly on chemoreceptor trigger zone and vomiting center

Adverse Reactions

Cardiovascular: Hypotension, peripheral edema

Central nervous system: Drowsiness, extrapyramidal effects, seizures, fever, headache

Gastrointestinal: Dry mouth, anorexia

Hepatic: Cholestatic jaundice

Ocular: Blurred vision

Respiratory: Dryness of nose

Miscellaneous: Porphyrinogenic

Signs & Symptoms of Acute Overdose Deep sleep, coma, extrapyramidal reaction, abnormal involuntary muscle movements, hypotension or hypertension, systemic lupus erythematosus (SLE), urine discoloration (pink), urine discoloration (red), urine discoloration (red-brown)

Toxicodynamics/Kinetics Following administration antiemetic effects occur within 30 minutes and continue for approximately 4 hours

Absorption: Oral: Well absorbed

Metabolism: Hepatic

Elimination: Renal

Usual Dosage Children >12 years and Adults:

Oral, I.M., rectal: 10 mg 1-3 times/day as needed

I.V. and S.C. routes of administration are not recommended

Dosing comments in hepatic impairment: Use with caution

Contraindications Comatose states, hypersensitivity to thiethylperazine or any component; pregnancy

Warnings Reduce or discontinue if extrapyramidal effects occur; safety and efficacy in children <12 years of age have not been established; hypotension (orthostatic) may occur after I.M. injection; the injectable form contains sulfite which may cause allergic reactions in some patients

Dosage Forms

Injection: 5 mg/mL (2 mL)

Suppository, rectal: 10 mg

Tablet: 10 mg

Overdosage Treatment

Decontamination: Lavage/activated charcoal; charcoal may need to be given in multiple doses for adequate decontamination

Supportive therapy: Initiate support with fluids, norepinephrine may be useful for hypotension; hypoperfusion states may respond to inotropic support with do-

(Continued)

Thiethylperazine Maleate *(Continued)*

butamine. Bradyarrhythmia or ventricular dysrhythmia may respond to sodium bicarbonate or phenytoin; must avoid class 1A and 1C antiarrhythmics. Torsade de pointes may respond to magnesium; seizures should be managed with benzodiazepines or barbiturates; extrapyramidal reactions should be managed with diphenhydramine or benztropine.

Enhancement of elimination: Multiple dosing of charcoal may not be effective

Drug Interactions CNS depressants

Pregnancy Risk Factor X

Patient Information May cause drowsiness, impair judgment and coordination; may cause photosensitivity; avoid excessive sunlight; notify physician of involuntary movements or feelings of restlessness

Nursing Implications Inject I.M. deeply into large muscle mass, patient should be lying down and remain so for at least 1 hour after administration; help with ambulation

Specific References

Khanderia U, "Recurrent Dystonic Reactions Induced by Thiethylperazine," *Drug Intell Clin Pharm*, 1985, 19(7-8):550-1.

Sulkava R, "Thiethylperazine and Tardive Dyskinesia," *Acta Neurol Scand*, 1984, 70(5):364-72.

Thimerosal (thye mer' oh sal)

CAS Number 54-64-8

Brand Names Aeroaid® [OTC]; Mersol® [OTC]

Use Organomercurial antiseptic with sustained bacteriostatic and fungistatic activity; 47% mercury by weight

Mechanism of Action Weakly bacteriostatic

Signs & Symptoms of Acute Overdose Elemental mercury is poorly absorbed orally with minimal adverse effects; inhalation acutely can cause chemical pneumonitis, noncardiogenic pulmonary edema, and gingivostomatitis; chronic exposure to mercury vapor will cause tremor, fatigue, insomnia, loss of memory, and acrodynia

Inorganic mercury: After oral administration, will develop abdominal pain, gastrointestinal irritation, gastrointestinal bleeding, shock, renal failure, and ATN; possible CNS toxicity

Organic mercury: Cause CNS toxicity including ataxia, dysarthria, paresthesias, hearing and visual loss, and gastrointestinal distress

Usual Dosage Apply 1-3 times/day

Contraindications Hypersensitivity to thimerosal

Warnings Prolonged administration can result in mercury toxicity; contains 49% mercury

Dosage Forms

Ointment, ophthalmic: 0.02% [0.2 mg/mL] (3.5 g)

Solution, topical: 0.1% [1 mg/mL = 1:1000] (120 mL, 480 mL, 4000 mL)

Spray, antiseptic: 0.1% [1 mg/mL = 1:1000] with alcohol 2% (90 mL)

Tincture: 0.1% [1 mg/mL = 1:1000] with alcohol 50% (120 mL, 480 mL, 4000 mL)

Overdosage Treatment

Decontamination: Lavage if ingested within 1 hour; charcoal has been shown to decrease inorganic mercury absorption in rats and should be used; milk or egg white may also be useful to bind mercury; whole bowel irrigation with GoLYTELY® may be beneficial if abdominal x-ray shows evidence of mercury; do not induce emesis for inorganic mercury ingestions as this agent has corrosive properties. Patients with inhalation exposures should be monitored for pulmonary edema and pneumonitis; give oxygen if necessary. Skin decontamination with soap and water

Supportive therapy:

Elemental mercury: Oral DMSA (succimer) 10 mg/kg every 8 hours for 5 days then 10 mg/kg every 12 hours for 2 or more weeks will enhance urinary mercury excretion

Inorganic mercury: BAL 5 mg/kg deep I.M. initially, then 2.5 mg/kg every 12 hours for 10 days; if given within the first 2 hours BAL may prevent renal toxicity; **do not given BAL I.V.**

Organic mercury: Oral DMSA (succimer) with dosing as above

BAL is not recommended for elemental and organic mercury poisoning since BAL may cause redistribution of mercury to the brain which is the primary target organ in these poisonings

Enhancement of elimination: Generally ineffective; BAL - mercury complex is dialyzable and is useful in patients with renal failure; it does not enhance elimination in those with good renal function

Specific References

Rohyans J, Walson PD, Wood GA, et al, "Mercury Toxicity Following Merthiolate® Ear Irrigations," *J Pediatr*, 1984, 104(2):311-73.

Thiophenicol *see* Thiamphenicol *on page 742*

Thioridazine Hydrochloride (thye oh rid' a zeen)

Related Information

Antipsychotic Agents Comparison *on page 1642*

CAS Number 50-52-2; 13-61-0

Brand Names Mallorol®; Meleretten®; Mellaril®; Mellaril-S®; Novoridazine®; Ridazine®

Use Management of manifestations of psychotic disorders; depressive neurosis; alcohol withdrawal; dementia in elderly; behavioral problems in children

Mechanism of Action Blocks postsynaptic mesolimbic dopaminergic receptors in the brain; exhibits a strong alpha-adrenergic blocking effect and depresses the release of hypothalamic and hypophyseal hormones

Adverse Reactions Anticholinergic toxidrome

Cardiovascular: Hypotension (especially with I.V. use), hypotension (orthostatic), edema, tachycardia, cardiac arrhythmias, QRS prolongation, T-wave abnormality, ectopy, torsade de pointes, prolonged Q-T interval

Central nervous system: Sedation, drowsiness, restlessness, Parkinson's, anxiety, extrapyramidal reactions, pseudoparkinsonian signs and symptoms, tardive dyskinesia, neuroleptic malignant syndrome, seizures, altered central temperature regulation

Dermatologic: Hyperpigmentation, pruritus, rash, photosensitivity

Endocrine & metabolic: Amenorrhea, galactorrhea, gynecomastia, syndrome of inappropriate antidiuretic hormone, weight gain

Gastrointestinal: gastrointestinal upset, dry mouth, constipation, abdominal distention

Genitourinary: Urinary retention, impotence

Hematologic: Agranulocytosis, leukopenia (usually in patients with large doses for prolonged periods), thrombocytopenia, hemolysis, eosinophilia, epistaxis, neutropenia, granulocytopenia

Hepatic: Cholestatic jaundice

Neuromuscular & skeletal: Myoclonus

Ocular: Retinal pigmentation, blurred vision, mydriasis

Miscellaneous: Anaphylactoid reactions

Signs & Symptoms of Acute Overdose Deep sleep, coma, impotence, tachycardia (ventricular), Q-T prolongation, hypertonia, hyponatremia, neuroleptic malignant syndrome, hepatic failure, hyperprolactinemia, ejaculatory disturbances, galactorrhea, gynecomastia, extrapyramidal reaction, dysphagia, abnormal involuntary muscle movements, Stevens-Johnson syndrome, hypotension or hypertension, nystagmus, hypothermia or hyperthermia, hirsutism, tachycardia (ventricular), hyperreflexia, myoclonus, QRS prolongation, first degree A-V block, vision color changes (brown tinge); priapism, systemic lupus erythematosus (SLE), urine discoloration (pink), urine discoloration (red), urine discoloration (red-brown)

Toxicodynamics/Kinetics

Onset of action: 30 minutes to 1 hour

Duration: 4-6 hours

Absorption: Absorbed well from gastrointestinal tract

Distribution: V_d: 18 L/kg

Protein binding: ≥90%

Metabolism: Hepatic; metabolized in liver

Half-life: 26-36 hours

Time to peak serum concentration: Within 1 hour

Elimination: Kidneys (up to 17%)

Usual Dosage Oral:

Children >2 years: Range: 0.5-3 mg/kg/day in 2-3 divided doses; usual: 1 mg/kg/day; maximum: 3 mg/kg/day

Behavior problems: Initial: 10 mg 2-3 times/day, increase gradually

Severe psychoses: Initial: 25 mg 2-3 times/day, increase gradually

Adults:

Psychoses: Initial: 50-100 mg 3 times/day with gradual increments as needed and tolerated; maximum: 800 mg/day in 2-4 divided doses; if >65 years, initial dose: 10 mg 3 times/day

Depressive disorders, dementia: Initial: 25 mg 3 times/day; maintenance dose: 20-200 mg/day

Contraindications Severe CNS depression, hypersensitivity to thioridazine or any component; cross-sensitivity to other phenothiazines may exist; avoid use in patients with narrow-angle glaucoma, blood dyscrasias, severe liver or cardiac disease; may enhance thyrotoxicosis

Warnings Use with caution in patients with severe cardiovascular disorder or seizures

Dosage Forms

Concentrate, oral: 30 mg/mL (120 mL); 100 mg/mL (3.4 mL, 120 mL)

Suspension, oral: 25 mg/5 mL (480 mL); 100 mg/5 mL (480 mL)

Tablet: 10 mg, 15 mg, 25 mg, 50 mg, 100 mg, 150 mg, 200 mg

(Continued)

Thioridazine Hydrochloride *(Continued)*

Stability Protect all dosage forms from light

Reference Range

Therapeutic: 1.0-1.5 μg/mL (SI: 2.7-4.1 μmol/L)

Toxic: >10.0 μg/mL (SI: >27.0 μmol/L); no relationship between serum levels and cardiac toxicity

Overdosage Treatment

Decontamination: Lavage/activated charcoal with cathartic

Supportive therapy: Following initiation of essential overdose management, toxic symptom treatment and supportive treatment should be initiated. Hypotension usually responds to I.V. fluids or Trendelenburg positioning. If unresponsive to these measures, the use of a parenteral inotrope may be required (eg, norepinephrine 0.1-0.2 mcg/kg/minute titrated to response). Seizures commonly respond to lorazepam or diazepam (I.V. 5-10 mg bolus in adults every 15 minutes if needed up to a total of 30 mg); I.V. 0.25-0.4 mg/kg/dose up to a total of 10 mg in children) or to phenytoin or phenobarbital. Also critical cardiac arrhythmias often respond to I.V. phenytoin (15 mg/kg up to 1 g), while other antiarrhythmics can be used. Neuroleptics often cause extrapyramidal reaction (eg, dystonic reactions) requiring management with diphenhydramine 1-2 mg/kg (adults) up to a maximum of 50 mg I.M. or I.V. slow push followed by a maintenance dose for 48-72 hours. When these reactions are unresponsive to diphenhydramine, benztropine mesylate I.V. 1-2 mg (adults) may be effective. These agents are generally effective within 2-5 minutes. Physostigmine can reverse central and peripheral life-threatening anticholinergic toxicity; do not use physostigmine if cardiac conduction abnormalities are present; sodium bicarbonate (1-3 mEq/kg I.V. can be used for cardiac conduction abnormalities.

Enhancement of elimination: Multiple dosing of activated charcoal may not be effective; forced diuresis is not effective; not dialyzable (0% to 5%)

Antidote(s)

Physostigmine *on page 1457*

Test Interactions False-positives for phenylketonuria, urinary amylase, uroporphyrins, urobilinogen; lowers testosterone levels and serum luteinizing hormone concentrations; may interfere with serum tricyclic levels

Diagnostic Tests/Procedures

Thioridazine, Quantitative *on page 1360*

Drug Interactions Additive effects with other CNS depressants; concurrent use with lithium has rarely caused acute encephalopathy-like syndrome; increased cardiac arrhythmias with tricyclic antidepressants; epinephrine may cause hypotension; beta-blockers may cause increased plasma levels of thioridazine

Pregnancy Risk Factor C

Pregnancy Implications Crosses the placenta; appears in breast milk

Monitoring Parameters For patients on prolonged therapy: CBC, ophthalmologic exam, blood pressure, liver function tests; cardiac monitoring for 48 hours in overdose setting

Patient Information Oral concentrate must be diluted in 2-4 oz of liquid (water, fruit juice, carbonated drinks, milk, or pudding); do not take antacid within 1 hour of taking drug; avoid alcohol; avoid excess sun exposure

Nursing Implications Dilute the oral concentrate with water or juice before administration; avoid skin contact with oral suspension or solution; may cause contact dermatitis

Additional Information Oral formulations may cause stomach upset; may cause thermoregulatory changes; extrapyramidal reactions are lower with thioridazine than with other phenothiazines due to high antimuscarinic potency

Thioridazine: Mellaril-S® oral suspension

Thioridazine hydrochloride: Mellaril® oral solution and tablet

Specific References

Appell RA, Shield DE, and McGuire EJ, "Thioridazine-Induced Priapism," *Br J Urol*, 1977, 49(2):160.

Baker PB, Merigian KS, Roberts JR, et al, "Hyperthermia, Hypertension, Hypertonia, and Coma in Massive Thioridazine Overdose," *Am J Emerg Med*, 1988, 6(4):346-9.

Buckley NA, Whyte IM, and Dawson AH, "Cardiotoxicity More Common in Thioridazine Overdose Than With Other Neuroleptics," *Clin Toxicol*, 1995, 33(3):199-204.

Burgess KR, Jefferis RW, and Stevenson IF, "Fatal Thioridazine Cardiotoxicity," *Med J Aust*, 1979, 2(4):177-8.

Cowen TD and Meythaler JM, "Hypotensive Effects of Thioridazine in an Elderly Patient With Traumatic Brain Injury," *Brain Inj*, 1994, 8(8):735-7.

Goss JB, "Concomitant Use of Thioridazine With Risperidone," *Am J Health-Syst Pharm*, 1995, 52:1012.

Oshika T, "Ocular Adverse Effects of Neuropsychiatric Agents: Incidence and Management," *Drug Saf*, 1995, 12:256-63.

Weisdorf D, Kramer J, Goldbarg A, et al, "Physostigmine for Cardiac and Neurologic Manifestations of Phenothiazine Poisoning," *Clin Pharmacol Ther*, 1978, 24(6):663-7.

Thiothixene (thye oh thix' een)

Related Information

Antipsychotic Agents Comparison *on page 1642*

CAS Number 5591-45-7; 58513-59-0; 49746-04-5; 22189-31-7; 49746-09-0

Brand Names Navane®; Orbinamon®

Synonyms Tiotixene

Use Management of psychotic disorders

Mechanism of Action Elicits antipsychotic activity by postsynaptic blockade of CNS dopamine receptors resulting in inhibition of dopamine-mediated effects; also has alpha-adrenergic blocking activity

Adverse Reactions

Cardiovascular: Hypotension (especially with I.V. use), hypotension (orthostatic), tachycardia, cardiac arrhythmias

Central nervous system: Sedation, drowsiness, restlessness, anxiety, extrapyramidal reactions, pseudoparkinsonian signs and symptoms, tardive dyskinesia, neuroleptic malignant syndrome, seizures, altered central temperature regulation, electroencephalogram abnormalities

Dermatologic: Hyperpigmentation, pruritus, rash, photosensitivity

Endocrine & metabolic: Amenorrhea, galactorrhea, gynecomastia, syndrome of inappropriate antidiuretic hormone, may cause hyponatremia due to inappropriate secretion of antidiuretic hormone, weight gain

Gastrointestinal: gastrointestinal upset, dry mouth, constipation

Genitourinary: Urinary retention, impotence

Hematologic: Agranulocytosis, leukopenia (usually in patients with large doses for prolonged periods), thrombocytopenia, hemolysis, eosinophilia

Hepatic: Cholestatic jaundice

Ocular: Retinal pigmentation, blurred vision

Miscellaneous: Anaphylactoid reactions

Signs & Symptoms of Acute Overdose Muscle myoclonus, priapism, eosinophilia, impotence, hyponatremia, gynecomastia, neuroleptic malignant syndrome, ejaculatory disturbances, extrapyramidal reaction, leukocytosis, drowsiness, galactorrhea, blood dyscrasias, Parkinson's-like symptoms, systemic lupus erythematosus (SLE), dizziness, rigidity, tremors, hypotension, urine discoloration (pink), urine discoloration (red), urine discoloration (red-brown), leukopenia; neutropenia; agranulocytosis; granulocytopenia

Toxicodynamics/Kinetics

Onset of action: I.M.: 10-30 minutes

Duration: Up to 12 hours

Absorption: Rapid

Distribution: Widely distributed into body

Protein binding: 91% to 99%

Metabolism: Extensive liver metabolism

Half-life: >24 hours with chronic use

Time to peak serum concentration: 1-3 hours

Elimination: Bile and feces

Usual Dosage

Children <12 years: Oral: 0.25 mg/kg/24 hours in divided doses (dose not well established)

Children >12 years and Adults: Mild to moderate psychosis:

- Oral: 2 mg 3 times/day, up to 20-30 mg/day; more severe psychosis: Initial: 5 mg 2 times/day, may increase gradually, if necessary; maximum: 60 mg/day
- I.M.: 4 mg 2-4 times/day, increase dose gradually; usual: 16-20 mg/day; maximum: 30 mg/day; change to oral dose as soon as able

Contraindications Hypersensitivity to thiothixene or any component; cross-sensitivity with other phenothiazines may exist; avoid use in patients with narrow-angle glaucoma, bone marrow depression, severe liver or cardiac disease

Warnings Watch for hypotension when administering I.M. or I.V.; safety in children <6 months of age has not been established; use with caution in patients with narrow-angle glaucoma, bone marrow depression, severe liver or cardiac disease, seizures

Dosage Forms

Capsule: 1 mg, 2 mg, 5 mg, 10 mg, 20 mg

Concentrate, oral, as hydrochloride: 5 mg/mL (30 mL, 120 mL)

Injection, as hydrochloride: 2 mg/mL (2 mL)

Powder for injection, as hydrochloride: 5 mg/mL (2 mL)

Stability Refrigerate

Reference Range At 2.5 hours after dosing of 15-60 mg/day, serum levels ranged from 10.0-22.5 ng/mL; therapeutic: 10-40 ng/mL

Overdosage Treatment

Decontamination: Lavage/activated charcoal with cathartic

Supportive therapy: Following initiation of essential overdose management, toxic symptom treatment and supportive treatment should be initiated. Hypotension

(Continued)

Thiothixene *(Continued)*

usually responds to I.V. fluids or Trendelenburg positioning. If unresponsive to these measures, the use of a parenteral inotrope may be required (eg, norepinephrine 0.1-0.2 mcg/kg/minute titrated to response). Seizures commonly respond to lorazepam or diazepam (I.V. 5-10 mg bolus in adults every 15 minutes if needed up to a total of 30 mg; I.V. 0.25-0.4 mg/kg/dose up to a total of 10 mg in children) or to phenytoin or phenobarbital. Also critical cardiac arrhythmias often respond to I.V. phenytoin (15 mg/kg up to 1 g), while other antiarrhythmics can be used. Neuroleptics often cause extrapyramidal reaction (eg, dystonic reactions) requiring management with diphenhydramine 1-2 mg/kg (adults) up to a maximum of 50 mg I.M. or I.V. slow push followed by a maintenance dose for 48-72 hours. When these reactions are unresponsive to diphenhydramine, benztropine mesylate I.V. 1-2 mg (adults) may be effective. These agents are generally effective within 2-5 minutes. Sodium bicarbonate (1-3 mEq/kg) can be used for cardiac conduction for abnormalities.

Enhancement of elimination: Multiple dosing of activated charcoal may not be effective; forced diuresis is not effective; not dialyzable (0% to 5%)

Test Interactions Increases cholesterol (S), glucose; decreases uric acid (S)

Diagnostic Tests/Procedures

Thiothixene, Blood *on page 1361*

Drug Interactions May potentiate the action of other CNS depressants, anticholinergics, or hypotensive agents; ethanol has an additive effect

Pregnancy Risk Factor C

Pregnancy Implications Crosses placenta

Monitoring Parameters Liver function tests; for patients on prolonged therapy: CBC, ophthalmologic exam

Patient Information May cause drowsiness; avoid alcoholic beverages

Nursing Implications Store injection in refrigerator; injection for I.M. use only

Specific References

Schneider SM, "Neuroleptic Malignant Syndrome: Controversies in Treatment," *Am J Emerg Med*, 1991, 9(4):360-2.

Thorazine® *see* Chlorpromazine Hydrochloride *on page 205*

Thrombran® *see* Trazodone Hydrochloride *on page 765*

Thyranon® *see* Thyroid *on next page*

Thyrar® *see* Thyroid *on next page*

Thyrax® *see* Levothyroxine Sodium *on page 465*

Thyreoid-Dispert® *see* Thyroid *on next page*

Thyreustat II® *see* Propylthiouracil *on page 660*

Thyroglobulin (thye roe glob' yoo lin)

CAS Number 9010-34-8

Brand Names Proloid®; Proloide®

Use Replacement or supplemental therapy in hypothyroidism

Mechanism of Action The primary active compound is T_3 (tri-iodothyronine), which may be converted from T_4 (thyroxine) and then circulates throughout the body to influence growth and maturation of various tissues; obtained through fractionation of hog (*Sus scrofa*) thyroid gland

Adverse Reactions

Cardiovascular: Tachycardia, palpitations, angina, hypertension
Central nervous system: Nervousness, insomnia
Endocrine & metabolic: Menstrual irregularities
Gastrointestinal: Diarrhea, vomiting, weight loss
Neuromuscular & skeletal: Tremors
Miscellaneous: Heat intolerance, sweating

Signs & Symptoms of Acute Overdose Weight loss, congestive heart failure, coma, nervousness, sweating, mydriasis, mild hypertension, pseudotumor cerebri, delayed tachycardia, insomnia, heat intolerance, menstrual irregularities, angina, nausea, vomiting, CHF, fever (within 12-24 hours), flushing

Toxicodynamics/Kinetics Absorption: Oral: Absorbed well from gastrointestinal tract

Usual Dosage

Children: See table on next page.

Adults: Oral: 30-180 mg/day; see table for approximate clinical equivalents which should be used in guiding dosage adjustment

Contraindications Acute myocardial infarction or thyrotoxicosis, hypersensitivity to thyroglobulin or any component

Warnings Ineffective for weight reduction; high doses may produce serious or even life-threatening toxic effects particularly when used with some anorectic drugs;

use with caution in patients with cardiovascular or coronary artery disease, diabetes, adrenal cortical insufficiency, myxedema; long-term therapy may cause decreased bone density

Recommended Pediatric Dosage for Congenital Hypothyroidism

Age	Daily Dose (mg)	Daily Dose/kg (mg)
0–6 mo	15–30	4.8–6
6–12 mo	30–45	3.6–4.8
1–5 y	45–60	3–3.6
6–12 y	60–90	2.4–3
>12 y	>90	1.2–1.8

Dosage Forms Tablet: 30 mg, 60 mg, 90 mg, 120 mg, 180 mg

Reference Range Therapeutic: ~1 up to 20 ng/mL; mean values 5.1-9.5 ng/mL; detectable in most healthy adults; slightly increased in the last trimester of gestation and in neonates

Overdosage Treatment

Decontamination: Ipecac or lavage/activated charcoal with cathartic

Supportive therapy: Propranolol may be used for hyperadrenergic signs (1 mg I.V. in adults, 0.01-0.1 mg/kg in pediatrics); sodium ipodate (3 g/1.7 m^2) has been used in acute ingestion to prevent T_4 to T_3 conversion

Enhancement of elimination: Plasmapheresis increases elimination 30-fold while charcoal hemoperfusion enhances T_4 elimination fivefold; multiple dosing of charcoal may be of benefit

Test Interactions ↑ calcium (S)

Drug Interactions Thyroglobulin may potentiate the hypoprothrombinemic effects of oral anticoagulants, the therapeutic need for oral hypoglycemics or insulin; cholestyramine can bind thyroglobulin and reduce its absorption

Pregnancy Risk Factor A

Monitoring Parameters Pulse rate and blood pressure

Patient Information Do not change brands, dose, or discontinue without physician's knowledge; report immediately to physician any chest pain, increased pulse palpitations, heat intolerances, excessive sweating; take as a single daily dose

Additional Information Contains levothyroxine and liothyronine in 2.5:1 ratio

Specific References

Lehrner LM and Weir MR, "Acute Ingestions of Thyroid Hormones," *Pediatrics*, 1984, 73(3):313-7.

Thyroid (thye' roid)

Brand Names Armour® Thyroid; Cinetic; S-P-T®; Thyranon®; Thyrar®; Thyreoid-Dispert®; Westhroid®

Synonyms Desiccated Thyroid; Dry Thyroid; Thyroid Extract

Use Replacement or supplemental therapy in hypothyroidism; pituitary TSH suppressants (thyroid nodules, thyroiditis, multinodular goiter, thyroid cancer), thyrotoxicosis, diagnostic suppression tests

Mechanism of Action The primary active compound is T_3 (tri-iodothyronine), which may be converted from T_4 (thyroxine) and then circulates throughout the body to influence growth and maturation of various tissues; exact mechanism of action is unknown; however, it is believed the thyroid hormone exerts its many metabolic effects through control of DNA transcription and protein synthesis; involved in normal metabolism, growth, and development; promotes gluconeogenesis, increases utilization and mobilization of glycogen stores and stimulates protein synthesis, increases basal metabolic rate

Adverse Reactions

Cardiovascular: Palpitations, tachycardia, cardiac arrhythmias

Central nervous system: Nervousness, insomnia, fever, headache

Dermatologic: Hair loss

Gastrointestinal: Weight loss, appetite (increased), diarrhea, abdominal cramps

Neuromuscular & skeletal: Tremors

Miscellaneous: Sweating

Signs & Symptoms of Acute Overdose Weight loss, nervousness, hyperthermia, sweating, mydriasis, mild hypertension, delayed tachycardia, insomnia, heat intolerance, menstrual irregularities, angina, nausea, vomiting, CHF, fever (within 12-24 hours), flushing

(Continued)

Thyroid *(Continued)*

Toxicodynamics/Kinetics

Absorption: T_4 is 48% to 79% absorbed; T_3 is 95% absorbed; desiccated thyroid contains thyroxine, liothyronine, and iodine (primarily bound); following absorption thyroxine is largely converted to liothyronine

Protein binding: 99% (bound to albumin, thyroxine-binding globulin, and thyroxin-binding prealbumin); desiccated thyroid contains thyroxine, liothyronine, and iodine (primarily bound)

Metabolism: Largely converted to liothyronine; liothyronine is metabolized in the liver to inactive compounds

Half-life:

Liothyronine: 1-2 days

Thyroxine: 6-7 days

Elimination: Excreted in urine as conjugated forms

Usual Dosage Oral:

Children: See table.

Recommended Pediatric Dosage for Congenital Hypothyroidism

Age	Daily Dose (mg)	Daily Dose/kg (mg)
0–6 mo	15–30	4.8–6
6–12 mo	30–45	3.6–4.8
1–5 y	45–60	3–3.6
6–12 y	60–90	2.4–3
>12 y	>90	1.2–1.8

Adults: Start at 15 mg/day and titrate by 15 mg/day in increments of 2- to 4-week intervals; usual maintenance dose: 60-120 mg/day

Contraindications Recent myocardial infarction or thyrotoxicosis uncomplicated by hypothyroidism uncorrected adrenal cortical insufficiency, hypersensitivity to beef or pork or any constituent

Warnings Ineffective for weight reduction; high doses may produce serious or even life-threatening toxic effects particularly when used with some anorectic drugs; use with caution in patients with cardiovascular or coronary artery disease, diabetes, adrenal cortical insufficiency, myxedema; long-term therapy may cause decreased bone density. Diabetes mellitus and insipidus may have symptoms exaggerated or aggravated. Chronic hypothyroidism predisposes patients to coronary artery disease. Desiccated thyroid contains variable amounts of T_3, T_4, and other tri-iodothyronine compounds which are more likely to cause cardiac signs and symptoms due to fluctuating levels; should avoid use in elderly for this reason; drug of choice is levothyroxine in the minds of many clinicians.

Dosage Forms

Capsule; 60 mg, 120 mg, 180 mg, 300 mg

Tablet: 15 mg, 30 mg, 60 mg, 90 mg, 120 mg, 180 mg, 240 mg, 300 mg

Reference Range See table.

Laboratory Teon

	Normal Values
Total T_4	5–11 mcg/dL
Serum T_3	85–185 ng/dL
T_3 resin uptake (RT_3U)	25%–35%
Free thyroxine index (FT_4I)	1.3–4.2
TSH	0.4–4.8 μU/mL

Overdosage Treatment

Decontamination: Gastric emptying indicated for ingestions >5 mg; ipecac or lavage with activated charcoal with cathartic

Supportive therapy: Propranolol may be used for hyperadrenergic signs (1 mg I.V. in adults, 0.01-0.1 mg/kg in pediatrics); sodium ipodate (3 g/1.7 m^2) has been used in acute ingestion to prevent T_4 to T_3 conversion

Enhancement of elimination: Plasmapheresis increases elimination 30-fold while charcoal hemoperfusion enhances T_4 elimination fivefold

Test Interactions Many drugs may have effects on thyroid function tests; para-aminosalicylic acid, aminoglutethimide, amiodarone, barbiturates, carbamazepine, chloral hydrate, clofibrate, colestipol, corticosteroids, danazol, diazepam, estrogens, ethionamide, fluorouracil, I.V. heparin, insulin, lithium, methadone, methimazole, mitotane, nitroprusside, oxyphenbutazone, phenylbutazone, PTU, perphenazine, phenytoin, propranolol, salicylates, sulfonylureas, and thiazides

Diagnostic Tests/Procedures

Thyroxine, Blood *on page 1361*

Drug Interactions

Increased effect: The therapeutic need for oral hypoglycemics or insulin; cholestyramine can bind thyroid and reduce its absorption

Increased toxicity: Thyroid may potentiate the hypoprothrombinemic effect of oral anticoagulants

Pregnancy Risk Factor A

Monitoring Parameters T_3, T_4, TSH, heart rate, blood pressure, clinical signs of hypo- and hyperthyroidism; in cases where T_4 remains low and TSH is within normal limits, an evaluation of "free" (unbound) T_4 is needed to evaluate further increase in dosage. Check levels of T_3 and T_4 after ingestion, and then every 3 days. Thyroid replacement requires periodic assessment of thyroid status; TSH is the most reliable guide for evaluating adequacy of thyroid replacement dosage. TSH may be elevated during the first few months of thyroid replacement despite patients being clinically euthyroid.

Patient Information Do not change brands, dose, or discontinue without physician's knowledge; report immediately to physician any chest pain, increased pulse, palpitations, heat intolerances, excessive sweating; take as a single daily dose

Nursing Implications Monitor pulse rate and blood pressure

Specific References

Bhasin S, Wallace W, Lawrence JB, et al, "Sudden Death Associated With Thyroid Hormone Abuse," *Am J Med*, 1981, 71(5):887-90.

Tunget CL, Clark RF, Turchen SG, et al, "Raising the Decontamination Level for Thyroid Hormone Ingestions," *Am J Emerg Med*, 1995, 13(1):9-13.

Tiagabine Hydrochloride

Use Investigational: Antiepileptic primarily used as an adjunct in resistant epilepsy (complex partial, simple partial, secondary generalized seizures)

Mechanism of Action Prolongs action of GABA by inhibiting its reuptake into presynaptic neurons

Adverse Reactions All adverse effects are dose related

Central nervous system: Dizziness, headache, somnolence, depression, asthenia

Neuromuscular & skeletal: Ataxia, tremors

Toxicodynamics/Kinetics

Absorption: Rapid (within 1 hour); food prolongs absorption

Protein binding: 96%

Half-life: 6.7 hours

Usual Dosage Therapeutic: 32-64 mg/day

Reference Range Maximal plasma level after a 24 mg/dose: 552 ng/mL

Overdosage Treatment

Decontamination: Lavage/activated charcoal

Enhancement of elimination: Due to this drug undergoing enterohepatic recirculation, multiple dosing of activated charcoal may be effective

Drug Interactions Carbamazepine, phenytoin, primidone, vigabatrin; can induce the metabolism of tiagabine

Specific References

Patsalos PN and Sander JW, "Newer Antiepileptic Drugs: Towards an Improved Risk-Benefit Ratio," *Drug Saf*, 1994, 11(1):37-67.

Tilidine Hydrochloride (til' i deen)

Related Information

Pharmacokinetics of Narcotic Agonist Analgesics *on page 1654*

CAS Number 20380-58-9; 2107-79-5; 24357-97-9

Brand Names Tilitrate®; Valoron®

Synonyms Tilidate; Tilidin

Use Treat moderate to severe pain

Mechanism of Action Binds to opiate receptors in the CNS, causing inhibition of ascending pain pathways, altering the perception of and response to pain; produces generalized CNS depression; a cogenor of atropine

Adverse Reactions

Central nervous system: Hallucinations, dizziness, confusion
Dermatologic: Pruritus
Gastrointestinal: Nausea, vomiting
Neuromuscular & skeletal: Tremors, hyperreflexia, hyperactive deep tendon reflexes
Ocular: Miosis
Respiratory: Apnea, respiratory depression
Miscellaneous: Porphyrinogenic, salivation, clonus

Toxicodynamics/Kinetics

Onset of action: Oral: 15-30 minutes
Duration of action: 4-6 hours
Distribution: V_d: 3.71 L/kg
Metabolism: Hepatic to nortilidine (active metabolite) and bis-nortilidine
Half-life: 5 hours

Usual Dosage

Oral:
- Children >2 years: 5 mg plus 2.5 mg per year, not to exceed 1 mg/kg
- Adults: 50-100 mg up to 4 times/day; maximum daily dose: 400 mg

Parenteral: Up to 400 mg
Rectal: 75 mg 4 times/day

Dosing adjustment in renal impairment: Reduce dose

Contraindications Hypersensitivity to tilidine, patients with porphyria, pregnancy, breast feeding, respiratory depression

Warnings Use with caution in patients with myasthenia gravis; may cause dependency

Reference Range Maximum tilidine plasma concentration of 907 ng/mL achieved after 50 mg dose (I.V.); nortilidine peak plasma level after a 50 mg dose: 69 ng/mL

Overdosage Treatment

Supportive therapy: Naloxone hydrochloride (0.4-2 mg I.V., S.C., or through an endotracheal tube); a continuous infusion (at ⅔ the response dose/hour) may be required

Antidote(s)

Naloxone Hydrochloride *on page 1447*

Drug Interactions Increased sedation with alcohol or other sedative agents

Additional Information Often combined orally with naloxone (ie, Valoron N®)

Specific References

Levenstein JH, "An Evaluation of Tilidine Hydrochloride in the Treatment of Pain Requiring Immediate Analgesia," *S Afr Med J*, 1975, 49:143-6.
McCormack CD, "Tilidine Hydrochloride – Dose by Weight and Not by Age," *S Afr Med J*, 1992, 82(6):476-7.

Tilitrate® *see* Tilidine Hydrochloride *on this page*

Timolol Maleate (tye' moe lole)

Related Information

Beta-Blockers Comparison *on page 1644-1645*
Therapeutic Drugs Associated With Hallucinations *on page 1558-1559*

CAS Number 26839-75-8; 26921-17-5

Brand Names Betim®; Blocadren®; Timoptic®

Use Ophthalmic dosage form used to treat elevated intraocular pressure such as glaucoma or ocular hypertension; orally for treatment of hypertension and angina and reduce mortality following myocardial infarction and prophylaxis of migraine; may exacerbate myasthenia gravis

Mechanism of Action Blocks both $beta_1$-adrenergic and $beta_2$-adrenergic receptors, reduces intraocular pressure by reducing aqueous humor production or possibly outflow; reduces blood pressure by blocking adrenergic receptors and decreasing sympathetic outflow, produces a negative chronotropic and inotropic activity through an unknown mechanism

Adverse Reactions

Cardiovascular: Bradycardia, arrhythmias, hypotension, syncope, palpitation
Central nervous system: Dizziness, headache, fatigue, disorientation, hallucinations

Endocrine & metabolic: Hypoglycemia episodes, decreased libido
Gastrointestinal: Diarrhea, nausea, dyspepsia, vomiting
Ocular: Irritation, conjunctivitis, keratitis, visual disturbances, diplopia, eyelid edema and erythema, dryness
Respiratory: Wheezing, respiratory distress
Miscellaneous: Retroperitoneal fibrosis

Signs & Symptoms of Acute Overdose Severe hypotension, dyspnea, ataxia, myasthenia gravis (exacerbation or precipitation of), hypertension, depression, impotence, hypoglycemia, bradycardia, heart failure, and wheezing, confusion

Toxicodynamics/Kinetics
Onset of action: Oral: Within 15-45 minutes
Peak effect: Oral: 30-150 minutes
Duration:
Oral: ~4 hours
Ophthalmic: Intraocular effects persist for 24 hours
Absorption: From gastrointestinal tract (90%)
Distribution: V_d: 1.3-3.6 L/kg; distributed throughout the body; low degree of lipid solubility
Protein binding: <10%
Metabolism: Extensive first-pass effect (50%); extensively metabolized in the liver (80%)
Half-life: 2-2.7 hours; prolonged with reduced renal function
Elimination: Urinary excretion (15% to 20% as unchanged drug)

Usual Dosage
Children and Adults:
Ophthalmic gel: Use once daily
Ophthalmic solution: Initial: 0.25% solution, instill 1 drop twice daily; increase to 0.5% solution if response not adequate; decrease to 1 drop/day if controlled; do not exceed 1 drop twice daily of 0.5% solution

Adults: Oral:
Hypertension: Initial: 10 mg twice daily, increase gradually every 7 days, usual dosage: 20-40 mg/day in 2 divided doses; maximum: 60 mg/day
Prevention of myocardial infarction: 10 mg twice daily initiated within 1-4 weeks after infarction
Migraine headache: Initial: 10 mg twice daily, increase to maximum of 30 mg/day

Contraindications Uncompensated congestive heart failure, cardiogenic shock, bradycardia or heart block, bronchial asthma, severe chronic obstructive pulmonary disease or history of asthma, congestive heart failure

Warnings Severe CNS, cardiovascular and respiratory adverse effects have been seen following ophthalmic use; patients with a history of asthma, congestive heart failure, or bradycardia appear to be at a higher risk; some products contain sulfites which can cause allergic reactions; diminished response over time; may increase muscle asthenia; use with a miotic in angle-closure glaucoma; similar to other beta-blockers; use with caution in patients with decreased renal or hepatic function (dosage adjustment required)

Dosage Forms
Gel, ophthalmic (Timoptic-XE®): 0.25% (2.5 mL, 5 mL); 0.5% (2.5 mL, 5 mL)
Solution, ophthalmic (Timoptic®): 0.25% (2.5 mL, 5 mL, 10 mL, 15 mL); 0.5% (2.5 mL, 5 mL, 10 mL, 15 mL)
Solution, ophthalmic, preservative free, single use (Timoptic® OcuDose®): 0.25%, 0.5%
Tablet (Blocadren®): 5 mg, 10 mg, 20 mg

Reference Range Following single 20 mg dose, levels may range from 60-114 ng/mL

Overdosage Treatment
Decontamination: Lavage/activated charcoal with cathartic; do not use ipecac
Supportive therapy: Sympathomimetics (eg, epinephrine or dopamine), glucagon, atropine or a pacemaker can be used to treat the toxic bradycardia, asystole, and/or hypotension; initially, fluids may be the best treatment for toxic hypotension
Enhancement of elimination: Multiple dosing of activated charcoal may be effective

Test Interactions Increases cholesterol (S), glucose

Drug Interactions May cause bradycardia and asystole when also giving verapamil or quinidine; has caused sinus bradycardia in one patient also taking quinidine; controversial when used with epinephrine

Pregnancy Risk Factor C

Pregnancy Implications Actively secreted in breast milk

Monitoring Parameters EKG, glucose

Patient Information Apply gentle pressure to lacrimal sac during and immediately following instillation (1 minute) to avoid systemic absorption; stop drug if breathing difficulty occurs

(Continued)

Timolol Maleate *(Continued)*

Nursing Implications Apply gentle pressure to lacrimal sac during and immediately following instillation (1 minute) to avoid systemic absorption; stop drug if breathing difficulty occurs

Additional Information First beta-blocker approved for treatment of the post-myocardial infarction patient; does not cause night blindness

Specific References

Botet C, Grau J, Benito P, et al, "Timolol Ophthalmic Solution and Respiratory Arrest," *Ann Intern Med*, 1986, 105(2):306-7.

Britman NA, "Cardiac Effects of Topical Timolol," *N Engl J Med*, 1979, 300(10):566.

Fraunfelder FT, "Ocular Beta Blockers and Systemic Effects," *Arch Intern Med*, 1986, 146(6):1073-4.

Wilkinson J, "Beta Blocker Overdoses," *Ann Emerg Med*, 1986, 15(8):982.

Timoptic® *see* Timolol Maleate *on page 752*

Tioclin® *see* Oxymetazoline Hydrochloride *on page 586*

Tiotil® *see* Propylthiouracil *on page 660*

Tiotixene *see* Thiothixene *on page 747*

Tirilazad Mesylate (tye ri' la zad)

Brand Names Freedox®

Synonyms U-74006F

Use Investigational: Subarachnoid hemorrhage, spinal cord injury, stroke, head traumas

Mechanism of Action A 21-aminosteroid with antioxidant effects similar to methylprednisolone; inhibits lipid peroxidation

Adverse Reactions

Cardiovascular: Supraventricular tachycardia, tachycardia (ventricular), palpitations

Central nervous system: Lightheadedness, drowsiness, headache

Gastrointestinal: Nausea, abdominal pain

Hepatic: Elevation of liver function tests

Local: Pain at injection site

Neuromuscular & skeletal: Muscle cramps

Toxicodynamics/Kinetics

Distribution: V_d:3 L/kg (single dose); 16-30 L/kg (multiple doses)

Protein binding: 99%

Metabolism: Hepatic

Half-life: 16 hours

Elimination: Feces

Usual Dosage

Subarachnoid hemorrhage: I.V.: 2-6 mg/kg/day up to 10 days

Spinal cord injury: 10 mg/kg/day for 2 days is being investigated

Contraindications Previous hypersensitivity to tirilazad

Warnings Use with caution in patients with hepatic or cardiovascular disease

Reference Range Peak serum levels after a 3 mg/kg dose: 11.2 µg/L in men and 7.4 µg/mL in women

Overdosage Treatment

Supportive therapy: Supportive and symptomatic treatment, including I.V. fluids and Trendelenburg positioning, should be initiated as intoxication may cause hypotension. Although calcium (calcium chloride I.V. 1-2 g in adults or 10-30 mg/kg in children over 5-10 minutes with repeats as needed) has been used as an "antidote" for acute intoxications, there is limited experience to support its routine use and should be reserved for those cases where definite signs of myocardial depression are evident. Heart block may respond to isoproterenol, glucagon, atropine and/or calcium, although a temporary pacemaker may be required; norepinephrine, dopamine, or amrinone for refractory hypotension.

Drug Interactions No interaction with nimodipine or cimetidine

Additional Information As of December 28, 1994, clinical trials of this agent were suspended in treatment of head trauma due to increase in mortality compared to placebo; no glucocorticoid activity; probably most effective when used within 4 hours postinjury

Specific References

Hall ED, "Lipid Antioxidants in Acute Central Nervous System Injury," *Ann Emerg Med*, 1993, 22(6):1022-7.

Hall ED, "The Role of Oxygen Radicals in Traumatic Injury: Clinical Implications," *J Emerg Med*, 1993, 11(Suppl 1):31-6.

Tirodril® *see* Methimazole *on page 512*

Tissue Plasminogen Activator, Recombinant *see* Alteplase, Recombinant *on page 100*

Ti-Tre® *see* Liothyronine Sodium *on page 471*

Titus® *see* Lorazepam *on page 482*

TMP-SMX *see* Co-trimoxazole *on page 242*

Tocainide Hydrochloride (toe kay' nide)

Related Information

Therapeutic Drugs Associated With Hallucinations *on page 1558-1559*

CAS Number 41708-72-9; 35891-93-1

Brand Names Tonocard®; Xylotocan®

Use Suppresses and prevents symptomatic ventricular arrhythmias; limited effectiveness in tachycardia (ventricular)

Mechanism of Action Suppresses automaticity of conduction tissue, by increasing electrical stimulation threshold of ventricle, HIS-Purkinje system, and spontaneous depolarization of the ventricles during diastole by a direct action on the tissues; blocks both the initiation and conduction of nerve impulses by decreasing the neuronal membrane's permeability to sodium ions, which results in inhibition of depolarization with resultant blockade of conduction

Adverse Reactions Similar to lidocaine and mexiletine

Cardiovascular: Hypotension, bradycardia, tachycardia, tachycardia (ventricular), palpitations, heart block

Central nervous system: Lightheadedness, dizziness, visual hallucinations, seizures, paranoid psychosis, ataxia

Dermatologic: Rash, skin lesions, Stevens-Johnson syndrome, erythema multiforme

Gastrointestinal: Nausea, vomiting, diarrhea

Hematologic: Agranulocytosis (0.1% to 0.2%), anemia, leukopenia, neutropenia, aplastic anemia, thrombocytopenia

Hepatic: Granulomatous hepatitis

Neuromuscular & skeletal: Tremors, paresthesia

Ocular: Nystagmus, diplopia

Otic: Tinnitus

Respiratory: Respiratory arrest, pulmonary fibrosis (0.03 to 0.11%)

Miscellaneous: Exacerbation of lupus erythematosus, sweating

Signs & Symptoms of Acute Overdose Leukopenia or neutropenia (agranulocytosis, granulocytopenia); diuresis, delirium, tinnitus, A-V block, metallic taste, tachycardia (ventricular), hematuria, systemic lupus erythematosus (SLE), pericarditis, heart block, exfoliative dermatitis, anorexia

Toxicodynamics/Kinetics

Absorption: Oral: Extensive (99% to 100%); delayed with food

Distribution: V_d: 3 L/kg

Protein binding: 10% to 15%

Metabolism: In the liver to inactive metabolites

Half-life: 11-23 hours, prolonged with renal and hepatic impairment, congestive heart failure

Time to peak serum concentration: Within 30-160 minutes

Elimination: Urine (40% as unchanged drug); clearance: 0.16 L/hour/kg

Usual Dosage Adults: Oral: 1200-1800 mg/day in 3 divided doses, up to 2400 mg/day

Dosing adjustment in renal impairment: Cl_{cr} <30 mL/minute: Administer 50% of normal dose or 600 mg once daily

Dosing adjustment in hepatic impairment: Maximum daily dose: 1200 mg

Minimal lethal dose: 16 g

Contraindications Second or third degree A-V block without a pacemaker, hypersensitivity to tocainide, amide-type anesthetics, or any component

Warnings May exacerbate some arrhythmias (ie, fibrillation (atrial)/flutter); use with caution in CHF patients; administer with caution in patients with pre-existing bone marrow failure, cytopenia, severe renal or hepatic disease

Dosage Forms Tablet: 400 mg, 600 mg

Reference Range Therapeutic: 5-12 μg/mL (SI: 22-52 μmol/L)

Overdosage Treatment

Decontamination: Lavage/activated charcoal with cathartic

Supportive therapy: Seizures can be treated with lorazepam or diazepam, phenytoin, or phenobarbital; do not use isoproterenol for arrhythmia treatment. Hypotension can be managed with isotonic saline, with placement in Trendelenburg position; dopamine or norepinephrine can also be used for refractory hypotension; pacemaker placement may need to be performed for heart block.

Enhancement of elimination: Hemodialysis or hemoperfusion are effective; moderately dialyzable (20% to 50%)

Diagnostic Tests/Procedures

Electrocardiography *on page 1253*

(Continued)

Tocainide Hydrochloride *(Continued)*

Complete Blood Count *on page 1236*
Chest Films *on page 1224*

Drug Interactions Decreased effect/levels with cimetidine and rifampin; same possible effect with phenobarbital or phenytoin

Pregnancy Risk Factor C

Patient Information Report any unusual bleeding, fever, sore throat, or any breathing difficulties; do not discontinue or alter dose without notifying physician; may cause drowsiness, dizziness, impair judgment, and coordination

Nursing Implications Monitor for tremor; titration of dosing and initiation of therapy require cardiac monitoring

Additional Information Response correlates with response to lidocaine

Specific References

Clarke CW and el-Mahdi EO, "Fatal Oral Tocainide Overdosage," *Br Med J*, 1984, 288:606-7, 760.
Denaro CP and Benowitz NL, "Poisoning Due to Class IB Antiarrhythmic Drugs: Lignocaine, Mexiletine, and Tocainide," *Med Toxicol Adverse Drug Exp*, 1989, 4(6):412-28.
Roden DM and Woosley RL, "Drug Therapy. Tocainide," *N Engl J Med*, 1986, 315(1):41-5.
Wiegers U, Hanrath P, Kuck KH, et al, "Pharmacokinetics of Tocainide in Patients With Renal Dysfunction and During Haemodialysis," *Eur J Clin Pharmacol*, 1983, 24(4):503-7.

Toco *see* Vitamin E *on page 798*

Tocoferolo Bioglan® *see* Vitamin E *on page 798*

Tocogen® *see* Vitamin E *on page 798*

Tofranil® *see* Imipramine *on page 422*

Tofranil-PM® *see* Imipramine *on page 422*

Tolamide® *see* Tolazamide *on this page*

Tolanase® *see* Tolazamide *on this page*

Tolazamide (tole az' a mide)

Related Information

Hypoglycemic Agents Comparison, Oral *on page 1650*

CAS Number 1156-19-0

Brand Names Diabewas®; Norglycin®; Ronase®; Tolamide®; Tolanase®; Tolinase®

Use Adjunct to diet for the management of mild to moderately severe, stable, noninsulin-dependent (type II) diabetes mellitus

Mechanism of Action Stimulates insulin release from the pancreatic beta cells; reduces glucose output from the liver; insulin sensitivity is increased at peripheral target sites

Adverse Reactions

Central nervous system: Headache, ataxia, dizziness, fasciculations
Dermatologic: Rash, hives, photosensitivity
Endocrine & metabolic: Disulfiram reactions, hypoglycemia
Gastrointestinal: Anorexia, nausea, vomiting, diarrhea, constipation, heartburn, epigastric fullness
Hematologic: Leukopenia, thrombocytopenia, aplastic anemia, hemolysis, bone marrow depression, thrombocytopenia, agranulocytosis, porphyria
Hepatic: Jaundice
Neuromuscular & skeletal: Weakness
Miscellaneous: Porphyrinogenic

Signs & Symptoms of Acute Overdose Leukopenia or neutropenia (agranulocytosis, granulocytopenia); hyponatremia, hypoglycemia, photophobia, lichenoid eruptions, diuresis

Toxicodynamics/Kinetics

Onset of action: Oral: Within 4-6 hours
Duration: 10-24 hours
Absorption: Slow
Distribution: V_d: 0.1-0.3 L/kg
Protein binding: 94%
Metabolism: Extensive in the liver to one active and three inactive metabolites
Half-life: 4-7 hours
Time to peak plasma concentration: 2-5 hours
Elimination: Renal (85%)

Usual Dosage Oral (doses >1000 mg/day normally do not improve diabetic control):

Adults: Initial: 100 mg/day, increase at 2- to 4-week intervals; maximum dose: 1000 mg; give as a single or twice daily dose
Conversion from insulin → tolazamide
10 units day = 100 mg/day
20-40 units/day = 250 mg/day
>40 units/day = 250 mg/day and 50% of insulin dose
Doses >500 mg/day should be given in 2 divided doses

Dosing comments in hepatic impairment: Initial and maintenance doses should be conservative

Contraindications Type I diabetes therapy (IDDM), hypersensitivity to sulfonylureas, diabetes complicated by ketoacidosis

Warnings False-positive response has been reported in patients with liver disease, idiopathic hypoglycemia of infancy, severe malnutrition, acute pancreatitis, renal dysfunction. Transferring a patient from one sulfonylurea to another does not require a priming dose; doses >1000 mg/day normally do not improve diabetic control. Has not been studied in older patients; however, except for drug interactions, it appears to have a safe profile and decline in renal function does not affect its pharmacokinetics. How "tightly" an elderly patient's blood glucose should be controlled is controversial; however, a fasting blood sugar of <150 mg/dL is now an acceptable end point. Such a decision should be based on the patient's functional and cognitive status, how well they recognize hypoglycemic or hyperglycemic symptoms, and how to respond to them and their other disease states.

Dosage Forms Tablet: 100 mg, 250 mg, 500 mg

Reference Range Fasting blood glucose: Adults: 80-140 mg/dL; Elderly: 100-180 mg/dL

Overdosage Treatment

Decontamination: Lavage/activated charcoal with cathartic

Supportive therapy: Glucose (25 g I.V.) is mainstay of therapy. Glucagon (1-5 mg I.V., I.M., or S.C.) (0.03-0.1 mg/kg in pediatrics) will have limited benefit; diazoxide is a third-line agent (3-8 mg/kg/24 hours).

Enhancement of elimination: Multiple dosing of activated charcoal may be effective; not dialyzable (0% to 5%)

Antidote(s)

Dextrose *on page 1409*

Glucagon *on page 1431*

Diagnostic Tests/Procedures

Complete Blood Count *on page 1236*

Electrolytes, Blood *on page 1254*

Glucose, Random *on page 1269*

Drug Interactions Increased toxicity: Monitor patient closely; large number of drugs interact with sulfonylureas including salicylates, anticoagulants, H_2 antagonists, TCA, MAO inhibitors, beta-blockers, thiazides

Pregnancy Risk Factor D

Pregnancy Implications Can cause neonatal hypoglycemia

Monitoring Parameters Signs and symptoms of hypoglycemia, (fatigue, sweating, numbness of extremities); urine for glucose and ketones; fasting blood glucose; hemoglobin A, C, or fructosamine

Patient Information Tablets may be crushed; take drug at the same time each day; avoid alcohol; recognize signs and symptoms of hyper- and hypoglycemia; report any persistent or severe sore throat, fever, malaise, unusual bleeding, or bruising; can take with food; do not skip meals; carry a quick sugar source; medical alert bracelet

Nursing Implications Patients who are anorexic or NPO may need to have their dose held to avoid hypoglycemia

Specific References

Rull JH and Lennhoff M, "Prolonged and Recurrent Tolazamide-Induced Hypoglycemia," *Diabetes*, 1967, 16(5):352-3.

Seger D, "Toxic Emergencies of Endocrine and Metabolic Therapeutic Agents," *J Emerg Med*, 1988, 6(6):527-37.

Tolbutamide (tole byoo' ta mide)

Related Information

Hypoglycemic Agents Comparison, Oral *on page 1650*

CAS Number 64-77-7; 473-41-6

Brand Names Oramide®; Orinase®

Use Adjunct to diet for the management of mild to moderately severe, stable, noninsulin-dependent (type II) diabetes mellitus

Mechanism of Action A sulfonylurea hypoglycemic agent; its ability to lower elevated blood glucose levels in patients with functional pancreatic beta cells is similar to the other sulfonylurea agents; stimulates synthesis and release of endogenous insulin from pancreatic islet tissue. The hypoglycemic effect is attributed to an increased sensitivity of insulin receptors and improved peripheral utilization of insulin. Suppression of glucagon secretion may also contribute to the hypoglycemic effects of tolbutamide.

Adverse Reactions

Cardiovascular: Venospasm

Central nervous system: Fasciculations, ataxia

Dermatologic: Pruritus

Endocrine & metabolic: Hypoglycemia, disulfiram-type reactions, syndrome of inappropriate antidiuretic hormone

(Continued)

Tolbutamide *(Continued)*

Gastrointestinal: Anorexia, nausea, vomiting, diarrhea
Hematologic: Leukopenia, thrombocytopenia
Hepatic: Jaundice
Local: Thrombophlebitis
Neuromuscular & skeletal: Weakness
Otic: Ototoxicity, tinnitus
Miscellaneous: Hypersensitivity reaction

Signs & Symptoms of Acute Overdose Leukopenia or neutropenia (agranulocytosis, granulocytopenia); hypothyroidism, eczema, photophobia, photosensitivity, hypoglycemia

Toxicodynamics/Kinetics

Peak hypoglycemic action:
- Oral: 1-3 hours
- I.V.: 30 minutes

Duration:
- Oral: 6-12 hours
- I.V.: 3 hours

Time to peak serum concentration: 2-5 hours
Absorption: Oral: Rapid
Distribution: V_d: 0.1-0.15 L/kg
Protein binding: 95% to 97% (principally to albumin) ionic/nonionic
Metabolism: Hepatic metabolism to hydroxymethyltolbutamide (mildly active) and carboxytolbutamide (inactive); metabolism does not appear to be affected by age
Increased plasma concentrations and volume of distribution secondary to decreased albumin concentrations and less protein binding have been reported.
Half-life, plasma: 4-6 hours
Elimination: Metabolites rapidly excreted renally (85%); less than 2% excreted in the urine unchanged; 9% excreted by biliary

Usual Dosage Divided doses may increase side effects

Adults:
- Oral: Initial: 500-1000 mg 1-3 times/day; usual dose should not be more than 2 g/day
- I.V. bolus: 1 g over 2-3 minutes

Elderly: Oral: Initial: 250 mg 1-3 times/day; usual: 500-2000 mg; maximum: 2 g/day

Dosing adjustment in hepatic impairment: Dose reduction is necessary

Contraindications Diabetes complicated by ketoacidosis, therapy of IDDM, hypersensitivity to sulfonylureas

Warnings False-positive response has been reported in patients with liver disease, idiopathic hypoglycemia of infancy, severe malnutrition, acute pancreatitis. Because of its low potency and short duration, it is a useful agent in the elderly if drug interactions can be avoided. How "tightly" an elderly patient's blood glucose should be controlled is controversial; however, a fasting blood sugar of <150 mg/dL is now an acceptable end point. Such a decision should be based on the patient's functional and cognitive status, how well they recognize hypoglycemic or hyperglycemic symptoms, and how to respond to them and their other disease states.

Dosage Forms

Injection, diagnostic, as sodium: 1 g (20 mL)
Tablet: 250 mg, 500 mg

Stability Use parenteral formulation within 1 hour following reconstitution

Reference Range Fasting blood glucose: Adults: 80-140 mg/dL; Elderly: 100-180 mg/dL

Overdosage Treatment

Decontamination: Lavage/activated charcoal with cathartic
Supportive therapy: Glucose (25 g I.V.) is mainstay of therapy. Glucagon (1-5 mg I.V., I.M., or S.C.) (0.03-0.1 mg/kg in pediatrics) will have limited benefit; diazoxide is a third-line agent (3-8 mg/kg/24 hours)
Enhancement of elimination: Multiple dosing of activated charcoal may be effective; not dialyzable (0% to 5%)

Antidote(s)

Dextrose *on page 1409*
Glucagon *on page 1431*

Diagnostic Tests/Procedures

Electrolytes, Blood *on page 1254*
Glucose, Random *on page 1269*
Kidney Profile *on page 1279*

Drug Interactions Increased toxicity: Phenylbutazone may potentiate hypoglycemic effect; chloramphenicol → ↑ half-life of tolbutamide

Pregnancy Risk Factor D

Monitoring Parameters Fasting blood glucose, hemoglobin A_{1c} or fructosamine

Patient Information Tablets may be crushed; take drug at the same time each day; avoid alcohol; recognize signs and symptoms of hyper- and hypoglycemia; report any persistent or severe sore throat, fever, malaise, unusual bleeding, or bruising; can take with food

Nursing Implications Patients who are anorexic or NPO may need to have their dose held to avoid hypoglycemia

Additional Information Sodium content of 1 g vial: 3.5 mEq

Specific References

Huupponen R, "Adverse Cardiovascular Effects of Sulphonylurea Drugs. Clinical Significance," *Med Toxicol*, 1987, 2(3):190-209.

Lazner J, "Fatal Hypoglycaemia From Tolbutamide in a Nondiabetic Patient," *Med J Aust*, 1970, 1:327-8.

Seger D, "Toxic Emergencies of Endocrine and Metabolic Therapeutic Agents," *J Emerg Med*, 1988, 6(6):527-37.

Seltzer HS, "Drug-Induced Hypoglycemia: A Review Based on 473 Cases," *Diabetes*, 1972, 21(9):955-66.

Tolectin® *see* Tolmetin Sodium *on this page*

Tolinase® *see* Tolazamide *on page 756*

Tolmetin Sodium (tole' met in)

Related Information

Nonsteroidal Anti-Inflammatory Comparison *on page 1655*

CAS Number 26171-23-3 (Base); 35711-34-3 (Anhydrous Sodium); 64490-92-2 (Dihydrate Sodium)

Brand Names Tolectin®

Use Treatment of rheumatoid arthritis and osteoarthritis, juvenile rheumatoid arthritis

Mechanism of Action Inhibits prostaglandin synthesis by decreasing the activity of the enzyme, cyclo-oxygenase, which results in decreased formation of prostaglandin precursors

Adverse Reactions

Cardiovascular: Fluid retention, circulatory collapse

Central nervous system: Headache, aseptic meningitis, psychosis, cognitive dysfunction, coma, seizures

Dermatologic: Rash, pruritus

Endocrine & metabolic: Hyperkalemia, anion gap metabolic acidosis

Gastrointestinal: Abdominal pain, nausea, vomiting, bleeding, ulceration, constipation, diarrhea, dyspepsia

Genitourinary: Albuminuria

Hematologic: Leukopenia, neutropenia, agranulocytosis, granulocytopenia; aplastic anemia (rare), platelet inhibition

Hepatic: Elevation of transaminases, fulminant hepatitis

Otic: Ototoxicity, tinnitus

Renal: Renal failure (acute), nephrotic syndrome, proteinuria, chronic renal failure

Respiratory: Wheezing, respiratory depression

Miscellaneous: Hypersensitivity

Signs & Symptoms of Acute Overdose Nausea, vomiting, wheezing, nephrotic syndrome, gastrointestinal bleeding, gastritis; thrombocytopenia, systemic lupus erythematosus (SLE), cognitive dysfunction, ototoxicity; tinnitus, drowsiness; severe poisoning can manifest with coma, seizures, renal and or hepatic failure, hypotension, respiratory depression

Toxicodynamics/Kinetics

Absorption: Oral: Well absorbed

Protein binding: 99%

Distribution: V_d: 0.1 L/kg

Metabolism: Oxidized in the liver to an inactive dicarboxylic acid metabolite

Half-life: 4.9 hours

Time to peak serum concentration: Within 30-60 minutes

Elimination: In urine within 24 hours as dicarboxylic acid metabolite (60%), unchanged tolmetin (20%), tolmetin conjugates (20%)

Usual Dosage Oral:

Children ≥2 years:

Anti-inflammatory: Initial: 20 mg/kg/day in 3 divided doses, then 15-30 mg/kg/day in 3 divided doses

Analgesic: 5-7 mg/kg/dose every 6-8 hours

Adults: 400 mg 3 times/day; usual dose: 600-1.8 g/day; maximum: 2 g/day

Contraindications Known hypersensitivity to tolmetin or any component, aspirin, or other nonsteroidal anti-inflammatory drugs (NSAIDs)

Warnings Use with caution in patients with upper gastrointestinal disease, impaired renal function, congestive heart failure, hypertension, and patients receiving anticoagulants

(Continued)

Tolmetin Sodium *(Continued)*

Dosage Forms

Capsule (Tolectin® DS): 400 mg

Tablet (Tolectin®): 200 mg, 600 mg

Overdosage Treatment

Decontamination: Ipecac or lavage/activated charcoal with cathartic

Supportive therapy: Hypotension/dehydration can be managed with intravenous fluid therapy; acidosis should be treated with bicarbonates, seizures with benzodiazepines; antacids, blood products are indicated, as appropriate, for hemorrhage

Enhancement of elimination: Dialysis or perfusion is indicated for secondary complications, acidosis, or renal failure and not toxin removal alone; multiple dosing of activated charcoal may be effective

Test Interactions Increases protein

Drug Interactions Aspirin decreases serum concentrations probably by protein-binding displacement; there is an increased bleeding potential with concomitant warfarin therapy; may increase lithium and methotrexate concentrations by decreasing renal clearance; may decrease diuretic and hypotensive effects of thiazides, loop diuretics, ACE inhibitors, and beta-blockers; may increase nephrotoxicity of cyclosporine

Pregnancy Risk Factor B (D at term)

Monitoring Parameters Occult blood loss, CBC, liver enzymes, BUN, serum creatinine, periodic liver function test

Nursing Implications Assess audiometric and ophthalmic exam before, during, and after treatment

Additional Information Sodium content of 200 mg: 0.8 mEq; only NSAID affected by food/milk, which decreases total bioavailability by 16%; if gastrointestinal upset occurs with tolmetin take with antacids other than sodium bicarbonate

Specific References

Court H and Volans GN, "Poisoning After Overdose With Nonsteroidal Anti-inflammatory Drugs," *Adverse Drug React Acute Poisoning Rev*, 1984, 3(1):1-21.

Hoppmann RA, Peden JG, and Ober SK, "Central Nervous System Side Effects of Nonsteroidal Anti-inflammatory Drugs. Aseptic Meningitis, Psychosis, and Cognitive Dysfunction," *Arch Intern Med*, 1991, 151(7):1309-13.

Smolinske SC, Hall AH, Vandenberg SA, et al, "Toxic Effects of Nonsteroid Anti-inflammatory Drugs in Overdose. An Overview of Recent Evidence on Clinical Effects and Dose-Response Relationships," *Drug Saf*, 1990, 5(4):252-74.

Vale JA and Meredith TJ, "Acute Poisoning Due to Nonsteroidal Anti-inflammatory Drugs," *Med Toxicol*, 1986, 1(1):12-31.

Verbeeck RK, "Pharmacokinetic Drug Interactions With Nonsteroidal Anti-inflammatory Drugs," *Clin Pharmacokinet*, 1990, 19(1):44-66.

Tolrestat

CAS Number 82964-04-03

Brand Names Alredase®; Lorestat®

Use Investigational: Decrease the adverse effects of diabetes mellitus, specifically diabetic, nephropathy, retinopathy, neuropathy, and cataract formation

Mechanism of Action Carboxylic acid; decreased amounts of sorbitol and fructose are formed from glucose; thus, less water is drawn into the lens (through osmosis) and neurons, thus possibly leading to less diabetic complications

Adverse Reactions Overdose experience has not been reported

Central nervous system: Dizziness (11%)

Dermatologic: Rash

Hepatic: Elevated liver enzymes

Miscellaneous: Hyperchloremic acidosis may occur

Toxicodynamics/Kinetics

Absorption: Within 2 hours

Protein binding: 99%

Half-life: 10-13 hours

Elimination: Renal (63% to 68%) and fecal (25% to 27%)

Usual Dosage 200 mg before breakfast or 100 mg twice daily

Contraindications Hypersensitivity to tolrestat

Reference Range Peak plasma level after a 100 mg oral dose: 5.3-8.8 μg/mL

Overdosage Treatment

Decontamination: Emesis or lavage if >1.2 g ingested; activated charcoal with cathartic can be given

Enhancement of elimination: Multiple dosing of activated charcoal may be effective

Drug Interactions Protein-binding displacement can occur with concomitant tolbutamide and salicylic acid therapy

Specific References

Clark Jr CM and Lee DA, "Prevention and Treatment of the Complications of Diabetes Mellitus," *N Engl J Med*, 1995, 332:1210-7.

Cogan DG, Kinoshita JH, Kador PF, et al, "Aldose Reductase and Complications of Diabetes," *Ann Intern Med*, 1984, 101(1):82-91.

Hicks DR, Kraml M, Cayen MN, et al, "Tolrestat Kinetics," *Clin Pharmacol Ther*, 1984, 36(4):493-9.
Masson EA and Boulton AJ, "Aldose Reductase Inhibitors in the Treatment of Diabetic Neuropathy: A Review of the Rationale and Clinical Evidence," *Drugs*, 1990, 39(2):190-202.

Tolvin® *see* Mianserin Hydrochloride *on page 529*

Tonocard® *see* Tocainide Hydrochloride *on page 755*

Topicycline® Topical *see* Tetracycline *on page 732*

Toprol XL® *see* Metoprolol Tartrate *on page 524*

Toradol® *see* Ketorolac Tromethamine *on page 455*

Torbetol® *see* Benzalkonium Chloride *on page 147*

Torecan® *see* Thiethylperazine Maleate *on page 743*

Torental® *see* Pentoxifylline *on page 607*

Torsemide (tore' se mide)

CAS Number 56211-40-6; 72810-59-4

Brand Names Demadex®

Synonyms AC-4464

Use Management of edema associated with congestive heart failure and hepatic or renal disease; used alone or in combination with antihypertensives in treatment of hypertension

Mechanism of Action Inhibits reabsorption of sodium and chloride in the ascending loop of Henle and distal renal tubule, interfering with the chloride-binding cotransport system, thus causing increased excretion of water, sodium, chloride, magnesium, and calcium; less potassium loss than furosemide

Adverse Reactions

Central nervous system: Dizziness, headache
Dermatologic: Urticaria, photosensitivity
Endocrine & metabolic: Hypokalemia, hyponatremia, hypochloremia, alkalosis, dehydration, hyperuricemia
Gastrointestinal: Pancreatitis, nausea, oral solutions may cause diarrhea due to sorbitol content
Genitourinary: Prerenal azotemia
Hematologic: Agranulocytosis, anemia, thrombocytopenia
Otic: Potential ototoxicity, tinnitus
Renal: Nephrocalcinosis, interstitial nephritis, hypercalciuria

Signs & Symptoms of Acute Overdose Hypotension, leukopenia, disorientation, nocturia, diuresis, hyponatremia, hypokalemia, hyperuricemia, neutropenia, agranulocytosis, granulocytopenia

Toxicodynamics/Kinetics

Onset of diuresis: 30-60 minutes
Peak effect: 1-4 hours
Duration: ~6 hours
Absorption: Oral: Rapid
Distribution: V_d: 0.16 L/kg
Protein binding: Plasma: ~97% to 99%
Metabolism: Hepatic by cytochrome P-450, 80%
Bioavailability: 80% to 90%
Half-life: 2-4; 7-8 hours in cirrhosis (dose modification appears unnecessary)
Elimination: 20% eliminated unchanged in urine (increases to 40% in cirrhotic/ascitic patients)

Usual Dosage Adults:

Oral: 5-10 mg once daily; if ineffective, may double dose until desired effect is achieved
I.V.: 10-20 mg/dose repeated in 2 hours as needed with a doubling of the dose with each succeeding dose until desired diuresis is achieved
Continues to be effective in patients with cirrhosis, no apparent change in dose is necessary

Contraindications Hypersensitivity to torsemide or any component or other sulfonylureas

Warnings Loop diuretics are potent diuretics, excess amounts can lead to profound diuresis with fluid and electrolyte loss; close medical supervision and dose evaluation is required

Dosage Forms

Injection: 10 mg/mL (2 mL, 5 mL)
Tablet: 5 mg, 10 mg, 20 mg, 100 mg

Reference Range Peak serum level:

Normal patient: 4 μg/mL 1 hour after 20 mg dose
Edematous patient: 3.7 μg/mL 1 hour after 20 mg dose

Overdosage Treatment

Decontamination: Lavage/activated charcoal with cathartic

(Continued)

Torsemide *(Continued)*

Supportive therapy: Crystalloid (normal saline) with Trendelenburg position for hypotension; dopamine or norepinephrine for refractory hypotension

Enhancement of elimination: Multiple dosing of activated charcoal may be effective; not dialyzable

Antidote(s)

Dopamine Hydrochloride *on page 1418*

Norepinephrine Bitartrate *on page 1451*

Test Interactions Increases uric acid, creatinine

Drug Interactions

Decreased effect with nonsteroidal anti-inflammatory drugs

Increased toxicity: Hypokalemia with lithium

Pregnancy Risk Factor C

Patient Information May be taken with food or milk; rise slowly from a lying or sitting position to minimize dizziness, lightheadedness, or fainting; also use extra care when exercising, standing for long periods of time, and during hot weather; take last dose of day early in the evening to prevent nocturia

Nursing Implications Monitor renal function, electrolytes, and fluid states closely including weight and I & O

Additional Information 10-20 mg torsemide is approximately equivalent to:

Furosemide: 40 mg

Bumetanide: 1 mg

Piretanide: 12 mg

Specific References

Friedel HA and Buckley MM, "Torsemide. A Review of Its Pharmacologic Properties and Therapeutic Potential," *Drugs*, 1991, 41(1):81-103.

Hariman RJ, Bremner S, Louie EK, et al, "Dose-Response Study of Intravenous Torsemide in Congestive Heart Failure," *Am Heart J*, 1994, 128(2):352-7.

Kramer WG, "Effect of Food on the Pharmacokinetics and Pharmacodynamics of Torsemide," *Am J Therapeut*, 1995, 2:499-503.

Krück F and Puschett JB, "Symposium on Torsemide: Pharmacology and Clinical Application of Loop Diuretics," *Drugs*, 1991, 41(Suppl 3):1-97.

Rudy DW, Gehr TW, Matzke GR, et al, "The Pharmacodynamics of Intravenous and Torsemide in Patients With Chronic Renal Insufficiency*Clin Pharmacol Ther*, 1994, 56(1):39-47.

Vargo DL, Kramer WG, Black PK, et al, "Bioavailability, Pharmacokinetics, and Pharmacodynamics of Torsemide and Furosemide in Patients With Congestive Heart Failure," *Clin Pharmacol Ther*, 1995, 57:601-9.

Totacillin® *see* Ampicillin *on page 125*

Totacillin®-N *see* Ampicillin *on page 125*

Touro Ex® *see* Guaifenesin *on page 390*

Tovon® *see* Mianserin Hydrochloride *on page 529*

Toxicities of Chemotherapeutic Agents *see page 1631*

Toxins Which Should be Lavaged With Solutions Other Than Water *see page 1635*

t-PA *see* Alteplase, Recombinant *on page 100*

Tracix® *see* Imipenem/Cilastatin *on page 420*

Tradon® *see* Pemoline *on page 598*

Tramadol Hydrochloride (tra' ma dole)

CAS Number 27203-92-5; 22204-88-2; 36282-47-0

Brand Names Crispin®; Tramal®; Trodon®; Ultram®

Use Relief of moderate to moderately severe pain

Mechanism of Action Centrally acting analgesic with selective (mu) opioid receptor agonist and norepinephrine and serotonin reuptake inhibition

Adverse Reactions

Cardiovascular: Orthostatic hypotension

Central nervous system: Headache, dizziness, lethargy, stimulation, euphoria

Dermatologic: Sweating, Pruritus, erythema

Gastrointestinal: Constipation, nausea, vomiting

Otic: Tinnitus

Respiratory: Respiratory depression

Signs & Symptoms of Acute Overdose Sleepiness, coma, seizures (at oral doses exceeding 700 mg or I.V. doses exceeding 300 mg), miosis, respiratory depression

Toxicodynamics/Kinetics

Duration of action: 9 hours

Peak serum levels: 2 hours

Absorption: Rapid and complete

Distribution: V_d: 2.5-3 L/kg

Protein binding:, plasma: 20%

Metabolism: Extensive in the liver via demethylation, glucuronidation, and sulfation; has pharmacologically active metabolite formed by P-450 oxidative reaction (CYP 2D6)

Half-life, elimination:

Tramadol: 6 hours

Active metabolite: 7 hours

Half-life prolonged in the elderly and/or hepatic/renal dysfunction

Bioavailability: 75%

Usual Dosage

Oral:

Children >1 year: 1-2 mg/kg

Adults: 50-100 mg every 4-6 hours, not to exceed 400 mg/day

Patients with cirrhosis: 50 mg every 12 hours

Dosing interval in renal impairment: Dosing interval should be 12 hours (maximum daily dose of 200 mg)

Rectal: 100 mg

Contraindications Previous hypersensitivity to tramadol or any components; concurrent use of monoamine oxidase inhibitors; acute alcohol intoxication; concurrent use of centrally acting analgesics, opioids, or psychotropic drugs

Warnings Concomitant CNS depressants, MAO inhibitors may predispose to additive toxicities

Dosage Forms Tablet: 50 mg

Reference Range Serum tramadol levels ranging from 100-300 ng/mL can be considered therapeutic

Overdosage Treatment

Decontamination: Activated charcoal/sorbitol

Supportive therapy: Treat seizures with benzodiazepines or barbiturates; naloxone is probably not effective in treating seizures but may be of some use in treating CNS depression

Elimination: Multiple doses of activated charcoal; hemodialysis or hemoperfusion not likely to be beneficial after absorption and distribution are completed

Antidote(s)

Naloxone Hydrochloride *on page 1447*

Test Interactions Does not generally interfere with urine opiate screens

Drug Interactions Carbamazepine induces tramadol metabolism; with its discontinuation, tramadol toxicity may occur; MAO inhibitors in combination with tramadol may result in serotonin syndrome

Pregnancy Risk Factor C

Pregnancy Implications Crosses placenta with umbilical/maternal venous concentration ratio of 80%

Additional Information Fatal dose: ~3 g; metoclopramide can be used to treat tramadol-induced nausea and vomiting

Specific References

Dayer P, Collart L, and Desmeules J, "The Pharmacology of Tramadol," *Drugs*, 1994, 47(Suppl 1):3-7.

Riedal F and Stockhausen HB, "Severe Cerebral Depression After Intoxication With Tramadol in a 6-Month-Old Infant," *Eur J Clin Pharmacol*, 1984, 26:631-2.

Sunshine A, "New Clinical Experience With Tramadol," *Drugs*, 1994, 47(Suppl 1):8-18.

Tramal® *see* Tramadol Hydrochloride *on previous page*

Trandate® *see* Labetalol Hydrochloride *on page 458*

Trangorex® *see* Amiodarone Hydrochloride *on page 113*

Tranilcipromina *see* Tranylcypromine Sulfate *on this page*

Trankimazin® *see* Alprazolam *on page 99*

Transamine *see* Tranylcypromine Sulfate *on this page*

Transannon® *see* Estrogens, Conjugated *on page 325*

Transdermal-NTG® *see* Nitroglycerin *on page 566*

Transderm-Nitro® *see* Nitroglycerin *on page 566*

Transderm Scop® *see* Scopolamine *on page 691*

Transene® *see* Clorazepate Dipotassium *on page 232*

Trans-Testosterone *see* Testosterone *on page 729*

Tranxene® *see* Clorazepate Dipotassium *on page 232*

Tranxilium® *see* Clorazepate Dipotassium *on page 232*

Tranylcypromine Sulfate (tran ill sip' roe meen)

CAS Number 13492-01-8; 155-09-9

Brand Names Parnate®

Synonyms Tranilcipromina; Transamine

(Continued)

Tranylcypromine Sulfate *(Continued)*

Use Symptomatic treatment of atypical, nonendogenous or neurotic depression

Mechanism of Action Thought to act by increasing endogenous concentrations of epinephrine, norepinephrine, dopamine and serotonin through inhibition of the enzyme (monoamine oxidase) responsible for the breakdown of these neurotransmitters

Adverse Reactions

Cardiovascular: Hypotension, edema, hypertensive crises
Central nervous system: Drowsiness, hyperexcitability, insomnia
Dermatologic: Skin rash
Endocrine & metabolic: Syndrome of inappropriate antidiuretic hormone
Gastrointestinal: Dry mouth, constipation
Genitourinary: Urinary retention, impotence
Hematologic: Leukopenia, thrombocytopenia, aplastic anemia, porphyria
Ocular: Blurred vision, photophobia, amblyopia, nystagmus
Otic: Tinnitus
Miscellaneous: Porphyrinogenic

Signs & Symptoms of Acute Overdose Fever, impotence, numbness, extrapyramidal reaction, leukopenia, insomnia, neutropenia, ptosis, hypertension, agranulocytosis, granulocytopenia, delirium, thrombocytopenia

Toxicodynamics/Kinetics

Distribution: V_d: 3.1 L/kg
Half-life: 1.5-2.5 hours (longer in overdose)

Usual Dosage Adults: Oral: 10 mg twice daily, increase by 10 mg increments at 1- to 3-week intervals; maximum: 60 mg/day

Minimum lethal dose: 170 mg

Contraindications Uncontrolled hypertension, known hypersensitivity to isocarboxazid, pheochromocytoma, congestive heart failure, severe renal or hepatic impairment

Warnings Avoid tyramine-containing foods: red wine, cheese (except cottage, ricotta, and cream), smoked or pickled fish, beef or chicken liver, dried sausage, fava or broad bean pods, yeast vitamin supplements; avoid use with patients <16 or >60 years of age

Dosage Forms Tablet: 10 mg

Reference Range Therapeutic blood level: 0.1 mg/L; serum level of 1 mg/L has been associated with coma

Overdosage Treatment

Decontamination: Lavage/activated charcoal with cathartic

Supportive therapy: Diazepam or lorazepam can be used for agitation/seizures; dantrolene (2.5 mg/kg every 6 hours) can be used for muscle rigidity and hyperthermia; labetalol may be useful for hypertension, while norepinephrine is the preferred agent for treatment of hypotension; avoid bretylium for ventricular dysrhythmia, lidocaine or procainamide are preferred

Enhancement of elimination: Hemodialysis may be useful

Diagnostic Tests/Procedures

Creatine Kinase, Blood *on page 1242*
Electrocardiography *on page 1253*
Electrolytes, Blood *on page 1254*
Kidney Profile *on page 1279*

Drug Interactions

Decreased effect of antihypertensives

Increased toxicity with disulfiram (possible seizures, delirium), fluoxetine (and other serotonin active agents), TCAs (cardiovascular instability), meperidine (cardiovascular instability), phenothiazines (hyperpyretic crisis), levodopa, sympathomimetics (hyperpyretic crisis), barbiturates, rauwolfia alkaloids (eg, reserpine), dextroamphetamine (psychoses), foods containing tyramine (hypertension, headache, seizures); theophylline/caffeine (hyperthermia), cyclobenzaprine (fever/seizures)

Potentiation of hypoglycemia with oral hypoglycemic agents

Pregnancy Risk Factor C

Additional Information Chronic overdosage, eventually a reported 550 mg/day, has resulted in only reversible thrombocytopenia and delirium

Specific References

Blansjaar BA and Egberts TC, "Delirium in a Patient Treated With Disulfiram and Tranylcypromine," *Am J Psychiatry*, 1995, 152(2):296.

Boniface PJ, "Two Cases of Fatal Intoxication Due to Tranylcypromine Overdose," *J Anal Toxicol*, 1991, 15(1):38-40.

Brady KT, Lydiard RB, and Kellner C, "Tranylcypromine Abuse," *Am J Psychiatry*, 1991, 148(9):1268-9.

Chatterjee A and Tosyali MC, "Thrombocytopenia and Delirium Associated With Tranylcypromine Overdose," *J Clin Psychopharmacol*, 1995, 15:143-5.

LeJoyeux M, et al, "Serotonin Syndrome: Incidence, Symptoms, and Treatment," *CNS Drugs*, 1994, 2:132-43.

Linden CH, Rumack BH, and Strehlke C, "Monoamine Oxidase Inhibitor Overdose," *Ann Emerg Med*, 1984, 13(12):1137-44.

Matter BJ, Donat PE, Brill ML, et al, "Tranylcypromine Sulfate Poisoning: Successful Treatment by Hemodialysis," *Arch Intern Med*, 1965, 116:18-20.

Quill TE, "Peak 'T' Waves With Tranylcypromine (Parnate) Overdose," *Int J Psychiatry Med*, 1981-82, 11(2):155-60.

Robertson JC, "Recovery After Massive MAOI Overdose Complicated by Malignant Hyperfever Treated With Chlorpromazine," *Postgrad Med J*, 1972, 48(555):64-5.

Sakkas P, Davis JM, Janicak PG, et al, "Drug Treatment of the Neuroleptic Malignant Syndrome," *Psychopharmacol Bull*, 1991, 27(3):381-4.

Trasylol® *see* Aprotinin *on page 130*

Traumacut® *see* Methocarbamol *on page 513*

Trazodone Hydrochloride (traz' oh done)

Related Information

Antidepressant Agents Comparison *on page 1639*

CAS Number 19794-93-5; 25332-39-2

Brand Names Deprax®; Desyrel®; Molipaxin®; Thrombran®; Trittico®

Use Treatment of depression

Mechanism of Action Inhibits reuptake of serotonin and norepinephrine; hypotension may be due to alpha-receptor blockade

Adverse Reactions

Cardiovascular: Postural hypotension, cardiac arrhythmias, dizziness, edema, prolongation of Q-T interval, decreases amplitude of T wave

Central nervous system: Drowsiness, sedation, asthenia, insomnia, confusion, agitation, seizures, extrapyramidal reactions, headache, mania

Dermatologic: Leukocytoclastic dermatitis, erythema multiforme, exacerbation of plaque, psoriasis

Endocrine & metabolic: Syndrome of inappropriate antidiuretic hormone, serotonin syndrome

Gastrointestinal: Dry mouth, constipation, nausea, vomiting

Genitourinary: Urinary retention, prolonged priapism

Hepatic: Hepatitis

Ocular: Blurred vision

Signs & Symptoms of Acute Overdose Drowsiness, delirium, photosensitivity, erythema multiforme, insomnia, dry mouth, myoclonus, hepatic failure, vomiting, ejaculatory disturbances, clitoral hypertrophy, extrapyramidal reaction, hypotension, drowsiness, heart block, ataxia, ototoxicity; tinnitus, incontinence, bradycardia, coma, priapism, seizures (rarely), bradycardia, first degree A-V block, respiratory depression, muscle asthenia, torsade de pointes

Toxicodynamics/Kinetics

Onset of action: 7 days

Peak effect: Maximum antidepressant effect usually occurs within 2 weeks; roughly 25% of patients require up to 4 weeks of therapy to reach optimum response

Absorption: Absorbed well; when taken after ingestion of food, there may be an increase in the amount of drug absorbed

Distribution: Wide in body; does not concentrate in any particular tissue but small amounts may appear in breast milk

Protein binding: 85% to 95%

Metabolism: In the liver to an active metabolite (m-chlorophenylpiperazine)

Half-life: 4-7.5 hours

Time to peak serum concentration: Within 30-100 minutes, prolonged in the presence of food (up to $2^1/_2$ hours)

Elimination: Primarily in urine and secondarily in feces

Usual Dosage Therapeutic effects may take up to 4 weeks to occur; therapy is normally maintained for several months after optimum response is reached to prevent recurrence of depression

Oral:

- Adolescents: Initial: 25-50 mg/day; increase to 100-150 mg/day in divided doses
- Adults: Initial: 150 mg/day in 3 divided doses (may increase by 50 mg/day every 3-7 days); maximum: 600 mg/day

Maximum tolerated dose:

- Children: 200 mg
- Adults: 9 g

Contraindications Hypersensitivity to trazodone or any component

Warnings Monitor closely and use with extreme caution in patients with cardiac disease, arrhythmias, epilepsy, or penile erection disorders; safety and efficacy in children <18 years of age have not been established

Dosage Forms Tablet: 50 mg, 100 mg, 150 mg, 300 mg

Reference Range Therapeutic: 0.5-2.5 μg/mL (SI: 1-6 μmol/L); overdoses of 4-5 g are associated with levels of 15-19 μg/mL

(Continued)

Trazodone Hydrochloride *(Continued)*

Overdosage Treatment

Decontamination: Lavage/activated charcoal with cathartic; multiple dosing of activated charcoal may be effective

Supportive therapy: Following initiation of essential overdose management, toxic symptoms should be treated. Ventricular arrhythmias often respond to phenytoin 15-20 mg/kg (adults) with concurrent systemic alkalinization (sodium bicarbonate 0.5-2 mEq/kg I.V.). Arrhythmias unresponsive to this therapy may respond to lidocaine 1 mg/kg I.V. followed by a titrated infusion. Treat bradycardia with atropine; benztropine may be useful to treat priapism. Seizures usually respond to lorazepam or diazepam I.V. boluses (5-10 mg for adults up to 30 mg or 0.25-0.4 mg/kg/dose for children up to 10 mg/dose). If seizures are unresponsive or recur, phenytoin or phenobarbital may be required. Priapism can be treated with alpha-adrenergic agonists

Diagnostic Tests/Procedures

Trazodone, Blood *on page 1367*

Drug Interactions Trazodone may antagonize the antihypertensive effects of clonidine and methyldopa; may increase the serum concentrations of phenytoin or digoxin; effects may be additive with other CNS depressants or ethanol; fluoxetine may increase trazodone serum concentration

Pregnancy Risk Factor C

Monitoring Parameters EKG for at least 4 hours

Patient Information Take shortly after a meal or light snack, can be taken as bedtime dose if drowsiness occurs; avoid alcohol; be aware of possible photosensitivity reaction; may cause painful erections

Nursing Implications Use side rails on bed if administered to the elderly; observe patient's activity and compare with admission level

Additional Information Therapeutic effects may take up to 4 weeks to occur; therapy is normally maintained for several months after optimum response is reached to prevent recurrence of depression

Specific References

Fishbain DA, "Priapism Associated With Trazodone Therapy," *J Urol*, 1989, 142(3):831.

LeJoyeux M, et al, "Serotonin Syndrome: Incidence, Symptoms, and Treatment," *CNS Drugs*, 1994, 2:132-43.

Lesar T, Kingston R, Dahms R, et al, "Trazodone Overdose," *Ann Emerg Med*, 1982, 12(4):221-3.

Reeves RR and Bullen JA, "Serotonin Syndrome Produced by Paroxetine and Low-Dose Trazodone," *Psychosomatics*, 1995, 36:159-60.

Zmitek A, "Trazodone-Induced Mania," *Br J Psychiatry*, 1987, 151:274-5.

Trecator®-SC *see* Ethionamide *on page 333*

Trendar® [OTC] *see* Ibuprofen *on page 418*

Trendinol® *see* Nitrendipine *on page 562*

Trental® *see* Pentoxifylline *on page 607*

Trepidan® *see* Prazepam *on page 637*

Trepiline® *see* Amitriptyline Hydrochloride *on page 116*

Tresortil® *see* Methocarbamol *on page 513*

Trexan™ *see* Naltrexone Hydrochloride *on page 548*

Tri® *see* Nitrazepam *on page 562*

Triadapin® *see* Doxepin Hydrochloride *on page 301*

Trialmin® *see* Gemfibrozil *on page 378*

Triamterene (trye am' ter een)

CAS Number 396-01-0

Brand Names Dyrenium®; Dytac®; Jatropur®; Teriam®; Urocaudal®

Use Alone or in combination with other diuretics to treat edema and hypertension; decreases potassium excretion caused by kaliuretic diuretics

Mechanism of Action Competes with aldosterone for receptor sites in the distal renal tubules, increasing sodium, chloride, and water excretion while conserving potassium and hydrogen ions; may block the effect of aldosterone on arteriolar smooth muscle as well

Adverse Reactions

Cardiovascular: Bradycardia

Central nervous system: Headache, hyperthermia

Dermatologic: Photosensitivity, purpura

Endocrine & metabolic: Hyperkalemia, hyperuricemia

Gastrointestinal: Nausea, vomiting, diarrhea

Hematologic: Pancytopenia, anemia (megaloblastic)

Renal: Reversible renal failure, renal stone formation, interstitial nephritis

Miscellaneous: Urine discoloration (blue), urine discoloration (fluorescent)

Toxicodynamics/Kinetics

Onset of action: Diuresis occurs within 2-4 hours

Duration: 7-9 hours

Absorption: Oral: Unreliable

Distribution: V_d: 2.5 L/kg

Protein binding: 55% (parent compound); 90% (active metabolite)

Metabolism: Hepatic to an active metabolite (hydroxytriamterene sulfate)

Bioavailability: 52%

Half-life: 1.5-2.5 hours

Usual Dosage Oral:

Children: 2-4 mg/kg/day in 1-2 divided doses; maximum: 300 mg/day

Adults: 100-300 mg/day in 1-2 divided doses; maximum: 300 mg/day

Dosing comments in renal impairment: Cl_{cr} <10 mL/minute: Avoid use

Dosing adjustment in hepatic impairment: Dose reduction is recommended in patients with cirrhosis

Contraindications Hyperkalemia, renal impairment, hypersensitivity to triamterene or any component; do not give to patients receiving spironolactone or amiloride

Warnings Use with caution in patients with severe hepatic encephalopathy, patients with diabetes, renal dysfunction, a history of renal stones, or those receiving potassium supplements or ACE inhibitors

Dosage Forms Capsule: 50 mg, 100 mg

Reference Range Peak plasma levels after a 50 mg oral dose: 25 ng/mL (of hydroxytriamterene sulfate - 770 ng/mL)

Overdosage Treatment

Decontamination: Ipecac or lavage/activated charcoal with cathartic

Supportive therapy: Hyperkalemia can be treated with glucose/insulin and sodium bicarbonate (1 mEq/kg); sodium polystyrene sulfonate can also be given; I.V. fluids administration of 0.45% sodium chloride with furosemide (1 mg/kg, up to 40 mg) can be used to promote urine flow

Test Interactions Interferes with fluorometric assay of quinidine

Drug Interactions

Increased risk of hyperkalemia if given together with amiloride, spironolactone, angiotensin-converting enzyme (ACE) inhibitors

Increased toxicity of amantadine (possibly by decreasing its renal excretion)

Pregnancy Risk Factor D

Monitoring Parameters Serum electrolytes, liver function tests, renal function

Additional Information Abrupt discontinuation of therapy may result in rebound kaliuresis; taper off gradually; can discolor urine to bluish color; has antifolate activity

Specific References

Hollenberg NK and Mickiewicz CW, "Postmarketing Surveillance in 70,898 Patients Treated With a Triamterene/Hydrochlorothiazide Combination (Maxzide®)," *Am J Cardiol*, 1989, 63(4):37B-41B.

Triatec® *see* Ramipril *on page 673*

Triavil® *see* Amitriptyline and Perphenazine *on page 115*

Triazolam (trye ay' zoe lam)

Related Information

Benzodiazepines Comparison *on page 1643*

Therapeutic Drugs Associated With Hallucinations *on page 1558-1559*

CAS Number 28911-01-5

Brand Names Halcion®; Novodorm®; Songar®

Synonyms Cloxazolam

Use Short-term treatment of insomnia

Mechanism of Action Depresses all levels of the CNS, including the limbic and reticular formation, probably through the increased action of gamma-aminobutyric acid (GABA), which is a major inhibitory neurotransmitter in the brain

Adverse Reactions

Central nervous system: Drowsiness, anterograde amnesia, confusion, dizziness, psychosis, agitation, auditory, visual, and tactile hallucinations, night terrors, memory impairment, headache, ataxia

Gastrointestinal: Dry mouth, nausea, vomiting

Hepatic: Intrahepatic cholestasis

Miscellaneous: Physical and psychological dependence may occur with prolonged use; noncardiogenic pulmonary edema

Signs & Symptoms of Acute Overdose Somnolence, confusion, night terrors, cognitive dysfunction, hypothermia, cholestatic jaundice, mania, coma, rhabdomyolysis, ataxia, myoglobinuria, slurred speech, diminished reflexes, respiratory depression, hypotension, visual or auditory hallucinations

(Continued)

Triazolam *(Continued)*

Toxicodynamics/Kinetics Studies have shown that the elderly are more sensitive to the effects of benzodiazepines as compared to younger adults

Onset of action: Hypnotic effects occur within 15-30 minutes

Duration: 6-7 hours

Absorption: Readily from gastrointestinal tract

Distribution: V_d: 0.8-1.8 L/kg; distributed widely throughout body

Protein binding: 89%

Metabolism: Extensive in the liver

Half-life: 1.7-5 hours

Time to peak plasma concentration: 42 minutes

Elimination: In urine as unchanged drug and metabolites; clearance: 6.5-10.1 mL/minute/kg

Usual Dosage Onset of action is rapid, patient should be in bed when taking medication. Oral:

Children <18 years: Dosage not established

Adults: 0.125-0.25 mg at bedtime

Dosing adjustment/comments in hepatic impairment: Reduce dose or avoid use in cirrhosis

Contraindications Hypersensitivity to triazolam, or any component, cross-sensitivity with other benzodiazepines may occur; severe uncontrolled pain; pre-existing CNS depression; narrow-angle glaucoma; not to be used in pregnancy or lactation

Warnings Anterograde amnesia has occurred with triazolam, generally it occurred with doses of 0.5 mg but it has also been reported with lower doses; prolonged clearance noted in obese patients; abrupt discontinuance of the drug should be avoided since manifestations of withdrawal can be precipitated or rebound insomnia can result

Dosage Forms Tablet: 0.125 mg, 0.25 mg

Reference Range Fatalities associated with postmortem levels >47 nmol/L

Overdosage Treatment

Decontamination: Lavage/activated charcoal with cathartic

Supportive therapy: Treatment for benzodiazepine overdose is supportive. Rarely is mechanical ventilation required. Flumazenil (Romazicon™) has been shown to selectively block the binding of benzodiazepines to CNS receptors, resulting in a reversal of benzodiazepine-induced CNS depression.

Enhancement of elimination: Multiple dose of activated charcoal may be effective

Antidote(s)

Flumazenil *on page 1428*

Test Interactions Visine®, Drano®, bleach may cause false-negative urine tests; oxazepam may interfere in giving falsely elevated glucose results

Drug Interactions CNS depressants may increase CNS adverse effects; cimetidine may decrease and enzyme inducers may increase the metabolism of triazolam; both ketoconazole and itraconazole can increase peak concentration and elimination half-life of triazolam; ketoconazole can increase the plasma levels of triazolam

Pregnancy Risk Factor X

Monitoring Parameters Respiratory and cardiovascular status

Patient Information May cause daytime drowsiness, avoid alcohol and drugs with CNS depressant effects; for short-term use only; do not exceed prescribed dose

Nursing Implications Provide safety measures (ie, side rails, night light, call button); remove smoking materials from area; supervise ambulation

Additional Information Onset of action is rapid, patient should be in bed when taking medication

Specific References

Chan TH, Ho SS, and Li PK, "Noncardiogenic Pulmonary Edema Associated With Triazolam," *J Toxicol Clin Toxicol*, 1995, 33(2):185-7.

Gillin JC and Byerley WF, "Drug Therapy: The Diagnosis and Management of Insomnia," *N Engl J Med*, 1990, 322(4):239-48.

Greenblatt DJ, von Moltke LL, Harmatz JS, et al, "Interaction of Triazolam and Ketoconazole," *Lancet*, 1995, 345(8943):191.

McKinnon NE, "Triazolam Intoxication," *Can Med Assoc J*, 1982, 126(8):893-4.

Neutel CI, Downey W, and Senft D, "Medical Events After a Prescription for a Benzodiazepine," *Pharmacoepidemiology and Drug Safety*, 1995, 4:63-73.

Olson KR, Yin L, Osterloh J, et al, "Coma Caused by Trivial Triazolam Overdose," *Am J Emerg Med*, 1985, 3(3):210-1.

Sullivan RJ Jr, "Respiratory Depression Requiring Ventilatory Support Following 0.5 mg of Triazolam," *J Am Geriatr Soc*, 1989, 37(5):450-2.

Sunter JP, Bal TS, and Cowan WK, "Three Cases of Fatal Triazolam Poisoning," *Br Med J (Clin Res)*, 1988, 297(6650):719.

Varhe A, Olkkola KT, and Neuvonen PJ, "Oral Triazolam is Potentially Hazardous to Patients Receiving Systemic Antimycotics Ketoconazole or Itraconazole," *Clin Pharmacol Ther*, 1994, 56(6 Pt 1):601-7.

Votey SR, Bosse GM, Bayer MJ, et al, "Flumazenil: A New Benzodiazepine Antagonist," *Ann Emerg Med*, 1991, 20(2):181-8.

Tribavirin *see* Ribavirin *on page 679*

Trichloroacetaldehyde Monohydrate *see* Chloral Hydrate *on page 193*

Tricodein *see* Codeine *on page 238*

Tricosal® *see* Choline Magnesium Trisalicylate *on page 211*

Tridil® *see* Nitroglycerin *on page 566*

Triflucan® *see* Fluconazole *on page 353*

Trifluoperazine Hydrochloride (trye floo oh per' a zeen)

Related Information

Antipsychotic Agents Comparison *on page 1642*

CAS Number 117-89-5; 440-17-5

Brand Names Calmazine®; Eskazina®; Novoflurazine®; Solazine®; Stelazine®; Terfluzin®

Use Treatment of psychoses and management of anxiety

Mechanism of Action Blocks postsynaptic mesolimbic dopaminergic receptors in the brain; exhibits a strong alpha-adrenergic blocking effect and depresses the release of hypothalamic and hypophyseal hormones

Adverse Reactions

Cardiovascular: Hypotension (especially with I.V. use), hypotension (orthostatic), tachycardia, cardiac arrhythmias

Central nervous system: Sedation, drowsiness, restlessness, anxiety, extrapyramidal reactions, pseudoparkinsonian signs and symptoms, tardive dyskinesia, neuroleptic malignant syndrome, seizures, altered central temperature regulation

Dermatologic: Hyperpigmentation, pruritus, rash, photosensitivity

Endocrine & metabolic: Amenorrhea, galactorrhea, gynecomastia, syndrome of inappropriate antidiuretic hormone, weight gain

Gastrointestinal: gastrointestinal upset, dry mouth, constipation

Genitourinary: Urinary retention, impotence

Hematologic: Agranulocytosis, leukopenia (usually in patients with large doses for prolonged periods), thrombocytopenia, hemolysis, eosinophilia, aplastic anemia

Hepatic: Cholestatic jaundice

Ocular: Retinal pigmentation, nystagmus, blurred vision, lenticular opacities

Miscellaneous: Anaphylactoid reactions

Signs & Symptoms of Acute Overdose Deep sleep, coma, impotence, Parkinson's-like symptoms, gynecomastia, galactorrhea, nystagmus, dysphagia, extrapyramidal reaction, abnormal involuntary muscle movements, neuroleptic malignant syndrome, hyperthermia, hepatic failure, hypotension or hypertension; generalized rigidity, torticollis, facial grimacing, slurred speech, stridor trismus, systemic lupus erythematosus (SLE), urine discoloration (pink), urine discoloration (red), urine discoloration (red-brown), vision color changes (brown tinge); leukopenia; neutropenia; agranulocytosis; granulocytopenia

Toxicodynamics/Kinetics

Onset of action: Rapid

Duration: ≥12 hours

Distribution: Widely distributed into body

Protein binding: ≥90%

Metabolism: Extensive liver metabolism

Half-life: >24 hours with chronic use; 7-18 hours with one dose

Time to peak plasma concentration: 1.5-4.5 hours

Elimination: Primarily excreted renally; biliary

Usual Dosage

Children 6-12 years: Psychoses:

- Oral: Hospitalized or well supervised patients: Initial: 1 mg 1-2 times/day, gradually increase until symptoms are controlled or adverse effects become troublesome; maximum: 15 mg/day
- I.M.: 1 mg twice daily

Adults:

- Psychoses:
  - Outpatients: Oral: 1-2 mg twice daily
  - Hospitalized or well supervised patients: Initial: 2-5 mg twice daily with optimum response in the 15-20 mg/day range; do not exceed 40 mg/day
  - I.M.: 1-2 mg every 4-6 hours as needed up to 10 mg/24 hours maximum
- Nonpsychotic anxiety: Oral: 1-2 mg twice daily; maximum: 6 mg/day; therapy for anxiety should not exceed 12 weeks; do not exceed 6 mg/day for longer than 12 weeks when treating anxiety; agitation, jitteriness, or insomnia may be confused with original neurotic or psychotic symptoms

Contraindications Hypersensitivity to trifluoperazine or any component, cross-sensitivity with other phenothiazines may exist; avoid use in patients with narrow-angle glaucoma, bone marrow depression, severe liver or cardiac disease

(Continued)

Trifluoperazine Hydrochloride *(Continued)*

Warnings Watch for hypotension when administering I.M. or I.V.; safety in children <6 months of age has not been established; use with caution in patients with cardiovascular disease or seizures

Dosage Forms

Concentrate, oral: 10 mg/mL (60 mL)
Injection: 2 mg/mL (10 mL)
Tablet: 1 mg, 2 mg, 5 mg, 10 mg

Stability Store injection at room temperature; protect from heat and from freezing; use only clear or slightly yellow solutions

Overdosage Treatment

Decontamination: Lavage/activated charcoal with cathartic

Supportive therapy: Following initiation of essential overdose management, toxic symptom treatment and supportive treatment should be initiated. Hypotension usually responds to I.V. fluids or Trendelenburg positioning. If unresponsive to these measures, the use of a parenteral inotrope may be required (eg, norepinephrine 0.1-0.2 mcg/kg/minute titrated to response). Seizures commonly respond to lorazepam or diazepam (adults: I.V.: 5-10 mg bolus every 15 minutes if needed up to a total of 30 mg; children: I.V.: 0.25-0.4 mg/kg/dose up to a total of 10 mg) or to phenytoin or phenobarbital. Also critical cardiac arrhythmias often respond to I.V. phenytoin (15 mg/kg up to 1 g), while other antiarrhythmics can be used. Neuroleptics often cause extrapyramidal reaction (eg, dystonic reactions) requiring management with diphenhydramine 1-2 mg/kg (adults) up to a maximum of 50 mg I.M. or I.V. slow push followed by a maintenance dose for 48-72 hours. When these reactions are unresponsive to diphenhydramine, benztropine mesylate I.V. 1-2 mg (adults) may be effective. These agents are generally effective within 2-5 minutes.

Enhancement of elimination: Multiple dosing of activated charcoal may be effective; not dialyzable (0% to 5%)

Test Interactions Increases cholesterol (S), glucose; decreases uric acid (S); may cross react with serum tricyclic assay

Drug Interactions Other CNS depressants, anticonvulsants, lithium, metrizamide

Pregnancy Risk Factor C

Pregnancy Implications Distributes into breast milk

Monitoring Parameters EKG for 24 hours

Patient Information Avoid alcohol ingestion; avoid exposure to sunlight or heat lamps; concentrate must be diluted in 2-4 oz of liquid (water, carbonated drinks, fruit juices, tomato juice, milk, or pudding)

Nursing Implications Give I.M. injection deep in upper outer quadrant of buttock; watch for hypotension when administering I.M. or I.V.

Additional Information Do not exceed 6 mg/day for longer than 12 weeks when treating anxiety; agitation, jitteriness or insomnia may be confused with original neurotic or psychotic symptoms; radiopaque

Specific References

Beighton PH and Wilkinson DJ, "Trifluoperazine Overdosage," *Practitioner*, 1967, 199(189):73-4.
FitzGerald MX and FitzGerald O, "Reaction to Trifluoperazine Abuse," *Lancet*, 1969, 1(605):1100.

Triflupromazine Hydrochloride (trye floo proe' ma zeen)

CAS Number 1098-60-8; 146-54-3

Brand Names Psyquil®; Siquil®; Vesprin®

Synonyms Fluopromazine

Use Treatment of psychoses, nausea, vomiting, and intractable hiccups

Adverse Reactions

Cardiovascular: Hypotension

Central nervous system: Neuroleptic malignant syndrome, extrapyramidal signs, sedation

Endocrine & metabolic: Syndrome of inappropriate antidiuretic hormone

Ocular: Nystagmus

Signs & Symptoms of Acute Overdose Deep sleep, euphoria, ejaculatory disturbances, priapism, insomnia, hyperglycemia, leukopenia, nystagmus, neuroleptic malignant syndrome, coma, extrapyramidal reaction, depression, neutropenia, abnormal involuntary muscle movements, hypotension or hypertension; vision color changes (brown tinge); generalized rigidity, torticollis, facial grimacing, slurred speech, stridor trismus, systemic lupus erythematosus (SLE)

Usual Dosage

Children: I.M.: 0.2-0.25 mg/kg

Adults:

- I.M.: 5-15 mg every 4 hours
- I.V.: 1 mg

Contraindications Hypersensitivity to triflupromazine or any component, cross-sensitivity with other phenothiazines may exist; avoid use in patients with narrow-angle glaucoma, bone marrow depression, severe liver or cardiac disease

Dosage Forms Injection: 20 mg/mL (1 mL)

Reference Range Therapeutic: 0.002-0.0600 mg/L

Overdosage Treatment

Decontamination: Lavage/activated charcoal with cathartic

Supportive therapy: Following initiation of essential overdose management, toxic symptom treatment and supportive treatment should be initiated. Hypotension usually responds to I.V. fluids or Trendelenburg positioning. If unresponsive to these measures, the use of a parenteral inotrope may be required (eg, norepinephrine 0.1-0.2 mcg/kg/minute titrated to response). Seizures commonly respond to lorazepam or diazepam (adults: I.V.: 5-10 mg bolus every 15 minutes if needed up to a total of 30 mg; children: I.V.: 0.25-0.4 mg/kg/dose up to a total of 10 mg) or to phenytoin or phenobarbital. Also critical cardiac arrhythmias often respond to I.V. phenytoin (15 mg/kg up to 1 g), while other antiarrhythmics can be used. Neuroleptics often cause extrapyramidal reaction (eg, dystonic reactions) requiring management with diphenhydramine 1-2 mg/kg (adults) up to a maximum of 50 mg I.M. or I.V. slow push followed by a maintenance dose for 48-72 hours. When these reactions are unresponsive to diphenhydramine, benztropine mesylate I.V. 1-2 mg (adults) may be effective. These agents are generally effective within 2-5 minutes.

Enhancement of elimination: Multiple dosing of activated charcoal may be effective

Test Interactions Increases cholesterol (S), glucose; decreases uric acid (S); may cross react with serum tricyclic assay

Pregnancy Risk Factor C

Monitoring Parameters Monitor EKG for 24 hours

Specific References

Bhugra DK and Low NC, "Neuroleptic Malignant Syndrome," *Br J Clin Pract*, 1986, 40(10):445-6.

Trilafon® *see* Perphenazine *on page 609*

Trilisate® *see* Choline Magnesium Trisalicylate *on page 211*

Triludan® *see* Terfenadine *on page 728*

Trimazide® *see* Trimethobenzamide Hydrochloride *on next page*

Trimepramine *see* Trimipramine Maleate *on page 775*

Trimetaphan Camsilate *see* Trimethaphan Camsylate *on this page*

Trimethaphan Camphorsulfonate *see* Trimethaphan Camsylate *on this page*

Trimethaphan Camsylate (trye meth' a fan)

CAS Number 7187-66-8; 68-91-7

Brand Names Arfonad®

Synonyms Methioplequim; Trimetaphan Camsilate; Trimethaphan Camphorsulfonate

Use Immediate and temporary reduction of blood pressure in patients with hypertensive emergencies; controlled hypotension during surgery

Mechanism of Action Blocks transmission in both adrenergic and cholinergic ganglia by blocking stimulation from presynaptic receptors to postsynaptic receptors mediated by acetylcholine; possesses direct peripheral vasodilatory activity and is a weak histamine releaser

Adverse Reactions

Cardiovascular: Hypotension (especially orthostatic), tachycardia, left bundle-branch block, first degree A-V block, reduced cardiac output

Central nervous system: Restlessness, asthenia

Dermatologic: Itching, rash, anhidrosis

Gastrointestinal: Anorexia, nausea, vomiting, dry mouth, adynamic ileus, constipation

Genitourinary: Urinary retention, impotence

Ocular: Mydriasis, cycloplegia

Respiratory: Apnea, respiratory arrest

Miscellaneous: Sodium and water retention

Signs & Symptoms of Acute Overdose Hypotension, respiratory arrest, A-V block, impotence, tachycardia

Toxicodynamics/Kinetics

Onset of action: I.V.: Immediate

Peak effect: 5 minutes

Duration: 10-30 minutes

Metabolism: Primarily by postganglionic pseudocholinesterase

Elimination: Urinary excretion

Usual Dosage Administration requires the use of an infusion pump

Severe hypertension and hypertensive emergencies: I.V.:

Children: 50-150 mcg/kg/minute; dilute 150 mg x weight (kg) to 250 mL in D_5W then dose in mcg/kg/minute = 10 x infusion rate in mL/hour

(Continued)

Trimethaphan Camsylate *(Continued)*

Adults: Initial rate: 0.5-1 mg/minute; titrate dose to the desired effect

Hypertension due to acute dissecting aneurysms: Initial rate: 1-2 mg/minute, adjusting as needed to keep systolic blood pressure of 100-120 mm Hg

Controlled hypotension during surgery: Initial rate: 3-4 mg/minute adjusted to maintain blood pressure at a desirable level; usual dosage needed 0.3-6 mg/minute

Contraindications Hypersensitivity to trimethaphan camsylate or any component; hypovolemia or shock; anemia; respiratory insufficiency

Warnings Use with caution in patients with allergies, cardiac, hepatic, renal, diabetes mellitus, or Addison's disease. Pupillary dilation does not necessarily indicate anoxia or the depth of anesthesia since the drug appears to have a specific effect on the pupil.

Dosage Forms Injection: 50 mg/mL (10 mL)

Stability Refrigerate; however, is stable for up to 14 days at room temperature

Overdosage Treatment Supportive therapy: Following initiation of essential overdose management, toxic symptoms should be treated. Seizures usually respond to lorazepam or diazepam I.V. boluses (5-10 mg for adults up to 30 mg or 0.25-0.4 mg/kg/dose for children up to 10 mg/dose). If seizures are unresponsive or recur, phenytoin or phenobarbital may be required. Hypotension usually responds to I.V. fluids or Trendelenburg positioning. If unresponsive to these measures, the use of a parenteral inotrope may be required (eg, norepinephrine 0.1-0.2 mcg/kg/minute titrated to response). Physostigmine or neostigmine 0.5-1 mg I.V. slow push reverses many of the drug's acute toxic effects, while bethanechol has proven useful in treating the drug-induced urinary retention.

Test Interactions Lowers serum potassium

Drug Interactions Anesthetics, procainamide, diuretics and other hypotensive agents may increase hypotensive effects of trimethaphan; effects of tubocurarine and succinylcholine may be prolonged by trimethaphan

Pregnancy Risk Factor C (can cause meconium ileus in neonates)

Pregnancy Implications Crosses placenta

Monitoring Parameters Blood pressure and heart rate

Nursing Implications Must be diluted; usually mixed as 1 mg/mL concentration in 5% dextrose; solution should be freshly prepared and any unused portion discarded

Additional Information Pupillary dilation does not necessarily indicate depth of anesthesia; discontinue drug before wound closure

Specific References

Dale RC and Schroeder ET, "Respiratory Paralysis During Treatment of Hypertension With Trimethaphan Camsylate," *Arch Intern Med*, 1976, 136(7):816-8.

Di Leo M, Dalmasso M, Libero L, et al, "Severe Electrocardiographic Abnormalities During Arfonad® Administration," *G Ital Cardiol*, 1984, 14(11):931-4.

Nakamura K, Koide M, Imanaga T, et al, "Prolonged Neuromuscular Blockade Following Trimethaphan Infusion," *Anaesthesia*, 1980, 35(12):1202-7.

Trimethobenzamide Hydrochloride (trye meth oh ben' za mide)

CAS Number 554-92-7

Brand Names Arrestin®; Bio-Gan®; Stemetic®; Tebamide®; T-Gen®; Ticon®; Tigan®; Tiject®; Trimazide®

Use Control of nausea and vomiting (especially for long-term antiemetic therapy)

Mechanism of Action Acts centrally to inhibit the medullary chemoreceptor trigger zone

Adverse Reactions

Cardiovascular: Hypotension

Central nervous system: Drowsiness, sedation, extrapyramidal reaction, dizziness, seizures, Parkinson syndrome

Gastrointestinal: Diarrhea

Hematologic: Blood dyscrasias

Ocular: Blurred vision

Miscellaneous: Hypersensitivity skin reactions

Signs & Symptoms of Acute Overdose Hypotension, seizures, CNS depression

Toxicodynamics/Kinetics

Onset of action:

Oral: Antiemetic effects occur within 10-40 minutes

I.M.: Within 15-35 minutes

Duration: 3-4 hours

Absorption: ~60%

Distribution: Unknown

Metabolism: Hepatic

Elimination: Renal, biliary

Usual Dosage Rectal use is contraindicated in neonates and premature infants

Children:

Rectal: <14 kg: 100 mg 3-4 times/day

Oral, rectal: 14-40 kg: 100-200 mg 3-4 times/day

Adults:
Oral: 250 mg 3-4 times/day
I.M., rectal: 200 mg 3-4 times/day

Contraindications Benzocaine, hypersensitivity to trimethobenzamide or any component; injection contraindicated in children and suppositories are contraindicated in premature infants or neonates

Warnings Use in patients with acute vomiting should be **avoided**; may mask emesis due to Reye's syndrome or mimic CNS effects of Reye's syndrome in patients with emesis of other etiologies

Dosage Forms
Capsule: 100 mg, 250 mg
Injection: 100 mg/mL (2 mL, 20 mL)
Suppository, rectal: 100 mg, 200 mg

Stability Store injection at room temperature; protect from heat and from freezing; use only clear solutions

Overdosage Treatment
Decontamination: Lavage/activated charcoal; charcoal may need to be given in multiple doses for adequate decontamination
Supportive therapy: Initiate support with fluids, norepinephrine may be useful for hypotension; hypoperfusion states may respond to inotropic support with dobutamine. Bradyarrhythmia or ventricular dysrhythmia may respond to sodium bicarbonate or phenytoin; must avoid class 1A and 1C antiarrhythmics. Torsade de pointes may respond to magnesium; seizures should be managed with benzodiazepines or barbiturates; extrapyramidal reactions should be managed with diphenhydramine or benztropine.
Enhancement of elimination: Multiple dosing of charcoal may not be effective

Drug Interactions May antagonize the anticoagulant effect of warfarin; phenothiazines, barbiturates, belladonna derivatives

Pregnancy Risk Factor C

Patient Information May cause drowsiness

Nursing Implications Use only clear solution

Additional Information Note: Less effective than phenothiazines but may be associated with fewer side effects; rectal is ~60% absorbed

Specific References
Kaan SK and Eshelman FN, "The Antiemetic Effects of Trimethobenzamide During Chemotherapy: A Controlled Study," *Curr Ther Res*, 1979, 26:210-3.
Ku LL, Ward CO, and Durgan JM, "A Clinical Study of Drug Interaction and Anticoagulant Therapy," *Drug Intell Clin Pharm*, 1970, 4:300-6.

Trimethoprim and Sulfamethoxazole *see* Co-trimoxazole *on page 242*

1,3,7-Trimethylxanthine *see* Caffeine *on page 175*

Trimetrexate Glucuronate (tri me trex' ate)

Related Information
Methotrexate *on page 515*
Toxicities of Chemotherapeutic Agents *on page 1631-1633*

CAS Number 52128-38-5; 82952-64-5

Brand Names Neutrexin™

Synonyms CI-898; JB-11

Use Alternative therapy for the treatment of moderate-to-severe *Pneumocystis carinii* pneumonia (PCP) in immunocompromised patients, including patients with acquired immunodeficiency syndrome (AIDS), who are intolerant of, or are refractory to, co-trimoxazole therapy or for whom co-trimoxazole is contraindicated

Cancers utilized in: Acute lymphocytic leukemia, breast cancer, colorectal, esophageal, nonsmall cell lung cancer, refractory squamous head and neck

Mechanism of Action Exerts an antimicrobial effect through potent inhibition of the enzyme dihydrofolate reductase (DHFR); similar to methotrexate

Adverse Reactions
Central nervous system: Convulsions, fever
Dermatologic: Rash, hyperpigmentation, radiation recall rash
Gastrointestinal: Stomatitis, nausea, vomiting
Hematologic: Neutropenia, thrombocytopenia, anemia
Hepatic: Elevated liver function tests
Neuromuscular & skeletal: Paresthesia
Renal: Serum creatinine (increased)
Miscellaneous: Flu-like illness, hypersensitivity reactions

Signs & Symptoms of Acute Overdose Leukopenia or neutropenia (agranulocytosis, granulocytopenia)

Toxicodynamics/Kinetics
Distribution: V_d: 0.62 L/kg (0.46 L/kg in pediatric patients)
(Continued)

Trimetrexate Glucuronate *(Continued)*

Protein binding: 98%
Bioavailability: 44%
Metabolism: Extensive in the liver
Half-life: 15-17 hours

Usual Dosage Adults: I.V.: 45 mg/m^2 once daily over 60 minutes for 21 days; it is necessary to reduce the dose in patients with liver dysfunction, although no specific recommendations exist

Administration Reconstituted solution should be filtered (0.22 μM) prior to further dilution; final solution should be clear, hue will range from colorless to pale yellow; trimetrexate forms a precipitate instantly upon contact with chloride ion or leucovorin, therefore it should not be added to solutions containing sodium chloride or other anions; trimetrexate and leucovorin solutions **must** be administered separately; intravenous lines should be flushed with at least 10 mL of D_5W between trimetrexate and leucovorin

Contraindications Previous hypersensitivity to trimetrexate or methotrexate, severe existing myelosuppression

Warnings Must be administered with concurrent leucovorin to avoid potentially serious or life-threatening toxicities; leucovorin therapy must extend for 72 hours past the last dose of trimetrexate; use with caution in patients with mild myelosuppression, severe hepatic or renal dysfunction, hypoproteinemia, hypoalbuminemia, or previous extensive myelosuppressive therapies

Dosage Forms Powder for injection: 25 mg

Stability Reconstituted I.V. solution is stable for 24 hours at room temperature or 7 days when refrigerated; intact vials should be refrigerated at 2°C to 8°C

Reference Range Peak plasma level:
Oral: 3 μg/L after 60 mg/m^2 dose
I.V.: 12 nmol/L after 30 mg/m^2 dose

Overdosage Treatment
Decontamination: Ipecac or lavage/activated charcoal with cathartic
Supportive therapy: Severe bone marrow toxicity can result from overdose; leucovorin rescue can reduce the toxicity; administer as quickly as possible 10 mg/m^2 (5-15 mg) every 6 hours for 72 hours
Enhancement of elimination: Multiple dosing of activated charcoal is effective; renal excretion is optimized at a urinary pH of 7.0. Charcoal hemoperfusion, hydration, and urinary alkalinization may enhance elimination and prevent precipitation in renal tubules; not dialyzable (0% to 5%)

Antidote(s)
Folic Acid *on page 1430*
Leucovorin Calcium *on page 1437*

Test Interactions Mild creatinine elevation, mild liver function test elevation

Drug Interactions
Decreased effect of pneumococcal vaccine
Increased toxicity (infection rates) of yellow fever vaccine

Pregnancy Risk Factor D

Monitoring Parameters Check and record patient's temperature daily
Lab tests:
- Hematology (absolute neutrophil counts (ANC)), platelets
- Renal functions (serum creatinine, BUN)
- Hepatic function (ALT, AST, alkaline phosphatase)

Patient Information Report promptly any fever, rash, flu-like symptoms, numbness or tingling in the extremities, nausea, vomiting, abdominal pain, mouth sores, increased bruising or bleeding, black tarry stools

Nursing Implications Notify primary physician if there is:
Fever ≥103°F
Generalized rash
Seizures
Bleeding from any site
Uncontrolled nausea/vomiting
Laboratory abnormalities which warrant dose modification
Any other clinical adverse event or laboratory abnormality occurring in therapy which is judged as serious for that patient or which causes unexplained effects or concern

Initiate "Bleeding Precautions" for platelet counts ≤50,000/mm^3

Initiate "Infection Control Measures" for absolute neutrophil counts (ANC) ≤1000/mm^3

Additional Information Not a vesicant; methotrexate derivative; incompatible with foscarnet

Specific References
Bertino JR, "Folate Antagonists: Toward Improving the Therapeutic Index and Development of New Analogs," *J Clin Pharmacol*, 1990, 30(4):291-5.
Donehower RC, "Understanding Trimetrexate Toxicity," *J Natl Cancer Inst*, 1988, 80(16):1268-9.

Levien TL and Baker DE, "Reviews of Trimetrexate and Oxadrolone," *Hosp Pharm*, 1994, 29:696-708.

Trimipramine Maleate (trye mi' pra meen)

CAS Number 521-78-8; 739-71-9

Brand Names Surmontil®

Synonyms Trimepramine

Use Treatment of various forms of depression, often in conjunction with psychotherapy

Mechanism of Action Increases the synaptic concentration of serotonin and/or norepinephrine in the central nervous system by inhibition of their reuptake by the presynaptic neuronal membrane

Adverse Reactions

Cardiovascular: Postural hypotension, cardiac arrhythmias, tachycardia, sudden death

Central nervous system: Sedation, asthenia, fatigue, anxiety, impaired cognitive function, seizures have occurred occasionally

Endocrine & metabolic: Syndrome of inappropriate antidiuretic hormone

Gastrointestinal: Dry mouth, constipation

Genitourinary: Urinary retention

Hematologic: Agranulocytosis, eosinophilia, may cause alterations in bleeding time, thrombocytopenia

Hepatic: Jaundice

Neuromuscular & skeletal: Tremors

Ocular: Blurred vision, intraocular pressure (increased), mydriasis, nystagmus

Miscellaneous: Allergic reactions

Signs & Symptoms of Acute Overdose Agitation, confusion, hallucinations, urinary retention, hypothermia, hypotension, intraocular pressure (increased), dementia, neuroleptic malignant syndrome, tachycardia, seizures, coma, leukopenia; neutropenia; agranulocytosis; granulocytopenia

Toxicodynamics/Kinetics

Absorption: Rapid from the gastrointestinal tract

Distribution: V_d: 17-48 L/kg; distributed widely in the body

Protein binding: 95%

Metabolism: Undergoes significant first-pass metabolism metabolized in the liver to desmethyl trimipramine

Half-life: 20-26 hours

Time to peak serum concentration: Within 6 hours

Elimination: Urine

Usual Dosage Adults: Oral: 50-150 mg/day as a single bedtime dose up to a maximum of 200 mg/day outpatient and 300 mg/day inpatient

Contraindications Narrow-angle glaucoma; avoid use during pregnancy and lactation

Warnings Use with caution in patients with cardiovascular disease, conduction disturbances, seizure disorders, urinary retention, hyperthyroidism or those receiving thyroid replacement; avoid use during lactation; use with caution in pregnancy; do not discontinue abruptly in patients receiving chronic high-dose therapy

Dosage Forms Capsule: 25 mg, 50 mg, 100 mg

Reference Range An oral dose of 50 mg yields a peak serum level of 260 nmol/L

Overdosage Treatment

Decontamination: Do **not** induce emesis; gastric lavage/activated charcoal with cathartic is useful; multiple dosing of activated charcoal may be useful

Supportive therapy: Following initiation of essential overdose management, toxic symptoms should be treated. Ventricular arrhythmias often respond to phenytoin 15-20 mg/kg (adults) with concurrent systemic alkalinization (sodium bicarbonate 0.5-2 mEq/kg I.V.). Arrhythmias unresponsive to this therapy may respond to lidocaine 1 mg/kg I.V. followed by a titrated infusion. Physostigmine (1-2 mg I.V. slowly for adults or 0.5 mg I.V. slowly for children) may be indicated in reversing anticholinergic-induced movement disorders or seizures, but only as **a last resort**. Seizures usually respond to lorazepam or diazepam I.V. boluses (5-10 mg for adults up to 30 mg or 0.25-0.4 mg/kg/dose for children up to 10 mg/dose). If seizures are unresponsive or recur, phenytoin or phenobarbital may be required.

Antidote(s)

Sodium Bicarbonate *on page 1467*

Test Interactions Increases glucose; may cross react with phenothiazine assay

Drug Interactions May not have similar interaction with phenelzine as imipramine

Pregnancy Risk Factor C

Monitoring Parameters Cardiac status/EKG

Patient Information To prevent dizziness, lie down for approximately 30 minutes after each dose and avoid abrupt changes of position

(Continued)

Trimipramine Maleate *(Continued)*

Additional Information May cause alterations in bleeding time

Specific References

Druid H and Holmgren P, "Fatal Seizures Associated With Trimipramine Overdose," *Forensic Sci Int*, 1991, 49(1):75-9.

Nebinger P and Koel M, "Specificity Data of the Tricyclic Antidepressants Assay by Fluorescent Polarization Immunoassay," *J Anal Toxicol*, 1990, 14(4):219-21.

Remy A-J, Larrey D, Pageaux G-P, et al, "Cross Hepatotoxicity Between Tricyclic Antidepressants and Phenothiazines," *Eur J Gastroenterol Hepatol*, 1995, 7:373-6.

Trimox® *see* Amoxicillin *on page 121*

Triniad® *see* Isoniazid *on page 443*

Trinitrin *see* Nitroglycerin *on page 566*

Trinosin® *see* Adenosine Triphosphate *on page 90*

Triostat™ *see* Liothyronine Sodium *on page 471*

Tripelennamine (tri pel enn' a meen)

Related Information

H1-Antihistamine Comparison *on page 1649*

CAS Number 91-81-6 (base); 6138-56-3 (citrate); 154-69-8 (hydrochloride)

Brand Names PBZ®; PBZ-SR®

Synonyms Pyribenzamine®; Super Blue; Tripelennamine Citrate; Tripelennamine Hydrochloride

Use Perennial and seasonal allergic rhinitis and other allergic symptoms including rash

Mechanism of Action Competes with histamine for H_1-receptor sites on effector cells in the gastrointestinal tract, blood vessels, and respiratory tract

Adverse Reactions

Central nervous system: Drowsiness
Gastrointestinal: Nausea, vomiting, dry mouth
Genitourinary: Urinary retention
Ocular: Nystagmus

Signs & Symptoms of Acute Overdose CNS stimulation or CNS depression; mydriasis, ataxia, athetosis, flushing

Toxicodynamics/Kinetics

Onset of action: Within 15-30 minutes
Duration: 4-6 hours (up to 8 hours with PBZ-SR®)
Metabolism: Almost completely in the liver
Elimination: Urine

Usual Dosage Oral:

Infants and Children: 5 mg/kg/day in 4-6 divided doses, up to 300 mg/day maximum

Adults: 25-50 mg every 4-6 hours, extended release tablets 100 mg morning and evening up to 100 mg every 8 hours

Contraindications Hypersensitivity to tripelennamine or any component, narrow-angle glaucoma, bladder neck obstruction, symptomatic prostate hypertrophy, asthmatic attacks, and stenosing peptic ulcer

Dosage Forms

Elixir, as citrate: 37.5 mg/5 mL (473 mL)
Tablet, as hydrochloride: 25 mg, 50 mg
Tablet, extended release, as hydrochloride: 100 mg

Reference Range Peak serum concentration: 60-200 μg/L

Overdosage Treatment There is no specific treatment for an antihistamine overdose, however, most of its clinical toxicity is due to anticholinergic effects. Anticholinesterase inhibitors may be useful by reducing acetylcholinesterase. Anticholinesterase inhibitors include physostigmine, neostigmine, pyridostigmine and edrophonium. For anticholinergic overdose with severe life-threatening symptoms, physostigmine 1-2 mg (0.5 or 0.02 mg/kg for children) I.V., slowly may be given to reverse these effects.

Pregnancy Risk Factor B

Patient Information Do not crush extended release tablets; urinary hesitancy can be reduced if patient voids just prior to taking drug; may cause drowsiness; swallow whole, do not crush or chew sustained release product; avoid alcohol, may impair coordination and judgment

Nursing Implications Raise bed rails, institute safety measures, assist with ambulation

Additional Information Do not crush extended release tablets; urinary hesitancy can be reduced if patient voids just prior to taking drug; occasionally associated with pentazocine abuse (Ts and blues)

Tripelennamine citrate: PBZ® elixir
Tripelennamine hydrochloride: PBZ® tablet, PBZ-SR® tablet

Specific References

Monforte JR, Gault R, Smialek J, et al, "Toxicological and Pathological Findings in Fatalities Involving Pentazocine and Tripelennamine," *J Forensic Sci*, 1983, 28(1):90-101.
Yeh SY, Todd GD, Johnson RE, et al, "The Pharmacokinetics of Pentazocine and Tripelennamine," *Clin Pharmacol Ther*, 1986, 39(6):669-76.

Tripelennamine Citrate *see* Tripelennamine *on previous page*

Tripelennamine Hydrochloride *see* Tripelennamine *on previous page*

Triphacycline® *see* Tetracycline *on page 732*

Triptazine® *see* Amitriptyline and Perphenazine *on page 115*

TripTone® Caplets® [OTC] *see* Dimenhydrinate *on page 289*

Tritace® *see* Ramipril *on page 673*

Trittico® *see* Trazodone Hydrochloride *on page 765*

Trocal® [OTC] *see* Dextromethorphan Hydrobromide *on page 270*

Trodon® *see* Tramadol Hydrochloride *on page 762*

Troglitazone

Synonyms CS-045

Use Investigational: Treatment of noninsulin-dependent diabetes mellitus

Mechanism of Action Thiazolidinedione agent which potentiates insulin sensitivity in liver, muscle, and fat; no change in insulin secretion occurs

Adverse Reactions

Cardiovascular: Palpitations
Dermatologic: Skin rash
Endocrine & metabolic: Hypoglycemia
Gastrointestinal: Nausea, vomiting, epigastric pain, diarrhea
Hematologic: Anemia (5%)

Toxicodynamics/Kinetics Onset of hypoglycemic effect: 2-6 weeks at steady-state levels

Usual Dosage Oral: 200 mg twice daily

Contraindications Hypersensitivity to troglitazone; diabetic ketoacidosis

Warnings Use with caution in elderly, renal or hepatic insufficiency, patients with infection or pregnancy

Overdosage Treatment

Decontamination: Lavage/activated charcoal with cathartic
Supportive therapy: Glucose (25 g I.V.) is mainstay of therapy; glucagon (1-5 mg I.V., I.M., or S.C.) (0.03-0.1 mg/kg in pediatrics) will have limited benefit; diazoxide is a third-line agent (3-8 mg/kg/24 hours)
Enhancement of elimination: Multiple dosing of activated charcoal may be more effective for this agent than for other oral hypoglycemics due to enterohepatic recirculation of glipizide; peritoneal dialysis has been used with some success; urine alkalinization is also useful

Antidote(s)

Dextrose *on page 1409*

Test Interactions Can cause an increase in serum lactate dehydrogenase levels; lowers plasma triglyceride levels

Monitoring Parameters Blood sugar

Additional Information May also lower blood pressure in nondiabetic obese patients

Specific References

Keen H, "Insulin Resistance and the Prevention of Diabetes Mellitus," *N Engl J Med*, 1994, 331(18):1226-7.
Nolan JJ, Ludvik B, Beerdsen P, et al, "Improvement in Glucose Tolerance and Insulin Resistance in Obese Subjects Treated With Troglitazone," *N Engl J Med*, 1994, 331(18):1188-93.

Tronolane® [OTC] *see* Pramoxine Hydrochloride *on page 636*

Tronothane® [OTC] *see* Pramoxine Hydrochloride *on page 636*

Tropium® *see* Chlordiazepoxide *on page 198*

Truphylline® *see* Aminophylline *on page 110*

Truxal® *see* Chlorprothixene *on page 209*

Truxaletter® *see* Chlorprothixene *on page 209*

Tryptizol® *see* Amitriptyline Hydrochloride *on page 116*

Tussigon® *see* Hydrocodone and Homatropine *on page 407*

Tylenol® [OTC] *see* Acetaminophen *on page 79*

Tylox® *see* Oxycodone and Acetaminophen *on page 584*

Urapidil Hydrochloride (Yu rap' i dil)

CAS Number 34661-75-1; 64887-14-5

Brand Names Ebrantil®; Eupressyl®; Uraprene®

Use Hypertension

Mechanism of Action Alpha$_1$-adrenoceptor antagonist (peripheral vasodilator); a phenylpiperazine derivative of 4-aminouracil

Adverse Reactions
- Cardiovascular: Palpitations, bradycardia, hypotension (orthostatic)
- Central nervous system: Headache, dizziness, fatigue
- Dermatologic: Allergic skin reactions, pruritus
- Gastrointestinal: Nausea
- Renal: Enuresis
- Respiratory: Nasal congestion

Signs & Symptoms of Acute Overdose Hypotension, enuresis, eosinophilia, diarrhea, drowsiness, coagulopathy

Toxicodynamics/Kinetics
- Protein binding: 80%
- Metabolism: Hepatic to p-hydroxylated urapidil – first pass (20%)
- Bioavailability: 70%
- Half-life:
  - Oral: 4.7 hours
  - I.V.: 2.7 hours
- Elimination: Urine (15% to 30% unchanged)

Usual Dosage
- Oral: 30-90 mg twice daily
- I.V.: 25 mg over 20 seconds

Dosage Forms Injection:
- Somatropin, Humatrope®: 5 mg ~13 units (5 mL)
- Somatrem, Protropin®: 5 mg ~13 units (10 mL)

Reference Range Dose of 120 mg can cause a urapidil blood level of 750 ng/mL 3-5 hours postingestion

Overdosage Treatment
- Decontamination: Ipecac or lavage/charcoal
- Supportive therapy: Treat hypotension with fluids or Trendelenburg positioning

Drug Interactions Cimetidine modifies pharmacokinetics such that dosage reduction is necessary

Additional Information 20% as potent as prazosin; may increase plasma renin and catecholamine level

Specific References

Culbertson VL, Bryant PJ, Cady WJ, et al, "Acute Effects of Increasing Doses of Urapidil in Patients With Hypertension," *Clin Pharmacol Ther*, 1986, 39(6):690-6.

Hirschl MM, Seidler D, Zeiner A, et al, "Intravenous Urapidil Versus Sublingual Nifedipine in the Treatment of Hypertensive Urgencies," *Am J Emerg Med*, 1993, 11(6):653-6.

Jonville AP, Echenberger J, Dutertre JP, et al, "Urapidil and Enuresis," *Lancet*, 1992, 339(8794):688.

Langtry HD, Mammen GJ, and Sorkin EM, "Urapidil. A Review of Its Pharmacodynamic and Pharmacokinetic Properties, and Therapeutic Potential in the Treatment of Hypertension," *Drugs*, 1989, 38(6):900-40.

van Zwieten PA, "Conclusions on the Position of Urapidil," *Am J Cardiol*, 1989, 64(7):38D-39D.

Uraprene® *see* Urapidil Hydrochloride *on previous page*

Urbadan® *see* Clobazam *on page 224*

Urbanol® *see* Clobazam *on page 224*

Urbanyl® *see* Clobazam *on page 224*

Urecholine® *see* Bethanechol Chloride *on page 154*

Urex® *see* Furosemide *on page 373*

Urfamycin® *see* Thiamphenicol *on page 742*

Uriben® *see* Nalidixic Acid *on page 547*

Uricovac® *see* Benzbromarone *on page 148*

Urinorm® *see* Benzbromarone *on page 148*

Uritol® *see* Furosemide *on page 373*

Urocarb® *see* Bethanechol Chloride *on page 154*

Urocaudal® *see* Triamterene *on page 766*

Urodil® *see* Nitrofurantoin *on page 564*

Urogram® *see* Nalidixic Acid *on page 547*

Urokinase (yoor oh kin' ase)

CAS Number 9039-53-6

Brand Names Abbokinase® Injection; Actosolv®; Alphakinase®; Kisolu®; Natel®; Persolu Richter®; Purochin®; Ukidan®; Uroquidan®; Uroquinasa®

Use Thrombolytic agent used in treatment of recent severe or massive deep vein thrombosis, pulmonary emboli, myocardial infarction, and occluded arteriovenous cannulas; more expensive than streptokinase; not useful on thrombi over 1 week old; useful in clearing clots due to eye hemorrhage (hyphaemia)

Mechanism of Action Promotes thrombolysis by directly activating plasminogen to plasmin, which degrades fibrin, fibrinogen, and other procoagulant plasma proteins

Adverse Reactions

Cardiovascular: Arrhythmias, hypotension

Central nervous system: Headache, chills, hyperthermia (2% to 3%)

Dermatologic: Rash

Gastrointestinal: Nausea, vomiting

Hematologic: Epistaxis, anemia, eye hemorrhage

Respiratory: Bronchospasm

Miscellaneous: Periorbital swelling, angioneurotic edema, anaphylaxis, bleeding at sites of percutaneous trauma, sweating

Signs & Symptoms of Acute Overdose Epistaxis, bleeding gums, hemoptysis, hematuria, gastrointestinal bleeding, coagulopathy, ocular hemorrhage, intracranial hemorrhage, hematoma, spontaneous ecchymoses, oozing at catheter site

Toxicodynamics/Kinetics

Onset of action: I.V.: Fibrinolysis occurs rapidly

Duration: 4 or more hours

Half-life: 10-20 minutes

Elimination: Cleared by the liver with a small amount excreted in urine and bile

Usual Dosage

Children and Adults: Deep vein thrombosis: I.V.: Loading: 4400 units/kg over 10 minutes, then 4400 units/kg/hour for 12 hours

Adults:

Myocardial infarction: Intracoronary: 750,000 units over 2 hours (6000 units/minute over up to 2 hours)

Occluded I.V. catheters:

5000 units (use only Abbokinase® Open Cath) in each lumen over 1-2 minutes, leave in lumen for 1-4 hours, then aspirate; may repeat with 10,000 units in each lumen if 5000 units fails to clear the catheter; **do not infuse into the patient**; volume to instill into catheter is equal to the volume of the catheter

I.V. infusion: 200 units/kg/hour in each lumen for 12-48 hours at a rate of at least 20 mL/hour

(Continued)

Urokinase *(Continued)*

Dialysis patients: 5000 units is administered in each lumen over 1-2 minutes; leave urokinase in lumen for 1-2 days, then aspirate

Clot lysis (large vessel thrombi): Loading: I.V.: 4400 units/kg over 10 minutes, increase to 6000 units/kg/hour; maintenance: 4400-6000 units/kg/hour adjusted to achieve clot lysis or patency of affected vessel; doses up to 50,000 units/kg/hour have been used. **Note:** Therapy should be initiated as soon as possible after diagnosis of thrombi and continued until clot is dissolved (usually 24-72 hours).

Anterior eye chamber clots: 5000 units dissolved in 2 mL of sodium chloride (0.9%) for clot irrigation

Intravitreous hemorrhage: 25,000 units in 0.3 mL water

Acute pulmonary embolism: Three treatment alternatives: 3 million unit dosage

Alternative 1: 12-hour infusion: 4400 units/kg (2000 units/lb) bolus over 10 minutes followed by 4400 units/kg/hour (2000 units/lb); begin heparin 1000 units/hour approximately 3-4 hours after completion of urokinase infusion or when PTT is <100 seconds

Alternative 2: 2-hour infusion: 1 million unit bolus over 10 minutes followed by 2 million units over 110 minutes; begin heparin 1000 units/hour approximately 3-4 hours after completion of urokinase infusion or when PTT is <100 seconds

Alternative 3: Bolus dose only: 15,000 units/kg over 10 minutes; begin heparin 1000 units/hour approximately 3-4 hours after completion of urokinase infusion or when PTT is <100 seconds

Administration I.V. infusion: Usual concentration: 1250-1500 units/mL; maximum concentration not yet defined

Contraindications Hypersensitivity to urokinase or any component; active internal bleeding; CVA (within 2 months); brain carcinoma, bacterial endocarditis, anticoagulant therapy, intracranial or intraspinal surgery, surgery or trauma within past 10 days

Warnings Use with caution in patients with severe hypertension, recent L.P., patients receiving I.M. administration of medications, patients with trauma or surgery in the last 10 days

Dosage Forms

Powder for injection: 250,000 units (5 mL)

Powder for injection, catheter clear: 5000 units (1 mL)

Stability Store in refrigerator; reconstitute by gently rolling and tilting; do not shake; contains no preservatives, should not be reconstituted until immediately before using, discard unused portion; stable at room temperature for 24 hours after reconstitution

Overdosage Treatment

Supportive therapy: Treat bleeding complications with transfusions of red blood cells, fresh frozen plasma, and cryoprecipitate; do not administer dextran; although human overdose data is lacking, administration of aminocaproic acid (Amicar®) at a dose of 3-5 g I.V. followed by an infusion rate of 1-1.25 g/hour may be useful

Test Interactions Earlier peaks of creatine phosphokinase isoenzyme can occur

Drug Interactions Increased toxicity (increased bleeding) with anticoagulants, antiplatelet drugs, aspirin, indomethacin, dextran; increased levels of thiotepa can occur

Pregnancy Risk Factor B

Monitoring Parameters CBC, reticulocyte, platelet count, DIC panel (fibrinogen, plasminogen, FDP, D Dimers, PT, PTT), thrombosis panel (AT-III, protein C), urinalysis, ACT

Nursing Implications Use 0.22 or 0.45 micron filter during I.V. therapy

Additional Information Abbokinase® Open Cath 5000 unit product is **not** for systemic administration; it must be aspirated out of the catheter

Specific References

de Boer A and van Griensven JMT, "Drug Interactions With Thrombolytic Agents," *Clin Pharmacokinet*, 1995, 28:315-26.

Dehmer GJ, Gresalfi N, Daly D, et al, "Impairment of Fibrinolysis by Streptokinase, Urokinase, and Recombinant Tissue-Type Plasminogen Activator in the Presence of Radiographic Contrast Agents," *J Am Coll Cardiol*, 1995, 25(5):1069-75.

Ejaz AA, Aijaz M, Nawab ZM, et al, "Hemorrhagic Bullas as a Complication of Urokinase Therapy for Hemodialysis Catheter Thrombosis," *Am J Nephrol*, 1995, 15:178-9.

Haire WD and Lieberman RP, "Thrombosed Central Venous Catheters: Restoring Function With 6-Hour Urokinase Infusion After Failure of Bolus Urokinase," *J Parenteral Enteral Nutr*, 1992, 16(2):129-32.

Panteghini M and Pagani F, "Isoforms of Creatine Kinase Isoenzymes in Serum in Acute Myocardial Infarction After Intracoronary Thrombolysis," *Clin Chem*, 1987, 33(11):2039-42.

Pavlou H, Panagiotopoulos A, Graham A, et al, "Urokinase-Induced Cytohepatolysis in a Patient With Acute Myocardial Infarction," *Eur Heart J*, 1995, 16:291-2.

Tenney RD and Sasahara AA, "Urokinase Dissolution of a Right Atrial Thrombus," *Arch Intern Med*, 1989, 149(2):475.

Urolin® *see* Chlorthalidone *on page 210*

Urolong® *see* Nitrofurantoin *on page 564*

Uronorm® *see* Cinoxacin *on page 214*

Uropan® *see* Nalidixic Acid *on page 547*

Uroplus® DS *see* Co-trimoxazole *on page 242*

Uroplus® SS *see* Co-trimoxazole *on page 242*

Uroquidan® *see* Urokinase *on page 779*

Uroquinasa® *see* Urokinase *on page 779*

Uroxacin® *see* Cinoxacin *on page 214*

Uvilon® *see* Piperazine Citrate *on page 629*

Vagilen *see* Metronidazole *on page 526*

Valaciclovir *see* Valacyclovir Hydrochloride *on this page*

Valacyclovir Hydrochloride

Related Information

Acyclovir *on page 88*

Brand Names Valtrex®

Synonyms Valaciclovir

Use Herpes simplex genital infections; may be effective in reducing postherpetic neuralgia in herpes zoster infections

Mechanism of Action Inhibits DNA synthesis and viral replication by competing with deoxyguanosine triphosphate for viral DNA polymerase (thymidine kinase) and being incorporated into viral DNA

Adverse Reactions

Central nervous system: Headache, drowsiness, delirium, coma, dizziness, seizures, mania, hyperacusis, pain, insomnia, visual and tactile hallucinations, confusion, agitation, encephalopathy, mental depression, fever, hyperthermia

Dermatologic: Skin rash

Gastrointestinal: Nausea, vomiting, anorexia, diarrhea, colitis

Hematologic: Bone marrow depression, thrombocytopenia, leukopenia

Hepatic: Elevation of liver enzymes

Local: Phlebitis at injection site, local pain and stinging with topical use

Neuromuscular & skeletal: Tremors, tremulousness, myoclonus

Renal: Can cause obstructive nephrotoxicity due to crystalluria at renal concentrations >2.5 mg/mL, impaired renal function (dose dependent)

Miscellaneous: Sore throat, sweating

Toxicodynamics/Kinetics

Absorption: Oral: Rapid

Metabolism: Converted to acyclovir rapidly

Half-life: Valacyclovir: 30 minutes; acyclovir: 3 hours

Elimination: Renal

Usual Dosage Herpes simplex: 1 g twice daily for 5 days

Warnings Use with caution in patients with pre-existing renal disease or in those receiving other nephrotoxic drugs concurrently; maintain adequate urine output during the first 2 hours after I.V. infusion; use with caution in patients with underlying neurologic abnormalities, serious hepatic or electrolyte abnormalities, or substantial hypoxia; appears to reduce the length and severity of chickenpox, but should not be used unless patient is immunosuppressed

Reference Range After a 1 g oral dose, peak serum acyclovir levels were ~5.65 μg/mL

Overdosage Treatment

Decontamination: Ipecac or lavage/activated charcoal with cathartic

Supportive therapy: Renal toxicity and crystalluria can be managed with intravenous fluid hydration

Enhancement of elimination: Multiple dosing of activated charcoal may be effective; hemodialysis can remove about 60% of total body burden; exchange transfusion is not useful

Additional Information Due to higher bioavailability than acyclovir, plasma acyclovir levels are 3-5 times higher with valacyclovir administration as compared with acyclovir administration

Specific References

Jacobson MA, "Valaciclovir (BW256U87): the L-Valyl Ester of Acyclovir," *J Med Virol*, 1993, Suppl 1:150-3.

Weller S, Blum MR, Doucette M, et al, "Pharmacokinetics of the Acyclovir Pro-Drug Valaciclovir After Escalating Single and Multiple-Dose Administration to Normal Volunteers," *Clin Pharmacol Ther*, 1993, 54(6):595-605.

Valeans® *see* Alprazolam *on page 99*

Valium® *see* Diazepam *on page 271*

Valkote® *see* Valproic Acid and Derivatives *on this page*

Valoron® *see* Tilidine Hydrochloride *on page 752*

Valproate Semisodium *see* Valproic Acid and Derivatives *on this page*

Valproate Sodium *see* Valproic Acid and Derivatives *on this page*

Valproic Acid *see* Valproic Acid and Derivatives *on this page*

Valproic Acid and Derivatives (val proe' ik)

Related Information

Drugs and Chemicals Proven to be Teratogenic in Humans *on page 1572-1575*

CAS Number 99-66-1; 76584-70-8; 1069-66-5; 77372-61-3; 2430-27-5

Brand Names Depakene®; Depakote®; Epilim®; Ergenyl®; Leptilan®; Valkote®

Synonyms Dipropylacetic Acid; Divalproex Sodium; DPA; 2-Propylpentanoic Acid; 2-Propylvaleric Acid; Sodium Valproate; Valproate Semisodium; Valproate Sodium; Valproic Acid

Use Management of simple and complex absence seizures; mixed seizure types; myoclonic and generalized tonic-clonic (grand mal) seizures; may be effective in partial seizures and infantile spasm; approved for migraine prophylaxis (after other traditional agents have failed); acute and maintenance therapy for bipolar disease

Mechanism of Action Causes increased availability of gamma-aminobutyric acid (GABA), an inhibitory neurotransmitter, to brain neurons or may enhance the action of GABA or mimic its action at postsynaptic receptor sites

Adverse Reactions

Central nervous system: Drowsiness, irritability, confusion, restlessness, hyperactivity, psychosis, malaise, visual hallucinations, extrapyramidal syndrome, headache, ataxia

Dermatologic: Alopecia, erythema multiforme

Endocrine & metabolic: Hyperammonemia, hypernatremia with sodium valproate, weight gain

Gastrointestinal: Nausea, vomiting, diarrhea, pancreatitis, abdominal cramps, anorexia, hemorrhage

Hematologic: Thrombocytopenia, prolongation of bleeding time, leukopenia, pancytopenia

Hepatic: Transient liver enzymes (increased), liver failure (especially noted in children <2 years of age), fatty degeneration of liver

Neuromuscular & skeletal: Tremors, chorea

Ocular: Nystagmus

Renal: Enuresis, anuria

Signs & Symptoms of Acute Overdose Coma, cholestatic jaundice, jaundice, photophobia, hypothyroidism, hyporeflexia, hyperglycemia, nephritis, myoclonus, night terrors, mania, dementia, ileus, Fanconi's syndrome, extrapyramidal reaction, pseudotumor cerebri, migraine headache (exacerbation of), enuresis, encephalopathy, coagulopathy, nystagmus, tremors, irritability, hyperactivity, confusion, cerebral edema, optic nerve atrophy, metabolic acidosis, miosis, hyperthermia, hypothermia, systemic lupus erythematosus (SLE), leukopenia; neutropenia; agranulocytosis; granulocytopenia

Toxicodynamics/Kinetics

Absorption: Rapid from gastrointestinal tract; slight delay when taken with food

Distribution: V_d: 0.1-0.4 L/kg; distributed rapidly throughout body

Protein binding: 80% to 90% (dose dependent)

Metabolism: Extensive in the liver to glucuronide salt

Half-life:

- Children: 4-14 hours, increased half-life in neonates and patients with liver disease
- Adults: 8-17 hours
- In overdose: 19-20 hours

Time to peak serum concentration: Within 1-4 hours; 3-5 hours after divalproex (enteric coated)

Elimination: 2% to 3% excreted unchanged in urine; clearance: 12.7 mL/minute

Usual Dosage Children and Adults:

Oral: Initial: 10-15 mg/kg/day in 1-3 divided doses; increase by 5-10 mg/kg/day at weekly intervals until therapeutic levels are achieved; maintenance: 30-60 mg/kg/day in 2-3 divided doses

Children receiving more than 1 anticonvulsant (ie, polytherapy) may require doses up to 100 mg/kg/day in 3-4 divided doses

Rectal: Dilute syrup 1:1 with water for use as a retention enema; loading dose: 17-20 mg/kg one time; maintenance: 10-15 mg/kg/dose every 8 hours

Dosing adjustment/comments in hepatic impairment: Reduce dose

Contraindications Hypersensitivity to valproic acid or derivatives or any component; hepatic dysfunction, spontaneous bleeding and bruising

Warnings Hepatic failure resulting in fatalities has occurred in patients; children <2 years of age especially those on polytherapy are at considerable risk; hepatitis has been reported after 3 days to 6 months of therapy; monitor patients closely for appearance of malaise, asthenia, facial edema, anorexia, jaundice, and vomiting; may cause severe thrombocytopenia, bleeding

Dosage Forms

Capsule, sprinkle, as divalproex sodium (Depakote® Sprinkle®): 125 mg

Capsule, as valproic acid (Depakene®): 250 mg

Syrup, as sodium valproate (Depakene®): 250 mg/5mL (5 mL, 50 mL, 480 mL)

Tablet, delayed release, as divalproex sodium (Depakote®): 125 mg, 250 mg, 500 mg

Reference Range

Therapeutic: 50-100 μg/mL (SI: 350-690 μmol/L); seizure control may improve at levels >100 μg/mL (SI: >690 μmol/L)

Toxic: Toxicity may occur at levels of 100-150 μg/mL (SI: 690-1040 μmol/L)

Overdosage Treatment

Decontamination: Emesis or lavage/activated charcoal with cathartic

Supportive therapy: Supportive treatment is necessary; naloxone has been used to reverse CNS depressant effects, but may block action of other anticonvulsants; carnitine (1 g 3 times/day) is useful in reducing ammonia level

Enhancement of elimination: Multiple dosing of activated charcoal is effective; hemoperfusion and/or hemodialysis may be effective; (0% to 5%); not hemodialyzed in a normal dose situation due to high protein-binding of valproic acid, but in an overdose situation, whereupon protein binding is decreased, hemodialysis may be effective. Simultaneous "in series" hemodialysis/hemoperfusion has been demonstrated to decrease valproate half-life to <2 hours.

Antidote(s)

Naloxone Hydrochloride *on page 1447*

Test Interactions False-positive result for urine ketones; causes high sodium, hypocalcemia, high glucose

Diagnostic Tests/Procedures

Valproic Acid, Blood *on page 1377*

Drug Interactions May cause increased levels of phenobarbital and either increased or decreased levels of effectiveness of phenytoin; levels of these drugs must be followed and dosages adjusted accordingly when valproic acid is added to the anticonvulsant regimen; increased prothrombin time may result with concomitant valproic acid and warfarin therapy

Pregnancy Risk Factor D (1st trimester use causally associated with neural tube defects)

Monitoring Parameters Liver enzymes, CBC with platelets, respiratory status

Patient Information Take with food or milk; do not chew, break, or crush the tablet or capsule; do not administer with carbonated drinks; report any sore throat, fever, or fatigue

Nursing Implications Do not crush enteric-coated drug product or capsules

Additional Information Tremors may indicate overdosage; monitor serum ammonium; may cause increase in alkaline phosphatase in pediatric patients

Sodium content of valproate sodium syrup (5 mL): 23 mg (1 mEq)

Divalproex sodium: Depakote®

Valproate sodium: Depakene® syrup

Valproic acid: Depakene® capsule

Specific References

Alberto G, Erickson T, Popiel R, et al, "Central Nervous System Manifestation of a Valproic Acid Overdose Responsive to Naloxone," *Ann Emerg Med*, 1989, 18(8):889-91.

Andersen GI and Ritland S, "Life Threatening Intoxication With Sodium Valproate," *Clin Toxicol*, 1995, 33(3):279-84.

Browne TR, "Drug Therapy: Valproic Acid," *N Engl J Med*, 1980, 302(12):661-6.

Costello LE and Suppes TA, "A Clinically Significant Interaction Between Clozapine and Valproate," *J Clin Psychopharmacol*, 1995, 15:139-41.

Evans RJ, Miranda RN, Jordan J, et al, "Fatal Acute Pancreatitis Caused by Valproic Acid," *Am J Forensic Med Pathol*, 1995, 16:62-5.

Guthrie SK, Stoysich AM, Bader G, et al, "Hypothesized Interaction Between Valproic Acid and Warfarin," *J Clin Psychopharmacol*, 1995, 15:138-9.

Kerrick JM, Wolff DL, and Graves NM, "Predicting Unbound Phenytoin Concentrations in Patients Receiving Valproic Acid: A Comparison of Two Prediction Methods," *Ann Pharmacother*, 1995, 29:470-4.

Kulick SK and Kramer DA, "Hyperammonemia Secondary to Valproic Acid as a Cause of Lethargy in a Postictal Patient," *Ann Emerg Med*, 1993, 22(3):610-2.

Leao M, "Valproate as a Cause of Hyperammonemia in Heterozygotes With Ornithine-Transcarbamylase Deficiency," *Neurology*, 1995, 45(3 Pt 1):593-4.

Marbury TC, Lee CS, Bruni J, et al, "Hemodialysis of Valproic Acid in Uremic Patients," *Dialysis and Transplantation*, 1980, 9:961.

Perrone J, Meyer R, Hoffman RS, et al, "Hypernatremia Associated With Chronic Sodium Valproate Therapy," *Vet Hum Toxicol*, 1994, 36:372.

Robinson D, Langer A, Casso D, et al, "Pancytopenia and Valproic Acid – A Possible Association," *J Am Geriatr Soc*, 1995, 43(2):198.

Schnabel R, Rambeck B, and Janssen F, "Fatal Intoxication With Sodium Valproate," *Lancet*, 1984, 1(8370):221-2. *Solahia Igaku*, 1995, 37:383-9.

(Continued)

Valproic Acid and Derivatives *(Continued)*

Tank JE and Palmer BF, "Simultaneous "In Series" Hemodialysis and Hemoperfusion in the Management of the Valproic Acid Overdose," *Am J Kidney Dis*, 1993, 22(2):341-4.

Tohen M, Castillo J, Baldessarini RJ, et al, "Blood Dyscrasias With Carbamazepine and Valproate: A Pharmacoepidemiological Study of 2,228 Patients at Risk," *Am J Psychiatry*, 1995, 152(3):413-8.

Valrelease® *see* Diazepam *on page 271*

Valsera® *see* Flunitrazepam *on page 354*

Valtrex® *see* Valacyclovir Hydrochloride *on page 781*

Vamate® *see* Hydroxyzine *on page 414*

Vancocin® *see* Vancomycin Hydrochloride *on this page*

Vancoled® Injection *see* Vancomycin Hydrochloride *on this page*

Vancomycin Hydrochloride (van koe mye' sin)

CAS Number 1404-93-9

Brand Names Lyphocin® Injection; Vancocin®; Vancoled® Injection

Use Treatment of patients with the following infections or conditions:

Infections due to documented or suspected methicillin-resistant *S. aureus* or beta-lactam resistant coagulase negative *Staphylococcus*

Serious or life-threatening infections (ie, endocarditis, meningitis) due to documented or suspected staphylococcal or streptococcal infections in patients who are allergic to penicillins and/or cephalosporins

Empiric therapy of infections associated with gram-positive organisms; used orally for staphylococcal enterocolitis or for antibiotic-associated pseudomembranous colitis produced by *C. difficile*

Mechanism of Action Inhibits bacterial cell wall synthesis by blocking glycopeptide polymerization through binding tightly to D-alanyl-D-alanine portion of cell wall precursor

Adverse Reactions Rapid infusion associated with redneck or redman syndrome: Erythema multiforme-like reaction with intense pruritus, tachycardia, hypotension, rash involving face, neck, upper trunk, back and upper arms

Cardiovascular: Cardiac arrest, hypotension

Central nervous system: Fever, chills, hyperthermia

Dermatologic: Redneck or redman syndrome, rash, macular skin rash

Gastrointestinal: Nausea

Hematologic: Neutropenia, eosinophilia

Local: Phlebitis

Neuromuscular & skeletal: Lower back pain

Otic: Ototoxicity, tinnitus associated with prolonged serum concentration >40 μg/mL

Renal: Nephrotoxicity (higher incidence with trough concentrations >10 μg/mL)

Miscellaneous: Hypersensitivity reactions

Signs & Symptoms of Acute Overdose Leukopenia or neutropenia (agranulocytosis, granulocytopenia); exfoliative dermatitis, lacrimation, thrombocytopenia, dermatitis, tubular necrosis, Stevens-Johnson syndrome, deafness, colitis

Toxicodynamics/Kinetics

Absorption:

- Oral: Poor
- I.M.: Erratic

Distribution: V_d: 0.47-1.25 L/kg; poor CSF penetration

Protein binding: 10%

Half-life, terminal (biphasic):

- Newborns: 6-10 hours
- 3 months to 4 years: 4 hours
- >3 years: 2.2-3 hours
- Adults: 6-8 hours, prolonged significantly with reduced renal function

Time to peak serum concentration: I.V.: Within 45-65 minutes

Elimination: Excreted as unchanged drug in urine (80% to 90%); oral doses excreted primarily in feces

Usual Dosage Initial dosage recommendation: I.V.:

Neonates:

- Postnatal age <7 days:
  - <1200 g: 7.5 mg/kg/dose given every 24 hours
  - 1200-2000 g: 10 mg/kg/dose given every 12 hours
  - >2000 g: 15 mg/kg/dose given every 12 hours
- Postnatal age >7 days:
  - <1200 g: 7.5 mg/kg/dose given every 24 hours
  - ≥1200 g: 10 mg/kg/dose given every 8 hours

Infants >1 month and Children: 40 mg/kg/day in divided doses every 6 hours

Infants >1 month and Children with staphylococcal central nervous system infection: 60 mg/kg/day in divided doses every 6 hours

Note: Some patients may require larger or more frequent doses if serum levels document the need (ie, febrile granulocytopenic patients)

Adults:

<60 kg: 750 mg every 12 hours
60-100 kg: 1 g every 12 hours
100-120 kg: 1.25 g every 12 hours
>120 kg: 1.5 g every 12 hours

Dosing interval in renal impairment: Following a usual loading dose, dosages and frequency of administration are best determined by measurement of serum levels and assessment of renal insufficiency

Dosing adjustments/comments in hepatic impairment: Reduce dose by 60%

Intrathecal:

Neonates: 5-10 mg/day
Children: 5-20 mg/day
Adults: 20 mg/day

Oral: Pseudomembranous colitis produced by *C. difficile*:

Neonates: 10 mg/kg/day in divided doses
Children: 40 mg/kg/day in divided doses, added to fluids
Adults: 250-500 mg 3 times/day in divided doses

Dosage Forms

Capsule: 125 mg, 250 mg
Powder for oral solution: 1 g, 10 g
Powder for injection: 500 mg, 1 g, 2 g, 5 g, 10 g

Reference Range Ototoxicity may occur at peak plasma levels >30 mg/L; nephrotoxicity may occur at trough plasma levels >10 mg/L

Overdosage Treatment

Decontamination: Ipecac or lavage/activated charcoal with cathartic

Supportive therapy: Hypotension can respond to fluids; has responded to diphenhydramine (12.5 mg I.V.) in one case

Enhancement of elimination: While hemodialysis or charcoal hemoperfusion are not helpful, peritoneal dialysis can remove 40% of drug in 15 hours; continuous arteriovenous or intermittent hemofiltration may also be useful; multiple dosing of activated charcoal may be useful

Drug Interactions Antibacterial synergy with other aminoglycosides; nephrotoxicity increases when combined with other aminoglycosides or amphotericin

Pregnancy Risk Factor C

Pregnancy Implications Can cause fetal bradycardia

Specific References

Ahkee S, Smith R, and Ritter GW, "Once-Daily Aminoglycoside Dosing in Lower Respiratory Tract Infections," *Pharm Therap*, 1995, 20:226-34.

Burkhart KK, Metcalf S, Shurnas E, et al, "Exchange Transfusion and Multidose Activated Charcoal Following Vancomycin Overdose," *J Toxicol Clin Toxicol*, 1992, 30(2):285-94.

Cunha BA, "Vancomycin," *Med Clin North Am*, 1995, 79(4):817-32.

DeVries E, van Rossum MAJ, Garritsen EJA, et al, "No Difference in Frequency of Adverse Reactions to Either Vancomycin or Teicoplanin in 70 Pediatric Bone Marrow Transplant Patients," *Bone Marrow Transplant*, 1995, 15(Suppl 2):124.

Duffull SB and Begg EJ, "Vancomycin Toxicity. What Is the Evidence for Dose Dependency?" *Adverse Drug React Toxicol Rev*, 1994, 13(2):103-14.

Frimat L, Hestin D, Hanesse B, et al, "Acute Renal Failure Due to Vancomycin Alone," *Nephrol Dial Transplant*, 1995, 10:550-1.

Geissmann C, Beylot-Barry M, Doutre M-S, et al, "Drug-Induced Linear IgA Bullous Dermatosis," *J Am Acad Dermatol*, 1995, 32(2 Pt 1):296.

Hill LM, "Fetal Distress Secondary to Vancomycin-Induced Maternal Hypotension," *Am J Obstet Gynecol*, 1985, 153(1):74-5.

Leader WG, Chandler MHH, and Castiglia M, "Pharmacokinetic Optimisation of Vancomycin Therapy," *Clin Pharmacokinet*, 1995, 28:327-42.

Lyon GD and Bruce DL, "Diphenhydramine Reversal of Vancomycin-Induced Hypotension," *Anesth Analg*, 1988, 67(11):1109-10.

Nielsen HE, Sorensen I, and Hansen HE, "Peritoneal Transport of Vancomycin During Peritoneal Dialysis," *Nephron*, 1979, 24(6):274-7.

Schenfeld LA and Pote HH Jr, "Diarrhea Associated With Parental Vancomycin Therapy," 1995, 20:1578-9.

Vascor® *see* Bepridil Hydrochloride *on page 152*

Vasocard® *see* Terazosin *on page 725*

Vasofirin *see* Pentoxifylline *on page 607*

Vaso-Pav® *see* Papaverine *on page 591*

Vasotec® *see* Enalapril *on page 311*

Vasoxine® *see* Methoxamine Hydrochloride *on page 518*

Vasoxyl® *see* Methoxamine Hydrochloride *on page 518*

Vatran® *see* Diazepam *on page 271*

VCR *see* Vincristine Sulfate *on page 792*

Velban® Injection *see* Vinblastine Sulfate *on page 790*

Velbe® *see* Vinblastine Sulfate *on page 790*

Velosef® *see* Cephradine *on page 191*

Velosulin® *see* Insulin Preparations *on page 426*

Velsar® Injection *see* Vinblastine Sulfate *on page 790*

Veltane® *see* Brompheniramine Maleate *on page 165*

Venlafaxine (ven' la fax een)

CAS Number 99300-78-4

Brand Names Effexor®

Use Treatment of depression in adults

Mechanism of Action Phenylethylamine antidepressant which inhibits norepinephrine, serotonin, and dopamine (weakly) reuptake in the central nervous system

Adverse Reactions

Cardiovascular: Palpitations, hypertension, sinus tachycardia, Q-T prolongation

Central nervous system: Dizziness (14%), insomnia (19%), somnolence (20%), headache (25%), asthenia (11%), nervousness (11%)

Endocrine & metabolic: Syndrome of inappropriate antidiuretic hormone

Gastrointestinal: Nausea (32%), dry mouth (20%), constipation (15%), weight loss, seizures (0.3%), vomiting

Genitourinary: Impotence, ejaculatory disturbances

Ocular: Blurred vision

Otic: Tinnitus

Miscellaneous: Sweating (13%), suicide attempts (1.1%)

Signs & Symptoms of Acute Overdose Sedation, sinus tachycardia; profound CNS depression can occur with concomitant ingestions of other CNS depressants

Toxicodynamics/Kinetics

Distribution: V_d: 7.5 L/kg; parent drug: 4-6 L/kg (ODV)

Protein binding: 27% to 30%

Metabolism: Hepatic to an active metabolite, O-desmethyl-venlafaxine (ODV)

Bioavailability: Oral: 92% to 100%

Half-life: 5 hours (venlafaxine); 11 hours (ODV); prolonged in renal impairment

Time to peak serum levels: Oral: 1-2 hours

Usual Dosage Adults: Oral: 75 mg/day, administered in 2 or 3 divided doses, taken with food; dose may be increased to 150 mg/day up to 225-375 mg/day; a daily maximum of 375 mg may be needed for severely depressed patients; reduce dosage by 25% in patients with mild renal impairment or 50% in patients with renal or hepatic impairment

Contraindications Do not use concomitantly with MAO inhibitors, contraindicated in patients with hypersensitivity to venlafaxine

Warnings Use with caution in patients with mania, high diastolic blood pressure, epilepsy, coronary heart disease, hyperlipidemia

Dosage Forms Tablet: 25 mg, 37.5 mg, 50 mg, 75 mg, 100 mg

Reference Range Peak serum level of 163 ng/mL (325 ng/mL of ODV metabolite) obtained after a 150 mg oral dose; 4-hour postingestion serum level of 6100 ng/mL (1800 ng/mL of ODV metabolite) associated with coma

Overdosage Treatment

Decontamination: Lavage/activated charcoal with cathartic

Enhancement of elimination: Multiple dosing of activated charcoal may be of some benefit; forced diuresis/extracorporeal removal is not expected to be of any benefit

Test Interactions Increases serum cholesterol

Drug Interactions Increased drug concentration with concomitant use of cimetidine

Pregnancy Risk Factor C

Specific References

Ahmad S, "Venlafaxine and Severe Tinnitus," *Am Fam Physician*, 1995, 51:1830.

Danjou P and Hackett D, "Safety and Tolerance Profile of Venlafaxine," *Int Clin Psychopharmacol*, 1995, 10(Suppl 2):15-20.

De Jonghe F and Swinkels JA, "The Safety of Antidepressants," *Drugs*, 1992, 43(Suppl 2):40-6.

Ellingrod VL and Perry PJ, "Venlafaxine: A Heterocyclic Antidepressant," *Am J Hosp Pharm*, 1994, 51(24):3033-46.

Fantaskey A and Burkhart KK, "A Case Report of Veniafaxine Toxicity," *J Toxicol Clin Toxicol*, 1995, 33(4):359-61.

Khan A, Fabre LF, and Rudolph R, "Venlafaxine in Depressed Outpatients," *Psychopharmacol Bull*, 1991, 27(2):141-4.

Klamerus KJ, Maloney K, Rudolph RL, et al, "Introduction of a Composite Parameter to the Pharmacokinetics of Venlafaxine and Its Active O-desmethyl Metabolite," *J Clin Pharmacol*, 1992, 32(8):716-24.

Zajecka JM, Fawcett J, and Guy C, "Coexisting Major Depression and Obsessive-Compulsive Disorder Treated With Venlafaxine," *J Clin Psychopharmacol*, 1990, 10(2):152-3.

Venocaina® *see* Procaine Hydrochloride *on page 644*

Ventolin® *see* Albuterol *on page 92*

Veramex® *see* Verapamil Hydrochloride *on this page*

Verapamil Hydrochloride (ver ap' a mill)

Related Information

Calcium Channel Blocking Agents Comparison *on page 1646-1647*

CAS Number 52-53-9; 152-11-4

Brand Names Azupamil®; Calan®; Cordilox®; Ikacor®; Isoptin®; Securon®; Veramex®; Verelan®

Synonyms Iproveratril Hydrochloride

Use Angina, hypertension; I.V. for supraventricular tachyarrhythmias (PSVT, fibrillation (atrial), flutter); hypertrophic cardiomyopathy

Mechanism of Action Inhibits calcium ion from entering the "slow channels" or select voltage-sensitive areas of vascular smooth muscle and myocardium during depolarization; produces a relaxation of coronary vascular smooth muscle and coronary vasodilation; increases myocardial oxygen delivery in patients with vasospastic angina

Adverse Reactions

Cardiovascular: Hypotension, bradycardia; first, second, or third degree A-V block; worsening heart failure

Central nervous system: Dizziness, psychosis, fatigue, seizures, (occasionally with I.V. use), headache (1%)

Gastrointestinal: Constipation (5%), nausea, abdominal discomfort, vomiting

Hepatic: Hepatic enzymes (increased), cholestasis

Respiratory: May precipitate insufficiency of respiratory muscle function in Duchenne muscular dystrophy

Signs & Symptoms of Acute Overdose Nausea, constipation, eosinophilia, gingival hyperplasia, flatulence, dyspnea, cholestatic jaundice, gynecomastia, extrapyramidal reaction, coma, coagulopathy, syncope, impotence, A-V block, asthenia, hypoglycemia, esophageal ulceration, rhabdomyolysis, myoglobinuria, drowsiness, confusion, acidosis, may result in bezoars with resultant bowel infarction, heart block, hypotension, asystole, cardiac arrhythmias, bundle-branch block, seizures, skin flushing, junctional bradycardia, hyperglycemia

Toxicodynamics/Kinetics

Onset of action:
- Oral: 1-2 hours
- I.V.:
  - Antiarrhythmic: Within 1-5 minutes
  - Hemodynamic: Within 3-5 minutes

Duration:
- Oral: 6-8 hours
- I.V.: 10-20 minutes

Peak effects:
- Oral (nonsustained tablets): 2 hours
- I.V.: 1-5 minutes;

Absorption: Rapid and complete from gastrointestinal tract (90%)

Distribution: V_d: 4.5-7 L/kg in healthy adults; 12.1 L/kg in cirrhotic patients

Protein binding: 90%

Metabolism: In the liver to norverapamil; extensive first-pass effect

Bioavailability: Oral: 20% to 35%

Half-life: (single dose):
- Infants: 4.4-6.9 hours
- Adults: 2-8 hours, increased up to 12 hours with multiple dosing; increased half-life with hepatic cirrhosis

Time to peak serum concentration: Oral:
- Extended-release tablets: 5-7 hours
- Tablets: 1-2 hours

Elimination: 70% of dose excreted in urine (3% to 4% as unchanged drug), and 16% in feces; clearance: 0.9 L/hour/kg

Usual Dosage

Children: SVT:
- I.V.:
  - <1 year: 0.1-0.2 mg/kg over 2 minutes; repeat every 30 minutes as needed
  - 1-16 years: 0.1-0.3 mg/kg over 2 minutes; maximum: 5 mg/dose, may repeat dose in 15 minutes if adequate response not achieved; maximum for second dose: 10 mg/dose
- Oral (dose not well established):
  - 1-5 years: 4-8 mg/kg/day in 3 divided doses **or** 40-80 mg every 8 hours

(Continued)

Verapamil Hydrochloride *(Continued)*

>5 years: 80 mg every 6-8 hours

Adults:

SVT: I.V.: 5-10 mg (approximately 0.075-0.15 mg/kg), second dose of 10 mg (approximately 0.15 mg/kg) may be given 15-30 minutes after the initial dose if patient tolerates, but does not respond to initial dose

Angina: Oral: Initial dose: 80-120 mg twice daily (elderly or small stature: 40 mg twice daily); range: 240-480 mg/day in 3-4 divided doses

Hypertension: Usual dose is 80 mg 3 times/day or 240 mg/day (sustained release); range 240-480 mg/day (no evidence of additional benefit in doses >360 mg/day)

Dosing adjustment in renal impairment: Cl_{cr} <10 mL/minute: Administer at 50% to 75% of normal dose

Dosing adjustment/comments in hepatic disease: Reduce dose in cirrhosis, reduce dose to 20% to 50% of normal and monitor EKG

Contraindications Sinus bradycardia; advanced heart block; tachycardia (ventricular); cardiogenic shock; hypersensitivity to verapamil or any component; fibrillation (atrial) or flutter associated with accessory conduction pathways; severe hypotension; Wolff-Parkinson-White or Lown-Ganong-Levine syndrome; severe CHF, concurrent (within a few hours) administration of I.V. beta-blocking agents

Warnings Avoid I.V. use in neonates and young infants due to severe apnea, bradycardia, or hypotensive reactions; monitor EKG and blood pressure closely in patients receiving I.V. therapy; sick sinus syndrome, severe left ventricular dysfunction, hepatic or renal impairment, hypertrophic cardiomyopathy (especially obstructive), concomitant therapy with beta-blockers or digoxin

Dosage Forms

Capsule, sustained release: 120 mg, 180 mg, 240 mg

Injection: 2.5 mg/mL (2 mL, 4 mL)

Tablet: 40 mg, 80 mg, 120 mg

Tablet, sustained release: 120 mg, 180 mg, 240 mg

Stability Store injection at room temperature; protect from heat and from freezing; use only clear solutions; is compatible in solutions of pH of 3-6, but may precipitate in solutions having a pH of ≥6

Reference Range A ratio of verapamil/norverapamil >2.3 may be a predictor for fatal outcome

Therapeutic: 50-200 ng/mL (SI: 100-410 nmol/L) for parent; under normal conditions norverapamil concentration is the same as parent drug

Toxic: >845 ng/mL

Fatal: >2000 ng/mL

Overdosage Treatment

Decontamination: Ipecac-induced emesis can hypothetically worsen calcium antagonist toxicity, since it can produce vagal stimulation. The potential for seizures precipitously following acute ingestion of large doses of a calcium antagonist may also contraindicate the use of ipecac. Lavage/activated charcoal with cathartic, whole bowel irrigation may be effective for sustained release preparations

Supportive therapy: Supportive and symptomatic treatment, including I.V. fluids and Trendelenburg positioning, should be initiated as intoxication may cause hypotension. Although calcium (calcium chloride I.V. 1-2 g in adults or 10-30 kg in children over 5-10 minutes with repeats as needed) has been used as an "antidote" for acute intoxications, amrinone or dopamine may be needed for hypotension. Heart block may respond to isoproterenol, glucagon, atropine and/or calcium, although a temporary pacemaker may be required; sodium bicarbonate should be given for acidosis. Glucagon may increase myocardial contractility. In an animal model, the therapy of hyperinsulinemia with euglycemia allowed for larger increases in myocardial contractility than calcium chloride, epinephrine, and glucagon.

Enhancement of elimination: Multiple dosing of activated charcoal may be effective; not dialyzable (0% to 5%)

Antidote(s)

Calcium Chloride *on page 1400*

Calcium Gluconate *on page 1401*

Glucagon *on page 1431*

Test Interactions Elevates glucose (S)

Drug Interactions Increased cardiovascular adverse effects with beta-adrenergic blocking agents (especially when administered intravenously), digoxin, quinidine, and disopyramide. Verapamil may increase serum concentrations of digoxin, quinidine, carbamazepine, and cyclosporine necessitating a decrease in dosage. Phenobarbital and rifampin may decrease verapamil serum concentrations by increased hepatic metabolism. Glucagon can exacerbate hyperglycemia caused by verapamil. Avoid combination with disopyramide, discontinue disopyramide 48 hours before starting therapy, do not restart until 24 hours after verapamil has been discontinued.

Pregnancy Risk Factor C

Pregnancy Implications Excreted in breast milk

Monitoring Parameters EKG, cardiac monitoring for at least 8 hours

Patient Information Sustained release products should be taken with food and not crushed; limit caffeine intake; avoid alcohol; notify physician if angina pain is not reduced when taking this drug

Nursing Implications Help patient with ambulation; monitor blood pressure closely; I.V. rate of infusion is over 2 minutes; do not crush sustained-release drug product

Additional Information Incidence of adverse reactions is most common with I.V. administration; discontinue disopyramide 48 hours before starting therapy, do not restart therapy until 24 hours after verapamil has been discontinued; response to atropine may not be observed until after I.V. calcium administration

Specific References

Buckley CD and Aronson JK, "Prolonged Half-Life of Verapamil in a Case of Overdose: Implications of Therapy," *Br J Clin Pharm*, 1995, 39:680-3.

Cobb MM, Johnson D, Gallo J, et al, "Large Scale Postmarketing Surveillance of Hypertensive Patients Treated With Verapamil," *Am J Therapeut*, 1995, 2:455-61.

Graumlich JF, Spyker DA, and Cantilena JR, "Predictors of Fatality After Oral Verapamil Overdose," *Vet Hum Toxicol*, 1993, 35:345.

Howarth DM, Dawson AH, Smith AJ, et al, "Calcium Channel Blocking Drug Overdose: An Australian Series," *Hum Exp Toxicol*, 1994, 13(3):161-6.

Kline JA, Leonova E, and Raymond RM, "Beneficial Myocardial Metabolic Effects of Insulin During Verapamil Toxicity in the Anesthetized Canine," *Crit Care Med*, 1995, 23(7):1251-68.

Kline JA, Williams TC, Quinn ME, et al, "Verapamil Shock Inhibits Myocardial Fatty Acid Uptake," *Acad Emerg Med*, 1995, 2:395-6.

Kumar KL and Colley CA, "Verapamil-Induced Hepatotoxicity," *West J Med*, 1994, 160(5):485-6.

MacDonald D and Alguire PC, "Case Report: Fatal Overdose With Sustained Release Verapamil," *Am J Med Sci*, 1992, 303(2):115-7.

Madsen CD, Pointer JE, and Lynch TG, "A Comparison of Adenosine and Verapamil for the Treatment of Supraventricular Tachycardia in the Prehospital Setting," *Ann Emerg Med*, 1995, 25:649-55.

Perkins CM, "Serious Verapamil Poisoning: Treatment With Intravenous Calcium Gluconate," *Br Med J*, 1978, 2(6145):1127.

Ramoska EA, Spiller HA, and Myers A, "Calcium Channel Blocker Toxicity," *Ann Emerg Med*, 1990, 19(6):649-53.

Sporer KA and Manning JJ, "Massive Ingestion of Sustained-Release Verapamil With a Concretion and Bowel Infarction," *Ann Emerg Med*, 1993, 22(3):603-5.

Stone CK, May WA, and Carroll R, "Treatment of Verapamil Overdose With Glucagon in Dogs," *Ann Emerg Med*, 1995, 25(3):369-74.

Stone CK, Thomas SH, Koury SI, et al, "Glucagon and Phenylephrine Combination Versus Glucagon Alone in Experimental Verapamil Overdose," *Acad Emerg Med*, 1995, 2:396.

Thomas SH, Stone CK, and May WA, "Exacerbation of Verapamil-Induced Hyperglycemia With Glucagon," *Am J Emerg Med*, 1995, 13(1):27-9.

Tom PA, Morrow CT, and Kelen GD, "Delayed Hypotension After Overdose of Sustained Release Verapamil," *J Emerg Med*, 1994, 12(5):621-5.

Verdiana® *see* Deslanoside *on page 264*

Verelan® *see* Verapamil Hydrochloride *on page 787*

Vericordin® *see* Atenolol *on page 137*

Vermi® *see* Piperazine Citrate *on page 629*

Vermizine® *see* Piperazine Citrate *on page 629*

Versed® *see* Midazolam Hydrochloride *on page 532*

Versola® *see* Tetracaine Hydrochloride *on page 731*

Verstadol® *see* Butorphanol Tartrate *on page 174*

Vesprin® *see* Triflupromazine Hydrochloride *on page 770*

V-Gan® *see* Promethazine Hydrochloride *on page 650*

Vibramycin® *see* Doxycycline *on page 305*

Vibra-Tabs® *see* Doxycycline *on page 305*

Vicemycetin *see* Thiamphenicol *on page 742*

Vicks Formula 44® [OTC] *see* Dextromethorphan Hydrobromide *on page 270*

Vicks Formula 44® Pediatric Formula [OTC] *see* Dextromethorphan Hydrobromide *on page 270*

Vicks Sinex® Long-Acting Nasal Solution [OTC] *see* Oxymetazoline Hydrochloride *on page 586*

Vicks® Vaporub® *see* Camphor *on page 179*

Vicks® Vaposteam® *see* Camphor *on page 179*

Vicks Vatronol® *see* Ephedrine Sulfate *on page 316*

Videne® *see* Povidone-Iodine *on page 635*

Videx® Oral *see* Didanosine *on page 278*

Vigabatrin (vye ga' ba trin)

CAS Number 60643-86-9

Brand Names Sabril®; Sabrilex®

Synonyms GVG; MDL-71754

Use Investigational: Partial/secondary generalized seizures; useful for spasticity or tardive dyskinesia

Mechanism of Action Irreversible inhibitor of GABA transaminase – a structural analog of GABA

Adverse Reactions Central nervous system: Lethargy, mania, confusion, dry mouth, depression, diplopia, myoclonus, insomnia, fatigue, dizziness, facial flushing, sedation (at onset of therapy), psychosis (especially in patients with behavioral abnormalities), headache, myoclonus

Toxicodynamics/Kinetics

Duration of effect: >24 hours

Absorption: 60% to 80%

Distribution: V_d: 0.6-0.8 L/kg

Protein binding: 0%

Metabolism: Hepatic and renal

Half-life: 5-7 hours

Elimination: Renal (60% to 70%); clearance: 1.3 mL/kg/minute

Usual Dosage

Initial dose: 1-2 g/day then titrate to maintenance dose of 2-4 g/day in 1-2 divided doses (lower initial doses in the elderly, patients with renal insufficiency, or patients with psychiatric illnesses)

Infantile spasm: 50-200 mg/kg/day

Spasticity: 2-3 g/day

Tardive dyskinesia: 2-8 g/day

Dosage Forms Tablet: 500 mg

Reference Range

Peak S+ enantiomer: 93 nmol/mL after 1.5 g dose

Peak R- enantiomer: 169 nmol/mL after 1.5 g dose

Overdosage Treatment

Decontamination: Lavage/activated charcoal with cathartic

Enhancement of elimination: Multiple dosing of activated charcoal may be useful; hemodialysis may be useful

Drug Interactions Decreases phenytoin level by 20% to 30%

Pregnancy Implications Cleft palate observed in rabbit studies

Additional Information Water soluble; may worsen myoclonic seizures; rodent studies showed intramyelinic edema (reversible on cessation of treatment)

Specific References

Betts T and Thomas L, "Vigabatrin and Behavior Disturbances," *Lancet*, 1990, 335(8689):605-6.

Campbell MM, "Focus on Vigabatrin," *Hosp Formul*, 1995, 30:143-7.

Grant SM and Heel RC, "Vigabatrin: A Review of Its Pharmacodynamic and Pharmacokinetic Properties and Therapeutic Potential in Epilepsy and Disorders of Motor Control," *Drugs*, 1991, 41(6):889-926.

Neufeld MY and Vishnevska S, "Vigabatrin and Multi-Focal Myoclonus in Adusts With Partial Seizures," *Clin Neuropharmacol*, 1995, 18:280-3.

Vikonon® *see* Yohimbine Hydrochloride *on page 805*

Vinblastine Sulfate (vin blas' teen)

Related Information

Toxicities of Chemotherapeutic Agents *on page 1631-1633*

CAS Number 865-21-4; 143-67-9

Brand Names Alkaban-AQ® Injection; Periblastine®; Velban® Injection; Velbe®; Velsar® Injection

Synonyms Vincaleukoblastine; VLB

Use Hodgkin's and non-Hodgkin's lymphoma, testicular, lung, head and neck, breast, and renal carcinomas, Kaposi's sarcoma, histiocytosis, choriocarcinoma, and idiopathic thrombocytopenic purpura

Mechanism of Action VLB binds to tubulin and inhibits microtubule formation, therefore, arresting the cell at metaphase by disrupting the formation of the mitotic spindle; it is specific for the M and S phases; binds to microtubular protein of the mitotic spindle causing metaphase arrest; extracted from *Vinca rosea* (periwinkle)

Adverse Reactions

Cardiovascular: Tachycardia, hypotension (orthostatic), exacerbation of Raynaud's phenomenon

Central nervous system: Depression, malaise, seizures, headache, dizziness
Dermatologic: Rash, mild alopecia, photosensitivity
Endocrine & metabolic: Hyperuricemia, syndrome of inappropriate antidiuretic hormone
Gastrointestinal: Nausea, hemorrhagic enterocolitis, vomiting, constipation, abdominal pain, paralytic ileus, stomatitis
Genitourinary: Urinary retention
Hematologic: Bone marrow depression
Local: Severe tissue burn if infiltrated
Neuromuscular & skeletal: Jaw pain, myalgia, paresthesia
Miscellaneous: Syndrome of inappropriate secretion of antidiuretic hormone

Signs & Symptoms of Acute Overdose Fever, diarrhea, deafness, ataxia, hyperuricemia, colitis, Parkinson's-like symptoms, ptosis, bleeding, thrombocytopenia, hypertension, tachycardia, paresthesia, leukopenia; neutropenia; agranulocytosis; granulocytopenia; hyponatremia

Toxicodynamics/Kinetics
Absorption: Not reliably absorbed from gastrointestinal tract and must be given I.V.
Distribution: V_d: 27.3 L/kg; binds extensively to tissues; does not penetrate CNS or other fatty tissues; distributes to the liver
Protein binding: 75%
Metabolism: Hepatic to a more active metabolite (desacetyl-vinblastine)
Half-life (biphasic): Initial 0.164 hours; terminal: 25 hours
Elimination: Biliary excretion (95%); <1% eliminated unchanged in urine

Usual Dosage Refer to individual protocol. Varies depending upon clinical and hematological response. Give at intervals of at least 7 days and only after leukocyte count has returned to at least 4000/mm^3; maintenance therapy should be titrated according to leukocyte count. Dosage should be reduced in patients with recent exposure to radiation therapy or chemotherapy; single doses in these patients should not exceed 5.5 mg/m^2.

Children and Adults: I.V.: 4-12 mg/m^2 every 7-10 days **or** 5-day continuous infusion of 1.4-1.8 mg/m^2/day **or** 0.1-0.5 mg/kg/week

Dosing adjustment in hepatic impairment:
Serum bilirubin 1.5-3.0 mg/dL or AST 60-180 units: Administer 50% of normal dose
Serum bilirubin 3.0-5.0 mg/dL: Administer 25% of dose
Serum bilirubin >5.0 mg/dL or AST >180 units: Omit dose

Administration May be administered IVP or into a free flowing I.V. over a 1-minute period at a concentration for administration of 1 mg/mL

Contraindications For I.V. use only; **I.T. use may result in death**; severe bone marrow suppression or presence of bacterial infection not under control prior to initiation of therapy

Warnings The U.S. Food and Drug Administration (FDA) currently recommends that procedures for proper handling and disposal of antineoplastic agents be considered. Avoid extravasation; dosage modification required in patients with impaired liver function and neurotoxicity. Using small amounts of drug daily for long periods may increase neurotoxicity and is therefore not advised. For I.V. use only. **Intrathecal administration may result in death**. Use with caution in patients with cachexia or ulcerated skin; monitor closely for dyspnea or wheezing in patients receiving mitomycin C

Dosage Forms
Injection: 1 mg/mL (10 mL)
Powder for injection: 10 mg

Stability Refrigerate; however, is stable for up to 1-3 months (depending on manufacturer) at room temperature; constituted solutions remain stable for 30 days when refrigerated; protect from light, must be dispersed in amber bag; **compatible** with doxorubicin, metoclopramide, dacarbazine, bleomycin

Overdosage Treatment
Supportive therapy: Seizures can be treated with diazepam, lorazepam, phenytoin, or barbiturates; extravasation can be treated with warm compresses with infiltration of hyaluronidase (150 units in saline in a concentration of 15 units/mL); surgical debridement may be necessary
Enhancement of elimination: Exchange transfusion (2 volume) has been performed in a child 3 years of age who received ten times the therapeutic dose; not removed by hemodialysis

Antidote(s)
Hyaluronidase *on page 1432*

Drug Interactions
Decreased effect: Phenytoin plasma levels may be reduced with concomitant combination chemotherapy with vinblastine; phenytoin may reduce plasma levels
Increased toxicity: Mitomycin-C in combination with administration of VLB may cause acute dyspnea and severe wheezing, onset may be within minutes or

(Continued)

Vinblastine Sulfate *(Continued)*

several hours after VLB injection; previous or simultaneous use with mitomycin-C has resulted in acute dyspnea and severe wheezing within minutes or several hours after *Vinca* alkaloid injection and may occur up to 2 weeks after the dose of mitomycin. Alpha interferon enhances interferon toxicity; neutropenia and muscle pain can result if vinblastine and erythromycin are used together.

Pregnancy Risk Factor D

Pregnancy Implications Microphthalmia, anophthalmia noted in rodents

Monitoring Parameters CBC with differential and platelet count, serum uric acid, hepatic function tests

Patient Information Hair may be lost during treatment but will regrow to its pretreatment extent even with continued treatment; report any bleeding; examine mouth daily and report soreness to a physician; jaw pain or pain in the organs containing tumor tissue; avoid constipation. Any signs of infection, easy bruising or bleeding, dyspnea, or painful or burning urination should be brought to physician's attention. Nausea, vomiting or hair loss sometimes occur. The drug may cause permanent sterility and may cause birth defects. The drug may be excreted in breast milk, therefore, an alternative form of feeding your baby should be used.

Nursing Implications May be administered by I.V. push or into a free flowing I.V.; monitor for life-threatening wheezing (most likely to occur if patient is also taking mitomycin); maintain adequate hydration; allopurinol may be given to prevent uric acid nephropathy; may cause sloughing upon extravasation

Extravasation treatment: Inject 3-5 mL of hyaluronidase (10 units/mL) S.C. clockwise into the infiltrated area using a 25-gauge needle; change the needle with each injection; apply heat immediately for 1 hour, repeat 4 times/day for 3-5 days (application of cold and injection of hydrocortisone is contraindicated)

Additional Information Urine (for 4 days) and feces (for 7 days) should be handled with care

Myelosuppressive effects:
- Onset (days): 4-7
- Nadir (days): 10
- Recovery (days): 17

Specific References

Dorr RT and Alberts DS, "Vinca Alkaloid Skin Toxicity: Antidote and Drug Disposition Studies in the Mouse," *J Natl Cancer Inst*, 1985, 74(1):113-20.

Rodrigues RL, "Pharmacology and Toxicology of Chemotherapeutic Agents," *Emerg Med Clin North Am*, 1993, 11(2):431-43.

Tobe SW, Siu LL, Jamal SA, et al, "Vinblastine and Erythromycin: An Unrecognized Serious Drug Interaction," *Cancer Chemother Pharmacol*, 1995, 35(3):188-90.

Winter SC and Arbus GS, "Syndrome of Inappropriate Secretion of Antidiuretic Hormone Secondary to Vinblastine Overdose," *Can Med Assoc J*, 1977, 117(10):1134.

Vincaleukoblastine *see* Vinblastine Sulfate *on page 790*

Vincasar® PFS™ Injection *see* Vincristine Sulfate *on this page*

Vincristine Sulfate (vin kris' teen)

Related Information

Therapeutic Drugs Associated With Hallucinations *on page 1558-1559*

Toxicities of Chemotherapeutic Agents *on page 1631-1633*

CAS Number 57-22-7; 2068-78-2

Brand Names Norcristine®; Oncovin® Injection; Pericristine®; Vincasar® PFS™ Injection; Vincrisul®

Synonyms LCR; Leurocristine; VCR

Use Treatment of leukemias, Hodgkin's disease, neuroblastoma, malignant lymphomas, Wilms' tumor, and rhabdomyosarcoma; may be useful to treat life-endangering infantile hemangiomas which are corticosteroid resistant

Mechanism of Action Binds to microtubular protein of the mitotic spindle causing metaphase arrest; cell-cycle phase specific in the M and S phases; extracted from *Vinca rosea* (periwinkle)

Adverse Reactions

Cardiovascular: Orthostatic hypotension

Central nervous system: Neurotoxicity, numbness, asthenia, seizures, CNS depression, psychosis, hallucinations, cranial nerve paralysis, visual hallucinations, ataxia

Dermatologic: Alopecia (occurs in 20% to 70% of patients and is reversible), rash

Endocrine & metabolic: Hyperuricemia, syndrome of inappropriate antidiuretic hormone

Gastrointestinal: Constipation (at doses of 12.5-75 mcg/kg), paralytic ileus secondary to neurologic toxicity (particularly in the elderly), nausea, vomiting, diarrhea, stomatitis

Local: Pain, cellulitis and tissue necrosis if infiltrated, phlebitis

Ocular: Optic atrophy with cortical blindness has been reported, ptosis/diplopia (32%)

Neuromuscular & skeletal: Jaw pain, leg pain, myalgias, cramping, motor difficulties

Neurologic: Effects of VCR may be additive with those of other neurotoxic agents and spinal cord irradiation. Dose related: Begins at 5-6 g and is significant at 15-20 g

Respiratory: Dyspnea

Signs & Symptoms of Acute Overdose Fever, deafness, thrombocytosis, thrombocytopenia, numbness, hyperuricemia, paresthesia, muscle atrophy, Mees' lines, leukopenia, myopathy, migraine headache (exacerbation of), confusion, hypertension, occipital headache, ascending paralysis, coma with intrathecal injection

Toxicodynamics/Kinetics

Absorption: Oral: Poor

Distribution: Poor penetration into the CSF; rapidly removed from the bloodstream and tightly bound to tissues; penetrates blood-brain barrier poorly; concentrates in platelets

Protein binding: 75%

Metabolism: Extensive in the liver

Half-life: Terminal: 24 hours

Elimination: Primarily in bile (~80%); <1% excreted unchanged in urine

Usual Dosage **Refer to individual protocol as dosages vary with protocol used**. Adjustments are made depending upon clinical and hematological response and upon adverse reactions.

Children: I.V. (maximum single dose: 2 mg):

≤10 kg or BSA <1 m^2: 0.05 mg/kg once weekly

1-2 mg/m^2; may repeat every week

Adults: I.V.: 0.4-1.4 mg/m^2, up to 2 mg maximum; may repeat every week

Dosing adjustment in hepatic impairment:

Serum bilirubin 1.5-3.0 mg/dL or AST 60-180 units: Administer 50% of normal dose

Serum bilirubin 3.0-5.0 mg/dL: Administer 25% of dose

Serum bilirubin >5.0 mg/dL or AST >180 units: Omit dose

Average total dose per course of treatment should be around 2-2.5 mg; some recommend capping the dose at 2 mg maximum to reduce toxicity; however, it is felt that this measure can reduce the efficacy of the drug

Administration Vincristine is administered IVP or into a free flowing I.V. over a period of 1 minute at a concentration for administration of 1 mg/mL

Contraindications Hypersensitivity to vincristine or any component; **for I.V. use only, fatal if given intrathecally**; patients with demyelinating form of Charcot-Marie-Tooth syndrome

Warnings The U.S. Food and Drug Administration (FDA) currently recommends that procedures for proper handling and disposal of antineoplastic agents be considered. Dosage modification required in patients with impaired hepatic function or who have pre-existing neuromuscular disease; avoid extravasation; use with caution in the elderly; avoid eye contamination; observe closely for dyspnea, wheezing, especially in patients treated with mitomycin C. For I.V. use only; **intrathecal administration results in death**; give allopurinol to prevent uric acid nephropathy; not to be used with radiation.

Dosage Forms Injection: 1 mg/mL (1 mL, 2 mL, 5 mL)

Stability Refrigerate; however, is stable for up to 1 month at room temperature; drug may be administered IVP or IVPB and is **compatible** with D_5W; should be protected from light; **compatible** with doxorubicin, bleomycin, cytarabine, fluorouracil, methotrexate, and metoclopramide

Reference Range 5-day continuous infusion (total dose: 4 mg/m^2) produced plasma level of 1.8-10.9 ng/mL at 1 hour and <0.25 ng/mL at 24 hours after discontinuation of therapy

Overdosage Treatment

Supportive therapy: Constipation resolves after 2 weeks; neurotoxicity can be decreased with pretreatment during induction period with glutamic acid (1.5 g/day); folinic acid has been utilized but efficacy is not known (100 mg every 3 hours for 1 day, then 100 mg every 6 hours for 2 days)

Enhancement of elimination: For intrathecal route, remove contaminated CNS fluid and flush with lactated Ringer's solution with fresh frozen plasma to maintain a protein level of 150 mg/dL; glutamic acid 10 g I.V. over 1 day followed by 500 mg/day orally until neurotoxicity is stabilized

Antidote(s)

Hyaluronidase *on page 1432*

Drug Interactions

Decreased effect: Phenytoin levels may decrease with combination chemotherapy

Increased toxicity: Digoxin plasma levels and renal excretion may decrease with combination chemotherapy including vincristine. Vincristine should be given

(Continued)

Vincristine Sulfate *(Continued)*

12-24 hours before asparaginase to minimize toxicity (may reduce the hepatic clearance of vincristine). Acute pulmonary reactions may occur with mitomycin-C. Previous or simultaneous use with mitomycin-C has resulted in acute dyspnea and severe wheezing within minutes or several hours after *Vinca* alkaloid injection and may occur up to 2 weeks after the dose of mitomycin.

Pregnancy Risk Factor D

Monitoring Parameters Serum electrolytes (sodium), hepatic function tests, neurologic examination, CBC, serum uric acid

Patient Information Maintain adequate fluid intake; rinse mouth with water 3-4 times/day, brush teeth with soft brush and floss with waxed floss; loss of hair occurs in approximately 70% of patients; report any nerve effects to physician; stool softener should be used for constipation prophylaxis; report to physician any persistent or severe fever, sore throat, bleeding, or bruising; dyspnea

Nursing Implications Maintain adequate hydration; allopurinol may be given to prevent uric acid nephropathy; observe for life-threatening wheezing after administration; use of rectal thermometer or rectal tubing should be avoided to prevent injury to rectal mucosa

Extravasation treatment: Inject 3-5 mL of hyaluronidase (10 units/mL) S.C. clockwise into the infiltrated area using a 25-gauge needle; change the needle with each injection; apply heat immediately for 1 hour, repeat 4 times/day for 3-5 days (application of cold and injection of hydrocortisone is contraindicated)

Additional Information Urine (for 4 days) and feces (for 1 week) must be handled with care

Specific References

Dyke RW, "Treatment of Inadvertent Intrathecal Injection of Vincristine," *N Engl J Med*, 1989, 321(18):1270-1.

Ghosh K, Sivakumaran M, Murphy P, et al, "Visual Hallucinations Following Treatment With Vincristine," *Clin Lab Haematol*, 1994, 16:355-7.

Grush OC and Morgan SK, "Folinic Acid Rescue for Vincristine Toxicity," *Clin Toxicol*, 1974, 14(1):71-8.

Jackson DV, Wells HB, Atkins JN, et al, "Amelioration of Vincristine Neurotoxicity by Glutamic Acid," *Am J Med*, 1988, 84(6):1016-22.

Kanwar VS, Albuquerque MLC, Ribeiro RC, et al, "Veno-occlusive Disease of the Liver After Chemotherapy for Rhabdomyosarcoma: Case Report With a Review of the Literature," *Med Pediatr Oncol*, 1995, 24:334-40.

Legha SS, "Vincristine Neurotoxicity. Pathophysiology and Management," *Med Toxicol*, 1986, 1(6):421-7.

Payarols JP, Masferrer JP, and Bellvert CG, "Treatment of Life-Threatening Infantile Hemangiomas With Vincristine," *N Engl J Med*, 1995, 333(1):69.

Rodrigues RL, "Pharmacology and Toxicology of Chemotherapeutic Agents," *Emerg Med Clin North Am*, 1993, 11(2):431-43.

Vincrisul® *see* Vincristine Sulfate *on page 792*

Vinorelbine Ditartrate

Related Information

Toxicities of Chemotherapeutic Agents *on page 1631-1633*

CAS Number 71486-22-1

Brand Names Navelbine®

Synonyms 3',4'-Didehydro-4'-Deoxy-8'-Norvinca Leukoblastine Ditartrate

Use Single agent (or in combination with cisplatin) for the therapy of unrejectable advanced nonsmall cell lung cancer

Investigational: Advanced breast cancer, ovarian cancer, and squamous cell carcinoma of head and neck

Mechanism of Action Inhibits polymerization of tubulin use for cellular microtubule or spindle formation thus inhibiting cellular mitosis (during metaphase)

Adverse Reactions

Central nervous system: Fatigue, delirium
Dermatologic: Vesicant formation, alopecia (12%)
Gastrointestinal: Nausea (34%), constipation, diarrhea, stomatitis
Hematologic: Myelosuppression (dose related), anemia, thrombocytopenia
Neuromuscular & skeletal: Peripheral neuropathy, myalgia, paresthesia
Respiratory: Dyspnea

Toxicodynamics/Kinetics

Absorption: Oral: 26% to 45%; not affected by food
Distribution: V_d: 27 L/kg
Protein binding: 50% to 80%
Metabolism: Hepatic to desacetyl-vinorelbine (active) and N-oxide vinorelbine (inactive)
Half-life:
- Oral: 24-56 hours
- I.V.: 42-45 hours

Elimination: Feces (70% to 80%) and renal (20% to 30%); clearance: 0.8 L/kg/hour

Usual Dosage I.V.: 30 mg/m^2/week (over 6-10 minutes); reduce dosage to 15 mg/m^2 if granulocyte count is 1000-1499 cells/m^3 or total bilirubin is between 2.1-3 mg/dL; further reduction in dose to 7.5 mg/m^2 should occur if total bilirubin is >3 mg/dL; do not administer if granulocyte count is <1000 cells/m^3

Contraindications Previous history of vinorelbine hypersensitivity

Warnings Use with caution in patients with vincristine, or vinblastine hypersensitivity; herpes infections, myelosuppression, previous nervous system disorders, bone marrow infiltration by tumor cells, or pretreated patients

Dosage Forms

Capsule, gelatin, oral (investigational): 40 mg

Injection: 10 mg/mL (single use vial); 50 mg/5 mL (single use vial)

Reference Range Peak serum level of 1130 ng/mL achieved 15 minutes after a 30 mg/m^2 I.V. dose

Overdosage Treatment

Supportive therapy: Seizures can be treated with diazepam, lorazepam, phenytoin, or barbiturates; extravasation can be treated with warm compresses with infiltration of hyaluronidase (150 units in saline in a concentration of 15 units/mL); surgical debridement may be necessary

Enhancement of elimination: Not dialyzable

Drug Interactions Increased pulmonary toxicity when used with mitomycin; increased incidence of granulocytopenia with cisplatin; may potentiate 5-FU induced mucositis

Monitoring Parameters Hematological/hepatic parameters

Additional Information Not useful in renal cell carcinoma; metoclopramide (20-40 mg) can be given prophylactically as an antiemetic agent; I.V. route usually utilized, although oral weekly doses of 50-160 mg have been used in patients with advanced breast cancer; less neurotoxic than vincristine or vinblastine

Specific References

Cvitkovic E and Izzo J, "The Current and Future Place of Vinorelbine in Cancer Therapy," *Drugs*, 1992, 44(Suppl 4):36-45.

Monnet I, Chariot P, Azli N, et al, "Severe Mucositis After Chemotherapy With Vinorelbine, 5-Fluorouracil, Leucovorin, and Cisplatin," *Eur J Cancer*, 1991, 27(12):1716-7.

Viosterol *see* Vitamin D *on page 797*

Viramid® *see* Ribavirin *on page 679*

Virazid® *see* Ribavirin *on page 679*

Virazide® *see* Ribavirin *on page 679*

Virazole® Aerosol *see* Ribavirin *on page 679*

Virilon® *see* Testosterone *on page 729*

Virormone® *see* Testosterone *on page 729*

Viscor® *see* Dipyridamole *on page 292*

Visine® *see* Oxymetazoline Hydrochloride *on page 586*

Viskaldix® *see* Pindolol *on page 627*

Visken® *see* Pindolol *on page 627*

Viskos® *see* Boric Acid *on page 160*

Vistacon-50® *see* Hydroxyzine *on page 414*

Vistaject-25® *see* Hydroxyzine *on page 414*

Vistaject-50® *see* Hydroxyzine *on page 414*

Vistaquel® *see* Hydroxyzine *on page 414*

Vistaril® *see* Hydroxyzine *on page 414*

Vistazine® *see* Hydroxyzine *on page 414*

Vitacin® *see* Vitamin E *on page 798*

Vita-C® [OTC] *see* Ascorbic Acid *on page 131*

Vitamin A (vye' ta min)

Related Information

Isotretinoin *on page 447*

CAS Number 68-26-8

Brand Names Aquasol A®; Arovit®; Avitina®; Ido A50®; Primavit®; Ro-A-Vit®; Vogan®

Synonyms Axerophtholum; Oleovitamin A

Use Treatment and prevention of vitamin A deficiency

Mechanism of Action Needed for bone development, growth, visual adaptation to darkness, testicular and ovarian function, and as a cofactor in many biochemical processes

Adverse Reactions Reactions are only seen with doses exceeding physiologic replacement

(Continued)

Vitamin A *(Continued)*

Central nervous system: Irritability, sedation, drowsiness, dizziness, delirium, headache due to increased intracranial pressure, coma

Dermatologic: Erythema, peeling skin, alopecia, increased yellow pigmentation

Gastrointestinal: Vomiting, diarrhea

Hematologic: Normochromic macrocytic anemia

Hepatic: Hepatomegaly

Ocular: Visual disturbances, papilledema

Otic: Ototoxicity, tinnitus

Miscellaneous: Perioral fissures

Signs & Symptoms of Acute Overdose Fatigue, anorexia, hypercalcemia, hypoprothrombinemia, diplopia, coagulopathy, nausea, vomiting, pseudotumor cerebri, rhabdomyolysis, myoglobinuria, ascites, low grade fever, dizziness, nystagmus, erythema, pruritus, skin desquamation over hands and feet, intracranial pressure (increased), portal hypertension

Toxicodynamics/Kinetics

Absorption: Oral: Dependent on bile salts, pancreatic lipase, and dietary fat

Distribution: Oral: Large amounts (90%) concentrate for storage in the liver

Metabolism: Hepatic transformation to retinal and retinoic acid and bound to a specific carrier protein (retinol-binding protein)

Half-life: 9.1 hours

Elimination: Feces (50%) and urine (20%)

Usual Dosage

RDA:
- 0-3 years: 400 mcg*
- 4-6 years: 500 mcg*
- 7-10 years: 700 mcg*
- >10 years: 800-1000 mcg*
- *mcg retinol equivalent (0.3 mcg retinol = 1 unit vitamin A)

Supplementation in measles: Children: Oral:
- <1 year: 100,000 units/day for 2 days
- >1 year: 200,000 units/day for 2 days

Severe deficiency with xerophthalmia:
- Children 1-8 years:
  - Oral: 5000-10,000 units/kg/day for 5 days or until recovery occurs
  - I.M.: 5000-15,000 units/day for 10 days
- Children >8 years and Adults:
  - Oral: 500,000 units/day for 3 days, then 50,000 units/day for 14 days, then 10,000-20,000 units/day for 2 months
  - I.M.: 50,000-100,000 units/day for 3 days, 50,000 units/day for 14 days

Deficiency (without corneal changes): Oral:
- Infants <1 year: 10,000 units/kg/day for 5 days, then 7500-15,000 units/day for 10 days
- Children 1-8 years: 5000-10,000 units/kg/day for 5 days, then 17,000-35,000 units/day for 10 days
- Children >8 years and Adults: 100,000 units/day for 3 days then 50,000 units/day for 14 days

Malabsorption syndrome (prophylaxis): Children >8 years and Adults: Oral: 10,000-50,000 units/day of water miscible product

Dietary supplement: Oral:
- Infants up to 6 months: 1500 units/day
- Children:
  - 6 months to 3 years: 1500-2000 units/day
  - 4-6 years: 2500 units/day
  - 7-10 years: 3300-3500 units/day
- Children >10 years and Adults: 4000-5000 units/day

Hepatotoxic dose: 600,000 units (acute); 25,000-50,000 units/day (chronic)

Contraindications Hypervitaminosis A, hypersensitivity to vitamin A or any component

Warnings Evaluate other sources of vitamin A while receiving this product; patients receiving >25,000 units/day should be closely monitored for toxicity

Dosage Forms

Capsule: 10,000 units, 25,000 units, 50,000 units

Drops, oral (water miscible): 5000 units/0.1 mL (30 mL)

Injection: 50,000 units/mL (2 mL)

Stability Protect from light

Reference Range

RDA: Male: 1000 μg retinol equivalent (RE); Female: 800 μg RE; 1 RE = 1 retinol equivalent; 1 RE = 1 μg retinol or 6 mg beta-carotene

Normal levels: >0.67 units/mL or 20-60 μg/dL; levels >100 μg/dL are associated with the toxic state

Overdosage Treatment

Decontamination: Emesis or lavage if ingestion is acute and >300,000 units in children or over 1,000,000 units in adults/cholestyramine or activated charcoal with cathartic

Supportive therapy: Hypercalcemia can be treated with furosemide (20-40 mg I.V.), saline hydration and prednisone (10-40 mg orally)

Drug Interactions Cholestyramine decreases absorption of vitamin A; neomycin and mineral oil may also interfere with vitamin A absorption

Pregnancy Risk Factor A (X if dose exceeds RDA recommendation)

Pregnancy Implications Craniofacial abnormalities may occur; appears in breast milk

Monitoring Parameters Monitor calcium; serum alkaline phosphatase, bilirubin, and prothrombin time may be elevated

Patient Information Avoid use of mineral oil when taking drug; take with food; notify physician if nausea, vomiting, anorexia, malaise, drying or cracking of skin or lips, irritability, headache, or loss of hair occurs

Nursing Implications Do not give by I.V. push; patients receiving >25,000 units/day should be closely monitored for toxicity

Additional Information 1 mg equals 3333 units

Specific References

Cetaruk EW and Aaron CK, "Hazards of Nonprescription Medications," *Emerg Med Clin North Am*, 1994, 12(2):483-510.

de Francisco A, Chakraborty J, Chowdhury HR, et al, "Acute Toxicity of Vitamin A Given With Vaccines in Infancy," *Lancet*, 1993, 342(8870):526-7.

Kowalski TE, Falestiny M, Furth E, et al, "Vitamin A Hepatotoxicity: A Cautionary Note Regarding 25,000 IU Supplements," *Am J Med*, 1994, 97(6):523-8.

LaMantia RS and Andrews CE, "Acute Vitamin A Intoxication," *South Med J*, 1981, 74(8):1012-4.

Nesher G and Zuckner J, "Rheumatologic Complications of Vitamin A and Retinoids," *Semin Arthritis Rheum*, 1995, 24:291-6.

Sanders TA, "Vitamin A and Pregnancy," *Lancet*, 1990, 336(8727):1375.

White JM, "Vitamin A-Induced Anaemia," *Lancet*, 1984, 2(8402):573.

Vitamin B_1 *see* Thiamine Hydrochloride *on page 741*

Vitamin B_3 *see* Niacin *on page 554*

Vitamin B_3 *see* Niacinamide *on page 555*

Vitamin B_{12} *see* Cyanocobalamin *on page 246*

Vitamin C *see* Ascorbic Acid *on page 131*

Vitamin D

CAS Number 41294-56-8; 19356-17-3; 63283-36-3; 32222-06-3; 67-97-0; 67-96-9; 50-14-6

Brand Names Calciferol™; Drisdol®

Synonyms Activated Ergosterol; Alfacalcidol; Calcifediol; Calcitriol; Cholecalciferol; Dihydrotachysterol; Ergocalciferol; Viosterol

Use Treatment of refractory rickets, hypophosphatemia, hypoparathyroidism; vitamin D-deficient states

Mechanism of Action Fat soluble vitamin; stimulates calcium and phosphate absorption from the small intestine, promotes secretion of calcium from bone to blood

Adverse Reactions

Cardiovascular: Hypertension, arrhythmias

Central nervous system: Drowsiness, irritability, headache

Endocrine & metabolic: Acidosis

Gastrointestinal: Nausea, diarrhea, vomiting, anorexia, dry mouth, metallic taste

Neuromuscular & skeletal: Weakness, muscle and bone pain

Renal: Polyuria, nephrocalcinosis

Signs & Symptoms of Acute Overdose Anorexia, drowsiness, hypomagnesemia, headache, confusion, nausea, anemia, vomiting, nystagmus, hypercalcemia, dysosmia, azotemia, albuminuria, pancreatitis, ectopic calcification, muscle asthenia, hypertension, renal failure, hyperphosphatemia

Toxicodynamics/Kinetics

Peak effect: In ~1 month following daily doses

Absorption: Readily absorbed from gastrointestinal tract; absorption requires intestinal presence of bile

Metabolism: Inactive until hydroxylated in the liver and the kidney to calcifediol and then to calcitriol (most active form)

Usual Dosage

Dietary supplementation: Oral:

- Infants, premature: 10-20 mcg/day (400-800 units), up to 750 mcg/day (30,000 units)
- Infants and healthy Children: 10 mcg/day (400 units)
- Adults:

(Continued)

Vitamin D *(Continued)*

<25 years: 400 units
>25 years: 200 units

Renal failure: Oral:
Children: 0.1-1 mg/day (4000-40,000 units)
Adults: 0.5 mg/day (20,000 units)

Hypoparathyroidism: Oral:
Children: 1.25-5 mg/day (50,000-200,000 units) and calcium supplements (500 mg elemental calcium 6 times/day)
Adults: 625 mcg to 5 mg/day (25,000-200,000 units) and calcium supplements (500 mg elemental calcium 6 times/day)

Vitamin D-dependent rickets: Oral:
Children: 75-125 mcg/day (3000-5000 units)
Adults: 250 mcg to 1.5 mg/day (10,000-60,000 units)

Nutritional rickets and osteomalacia:
Children and Adults (with normal absorption): Oral: 25 mcg/day (1000 units)
Children with malabsorption: Oral: 250-625 mcg/day (10,000-25,000 units)
Adults: I.M.: 250 mcg/day

Dosage Forms
Capsule (Drisdol®): 50,000 units [1.25 mg]
Injection (Calciferol™): 500,000 units/mL [12.5 mg/mL] (1 mL)
Liquid (Calciferol™, Drisdol®): 8000 units/mL [200 mcg/mL] (60 mL)
Tablet (Calciferol™): 50,000 units [1.25 mg]

Reference Range
Normal serum range of vitamin D and 25-hydroxy D_3: 10-50 pg/mL
Normal serum range of 1.25-hydroxy D_3: 10-20 pg/mL; free 1,25 dihydroxy vitamin D levels that are elevated (mean level 852 fmol/L with a reference range of 305-523 fmol/L) may contribute to pathogenesis of hypercalcemia
Toxicity is associated with serum 25-hydroxyD_3 >850 nmol/L and free 1,25 dihydroxyD_3 >280 fmol/L; overdosage is associated with normal serum total 1,25 dihydroxyD_3 and elevated serum 25-hydroxyD_3 and free 1,25 dihydroxyD_3 due to protein binding interaction

Overdosage Treatment Supportive therapy: Hypercalcemia can be treated with saline, diuresis, furosemide (20-40 mg I.V.) and hydrocortisone (100 mg I.V. every 6 hours); calcitonin (4-8 IU/kg I.M. every 6-12 hours) can be used for persistent or severe hypercalcemia; hemodialysis can also be used for severe hypercalcemia

Test Interactions Serum cholesterol can be falsely elevated by vitamin D

Drug Interactions Hepatic metabolism is increased with glutethimide/phenytoin; effects of vitamin D are decreased with concomitant administration of phenobarbital

Pregnancy Risk Factor A (D if dose exceeds RDA recommendation)

Pregnancy Implications Large doses (10,000 IU/kg) can produce arterial stenosis, abnormal bone mineralization, elfin facies, and nephrocalcinosis in the neonate

Monitoring Parameters Serum calcium and phosphorous levels, BUN, renal status

Additional Information Cholecalciferol (vitamin D_3) is a potent rodenticide containing 13,000 IU of vitamin D per g; marketed as Rampage or Quintox; present in fish, cod liver oils, butter, eggs, liver; 1.25 mg ergocalciferol provides 50,000 units of vitamin D activity; elimination of vitamin D metabolites delayed in hypothyroid individuals; insoluble in water

Specific References

Cardella CJ, Birkin BL, and Rapoport A, "Role of Dialysis in the Treatment of Severe Hypercalcemia: Report of Two Cases Successfully Treated With Hemodialysis and Review of the Literature," *Clin Nephrol*, 1979, 12(6):285-90.

Cetaruk EW and Aaron CK, "Hazards of Nonprescription Medications," *Emerg Med Clin North Am*, 1994, 12(2):483-510.

Pettifor JM, Bikle DD, Cavaleros M, et al, "Serum Levels of Free 1,25-Dihydroxyvitamin D in Vitamin D Toxicity," *Ann Intern Med*, 1995, 122(7):511-3.

Vitamin E

CAS Number 59-02-9; 10191-41-0; 58-95-7; 7695-91-2; 4345-03-3; 17407-37-3

Brand Names Amino-Opti-E® Oral [OTC]; Aquasol E® Oral [OTC]; Auxina E®; Bio E®; Dal-E®; E-Caps®; E-Vimin®; Evion®; Ido-E®; Invite E®; Prairie Gold®; Spondyvit®; Taxofit Vitamin E®; Tocoferolo Bioglan®; Tocogen®; Vitacin®; Vitec® Topical [OTC]; Viteril®

Synonyms *d*-Alpha Tocopherol; *dl*-Alpha Tocopherol; Toco

Use Prevention and treatment of hemolytic anemia secondary to vitamin E deficiency, dietary supplement

Mechanism of Action Prevents oxidation of vitamin A and C; protects polyunsaturated fatty acids in membranes from attack by free radicals and protects red blood cells against hemolysis

Adverse Reactions

Central nervous system: Headache

Dermatologic: Rash, contact dermatitis and erythema multiforme with topical preparation

Endocrine & metabolic: Gonadal dysfunction; decreased serum thyroxine and triiodothyronine

Gastrointestinal: Nausea, diarrhea, intestinal cramps

Hepatic: Cholesterol (increased) and hypertriglyceridemia

Neuromuscular & skeletal: Weakness

Ocular: Blurred vision

Renal: Creatinuria and increased serum creatinine kinase; increased urinary estrogens and androgens

Signs & Symptoms of Acute Overdose Diarrhea, cholestatic jaundice, abdominal pain, asthenia, nausea, azotemia

Toxicodynamics/Kinetics

Absorption: Complete

Distribution: Distributes to all body tissues, especially adipose tissue, where it is stored

Metabolism: In the liver to tocopheronic acid

Elimination: Feces

Usual Dosage

RDA: Oral:

- Infants:
  - Premature, ≤3 months: 25 units/day
  - ≤6 months: 4.5 units/day
  - 6-12 months: 6 units/day
- Children:
  - 1-3 years: 9 units/day
  - 4-10 years: 10.5 units/day
- Children >11 years and Adults:
  - Male: 15 units/day
  - Female: 12 units/day

Prevention of vitamin E deficiency: Neonates, premature, low birthweight (results in normal levels within 1 week): Oral: 25-50 units/24 hours until 6-10 weeks of age or 125-150 units/kg total in 4 doses on days 1, 2, 7, and 8 of life

Vitamin E deficiency treatment: Adults: Oral: 50-200 units/24 hours for 2 weeks

Topical: Apply a thin layer over affected areas as needed

Contraindications Should not be given I.V., hypersensitivity to drug or any components

Warnings May induce vitamin K deficiency

Dosage Forms

Capsule: 100 units, 200 units, 400 units, 500 units, 600 units, 1000 units

Capsule, water miscible: 73.5 mg, 147 mg, 165 mg, 330 mg, 400 units

Cream: 50 mg/g (15 g, 30 g, 60 g, 75 g, 120 g, 454 g)

Drops, oral: 50 mg/mL

Liquid, topical: 10 mL, 15 mL, 30 mL, 60 mL

Oil: 15 mL, 30 mL, 60 mL

Ointment, topical: 30 mg/g (45 g, 60 g)

Tablet: 200 units, 400 units

Stability Protect from light

Reference Range

Therapeutic: 0.8-2.5 mg/dL (SI: 19-35 μmol/L), some method variation

Toxic: >3.5 mg/dL; levels >4.5 mg/dL associated with necrotizing enterocolitis

Overdosage Treatment Decontamination: Oral: Emesis or lavage/activated charcoal with cathartic

Drug Interactions

Decreased absorption with mineral oil

Delayed absorption of iron

Increased effect of oral anticoagulants; antagonizes effect of vitamin K

Pregnancy Risk Factor A (C if dose exceeds RDA recommendation)

Monitoring Parameters Plasma tocopherol concentrations (normal range: 6-14 μg/mL)

Patient Information Drops can be placed directly in the mouth or mixed with cereal, fruit juice, or other food; take only the prescribed dose. Vitamin E toxicity appears as blurred vision, diarrhea, dizziness, flu-like symptoms, nausea, headache; swallow capsules whole, do not crush or chew.

Additional Information Cluster of deaths in low birthweight infants in 1984 (about 38) secondary to injectable vitamin E (E-Ferol); ascribed to large amount of polysorbates injected; found in sunflower oil, vegetable oils, eggs, wheat germ oil

Specific References

Bieri JG, Corash L, and Hubbard VS, "Medical Uses of Vitamin E," *N Engl J Med*, 1983, 308(18):1063-71.

(Continued)

Vitamin E *(Continued)*

Hale TW, Rais-Bahrami K, Montgomery DL, et al, "Vitamin E Toxicity in Neonatal Piglets," *J Toxicol Clin Toxicol*, 1995, 33(2):123-30.

Hodis HN, Mack WJ, LaBree L, et al, "Serial Coronary Angiographic Evidence That Antioxidant Vitamin Intake Reduces Progression of Coronary Artery Artherosclerosis," *JAMA*, 1995, 273:1849-54.

Johnson L, Bowen FW Jr, Abbasi S, et al, "Relationship of Prolonged Pharmacologic Serum Levels of Vitamin E to Incidence of Sepsis and Necrotizing Enterocolitis in Infants With Birth Weight 1500 Grams or Less," *Pediatrics*, 1985, 75(4):619-38.

Karp WB and Robertson AF, "Vitamin E in Neonatology," *Adv Pediatr*, 1986, 33:127-47.

Saperstein H, Rapaport M, and Rietschel RL, "Topical Vitamin E as a Cause of Erythema Multiforme-Like Eruption," *Arch Dermatol*, 1984, 120(7):906-8.

Vitantial® *see* Thiamine Hydrochloride *on page 741*

Vitec® Topical [OTC] *see* Vitamin E *on page 798*

Viteril® *see* Vitamin E *on page 798*

Vivarin® [OTC] *see* Caffeine *on page 175*

Vivol® *see* Diazepam *on page 271*

VLB *see* Vinblastine Sulfate *on page 790*

Vogan® *see* Vitamin A *on page 795*

Volital® *see* Pemoline *on page 598*

Voltaren® *see* Diclofenac Sodium *on page 276*

Vorigeno® *see* Scopolamine *on page 691*

VoSol® *see* Acetic Acid *on page 85*

Waran® *see* Warfarin Sodium *on this page*

Warfarin Sodium (war' far in)

Related Information

Dicumarol *on page 277*

Drugs and Chemicals Proven to be Teratogenic in Humans *on page 1572-1575*

CAS Number 81-81-2; 129-06-6; 2610-86-8

Brand Names Aldocumar®; Coumadin®; Marevan®; Panwarfarin®; Sofarin®; Waran®; Warfilione®

Synonyms Brumolin; Sodium Warfarin

Use Prophylaxis and treatment of thromboembolic disorders; prevention of recurrent myocardial infarction and thromboembolic events in postmyocardial infarction patients

Mechanism of Action Interferes with hepatic synthesis of vitamin K-dependent coagulation factors (II, VII, IX, X)

Adverse Reactions

Central nervous system: Fever
Dermatologic: Skin lesions, pruritus, purpura, skin necrosis
Gastrointestinal: Anorexia, nausea, vomiting, diarrhea
Hematologic: Hemorrhage, cholestasis
Respiratory: Hemoptysis

Signs & Symptoms of Acute Overdose Alopecia, coagulopathy, pericardial effusion/pericarditis, cholelithiasis, esophageal ulceration, ocular hemorrhage, intracranial hemorrhage, hepatitis, eosinophilia, circulatory collapse, hematuria, numbness, bleeding gums, urine discoloration (orange), feces discoloration (black), feces discoloration (light brown), feces discoloration (pink), feces discoloration (red), feces discoloration (tarry)

Toxicodynamics/Kinetics

Onset of anticoagulation effect: Oral: Within 36-72 hours
Peak effect: Within 5-7 days
Absorption: Oral: Rapid
Distribution: V_d: 0.14-0.17 L/kg
Protein binding: 99%
Metabolism: In the liver
Half-life: 37-42 hours, highly variable among individuals
Elimination: Urine (reabsorbed in the bile); clearance: 0.04-0.36 mL/min/kg

Usual Dosage Oral:

Infants and Children: 0.05-0.34 mg/kg/day; infants <12 months of age may require doses at or near the high end of this range; consistent anticoagulation may be difficult to maintain in children <5 years of age

Adults: 5-15 mg/day for 2-5 days, then adjust dose according to results of prothrombin time; usual maintenance dose ranges from 2-10 mg/day

Target international normalized ratios for:

Patients with nonrheumatic atrial fibrillation and recent cerebral ischemia: 2-3.9

Prosthetic heart valves: 3-4; caged ball/tilting-disk valves: 4-4.9; bileaflet valves: 2-3.9

Dosing adjustment/comments in hepatic disease: Monitor effect at usual doses; the response to oral anticoagulants may be markedly enhanced in obstructive jaundice (due to reduced vitamin K absorption) and also in hepatitis and cirrhosis (due to decreased production of vitamin K-dependent clotting factors); prothrombin index should be closely monitored

Contraindications Hypersensitivity to warfarin or any component; severe liver or kidney disease; open wounds; uncontrolled bleeding; gastrointestinal ulcers; neurosurgical procedures; malignant hypertension, pregnancy

Warnings Do not switch brands once desired therapeutic response has been achieved; use with caution in patients with active tuberculosis or diabetes; concomitant use with vitamin K may decrease anticoagulant effect; monitor carefully; concomitant use with NSAIDs; aspirin increases warfarin's effect on clotting time and may cause severe gastrointestinal irritation

Dosage Forms

Injection: 5 mg vial

Tablet: 1 mg, 2 mg, 2.5 mg, 4 mg, 5 mg, 7.5 mg, 10 mg

Stability Protect from light

Reference Range

Therapeutic: 2-5 μg/mL (SI: 6.5-16.2 μmol/L); free warfarin level: 5-23 ng/mL

Prothrombin time should be 1½ to 2 times the control or INR (international normalized ratio) should be increased 2-3 times based upon indication; if it is between 4.5-7, withhold warfarin for 1 or 2 days; if it is >7, vitamin K should be given

Normal prothrombin time: 10-13 seconds

Lee-White clotting time: 8-15 minutes

Target INR range:

2-3: Treatment of proximal DVT and PE. Prophylaxis for fibrillation (atrial), valvular heart disease, bioprosthetic heart valves

3-4.5: Prophylaxis in patients with mechanical heart valves or recurrent systemic embolism

Overdosage Treatment

Decontamination: Activated charcoal with cathartic should be given; lavage can be performed within 2 hours of ingestion

Supportive therapy: Vitamin K_1 should be given in doses as outlined in phytonadione; monitor PT and INR until normalization

Enhancement of elimination: Cholestyramine or multiple dosing of activated charcoal may be useful

Antidote(s)

Cholestyramine Resin *on page 1405*

Phytonadione *on page 1458*

Test Interactions Warfarin ↑ PTT

Diagnostic Tests/Procedures

Warfarin, Blood *on page 1379*

Drug Interactions Several drugs have been documented to alter the effect of warfarin; caution must be observed when any drug is added to or deleted from a therapeutic regimen of a patient receiving warfarin. The following is only a partial list of interacting drugs. Warfarin may enhance the effects of sulfonylurea agents.

Decreased effect: Barbiturates, carbamazepine, cholestyramine, carbamazepine, glutethimide, griseofulvin, phenytoin, rifampin, sucralfate, acetaminophen, ethchlorvynol, nafcillin

Increased effect: Anabolic steroids, allopurinol, chloral hydrate, chloramphenicol, cimetidine, ciprofloxacin, clofibrate, alcohol, danazol, disulfiram, erythromycin, felbamate, fluconazole, gemfibrozil, glucagon, thyroid, ketoconazole, metronidazole, NSAIDs, miconazole, quinidine, sulfonamides, tamoxifen, tienilic acid, amiodarone, azapropazone, cefamandole, dipyridamole, ethacrynic acid, phenylbutazone, cotrimoxazole, isoniazid, piroxicam; increased bleeding with fluoxetine; increased prothrombin time may result with concomitant valproic acid and warfarin therapy

Pregnancy Risk Factor D

Pregnancy Implications First trimester usage may cause fetal bone stippling and nasal hypoplasia. Can cause CNS abnormalities. Stillbirth also noted with higher frequency.

Monitoring Parameters Prothrombin time, hematocrit, INR

Patient Information Do not take with food; report any signs of bleeding; avoid hazardous activities; use soft tooth brush; urine may turn red/orange; carry Medi-Alert® ID identifying drug usage; be sure of other drugs and foods to avoid; report any bleeding to physician at once; notify physician if urine turns dark brown or if red or tar black stools occur

Nursing Implications Avoid all I.M. injections

Additional Information High intensity warfarin therapy (titrated to an internal nor-

(Continued)

Warfarin Sodium *(Continued)*

malized ratio ≥3) can prevent thrombosis in patients with antiphospholipid-antibody syndrome; for I.V. injection, reconstitute with 2.7 mL of sterile water to yield 2 mg/mL; see table. Further information can be obtained by calling DuPont Pharma at 800-474-2762.

TLV-TWA: 0.1 mg/m^3

IDLH: 200 mg/m^3

The chart provides information about the amount of reconstituted solution of Coumadin® for injection that corresponds to a specific dose

Desired Dose of Coumadin® (mg)	Coumadin® for Injection Administration Volume (mL)
0.5	0.25
1	0.50
1.5	0.75
2	1
2.5	1.25
3	1.50
3.5	1.75
4	2
4.5	2.25
5	2.50
5.5	2.75*
6	3*
6.5	3.25*
7	3.50*
7.5	3.75*
8	4*
8.5	4.25*
9	4.50*
9.5	4.75*
10	5*

*More than 1 vial required for this dose.

Specific References

Cannegieter SC, Rosendaal FR, Wintzen AR, et al, "Optimal Oral Anticoagulant Therapy in Patients With Mechanical Heart Valves," *N Engl J Med*, 1995, 333:11-17.

Chan TY, Lui SF, Chung SY, et al, "Adverse Interaction Between Warfarin and Indomethacin," *Drug Saf*, 1994, 10(3):267-9.

Chaudhry S and Oelsner D, "Cholestatic Reaction to Warfarin," *Am J Gastroenterol*, 1995, 90:853.

Fihn SD, "Aiming for Safe Anticoagulation," *N Engl J Med*, 1995, 333:54-5.

Fihn SD, McDonell M, Martin D, et al, "Risk Factors for Complications of Chronic Anticoagulation," *Ann Intern Med*, 1993, 118(7):511-20.

Fiske WD, Connell JM, and Benedek IH, "Lack of Pharmacokinetic Interaction Between Aspirin and Warfarin," *Am J Therapeut*, 1995, 2:407-13.

Ginsberg JS and Hirsh J, "Optimum Use of Anticoagulants in Pregnancy," *Drugs*, 1988, 36(4):505-12.

Guthrie SK, Stoysich AM, Bader G, et al, "Hypothesized Interaction Between Valproic Acid and Warfarin," *J Clin Psychopharmacol*, 1995, 15:138-9.

Hanger HC and Thomas F, "Fluoxetine and Warfarin Interactions," *N Z Med J*, 1995, 108:157.

Harrington R and Ansell J, "Risk-Benefit Assessment of Anticoagulant Therapy," *Drug Saf*, 1991, 6(1):54-69.

Khamashta MA, Cuadrado MJ, Mujic F, et al, "The Management of Thrombosis in the Antiphospholipid-Antibody Syndrome," *N Engl J Med*, 1995, 332(15):993-7.

Lal LS and Anassi E, "Diagnosing a Covert Ingestion of Warfarin Using Warfarin Levels," *Hosp Pharm*, 1995, 30:381-3.

Mathiesen T, Benediktadottir K, Johnsson H, et al, "Intracranial Traumatic and Non-traumatic Haemorrhagic Complications of Warfarin Treatment," *Acta Neurol Scand*, 1995, 91:208-14.

Schulman S, Rhedin A-S, Lindmarker P, et al, "A Comparison of Six Weeks With Six Months of Oral Anticoagulant Therapy After a First Episode of Venous Thromboembolism," *N Engl J Med*, 1995, 332:1661-5.

Sternberg ML and Pettyjohn FS, "Warfarin Sodium-Induced Skin Necrosis," *Ann Emerg Med*, 1995, 26(1):94-7.

The European Atrial Fibrillation Trial Study Group, "Optimal Oral Anticoagulant Therapy in Patients With Nonrheumatic Atrial Fibrillation and Recent Cerebral Ischemia," *N Engl J Med*, 1995, 333:5-10.

The following factors, alone or in combination, may be responsible for **increased** PT response:

Endogenous Factors

Cancer
Collagen disease
Congestive heart failure
Diarrhea
Elevated temperature
Hepatic disorders
  Infectious hepatitis, jaundice
Hyperthyroidism
Poor nutritional state
Steatorrhea
Vitamin K deficiency

Exogenous Factors

Acetaminophen
Alcohol*
Allopurinol
Aminosalicylic acid
Amiodarone HCl
Anabolic steroids
Anesthetics, inhalation
Antibiotics
Bromelains
Chenodiol
Chloral hydrate*
Chlorpropamide
Chymotrypsin
Cimetidine
Clofibrate
Coumadin® overdosage
Danshen
Dextran
Dextrothyroxine
Diazoxide
Diflunisal
Diuretics*
Disulfiram
Ethacrynic acid
Fenoprofen
Fluoroquinolone antibiotics
Glucagon
Hepatotoxic drugs
Ibuprofen
Indomethacin
Influenza virus vaccine
Lovastatin
Mefenamic acid
Methyldopa
Methylphenidate
Metronidazole
Miconazole
Monoamine oxidase inhibitors
Moricizine hydrochloride*
Nalidixic acid
Naproxen
Narcotics, prolonged
Omeprazole
Pentoxifylline
Phenylbutazone
Phenytoin
Propafenone
Propranolol
Pyrazolones
Quinidine
Quinine
Ranitidine*
Salicylates
Sulfinpyrazone
Sulfonamides, long-acting
Sulindac
Tamoxifen
Thyroid drugs
Tolbutamide
Trimethoprim/sulfamethoxazole

Also:
Other medications affecting blood elements which may modify hemostasis
Dietary deficiencies
Prolonged hot weather
Unreliable PT determinations

*Increased and decreased PT responses have been reported.

The following factors, alone or in combination, may be responsible for **decreased** PT response:

Endogenous Factors
Edema
Hereditary Coumadin® resistance
Hyperlipemia
Hypothyroidism

Exogenous Factors
Adrenocortical steroids
Alcohol*
Aminoglutethimide
Antacids
Antihistamines
Barbiturates
Carbamazepine
Chloral hydrate*
Chlordiazepoxide
Cholestyramine
Coumadin® underdosage
Diuretics*
Ethchlorvynol
Glutethimide
Griseofulvin
Haloperidol
Meprobamate
Moricizine hydrochloride*
Nafcillin
Oral contraceptives
Paraldehyde
Primidone
Ranitidine*
Rifampin
Sucralfate
Toxaphene
Trazodone
Vitamin C

Also:
Diet high in vitamin K
Unreliable PT determinations

*Increased and decreased PT responses have been reported.

Warfilione® *see* Warfarin Sodium *on page 800*
WariActiv® *see* Ethyl Chloride *on page 337*

4-Way® Long Acting Nasal Solution [OTC] *see* Oxymetazoline Hydrochloride *on page 586*

Wehamine® *see* Dimenhydrinate *on page 289*
Wellbutrin® *see* Bupropion *on page 170*

Wesfalin® *see* Acebutolol Hydrochloride *on page 77*
Westhroid® *see* Thyroid *on page 749*
Westrim® LA [OTC] *see* Phenylpropanolamine Hydrochloride *on page 622*

White Copperas *see* Zinc *on page 811*
White Mineral Oil *see* Mineral Oil *on page 534*
White Vitriol *see* Zinc *on page 811*

Whole Root Rauwolfia *see* Rauwolfia Serpentina *on page 677*
Wigraine® *see* Ergotamine *on page 317*
Wincoram® *see* Amrinone Lactate *on page 127*

Winobanin® *see* Danazol *on page 257*
Wolfina® *see* Rauwolfia Serpentina *on page 677*
Wormex® *see* Piperazine Citrate *on page 629*

Wy-3498 *replaced by* Oxazepam *on page 582*
WY-8678 *see* Guanabenz Acetate *on page 391*
Wyamycin® S Oral *see* Erythromycin *on page 319*

Wygesic® *see* Propoxyphene and Acetaminophen *on page 656*
Wymox® *see* Amoxicillin *on page 121*
Wytensin® *see* Guanabenz Acetate *on page 391*

Xanax® *see* Alprazolam *on page 99*

Xanef® *see* Enalapril *on page 311*

Xanor® *see* Alprazolam *on page 99*

Xylocaine® *see* Lidocaine Hydrochloride *on page 468*

Xylocaine® With Epinephrine *see* Lidocaine and Epinephrine *on page 467*

Xylotocan® *see* Tocainide Hydrochloride *on page 755*

Yobinol® *see* Yohimbine Hydrochloride *on this page*

Yocon® *see* Yohimbine Hydrochloride *on this page*

Yohimbine Hydrochloride (yo him' bine)

CAS Number 146-48-5; 65-19-0

Brand Names Afrodex®; Aphrodyne™; Dayto Himbin®; Potensan®; Vikonon®; Yobinol®; Yocon®; Yohimex™

Synonyms Aphrodine Hydrochloride; Corynathe Yohimbe; Corynine Hydrochloride

Use No FDA sanctioned indications; has been used to treat male erectile impotence; allegedly has aphrodisiac properties; has been used in veterinary medicine as a reversal agent for xylazine

Mechanism of Action Derived from the bark of the yohimbe tree (Pausingstalia yohimbe), this indole alkaloid produces an alpha$_2$-adrenergic blockade; also is a weak MAO inhibitor; parasympathetic tone is also decreased

Adverse Reactions

Cardiovascular: Tachycardia, bradycardia, hypertension, hypotension (orthostatic), flushing

Central nervous system: Anxiety, mania, hallucinations, irritability, dizziness, psychosis, insomnia, headache

Gastrointestinal: Nausea, vomiting, anorexia

Neuromuscular & skeletal: Tremors, paresthesia

Ocular: Lacrimation, mydriasis

Respiratory: Bronchospasm

Miscellaneous: Antidiuretic action, salivation, sweating

Toxicodynamics/Kinetics

Duration of action: Usually 3-4 hours, but may last 36 hours

Absorption: Oral: 33%

Distribution: V_d: 0.3-3 L/kg

Half-life: 0.6 hours

Usual Dosage Adults: Oral: Impotence: 5.4 mg 3 times/day

Contraindications Hepatic/renal disease, hypersensitivity to yohimbine

Warnings Do not use in pregnancy; do not use in children; not for use in geriatric, psychiatric, or cardio-renal patients with a history of gastric or duodenal ulcer; generally not for use in females

Dosage Forms Tablet: 5.4 mg

Reference Range After a 10 mg oral dose, peak plasma yohimbine level achieved was ~75 μg/L after 45 minutes

Overdosage Treatment

Decontamination: Lavage/activated charcoal

Supportive therapy: For hypertension, nifedipine or labetalol may be useful; for hypertensive emergencies, phentolamine with nitroprusside is useful; benzodiazepines can be used for agitation; clonidine (5 mcg/kg) may be particularly useful in treating hypertension or anxiety; phenothiazines and tricyclic antidepressants can potentiate psychic effects and thus should be avoided

Test Interactions Elevation of serum catecholamine levels can occur

Drug Interactions Antidepressants, other mood-modifying drugs

Additional Information Also a street drug of abuse that can be smoked; has a bitter taste; dissociative state may resemble phencyclidine intoxication

Specific References

Charney DS, Heninger GR, and Redmond DE, "Yohimbine-Induced Anxiety and Increased Noradrenergic Function in Humans: Effects of Diazepam and Clonidine," *Life Sci*, 1983, 33:19-29.

Landis E and Shore E, "Yohimbe-Induced Bronchospasm," *Chest*, 1989, 96(6):1424.

Linden CH, Vellman WP, and Rumack B, "Yohimbine: A New Street Drug," *Ann Emerg Med*, 1985, 14(10):1002-4.

Owen JA, Nakatsu SL, Fenemore J, et al, "The Pharmacokinetics of Yohimbine in Man," *Eur J Clin Pharmacol*, 1987, 32(6):577-82.

Yohimex™ *see* Yohimbine Hydrochloride *on this page*

Yurelax® *see* Cyclobenzaprine Hydrochloride *on page 248*

Yutopar® *see* Ritodrine Hydrochloride *on page 687*

Zalcitabine

CAS Number 7481-89-2

Brand Names Hivid®

Synonyms ddC; ddCyd; Dideoxycytidine

(Continued)

Zalcitabine *(Continued)*

Use Orphan drug use in the treatment of AIDS

Mechanism of Action Potent synthetic, pyrimidine nucleoside inhibitor of viral reverse transcriptase of DNA; ~10 times as potent as zidovudine

Adverse Reactions

Central nervous system: Fever, malaise

Dermatologic: Pruritus, urticaria

Endocrine & metabolic: Hypoglycemia, hyperglycemia, hypophosphatemia, hypernatremia, hyponatremia, hypocalcemia, hypomagnesemia

Gastrointestinal: Anorexia, pancreatitis, diarrhea, nausea, vomiting

Hematologic: Anemia (6% to 8%), neutropenia (15% to 17%), eosinophilia (2% to 6%), thrombocytopenia (1% to 3%)

Hepatic: Hepatotoxicity

Neuromuscular & skeletal: Distal neuropathy (peripheral) (22% to 35%), arthralgias

Otic: Tinnitus

Miscellaneous: Night sweats

Toxicodynamics/Kinetics

Protein binding: Low

Metabolism: Not significant

Distribution:

V_d:

Children: 9.3 L/m^3

Adults: 0.54 L/kg

Half-life:

Children: 0.8 hours

Adults: 1-3 hours

Bioavailability (reduced by 14% with food):

Children: 29% to 100%

Adults: 80% to 88%

Peak serum levels: 1-2 hours

Elimination: Renal: Urinary metabolite is 2',3'-dideoxyuridine (ddU)

Usual Dosage Oral:

Children: 0.015-0.04 mg/kg every 6 hours

Adults: 0.75 mg every 8 hours

Contraindications Hypersensitivity to zalcitabine

Warnings Reduce dosage in renal or hepatic insufficiency; use with caution in patients with pancreatitis, myelosuppression, pre-existing signs of neuropathy (peripheral), or congestive heart failure; use with caution in patients concomitantly taking drugs that cause neuropathy (peripheral) (didanosine, dapsone, disulfiram, isoniazid, lithium, metronidazole, pentamidine, phenytoin, ribavirin, or vincristine), or renal insufficiency (amphotericin B, aminoglycosides, or foscarnet)

Dosage Forms Tablet: 0.375 mg, 0.75 mg

Reference Range Therapeutic blood level: ~0.5 μmol/L

Overdosage Treatment

Decontamination: Lavage/activated charcoal with cathartic

Enhancement of elimination: Multiple dosing of activated charcoal may be effective; dialysis may be effective, although there is no data in an overdosage setting

Drug Interactions Additive or synergistic peripheral neurotoxicity with didanosine; synergism with interferon alpha, heparin, and rifabutine

Pregnancy Risk Factor C

Monitoring Parameters Complete blood counts

Additional Information Can be combined with zidovudine (at a zidovudine dose of 200 mg every 8 hours); limiting dosage for distal, symmetrical neuropathy (peripheral) is 0.01 mg/kg every 8 hours; less bone marrow suppression than with zidovudine

Specific References

Devineni D and Gallo JM, "Zalcitabine: Clinical Pharmacokinetics and Efficacy," *Clin Pharmacokinet*, 1995, 28(5):351-60.

Zantac® *see* Ranitidine Hydrochloride *on page 675*

Zantan® *see* Ranitidine Hydrochloride *on page 675*

Zantryl® *see* Phentermine Hydrochloride *on page 619*

Zarontin® *see* Ethosuximide *on page 333*

Zeasorb-AF® Powder [OTC] *see* Miconazole *on page 530*

Zebeta® *see* Bisoprolol Fumarate *on page 157*

Zephiran® [OTC] *see* Benzalkonium Chloride *on page 147*

Zephirol *see* Benzalkonium Chloride *on page 147*

Zergamet® *see* Cimetidine *on page 212*

Zerit® *see* Stavudine *on page 706*

Zestril® *see* Lisinopril *on page 475*

Zetran® *see* Diazepam *on page 271*

Zidovudine (zye doe' vue deen)

CAS Number 30516-87-1

Brand Names Retrovir®

Synonyms 3'-azido-2',3'-dideoxythymidine; Azidothymidine; AZT; Compound S

Use Management of patients with HIV infections who have had at least one episode of *Pneumocystis carinii* pneumonia or who have CD4 cell counts of ≤500/mm^3; patients who have HIV-related symptoms or who are asymptomatic with abnormal laboratory values indicating HIV-related immunosuppression; does not reduce risk of transmitting HIV infections; can reduce perinatal HIV transmission by 20% to 50%; has been used to treat adult T cell leukemia-lymphoma with interferon alfa; possible antineoplastic role to treat solid tumors such as colon cancer

Mechanism of Action Zidovudine is a thymidine analog which interferes with the HIV viral RNA dependent DNA polymerase by competing with thymidine triphosphate resulting in inhibition of viral replication

Adverse Reactions

Central nervous system: Malaise, dizziness, asthenia, manic syndrome, seizures, psychosis, confusion, fever, severe headache, insomnia

Dermatologic: Rash, pigmentation of nails (blue)

Gastrointestinal: Nausea (46%), diarrhea, dyspepsia, vomiting

Hematologic: Granulocytopenia, thrombocytopenia, leukopenia, anemia (macrocytic)

Hepatic: Cholestatic hepatitis

Neuromuscular & skeletal: Tremors, myalgia, arthropathy, polymyositis syndrome

Signs & Symptoms of Acute Overdose Generalized seizures, drowsiness (after 20 g ingestion), ataxia, nystagmus, leukopenia; cardiomyopathy; insomnia, mania, lymphoma, gynecomastia, cholestatic jaundice; neutropenia; agranulocytosis; granulocytopenia; headache, nausea

Toxicodynamics/Kinetics

Absorption: Oral: Well absorbed, 66% to 70% (reduced when ingesting high-fat meal)

Distribution: V_d: 1.6 L/kg; significant penetration into the CSF (60% of plasma)

Protein binding: 30% to 38%

Metabolism: Extensive first-pass metabolism; metabolized in the liver via glucuronidation to inactive metabolites (D-glycopyranuronosylthymidine) or GAZT

Half-life:

- Terminal: 1 hour
- Parent compound: 0.6-1.7 hours (GAZT)
- Uremia: 1.4 hours
- Cirrhosis: 2.4 hours

Time to peak serum concentration: Within 0.5-1.5 hours

Elimination: Urinary excretion (63% to 95%); following oral administration, 72% to 74% of drug is excreted in urine as metabolites and 14% to 18% as unchanged drug; following I.V. administration, 45% to 60% excreted in urine as metabolites and 18% to 29% as unchanged drug; renal clearance: 0.2-0.3 L/kg/hour

Usual Dosage

Children 3 months to 12 years:

- Oral: 90-180 mg/m^2/dose every 6 hours; maximum: 200 mg every 6 hours
- I.V. continuous infusion: 0.5-1.8 mg/kg/hour
- I.V. intermittent infusion: 100 mg/m^2/dose every 6 hours

Adults:

- Oral:
  - Asymptomatic infection: 100 mg every 4 hours while awake (500 mg/day)
  - Symptomatic HIV infection: Initial: 200 mg every 4 hours (1200 mg/day), then after 1 month, 100 mg every 4 hours (600 mg/day)
- I.V.: 1-2 mg/kg/dose every 4 hours

Dosing interval in renal impairment: Cl_{cr} <10 mL/minute: Administer 100 mg every 4 hours

Dosing adjustment in hepatic impairment: Reduce dose by 50% or double dosing interval in patients with cirrhosis

Administration Infuse I.V. zidovudine over 1 hour at a final concentration not to exceed 4 mg/mL in D_5W

Contraindications Life-threatening hypersensitivity to zidovudine or any component

Warnings Use with caution in patients with impaired renal or hepatic function; reduce dosage or interrupt therapy in patients with anemia and/or granulocytopenia

(Continued)

Zidovudine *(Continued)*

and myopathy; often associated with hematologic toxicity including granulocytopenia, thrombocytopenia, and severe anemia requiring transfusions; zidovudine has been shown to be carcinogenic in rats and mice

Dosage Forms

Capsule: 100 mg

Injection: 10 mg/mL (20 mL)

Syrup (strawberry flavor): 50 mg/5 mL (240 mL)

Reference Range Peak serum level after 200 mg dose: ~0.9 μg/mL; serum level taken 12 hours after a 20 g overdose: 49.4 μg/mL

Overdosage Treatment

Decontamination: Lavage/activated charcoal with cathartic

Supportive therapy: Transfusions with blood component; vitamin B_{12} administration may assist in preventing anemia

Enhancement of elimination: Multiple dosing of activated charcoal may be effective; while hemodialysis may remove its metabolites, it has no effect on the parent compound and cannot be routinely recommended

See tables.

Demographic Summary of Zidovudine Overdoses 1988–1994

Age/Sex	Amount Ingested	Coingestants
27 mo/male	130 mg 10.2 mg/kg	None
26 y/male*	10–20 g 110–220 mg/kg	Phenobarbs and benzodiazepines
28 y/male	10 g, then additional 10 g	Marijuana
32 y/female	7–8 g	None
34 y/male	10 g	Temazepam
35 y/male	36 g	Anti-TB meds
36 y/male	2.5 g x 16 d 33 mg/kg	Marijuana, benzodiazepines
37 y/male	3.6 g	None
Patient A: 35 y/male	10 g 164 mg/kg	None
Patient B: 7 y/male	25 g 454 mg/kg	None
24 y/male	6 g	2 g acyclovir
25 y/male	3 g	None
34 y/male	22.5 g	None
36 y/male		Ketoconazole

*This patient weighed 91.6 kg.

Antidote(s)

Filgrastim *on page 1425*

Diagnostic Tests/Procedures

Zidovudine, Blood *on page 1381*

Drug Interactions

Dapsone; pentamidine and amphotericin B impair renal excretion of zidovudine; flucytosine, vincristine, vinblastine, doxorubicin, interferon

Increased toxicity: Coadministration with drugs that are nephrotoxic, cytotoxic, or interfere with RBC/WBC number or function; coadministration with acetaminophen can increase incident of anemia; morphine, salicylic acid, nonsteroidal anti-inflammatory agents, probenecid; possible increase antineoplastic efficacy when combined with 5-fluorouracil and methotrexate

Pregnancy Risk Factor C

Pregnancy Implications May be associated with fetal anemia or intrauterine growth retardation; crosses the placenta

Monitoring Parameters CBC, hemoglobin, MCV, serum creatinine kinase

Patient Information Take 30 minutes before or 1 hour after a meal with a glass of water; take zidovudine exactly as prescribed and that administration every 4 hours means dosing around-the-clock

Nursing Implications Monitor complete blood count and platelet count at least every 2 weeks; observe for appearance of opportunistic infections; give around-the-clock to promote less variation in peak and trough serum levels

Physical and Laboratory Findings of Zidovudine Overdoses, 1988–1994

Time After Ingestion	Symptoms	Physical Exam Results	Abnormal Lab Values	Treatment	Outcome
Unknown	Lethargy, fatigue	Normal	WBC 3.8 x 10^9/L to 2.3 x 10^9/L, Hgb 9.9–8.7 g/dL, Hct 29.7%–26.6%, platelets 181 x 10^9/L to 127 x 10^9/L at 48 h after ingestion	None	No sequelae
Unknown	None	NA	Aspartate transaminase 9–28 IU/L, alanine transaminase 14–68 IU/L, CD4 299, CD8 1657	None	CD4 200, CD8 1155 LFTs normal after dose change
Unknown (Patient A)	None	NA	Hgb 15.2–13.7 g/dL, WBC 10.4 x 10^9/L to 5.2 x 10^9/L, platelets 222 x 10^9/L to 195 x 10^9/L over 1 week	None	No sequelae
30 min	None	NA	NA	Ipecac	No sequelae
75 min	None	Hepatosplenomegaly (present before overdose)	None (CBC, LFTs same as baseline at 1, 4, 56 days after)	Ipecac	No sequelae
2 h	Lethargy	Normal	None	Ipecac, activated charcoal	No sequelae
3 h	Grand mal seizure	No focal deficit	CSF, 8 RBC, 15 WBC, glucose 3.8 mmol/L, protein 60 mg/dL	None	Computed tomography, electroencephalogram normal after 3 d, no sequelae

(Continued)

(continued)

Time After Ingestion	Symptoms	Physical Exam Results	Abnormal Lab Values	Treatment	Outcome
3 h	Muscle ache, dizziness, sweating, diarrhea	Normal	None	NA	No sequelae
4 h	Headache, fatigue, tinnitus	Lymphadenopathy	None	Activated charcoal	No sequelae
6 h	Drowsy	Normal	Hgb 14.2–12.5 g/dL over 3 d	None	No sequelae
8 h	Headache, nausea	Nystagmus Upper and lower extremity ataxia	CSF, 2 WBC, 2 RBC; CO_2 21 mmol/L; elevated bilirubin, alanine transaminase, alkaline phosphatase	I.V. fluids	Lab abnormalities resolved in 48 h
8 h (Patient B)	None	NA	NA	None	No sequelae
10 h	None	Normal	None	None	No sequelae
Several h	Abdominal pain	Normal	Hgb 11–8.8 g/dL, WBC 2.4 x 10^9/L to 0.9 x 10^9/L, platelets 213 x 10^9/L to 27 x 10^9/L; nadir day 8	None	Bone marrow biopsy day 8; toxic hypoplasia; CBC normal by day 20

LFTs = liver function tests.

Specific References

Bendayan R, Georgis W, and Shahryar R-T, "Interaction of 3'-Axido-3'-Deoxythymidine With the Organic Base Transporter in a Cultured Renal Epithelium," *Pharmacotherapy*, 1995, 15:338-44.

Collins JM and Unadkat JD, "Clinical Pharmacokinetics of Zidovudine: An Overview of Current Data," *Clin Pharmacokinet*, 1989, 17(1):1-9.

Gill PS, Harrington W, Kaplan MH, et al, "Treatment of Adult T-Cell Leukemia-Lymphoma With a Combination of Interferon Alfa and Zidovudine," *N Engl J Med*, 1995, 332:1744-8.

Gorman SE, Dela Cruz F, and Paloucek F, "Ketoconazole and Zidovudine Overdose," *Am J Emerg Med*, 1995, 13(1):115-6.

Hagler DN and Frame PT, "Azidothymidine Neurotoxicity," *Lancet*, 1986, 2(8520):1392-3.

Hermine O, Bouscary D, Gessain A, et al, "Brief Report: Treatment of Adult T-Cell Leukemia-Lymphoma With Zidovudine and Interferon Alfa," *N Engl J Med*, 1995, 332(26):1749-51.

Ioannidis JPA, Cappelleri JC, Lau J, et al, "Early or Deferred Zidovudine Therapy in HIV-Infected Patients Without an AIDS-Defining Illness: A Meta Analysis," *Ann Intern Med*, 1995, 122:856-66.

Marchbanks K, Dudley MN, Posner MR, et al, "Pharmacokinetics and Pharmacodynamics of High-Dose Zidovudine Administered as a Continuous Infusion in Patients With Cancer," *Pharmacotherapy*, 1995, 15(4):451-7.

Morris DJ, "Adverse Effects and Drug Interactions of Clinical Importance With Antiviral Drugs," *Drug Saf*, 1994, 10(4):281-91.

Newell M-L and Gibb DM, "A Risk-Benefit Assessment of Zidovudine in the Prevention of Perinatal HIV Transmission," *Drug Saf*, 1995, 12:274-82.

Rachlis A and Fanning MM, "Zidovudine Toxicity: Clinical Features and Management," *Drug Saf*, 1993, 8(4):312-20.

Zienam® *see* Imipenem/Cilastatin *on page 420*

Zilden® *see* Diltiazem *on page 287*

Zileuton

CAS Number 11406-87-2

Brand Names Leutrol®

Synonyms A-64077

Use Investigational: Treatment of ulcerative colitis, asthma, allergic rhinitis, psoriasis, and rheumatoid arthritis

Mechanism of Action Benzothiphene hydroxyurea derivative which inhibits 5-lipoxygenase thus inhibiting cysteinyl leukotriene synthesis

Adverse Reactions Urticaria, diarrhea, dyspepsia, intraocular pressure (increased), reversible transaminase increases

Toxicodynamics/Kinetics Half-life: 90-180 minutes

Usual Dosage Asthma: Oral: 400-600 mg 4 times/day

Overdosage Treatment

Decontamination: Ipecac or lavage/activated charcoal with cathartic

Supportive therapy: Urticaria can be treated with epinephrine and antihistamines

Antidote(s)

Epinephrine *on page 1422*

Additional Information No effect on release of prostaglandin D_2 or histamine; in April, 1995, the Advisory Committee of the FDA Division of Pulmonary and Allergy Drugs unanimously voted to recommend that zileuton be approved for marketing

Specific References

Harris RR, Carter GW, Bell RL, et al, "Clinical Activity of Leukotriene Inhibitors," *Int J Immunopharmacol*, 1995, 17:147-56.

Israel E, Rubin P, Kemp JP, et al, "The Effect of Inhibition of 5-Lipoxygenase by Zileuton in Mild-to-Moderate Asthma," *Ann Intern Med*, 1993, 119(11):1059-66.

Knapp HR, "Reduced Allergen-Induced Nasal Congestion and Leukotriene Synthesis With an Orally Active 5-Lipoxygenase Inhibitor," *N Engl J Med*, 1990, 323(25):1745-8.

Stechschulte DJ, "Leukotrienes in Asthma and Allergic Rhinitis," *N Engl J Med*, 1990, 323(25):1769-70.

St Peter JV, Braeckman RA, Granneman GR, et al, "The Effect of Zileuton on Antipyrine and Indocyanine Green Disposition," *Clin Pharmacol Ther*, 1995, 57:299-308.

Zinaderm® *see* Zinc Oxide *on page 813*

Zinamide® *see* Pyrazinamide *on page 663*

Zinc (zink)

CAS Number 7440-66-6; 4468-02-4 (zinc gluconate); 7733-02-0 (zinc sulfate); 7446-20-0 (zinc sulfate)

Brand Names Zincaps®

Synonyms White Copperas; White Vitriol; Zn

Use Supplement for correction of zinc deficiency; used in treatment of acrodermatitis enteropathica

Mechanism of Action Needed for DNA and RNA synthesis and other enzyme symptoms

Adverse Reactions

Central nervous system: Lethargy, chills

(Continued)

Zinc *(Continued)*

Gastrointestinal: Vomiting, pancreatitis
Hematologic: Sideroblastic anemia (due to zinc-induced copper deficiency), thrombocytopenia, leukopenia

Toxicodynamics/Kinetics
Absorption: Zinc sulfate: 20% to 30%
Protein binding: 99%
Half-life: 3 hours
Elimination: Through small bowel excretion

Usual Dosage
Maximum daily dose:
Zinc gluconate: 230 mg
Zinc sulfate: 660 mg
Lethal dose of zinc sulfate: I.V.: 7.4 g

Contraindications Hypersensitivity to any component

Warnings Excessive dose may increase HDL and impair immune system function

Dosage Forms
Capsule: 110 mg [elemental zinc 25 mg]; 220 mg [elemental zinc 50 mg]
Injection: 1 mg/mL (10 mL, 30 mL); 4 mg/mL (10 mL); 5 mg/mL (5 mL, 10 mL, 50 mL)
Tablet: 66 mg [elemental zinc 15 mg]; 200 mg [elemental zinc 46 mg]

Stability Store oral liquid (injectable used orally) in refrigerator

Reference Range Normal serum zinc: 9.2-23.0 μmol/L; levels >30.0 μmol/L associated with bone marrow suppression; normal urinary zinc levels: 0.3-0.4 mg/day (increased to 2.1 mg/day in patients with proteinuria)

Overdosage Treatment
Decontamination:
Dermal: Wash with soap and water
Ocular: Irrigate copiously with saline
Oral: Lavage may be useful; dilute with milk; whole bowel irrigation has been utilized
Supportive therapy: Removal of excess zinc will eventually lead to normal hematopoiesis, although copper levels should be monitored and copper replaced as needed
Enhancement of elimination: Calcium disodium, ethylene diamine tetra-acetate, dimercaprol or BAL has been used with some success; acetylcysteine has been used to increase the urinary excretion of zinc sulfate

Drug Interactions Decreased absorption with penicillamine, iron, tetracyclines, caffeine; zinc decreased absorption of ciprofloxacin, tetracyclines, norfloxacin

Pregnancy Risk Factor C

Pregnancy Implications Zinc deficiency during pregnancy can lead to intrauterine growth retardation during last trimester of pregnancy; has been associated with increased incidence of premature deliveries and stillborns at zinc ingestion of 0.6 mg/kg/day

Monitoring Parameters Patients on TPN therapy should have periodic serum copper and serum zinc levels

Patient Information Take with food if gastrointestinal upset occurs, but avoid foods high in calcium, phosphorous, or phytate; do not exceed recommended dose; notify physician if irritation persists or continues with ophthalmic use

Nursing Implications Do not give undiluted by direct injection into a peripheral vein because of potential for phlebitis, tissue irritation, and potential to increase renal loss of minerals from a bolus injection

Additional Information Daily consumption of 100-150 mg of zinc results in a negative copper balance; can cause a decrease in HDL cholesterol
RDA requirement of zinc:
Infants: 5 mg
Children: 10 mg
Adults:
Male: 15 mg
Female: 12 mg
During pregnancy: 15 mg
Lactating females: 16-19 mg
Historically, zinc sulfate was used as an emetic agent and is radiopaque; elevated zinc levels can occur from chronic ingestion of coins (especially pennies)

Specific References

Banner W, Koch M, Hopf S, et al, "N-Acetylcysteine in the Chelation of Zinc Sulfate," *Vet Hum Toxicol*, 1985, 28:293.

Brocks A, Reid H, and Glazer G, "Acute Intravenous Zinc Poisoning," *Br Med J*, 1977, 1:1390.

Broun ER, Greist A, Tricot G, et al, "Excessive Zinc Ingestion. A Reversible Cause of Sideroblastic Anemia and Bone Marrow Depression," *JAMA*, 1990, 264(11):1441-3.

Burkhart KK, Kulig KW, and Rumack B, "Whole Bowel Irrigation as Treatment for Zinc Sulfate Overdose," *Ann Emerg Med*, 1990, 19(10):1167-70.

Goldenberg RL, Tamura T, Neggers Y, et al, "The Effect of Zinc Supplementation on Pregnancy Outcome," *JAMA*, 1995, 274:463-8.

Hjortso E, Qvist J, Bud MI, et al, "ARDS After Accidental Inhalation of Zinc Chloride Smoke," *Intensive Care Med*, 1988, 14(1):17-24.
Kumar S, "Effect of Zinc Supplementation on Rats During Pregnancy," *Nutr Rep Int*, 1976, 13:33-6.

Zincaps® *see* Zinc *on page 811*

Zinc Oxide

CAS Number 1314-13-2; 8051-03-4
Brand Names Desitin®; Herisan®; Zinaderm®
Synonyms Base Ointment; Blanc de Zinc; Lassar's Zinc Paste
Use Protective coating for mild skin irritations and abrasions, soothing and protective ointment to promote healing of chapped skin, diaper rash, and superficial (but not deep) skin ulcers; used with coal tar in treatment of eczema; also used in sunscreens; used in dental cements as a temporary filling
Mechanism of Action Mild astringent with weak antiseptic properties; blocks ultraviolet A and B along with long-wave light
Adverse Reactions
Dermatologic: Skin sensitivity, irritation
Miscellaneous: Solitary aspergillosis of maxillary sinus associated with zinc oxide from overfilled teeth
Toxicodynamics/Kinetics Absorption: May be absorbed dermally in burns
Usual Dosage Infants, Children, and Adults: Topical: Apply as required to affected areas several times/day
Contraindications Hypersensitivity to any component
Warnings Do not use in eyes; for external use only
Dosage Forms
Ointment, topical: 20% in white ointment (480 g)
Paste, topical: 25% in white petrolatum (480 g)
Stability Avoid prolonged storage at temperatures >30°C
Overdosage Treatment
Decontamination: For maxillary sinus aspergillosis, treatment consists of removal of fungal ball; antifungal therapy is usually not required
Patient Information If irritation develops, discontinue use and consult a physician; paste is easily removed with mineral oil; for external use only; do not use in the eyes
Additional Information Black discoloration when exposed to light can accelerate growth of *Aspergillus fumigatus*, calamine is a combination of zinc oxide with ferric oxide
Specific References

Agren MS, "Percutaneous Absorption of Zinc From Zinc Oxide Applied Topically to Intact Skin in Man," *Dermatologica*, 1990, 180(1):36-9.
Beck-Mannagetta J, "Solitary Aspergillosis of Maxillary Sinus, A Complication of Dental Treatment," *Lancet*, 1983, ii:1260.
Gordon EF, Gordon RC, and Passal DB, "Zinc Metabolism: Basic, Clinical, and Behavioral Aspects," *J Pediatr*, 1981, 99:L341-9.
Preston SL and Bryant BG, "Etiology and Treatment of Diaper Dermatitis," *Hosp Pharm*, 1994, 28(12):1086-9.

Zipeprol Hydrochloride (zi' pa prole)

Related Information
Therapeutic Drugs Associated With Hallucinations *on page 1558-1559*
CAS Number 34758-83-3; 34758-84-4
Brand Names Antituxil-Z®; Bechizolo®; Bronocozina®; Bronx®; Mirsol®; Respirase®; Respirex®; Zitoxil®
Use Antitussive agent
Mechanism of Action Central nervous system activity with antihistaminic, antiserotonin, anticholinergic, and antibradykinin effects
Adverse Reactions
Central nervous system: Drowsiness, dizziness, auditory and visual hallucinations, ataxia
Neuromuscular & skeletal: Opisthotonos, chorea
Miscellaneous: Abuse potential
Signs & Symptoms of Acute Overdose Seizures, cerebral edema, pseudotumor cerebri, coma, respiratory depression
Usual Dosage
Children:
Oral: 3-5 mg/kg/day in divided doses
Rectal: 100-150 mg/day
Adults:
Oral: 150-300 mg/day in divided doses
Rectal: 150 mg 1-2 times/day
Contraindications Hypersensitivity to zipeprol

(Continued)

Zipeprol Hydrochloride *(Continued)*

Warnings Use with caution in patients with a seizure history, history of drug abuse, pregnancy

Reference Range Postmortem blood level in fatal overdose: 5.8 μg/mL and 10.6 μg/mL

Overdosage Treatment

Decontamination: Lavage/activated charcoal with cathartics

Supportive therapy: High doses of naloxone may be required

Antidote(s)

Naloxone Hydrochloride *on page 1447*

Specific References

Crippa O, Polettini A, and Avato FM, "Lethal Poisoning by Zipeprol in Drug Addicts," *J Forensic Sci*, 1990, 35(4):992-9.

Moroni C, Cerchiari EL, Gasparinin, et al, "Overdosage of Zipeprol, a Non-Opiod Antitussive Agent," *Lancet*, 1984, 1(8367):45.

Perraro F and Beorchia A, "Convulsions and Cerebral Oedema Associated With Zipeprol Abuse," *Lancet*, 1984, 1(8367):45-6.

Zithromax™ *see* Azithromycin *on page 140*

Zitoxil® *see* Zipeprol Hydrochloride *on previous page*

Zn *see* Zinc *on page 811*

Zocor™ *see* Simvastatin *on page 697*

Zocord® *see* Simvastatin *on page 697*

Zofran® Injection *see* Ondansetron *on page 578*

Zofran® Oral *see* Ondansetron *on page 578*

Zolin® *see* Oxymetazoline Hydrochloride *on page 586*

Zoloft™ *see* Sertraline Hydrochloride *on page 695*

Zolpidem Tartrate (zole pi' dem)

CAS Number 82626-48-0; 99294-93-6

Brand Names Ambien™; Bikalm®; Niotal®; Stilnox®

Use Hypnotic for short-term management of insomnia

Mechanism of Action Selective agonist of the omega-1 receptor at the CNS gamma amino butyric acid (GABA)/chloride channel complex; not a benzodiazepine, but an imidazopyridin

Adverse Reactions

Central nervous system: Headache, drowsiness, dizziness, slurred speech, hallucinations, anterograde amnesia, headache, night terrors, confusion, drowsiness, coma, ataxia

Dermatologic: Pruritus

Gastrointestinal: Nausea, vomiting, diarrhea

Hepatic: Hepatitis

Neuromuscular & skeletal: Myalgia

Ocular: Miosis

Respiratory: Apnea, respiratory depression

Signs & Symptoms of Acute Overdose Miosis, coma, diplopia, esophageal ulceration, night terrors, respiratory depression, hypotension

Toxicodynamics/Kinetics

Onset of action: 7-27 minutes

Peak oral plasma levels: 2 hours

Duration: 6-8 hours

Absorption: Rapid

Distribution: V_d: 0.54 L/kg

Protein binding: 92% (reduced in renal failure)

Metabolism: Hepatic to inactive metabolites

Bioavailability: 70%

Half-life: 2 hours, (4 hours in renal failure, 10 hours in cirrhosis)

Elimination: Urine and feces; clearance: 0.26 L/hour/kg

Usual Dosage Adults: Oral: 10 mg immediately before bedtime; 5 mg in elderly patients or patients with renal/liver disease; maximum dose: 20 mg

Contraindications Lactation

Warnings Elderly, debilitated, depression, behavior changes, not recommended for use in children <18 years of age

Dosage Forms Tablet: 5 mg, 10 mg

Reference Range Therapeutic: 80-150 ng/mL; serum levels of 500 ng/mL associated with coma

Overdosage Treatment

Decontamination: Lavage/activated charcoal with cathartic for adults ingestions >100 mg

Supportive therapy: Flumazenil effectively antagonizes CNS depressant effects
Enhancement of elimination: Not dialyzable; multiple dosing of activated charcoal may be effective

Antidote(s)

Flumazenil *on page 1428*

Drug Interactions Increased effect/toxicity with alcohol, CNS depressants; increases half-life of chlorpromazine

Pregnancy Risk Factor B

Pregnancy Implications Incomplete calcification of fetal skull bones in rats at levels of 20-100 mg/kg; very low amounts secreted in breast milk

Monitoring Parameters Respiratory and cardiac status

Patient Information Avoid alcohol and other CNS depressants while taking this medication

Nursing Implications Patients may require assistance with ambulation; lower doses in the elderly are usually effective; institute safety measures

Specific References

Garnier R, Guerault E, Muzard D, et al, "Acute Zolpidem Poisoning - Analysis of 344 Cases," *J Toxicol Clin Toxicol*, 1994, 32(4):391-404.

Langtry HD and Benfield P, "Zolpidem: A Review of Its Pharmacodynamic and Pharmacokinetic Properties and Therapeutic Potential," *Drugs*, 1990, 40(2):291-313.

Lheureux P, Debailleul G, De Witte O, et al, "Zolpidem Intoxication Mimicking Narcotic Overdose: Response to Flumazenil," *Hum Exp Toxicol*, 1990, 9(2):105-7.

Meram D and Descotes J, "Acute Poisoning By Zolpidem," *Rev Med Interne*, 1989, 10(5):466.

Mercurio M, De Roos F, and Hoffman RS, "Zolpidem (Ambien™): Exposure Assessment of a New Nonbenzodiazepine GABA Agonist," *Vet Hum Toxicol*, 1994, 36:371.

Pacifici GM, Viani A, Rizzo G, et al, "Plasma Protein Binding of Zolpidem in Liver and Renal Insufficiency," *Int J Clin Pharmacol Ther Toxicol*, 1988, 26(9):439-43.

Queneau PE, Koch S, Hrusovsky S, et al, "Cytolytic Hepatitis Related to Zolpidem," 1st International Symposium on Hepatology and Clinical Pharmacology Liver and Drugs, Abstract, 1994, 39.

Zorkaptil® *see* Captopril *on page 181*

ZORprin® *see* Aspirin *on page 133*

Zosyn™ *see* Piperacillin Sodium and Tazobactam Sodium *on page 628*

Zovirax® *see* Acyclovir *on page 88*

Zurinol® *see* Allopurinol *on page 97*

Zyloprim® *see* Allopurinol *on page 97*

Zymenol® [OTC] *see* Mineral Oil *on page 534*

NONMEDICINAL AGENTS

APPROACH TO INDUSTRIAL TOXINS

SCOPE OF PROBLEM

Chemicals are an inextricable part of modern life and its industrial processes. Over 2 million distinct compounds have been generated, and 50,000-70,000 are part of common commerce. The health effects of most of these more common compounds remain incompletely characterized, particularly for lower level exposures.[1]

The potential for serious incidents with industrial toxins affecting public health is clear, though exposures may occur in unexpected ways. In the extreme, a Union Carbide pesticide plant in Bhopal, India released about 25,000 kg of a production intermediate, methyl isocyanate, over 90 minutes in December 1984. At least 2500 people died, and perhaps 200,000 were injured.[2] In May 1981, distribution of adulterated cooking oil near Madrid, Spain caused 11,000 hospitalizations and 330 deaths from severe pneumonitis. About 30% of those affected developed long-term sequelae, including neuropathy, myopathy, and a form of scleroderma. Industrial contamination of the oil was suspected but the exact agent was never confirmed. More recently in the United States in 1992-93, a change in formula of a nationally distributed leather conditioner was associated with over 500 cases of illness in 17 states, typically cough, dyspnea, and pleuritic chest pain.[3]

The number of individuals injured or killed in incidents involving industrial toxins is uncertain. Surveys during the 1980s suggested perhaps only a dozen individuals per year were injured, but more recent work has shown that these figures are seriously flawed due to inadequate reporting.[4] Some issues are definitional. For instance, industrial toxins may do more harm by their contribution to fires and explosions, than through a direct toxic effect on workers or bystanders. The death of individuals killed in an accident involving transport of toxic chemicals may have far more to do with traumatic injury than toxic exposure. Finally, incidents may not be reported because they involve fuels, regulated toxins in quantities below reporting thresholds, or substances which can be hazardous but not subject to mandatory reporting. Flammable liquids and gases were involved in 70% of incidents in a recent careful national survey from Australia.[5]

While many incidents involve small releases of known compounds in a fixed industrial setting where identification and reporting tends to be better, others may occur in transport, in small business, in high school chemistry labs, or even in homes. Toxins encountered in nonindustrial settings usually are present in smaller quantities and in less lethal concentrations, but proper labeling is often absent. Diagnosis of exposures may be easily missed without detailed history and clinical vigilance. A contaminated victim may also be brought to the emergency department by unsuspecting paramedics, family, or neighbors. For some substances, such contamination may pose a threat to medical personnel, and in unusual circumstances even temporarily close emergency departments for cleanup.

IDENTIFYING A HAZARDOUS MATERIALS (HAZMAT) INCIDENT

Paramedics and emergency medical technicians responding to emergency medical calls today generally have more training and awareness of the acute hazards of industrial toxins thanks to professional and governmental efforts of the past decade. In larger cities, organized hazardous materials units are increasingly common, with specialized training, databases, and equipment. Federal legislation, notably the Superfund Amendments and Reauthorization Act (SARA) Title III of 1986, included chemical emergency training, community planning, toxics inventory, and right-to-know provisions. In theory, these efforts have made it easier to identify the industrial toxins involved in an incident through material safety data sheets and information on file with fire departments and emergency agencies.

While budgetary and organizational constraints have kept this vision from being fulfilled, progress has been made. Material safety data sheets (MSDS) are available in most larger workplaces, though compliance is spottier in smaller operations. These sheets typically include at least cursory information on a substance's physical properties, acute health effects, and simple first aid measures, though they are often insufficient for the purposes of a treating physician.[6] Copies are often kept on file with fire services, at poison control centers, or in lock boxes on industrial premises, accessible to first responders. Trade secret ingredients may not be listed on such sheets, but must be revealed to physicians with a reasonable need to know for a given case, and who agree to respect confidentiality.

Computerization has advanced the cause in some fortunate areas with operating programs such as CAMEO, which electronically maintains the locations and quantities of toxic substances in local industries, and CD-ROM and telephone database links. Larger manufacturers will often have safety personnel who can identify the industrial toxin involved in an incident onsite, or when shipped offsite. With the assistance of CHEMTREC (Chemical Transportation Emergency Center — 800-424-9300 or (202)-887-1255), an industry-supported informational clearinghouse in operation since 1971, medical personnel can receive help in identifying substances through their markings or papers, and can be placed in touch with industrial experts. The Canadian counterpart is known as the Canadian Transportation Emergency Center (CANUTEC 613-996-6666).

Setting

Industrial plants, laboratories, warehouses, hardware and garden outlets, grain silos, and dry cleaners are examples of settings where an injured or unconscious victim may be suffering from a toxic exposure. Events at some sites may seem surprising (ie, significant chlorine gas exposures from a tank rupture at a community swimming pool) and community preplanning is crucial. "Confined space" environments such as sealed rooms, storage tanks, and even ditches filled with a heavier than air gas, kill nearly 90 U.S workers each year, 25% of whom are would-be rescuers.[7] Remember, even residential basements may contain significant toxic hazards.

Container and Content Appearance

In transport incidents, the size, shape, paint schemes, and markings of a truck or rail car can help identify its contents or shipper. In laboratories or factories, characteristic barrels, bottles, or vessels may provide identification clues that a coworker or supervisor can help decipher. The odor, color, and consistency of spilled contents, escaping fumes, or flames may be useful to knowledgeable persons, but cannot be counted on to warn responders of serious toxic hazards. Field personnel should note these things to the extent safely possible when suspicions of a toxic exposure exists.

Placards and Labels

These can provide general and specific information. These should be examined at an appropriate distance, and with alertness to the possible presence of a toxic or other threat to rescuers. For instance, a freight train derailment may involve large quantities of industrial toxins with consequent risk of explosion; binoculars should be used for reading placards. Several common types of placards and labels exist.

- U.S. Department of Transportation (DOT) placards with colors, North American class numbers, and symbols for general hazard classes, are outlined in the following table. The simple placard "dangerous" is used to indicate mixed loads. It must be recognized that federal regulations do not require vehicle placards when toxins are carried in quantities less than 1000 pounds, the only exceptions being explosives, higher level poisons, radioactives, and water-reactive flammable solids.
- National Fire Protection Association (NFPA) diamond (704) system divides the diamond-shaped placard into four quadrants: top (red) is flammability, the right (yellow) is instability, the left (blue) is general health hazard, and bottom (white) contains special information, for instance, water reactivity. The top three quadrants are labeled 0-4, 4 being most hazardous. This system may be used on buildings, terminals, or in labeling containers and packages.
- Four-digit United Nations or North America numbers (UN/NA) are often placed in the center of DOT placards. Such numbers are fairly, but not completely specific, as one may apply to several related compounds. Using these numbers with the index in the DOT guidebook, or by other authors, can provide basic guidelines on first aid and very simple medical management.[8,9]
- Small end-use container labels. Be very certain of your own safety if you are close enough to read these! Other obvious problems are substances placed in another product's container. Note the concentration and expiration date, since some products convert with time to more toxic byproducts.

International Classification System for Shipping of Hazardous Materials
(usually displayed at the bottom of the placard)

CLASS 1	**Explosives** (instantaneous release of gas or heat)
Division	
1.1	Explosive with a mass explosion hazard (ie, dynamite, TNT, black powder, military ammunition)
1.2	Explosives with a projection hazard
1.3	Explosives with a predominantly fire hazard (ie, fireworks, rocket motors, military ammunition)
1.4	Explosives with no significant blast hazard
1.5	Very insensitive explosives
1.6	Extremely insensitive explosive articles
CLASS 2	**Gases**
Division	
2.1	Flammable gases (ie, hydrogen, acetylene, propane, methane, butane)
2.2	Nonflammable gases — may support combustion (ie, carbon dioxide, oxygen, anhydrous ammonia, chlorine)
2.3	Poison gases
2.4	Corrosive gases (Canadian)
CLASS 3	**Flammable Liquids**
Division	
3.1	Flashpoint below -18°C (0°F) (ie, n-pentane, propylene oxide, petroleum distillates)
3.2	Flashpoint at -18°C and above but less than 23°C (73°F) (ie, triethylamine, toluene, tetrahydroforan, pyridine, methyl alcohol)
3.3	Flashpoint of 23°C and up to 61°C (141°F) (ie, turpentine, trichloroethylene, tetramethyl lead, styrene, nitroethane)

CLASS 4 **Flammable Solids, Spontaneously Combustible Materials, and Materials That Are Dangerous When Wet**

Division

4.1 Flammable solid (ie, white phosphorous, phosphorus pentasulfide)

4.2 Spontaneously combustible materials (ie, oily cotton waste, burnt fibers)

4.3 Materials that are dangerous when wet (ie, metallic sodium, sodium hydroxide, calcium carbide)

CLASS 5 **Oxidizers and Organic Peroxides**

Division

5.1 Oxidizers (ie, nitric acid, calcium hypochlorite, potassium permanganate, ammonium persulfate, sodium nitrate)

5.2 Organic peroxides (ie, benzoyl peroxide, lauroyl peroxide, peracetic acid, bleaching peroxides)

CLASS 6 **Poisonous and Etiologic (infectious) Materials**

Division

6.1 Poisonous materials (ie, hydrogen cyanide, phosgene, nitrogen tetroxide, aniline, tetraethyl lead, parathion)

6.2 Etiologic/infectious agent (ie, measles, rabies virus)

CLASS 7 **Radioactive Materials**

CLASS 8 **Corrosives**

CLASS 9 **Miscellaneous Hazardous Materials**

Shipping Papers

These should accompany hazardous material shipments and provide more precise detail about contents, their location in the shipment, packaging, and quantities. These may also provide the names and possibly emergency phone numbers for the originating manufacturer and some information about the shipment's destination. Commonly, these papers also include the UN number used on placards, clues to hazards (marked by occurring first, being in a distinctive color, or marked with an "X" or "RQ" in the "HM" column). CHEMTREC can provide help with using the information in such papers.

Behavior and Symptoms

Burning eyes and skin irritation may warn of the presence of an industrial toxin. "Toxidromes", such as the cholinergic syndrome associated with organophosphate poisoning, can alert an observant clinician. Giddiness or ataxia can suggest solvent intoxication. Unfortunately, the lack of sensory warning or symptoms does not assure safety. Some persons are genetically unable to detect the almond odor of cyanide, and other toxins may have no odor (eg, carbon monoxide) or quickly extinguish perception (eg, hydrogen sulfide). Still other toxins have treacherous delayed effects. For instance, nitrogen oxide gases may initially cause only nonspecific symptoms of hypoxia without eye and throat irritation. These symptoms may resolve into 4-12 hours of relative well-being, only then followed by fatal pulmonary edema. At the opposite end of the spectrum, many symptoms can be produced simply by anxiety, and outbreaks of mass psychogenic illness are well-reported, particularly in school settings when an unusual odor is noted. This diagnosis is one of exclusion and should be made with great wariness for organic etiologies.[10]

Several caveats about identification must be emphasized. Rescuers should not place themselves in harm's way to gather such data. Placards and papers may not be present, may be destroyed, or may be overlooked in accidents. As the costs of appropriate hazardous waste disposal increase, the potential for illegal and unmarked storage, transport, and disposal may increase. Placards and guidebooks may identify only the most salient hazard associated with a substance, such as flammability, but omit important clinical effects such as central nervous system toxicity.

Precise identification of the agent(s) in an incident is important, but must be kept in perspective for at least several reasons. Regardless of the exact identity, ending ongoing exposure and basic supportive care are needed. Simply by knowing the general class of an agent, such as a solvent, treating physicians will have some useful guidance on expected effects and management. Finally, clinicians must always be alert when a given patient's illness and course are not well explained by the agent initially blamed. The "accident" may represent a suicide attempt or be a manifestation of ethanol or other substance abuse. While seizures or syncope may represent an unsuspected toxic exposure, it is also perilous for unrelated medical conditions to be missed or ignored through false attribution to an otherwise trivial contamination.

RESCUER AND BYSTANDER SAFETY

Once an event is thought to possibly involve industrial toxins and exposed individuals, several important issues beyond medical management must be addressed. These concerns are particularly true for field responders, for instance, paramedics working under the medical control of an emergency department (ED), but also apply to patients arriving unannounced to an ED or office.

Industrial toxins may be more dangerous because of their flammability, explosiveness, or cryogenic properties, rather than their inherent toxicity. A train wreck or fire may create hazards of chemical mixtures and pyrolytic products with risks considerably beyond those of the individual constituents. Ambulances should park uphill and upwind of accident scenes. Hot vehicle catalytic converters can ignite spilled fuel or product at the scene of an industrial toxin spill. Placards should be read with binoculars, and rescuers should not enter situations without adequate precautions in the manner of proper protective gear, and backup for the threat likely present. Even inert agents, like noble gases, can be hazardous if they displace air and oxygen from a confined space.

Police and fire personnel need to establish adequate zones to control bystanders and media, permit efficient staging and flow of rescue vehicles and personnel, and facilitate extrication and decontamination of victims. Individuals should move at least 150 feet up or crosswind from a spill, and further in the presence of fire because of the uncertainties of toxic combustion products and explosion hazard. In occasional events, industrial toxins are present in sufficient toxicity and quantity that evacuation of buildings and neighborhoods within 1000 feet or more becomes necessary to consider. This is an extreme measure, and runs the risk of exposing individuals in transit to higher levels of toxin than they would face secured in their own home or workplace. Sheltering in place makes more sense for above ground structures which can limit entrance of outside air, for substances with peak rather than cumulative toxicity, and for events with short warning times and rapid toxin dispersion.[11]

Patients presenting acutely exposed to an industrial first aid station, emergency department, or clinic may not have had the benefit of field decontamination. They will not present the hazards of the scene with its potentially large quantities of a toxin, but they may still have sufficient quantities of a toxin in their clothes, hair, and skin to pose some risk to unwary emergency personnel. At the very least, contaminated individuals should remain within a restricted area in the receiving facility, have their clothes expeditiously removed, bagged, and labeled, and have obvious contamination gently blotted or brushed off. With improvised barriers and climate permitting, this may be done outdoors, and to the extent possible, by the patient.

Requirements for personal protective gear can be controversial. In the field, an experienced hazardous materials team will have air-tight suits and positive pressure self-contained breathing apparatus (SCBA) equipment which may permit trained personnel to enter highly toxic environments for rescue purposes. In an office or ED, this level of protection is not generally possible because of the expense, staff turnover, and training essential to make safe use of such equipment. Vision, communication, and clinical examination and procedural skills of medical staff in such protective gear is also severely hindered. Gowning with Saranex coated Tyvek material and double-gloving with thicker surgical gloves are generally a minimum for responders faced with a patient with evident or likely contamination. In areas where preplanning would indicate a higher risk of receiving such patients (ie, industrial zones), cartridge respirators and more chemical resistant gloves may be worthwhile investments. The four basic levels of protective suits are as follows.

Protective Clothing — EPA Designated Classification

Level A

Maximum skin protection
Maximum respiratory protection

Level B

Maximum respiratory protection (same as Level A)
Moderate skin protection

Level C

Minimum respiratory protection (ie, air purifying respirator)
Moderate/minimum skin protection

Level D

No respiratory protection
Minor skin protection

HEALTH IMPLICATIONS OF AN EXPOSURE

Once an identification has been made and reasonable safety precautions taken, just as with a pharmaceutical adverse reaction or overdose, the clinician will need to take the next logical steps of learning more about the substance, its health effects at different doses, and immediate management. Central to all of these is the concept of "dose", since even the world's most deadly substance will not hurt a patient who fails to come into contact with it. Proximity alone does not equal prognosis.

Exposure Assessment

Estimating exposure in a pharmaceutical overdose is often a simple matter of multiplication — knowing the medicine, its strength, and using an estimate of the number of pills ingested to calculate a total dosage. Exposure to industrial toxins poses additional challenges because the routes of absorption can vary, field measurements of exposures are usually not available, and biomarkers (ie, serum drug levels) are not consistently available, particularly for use in initial management. Despite these obstacles, history is often quite useful in establishing a reasonably accurate idea of exposure, which in turn will provide guidance for the clinician in triage and management.

The following are questions essential to address when assessing patient exposure:

- toxin, form, concentration, vehicle, potential routes of exposure
- quantity present, degree of release, and warning properties
- patient proximity, activity, and duration of exposure
- modifying factors: closed space, engineering controls, temperature and weather, personal protective equipment (PPE), decontamination
- presence and time course of symptoms and signs

Industrial chemicals exist in widely differing concentrations and formulations, and their physical state and properties will be affected by the conditions of their storage and release. Melting point, boiling point, vapor pressure, storage techniques, and accident conditions will determine the physical form of the substance. Density relative to air and water will help determine whether gases or liquids will float, dissipate, or collect in low places. Storage under pressure or cryogenic conditions may alter the circumstances and degree of exposure, as will the quantities stored and the rate and totality of release.

Reconstructing the activity of the patient is an important element, especially when reviewed with knowledge of the toxin's most relevant routes of exposure. In general, inhalation is the most significant. Substances absorbed in this manner include not only the gases or vapors of volatile liquids, but also the aerosols and dusts of nonvolatile liquids and solids. Dermal absorption is next in importance, especially for fat soluble substances, though water soluble agents can be absorbed through mucus membranes or open wounds. A substance's vehicle can also affect dermal absorption. Ingestion may occur through error or suicidal attempt. Lesser amounts may be swallowed through smoking, drinking or eating in a contaminated area, or swallowing dust-impregnated mucus. Occasional accidents can involve very significant systemic absorption through trauma or high pressure hydraulic injection into soft tissue.

A patient's knowledge of the duration of exposure depends in part on the warning properties of the toxin through symptoms like coughing, or burning of the skin and eyes. A patient trapped or working in a confined space (a poorly ventilated area) or standing in spilled chemicals is obviously at risk for greater exposure.[7,12] However, in incidents where rescue personnel have adequate and unbreached protective clothing and respiratory equipment, higher exposures may occur to more distant response personnel such as police involved in traffic control without the benefit of respirators. Weather conditions may exacerbate exposure through wind shifts, or heat which may volatilize more of the toxin and increase skin blood flow, sweating, and absorption. In indoor events, proper engineering controls (if operational) such as exhaust systems, protective gear, emergency showers, and alarms can mitigate exposure. Prompt and thorough decontamination is a similar plus in limiting exposure.

Occupational Exposure Limits

Value	Abbreviation	Definition
Threshold limit value (3 types) (ACGIH)*	TVL	Refers to airborne concentrations of substances and represents conditions under which it is believed that nearly all workers may be repeatedly exposed day after day without adverse effect.
1. Threshold limit value — time-weighted average (ACGIH)*	TLV-TWA	The time-weighted average concentration for a normal 8-hour workday and a 40-hour workweek, to which nearly all workers may be repeatedly exposed, day after day, without adverse effect.
2. Threshold limit value — short-term exposure limit (ACGIH)*	TLV-STEL	The concentration to which workers can be exposed continuously for a short period of time without suffering from irritation, chronic or irreversible tissue damage, or narcosis of sufficient degree to increase the likelihood of accidental injury, impair self-rescue or materially reduce work efficiency, and provided that the daily TLV-TWA is not exceeded.
3. Threshold limit value — ceiling (ACGIH)*	TLV-C	The concentration that should not be exceeded during any part of the working exposure.
Permissible exposure limit (OSHA)†	PEL	Same as TLV-TWA.
Immediately dangerous to life and health (OSHA)†	IDLH	A maximum concentration (in air) from which one could escape within 30 minutes without any escape-impairing symptoms or any irreversible health effects.
Recommended exposure limit (NIOSH)‡	REL	Highest allowable airborne concentration that is not expected to injure a worker; expressed as a ceiling limit or time-weighted average for an 8- or 10-hour workday.

*American Conference of Governmental Industrial Hygienists.
†Occupational Safety and Health Administration.
‡National Institute for Occupational Safety and Health.

In some situations, portable or fixed monitoring devices can provide actual ambient environmental levels of toxins to which patients may have been exposed. While toxin concentrations in liquids or surface contaminant levels can be assessed, the airborne contaminants (gas, vapor, or particulate) are generally most applicable to an individual patient's exposure. Interpreting standards for the toxins can be problematic since any given value may not reflect the actual exposure experience of the individual under consideration, and individual sensitivity to an acute exposure may occur considerably below the most common standards, those designed to protect a healthy worker in occupational settings. Age, medical conditions, and medications are among a number of factors which may make a "safe" level (ie, less than the standard), in fact hazardous for a given person. The most common occupational standards for airborne contaminants in U.S. are as follows.

Threshold limit values (TLV) — Set by the American Conference of Governmental Industrial Hygiene, these specify limits of worker exposure to ambient substances, not absorbed dose. There are three general types of TLV. The first is an 8 hours per day, 40 hours per week occupational time weighted average exposure (TLV-TWA) "to which nearly all workers can be repeatedly exposed day after day without adverse effect." These were adopted by Occupational Safety and Health Administration in 1972 and renamed PELs (permissible exposure limits), though with two decades of modification TLV and PEL may not precisely correspond today. RELs (recommended exposure limits) are similar standards set by NIOSH. These are generally set for a 10-hour workday and tend to be stricter than the PELs and RELs, but are not set for as many substances.

A second form of TLV is the short-term exposure limit (TLV-STEL), a 15-minute time weighted average to which workers can be exposed without suffering irritation, chronic or irreversible tissue damage, or narcosis which threatens safety or work efficiency. Ceiling values can be applied as a modification of TLVs, PELs, or RELs, and indicate instantaneous concentrations of a substance which should never be exceeded in the workplace. The biological exposure indices (BEI) are levels of agents collected from biological fluids from a healthy worker who had been exposed to that agent (through inhalation) at an exposure equivalent to the TLV. Examples of BEI are found in the following table.

Agent	BEI (end of work-shift, unless otherwise noted)
Acetone	Urine: 100 mg/L
Arsenic (inorganic)	Urine: 50 mcg/g creatinine
Benzene	Urine: Total urine phenol: 50 mg/g creatinine
Carbon disulfide	Urine: 5 mg of 2-thiothiazolidine-4-carboxylic acid/g of creatinine
Carbon monoxide	Blood carboxyhemoglobin: 3.5%
Ethylbenzene	Urine (end of work week): 1.5 g mandelic acid/g creatinine
n-Hexane	Urine: 5 mg 2.5-hexanedione/g creatinine
Mercury	Blood (end of work week): 15 mcg/L
Methanol	Urine: 15 mg/L
Methyl ethyl ketone (2-butanone)	Urine: 2 mg/L
Methyl isobutyl ketone	Urine: 2 mg/L
Parathion	Urine: Para-nitrophenol 5 mg/g creatinine
Pentachlorophenol	Plasma: 5 mg/L
Phenol	Urine: 250 mg/g creatinine
Styrene (vinylbenzene)	Urine: 800 mg mandelic acid/g creatinine or 240 mg phenylglyoxylic acid/g creatinine
Toluene	Blood: 1 mg/L Urine: 2.5 g of hippuric acid/g creatinine
Xylene	Urine: 1.5 g methylhippuric acid/g creatinine

Finally, there are a variety of air pollution standards set by the U.S. Environmental Protection Agency which regulate air pollution and emissions. Since these apply to the chronic outdoor exposures of the general public, levels are usually several orders of magnitude lower than occupational standards.

Shorter-term emergency exposure standards are more relevant to the situations patients brought ill to emergency departments have faced, but even here, standards may differ by an order of magnitude or more, and they may inconsistently reflect toxicity.[13,14] The best known emergency standard is the immediately dangerous to life or health (IDLH), set by EPA and NIOSH. IDLH situations include conditions of oxygen deficiency and risk from radiation and explosion, or high acutely toxic airborne chemical levels which mandate adequate respirator use. Other emergency standards include the emergency exposure guidance level (EEGL), a 1-hour exposure standard set for military personnel by the National Academy of Sciences, and the emergency response planning guidelines (ERPGs) developed through the American Industrial Hygiene Association which are also 1-hour exposure guidelines. These range from "level of concern" up through ERPG-1 (mild transient health effects), and ERPG-2 (irreversible or serious health effects), to ERPG-3 (life-threatening health effects). Forty-three of these had been approved through 1992.[15] Some of the most important are listed in the following table. Finally, community emergency exposure levels (CEELs) are being developed for the EPAs 366 extremely hazardous substances. These are ceiling values which should not be exceeded for the general public over a 1- to 8-hour period.

Selected Currently Approved ERPGs (1992)

Chemical	ERPG-1	ERPG-2	ERPG-3
Ammonia	25 ppm	200 ppm	1000 ppm
1,3 Butadiene	10 ppm	50 ppm	5000 ppm
Chlorine	1 ppm	3 ppm	20 ppm
Epichlorhydrin	2 ppm	20 ppm	100 ppm
Formaldehyde	1 ppm	10 ppm	25 ppm
Hydrogen chloride	3 ppm	20 ppm	100 ppm
Hydrogen fluoride	5 ppm	20 ppm	50 ppm
Hydrogen sulfide	0.1 ppm	30 ppm	100 ppm
Methyl mercaptan	0.005 ppm	25 ppm	100 ppm
Phosphorus pentoxide	5 mg/m^3	25 mg/m^3	100 mg/m^3
Sulphur dioxide	0.3 ppm	3 ppm	15 ppm
Sulphuric acid	2 mg/m^3	10 mg/m^3	30 mg/m^3
Vinyl acetate	5 ppm	75 ppm	500 ppm

It must be emphasized that the actual level of chemicals at an emergency site is generally unknown, and even when known, does not take into account mixtures, combustion, reaction products, or the special vulnerabilities of individual victims. Moreover, few chemicals have guidelines in all of the above categories, and most have not had standards set at all. Release plume computer modeling software, such as CAMEO, is increasingly available to more organized hazardous materials accident response teams. Such techniques use wind speed and estimated release quantities to suggest in real time the range and area downwind that dangerous chemical concentrations will be found. Such models cannot account for microenvironments such as ditches, courtyards, and stairwells which may have concentrations significantly exceeding predictions. In the final analysis, no level can substitute for cautious response to an incident and repeated clinical evaluation of an exposed patient.

Interrupting Further Exposure and Decontamination

Stopping further exposure is an obvious but often overlooked therapy. In the field, patients under their own power should be removed from the immediate area of toxin (the hot zone) by directing them to safer areas. If rescuers have adequate training and protection for the situation, removing incapacitated victims to a decontamination area will permit field medical personnel to begin simple decontamination and simple supportive care. In the hot zone, only the simplest resuscitation is generally indicated, such as opening the airway and protecting the cervical spine, and early rescuers should not take on the risk of removing obviously dead victims.

In the decontamination (or warm zone), clothes should be stripped to the extent made possible by weather conditions. Modesty and shelter from wind can be improved with the use of tarpaulins or portable shelters. Shoes can be significant sources of ongoing exposure, and should be removed wherever possible. If the patient's only exposure is to gas or vapors, no other decontamination, other than a simple washing of exposed skin, may be needed. Dry or particulate material should be gently brushed or shaken off with attention to minimizing dust. Copious warm water is almost always appropriate for eye and dermal irrigation; the exothermia of the few water reactive substances should be manageable with adequate water flow. Acids and especially bases may require prolonged irrigation of eyes and skin (30 minutes to hours). Attention to the possibility of iatrogenic hypothermia is warranted. Decontaminating personnel should be trained, should have splash protection, may require cartridge respirators or more, and will require decontamination themselves. Expert opinion should be sought promptly from pre-arranged sources such as the U.S. Agency for Toxic Substances and Disease Registry or an industrial toxin savvy poison control center. The patient should be wrapped and transferred to the support (clean or cold) zone; intravenous lines, oxygen, and other stabilization can be performed. Transportation and communication with receiving hospitals should be arranged. Preparation of ambulances and other transport vehicles with polyvinyl chloride sheets can reduce contamination by residual toxins.

In the emergency department, the adequacy of field decontamination should be reviewed. Few hospitals have great experience with managing grossly contaminated patients, and prior agreements with fire departments or HAZMAT units to assist EDs in decontamination can be useful. Essential aspects of personnel protection have been discussed previously. There are now explicit JCAHO accreditation standards for hospital ED emergency preparedness to "environmental or man-made events". Key elements include current toxicologic reference materials and antidote information, a list of referral and consultation services, and equipment for chemical incidents.[16] Great care should be taken to avoid contaminating expensive, nondisposable hospital equipment. Not only may it spread toxins to other staff and patients, but it may be placed out of commission. Even after apparently thorough decontamination, continued absorption may take place under watchbands, underwear, or through residual material in body folds or ear canals. A final method of preventing absorption is through methods of enhancing elimination. These are generally more appropriate for ingestion exposures, and would include activated charcoal, saline diuresis, and high flow or hyperbaric oxygen. Inducing emesis is generally not advised because of the frequency of corrosives and solvents in industrial toxins, both of which contraindicate this approach.

DETAILED CLINICAL INFORMATION ABOUT AN INDUSTRIAL TOXIN

Clinical management of industrial toxin exposure is usually supportive; antidotes are generally not available. The notable exceptions are the cyanide containing compounds, hydrogen sulfide, hydrogen fluoride, cholinergic poisoning, metals, and methemoglobin-forming agents. These are discussed in detail elsewhere in the handbook. The toxic entity may not be readily apparent in the product names and "sound alikes" are common in chemical terminology. Names should be spelled out over the phone and Chemical Abstract Service registry numbers repeated. An excellent source of detailed information about a known product is the 24-hour hotline sponsored by the Chemical Manufacturers' Association (CHEMTREC, 800-424-9300). Staff there can help identify products through train and truck markings, and can often place callers in touch with industrial personnel knowledgable about a substance's properties. For more clinically relevant information, a fine 24-hour information source is the Agency for Toxic Substances and Disease Registry's emergency division (404-639-0615) with on-call access to physicians and toxicologists experienced in toxic exposures. Poison control centers can also be extremely valuable, particularly those with the CD-ROM resource TOMES Plus which includes Meditext. For agricultural and animal toxins, the National Animal Poison Control Center (217-333-3611) is an excellent resource. Less acute information can be provided by NIOSH, EPA, and a variety of National Library of Medicine databases, most notably TOXNET (301-496-6531). The Registry of Toxic Effects and Chemical Substances (RTECS) identification number found in the NIOSH Guidebook, among other places, is especially useful for searching databases in the U.S. National Library of Medicine. It should be noted that U.S. federal law requires notification of the National Response Center (800-424-8802) for releases of certain hazardous substances which exceed a certain threshold.

MEDICAL MANAGEMENT

Detailed discussion of management for thousands of substances is obviously beyond the scope of this chapter and handbook. A few generalizations may be useful. Unconsciousness should not be attributed to the toxin without attention to the possibility of head trauma, seizures, and hypoxia. Hypotension usually responds to fluid resuscitation; adrenergic agents such as dopamine may induce fatal dysrhythmias in patients whose myocardium has been sensitized by halogenated hydrocarbons. Heat stress is an important issue in rescuers who have been working in encapsulated suits, even in cool weather. The issue of delayed toxicity should be explicitly considered in victims of industrial poisoning; observational units may help in appropriate management.

LONG-TERM EFFECTS OF EXPOSURE

Once someone has been stabilized, treated, observed, and released from the ED or hospital, there remain a number of important health issues. These include the sequelae of burns and chronic dermatitis, a variety of respiratory and other target organ effects, such as reactive airways disease, and psychological issues such as post-traumatic stress disorder. Some patients experience disabling fatigue or more generalized sensitivity to formerly innocuous substances like perfumes, the so-called multiple chemical sensitivity syndrome.[17]

Other patients fear that their immune system has been seriously affected by an exposure. Immune effects can include inflammation, hypersensitivity, autoimmunity, proliferation, and deficiency. All these effects can be conditioned by prior exposure, neuroendocrine modulators, and stress.

Relatively few clinically relevant immunotoxins have been well characterized and validated laboratory parameters rarely exist to establish immunotoxicity and prognosis following an exposure. A basic investigative panel would comprise a CBC, 5-part leukocyte differential, absolute lymphocyte count, serum total protein, albumin, globulin, ESR, and ANA. A more detailed approach has been recently published.

Perhaps the long-term effect of greatest concern to most people is the threat of cancer after exposure to a putative carcinogen. Cancer kills about 20% of Americans, and affects >30% at some time in their life. Because a substance's carcinogenicity engenders such fears and has important implications for regulation and reporting, industrial toxins with such properties deserve special discussion. Despite the cynical popular wisdom that "everything gives you cancer", surprisingly few substances are well documented to do so. Proof of carcinogenesis rests on five general pillars.[18] The most conclusive are well-designed human epidemiologic studies, but these are daunting to execute and fund, and available for relatively few toxins. The four other elements include animal studies, pathological reports, Ames testing, and increasingly, molecular modeling. Adverse reproductive consequences are another area of high patient concern. Pragmatic guidelines in this area have recently been published, and reproductive hotlines exist in many areas of the country.[19] The following tables list those toxins which have been best documented to be carcinogenic.

Potential Human Carcinogens*

2-Acetylaminofluorene (CAS #53-96-3)	Urinary pancreas
4-Aminodiphenyl (CAS #92-67-1)	Bladder
Benzidine (UN #1885; CAS #92-87-5)	Urinary, liver, skin
Bis-chloromethyl ether (2249: 542-88-1)	Lungs
3,3′-Dichlorbenzidine (and its salts) (CAS #91-94-1)	
4-Dimethylaminoazobenzene (CAS #60-11-7)	Urinary
Ethyleneimine (1185; 151-56-4)	
Methyl chloromethyl ether (UN #1239; CAS #07-30-2)	
α-Naphthylamine (2077; 134-32-7)	Bladder
β-Naphthylamine (1650; 91-59-8)	Bladder
4-Nitrobiphenyl (PNB) (CAS #92-93-3)	Bladder
N-Nitrosodimethylamine (CAS #62-75-9)	
β-Propiolactone (BPL) (CAS #57-57-8)	

*OSHA regulated carcinogens (outlined in 29 CFR 1910.1003-1910.1016)

NIOSH Occupational Carcinogens

(as identified in rule 29 CFR 1990.0103)

	UN #	CAS #	Neoplasm Site
Acetaldehyde	1089	75-07-0	Squamous cell/adenocarcinomas in rodents at 735 ppm or higher
2-Acetylaminofluorene*		53-96-3	Urinary, pancreas
Acrylamide	2074	79-06-01	Skin
Acrylonitrile	1093	107-13-1	Prostate, colon, lung, stomach, and lymphatic cancer suspected
Aldrin	2761	309-00-2	Liver
4-Aminodiphenyl*		92-67-1	Bladder
Aniline	1547	62-53-3	Bladder
Ansidine (O-,p-isomers)	2431	90-04-0 104-94-9	
Arsenic	1554	7740-38-2	Basal cell/squamous cell of skin; lung, (RR 208) lymphoma, bone marrow
Arsine	2188	7784-42	
Asbestos	2213, 2590	1332-21-4	Bronchial (RR = 1.5-12), carcinoma/mesothelioma
Benzene	1114	71-43-2	Leukemia (RR = 2.5)
Benzidine*	1885	92-87-5	Bladder (RR = 14)
Beryllium (Be)	1566, 1567	7440-41-7	Lungs
1,3-Butadiene	1010	106-99-0	Lymphoma, lung, hemangiosarcoma
Tert-butyl chromate		1189-85-1	
Cadmium (dust or fume)	2570	7440-43-9 1306-19-0	Lung/prostate
Calcium arsenate	1573	7778-44-1	See arsenic
Carbon black		1333-86-4	
Carbon tetrachloride	1846	56-23-5	Brain, lymphocytic leukemia, liver
Chlordane	2762	57-74-9	Liver
Chlorinated camphene	2761	8001-350-2	Skin
Chlorodiphenyl (42% chlorine)	2315	53469-21-9	Liver, renal
Chlorodiphenyl (54% chlorine)	2315	11097-69-1	Liver, renal
Chloroform	1888	67-66-3	Liver, renal
Chloromethyl methyl ether	1239	107-30-2	
Bis-chloromethyl ether*	2249	542-88-1	Lungs (RR = 100)
β-Chloroprene	1991	126-99-8	
Chromic acid and chromates	1755, 1463	7738-94-5	Lung, nasal sinuses (RR = 4-20)
Coal tar pitch volatiles (not asphalt)		65996-93-2	
DDT	2761	50-29-3	Breast, leukemia, lymphoma, lung
1,2-Dibromo-3-chloropropane	2872	96-12-8	Stomach, liver, skin, kidney, lung, testes
Para-dichlorobenzene	1592	106-46-7	Leukemia

(continued)

	UN #	CAS #	Neoplasm Site
3-3′-Dichlorbenzidine (and its salts)*		91-94-1	
Dichloroethyl ether	1916	111-44-4	Liver
Dieldrin	2761	60-57-1	Liver
Diglycidyl ether		2238-07-5	
1-1-Dimethylhydrazine	1163	57-14-7	Nasal, lung
4-Dimethylaminoazobenzene*		60-11-7	Urinary
Dimethyl sulfate	1595	77-78-1	
Dinitrotoluene (DNT)	1600, 2038	25321-14-9	
Di-sec octyl phthalate		117-81-7	
Dioxane	1165	123-91-1	Nasal, respiratory
Epichlorohydrin	2023	106-89-8	
Ethyl acrylate	1917	140-88-5	Nasal, thyroid
Ethylene dibromide	1605	106-93-4	Nasal, mesothelioma
Ethylene dichloride	1184	107-06-02	
Ethyleneimine*	1185	151-56-4	
Ethylene oxide	1040	75-21-8	Leukemia, Hodgkin's disease, stomach, pancreas
Formaldehyde (aqueous or gaseous)	1198, 2209	50-00-0	Nasal
Heptachlor	2761	76-44-8	Liver
Hexachloroethane	9037	67-72-1	
Hydrazine	2029, 2030	302-01-2	Lung
Methoxychlor	2761	72-43-5	Liver
Methyl bromide	1062	74-83-9	Stomach, testes
Methyl chloride	1063	74-87-3	Renal
Methylene chloride	1593	75-09-2	
Methyl chloromethyl ether*	1239	07-30-2	
Methyl hydrazine (MMH)	1244	60-34-4	Lung, colon
Methyl iodide	2644	74-88-4	
α-Naphthylamine*	2077	134-32-7	Bladder
β-Naphthylamine*	1650	91-59-8	Bladder (RR = 87)
Nickel (metal and other compounds)		7440-02-0	Lung
Nickel carbonyl	1259	13463-39-3	Nasal, lung
4-Nitrobiphenyl (PNB)*		92-93-3	Bladder
Para-nitrochlorobenzene	1578	100-00-5	
2-Nitropropane (2-NP)	2608	79-46-9	Liver
N-nitrosodimethylamine*		62-75-9	
Phenyl glycidyl ether (PGE)		122-60-01	
Phenylhydrazine	2572	100-63-0	Lung
β-Propiolactone (BPL)*		57-57-8	
Propylene dichloride	1279	78-87-5	Liver
Propylene imine	1921	75-55-8	
Propylene oxide	1280	75-56-9	Nasal, sarcoma, pheochromocytoma
Silica (crystalline)		14808-60-7 1317-79-9	
1,1,2,2-Tetrachloroethane	1702	79-34-5	Liver, leukemia
Tetrachloroethylene	1897	127-18-4	Liver, leukemia
Titanium dioxide (Rutile)		13463-67-7	Lung
O-Toluidine	1708	95-53-4	
1,1,2-Trichloroethane	2831	79-00-5	
Trichloroethylene	1710	79-01-6	
1,2,3-Trichloropropane		96-18-4	
Uranium (soluble and insoluble compounds)	2979, 9175	7440-61-1	Leukemia
Vinyl chloride	1086	75-01-4	Liver (angiosarcoma), brain, digestive, melanoma

*OSHA regulated carcinogens (outlined in 29 CFR 1910.1003-1910.1016)

RR = Relative risk to exposed workers

The past decade has been marked by increasing assault on the validity of animal testing[20,21] as a predictor of human health consequences. Even intensely studied compounds such as dioxins and asbestos continue to generate enormous debate about their potency as carcinogens. Controversy in the U.S. has also been abetted by public environmental awareness and concerns about the social justice of the current patterns of community toxin exposures. Such sentiments often clash with antiregulatory ideology and concerns that global competitiveness has been hurt by burdensome regulation of dubious public health merit. Adding to the controversy is a broader, but still very incomplete understanding of molecular biology and mechanisms of carcinogenesis.[22] This newer understanding often defies simple modeling of a substance's potential for harm, as it may implicate a complex interaction between direct DNA damage, and a variety of immunological, neuroendocrine, nutritional, and behavioral epigenetic factors influencing receptor function, protein-protein interactions, tumor initiation, growth, and metastasis.

SUMMARY

Clinicians are less familiar with the ill effects of industrial toxins than those of medications, but many of the same principles in patient assessment apply. The major differences are the possible threat of the toxin to medical staff, especially in the field, and different measures of exposure assessment. Patients will often have more concerns about sequelae, especially cancer, than after better known toxin exposures. Fortunately, the vast majority of industrial toxin exposures cause no evident harm to the patient, and standard emergency medical supportive strategies are usually successful. Information and referral resources are increasing in number and quality, and can provide valuable support for emergency and primary care providers.

FOOTNOTES

1. National Research Council, "Toxicity Testing, Strategies to Determine Needs and Priorities," *National Research Council, (U.S.), Steering Committee on Identification of Toxic and Potentially Toxic Chemicals for Consideration by the National Toxicology Program*, 1984.
2. Mehta PS, Mehta AS, Mehta SJ, et al, "Bhopal Tragedy's Health Effects: A Review of Methyl Isocyanate Toxicity," *JAMA*, 1990, 264(21):2781-7.
3. "Acute Respiratory Illness Linked to Use of Aerosol Leather Conditioner," *MMWR Morb Mortal Wkly Rep*, 1993, 41(52-53):965-7.
4. Binder S, "Deaths, Injuries and Evacuations From Hazardous Materials Releases," *Am J Public Health*, 1989, 79(8):1042-4.
5. Winder C, Tottszer A, Navratil J, et al, "Hazardous Materials Incidents Reporting: Results of a Nationwide Trial," *J Hazardous Materials*, 1992, 31:119-34.
6. Lerman SE and Kipen HM, "Material Safety Data Sheets: Caveat Emptor," *Arch Intern Med*, 1990, 150(5):981-4.
7. Suruda AJ, Pettit TA, Noonan GP, et al, "Deadly Rescue: The Confined Space Hazard", *J Hazardous Materials*, 1994, 36:45-53.
8. Bronstein A and Currance P, *Emergency Care for Hazardous Materials Exposure*, St Louis, MO: CV Mosby Yearbook Inc, 1988, 379.
9. Stutz D and Janusz S, ed, *Hazardous Materials Injuries: A Handbook for Prehospital Care*, 2nd ed, Beltsville, MD: Bradford Communications Corp, 1988, 472.
10. "Mass Sociogenic Illness in a Day Care Center," *MMWR Morb Mortal Wkly Rep*, 1990, 39(18):301-4.
11. Glickman TS and Ujuhara AM, "Deciding Between In-Place Protection and Evacuation in Toxic Vapor Cloud Emergencies," *J Hazardous Materials*, 1990, 23:57-72.
12. Leikin JB, Kaufman D, Lipscomb JW, et al, "Methylene Chloride: Report of Five Exposures and Two Deaths," *Am J Emerg Med*, 1990, 8(6):534-7.

13. Alexeff GV, Lewis DC, and Lipsett M, "Use of Toxicity Information in Risk Assessment for Accidental Releases of Toxic Gases," *J Hazardous Materials*, 1992, 29:387-403.

14. Alexeff GV, Lewis DC, and Ragle NL, "Estimation of Potential Health Effects From Acute Exposure to Hydrogen Fluoride Using a "Benchmark Dose" Approach," *Risk Anal*, 1993: 13(1):63-9.

15. Rusch GM, "The History and Development of Emergency Response Planning Guidelines," *J Hazardous Materials*, 1993, 33:193-202.

16. ATSDR, "Managing Hazardous Materials Incidents: Volume I. Emergency Medical Services: Volume II. Hospital Emergency Departments: Volume III. Medical Management Guidelines for Acute Chemical Exposures," *U.S. Department of Health and Human Services, Public Health Service*, 1992, 1:78, 2:76, 3:in prep.

17. Rest K, "Advancing the Understanding of Multiple Chemical Sensitivity (MCS): Overview and Recommendations From an AOEC Workshop," *Toxicol Ind Health*, 1992, 8(4):1-13.

18. Egilman DS, "Public Health and Epistemology," *Am J Ind Med*, 1992, 22(3):457-9.

19. Paul ME, *Occupational and Environmental Reproductive Hazards: A Guide for Clinicians*, Baltimore, MD: Williams and Wilkins, 1993.

20. Marx J, "Animal Carcinogen Testing Challenged," *Science*, 1990, 250(4982):743-5.

21. Marwick C, "What Constitutes an Expert Witness?" *JAMA*, 1993, 269(16):2057.

22. Marshall E, "Toxicology Goes Molecular," *Science*, 1993, 259(5100):1394-8.

— This introductory text was written by Andrew M. Davis, MD
Rush-Presbyterian-St Luke's Medical Center

How to Use the Table of Initial Isolation and Protective Action Distances

Adapted from the *1993 Emergency Response Guidebook*, prepared by the Staff of the Associate Administrator for Hazardous Materials, Safety, Research and Special Programs Administration, U.S. Department of Transportation (DOT), 1993.

1. You should already have:
   - identified the material by its ID number and name
   - read the 2-digit guide for that material and taken the emergency actions it recommends
   - noted the wind direction
2. Now you should look in this table for the ID number and name of the material involved in this incident. Some ID numbers have more than one shipping name listed - look for the specific name of the material.
3. Determine if the incident involves a small or large spill and if DAY or NIGHT. Generally, a small spill is one which involves a single, small package (ie, up to a 55 gallon drum), small cylinder, or a small leak from a large package. A large spill is one which involves a spill from a large package or multiple spills from many small packages. Day is any time after sunrise and before sunset. Night is any time between sunset and sunrise.
4. Look up the initial isolation distance. Direct all persons to move, in an upwind or crosswind direction, away from the spill to the specified distance - in feet.

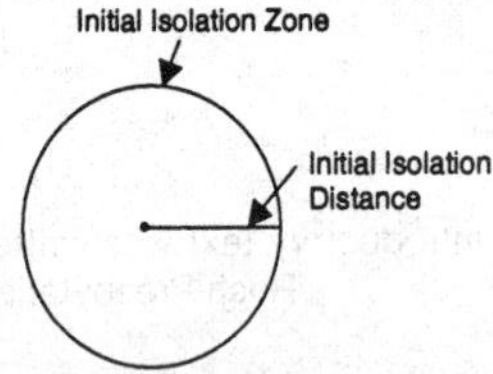

5. Next, look up the initial protective action distance shown in the table. For a given hazardous material, spill size, and whether day or night, the table gives the distance - in miles - downwind for which protective actions should be considered. For practical purposes, the protective action zone (ie, the area in which people are at risk of harmful exposure) is a square whose length and width are the same as the downwind distance shown in the table.
6. Initiate protection actions to the extent you can, beginning with those closest to the spill site and working away from the site in the downwind direction.

The shape of the area in which protective actions should be taken (the protective action zone) is shown in the following figure. The spill is located at the center of the small circle. The larger circle represents the initial isolation zone around the spill.

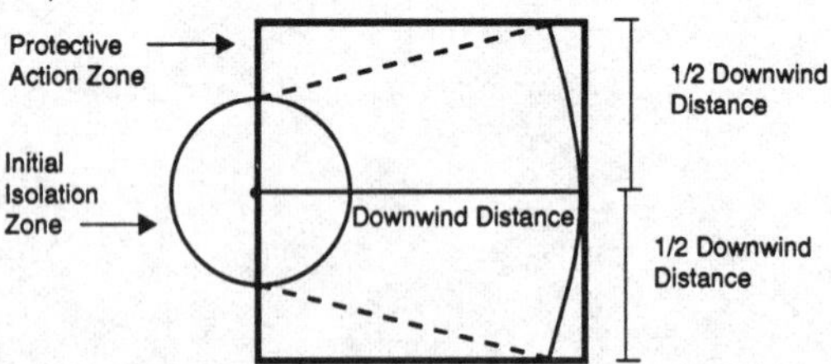

Call the emergency response telephone number listed on the shipping paper, or CHEMTREC (1-800-424-9300), as soon as possible for additional information on the material, safety precautions, and mitigation procedures.

Table of Initial Isolation and Protective Action Distances

ID#	Name of Material	Small Spills (From a small package or small leak from a large package)			Large Spills (From a large package or from many small packages)		
		First ISOLATE in all directions (feet)	Then, protect persons DOWNWIND DAY (miles)	NIGHT (miles)	First ISOLATE in all directions (feet)	Then, protect persons DOWNWIND DAY (miles)	NIGHT (miles)
1005	AMMONIA	500	0.1	0.6	500	0.3	2.2
1005	AMMONIA, ANHYDROUS, liquefied	500	0.1	0.6	500	0.3	2.2
1005	AMMONIA SOLUTIONS with more than 50% ammonia	500	0.1	0.6	500	0.3	2.2
1005	ANHYDROUS AMMONIA	500	0.1	0.6	500	0.3	2.2
1008	BORON TRIFLUORIDE	500	0.3	2.0	500	0.8	2.9
1016	CARBON MONOXIDE	500	0.3	2.0	500	0.7	2.8
1017	CHLORINE	500	0.7	2.8	1500	2.4	4.6
1023	COAL GAS	500	0.1	1.2	500	0.7	2.8
1026	CYANOGEN	500	0.1	1.1	500	0.7	2.8
1026	CYANOGEN, liquefied	500	0.1	1.1	500	0.7	2.8
1026	CYANOGEN GAS	500	0.1	1.1	500	0.7	2.8
1040	ETHYLENE OXIDE	500	0.1	0.9	500	0.2	1.5
1040	ETHYLENE OXIDE with nitrogen	500	0.1	0.9	500	0.2	1.5
1045	FLUORINE, compressed	1000	1.7	3.8	1500	3.9	6.5
1048	HYDROGEN BROMIDE, anhydrous	500	0.1	0.7	500	0.3	2.2
1050	HYDROCHLORIC ACID, anhydrous	500	0.3	1.9	1000	1.1	3.2
1050	HYDROGEN CHLORIDE, anhydrous	500	0.3	1.9	1000	1.1	3.2
1051	HYDROCYANIC ACID	500	0.2	1.4	500	0.3	2.2
1051	HYDROGEN CYANIDE, anhydrous, stabilized	500	0.2	1.4	500	0.3	2.2
1051	HYDROGEN CYANIDE, stabilized, containing less than 3% water	500	0.2	1.4	500	0.3	2.2
1052	HYDROFLUORIC ACID, anhydrous	500	0.1	0.5	500	0.3	2.2
1052	HYDROGEN FLUORIDE, anhydrous	500	0.1	0.5	500	0.3	2.2
1053	HYDROGEN SULFIDE	500	0.2	1.8	1000	1.3	3.4
1053	HYDROGEN SULFIDE, liquefied	500	0.2	1.8	1000	1.3	3.4
1062	METHYL BROMIDE	500	0.1	0.4	500	0.3	2.1
1064	METHYL MERCAPTAN	500	0.1	0.4	500	0.3	2.0
1067	DINITROGEN TETROXIDE, liquefied	500	0.1	0.4	500	0.7	2.8
1067	NITROGEN DIOXIDE, liquefied	500	0.1	0.4	500	0.7	2.8
1067	NITROGEN PEROXIDE	500	0.1	0.4	500	0.7	2.8
1067	NITROGEN TETROXIDE	500	0.1	0.4	500	0.7	2.8
1069	NITROSYL CHLORIDE	500	0.3	2.1	1000	1.8	3.9
1071	OIL GAS	500	0.3	2.1	1500	2.2	4.3
1076	PHOSGENE	500	0.6	2.6	1500	3.2	5.5
1079	SULFUR DIOXIDE	500	0.5	2.5	1500	2.0	4.1
1079	SULFUR DIOXIDE, liquefied	500	0.5	2.5	1500	2.0	4.1
1082	TRIFLUORO-CHLOROETHYLENE	500	0.1	0.4	500	0.3	2.1
1082	TRIFLUORO-CHLOROETHYLENE, inhibited	500	0.1	0.4	500	0.3	2.1
1092	ACROLEIN, inhibited	500	1.0	3.1	1000	1.8	3.9
1098	ALLYL ALCOHOL	500	0.1	0.8	500	0.3	2.2
1135	ETHYLENE CHLOROHYDRIN	500	0.1	0.5	500	0.1	1.0
1143	CROTONALDEHYDE, inhibited	500	0.1	0.1	500	0.1	0.6
1143	CROTONALDEHYDE, stabilized	500	0.1	0.1	500	0.1	0.6
1163	DIMETHYLHYDRAZINE, unsymmetrical	500	0.1	1.4	1500	2.1	4.2
1182	ETHYL CHLOROFORMATE	500	0.1	1.2	500	0.2	1.5
1185	ETHYLENIMINE, inhibited	500	0.5	2.5	500	0.7	2.8
1238	METHYL CHLOROCARBONATE	500	0.2	1.4	500	0.2	1.8
1238	METHYL CHLOROFORMATE	500	0.2	1.4	500	0.2	1.8
1239	METHYL CHLOROMETHYLETHER	500	0.1	1.1	500	0.3	2.1
1244	METHYLHYDRAZINE	500	0.8	3.0	1500	3.1	5.3
1251	METHYL VINYL KETONE	1000	1.3	3.4	1500	2.0	4.1
1259	NICKEL CARBONYL	1500	2.1	4.2	1500	4.4	7.0+
1380	PENTABORANE	1000	1.2	3.3	1500	3.3	5.6
1510	TETRANITROMETHANE	500	0.1	0.1	500	0.1	0.9
1541	ACETONE CYANOHYDRIN, stabilized	500	0.1	0.1	500	0.1	0.5

(continued)

ID#	Name of Material	Small Spills (From a small package or small leak from a large package): First ISOLATE in all directions (feet)	Small Spills: Then, protect persons DOWNWIND DAY (miles)	Small Spills: Then, protect persons DOWNWIND NIGHT (miles)	Large Spills (From a large package or from many small packages): First ISOLATE in all directions (feet)	Large Spills: Then, protect persons DOWNWIND DAY (miles)	Large Spills: Then, protect persons DOWNWIND NIGHT (miles)
1545	ALLYL ISOTHIOCYANATE, inhibited	500	0.1	0.1	500	0.1	0.2
1545	ALLYL ISOTHIOCYANATE, stabilized	500	0.1	0.1	500	0.1	0.2
1556	METHYLDICHLOROARSINE	500	0.2	1.9	1000	1.0	3.2
1560	ARSENIC CHLORIDE	1500	2.9	5.1	1500	3.5	5.8
1560	ARSENIC TRICHLORIDE	1500	2.9	5.1	1500	3.5	5.8
1569	BROMOACETONE	500	0.1	1.4	1000	1.4	3.5
1580	CHLOROPICRIN	500	0.5	2.6	500	0.8	2.9
1581	CHLOROPICRIN and METHYL BROMIDE MIXTURES	500	0.5	2.6	500	0.8	2.9
1581	METHYL BROMIDE and CHLOROPICRIN MIXTURES	500	0.5	2.6	500	0.8	2.9
1582	CHLOROPICRIN and METHYL CHLORIDE MIXTURES	500	0.5	2.6	500	0.8	2.9
1582	METHYL CHLORIDE and CHLOROPICRIN MIXTURES	500	0.5	2.6	500	0.8	2.9
1583	CHLOROPICRIN MIXTURES, n.o.s. (When "Inhalation Hazard" is on a package or shipping paper.)	500	0.5	2.6	500	0.8	2.9
1589	CYANOGEN CHLORIDE, inhibited	500	0.5	2.4	500	0.9	3.1
1595	DIMETHYL SULFATE	500	0.1	0.2	500	0.1	0.4
1595	METHYL SULFATE	500	0.1	0.2	500	0.1	0.4
1605	1,2-DIBROMOETHANE	500	0.1	0.2	500	0.1	0.2
1605	ETHYLENE DIBROMIDE	500	0.1	0.2	500	0.1	0.2
1612	HEXAETHYL TETRAPHOSPHATE and COMPRESSED GAS MIXTURES	500	0.6	2.6	1500	3.2	5.5
1613	HYDROCYANIC ACID, aqueous solution, with not more than 20% hydrogen cyanide (When "Inhalation Hazard" is on a package or shipping paper.)	500	0.2	1.4	500	0.3	2.2
1613	HYDROGEN CYANIDE, aqueous solution, with not more than 20% hydrogen cyanide (When "Inhalation Hazard" is on a package or shipping paper.)	500	0.2	1.4	500	0.3	2.2
1614	HYDROGEN CYANIDE, stabilized (absorbed)	500	0.2	1.4	500	0.3	2.2
1614	HYDROGEN CYANIDE anhydrous, stabilized, containing less than 3% water (absorbed in a porous inert material)	500	0.2	1.4	500	0.3	2.2
1647	METHYL BROMIDE and ETHYLENE DIBROMIDE MIXTURES, liquid	500	0.1	0.4	500	0.3	2.1
1660	NITRIC OXIDE	500	0.1	0.1	500	0.3	1.9
1670	PERCHLOROMETHYL MERCAPTAN	500	0.1	1.0	500	0.1	1.4
1672	PHENYLCARBYLAMINE CHLORIDE	500	0.2	1.9	1500	3.2	5.4
1695	CHLOROACETONE, stabilized	500	0.1	0.1	500	0.1	0.3
1695	MONOCHLOROACETONE, inhibited	500	0.1	0.1	500	0.1	0.3
1695	MONOCHLOROACETONE, stabilized	500	0.1	0.1	500	0.1	0.3
1703	TETRAETHYL DITHIOPYROPHOSPHATE and compressed gas mixture	500	0.6	2.6	1500	3.2	5.5
1703	TETRAETHYL DITHIOPYROPHOSPHATE and gases, mixtures, or in solution (LC50 more than 200 ppm but not more than 5000 ppm)	500	0.6	2.6	1500	3.2	5.5
1703	TETRAETHYL DITHIOPYROPHOSPHATE and gases, mixtures, or in solution (LC50 not more than 200 ppm)	500	0.6	2.6	1500	3.2	5.5
1705	TETRAETHYL PYROPHOSPHATE and compressed gas mixture	500	0.6	2.6	1500	3.2	5.5
1705	TETRAETHYL PYROPHOSPHATE and compressed gas mixtures (LC50 more than 200 ppm but not more than 5000 ppm)	500	0.6	2.6	1500	3.2	5.5
1705	TETRAETHYL PYROPHOSPHATE and compressed gas mixtures (LC50 not more than 200 ppm)	500	0.6	2.6	1500	3.2	5.5
1722	ALLYL CHLOROCARBONATE	500	0.1	1.3	500	0.2	1.6

(continued)

ID#	Name of Material	Small Spills (From a small package or small leak from a large package): First ISOLATE in all directions (feet)	Small Spills: Then, protect persons DOWNWIND DAY (miles)	Small Spills: Then, protect persons DOWNWIND NIGHT (miles)	Large Spills (From a large package or from many small packages): First ISOLATE in all directions (feet)	Large Spills: Then, protect persons DOWNWIND DAY (miles)	Large Spills: Then, protect persons DOWNWIND NIGHT (miles)
1722	ALLYL CHLOROFORMATE	500	0.1	1.3	500	0.2	1.6
1741	BORON TRICHLORIDE	500	0.1	0.1	500	0.1	1.1
1744	BROMINE	500	0.7	2.8	1000	1.1	3.2
1744	BROMINE SOLUTIONS (When "Inhalation Hazard" is on a package or shipping paper.)	500	0.2	1.6	500	0.3	1.9
1745	BROMINE PENTAFLUORIDE	500	0.7	2.8	1500	2.3	4.4
1746	BROMINE TRIFLUORIDE	500	0.1	1.2	500	0.1	1.4
1749	CHLORINE TRIFLUORIDE	500	0.2	1.9	1000	1.7	3.8
1752	CHLOROACETYL CHLORIDE	500	0.2	1.9	500	0.3	2.1
1754	CHLOROSULFONIC ACID	500	0.1	0.2	500	0.1	1.2
1754	CHLOROSULFONIC ACID and SULFUR TRIOXIDE MIXTURE	500	0.1	0.2	500	0.1	1.2
1809	CHLORIDE OF PHOSPHORUS	500	0.5	2.5	500	0.8	2.9
1809	PHOSPHORUS TRICHLORIDE	500	0.5	2.5	500	0.8	2.9
1810	PHOSPHORUS OXYCHLORIDE	500	0.4	2.3	500	0.6	2.6
1810	PHOSPHORYL CHLORIDE	500	0.4	2.3	500	0.6	2.6
1828	CHLORIDE OF SULFUR	500	0.1	0.1	500	0.1	0.5
1828	SULFUR CHLORIDES	500	0.1	0.1	500	0.1	0.5
1829	SULFURIC ANHYDRIDE	500	0.1	0.5	500	0.3	1.9
1829	SULFUR TRIOXIDE	500	0.1	0.5	500	0.3	1.9
1829	SULFUR TRIOXIDE, inhibited	500	0.1	0.5	500	0.3	1.9
1829	SULFUR TRIOXIDE, uninhibited	500	0.1	0.5	500	0.3	1.9
1831	OLEUM, with not less than 30% free sulfur trioxide	500	0.1	0.1	500	0.1	0.2
1831	SULFURIC ACID, fuming, with not less than 30% free sulfur trioxide	500	0.1	0.1	500	0.1	0.2
1834	SULFURYL CHLORIDE	500	0.2	1.8	500	0.3	2.1
1838	TITANIUM TETRACHLORIDE	500	0.1	0.9	500	0.1	1.3
1859	SILICON TETRAFLUORIDE	1500	2.0	4.1	1500	4.3	6.9
1892	ETHYLDICHLOROARSINE	500	0.1	0.2	500	0.1	1.4
1911	DIBORANE	1000	2.0	4.1	1500	4.3	6.9
1953	COMPRESSED GAS, toxic, flammable, n.o.s. (Inhalation Hazard Zone A)	1000	1.0	3.2	1500	5.9	6.9
1953	COMPRESSED GAS, toxic, flammable, n.o.s. (Inhalation Hazard Zone B)	500	0.8	2.9	1500	2.4	4.6
1953	COMPRESSED GAS, toxic, flammable, n.o.s. (Inhalation Hazard Zone C)	500	0.2	1.7	1000	1.7	3.8
1953	COMPRESSED GAS, toxic, flammable, n.o.s. (Inhalation Hazard Zone D)	500	0.2	1.7	1000	1.7	3.8
1953	COMPRESSED GASES, flammable, poisonous, n.o.s.	1000	1.0	3.2	1500	5.9	6.9
1953	COMPRESSED GASES, flammable, toxic, n.o.s. (Inhalation Hazard Zone A)	1000	1.0	3.2	1500	5.9	6.9
1953	COMPRESSED GASES, flammable, toxic, n.o.s. (Inhalation Hazard Zone B)	500	0.8	2.9	1500	2.4	4.6
1953	COMPRESSED GASES, flammable, toxic, n.o.s. (Inhalation Hazard Zone C)	500	0.3	2.1	1500	2.2	4.3
1953	COMPRESSED GASES, flammable, toxic, n.o.s. (Inhalation Hazard Zone D)	500	0.2	1.7	1000	1.7	3.8
1953	LIQUEFIED GASES, flammable, poisonous, n.o.s.	1000	1.0	3.2	1500	5.9	7.0+
1953	LIQUEFIED GASES, flammable, toxic, n.o.s. (Inhalation Hazard Zone A)	1000	1.0	3.2	1500	5.9	7.0+
1953	LIQUEFIED GASES, flammable, toxic, n.o.s. (Inhalation Hazard Zone B)	500	0.8	2.9	1500	2.4	4.6
1953	LIQUEFIED GASES, flammable, toxic, n.o.s. (Inhalation Hazard Zone C)	500	0.3	2.1	1500	2.2	4.3
1953	LIQUEFIED GASES, flammable, toxic, n.o.s. (Inhalation Hazard Zone D)	500	0.2	1.7	1000	1.7	3.8
1955	CHLOROPICRIN and NONFLAMMABLE COMPRESSED GAS MIXTURES	500	0.5	2.6	500	0.8	2.9
1955	COMPRESSED GASES, poisonous, n.o.s.	1000	1.0	3.2	1500	5.9	6.9
1955	COMPRESSED GASES, toxic, n.o.s. (Inhalation Hazard Zone A)	1000	1.0	3.2	1500	5.9	6.9
1955	COMPRESSED GASES, toxic, n.o.s. (Inhalation Hazard Zone B)	500	0.8	2.9	1500	2.4	4.6

(continued)

ID#	Name of Material	Small Spills (From a small package or small leak from a large package) First ISOLATE in all directions (feet)	Small Spills Then, protect persons DOWNWIND DAY (miles)	Small Spills NIGHT (miles)	Large Spills (From a large package or from many small packages) First ISOLATE in all directions (feet)	Large Spills Then, protect persons DOWNWIND DAY (miles)	Large Spills NIGHT (miles)
1955	COMPRESSED GASES, toxic, n.o.s. (Inhalation Hazard Zone C)	500	0.3	2.1	1500	2.2	4.3
1955	COMPRESSED GASES, toxic, n.o.s. (Inhalation Hazard Zone D)	500	0.2	1.7	1000	1.7	3.8
1955	LIQUEFIED GASES, poisonous, n.o.s.	1000	1.0	3.2	1500	5.9	7.0+
1955	LIQUEFIED GASES, toxic, n.o.s. (Inhalation Hazard Zone A)	1000	1.0	3.2	1500	5.9	7.0+
1955	LIQUEFIED GASES, toxic, n.o.s. (Inhalation Hazard Zone B)	500	0.8	2.9	1500	2.4	4.6
1955	LIQUEFIED GASES, toxic, n.o.s. (Inhalation Hazard Zone C)	500	0.3	2.1	1500	2.2	4.3
1955	LIQUEFIED GASES, toxic, n.o.s. (Inhalation Hazard Zone D)	500	0.2	1.7	1000	1.7	3.8
1955	METHYL BROMIDE and NONFLAMMABLE COMPRESSED GAS MIXTURE	500	0.1	0.4	500	0.3	2.1
1955	ORGANIC PHOSPHATE, mixed with COMPRESSED GAS	500	0.6	2.6	1500	3.2	5.5
1955	ORGANIC PHOSPHATE COMPOUND, mixed with COMPRESSED GAS	500	0.6	2.6	1500	3.2	5.5
1955	ORGANIC PHOSPHORUS COMPOUND, mixed with COMPRESSED GAS	500	0.6	2.6	1500	3.2	5.5
1967	INSECTICIDE GASES, toxic n.o.s.	500	0.1	0.6	1000	1.0	3.2
1967	METHYL PARATHION and COMPRESSED GAS MIXTURE	500	0.1	0.6	1000	1.0	3.2
1967	PARATHION and COMPRESSED GAS MIXTURE	500	0.1	0.6	1000	1.0	3.2
1975	NITRIC OXIDE and DINITROGEN TETROXIDE MIXTURES	500	0.1	0.1	500	0.3	1.9
1975	NITRIC OXIDE and NITROGEN DIOXIDE MIXTURES	500	0.1	0.1	500	0.3	1.9
1975	NITRIC OXIDE and NITROGEN TETROXIDE MIXTURES	500	0.1	0.1	500	0.3	1.9
1994	IRON PENTACARBONYL	500	0.1	1.3	1000	1.4	3.5
2032	NITRIC ACID, fuming	500	0.1	1.2	500	0.2	1.6
2032	NITRIC ACID, red fuming	500	0.1	1.2	500	0.2	1.6
2186	HYDROGEN CHLORIDE, refrigerated liquid (cryogenic liquid)	500	0.3	1.9	1000	1.1	3.2
2188	ARSINE	1500	2.5	4.7	1500	7.0+	7.0+
2189	DICHLOROSILANE	500	0.1	0.3	500	0.3	2.2
2190	OXYGEN DIFLUORIDE	1500	4.2	7.0+	1500	7.0+	7.0+
2191	SULFURYL FLUORIDE	500	0.2	1.7	1000	1.7	3.8
2192	GERMANE (germanium hydride)	1000	1.9	4.0	1500	5.3	7.0+
2194	SELENIUM HEXAFLUORIDE	1500	2.8	5.0	1500	5.4	7.0+
2195	TELLURIUM HEXAFLUORIDE	500	0.3	2.1	1500	3.6	6.1
2196	TUNGSTEN HEXAFLUORIDE	500	0.2	1.4	500	0.5	2.5
2197	HYDROGEN IODIDE, anhydrous	500	0.1	0.4	500	0.3	2.0
2198	PHOSPHOROUS PENTAFLUORIDE	1000	1.6	3.7	1500	3.8	6.2
2199	PHOSPHINE	1500	2.0	4.1	1500	4.1	6.7
2202	HYDROGEN SELENIDE, anhydrous	1500	2.6	4.8	1500	6.7	7.0+
2204	CARBONYL SULFIDE	500	0.1	1.2	500	0.7	2.8
2232	CHLOROACETALDEHYDE	500	0.1	0.3	500	0.2	1.6
2232	2-CHLOROETHANAL	500	0.1	0.3	500	0.2	1.6
2334	ALLYLAMINE	500	0.1	1.1	500	0.2	1.6
2337	PHENYL MERCAPTAN	500	0.1	0.1	500	0.1	0.2
2382	DIMETHYLHYDRAZINE, symmetrical	500	0.1	0.2	500	0.2	1.4
2407	SOPROPYL CHLOROFORMATE	500	0.1	0.1	500	0.1	0.5
2417	CARBONYL FLUORIDE	500	0.6	2.7	1500	2.4	4.6
2418	SULFUR TETRAFLUORIDE	1500	1.4	3.5	1500	4.9	7.0+
2420	HEXAFLUOROACETONE	500	0.8	2.9	1500	4.3	6.9
2421	NITROGEN TRIOXIDE	500	0.9	3.1	1500	4.4	6.9
2438	TRIMETHYLACETYL CHLORIDE	500	0.1	0.1	500	0.3	2.0
2442	TRICHLOROACETYL CHLORIDE	500	0.1	0.9	500	0.1	1.3

(continued)

ID#	Name of Material	Small Spills (From a small package or small leak from a large package) First ISOLATE in all directions (feet)	Small Spills Then, protect persons DOWNWIND DAY (miles)	Small Spills Then, protect persons DOWNWIND NIGHT (miles)	Large Spills (From a large package or from many small packages) First ISOLATE in all directions (feet)	Large Spills Then, protect persons DOWNWIND DAY (miles)	Large Spills Then, protect persons DOWNWIND NIGHT (miles)
2474	THIOPHOSGENE	1000	1.6	3.6	1500	2.2	4.3
2477	METHYL ISOTHIOCYANATE	500	0.1	0.2	500	0.3	2.1
2480	METHYL ISOCYANATE	1000	1.2	3.3	1500	3.5	5.9
2481	ETHYL ISOCYANATE	500	0.2	1.9	1500	3.2	5.4
2482	n-PROPYL ISOCYANATE	500	0.1	0.2	500	0.1	1.3
2483	ISOPROPYL ISOCYANATE	500	0.2	1.9	1500	3.2	5.4
2484	tert-BUTYL ISOCYANATE	500	0.1	0.4	500	0.2	1.8
2485	n-BUTYL ISOCYANATE	1000	1.0	3.2	1000	1.8	3.9
2486	ISOBUTYL ISOCYANATE	1000	1.2	3.3	1500	3.5	5.9
2487	PHENYL ISOCYANATE	500	0.1	0.1	500	0.1	0.8
2488	CYCLOHEXYL ISOCYANATE	500	0.1	0.6	500	0.1	1.3
2521	DIKETENE	500	0.1	0.1	500	0.1	0.7
2534	METHYLCHLOROSILANE	500	0.2	1.6	500	0.3	2.1
2548	CHLORINE PENTAFLUORIDE	500	0.3	1.9	1500	2.6	4.8
2600	CARBON MONOXIDE and HYDROGEN MIXTURE	500	0.3	2.0	500	0.7	2.8
2605	METHOXYMETHYL ISOCYANATE	500	0.2	1.9	1500	3.2	5.4
2606	METHYL ORTHOSILICATE	500	0.1	0.1	500	0.1	0.8
2644	METHYL IODIDE	500	0.1	0.1	500	0.1	1.1
2646	HEXACHLOROCYCLO-PENTADIENE	500	0.1	0.5	500	0.1	0.8
2668	CHLOROACETONITRILE	500	0.1	0.1	500	0.1	0.4
2676	STIBINE	500	0.5	2.5	1500	2.1	4.2
2692	BORON TRIBROMIDE	500	0.1	0.5	500	0.1	0.7
2740	n-PROPYL CHLOROFORMATE	500	0.1	0.1	500	0.1	0.4
2742	sec-BUTYL CHLOROFORMATE	500	0.1	0.2	500	0.3	2.2
2742	ISOBUTYL CHLOROFORMATE	500	0.1	1.3	1000	2.0	4.1
2743	n-BUTYL CHLOROFORMATE	500	0.1	1.3	1000	2.0	4.1
2810	POISONOUS LIQUIDS, n.o.s. (Inhalation Hazard Zone A)	1500	2.1	4.2	1500	4.4	6.9
2810	POISONOUS LIQUIDS, n.o.s. (Inhalation Hazard Zone B)	500	0.1	1.3	1000	2.0	4.1
2810	TOXIC LIQUID, organic, n.o.s. (When "Inhalation Hazard" is on a package or shipping paper.)	500	0.5	2.5	1500	4.4	6.9
2826	ETHYL CHLOROTHIOFORMATE	500	0.1	0.1	500	0.1	0.2
2845	ETHYL PHOSPHONOUS DICHLORIDE, anhydrous	500	0.1	1.4	1500	2.1	4.2
2845	METHYL PHOSPHONOUS DICHLORIDE	500	0.1	1.4	1500	2.1	4.2
2901	BROMINE CHLORIDE	500	0.1	0.2	500	0.4	2.3
2927	ETHYL PHOSPHONOTHIOIC DICHLORIDE, anhydrous	500	0.1	1.4	1500	2.1	4.2
2927	ETHYL PHOSPHORO-DICHLORIDATE	500	0.3	2.2	500	0.6	2.7
2927	POISONOUS LIQUIDS, corrosive, n.o.s. (Inhalation Hazard Zone A)	1000	1.2	3.3	1500	3.5	5.9
2927	POISONOUS LIQUIDS, corrosive, n.o.s. (Inhalation Hazard Zone B)	500	0.1	1.3	1000	2.0	4.1
2927	TOXIC LIQUID, corrosive, organic, n.o.s. (When "Inhalation Hazard" is on a package or shipping paper.)	500	0.5	2.5	1500	4.4	6.9
2929	POISONOUS LIQUIDS, flammable, n.o.s. (Inhalation Hazard Zone A)	1000	1.2	3.3	1500	3.5	5.9
2929	POISONOUS LIQUIDS, flammable, n.o.s. (Inhalation Hazard Zone B)	500	0.1	1.3	1000	2.0	4.1
2929	TOXIC LIQUID, flammable, organic, n.o.s. (When "Inhalation Hazard" is on a package or shipping paper.)	1000	1.2	3.3	1500	3.5	5.9
3023	tert-OCTYL MERCAPTAN	500	0.1	0.3	500	0.1	0.6
3057	TRIFLUOROACETYL CHLORIDE	500	0.1	0.2	500	0.3	2.2
3079	METHACRYLONITRILE, inhibited	500	0.1	0.2	500	0.2	1.5
3083	PERCHLORYL FLUORIDE	500	0.3	2.1	1500	2.2	4.3

(continued)

ID#	Name of Material	Small Spills (From a small package or small leak from a large package) First ISOLATE in all directions (feet)	Small Spills Then, protect persons DOWNWIND DAY (miles)	Small Spills Then, protect persons DOWNWIND NIGHT (miles)	Large Spills (From a large package or from many small packages) First ISOLATE in all directions (feet)	Large Spills Then, protect persons DOWNWIND DAY (miles)	Large Spills Then, protect persons DOWNWIND NIGHT (miles)
3122	POISONOUS LIQUIDS, oxidizing, n.o.s. (Inhalation Hazard Zone A)	1000	1.2	3.3	1500	3.5	5.9
3122	POISONOUS LIQUIDS, oxidizing, n.o.s. (Inhalation Hazard Zone B)	500	0.1	1.3	1000	2.0	4.1
3122	TOXIC LIQUID, oxidizing, n.o.s. (When "Inhalation Hazard" is on a package or shipping paper.)	1000	1.2	3.3	1500	3.5	5.9
3123	POISONOUS LIQUIDS, which in contact with water emit FLAMMABLE GASES, n.o.s. (Inhalation Hazard Zone A)	1000	1.2	3.3	1500	3.5	5.9
3123	POISONOUS LIQUIDS, which in contact with water emit FLAMMABLE GASES, n.o.s. (Inhalation Hazard Zone B)	500	0.1	1.3	1000	2.0	4.1
3123	TOXIC LIQUID, water-reactive, n.o.s. (When "Inhalation Hazard" is on a package or shipping paper.)	1000	1.2	3.3	1500	3.5	5.9
3160	LIQUEFIED GAS, toxic. flammable, n.o.s.	1000	1.0	3.2	1500	5.9	7.0+
3246	METHANESULFONYL CHLORIDE	500	0.1	0.2	500	0.1	1.3
3275	NITRILES, toxic, flammable, n.o.s. (When "Inhalation Hazard" is on a package or shipping paper.)	1000	1.2	3.3	1500	3.5	5.9
3279	ORGANOPHOSPHORUS COMPOUND, toxic, flammable, n.o.s. (When "Inhalation Hazard" is on a package or shipping paper.)	1000	1.2	3.3	1500	3.5	5.9
3289	TOXIC LIQUID, corrosive, inorganic, n.o.s.(When "Inhalation Hazard" is on a package or shipping paper.)	1000	1.2	3.3	1500	3.5	5.9
3294	HYDROGEN CYANIDE, solution in alcohol with not more than 45% hydrogen cyanide (When "Inhalation Hazard" is on a package or shipping paper.)	500	0.2	1.4	500	0.3	2.2
3300	ETHYLENE OXIDE and CARBON DIOXIDE MIXTURE, with more than 87% ethylene oxide	500	0.1	0.9	500	0.2	1.5
9192	FLUORINE, refrigerated liquid (cryogenic liquid)	1000	1.7	3.8	1500	3.9	6.5
9202	CARBON MONOXIDE, refrigerated liquid (cryogenic liquid)	500	0.3	2.0	500	0.7	2.8
9206	METHYL PHOSPHONIC DICHLORIDE	500	0.1	0.7	1000	1.2	3.3
9263	CHLOROPIVALOYL CHLORIDE	500	0.1	0.3	500	0.5	2.6
9264	3,5-DICHLORO-2,4,6-TRIFLUOROPYRIDINE	500	0.1	0.7	1000	1.3	3.4
9269	TRIMETHOXYSILANE	500	0.1	0.2	500	0.4	2.4

CARBON MONOXIDE DETECTORS: PROTECTION AGAINST THE SILENT KILLER

Carbon monoxide (CO) poisoning is the leading cause of deaths by poisoning in the United States. A survey of death certificates nationally from 1979 through 1988 indicated that carbon monoxide may have contributed to over 56,133 deaths with 11,547 considered as unintentional. As an odorless, colorless, nonirritating gas, its onset can be quite insidious with multiple cohabitants often being involved in a single exposure. Until recently, it was nearly impossible to detect before its victims experienced signs of poisoning. Accidental CO poisoning is usually the result of incomplete combustion; sources include malfunctioning or unvented fuel-burning appliances, blocked chimneys, rusted vent pipes, vehicle exhaust, or the use of cooking appliances for heating purposes.

Some people will not experience any serious health effects when exposed to CO at very low levels - under 15 parts per million (ppm). Symptoms of CO poisoning get progressively worse as the exposure increases in amount or time. Initial signs include bifrontal headache, nausea, or dizziness and can lead to tightness of chest, brain damage, coma, and even death.

What makes CO particularly hard to combat is that its effect on individuals is based not only on the concentration of CO present, but also on the duration of exposure. If exposed to CO at 100 ppm, a person will not reach a 10% carboxyhemoglobin (COHb) level until 90 minutes have elapsed. But at exposure to CO at 400 ppm, a person will reach 10% COHb within 15 minutes.

On October 1, 1994, a city of Chicago ordinance went into effect requiring an Underwriters Laboratory (UL; Northbrook, IL) Listed CO detector in any home where fuel-burning appliances were used. With national media focused on the Chicago ordinance, CO detectors were being snapped up at hardware and retail stores across the country.

CO detectors for industrial use have been manufactured and distributed for decades. Only recently did CO detectors become available for home and recreational vehicle use. Advancements in microprocessor and sensor technologies enabled CO detectors to be made for residential use at a relative inexpensive cost.

In 1989, the Consumer Product Safety Commission (CPSC) urged UL to write a standard governing CO detectors. After researching the subject and receiving suggestions from the industry, UL published UL 2034 - Standard for Single and Multiple Station Carbon Monoxide Detectors in April, 1992. Six months later, UL Listed the first two CO detectors.

UL's primary concerns for CO detectors relate to performance requirements: at what level should the detector sound an alarm? UL 2034 requires Listed CO detectors to sound an 85-decibel alarm if elevated concentrations of CO are present, using test points based on the 10% COHb level. The chart below indicates the concentration and maximum response time which UL Listed CO detectors are required to meet.

Concentration (PPM)	Maximum Response Time (Minutes)
100	90
200	35
400	15

Detectors are placed inside a test chamber that is conditioned to maintain an ambient temperature of 23±3°C or a higher temperature if specified by the manufacturer; a relative humidity of 50±20% and an oxygen concentration of 20±1%. CO is introduced into the test chamber and slowly circulated until a uniform concentration of 100±5 ppm is achieved. Once the specified CO level has been established, the detectors must alarm within the time range specified by the manufacturer but not to exceed 90 minutes. This test is repeated for the sensitivity requirements of 200 ppm and 400 ppm CO exposures at appropriate durations.

There are two types of technologies that are used in UL Listed CO detectors. "Gel Cell" technology-based detectors monitor CO by sending a beam of light through a biomimetic sensor to a photosensitive component. The sensor becomes obscure. An electronic device in the detector reads the obscuration and will alarm at the appropriate set points. The sensor is normally a yellow or amber color, but will become brown or black if it has absorbed a high level of CO. "Gel Cell" sensors must be replaced every two years.

A detector using a tin-oxide sensor will detect CO by measuring the resistivity of a metal component which changes upon the presence of CO. The detector then measures the resistivity and actuates the alarm at the product's set point.

UL does not specify which technology a CO detector must use. Other technologies beside the "Gel Cell" and tin-oxide sensors are currently being researched by industry groups.

CO detectors gained a certain notoriety in late 1994 when fire departments, responding to CO alarms, found low levels of the gas in some homes (<15 ppm). These calls were termed "nuisance alarms" by area fire departments. Response personnel cannot always find the source of the CO which causes an alarm. UL has received reports indicating that the number of CO alarms was significantly higher on days when wind was gusty or downdrafts occurred. CO that normally vents through chimneys is often pushed back into the home. Some unvented fuel-burning appliances such as ranges and stoves can emit high levels of CO (up to 800 ppm) if used over an extended period of time. CO levels can also increase if fuel-burning appliances are used to heat the home. A CO detector goes into alarm because it registers elevated levels of CO.

New studies on indoor air quality indicate that CO exists in transient, low concentrations within the household. In December, 1994, the city of Chicago reported 1800 alarms in one day because of a temperature inversion which trapped elevated levels of CO in the atmosphere for over 24 hours. Atmospheric ambient CO levels >15 ppm were recorded during this period as opposed to a baseline of <4 ppm which is noted in normal weather conditions in Chicago. Thus, alarms that were set to ignore low levels after 8 hours were responding to the elevated CO by sounding an alarm. Previously, UL 2034 required Listed CO detectors to ignore a low level concentration of CO (15 ppm) for 8 hours before they could sound an alarm. UL has revised that requirement and effective October 1, 1995, Listed CO detectors must ignore 15 ppm for a period of 30 days.

Other stability tests require the unit to ignore 100 ppm for at least 16 minutes without sounding the alarm. The unit is also exposed to a simulated "rush hour" test whereby the detector must ignore 35 ppm CO for at least 1 hour; followed by 6 hours of fresh air, followed by another hour at 35 ppm. UL Listed CO detectors must not alarm anytime during this test.

UL Listed detectors manufactured after October 1, 1995 also will be required to have a reset button, which allows consumers to turn off the alarm while investigating the source of the CO. If dangerous levels of CO exist in the residence, then the alarm will automatically sound again within 6 minutes. Some detectors respond to lower levels of CO; if a reset button is activated, these units may take up to 30 minutes to re-alarm.

UL evaluates CO detectors not only for performance requirements, but also for construction specifications. Enclosures of the detector must be constructed to resist the abuses likely to be encountered in normal operation. All electrical parts of the detector, except for plug-in blades, must be enclosed to provide protection against contact with uninsulated live parts. CO detectors can operate from an electrical power source, battery, or electrical supply source with a battery backup. Batteries must be located so that no one will come in contact with uninsulated live parts while replacing them. Batteries must operate for 12 months continuously, provide 7 days of a low battery trouble signal, then operate the detector for a minimum of 4 minutes of alarm.

UL Listed CO detectors must not alarm when subjected to the following concentration of gases for a 2-hour period: 500 ppm methane, 300 ppm butane, 500 ppm heptane, 200 ppm ethyl acetate, 200 ppm isopropyl alcohol, and 1000 ppm carbon dioxide. UL 2034 also sets requirements for an overload test, endurance test, humidity test, dielectric voltage-withstand test, abnormal operation test, undervoltage test, static discharge test, drop test, paint test, corrosion test, battery replacement test, and more.

Similar to smoke detectors, UL Listed CO detectors must sound an alarm that is loud enough to wake most people when sounding outside a bedroom through a closed door. Listed CO detectors must emit an 85 decibel alarm at 10 feet to meet this requirement.

CO is nearly the same weight as air. Unlike smoke, which rises quickly to the ceiling, CO will mix evenly with air. Detectors can be placed near the ceiling or near the floor. Depending upon the model, CO detectors can plug directly into an electrical receptacle, operate off a battery, or be wired directly into a home's electrical system. CO detectors are also manufactured for use in recreational vehicles and are subject to slightly different requirements.

Sensors which measure CO are sensitive to common household chemicals and gases such as cleaners and bleach. These chemicals should not be placed near a detector, as low exposure over an extended period of time could damage the sensing device and cause the detector to sound a false alarm.

If a consumer can only afford one detector, UL suggests that they install the detector near sleeping areas. Additional detectors can be placed in rooms where fuel-burning appliances are operated. CO detectors should never be placed directly on top of or across from fuel-burning appliances as they emit elevated levels of CO when initially turned on. When installing a CO detector, carefully follow the manufacturer's instructions as outlined in the use and care booklet.

A CO alarm should never be ignored. If an alarm sounds and anyone in the home is experiencing flu-like symptoms, including nausea, fatigue, headaches, dizziness, confusion, and breathing difficulty, the fire department should be contacted and the residence evacuated. Young children and infants who have trouble explaining their symptoms should be thoroughly examined. No one should re-enter the home until the problem is addressed and corrected. Because ventilation has been provided by leaving windows and doors open, the CO buildup may have dissipated by the time help responds. Although the problem may appear to be temporarily solved, it is crucial that the source of the CO is determined and appropriate action is taken.

CO detectors are like any other appliance - they require proper use and maintenance. CO detectors should be tested regularly and cleaned as indicated in the manufacturer's use and care booklet. If the product is wired directly into the home's electrical system, it should be tested monthly. If the product operates off a battery, it should be tested weekly and the battery replaced at least once a year or when the low battery audible signal is energized.

CO detectors are life-saving devices that can warn residents of elevated levels of CO in the home. Installing a UL Listed CO detector in the home, near sleeping areas, can warn residents of this potentially deadly gas. UL, in cooperation with the CPSC, set initial requirements for the detectors that were designed to provide an early warning to a potential problem. Revisions to UL 2034 were made after UL received reports from consumers, fire departments, and other groups concerning the stability of the detectors. Detectors meeting the new requirements will be available to consumers for the 1995-96 heating season.

UL evaluates other types of gas detectors for residential and recreational vehicle use. These gas detectors are intended to detect natural gas and LP gas (propane) which may be present in residential buildings or recreational vehicles as a result of leaks from a gas-fired appliance. UL Listed gas detectors will sound an alarm at or below 25% of the lower flammable limit of natural gas or propane. UL Listed gas detectors are not evaluated as heat, fire, or smoke detectors. The standard used to evaluate these products is UL 1484 - Residential Gas Detectors.

UL has also developed an outline for UL 2075 - Gas and Vapor Detectors and Sensors. These detectors will be investigated to ensure that they consistently trip at levels within 5% of the gas concentration levels indicated by the manufacturer. Products used to detect ignitable air-vapor mixtures must activate an alarm signal at 25% or less of the Lower Explosive Limit (LEL). Products designed to detect toxic vapors and gases which present a health hazard to the user will alarm at 50% of the immediately Dangerous for Life and Health (DHL) level or less as determined by Federal Register, Code of Federal Regulations 29. CFR, subpart Z, "Threshold Limit Values for Chemical Substances and Physical Agents and Biological Exposures Indices," and "Ventilation for Acceptable Indoor Air Quality."

UL 2075 was written to include gas detectors, gas sensors, and CO detectors for industrial and commercial uses. Requirements for these sensors and detectors vary considerably from those in UL 2034 and UL 1484. At this date, UL 2075 is an outline of tests only, and has not been published as a UL Standard for Safety.

— This introductory text was written by
Teresa L. Hrones, Media Relations Associate
and
Paul E. Patty, PE, Associate Managing Engineer
Underwriters Laboratories Inc (UL), Northbrook, IL

SELECTED REFERENCES

Cobb N and Etzel RA, "Unintentional Carbon Monoxide - Related Deaths in the United States, 1979 through 1988" *JAMA*, 1991, 266:659-63.

Federal Register, Code of Federal Regulations 29 - CFR, Subpart Z, Published 7-1-94 (annually, every July).

Hardy KR and Thom SR, "Pathophysiology and Treatment of Carbon Monoxide Poisoning," *J Toxicol Clin Toxicol*, 1994, 32:613-29.

Heckerling PS, Leikin JB, and Maturen A, "Occult Carbon Monoxide Poisoning: Validation of a Predication Model," *Am J Med*, 1988, 84:251-6.

Hexter AC and Goldsmith JR, "Carbon Monoxide: Association of Community Air Pollution With Mortality," *Science*, 1971, 172:265-6.

Longo LD, "The Biologic Effects of Carbon Monoxide on the Pregnant Woman, Fetus, and Newborn," *Am J Obstet Gynecol*, 1977, 129:69-103.

Outline of Tests, UL 2075 - Gas and Vapor Detectors and Sensors.

Standard for Safety, UL 2034 - Single and Multiple Station Carbon Monoxide Detectors, First Edition, April 30, 1992.

Standard for Safety, UL1484 - Gas Detectors, Residential and Recreational Vehicles, First Edition, October 13, 1989.

"Threshold Limit Values for Chemical Substances and Physical Agents and Biological Indices," American Conference of Governmental Industrial Hygienistry, Published annually (1994-1995).

"Ventilation for Acceptable Indoor Air Quality," American Society of Heating and Refrigeration Engineers (A.S.H.R.E), 1989.

CARBON MONOXIDE

REVIEW OF THE CHICAGO FIRE DEPARTMENT EXPERIENCE

Carbon monoxide has long been recognized by public safety officials as one of the most deadly gases known to man. Undetectable by any of the human senses, the gas is responsible for hundreds of deaths in America each year. A family of ten were found dead in their south side Chicago home in 1991 as a result of leaking carbon monoxide gas. An investigation revealed that the vent from a furnace to the chimney had corroded and allowed the gas to infiltrate the entire house during a cold November night.

Officials of the City Council were alarmed and enacted an ordinance to protect residents of the city by requiring carbon monoxide detectors in all residential structures heated by fossil fuels or where fossil fuels were used for cooking. The ordinance became effective October 1, 1994.

The Chicago Department of Buildings was the agency responsible for monitoring compliance with the ordinance and much like the smoke detector ordinance passed in 1985, enforcement depended largely on the cooperation of the average citizens concern for their family's safety.

The Chicago Fire Department {CFD) had traditionally responded to emergencies related to carbon monoxide poisoning and reports of other dangerous conditions related to "gas investigations" and began receiving many calls for investigations regarding the new carbon monoxide detectors activating. The CFD was equipped with 15 hazardous gas detectors, including CO, that were strategically located throughout the city. Calls for carbon monoxide detectors activating increased on a daily basis, and although the overwhelming majority of investigations determined nonlife-threatening incidents, it was obvious that additional CO meters were necessary to handle the volume. The Fire Commissioner, Raymond E. Orozco, made an order for CO meters for all fire companies and 60 new meters were added to the 15 in use by mid-November.

On December 21, 1994 Chicago experienced a somewhat rare weather condition known among meterologists as a "thermal inversion." The unusual weather condition lasted for nearly 48 hours and was described by meterologists as a condition in which warmer air is trapped near ground level allowing levels of carbon monoxide to accumulate without dissipating in the atmosphere. During the 48-hour period, the CFD responded to 3,464 CO investigations. A total of 14 residents were treated and transported to area hospitals, but no fatalities occurred as a result of this unusual weather-related event.

By mid-January of 1995, every fire apparatus (98 engines, 58 trucks, and 3 rescue squads) were equipped with the CO meter and available throughout the city for CO investigations.

— This introductory text was written by John M. Eversole
Hazardous Materials Coordinator, Chicago Fire Department

CHICAGO FIRE DEPARTMENT PROTOCOL

I. PURPOSE

This Order:

A. establishes a procedure for the Chicago Fire Department's response to reports of carbon monoxide (CO) incidents.

B. rescinds General Order 94-006 and supercedes all memos and directives pertaining to carbon monoxide incident response.

C. becomes effective immediately.

II. GENERAL

Carbon monoxide is an odorless, tasteless, colorless gas that is deadly. It is a byproduct of a fuel burning process. Many appliances such as furnaces, kitchen stoves, hot water heaters, automobiles, etc, can produce carbon monoxide. When a faulty or unusual condition exists, carbon monoxide may be vented into areas where people are present.

Carbon monoxide poisoning may be difficult to diagnose. Its symptoms are similar to the flu, which may include headache, nausea, fatigue, and dizzy spells.

The Occupational Safety and Health Administration has established a maximum safe working level for carbon monoxide at 35 parts per million (ppm) over an 8-hour period, in the general workplace. The U.S. Environmental Protection Agency has established that residential levels are not to exceed 9 ppm over an 8-hour average.

The gas company will no longer respond automatically to all carbon monoxide (CO) investigations. They will respond only if the initial call received by them indicates that someone is ill or if the Fire Department requests that they respond to the scene.

III. PROCEDURES

A. Issuance and Maintenance of Meters:

1. The Department will issue a carbon monoxide meter to each company designated as a meter company.

2. Company commanders shall enter the meter onto their company inventory as per current Department procedure.

3. This meter shall be used to monitor the atmosphere during any suspected carbon monoxide investigation.

4. Each morning the CO gas meter shall be examined, tested, and the results entered in the company journal.

5. Should any problem be noted, the company officer shall immediately contact the Hazardous Incident Team (ML 9222) who will take steps to correct the problem or issue a replacement meter. The Hazardous Incident Team will also provide periodic recalibration and maintenance of all CO gas meters, as per the manufacturer's recommendations.

6. Company officers shall see that their assigned meter is stored in a secured location on their apparatus.

B. Fire Alarm Office Shall Attempt to Verify if Mechanism That Is Sounding the Alarm Is a Smoke Detector or a Carbon Monoxide Detector

1. If it is a smoke detector, the Fire Alarm Office will determine what, if any, fire response is necessary.

2. If it is a carbon monoxide detector:

   a. Determine if any persons at the scene are exhibiting symptoms of carbon monoxide poisoning.

      (1) If yes, dispatch the closest meter company and ambulance;

      (2) If no, dispatch the closest meter company to conduct an investigation.

C. The First Arriving Company Shall Establish Scene Control - As Per C.F.D. Incident Command Procedure

   1. Verification shall be made if the alarm is coming from a smoke detector or carbon monoxide detector. The cause of the alarm shall be determined, ie, true alarm, low battery indication, poor location of device, etc.

      a. If it is a smoke detector alarm they shall:

         (1) investigate the cause of the alarm;

         (2) take the necessary action to mitigate the situation;

         (3) advise the fire alarm office of the situation.

      b. If it is a CO detector they shall:

         (1) determine if anyone is exhibiting any symptoms of possible carbon monoxide poisoning; if so, immediately evacuate and ventilate the premises;

         (2) request necessary E.M.S. response;

         (2) begin the investigative procedure.

      c. If no one exhibits any symptoms of carbon monoxide poisoning, it will not be necessary to evacuate or ventilate the premises unless a level of over 9 ppm is detected by a meter as described below.

      d. The incident commander shall request that the gas company respond to the scene through the appropriate Fire Alarm Office if:

         (1) a CO level of over 9 ppm is indicated on their meters,

         (2) or the responding company shuts off gas appliance,

         (3) or someone is showing signs of being ill due to carbon monoxide,

         (4) or the incident commander feels a response by the gas company is needed.

D. Carbon Monoxide Investigations (Procedure)

   1. Zero their meter in fresh air and comply with all other start up procedures as recommended by the manufacturer of the metering equipment.

   2. Initiate a survey of the premises to determine if there are any amounts above 9 ppm of carbon monoxide present.

   3. All members shall make complete use of the SCBA in any atmosphere that is in excess of 35 ppm of CO.

4. Reading of 9 ppm or less:
   (1) Inform the occupants that our instrument did not detect an elevated level of CO at this time.
   (2) Recommend occupants check their CO detector per manufacturer recommendations.
   (3) Attempt to reset detector.
   (4) Inform occupants that if it activates again, call 9-1-1.
5. Readings of more than 9 ppm but less than 100 ppm:
   (1) Any reading above 9 ppm shall be considered above normal reading.
   (2) Occupants shall be informed that we have detected a potentially dangerous level of CO.
   (3) Recommend that all persons leave the premises and begin ventilation.
   (4) If it is determined that an appliance is malfunctioning and thereby producing CO, it shall be shut down.
   (5) Once the premises have been reduced to a safe level of CO, the premises may be occupied - at the discretion of the occupant.
   (6) Attempt shall be made to reset the detector.
   (7) Inform occupants that if it activates again, call 9-1-1.
   (8) The occupants shall be informed of the action that has taken place and that Peoples Gas Company has been requested to respond by the Fire Department.
6. Readings of 100 ppm or greater:
   (1) Any reading of 100 ppm or greater - inform the occupants that we have detected a potentially lethal level of CO.
   (2) Order the occupants to leave the premises immediately.
   (3) If it is determined that an appliance is malfunctioning and thereby producing CO, it shall be shut down.
   (4) Once the premises have been reduced to a safe level of CO, the premises may be occupied at the discretion of the occupant.
   (5) Attempt shall be made to reset the detector.
   (6) Inform occupants that if it activates again, call 9-1-1.
   (7) The occupants shall be informed of the action that has taken place and that Peoples Gas Company has been requested to respond by the Fire Department.

By order of:
Raymond E. Orozco
Fire Commissioner

A-200™ Pyrinate [OTC] *see* Pyrethrins *on page 1003*

Acenaphthylene *see* Polycyclic Aromatic Hydrocarbons *on page 997*

Acetic Acid *see* Vinyl Acetate *on page 1037*

Acetone

CAS Number 67-64-1

UN Number 1090

Synonyms Dimethyl Formaldehyde; Dimethyl Ketone; 2-Propanone

Use Volatile solvent (ie, fingernail polish remover, glues, rubber cement); defatting agent in semiconductor industry

Mechanism of Toxic Action Release of norepinephrine on heart; narcotic properties

Adverse Reactions

Cardiovascular: Tachycardia
Central nervous system: Depression
Ocular: Eye irritation, lacrimation
Respiratory: Respiratory depression

Signs & Symptoms of Acute Overdose Sedation, vomiting, cough, ataxia, coma, seizures (in children), bronchial irritation, hyperglycemia, hypoglycemia, hypotension, narcosis, headache

Toxicodynamics/Kinetics

Absorption: Readily through the lungs (75% to 80%) and skin (more slowly) and gastrointestinal tract (74% to 83%)
Distribution: V_d: 0.8 L/kg
Metabolism: Hepatic oxidation to acetate and formate at a rate of 1-3 mg/kg/hour
Half-life, elimination: 25 hours
Elimination: Excreted through the lungs and urine

Reference Range Toxic: Blood levels >330 mg/L; urinary acetone levels correlating to air acetone levels of 200 ppm and 750 ppm are 21.6 mg/L and 76.6 mg/L respectively; blood acetone levels associated with air acetone levels of 200 ppm and 750 ppm are 41.4 mg/L and 118 mg/L respectively; average amount of acetone in expired air of a healthy subject is ~1 μg/L

Overdosage Treatment

Decontamination: Ingestion: Do not induce vomiting; activated charcoal with cathartic can adsorb 42% to 44% of acetone
Supportive therapy: Inhalation: Airway support and 100% humidified oxygen

Diagnostic Tests/Procedures

Glucose, Random *on page 1269*
Ketone Bodies, Blood *on page 1277*
Ketones, Urine *on page 1278*
pH, Blood *on page 1318*

Monitoring Parameters Blood glucose, serum/urine acetone, arterial pH

Pregnancy Implications Shortening of menstrual cycle noted in women exposed to acetone: 1000 ppm for 7.5 hours; exposure to acetone at levels of 14-126 ppm reported to have higher incidences of miscarriage, decreased birth weight and length

Additional Information Fruity odor, sweet taste; acetone is a metabolite of isopropyl alcohol; cigarette smoke contains <0.5 mg acetone per cigarette; no increased cancer risk; very water soluble; potentiates CNS toxicity of ethanol

Odor threshold: 13-20 ppm
Ingestion: Toxic dose: 2-3 mL/kg
Inhalation:
  TLV-TWA: 750 ppm
  IDLH: 20,000 ppm
  PEL-TWA: 1000 ppm
Atmospheric half-life: ~22 days
Average acetone levels in urban areas: ~7 ppb in the troposphere
Average amount in drinking water: ~1 ppb
Estimated inhalational dose of acetone in an adult: ~0.37 mg/day

Specific References

Burkhart KK and Martinez MA, "The Adsorption of Isopropanol and Acetone by Activated Charcoal," *J Toxicol Clin Toxicol*, 1992, 30(3):371-5.
Gamis AS and Wasserman GS, "Acute Acetone Intoxication in a Pediatric Patient," *Pediatr Emerg Care*, 1988, 4(1):24-6.
Ramu A, Rosenbaum J, and Blaschke TF, "Disposition of Acetone Following Acute Acetone Intoxication," *West J Med*, 1978, 129(5):429-32.
U.S. Department of Health and Human Services, "Toxicological Profile for Acetone TP-93/01," Agency for Toxic Substances and Diseases Registry, May 1994.

Acetonitrile

CAS Number 75-05-8

UN Number 1648

Synonyms Cyanomethane; Methyl Cyanide

Brand Names Ardell Instant Glue Remover®; Artificial Nail Tip and Glue Remover®; Super Nail Glue Off®; Super Nail Off®

Use Highly polar solvent used in cosmetic nail remover

Mechanism of Toxic Action Converts to cyanide by hepatic metabolism

Signs & Symptoms of Acute Overdose Myocardial depression, CNS stimulation followed by CNS depression, seizures, respiratory depression

Toxicodynamics/Kinetics

Absorption: Dermal, oral, and inhalation

Distribution: V_d: 0.7 L/kg

Protein binding: 0%

Metabolism: Hepatic hydrolysis to hydrogen cyanide

Half-life:

Acetonitrile: 32 hours

Cyanide: 15 hours

Reference Range Whole blood cyanide level of 6 μg/mL (2310 μmol/L) reported 12 hours after exposure in a 16-month of age boy

Overdosage Treatment

Decontamination: Basic poison management; emesis is contraindicated due to rapid course of the neurologic symptoms; give 100% oxygen

Supportive therapy: Give sodium bicarbonate for acidosis

Enhancement of elimination: Hemodialysis and charcoal hemoperfusion have been utilized; hyperbaric oxygen may also be utilized; hydroxocobalamin and dicobalt-EDTA used for chelation in Europe

Antidote(s)

Amyl Nitrite *on page 1390*

Sodium Nitrite *on page 1469*

followed by

Sodium Thiosulfate *on page 1470*

Diagnostic Tests/Procedures

Anion Gap, Blood *on page 1193*

Blood Gases, Arterial *on page 1207*

Electrolytes, Blood *on page 1254*

Methemoglobin, Blood *on page 1296*

Additional Information Decomposes to hydrogen cyanide gas at 120°C

Specific References

Caravati EM and Litovitz TL, "Pediatric Cyanide Intoxication and Death From an Acetonitrile-Containing Cosmetic," *JAMA*, 1988, 260(23):3470-3.

Geller RJ, Ekins BR, and Iknoian RC, "Cyanide Toxicity From Acetonitrile-Containing False Nail Remover," *Am J Emerg Med*, 1991, 9(3):268-70.

Kurt TL, Day LC, Reed WG, et al, "Cyanide Poisoning From Glue-On Nail Remover," *Am J Emerg Med*, 1991, 9(3):271-2.

Losek JD, Rock AL, and Boldt RR, "Cyanide Poisoning From a Cosmetic Nail Remover," *Pediatrics*, 1991, 88(2):337-40.

1-Acetoxy-Ethylene *see* Vinyl Acetate *on page 1037*

Acetylene Dichloride

CAS Number 540-59-0; 156-59-2 (cis); 156-60-5 (trans)

UN Number 1150

Synonyms 1,2 DCE; 1,2-Dichloroethene

Brand Names Dioform®

Use Chemical intermediate in the production of chlorinated solvents; used in production of dyes, perfumes, and thermoplastics

Mechanism of Toxic Action Mucosal irritant and CNS depressant

Adverse Reactions

Central nervous system: CNS depression

Dermatologic: Irritation

Ocular: Eye irritation at concentrations of 1000 ppm

Signs & Symptoms of Acute Overdose Lethargy, dizziness, nausea (at concentrations of ~2000 ppm), tremor, muscle cramps

Toxicodynamics/Kinetics

Absorption: Through inhalation (75%)

Metabolism: Hepatic (cytochrome P-450) epoxidation to dichloroethanol and dichloroacetic acid

Overdosage Treatment

Decontamination:

Dermal: Wash with soap and water

Inhalation: Remove from source and administer 100% humidified oxygen

Oral: Lavage within 1 hour of ingestion

Supportive therapy: Calcium gluconate may relieve muscle cramping

Additional Information Very flammable

Odor threshold: 17 ppm (acrid)

(Continued)

Acetylene Dichloride *(Continued)*

Half-life:

Atmospheric: 8.3 days (cis-isomer); 3.6 days (trans-isomer)

Water: 3-6 hours

Usual general population exposure: 0.013 to 0.076 ppb (1-6 mcg/day)

TLV-TWA: 200 ppm

EPA water maximum containment level: 0.07 mg/L (cis-isomer); 0.1 mg/L (trans-isomer)

Specific References

Brock WJ, "Acute Toxicity Studies With Trans 1,2-Dichloroethylene (DCE)," *J Am Coll Toxicol*, 1990, 1:10-1.

Acetylene Tetrachloride *see* Tetrachloroethane *on page 1022*

Acetylene Trichloride *see* Trichloroethylene *on page 1033*

Acrolein

CAS Number 100-73-2; 107-02-8; 869-29-4

UN Number 2607; 1092

Synonyms Propylene Aldehyde; Pyran Aldehyde

Brand Names Aqualin®; Magnacide H®

Use Manufacture of pharmaceuticals, herbicides, textiles, and as a tear gas; found as an irritant gas generated by fire; production of acrylic acid; as a tissue fixative, biocide, and slimicide in paper industry

Mechanism of Toxic Action Irritation of mucous membranes; suppresses glycolysis and reacts with sulfhydryl groups of proteins; release of catecholamines is noted; high water stability can lead to primary upper airway damage

Adverse Reactions Respiratory: Pulmonary edema

Signs & Symptoms of Acute Overdose Lacrimation, erythema, bronchial constriction, dyspnea, hypertension, coma, tachycardia, cough, tachypnea at air levels of 0.6 ppm

Toxicodynamics/Kinetics

Absorption: Through ingestion and inhalation

Metabolism: Hepatic to S-carboxy ethyl mercapturic acid methyl ester

Overdosage Treatment

Decontamination: Ingestion: Lavage/activated charcoal with cathartic

Supportive therapy: Inhalation: Humidified oxygen, inhaled beta-agonist agents for wheezing; treat for pulmonary edema

Diagnostic Tests/Procedures

Alkaline Phosphatase, Serum *on page 1184*

Liver Profile *on page 1286*

Pregnancy Implications None known by inhalation route; teratogenicity and embryotoxicity produced when directly injected

Additional Information One of the major irritants in smog; yellow liquid with pungent odor (acrid)

Acrolein is present in cigarette smoke: 3-220 μg/cigarette and marijuana : 92-145 μg/joint

Odor threshold

Water: 0.11 ppm

Air: 0.16 ppm

Toxic dose for irritation: 10 ppm

TLV-TWA: 0.1 ppm

IDLH: 5 ppm

PEL-TWA: 0.1 ppm

Atmospheric half-life: 15-20 hours

Ambient air level: ~0.3 ppb

Newer concepts: N-acetylcysteine protected against hepatitis in laboratory animals

Specific References

Leach CL, Hatoum NS, Ratajczak HV, et al, "The Pathologic and Immunologic Effects of Inhaled Acrolein in Rats," *Toxicol Lett*, 1987, 39(2-3):189-98.

Nielsen GD, Bakbo JC, and Holst E, "Sensory Irritation and Pulmonary Irritation by Airborne Allyl Acetate, Allyl Alcohol, and Allyl Ether Compared to Acrolein," *Acta Pharmacol Toxicol (Copenh)*, 1984, 54(4):292-8.

U.S. Department of Health and Human Services, "Toxicological Profile for Acrolein TP-90/01," Agency for Toxic Substances and Diseases Registry, December 1990.

Acrylamide

CAS Number 79-06-1

UN Number 2074

Synonyms Acrylic Amide; Ethylene Carboxamide; Propenamide; 2-Propenamide

Brand Names Nyloprint®

Use Vinyl monomer synthesized from acetonitrile; it is polymerized to produce flocculators used in waste water treatment, paper strengtheners, grouting agents, gels, and adhesive agents

Mechanism of Toxic Action Causes progressive degeneration by sensory neurons ("dying back"), starting distally and progressing proximally; thought to be due to activation of activity of sulfhydryl-dependent glycolytic enzymes inhibiting axonal energy production

Adverse Reactions

Central nervous system: Ataxia, paresthesia

Dermatologic: Irritation, desquamation of palms and soles

Gastrointestinal: Anorexia

Neuromuscular & skeletal: Hyporeflexia, neuritis

Respiratory: Cough

Miscellaneous: Palm sweating

Signs & Symptoms of Acute Overdose Dependent on time and duration, total dose, and rate of exposure

High-dose:

Acute: Somnolence, hypothermia, confusion, hallucinations, disorientation, ataxia, tremor, and possible seizures, with cardiovascular collapse

Subacute (days/weeks): Drowsiness, somnolence, decreased concentration, truncal ataxia, dysarthria, nystagmus, urinary retention, paresthesia may follow in 2-3 weeks

Chronic: Sensorimotor and proprioceptive neuropathy

Complete recovery over weeks to months in mild, but in severe, may have incomplete recovery; elevated liver transaminases and decreased urinary output have been reported; severe thrombocytopenia has been reported; exfoliated, erythematous rash, especially on hands, occurs with chronic exposure

Toxicodynamics/Kinetics

Absorption: Rapid through oral, dermal, and inhalation

Distribution: Rapid to blood and then tissue

Metabolism: Hepatic

Half-life: 2 hours

Time to peak blood levels: 1 hour

Elimination: Renal

Warnings When vapors are present, must use impervious body protector as significant toxicity may occur through dermal absorption

Overdosage Treatment

Decontamination: Lavage/activated charcoal with cathartic

Supportive therapy: Pyridoxine (vitamin B_6) 3-10 g of 10% solution in D_5W over 30-60 minutes; may delay neurotoxic effect; N-acetylcysteine has been utilized, but it is of unproven benefit

Antidote(s)

Pyridoxine Hydrochloride *on page 1465*

Test Interactions Sensory nerve action potentials appear the most sensitive indicator, showing decreases in action potential and velocity

Pregnancy Implications Animal data: No neurologic effect on offspring was noted with prenatal exposure; it does cross placenta barrier and may cause decrease in birth weight; may pass through breast milk

Additional Information Acrylamide may be measured in tissue and blood by HPLC; considered a suspected human skin carcinogen; odorless, colorless, white flake-like powder

Specific References

Donovan JW and Pearson TO, "Ingestion of Acrylamide With Severe Encephalopathy, Neurotoxicity and Hepatotoxicity," *Vet Hum Toxicol*, 1987, 29:462.

He FS, Zhang SL, Wang HL, et al, "Neurological and Electroneuromyographic Assessment of the Adverse Effects of Acrylamide on Occupationally Exposed Workers," *Scand J Work Environ Health*, 1989, 15(2):125-9.

Howland RD, "Biochemical Studies of Acrylamide Neuropathy," *Neurotoxicology*, 1985, 6(4):7-16.

Kesson CM, Baird AW, and Lawson DH, "Acrylamide Poisoning," *Postgrad Med J*, 1977, 53(615):16-7.

Le Quesne PM, "Clinical and Morphological Findings in Acrylamide Toxicity," *Neurotoxicology*, 1985, 6(4):17-24.

Le Quesne PM, "Neurophysiological Investigation of Subclinical and Minimal Toxic Neuropathies," *Muscle Nerve*, 1978, 1(5):392-5.

Acrylic Amide *see* Acrylamide *on previous page*

Acrylonitrile

CAS Number 107-13-1

UN Number 1093

Synonyms Cyanoethylene; 2-Propenenitrile; Vinyl Cyanide

Use Raw material in acrylic/modacrylic fibers; also used in the manufacture of plastics, rubber, acrylics, and adhesives; used as a fumigant and pesticide

(Continued)

Acrylonitrile *(Continued)*

Mechanism of Toxic Action Produced through the process of propylene amoxidation; hepatic conversion to cyanide can produce signs and symptoms of cyanide

Adverse Reactions

Cardiovascular: Tachycardia
Central nervous system: Dizziness, headache, seizures
Dermatologic: Irritation, desquamation, toxic epidermal necrosis may develop in 3 weeks
Endocrine & metabolic: Lactic acidosis
Gastrointestinal: Nausea, diarrhea, vomiting
Hematologic: Anemia
Hepatic: Jaundice, hepatic injury
Neuromuscular & skeletal: Limb asthenia
Ocular: Conjunctivitis
Respiratory: Irregular breathing, dyspnea

Toxicodynamics/Kinetics

Absorption:
Inhalation: 52%
Dermal: 0.6 $mg/cm^2/hour$
Metabolism: To 2-cyanoethylene oxide then converted to cyanide
Half-life: 7-8 hours
Elimination: Renal (68%)

Reference Range Plasma thiocyanate levels >20 mg/L in nonsmokers or 30 mg/L in smokers is consistent with exposure to acrylonitrile; exposure to an average air level of 4.2 ppm of acrylonitrile over an 8-hour day produces a urinary acrylonitrile level of 360 μg/L and a urinary thiocyanate level of 11.4 mg/L

Overdosage Treatment

Decontamination: Basic poison management (lavage/activated charcoal with cathartic); emesis is contraindicated due to rapid course of the neurologic symptoms; give 100% oxygen

Supportive therapy: Give sodium bicarbonate for acidosis; cyanide antidote kit (amyl nitrate, sodium nitrate followed by sodium thiosulfate); N-acetylcysteine has been effective in rodent models

Enhancement of elimination: Hemodialysis and charcoal hemoperfusion have been utilized; hyperbaric oxygen may also be utilized; hydroxocobalamin, dicobalt-EDTA, and 4-dimethylaminophenol used for chelation in Europe

Antidote(s)

Amyl Nitrite *on page 1390*
Cyanide Antidote Kit *on page 1406*
Hydroxocobalamin *on page 1433*
Oxygen (Hyperbaric) *on page 1453*
Sodium Nitrite *on page 1469*
followed by
Sodium Thiosulfate *on page 1470*

Diagnostic Tests/Procedures

Anion Gap, Blood *on page 1193*
Blood Gases, Arterial *on page 1207*
Cyanide, Blood *on page 1246*
Electrolytes, Blood *on page 1254*
Methemoglobin, Blood *on page 1296*
Thiocyanate, Blood or Urine *on page 1360*

Pregnancy Implications Teratogenic in rodents (little maternal toxicity)

Additional Information Levels of 16-100 ppm for 20-45 minutes can produce symptoms; odor is pungent (onion/garlic-like); children are more susceptible than adults; will be absorbed through leather products; associated with increase in prostate, colon, lung, and stomach cancer; full recovery will usually occur if patient survives for 4 hours

TLV-TWA: 2 ppm
IDLH: 4000 ppm
Odor threshold in water: 19 ppm
Typical acrylonitrile level in margarine: 25 μg/kg; in cigarettes: 1-2 mg/cigarette
Atmospheric half-life: 12 hours

Specific References

U.S. Department of Health and Human Services, "Public Health Service Toxicological Profile for Acrylonitrile TP-90/02," Agency for Toxic Substances and Diseases Registry, December 1990

Activator-M® *see* 4,4'-Methylenebis (2-Chloroaniline) *on page 965*

Agricide Maggot Killer® *see* Toxaphene *on page 1031*

A-Gro® *see* Methyl Parathion *on page 969*

Alcojel *see* Isopropyl Alcohol *on page 943*

Aldicarb

CAS Number 116-06-3

Brand Names Temik®

Use Marketed in solutions of up to 100% aldicarb; insecticide

Mechanism of Toxic Action Potent, reversible inhibition of acetylcholinesterase and plasma cholinesterase, resulting in excess accumulation of acetylcholine at muscarinic and nicotinic receptors, and in the central nervous system

Adverse Reactions

Cardiovascular: Hyperdynamic (~18% to 21%) or hypodynamic (~7% to 10%) states, edema

Central nervous system: Toxicity is limited because carbamates do not significantly cross the blood-brain barrier; CNS changes occur with most severe intoxications, hyperactivity

Genitourinary: Incontinence

Neuromuscular & skeletal: Weakness, paralysis

Respiratory: Respiratory depression

General: Flu-like symptoms (especially with chronic exposure)

Signs & Symptoms of Acute Overdose Miosis (unreactive to light), mydriasis (rarely), lacrimation, pallor, excessive sweating, confusion, agitation, headache, dysarthria, generalized asthenia, seizures, A-V block, coma, decreased hemoglobin/red blood cell count/platelet count, metabolic acidosis and hyperglycemia (severe intoxication), hypotension, hypertension, bradycardia, tachycardia, Q-T prolongation, heart block, asystole, salivation, bronchorrhea, tachypnea, pulmonary edema, respiratory depression, diaphragmatic paralysis, skeletal muscle fasciculation and flaccid paralysis, nausea, vomiting, abdominal pain, fecal and urinary incontinence, cranial nerve palsies

Toxicodynamics/Kinetics

Absorption: Readily through oral, dermal, or respiratory exposure

Metabolism: Rapidly metabolized to weakly active compounds through hepatic hydrolysis and other pathways, and may undergo enterohepatic recirculation

Elimination: Metabolites are excreted in urine

Warnings Aldicarb translocates from soil into food sources in significant quantity; readily absorbed through intact skin; risk of aspiration pneumonitis exists with agents having a hydrocarbon vehicle

Overdosage Treatment

Decontamination: Isolation, bagging, and disposal of all contaminated clothing and other articles; all emergency medical workers and hospital staff should follow appropriate precautions regarding exposure to hazardous material including the use of protective clothing, masks, goggles, and respiratory equipment

- Dermal: Prompt thorough scrubbing of all affected areas with soap and water, including hair and nails
- Gastric: Activated charcoal can be administered either orally or via a nasogastric tube; do not induce emesis because of danger of sudden respiratory compromise, alterations in mental status, seizures, coma, and possible aspiration of hydrocarbon vehicles
- Ocular: Irrigation with copious tepid sterile water or saline

Supportive therapy: Including airway management, ventilatory assistance, humidified oxygen administration, and close monitoring for sudden respiratory failure

Antidote:

- Atropine: Administration should be guided by respiratory status, starting at 1-5 mg I.V. every 5-10 minutes as needed, and should be titrated to the resolution of excess pulmonary secretions; frequent administration of large doses (cumulative doses >100 mg) may be necessary in massive exposures
- Glycopyrrolate: May be administered if atropine is unavailable
- 2-PAM: Although not specifically indicated, 2-PAM may be considered in the following situations:
  - Life-threatening symptoms such as respiratory paralysis
  - Continued excessive atropine requirements
  - Concomitant organophosphate and carbamate exposure

Enhancement of elimination: Dialysis and hemoperfusion are not indicated due to effectiveness of the prescribed treatment, large volumes of distribution of organophosphates

Antidote(s)

Atropine Sulfate *on page 1395*

Diagnostic Tests/Procedures

Blood Gases, Arterial *on page 1207*

Chest Films *on page 1224*

Complete Blood Count *on page 1236*

Creatinine, Serum *on page 1243*

Electrocardiography *on page 1253*

(Continued)

Aldicarb *(Continued)*

Liver Profile *on page 1286*

Pseudocholinesterase, Serum *on page 1340*

Pregnancy Implications Human data regarding organophosphate exposure in pregnancy is limited and anecdotal; teratogenesis and fetal death have been produced in animal models at exposure levels that cause obvious toxicity to the pregnant animal

Additional Information Spray solutions are balanced to pH = 7.0 and also contain dichloromethane and methyl isocyanate; red blood cell cholinesterase and serum pseudocholinesterase may be depressed following acute or chronic organophosphate exposure and are theoretically useful for differentiating between carbamate and organophosphate exposures; RBC cholinesterase is typically not analyzed by in-house laboratories and is usually not available for consideration during acute management. Pseudocholinesterase levels may be rapidly available from some in-house laboratories, but are not as reliable a marker of organophosphate exposure because of variability secondary to variant genotypes, hepatic disease, oral estrogen use, or malnutrition, thus they may not be useful in ruling out carbamate exposure.

Other information concerning pesticide exposures is available through the EPA-funded National Pesticide Telecommunications Network: 1-800-858-7378 (weekdays, 8 AM to 6 PM, Central Standard time)

Specific References

Green MA, Heumann MA, Wehr HM, et al, "An Outbreak of Watermelon-Borne Pesticide Toxicity," *Am J Public Health*, 1987, 77(11):1431-4.

Lifshitz M, Rotenberg M, Sofer S, et al, "Carbamate Poisoning and Oxime Treatment in Children, A Clinical and Laboratory Study," *Pediatrics*, 1994, 93(4):652-5.

Montesissa C, DeLiguoro M, Amorena M, et al, "*In Vitro* Comparison of Aldicarb Oxidation in Various Food-Producing Animal Species," *Vet Hum Toxicol*, 1995, 37(4):333-6.

Zwiener RJ and Ginsburg CM, "Organophosphate and Carbamate Poisoning in Infants and Children," *Pediatrics*, 1988, 81(1):121-6.

Aldrec® *see* Aldrin *on this page*

Aldrex® *see* Aldrin *on this page*

Aldrin

Related Information

Dieldrin *on page 911*

Organochlorines *on page 983*

CAS Number 309-00-2

Synonyms HHDN

Brand Names Aldrec®; Aldrex®; Aldrite®; Compound 118®; Drinox®; Octalene®; Seedrin®

Use Insecticide – general crop protection, used against termites, EPA discontinued use in 1970s

Mechanism of Toxic Action Cyclodiene organochlorine agent which may be a competitive inhibitor of the inhibitory neurotransmitter GABA at the GABA A receptor

Adverse Reactions

Central nervous system: Convulsions, headache, dizziness, seizures

Gastrointestinal: Nausea, vomiting, anorexia

Neuromuscular & skeletal: Muscle twitching

Renal: Hematuria, albuminuria

Miscellaneous: Elevated blood urea nitrogen, hemolysis

Toxicodynamics/Kinetics

Absorption: Absorbed by oral or dermal routes; also by inhalation

Metabolism: Epoxidized to dieldrin (by mono-oxygenase) then to pentachloroketone and aldrin dicarboxylic acid (among other metabolites)

Elimination: Feces

Reference Range Blood aldrin levels taken from general population in El Paso, TX (1982-3) demonstrated presence of Aldrin in 34% of subjects at a mean level of 4.6 ppb

Overdosage Treatment

Decontamination:

- Dermal: Soap and water wash
- Ocular: Irrigate with saline
- Oral: Activated charcoal with cathartic

Supportive therapy: Beta-adrenergic blocking agents may be used for tachycardia or hypertension; benzodiazepines, phenobarbital, or phenytoin can be used for seizures

Enhancement of elimination: Multiple dosing of activated charcoal may be effective

Pregnancy Implications May be associated with premature labor or spontaneous abortions; placental transfer can occur

Additional Information

Oral lethal dose: 71 mg/kg

Odor threshold: 0.02 mg/kg

Specific References

Amoateng-Adjepong Y, Sathiakumar N, Delzell E, et al, "Mortality Among Workers at a Pesticide Manufacturing Plant," *J Emerg Med*, 1995, 37:471-8.

Mossing ML, Redetzke KA, and Applegate HG, "Organochlorine Pesticides in Blood of Persons From El Paso, Texas," *J Environ Health*, 1985, 47:312-3.

U.S. Department of Health and Human Services, "Toxicological Profile in Aldrin/Dieldrin, TP-92/01," Agency for Toxic Substances and Diseases Registry, April, 1993.

Aldrite® *see* Aldrin *on previous page*

Alfadex® *see* Pyrethrins *on page 1003*

Alfa-Tox® *see* Diazinon *on page 904*

Algistat® *see* Dichloronaphthoquinone *on page 908*

Alkylene Oxide Adducts *see* Glycol Ethers *on page 934*

Alltox® *see* Toxaphene *on page 1031*

Allyl Trichloride *see* 1,2,3-Trichloropropane *on page 1034*

Alpha TNT *see* 2,4,6-Trinitrotoluene *on page 1035*

Al-Phos® *see* Aluminum Phosphide *on this page*

Aluminum Monophosphide *see* Aluminum Phosphide *on this page*

Aluminum Phosphide

Related Information

Phosphine *on page 993*

Toxins Which Should be Lavaged With Solutions Other Than Water *on page 1635*

CAS Number 20859-73-8; 7803-51-2

UN Number 1397; 3048

Synonyms Aluminum Monophosphide

Brand Names Al-Phos®; Celphos®; Delicia®; Detia®; Phostoxin®; Quickphos®

Use Fumigation of grain, rodenticide

Mechanism of Toxic Action Liberates phosphine gas in the gastrointestinal tract which blocks cytochrome C thus uncoupling oxidative phosphorylation and electron transport in the mitochondria

Adverse Reactions

Cardiovascular: Hypotension (within 6 hours), myocardial injury with widening of QRS complex on EKG, atrial fibrillation, tachycardia (ventricular), cyanosis

Central nervous system: Headache, ataxia, dizziness, paresthesia

Endocrine & metabolic: Hyperkalemia, metabolic acidosis, adrenal dysfunction may occur, hypomagnesemia and hypermagnesemia have been reported

Gastrointestinal: Epigastric pain, vomiting, watery diarrhea

Genitourinary: Oliguria

Ocular: Diplopia

Neuromuscular & skeletal: Tremors

Renal: Renal failure

Respiratory: Tachypnea, pulmonary edema

Miscellaneous: Pericarditis, bleeding, diathesis

Toxicodynamics/Kinetics Protein binding: 60% to 70%

Overdosage Treatment

Decontamination: Gastric lavage with 1:5000 potassium permanganate to oxidize unabsorbed toxin; sodium bicarbonate (2% solution) can also be utilized to neutralize gastric hydrochloric acid thus inhibiting release of phosphine

Supportive therapy: Sodium bicarbonate should be used to treat acidosis; dopamine can be used to treat hypotension; if hypotension does not respond to vasopressors, hydrocortisone (400 mg every 4-6 hours) or dexamethasone (4 mg I.V. every 4 hours) can be used to treat adrenal dysfunction; magnesium needs to be monitored and supplemented if low high doses (up to 14 g/day) may be required

Additional Information Decomposes in water; dark gray or dark yellow crystals; oral estimate of daily human exposure that is likely to be without risk of deleterious effects during a lifetime: 0.0004 mg/kg/day

Specific References

Gupta S and Ahlawat SK, "Aluminum Phosphide Poisoning – A Review," *J Toxicol Clin Toxicol*, 1995, 33(1):19-24.

Khosla SN, Nand N, and Khosla P, "Aluminum Phosphide Poisoning," *J Trop Med Hyg*, 1988, 91(4):196-8.

Alvit® *see* Dieldrin *on page 911*

Amatin® *see* Hexachlorobenzene *on page 936*

Ambush *see* Pyrethrins *on page 1003*

Aminobenzene *see* Aniline *on this page*

Aminophen *see* Aniline *on this page*

Ammonia

CAS Number 7664-41-7

UN Number 2073; 2672; 1005

Synonyms Spirit of Hartshorn

Commonly Found In Household cleaners (5% to 10%) and bleach

Use Primarily in fertilizers; manufacture of nitrous oxide; petroleum refining

Mechanism of Toxic Action Tissue injury of moist mucosal membranes caused by reaction with water to form ammonia hydroxide; can cause burns by liquefaction necrosis

Adverse Reactions Miscellaneous: Mucosal irritation, salivation

Signs & Symptoms of Acute Overdose Conjunctivitis, corneal defects, chest pain, upper airway irritation, burns, dyspnea, pulmonary edema, urticaria, gastrointestinal irritant, coma, headache, salivation, lacrimation, swelling, cough, wheezing, nausea, vomiting. Long-term sequelae include bronchiolitis obliterans, peribronchial fibrosis.

Toxicodynamics/Kinetics

Absorption: Not well absorbed

Metabolism: Hepatic to urea and glutamine

Reference Range Serum: 80-110 μg/dL

Overdosage Treatment

Decontamination: Do not induce emesis or perform gastric lavage; dilute with water or milk (4 oz in children, 8 oz in adults); irrigate eyes copiously with normal saline

Supportive therapy: Flush injured surfaces with water; treat for pulmonary edema; use steroids for third degree esophageal burns

Diagnostic Tests/Procedures

Amylase, Serum *on page 1191*

Blood Gases, Arterial *on page 1207*

Chest Films *on page 1224*

Additional Information Colorless liquid; penetrating pungent odor; stable, colorless gas; highly water soluble; alkali (pH 11.6); irritation can occur at 400 ppm; stomatitis can occur at ammonia concentrations of 50 ppm; the mixture of ammonia with hypochlorite bleach can result in chloramine which can produce pulmonary edema

Odor threshold: 25-48 ppm (air); 1.5 ppm (water)

Atmospheric half-life: 2-3 days

TLV-TWA: 25 ppm

IDLH: 500 ppm

Specific References

Arwood R, Hammond J, and Ward GG, "Ammonia Inhalation," *J Trauma*, 1985, 25(5):444-7.

Howell JM, "Alkaline Ingestions," *Ann Emerg Med*, 1987, 15(7):820-5.

Klein J, Olson KR, and McKinney HE, "Caustic Injury From Household Ammonia," *Am J Emerg Med*, 1985, 3(4):320.

U.S. Department of Health and Human Services, "Toxicological Profile for Ammonia TP-90/03," Agency for Toxic Substances and Diseases Registry, December 1990.

Analine *see* Aniline *on this page*

Anhydrous Hydrazine *see* Hydrazine *on page 939*

Aniline

CAS Number 62-53-3

UN Number 1547

Synonyms Aminobenzene; Aminophen; Analine; Aniline Oil; Benzeneamine; Blue Oil; Krystalline; Kyanor; Phenylamine

Use Prepared from indigo and potash; used in manufacture of dyes, resins, varnishes, perfumes, shoe blacks, vulcanizing rubber, paint removers, herbicides, fungicides, explosives, photographic chemicals, isocyanates, rigid polyurethane, and as a solvent

Signs & Symptoms of Acute Overdose Mild skin and eye irritant; inducement of methemoglobinemia causing headache, tinnitus, confusion, seizures, dizziness, drowsiness, loss of consciousness, and coma in the absence of respiratory compromise; central cyanosis is evident which does not improve with 100% oxygen. Blood is noted to be "chocolate brown" and will not become red while bubbling in 100% oxygen; hemolysis may also occur, causing heart, kidney, and liver damage; renal failure may ensue.

Toxicodynamics/Kinetics

Absorption: Readily through all routes; delay rate up to 4 hours, the development of methemoglobinemia; methemoglobin is caused by oxidation of iron in hemoglobin Fe^{+2} to Fe^{+3} which is incapable of transporting oxygen; hemolysis then occurs 2-7 days after exposure

Metabolism: By ring hydroxylation and then conjugated to glucuronides and sulfates

Half-life: 2-7 hours

Elimination: Metabolites are renally cleared

Warnings Persons with hemoglobin M, G-6-PD deficiency or NADH-cytochrome B_5 reductase deficiency may be more sensitive; patients exposed to other methemoglobin inducers are at increased risks; patients with cardiovascular disease are at greater risk from consequences; when vapors are present, must use impervious body protector as significant toxicity may occur through dermal absorption

Reference Range Urinary p-aminophenol >10 mg/L may indicate potential toxic dose with 20 mg/L indicating the need for medical intervention; as little as 1 g can be fatal in human; lethal dose has been estimated at 15-30 g; aniline vapor concentrations >100-160 ppm cause serious disturbances

Overdosage Treatment

Decontamination: Emesis, lavage/activated charcoal with cathartic; remove patient from inhalation and administer 100% humidified air; exposed skin and eyes should be irrigated with water

Supportive therapy: Methemoglobinemia: Treat symptomatic patients or if level is >20%, administer 100% oxygen; if required, methylene blue: 1-2 mg/kg/dose I.V. over a few minutes; may repeat in 4 hours if needed; doses >15 mg/kg may cause hemolysis. High doses of methylene blue may precipitate Heinz body formation and hemolysis. Transfusion of PRBCs may be needed; treatment for myoglobinuria may require urine alkalinization and maintenance of adequate urinary output to prevent renal damage.

Enhanced elimination: One reported case of hemodialysis used in an aniline exposure, refractory to supportive care; hemodialysis should be instituted for those who develop renal failure; exchange transfusion has been used after unsuccessful treatment with methylene blue

Antidote(s)

Methylene Blue *on page 1444*

Diagnostic Tests/Procedures

Methemoglobin, Blood *on page 1296*

Monitoring Parameters Methemoglobin levels; aniline levels have not been measured in blood or serum; urinary p-aminophenol can be measured by colorimetry; CBC, WBC smear, renal function, myoglobin, urinalysis and other indices of hemolysis may be required

Pregnancy Implications Fetus is at special risk for methemoglobinemia; aniline hydrochloride is not teratogenic in rats; aniline crosses placental barrier; fetal liver has the capacity to metabolize to metabolites thought to induce methemoglobinemia

Additional Information Inadequate information concerning human carcinogenicity (bladder cancer); limited evidence that has been carcinogenic in animals (splenic sarcomas, bladder carcinoma)

Specific References

Diggle GE, "The Toxic Oil Syndrome: A Continuing Challenge," *Advance Drug React Toxicol Rev*, 1995, 14(1):11-35.

Harvey JW and Keitt AS, "Studies of the Efficacy and Potential Hazards of Methylene Blue Therapy in Aniline-Induced Methaemoglobinemia," *Br J Haematol*, 1983, 54(1):29-41.

Kearney TE, Manoguerra AS, and Dunford JV Jr, "Chemically Induced Methemoglobinemia From Aniline Poisoning," *West J Med*, 1984, 140(2):282-6.

Labash GD, Phillips RE, Shields JD 3d, et al, " Acute Aniline Poisoning Treated by Hemodialysis," *Arch Intern Med*, 1964, 114:530-2.

Mier RJ, "Treatment of Aniline Poisoning With Exchange Transfusions," *J Toxicol Clin Toxicol*, 1988, 26(5-6):357-64.

Phillips D, Gradisek R, and Heiselman DE, "Methemoglobinemia Secondary to Aniline Exposure," *Ann Emerg Med*, 1990, 19(4):425-9.

Aniline Oil *see* Aniline *on previous page*

(6)-Annulene *see* Benzene *on page 867*

Anofex® *see* DDT *on page 903*

Anozol® *see* Diethyl Phthalate *on page 912*

Anprolene® *see* Ethylene Oxide *on page 927*

Anthracene *see* Polycyclic Aromatic Hydrocarbons *on page 997*

Anti-Carie® *see* Hexachlorobenzene *on page 936*

Anticoagulant Rodenticide

CAS Number 56073-10-1; 56073-07-5; 82-66-6; 83-26-1; 117-52-2

Synonyms Brodifacoum; Bromadiolone; Chlorphacinone; Coumafuryl; Coumatetralyl; Difenacoum; Diphacinone; Hydroxycoumarin; Indanedione; Phytonadione; Pindone; Pivaldione

(Continued)

Anticoagulant Rodenticide *(Continued)*

Brand Names Bromone®; Caid®; d-Con®; Dipazin®; Diphacin®; Drat®; Endox®; Endrocide®; Foumarin®; Havoc®; Krumkil®; Lurat®; Maki®; Microzul®; Pivacin®; Pival®; Racumin®; Ramucide®; Ratafin®; Ratak®; Ratimus®; Ratindan®; Raviac®; Rodentin®; SuperCaid®; Talon®; Talon-G®; Topitox®; Tri-Ban®

Mechanism of Toxic Action Inhibition of synthesis of vitamin K_1-dependent clotting factors II, VII, IX, and X through potent inhibition of vitamin K_1-2,3-epoxide reductase; resulting hypoprothrombinemia and decreased coagulability predisposes toward hemorrhage; benzylacetone metabolite of hydroxycoumarins also induces direct capillary injury, further predisposing toward hemorrhage

Adverse Reactions

Cardiovascular: Hypovolemic/hemorrhagic hypotension and shock

Central nervous system: Dizziness, subarachnoid, intracerebral and intraventricular hemorrhage

Dermatologic: Easy bruising, petechial rash, ecchymoses, skin necrosis, "purple toe" syndrome

Gastrointestinal: Bleeding gums, punctate or frank hemorrhage of mucosal surfaces, abdominal pain, hematemesis, hematochezia, melena

Genitourinary: Uterine bleed

Hepatic: Cholestasis

Renal: Cystitis, hematuria

Respiratory: Hemoptysis

Miscellaneous: Epistaxis

Signs & Symptoms of Acute Overdose Easy bruising, ecchymoses, bleeding gums, epistaxis, and mucosal hemorrhage progressing to symptoms of upper and lower gastrointestinal bleeding; hypotension and hypovolemic shock may follow hemorrhage; intracranial hemorrhage may occur, especially following trauma; indanediones may also cause neurologic and cardiopulmonary symptoms independent of anticoagulant activity

Toxicodynamics/Kinetics

Onset of anticoagulation: Typically within 24-48 hours

Maximum effect: 36-72 hours

Duration: Following repeated doses, may persist up to 45-300 days

Absorption: Complete and rapid following oral exposure

Distribution: Rapid tissue distribution with V_d of 0.12-0.9 L/kg

Protein binding: Extensive plasma protein binding (97% to 99%)

Metabolism: Hepatic microsomal hydroxylation and conjugation of the inactive metabolites

Elimination: Extensive renal elimination of metabolites, with some biliary excretion

Overdosage Treatment Decontamination is usually not required for one-time acute ingestions in pediatric patients; in suicide attempts, decontamination should be performed

Decontamination:

- Emesis is contraindicated in patients who may experience alterations in consciousness, or who have prolonged PT values; intracranial hemorrhage may follow vomiting-induced elevations in intracranial pressures, in anticoagulated patients
- Activated charcoal administration or gastric lavage should follow large ingestions of long-acting anticoagulants, unless otherwise contraindicated

Supportive therapy:

- Obtain PT values immediately postingestion, then 24 and 48 hours postingestion; if significant prolongation occurs, obtain PT values every 6-12 hours thereafter; repeat PT may be obtained 4-5 days postevent; the patient should be closely monitored for signs and symptoms of bleeding for several weeks postingestion
- Vitamin K_1: Oral, S.C., I.M., I.V.: Children: 1-5 mg; Adults: 10 mg
  - I.V. doses of up to 0.6 mg/kg diluted in saline or dextrose may be administered to refractory cases. I.V. infusion rates should not exceed 1 mg/minute or 5% of total dose/minute. I.M. administration of phytonadione may lead to significant hematoma formation. I.V. administration may elicit a hypotensive anaphylactoid reaction, and steps should be taken to anticipate hemodynamic and ventilatory support, as well as decreasing or discontinuation of the infusion.
- Prophylactic oral vitamin K_1 is not indicated for accidental nonsuicidal ingestions because it may further delay the onset of PT prolongation thereby masking the need for long-term vitamin K_1 therapy
- Packed red blood cells (PRBCs) and intravenous crystalloids and colloids will provide immediate hemodynamic support in hypovolemia and hemorrhage. Fresh frozen plasma (FFP), and in extreme cases pooled clotting factors, may be used for cases of refractory hemorrhage.

Enhancement of elimination: Plasmapheresis has been used to increase brodifacoum clearance

Antidote(s)

Charcoal *on page 1403*

Ipecac Syrup *on page 1435*

Phytonadione *on page 1458*

Diagnostic Tests/Procedures

Complete Blood Count *on page 1236*

Urinalysis *on page 1373*

Monitoring Parameters Hemoglobin, hematocrit, INR, partial thromboplastin time (PTT), prothrombin time (PT), stool guaiac

Pregnancy Implications Nasal, laryngeal, and bony malformation, known as warfarin embryopathy, may follow first trimester exposure. Ophthalmologic and neurologic dysfunction and malformation may follow second and third trimester exposure. Third trimester exposure may lead to prenatal, perinatal, and postnatal hemorrhage. Spontaneous abortion may follow any significant ingestion.

Additional Information Single small ingestions of long-acting agents rarely lead to clinically significant anticoagulation and bleeding. Prolonged PT values will identify chronic ingestions, massive ingestions, or patients who were previously anticoagulated. Anticoagulant ingestion may exacerbate underlying diseases such as peptic ulceration. These agents may be absorbed through intact skin, or by inhalation of powders, sprays, or concentrates. Rodent baits and pellets are usually colored with water-soluble blue or green dye to facilitate recognition of oral exposure. NO deaths reported in the American Association of Poison Control Centers annual data reports from 1987 to 1993 among children <6 years of age (encompassing about 72,060 warfarin-related exposures in rodenticides)

See table for comparison

Anticoagulant Rodenticides

Class	Drug	Notes
Hydroxycoumarins Short-acting	Coumafuryl (Foumarin®, Lurat®, Krumkil®, Ratafin®)	0.5% concentrate often used in a 0.025% solution odorless and tasteless
Long-acting	Brodifacoum (d-Con®, Talon®, Talon-G®, Havoc®)	$t_{1/2}$= 120 d (dogs) $t_{1/2}$= 156 h (rats) 0.005% grain-based pellets
	Bromadiolone (Bromone®, Super-Caid®, Ratimus®, Maki®)	Grain-based pellets
	Coumatetralyl (Endox®, Endrocide®, Racumin®, Rodentin®)	Little human experience
	Difenacoum (Ratak®)	0.005% grain-based pellets
Indanediones (may be considered long-acting)	Chlorphacinone (Caid®, Drat®, Microzul®, Ramucide®, Raviac®, Topitox®)	$t_{1/2}$= 5.9-11 d (human) 0.005%, 0.25%, or 2.5% bait, solution, or concentrate
	Diphacinone (Dipazin®, Diphacin®, Ratindan®)	0.005%, 0.05%, 0.1%, 0.2%, or 2% cake, bait, or concentrate
	Pindone/pivaldione (Pival®, Pivacin®, Tri-Ban®)	0.025%, 0.1%, 0.2%, 0.5%, 1.5%, or 2% powder or concentrate

Morrissey B, Burgess JL, and Robertson WO, "Washington's Experience and Recommendations Re: Anticoagulant Rodenticides," *Hum Toxicol*, 1995, 37(4):362-3.

Specific References

Jones EC, Growe GH, and Naiman SC, "Prolonged Anticoagulation in Rat Poisoning," *JAMA*, 1984, 252(21):3005-7.

MacCallum SJ, Nicholls MD, and Motum PI, "Plasmapheresis in the Management of Superwarfarin Poisoning," *Aust N Z J Med*, 1994, 24(2):242.

Sheen SR, Spiller HA, and Grossman D, "Symptomatic Brodifacoum Ingestion Requiring High-Dose Phytonadione Therapy," *Vet Hum Toxicol*, 1994, 36(3):216-7.

Smolinske SC, Scherger DL, Kearns PS, et al, "Superwarfarin Poisoning in Children: A Prospective Study," *Pediatrics*, 1989, 84(3):490-4.

Antimony

CAS Number 7440-36-0; 1315-04-4; 1314-60-9; 28300-74-5; 10025-91-9; 1309-64-4; 1345-04-6; 7803-52-3

UN Number 2871; 1551; 1733; 1549; 2676

Synonyms Sb(0); Sb(-3); Sb(+3); Sb(+5)

Use Naturally brittle metal usually alloyed with lead or other metals; used in grid metal for lead storage batteries, solder, sheet/pipe metal, castings, ammunition, cable sheathing, pewter; antimony trioxide is used as a fire retardant; trivalent organic antimony was used in therapy for schistosomiasis

Mechanism of Toxic Action Primarily an irritant, inhibits the enzyme phosphofructokinase

Adverse Reactions

Cardiovascular: High blood pressure, A-V block

Dermatological: Dermal irritation

Gastrointestinal: Abdominal pain, vomiting, diarrhea, peptic ulceration

Hematologic: Hemolytic anemia

Ocular: Eye irritation

Miscellaneous: Menstruation disturbances; inhalation can cause pneumoconiosis

Signs & Symptoms of Acute Overdose EKG abnormalities (elevation of S-T segment, flat T waves); vomiting can occur with oral ingestion of 0.5 mg/kg antimony tartrate

Toxicodynamics/Kinetics

Absorption: Oral: 2% to 7% (antimony tartrate/antimony trichloride)

Half-life: 38 days

Elimination: Renal (faster with pentavalent than trivalent compounds)

Reference Range Baseline antimony levels: 0.4 µg/L (blood); 0.096-0.12 µg/g (hair); 0.6 µg/L (urine)

Overdosage Treatment

Decontamination: Oral: Dilute with milk or water

Enhancement of elimination: Chelation therapy with BAL may mitigate to toxicity of trivalent antimony compounds; hemodialysis may be useful in increasing clearance of pentavalent (but not trivalent) antimony although human experience in this modality is lacking

Antidote(s)

Dimercaprol *on page 1414*

Pregnancy Implications Increased rate of spontaneous abortions related to airborne antimony

Additional Information Silvery white powder

OSHA-PEL-TWA: 0.5 mg/m^3 (air)

Water standard: 145 mcg/L

Average daily intake:

- Ingestion: ~5 mcg
- Inhalation: ~0.04 mcg

Specific References

Katz M, "Anthelmintics," *Drugs*, 1977, 13(2):124-36.

U.S. Department of Health and Human Services, "Toxicological Profile for Antimony TP-91/02," Agency for Toxic Substances and Diseases Registry, September, 1992.

Antinonnin® *see* Dinitrocresol *on page 915*

Apachlor® *see* Chlorfenvinphos *on page 886*

API 79-7 *see* Mineral-Based Crankcase Oil *on page 971*

Aqualin® *see* Acrolein *on page 852*

Arasan® *see* Thiram *on page 1027*

Ardell Instant Glue Remover® *see* Acetonitrile *on page 850*

Argentum *see* Silver *on page 1012*

Arilate® *see* Carbaryl *on page 877*

Aroclor *see* Polychlorinated Biphenyls *on page 995*

Arsenate *see* Arsenic *on this page*

Arsenic

Related Information

Copper *on page 896*

Radiation: Basics of Exposure *on page 1594-1600*

CAS Number 7440-38-2

UN Number 1554; 1558; 1573

Synonyms Arsenate; Arsenite; Arsine

Commonly Found In Pesticides, rodenticides, ant pastes, wood preservative, microchips

Mechanism of Toxic Action Multisystem disease secondary to inhibition of oxidative phosphorylation

Adverse Reactions

Cardiovascular: Cardiotoxicity, tachycardia

Central nervous system: Neurotoxicity, peripheral axonopathy

Hematologic: Bone marrow depression, neutropenia, pancytopenia (leukopenia, thrombocytopenia, aplastic anemia)

Gastrointestinal: Gastrointestinal pathology, nausea, vomiting, metallic taste

Renal: Tubular necrosis (acute), hematuria

Miscellaneous: Salivation, feces discoloration (black), hyperthermia

Signs & Symptoms of Acute Overdose Torsade de pointes, neuritis, lacrimation, pancytopenia, encephalopathy, stocking glove sensory neuropathy, Mees' lines (on nail beds forms at 4-6 weeks postexposure), nystagmus, hematuria, leukopenia, garlic-like breath, blindness, fasciculations, agranulocytosis, hypotension, tachycardia, seizures, fever, paresthesia, radiopaque, tremor, myoglobinuria, alopecia, sweating, cough, hemolytic anemia

Toxicodynamics/Kinetics

Absorption: Orally, inhalation, and dermally

Distribution: V_d: 0.2 L/kg

Half-life: 42-48 hours

Elimination: Renal, degree of metabolism is ingestant dependent

Reference Range Urine concentrations in nonexposured individuals $\leq$50 μg/L; hair concentrations detectable 30 hours postingestion; urine $\geq$100 μg/L is suggestive for chronic exposure; blood not usually helpful, although blood arsenic levels >1000 μg/L usually associated with fatality; background blood arsenic level is usually <1 μg/L

Overdosage Treatment

Decontamination:

- Oral: Lavage/activated charcoal with cathartic; aluminum hydroxide may prevent absorption of pentavalent arsenic compounds (due to its phosphate-binding abilities), although this has not been investigated in humans; whole bowel irrigation is effective in radiopaque arsenic
- Dermal: Remove contaminated clothing, wash with soap and water
- Ocular: Copious irrigation with saline

Supportive therapy: 2,3-Dimercaptopropane-sulphonate (DMPS), a water soluble derivative of dimercaprol, has been recently demonstrated to prevent polyneuropathy when started within 48 hours of exposure at a dose of 5 mg/kg I.V. every 4 hours for 24 hours and then 400 mg orally every 4 hours for 5-7 days; BAL should be utilized for severe acute exposures except for arsine gas; penicillamine and succimer provide long-term therapy or alternatives to BAL

Antidote(s)

Dimercaprol *on page 1414*

Penicillamine *on page 1454*

Succimer *on page 1473*

Diagnostic Tests/Procedures

Arsenic, Blood *on page 1197*

Arsenic, Hair, Nails *on page 1197*

Arsenic, Urine *on page 1197*

Complete Blood Count *on page 1236*

Electrolytes, Blood *on page 1254*

Heavy Metal Screen, Blood *on page 1271*

Kidney Profile *on page 1279*

Pregnancy Implications Inorganic arsenic is teratogenic in rats

Additional Information Causes garlic odor; present in seafood; dietary history is important; found in some homeopathic medications; radiopaque compound but rapid absorption makes observation unlikely; arsine gas most toxic, then trivalent arsenite, then pentavalent arsenate; acute exposure can cause chronic symptoms; bone marrow, skin, and peripheral nerve system usual targets of chronic exposure; found in earth's crust at an arsenic level of 2 ppm

TLV-TWA: 0.2 mg/m^3

Urban arsenic levels of ambient air: 20-30 ng/m^3

Arsenic levels in groundwater: 1-2 ppb

Arsenic levels in selected media:

- Grains: 0.22 ppm
- Meat: 0.14 ppm
- Seafood: 4-5 ppm
- Cigarette: 1.5 ppm

Estimated daily intake of arsenic (adult):

- Nonsmoke: 51.5 mcg
- Smoker (2 packs/day): 63.5 mcg

Specific References

Franzblau A and Lilis R, "Acute Arsenic Intoxication From Environmental Arsenic Exposure," *Arch Environ Health*, 1989, 44(6):385-90.

Gorby MS, "Arsenic Poisoning," *West J Med*, 1988, 149(3):308-15.

(Continued)

Arsenic *(Continued)*

Lagerkvist BJ and Zetterlund B, "Assessment of Exposure to Arsenic Among Smelter Workers: A Five Year Follow-up," *Am J Ind Med*, 1994, 25(4):477-88.

Lee DC, Roberts JR, Kelly JJ, et al, "Whole Bowel Irrigation as an Adjunct in the Treatment of Radiopaque Arsenic," *Am J Emerg Med*, 1995, 13(2):244-5.

Martin DS, Willis SE, and Cline DM, "N-Acetylcysteine in the Treatment of Human Arsenic Poisoning," *J Am Board Fam Pract*, 1990, 3(4):293-6.

Moore DF, O'Callaghan CA, Berlyne G, et al, "Acute Arsenic Poisoning: Absence of Polyneuropathy After Treatment With 2,3-Dimercaptopropanesulphonate (DMPS)," *J Neurol Neurosurg Psychiatry*, 1994, 57(9):1133-5.

Sheerin NS, Monk PN, Aslam M, et al, "Simultaneous Exposure to Lead, Arsenic, and Mercury From Indian Ethnic Remedies," *Br J Clin Pract*, 1994, 48(6):332-3.

Shum S, Whitehead J, Vaughn L, et al, "Chelation of Organoarsenate With Dimercaptosuccinic Acid," *Vet Hum Toxicol*, 1995, 37(3):239-42.

Szeimies R-M, Karrer S, Heine A, et al, "Arsenic-Induced Skin Tumors Treated With Topical Photodynamic Therapy After Application of 5-Aminolevulinic Acid," *Eur J Dermatol*, 1995, 5:208-11.

U.S. Department of Health and Human Services, "Toxicological Profile for Arsenic TP-92/02," Agency for Toxic Substances and Diseases Registry, April 1993.

Arsenic Trihydride *see* Arsine *on this page*

Arsenite *see* Arsenic *on page 862*

Arsenous Hydride *see* Arsine *on this page*

Arsine

CAS Number 7784-42-1

UN Number 2188

Synonyms Arsenic Trihydride; Arsenous Hydride; Hydrogen Arsenide

Use Produced when water comes into contact with molten arsenic; used in the semiconductor industry; also found in jewelry, lead burners, etchers, silicone chips, fertilizer makers, aniline workers

Mechanism of Toxic Action Decline of erythrocyte glutathione concentrations after arsine binds to hemoglobin

Adverse Reactions Hematologic: Hemolysis

Signs & Symptoms of Acute Overdose Headache, hypotension, shivering, painless hemoglobinuria, dizziness, asthenia, seizures, nausea, vomiting, abdominal cramping, abdominal tenderness; jaundice, oliguria may also occur later

Toxicodynamics/Kinetics

Absorption: Inhalation: Well absorbed

Metabolism: To arsenic and trimethylarsine

Elimination: Excreted as arsenic in urine, feces, hair, fingernails, and by the lungs

Reference Range

Toxic: Blood: >200 µg/dL; urine: >1000 µg/L

A plasma free hemoglobin level >1.5 g/dL indicates a need for definitive treatment (possibly exchange transfusion)

Overdosage Treatment

Decontamination:

Inhalation: Administer 100% humidified oxygen

Dermal: Wash with soap and water

Supportive therapy: Immediate removal from victim; alkalinization of urine to prevent renal failure; exchange transfusions helpful in severe hemolysis; heavy metal chelators are ineffective

Elimination: Hemodialysis may be required for renal failure but will not remove the arsine-hemoglobin complex

Diagnostic Tests/Procedures

Complete Blood Count *on page 1236*

Electrocardiography *on page 1253*

Hemoglobin, Qualitative, Urine *on page 1272*

Reticulocyte Count *on page 1346*

Additional Information One of the most potent hemolytic toxins known; colorless; nonirritating at low concentrations; garlic-like odor at higher concentrations; potential human carcinogen

TLV-TWA: 0.05 ppm

IDLH: 6 ppm

PEL-TWA: 0.05 ppm

1 hour exposure: 5 ppm

Specific References

Fowler BA and Weissberg JB, "Arsine Poisoning," *N Engl J Med*, 1974, 291(22):1171-4.

Nau CA, "The Accidental Generation of Arsine Gas in an Industry," *South Med J*, 1985, 41:341-4.

Pinto SS, "Arsine Poisoning: Evolution of the Acute Phase," *J Occup Med*, 1976, 18(9):633-5.

Arsine *see* Arsenic *on page 862*

Artic® *see* Chloromethane *on page 891*

Artificial Nail Tip and Glue Remover® *see* Acetonitrile *on page 850*

Asbestos

CAS Number 1332-21-4

UN Number 2212; 2590

Synonyms Magnesium Silicate

Brand Names Avibest® (Chrysotile type)

Use Found in manufacture of cement pipe or panels, electrical insulation, fireproof clothing, locomotive repair, power plants, building demolition, car repair, chemical filters, gaskets, brake/clutch linings, transmission component

Mechanism of Toxic Action Not well delineated; asbestos is fibrogenic with accumulation of macrophage and fiber phagocytosis occurring; it is unclear whether asbestos fibers induce carcinogenesis or are tumor promoting agents; lipid peroxidation can occur with chrysotile agents

Signs & Symptoms of Acute Overdose Asbestosis: Bilateral interstitial fibrosis affecting lower $^{2}/_{3}$ of lung; symptoms include dyspnea, rales (usually occur 10-40 years after exposure), renal failure, acute myelocytic leukemia, and skin warts

Toxicodynamics/Kinetics Fibers $>3\ \mu m$ in diameter or longer than 100 μm are not rapidly cleared from pulmonary tract

Absorption: No dermal or gastrointestinal absorption

Elimination: Mucociliary transport through lung

Clearance:

- Upper airways: 2-3 hours
- Lower airways: 10-160 days

Overdosage Treatment

Supportive therapy: No specific treatment for asbestosis; traditional antineoplastic therapy for tumors are mainstay of treatment; certainly, patients with asbestos exposure should avoid cigarette smoking

Diagnostic Tests/Procedures

Chest Films *on page 1224*

Pregnancy Implications Placental transfer of fibers can occur

Additional Information Levels of airborne asbestos (fibers measured by phase contrast microscopy/L of air):

School: 0.00024
Rural: 0.000002
Urban: 0.003-0.000003
Industrial operations: 0.15-0.0015

Serpentine asbestos (extended sheet polysilicate structure)
- Chrysotile (white asbestos)* – TLV: 2 fibers/mL of air

Amphibole group (linear double chain polysilicate structure)
- Actinolite TLV: 2 fibers/mL of air
- Amosite (brown asbestos*) – TLV: 0.5 fibers/mL of air
- Anthophyllite (gray asbestos)* – TLV: 2 fibers/mL of air
- Crocidolite (blue asbestos)* – TLV: 0.2 fibers/mL of air
- Mullite – TLV: 2 fibers/mL of air
- Tremolite (silicic acid: calcium magnesium salt) – TLV: 2 fibers/mL of air
- * Associated with high fibrogenic potential

OSHA-PEL: 0.2 fibers/nL of air

Carcinomas associated with asbestos include lung (especially in smokers), pleural mesothelioma (not increased in smokers), peritoneum mesothelioma, laryngeal carcinoma; carcinomas of questionable association with asbestos include colon, renal, pancreas, ovary, esophagus, and lymphomas

While all types of fibers can cause lung cancer, amphibole group fibers are more potent for inducing mesotheliomas than serpentine fibers; EPA estimates that lifetime exposure of asbestos dust (0.001 fiber $>5\ \mu m$ in length per mL of air) could result in 2-4 excess lung cancer or mesothelioma deaths per 100,000 individuals.

Pulmonary function tests may show restrictive pattern; open lung biopsy may be required; gallium scanning or bronchoalveolar lavage may be helpful

In older homes (built from 1920s to 1970s), asbestos may be located around boilers, steam pipes, ductwork, floor coverings (especially 9" vinyl tiles), "popcorn" ceiling finishes, exterior siding, roofing shingles, and acoustical ceiling tiles

Specific References

Becklake MR, "Asbestos and Other Fiber-Related Diseases of the Lungs and Pleura. Distribution and Determinants in Exposed Populations," *Chest*, 1991, 100(1):248-54.

Omenn GS, "A Double-Blind Randomized Trial With Beta-Carotene and Retinol in Persons at High Risk of Lung Cancer Due to Occupational Asbestos Exposures and/or Cigarette Smoking," *Public Health Rev*, 1988, 16(1-2):99-125.

"Safe at Home," *Consumer Reports*, 1995, 60(7):459-69.

Shih JF, Wilson JS, Broderick A, et al, "Asbestos-Induced Pleural Fibrosis and Impaired Exercise Physiology," *Chest*, 1994, 105(5):1370-6.

(Continued)

Asbestos (Continued)

U.S. Department of Health and Human Services, "Public Health Service: Toxicological Profile for Asbestos," Agency for Toxic Substances and Diseases Registry, October, 1993.

Asex *see* Chlorate Salts *on page 884*

Atonik® *see* Nitrophenol *on page 980*

Automotive Motor Oil *see* Mineral-Based Crankcase Oil *on page 971*

Avibest® (Chrysotile type) *see* Asbestos *on previous page*

Avlothane® *see* Hexachloroethane *on page 937*

Azabenzine *see* Pyridine *on page 1005*

Azine *see* Pyridine *on page 1005*

Azofos® *see* Methyl Parathion *on page 969*

Ba *see* Barium *on this page*

Barium

Related Information

Radiation: Basics of Exposure *on page 1594-1600*

Toxins Which Should be Lavaged With Solutions Other Than Water *on page 1635*

CAS Number 7440-39-3

UN Number 1400; 1339; 1854

Synonyms Ba

Mechanism of Toxic Action Barium can sequester potassium within muscle cells resulting in paralysis

Adverse Reactions

Cardiovascular: Hypertension, tachycardia (ventricular)

Central nervous system: Paresthesia

Dermatologic: Angioedema

Endocrine & metabolic: Hypokalemia, hypophosphatemia, hypothermia

Gastrointestinal: Abdominal pain, diarrhea, nausea, vomiting, feces discoloration (black), feces discoloration (clay/putty), feces discoloration (red), feces discoloration (white/speckling)

Neuromuscular & skeletal: Rhabdomyolysis, muscle paralysis, myopathy

Ocular: Mydriasis

Respiratory: Wheezing, apnea, allergic rhinitis

Signs & Symptoms of Acute Overdose Hypertension, fasciculations, tachycardia (ventricular), angioedema, paresthesia, abdominal pain, A-V block, diarrhea, nausea, vomiting, rhabdomyolysis, muscle paralysis, mydriasis, dermal burns, wheezing, apnea, feces discoloration (black), feces discoloration (clay/putty), feces discoloration (red), feces discoloration (white/speckling), hypokalemia, hypophosphatemia, allergic rhinitis, hypothermia

Toxicodynamics/Kinetics

Absorption: Oral absorption from food sources: 1% to 15% (average 6%)

Distribution: Primarily to skeleton and teeth

Half-life: 3.6 days

Elimination: Primarily fecal

Reference Range Ingestion of barium carbonate resulting in muscle paralysis was associated with a peak barium level of 150 mEq/L

Overdosage Treatment

Decontamination: Lavage/activated charcoal will not bind barium; magnesium sulfate or sodium sulfate is the preferred cathartic in order to convert barium to inabsorbable barium sulfate

Supportive therapy: Monitor potassium, paralysis and ventricular arrhythmia will respond to potassium; avoid the use of sulfate salts since this may cause precipitation of barium in the kidneys; atropine and naloxone have been demonstrated in rodents to decrease mortality but his has not been used in humans

Enhancement of elimination: Forced diuresis with intravenous saline solution with furosemide (1 mg/kg I.V.) to keep a urine flow of 3-6 mL/kg/hour will hasten elimination; hemodialysis with a sodium bicarbonate/potassium dialysate may also be useful

Diagnostic Tests/Procedures

Potassium, Blood *on page 1328*

Additional Information Found in most soils ranging from 15-3000 ppm; average atmospheric barium concentration in North America is 0.012 mcg/m^3; in seawater it is about 13 mcg/L; Brazil nuts have high concentrations of barium (3000-4000 ppm)

TLV-TWA:

Barium: 0.5 mg/m^3

Barium sulfate: 10 mg/m^3

Total daily barium intake: 650-1770 mg

Average amount of barium ingested through drinking water: 1-2 mg/kg/day

Average amount of barium intake through inhalation: 1-30 mg/day (75% absorbed)

Specific References

Aks S, Vanden Hoek T, Hryhorczuk DO, et al, "Barium Sulfide Ingestions in a Prison Population," *Vet Hum Toxicol*, 1991, 33:370.

Schorn TF, Olbricht C, Schuler A, et al, "Barium Carbonate Intoxication," *Intensive Care Med*, 1991, 17(1):60-2.

Shankle R and Keane JR, "Acute Paralysis From Inhaled Barium Carbonate," *Arch Neurol*, 1988, 45(5):579-80.

U.S. Department of Health and Human Services, "Toxicological Profile for Barium TP-91/03," Agency for Toxic Substances and Diseases Registry, July, 1992.

Base Engine Oil *see* Mineral-Based Crankcase Oil *on page 971*

Battery Acid *see* Sulfuric Acid *on page 1019*

Bay E-605® *see* Parathion *on page 988*

Baygon® *see* Propoxur *on page 1000*

Baytex® *see* Fenthion *on page 929*

Bazinon® *see* Diazinon *on page 904*

BBC12 *see* 1,2-Dibromo-3-Chloropropane *on page 906*

Bent-Cure® *see* Hexachlorobenzene *on page 936*

Bent-No-More® *see* Hexachlorobenzene *on page 936*

Benzamide *see* Diethyltoluamide *on page 912*

Benz[*a*]anthracene *see* Polycyclic Aromatic Hydrocarbons *on page 997*

Benzene

Related Information

Gasoline *on page 932*

CAS Number 71-43-2

UN Number 1114

Synonyms (6)-Annulene; Carbon Oil; Mineral Naphtha; Phene; Phenyl Hydride

Brand Names Polystream®

Commonly Found In Industrial solvent, gasoline (0.81% to 1.35%, higher percentage in Europe)

Use In lacquers, manufacture of dyes, oil cloths, varnishes

Mechanism of Toxic Action Hematotoxicity, CNS depression, leukemogenic

Adverse Reactions

Cardiovascular: Cardiac toxicity

Central nervous system: CNS depression, euphoria

Hematologic: Leukemia usually after chronic exposure, aplastic anemia, neutropenia

Hepatic: Hepatotoxicity

Respiratory: Bronchial irritation, pulmonary edema

Miscellaneous: Burning sensation of mucous membranes, feces discoloration (black)

Signs & Symptoms of Acute Overdose Cough, hoarseness, aspiration, dementia, blistering, headache, coma, seizures, dizziness, hematuria, ataxia, mydriasis, leukopenia, paresthesia, ototoxicity, tinnitus

Toxicodynamics/Kinetics

Absorption:

Inhalation: Rapid (70% to 80% within first 5 minutes)

Oral: 90% to 97% of dose in rodent models

Dermal: <1%; absorption rate: 0.4 mg/cm^2/hour

Metabolism: Hepatic via cytochrome P-450-dependent mixed function oxidase through two detoxification pathways: 1) via glutathione to mercapturic acid, and 2) through sulfate/glucuronide conjugation. Hematotoxic metabolites include hydroquinone, phenol, muconic dialdehyde, and catechol.

Half-life: 8 hours

Elimination: Renal (<1%) and by inhalation (16% to 42%); through dermal absorption as much as 30% can be excreted through the kidneys as phenol. Oral ingestion (rabbit model), 43% was eliminated through the lungs (1.5% as carbon dioxide), with urinary excretion accounting for 33%.

Reference Range Urine phenol level >10 mg/L, blood benzene level of 0.2 mg/L is consistent with exposure of 25 ppm

Overdosage Treatment

Supportive therapy: Move patient to fresh air; give 100% humidified oxygen; avoid epinephrine; ingestion – basic poison management

(Continued)

Benzene *(Continued)*

Enhancement of elimination: Although there is no experience in its use, acetylcysteine has a theoretical role in increasing glutathione stores and enhance elimination

Diagnostic Tests/Procedures

Benzene, Blood *on page 1201*
Complete Blood Count *on page 1236*
Liver Profile *on page 1286*

Additional Information Daily benzene intake of a smoker (32 cigarettes daily) is about 10 times (1.8 mg/day) than that of a nonsmoker. Median benzene levels in homes with smokers is about 50% greater than that of nonsmokers (3.3 ppb vs 2.2 ppb). Atmospheric half-life of benzene is ~5.6 days. In water, it is ~17 days, although the half-life of its hydroxyl radicals in water may be 8-9 months.

Benzene has been substantially reduced in automotive gasoline after 1995 (see Gasoline monograph). It has been estimated that benzene exposure to pumping gasoline at service stations is ~1 ppm; ambient median benzene levels in urban areas is ~12.6 ppb while California's median benzene level is much lower (3.3 ppb) due to stricter gasoline requirements.

Lethal dose: 100 mL
TLV-TWA: 1 ppm
IDLH: 2000 ppm
PEL-TWA: 1-10 ppm

Specific References

Aksoy M, "Benzene as a Leukemogenic and Carcinogenic Agent," *Am J Ind Med*, 1985, 8(1):9-20.

U.S. Department of Health and Human Services, "Toxicological Profile for Benzene TP-92/03," Agency for Toxic Substances and Diseases Registry, April, 1993.

Benzeneamine *see* Aniline *on page 858*

Benzene Chloride *see* Chlorobenzene *on page 889*

Benzidin *see* Benzidine *on this page*

Benzidine

CAS Number 92-87-5

UN Number 1885

Synonyms Benzidin; 4,4'-Diphenylediamine

Brand Names Fast Corinth Base B

Use In the production of azo dyes for leathers, textiles, and paper; not produced in the U.S. for dye manufacture

Mechanism of Toxic Action Intermediate metabolites through hepatic degradation; may be carcinogenic

Adverse Reactions Dermal exposure: Allergic eczematous dermatitis

Toxicodynamics/Kinetics

Absorption: Through intact skin, lungs, intestine
Metabolism: Hepatic to N-acetylbenzidine; undergoes enterohepatic recirculation
Half-life: 5 hours
Elimination: Renal and bile

Reference Range Urinary levels in workers exposed to benzidine based dyes ranged from:

Benzidine: 0-363 μg/L
Monoacetylbenzidine: 6-1117 μg/L
Diacetylbenzidine: 4-160 μg/L

Overdosage Treatment

Decontamination:

- Dermal: Irrigate with soap and water; remove contaminated clothing
- Ocular: Irrigate with saline
- Oral: Lavage/activated charcoal; do not use mineral oil as a cathartic in that oils may enhance intestinal absorption

Supportive therapy: While no human treatment data exists, interruption of benzidine metabolism by such agents as aspirin or indomethacin (through inhibition of cyclo-oxygenase) may reduce peroxide formation; similarly, a reducing agent such as ascorbic acid may decrease levels of toxic oxidized reactive metabolites which can be carcinogenic

Enhancement of elimination: Due to enterohepatic recirculation, multiple dosing of activated charcoal may be effective

Additional Information Occupationally exposed workers may have higher incidence of bladder (transitional cell) carcinoma; may alter natural killer cell activity

Atmospheric half-life: 12 hours
Water half-life: 100 days

Specific References

Tanigawa T, Araki S, Ishizu S, et al, "Natural Killer Cell Activity in Workers Exposed to Benzidine and Beta-Naphthylamine," *Br J Ind Med*, 1990, 47(5):338-41.

U.S. Department of Health and Human Services, "Toxicological Profile for Benzidine," Agency for Toxic Substances and Diseases Registry, October, 1993.

Benzin *see* Petroleum Distillates – Naphtha *on page 991*

Benzinoform® *see* Carbon Tetrachloride *on page 882*

Benzo[*b*]fluoranthene *see* Polycyclic Aromatic Hydrocarbons *on page 997*

Benzo[*j*]fluoranthene *see* Polycyclic Aromatic Hydrocarbons *on page 997*

Benzo[*k*]fluoranthene *see* Polycyclic Aromatic Hydrocarbons *on page 997*

Benzofuran *see* 2,3-Benzofuran *on this page*

2,3-Benzofuran

CAS Number 271-89-6

Synonyms Benzofuran; Benzofurfuran; Coumarone; Cumaron

Use Found in cigarette smoke, as a coating on citrus fruits, asphalt floor tiles, food container adhesives; used in paint production

Mechanism of Toxic Action Produced by destructive distillation of coal (naphtha fraction) and fossil fuels

Adverse Reactions Little human adverse effect experience

Overdosage Treatment

Decontamination: Flush skin or eyes with copious amounts of water

Supportive therapy: Give oxygen if patient is exposed to heated decomposition products; monitor pulmonary status

Additional Information Aromatic odor, colorless liquid, insoluble in water; found in breast milk; FDA regulation for protective coating on citrus fruits: maximum: 200 ppm; when heated, can emit acrid fumes

Specific References

Pellizzari ED, Hartwell TD, Harris BS 3d, et al, "Purgeable Organic Compounds in Mother's Milk," *Bull Environ Contam Toxicol*, 1982, 28(3):322-8.

U.S. Department of Health and Human Services, "Toxicological Profile for 2,3-Benxofuran TP-91/04," Agency for Toxic Substances and Diseases Registry, September, 1992.

Benzofurfuran *see* 2,3-Benzofuran *on this page*

Benzo[*ghi*]perylene *see* Polycyclic Aromatic Hydrocarbons *on page 997*

Benzo[*e*]pyrene *see* Polycyclic Aromatic Hydrocarbons *on page 997*

Benzo[*a*]pyrene (BaP) *see* Polycyclic Aromatic Hydrocarbons *on page 997*

Benzoyl Peroxide *see* Dibenzoyl Peroxide *on page 906*

Beosit® *see* Endosulfan *on page 921*

Bercema *see* Methyl Bromide *on page 964*

Bertholite *see* Chlorine *on page 888*

Beryl *see* Beryllium *on this page*

Beryllium

CAS Number 7440-41-7; 7787-47-5; 7787-49-7; 1304-56-9; 13327-32-7; 35089-00-0; 13597-99-4; 13510-48-0; 13510-49-1; 14215-00-0; 7787-56-6; 66104-24-3

UN Number 1566; 1567; 2464

Synonyms Beryl; Glucinium

Commonly Found In Ore processing, aircraft disc brakes, space vehicles, optics, microwave oven components, automotive electronics, fuel containers

Mechanism of Toxic Action Acute (rare) and chronic toxicities most commonly seen with inhalation exposure of soluble compounds in occupational setting; inhibits phosphatases, hexokinase, lactate dehydrogenase

Adverse Reactions

Dermatologic: Skin ulceration, granulomas

Renal: Kidney stones, nephritis

Respiratory: Chronic "sarcoid-like" pulmonary disease

Signs & Symptoms of Acute Overdose Acute conjunctivitis, pneumonitis, right-sided heart failure, dermatotoxic, pulmonary fibronodular disease, seizures, nausea, vomiting

Toxicodynamics/Kinetics

Absorption: Inhalation (primarily); oral and dermal (poorly absorbed)

Protein binding: 70%

Metabolism: Not biotransformed

(Continued)

Beryllium *(Continued)*

Half-life: 2-8 weeks

Reference Range Urine concentrations: 0.4-1.0 μg/L in controls

Overdosage Treatment

Decontamination: Remove from exposure source; oxygen indicated for symptomatic inhalation exposure

Supportive therapy: Chronic pulmonary symptoms may respond to corticosteroids; oral exposure should be treated with diluting with milk or water; chelation is not effective; high calcium diet might displace beryllium from bones

Pregnancy Implications No known teratogenicity; has been found in neonates of exposure mother

Additional Information Beryllium is odorless; chronic beryllium poisoning requires at least four of these findings:

1. Exposure
2. Beryllium in lung/granulomas
3. Respiratory disease
4. Radiograph of fibronodular disease
5. Restrictive pulmonary function
6. Consistent lung/lymph pathology

Average concentration of beryllium:

Atmospheric air: <0.1 ng/m^3

Fresh water: 10-1000 ng/L

Soil: 2.8-5 mg/kg

Cigarette smoke: 2% to 10%

Idiosyncratically affects 5% of heavily exposed workers after 1- to 20-year latency

TLV: 0.002 mg/m^3

Beryllium measurable in lung and granulomas of chronic beryllium disease patients; also useful in lymphoblast transformation test from bronchoalveolar lavage fluid

Specific References

Cullen MR, Cherniack MG, and Kominsky JR, "Chronic Beryllium Disease in the United States," *Semin Respir Med*, 1986, 7:203-9.

Hardy HL, "Beryllium Disease: A Clinical Perspective," *Environ Res*, 1980, 21(1):1-9.

U.S. Department of Health and Human Services, "Toxicological Profile for Beryllium TP-92/04," Agency for Toxic Substances and Diseases Registry, April, 1993.

Betanal *see* Phenmedipham *on page 992*

B-Herbtox *see* Chlorate Salts *on page 884*

1,2-Bichlorethane *see* Ethylene Dichloride *on page 924*

Bidrin® *see* Dicrotophos *on page 909*

Biethylene *see* 1,3-Butadiene *on page 874*

Birlane® *see* Chlorfenvinphos *on page 886*

Bis(2-Chloroethyl) Sulfide *see* Mustard Gas *on page 972*

1,1-Bis(4-Chlorophenyl)-2 *see* DDD *on page 902*

Bis-Amine A® *see* 4,4'-Methylenebis (2-Chloroaniline) *on page 965*

Bivinyl *see* 1,3-Butadiene *on page 874*

"Blackstones" *see* Paraphenylenediamine *on page 986*

Bladan F® *see* Parathion *on page 988*

Bladan-M® *see* Methyl Parathion *on page 969*

"Blue Heaven" *see* Isopropyl Alcohol *on page 943*

Blue Oil *see* Aniline *on page 858*

Bonoform® *see* Tetrachloroethane *on page 1022*

Borates

CAS Number 7440-42-8; 1303-86-2; 10043-35-3; 1303-96-4; 10294-33-4; 7637-07-2

UN Number 1458; 2692; 1008

Synonyms Boric Anhydride; Boron Oxide; Boron Sesquioxide; Boron Trioxide; Magnesium Perborate; Sodium Biborate; Sodium Borate; Sodium Metaborate; Sodium Perborate; Sodium Pyroborate; Sodium Tetraborate

Brand Names Borax®; Dobill's Solution®

Use Various; used in herbicides; common ingredient of medicated powders, skin lotions, mouthwashes, toothpastes, powders, water softeners, topical astringents and antiseptics; also used in making glass fibers, enamels, glazes, fire-resistant materials, pigments, paints, catalysts, photographic agents, and insecticides; found in rodent and ant poisons

Signs & Symptoms of Acute Overdose Toxicity may be delayed for hours; gastrointestinal upset and vomiting (emesis has been described as blue-green), and retching, CNS depression, restlessness, irritability, and seizures occur from chronic exposure; death results from dehydration, shock, circulatory collapse and renal failure. Renal failure, oliguria, anuria occur several days after exposure; metabolic acidosis may occur; erythematous rash, usually on buttocks and scrotum, with desquamation occurring where rash is persistent and mucous membranes, perianal and anal surfaces. Alopecia totalis can occur with acute or chronic poisoning.

Toxicodynamics/Kinetics

Absorption: Through gastrointestinal tract, mucous membranes, and abraded and denuded skin

Distribution: V_d: 0.17-0.5 L/kg; distributes to all tissues except brain in 30 minutes

Half-life: 5-27 hours

Peak CNS concentration: In 3 hours

Elimination: 50% excreted in urine within 12 hours and 80% to 100% over 5-7 days

Warnings High affinity for brain, liver, and kidney; damage to tissues, especially renal tubular epithelium may be irreversible

Reference Range Normal: 0.0-0.72 mg/dL in children; 0.0-0.2 mg/dL in adults; levels do not seem to correlate well with severity of symptoms; levels >40 mg/dL associated with fatality in infants

Overdosage Treatment

Decontamination:

- Dermal: Wash skin with soap and water
- Ocular: Irrigate with saline
- Oral: Ipecac or lavage; activated charcoal will probably not be useful

Supportive therapy: Monitor for hypotension, shock, seizures

Enhancement of elimination: Hemodialysis or exchange transfusion may enhance elimination; saline diuresis may be of some benefit; early institution of peritoneal dialysis in asymptomatic patients ingesting a large dose has been advocated

Test Interactions While tumeric acid strips can detect boric acid in the urine, false-positives can occur

Monitoring Parameters Serum boric acid levels may be sent to:

U.S. Borax and Chemical Co
U.S. Borax Laboratories
412 Crescent Way
Anaheim, CA 92801
Telephone: (714) 774-2673

Send 10 mL of heparinized blood in a polyethylene bottle accompanied by case summary

Additional Information

Average amount of boron in surface water: ~0.1 mg/L

Mean boron level in soil in U.S.: 26 mg/kg

FDA tolerance limit for boron in citrus fruit: 8 ppm

Average daily intake in humans of boron: 10-25 mg

Concentration of boron in sea water: ~4.5 mg/L

Specific References

Baliah T, MacLeish H, and Drummond KN, "Acute Boric Acid Poisoning: Report of an Infant Successfully Treated by Peritoneal Dialysis," *Can Med Assoc J*, 1969, 101(3):166-8.

Goldbloom RB and Goldbloom A, "Boric Acid Poisoning: Report of 4 Cases and a Review of 109 Cases From the World Literature," *J Pediatr*, 1953, 43(6):631-43.

Litovitz TL, Klein-Schwartz W, Oderda GM, et al, "Clinical Manifestations of Toxicity in a Series of 784 Boric Acid Ingestions," *Am J Emerg Med*, 1988, 6(3):209-13.

Siegel E and Wason S, "Boric Acid Toxicity," *Pediatr Clin North Am*, 1986, 33(2):363-7.

U.S. Department of Health and Human Services, "Toxicological Profile for Boron TP-91/05," Agency for Toxic Substances and Diseases Registry, July 1992.

Wong LC, Heimbach MD, Truscott DR, et al, "Boric Acid Poisoning: Report of 11 Cases," *Can Med Assoc J*, 1964, 90:1018-23.

Borax® *see* Borates *on previous page*

Borer Sol *see* Ethylene Dichloride *on page 924*

Boric Anhydride *see* Borates *on previous page*

Boron Oxide *see* Borates *on previous page*

Boron Sesquioxide *see* Borates *on previous page*

Boron Trioxide *see* Borates *on previous page*

Brass Chills *see* Metal Fume Fever *on page 956*

Brocide *see* Ethylene Dichloride *on page 924*

Brodifacoum *see* Anticoagulant Rodenticide *on page 859*

Brofene® *see* Bromophos *on page 873*

Bromadiolone *see* Anticoagulant Rodenticide *on page 859*

Bromates

Related Information

Toxins Which Should be Lavaged With Solutions Other Than Water *on page 1635*

CAS Number 7758-01-2; 7789-38-0

UN Number 3213; 1450

Use Found in permanent wave hair neutralizers as potassium bromate (2%) or sodium bromate (10%), and bread preservatives

Mechanism of Toxic Action Mucosal irritant; oxidizing effect on renal tubule can cause renal failure; potassium bromate may be more toxic than sodium bromate

Signs & Symptoms of Acute Overdose Nausea, vomiting, deafness, diarrhea, hemolysis, hypotension, seizures, renal failure, ototoxicity, tinnitus (more common in adults than children), tachypnea, albuminuria, albuminuria, hiccups, hemolysis, dizziness

Toxicodynamics/Kinetics Distribution: V_d: 0.24 L/kg

Overdosage Treatment

Decontamination: Lavage with sodium bicarbonate (2% to 5%) to prevent formation of hydrobromic acid

Supportive therapy: Give sodium thiosulfate (10-50 mL of a 10% solution over 30-60 minutes) to convert bromate to less toxic bromide; monitor with audiograms

Enhancement of elimination: Hemodialysis can be used if renal failure ensues, but is not effective in reducing bromide levels

Specific References

Lue JN, Johnson CE, and Edwards DC, "Bromate Poisoning From Ingestion of Professional Hair-Care Neutralizer," *Clin Pharm*, 1988, 7(1):66-70.

Warshaw BL, "Treatment of Bromate Poisoning," *J Pediatr*, 1989, 115(4):660-1.

Bromoform

Related Information

Dibromochloromethane *on page 907*

CAS Number 75-25-2

UN Number 2515

Synonyms Methenyl Tribromide; Tribromomethane

Use Not produced in the U.S.; used as a fluid for mineral ore separation, a laboratory reagent and used in quality control in the electronics industry; formerly used medicinally as a sedative or antitussive agent

Mechanism of Toxic Action Central nervous depressant; can be generated during water chlorination when water reacts with organic acids; thus, exposure can occur through drinking water (levels usually ~5 mcg/L)

Adverse Reactions

Central nervous system: Depression

Miscellaneous: On inhalation, can be a mucosal irritant and lacrimator

Signs & Symptoms of Acute Overdose Coma, stupor, respiratory depression, miosis, tremor; may be hepatotoxic and nephrotoxic

Toxicodynamics/Kinetics

Absorption: Absorbed by inhalation and oral routes (60% to 90%)

Metabolism: Oxidation in liver

Elimination: Pulmonary hepatotoxic in animal models

Reference Range Background blood levels in individuals exposed to bromoform only through drinking water is ~0.6 ppb

Overdosage Treatment

Decontamination (oral overdose): Lavage/activated charcoal

Supportive therapy: Although human overdose experience is virtually nonexistent over the past 90 years, respiratory support appears to be a crucial modality; naloxone may be of some benefit; otherwise would treat as for bromides

Pregnancy Implications Low toxicity

Additional Information Colorless liquid with a sweet odor; not flammable; prepared by mixing acetone with sodium hypobromite or by treating chloroform with aluminum bromide; anesthetic properties similar to chloroform; upon heating, it decomposes to bromide ion fumes

OSHA: PEL-TWA: 0.5 ppm

TLV-TWA: 0.5 ppm

FDA: Bottled water regulation for total trihalomethanes: 0.1 mg/L

Atmospheric half-life: Possibly 1-2 months; estimated daily dose to an average adult: <1 mcg

Fatal oral dose: 250-500 mg/kg

Odor threshold:

- Air: 13.45 mg/m^3
- Water: 0.5 mg/L

Mean urban ambient air concentration of bromoform: 3.6 ppt

Specific References

Antoine SR, DeLeon IR, and O'Dell-Smith RM, "Environmentally Significant Volatile Organic Pollutants in Human Blood," *Bull Environ Contam Toxicol*, 1986, 36(3):364-71.

U.S. Department of Health and Human Services, "Bromoform, Chlorodibromomethane," Public Health Service, Agency for Toxic Substances and Diseases Registry, December 1990.

Bromofume® *see* Ethylene Bromide *on page 924*

Bromomethane *see* Methyl Bromide *on page 964*

Bromone® *see* Anticoagulant Rodenticide *on page 859*

Bromophos

CAS Number 2104-96-3

Synonyms O,O-Dimethyl-O-(2,5-Dichloro-4-Bromophenyl) Phosphorothioate

Brand Names Brofene®; Nexion®

Use Marketed as insecticide granules, dusting agent, or spray liquid with or without petroleum derivative as a solvent

Mechanism of Toxic Action Irreversible inhibition of acetylcholinesterase and plasma cholinesterase, resulting in excess accumulation of acetylcholine at muscarinic and nicotinic receptors, and in the central nervous system

Adverse Reactions

Cardiovascular: Hyperdynamic (~18% to 21%) or hypodynamic (~7% to 10%) states

Central nervous system: Depression, seizures, hyperactivity

Genitourinary: Incontinence

Neuromuscular & skeletal: Weakness, paralysis

Respiratory: Depression, edema

General: Flu-like symptoms (especially with chronic exposure)

Delayed: Muscle asthenia and paresthesia

Signs & Symptoms of Acute Overdose Miosis (unreactive to light), mydriasis (rarely), lacrimation, pallor, excessive sweating, confusion, agitation, headache, dysarthria, generalized asthenia, seizures, coma, cranial nerve palsies, decreased hemoglobin/red blood cell count/platelet count, metabolic acidosis and hyperglycemia (severe intoxication), hypotension, hypertension, bradycardia, tachycardia, Q-T prolongation, A-V block, heart block, asystole, salivation, bronchorrhea, tachypnea, pulmonary edema, respiratory depression, diaphragmatic paralysis, skeletal muscle fasciculation and flaccid paralysis, nausea, vomiting, abdominal pain, fecal and urinary incontinence; an "intermediate syndrome" of limb asthenia and respiratory paralysis has been reported to occur between 24 and 96 hours postorganophosphate exposure, and is independent of the acute cholinergic crisis; late paresthesia characterized by stocking and glove paresthesia, anesthesia, and asthenia is infrequently observed weeks to months following acute exposure to certain organophosphates

Toxicodynamics/Kinetics

Absorption: Readily through oral, dermal, or respiratory exposure

Metabolism: Rapid to weakly active compounds through hepatic hydrolysis and other pathways

Elimination: Metabolites are excreted in urine

Warnings Risk of aspiration pneumonitis exists following oral exposure to agents having a hydrocarbon vehicle; severe laryngeal irritation and violent coughing may result from exposure to dusting powders; exposure to dusting powders and insecticide granules may cause contact dermatitis

Overdosage Treatment

Decontamination: Isolation, bagging, and disposal of all contaminated clothing and other articles; all emergency medical workers and hospital staff should follow appropriate precautions regarding exposure to hazardous material including the use of protective clothing, masks, goggles, and respiratory equipment

Dermal: Prompt thorough scrubbing of all affected areas with soap and water, including hair and nails

Gastric: Activated charcoal can be administered either orally or via a nasogastric tube; do not induce emesis because of danger of sudden respiratory compromise, alterations in mental status, seizures, coma, and possible aspiration of hydrocarbon vehicles

Ocular: Irrigation with copious tepid sterile water or saline

Supportive therapy: Including airway management, ventilatory assistance, humidified oxygen administration, and close monitoring for sudden respiratory failure

Antidote:

Atropine: Administration should be guided by respiratory status, starting at 1-5 mg I.V. every 5-10 minutes as needed, and should be titrated to the resolution of excess pulmonary secretions; frequent administration of large doses (cumulative doses >100 mg) may be necessary in massive exposures

Glycopyrrolate: May be administered if atropine is unavailable

2-PAM: For more significant exposures (ie, exposures requiring large doses of atropine, or with recurring symptoms, or exposures to more lipid soluble agents), administration should follow: 1-2 g I.V. over 5-10 minutes, repeated in 1 hour if asthenia reoccurs, then every 4-12 hours for recurring symptoms

(Continued)

Bromophos *(Continued)*

Enhancement of elimination: Dialysis and hemoperfusion are not indicated due to effectiveness of the prescribed treatment, large volumes of distribution of organophosphates

Antidote(s)

Atropine Sulfate *on page 1395*
Pralidoxime Chloride *on page 1461*

Diagnostic Tests/Procedures

Blood Gases, Arterial *on page 1207*
Chest Films *on page 1224*
Complete Blood Count *on page 1236*
Creatinine, Serum *on page 1243*
Electrocardiography *on page 1253*
Liver Profile *on page 1286*
Pseudocholinesterase, Serum *on page 1340*

Pregnancy Implications Human data regarding organophosphate exposure in pregnancy is limited and anecdotal; teratogenesis and fetal death have been produced in animal models at exposure levels that cause obvious toxicity to the pregnant animal

Additional Information Red blood cell cholinesterase and serum pseudocholinesterase may be depressed following acute or chronic organophosphate exposure; RBC cholinesterase is typically not analyzed by in-house laboratories and is usually not available for consideration during acute management. Pseudocholinesterase levels may be rapidly available from some in-house laboratories, but are not as reliable a marker of organophosphate exposure because of variability secondary to variant genotypes, hepatic disease, oral estrogen use, or malnutrition. Because of this variability, true indication of suppression of either of these enzymes can only be estimated through comparison to pre-exposure values; these enzymes may be useful in measuring a patient's recovery postexposure, especially if the recovery is not progressing as expected.

Other information concerning pesticide exposures is available through the EPA-funded National Pesticide Telecommunications Network: 1-800-858-7378 (weekdays, 8 AM to 6 PM, Central Standard time)

Specific References

Minton NA and Murray VS, "A Review of Organophosphate Poisoning," *Med Toxicol Adverse Drug Exp*, 1988, 3(5):350-75.

Namba T, Nolte CT, Jackrel J, et al, "Poisoning Due to Organophosphate Insecticides. Acute and Chronic Manifestations," *Am J Med*, 1971, 50(4):475-92.

Buhach *see* Pyrethrins *on page 1003*

1,3-Butadiene

CAS Number 106-99-0

UN Number 1010

Synonyms Biethylene; Bivinyl; Butadiene Divinyl

Use In the manufacture of foams, carpet backing, paper coating, production of fungicides

Mechanism of Toxic Action Asphyxiant – anesthesia at high concentrations; no cumulative toxicity

Adverse Reactions

Cardiovascular: Bradycardia, hypotension
Central nervous system: CNS depression
Hematologic: Possibly leukemogenic

Signs & Symptoms of Acute Overdose Headache, irritation of upper airway, blurred vision, coughing, drowsiness, skin irritation, hallucinations

Toxicodynamics/Kinetics

Metabolism: Though not studies in humans, major metabolites appear to be diepoxybutane and 3,4-epoxy-1,2-butanediol; glutathione-S-tranferase appears to be one detoxifying pathway

Half-life (animal model): 2-10 hours

Overdosage Treatment Although there is no experimental data, there is a theoretical basis to utilize acetylcysteine to help detoxify this substance

Decontamination:

Ingestion: Basic poison management
Inhalation: Move patient to fresh air; treat with 100% humidified oxygen

Test Interactions Gas chromatography

Diagnostic Tests/Procedures

Glucose, Random *on page 1269*

Monitoring Parameters Blood glucose

Pregnancy Implications Animal teratogen - possible adverse effects on testes, ovaries, and musculoskeletal system

Additional Information Colorless; mild aromatic odor at >1.3 ppm; carcinogenic and genotoxic; metabolites are active alkylating agents

TLV-TWA: 10 ppm

IDLH: 20,000 ppm

PEL-TWA: 1000 ppm

Organic vapor cartridges can adsorb up to 1000 ppm of butadiene

Atmospheric half-life: 6 hours

Median 1,3-butadiene concentration in ambient air: 0.3 ppb in urban areas and 0.1 ppb in rural areas; indoor air concentrations may be higher (1-9 ppb) due to cigarette smoke, thus leading to an estimated daily intake of ~13 mcg per person

Specific References

Acquavella JF, "The Paradox of Butadiene Epidemiology," *Exp Pathol*, 1989, 37(1-4):114-8.

Downs TD, Crane MM, and Kim KW, "Mortality Among Workers at a Butadiene Facility," *Am J Ind Med*, 1987, 12(3):311-29.

U.S. Department of Health and Human Services, "Toxicological Profile for 1,3-Butadiene TP-91/07," Agency for Toxic Substances and Diseases Registry, July, 1992.

Butadiene Divinyl *see* 1,3-Butadiene *on previous page*

Butan-l-ol *see* Butyl Alcohol *on this page*

Butanol *see* Butyl Alcohol *on this page*

2-Butanone *see* Methyl Ethyl Ketone *on page 967*

Button Batteries (Disc)

Synonyms Disc Battery; Watch Battery

Mechanism of Toxic Action Leakage of mercury, potassium, lithium thionyl chloride, or sodium hydroxide at the site of the battery seal can cause gastrointestinal burns; electrical burns or pressure necrosis can occur in the gastrointestinal tract

Adverse Reactions

Gastrointestinal: Esophageal impaction for larger cells (>20 mm in diameter); can also occur in infants <1 year of age for cells >16 mm in diameter: dysphagia, odynophagia, intestinal obstruction

Respiratory: Tachypnea, tracheoesophageal fistula, nasal septal perforation

Signs & Symptoms of Acute Overdose Tachypnea, dysphagia, esophageal ulceration, abdominal pain, fever

Overdosage Treatment

Decontamination: Lavage or activated charcoal (avoid emesis)

Supportive therapy: Withhold nasal or otic drops for exposure to nose or ear; remove promptly; obtain plain radiographs; mercury level for mercury-containing cells may be required; endoscopic removal for esophageal impaction. If battery is beyond the esophagus, it is likely (85%) to pass within 72 hours. Indications for laparotic include failure of endoscopic removal, signs of peritonitis, or lodging proximal to pylorus within 48 hours. Cimetidine can be used to reduce corrosion.

Enhancement of elimination: Metoclopramide may be utilized when there are no signs for obstruction or peritonitits; similarly, one dose of a saline cathartic or sorbitol can be utilized, although these modalities have not been proven to be of value

Monitoring Parameters Mercury levels (for mercury-based batteries) and radiographs

Additional Information Button battery hotline: 202-625-3333

Specific References

Bass DH and Millar AJ, "Mercury Absorption Following Button Battery Ingestion," *J Pediatr Surg*, 1992, 27(12):1541-2.

Kuhns DW and Dire DJ, "Button Battery Ingestions," *Ann Emerg Med*, 1989, 18(3):293-300.

Litovitz T and Schmitz BF, "Ingestion of Cylindrical and Button Batteries: An Analysis of 2382 Cases," *Pediatrics*, 1992, 89(4 Pt 2):747-57.

Rauber A, "Button Batteries: Letting the Skeleton Out of Our Closet," *Vet Hum Toxicol*, 1990, 32(5):460-4.

Butyl Alcohol

CAS Number 71-36-3

UN Number 1120

Synonyms Butan-l-ol; Butanol; Butyl Hydroxide; Propylcarbinol; Propylmethanol

Use In solvents in paints, lacquers, and resins; also used as extractants in the manufacture of pharmaceuticals; has been used as a sedative

Mechanism of Toxic Action Central nervous system depression

Adverse Reactions

Central nervous system: Depression

Miscellaneous: Irritant to mucous membranes

Signs & Symptoms of Acute Overdose Eye irritation (at 50 ppm), porphyria, cornea abnormalities, respiratory depression, feces discoloration (black), dizziness, drowsiness, fatigue, dermal erythema, slight headache, keratitis, cough, headache, ataxia, confusion, coma, vomiting, diarrhea

(Continued)

Butyl Alcohol *(Continued)*

Toxicodynamics/Kinetics

Absorption: Rapid from the gastrointestinal tract and dermally

Elimination: By the kidneys faster than ethanol

Overdosage Treatment

Decontamination: Ipecac/activated charcoal with cathartic may be useful

Enhancement of elimination: Use hemodialysis for persistent coma

Diagnostic Tests/Procedures

Blood Gases, Arterial *on page 1207*

Electrolytes, Blood *on page 1254*

Glucose, Random *on page 1269*

Kidney Profile *on page 1279*

Liver Profile *on page 1286*

Osmolality, Serum *on page 1310*

Additional Information Fusel oil odor is irritating; in pregnancy, tert-butyl alcohol may be fetotoxic

Odor threshold: 50 ppm

TLV-TWA: 100 ppm

Minimum toxic dose: 3-7 oz

Specific References

Kristiansen U, Vinggaard AM, and Nielsen GD, "The Effects of n-Butanol Vapour on Respiratory Rate and Tidal Volume," *Arch Toxicol*, 1988, 61(3):229-36.

Butyl Hydroxide *see* Butyl Alcohol *on previous page*

Butyl Methyl Ketone *see* 2-Hexanone *on page 938*

Butylphthalate *see* Di-n-Butyl Phthalate *on page 914*

BW-21-Z *see* Pyrethrins *on page 1003*

CA-800® *see* 4,4'-Methylenebis (2-Chloroaniline) *on page 965*

Cadmium

CAS Number 7440-43-9

UN Number 2570

Commonly Found In Solder, metal ores, amalgams, alkaline storage batteries, polyvinyl chloride pigments, electroplating processes, cigarette smoke

Mechanism of Toxic Action Local irritation with system toxic effects, primarily renal

Adverse Reactions

Cardiovascular: Hypertension

Hematologic: Anemia

Neuromuscular & skeletal: Osteomalacia

Renal: Nephrotoxicity

Respiratory: Emphysema, bronchitis

Miscellaneous: Salivation

Signs & Symptoms of Acute Overdose Acute inhalational exposure resembles metal fume fever; acute oral causes vomiting, photosensitivity, nephritis, diarrhea, metallic taste, hypotension, respiratory arrest, hypokalemia, myoclonus, seizures, albuminuria, glycosuria, hepatic necrosis, hypochromic anemia, chemical pneumonitis can be progressive

Toxicodynamics/Kinetics Potential carcinogen

Absorption: 10% either pulmonary or gastrointestinal

Distribution: Concentrates in liver and kidney; does not cross placenta; low concentrations in breast milk

Protein binding: Bound primarily to metallothionein and albumin in the +2 valence

Half-life, elimination: 16 years

Reference Range Suggested significant exposure with urinary levels >10 μg/L (concentrations fourfold higher in smokers than nonsmokers) or blood levels >15 μg/L

Overdosage Treatment

Decontamination: Ipecac or lavage; whole bowel irrigation may be helpful; can dilute with milk or water; activated charcoal does not appear to be effective

Supportive therapy: Charcoal is ineffective; no treatment for chronic intoxication; BAL and calcium disodium EDTA are contraindicated due to increased incidence of cadmium-induced renal disease; dimercaptosuccinic acid (150 mg 3 times/day for 5 days, then twice daily for 14 days) has been shown to increase cadmium excretion by about 30%

Enhancement of elimination: Hemoperfusion would not be expected to be effective

Antidote(s)

Succimer *on page 1473*

Diagnostic Tests/Procedures
Cadmium, Blood *on page 1213*
Cadmium, Hair *on page 1213*
Cadmium, Urine *on page 1214*

Additional Information Environmental exposure in Japan resulted in Itai-Itai disease; increased beta$_2$-migroglobulin excretion is a nonspecific marker for cadmium renal toxicity; diabetic patients appear to be particularly prone to the adverse renal effects of cadmium. Foods which contain the highest levels of cadmium include potatoes (0.04 ppm), leafy vegetables (0.03 ppm), grain and cereal products (0.02 ppm); total daily intake from food is ~30 mcg of cadmium. Content in cigarettes averages from 1-2 mcg per cigarette. Zinc deficiency may exacerbate cadmium-induced nephrotoxicity.

Specific References

Britt A, Burkhart K, and Petrini G, "Treatment of a Child Intoxicated With Cadmium Using Succimer: A Case Report," *Vet Hum Toxicol*, 1994, 31:341.
Payette Y, Lachapelle M, Daniel C, et al, "Decreased Interleukin-2 Receptor and Cell Cycle Changes in Murine Lymphocytes Exposed *In Vitro*, to Low Doses of Cadmium Chloride," *Int J Immunopharmacol*, 1995, 17(3):235-46.
Tanaka M, Yanagi M, Shirota K, et al, "Effect of Cadmium in the Zinc Deficient Rat," *Vet Hum Toxicol*, 1995, 37(3):203-8.
U.S. Department of Health and Human Services, "Toxicological Profile for Cadmium TP-92/06," Agency for Toxic Substances and Diseases Registry, April, 1993.

CAF *see* Chloroacetophenone *on page 889*

Caid® *see* Anticoagulant Rodenticide *on page 859*

Campheclor *see* Toxaphene *on page 1031*

Camphofene® *see* Toxaphene *on page 1031*

Camphor Tar *see* Naphthalene *on page 973*

Captan

CAS Number 133-06-2
Synonyms Captane; Captano
Brand Names Orthocide®; Orthocide® 406; Vancide® 89
Use Foliage protection
Mechanism of Toxic Action A phthalimide (chloroalkyl thio) fungicide which is not phytotoxic
Signs & Symptoms of Acute Overdose Conjunctivitis, dermatitis, persistent erythema, desquamation, photosensitivity
Toxicodynamics/Kinetics
Absorption: Poor through gastrointestinal tract (60%)
Metabolism: Hepatic
Elimination: Urine (52%), feces (16%), air (23%)
Overdosage Treatment Decontamination: Emesis or lavage/activated charcoal with cathartic; irrigate skin with soap and water
Pregnancy Implications Induces uterine abnormalities in pregnant rats; craniofacial and CNS abnormalities in pregnant rodents
Specific References

Rudner EJ, "North American Group Results," *Contact Dermatitis*, 1977, 3(4):208-9.
Zweig G, Gao R, and Popendorf W, "Simultaneous Dermal Exposure to Captan and Benomyl by Strawberry Harvesters," *J Agric Food Chem*, 1983, 31(5):1109-13.

Captane *see* Captan *on this page*

Captano *see* Captan *on this page*

Carbaryl

CAS Number 63-25-2
UN Number 2757
Synonyms 1-Naphthyl N-Methylcarbamate
Brand Names Arilate®; Carbatox®; Crunch®; Hexavin®; Sevin®; Vioxan®
Use Marketed as an insecticide dusting agent or spray liquid
Mechanism of Toxic Action Reversible inhibition of acetylcholinesterase and plasma cholinesterase, resulting in excess accumulation of acetylcholine at muscarinic and nicotinic receptors, and in the central nervous system
Adverse Reactions
Cardiovascular: Hyperdynamic (~18% to 21%) or hypodynamic (~7% to 10%) states
Central nervous system: Toxicity is limited because carbamates do not significantly cross the blood-brain barrier; CNS changes occur with most severe intoxications, hyperactivity
Genitourinary: Incontinence
Neuromuscular & skeletal: Weakness, paralysis
(Continued)

Carbaryl *(Continued)*

Respiratory: Depression, edema

General: Flu-like symptoms (especially with chronic exposure)

Signs & Symptoms of Acute Overdose Miosis (unreactive to light), mydriasis (rarely), lacrimation, pallor, cranial nerve palsies, excessive sweating, confusion, agitation, headache, dysarthria, generalized asthenia, A-V block, seizures, coma, decreased hemoglobin/red blood cell count/platelet count, metabolic acidosis and hyperglycemia (severe intoxication), hypotension, hypertension, bradycardia, tachycardia, Q-T prolongation, heart block, asystole, salivation, bronchorrhea, tachypnea, pulmonary edema, respiratory depression, diaphragmatic paralysis, skeletal muscle fasciculation and flaccid paralysis, nausea, vomiting, abdominal pain, fecal and urinary incontinence; delayed neurotoxicity manifesting as limb asthenia has been reported following a massive ingestion of carbaryl (~500 mg/kg)

Overdosage Treatment

Decontamination: Isolation, bagging, and disposal of all contaminated clothing and other articles; all emergency medical workers and hospital staff should follow appropriate precautions regarding exposure to hazardous material including the use of protective clothing, masks, goggles, and respiratory equipment

- Dermal: Prompt thorough scrubbing of all affected areas with soap and water, including hair and nails
- Gastric: Activated charcoal can be administered either orally or via a nasogastric tube; do not induce emesis because of danger of sudden respiratory compromise, alterations in mental status, seizures, coma, and possible aspiration of hydrocarbon vehicles
- Ocular: Irrigation with copious tepid sterile water or saline

Supportive therapy: Including airway management, ventilatory assistance, humidified oxygen administration, and close monitoring for sudden respiratory failure

Antidote:

- Atropine: Administration should be guided by respiratory status, starting at 1-5 mg I.V. every 5-10 minutes as needed, and should be titrated to the resolution of excess pulmonary secretions; frequent administration of large doses (cumulative doses >100 mg) may be necessary in massive exposures
- Glycopyrrolate: May be administered if atropine is unavailable
- 2-PAM: Experimental data has indicated that carbaryl toxicity may be potentiated by oxime therapy; do not use 2-PAM for a known or strongly suspected single ingestion of carbaryl

Enhancement of elimination: Dialysis and hemoperfusion are not indicated due to effectiveness of the prescribed treatment, large volumes of distribution of organophosphates

Antidote(s)

Atropine Sulfate *on page 1395*

Diagnostic Tests/Procedures

Blood Gases, Arterial *on page 1207*
Chest Films *on page 1224*
Complete Blood Count *on page 1236*
Creatinine, Serum *on page 1243*
Electrocardiography *on page 1253*
Liver Profile *on page 1286*
Pseudocholinesterase, Serum *on page 1340*

Pregnancy Implications Human data regarding organophosphate exposure in pregnancy is limited and anecdotal; teratogenesis and fetal death have been produced in animal models at exposure levels that cause obvious toxicity to the pregnant animal

Additional Information Odorless and colorless, white, or gray solid; vapor pressure: 0.005 mm Hg at 20°C; red blood cell cholinesterase, and serum pseudocholinesterase may be depressed following acute or chronic organophosphate exposure and are theoretically useful for differentiating between carbamate and organophosphate exposures; RBC cholinesterase is typically not analyzed by inhouse laboratories and is usually not available for consideration during acute management. Pseudocholinesterase levels may be rapidly available from some inhouse laboratories, but are not as reliable a marker of organophosphate exposure because of variability secondary to variant genotypes, hepatic disease, oral estrogen use, or malnutrition, thus they may not be useful in ruling out carbamate exposure.

ACGIH TLV: 5 mg/m^3
PEL-TWA: 5 mg/m^3
IDLH: 625 mg/m^3

Other information concerning pesticide exposures is available through the EPA-funded National Pesticide Telecommunications Network: 1-800-858-7378 (weekdays, 8 AM to 6 PM, Central Standard time)

Specific References

Dickoff DJ, Gerber O, and Turovsky Z, "Delayed Neurotoxicity After Ingestion of Carbamate Pesticide," *Neurology*, 1987, 37(7):1229-31.

Harris LW, Talbot BG, Lennox WJ, et al, "The Relationship Between Oxime-Induced Reactivation of Carbamylated Acetylcholinesterase and Antidotal Efficacy Against Carbamate Intoxication," *Toxicol Appl Pharmacol*, 1989, 98(1):128-33.

Natoff IL and Reiff B, "Effect of Oximes on the Acute Toxicity of Anticholinesterase Carbamates," *Toxicol Appl Pharmacol*, 1973, 25(4):569-75.

Zwiener RJ and Ginsburg CM, "Organophosphate and Carbamate Poisoning in Infants and Children," *Pediatrics*, 1988, 81(1):121-6.

Carbatox® *see* Carbaryl *on page 877*

Carbinol *see* Methanol *on page 957*

Carbofos® *see* Malathion *on page 950*

Carbon Bisulfide *see* Carbon Disulfide *on this page*

Carbon Chloride *see* Carbon Tetrachloride *on page 882*

Carbon Disulfide

CAS Number 75-15-0

UN Number 1131

Synonyms Carbon Bisulfide; Carbon Sulfide; Dithiocarbonic Anhydride

Brand Names Caswell No 162; Weeviltox®

Use Organic solvent used in gums and resins; used in manufacture of matches, instant color photography, corrosion inhibitors, gold and nickel plating, and rayon

Mechanism of Toxic Action Reacts with amino and thiols to inhibit cellular functions; damages the hepatic enzyme systems

Adverse Reactions

Cardiovascular: May be atherosclerogenic, angina, paresthesia

Central nervous system: CNS depression, polyneuropathy, parkinsonism, hypothermia, seizures

Dermatologic: Burns on dermal contact

Hepatic: Fatty degeneration of liver

Respiratory: Dyspnea

Signs & Symptoms of Acute Overdose Headache, tremor, neuritis, nausea, vomiting, burning of upper airway, cranial nerve palsies, hypertension, rotten egg breath, dyspnea, dizziness, nystagmus, diplopia, seizures, psychosis, possibly diabetogenic; death can occur from respiratory paralysis

Toxicodynamics/Kinetics

Absorption: Dermal absorption does occur; lipid soluble

Metabolism: Hepatic cytochrome P-450 to carbonyl sulfide; also detoxified by glutathione pathway

Half-life: <1 hour

Elimination: Excreted by the lungs

Reference Range Monitor urine level of 2-thiothiazolidine-4-carboxylic acid; blood carbon disulfide levels ranging from 0.1-0.78 mg/L associated with air levels of ~80 ppm

Overdosage Treatment

Decontamination: Emesis or lavage/activated charcoal with cathartic

Supportive therapy: Avoid catecholamines due to probable monoamine oxidase inhibition; diazepam/lorazepam can be used for seizures; pyridoxine use for neurologic toxicity is unproven; although its use is unproven, there is a theoretical basis in which to use acetylcysteine to help detoxify carbon disulfide

Pregnancy Implications Spontaneous abortions and prematurity have been reported

Additional Information Colorless liquid; may have aromatic, sweet odor; similar effect of disulfiram; parkinsonism has been described

Fatal oral dose: 15 mL

TLV-TWA: 10 ppm

IDLH: 500 ppm

PEL-TWA: 4 ppm

Odor threshold: 0.1 ppm

Atmospheric half-life: 12 days

Water half-life: ~1 year

Ambient carbon disulfide levels average 65 ppt in urban areas and 41 ppt in rural areas

Specific References

Bleecker ML, "Parkinsonism: A Clinical Marker of Exposure to Neurotoxins," *Neurotoxicol Teratol*, 1988, 10(5):475-8.

MacMahon B and Monson RR, "Mortality in the U.S. Rayon Industry," *J Occup Med*, 1988, 30(9):698-705.

Spyker DA, Gallanosa AG, and Suratt PM, "Health Effects of Acute Carbon Disulfide Exposure," *J Toxicol Clin Toxicol*, 1982, 19(1):87-93.

U.S. Department of Health and Human Services, "Toxicological Profile for Carbon Disulfide," Agency for Toxic Substances and Diseases Registry, July, 1994.

Carbon Hexachloride *see* Hexachloroethane *on page 937*

Carbonic Dichloride *see* Phosgene *on page 992*

Carbonic Oxide *see* Carbon Monoxide *on this page*

Carbon Monoxide

Related Information

Drugs and Chemicals Proven to be Teratogenic in Humans *on page 1572-1575*

CAS Number 630-08-0

UN Number 1016

Synonyms Carbonic Oxide; Carbon Oxide; CO; Exhaust Gas; Flue Gas

Commonly Found In Auto exhaust, byproduct of methylene chloride; produced in a closed space fire due to incomplete combustion of materials

Mechanism of Toxic Action Causes tissue hypoxia and inhibition of cellular respiration

Adverse Reactions

Cardiovascular: Cardiac abnormalities most pronounced, syncope

Central nervous system: CNS effects, acute neurological abnormalities including dementia, drowsiness, coma, seizures, headache, chorea, amnesia, confabulation, apraxia, deafness, Parkinson-like syndrome, cortical blindness, and neuropathy (peripheral)

Delayed neurological sequelae observed within 40 days of significant carbon monoxide poisoning (12% to 43% incidence) including disorientation, bradykinesia, chorea (extrapyramidal), equilibrium disturbances, apathy, cogwheel rigidity, aphasia, incontinence, personality changes, short-term memory deficit, seizure disorders, and chronic headaches

Signs & Symptoms of Acute Overdose Frontal headache, ataxia, tremor, nausea, vomiting, blurred vision, aspiration, dementia, A-V block, arrhythmias, angina, visual changes, dyspnea with hyperventilation, nystagmus, dizziness, encephalopathy, seizures, disorientation, hypothermia, drowsiness, hyperglycemia, hypotension, mydriasis, tachycardia, ototoxicity, tinnitus, bradycardia, myoglobinuria

Toxicodynamics/Kinetics

Absorption: Readily through the lungs; does not accumulate over time

Half-life: 5-6 hours in room air; 30-90 minutes in 100% oxygen; 30 minutes in hyperbaric oxygen

Elimination: Through the lungs; see figure.

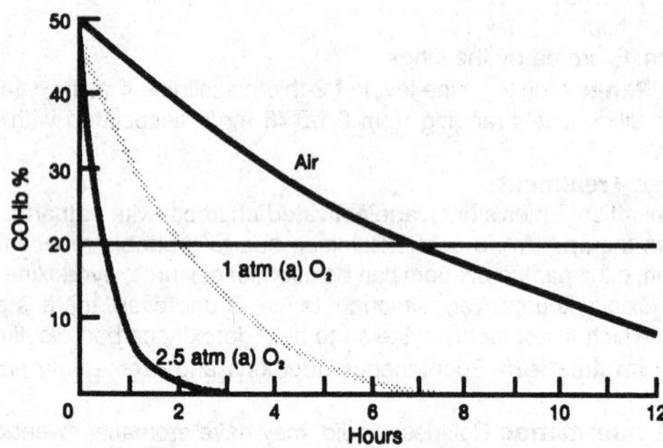

Carbon monoxide elimination. Used with permission and adapted from Winter PM and Miller JN, "Carbon Monoxide Poisoning," *JAMA*, 1976, 236:1502-4.

Effect of anemia and carboxyhemoglobin on oxyhemoglobin dissociation curve. Note that 60% carboxyhemoglobin has a greater affinity for oxygen than an equivalent physiological anemia which indicates that carbon monoxide shifts the oxygen dissociation curve leftward; see figure.

Reference Range Carboxyhemoglobin level by CO-Oximeter™: Endogenous level: ≤0.65; smokers may have from 3% to 8%

Severe symptoms may start at 10%; >35% is associated with fatalities from acute exposure; BEI is <8%; venous and arterial samples are equivalent

Overdosage Treatment

Decontamination: 100% humidified oxygen; hyperbaric oxygen for patients with acute neurotoxicity, patients with angina, maternal carboxyhemoglobin of 20% in pregnant patients, or asymptomatic carboxyhemoglobin of 30%. Do not consider hypothermia or exchange transfusion.

Supportive therapy: Dopamine (17 mcg/kg/minute) has been shown in a case report to reverse carbon monoxide-induced blindness

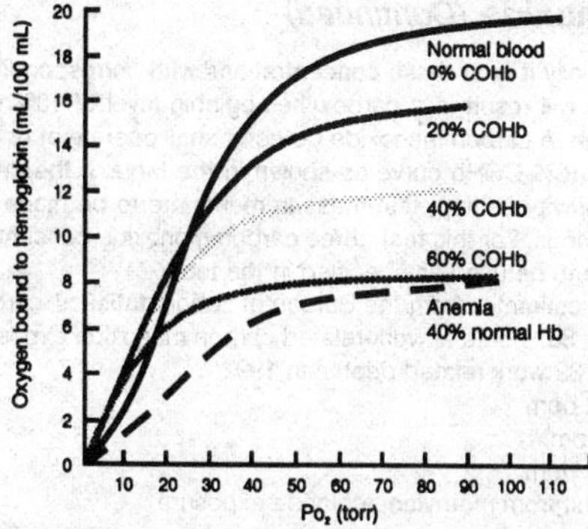

Effect of anemia and carboxyhemoglobin on oxyhemoglobin dissociation curve. Note that 60% carboxyhemoglobin has a greater affinity for oxygen than an equivalent physiological anemia which indicates that carbon monoxide shifts the oxygen dissociation curve leftward. Used with permission and adapted from Fein A, Leff A and Hopewell PC, "Pathophysiology and Management of the Complications Resulting From Fire and the Inhaled Products of Combustion. A Review of the Literature," *Crit Care Med*, 1980, 8:95.

Antidote(s)

Oxygen (Hyperbaric) *on page 1453*

Diagnostic Tests/Procedures

Blood Gases, Arterial *on page 1207*
Carboxyhemoglobin, Blood *on page 1221*
Complete Blood Count *on page 1236*
Computed Transaxial Tomography, Head Studies *on page 1240*
Creatine Kinase, Blood *on page 1242*
Electrolytes, Blood *on page 1254*
Glucose, Random *on page 1269*
Urea Nitrogen, Blood *on page 1370*

Monitoring Parameters Arterial blood gases, carboxyhemoglobin

Pregnancy Implications Embryotoxic, telencephalic dysgenesis noted; readily crosses the placenta with stillbirths, mental retardation, and microcephalus all noted

Additional Information Colorless, odorless gas; delayed neurotoxicity consisting of short-term memory deficit, ataxia, cognitive impairment may occur 2-3 weeks after an acute exposure; Parkinson syndrome may occur; carbon monoxide detectors are usually set to alarm at indoor carbon monoxide air concentrations of 100 ppm (within 90 minutes), 200 ppm (within 35 minutes), or 400 ppm (within 15 min-

CARBON MONOXIDE CONCENTRATION (ppm CO)
VS.
TIME (minutes)

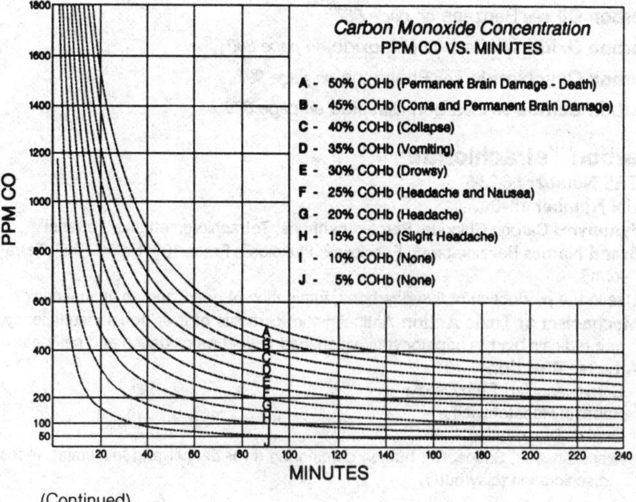

(Continued)

Carbon Monoxide *(Continued)*

utes); essentially it is at these concentrations with corresponding time exposure duration that will result in a carboxyhemoglobin level of 10% during periods of heavy exertion. A carbon monoxide detector shall operate at or below the plotted limits for the 10% COHb curve as shown in the table. If the detector employs a variable sensitivity setting, test measurements are to be made at maximum and minimum settings. For this test, three carbon monoxide concentrations (100, 200, 400 ppm) are to be used as specified in the table.

According to estimates from the Bureau of Labor statistics, carbon monoxide accounted for 867 nonfatal work-related carbon monoxide exposures in private industry and 32 work-related deaths in 1992

TLV-TWA: 50 ppm

IDLH: 1500 ppm

PEL-TWA: 35 ppm

May also result from methylene chloride exposure

Specific References

Balzan MV and Cacciottolo JM, "The Dangers of Carbon Monoxide," *N Engl J Med*, 1995, 332(13):894.

Barrett L, Danel V, and Faure J, "Carbon Monoxide Poisoning, a Diagnosis Frequently Overlooked," *J Toxicol Clin Toxicol*, 1985, 23(4-6):309-13.

CDC, "Carbon Monoxide Poisoning From Use of Gasoline-Fueled Power Washers in an Underground Parking Garage - District of Columbia - 1994," *MMWR*, 1995, 44(18):356-9.

Crocker PJ and Walker JS, "Pediatric Carbon Monoxide Toxicity," *J Emerg Med*, 1985, 3(6):443-8.

Dean BS, Verdile VP, and Krenzelok EP, "Coma Reversal With Cerebral Dysfunction Recovery After Repetitive Hyperbaric Oxygen Therapy for Severe Carbon Monoxide Poisoning," *Am J Emerg Med*, 1993, 11(6):616-8.

Duncan JS and Gumpert J, "A Case of Blindness Following Carbon Monoxide Poisoning, Treated With Dopamine," *J Neurol Neurosurg Psychiatry*, 1982, 46:459-60.

Ely EW, Moorehead B, and Haponik EF, "Warehouse Workers' Headache: Emergency Evaluation and Management of 30 Patients With Carbon Monoxide Poisoning," *Am J Med*, 1995, 98(2):145-6.

Hardy KR and Thom SR, "Pathophysiology and Treatment of Carbon Monoxide Poisoning," *J Toxicol Clin Toxicol*, 1994, 32(6):613-29.

Heckerling PS, Leikin JB, and Maturen A, "Occult Carbon Monoxide Poisoning: Validation of a Prediction Model," *Am J Med*, 1988, 84(2):251-6.

McMurray B, Seger D, Bonfiglio F, et al, "Criteria Used to Recommend HBO in Carbon Monoxide Poisoning: A Survey of Poison Centers, Burn Centers, and HBO Centers," *Vet Hum Toxicol*, 1994, 36:344.

Myers RA, "Carbon Monoxide Poisoning," *J Emerg Med*, 1984, 1(3):245-8.

Olson KR and Seger D, "Hyperbaric Oxygen for Carbon Monoxide Poisoning: Does it Really Work?" *Ann Emerg Med*, 1995, 25:535-7.

"Safe at Home," *Consumer Reports*, 1995, 60(7):459-69.

Thom SR, Taber RL, Mendiguren I, et al, "Delayed Neuropsychologic Sequelae After Carbon Monoxide Poisoning: Prevention by Treatment With Hyperbaric Oxygen," *Ann Emerg Med*, 1995, 25:474-80.

Touger M, Gallagher EJ, and Tyrell J, "Relationship Between Venous and Arterial Carboxyhemoglobin Levels in Patients With Suspected Carbon Monoxide Poisoning," *Ann Emerg Med*, 1995, 25:481-3.

Winter PM and Miller JN, "Carbon Monoxide Poisoning," *JAMA*, 1976, 236(13):1502.

Carbon Nitride Ion *see* Cyanide *on page 899*

Carbon Oil *see* Benzene *on page 867*

Carbon Oxide *see* Carbon Monoxide *on page 880*

Carbon Oxychloride *see* Phosgene *on page 992*

Carbon Sulfide *see* Carbon Disulfide *on page 879*

Carbon Tetrachloride

CAS Number 56-23-5

UN Number 1846

Synonyms Carbon Chloride; Perchlormethane; Tetrachloromethane; Tetrasol

Brand Names Benzinoform®; Fasciolin®; Flukoids®; Freon 10®; Halon 104®; Tetraform®

Use In the production of fluorocarbons, fumigation of grain, and as an insecticide

Mechanism of Toxic Action Antihelmintic; cirrhosis of liver, renal insufficiency; free radicals bind to hepatocytes which lead to lipid peroxidation and cell death

Adverse Reactions

Cardiovascular: Tachycardia

Hepatic: Hepatotoxicity

Ocular: Eye irritation

Miscellaneous: Suspected human carcinogen (liver cancer and leukemia), feces discoloration (clay/putty)

Signs & Symptoms of Acute Overdose Confusion, delirium, coma, dementia, ataxia, tremor (intention), vomiting, nausea, jaundice, anuria, aplastic anemia, hematuria, erythema of skin, seizures

Toxicodynamics/Kinetics

Absorption: Readily from the skin, lungs, and gastrointestinal tract (85%; rapid, within 10 minutes); can produce renal or hepatic toxicity from any of these sites

Metabolism: In the liver, metabolites include hexachloroethane, carbon dioxide, and phosgene

Half-life:

Oral: 40-85 hours

Inhalation: 1-40 hours

Elimination: Excreted through the lungs (50% to 80%) as carbon dioxide

Reference Range Toxic: 2.0-5.0 mg/dL

Overdosage Treatment

Decontamination: Administer 100% humidified oxygen; for ingestion – basic poison management; avoid ipecac; do not use catecholamines due to enhancement of ventricular arrhythmia; avoid enzyme-inducing agents such as phenobarbital

Supportive therapy: Hyperbaric oxygen may be of benefit to prevent hepatitis; N-acetylcysteine may be of benefit to prevent hepatitis; due to the face that these agents induce cytochrome P-450, avoid the use of ethanol or phenobarbital

Antidote(s)

Acetylcysteine *on page 1388*

Oxygen (Hyperbaric) *on page 1453*

Diagnostic Tests/Procedures

Ammonia, Blood *on page 1188*

Blood Gases, Arterial *on page 1207*

Complete Blood Count *on page 1236*

Electrolytes, Blood *on page 1254*

Electrolytes, Urine *on page 1254*

Kidney Profile *on page 1279*

Liver Profile *on page 1286*

Pregnancy Implications Fetotoxic, teratogenic (musculoskeletal abnormalities)

Additional Information Colorless liquid with odor of chloroform; N-acetylcysteine may be of benefit (research studies); radiopaque

Lethal dose: 43 mg/kg

TLV-TWA: 5 ppm

IDLH: 300 ppm

PEL-TWA: 2 ppm

Atmospheric half-life: Over 30 years

Water half-life: ~6-12 months

Soil half-life: 6-12 months

Average urban ambient carbon tetrachloride levels: 0.1-0.3 ppb; average indoor carbon tetrachloride level: 0.2-0.4 ppb; median drinking water carbon tetrachloride level: 0.3-0.7 mcg/L; average daily exposure of carbon tetrachloride: ~0.11 mcg/kg

Specific References

Burkhart KK, Hall AH, Gerace R, et al, "Hyperbaric Oxygen Treatment for Carbon Tetrachloride Poisoning," *Drug Saf*, 1991, 6(5):332-8.

Hadi SF and El-Mikatti N, "Acute Carbon Tetrachloride Poisoning," *Intensive Care Med*, 1981, 7(4):203-4.

Kalf GF, Post GB, and Snyder R, "Solvent Toxicology: Recent Advances in the Toxicology of Benzene, the Glycol Ethers, and Carbon Tetrachloride," *Annu Rev Pharmacol Toxicol*, 1987, 27:399-427.

Ruprah M, Mant TG, and Flanagan RJ, "Acute Carbon Tetrachloride Poisoning in 19 Patients: Implications for Diagnosis and Treatment," *Lancet*, 1985, 1(8436):1027-9.

Truss C and Killenberg P, "Treatment of Carbon Tetrachloride Poisoning With Hyperbaric Oxygen," *Gastroenterology*, 1982, 82(4):767-9.

U.S. Department of Health and Human Services, "Toxicological Profile for Carbon Tetrachloride TP-93/02," Agency for Toxic Substances and Diseases Registry, May, 1994.

Carbonyl Chloride *see* Phosgene *on page 992*

Carbonyl Nickel Powder *see* Nickel *on page 976*

Carrel-Dakin Solution *see* Sodium Hypochlorite *on page 1013*

Caswell No 66 *see* Nitrobenzene *on page 979*

Caswell No 162 *see* Carbon Disulfide *on page 879*

Caswell No 183A *see* Chlorobenzene *on page 889*

Caswell No 292 *see* Di-n-Butyl Phthalate *on page 914*

Caswell No 880C® *see* 2,4,6-Trichlorophenol *on page 1034*

CE *see* Tetryl *on page 1025*

Cellon® *see* Tetrachloroethane *on page 1022*

Cellosolves *see* Glycol Ethers *on page 934*

Celluflux DOP® *see* Di-n-Octylphthalate *on page 916*

Celphos® *see* Aluminum Phosphide *on page 857*

Certox® *see* Strychnine *on page 1016*

CF 2 *see* Trichloroethane *on page 1032*

Chenopodium Oils

CAS Number 8006-99-3

Synonyms Oil of American Wormseed; Volatile Oil

Signs & Symptoms of Acute Overdose Nausea, vomiting, abdominal pain, headache, flushing, dizziness, tinnitus, salivation; start several hours after ingestion; this is followed by drowsiness, tinnitus, deafness, and in some cases progress to ataxia, coma, tachycardia, seizures, and death. Respiratory depression is seen with large ingestions with pulmonary edema being a common finding in fatal cases; renal and hepatitis. Primarily mucous membrane irritants, CNS depressants or CNS stimulants; camphor causes mydriasis while eucalyptus oil may cause miosis; tachycardia and bradycardia have been reported; chemical pneumonitis and pulmonary edema are possible; CNS depression may be rapid (30 minutes) or delayed (up to 4 hours) and may continue for up to 3 days; seizures may occur with eucalyptus oil; camphor causes sudden seizures, abdominal pain, vomiting, diarrhea; mild elevation of liver enzymes

Toxicodynamics/Kinetics

Absorption: Well absorbed through mucous membranes

Metabolism: By the liver

Elimination: Excreted primarily through kidney

Reference Range No toxic levels established

Overdosage Treatment

Decontamination: Emesis is not recommended because as an essential oil, *Chenopodium* oil may be aspirated and potential for CNS depression and seizures; gastric lavage is preferred; activated charcoal with sorbitol is recommended; for products with a thick hydrocarbon base, gastric lavage may decrease systemic effects

Supportive therapy: Liver function and renal function should be monitored; cardiac and respiratory systems should be supported; CNS and electrolytes should be followed closely

Enhancement of elimination: Eucalyptus oil has been successfully treated with mannitol, peritoneal and hemodialysis; camphor has been reported to be extracted with amberlite resin hemoperfusion. Use of enhanced elimination techniques for these overdoses should be based on amount ingested, clinical picture, and/or symptoms that are failing to respond to supportive care.

Pregnancy Implications Contraindicated in pregnancy

Additional Information Volatile oils: Camphor, cedar leaf, cinnamon oil, eucalyptus, lavender, menthol, myristica, peppermint oil, sandalwood oil, sassafras oil, thymol, turpentine oil; may explode when heated

Specific References

Stentoft J, "The Toxicity of Cytarabine," *Drug Saf*, 1990, 5(1):7-27.

Williams AC and Barry BW, "Essential Oils as Novel Human Skin Penetration Enhancers," *Int J Pharmaceutics*, 1989, 57:R7-9.

Chlon® *see* Pentachlorophenol *on page 990*

Chlorate of Soda *see* Chlorate Salts *on this page*

Chlorate Salt of Sodium *see* Chlorate Salts *on this page*

Chlorate Salts

CAS Number 7775-09-0

UN Number 3210; 1461

Synonyms Asex; B-Herbtox; Chlorate of Soda; Chlorate Salt of Sodium; Chlorax; Chloric Acid-Sodium Salt; De-fol-ate; Desolat; Drexel Acetol; Evalu-Super; Grain Sorghum Harvest Aid; Granex O; Harvest-Aid; Klorex; Kusa-Tohru; Ortho C-1 Defoliant and Weed Killer; Rasikal; Shed-a-Leaf; Sodium Chlorate; Travex; Tumbleaf; Val-Drop

Signs & Symptoms of Acute Overdose Cyanosis resistant to oxygen therapy; nausea, vomiting, and abdominal cramping; diarrhea or colic usually precede pallor; methemoglobinemia and hemolysis may occur; drowsiness, coma, and seizures have been reported. Moderate elevations of LFT with hepatomegaly and jaundice have been reported; chlorates are nephrotoxic and acute renal insufficiency with oliguria or anuria is common; severe exposure may cause subacute intravascular coagulation and leukocytosis lasting 40 days; chronic exposure of 5-10 days to chlorates will also follow similar pattern.

Toxicodynamics/Kinetics

Absorption: Good through respiratory and gastrointestinal tract; poor through skin

Elimination: Slow through the kidneys

Overdosage Treatment

Decontamination: Emesis, lavage/activated charcoal with sorbitol

Supportive therapy: Obtain baseline hemoglobin, hematocrit, and methemoglobin; monitor urinalysis, BUN, creatinine, CBC, and methemoglobin; transfuse if needed. Alkaline diuresis may be required if significant hemoglobinuria; methylene blue 1-2 mg/kg/dose of 1% slow I.V. to those patients who are symptomatic or methemoglobin >30%; additional doses may be required. A DIC profile may be needed; sodium thiosulfate should be considered (2-5 g oral or in 100 mL of 5% sodium hydrochloride) to symptomatic patients to attempt to inactivate the chlorate ion; methemoglobinemia produced by chlorates may be refractory to methylene blue.

Enhancement of elimination: Exchange transfusion combined with hemodialysis or peritoneal dialysis should be considered in severely intoxicated patients

Antidote(s)

Methylene Blue *on page 1444*

Sodium Thiosulfate *on page 1470*

Test Interactions Other oxidizing agents may interfere

Monitoring Parameters When 1 mL of a 1% (w/v) solution of diphenylamine in concentrated sulfuric acid is added to material containing chlorates, a blue color is produced; urine is probably the fluid of choice, but blood can also be measured through spectrophotometry for chlorate

Specific References

Helliwell M and Nunn J, "Mortality in Sodium Chlorate Poisoning," *Br Med J*, 1979, 1(6171):1119.

Knight RK, Trounce JR, and Cameron JS, "Suicidal Chlorate Poisoning Treated With Peritoneal Dialysis," *Br Med J*, 1967, 3:601-2.

Lee DB, Brown DL, Baker LR, et al, "Haematological Complications of Chlorate Poisoning," *Br Med J*, 1970, 2(700):31-2.

O'Grady J and Jarecsni E, "Sodium Chlorate Poisoning," *Br J Clin Pract*, 1971, 25(1):38-9.

Singelmann E, and Stetten C, "Increased Erythrocyte Rigidity in Chlorate Poisoning," *J Clin Pathol*, 1983, 36(6):719.

Chlorax *see* Chlorate Salts *on previous page*

Chlorbenzilate *see* Organochlorines *on page 983*

Chlorbipheny *see* Polychlorinated Biphenyls *on page 995*

Chlordan® *see* Chlordane *on this page*

Chlordane

Related Information

Heptachlor *on page 935*

Organochlorines *on page 983*

CAS Number 12789-03-6; 57-74-9; 5103-71-9; 5103-74-2

Brand Names Chlordan®; Niran®; Octachlor®; Ortho-Klor®; Velsicol® 1068

Use Organochlorine subterranean termiticide by which all commercial use was discontinued by the EPA in April, 1988

Mechanism of Toxic Action Neurotoxic mechanism unknown; may involve competitive inhibition of GABA or reduced levels of norepinephrine involved in neuronal transmission

Adverse Reactions

Cardiovascular: Tachycardia

Central nervous system: Headache, dizziness, irritability, seizures (usually within 3 hours of exposure), paresthesia

Gastrointestinal: Nausea, diarrhea, anorexia

Genitourinary: Oliguria

Hepatic: Jaundice, elevated liver function tests

Ocular: Blurred vision, diplopia

Respiratory: Dyspnea

Toxicodynamics/Kinetics

Absorption: By inhalation (76%), oral, and dermal routes

Metabolism: Hepatic; active metabolites include heptachlor and oxychlordane

Half-life: 88 days

Elimination: Primarily fecal

Reference Range Ingestion of 215 g (3 g/kg) of chlordane resulted in a chlordane blood level of 5 mg/L (patient recovered); seizures can occur at chlorane serum levels of 2-4 μg/L

Overdosage Treatment

Decontamination:

Dermal: Repeated and copious scrubbing with soap and water

Oral: Lavage/activated charcoal or cholestyramine; do not use oil-based cathartics

Supportive therapy: Since barbiturates hasten the elimination of oxychlordane, this may be the antiseizure drug of choice; benzodiazepines can also be used

Enhancement of elimination: Multiple doses of activated charcoal or cholestyramine may be useful

(Continued)

Chlordane *(Continued)*

Additional Information Lethal oral dose: 25 mg/kg

Can cause sclerodermatous changes of the hands

TWA-TLV: 0.5 mg/m^3

World Health Organization guideline limit for drinking water: 0.3 μg/L

Specific References

Aldrich FD and Holmes JH, "Acute Chlordane Intoxication in a Child," *Arch Environ Health*, 1969, 19(1):129-32.

Garrettson LK, Guzelian PS, and Blanke RV, "Subacute Chlordane Poisoning," *J Toxicol Clin Toxicol*, 1984-85, 22(6):565-71.

Olanoff LS, Bristow WJ, Cololough J, et al, "Acute Chlordane Intoxication," *Clin Toxic*, 1983, 20:291-306.

Smith TJ, Wilcock RJ, Pridmore RD, et al, "Persistence of Chlordane Applied to an Intertidal Sandflat," *Bull Environ Contam Toxicol*, 1992, 49(1):129-36.

Wester RC, Maibach HI, Sedik L, et al, "Percutaneous Absorption of [14C]Chlordane From Soil," *J Toxicol Environ Health*, 1992, 35(4):269-77.

Chlordecone

Related Information

Organochlorines *on page 983*

CAS Number 143-50-0

Synonyms Decachloroketone

Brand Names Compound 1189®; Kepone®; Merex®

Use Insecticide (fire ant, slugs, grass mole cricket, tobacco fireworm) on tobacco, shrubs, and banana plants

Mechanism of Toxic Action Increases permeability of neuronal membrane; has estrogenic properties

Adverse Reactions

Central nervous system: Auditory and visual hallucinations, headache, slurred speech, ataxia

Dermatologic: Rash, maculopapular rash

Gastrointestinal: Nausea

Genitourinary: Oligospermia

Neuromuscular & skeletal: Tremors, arthralgia, neuropathy (peripheral)

Ocular: Cataracts, nystagmus

Miscellaneous: Increased intracranial pressure, papilledema, pleuritic chest pain, elevation of alkaline phosphatase

Toxicodynamics/Kinetics

Absorption: Inhalation, oral (90%), and dermal

Metabolism: Hepatic reduction to chlordecone alcohol

Half-life: 63-148 days

Elimination: Primarily fecal (biliary)

Reference Range Blood chlordecone levels >1 ppm associated with neurotoxicity; blood levels >2000 ng/mL associated with tremor

Overdosage Treatment

Decontamination:

Dermal: Wash with soap and water

Ocular: Copious irrigation with saline

Oral: Lavage/activated charcoal or cholestyramine

Supportive therapy: Do not use phenytoin for tremor since it may exacerbate tremor; propranolol may be effective to alleviate tremor; prednisolone has been used to alleviate headache due to increased intracerebral pressure

Enhancement of elimination: Due to enterohepatic recirculation, multiple dosing with cholestyramine (4 g every 8 hours) has been shown to be effective

Monitoring Parameters Alkaline phosphatase

Additional Information FDA action level for oysters, clams, mussels, and fin fish: 0.03 ppm; crabs: 0.4 ppm; high bioaccumulation potential in fish

Specific References

Boylan JJ, Egle JL, and Guzelian PS, "Cholestyramine: Use as a New Therapeutic Approach for Chlordecone (Kepone) Poisoning," *Science*, 1978, 199(4331):893-5.

Taylor JR, "Neurological Manifestations in Humans Exposed to Chlordecone: Follow-up Results," *Neurotoxicology*, 1985, 6(1):231-6.

Chlorfenvinphos

CAS Number 470-90-6; 18708-87-7

Synonyms O,O-Diethyl O-(2-Chloro-1(2',4'-Dichlorophenyl)Vinyl)Phosphate

Brand Names Apachlor®; Birlane®; Supone®; Unitox®

Use Marketed as insecticide granules, dusting agent, or spray liquid with or without petroleum derivative as a solvent

Mechanism of Toxic Action Potent, irreversible inhibition of acetylcholinesterase and plasma cholinesterase, resulting in excess accumulation of acetylcholine at muscarinic and nicotinic receptors, and in the central nervous system

Adverse Reactions

Cardiovascular: Hyperdynamic (~18% to 21%) or hypodynamic (~7% to 10%) states

Central nervous system: Depression, seizures, hyperactivity
Genitourinary: Incontinence
Neuromuscular & skeletal: Weakness, paralysis
Respiratory: Depression, edema
General: Flu-like symptoms (especially with chronic exposure)
Delayed: Muscle asthenia and paresthesia

Signs & Symptoms of Acute Overdose Miosis (unreactive to light), mydriasis (rarely), lacrimation, pallor, excessive sweating, confusion, agitation, headache, dysarthria, generalized asthenia, seizures, A-V block, coma, cranial nerve palsies, decreased hemoglobin/red blood cell count/platelet count, metabolic acidosis and hyperglycemia (severe intoxication), hypotension, hypertension, bradycardia, tachycardia, Q-T prolongation, heart block, asystole, salivation, bronchorrhea, tachypnea, pulmonary edema, respiratory depression, diaphragmatic paralysis, skeletal muscle fasciculation and flaccid paralysis, nausea, vomiting, abdominal pain, fecal and urinary incontinence; an "intermediate syndrome" of limb asthenia and respiratory paralysis has been reported to occur between 24 and 96 hours postorganophosphate exposure, and is independent of the acute cholinergic crisis; late paresthesia characterized by stocking and glove paresthesia, anesthesia, and asthenia is infrequently observed weeks to months following acute exposure to certain organophosphates

Toxicodynamics/Kinetics

Absorption: Readily through oral, dermal, or respiratory exposure
Metabolism: Rapidly metabolized to weakly active compounds through hepatic hydrolysis and other pathways
Elimination: Metabolites are excreted in urine

Warnings Environmentally persistent; chlorfenvinphos is a soil applied insecticide used for arable crops, and may translocate into plants, fruits, and vegetables grown in treated soil; risk of aspiration pneumonitis exists with agents having a hydrocarbon vehicle; severe laryngeal irritation and violent coughing may result from exposure to dusting powders; exposure to dusting powders and insecticide granules may cause contact dermatitis

Overdosage Treatment

Decontamination: Isolation, bagging, and disposal of all contaminated clothing and other articles; all emergency medical workers and hospital staff should follow appropriate precautions regarding exposure to hazardous material including the use of protective clothing, masks, goggles, and respiratory equipment
- Dermal: Prompt thorough scrubbing of all affected areas with soap and water, including hair and nails
- Gastric: Activated charcoal can be administered either orally or via a nasogastric tube; do not induce emesis because of danger of sudden respiratory compromise, alterations in mental status, seizures, coma, and possible aspiration of hydrocarbon vehicles
- Ocular: Irrigation with copious tepid sterile water or saline

Supportive therapy: Including airway management, ventilatory assistance, humidified oxygen administration, and close monitoring for sudden respiratory failure

Antidote:
- Atropine: Administration should be guided by respiratory status, starting at 1-5 mg I.V. every 5-10 minutes as needed, and should be titrated to the resolution of excess pulmonary secretions; frequent administration of large doses (cumulative doses >100 mg) may be necessary in massive exposures
- Glycopyrrolate: May be administered if atropine is unavailable
- 2-PAM: For more significant exposures (ie, exposures requiring large doses of atropine, or with recurring symptoms, or exposures to more lipid soluble agents), administration should follow: 1-2 g I.V. over 5-10 minutes, repeated in 1 hour if asthenia reoccurs, then every 4-12 hours for recurring symptoms

Enhancement of elimination: Dialysis and hemoperfusion are not indicated due to effectiveness of the prescribed treatment, large volumes of distribution of organophosphates

Antidote(s)

Atropine Sulfate *on page 1395*
Pralidoxime Chloride *on page 1461*

Diagnostic Tests/Procedures

Blood Gases, Arterial *on page 1207*
Chest Films *on page 1224*
Complete Blood Count *on page 1236*
Creatinine, Serum *on page 1243*
Electrocardiography *on page 1253*
Liver Profile *on page 1286*
Pseudocholinesterase, Serum *on page 1340*

Pregnancy Implications Human data regarding organophosphate exposure in pregnancy is limited and anecdotal; teratogenesis and fetal death have been produced in animal models at exposure levels that cause obvious toxicity to the pregnant animal

(Continued)

Chlorfenvinphos *(Continued)*

Additional Information Red blood cell cholinesterase, and serum pseudocholinesterase may be depressed following acute or chronic organophosphate exposure; RBC cholinesterase is typically not analyzed by in-house laboratories, and is usually not available for consideration during acute management. Pseudocholinesterase levels may be rapidly available from some in-house laboratories, but are not as reliable a marker of organophosphate exposure because of variability secondary to variant genotypes, hepatic disease, oral estrogen use, or malnutrition. Because of this variability, true indication of suppression of either of these enzymes can only be estimated through comparison to pre-exposure values; these enzymes may be useful in measuring a patient's recovery postexposure, especially if the recovery is not progressing as expected.

Other information concerning pesticide exposures is available through the EPA-funded National Pesticide Telecommunications Network: 1-800-858-7378 (weekdays, 8 AM to 6 PM, Central Standard time)

Specific References

Minton NA and Murray VS, "A Review of Organophosphate Poisoning," *Med Toxicol Adverse Drug Exp*, 1988, 3(5):350-75.

Namba T, Nolte CT, Jackrel J, et al, "Poisoning Due to Organophosphate Insecticides. Acute and Chronic Manifestations," *Am J Med*, 1971, 50(4):475-92.

Chloric Acid-Sodium Salt *see* Chlorate Salts *on page 884*

Chlorinated Camphene *see* Toxaphene *on page 1031*

Chlorinated Hydrocarbon Insecticides *see* Organochlorines *on page 983*

Chlorine

Related Information

Sodium Hypochlorite *on page 1013*

CAS Number 7782-50-5

UN Number 1017

Synonyms Bertholite

Commonly Found In War gas used in World War I; can be produced by mixing bleach with acid

Use In pulp mills and for swimming pools; also used in bleaching

Mechanism of Toxic Action Converted to hydrogen chloride in lung parenchyma, strong irritant; free radical generation may be present

Adverse Reactions

Cardiovascular: Cardiovascular collapse

Respiratory: Pulmonary edema, bronchoconstriction

Miscellaneous: Increased risk for lymphoma, lacrimation

Signs & Symptoms of Acute Overdose Eye irritation, airway irritation, hypotension, dyspnea, headache, vomiting, dermal burns, hypertension, cough, stomatitis, wheezing, chest pain, hyperchloremic metabolic acidosis

Toxicodynamics/Kinetics Absorption: Not well absorbed, low solubility

Reference Range Not measurable

Overdosage Treatment

Supportive therapy: Administer 100% humidified oxygen; a 3.75% to 5% sodium bicarbonate solution by nebulization may be helpful for acute respiratory symptoms; wheezing can be treated with beta-adrenergic agonists; steroids of no proven benefit

Diagnostic Tests/Procedures

Blood Gases, Arterial *on page 1207*

Chest Films *on page 1224*

Lung Scan, Ventilation *on page 1288*

Pulmonary Compliance (Dynamic) *on page 1342*

Additional Information Green-yellow gas; mixing hypochlorite (bleach) with an acid can release chlorine gas; mixing hypochlorite (bleach) with ammonia can release chloramine gas

Odor threshold: 3.5 ppm

TLV-TWA: 0.5 ppm

IDLH: 30 ppm

PEL-TWA: 0.5 ppm

Specific References

Bosse GM, "Nebulized Sodium Bicarbonate in the Treatment of Chlorine Gas Inhalation," *J Toxicol Clin Toxicol*, 1994, 32(3):233-41.

Deschamps D, Soler P, Rosenberg N, et al, "Persistent Asthma After Inhalation of a Mixture of Sodium Hypochlorite and Hydrochloric Acid," *Chest*, 1994, 105(6):1895-6.

Done AK, "The Toxic Emergency: It's a Gas," *J Emerg Med*, 1976, 305-14.

Hryhorczuk DO, "Ammonia and Chlorine," *Clin Toxicol Rev*, 1986, 9:1-3.

Krenzelok E and Mrvos R, "Chlorine/Chloramine," *J Toxicol Clin Toxicol*, 1995, 33(4):355-7.

Maddy KT and Edmiston S, "Selected Incidents of Illnesses and Injuries Related to Exposure to Pesticides Reported by Physicians in California in 1986," *Vet Hum Toxicol*, 1988, 30(3):246-54.

Martinez TT and Long C, "Explosion Risk From Swimming Pool Chlorinators and Review of Chlorine Toxicity," *J Toxicol Clin Toxicol*, 1995, 33(4):349-54.

Schwartz DA, Smith DD, and Lakshminarayan S, "The Pulmonary Sequelae Associated With Accidental Inhalation of Chlorine Gas," *Chest*, 1990, 97(4):820-5.

Vinsel PJ, "Treatment of Acute Chlorine Gas Inhalation With Nebulized Sodium Bicarbonate," *J Emerg Med*, 1990, 8(3):327-9.

Chloroacetophenone

CAS Number 532-27-4

UN Number 1697

Synonyms CAF; CN; MACE; Phenacyl Chloride

Use Active ingredient in tear gas

Mechanism of Toxic Action Lacrimator – irritation due to the active halogen group reacting with sulfhydryl groups

Adverse Reactions Ocular: Ocular burning, blepharospasms, cataract

Signs & Symptoms of Acute Overdose Rhinorrhea, sneezing, pharyngitis, agitation, tearing, eye pain, skin irritation, broncho- and laryngospasm, nausea, vomiting, coughing

Toxicodynamics/Kinetics

Onset of effect: Rapid

Duration: Usually resolves in 30 minutes, skin effects may last for 2-3 hours

Absorption: Not absorbed

Overdosage Treatment

Decontamination: Move patient to fresh air and monitor for wheezing; personnel should avoid contaminating themselves; wash skin with soap and water; avoid rubbing of eyes as it may prolong effect; copious irrigation needed

Diagnostic Tests/Procedures

Blood Gases, Arterial *on page 1207*

Chest Films *on page 1224*

Complete Blood Count *on page 1236*

Pulmonary Compliance (Dynamic) *on page 1342*

Additional Information Fragrant odor of apple blossom; can be detected using gas chromatography/mass spectrophotometry (GC/MS)

TLV-TWA: 0.05 ppm

IDLH: 100 mg/m^3

PEL-TWA: 0.05 ppm

Specific References

Beswick FW, "Chemical Agents Used in Riot Control and Warfare," *Hum Toxicol*, 1983, 2(2):247-56.

Chapman AG and White C, "Death Resulting From Lacrimatory Agents," *J Forensic Sci*, 1978, 23(3):527-30.

Hu H, Fine J, Epstein P, et al, "Tear Gas – Harrassing Agent or Toxic Chemical Weapon?" *JAMA*, 1989, 262(5):660-3.

Chlorobenzene

CAS Number 108-90-7

UN Number 1134

Synonyms Benzene Chloride; MCB; Monochlorobenzene

Brand Names Caswell No 183A

Use Solvent used in production of DDT, phenol compounds (replaced primarily by cumene), diisocyanate, nitrochlorobenzene, and degreasing car parts

Adverse Reactions

Cardiovascular: Cyanosis

Central nervous system: CNS depression, seizures, coma, hyperesthesia

Neuromuscular & skeletal: Muscle spasms, neuritis, myoclonus

Miscellaneous: Mucosal irritant (at levels >200 ppm)

Toxicodynamics/Kinetics

Absorption:

- Inhalation: 38% to 45%
- Gastrointestinal: 31%

Metabolism: Hepatic transition to 4-chlorophenol and through glutathione conjugation to parachlorophenyl mercapturic acid

Reference Range Levels of residents living near a former toxic chemical dump ranged from 25-120 μg/L of chlorobenzene in the urine and 0.05-17 ng/L of chlorobenzene in blood

Overdosage Treatment

Decontamination:

- Ocular: Irrigate with normal saline
- Dermal: Wash with soap and water

Supportive therapy: Respiratory support with administration of 100% humidified oxygen

(Continued)

Chlorobenzene *(Continued)*

Additional Information This compound can decompose through heating to chlorine gas

Odor threshold: 0.21 ppm

IDLH: 2400 ppm

PEL-TWA: 75 ppm

Specific References

Ogata M and Shimada Y, "Differences in Urinary Monochlorobenzene Metabolites Between Rats and Humans," *Int Arch Occup Environ Health*, 1983, 53:51-7.

U.S. Department of Health and Human Services, "Toxicological Profile for Chlorobenzene TP-90-06," Agency for Toxic Substances and Diseases Registry, December 1990.

Chlorodibenzofurans *see* Polychlorinated Dibenzofurans *on page 996*

Chlorodibromomethane *see* Dibromochloromethane *on page 907*

Chloroethylene *see* Vinyl Chloride *on page 1038*

Chloroform

CAS Number 67-66-3

UN Number 1888

Synonyms Formyl Trichloride; Freon 20; Methane Trichloride; TCM; Trichloroform; Trichloromethane

Use Solvent, grain fumigant, found in emulsions, spirits, tinctures; has been used as an anesthetic agent, refrigerant, and aerosol propellant

Mechanism of Toxic Action A direct depressant on the respiratory center in the brainstem; interferes with gangliosides in neuronal membranes and phospholipids on surfactant layer in lungs; can cause lipid peroxidation

Adverse Reactions Gastrointestinal: Nausea and vomiting can occur at doses of 22-237 ppm

Signs & Symptoms of Acute Overdose Burning, corneal injury, urticaria, conjunctivitis may occur with eye exposure; cardiac arrhythmias, mydriasis, nystagmus, acetone breath, cardiac arrest have been reported; respiratory depression, chemical pneumonitis, and pulmonary edema may occur; CNS depression occurs; chronic use may produce degenerative brain changes and psychotic behavior; nausea, hemolysis, hepatitis, hepatomegaly, vomiting, headache, drowsiness, dizziness, hypotension, dry mouth, fibrillation, bradycardia, tachycardia (ventricular)

Toxicodynamics/Kinetics

Absorption: Well through inhalation, oral, and dermal exposure

Distribution: V_d: 2.6 L/kg; throughout and soluble in adipose tissue

Metabolism: To chlormethanol, hydrochloric acid, phosgene, chloride, and CO_2

Half-life: 1.5 hours

Elimination: Primarily from lungs in the form of chloroform and carbon dioxide; <1% excreted in urine

Reference Range Blood chloroform levels with anesthesia: 0.07-0.165 mg/mL

Overdosage Treatment

Decontamination: Emesis, lavage/activated charcoal with cathartic; remove from area of exposure and remove clothing; wash thoroughly

Supportive therapy: Treatment of cardiac and respiratory status; lidocaine, propranolol, bretylium, phenytoin, disopyramide, or overdrive pacing has been used in treatment of PVCs; atropine may be used if severe bradycardia is present. If oral ingestion, radiograph may show radio-opacity; monitor blood glucose, urinalysis, LFTs and renal function; administration of N-acetylcysteine for treatment of hepatitis is still theoretical.

Antidote(s)

Atropine Sulfate *on page 1395*

Diagnostic Tests/Procedures

Liver Profile *on page 1286*

Monitoring Parameters Gas chromatograph and flame ionization detector as well as HPLC have been used to determine levels in blood; blood levels in fatalities range from 1-12 mg/dL

Pregnancy Implications May be embryotoxic; diffuses readily across placenta, but no increased frequency of congenital malformations noted with 1st trimester exposure; strong evidence that chloroform may be mutagenic and carcinogenic

Additional Information Listed as a suspected carcinogen/radiopaque

TLV-TWA: 10 ppm

Anesthetic dose: 8000-10,000 ppm

Fatal dose: 40,000 ppm

Odor threshold:

- Air: 85 ppm
- Water: 2.4 ppm

Average daily intake of chloroform through drinking water: 4-88 mcg; from urban ambient atmosphere: 6-200 mcg

Atmospheric half-life: 80 days
Water (pH 9) half-life: 25-37 years

Specific References

Axelsson G, Lutz C, and Rylander R, "Exposure to Solvents and Outcome of Pregnancy in University Laboratory Employees," *Br J Ind Med*, 1984, 41(3):305-12.

Schroeder HG, "Acute and Delayed Chloroform Poisoning," *Br J Anaesth*, 1965, 37:972-5.

Timms RM and Moser KM, "Toxicity Secondary to Intravenous Administrated Chloroform in Humans," *Arch Intern Med*, 1975, 135(12):1601-3.

U.S. Department of Health and Human Services, "Toxicological Profile for Chloroform TP-92/07," Agency for Toxic Substances and Diseases Registry, April, 1993.

Chloroformyl Chloride *see* Phosgene *on page 992*

Chlorohydric Acid *see* Hydrogen Chloride *on page 940*

Chloromethane

CAS Number 74-87-3

UN Number 1063

Synonyms Methyl Chloride; Monochloromethane

Brand Names Artic®; Freon 40; R40

Use Chlorinated hydrocarbon used in the production of silicones, butyl rubber, methyl cellulose; was also used as a refrigerant (although this use has declined over the past 30 years), as a propellant, and as a herbicide; also used in molding polystyrene and polyurethane foams and as an oil extractant

Mechanism of Toxic Action Narcotic effect causing central nervous system depression

Adverse Reactions Primarily from inhalation with a latent period of up to 2 days postinhalation; respiratory depression, nephritis

Signs & Symptoms of Acute Overdose Diplopia, blurred vision, mydriasis, tachycardia, hypotension, wheezing, dizziness, drowsiness, headache, ataxia, seizures, slurred speech, tremor, coma, asthenia, nausea, vomiting, diarrhea, albuminuria, hematuria, oliguria, anemia, dermal erythema, elevated BUN and creatinine

Toxicodynamics/Kinetics

Absorption: Not absorbed through intact skin
Protein binding: 0%
Metabolism: Hepatic to formaldehyde and carbon dioxide
Half-life: 50-90 minutes
Elimination: Renal (N-acetyl-S-methylcysteine)

Reference Range After exposure to 50 ppm, chloromethane breath levels range from 50-80 μg/L; while chloromethane blood levels range from 35-100 μg/L

Overdosage Treatment

Decontamination: Inhalation: Move patient out of environment; administer 100% humidified oxygen

Supportive therapy: Benzodiazepines for seizure control; symptoms usually abate after 6 hours

Monitoring Parameters CBC, liver enzymes, renal tests, urine analysis

Pregnancy Implications Birth defects with retarded development in rodents; implicated (though not proven) to be a cause for sacral agenesis in humans

Additional Information Colorless gas with a sweet odor

Lethal concentration: 20,000 ppm
Toxic symptoms: 200 ppm
IDLH: 10,000 ppm
TLV-TWA: 50 ppm

Specific References

Kucera J, "Exposure to Fat Solvents: A Possible Cause of Sacral Agenesis in Man," *J Pediatr*, 1968, 72(6):857-9.

Repko JD, "Neurotoxicity of Methyl Chloride," *Neurobehav Toxicol Teratol*, 1981, 3(4):425-9.

U.S. Department of Health and Human Services, "Toxicological Profile for Chloromethane TP-90/07," Agency for Toxic Substances and Diseases Registry, December 1990.

Chlorophenothane® *see* DDT *on page 903*

Chlorphacinone *see* Anticoagulant Rodenticide *on page 859*

Chlorpyrifos

CAS Number 2921-88-2

UN Number 2783

Synonyms O,O-Diethyl-O-(3,5,6-Trichloro-2-Pyridyl) Phosphorothioate; Phosphorothioic Acid; Trichlorpyriphos (Discontinued)

Brand Names Dursban®; Dursban TC®; Lorsban®; Pyrinex®

Use Broad spectrum insecticide for control of mosquitoes, flies, cockroaches, fleas, and termites (TC formulation); has been used as an ascaricide and a veterinary ectoparasiticide

(Continued)

Chlorpyrifos *(Continued)*

Adverse Reactions

Central nervous system: Chloreoathetosis, anxiety, restlessness, dizziness

Dermatologic: Milk skin irritant

Ocular: Miosis (82%), mydriasis can be present in severely affected individuals; conjunctivitis, photophobia, opsoclonus

Respiratory: Rhinorrhea

Miscellaneous: Sweating

Signs & Symptoms of Acute Overdose Miosis (unreactive to light), mydriasis (rarely), lacrimation, pallor, excessive sweating, confusion, agitation, headache, dysarthria, generalized asthenia, seizures, A-V block, coma, decreased hemoglobin/red blood cell count/platelet count, metabolic acidosis and hyperglycemia (severe intoxication), hypotension, hypertension, bradycardia, tachycardia, Q-T prolongation, heart block, asystole, salivation, bronchorrhea, tachypnea, pulmonary edema, respiratory depression, diaphragmatic paralysis, skeletal muscle fasciculation and flaccid paralysis, nausea, vomiting, abdominal pain, fecal and urinary incontinence; an "intermediate syndrome" of limb asthenia and respiratory paralysis has been reported to occur between 24 and 96 hours postorganophosphate exposure, and is independent of the acute cholinergic crisis; late paresthesia characterized by stocking and glove paresthesia, anesthesia, and asthenia is infrequently observed weeks to months following acute exposure to certain organophosphates; cases of delayed neurotoxicity have been described

Toxicodynamics/Kinetics

Absorption: Oral: 70%; Dermal: <3%

Metabolism: Hepatic to diethylphosphate, diethylthiophosphate, and 3,5,6-trichloro-2-pyridinol (TCP)

Half-life: 27 hours

Reference Range Oral dose of 5 mg/kg followed by dermal exposures between 0.5-5 mg/kg 2 weeks later produced blood chlorpyrifos levels <30 μg/L (blood TCP levels were 0.9 mg/L 6 hours after oral ingestion and 0.06 mg/L 24 hours after dermal administration); a single oral dose of 0.5 mg/kg can depress plasma cholinesterase levels by 85%

Overdosage Treatment

Decontamination: Isolation, bagging, and disposal of all contaminated clothing and other articles; all emergency medical workers and hospital staff should follow appropriate precautions regarding exposure to hazardous material including the use of protective clothing, masks, goggles, and respiratory equipment

Dermal: Prompt thorough scrubbing of all affected areas with soap and water, including hair and nails

Gastric: Activated charcoal can be administered either orally or via a nasogastric tube; do not induce emesis because of danger of sudden respiratory compromise, alterations in mental status, seizures, coma, and possible aspiration of hydrocarbon vehicles

Ocular: Irrigation with copious tepid sterile water or saline

Supportive therapy: Including airway management, ventilatory assistance, humidified oxygen administration, and close monitoring for sudden respiratory failure

Antidote:

Atropine: Administration should be guided by respiratory status, starting at 1-5 mg I.V. every 5-10 minutes as needed, and should be titrated to the resolution of excess pulmonary secretions; frequent administration of large doses (cumulative doses >100 mg) may be necessary in massive exposures

Glycopyrrolate: May be administered if atropine is unavailable

2-PAM: For more significant exposures (ie, exposures requiring large doses of atropine, or with recurring symptoms, or exposures to more lipid soluble agents), administration should follow: 1-2 g I.V. over 5-10 minutes, repeated in 1 hour if asthenia reoccurs, then every 4-12 hours for recurring symptoms

Enhancement of elimination: Dialysis and hemoperfusion are not indicated due to effectiveness of the prescribed treatment, large volumes of distribution of organophosphates

Antidote(s)

Atropine Sulfate *on page 1395*

Pralidoxime Chloride *on page 1461*

Diagnostic Tests/Procedures

Blood Gases, Arterial *on page 1207*

Chest Films *on page 1224*

Complete Blood Count *on page 1236*

Creatinine, Serum *on page 1243*

Electrocardiography *on page 1253*

Liver Profile *on page 1286*

Pseudocholinesterase, Serum *on page 1340*

Pregnancy Implications No evidence for embryo or fetal toxicity in rodents at doses which can cause maternal toxicity (>15 mg/kg/day oral ingestion)

Additional Information Red blood cell cholinesterase, and serum pseudocholinesterase may be depressed following acute or chronic organophosphate exposure; RBC cholinesterase is typically not analyzed by in-house laboratories, and is usually not available for consideration during acute management. Pseudocholinesterase levels may be rapidly available from some in-house laboratories, but are not as reliable a marker of organophosphate exposure because of variability secondary to variant genotypes, hepatic disease, oral estrogen use, or malnutrition. Because of this variability, true indication of suppression of either of these enzymes can only be estimated through comparison to pre-exposure values; these enzymes may be useful in measuring a patient's recovery postexposure, especially if the recovery is not progressing as expected. Emits a sulfur (garlic) odor at airborne concentrations exceeding 1 ppb.

Other information concerning pesticide exposures is available through the EPA-funded National Pesticide Telecommunications Network: 1-800-858-7378 (weekdays, 8 AM to 6 PM, Central Standard time)

Toxic dose: 300 mg/kg

Specific References

Aiuto LA, Pavlakis SG, and Boxer RA, "Life-Threatening Organophosphate-Induced Delayed Polyneuropathy in a Child After Accidental Chlorpyrifos Ingestion," *J Pediatr*, 1993, 122(4):658-60.

Brenner FE, Bond GG, McLaren EA, et al, "Morbidity Among Employees Engaged in the Manufacture or Formulation of Chlorpyrifos," *Br J Ind Med*, 1989, 46(2):133-7.

Lotti M, Moretto A, Zopellari R, et al, "Inhibition of Lymphocytic Neuropathy Target Esterase Predicts the Development of Organophosphate-Induced Delayed Polyneuropathy," *Arch Toxicol*, 1986, 59(3):176-9.

Nolan RJ, Rick DL, Freshour NL, et al, "Chlorpyrifos: Pharmacokinetics in Human Volunteers," *Toxicol Appl Pharmacol*, 1984, 73(1):8-15.

Chromar *see* Isopropyl Alcohol *on page 943*

Chrometrace® *see* Chromium *on this page*

Chromium

Related Information

Radiation: Basics of Exposure *on page 1594-1600*

Toxins Which Should be Lavaged With Solutions Other Than Water *on page 1635*

CAS Number 7778-50-9; 7775-11-3; 7789-12-0; 13530-65-9; 7789-09-5; 12018-01-8; 7778-50-9; 10025-73-7; 10060-12-5; 7440-47-3; 25013-82-5; 7789-02-8; 10101-53-8; 12314-42-0

UN Number 1463; 1758; 2720; 1439

Synonyms Cr; Hexaquachromium Chloride

Brand Names Chrometrace®

Commonly Found In Chromium exposure may be found in battery manufacturers, painters, printers, welders, jewelers, steel workers, oil drillers, match manufacturers, leather workers, lithographers, tanners, cement workers

Mechanism of Toxic Action Dermatologic and pulmonary sensitizers; possibly carcinogenic with compounds of valence +6 (hexavalent)

Adverse Reactions

Dermatologic: Dermal sensitization

Gastrointestinal: Gastroenteritis

Hematologic: Hemolysis

Hepatic: Necrosis, tubular necrosis (acute)

Signs & Symptoms of Acute Overdose Acute nausea, vomiting, dark red urine and stool, thrombocytopenia, hypotension, skin burns, coma

Reference Range Serum: 0.05-0.15 ng/mL (SI: 1-3 nmol/L); normal population urine range: 0.24-1.80 μg/L.

Some laboratories report much higher "normals" because the methods they use or the collection technique is not adequate to prevent substantial contamination. If a laboratory reports "<1 ng/mL" or some similar figure without a lower level for normal, the value can be relied upon to discover toxic states, perhaps, but not deficiency states. Serum levels of 10 ng/mL correspond to short-term atmospheric exposure limit of 0.1 mg/m^3 of chromium trioxide. Serum levels even higher would be expected in acute systemic toxicity. Almost a twofold diurnal variation is noted in serum chromium levels, with the level highest in the morning and falling after each meal as insulin levels rise. Serum chromium levels are about 60% of normal in diabetic patients, which overlaps the normal range.

Less than 1 μg/24 hours. Levels vary with the laboratory and have declined with improved methods of avoiding contamination. Levels two- to threefold above this may reflect supplementation or excess losses. Levels elevated tenfold and higher have been seen in exposed asymptomatic tannery workers. Spot levels of chromium in urine of 30 ng/g creatinine correspond to the short-term atmospheric exposure limit of 0.1 mg/m^3 of chromium trioxide in industrial exposure situations.

(Continued)

Chromium *(Continued)*

Overdosage Treatment

Decontamination:

Dermal: Copious irrigation; use 10% ascorbic acid topically to convert hexavalent chromium to a less toxic trivalent form

Oral: Lavage with 1% ascorbic acid solution (10 g ascorbic acid orally for every L of lavage fluid); do not use antacids since antacids may increase absorption

Supportive therapy: Nephrotoxicity can be managed with ascorbic acid (1 g I.V. every 10-20 minutes up to 3 g) and calcium disodium EDTA; monitor serum/urine pH during treatment with ascorbic acid

Enhancement of elimination: Acetylcysteine may be an effective therapy in enhancing chromium elimination; hemodialysis should also be employed especially if renal insufficiency is present; hemodialysis or exchange transfusions

Diagnostic Tests/Procedures

Chromium, Serum *on page 1230*
Chromium, Urine *on page 1231*

Pregnancy Implications Significant decreases in fetal weight, length, and other fetotoxic effects noted to high concentrations of chromium (VI) in a rodent model

Additional Information Determination of the amount of chromium in the serum or urine of normal persons is extremely difficult, due to the very low levels present. Levels observed are in the 0.1 ng/mL range, equivalent to one part in 10 billion. Extreme caution must be taken to avoid contamination by dust (from skin, leather, cloth) and contact with steel (which contains chromium). Chromium is felt to be an essential element in the human, with chromium III purported to be an integral part of "glucose tolerance factor," a partially characterized complex that has been suggested to contain two molecules of nicotinic acid and a small oligopeptide complexed to chromium III. This organic moiety is thought necessary for insulin action on the cell surface. Deficiency of chromium can cause an acquired insulin resistance or diabetes mellitus with associated hyperlipidemia in otherwise well-nourished patients. The classic cases, however, were reported prior to the availability of accurate serum levels of chromium, and reported levels then in "deficiency" were tenfold or more higher than we now know to be "normal". Chromium deficiency with associated glucose intolerance and fasting hypoglycemia has been most often observed during refeeding of malnourished individuals after famine starvation in relief programs. In infants, one or more oral doses of chromium, 250 mcg, have been curative. Chromium deficiency with associated glucose intolerance has also been observed in long-term parenteral nutrition when inadequate chromium was included. Neuropathy, encephalopathy, and abnormalities of amino acid profile (serum low in branched-chain amino acids and high in aromatic amino acids) have been noted in conjunction with this condition.

With regard to toxicity, pure metallic chromium is nontoxic. Chromium III is poorly absorbed, and much less toxic than chromium VI. Industrial monitoring for toxicity in the past has relied on air samples largely for total and hexavalent chromium, the major species of concern. Workers are potentially exposed in tanneries, mines, and industries for metal plating, welding, photography, paint, dye, and explosives. Skin exposure may lead to dermatitis, and respiratory exposure to bronchitis, asthma, and lung cancer. Hair contains 1000-fold more chromium than serum or urine, and hair chromium content does correlate with industrial exposure; but more data are needed before hair chromium monitoring can replace industrial air monitoring and samples of blood and urine in cases of suspected toxicity or deficiency. Acute systemic chromate toxicity may cause acute tubular necrosis, acute hepatitis, seizures, and coma. Acute respiratory or gastrointestinal symptoms relate to the locus of absorption. Intermediate levels of long-term exposure may cause tubular albuminuria in industrial workers.

Chromium supplementation has been shown by some workers to improve glucose tolerance and improve insulin efficiency in glucose intolerant (but not in normal or overtly diabetic) patients on diets equivalent to the lower quartile of ordinary chromium intake in the United States. The implication is that many individuals in the U.S. population have a marginal chromium intake. We may, therefore, anticipate increased self-medication and supplementation in the future, and greater medical interest in this trace metal. The literature regarding chromium was for many years confused due to difficulties with analysis and contamination. Much old work needs to be repeated, and this field is still very much in flux.

The main excretory pathway for chromium III is renal. Estimated safe and adequate, oral intake recommended by the U.S. National Academy of Sciences range from 50-200 mcg/day, but in the U.S. 90% of people eat less, the mean intake being 25-33 mcg/day. Such intake recommendations likely derive from the 1980s when average estimated intake was determined to be 50-100 mcg/day. With increasingly accurate assays, new recommended ranges may be set lower. Absorption of chromium III is on the order of 0.5%, by radioisotope studies. One hospital pharmacy supplies 12 mcg of chromium from MTE5® trace mineral parenteral nutrition supplement per day. We are unaware of a large survey.

Specific References

Junaid M, Murthy RC, and Saxena DK, "Chromium Fetotoxicity in Mice During Late Pregnancy," *Vet Hum Toxicol*, 1995, 37(4):320-3.

U.S. Department of Health and Human Services, "Toxicological Profile for Chromium TP-92/08," Agency for Toxic Substances and Diseases Registry, 1993.

Chrysanthemum cinerareaefolium *see* Pyrethrins *on page 1003*

Chrysene *see* Polycyclic Aromatic Hydrocarbons *on page 997*

Cinerin *see* Pyrethrins *on page 1003*

Cinnamene *see* Styrene *on page 1017*

Clophen *see* Polychlorinated Biphenyls *on page 995*

Clorox *see* Sodium Hypochlorite *on page 1013*

CN *see* Chloroacetophenone *on page 889*

CO *see* Carbon Monoxide *on page 880*

Coal Tar Creosote (Creosote Oil, Brick Oil) *see* Creosote *on page 898*

Cobalt

Related Information

Radiation: Basics of Exposure *on page 1594-1600*

CAS Number 7440-48-4; 7646-79-9; 1307-96-6; 10724-43-4; 1308-04-9; 1308-06-1; 10026-22-9; 513-79-1

UN Number 1318; 2001

Synonyms Cobalt Chloride; Cobalt Oxide; Cobalt Sulfate

Commonly Found In Superalloys as a paint drier, magnets, in pigment manufacture, glass decolorizer; industries with significant exposure to cobalt include tool sharpeners, miners, grinders; component in hard metal

Mechanism of Toxic Action Essential element in vitamin B_{12} which acts as a coenzyme in hemopoiesis

Adverse Reactions

Cardiovascular: Cardiomyopathy

Dermatologic: Contact dermatitis, allergic dermatitis, eczema

Endocrine & metabolic: Metabolic acidosis

Gastrointestinal: Nausea, vomiting, diarrhea

Hematologic: Anemia or polycythemia (not noted after inhalation exposure)

Ocular: Optic atrophy, conjunctivitis

Respiratory: Wheezing, interstitial fibrosis, and giant cell pneumonitis, pulmonary fibrosis

Miscellaneous: Hypothyroidism, Goodpasture's syndrome, hyperlipidemia, neutropenia, goiter

Signs & Symptoms of Acute Overdose Hypothyroid goiter, hypertension, cardiomegaly, cyanosis, polycythemia, pruritus

Toxicodynamics/Kinetics

Absorption: Variable gastrointestinal absorption (18% to 97%); absorbed through skin and also by inhalation

Half-life: 5-10 years

Elimination: Through lungs and feces

Reference Range Normal levels of urine: Up to 2.2 μg/L; Plasma: Up to 1.2 μg/L; Hair: 0.047 mg/kg; Nails: 0.06 mg/kg

Overdosage Treatment

Decontamination: Lavage/activated charcoal with cathartic; in oral ingestion, iron can decrease cobalt absorption

Supportive therapy: Sodium bicarbonate for metabolic acidosis

Enhancement of elimination: Calcium disodium EDTA (50 mg/kg/day for 5 days); can increase cobalt excretion fourfold; BAL, acetylcysteine, or succimer have been shown experimentally to increase fecal excretion of cobalt; hemodialysis may be of some value

Antidote(s)

Acetylcysteine *on page 1388*

Dimercaprol *on page 1414*

Edetate Calcium Disodium *on page 1419*

Succimer *on page 1473*

Test Interactions Increases levels of erythropoietin

Diagnostic Tests/Procedures

Cobalt, Serum *on page 1233*

Cobalt, Urine *on page 1233*

Additional Information Cobalt, a metallic element, is a component of vitamin B_{12} and is found in most foods. The daily requirement is unknown, as is deficiency in humans. Cobalt has the capacity to cause polycythemia, and for that reason, co-

(Continued)

Cobalt *(Continued)*

baltous chloride is used to successfully treat certain types of anemia. Accidental overdose of cobaltous chloride, especially in children, may lead to cyanosis, coma, and death. Cobalt dust inhaled in industrial settings may produce asthma and pulmonary symptoms. Long-term exposure may result in accumulation and cause polycythemia, goiter, cardiomyopathy, and nerve damage. Epidemic of lethal cardiomyopathy due to ingestion of 0.04-0.14 mg/kg/day of cobalt which was added as a foam stabilizer, occurred in the U.S. and Canada in the 1960s.

IDLH: 20 mg/m^3

PEL-TWA: 0.05 mg/m^3

TLV-TWA: 0.05 mg/m^3

Total body content of cobalt: 1-1.5 mg

Normal amounts of cobalt ingested from food amount: 50-40 mcg/day

Specific References

Henretig F, Joffe M, Baffa G, et al, "Elemental Cobalt Toxicity and Effects of Chelation Therapy," *Vet Hum Toxicol*, 1988, 30:372.

Jarvis JQ, Hammond E, Meier R, et al, "Cobalt Cardiomyopathy. A Report of Two Cases From Mineral Assay Laboratories and a Review of the Literature," *J Occup Med*, 1992, 34(6):620-6.

Lins LE and Pehrsson K, "Cobalt Intoxication in Uraemic Myocardiopathy?" *Lancet*, 1976, 1(7970):1191-2.

Llobet JM, Domingo JL, and Corbella J, "Comparative Effects of Repeated Parenteral Administration of Several Chelators on the Distribution and Excretion of Cobalt," *Res Commun Chem Pathol Pharmacol*, 1988, 60(2):225-33.

U.S. Department of Health and Human Services, "Toxicological Profile for Cobalt," Agency for Toxic Substances and Diseases Registry, 1992.

Cobalt Chloride *see* Cobalt *on previous page*

Cobalt Oxide *see* Cobalt *on previous page*

Cobalt Sulfate *see* Cobalt *on previous page*

Composition C-4 *see* RDX *on page 1009*

Compound 118® *see* Aldrin *on page 856*

Compound 605® *see* Dichloronaphthoquinone *on page 908*

Compound 1080® *see* Sodium Monofluoroacetate *on page 1014*

Compound 1189® *see* Chlordecone *on page 886*

Compound 4049® *see* Malathion *on page 950*

Copper

Related Information

Arsenic *on page 862*

Cyanide *on page 899*

Organochlorines *on page 983*

Selenium *on page 1011*

CAS Number 142-71-2; 544-92-3; 866-82-0; 1317-39-1; 1332-40-7; 3251-23-8; 7288-92-0; 7440-50-8; 7758-89-6; 7758-99-8; 10290-12-7; 12002-03-8; 12069-69-1; 12258-96-7; 20427-59-2; 26506-47-8

UN Number 1479; 1578; 1585; 1586; 2630; 2721; 2775; 2776; 3009; 3010

Commonly Found In Elemental copper, and as the following hydrated or anhydrous salts: acetate, arsenate, chlorate, chloride, citrate, cyanide, dinitrate, fluoroborate, hydrate, hydroxide, malonate, oxide, oxychloride, selenate, silicate, sulfate, and copper in association with organochlorine (DDT), or carbamate insecticide; used in electrical industry, plumbing, industrial valves and fittings, pigments, furniture polish

Mechanism of Toxic Action Copper is a cofactor for ascorbic acid oxidase, catalase, peroxidase, lactase, and tyrosinase; copper may induce hemolysis through oxidation of hemoglobin sulfhydryl groups, thereby increasing permeability of the red blood cell. Copper also inhibits the sulfhydryl moieties of G-6-PD and glutathione, thereby reducing their free radical scavenging activities.

Adverse Reactions

Cardiovascular: Shock and cardiovascular collapse

Central nervous system: Lethargy, confusion, coma, drowsiness

Dermatologic: Delayed allergic contact dermatitis

Gastrointestinal: Oral thermal injury, ulceration, gastroenteritis

Hematologic: Hemolysis, methemoglobinemia

Hepatic: Hepatitis

Ocular: Corneal discoloration (chalcosis), irritation, conjunctivitis, ulceration

Renal & genitourinary: Renal tubular necrosis, renal failure

Respiratory: Irritation, nasal ulceration, wheezing, rales

Miscellaneous: Metal fume fever

Signs & Symptoms of Acute Overdose Mucous membrane irritation, ulceration and burns, green hair, nausea, vomiting, metallic taste, blue-green vomitus, diarrhea, gastroenteritis, corneal discoloration and ulceration, hair discoloration (green), nasal ulceration, oral ulceration, allergic contact dermatitis, urticaria, hemolysis, feces discoloration (black), methemoglobinemia, acute tubular necrosis and renal failure, hepatomegaly and hepatitis with centrilobular necrosis and biliary stasis, jaundice, pulmonary edema, fibrosis, hypotension, shock, and cardiovascular collapse

Toxicodynamics/Kinetics

Onset of reaction: Hemorrhagic gastritis, diarrhea, hemolytic anemia, and renal tubule necrosis may follow 36-48 hours after exposure

Absorption: Oral: ~30%

Distribution: V_d: 2 L/kg; found extensively in red blood cells, kidney, liver, and lungs

Protein binding: 95% to ceruloplasmin

Half-life: 26 days

Elimination: Urine: 4%; bile and feces: 80%

Reference Range Serum copper concentrations average 1 mg/L in normal patients, and 2 mg/L in pregnant patients (10.5-23 μmol/L); serum copper concentrations >5 mg/mL are usually accompanied by signs of toxicity; whole blood copper concentrations correlate more closely with toxicity, but are usually not available; normal urinary copper excretion: 33 μg/L (602 μg/L in Wilson's disease); normal hair level: 8.9 mg/g

Overdosage Treatment

Decontamination:

Dermal: Prompt, thorough scrubbing of all affected areas with soap and water

Gastric: Lavage cautiously, but because of gastrointestinal ulceration and erosion, do not induce emesis; activated charcoal does not bind copper

Ocular: Irrigation with copious tepid water or saline

Respiratory: Remove from exposure, give supplemental oxygen, and treat wheezing

Supportive therapy: Including airway management, treatment of wheezing, humidified oxygen administration and close monitoring for renal compromise; BAL (dimercaprol), EDTA, or penicillamine should be considered for massive ingestions, persistent symptomatology, or persistently elevated serum copper concentrations; BAL and EDTA are preferred agents for severe intoxication; penicillamine may be used in patients that will tolerate oral therapy; trientine might be an effective copper chelator in an overdose setting, although it has not been studied for this use

Shock: Treat blood loss aggressively with I.V. fluids and vasopressors such as dopamine or norepinephrine; consider endoscopy to rule out corrosive gastrointestinal injury and blood loss

Enhancement of elimination: Dialysis or hemoperfusion has not been demonstrated to increase the elimination of copper

Antidote(s)

Dimercaprol *on page 1414*

Dopamine Hydrochloride *on page 1418*

Edetate Calcium Disodium *on page 1419*

Norepinephrine Bitartrate *on page 1451*

Penicillamine *on page 1454*

Trientine Dihydrochloride *on page 1474*

Diagnostic Tests/Procedures

Aspartate Aminotransferase *on page 1199*

Blood Gases, Arterial *on page 1207*

Chest Films *on page 1224*

Creatinine, Serum *on page 1243*

Electrolytes, Blood *on page 1254*

Methemoglobin, Blood *on page 1296*

Urea Nitrogen, Blood *on page 1370*

Pregnancy Implications Fetal risk relates directly to metabolic and respiratory abnormalities experienced by the mother

Additional Information Metal fume fever has been reported at copper dust concentrations of 0.075-0.12 mg/m^3. Copper salts were previously used as medicinal agents. Exposure may also follow the use of older vending machines, and brass or copper cooking or drinking vessels. Copper metal is radiopaque, but copper salts are not; elemental copper is poorly absorbed orally, but dusts or fumes may cause pneumonitis and metal fume fever. Copper salts may be irritating to the gastrointestinal tract, and may possess other toxicities due to salts such as arsenate or cyanide. Anhydrous compounds may produce thermal injury following contact with water or mucous membranes. Most U.S. coins contain 75% copper; diethyldithiocarbonate (intraocular use) is not useful to prevent ocular opacification due to copper nitrate.

ACGIH TLV: 1 mg/m^3 (dusts/mists), 0.2 mg/m^3 (fumes)

PEL-TWA: 1 mg/m^3 (dusts/mists), 0.1 mg/m^3 (fumes)

(Continued)

Copper *(Continued)*

Specific References

Chugh KS, Sharma BK, Singhal PC, et al, "Acute Renal Failure Following Copper Sulfate Intoxication," *Postgrad Med*, 1977, 53:18.

Schwartz E and Schmidt E, "Refractory Shock Secondary to Copper Sulfate Ingestion," *Ann Emerg Med*, 1986, 15(8):952-4.

Copper Fever *see* Metal Fume Fever *on page 956*

Coumafuryl *see* Anticoagulant Rodenticide *on page 859*

Coumarone *see* 2,3-Benzofuran *on page 869*

Coumatetralyl *see* Anticoagulant Rodenticide *on page 859*

Counter® *see* Terbufos *on page 1020*

Cr *see* Chromium *on page 893*

Creolina® *see* Cresols *on this page*

Creosote

Related Information

Toxins Which Should be Lavaged With Solutions Other Than Water *on page 1635*

CAS Number 8021-39-4 (wood); 8001-58-9 (coal tar)

Synonyms Coal Tar Creosote (Creosote Oil, Brick Oil); Wood Creosote (Beechwood Creosote)

Brand Names Sakresote® 100 (Coal Tar Creosote)

Use

Wood creosote: Disinfectant, carbonate, laxative, and expectorant (rarely used in U.S.)

Coal tar creosote: Carbonization of coal (bituminous) to produce natural gas (coking procedure); also used as a timber preservative

Mechanism of Toxic Action Mucosal irritant

Adverse Reactions

Cardiovascular: Increased diastolic pressure, hypertension

Dermal: Burns/irritation, phototoxic

Gastrointestinal: Oropharyngeal ulceration, esophageal corrosion

Hepatic: Hepatic degeneration

Ocular: Keratoconjunctivitis, photophobia, hyperemia

Renal: Renal failure, albuminuria

Signs & Symptoms of Acute Overdose Dyspnea, nasal irritation on inhalation, dizziness, lightheadedness, anuria, myoclonus

Toxicodynamics/Kinetics

Absorption: Dermal absorption may occur

Metabolism: Hepatic to 1-hydroxypyrene

Reference Range Workers of coal tar creosote excrete from 1-40 μg of creosote/g creatinine in urine

Overdosage Treatment

Decontamination:

- Ingestion: Do not induce emesis; lavage with olive oils may be effective; activated charcoal with cathartic (not castor oil) should be given
- Ocular: Copious irrigation with saline should be performed

Supportive therapy: Inhalation: Give 100% humidified oxygen

Enhancement of elimination: Charcoal hemoperfusion may be effective

Additional Information

Fatal oral dose of coal tar creosote:

- Children: 1-2 g
- Adults: 7 g

Exposure to coal tar creosote was possibly related in increased incidence of bladder cancer and squamous papillomas and carcinomas; phototoxicity of coal tar creosote may be enhanced with tetracycline

Specific References

Bowman CE, Muhleman MF, and Walters E, "A Fatal Case of Creosote Poisoning," *Postgrad Med J*, 1984, 60(705):499-500.

"Chaparral-Induced Toxic Hepatitis – California and Texas – 1992," *MMWR Morb Mortal Wkly Rep*, 1992, 41(43):812-4.

Cresols

CAS Number 95-48-7 (ortho); 106-445-5 (para); 108-39-4 (meta); 1319-77-3

UN Number 2076; 2022

Synonyms Cresylic Acid; Hydroxytoluene; Methylphenol; Tar Acids

Brand Names Creolina®

Use Organic acid which occurs naturally in mammals and plants (Easter lily, jasmine, camphor, eucalyptus); also found as a byproduct of natural fires (volcano lightning), through the combustion of petroleum fuels, wood, or coal (fly-ash); ortho cresol has been used as an antiseptic; a metabolic breakdown product of toluene

Mechanism of Toxic Action Mucosal irritant and a central nervous system depressant

Adverse Reactions

Cardiovascular: Premature ventricular contractions, tachycardia
Dermatologic: Burns
Gastrointestinal: Oropharyngeal burns, hemorrhagic pancreatitis
Hematologic: Methemoglobinemia, intravascular hemolysis, Heinz body anemia
Hepatic: Fatty degeneration
Neurologic: Cerebral edema
Ocular: Lacrimation, corneal burns, optic atrophy
Renal: Hematuria, eosinophilic necrosis, renal failure
Respiratory: Necrosis of bronchial epithelium, pulmonary edema

Signs & Symptoms of Acute Overdose Abdominal pain, coma, aspiration, dyspnea, hypoactivity, drowsiness, tremor, cough with bloody sputum, facial paralysis, seizures, vomiting

Toxicodynamics/Kinetics

Absorption: Dermal: May be absorbed (fatalities can occur)
Elimination: Renal

Reference Range Para-cresol concentration in urine normally averages about 90 mg/L (range: 20-200 mg/L); serum cresol level >90 mg/L associated with lethality

Overdosage Treatment

Decontamination:
- Dermal: Wash with soap and water copiously
- Ocular: Irrigate copiously with saline
- Oral: Dilute with water or milk; activated charcoal may be useful with a cathartic; do not induce emesis

Supportive therapy: Convulsions can be treated with a benzodiazepine or phenobarbital; significant methemoglobinemia should be treated with methylene blue

Antidote(s)

Methylene Blue *on page 1444*

Diagnostic Tests/Procedures

Methemoglobin, Blood *on page 1296*

Additional Information Individuals with glucose-6-phosphate deficiency may be at higher risk for methemoglobin formation; toxicity may be enhanced when patient is exposed concomitantly to oxidizing compounds (ie, hydroquinone); cigarette smokers may inhale as much as 3 mcg/day of cresols; not to be used for dermal disinfection

Lethal oral dose: 2 g/kg
Lethal dermal dose: 2 g/kg

Specific References

Arthurs GJ, Wise CC, and Coles GA, "Poisoning by Cresol," *Anaesthesia*, 1977, 32(7):642-3.

Cote MA, Lyonnais J, and Leblond PF, "Acute Heinz-Body Anemia Due to Severe Cresol Poisoning: Successful Treatment With Erythrocytapheresis," *Can Med Assoc J*, 1984, 130(10):1319-22.

U.S. Department of Health and Human Services, "Toxicological Profile for Cresols TP-91/11," Agency for Toxic Substances and Diseases Registry, July, 1992.

Cresylic Acid *see* Cresols *on previous page*

Crunch® *see* Carbaryl *on page 877*

Cuamine-M® *see* 4,4'-Methylenebis (2-Chloroaniline) *on page 965*

Cumaron *see* 2,3-Benzofuran *on page 869*

Curacron® *see* Profenofos *on page 998*

Curene® 442 *see* 4,4'-Methylenebis (2-Chloroaniline) *on page 965*

Curetard A® *see* N-Nitrosodiphenylamine *on page 982*

Cyanide

Related Information

Copper *on page 896*

CAS Number 57-12-5

UN Number 1588

Synonyms Carbon Nitride Ion; Isocyanide

Commonly Found In Gold and silver ore extraction, electroplating, fumigant, stainless steel manufacture, petroleum refining, rodenticide; plant sources include amygdalin glycodes (such as peach pits), cassava, linium, prunus, sorghum, and bamboo sprouts; also a byproduct of nitroprusside and succinonitrile along with laetrile

Mechanism of Toxic Action Forms a stable complex with ferric ion of cytochrome oxidase enzymes inhibiting cellular respiration; then converted to thiocyanate (less toxic form) by rhodanase enzyme

(Continued)

Cyanide *(Continued)*

Adverse Reactions

Cardiovascular: Myocardial depression, hypotension
Central nervous system: CNS stimulation followed by CNS depression
Ocular: Blurred vision
Respiratory: Respiratory depression
Miscellaneous: Bitter almond, burning taste

Signs & Symptoms of Acute Overdose Tachycardia followed by bradycardia, hypotension, tachypnea, pruritus, headache, nystagmus, metabolic acidosis, hyperventilation, cyanosis, flushing, dizziness, progressing to agitation, bitter almond breath, myoglobinuria, hypothermia, coma, seizures, apnea, mydriasis, pulmonary edema, nausea, vomiting, skin irritation, ototoxicity, tinnitus

Toxicodynamics/Kinetics

Absorption: By inhalation (58% to 77%), oral (~50%), dermally, and ocular
Distribution: V_d: 0.4 L/kg
Metabolism: Hepatic by rhodanese or 3-mercaptopyruvate to thiocyanate; also combines with hydroxocobalamin to form cyanocobalamin (vitamin B_{12})
Half-life: 0.7-2.1 hours
Elimination: Excreted through the lungs and the kidneys

Reference Range

Whole blood levels: Smoker: ≤0.5 mg/L
Flushing and tachycardia seen at 0.5-1.0 mg/L; obtundation at 1.0-2.5 mg/L
Coma and death occur at >2.5 mg/L
Plasma cyanide:
Normal: 4-5 μg/L
Asymptomatic (with metabolic acidosis): 80 μg/L
Death: >260 μg/L
Red blood cell cyanide:
Normal: <26 μg/L
Metabolic acidosis: 1040 μg/L
Symptomatic: 5200 μg/L
Fatal: >10,400 μg/L

Overdosage Treatment

Decontamination: Basic poison management (lavage/activated charcoal with cathartic); emesis is contraindicated due to rapid course of the neurologic symptoms; give 100% oxygen
Supportive therapy: Give sodium bicarbonate for acidosis; cyanide antidote kit (amyl nitrate, sodium nitrate followed by sodium thiosulfate)
Enhancement of elimination: Hemodialysis and charcoal hemoperfusion have been utilized; hyperbaric oxygen may also be utilized; hydroxocobalamin, dicobalt-EDTA, and 4-dimethylaminophenol used for chelation in Europe

Antidote(s)

Amyl Nitrite *on page 1390*
Cyanide Antidote Kit *on page 1406*
Hydroxocobalamin *on page 1433*
Oxygen (Hyperbaric) *on page 1453*
Sodium Nitrite *on page 1469*
followed by
Sodium Thiosulfate *on page 1470*

Diagnostic Tests/Procedures

Anion Gap, Blood *on page 1193*
Blood Gases, Arterial *on page 1207*
Cyanide, Blood *on page 1246*
Electrolytes, Blood *on page 1254*
Methemoglobin, Blood *on page 1296*
Thiocyanate, Blood or Urine *on page 1360*

Pregnancy Implications Teratogenicity not noted

Additional Information Bitter almond odor, zinc cyanide is odorless; up to 60% of the population may be unable to smell cyanide; parkinsonism has been noted after ingestion of sodium or potassium cyanide; hydroxocobalamin and dicobalt-EDTA used for chelation in Europe; ratio of red blood cell to plasma cyanide concentrations is 60:1; nut and nut products (especially unsalted pecans) contain the highest amount of copper (0.067-1.245 mg of copper per 100 g/nut); most U.S. coins contain 75% copper. Diethyldithiocarbamate (intraocular use) is not useful to prevent ocular opacification due to copper nitrate.

Average daily intake of copper by inhalation: 600 mcg
Average daily intake of copper through drinking water: 0.15 mg
Fatal dose of cyanide: 200-300 mg (adult)
ACGIH-TLV-TWA: 5 mg/m^3
IDLH: 50 mg/m^3
PEL-TWA: 5 mg/m^3

Fatal dose (hydrogen cyanide):
Dermal: 100 mg/kg
Inhalation for <1 hour: 110-135 ppm
Oral: 0.6-1.5 mg/kg

Residence time in atmosphere of hydrogen cyanide: 2 years; in natural rivers, half-life of cyanide: 10-24 days; daily intake of hydrogen cyanide by inhalation: ~3.8 mcg; through drinking water: 0.4-0.7 mcg; allowable daily intake: ~0.6 mg

Fruit juice typically contains from 1.9-5.3 mg/L of hydrogen cyanide while apricot pits contain 89-2,170 mg/kg (wet weight); inhaled smoke from cigarettes contain from 10-400 mcg/cigarette while sidestream smoke usually runs <27% of main-stream smoke concentrations. Average cyanide emission rate in automobiles varies from 11-14 mg/mile in cars; catalytic converters can reduce cyanide emissions by 90%.

Specific References

Blanc P, Hogan M, Mallin K, et al, "Cyanide Intoxication Among Silver-Reclaiming Workers," *JAMA*, 1985, 253(3):367-71.

Graham DL, Laman D, Theodore J, et al, "Acute Cyanide Poisoning Complicated by Lactic Acidosis and Pulmonary Edema," *Arch Intern Med*, 1977, 137(8):1051-5.

Hall AH and Rumack BH, "Clinical Toxicology of Cyanide," *Ann Emerg Med*, 1986, 15(9):1067-74.

Hall AH and Rumack BH, "Hydroxocobalamin/Sodium Thiosulfate as a Cyanide Antidote," *J Emerg Med*, 1987, 5(2):115-21.

Kruszyna R, Kruszyna HG, and Smith RP, "A Spectrophotometric Method for Estimating Methemoglobin Concentration in the Presence of Cyanide," *Am J Emerg Med*, 1993, 11(6):642-3.

Lopez BL, Birenban DS, Snyder J, et al, "Chlorpromazine, A Protectant Against Cyanide Toxicity, Inhibits the Generation of Endothelium-Derived Nitric Oxide," *Acad Emerg Med*, 1995, 2:397.

Salkowski AA and Penney DG, "Cyanide Poisoning in Animals and Humans," *Vet Hum Toxicol*, 1994, 36(5):455-66.

U.S. Department of Health and Human Services, "Toxicological Profile for Cyanide TP-92/09," Agency for Toxic Substances and Diseases Registry, April, 1993.

Cyanoethylene *see* Acrylonitrile *on page 853*

Cyanomethane *see* Acetonitrile *on page 850*

Cyclonite *see* RDX *on page 1009*

Cyclopropanecarboxylic Acid *see* Pyrethrins *on page 1003*

Cyclotetramethylenetetranitramine *see* HMX *on page 939*

Cythion® *see* Malathion *on page 950*

2,4-D

CAS Number 94-75-7

Synonyms 2,4-Dichlorophenoxyacetic Acid

Commonly Found In Choroxone®; Esteron®; Salvo®; Weedar®; Weedone®

Mechanism of Toxic Action A chlorophenoxy herbicide used to control broad-leaf weeds; an auxin which causes abnormal plant growth

Adverse Reactions

Cardiovascular: Cardiac arrhythmias, bradycardia
Dermatologic: Concentrated solutions (>12%) can cause dermal burns
Endocrine & genitourinary: Hypokalemia
Gastrointestinal: Acute nausea, diarrhea, vomiting
Hematologic: Thrombocytopenia
Neuromuscular & skeletal: Myoclonus, peripheral (sensory) neuropathy
Respiratory: Pulmonary edema

Signs & Symptoms of Acute Overdose Myoglobinuria, rhabdomyolysis, elevated liver function tests, hypophosphatemia, miosis, tachycardia, myotonia is rare

Toxicodynamics/Kinetics

Absorption: Absorbed through skin/oral/inhalation routes
Distribution: V_d: 0.1 L/kg; 10 L/kg in overdose
Protein binding: Extensive
Half-life: 4-140 hours
Peak effect: 4-24 hours
Elimination: Urine; does not bioaccumulate

Reference Range At an oral ingested dose of 5 mg/kg, peak plasma level was 35 mg/L at 24 hours; plasma levels >100 mg/L associated with coma
Minimum lethal dose: 80 mg/kg

Overdosage Treatment

Decontamination: Irrigate with saline; lavage/activated charcoal with cathartic for ingestions exceeding 400 mg/kg

Supportive therapy: Hypotension can be treated with 10-20 mL/kg of isotonic saline and Trendelenburg positioning; dopamine or norepinephrine can be used; quinidine may be helpful for cardiac arrhythmias

Enhancement of elimination: Alkaline diuresis for patients with metabolic acidosis, mental status changes, or a serum level >500 mg/L; keep urine pH between 7.6-8.8; furosemide can be given to maintain diuresis

(Continued)

2,4-D *(Continued)*

Pregnancy Implications Teratogenic

Additional Information Slight phenol odor when heated; does not contain tetrachlorodibenzoparadioxin (TCDD); does not accumulate in food chain

Specific References

Berwick P, "2,4-Dichlorophenoxyacetic Acid Poisoning in Man," *JAMA*, 1970, 214(6):1114-7.

Kancir CB, Andersen C, and Olesen AS, "Marked Hypocalcemia in a Fatal Poisoning With Chlorinated Phenoxy Acid Derivatives," *J Toxicol Clin Toxicol*, 1988, 26(3-4):257-64.

Oliveira GH and Palermo-Neto J, "Toxicology of 2,4-Dichlorophenoxyacetic Acid (2,4-D) and its Determination in Serum and Brain Tissue Using Gas Chromatography-Electron Capture Detection," *J Anal Toxicol*, 1995, 19:251-5.

Paulino CA and Palermo-Neto J, "Effects of Acute 2,4-Dichlorophenoxyacetic Acid on Cattle Serum Components and Enzyme Activities," *Vet Hum Toxicol*, 1995, 37(4):329-32.

Smith RA and Lewis D, "Suicide by Ingestion of 2,4-D: A Case History Demonstrating the Prudence of Using GC/MS as an Investigative Rather Than Confirmatory Tool," *Vet Hum Toxicol*, 1987, 29(3):259-61.

DAC *see* 4,4'-Methylenebis (2-Chloroaniline) *on page 965*

DACPM *see* 4,4'-Methylenebis (2-Chloroaniline) *on page 965*

Dalf® *see* Methyl Parathion *on page 969*

Dalmation-Insect Flowers *see* Pyrethrins *on page 1003*

Dalmation-Insect Powder *see* Pyrethrins *on page 1003*

Dansit® *see* Fensulfothion *on page 928*

DBCP *see* 1,2-Dibromo-3-Chloropropane *on page 906*

DBP *see* Di-n-Butyl Phthalate *on page 914*

DCE *see* Ethylene Dichloride *on page 924*

1,1 DCE *see* 1,1-Dichloroethene *on page 907*

1,2 DCE *see* Acetylene Dichloride *on page 851*

d-Con® *see* Anticoagulant Rodenticide *on page 859*

2,4-DCP *see* 2,4-Dichlorophenol *on page 908*

DD-92 *see* 1,3-Dichloropropene *on page 909*

DDD

Related Information

DDT *on next page*

Organochlorines *on page 983*

CAS Number 72-54-8

Synonyms 1,1-Bis(4-Chlorophenyl)-2; 2-Dichloroethane; TDE

Brand Names Dilene®; Rothane®

Use Primarily as a pesticide; one form (ortho, para DDD) was used as a medicinal agent for the treatment of adrenal gland carcinoma

Mechanism of Toxic Action Organochlorine agent, interferes with sodium, potassium, and calcium ion movement along neuronal membranes; may be related to serotonin deficiency in the brain

Adverse Reactions Not well described in humans, but probably very similar to DDT; nervous system would appear to be target organ

Toxicodynamics/Kinetics

Absorption: Inhalation, oral, and dermal

Metabolism: Hepatic to 1,1-bis(parachlorophenyl) ethane (DDNU)

Elimination: Renal

Overdosage Treatment

Decontamination:

- Dermal: Wash with soap and water
- Ocular: Irrigate copiously with saline
- Oral: Do not induce emesis; lavage (with water or mannitol)/activated charcoal is effective; do not use an oil-based cathartic in that absorption may increase

Supportive therapy: Seizures may be treated with a benzodiazepine, phenobarbital, or phenytoin

Enhancement of elimination: Multiple dosing of activated charcoal or cholestyramine (4 g every 8 hours) may be effective after recent oral exposure

Additional Information Metabolite of DDT; degrades slowly by solar radiation in the atmosphere to carbon dioxide and hydrochloric acid

Specific References

U.S. Department of Health and Human Services, "Toxicological Profile for 4,4'DDT, 4,4'-DDE, 4,4' DDD TP-93/05," Agency for Toxic Substances and Diseases Registry, May, 1994.

DDM *see* Methylene Dianiline *on page 966*

DDT

Related Information

DDD *on previous page*
Organochlorines *on page 983*
Toxins Which Should be Lavaged With Solutions Other Than Water *on page 1635*

CAS Number 50-29-3

UN Number 2761

Synonyms 4,4' DDT; Dichlorodiphenyltrichloroethane

Brand Names Anofex®; Chlorophenothane®; Detoxan®; Dicophane®; Genitox®; Pentachlorin®

Use Primarily as an insecticide on cotton, peanut, and soybean crops; not imported into the U.S. since 1972; contaminant of dicofol

Mechanism of Toxic Action Organochlorine agent, interferes with sodium, potassium, and calcium ion movement along neuronal membranes; may be related to serotonin deficiency in the brain; estrogenic action has been described

Adverse Reactions

Cardiovascular: Tachycardia
Central nervous system: Headache, dizziness
Gastrointestinal: Nausea noted at oral doses of 6 mg/kg; vomiting noted at a dose of 10 mg/kg while seizures can occur at oral doses >16 mg/kg
Hepatic: Elevation of liver enzymes can occur
Neuromuscular & skeletal: Tremors
Miscellaneous: Stomatitis, opsoclonus, hypomagnesemia; sclerodermatous changes on hands have been described; sweating; myoclonus

Toxicodynamics/Kinetics

Absorption: Through inhalation, oral, and dermal exposure
Distribution: Concentrated in fat
Metabolism: Hepatic to 2,2-bis(parachlorophenyl) acetic acid (DDA)
Elimination: Urine (feces at high doses)

Reference Range DDT blood levels in asymptomatic individuals not occupationally exposed to DDT was <15 μg/L (0.04 μmol/L); in those individuals occupationally exposed, average blood DDT level was 57 μg/L (0.16 μmol/L); average daily intake of 18 mg by occupational exposure results in DDA urine levels of ~1.27 mg/L (3.59 μmol/L)

Overdosage Treatment

Decontamination:
- Dermal: Wash with soap and water
- Ocular: Irrigate copiously with saline
- Oral: Do not induce emesis; lavage (with water or mannitol)/activated charcoal is effective; do not use an oil-based cathartic in that absorption may increase

Supportive therapy: Seizures may be treated with a benzodiazepine, phenobarbital, or phenytoin
Enhancement of elimination: Multiple dosing of activated charcoal or cholestyramine (4 g every 8 hours) may be effective after recent oral exposure

Additional Information Carcinogenic in animals (primarily liver)

Atmospheric half-life: 2 days (to carbon dioxide and hydrochloric acid)
Soil half-life: 2-15 years
Estimated dietary intake of DDT in the U.S. (per person)
- 1970: 240 mcg
- 1974: 8 mcg
- 1980: 2.4 mcg
- 1981: 2.2 mcg

Acceptable daily DDT intake established by WHO: 20 mcg/kg; root and leafy vegetables have highest amount of DDT (0.4-0.6 ppb)
PEL-TWA (skin designation): 1 mg/m^3
TLV-TWA: 1 mg/m^3

Specific References

U.S. Department of Health and Human Services, "Toxicological Profile for 4,4'DDT, 4,4'-DDE, 4,4' DDD TP-93/05," Agency for Toxic Substances and Diseases Registry, May, 1994.

4,4' DDT *see* DDT *on this page*

Decachloroketone *see* Chlordecone *on page 886*

Dechlorane® 4070 *see* Mirex *on page 971*

DEET *see* Diethyltoluamide *on page 912*

De-fol-ate *see* Chlorate Salts *on page 884*

Delac J® *see* N-Nitrosodiphenylamine *on page 982*

Delicia *see* Phosphine *on page 993*

Delicia® *see* Aluminum Phosphide *on page 857*

Delnatex® *see* Dioxathion *on page 916*

Delnav® *see* Dioxathion *on page 916*

Delta-keto® 153 *see* Endrin *on page 922*

Deltic® *see* Dioxathion *on page 916*

DEP *see* Diethyl Phthalate *on page 912*

Desolat *see* Chlorate Salts *on page 884*

Detal® *see* Dinitrocresol *on page 915*

Detia® *see* Aluminum Phosphide *on page 857*

Detia Gas EX-B *see* Phosphine *on page 993*

Detoxan® *see* DDT *on previous page*

Diamide *see* Hydrazine *on page 939*

Diamine *see* Hydrazine *on page 939*

Diazinon

CAS Number 333-41-5

UN Number 2783

Synonyms O,O-Diethyl O-2-Isopropyl-4-Methyl-6-Pyrimidinyl Thiophosphate

Brand Names Alfa-Tox®; Bazinon®; Diazol®; Gardentox®; Knox-Out®; Spectracide®

Use Marketed as insecticide granules, dusting agent, or spray liquid with or without petroleum derivative as a solvent

Mechanism of Toxic Action Irreversible inhibition of acetylcholinesterase and plasma cholinesterase, resulting in excess accumulation of acetylcholine at muscarinic and nicotinic receptors, and in the central nervous system

Adverse Reactions

Cardiovascular: Hyperdynamic (~18% to 21%) or hypodynamic (~7% to 10%) states, tachycardia, hypertension

Central nervous system: Depression, seizures, hyperactivity

Gastrointestinal: Pancreatitis (after ingestion of 1.5 mg/kg), diarrhea

Genitourinary: Incontinence

Neuromuscular & skeletal: Weakness, paralysis

Ocular: Miosis

Respiratory: Depression, edema

General: Flu-like symptoms (especially with chronic exposure), sweating, hypokalemia

Delayed: Muscle asthenia and paresthesia

Signs & Symptoms of Acute Overdose Miosis (unreactive to light), mydriasis (rarely), nystagmus, lacrimation, pallor, excessive sweating, confusion, dementia, agitation, headache, dysarthria, generalized asthenia, seizures, A-V block, coma, decreased hemoglobin/red blood cell count/platelet count, metabolic acidosis and hyperglycemia (severe intoxication), cranial nerve palsies, hypotension, hypertension, bradycardia, tachycardia, Q-T prolongation, heart block, asystole, salivation, bronchorrhea, tachypnea, pulmonary edema, respiratory depression, diaphragmatic paralysis, skeletal muscle fasciculation and flaccid paralysis, nausea, vomiting, abdominal pain, fecal and urinary incontinence; an "intermediate syndrome" of limb asthenia and respiratory paralysis has been reported to occur between 24 and 96 hours postorganophosphate exposure and is independent of the acute cholinergic crisis. Late paresthesia characterized by stocking and globe paresthesia, anesthesia and asthenia is infrequently observed weeks to months following acute exposure to certain organophosphates.

Toxicodynamics/Kinetics

Absorption: Readily through gastrointestinal (~85%), dermal (3% to 4%), or inhalation

Metabolism: Rapidly metabolized to weakly active compounds through hepatic hydrolysis and other pathways

Half-life: 15 hours

Elimination: Metabolites are excreted in urine

Warnings Significant dermal absorption may occur across intact skin; risk of aspiration pneumonitis exists following oral exposure to agents having a hydrocarbon vehicle; severe laryngeal irritation and violent coughing may result from exposure to dusting powders; exposure to dusting powders and insecticide granules may cause contact dermatitis

Reference Range Peak plasma diazinon levels in symptomatic patients (who survived) ranged from 0.1-1.7 mg/L

Mild poisoning: Serum cholinesterase is 20% to 50% of normal

Moderate poisoning: Serum cholinesterase is 10% to 20% of normal

Severe poisoning (respiratory distress and coma): Serum cholinesterase is <10%

Overdosage Treatment

Decontamination: Isolation, bagging, and disposal of all contaminated clothing and other articles; all emergency medical workers and hospital staff should follow appropriate precautions regarding exposure to hazardous material including the use of protective clothing, masks, goggles, and respiratory equipment. Gastric lavage with water, 5% sodium bicarbonate or 2% potassium permanganate can be considered within 1 hour of ingestion; do not use cathartic with activated charcoal.

Dermal: Prompt thorough scrubbing of all affected areas with soap and water, including hair and nails

Gastric: Activated charcoal can be administered either orally or via a nasogastric tube; do not induce emesis because of danger of sudden respiratory compromise, alterations in mental status, seizures, coma, and possible aspiration of hydrocarbon vehicles

Ocular: Irrigation with copious tepid sterile water or saline

Supportive therapy: Including airway management, ventilatory assistance, humidified oxygen administration, and close monitoring for sudden respiratory failure

Antidote:

Atropine: Administration should be guided by respiratory status, starting at 1-5 mg I.V. every 5-10 minutes as needed, and should be titrated to the resolution of excess pulmonary secretions; frequent administration of large doses (cumulative doses >100 mg) may be necessary in massive exposures

Glycopyrrolate: May be administered if atropine is unavailable

2-PAM: For more significant exposures (ie, exposures requiring large doses of atropine, or with recurring symptoms, or exposures to more lipid soluble agents), administration should follow: 1-2 g I.V. over 5-10 minutes, repeated in 1 hour if asthenia reoccurs, then every 4-12 hours for recurring symptoms

Enhancement of elimination: Dialysis and hemoperfusion are not indicated due to effectiveness of the prescribed treatment, large volumes of distribution of organophosphates

Antidote(s)

Atropine Sulfate *on page 1395*

Pralidoxime Chloride *on page 1461*

Diagnostic Tests/Procedures

Blood Gases, Arterial *on page 1207*

Chest Films *on page 1224*

Complete Blood Count *on page 1236*

Creatinine, Serum *on page 1243*

Electrocardiography *on page 1253*

Liver Profile *on page 1286*

Pseudocholinesterase, Serum *on page 1340*

Pregnancy Implications Human data regarding organophosphate exposure in pregnancy is limited and anecdotal; teratogenesis and fetal death have been produced in animal models at exposure levels that cause obvious toxicity to the pregnant animal; diazinon has demonstrated significant teratogenicity in an avian embryo model

Additional Information Yellow to brown liquid; vapor pressure of 0.00014 mm Hg at 20°C; thermal breakdown products include nitrogen and sulfur oxides; red blood cell cholinesterase and serum pseudocholinesterase may be depressed following acute or chronic organophosphate exposure; RBC cholinesterase is typically not analyzed by in-house laboratories, and is usually not available for consideration during acute management. Pseudocholinesterase levels may be rapidly available from some in-house laboratories, but are not as reliable a marker of organophosphate exposure because of variability secondary to variant genotypes, hepatic disease, oral estrogen use, or malnutrition. Because of this variability, true indication of suppression of either of these enzymes can only be estimated through comparison to pre-exposure values; these enzymes may be useful in measuring a patient's recovery postexposure, especially if the recovery is not progressing as expected.

ACGIH TLV: 0.1 mg/m^3

PEL-TWA: 0.1 mg/m^3

Water solubility: 40 ppm

Water half-life: 3 days to 7.7 weeks (shorter in acidic conditions)

Mean atmospheric diazinon levels in urban areas: 2.1 ng/m^3

Oral ingestion of 294 mg/kg of a 10% diazinon formulation associated with fatality; diazinon may prolong the effects of succinylcholine

Other information concerning pesticide exposures is available through the EPA-funded National Pesticide Telecommunications Network: 1-800-858-7378 (weekdays, 8 AM to 6 PM, Central Standard time)

Specific References

Martinez-Chuecos J, Del Carmen Jurado M, Gimenez MP, et al, "Experience With Hemoperfusion for Organophosphate Poisoning," *Med Toxicol Adverse Drug Exp*, 1988, 3(5):350-75.

Minton NA and Murray VS, "A Review of Organophosphate Poisoning," *Med Toxicol Adverse Drug Exp*, 1988, 3(5):350-75.

Namba T, Nolte CT, Jackrel J, et al, "Poisoning Due to Organophosphate Insecticides. Acute and Chronic Manifestations," *Am J Med*, 1971, 50(4):475-92.

(Continued)

Diazinon *(Continued)*

Poklis A, Kutz FW, Sperling JF, et al, "A Fatal Diazinon Poisoning," *Forensic Sci Int*, 1980, 15(2):135-40.

Diazol® *see* Diazinon *on page 904*

Dibenz[*a,h*]anthracene *see* Polycyclic Aromatic Hydrocarbons *on page 997*

Dibenzo-p-Dioxins *see* Polychlorinated Dibenzofurans *on page 996*

Dibenzoyl Peroxide

CAS Number 94-36-0

UN Number 2085; 2086; 2087; 2088; 2089; 2090

Synonyms Benzoyl Peroxide; Lucidol

Use In concentrations of 5% to 10% topically for the treatment of acne, ulcers, bed sores, and pyoderma gangrenosum

Mechanism of Toxic Action Allergen for skin sensitization, enhances platelet aggregation

Adverse Reactions Miscellaneous: Irritation of nose, throat, eyes, and skin; may be a tumor promoter; can cause platelet aggregation (vitamin E may be of some use in preventing platelet aggregation)

Signs & Symptoms of Acute Overdose Erythema, edema of skin, conjunctivitis

Toxicodynamics/Kinetics

Absorption: Not well absorbed

Elimination: Metabolized to and excreted as benzoic acid (95%)

Overdosage Treatment

Decontamination:

- Oral: Irrigation with 4-8 oz of milk or water
- Inhalation: Give 100% humidified oxygen
- Dermal: Irrigate with soap and water

Additional Information Odorless gas, flammable and explosive

TLV-TWA: 5 mg/m^3

IDLH: 1000 mg/m^3

PEL-TWA: 5 mg/m^3

Specific References

Bonnekoh B and Merk HF, "Airborne Allergic Contact Dermatitis From Benzoyl Peroxide as a Bleaching Agent of Candle Wax," *Contact Dermatitis*, 1991, 24(5):367-8.

Gwebu ET, Holness P, Coopwood R, et al, "Benzoyl Peroxide, A Potent Human Platelet Aggregating Agent," *Cent Afr J Med*, 1983, 29(9):178-80.

Hogan DJ, "Benzoyl Peroxide. Carcinogenicity and Allergenicity," *Int J Dermatol*, 1991, 30(7):467-70.

Yeung D, Nacht S, Bucks D, et al, "Benzoyl Peroxide: Percutaneous Penetration and Metabolic Disposition. II. Effect of Concentration," *J Am Acad Dermatol*, 1983, 9(6):920-4.

1,2-Dibromo-3-Chloropropane

CAS Number 96-12-8

UN Number 2872

Synonyms BBC12; DBCP

Brand Names Fumagon®; Fumazone®; Nemafume®; Nemagon®; Nemapax®; Nemazon®

Use Soil fumigant and nematocide to protect field crops; also used as an intermediate in organic chemical synthesis; was the preferred fumigant for pineapples in Hawaii, although this practice was stopped by the EPA in 1985

Mechanism of Toxic Action Possibly inhibits carbohydrate metabolism of sperm at the level of nicotinamide adenine dinucleotide dehydrogenase

Adverse Reactions

Endocrine: Decreased; spermatogenesis preponderate of female offspring to male workers

Ocular: Irritant

Respiratory: Pulmonary edema

Signs & Symptoms of Acute Overdose Eye irritation, nausea, headache, azoospermia, lightheadedness, epigastric pain

Toxicodynamics/Kinetics

Absorption: Can be absorbed by dermal, gastrointestinal, or inhalation

Elimination: Inhalation: Feces (14%)

Overdosage Treatment

Decontamination:

- Dermal: Wash with soap and water
- Ocular: Irrigate with saline
- Oral: Dilute with milk or water; do not induce emesis; activated charcoal may be useful

Additional Information FSH and LH elevations may occur; pungent odor

TLV: 0.01 ppm

Taste threshold: 0.01 mg/L

Specific References

U.S. Department of Health and Human Services, "Toxicological Profile for 1,2-Dibromo-3-Chloropropane TP-91/12," Agency for Toxic Substances and Diseases Registry, September, 1992.

Dibromochloromethane

Related Information

Bromoform *on page 872*

CAS Number 124-48-1

Synonyms Chlorodibromomethane

Use Inadvertently generated during water chlorination process (usually <5 mcg/L; median: 1.2 mcg/L)

Mechanism of Toxic Action CNS depressant

Adverse Reactions No human data; hepatotoxic (centrilobular necrosis) in animal models; a central nervous system depressant with little long lasting behavioral effect

Toxicodynamics/Kinetics

Absorption: Absorbed by inhalation and oral routes

Metabolism: Hepatic oxidation

Elimination: Pulmonary

Overdosage Treatment

Decontamination (oral overdose): Lavage/activated charcoal

Supportive therapy: Although human overdose experience is virtually nonexistent over the past 90 years, respiratory support appears to be a crucial modality; naloxone may be of some benefit; otherwise would treat as for bromides

Additional Information Not flammable; a colorless to pale yellow liquid;

Mean ambient air chlorodibromomethane urban values: 3.8 ppt

Average daily dose: <1 mcg/kg

PEL-TWA: 0.5 ppm

Specific References

U.S. Department of Health and Human Services, "Toxicological Profile for Bromoform/Chlorodibromomethane TP-90/05," Agency for Toxic Substances and Diseases Registry, December 1990.

Dibromoethane *see* Ethylene Bromide *on page 924*

1,2-Dibromoethane *see* Ethylene Bromide *on page 924*

Dibutyl Ester *see* Di-n-Butyl Phthalate *on page 914*

Dichlone *see* Dichloronaphthoquinone *on next page*

Dichloricide *see* Para-Dichlorobenzene *on page 985*

1,4-Dichlorobenzene *see* Para-Dichlorobenzene *on page 985*

Dichlorodifluoromethane *see* Freon *on page 932*

Dichlorodiphenyltrichloroethane *see* DDT *on page 903*

2-Dichloroethane *see* DDD *on page 902*

1,1-Dichloroethene

CAS Number 75-35-4

UN Number 1303

Synonyms 1,1 DCE; VCD; Vinylidene Chloride

Use Chemical intermediate in polyvinylidene chloride production; found in food wraps and other packaging materials; also as a coating for steel pipes, retardant coating in carpet backing, and adhesives

Mechanism of Toxic Action Mucosal irritant and CNS depressant

Adverse Reactions

Central nervous system: Narcosis, cranial nerve palsies

Dermal: Leucoderma

Hepatic: Elevation of liver enzymes

Ocular: Irritant

Signs & Symptoms of Acute Overdose Lethargy

Toxicodynamics/Kinetics

Metabolism: By way of oxidation

Elimination: Renal

Overdosage Treatment

Decontamination: Do not induce emesis; lavage/activated charcoal; dilute with water or milk

Enhancement of elimination: Forced diuresis may be beneficial (although there is no human data)

Pregnancy Implications Possible association with neural tube defects though ingestion of contaminated water

(Continued)

1,1-Dichloroethene *(Continued)*

Additional Information Levels of 4000 ppm associated with narcosis; possible increased toxicity with acetaminophen, ethanol, or phenobarbital

TLV-TWA: 5 ppm

Specific References

Chivers CP, "Two Cases of Occupational Leucoderma Following Contact With Hydroquinone Monomethyl Ether," *Br J Ind Med*, 1972, 29(1):105-7.

D'Souza RW and Andersen ME, "Physiologically Based Pharmacokinetic Model for Vinylidene Chloride," *Toxicol Appl Pharmacol*, 1988, 95(2):230-40.

Haley TJ, "Vinylidene Chloride: A Review of the Literature," *Clin Toxicol*, 1975, 8(6):633-43.

1,2-Dichloroethene *see* Acetylene Dichloride *on page 851*

Dichloromethane *see* Methylene Chloride *on page 966*

Dichloronaphthoquinone

CAS Number 117-80-6

Synonyms Dichlone; Quintar; Sanquinon

Brand Names Algistat®; Compound 605®; Phygon®

Use Vegetable seed disinfectant; foliage/textile fungicide; aquatic herbicide

Adverse Reactions

Dermatologic: Skin irritation

Gastrointestinal: Nausea, vomiting

Ocular: Conjunctivitis

Signs & Symptoms of Acute Overdose Coma, emesis

Toxicodynamics/Kinetics Absorption: Poor from gastrointestinal tract

Overdosage Treatment

Decontamination: Lavage/charcoal; irrigate skin with soap and water; irrigate eyes with saline with a Morgan lens

Supportive therapy: Endoscopy for oral ingestion to evaluate gastrointestinal mucosal injury

Additional Information Heating dichloronaphthoquinone can emit chloride fumes

Specific References

Pritsos CH, Pisani DE, and Pardini RS, "Inhibition of Liver Glycolysis in Rats by Dietary Dichlone (2,3-dichloro-1,4-naphthoquinone)," *Bull Environ Contam Toxicol*, 1985, 35(1):23-8.

2,4-Dichlorophenol

CAS Number 120-83-2

UN Number 2020

Synonyms 2,4-DCP; 4,6-Dichlorophenol

Use Intermediate in production of 2,4-dichlorophenoxy acetic acid (2,4-D), bifenox, and dichloroprop herbicides; also used in production of pentachlorophenol and other disinfectants, fungicides, bactericides, and antiseptics; a waterborne contaminant of the kraft pulping process

Mechanism of Toxic Action Interferes with cell division by disrupting spindle formation and interfering with oxidative phosphorylation

Adverse Reactions

Dermal: Chloracne, hyperpigmentation, hirsutism, cutanea tarda

Miscellaneous: Porphyria

Toxicodynamics/Kinetics

Absorption: Dermally and orally

Half-life: ~10 minutes

Overdosage Treatment

Decontamination:

- Dermal: Wash with soap and water
- Inhalation: Give 100% humidified oxygen
- Ocular: Irrigate with saline
- Oral: Do not induce emesis; lavage/activated charcoal

Diagnostic Tests/Procedures

Liver Profile *on page 1286*

Additional Information Human exposure may occur from drinking contaminated water; half-life in water: 62 hours at a pH of 8 with a mean concentration of 0.2 mcg/L; combustion products can contain hydrochloric acid

Average daily intake of 2,3-dichlorophenol: ~0.4 mcg

Taste threshold (medicinal): ~2-8 mcg/L

Odor threshold in water: 0.0003 to 0.04 mg/L

Specific References

U.S. Department of Health and Human Services, "Toxicological Prodile for 2,4-Dichlorophenol TP-91/14," Agency for Toxic Substances and Diseases Registry, July, 1992.

4,6-Dichlorophenol *see* 2,4-Dichlorophenol *on this page*

2,4-Dichlorophenoxyacetic Acid *see* 2,4-D *on page 901*

1,3-Dichloropropene

CAS Number 542-75-6; 10061-01-5 (cis); 10061-02-6 (trans)

Synonyms 1,3-Dichloropropylene

Brand Names DD-92; Telone®; Terr-o-cide® 15-D; Terr-O-Gas® 57/43T

Use Soil fumigant for nematodes used primarily on soil of vegetable or tobacco crops (preplanting); also used as a solvent

Mechanism of Toxic Action Mucous membrane irritant; chemical structure is similar to vinyl chloride

Adverse Reactions

Dermatologic: Skin vesicant; delayed hypersensitivity

Respiratory: Respiratory irritant

Signs & Symptoms of Acute Overdose Pruritus (dermal contact), dyspnea, headache, dizziness, nausea, vomiting, malaise, cough, neck pain, pleuritic chest pain, diarrhea, metabolic acidosis, pancreatitis, hypotension

Toxicodynamics/Kinetics

Absorbed by inhalation and/or dermal exposure

Metabolism: Hepatic to an N-acetyl cysteine conjugate through glutathione pathway

Reference Range Excretion of n-acetyl glucosaminidase (NAG) >1.5 mg/day is considered elevated

Overdosage Treatment

Decontamination:

Dermal: Wash with soap and water

Ocular: Irrigate with normal saline

Gastric: Do not induce emesis; dilute with milk or water; lavage/activated charcoal

Additional Information Possible association with development of histiocytic lymphoma and acute myelomonocytic leukemia; lung tumors noted in rodents; penetrates rubber protective gear

PEL-TWA (skin): 1 ppm

TWA-TLV: 1 ppm

Odor threshold: 1-3 ppm (garlic-like)

Specific References

Hernandez AF, Martin-Rubi JC, Ballestros JL, et al, "Clinical and Pathological Findings in Fatal 1,3-Dichloropropene Intoxication," *Hum Exp Toxicol*, 1994, 13(5):303-6.

Markovitz A and Crosby WH, "Chemical Carcinogenesis. A Soil Fumigant, 1,3-Dichloropropene, as Possible Cause of Hematologic Malignancies," *Arch Intern Med*, 1984, 144(7):1409-11.

Osterloh JD, Wang R, Schneider F, et al, "Biological Monitoring of Dichloropropene: Air Concentrations, Urinary Metabolite and Renal Enzyme Excretion," *Arch Environ Health*, 1989, 44(4):207-13.

U.S. Department of Human Services, "Toxicological Profile for 1,3-Dichloropropene TP-91/15," Agency for Toxic Substances and Diseases Registry, September, 1992.

1,3-Dichloropropylene *see* 1,3-Dichloropropene *on this page*

Dicophane® *see* DDT *on page 903*

Dicrotophos

CAS Number 141-66-2

Synonyms Dimethyl Cis-2-Dimethylcarbamoyl-1-Methylvinyl Phosphate

Brand Names Bidrin®; Ektofos®

Use Marketed as insecticide granules, dusting agent, or spray liquid with or without petroleum derivative as a solvent

Mechanism of Toxic Action Potent, irreversible inhibition of acetylcholinesterase and plasma cholinesterase, resulting in excess accumulation of acetylcholine at muscarinic and nicotinic receptors, and in the central nervous system

Adverse Reactions

Cardiovascular: Hyperdynamic (~18% to 21%) or hypodynamic (~7% to 10%) states

Central nervous system: Depression, seizures, hyperactivity

Genitourinary: Incontinence

Neuromuscular & skeletal: Weakness, paralysis

Respiratory: Depression, edema

General: Flu-like symptoms (especially with chronic exposure)

Delayed: Muscle asthenia and paresthesia

Signs & Symptoms of Acute Overdose Miosis (unreactive to light), mydriasis (rarely), lacrimation, pallor, excessive sweating, confusion, agitation, headache, dysarthria, generalized asthenia, seizures, coma, cranial nerve palsies, decreased hemoglobin/red blood cell count/platelet count, metabolic acidosis and hyperglycemia (severe intoxication), A-V block, hypotension, hypertension, bradycardia, tachycardia, Q-T prolongation, heart block, asystole, salivation, bronchorrhea, tachypnea, pulmonary edema, respiratory depression, diaphragmatic paralysis, skeletal muscle fasciculation and flaccid paralysis, nausea, vomiting, abdominal pain, fecal and urinary incontinence; an "intermediate syndrome" of limb asthenia

(Continued)

Dicrotophos *(Continued)*

and respiratory paralysis has been reported to occur between 24 and 96 hours postorganophosphate exposure, and is independent of the acute cholinergic crisis; late paresthesia characterized by stocking and glove paresthesia, anesthesia, and asthenia is infrequently observed weeks to months following acute exposure to certain organophosphates

Toxicodynamics/Kinetics

Absorption: Readily through oral, dermal, or respiratory exposure

Metabolism: Rapidly metabolized to weakly active compounds through hepatic hydrolysis and other pathways

Elimination: Metabolites are excreted in urine

Warnings Significant absorption through intact skin may occur; risk of aspiration pneumonitis exists with agents having a hydrocarbon vehicle; severe laryngeal irritation and violent coughing may result from exposure to dusting powders; exposure to dusting powders and insecticide granules may cause contact dermatitis

Overdosage Treatment

Decontamination: Isolation, bagging, and disposal of all contaminated clothing and other articles; all emergency medical workers and hospital staff should follow appropriate precautions regarding exposure to hazardous material including the use of protective clothing, masks, goggles, and respiratory equipment

- Dermal: Prompt thorough scrubbing of all affected areas with soap and water, including hair and nails
- Gastric: Activated charcoal can be administered either orally or via a nasogastric tube; do not induce emesis because of danger of sudden respiratory compromise, alterations in mental status, seizures, coma, and possible aspiration of hydrocarbon vehicles
- Ocular: Irrigation with copious tepid sterile water or saline

Supportive therapy: Including airway management, ventilatory assistance, humidified oxygen administration, and close monitoring for sudden respiratory failure

Enhancement of elimination: Dialysis and hemoperfusion are not indicated due to effectiveness of the prescribed treatment, large volumes of distribution of organophosphates

Antidote:

- Atropine: Administration should be guided by respiratory status, starting at 1-5 mg I.V. every 5-10 minutes as needed, and should be titrated to the resolution of excess pulmonary secretions; frequent administration of large doses (cumulative doses >100 mg) may be necessary in massive exposures
- Glycopyrrolate: May be administered if atropine is unavailable
- 2-PAM: For more significant exposures (ie, exposures requiring large doses of atropine, or with recurring symptoms, or exposures to more lipid soluble agents), administration should follow: 1-2 g I.V. over 5-10 minutes, repeated in 1 hour if asthenia reoccurs, then every 4-12 hours for recurring symptoms

Antidote(s)

Atropine Sulfate *on page 1395*

Pralidoxime Chloride *on page 1461*

Diagnostic Tests/Procedures

Blood Gases, Arterial *on page 1207*

Chest Films *on page 1224*

Complete Blood Count *on page 1236*

Creatinine, Serum *on page 1243*

Electrocardiography *on page 1253*

Liver Profile *on page 1286*

Pseudocholinesterase, Serum *on page 1340*

Pregnancy Implications Human data regarding organophosphate exposure in pregnancy is limited and anecdotal; teratogenesis and fetal death have been produced in animal models at exposure levels that cause obvious toxicity to the pregnant animal; dicrotophos has demonstrated significant teratogenicity in an avian embryo model

Additional Information Brown liquid with mild ester odor; red blood cell cholinesterase, and serum pseudocholinesterase may be depressed following acute or chronic organophosphate exposure; RBC cholinesterase is typically not analyzed by in-house laboratories, and is usually not available for consideration during acute management. Pseudocholinesterase levels may be rapidly available from some in-house laboratories, but are not as reliable a marker of organophosphate exposure because of variability secondary to variant genotypes, hepatic disease, oral estrogen use, or malnutrition. Because of this variability, true indication of suppression of either of these enzymes can only be estimated through comparison to pre-exposure values; these enzymes may be useful in measuring a patient's recovery postexposure, especially if the recovery is not progressing as expected.

ACGIH TLV: 0.25 mg/m^3

PEL-TWA: 0.25 mg/m^3

Other information concerning pesticide exposures is available through the EPA-funded National Pesticide Telecommunications Network: 1-800-858-7378 (weekdays, 8 AM to 6 PM, Central Standard time)

Specific References

Minton NA and Murray VS, "A Review of Organophosphate Poisoning," *Med Toxicol Adverse Drug Exp*, 1988, 3(5):350-75.

Namba T, Nolte CT, Jackrel J, et al, "Poisoning Due to Organophosphate Insecticides. Acute and Chronic Manifestations," *Am J Med*, 1971, 50(4):475-92.

Dieldrin

Related Information

Aldrin *on page 856*

Organochlorines *on page 983*

CAS Number 60-57-1

Synonyms HEOD

Brand Names Alvit®; Dieldrix®; Octalox®; Quintox®; Red Shield®

Use Termiticide; banned by EPA in 1970s

Mechanism of Toxic Action Organochlorine agent which may be a competitive inhibitor of the inhibitory neurotransmitter GABA at the GABA A receptor

Adverse Reactions

Cardiovascular: Tachycardia, hypertension

Central nervous system: Convulsions, headache, dizziness

Gastrointestinal: Nausea, vomiting, anorexia

Hepatic: Elevation of liver enzymes

Neuromuscular & skeletal: Muscle twitching

Ocular: Nystagmus

Miscellaneous: May increase serum cholesterol levels, contact dermatitis, hemolysis

Toxicodynamics/Kinetics

Absorption: Absorbed by oral and dermal routes

Distribution: V_d: 13-69 L/kg

Metabolism: By epoxide hydrase to 6,7-trans-dihydroxydihydroaldrin glucuronide; aldrin dicarboxylic acid; also metabolized to pentachloroketone (Klein's metabolite) and 9-hydroxydieldrin glucuronide

Half-life: 2-12 months

Elimination: Feces

Overdosage Treatment

Decontamination:

Dermal: Soap and water wash

Ocular: Irrigate with saline

Oral: Activated charcoal with cathartic

Supportive therapy: Beta-adrenergic blocking agents may be used for tachycardia or hypertension; benzodiazepines, phenobarbital, or phenytoin can be used for seizures

Enhancement of elimination: Multiple dosing of activated charcoal may be effective

Additional Information Highest amount of dietary intake is in garden fruits (0.0021 mcg/day) and fish, poultry, and meat (0.0012 mcg/day)

Oral lethal dose: 71 mg/kg

Odor threshold: 0.047 mg/kg

Estimated atmospheric lifetime: 1 day

Specific References

Mossing ML, Redetzke KA, and Applegate HG, "Organochlorine Pesticides in Blood of Persons From El Paso, Texas," *J Environ Health*, 1985, 47:312-3.

U.S. Department of Health and Human Services, "Toxicological Profile in Aldrin/Dieldrin, TP-92/01," Agency for Toxic Substances and Diseases Registry, April, 1993.

Dieldrix® *see* Dieldrin *on this page*

Diethylamide *see* Diethyltoluamide *on next page*

Diethylene Glycol

CAS Number 111-46-6

Synonyms Diglycol; Ethylene Diglycol; Glycol Ether

Commonly Found In Industrial solvents and antifreeze; softening agent in cellophane; in silver sulfadiazine

Mechanism of Toxic Action Central nervous system depression and nephrotoxicity with intravascular hemolysis, mechanism unknown

Adverse Reactions

Cardiovascular: Bradycardia

Hepatic: Hepatotoxicity

Renal: Renal tubular necrosis (acute); renal failure due to bilateral cortical necrosis

Signs & Symptoms of Acute Overdose Nausea, vomiting, headaches, severe abdominal pain, back pain, seizures, drowsiness; coma and pulmonary edema can develop, porphyria, feces discoloration (black), leukocytosis, jaundice, tachypnea, diarrhea; metabolic acidosis is less common than with ethylene glycol

(Continued)

Diethylene Glycol *(Continued)*

Toxicodynamics/Kinetics

Absorption: Small amount may be absorbed dermally; not absorbed by inhalation

Metabolism: Oxidized by alcohol dehydrogenase and aldehyde dehydrogenase to 2-hydroxyethoxy-acetaldehyde and then to 2-hydroxy-ethoxyacetic acid (2-HEAA)

Half-life: 3 hours

Elimination: 70% excreted unchanged; major metabolite is (2-hydroxyethoxy) acetic acid

Overdosage Treatment

Decontamination: Do not induce emesis; lavage (within 2 hours/activated charcoal)

Supportive therapy: Ethanol therapy may be theoretically useful to block conversion to toxic metabolites, but there is not human experience; treat acidosis with I.V. sodium bicarbonate (1-2 mEq/kg)

Enhancement of elimination: Hemodialysis for severe metabolic disturbance or renal failure

Antidote(s)

Sodium Bicarbonate *on page 1467*

Diagnostic Tests/Procedures

Blood Gases, Arterial *on page 1207*

Kidney Profile *on page 1279*

Osmolality, Serum *on page 1310*

Protein, Quantitative, Urine *on page 1335*

White Blood Count *on page 1380*

Pregnancy Implications None known

Additional Information Can cause centrilobular necrosis of the liver; diethylene glycol is odorless but has a sweet taste; more toxic than ethylene glycol; radiopaque compound with rapid absorption

Lethal dose: 1 mL/kg

Specific References

Cantarell MC, Fort J, Camps J, et al, "Acute Intoxication Due to Topical Application of Diethylene Glycol," *Ann Intern Med*, 1987, 106(3):478-9.

Hanif M, Mobarak MR, Ronan A, et al, "Fatal Renal Failure Caused by Diethylene Glycol in Paracetamol Elixir: The Bangladesh Epidemic," *Br Med J*, 1995, 311:88-91.

Wilkinson DP, "Diethylene Glycol Poisoning," *Med J Aust*, 1967, 2:403-4.

Diethyl Phthalate

CAS Number 84-66-2

Synonyms DEP; Ethyl Phthalate

Brand Names Anozol®; Neantine®; Palatinol® A; Phthalol®; Placidol® E; Solvanol®

Use Plasticizer (photographic applications, toothbrushes, toys, tool handles) and in cosmetics (nail polish, hair spray, perfume, bath products)

Mechanism of Toxic Action Irritant

Adverse Reactions Dermatologic: Irritant, allergic contact dermatitis

Toxicodynamics/Kinetics

Absorption: Slightly through intact human skin

Overdosage Treatment

Decontamination:

- Dermal: Wash with soap and water
- Ocular: Irrigate copiously with water

Specific References

Vidovic R and Kansky A, "Contact Dermatitis in Workers Processing Polyvinyl Chloride Plastics," *Derm Beruf Umwelt*, 1985, 33(3):104-5.

Diethyltoluamide

CAS Number 134-62-3

Synonyms Benzamide; DEET; Diethylamide; M-delphene; M-det; M-deta; Metadelphene; 3-Methyl-N,N-Diethylbenzamide; MGK Diethyltoluamide; M-Toluamide; M-Toluic Acid Diethylamide; N,N-Diethyl-3-Methyl-Diethyl-M-Toluamide; N,N-Diethyl-M-Toluamide; N,N-Diethyl-M-Toluic Acid

Brand Names OFF®

Commonly Found In Some formulations use as vehicles ethyl and isopropyl alcohols and freon, which may contribute significantly to toxicity

Use Insect repellent against mosquitoes, ticks, fleas, leeches, blackflies; used since 1957

Adverse Reactions

Cardiovascular: Hypotension, bradycardia

Central nervous system: Psychosis, anaphylactic shock, seizures, coma, hypertonicity, drowsiness, headache, athetosis, mania, slurred speech, ataxia

Dermatologic: Urticaria, skin necrosis, bullous eruption

Gastrointestinal: Nausea, vomiting

Neuromuscular & skeletal: Tremors, myoclonus

Signs & Symptoms of Acute Overdose Coma and seizures may occur rapidly within 30-60 minutes after ingestion; hypotension, bradycardia, confusion, ataxia, hypertonicity, clonic jerking, coma, urticaria, seizures, abdominal pain, nausea, vomiting, toxic hepatitis, renal damage, skin irritation, contact rash, bullous eruption/skin necrosis, acute psychosis, cerebral edema, anaphylactic shock; burning sensation of eyes, lips, tongue, and mouth

Toxicodynamics/Kinetics

Onset of action: Oral: Rapid

Absorption:

Oral: Rapid

Topical: Within 6 hours

Distribution: Skin and fatty tissues retain DEET and its metabolites for 1-2 months after topical application and may act as reservoirs for DEET

Metabolism: Occurs in the liver by oxidative enzymes

Peak plasma concentration: 1 hour

Warnings Significant and severe toxicity has occurred following both dermal and oral exposures to large amounts of DEET

Reference Range DEET serum level 8 hours after dermal application: 0.3 mg/dL (0.016 mmol/L) in asymptomatic patient; serum concentration of DEET of 63 mg/L associated with hypotension, lethargy, and EKG changes (S-T abnormalities); serum DEET level of 239 mg/L associated with fatality

Overdosage Treatment

Decontamination: Syrup of ipecac/emesis is contraindicated following oral ingestions due to rapid onset of coma and seizures; cautious gastric lavage followed by activated charcoal/cathartic

Supportive therapy: Diazepam or lorazepam for seizures; phenobarbital for recurrent seizures; for dermal exposures, wash twice with copious amounts of soap and water, preferably using alcohol-detergent solutions such as "green soap". If irritation or pain persists after washing, consult physician to examine affected area. For eye exposure, irrigate with copious amounts of tepid water for at least 15 minutes; patients should seek medical advice if irritation, pain, swelling, lacrimation, or photophobia persists.

Enhancement of elimination: Lipid based hemodialysis may be helpful although there is no data on this modality

Monitoring Parameters Monitor for renal and hepatic dysfunction with chronic oral and dermal exposures; consider CT and LP to rule out other causes for neurologic effects; sterile CSF pleocytosis, usually with lymphocytic predominance, has been associated with DEET

Additional Information Severe toxicity occurred in a child 1 year of age following oral ingestion of 25 mL of 50% DEET. Severe toxicity and death occurred following oral ingestion of 50 mL of 100% DEET in adolescents or adults. Extensive daily dermal applications of 10% to 15% solutions for 2 days to 3 months have resulted in encephalopathy in children.

National DEET Registry (Pegus Research, Inc), Salt Lake City, UT, (800)-949-0089

Specific References

Clem JR, Havemann DF, and Raebel MA, "Insect Repellent (N,N-Diethyl-m-toluamide) Cardiovascular Toxicity in an Adult," *Ann Pharmacother*, 1993, 27(3):289-93.

Fraser AD, MacNeil A, Theriault M, et al, "Analysis of Diethyltoluamide (DEET) Following Intentional Oral Ingestion of Muscol®," *J Anal Toxicol*, 1995, 19:197-9.

Lipscomb JW, Kramer JE, Leikin JB, "Seizure Following Brief Exposure to the Insect Repellent N,N-diethyl-m-toluamide," *Ann Emerg Med*, 1992, 21(3):315-7.

Miller JD, "Anaphylaxis Associated With Insect Repellent," *N Engl J Med*, 1982, 307(21):1341-2.

National DEET Registry (Pegus Research, Inc): Salt Lake City, UT, 800-949-0089

Tenenbein M, "Severe Toxic Reactions and Death Following the Ingestion of Diethyltoluamide-Containing Insect Repellents," *JAMA*, 1987, 258(11):1509-11.

Difenacoum *see* Anticoagulant Rodenticide *on page 859*

Diglycol *see* Diethylene Glycol *on page 911*

Dihydroacenapthylene *see* Polycyclic Aromatic Hydrocarbons *on page 997*

Dihydrooxirene *see* Ethylene Oxide *on page 927*

Dilene® *see* DDD *on page 902*

Dimax® *see* Disulfoton *on page 919*

1,1'-Dimethyl-4,4'-Dipyridilium Ion *see* Paraquat *on page 987*

3,5-Dimethyl-4-Methylthiophenyl N-Methylcarbamate *see* Methiocarb *on page 961*

Dimethylane Oxide *see* Ethylene Oxide *on page 927*

Dimethyl Benzene *see* Xylene *on page 1040*

Dimethyl Carbinol *see* Isopropyl Alcohol *on page 943*

Dimethyl Cis-2-Dimethylcarbamoyl-1-Methylvinyl Phosphate *see* Dicrotophos *on page 909*

Dimethyl Formaldehyde *see* Acetone *on page 850*

Dimethyl Ketone *see* Acetone *on page 850*

Dimethylmethane *see* Propane *on page 999*

Dimethyl Viologen *see* Paraquat *on page 987*

Di-n-Butyl Phthalate

CAS Number 84-74-2

UN Number 9095

Synonyms Butylphthalate; DBP; Dibutyl Ester

Brand Names Caswell No 292; Staflex® DBP; Uniflex® DBP

Use Plasticizer for polyvinyl chloride; insect repellant, also used as a solvent for perfume oils; concrete additive; in plastisol formulations for carpets; a solvent for nail polish

Mechanism of Toxic Action Uncouples oxidative phosphorylation

Adverse Reactions

Cardiovascular: Hypertension
Dermatologic: Allergic dermatitis
Gastrointestinal: Nausea
Neuromuscular & skeletal: Polyneuritis
Ocular: Keratitis
Renal: Nephritis

Signs & Symptoms of Acute Overdose Spasms, asthenia, ocular irritation, photophobia, lacrimation, dizziness (to 10 g ingestion)

Toxicodynamics/Kinetics

Absorption: Inhalation; absorbed slowly through intact skin
Metabolism: Hepatic hydrolysis to phthalic acid and butanol

Overdosage Treatment

Decontamination: Oral: Dilute with water; lavage/activated charcoal

Specific References

Calan CD, "Dibutyl Phthalate," *Contact Dermatitis*, 1975, 1:388.

Daniel JW, "Toxicity and Metabolism of Phthalate Esters," *Clin Toxicol*, 1978, 13(2):257-68.

U.S. Department of Health and Human Services, "Toxicological Profile for Di-n-Butyl Phthalate TP-90/10," Agency for Toxic Substances and Diseases Registry, December 1990.

Dinitrobenzene *see* 1,3-Dinitrobenzene *on this page*

1,3-Dinitrobenzene

CAS Number 99-65-0

UN Number 1597

Synonyms Dinitrobenzene; 1,3 DNB; Meta-Dinitrobenzene

Use Primarily used as an explosive, as a camphor substitute in nitrocellulose; medicinally, has been used as an indicator for 17-ketosteroid detection

Mechanism of Toxic Action Causes methemoglobinemia through oxidation of ferrous hemoglobin to ferric derivative

Adverse Reactions No apparent long-term effects

Cardiovascular: Hypotension, tachycardia, cyanosis
Central nervous system: Dizziness, headache, fatigue, ataxia
Gastrointestinal: Nausea, vomiting
Hematologic: Anemia, methemoglobinemia
Ocular: Nystagmus
Respiratory: Dyspnea
Miscellaneous: Hyperthermia

Toxicodynamics/Kinetics

Absorption: Oral, inhalation, and dermal

Overdosage Treatment

Decontamination:
Dermal: Wash with soap and water
Ocular: Irrigate copiously with saline

Supportive therapy: Treat symptomatic methemoglobinemia with methylene blue; ascorbic acid (3 g/day during periods of cyanosis) has been used to improve oxygen delivery, although its efficacy is not proven; administer 100% humidified oxygen

Antidote(s)

Methylene Blue *on page 1444*

Monitoring Parameters Methemoglobinemia

Additional Information Penetrates latex gloves; odor of bitter almonds in vomitus or urine may be noted

Specific References

Ishihara N and Ikeda M, "Effects of Solvents and Solutes on the Percutaneous Absorption of M-Dinitrobenzene," *Int Arch Occup Environ Health*, 1979, 44(2):91-8.

Okubo T and Shigeta S, "Anemia Causes After Acute M-Dinitrobenzene Intoxication Due to an Occupational Exposure," *Ind Health*, 1982, 20(4):297-304.

Dinitrocresol

CAS Number 616-73-9; 534-52-1; 497-56-3; 609-93-8

UN Number 1598

Synonyms DNC; DNOC; DNPC

Brand Names Antinonnin®; Detal®; Dinitrol®; Ditrosol®; Elgetol®; Selinon®; Sinox®; Victoria Orange®

Use Contact herbicide (for broad leaf weeds); insecticide useful against locusts; fungicide; unapproved for weight reduction earlier this century

Mechanism of Toxic Action Uncouples oxidative phosphorylation

Adverse Reactions

Cardiovascular: Tachycardia
Central nervous system: Lethargy, seizures, headaches, hyperthermia
Dermatologic: Yellow stains on skin, rash, mild dermal irritant
Gastrointestinal: Nausea
Ocular: Cataracts
Respiratory: Tachypnea, dyspnea
Miscellaneous: Sweating

Toxicodynamics/Kinetics

Absorption: Inhalation, oral (40%), and by dermal routes
Metabolism: Hepatic
Half-life: 5-6 days

Reference Range Serum dinitrocresol (ortho) level of 1000 μg/mL associated with fatality; toxic blood levels if exposed to >30 ppm

Overdosage Treatment

Decontamination:

Dermal: Wash with soap and water
Ocular: Irrigate with copious amounts of saline
Oral: Do not induce emesis; lavage/activated charcoal; castor oil (nonpurgative dose) may reduce absorption by almost 50%

Supportive therapy: Benzodiazepine for seizure control; chlorpromazine (high doses), salicylates, barbiturates, or anticholinergic agents can potentiate toxicity of dinitrocresol; reduce body temperature by means of sponge baths or lavage with cold solutions; haloperidol use (in competing with binding sites) is experimental; 10 mL of a 2.5% solution (intravenous) of sodium methyl thiouracil has been claimed to reduce metabolic rate induced by dinitrocresol although this is unproven

Enhancement of elimination: Dialysis or forced diuresis is not helpful

Pregnancy Implications Possible effect of induction of labor after dermal exposure

Additional Information After death, rigor mortis develops rapidly

Toxic oral dose: >0.75 mg/kg/day

Specific References

Bidstrup PL and Payne DJH, "Poisoning by Dinitro-Ortho-Cresol," *Br Med J*, 1951, 2:16-9.
Steer C, "Death From Dinitro-Ortho-Cresol," *Lancet*, 1951, 1:1419.

Dinitrol® *see* Dinitrocresol *on this page*

Dinitrophenols

CAS Number 66-56-8; 51-28-5; 329-71-5; 573-56-8; 577-71-9; 586-11-8; 25550-58-7

UN Number 1599; 1320

Use In synthesis of dyes and organic chemicals; pesticide, herbicide, fungicide, and acaricide; pH reagent; potassium and ammonium ion detection; wood preservative; World War I explosive agent; had been used against lice; also used in weight control (100 mg 3 times/day) in the 1930s

Mechanism of Toxic Action Uncouples oxidative phosphorylation

Adverse Reactions

Cardiovascular: Tachycardia
Central nervous system: Lethargy, seizures, headache, hyperthermia
Dermatologic: Yellow stains on skin, rash, mild dermal irritant
Endocrine & metabolic: Acidosis
Gastrointestinal: Nausea, vomiting
Hematologic: Neutropenia, hemolytic anemia, methemoglobinemia (by 2,4 dinitrophenol only)
Hepatic: Hepatic injury, jaundice
Neuromuscular & skeletal: Peripheral neuritis
Ocular: Cataracts, intraocular pressure (increased), nystagmus, blurred vision
Respiratory: Tachypnea, dyspnea, hyperventilation
Miscellaneous: Agranulocytosis, yellow stools, oliguria, sweating, hyperthermia

Toxicodynamics/Kinetics

Absorption: Dermal and oral routes
Metabolism: Hepatic to aminonitrophenols

(Continued)

Dinitrophenols *(Continued)*

Half-life: 5-14 days
Elimination: Hepatic

Reference Range Blood dinitrophenol level >10 μg/mL associated with toxicity

Overdosage Treatment

Decontamination:

Dermal: Wash with soap and water

Ocular: Irrigate with copious amounts of saline

Oral: Do not induce emesis; lavage/activated charcoal; castor oil (nonpurgative dose) may reduce absorption by almost 50%

Supportive therapy: Benzodiazepine for seizure control; chlorpromazine (high doses), salicylates, barbiturates, or anticholinergic agents can potentiate toxicity of dinitrocresol; reduce body temperature by means of sponge baths or lavage with cold solutions; haloperidol use (in competing with binding sites) is experimental; 10 mL of a 2.5% solution (intravenous) of sodium methyl thiouracil has been claimed to reduce metabolic rate induced by dinitrocresol although this is unproven; methemoglobinemia can be treated with methylene blue

Enhancement of elimination: Dialysis or forced diuresis is not helpful

Additional Information Atmospheric half-life: Probably exceeds 1 month; does not accumulate in the body

Toxic oral dose: 3-5 mg/kg

Specific References

Kurt TL, Anderson R, Petty C, et al, "Dinitrophenol in Weight Loss. The Poison Center and Public Health Safety," *Vet Hum Toxicol*, 1986, 28(6):574-5.

Di-n-Octylphthalate

CAS Number 117-84-0

Synonyms DNOP; DOP; Phthalic Acid, Dioctyl Ester

Brand Names Celluflux DOP®; Dinopol NOP®; Polycizer 162®; PX-138®; Vinicizer 85®

Use Colorless, odorless chemical primarily used as a plasticizer in plastics and PVC resin production; active ingredient in pesticides and can be found in electrical capacitor fluid and plastisols for carpetback coating

Mechanism of Toxic Action Hepatotoxin which causes centrilobular necrosis and accumulation of fat; loss of glycogen has also been noted

Adverse Reactions No human health effects noted while this agent is a skin and eye irritant, the liver appears to be the target organ of toxicity with centrilobular fat accumulation and glycogen loss; can also serve as a promoter that results in hepatic adenomas and carcinomas

Toxicodynamics/Kinetics

Absorption: Primarily oral; not significantly absorbed by dermal or inhalation route

Metabolism: Hepatic hydrolysis to mono-n-octylphthalate beta oxidation then occurs to form phthalate monoesters

Half-life: 20 minutes (I.V. administration)

Elimination: Renal

Overdosage Treatment

Decontamination:

Dermal: Wash with soap and water

Ocular: Copious irrigation with saline

Oral: Dilute with milk or water; activated charcoal with a cathartic can be utilized

Monitoring Parameters Liver function tests, glucose

Pregnancy Implications Teratogenic in animals

Additional Information

Atmospheric half-life: 4.5-4.8 hours

Levels of di-n-octylphthalate in drinking water: <0.5 ppb

Lethal oral dose: ~0.5-15 g/kg

TLV-TWA: 5 mg/m^3

Specific References

U.S. Department of Health and Human Services, "Toxicological Profile for Di-n-octylphthalate," Agency for Toxic Substances and Diseases Registry, June, 1994.

Dinopol NOP® *see* Di-n-Octylphthalate *on this page*

Dioform® *see* Acetylene Dichloride *on page 851*

Dioxathion

CAS Number 78-34-2

Brand Names Delnatex®; Delnav®; Deltic®

Use Marketed as insecticide granules, dusting agent, or spray liquid with or without petroleum derivative as a solvent

Mechanism of Toxic Action Irreversible inhibition of acetylcholinesterase and plasma cholinesterase, resulting in excess accumulation of acetylcholine at muscarinic and nicotinic receptors, and in the central nervous system

Adverse Reactions

Cardiovascular: Hyperdynamic (~18% to 21%) or hypodynamic (~7% to 10%) states

Central nervous system: Depression, seizures, hyperactivity

Genitourinary: Incontinence

Neuromuscular & skeletal: Weakness, paralysis

Respiratory: Depression, edema

General: Flu-like symptoms (especially with chronic exposure)

Delayed: Muscle asthenia and paresthesia

Signs & Symptoms of Acute Overdose Miosis (unreactive to light), mydriasis (rarely), lacrimation, pallor, excessive sweating, confusion, agitation, headache, dysarthria, generalized asthenia, seizures, A-V block, coma, decreased hemoglobin/red blood cell count/platelet count, metabolic acidosis and hyperglycemia (severe intoxication), hypotension, hypertension, bradycardia, tachycardia, cranial nerve palsies, Q-T prolongation, heart block, asystole, salivation, bronchorrhea, tachypnea, pulmonary edema, respiratory depression, diaphragmatic paralysis, skeletal muscle fasciculation and flaccid paralysis, nausea, vomiting, abdominal pain, fecal and urinary incontinence; an "intermediate syndrome" of limb asthenia and respiratory paralysis has been reported to occur between 24 and 96 hours postorganophosphate exposure, and is independent of the acute cholinergic crisis; late paresthesia characterized by stocking and glove paresthesia, anesthesia, and asthenia is infrequently observed weeks to months following acute exposure to certain organophosphates

Toxicodynamics/Kinetics

Absorption: Readily through oral, dermal, or respiratory exposure

Metabolism: Rapidly metabolized to weakly active compounds through hepatic hydrolysis and other pathways

Elimination: Metabolites are excreted in urine

Warnings Risk of aspiration pneumonitis exists with agents having a hydrocarbon vehicle; severe laryngeal irritation and violent coughing may result from exposure to dusting powders; exposure to dusting powders and insecticide granules may cause contact dermatitis

Overdosage Treatment

Decontamination: Isolation, bagging, and disposal of all contaminated clothing and other articles; all emergency medical workers and hospital staff should follow appropriate precautions regarding exposure to hazardous material including the use of protective clothing, masks, goggles, and respiratory equipment

Dermal: Prompt thorough scrubbing of all affected areas with soap and water, including hair and nails

Gastric: Activated charcoal can be administered either orally or via a nasogastric tube; do not induce emesis because of danger of sudden respiratory compromise, alterations in mental status, seizures, coma, and possible aspiration of hydrocarbon vehicles

Ocular: Irrigation with copious tepid sterile water or saline

Supportive therapy: Including airway management, ventilatory assistance, humidified oxygen administration, and close monitoring for sudden respiratory failure

Enhancement of elimination: Dialysis and hemoperfusion are not indicated due to effectiveness of the prescribed treatment, large volumes of distribution of organophosphates

Antidote:

Atropine: Administration should be guided by respiratory status, starting at 1-5 mg I.V. every 5-10 minutes as needed, and should be titrated to the resolution of excess pulmonary secretions; frequent administration of large doses (cumulative doses >100 mg) may be necessary in massive exposures

Glycopyrrolate: May be administered if atropine is unavailable

2-PAM: For more significant exposures (ie, exposures requiring large doses of atropine, or with recurring symptoms, or exposures to more lipid soluble agents), administration should follow: 1-2 g I.V. over 5-10 minutes, repeated in 1 hour if asthenia reoccurs, then every 4-12 hours for recurring symptoms

Antidote(s)

Atropine Sulfate *on page 1395*

Pralidoxime Chloride *on page 1461*

Diagnostic Tests/Procedures

Blood Gases, Arterial *on page 1207*

Chest Films *on page 1224*

Complete Blood Count *on page 1236*

Creatinine, Serum *on page 1243*

Electrocardiography *on page 1253*

Liver Profile *on page 1286*

Pseudocholinesterase, Serum *on page 1340*

Pregnancy Implications Human data regarding organophosphate exposure in pregnancy is limited and anecdotal; teratogenesis and fetal death have been pro-

(Continued)

Dioxathion *(Continued)*

duced in animal models at exposure levels that cause obvious toxicity to the pregnant animal

Additional Information Poorly volatile amber liquid; thermal degradation products include sulfur oxides; red blood cell cholinesterase, and serum pseudocholinesterase may be depressed following acute or chronic organophosphate exposure; RBC cholinesterase is typically not analyzed by in-house laboratories, and is usually not available for consideration during acute management. Pseudocholinesterase levels may be rapidly available from some in-house laboratories, but are not as reliable a marker of organophosphate exposure because of variability secondary to variant genotypes, hepatic disease, oral estrogen use, or malnutrition. Because of this variability, true indication of suppression of either of these enzymes can only be estimated through comparison to pre-exposure values; these enzymes may be useful in measuring a patient's recovery postexposure, especially if the recovery is not progressing as expected.

ACGIH TLV: 0.2 mg/m^3
PEL-TWA: 0.2 mg/m^3

Other information concerning pesticide exposures is available through the EPA-funded National Pesticide Telecommunications Network: 1-800-858-7378 (weekdays, 8 AM to 6 PM, Central Standard time)

Specific References

Minton NA and Murray VS, "A Review of Organophosphate Poisoning," *Med Toxicol Adverse Drug Exp*, 1988, 3(5):350-75.

Namba T, Nolte CT, Jackrel J, et al, "Poisoning Due to Organophosphate Insecticides. Acute and Chronic Manifestations," *Am J Med*, 1971, 50(4):475-92.

Dipazin® *see* Anticoagulant Rodenticide *on page 859*

Diphacin® *see* Anticoagulant Rodenticide *on page 859*

Diphacinone *see* Anticoagulant Rodenticide *on page 859*

4,4'-Diphenylediamine *see* Benzidine *on page 868*

Diphenylnitrosamine *see* N-Nitrosodiphenylamine *on page 982*

Diphosgene *see* Phosgene *on page 992*

Dipropyl *see* Hexane *on page 938*

Diquat Dibromide

Related Information

Paraquat *on page 987*

CAS Number 2764-72-9; 85-00-7

Commonly Found In Ethylene bipyridylium

Adverse Reactions

Renal: Renal failure
Respiratory: Pulmonary fibrosis less likely to occur than with paraquat
Miscellaneous: Third spacing of gastrointestinal fluid

Signs & Symptoms of Acute Overdose Coma, hypotension, fingernail loss, Mees' lines, dermal burns, drowsiness (72-96 hours postingestion), parkinsonism may occur, paralytic ileus, seizures

Reference Range Minimal lethal dose: 20 mL of a 20% solution (6-12 g)

Overdosage Treatment

Decontamination: Emesis/lavage with activated charcoal with cathartic; Fuller's earth or 7% bentonite; sodium polystyrene sulfonate may also be effective

Supportive therapy: Do not utilize oxygen in that it may promote pulmonary fibrosis; monitor for hypercalcemia if Fuller's earth used

Enhancement of elimination: Multiple dosing of activated charcoal, Fuller's earth (100-150 g in adults or 2 g/kg in children) or bentonite may be given every 2-4 hours; charcoal hemoperfusion for prolonged periods of time (up to 10 hours) may be helpful if instituted within 2 hours; forced diuresis is not helpful

Additional Information Does not produce pulmonary fibrosis; dithionate test: 1 part urine, 0.5 part sodium dithionate in IN NaOH: Deep blue color indicates presence of paraquat or diquat

Specific References

Manoguerra AS, "Full Thickness Skin Burns Secondary to an Unusual Exposure to Diquat Dibromide," *J Toxicol Clin Toxicol*, 1990, 28(1):107-10.

McCarthy LG and Speth CP, "Diquat Intoxication," *Ann Emerg Med*, 1983, 12(6):394-6.

Sechi GP, Agnetti V, Piredda M, et al, "Acute and Persistent Parkinsonism After Use of Diquat," *Neurology*, 1992, 42(1):261-3.

Disc Battery *see* Button Batteries (Disc) *on page 875*

Distilled Mustard *see* Mustard Gas *on page 972*

Distokal® *see* Hexachloroethane *on page 937*

Distopan® *see* Hexachloroethane *on page 937*

Disulfoton

CAS Number 298-04-4

UN Number 2783

Synonyms Ethylthiodemeton; Thiodemeton

Brand Names Dimax®; Di-Syston®; Dithiosystox®; Solvirex®

Use Crop systemic organophosphate insecticide and acaricide; useful for mosquito abatement

Mechanism of Toxic Action Highly toxic organophosphate agent which causes irreversible inhibition of acetylcholinesterase and plasma cholinesterase, resulting in excess accumulation of acetylcholine at muscarinic and nicotinic receptors, and in the central nervous system

Adverse Reactions

Cardiovascular: Hyperdynamic (~18% to 21%) or hypodynamic (~7% to 10%) states, tachycardia, hypertension

Central nervous system: Depression, seizures, hyperactivity

Gastrointestinal: Pancreatitis (after ingestion of 1.5 mg/kg), diarrhea

Genitourinary: Incontinence

Neuromuscular & skeletal: Weakness, paralysis

Ocular: Can cause myopia in children, miosis

Respiratory: Depression, edema

General: Flu-like symptoms (especially with chronic exposure), sweating, hypokalemia

Delayed: Muscle asthenia and paresthesia

Signs & Symptoms of Acute Overdose Miosis (unreactive to light), mydriasis (rarely), lacrimation, pallor, excessive sweating, confusion, agitation, headache, dysarthria, generalized asthenia, seizures, A-V block, coma, decreased hemoglobin/red blood cell count/platelet count, metabolic acidosis and hyperglycemia (severe intoxication), cranial nerve palsies, hypotension, hypertension, bradycardia, tachycardia, Q-T prolongation, heart block, asystole, salivation, bronchorrhea, tachypnea, pulmonary edema, respiratory depression, diaphragmatic paralysis, skeletal muscle fasciculation and flaccid paralysis, nausea, vomiting, abdominal pain, fecal and urinary incontinence; an "intermediate syndrome" of limb asthenia and respiratory paralysis has been reported to occur between 24 and 96 hours postorganophosphate exposure and is independent of the acute cholinergic crisis. Late paresthesia characterized by stocking and globe paresthesia, anesthesia and asthenia is infrequently observed weeks to months following acute exposure to certain organophosphates.

Toxicodynamics/Kinetics

Absorption: Easily absorbed orally and possibly dermally

Metabolism: To phosphorothiolate sulfone (active metabolite)

Warnings Risk of aspiration pneumonitis exists following oral exposure to agents having a hydrocarbon vehicle; severe laryngeal irritation and violent coughing may result from exposure to dusting powders; exposure to dusting powders and insecticide granules may cause contact dermatitis

Reference Range Blood disulfoton level of 1.45 nmol/g associated with fatality; peak plasma phosphorodithioate sulfone concentration of 1322 ng/mL 56 hours postingestion resulted in severe toxicity, but survival levels may rebound in first 2-3 days

Overdosage Treatment

Decontamination: Isolation, bagging, and disposal of all contaminated clothing and other articles; all emergency medical workers and hospital staff should follow appropriate precautions regarding exposure to hazardous material including the use of protective clothing, masks, goggles, and respiratory equipment. Gastric lavage with water, 5% sodium bicarbonate or 2% potassium permanganate can be considered within 1 hour of ingestion; do not use cathartic with activated charcoal.

Dermal: Prompt thorough scrubbing of all affected areas with soap and water, including hair and nails

Gastric: Activated charcoal can be administered either orally or via a nasogastric tube; do not induce emesis because of danger of sudden respiratory compromise, alterations in mental status, seizures, coma, and possible aspiration of hydrocarbon vehicles; prolonged or repetitive gastric lavage (with activated charcoal) may be beneficial to prevent rebound of plasma levels due to delayed absorption

Ocular: Irrigation with copious tepid sterile water or saline

Supportive therapy: Including airway management, ventilatory assistance, humidified oxygen administration, and close monitoring for sudden respiratory failure

Antidote:

Atropine: Administration should be guided by respiratory status, starting at 1-5 mg I.V. every 5-10 minutes as needed, and should be titrated to the resolution

(Continued)

Disulfoton *(Continued)*

of excess pulmonary secretions; frequent administration of large doses (cumulative doses >100 mg) may be necessary in massive exposures

Glycopyrrolate: May be administered if atropine is unavailable

2-PAM: For more significant exposures (ie, exposures requiring large doses of atropine, or with recurring symptoms, or exposures to more lipid soluble agents), administration should follow: 1-2 g I.V. over 5-10 minutes, repeated in 1 hour if asthenia reoccurs, then every 4-12 hours for recurring symptoms

Enhancement of elimination: Dialysis and hemoperfusion are not indicated due to effectiveness of the prescribed treatment, large volumes of distribution of organophosphates; due to enterohepatic recirculation, multiple dosing of activated charcoal may be effective

Antidote(s)

Atropine Sulfate *on page 1395*

Pralidoxime Chloride *on page 1461*

Diagnostic Tests/Procedures

Blood Gases, Arterial *on page 1207*

Chest Films *on page 1224*

Complete Blood Count *on page 1236*

Creatinine, Serum *on page 1243*

Electrocardiography *on page 1253*

Liver Profile *on page 1286*

Pseudocholinesterase, Serum *on page 1340*

Pregnancy Implications Fetotoxic effects (incomplete ossification) in rodents at doses >1 mg/kg/day

Additional Information Not carcinogenic; cross tolerance with chlorpyrifos noted in rodents

Lethal adult dose: 500 mg

Specific References

Futagami K, Otsubo K, Nakao Y, et al, "Acute Organophosphate Poisoning After Disulfoton Ingestion," *J Toxicol Clin Toxicol*, 1995, 33(2):151-5.

Watson M, Benson WW, and Gabica J, "Accidental Organophosphate Poisoning in Cattle, Two Case Histories," *Arch Environ Health*, 1971, 22:582-3.

Yashiki M, Kojima T, Ohtani M, et al, "Determination of Disulfoton and its Metabolites in the Body Fluids of a Di-Syston Intoxication Case," *Forensic Sci Int*, 1990, 48(2):145-54.

Di-Syston® *see* Disulfoton *on previous page*

Dithiocarbonic Anhydride *see* Carbon Disulfide *on page 879*

Dithiosystox® *see* Disulfoton *on previous page*

Ditrosol® *see* Dinitrocresol *on page 915*

Diuron

CAS Number 330-54-1

Commonly Found In Dailon®; Diater®; Di-On®; Direx 4L®; Diurex®; Diurol®; Rout®

Mechanism of Toxic Action Inhibitor of plant photosynthesis, a urea substituted herbicide

Signs & Symptoms of Acute Overdose Can cause methemoglobinemia

Toxicodynamics/Kinetics

Metabolism: To 1-(3,4-dichlorophenyl)-3-methyl urea and to 1-(3,4-dichlorophenyl) urea

Elimination: Urine

Reference Range Maximum tolerated dose: 38 mg/kg

Overdosage Treatment Supportive therapy: Methylene blue 1-2 mg/kg/dose if methemoglobinemia is noted

Antidote(s)

Methylene Blue *on page 1444*

Pregnancy Implications No known adverse effects

Additional Information Available as a 80% powder/40% suspension in water; or can be combined with bramacil or sodium metaborate

Specific References

Geldmacher-von Mallinck and Schussler F, "The Metabolism and Toxicity of 1-(3,4-dichlorophenyl)-3,3-dimethyl urea (diuron) by Man," *Arch Toxicol*, 1971, 27(3):187-92 (German).

DMDT *see* Methoxychlor *on page 963*

1,3 DNB *see* 1,3-Dinitrobenzene *on page 914*

DNC *see* Dinitrocresol *on page 915*

DNOC *see* Dinitrocresol *on page 915*

DNOP *see* Di-n-Octylphthalate *on page 916*

DNPC *see* Dinitrocresol *on page 915*

Dobill's Solution® *see* Borates *on page 870*

Dolco Mouse Ceral® *see* Strychnine *on page 1016*

Dolen-Pur *see* Hexachlorobutadiene *on page 937*

DOP *see* Di-n-Octylphthalate *on page 916*

Dowfume® EDB *see* Ethylene Bromide *on page 924*

Dowicide 2S® *see* 2,4,6-Trichlorophenol *on page 1034*

Dowicide® 7 *see* Pentachlorophenol *on page 990*

Drat® *see* Anticoagulant Rodenticide *on page 859*

Draza® *see* Methiocarb *on page 961*

Drexel Acetol *see* Chlorate Salts *on page 884*

Drinox® *see* Aldrin *on page 856*

Drinox® *see* Heptachlor *on page 935*

Drugs and Chemicals Proven to be Teratogenic in Humans *see page 1572*

Dry Cleaning Safety Solvent *see* Stoddard Solvent *on page 1015*

Dura Treet® II *see* Pentachlorophenol *on page 990*

Dursban® *see* Chlorpyrifos *on page 891*

Dursban TC® *see* Chlorpyrifos *on page 891*

Dutch Oil *see* Ethylene Dichloride *on page 924*

EB *see* Ethylbenzene *on page 923*

Ectiban *see* Pyrethrins *on page 1003*

EDB *see* Ethylene Bromide *on page 924*

EDC *see* Ethylene Dichloride *on page 924*

Egitol® *see* Hexachloroethane *on page 937*

Ektofos® *see* Dicrotophos *on page 909*

Elgetol® *see* Dinitrocresol *on page 915*

Embafume® *see* Methyl Bromide *on page 964*

Endocide® *see* Endosulfan *on this page*

Endosulfan

CAS Number 115-29-7; 33213-65-9; 1031-07-8

UN Number 2761

Synonyms Hoe-2671

Brand Names Beosit®; Endocide®; Endosulphan®; Malix®; Thifor®; Thiodan®; Thionex®

Use Crop pesticide usually applied before harvest on tobacco and fruit trees; used as a wood preservative

Mechanism of Toxic Action No mechanism proven although decrease of brain acetylcholinesterase, serotonin, norepinephrine has been hypothesized; also acts as a GABA antagonist; chlorinated hydrocarbon (sulfurous acid ester)

Adverse Reactions

Cardiovascular: Tachycardia, cyanosis

Central nervous system: Seizures, dizziness, confusion, loss of consciousness, agitation, ataxia

Endocrine & metabolic: Metabolic acidosis, hyperglycemia

Gastrointestinal: Nausea, vomiting, diarrhea

Hematologic: Thrombocytopenia, leukocytosis

Neuromuscular & skeletal: Tremors

Ocular: Miosis

Respiratory: Dyspnea, pulmonary edema

Miscellaneous: Acute tubular necrosis

Toxicodynamics/Kinetics

Absorption: By inhalation, oral (65%) and dermal (25%) routes

Metabolism: Hepatic to endosulfan lactone, hydroxyether, and ether

Elimination: Primarily fecal

Overdosage Treatment

Decontamination: Do not induce emesis; lavage/activated charcoal or cholestyramine; do not use on oil based cathartic

Supportive therapy: Diazepam or phenobarbital for seizure control

Enhancement of elimination: Multiple dosing of activated charcoal or cholestyramine (4 g every 8 hours) may be useful in increasing clearance

(Continued)

Endosulfan *(Continued)*

Additional Information Ethanol may enhance toxicity

Specific References

Blanco-Coronado JL, Repetto M, Ginestal RJ, et al, "Acute Intoxication by Endosulfan," *J Toxicol Clin Toxicol*, 1992, 30(4):575-83.

Garnier R and Chataigner R, "Acute Tubular Necrosis Following Endosulfan Insecticide Poisoning," *J Toxicol Clin Toxicol*, 1995, 33(4):375.

Lo RS, Chan JC, Cockram CS, et al, "Acute Tubular Necrosis Following Endosulphan Insecticide Poisoning," *J Toxicol Clin Toxicol*, 1995, 33(1):67-9.

Shemesh Y, Bourvine A, Gold D, et al, "Survival After Acute Endosulfan Intoxication," *J Toxicol Clin Toxicol*, 1988, 26(3-4):265-8.

Endosulphan® *see* Endosulfan *on previous page*

Endothall

CAS Number 145-73-3

Commonly Found In Endothall; Aquathol; Hydout; Hydrothol 47; Tri-Endothall; Niagrathal; 3,6-Endoxohexahydrophthalic Acid

Mechanism of Toxic Action Water herbicide (organic acid)

Signs & Symptoms of Acute Overdose Irritant to mucous membrane/skin; can cause hypotension, hematemesis, abdominal pain, disseminated intravascular coagulation, diarrhea, anuria, acidosis

Toxicodynamics/Kinetics Absorption: Dermal: Slight

Reference Range Postmortem blood level of 1 mg/dL documented

Minimum lethal dose: 130 mg/kg

Overdosage Treatment

Decontamination: Activated charcoal with cathartic; dilute with 4-8 oz of milk or water

Supportive therapy: Avoid adrenergic amines

Additional Information Emits acrid fumes when heated

Specific References

Allender WJ, "Suicidal Poisoning by Endothall," *J Anal Toxicol*, 1983, 7(2):79-82.

Day LC, "Delayed Death by Endothall, an Herbicide," *Vet Hum Toxicol*, 1988, 30:366.

Endox® *see* Anticoagulant Rodenticide *on page 859*

Endrin

Related Information

Organochlorines *on page 983*

CAS Number 72-20-8; 7421-93-4; 53494-70-5

UN Number 2811

Brand Names Delta-keto® 153; Hexadrin®; Medrin®

Use Chlorinated hydrocarbon pesticide, rodenticide, and avicide used on tobacco, apple trees, cotton, sugar cane, and grain; not used in U.S. since 1986

Mechanism of Toxic Action Interferes with normal flux of sodium and potassium ions over axonal membrane

Adverse Reactions

Cardiovascular: Hypotension

Central nervous system: Seizures, dizziness, hyperthermia

Gastrointestinal: Nausea, vomiting

Hematologic: Thrombocytopenia

Neuromuscular & skeletal: Tremors

Otic: Temporary deafness

Respiratory: Respiratory depression

Miscellaneous: Hypersalivation

Toxicodynamics/Kinetics

Absorption: By inhalation, oral, and dermal (1.5%) routes

Metabolism: Hepatic oxidation and hydroxylation occurs to 12-hydroxyedrin and 12-ketoedrin

Elimination: Urine

Reference Range Blood endrin level of 0.05 mg/L associated with seizures

Overdosage Treatment

Decontamination: Do not induce emesis; lavage/activated charcoal or cholestyramine; do not use on oil based cathartic

Supportive therapy: Diazepam or phenytoin may be used for seizure control; try to avoid catecholamine as arrhythmias can be induced; assisted ventilation with succinylcholine (0.5-1 mg/minute for 1 day) for seizure control may be necessary; atropine can be used to control bronchial secretions

Enhancement of elimination: Multiple dosing of activated charcoal or cholestyramine (4 g every 8 hours) may be useful in increasing clearance

Additional Information Edrin concentration in foods (contaminated flour) exceeding 150 ppm can cause seizures upon ingestion

Seizuregenic oral dose: 0.25 mg/kg
Fatal oral dose: 12 g (100 mg/kg)
IDLH: 200 mg/m^3
Milk or ethanol can increase toxicity of endrin by enhancing its absorption; onset of seizures is usually within 4 hours postingestion; bioaccumulation does not occur

Specific References

Rowley DL, Rab MA, Hardjotanojo W, et al, "Convulsions Caused by Endrin Poisoning in Pakistan," *Pediatrics*, 1987, 79(6):928-34.
Runhaar EA, Sangster B, Greve PA, et al, "A Case of Fatal Endrin Poisoning," *Hum Toxicol*, 1985, 4(3):241-7.
Waller K, Prendergast TJ, Slagle A, et al, "Seizures After Eating a Snack Food Contaminated With the Pesticide Endrin. The Tale of Toxic Taquitos," *West J Med*, 1992, 157(6):648-51.

Endrocide® *see* Anticoagulant Rodenticide *on page 859*
Entex® *see* Fenthion *on page 929*
EP-452 *see* Phenmedipham *on page 992*
Ethanoic Acid *see* Vinyl Acetate *on page 1037*
Ethenylbenzene *see* Styrene *on page 1017*
Ethenyl Ester *see* Vinyl Acetate *on page 1037*

Ethylbenzene

CAS Number 100-41-4
UN Number 1175
Synonyms EB; Ethylbenzol; Phenylethane
Use Solvent which is found in asphalt, fuels, and naphtha; used in the products of styrene and other organic chemicals; used in paint thinners and as a degreaser
Mechanism of Toxic Action Aromatic hydrocarbon with mucosal irritant effects; central nervous system depression can occur at very high concentrations

Adverse Reactions

Central nervous system: Dizziness at levels >2000 ppm
Dermatologic: Dermal irritant at levels of 200 ppm
Hematologic: Anemia (long-term exposure)
Hepatic: Hepatotoxicity
Ocular: Irritation with lacrimation at levels >1000 ppm
Respiratory: Upper respiratory tract irritation at levels >2000 ppm

Toxicodynamics/Kinetics

Absorption: Rapid from inhalation (57%) and skin (rate of 20-33 mg/cm^2/hour)
Metabolism: Hepatic to mandelic acid and phenylglyoxylated acid
Elimination: Renal

Reference Range Ethylbenzene blood levels of 61 μg/L associated with anemia; at 100 ppm exposure of ethylbenzene, it has been estimated that urinary phenylglyoxylic acid and mandelic acid concentrations would be 95 mg/L and 395 mg/L respectively

Overdosage Treatment

Decontamination: Do not induce emesis or lavage due to risk of aspiration pneumonia; activated charcoal can adsorb benzene
Supportive therapy: Benzodiazepines for seizure control; avoid use of catecholamines due to risk of ventricular arrhythmia

Additional Information Not associated with cancer; carbon monoxide and ethanol inhibit metabolism of ethylbenzene in rodents; does not bioaccumulate
IDLH: 2000 ppm; TLV-PEL: 100 ppm
BEI (urinary mandelic acid) at the end of shift at the end of work week: 2 g/L or 1.5 g/g creatinine
Frequently found in ground water at hazardous waste sites (average concentration: 0.65 ppm)
Minimal uptake of fluorescein on ocular exposure

Specific References

Angerer J and Wulf H, "Occupational Chronic Exposure to Organic Solvents. XI. Alkylbenzene Exposure of Varnish Workers: Effects on Hematopoietic System," *Int Arch Occup Environ Health*, 1985, 56(4):307-21.
Inove O, Seiji K, Kudo S, et al, "Urinary Phenylglyoxylic Acid Excretion After Exposure to Ethylbenzene Among Solvent-Exposed Chinese Workers," *Int J Occup Med Environ Health*, 1995, 1:1-8.
Upton AC, Kneip T, and Toniolo P, "Public Health Aspects of Toxic Chemical Disposal Sites," *Annu Rev Public Health*, 1989, 10:1-25.
U.S. Department of Health and Human Services, "Toxicological Profile for Ethylbenzene TP-90/15," Agency for Toxic Substances and Diseases Registry, December 1990.

Ethylbenzol *see* Ethylbenzene *on this page*
Ethylene Alcohol *see* Ethylene Glycol *on page 925*

Ethylene Bromide

CAS Number 106-93-4

UN Number 1605

Synonyms Dibromoethane; 1,2-Dibromoethane; EDB; Glycol Dibromide

Brand Names Bromofume®; Dowfume® EDB; Fumogas®; Nephis®; Soilfume®

Use Additive (as a lead scavenger to gasoline); soil and grain fumigant (banned by the EPA in 1984); manufacture for dyes, waxes, and resins

Mechanism of Toxic Action CNS depression; antispermatogenic effects; binds directly to DNA

Adverse Reactions

Central nervous system: CNS depression
Dermal: Local inflammation, vesiculation, rash
Endocrine & metabolic: Metabolic acidosis
Gastrointestinal: Ulceration
Hepatic: Hepatic failure within 2 days
Neuromuscular & skeletal: Muscle necrosis
Renal: Renal failure within 2 days
Respiratory: Pulmonary edema, respiratory depression

Signs & Symptoms of Acute Overdose Headache, urticaria, dizziness, asthenia, vomiting, diarrhea, erythema, ocular irritation, drowsiness, mydriasis, nystagmus, hypoglycemia, skin necrosis, burning of eyes

Toxicodynamics/Kinetics

Absorption: Well through intact skin
Metabolism: Hepatic through oxidation and conjugation through glutathione

Reference Range Serum bromide levels of 830 mg/L and 380 mg/L have been correlated with fatalities

Overdosage Treatment

Decontamination: Emesis is contraindicated; dilute with milk or water; activated charcoal may be useful
Supportive therapy: Supplemental oxygen

Diagnostic Tests/Procedures

Blood Gases, Arterial *on page 1207*
Bromide, Serum *on page 1212*
Chest Films *on page 1224*
Glucose, Random *on page 1269*

Additional Information Chloroform odor; penetrates clothing

IDLH: 400 ppm
PEL-TWA: 20 ppm

Specific References

"1,2-Dibromoethane," *Environ Health Perspect*, 1983, 47:359-63.
U.S. Department of Health and Human Services, "Toxicological Profile for 1,2-Dibromethane TP-91/13," Agency for Toxic Substances and Diseases Registry, July, 1992.

Ethylene Carboxamide *see* Acrylamide *on page 852*

Ethylene Dichloride

CAS Number 107-06-2

UN Number 1184

Synonyms 1,2-Bichlorethane; Borer Sol; Brocide; DCE; Dutch Oil; EDC; Freon 150; Glycol Dichloride

Use Fat solvent; soil fumigant

Mechanism of Toxic Action CNS depression; also can cause increased myocardial irritability and mucosal injury

Adverse Reactions

Cardiovascular: Cardiovascular failure, ventricular fibrillation
Central nervous system: CNS depression, delirium
Hepatic: Elevated liver enzymes
Renal & genitourinary: Tubular necrosis (acute)
Respiratory: Pulmonary edema, respiratory failure

Signs & Symptoms of Acute Overdose Vomiting, dyspnea, headache, asthenia, tremor, dizziness, corneal lesions, throat burning, diarrhea, abdominal pain

Toxicodynamics/Kinetics

Absorption: Well absorbed dermally, through lung (90%), and gastrointestinal tract (90%)
Elimination: Through lungs

Reference Range Oral dose of 25 mg/kg or inhalation dose >150 ppm correspond to blood level of 5-10 μg/mL

Overdosage Treatment

Decontamination: Emesis is contraindicated; dilute with milk or water
Supportive therapy: Supplemental oxygen

Diagnostic Tests/Procedures

Blood Gases, Arterial *on page 1207*

Chest Films *on page 1224*

Pregnancy Implications Cardiac defects in fetus suggested after maternal exposure to contaminated water

Additional Information Pleasant odor

Odor threshold: 50-100 ppm
ILV-TWA: 10 ppm
IDLH: 1000 ppm
PEL-TWA: 50 ppm
Fatalities have occurred at doses of 30-70 g

Specific References

Hubbs RS and Prusmack JJ, "Ethylene Dichloride Poisoning," *JAMA*, 1955, 159(7):673-5.

Ethylene Diglycol *see* Diethylene Glycol *on page 911*

Ethylene Dihydrate *see* Ethylene Glycol *on this page*

Ethylene Glycol

CAS Number 107-21-1

Synonyms Ethylene Alcohol; Ethylene Dihydrate; Glycol Alcohol; Monoethylene Glycol

Use Automotive antifreeze and coolants, solvent

Mechanism of Toxic Action Metabolized into glycolic acid and oxalate via the alcohol dehydrogenase pathway (ADH), thus producing profound metabolic acidosis

Adverse Reactions

Central nervous system: Cranial nerve palsies, ataxia, anisocoria, hyperreflexia, slurred speech, seizures, coma, headache
Endocrine & metabolic: Metabolic acidosis, hypocalcemia
Ocular: Mydriasis, diplopia, optic neuropathy, nystagmus
Renal: Renal tubular damage progressing to renal insufficiency
Respiratory: Respiratory irritation/cough on inhalation; hyperventilation
Miscellaneous: Porphyria, myoglobinuria, feces discoloration (black), osmolal gap

Signs & Symptoms of Acute Overdose Similar to methanol ingestion, ethylene glycol can initially result in inebriation; the toxicity of ethylene glycol can be divided into three stages:

Stage I (30 minutes to 12 hours after ingestion): Inebriation, ataxia, and metabolic acidosis with resulting respiratory compensation (Kussmaul's breathing), seizures, hypocalcemia, cranial nerve palsies, calcium oxaluria (4-8 hours after ingestion), and myoclonus; coma can occur, and death is usually due to cerebral edema during this stage

Stage II (12-36 hours after ingestion): Respiratory status deteriorates, with tachypnea, tachycardia, cyanosis, dyspnea, and pulmonary edema with cardiomegaly developing; death is usually due to cardiovascular causes or bronchopneumonia during this stage

Stage III (36-72 hours after ingestion): Renal failure dominates this phase, with acute tubular necrosis, hematuria, oliguria, albuminuria, or anuria occurring; noncardiogenic pulmonary edema may occur in this stage

Toxicodynamics/Kinetics

Specific gravity: 1.11 g/mL
Absorption:
- Oral, percutaneous: Rapid
- Inhalation: Not well absorbed

Distribution: V_d: 0.83 L/kg
Metabolism: Liver with principle toxic metabolites including glycolic acid (96%) and oxalic acid (2.3%); see figure on next page.
Half-life, elimination:
- No ethanol therapy: 3 hours
- During ethanol therapy: 17 hours
- During ethanol therapy and hemodialysis: $2^1/_2$ hours
- During 4-methylpyrazole therapy: 13 hours

Elimination: Renal clearance 3.2 mL/kg/minute

Reference Range

Toxic: Plasma level of 50 mg/dL
Fatal: Levels >85 mg/dL

Overdosage Treatment

Decontamination: Avoid emesis with ipecac; activated charcoal is not effective at a 5:1 ratio (charcoal:toxin)

Supportive therapy: Ethanol therapy should be initiated at 20 mg/dL, severe acidosis or electrolyte abnormality present, or renal failure; treat acidosis with I.V. sodium bicarbonate; administer thiamine and pyridoxine, 100 mg once a day for 2 days for both drugs. Calcium chloride can be given for hypocalcemia.

Enhancement of elimination: Hemodialysis should be considered if ethylene glycol level is >20 mg/dL or if metabolite acidosis is present; continuous arteriovenous hemofiltration; dialysis may also be effective

(Continued)

Ethylene Glycol *(Continued)*

Metabolic Pathway for Oxidation of Ethylene Glycol*

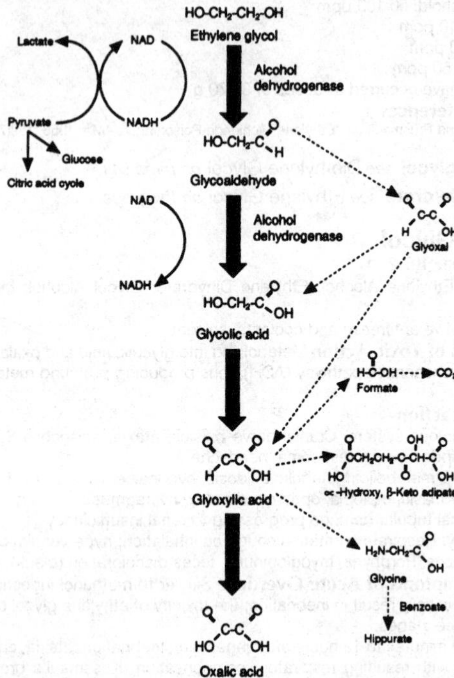

Adapted from the U.S. Department of Health and Human Services, "Technical Report for Ethylene Glycol/Propylene Glycol," Agency for Toxic Substances and Disease Registry, May 1993.

Antidote(s)
- Calcium Chloride *on page 1400*
- Ethanol *on page 1424*
- 4-Methylpyrazole *on page 1446*
- Pyridoxine Hydrochloride *on page 1465*
- Sodium Bicarbonate *on page 1467*

Test Interactions May interfere with methanol when fluorometrically measured; glycolaldehyde and glycerol may interfere with enzymatic assays; 4-methylpyrazole as a competitive inhibitor of alcohol dehydrogenase use is investigational

Diagnostic Tests/Procedures
- Anion Gap, Blood *on page 1193*
- Calcium, Serum *on page 1214*
- Crystals, Urine *on page 1246*
- Electrolytes, Blood *on page 1254*
- Kidney Profile *on page 1279*
- Osmolality, Serum *on page 1310*
- Osmolality, Urine *on page 1311*

Pregnancy Implications Facial anomalies, neural tube defects, and increased neonatal fatalities have been documented in laboratory animals

Additional Information Sweet tasting liquid

Atmospheric half-life: 24-50 hours
Water half-life: 3-5 days
Lethal dose: 100 mL (1.5 mL/kg)
Contribution of a serum concentration level of 100 mg/dL to elevation of osmolar gap: 16

Specific References

Baud FJ, Galliot M, Astier A, et al, "Treatment of Ethylene Glycol Poisoning With Intravenous 4-Methylpyrazole," *N Engl J Med*, 1988, 319(2):97-100.

Christiansson LK, Kaspersson KE, Kulling EJ, et al, "Treatment of Severe Ethylene Glycol Intoxication With Continuous Arteriovenous Hemofiltration Dialysis," *J Toxicol Clin Toxicol*, 1995, 33(3):267-70.

Jackson MH and Payne HA, "Bittering Agents: Their Potential Application in Reducing Ingestions of Engine Coolants and Windshield Wash," *Vet Hum Toxicol*, 1995, 37(4):323-6.

Jacobsen D and McMartin KE, "Methanol and Ethylene Glycol Poisonings. Mechanism of Toxicity, Clinical Course, Diagnosis, and Treatment," *Med Toxicol*, 1986, 1(5):309-34.

Peterson CD, Collins AJ, Himes JM, et al, "Ethylene Glycol Poisoning. Pharmacokinetics During Therapy With Ethanol and Hemodialysis," *N Engl J Med*, 1981, 304(1):21-3.

U.S. Department of Health and Human Services, "Technical Report for Ethylene Glycol/ Propylene Glycol," Agency for Toxic Substances and Diseases Registry, May 1993.

Walder AD and Tyler CKG, "Ethylene Glycol Antifreeze Poisoning," *Anesthesia*, 1994, 49:964-7.

Ethylene Monochloride *see* Vinyl Chloride *on page 1038*

Ethylene Oxide

CAS Number 75-21-8

UN Number 1040

Synonyms Dihydrooxirene; Dimethylane Oxide; Merpol; Oxidoethane; Oxirane; T-Gas

Brand Names Anprolene®; Oxyfume®

Use Gas sterilization agent (can inactivate all organisms); used in the production of ethylene glycol, cosmetics, detergents, inks, brake fluids, plasticizers, fumigant

Mechanism of Toxic Action Alkylating agent

Adverse Reactions

Cardiovascular: Cardiovascular collapse

Central nervous system: CNS depression

Neuromuscular & skeletal: Motor and sensory neuropathy (axonopathy)

Miscellaneous: Mucous membrane irritation

Signs & Symptoms of Acute Overdose Cough, dyspnea, pulmonary edema, headache, conjunctivitis, pulmonary edema, polyneuropathy, dermal burns, dizziness, myoclonus, vomiting, coma, nystagmus, seizures, contact dermatitis, bradycardia, possible excess risk for leukemia or gastric cancer

Toxicodynamics/Kinetics

Absorption: Orally and by inhalation

Metabolism: Hepatic; two pathways: hydrolysis to ethylene glycol and glutathione conjugation to mercapturic acid

Overdosage Treatment Decontamination: Basic poison management; do not induce emesis; irrigate skin with high pressure water

Diagnostic Tests/Procedures

Chest Films *on page 1224*

Pregnancy Implications Considered as an animal teratogen and a possible human teratogen; increased risk of spontaneous abortions

Additional Information Ether-like odor (delete limit 50 ppm); air levels in a hospital sterilizing unit: 0.1-7.8 ppm

TLV-TWA: 1 ppm

IDLH: 800 ppm

PEL-TWA: 1 ppm

Odor threshold: 430 ppm (air); 140 mg/L (water)

Atmospheric half-life: 69-149 days

Water half-life: 9-14 days

Specific References

Austin SG and Sielken RL Jr, "Issues in Assessing the Carcinogenic Hazards of Ethylene Oxide," *J Occup Med*, 1988, 30(3):236-45.

Crystal HA, Schaumburg HH, Grober E, et al, "Cognitive Impairment and Sensory Loss Associated With Chronic Low-Level Ethylene Oxide Exposure," *Neurology*, 1988, 38(4):567-9.

Landrigan PJ, Meinhardt TJ, Gordon J, et al, "Ethylene Oxide: An Overview of Toxicologic and Epidemiologic Research," *Am J Ind Med*, 1984, 6(2):103-15.

Schulte PA, Walker JT, and Boeniger MF, "Molecular, Cytogenetic and Hematologic Effects of Ethylene Oxide on Female Hospital Workers," *JOEM*, 1995, 37(3):313-20.

Ethyl Methyl Ketone *see* Methyl Ethyl Ketone *on page 967*

Ethyl Phthalate *see* Diethyl Phthalate *on page 912*

Ethylthiodemeton *see* Disulfoton *on page 919*

Evalu-Super *see* Chlorate Salts *on page 884*

Exhaust Gas *see* Carbon Monoxide *on page 880*

Factitious Air *see* Nitrous Oxide *on page 981*

Fannoform *see* Formaldehyde *on page 931*

Fasciolin® *see* Carbon Tetrachloride *on page 882*

Fast Corinth Base B *see* Benzidine *on page 868*

Fenclor *see* Polychlorinated Biphenyls *on page 995*

Fenmedifam *see* Phenmedipham *on page 992*

Fensulfothion

CAS Number 115-90-2

Brand Names Dansit®

Use Marketed as insecticide granules, dusting agent, or spray liquid with or without petroleum derivative as a solvent

Mechanism of Toxic Action Potent, irreversible inhibition of acetylcholinesterase and plasma cholinesterase, resulting in excess accumulation of acetylcholine at muscarinic and nicotinic receptors, and in the central nervous system

Adverse Reactions

Cardiovascular: Hyperdynamic (~18% to 21%) or hypodynamic (~7% to 10%) states

Central nervous system: Depression, seizures, hyperactivity

Genitourinary: Incontinence

Neuromuscular & skeletal: Weakness, paralysis

Respiratory: Depression, edema

General: Flu-like symptoms (especially with chronic exposure)

Delayed: Muscle asthenia and paresthesia

Signs & Symptoms of Acute Overdose Miosis (unreactive to light), mydriasis (rarely), lacrimation, pallor, excessive sweating, confusion, agitation, headache, dysarthria, generalized asthenia, seizures, A-V block, coma, decreased hemoglobin/red blood cell count/platelet count, metabolic acidosis and hyperglycemia (severe intoxication), hypotension, hypertension, bradycardia, tachycardia, Q-T prolongation, heart block, asystole, salivation, bronchorrhea, tachypnea, pulmonary edema, respiratory depression, cranial nerve palsies, diaphragmatic paralysis, skeletal muscle fasciculation and flaccid paralysis, nausea, vomiting, abdominal pain, fecal and urinary incontinence; an "intermediate syndrome" of limb asthenia and respiratory paralysis has been reported to occur between 24 and 96 hours postorganophosphate exposure, and is independent of the acute cholinergic crisis; late paresthesia characterized by stocking and glove paresthesia, anesthesia, and asthenia is infrequently observed weeks to months following acute exposure to certain organophosphates

Toxicodynamics/Kinetics

Absorption: Readily through oral, dermal, or respiratory exposure

Metabolism: Rapidly metabolized to weakly active compounds through hepatic hydrolysis and other pathways

Elimination: Metabolites are excreted in urine

Warnings Risk of aspiration pneumonitis exists with agents having a hydrocarbon vehicle; severe laryngeal irritation and violent coughing may result from exposure to dusting powders; exposure to dusting powders and insecticide granules may cause contact dermatitis

Overdosage Treatment

Decontamination: Isolation, bagging, and disposal of all contaminated clothing and other articles; all emergency medical workers and hospital staff should follow appropriate precautions regarding exposure to hazardous material including the use of protective clothing, masks, goggles, and respiratory equipment

Dermal: Prompt thorough scrubbing of all affected areas with soap and water, including hair and nails

Gastric: Activated charcoal can be administered either orally or via a nasogastric tube; do not induce emesis because of danger of sudden respiratory compromise, alterations in mental status, seizures, coma, and possible aspiration of hydrocarbon vehicles

Ocular: Irrigation with copious tepid sterile water or saline

Supportive therapy: Including airway management, ventilatory assistance, humidified oxygen administration, and close monitoring for sudden respiratory failure

Antidote:

Atropine: Administration should be guided by respiratory status, starting at 1-5 mg I.V. every 5-10 minutes as needed, and should be titrated to the resolution of excess pulmonary secretions; frequent administration of large doses (cumulative doses >100 mg) may be necessary in massive exposures

Glycopyrrolate: May be administered if atropine is unavailable

2-PAM: For more significant exposures (ie, exposures requiring large doses of atropine, or with recurring symptoms, or exposures to more lipid soluble agents), administration should follow: 1-2 g I.V. over 5-10 minutes, repeated in 1 hour if asthenia reoccurs, then every 4-12 hours for recurring symptoms

Enhancement of elimination: Dialysis and hemoperfusion are not indicated due to effectiveness of the prescribed treatment, large volumes of distribution of organophosphates

Antidote(s)

Atropine Sulfate *on page 1395*

Pralidoxime Chloride *on page 1461*

Diagnostic Tests/Procedures

Blood Gases, Arterial *on page 1207*

Chest Films *on page 1224*
Complete Blood Count *on page 1236*
Creatinine, Serum *on page 1243*
Electrocardiography *on page 1253*
Liver Profile *on page 1286*
Pseudocholinesterase, Serum *on page 1340*

Pregnancy Implications Human data regarding organophosphate exposure in pregnancy is limited and anecdotal; teratogenesis and fetal death have been produced in animal models at exposure levels that cause obvious toxicity to the pregnant animal

Additional Information Yellow/tan viscous/oily liquid with a garlic odor; noncombustible, with a vapor pressure of 0.00003 mm Hg at 20°C; red blood cell cholinesterase, and serum pseudocholinesterase may be depressed following acute or chronic organophosphate exposure; RBC cholinesterase is typically not analyzed by in-house laboratories, and is usually not available for consideration during acute management. Pseudocholinesterase levels may be rapidly available from some in-house laboratories, but are not as reliable a marker of organophosphate exposure because of variability secondary to variant genotypes, hepatic disease, oral estrogen use, or malnutrition. Because of this variability, true indication of suppression of either of these enzymes can only be estimated through comparison to pre-exposure values; these enzymes may be useful in measuring a patient's recovery postexposure, especially if the recovery is not progressing as expected.

ACGIH TLV: 0.2 mg/m^3
PEL-TWA: 0.2 mg/m^3

Other information concerning pesticide exposures is available through the EPA-funded National Pesticide Telecommunications Network: 1-800-858-7378 (weekdays, 8 AM to 6 PM, Central Standard time)

Specific References

Minton NA and Murray VS, "A Review of Organophosphate Poisoning," *Med Toxicol Adverse Drug Exp*, 1988, 3(5):350-75.
Namba T, Nolte CT, Jackrel J, et al, "Poisoning Due to Organophosphate Insecticides. Acute and Chronic Manifestations," *Am J Med*, 1971, 50(4):475-92.

Fenthion

CAS Number 55-38-9

Brand Names Baytex®; Entex®; Lysoff®; Spotton®; Tiguvon®

Use Marketed as insecticide granules, dusting agent, or spray liquid with or without petroleum derivative as a solvent

Mechanism of Toxic Action Irreversible inhibition of acetylcholinesterase and plasma cholinesterase, resulting in excess accumulation of acetylcholine at muscarinic and nicotinic receptors, and in the central nervous system

Adverse Reactions

Cardiovascular: Hyperdynamic (~18% to 21%) or hypodynamic (~7% to 10%) states
Central nervous system: Depression, seizures, hyperactivity
Genitourinary: Incontinence
Neuromuscular & skeletal: Weakness, paralysis
Respiratory: Depression, edema
General: Flu-like symptoms (especially with chronic exposure)
Delayed: Muscle asthenia and paresthesia

Signs & Symptoms of Acute Overdose Miosis (unreactive to light), mydriasis (rarely), lacrimation, pallor, excessive sweating, confusion, agitation, headache, dysarthria, generalized asthenia, seizures, A-V block, coma, decreased hemoglobin/red blood cell count/platelet count, metabolic acidosis and hyperglycemia (severe intoxication), hypotension, hypertension, cranial nerve palsies, bradycardia, tachycardia, Q-T prolongation, heart block, asystole, salivation, bronchorrhea, tachypnea, pulmonary edema, respiratory depression, diaphragmatic paralysis, skeletal muscle fasciculation and flaccid paralysis, nausea, vomiting, abdominal pain, fecal and urinary incontinence; an "intermediate syndrome" of limb asthenia and respiratory paralysis has been reported to occur between 24 and 96 hours postorganophosphate exposure, and is independent of the acute cholinergic crisis; late paresthesia characterized by stocking and glove paresthesia, anesthesia, and asthenia is infrequently observed weeks to months following acute exposure to certain organophosphates; symptomatology may be delayed over 12 hours due to high lipid solubility

Toxicodynamics/Kinetics

Absorption: Readily through oral, dermal, or respiratory exposure
Metabolism: Rapidly metabolized to weakly active compounds through hepatic hydrolysis and other pathways
Elimination: Metabolites are excreted in urine

Warnings Rapid dermal absorption may occur across intact skin; toxicity may be prolonged due to the high lipid solubility exhibited by fenthion; a risk of aspiration

(Continued)

Fenthion *(Continued)*

pneumonitis exists following oral exposure to agents having a hydrocarbon vehicle; severe laryngeal irritation and violent coughing may result from exposure to dusting powders; exposure to dusting powders and insecticide granules may cause contact dermatitis

Overdosage Treatment

Decontamination: Isolation, bagging, and disposal of all contaminated clothing and other articles; all emergency medical workers and hospital staff should follow appropriate precautions regarding exposure to hazardous material including the use of protective clothing, masks, goggles, and respiratory equipment

Dermal: Prompt thorough scrubbing of all affected areas with soap and water, including hair and nails

Gastric: Activated charcoal can be administered either orally or via a nasogastric tube; do not induce emesis because of danger of sudden respiratory compromise, alterations in mental status, seizures, coma, and possible aspiration of hydrocarbon vehicles

Ocular: Irrigation with copious tepid sterile water or saline

Supportive therapy: Including airway management, ventilatory assistance, humidified oxygen administration, and close monitoring for sudden respiratory failure

Enhancement of elimination: Dialysis and hemoperfusion are not indicated due to effectiveness of the prescribed treatment, large volumes of distribution of organophosphates

Antidote:

Atropine: Administration should be guided by respiratory status, starting at 1-5 mg I.V. every 5-10 minutes as needed, and should be titrated to the resolution of excess pulmonary secretions; frequent administration of large doses (cumulative doses >100 mg) may be necessary in massive exposures

Glycopyrrolate: May be administered if atropine is unavailable

2-PAM: For more significant exposures (ie, exposures requiring large doses of atropine, or with recurring symptoms, or exposures to more lipid soluble agents), administration should follow: 1-2 g I.V. over 5-10 minutes, repeated in 1 hour if asthenia reoccurs, then every 4-12 hours for recurring symptoms

Antidote(s)

Atropine Sulfate *on page 1395*
Pralidoxime Chloride *on page 1461*

Diagnostic Tests/Procedures

Blood Gases, Arterial *on page 1207*
Chest Films *on page 1224*
Complete Blood Count *on page 1236*
Creatinine, Serum *on page 1243*
Electrocardiography *on page 1253*
Liver Profile *on page 1286*
Pseudocholinesterase, Serum *on page 1340*

Pregnancy Implications Human data regarding organophosphate exposure in pregnancy is limited and anecdotal; teratogenesis and fetal death have been produced in animal models at exposure levels that cause obvious toxicity to the pregnant animal

Additional Information Yellow to tan viscous liquid with a mild garlic odor; red blood cell cholinesterase and serum pseudocholinesterase may be depressed following acute or chronic organophosphate exposure; RBC cholinesterase is typically not analyzed by in-house laboratories, and is usually not available for consideration during acute management. Pseudocholinesterase levels may be rapidly available from some in-house laboratories, but are not as reliable a marker of organophosphate exposure because of variability secondary to variant genotypes, hepatic disease, oral estrogen use, or malnutrition. Because of this variability, true indication of suppression of either of these enzymes can only be estimated through comparison to pre-exposure values; these enzymes may be useful in measuring a patient's recovery postexposure, especially if the recovery is not progressing as expected.

ACGIH TLV: 0.2 mg/m^3
PEL-TWA: 0.2 mg/m^3
Vapor pressure is 0.00003 mm Hg at 20°C

Other information concerning pesticide exposures is available through the EPA-funded National Pesticide Telecommunications Network: 1-800-858-7378 (weekdays, 8 AM to 6 PM, Central Standard time)

Specific References

Borowitz SM, "Prolonged Organophosphate Toxicity in a Twenty-Six Month Old Child," *J Pediatr*, 1988, 112(2):302-4.

Martinez-Chuecos J, Del Carmen Jurado M, Gimenez MP, et al, "Experience With Hemoperfusion for Organophosphate Poisoning," *Med Toxicol Adverse Drug Exp*, 1988, 3(5):350-75.

Minton NA and Murray VS, "A Review of Organophosphate Poisoning," *Med Toxicol Adverse Drug Exp*, 1988, 3(5):350-75.

Namba T, Nolte CT, Jackrel J, et al, "Poisoning Due to Organophosphate Insecticides. Acute and Chronic Manifestations," *Am J Med*, 1971, 50(4):475-92.
Senanayake N and Karalliedde L, "Neurotoxic Effects of Organophosphorus Insecticides. An Intermediate Syndrome," *N Engl J Med*, 1987, 316(13):761-3.

Ferriamicide® *see* Mirex *on page 971*

Fire Ant Bait *see* Mirex *on page 971*

Fire Damp *see* Methane *on page 957*

Firemaster BP-6 *see* Hexabromobiphenyl *on page 935*

Firemaster FF-1 *see* Hexabromobiphenyl *on page 935*

Firmotox *see* Pyrethrins *on page 1003*

Flue Gas *see* Carbon Monoxide *on page 880*

Flukoids® *see* Carbon Tetrachloride *on page 882*

Fluohydric Acid *see* Hydrogen Fluoride *on page 941*

Fluoranthene *see* Polycyclic Aromatic Hydrocarbons *on page 997*

Fluorene *see* Polycyclic Aromatic Hydrocarbons *on page 997*

Fluorinated Hydrocarbons *see* Freon *on next page*

Fluoroacetic Acid (Sodium Salt) *see* Sodium Monofluoroacetate *on page 1014*

FMX 33297 *see* Pyrethrins *on page 1003*

Formaldehyde

CAS Number 50-00-0

UN Number 1198 (solution); 2209 (formalin)

Synonyms Fannoform; Formic Aldehyde, Formalin; Fyde; Hoch; Morbicid; Paraform; Trioxane; Veracur

Use In embalming, fireproofing, glues/adhesives, lacquers, electrical insulation, tannery products

Mechanism of Toxic Action Covalently binds to proteins and causes cell necrosis; mucous membrane irritant

Adverse Reactions

Cardiovascular: Cardiovascular collapse, hypotension
Central nervous system: CNS depression
Dermatologic: Contact dermatitis, dermal irritation
Endocrine & metabolic: Metabolic acidosis
Gastrointestinal: Coagulation necrosis on ingestion, vomiting, diarrhea, feces discoloration (black)
Renal: Nephritis, renal failure
Respiratory: Wheezing, tachypnea
Miscellaneous: Throat irritation

Signs & Symptoms of Acute Overdose Dizziness, urticaria, dyspnea, hyposmia, cough, drowsiness, ataxia, coma, gastritis

Toxicodynamics/Kinetics

Absorption: Well absorbed from the gastrointestinal tract and by inhalation; to a lesser extent, absorbed through the skin
Metabolism: Rapidly (within 1.5 minutes) to formic acid which is then metabolized to carbon dioxide and water
Half-life: Formate: 1.5 hours

Reference Range Blood formaldehyde levels of 4.8 mg/L and 11 mg/L associated with fatality due to ingestion

Overdosage Treatment

Decontamination: Lavage; basic poison management; do not induce emesis; dilute with water
Supportive therapy: Correct acidosis with sodium bicarbonate; endoscopy to evaluate mucosal injury
Enhancement of elimination: Consider hemodialysis if acidosis develops or if methanol level is elevated

Antidote(s)

Sodium Bicarbonate *on page 1467*

Diagnostic Tests/Procedures

Anion Gap, Blood *on page 1193*
Blood Gases, Arterial *on page 1207*
Electrolytes, Blood *on page 1254*
Liver Profile *on page 1286*
Methanol, Blood *on page 1295*

Pregnancy Implications Suggestion of low birthweight children but no documentation of animal or human teratogenesis

Additional Information Implicated in squamous cell carcinoma of the nasopharynx (probable human carcinogen)

(Continued)

Formaldehyde *(Continued)*

30 mL (of a 37% solution) may cause fatalities
TLV-TWA: 1 ppm
IDLH: 100 ppm
PEL-TWA: 3 ppm
Formalin contains 37% formaldehyde and 12% to 15% methanol

Specific References

Andjelkovich DA, Janszen DB, Brown MH, et al, "Mortality of Iron Foundry Workers: I.V. Analysis of a Subcohort Exposed to Formaldehyde," *J Occup Med*, 1995, 37(7):826-37.

Bardana EJ Jr and Montanaro A, "Formaldehyde Asthma," *J Allergy Clin Immunol*, 1986, 77(2):384-5.

Burkhart KK, Kulig KW, and McMartin KE, "Formate Levels Following a Formalin Ingestion," *Vet Hum Toxicol*, 1990, 32(2):135-7.

Council on Scientific Affairs, "Formaldehyde," *JAMA*, 1989, 261(8):1183-7.

Kilburn KH, Warshaw R, Boylen CT, et al, "Pulmonary and Neurobehavioral Effects of Formaldehyde Exposure," *Arch Environ Health*, 1985, 40(5):254-60.

Formic Aldehyde, Formalin *see* Formaldehyde *on previous page*

Formyl Trichloride *see* Chloroform *on page 890*

Fosfothion® *see* Malathion *on page 950*

Fosvex® *see* Tetraethyl Pyrophosphate *on page 1024*

Foumarin® *see* Anticoagulant Rodenticide *on page 859*

Freon

Synonyms Dichlorodifluoromethane; Fluorinated Hydrocarbons; Halon

Use Refrigerant and in fire extinguishers/propellant

Mechanism of Toxic Action Can cause cold injury to surface on contact, sensitizer of myocardium to catecholamines

Adverse Reactions

Cardiovascular: Myocardial depression, arrhythmias
Dermatologic: Contact dermatitis
Respiratory: Pulmonary edema, bronchoconstriction

Signs & Symptoms of Acute Overdose Conjunctivitis, dyspnea, dizziness, hemoptysis, ataxia, slurred speech, drowsiness, coma, seizures, tremor, bradycardia, diarrhea

Toxicodynamics/Kinetics

Absorption: Immediate
Half-life: 75 minutes

Overdosage Treatment Decontamination: Basic poison management, avoid emesis, avoid catecholamines

Additional Information Odor of "fresh cut grass;" levels peak almost immediately after inhalation; heating may produce phosgene

Specific References

Thyrum PT, "Fluorinated Hydrocarbons and the Heart," *Anesthesiology*, 1972, 36(2):103-4.

Voge VM, "Freon: An Unsuspected Problem," *Aviat Space Environ Med*, 1989, 60(10 Pt 2):B27-8.

Freon 10® *see* Carbon Tetrachloride *on page 882*

Freon 20 *see* Chloroform *on page 890*

Freon 30 *see* Methylene Chloride *on page 966*

Freon 40 *see* Chloromethane *on page 891*

Freon 150 *see* Ethylene Dichloride *on page 924*

Fumagon® *see* 1,2-Dibromo-3-Chloropropane *on page 906*

Fumazone® *see* 1,2-Dibromo-3-Chloropropane *on page 906*

Fume Fever *see* Metal Fume Fever *on page 956*

Fumogas® *see* Ethylene Bromide *on page 924*

Fungifen® *see* Pentachlorophenol *on page 990*

Fyde *see* Formaldehyde *on previous page*

Gamoxone *see* Paraquat *on page 987*

Gardentox® *see* Diazinon *on page 904*

Gasoline

CAS Number 8006-61-9

UN Number 1203; 1257

Synonyms Mogas; Motor Fuel; Motor Spirit; Natural Gasoline; Petrol

Use Fuel for internal combustion engines

Mechanism of Toxic Action A volatile hydrocarbon with central nervous system depressant and arrhythmogenic effects

Signs & Symptoms of Acute Overdose Death due to ingestion usually due to aspiration; symptoms occur at 1000 ppm after 1 hour

Inhalation: Pulmonary edema, intra-alveolar hemorrhage, cardiac arrhythmia, muscle cramps, nausea, vomiting, drowsiness, dizziness, hallucinations, ataxia, myoclonus, paresthesias, insomnia

Ingestion: Pulmonary congestion, belching, hypotension, hemolysis, elevated hepatic enzymes, oliguria, aspiration, hematuria, disseminated intravascular coagulation can occur

Toxicodynamics/Kinetics

Protein binding: None

Half-life: 17 hours

Elimination: Pulmonary/renal

Reference Range Urinary phenol (for benzene measurement) >40 mg/L consistent with gasoline exposure in gasoline pump workers; blood 2 methylpentane levels >50 mg/L associated with fatality

Overdosage Treatment

Decontamination: Do not induce emesis or lavage due to risk of aspiration pneumonia; activated charcoal can adsorb benzene

Supportive therapy: Benzodiazepines for seizure control; avoid use of catecholamines due to risk of ventricular arrhythmia

Diagnostic Tests/Procedures

Chest Films *on page 1224*

Lead, Urine *on page 1283*

Creatine Kinase, Blood *on page 1242*

Liver Profile *on page 1286*

Additional Information Highly lipid soluble; gasoline contains a mixture of benzene (0.5%-2.5%), toluene, xylene, ethyl benzene, and possible lead (tetraethyl lead); other additives include ethylene dichloride and ethylene dibromide; lead poisoning is unusual from inhalation of gasoline containing tetraethyl lead

Odor threshold of gasoline: 0.25 ppm

Lethal inhalation concentration: 5000 ppm

Lethal ingestion concentration: 5 g/kg (12 oz)

Ambient level of gasoline at service stations is usually <100 ppm

OSHA – PEL-TWA: 300 ppm

TLV-TWA: 300 ppm

Lead in agriculture gasoline use should be phased out in 1995; goal of phase I toxic reductions is 15% and phase II toxic reduction is 20% to 22%; see table.

Automotive Gasoline

Fuel Parameter	Conventional Gasoline (prior to 1995)	Reformulated Gasoline		
		Phase I (1995–1999)	Phase II (2000–)	California
Reid vapor pressure (psi)	8.7/7.8	8.0/7.1	6.7	6.8
Sulfur (ppm)	339	305	140	30
Oxygen (w%)*	<0.5	2.1	2.1	2
Aromatics (vol%)	32	27	25	22
Olefins (vol%)	13	12	12	4
E200 (%)†	41	49	49	49
E300 (%)‡	83	87	87	91
Benzene (vol%)	1.5	0.95	0.95	0.8

*Increased oxygen percentage obtained by addition of ethanol or methanol.

†Of fuel evaporated at 200°F.

‡Of fuel evaporated at 300° F.

Adapted from the Environmental Protection Agency (EPA).

Specific References

Banner W and Walson PD, "Systemic Toxicity Following Gasoline Aspiration," *Am J Emerg Med*, 1983, 1:292-4.

Janssen S, van der Geest S, Meijer S, et al, "Impairment of Organ Function After Oral Ingestion of Refined Petrol," *Intensive Care Med*, 1988, 14(3):238-40.

Scala RA, "Motor Gasoline Toxicity," *Fundam Appl Toxicol*, 1988, 10(4):533-62.

Geniphene® *see* Toxaphene *on page 1031*

Genitox® *see* DDT *on page 903*

Glucinium *see* Beryllium *on page 869*

Glycerol Trichlorohydrin *see* 1,2,3-Trichloropropane *on page 1034*

Glycol Alcohol *see* Ethylene Glycol *on page 925*

Glycol Dibromide *see* Ethylene Bromide *on page 924*

Glycol Dichloride *see* Ethylene Dichloride *on page 924*

Glycol Ether *see* Diethylene Glycol *on page 911*

Glycol Ethers

Synonyms Alkylene Oxide Adducts; Cellosolves

Use In the production of photoresists of the microelectronic industry, industrial solvents, varnish removers, leather treatment products, anti-icing agents

Mechanism of Toxic Action Hemolysis, bone marrow depression by metabolites by interfering with RNA and DNA synthesis

Adverse Reactions

Central nervous system: Encephalopathy, coma

Hematologic: Bone marrow depression, hemolytic anemia

Hepatic: Fatty degeneration of the liver (methyl ether)

Renal: Tubular necrosis (acute), renal failure

Signs & Symptoms of Acute Overdose Hyperventilation, hypotension, ataxia, tremor, drowsiness, headache, confusion, coma, hypokalemia, metabolic acidosis, hypocalcemia, tachycardia (ventricular), hemorrhagic gastritis; symptoms may be delayed up to 18 hours

Toxicodynamics/Kinetics

Absorption: Readily through the skin, lungs, and gastrointestinal tract

Elimination: Oxidized by alcohol dehydrogenase and excreted in urine

Overdosage Treatment

Decontamination: Emesis or lavage/activated charcoal with cathartic

Supportive therapy: Treat acidosis with sodium bicarbonate; ethanol administration may be of some use

Enhancement of elimination: Hemodialysis is useful for renal failure or acid abnormalities

Antidote(s)

Sodium Bicarbonate *on page 1467*

Diagnostic Tests/Procedures

Blood Gases, Arterial *on page 1207*

Calcium, Serum *on page 1214*

Complete Blood Count *on page 1236*

Crystals, Urine *on page 1246*

Electrolytes, Blood *on page 1254*

Potassium, Blood *on page 1328*

Pregnancy Implications Fetotoxic at high doses; 2-methoxyethanol and 2-ethoxyethanol are teratogenic

Additional Information Mild ethereal odor

Minimum lethal dose: 8 mL (methoxyethanol)

Order of toxicity: Methoxyethanol > ethoxyethanol > butoxyethanol; may give a positive ethylene glycol level on laboratory testing

Diagnostic effects caused by glycol ethers include hypocalcemia (methyl ether), hypokalemia (methyl ether and butyl ether), pancytopenia, metabolic acidosis with high anion gap, and oxalate crystals may be seen in urine; does not affect osmolar gap

Specific References

Ballantyne B and Myers RC, "The Comparative Acute Toxicity and Primary Irritancy of the Monohexyl Ethers of Ethylene and Diethylene Glycol," *Vet Hum Toxicol*, 1987, 29(5):361-6.

Welch LS and Cullen MR, "Effect of Exposure to Ethylene Glycol Ethers on Shipyard Painters: III. Hematologic Effects," *Am J Ind Med*, 1988, 14(5):527-36.

Grain Sorghum Harvest Aid *see* Chlorate Salts *on page 884*

Granex O *see* Chlorate Salts *on page 884*

Grisol® *see* Tetraethyl Pyrophosphate *on page 1024*

Gum Spirits *see* Turpentine Oil *on page 1035*

Halizan® *see* Metaldehyde *on page 955*

Halon *see* Freon *on page 932*

Halon 104® *see* Carbon Tetrachloride *on page 882*

Harvest-Aid *see* Chlorate Salts *on page 884*

Havoc® *see* Anticoagulant Rodenticide *on page 859*

HCB *see* Hexachlorobenzene *on page 936*

HCE *see* Hexachloroethane *on page 937*

HD *see* Mustard Gas *on page 972*

HEOD *see* Dieldrin *on page 911*

Hepatic Gas *see* Hydrogen Sulfide *on page 942*

Heptachlor

Related Information

Organochlorines *on page 983*

CAS Number 76-44-8; 1024-57-3

Brand Names Drinox®; Heptagran®; Heptamul®; Soleptax®; Termide®; Velsicol 104®

Use While it had been used as a dermal insecticide and for control of crop pests and termites, its use has been sharply curtailed in the U.S. by the EPA since 1988; primarily currently used as a termiticide for domestic use and in fire ant control in power transformers

Mechanism of Toxic Action In the cyclodiene class of organochlorine pesticides; interferes with axonal transmembrane flux of sodium and potassium; also inhibits oxidative phosphorylation

Adverse Reactions

Gastrointestinal: Nausea, vomiting
Hematologic: Thrombocytopenia
Neuromuscular & skeletal: Tremors
Ocular: Mydriasis

Toxicodynamics/Kinetics

Absorption: Oral
Metabolism: Hepatic epoxidation to heptachlor epoxide and oxychlordane

Reference Range Heptachlor exposed dairy farm workers from raw milk (levels up to 89 ppm) had elevated blood heptachlor epoxide levels (0.84 ± 1.0 ppb) and oxychlordane levels (0.71 ± 0.8 ppb); U.S. sampling of adipose tissue averages about 0.1 ppm (FDA "action level")

Overdosage Treatment

Decontamination:

- Dermal: Wash with soap and water; avoid oils as they can enhance absorption
- Inhalation: Administer 100% humidified oxygen
- Oral: Lavage/activated charcoal or cholestyramine; do not administer milk or cream as it can enhance absorption

Enhancement of elimination: Multiple dosing of activated charcoal or cholestyramine may be effective

Additional Information Usually found in conjunction with chlordane exposure; heptachlor can be formed as a chlordane metabolite; some association with leukemia noted; leather clothing absorbs heptachlor; can cause sclerodermatous changes of the hands

TLV-TWA: 0.5 mg/m^3
IDLH: 100 mg/m^3
Odor threshold: 0.3 mg/m^3

Specific References

Epstein SS and Ozonoff D, "Leukemias and Blood Dyscrasias Following Exposure to Chlordane and Heptachlor," *Teratog Carcinog Mutagen*, 1987, 7(6):527-40.

Stehr-Green PA, Wohlleb JC, Royce W, et al, "An Evaluation of Serum Pesticide Residue Levels and Liver Function in Persons Exposed to Dairy Products Contaminated With Heptachlor," *JAMA*, 1988, 259(3):374-7.

U.S. Department of Health and Human Services, "Toxicological Profile of Heptachlor/Heptachlor Epoxide TP-92/11," Agency for Toxic Substances and Diseases Registry, April, 1993.

Heptagran® *see* Heptachlor *on this page*

Heptamul® *see* Heptachlor *on this page*

Hexabromobiphenyl

CAS Number 59536-65-1; 67774-32-7; 36355-01-8

Synonyms Firemaster BP-6; Firemaster FF-1

Use Fire retardant in thermoplastics for use in motor housing, electrical products, and auto upholstery; not imported or produced in the U.S. since 1979

Mechanism of Toxic Action Binds to a cellular receptor (Ah receptor) which alters protein and enzyme synthesis

Adverse Reactions Similar to polychlorinated biphenyl agents; halogen acne (bromacne), hypothyroidism, impairment of memory upon inhalation; elevated liver function tests and hepatomegaly have been noted after oral ingestion; hepatocellular carcinomas have been noted in animal models

Toxicodynamics/Kinetics

Absorption: By dermal contact, oral, or inhalation routes
Protein binding: 80%
Metabolism: Hepatic debromination and hydroxylation
Elimination: Fecal and urinary routes

Reference Range General population adipose tissue concentration: Ranges from 1.0-2.0 μg/kg; baseline serum level of polybrominated biphenyls: ~0.2 μg/L

(Continued)

Hexabromobiphenyl *(Continued)*

Overdosage Treatment

Decontamination:

Dermal: Wash with soap and water

Ocular: Irrigate with saline

Oral: Lavage/activated charcoal or cholestyramine

Additional Information Exposure can occur via ingestion of contaminated food; one such episode occurred in Michigan involving contaminated feed from polybrominated biphenyls (PBB) in May 1973; dairy products were involved. While spray drying of milk reduced PBB levels in milk, there was no effect when pasteurization, aging of cheese, or freeze drying occurred; pressure cooking meat also reduces meat PBB content.

Atmospheric half-life: 182 days

Specific References

U.S. Department of Health and Human Services, "Toxicological Profile for Polybrominated Biphenyls (PBBs)," Agency for Toxic Substances and Diseases Registry, October, 1993.

Hexachlorobenzene

CAS Number 118-74-1

UN Number 2729

Synonyms HCB; Perchlorobenzene; Phenyl Perchloryl

Brand Names Amatin®; Anti-Carie®; Bent-Cure®; Bent-No-More®; No Bent®; Sanocide®

Use Waste product of perchlorethylene used for seed treatment

Mechanism of Toxic Action Induction of porphyria can occur by inhibition of the enzyme uroporphyrinogen decarboxylase and increased d-ALA-synthetase, thus increasing uroporphyrin III levels; lipid peroxidation and mitochondrial inhibition can also occur

Adverse Reactions In children, diarrhea, fever, pink skin papules are noted; hypochromic anemia

Central nervous system: Paresthesia in children

Dermatologic: Skin blisters, epidermolysis, increased pigmentation, porphyria cutanea tarda syndrome ("pink sore disease") from estimated ingestion of 0.05-0.2 g/day

Endocrine & metabolic: Thyromegaly

Gastrointestinal: Anorexia

Hematologic: Porphyria

Hepatic: Hepatomegaly

Neuromuscular & skeletal: Hand atrophy, muscle weakness

Respiratory: Pulmonary irritant

Miscellaneous: Hypothermia, dark-colored (port wine) urine

Signs & Symptoms of Acute Overdose Porphyria, alopecia, hirsutism, hyperthermia, ataxia

Toxicodynamics/Kinetics

Distribution: Very lipophilic; found in breast milk

Metabolism: Hepatic to pentachlorophenol, pentachlorobenzene, and tetrachlorobenzene

Half-life: 60 days

Reference Range Whole blood hexachlorobenzene levels of 0.41 ppb not associated with adverse health effects

Overdosage Treatment

Decontamination: Lavage/activated charcoal with cathartic; do not use oil based cathartics

Supportive therapy: Avoid sunlight; calcium disodium ethyl-enediaminetetracetic acid (EDTA) at 1.5 g I.V. for 5 days or 500 mg to 1.5 g/day orally has been shown to be useful; barbiturates should be used for seizure control

Enhancement of elimination: Multiple dosing of activated charcoal or cholestyramine may be effective

Antidote(s)

Cholestyramine Resin *on page 1405*

Edetate Calcium Disodium *on page 1419*

Additional Information Insoluble in water; little CNS toxicity; increased death rate in children with maternal hexachlorobenzene-induced porphyria during first 2 years of life, probably through contaminated breast milk; pentachlorophenol can increase toxicity (porphyringenicity) of hexachlorobenzene

Atmospheric half-life: 90 days

Soil half-life: 3-6 years

Specific References

Chu TC and Chu EJ, "Effect of Various Additives on Porphyrin Biosynthesis," *Biochim Biophys Acta*, 1970, 215(2):377-92.

Peters HA, Gocmen A, Cripps DJ, et al, "Epidemiology of Hexachlorobenzene-Induced Porphyria in Turkey: Clinical and Laboratory Follow-up After 25 Years," *Arch Neurol*, 1982, 39(12):744-9.

Peters HA, Johnson SA, Cam S, et al, "Hexachlorobenzene-Induced Porphyria: Effect on Chelation on the Disease, Porphyrin and Metal Metabolism," *Am J Med Sci*, 1966, 251(3):314-22.

Hexachlorobutadiene

Related Information

Organochlorines *on page 983*

CAS Number 87-68-3

UN Number 2279

Synonyms Dolen-Pur; Perchlorobutadiene

Use Solvent in the manufacture of rubber, lubricants, and chlorofluorocarbons; fumigant; fluid in gyroscopes

Mechanism of Toxic Action Cysteine metabolite causes uncoupling of oxidative phosphorylation and inhibition of cytochrome oxidase activity and electron transport in the mitochondria

Adverse Reactions Increased serum bile acids with chronic inhalation exposure (0.005-0.02 ppm)

Toxicodynamics/Kinetics

Absorption: After inhalation

Metabolism: Conjugation with glutathione (toxic metabolite)

Elimination: Biliary

Reference Range Range noted in human adipose tissue 0.8-8.0 µg/kg wet weight

Overdosage Treatment

Decontamination: Lavage/activated charcoal; do not use oil-based cathartic

Supportive therapy: In animal studies, probenecid decreased levels of mercapturic acid derivative and decreased renal toxicity

Enhancement of elimination: Due to enterohepatic recirculation, multiple dosing of activated charcoal may be effective

Additional Information

PEL-TWA: 0.02 ppm

TLV-TWA: 0.02 ppm

Range of urban ambient air hexachlorobutadiene levels: 2-11 ppt

Drinking water contains <3 ppt; not found in sewage samples

Specific References

Driscoll TR, Hamdan HH, Wang G, et al, "Concentrations of Individual Serum or Plasma Bile Acids in Workers Exposed to Chlorinated Aliphatic Hydrocarbons," *Br J Ind Med*, 1992, 49(10):700-5.

Lock EA and Ishmael J, "Effect of the Organic Acid Transport Inhibitor Probenecid on Renal Cortical Uptake and Proximal Tubular Toxicity of Hexachloro-1,3-Butadiene and Its Conjugates," *Toxicol Appl Pharmacol*, 1985, 81(1):32-42.

Mes J, Davies DJ, and Turton D, "Polychlorinated Biphenyl and Other Chlorinated Hydrocarbon Residues in Adipose Tissues of *Canadians*," *Bull Environ Contam Toxicol*, 1982, 28(1):97-104.

Hexachloroethane

CAS Number 67-72-1

UN Number 9037

Synonyms Carbon Hexachloride; HCE; Perchloroethane

Brand Names Avlothane®; Distokal®; Distopan®; Egitol®; Phenohep®

Use Moth repellant; antihelmintic agent in sheep; used in the military in smoke screens and pyrotechnic devices

Mechanism of Toxic Action Mucosal irritant; this chlorinated hydrocarbon can cause a tubular nephropathy and hepatic toxicity through free radical-induced lipid peroxidation

Adverse Reactions No systemic adverse effects described in humans although there is one report of a liver tumor associated with a 6-year hexachloroethane exposure; liver and kidneys are target organs for pathology in animals; neurotoxicity (ataxia and tremor) has also been noted; not fetotoxic in rodent models; blepharospasm, lacrimation, and photophobia noted to fume exposure

Toxicodynamics/Kinetics

Absorption: Limited from inhalation or dermal routes; Oral absorption: 50% to 88%

Metabolism: Hepatic to tetrachloroethane and pentachloroethane

Overdosage Treatment

Decontamination:

Dermal: Wash with soap and water; remove contaminated clothing

Ocular: Irrigate copiously with saline

Oral: Do not induce emesis, lavage/activated charcoal; do not administer milk or cream in that it can increase absorption

Supportive therapy: Although there is no experience in this toxicity, N-acetylcysteine may have a theoretical role in reducing hepatotoxic effects

Enhancement of elimination: Although there is no experience in this toxicity, hemodialysis may play a role in enhancing elimination of hexachloroethane in patients developing renal failure

Additional Information Hexachloroethane is a metabolite of carbon tetrachloride

Odor threshold:

(Continued)

Hexachloroethane *(Continued)*

Air: 0.015 ppm (camphoraceous)
Water: 0.01 mg/L

Background air level in northern hemisphere: 5-7 ppt
TLV-TWA: 1 ppm
Water half-life: 1 year

Specific References

Scherling SS and Blondis RR, "The Effect of Chemical Warfare Agents on the Human Eye," *Mil Surgeon*, 1945, 96:70-8.

Selden A, Jacobson G, Berg P, et al, "Hepatocellular Carcinoma and Exposure to Hexachlorobenzene: A Case Report," *Br J Ind Med*, 1989, 46(2):138-40.

Weeks MH, Angerhofer RA, Bishop R, et al, "The Toxicity of Hexachloroethane in Laboratory Animals," *Am Ind Hyg Assoc J*, 1979, 40(3):187-99.

Hexadrin® *see* Endrin *on page 922*

Hexamite® *see* Tetraethyl Pyrophosphate *on page 1024*

Hexane

CAS Number 110-54-3

UN Number 1208

Synonyms Dipropyl; Skellysolve B

Commonly Found In Production of glues, adhesives, paints, shoes, and furniture; component of crude oil

Mechanism of Toxic Action Metabolite 2,5-hexanedione is neurotoxic; 2-methyl pentone leads to hexone

Adverse Reactions

Cardiovascular: Tachycardia
Central nervous system: CNS depression
Respiratory: Respiratory depression

Signs & Symptoms of Acute Overdose Lacrimation, upper airway irritation, dyspnea, muscle cramps, ototoxicity, tinnitus, blurred vision; peripheral muscles are affected first; peripheral sensorimotor neuropathy

Toxicodynamics/Kinetics

Absorption: Through the skin (within 30 minutes), gastrointestinal tract, and lungs
Metabolism: To 2,5-hexanedione
Half-life: 1.5-2 hours
Elimination: Excreted renally

Reference Range Urine concentration of 2,5-hexanedione should be <5 mg/L; background blood hexane concentrations in unexposed adults range from 0.02-7.7 μg/L (average: 0.6 μg/L)

Overdosage Treatment Decontamination: Lavage; dilute with 4-8 oz of milk or water; irrigate skin with soap and water

Diagnostic Tests/Procedures

Nerve Conduction Studies *on page 1304*

Additional Information Parkinsonism may occur with chronic exposure along with a sensory polyneuropathy and memory deficits

TLV-TWA: 50 ppm

Specific References

Brugnone F, Maranelli G, Romeo L, et al, "Ubiquitous Pollution by N-Hexane and Reference Biological Levels in the General Population," *Int Arch Occup Environ Health*, 1991, 63(3):157-60.

Couri DC and Milks MM, "Hexacarbon Neuropathy: Tracking a Toxin," *Neurotoxicology*, 1985, 6(4):65-72.

Huang CC and Chu NS, "Evoked Potentials in Chronic n-Hexane Intoxication," *Clin Electroencephalogr*, 1989, 20(3):162-8.

Paulson GW and Waylonis GW, "Polyneuropathy Due to n-Hexane," *Arch Intern Med*, 1976, 136(8):880-2.

Pezzoli G, Barbieri S, Ferrante C, et al, "Parkinsonism Due to n-Hexane Exposure," *Lancet*, 1989, 2(8667):874.

2-Hexanone

CAS Number 591-78-6

Synonyms Butyl Methyl Ketone; MBK; Methyl-n-Butyl Ketone; 2-Oxohexane; Propylacetone

Commonly Found In Coated fabrics, paints, solvents

Mechanism of Toxic Action Metabolite 2,5-hexanedione can cause distal neuronal swelling and axonal degeneration

Adverse Reactions

Cardiovascular: Tachycardia
Central nervous system: Polyneuropathy (distal sensory), CNS depression
Respiratory: Respiratory depression

Signs & Symptoms of Acute Overdose Lacrimation, ocular irritation, upper airway irritation, dyspnea, paresthesia, nausea and vomiting, asthenia

Toxicodynamics/Kinetics

Absorption: Through lungs (75% to 92%), oral (66%), and dermal (rate of 4.8-8.0 mcg/minute/cm^2)

Metabolism: To 2,5-hexanedione (neurotoxic agent)
Elimination: Through lungs, in urine

Reference Range 2,5-hexanedione: urine: <5.0 mg/L; blood: <10.0 μg/L

Overdosage Treatment Decontamination: Lavage; dilute with 4-8 oz milk or water; irrigate skin with soap and water

Diagnostic Tests/Procedures
Nerve Conduction Studies *on page 1304*

Additional Information Very soluble in water; has been found in milk and cream at levels of 7-18 ppb
Odor threshold: 0.076 ppm (acetone)
TLV-TWA: 5 ppm
PEL-TWA: 5 ppm
IDLH: 1000 ppm
Atmospheric half-life: 36 hours
River water half-life: 10-15 days

Specific References

Allen N, Mendell JM, Billmaier DJ, et al, "Toxic Polyneuropathy Due to Methyl-n-Butyl Ketone," *Arch Neurol*, 1975, 32(4):209-18.
Mullov JS, "MBK Neuropathy Among Spray Painters," *JAMA*, 1976, 235(14):1455-7.
U.S. Department of Health and Human Services, "Toxicological Profile for 2-Hexanone TP-91/18," Agency for Toxic Substances and Diseases Registry, TP-91/11, September, 1992.

Hexaquachromium Chloride *see* Chromium *on page 893*

Hexavin® *see* Carbaryl *on page 877*

Hexogen *see* RDX *on page 1009*

Hexolite *see* RDX *on page 1009*

HHDN *see* Aldrin *on page 856*

High Melting Explosive *see* HMX *on this page*

HMX

CAS Number 2691-41-0

UN Number 0226

Synonyms Cyclotetramethylenetetranitramine; High Melting Explosive; Octogen

Use Explosive polynitramine which is primarily used in nuclear devices to implode fissionable material; also used as a solid rocket fuel propellant and in plastic explosives; primarily produced in the U.S. at the Holston Army Ammunition Plant in Kingsport, Tennessee

Mechanism of Toxic Action Essentially not known but may involve its toxic metabolites nitrite, hydrazines, and formaldehyde

Adverse Reactions No documented adverse effects to exposure in humans have been described; in animals, this toxin appears to act as a neurological stimulant

Toxicodynamics/Kinetics
Absorption: Poor orally (<5% in animals)
Metabolism: To nitrites and then nitroreduction to hydrazines
Elimination: Primarily renal

Additional Information A high explosive; not usually found in air; essentially insoluble in water
Photolytic half-life in water: 1-70 days

Specific References

Hathaway JA and Buck CR, "Absence of Health Hazards Associated With RDX Manufacture and Use," *J Occup Med*, 1977, 19(4):269-72.

Hoch *see* Formaldehyde *on page 931*

Hoe-2671 *see* Endosulfan *on page 921*

Huilex® *see* Toxaphene *on page 1031*

Hydrazine

CAS Number 302-01-2

UN Number 2029; 2030

Synonyms Anhydrous Hydrazine; Diamide; Diamine

Brand Names Levoxin®; Oxytreat 35®; Zerox®

Use Commonly used as a rocket fuel, laboratory reagent, soldering flux, photography, silvering of mirrors and inhibitor of corrosion; also used in preparation of pharmaceutical agents, pesticides, and as a scavenging agent for oxygen; had been used (unapproved) as medication for sickle cell disease and cancer

Mechanism of Toxic Action Hydrazines are direct cellular toxins which also produce a pyridoxine deficiency by binding to vitamin B_6 derivatives and thus inhibiting reactions that require vitamin B_6 as a cofactor

Adverse Reactions
Cardiovascular: Hypotension (due to myocardial depression), atrial fibrillation

(Continued)

Hydrazine *(Continued)*

Central nervous system: Fever, coma, headache, ataxia
Dermatologic: Facial edema, dermal irritant, lupus, eczema, photosensitivity
Gastrointestinal: Anorexia, vomiting, nausea
Hematologic: Hemolysis, methemoglobinemia (monomethylhydrazine)
Hepatic: Hepatotoxicity (fatty degeneration)
Neuromuscular & skeletal: Arthralgia, tremor
Ocular: Eye irritation, nystagmus, mydriasis
Respiratory: Dyspnea, pulmonary edema, rhinitis, cough
Miscellaneous: Salivation

Toxicodynamics/Kinetics

Absorption: By oral, inhalation, and dermal routes
Half-life: 2 hours
Metabolism: Hepatic to acetyl hydrazine, diacetyl hydrazine, and pyruvate hydrazine (through binding with ketoacids)
Elimination: Renal

Overdosage Treatment

Decontamination:

Oral: Do **not** induce emesis; lavage/activated charcoal
Ocular: Hydrazine hydrate is a strong corrosive alkali agent, need to irrigate copiously with saline

Supportive therapy: Pyridoxine hydrochloride (25 mg/kg I.V.) may be antidotal for coma or seizures; methylene blue can be used for symptomatic methemoglobinemia

Enhancement of elimination: Force urine diuresis (with the addition of mannitol); may increase the clearance of hydrazine

Antidote(s)

Pyridoxine Hydrochloride *on page 1465*
Methylene Blue *on page 1444*

Additional Information Symptoms may be delayed for 14 hours following skin exposure

Odor threshold: 3.7 ppm (ammonia gas odor)
TLV-TWA: 0.1 ppm
IDLH: 80 ppm
Water and atmospheric half-life: <2 hours

Specific References

Albert DM and Puliafito CA, "Choroidal Melanoma. Possible Exposure to Industrial Toxins," *N Engl J Med*, 1977, 296(11):634-5.
Durant PJ and Harris RA, "Hydrazine and Lupus," *N Engl J Med*, 1980, 303(10):584-5.
Harati Y and Niakan E, "Hydrazine Toxicity, Pyridoxine Therapy, and Peripheral Neuropathy," *Ann Intern Med*, 1986, 104(5):728-9.
Reid FJ, "Hydrazine Poisoning," *Br Med J*, 1965, 2:5472.
Wrangsio K and Martensson A, "Hydrazine Contact Dermatitis From Gold Plating," *Contact Dermatitis*, 1986, 15(4):244-5.

Hydrochloride *see* Hydrogen Chloride *on this page*
Hydrofluoric Acid *see* Hydrogen Fluoride *on next page*
Hydrogen Arsenide *see* Arsine *on page 864*

Hydrogen Chloride

CAS Number 7647-01-0

UN Number 1789; 1050

Synonyms Chlorohydric Acid; Hydrochloride; Muriatic Acid; Spirits of Salt

Use In the manufacture of vinyl chloride and rubber; a combustible product of vinyl chloride (PVC)

Mechanism of Toxic Action Corrosive to the skin, eyes, nose, respiratory and gastrointestinal tract; primarily local effects, minimal systemic effects; high water solubility leading to upper airway edema

Adverse Reactions

Ocular: Corneal injury
Respiratory: Laryngeal spasms, pulmonary edema, reactive airways disease syndrome (RADS)

Signs & Symptoms of Acute Overdose Conjunctivitis, nasal ulcerations, choking sensation, cough, dyspnea, hemoptysis, dermal burns, chest tightness, headache, dizziness, and nausea

Toxicodynamics/Kinetics

Absorption: Not absorbed
Metabolism: Ionized to hydronium and chloride ions

Overdosage Treatment Supportive therapy: Give 100% humidified oxygen, treat wheezing with inhaled beta agonists; corticosteroids may be helpful

Test Interactions Hypothesized to cause elevated chloride levels

Diagnostic Tests/Procedures
Chest Films *on page 1224*
Complete Blood Count *on page 1236*

Pregnancy Implications Fetotoxic in animals

Additional Information Pungent odor; clear, colorless
Odor threshold: 1-5 ppm
TLV-ceiling: 5 ppm
IDLH: 100 ppm

Specific References

Dyer RF and Esch VH, "Polyvinyl Chloride Toxicity in Fires. Hydrogen Chloride Toxicity in Fire Fighters," *JAMA*, 1976, 235(4):393-7.
Finnegan MJ and Hodson ME, "Prolonged Hypoxaemia Following Inhalation of Hydrogen Chloride Vapour," *Thorax*, 1989, 44(3):238-9.
Goldstein DA, "Reactive Airways Disease Syndrome Following Inhalational Exposure to Hydrochloric Acid Mist or Vapors," *Vet Hum Toxicol*, 1994, 36:345.
Penner GE, "Acid Ingestion: Toxicology and Treatment," *Ann Emerg Med*, 1980, 9(7):374-9.

Hydrogen Fluoride

CAS Number 7664-39-3

UN Number 1052; 1786; 1790

Synonyms Fluohydric Acid; Hydrofluoric Acid

Commonly Found In Automotive cleaning products; production of integrated circuits

Use In etching and cleaning of glass and porcelain; produce computer screen, fluorescent bulbs; refine high octane gasoline

Mechanism of Toxic Action Corrosive, produces heat when exposed to water; binds calcium, potassium, and magnesium; dissociates in tissue to free H^+ and F^- ions; fluoride anion inhibits Na^+/K^+ ATPase enzyme

Adverse Reactions
Cardiovascular: Ventricular fibrillation
Dermatologic: Dermal burns, onycholysis
Gastrointestinal: Vomiting (with ingestion)
Respiratory: Pneumonitis, hemorrhagic pulmonary edema

Signs & Symptoms of Acute Overdose Erythema of skin, blistering, pain, burns, vomiting (with ingestion), pulmonary edema, nausea (22%), diarrhea (22%), bone pain, vomiting

Toxicodynamics/Kinetics
Onset of action: Immediate corrosive effects although symptoms may be delayed 12-24 hours
Absorption: Inhalation and dermal routes
Half-life: 2-9 hours
Elimination: Renal

Reference Range Normal plasma fluoride levels are <0.1 μg/L

Overdosage Treatment
Decontamination: Dilute with milk or water; emesis is contraindicated. As first aid, affected extremity can be irrigated with water and bathed in an iced solution of 25% magnesium sulfate; give 300 mL of magnesium citrate orally for oral ingestion; give 20 mL 10% calcium gluconate I.V. for oral ingestion; nebulized calcium gluconate (2.5%) for inhalation or infiltrate with subcutaneous injection of 0.5 mL of 10% calcium gluconate or 10% magnesium sulfate with a 30-gauge needle not greater than 0.5 mL/cm^2; magnesium sulfate may also given I.V. (Do not use calcium chloride for injection.) 2.5% calcium gluconate gel can also be utilized.
Supportive therapy: Arterial infusion for distal extremity burns may be useful
Enhancement of elimination: Hemodialysis may be used to remove fluoride anions

Antidote(s)
Calcium Chloride *on page 1400*
Calcium Gluconate *on page 1401*
Magnesium Sulfate *on page 1440*

Diagnostic Tests/Procedures
Blood Gases, Arterial *on page 1207*
Calcium, Serum *on page 1214*
Chest Films *on page 1224*
Electrocardiography *on page 1253*
Electrolytes, Blood *on page 1254*
Magnesium, Serum *on page 1289*

Additional Information Latex gloves are not protective; as little as 7 mL of anhydrous topical hydrogen fluoride can cause profound hypocalcemia; a 2.5% total body surface burn can be fatal; colorless
Odor threshold: 0.03 mg/m^3
Minimum lethal exposure: 1.5 g
TLV-ceiling: 3 ppm
IDLH: 20 ppm

(Continued)

Hydrogen Fluoride *(Continued)*

PEL-TWA: 3 ppm

Specific References

Braun J, Stoss H, and Zober A, "Intoxication Following the Inhalation of Hydrogen Fluoride," *Arch Toxicol*, 1984, 56(1):50-4.
Cox RD and Osgood KA, "Evaluation of Intravenous Magnesium Sulfate for the Treatment of Hydrofluoric Acid Burns," *J Toxicol Clin Toxicol*, 1994, 32(2):123-36.
Daniel CR 3d, "Onycholysis: An Overview," *Semin Dermatol*, 1992, 10(1):34-40.
el Saadi MS, Hall AH, Hall PK, et al, "Hydrofluoric Acid Dermal Exposure," *Vet Hum Toxicol*, 1989, 31(3):243-7.
Henry JA and Hla KK, "Intravenous Regional Calcium Gluconate Perfusion for Hydrofluoric Acid Burns," *J Toxicol Clin Toxicol*, 1992, 30(2):203-7.
O'Neil K, "A Fatal Hydrogen Fluoride Exposure," *J Emerg Nurs*, 1994, 20:451-3.
Stremski ES, Grande GA, and Ling LJ, "Survival Following Hydrofluoric Acid Ingestion," *Ann Emerg Med*, 1992, 21(11):1396-9.
Velvart J, "Arterial Perfusion for Hydrofluoric Acid Burns," *Hum Toxicol*, 1983, 2(2):233-8.

Hydrogen Phosphide *see* Phosphine *on page 993*

Hydrogen Sulfide

CAS Number 7783-06-4

UN Number 1053

Synonyms Hepatic Gas; Hydrosulfuric Acid; Sewer Gas; Stink Damp; Sulfureted Hydrogen

Commonly Found In Volcanoes, manure

Use In farming, brewing, tanning, glue making, lithography, rayon manufacture

Mechanism of Toxic Action Inhibition of cytochrome oxidase; irritant

Adverse Reactions

Central nervous system: CNS depression, subacute encephalopathy
Dermatologic: Skin irritation
Respiratory: Pulmonary edema, respiratory depression, hyperventilation

Signs & Symptoms of Acute Overdose Lacrimation, conjunctivitis, hyposmia, cough, dementia, hypothermia, myoglobinuria, hypertension, extrapyramidal symptoms, dyspnea, nausea, vomiting; higher concentrations may cause headache, dizziness, confusion, bradycardia, hypotension, coma, seizures, rotten egg breath, paresthesia, bradycardia

Toxicodynamics/Kinetics

Absorption: Readily as a systemic toxicant through the lungs/gastrointestinal tract
Metabolism: To thiosulfate
Elimination: Oxidized by hemoglobin and liver and renally excreted

Reference Range Normal whole blood sulfide is <0.05 mg/L; >0.9 mg/L has been correlated with death; serum thiosulfate >1.3 µg/mL associated with toxicity; serum thiosulfate level >12 µg/mL associated with immediate fatality

Normal levels of thiosulfate:
Blood: Not detectable
Urine: <8 µg/mL

Overdosage Treatment

Supportive therapy: 100% humidified oxygen; hyperbaric oxygen if symptoms do not improve with supplemental oxygen; amyl nitrate and sodium nitrite (10 mg/kg up to 300 mg) can be given (monitor for methemoglobinemia). Do not give sodium thiosulfate. Wash surfaces with soap and water.
Enhancement of elimination: For infants, consider exchange transfusion

Antidote(s)

Amyl Nitrite *on page 1390*
Oxygen (Hyperbaric) *on page 1453*
Sodium Nitrite *on page 1469*

Diagnostic Tests/Procedures

Blood Gases, Arterial *on page 1207*
Lactic Acid, Blood *on page 1281*
Methemoglobin, Blood *on page 1296*
Sulfhemoglobin *on page 1358*
Urinalysis *on page 1373*

Monitoring Parameters Albuminuria and hematuria; methemoglobin if giving nitrite therapy; sulfhemoglobin levels are of no use

Pregnancy Implications Increased rates of spontaneous abortions

Additional Information Produced by decaying organic matter; heavier than air; colorless; rotten egg odor at levels of 0.0047 ppm; note that olfactory fatigue occurs at 50-150 ppm; neurologic sequelae of survivors include intention tremor, amnesia, ataxia; heavier than air (density: 1.2); air levels >700 ppm can be fatal; overall mortality: 2% to 6%

TLV-TWA: 10 ppm
IDLH: 300 ppm

PEL-TWA: 10 ppm

Specific References

Done AK, "The Toxic Emergency: The Perils Under the City," *J Emerg Med*, 1979, 70-7.
Hoffman RS, "Hydrogen Sulfide," *Emerg Med Clin North Am*, 1995, 27(7):45.
Jappinen P and Tenhunen R, "Hydrogen Sulphide Poisoning: Blood Sulphide Concentration and Changes in Haem Metabolism," *Br J Ind Med*, 1990, 47(4):283-5.
Ravizza AG, Carugo D, and Cerchiari EL, "The Treatment of Hydrogen Sulfide Intoxication, Oxygen Vs Nitrites," *Vet Hum Toxicol*, 1982, 24(4):241-2.
Snyder JW, Safir EF, Summerville GP, et al, "Occupational Fatality and Persistent Neurological Sequelae After Mass Exposure to Hydrogen Sulfide," *Am J Emerg Med*, 1995, 13(2):199-203.

Hydrosulfuric Acid *see* Hydrogen Sulfide *on previous page*

Hydroxycoumarin *see* Anticoagulant Rodenticide *on page 859*

Hydroxytoluene *see* Cresols *on page 898*

Hypochlorous Acid *see* Sodium Hypochlorite *on page 1013*

Indanedione *see* Anticoagulant Rodenticide *on page 859*

Insect Powder *see* Pyrethrins *on page 1003*

Isocarb® *see* Propoxur *on page 1000*

Isocyanate *see* Methyl Isocyanate *on page 968*

Isocyanatomethane *see* Methyl Isocyanate *on page 968*

Isocyanide *see* Cyanide *on page 899*

Isopropanol *see* Isopropyl Alcohol *on this page*

Isopropyl Alcohol

CAS Number 67-63-0

UN Number 1219

Synonyms Alcojel; "Blue Heaven"; Chromar; Dimethyl Carbinol; Isopropanol; Propol

Commonly Found In Rubbing alcohol, secondary propyl alcohol, solvents in perfumes, paint thinners, cleaners, disinfectants, racing fuels

Mechanism of Toxic Action Metabolized by alcohol dehydrogenase to acetone which contributes to central nervous system depression

Adverse Reactions Central nervous system: Depression, drowsiness, ataxia, areflexia, headache

Signs & Symptoms of Acute Overdose Lethargy, aplastic anemia, coma, vomiting, myoglobinuria, hypotension, tachycardia, hypothermia, hyperglycemia, porphyria, feces discoloration (black), hypotension due to myocardial depression, hemolytic anemia, rhabdomyolysis

Toxicodynamics/Kinetics

Specific gravity: 0.79 g/mL

Absorption: Rapid from gastrointestinal tract or by inhalation; little absorption through intact skin

Distribution: V_d: 0.5-0.7 L/kg

Metabolism: In the liver; 15% metabolized to acetone

Half-life:

- Isopropyl alcohol: 2.9-16.2 hours
- Acetone: 7.6-26.2 hours

Peak plasma level: 1 hour postingestion

Elimination: Excreted renally, 25% to 50% unchanged

Reference Range Toxic: >50 mg/dL; death can occur at 150 mg/dL

Overdosage Treatment

Decontamination: Activated charcoal with cathartic may be useful when used in a charcoal solvent ratio of 20:1; do not induce emesis with ipecac

Enhancement of elimination: Hemodialysis in those patients who do not respond to supportive therapy or whose levels exceed 400 mg/dL

Test Interactions Do not use breathalyzer; creatinine may be falsely elevated when colorimetric methods are used in presence of acetone concentrations >40 mg/dL

Diagnostic Tests/Procedures

Glucose, Random *on page 1269*
Isopropanol, Blood *on page 1277*
Ketone Bodies, Blood *on page 1277*
Liver Profile *on page 1286*
Myoglobin, Qualitative, Urine *on page 1302*
Osmolality, Serum *on page 1310*
Osmolality, Urine *on page 1311*

Pregnancy Implications Increased skeletal malformations with decreased fetal weight have been noted in pregnant laboratory animals

Additional Information No long-term sequelae; twice as lethal as ethanol; spirituous odor but a clean colorless liquid; bitter taste; can cause skin burns when used topically on premature infants

(Continued)

Isopropyl Alcohol *(Continued)*

Contribution of a serum concentration level of 100 mg/dL to elevation of osmolar gap: 17

Lethal dose in adults: 250 mL; serious illness can occur with ingestion of 10 mL

Specific References

Burkhart KK and Martinez MA, "The Absorption of Isopropanol and Acetone by Activated Charcoal," *J Toxicol Clin Toxicol*, 1992, 30(3):371-5.

Lacouture PG, Heldreth DD, Shannon M, et al, "The Generation of Acetonemia/Acetonuria Following Ingestion of Subtoxic Dose of Isopropyl Alcohol," *Am J Emerg Med*, 1989, 7(1):38-40.

Martinez TT, Jaeger RW, deCastro FJ, et al, "A Comparison of the Absorption and Metabolism of Isopropyl Alcohol by Oral, Dermal, and Inhalation Routes," *Vet Hum Toxicol*, 1986, 28(3):233-6.

Monaghan MS, Olsen KM, Ackerman BH, et al, "Measurement of Serum Isopropanol and the Acetone Metabolite by Proton Nuclear Magnetic Resonance: Application to Pharmacokinetic Evaluation in a Simulated Overdose Model," *J Toxicol Clin Toxicol*, 1995, 33(2):141-9.

Rich J, Scheife RT, Katz N, et al, "Isopropyl Alcohol Intoxication," *Arch Neurol*, 1990, 47(3):322-4.

Isopropylene Dinitrate *see* Propylene Glycol Dinitrate *on page 1003*

Jasmolin *see* Pyrethrins *on page 1003*

Jet Fuel-4

CAS Number 50815-00-4

UN Number 1863

Synonyms Jet Fuel: JP-4; JP-4

Brand Names MIL-T-5624-L-Amd 1

Use Aviation turbine fuel used by the U.S. military (constitutes 85% of turbine fuel used by Department of Defense)

Mechanism of Toxic Action A mixture of alkanes (43%), cycloalkanes (11%), alkylbenzenes (12%), and naphthalenes (2%) which can cause CNS depression

Adverse Reactions

Dermatologic: Dermal irritant

Central nervous system: Neurologic, headache, dizziness, polyneuropathy (on long-term exposure), ataxia

Gastrointestinal: Nausea

Neuromuscular & skeletal: Muscle asthenia (at inhalation levels between 3000-7000 ppm)

Overdosage Treatment

Decontamination: Do not induce emesis or lavage due to risk of aspiration pneumonia; activated charcoal can adsorb benzene

Supportive therapy: Benzodiazepines for seizure control; avoid use of catecholamines due to risk of ventricular arrhythmia

Additional Information

Odor threshold: 1 ppm

PEL-TWA: 400 ppm

Specific References

Davis NE, "Jet Fuel Intoxication," *Aerospace Med*, 1964, 35:481-2.

U.S. Department of Health and Human Services, "Toxicological Profile for Jet Fuels JP-4 and JP-7," Agency for Toxic Substances and Diseases Registry, May, 1993.

Jet Fuel: JP-4 *see* Jet Fuel-4 *on this page*

JP-4 *see* Jet Fuel-4 *on this page*

Kanechlor *see* Polychlorinated Biphenyls *on page 995*

Kelthane *see* Organochlorines *on page 983*

Kemifan *see* Phenmedipham *on page 992*

Kepone® *see* Chlordecone *on page 886*

Klorex *see* Chlorate Salts *on page 884*

Knox-Out® *see* Diazinon *on page 904*

Krumkil® *see* Anticoagulant Rodenticide *on page 859*

Krystalline *see* Aniline *on page 858*

Kusa-Tohru *see* Chlorate Salts *on page 884*

Kwik-kil® *see* Strychnine *on page 1016*

Kyanor *see* Aniline *on page 858*

Lannate® *see* Methomyl *on page 962*

Laughing Gas *see* Nitrous Oxide *on page 981*

Lauxtol® *see* Pentachlorophenol *on page 990*

Lead

Related Information

Drugs and Chemicals Proven to be Teratogenic in Humans *on page 1572-1575*

Gasoline *on page 932*

Radiation: Basics of Exposure *on page 1594-1600*

CAS Number 7439-92-1; 301-04-2; 13424-46-9; 13814-96-5; 10031-22-8; 10101-63-0; 7758-95-4; 7758-97-6

UN Number 1616; 2291; 2811

Use Lead is available in 19 inorganic and 2 organic compounds; common sources (especially for children) are air, water, soil, and leaded paint chips. Use of tap water (as "first-drawn" or with excessive boiling or stored in lead-based kettles) in reconstituting infant formulas for infants; additional sources/uses include leaded foreign bodies such as bullet fragments, numerous imported Asian products, herbal/folk remedies, Mexican remedies for "empacho" and home abortifacients; recreational sources include lead-based cosmetics, contamination of illicitly distilled alcohols or illicit intravenous drug products, leaded gasoline "sniffing", and even chewing colored plastic wires.

Mechanism of Toxic Action Lead's effects are mediated by its ability to complex sulfhydryl groups and other ligands, in enzyme systems throughout the body

Adverse Reactions Lead toxicity occurs in the acute, acute-on-chronic, or chronic

Effects of Inorganic Lead on Children and Adults– Lowest Observable Adverse Effect Levels

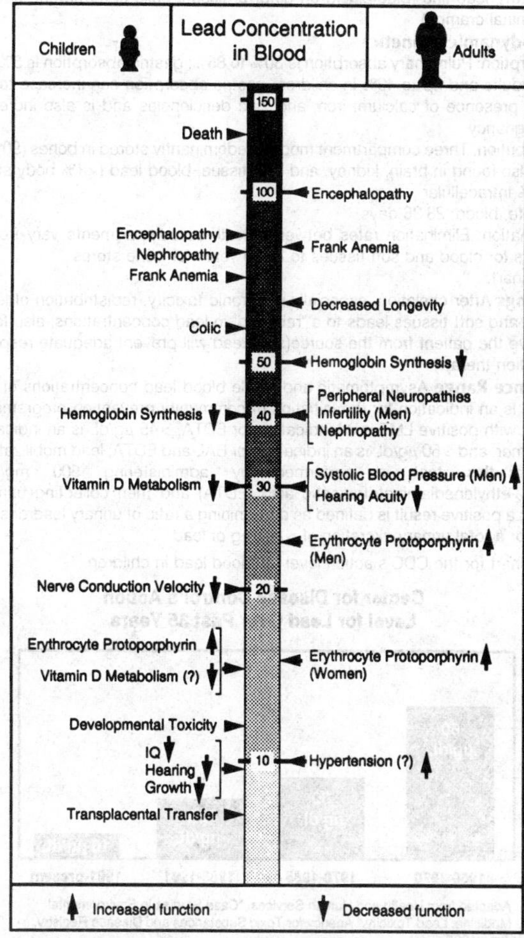

Adapted from U.S. Department of Health and Human Services, "Case Studies in Environmental Medicine: Lead Toxicity," Agency for Toxic Substances and Disease Registry, June 1990.

settings secondary to environmental, occupational, intentional, or recreational activities. Acute exposures are commonly associated with symptoms of malaise, nausea, vomiting, myoclonus, metallic taste, fasciculations, abdominal pain; severe exposures can result in encephalopathy, and death; chronic exposures manifest with neuropsychiatric symptoms, anemia, renal dysfunction/chronic failure, hypertension, arthralgias, teratogenesis, and impotence. See chart.

Central nervous system: Ataxia, encephalopathy, headache, learning disabilities, drowsiness, dementia, mood and/or mental status changes, seizures, paresthesia

Gastrointestinal: Abdominal pain, colic, constipation, nausea, vomiting

Hematologic: Anemia, hemolysis

Hepatic: Hepatitis

Neuromuscular & skeletal: Hypermineralization, arthralgia

Ocular: Blurred vision, diplopia, optic neuropathy

Renal & genitourinary: Proteinuria, hematuria, chronic renal failure due to interstitial nephritis

Signs & Symptoms of Acute Overdose

Mild toxicity: Myalgia or parasthesia, mild fatigue, irritability, drowsiness, occasional abdominal discomfort

Moderate toxicity: Arthralgia, general fatigue, difficulty concentrating, muscular exhaustibility, deafness, tremor, headache, diffuse abdominal pain, vomiting, weight loss, constipation

Severe toxicity: Paresis or paralysis, cranial nerve palsies, blindness, encephalopathy (may abruptly lead to seizures, changes in consciousness, coma, and death), lead line (blue-black) on gingival tissue, colic (intermittent, severe abdominal cramps)

Toxicodynamics/Kinetics

Absorption: Pulmonary absorption is 30% to 85%; gastric absorption is 5% to 15% in adults and up to 40% in children; gastric absorption can increase to 50% in the presence of calcium, iron, and zinc deficiencies and is also increased in pregnancy

Distribution: Three compartment model predominantly stored in bones (90%), lead is also found in brain, kidney, and liver tissue; blood lead (<1% body stores) is 95% intracellular

Half-life, blood: 28-36 days

Elimination: Elimination rates between the three compartments vary from ~40 days for blood and soft tissues to 20-30 years for bone stores

See chart.

Warnings After chelation, especially in chronic toxicity, redistribution of lead into blood and soft tissues leads to a "rebound" in lead concentrations; also failure to remove the patient from the source(s) of lead will prevent adequate response to chelation therapy

Reference Range Asymptomatic and whole blood lead concentrations of >10-25 μg/dL is an indication for the initiation of community prevention programs, 25-50 μg/dL with positive LMT is an indication for EDTA, >45 μg/dL is an indication for succimer, and >50 μg/dL is an indication for BAL and EDTA; lead mobilization test (LMT); this test is performed by administering 500 mg/m² of $CaNA_2$-ethylenediaminetetraacetic acid (EDTA) and then collecting urine for 8 hours; a positive result is defined as determining a ratio of urinary lead/dose EDTA >0.6 or a total urinary excretion of >200 μg of lead

See chart for the CDC's action level for blood lead in children.

Center for Disease Control's Action Level for Lead Over Past 35 Years

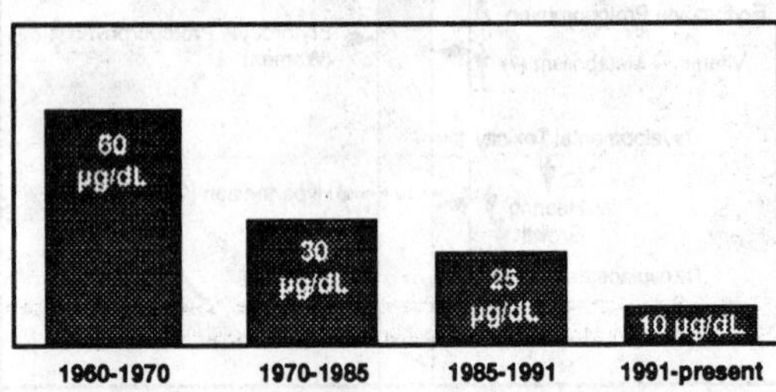

Adapted from Health and Human Services, "Case Studies in Environmental Medicine: Lead Toxicity," Agency for Toxic Substances and Disease Registry, June 1990.

Overdosage Treatment

Decontamination: Prehospital ipecac, otherwise gastric lavage or whole bowel irrigation

Multiorgan Impact of Reduction of Heme Body Pool by Lead
(Derived from EPA 1986a)

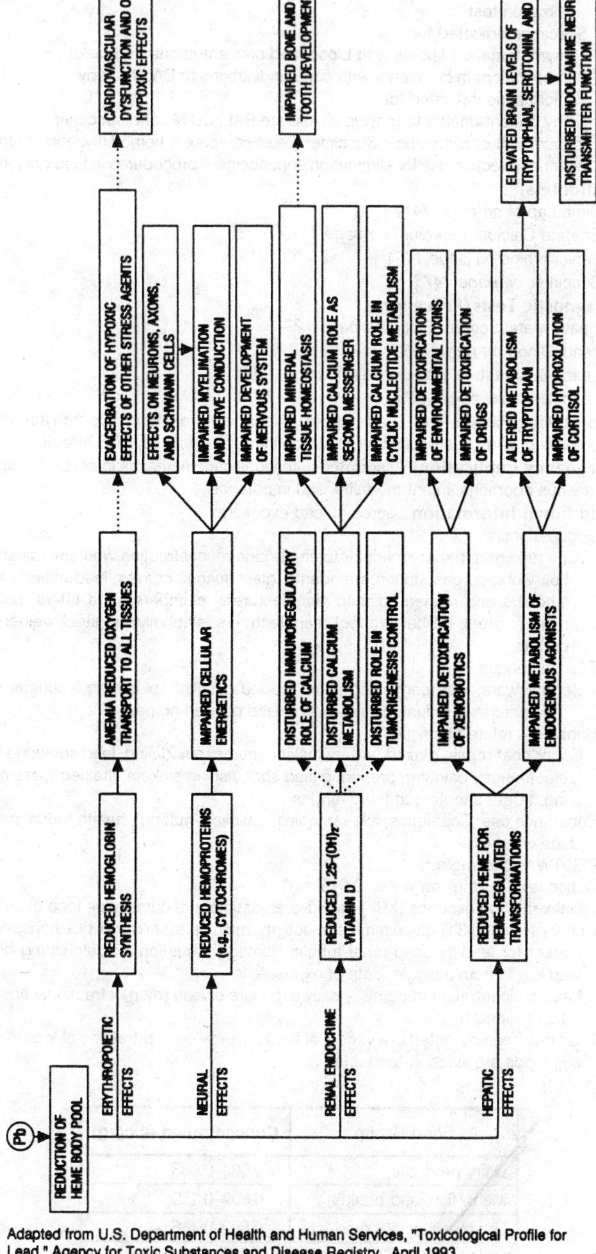

Adapted from U.S. Department of Health and Human Services, "Toxicological Profile for Lead," Agency for Toxic Substances and Disease Registry, April 1993.

Antidotes:

BAL indicated for:

any encephalopathic patient for at least one 5-day treatment course
any other symptomatic patient for at least one 3-day treatment course
any asymptomatic patient with a lead concentration of 70 μg/dL

(Continued)

Lead *(Continued)*

EDTA indicated for:

any patient receiving BAL at least 4 hours after the initial BAL dose

as single agent, for any asymptomatic patient with a lead concentration of >45 μg/dL

any patient with lead concentrations between 25-55 μg/dL with the lead mobilization test

Succimer indicated for:

asymptomatic patients with blood lead concentrations >45 μg/dL

encephalopathic patients with contraindications to BAL therapy

Penicillamine indicated for:

any patient unable to receive or tolerate BAL, EDTA, and succimer

Enhancement of elimination: Succimer: Lead complex is hemodialyzable, there is no other effective use for elimination enhancement procedures in lead poisoning

Antidote(s)

Dimercaprol *on page 1414*
Edetate Calcium Disodium *on page 1419*
Penicillamine *on page 1454*
Succimer *on page 1473*

Diagnostic Tests/Procedures

Heavy Metal Screen, Blood *on page 1271*
Lead, Blood *on page 1282*
Lead, Quantitative, Hair or Nails *on page 1283*
Lead, Urine *on page 1283*

Monitoring Parameters Lead concentrations, erythrocyte protoporphyrin, KUB, potassium x-ray fluorescence, CBC, creatinine, electrolytes, CNS effects

Pregnancy Implications Associated with significant increases in stillbirths, spontaneous abortions, infant mortality, and impotence

Additional Information Source of lead exposure:

Occupational:

Auto repairers, battery manufacturers, bridge reconstruction workers, construction workers, gas station attendants, glass manufacturers, lead miners, lead smelters and refiners, plastic manufacturers, plumbers, pipe fitters, policemen, printers, rubber product manufacturers, shipbuilders, steel welders or cutters

Environmental:

Ceramicware, lead containing paint, leaded gasoline, plumbing leachate, soil/dust near lead industries, roadways, lead painted homes

Hobbies & related activities:

Car or boat repair, glazed pottery making, home remodeling, lead soldering (eg, electronics), painting, preparing lead shot, fishing sinkers, stained glass making, target shooting at firing ranges

Substance use: Cosmetics, folk remedies, gasoline "huffing", health foods, moonshine whiskey

PEL-TWA: 0.05 mg/m^3

Action level in drinking water: 0.015 mg/L

Tibial x-ray fluorescence (XRF) provides an estimate of cumulative lead exposure

Urinary N-acetyl-3-D-glucosamidase activity may be a sensitive but nonspecific marker for lead-induced renal tubular damage. Equation for calculating blood lead levels from a single route of exposure is:

Lead concentration (mcg/dL = daily exposure of lead (mcg) x fractional absorption divided by 3.3)

Lead has been detected in a variety of foods; typical concentrations of lead in various foods are listed in the table.

Food Group	Concentration (mcg/g)
Dairy products	0.003–0.083
Meat, fish, and poultry	0.002–0.159
Grain and cereal products	0.002–0.136
Vegetables	0.005–0.649
Fruit and fruit juices	0.005–0.223
Oils, fats, and shortenings	0.002–0.028
Sugar and adjuncts	0.006–0.073
Beverages	0.002–0.041 (mcg/L)

The following table shows the average daily intakes of lead for adults, based on an analysis of 27 market basket samples taken nationwide for a 1980-82 Total Diet Study

Food Group	Average Adult Intake (mcg/d)
Dairy products	4.54
Meat, fish, and poultry	4.09
Grain and cereal products	9.84
Potatoes	1.39
Leafy vegetables	0.94
Legume vegetables	9.18
Root vegetables	1.39
Garden fruits	4.44
Fruits	10
Oils and fats	1.23
Sugar and adjuncts	2.34
Beverages	6.86
Total lead intake per day	56.5

Lead intoxication has been observed in children but rarely in adults in a residential setting (Sedman 1989). The following table shows the average daily intake of lead over a 10-year span in children and adults.

Daily Average Intake of Lead*
(mcg Lead/Day)

Age	Year					
	1980	1982	1984	1986	1988	1990
6–11 mo	~34	20	16.7	10	5	3.8
2 y female	No data	No data	No data	No data	No data	No data
male	~45	25.1	23	12.8	5	4.3
14–16 y female	No data	No data	28.7	15.2	6.1	6.1
male	No data	No data	40.9	21.8	8.2	8.5
25–30 y female	No data	32	28.7	14.8	7.9	6.7
male	84	45.2	40.9	21.2	10	8.5
60–65 y female	No data	No data	30.4	15.6	No data	2.2
male	No data	No data	37.6	19.1	No data	8.1

Lead dust can be removed by scrubbing with water plus a phosphate detergent or powdered dishwasher detergent. Vacuuming lead dust should be performed with a high efficiency particle arresting (HEPA) vacuum cleaner. Since lead is more soluble in acidic solutions, vinegar can cause leaching of lead from leaded containers or bottles.

Action level for home water lead amounts are 15 ppb for first draw water and 5 ppb for purged-line water (water that has run for at least 1 minute)

Specific References

Bayly GR, Braithwaite RA, Sheehan TMT, et al, "Lead Poisoning From Asian Traditional Remedies in the West Midlands – Report of a Series of Five Cases," *Hum Exp Toxicol*, 1995, 14:24-8.

Chau TT, Chen WY, Hsiao TM, et al, "Chronic Lead Intoxication at an Indoor Firing Range in Taiwan," *J Toxicol Clin Toxicol*, 1995, 33:371-2.

Chisolm JJ Jr, "BAL, EDTA, DMSA, DMPS in the Treatment of Lead Poisoning in Children," *J Toxicol Clin Toxicol*, 1992, 30(4):493-504.

Committee on Drugs, American Academy of Pediatrics, "Treatment Guidelines for Lead Exposure in Children," *Pediatrics*, 1995, 96:155-60.

Cory-Slechta DA, "Relationships Between Lead-Induced Learning Impairments and Changes in Dopaminergic, Cholinergic, and Glutanergic Neurotransmitter System Functions," *Annu Rev Pharmacol Toxicol*, 1995, 35:391-416.

(Continued)

Lead (Continued)

Ellin RI, "A Simple Means of Calculating Blood Lead Concentrations," *J Toxicol Clin Toxicol*, 1995, 33:385-7.

Glotzer DE and Bauchner H, "Management of Childhood Lead Poisoning: A Survey," *Pediatrics*, 1992, 89(4 Pt 1):614-8.

Kumar D and Krishnaswamy K, "Defection of Occupational Lead Nephropathy Using Early Renal Markers," *J Toxicol Clin Toxicol*, 1995, 33:331-5.

Meggs WJ, Gerr F, Aly MH, et al, "The Treatment of Lead Poisoning From Gunshot Wounds With Succimer," *J Toxicol Clin Toxicol*, 1994, 32(4):377-87.

Needleman HL and Gatsonis CA, "Low-Level Lead Exposure and the IQ of Children," *JAMA*, 1990, 263(5):673-8.

Paloucek FP, "Lead Poisoning," *Am Pharm*, 1993, NS33(11):81-8.

"Safe at Home," *Consumer Reports*, 1995, 60(7):459-69.

Sheerin NS, Monk PN, Aslam M, et al, "Simultaneous Exposure to Lead, Arsenic, and Mercury From Indian Ethnic Remedies," *Br J Clin Pract*, 1994, 48(6):332-3.

Staessen JA, Lauwerys RR, Buchet JP, et al, "Impairment of Renal Function With Increasing Blood Lead Concentrations in the General Population," *N Engl J Med*, 1992, 327(3):151-6.

Levoxin® *see* Hydrazine *on page 939*

Lindane *see* Organochlorines *on page 983*

Liquid Bright Platinum *see* Platinum *on page 994*

Liquid Nitrogen Tetroxide *see* Nitrogen Oxide *on page 980*

Lorsban® *see* Chlorpyrifos *on page 891*

Lucidol *see* Dibenzoyl Peroxide *on page 906*

Lurat® *see* Anticoagulant Rodenticide *on page 859*

Lysoff® *see* Fenthion *on page 929*

MACE *see* Chloroacetophenone *on page 889*

Magnacide H® *see* Acrolein *on page 852*

Magnesium Perborate *see* Borates *on page 870*

Magnesium Silicate *see* Asbestos *on page 865*

Maki® *see* Anticoagulant Rodenticide *on page 859*

Malathion

CAS Number 121-75-5

UN Number 2783

Synonyms O,O-Dimethyldithiophosphate Diethylmercaptosuccinate

Brand Names Carbofos®; Compound 4049®; Cythion®; Fosfothion®; Mercaptothion®

Use Marketed as insecticide granules, powder or dusting agent, or spray liquid concentrate with or without petroleum derivative as a solvent

Mechanism of Toxic Action Irreversible inhibition of acetylcholinesterase and plasma cholinesterase, resulting in excess accumulation of acetylcholine at muscarinic and nicotinic receptors, and in the central nervous system

Adverse Reactions

Cardiovascular: Hyperdynamic (~18% to 21%) or hypodynamic (~7% to 10%) states

Central nervous system: Depression, seizures, hyperactivity

Genitourinary: Incontinence

Neuromuscular & skeletal: Weakness, paralysis, sclerodermatous changes accompanied by Raynaud's phenomena

Respiratory: Depression, edema

General: Flu-like symptoms (especially with chronic exposure)

Delayed: Muscle asthenia and paresthesia

Signs & Symptoms of Acute Overdose Miosis (unreactive to light), mydriasis (rarely), lacrimation, pallor, excessive sweating, confusion, agitation, headache, dysarthria, generalized asthenia, cranial nerve palsies, A-V block, dementia, seizures, coma, decreased hemoglobin/red blood cell count/platelet count, metabolic acidosis and hyperglycemia (severe intoxication), hypotension, hypertension, bradycardia, tachycardia, Q-T prolongation, heart block, asystole, salivation, bronchorrhea, tachypnea, garlic-like breath, pulmonary edema, respiratory depression, diaphragmatic paralysis, skeletal muscle fasciculation and flaccid paralysis, nausea, vomiting, abdominal pain, fecal and urinary incontinence; an "intermediate syndrome" of limb asthenia and respiratory paralysis has been reported to occur between 24 and 96 hours postorganophosphate exposure, and is independent of the acute cholinergic crisis; late paresthesia characterized by stocking and glove paresthesia, anesthesia, and asthenia is infrequently observed weeks to months following acute exposure to certain organophosphates

Toxicodynamics/Kinetics

Absorption: Readily through oral, dermal, or respiratory exposure

Metabolism: Rapid to weakly active compounds through hepatic hydrolysis and other pathways

Half-life: 2.9 hours
Elimination: Metabolites excreted in urine

Warnings Significant dermal absorption may occur across intact skin; risk of aspiration pneumonitis exists following oral exposure to agents having a hydrocarbon vehicle; severe laryngeal irritation and violent coughing may result from exposure to dusting powders; exposure to dusting powders and insecticide granules may cause contact dermatitis

Reference Range A 1.8 g ingestion with undetectable pseudocholinesterase resulted in a serum malathion level of 0.35 mg/L 2 hours postingestion
Mild poisoning: Serum cholinesterase is 20% to 50% of normal;
Moderate poisoning: Serum cholinesterase is 10% to 20% of normal
Severe poisoning (respiratory distress and coma): Serum cholinesterase is $<10\%$

Overdosage Treatment
Decontamination: Isolation, bagging, and disposal of all contaminated clothing and other articles; all emergency medical workers and hospital staff should follow appropriate precautions regarding exposure to hazardous material including the use of protective clothing, masks, goggles, and respiratory equipment
Dermal: Prompt thorough scrubbing of all affected areas with soap and water, including hair and nails
Gastric: Activated charcoal can be administered either orally or via a nasogastric tube; do not induce emesis because of danger of sudden respiratory compromise, alterations in mental status, seizures, coma, and possible aspiration of hydrocarbon vehicles
Ocular: Irrigation with copious tepid sterile water or saline
Supportive therapy: Including airway management, ventilatory assistance, humidified oxygen administration, and close monitoring for sudden respiratory failure
Enhancement of elimination: Dialysis and hemoperfusion are not indicated due to effectiveness of the prescribed treatment, large volumes of distribution of organophosphates
Antidote:
Atropine: Administration should be guided by respiratory status, starting at 1-5 mg I.V. every 5-10 minutes as needed, and should be titrated to the resolution of excess pulmonary secretions; frequent administration of large doses (cumulative doses >100 mg) may be necessary in massive exposures
Glycopyrrolate: May be administered if atropine is unavailable
2-PAM: For more significant exposures (ie, exposures requiring large doses of atropine, or with recurring symptoms, or exposures to more lipid soluble agents), administration should follow: 1-2 g I.V. over 5-10 minutes, repeated in 1 hour if asthenia reoccurs, then every 4-12 hours for recurring symptoms

Antidote(s)
Atropine Sulfate *on page 1395*
Pralidoxime Chloride *on page 1461*

Diagnostic Tests/Procedures
Blood Gases, Arterial *on page 1207*
Chest Films *on page 1224*
Complete Blood Count *on page 1236*
Creatinine, Serum *on page 1243*
Electrocardiography *on page 1253*
Liver Profile *on page 1286*
Pseudocholinesterase, Serum *on page 1340*

Pregnancy Implications Human data regarding organophosphate exposure in pregnancy is limited and anecdotal; teratogenesis and fetal death have been produced in animal models at exposure levels that cause obvious toxicity to the pregnant animal

Additional Information Colorless to brown liquid with foul, skunk-like odor; thermal degradation products include sulfur and phosphorus oxides; red blood cell cholinesterase and serum pseudocholinesterase may be depressed following acute or chronic organophosphate exposure; RBC cholinesterase is typically not analyzed by in-house laboratories, and is usually not available for consideration during acute management. Pseudocholinesterase levels may be rapidly available from some in-house laboratories, but are not as reliable a marker of organophosphate exposure because of variability secondary to variant genotypes, hepatic disease, oral estrogen use, or malnutrition. Because of this variability, true indication of suppression of either of these enzymes can only be estimated through comparison to pre-exposure values; these enzymes may be useful in measuring a patient's recovery postexposure, especially if the recovery is not progressing as expected.

ACGIH TLV: 10 mg/m^3
PEL-TWA: 10 mg/m^3 (total dust); 5 mg/m^3 (respirable fraction of dust)
IDLH: 5000 mg/m^3
Water solubility: 143 ppm

(Continued)

Malathion *(Continued)*

vapor pressure is 0.00004 mm Hg at 20°C

Other information concerning pesticide exposures is available through the EPA-funded National Pesticide Telecommunications Network: 1-800-858-7378 (weekdays, 8 AM to 6 PM, Central Standard time)

Specific References

Chaturvedi AK, Singh G, Rao NG, et al, "Toxicological Evaluation of a Poisoning Attributed to Ingestion of Malathion Insect Spray and Correlation With In Vitro Inhibition of Cholinesterases," *Hum Toxicol*, 1989, 8(1):11-8.

Dive A, Mahieu P, Van Binst R, et al, "Unusual Manifestations After Malathion Poisoning," *Hum Exp Toxicol*, 1994, 13(4):271-4.

Garcia-Repetto R, Martinez D, and Repetto M, "Malathion and Dichlorvos Toxicokinetics After the Oral Administration of Malathion and Trichlorfon," *Vet Hum Toxicol*, 1995, 37(4):306-9.

Minton NA and Murray VS, "A Review of Organophosphate Poisoning," *Med Toxicol Adverse Drug Exp*, 1988, 3(5):350-75.

Namba T, Nolte CT, Jackrel J, et al, "Poisoning Due to Organophosphate Insecticides. Acute and Chronic Manifestations," *Am J Med*, 1971, 50(4):475-92.

Malix® *see* Endosulfan *on page 921*

Manganese

CAS Number 1313-13-1; 1317-34-6; 6156-78-1; 7439-96-5; 7773-01-5; 7785-87-7; 14024-58-9

UN Number 1490

Commonly Found In Elemental manganese metal, and as the following salts: acetate, chloride, dioxide, and sulfate; found in fertilizer, welding rods, ceramics, electrical coils, matches, animal food additives

Mechanism of Toxic Action Catalyses dopamine depletion and free radical production within the central nervous system; results in diffuse cortical and cerebellar degeneration

Adverse Reactions

Central nervous system: Parkinson-like syndrome, nervousness, dementia, ataxia, impotence, irritability, "manganese psychosis", gait instability, chorea (extrapyramidal)

Neuromuscular & skeletal: Bradykinesia

Respiratory: Pleuritis, pneumonia

Miscellaneous: Metal fume fever

Signs & Symptoms of Acute Overdose Symptoms correlate with duration of exposure, either acute or chronic. Acute exposure primarily results in respiratory symptoms such as cough, pleuritis, pneumonia, and in gastrointestinal irritation and pancreatitis. Chronic exposure primarily results in CNS symptoms such as nervousness, irritability, Parkinson-like symptoms, nystagmus, tremor, fasciculations, slurred speech, feces discoloration (dark brown); diminished libido, "manganese psychosis" (*Locura manganical*), limb asthenia, and insomnia may persist for several months.

Toxicodynamics/Kinetics

Absorption: Oral: Poor (3% to 7.5%); poorly absorbed through intact skin and mucosal surfaces; increased with accompanying iron deficiency

Distribution: Highest tissue concentrations are found in liver, pancreas, bone, and intestinal wall

Half-life: 12-36 days

Elimination: Primarily excreted through biliary tract

Reference Range

Typical normal ranges in adults:

- Blood: 2.0-8.0 µg/100 mL
- Urine: 0.1-0.8 µg/100 mL
- CSF: 0.4-1.2 µg/100 mL

Overdosage Treatment

Decontamination:

- Dermal: Prompt thorough scrubbing of all affected areas with soap and water
- Gastric: Since most symptomatic exposures are chronic, emesis with ipecac or gastric lavage may be used to eliminate large acute ingestions. Chronically exposed patients may become obtunded or may develop acute respiratory symptoms, and should not receive lavage or ipecac. Single dose activated charcoal will not adsorb manganese, but is useful for coingestants.
- Ocular: Irrigation with copious tepid water or saline
- Inhalation: Remove patient from source of exposure

Supportive therapy: Including airway management, ventilatory assistance, humidified oxygen administration, and close monitoring for renal compromise, respiratory decompensation, or further convulsive activity

- Chelation: EDTA therapy instituted early into the manganese intoxication is most promising; BAL has not demonstrated utility in chronic toxicity
- Intention tremor: Trihexyphenidil 1-5 mg/day orally in divided doses
- Anti-Parkinson's therapy: Improvement in neurologic toxicity may result with therapy using anti-Parkinson's therapy of levodopa 3.5-12 g/day orally or levo-

dopa/carbidopa (Sinemet®) 100 mg/25 mg 2-3 times/day orally, up to 6 tablets/day for 8 weeks

Antidote(s)

Charcoal *on page 1403*

Edetate Calcium Disodium *on page 1419*

Diagnostic Tests/Procedures

Aspartate Aminotransferase *on page 1199*

Blood Gases, Arterial *on page 1207*

Calcium, Serum *on page 1214*

Complete Blood Count *on page 1236*

Creatinine, Serum *on page 1243*

Electrolytes, Blood *on page 1254*

Glucose, Random *on page 1269*

Urea Nitrogen, Blood *on page 1370*

Pregnancy Implications Manganese has documented deleterious effects on the fetus, namely disturbance in gait and coordination, cleft palate, cardiac defects, and deafness; it also presents metabolic abnormalities to the fetus through its effects on the metabolism of the mother

Additional Information

Urine or plasma concentrations of manganese do not correlate with severity of symptoms. Toxicity following ingestion of inorganic salts is unlikely because of poor gastrointestinal absorption; neurologic manifestations may be permanently established after 1-2 years for chronic exposure. Magnetic resonance imaging may be useful for manganese encephalopathy.

TLV-TWA: Dust: 5 mg/m^3; Fumes: 1 mg/m^3

IDLH: 10,000 mg/m^3

PEL-TWA: 1 mg/m^3 (fumes)

Average ambient atmospheric manganese levels:

Urban: 33 ng/m^3

Nonurban: 5 ng/m^3

Mean level in drinking water: 4-32 mcg/L

Safe infant daily dose: 0.7-1 mg

Foods with the highest amount of manganese concentrations are nuts and nut products (18-47 ppm); average amount of ingestion of manganese from food: 3.8 mg/day; average cup of tea may contain from 0.4-1.3 mg of manganese; legumes may contain from 2-7 ppm of manganese

Specific References

Angle C and Nelson K, "Manganese Encephalopathy. Utility of Early Magnetic Resonance Imaging," *Vet Hum Toxicol*, 1992, 34:355.

Huang CC, Chu NS, Lu CS, et al, "Chronic Manganese Intoxication," *Arch Neurol*, 1989, 46(10):1104-6.

Lesser SH and Weiss SJ, "Art Hazards," *Am J Emerg Med*, 1995, 13(4):451-8.

Parenti M, Flauto C, Parati E, et al, "Manganese Neurotoxicity: Effects of L-dopa and Pargyline Treatments," *Brain Res*, 1986, 367(1-2):8-13.

U.S. Department of Health and Human Services, "Toxicological Profile for Manganese TP-91/19," Agency for Toxic Substances and Diseases Registry, July, 1992.

Marine Diesel Oil *see* Mineral-Based Crankcase Oil *on page 971*

Marlate® *see* Methoxychlor *on page 963*

Marsh Gas *see* Methane *on page 957*

Mat Powder *see* Tin *on page 1028*

MBE *see* Methyl Tert-Butyl Ether *on page 970*

MBK *see* 2-Hexanone *on page 938*

MCB *see* Chlorobenzene *on page 889*

MCOVA *see* 4,4'-Methylenebis (2-Chloroaniline) *on page 965*

MDA *see* Methylene Dianiline *on page 966*

M-delphene *see* Diethyltoluamide *on page 912*

M-det *see* Diethyltoluamide *on page 912*

M-deta *see* Diethyltoluamide *on page 912*

Medrin® *see* Endrin *on page 922*

Meetco® *see* Methyl Ethyl Ketone *on page 967*

MEK *see* Methyl Ethyl Ketone *on page 967*

ME-Parathion® *see* Methyl Parathion *on page 969*

Mercaptothion® *see* Malathion *on page 950*

Mercury

Related Information

Drugs and Chemicals Proven to be Teratogenic in Humans *on page 1572-1575*

Radiation: Basics of Exposure *on page 1594-1600*

Toxins Which Should be Lavaged With Solutions Other Than Water *on page 1635*

CAS Number 7439-97-6

UN Number 2809; 2024; 2025; 1629

Commonly Found In Inorganic mercury salts; organic mercury; elemental mercury; found in thimerosal; used by amalgam makers, jewelers, paint manufacturers, laboratorians, taxidermists, fireworks, embalmers, button batteries, dye makers, fur processors, photographers, electroplaters

Mechanism of Toxic Action Causes cell membrane damage; elemental and organic mercury are CNS toxins; inorganic is a corrosive; organic mercury causes teratogenicity; high-binding affinity of divalent cation form of mercury to thiol or sulfhydryl protein groups occur

Adverse Reactions

Cardiovascular: Hypertension, tachycardia, hypotension

Central nervous system: Dementia, neuritis, cranial nerve palsies, hyperthermia, encephalopathy

Gastrointestinal: Salivation

Neuromuscular & skeletal: Tremor, myoclonus

Ocular: Nystagmus, diplopia, photophobia

Otic: Deafness

Signs & Symptoms of Acute Overdose Elemental mercury is poorly absorbed orally with minimal adverse effects; inhalation acutely can cause chemical pneumonitis, noncardiogenic pulmonary edema, and gingivostomatitis; chronic exposure to mercury vapor will cause tremor, hematuria, leukocytosis, fatigue, proteinuria, alopecia, fasciculations, insomnia, loss of memory, and acrodynia

Inorganic mercury: After oral administration, will develop abdominal pain, gastrointestinal irritation, gastrointestinal bleeding, shock, renal failure, and ATN; possible CNS toxicity

Organic mercury: Causes CNS toxicity including ataxia, dysarthria, paresthesias, hearing and visual loss, and gastrointestinal distress

Toxicodynamics/Kinetics

Absorption: Elemental mercury is poorly absorbed orally and well absorbed by inhalation while inorganic and organic mercury are well absorbed orally; metallic mercury is minimally absorbed dermally (0.024 ng of mercury absorbed per cm^2 of skin)

Distribution: Elemental to CNS, kidney, liver, and heart; inorganic mercury concentrates in the kidney; organic mercury (alkyl mercury groups) distribute throughout the body while methylmercury concentrates in blood and CNS

Metabolism: Metallic/inorganic mercury: Oxidized to an inorganic divalent form in the red blood cells (note that ethanol can inhibit this step)

Half-life:

Elemental and inorganic: 40-60 days; organic: 70 days

Organic: Converted to divalent cation form in tissues

Elimination:

Metallic: Urine, feces, and lung

Inorganic: Urine, feces

Organic: Primarily feces

Reference Range Urinary and whole blood levels can be obtained; normally urinary values are <10 µg/dL and whole blood <2 µg/dL; whole blood levels <50 µg/dL are usually associated with gastroenteritis and acute tubular necrosis; urinary levels for organic mercury are not useful since 90% is eliminated through bile in the feces

Overdosage Treatment

Decontamination:

Oral: Lavage if ingested within 1 hour; charcoal has been shown to decrease inorganic mercury absorption in rats and should be used; milk or egg white may also be useful to bind mercury as is 5% sodium formaldehyde or 2% to 5% sodium bicarbonate solution; whole bowel irrigation with GoLYTELY® may be beneficial if abdominal x-ray shows evidence of mercury; do not induce emesis for inorganic mercury ingestions as this agent has corrosive properties.

Inhalation: Patients should be monitored for pulmonary edema and pneumonitis; give oxygen if necessary

Dermal: Wash with tincture of green soap and water

Ocular: Copious irrigation with saline

Supportive therapy: D-penicillamine can be administered orally in 4 divided doses totalling 20-30 mg/kg (250 mg 4 times/day in adults) if prolonged therapy is required, especially for short-chain alkyl organic mercury compounds; another less toxic form of penicillamine (N-acetyl-D-L-penicillamine from Aldrich Chemical Co, Milwaukee, WI) is a specific chelator for mercury. Both are also effective for long-chain alkyl, aryl mercurials, or for treatment of acrodynia.

Elemental mercury: Oral DMSA (succimer) 10 mg/kg every 8 hours for 5 days then 10 mg/kg every 12 hours for 2 or more weeks will enhance urinary mercury excretion

Inorganic mercury: BAL 5 mg/kg deep I.M. initially, then 2.5 mg/kg every 12 hours for 10 days; if given within the first 2 hours BAL may prevent renal toxicity; **do not give BAL I.V.**

Organic mercury: Oral DMSA (succimer) with dosing as above

BAL is not recommended for elemental and organic mercury poisoning since BAL may cause redistribution of mercury to the brain which is the primary target organ in these poisonings

Enhancement of elimination: Generally ineffective; BAL, mercury complex is dialyzable and is useful in patients with renal failure; it does not enhance elimination in those with good renal function; some clinical improvement with increased clearance noted after exchange transfusion

Antidote(s)

Dimercaprol *on page 1414*
Succimer *on page 1473*

Diagnostic Tests/Procedures

Aspartate Aminotransferase *on page 1199*
Blood Gases, Arterial *on page 1207*
Chest Films *on page 1224*
Mercury, Blood *on page 1292*
Mercury, Urine *on page 1292*
Urinalysis *on page 1373*

Additional Information

Ambient atmospheric mercury levels range from 10-20 ng/m^3
Surface water levels: <5 ng/L
Soil levels: 20-625 ng/g
IDLH: Mercury vapor: 28 mg/m^3
Alkyl mercury compounds: 10 mg/m^3
WHO guideline for drinking water: 1 mcg/L
Permissible tolerable weekly intake: 5 mcg/kg
Mean mercury levels in fish: ~0.4 mcg/g
Other foods: ~0.004 mcg/g
Cigarette smoke: ~0.004 mcg/cigarette
Estimated daily intake of mercury from air: 0.2 mcg; from drinking water: 0.1 mcg
Residence atmospheric time of elemental mercury: 6-24 months
Average methyl mercury content in tuna: 0.17 ppm

Specific References

Aks SE, Erickson T, Branches FJ, et al, "Fractional Mercury Levels in Brazilian Gold Refiners and Miners," *J Toxicol Clin Toxicol*, 1995, 33(1):1-10.

Florentine MJ and Sanfilippo DJ 2d, "Elemental Mercury Poisoning," *Clin Pharm*, 1991, 10(3):213-21.

Fung YK, Meade AG, Rack EP, et al, "Determination of Blood Mercury Concentrations in Alzheimer's Patients," *J Toxicol Clin Toxicol*, 1995, 33(3):243-7.

Hryhorczuk DO, Meyers L Jr, and Chen G, "Treatment of Mercury Intoxication in a Dentist With N-Acetyl-D,L-Penicillamine," *J Toxicol Clin Toxicol*, 1982, 19(4):401-8.

Laundy T, Adam AE, Kershaw JB, et al, "Deaths After Peritoneal Lavage With Mercuric Chloride Solutions: Case Report and Review of the Literature," *Br Med J (Clin Res)*, 1984, 289(6437):96-8.

Sheerin NS, Monk PN, Aslam M, et al, "Simultaneous Exposure to Lead, Arsenic, and Mercury From Indian Ethnic Remedies," *Br J Clin Pract*, 1994, 48(6):332-3.

U.S. Department of Health and Human Services, "Toxicological Profile for Mercury TP-93/10," Agency for Toxic Substances and Diseases Registry, May, 1994.

Merex® *see* Chlordecone *on page 886*

Merpol *see* Ethylene Oxide *on page 927*

Mesurol® *see* Methiocarb *on page 961*

Metadelphene *see* Diethyltoluamide *on page 912*

Meta-Dinitrobenzene *see* 1,3-Dinitrobenzene *on page 914*

Meta-Fuel® *see* Metaldehyde *on this page*

Metaldehyde

CAS Number 108-62-3; 9002-91-9

UN Number 1332

Brand Names Halizan®; Meta-Fuel®; Metason®; Slug Death®; Slugit® Pellets

Use Snail/slug bait, heating fuel, ingredient in fire lighters

Mechanism of Toxic Action Acyclic tetramer of acetaldehyde with direct effects on neurotransmitters (ie, decreases gamma-aminobutyric acid, noradrenaline, 5-hydroxytrytamine); mucosal irritant

(Continued)

Metaldehyde *(Continued)*

Adverse Reactions

Cardiovascular: Hypotension, flushing

Central nervous system: Lethargy, seizures, ataxia, coma, hypertonia, fever, confusion

Dermatologic: Pruritus

Endocrine & metabolic: Metabolic acids

Gastrointestinal: Salivation, nausea, diarrhea, abdominal pain, vomiting

Ocular: Mydriasis

Neuromuscular & skeletal: Tremors, opisthotonos

Respiratory: Bronchial secretions, cough

Toxicodynamics/Kinetics

Metabolism: Hydrolyzed in the stomach (by gastric acid) to acetaldehyde

Half-life: 27 hours

Reference Range Serum acetaldehyde level of 1 mg/dL (and urine metaldehyde level of 3 mg/dL) associated with seizures and acidosis

Overdosage Treatment

Decontamination: Lavage/activated charcoal with cathartic

Supportive therapy: Seizures should be treated with benzodiazepine, phenobarbital, or phenytoin; sodium bicarbonate for acidosis

Enhancement of elimination: Diuresis or hemodialysis is not expected to be useful

Additional Information Very flammable; memory loss may occur and last for several months; usual concentration in U.S. is <4%; but in Europe, metaldehyde concentration in molluscicides may approach 50%

Adverse reactions often related to dose ingested:

- <50 mg/kg: Spasms, tachycardia, nausea
- 50-100 mg/kg: Ataxia, hypertonia
- 100-200 mg/kg: Seizures, tremor
- >400 mg/kg: Coma, death

Minimal lethal dose (child): 4 g

Specific References

Booze TF and Oehme FW, "Metaldehyde Toxicity: A Review," *Vet Hum Toxicol*, 1985, 27(1):11-9.

Jay MS, Kearns GL, Stone V, et al, "Toxic Pneumonitis in an Adolescent Following Exposure to Snow Storm Tablets," *J Adolescent Health Care*, 1988, 9:431-3.

Keller KH, Shimizu G, Walter FG, et al, "Acetaldehyde Analysis in Severe Metaldehyde Poisoning," *Vet Hum Toxicol*, 1991, 33:374.

Longstreet WT and Pierson DJ, "Metaldehyde Poisoning from Slug Bait Ingestion," *West J Med*, 1982, 137:134-37.

Metal Fume Fever

Synonyms Brass Chills; Copper Fever; Fume Fever; Metal Shakes; Welding Fume Fever; Zinc Shakes

Commonly Found In Produced when inhaling metal oxides such as zinc oxide, elemental mercury, copper, brass, cadmium, tin, iron, nickel, manganese, chromium, cobalt, magnesium; encountered with welding or torch cutting

Mechanism of Toxic Action Unknown

Adverse Reactions Miscellaneous: Respiratory and gastrointestinal symptoms about 5 hours postexposure

Signs & Symptoms of Acute Overdose Sudden onset of thirst, flushing, tachypnea, headache, blurred vision, sore throat, metallic taste, dyspnea, nonproductive cough, myalgia, abdominal pain, nausea, vomiting, mild fever, sweating; usually occurs 4-8 hours after exposure

Toxicodynamics/Kinetics Absorption: Primary route is inhalation

Reference Range Zinc levels >2 mg/L are above normal

Overdosage Treatment Supportive therapy: Humidified oxygen; chelation not effective; course is usually benign; symptoms usually resolve in 1-2 days

Diagnostic Tests/Procedures

Chest Films *on page 1224*

Heavy Metal Screen, Blood *on page 1271*

Lactate Dehydrogenase, Blood *on page 1279*

White Blood Count *on page 1380*

Specific References

Malo JL and Cartier A, "Occupational Asthma Due to Fumes of Galvanized Metal," *Chest*, 1987, 92(2):375-7.

Mueller EJ and Seger DL, "Metal Fume Fever – A Review," *J Emerg Med*, 1985, 2(4):271-4.

Metal Shakes *see* Metal Fume Fever *on this page*

Metapon® *see* Methyl Parathion *on page 969*

Metason® *see* Metaldehyde *on previous page*

Meta-Toluene Diisocyanate *see* Toluene Diisocyanate *on page 1031*

Methacrylate Monomer *see* Methacrylates *on this page*

Methacrylates

CAS Number 80-62-6

Synonyms Methacrylate Monomer; Methyl Ester of Methacrylic Acid; Methyl Methacrylate Monomer; MMA; "Monocite" Methacrylate Monomer; Pegalan

Use In bone cements; artificial fingernail extender

Mechanism of Toxic Action Not well known

Adverse Reactions Moderate irritant and sensitizer, once polymerized becomes inert and nontoxic; vasodilation and transient hypotension have been reported following use as a bone cement; direct cardiotoxicity has been noted; oral ingestion can produce vomiting, gastrointestinal ulceration

Signs & Symptoms of Acute Overdose Headache and irritability, hepatic metabolism disturbances, allergic dermatitis; occupational asthma has been associated with various methyl methacrylates

Toxicodynamics/Kinetics Metabolism: Possible in liver and hydroxylated to an alcohol, then oxidized to aldehyde and deformulated to pyruvic acid where it enters Kreb cycle

Overdosage Treatment

Decontamination: Lavage/activated charcoal with cathartic

Supportive therapy: Parenteral nutrition for severe gastrointestinal burns

Pregnancy Implications No adverse effects on humans reported

Additional Information Monomer has an acrid odor until polymerizes; the colorless liquid form has a fruity smell; may polymerize and cause an exothermic reaction

Specific References

Dowsett R and Woolf A, "Gastrointestinal Corrosive Injury Due to Ingestional of Methacrylic Acid," *Vet Hum Toxicol*, 1994, 36:373.

Methane

CAS Number 74-82-8

UN Number 1971

Synonyms Fire Damp; Marsh Gas; Methyl Hydride; Natural Gas (85% Methane)

Commonly Found In Sludge digestion; produced through natural breakdown of sewage; raw material for hydrogen, ammonia, or acetylene production; found in mining industry

Mechanism of Toxic Action Asphyxiant – Displaces oxygen from the atmosphere

Adverse Reactions Respiratory: Hypoxia, hyperventilation; no direct lung damage

Signs & Symptoms of Acute Overdose Tachypnea, cough, tachycardia, blurred or decreased vision, unconsciousness, CNS depression

Overdosage Treatment Supportive therapy: 100% humidified oxygen

Diagnostic Tests/Procedures

Blood Gases, Arterial *on page 1207*

Pregnancy Implications Fetal hypoxia may occur

Additional Information Colorless, odorless

TLV-TWA: No limits as long as sufficient atmospheric oxygen is available. Usually when asphyxiant is 33% of atmosphere, symptoms will develop; methane is flammable at concentrations of 5%

Death can occur at 75% concentration

Specific References

Kizer KW, "Toxic Inhalations," *Emerg Med Clin North Am*, 1984, 2(3):649-66.

Methane Dichloride *see* Methylene Chloride *on page 966*

Methanethiol *see* Methyl Mercaptan *on page 968*

Methane Trichloride *see* Chloroform *on page 890*

Methanol

CAS Number 67-56-1

UN Number 1230

Synonyms Carbinol; Methyl Alcohol; Wood Alcohol; Wood Naphtha

Commonly Found In Industrial and household solvent

Use Fuel, paint remover; also is an additive to gasoline

Mechanism of Toxic Action Slowly metabolized to formaldehyde and then converted rapidly to formic acid which accounts for the acidosis and ocular toxicity

Adverse Reactions

Ocular: Visual abnormalities, blindness with edematous optic disk, photophobia, optic neuropathy

Endocrine & metabolic: Anion gap metabolic acidosis (lactic acidosis)

Renal: Hematuria

Miscellaneous: Osmolal gap

Signs & Symptoms of Acute Overdose Blurred vision or diplopia progressing to

(Continued)

Methanol *(Continued)*

blindness in about 33% of patients, feces discoloration (black), porphyria, headache, dyspnea, coma, seizures, hypomagnesemia, extrapyramidal symptoms, visual changes, hyperventilation, bilateral basal ganglia, metabolic acidosis, nystagmus, hemorrhage, and renal failure can develop, parkinsonism, hypotension, paresthesia, myoglobinuria, ototoxicity, dementia, tinnitus, hypophosphatemia, bradycardia; symptoms may not occur for 24 hours

Toxicodynamics/Kinetics

Specific gravity: 0.79 g/mL

Absorption: Dermally (enhanced with gasoline mixtures), by inhalation (58%), and through the gastrointestinal tract (~100%)

Distribution: V_d: 0.6 L/kg

Metabolism: Slowly in the liver by alcohol dehydrogenase to formaldehyde and then to formic acid; see figure

Methanol metabolism to toxic intermediates—formaldehyde and formic acid (formate)

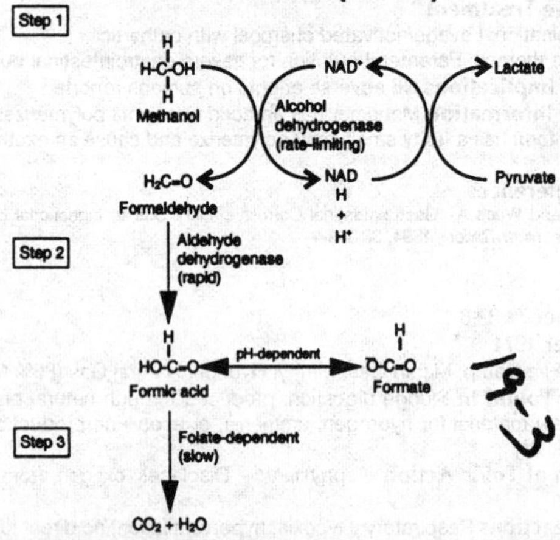

Discovery of methanol's metabolic pathway has led to several practical treatments; among them are the therapeutic administration of ethanol and folic acid. Alcohol dehydrogenase, the enzyme responsible for the first step of methanol metabolism, has an approximately ninefold greater affinity for ethanol than for methanol. Administration of ethanol blocks the oxidation of methanol, preventing the lethal synthesis of formaldehyde and formic acid and increasing the amount of methanol that is eliminated unchanged (now approximately equal amounts in urine and exhaled breath). Administration of folic acid and its analogues, which affect Step 3, enhances the conversion of toxic formic acid to carbon dioxide and water.

Adapted from Shusterman D and Osterloh JD, "Methanol Toxicity," *Case Studies in Environmental Medicine*, U.S. Department of Health and Human Services, Agency for Toxic Substances and Disease Registry, July 1992.

Peak serum concentration: Within 1 hour; found in higher concentrations in ocular and cerebrospinal fluids

Half-life, elimination: 8-28 hours (8 mg/dL/hour); with hemodialysis: 2 hours

Elimination: ~3% excreted unchanged renally and 12% by the lungs

Reference Range

Blood methanol level >50 mg/dL is associated with severe toxicity; minimal lethal level without treatment: 80 mg/dL

Central nervous system toxicity usually appears at methanol blood levels of 20 mg/dL; ocular symptoms occur at 100 mg/dL; fatalities can occur at blood methanol levels >150 mg/dL; serum formate levels >20 mg/dL are consistent with ocular symptoms and metabolic acidosis

Overdosage Treatment

Decontamination: Lavage/activated charcoal with cathartic in a 5:1 ratio (charcoal:methanol); do not induce emesis by ipecac if initiated longer than 30 minutes after ingestion

Supportive therapy: Treat acidosis with sodium bicarbonate (I.V.). Leucovorin calcium, 1 mg/kg up to 50 mg, followed by folic acid, 1 mg/kg up to 50 mg (every 4 hours), should be given in symptomatic patients. Folic acid, at the same dose, may be given alone in asymptomatic patients. Treat acidosis aggressively with I.V. sodium bicarbonate; ethanol therapy should be initiated if methanol level is >20 mg/dL, patient has anion-gap acidosis, or other symptoms develop.

Enhancement of elimination: Hemodialysis (with ethanol) should be utilized for methanol levels >20 mg/dL or if metabolic acidosis is present; 4-methyl pyrazole as an inhibitor of alcohol dehydrogenase is investigational

Antidote(s)

Ethanol *on page 1424*
Folic Acid *on page 1430*
Leucovorin Calcium *on page 1437*
4-Methylpyrazole *on page 1446*
Sodium Bicarbonate *on page 1467*

Diagnostic Tests/Procedures

Anion Gap, Blood *on page 1193*
Electrolytes, Blood *on page 1254*
Kidney Profile *on page 1279*
Methanol, Blood *on page 1295*
Osmolality, Serum *on page 1310*
Osmolality, Urine *on page 1311*

Pregnancy Implications Skeletal, urinary, and cardiovascular defects noted in pregnant rats

Additional Information Parkinson syndrome has been described; methanol has $\frac{1}{3}$ the intoxicating effect of ethanol; discontinue ethanol therapy if methanol level is <10 mg/dL, or acidosis or central nervous system abnormalities have resolved; headaches can occur at air methanol levels in the range of 200-375 ppm; 4-Methylpyrazole has been used to treat methanol poisoning in Europe; bilateral basal ganglion lesions along with symmetrical putamen necrosis may be noted on CT scan or MRI

Minimum oral lethal exposure: ~50 mL with blindness occurring at 10 mL

Contribution of a serum concentration level of 100 mg/dL to elevation of osmolar gap: 31

Odor threshold: 100-250 ppm

TLV-TWA: 200 ppm

Specific References

Berendt RC, Passerini L, LeGatt D, et al, "Severe Methanol Intoxication: Methanol Pharmacokinetics and Serum Osmolality," *J Crit Care*, 1987, 2:181-6.

Burkhart KK and Kulig KW, "The Other Alcohols: Methanol Ethylene Glycol, and Isopropanol," *Emerg Med Clin North Am*, 1990, 8(4):913-28.

Haines JD Jr, "Methanol Poisoning: How to Recognize and Treat a Deadly Intoxication," *Postgrad Med*, 1987, 82(8):149-51.

Harchelroad F, "Hypomagnesemia During Methanol Intoxication," *Vet Hum Toxicol*, 1993, 35:364.

Jackson MH and Payne HA, "Bittering Agents: Their Potential Application in Reducing Ingestions of Engine Coolants and Windshield Wash," *Vet Hum Toxicol*, 1995, 37(4):323-6.

Naeser P, "Optic Nerve Involvement in a Case of Methanol Poisoning," *Br J Ophthalmol*, 1988, 72(10):778-81.

Nanji AA, "Absence of Symptoms and Acidosis in Potentially Lethal Methanol Poisoning," *Ann Emerg Med*, 1984, 13(6):487.

Palatnick W, Redman LW, Sitar DS, et al, "Methanol Half-life During Ethanol Administration: Implications for Management of Methanol Poisoning," *Ann Emerg Med*, 1995, 26:202-7.

Shusterman D and Osterloh JD, "Case Studies in Environmental Medicine: Methanol Toxicity," Agency for Toxic Substances and Diseases Registry, U.S. Department of Health and Human Services, July, 1992.

Yu FC, Lin SH, Lin YF, et al, "Double Gaps Metabolic Acidosis and Bilateral Basal Ganglion Lesions in Methanol Intoxication," *Am J Emerg Med*, 1995, 13:369-71.

Methenyl Tribromide *see* Bromoform *on page 872*

Methidathion

CAS Number 950-37-8

Brand Names Sumonil®; Supracide®; Ultracide®

Use Marketed as insecticide granules, dusting agent, or spray liquid with or without petroleum derivative as a solvent

Mechanism of Toxic Action Potent, irreversible inhibition of acetylcholinesterase and plasma cholinesterase, resulting in excess accumulation of acetylcholine at muscarinic and nicotinic receptors, and in the central nervous system

Adverse Reactions

Cardiovascular: Hyperdynamic (~18% to 21%) or hypodynamic (~7% to 10%) states

Central nervous system: Depression, seizures, hyperactivity

Genitourinary: Incontinence

Neuromuscular & skeletal: Weakness, paralysis

Respiratory: Depression, edema

General: Flu-like symptoms (especially with chronic exposure)

Delayed: Muscle asthenia and paresthesia

Signs & Symptoms of Acute Overdose Miosis (unreactive to light), mydriasis (rarely), lacrimation, pallor, excessive sweating, confusion, agitation, headache, dysarthria, generalized asthenia, seizures, A-V block, coma, decreased hemoglo-

(Continued)

Methidathion *(Continued)*

bin/red blood cell count/platelet count, metabolic acidosis and hyperglycemia (severe intoxication), hypotension, hypertension, cranial nerve palsies, bradycardia, tachycardia, Q-T prolongation, heart block, asystole, salivation, bronchorrhea, tachypnea, pulmonary edema, respiratory depression, diaphragmatic paralysis, skeletal muscle fasciculation and flaccid paralysis, nausea, vomiting, abdominal pain, fecal and urinary incontinence; an "intermediate syndrome" of limb asthenia and respiratory paralysis has been reported to occur between 24 and 96 hours postorganophosphate exposure, and is independent of the acute cholinergic crisis; late paresthesia characterized by stocking and glove paresthesia, anesthesia, and asthenia is infrequently observed weeks to months following acute exposure to certain organophosphates

Toxicodynamics/Kinetics

Absorption: Readily through oral, dermal, or respiratory exposure

Metabolism: Rapidly metabolized to weakly active compounds through hepatic hydrolysis and other pathways

Elimination: Metabolites are excreted in urine

Warnings Risk of aspiration pneumonitis exists with agents having a hydrocarbon vehicle; severe laryngeal irritation and violent coughing may result from exposure to dusting powders; exposure to dusting powders and insecticide granules may cause contact dermatitis

Overdosage Treatment

Decontamination: Isolation, bagging, and disposal of all contaminated clothing and other articles; all emergency medical workers and hospital staff should follow appropriate precautions regarding exposure to hazardous material including the use of protective clothing, masks, goggles, and respiratory equipment

Dermal: Prompt thorough scrubbing of all affected areas with soap and water, including hair and nails

Gastric: Activated charcoal can be administered either orally or via a nasogastric tube; do not induce emesis because of danger of sudden respiratory compromise, alterations in mental status, seizures, coma, and possible aspiration of hydrocarbon vehicles

Ocular: Irrigation with copious tepid sterile water or saline

Supportive therapy: Including airway management, ventilatory assistance, humidified oxygen administration, and close monitoring for sudden respiratory failure

Enhancement of elimination: Dialysis and hemoperfusion are not indicated due to effectiveness of the prescribed treatment, large volumes of distribution of organophosphates

Antidote:

Atropine: Administration should be guided by respiratory status, starting at 1-5 mg I.V. every 5-10 minutes as needed, and should be titrated to the resolution of excess pulmonary secretions; frequent administration of large doses (cumulative doses >100 mg) may be necessary in massive exposures

Glycopyrrolate: May be administered if atropine is unavailable

2-PAM: For more significant exposures (ie, exposures requiring large doses of atropine, or with recurring symptoms, or exposures to more lipid soluble agents), administration should follow: 1-2 g I.V. over 5-10 minutes, repeated in 1 hour if asthenia reoccurs, then every 4-12 hours for recurring symptoms

Antidote(s)

Atropine Sulfate *on page 1395*
Pralidoxime Chloride *on page 1461*

Diagnostic Tests/Procedures

Blood Gases, Arterial *on page 1207*
Chest Films *on page 1224*
Complete Blood Count *on page 1236*
Creatinine, Serum *on page 1243*
Electrocardiography *on page 1253*
Liver Profile *on page 1286*
Pseudocholinesterase, Serum *on page 1340*

Pregnancy Implications Human data regarding organophosphate exposure in pregnancy is limited and anecdotal; teratogenesis and fetal death have been produced in animal models at exposure levels that cause obvious toxicity to the pregnant animal

Additional Information Red blood cell cholinesterase, and serum pseudocholinesterase may be depressed following acute or chronic organophosphate exposure; RBC cholinesterase is typically not analyzed by in-house laboratories, and is usually not available for consideration during acute management. Pseudocholinesterase levels may be rapidly available from some in-house laboratories, but are not as reliable a marker of organophosphate exposure because of variability secondary to variant genotypes, hepatic disease, oral estrogen use, or malnutrition. Because of this variability, true indication of suppression of either of these enzymes can only be estimated through comparison to pre-exposure values; these enzymes may be useful in measuring a patient's recovery postexposure, especially if the recovery is not progressing as expected.

Other information concerning pesticide exposures is available through the EPA-funded National Pesticide Telecommunications Network: 1-800-858-7378 (weekdays, 8 AM to 6 PM, Central Standard time)

Specific References

Minton NA and Murray VS, "A Review of Organophosphate Poisoning," *Med Toxicol Adverse Drug Exp*, 1988, 3(5):350-75.

Namba T, Nolte CT, Jackrel J, et al, "Poisoning Due to Organophosphate Insecticides. Acute and Chronic Manifestations," *Am J Med*, 1971, 50(4):475-92.

Methiocarb

CAS Number 2032-65-7

Synonyms 3,5-Dimethyl-4-Methylthiophenyl N-Methylcarbamate

Brand Names Draza®; Mesurol®

Use Marketed as an insecticide dusting powder or a colorless spray liquid

Mechanism of Toxic Action Reversible inhibition of acetylcholinesterase and plasma cholinesterase, resulting in excess accumulation of acetylcholine at muscarinic and nicotinic receptors, and in the central nervous system

Adverse Reactions

Cardiovascular: Hyperdynamic (~18% to 21%) or hypodynamic (~7% to 10%) states

Central nervous system: Toxicity is limited because carbamates do not significantly cross the blood-brain barrier; CNS changes occur with most severe intoxications, hyperactivity

Genitourinary: Incontinence

Neuromuscular & skeletal: Weakness, paralysis

Respiratory: Depression, edema

General: Flu-like symptoms (especially with chronic exposure)

Signs & Symptoms of Acute Overdose Miosis (unreactive to light), mydriasis (rarely), lacrimation, pallor, excessive sweating, confusion, agitation, headache, dysarthria, generalized asthenia, seizures, A-V block, coma, decreased hemoglobin/red blood cell count/platelet count, cranial nerve palsies, metabolic acidosis and hyperglycemia (severe intoxication), hypotension, hypertension, bradycardia, tachycardia, Q-T prolongation, heart block, asystole, salivation, bronchorrhea, tachypnea, pulmonary edema, respiratory depression, diaphragmatic paralysis, skeletal muscle fasciculation and flaccid paralysis, nausea, vomiting, abdominal pain, fecal and urinary incontinence

Toxicodynamics/Kinetics

Absorption: Readily through oral, dermal, or respiratory exposure

Metabolism: Rapidly metabolized to weakly active compounds through hepatic hydrolysis and other pathways

Elimination: Metabolites are excreted in urine

Warnings Risk of aspiration pneumonitis exists following oral exposure to agents having a hydrocarbon vehicle; severe laryngeal irritation and violent coughing may result from exposure to dusting powders; exposure to dusting powders and insecticide granules may cause contact dermatitis

Overdosage Treatment

Decontamination: Isolation, bagging, and disposal of all contaminated clothing and other articles; all emergency medical workers and hospital staff should follow appropriate precautions regarding exposure to hazardous material including the use of protective clothing, masks, goggles, and respiratory equipment

Dermal: Prompt thorough scrubbing of all affected areas with soap and water, including hair and nails

Gastric: Activated charcoal can be administered either orally or via a nasogastric tube; do not induce emesis because of danger of sudden respiratory compromise, alterations in mental status, seizures, coma, and possible aspiration of hydrocarbon vehicles

Ocular: Irrigation with copious tepid sterile water or saline

Supportive therapy: Including airway management, ventilatory assistance, humidified oxygen administration, and close monitoring for sudden respiratory failure

Antidote:

Atropine: Administration should be guided by respiratory status, starting at 1-5 mg I.V. every 5-10 minutes as needed, and should be titrated to the resolution of excess pulmonary secretions; frequent administration of large doses (cumulative doses >100 mg) may be necessary in massive exposures

Glycopyrrolate: May be administered if atropine is unavailable

2-PAM: Although not specifically indicated, 2-PAM may be considered in the following situations:

Life-threatening symptoms such as respiratory paralysis

Continued excessive atropine requirements

Concomitant organophosphate and carbamate exposure

Enhancement of elimination: Dialysis and hemoperfusion are not indicated due to effectiveness of the prescribed treatment, large volumes of distribution of organophosphates

(Continued)

Methiocarb *(Continued)*

Antidote(s)
Atropine Sulfate *on page 1395*

Diagnostic Tests/Procedures
Blood Gases, Arterial *on page 1207*
Chest Films *on page 1224*
Complete Blood Count *on page 1236*
Creatinine, Serum *on page 1243*
Electrocardiography *on page 1253*
Liver Profile *on page 1286*
Pseudocholinesterase, Serum *on page 1340*

Pregnancy Implications Human data regarding organophosphate exposure in pregnancy is limited and anecdotal; teratogenesis and fetal death have been produced in animal models at exposure levels that cause obvious toxicity to the pregnant animal

Additional Information Red blood cell cholinesterase, and serum pseudocholinesterase may be depressed following acute or chronic organophosphate exposure and are theoretically useful for differentiating between carbamate and organophosphate exposures; RBC cholinesterase is typically not analyzed by in-house laboratories, and is usually not available for consideration during acute management. Pseudocholinesterase levels may be rapidly available from some in-house laboratories, but are not as reliable a marker of organophosphate exposure because of variability secondary to variant genotypes, hepatic disease, oral estrogen use, or malnutrition, thus they may not be useful in ruling out carbamate exposure.

Other information concerning pesticide exposures is available through the EPA-funded National Pesticide Telecommunications Network: 1-800-858-7378 (weekdays, 8 AM to 6 PM, Central Standard time)

Specific References
Zwiener RJ and Ginsburg CM, "Organophosphate and Carbamate Poisoning in Infants and Children," *Pediatrics*, 1988, 81(1):121-6.

Methomyl

CAS Number 16752-77-5

Brand Names Lannate®; Nudrin®

Use Marketed as an insecticide dusting agent

Mechanism of Toxic Action Potent, reversible inhibition of acetylcholinesterase and plasma cholinesterase, resulting in excess accumulation of acetylcholine at muscarinic and nicotinic receptors, and in the central nervous system

Adverse Reactions
Cardiovascular: Hyperdynamic (~18% to 21%) or hypodynamic (~7% to 10%) states
Central nervous system: Toxicity is limited because carbamates do not significantly cross the blood-brain barrier; CNS changes occur with most severe intoxications, paresthesia, hyperactivity
Genitourinary: Incontinence
Neuromuscular & skeletal: Weakness, paralysis
Respiratory: Depression, edema
General: Flu-like symptoms (especially with chronic exposure)

Signs & Symptoms of Acute Overdose Miosis (unreactive to light), mydriasis (rarely), lacrimation, pallor, excessive sweating, confusion, agitation, headache, dysarthria, generalized asthenia, seizures, A-V block, coma, decreased hemoglobin/red blood cell count/platelet count, cranial nerve palsies, metabolic acidosis and hyperglycemia (severe intoxication), hypotension, hypertension, bradycardia, tachycardia, Q-T prolongation, heart block, asystole, salivation, bronchorrhea, tachypnea, pulmonary edema, respiratory depression, diaphragmatic paralysis, skeletal muscle fasciculation and flaccid paralysis, nausea, vomiting, abdominal pain, fecal and urinary incontinence; an "intermediate syndrome" of limb asthenia and respiratory paralysis has been reported to occur between 24 and 96 hours postorganophosphate exposure, and is independent of the acute cholinergic crisis; late paresthesia characterized by stocking and glove paresthesia, anesthesia, and asthenia is infrequently observed weeks to months following acute exposure to certain organophosphates

Toxicodynamics/Kinetics
Absorption: Readily through oral, dermal, or respiratory exposure
Metabolism: Rapidly metabolized to weakly active compounds through hepatic hydrolysis and other pathways
Elimination: Metabolites are excreted in urine

Warnings Severe laryngeal irritation and violent coughing may result from exposure to dusting powders; exposure to dusting powders and insecticide granules may cause contact dermatitis

Overdosage Treatment

Decontamination: Isolation, bagging, and disposal of all contaminated clothing and other articles; all emergency medical workers and hospital staff should follow appropriate precautions regarding exposure to hazardous material including the use of protective clothing, masks, goggles, and respiratory equipment

Dermal: Prompt thorough scrubbing of all affected areas with soap and water, including hair and nails

Gastric: Activated charcoal can be administered either orally or via a nasogastric tube; do not induce emesis because of danger of sudden respiratory compromise, alterations in mental status, seizures, coma, and possible aspiration of hydrocarbon vehicles

Ocular: Irrigation with copious tepid sterile water or saline

Supportive therapy: Including airway management, ventilatory assistance, humidified oxygen administration, and close monitoring for sudden respiratory failure

Antidote:

Atropine: Administration should be guided by respiratory status, starting at 1-5 mg I.V. every 5-10 minutes as needed, and should be titrated to the resolution of excess pulmonary secretions; frequent administration of large doses (cumulative doses >100 mg) may be necessary in massive exposures

Glycopyrrolate: May be administered if atropine is unavailable

2-PAM: Although not specifically indicated, 2-PAM may be considered in the following situations:

Life-threatening symptoms such as respiratory paralysis

Continued excessive atropine requirements especially nicotinic symptoms

Concomitant organophosphate and carbamate exposure

Enhancement of elimination: Dialysis and hemoperfusion are not indicated due to effectiveness of the prescribed treatment, large volumes of distribution of organophosphates

Antidote(s)

Atropine Sulfate *on page 1395*

Diagnostic Tests/Procedures

Blood Gases, Arterial *on page 1207*

Chest Films *on page 1224*

Complete Blood Count *on page 1236*

Creatinine, Serum *on page 1243*

Electrocardiography *on page 1253*

Liver Profile *on page 1286*

Pseudocholinesterase, Serum *on page 1340*

Pregnancy Implications Human data regarding organophosphate exposure in pregnancy is limited and anecdotal; teratogenesis and fetal death have been produced in animal models at exposure levels that cause obvious toxicity to the pregnant animal

Additional Information Possesses a slight sulfur odor; thermal breakdown products include nitrogen oxides and sulfur oxides; red blood cell cholinesterase, and serum pseudocholinesterase may be depressed following acute or chronic organophosphate exposure; RBC cholinesterase is typically not analyzed by in-house laboratories, and is usually not available for consideration during acute management. Pseudocholinesterase levels may be rapidly available from some in-house laboratories, but are not as reliable a marker of organophosphate exposure because of variability secondary to variant genotypes, hepatic disease, oral estrogen use, or malnutrition, thus they may not be useful in ruling out carbamate exposure.

ACGIH TLV: 2.5 mg/m^3

PEL-TWA: 2.5 mg/m^3

Vapor pressure is 0.00005 mm Hg at 20°C

Other information concerning pesticide exposures is available through the EPA-funded National Pesticide Telecommunications Network: 1-800-858-7378 (weekdays, 8 AM to 6 PM, Central Standard time)

Specific References

Ekins BR and Geller RJ, "Methomyl-Induced Carbamate Poisoning Treated With Pralidoxime Chloride," *West J Med*, 1994, 161(1):68-70.

Lifshitz M, Rotenberg M, Sofer S, et al, "Carbamate Poisoning and Oxime Treatment in Children, A Clinical and Laboratory Study," *Pediatrics*, 1994, 93(4):652-5.

Zwiener RJ and Ginsburg CM, "Organophosphate and Carbamate Poisoning in Infants and Children," *Pediatrics*, 1988, 81(1):121-6.

Methoxcide® *see* Methoxychlor *on this page*

Methoxychlor

Related Information

Organochlorines *on page 983*

CAS Number 72-43-5

UN Number 2761

(Continued)

Methoxychlor *(Continued)*

Synonyms DMDT; Methoxy-DDT

Brand Names Marlate®; Methoxcide®; Metox®; Metron®; Prentox®

Use Essentially has replaced DDT (dichlorodiphenyltrichloroethane); methoxychlor is an effective insecticide used on crops, stored grain, livestock, pets, garbage containers, and sewage areas; also used in aerial operations regarding mosquito abatement

Mechanism of Toxic Action Metabolites of methoxychlor essentially act as estrogen analogues; also may deactivate the sodium channel after neuronal activation thus leading to neuronal hyperexcitability

Adverse Reactions While no systemic adverse effects have been attributed solely to methoxychlor to date, the central nervous system and reproductive system (as an estrogen analogue) have been target organs in animal studies

Toxicodynamics/Kinetics

Metabolism: Hepatic demethylation to metabolites conjugated to glucuronic acid

Elimination: Primarily fecal

Overdosage Treatment

Decontamination:

Dermal: Wash with soap and water; remove contaminated clothing

Ocular: Copious irrigation with saline

Oral: Lavage/activated charcoal; do not use oil-based cathartics in that increased absorption of methoxychlor can result

Supportive therapy: Benzodiazepines or phenobarbital can be used for seizure control

Enhancement of elimination: Due to its high lipid solubility and low rate of enterohepatic recirculation (5% to 10%), multiple dosing of activated charcoal is not expected to be effective

Additional Information No adverse effects noted in human volunteers ingesting 2 mg/kg/day for 8 weeks; average daily intake is estimated to be from 0.15 mcg in infants to 0.28 mcg in adults

TLV-TWA: 10 mg/m^2

Odor threshold in water: 4.7 ppm (fruity)

Half-life:

Atmospheric: 1-11 hours

Water: 1 year

Soil: 30-100 days

Specific References

Kupfer D and Bulger WH, "Metabolic Activation of Pesticides With Proestrogenic Activity," *Fed Proc*, 1987, 46(5):1864-9.

U.S. Department of Health and Human Services, "Toxicological Profile for Methoxychlor TP-93/11", Agency for Toxic Substances and Diseases Registry, May, 1994.

Methoxy-DDT *see* Methoxychlor *on previous page*

Methyl-3-Metatolycarbamoloxyphenyl Carbamate *see* Phenmedipham *on page 992*

Methyl Acetone *see* Methyl Ethyl Ketone *on page 967*

Methyl Alcohol *see* Methanol *on page 957*

Methyl Benzene *see* Toluene *on page 1029*

Methyl Bromide

CAS Number 74-83-9

UN Number 1062

Synonyms Bercema; Bromomethane; Monobromomethane

Brand Names Embafume®; Terabol®

Use Degreasing wool, extracting oils, insect fumigant, fire extinguishers

Mechanism of Toxic Action Intense vesicant; alkylating agent/sulfhydryl enzyme inhibitors

Adverse Reactions

Cardiovascular: Myocardial irritability

Central nervous system: CNS depression, extrapyramidal signs, cerebellar ataxia, headache, confusion, seizures

Hepatic: Liver injury, hepatomegaly

Neuromuscular & skeletal: Tremors

Ocular: Blurred vision, diplopia, mydriasis

Renal & genitourinary: Nephritis, oliguria, albuminuria

Respiratory: Pulmonary edema, pulmonary hemorrhage

Miscellaneous: Potentially carcinogenic

Signs & Symptoms of Acute Overdose Dermal burns, myoclonus, acetone breath, coma, seizures, difficulty in focusing, hyperthermia, nystagmus, dyspnea, dizziness, hyposmia, drowsiness, headache, nausea, vomiting, anorexia, distal neuritis, loss of ankle reflexes

Toxicodynamics/Kinetics
Absorption: By inhalation or through the skin
Metabolism: Hepatic, metabolites to methanol and bromide ion
Half-life: Probably <1 hour

Reference Range Bromide level >5 mg/100 mL is toxic

Overdosage Treatment Decontamination: Basic poison management; do not induce vomiting; dilute with 4-8 oz of milk or water. For inhalation, give 100% humidified oxygen.

Antidote(s)
Dimercaprol *on page 1414*

Diagnostic Tests/Procedures
Aspartate Aminotransferase *on page 1199*
Blood Gases, Arterial *on page 1207*
Chest Films *on page 1224*
Electrocardiography *on page 1253*
Lactate Dehydrogenase, Blood *on page 1279*
White Blood Count *on page 1380*

Additional Information Permanent neurological sequelae include depression, paralysis, ataxia, myoclonus; colorless, odorless gas; burning taste; readily penetrates leather; average daily inhalation dose in U.S. urban areas: 4.5-24.5 mcg/adult
TLV-TWA: 5 ppm
IDLH: 2000 ppm
PEL-TWA: 5 ppm

Specific References
Anger WK, Moody L, Burg J, et al, "Neurobehavioral Evaluation of Soil and Structural Fumigators Using Methyl Bromide and Sulfuryl Fluoride," *Neurotoxicology*, 1986, 7(3):137-56.
Goldman LR, Mengle D, Epstein DM, et al, "Acute Symptoms in Persons Residing Near a Field Treated With the Soil Fumigants Methyl Bromide and Chloropicrin," *West J Med*, 1987, 147(1):95-8.
Hezemans-Boer M, Toonstra J, Meulenbelt J, et al, "Skin Lesions Due to Exposure to Methyl Bromide," *Arch Dermatol*, 1988, 124(6):917-21.
Zwaveling JH, de Kort WL, Meulenbelt J, et al, "Exposure of the Skin to Methyl Bromide: A Study of Six Cases Occupationally Exposed to High Concentrations During Fumigation," *Hum Toxicol*, 1987, 6(6):491-5.

Methyl Chloride *see* Chloromethane *on page 891*

Methyl Chloroform *see* Trichloroethane *on page 1032*

Methyl Cyanide *see* Acetonitrile *on page 850*

4,4'-Methylenebis (2-Chloroaniline)

Related Information
Benzidine *on page 868*

CAS Number 191-14-4

Synonyms DACPM; MCOVA

Brand Names Activator-M®; Bis-Amine A®; CA-800®; Cuamine-M®; Curene® 442; DAC; MOCA

Use Primarily as a curing agent in polymers containing isocyanate; also used in manufacture of epoxy resins; involved in manufacture of belt drives in computers, elevator or escalator wheels, gun mounts, radar systems, and shoe soles

Mechanism of Toxic Action Forms adducts with hemoglobin, serum albumin, and tissue DNA; may be tumor promotor similar to benzidine

Adverse Reactions Proteinuria in humans; carcinogenic in animals (not demonstrated in humans) with lungs, liver, breast, and bladder being the target organs in a dose-dependent manner

Toxicodynamics/Kinetics
Absorption: Inhalation, oral (40% in animal models), and dermal
Metabolism: Hepatic N-hydroxylation and N-acetylatoin to toxic metabolites
Half-life: 23 hours
Elimination: Renal and fecal

Overdosage Treatment
Decontamination:
Dermal: Wash with soap and water; remove contaminated clothing; penetration of gloves is concentration-dependent and can occur from 2-35 hours with natural latex gloves appearing to be most effective
Ocular: Irrigate copiously with saline

Additional Information
Atmospheric half-life: 0.3-2.9 hours (photoxidation)
Water half-life: 1-72 days (surface); 8 weeks to 1 year (groundwater)
PEL-TWA (skin designation): 0.2 ppm
TLV-TWA (skin designation): 0.2 ppm

Specific References
U.S. Department of Health and Human Services, "Toxicological Profile for 4,4'-Methylenebis (2-

(Continued)

4,4'-Methylenebis (2-Chloroaniline) *(Continued)*

Chloroaniline) (MBOCA) TP-93/12," Agency for Toxic Substances and Diseases Registry, May, 1994.

Methylene Chloride

CAS Number 75-09-2

UN Number 1593

Synonyms Dichloromethane; Freon 30; Methane Dichloride

Commonly Found In Paint and varnish removers, fire extinguishers, and fumigants

Mechanism of Toxic Action Solvent-induced depression/carbon monoxide effects

Adverse Reactions

Central nervous system: Anesthesia

Renal & genitourinary: Tubular necrosis (acute)

Signs & Symptoms of Acute Overdose Eye irritation, skin irritation, dyspnea, encephalopathy, dermal burns, lightheadedness, dizziness, tremor

Toxicodynamics/Kinetics

Absorption: Inhalation (70% to 75%), oral (98% within 20 minutes), and dermal

Metabolism: Converted hepatically to carbon monoxide (30%) and carbon dioxide (70%)

Half-life: 40 minutes

Elimination: Primarily pulmonary (carbon monoxide/carbon dioxide)

Reference Range Blood levels of 2 mg/L correlate with exposure of 200 ppm; carboxyhemoglobin levels usually in the range of 8% to 20%

Overdosage Treatment

Decontamination: Basic poison management; induce vomiting only in large ingestions

Supportive therapy: 100% humidified oxygen; hyperbaric oxygen has been advocated for patients with neurological abnormalities

Enhancement of elimination: Inhalation

Diagnostic Tests/Procedures

Carboxyhemoglobin, Blood *on page 1221*

Liver Profile *on page 1286*

Pregnancy Implications Embryotoxic, telencephalic dysgenesis noted; readily crosses the placenta with stillbirths, mental retardation, and microcephalus all noted

Additional Information Colorless fluid, pleasant odor; not flammable nor explosive

TLV-TWA: 50 ppm

IDLH: 5000 ppm

PEL-TWA: 500 ppm

Atmospheric half-life: 100-500 days

Ambient atmospheric concentrations of methylene chloride in U.S. urban areas range from 0.8-6.7 ppt; in rural/suburban areas, the range is from 0.18-2.1 ppt; hair spray can cause levels as high as 50 ppm (TWA: 0.17 ppm) of methylene chloride

Mean concentrations in drinking water: Usually <1 mcg/L

Odor threshold (sweet): Water: 9.1 ppm; air: 160-620 ppm

Minimum lethal oral dose: 0.5-5.0 mL/kg

Specific References

Buie SE, Pratt DS, and May JJ, "Diffuse Pulmonary Injury Following Paint Remover Exposure," *Am J Med*, 1986, 81(4):702-4.

Langehennig PL, Seeler RA, and Berman E, "Paint Removers and Carboxyhemoglobin," *N Engl J Med*, 1976, 295(20):1137.

Leikin JB, Kaufman D, Lipscomb JW, et al, "Methylene Chloride: Report of Five Exposures and Two Deaths," *Am J Emerg Med*, 1990, 8(6):534-7.

Rioux JP and Myers RA, "Hyperbaric Oxygen for Methylene Chloride Poisoning: Report on Two Cases," *Ann Emerg Med*, 1989, 18(6):691-5.

Wells GG and Waldron HA, "Methylene Chloride Burns," *Br J Ind Med*, 1984, 41(3):420.

U.S. Department of Health and Human Services, "Toxicological Profile for Methylene Chloride TP-92/13," Agency for Toxic Substances and Diseases Registry, April, 1993.

Methylene Dianiline

CAS Number 101-77-9

UN Number 2651

Synonyms DDM; MDA; 4,4-Methylene Dianiline

Use Curing agent for polyurethane; corrosive inhibitor; used in preparation of A_{30} dyes; epoxy resin-hardening agent

Mechanism of Toxic Action Contact allergen, hepatotoxin; possibly carcinogenic in humans (urinary tract)

Adverse Reactions

Hepatic: Toxic hepatitis ("epping jaundice"), cholestasis

Ocular: Optic neuritis

Respiratory: Bronchoconstriction

Signs & Symptoms of Acute Overdose Jaundice, epigastric pain, nausea, dyspnea, myalgia, hepatomegaly, yellow discoloration of skin, fingernails, and hair; ocular irritation, visual dysfunction

Toxicodynamics/Kinetics Absorption: Dermal

Reference Range Can be measured in urine to a detection level of 2 μg/L

Overdosage Treatment Supportive therapy: Beta agonists (nebulized) can be utilized for bronchoconstriction

Diagnostic Tests/Procedures

Alkaline Phosphatase, Serum *on page 1184*

Liver Profile *on page 1286*

Additional Information Faint amine-like odor; irritating at levels of 1 ppm; causative agent in "epping jaundice" due to flour contamination in Epping, England in 1965

TLV-TWA: 0.1 ppm

Specific References

Bastian PG, "Occupational Hepatitis Caused by Methylenedianiline," *Med J Aust*, 1984, 141(8):533-5.

Kopelman H, Robertson MH, and Sanders PG, "The Epping Jaundice," *Br Med J*, 1966, 1(5486):514-6.

McQueen CA and Williams GM, "Review of the Genotoxicity and Carcinogenicity of 4,4'-Methylene-Dianiline and 4,4'-Methylene-Bis-2-Chloroaniline," *Mutat Res*, 1990, 239(2):133-42.

Selden A, Berg P, Jakobsson R, et al, "Methylene Dianiline: Assessment of Exposure and Cancer Morbidity in Power Generator Workers," *Int Arch Occup Environ Health*, 1992, 63(6):403-8.

4,4-Methylene Dianiline *see* Methylene Dianiline *on previous page*

Methyl Ester of Methacrylic Acid *see* Methacrylates *on page 957*

Methyl Ethyl Ketone

CAS Number 78-93-3

UN Number 1193; 1232

Synonyms 2-Butanone; Ethyl Methyl Ketone; MEK; Methyl Acetone; 2-Oxobutane

Brand Names Meetco®

Use In production of drugs of abuse; used as a solvent for coatings, adhesives, magnetic tapes, printing inks, paint remover, vinyl films, polystyrene, polyurethane; also used in manufacture of aluminum foil and synthetic leather

Mechanism of Toxic Action Mucosal irritant and central nervous system depressant

Adverse Reactions

Cardiovascular: Hypotension, tachycardia

Central nervous system: Headache at 300 ppm; coma, dizziness, fatigue, paresthesia

Dermatologic: Urticaria

Endocrine & metabolic: Metabolic acidosis, hyperglycemia

Gastrointestinal: Nausea

Ocular: Irritant at 200 ppm; can cause conjunctival irritation

Respiratory: Irritant at 100 ppm; hyperventilation

Toxicodynamics/Kinetics

Absorption: Inhalation: 41% to 56%

Protein binding: 0%

Metabolism: Hepatic to 3-hydroxy-2-butanone and 2,3-butanediol

Half-life: 49-96 minutes

Elimination: Lungs

Reference Range Plasma 2-butanone level of 95 mg/100 mL consistent with coma in an oral ingestion

Overdosage Treatment

Decontamination: Do not use ipecac; lavage (preferably with a cuffed endotracheal tube in place to prevent aspiration) for large ingestions within 2 hours; activated charcoal may be useful

Supportive therapy: Sodium bicarbonate for acidosis

Pregnancy Implications Slightly fetotoxic in rodents (delayed development) at concentrations >1000 ppm

Additional Information Colorless liquid with acetone odor

Odor threshold: <10 ppm

OSHA-PEL: 200 ppm

OSHA-STEL: 300 ppm

BEI: 2 mg MEK/L

Specific References

Kopelman P and Kalfayan P, "Severe Metabolic Acidosis After Ingestion of Butanone," *Br Med J*, 1983, 286:21-2.

Varigos GA and Nurse DS, "Contact Urticaria From Methyl Ethyl Ketone," *Contact Dermatitis*, 1986, 15(4):259-60.

Methyl Glycol *see* Propylene Glycol *on page 1002*

Methyl Hydride *see* Methane *on page 957*

Methyl Isocyanate

Related Information

Toluene *on page 1029*

CAS Number 624-83-9

UN Number 2480

Synonyms Isocyanate; Isocyanatomethane; MIC

Use Intermediate agent in the production of carbaryl (Sevin®, a carbamate pesticide) and herbicides

Mechanism of Toxic Action Mucosal irritant; reacts with water to form exothermic reaction; hydrolyzes to form methylamine and CO_2

Adverse Reactions

Central nervous system: Fatigue, vertigo, ataxia

Gastrointestinal: Vomiting

Ocular: Burning, lacrimation, blepharospasm, photophobia, corneal ulceration, lid edema

Neuromuscular & skeletal: Muscle weakness, tremor

Renal: Renal tubular acidosis

Respiratory: Cough, chest pain, dyspnea, bronchospasm (wheezing), throat irritation, interstitial edema

Toxicodynamics/Kinetics

Absorption: By inhalation and dermal routes

Reference Range Leukocytosis, lymphocytosis and elevated erythrocyte sedimentation rate noted; blood carboxyhemoglobin, methemoglobin, and thiocyanate levels may be high, but this may be due to contaminants

Overdosage Treatment

Decontamination: Give 100% humidified oxygen

Supportive therapy: Beta agonist agents with theophylline may be helpful; steroids may be useful; thiosulfate does not appear to be helpful

Pregnancy Implications Fetotoxic; increased fetal mortality may be related either to maternal hypoxia or direct toxic effect

Additional Information Toxic agent responsible for 3,828 deaths in December 1984 in Bhopal, India; pyrolysis decomposition products include hydrogen cyanide and carbon dioxide; very flammable; involved in the recall of over 8 billion cigarettes by the Philip Morris Co in May 1995 due to contaminated plasticizer compound in the cigarette filter

TLV-TWA: 0.02 ppm

Mucous membrane irritant threshold: 0.2 ppm

Odor threshold: 2 ppm

Unbearable exposure: 21 ppm

Specific References

Alexeeff GV, Shusterman DJ, Howd RA, et al, "Dose Response Assessment of Airborne Methyl Isothiocyanate Following a Metam Sodium Spill," *Risk Assessment*, 1994, 14(2):191-8.

Dhara R and Dhara VR, "Bhopal – A Case Study of International Disaster," *Int J Occup Med Environ Health*, 1995, 1:58-9.

Mehta PS, Mehta AS, Mehta SJ, et al, "Bhopal: Tragedy's Health Effects," *JAMA*, 1990, 264(21):2781-7.

Methyl Mercaptan

CAS Number 74-93-1

UN Number 1064

Synonyms Methanethiol; Thiomethanol; Thiomethyl Alcohol

Use Production of jet fuel, pesticides, and plastics; used as an agent to add odor to odorless hazardous gases (not natural gas)

Mechanism of Toxic Action Can cause oxidative stress to red blood cell membranes (especially in patients with glucose-6-phosphate dehydrogenase deficiency) thus resulting in hemolysis

Adverse Reactions

Cardiovascular: Tachycardia, hypertension

Central nervous system: Seizures, coma

Hematologic: Hemolytic anemia, methemoglobinemia

Miscellaneous: Mucosal irritation

Toxicodynamics/Kinetics

Absorption: By inhalation

Metabolism: To dimethyl sulfide

Elimination: Primarily by lungs

Overdosage Treatment

Decontamination:

- Dermal: Wash with soap and water
- Inhalation: Give 100% humidified oxygen

Ocular: Irrigate copiously with saline

Supportive therapy: Treat symptomatic methemoglobinemia with methylene blue (monitor closely in G-6-PD-deficient patients); promote an alkaline diuresis to avoid adverse renal effects of hemolysis

Antidote(s)

Methylene Blue *on page 1444*

Diagnostic Tests/Procedures

Methemoglobin, Blood *on page 1296*

Additional Information Very soluble in water; a flammable gas which can be explosive; a reduced sulfur gas from pulp air emissions

Odor threshold: 1.6 ppb (rotten cabbage)
TLV-TWA: 0.5 ppm
IDLH: 400 ppm
Atmospheric half-life: 0.2-30 hours

Specific References

Shults WT, Fountain EN, and Lynch EC, "Methanethiol Poisoning: Irreversible Coma and Hemolytic Anemia Following Inhalation," *JAMA*, 1970, 211(13):2153-4.

U.S. Department of Health and Human Services, "Toxicological Profile for Methyl Mercaptan TP-91/20," Agency for Toxic Substances and Diseases Registry, September, 1992.

Methyl Methacrylate Monomer *see* Methacrylates *on page 957*

Methyl-n-Butyl Ketone *see* 2-Hexanone *on page 938*

Methyl Nitroglycol *see* Propylene Glycol Dinitrate *on page 1003*

3-Methyl-N,N-Diethylbenzamide *see* Diethyltoluamide *on page 912*

Methyl Parathion

CAS Number 298-00-0

UN Number 3017

Brand Names A-Gro®; Azofos®; Bladan-M®; Dalf®; ME-Parathion®; Metapon®; Wofatox®

Use Insecticide which is applied to crops, cotton, and fruit trees

Mechanism of Toxic Action Potent, irreversible inhibition of acetylcholinesterase and plasma cholinesterase, resulting in excess accumulation of acetylcholine at muscarinic and nicotinic receptors, and in the central nervous system; this is in the class of a phosphorthioate organophosphate

Adverse Reactions

Cardiovascular: Hyperdynamic (~18% to 21%) or hypodynamic (~7% to 10%) states
Central nervous system: Depression, seizures, hyperactivity
Genitourinary: Incontinence
Neuromuscular & skeletal: Weakness, paralysis
Respiratory: Depression, pulmonary edema
General: Flu-like symptoms (especially with chronic exposure)
Delayed: Muscle asthenia and paresthesia

Toxicodynamics/Kinetics

Absorption: Inhalation, oral, and dermal routes
Metabolism: Enzymatic hydrolysis to dimethylphosphoric acid and 4-nitrophenol
Elimination: Renal

Reference Range

Mild poisoning: Serum cholinesterase is 20% to 50% of normal
Moderate poisoning: Serum cholinesterase is 10% to 20% of normal
Severe poisoning (respiratory distress and coma): Serum cholinesterase is <10%

Overdosage Treatment

Decontamination: Isolation, bagging, and disposal of all contaminated clothing and other articles; all emergency medical workers and hospital staff should follow appropriate precautions regarding exposure to hazardous material including the use of protective clothing, masks, goggles, and respiratory equipment

Dermal: Prompt thorough scrubbing of all affected areas with soap and water, including hair and nails

Gastric: Activated charcoal can be administered either orally or via a nasogastric tube; do not induce emesis because of danger of sudden respiratory compromise, alterations in mental status, seizures, coma, and possible aspiration of hydrocarbon vehicles

Ocular: Irrigation with copious tepid sterile water or saline

Supportive therapy: Including airway management, ventilatory assistance, humidified oxygen administration, and close monitoring for sudden respiratory failure

Enhancement of elimination: Dialysis and hemoperfusion are not indicated due to effectiveness of the prescribed treatment, large volumes of distribution of organophosphates

Antidote:

Atropine: Administration should be guided by respiratory status, starting at 1-5 mg I.V. every 5-10 minutes as needed, and should be titrated to the resolution

(Continued)

Methyl Parathion *(Continued)*

of excess pulmonary secretions; frequent administration of large doses (cumulative doses >100 mg) may be necessary in massive exposures

Glycopyrrolate: May be administered if atropine is unavailable

2-PAM: For more significant exposures (ie, exposures requiring large doses of atropine, or with recurring symptoms, or exposures to more lipid soluble agents), administration should follow: 1-2 g I.V. over 5-10 minutes, repeated in 1 hour if asthenia reoccurs, then every 4-12 hours for recurring symptoms

Additional Information Estimated oral lethal dose: Adults: 5-50 mg/kg (7 drops to 1 teaspoon); no neurologic effect at oral daily doses of up to 19 mg; toxicity is lower than that of parathion

Odor threshold: 0.012 ppm

Depression of cholinesterase can occur with daily dosage exceeding 0.43 mg/kg

Estimated daily intake in adults:

- Inhalation: In agricultural areas: 0.1-2.6 mcg
- Ingestion:
  - Food: 0.01-2 mcg
  - Drinking water: 0.4 mcg

Soil half-life (degrades faster in nonsterile soil):

- Aerobic: 64 days
- Anaerobic: 7 days

Water half-life:

- pH <8: 72-89 days (40°C)
- pH >8: 4 days (40°C)

Specific References

U.S. Department of Health and Human Services, "Toxicological Profile for Methyl Parathion TP-91/21," Agency for Toxic Substances and Diseases Registry, September, 1992.

Methylphenol *see* Cresols *on page 898*

Methyl Tert-Butyl Ether

CAS Number 1634-04-4

UN Number 2398

Synonyms MBE; MTBE; Tert-Butyl Methyl Ether

Use Reformulated gasoline; pharmaceutical agent to dissolve gallstones through an intraductal route via a thistle catheter; to increase octane (up to 15%) and reduce levels of carbon monoxide emissions; oxygenate agent in motor gasoline

Investigational use: Cholesterol gallstones

Mechanism of Toxic Action Lipophilic, volatile solvent which acts as a central nervous system depressant (through changes in neuronal membrane fluidity)

Adverse Reactions

- Central nervous system: Headache, dizziness, sedation, ataxia, coma
- Gastrointestinal: Nausea, vomiting
- Hematologic: Hemolysis
- Ocular: Ocular irritation, lacrimation
- Respiratory: Coughing, nasal irritation

Toxicodynamics/Kinetics

- Absorption: Inhalation, orally, and dermally
- Metabolism: Hepatic to tert-butanol, formaldehyde, methanol, and carbon dioxide
- Half-life (rodents): 1-2 hours
- Elimination: Lungs, feces, and urine

Reference Range

Median blood levels of MTBE:

- Commuters: 0.1 µg/L
- Car repairers: 2.0 µg/L
- Gas station attendants: 15.0 µg/L

Healthy volunteers exposed for 1 hour at 1.7 ppm: 17.0 µg/L

After intracystic administration, mean tert-butanol blood levels were 0.04 mg/mL and 0.02-0.03 mg/mL in urine

Overdosage Treatment

Decontamination:

- Dermal: Wash with soap and water
- Ocular: Copious irrigation with saline
- Oral: Do not induce emesis; activated charcoal is not recommended since it is poorly absorbed to activated charcoal; dilute with milk or water
- Inhalation: 100% humidified oxygen

Monitoring Parameters Liver function tests, chest x-ray

Pregnancy Implications Fetotoxic in rodents (increased incidence of cleft palate, fused sternebrae, reduced birth rate)

Additional Information Methanol is only detected in trace amounts and is not considered to be a major problem

Intraductal dose of MTBE for treatment of gallstones: 1-15 mL (up to 140 mL) instilled 3-6 times/minute and then reaspirated

Odor threshold in water: 680 ppb
Workplace environmental exposure level (8-hour weighted average): 100 ppm
Atmospheric lifetime: 4 days
Ambient water level of MTBE: 15-81 mcg/L

Specific References

Allen MJ, Borody TJ, Bugliosi TF, et al, "Cholelitholysis Using Methyl Tertiary Butyl Ether," *Gastroenterology*, 1985, 88(1 Pt 1):122-5.

Allen MJ, Borody TJ, Bugliosi TF, et al, "Rapid Dissolution of Gallstones by Methyl Tert-Butyl Ether. Primary Observations," *N Engl J Med*, 1985, 312(4):217-20.

Bonin MA, Ashley DL, Cardinali FL, et al, "Measurement of Methyl *tert*-Butyl Ether and *tert*-Butyl Alcohol in Human Blood by Purge-and-Trap Gas Chromatography-Mass Spectrometry Using an Isotope-Dilution Method," *J Anal Toxicol*, 1995, 19:187-91.

U.S. Department of Health and Human Services, "Toxicological Profile for Methyl T-Butyl Ether," Agency for Toxic Substances and Diseases Registry, August, 1994.

Methyltoluene *see* Xylene *on page 1040*

Metox® *see* Methoxychlor *on page 963*

Metron® *see* Methoxychlor *on page 963*

Mezotox® *see* Nitrofen *on page 980*

MG *see* Mustard Gas *on next page*

MGK Diethyltoluamide *see* Diethyltoluamide *on page 912*

MIC *see* Methyl Isocyanate *on page 968*

Microzul® *see* Anticoagulant Rodenticide *on page 859*

MIL-T-5624-L-Amd 1 *see* Jet Fuel-4 *on page 944*

Mineral-Based Crankcase Oil

CAS Number 8002-05-9

UN Number 1267; 1270

Synonyms API 79-7; Automotive Motor Oil; Base Engine Oil; Marine Diesel Oil; Petroleum

Use Supplemental fuel in engines, steam boilers, and domestic oil burners; incorporated into asphalt and as a dust suppressant on rural roads

Mechanism of Toxic Action Mixture of low and high molecular weight hydrocarbons (aliphatic, aromatic, naphthenic, and paraffinic); sulfur, oxygen, nitrogen compounds, and metals (lead, zinc, cadmium, nickel) may be present

Adverse Reactions

Central nervous system: Headache
Dermatologic: Rash
Neuromuscular & skeletal: Tremors
Miscellaneous: Stomatitis and ocular irritation at levels of 18.9 mg/m^3

Toxicodynamics/Kinetics

Absorption: Some dermally
Elimination: Primarily fecal

Overdosage Treatment

Decontamination:
- Dermal: Wash skin with water and mild green (lipophilic) soap
- Ocular: Copious irrigation with normal saline
- Oral: Dilute with water

Additional Information Monitor for toxicity of lead or molybdenum in used oil; oil from engines emitted directly with auto exhaust at concentrations of 0.1-0.3 L/1000 km; lead levels on road surfaces treated with this compound are over 5 times higher than background lead levels (209 mg/kg vs 39 mg/kg respectively); hydrocarbon levels at the surface of treated roads range from 5880-13,441 mg/kg; background concentration of hydrocarbons in road soil near industrial area is ~856 mcg/g; near highways it is 265 mcg/g

Specific References

U.S. Department of Health and Human Services, "Toxicological Profile for Mineral-Based Crankcase Oil," Agency for Toxic Substances and Diseases Registry, June, 1994.

Mineral Naphtha *see* Benzene *on page 867*

Mirex

Related Information

Organochlorines *on page 983*

CAS Number 2385-85-5

Synonyms Fire Ant Bait

Brand Names Dechlorane® 4070; Ferriamicide®

Use Primarily an insecticide to control fire ants and Western harvester ants; control leaf cutters, mealy bugs, and yellow jackets; historical use (until 1972) as a fire retardant

(Continued)

Mirex *(Continued)*

Mechanism of Toxic Action In animal models, mirex induces liver growth possibly mediated by corticosterone

Adverse Reactions None described in humans; target organ in animal models for toxicity is liver and thyroid

Toxicodynamics/Kinetics

Metabolism: Not metabolized

Half-life: >1 year

Elimination: Primarily fecal and through breast milk

Reference Range Mirex blood levels in asymptomatic unexposed individuals should be <0.04 ng/g whole blood

Pregnancy Implications Not fetotoxic in animals

Additional Information

FDA action level for fish: 0.1 ppm

Water half-life: 48 hours

Specific References

Gaines TB and Kimbrough RD, "Oral Toxicity of Mirex in Adult and Suckling Rats," *Arch Environ Health*, 1970, 21(1):7-14.

MMA *see* Methacrylates *on page 957*

MOCA *see* 4,4'-Methylenebis (2-Chloroaniline) *on page 965*

Mogas *see* Gasoline *on page 932*

Monobromomethane *see* Methyl Bromide *on page 964*

Monochlorobenzene *see* Chlorobenzene *on page 889*

Monochloromethane *see* Chloromethane *on page 891*

"Monocite" Methacrylate Monomer *see* Methacrylates *on page 957*

Monoethylene Glycol *see* Ethylene Glycol *on page 925*

Morbicid *see* Formaldehyde *on page 931*

Moth Balls *see* Naphthalene *on next page*

Moth Flakes *see* Naphthalene *on next page*

Motor Fuel *see* Gasoline *on page 932*

Motor Spirit *see* Gasoline *on page 932*

Motox® *see* Toxaphene *on page 1031*

Mouse-Rid® *see* Strychnine *on page 1016*

Mouse-Tox® *see* Strychnine *on page 1016*

MTBE *see* Methyl Tert-Butyl Ether *on page 970*

M-Toluamide *see* Diethyltoluamide *on page 912*

M-Toluic Acid Diethylamide *see* Diethyltoluamide *on page 912*

Muriatic Acid *see* Hydrogen Chloride *on page 940*

Mustard Gas

CAS Number 505-60-2

Synonyms Bis(2-Chloroethyl) Sulfide; Distilled Mustard; HD; MG; S-Mustard; Yperite

Use Primarily of historical use during World War I as a vesicant chemical warfare agent; most recently used for this purpose during the Iran-Iraq War in the 1980s; derivative of this chemical has been used as an antineoplastic agent (an alkylating agent – nitrogen mustard)

Mechanism of Toxic Action Dermal, ocular, and respiratory corrosive agent; this agent combines with DNA thus preventing cell replication

Adverse Reactions

Dermal: Erythema and pruritus; may be delayed for up to 8 hours, then dermal burns and blisters can result

Inhalation: Dyspnea, cough, vomiting

Ocular: Lacrimation, photophobia, blepharospasm, ocular irritation

Miscellaneous: Bone marrow depression

Toxicodynamics/Kinetics

Absorption: Lungs or skin (at a rate of 1-4 mcg/cm^2/minute)

Metabolism: Hepatic through hydrolysis and glutathione pathways

Elimination: Renal accounts for about 21% of excretion

Overdosage Treatment

Decontamination:

Dermal: Remove all contaminated clothing; towels soaked in 0.2% chloramine-T in water (Dakin solution) placed over wounds for first 2 hours may be helpful;

wash with soap and water (not hot); if no water is available, dry decontamination with Fuller's earth can be utilized; treat wounds as burns with use of 1% silver sulfadiazine (twice daily)

Ocular: Copious irrigation with saline

Oral: Activated charcoal with cathartic

Supportive therapy: N-acetylcysteine 4 times/day (up to 150 mg/kg) along with ascorbic acid (3 g), thienamycin (2 g twice daily), L-carnitine (3 g), and sodium thiosulfate (3 g/day) have been used to ameliorate effects, but is unproven in its efficacy

Additional Information

Toxic dermal dose: 0.1% solution; fair skinned individuals are more at risk for adverse dermal effects than dark skinned individuals

Higher wind speeds, higher temperature and humidity increase the atmospheric vaporization rate; may persist in soil for weeks

Combat zones atmospheric concentration of mustard gas during WWI was estimated to be from 3-5 ppm; case fatality rate: 2% to 4%; since mustard gas binds rapidly and avidly to tissue proteins, decontamination must begin immediately and increasing elimination of absorbed chemical is difficult

Specific References

Borak J and Sidell FR, "Agents of Chemical Warfare: Sulfur Mustard," *Ann Emerg Med*, 1992, 21(3):303-8.

Fouyn Th, Lison D, and Wouters M, "Management of Chemical Warfare Injuries," *Lancet*, 1991, 337:121-2.

Heyndrickx A and Heyndrickx B, "Management of War Gas Injuries," *Lancet*, 1990, 336(8725):1248-9.

Maynard RL, Meredith TJ, Marrs TC, et al, "Management of Chemical Warfare Injuries," *Lancet*, 1991, 337:122.

Naphthalene

CAS Number 91-20-3

UN Number 1334; 2304

Synonyms Camphor Tar; Moth Balls; Moth Flakes; Naphthalin; Naphthene; White Tar

Use Moth repellents, toilet bowel deodorizers, in scintillation counters, in the manufacture of phallic anhydride, naphthol, hydrogenated naphthalenes, and halogenated naphthalenes; formerly used as an antihelmintic

Mechanism of Toxic Action Hemolysis caused by oxidation products of naphthalene; in patients with G-6-PD deficiency, metabolites cause instability of erythrocyte glutathione

Signs & Symptoms of Acute Overdose Headache, restlessness, drowsiness, vomiting, hemolysis, methemoglobinemia, hyperkalemia, fever, hematuria, anemia, seizures, and coma may develop in severe intoxications; tachycardia or hypotension may occur; hepatocellular injury is rare, but may occur 3-5 days after; urine discoloration (black)

Toxicodynamics/Kinetics

Absorption:

Dermal: Also enhanced by oil

Inhalation: Rapid

Oral: Erratic; soluble in oil so coadministration will enhance absorption

Metabolism: Through liver; oxidation to naphthol and naphthoquinone; glutathione conjugated to thioethers are also noted

Elimination: Excreted in kidney as a 1,4-naphthoquinone metabolite over a 2-week period; fecal excretion accounts for <10%

Reference Range Adipose tissue levels up to 63 μg/kg have been detected in asymptomatic individuals

Overdosage Treatment

Decontamination:

Oral: Emesis or lavage within 2 hours; activated charcoal with cathartics; avoid milk for 2-3 hours in that absorption may increase

Dermal: Wash with soap and water; avoid oil-based compounds

Ocular: Copious irrigation with saline

Supportive therapy: Alkaline diuresis may be needed if hemolysis occurs; methylene blue 1-2 mg/kg of 1% if the patient is symptomatic or a methemoglobin level >30%. Transfusion for severe anemia; dialysis has been used for supportive care; exchange transfusion has been used for supportive care, but is not routinely recommended.

Antidote(s)

Methylene Blue *on page 1444*

Pregnancy Implications Hemolytic anemia and jaundice have developed in neonates following *in utero* exposure

Additional Information Detection and quantitation of naphthalene and metabolites through TLC, HPLC, gas chromatography with mass spectrometry, and high resolution proton magnetic resonance. CBC with smear to detect for schistocytes

(Continued)

Naphthalene *(Continued)*

and cell fragments, BUN, creatinine, electrolytes, methemoglobin, urinalysis (check for hemoglobinuria), G-6-PD, LFTs; urine may be sent for 1-naphthol. See table.

Distinguishing Characteristics of Mothballs

	PDB	Naphtha	Camphor
Physical	Wet and oily	Dry	
Water	Sink	Sink	Float
4 oz water + 3 heaping tsp salt	Sink	Float	Float
Drop of turpentine	Soluble	Moderately soluble	
Heating	Green color	No color	

PDB = paradichlorobenzene.
Naphtha = naphthalene.

Odor threshold:
Water: 0.021 mg/L
Air: 0.44 mg/m^3
PEL-TWA: 10 ppm (50 mg/m^3)
TLV-TWA: 10 ppm (52 mg/m^3)
IDLH: 500 ppm
Water half-life (photolysis): 71 hours (surface water); 550 days (deep water >5 meters)
Ambient atmospheric concentration in U.S. is ~1 ppm
In drinking water, concentrations as high as 1.5 mcg/L have been noted
Average daily intake of naphthalene is ~19 mcg by inhalation and from 0.002-4 mcg from drinking water

Specific References

Anziulewicz JA, Dick HJ, and Chiarulli EE, "Transplacental Naphthalene Poisoning," *Am J Obstet Gynecol*, 1959, 78(3):519-21.

Kucharski E, Gorman R, and Kein-Schwartz W, "A Prospective Evaluation of Naphthalene Moth Repellent Toxicity," *Vet Hum Toxicol*, 1992, 34:340.

Shah BR and Santucci KA, "Naphthalene-Induced Acute Hemolytic Anemia in Children With Glucose-6-Phosphate Dehydrogenase (G-6-PD) Deficiency - An Overlooked Inner-City Toxin," *Acad Emerg Med*, 1995, 2:396.

Siegel E and Wason S, "Mothball Toxicity," *Pediatr Clin North Am*, 1986, 33(2):369-74.

U.S. Department of Health and Human Services, "Toxicological Profile for Naphthalene," Agency for Toxic Substances and Diseases Registry, October, 1993.

Naphthalin *see* Naphthalene *on previous page*

Naphthene *see* Naphthalene *on previous page*

1-Naphthyl N-Methylcarbamate *see* Carbaryl *on page 877*

Natural Gas (85% Methane) *see* Methane *on page 957*

Natural Gasoline *see* Gasoline *on page 932*

Naugard TJB® *see* N-Nitrosodiphenylamine *on page 982*

NDPA *see* N-Nitrosodiphenylamine *on page 982*

NDPHA *see* N-Nitrosodiphenylamine *on page 982*

Neantine® *see* Diethyl Phthalate *on page 912*

Nemafume® *see* 1,2-Dibromo-3-Chloropropane *on page 906*

Nemagon® *see* 1,2-Dibromo-3-Chloropropane *on page 906*

Nemapax® *see* 1,2-Dibromo-3-Chloropropane *on page 906*

Nemazon® *see* 1,2-Dibromo-3-Chloropropane *on page 906*

Nephis® *see* Ethylene Bromide *on page 924*

Nerve Gases

CAS Number 107-44-8 (sarin); 96-64-0 (soman); 77-81-6 (tabun); 50782-69-9 (VX)

Synonyms Sarin (GB or Isopropyl Methylphosphonofluoridate); Soman (GD or Pinacolyl Methylphosphonofluoridate); Tabun (Ethyl N-Dimethylphophoramidocyanidate or GA); VX (Methylphosphonothioic Acid S-(2-(bis(1-Methyl-Ethyl)Amino)Ethyl) O-Ethyl Ester or V)

Use Chemical warfare weapon

Mechanism of Toxic Action Similar to organophosphate agent; inhibits the enzyme acetylcholinesterase thus resulting in acetylcholine excess at the neuronal synapse; may penetrate blood brain barrier and thus affect GABA transmission

Adverse Reactions

Central nervous system: Insomnia, fatigue, memory loss, seizures, ataxia, coma

Gastrointestinal: Diarrhea

Ocular: Lacrimation, miosis

Respiratory: Rhinorrhea; death is usually due to respiratory failure

Miscellaneous: Excess muscarinic activity (bronchial secretion, salivation, sweating, miosis, bronchospasm, bradycardia) and nicotinic activity (muscle twitching, weakness, paralysis)

Toxicodynamics/Kinetics

Onset of action: Inhalation: Within 5 minutes

Half-time:

Aging of sarin-acetylcholine complex: 5 hours

Aging of soman-acetylcholine complex: 2 minutes

Reference Range Cholinesterase activity <10% of normal is consistent with severe poisoning

Overdosage Treatment

Decontamination:

Dermal: Remove all contaminated clothing; wash with 5% hypochlorite solution (household bleach) followed by copious water irrigation; if bleach is not available, a gentle blotting with an alkaline soap can be used

Inhalation: Administer 100% humidified oxygen

Ocular: Irrigate with saline

Supportive therapy: Atropine is the mainstay of treatment with doses from 10-20 mg cumulatively over the first 2-3 hours usually required; this should be titrated to bronchial secretions and not to ocular signs; pralidoxime (1-2 g I.V. over 10 minutes, repeat in 1 hour if weakness occurs, then every 4-12 hours as needed) should be administered; diazepam or midazolam has been effective anticonvulsant in primate models; since aging is longer for tabun or VX, pralidoxime may be particularly useful; administer oxygen. Seizures often respond to atropine or pralidoxime; for refractory seizures, diazepam can be used; in fact, 5-10 mg of diazepam is often given as pretreatment in severely affected patients. Hemodialysis/hemoperfusion has been noted to increase cholinesterase levels and improve clinical symptomatology in one patient

Antidote(s)

Atropine Sulfate *on page 1395*

Pralidoxime Chloride *on page 1461*

Pyridostigmine Bromide *on page 1463*

Pregnancy Implications Does not appear to be teratogenic

Additional Information Sarin has been implicated in the Tokyo subway terrorist incident occurring in March, 1995. It has been estimated that 800 kg of sarin will cause heavy casualties over 1 square mile area. Sarin is 4000 times more potent than parathion. Lethal inhaled dose of tabun, sarin, and soman is ~1 mg; VX has highest lethality in dermal applications (as an oily liquid) rather than through inhalation; while sarin and tabun may cause a delayed neuropathy, VX is not known to cause a delayed neuropathy. Emergency medical ambulances in New York City now stock up to 52 mg of atropine; this is up from 4 mg which was a typical ambulance stock of atropine before the March, 1995 Tokyo subway sarin attack.

See table for maximum control limits:

Maximum Agent Control Limits

	Workplace (8 h in mg/m^3)	General Population (72 h TWA mg/m^3)
Sarin and tabun	1 x 10^{-5}	3 x 10^{-3}
VX	1 x 10^{-4}	3 x 10^{-6}

Rescuers should wear protective masks (ie, charcoal filter of self-contained breathing apparatus) with heavy rubber gloves

Pretreatment with pyridostigmine bromide (30 mg orally every 8 hours) may be effective (especially for soman)

Lethal dermal dose (70 kg adult):

Sarin: 1.7 g

Tabun: 1 g

Soman: 100 mg

VX: 6 mg

These agents are 4-6 times denser than air and thus remain close to the ground; they are soluble in water, but hydrolyze in alkaline solutions (see Treatment); contaminated vegetation with VX can cause toxic effects upon ingestion

Specific References

Carnes SA and Watson AP, "Disposing of the U.S. Chemical Weapons Stockpile: An Approaching Reality," *JAMA*, 1989, 262(5):653-9.

(Continued)

Nerve Gases *(Continued)*

Dunn MA and Sidell FR, "Progress in Medical Defense Against Nerve Agents," *JAMA*, 1989, 262(5):649-52.

Grob D and Harvey JC, "Effects in Man of the Anticholinesterase Compound Sarin (Isopropyl Methyl Phosphonofluoridate)," *J Clin Invest*, 1958, 37:350.

Jamal GA, "Long Term Neurotoxic Effects of Chemical Warfare Organophophate Compounds (Sarin)," *Adverse Drug React Toxicol Rev*, 1995, 14(2):83-4.

Nelan BW, "The Price of Fanaticism," *TIME*, 1995, 145(14):38-41.

Sidell FR and Borak J, "Chemical Warfare Agents: II. Nerve Agents," *Ann Emerg Med*, 1992, 21(7):865-71.

Yokoyama K, Ogura Y, Kishimoto M, et al, "Blood Purification for Severe Sarin Poisoning After the Tokyo Subway Attack," *JAMA*, 1995, 274(5):379.

Nexion® *see* Bromophos *on page 873*

Nickel

Related Information

Nickel Carbonyl *on next page*

CAS Number 7440-02-0

UN Number 2881;1325

Synonyms Carbonyl Nickel Powder; Nickel Sponge; Raney Alloy; Raney Nickel

Mechanism of Toxic Action In nickel refiners, nickel is a respiratory tract carcinogen

Adverse Reactions Nickel carbonyl is much more toxic than nickel metal or alloys; nose, throat, cardiovascular, neurologic, gastrointestinal, hepatic, hematologic, dermatologic

Signs & Symptoms of Acute Overdose Nasal carcinoma, sore throat, EKG changes, dyspnea, cough, giddiness, CNS stimulation followed by cold, clammy skin; sleeplessness, nausea, vomiting, diarrhea, hematuria, urticaria, coma, seizures, transient increase in ALT, bilirubin, leukocytosis, erythrocytosis, contact dermatitis (nickel itch), hypothermia, impaired thermoregulation

Toxicodynamics/Kinetics

Absorption:

- Inhalation: 35%
- Oral: 1% to 27% (reduced by food)
- Dermal: Nickel sulfate: 55% to 77%

Distribution: Nickel carbonyl crosses the alveolar membrane and dissociates to nickel and carbon monoxide; wide volume of distribution

Protein binding: 59%

Half-life: 11 hours

Elimination: Excreted primarily in urine; oral ingestion results in a large amount excreted through gastrointestinal tract

Reference Range Normal blood levels: 1.1-4.6 μg/L; normal urine level is about 50 μg/L; an 8-hour urine level of <100 μg/L associated with mild exposure, 100-500 μg/L associated with moderate exposure, and >500 μg/L associated with severe exposure

Overdosage Treatment

Decontamination:

- Dermal: Wash with soap and water
- Inhalation: Give 100% humidified oxygen
- Ocular: Copious irrigation with saline
- Oral: Dilute with milk

Supportive therapy: Diethyldithiocarbamate (DDC) is the preferred chelating agent; it is available through Dr Sunderman (215) 922-6554; disulfiram can enhance the elimination of nickel and has been used to treat nickel dermatitis, although its efficacy is questionable; oxygen, bronchodilators, and steroids (for adrenocortical insufficiency) may be required

Enhancement of elimination: Forced saline diuresis can decrease half-life of nickel sulfate and nickel chloride by >50%

Antidote(s)

Diethyldithiocarbamate Trihydrate *on page 1410*

Test Interactions Increased levels of erythropoietin have been noted after nickel subsulfide exposure

Diagnostic Tests/Procedures

Nickel, Urine *on page 1308*

Pregnancy Implications Crosses the placenta; enters breast milk

Additional Information

TWA-TLV: 15 mcg/m^3

Average daily intake of nickel from food: ~168 mcg; from drinking water: ~2 mcg; from inhalation: 0.1-1 mcg

Cigarette smoking accounts for 2-12 mcg of nickel inhaled per cigarette pack; skin application of 1:10,000 dose of nickel salts can elicit a sensitivity reaction. Baking powder (13.4 ppm), orange pekoe tea (7.6 ppm), buckwheat (6.5 ppm), and cocoa (5 ppm) contain the highest amount of nickel. Most U.S. coins contain about 25% nickel; range of atmospheric nickel concentration in urban U.S. areas is from 1-328 ng/m^3; in rural areas, the range is 0.6-78 ng/m^3.

Specific References

Sunderman FW Jr, Aitio A, Morgan LG, et al, "Biological Monitoring of Nickel," *Toxicol Ind Health*, 1986, 2(1):17-78.

Sunderman FW Jr, Dingle B, Hopfer SM, et al, "Acute Nickel Toxicity in Electroplating Workers Who Accidentally Ingested a Solution of Nickel Sulfate and Nickel Chloride," *Am J Ind Med*, 1988, 14(3):257-66.

U.S. Department of Health and Human Services, "Toxicological Profile for Nickel TP-92/14," Agency for Toxic Substances and Diseases Registry, April, 1993.

Vyskocil A, Senft V, Viau C, et al, "Biochemical Renal Changes in Workers Exposed to Soluble Nickel Compounds," *Hum Exp Toxicol*, 1994, 13(4):257-61.

Nickel Carbonyl

Related Information

Nickel *on previous page*

CAS Number 13463-39-3

UN Number 1259

Synonyms Nickel Tetracarbonile

Use Catalyst in petroleum and rubber industries; used in electroplating; formed as an intermediate (by a reaction with carbon monoxide) in nickel ore purification

Mechanism of Toxic Action Inhibits ribonucleic acid synthesis; mucosal irritant

Adverse Reactions Symptoms may be delayed 12-24 hours

Cardiovascular: Tachycardia, bradycardia, Q-T prolongation, chest pain

Central nervous system: Headache, dizziness, delirium, hyperthermia, chills

Hematologic: Leukocytosis

Respiratory: Pulmonary edema, dyspnea, interstitial pneumonitis

Miscellaneous: Diaphoresis

Toxicodynamics/Kinetics

Absorption: By inhalation

Metabolism: Metabolized to carbon monoxide and nickel

Elimination: Urine

Reference Range Normal blood levels: 1.1-4.6 μg/L; an 8-hour urine level of <100 μg/L associated with mild exposure, 100-500 μg/L associated with moderate exposure, and >500 μg/L associated with severe exposure

Overdosage Treatment

Decontamination:

Dermal: Wash with soap and water

Inhalation: Give 100% humidified oxygen

Ocular: Copious irrigation with saline

Supportive therapy: Diethyldithiocarbamate (DDC) is the preferred chelating agent; it is available through Dr Sunderman (215) 922-6554; disulfiram can enhance the elimination of nickel and has been used to treat nickel dermatitis; disulfiram (250-750 mg every 8 hours or half the DDC dose) is second choice therapy to diethyldithiocarbamate; oxygen, bronchodilators, and steroids (for adrenocortical insufficiency) may be required

Enhancement of elimination: Forced saline diuresis can decrease half-life

Antidote(s)

Diethyldithiocarbamate Trihydrate *on page 1410*

Pregnancy Implications Ocular abnormalities (anophthalmia/microphthalmia) noted in rodent offspring during exposure in early pregnancy

Additional Information Nickel carbonyl is the most toxic of nickel compounds; nickel carbonyl is formed when nickel is in contact with carbon monoxide; toxicity from nickel carbonyl results from inhalation, whereas toxicity from Ni^{2+} results from oral/parenteral exposure; in nickel carbonyl poisoning after the acute symptoms subside, delayed pulmonary, cardiac, and neurologic symptoms occur after 1-5 days

Potentially carcinogenic (nasal and lung cancer)

Cigarette smoke contains ~3.5 ppm of nickel carbonyl

Colorless gas with a "sooty" or musty odor with an odor threshold of 1 ppm

Lethal air concentration: 30 ppm at 30 minutes

Heavier than air (vapor density is almost 6)

Highly explosive

Specific References

Kurta DL, Dean BS, and Krenzelok EP, "Acute Nickel Carbonyl Poisoning," *Am J Emerg Med*, 1993, 11(1):64-5.

Shi ZC, "Acute Nickel Carbonyl Poisoning: A Report of 179 Cases," *Br J Ind Med*, 1986, 43(6):422-4.

Sunderman Jr FW and Allpass PR, "Eye Malformations in Rats: Induction by Prenatal Exposure to Nickel Carbonyl," *Science*, 1979, 203:550-3.

Sunderman Sr FW, "Efficacy of Sodium Diethyldithiocarbamate (Dithiocarb) in Acute Nickel Carbonyl Poisoning," *Ann Clin Lab Sci*, 1979, 9:1-10.

Nickel Sponge *see* Nickel *on page 976*

Nickel Tetracarbonile *see* Nickel Carbonyl *on previous page*

Niclofen® *see* Nitrofen *on page 980*

Nip® *see* Nitrofen *on page 980*

Niran® *see* Chlordane *on page 885*

Nitramine *see* Tetryl *on page 1025*

Nitrates

UN Number 1477

Commonly Found In Munition and explosives (dynamite is 60% nitrates); may be found in well water

Use Ammonium nitrates are in cold packs

Mechanism of Toxic Action Accelerates atherosclerosis

Adverse Reactions

Cardiovascular: Hypotension, tachycardia, atrial fibrillation, bigeminy

Gastrointestinal: Gastritis

Miscellaneous: Nitrate withdrawal syndrome includes vasodilatory effects (flushing, headaches); can produce sulfhemoglobin, feces discoloration (black)

Signs & Symptoms of Acute Overdose Headaches, fatigue, nausea, hematuria, vomiting, dyspnea within 2 hours, coma, cyanosis, and pallor may develop later

Toxicodynamics/Kinetics Absorption: Readily through the skin and lungs

Reference Range Toxic: >5 mg/kg

Overdosage Treatment Decontamination: Do not induce emesis for ammonium nitrate ingestion; methylene blue (1-2 mg/kg per dose) for elevated methemoglobin as needed every 4 hours

Antidote(s)

Methylene Blue *on page 1444*

Test Interactions Falsely elevates serum bicarbonate levels

Diagnostic Tests/Procedures

Blood Gases, Arterial *on page 1207*

Complete Blood Count *on page 1236*

Electrocardiography *on page 1253*

Methemoglobin, Blood *on page 1296*

Oxygen Saturation, Blood *on page 1313*

Potassium, Blood *on page 1328*

Sulfhemoglobin *on page 1358*

Pregnancy Implications Neural tube defects have been suggested with high levels of nitrates in drinking water

Additional Information Can penetrate gloves

Specific References

Comly HH, "Cyanosis in Infants Caused by Nitrates in Well-Water," *JAMA*, 1987, 257(20):2788-92.

Gao L and Guo YS, "Acute Nitrate Poisoning: A Report of 80 Cases," *Am J Emerg Med*, 1991, 9(2):200-1.

Morton WE, "Occupational Habituation to Aliphatic Nitrates and the Withdrawal Hazards of Coronary Disease and Hypertension," *J Occup Med*, 1977, 19(3):197-200.

Nitrites

UN Number 2627

Synonyms Poppers; Snappers; Thrust

Commonly Found In Inhalation abuse of volatile nitrates

Use In cyanide antidote kits; used in the manufacture of dyes, fabrics, and linen; photography; corrosive inhibition

Mechanism of Toxic Action Peripheral vasodilation; produces methemoglobin; is an oxidizing agent

Adverse Reactions

Cardiovascular: Paradoxical bradycardia, hypotension

Hematologic: Methemoglobinemia followed by hemolysis

Ocular: Visual disturbances

Respiratory: Tachypnea

Miscellaneous: Infants, pregnant women, and patients with malignancy may be especially sensitive

Signs & Symptoms of Acute Overdose Blurred vision, dyspnea, light headedness (postural), nausea, vomiting, flushing, seizures, cyanosis, headache, diarrhea, abdominal pain, skin irritation

Toxicodynamics/Kinetics

Metabolism: 60% metabolized – most to ammonia

Elimination: Excreted renally (40% unchanged)

Reference Range Fatal nitrite serum range: 0.5-350 mg/L

Overdosage Treatment

Decontamination: Basic poison management. Methylene blue for symptomatic methemoglobinemia

Supportive therapy: Hyperbaric oxygen may be of use, though controlled human data are lacking

Antidote(s)

Methylene Blue *on page 1444*

Diagnostic Tests/Procedures

Blood Gases, Arterial *on page 1207*

Methemoglobin, Blood *on page 1296*

Oxygen Saturation, Blood *on page 1313*

Monitoring Parameters Obtain methemoglobin levels – cyanosis may occur at levels >20%

Pregnancy Implications Can pass through the placenta and cause fetal methemoglobin; animal auditory and visual defects were noted

Additional Information Ingestion of 10 mL of isobutyl or amyl nitrate may be toxic; oral ingestion produces more rapid methemoglobin than inhalation

May be toxic at >0.4 mg/kg

Specific References

Curry S, "Methemoglobinemia," *Ann Emerg Med*, 1982, 11(4):214-21.

Laaban JP, Bodenan P, and Rochemaure J, "Amyl Nitrite Poppers and Methemoglobinemia," *Ann Intern Med*, 1985, 103(5):804-5.

Nitrito *see* Nitrogen Oxide *on next page*

Nitrobenzene

CAS Number 98-95-3

UN Number 1662

Synonyms Nitrobenzol Oil of Mirbane

Brand Names Caswell No 66

Use Production of aniline, cellulose ethers, and acetaminophen; perfume agent in soaps; solvent in shoe dyes (preservative) and floor polishes

Mechanism of Toxic Action Binds to hemoglobin which results in methemoglobin formation; resembles aniline in its action

Adverse Reactions

Cardiovascular: Tachycardia, hypotension

Central nervous system: Headache, coma, seizures, paresthesia, dizziness

Gastrointestinal: Nausea

Hepatic: Hepatomegaly, elevated liver function tests

Respiratory: Respiratory failure, bitter almond breath, apnea

Miscellaneous: Methemoglobin formation (postexposure from 30 minutes to 12 hours), hemolytic anemia

Toxicodynamics/Kinetics

Absorption:

- Inhalation: 80% to 87%
- Oral, dermal: ~50%

Half-life: 84 hours (of metabolites)

Metabolism: Primarily intestinal reduction to nitrosobenzene, phenylhydroxylamine, and aniline

Elimination: Primarily renal (within first 2 hours) in the forms of para-aminophenol and para-nitrophenol (most toxic metabolite)

Overdosage Treatment

Decontamination:

- Dermal: Wash with soap and water
- Ocular: Irrigate copiously with saline
- Oral: Lavage/activated charcoal

Supportive therapy: Treat symptomatic methemoglobinemia with methylene blue; seizures can be treated with benzodiazepines or phenobarbital

Enhancement of elimination: Exchange transfusion has been utilized in an adult for 6 hours to reduce severe methemoglobinemia from 65% to 25% levels

Additional Information Higher airborne concentrations of nitrobenzene (up to 0.1 ppb) are noted in summer than in winter; methemoglobinemia can develop after exposure of 3-6 ppm for several hours

Odor threshold (almond-like): Water: 0.11 mg/L; Air: 0.092 mg/m^3

PEL-TWA: 1 ppm

TLV-TWA: 1 ppm

IDLH: 200 ppm

Atmospheric half-life: 6 months to 6 years

Fatal oral dose: 1 g

Specific References

Harrison MR, "Toxic Methaemoglobinaemia: A Case of Acute Nitrobenzene and Aniline Poisoning Treated by Exchange Transfusion," *Anaesthesia*, 1977, 32(3):270-2.

U.S. Department of Health and Human Services, "Toxicological Profile for Nitrobenzene TP-90/19," Agency for Toxic Substances and Diseases Registry, December 1990.

Nitrobenzol Oil of Mirbane *see* Nitrobenzene *on this page*

Nitrochlor® *see* Nitrofen *on this page*

Nitrofen

CAS Number 1836-75-7

Synonyms Nitrofene

Brand Names Mezotox®; Niclofen®; Nip®; Nitrochlor®; Tok®; Tokkorn®; Trixilin®

Mechanism of Toxic Action A diphenyl ether which can cause photobleaching and has phytotoxic effects by interfering with ATP synthesis

Signs & Symptoms of Acute Overdose Irritant to eyes, skin, and lungs; headache, dizziness, nausea, vomiting, diarrhea

Overdosage Treatment Decontamination: Remove contaminated clothing (especially leather); wash thoroughly with soap and water; irrigate eyes with normal saline for ocular exposure

Pregnancy Implications Teratogenic in rodents

Specific References

Shusterman D, "Problem-Solving Techniques in Occupational Medicine," *J Fam Pract*, 1985, 21(3):195-9.

Nitrofene *see* Nitrofen *on this page*

Nitrogen Di-Dioxide *see* Nitrogen Oxide *on this page*

Nitrogen Monoxide *see* Nitrous Oxide *on next page*

Nitrogen Oxide

CAS Number 10102-44-0; 10544-72-6

UN Number 1067

Synonyms Liquid Nitrogen Tetroxide; Nitrito; Nitrogen Di-Dioxide; Nitrous Fumes; Nox; Silo-Filler's Disease

Commonly Found In Exhaust from metal cleaning, electric arc welding

Use As an anesthetic

Mechanism of Toxic Action Reacts with water in respiratory tract to form nitric acid; lipid auto-oxidation may occur; suspected carcinogen

Adverse Reactions

Cardiovascular: Weak, rapid pulse; cardiovascular collapse

Respiratory: Pulmonary edema, asphyxia

Signs & Symptoms of Acute Overdose Eye irritation, cough, dyspnea, tachypnea, wheezing (nitrogen dioxide), fatigue, confusion, nausea, methemoglobin possible

Toxicodynamics/Kinetics Absorption: By the lungs

Overdosage Treatment

Decontamination: Treat inhalation exposure; steroids may be of benefit

Supportive therapy: treat symptomatic methemoglobinemia with methylene blue

Antidote(s)

Methylene Blue *on page 1444*

Diagnostic Tests/Procedures

Blood Gases, Arterial *on page 1207*

Methemoglobin, Blood *on page 1296*

Pregnancy Implications Documented in animals (nitrogen oxide)

Additional Information Odor of nitrogen dioxide detected at 1-3 ppm; pungent/acrid odor; bronchiolitis obliterans may develop 2-4 weeks postexposure

Nitrogen dioxide: TLV-TWA: 3 ppm

Nitric oxide: TLV-TWA: 25 ppm

IDLH: 100 ppm

PEL-TWA: 25 ppm

Specific References

Douglas WW, Hepper NG, and Colby TV, "Silo-Filler's Disease," *Mayo Clin Proc*, 1989, 64(3):291-304.

Hedberg K, Hedberg CW, Iber C, et al, "An Outbreak of Nitrogen Dioxide-Induced Respiratory Illness Among Ice Hockey Players," *JAMA*, 1989, 262(21):3014-7.

Kim SU, Koenig JQ, Pierson WE, et al, "Acute Pulmonary Effects of Nitrogen Dioxide Exposure During Exercise in Competitive Athletes," *Chest*, 1991, 99(4):815-9.

Maurer WJ, "Silo-Filler's Disease: A Historical Perspective and Report of a Case," *Wis Med J*, 1985, 84(8):13-6.

Nitrophenol

CAS Number 88-75-5 (2-Nitrophenol); 100-02-7 (4-Nitrophenol)

UN Number 1663

Brand Names Atonik®

Use Primarily as a laboratory reagent, fungicide, and in production of dye stuffs and pigments; 4-nitrophenol is a metabolite of nitrobenzene

Mechanism of Toxic Action Formation of methemoglobinemia

Adverse Reactions No experience in humans; animals develop methemoglobinemia; stomatitis is also noted

Toxicodynamics/Kinetics
Absorption: Probably by inhalation, oral, or dermal exposure
Metabolism: Hepatic to glucuronide or sulfate conjugates
Elimination: Renal within 48 hours

Reference Range Urinary 4-nitrophenol levels in general population is $<10\ \mu g/L$; may also be noted in nitrobenzene, methyl, or ethyl parathione exposures

Overdosage Treatment
Decontamination:
- Dermal: Wash with soap and water
- Ocular: Irrigate with saline
- Oral: Lavage/activated charcoal

Supportive therapy: Methylene blue for symptomatic methemoglobinemia

Additional Information 4-nitrophenol is more toxic than 2-nitrophenol; vehicular exhaust contains 3.1 ppb of 2-nitrophenol

Atmospheric half-life: 18 days
Water half-life (photolysis): 1-13 days (longer with high pH)

Specific References

U.S. Department of Health and Human Services, "Toxicological Profile for Nitrophenols TP-91/23," Agency for Toxic Substances and Diseases Registry, July, 1992.

Nitrophenolurea

Synonyms PNU; Pyriminil; Vacor

Mechanism of Toxic Action Interferes with nicotinamide metabolism resulting in pancreatic beta-cell destruction

Adverse Reactions
Central nervous system: Neuropathic
Endocrine & metabolic: Diabetes mellitus

Signs & Symptoms of Acute Overdose gastrointestinal irritant, hypotension, hyperglycemia with or without ketoacidosis

Overdosage Treatment
Decontamination: Emesis or lavage, followed by oral activated charcoal with cathartic
Supportive therapy: Nicotinamide (also known as niacinamide) (I.M., I.V.): 500 mg loading dose followed by doses of 100-200 mg I.M. or I.V. every 4 hours for 48 hours. Orally, patient may take 100 mg nicotinamide 3-5 times/day for 2 weeks; children can be given half the adult dose; insulin may be needed for hyperglycemia
Supportive therapy: Diabetes: Insulin and fluids

Diagnostic Tests/Procedures

Amylase, Serum *on page 1191*
Anion Gap, Blood *on page 1193*
Ketones, Urine *on page 1278*
Liver Profile *on page 1286*

Additional Information Withdrawn in U.S. as general use pesticide in 1979; smells like peanuts; yellow color appears like cornmeal

Specific References

LeWitt PA, "The Neurotoxicity of the Rat Poison, Vacor. A Clinical Study of 12 Cases," *N Engl J Med*, 1980, 302(2):73-7.
Pont A, Rubino JM, Bishop D, et al, "Diabetes Mellitus and Neuropathy Following Vacor Ingestion in Man," *Arch Intern Med*, 1979, 139(2):185-7.
Prosser PR and Karam JH, "Diabetes Mellitus Following Rodenticide Ingestion in Man," *JAMA*, 1978, 239(12):1148-50.

Nitrous Fumes *see* Nitrogen Oxide *on previous page*

Nitrous Oxide

CAS Number 10024-97-2
UN Number 1020
Synonyms Factitious Air; Laughing Gas; Nitrogen Monoxide; Whippet
Use As an anesthetic, foaming agent, and rocket fuel

Mechanism of Toxic Action Asphyxiant; oxidizes cobalt in vitamin B_{12}; partial agonist of opioid receptors

Adverse Reactions
Cardiovascular: Hypotension, arrhythmias, A-V dissociation, myeloneuropathies
Central nervous system: CNS depression, ataxia
Hematologic: Bone marrow depression, methemoglobin formation, aplastic anemia (chronic use)
Neuromuscular & skeletal: Peripheral neuropathy
Miscellaneous: Potential carcinogen, cerebral edema

Signs & Symptoms of Acute Overdose Dyspnea, neuritis, headache, dizziness, euphoria, nausea and vomiting (rarely), mood disorder, leukopenia, agranulocytosis; can cause a pneumothorax by barotrauma

(Continued)

Nitrous Oxide *(Continued)*

Toxicodynamics/Kinetics
Absorption: Readily through the lungs
Elimination: Through the lungs

Reference Range Arterial blood nitrous oxide concentrations associated with surgical anesthesia range from 170-220 mL/L

Overdosage Treatment Supportive therapy: Give 100% humidified oxygen; hyperventilation and 20% mannitol for cerebral edema; dexamethasone may be useful. Naloxone may reverse analgesic action; avoid epinephrine; treat symptomatic methemoglobinemia with methylene blue. Replace vitamin B_{12} as needed for chronic exposures; do not administer hyperbaric oxygen; pretreatment with methylcobalamin (5 mg I.V.) 2 hours postanesthesia induction and folinic acid (15 mg I.V.) at end of anesthesia was hematoprotective.

Antidote(s)
Methylene Blue *on page 1444*
Naloxone Hydrochloride *on page 1447*

Diagnostic Tests/Procedures
Complete Blood Count *on page 1236*

Pregnancy Implications While a single course of nitrous oxide is considered safe during pregnancy, occupational exposure has been associated with reduced fertility; teratogenic in rodents

Additional Information Colorless, sweet odor; chronic inhalation may result in pancytopenia including anemia (megaloblastic); nitrous oxide cylinders are painted blue; anemia (megaloblastic) (vitamin B_{12} deficiency)
TLV-TWA: 50 ppm
Minimal toxic dose by inhalation: 24 mg/kg over 2 hours

Specific References

Brodsky JB and Cohen EN, "Adverse Effects of Nitrous Oxide," *Med Toxicol*, 1987, 1(5):362-74.
Crawford JS and Lewis M, "Nitrous Oxide in Early Human Pregnancy," *Anaesthesia*, 1986, 41(9):900-5.
Joseph WL, Fletcher HS, and Giordano JM, "Pulmonary and Cardiovascular Implications of Drug Addiction," *Ann Thorac Surg*, 1973, 15(3):263-74.
Kunkel DB, "Nitrous Oxide: Not a Laughing Matter Anymore," *J Emerg Med*, 1987, 19:79-84.
Louis-Ferdinand RT, "Myelotoxic, Neurotoxic, and Reproductive Adverse Effects of Nitrous Oxide," *Adverse Drug React Toxicol Rev*, 1994, 13(4):193-206.
Rowland AS, Baird DD, Weinberg CR, et al, "Reduced Fertility Among Women Employed as Dental Assistants Exposed to High Levels of Nitrous Oxide," *N Engl J Med*, 1992, 327(14):993-7.

N-Methyl-2-Isopropoxyphenylcarbamate *see* Propoxur *on page 1000*

N-Methyl-N,2,4,6-Tetranitroaniline *see* Tetryl *on page 1025*

N,N-Diethyl-3-Methyl-Diethyl-M-Toluamide *see* Diethyltoluamide *on page 912*

N,N-Diethyl-M-Toluamide *see* Diethyltoluamide *on page 912*

N,N-Diethyl-M-Toluic Acid *see* Diethyltoluamide *on page 912*

N-Nitrosodiphenylamine

CAS Number 86-30-6

Synonyms Diphenylnitrosamine; NDPA; NDPHA

Brand Names Curetard A®; Delac J®; Naugard TJB®; Redax®; Retarder J®; TJB; Vulcatard A®

Use Retardant (to prevent premature vulcanization of rubber) in rubber processing industry

Mechanism of Toxic Action DNA adduct formation in bladder may be the mechanism for urinary bladder cancer

Adverse Reactions No human toxic effects described; toxic effects in animals appear to be carcinogenesis (bladder) and skin ulcerations on dermal contact (0.1 mL of 0.1% solution for 20 weeks); nephrotoxicity has also been noted; does not bioaccumulate

Toxicodynamics/Kinetics
Absorption: Oral and dermal
Metabolism: Hepatic denitrosation to diphenylamine and nitric oxide
Elimination: Primarily renal within 2 days

Overdosage Treatment
Decontamination:
- Dermal: Wash with soap and water
- Ocular: Irrigate with saline
- Oral: Lavage/activated charcoal

Additional Information Soluble in water (40 mg/L); adding wheat straw in soil to increase microbial activity reduces soil residence time from 30 days to 10 days; tire chemical factories may have workplace air levels as high as 6 ppm (47 mcg/m^3)

Atmospheric half-life: ~7 hours

Specific References

Fajen JM, Carson GA, Rounbehler DP, et al, "N-Nitrosamines in the Rubber and Tire Industry," *Science*, 1979, 205(4412):1262-4.

U.S. Department of Health and Human Services, "Toxicological Profile for N-Nitrosodiphenylamine TP-92/15," Agency for Toxic Substances and Diseases Registry, April, 1993.

No Bent® *see* Hexachlorobenzene *on page 936*

Nox *see* Nitrogen Oxide *on page 980*

n-Propyl Alcohol *see* 1-Propanol *on page 1000*

Nudrin® *see* Methomyl *on page 962*

Nyloprint® *see* Acrylamide *on page 852*

O-(4-Bromo-2-Chlorophenyl)-O-Ethyl-S-Propylphospharathioate *see* Profenofos *on page 998*

Octachlor® *see* Chlordane *on page 885*

Octalene® *see* Aldrin *on page 856*

Octalox® *see* Dieldrin *on page 911*

Octogen *see* HMX *on page 939*

OFF® *see* Diethyltoluamide *on page 912*

Oil of American Wormseed *see Chenopodium* Oils *on page 884*

Oil of Vitrial *see* Sulfuric Acid *on page 1019*

Omal® *see* 2,4,6-Trichlorophenol *on page 1034*

O,O-Diethyl O-(2-Chloro-1(2',4'-Dichlorophenyl)Vinyl)Phosphate *see* Chlorfenvinphos *on page 886*

O,O-Diethyl O-2-Isopropyl-4-Methyl-6-Pyrimidinyl Thiophosphate *see* Diazinon *on page 904*

O,O-Diethyl-O-(3,5,6-Trichloro-2-Pyridyl) Phosphorothioate *see* Chlorpyrifos *on page 891*

O,O-Diethyl O-p-Nitrophenyl Phosphorothioate *see* Parathion *on page 988*

O,O-Dimethyldithiophosphate Diethylmercaptosuccinate *see* Malathion *on page 950*

O,O-Dimethyl-O-(2,5-Dichloro-4-Bromophenyl) Phosphorothioate *see* Bromophos *on page 873*

Optal *see* 1-Propanol *on page 1000*

Organochlorines

Related Information

Aldrin *on page 856*
Chlordane *on page 885*
Chlordecone *on page 886*
Copper *on page 896*
DDD *on page 902*
DDT *on page 903*
Dieldrin *on page 911*
Endrin *on page 922*
Heptachlor *on page 935*
Hexachlorobutadiene *on page 937*
Methoxychlor *on page 963*
Mirex *on page 971*
Toxaphene *on page 1031*

UN Number 2761; 2762; 2995; 2996

Synonyms Chlorbenzilate; Chlorinated Hydrocarbon Insecticides; Kelthane; Lindane; Orthodichlorobenzene; Perthane

Mechanism of Toxic Action Interferes with axonal transmembrane flux of sodium and potassium

Adverse Reactions CNS stimulation, respiratory depression, gastrointestinal, blood dyscrasias

Signs & Symptoms of Acute Overdose Aspiration pneumonitis (aspiration of petroleum distillates), seizures, tremor (may be first symptom), fever, headache, ataxia, agitation, nervousness, amnesia, nausea, vomiting, diarrhea, anemia, leukemia, dermal irritation; respiratory depression is more common with aldrin, chlordane, DDT, dieldrin, endrin, and toxaphene; seizures common with aldrin, chlor-

(Continued)

Organochlorines *(Continued)*

dane, DDT, dieldrin, endrin, heptachlor, lindane, strobane, and toxaphene; opsoclonus occurs with chlordecone; hepatic failure has been associated with orthodichlorobenzene; possible association with anemia and leukemia

Toxicodynamics/Kinetics

Absorption: Well absorbed through the gastrointestinal tract, especially in presence of absorbable lipid fat

Metabolism: Aldrin is metabolized to dieldrin in the skin; the following are metabolized in a few hours to days: chlorbenzilate, chlordane, endosulfan, endrin, kelthane, methoxychlor, perthane, and toxaphene

Elimination: Aldrin, dieldrin, heptachlor, and hexachlorobenzene are excreted in several weeks to a few months; the beta isomer of benzene hexachloride, DDT, kepone, and mirex is excreted over several months or years; kepone and chlordane are enterohepatically recycled

Reference Range Blood levels are not clinically useful for acute exposures; blood, urine, and tissue levels may indicate long-term exposure

Overdosage Treatment

Decontamination: Gastric with lavage followed by activated charcoal with cathartic or cholestyramine; syrup of ipecac/emesis contraindicated due to seizures and CNS depression

Supportive therapy: Diazepam or lorazepam for seizures; phenobarbital for recurrent seizures. Avoid administration of oils by mouth and administration of adrenergic agents; cholestyramine may be given to bind enterohepatically recycled kepone and chlordane; remove contaminated clothing and wash skin using three stages of soap followed by alcohol washing then soap washing; discard contaminated leather.

Enhancement of elimination: Multiple dosing of cholestyramine (16 g/day) may be effective

Antidote(s)

Cholestyramine Resin *on page 1405*

Monitoring Parameters Respiratory distress and seizures; consider liver function tests and CBC; abdominal x-ray may detect presence of chlorinated pesticide

Pregnancy Implications Crosses placenta; blood levels in newborns are $\frac{1}{3}$ that of mother's; weak estrogenic effects of organochlorines may induce labor; passes into milk of breast-feeding mothers

Additional Information Probably carcinogenic to man, however, inadequately studied; chronic exposure to hexachlorobenzene over a long period of time may result in cutaneous porphyria; radiopaque

Specific References

Cohn WJ, Boylan JJ, Blanke RV, et al, "Treatment of Chlordecone (Kepone) Toxicity With Cholestyramine. Results of a Controlled Clinical Trial," *N Engl J Med*, 1978, 298(5):243-8.

Garrettson LK, Guzelian PS, and Blanke RV, "Subacute Chlordane Poisoning," *J Toxicol Clin Toxicol*, 1984-85, 22(6):565-71.

Taylor JR, "Neurological Manifestations in Humans Exposed to Chlordecone: Follow-Up Results," *Neurotoxicology*, 1985, 6(1):231-6.

Ortho C-1 Defoliant and Weed Killer *see* Chlorate Salts *on page 884*

Orthocide® *see* Captan *on page 877*

Orthocide® 406 *see* Captan *on page 877*

Orthodichlorobenzene *see* Organochlorines *on previous page*

Ortho-Klor® *see* Chlordane *on page 885*

Orthophos® *see* Parathion *on page 988*

Osmic Acid *see* Osmium *on this page*

Osmium

CAS Number 20816-12-0

UN Number 2471

Synonyms Osmic Acid; Osmium Tetroxide; Parosmic Acid

Mechanism of Toxic Action Direct irritant to mucous membranes, skin, eyes

Adverse Reactions Eyes, nose, throat, neurologic, gastrointestinal, dermatologic

Signs & Symptoms of Acute Overdose Visual changes, conjunctivitis, irritation of respiratory tract, wheezing, pulmonary edema, headache, dermatitis, rhinitis, cough, chest pain

Toxicodynamics/Kinetics No human ingestions reported

Overdosage Treatment

Decontamination: Remove patient from toxic environment, administer 100% humidified O_2; provide ventilatory assistance if needed; decontaminate skin and eyes with water

Supportive therapy: Treat wheezing with bronchodilators; equivocal what the role of steroids is in prevention of pulmonary edema

Additional Information Direct contact may cause green-black discoloration of skin; no harmful effects at 0.001 mg/m^3 for 6 hours (ACGIH 1986); concentration of 0.1 mg/m^3 associated with ocular irritation; TCLO (human): 133 mcg/m^3 lacrimation; 1 ppm = 10 mg/m^3

TLV-TWA: 0.002 ppm

TLV-STEL: 0.0006 ppm

OSHA PEL-TWA: 0.002 mg/m^3

Specific References

ACGIH, *Documentation of Threshold Limit Values,* 5th ed, Cincinnati, OH: American Conference of Government Industrial Hygiene, Inc, 1986, 450.

Osmium Tetroxide *see* Osmium *on previous page*

Oxidoethane *see* Ethylene Oxide *on page 927*

Oxirane *see* Ethylene Oxide *on page 927*

2-Oxobutane *see* Methyl Ethyl Ketone *on page 967*

2-Oxohexane *see* 2-Hexanone *on page 938*

Oxyfume® *see* Ethylene Oxide *on page 927*

Oxytreat 35® *see* Hydrazine *on page 939*

PAH *see* Polycyclic Aromatic Hydrocarbons *on page 997*

Painters' Naphtha *see* Petroleum Distillates – Naphtha *on page 991*

Palatinol® A *see* Diethyl Phthalate *on page 912*

Palladium

CAS Number 7440-05-3

Mechanism of Toxic Action Colloidal palladium hydroxides cause RBC hemolysis; chronic intoxication results in malignant lung tumor and decreased growth

Adverse Reactions

Dermatologic: Irritant dermatitis

Respiratory: Inhalation: Wheezing

Signs & Symptoms of Acute Overdose Classic signs/symptoms of allergic reaction; urticaria, rash, rhinorrhea, cough, dyspnea, wheezing, eczema, eosinophilia, lymphocytosis

Toxicodynamics/Kinetics Absorption: Poor from gastrointestinal tract

Reference Range No TLV recommended

Overdosage Treatment

Decontamination: Irrigation

Supportive therapy: Beta agonists can be used for wheezing

Additional Information Causes black discoloration at site of injection; water soluble

Specific References

van Ketel WG and Niebber C, "Allergy to Palladium in Dental Alloys," *Contact Dermatitis*, 1981, 7(6):331.

Paracide® *see* Para-Dichlorobenzene *on this page*

Paradiaminobenzene *see* Paraphenylenediamine *on next page*

Para-Dichlorobenzene

CAS Number 106-46-7

UN Number 1592

Synonyms Dichloricide; 1,4-Dichlorobenzene; PDB

Brand Names Paracide®

Use Toilet/refuse deodorant; mold and mildew fumigant; moth repellant; diaper pail repellant

Mechanism of Toxic Action Mucosal irritant due to necrosis of tissue proteins by epoxide intermediates

Adverse Reactions

Central nervous system: Cerebellar ataxia

Dermal: Allergic purpura, burns, skin edema, hyperpigmentation

Hematological: Hemolysis/methemoglobin formation (especially in children)

Hepatic: Hepatitis and hepatic necrosis with cirrhosis

Ocular: Irritation

Renal: Glomerulonephritis

Respiratory: Granuloma development

Signs & Symptoms of Acute Overdose Jaundice, dyspnea, ataxia, headache, nausea, vomiting, diarrhea, slurred speech, oral burning

Toxicodynamics/Kinetics

Absorption: By dermal routes and:

(Continued)

Para-Dichlorobenzene *(Continued)*

Inhalation: 20%
Oral: 100%
Metabolism: Hepatic: Oxidation to 2,5 dichlorophenol and 2,3-dichloroquinol
Elimination: Renal and biliary

Reference Range Urinary 2,5 dichlorophenol level range of 90-100 mg/L associated with air para-dichlorobenzene levels of 33 ppm; whole blood paradichlorobenzene levels averaging 10 μg/L associated with Tokyo residents

Overdosage Treatment

Decontamination: Emesis (>5 g ingestion) or lavage in conjunction with activated charcoal may be utilized; do not dilute with milk
Dermal: Wash with soap and water; remove contaminated clothing
Ocular: Irrigate with saline
Supportive therapy: Treat symptomatic methemoglobinemia with methylene blue

Diagnostic Tests/Procedures

Complete Blood Count *on page 1236*
Liver Profile *on page 1286*
Methemoglobin, Blood *on page 1296*

Monitoring Parameters Methemoglobin level, CBC, liver function test

Additional Information Milk or fatty foods promote oral absorption; nasal irritant at level >50 ppm
TLV-TWA: 75 ppm
IDLH: 1000 ppm
Odor threshold: 15-30 ppm
Average adult exposure: 35 mcg/day by inhalation and 0.2 mcg/day through drinking water

Specific References

Ambre J, Ruo TI, and Smith-Coggins R, "Mothball Composition: Three Simple Tests for Distinguishing Paradichlorobenzene From Naphthalene," *Ann Emerg Med*, 1986, 15(6):724-6.
Morita M and Ohi G, "Para-Dichlorobenzene in Human Tissue and Atmosphere in Tokyo Metropolitan Area," *Environ Pollut*, 1975, 8:269-79
U.S. Department of Health and Human Services, "Toxicological Profile for 1,4-Dichlorobenzene TP-92/10," Agency for Toxic Substances and Diseases Registry, April, 1993.
Winkler JV, Kulig K, and Rumack BH, "Mothball Differentiation: Naphthalene From Paradichlorobenzene," *Ann Emerg Med*, 1985, 14(1):30-2.

Paraform *see* Formaldehyde *on page 931*

Paraphenylenediamine

CAS Number 106-50-3; 624-18-0

UN Number 1673

Synonyms "Blackstones"; Paradiaminobenzene; PPD

Use Black dye used on fur or as a hair dye, photographic developer, and as a chemical intermediate in the production of polyparaphenylene terephthalamide

Mechanism of Toxic Action Aniline derivative; can cause muscle necrosis through free radical production; ~4% of individuals can develop allergic reactions

Adverse Reactions

Cardiovascular: Hypotension
Central nervous system: Vertigo
Dermatologic: Erythema multiforme
Gastrointestinal: Vomiting, abdominal pain
Hepatic: Hepatic necrosis
Neuromuscular & skeletal: Rhabdomyolysis, tremor
Ocular: Lacrimation, exophthalmos, proptosis, iritis, optic neuritis, cataract
Renal: Acute tubular necrosis, oliguria
Respiratory: Dyspnea, bronchospasm/wheezing
Miscellaneous: Facial edema, laryngeal edema, anaphylaxis

Toxicodynamics/Kinetics Absorption: Orally; <1% absorbed by dermal route

Overdosage Treatment

Decontamination:
Oral: Do not administer ipecac on oral ingestion; activated charcoal with cathartic can be administered
Ocular: Irrigate copiously with saline
Dermal: Wash with soap and water
Supportive therapy: Intravenous fluid hydration and diuretics should be given for treatment of myoglobinuria; standard antianaphylaxis therapy can be administered

Monitoring Parameters Urinalysis, CPK, renal function tests

Pregnancy Implications Does not appear to be teratogenic in rodent models

Additional Information

IDLH: 25 mg/m^3
TLV-TWA: 0.1 mg/m^3
White to light purple crystals; cosmetic use is common in Sudan, India, Israel, Pakistan, and Morocco, but is not permitted in the U.S.

Ingestion of 1.8 g associated with acute renal failure in an adult

Specific References

Ashraf W, Dawling S, and Farrow LJ, "Systemic Paraphenylenediamine (PPD) Poisoning: A Case Report and Review," *Hum Exp Toxicol*, 1994, 13(3):167-70.

El-Ansary EH, Ahmed ME, and Clague HW, "Systemic Toxicity of Paraphenylenediamine," *Lancet*, 1983, 1:1341.

Shemesh IY, Mishal Y, Baruchin AM, et al, "Rhabdomyolysis in Paraphenylenediamine Intoxication," *Vet Hum Toxicol*, 1995, 37:244-5.

Paraquat

Related Information

Diquat Dibromide *on page 918*

Toxins Which Should be Lavaged With Solutions Other Than Water *on page 1635*

CAS Number 4685-14-7; 2074-50-2; 1910-42-5

Synonyms 1,1'-Dimethyl-4,4'-Dipyridilium Ion; Dimethyl Viologen; Gamoxone; PP-148; PP-190

Commonly Found In Crisquat; Dextrone; Dexuron; Esgran; Goldquat 276; Gramoxone; Hebaxon; Osaquat Super; Sweep

Mechanism of Toxic Action Usually in a 20% solution; a quaternary nitrogen compound which can produce photobleaching by destroying plant cellular membrane; can also inhibit photosynthesis

Adverse Reactions

Dermatologic: Skin irritation, fingernail atrophy, fingernail loss, Mees' lines

Gastrointestinal: Nausea, vomiting, gastrointestinal ulceration, pancreatitis

Ocular: Corneal edema (by ocular contact)

Respiratory: Cough, pulmonary fibrosis

Miscellaneous: Nasal bleeding with inhalation, myoglobinuria, no acute neurological signs, hyperthermia, dysphagia

Signs & Symptoms of Acute Overdose

Group I, mild poisoning (<20 mg/kg): Nausea, vomiting, diarrhea

Group II, moderate poisoning (20-40 mg/kg): Vomiting, diarrhea, pulmonary fibrosis, renal/hepatic failure – death in 2 weeks

Group III, severe poisoning (>40 mg/kg): Vomiting, diarrhea, oropharyngeal ulceration with cardiac, respiratory, hepatic, renal failure – death usually within 1 day

Toxicodynamics/Kinetics

Absorption: Dermal absorption can occur through skin that is not intact; oral absorption: 30%

Distribution: V_d: 1.2-1.6 L/kg

Half-life: 12-120 hours

Elimination: Renal

Reference Range Plasma level of 3 mg/L associated with death; see graph

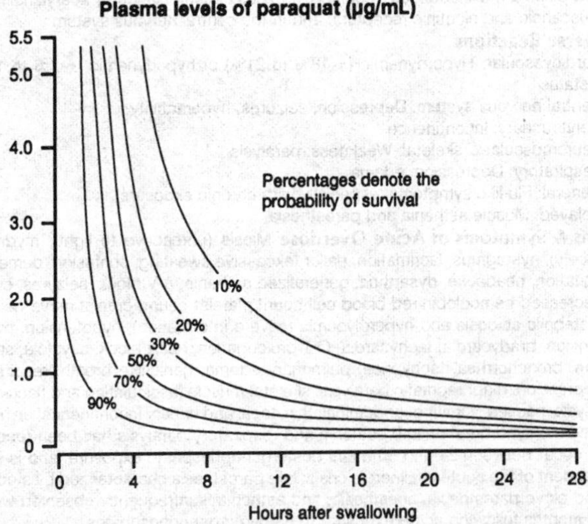

The relationship between the plasma concentrations of paraquat on the ordinate (µg/mL), time after ingestion on the abscissa, and the probability of survival. (Reproduced with permission from Hart RB, Nevitt A, Whitehead A; "A New Statistical Approach to the Prognostic Significance of Plasma Paraquat Concentration" (letter), *Lancet 2:* 1984, 1147.)

(Continued)

Paraquat *(Continued)*

Overdosage Treatment

Decontamination: Emesis/lavage with activated charcoal with cathartic; Fuller's earth (15%) or 7% bentonite; sodium polystyrene sulfonate may also be effective

Supportive therapy: Do not utilize oxygen in that it may promote pulmonary fibrosis; monitor for hypercalcemia if Fuller's earth used; inhaled nitric oxide (at 25 ppm) has been used to treat ARDS; vitamin C (4000 mg/day) and vitamin E (250 mg/day), dexamethasone, cyclophosphamide, and acetylcysteine have been used to treat lung toxicity, but are of unproven benefit

Enhancement of elimination: Multiple dosing of activated charcoal, Fuller's earth (100-150 g in adults or 2 g/kg in children) or bentonite may be given every 2-4 hours; charcoal hemoperfusion for prolonged periods of time (up to 10 hours) may be helpful if instituted within 2 hours; forced diuresis is not helpful

Diagnostic Tests/Procedures

Paraquat, Blood *on page 1316*

Additional Information Not well absorbed through intact skin but prolonged contact can cause systemic toxicity; faint ammonia-like odor; dithionate test: 1 part urine, 0.5 part sodium dithionate in IN NaOH: Deep blue color indicates presence of paraquat or diquat

Specific References

Garnier R, Chataigner D, Efthymiou ML, et al, "Paraquat Poisoning by Skin Absorption: Report of Two Cases," *Vet Hum Toxicol*, 1994, 36(4):313-5.

Honore P, Hantson P, Fauville JP, et al, "Paraquat Poisoning – State of the Art," *Acta Clin Belg*, 1994, 49(5):220-8.

Houze P, Baud FJ, Mouy R, et al, "Toxicokinetics of Paraquat in Humans," *Hum Exp Toxicol*, 1990, 9(1):5-12.

Kaojarern S and Ongphiphadhanakul B, "Predicting Outcomes in Paraquat Poisoning," *Vet Hum Toxicol*, 1991, 33(2):115-8.

Koppel C, Wissmann CV, Barchow D, et al, "Inhaled Nitric Oxide in Advanced Paraquat Intoxication," *J Toxicol Clin Toxicol*, 1994, 32:205-14.

Perriens JH, Benimadho S, Kiauw IL, et al, "High-Dose Cyclophosphamide and Dexamethasone in Paraquat Poisoning: A Prospective Study," *Hum Exp Toxicol*, 1992, 11(2):129-34.

Suzuki K, Takasu N, Okabe T, et al, "Effect of Aggressive Hemoperfusion on the Clinical Course of Patients with Paraquat Poisoning," *Hum Exp Toxicol*, 1993, 12(4):323-7.

Talbot AR, Barnes MR, and Ting RS, "Early Radiotherapy in the Treatment of Paraquat Poisoning," *Br J Radiol*, 1988, 61(725):405-8.

Tinoco R, Parsonnet J, and Halperin D, "Paraquat Poisoning in Southern Mexico: A Report of 25 Cases," *Arch Environ Health*, 1993, 48(2):78-80.

Parathion

CAS Number 56-38-2

UN Number 2783; 2784

Synonyms O,O-Diethyl O-p-Nitrophenyl Phosphorothioate

Brand Names Bay E-605®; Bladan F®; Orthophos®; Parathion®

Mechanism of Toxic Action Potent, irreversible inhibition of acetylcholinesterase and plasma cholinesterase, resulting in excess accumulation of acetylcholine at muscarinic and nicotinic receptors, and in the central nervous system

Adverse Reactions

Cardiovascular: Hyperdynamic (~18% to 21%) or hypodynamic (~7% to 10%) states

Central nervous system: Depression, seizures, hyperactivity

Genitourinary: Incontinence

Neuromuscular & skeletal: Weakness, paralysis

Respiratory: Depression, edema

General: Flu-like symptoms (especially with chronic exposure)

Delayed: Muscle asthenia and paresthesia

Signs & Symptoms of Acute Overdose Miosis (unreactive to light), mydriasis (rarely), nystagmus, lacrimation, pallor, excessive sweating, confusion, dementia, agitation, headache, dysarthria, generalized asthenia, A-V block, seizures, coma, decreased hemoglobin/red blood cell count/platelet count, cranial nerve palsies, metabolic acidosis and hyperglycemia (severe intoxication), hypotension, hypertension, bradycardia, tachycardia, Q-T prolongation, heart block, asystole, salivation, bronchorrhea, tachypnea, pulmonary edema, garlic-like breath, respiratory depression, diaphragmatic paralysis, skeletal muscle fasciculation and flaccid paralysis, nausea, vomiting, abdominal pain, fecal and urinary incontinence; an "intermediate syndrome" of limb asthenia and respiratory paralysis has been reported to occur between 24 and 96 hours postorganophosphate exposure, and is independent of the acute cholinergic crisis; late paresthesia characterized by stocking and glove paresthesia, anesthesia, and asthenia is infrequently observed weeks to months following acute exposure to certain organophosphates

Toxicodynamics/Kinetics

Absorption: Readily through oral, dermal, or respiratory exposure

Metabolism: Rapidly metabolized to weakly active compounds through hepatic hydrolysis and other pathways

Elimination: Metabolites are excreted in urine (p-nitrophenol)

Warnings Risk of aspiration pneumonitis exists with agents having a hydrocarbon vehicle; severe laryngeal irritation and violent coughing may result from exposure to dusting powders; exposure to dusting powders and insecticide granules may cause contact dermatitis

Reference Range Serum parathion levels in asymptomatic occupationally exposed worker range from 0.004-0.2 mg/L: urinary para-nitrophenol levels in these individuals ranged from 0.4-13.2 mg/L; no correlation in cholinesterase (plasma or red blood cell) noted

Mild poisoning: Serum cholinesterase is 20% to 50% of normal;

Moderate poisoning: Serum cholinesterase is 10% to 20% of normal

Severe poisoning (respiratory distress and coma): Serum cholinesterase is <10%

Overdosage Treatment

Decontamination: Isolation, bagging, and disposal of all contaminated clothing and other articles; all emergency medical workers and hospital staff should follow appropriate precautions regarding exposure to hazardous material including the use of protective clothing, masks, goggles, and respiratory equipment

Dermal: Prompt thorough scrubbing of all affected areas with soap and water, including hair and nails

Gastric: Activated charcoal can be administered either orally or via a nasogastric tube; do not induce emesis because of danger of sudden respiratory compromise, alterations in mental status, seizures, coma, and possible aspiration of hydrocarbon vehicles

Ocular: Irrigation with copious tepid sterile water or saline

Supportive therapy: Including airway management, ventilatory assistance, humidified oxygen administration, and close monitoring for sudden respiratory failure

Enhancement of elimination: Dialysis and hemoperfusion are not indicated due to effectiveness of the prescribed treatment, large volumes of distribution of organophosphates

Antidote:

Atropine: Administration should be guided by respiratory status, starting at 1-5 mg I.V. every 5-10 minutes as needed, and should be titrated to the resolution of excess pulmonary secretions; frequent administration of large doses (cumulative doses >100 mg) may be necessary in massive exposures

Glycopyrrolate: May be administered if atropine is unavailable

2-PAM: For more significant exposures (ie, exposures requiring large doses of atropine, or with recurring symptoms, or exposures to more lipid soluble agents), administration should follow: 1-2 g I.V. over 5-10 minutes, repeated in 1 hour if asthenia reoccurs, then every 4-12 hours for recurring symptoms

Antidote(s)

Atropine Sulfate *on page 1395*

Pralidoxime Chloride *on page 1461*

Diagnostic Tests/Procedures

Blood Gases, Arterial *on page 1207*

Chest Films *on page 1224*

Complete Blood Count *on page 1236*

Creatinine, Serum *on page 1243*

Electrocardiography *on page 1253*

Liver Profile *on page 1286*

Pesticide Screen, Chlorinated *on page 1317*

Pesticide Screen, Organophosphate *on page 1317*

Pseudocholinesterase, Serum *on page 1340*

Pregnancy Implications Human data regarding organophosphate exposure in pregnancy is limited and anecdotal; teratogenesis and fetal death have been produced in animal models at exposure levels that cause obvious toxicity to the pregnant animal; parathion has demonstrated significant teratogenicity in an avian embryo model

Additional Information Yellow to brown liquid with a garlic odor; thermal degradation products include sulfur, nitrogen, and phosphorus oxides; red blood cell cholinesterase, and serum pseudocholinesterase may be depressed following acute or chronic organophosphate exposure; RBC cholinesterase is typically not analyzed by in-house laboratories, and is usually not available for consideration during acute management. Pseudocholinesterase levels may be rapidly available from some in-house laboratories, but are not as reliable a marker of organophosphate exposure because of variability secondary to variant genotypes, hepatic disease, oral estrogen use, or malnutrition. Because of this variability, true indication of suppression of either of these enzymes can only be estimated through comparison to pre-exposure values; these enzymes may be useful in measuring a patient's recovery postexposure, especially if the recovery is not progressing as expected.

ACGIH TLV: 0.1 mg/m^3

PEL-TWA: 0.1 mg/m^3

(Continued)

Parathion *(Continued)*

IDLH: 20 mg/m^3
Water solubility: 12 ppm
Odor threshold: 0.04 ppm
Vapor pressure of 0.0004 mm Hg at 20°C

Other information concerning pesticide exposures is available through the EPA-funded National Pesticide Telecommunications Network: 1-800-858-7378 (weekdays, 8 AM to 6 PM, Central Standard time)

Specific References

Clifford NJ and Nies AS, "Organophosphate Poisoning From Wearing a Laundered Uniform Previously Contaminated With Parathion," *JAMA*, 1989, 262(21):3035-6.

Minton NA and Murray VS, "A Review of Organophosphate Poisoning," *Med Toxicol Adverse Drug Exp*, 1988, 3(5):350-75.

Namba T, Nolte CT, Jackrel J, et al, "Poisoning Due to Organophosphate Insecticides. Acute and Chronic Manifestations," *Am J Med*, 1971, 50(4):475-92.

Roan CC, Morgan DP, Cook N, et al, "Blood Cholinesterases, Serum Parathion Concentrations and Urine p-Nitrophenol Concentrations in Exposed Individuals," *Bull Environ Contam Toxicol*, 1969, 4:362-9.

Parathion® *see* Parathion *on page 988*

Parosmic Acid *see* Osmium *on page 984*

PBX *see* RDX *on page 1009*

PCB *see* Polychlorinated Biphenyls *on page 995*

PCDF *see* Polychlorinated Dibenzofurans *on page 996*

PCE *see* Tetrachloroethylene *on page 1022*

PCP *see* Pentachlorophenol *on this page*

PDB *see* Para-Dichlorobenzene *on page 985*

Pegalan *see* Methacrylates *on page 957*

Penchlorol *see* Pentachlorophenol *on this page*

Penphene® *see* Toxaphene *on page 1031*

Pentachlorin® *see* DDT *on page 903*

Pentachlorophenol

Related Information

Hexachlorobenzene *on page 936*

CAS Number 87-86-5

UN Number 3155

Synonyms PCP; Penchlorol

Brand Names Chlon®; Dowicide® 7; Dura Treet® II; Fungifen®; Lauxtol®; Penta Ready®; Permasan®; Santophen® 20; Woodtreat®

Use Termiticide, fungicide, herbicide, and disinfectant; primarily used as a wood preservative; restricted use pesticide

Mechanism of Toxic Action Uncouples oxidative phosphorylation; hexachlorobenzene, pentachlorobenzene, and hexachlorocyclobenzene all metabolize to pentachlorophenol

Adverse Reactions

Cardiovascular: Tachycardia
Central nervous system: Seizures, hyperthermia
Dermatologic: Alopecia
Endocrine & metabolic: Acidosis
Gastrointestinal: Nausea, vomiting
Hematologic: Hemolysis, aplastic anemia
Hepatic: Hepatotoxicity with elevation of liver function tests
Neuromuscular & skeletal: Tremors, muscle spasms
Ocular: Mydriasis
Renal: Nephrotoxicity (reduced glomerular filtration rate and tubular function)
Respiratory: Hyperventilation
Miscellaneous: Pulmonary irritation, dermal and ocular irritant (at levels in air >0.1 ppm), intense thirst, sweating, hyperthermia

Toxicodynamics/Kinetics

Absorption:
- Dermal: 62% in oil-based solution and 16% in aqueous based
- Inhalation: 76% to 88%
- Oral: Within 1.3 hours

Distribution: V_d: 0.35 L/kg
Protein binding: 99% in animal models
Metabolism: Hepatic conjugation to form a glucuronide and oxidative dechlorination to form tetrachloro-para-hydroquinone (TCHQ)

Half-life: 13-19 days (ethanol solution); 30 hours (sodium salt)
Elimination: Renal (~78% as pentachlorophenol and 12% as pentachlorophenol glucuronide)

Reference Range Mean blood pentachlorophenol level in patients with neurological symptoms: 22 μg/L (range: 4-60 μg/L); people living in log homes can have 10 times the blood levels than general population (420 ppb vs 40 ppb respectively); adipose tissue levels in general population: 26.3 μg/kg; baseline urine pentachlorophenol level in general population: 3.4 ppb; for residents of log homes: 69 ppb

Overdosage Treatment

Decontamination:

- Dermal: Wash with soap and water; remove all contaminated clothing
- Ocular: Copious irrigation with saline
- Oral: Lavage within 1 hour of exposure; cholestyramine can be effective in adsorbing this agent

Supportive: Cool with external methods; avoid use of aspirin or atropine; diazepam can be used for muscle spasm

Enhancement of elimination: Exchange transfusion may be effective in infants; due to enterohepatic recirculation, multiple dosing of cholestyramine (4 g every 8 hours) may be effective; dialysis, forced diuresis, or hemoperfusion is not useful

Pregnancy Implications While animal studies do not reveal any teratogenesis, pentachlorophenol is fetotoxic and can produce maternal toxicity

Additional Information Usually contaminated with chlorinated dibenzo-paradioxins; WHO guidelines for drinking water is 10 mcg/L; dairy products, grains, and cereals have highest levels of this agent; concentrations >10% can cause dermal irritation

Daily dietary intake: ~1.5 mg
Daily drinking water intake: 0.02-24 mcg
Inhalation exposure of general U.S. population: 12-136 mcg/day; residents of log homes: 140-157 mcg/day due primarily to treated logs (although this agent is no longer used for this purpose); sealers decrease this concentration significantly
Soil samples within one foot of treated utility poles: 3-654 ppm
PEL-TWA (skin): 0.5 mg/m^3
IDLH: 150 mg/m^3
Half-life in soil: 2-4 weeks
Lethal oral dose: 1 g (~17 mg/kg)

Specific References

Roberts HS, "Aplastic Anemia Due to Pentachlorophenol," *N Engl J Med*, 1981, 305(27):1650-1.
U.S. Department of Health and Human Services, "Toxicological Profile for Pentachlorophenol TP-93/13," Agency for Toxic Substances and Diseases Registry, May, 1994.

Penta Ready® *see* Pentachlorophenol *on previous page*

Perchlor *see* Tetrachloroethylene *on page 1022*

Perchlormethane *see* Carbon Tetrachloride *on page 882*

Perchlorobenzene *see* Hexachlorobenzene *on page 936*

Perchlorobutadiene *see* Hexachlorobutadiene *on page 937*

Perchloroethane *see* Hexachloroethane *on page 937*

Perclene *see* Tetrachloroethylene *on page 1022*

Permasan® *see* Pentachlorophenol *on previous page*

Permethrin *see* Pyrethrins *on page 1003*

Permetrina (Portuguese) *see* Pyrethrins *on page 1003*

Persian-Insect Powder *see* Pyrethrins *on page 1003*

Perthane *see* Organochlorines *on page 983*

Petrol *see* Gasoline *on page 932*

Petroleum *see* Mineral-Based Crankcase Oil *on page 971*

Petroleum Distillates – Naphtha

CAS Number 8030-30-6

UN Number 2553

Synonyms Benzin; Painters' Naphtha; Petroleum Spirit; Stoddard Solvent; White Spirit

Commonly Found In Coal tar, solvent for oils, lacquers, paints, rubber cement

Mechanism of Toxic Action Aspiration pneumonia related to low viscosity agents

Adverse Reactions

- Central nervous system: CNS depressant
- Respiratory: Aspiration pneumonitis
- Miscellaneous: Intravenous administration produces fever and local tissue damage; irritant of mucous membranes

(Continued)

Petroleum Distillates – Naphtha *(Continued)*

Signs & Symptoms of Acute Overdose Headache, dizziness, nausea, hematuria, dyspnea, dermatitis, coughing (persistent), fever, hemoptysis, erythema, unlikely to produce systemic signs

Toxicodynamics/Kinetics Absorption: Not well absorbed in the gastrointestinal tract

Overdosage Treatment Decontamination: Do not induce emesis or lavage; basic poison management; avoid positive net fluid balance; avoid catecholamines due to sensitivity of myocardium

Diagnostic Tests/Procedures

Blood Gases, Arterial *on page 1207*

Chest Films *on page 1224*

Complete Blood Count *on page 1236*

Additional Information

IDLH: 10,000 ppm

PEL-TWA: 500 ppm

Specific References

Banner W Jr and Walson PD, "Systemic Toxicity Following Gasoline Aspiration," *Am J Emerg Med*, 1983, 1(3):292-4.

Case ME, Poklis A, and Mackell MA, "Homicide by Intravenous Injection of Naphtha," *J Forensic Sci*, 1985, 30(1):208-12.

Petroleum Spirit *see* Petroleum Distillates – Naphtha *on previous page*

PG 12 *see* Propylene Glycol *on page 1002*

PGDN *see* Propylene Glycol Dinitrate *on page 1003*

Phenachlor® *see* 2,4,6-Trichlorophenol *on page 1034*

Phenacyl Chloride *see* Chloroacetophenone *on page 889*

Phenanthrene *see* Polycyclic Aromatic Hydrocarbons *on page 997*

Phenatox® *see* Toxaphene *on page 1031*

Phene *see* Benzene *on page 867*

Phenicide® *see* Toxaphene *on page 1031*

Phenmedipham

CAS Number 13684-63-4

Synonyms Methyl-3-Metatolycarbamoloxyphenyl Carbamate

Brand Names Betanal; EP-452; Fenmedifam; Kemifan; Spin-Aid

Use Control weeds of sugar beet crops

Mechanism of Toxic Action Inhibitor of photosynthesis

Signs & Symptoms of Acute Overdose Photosensitivity reaction, bullous dermatitis

Overdosage Treatment Decontamination: Remove contaminated clothing (especially leather); wash thoroughly with soap and water; irrigate eyes with normal saline for ocular exposure

Additional Information Does not affect cholinesterase; leather absorbs phenmedipham

Specific References

Nater JP and Grosfeld JC, "Allergic Contact Dermatitis From Betanol (Phenmedipham)," *Contact Dermatitis*, 1979, 5(1):59-60.

Phenochlor *see* Polychlorinated Biphenyls *on page 995*

Phenohep® *see* Hexachloroethane *on page 937*

Phenylamine *see* Aniline *on page 858*

Phenylethane *see* Ethylbenzene *on page 923*

Phenylethylene *see* Styrene *on page 1017*

Phenyl Hydride *see* Benzene *on page 867*

Phenyl Perchloryl *see* Hexachlorobenzene *on page 936*

Phosgen *see* Phosgene *on this page*

Phosgene

CAS Number 75-44-5

UN Number 1076

Synonyms Carbonic Dichloride; Carbon Oxychloride; Carbonyl Chloride; Chloroformyl Chloride; Diphosgene; Phosgen

Use In the manufacture of isocyanates, aniline dyes, plastics, and insecticides; World War I gas warfare; product of combustion of volatile chlorine compounds

Mechanism of Toxic Action Direct cytotoxicity. Reacts readily with hydroxyl, sulfhydryl, and ammonia groups found in albumin, amino acids, and vitamins; pulmonary irritant with low water solubility thus primarily affecting lung parenchyma on inhalation (delayed alveolar injury)

Adverse Reactions

Cardiovascular: Hypotension, bradycardia

Endocrine & metabolic: Hypovolemia

Respiratory: Respiratory distress, pulmonary edema

Signs & Symptoms of Acute Overdose Dyspnea, ocular irritation, throat burning, headache, nausea, vomiting, cough, hemoptysis, asthenia, chest pain, dermal burns

Toxicodynamics/Kinetics Metabolism: Hydrolyzes slowly to produce carbon dioxide and hydrochloric acids

Overdosage Treatment

Decontamination:

Oral: Lavage; irrigate exposed areas; steroids may be helpful; do not use diuretics

Dermal: Irrigate copiously with water (especially with diphosgene exposure)

Diagnostic Tests/Procedures

Blood Gases, Arterial *on page 1207*

Chest Films *on page 1224*

Electrolytes, Blood *on page 1254*

Pulse Oximetry *on page 1342*

Additional Information Colorless gas; latent period may last 3 days. Odor threshold: 0.5 ppm; at low doses, it has a freshly mowed grass odor; higher doses give a pungent odor. Olfactory paralysis may occur after a short time of initial exposure. Blindness may occur; rescuer contamination possibility from affected patients is low.

TLV-TWA: 0.1 ppm

IDLH: 2 ppm

PEL-TWA: 0.1 ppm

On chest x-ray, blurred enlargement of hilar area may be earliest finding

Specific References

Diller WF, "Medical Phosgene Problems and Their Possible Solution," *J Occup Med*, 1978, 20(3):189-93.

Phosphine

Related Information

Aluminum Phosphide *on page 857*

CAS Number 7803-51-2

UN Number 2199

Synonyms Delicia; Detia Gas EX-B; Hydrogen Phosphide; Phosphoreted Hydrogen; Phosphorus Trihydride

Use Silicon crystal treatment in semiconductor industry, contaminant in acetylene, grain fumigation, and rat poisons

Mechanism of Toxic Action Protoplasmic toxicity inhibits cytochrome C oxidase pathway primarily in myocardium

Adverse Reactions

Cardiovascular: Tachycardia, cardiovascular collapse, hypotension

Hepatic: Hepatic toxicity (late)

Renal & genitourinary: Oliguria, renal failure

Respiratory: Pulmonary edema

Signs & Symptoms of Acute Overdose Irritability, drowsiness, tremor, dizziness, vomiting, diplopia, ataxia, dyspnea, garlic-like breath, cough, chest pain, abdominal pain, seizures, jaundice, cardiac arrhythmia (atrial fibrillation, tachycardia (ventricular))

Toxicodynamics/Kinetics Onset of action: Rapid, within 3 hours of exposure

Reference Range Blood and urine phosphorus levels are not reliable

Overdosage Treatment

Decontamination: Oxygenation; if ingested, lavage with 1:10,000 dilution of potassium permanganate to reduce availability of phosphine within 1 hour

Supportive therapy: Calcium gluconate and magnesium sulfate may be useful for cardiac arrhythmia. May be unresponsive to vasopressin.

Enhancement of elimination: Hemodialysis may be useful in cases of renal damage

Antidote(s)

Calcium Gluconate *on page 1401*

Magnesium Sulfate *on page 1440*

Diagnostic Tests/Procedures

Blood Gases, Arterial *on page 1207*

Chest Films *on page 1224*

Electrocardiography *on page 1253*

Kidney Profile *on page 1279*

Liver Profile *on page 1286*

(Continued)

Phosphine *(Continued)*

Magnesium, Serum *on page 1289*
Potassium, Blood *on page 1328*
Protein, Semiquantitative, Urine *on page 1337*

Additional Information Colorless gas; flammable; garlic odor
Odor threshold: 2 ppm
TLV-TWA: 0.3 ppm
IDLH: 200 ppm
PEL-TWA: 0.3 ppm
Adult deaths have been described with ingestion of 4 g of zinc phosphide or 500 mg aluminum phosphide

Specific References

Chopra JS, Kalra OP, Malik VS, et al, "Aluminum Phosphide Poisoning: A Prospective Study of 16 Cases in One Year," *Postgrad Med J*, 1986, 62(734):1113-5.
Rodenberg HD, Chang CC, and Watson WA, "Zinc Phosphide Ingestion: A Case Report and Review," *Vet Hum Toxicol*, 1989, 31(6):559-62.
Singh S, Dilawari JB, Vashist R, et al, "Aluminum Phosphide Ingestion," *Br Med J Clin Res Ed*, 1985, 290(6475):1110-1.

Phosphoreted Hydrogen *see* Phosphine *on previous page*
Phosphorodithioic Acid S-((Tert-Butylthio)methyl) O,O-Diethyl Ester *see* Terbufos *on page 1020*
Phosphorothioic Acid *see* Chlorpyrifos *on page 891*
Phosphorus Tetramen *see* White Phosphorus *on page 1039*
Phosphorus Trihydride *see* Phosphine *on previous page*
Phostoxin® *see* Aluminum Phosphide *on page 857*
Phthalic Acid, Dioctyl Ester *see* Di-n-Octylphthalate *on page 916*
Phthalol® *see* Diethyl Phthalate *on page 912*
Phygon® *see* Dichloronaphthoquinone *on page 908*
Phytonadione *see* Anticoagulant Rodenticide *on page 859*
Pied Piper Mouse Seed® *see* Strychnine *on page 1016*
Pindone *see* Anticoagulant Rodenticide *on page 859*
Pivacin® *see* Anticoagulant Rodenticide *on page 859*
Pival® *see* Anticoagulant Rodenticide *on page 859*
Pivaldione *see* Anticoagulant Rodenticide *on page 859*
Placidol® E *see* Diethyl Phthalate *on page 912*
Platin *see* Platinum *on this page*

Platinum

CAS Number 7440-06-4

Synonyms Liquid Bright Platinum; Platin; Platinum Black; Platinum Sponge

Adverse Reactions Eyes, nose, respiratory, dermatologic

Signs & Symptoms of Acute Overdose Classic signs/symptoms of allergic reaction; urticaria, rash, neuritis, rhinorrhea, cough, dyspnea, urticaria, wheezing, eczema, eosinophilia, lymphocytosis

Toxicodynamics/Kinetics
Absorption:
Oral: Poor
Inhalation: Readily absorbed
Distribution: To soft tissue
Protein binding: 90% to 95%
Half-life: 59-73 hours

Reference Range TLV-TWA metallic platinum dust: 1 mg/m^3; for soluble platinum salts: 0.002 mg/m^3

Overdosage Treatment
Decontamination: Irrigation
Supportive therapy: Beta agonists can be used for wheezing

Diagnostic Tests/Procedures
Platinum, Blood *on page 1325*
Platinum, Urine *on page 1325*

Pregnancy Implications No information available; not thought to be teratogenic

Additional Information Platinum metal is biologically inert; parenteral administration of platinum salts in animal model produces seizures, coma, and death; simple platinum salts are toxic to the gastrointestinal tract; complex platinum salts are toxic to the nervous system; an allergic response to complex platinum salts is known as platinosis

Specific References

Luckey TD and Venugopal B, eds, *Metal Toxicity in Mammals*, New York, NY: Plenum Press, 1977.

Platinum Black *see* Platinum *on previous page*

Platinum Sponge *see* Platinum *on previous page*

Plutonium

Related Information

Radiation: Basics of Exposure *on page 1594-1600*

CAS Number 7440-07-5

UN Number 2918

Synonyms Plutonium-236 Isotope; Plutonium-237 Isotope; Plutonium-238 Isotope; Plutonium-239 Isotope; Plutonium-240 Isotope; Plutonium-241 Isotope; Plutonium-242 Isotope; Plutonium-243 Isotope; Plutonium Metal; Pu

Use Primarily in the production of nuclear weapons (plutonium-239 isotope); also used as a heat source for thermoelectric power devices (plutonium-238 isotope) (especially the breeder type of reactor)

Adverse Reactions Causes tissue necrosis on contact; dermal burns

Toxicodynamics/Kinetics

Absorption: By inhalation (especially more soluble forms of plutonium such as plutonium citrate or plutonium nitrate); very limited absorption by oral or dermal routes (0.0002% per hour of plutonium nitrate)

Distribution: Highest concentration after inhalation in tracheal-bronchial lymph nodes and liver

Half-life: 180-200 years

Elimination: By feces and urine

Overdosage Treatment

Decontamination: Remove contaminated clothing; isolate all run-off

Dermal: Irrigate with water; scrub gently with soft sponge or brush (avoid abrading skin); a 50% powdered detergent solution followed by a 5% sodium hypochlorite solution can be used for persistent contamination

Ocular: Wash copiously with saline

Supportive therapy: DTPA (diethylenetriamine pentacetic acid) which is available from the Radiation Emergency Assistance Center (615-576-1004) is an effective chelator; the calcium salt should be used as follows: 1 g of Ca^{++} DTPA diluted in 250 mL of 5% dextrose in water should be infused over a 1- to 1½-hour time period daily for 5 days; $CaNa_2$ EDTA (calcium Versenate®) can also be used, but is less effective; DTPA should be used for dermal exposure with open wounds as well as inhalation or oral ingestion

Antidote(s)

Diethylene Triamine Penta-acetic Acid *on page 1411*

Diagnostic Tests/Procedures

Complete Blood Count *on page 1236*

Additional Information Background radiation to an individual in U.S. is estimated to be 360 mrem (2.6 mSv); cigarettes can accentuate plutonium toxicity; odorless and tasteless; carcinogenic in animals (squamous cell)

Physical half-life: 24,900 years

Decontamination should be monitored by use of a Geiger-Mueller counter

Specific References

Saenger EL, "Radiation Accidents," *Ann Emerg Med*, 1986, 15(9):1061-6.

U.S. Department of Health and Human Services, "Toxicological Profile for Plutonium TP-90/21," Agency for Toxic Substances and Diseases Registry, December 1990.

Plutonium-236 Isotope *see* Plutonium *on this page*

Plutonium-237 Isotope *see* Plutonium *on this page*

Plutonium-238 Isotope *see* Plutonium *on this page*

Plutonium-239 Isotope *see* Plutonium *on this page*

Plutonium-240 Isotope *see* Plutonium *on this page*

Plutonium-241 Isotope *see* Plutonium *on this page*

Plutonium-242 Isotope *see* Plutonium *on this page*

Plutonium-243 Isotope *see* Plutonium *on this page*

Plutonium Metal *see* Plutonium *on this page*

PNU *see* Nitrophenolurea *on page 981*

Polychlorinated Biphenyls

Related Information

Hexabromobiphenyl *on page 935*

Polychlorinated Dibenzofurans *on next page*

(Continued)

Polychlorinated Biphenyls *(Continued)*

CAS Number 12674-11-2; 11104-28-2; 11141-16-5; 53469-21-9; 12672-29-6; 11097-69-1; 11096-82-5; 37324-23-5; 11100-14-4; 1336-36-3; 37317-41-2; 12737-87-0

UN Number 2315

Synonyms Aroclor; Chlorbipheny; Clophen; Fenclor; Kanechlor; PCB; Phenochlor

Use Was used (up until 1979) as a coolant in capacitors and transformers; also had been used as a lubricant for gas turbine engines

Mechanism of Toxic Action Binds to a cellular receptor (Ah receptor) which alters protein and enzyme synthesis

Adverse Reactions

Central nervous system: Headache, fatigue

Dermatologic: Hyperpigmentation, chloracne, orbital swelling, pruritus

Gastrointestinal: Nausea, vomiting, diarrhea

Hepatic: Hepatitis

Miscellaneous: Elevated serum triglycerides and hyperthyroxinemia (with normal TSH levels) have been noted; clearly carcinogenic in animals (hepatocellular), not well described in humans

Toxicodynamics/Kinetics

Absorption: By inhalation (80%), oral, and dermal (15% to 56%)

Distribution: Accumulates in fat

Metabolism: Hepatic hydroxylation and conjugation with glucuronic acid; as rate of chlorination of biphenyl rings increases, metabolic rate decreases

Half-life: 4 months to 2 years

Elimination: Primarily fecal

Reference Range Blood level of general unexposed population: ~20 ppb; in adipose tissue: 1-2 ppm

Overdosage Treatment

Decontamination:

Dermal: Wash with soap and water; remove contaminated clothing; acetone can also be used for dermal washing

Inhalation: Administer 100% humidified oxygen

Oral: Lavage/activated charcoal

Pregnancy Implications Fetotoxicity with abnormal fetal pigmentation and low birth weight have been noted

Additional Information Usually mixed with chlorine; high food concentration is in fish (almost 1 ppm)

Average daily intake of PCB by inhalation: ~100 ng; by drinking water: <200 ng

Trophospheric water half-life: 3.5-83.2 days

Water half-life: 27-82 days

Urban atmospheric concentrations of PCB in the U.S. range from 0.5-30 ng/m^3 (mean: 5-10 ng/m^3); Lake Michigan average PCB level: 1.8 ng/L; Lake Huron: 0.5 ng/L; low water solubility inducer of hepatic microsomal enzymes

Toxic oral dose: 500 mg

Specific References

Letz G, "The Toxicology of PCBs - An Overview for Clinicians," *West J Med*, 1983, 138:534-40.

U.S. Department of Health and Human Services, "Toxicological Profile for Selected PCBs TP-92/16," Agency for Toxic Substances and Diseases Registry, April, 1993.

Polychlorinated Dibenzofurans

Related Information

Polychlorinated Biphenyls *on previous page*

CAS Number 57117-35-8; 57117-37-0; 51207-31-9; 67517-48-0; 57117-41-6; 57117-31-4; 70648-26-9; 57117-44-9; 72918-21-9; 75627-02-0; 60851-34-5; 67562-39-4; 70648-25-8; 69698-58-4; 55673-89-7; 39001-02-0

Synonyms Chlorodibenzofurans; Dibenzo-p-Dioxins; PCDF

Use No commercial use; primarily produced as byproducts during the production of polychlorinated biphenyl agents (PCBs) (ie, Agent Orange), polychlorinated phenols, herbicides, and chlorine bleaching at paper and pulp mills; formed from the photolysis of PCBs and from PCB transformer fires or incineration

Mechanism of Toxic Action Binds to a cellular receptor (Ah receptor) which alters protein and enzyme synthesis

Adverse Reactions

Central nervous system: Headache, paresthesia

Dermatologic: Dermal changes include comedo formatting, hyperpigmentation, hyperkeratosis, acneform eruptions on face, head, and trunk

Gastrointestinal: Vomiting (25% on oral exposure), diarrhea (18%)

Genitourinary: Increased urinary excretion of uroporphyrin

Hematologic: Normocytic anemia, leukocytosis

Neuromuscular & skeletal: Limb neuralgia, neuropathy (peripheral)

Miscellaneous: Increased serum triglycerides

Toxicodynamics/Kinetics

Absorption: Through ingestion, inhalation, or dermal routes

Metabolism: Hepatic hydroxylation followed by glucuronidation
Half-life: >7 years of 2,3,7,8-tetrachlorodibenzoparadioxin
Elimination: Feces

Reference Range Whole blood level of total PCDFs in occupationally exposed individuals is over double that of nonexposed subjects (103 ppt vs 47 ppt respectively)

Overdosage Treatment
Decontamination:
Dermal: Remove contaminated clothing; wash with soap and water
Ocular: Irrigate copiously with saline
Oral: Lavage/activated charcoal
Enhancement of elimination: Multiple dosing of cholestyramine (4 g 3 times/day) has been inconclusive

Pregnancy Implications Increased prevalence of neural tube defects described in humans; fetotoxic in rodents with daily doses as low as 0.25 mcg/kg over 10-day period

Additional Information 2,3,7,8-substituted PCDFs seem to be the most hepatotoxic agent of CDF; Tetra CDF, Penta CDF, and Hexa CDF have skin tumor promotor activity; tropospheric lifetime of PCDFs: 1.9-39 days (higher chlorinated congeners have longer lifetimes); foods (especially meat and shellfish) account for the highest amount of CDF ingested daily; inhalation accounts for only 3% of total daily CDF intake. These chemicals are solid at room temperature; possible increased risk in soft tissue, sarcoma; carcinogenic in mice models at doses of 0.5-2 mcg/kg/week.

Specific References

Centers for Disease Control Veteran's Health Studies, "Serum 2,3,7,8-Tetrachlorodibenzo-p-Dioxin Levels in U.S. Army Vietnam-Era Veterans," *JAMA*, 1988, 260(9):1249-54.

Field B and Kerr C, "Herbicide Use and Incidence of Neural Tube Defects," *Lancet*, 1979, 1(8130):1341-2.

Hryhorczuk DO, Orris P, Kominsky JR, et al, "PCB, PCDF, and PCDD Exposure Following a Transformer Fire: Chicago," *Chemosphere*, 1986, 15:1297-303.

Schecter A, Furst P, Furst C, et al, "Dioxins, Dibenzofurans, and Selected Chlorinated Organic Compound in Human Milk and Blood From Cambodia, Germany, Thailand, the USA, the USSR, and Vietnam," *Chemosphere*, 1991, 23:1903-12.

U.S. Department of Health and Human Services, "Toxicological Profile for Chlorodibenzofurans TP-93/04," Agency for Toxic Substances and Diseases Registry, May, 1994.

Polycizer 162® *see* Di-n-Octylphthalate *on page 916*

Polycron® *see* Profenofos *on next page*

Polycyclic Aromatic Hydrocarbons

CAS Number 83-32-9; 208-96-8; 120-12-7; 56-55-3; 50-32-8; 205-99-2; 192-97-2; 207-08-9; 191-24-2; 205-82-3; 218-01-9; 53-70-3; 206-44-0; 86-73-7; 193-39-5; 85-01-8; 129-00-00

Synonyms Acenaphthylene; Anthracene; Benz[*a*]anthracene; Benzo[*b*]fluoranthene; Benzo[*j*]fluoranthene; Benzo[*k*]fluoranthene; Benzo[*ghi*]perylene; Benzo[*e*]pyrene; Benzo[*a*]pyrene (BaP); Chrysene; Dibenz[*a,h*]anthracene; Dihydroacenapthylene; Fluoranthene; Fluorene; PAH; Phenanthrene; Polycyclic Organic Matter; POM; Pyrene

Commonly Found In Tobacco smoke, tar oil, automobile exhaust, flue gases, smoked foods, coke production

Use In rubber industry as a plasticizer; anthracene is used in dye production

Mechanism of Toxic Action Fused benzene ring compounds (usually 3 rings) which bind to DNA (especially diol-epoxide metabolites) leading to tumor initiation; can also cause decrease in brain dopamine and norepinephrine in the corpus striatum and hypothalamus

Adverse Reactions Anthracene laxatives can cause melanosis of colon and rectum; lung (upon inhalation) and skin cancers can occur; warts can occur upon dermal exposure as can pemphigus vulgaris

Benz(a)anthracene, benzo(b)fluoranthene, benzo(k)fluoranthene, benzo(a)pyrene, chrysene, and indeno(1,2,3-c,d)pyrene are considered a probable human carcinogen (EPA classification B_2)

Toxicodynamics/Kinetics
Absorption: Orally, by inhalation, and dermal exposure
Metabolism: Hepatic, epoxidation and epoxide conversion
Elimination: Renal

Overdosage Treatment
Decontamination:
Dermal: Wash with soap and water
Ocular: Copious irrigation with saline
Oral: Do not induce emesis; activated charcoal may be useful

Additional Information Formed after incomplete pyrolysis of fossil fuel; furnaces, coal refuse fires, and coke production account for a large amount of emissions

(Continued)

Polycyclic Aromatic Hydrocarbons *(Continued)*

Spinach, tea, meat, and fish have the highest amount of PAH levels; surface water concentrations of BaP range from 0.6-114 ng/L; skin carcinogen in animals; formed when tars and mineral oils are heated; retinoids, dietary plant phenols (ie, tannic acid) and N-acetylcysteine (NAC) may be effective in animal models in antagonizing the tumorigenic effect of benzo(a)pyrene

Daily intake of carcinogenic PAHs by an adults is estimated to be 1-5 mcg (6-9 mcg for individuals ingesting a large amount of meat); inhalation daily dose is estimated to be 0.2 mcg/day; drinking water is estimated to contribute 0.006 mcg/day of PAHs. Smoking three packs of cigarettes daily can increase exposure of PAH to 6-15 mcg/day.

Atmospheric half-life: Usually about 1 month
Soil half-life: 2 days to 2 months

Specific References

De Flora S, D'Agostini F, Izzotti A, et al, "Prevention by N-Acetylcysteine of Benzo(a)pyrene Clastogenicity and DNA Adducts in Rats," *Mutat Res*, 1991, 250(1-2):87-93.

U.S. Department of Health and Human Services, "Toxicological Profile of Polycyclic Aromatic Hydrocarbons (PAHs)," Agency for Toxic Substances and Diseases Registry, October 1993.

Polycyclic Organic Matter *see* Polycyclic Aromatic Hydrocarbons *on previous page*

Polystream® *see* Benzene *on page 867*

POM *see* Polycyclic Aromatic Hydrocarbons *on previous page*

Pomarsol® *see* Thiram *on page 1027*

Poppers *see* Nitrites *on page 978*

Pounce *see* Pyrethrins *on page 1003*

PP-148 *see* Paraquat *on page 987*

PP-190 *see* Paraquat *on page 987*

PPD *see* Paraphenylenediamine *on page 986*

Prentox® *see* Methoxychlor *on page 963*

Profenofos

CAS Number 41198-08-7

Synonyms O-(4-Bromo-2-Chlorophenyl)-O-Ethyl-S-Propylphospharathioate

Brand Names Curacron®; Polycron®; Selecron®

Use Marketed as insecticide granules, dusting agent, or spray liquid with or without petroleum derivative as a solvent

Mechanism of Toxic Action Irreversible inhibition of acetylcholinesterase and plasma cholinesterase, resulting in excess accumulation of acetylcholine at muscarinic and nicotinic receptors, and in the central nervous system

Adverse Reactions

Cardiovascular: Hyperdynamic (~18% to 21%) or hypodynamic (~7% to 10%) states
Central nervous system: Depression, seizures, hyperactivity
Genitourinary: Incontinence
Neuromuscular & skeletal: Weakness, paralysis
Respiratory: Depression, edema
General: Flu-like symptoms (especially with chronic exposure)
Delayed: Muscle asthenia and paresthesia

Signs & Symptoms of Acute Overdose Miosis (unreactive to light), mydriasis (rarely), lacrimation, pallor, excessive sweating, confusion, agitation, headache, dysarthria, generalized asthenia, seizures, A-V block, coma, decreased hemoglobin/red blood cell count/platelet count, cranial nerve palsies, metabolic acidosis and hyperglycemia (severe intoxication), hypotension, hypertension, bradycardia, tachycardia, Q-T prolongation, heart block, asystole, salivation, bronchorrhea, tachypnea, pulmonary edema, respiratory depression, diaphragmatic paralysis, skeletal muscle fasciculation and flaccid paralysis, nausea, vomiting, abdominal pain, fecal and urinary incontinence; an "intermediate syndrome" of limb asthenia and respiratory paralysis has been reported to occur between 24 and 96 hours postorganophosphate exposure, and is independent of the acute cholinergic crisis; late paresthesia characterized by stocking and glove paresthesia, anesthesia, and asthenia is infrequently observed weeks to months following acute exposure to certain organophosphates

Toxicodynamics/Kinetics

Absorption: Readily through oral, dermal, or respiratory exposure
Metabolism: Rapidly metabolized to weakly active compounds through hepatic hydrolysis and other pathways
Elimination: Metabolites are excreted in urine

Warnings Risk of aspiration pneumonitis exists with agents having a hydrocarbon vehicle; severe laryngeal irritation and violent coughing may result from exposure to dusting powders; exposure to dusting powders and insecticide granules may cause contact dermatitis

Overdosage Treatment

Decontamination: Isolation, bagging, and disposal of all contaminated clothing and other articles; all emergency medical workers and hospital staff should follow appropriate precautions regarding exposure to hazardous material including the use of protective clothing, masks, goggles, and respiratory equipment

Dermal: Prompt thorough scrubbing of all affected areas with soap and water, including hair and nails

Gastric: Activated charcoal can be administered either orally or via a nasogastric tube; do not induce emesis because of danger of sudden respiratory compromise, alterations in mental status, seizures, coma, and possible aspiration of hydrocarbon vehicles

Ocular: Irrigation with copious tepid sterile water or saline

Supportive therapy: Including airway management, ventilatory assistance, humidified oxygen administration, and close monitoring for sudden respiratory failure

Enhancement of elimination: Dialysis and hemoperfusion are not indicated due to effectiveness of the prescribed treatment, large volumes of distribution of organophosphates

Antidote:

Atropine: Administration should be guided by respiratory status, starting at 1-5 mg I.V. every 5-10 minutes as needed, and should be titrated to the resolution of excess pulmonary secretions; frequent administration of large doses (cumulative doses >100 mg) may be necessary in massive exposures

Glycopyrrolate: May be administered if atropine is unavailable

2-PAM: For more significant exposures (ie, exposures requiring large doses of atropine, or with recurring symptoms, or exposures to more lipid soluble agents), administration should follow: 1-2 g I.V. over 5-10 minutes, repeated in 1 hour if asthenia reoccurs, then every 4-12 hours for recurring symptoms

Antidote(s)

Atropine Sulfate *on page 1395*

Pralidoxime Chloride *on page 1461*

Diagnostic Tests/Procedures

Blood Gases, Arterial *on page 1207*

Chest Films *on page 1224*

Complete Blood Count *on page 1236*

Creatinine, Serum *on page 1243*

Electrocardiography *on page 1253*

Liver Profile *on page 1286*

Pseudocholinesterase, Serum *on page 1340*

Pregnancy Implications Human data regarding organophosphate exposure in pregnancy is limited and anecdotal; teratogenesis and fetal death have been produced in animal models at exposure levels that cause obvious toxicity to the pregnant animal

Additional Information Red blood cell cholinesterase, and serum pseudocholinesterase may be depressed following acute or chronic organophosphate exposure; RBC cholinesterase is typically not analyzed by in-house laboratories, and is usually not available for consideration during acute management. Pseudocholinesterase levels may be rapidly available from some in-house laboratories, but are not as reliable a marker of organophosphate exposure because of variability secondary to variant genotypes, hepatic disease, oral estrogen use, or malnutrition. Because of this variability, true indication of suppression of either of these enzymes can only be estimated through comparison to pre-exposure values; these enzymes may be useful in measuring a patient's recovery postexposure, especially if the recovery is not progressing as expected.

Other information concerning pesticide exposures is available through the EPA-funded National Pesticide Telecommunications Network: 1-800-858-7378 (weekdays, 8 AM to 6 PM, Central Standard time)

Specific References

Minton NA and Murray VS, "A Review of Organophosphate Poisoning," *Med Toxicol Adverse Drug Exp*, 1988, 3(5):350-75.

Namba T, Nolte CT, Jackrel J, et al, "Poisoning Due to Organophosphate Insecticides. Acute and Chronic Manifestations," *Am J Med*, 1971, 50(4):475-92.

Propane

CAS Number 74-98-6

UN Number 1978

Synonyms Dimethylmethane; Propyl Hydride

Commonly Found In Component in fuels, solvent

Use In the manufacture of ethylene

(Continued)

Propane *(Continued)*

Mechanism of Toxic Action Displaces oxygen resulting in hypoxia

Adverse Reactions

Cardiovascular: Tachycardia, myocardial ischemia
Ocular: Decreased visual acuity
Respiratory: Tachypnea

Signs & Symptoms of Acute Overdose Chest pain, dyspnea, cyanosis, headache, dizziness, seizures

Overdosage Treatment Supportive therapy: Oxygen therapy - 100% humidified oxygen

Diagnostic Tests/Procedures

Blood Gases, Arterial *on page 1207*
Oxygen Saturation, Blood *on page 1313*

Pregnancy Implications Fetal hypoxia

Additional Information Colorless gas; petroleum-like odor; heavier than air; may form a vapor cloud as a result from refrigeration effect of liquified propane
IDLH: 20,000 ppm

Specific References

Kizer KW, "Toxic Inhalations," *Emerg Med Clin North Am*, 1984, 2(3):649-66.
Siegel E and Wason S, "Sudden Death Caused by Inhalation of Butane and Propane," *N Engl J Med*, 1990, 323(23):1638.

Propane-1,2-Diol *see* Propylene Glycol *on page 1002*

Propanol *see* 1-Propanol *on this page*

1-Propanol

CAS Number 71-23-8

UN Number 1274

Synonyms n-Propyl Alcohol; Optal; Propanol; Propyl Alcohol; Propylic Alcohol

Use In lacquers, cosmetics, cleaners, polishes, and antiseptic agents

Mechanism of Toxic Action Central nervous system depression

Adverse Reactions

Central nervous system: Delirium, coma
Gastrointestinal: Nausea, vomiting
Miscellaneous: Eye, skin, mucous membrane irritation

Signs & Symptoms of Acute Overdose Cutaneous erythema, porphyria, hypotension, nausea, vomiting, diarrhea, gastrointestinal irritation, feces discoloration (black); seizures and coma may develop

Toxicodynamics/Kinetics Absorption: Quick from gastrointestinal tract; can be absorbed dermally

Overdosage Treatment

Decontamination: Lavage/activated charcoal with cathartic
Enhancement of elimination: Hemodialysis for patients in deep and persistent coma

Diagnostic Tests/Procedures

Glucose, Random *on page 1269*
Osmolality, Serum *on page 1310*
pH, Blood *on page 1318*

Pregnancy Implications No effect noted

Additional Information More toxic than isopropyl alcohol; 20 mL of 1-propanol with water can cause hypotension

Specific References

Wallgren H, "Relative Intoxicating Effects on Rats of Ethyl, Propyl, and Butyl Alcohols," *Acta Pharmacol Toxicol (Copenh)*, 1960, 16:217-22.

2-Propanone *see* Acetone *on page 850*

Propenamide *see* Acrylamide *on page 852*

2-Propenamide *see* Acrylamide *on page 852*

2-Propenenitrile *see* Acrylonitrile *on page 853*

Propol *see* Isopropyl Alcohol *on page 943*

Propoxur

CAS Number 114-26-1

Synonyms N-Methyl-2-Isopropoxyphenylcarbamate

Brand Names Baygon®; Isocarb®

Use Marketed as insecticide granules, dusting agent, or spray liquid with or without petroleum derivative as a solvent

Mechanism of Toxic Action Reversible inhibition of acetylcholinesterase and plasma cholinesterase, resulting in excess accumulation of acetylcholine at muscarinic and nicotinic receptors, and in the central nervous system

Adverse Reactions

Cardiovascular: Hyperdynamic (~18% to 21%) or hypodynamic (~7% to 10%) states

Central nervous system: Toxicity is limited because carbamates do not significantly cross the blood-brain barrier; CNS changes occur with most severe intoxications, hyperactivity

Genitourinary: Incontinence

Neuromuscular & skeletal: Weakness, paralysis

Respiratory: Depression, edema

General: Flu-like symptoms (especially with chronic exposure)

Signs & Symptoms of Acute Overdose Miosis (unreactive to light), mydriasis (rarely), lacrimation, pallor, excessive sweating, confusion, agitation, headache, dysarthria, generalized asthenia, seizures, A-V block, coma, decreased hemoglobin/red blood cell count/platelet count, metabolic acidosis and hyperglycemia (severe intoxication), hypotension, hypertension, cranial nerve palsies, bradycardia, tachycardia, Q-T prolongation, heart block, asystole, salivation, bronchorrhea, tachypnea, pulmonary edema, respiratory depression, diaphragmatic paralysis, skeletal muscle fasciculation and flaccid paralysis, nausea, vomiting, abdominal pain, fecal and urinary incontinence; disseminated intravascular coagulation has been reported following massive exposure to propoxur

Toxicodynamics/Kinetics

Absorption: Readily through oral, dermal, or respiratory exposure

Metabolism: Rapidly metabolized to weakly active compounds through hepatic hydrolysis and other pathways, and may undergo enterohepatic recirculation

Elimination: Metabolites are excreted in urine

Warnings Risk of aspiration pneumonitis exists following oral exposure to agents having a hydrocarbon vehicle; severe laryngeal irritation and violent coughing may result from exposure to dusting powders; exposure to dusting powders and insecticide granules may cause contact dermatitis

Overdosage Treatment

Decontamination: Isolation, bagging, and disposal of all contaminated clothing and other articles; all emergency medical workers and hospital staff should follow appropriate precautions regarding exposure to hazardous material including the use of protective clothing, masks, goggles, and respiratory equipment

- Dermal: Prompt thorough scrubbing of all affected areas with soap and water, including hair and nails
- Gastric: Activated charcoal can be administered either orally or via a nasogastric tube; do not induce emesis because of danger of sudden respiratory compromise, alterations in mental status, seizures, coma, and possible aspiration of hydrocarbon vehicles
- Ocular: Irrigation with copious tepid sterile water or saline

Supportive therapy: Including airway management, ventilatory assistance, humidified oxygen administration, and close monitoring for sudden respiratory failure

Antidote:

- Atropine: Administration should be guided by respiratory status, starting at 1-5 mg I.V. every 5-10 minutes as needed, and should be titrated to the resolution of excess pulmonary secretions; frequent administration of large doses (cumulative doses >100 mg) may be necessary in massive exposures
- Glycopyrrolate: May be administered if atropine is unavailable
- 2-PAM: Although not specifically indicated, 2-PAM may be considered in the following situations:
  - Life-threatening symptoms such as respiratory paralysis
  - Continued excessive atropine requirements
  - Concomitant organophosphate and carbamate exposure

Enhancement of elimination: Dialysis and hemoperfusion are not indicated due to effectiveness of the prescribed treatment, large volumes of distribution of organophosphates

Antidote(s)

Atropine Sulfate *on page 1395*

Diagnostic Tests/Procedures

Blood Gases, Arterial *on page 1207*

Chest Films *on page 1224*

Complete Blood Count *on page 1236*

Creatinine, Serum *on page 1243*

Electrocardiography *on page 1253*

Liver Profile *on page 1286*

Pseudocholinesterase, Serum *on page 1340*

Pregnancy Implications Human data regarding organophosphate exposure in pregnancy is limited and anecdotal; teratogenesis and fetal death have been produced in animal models at exposure levels that cause obvious toxicity to the pregnant animal

Additional Information Red blood cell cholinesterase, and serum pseudocholinesterase may be depressed following acute or chronic organophosphate expo-

(Continued)

Propoxur *(Continued)*

sure and are theoretically useful for differentiating between carbamate and organophosphate exposures; RBC cholinesterase is typically not analyzed by inhouse laboratories, and is usually not available for consideration during acute management. Pseudocholinesterase levels may be rapidly available from some inhouse laboratories, but are not as reliable a marker of organophosphate exposure because of variability secondary to variant genotypes, hepatic disease, oral estrogen use, or malnutrition, thus they may not be useful in ruling out carbamate exposure.

Other information concerning pesticide exposures is available through the EPA-funded National Pesticide Telecommunications Network: 1-800-858-7378 (weekdays, 8 AM to 6 PM, Central Standard time)

Specific References

Zwiener RJ and Ginsburg CM, "Organophosphate and Carbamate Poisoning in Infants and Children," *Pediatrics*, 1988, 81(1):121-6.

Propylacetone *see* 2-Hexanone *on page 938*

Propyl Alcohol *see* 1-Propanol *on page 1000*

Propylcarbinol *see* Butyl Alcohol *on page 875*

Propylene Aldehyde *see* Acrolein *on page 852*

Propylene Glycol

CAS Number 57-55-6

Synonyms Methyl Glycol; PG 12; Propane-1,2-Diol; Trimethyl Glycol

Use In cosmetics and as a solvent in pharmaceuticals; also used as a deicer

Mechanism of Toxic Action Metabolized to lactic acid, pyruvic acid, acetic acid, and propionaldehyde

Adverse Reactions

Cardiovascular: Bradycardia, ventricular arrhythmias

Endocrine & metabolic: Hypoglycemia, lactic acidosis, hyperosmolality

Hematologic: Hemolysis

Renal: Renal failure

Signs & Symptoms of Acute Overdose Stupor, seizures, porphyria, feces discoloration (black), lacrimation, hypotension, central nervous system depression

Toxicodynamics/Kinetics

Distribution: V_d: 0.55 L/kg

Metabolism: To lactic acid and pyruvic acid

Half-life: Adults: 2-5 hours

Peak serum concentration: 1 hour postingestion

Elimination: 12% to 45% excreted unchanged renally; total body elimination: 0.1 L/kg/hour

Reference Range Propylene glycol level (mg/dL): 84.6 + (7.8 x osmolar gap in mOsm/kg); serum levels of 6-1000 mg/L have been noted following intravenous administration

Overdosage Treatment

Decontamination: Do not use ipecac

Supportive therapy: Sodium bicarbonate (I.V.) for metabolic acidosis; ethanol therapy is not useful

Enhancement of elimination: Hemodialysis is effective

Antidote(s)

Sodium Bicarbonate *on page 1467*

Diagnostic Tests/Procedures

Glucose, Random *on page 1269*

Ketone Bodies, Blood *on page 1277*

Kidney Profile *on page 1279*

Lactic Acid, Blood *on page 1281*

Osmolality, Serum *on page 1310*

pH, Blood *on page 1318*

Pregnancy Implications Not teratogenic

Additional Information 60 mL of propylene glycol can cause stupor in infants; clear, colorless, and odorless; found in intravenous preparations of diazepam and phenytoin; added to foods at concentrations up to 15% to food seasoning

Atmospheric half-life: 20-32 hours

Water half-life: 1.3-2.3 years

Specific References

Arulanantham K and Genel M, "Central Nervous System Toxicity Associated With Ingestion of Propylene Glycol," *J Pediatr*, 1978, 93(3):515-6.

Fisher AA, "Systemic Contact Dermatitis Due to Intravenous Valium in a Person Sensitive to Propylene Glycol," *Cutis*, 1995, 55:327-8.

Hardin BD and Lyon JP, "Summary and Overview of NIOSH Symposium on Toxic Effects of Glycol Ethers," *Environ Health Perspect*, 1984, 57:273.

Kelner MJ and Bailey DN, "Propylene Glycol as the Cause of Lactic Acidosis," *J Anal Toxicol*, 1985, 9(1):40-2.

Lolin Y, Francis DA, Flanagan RJ, et al, "Cerebral Depression Due to Propylene Glycol in a Patient With Chronic Epilepsy - The Value of the Plasma Osmolol Gap in Diagnosis," *Postgrad Med J*, 1988, 64(754):610-3.

Propylene Glycol Dinitrate

Related Information

Nitrates *on page 978*

CAS Number 6423-43-4; 106602-80-6 (Otto Fuel II)

Synonyms Isopropylene Dinitrate; Methyl Nitroglycol; PGDN

Use Nitrated ester primarily used as a propellant in Oto Fuel II (a liquid monopropellant used by the U.S. Navy in torpedoes and other weapons); has been used in explosives

Adverse Reactions

Central nervous system: Ataxia at air levels of 1.5 ppm; headaches

Gastrointestinal: Nausea/dizziness at levels of 0.5 ppm

Miscellaneous: Methemoglobin levels as high as 24% noted in rodents exposed to 200 ppm for 4 hours

Toxicodynamics/Kinetics

Absorption: Inhalation and dermal

Metabolism: Broken down in erythrocytes to nitrate

Elimination: Urinary

Reference Range Blood propylene glycol dinitrate level of 5 ppb noted after 3.2 hours exposure to 1.5 ppm air concentration

Overdosage Treatment

Decontamination:

- Inhalation: Administer 100% oxygen
- Dermal: Wash with soap and water
- Ocular: Irrigate with saline
- Oral: Dilute with milk or water; activated charcoal may be given

Supportive therapy: Methylene blue for symptomatic methemoglobinemia

Antidote(s)

Methylene Blue *on page 1444*

Monitoring Parameters Methemoglobin

Additional Information High explosive agent; slightly soluble in water (1.3 g/L) and does not persist in water for more than a few days; air levels near U.S. torpedo facilities of propylene glycol dinitrate range from 0-2.2 ppm

PEL-TWA: 0.05 ppm

TLV-TWA (skin designation): 0.05 ppm

Specific References

Horvath EP, Ilka RA, Boyd J, et al, "Evaluation of Neurophysiologic Effects of 1,2-Propylene Glycol Dinitrate by Quantitative Ataxia and Oculomotor Function Tests," *Am J Ind Med*, 1981, 2(4):365-8.

Stewart RD, Peterson JE, Newton PE, et al, "Experimental Human Exposure to Propylene Glycol Dinitrate," *Toxicol Appl Pharmacol*, 1974, 30(3):377-95.

U.S. Department of Health and Human Services, "Toxicological Profile for Otto Fuel II and its Components," Agency for Toxic Substances and Diseases Registry, May, 1993.

Propyl Hydride *see* Propane *on page 999*

Propylic Alcohol *see* 1-Propanol *on page 1000*

Propylmethanol *see* Butyl Alcohol *on page 875*

Pu *see* Plutonium *on page 995*

Puralin® *see* Thiram *on page 1027*

PX-138® *see* Di-n-Octylphthalate *on page 916*

Pyran Aldehyde *see* Acrolein *on page 852*

Pyrene *see* Polycyclic Aromatic Hydrocarbons *on page 997*

Pyrethrins (pye ree' thrins)

CAS Number 8003-34-7; 121-21-1; 121-29-9; 25402-06-6; 121-20-0; 52645-53-1

Synonyms Ambush; Buhach; BW-21-Z; *Chrysanthemum cinerareaefolium*; Cinerin; Cyclopropanecarboxylic Acid; Dalmation-Insect Flowers; Dalmation-Insect Powder; Ectiban; Firmotox; FMX 33297; Insect Powder; Jasmolin; Permethrin; Permetrina (Portuguese); Persian-Insect Powder; Pounce; Pyrethrum Esters; Trieste Flowers

Brand Names A-200™ Pyrinate [OTC]; Alfadex®; RID® [OTC]; Tisit® [OTC]

Commonly Found In Pyrethrins include pyrethrum extract and the pyrethrum esters: cinerin I and II, jasmolin I and II, and pyrethrin I and II; semisynthetic derivatives (pyrethroids) include allethrin, barthrin, bioallethrin, bioresmethrin, cyclethrin, cypermethrin, decamethrin, dimethrin, fenvalerate, flucythrinate, permethrin, phenothrin, and resmethrin; preparations often contain a synergist which increases

(Continued)

Pyrethrins *(Continued)*

stability and insecticidal activity, such as N-isobutyldecylenamidepiperonyl butoxide, piperonyl cyclonene, n-octyl sulfoxide of isosafrole, n-propylisome, and sesamex; sprays often formulated in petroleum solvent bases, such as kerosene and naphtha, which are generally more hazardous than the pyrethrins

Use Treatment of *Pediculus humanus* infestations

Mechanism of Toxic Action Delay closure of sodium channel by holding activation gate in the open position, producing a prolonged sodium current during the end of depolarization; sodium tail currents are more prolonged with pyrethroids with an alpha-cyano group (eg, cypermethrin, fenvalerate, flucythrinate) than with other pyrethroids. Derived from flowers that belong to the chrysanthemum family. The mechanism of action on the neuronal membranes of lice is similar to that of DDT. Piperonyl butoxide is usually added to pyrethrin to enhance the product's activity by decreasing the metabolism of pyrethrins in arthropods.

Adverse Reactions

Dermatologic: Pruritus, erythema

Local: Burning, stinging

Respiratory: Oropharyngeal irritation, wheezing, sneezing, rhinitis, chest pain, hypersensitivity pneumonitis

Signs & Symptoms of Acute Overdose Generally of very low order of toxicity in man due to low bioavailability and high first-pass metabolism; pyrethrins are potent sensitizers, therefore, most common complications are hypersensitivity reactions, including erythematous, vesicular, papular, bullous contact dermatitis (occurs in 50% of those sensitive to ragweed, sometimes with eosinophilia), wheezing, asthma, and anaphylactic shock. Dizziness, headache, nausea, vomiting, and asthenia are commonly seen with oral ingestions; other symptoms that may occur are pneumonitis, seizures, pulmonary edema, cough, and chest pain. Ingestion of massive quantities or concentrated formulations may cause CNS stimulation, tremor, ataxia, and cardiopulmonary arrest. Nasal congestion, rhinorrhea, scratchy throat, and hypersensitivity reactions including wheezing, sneezing, dyspnea, and wheezing may be seen with inhalational exposure; corneal abrasions may occur with eye exposure; paresthesia and erythema are common following dermal exposure. In general, pyrethroids or synthetic derivatives are neither cutaneous sensitizers nor irritants and are less toxic than natural pyrethrins; however, they may cause paresthesias following dermal exposure. Synergists appear to be of even lower toxicity based on experiments with laboratory mammals, despite their ability to enhance insecticidal activity. However, it has been postulated that they might have the potential to inhibit the microsomal enzyme metabolism of pyrethrins and perhaps increase their toxicity in man.

Toxicodynamics/Kinetics

Onset of action: ~30 minutes

Absorption: Rapid; pyrethrins and pyrethroids are believed to be poorly absorbed through intact skin

Distribution: Through body tissues and brain

Metabolism: Rapid, however pathways of metabolism are somewhat controversial; pyrethrins I and II are metabolized rapidly by hydrolysis to chrysanthemumic acid and an alcohol, which is oxidized to the aldehyde and acid or conjugated with glucuronide; more recent evidence in rats indicates that the principal metabolites are oxidation products; pyrethroids are primarily metabolized by ester hydrolysis

Elimination: Slowly excreted in bile and urine and may remain detectable in body tissues for up to 3 weeks after ingestion

Contraindications Known hypersensitivity to pyrethrins

Reference Range Pyrethrin plasma levels are not clinically useful

Overdosage Treatment

Decontamination: Usually sufficient for most causal exposures; for oral ingestions, gastric emptying should be performed with lavage, avoiding syrup of ipecac/emesis due to risk of seizures; follow with administration of activated charcoal/cathartic; the principal concern with most solutions and sprays is the hydrocarbon solvent. For preparations containing a hydrocarbon, refer to appropriate monograph; avoid administration of fats and oils, which increase intestinal absorption of pyrethrins; diazepam or lorazepam for seizures; atropine may be effective for diarrhea; irrigate eye exposures promptly with copious amounts of water. Wash contaminated skin promptly with copious amounts of soap and water.

Supportive therapy: Topical vitamin E may relieve paresthesias; symptomatic and supportive treatment for allergic reactions; epinephrine or diphenhydramine for allergic reactions; nebulized bronchodilators for wheezing

Monitoring Parameters Seizures, respiratory distress, and hypersensitivity reactions

Additional Information Patients with allergy to ragweed may develop cross-allergy to pyrethrins

IDLH: 5000 mg/m^3
TLV-TWA: 5 mg/m^3
PEC-TWA: 5 mg/m^3

Specific References

Coats JR, "Mechanisms of Toxic Action and Structure-Activity Relationships for Organochlorine and Synthetic Pyrethroids Insecticide," *Environ Health Perspect*, 1990, 87:255-62.

Culver CA, Malina JJ, and Talbert RL, "Probable Anaphylactoid Reaction to a Pyrethrin Pediculicide Shampoo," *Clin Pharm*, 1988, 7(11):846-9.

Dorman DC and Beasley VR, "Neurotoxicity of Pyrethrin and the Pyrethroid Insecticides," *Vet Hum Toxicol*, 1991, 33(3):238-43.

Wax PM and Hoffman RS, "Fatality Associated With Inhalation of a Pyrethrin Shampoo," *J Toxicol Clin Toxicol*, 1994, 32(4):457-60.

Pyrethrum Esters *see* Pyrethrins *on page 1003*

Pyridine

CAS Number 110-86-1

UN Number 1282

Synonyms Azabenzine; Azine

Use Primarily in production of pesticides, herbicides, antihistamines, steroids, sulfa antibiotics, water repellants, dyes, paint, and rubber; flavoring agent and as an agent to denature alcohol

Mechanism of Toxic Action Lipid peroxidation of the brain can occur

Adverse Reactions

Cardiovascular: Tachycardia
Central nervous system: Lethargy, headaches, slurred speech, insomnia, fatigue
Dermatologic: Dermatitis
Gastrointestinal: Nausea, vomiting
Hepatic: Cirrhosis
Respiratory: Tachypnea

Toxicodynamics/Kinetics

Absorption: With oral ingestion
Metabolism: Hepatic to N-methylpyridinium
Elimination: Renal

Overdosage Treatment

Decontamination:
- Dermal: Wash with soap and water
- Ocular: Irrigate with saline
- Oral: Lavage/activated charcoal; do not induce emesis

Pregnancy Implications Skeletal abnormalities noted in chickens

Additional Information Central nervous symptoms can occur with exposures of 6-12 ppm; inhibits metabolism of benzene; not usually detected in ambient air

Lethal dose: 125 mL
Odor threshold: Air: 0.17 ppm; water: 0.95 mg/L
Atmospheric half-life: 23-46 days
Water half-life: 1.2 years
Soil half-life: 3 days
Yearly total pyridine intake: ~500 mg
PEL-TWA: 5 ppm
TLV-TWA: 5 ppm
IDLH: 3600 ppm

Specific References

U.S. Department of Health and Human Services, "Toxicological Profile for Pyridine TP-91/24," Agency for Toxic Substances and Diseases Registry, September 1992.

Pyriminil *see* Nitrophenolurea *on page 981*

Pyrinex® *see* Chlorpyrifos *on page 891*

Pyrophoric *see* Thorium *on page 1027*

Quickphos® *see* Aluminum Phosphide *on page 857*

Quintar *see* Dichloronaphthoquinone *on page 908*

Quintox® *see* Dieldrin *on page 911*

R40 *see* Chloromethane *on page 891*

Racumin® *see* Anticoagulant Rodenticide *on page 859*

Radiation: Basics of Exposure *see page 1594*

Radium

Related Information

Radiation: Basics of Exposure *on page 1594-1600*
Radon *on next page*

CAS Number 7440-14-4

Synonyms Radium-223; Radium-224; Radium-226; Radium-228

(Continued)

Radium *(Continued)*

Use Radiation source in treating neoplasms

Adverse Reactions

Hematologic: Leukopenia
Hepatic: Cirrhosis
Ocular: Cataracts

Toxicodynamics/Kinetics

Absorption: Inhalation and oral (~20%)
Elimination: Primarily fecal

Overdosage Treatment

Decontamination:
Dermal: Wash with soap and water; monitor with a Geiger-Mueller counter
Ocular: Irrigate with saline

Additional Information Bone sarcomas, breast cancer, and liver cancer have been associated with radium exposure; chronic myeloid leukemia also noted
Oral lethal dose: 56 uCi/kg (2.074 kBq/kg)
Malignancy can occur at a dose of 1.03 uCi/kg (38 kBq/kg)
Residence atmosphere time: 1-10 days
Radium-223:
Decay mode: Alpha
Soil half-life: 11 days
Radium-224:
Decay mode: Alpha
Soil half-life: 4 days
Radium-226:
Decay mode: Alpha
Soil half-life: 1620 years
Radium-228:
Decay mode: Beta
Soil half-life: 6 years

Specific References

Polednak AP, Stehney AF, and Rowland RE, "Mortality in Women First Employed Before 1930 in the U.S. Radium Dial-Painting Industry," *Am J Epidemiol*, 1978, 107(3):179-95.

Radium-223 *see* Radium *on previous page*

Radium-224 *see* Radium *on previous page*

Radium-226 *see* Radium *on previous page*

Radium-228 *see* Radium *on previous page*

Radon

Related Information

Radium *on previous page*

CAS Number 10043-92-2; 14859-67-7

Synonyms Radon 222; Rn

Use Product of natural decay of uranium which is then converted to radium 222 and finally as a sixth decay product as uranium 238; miners can be exposed in uranium or phosphate mines; also used as a gas tracer in detecting leaks and in the study of atmospheric transport; building materials made of vanadium or concrete produced from phosphate slag may have elevated radon content; see figure.

Mechanism of Toxic Action Attaches to bronchial epithelium which can lead to malignant transformation

Adverse Reactions

Dermal: Radiation dermatitis
Ocular: Cataracts
Renal: Nephritis
Respiratory: Lung cancer (additive effect with smoking), emphysema, pulmonary fibrosis at high doses

Toxicodynamics/Kinetics

Absorption:
Inhalation: 30% to 40%
Oral: 90%
Dermal: 5%
Half-life:
Air: 4 days
Lungs: 6-60 hours
Fat: 21-130 minutes
Oral ingestion: 18-180 minutes
Metabolism: Radon daughters include polonium 218, lead 214, bismuth 214, and polonium 214; does not undergo biological metabolism
Elimination: Exhalation primarily

Overdosage Treatment

Decontamination: Affected homes may require subslab depressurization; open windows can reduce indoor radon levels by 50% to 70%; see figure.

Sources of Radon and Common Entry Points

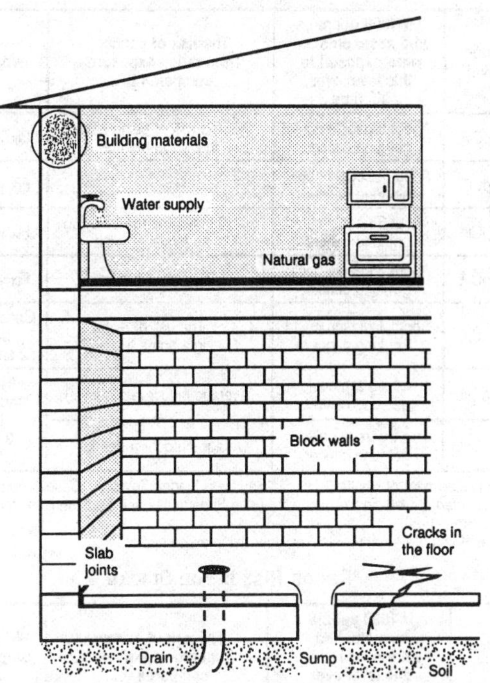

Subslab Depressurization

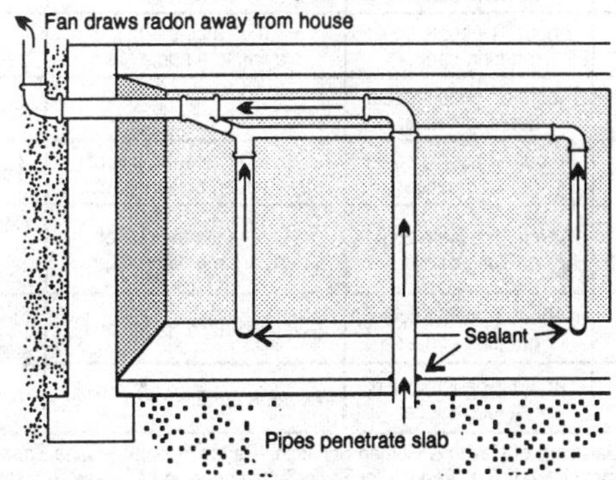

Supportive therapy: Cataracts and lung carcinoma are treated with standard therapies; affected individuals should stop smoking

Diagnostic Tests/Procedures

Chest Films *on page 1224*

Pregnancy Implications Increased incidence of spontaneous abortions

Additional Information For risk assessment, see tables on next page.

Ambient, outdoor air concentration of 0.2-0.7 pCi/L; radon is odorless, inert, and colorless; EPA action level: 4 pCi/L (0.02 working level of radon); levels exceeding the EPA action level may be present in ~25% of homes in the U.S.

Specific References

American College of Occupational and Environmental Medicine, "ACOEM Position Statement on Residential Radon Exposure," *J Occup Med*, 1992, 34(10):1028-30.

Council on Scientific Affairs, "Radon in Homes," *JAMA*, 1987, 258(5):668-72.

Pershagen G, Akerblom G, Axelson O, et al, "Residential Radon Exposure and Lung Cancer in Sweden," *N Engl J Med*, 1994, 330(3):159-64.

U.S. Department of Health and Human Services, "Case Studies in Environmental Medicine Radon Toxicity," Agency for Toxic Substances and Diseases Registry, September, 1992.

Radon Risk if You Have Never Smoked

Radon Level	If 1000 people who never smoked were exposed to this level over a lifetime...	The risk of cancer from radon exposure compares to...	What to Do:
20 pCi/L	About 8 people could get lung cancer	← The risk of being killed in a violent crime	Fix your home
10 pCi/L	About 4 people could get lung cancer		Fix your home
8 pCi/L	About 3 people could get lung cancer	← 10 times the risk of dying in an airplane crash	Fix your home
4 pCi/L	About 2 people could get lung cancer	← The risk of drowning	Fix your home
2 pCi/L	About 1 person could get lung cancer	← The risk of dying in a home fire	Consider fixing between 2 and 4 pCi/L
1.3 pCi/L	<1 person could get lung cancer	(Average indoor radon level)	(Reducing radon levels below 2 pCi/L is difficult)
0.4 pCi/L	<1 person could get lung cancer	(Average outdoor radon level)	

U.S. Department of Health & Human Services, "Radon Toxicity," *Case Studies in Environmental Medicine,* Agency for Toxic Substances and Disease Registry, September 1992.
Note: If you are a former smoker, your risk may be higher.

Radon Risk if You Smoke

Radon Level	If 1000 people who smoked were exposed to this level over a lifetime...	The risk of cancer from radon exposure compares to...	What to Do: Stop smoking and...
20 pCi/L	About 135 people could get lung cancer	← 100 times the risk of drowning	Fix your home
10 pCi/L	About 71 people could get lung cancer	← 100 times the risk of dying in a home fire	Fix your home
8 pCi/L	About 57 people could get lung cancer		Fix your home
4 pCi/L	About 29 people could get lung cancer	← 100 times the risk of dying in an airplane crash	Fix your home
2 pCi/L	About 15 people could get lung cancer	← 2 times the risk of dying in a car crash	Consider fixing between 2 and 4 pCi/L
1.3 pCi/L	About 9 people could get lung cancer	(Average indoor radon level)	(Reducing radon levels below 2 pCi/L is difficult)
0.4 pCi/L	About 3 people could get lung cancer	(Average outdoor radon level)	

U.S. Department of Health & Human Services, "Radon Toxicity," *Case Studies in Environmental Medicine,* Agency for Toxic Substances and Disease Registry, September 1992.
Note: If you are a former smoker, your risk may be lower.

Radon 222 *see* Radon *on page 1006*

Ramucide® *see* Anticoagulant Rodenticide *on page 859*

Raney Alloy *see* Nickel *on page 976*

Raney Nickel *see* Nickel *on page 976*

Rasikal *see* Chlorate Salts *on page 884*

Ratafin® *see* Anticoagulant Rodenticide *on page 859*

Ratak® *see* Anticoagulant Rodenticide *on page 859*

Ratimus® *see* Anticoagulant Rodenticide *on page 859*

Ratindan® *see* Anticoagulant Rodenticide *on page 859*

Raviac® *see* Anticoagulant Rodenticide *on page 859*

RDX

Related Information

HMX *on page 939*

CAS Number 121-82-4

Synonyms Cyclonite; Hexogen; Hexolite; PBX

Brand Names Composition C-4

Use Class A explosive; nitrate compound used in plastic explosives, fireworks, and as a detonator; rodenticide

Mechanism of Toxic Action Causes fatty degeneration of liver; seizure mechanism of action is unknown

Adverse Reactions

Cardiovascular: Tachycardia
Central nervous system: Seizures, irritability, amnesia, confusion, hyperthermia
Dermatologic: Dermal irritant
Gastrointestinal: Nausea, vomiting
Hematologic: Anemia
Hepatic: Liver tumors (adenomas and carcinomas) produced in rodent models
Neuromuscular & skeletal: Muscle twitching, myoclonus
Renal: Hematuria

Toxicodynamics/Kinetics

Absorption: Oral (slowly) and inhalation; not readily absorbed by dermal route
Distribution: V_d: 2.2 L/kg
Half-life: 15 hours
Elimination: Feces (primarily) and urine

Reference Range Serum RDX level of 10.7 mg/L associated with seizures

Overdosage Treatment

Decontamination:
Dermal: Wash hands with soap and water
Ocular: Irrigate with saline
Oral: Activated charcoal may be used
Supportive therapy: Seizures can be treated with benzodiazepines or phenobarbital

Additional Information Oral dose of 85 mg/kg has caused seizures in a child

Atmospheric half-life: 1.5 hours
Water half-life: 9-13 hours (by photolysis)
PEL-TWA: 1.5 mg/m^3 (skin designation)
TLV-TWA: 1.5 mg/m^3 (skin designation)
Toxic oral dose: 15 mL

Specific References

Twibell JD, Turner SL, Smalldon KW, et al, "The Persistence of Military Explosives on Hands," *J Forensic Sci*, 1984, 29:284-90.

U.S. Department of Health and Human Services, "Toxicological Profile of RDX," Agency for Toxic Substances and Diseases Registry, May 1993.

Woody RC, Kearns GL, Brewster MA, et al, "The Neurotoxicity of Cyclotrimethylenetrinitramine (RDX) in a Child: A Clinical and Pharmacokinetic Evaluation," *J Toxicol Clin Toxicol*, 1986, 24(4):305-19.

Redax® *see* N-Nitrosodiphenylamine *on page 982*

Red Phosphorus *see* White Phosphorus *on page 1039*

Red Shield® *see* Dieldrin *on page 911*

Retarder J® *see* N-Nitrosodiphenylamine *on page 982*

Rezifilm® *see* Thiram *on page 1027*

Rhodium

CAS Number 7440-16-6

Mechanism of Toxic Action Some reaction with rhodium and DNA/RNA is apparent; it is not known what the clinical implication of this is

Adverse Reactions Likely that soluble rhodium is toxic, but there is no human literature to support this; mice have shown both respiratory and CNS depression

Signs & Symptoms of Acute Overdose Mild ocular irritation; urticaria

Toxicodynamics/Kinetics Absorption: Elemental rhodium is poorly soluble and minimally absorbed; organic rhodium and rhodium trichloride are more readily absorbed

Reference Range No established toxic levels; TWA (metal): 1 mg/m^3; TWA (insoluble compound): 1 mg/m^3; TWA (soluble compound): 0.01 mg/m^3

Overdosage Treatment Decontamination: Irrigate eyes with normal saline using a Morgan's lens

Specific References

Proctor NH, Hughes JP, and Fischman ML, *Chemical Hazards of the Workplace*, 2nd ed, Philadelphia, PA: Lippincott Co, 1988.

RID® [OTC] *see* Pyrethrins *on page 1003*

Rn *see* Radon *on page 1006*

Rodentin® *see* Anticoagulant Rodenticide *on page 859*

Ro-Dex® *see* Strychnine *on page 1016*

Rothane® *see* DDD *on page 902*

Ruthenium

Related Information

Radiation: Basics of Exposure *on page 1594-1600*

CAS Number 7440-18-8

Signs & Symptoms of Acute Overdose Fumes may be injurious to eyes and lungs

Reference Range No TLV recommended

Overdosage Treatment

Decontamination: Irrigate eyes with normal saline using a Morgan's lens

Supportive therapy: Humidified oxygen for fume exposure

Specific References

Browning E, *Toxicity of Industrial Metals*, 2nd ed, London: Butlerworths, 1969.

Sakresote® 100 (Coal Tar Creosote) *see* Creosote *on page 898*

Sanocide® *see* Hexachlorobenzene *on page 936*

Sanquinon *see* Dichloronaphthoquinone *on page 908*

Santophen® 20 *see* Pentachlorophenol *on page 990*

Sarin (GB or Isopropyl Methylphosphonofluoridate) *see* Nerve Gases *on page 974*

Sb(0) *see* Antimony *on page 862*

Sb(-3) *see* Antimony *on page 862*

Sb(+3) *see* Antimony *on page 862*

Sb(+5) *see* Antimony *on page 862*

Seedrin® *see* Aldrin *on page 856*

Selecron® *see* Profenofos *on page 998*

Selenate *see* Selenium *on next page*

Selenious Acid

CAS Number 7783-00-8

Synonyms Selenous Acid, Monohydrated Selenium Dioxide

Commonly Found In Component of compound for gun blueing agent, reagent for alkaloids

Mechanism of Toxic Action Inhibition of sulfhydryl-containing enzymes

Adverse Reactions

Cardiovascular: Hypertension, tachycardia, cardiomyopathy

Central nervous system: Convulsions

Dermatologic: Alopecia

Gastrointestinal: Pharyngeal edema, intestinal distention, hypersalivation, garlic odor, vomiting, watery diarrhea

Miscellaneous: Burns to the esophagus, pharyngeal, and gastrointestinal tract

Signs & Symptoms of Acute Overdose Hypersalivation, vomiting, diarrhea, seizures, muscle spasms, dermal irritant, garlic odor

Toxicodynamics/Kinetics

Absorption:
- Inhalation: 97%
- Ingestion: 87%
- Dermal

Half-life: 1.2 days

Elimination: 50% excreted renally

Reference Range

Normal range:
- Urine: 7.0-160.0 μg/L
- Blood: 100.0-340.0 μg/L
- Serum: 86.0-125.0 μg/L

Toxic range:
- Urine: >400.0 μg/L
- Postmortem serum level of 18.4 mg/L and urine level of 2.11 mg/L described in one case report

Overdosage Treatment

Decontamination: Emesis is contraindicated; basic poison management with lavage/activated charcoal with cathartic

Supportive therapy: British anti-Lewisite (BAL), calcium sodium EDTA, D-penicillamine is contraindicated since it can increase renal injury

Diagnostic Tests/Procedures

Blood Gases, Arterial *on page 1207*

Complete Blood Count *on page 1236*

Glucose, Random *on page 1269*

Liver Profile *on page 1286*

Monitoring Parameters Thrombocytopenia, leukocytosis, metabolic acidosis, hyperglycemia, transient elevation of hepatic enzymes

Additional Information Garlic odor; vapors are pink; bitter taste

Odor threshold: 0.002 mg/m^3

TLV-TWA: 0.2 mg/m^3

IDLH: 100 mg/m^3

PEL-TWA: 0.2 mg/m^3

Ingestion of 15 mL of 2% solution has been fatal in a 2 year old; 30-60 mL fatal in adults

Specific References

Nantel AJ, Brown M, Dery P, et al, "Acute Poisoning by Selenious Acid," *Vet Hum Toxicol*, 1985, 27(6):531-3.

Selenium

Related Information

Copper *on page 896*

CAS Number 7782-49-2

UN Number 2658

Synonyms Selenate

Use Blasting caps, rectifiers, photoelectric cells, nutritional food additive for poultry and livestock

Mechanism of Toxic Action Inactivates sulfhydryl groups of enzymes; selenium is a component of glutathione peroxidase enzyme

Adverse Reactions Eyes, nose, throat, cardiovascular, respiratory, neurologic, gastrointestinal, hepatic, genitourinary, dermatologic

Signs & Symptoms of Acute Overdose Redness of eye, nasal irritation, tremor, myoglobinuria, sore throat, garlic-like breath, T-wave flattening → inversion, prolonged Q-T, pulmonary edema, fingernail loss, metal fume fever, CNS depression → coma, paresthesia, nausea, vomiting, salivation, hair discoloration (red), increased LFTs, fatty degeneration of liver, tubular degeneration, photocontact dermatitis, pruritus

Toxicodynamics/Kinetics

Absorption: Orally (80%) and by inhalation

Distribution: To all soft tissue, especially liver and kidney

Protein binding: 95%

Half-life: 116 days

Elimination: Primarily by kidney, also through breath and feces

Reference Range

Normal range:

Serum: 95-165 ng/mL

Urine: 15-150 μg/L

Overdosage Treatment

Decontamination:

Dermal: Remove contaminated clothing; wash with soap and water

Ocular: Irrigate with saline

Oral: Emesis is contraindicated; basic poison management with lavage/activated charcoal with cathartic

Supportive therapy: British anti-Lewisite (BAL), calcium sodium EDTA, D-penicillamine is contraindicated since it can increase renal injury; humidified oxygen for fume exposure; ascorbic acid can increase toxic effects and should be avoided

Diagnostic Tests/Procedures

Selenium, Serum *on page 1349*

Selenium, Urine *on page 1350*

Pregnancy Implications Selenium readily crosses placenta; at term, maternal and fetal levels are similar; there has been an unconfirmed association with abortion

Additional Information Soluble selenites, selenates, and organic selenium compounds are more toxic than the insoluble (ie, selenium sulfide)

24-hour urine level: <30 μg/L

Average hair levels in U.S.: 0-0.5 ppm

Average air concentrations: >10 ng/m^3

Average concentration in earth's crust: 0.05-0.09 mg/kg; highest concentrations are found in volcanic rocks in Western and Midwest U.S. and may be as high as 120 mg/kg; coal contains 2 mg/kg, while crude petroleum contains as high as 950 mg/kg

Raw beef kidney (average 1.7 mg selenium/kg weight), swordfish (2.8 mg/kg), and Brazilian nuts (14.7 mg/kg) are foods containing highest amount of selenium

(Continued)

Selenium *(Continued)*

Daily intake: ~0.07-0.15 mg
TLV-TWA: 0.2 mg/m^3

Specific References

Barlow SM and Sullivan FM, eds, *Reproductive Hazards of Industrial Chemicals: An Evaluation of Animal and Human Studies*, London: Academic Press, 1982.

Longnecker MP, "Selenium: The Public Health Connection," *Health Environ Dig*, 1989, 3:1-3.

U.S. Department of Health and Human Services, "Toxicological Profile for Selenium," Agency for Toxic Substances and Diseases Registry, August, 1994.

Selenium Dioxide

CAS Number 7746-08-4

UN Number 2811

Synonyms Selenium Oxide

Commonly Found In Gun-blueing solution

Use Catalyst in production of organic compounds

Mechanism of Toxic Action Inhibition of sulfhydryl-containing enzymes; selenium is a component of glutathione peroxidase enzyme

Adverse Reactions

Central nervous system: Coma
Respiratory: Wheezing
Miscellaneous: Fingernails, teeth, and hair may stain red

Signs & Symptoms of Acute Overdose Cough, dyspnea, transient loss of consciousness, tachypnea, fever, throat irritation, sternal pain, dermal burns, gagging, headache, dizziness

Toxicodynamics/Kinetics Absorption: Inhalation: Well absorbed

Reference Range

Normal range:
Serum: 95-165 ng/mL
Urine: 15-150 μg/L

Overdosage Treatment

Decontamination: Oxygenation; 10% ointment of sodium thiosulfate may be useful; British anti-Lewisite (BAL) is contraindicated
Dermal: Remove contaminated clothing; wash with soap and water
Ocular: Irrigate with saline

Supportive therapy: British anti-Lewisite (BAL), calcium sodium EDTA, D-penicillamine is contraindicated since it can increase renal injury; ascorbic acid can increase toxic effects and should be avoided

Diagnostic Tests/Procedures

Blood Gases, Arterial *on page 1207*
Chest Films *on page 1224*

Specific References

Hamilton and Hardy, *Industrial Toxicology*, 4th edition, Finkel AF, ed, Boston, MA: John Wright, PSG Inc, 1983, 123-5.

Koppel C, Baudisch H, and Beyer KH, "Fatal Poisoning With Selenium Dioxide," *J Toxicol Clin Toxicol*, 1986, 24(1):21-35.

U.S. Department of Health and Human Services, "Toxicological Profile for Selenium," Agency for Toxic Substances and Diseases Registry, August 1994.

Selenium Oxide *see* Selenium Dioxide *on this page*

Selenous Acid, Monohydrated Selenium Dioxide *see* Selenious Acid *on page 1010*

Selinon® *see* Dinitrocresol *on page 915*

Sevin® *see* Carbaryl *on page 877*

Sewer Gas *see* Hydrogen Sulfide *on page 942*

Shed-a-Leaf *see* Chlorate Salts *on page 884*

Shell Silver *see* Silver *on this page*

Silber *see* Silver *on this page*

Silo-Filler's Disease *see* Nitrogen Oxide *on page 980*

Silver

CAS Number 7440-22-4

Synonyms Argentum; Shell Silver; Silber

Use Primarily in photography and electronic products (ie, batteries); coinage use was discontinued in 1970

Mechanism of Toxic Action Silver has a strong affinity for sulfhydryl groups and proteins; systemic toxicity is rare due to rapid binding to proteins; argyria is a blue-gray discoloration of skin, mucous membrane, and eye which results from silver deposition

Adverse Reactions HEENT, respiratory, photocontact dermatitis

Signs & Symptoms of Acute Overdose Blue-gray discoloration of conjunctivitis, cornea, and lens; bronchitis, cough, throat irritation, feces discoloration (black), abdominal pain, wheezing, skin burns, proteinuria, hypertension, bradycardia, nail bed pigmentation

Toxicodynamics/Kinetics

Absorption: From the respiratory tract and gastrointestinal tract occurs with soluble silver salts; complex salts are dermally absorbed; burn patients absorb silver from silver sulfadiazine

Distribution: Widely distributed

Half-life, biological: Human lung: ~1 day

Elimination: Primarily excreted through bile

Reference Range

Normal blood levels: Undetectable

Mean blood silver levels: 0.11 μg/mL documented in workers of a photographic materials manufacturer exposed to 0.001-0.1 mg/m^3 of silver

Overdosage Treatment

Decontamination: Do not induce emesis, activated charcoal with cathartic may be utilized

Supportive therapy: Wheezing can be treated with nebulized beta agonist agents

Diagnostic Tests/Procedures

Silver, Serum *on page 1351*

Silver, Urine *on page 1351*

Additional Information Argyria is the development of a slate gray or blue gray irreversible pigmentation of skin due to deposition of silver sulfide in the dermis; argyria generally occurs after injection of 1 g of elemental silver or ingestion of 3.8 g; average dietary intake of silver: 70-88 mcg with drinking water providing ~20 mcg of silver

OSHA TWA: 0.01 mg/m^3

PEL-TWA: 0.01 mg/m^3

Background atmospheric silver levels: <1 ng/m^3

Background water silver levels: ~0.2 μg/L in freshwater and 0.25 μg/L in salt water

Average silver concentration in earth's crust: 0.1 ppm

Cigarettes contain from 0.2 mg/kg (nonfilter) to 0.3 mg/kg (filter) of silver

Shellfish (particularly oysters) may contain as much as 5.5 mg/kg of silver

Permissible amount of silver in bottled water: 0.05 mg/L

Specific References

OSHA: Department of Labor, Occupational Safety and Health Administration, 29 CFR, Part 1910, Air Contaminants, Final Rule, Federal Register 1989, 54(12):2332-983.

"Patty's Industrial Hygiene and Toxicology," Vol 2, *Toxicology*, 3rd ed, Clayton GD and Clayton FE, eds, New York, NY: John Wiley & Sons, 1982.

U.S. Department of Health and Human Services, "Toxicological Profile for Silver TP-90/24," Agency for Toxic Substances and Diseases Registry, December 1990.

Sinox® *see* Dinitrocresol *on page 915*

Skellysolve B *see* Hexane *on page 938*

Slug Death® *see* Metaldehyde *on page 955*

Slugit® Pellets *see* Metaldehyde *on page 955*

SMFA *see* Sodium Monofluoroacetate *on next page*

S-Mustard *see* Mustard Gas *on page 972*

Sn *see* Tin *on page 1028*

Snappers *see* Nitrites *on page 978*

Sodium Biborate *see* Borates *on page 870*

Sodium Borate *see* Borates *on page 870*

Sodium Chlorate *see* Chlorate Salts *on page 884*

Sodium Fluoacetate *see* Sodium Monofluoroacetate *on next page*

Sodium Hypochlorite

Related Information

Chlorine *on page 888*

Radiation: Basics of Exposure *on page 1594-1600*

CAS Number 7681-52-9

Synonyms Carrel-Dakin Solution; Clorox; Hypochlorous Acid; Sodium Salt

Commonly Found In Bleach, disinfectants, deodorizers, water purifiers

Mechanism of Toxic Action Corrosive – oxidizing agent directly related to concentration of chlorine

Adverse Reactions

Cardiovascular: Hypotension, bradycardia, cardiac arrest

Dermatologic: Dermal burns, blistering, onycholysis

Gastrointestinal: Esophageal perforation

(Continued)

Sodium Hypochlorite *(Continued)*

Hematologic: Hemolysis

Signs & Symptoms of Acute Overdose Local edema, pain, erythema, chest pain, vomiting, sore throat, dyspnea

Toxicodynamics/Kinetics Metabolism: In the stomach, acid solution forms hypochlorous acid and HCl

Overdosage Treatment Decontamination: Do not induce vomiting; do not use gastric lavage; dilute with milk or water; irrigate eyes and skin with saline; early endoscopy may be useful for oral ingestions; do not neutralize

Diagnostic Tests/Procedures

Blood Gases, Arterial *on page 1207*

Electrolytes, Blood *on page 1254*

Osmolality, Serum *on page 1310*

Monitoring Parameters Produces high osmolal gap (I.V. use). May cause hypernatremia and hyperchloremia.

Additional Information Odor of liquid bleach; chloramine gas is liberated when ammonia and bleach are mixed; chlorine gas is emitted when sodium hypochlorite decomposes in a fire

Specific References

Daniel CR 3d, "Onycholysis: An Overview," *Semin Dermatol*, 1992, 10(1):34-40.

Morgan DL, "Intravenous Injection of Household Bleach," *Ann Emerg Med*, 1992, 21(11):1394-5.

Ward MJ and Routledge PA, "Hypernatremia and Hyperchloraemic Acidosis After Bleach Ingestion," *Hum Toxicol*, 1988, 7(1):37-8.

Sodium Metaborate *see* Borates *on page 870*

Sodium Monofluoroacetate

Related Information

Radiation: Basics of Exposure *on page 1594-1600*

Toxins Which Should be Lavaged With Solutions Other Than Water *on page 1635*

CAS Number 62-74-8

UN Number 2629

Synonyms Fluoroacetic Acid (Sodium Salt); SMFA; Sodium Fluoacetate

Brand Names Compound 1080®

Use Rodenticide

Mechanism of Toxic Action Metabolized to fluorocitrate which then blocks Kreb cycle metabolism by inhibiting the mitochondrial enzyme aconitase

Adverse Reactions

Cardiovascular: Prolonged Q-T intervals on EKG, ventricular fibrillation, hypotension

Central nervous system: Salivation, auditory hallucinations, seizures, paresthesia, hypertonicity, carpopedal spasms, tetany, coma, ataxia

Endocrine & metabolic: Hypocalcemia

Gastrointestinal: Vomiting

Ocular: Nystagmus

Renal & genitourinary: Renal failure (acute)

Respiratory: Hemorrhagic pulmonary edema, hyperventilation

Signs & Symptoms of Acute Overdose Hallucinations, paresthesia, myoglobinuria, muscle spasms, stupor, seizures, coma, mydriasis, sinus tachycardia, hypotension; late findings include renal and/or hepatic necrosis; typically begin 30-90 minutes after exposure

Toxicodynamics/Kinetics Absorption: Orally and in lungs; dermal absorption does not appear to occur if skin is intact

Reference Range Autopsy urinary levels of 368 mg/L associated with lethality 17 hours after exposure to 465 mg of sodium fluoroacetate

Overdosage Treatment

Decontamination: Lavage with magnesium sulfate/activated charcoal with cathartic; remove contaminated clothing and irrigate skin with soap and water with dermal contact

Supportive therapy: Treat seizures with phenobarbital or diazepam, intravenous calcium (10-20 mL of 10% calcium chloride in adults or 10-20 mL/kg in children); or 0.1-0.2 mL/kg of 10% calcium gluconate up to 20 mL should be given for evidence of hypocalcium (prolonged Q-T interval, tetany); mephentermine may be more effective than levarterenol in treating hypotension; digitalis can be utilized in pulmonary edema results; procainamide may be useful for ventricular arrhythmias; glycerol monoacetate effective in animals, clinical use not as promising; ethanol use is also controversial

Enhancement of elimination: Multiple dose of activated charcoal may be effective

Diagnostic Tests/Procedures

Blood Gases, Arterial *on page 1207*

Calcium, Serum *on page 1214*

Glucose, Random *on page 1269*
Kidney Profile *on page 1279*
Liver Profile *on page 1286*

Additional Information Odorless, tasteless, water soluble; initially developed for chemical warfare; available only for commercially licensed rodenticide use; when heated, toxic sodium oxide and fluoride fumes are emitted; a white odorless powder usually associated with a blue dye; approximately 5 mg/kg is fatal; fluoroacetamide less toxic; trifluoroacetic acid used in high performance liquid chromatography is an irritant and can be dermally absorbed, but is not as toxic

Specific References

Chung HM, "Acute Renal Failure Cause by Acute Monofluoroacetate Poisoning," *Vet Hum Toxicol*, 1984, 26(Suppl 2):29-32.
Egekeze JO and Oehme FW, "Sodium Monofluoroacetate (SMFA, Compound 1080): A Literature Review," *Vet Hum Toxicol*, 1979, 21(6):411-6.
Harrisson JW, Ambrus JL, Ambrus CM, et al, "Acute Poisoning With Sodium Fluoroacetate (Compound 1080)," *JAMA*, 1952, 149(17):1520-2.
McTaggart DR, "Poisoning Due to Sodium Fluoroacetate," *Med J Aust*, 1970, 2(14):641-2.
Shapira AR, Taitelman U, and Bursztein S, "Evaluation of the Role of Ionized Calcium in Sodium Fluoroacetate (1080) Poisoning," *Toxicol Appl Pharmacol*, 1980, 56(2):216-20.

Sodium Perborate *see* Borates *on page 870*
Sodium Pyroborate *see* Borates *on page 870*
Sodium Salt *see* Sodium Hypochlorite *on page 1013*
Sodium Tetraborate *see* Borates *on page 870*
Soilfume® *see* Ethylene Bromide *on page 924*
Soleptax® *see* Heptachlor *on page 935*
Solvanol® *see* Diethyl Phthalate *on page 912*
Solvirex® *see* Disulfoton *on page 919*
Soman (GD or Pinacolyl Methylphosphonofluoridate) *see* Nerve Gases *on page 974*
Spectracide® *see* Diazinon *on page 904*
Spin-Aid *see* Phenmedipham *on page 992*
Spirit of Hartshorn *see* Ammonia *on page 858*
Spirits of Salt *see* Hydrogen Chloride *on page 940*
Spirits of Turpentine *see* Turpentine Oil *on page 1035*
Spotrete® *see* Thiram *on page 1027*
Spotting Naphtha *see* Stoddard Solvent *on this page*
Spotton® *see* Fenthion *on page 929*
Staflex® DBP *see* Di-n-Butyl Phthalate *on page 914*
Stink Damp *see* Hydrogen Sulfide *on page 942*

Stoddard Solvent

CAS Number 8052-41-3; 8030-30-6
UN Number 1271; 1255; 1256; 2553
Synonyms Dry Cleaning Safety Solvent; Spotting Naphtha; White spirits
Brand Names Texsolve S®; Varsol 1®
Use Petroleum solvent which is used as a paint thinner, printing ink, adhesive, in liquid photocopier toners, degreaser used in dry cleaning plants
Mechanism of Toxic Action Mixture of hydrocarbons (alkanes, cycloalkanes, and aromatics), this solvent can cause central nervous system depression and cerebral atrophy and axonal prenodal swellings

Adverse Reactions

Central nervous system: Dizziness, headache, ataxia
Gastrointestinal: Nausea
Hepatic: Elevated liver function tests
Ocular: Ocular irritation
Renal: Glomerulonephritis

Toxicodynamics/Kinetics

Absorption: From lungs, orally, and dermally
Distribution: V_d: 10-11 L/kg
Metabolism: Hepatic to dimethylbenzoic acid
Elimination: Urine/feces (clearance: 263 mL/minute)

Reference Range Mean blood level after an exposure (airborne) of 600 mg/m^3 for 5 days (6 hours/day): ~2-2.5 mg/L

Overdosage Treatment

Decontamination:
Dermal: Wash with soap and water

(Continued)

Stoddard Solvent *(Continued)*

Ocular: Irrigate with saline
Oral: Dilute with water

Additional Information

Odor threshold: 0.9 ppm; insoluble in water
TLV-TWA: 100 ppm
PEL-TWA: 100 ppm

Specific References

U.S. Department of Health and Human Services, "Toxicological Profile of Stoddard Solvent," Agency for Toxic Substances and Diseases Registry, May 1993.

Stoddard Solvent *see* Petroleum Distillates – Naphtha *on page 991*
Strobane *see* Trichloroethane *on page 1032*

Strychnine

Related Information

Toxins Which Should be Lavaged With Solutions Other Than Water *on page 1635*

CAS Number 57-24-9; 60-41-3; 66-32-1; 509-42-2; 60491-10-3

UN Number 1692

Synonyms *Strychnos ignatii*; *Strychnos nux-vomica*; *Strychnos tiente*

Brand Names Certox®; Dolco Mouse Ceral®; Kwik-kil®; Mouse-Rid®; Mouse-Tox®; Pied Piper Mouse Seed®; Ro-Dex®

Use Rodenticide; also used as an adulterant in production of illicit cocaine, heroin, and amphetamine; an antiquated antidote historically used in analeptic treatment for barbiturate overdose; unapproved use for nonketotic hyperglycinemia and sleep apnea (100 mcg/kg)

Mechanism of Toxic Action Strychnine competitively antagonizes the inhibitory action of glycine at the postsynaptic receptors in the spinal cord; this loss of post-synaptic inhibition results in excessive motor neuron activity; binding within the CNS may also be responsible for exaggerated responses to visual, auditory, and tactile stimulation

Adverse Reactions

Central nervous system: Anxiety and seizures without loss of consciousness, dysphagia
Neuromuscular & skeletal: Rigidity, cramps, hypertonicity, dysesthesia
Respiratory: Tachypnea, apnea, respiratory paralysis
Miscellaneous: Hypersensitivity to external stimuli, nystagmus

Signs & Symptoms of Acute Overdose Prodromal syndrome of muscular cramps and pain; neck and back stiffness; limb rigidity; agitation and anxiety, followed by excessive muscular activity and hypertonicity; seizures during which the patients remain awake and lucid; opisthotonos; trismus; tachycardia, metabolic acidosis; hypertension, hypomagnesemia, tachypnea and hyperthermia accompanying muscular activity; risus sardonicus (sardonic grinning); respiratory paralysis, fasciculations, apnea and cyanosis; acidosis; rhabdomyolysis and myoglobinuria; leukocytosis; death from respiratory and cardiac arrest

Toxicodynamics/Kinetics

Onset of symptoms:
- Oral: 15-30 minutes
- Intranasal, parenteral: <5 minutes

Absorption: Complete and rapid absorption following oral or parenteral exposure; readily absorbed through intact skin and mucosal surfaces
Distribution: V_d: 13 L/kg; rapid tissue distribution
Metabolism: Hepatic microsomal oxidation through P-450 pathways; evidence of saturable metabolism at higher concentrations with V_{max} = 3.7 mg/kg/hour and K_m = 1.46 mg/L
Half-life: 10 hours
Elimination: ~10% to 20% excreted unchanged in liver within 24 hours

Warnings Any external visual, auditory, or tactile stimuli may precipitate muscle hyperactivity and seizures; minimize any external stimuli

Overdosage Treatment

Decontamination:
- Dermal exposure: Prompt thorough scrubbing of all affected areas with soap and water
- Gastric: Do not induce emesis because of danger of sudden respiratory compromise or aspiration following seizures or muscle spasms; gastric lavage should be approached cautiously and only after aggressive control of muscular dysphoria; activated charcoal should be administered as soon as possible; the efficacy of repeated-dose activated charcoal has not been documented
- Ocular exposure: Irrigation with copious tepid water or saline

Supportive therapy: Airway management, ventilatory assistance, and humidified oxygen administration

Hyperthermia: Treat with cooling blankets, cool water sponging, and cold water lavage; antipyretics are not effective

Rhabdomyolysis: Vigorously hydrate to a urine output of 100-200 mL/hour

Metabolic acidosis: Treat with sodium bicarbonate

Hyperkalemia: Consider insulin and sodium polystyrene sulfonate for significant hyperkalemia; also consider urinary alkalinization or parenteral mannitol administration 0.5-1 g/kg I.V. every 4-6 hours to enhance elimination

Convulsions: Minimize external stimuli and treat with benzodiazepines or barbiturates; consider neuromuscular blockade and barbiturate coma with status epilepticus

Enhancement of elimination: Rapid metabolism and early onset and resolution of symptoms reduce the utility of dialysis or hemoperfusion

Antidote(s)

Charcoal *on page 1403*

Mannitol *on page 1442*

Sodium Bicarbonate *on page 1467*

Pregnancy Implications Fetal risk relates directly to metabolic and respiratory abnormalities experienced by the mother

Additional Information Any exposure to strychnine should be considered potentially life-threatening; intensive care unit admission criteria include seizures, acidosis, and hypoxia; observation care unit admission criteria include evidence of hyperreflexia or neuromuscular irritability, hypertension or tachycardia, that persists longer than 4 hours for onset; patients who remain asymptomatic for at least 6 hours, or who become asymptomatic and remain so for at least 6 hours, may be considered for medical clearance; has a bitter taste

Lethal dose: 5-10 mg

Specific References

Edmunds M, Sheehan TM, and Van't Hoff W, "Strychnine Poisoning: Clinical and Toxicological Observations on a Non-Fatal Case," *J Toxicol Clin Toxicol*, 1986, 24(3):245-55.

Heiser JM, Daya MR, Magnussen AR, et al, "Massive Strychnine Intoxication: Serial Blood Levels in a Fatal Case," *J Toxicol Clin Toxicol*, 1992, 30(2):269-83.

Nishiyama T and Nagase M, "Strychnine Poisoning: Natural Course of a Nonfatal Case," *Am J Emerg Med*, 1995, 13(2):172-3.

Woolf A, Prescott K, and Katz J, "Strychnine Poisoning From the Use of a Cambodian Traditional Remedy," *Vet Hum Toxicol*, 1994, 36:360.

Strychnos ignatii *see* Strychnine *on previous page*

Strychnos nux-vomica *see* Strychnine *on previous page*

Strychnos tiente *see* Strychnine *on previous page*

Styrene

CAS Number 100-42-5

UN Number 2055

Synonyms Cinnamene; Ethenylbenzene; Phenylethylene; Vinylbenzene

Use Production of polystyrene plastics for use in insulation or fiberglass materials

Mechanism of Toxic Action Essentially unknown; may cause increase in brain serotonin and noradrenaline levels; can cause central nervous system depression

Adverse Reactions

Central nervous system: Air styrene levels >30 ppm can cause changes in EEG and psychomotor changes

Gastrointestinal: Nausea (at 376 ppm after 1 hour), metallic taste, stomatitis

Neuromuscular & skeletal: Peripheral neuropathy

Ocular: Irritation (at 376 ppm after 1 hour exposure), rotatory nystagmus

Respiratory: Sore throat, rhinorrhea, bronchospasm, cough

Toxicodynamics/Kinetics

Absorption:

Inhalation: 63%

Oral/dermal: LImited with absorption rate being 1 mcg/cm^2/minute or ~0.1% to 2% of inhalation absorption amount

Distribution: V_d: 1.2-1.7 L/kg Adipose tissue

Metabolism: Hepatic to hippuric acid, mandelic acid (MA) and phenylglyoxilic acid (PGA)

Elimination: Urine as MA (57%), PGA (33%), and hippuric acid (8%)

Half-life: 2-4 days

Reference Range

Workers exposed to TWA levels of inhalation of styrene (biological exposure indices or BEI):

Before shift: 0.02 mg/L

End shift: 1 mg/L

Urinary levels of MA (1 g/L) and PGA (250 mcg/L); urine level of AA of 0.8 g/L has been associated with some central nervous system depression

An exposure of 80 ppm of styrene has been associated with a blood styrene level of ~1 mcg/mL; general population blood styrene level: 0.4 mcg/L

(Continued)

Styrene *(Continued)*

Fat levels range from 8-350 ng/g

Overdosage Treatment

Decontamination:

Dermal: Remove contaminated clothing; wash with soap and water

Ocular: Irrigate with saline

Oral: Dilute with water; do not induce emesis; activated charcoal may be effective

Supportive therapy: Inhaled beta agonist agents may be used for bronchospasm

Pregnancy Implications Menstrual disorders noted, though no increase in birth defects documented

Additional Information Increased cholinesterase activity noted

Relationship between workplace styrene air levels and urinary MA concentration is expressed as:

In (styrene air concentration in PPM equals - 3.4915 + 1.0568) times In (urinary MA level in mg/L)

PEL-TWA: 50 ppm

TLV-TWA: 50 ppm

IDLH: 5000 ppm

Indoor air exposure daily of styrene: 14-151 mcg

Exposure from drinking water: 0-0.5 mcg/day

Exposure from food: ~30 mcg/day

Urban ambient air styrene levels: 0.6-21 mcg/m^3

Half-life in groundwater: 6 weeks to 7.5 months

Atmospheric half-life: 0.5-17 hours

Atmospheric half-life by photolysis: 50 years

Styrene is found in cigarette smoke at the level of 18 mcg/cigarette

Specific References

Lemasters GK, Hagen A, and Samuels SJ, "Reproductive Outcomes in Women Exposed to Solvent in 36 Reinforced Plastics Companies. I. Menstrual Dysfunction," *J Occup Med*, 1985, 27(7):490-4.

U.S. Department of Health and Human Services, "Toxicological Profile for Styrene TP-91/25," Agency for Toxic Substances and Diseases Registry, September 1992.

Sulfur Acid *see* Sulfuric Acid *on next page*

Sulfur Dioxide

CAS Number 7446-09-5

UN Number 1079

Synonyms Sulfurous Anhydride; Sulfur Oxide

Commonly Found In Disinfectant, fumigant, food preservative, Portland cement manufacture, antioxidant; air pollutant near smelters; associated with kerosene space heaters

Use In the manufacture of sulfites, thiosulfates, and sulfonation of oils

Mechanism of Toxic Action Irritation to mucous membranes, highly soluble

Adverse Reactions

Ocular: Eye irritation with corneal injury

Respiratory: Upper respiratory tract edema and obstruction, pulmonary edema, bronchoconstriction

Signs & Symptoms of Acute Overdose Chest pain, dyspnea, cough, cyanosis, lacrimation, rhinorrhea, choking sensation, caustic dermal burns

Toxicodynamics/Kinetics

Metabolism: With ambient air, it is oxidized to sulfur trioxide then hydrated to sulfuric acid

Elimination: Excreted in urine as inorganic sulfate

Reference Range Sulfhemoglobin formation has been associated with exposure; levels of 6% to 12% associated with death

Overdosage Treatment

Decontamination: Oxygenation/respiratory support – 100% humidified oxygen; irrigate eyes

Supportive therapy: Aerosolized sodium bicarbonate (5%) may alleviate respiratory mucous membrane irritation (although this is not proven); beta-adrenergic agents for wheezing

Diagnostic Tests/Procedures

Blood Gases, Arterial *on page 1207*

Chest Films *on page 1224*

Sulfhemoglobin *on page 1358*

Pregnancy Implications Embryotoxic in laboratory rodents; no reproductive risk below concentrations of 5 ppm

Additional Information Colorless; sulfur odor

Odor threshold: 1 ppm

TLV-TWA: 2 ppm

IDLH: 100 ppm

PEL-TWA: 2 ppm

Bronchoconstriction may progress to reactive airway disease

Specific References

Charan NB, Myers CG, Lakshminarayan S, et al, "Pulmonary Injuries Associated With Acute Sulfur Dioxide Inhalation," *Am Rev Respir Dis*, 1979, 119(4):555-60.

Harkonen H, Nordman H, Korhonen O, et al, "Long Term Effects of Exposure to Sulfur Dioxide. Lung Function Four Years After a Pyrite Dust Explosion," *Am Rev Respir Dis*, 1983, 128(5):890-3.

Sulfureted Hydrogen *see* Hydrogen Sulfide *on page 942*

Sulfuric Acid

CAS Number 7664-93-9

UN Number 1832

Synonyms Battery Acid; Oil of Vitrial; Sulfur Acid; Vitriol Brown Oil

Commonly Found In Automotive batteries; used in fur and leather industries; component in smog; major component in acid rain; formed from sulfur trioxide and water

Use In the manufacture of acetic acid, hydrochloric acid, hydrolysis of cellulose; used for metal cleaning

Mechanism of Toxic Action Acid oxidizer; corrosive to the skin, eyes, mucous membranes, gastrointestinal and respiratory tract; chars tissue by removing water

Adverse Reactions

Cardiovascular: Shock, vascular collapse

Gastrointestinal: Gastritis, throat irritation

Renal: Renal failure

Respiratory: Tachypnea, bronchoconstriction, ARDS, laryngeal edema

Signs & Symptoms of Acute Overdose Dyspnea, discoloration of teeth, corneal or dermal burns, cough, choking, hemoptysis/hematemesis; esophageal/gastric burns are rare

Toxicodynamics/Kinetics

Absorption: Can be absorbed

Metabolism: Dissociates into hydronium and sulfate

Overdosage Treatment

Decontamination: Do not induce emesis. Treat inhalation injuries with supplemental oxygen; activated charcoal is not effective. Dilute with cold milk, cornstarch, or large amounts of cold water. Endoscopy for severe mouth burns.

Enhancement of elimination: Hemodialysis if renal failure develops

Diagnostic Tests/Procedures

Blood Gases, Arterial *on page 1207*

Chest Films *on page 1224*

White Blood Count *on page 1380*

Pregnancy Implications Possible increased risk of spontaneous abortion

Additional Information Clear, colorless gas; odorless except when heating (choking odor)

Lethal dose: 135 mg/kg

TLV-TWA: 1 mg/m^3

IDLH: 80 mg/m^3

PEL-TWA: 1 mg/m^3

Specific References

el-Sadik YM, Osman HA, and el-Gazzar RM, "Exposure to Sulfuric Acid in Manufacture of Storage Batteries," *J Occup Med*, 1972, 14(3):224-6.

Maull KI, Osmand AP, and Maull CD, "Liquid Caustic Ingestions: An *In Vitro* Study of the Effects of Buffer, Neutralization, and Dilution," *Ann Emerg Med*, 1985, 14(12):1160-2.

Penner GE, "Acid Ingestion: Toxicology and Treatment," *Ann Emerg Med*, 1980, 9(7):374-9.

Sulfurous Anhydride *see* Sulfur Dioxide *on previous page*

Sulfur Oxide *see* Sulfur Dioxide *on previous page*

Sumonil® *see* Methidathion *on page 959*

SuperCaid® *see* Anticoagulant Rodenticide *on page 859*

Super Nail Glue Off® *see* Acetonitrile *on page 850*

Super Nail Off® *see* Acetonitrile *on page 850*

Supone® *see* Chlorfenvinphos *on page 886*

Supracide® *see* Methidathion *on page 959*

2,4,5-T

CAS Number 93-76-5

Synonyms 2,4,5-Trichlorophenoxyacetic Acid

Mechanism of Toxic Action Has been banned by the EPA in 1979

Adverse Reactions

Central nervous system: Paresthesia

(Continued)

2,4,5-T *(Continued)*

Dermatologic: More irritating to the skin and mucous membranes than 2,4-D

Signs & Symptoms of Acute Overdose Paresthesia

Toxicodynamics/Kinetics Half-life: 23-33 hours

Contraindications Estron; Brush Killer; Shellstar; Weedar® 2,4,5-T; Weedone® 2,4,5-T

Overdosage Treatment

Decontamination: Irrigate with saline; lavage/activated charcoal with cathartic for ingestions exceeding 400 mg/kg

Supportive therapy: Hypotension can be treated with 10-20 mL/kg of isotonic saline and Trendelenburg positioning; dopamine or norepinephrine can be used; quinidine may be helpful for cardiac arrhythmias

Enhancement of elimination: Alkaline diuresis for patients with metabolic acidosis, mental status changes, or a serum level >500 mg/L; keep urine pH between 7.6-8.8; furosemide can be given to maintain diuresis

Pregnancy Implications Teratogenic and fetotoxic

Additional Information 2,3,7,8-tetrachlorodibenzoparadioxin (TCDD) is a contaminant of 2,4,5-T; 2,3,5-T and 2,3-D was used as a 50:50 mixture in agent orange; 2,4,5-T alone usually contains <0.1 ppm of TCDD; does not affect cholinesterase level

Specific References

Dickson LC and Buzik SC, "Health Risks of Dioxins: A Review of Environmental and Toxicological Considerations," *Vet Hum Toxicol*, 1993, 35(1):68-77.

Fox JL, "Dioxins' Health Effects Remain Puzzling. *In vitro* Tests Suggest it Causes Cancer, Medical Results Remain Ambiguous," *Science*, 1983, 221(4616):1161-2.

Smith EA and Oehme FW, "A Review of Selected Herbicides and Their Toxicities," *Vet Hum Toxicol*, 1991, 33(6):596-60.

Tabun (Ethyl N-Dimethylphophoramidocyanidate or GA) *see* Nerve Gases *on page 974*

Talon® *see* Anticoagulant Rodenticide *on page 859*

Talon-G® *see* Anticoagulant Rodenticide *on page 859*

Tar Acids *see* Cresols *on page 898*

TCA *see* Trichloroethane *on page 1032*

TCE *see* Trichloroethane *on page 1032*

TCM *see* Chloroform *on page 890*

TDE *see* DDD *on page 902*

TDI *see* Toluene Diisocyanate *on page 1031*

Telone® *see* 1,3-Dichloropropene *on page 909*

Temik® *see* Aldicarb *on page 855*

TEPP *see* Tetraethyl Pyrophosphate *on page 1024*

Terabol® *see* Methyl Bromide *on page 964*

Terbufos

CAS Number 13071-79-9

Synonyms Phosphorodithioic Acid S-((Tert-Butylthio)methyl) O,O-Diethyl Ester

Brand Names Counter®

Use Commonly marketed as insecticide granules, or spray liquid with or without petroleum derivative as a solvent

Mechanism of Toxic Action Potent, irreversible inhibition of acetylcholinesterase and plasma cholinesterase, resulting in excess accumulation of acetylcholine at muscarinic and nicotinic receptors, and in the central nervous system

Adverse Reactions

Cardiovascular: Hyperdynamic (~18% to 21%) or hypodynamic (~7% to 10%) states

Central nervous system: Depression, seizures, hyperactivity

Genitourinary: Incontinence

Neuromuscular & skeletal: Weakness, paralysis

Respiratory: Depression, edema

General: Flu-like symptoms (especially with chronic exposure)

Delayed: Muscle asthenia and paresthesia

Signs & Symptoms of Acute Overdose Miosis (unreactive to light), mydriasis (rarely), lacrimation, pallor, excessive sweating, confusion, agitation, headache, dysarthria, generalized asthenia, seizures, A-V block, coma, decreased hemoglobin/red blood cell count/platelet count, metabolic acidosis and hyperglycemia (severe intoxication), hypotension, hypertension, bradycardia, tachycardia, Q-T prolongation, heart block, asystole, salivation, cranial nerve palsies, bronchorrhea, tachypnea, pulmonary edema, respiratory depression, diaphragmatic paralysis, skeletal muscle fasciculation and flaccid paralysis, nausea, vomiting, abdominal pain, fecal and urinary incontinence; an "intermediate syndrome" of limb asthenia and respiratory paralysis has been reported to occur between 24 and 96 hours postorganophosphate exposure and is independent of the acute cholinergic crisis. Late paresthesia characterized by stocking and globe paresthesia, anesthesia and asthenia is infrequently observed weeks to months following acute exposure to certain organophosphates.

Toxicodynamics/Kinetics

Absorption: Readily through oral, dermal, or respiratory exposure

Metabolism: Rapidly metabolized to weakly active compounds through hepatic hydrolysis and other pathways

Elimination: Metabolites are excreted in urine

Warnings Risk of aspiration pneumonitis exists with agents having a hydrocarbon vehicle; severe laryngeal irritation and violent coughing may result from exposure to dusting powders; exposure to dusting powders and insecticide granules may cause contact dermatitis

Overdosage Treatment

Decontamination: Isolation, bagging, and disposal of all contaminated clothing and other articles; all emergency medical workers and hospital staff should follow appropriate precautions regarding exposure to hazardous material including the use of protective clothing, masks, goggles, and respiratory equipment

Dermal: Prompt thorough scrubbing of all affected areas with soap and water, including hair and nails

Gastric: Activated charcoal can be administered either orally or via a nasogastric tube; do not induce emesis because of danger of sudden respiratory compromise, alterations in mental status, seizures, coma, and possible aspiration of hydrocarbon vehicles

Ocular: Irrigation with copious tepid sterile water or saline

Supportive therapy: Including airway management, ventilatory assistance, humidified oxygen administration, and close monitoring for sudden respiratory failure

Enhancement of elimination: Dialysis and hemoperfusion are not indicated due to effectiveness of the prescribed treatment, large volumes of distribution of organophosphates

Antidote:

Atropine: Administration should be guided by respiratory status, starting at 1-5 mg I.V. every 5-10 minutes as needed, and should be titrated to the resolution of excess pulmonary secretions; frequent administration of large doses (cumulative doses >100 mg) may be necessary in massive exposures

Glycopyrrolate: May be administered if atropine is unavailable

2-PAM: For more significant exposures (ie, exposures requiring large doses of atropine, or with recurring symptoms, or exposures to more lipid soluble agents), administration should follow: 1-2 g I.V. over 5-10 minutes, repeated in 1 hour if asthenia reoccurs, then every 4-12 hours for recurring symptoms

Antidote(s)

Atropine Sulfate *on page 1395*

Pralidoxime Chloride *on page 1461*

Diagnostic Tests/Procedures

Blood Gases, Arterial *on page 1207*

Chest Films *on page 1224*

Complete Blood Count *on page 1236*

Creatinine, Serum *on page 1243*

Electrocardiography *on page 1253*

Liver Profile *on page 1286*

Pseudocholinesterase, Serum *on page 1340*

Pregnancy Implications Human data regarding organophosphate exposure in pregnancy is limited and anecdotal; teratogenesis and fetal death have been produced in animal models at exposure levels that cause obvious toxicity to the pregnant animal

Additional Information Red blood cell cholinesterase and serum pseudocholinesterase may be depressed following acute or chronic organophosphate exposure; RBC cholinesterase is typically not analyzed by in-house laboratories, and is usually not available for consideration during acute management. Pseudocholinesterase levels may be rapidly available from some in-house laboratories, but are not as reliable a marker of organophosphate exposure because of variability secondary to variant genotypes, hepatic disease, oral estrogen use, or malnutrition. Because of this variability, true indication of suppression of either of these enzymes can only be estimated through comparison to pre-exposure values; these enzymes may be useful in measuring a patient's recovery postexposure, especially if the recovery is not progressing as expected.

Water solubility: 6 ppm

Other information concerning pesticide exposures is available through the EPA-funded National Pesticide Telecommunications Network: 1-800-858-7378 (weekdays, 8 AM to 6 PM, Central Standard time)

(Continued)

Terbufos *(Continued)*

Specific References

Minton NA and Murray VS, "A Review of Organophosphate Poisoning," *Med Toxicol Adverse Drug Exp*, 1988, 3(5):350-75.

Namba T, Nolte CT, Jackrel J, et al, "Poisoning Due to Organophosphate Insecticides. Acute and Chronic Manifestations," *Am J Med*, 1971, 50(4):475-92.

Termide® *see* Heptachlor *on page 935*

Terr-o-cide® 15-D *see* 1,3-Dichloropropene *on page 909*

Terr-O-Gas® 57/43T *see* 1,3-Dichloropropene *on page 909*

Tersan-75® *see* Thiram *on page 1027*

Tert-Butyl Methyl Ether *see* Methyl Tert-Butyl Ether *on page 970*

Tetra *see* Tetrachloroethylene *on this page*

Tetrachloroethane

CAS Number 79-34-5

UN Number 1702

Synonyms Acetylene Tetrachloride; 1,1,2,2-Tetrachloroethane

Brand Names Bonoform®; Cellon®; Westron®

Use Primarily as a solvent in metal cleaning procedures, paint removers, varnishes, photographic films, and oil or fat extractant; production of trichloroethylene, tetrachloroethylene, and 1,2-dichloroethylene

Mechanism of Toxic Action Central nervous system depression; direct effect on neuronal membrane and hepatotoxic effects can occur through lipid peroxidation

Adverse Reactions

Cardiovascular: Hypotension

Central nervous system: Confusion, delirium, coma

Gastrointestinal: Nausea, vomiting, anorexia (gastrointestinal effects seen with exposure levels of 116 ppm for 10-30 minutes), diarrhea

Hepatic: Fatty degeneration of liver

Ocular: Lacrimation, irritation

Miscellaneous: Leukocytosis

Toxicodynamics/Kinetics

Absorption: Through inhalation (97%), oral, and dermal routes

Metabolism: Hepatic to glyoxylic acid and oxyalic acid, tetrachloroethylene is also a metabolite

Elimination: Through lungs, feces, and urine

Reference Range Toxic effects are predicted to occur at blood tetrachloroethane levels >1.1 ng/mL (1.1 ppt)

Overdosage Treatment

Decontamination:

- Dermal: Remove contaminated clothing; wash with soap and water
- Ocular: Irrigate with saline
- Oral: Dilute with milk or water

Additional Information Nonflammable

Minimal lethal dose (oral): 357 mg/kg

Toxic oral dose (causing coma): 100 mg/kg

Odor threshold:

- Air: 3-5 ppm (chloroform-like)
- Water: 0.5 ppm

Atmospheric half-life: >800 days

Atmospheric concentrations in U.S. (urban/suburban)

- Mean level: 5.4 ppt
- Drinking water: <0.5 ppb

PEL-TWA: 1 ppm

TLV-TWA (skin): 1 ppm

IDLH: 150 ppm

Specific References

U.S. Department of Health and Human Services, "Toxicological Profile of 1,1,2,2-Tetrachloroethane," Agency for Toxic Substances and Diseases Registry, August 1994.

1,1,2,2-Tetrachloroethane *see* Tetrachloroethane *on this page*

Tetrachloroethylene

CAS Number 127-18-4

UN Number 1897

Synonyms PCE; Perchlor; Perclene; Tetra; 1,1,2,2-Tetrachloroethylene

Use In textile industry for dry cleaning fabric; degreasing; used in the manufacture of freons, antihelminth for animals

Mechanism of Toxic Action CNS depressant, irritant; probable human carcinogen

Adverse Reactions

Central nervous system: CNS depression

Ocular: Irritation at air levels >1000 ppm

Respiratory: Respiratory depression, irritation

Signs & Symptoms of Acute Overdose Headache, irritability, conjunctival injection, epistaxis, dermatitis, short-term memory deficiency, hepatomegaly, euphoria, ataxia, nausea, cough, sweating

Toxicodynamics/Kinetics

Absorption: Well absorbed in the lungs and gastrointestinal tract; not well absorbed dermally; highly lipid soluble

Distribution: V_d: 8.2 L/kg

Half-life:

Oral: 144 hours

Inhalation: 33-72 hours

In adipose tissues: 72 hours

Metabolism: In the liver to trichloroacetic acid and trichloroethanol

Elimination: 80% excreted through the lungs, metabolites excreted renally

Reference Range Tetrachloroethylene serum level of 100 µg/dL and trichloroacetic acid levels in urine of 7 mg/L correlate with weekly exposure of 50 ppm; BEI of 1 mg/L; an oral ingestion of 12-16g in a 6-year-old boy resulted in a blood tetrachloroethylene level of 21 µg/dL 1-hour postingestion

Overdosage Treatment

Decontamination:

Inhalation: Give 100% humidified oxygen

Ocular: Irrigate with saline

Dermal: Remove contaminated clothing; wash with soap and water

Supportive therapy: Controlled hyperventilation (volume 10 L/min) may be useful; epinephrine may predispose patient to cardiac arrhythmia

Diagnostic Tests/Procedures

Blood, Urine *on page 1210*

Kidney Profile *on page 1279*

Liver Profile *on page 1286*

Protein, Semiquantitative, Urine *on page 1337*

Additional Information Clear, colorless; fruity odor of chloroform

Odor threshold: 5-50 ppm

TLV-TWA: 50 ppm; radiopaque. Symptoms occur at 75 ppm.

See table for duration and effect of inhaling vapors.

Dose-Response Relationship for Humans Inhaling Tetrachlorothylene Vapors

Levels in Air	Duration of Exposure	Effect on Nervous System
50 ppm		Odor threshold
100 ppm	7 h	Headache, drowsiness
200 ppm	2 h	Dizziness, uncoordination
600 ppm	10 min	Dizziness, loss of inhibitions
1000 ppm	1–2 min	Marked dizziness, intolerable eye and respiratory tract irritation
1500 ppm	30 min	Coma

U.S. Department of Health & Human Services, "Hospital Emergency Departments: A Planning Guide for the Management of Contaminated Patients," *Managing Hazardous Materials Incidents,* Agency for Toxic Substances and Disease Registry, 1995, 2:796.

Estimated daily intake:

Inhalation: 41-204 mcg

Drinking water: 0.6-6 mcg

Ambient atmospheric urban concentrations: ~0.8 ppb

Drinking water tetrachloroethylene: 0.3-3 ppb

Dairy products contain 0.3-13 mcg/kg; beverages average 2-3 mcg/kg

Atmospheric half-life: 96-251 days

Water half-life at pH 7 (25°C): ~9 months (by hydrolysis)

Specific References

Koppel C, Arndt I, Arendt U, et al, "Acute Tetrachloroethylene Poisoning: Blood Elimination Kinetics During Hyperventilation Therapy," *J Toxicol Clin Toxicol*, 1985, 23(2-3):103-15.

U.S. Department of Health and Human Services, "Toxicological Profile for Tetrachloroethylene TP-92/18," Agency for Toxic Substances and Diseases Registry, April 1993.

1,1,2,2-Tetrachloroethylene *see* Tetrachloroethylene *on previous page*

Tetrachloromethane *see* Carbon Tetrachloride *on page 882*

Tetraethyl Pyrophosphate

CAS Number 107-49-3

UN Number 3018

Synonyms TEPP

Brand Names Fosvex®; Grisol®; Hexamite®; Tetron®

Use Marketed as insecticide spray liquid with or without petroleum derivative as a solvent

Mechanism of Toxic Action Potent, irreversible inhibition of acetylcholinesterase and plasma cholinesterase, resulting in excess accumulation of acetylcholine at muscarinic and nicotinic receptors, and in the central nervous system

Adverse Reactions

Cardiovascular: Hyperdynamic (~18% to 21%) or hypodynamic (~7% to 10%) states

Central nervous system: Depression, seizures, hyperactivity

Genitourinary: Incontinence

Neuromuscular & skeletal: Weakness, paralysis

Respiratory: Depression, edema

General: Flu-like symptoms (especially with chronic exposure)

Delayed: Muscle asthenia, paresthesia

Signs & Symptoms of Acute Overdose Miosis (unreactive to light), mydriasis (rarely), lacrimation, pallor, excessive sweating, confusion, agitation, headache, dysarthria, generalized asthenia, A-V block, seizures, coma, decreased hemoglobin/red blood cell count/platelet count, metabolic acidosis and hyperglycemia (severe intoxication), hypotension, hypertension, cranial nerve palsies, bradycardia, tachycardia, Q-T prolongation, heart block, asystole, salivation, bronchorrhea, tachypnea, pulmonary edema, respiratory depression, diaphragmatic paralysis, skeletal muscle fasciculation and flaccid paralysis, nausea, vomiting, abdominal pain, fecal and urinary incontinence; an "intermediate syndrome" of limb asthenia and respiratory paralysis has been reported to occur between 24 and 96 hours postorganophosphate exposure and is independent of the acute cholinergic crisis. Late paresthesia characterized by stocking and globe paresthesia, anesthesia and asthenia is infrequently observed weeks to months following acute exposure to certain organophosphates.

Toxicodynamics/Kinetics

Absorption: Readily through oral, dermal, or respiratory exposure

Metabolism: Rapidly metabolized to weakly active compounds through hepatic hydrolysis and other pathways

Elimination: Metabolites are excreted in urine

Warnings Risk of aspiration pneumonitis exists with agents having a hydrocarbon vehicle; severe laryngeal irritation and violent coughing may result from exposure to dusting powders; exposure to dusting powders and insecticide granules may cause contact dermatitis

Overdosage Treatment

Decontamination: Isolation, bagging, and disposal of all contaminated clothing and other articles; all emergency medical workers and hospital staff should follow appropriate precautions regarding exposure to hazardous material including the use of protective clothing, masks, goggles, and respiratory equipment

- Dermal: Prompt thorough scrubbing of all affected areas with soap and water, including hair and nails
- Gastric: Activated charcoal can be administered either orally or via a nasogastric tube; do not induce emesis because of danger of sudden respiratory compromise, alterations in mental status, seizures, coma, and possible aspiration of hydrocarbon vehicles
- Ocular: Irrigation with copious tepid sterile water or saline

Supportive therapy: Including airway management, ventilatory assistance, humidified oxygen administration, and close monitoring for sudden respiratory failure

Enhancement of elimination: Dialysis and hemoperfusion are not indicated due to effectiveness of the prescribed treatment, large volumes of distribution of organophosphates

Antidote:

- Atropine: Administration should be guided by respiratory status, starting at 1-5 mg I.V. every 5-10 minutes as needed, and should be titrated to the resolution of excess pulmonary secretions; frequent administration of large doses (cumulative doses >100 mg) may be necessary in massive exposures
- Glycopyrrolate: May be administered if atropine is unavailable
- 2-PAM: For more significant exposures (ie, exposures requiring large doses of atropine, or with recurring symptoms, or exposures to more lipid soluble agents), administration should follow: 1-2 g I.V. over 5-10 minutes, repeated in 1 hour if asthenia reoccurs, then every 4-12 hours for recurring symptoms

Antidote(s)

Atropine Sulfate *on page 1395*

Pralidoxime Chloride *on page 1461*

Diagnostic Tests/Procedures

Blood Gases, Arterial *on page 1207*
Chest Films *on page 1224*
Complete Blood Count *on page 1236*
Creatinine, Serum *on page 1243*
Electrocardiography *on page 1253*
Liver Profile *on page 1286*
Pseudocholinesterase, Serum *on page 1340*

Pregnancy Implications Human data regarding organophosphate exposure in pregnancy is limited and anecdotal; teratogenesis and fetal death have been produced in animal models at exposure levels that cause obvious toxicity to the pregnant animal

Additional Information Colorless/light amber liquid with faint fruity odor; noncombustible; slowly hydrolyses in water, and is therefore environmentally persistent; thermal breakdown products include phosphoric acid; red blood cell cholinesterase and serum pseudocholinesterase may be depressed following acute or chronic organophosphate exposure; RBC cholinesterase is typically not analyzed by in-house laboratories, and is usually not available for consideration during acute management. Pseudocholinesterase levels may be rapidly available from some in-house laboratories, but are not as reliable a marker of organophosphate exposure because of variability secondary to variant genotypes, hepatic disease, oral estrogen use, or malnutrition. Because of this variability, true indication of suppression of either of these enzymes can only be estimated through comparison to pre-exposure values; these enzymes may be useful in measuring a patient's recovery postexposure, especially if the recovery is not progressing as expected.

ACGIH TLV: 0.0004 ppm
IDLH: 10 mg/m^3

Other information concerning pesticide exposures is available through the EPA-funded National Pesticide Telecommunications Network: 1-800-858-7378 (weekdays, 8 AM to 6 PM, Central Standard time)

Specific References

Minton NA and Murray VS, "A Review of Organophosphate Poisoning," *Med Toxicol Adverse Drug Exp*, 1988, 3(5):350-75.
Namba T, Nolte CT, Jackrel J, et al, "Poisoning Due to Organophosphate Insecticides. Acute and Chronic Manifestations," *Am J Med*, 1971, 50(4):475-92.

Tetraform® *see* Carbon Tetrachloride *on page 882*

Tetralite *see* Tetryl *on this page*

Tetramethyl Thiuram Disulfide *see* Thiram *on page 1027*

Tetrasol *see* Carbon Tetrachloride *on page 882*

Tetril *see* Tetryl *on this page*

Tetron® *see* Tetraethyl Pyrophosphate *on previous page*

Tetryl

CAS Number 479-45-8
UN Number 0208
Synonyms CE; Nitramine; N-Methyl-N,2,4,6-Tetranitroaniline; Tetralite; Tetril
Use Primarily as a military explosive (detonator and primer)
Mechanism of Toxic Action Essentially unknown; can cause an allergic reaction
Adverse Reactions

Central nervous system: Fatigue, headache
Dermatologic: Yellow staining of skin, rash, urticaria
Gastrointestinal: Nausea, vomiting, abdominal pain; anorexia
Hepatic: Liver failure, jaundice
Respiratory: Bronchospasm, cough
Miscellaneous: Leukocytosis, epistaxis, stomatitis

Toxicodynamics/Kinetics

Absorption: By inhalation, dermal, and oral routes
Metabolism: Hepatic to picramic acid
Elimination: Probably renal

Overdosage Treatment

Decontamination:
Dermal: Wash with soap and water; calamine lotion or zinc oxide may be used to treat dermatitis
Ocular: Irrigate with saline

Additional Information Odorless but highly explosive

Atmospheric half-life: 11 days
Water half-life: 302 days (lower at higher pH)
Soil half-life: 1.2 weeks
PEL-TWA (skin designation): 1.5 mg/m^3

(Continued)

Tetryl *(Continued)*

Specific References

U.S. Department of Health and Human Services, "Toxicological Profile of Tetryl," Agency for Toxic Substances and Diseases Registry, May 1993.

Texsolve S® *see* Stoddard Solvent *on page 1015*

T-Gas *see* Ethylene Oxide *on page 927*

Thallium

Related Information

Toxins Which Should be Lavaged With Solutions Other Than Water *on page 1635*

CAS Number 7440-28-0

Use Primarily in semiconduction industry in manufacture of switches and closures; radiopharmaceutical agent banned by the EPA as a pesticide in 1972

Mechanism of Toxic Action Thallium distributes intracellularly like potassium; it is a cellular toxin; inhibits mitochondrial oxidative phosphorylation, disrupts protein synthesis, alters heme metabolism

Adverse Reactions Neurologic, dysphagia, cardiac, hepatic, renal, dermatologic, gastrointestinal, pulmonary, salivation, chorea (extrapyramidal)

Signs & Symptoms of Acute Overdose Degeneration of central and peripheral nervous systems, tremor, disorientation, drowsiness, lacrimation, seizures, coma, cerebral edema, motor/sensory neuropathy, hyperesthesia of palm and sole, alopecia, optic neuropathy, Mees' lines, garlic-like breath, fatty infiltration, necrosis of liver, mydriasis, feces discoloration (black), dementia, nephritis, gastroenteritis, pulmonary edema, tachycardia, bradycardia, cardiac arrhythmias, nausea, vomiting, paresthesia, ataxia

Toxicodynamics/Kinetics

Absorption: Through skin and gastrointestinal tract

Distribution: V_d: 1-5 L/kg; following intoxication, highest concentration found in kidney and urine with lesser amounts in intestine, thyroid, testes, pancreas, skin, bone, spleen

Half-life: 2-4 days

Elimination: Large amount excreted in urine within first 24 hours after which fecal elimination predominates

Reference Range Serum <10 ng/mL; blood levels >30 μg/dL are indicative of severe exposure; toxicity associated with blood levels of ≥ 10 μg/dL or urine levels >20 μg/dL

Overdosage Treatment

Decontamination:

- Dermal: Remove contaminated clothing; wash with soap and water
- Ocular: Irrigate with saline
- Oral: Lavage preferable over ipecac, activated charcoal may be effective; Prussian blue (not commercially available for therapeutic use and not FDA approved) exchanges thallium for potassium and is fecally excreted; dosage: 250 mg/kg orally in 4 divided doses; continue therapy until thallium urinary levels falls to <0.5 μg/24 hours; acetylcysteine treatment is investigational

Enhancement of elimination: Multiple dosing of activated charcoal may be effective; potassium chloride administration also may enhance elimination when given after 48-72 hours; forced saline diuresis is recommended, hemodialysis or hemoperfusion may be effective; furosemide can enhance urinary thallium excretion in animal models

Pregnancy Implications Crosses placenta, fetal exposure in 3rd trimester resulted in fetal alopecia and nail changes

Additional Information Odorless, tasteless; chelating agents are not effective; dithiocarb worsens symptoms by causing central redistribution of thallium; assay blood by flame atomic absorption; monitor for hypocalcemia in acute phase; the water soluble salts of thallium (sulfate, acetate, malonate, and carbonate) are more toxic than the sulfide and iodide (less water soluble)

Estimated lethal dose in humans: 8-12 mg/kg

Estimated daily thallium intake in a 70 kg adult:

- From drinking water: 2 mcg
- From food: 5 mcg
- From inhalation: 3.4 ng

Thallium is present in concentrations of 0.024 mcg/g of cigarettes and 0.06-0.17 mcg/g in cigar stubs

Average ambient urban air concentration of thallium: 0.04 ng/m^3; thallium is present in earth's crust at concentrations of 0.3-0.7 ppm

PEL-TWA: 0.1 mg/m^3

TLV-TWA: 0.1 mg/m^3

IDLH: 20 mg/m^3

Specific References

Herrero F, Fernandez E, Gomez J, et al, "Thallium Poisoning Presenting With Abdominal Colic, Paresthesia, and Irritability," *J Toxicol Clin Toxicol*, 1995, 33(3):261-4.

Lovejoy FH, "Thallium," *Clin Toxicol Rev*, 1982, 4:1-2.
Meggs WJ, Hoffman RS, Shih RD, et al, "Thallium Poisoning From Maliciously Contaminated Food," *J Toxicol Clin Toxicol*, 1994, 32(6):723-30.
Meggs WJ, Morasco R, Shih RD, et al, "Effects of Prussian Blue and N-Acetylcysteine on Thallium Toxicity in Mice," *Vet Hum Toxicol*, 1994, 36:364.
Moeschlin S, "Thallium Poisoning," *Clin Toxicol*, 1980, 17(1):133-46.
U.S. Department of Health and Human Services, "Toxicological Profile for Thallium TP-91/26", Agency for Toxic Substances and Diseases Registry, July 1992.
Wax PM, "Tortilla Thallotoxicosis," *J Toxicol Clin Toxicol*, 1995, 33(3):265.

Thifor® *see* Endosulfan *on page 921*

Thiodan® *see* Endosulfan *on page 921*

Thiodemeton *see* Disulfoton *on page 919*

Thiomethanol *see* Methyl Mercaptan *on page 968*

Thiomethyl Alcohol *see* Methyl Mercaptan *on page 968*

Thionex® *see* Endosulfan *on page 921*

Thiram

CAS Number 137-26-8

Synonyms Tetramethyl Thiuram Disulfide; Thirame; Thiuram

Brand Names Arasan®; Pomarsol®; Puralin®; Rezifilm®; Spotrete®; Tersan-75®; Thiurad®; Tuads®; Tulisan®

Use Foliage disinfectant for fruits, mushrooms; rubber accelerator (volcanizing agent); seed disinfectant

Mechanism of Toxic Action Antioxidant and bisdithiocarbamate

Adverse Reactions

Dermatologic: Irritating to skin, eczema
Ocular: Conjunctivitis
Respiratory: Sneezing, rhinitis, cough
Miscellaneous: Disulfiram-like reaction with ethanol may occur

Signs & Symptoms of Acute Overdose Cholinergic symptoms do not occur; ataxia, dizziness, confusion, drowsiness, paralysis, nausea, vomiting, diarrhea

Toxicodynamics/Kinetics Metabolism: To carbon disulfide

Overdosage Treatment

Decontamination: Lavage/activated charcoal with cathartic for ingestion; irrigate for skin exposure
Supportive therapy: Oxygen for antabuse-like reaction; crystalloid solution for hypotension

Monitoring Parameters May increase urinary xanthurenic acid levels

Pregnancy Implications Teratogenic in rats

Additional Information No effect on cholinesterase; acceptable daily intake: 5 mcg/kg affects acetylaldehyde dehydrogenase for 10-14 days

Specific References

Dalvi R, "Toxicology of Thiram (Tetramethylthiuram Disulfide) - A Review," *Vet Hum Toxicol*, 1988, 30(5):480-2.
Shelley WB, "Golf Course Dermatitis Due to Thiram Fungicide - Cross Hazards of Alcohol, Disulfiram, and Rubber," *JAMA*, 1964, 188(5):415-7.

Thirame *see* Thiram *on this page*

Thiurad® *see* Thiram *on this page*

Thiuram *see* Thiram *on this page*

Thorium

CAS Number 7440-29-1

UN Number 2975

Synonyms Pyrophoric; Thorium 232

Use Refractory applications, welding electrodes, lamp mantles, and in nuclear weapon production, portable gas lighters

Mechanism of Toxic Action Most toxic effects are through alpha-radiation effects

Adverse Reactions

Hematologic: Aplastic anemia, leukopenia
Hepatic: Elevated liver function tests
Miscellaneous: Increased incidence of pancreatic cancers and hematopoietic tissue malignancies

Toxicodynamics/Kinetics

Absorption: By inhalation (5%); limited absorption by oral route (0.02% to 1%)
Distribution: Bone and soft tissue
Half-life: 2.6 years
Elimination: Feces

Reference Range

General population blood level in the United Kingdom: 2.4 mcg/L
Background urine level: <0.001 mcg/L

(Continued)

Thorium *(Continued)*

Overdosage Treatment

Decontamination: Remove contaminated clothing; isolate all run-off

Dermal: Irrigate with water; scrub gently with soft sponge or brush (avoid abrading skin); a 50% powdered detergent solution followed by a 5% sodium hypochlorite solution can be used for persistent contamination

Supportive therapy: DTPA (diethylenetriamine pentacetic acid) which is available from the Radiation Emergency Assistance Center (615-576-1004) is an effective chelator; the calcium salt should be used as follows: 1 g of calcium DTPA diluted in 250 mL of 5% dextrose in water should be infused over a 1- to 1.5-hour time period daily for 5 days; $CaNa_2$ EDTA (calcium Versenate®) can also be used, but is less effective; DTPA should be used for dermal exposure with open wounds as well as inhalation or oral ingestion

Ocular: Wash copiously with saline

Additional Information Sesame seeds are foods with highest thorium concentration (0.01 pCi/g wet weight); thorotrast is a colloid consisting of thorium-232 dioxide (25%) and dextran used as an I.V. contrast agent up to 1955; granulomas, blood disorders, and hemangiosarcoma of the liver has been associated with its use (after a delay of 20 years)

Thorium 232 rarely exceeds 0.1 pCi/L in natural waters; in soil, average soil concentration: 6 mcg/g

Estimated daily intake in U.S.: <0.02 pCi

Specific References

U.S. Department of Health and Human Services, "Toxicological Profile of Thorium TP-90/25," Agency for Toxic Substances and Diseases Registry, October 1990.

Thorium 232 *see* Thorium *on previous page*

Thrust *see* Nitrites *on page 978*

"Tickle" *see* Titanium *on next page*

Tiguvon® *see* Fenthion *on page 929*

Tin

CAS Number 7440-31-5; 7772-99-8 (Stannous Chloride); 18282-10-5 (Stannic Oxide); 683-18-1 (Dibutyltin Chloride)

UN Number 1759 (Stannous Chloride)

Synonyms Mat Powder; Sn; Tin Flake

Use Primarily in the manufacture of containers (particularly aerosol cans); used to coat copper wire and as a soldering agent

Mechanism of Toxic Action Possible toxic mechanism may involve uncoupling of oxidative phosphorylation

Adverse Reactions

Inorganic tin:

Gastrointestinal: Nausea, vomiting, diarrhea

Miscellaneous: Pneumoconiosis, mucosal/skin irritation

Organic tin:

Central nervous system: Headache, disorientation, dizziness, seizures

Dermal: Dermal burns on contact with phenyltin

Hepatic: Fatty degeneration of liver

Ocular: Photophobia, nystagmus

Otic: Tinnitus, ototoxicity

Renal: Renal tubule injury

Respiratory: Respiratory depression

Miscellaneous: Stomatitis, hyporeflexia, polyneuropathy

Toxicodynamics/Kinetics

Absorption: Inorganic tin is not readily absorbed by any route; organic tin is readily absorbed by inhalation, dermal, and oral routes

Half-life: 4-400 days

Elimination: Feces and urine

Reference Range General population adipose tissue level: 8.7-15 μg/g; normal mean urine tin concentration: 17 μg/mL; average blood tin level: ~0.14 mg/L

Overdosage Treatment

Decontamination:

Dermal: Wash with soap and water

Ocular: Irrigate with saline

Oral: Dilute with water

Supportive therapy: Chelation therapy is not effective

Additional Information Radiopaque; a cause of metal fume fever

Toxic oral dose: Triethyltin: 70 mg (>8 days)

Half-life in water: >89 days (photolysis)

Ambient air concentrations of tin in U.S. cities: <0.8 mcg/m^3

Mean soil background tin levels in U.S.: 0.89 mg tin/kg soil

TLV-TWA:

Inorganic metal tin: 2 mg/m^3

Organic tin (skin exposure): 0.1 mg/m^3

Canned food may contain from 1.8-500 mg/kg with all-lacquered cans having lower tin concentrations

Estimated daily intake of tin in U.S. by an adult: 4 mg from food and 0.003 mg by inhalation (virtually none from drinking water)

Specific References

Wax PM and Dockstader L, "Tributyltin Use in Interior Paints: A Continuing Health Hazard," *J Toxicol Clin Toxicol*, 1995, 33(3):239-41.

U.S. Department of Health and Human Services, "Toxicological Profile for Tin TP-91/27," Agency for Toxic Substances and Diseases Registry, September 1992.

Tin Flake *see* Tin *on previous page*

Tisit® [OTC] *see* Pyrethrins *on page 1003*

Titanic Chloride *see* Titanium *on this page*

Titanium

CAS Number 7550-45-0

UN Number 1838

Synonyms "Tickle"; Titanic Chloride; Titanium Tetrachloride; Titanocene

Use Production of iridescent glass and artificial pearls; production of inorganic titanium compounds; has been used by the military as a smoke-producing screen

Mechanism of Toxic Action Respiratory irritant

Adverse Reactions Respiratory, eye, nose, throat, gastrointestinal, temperature regulation, dermatologic (including dermal burns), fever

Signs & Symptoms of Acute Overdose Eye exposure may result in cataract; suppurative conjunctivitis and keratitis; irritation of mouth, nose, throat; chemical pneumonitis, pulmonary edema, edema of pharynx, vocal cord, stenosis of larynx, trachea, upper bronchia, vomiting, burns of gastrointestinal tract may lead to strictures, fever

Toxicodynamics/Kinetics

Absorption: Oral: ~3%

Elimination: In urine

Reference Range Normal urine concentration: 10 μg/L

Overdosage Treatment

Decontamination:

Dermal: Do **not** immediately wash with water; first dry wipe (with towels or gauze before irrigating with water to prevent hydrochloric acid burns) whereupon a yellow or white granular deposit is noted; at this point, wash the deposit off with cool water; dermal burns can be treated by traditional methods

Ocular: Wipe eyelids preliminarily with a dry cloth or gauze, then irrigate copiously with water (3-4 L over 20 minutes); do not use neutralizing solutions

Oral: Do not evacuate gastric contents; following oral exposure, dilute with water or milk; do not use neutralizing solution because of exothermic reaction

Supportive therapy: Unclear what the utility of corticosteroids is in the prevention/treatment of noncardiogenic pulmonary edema

Additional Information Colorless, fuming liquid; titanium tetrachloride in the presence of moisture decomposes to hydrochloric acid and titanium dioxide; heat is liberated; soluble in cold water; has a penetrating acid odor; titanium forms four oxides: titanium monoxide, titanium trioxide, titanium dioxide, and titanium trioxide

ACGIH TLV: 10 mg/m^3

OSHA TWA: 15 mg/m^3 dust

Specific References

Kazantzis G, "Role of Cobalt, Iron, Lead, Manganese, Mercury, Platinum, Selenium, and Titanium in Carcinogenesis," *Environ Health Perspect*, 1981, 40:143-61.

Lawson JJ, "The Toxicity of Titanium Tetrachloride," *J Occup Med*, 1961, 3(1):7-12.

U.S. Department of Health and Human Services, "Toxicological Profile for Titanium Tetrachloride," Agency for Toxic Substances and Diseases Registry, June 1994.

Titanium Tetrachloride *see* Titanium *on this page*

Titanocene *see* Titanium *on this page*

TJB *see* N-Nitrosodiphenylamine *on page 982*

TNT *see* 2,4,6-Trinitrotoluene *on page 1035*

Tok® *see* Nitrofen *on page 980*

Tokkorn® *see* Nitrofen *on page 980*

Tolit *see* 2,4,6-Trinitrotoluene *on page 1035*

Toluene

Related Information

Gasoline *on page 932*

Methyl Isocyanate *on page 968*

(Continued)

Toluene *(Continued)*

CAS Number 108-88-3

UN Number 1294

Synonyms Methyl Benzene; Tolu-Sol

Commonly Found In Glues, paint removers, pesticides, degreasers

Mechanism of Toxic Action

Three mechanisms proposed:

- Alters lipid structure of cell membranes
- Alters membrane-bound enzyme or receptor-site specificity
- Toxic metabolite modifies function of cell microsomal proteins and RNA

Adverse Reactions

Central nervous system: CNS depression following early CNS stimulation

Hepatic: Transient liver injury

Renal: Renal tubular acidosis

Respiratory: Bronchitis/wheezing; pulmonary edema

Signs & Symptoms of Acute Overdose Eye irritation, asthenia, dementia, chorea (extrapyramidal), skin irritation, myoglobinuria, metabolic acidosis, hypokalemia, ototoxicity, tinnitus, euphoria, memory loss, fatigue, irritability, vomiting, mydriasis, burns, nonoliguric renal failure

Toxicodynamics/Kinetics

Absorption: Readily by inhalation (within 30 minutes) or ingestion (within 2 hours); slowly by dermal route (14-23 mg/cm^2/hour); accumulates in adipose tissue

Metabolism: Hepatic to hippuric acid (60% to 70%), benzoyl glucuronide (10% to 20%), and ortho or para cresol (<1%)

Half-life: 3 days

Elimination: Hippuric acid excreted in urine, 20% excreted through the lungs, unchanged

Reference Range Determined by measurement of urine hippuric acid. Blood toluene levels of 1.0-2.5 mg/L are associated with intoxication. Coma and death occur at levels of 2.5-10.0 mg/L. Blood toluene BEI is 1.0 mg/L. S-benzyl-N-acetyl-L-cysteine can be measured by HPLC and GC/MS at a lower urinary detection limit of 0.01 mg/L.

Overdosage Treatment

Decontamination:

- Dermal: Wash with soap and water
- Inhalation: Administer 100% humidified oxygen
- Ocular: Irrigate with saline
- Oral: Emesis is contraindicated; lavage is not to be used unless there is a large ingestion

Supportive therapy: Avoid epinephrine because of myocardial sensitization; avoid haloperidol (which can further deplete dopamine concentration of the brain); avoid aspirin due to increased ototoxicity and decreased toluene clearance

Diagnostic Tests/Procedures

Blood Gases, Arterial *on page 1207*

Chest Films *on page 1224*

Complete Blood Count *on page 1236*

Electrolytes, Blood *on page 1254*

Phosphorus, Serum *on page 1322*

Monitoring Parameters Monitor for benzene contamination

Pregnancy Implications Animal teratogenesis (cleft palate, skeletal malformations); human studies have indicated developmental delay, microcephaly, and growth retardation; neonatal acidosis (renal tubular) may occur (usually resolves in 3 days)

Additional Information Sweet odor; largest source of airborne emissions is through combustion of gasoline (5% to 7% toluene by weight); levels in drinking water is usually <3 mcg/L

Lethal oral dose: 625 mg/kg

Estimated daily dose by inhalation: 300 mcg

Cigarette smoking can cause a daily increase in toluene inhalation of 1000 mcg

Drinking water contributes 0.3-0.5 mcg/day of toluene exposure

Mean toluene level in ambient air: 2.8 ppb in urban areas; 0.4 ppb in rural areas

Atmospheric half-life: 10-104 hours

Soil half-life: 1-7 days

Odor threshold: 0.17 ppm

TLV-TWA: 100 ppm

PEL-TWA: 200 ppm

Urinary BEI of O-cresol: 1 mg/g creatinine

Specific References

Mizutani T, Oohashi N, and Naito H, "Myoglobinemia and Renal Failure in Toluene Poisoning: A Case Report," *Vet Hum Toxicol*, 1989, 31(5):448-50.

Shibata K, Yoshita Y, and Matsumoto H, "Extensive Chemical Burns From Toluene," *Am J Emerg Med*, 1994, 12(3):353-5.

Streicher HZ, Gabow PA, Moss AH, et al, "Syndromes of Toluene Sniffing in Adults," *Ann Intern Med*, 1981, 94(6):758-62.

Takahashi S, Kagawa M, Shiwaku K, et al, "Determination of S-Benzyl-N-Acetyl-L-Cysteine by Gas Chromatography/Mass Spectrometry as a New Marker of Toluene Exposure," *J Anal Toxicol*, 1994, 18(2):78-80.

U.S. Department of Health and Human Services, "Toxicological Profile for Toluene TP-93/14," Agency for Toxic Substances and Diseases Registry, May 1994.

Toluene Diisocyanate

CAS Number 584-84-9

UN Number 2078

Synonyms Meta-Toluene Diisocyanate; TDI

Use In the manufacture of polyurethane foams, elastomers

Mechanism of Toxic Action Irritation to mucous membranes/sensitizer as an allergen

Adverse Reactions Respiratory: Respiratory irritation and sensitization, wheezing, hemorrhagic alveolitis

Signs & Symptoms of Acute Overdose Eye irritation, burning of throat and nose, choking, cough, hemoptysis, chest pain, nystagmus, dyspnea, retrosternal chest pain, euphoria, ataxia, nausea, vomiting, impotence, decreased libido

Toxicodynamics/Kinetics Metabolism: May be metabolized to 2,4-toluene diamine (a carcinogen)

Overdosage Treatment

Decontamination: Emesis is contraindication

Inhalation exposure: Give supplemental oxygen, bronchodilators

Oral exposure: Dilute with milk or water; basic poison management

Additional Information Fruity, pungent odor

Odor threshold: 2 ppm

TLV-TWA: 0.005 ppm

IDLH: 10 ppm

Asthma, chronic bronchitis are long-term sequelae; acute pulmonary pathology will be evident within 8 hours

Specific References

Banks, DE, Butcher BT, and Salvaggio JE, "Isocyanate-Induced Respiratory Diseases," *Ann Allergy*, 1986, 57(6):389-96.

Tolu-Sol *see* Toluene *on page 1029*

Topitox® *see* Anticoagulant Rodenticide *on page 859*

Toxakil® *see* Toxaphene *on this page*

Toxaphene

Related Information

Organochlorines *on page 983*

CAS Number 8001-35-2

UN Number 2761

Synonyms Campheclor; Chlorinated Camphene

Brand Names Agricide Maggot Killer®; Alltox®; Camphofene®; Geniphene®; Huilex®; Motox®; Penphene®; Phenatox®; Phenicide®; Toxakil®; Tox-Sol®

Use Chlorinated hydrocarbon insecticide used on livestock to control lice, flies, ticks, mange, and mites; used in treating flowering plants; not used on agricultural commodities as of 1993

Mechanism of Toxic Action Blocks GABA-regulated chloride ionophore of the neuronal synapse

Adverse Reactions Salivation

Signs & Symptoms of Acute Overdose Seizures, respiratory failure, elevated liver function tests, nausea, tremor, ataxia, hyperthermia

Toxicodynamics/Kinetics

Absorption: Oral and dermal

Metabolism: Hepatic dechlorination, oxidation, and dehydrodechlorination

Elimination: Urine and feces

Overdosage Treatment

Decontamination:

Dermal: Remove contaminated clothing (especially leather); wash with soap and water

Inhalation: Administer 100% humidified oxygen

Ocular: Irrigate with saline copiously

Oral: Do not induce emesis; lavage/activated charcoal

Supportive therapy: Benzodiazepines, phenobarbital, or phenytoin may be used for seizure control; to to avoid catecholamine in that it may increase myocardial irritability and result in ventricular arrhythmias

Enhancement of elimination: Multiple dosing of activated charcoal or cholestyramine may be effective; hemodialysis or hemoperfusion is not likely to be beneficial

(Continued)

Toxaphene *(Continued)*

Additional Information Adrenal-based corticosteroid synthesis may be decreased; contains 67% to 69% chlorine; may decrease effect of warfarin

Minimum lethal dose: Oral: 2-7 g
Seizuregenic oral dose: 10 mg/kg
Toxic dermal dose: 660 mg/kg
Average dietary intake for an adult: <0.01 mcg/kg/day
Average inhalation exposure: ~0.0004-0.0033 mcg/day
Atmospheric residence time: 46-70 days
Water half-life: >10 years
PEL-TWA: 0.5 mg/m^3
TLV-TWA: 0.5 mg/m^3

Specific References

U.S. Department of Health and Human Services, "Toxicological Profile for Toxaphene," Agency for Toxic Substances and Diseases Registry, August 1994.

Toxins Which Should be Lavaged With Solutions Other Than Water *see page 1635*

Tox-Sol® *see* Toxaphene *on previous page*

Travex *see* Chlorate Salts *on page 884*

TRI *see* Trichloroethylene *on next page*

Tri-Ban® *see* Anticoagulant Rodenticide *on page 859*

Tribromomethane *see* Bromoform *on page 872*

Trichloren *see* Trichloroethylene *on next page*

Trichloroethane

CAS Number 71-55-6

UN Number 2831

Synonyms CF 2; Methyl Chloroform; Strobane; TCA; TCE

Commonly Found In Cleaning solvent lubricant, ink, typewriter correction fluid; also is frequently used in an abused setting ("bagging")

Mechanism of Toxic Action CNS depression, rapid anesthetic action

Adverse Reactions

Cardiovascular: Hypotension, cardiovascular collapse, ventricular fibrillation
Central nervous system: Anesthesia
Neuromuscular & skeletal: Peripheral neuropathy (axonopathy)
Ocular: Eye irritation
Respiratory: Respiratory depression, pulmonary edema

Signs & Symptoms of Acute Overdose Diplopia, dizziness, acetone breath, coma, ataxia, agitation, drowsiness, hallucinations, nausea, vomiting, diarrhea, erythema, seizures

Toxicodynamics/Kinetics

Absorption: Rapid dermally, through inhalation, or through ingestion
Metabolism: Hepatic (<10%) to trichloroacetic acid
Half-life: 53 hours
Elimination: Primarily by the lungs (91%)

Reference Range Fatal serum levels range from 1.7-42.0 mg/L of trichloroethane concentration. Blood level of 1.4 mg/L consistent with exposure of 250 ppm.

Overdosage Treatment

Decontamination:
- Dermal: Wash with soap and water; isopropyl alcohol can be used
- Inhalation: Administer 100% humidified oxygen
- Ocular: Irrigate with saline
- Oral: Emesis is contraindicated; dilute with milk

Supportive therapy: Propranolol may be beneficial for tachycardia; avoid catecholamines as it can sensitize the myocardium; calcium gluconate or phenylephrine has been useful to treat hypotension in the dog model

Diagnostic Tests/Procedures

Electrocardiography *on page 1253*
Liver Profile *on page 1286*
Urobilinogen, 2-Hour Urine *on page 1376*

Additional Information Pleasant odor; door spray lubricants, VCR cleaners, typewriter correction fluid, and nonacid drain cleaners have highest amount of 1,1,1-trichloroethane

Odor threshold: 120-500 ppm
Estimated daily intake: 50-1000 mg by all routes of exposure
Foods with highest levels include allspice (16,000 ppb), celery seed (909 ppb), and pickling spice (549 ppb)
Atmospheric half-life: 2.7-6 years
Soil half-life (aerobic degradation): ~1 week
Urban atmospheric concentration in U.S.: 0.1-1 ppb

TLV-TWA: 350 ppm
PEL-TWA: 350 ppm
Levels of 1000 ppm will cause ataxia; BEI of urinary trichloroacetic acid is 10 mcg/L

Specific References

Bass M, "Sudden Sniffing Death," *JAMA*, 1970, 212(12):2075-9.
Gerace RV, "Near Fatal Intoxication by 1, 1, 1-Trichloroethane," *Ann Emerg Med*, 1981, 10(10):533-4.
House RA, Liss GM, and Wills MC, "Peripheral Sensory Neuropathy Associated With 1,1,1-Trichloroethane," *Arch Environ Health*, 1994, 49(3):196-9.
Kelafant GA, Berg RA, and Schleenbaker R, "Toxic Encephalopathy Due to 1,1,1-Trichloroethane Exposure," *Am J Ind Med*, 1994, 25(3):439-46.
King GS, Smialek JE, and Troutman WG, "Sudden Death in Adolescents Resulting From the Inhalation of Typewriter Correction Fluid," *JAMA*, 1985, 253(111):1604-6.
Troutman WG, "Additional Deaths Associated With the Intentional Inhalation of Typewriter Correction Fluid," *Vet Hum Toxicol*, 1988, 30(2):130-2.
U.S. Department of Health and Human Services, "Toxicological Profile for 1,1,1-Trichloroethane," Agency for Toxic Substances and Diseases Registry, October 1993.

Trichloroethylene

CAS Number 79-01-6

UN Number 1710

Synonyms Acetylene Trichloride; TRI; Trichloren; Trilene

Use Industrial degreaser, fire retardant, lacquer/adhesive, house cleaning solvent, typewriter correction fluid

Mechanism of Toxic Action CNS depressant; may induce peroxisome proliferation

Adverse Reactions

Cardiovascular: Ventricular fibrillation, bradycardia
Central nervous system: CNS depression
Hepatic: Hepatitis
Ocular: Diplopia, blurred vision progressing to blindness, optic neuropathy
Renal & genitourinary: Tubular necrosis (acute)
Respiratory: Respiratory depression, pulmonary edema

Signs & Symptoms of Acute Overdose Mydriasis, salivation, slurred speech, loss of taste, cyanosis, dyspnea, ataxia, nystagmus, dizziness, dementia, cranial nerve palsies, fatigue, resting tremor, headache, vomiting, impotence, seizures, bradycardia

Toxicodynamics/Kinetics

Absorption: Rapid by ingestion and inhalation; minimal dermal exposure
Metabolism: In the liver; fat soluble
Half-life: 30-38 hours
Excretion: Excreted in urine, feces, and lung (16%)

Reference Range Blood concentrations of 5.0-10.0 mg/dL related to anesthetic action; levels of 0.3-11.0 mg/dL are associated with fatalities; blood level of 0.1 mg/dL is consistent with exposure of 100 ppm

Overdosage Treatment

Decontamination:
Dermal: Wash with soap and water
Ocular: Irrigate with saline
Oral: Do not induce emesis; activated charcoal with cathartic may be used
Supportive therapy: Avoid catecholamines in that they may sensitize the myocardium; propranolol may be useful for treatment

Diagnostic Tests/Procedures

Electrocardiography *on page 1253*

Pregnancy Implications Fetotoxic in rodents; possible relationship to congenital heart disease

Additional Information Chloroform odor; degreaser's flush occurs in workers who ingest ethanol following exposure to trichloroethylene

BEI of urinary trichloroacetic acid: 100 mg/g creatinine
Odor threshold: 20 ppm
TLV-TWA: 50 ppm
PEL-TWA: 100 ppm
Toxic ingestion: 0.5 mL/kg
Atmospheric half-life: 6.8 days
Average air intake: 11-33 mcg/day
Ambient atmospheric levels in urban areas: 0.46 ppb
Average intake through drinking water: 2-20 mcg/day

Specific References

Barceloux DG and Rosenberg J, "Trichloroethylene Toxicity," *J Toxicol Clin Toxicol*, 1990, 28:479-504.
Ford ES, Rhodes S, McDiarmid M, et al, "Deaths From Acute Exposure to Trichloroethylene," *JOEM*, 1995, 37:749-54.
Perbellini L, Olivato D, Zedde A, et al, "Acute Trichloroethylene Poisoning by Ingestion: Clinical and Pharmacokinetic Aspects," *Intensive Care Med*, 1991, 17(4):234-5.

(Continued)

Trichloroethylene *(Continued)*

U.S. Department of Health and Human Services, "Toxicological Profile for Trichloroethylene TP-92/19," Agency for Toxic Substances and Diseases Registry, April 1993.

Trichloroform *see* Chloroform *on page 890*

Trichlorohydrin *see* 1,2,3-Trichloropropane *on this page*

Trichloromethane *see* Chloroform *on page 890*

2,4,6-Trichlorophenol

CAS Number 88-06-2; 25167-82-2

UN Number 2020

Brand Names Caswell No 880C®; Dowicide 2S®; Omal®; Phenachlor®

Use Antiseptic and pesticide; used as a wood and glue preservative; antimildew agent in textile manufacture

Mechanism of Toxic Action Chemical which is actually a metabolite of lindane, 2,4,6-trichlorophenol is a respiratory irritant

Adverse Reactions

Respiratory: Bronchospasm and cough on inhalation

Miscellaneous: Chronic oral exposure has produced liver cancer and leukemia in rodent models

Toxicodynamics/Kinetics

Absorption: Probably by oral or dermal (9.9 x 10^{-4} cm/minute) routes

Metabolism: Hepatic

Elimination: Urine

Overdosage Treatment

Decontamination:

Dermal: Wash with soap and water

Inhalation: Administer 100% humidified oxygen

Ocular: Irrigate with saline

Additional Information Fish and shellfish may concentrate 2,4,6-trichlorophenol and it has been estimated that a daily ingestion of 21 g of fish can result in an intake of 95 mcg of this agent

Taste threshold: 2 ppb

Odor threshold: 2.6 ppb

Daily intake from drinking water: 0.4-100 mcg

Atmospheric half-life: 1 day to 3 weeks

Water half-life: 1-19 days

Specific References

U.S. Department of Health and Human Services, "Toxicological Profile for 2,4,6-Trichlorophenol TP-90/28," Agency for Toxic Substances and Diseases Registry, December 1990.

2,4,5-Trichlorophenoxyacetic Acid *see* 2,4,5-T *on page 1019*

1,2,3-Trichloropropane

CAS Number 96-18-4

Synonyms Allyl Trichloride; Glycerol Trichlorohydrin; Trichlorohydrin

Use Primarily as a paint or varnish remover, cleaning or degreasing agent

Mechanism of Toxic Action Metabolites may lead to DNA/protein adducts or lipid peroxidation; a respiratory irritant

Adverse Reactions Throat and ocular irritation at levels ~100 ppm; has caused squamous cell carcinomas in rodent models

Toxicodynamics/Kinetics

Absorption: Probably by inhalation, oral (up to 80%), and dermal routes

Metabolism: To carbon dioxide (which is expired) and glutathione conjugated (mercapturic acid)

Elimination: Urine and fecal

Overdosage Treatment

Decontamination:

Dermal: Wash with soap and water

Ocular: Irrigate with saline

Oral: Dilute with milk or water; activated charcoal may be used with cathartic

Additional Information Found in soil in California and Hawaii at levels ranging from 0.2-2 ppb; combustion products include chloride fumes

TLV-TWA (skin): 10 ppm

Drinking water concentrations: <0.2 mcg/L

Atmospheric half-life: 15.3 days

Water half-life: 44 days (hydrolysis)

Specific References

U.S. Department of Health and Human Services, "Toxicological Profile for 1,2,3-Trichloropropane TP-91/28", Agency for Toxic Substances and Diseases Registry, September 1992.

Trichlorpyriphos (Discontinued) *see* Chlorpyrifos *on page 891*

Trieste Flowers *see* Pyrethrins *on page 1003*

Trilene *see* Trichloroethylene *on page 1033*

Trilit *see* 2,4,6-Trinitrotoluene *on this page*

Trimethyl Glycol *see* Propylene Glycol *on page 1002*

2,4,6-Trinitrotoluene

CAS Number 118-96-7

UN Number 0209 (<30% water); 1356 (>30% water)

Synonyms Alpha TNT; TNT; Tolit; Trilit; Tritol

Use High explosive agent used in military or civilian blasting procedures; chemical intermediate in production of dyes and photographic chemicals

Mechanism of Toxic Action Cause of methemoglobin; dermal irritant

Signs & Symptoms of Acute Overdose Anemia (aplastic anemia), toxic hepatitis, elevated liver enzymes, cataract, altered taste, paresthesia, red color to urine, hemolytic anemia (especially in individuals deficient in glucose-6-phosphate dehydrogenase enzyme), dermal burns, methemoglobinemia

Toxicodynamics/Kinetics

Absorption: Inhalation, oral, and dermal exposure

Metabolism: Hepatic

Elimination: Renal

Overdosage Treatment

Decontamination:

Dermal: Wash with soap and water

Ocular: Irrigate with saline

Supportive therapy: Methylene blue for symptomatic methemoglobinemia

Antidote(s)

Methylene Blue *on page 1444*

Additional Information Combustible, pale yellow solid

Atmospheric half-life: 18-184 days

Water half-life: 14-84 hours

PEL-TWA (skin designation): 0.5 mg/m^3

TLV-TWA (skin designation): 0.5 mg/m^3

Specific References

Thierfelder W and Masihi KN, "Effects of Trinitrotoluene (TNT) Metabolites on Chemiluminescence Response of Phagocytic Cells," *Int J Immunopharmacol*, 1995, 17:453-6.

U.S. Department of Health and Human Services, "Toxicological Profile for 2,4,6-Trinitrotoluene," Agency for Toxic Substances and Diseases Registry, May 1993.

Trioxane *see* Formaldehyde *on page 931*

Tritol *see* 2,4,6-Trinitrotoluene *on this page*

Trixilin® *see* Nitrofen *on page 980*

Tuads® *see* Thiram *on page 1027*

Tulisan® *see* Thiram *on page 1027*

Tumbleaf *see* Chlorate Salts *on page 884*

Turpentine Oil

CAS Number 8006-64-2; 9005-90-7

UN Number 1299

Synonyms Gum Spirits; Spirits of Turpentine

Commonly Found In Oleoresin solvent, paint vehicle, deodorizer fragrance, rubefacient

Mechanism of Toxic Action CNS depressant, irritant to mucous membranes; high volatility with low viscosity

Adverse Reactions

Cardiovascular: Tachycardia

Central nervous system: Ataxia

Dermatologic: Contact dermatitis

Gastrointestinal: Hemorrhagic gastritis and cystitis, diarrhea

Ocular: Conjunctivitis

Renal & genitourinary: Glomerulonephritis

Respiratory: Pulmonary edema, aspiration pneumonitis, wheezing

Signs & Symptoms of Acute Overdose Eye pain, vomiting, aspiration, fever, chills, cough, dyspnea, seizures

Toxicodynamics/Kinetics

Absorption: Well absorbed through the gastrointestinal tract, by inhalation, and dermally; high fat solubility

Metabolism: In the liver

Elimination: Renally and through the lungs

Overdosage Treatment Decontamination: Emesis indicated only for large ingestions and within 30 minutes of ingestion; lavage only after patient is intubated; activated charcoal with cathartic is useful; steroids not beneficial

(Continued)

Turpentine Oil *(Continued)*

Diagnostic Tests/Procedures
Blood Gases, Arterial *on page 1207*
Blood, Urine *on page 1210*
Chest Films *on page 1224*
Complete Blood Count *on page 1236*

Additional Information Pungent odor, although an odor of violets may be noted in overdose settings; combustible
TLV-TWA: 100 ppm
IDLH: 1900 ppm
PEL-TWA: 100 ppm
Minimum lethal dose:
Children: 15 mL
Adults: 140 mL

Specific References
Falk AA, Hagberg MT, Lof AE, et al, "Uptake, Distribution, and Elimination of Alpha-Pinene in Man After Exposure by Inhalation," *Scand J Work Environ Health*, 1990, 16(5):372-8.

Ultracide® *see* Methidathion *on page 959*

Uniflex® DBP *see* Di-n-Butyl Phthalate *on page 914*

Unitox® *see* Chlorfenvinphos *on page 886*

Uranium

Related Information
Radiation: Basics of Exposure *on page 1594-1600*

CAS Number 7440-61-1

UN Number 2979

Use Primarily in nuclear power plants, radiation shielding material, x-ray targets, gyro compasses, and in large incandescent lamps; mordant in silk and wood industry

Mechanism of Toxic Action Uranyl ion complexes with bicarbonate and produces acute renal proximal tubular damage/failure

Adverse Reactions
Renal: Renal tubular damage with a dose >0.1 mg/kg
Miscellaneous: Possible increase in skin cancer rate

Signs & Symptoms of Acute Overdose Albuminuria, elevated BUN, weight loss, pulmonary edema, wheezing

Toxicodynamics/Kinetics
Absorption: Uranyl ion is rapidly absorbed from gastrointestinal tract
Distribution: Lung retains insoluble salts following inhalation
Half-life: 1500 days
Elimination: 60% excreted within 24 hours

Reference Range Average uranium concentration in N.Y. human blood donors: 0.14 μg uranium/kg wet weight of both whole blood and red blood cells

Overdosage Treatment
Decontamination: Irrigate with soap and water; waste should be kept in separate receptacles; use a Geiger-Mueller meter to survey extent of contamination
Supportive therapy: Give 1-3 mEq/kg of I.V. sodium bicarbonate to cause a forced alkaline diuresis which can be nephroprotective

Additional Information Soluble uranium compound in known as uranyl ion; radon decays and forms radon daughters (isotopes of lead, bismuth, and polonium); the radon daughters attach to dust particles and are inhaled by uranium miners; uranium tetrafluoride and uranyl fluoride are hydrolyzed to HF; can call U.S. Department of Energy Regional Coordinating Office at 615-576-1004

Average daily intake from food and water: 1 mcg
Atmospheric half-life of uranyl fluoride: 35 minutes
Rock levels of uranium range from 0.5-4.7 mcg/g
Soil levels average ~1.8 mcg/g in the U.S.
Root crops (potatoes, parsnips, turnips) have the highest uranium levels, and thus dietary daily uranium intake may range from 3.3-4.2 mcg
Estimated intake due to drinking water: 0.6-2 pCi/day (0.02-0.07 Bq/day); essentially insoluble in water

Specific References
Moore RH and Kathren RL, "A World War II Uranium Hexafluoride Inhalation Event With Pulmonary Implications for Today," *J Occup Med*, 1985, 27(10):753-6.
U.S. Department of Health and Human Services, "Toxicological Profile for Uranium TP-90/29," Agency for Toxic Substances and Diseases Registry, December 1990.

VAC® *see* Vinyl Acetate *on next page*

Vacor *see* Nitrophenolurea *on page 981*

Val-Drop *see* Chlorate Salts *on page 884*

Vanadium

CAS Number 7440-62-2

UN Number 3285

Use Primarily as an alloying agent in steel; jet engine manufacture; pesticide production, inks, dyes and pigments

Mechanism of Toxic Action Vanadium reduces alveolar macrophage viability; this may account for vanadium's respiratory irritant effect; vanadium also causes redistribution of iron, chromium, copper, manganese, and zinc; it also has positive inotropic effects on the heart

Adverse Reactions HEENT, cardiovascular, respiratory, neurologic, gastrointestinal, dermatologic, salivation

Signs & Symptoms of Acute Overdose Headache, CNS depression, dry mouth, metallic taste, green tongue, abdominal pain, diarrhea, black stools, ocular irritation, occupational asthma, pulmonary edema, tracheitis, rhinitis, epistaxis, peripheral vasoconstriction of lungs, spleen, kidney, intestine, dermatitis

Toxicodynamics/Kinetics

Absorption: Primarily through inhalation; oral and dermal absorption is poor

Distribution: Although vanadium is found throughout tissues, majority is found in fat

Elimination: Excreted in both urine and feces

Reference Range Normal urine levels: <8 μg/24 hours; total body burden considered to be safe in U.S.: 0.5 mg/L; normal serum concentrations range from 0.26-1.3 ng/mL; normal serum levels: 2-4 μg/L

Overdosage Treatment

Decontamination:

Dermal: Wash with soap and water

Ocular: Irrigate with saline

Oral: Lavage followed by dilution with milk or water; give a cathartic

Enhancement of elimination: BAL is not useful; deferoxamine mesylate or ethylene diamine tetracetate has had some success in animal models

Test Interactions Urine levels performed by atomic absorption spectrometry and adjusted for creatinine are reliable

Additional Information Pentavalent vanadium is more toxic than other forms; the parenteral form is most toxic, followed by inhalation and oral; U.S. coal can contain as much as 10 g/kg of vanadium

Drinking water concentrations: Average 4.3 mcg/L

Daily adult intake by inhalation: ~ 1 mcg

Atmospheric residence time: 1 day

Vanadium concentration in earth's crust: 150 mg/kg

Average content in U.S. soil: 200 mg/kg

Food items with highest levels include ground parsley (1800 ng/g), freeze-dried spinach (533-840 ng/g), wild mushrooms (50-2000 ng/g), and oysters (450 ng/g)

ACGIH TLV: 0.05 mg/m^3 respirable dust or fumes

OSHA TWA: 0.5 mg/m^3 dust, 0.1 mg/m^3 fumes

Specific References

Gomez M, Domingo JL, Llobet JM, et al, "Effectiveness of Chelation Therapy With Time After Acute Vanadium Intoxication," *J Appl Toxicol*, 1988, 8(6):439-44.

Gylseth B, Leira H, Steines E, et al, "Vanadium in the Blood and Urine of Workers in a Ferroalloy Plant," *Scand J Work Environ Health*, 1979, 5:188-94.

U.S. Department of Health and Human Services, "Toxicological Profile for Vanadium TP-91/29," Agency for Toxic Substances and Diseases Registry, July 1992.

Vancide® 89 *see* Captan *on page 877*

Varsol 1® *see* Stoddard Solvent *on page 1015*

VCD *see* 1,1-Dichloroethene *on page 907*

Velsicol 104® *see* Heptachlor *on page 935*

Velsicol® 1068 *see* Chlordane *on page 885*

Veracur *see* Formaldehyde *on page 931*

Victoria Orange® *see* Dinitrocresol *on page 915*

Vinicizer 85® *see* Di-n-Octylphthalate *on page 916*

Vinyl Acetate

CAS Number 108-05-4

UN Number 1301

Synonyms Acetic Acid; 1-Acetoxy-Ethylene; Ethanoic Acid; Ethenyl Ester; Vinyl Ethanoate

Brand Names VAC®; VYAC®; Zeset T®

Use Production of polyvinyl acetate (adhesives, wood gluing, paints) and polyvinyl alcohol (adhesives, textiles, automobile glass)

(Continued)

Vinyl Acetate *(Continued)*

Mechanism of Toxic Action Primarily a respiratory irritant

Adverse Reactions

Central nervous system: Insomnia, dizziness
Dermatologic: Dermatitis, blisters
Hepatic: Elevated liver function tests
Respiratory: Cough, hoarseness, bronchospasm
Miscellaneous: Mucous membrane irritation, throat and ocular irritation, polyneuritis

Toxicodynamics/Kinetics

Absorption: Probably through inhalation, oral, and dermal routes
Metabolism: Plasma and liver esterases hydrolyze vinyl acetate to acetaldehyde and acetic acid along with carbon dioxide

Overdosage Treatment

Decontamination:
Dermal: Wash with soap and water
Inhalation: Administer 100% humidified oxygen
Ocular: Irrigate with saline
Oral: Dilute with milk or water

Additional Information Irritation can occur at air concentrations >20 ppm

TLV-TWA: 10 ppm
Odor threshold: 0.12 ppm
Half-life in water: 7.3 days
Atmospheric half-life: 4-6.5 hours
Amount of vinyl acetate in a cigarette: 400 ng

Specific References

U.S. Department of Health and Human Services, "Toxicological Profile for Vinyl Acetate TP-91/30," Agency for Toxic Substances and Diseases Registry, July 1992.

Vinylbenzene *see* Styrene *on page 1017*

Vinyl Chloride

CAS Number 75-01-4

UN Number 1086

Synonyms Chloroethylene; Ethylene Monochloride

Commonly Found In Adhesives, propellants

Use As a refrigerant, used in production of methylchloroform and in manufacture of polyvinyl chloride (PVC)

Mechanism of Toxic Action Dermal exposure to escaping pressurized gas may cause injury or frostbite due to rapid evaporation; narcotic properties; metabolite (chloroethylene epoxide) is toxic; human carcinogen – angiosarcoma of the liver

Adverse Reactions

Cardiovascular: Ventricular fibrillation
Central nervous system: CNS depression
Respiratory: Respiratory irritation, respiratory depression

Signs & Symptoms of Acute Overdose Inhalation of high concentrations may result in narcotic-like CNS and apnea; chronic exposure may result in angiosarcoma, cancers of the brain, liver, and lung have also been documented; in addition, chronic exposure may result in "vinyl chloride disease" which consists of a scleroderma-like condition of the connective tissue of the fingers and a thickening of the dermas, acro-osteolysis and a Raynaud's-type phenomenon; thrombocytopenia may also occur; ocular irritation, dyspnea, headache, fatigue, seizures, euphoria, ataxia, fingernail clubbing, epigastric pain, hepatomegaly, loss of libido, arthralgia

Toxicodynamics/Kinetics

Absorption: Inhalation or dermal exposure; 42% retained in the lungs; concentrated in the liver and kidneys
Metabolism: In the liver, thiodiglycolic acid is the major metabolite
Elimination: Excreted renally

Reference Range Urinary thiodiglycolic acid level of 0.3-4.0 mg/L may indicate recent exposure

Overdosage Treatment

Decontamination:
Dermal: Remove and discard all contaminated clothing as hazardous waste; wash exposed areas twice with soap and water and rinse well; wash water should be contained and appropriately discarded
Ocular: Irrigate with saline
Oral: Do **not** induce emesis; lavage/activated charcoal with cathartic
Supportive therapy: Symptomatic and supportive care are the mainstay of treatment; administer 100% humidified oxygen as needed; frostbite should be treated with rapid rewarming in a 42°C water bath

Diagnostic Tests/Procedures

Complete Blood Count *on page 1236*

Kidney Profile *on page 1279*
Liver Profile *on page 1286*
Porphyrins, Quantitative, Urine *on page 1326*

Pregnancy Implications Conclusive studies have not been performed; increases in CNS, genital tract, upper alimentary tract defects, and clubfoot have been reported

Additional Information Liver and renal function tests should be performed and repeated annually. Rescue and treatment personnel should take care not to become exposed; this may include self-contained breathing apparatus, chemical protective gloves and goggles, and fluorocarbon rubber protective clothing. Colorless, pleasant sweet ether odor.

Odor threshold: 260 ppm
TLV-TWA: 5 ppm
Cigarette smoke contains 5.6-27 ng/cigarette
Atmospheric half-life: 1.2-1.8 days
Daily intake by an average U.S. adult by inhalation, ingestion, or dermal route is essentially zero

Specific References

"ATSDR Case Studies in Environmental Medicine, Vinyl Chloride Toxicity," *J Toxicol Clin Toxicol*, 1990, 28(3):267-86.
Doll R, "Effects of Exposure to Vinyl Chloride. An Assessment of the Evidence," *Scand J Work Environ Health*, 1988, 14(2):61-78.
U.S. Department of Health and Human Services, "Toxicological Profile for Vinyl Chloride TP-92/20," Agency for Toxic Substances and Diseases Registry, April 1993.
Walker AE, "Vinyl Chloride Disorder," *Br J Dermatol*, 1981, 105(Suppl 21):19-21.
Wu W, Steenland K, Brown D, et al, "Cohort and Case-Control Analyses of Workers Exposed to Vinyl Chloride: An Update," *J Occup Med*, 1989, 31(6):518-23.

Vinyl Cyanide *see* Acrylonitrile *on page 853*

Vinyl Ethanoate *see* Vinyl Acetate *on page 1037*

Vinylidene Chloride *see* 1,1-Dichloroethene *on page 907*

Violet 3 *see* Xylene *on next page*

Vioxan® *see* Carbaryl *on page 877*

Vitriol Brown Oil *see* Sulfuric Acid *on page 1019*

Volatile Oil *see* *Chenopodium* Oils *on page 884*

Vulcatard A® *see* N-Nitrosodiphenylamine *on page 982*

VX (Methylphosphonothioic Acid S-(2-(bis(1-Methyl-Ethyl)Amino)Ethyl) O-Ethyl Ester or V) *see* Nerve Gases *on page 974*

VYAC® *see* Vinyl Acetate *on page 1037*

Watch Battery *see* Button Batteries (Disc) *on page 875*

Weeviltox® *see* Carbon Disulfide *on page 879*

Welding Fume Fever *see* Metal Fume Fever *on page 956*

Westron® *see* Tetrachloroethane *on page 1022*

Whippet *see* Nitrous Oxide *on page 981*

White Phosphorus

CAS Number 7723-14-0; 12185-10-3

UN Number 1381 (Dry or in Water); 2447 (molten)

Synonyms Phosphorus Tetramen; Red Phosphorus; Yellow Phosphorus

Commonly Found In Phosphorus sesquisulfide, phosphine gas

Use Fertilizers, roach poisons, rodenticides, water treatment; used in military as ammunition in motor/artillery shells

Mechanism of Toxic Action Damages endoplasmic reticulum; inhibits fatty acid oxidation

Adverse Reactions

Cardiovascular: Hypotension, tachycardia, atrial fibrillation
Central nervous system: Lethargy, irritability, coma, hyperthermia
Dermatologic: Dermal burns
Endocrine & metabolic: Hypoglycemia can occur on chronic exposure
Gastrointestinal: Irritant, vomiting, abdominal cramps
Hematologic: Anemia, leukopenia, hemolysis
Hepatic: Degeneration and necrosis
Neuromuscular & skeletal: Degeneration and osteoporosis, fasciculations, asterixis, hemiplegia
Renal: Tubular necrosis (acute) and cortical necrosis
Respiratory: Cough on inhalation, tachypnea, dyspnea
Miscellaneous: "Phossy jaw" (degeneration and necrosis of soft tissue and teeth in oral cavity resulting in life-threatening infections); fatty deposition of muscles

(Continued)

White Phosphorus *(Continued)*

and liver, decreases in serum calcium, potassium, and sodium; liver/renal toxicity along with cerebral edema may occur after 5-10 days

Signs & Symptoms of Acute Overdose Gastrointestinal irritant, dermal burns, seizures, coma, breath odor, luminescent stool, flatulence, hypocalcemia, vomiting followed by asymptomatic phase of <12 to 3 days; subsequent signs/symptoms of hepatic or renal failure develop; chronic exposure (5+ years) results in osteoporosis and bone degeneration, commonly of jaw ("phossy jaw"), feces discoloration (black)

Toxicodynamics/Kinetics

Absorption: By oral routes; yellow phosphorus well absorbed dermally and orally; phosphine gas absorbable in lungs; red phosphorus nonabsorbable

Metabolism: Oxidation and hydrolysis to hypophosphites

Elimination: Urine and feces

Reference Range Normal serum phosphate concentrations: 3.0-4.5 mg/100 mL

Overdosage Treatment

Decontamination:

Dermal: Remove contaminated clothing; brush off phosphorus from skin and then continuously irrigate skin with water; apply saline soaked dressings to affected area; phosphorus will fluoresce under a Wood's lamp; 1% copper sulfate solution or silver nitrate has been advocated to aid in decontamination of dermal burns, although its use is controversial

Ocular: Irrigate with saline

Inhalation: Administer 100% humidified oxygen

Oral: Do not induce emesis; lavage within 2-3 hours with 1:5000 to 1:10,000 potassium permanganate or water; activated charcoal may be used

Supportive therapy: Treat dermal burns in traditional method; monitor calcium; steroids are of no benefit in preventing liver injury

Enhancement of elimination: Mineral oil (200-250 mL) can be used as a cathartic; exchange transfusion may be helpful

Diagnostic Tests/Procedures

Liver Profile *on page 1286*

Kidney Profile *on page 1279*

Pregnancy Implications Uterine hemorrhage has occurred in first trimester after a 2 mg/kg dose (an abortifacient)

Additional Information Garlic breath odor and luminescent vomitus, flatus, or stool is pathognomonic although not frequent; phosphine gas has garlic odor; gas release occurs in industrial use or with moisture contamination of aluminum or zinc phosphide rodenticides; match phosphorus content essentially nontoxic; match toxicities are secondary to potassium chlorate content; vomiting can occur after oral ingestion of 2-23 mg/kg; red phosphorus is not soluble and essentially not absorbed through the gastrointestinal tract and is, therefore, considered nontoxic

Lethal oral dose: >1.5 g

Atmospheric half-life: 5 minutes

PEL-TWA: 0.1 mg/m^3

TLV-TWA: 0.1 mg/m^3

Specific References

Simon FA and Pickering LK, "Acute Yellow Phosphorus Poisoning. 'Smoking Stool Syndrome'," *JAMA*, 1976, 235(13):1343-4.

U.S. Department of Health and Human Services, "Toxicological Profile for White Phosphorus," Agency for Toxic Substances and Diseases Registry, June 1994.

Zong-Yue S, Yao-Ping L, and Xue-qi G, "Treatment of Yellow Phosphorus Skin Burns With Silver Nitrate Instead of Copper Sulfate," *Scan J Environ Health*, 1985, 11(Suppl 4):33.

White Spirit *see* Petroleum Distillates – Naphtha *on page 991*

White spirits *see* Stoddard Solvent *on page 1015*

White Tar *see* Naphthalene *on page 973*

Wofatox® *see* Methyl Parathion *on page 969*

Wood Alcohol *see* Methanol *on page 957*

Wood Creosote (Beechwood Creosote) *see* Creosote *on page 898*

Wood Naphtha *see* Methanol *on page 957*

Woodtreat® *see* Pentachlorophenol *on page 990*

Xylene

CAS Number 1330-20-7; 106-42-3; 108-38-3; 95-47-6

UN Number 1307

Synonyms Dimethyl Benzene; Methyltoluene; Violet 3; Xylol

Use In histology laboratories (M-xylene), manufacture of polymers, glues, paints, and as a vehicle for pesticides

Mechanism of Toxic Action Anesthetic at high doses (>5000 ppm)

Adverse Reactions

Central nervous system: CNS depression
Hepatic: Liver necrosis
Respiratory: Irritation to upper airway

Signs & Symptoms of Acute Overdose Dizziness, headache, fatigue, dementia, nausea, ocular irritation, syncope, throat burning, nystagmus, skin irritation, cough

Toxicodynamics/Kinetics

Absorption: By inhalation, dermally, or through the gastrointestinal tract
Protein binding: 90%
Metabolism: In the liver
Half-life: 20-30 hours
Elimination: 2,4-Xylenol and methyl hippuric acid are excreted renally; xylene is protein bound

Reference Range BEI of methyl hippuric acid (urine) is 1.5 g/g creatinine; blood level of 1 mg/L is consistent with exposure of 100 ppm

Overdosage Treatment

Decontamination:
- Dermal: Wash with soap and water
- Ocular: Irrigate with saline
- Oral: Do not induce emesis; dilute with milk or water

Supportive therapy: Avoid use of catecholamines since they may exacerbate myocardial irritability

Diagnostic Tests/Procedures

Chest Films *on page 1224*
Electrolytes, Blood *on page 1254*
Kidney Profile *on page 1279*
Liver Profile *on page 1286*

Pregnancy Implications Fetotoxic in animals

Additional Information Patients may be more sensitive to ethanol; sweet odor; aspirin or ethanol can produce a false-positive urine test result for hippuric acid; air xylene concentrations >10,000 ppm can result in unconsciousness and death; xylene may be present in the gas phase delivery in cigarettes at a concentration of up to 20 mcg/cigarette

Lethal oral dose: 15 mL
Odor threshold: 0.05 ppm
TLV-TWA: 100 ppm
PEL-TWA: 100 ppm
Average daily intake by inhalation: ~353 mcg
Average daily intake through drinking water: ~39.4 mcg/kg/day
Average amount in drinking water: ~2 mcg/L
Median urban atmospheric level: 7.2 ppb
Atmospheric half-life: 0.5-1 day
Water half-life (by biodegradation) 10.3 days; by volatilization: 5.6 hours
Soil half-life: 1-2 days (photo-oxidation)

Specific References

Riihimaki V and Savolainen K, "Human Exposure to M-Xylene Kinetics and Acute Effects on the Central Nervous System," *Ann Occup Hyg*, 1980, 23(4):411-22.

U.S. Department of Health and Human Services, "Toxicological Profile for Xylenes," Agency for Toxic Substances and Diseases Registry, October 1993.

Xylol *see* Xylene *on previous page*

Yellow Phosphorus *see* White Phosphorus *on page 1039*

Yperite *see* Mustard Gas *on page 972*

Zerox® *see* Hydrazine *on page 939*

Zeset T® *see* Vinyl Acetate *on page 1037*

Zinc (Chloride and Oxide)

Related Information

Radiation: Basics of Exposure *on page 1594-1600*
Toxins Which Should be Lavaged With Solutions Other Than Water *on page 1635*

CAS Number 7440-66-6

UN Number 1436

Adverse Reactions Respiratory, gastrointestinal, ocular, pancreatic

Signs & Symptoms of Acute Overdose Inhalation of zinc chloride fumes from soldering has caused asthma; ingestion of zinc salts has produced gastritis, vomiting, diarrhea, hyperthermia, shock, and death; eye exposure may result in corneal damage, cough, lens opacification; metal fume fever, pancreatitis; zinc chloride is highly corrosive, hypertension, nephritis (hematuria), pancreatic insufficiency

(Continued)

Zinc (Chloride and Oxide) *(Continued)*

Toxicodynamics/Kinetics

Absorption: In small intestine (20% to 30%); iron and dairy products decrease absorption

Protein binding: Highly protein bound

Elimination: Primarily fecal; urinary excretion is 0.3-0.4 mg/day

Reference Range Normal blood levels of zinc: 68-136 μg/dL

Overdosage Treatment

Decontamination: Do not evacuate gastric contents with zinc chloride or phosphide because they are corrosive; dilute with milk

Enhancement elimination: Calcium disodium, ethylene diaminetetra-acetate, of dimercaprol has been used with success; N-acetylcysteine has been used to increase urinary excretion of zinc sulfate

Additional Information Radiopaque

Zinc chloride fume: TLV-TWA: 1 mg/m^3; TLV-STEL: 2 mg/m^3

Zinc oxide fume: TLV-TWA: 5 mg/m^3; TLV-STEL: 10 mg/m^3

Zinc oxide dust: TLV-TWA: 10 mg/m^3

Zinc chloride is most toxic form

Specific References

Chobanian SJ, "Accidental Ingestion of Liquid Zinc Chloride: Local and Systemic Effects," *Ann Emerg Med*, 1981, 10(2):91-3.

Hedtke J, Daya MR, Neace G, et al, "Local and Systemic Toxicity Following Zinc Chloride ($ZnCl_2$) Ingestion," (Abstract 50), *Vet Hum Toxicol*, 1989, 31:342.

Hjortso E, Qvist J, Bud MI, et al, "ARDS After Accidental Inhalation of Zinc Chloride Smoke," *Intensive Care Med*, 1988, 14(1):17-24.

McKinney PE, Brent J, and Kulig K, "Acute Zinc Chloride Ingestion in a Child: Local and Systemic Effects," *Ann Emerg Med*, 1994, 23(6):1383-7.

McKinney PE, Brent J, and Kulig K, "Zinc Chloride Ingestion in a Child: Exocrine Pancreatic Insufficiency," *Ann Emerg Med*, 1995, 25:562.

Zinc Shakes *see* Metal Fume Fever *on page 956*

BIOLOGICAL AGENTS

GENERAL CONSIDERATIONS REGARDING BIOLOGICAL POISONINGS

Some of the most interesting and challenging poisonings for the toxicologist or poison information specialist are those that can be classified as "biological intoxications." Specifically included in this category are a myriad of naturally occurring chemical toxins, alkaloids, venoms, and microbial contaminants. Representative sources for these biological toxins are poisonous plants (plants), fungi (mushrooms), spoiled or tainted food (food-borne toxins), venomous fish, arthropods, and reptiles (envenomations).

The incidence and significance of biological intoxications can best be illustrated through data extracted from the 1993 annual report of the American Associations of Poison Control Centers toxic exposure surveillance system (Table 1). Figures given in this collection system were compiled from 64 poison control centers with a population base of 181.3 million.

Table 1. Known Outcomes of Biological Toxins

Adapted from the *American Journal of Emergency Medicine*, 1994, 12(5):546-99.

Biological Toxin	1993 Exposures	No Effect	Minor Effect	Moderate Effect	Major Effect	Death
Snake Bites	4736	314	1840	591	86	0
Other/Unknown Reptiles	919	77	267	24	1	0
Insect Bites/Stings	38,558	990	16,028	1704	47	1
Spider/Unknown Insect	21,958	443	8230	1594	243	0
Fish Stings	1164	13	449	124	0	0
Mushroom Ingestions	7976	4625	772	312	17	1
Plant Exposures	94,725	26,270	10,860	1252	45	1
Food Contamination	59,997	6132	11,103	1883	54	3
Totals	230,033	38,864	49,549	7484	493	6

Out of 1,751,476 human exposure cases for 1993, 230,033 involved poisonings with biological agents. Therefore, it is very significant to note that 13.4% of all poisoning episodes handled by clinicians will involve a substance in this group. Accordingly, with a greater than 1 in 10 chance that a poisoning will be caused by a biological toxin, it is incumbent upon physicians and poison control center specialists to be familiar with toxicity and treatment approaches.

Although the incidence of these poisonings is high, morbidity and mortality are surprisingly low. Only 5% of the outcomes were reported having a moderate or serious outcome. Fatalities were rare with only 6 reported deaths (0.003%). This figure accounts for only 1% of the 626 fatal cases reported to the data collection system.

There are at least 5 important considerations or dilemmas for the more challenging aspects for the clinician managing a poisoning episode involving a substance from this group. Atypical problems which are encountered may include any of the following: identification of the poison, quantification of the dose, lack of specific laboratory analysis, lack of specific antidotes, and use of nonmedical consultants. Although these potential problems may add to the complexities of patient management, they are by no means insurmountable. Chances for a positive outcome are improved when available resources are combined with consultations with the geographically nearest regional poison control center and skilled toxicologist.

IDENTIFICATION OF THE POISON

In most cases of accidental poisoning or intentional overdose, the identification of the offending medication or chemical can be determined with little difficulty. A good patient or family history, OTC and prescription bottles retrieved from the scene, ingredient listings on containers, or a material safety data sheet (MSDS) on file at the work site provide immediate clues as to the toxin(s) involved.

When triaging exposures involving biological toxins, however, the above methods of identification may be of little or no value. Mother Nature has not conveniently tagged plants, mushrooms, spiders, and snakes with their unique botanical, mycological, or zoological nomenclature for the medical expediency of exacting healthcare professionals. Accurate identification may hinge on a combination of piecing together a fragmented exposure history, recognizing a constellation of signs and symptoms as a particular toxidrome, and/or utilizing the expertise of a non-healthcare professional such as a botanist or mycologist.

Consider the problem of substance identification inherent in each of the following not-so-uncommon scenarios:

1. A small child arrives home to admit he/she "ate a small handful of those little red berries on a bush out in the prairie."
2. A mother calls to state that her toddler ingested a few bites of a household plant she can only best describe as "it's green and has leaves."
3. The weekend trail hiker clad in shorts and sandals who arrives in the ED after being bitten by a snake but was too stunned to recall any pertinent identifying characteristics.
4. The amateur mushroom picker who experiences cramping, vomiting, and diarrhea 1 hour after consuming his gatherings with no intact specimens which would allow you to compare the mushrooms to ones pictured in reference manuals.
5. An adult who presents with a festering lesion on the leg several days after being bitten or stung by an unknown insect while sleeping in a basement apartment.
6. An otherwise healthy adult complains of gastritis and malaise after lavishly indulging at a smorgasbord dinner. Suspected causes may include, but not be limited to, *Salmonella* in poultry, a seafood toxin, *Staphylococcus* in a creamed dressing, a food additive or preservative, *Clostridium perfringens* in a gravy, or a drug-alcohol interaction.

QUANTIFICATION OF A DOSE

In most cases of biological poisoning, the exact dose of the pharmacologically active toxin may never be known. Nature is under no jurisdiction to provide standardization or quality control for the constituents of any given plant, mushroom, or envenomation. Marked variation exists inter- and intraspecies, between geographic or structural location, and even seasonally. Problems with laboratory analysis discussed below preclude routine use of objective tests and their results to retroactively determine dose ingested or extrapolation to future outcomes.

Under these circumstances, the severity of the event is best judged by the nature and extent of the symptoms, complications, or laboratory derangements.

The following are a few examples.

1. It may be well documented that a small child ingested exactly six unripe black nightshade (*Solanum nigrum*) berries. It is unknown how many milligrams of solanine alkaloid comprised the actual ingested dose.
2. In some instances of exposure, the dose involved may be zero. For instance, a person may show fang marks as proof of a rattlesnake bite yet show no local or systemic toxicity since approximately 20% of all snake bites are described as "dry bites."
3. With regard to foodborne microbial toxins, quantification may be performed in some laboratories (ie, public health departments). This process is slow, not routinely ordered, and is of little clinical value in treating individual cases of food poisoning.
4. Individual susceptibility may play a major role in determining a response to a given dose of biological agent. For example, several people may be exposed to dusts and pollens of the common chrysanthemum flowers (*Chrysanthemum morifolium*). However, only one may require ED treatment to correct bronchospasm and wheezing secondary to hypersensitivity to the naturally occurring pyrethrum in the plant.

NONSPECIFICITY OF LABORATORY ANALYSIS

When confronted with the biologically intoxicated patient, however, typical laboratory analytical procedures and their subsequent interpretation simply do not exist. In these cases, treatment plans will be influenced more by exposure history, clinical presentation, and other laboratory indices. These factors taken together will give a much clearer picture of the severity of these toxic events.

Examples where nonspecific laboratory tests are valuable in the monitoring and management of patients exposed to biological toxins are

- serial serum potassium measurements and continuous EKG monitoring in cases of ingestions involving Oleander (*Nerium oleander*), a cardiac glycoside-containing plant
- frequent coagulation profiles and CBCs following *Crotalidae* snake envenomations
- frequent liver and kidney function tests following ingestion of death cap (*Amanita phalloides*), a cyclopeptide-containing mushroom
- a stat CBC, electrolyte, and urinalysis in evaluating a debilitated food poison patient
- platelet count, PT, PTT, BUN, and creatinine in suspected bites of the brown recluse (*loxosceles reclusa*) spider

FEW SPECIFIC ANTIDOTES

Biological toxins possess few specific antidotes. In a vast majority of these cases, cautious observation and conservative symptomatic and supportive care are the mainstay of therapy.

A high percentage of poisoning inquiries, especially those originating from the home environment, can be safely handled with nothing more than calm reassurance to the parent and simple over-the-counter remedies such as:

- the BRATT diet with glucose/electrolyte solutions for mild food poisoning cases

- application of ice and antipruritics (ie, diphenhydramine, hydrocortisone, or benzocaine) for nonvenomous insect bites and stings
- antiseptics and wound care for nonpoisonous snake bites
- syrup of ipecac induced emesis and telephone follow-up for ingestion of mouthful amounts of lawn mushrooms
- antihistamines (eg, diphenhydramine) may ameliorate mild histamine reactions (eg, flushing, pruritis, headache, and palpitations) associated with scromboid fish poisoning

A few notable antidotes for biologic toxins do exist. Their use is generally reserved for serious and life-threatening poisoning incidents. Examples of these antidotes are

- rattlesnake or pit viper (polyvalent Crotalidae) antivenin
- Eastern coral snake (*Micrurus fulvius*) antivenin (Note: No antivenin for Arizona coral snake (*Micruoides euryxantus*))
- black widow spider (*Latrodectus mactans*) antivenin
- scorpion (*Centruroides exilcauda*) antivenin (Note: Available in Arizona only)
- botulism (trivalent types A, B, and E) for botulism (*Clostridium botulinum*)
- physostigmine for severe anticholinergic complications from Jimson weed (*Datura stramonium*) or Deadly Nightshade (*Atropa belladonna*)
- pyridoxine for symptomatic poisonings from monomethyl hydrazine mushrooms like the false morel (*Gyromitra esculenta*)
- atropine to reverse cholinergic symptoms following muscarine-containing mushrooms (ie, *Boletus calopus*)
- digoxin-specific Fab fragments to reverse toxicity associated with oleander (*Nerium oleander*) and Foxglove (*Digitalis purpurea*) plant poisoning
- although more of an infectious disease issue, various antimicrobial agents may be indicated for specific illnesses attributed to food-borne pathogens (eg, sulfamethoxazole/trimethoprim in all documented cases of shigellosis and ampicillin with gentamicin for severe cases of listeriosis)
- cyanide-antidote kit for plants containing amygdalin (a cyanogenic glycoside)

Regional poison control centers often serve as antidote depots. Rarely used antidotes such as antivenin along with protocols for their safe use are available on a 24-hour basis. If a particular agent is not stored in the center, referrals for emergency access from other sources such as pharmaceutical companies, zoos, aquariums, or botanical gardens can be quickly made.

NEED FOR NONMEDICAL CONSULTANTS

In providing optimal care to the patient intoxicated by more commonly encountered medications and chemicals, the clinician may call upon the services of a number of other physician specialists or medical consultants.

Biological intoxications are rather unique in that identification of the toxic specimen may require consultation with a variety of other nonmedical, yet highly skilled, professionals. Accordingly, these professionals and scientists are located in diverse nonhealthcare facility settings such as museums, zoos, aquariums, arboretums, botanical gardens, greenhouses, florist shops, universities, cooperative extension services, and mycological societies.

Consider the indispensable value of the expertise and service rendered by a nonmedical consultant in the following scenarios:

- a herpetologist to identify an unknown snake
- a mycologist to identify an unknown mushroom
- an entomologist to identify a spider or other unknown insect
- a botanist to identify an unknown wild plant specimen
- a florist or horticulturist to identify an unknown household plant

Regional poison control centers often maintain updated consultant files and are an excellent source for these referrals.

Until such time as the biological specimen is identified precisely, the poison control center can formulate a management strategy. The treatment regimen can then be modified once the identity of the substance is accurately made.

— This introductory text was written by
Anthony M. Burda, RPh, CSPI
Rush-Presbyterian-St Luke's Medical Center

REGARDING MUSHROOMS

When locating a specific mushroom in this biological section alphabetically, either by scientific or common name, refer to the appropriate toxic mushroom group (I-VIII) as identified in the boxes below. If the mushroom's identity is not known or verified, then the reader should use the following figure as a guide to accessing the appropriate toxic mushroom group.

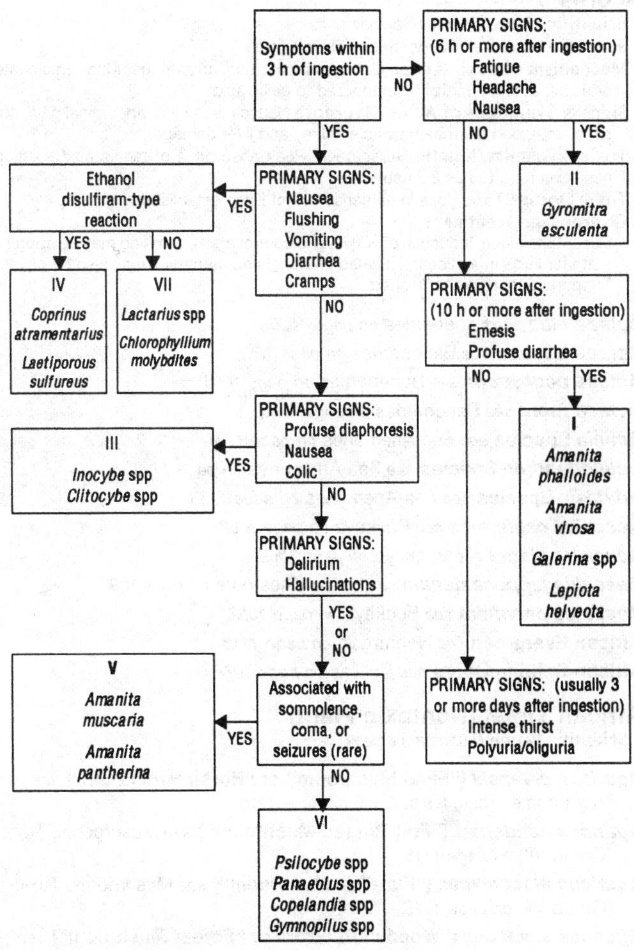

Clinical differentation of mushroom poisoning. (Modified from Lampe KF, "Mushroom Poisoning in Children, Updated". *Pediatrician*, 1977, 6:289-299) Goldfrank LR, Flomenbaum NE, Lewin NA, et al, *Goldfrank's Toxicologic Emergencies*, 5th ed, 1994, 954.

Abrus precatorius *see* Jequirity Bean *on page 1093*

Acid Yellow T *see* Tartrazine Food Poisoning *on page 1149*

Acilan Yellow GG *see* Tartrazine Food Poisoning *on page 1149*

Aconite *see* Monkshood *on page 1108*

Aconitine *see* Monkshood *on page 1108*

Aconitum napellus *see* Monkshood *on page 1108*

Aconitum uncinatum *see* Monkshood *on page 1108*

Acorns

Scientific Name *Quercus* Species

Synonyms Oak Tree Seeds; Seeds of Oak Trees

Mechanism of Toxic Action Contains tannic acid, an astringent that precipitates proteins; at least partially metabolized to gallic acid

Signs & Symptoms of Acute Overdose Nausea, vomiting, abdominal pain, constipation, blood diarrhea, possible kidney and liver damage

Toxicodynamics/Kinetics Absorption: Peak absorption of tannic acid solutions has been reported as 2-3 hours

Toxic Dosage Toxic dose in humans has not been established

Overdosage Treatment

Decontamination: Induction of vomiting is controversial, vomiting may be appropriate for large ingestions; activated charcoal and cathartics may also be of value

Supportive therapy: As needed

Actaea alba *see* Baneberries *on page 1056*

Actaea apgerta *see* Baneberries *on page 1056*

Actaea pachypoda *see* Baneberries *on page 1056*

Actaea rubra *see* Baneberries *on page 1056*

***Actinia* Species** *see* Sea Anemones *on page 1138*

***Actinodendron* Species** *see* Sea Anemones *on page 1138*

***Adamsia* Species** *see* Sea Anemones *on page 1138*

Aesculus californica *see* Buckeye *on page 1062*

Aesculus glabra *see* Buckeye *on page 1062*

Aesculus hippocastanum *see* Horse Chestnuts *on page 1090*

Aesculus parviflora *see* Buckeye *on page 1062*

African Evergreen *see* Nephthytis *on page 1118*

African Spitting Cobra *see* Cobras *on page 1072*

African Violet (Nontoxic Plant)

Scientific Name *Prunus armeniaca*

***Agaricus arvensis* ("Field Mushroom" or "Horse Mushroom")** *see* Mushrooms, Toxic (Group VII) *on page 1116*

***Agaricus hondensis* ("Felt-Ringed Mushroom")** *see* Mushrooms, Toxic (Group VII) *on page 1116*

***Agaricus placomyces* ("Flat-Top Mushroom")** *see* Mushrooms, Toxic (Group VII) *on page 1116*

***Agaricus silvaticus* ("Woods" *Psalliota* or "Forest Mushroom")** *see* Mushrooms, Toxic (Group VII) *on page 1116*

***Agaricus sylvicola* ("Wood-Loving Mushroom" or "Sylvan Mushroom")** *see* Mushrooms, Toxic (Group VII) *on page 1116*

Agave americana *see* Century Plant *on page 1067*

Agkistrodon contortrix *see* Copperhead Snake *on page 1074*

***Agkistrodon contortrix* (Copperhead)** *see Crotalidae on page 1075*

***Agkistrodon piscivorus* (Cottonmouth)** *see Crotalidae on page 1075*

Air Fern (Nontoxic Plant)

Akee Fruit Food Poisoning

Synonyms Jamaican Vomiting Sickness

Commonly Found in Unripe akee fruit in Jamaica, West Africa, Central America, and South Florida

Mechanism of Toxic Action Contains hypoglycin A and B which are CNS depressants; incubation period: 1-3 hours

Signs & Symptoms of Acute Overdose Vomiting, hypothermia, hypoglycemia; can lead to seizures and coma; hypokalemia may occur

Overdosage Treatment Supportive therapy: Intravenous fluids/electrolyte replacement including glucose

Antidote(s)

Dextrose *on page 1409*

Diagnostic Tests/Procedures

Electrolytes, Blood *on page 1254*

Additional Information Hypoglycin is water soluble

Specific References

McTague JA and Forney R Jr, "Jamaican Vomiting Sickness in Toledo, Ohio," *Ann Emerg Med*, 1994, 23(5):1116-8.

Tanaka K, Kean EA, and Johnson B, "Jamaican Vomiting Sickness," *N Engl J Med*, 1976, 295(9):461-7.

Alder Buckthorn *see* Buckthorn *on page 1062*

Alleluia *see* Shamrock *on page 1140*

Alocasia *see* Caladium *on page 1063*

Aloe (Nontoxic Plant)

Adverse Reactions May cause contact dermatitis or catharsis

Aluminum Plant (Nontoxic Plant)

***Amanita bisporigera* ("Destroying Angel")** *see* Mushrooms, Toxic (Group I) *on page 1111*

***Amanita brunnescens* ("Cleft-Foot Deathcap")** *see* Mushrooms, Toxic (Group VII) *on page 1116*

***Amanita citrina* ("False Deathcap")** *see* Mushrooms, Toxic (Group III) *on page 1112*

***Amanita citrina* ("False Deathcap")** *see* Mushrooms, Toxic (Group V) *on page 1114*

***Amanita cokeri* ("Solitary Lepidella")** *see* Mushrooms, Toxic (Group III) *on page 1112*

***Amanita cothurnata* ("Booted" *Amanita*)** *see* Mushrooms, Toxic (Group V) *on page 1114*

***Amanita frostiana* ("Frost's" *Amanita*)** *see* Mushrooms, Toxic (Group V) *on page 1114*

***Amanita gemmata* ("Jeweled Deathcap" or "Jonquil" *Amanita*)** *see* Mushrooms, Toxic (Group V) *on page 1114*

***Amanita muscaria* ("Fly Agaric")** *see* Mushrooms, Toxic (Group III) *on page 1112*

***Amanita muscaria* ("Fly Agaric")** *see* Mushrooms, Toxic (Group V) *on page 1114*

Amanita ocreata *see* Mushrooms, Toxic (Group I) *on page 1111*

***Amanita pantherina* ("Panther" *Amanita*)** *see* Mushrooms, Toxic (Group III) *on page 1112*

***Amanita pantherina* ("Panther" *Amanita*)** *see* Mushrooms, Toxic (Group V) *on page 1114*

***Amanita phalloides* ("Deathcap")** *see* Mushrooms, Toxic (Group I) *on page 1111*

***Amanita smithiana* ("Smith's" *Amanita*)** *see* Mushrooms, Toxic (Group III) *on page 1112*

Amanita strobiliformis *see* Mushrooms, Toxic (Group III) *on page 1112*

Amanita suballiacea *see* Mushrooms, Toxic (Group I) *on page 1111*

***Amanita tenuifolia* ("Slender Death Angel")** *see* Mushrooms, Toxic (Group I) *on page 1111*

***Amanita verna* ("Deadly Agaric" or "Death Angel")** *see* Mushrooms, Toxic (Group I) *on page 1111*

Amanita virosa *see* Mushrooms, Toxic (Group I) *on page 1111*

Amaryllis

Related Information

Star-of-Bethlehem (*Ornithogalum pyrenaicum*) *on page 1145*
Star-of-Bethlehem (*Ornithogalum umbellatum*) *on page 1146*

Synonyms Belladonna Lily; St Joseph's Lily

Mechanism of Toxic Action Contains lycorine (an *Amaryllidaceae* alkaloid) a centrally acting emetic

Signs & Symptoms of Acute Overdose Usually nausea, vomiting, abdominal pain, diarrhea, and salivation; symptoms develop soon after oral ingestion (within 30 minutes) and resolve within 3 hours (according to one report)

Adverse Reactions Dermatologic: May cause dermatitis

Overdosage Treatment Decontamination: Ipecac relatively contraindicated; may be useful, if given soon after ingestion; vomiting has not occurred with ingestion of more than one bulb; activated charcoal with cathartic/lavage may be beneficial depending on amount ingested and time elapsed since ingestion

Additional Information All parts contain alkaloid; bulb is most toxic

Specific References

Litovitz TL and Fahey BA, "Please Don't Eat the Daffodils," *N Engl J Med*, 1982, 306(9):547.

American Aloe *see* Century Plant *on page 1067*

American Elder *see* Elderberry *on page 1081*

American Hellebore *see* Corn Lily *on page 1074*

American Laurel *see* Mountain Laurel *on page 1110*

American Mandrake *see* Mayapple *on page 1105*

American Mistletoe *see* Mistletoe *on page 1107*

American Nightshade *see* Pokeweed *on page 1127*

American Red Elder *see* Elderberry *on page 1081*

American Yew *see* Yew *on page 1159*

Ammonium Sulfite *see* Sulfite Food Poisoning *on page 1148*

Anacardium occidentale *see* Cashew *on page 1066*

***Anemonia* Species** *see* Sea Anemones *on page 1138*

Angel's Trumpet *see* Jimson Weed *on page 1094*

Angel Wings *see* Caladium *on page 1063*

Anopheles freeborni *see* Mosquitoes *on page 1110*

Anopheles quadrimaculatus *see* Mosquitoes *on page 1110*

***Anthea* Species** *see* Sea Anemones *on page 1138*

***Anthoptreura* Species** *see* Sea Anemones *on page 1138*

Appalachian Tea *see* Holly *on page 1089*

Apple of Peru *see* Jimson Weed *on page 1094*

Apricot

Mechanism of Toxic Action Amygdalin (a cyanogenic glycoside) is hydrolyzed in the gut to release hydrocyanic acid, cellular hypoxia occurs after absorption and complexation with cytochrome oxidase

Signs & Symptoms of Acute Overdose Symptoms delayed 30 minutes to 2 hours or longer due to hydrolysis preferentially occurring in alkaline duodenum plus intestinal flora hydrolyzing amygdalin

Adverse Reactions

Central nervous system: Lethargy, drowsiness, headache, coma, seizures, sweating
Gastrointestinal: Abdominal pain, vomiting
Respiratory: Dyspnea
Miscellaneous: Cyanosis, paralysis

Toxic Dosage 1-2 pits likely nontoxic; toxicity unusual with accidental ingestion

Overdosage Treatment

Decontamination: Basic poison management; vomiting is contraindicated due to rapid course of the neurologic symptoms; give 100% oxygen

Supportive therapy: Give sodium bicarbonate for acidosis; cyanide antidote kite should be used for patients symptomatic from cyanide toxicity

Enhancement of elimination: Hemodialysis and charcoal hemoperfusion have been utilized; hyperbaric oxygen may also be utilized; hydroxocobalamin and dicobalt-EDTA used for chelation in Europe

Antidote(s)

Cyanide Antidote Kit *on page 1406*

Diagnostic Tests/Procedures
Anion Gap, Blood *on page 1193*
Blood Gases, Arterial *on page 1207*
Cyanide, Blood *on page 1246*
Electrolytes, Blood *on page 1254*
Methemoglobin, Blood *on page 1296*

Pregnancy Implications Teratogenicity not noted

Additional Information Amygdalin is also found in leaves, flowers, bark, seeds; young leaves have highest concentration; intact pit does not release chemical; apricot most toxic within species

Arabian Cobra *see* Cobras *on page 1072*

Arachnida *see* Mites *on page 1107*

Aralia, False (Nontoxic Plant)

Arbacia punctulata *see* Sea Urchins *on page 1139*

Arborrescent *see* Hydrangea *on page 1090*

Arisaema triphyllum *see* Jack-in-the-Pulpit *on page 1093*

Arizona Bark Scorpion

Scientific Name *Centruroides sculpturatus*

Synonyms Scorpion

Mechanism of Toxic Action Neurotoxin which is heat stable; neurotoxin increases sodium transfer

Signs & Symptoms of Acute Overdose Pain, salivation, muscle myoclonus, gastric/pancreatic hypersecretion, vomiting, fasciculations, sweating, pain at site of bite, tachycardia, restlessness, hypertension, tachypnea, stridor, blurred vision, slurred speech

Grading for *Centruroides sculpturatus* envenomation:
Grade I: Local pain and/or paresthesia
Grade II: Pain and/or paresthesias remote from envenomation site with local signs present
Grade III: Either cranial nerve or somatic skeletal neuromuscular dysfunction
Grade IV: Both cranial nerve and somatic skeletal neuromuscular dysfunction

Overdosage Treatment
Decontamination: Pressure tourniquet (50-70 mm Hg) to slow systemic absorption on affected limb
Supportive therapy: Antivenom from goat serum (I.V.); propranolol or phentolamine can be used for hypertension; bradycardia can respond to atropine
Antivenin is available from the Arizona Poison Center (602-253-3334, 602-253-0813) or Good Samaritan Poison Center in Phoenix, Arizona (602-626-6016)

Antidote(s)
Centruroides Scorpion Venom Antisera *on page 1403*

Drug Interactions Avoid phenothiazines in that they can lower the seizure threshold

Additional Information Antivenom dose is one vial; give second vial at 1 hour if symptoms not improved; allergic effects can occur

Specific References
Amitai Y, Mines Y, Aker M, et al, "Scorpion Sting in Children: A Review of 51 Cases," *Clin Pediatr (Phila)*, 1985, 24(3):136-40.
Amitai Y, "Venomous Scorpions," *Clin Toxicol Rev*, 1987, 10:2.
Bernstein JN, Dart RC, Garcia R, et al, "Efficacy of Antiscorpion (*Centruroides exilicauda*) Fab in a Mouse Model," *Vet Hum Toxicol*, 1994, 36:346.
Curry SC, Vance MV, Ryan PJ, et al, "Envenomation by the Scorpion *Centruroides sculpturatus*," *J Toxicol Clin Toxicol*, 1983-84, 21(4-5):417-49.

Armillariella mellea **("Stumper" or "Honey Mushroom")** *see* Mushrooms, Toxic (Group VII) *on page 1116*

Arrow Head Vine *see* Nephthytis *on page 1118*

Arrow Wood *see* Buckthorn *on page 1062*

Artillery Plant (Nontoxic Plant)

Asian Cobra *see* Cobras *on page 1072*

Asparagus (Berries and Young Shoots)

Scientific Name *Asparagus officinalis*

Signs & Symptoms of Acute Overdose Allergic dermatitis after repeated exposure; berries may possibly cause GI irritation

(Continued)

Asparagus (Berries and Young Shoots) *(Continued)*

Adverse Reactions

Dermatologic: Pruritus, vesiculation

Gastrointestinal: Gastrointestinal irritation, gastrointestinal upset

Overdosage Treatment

Decontamination: Wash thoroughly

Supportive therapy: Treat symptoms

Asparagus officinalis *see* Asparagus (Berries and Young Shoots) *on previous page*

Assassin Bugs *see* Reduvids *on page 1133*

Asthma Weed *see* Indian Tobacco *on page 1091*

Aurelia aurita *see* Jellyfish *on page 1093*

Australian Blue-Ringed Octopus *see* Blue-Ringed Octopus *on page 1059*

Australian Jellyfish (*Chiropsalmus quadrigatus*) *see* Box Jellyfish *on page 1060*

"Autumnal" *Galerina* Mushroom *see* Mushrooms, Toxic (Group I) *on page 1111*

Autumn Crocus

CAS Number 64-86-8

Scientific Name *Colchicum autumnale*

Synonyms Crocus; Fall Crocus; Meadow Crocus; Meadow Saffron; Mysteria; Wonderbulb

Use Colchicine has been used for centuries to treat gout and rheumatism

Mechanism of Toxic Action Inhibits cell division by blocking spindle formation and inhibiting mitosis; cells with high turnover rates are most affected

Signs & Symptoms of Acute Overdose Toxic:

1st phase: 2-24 hours postexposure: Abdominal pain, nausea, vomiting, and diarrhea resulting in hypovolemia, hypotension, electrolyte abnormalities, also peripheral leukocytosis has been reported

2nd phase: 1-7 days postexposure: Multisystem failure, mental status changes, bone marrow depression, proteinuria, oliguric renal failure, coagulopathy, paresthesia, pulmonary edema, respiratory failure, and sudden asystole

3rd phase: 7 or more days: Rebound leukocytosis and alopecia

Toxicodynamics/Kinetics

Absorption: Rapid with peak levels occurring in 30 minutes to 2 hours

Distribution: V_d: 2 L/kg; distributed within 30 minutes; deacetylated in the liver and both colchicine and its metabolites undergo enterohepatic recirculation

Protein binding: Weak, 10% to 30%

Toxic Dosage As little as 7-8 mg of colchicine have resulted in fatalities; ingestion of 12 flowers of *Colchicum autumnale* has caused death; colchicine ingestions ≥0.5 mg/kg are associated with severe poisoning and death

Overdosage Treatment

Decontamination: Lavage may be indicated if performed prior to the onset of symptoms; multiple dose activated charcoal should be of value; one dose of a cathartic may be used if administered prior to the onset of symptoms; due to the delay in the onset of toxicity, asymptomatic patients should be observed for at least 12 hours

Supportive therapy: Aggressive supportive therapy may be required in symptomatic patients; this includes fluid and electrolyte replacement and respiratory support. Hypotension unresponsive to fluids should be treated with dopamine or norepinephrine.

Enhancement of elimination: Hemodialysis and exchange transfusions have not been useful and are not recommended

Antidote(s)

Dopamine Hydrochloride *on page 1418*

Epinephrine *on page 1422*

Test Interactions Colchicine decreases serum cholesterol levels, may interfere with some urine steroid tests

Drug Interactions Colchicine therapy can increase cyclosporine levels

Pregnancy Implications Colchicine is considered a potent teratogen in animals and should be avoided in pregnancy

Additional Information

Family: Liliaceae

Toxin: Colchicine and related alkaloids

Range: Native to Europe, widely cultivated in the U.S.

Toxic parts: Entire plant; colchicine concentrations range from 0.1% in the flowers to 0.8% in the seeds

Specific References

Ellwood MG and Robb GH, "Self-Poisoning With Colchicine," *Postgrad Med J*, 1971, 47(544):129-31.

Levy M, Spino M, and Read SE, "Colchicine: A State-of-the-Art Review," *Pharmacotherapy*, 1991, 11(3):196-211.

Naidus RM, Rodvien R, and Mielke CH Jr, "Colchicine Toxicity: A Multisystem Disease," *Arch Intern Med*, 1977, 137(3):394-6.

Stahl N, Weinberger A, Benjamin D, et al, "Fatal Colchicine Poisoning in a Boy With Familial Mediterranean Fever," *Am J Med Sci*, 1979, 278(1):77-81.

Stapczynski JS, Rothstein RJ, Gaye WA, et al, "Colchicine Overdose: Report of Two Cases and Review of the Literature," *Ann Emerg Med*, 1981, 10(7):364-9.

Azalea

Scientific Name *Rhododendron nudiflorum*

Synonyms Mountain Rosebay; Pinxter Flower; Purple Laurel; Rhododendron

Mechanism of Toxic Action Contains grayanotoxin which binds to a subset of sodium channels causing structural modifications which cause slow opening of these channels which leads to cell depolarization

Signs & Symptoms of Acute Overdose Hypotension, bradycardia; sweating, seizures, asthenia; dermatitis; nausea, vomiting, oral numbness or burning, paresthesia, transient blindness and visual changes

Toxic Dosage Three whole leaves or flowers likely nontoxic; consider decontamination if more

Overdosage Treatment

Decontamination: Avoid ipecac, vagal stimulation increases toxicity; lavage/activated charcoal with cathartic

Supportive therapy: Atropine for bradycardia, I.V. fluids should be sufficient for hypotension

Antidote(s)

Atropine Sulfate *on page 1395*

Additional Information Toxicity is unpredictable, variable among rhododendron types; whole plant toxic, foliage especially; contaminated honey may cause systemic symptoms

Baby's Tears (Nontoxic Plant)

Bacillus cereus Food Poisoning (Type I and II)

Commonly Found in Fried rice (Type I), cereals (Type II), vegetables (Type II), milk (Type II), meat (Type II), turkey (Type II)

Mechanism of Toxic Action

Type I: Heat and pH stable toxin; incubation period: 1-6 hours (emetic form)

Type II: Heat labile enterotoxin; incubation period: 10-12 hours (diarrheal form)

Signs & Symptoms of Acute Overdose Fever is uncommon

Type I: Vomiting is prominent, abdominal cramps, diarrhea can occur

Type II: Watery diarrhea, abdominal cramps, can cause more volume depletion than Type I

Overdosage Treatment *Bacillus cereus* food poisoning does not respond to antimicrobial therapy. Attention should instead be focused on supportive measures such as hydration and electrolyte balance. Clinically significant infections with this organism should be treated with vancomycin intravenously. Unlike other *Bacillus* species (eg, *Bacillus alvei*, *B. subtilis*, *B. circulans*, etc.), *Bacillus cereus* is often resistant to beta-lactam antibiotics such as the penicillins and cephalosporins. Vancomycin should be used until the antimicrobial susceptibility pattern is finalized; limited data suggests the addition of an aminoglycoside to vancomycin may have some minor benefit in serious infections.

Diagnostic Tests/Procedures

Electrolytes, Blood *on page 1254*

Stool Culture *on page 1356*

Additional Information

Microbiology: *Bacillus cereus* is an aerobic, gram-positive bacillus associated with a variety of disease states including food poisoning, ocular infections, bacteremia, and septicemia. *Bacillus cereus* is a spore-forming aerobe which stains gram-positive or gram-variable. It grows readily on standard laboratory media and does not need special culturing techniques.

Epidemiology: *Bacillus cereus* is ubiquitous in the environment, growing readily in such diverse areas as soil, water, vegetables, decaying matter, and dust. In certain individuals, it can be part of the normal human flora, explaining in part its tendency to colonize surgical wounds and serious burn injuries. The needles and syringes of heroin addicts in the United States have also been found to be contaminated with this bacterium. *Bacillus cereus* food poisoning, caused by ingestion of a toxin elaborated by this organism, has been reported from several countries around the world, including the United States and Canada.

(Continued)

Bacillus cereus Food Poisoning (Type I and II) *(Continued)*

Clinical Syndromes:

- **The "emetic form" of *Bacillus cereus* food poisoning:** This results from the ingestion of a preformed toxin produced by this organism. Nausea, vomiting, and abdominal cramping usually occur soon (1-6 hours) following the ingestion of contaminated foods. In particular, this emetic toxin has been associated with fried rice served in Chinese food restaurants. The spores of *B. cereus* can survive the process of boiling rice followed by quick frying.
- **The "diarrheal form" of *Bacillus cereus* food poisoning:** This results from ingestion of a different, heat-labile enterotoxin. The incubation period is longer than for the emetic form, usually more than 9 hours. Profuse watery diarrhea is the predominant symptom, along with abdominal cramping.

Diagnosis: *Bacillus cereus* is readily identified in the laboratory from cultures of blood and other sterile body fluids. In cases of suspected *Bacillus* food poisoning, the implicated foods should be cultured for this organism. There is little benefit in culturing the patient's stool since gastrointestinal tract colonization is not uncommon. As mentioned previously, isolation of *Bacillus cereus* from the blood need not be treated in every case, and clinical judgment is required.

Specific References

"*Bacillus cereus* Food Poisoning Associated With Fried Rice at Two Child Day Care Centers – Virginia, 1993," *MMWR Morb Mortal Wkly Rep*, 1994, 43(10):177-8.

Bean NH, Griffin PM, Goulding JS, et al, "Foodborne Disease Outbreaks, 5-Year Summary, 1973-1987," *MMWR CDC Surveill Summ*, 1990, 39(1):15-57.

Davey RT Jr and Tauber WB, "Post-traumatic Endophthalmitis: The Emerging Role of *Bacillus cereus* Infection," *Rev Infect Dis*, 1987, 9(1):110-23.

Schricker ME, Thompson GH, and Schreiber JR, "Osteomyelitis Due to *Bacillus cereus* in an Adolescent: Case Report and Review," *Clin Infect Dis*, 1994, 18(6):863-7.

Sliman R, Rehm S, and Shlaes DM, "Serious Infections Caused by *Bacillus* Species," *Medicine (Baltimore)*, 1987, 66(3):218-23.

Terranova W and Blake PA, "*Bacillus cereus* Food Poisoning," *N Engl J Med*, 1978, 298(3):143-4.

Tuazon CU, "Other *Bacillus* Species," *Principles and Practice of Infectious Diseases*, 3rd ed, Mandell GL, Douglas RG Jr, Bennett JE, eds, New York, NY: Churchill Livingstone, 1990, 1595-9.

Turnbull PC, "*Bacillus cereus* Toxins," *Pharmacol Ther*, 1981, 13(3):453-505.

Banded Rock Rattlesnake *see* Rattlesnakes *on page 1132*

Banded Water Cobra *see* Cobras *on page 1072*

Baneberries

Scientific Name *Actaea alba*; *Actaea apgerta*; *Actaea pachypoda*; *Actaea rubra*

Synonyms Cohosh

Mechanism of Toxic Action GI is unclear; dermatitis is contact type; protoanemonin reacts with SH groups and inactivates enzymes

Signs & Symptoms of Acute Overdose Oral irritation, gastroenteritis, bloody diarrhea, headache, dizziness, dysuria, hematuria, circulatory failure, tachycardia, visual hallucinations, confusion, seizures

Adverse Reactions Dermatitis, conjunctivitis, and vesiculation may occur

Toxicodynamics/Kinetics

Onset of effect: Oral: Within 30 minutes

Duration:

Dermal: May take several weeks to resolve

Oral: Within 3 hours

Overdosage Treatment

Decontamination: Ipecac relatively contraindicated due to rapid onset of symptoms, lavage recommended in large ingestion; activated charcoal with cathartic may be beneficial; do not give cathartic if diarrhea has developed

Supportive therapy: Maintain hydration and electrolyte balance; hydration also decreases protoanemonin concentration in urine; for dermal, wash thoroughly

Supportive therapy: Antihistamine and corticosteroid therapy as indicated; monitor fluid and electrolyte status

Additional Information Oral symptoms of pain and burning usually limit potential for systemic toxicity; root, berries, and sap are toxic

Basam *see* Scotch Broom *on page 1138*

Bayberry (Nontoxic Plant)

Bead Plant *see* Jequirity Bean *on page 1093*

Bean Tree *see* Golden Chain Tree *on page 1087*

Beauty Bush (Nontoxic Plant)

"Beefsteak Fungus" *see* Mushrooms, Toxic (Group II) *on page 1112*

Begonia (Nontoxic Plant)

Belladonna Lily *see* Amaryllis *on page 1052*

"Bell Mottlegill" Mushroom *see* Mushrooms, Toxic (Group VI) *on page 1115*

"Bell-Shaped" *Panaeolus* Mushroom *see* Mushrooms, Toxic (Group VI) *on page 1115*

Berry Alder *see* Buckthorn *on page 1062*

"Big Laughing" Mushroom *see* Mushrooms, Toxic (Group VI) *on page 1115*

Big Leaf Ivy *see* Mountain Laurel *on page 1110*

Bigroot *see* Wild Cucumber *on page 1157*

Bird of Paradise

Mechanism of Toxic Action Seeds contain tannins, leaves may contain hydrocyanic acid

Signs & Symptoms of Acute Overdose Vomiting, diarrhea, gastrointestinal irritation, drowsiness, dizziness

Toxicodynamics/Kinetics

Onset of effect: Within 30 minutes

Duration: Within 24 hours

Toxic Dosage Ingestion of 5 seed pods has caused poisoning

Overdosage Treatment

Decontamination: Emesis or lavage recommended if asymptomatic and more than small amount ingested

Supportive therapy: Fluid and electrolyte replacement as needed

Additional Information Not a cyanide risk; seeds, pods, leaves, and roots are toxic

Bird Snake *see* Colubrids *on page 1073*

Bisom *see* Scotch Broom *on page 1138*

Bittersweet Nightshade *see* Deadly Nightshade *on page 1078*

Bizzom *see* Scotch Broom *on page 1138*

Black Dogwood *see* Buckthorn *on page 1062*

Black Eyed Susan *see* Jequirity Bean *on page 1093*

Black Locust

Scientific Name *Robinia pseudoacacia*

Mechanism of Toxic Action Ricin, a toxalbumin inhibits protein synthesis

Signs & Symptoms of Acute Overdose Acutely causes irritation to oropharynx, esophagus, and GI tract; may cause hemorrhage and tissue sloughing

Adverse Reactions In addition to vomiting and diarrhea, late phase toxicity due to cytotoxic effects on liver, CNS, kidney, and adrenal system

Toxicodynamics/Kinetics Acute effects occur within 8 hours; late phase complications delayed by 2-5 days possibly with asymptomatic phase in between

Toxic Dosage Toxicity may occur with as little as one bean

Overdosage Treatment Decontamination: Consider ipecac if asymptomatic, activated charcoal may be useful; consider using osmotic cathartic despite hyperactive bowel as decreased exposure to mucosa may be beneficial, follow fluid and electrolyte status closely if symptomatic; if symptomatic, maintain high urine flow; consider alkalinization to prevent hemoglobin crystallization in severe poisonings; guaiac emesis, stool, follow fluid and electrolyte status; check hematologic parameters in severe poisoning, hepatic enzymes

Additional Information Toxicity is variable; related to variations within plants and GI absorption, seed has hard coat; rupture makes toxin available; symptomatic patients should be hospitalized; asymptomatic patients that have received early thorough decontamination may be observed at home; bark, seeds, and leaves are toxic; honey locust is nontoxic

Black Nightshade

Scientific Name *Solanum nigrum*

Synonyms Common Nightshade; Deadly Nightshade; Morelle Noire; Wonderberry

Mechanism of Toxic Action Contains toxic alkaloids; some plants may also contain alpha-cholinergic alkaloids

Signs & Symptoms of Acute Overdose Nausea, vomiting, diarrhea, headache, visual changes, drowsiness, fever, sweating, asthenia, hallucinations, anticholinergic effects may or may not be present to varying degrees

(Continued)

Black Nightshade *(Continued)*

Toxicodynamics/Kinetics Toxicity occurs within 2-24 hours, diarrhea may last 3-6 days, anticholinergic effects may delay GI emptying and produce delayed effects

Toxic Dosage 2-3 green berries or 6 red or black berries should not cause significant toxicity (fatal dose reported as: 200 berries)

Overdosage Treatment

Decontamination: Ipecac if vomiting has not already occurred, lavage and/or charcoal may be beneficial if patient presents symptomatic

Supportive therapy: Maintain fluid and electrolyte balance as necessary, support vital signs; physostigmine will reverse anticholinergic toxicity that may be associated with exposure

Antidote(s)

Physostigmine *on page 1457*

Drug Interactions Solanine poorly absorbed, delayed decontamination may be effective

Additional Information

Toxic parts: Green or yellow berries more toxic than red or black; toxicity may be mistaken for food poisoning; plants may also contain varying amounts of anticholinergic alkaloids

Specific References

Dalvi RR and Bowie WC, "Toxicology of Solanine: An Overview," *Vet Hum Toxicol*, 1983, 25(1):13-5.

Black Snakeroot *see* Death Camas *on page 1078*

Black-Tailed Rattlesnake *see* Rattlesnakes *on page 1132*

Black Widow Spider

Scientific Name *Latrodectus mactans*

Mechanism of Toxic Action Envenomation (neurotoxin and alpha-latrotoxin)

Signs & Symptoms of Acute Overdose Initial bite may be sharply painful or unrecognized; possible papule or punctum on exam with surrounding skin slightly erythematous and indurated; within 30-60 minutes of the bite, however, involuntary spasm and rigidity affect the large muscle groups of the abdomen and limbs

Adverse Reactions

Cardiovascular: Hypertension

Central nervous system: Fasciculations, ptosis

Renal & genitourinary: Priapism

Respiratory: Muscle asthenia/arrest

Overdosage Treatment

Decontamination: Wound care including tetanus prophylaxis; pain and muscle spasm may be managed initially with calcium gluconate 10% solution at 10 mL/dose; may start calcium infusion

Antivenin is available and should be reserved for cases involving respiratory arrest, seizures, uncontrolled hypertension, or pregnancy; usual therapeutic dose: I.V. infusion: 1-2 vials

Supportive therapy: Alternative muscle relaxants including methocarbamol or benzodiazepines

Antidote(s)

Antivenin *(Latrodectus)* *on page 1393*

Calcium Chloride *on page 1400*

Calcium Gluconate *on page 1401*

Pregnancy Implications May be complicated by uterine contractions and potentially, premature delivery; although pregnancy is usually not affected

Additional Information Female responsible for all envenomations

Range: Found throughout the U.S.; web found in corners of buildings, gardens, and fields

Specific References

Handel CC, Izquierdo LA, and Curet LB, "Black Widow Spider (*Latrodectus mactans*) Bite During Pregnancy," *West J Med*, 1994, 160(3):261-2.

Hassen LB, "Reptile and Arthropod Envenomations," *Occup Med*, 1991, 6(3):447-61.

Suntorntham S, Roberts JR, and Nilsen GJ, "Dramatic Clinical Response to the Delayed Administration of Black Widow Spider Antivenin," *Ann Emerg Med*, 1994, 24(6):1198-9.

Bladder Pod *see* Indian Tobacco *on page 1091*

Bleeding Heart

Scientific Name *Dicentra cucullaria*; *Dicentra formosa*

Synonyms Dutchman's Breeches; Stagger Weed

Mechanism of Toxic Action Isoquinoline-type alkaloids may cause dermatitis

Signs & Symptoms of Acute Overdose Burning sensation, pruritus, erythema

Overdosage Treatment

Decontamination: Wash thoroughly

Supportive therapy: Antihistamines and corticosteroids as needed

Additional Information Do not confuse with nontoxic hemorrhage heart vine; all parts are toxic; foliage and roots are most toxic; systemic toxicity not seen in humans

Blood Leaf (Nontoxic Plant)

Blue Blindweed *see* Deadly Nightshade *on page 1078*

Blue Bonnet *see* Lupine *on page 1102*

Blue Elder *see* Elderberry *on page 1081*

"Blue Foot" Mushroom *see* Mushrooms, Toxic (Group VI) *on page 1115*

"Blueing" *Psilocybe* Mushroom *see* Mushrooms, Toxic (Group VI) *on page 1115*

Blue Nightshade *see* Deadly Nightshade *on page 1078*

Blue-Ringed Octopus

Synonyms Australian Blue-Ringed Octopus; Spotted Octopus

Mechanism of Toxic Action Bite – envenomation; autonomic ganglia blockade; maculotoxin (tetrodotoxin)

Signs & Symptoms of Acute Overdose Pain, burning sensation, numbness, local ischemia, paresthesia, aphonia, slurred speech, blurred vision, coma, respiratory collapse

Adverse Reactions

Central nervous system: Ataxia, perioral and intra-oral anesthesia, paresthesia

Neuromuscular & skeletal: Flaccid muscular paralysis

Respiratory: Respiratory depression

Overdosage Treatment

Decontamination: No antivenin

Supportive therapy: Symptomatic and supportive; for serious envenomations, be prepared to provide artificial ventilation, wound care

Additional Information Range: Waters off the coast of Australia

Specific References

Auerbach PS, Halstead BW, Bush RK, et al, "Hazardous Aquatic Life," *Management of Wilderness and Environmental Emergencies*, 2nd ed, Auerbach PS and Geehr EC, eds, St Louis, MO: CV Mosby Co, 1989, 933-1028.

Kizer KW, "Marine Envenomations," *J Toxicol Clin Toxicol*, 1983-84, 21(4-5):527-55.

Blue Star *see* Morning Glory *on page 1109*

"Blushing Bowlcap" Mushroom *see* Mushrooms, Toxic (Group VII) *on page 1116*

"Blushing" *Inocybe* Mushroom *see* Mushrooms, Toxic (Group III) *on page 1112*

"Blushing" *Inocybe* Mushroom *see* Mushrooms, Toxic (Group V) *on page 1114*

Body Louse *see* Lice *on page 1097*

Bog Onion *see* Jack-in-the-Pulpit *on page 1093*

Bois Gentil *see* Daphne Mezereum *on page 1077*

Bois Joli *see* Daphne Mezereum *on page 1077*

Boletus calopus *see* Mushrooms, Toxic (Group III) *on page 1112*

Boletus calopus *see* Mushrooms, Toxic (Group VII) *on page 1116*

***Boletus erythropus* ("Red-Footed Bolete")** *see* Mushrooms, Toxic (Group VII) *on page 1116*

***Boletus luridus* ("Lurid" *Boletus*)** *see* Mushrooms, Toxic (Group III) *on page 1112*

***Boletus luridus* ("Lurid" *Boletus*)** *see* Mushrooms, Toxic (Group V) *on page 1114*

***Boletus luridus* ("Lurid" *Boletus*)** *see* Mushrooms, Toxic (Group VII) *on page 1116*

***Boletus pulcherrimus* ("Red-Pored Bolete")** *see* Mushrooms, Toxic (Group III) *on page 1112*

***Boletus pulcherrimus* ("Red-Pored Bolete")** *see* Mushrooms, Toxic (Group VII) *on page 1116*

***Boletus satanus* ("Satan's Bolete")** *see* Mushrooms, Toxic (Group III) *on page 1112*

***Boletus satanus* ("Satan's Bolete")** *see* Mushrooms, Toxic (Group VII) *on page 1116*

***Boletus sensibilis* ("Sensitive" *Boletus*)** *see* Mushrooms, Toxic (Group VII) *on page 1116*

Boomslang (Tree Snake of Africa) *see* Colubrids *on page 1073*

"Booted" *Amanita* Mushroom *see* Mushrooms, Toxic (Group III) *on page 1112*

"Booted" *Amanita* Mushroom *see* Mushrooms, Toxic (Group V) *on page 1114*

Boston Fern (Nontoxic Plant)

Boston Ivy

Scientific Name *Parthenocissus*

Mechanism of Toxic Action Leaves are toxic and contain soluble and insoluble oxalates

Signs & Symptoms of Acute Overdose

Dermal: Pain, irritation, swelling; may also cause dermatitis reaction

Ocular: Sap may cause pain, lacrimation, photophobia, corneal abrasion;

Oral: Edema, vomiting, diarrhea, salivation, dysphonia

Miscellaneous: Hypocalcemia, renal injury due to calcium oxalate precipitation

Overdosage Treatment

Decontamination: Oral: Dilute; ipecac/lavage/activated charcoal not likely necessary; milk/water to rinse crystals

Supportive therapy: For treatment of soluble oxalates, which may cause systemic oxalate toxicity, keep well hydrated, monitor renal function, fluid/electrolytes; hypocalcemia may occur which can be treated with calcium gluconate, monitor urine for crystals; treat other symptoms supportively

Botulism *see Clostridium botulinum* Food Poisoning *on page 1070*

***Boulengerina annulata* (Banded Water Cobra)** *see* Cobras *on page 1072*

Box Jellyfish

Related Information

Sea Wasp *on page 1139*

Scientific Name *Carybdea rastonii* (Jimble); *Chironex fleckeri*; *Chiropsalmus marsupialis*; *Chiropsalmus quadrigatus*; *Chiropsalmus quadrumanus*; *Scyphozoa* Class

Synonyms Australian Jellyfish (*Chiropsalmus quadrigatus*); *Chironex* Sea Wasp; Indo-Pacific Box Jellyfish

Mechanism of Toxic Action Sting, venom; lethal fraction and lethal hemolytic-dermatonecrotic fraction

Signs & Symptoms of Acute Overdose Pain, erythema, nausea, vomiting, cardiovascular collapse, respiratory depression, coma

Adverse Reactions

Cardiovascular: Hypotension, cardiovascular collapse

Central nervous system: Depression, coma

Respiratory: Wheezing, pulmonary edema, respiratory depression/collapse

Overdosage Treatment

Decontamination: Rapidly assess airway; support with artificial ventilation, if necessary; immediately rinse with seawater, should then prevent further envenomation by applying acetic acid 5% (vinegar) to any tentacles still adhering to tissue; if acetic acid is not available, use isopropyl alcohol 40% to 70% or finally may use aluminum sulfate; shave envenomated area after initial treatment, then repeat local decontamination therapy. Ocular exposures are to be decontaminated by water irrigation only. Do not rub affected area. Wear gloves during decontamination. Meat tenderizers have been used, however they are not preferred decontamination measures and should not have prolonged contact times (>10 minutes).

Antivenin should be administered I.V. diluted 1:5 with isotonic crystalloid; dose equals 1 ampul or 20,000 units over 5 minutes; if administered I.M., use 3 ampuls or 60,000 units

Antivenin available in Australia through Commonwealth Serum Laboratories, Melbourne.

Additional Information Most venomous of all sea creatures; use of verapamil is still controversial

Range: Found chiefly in the waters off Northern Queensland, Australia; may be found in the open ocean

Specific References

Beadnell CE, Rider TA, Williamson JA, et al, "Management of a Major Box Jellyfish (*Chironex fleckeri*) Sting. Lessons From the First Few Minutes and Hours," *Med J Aust*, 1992, 156(9):655-8.

Currie B, "Clinical Implications of Research on the Box Jellyfish *Chironex Fleckeri*," *Toxicon*, 1994, 32(11):1305-13.

Kizer KW, "Marine Envenomations," *J Toxicol Clin Toxicol*, 1983-84, 21(4-5):527-55.

Box Thorn

Scientific Name *Lycium halmifolium*

Synonyms Matrimony Vine

Mechanism of Toxic Action The whole plant may contain atropine and other anticholinergic compounds

Signs & Symptoms of Acute Overdose Dry mouth, mydriasis, tachycardia, delirium, constipation

Toxic Dosage Not established, may vary from plant to plant

Overdosage Treatment

Decontamination: Ipecac/lavage, activated charcoal, cathartic may be considered in large ingestions

Supportive therapy: Propranolol may be used for tachyarrhythmias

Antidote(s)

Physostigmine *on page 1457*

"Brain" *Gyromitra* Mushroom *see* Mushrooms, Toxic (Group II) *on page 1112*

***Brassica* Species** *see* Wild Mustard *on page 1157*

Breeam *see* Scotch Broom *on page 1138*

Bridal Veil (Nontoxic Plant)

Broom Tops *see* Scotch Broom *on page 1138*

Browme *see* Scotch Broom *on page 1138*

Brown Dragon *see* Jack-in-the-Pulpit *on page 1093*

"Brown False Morel" Mushroom *see* Mushrooms, Toxic (Group II) *on page 1112*

Brown Recluse Spider

Scientific Name *Loxosceles reclusa*

Synonyms "Fiddle Back" Spider; Violin Brown Recluse Spider

Mechanism of Toxic Action Toxin has sphingomyelinase activity which has lytic action on red blood cells

Signs & Symptoms of Acute Overdose Mild erythema and pruritus can progress to severe skin ulceration; systemic findings occur at 1-3 days and can include hypotension, severe vomiting, myalgias, myopathy, hemolysis, anemia, hemolytic anemia, dark urine, fever, nausea, thrombocytopenia; bite site may have a "halo" appearance with a small pustule surrounded by pallor; wound can become necrotic in 3 days; death may be related to disseminated intravascular coagulation or renal failure

Overdosage Treatment

Supportive therapy: Elevate affected limb; antihistamine may be given for pruritus; dexamethasone (4 mg I.M. 4 times/day) can be helpful if given early in the course; dapsone (50-200 mg orally divided into twice daily dosing) or colchicine (1.2 mg orally, then 0.6 mg every 2 hours for 2 days, then 0.6 mg every 4 hours for 2 days) may be helpful to avoid cutaneous necrosis; ice packs may relieve pain/heat may exacerbate pain; hyperbaric oxygen has been used (2-6 days postbite) in order to improve necrotic lesions. A recent rabbit study did not reveal any benefit of hyperbaric oxygen, dapsone, or cyproheptadine in the treatment of brown recluse spider envenomation.

Antidote(s)

Oxygen (Hyperbaric) *on page 1453*

Additional Information Bites usually occur at night; dorsal cephalothorax has characteristic fiddle-shaped marking

Range: South/Southwestern U.S.: Illinois, Iowa, Ohio

Specific References

Alario A, Price G, Stahl R, et al, "Cutaneous Necrosis Following a Spider Bite: A Case Report and Review," *Pediatrics*, 1987, 79(4):618-21.

Berger RS, "Management of Brown Recluse Spider Bite," *JAMA*, 1984, 251(7):889-90.

Bernstein B and Ehrlich F, "Brown Recluse Spider Bites," *J Emerg Med*, 1986, 4(6):457-62.

Erickson T, Hryhorczuk DO, Lipscomb JW, et al, "Brown Recluse Spider Bites in an Urban Wilderness," *J Wilderness Medicine*, 1990, 1:258-64.

Knapp JF, Thomas KR, Mathews R, et al, "Case 06-1994: A Ten Year-Old Female With Fever, Jaundice, and Orthostatic Hypotension," *Pediatr Emerg Care*, 1994, 10(6):364-8.

Phillips S, Kohn M, Baker D, et al, "Therapy of Brown Spider Envenomation: A Controlled Trial of Hyperbaric Oxygen, Dapsone, and Cyproheptadine," *Ann Emerg Med*, 1995, 25(3):363-8.

(Continued)

Brown Recluse Spider *(Continued)*

Tomaszewski CA and Thom SR, "Use of Hyperbaric Oxygen in Toxicology," *Emerg Med Clin North Am*, 1994, 12(2):437-59.

Brum *see* Scotch Broom *on page 1138*

Buckeye

Scientific Name *Aesculus californica*; *Aesculus glabra*; *Aesculus parviflora*

Synonyms Horse Chestnut

Mechanism of Toxic Action Contains aescin which is a mixture of saponeus and is cytotoxic

Signs & Symptoms of Acute Overdose Vomiting, diarrhea, oral irritation; repeat exposure or large amounts in small children may also produce CNS depression, paralysis, muscle asthenia, ataxia, and myoclonus

Toxic Dosage 1-2 seeds may cause gastroenteritis only; repeat exposures allow saponin absorption through irritated mucous membranes

Overdosage Treatment

Decontamination: 1-2 berries: Activated charcoal alone may be more beneficial than vomiting since effects of ipecac are similar to toxicity; more than 1-2 berries may cause more severe GI effects and systemic effects, therefore, use of ipecac may be worthwhile to prevent more serious effects; cathartics should be avoided

Supportive therapy: Maintain proper electrolyte and fluid balance, support cardiac and respiratory function if necessary; monitor fluid and electrolytes

Additional Information Young leaves, flowers, and bark are most toxic; aescin content in seeds varies with growth and peaks in mid-July to mid-August

Buckthorn

Scientific Name *Rhamnus cathartica*

Synonyms Alder Buckthorn; Arrow Wood; Berry Alder; Black Dogwood; Cascara; Harts Horn; Maythorn; Persian Berry; Purging Buckthorn

Mechanism of Toxic Action Contains frangula, an anthraquinone which stimulates the colon

Signs & Symptoms of Acute Overdose Nausea, abdominal pain, vomiting, cramping, diarrhea; could potentially cause kidney damage with large enough ingestion

Toxicodynamics/Kinetics Onset is likely soon after ingestion

Toxic Dosage Mild intoxication upon ingestion of berries by children; apparently ingestion of about 20 berries or chewing the fresh bark is necessary to induce pronounced symptoms

Overdosage Treatment

Decontamination: Ipecac/cathartic not recommended, activated charcoal/lavage may be useful

Supportive therapy: Treat any fluid or electrolyte imbalance

Additional Information Fruit, leaves, and bark are poisonous; may color alkaline urine red; do not confuse with hematuria

Buddhist Rosary Bead *see* Jequirity Bean *on page 1093*

Bufotenine

CAS Number 487-93-4

Synonyms Bufox® (France); Ch'an Su; Hallucinogenic Snuff

Commonly Found in Skin glands (parotid glands) of toads (*Bufo alvarius*, Colorado river toad) and *Bufo marinus* (cane toad); in the seeds and leaves of *Piptadenia peregrina* and *Piptadenia macrocarpa*; found in the Chinese preparation Yixin Wan, Kyushin, and Lu-Shen Wan; also found in the mushrooms *Amanita citrina, Amanita porphyria*, and *Amanita tomentella*

Mechanism of Toxic Action Indole alkaloid with serotonergic activity; also inhibits sodium, potassium, and muscle ATP, ACE activity in muscle similar to digoxin

Signs & Symptoms of Acute Overdose Salivation, seizures, cardiac arrhythmias similar to digitalis toxicity, hypokalemia, dyspnea

Overdosage Treatment

Decontamination: Activated charcoal with cathartic may be effective in ingestions; mucous membranes should be flushed with water

Supportive therapy: Diazepam or lorazepam may be utilized for agitation or seizures; phenobarbital is also effective for seizures; although it is unproven in a clinical setting, digoxin specific Fab antibodies can be considered if a toxic arrhythmia develops; atropine can be utilized for bradyarrhythmias while phenytoin can be used for ventricular arrhythmias

Enhancement of elimination: Multiple dosing of activated charcoal may be effective

Test Interactions Cross reacts to give a positive digoxin reading in immunoreactive assays

Pregnancy Implications Stimulates uterine musculature

Additional Information Usual mechanism of abuse is through licking the skin of the toad, although "toad smoking" and ingestions have occurred; the Colorado river toad is found in the Sonoran desert of Northern Mexico along with Southern California and Arizona; while the toads primarily live underground, they do emerge during the rainy season in midsummer; not centrally active at oral doses of 50 mg or I.V. doses of 20 mg or I.M. doses of 40 mg; 100 kg of *Amanita citrina* contains only 7 g of bufotenine

Specific References

Hitt M and Ettinger DD, "Toad Toxicity," *N Engl J Med*, 1986, 314(23):1517-8.

Kwan T, Paiusco AD, and Kohl L, "Digitalis Toxicity Caused by Toad Venom," *Chest*, 1992, 102(3):949-50.

Bufox® (France) *see* Bufotenine *on previous page*

Bull Flower *see* Marsh Marigold *on page 1105*

"Bull Nose" Mushroom *see* Mushrooms, Toxic (Group II) *on page 1112*

Bunch Berry *see* Lantana *on page 1096*

Burros Tail (Nontoxic Plant)

Bushmaster

Scientific Name *Lachesis mutus*

Signs & Symptoms of Acute Overdose Coagulopathy

Overdosage Treatment

Decontamination: Rapid transport to medical facility; immobilize area; if negative pressure suction device is available, this may be used; do not incise the wound; constriction band may be applied, not a tourniquet; ABC assessment, physical exam; mark extent of local edema with skin-marking pen

Supportive therapy: Repeat lab testing every 3-4 hours for first 12 hours; I.V. fluids, tetanus prophylaxis and analgesics may need to be given; antibiotics may be indicated for infected wound sites; antivenin indicated for moderate to severe envenomation

Antidote: Wyeth crotalid polyvalent antivenin: Treat moderate to severe envenomations with increments of 5-10 vials at a time; skin test per manufacturer's instructions; if positive, may prophylax with H_1- and H_2-histamine receptor blockers; give until local injury has stopped and coagulopathy is reversed; complications include allergic reaction, anaphylaxis, and delayed serum sickness

Antidote(s)

Antivenin (Crotalidae) Polyvalent *on page 1392*

Additional Information Largest American poisonous snake (length to 12 feet); unlike other pit vipers, lays eggs from which young are hatched

Buttercup

Scientific Name *Ranunculus aquatilis*

Synonyms Crowfoot; Water Buttercup

Mechanism of Toxic Action Contains protoanemonin, which reacts with SH groups to produce irritation and vesication, excreted unchanged in urine

Signs & Symptoms of Acute Overdose Salivation, vomiting, bloody diarrhea, abdominal cramps, pain and swelling, blistering, ulceration, contact dermatitis; potential renal irritation or damage if large enough amount is ingested

Toxicodynamics/Kinetics Significant dermal symptoms may take several weeks to resolve

Toxic Dosage Not established, but overdose producing systemic effects is unlikely due to painful skin contact

Overdosage Treatment

Decontamination: Avoid use of ipecac or cathartics, consider lavage and/or activated charcoal with large ingestion to prevent systemic absorption and possibility of subsequent renal irritation

Supportive therapy: Maintain fluid and electrolytes, maintain adequate urine flow in large overdose; monitor symptomatic patients for fluid or electrolyte deficiencies

Additional Information Sap is toxic; plant is most toxic during flowering stage

Butterflies *see* Lepidoptera *on page 1097*

Butterfly Cod *see* Lionfish *on page 1099*

Cake Yellow *see* Tartrazine Food Poisoning *on page 1149*

Caladium

Synonyms Alocasia; Angel Wings; Candidum Exposition; Cocoyam; Colcasia; Dasheen; Eddo; Elephant Ear; Heart of Jesus; Kalo; Mother-in-Law Plant; Pink Cloud; Seagull; Stoplight; Taro; Texas Wonder

(Continued)

Caladium *(Continued)*

Mechanism of Toxic Action Contains insoluble calcium oxalate crystals which cause mechanical injury

Signs & Symptoms of Acute Overdose

Ocular: Contact with sap may produce pain, lacrimation, photophobia, corneal abrasion, and deposit of calcium oxalate crystals on corneal epithelium

Oral: Pain, swelling, irritation, dysphonia, vomiting

Toxicodynamics/Kinetics Irritation is immediate

Toxic Dosage Contact with sap or mouthful ingestions may produce symptoms

Overdosage Treatment

Decontamination:

Oral: Dilute; ipecac/lavage/activated charcoal/cathartic not likely necessary; milk/water to rinse crystals

Dermal: Wash thoroughly

Ocular: Irrigate with tepid water for 15 minutes

Supportive therapy: Cool compresses may minimize pain and swelling

Additional Information Whole plant is toxic including sap; ice or popsicles may help oral irritation, especially in children

Calcium Sulfite *see* Sulfite Food Poisoning *on page 1148*

Calf Kill *see* Mountain Laurel *on page 1110*

Calico Bush *see* Mountain Laurel *on page 1110*

"California False Morel" Mushroom *see* Mushrooms, Toxic (Group II) *on page 1112*

California Ivy *see* English Ivy *on page 1081*

California Rape *see* Wild Mustard *on page 1157*

Calla

Scientific Name *Zantedeschia aethiopica*

Synonyms Common Calla; Florist's Calla; Garden Calla

Mechanism of Toxic Action Contains insoluble calcium oxalate crystals which cause mechanical irritation

Signs & Symptoms of Acute Overdose

Dermal: Pain, irritation, swelling

Ocular: Sap may cause pain, lacrimation, photophobia, corneal abrasion; oxalate crystals may be deposited on cornea; may also cause dermatitis reaction

Oral: Edema, vomiting, diarrhea, salivation, dysphonia

Toxicodynamics/Kinetics Rapid onset of local symptoms

Overdosage Treatment

Decontamination:

Dermal: Wash thoroughly

Ocular: Irrigate

Oral: Dilute; ipecac/lavage/activated charcoal with cathartic not likely necessary; milk/water to rinse crystals

Supportive therapy: Cool compresses may minimize pain and swelling

Additional Information Whole plant is toxic, symptoms dependent on liberation of oxalate crystals or contact with sap, dried plant will not liberate crystals; wide variation in potential for toxicity between plants; treat symptoms

Caltha palustris *see* Marsh Marigold *on page 1105*

Campylobacter jejuni Food Poisoning

Commonly Found in Poultry, meat, dairy products

Mechanism of Toxic Action Heat labile enterotoxin; incubation period: 1-7 days

Signs & Symptoms of Acute Overdose Diarrhea, fever, bloody diarrhea, malaise, cramping, abdominal pain, vomiting, feces discoloration (red)

Overdosage Treatment The organism is sensitive *in vitro* to many common antimicrobial agents including erythromycin, ciprofloxacin, tetracyclines, aminoglycosides, and others. Ampicillin or penicillin should usually be avoided, and the susceptibility to co-trimoxazole is variable. Most patients with *Campylobacter* enteritis do not require antibiotics; they recover quickly without sequelae. Antimicrobial therapy should be targeted towards the more acutely ill patient. Limited clinical trials suggest that the following groups may benefit from the prompt use of antibiotics: children with severe dysentery, adults with severe bloody diarrhea and fever, individuals with worsening symptoms when seeking medical attention, and prolonged diarrhea (more than 1 week). Treatment with antibiotics does not prolong the fecal carriage of *C. jejuni* (as opposed to *Salmonella*). The drug of choice is erythromycin. For the toxic patient, combination therapy may be useful, but consultation should be made with an Infectious Disease specialist.

Diagnostic Tests/Procedures

Blood Culture, Aerobic and Anaerobic *on page 1204*

Fecal Leukocyte Stain *on page 1263*

Stool Culture *on page 1356*

Pregnancy Implications May cause septic abortion

Additional Information Febrile seizures may occur in children; meningitis or endocarditis may occur as may Guillain-Barré syndrome

Microbiology:

Campylobacter jejuni is a curved, gram-negative bacillus which is the most common cause of bacterial diarrhea in the United States. On Gram's stain, *Campylobacter jejuni* appears as a curved, comma-shaped, gram-negative rod which often has a distinctive "seagull wing" appearance.

Campylobacter jejuni is a microaerophilic organism and fails to grow under routine aerobic and anaerobic conditions. The laboratory should be informed that *C. jejuni* is suspected clinically and a special request made for *Campylobacter* culture. A 5% to 10% oxygen, 5% to 10% carbon dioxide, and 80% to 90% nitrogen atmosphere is generally used to facilitate growth.

Epidemiology: Infection with this agent occurs worldwide. With over 2 million cases per year in the U.S., *Campylobacter*-induced enteritis is more common than *Salmonella* and *Shigella* combined. The organism is found in the gastrointestinal flora of a number of wild and domestic animals, most notably in chickens. Transmission to humans generally occurs by consumption of the meat or milk of an infected animal, consumption of water contaminated with the feces of infected animals (eg, mountain streams), or fecal-oral transmission from an infected human or household pet. Undercooked chicken is notorious for transmission of *C. jejuni*, accounting for >50% of the cases of campylobacteriosis. Outbreaks have been linked to unpasteurized goat's cheese, clams, and untreated stream water in Wyoming. Infection occurs year-round but is most common in the summer months.

Clinical Syndromes:

- **Acute enteritis:** The organism can cause destructive, ulcerative changes in the mucosal surfaces of the small intestine (especially jejunum and distal ileum) and colon. Invasion of the organism causes inflammation of the lamina propria, bowel wall edema, and crypt abscesses. Patients initially present with nonspecific symptoms such as fever, headache, and myalgias. One to 2 days later, there is crampy abdominal pain and diarrhea. The quality and severity of the diarrhea is variable (although usually mild), and stools may be frequent and watery or visibly bloody. Most cases resolve spontaneously without antimicrobial therapy within 1 week. Less commonly, a fulminant acute colitis may occur. Again, a nonspecific prodrome of fever and malaise precedes any gastrointestinal complaints. However, the diarrhea which follows is voluminous and bloody with large amounts of mucous. Tenesmus is common and further suggests involvement of the colon. Fevers can reach 40°C and occasionally the patient can appear in extremis. This syndrome may be confused with bacillary dysentery from *Shigella* species, severe salmonellosis, or even the initial presentation of inflammatory bowel disease (particularly if it is in a young adult). Toxic megacolon may complicate the hospital course.
- **Appendicitis-like syndrome:** Occasionally, *C. jejuni* can cause right lower quadrant pain mimicking appendicitis, without diarrhea. This "pseudoappendicitis" has been seen in association with other enteric pathogens including *Yersinia enterocolitica.*
- **Bacteremia:** This is an unusual finding in *C. jejuni* infection (even when the patient is febrile), unlike *Campylobacter fetus* which is commonly recovered from the blood. Blood cultures may turn positive several days after a mild diarrheal illness has already resolved; in such cases, antibiotic therapy is usually unnecessary. In other cases, bacteremia may be sustained, particularly in immunocompromised hosts, and this may suggest a deep focus of infection. Infectious disease consultation is appropriate in such cases since prolonged antimicrobial therapy may be necessary.
- **Septic abortion:** *C. jejuni* infection in the pregnant female may lead to this complication. However, *Campylobacter* bacteremia during pregnancy does not automatically justify a therapeutic abortion since the outcome is not uniformly poor.

Diagnosis: *Campylobacter jejuni* should be suspected in any case of acute gastroenteritis or fulminant colitis. The findings of fecal leukocytes and occult blood in the stool are suggestive of campylobacteriosis and other gastrointestinal infections such as those caused by *Salmonella* sp, *Shigella* sp, enteroinvasive *E. coli*, enterohemorrhagic *E. coli* (0157:H7), Crohn's disease or ulcerative colitis, and others. The diagnosis is confirmed by a positive stool culture for *C. jejuni* or positive blood cultures for the organism.

Specific References

Blaser MJ and Reller LB, "*Campylobacter* Enteritis," *N Engl J Med*, 1981, 305(24):1444-52.

(Continued)

Campylobacter jejuni Food Poisoning *(Continued)*

Blaser MJ, Wells JG, Feldman RA, et al, "*Campylobacter* Enteritis in the United States. A Multicenter Study," *Ann Intern Med*, 1983, 98(3):360-5.

Johnson RJ, Nolan C, Wang SP, et al, "Persistent *Campylobacter jejuni* Infection in an Immunocompromised Patient," *Ann Intern Med*, 1984, 100(6):832-4.

Peterson MC, Farr RW, and Castiglia M, "Prosthetic Hip Infection and Bacteremia Due to *Campylobacter jejuni* in a Patient With AIDS," *Clin Infect Dis*, 1993, 16(3):439-40.

Sorvillo FJ, Lieb LE, and Waterman SH, "Incidence of Campylobacteriosis Among Patients With AIDS in Los Angeles County," *J Acquir Immune Defic Syndr*, 1991, 4(6):598-602.

Candidum Exposition *see* Caladium *on page 1063*

Canebrake Rattlesnake *see* Rattlesnakes *on page 1132*

Cannabis sativa *see* Marijuana (Cannabis) *on page 1103*

Cape Cobra *see* Cobras *on page 1072*

Capsicum annuum cenoides *see* Pepper *on page 1123*

"Carolina False Morel" Mushroom *see* Mushrooms, Toxic (Group II) *on page 1112*

Carolina Pygmy Rattlesnake *see* Rattlesnakes *on page 1132*

***Carybdea rastonii* (Jimble)** *see* Box Jellyfish *on page 1060*

Cascara *see* Buckthorn *on page 1062*

Cashew

Scientific Name *Anacardium occidentale*

Mechanism of Toxic Action Shell contains anacardic acid, cardol, anacardol, irritants that can precipitate type IV cell-mediated allergic reaction (allergic contact dermatitis)

Signs & Symptoms of Acute Overdose Dermatitis, nausea, vomiting

Toxicodynamics/Kinetics

Onset of effect: Variable, but effects usually seen within 24-48 hours
Peak dermal effect: After 3-5 days

Overdosage Treatment

Decontamination: Soap and water washing likely ineffective unless done within 5-15 minutes after exposure

Supportive therapy: Cool compresses or showers, Burow's solution, topical/oral steroids

Additional Information Shell contains toxin; raw nut should not be eaten

Cassena *see* Holly *on page 1089*

Cast Iron Plant (Nontoxic Plant)

Cathinone

Related Information

Methcathinone *on page 1106*

CAS Number 71031-15-7

Mechanism of Toxic Action Derived from the leaves of the *Catha edulis* plant (an evergreen bush which grows up to 5 meters in Eastern Africa at high altitudes) this stimulant possesses local anesthetic, anorectic, and neuromuscular junction blocking activities; may have some monoamine oxidase inhibition properties; similar in action to cocaine or amphetamines

Adverse Reactions

Cardiovascular: Tachycardia, hypertension, palpitations, flushing
Central nervous system: Fever, insomnia, headache, mania, visual/auditory hallucinations, euphoria
Gastrointestinal: Dry mouth, anorexia, constipation
Genitourinary: Urinary retention, impotence
Neuromuscular & skeletal: Tremors, rhabdomyolysis
Ocular: Mydriasis
Respiratory: Tachypnea, dyspnea
Miscellaneous: Diaphoresis

Toxicodynamics/Kinetics

Onset of action: 20 minutes
Duration of action: 2 hours
Metabolism: To norephedrine and norpseudoephedrine
Elimination: Renal

Toxic Dosage

Khat (0.1% to 0.3% cathinone): 100-200 g
Anorexiant: 15-60 mg

Overdosage Treatment

Decontamination: Emesis or lavage/activated charcoal with cathartic

Supportive therapy: Agitation can be treated with chlorpromazine, benzodiazepines, or haloperidol; ventricular arrhythmias can be treated with lidocaine, procaine, or bretylium; hyperthermia can be treated with standard cooling techniques (avoid salicylates)

Enhancement of elimination: Multiple dosing of activated charcoal may be effective; although acid diuresis may enhance its elimination, this modality is not recommended due to its danger in exacerbating renal failure due to rhabdomyolysis

Test Interactions May give false-positive urinary amphetamine orphenypropanolamine radioimmunoassay test

Pregnancy Implications Low birthweight infants have been noted

Additional Information Khat is usually utilized by chewing the leaves and swallowing its juice; red khat has a higher cathinone content than white khat; khat addiction can be treated with bromocriptine mesylate (1.25 mg every 6 hours as an initial dose); for medicinal purposes (as an anorexiant): 15-60 mg

Specific References

Critchlow S and Seifert R, "Khat-Induced Paranoid Psychosis," *Br J Psychiatry*, 1987, 150:247-9.

Drake PH, "Khat-Chewing in the Near East," *Lancet*, 1988, 1(8584):532-3.

Giannini AJ and Nakoneczie AM, "Treatment of Khat Addiction With Bromocriptine Mesylate: A Case Report and Review of Cocaine- and Amphetamine-Like Effects," *Am J Therapeutics*, 1995, 2:487-9.

Louman W and Danouske MD, "The Use of Khat (*Catha edulis*) in Yemen: Social and Medical Observations," *Ann Intern Med*, 1976, 85:246-9.

Centruroides sculpturatus *see* Arizona Bark Scorpion *on page 1053*

Century Plant

Scientific Name *Agave americana*

Synonyms American Aloe; Henequen; Maguey; Mescal; Potosina; Sisal; Yaxci

Mechanism of Toxic Action Contains insoluble calcium oxalate crystals which cause mechanical irritation; may also cause dermatitis

Signs & Symptoms of Acute Overdose

Dermal: Pain, irritation, swelling

Ocular: Sap may cause pain, lacrimation, photophobia, corneal abrasion; oxalate crystals may be deposited on cornea; may also cause dermatitis reaction

Oral: Edema, vomiting, diarrhea, salivation, dysphonia

Toxicodynamics/Kinetics Onset of action: Rapid onset of local symptoms due to oxalate; dermatitis reaction may develop within a few hours

Overdosage Treatment

Decontamination:

Dermal: Wash thoroughly; antihistamines/steroids may be useful

Ocular: Irrigate

Oral: Dilute; ipecac/lavage/activated charcoal with cathartic not likely necessary

Supportive therapy: Cool compresses may minimize pain and swelling

Additional Information Sap toxic, other parts may be also (especially thorns)

Ch'an Su *see* Bufotenine *on page 1062*

Charlock *see* Wild Mustard *on page 1157*

Cherry

Scientific Name *Prunus*

Mechanism of Toxic Action Contains amygdalin, a cyanogenic glycoside hydrolyzed to hydrocyanic acid in the gut, complexes with cytochrome oxidase to produce cellular hypoxia after absorption

Signs & Symptoms of Acute Overdose Lethargy, drowsiness, headache, coma, seizures, sweating, abdominal pain, vomiting, dyspnea, cyanosis, paralysis

Toxic Dosage 1-2 pits likely nontoxic, toxicity uncommon after accidental ingestion

Overdosage Treatment

Decontamination: Basic poison management; vomiting is contraindicated due to rapid course of the neurologic symptoms; give 100% oxygen

Supportive therapy: Give sodium bicarbonate for acidosis; cyanide antidote kite should be used for patients symptomatic from cyanide toxicity

Enhancement of elimination: Hemodialysis and charcoal hemoperfusion have been utilized; hyperbaric oxygen may also be utilized; hydroxocobalamin and dicobalt-EDTA used for chelation in Europe

Additional Information Intact pit does not release CN

Chiggers-Harvestmites (*Trombicula irritans*) *see* Mites *on page 1107*

Chinese Evergreen (Nontoxic Plant)

Chinese Restaurant Syndrome *see* Monosodium Glutamate Food Poisoning *on page 1109*

Chinese Seasoning *see* Monosodium Glutamate Food Poisoning *on page 1109*

Chinese Yew *see* Yew *on page 1159*

Chironex fleckeri *see* Box Jellyfish *on page 1060*

Chironex fleckeri *see* Sea Wasp *on page 1139*

***Chironex* Sea Wasp** *see* Box Jellyfish *on page 1060*

Chiropsalmus marsupialis *see* Box Jellyfish *on page 1060*

Chiropsalmus quadrigatus *see* Box Jellyfish *on page 1060*

Chiropsalmus quadrumanus *see* Box Jellyfish *on page 1060*

***Chlorophyllum molybdites* ("Green Parasol")** *see* Mushrooms, Toxic (Group VII) *on page 1116*

***Chlorophyllum* Mushrooms** *see* Mushrooms, Toxic (Group VII) *on page 1116*

Chocolate Soldier (Nontoxic Plant)

***Chondylactis* Species** *see* Sea Anemones *on page 1138*

Christmas Begonia (Nontoxic Plant)

Christmas Cactus (Nontoxic Plant)

Christmas Cheer *see Sedum on page 1140*

Christmas Cherry

Scientific Name *Solanum*

Synonyms Jerusalem Cherry; Natal Cherry; Ornamental Pepper; Tom Thumb; Winter Cherry

Mechanism of Toxic Action Contains solanocapsine, an alkaloid related to salanine that is structurally similar to cardiac glycoside and has irritant effect similar to saponins

Signs & Symptoms of Acute Overdose Nausea, vomiting, diarrhea, headache, drowsiness, bradycardia, hypotension

Toxicodynamics/Kinetics Effects expected within 2-24 hours

Toxic Dosage Unclear, but large amount likely necessary for toxicity

Overdosage Treatment

Decontamination: If necessary due to large ingestion, use ipecac if soon after ingestion; otherwise, consider activated charcoal with cathartic or lavage

Supportive therapy: Maintain proper fluid and electrolyte balance

Additional Information Potential for solamine toxicity but no cases on record

Christmas Dagger Fern (Nontoxic Plant)

Christmas Flower *see* Poinsettia *on page 1126*

Christmas Kalanchoe (Nontoxic Plant)

Christmas Orchid (Nontoxic Plant)

Christmas Palm (Nontoxic Plant)

Christmas Pride (Nontoxic Plant)

Christmas Rose

Mechanism of Toxic Action Primary toxicity relates to proteoanemonin which reacts with SH groups to produce vesicant action; also contains saponins that act as irritants

Signs & Symptoms of Acute Overdose Oral numbness, seizures, abdominal pain, vomiting, bloody diarrhea

Toxicodynamics/Kinetics Significant dermal symptoms may take several weeks to resolve

Toxic Dosage Small amounts likely to produce symptoms

Overdosage Treatment

Decontamination: Avoid use of ipecac or cathartics, consider lavage and/or activated charcoal with large ingestion to prevent systemic absorption and possibility of subsequent renal irritation

Supportive therapy: Maintain fluid and electrolytes, maintain adequate urine flow in large overdose; monitor symptomatic patients for fluid or electrolyte deficiencies

Additional Information

Family: Hellebore

Toxic parts: Entire plant; digitalis toxicity; varies within the species and is not seen in *Helleborus niger*

Christmas Star *see* Poinsettia *on page 1126*

Christ Plant *see* Crown of Thorns *on page 1076*

Chrysanthemum

Scientific Name *Chrysanthemum*

Synonyms Mum; Ox-Eye Daisy

Signs & Symptoms of Acute Overdose Allergenic dermatitis, pruritus, erythema, hives, localized edema

Overdosage Treatment

Decontamination: Wash skin with soap and water

Supportive therapy: Oral or topical corticosteroids or diphenhydramine may be beneficial

Additional Information Ingestion of large amounts of flowers may cause pyrethrin-type toxicity

Chrysanthemum *see* Chrysanthemum *on this page*

Cicuta bulbifera *see* Water Hemlock *on page 1156*

Cicuta douglasii *see* Water Hemlock *on page 1156*

Cicuta maculata *see* Water Hemlock *on page 1156*

Ciguatera Food Poisoning

Synonyms Ichthyosarcotoxism

Commonly Found in Amberjack, barracuda, dolphin, eel, emperor fish, red snapper, sea bass, surgeon fish in Caribbean or South Pacific oceans; especially related to larger fish (>3 kg)

Mechanism of Toxic Action Due to ingestion of dinoflagellates, ciguatoxin accumulates in larger fish; affects membranes and ionic flux of nervous tissue

Signs & Symptoms of Acute Overdose Three phases:

Phase I (1-6 hours postingestion): Gastrointestinal symptoms, abdominal pain, watery diarrhea, headache, vomiting, nausea

Phase II (6-12 hours postingestion): Neurologic symptoms – paresthesia in extremities, adynamic ileus, heat-cold reversal; metallic taste in mouth, pruritus, myalgia, and sinus bradycardia are also common as is blurred vision

Phase III (more than 12 hours postingestion): Weakness, ataxia, hypotension, hypothermia, dysaethesias. Respiratory complications are rare.

Overdosage Treatment

Decontamination: Activated charcoal (a cathartic is usually not required)

Supportive therapy: Atropine is useful for sinus bradycardia; amitriptyline (25 mg twice daily), nifedipine, or mannitol (1 g/kg over 30-45 minutes) has been used for paresthesias with some effect; fluid/electrolyte replacement

Antidote(s)

Mannitol *on page 1442*

Diagnostic Tests/Procedures

Electrocardiography *on page 1253*

Electrolytes, Blood *on page 1254*

Pregnancy Implications Can cause premature labor or spontaneous abortion

Additional Information Ciguatoxin is odorless and tasteless. May be transmitted during breast-feeding. Minimum pathogenic dose of ciguatoxin is 0.6 ng/kg; stable in heat and gastric acid. Can be transmitted by vaginal secretions thus causing penile irritation through sexual intercourse. May occur in farm-raised salmon.

Specific References

Bowman PB, "Amitriptyline and Ciguatera," *Med J Aust*, 1984, 140(13):802.

Calvert GM, Hryhorczuk DO, and Leikin JB, "Treatment of Ciguatera Fish Poisoning With Amitriptyline and Nifedipine," *J Toxicol Clin Toxicol*, 1987, 25(5):423-8.

Davis RT and Villar LA, "Symptomatic Improvement With Amitriptyline in Ciguatera Fish Poisoning," *N Engl J Med*, 1986, 315(1):65.

Di Nubile MJ and Hokama Y, "The Ciguatera Poisoning Syndrome From Farm-Raised Salmon," *Ann Intern Med*, 1995, 122(2):113-4.

Glaziou P and Legrand AM, "The Epidemiology of Ciguatera Fish Poisoning," *Toxicon*, 1994, 32(8):863-73.

Lange WR, "Ciguatera Fish Poisoning," *Am Fam Physician*, 1994, 50(3):579-84.

Palafox NA, Jain LG, Pinano AZ, et al, "Successful Treatment of Ciguatera Fish Poisoning With Intravenous Mannitol," *JAMA*, 1988, 259(18):2740-2.

Swift AE and Swift TR, "Ciguatera," *J Toxicol Clin Toxicol*, 1993, 31(1):1-29.

Cipril *see* Star-of-Bethlehem (*Hippobroma longiflora*) *on page 1145*

Clavate-Stalked *Clitocybe* *see* Mushrooms, Toxic (Group III) *on page 1112*

"Cleft-Foot Deathcap" Mushroom *see* Mushrooms, Toxic (Group VII) *on page 1116*

Climbing Nightshade *see* Deadly Nightshade *on page 1078*

Clitocybe cerussata *see* Mushrooms, Toxic (Group III) *on page 1112*

***Clitocybe clavipes* ("Clubfoot Funnelcap" Mushroom)** *see* Mushrooms, Toxic (Group III) *on page 1112*

***Clitocybe dealbata* ("Sweat" Mushroom)** *see* Mushrooms, Toxic (Group III) *on page 1112*

***Clitocybe dilatata* ("Crowded-White" *Clitocybe*)** *see* Mushrooms, Toxic (Group III) *on page 1112*

***Clitocybe irina* ("Blushing Bowlcap")** *see* Mushrooms, Toxic (Group VII) *on page 1116*

***Clitocybe nebularis* ("Gray Cap" or "Cloudy Funnelcap")** *see* Mushrooms, Toxic (Group VII) *on page 1116*

Clitocybe rivulosa *see* Mushrooms, Toxic (Group III) *on page 1112*

Clostridium botulinum Food Poisoning

Synonyms Botulism; Oculinum® (Botulinum A Toxin); Sysport

Commonly Found in Poorly preserved meat, sausage, fruit, or vegetables (type A or B), marine products (type E); liver pate, venison jerky (type F)

Mechanism of Toxic Action An anaerobic, spore-forming, gram-positive bacteria; ingestion of the toxin or wound contamination are likely routes of exposure; a heat labile neurotoxin which causes irreversible neuromuscular blockade and prevents acetylcholine release; the spores are heat-resistant

Signs & Symptoms of Acute Overdose May be delayed 12-36 hours; ptosis, slurred speech, blurred vision, mydriasis, dry mouth, dry skin, adynamic ileus, constipation followed by descending paralysis and respiratory failure, aspiration, dysphagia, hyporeflexia, fasciculations, cranial nerve palsies

Toxic Dosage Human lethal dose: 1 pg/kg

Overdosage Treatment

Decontamination: Do not induce vomiting, lavage with activated charcoal (sorbitol as a cathartic) may be useful to remove spores; activated charcoal avidly bind to *C. botulinum*, type A neurotoxin

Supportive therapy: Primarily respiratory: Mechanical ventilation may be necessary; "tensilon test" up to 10 mg of edrophonium I.V. over 5 minutes; may show improvement in muscle strength in botulism; guanidine (15-50 mg/kg/day orally) may be given (although its use is not proven). Trivalent (A, B, E) (Liosiero) antitoxin should precede administration; give 2 mL of antitoxin diluted in 100 mL of 0.9% saline over 30 minutes; 10 mL of antitoxin may be given in another 2-4 hours, then at 12- to 24-hour intervals as necessary. Sensitivity skin testing should proceed antitoxin administration. Give 20 mL of antitoxin diluted in 100 mL of 0.9% saline over 30 minutes intravenously. 10 mL of antitoxin may be given in another 2-4 hours, then at 12- to 24-hour intervals as necessary.

Antidote(s)

Antitoxin Botulinin Types A, B, and E *on page 1391*

Diagnostic Tests/Procedures

Botulism Diagnostic Procedure *on page 1211*

Electromyography *on page 1255*

Stool Culture *on page 1356*

Pregnancy Implications Therapeutically used for blepharospasm or strabismus

Additional Information

Stools or gastric contents may be contagious. Infantile botulism has been related to honey ingestion. Symptoms may be delayed for 1 week. Antitoxin can be obtained from the CDC (404-639-3753 [days], 404-639-2888 [nights]).

Electromyogram shows decreased evoked action potential at 2 Hz/sec and an increased evoked action potential at 50 Hz/sec. Up to 15% of affected individuals will have normal electromyograms.

34 cases of foodborne botulism has been reported to the CDC in 1994. Boiling food for 10 minutes (>100°C) destroys the toxin; cooked foods should not be kept at room temperature (4°C to 60°C) for longer than 4 hours; recent cases have been associated with commercial pot pies, home-canned foods, asparagus, green beans, peppers, and onions sauteed in margarine.

Specific References

Center for Disease Control, "Foodborne Botulism - Oklahoma - 1994," 1995, 44(11):200-2.

Cherington M, "Botulism: Ten Year Experience," *Arch Neurol*, 1974, 30(6):432-7.

Gomez HF, Johnson R, Guven H, et al, "Adsorption of Botulinum Toxin to Activated Charcoal With a Mouse Bioassay," *Ann Emerg Med*, 1995, 25:818-22.

Sanders AB, Seifert S, and Kobernick M, "Botulism," *J Fam Pract*, 1983, 16(5):987-8, 993-4, 999-1000.

Schmidt RD and Schmidt TW, "Infant Botulism: A Case Series and a Review of the Literature," *J Emerg Med*, 1992, 10(6):713-8.

Clostridium perfringens Food Poisoning

Commonly Found in Meat, poultry, dairy products, fruits, vegetables, meat-based gravies

Mechanism of Toxic Action Anaerobic, gram-positive, spore-forming organism; 12 toxins have been associated with toxin A and C causing disease in humans. Enterotoxin causes fluid secretion; incubation period: 12-24 hours; rarely lasts more than 1 day.

Signs & Symptoms of Acute Overdose Diarrhea and abdominal cramps, myopathy; vomiting and fever are rare

Overdosage Treatment In general, the treatment of clostridial infection is high-dose penicillin G, to which the organism has remained susceptible. For skin and soft tissue infections, the extent of infection determines the need for surgical debridement. When wounds are simply colonized with clostridia, neither antibiotics nor surgery are indicated. Localized soft tissue infections can often be managed by surgical debridement alone, without antibiotics. When systemic symptoms are present and there is extension of infection into deeper tissues, antibiotics and surgical intervention are required. In fulminant cases of gas gangrene with myonecrosis, immediate surgical intervention (debridement, amputation) is the primary treatment of choice, and antibiotics have little effect.

Diagnostic Tests/Procedures

Electrolytes, Blood *on page 1254*

Stool Culture *on page 1356*

Additional Information Heat labile; destroyed by cooking at 100°C

Microbiology:

Clostridium perfringens is an anaerobic gram-positive rod; occasionally it can appear gram-negative or gram-variable. It is a spore-forming organism, but the spores are not usually seen on Gram's stain. It has been termed "aerotolerant" because of its ability to survive when exposed to oxygen for limited periods of time.

The organism produces 12 toxins active in tissues and several enterotoxins which cause severe diarrhea. Four toxins can be lethal. The toxins separate the species into five types, A-E.

- Alpha toxin: A lecithinase which damages cell membranes. It is produced by *C. perfringens* type A. It is the major factor causing tissue damage in *C. perfringens*-induced gas gangrene (myonecrosis). The toxin is a phospholipase which hydrolyzes phosphatidylcholine and sphingomyelin and leads to increased vascular permeability, myocardial depression, hypotension, bradycardia, and shock.
- Enterotoxin: Produced mainly by *C. perfringens* type A but also by types C and D. This toxin is responsible for the diarrheal syndromes classically ascribed to this organism. The enterotoxin binds to intestinal epithelial cells after the human ingests food contaminated with *C. perfringens*. The small bowel (ileum) is primarily involved. The toxin inhibits glucose transport and causes protein loss.
- Beta toxin: Produced by *C. perfringens* type B and C. This toxin causes enteritis necroticans or pigbel. This disease is seen in New Guinea where some natives ingest massive amounts of pork at feasts after first gorging on sweet potatoes. The sweet potatoes have protease inhibitors which prevent the person from degrading the beta toxin which is ingested in the contaminated pork.

Epidemiology: *C. perfringens* is ubiquitous in the environment, being found in soil and decaying vegetation. The organism has been isolated from nearly every soil sample ever examined except in the sand of the Sahara desert. In the human, *C. perfringens* is common in the human gastrointestinal tract. In one study, it was found in 28 of 40 adults. It can also be commonly recovered from many mammals including cats, dogs, whales, and others.

Clinical Syndromes:

The organism can be pathogenic, commensal, or symbiotic. Important diseases caused by *C. perfringens* include the following:

- **Food poisoning:** *C. perfringens* is one of the most common causes of food poisoning in the United States. Foods commonly contaminated with *C. perfringens* are meat, poultry, and meat products such as gravies, hash, and stew. Human disease is caused by ingestion of heat-labile toxin. The highest risk comes from meats which are partially cooked, cooled, then reheated. Spores present in the food germinate during the reheating process. Symptoms include watery diarrhea and abdominal cramps, which occur about 12 hours after the meal. Fever is generally not part of this illness. Vomiting is unusual.

(Continued)

Clostridium perfringens Food Poisoning *(Continued)*

Duration of symptoms is about 24 hours. The diagnosis is made by culturing the stools and, for epidemiological purposes, the food.

- **Pigbel:** See description under Microbiology above. This follows massive ingestion of contaminated pork and sweet potatoes. Incubation period is 24 hours. There is intense abdominal pain, bloody diarrhea, vomiting, shock, and intestinal perforation in some cases. A vaccine is available for travelers.

Diagnosis:

The diagnosis of infection by *C. perfringens* begins with a high index of suspicion when a patient presents with one of the clinical syndromes described above. One important caveat is that the laboratory isolation of *C. perfringens* from a necrotic wound does not necessarily imply disease from this organism; many wounds can be colonized. In the right clinical setting, however, a positive *C. perfringens* culture and a compatible clinical presentation are highly suggestive of disease caused by this agent. Gram's stain preparations of wound material, uterine tissue, cervical discharge, muscle tissues, and other relevant materials should be made; a predominance of gram-positive rods should bring anaerobic infection, including *C. perfringens*, to mind.

In patients with clostridial septicemia, accompanying abnormalities may be a clue to clostridial disease before culture confirmation is made. Patients may have disseminated intravascular coagulation with a brisk hemolysis, hemoglobinuria, and proteinuria. X-rays of diseased areas may reveal the presence of gas in muscle or soft tissue; this is suggestive of clostridial infection, although other anaerobes (and aerobes) can cause gas formation. If clostridial myonecrosis is suspected, a muscle biopsy usually performed at the time of tissue debridement, can be diagnostic.

Specific References

Barlett JG, "Gas Gangrene (Other *Clostridium*-Associated Diseases)," *Principles and Practice of Infectious Diseases*, 3rd ed, Mandell GL, Douglas RG Jr, Bennett JE, eds, New York, NY: Churchill Livingstone, 1990, 1850-60.

"*Clostridium perfringens* Gastroenteritis Associated With Corned Beef Served at St Patrick's Day Meals – Ohio and Virginia, 1993," *MMWR Morb Mortal Wkly Rep*, 1994, 43(8):137, 143-4.

Loewenstein MS, "Epidemiology of *Clostridium perfringens* Food Poisoning," *N Engl J Med*, 1972, 286(19):1026-8.

Shandera WX, Tacket CO, and Blake PA, "Food Poisoning Due to *Clostridium perfringens* in the United States," *J Infect Dis*, 1983, 147(1):167-70.

"Cloudy Funnelcap" Mushroom *see* Mushrooms, Toxic (Group VII) *on page 1116*

"Clubfoot Funnelcap" Mushroom *see* Mushrooms, Toxic (Group III) *on page 1112*

Cobras

Scientific Name *Boulengerina annulata* (Banded Water Cobra); *Dendraspis* Species; *Naja naja arabicus* (Arabian Cobra); *Naja naja naja* (Indian Cobra, Asian Cobra); *Naja nigricollis* (African Spitting Cobra); *Naja nivea* (Cape Cobra)

Synonyms African Spitting Cobra; Arabian Cobra; Asian Cobra; Banded Water Cobra; Cape Cobra; Indian Cobra; Mambra; Tree Cobra

Mechanism of Toxic Action Venom: Antitoxins that are neuromuscular depolarizing agents; also may contain phospholipases and cardiotoxins

Signs & Symptoms of Acute Overdose Coagulopathy

Adverse Reactions

Cardiovascular: Hypotension, collapse

Central nervous system: Ptosis, paresthesias, paralysis, coma, seizures, ophthalmoloplegia

Dermatologic: Tissue necrosis, local edema

Ocular: Pain, conjunctivitis, blindness, corneal injury (with spitting cobra spit)

Overdosage Treatment

Decontamination: Rapid transport to medical facility; immobilize area; if negative pressure suction device is available, this may be used; do not incise the wound; constriction band may be applied, not a tourniquet; ABC assessment, physical exam; mark extent of local edema with skin-marking pen

Supportive therapy: Repeat lab testing every 3-4 hours for first 12 hours; I.V. fluids, tetanus prophylaxis and analgesics may need to be given; antibiotics may be indicated for infected wound sites; antivenin indicated for moderate to severe envenomation; neurologic findings may respond to intravenous edrophonium. For antidote, in U.S., contact nearest regional poison center for availability. France, India, and South Africa are international sources for antivenin.

Additional Information Family: Elapidae; neck flares to form characteristic hood

Specific References

Coppola M and Hogan DE, "Venomous Snakes of Southwest Asia," *Am J Emerg Med*, 1992, 10(3):230-6.

Nelson BK, "Snake Envenomation. Incidence, Clinical Presentation, and Management," *Med Toxicol Adverse Drug Exp*, 1989, 4(1):17-31.

Watt G, Theakston RD, Hayes CG, et al, "Positive Response to Edrophonium in Patients With Neurotoxic Envenomation by Cobras (*Naja naja philippinensis*). A Placebo-Controlled Study," *N Engl J Med*, 1986, 315(23):1444-8.

Cocoyam *see* Caladium *on page 1063*

Cohosh *see* Baneberries *on page 1056*

Colcasia *see* Caladium *on page 1063*

Colchicum autumnale *see* Autumn Crocus *on page 1054*

Coleus (Nontoxic Plant)

Collybia dryophila **("Nut-Brown"** ***Collybia*** **or "Forest Friend" or "Oak-Loving"** ***Collybia*****)** *see* Mushrooms, Toxic (Group VII) *on page 1116*

Colubrids

Scientific Name *Dispholidus typhus*; *Thelotornis kirtlandi*

Synonyms Bird Snake; Boomslang (Tree Snake of Africa)

Signs & Symptoms of Acute Overdose Venoms may cause fatality; venom of *Dispholidus typhus* may contain a prothrombin-activating enzyme that can cause a prolonged coagulation defect; coagulopathy

Overdosage Treatment Supportive therapy: Monitor blood counts and replace with blood products as necessary; monitor for occult hemorrhage

Additional Information

Family: Colubridae; *Opisthoglypha* (grooved fangs under eyes)

Range: (Boomslang): African rain forest, Southern African rain forest; *Thelotornis kirtlandi* (Bird Snake): Central and Southern African rain forest

Adults average 4-6 feet in length

Specific References

Gomperts ED and Demetriou D, "Laboratory Studies and Clinical Features in a Case of Boomslang Envenomation," *S Afr Med J*, 1977, 51(6):173-5.

Common Calla *see* Calla *on page 1064*

Common Hyacinth *see* Hyacinth *on page 1090*

Common Ivy *see* English Ivy *on page 1081*

Common Nightshade *see* Black Nightshade *on page 1057*

Common Oleander *see* Oleander *on page 1120*

Cone Shells

Scientific Name *Conus aulicus*; *Conus geographus*; *Conus gloriamaris*; *Conus omaria*; *Conus strictus*; *Conus textile*; *Conus tulipa*

Synonyms Court Cone; Geographer Cone; Glory of the Sea; Marbled Cone; Stricted Cone; Textile Cone; Tulip Cone

Mechanism of Toxic Action Venom; neurotoxin (may have a curare effect)

Signs & Symptoms of Acute Overdose Pain, burning sensation, numbness, local ischemia, paresthesia, aphonia, slurred speech, blurred vision, coma, respiratory collapse

Adverse Reactions

Cardiovascular: Cardiac failure

Central nervous system: Coma, cerebral edema

Hematologic: Disseminated intravesicular coagulopathy

Respiratory: Respiratory arrest

Overdosage Treatment Decontamination: Place involved area in hot water (110°F to 115°F) to relieve pain; tetanus toxoid and immune globulin should be administered if not current; no antivenin available

Additional Information Range: Shallow Indo-Pacific waters

Specific References

Hughes JM and Merson MH, "Current Concepts Fish and Shellfish Poisoning," *N Engl J Med*, 1976, 295(20):1117-20.

Kizer KW, "Marine Envenomations," *J Toxicol Clin Toxicol*, 1983-84, 21(4-5):527-55.

"Conic Fiberhead" Mushroom *see* Mushrooms, Toxic (Group III) *on page 1112*

Conium maculatum *see* Poison Hemlock *on page 1126*

Conocybe cyanopus *see* Mushrooms, Toxic (Group VI) *on page 1115*

Conus aulicus *see* Cone Shells *on this page*

Conus geographus *see* Cone Shells *on this page*

Conus gloriamaris *see* Cone Shells *on this page*

Conus omaria *see* Cone Shells *on previous page*

Conus strictus *see* Cone Shells *on previous page*

Conus textile *see* Cone Shells *on previous page*

Conus tulipa *see* Cone Shells *on previous page*

Convallaria majalis *see* Lily-of-the-Valley *on page 1099*

Copperhead *see Crotalidae on next page*

Copperhead Snake

Scientific Name *Agkistrodon contortrix*

Mechanism of Toxic Action Venom; quality and potency vary among species; composition: 90% water with 5-15 enzymes, 3-12 nonenzymatic proteins, as well as other unidentified substances

Signs & Symptoms of Acute Overdose Local signs include tenderness, edema, erythema, ecchymoses, hemorrhage, bullae, lymphangitis, and rarely a compartment syndrome. Systemic signs and symptoms include hypotension, asthenia, sweating, chills, paresthesia, nausea, vomiting, coagulopathy, fasciculations, and CNS depression; coagulopathies can occur including thrombocytopenia, hypofibrinogenemia, increased PT and PTT. Shock, hypotension, lactic acidosis, hemoconcentration, hypoproteinemia, proteinuria, and hematuria are also potential complications.

Overdosage Treatment

Decontamination: Immobilize the area, rapid transport to medical facility. Use negative pressure device to remove venom if available, do not incise the wound; constriction band may be applied, **not** a tourniquet

Wyeth Crotalid Polyvalent antivenin; treat moderate to severe envenomations with increments of 5-10 vials at a time; skin test per manufacturer's instructions; if positive skin test develops, may prophylax with H_1- and H_2-receptor blockers; give until local injury has stopped and coagulopathy is reversed; complications include allergic reactions, anaphylaxis, and delayed serum sickness

Supportive therapy: ABC assessment, physical exam; mark the extent of local edema with skin marking pen; repeat CBC, platelets, PT, PTT, fibrinogen, CPK, UA every 3-4 hours for at least first 12 hours; I.V. fluids, tetanus prophylaxis, and analgesics may be given as needed; treat infected wounds with antibiotics. Snakes' mouths contain primarily gram-negative and anaerobic organisms.

Antidote(s)

Antivenin (Crotalidae) Polyvalent *on page 1392*

Additional Information

Family: Crotalidae (Pit Viper)

Range: Eastern U.S. to Southern Texas

Distinguishing characteristics: Facial pits, vertical elliptical pupils, triangular head, single row of subcaudal scales

Specific References

Hassen LB, "Reptile and Arthropod Envenomations," *Occup Med*, 1991, 6(3):447-61.

Sullivan JB Jr and Wingert WA, "Reptile Bites," *Management of Wilderness and Environmental Emergencies*, 2nd ed, Auerbach PS and Geehr EC, eds, St Louis, MO: CV Mosby Co, 1989, 479-511.

Coprine-Containing Mushrooms *see* Mushrooms, Toxic (Group IV) *on page 1114*

Coprinus atramentarius **("Inky Cap")** *see* Mushrooms, Toxic (Group IV) *on page 1114*

Coprinus insignis *see* Mushrooms, Toxic (Group IV) *on page 1114*

Coral Bead Plant *see* Jequirity Bean *on page 1093*

Coral Bells (Nontoxic Plant)

Corn Flag *see* Iris *on page 1092*

Corn Lily

Synonyms American Hellebore; European Hellebore; False Hellebore; Green Hellebore; Indian Poke; Itch Weed; Langwort; Pepper Root; Rattlesnake Weed; Skunk Cabbage; Swamp Hellebore; Tickleweed; White Hellebore

Mechanism of Toxic Action Contains veratrum alkaloids which act on nerve cells lowering the stimulus threshold, thus resulting in repetitive nerve firing after a single stimulus

Signs & Symptoms of Acute Overdose Nausea, vomiting, bradycardia, hypotension, hypertension (uncommon), oral burning, abdominal pain, sweating, blurred vision, confusion, mydriasis, vertigo; these alkaloids produce different effects in various nerve groups depending on their baseline stimulus threshold (afferent vagal fibers of coronary sinus and left ventricle most affected)

Toxicodynamics/Kinetics
Onset: Within 30 minutes to 4 hours
Duration: 12-15 hours

Toxic Dosage Unclear; likely 1-2 bulbs in a child

Overdosage Treatment
Decontamination: Avoid ipecac due to vagal stimulation, potentiating rapid onset of symptoms; activated charcoal with cathartic may be useful, but might not be tolerated if patient is vomiting
Supportive therapy: Atropine for bradycardia, hypotension may require I.V. fluids or vasopressors

Additional Information All parts are toxic

Specific References
Jaffe AM, Gephardt D, Courtemanche L, et al, "Poisoning Due to Ingestion of *Veratrum viride* (False Hellebore)," *J Emerg Med*, 1990, 8(2):161-7.
Nelson DA, "Accidental Poisoning by *Veratrum japonicum*," 1954, *JAMA*, 156(1):33-5.

"Corn Silk" *Inocybe* Mushroom *see* Mushrooms, Toxic (Group III) *on page 1112*

***Cortinarius gentilis* ("Deadly Cort" or "Goldband Webcap")** *see* Mushrooms, Toxic (Group VIII) *on page 1117*

***Cortinarius orellanus* ("Poznan Cort")** *see* Mushrooms, Toxic (Group VIII) *on page 1117*

Cortinarius rainierensis *see* Mushrooms, Toxic (Group VIII) *on page 1117*

Cortinarius speciosissimus *see* Mushrooms, Toxic (Group VIII) *on page 1117*

***Cortinarius splendicus* ("Splendid Webcap")** *see* Mushrooms, Toxic (Group VIII) *on page 1117*

Cortinarius venenosus *see* Mushrooms, Toxic (Group VIII) *on page 1117*

Cotoneaster [NT]

Overdosage Treatment dicobalt-EDTA used for chelation in Europe

"Cotton Milkcap" Mushroom *see* Mushrooms, Toxic (Group VII) *on page 1116*

Cottonmouth *see Crotalidae on this page*

Court Cone *see* Cone Shells *on page 1073*

Cowbane *see* Water Hemlock *on page 1156*

Cowslip *see* Marsh Marigold *on page 1105*

Crab Louse *see* Lice *on page 1097*

Crab's Eyes *see* Jequirity Bean *on page 1093*

Creeping Charlie (Nontoxic Plant)

Crocus *see* Autumn Crocus *on page 1054*

Crotalidae

Scientific Name *Agkistrodon contortrix* (Copperhead); *Agkistrodon piscivorus* (Cottonmouth); *Sistrurus catenatus* (Pygmy Rattler, Massasauga)

Synonyms Copperhead; Cottonmouth; Massasauga; Pygmy Rattler

Mechanism of Toxic Action Venom, quality and potency vary among species; composition is 90% water with 5-15 enzymes, 3-12 nonenzymatic proteins, as well as other unidentified substances

Signs & Symptoms of Acute Overdose
Systemic signs and symptoms include hypotension, asthenia, sweating, chills, paresthesia, nausea, vomiting, fasciculations, and CNS depression; coagulopathy can occur including thrombocytopenia, hypofibrinogenemia, increased PT and PTT; shock, myopathy, lactic acidosis, hemoconcentration, hypoproteinemia, proteinuria, and hematuria are also potential complications
Local signs include tenderness, edema, erythema, ecchymoses, hemorrhage, bullae, lymphangitis, and rarely a compartment syndrome

Overdosage Treatment
Decontamination: Rapid transport to medical facility; immobilize area; if negative pressure suction device is available, this may be used; do not incise the wound; constriction band may be applied, not a tourniquet; ABC assessment, physical exam; mark extent of local edema with skin-marking pen
Supportive therapy: Repeat lab testing every 3-4 hours for first 12 hours; I.V. fluids, tetanus prophylaxis and analgesics may need to be given; antibiotics may be in-

(Continued)

Crotalidae (Continued)

dicated for infected wound sites; antivenin indicated for moderate to severe envenomation

Antidote: Wyeth crotalid polyvalent antivenin: Treat moderate to severe envenomations with increments of 5-10 vials at a time; skin test per manufacturer's instructions; if positive, may prophylax with H_1- and H_2-histamine receptor blockers; give until local injury has stopped and coagulopathy is reversed; complications include allergic reaction, anaphylaxis, and delayed serum sickness

Antidote(s)

Antivenin (Crotalidae) Polyvalent *on page 1392*

Additional Information Distinguishing characteristics: Facial pits, vertical elliptical pupils, triangular head, single row of subcaudal scales; 6-12 foot brown/tan snake with dark rhomboid markings indigenous to Central and South America

Specific References

Clark RF, Selden BS, and Furbee B, "The Incidence of Wound Infection Following Crotalid Envenomation," *J Emerg Med*, 1993, 11(5):583-6.

Hassen LB, "Reptile and Arthropod Envenomations," *Occup Med*, 1991, 6(3):447-61.

Simon TL and Grace TG, "Envenomation Coagulopathy in Wounds From Pit Vipers," *N Engl J Med*, 1981, 305(8):443-7.

Crotalus adamanteus *see* Rattlesnakes *on page 1132*

Crotalus atrox *see* Rattlesnakes *on page 1132*

Crotalus horridus *see* Rattlesnakes *on page 1132*

Crotalus lepidus *see* Rattlesnakes *on page 1132*

Crotalus molossus *see* Rattlesnakes *on page 1132*

Crotalus scutulatus *see* Rattlesnakes *on page 1132*

Crotalus viridis *see* Rattlesnakes *on page 1132*

Crowfoot *see* Buttercup *on page 1063*

Crown of Thorns

Related Information

Milkbush *on page 1107*

Scientific Name *Euphorbia*; *Euphorbia millii*

Synonyms Christ Plant

Mechanism of Toxic Action Contact dermatitis

Signs & Symptoms of Acute Overdose Swelling, erythema, blistering, vesication, potentially severe ocular pain, irritation, swelling, ulceration, and temporary blindness

Toxicodynamics/Kinetics Symptoms are delayed 2-8 hours with peak effects at 8-24 hours; blisters heal in several days; ocular symptoms may take a month to resolve

Overdosage Treatment

Decontamination: Dermal: Wash thoroughly with soap and water

Supportive therapy: Antibiotics if infected, oral corticosteroids may be useful for severe reactions; no antidote; antihistamines are not likely to be beneficial

Additional Information Toxicity varies within species; blisters should heal without scarring

"Crown" Toadstool *see* Mushrooms, Toxic (Group VI) *on page 1115*

Cryptostegia grandiflora *see* Rubber Vine *on page 1134*

Cuckoo's Meat *see* Shamrock *on page 1140*

Cultivated Tobacco *see* Tobacco *on page 1150*

Cyclopeptide Mushrooms *see* Mushrooms, Toxic (Group I) *on page 1111*

Cytisus *see* Scotch Broom *on page 1138*

Daffodil

Scientific Name *Narcissus pseudo-narcissus*

Synonyms Lycorine; Narcissus

Mechanism of Toxic Action Contains lycorine alkaloid

Signs & Symptoms of Acute Overdose In humans, allergic and contact dermatitis; nausea, vomiting, abdominal pain

Toxicodynamics/Kinetics All parts of plant are toxic, especially the bulb; contains crinine, narcissine, licorine, and other

Toxic Dosage Not established

Overdosage Treatment

Decontamination: Ipecac relatively contraindicated; may be useful, if given soon after ingestion; vomiting has not occurred with ingestion of more than one bulb;

activated charcoal with cathartic/lavage may be beneficial depending on amount ingested and time elapsed since ingestion

Supportive therapy: Wash skin extremely thoroughly with soap and water

Additional Information All parts contain alkaloid, bulb is most toxic; bulbs have been mistaken for onions

"Damp Milkcap" Mushroom *see* Mushrooms, Toxic (Group VII) *on page 1116*

Dandelion (Nontoxic Plant)

Daphne

Scientific Name *Daphne mezereum*

Synonyms Dwarf Bay; February Daphne; Flax Olive; Garland Flower; Lady Laurel; Spurge Laurel; Spurge Olive; Thymelaeaceae

Mechanism of Toxic Action Contains mezerein and daphne toxin which are extremely irritating

Signs & Symptoms of Acute Overdose Mild to severe dermal irritation which may include pruritus, edema, erythema, vesiculation; ocular irritation, inflammation, possibly temporary blindness; nausea, vomiting, diarrhea, possibility of severe gastroenteritis

Toxicodynamics/Kinetics Few reports of exposure available, unclear; dermal symptoms may be immediate or delayed by several hours and resolve within 4-7 days

Toxic Dosage A single berry or leaf may produce symptoms; 2-3 may be fatal in a child; 12 may cause significant toxicity in an adult

Overdosage Treatment

Decontamination: Ipecac relatively contraindicated, may be useful if given soon after ingestion if patient is asymptomatic, activated charcoal with cathartic may be of benefit, lavage may be beneficial in large overdose or in asymptomatic patients presenting later

Dermal: Wash thoroughly even if asymptomatic

Ocular: Irrigate

Supportive therapy: Monitor fluid and electrolyte balance in patients with vomiting and diarrhea

Dermal: Antihistamines and steroids have not clearly been beneficial

Ocular: Supportive care

Oral: Maintain proper fluid and electrolyte balance in symptomatic patients

Additional Information All parts are toxic

Daphne Mezereum

Synonyms Bois Gentil; Bois Joli; Dwarf Bay; Flax Olive; Lady Laurel; Wild Pepper

Mechanism of Toxic Action Contains mezerein (in the bark) and daphnetoxin; seeds contain acrid resin; drying does not decrease toxicity; a very strong irritant

Adverse Reactions

Central nervous system: Fever, headache, delirium, seizures, lethargy, shock

Gastrointestinal: Nausea, vomiting, abdominal pain, watery diarrhea, thirst, dysphagia

Hematologic: Hematuria, proteinuria

Neuromuscular & skeletal: Muscle twitching

Miscellaneous: Facial edema, blisters

Toxicodynamics/Kinetics Absorption: Orally and through intact skin

Toxic Dosage Toxicity may occur following ingestion of 1 leaf or 1 berry in a child or 12 berries in an adult

Overdosage Treatment

Decontamination:

Oral: Lavage/activated charcoal with cathartic

Ocular: Irrigate copiously with saline

Dermal: Wash with water

Supportive therapy: Seizures can be treated with benzodiazepines, phenobarbital, or phenytoin

Additional Information

About 4-5 feet in height; leaves are elliptic and vivid green; flowers are lilac purple or while and about 1 cm in length; fruits are scarlet or yellow

Family: *Thymelaeaceae*

Range: Common hedge if United States, Eastern Canada, and Europe

Toxic parts: Whole plant is poisonous

Specific References

Nyborg J and La Cour T, "X-ray Diffraction Study of Molecular Structure and Conformation of Mezerein," *Nature*, 1975, 257:824-5.

Daphne mezereum *see* Daphne *on this page*

"Dark-Centered" *Hebeloma* Mushroom *see* Mushrooms, Toxic (Group VII) *on page 1116*

Dasheen *see* Caladium *on page 1063*

Datura stramonium *see* Jimson Weed *on page 1094*

"Deadly Agaric" Mushroom *see* Mushrooms, Toxic (Group I) *on page 1111*

"Deadly Cort" Mushroom *see* Mushrooms, Toxic (Group VIII) *on page 1117*

"Deadly" *Galerina* Mushroom *see* Mushrooms, Toxic (Group I) *on page 1111*

Deadly Hemlock *see* Poison Hemlock *on page 1126*

"Deadly Lawn" *Galerina* Mushroom *see* Mushrooms, Toxic (Group I) *on page 1111*

Deadly Nightshade

Scientific Name *Solanum dulcamara*

Synonyms Bittersweet Nightshade; Blue Blindweed; Blue Nightshade; Climbing Nightshade; Devil's Soda Apple; European Bittersweet; Felonwort; Poisonous Nightshade; Scarlet Berry; Violet Bloom; Weedy Nightshade

Mechanism of Toxic Action Contains toxic alkaloids, solanine most significant structurally similar to cardioglycoside, causes hemolytic and hemorrhagic damage to GI tract similar to saponins; some plants may also contain alpha-cholinergic alkaloids

Signs & Symptoms of Acute Overdose Nausea, seizures, vomiting, diarrhea, headache, visual changes, drowsiness, fever, sweating, asthenia, hallucinations, anticholinergic effects may or may not be present to varying degrees

Toxicodynamics/Kinetics Toxicity occurs within 2-24 hours, diarrhea may last 3-6 days, anticholinergic effects may delay GI emptying and produce delayed effects

Toxic Dosage 2-3 green berries or 6 red or black berries should not cause significant toxicity (fatal dose: 200 berries)

Overdosage Treatment

Decontamination: Ipecac if vomiting has not already occurred, lavage and/or charcoal may be beneficial if patient presents symptomatic

Supportive therapy: Maintain fluid and electrolyte balance as necessary, support vital signs; physostigmine will reverse anticholinergic toxicity that may be associated with exposure

Antidote(s)

Physostigmine *on page 1457*

Additional Information Toxic parts: All parts of plant contain solanum and are regarded as toxic

Deadly Nightshade *see* Black Nightshade *on page 1057*

"Deadly Parasol" Mushroom *see* Mushrooms, Toxic (Group I) *on page 1111*

"Death Angel" Mushroom *see* Mushrooms, Toxic (Group I) *on page 1111*

Death Camas

Scientific Name *Zigadenus nuttrallii*; *Zigadenus paniculatus*; *Zigadenus venenosus*

Synonyms Black Snakeroot; Poison Sego; Sand Corn

Mechanism of Toxic Action Contains an alkaloid of the veratrine group which increases muscle and nerve excitability; younger plants are more toxic

Signs & Symptoms of Acute Overdose Vomiting, hypotension, bradycardia, diarrhea, ataxia, muscle spasticity, hyperactive deep tendon reflexes, coma, respiratory depression, muscle fasciculation

Overdosage Treatment

Decontamination: Gastric lavage within 2 hours; activated charcoal

Supportive therapy: While bradycardia may respond to atropine, hypotension will not; give isotonic saline I.V. and supplement with vasopressors (dopamine or norepinephrine) as needed; recovery usually noted within 2 days

Additional Information An onion-like bulb plant of the lily family found in the dry soil of the Western U.S.; flowers appear in summer; 1-2 bulbs (10-15 g) can produce symptoms

Specific References

Heilpern KL, "*Zigadenus* Poisoning," *Ann Emerg Med*, 1995, 25(2):259-62.

Quatrehomme G, Bertrand F, Chauvet C, et al, "Intoxication From Veratrum Album," *Hum Exp Toxicol*, 1993, 12(2):111-5.

Spoerke DG and Spoerke SE, "Three Cases of *Zigadenus* (Death Camas) Poisoning," *Vet Hum Toxicol*, 1979, 21(5):346-7.

Wagstaff DJ and Case AA, "Human Poisoning by *Zigadenus*," *J Toxicol Clin Toxicol*, 1987, 25(4):361-7.

"Deathcap" Mushroom *see* Mushrooms, Toxic (Group I) *on page 1111*

"Deceptive" *Lactarius* Mushroom *see* Mushrooms, Toxic (Group VII) *on page 1116*

Deer Berry *see* Holly *on page 1089*

Delphinium

Synonyms Larkspur

Signs & Symptoms of Acute Overdose No reports of human toxicity; may contain alkaloids with effects similar to monkshood; tingling and burning of toes, fingers, lips, and tongue are seen first, then sweats, hypothermia, chills, paresthesia, numbness, dry mouth; later: diarrhea, paralysis, pain, hypotension, seizures, arrhythmias (supraventricular), bradycardia, ventricular fibrillation

Overdosage Treatment

Decontamination: Ipecac is questionable due to inducing rapid onset of symptoms; lavage may be beneficial, activated charcoal with cathartic

Supportive therapy: Fluid and electrolyte replacement; arrhythmias are relatively refractory to drug therapy

Demodex folliculorum *see* Mites *on page 1107*

***Dendraspis* Species** *see* Cobras *on page 1072*

"Destroying Angel" Mushroom *see* Mushrooms, Toxic (Group I) *on page 1111*

Devilfish *see* Octopus *on page 1119*

Devil's Apple *see* Jimson Weed *on page 1094*

Devil's Ear *see* Jack-in-the-Pulpit *on page 1093*

Devil's Ivy

Scientific Name *Epipremnum aureum*

Synonyms Golden Ceylon Creeper; Golden Hunter's Robe; Golden Pothos; Hunter's Robe; Ivy Arum; Marble Queen Pothos; Pothos Plant; Pothos Vine; Solomon Island Ivy; Taro Vine; Variegated Philodendron

Mechanism of Toxic Action Contains insoluble calcium oxalate crystals which cause mechanical irritation; also may cause irritant dermatitis

Signs & Symptoms of Acute Overdose Dermal pain, irritation, and swelling; sap may cause ocular pain, lacrimation, photophobia, corneal abrasion, oxalate crystals may be deposited on cornea; edema, dysphonia, vomiting, diarrhea, salivation

Toxicodynamics/Kinetics Rapid onset of local symptoms

Overdosage Treatment

Decontamination:

Dermal: Wash thoroughly

Ocular: Irrigate

Oral: Dilute; ipecac, lavage, activated charcoal not likely necessary

Supportive therapy:

Dermal, ocular: Cool compresses may minimize pain

Oral: Ice cream may provide some relief

Additional Information Whole plant is toxic; symptoms dependent on liberation of oxalate crystals or contact with sap; dried plant will not liberate crystals; insoluble calcium oxalates will not cause systemic symptoms

Devil's Soda Apple *see* Deadly Nightshade *on previous page*

Devil's Trumpet *see* Jimson Weed *on page 1094*

Devil's Weed *see* Jimson Weed *on page 1094*

Diarrheic Shellfish Poisoning (DSP) *see* Shellfish Food Poisoning *on page 1141*

Dicentra cucullaria *see* Bleeding Heart *on page 1058*

Dicentra formosa *see* Bleeding Heart *on page 1058*

Dieffenbachia

Synonyms Dumbcane; Leopard Lily; Mother-in-Law's Tongue; Tuft Root

Mechanism of Toxic Action Contains insoluble calcium oxalate crystals which cause mechanical irritation; may also cause irritation through an unclear enzymatic process

Signs & Symptoms of Acute Overdose Dermal pain, irritation, swelling; sap may cause ocular pain, lacrimation, photophobia, corneal abrasion; oxalate crys-

(Continued)

Dieffenbachia *(Continued)*

tals may be deposited on cornea; may also cause dermatitis reaction; edema, vomiting, diarrhea, salivation, dysphonia

Toxicodynamics/Kinetics Rapid onset of local symptoms

Overdosage Treatment

Decontamination:

Dermal: Wash thoroughly

Ocular: Irrigate

Oral: Dilute; ipecac/lavage/activated charcoal not likely necessary

Supportive therapy: Cool compresses may minimize pain and swelling; dexamethasone ophthalmic ointment can be used for eye exposure

Additional Information Whole plant is toxic, symptoms dependent on liberation of oxalate crystals or contact with sap, dried plant will not liberate crystals; wide variation in potential for toxicity between plants; treat symptoms; insoluble calcium oxalate will not cause systemic symptoms; ingestion of stems or stalk may cause upper airway obstruction

Specific References

Ellis W, Barfort P, and Mastman GJ, "Keratoconjunctivitis With Corneal Crystals Caused by Dieffenbachia Plant," *Am J Ophthalmol*, 1973, 76:143.

Digitalis purpurea *see* Foxglove *on page 1085*

Dispholidus typhus *see* Colubrids *on page 1073*

Domoic Acid Poisoning *see* Shellfish/Atlantic Mussel Food Poisoning *on page 1140*

Donkey's Tail (Nontoxic Plant)

Dove's Dung *see* Star-of-Bethlehem (*Ornithogalum umbellatum*) *on page 1146*

Dracaena (Nontoxic Plant)

Dragonroot *see* Jack-in-the-Pulpit *on page 1093*

DSP *see* Shellfish Food Poisoning *on page 1141*

Dumbcane *see* Dieffenbachia *on previous page*

Dusky Pygmy Rattlesnake *see* Rattlesnakes *on page 1132*

Dutch Hyacinth *see* Hyacinth *on page 1090*

Dutchman's Breeches *see* Bleeding Heart *on page 1058*

Dwarf Bay *see* Daphne *on page 1077*

Dwarf Bay *see* Daphne Mezereum *on page 1077*

Dwarf Laurel *see* Mountain Laurel *on page 1110*

Eastern Coral Snake (*Micrurus fulvius*) *see* Elapids *on this page*

Eastern Diamondback Rattlesnake *see* Rattlesnakes *on page 1132*

Eastern Massasauga *see* Rattlesnakes *on page 1132*

Ecballium elaterium *see* Squirting Cucumber *on page 1144*

Echinocystis oregana *see* Wild Cucumber *on page 1157*

***E. coli* 0157:H7** *see Escherichia coli* Food Poisoning *on page 1082*

Eddo *see* Caladium *on page 1063*

Eggplant (Nontoxic)

EHEC *see Escherichia coli* Food Poisoning *on page 1082*

Elapids

Scientific Name *Micrurus euryxanthus*; *Micrurus fulvius*

Synonyms Eastern Coral Snake (*Micrurus fulvius*); Harlequin Snake; Western Coral Snake (*Micrurus euryxanthus*)

Mechanism of Toxic Action Neurotoxin – average amount of dry venom injected: 2-6 mg; significant envenomations occur in 60% of cases

Signs & Symptoms of Acute Overdose

Western coral snake: Local injury

Eastern coral snake: Nausea, vomiting, diplopia, asthenia (within 1-2 hours), fasciculations, coagulopathy, paresthesias, complete paralysis within 36 hours may occur

Overdosage Treatment

Decontamination: Incision and suction can be performed within 30 minutes (1 hour if a tourniquet is in place); wide excision and suction should be reserved for severe envenomations on the trunk

Supportive therapy: Antivenin should be administered as soon as possible for Eastern coral snake envenomation (usual dose: 4-6 vials); horse-derived antivenin is available (Wyeth)

Antidote(s)

Antivenin *(Micrurus fulvius) on page 1394*

Additional Information

Family: Elapidae

Range: Western coral snake is found in Arizona and New Mexico, while Eastern coral snake is found in North Carolina, Florida, and the gulf states; average length is 16-28 inches

Specific References

Gold BS and Barish RA, "Venomous Snake Bites. Current Concepts in Diagnosis, Treatment, and Management," *Emerg Med Clin North Am*, 1992, 10(2):249-67.

Elderberry

Scientific Name *Sambucus*

Synonyms American Elder; American Red Elder; Blue Elder; European Elder; European Red Elder; Red Berried Elder; Stinking Elder

Mechanism of Toxic Action Laxative effect unclear; also contains cyanogenic glycoside

Signs & Symptoms of Acute Overdose Diarrhea, nausea; effects of cyanogenic glycoside include abdominal pain, vomiting, drowsiness, headache, dyspnea, sweating, cyanosis, coma, seizures

Toxic Dosage Unclear, variable

Overdosage Treatment

Decontamination: Ipecac recommended in ingestions of leaves, roots, bark, unripe fruit; activated charcoal with cathartic may be useful; do not give cathartic if diarrhea has developed

Supportive therapy: Maintain fluid and electrolyte balance

Additional Information Ripe fruit is edible when cooked; raw fruit may cause nausea or diarrhea if eaten in large amounts; leaves, roots, bark, unripe fruit may cause more severe diarrhea, although roots, stems, and leaves contain cyanogenic glycosides; there are no documented reports of cyanide toxicity

Elephant Ear *see* Caladium *on page 1063*

"Elfin Saddle" Mushroom *see* Mushrooms, Toxic (Group VII) *on page 1116*

Emerald Gem *see* English Ivy *on this page*

English Ivy

Scientific Name *Hedera helix*

Synonyms California Ivy; Common Ivy; Emerald Gem; Irish Ivy; Pin Oak Ivy

Mechanism of Toxic Action Falcarinol which is an irritant and sensitizer, is a potent alkylating agent; polyacetylenes cause direct contact irritation

Signs & Symptoms of Acute Overdose Irritant contact dermatitis is the most common finding; linear and streaked vesicles may be seen; ingestion may cause a burning sensation in the throat, rash, nausea, vomiting, diarrhea, mydriasis, ataxia, difficulty breathing, and coma

Toxic Dosage Low concentrations of falcarinol have been found to be irritating; specific amounts of plant material required to produce systemic symptoms are unknown, but poisonings are rare

Overdosage Treatment

Decontamination: Oral: Corticosteroids are used to treat the irritant dermatitis, but the reaction may not subside for 3-4 weeks

Supportive therapy: Systemic symptoms require symptomatic and supportive treatment

Additional Information

Range: Native to Europe; commonly found throughout the U.S. and Southern Canada

Toxic parts: All of the plant, especially leaves and berries

English-Oregon-American-Christmas-Indian Holly *see* Holly *on page 1089*

English Yew *see* Yew *on page 1159*

***Entoloma lividum* ("Gray Pinkgill")** *see* Mushrooms, Toxic (Group VII) *on page 1116*

Ephedrone *see* Methcathinone *on page 1106*

***Epicauta* Species (*Meloidae*)** *see* Striped Blister Beetles *on page 1148*

Epipremnum aureum *see* Devil's Ivy *on page 1079*

Escherichia coli Food Poisoning

Synonyms *E. coli* 0157:H7; EHEC; Travelers' Diarrhea (Enterotoxin); Weanling Diarrhea

Commonly Found in Contaminated water

Mechanism of Toxic Action Can produce heat labile and heat stable enterotoxins. Enteropathogenic *E. coli* and enterohemorrhagic *E. coli* (serogroup 0157) produce shiga toxin; incubation period: 1-3 days. Enterohemorrhagic *E. coli* produces hemorrhagic colitis and hemolytic uremia syndrome.

Signs & Symptoms of Acute Overdose Watery diarrhea (enterotoxin); fever and vomiting are unlikely

Overdosage Treatment Supportive therapy: Ampicillin or co-trimoxazole are effective for enterohemorrhagic *E. coli*; fluid/electrolyte replacement

Diagnostic Tests/Procedures

Stool Culture *on page 1356*

Additional Information Can cause necrotizing enterocolitis in the newborn or weanling diarrhea (in poor sanitation areas)

Escherichia coli, enterohemorrhagic:

Microbiology: Enterohemorrhagic *E. coli* causes a distinct form of hemorrhagic colitis in humans. Like other *E. coli* strains, enterohemorrhagic *E. coli* is a facultative, gram-negative bacillus. The most common serotype is 0157:H7. Essentially all published information regarding enterohemorrhagic *E. coli* refers only to this serotype.

Epidemiology:

In 1982, the first large-scale outbreak of *E. coli* 0157:H7 colitis was described. Multiple cases of severe bloody diarrhea were found to be epidemiologically linked to ingestion of contaminated hamburger meat. Since then, the organism has been recognized as an important cause of bloody diarrhea and the hemolytic uremic syndrome. Over 12 major outbreaks have been reported, along with numerous sporadic cases. The majority of cases have been traced to contaminated ground beef, although other potential sources have been cited, including unpasteurized milk, apple cider, municipal water, and roast beef. The organism inhabits the gastrointestinal tract of some healthy cattle and is thought to contaminate meat during slaughter and the processing of ground beef ("internal contamination"). If the ground beef is undercooked, the organism remains viable; undercooking of hamburger patties has proven important in several outbreaks.

In 1993, a well-publicized multistate outbreak of *E. coli* 0157:H7 took place in the Western United States (Washington, California, Idaho, and Nevada). Over 500 infections and four deaths were documented. The vast majority of cases were ultimately linked to contaminated hamburger meat from a particular restaurant chain. Further investigation by the Centers for Disease Control identified several slaughter plants in the United States and one in Canada as the probable source. Thousands of contaminated patties not yet consumed were discovered. In March, 1994, the USDA Food Safety and Inspection Service recommended that all raw meat should be cooked thoroughly, with an increase in the internal temperature for cooked hamburgers to 155°F.

A 2-year nationwide surveillance study by the Centers for Disease Control has found *E. coli* 0157:H7 to be the most commonly identified pathogen associated with bloody diarrhea. In many parts of the U.S., *E. coli* 0157:H7 is the second most common cause of bacterial diarrhea.

Acquisition of disease is usually by ingestion of contaminated food, but person-to-person transmission has been documented, especially in day care centers. Children and elderly individuals are at highest risk for severe infections. Simple and careful hand washing essentially eliminates the probability of person-to-person transmission.

Clinical Syndromes:

- **Hemorrhagic colitis:** *E. coli* 0157:H7 causes a bloody diarrhea associated with abdominal cramps. Pathologically, there is no invasion or inflammation of the intestinal mucosa, and thus fever is often absent. The diarrhea is caused by shiga-like toxins. In most cases, the illness resolves within 7 days, but death can occur in the elderly.
- **Hemolytic uremic syndrome:** Approximately 5% to 10% of patients with *E. coli* 0157:H7 diarrhea develop a syndrome characterized by acute renal failure, thrombocytopenia, and evidence of hemolysis on a peripheral blood smear. Children are at high risk for this syndrome. The patient may be toxic-appearing, and the presentation may be confused with a variety of diseases including sepsis with disseminated intravascular coagulation, vasculitis, thrombotic thrombocytopenia purpura, and others. The estimated mortality is 3% to 5%.

Diagnosis:

Enterohemorrhagic *E. coli* should be strongly considered in any patient presenting with bloody diarrhea, whether or not hemolytic uremic syndrome is present. It is likely that many sporadic cases of *E. coli* 0157:H7 diarrhea occur in the community and go unrecognized for two reasons: many clinicians do not order stool cultures for stable patients with diarrhea; many microbiology laboratories do not routinely culture stools for *E. coli* 0157:H7 unless there is a specific order from the physician.

Diagnosis is confirmed by isolation of *E. coli* 0157:H7 from stool specimens and subsequent serological confirmation. This requires special media in the microbiology laboratory (sorbitol-MacConkey medium). Other methods for the rapid detection of this organism are currently under study.

Escherichia coli, nonenterohemorrhagic:

Microbiology: *Escherichia coli* is a lactose-positive, gram-negative, facultative bacillus with variable motility. A member of the Enterobacteriaceae family, *E. coli* is probably the most widely studied free-living organism. Most *E. coli* are nonpigmented, produce lysine decarboxylase, utilize acetate as a carbon source, and hydrolyze tryptophan to indole. Serologic typing is based on three surface antigens (O, H, K). The lipopolysaccharide of the cell wall is known as endotoxin and is a factor in sepsis and septic shock in infected individuals.

Epidemiology: *E. coli*, as well as other Enterobacteriaceae, are normal colonizers of the human and animal gastrointestinal tract. It is often considered an opportunistic pathogen in hospitalized or debilitated patients but is the most common cause of urinary tract infections among "normal" hosts.

Diagnosis: *E. coli* infection diagnosis can be made by identification through Gram's stain and culture in patients with relevant clinical syndromes. No special media or conditions are necessary to grow this organism. *E. coli* should always be one of several suspected organisms in patients with peritonitis.

Escherichia coli 0157:H7 causes an estimated 20,000 cases of diarrhea in the U.S. of which 6% result in the hemolytic-uremic syndrome. As of March, 1995, 33 states have enacted legislation designating *E. coli* 0157:H7 infection as a reportable disease.

Specific References

Boyce TG, Swerdlow DL, and Griffin PM, "*Escherichia coli* 0157:H7 and the Hemolytic-Uremic Syndrome," *N Engl J Med*, 1995, 333(6):364-8.

CDC, "Enhanced Detection of Sporadic *Escherichia coli* 0157:H7 Infections; New Jersey, July 1994," *MMWR Morb Mortal Wkly Rep*, 1995, 44:417-8.

CDS, "*Escherichia coli* 0157:H7 Outbreak at a Summer Camp, Virginia, 1994," *MMWR Morb Mortal Wkly Rep*, 1995, 44:419-21.

Eisenstein BI, "*Enterobacteriaceae*," *Principles and Practice of Infectious Diseases*, 3rd ed, Mandell GL, Douglas RG Jr, and Bennett JE, eds, New York, NY: Churchill Livingston, 1990, 1658-73.

"*Escherichia coli* 0157:H7 Outbreak Linked to Home-Cooked Hamburger – California, July 1993," *MMWR Morb Mortal Wkly Rep*, 1994, 43(12):213-6.

Gorbach SL and Khurana CM, "Toxigenic *Escherichia coli*: A Cause of Infantile Diarrhea in Chicago," *N Engl J Med*, 1972, 287(16):791-5.

Griffin PM, Ostroff SM, Tauxe RV, et al, "Illnesses Associated With *Escherichia coli* 0157:H7 Infections: A Broad Clinical Spectrum," *Ann Intern Med*, 1988, 109(9):705-12.

Johnson WM, Lior H, and Bezanson GS, "Cytotoxic *Escherichia coli* 0157:H7 Associated With Hemorrhagic Colitis in Canada," *Lancet*, 1983, 1(8314-5):76.

Riley LW, Remis RS, Helgerson SD, et al, "Hemorrhagic Colitis Associated With a Rare *Escherichia coli* Serotype," *N Engl J Med*, 1983, 308(12):681-5.

"Update: Multistate Outbreak of *Escherichia coli* 0157:H7 Infections From Hamburgers – Western United States, 1992-1993," *MMWR Morb Mortal Wkly Rep*, 1993, 42(14):258-63.

Zwadyk P, "*Enterobacteriaceae*: General Characteristics," *Zinsser Microbiology*, 20th ed, Joklik WK, Willett HP, Amos DB, et al, eds, Norwalk, CT: Appleton & Lange, 1992, 538-43.

Zwadyk P, "Opportunistic *Enterobacteriaceae*," *Zinsser Microbiology*, 20th ed, Joklik WK, Willett HP, Amos DB, et al, eds, Norwalk, CT: Appleton & Lange, 1992, 544-55.

Euphorbia *see* Crown of Thorns *on page 1076*

Euphorbia *see* Milkbush *on page 1107*

Euphorbia millii *see* Crown of Thorns *on page 1076*

Euphorbia pulcherrima *see* Poinsettia *on page 1126*

European Bittersweet *see* Deadly Nightshade *on page 1078*

European Elder *see* Elderberry *on page 1081*

European Hellebore *see* Corn Lily *on page 1074*

European Mistletoe (*Viscum album*) *see* Mistletoe *on page 1107*

European Red Elder *see* Elderberry *on page 1081*

Exhirud® *see* Leeches *on page 1096*

Eye Bright *see* Indian Tobacco *on page 1091*

Fall Crocus *see* Autumn Crocus *on page 1054*

False Aralia (Nontoxic Plant)

"False Deathcap" Mushroom *see* Mushrooms, Toxic (Group III) *on page 1112*

"False Deathcap" Mushroom *see* Mushrooms, Toxic (Group V) *on page 1114*

False Hellebore *see* Corn Lily *on page 1074*

"False Morel" Mushroom *see* Mushrooms, Toxic (Group II) *on page 1112*

False Parsley *see* Water Hemlock *on page 1156*

February Daphne *see* Daphne *on page 1077*

Felonwort *see* Deadly Nightshade *on page 1078*

"Felt-Ringed" Mushroom *see* Mushrooms, Toxic (Group VII) *on page 1116*

Feuilles Crabe *see* Star-of-Bethlehem (*Hippobroma longiflora*) *on page 1145*

Ficus benjamina (Nontoxic Plant)

"Fiddle Back" Spider *see* Brown Recluse Spider *on page 1061*

Fiddlehead Fern *see* Ostrich Fern *on page 1121*

"Field" Mushroom *see* Mushrooms, Toxic (Group VII) *on page 1116*

Finger Tree *see* Milkbush *on page 1107*

Fire Ants

Scientific Name *Solenopsis invicta*; *Solenopsis richteri*

Mechanism of Toxic Action Venom (average amount injection: 0.04-0.11 μL), piperidine alkaloids causing histamine release and necrosis in human skin; similar toxin to the brown recluse spider; also contains phospholipase and hyaluronidase

Signs & Symptoms of Acute Overdose Characteristic signs of pain, erythema, wheal formation, and edema at the site of sting; classic allergic reaction symptoms may be seen; 2-3 mm sterile pustule may be noted although occasionally this may be hemorrhagic; pustules may last 3-8 days; hypertension, tachycardia, dyspnea, seizures, nausea, fever (for 1-2 days)

Adverse Reactions Allergic reaction symptoms; anaphylaxis in 0.6% to 1% of stings

Overdosage Treatment Supportive therapy: Urticaria can be treated with epinephrine and antihistamines (H_1- and H_2-blocking agents); oral corticosteroids can be given; local pain can be treated with local injections of lidocaine

Antidote(s)

Epinephrine *on page 1422*

Additional Information Infestations found as far north as Virginia Beach, Virginia; during the winter of 1993-94, 7% of the ant population survived in Eastern Tennessee; attracted to electric current, about 2% of fire ant bites result in severe consequences

Family: Formicidae

Range: Southern U.S.; native to South America

Specific References

Bjerklie D and Norville S, "Ants in Our Pants," *Time*, 1995, 145(23):57.

de Shazo RD, Butcher BT, and Banks WA, "Reactions to the Stings of the Imported Fire Ants," *N Engl J Med*, 1990, 323(7):462-6.

Read FW, Lind NK, and Oda CS, "Histamine Release by Fire Ant (*Solenopsis*) Venom," *Toxicon*, 1978, 16(4):361-7.

Rhoades RB, Schafer WL, Schmid WH, et al, "Hypersensitivity to the Imported Fire Ant: A Report of 49 Cases," *J Allergy Clin Immunol*, 1975, 56(2):85-93.

Stablein JJ and Lockey RF, "Adverse Reactions to Ant Stings," *Clin Rev Allergy*, 1987, 5(2):161-75.

Stafford CT, Hoffman DR, and Rhoades RB, "Allergy to Imported Fire Ants," *South Med J*, 1989, 82(12):1520-7.

Stafford CT, Hutto LS, Rhoades RB, et al, "Imported Fire Ant as a Health Hazard," *South Med J*, 1989, 82(12):1515-9.

Fire Coral

Scientific Name *Hydrozoa millepor*

Mechanism of Toxic Action Nematocysts bear tentacles which cause intense local reaction

Signs & Symptoms of Acute Overdose Pain/burning; severe abrasions from sharp exoskeletons; rash, erythema can also occur; abdominal pain, chills, fever can occur less commonly; full thickness skin burns may result; rubbing affected area worsens the envenomation; blisters can be seen within 6 hours; resolution of symptoms within 1 week

Overdosage Treatment
Decontamination: Soak affected area in hot water (110°F to 115°F); sea water rather than freshwater is preferred. Coral cuts should be cleansed (with acetic acid 5% or isopropyl alcohol 40% to 70%) and debrided. Do not rub affected area.
Supportive therapy: Treat rash with epinephrine and antihistamines; dermatitis can be treated with a topical steroid cream

Additional Information
Family: Milleporidae
Millepora alcicornis: Found in Caribbean
Millepora dichotoma: Found in Red Sea, Pacific

Specific References

Addy JH, "Red Sea Coral Contact Dermatitis," *Int J Dermatol*, 1991, 30(4):271-3.
McGoldrick J and Marx JA, "Marine Envenomations, Part 2: Invertebrates," *J Emerg Med*, 1992, 10(1):71-7.
Rosco MD, "Cutaneous Manifestations of Marine Animal Injuries Including Diagnosis and Treatment," *Cutis*, 1977, 19(4):507-10.
Sagi A, Rosenberg L, Ben-Meir P, et al, "The Fire Coral (*Millepora dichotoma*) as a Cause of Burns: A Case Report," *Burns Incl Therm Inj*, 1987, 13(4):325-6.

Fire Fern *see* Shamrock *on page 1140*

Fittonia (Nontoxic Plant)

Flame Violet (Nontoxic Plant)

"Flat-Top" Mushroom *see* Mushrooms, Toxic (Group VII) *on page 1116*

Flax Olive *see* Daphne *on page 1077*

Flax Olive *see* Daphne Mezereum *on page 1077*

"Fleecy Milkcap" Mushroom *see* Mushrooms, Toxic (Group VII) *on page 1116*

Fleur-de-lis *see* Iris *on page 1092*

Florida Yew *see* Yew *on page 1159*

Florist's Calla *see* Calla *on page 1064*

Flowering Maple (Nontoxic Plant)

Adverse Reactions May cause dermatitis; allergic skin reactions have been reported

"Fly Agaric" Mushroom *see* Mushrooms, Toxic (Group III) *on page 1112*

"Fly Agaric" Mushroom *see* Mushrooms, Toxic (Group V) *on page 1114*

Flying Saucers *see* Morning Glory *on page 1109*

Food and Drug Coloring No. 5 *see* Tartrazine Food Poisoning *on page 1149*

"Forest Friend" Mushroom *see* Mushrooms, Toxic (Group VII) *on page 1116*

"Forest" Mushroom *see* Mushrooms, Toxic (Group VII) *on page 1116*

Four-O'Clock

Scientific Name *Mirabilis jalapa*

Synonyms Mirakelblomst

Signs & Symptoms of Acute Overdose Handling the roots or seeds may result in dermatitis; ingestion may cause nausea, vomiting, diarrhea, and abdominal pain; smoking or eating the seeds is rumored to result in hallucinogenic effects

Toxic Dosage Not established

Overdosage Treatment Decontamination: Charcoal may be of value, one dose of cathartic may be considered if symptoms have not begun

Additional Information
Toxin: Trigonelline
Range: Native to Mexico and Central and South America, cultivated throughout the U.S.
Toxic part: Roots and seeds

Foxglove

CAS Number 17575-20-1

Scientific Name *Digitalis purpurea*

Synonyms Revebjelle; Willow-Leaves Foxglove

(Continued)

Foxglove *(Continued)*

Mechanism of Toxic Action Leaves and seeds contain digitalis glycosides which inhibit the sodium - potassium ATPase pump causing decreased intracellular potassium and increased intracytoplasmic calcium

Signs & Symptoms of Acute Overdose GI effects (nausea and vomiting) usually precede the cardiovascular effects by several hours; bradycardia; first, second, and third degree heart block; asystole, A-V block, hypotension, ventricular arrhythmias, atrial fibrillation, decreased Q-T interval and prolonged P-R interval; fatigue, confusion, delirium, headache, dizziness, contact dermatitis, seeing yellow halos, and hyperkalemia have also been reported

Toxicodynamics/Kinetics Upper limit of peak toxicity: 12 hours; all symptomatic patients should be observed for a minimum of 24 hours

Toxic Dosage One cup of foxglove tea produced junctional rhythm in the 40s with frequent PVCs in an adult; in accidental ingestion in children, ipecac and home observation are recommended for ingestion of one leaf or less; if greater than one leaf is ingested, decontamination and observation in the emergency room are recommended

Overdosage Treatment

Decontamination: Lavage and multidose activated charcoal with cathartic enhance total body clearance of digitalis; whole bowel irrigation is also beneficial in removing plant debris from the GI tract and is recommended for ingestions of large amounts of plant material

Supportive therapy: Monitor cardiac status and serum potassium levels; bradycardia will frequently respond to atropine; phenytoin is the recommended treatment for ventricular arrhythmias because it will also improve conduction through the A-V node; lidocaine can also be used to treat ventricular arrhythmias, but will not have an effect on A-V conduction; other antiarrhythmics which have been used in arrhythmias resistant to the above therapy include magnesium, amiodarone, and bretylium; a pacemaker should be considered for bradycardia and A-V nodal blocks resistant to medical management

Antidote: Digoxin immune Fab has been shown to interact with several different plant cardiac glycosides and may be beneficial in cases resistant to conventional treatment; indications for its use include ventricular arrhythmias resistant to conventional treatment, severe bradycardia and/or second or third degree heart block resistant to atropine and phenytoin

Antidote(s)

Digoxin Immune Fab *on page 1411*

Diagnostic Tests/Procedures

Digitoxin, Blood *on page 1249*

Additional Information Persons taking digoxin, beta-blockers, and calcium channel blockers are more susceptible to the toxin; digitoxin assay has been shown to cross-react with the digitalis glycoside and thus may be beneficial in documenting ingestion, however, serum levels and toxicity do not necessarily correlate

Family: Scophylariaceae

Range: Native to Europe, but commonly found in the U.S.

Toxin: Digitalis, digitoxin, cardiac glycosides

Friar's Cap *see* Monkshood *on page 1108*

Friar's Cowl *see* Monkshood *on page 1108*

"Frost's" *Amanita* Mushroom *see* Mushrooms, Toxic (Group V) *on page 1114*

Fuchsia (Nontoxic Plant)

Fuglestjerne *see* Star-of-Bethlehem (*Ornithogalum umbellatum*) *on page 1146*

***Galerina autumnalis* ("Deadly" *Galerina* or "Autumnal" *Galerina*)** *see* Mushrooms, Toxic (Group I) *on page 1111*

***Galerina marginata* (Marginate *Pholiota*)** *see* Mushrooms, Toxic (Group I) *on page 1111*

***Galerina venenata* ("Deadly Lawn" *Galerina*)** *see* Mushrooms, Toxic (Group I) *on page 1111*

Garden Calla *see* Calla *on page 1064*

Garden Hyacinth *see* Hyacinth *on page 1090*

Gardenia (Nontoxic Plant)

Adverse Reactions Odor may illicit hay fever reaction

Garland Flower *see* Daphne *on page 1077*

Gastrointestinal Irritant Mushrooms *see* Mushrooms, Toxic (Group VII) *on page 1116*

Genista scopafia *see* Scotch Broom *on page 1138*

Geographer Cone *see* Cone Shells *on page 1073*

German Iris *see* Iris *on page 1092*

"Giant False Morel" Mushroom *see* Mushrooms, Toxic (Group II) *on page 1112*

"Giant" *Hebeloma* Mushroom *see* Mushrooms, Toxic (Group VII) *on page 1116*

Gila Monster

Scientific Name *Helderma cinctum*; *Heloderma suspectum*

Mechanism of Toxic Action Venom contains hyaluronidase gilatoxin, helothermine, phospholipase A, kallikrein, and serotonin; venom is proteolytic with minimal tissue breakdown seen

Signs & Symptoms of Acute Overdose Hypotension, tachycardia, generalized asthenia, nausea, vomiting, localized erythema and edema, sweating, leukocytosis may occur; localized pain may be severe; regional lymphadenopathy may occur; tinnitus, exophthalmus, tachypnea, thrombocytopenia

Adverse Reactions Coagulopathy

Toxic Dosage Lethal dose: 5-8 mg

Overdosage Treatment

Decontamination: Avoid breaking off teeth when removing lizard; flame, cold water immersion, and handheld cast spreaders can assist in disengaging lizard

Supportive therapy: Local wound care with broad spectrum antibiotics should be administered; monitor tetanus immunization status; patient should be observed for at least 6 hours for systemic reactions; antivenom therapy (through the Poisonous Animal Research Laboratory at Arizona State University or the Venom Poisoning Center at the University of Southern California) is experimental

Additional Information Endemic in Southwestern United States, these lizards are 30-50 cm long; usually docile but will bite and hang on tenaciously when provoked; teeth may break and be left in the wound (teeth are not radiopaque); venom glands are located in lower anterior jaw; 30% of bites have no venom injected; *Heloderma horridum* (the beaded lizard) found in Mexico has a similar type of venom; submerging the animal in cold water may subdue the lizard thus allowing for disengagement; a handheld cast spreader can also be used to disengage the reptile's mandible

Specific References

Heitschel S, "Near Death From a Gila Monster Bite," *J Emerg Nurs*, 1986, 12(5):259-62.
Hooker KR and Caravati EM, "Gila Monster Envenomation," *Ann Emerg Med*, 1994, 24(4):731-5.
Kunkel DB, "Bites of Venomous Reptiles," *Emerg Med Clin North Am*, 1984, 2(3):563-77.
Miller MF, "Gila Monster Envenomation,"*Ann Emerg Med*, 1995, 25:720.

Ginbey *see* Star-of-Bethlehem (*Hippobroma longiflora*) *on page 1145*

"Girdled" *Panaeolus* Mushroom *see* Mushrooms, Toxic (Group VI) *on page 1115*

Glory of the Sea *see* Cone Shells *on page 1073*

Gloxinia (Nontoxic Plant)

Glycocome *see* Licorice *on page 1098*

Glycyrrhiza glabra *see* Licorice *on page 1098*

Glycyrrhiza lepidota *see* Licorice *on page 1098*

Glycyrrhiza uralensis *see* Licorice *on page 1098*

Gold Apple *see* Tomato (Leaves and Stems) *on page 1150*

"Goldband Webcap" Mushroom *see* Mushrooms, Toxic (Group VIII) *on page 1117*

"Gold-Drop Milkcap" Mushroom *see* Mushrooms, Toxic (Group VII) *on page 1116*

Golden Ceylon Creeper *see* Devil's Ivy *on page 1079*

Golden Chain Tree

Synonyms Bean Tree; Gullregn; Scotch Lanburnum

Mechanism of Toxic Action Contains cytisine which has effects similar to nicotine

Signs & Symptoms of Acute Overdose Nausea, vomiting, asthenia, headache, pallor, drowsiness, ataxia, mydriasis, tachycardia, hypotension, paralysis, seizures

(Continued)

Golden Chain Tree *(Continued)*

Toxicodynamics/Kinetics Onset of symptoms: Within 15 minutes to 4 hours

Overdosage Treatment

Decontamination: Ipecac relatively contraindicated because of risk of seizures occurring rapidly with large ingestion; lavage/activated charcoal with cathartic if large amounts ingested

Supportive care: Maintain respiration and blood pressure in symptomatic patient

Additional Information All parts toxic, no reports of toxic exposure to this plant exist in the U.S., however, British literature reports poisonings

Golden Hunter's Robe *see* Devil's Ivy *on page 1079*

Golden Pothos *see* Devil's Ivy *on page 1079*

Goldfish Plant (Nontoxic Plant)

***Gomphus floccosus* ("Woolly Chanterelle" or "Scaly Chanterelle")** *see* Mushrooms, Toxic (Group VII) *on page 1116*

Good Luck Leaf *see* Shamrock *on page 1140*

Good Luck Plant *see* Shamrock *on page 1140*

Gools *see* Marsh Marigold *on page 1105*

"Grape-Colored" *Lactarius* Mushroom *see* Mushrooms, Toxic (Group VII) *on page 1116*

Grape Ivy (Nontoxic Plant)

Adverse Reactions Report of dermal irritation (blisters, dermatitis)

"Gray Cap" Mushroom *see* Mushrooms, Toxic (Group VII) *on page 1116*

"Gray Pinkgill" Mushroom *see* Mushrooms, Toxic (Group VII) *on page 1116*

Green Broom *see* Scotch Broom *on page 1138*

Green Dragon *see* Jimson Weed *on page 1094*

Green Hellebore *see* Corn Lily *on page 1074*

"Green Parasol" Mushroom *see* Mushrooms, Toxic (Group VII) *on page 1116*

"Green" *Pholiota* Mushroom *see* Mushrooms, Toxic (Group VI) *on page 1115*

Ground Hemlock *see* Yew *on page 1159*

Gullregn *see* Golden Chain Tree *on previous page*

***Gymnopilus aeruginosa* ("Green" *Pholiota*)** *see* Mushrooms, Toxic (Group VI) *on page 1115*

Gymnopilus luteus *see* Mushrooms, Toxic (Group VI) *on page 1115*

***Gymnopilus spectabilis* ("Showy Flamecap" or "Big Laughing" Mushroom)** *see* Mushrooms, Toxic (Group VI) *on page 1115*

Gymnopilus validipes *see* Mushrooms, Toxic (Group VI) *on page 1115*

Gymnopilus viridans *see* Mushrooms, Toxic (Group VI) *on page 1115*

Gyromitra ambigua *see* Mushrooms, Toxic (Group II) *on page 1112*

***Gyromitra brunnea* ("Brown False Morel")** *see* Mushrooms, Toxic (Group II) *on page 1112*

***Gyromitra californica* ("California False Morel" Mushroom)** *see* Mushrooms, Toxic (Group II) *on page 1112*

***Gyromitra caroliniana* ("Carolina False Morel")** *see* Mushrooms, Toxic (Group II) *on page 1112*

Gyromitra esculenta *see* Mushrooms, Toxic (Group II) *on page 1112*

***Gyromitra esculenta* ("Beefsteak" or "Brain" *Gyromitra* or "False Morel" or "Turban Fungus")** *see* Mushrooms, Toxic (Group II) *on page 1112*

Gyromitra fastigiata *see* Mushrooms, Toxic (Group II) *on page 1112*

***Gyromitra gigas* ("Snow Morel" or "Giant False Morel")** *see* Mushrooms, Toxic (Group II) *on page 1112*

Gyromitra infula **("Hooded False Morel")** *see* Mushrooms, Toxic (Group II) *on page 1112*

Gyromitra korfii **("Bull Nose")** *see* Mushrooms, Toxic (Group II) *on page 1112*

Gyromitra sphaerospora *see* Mushrooms, Toxic (Group II) *on page 1112*

"Halfglobe" Mushroom *see* Mushrooms, Toxic (Group VI) *on page 1115*

Hallucinogenic Snuff *see* Bufotenine *on page 1062*

Harlequin Snake *see* Elapids *on page 1080*

Harts Horn *see* Buckthorn *on page 1062*

Head Louse *see* Lice *on page 1097*

Heart of Jesus *see* Caladium *on page 1063*

Heavenly Blue *see* Morning Glory *on page 1109*

Hebeloma crustuliniforme **("Poison Pie")** *see* Mushrooms, Toxic (Group VII) *on page 1116*

Hebeloma mesophaeum **("Dark-Centered"** ***Hebeloma*****)** *see* Mushrooms, Toxic (Group VII) *on page 1116*

Hebeloma sinapizans **("Giant"** ***Hebeloma*****)** *see* Mushrooms, Toxic (Group VII) *on page 1116*

Hedera helix *see* English Ivy *on page 1081*

Helderma cinctum *see* Gila Monster *on page 1087*

Hell's Fire Anemone *see* Sea Anemones *on page 1138*

Helmet Flower *see* Monkshood *on page 1108*

Heloderma suspectum *see* Gila Monster *on page 1087*

Helvella lacunosa **("Elfin Saddle")** *see* Mushrooms, Toxic (Group VII) *on page 1116*

Henequen *see* Century Plant *on page 1067*

Hens and Chickens (Nontoxic Plant)

Hills-of-Snow *see* Hydrangea *on next page*

Hippobroma longiflora *see* Star-of-Bethlehem (*Hippobroma longiflora*) *on page 1145*

Hirudo medicinalis *see* Leeches *on page 1096*

Holly

Scientific Name *Ilex aquifolium*; *Ilex opaca*; *Ilex vomitoria*

Synonyms Appalachian Tea; Cassena; Deer Berry; English-Oregon-American-Christmas-Indian Holly; Indian Black Drink; Kristtorn; Yanpon

Use Native Americans used the plant as an emetic and cardiac stimulant

Mechanism of Toxic Action Irritation of the gastrointestinal tract

Signs & Symptoms of Acute Overdose Nausea, vomiting, and diarrhea

Toxic Dosage Not well established; apparently berries must be eaten in quantity to produce toxic symptoms

Overdosage Treatment

Decontamination: Charcoal may be of value; one dose of cathartic may be given if symptoms have not begun

Supportive therapy: Replace fluids and electrolytes as needed to prevent dehydration

Additional Information

Range: Found throughout the Eastern and Southern U.S.

Toxin: Ilexanthin, ilex acid, tannic acid, ilicin

Toxic part: Berries are toxic in quantity

Specific References

Rodrigues TD, Johnson PN, and Jeffrey LP, "Holly Berry Ingestion: Case Report," *Vet Hum Toxicol*, 1984, 26(2):157-8.

"Honey" Mushroom *see* Mushrooms, Toxic (Group VII) *on page 1116*

Honeysuckle (Nontoxic Plant)

"Hooded False Morel" Mushroom *see* Mushrooms, Toxic (Group II) *on page 1112*

Horse Chestnut *see* Buckeye *on page 1062*

Horse Chestnuts

Scientific Name *Aesculus hippocastanum*

Mechanism of Toxic Action Contains frangula, an anthraquinone which stimulates the colon

Signs & Symptoms of Acute Overdose Nausea, abdominal pain, vomiting, cramping, diarrhea; could potentially cause kidney damage with large enough ingestion

Toxicodynamics/Kinetics Onset is likely to be soon after ingestion

Toxic Dosage Mild intoxication upon ingestion of berries by children; apparently ingestion of about 20 berries or chewing the fresh bark is necessary to induce pronounced symptoms

Overdosage Treatment

Decontamination: Ipecac/cathartic not recommended, activated charcoal/lavage may be useful

Supportive therapy: Treat any fluid or electrolyte imbalance

Additional Information Fruit, leaves, and bark are poisonous; may color alkaline urine red; do not confuse with hematuria

"Horse" Mushroom *see* Mushrooms, Toxic (Group VII) *on page 1116*

Horse Poison *see* Star-of-Bethlehem (*Hippobroma longiflora*) *on page 1145*

Hot Pepper *see* Pepper *on page 1123*

House Bane *see* Monkshood *on page 1108*

Hoya (Nontoxic Plant)

Hunter's Robe *see* Devil's Ivy *on page 1079*

Hyacinth

Scientific Name *Hyacinthus orientalis*

Synonyms Common Hyacinth; Dutch Hyacinth; Garden Hyacinth

Signs & Symptoms of Acute Overdose Predominantly gastrointestinal irritation, nausea, vomiting, diarrhea, stomach cramps; contact dermatitis has also been reported; may also cause rhinitis or trigger an asthma attack in sensitive individuals

Toxic Dosage Not well quantified; symptoms have been reported after small ingestions

Overdosage Treatment Supportive therapy: Maintain fluid and electrolyte balance as needed

Additional Information

Range: Common garden plant throughout U.S.

Toxin: Thought to be narcissine-like alkaloids

Toxic part: Bulb

Hyacinthus orientalis *see* Hyacinth *on this page*

Hydrangea

Scientific Name *Hydrangea paniculata*

Synonyms Arborrescent; Hills-of-Snow

Mechanism of Toxic Action Amygdalin (a cyanogenic glycoside) is hydrolyzed in the gut to release hydrocyanic acid, cellular hypoxia occurs after absorption and complexation with cytochrome oxidase

Signs & Symptoms of Acute Overdose Reported poisonings have shown hydrangea to cause nausea and gastroenteritis; may also cause contact dermatitis

Overdosage Treatment

Decontamination: Consider ipecac early after exposure if patient asymptomatic and large amount ingested; ipecac is not used to treat cyanogenic effects; activated charcoal with cathartic may be beneficial; lavage would be indicated if patient exhibited cyanogenic effects

Supportive therapy: Maintain fluid and electrolyte balance; give sodium bicarbonate for acidosis

Antidote(s)

Cyanide Antidote Kit *on page 1406*

Diagnostic Tests/Procedures

Anion Gap, Blood *on page 1193*

Blood Gases, Arterial *on page 1207*

Electrolytes, Blood *on page 1254*

Methemoglobin, Blood *on page 1296*

Additional Information Buds, flowers, and leaves are toxic; no cases of cyanogenic toxicity on record

Hydrangea paniculata *see* Hydrangea *on previous page*

Hydroids (Coral)

Mechanism of Toxic Action Nematocysts cause intense local reaction

Signs & Symptoms of Acute Overdose Stings produce painful stinging sensation; rarely abdominal pain, fever, diarrhea have occurred; rash, erythema is likely for free floating Portuguese Man-of-War, orange-striped jellyfish, and the stinging medusa may cause generalized symptoms including intense local pain (electric shock-like), arthralgia, myalgias, coagulopathy, lymphadenopathy with headache, fever, asthenia also present

Overdosage Treatment Supportive therapy: Epinephrine or antihistamines can be used for rash; muscle spasms can be treated with calcium gluconate I.V.; coral cuts should be cleansed and debrided; dermatitis can be treated with a topical corticosteroid cream. Meat tenderizer solution neutralizes protein toxin and thus can be sprinkled over wound of Portuguese Man-of-War; irrigate with sea water (not fresh water); apply 5% acetic acid or 40% to 70% isopropyl alcohol to inactivate nematocysts; diluted ammonia hydroxide may also be used; remove remaining nematocysts by shaving the area.

Additional Information Exoskeleton of calcium carbonate; an encrustation

Family: Hydrozoa

Millepora (Florida Keys and Caribbean)

Phylum: Coelenterata

Range: Found attached to rocks in shallow water in temperate zones

Specific References

Auerbach PS, "Hazardous Marine Animals," *Emerg Med Clin North Am*, 1984, 2(3):531-44.

McGoldrick J and Marx JA, "Marine Envenomations, Part 2: Invertebrates," *J Emerg Med*, 1992, 10(1):71-7.

Hydrozoa millepor *see* Fire Coral *on page 1084*

Ibotenic Acid-Containing Mushrooms *see* Mushrooms, Toxic (Group V) *on page 1114*

Ichthyosarcotoxism *see* Ciguatera Food Poisoning *on page 1069*

Ilex aquifolium *see* Holly *on page 1089*

Ilex opaca *see* Holly *on page 1089*

Ilex vomitoria *see* Holly *on page 1089*

Impatiens (Nontoxic Plant)

Indian Apple *see* Mayapple *on page 1105*

Indian Bean *see* Jequirity Bean *on page 1093*

Indian Black Drink *see* Holly *on page 1089*

Indian Cobra *see* Cobras *on page 1072*

Indian Licorice *see* Jequirity Bean *on page 1093*

Indian Poke *see* Corn Lily *on page 1074*

Indian Rubber Vine *see* Rubber Vine *on page 1134*

Indian Spurge Tree *see* Milkbush *on page 1107*

Indian Tobacco

Related Information

Star-of-Bethlehem (*Ornithogalum pyrenaicum*) *on page 1145*

Star-of-Bethlehem (*Ornithogalum umbellatum*) *on page 1146*

Scientific Name *Lobelia inflata*

Synonyms Asthma Weed; Bladder Pod; Eye Bright; "Puke Weed"; "Vomit Wort"; Wild Tobacco

Use Variety of purposes over the years; the extract has been used as an emetic; lobeline sulfate has been used as an aid to stop smoking

Mechanism of Toxic Action Contains lobeline alkaloids which have nicotinic-like action and other piperidine alkaloids

Signs & Symptoms of Acute Overdose Nausea, vomiting, diarrhea, abdominal pain, hypertension, bradycardia, paralysis, tremor, seizures, coma, and euphoria; dermatitis has also been reported

Toxic Dosage Lobeline content may vary, specific toxic amounts of plant material is unknown most poisonings have been from herbal preparations

Overdosage Treatment Decontamination: Emesis or lavage may be useful in large, recent ingestions if the patient has not started vomiting; activated charcoal

(Continued)

Indian Tobacco *(Continued)*

with cathartic should be administered; seizures should be managed by benzodiazepines

Additional Information Other related toxic species are *Lobelia cardinalis*, *Lobelia siphilotica*, and *Lobelia berlandieri*; *Eriogonum umbellatum* is also known as Indian tobacco and is considered nontoxic

Family: Campanulaceae

Range: Grows extensively throughout the U.S.

Toxic parts: All parts, especially roots and seeds

Specific References

Siegel RK, "Herbal Intoxication. Psychoactive Effects From Herbal Cigarettes, Tea, and Capsules," *JAMA*, 1976, 236(5):473-6.

Indian Turnip *see* Jack-in-the-Pulpit *on next page*

Indole-Containing Mushrooms *see* Mushrooms, Toxic (Group VI) *on page 1115*

Indo-Pacific Box Jellyfish *see* Box Jellyfish *on page 1060*

Inkberry *see* Pokeweed *on page 1127*

"Inky Cap" Mushroom *see* Mushrooms, Toxic (Group IV) *on page 1114*

Inocybe fastigiata **("Straw-Colored Fiberhead" or "Conic Fiberhead")** *see* Mushrooms, Toxic (Group V) *on page 1114*

Inocybe geophylla **("Earthblade Fiberhead")** *see* Mushrooms, Toxic (Group V) *on page 1114*

Inocybe godeyi *see* Mushrooms, Toxic (Group V) *on page 1114*

Inocybe lacera **("Torn-Capped Fiberhead")** *see* Mushrooms, Toxic (Group V) *on page 1114*

Inocybe lilacina *see* Mushrooms, Toxic (Group V) *on page 1114*

Inocybe patouillardi *see* Mushrooms, Toxic (Group V) *on page 1114*

Inocybe pudica **("Blushing"** ***Inocybe*****)** *see* Mushrooms, Toxic (Group V) *on page 1114*

Inocybe sororia **("Corn Silk"** ***Inocybe*****)** *see* Mushrooms, Toxic (Group V) *on page 1114*

Ipomoea purpurea *see* Morning Glory *on page 1109*

Iris

Scientific Name *Iris germanica*

Synonyms Corn Flag; Fleur-de-lis; German Iris; Poison Flag; Snake Lily

Mechanism of Toxic Action Resinous substance irisin which acts as an irritant

Signs & Symptoms of Acute Overdose Nausea, vomiting, diarrhea, abdominal pain, burning sensation in mouth and throat; dermal contact may result in a burning sensation and dermatitis

Toxic Dosage Specific quantities have not been determined

Overdosage Treatment

Decontamination: Gastrointestinal decontamination may be of value in large recent ingestions

Supportive therapy: Replace fluids and electrolytes as necessary

Additional Information There are many species of iris with similar toxicities

Family: Iridaceae

Range: Common garden flower cultivated throughout the U.S.

Toxic parts: Mainly the bulb, but possibly all parts

Iris germanica *see* Iris *on this page*

Irish Ivy *see* English Ivy *on page 1081*

Irish Shamrock *see* Shamrock *on page 1140*

Irish Tops *see* Scotch Broom *on page 1138*

Isotoma longiflora *see* Star-of-Bethlehem (*Hippobroma longiflora*) *on page 1145*

Itch Mite (*Sarcoptes scabiei*) *see* Mites *on page 1107*

Itch Weed *see* Corn Lily *on page 1074*

Ivy Arum *see* Devil's Ivy *on page 1079*

Ivy Bush *see* Mountain Laurel *on page 1110*

Jack-in-the-Pulpit

Scientific Name *Arisaema triphyllum*

Synonyms Bog Onion; Brown Dragon; Devil's Ear; Dragonroot; Indian Turnip; Memory Root; Pepper Turnip; Starch Wort; Three-Leaved Indian Turnip; Wake Robin; Wild Turnip

Mechanism of Toxic Action Entire plant contains calcium oxalate crystals which cause oral irritation, swelling, pain, and slurred speech; large ingestions necessary for systemic toxicity are unlikely to occur due to oral irritation seen with ingestion

Signs & Symptoms of Acute Overdose

Dermal: Pain, irritation, swelling

Ocular: Sap may cause pain, lacrimation, photophobia, corneal abrasion; oxalate crystals may be deposited on cornea; may also cause dermatitis reaction

Oral: Edema, vomiting, diarrhea, salivation, dysphonia

Overdosage Treatment

Decontamination:

Dermal: Wash thoroughly

Ocular: Irrigate with tepid water for 15 minutes

Oral: Dilute; ipecac/lavage/activated charcoal not likely necessary; milk/water to rinse crystals

Supportive therapy: Cool compresses may minimize pain and swelling

Additional Information Toxin: Calcium oxalate crystals

"Jack-O'-Lantern" Mushroom *see* Mushrooms, Toxic (Group III) *on page 1112*

Jade Plant (Nontoxic Plant)

Jalapeno Pepper *see* Pepper *on page 1123*

Jamaican Vomiting Sickness *see* Akee Fruit Food Poisoning *on page 1050*

Jamestown Weed *see* Jimson Weed *on next page*

Japanese Yew *see* Yew *on page 1159*

Jellyfish

Scientific Name *Aurelia aurita*

Mechanism of Toxic Action Stings

Signs & Symptoms of Acute Overdose Pain, burning, urticaria, regional lymph node involvement, skin ulceration, anaphylactic shock (rare)

Adverse Reactions Severe stings may include hematuria, syncope, paralysis, renal insufficiency, hypotension, cardiorespiratory failure

Central nervous system: Fever, chills

Neuromuscular & skeletal: Muscle spasms

Overdosage Treatment

Decontamination: Immediately rinse with seawater, should then prevent further envenomation by applying acetic acid 5% (vinegar) to any tentacles still adhering to tissue; if acetic acid is not available, use isopropyl alcohol 40% to 70% or finally may use aluminum sulfate; shave envenomated area after initial treatment, then repeat local decontamination therapy. Ocular exposures are to be decontaminated by water irrigation only. Do not rub affected area. Wear gloves during decontamination. Meat tenderizers have been used, however, they are not preferred decontamination measures and should not have prolonged contact times (>10 minutes).

Supportive therapy: Local symptoms persisting after the initial treatment may be treated with antihistamines, local anesthetics, or steroid lotion; tetanus prophylaxis should be given according to patient's immunization status

Additional Information

Class: Scyphozoa

Range: All oceans

Specific References

Auerbach PS, "Marine Envenomations," *N Engl J Med*, 1991, 325(7): 486-93.

Kizer KW, "Marine Envenomations," *J Toxicol Clin Toxicol*, 1983-84, 21(4-5):527-55.

Jequirity Bean

Scientific Name *Abrus precatorius*

Synonyms Bead Plant; Black Eyed Susan; Buddhist Rosary Bead; Coral Bead Plant; Crab's Eyes; Indian Bean; Indian Licorice; Jumble Bead; Licorice Plant; Love Bean; Love Pea; Lucky Bean; Mienie-Mienie; Ojode Pajaro; Prayer Bead; Prayer Bean; Precatory Bean; Precatory Pea; Rosary Bean; Seminole Bead; Weather Plant; Wild Licorice

Mechanism of Toxic Action Ricin, a toxalbumin, inhibits protein synthesis

Signs & Symptoms of Acute Overdose Acutely causes irritation to oropharynx, esophagus, and GI tract; may cause hemorrhage and tissue sloughing

(Continued)

Jequirity Bean *(Continued)*

Toxicodynamics/Kinetics Acute effects occur within 8 hours; late phase complications delayed by 2-5 days possibly with asymptomatic phase in between

Toxic Dosage Toxicity may occur with as little as one bean

Overdosage Treatment Decontamination: Consider ipecac if asymptomatic, activated charcoal may be useful; consider using osmotic cathartic despite hyperactive bowel as decreased exposure to mucosa may be beneficial, follow fluid and electrolyte status closely if symptomatic; if symptomatic, maintain high urine flow; consider alkalinization to prevent hemoglobin crystallization in severe poisonings; guaiac vomiting, stool, follow fluid and electrolyte status; check hematologic parameters in severe poisoning, hepatic enzymes

Additional Information Scarlet bean-shaped seed with a black spot where attached inside pod; used in necklaces and as good luck charms; toxicity will not occur unless seed coat is broken; toxicity is variable; related to variations within plants and GI absorption, seed has hard coat; rupture makes toxin available; symptomatic patients should be hospitalized; asymptomatic patients that have received early thorough decontamination may be observed at home; bark, seeds, and leaves are toxic; honey locust is nontoxic

Jerusalem Cherry *see* Christmas Cherry *on page 1068*

"Jeweled Deathcap" Mushroom *see* Mushrooms, Toxic (Group V) *on page 1114*

Jimson Weed

Scientific Name *Datura stramonium*

Synonyms Angel's Trumpet; Apple of Peru; Devil's Apple; Devil's Trumpet; Devil's Weed; Green Dragon; Jamestown Weed; Loco Weed; Mad Apple; Moon Weed; Stink Weed; Thorn Apple; Tolguacha; Trumpet Lily

Mechanism of Toxic Action The whole plant, especially the foliage and seeds, contains anticholinergic compounds like atropine, hyoscyamine, and scopolamine; seeds contain highest amount of atropine (0.1 mg atropine per seed); ~50-100 seeds may cause severe intoxication and hallucinations. **Note:** Seeds are often ingested for their deliriant effect.

Signs & Symptoms of Acute Overdose Usually occur within 1 hour and may last for 2 days; mydriasis, pruritus, visual hallucinations, hypertension, tachycardia, seizures, nausea, vomiting, dizziness, delirium, auditory hallucinations, decreased bowel sounds, disorientation, urinary retention, seizures

Toxicodynamics/Kinetics May decrease GI motility and, therefore, slow absorption

Overdosage Treatment

Decontamination: Due to decreased GI motility, vomiting/lavage may be useful later in the course of the ingestion unless oral/esophageal irritation, decreased gag reflex, or CNS depression is present where vomiting is therefore contraindicated

Supportive therapy: Physostigmine may be useful to treat life-threatening anticholinergic symptoms; physostigmine should not be used in this ingestion if tricyclic antidepressants are a suspected coingestant due to the potential for seizures; propranolol can be used to help in treating cardiovascular complications

Additional Information Toxin: Anticholinergic compounds

Specific References

"Jimson Weed Poisoning – Texas, New York, and California 1994," *MMWR Morb Mortal Wkly Rep*, 1995, 44(3):41-4.

Jonquil

Scientific Name *Narcissus jonquilla*

Mechanism of Toxic Action Contains lycorine (an *Amaryllidaceae* alkaloid) a centrally acting emetic

Signs & Symptoms of Acute Overdose Usually nausea, vomiting, abdominal pain, diarrhea, and salivation; symptoms develop soon after oral ingestion (within 30 minutes) and resolve within 3 hours (according to one report)

Toxic Dosage Not established

Overdosage Treatment Decontamination: Ipecac relatively contraindicated; may be useful, if given soon after ingestion; vomiting has not occurred with ingestion of more than one bulb; activated charcoal with cathartic/lavage may be beneficial depending on amount ingested and time elapsed since ingestion

Additional Information All parts contain alkaloid; bulb is most toxic

"Jonquil" *Amanita* Mushroom *see* Mushrooms, Toxic (Group III) *on page 1112*

"Jonquil" *Amanita* Mushroom *see* Mushrooms, Toxic (Group V) *on page 1114*

Julestjerne *see* Poinsettia *on page 1126*

Julicla *see* Shamrock *on page 1140*

Jumble Bead *see* Jequirity Bean *on page 1093*

Kalmia *see* Mountain Laurel *on page 1110*

Kalmia latifolia *see* Mountain Laurel *on page 1110*

Kalo *see* Caladium *on page 1063*

Kava Kava

CAS Number 500-64-1; 495-85-2; 500-62-9

Scientific Name Kavosporal Forte

Synonyms Kev; Piper Methysticum

Mechanism of Toxic Action Contains alpha-pyrones in root extracts; may possess central dopaminergic antagonistic properties

Signs & Symptoms of Acute Overdose Ataxia, deafness, yellow skin discoloration, sedation, extrapyramidal effects

Adverse Reactions Central nervous system: Euphoria

Overdosage Treatment

Decontamination: Lavage/activated charcoal with cathartic

Supportive therapy: Can treat extrapyramidal reactions with benztropine and/or diphenhydramine

Additional Information Social and ceremonial drink in South Pacific islands; has medicinal use as a G.U. antiseptic, antipyretic, diuretic, local anesthetic, and muscle relaxant agent; shrubs can grow 8-20 feet tall with green stems and rounded fruit; characteristic yellow discoloration rash resembles pellegra, but does not respond to nicotinamide

Specific References

Brown JL and Malone MH, "Legal Highs-Constituents Activity, Toxicology, and Herbal Folklore," *Clin Toxicol*, 1978, 12:1.

Cawte J, "Psychoactive Substances of the South Seas: Betel, Kava, and Pituri," *Aust N Z J Psychiatry*, 1985, 19(1):83-7.

Mathews JD, Riley MD, Fejo L, et al, "Effects of the Heavy Usage of Kava on Physical Health: Summary of a Pilot Survey in an Aboriginal Community," *Med J Aust*, 1988, 148(11):548-55.

Ruze P, "Kava-Induced Dermopathy: A Niacin Deficiency?," *Lancet*, 1990, 335(8703):1442-5.

Schelosky L, Ruffauf C, Jendroska K, et al, "Kava and Dopamine Antagonism," *J Neurol, Neurosurg, Psychiatry*, 1995, 58:639-40.

Kavosporal Forte *see* Kava Kava *on this page*

Kev *see* Kava Kava *on this page*

Kid Kill *see* Mountain Laurel *on page 1110*

Kidney Bean Tree *see* Wisteria *on page 1157*

Kingcup *see* Marsh Marigold *on page 1105*

"Kissing Bugs" *see* Reduvids *on page 1133*

Kristtorn *see* Holly *on page 1089*

Lachesis mutus *see* Bushmaster *on page 1063*

Lactarius chrysorrheus **("Yellow-Juiced"** ***Lactarius*** **or "Gold-Drop Milkcap")** *see* Mushrooms, Toxic (Group VII) *on page 1116*

Lactarius deceptivus **("Deceptive"** ***Lactarius*** **Mushroom or "Cotton Milkcap")** *see* Mushrooms, Toxic (Group VII) *on page 1116*

Lactarius piperatus **("Pepper Milkcap")** *see* Mushrooms, Toxic (Group VII) *on page 1116*

Lactarius repraesentaneus **("Shaggy Bear")** *see* Mushrooms, Toxic (Group VII) *on page 1116*

Lactarius rufus **("Red Milkcap")** *see* Mushrooms, Toxic (Group VII) *on page 1116*

Lactarius scrobiculatus **("Spotted-Stemmed"** ***Lactarius*** **or "Pitted Milkcap")** *see* Mushrooms, Toxic (Group VII) *on page 1116*

Lactarius subvellereus *see* Mushrooms, Toxic (Group VII) *on page 1116*

Lactarius torminosus **("Wooly Milkcap")** *see* Mushrooms, Toxic (Group VII) *on page 1116*

Lactarius uvidus **("Grape-Colored"** ***Lactarius*** **or "Damp Milkcap")** *see* Mushrooms, Toxic (Group VII) *on page 1116*

Lactarius vellereus **("Fleecy Milkcap")** *see* Mushrooms, Toxic (Group VII) *on page 1116*

Lady Laurel *see* Daphne *on page 1077*

Lady Laurel *see* Daphne Mezereum *on page 1077*

Lakriment Neu *see* Licorice *on page 1098*

Lamb Kill *see* Mountain Laurel *on page 1110*

Langwort *see* Corn Lily *on page 1074*

Lantana

Scientific Name *Lantana camara*

Synonyms Bunch Berry; Red Sage; Wild Sage; Yellow Sage

Signs & Symptoms of Acute Overdose Mydriasis, vomiting, diarrhea, photophobia, cyanosis, dyspnea, ataxia, drowsiness, coma, and death

Toxic Dosage Specific quantities are unknown, any amount of unripe berries should be considered potentially hazardous

Overdosage Treatment Decontamination: If the patient is not already vomiting, then vomiting or lavage should be initiated, followed by activated charcoal with cathartic

Additional Information Animal toxicity from grazing on leaves is well known

Family: Verbenaceae

Toxin: Leaves contain triterpenes, lantadene A or B; toxic component of berry is unknown

Range: Tropical plant found in Florida and Texas

Toxic parts: Unripe berries, toxicity of other parts is unknown

Specific References

Wolfson SL and Solomons TW, "Poisoning by Fruit of *Lantana camara*: An Acute Syndrome Observed in Children Following Ingestion of the Green Fruit," *Am J Dis Child*, 1964, 107:173-6.

Lantana camara *see* Lantana *on this page*

Larkspur *see* Delphinium *on page 1079*

Lathyrus odoratus *see* Sweet Pea *on page 1149*

Latrodectus mactans *see* Black Widow Spider *on page 1058*

Laurentia longiflora *see* Star-of-Bethlehem (*Hippobroma longiflora*) *on page 1145*

Leeches

Scientific Name Exhirud®

Synonyms *Hirudo medicinalis*

Use Blood evacuation; used in skin graft repair, breast reconstruction, periorbital hematomas, digital reimplantations, ring avulsion injuries; useful in areas where there is good arterial flow but no venous outflow

Mechanism of Toxic Action Contains several anticoagulants in its salivary glands including hirudin, hementin, hyaluronidase, lodellins, eglins, cathepsin G, subtilisin, and fibrinases

Adverse Reactions

Hematologic: Ecchymosis, hemorrhage, anemia, hemorrhage

Local: Wound infection, scarring at wound site

Toxicodynamics/Kinetics Elimination: Hirudin: Renal

Overdosage Treatment

Decontamination:

Skin: Do not pull leech off since its jaws may break off resulting in an ulcer or wound infection; salt, salt water, or vinegar can aid in topical leech removal

Pharyngeal: Gargle with salt water or vinegar

Supportive therapy: Wound infection rate is ~20%; wound infections can be treated with amoxicillin (with or without clavulanic acid) or cefuroxime; tetanus prophylaxis should be performed; localized hemorrhage can be controlled with firm pressure

Additional Information A black freshwater annelid which is 25-40 mm in length, each leech can ingest ~5-15 mL of blood; leeches should never be reused; disposal can be accomplished by narcotization of the leech in 70% alcohol for 5 minutes and then incinerate; leeches may be a vector for *Aeromonas hydrophila* and *Trypanosoma cruzi*; erysipelas and puerperal fevers have been known to be transmitted by leeches; localized wound hemorrhage may continue for up to one day; contraindications include hemorrhage diathesis, croup, and erysipelas. Leech therapy is usually needed for 3-7 days.

Medicinal leeches may be obtained from Leeches USA, 300 Shames Dr, Westbury, NY 11590 (516) 333-2570

Emergency delivery: (800) 488-4400, ext 475

Specific References

Abrutyn E, "Hospital-Associated Infection From Leeches," *Ann Intern Med*, 1988, 109(5):356-8.

Adams SL, "The Medicinal Leech: A Page From the Annelides of Internal Medicine," *Ann Intern Med*, 1988, 109(5):399-405.

Braidwood PS, "The Medicinal Leech," *Pharm J*, 1987, 239:766-7.
Menage MJ and Wright G, "Use of Leeches in a Case of Severe Periorbital Haematoma," *Br J Ophthalmol*, 1991, 75(12):755-6.

Leopard Lily *see* Dieffenbachia *on page 1079*

Lepidoptera

Scientific Name *Megalopyge opercularis*

Synonyms Butterflies; Moths; Puss Caterpillar (*Megalopyge opercularis*)

Mechanism of Toxic Action Toxin found on spines that break off into skin – "passive stinging"; irritant; may also contain histamine

Signs & Symptoms of Acute Overdose Pain at injury site, vomiting, rash, paralysis, seizures, headache, pruritus, lymphadenopathy (lepidopterism), muscle cramps, blindness, fever, dyspnea, coughing can occur on inhalation

Overdosage Treatment

Decontamination: Wash skin with warm water, hairs or broken spines can be removed by applying and then peeling Scotch® tape on the surface of the skin

Supportive therapy: Antihistamines/analgesics

Specific References

Allen VT, Miller OF 3d, and Tyler WB, "Gypsy Moth Caterpillar Dermatitis - Revisited," *J Am Acad Dermatol*, 1991, 24(6 Pt 1):979-81.
Everson GW, Chapin JB, and Normann SA, "Caterpillar Envenomations: A Prospective Study of 112 Cass," *Vet Hum Toxicol*, 1990, 32(2):114-9.

Lepiota helveola *see* Mushrooms, Toxic (Group I) *on page 1111*

***Lepiota josserandii* ("Deadly Parasol")** *see* Mushrooms, Toxic (Group I) *on page 1111*

***Lepiota molybdites* ("Morgan's" *Lepiota*)** *see* Mushrooms, Toxic (Group VII) *on page 1116*

Lepiota morgani *replaced by* Mushrooms, Toxic (Group VII) *on page 1116*

***Lepiota naucina* ("Smooth" *Lepiota* or "White" *Lepiota*)** *see* Mushrooms, Toxic (Group VII) *on page 1116*

Lepiota subincarnata *see* Mushrooms, Toxic (Group I) *on page 1111*

"Liberty Cap" Mushroom *see* Mushrooms, Toxic (Group VI) *on page 1115*

Lice

Scientific Name *Pediculus humanus*; *Phthirus pubis*

Synonyms Body Louse; Crab Louse; Head Louse

Mechanism of Toxic Action Requires human blood to survive; an ectoparasite

Signs & Symptoms of Acute Overdose Pruritus, erythema: Secondary impetiginization can occur; small macules may be seen in *Phthirus pubis* (maculae cerulea)

Overdosage Treatment General principles of treating pediculosis include discarding or carefully laundering clothing, discarding infested combs or hats, and laundering bedsheets. In general, clothes and bedsheets can be effectively decontaminated by dry cleaning or by machine washing and drying in a hot cycle. Secondary bacterial infections of the skin are common and generally respond to antibiotics effective against *Staphylococcus aureus* (dicloxacillin, erythromycin, and others). Pruritus is typically quite severe and may be alleviated by hydroxyzine (Atarax®), diphenhydramine (Benadryl®), and/or topical steroid creams. Treatment guidelines are as follows:

1. Pediculosis corporis: Since the louse resides mainly in the creases of clothes and not on the host, the infection can often be eradicated by delousing contaminated items and maintaining careful hygiene.
2. Pediculosis capitis: Several agents are effective: 1% lindane (Kwell®) shampoo to the scalp, pyrethrin liquid (RID), or permethrin creme rinse (Nix™) These insecticides are probably equal in efficacy. Only lindane requires a prescription. **Caution:** Lindane has been associated with seizures and other nervous system toxicities. However, the risk of serious adverse effects during treatment for pediculosis is small due to its minimal systemic absorption. Nevertheless, lindane should be avoided in pregnancy and in lactating women.
3. Pediculosis pubis: The treatment recommendations are the same as for *P. capitis*. In addition, sexual partners should be identified and treated in the same manner. Pediculosis involving the eyelashes should **not** be treated with insecticides. Instead, occlusive ophthalmic ointment should be applied to the eyelashes twice daily for at least 8 days in an attempt to smother the parasites.

Patients should be seen in follow-up if symptoms persist 1 week after treatment. A second application may be necessary. Some clinicians routinely instruct patients to reapply the insecticide at the 1 week point.

(Continued)

Lice *(Continued)*

Diagnostic Tests/Procedures
Arthropod Identification *on page 1198*

Additional Information Transmitted through body contact

Family: *Anoplura*

Pediculus humanus corporis (head louse, body louse); *Phthirus pubis* (crab louse)

Microbiology: Human lice are ectoparasites and thus tend to live on or in the skin of the host. They belong to the insect class *Hexapoda*. There are three species important in human infection. *Pediculus humanus* var. *corporis* is the human body louse, *Pediculus humanus* var. *capitis* is the human head louse, and *Phthirus pubis* is the crab louse. The body and head louse have similar appearances and are about 4 mm long. The pubic louse is much wider and has a crab-like appearance from which its name is derived. The eggs adhere to human hair and to clothing, and are termed nits.

Epidemiology: Humans are the reservoir for lice. Infestations have been described worldwide especially in areas of overcrowding. The incubation period is about 1-4 weeks following exposure. Individuals are communicable until all the lice and eggs have been treated and destroyed. Pediculosis capitis is a particular problem with school-aged children, where the practice of sharing combs or brushes facilitates epidemic transmission. All socioeconomic backgrounds are at risk for head lice. In contrast, pediculosis corporis is seen mainly in areas of poor sanitation. The body louse resides almost exclusively in soiled clothing, rather than the skin, and only leaves the clothing for a blood meal from the host. Pediculosis corporis also transmits the rickettsial infection epidemic typhus, as well a several others. *Phthirus pubis* is usually sexually transmitted, although spread via infested bedding or clothing can occur.

Clinical Syndromes:

- **Pediculosis corporis:** Typically, the patient complains of severe pruritus, and small, erythematous papules are found on the body. Often extensive self-induced excoriations across the trunk are noted If left untreated for long periods, hyperpigmentation and scarring may occur, called "vagabond's disease."
- **Pediculosis capitis:** The most common presentation is intractable scalp pruritus. On examination there may be evidence of secondary bacterial infection of the scalp from excoriations. At times, an "id reaction" occurs, characterized by a dramatic skin eruption over the arms and trunk, felt to be a hypersensitivity reaction.
- ***Pediculus pubis***: Most patients present with pruritus in the region of the pubic hairs, but other areas may be involved including the eyelashes and hairs in the axilla. Secondary bacterial infections are less common.

Diagnosis: The diagnosis of pediculosis is often suspected when an individual presents with severe pruritus. On some occasions, the patient may have identified lice themselves or have had a recent contact history. The diagnosis is confirmed by finding lice (1-4 mm long, depending on species) and/or the "nits" (usually 1 mm or less, attached to hairs).

Specific References

Honig PJ, "Arthropod Bites, Stings, and Infestations: Their Prevention and Treatment," *Pediatr Dermatol*, 1986, 3(3):189-97.

Meinking TL, Taplin D, Kalter DC, et al, "Comparative Efficacy of Treatments for Pediculosis Capitis Infestations," *Arch Dermatol*, 1986, 122(3):267-71.

Licorice

Scientific Name *Glycyrrhiza glabra*; *Glycyrrhiza lepidota*; *Glycyrrhiza uralensis*

Synonyms Glycocome; Lakriment Neu; Liquorice; Sweet Root; Ulgastrin Neo

Use Foodstuff in chewing gum, chewing tobacco, cough preparations

Mechanism of Toxic Action From the root of the plant *Glycyrrhiza glabra*, *Glycyrrhiza lepidota*, *Glycyrrhiza uralensis*; the toxic component is glycyrrhizic acid which inhibits enzymes in the degradation of mineralocorticoids hormones (aldosterone); also may act as a mineralocorticoid; inhibits steroid dehydrogenase and release enzymes

Adverse Reactions

Cardiovascular: Hypertension

Central nervous system: Headache, seizures

Endocrine & metabolic: Amenorrhea, hyponatremia, hypokalemia, hypomagnesemia

Neuromuscular & skeletal: Myopathy, rhabdomyolysis

Renal & genitourinary: Myoglobinuria

Miscellaneous: Bilateral ptosis, carpopedal spasms, tetany

Toxicodynamics/Kinetics

Metabolism: Glycyrrhizic acid is converted to glycyrrhetic acid

Half-life: Glycyrrhizic acid: 5 hours
Elimination: Fecal: 53% to 61%

Toxic Dosage 100 g (equivalent to 700 mg of glycyrrhizinic acid) of licorice found in 2-4 licorice twists; toxic effect can be seen if ingested daily (2-3 twists) for 2-4 weeks

Overdosage Treatment Supportive therapy: Fluid/electrolyte (especially potassium) replacement; spironolactone (1 g/day in divided doses) also may be useful in reversing electrolyte abnormalities; tetany can be treated with magnesium sulfate

Drug Interactions Attenuated effect of strychnine, tetrodoxine, nicotine, cocaine, barbiturates, pilocarpine, urethane, epinephrine, and ephedrine through glucuronic-like conjugation action; traditional emmenagogue and abortifacient; increases progesterone and cortisol half-life; concomitant use of furosemide can exacerbate hypokalemia

Additional Information Syndrome of pseudoprimary hyperaldosteronism is a complication of chronic licorice ingestion; serum potassium as low as 0.9 mmol/L have been noted

Specific References

Blachley JD and Knochel JP, "Tobacco Chewer's Hypokalemia: Licorice Revisited," *N Engl J Med*, 1980, 302(14):784-5.

Brayley J and Jones J, "Life-Threatening Hypokalemia Associated With Excessive Licorice Ingestion," *Am J Psychiatry*, 1994, 151(4):617-8.

Nielsen I and Pedersen RS, "Life-Threatening Hypokalaemia Caused by Liquorice Ingestion," *Lancet*, 1984, 1(8389):1305.

Woolf A, "Licorice Root Poisoning," *Clin Toxicol Rev*, 1994, 16(9):1-2.

Licorice Plant *see* Jequirity Bean *on page 1093*

Ligustrum vulgare *see* Privet (Berries and Leaves) *on page 1129*

Lilac (Nontoxic Plant)

Liljekonvall *see* Lily-of-the-Valley *on this page*

Lily-of-the-Valley

Scientific Name *Convallaria majalis*

Synonyms Liljekonvall

Mechanism of Toxic Action Whole plant contains cardiac glycosides convallamatian and convallarin

Signs & Symptoms of Acute Overdose GI effects (nausea and vomiting) usually precede the cardiovascular effects by several hours; bradycardia; first, second, and third degree heart block; asystole, hypotension, A-V block, ventricular arrhythmias, atrial fibrillation, decreased Q-T interval and prolonged P-R interval; fatigue, confusion, headache, dizziness, contact dermatitis, seeing yellow halos, and hyperkalemia have also been reported

Overdosage Treatment

Decontamination: Lavage and multidose activated charcoal enhance total body clearance of digitalis; whole bowel irrigation is also beneficial in removing plant debris from the GI tract and is recommended for ingestions of large amounts of plant material

Supportive therapy: Monitor cardiac status and serum potassium levels; bradycardia will frequently respond to atropine; phenytoin is the recommended treatment for ventricular arrhythmias because it will also improve conduction through the A-V node; lidocaine can also be used to treat ventricular arrhythmias, but will not have an effect on A-V conduction; other antiarrhythmics which have been used in arrhythmias resistant to the above therapy include magnesium, amiodarone, and bretylium; a pacemaker should be considered for bradycardia and A-V nodal blocks resistant to medical management

Digoxin immune Fab has been shown to interact with several different plant cardiac glycosides and may be beneficial in cases resistant to conventional treatment; indications for its use include ventricular arrhythmias resistant to conventional treatment, severe bradycardia, and/or second or third degree heart block resistant to atropine and phenytoin

Antidote(s)

Digoxin Immune Fab *on page 1411*

Additional Information Toxin: Cardiac glycosides

Specific References

Hollman A, "Plants and Cardiac Glycosides," *Br Heart J*, 1985, 54(3):258-61.

Lionfish

Synonyms Butterfly Cod; Turkeyfish (*Pterois*); Zebrafish

Signs & Symptoms of Acute Overdose Burning, pain, swelling in wound; numbness, paresthesia, erythema, nausea, or vomiting lasts 8-12 hours. Systemic symptoms are rare and include sweating, bradycardia, tachycardia, dyspnea, abdominal cramps, headache, syncope, hypotension.

(Continued)

Lionfish *(Continued)*

Overdosage Treatment Decontamination: Soak affected limb in hot water for 30-90 minutes (110°F to 115°F); provides relief in 94% of patients; antivenin is rarely needed (may be available in seaquariums)

Additional Information Venom has vasodilatory effect

Range: Found in Pacific/Indian Oceans; bottom-dwelling fish

Specific References

Kizer KW, McKinney HE, and Auerbach PS, "*Scorpaenidae* Envenomation. A Five-Year Poison Center Experience," *JAMA*, 1985, 253(6):807-10.

Lipstick Plant (Nontoxic Plant)

Liquorice *see* Licorice *on page 1098*

Listeria monocytogenes Food Poisoning

Commonly Found in Unpasteurized milk, feta cheese, undercooked chicken

Mechanism of Toxic Action *Listeria monocytogenes* is a gram-positive bacillus which causes sporadic cases of meningoencephalitis, neonatal infection, septicemia, and several less common syndromes. It is a leading cause of meningitis in immunocompromised individuals, especially renal transplant patients.

The organism is an aerobic, gram-positive rod which does not produce spores. At times it may assume a more coccoid appearance on Gram's stain of clinical samples (eg, cerebrospinal fluid) and may thus be mistaken for gram-positive cocci such as *Streptococcus pneumoniae. Listeria* can also be confused morphologically with the more commonly seen *Corynebacterium* species, which are also gram-positive bacilli (but are often contaminants). *Listeria* is primarily an intracellular pathogen, and tends to reside within mononuclear phagocytes of the host. This feature is thought to contribute to its pathogenicity, since the organism can spread from cell to cell in a somewhat protected fashion.

When *Listeria monocytogenes* meningitis is suspected, the clinician should try to submit at least 10 mL of cerebrospinal fluid for bacterial culture, since only a few *Listeria* organisms may be present. The organism generally grows well on most routine media used in the laboratory, and special requests for selective or enrichment cultures for *Listeria* are usually not necessary. It is important that the clinician does not automatically dismiss a report of a "gram-positive rod" isolated from multiple blood or a sterile body site as a contaminant, particularly in an immunocompromised host in whom *Listeria* infection is possible.

Signs & Symptoms of Acute Overdose Foodborne listeriosis: A prodromal illness of fever with nausea, vomiting, headache, or backache may precede the clinical syndrome (as described below) by as long as one week

Overdosage Treatment Supportive therapy: No randomized comparison trials have been performed to determine the drug(s) of choice for listeriosis. *In vitro* data show the organism is susceptible to many antibiotics. The most clinical experience has been limited to penicillin and ampicillin, and they are probably equivalent. Occasionally, penicillin-resistant strains of *Listeria* have been reported, and thus results of susceptibility testing should be followed up on. There is some *in vitro* evidence to suggest the combination of penicillin (or ampicillin) with an aminoglycoside may be synergistic against *Listeria*, and this combination has been used in serious, life-threatening infections; trimethoprim-sulfamethoxazole may also be effective. Cephalosporins do not reliably cover this organism and should not be used for cases of *Listeria* meningitis. Consultation with an infectious disease specialist is appropriate in complicated cases or in the patient with a penicillin allergy.

Diagnostic Tests/Procedures

Blood Culture, Aerobic and Anaerobic *on page 1204*

Additional Information Incidence of listeriosis has decreased by 44% in the U.S. from 1989 to 1993.

Epidemiology:

The epidemiology of listeriosis can be important in certain cases, since clinical presentations may be nonspecific. The precise prevalence of human infection is unclear, but the attack rate appears to be increasing (perhaps due to better reporting or laboratory recognition). Asymptomatic carriage of *Listeria* in stools is relatively frequent; some studies suggest a fecal excretion rate of 1% or more in healthy humans. Humans may be exposed to *Listeria* by one of several routes: consumption of contaminated food, direct exposure to infected animals, or exposure to environmental reservoirs (soil, water, etc).

Cases of listeriosis tend to be sporadic and difficult to predict. Most infections occur in the summer months and are more common in urban than rural settings, despite its reputation as a zoonotic infection. Often, the source of the *Listeria* remains unknown. Increasing attention has been given to foodborne transmission, particularly in the setting of a traceable outbreak. Mexican-style cheese, coleslaw, undercooked chicken, hot dogs, dairy products, and other foods have caused outbreaks. The ability of the organism to survive (and even multiply) during refrigeration probably contributes to food-related transmission.

Infection with *Listeria* usually occurs in definable groups in the community. Cell mediated immunity is critically important in defense against *Listeria*, whereas neutropenia is not clearly a risk factor. Those at highest risk include patients with solid organ transplants, malignancies (particularly lymphoma), and patients receiving corticosteroids. Pregnant females, neonates, and alcoholics are additional groups at risk for infection. Interestingly, listeriosis does not appear to be a common pathogen in patients with AIDS, despite the deficiencies in T-cell function. Although uncommon, serious infections with *Listeria* have been described in otherwise healthy individuals.

Diagnosis: Except for granulomatosis infantiseptica, the clinical presentations of listeriosis are not unique and microbiological confirmation is necessary. Depending on the clinical site of infection, specimens of blood and body fluids should be sent, as described above. Agglutination studies for antibodies directed against *L. monocytogenes* have little value. Stool culture or serologic testing is not useful.

Clinical Syndromes:

- **Adult meningoencephalitis:** *Listeria* is the most common cause of community-acquired meningitis in immunosuppressed individuals. *Listeria* meningitis can be quite variable in its presentation and can range from a subacute course to a rapid and fulminant one. In some cases the diagnosis may be quite difficult when high fevers and nuchal rigidity are absent. There are no pathognomonic features of *Listeria* meningitis which allow diagnosis on clinical grounds alone. CSF chemical analysis is variable and frequently nondiagnostic. The degree of CSF pleocytosis can range from several cells to $>12,000$ cells/mm^3. Differential cell counts vary from nearly 100% polymorphonuclear cells to 100% mononuclear cells. Often a modest elevation of CSF protein is seen, along with a minor decrease in CSF glucose. The differential diagnosis of a subacute meningitis in an immunosuppressed host must also include *Cryptococcus neoformans*. The finding of focal brain lesions by CT scan or MRI broadens the differential to include toxoplasmosis, *Nocardia asteroides*, bacterial brain abscess, fungal meningitis, and others. Meningoencephalitis has also been sporadically reported in otherwise healthy individuals and should be considered in the differential diagnosis of any community-acquired meningitis.
- **Meningoencephalitis of the neonate:** This is a "late-onset" neonatal disease, occurring several days to weeks postpartum. As with adult cases, isolated neonatal meningitis from *Listeria* can be variable in its presentation. Fever may be low grade or absent, and irritability and failure to thrive may be the only clues. CSF findings in the neonate are similar to those in the adult. It is important to review the Gram's stain of CSF carefully to avoid confusing *Listeria* with Group B streptococci, a common cause of neonatal meningitis.
- **Cerebritis:** This form of nonmeningeal central nervous system infection is gaining increased recognition. Patients may complain of fever, cephalgia, and hemiparesis. This form of listeriosis may be mistaken for a stroke, vasculitis, brain tumor, or abscess. CT and MRI scans suggest focal inflammation without a discrete abscess or ring enhancement. Cerebrospinal fluid is usually normal and CSF cultures are negative for *Listeria*. The diagnosis is usually made when *Listeria* is isolated from blood cultures.
- **Listeriosis in pregnancy:** Unfortunately, this is often difficult to diagnose, since the woman may be asymptomatic or complain of only a mild fever and malaise. Other symptoms variably present include diarrhea and flank pain. The differential diagnosis is usually broad and listeriosis may be mistaken for pyelonephritis, lower urinary tract infection, and viral syndromes (eg, influenza). Blood cultures may be positive and should be performed. Complications include premature delivery, septic abortion, and *in utero* fetal infection.
- **Granulomatosis infantiseptica:** This unique, transplacentally acquired infection is severe and often lethal. It is an "early onset" neonatal infection apparent within hours of birth. Typically, the infants are seriously ill. There are widespread abscesses involving visceral organs such as the liver, spleen, lungs, intestinal tract, and brain. The lesions are usually abscesses with polymorphonuclear leukocytes, but granulomas have also been seen (referred to as "miliary granulomatosis"). Dark papular skin lesions may be present on the trunk and lower extremities, suggesting the diagnosis. Gram's stain and culture of meconium, amniotic fluid, conjunctival exudates, CSF, throat, blood, or skin lesions frequently are positive for *L. monocytogenes*. Antibiotic therapy should be started immediately if this diagnosis is suspected, since death may occur if treatment is withheld until cultures are finalized.
- **Septicemia:** *Listeria* can be isolated from the blood in adults and neonates who present from the community with nonspecific fever and chills. Bacteremias are more likely in profoundly immunosuppressed hosts but have been seen in alcoholics, diabetics, pregnancy, and normal healthy individuals. The

(Continued)

Listeria monocytogenes Food Poisoning *(Continued)*

clinical presentation can be indistinguishable from gram-negative sepsis, with high fevers and hypotension (so-called "typhoidal listeremia"). On rare occasion, the diagnosis is suggested by the finding of a monocytosis on the peripheral blood smear, but blood cultures remain the highest yield.

- **Miscellaneous:** Endocarditis, ocular infections, lymphadenitis, osteomyelitis, brain abscess, peritonitis, and other focal infections have been rarely reported.

Specific References

Armstrong D, "*Listeria monocytogenes*," *Principles and Practice of Infectious Diseases*, 3rd ed, Mandell GL, Douglas RG Jr, Bennett JE, eds, New York, NY: Churchill Livingstone, 1990, 1587-93.

Gellin BG and Broome CV, "Listeriosis," *JAMA*, 1989, 261(9):1313-20.

Linnan MJ, Mascola L, Lou XD, et al, "Epidemic Listeriosis Associated With Mexican-Style Cheese," *N Engl J Med*, 1988, 319(13):823-8.

Nieman RE and Lorber B, "Listeriosis in Adults: A Changing Pattern. Report of Eight Cases and Review of the Literature, 1968-1978," *Rev Infect Dis*, 1980, 2(2):207-27.

Pinner RW, Schuchat A, Swaminathan B, et al, "Role of Foods in Sporadic Listeriosis. II. Microbiologic and Epidemiologic Investigation," *JAMA*, 1992, 267(15):2046-50.

Tappero JW, Schuchat A, Deaver KA, et al, "Reduction in the Incidence of Human Listeriosis in the United States: Effectiveness of Prevention Efforts?" *JAMA*, 1995, 273:1118-22.

Live Forever *see Sedum on page 1140*

Lobelia inflata *see* Indian Tobacco *on page 1091*

Lobster Plant *see* Poinsettia *on page 1126*

Loco Weed *see* Jimson Weed *on page 1094*

Lophophora williamsii *see* Mescaline *on page 1106*

Lophophora williamsii *see* Peyote *on page 1124*

Love Apple *see* Tomato (Leaves and Stems) *on page 1150*

Love Bean *see* Jequirity Bean *on page 1093*

Love Pea *see* Jequirity Bean *on page 1093*

Loxosceles reclusa *see* Brown Recluse Spider *on page 1061*

L-Sodium Glutamate *see* Monosodium Glutamate Food Poisoning *on page 1109*

Lucky Bean *see* Jequirity Bean *on page 1093*

Lucky Clover *see* Shamrock *on page 1140*

Lupine

Scientific Name *Lupinus* Species

Synonyms Blue Bonnet; Texas Blue Bonnet

Mechanism of Toxic Action All parts of the plants, especially the ripe seeds, contain quinolizidine alkaloids, lupanine, and some piperidine compounds; different species have varying concentrations of these alkaloids, and therefore, produce various effects; not all species are toxic; toxin is inactivated if the plant is dried

Signs & Symptoms of Acute Overdose Difficulty breathing, nervousness, muscle myoclonus, loss of motor control, frothing of the mouth, seizures, coma, asthenia, jaundice, tachycardia, PVCs, and mydriasis; amyotrophy and spasticity have been reported from chronic ingestions; death generally occurs from respiratory paralysis

Toxicodynamics/Kinetics Onset of symptoms: Within 1 hour, but can be delayed up to one day

Toxic Dosage Accidental ingestion of one plant leaf or a few seeds should be considered basically nontoxic; ingestion of 3 g of seeds per month for 8 years was associated with amyotrophy and spasticity; ingestion of 500 mL of water used to "debitter" lupine seeds resulted in mydriasis, tachycardia, PVCs, and urinary retention which resolved in 48 hours

Overdosage Treatment

Decontamination: Ipecac is probably not necessary in accidental ingestions and relatively contraindicated in large ingestions; lavage and activated charcoal with cathartic are probably beneficial for large ingestions

Supportive therapy: Required with particular attention to respiratory status

Additional Information Toxin: Lupine

***Lupinus* Species** *see* Lupine *on this page*

"Lurid" *Boletus* Mushroom *see* Mushrooms, Toxic (Group III) *on page 1112*

"Lurid" *Boletus* Mushroom *see* Mushrooms, Toxic (Group VII) *on page 1116*

Lycium halmifolium *see* Box Thorn *on page 1061*

Lycopersicon *see* Tomato (Leaves and Stems) *on page 1150*

Lycopersicon lycopersicum *see* Tomato (Leaves and Stems) *on page 1150*

Lycorine *see* Daffodil *on page 1076*

Madame Fate *see* Star-of-Bethlehem (*Hippobroma longiflora*) *on page 1145*

Mad Apple *see* Jimson Weed *on page 1094*

Maguey *see* Century Plant *on page 1067*

Mahi Mahi Flush *see* Scombroid Food Poisoning *on page 1137*

Malabar Tree *see* Milkbush *on page 1107*

Malaria Mosquito *see* Mosquitoes *on page 1110*

Malu-Malu *see* Sea Anemones *on page 1138*

Mambra *see* Cobras *on page 1072*

Mangifera indica *see* Mango *on this page*

Mango

Scientific Name *Mangifera indica*

Mechanism of Toxic Action Shell contains anacardic acid, cardol, anacardol, irritants that can precipitate type IV cell-mediated allergic reaction (allergic contact dermatitis)

Signs & Symptoms of Acute Overdose Dermatitis, nausea, vomiting, orange discoloration to skin

Toxicodynamics/Kinetics

Onset of effect: Variable, but effects usually seen within 24-48 hours

Peak effect: After 3-5 days

Overdosage Treatment

Decontamination: Soap and water washing likely ineffective unless done within 5-15 minutes after exposure

Supportive therapy: Cool compresses or showers, Burow's solution, topical/oral steroids

Additional Information An evergreen found in India; remove skin before eating, fruit; fruit weighs 4-5 lbs; fruit skin, sap, and shell contains toxin

Specific References

Palevsky S and Leung J, "Mangoism," *Am J Dis Child*, 1989, 143(10):1131-2.

"Manure Roundhead" Mushroom *see* Mushrooms, Toxic (Group VI) *on page 1115*

Marah oreganus *see* Wild Cucumber *on page 1157*

Marasmius urens *see* Mushrooms, Toxic (Group VII) *on page 1116*

Marbled Cone *see* Cone Shells *on page 1073*

Marble Queen Pothos *see* Devil's Ivy *on page 1079*

"Marginate" *Pholiota* Mushroom *see* Mushrooms, Toxic (Group I) *on page 1111*

Marigold (Nontoxic Plant)

Marijuana (Cannabis)

Related Information

Principal Pharmacological Properties of Hallucinogenic Drugs *on page 1557*

CAS Number 8063-14-7

Scientific Name *Cannabis sativa*

Mechanism of Toxic Action Antiemetic for therapeutic uses/hallucinogen; derived from the hemp plant *Cannabis sativa* (which contains 2% to 6% tetrahydrocannabinol) and which is psychotropically active in the (-) enantiometric form; affects serotonin release along with increasing catecholaminergic effect while inhibiting parasympathetic effects

Signs & Symptoms of Acute Overdose I.V. administration can cause nausea, vomiting, diarrhea, fevers progressing in 12 hours to cyanosis, hypotension, renal failure, thrombocytopenia, rhabdomyolysis

Mild cannabis intoxication (10 g/month): Relaxation, fatigue, sense of well being, perceptual alterations, impaired recall

Moderate intoxication (30 g/month): Mood swings, memory deficits, depersonalization

Excessive intoxication (60 g/month): Slurred speech, impaired coordination, hallucinations, delusions, paranoia

(Continued)

Marijuana (Cannabis) *(Continued)*

Adverse Reactions

Cardiovascular: Dose-related tachycardia

Central nervous system: Irritability, disorientation, euphoria, short-term memory loss, impotence, fine tremor, distortion of time and space

Gastrointestinal: Constipation

Genitourinary: Urinary retention

Ocular: Lateral gaze nystagmus, mydriasis, injected conjunctival vessels

Respiratory: Bronchial irritation

Miscellaneous: hypothermia, thirst

Toxicodynamics/Kinetics

Onset of action:

Inhalation: 6-12 minutes

Oral: 30-120 minutes

Duration of acute effect: 0.5-3 hours

Absorption:

Smoking: 18% to 50%

Ingestion: 5% to 20%

Distribution: V_d: 10 L/kg; increases with chronic use

Metabolism: Major metabolite is 11-hydroxy-tetrahydrocannabinol

Protein binding: 97% to 99%

Half-life: 28 hours (first-time users); 56 hours (chronic users)

Elimination: Feces (30% to 35%); renal (15% to 20%)

Toxic Dosage One "joint" weighs 0.5-1 g with an average THC content of 1% to 2% (5-20 mg); hash oil contains 30% to 50% THC; hashish is 3% to 6% THC; toxic dose is 15 mg/kg THC; lethal dose: 30 mg/kg

Overdosage Treatment

Decontamination: Ingestion: Lavage/activated charcoal with cathartic

Supportive therapy: Benzodiazepines for agitation; hypotension can be treated with Trendelenburg/crystalloid infusion; tachycardia can be treated with beta-blockers

Test Interactions Alkaline/acidic urine (or dilute urine) may cause false-negative urinary immunoassay tests; Visine® adulteration may also cause false-negative tests; bleach may cause a 14% to 45% decrease in THC concentrations in urine immunoassay results; urine drug screen is positive for 6 days with one time use; may be positive for weeks with chronic use

Drug Interactions Attenuation of drowsiness can occur with concomitant administration of CNS depressants; pretreatment with indomethacin may cause attenuation of the euphoria with decreased cardiac effects; cocaine, atropine along with tricyclic antidepressants may cause additive increase in heart rate; disulfiram may produce hypomanic state; may cause additive increase in blood pressure when given with amphetamines

Pregnancy Implications Increased incidence of protracted labor, fetal distress, stillbirths, low birth rate, small for gestational age infants; no associated congenital abnormalities

Additional Information Decreases intraocular pressure; can cause bronchodilatation; urine immunoassays may remain positive for up to 6 days in a one-time user to several weeks in a chronic user. Higher THC levels are associated with higher puff amount and higher potency; levels are not associated with how long puffs are held. THC levels can range from 33 ng/mL (with a 30 mL puff, 1.75% THC) to 167 ng/mL (90 mL puff, 3.55% THC concentration). Potential for medicinal uses of cannabinoids include to alleviate chemotherapy-induced nausea and vomiting, lowering intraocular pressure, antiseizure medication, muscle relaxation in spastic disorders, appetite stimulation, relief of phantom limb pain, menstrual cramps, and migraine therapy.

Specific References

Azorlosa JL, Greenwald MK, and Stitzer ML, "Marijuana Smoking: Effects of Varying Puff Volume and Breathhold Duration," *J Pharmacol Exp Ther*, 1995, 272(2):560-9.

Brandenburg D and Wernick R, "Intravenous Marijuana Syndrome," *West J Med*, 1986, 145(1):94-6.

Cone EJ and Huestis MA, "Relating Blood Concentrations of Tetrahydrocannabinol and Metabolites to Pharmacologic Effects and Time of Marijuana Usage," *Ther Drug Monit*, 1993, 15(6):527-32.

Grinspoon L and Bakalar JB, "Marijuana as Medicine. A Plea for Reconsideration," *JAMA*, 1995, 273:1875-6.

Howlett AC, "Pharmacology of Cannabinoid Receptors," *Annu Rev Pharmacol Toxicol*, 1995, 35:607-34.

Johnson BA, "Psychopharmacological Effects of Cannabis," *Br J Hosp Med*, 1990, 43(2):114-22.

Leikin JB, Krantz AJ, Zell-Kanter M, et al, "Clinical Features and Management of Intoxication Due to Hallucinogenic Drugs," *Med Toxicol Adverse Drug Exp*, 1989, 4(5):324-50.

Macnab A, Anderson E, and Susak L, "Ingestion of Cannabis: A Cause of Coma in Children," *Pediatr Emerg Care*, 1989, 5(4):238-9.

Manno JE, Kemp PM, Manno BR, et al, "Differentiation Between Recent (<24 hours) and Past Use of Marijuana by Urinalysis;" *Vet Hum Toxicol*, 1994, 36:343.

Rowland BJ, Irving J, and Keith S, "Increased Detection of Marijuana Use with a 50 mcg/L Urine Screening Cutoff," *Clin Chem*, 1994, 40(11 Pt 1):2114-5.

Marsh Marigold

Scientific Name *Caltha palustris*

Synonyms Bull Flower; Cowslip; Gools; Kingcup; May-Hurse Blob; Meadow Bright; Meadow-Gowan; Populage; Soldier's Buttons; Water Goggles

Mechanism of Toxic Action Contains protoanemonin, which reacts with SH groups to produce irritation and vesication; chemical is excreted unchanged in urine

Signs & Symptoms of Acute Overdose Salivation, hematovomiting, bloody diarrhea, abdominal cramps, pain and swelling, blistering, ulceration, contact dermatitis; has potential to cause renal irritation or damage if large enough amount is ingested

Toxicodynamics/Kinetics Significant dermal symptoms may take several weeks to resolve

Toxic Dosage Not established, but overdose producing systemic effects is unlikely due to painful skin contact

Overdosage Treatment

Decontamination: Avoid use of ipecac or cathartics, consider lavage and/or activated charcoal with large ingestion to prevent systemic absorption and possibility of subsequent renal irritation

Supportive therapy: Maintain fluid and electrolytes, maintain adequate urine flow in large overdose; monitor symptomatic patients for fluid or electrolyte deficiencies

Additional Information Toxic parts: All parts are toxic, young plants prior to flowering probably not toxic

Massasauga *see Crotalidae on page 1075*

Maternity Plant (Nontoxic Plant)

Matrimony Vine *see* Box Thorn *on page 1061*

Matteuccia Struthiopteris *see* Ostrich Fern *on page 1121*

Mayapple

Scientific Name *Podophyllum peltatum*

Synonyms American Mandrake; Indian Apple; Umbrella Leaf

Use Podophyllum has been used for treatment of venereal warts; podophyllotoxin appears to have anticancer activity

Mechanism of Toxic Action Podophyllum and podophyllotoxin block cell division in the metaphase; they have a direct effect on mitochondria and are spindle poisons

Signs & Symptoms of Acute Overdose Nausea, vomiting, severe diarrhea are typically early toxic manifestations; tachycardia, hypotension, tachypnea, dyspnea are frequently seen; ataxia, dizziness, drowsiness, stupor, coma, paresthesia, and paralysis have been reported; liver injury, oliguria, and renal failure, leukopenia, neutropenia, granulocytopenia, agranulocytopenia, and thrombocytopenia and death have all been reported. Hypokalemia and metabolic alkalosis have been reported from chronically using podophyllum as a purgative; conjunctivitis, keratitis, and ulcerative skin lesions have been reported in workers handling the powdered rhizome

Toxicodynamics/Kinetics Absorption: Well absorbed both orally and dermally

Toxic Dosage Not well established, 350 mg of podophyllum has been reported to cause death

Overdosage Treatment

Decontamination: Emesis or lavage may be useful in patients with large ingestions that have not developed vomiting yet; activated charcoal with cathartic should be administered

Elimination: Hemodialysis is ineffective in removing podophyllum but may be required in patients experiencing renal failure

Pregnancy Implications Podophyllum is considered teratogenic

Additional Information European Mandrake (*Mandragora officinarum*) is unrelated to Mayapple or American Mandrake

Family: Podophyllaceae (formerly *Berberidaceae*)

Toxin: Podophyllin resin, podophyllotoxin

Range: Throughout the U.S.

Toxic parts: Leaves, roots, and unripe fruit; ripe fruit is edible

Specific References

Cassidy DE, Drewry J, and Fanning JP, "Podophyllum Toxicity: A Report of a Fatal Case and Review of the Literature," *J Toxicol Clin Toxicol*, 1982, 19(1):35-44.

May-Hurse Blob *see* Marsh Marigold *on this page*

Maythorn *see* Buckthorn *on page 1062*

Meadow Bright *see* Marsh Marigold *on previous page*

Meadow Crocus *see* Autumn Crocus *on page 1054*

Meadow-Gowan *see* Marsh Marigold *on previous page*

Meadow Saffron *see* Autumn Crocus *on page 1054*

Megalopyge opercularis *see* Lepidoptera *on page 1097*

Memory Root *see* Jack-in-the-Pulpit *on page 1093*

Menispermum canadense *see* Moonseed *on page 1109*

Mescal *see* Century Plant *on page 1067*

Mescal Buttons *see* Mescaline *on this page*

Mescaline

Related Information

Peyote *on page 1124*

Principal Pharmacological Properties of Hallucinogenic Drugs *on page 1557*

CAS Number 54-04-6

Scientific Name *Lophophora williamsii*

Synonyms Mescal Buttons

Mechanism of Toxic Action Hallucinogenic methoxylated amphetamine stimulating both serotonin and dopamine receptors in the central nervous system

Signs & Symptoms of Acute Overdose Hypertension, chest pain, bradycardia, psychosis, hallucinations, headache, dizziness, ataxia, tremor, coma, fever, flushing, sweating, flashbacks, vomiting, mydriasis, tachypnea, hyperreflexia, myoglobinuria, rhabdomyolysis

Toxicodynamics/Kinetics

Duration of effect: Psychic effects last 6-12 hours

Protein binding: No binding

Metabolism: Hepatic to inactive metabolites

Half-life: 6 hours

Elimination: Renal (55% to 60% unchanged)

Toxic Dosage Hallucinogenic dose: Oral: 5 mg/kg

Dosage Forms Available as whole dried cactus tops ("buttons"); peyote contains 1% to 6% mescaline; each "button" contains about 45 mg of mescaline

Overdosage Treatment

Decontamination: Lavage/activated charcoal with cathartic

Supportive therapy: Benzodiazepines are useful for agitation; haloperidol or chlorpromazine can be used if psychiatric symptoms are not responsive to benzodiazepines; do not use phenothiazines for treatment of flashback

Drug Interactions Flashbacks may be exacerbated by phenothiazines

Pregnancy Implications Increased spontaneous abortions and low birth weight infants

Additional Information

Active ingredient in the peyote cactus (*Lophophora williamsii*)

Range: Found in the Southwestern U.S. and Mexico

Hallucinogenic effects occur at blood levels of mescaline of 1.5-14.8 µg/mL; peak blood level after an oral 500 mg dose: 3.8 mg/mL at 2 hours postingestion and 1.5 mg/L at 7 hours postingestion; after a 5 mg/kg intravenous dose, peak blood mescaline level was 14.8 µg/mL 15 minutes postdose

Specific References

Charalampous KD, Walker KE, and Kinross-Wright J, "Metabolic Fate of Mescaline in Man," *Psychopharmacologia*, 1966, 9:48-63.

Kulberg A, "Substance Abuse: Clinical Identification and Management," *Pediatr Clin North Am*, 1986, 33(2):325-61.

Reynolds PC and Jindrich EJ, "A Mescaline Associated Fatality," *J Anal Toxicol*, 1985, 9(4):183-4.

Schwartz RH, "Mescaline: A Survey," *Am Fam Physician*, 1988, 37(4):122-4.

Metabisulfites *see* Sulfite Food Poisoning *on page 1148*

Methcathinone

Related Information

Cathinone *on page 1066*

CAS Number 71031-15-7

Synonyms Ephedrone; N-Methyl-Cathinone

Mechanism of Toxic Action Related to cathinone (khat) found naturally in catha edulis; found primarily in production of clandestine labs in Washington, Illinois, Missouri, and upper Michigan peninsula; derived from ephedrine with amphetamine-like actions; causes release of dopamine from caudate nucleus

Signs & Symptoms of Acute Overdose Tachycardia (dose-related), hypertension (dose related), agitation, tremor, slurred speech, paranoia, auditory hallucinations, back pain, headache, abdominal pain, leukocytosis, anorexia, constipation, visual hallucinations, sweating, fever, myoglobinuria, rhabdomyolysis

Toxicodynamics/Kinetics Metabolism: To ephedrine and phenylpropanolamine (norephedrine)

Toxic Dosage Estimated to be 80-250 mg by intranasal use (can be used I.V.); typical daily dose: 500-1000 mg

Overdosage Treatment

Decontamination: GI lavage/activated charcoal with cathartic or phenothiazines

Supportive therapy: Benzodiazepines for agitation

Test Interactions Does not cause a positive amphetamine result on urine immunoassays

Additional Information Ephedrine, pseudoephedrine, and phenylpropanone may turn up positive in drug testing in that these chemicals are used in the production of methcathinone

Specific References

Emerson TS and Cisek JE, "Methcathinone: A Russian Designer Amphetamine Infiltrates the Rural Midwest," *Ann Emerg Med*, 1993, 22(12):1897-903.

Goldstone MS, "Cat: Methcathinone - A New Drug of Abuse," *JAMA*, 1993, 269(19):2508.

Zhingel YK, Dovensky BS, Crossman A, et al, "Ephedrone: 2-Methylamino-a-Phenylpropan-1-One (Jeff)," *J Forensic Sci*, 1991, 36:915-20.

Mexican Bed Bug *see* Reduvids *on page 1133*

Mexican Flameleaf *see* Poinsettia *on page 1126*

Micrurus euryxanthus *see* Elapids *on page 1080*

Micrurus fulvius *see* Elapids *on page 1080*

Mienie-Mienie *see* Jequirity Bean *on page 1093*

Milkbush

Related Information

Crown of Thorns *on page 1076*

Scientific Name *Euphorbia*

Synonyms Finger Tree; Indian Spurge Tree; Malabar Tree; Monkey Fiddle; Pencil Tree

Mirabilis jalapa *see* Four-O'Clock *on page 1085*

Mirakelblomst *see* Four-O'Clock *on page 1085*

Mistletoe

Scientific Name *Phoradendron flavescens*; *Phoradendron macrophyllum*; *Phoradendron rubrum*; *Phoradendron serotinum*; *Phoradendron tomentosum*; *Viscum album*

Synonyms American Mistletoe; European Mistletoe (*Viscum album*)

Signs & Symptoms of Acute Overdose Nausea, vomiting, diarrhea, abdominal pain may be seen; bradycardia, hypotension, seizures, and cardiovascular collapse have all been reported

Toxic Dosage Specific quantities are unknown; it is generally thought that ingestion of more than 2-3 berries is required for poisoning; most serious poisonings are from ingestion of teas or extracts of mistletoe

Overdosage Treatment

Decontamination: Ipecac or lavage may be of value in recent, large ingestions where vomiting has not yet occurred; activated charcoal should be administered; because of the probable diarrhea from substantial mistletoe ingestion, activated charcoal should be given as a water slurry

Supportive therapy: Replace fluids and electrolytes as needed

Additional Information

Family: Loranthaceae

Toxin: Phoratoxin and viscotoxin

Range: All mistletoes are parasitic plants and typically grow on deciduous trees such as oak; *P. rubrum* grows only on mahogany trees; in the U.S., *Viscum album* is found only in California

Toxic parts: All parts are considered toxic except for the berries of *Viscum album*

Specific References

Hall AH, Spoerke DG, and Rumack BH, "Assessing Mistletoe Toxicity," *Ann Emerg Med*, 1986, 105(11):1320-3.

Moore HW, "Mistletoe Poisoning: A Review of the Available Literature and the Report of a Case of Probable Fatal Poisoning," *J S C Med Assoc*, 1969, 59:269-71.

Stirpe F, "Mistletoe Toxicity," *Lancet*, 1983, 1(8319):295.

Mites

Scientific Name *Arachnida*; *Demodex folliculorum*; *Sarcoptes scabiei*; *Trombicula irritans*

Synonyms Chiggers-Harvestmites (*Trombicula irritans*); Itch Mite (*Sarcoptes scabiei*)

(Continued)

Mites *(Continued)*

Signs & Symptoms of Acute Overdose Pruritic, erythematous papules; fever, eczematous eruption, erythema multiforme

Overdosage Treatment Supportive therapy: Oral antihistamines and topical steroid cream (ie, fluocinonide cream) for relief of pruritus

Additional Information May transmit rickettsial pox, murine typhus, Q fever, tularemia, plague; the follicle mite (*Demodex folliculorum*) may be implicated in Kawasaki syndrome. Family: Acarina

Microbiology: *Sarcoptes scabiei*, or the human mite, is the causative agent of scabies, a common parasitic infestation of the skin. *Sarcoptes scabiei* is an ectoparasite of humans belonging to the class *Arachnida*. It tends to form skin "burrows" several millimeters wide within the stratum corneum of the epidermis. The fertilized female deposits its eggs in these skin burrows, and the larvae exit after several days to become adults weeks later. The adult is about 0.3 mm long.

Epidemiology: Scabies is distributed world wide. The incidence in the United States has been increasing since the 1970s. The reservoir resides in humans, although animal mites can sometimes cause brief human disease. Transmission is person to person by direct contact. Occasionally, transmission may occur when there is contact with heavily contaminated clothing or bedsheets. The incubation period varies from several days to weeks. Infected individuals remain communicable until all the ova and mites are eradicated from the skin.

Clinical Syndromes:

- **Human scabies:** Patients present with intense itching, usually in the interdigital web spaces, along the "belt line," the genital region, the periumbilical area, and also on the wrists, elbows, knees, and feet. Additional areas are common in children, including the hands and face. On physical examination, the characteristic burrows may be seen, appearing linear and several millimeters wide, often in the interdigital spaces. Atypical presentations of scabies may occur, including vesicles and bullae in infants, eczema, and rash. A variant known as "nodular scabies" has been described in which there are small, brown, intensely pruritic nodules usually on the penis and scrotum. An unusual manifestation of severe scabies called "Norwegian scabies" has been seen in immunocompromised individuals and patients with Down syndrome. The skin is diffusely scaling and thickened as a result of infestation of thousands of mites. Secondary bacterial infections of the skin may occur in all forms of scabies.
- **Animal scabies:** This is due to *Sarcoptes scabiei* var. *Canis*, carried on some dogs. The clinical presentation is similar to human scabies although burrows are not present.

Diagnosis: Infestation with scabies is often suspected when an individual presents with pruritic papules, or an otherwise compatible clinical history. Some patients may present because of a recent history of contact. It should be noted that scabies often imitates other skin lesions, and thus a broad differential diagnosis should be entertained if the linear burrows are not demonstrated. Other diagnostic considerations include impetigo, insect bites, drug eruptions, varicella, eczema, and others.

The linear burrows of the mite can be further demonstrated by applying blue ink over a possible burrow. The ink is drawn into the defect and when excess ink is wiped off with an alcohol pad, the ink within the burrow remains. This and other suspicious areas should be covered with oil, the area should be scraped with a sterile blade, the scrapings should be placed into oil on a microscope slide, and the preparation should be examined with a microscope.

Specific References

Glode MP, Brogden R, Joffe LS, et al, "Kawasaki Syndrome and House Dust Mite Exposure," *Pediatr Infect Dis*, 1986, 5(6):644-8.

Hewitt M, Barrow GI, Miller DC, et al, "Mites in the Personal Environment and Their Role in Skin Disorders," *Br J Dermatol*, 1973, 89(4):401-9.

Mock Cucumber *see* Wild Cucumber *on page 1157*

Mojave Rattlesnake *see* Rattlesnakes *on page 1132*

Monkey Fiddle *see* Milkbush *on previous page*

Monkey Plant (Nontoxic Plant)

Monkshood

Scientific Name *Aconitum napellus*; *Aconitum uncinatum*

Synonyms Aconite; Aconitine; Friar's Cap; Friar's Cowl; Helmet Flower; House Bane; Old Wife's Hood; Soldier's Cap; Storkjelm; Venusvogn; Wolfsbane

Mechanism of Toxic Action Aconite has a vagal action on the heart and also a more direct action on the heart muscle; death usually occurs; 2 hours to respiratory failure or heart failure usually 1-6 hours but can be from minutes to 4 days

Signs & Symptoms of Acute Overdose Symptoms occur in 10-20 minutes; tingling and burning of toes, fingers, lips, and tongue are seen first, then sweating, hypothermia, chills, paresthesia, numbness, dry mouth; later: diarrhea, paralysis, pain, hypotension, seizures, arrhythmias (supraventricular), bradycardia, ventricular fibrillation

Adverse Reactions Lack of CNS depression; poor prognosis

Toxic Dosage Fatalities have occurred with ingestion of 2-4 g root; estimated lethal dose of plant: 1 g

Overdosage Treatment

Decontamination: Ipecac is questionable due to inducing rapid onset of symptoms; lavage may be beneficial, activated charcoal with cathartic

Supportive therapy: Fluid and electrolyte replacement; arrhythmias are relatively refractory to drug therapy

Additional Information

Toxin: *Aconitum*

Toxic parts: All parts, especially seeds and roots

Monomethylhydrazine Containing Mushrooms *see* Mushrooms, Toxic (Group II) *on page 1112*

Monosodium Glutamate Food Poisoning

CAS Number 142-47-2

Synonyms Chinese Restaurant Syndrome; Chinese Seasoning; L-Sodium Glutamate; MSG; Sodium Glutamate

Commonly Found in Chinese food, sausage, canned soup, Accent®

Signs & Symptoms of Acute Overdose Flushing, wheezing, chest pain, burning sensation, tremor, angioedema, headache, paresthesia, syncope; occurs within 30 minutes postingestion and may last for 1-3 hours; minimal gastrointestinal symptoms

Overdosage Treatment Supportive therapy: Diphenhydramine may be useful, usually self-limited

Antidote(s)

Diphenhydramine Hydrochloride *on page 1415*

Diagnostic Tests/Procedures

Electrolytes, Blood *on page 1254*

Additional Information Salty or sweet to taste; soluble in water; a flavor enhancer. Intravenous doses can cause hypokalemia or alkalosis. Absorption is most rapid in a fasting state.

Specific References

Allen DH and Baker GJ, "Chinese Restaurant Asthma," *N Engl J Med*, 1981, 305(19):1154-5.

Schaumburg HH, Byck R, Gerstl R, et al, "Monosodium L-Glutamate: Its Pharmacology and Role in the Chinese Restaurant Syndrome," *Science*, 1969, 163(869):826-8.

Squire EN Jr, "Angio-Oedema and Monosodium Glutamate," *Lancet*, 1987, 1(8539):988.

Moonseed

Scientific Name *Menispermum canadense*

Synonyms Yellow Parilla

Signs & Symptoms of Acute Overdose Reportedly a stimulant action similar to water hemlock; seizures are the major concern

Overdosage Treatment Decontamination: Activated charcoal with cathartic may be of value in recent ingestions; manage seizures with diazepam

Additional Information

Family: Menispermum

Toxin: Dauricine and other isoquinoline alkaloids

Range: Found in the Eastern U.S.

Toxic part: Probably the whole plant, but especially the fruit

Moon Weed *see* Jimson Weed *on page 1094*

Morelle Noire *see* Black Nightshade *on page 1057*

"Morgan's" *Lepiota* Mushroom *see* Mushrooms, Toxic (Group VII) *on page 1116*

Morning Glory

CAS Number 2889-26-1; 478-94-4; 2390-99-0; 548-43-6; 602-85-7

Scientific Name *Ipomoea purpurea*; *Rivea corymbosa*

Synonyms Blue Star; Flying Saucers; Heavenly Blue; *Ololiuqui*; Pearly Gates

Mechanism of Toxic Action Source of lysergic acid amide which is ~10% as potent as lysergic acid diethylamide (LSD)

Signs & Symptoms of Acute Overdose Diarrhea, anxiety, drowsiness, mydriasis, flushing, depersonalization, hypotension, tachycardia

(Continued)

Morning Glory *(Continued)*

Toxic Dosage 300 seeds contain the equivalent of 200-300 mcg of LSD

Overdosage Treatment

Decontamination: Activated charcoal with cathartic with oral ingestion

Supportive therapy: Dantrolene (25 mg 2-4 times/day) should be given for neuroleptic malignant syndrome; diazepam or lorazepam can be used for agitation; haloperidol can be given for hallucinations

Additional Information Often a contaminant in soy bean crops

Specific References

Hoffer A, "D-Lysergic Acid Diethylamide (LSD): A Review of Its Present Status," *Clin Pharmacol Ther*, 1965, 6(2):183-255.

Schultes RE, "Hallucinogens of Plant Origin," *Science*, 1969, 163(864):245-54.

Mosquitoes

Scientific Name *Anopheles freeborni*; *Anopheles quadrimaculatus*

Synonyms Malaria Mosquito

Signs & Symptoms of Acute Overdose Urticarial reaction (rash)

Overdosage Treatment Supportive therapy: Local application of calamine lotion or aluminum acetate (Burow's solution); parenteral corticosteroids can also be given for systemic symptoms

Additional Information Anopheline (*A. quadrimaculatus* and *A. freeborni*) are the vectors for malaria (*Plasmodium*); N,N-diethyl-m-toluamides or DEET is an effective repellent

Order: Diptera

Family: Culicidae

Specific References

McKiel JA and West AS, "Nature and Causation of Insect Bite Reactions," *Pediatr Clin North Am*, 1961, 8(3):795-816.

Singal M, Shaw PK, Lindsay RC, et al, "An Outbreak of Introduced Malaria in California Possibly Involving Secondary Transmission," *Am J Trop Med Hyg*, 1977, 26(1):1-9.

Moss (Nontoxic Plant)

Mother-in-Law Plant *see* Caladium *on page 1063*

Mother-in-Law's Tongue *see* Dieffenbachia *on page 1079*

Moths *see* Lepidoptera *on page 1097*

Mottled Rock Rattlesnake *see* Rattlesnakes *on page 1132*

Mountain Ash [berries] (Nontoxic Plant)

Mountain Ivy Spoonwood *see* Mountain Laurel *on this page*

Mountain Laurel

Scientific Name *Kalmia*; *Kalmia latifolia*

Synonyms American Laurel; Big Leaf Ivy; Calf Kill; Calico Bush; Dwarf Laurel; Ivy Bush; Kid Kill; Lamb Kill; Mountain Ivy Spoonwood; Sheep Laurel; Spoonwood Ivy; Wicky; Wood Laurel

Mechanism of Toxic Action Contains grayanotoxin which binds to a subset of sodium channels causing structural modifications thereby causing slow opening of these channels which leads to cell depolarization

Signs & Symptoms of Acute Overdose Hypotension, bradycardia; seizures; sweating, asthenia; dermatitis; nausea, vomiting, oral numbness or burning, paresthesia, transient blindness, visual changes

Toxic Dosage Three whole leaves or flowers likely nontoxic; consider decontamination if more; toxicity is unpredictable, variable among azalea types

Overdosage Treatment

Decontamination: Avoid ipecac, vagal stimulation increases toxicity; lavage/activated charcoal with cathartic

Supportive therapy: Atropine for bradycardia, I.V. fluids should be sufficient for hypotension

Additional Information Toxic parts: Leaves and honey

Mountain Rosebay *see* Azalea *on page 1055*

"Mowers" Mushroom *see* Mushrooms, Toxic (Group VI) *on page 1115*

MSG *see* Monosodium Glutamate Food Poisoning *on previous page*

Mum *see* Chrysanthemum *on page 1069*

Muscarine-Containing Mushrooms *see* Mushrooms, Toxic (Group V) *on page 1114*

Mushrooms, Toxic (Group I)

CAS Number 23109-05-9; 21150-22-1; 21150-23-2; 17466-45-4 (phalloidin); 28227-92-1 (phalloin); 39412-56-1 (phallolysin)

Scientific Name *Amanita bisporigera* ("Destroying Angel"); *Amanita ocreata*; *Amanita phalloides* ("Deathcap"); *Amanita suballiacea*; *Amanita tenuifolia* ("Slender Death Angel"); *Amanita verna* ("Deadly Agaric" or "Death Angel"); *Amanita virosa*; *Galerina autumnalis* ("Deadly" *Galerina* or "Autumnal" *Galerina*); *Galerina marginata* (Marginate *Pholiota*); *Galerina venenata* ("Deadly Lawn" *Galerina*); *Lepiota helveola*; *Lepiota josserandii* ("Deadly Parasol"); *Lepiota subincarnata*

Synonyms "Autumnal" *Galerina* Mushroom; Cyclopeptide Mushrooms; "Deadly Agaric" Mushroom; "Deadly" *Galerina* Mushroom; "Deadly Lawn" *Galerina* Mushroom; "Deadly Parasol" Mushroom; "Death Angel" Mushroom; "Deathcap" Mushroom; "Destroying Angel" Mushroom; "Marginate" *Pholiota* Mushroom; "Slender Death Angel" Mushroom

Mechanism of Toxic Action May contain one of three types of cyclopeptides: phallotoxins, amatoxins, and virotoxins. Phallotoxins are rapid-acting agents inhibiting action formation and cell membrane function. Amatoxins (a cyclic octapeptide) cause liver necrosis through inhibition of RNA polymerase (II).

Adverse Reactions Three phases:

I: Gastroenteritis: up to 24 hours postingestion
II: Remission: up to 72 hours postingestion
III: Hepatic/renal effects: 3-6 days postingestion

Cardiovascular: Hypotension
Central nervous system: Coma, seizures, encephalopathy
Gastrointestinal: Gastroenteritis initially with colicky abdominal pain, vomiting, diarrhea, pancreatitis
Hematologic: Coagulopathy
Hepatic: Hepatic failure
Renal: Renal failure

Toxicodynamics/Kinetics

Absorption: Phallotoxin not well absorbed though the gastrointestinal tract
Distribution: V_d: 160-290 mL/kg
Protein binding: Not protein bound
Excretion: Excreted in urine, feces, and bile; enterohepatic recirculation may occur

Toxic Dosage

Toxic at doses of 0.1 mg/kg
Lethal at 50 g (about 3 mushrooms)

Overdosage Treatment

Decontamination: Lavage/activated charcoal with cathartic
Supportive therapy: Fluid with glucose; high-dose penicillin G (300,000-1,000,000 units/kg/day) may be effective. Silymarin (20-50 mg/kg/day) may also be hepatoprotective. Lactulose and neomycin should be utilized if hepatic encephalopathy develops. Successful orthotopic liver transplantation has been reported.
Enhancement of elimination: Charcoal hemoperfusion necessary within 24 hours of ingestion; multiple dosing of activated charcoal may be effective; the efficacy of hyperbaric oxygen is not known

Antidote(s)

Oxygen (Hyperbaric) *on page 1453*

Test Interactions Monitor for hypochloronatremia and hypokalemia during gastroenteritis phase. Insulin, calcitonin, and parathyroid hormone levels are increased. Serum thyroxine levels are decreased. Hypoglycemia may also develop.

Diagnostic Tests/Procedures

Factor V, Plasma *on page 1262*
Fibrinogen, Plasma *on page 1265*
Kidney Profile *on page 1279*
Liver Profile *on page 1286*

Pregnancy Implications Alpha-amanitine does not cross placental barrier

Additional Information Unfavorable prognostic signs include a fall in thromboplastin time (after 48 hours), elevated bilirubin levels (>3 mg/dL) on admission or elevated creatinine within 48 hours

Amanita: Spore print: White; mushroom flourishes from late summer to early winter; grows in proximity of oak trees; heat stable; insoluble in water; orthotopic. Liver transplantation may be necessary. Ninety percent of the deaths due to *A. phalloides* or *A. verna*. Chronic active hepatitis may be a long-term sequelae. Cimetidine and thioctic acid has not been proven to be clinically effective.

Galerina: Spore print: Rust brown; grows in fall/winter seasons

Specific References

Belliardo F, Massano G, and Accomo S, "Amatoxins Do Not Cross the Placental Barrier," *Lancet*, 1983, 1(8338):1381.

Feinfeld DA, Mofenson HC, Caraccio T, et al, "Poisoning by Amatoxin-Containing Mushrooms in Suburban New York - Report of Four Cases," *J Toxicol Clin Toxicol*, 1994, 32(6):715-21.

Floersheim GL, "Treatment of Human Amatoxin Mushroom Poisoning: Myths and Advances in Therapy," *Med Toxicol*, 1987, 2(1):1-9.

(Continued)

Mushrooms, Toxic (Group I) *(Continued)*

Hanrahan JP and Gordon MA, "Mushroom Poisoning. Case Reports and a Review of Therapy," *JAMA*, 1984, 251(8):1057-61.
Hoffman R, "Mushroom Poisoning," *Emergency Medicine*, 1995, 27(6):66.
Klein AS, Hart J, Brems JJ, et al, "*Amanita* Poisoning: Treatment and the Role of Liver Transplantation," *Am J Med*, 1989, 86(2):187-93.
McClain JL, Hause DW, and Clark MA, "*Amanita phalloides* Mushroom Poisoning: A Cluster of Four Fatalities," *J Forensic Sci*, 1989, 34(1):83-7.
Meunier BC, Camus CM, Houssin DP, et al, "Liver Transplantation After Severe Poisoning Due to Amatoxin-Containing Lepiota – Report of Three Cases," *Clin Toxicol*, 1995, 33:165-71.
Wauters JP, Rossel C, and Farquet JJ, "*Amanita phalloides* Poisoning Treated by Early Charcoal Haemoperfusion," *Br Med J*, 1978, 2(6150):1465.

Mushrooms, Toxic (Group II)

CAS Number 16568-02-8; 60-34-4 (MMH); 69349-96-8

Scientific Name *Gyromitra ambigua*; *Gyromitra brunnea* ("Brown False Morel"); *Gyromitra californica* ("California False Morel" Mushroom); *Gyromitra caroliniana* ("Carolina False Morel"); *Gyromitra esculenta*; *Gyromitra esculenta* ("Beefsteak" or "Brain" *Gyromitra* or "False Morel" or "Turban Fungus"); *Gyromitra fastigiata*; *Gyromitra gigas* ("Snow Morel" or "Giant False Morel"); *Gyromitra infula* ("Hooded False Morel"); *Gyromitra korfii* ("Bull Nose"); *Gyromitra sphaerospora*

Synonyms "Beefsteak Fungus"; "Brain" *Gyromitra* Mushroom; "Brown False Morel" Mushroom; "Bull Nose" Mushroom; "California False Morel" Mushroom; "Carolina False Morel" Mushroom; "False Morel" Mushroom; "Giant False Morel" Mushroom; "Hooded False Morel" Mushroom; Monomethylhydrazine Containing Mushrooms; "Snow Morel" Mushroom; "Turban Fungus" Mushroom

Use Monomethylhydrazine is used as rocket fuel; it is a strong reducing agent in industry (DOT/UN: 1244) and a corrosive inhibitor

Mechanism of Toxic Action Gyromithrins, a hydrazone, decompose to release methylhydrazine (MMH) which is an inhibitor of the hepatic coenzyme pyridoxal phosphate and gamma-aminobytyric acid (GABA) in the brain

Adverse Reactions

Central nervous system: Seizures, coma, dizziness, delirium
Gastrointestinal: Nausea, vomiting, abdominal pain, cramps, gastroenteritis, watery diarrhea
Hematologic: Hemolysis, anemia, hemolytic anemia
Hepatic: Elevated liver enzymes, jaundice
Renal & genitourinary: Intestinal nephritis may develop within 24 hours (latent period may be up to 24 hours)
Miscellaneous: Fever

Toxicodynamics/Kinetics

Absorption: Via inhalation of fumes from cooking occurs
Metabolism: 25% hydrolyzed to methylhydrazine

Toxic Dosage Lethal dose:

Children: 10-30 mg/kg
Adults: 20-50 mg/kg

Overdosage Treatment

Decontamination: Lavage/activated charcoal with cathartic
Supportive therapy: Pyridoxine (25 mg/kg I.V.) may prevent seizures; methylene blue used to treat methemoglobinemia

Antidote(s)

Methylene Blue *on page 1444*
Pyridoxine Hydrochloride *on page 1465*

Diagnostic Tests/Procedures

Glucose, Random *on page 1269*
Hemoglobin, Qualitative, Urine *on page 1272*
Methemoglobin, Blood *on page 1296*

Drug Interactions Phenobarbital may have an enhanced effect due to interference of hepatic metabolism

Pregnancy Implications May be teratogenic along with tumorigenic

Additional Information Mushrooms found on the ground; common in the spring; may be detoxified in boiling water, but fumes can cause vomiting; a nongilled fungus; spore print: brown; heat-labile toxin; MMH is volatile and water soluble. Mortality may exceed 40%; "brain-like" appearance.

Specific References

Giusti GV and Carnevale A, "A Case of Fatal Poisoning by *Gyromitra esculenta*," *Arch Toxicol*, 1974, 33(1):49-54.
Michelot D and Toth B, "Poisoning by *Gyromitra esculenta* – A Review," *J Appl Toxicol*, 1991, 11(4):235-43.

Mushrooms, Toxic (Group III)

CAS Number 2552-55-8 (ibotenic acid); 2763-96-4 (muscimol)

Scientific Name *Amanita citrina* ("False Deathcap"); *Amanita cokeri* ("Solitary Lepidella"); *Amanita muscaria* ("Fly Agaric"); *Amanita pantherina* ("Panther" *Amanita*);

Amanita smithiana ("Smith's" *Amanita*); *Amanita strobiliformis*; *Boletus calopus*; *Boletus luridus* ("Lurid" *Boletus*); *Boletus pulcherrimus* ("Red-Pored Bolete"); *Boletus* satanus ("Satan's Bolete"); *Clitocybe cerussata*; *Clitocybe clavipes* ("Clubfoot Funnelcap" Mushroom); *Clitocybe dealbata* ("Sweat" Mushroom); *Clitocybe dilatata* ("Crowded-White" *Clitocybe*); *Clitocybe rivulosa*; *Mycena pura* ("Lilac Fairy Helmet"); *Omphalotus illudens* ("Jack-O'-Lantern"); *Omphalotus olearius* ("Jack-O'-Lantern")

Synonyms "Blushing" *Inocybe* Mushroom; "Booted" *Amanita* Mushroom; Clavate-Stalked *Clitocybe*; "Clubfoot Funnelcap" Mushroom; "Conic Fiberhead" Mushroom; "Corn Silk" *Inocybe* Mushroom; "False Deathcap" Mushroom; "Fly Agaric" Mushroom; "Jack-O'-Lantern" Mushroom; "Jonquil" *Amanita* Mushroom; "Lurid" *Boletus* Mushroom; "Panther" *Amanita* Mushroom; "Red-Pored Bolete" Mushroom; "Satan's Bolete" Mushroom; "Straw-Colored Fiberhead" Mushroom; "Sweater" Mushroom; "Torn-Capped Fiberhead" Mushroom

Mechanism of Toxic Action

Amanita: Contains the toxin ibotenic acid-muscimol with primary anticholinergic effects (an isoxazole derivative); competes with gamma-aminobutyric acid (GABA)

Clitocybe: Contains muscarine which can produce a peripheral cholinergic effect (no central effect) also contains the toxin coprine which inhibits acetaldehyde dehydrogenase, thus, inhibiting the metabolism of ethanol (similar to disulfiram); reaction may last 1 week; when ingested with ethanol, vasodilative and hypotensive effect

Adverse Reactions

Cardiovascular: Bradycardia, hypotension, hypertension, arrhythmias

Central nervous system: Delirium, dizziness, ataxia, somnolence, seizures, psychosis, euphoria, residual headaches, fever, coma

Dermatological: Sweating

Gastrointestinal: Vomiting is rare, watery diarrhea, salivation

Neuromuscular & skeletal: Muscle myoclonus

Ocular: Miosis, visual hallucinations, lacrimation, teichopsia

Miscellaneous: Hyperthermia

Toxicodynamics/Kinetics

Onset of action: 1 hour

Duration: 24 hours

Toxic Dosage Maximum tolerable dose: 20 *Amanita muscaria* mushrooms; muscarine: 0.5 mg parenterally will give cholinergic effects

Overdosage Treatment

Amanita:

Decontamination: Lavage/activated charcoal with cathartic

Supportive therapy: Atropine (1-2 mg I.V. in adults or 0.05 mg/kg in children) is the specific antidote for muscarine poisoning; treat seizures with diazepam

Clitocybe clavipes:

Decontamination: Lavage/charcoal; ipecac is **not** indicated

Supportive therapy: Isotonic saline; atropine (1-2 mg I.V. in adults or 0.05 mg/kg in children) is the specific antidote for muscarine poisoning; treat seizures with diazepam

Clitocybe:

Decontamination: Emesis or lavage/charcoal

Supportive therapy: I.V. hydration; atropine (1-2 mg I.V. in adults or 0.05 mg/kg in children) is the specific antidote for muscarine poisoning; treat seizures with diazepam

Antidote(s)

Atropine Sulfate *on page 1395*

Dopamine Hydrochloride *on page 1418*

Norepinephrine Bitartrate *on page 1451*

Physostigmine *on page 1457*

Diagnostic Tests/Procedures

Electrolytes, Blood *on page 1254*

Liver Profile *on page 1286*

Additional Information

Amanita: Seen in conifer forests in the spring to fall; spore print: white

While *A. pantherina* and *A. muscaria* may also have muscarine, anticholinergic effects usually predominate; toxic effects may be retained in dried mushrooms

Clitocybe clavipes: 4-Methylpyrazole (5 mg/kg I.V. over 2-3 minutes) has been utilized to stop antabuse-alcohol reaction. Not approved for mushroom use. Dopamine may (coprine does not inhibit dopamine beta-hydroxylase) be useful for hypotension; also use norepinephrine for hypotension.

No toxicity when ingested alone; symptoms may last for 5 days; fatalities are rare. Found in Japan.

(Continued)

Mushrooms, Toxic (Group III) *(Continued)*

Clitocybe: Grows in lawns and parks; spore print: white; flesh: central stalks with gray caps; muscarine is heat stable

Atropine sulfate is useful for muscarinic symptoms; give as much as necessary to relieve bronchorrhea

Specific References

Caley MJ and Clark RA, "Cardiac Arrhythmia After Mushroom Ingestion," *Br Med J*, 1977, 2(6103):1633.

Johnston GA, "Muscimol and the Uptake of Gamma-Aminobutyric Acid by Rat Brain Slices," *Psychopharmacologia*, 1971, 22(3):230-3.

McDonald A, "Mushrooms and Madness. Hallucinogenic Mushrooms and Some Psychopharmacological Implications," *Can J Psychiatry*, 1980, 25(7):586-94.

Mushrooms, Toxic (Group IV)

Scientific Name *Coprinus atramentarius* ("Inky Cap"); *Coprinus insignis*

Synonyms Coprine-Containing Mushrooms; "Inky Cap" Mushroom

Mechanism of Toxic Action Contains the toxin coprine which inhibits acetaldehyde dehydrogenase. Thus, when taken concomitantly with alcohol, there is an increase in serum acetaldehyde levels. High acetaldehyde causes uncomfortable symptoms, including flushing, nausea, thirst, palpitations, chest pain, dizziness, and hypotension. This reaction is the basis for disulfiram use in postwithdrawal long-term care of alcoholism. May also boost the immune function in HIV patients.

Adverse Reactions

Cardiovascular: Flushing, cardiovascular collapse, myocardial infarction, death

Central nervous system: Dizziness, headache, seizures, paresthesia, headache, sweating

Gastrointestinal: Nausea, vomiting, metallic taste

Hepatic: Hepatitis

Ocular: Retrobulbar neuritis, nystagmus

Respiratory: Dyspnea, chest pain

Toxicodynamics/Kinetics

Onset of action: 0.5-2 hours

Duration of effects: 3-6 hours

Overdosage Treatment Management of disulfiram reaction: Institute support measures to restore blood pressure (pressors and fluids); monitor for hypokalemia; metoclopramide or prochlorperazine can be used for vomiting; dopamine is not useful to treat disulfiram-ethanol induced hypotension; norepinephrine is the preferred agent; use of 4-methylpyrazole is investigational

Antidote(s)

Norepinephrine Bitartrate *on page 1451*

Drug Interactions INH, metronidazole, phenytoin, alcohol, warfarin, diazepam, chlordiazepoxide; can cause elevation of theophylline

Additional Information Spore print: black; found in the summer and fall; no toxicity when ingested alone; toxicity with *C. atramentarius* can occur after drinking coffee; avoid ethanol-containing products for 72 hours

Specific References

Radford AP, "Ink Caps and Alcohol," *Br Med J*, 1978, 1(6105):112.

Mushrooms, Toxic (Group V)

CAS Number 2552-55-8 (ibotenic acid); 2763-96-4 (muscimol)

Scientific Name *Amanita citrina* ("False Deathcap"); *Amanita cothurnata* ("Booted" *Amanita*); *Amanita frostiana* ("Frost's" *Amanita*); *Amanita gemmata* ("Jeweled Deathcap" or "Jonquil" *Amanita*); *Amanita muscaria* ("Fly Agaric"); *Amanita pantherina* ("Panther" *Amanita*); *Boletus luridus* ("Lurid" *Boletus*); *Inocybe fastigiata* ("Straw-Colored Fiberhead" or "Conic Fiberhead"); *Inocybe geophylla* ("Earthblade Fiberhead"); *Inocybe godeyi*; *Inocybe lacera* ("Torn-Capped Fiberhead"); *Inocybe lilacina*; *Inocybe patouillardi*; *Inocybe pudica* ("Blushing" *Inocybe*); *Inocybe sororia* ("Corn Silk" *Inocybe*); *Mycena pura* ("Lilac Fairy Helmet")

Synonyms "Blushing" *Inocybe* Mushroom; "Booted" *Amanita* Mushroom; "False Deathcap" Mushroom; "Fly Agaric" Mushroom; "Frost's" *Amanita* Mushroom; Ibotenic Acid-Containing Mushrooms; "Jeweled Deathcap" Mushroom; "Jonquil" *Amanita* Mushroom; Muscarine-Containing Mushrooms; "Panther" *Amanita* Mushroom; "Straw-Colored Fiberhead" Mushroom; "Torn-Capped Fiberhead" Mushroom

Mechanism of Toxic Action Contains the toxin ibotenic acid-muscimol with primary anticholinergic effects (an isoxazole derivative); competes with gamma-aminobutyric acid (GABA)

Adverse Reactions

Cardiovascular: Tachycardia, hypotension

Central nervous system: Delirium, dizziness, ataxia, somnolence, seizures, psychosis, euphoria, residual headaches, fever, coma, fasciculations

Endocrine & metabolic: Hyperthermia

Gastrointestinal: Vomiting is rare, dry mouth

Neuromuscular & skeletal: Muscle myoclonus
Ocular: Mydriasis, visual hallucinations

Toxicodynamics/Kinetics
Onset of action: 1 hour
Duration of action: 24 hours

Toxic Dosage
Toxic dose:
Ibotenic acid: 30-60 mg
Muscimol: 6 mg
Sensory derangement can be produced at a dose of 2-4 mushrooms; maximum survivable ingestion: 20 mushrooms

Overdosage Treatment
Decontamination: Lavage/activated charcoal with cathartic; ipecac can be utilized if within 90 minutes of ingestion
Supportive therapy: Diazepam can be utilized for delirium; while physostigmine can be used for life-threatening anticholinergic crisis (0.5-2 mg I.V. over a 5-minute time period), it should not be routinely used. Likewise, atropine (0.05 mg/kg I.V. in children or 0.5-2 mg in adults), can be used for severe cholinergic crisis due to ibotenic acid or muscimol but is not for routine use; treat seizures with diazepam

Antidote(s)
Physostigmine *on page 1457*

Additional Information
Seen in conifer forests in the spring to fall; spore print: white
While *A. pantherina* and *A. muscaria* may also have muscarine, anticholinergic effects usually predominate; toxic effects may be retained in dried mushrooms

Specific References
Johnston GA, "Muscimol and the Uptake of Gamma-Aminobutyric Acid by Rat Brain Slices," *Psychopharmacologia*, 1971, 22(3):230-3.
McDonald A, "Mushrooms and Madness. Hallucinogenic Mushrooms and Some Psychopharmacological Implications," *Can J Psychiatry*, 1980, 25(7):586-94.

Mushrooms, Toxic (Group VI)

Scientific Name *Conocybe cyanopus*; *Gymnopilus aeruginosa* ("Green" *Pholiota*); *Gymnopilus luteus*; *Gymnopilus spectabilis* ("Showy Flamecap" or "Big Laughing" Mushroom); *Gymnopilus validipes*; *Gymnopilus viridans*; *Paneolus alter*, *Paneolus campanulatus* ("Bell-Shaped" *Panaeolus* or "Bell Mottlegill"); *Paneolus foenisecii* ("Mowers Mushroom"); *Paneolus sphinetrinus*; *Paneolus subbalteatus* ("Girdled" *Panaeolus*); *Paneolus tropicalis*; *Psilocybe baeocystis* ("Potent" *Psilocybe*); *Psilocybe caerulipes* ("Blue Foot"); *Psilocybe cubensis*; *Psilocybe cyanescens* ("Blueing" *Psilocybe*); *Psilocybe mexicana*; *Psilocybe pelliculosa*; *Psilocybe semilanceata* ("Liberty Caps"); *Psilocybe stuntzii* ("Stuntz's Blue Legs"); *Stropharia coronilla* ("Crown" Toadstool); *Stropharia semiglobata* ("Halfglobe Mushroom" or "Manure Roundhead")

Synonyms "Bell Mottlegill" Mushroom; "Bell-Shaped" *Panaeolus* Mushroom; "Big Laughing" Mushroom; "Blue Foot" Mushroom; "Blueing" *Psilocybe* Mushroom; "Crown" Toadstool; "Girdled" *Panaeolus* Mushroom; "Green" *Pholiota* Mushroom; "Halfglobe" Mushroom; Indole-Containing Mushrooms; "Liberty Cap" Mushroom; "Manure Roundhead" Mushroom; "Mowers" Mushroom; "Potent" *Psilocybe* Mushroom; "Showy Flamecap" Mushroom; "Silly Putty"; "Stuntz's Blue Legs" Mushroom

Mechanism of Toxic Action Contains psilocybin and psilocin which are indole alkaloids similar to LSD and/or serotonin

Adverse Reactions
Cardiovascular: Tachycardia, flushing, hypertension
Central nervous system: Paresthesia, ataxia, hyperkinesis, chills, rigors, headache, asthenia, dizziness, fever, seizures
Endocrine & metabolic: Methemoglobinemia
Gastrointestinal: Vomiting
Genitourinary: Urinary incontinence
Neuromuscular & skeletal: Myalgias
Ocular: Mydriasis, visual hallucinogens (colored patterns, impaired distanced perception)

Toxicodynamics/Kinetics
Onset of action: Within 20 minutes
Duration: 6-15 hours
Absorption: Oral: 50%
Metabolism: Hepatic
Elimination: Renal

Overdosage Treatment
Decontamination: Lavage/activated charcoal with cathartic; ipecac can be utilized
Supportive therapy: Diazepam for panic attacks; chlorpromazine may be useful for treatment of hallucinations; flashback may occur 4 months later

(Continued)

Mushrooms, Toxic (Group VI) *(Continued)*

Additional Information

Gymnopilus: Hallucinogenic dose: 20-100 mushrooms

Psilocybe: Hallucinogenic dose: 20-30 mushrooms (115-160 mcg/kg of psilocybin) Found in Southern U.S.; grows on buried logs in wooded areas. Spore print: rusty-orange. Indoles are heat stable; not removed by cooking.

Specific References

Curry SC and Rose MC, "Intravenous Mushroom Poisoning," *Ann Emerg Med*, 1985, 14(9):900-2.

Peden NR, Pringle SD, and Crooks J, "The Problem of *Psilocybin* Mushroom Abuse," *Hum Toxicol*, 1982, 1(4):417-24.

Schwartz RH and Smith BM, "Hallucinogenic Mushrooms," *Clin Pediatr (Phila)*, 1988, 27(2):70-3.

Mushrooms, Toxic (Group VII)

Scientific Name *Agaricus arvensis* ("Field Mushroom" or "Horse Mushroom"); *Agaricus hondensis* ("Felt-Ringed Mushroom"); *Agaricus placomyces* ("Flat-Top Mushroom"); *Agaricus silvaticus* ("Woods" *Psalliota* or "Forest Mushroom"); *Agaricus sylvicola* ("Wood-Loving Mushroom" or "Sylvan Mushroom"); *Amanita brunnescens* ("Cleft-Foot Deathcap"); *Armillariella mellea* ("Stumper" or "Honey Mushroom"); *Boletus calopus*; *Boletus erythropus* ("Red-Footed Bolete"); *Boletus luridus* ("Lurid" *Boletus*); *Boletus pulcherrimus* ("Red-Pored Bolete"); *Boletus satanus* ("Satan's Bolete"); *Boletus sensibilis* ("Sensitive" *Boletus*); *Chlorophyllum molybdites* ("Green Parasol"); *Clitocybe irina* ("Blushing Bowlcap"); *Clitocybe nebularis* ("Gray Cap" or "Cloudy Funnelcap"); *Collybia dryophila* ("Nut-Brown" *Collybia* or "Forest Friend" or "Oak-Loving" *Collybia*); *Entoloma lividum* ("Gray Pinkgill"); *Gomphus floccosus* ("Woolly Chanterelle" or "Scaly Chanterelle"); *Hebeloma crustuliniforme* ("Poison Pie"); *Hebeloma mesophaeum* ("Dark-Centered" *Hebeloma*); *Hebeloma sinapizans* ("Giant" *Hebeloma*); *Helvella lacunosa* ("Elfin Saddle"); *Lactarius chrysorrheus* ("Yellow-Juiced" *Lactarius* or "Gold-Drop Milkcap"); *Lactarius deceptivus* ("Deceptive" *Lactarius* Mushroom or "Cotton Milkcap"); *Lactarius piperatus* ("Pepper Milkcap"); *Lactarius repraesentaneus* ("Shaggy Bear"); *Lactarius rufus* ("Red Milkcap"); *Lactarius scrobiculatus* ("Spotted-Stemmed" *Lactarius* or "Pitted Milkcap"); *Lactarius subvellereus*; *Lactarius torminosus* ("Wooly Milkcap"); *Lactarius uvidus* ("Grape-Colored" *Lactarius* or "Damp Milkcap"); *Lactarius vellereus* ("Fleecy Milkcap"); *Lepiota molybdites* ("Morgan's" *Lepiota*); *Lepiota naucina* ("Smooth" *Lepiota* or "White" *Lepiota*); *Marasmius urens*; *Naematoloma fasciculare* ("Sulphur Tuft"); *Paxillus involutus*; *Paxillus involutus* ("Naked Brimcap"); *Pholiota squarrosa* ("Shaggy Scalecap"); *Ramaria formosa*; *Ramaria gelantinosa* ("Oregon Gelatinous Coral"); *Russula emetica*; *Tricholoma pardinum*; *Tricholoma pessundatum*

Synonyms "Blushing Bowlcap" Mushroom; *Chlorophyllum* Mushrooms; "Cleft-Foot Deathcap" Mushroom; "Cloudy Funnelcap" Mushroom; "Cotton Milkcap" Mushroom; "Damp Milkcap" Mushroom; "Dark-Centered" *Hebeloma* Mushroom; "Deceptive" *Lactarius* Mushroom; "Elfin Saddle" Mushroom; "Felt-Ringed" Mushroom; "Field" Mushroom; "Flat-Top" Mushroom; "Fleecy Milkcap" Mushroom; "Forest Friend" Mushroom; "Forest" Mushroom; Gastrointestinal Irritant Mushrooms; "Giant" *Hebeloma* Mushroom; "Gold-Drop Milkcap" Mushroom; "Grape-Colored" *Lactarius* Mushroom; "Gray Cap" Mushroom; "Gray Pinkgill" Mushroom; "Green Parasol" Mushroom; "Honey" Mushroom; "Horse" Mushroom; "Lurid" *Boletus* Mushroom; "Morgan's" *Lepiota* Mushroom; "Naked Brimcap" Mushroom; "Nut-Brown" *Collybia* Mushroom; "Oak-Loving" *Collybia* Mushroom; "Pepper Caps" Mushroom; "Pepper Milkcap" Mushroom; "Pitted Milkcap" Mushroom; "Poison Pie" Mushroom; "Red-Footed Bolete" Mushroom; "Red Milkcap" Mushroom; "Red-Pored Bolete" Mushroom; "Satan's Bolete" Mushroom; "Scaly Chanterelle" Mushroom; "Sensitive" *Boletus* Mushroom; "Shaggy Bear" Mushroom; "Shaggy Scalecap" Mushroom; "S-mooth" *Lepiota* Mushroom; "Spotted-Stemmed" Mushroom; "Stumper" Mushroom; "Sulphur Tuft" Mushroom; "Sylvan" Mushroom; "White" *Lepiota* Mushroom; "Wood-Loving" Mushroom; "Woods" *Psalliota* Mushroom; "Wooly Chanterelle" Mushroom; "Wooly Milkcap" Mushroom; "Yellow-Juiced" *Lactarius* Mushroom

Replaces *Lepiota morgani*

Mechanism of Toxic Action Gastrointestinal irritant; toxins have not been identified

Adverse Reactions

Central nervous system: Fatigue, drowsiness, paresthesia, headache (*Entoloma lividum*), pallor, chills

Gastrointestinal (within 3 hours): Nausea, vomiting, watery diarrhea progressing to bloody diarrhea, abdominal pain

Neuromuscular & skeletal: Myalgias occur within 3 hours but usually resolve in 48 hours

Overdosage Treatment

Decontamination: Activated charcoal with cathartic

Supportive therapy: Fluids for rehydration

Diagnostic Tests/Procedures

Blood, Urine *on page 1210*

Protein, Semiquantitative, Urine *on page 1337*
White Blood Count *on page 1380*

Additional Information Green gills; spore print: green; proteinuria, hematuria, and leukocytosis are common

Specific References

Blayney D, Rosenkranz E, and Zettner A, "Mushroom Poisoning From *Chlorophyllum molybdites*," *West J Med*, 1980, 132(1):74-7.
Levitan D, Macy JI, and Weissman J, "Mechanism of Gastrointestinal Hemorrhage in a Case of Mushroom Poisoning by *Chlorophyllum molybdites*," *Toxicon*, 1981, 19(1):179-80.
Vanden Hoek TL, Erickson T, Hryhorczuk DO, et al, "Jack O'Lantern Mushroom Poisoning," *Ann Emerg Med*, 1991, 20(5):559-61.

Mushrooms, Toxic (Group VIII)

CAS Number 37338-80-0 (Orellanine)

Scientific Name *Cortinarius gentilis* ("Deadly Cort" or "Goldband Webcap"); *Cortinarius orellanus* ("Poznan Cort"); *Cortinarius rainierensis*; *Cortinarius speciosissimus*; *Cortinarius splendicus* ("Splendid Webcap"); *Cortinarius venenosus*

Synonyms "Deadly Cort" Mushroom; "Goldband Webcap" Mushroom; Oreline and Orellanine-Containing Mushrooms; "Poznan Cort" Mushroom; "Splendid Webcap" Mushroom

Mechanism of Toxic Action Contains orelline and orellanine which can cause interstitial nephritis, renal tubular damage

Adverse Reactions

Central nervous system: Chills, headaches, paresthesias (15%)
Dermatologic: Skin rash (12%)
Gastrointestinal: Intense thirst, nausea, vomiting, diarrhea (20%), anorexia, constipation
Neuromuscular & skeletal: Muscle aches, myalgias
Otic: Ototoxicity, tinnitus
Renal & genitourinary: Oliguria, renal failure (30% to 46%), polyuria (30%)
Miscellaneous: Coldness, cold feeling

Toxicodynamics/Kinetics Onset of action: Delay of symptoms may occur as long as 2 weeks later

Toxic Dosage Lethal dose: 100-200 g/kg of fresh mushrooms

Overdosage Treatment

Decontamination: Lavage/activated charcoal with cathartic
Supportive therapy: Isotonic fluids for rehydration; renal transplant may be required for renal failure; forced diuresis is not effective; avoid use of furosemide in that it may aggravate renal dysfunction
Enhanced elimination: Hemodialysis and/or charcoal hemoperfusion should be started as soon as possible to prevent renal failure

Diagnostic Tests/Procedures

Blood, Urine *on page 1210*
Kidney Profile *on page 1279*
Protein, Semiquantitative, Urine *on page 1337*

Drug Interactions Increased toxicity may occur with phenobarbital or furosemide

Additional Information Bright orange; mainly occurs in Europe and Japan. The bipyridyl toxins are related to the herbicide diquat. Cooking or drying does not reduce toxicity. Renal transplantation may be necessary. Mortality rate is 15%.

Specific References

Bouget J, Bousser J, Pats B, et al, "Acute Renal Failure Following Collective Intoxication by Cortinarius Orellanus," *Intensive Care Med*, 1990, 16(8):506-10.
Holmdahl J, Mulec H, and Ahlmen J, "Acute Renal Failure After Intoxication With *Cortinarius* Mushrooms," *Hum Toxicol*, 1984, 3(4):309-13.
Moore B, Burton BT, Lindgren J, et al, "*Cortinarius* Mushroom Poisoning Resulting in Anuric Renal Failure," *Vet Hum Toxicol*, 1991, 33:369.
Short AK, Watling R, MacDonald MK, et al, "Poisoning by *Cortinarius speciosissimus*," *Lancet*, 1980, 2(8201):942-4.

Mustard Tree

Scientific Name *Nicotiana glauca*

Synonyms Tree Tobacco

Mechanism of Toxic Action All parts of the plant contain nicotine and are considered toxic

Signs & Symptoms of Acute Overdose Low doses can cause nausea, vomiting, oral irritation, headache, thirst, sweating, and asthenia; higher doses can cause hallucinations, confusion; CNS stimulation followed by depression, seizures, hyperthermia, hypertension, and tachycardia followed by hypotension, bradycardia, and an irregular pulse

Overdosage Treatment

Decontamination: Emesis not recommended due to potential for seizures; lavage with 1:10,000 potassium permanganate (100 mg/L) is recommended in ingestions after control of seizures; activated charcoal with cathartic use in acute ingestions not well established

(Continued)

Mustard Tree *(Continued)*

For dermal exposures, wash area well with cool water and dry; soap (especially alkaline soaps) may increase absorption; remove any remaining transdermal systems; nicotine will continue to be absorbed several hours after removal due to depot in skin

Supportive therapy: Control seizures with benzodiazepines; if continuous, use phenytoin or phenobarbital; atropine can be utilized for cholinergic toxicity while phentolamine can be used for hypertension

Enhancement of elimination: Hemodialysis/hemoperfusion of unknown value; multiple doses probably necessary in ingestions of transdermal systems due to slow release of nicotine. While acidifying the urine may enhance elimination, this modality is not recommended due to inherent dangers; would proceed with forced diuresis.

Additional Information Range: Arizona, Texas, Mexico, California, Hawaii

***Mycena pura* ("Lilac Fairy Helmet")** *see* Mushrooms, Toxic (Group III) *on page 1112*

***Mycena pura* ("Lilac Fairy Helmet")** *see* Mushrooms, Toxic (Group V) *on page 1114*

Myristica fragrans *see* Nutmeg *on next page*

Mysteria *see* Autumn Crocus *on page 1054*

***Naematoloma fasciculare* ("Sulphur Tuft")** *see* Mushrooms, Toxic (Group VII) *on page 1116*

***Naja naja arabicus* (Arabian Cobra)** *see* Cobras *on page 1072*

***Naja naja naja* (Indian Cobra, Asian Cobra)** *see* Cobras *on page 1072*

***Naja nigricollis* (African Spitting Cobra)** *see* Cobras *on page 1072*

***Naja nivea* (Cape Cobra)** *see* Cobras *on page 1072*

"Naked Brimcap" Mushroom *see* Mushrooms, Toxic (Group VII) *on page 1116*

Nap-at-Noon *see* Star-of-Bethlehem (*Ornithogalum umbellatum*) *on page 1146*

Narcissu Pseudo-Narcissus *see* Narcissus *on this page*

Narcissus

Scientific Name *Narcissu Pseudo-Narcissus*

Mechanism of Toxic Action Contains lycorine (an *Amaryllidaceae* alkaloid), a centrally acting emetic

Signs & Symptoms of Acute Overdose Usually nausea, vomiting, abdominal pain, diarrhea, and salivation; symptoms develop soon after oral ingestion (within 30 minutes) and resolve within 3 hours (according to one report)

Overdosage Treatment

Decontamination: Ipecac relatively contraindicated; may be useful, if given soon after ingestion; vomiting has not occurred with ingestion of more than one bulb; activated charcoal with cathartic/lavage may be beneficial depending on amount ingested and time elapsed since ingestion

Supportive therapy: Wash skin extremely thoroughly with soap and water

Additional Information All parts contain alkaloid; bulb is most toxic

Narcissus *see* Daffodil *on page 1076*

Narcissus jonquilla *see* Jonquil *on page 1094*

Narcissus pseudo-narcissus *see* Daffodil *on page 1076*

Natal Cherry *see* Christmas Cherry *on page 1068*

Nephthytis

Scientific Name *Syngonium*; *Syngonium podophyllum*

Synonyms African Evergreen; Arrow Head Vine

Mechanism of Toxic Action Contains insoluble calcium oxalate crystals which cause mechanical irritation; may also cause irritation through an unclear enzymatic process

Signs & Symptoms of Acute Overdose

Dermal: Pain, irritation, swelling

Ocular: Sap may cause pain, lacrimation, photophobia, corneal abrasion; oxalate crystals may be deposited on cornea; may also cause dermatitis reaction

Oral: Edema, vomiting, diarrhea, salivation, dysphonia

Toxicodynamics/Kinetics Rapid onset of local symptoms

Overdosage Treatment
Decontamination:
Dermal: Wash thoroughly
Ocular: Irrigate
Oral: Dilute; ipecac/lavage/activated charcoal not likely necessary
Supportive therapy: Cool compresses may minimize pain and swelling

Nerium odorum *see* Oleander *on next page*

Nerium oleander *see* Oleander *on next page*

Nicotiana glauca *see* Mustard Tree *on page 1117*

Nicotiana tabacum *see* Tobacco *on page 1150*

N-Methyl-Cathinone *see* Methcathinone *on page 1106*

"Nut-Brown" *Collybia* Mushroom *see* Mushrooms, Toxic (Group VII) *on page 1116*

Nutmeg

Scientific Name *Myristica fragrans*

Use In folk medicine for delayed menses

Mechanism of Toxic Action One theory for nutmeg's pharmacologic properties is that myristicin and elemicin are metabolized to psychoactive amphetamine derivatives, MMDA (3-methoxy-4,5 dimethylenedioxyamphetamine) and TMA (3,4,5-trimethoxyamphetamine); geraniol is a potent emetic

Signs & Symptoms of Acute Overdose The most prominent effects of significant ingestions appear to be hallucinations, nausea, and profound vomiting; miosis, tachycardia, mydriasis, hypothermia, dry skin, hypotension, and a feeling of impending doom may also be seen; symptoms may be delayed up to 8 hours after ingestion

Toxic Dosage It is estimated that 2 tablespoons of ground nutmeg will produce toxicity; however, amounts may vary depending on the content of volitile oil

Overdosage Treatment
Decontamination: Administer activated charcoal with cathartic for recent substantial ingestions
Supportive therapy: Symptomatic and supportive treatment as needed

Pregnancy Implications Nutmeg ingestion has been reported to increase fetal heart rate

Additional Information Nutmeg is the seed of *Myristica fragrans*; the spice mace is from the seed coat of *Myristica fragrans*
Family: Myristicaceae
Toxin: Myristicin, elemicin, geraniol
Range: Grows in India, Ceylon, and Granada
Toxic parts: Volitile oil in seed and seed coat appears to be responsible for pharmacologic effects

Specific References

Abernethy MK and Becker LB, "Acute Nutmeg Intoxication," *Am J Emerg Med*, 1992, 10(5):429-30.
Lavy G, "Nutmeg Intoxication in Pregnancy. A Case Report," *J Reprod Med*, 1987, 32(1):63-4.
Shafran I, "Letter: Nutmeg Toxicology," *N Engl J Med*, 1976, 294(15):849.

Oak

Scientific Name *Quercus*

Signs & Symptoms of Acute Overdose Nausea, vomiting, abdominal pain, constipation, blood diarrhea, possible kidney and liver damage

Overdosage Treatment
Decontamination: Induction of vomiting is controversial, vomiting may be appropriate for large ingestions; activated charcoal and cathartics may also be of value
Supportive therapy: As needed

"Oak-Loving" *Collybia* Mushroom *see* Mushrooms, Toxic (Group VII) *on page 1116*

Oak Tree Seeds *see* Acorns *on page 1050*

Octopus

Scientific Name *Octopus bairdi*

Synonyms Devilfish

Mechanism of Toxic Action Bite – envenomation

Signs & Symptoms of Acute Overdose Pain, burning sensation, numbness, local ischemia, paresthesia, aphonia, slurred speech, blurred vision, coma, cardiovascular collapse

Adverse Reactions Local: Erythema

Overdosage Treatment Symptomatic/supportive/wound care; no antidote available

(Continued)

Octopus *(Continued)*

Additional Information Octopus bites are rare, but can result in severe envenomations if due to blue-ringed octopus

Range: Warm/shallow waters including rock pools in the intertidal zones

Specific References

Auerbach PS, Halstead BW, Bush RK, et al, "Hazardous Aquatic Life," *Management of Wilderness and Environmental Emergencies*, 2nd ed, Auerbach PS and Geehr EC, eds, St Louis, MO: CV Mosby Co, 1989, 933-1028.

Kizer KW, "Marine Envenomations," *J Toxicol Clin Toxicol*, 1983-84, 21(4-5):527-55.

Octopus bairdi *see* Octopus *on previous page*

Oculinum® (Botulinum A Toxin) *see Clostridium botulinum* Food Poisoning *on page 1070*

Ojode Pajaro *see* Jequirity Bean *on page 1093*

Old Wife's Hood *see* Monkshood *on page 1108*

Oleander

Scientific Name *Nerium odorum*; *Nerium oleander*

Synonyms Common Oleander; Rosebay; *Thevitia*; Yellow Oleander

Mechanism of Toxic Action Entire plant contains cardiac glycosides oleandrin, oleandroside, and neriin

Signs & Symptoms of Acute Overdose GI effects (nausea and vomiting) usually precede the cardiovascular effects by several hours; bradycardia; first, second, and third degree heart block; asystole, hypotension, A-V block, ventricular arrhythmias, atrial fibrillation, decreased Q-T interval and prolonged P-R interval; fatigue, confusion, headache, dizziness, delirium, contact dermatitis, seeing yellow halos, and hyperkalemia have also been reported

Toxic Dosage Variable toxicity of leaves depending on growing conditions and time of year; seven leaves have produced bradycardia, nausea, vomiting, and abdominal cramps

Overdosage Treatment

Decontamination: Lavage and multidose activated charcoal enhance total body clearance of digitalis; whole bowel irrigation is also beneficial in removing plant debris from the GI tract and is recommended for ingestions of large amounts of plant material

Supportive therapy: Monitor cardiac status and serum potassium levels; bradycardia will frequently respond to atropine; phenytoin is the recommended treatment for ventricular arrhythmias because it will also improve conduction through the A-V node; lidocaine can also be used to treat ventricular arrhythmias, but will not have an effect on A-V conduction; other antiarrhythmics which have been used in arrhythmias resistant to the above therapy include magnesium, amiodarone, and bretylium; a pacemaker should be considered for bradycardia and A-V nodal blocks resistant to medical management

Antidote: Digoxin immune Fab has been shown to interact with several different plant cardiac glycosides and may be beneficial in cases resistant to conventional treatment; indications for its use include ventricular arrhythmias resistant to conventional treatment, severe bradycardia and/or second or third degree heart block resistant to atropine and phenytoin

Antidote(s)

Digoxin Immune Fab *on page 1411*

Additional Information Toxin: Cardiac glycosides

Ololiuqui *see* Morning Glory *on page 1109*

***Omphalotus illudens* ("Jack-O'-Lantern")** *see* Mushrooms, Toxic (Group III) *on page 1112*

***Omphalotus olearius* ("Jack-O'-Lantern")** *see* Mushrooms, Toxic (Group III) *on page 1112*

Oncolea Stuthiopteris *see* Ostrich Fern *on next page*

Oregon Grape (Nontoxic Plant)

Oreline and Orellanine-Containing Mushrooms *see* Mushrooms, Toxic (Group VIII) *on page 1117*

Ornamental Pepper *see* Christmas Cherry *on page 1068*

Ornithogalum pyrenaicum *see* Star-of-Bethlehem (*Ornithogalum pyrenaicum*) *on page 1145*

Ornithogalum umbellatum *see* Star-of-Bethlehem (*Ornithogalum umbellatum*) *on page 1146*

Orphine *see Sedum on page 1140*

Ostrich Fern

Scientific Name Matteuccia Struthiopteris; Oncolea Stuthiopteris; Pteretis Struthiopteris

Synonyms Fiddlehead Fern

Mechanism of Toxic Action Essentially unknown; may contain a heat-labile toxin that can cause gastroenteritis

Signs & Symptoms of Acute Overdose Usually begins within 12 hours of ingestion (incubation mean: 6 hours); diarrhea, nausea, vomiting, abdominal pain, headache; symptoms usually last about 1 day

Overdosage Treatment

Supportive therapy: Primarily symptomatic; replace fluid loss either orally or with intravenous hydration

Additional Information Spring vegetable found in Eastern North America; a large fern with oblong shaped leaves found along rivers, streams, and coastal waters; usually nontoxic, but a gastroenteritis syndrome has recently been described; recommendation is to boil the plant for 15 minutes or steam for 10-12 minutes before eating

Specific References

"Ostrich Fern Poisoning – New York and Western Canada," *MMWR Morb Mortal Wkly Rep*, 1994, 43(37):677, 683-4.

Oxalis hedysaroides *see* Shamrock *on page 1140*

Ox-Eye Daisy *see* Chrysanthemum *on page 1069*

Pacific Yew *see* Yew *on page 1159*

***Paeonia* Species** *see* Peony (Common) *on page 1123*

Paeony *see* Peony (Common) *on page 1123*

Painted Leaf *see* Poinsettia *on page 1126*

Paneolus alter *see* Mushrooms, Toxic (Group VI) *on page 1115*

***Paneolus campanulatus* ("Bell-Shaped" *Panaeolus* or "Bell Mottlegill")** *see* Mushrooms, Toxic (Group VI) *on page 1115*

***Paneolus foenisecii* ("Mowers Mushroom")** *see* Mushrooms, Toxic (Group VI) *on page 1115*

Paneolus sphinetrinus *see* Mushrooms, Toxic (Group VI) *on page 1115*

***Paneolus subbalteatus* ("Girdled" *Panaeolus*)** *see* Mushrooms, Toxic (Group VI) *on page 1115*

Paneolus tropicalis *see* Mushrooms, Toxic (Group VI) *on page 1115*

Pansy

Scientific Name *Viola* Species

Mechanism of Toxic Action Myosin and glucosides produce a cathartic effect, but large ingestions are required

Signs & Symptoms of Acute Overdose Nausea, vomiting, diarrhea

Overdosage Treatment Supportive therapy: Fluid replacement is seldom required; home observation is the treatment of choice

Additional Information Toxin: Seeds contain myosin and glucosides

"Panther" *Amanita* Mushroom *see* Mushrooms, Toxic (Group III) *on page 1112*

"Panther" *Amanita* Mushroom *see* Mushrooms, Toxic (Group V) *on page 1114*

Parson Parsley *see* Poison Hemlock *on page 1126*

Parthenocissus *see* Boston Ivy *on page 1060*

Pasteurella multocida

Signs & Symptoms of Acute Overdose

* **Animal bite-wound infections:** Patients who have *Pasteurella* inoculated via a bite wound develop rapid onset of pain, erythema, and edema locally. This may occur within hours of the bite or may be delayed by several days. Common sites include the upper extremities (in particular, hands), legs, and the head and neck region. An important complication is the development of regional lymphadenopathy. Occasionally, *Pasteurella* infection may be the cause of lymph node enlargement of unknown etiology; such patients should be questioned about seemingly minor animal scratches as well. Bite-wound infections are often limited to soft tissue cellulitis or focal abscesses. At times,

(Continued)

Pasteurella multocida (Continued)

the course may be complicated by tenosynovitis and osteomyelitis, which can be particularly difficult to treat when involving the hand. Note that the specific entity known as "cat scratch disease" is not caused by *Pasteurella multocida*. The exact cause of this lymphadenopathy syndrome is still being debated.

* **Upper and lower respiratory infections:** This unusual presentation of *Pasteurella* infection may be seen in patients who have had a significant exposure to animals but lack a history of an animal bite. *Pasteurella* has been implicated as a rare cause of bronchitis, sinusitis, and pneumonia in both healthy individuals and those with underlying chronic bronchitis.
* **Infection in the immunocompromised host:** Serious and life-threatening *Pasteurella* infections have been reported in patients with underlying malignancies, organ transplantations, and HIV infection.
* **Miscellaneous infections:** Meningitis, arthritis, peritonitis (particularly patients undergoing peritoneal dialysis), corneal ulcers, ophthalmitis, and urinary tract infections are rarely reported.

Overdosage Treatment Supportive therapy: Drug of choice for pasteurellosis is penicillin. If the infection is minor and limited to soft tissue, a trial of oral penicillin may be attempted (eg, penicillin V, 500 mg orally every 6 hours). If the infection is more serious, parenteral penicillin should be used. This includes deep wound infections of the extremities, osteomyelitis, septic arthritis, tenosynovitis, and pneumonia. Consultation with an infectious disease specialist may be useful in complicated cases, where therapy may be prolonged and surgical debridement necessary. Other antimicrobial agents are probably effective but the clinical experience is more limited: tetracycline, ampicillin, possibly ciprofloxacin, and the cephalosporins. Infectious disease consultation may be helpful for therapy with alternative agents.

Additional Information

Microbiology: *Pasteurella multocida* is a gram-negative rod which is primarily a pathogen in wild and domestic animals, but is also capable of causing sporadic human diseases such as animal bite infection, osteomyelitis, pneumonia, and sepsis. *P. multocida* is an aerobic, gram-negative coccobacillus which does not form spores. It belongs to the family *Pasteurellaceae* and is thus related to *Haemophilus* species. There are six distinct species of *Pasteurella*, but the most common to cause human disease is *Pasteurella multocida*. Special requests for identification for this organism are helpful for the microbiology laboratory but are usually not necessary; the organism grows readily on several standard culture media such as blood agar or chocolate agar.

Epidemiology:

*P. multocida*is a normal commensal of the oropharynx and the gastrointestinal tract of several kinds of animals. However, it is only rarely recovered from the respiratory tract of humans, and has been found to be part of the normal oral flora only in individuals with significant animal contact (eg, veterinarians). The frequency of recovery of this organism from a healthy animal depends on the particular animal species, as follows: cats, 50% to 75%; dogs, 10% to 60%; pigs, 50%; and rats, 15%.

Pasteurella has been reported in all age groups. Human infection usually occurs following an animal bite or scratch. One study found that up to 17% of patients being treated in an emergency room for an animal bite ultimately developed a *Pasteurella* infection. Cat scratches or bites cause the majority of *Pasteurella* infections (about 65% of cases). Dog bites are responsible for about 35% of cases. A smaller number of cases of *Pasteurella* infections are due to animal exposures without a clear history of an animal bite or scratch. The patient tends to be frequently exposed to animals (such as a veterinarian, livestock handler, pet shop worker), and the infections are generally in the respiratory tract, although cases of intra-abdominal infection have also been described. A small percentage of patients are infected with *P. multocida* without any significant animal exposure.

Diagnosis: *P. multocida* infection should be included in the differential diagnosis of any wound infection following an animal bite or deep scratch. The diagnosis strongly suggested if the onset of local inflammation is within 3-24 hours of the bite, and if the animal involved was a cat. Longer periods of incubation are more suggestive of streptococcal or staphylococcal infection, although certainly cases of pasteurellosis may have a delayed onset. The diagnosis is more difficult for nonbite *Pasteurella* infections; the clinician must carefully inquire about unusual or prolonged animal exposures in the workplace and at home.

Paxillus involutus *see* Mushrooms, Toxic (Group VII) *on page 1116*

***Paxillus involutus* ("Naked Brimcap")** *see* Mushrooms, Toxic (Group VII) *on page 1116*

Peach

Scientific Name *Prunus persica* Species

Mechanism of Toxic Action Amygdalin (a cyanogenic glycoside) is hydrolyzed in the gut to release hydrocyanic acid; cellular hypoxia occurs after absorption and complexation with cytochrome oxidase

Signs & Symptoms of Acute Overdose Symptoms delayed 30 minutes to 2 hours or longer due to hydrolysis preferentially occurring in alkaline duodenum plus intestinal flora hydrolyzing amygdalin

Toxic Dosage 1-2 pits likely nontoxic; toxicity unusual with accidental ingestion

Overdosage Treatment

Decontamination: Basic poison management; vomiting is contraindicated due to rapid course of the neurologic symptoms. Give 100% oxygen.

Supportive therapy: Give sodium bicarbonate for acidosis

Enhancement of elimination: Hemodialysis and charcoal hemoperfusion have been utilized; hyperbaric oxygen may also be utilized; hydroxocobalamin and dicobalt-EDTA used for chelation in Europe

Antidote(s)

Cyanide Antidote Kit *on page 1406*

Diagnostic Tests/Procedures

Anion Gap, Blood *on page 1193*

Blood Gases, Arterial *on page 1207*

Electrolytes, Blood *on page 1254*

Methemoglobin, Blood *on page 1296*

Additional Information Amygdalin is also found in leaves, flowers, bark, seeds; young leaves have highest concentration; intact pit does not release chemical; apricot most toxic within species

Pearly Gates *see* Morning Glory *on page 1109*

Pear Tomato *see* Tomato (Leaves and Stems) *on page 1150*

Pediculus humanus *see* Lice *on page 1097*

Pencil Tree *see* Milkbush *on page 1107*

Peon *see* Peony (Common) *on this page*

Peony (Common)

Scientific Name *Paeonia* Species

Synonyms Paeony; Peon; Pion

Mechanism of Toxic Action Toxin is located in plant's roots and the site of action is unknown

Signs & Symptoms of Acute Overdose Contact dermatitis with dermal exposure; oral exposure based on rat data: low dose (62.5 mg/kg) produces a diuretic effect; medium dose (125-500 mg/kg) has anti-inflammatory activity and decreased GI secretions; high dose (>500 mg/kg) causes CNS depression

Toxicodynamics/Kinetics

Absorption: Rapid

Half-life: 30 minutes

Toxic Dosage Minimal clinical symptoms are expected with accidental plant ingestion; clinically significant doses may be seen in ingestions of many Oriental medicines which contain this ingredient; paeonol 250 mg/kg is about as effective of a diuretic as hydrochlorothiazide 10 mg/kg; LD_{50} (based on rat data): 3430 mg/kg

Overdosage Treatment Topical steroids are probably beneficial for contact dermatitis

Decontamination: Ipecac is of questionable benefit due to the rapid absorption and onset of action; activated charcoal with sorbitol will aid in clearance of the toxin

Supportive therapy: Respiratory support is most critical intervention; maintain fluid and electrolyte replacement during diuretic phase, however, electrolyte depletion is not as severe as with hydrochlorothiazide

Additional Information Monitor electrolytes during the diuretic phase

Toxin: Paeonol

Peperomia (Nontoxic Plant)

Pepper

Scientific Name *Capsicum annuum cenoides*

Synonyms Hot Pepper; Jalapeno Pepper

Mechanism of Toxic Action Contains capsaicin which is a mucous membrane irritant; may also stimulate pain fibers and interact with nerve axons

Signs & Symptoms of Acute Overdose Cough, vomiting, diarrhea; blistering and rash with topical exposure

(Continued)

Pepper *(Continued)*

Overdosage Treatment

Decontamination:

Oral: Emesis generally contraindicated in GI irritant ingestions; oxygen may help pulmonary irritation; with topical exposure, cold water and/or vinegar washes have been helpful as have soaks in vegetable oil; for extremely painful exposures, lidocaine and prilocaine (Emla®) may be of benefit

Ocular exposure: Irrigate with saline

Specific References

Burnett JW, "Capsicum Pepper Dermatitis," *Cutis*, 1989, 43(6):534.

"Pepper Caps" Mushroom *see* Mushrooms, Toxic (Group VII) *on page 1116*

"Pepper Milkcap" Mushroom *see* Mushrooms, Toxic (Group VII) *on page 1116*

Pepper Root *see* Corn Lily *on page 1074*

Pepper Turnip *see* Jack-in-the-Pulpit *on page 1093*

Persian Berry *see* Buckthorn *on page 1062*

Peyote

Related Information

Mescaline *on page 1106*

Scientific Name *Lophophora williamsii*

Synonyms Peyotyl

Mechanism of Toxic Action Mescaline - structurally similar to amphetamines producing CNS and sympathetic stimulation and hallucinations

Signs & Symptoms of Acute Overdose Hypertension, pulse, fever, respiratory rate, salivation, mydriasis, blurred vision, headache, dizziness, ataxia, drowsiness, tremor, asthenia, nausea/vomiting preceding hallucinations, hunger, polyuria, flushing, visual hallucinations, auditory hallucinations, anxiety, suicide, flashbacks, paranoia

Toxicodynamics/Kinetics Urine, blood levels not correlated with clinical effects

Overdosage Treatment

Decontamination: Ipecac may cause increased agitation especially in paranoid individuals and is unlikely to be of benefit once clinical symptoms present; activated charcoal with cathartic preferred

Supportive therapy: Symptoms may need to be treated with benzodiazepines and/or haloperidol/chlorpromazine; flashbacks may be worsened by phenothiazines; no deaths reported from overdosage of mescaline/peyote

Additional Information May be contaminated; consider coingestants; "microdots" may also contain LSD

Specific References

Kapadia GJ and Fayez BN, "Peyote Constituents: Chemistry, Biogenesis, and Biological Effects," *J Pharm Sci*, 1970, 59:1699-727.

Peyotyl *see* Peyote *on this page*

Philodendron

Scientific Name *Philodendron* Species

Mechanism of Toxic Action Entire plant contains calcium oxalate crystals which cause oral irritation, swelling, pain, and slurred speech; large ingestions necessary for systemic toxicity are unlikely to occur due to oral irritation seen with ingestion

Signs & Symptoms of Acute Overdose Oral irritation, swelling, pain, vomiting, and slurred speech

Overdosage Treatment

Decontamination: Emesis or lavage/activated charcoal not usually necessary unless massive ingestion is suspected; dilution may be beneficial; milk/water to rinse crystals

Supportive therapy: I.V. hydration may be needed

Additional Information

Toxin: Calcium oxalate crystals concentration is <1%

Fatal dose due to oxalates is estimated to be 700 g of leaves (5 g of oxalate)

Specific References

Mrvos R, Dean BS, and Krenzelok EP, "Philodendron/Dieffenbachia Ingestions: Are They a Problem?" *J Toxicol Clin Toxicol*, 1991, 29(4):485-91.

McIntire MS, Guest JR, and Porterfield JF, "Philodendron – Infant Death," *J Toxicol Clin Toxicol*, 1990, 28(2):177-83.

***Philodendron* Species** *see* Philodendron *on this page*

***Pholiota squarrosa* ("Shaggy Scalecap")** *see* Mushrooms, Toxic (Group VII) *on page 1116*

Phoradendron flavescens *see* Mistletoe *on page 1107*

Phoradendron macrophyllum *see* Mistletoe *on page 1107*

Phoradendron rubrum *see* Mistletoe *on page 1107*

Phoradendron serotinum *see* Mistletoe *on page 1107*

Phoradendron tomentosum *see* Mistletoe *on page 1107*

Phthirus pubis *see* Lice *on page 1097*

Physalia pelagica *see* Portuguese Man-of-War *on page 1128*

Physalia utriculus *see* Portuguese Man-of-War *on page 1128*

***Physobrachia* Species** *see* Sea Anemones *on page 1138*

Phytolacca americana *see* Pokeweed *on page 1127*

Pigeon Berry *see* Pokeweed *on page 1127*

Piggy-Back Plant (Nontoxic Plant)

Pilea (Nontoxic Plant)

Pine Cone [seed] (Nontoxic Plant)

Pink *Allamanda* *see* Rubber Vine *on page 1134*

Pink Cloud *see* Caladium *on page 1063*

Pink Polka Dot Plant (Nontoxic Plant)

Pin Oak Ivy *see* English Ivy *on page 1081*

Pinxter Flower *see* Azalea *on page 1055*

Pion *see* Peony (Common) *on page 1123*

Piper Methysticum *see* Kava Kava *on page 1095*

"Pitted Milkcap" Mushroom *see* Mushrooms, Toxic (Group VII) *on page 1116*

Pit Vipers

Commonly Found in *Genera crotalus* (rattlesnake), *Agkistrodon* (copperhead, cottonmouth), *Sistrurus* (pygmy rattler, massasauga)

Mechanism of Toxic Action Venom; quality and potency vary among species; composition: 90% water with 5-15 enzymes, 3-12 nonenzymatic proteins, as well as other unidentified substances

Signs & Symptoms of Acute Overdose Local signs include tenderness, edema, erythema, ecchymoses, hemorrhage, bullae, lymphangitis, and rarely a compartment syndrome. Systemic signs and symptoms include hypotension, asthenia, sweating, chills, paresthesia, nausea, vomiting, fasciculations, and CNS depression; coagulopathy can occur including thrombocytopenia, hypofibrinogenemia, increased PT and PTT. Shock, hypotension, lactic acidosis, hemoconcentration, hypoproteinemia, proteinuria, and hematuria are also potential complications.

Overdosage Treatment

Decontamination: Rapid transport to medical facility; immobilize area; if negative pressure suction device is available, this may be used; do not incise the wound; constriction band may be applied, **not** a tourniquet

Wyeth crotalid polyvalent antivenin; treat moderate to severe envenomations with increments of 5-10 vials at a time; skin test per manufacturer's instructions; if positive skin test develops, may prophylax with H_1- and H_2-receptor blockers; give until local injury has stopped and coagulopathy is reversed; complications include allergic reactions, anaphylaxis, and delayed serum sickness

Supportive therapy: ABC assessment, physical exam; mark the extent of local edema with skin marking pen; repeat CBC, platelets, PT, PTT, fibrinogen, CPK, UA every 3-4 hours for at least first 12 hours; I.V. fluids, tetanus prophylaxis, and analgesics may be given as needed; treat infected wounds with antibiotics. Snakes' mouths contain primarily gram-negative and anaerobic organisms.

Additional Information

Family: Viperidae; subfamily: Crotalidae

Distinguishing characteristics: Facial pits, vertical elliptical pupils, triangular head, single row of subcaudal scales

All poisonous serpents except coral snakes belong to this group; copperheads, cottonmouths, and rattlesnakes are members

Specific References

Hassen LB, "Reptile and Arthropod Envenomations," *Occup Med*, 1991, 6(3):447-61.

Simon TL and Grace TG, "Envenomation Coagulopathy in Wounds From Pit Vipers," *N Engl J Med*, 1981, 305(8):443-7.

(Continued)

Pit Vipers *(Continued)*

Sullivan JB Jr and Wingert WA, "Reptile Bites," *Management of Wilderness and Environmental Emergencies*, 2nd ed, Auerbach PS and Geehr EC, eds, St Louis, MO: CV Mosby Co, 1989, 479-511.

Plectranthus (Nontoxic Plant)

Adverse Reactions *Fruticosus* species contains a volatile with pharmacologic and teratogenic properties

Podophyllum peltatum *see* Mayapple *on page 1105*

Poinsettia

Related Information

Star-of-Bethlehem (*Ornithogalum pyrenaicum*) *on page 1145*
Star-of-Bethlehem (*Ornithogalum umbellatum*) *on page 1146*

Scientific Name *Euphorbia pulcherrima*

Synonyms Christmas Flower; Christmas Star; Julestjerne; Lobster Plant; Mexican Flameleaf; Painted Leaf

Signs & Symptoms of Acute Overdose Frequently believed to be a toxic, even lethal plant, the poinsettia has little toxicity; nausea, vomiting, and skin irritation are rarely reported to Poison Control Centers; gastrointestinal symptoms are mild, self limited, and seldom require fluid replacement. Estimates, based on animal data, indicated that a 50-pound child would have to ingest 500-600 leaves to cause symptoms.

Overdosage Treatment Wash off patient if irritation is experienced; dilute with water, milk, or juice for ingestions

Additional Information

Family: Euphorbiaceae
Toxin: Acrid principle, not fully defined chemically
Range: Tropical plant widely distributed as a Christmas decoration

Specific References

D'Arcy WG, "Severe Contact Dermatitis From Poinsettia," *Arch Dermatol*, 1974, 109(6):909-10.
Klug S, Saleem G, Honcharuk L, et al, "Toxicity Potential of Poinsettia: Is a Plant Really Toxic?" *Vet Hum Toxicol*, 1990, 32:368.
Winek CL, Butala J, Shanor SP, et al, "Toxicology of Poinsettia," *Clin Toxicol*, 1978, 13(1):27-45.

Poison Flag *see* Iris *on page 1092*

Poison Hemlock

Scientific Name *Conium maculatum*

Synonyms Deadly Hemlock; Parson Parsley; Spotted Hemlock; Winter Fern

Mechanism of Toxic Action Coniine toxicity resembles that of nicotine; there is initial stimulation of autonomic ganglia, followed by depression

Signs & Symptoms of Acute Overdose Nausea, ataxia, vomiting, and burn sensation in the throat; tachycardia, followed by bradycardia, seizures, slurred speech, paralysis of skeletal muscles, myoglobinuria, rhabdomyolysis, apnea, renal failure, respiratory paralysis

Overdosage Treatment

Decontamination: Lavage may be performed, administer activated charcoal with cathartic; manage seizures with diazepam

Supportive therapy: Be prepared to support respirations; provide symptomatic and supportive treatment

Pregnancy Implications Coniine is teratogenic in animals

Additional Information Reportedly used by the Greeks to execute Socrates; human toxicity has been reported from eating birds that feed on poison hemlock

Family: Umbelliferae
Range: Found in the Eastern U.S., the West coast, and the Rocky Mountains
Toxin: Coniine
Toxic parts: Whole plant

Specific References

Bowman WC and Sanghvi IS, "Pharmacological Actions of Hemlock (*Conium maculatum*) Alkaloids," *J Pharm Pharmacol*, 1963, 15(1):1-25.
Rizzi D, Basile C, Di Maggio A, et al, "Rhabdomyolysis and Acute Tubular Necrosis in Coniine (Hemlock) Poisoning," *Lancet*, 1989, 2(8677):1461-2.

Poison Ivy

Scientific Name *Toxicodendron radicans*

Mechanism of Toxic Action Contains urushiol; shell contains anacardic acid, cardol, anacardol, irritants that can precipitate type IV cell-mediated allergic reaction (allergic contact dermatitis)

Signs & Symptoms of Acute Overdose Dermatitis, proteinuria

Toxicodynamics/Kinetics

Onset of effect: Variable, but effects usually seen within 24-48 hours

Peak effect: After 3-5 days

Overdosage Treatment

Decontamination: Soap and water washing likely ineffective unless done within 5-15 minutes after exposure

Supportive therapy: Cool compresses or showers, Burow's solution, topical/oral steroids

Additional Information Sap of entire plant is toxic

Poison Oak

Scientific Name *Toxicodendron guercifolium*

Mechanism of Toxic Action Contains urushiol; shell contains anacardic acid, cardol, anacardol, irritants that can precipitate type IV cell-mediated allergic reaction (allergic contact dermatitis)

Signs & Symptoms of Acute Overdose Dermatitis

Toxicodynamics/Kinetics

Onset of effect: Variable, but effects usually seen within 24-48 hours

Peak effect: After 3-5 days

Overdosage Treatment

Decontamination: Soap and water washing likely ineffective unless done within 5-15 minutes after exposure

Supportive therapy: Cool compresses or showers, Burow's solution, topical/oral steroids

Additional Information Sap of entire plant is toxic

Poisonous Nightshade *see* Deadly Nightshade *on page 1078*

"Poison Pie" Mushroom *see* Mushrooms, Toxic (Group VII) *on page 1116*

Poison Sego *see* Death Camas *on page 1078*

Poison Sumac

Scientific Name *Toxicodendron vernex*

Mechanism of Toxic Action Contains urushiol, shell contains anacardic acid, cardol, anacardol, irritants that can precipitate type IV cell-mediated allergic reaction (allergic contact dermatitis)

Signs & Symptoms of Acute Overdose Dermatitis

Toxicodynamics/Kinetics

Onset of effect: Variable, but effects usually seen within 24-48 hours

Peak effect: After 3-5 days

Overdosage Treatment

Decontamination: Soap and water washing likely ineffective unless done within 5-15 minutes after exposure

Supportive therapy: Cool compresses or showers, Burow's solution, topical/oral steroids

Additional Information Sap of entire plant is toxic

Pokeberry *see* Pokeweed *on this page*

Pokeweed

Scientific Name *Phytolacca americana*

Synonyms American Nightshade; Inkberry; Pigeon Berry; Pokeberry

Use In folk medicine for rheumatism, arthritis, ringworm, and purgative, etc

Signs & Symptoms of Acute Overdose Abdominal pain, nausea, A-V block, vomiting, diarrhea, dyspnea, seizures, and death

Adverse Reactions Cardiovascular: Mobitz type 1 heart block

Overdosage Treatment

Decontamination: Administer activated charcoal (in aqueous slurry) for recent ingestions

Supportive therapy: Replace fluids and electrolytes as needed

Additional Information Young leaves may be rendered nontoxic if boiled, rinsed, and boiled again; berries also appear to be edible if cooked

Family: Phytolaccaceae

Toxin: Triterpene saponins, pokeweed mitogen

Range: Eastern half of the U.S., California, and Hawaii

Toxic part: Whole plant, especially the root

Specific References

Hamilton RG, Shih RD, and Hoffman RS, "Mobitz Type I Heart Block After Pokeweed Ingestion," *Vet Hum Toxicol*, 1995, 27(1):66-7.

Lewis WG and Smith PR, "Poke Root Herbal Tea Poisoning," *JAMA*, 1979, 242(25):2759-60.

Populage *see* Marsh Marigold *on page 1105*

Portuguese Man-of-War

Scientific Name *Physalia pelagica; Physalia utriculus*

Commonly Found in Atlantic Portuguese Man-of-War (*Physalia physalis*); Pacific Portuguese Man-of-War (*Physalia utriculus*)

Signs & Symptoms of Acute Overdose Macular papular rash with intense pain; may progress to hyperpigmented vesicles and pustules; systemic reaction includes asthenia, nausea, vomiting, muscle spasms, pain, paresthesia, in rare cases, respiratory and cardiovascular depression; systemic effects are more common with the Atlantic Portuguese Man-of-War; symptoms can occur for up to 48 hours

Overdosage Treatment

Decontamination: Immobilize area to avoid further discharge of nematocysts; inactivate nematocysts with alcohol or vinegar; remove remaining tentacles by applying flour or shave cream and scraping with a sharp instrument

Supportive therapy: Pain control, oral antihistamine, local anesthetics, steroid cream, and tetanus prophylaxis as indicated; systemic effects may require respiratory and circulatory support

Additional Information Invertebrate, contains a nitrogen and carbon monoxide flotation device which functions as a sail similar to a Portuguese admiral's hat; venom consists of a protein neurotoxin

Specific References

Auerbach PS, "Coelenterate (Man-of-War) Envenomations," *West J Med*, 1983, 138:85.

Kaufman MB, "Portuguese Man-of-War Envenomation," *Pediatr Emerg Care*, 1992, 8(1):27-8.

Kizer KW, "Marine Envenomations," *J Toxicol Clin Toxicol*, 1983-84, 21(4-5):527-55.

Stein MR, Marraccini JV, Rothschild NE, et al, "Fatal Portuguese Man-of-War (*Physalia physalis*) Envenomation," *Ann Emerg Med*, 1989, 18(3):312-5.

Potassium Metabisulfite *see* Sulfite Food Poisoning *on page 1148*

Potato (Leaves, Stems, Tubercles)

Scientific Name *Solanum tuberosum*

Mechanism of Toxic Action Contains toxic alkaloids, solanine most significant structurally similar to cardioglycoside, causes hemolytic and hemorrhagic damage to GI tract similar to saponins; some plants may also contain alpha-cholinergic alkaloids

Signs & Symptoms of Acute Overdose Nausea, vomiting, diarrhea, headache, visual changes, drowsiness, fever, sweating, asthenia, hallucinations, anticholinergic effects may or may not be present to varying degrees

Toxicodynamics/Kinetics Unclear

Toxic Dosage Variable

Overdosage Treatment

Decontamination: Ipecac if vomiting has not already occurred, lavage and/or charcoal may be beneficial if patient presents symptomatic

Supportive therapy: Maintain fluid and electrolyte balance as necessary, support vital signs; physostigmine will reverse anticholinergic toxicity that may be associated with exposure

Antidote(s)

Physostigmine *on page 1457*

Additional Information Mature, properly stored tuber is edible; green foliage, immature tuber, improperly stored tuber (exposed to light) may be toxic

Specific References

Dalvi RR and Bowie WC, "Toxicology of Solanine: An Overview," *Vet Hum Toxicol*, 1983, 25(1):13-5.

"Potent" *Psilocybe* Mushroom *see* Mushrooms, Toxic (Group VI) *on page 1115*

Pothos Plant *see* Devil's Ivy *on page 1079*

Pothos Vine *see* Devil's Ivy *on page 1079*

Potosina *see* Century Plant *on page 1067*

"Poznan Cort" Mushroom *see* Mushrooms, Toxic (Group VIII) *on page 1117*

Prairie Rattlesnake *see* Rattlesnakes *on page 1132*

Prayer Bead *see* Jequirity Bean *on page 1093*

Prayer Bean *see* Jequirity Bean *on page 1093*

Prayer Plant (Nontoxic Plant)

Precatory Bean *see* Jequirity Bean *on page 1093*

Precatory Pea *see* Jequirity Bean *on page 1093*

Principal Pharmacological Properties of Hallucinogenic Drugs
see page 1557

Privet (Berries and Leaves)

Scientific Name *Ligustrum vulgare*

Signs & Symptoms of Acute Overdose Symptoms develop shortly after ingestion and include gastrointestinal irritation, abdominal tenderness, nausea, vomiting, diarrhea

Overdosage Treatment

Decontamination: Emesis/lavage usually not necessary due to vomiting which commonly occurs when the plant is ingested

Supportive therapy: Replace fluid/electrolyte losses

Additional Information Toxin: Ligon glycosides, saponins, and seco-iridoid bitter agents

Purple Passion (Nontoxic Plant)

Pussywillow (Nontoxic Plant)

Adverse Reactions Dermatitis has been reported with some species

Pyracantha (Nontoxic Plant)

Adverse Reactions May cause gastrointestinal upset

Rabies Virus

Mechanism of Toxic Action Rabies virus is a bullet-shaped single-stranded RNA virus which belongs to the family Rhabdoviridae. A number of important viral proteins have been identified such as viral polymerase, nucleocapsid protein, glycoprotein, and others. Some of these proteins have been used to develop specific di-

(Continued)

Rabies Virus *(Continued)*

agnostic monoclonal antibodies. Rabies virus can be isolated under the proper conditions in tissue culture. During active rabies infection, the virus can be cultured from a variety of human (and animal) tissues including saliva, brain tissue, respiratory secretions, and urine; the virus is most easily recovered from brain tissue.

The virus is highly neurotropic. When a human is inoculated with rabies virus, the viral glycoprotein attaches to the plasma membrane of cells, possibly the nicotinic acetylcholine receptor. The virus then replicates in skeletal muscle, and when the titer is high enough, it invades nearby sensory and motor nerves and enters the nervous system. It travels along the axon at speeds up to 20 mm/day and eventually reaches the spinal cord. From there, dissemination through the central nervous system occurs rapidly and encephalitis ensues. Other peripheral nerves become involved; the organism can be recovered from the saliva due to infection of nerves in the salivary glands.

Signs & Symptoms of Acute Overdose

Clinical rabies: There is a variable period of incubation before the onset of symptoms (4 days to 19 years), but most cases occur within 1 year of exposure. The initial prodrome of rabies is nonspecific with malaise, fatigue, and fever. In many patients, there may be pain at the initial exposure site. After about 10 days, the patient enters an acute neurologic phase, characterized by bizarre behavior, hyperactivity, and confusion. Photophobia, anisocoria, areflexia, and paresthesia may be noted. A small stimulus can elicit short periods of thrashing, biting, and other behaviors. Many patients will display hydrophobia (fear of water); there is often severe laryngospasm and choking when trying to drink water. This will progress to paralysis, which dominates the clinical picture for some days. Patients typically lapse into coma and develop respiratory failure or arrhythmias, leading to death in most cases despite full support in intensive care units. Occasional cases of recovery from rabies have been reported.

Overdosage Treatment

Supportive therapy: There is currently no treatment for rabies once it has become clinically established. Mortality approaches 100%. Thus, the main treatment issues involve rabies prevention, particularly postexposure prophylaxis. The physician deciding whether or not to initiate rabies treatment (rabies vaccine, rabies immunoglobulin) must answer the following questions: Has a significant exposure occurred, and what is the risk that an animal is rabid?

A significant exposure includes the following.

- An animal bite, defined as penetration of the person's skin by teeth with contamination of the wound with saliva
- Contamination of the mucous membranes with saliva or other potentially infectious tissue from an infected animal
- Certain nonbite exposures, including contamination of scratches, scrapes, wounds, or mucous membranes with saliva or other infectious tissues. The risk of rabies after nonbite exposures is extremely rare, although scattered cases have been reported.

Petting a rabid animal or contacting its blood or body fluids is not an exposure. If it appears that a significant exposure has taken place, the physician must determine whether or not the animal was rabid. As outlined by Fishbein and Robinson, this depends on the percentage of animals found to be rabid in the species in the particular geographical area.

Group 1: Rabies is endemic in animal species involved in exposure. This includes:

* bats – anywhere in the United States (3% to 20% positive for rabies); almost 50% of the rabies cases in the U.S. since 1980 were associated with bat vectors
* terrestrial animals – skunks, raccoons, foxes in areas of United States where rabies is endemic
* dogs in developing countries
* dogs in the United States along the Mexican border.

For Group 1 exposure, treatment should be initiated for both bite and nonbite exposures.

Group 2: Rabies is not endemic in species involved but is endemic in other wild animals in the area. The risk of rabies is about ten times lower in these animals compared with the predominant species. These animals include:

* wild carnivores such as wolves, bobcats, bears, and groundhogs. Up to 20% may have rabies. Bite exposures from these should be treated. Nonbite exposures should either be treated or the local health department consulted.
* rodents (squirrels, hamsters, guinea pigs, gerbils, rats, mice) have a low incidence of rabies, 0.01%. Bite exposures should not be treated (or in exceptional cases, the local health department could be consulted). Nonbite exposures should not be treated.
* dogs and cats – in the United States, the risk of rabies in dogs is less than 1% (except along the Mexican border) in areas where rabies is common in other

land animals. In addition, dogs almost always show signs of clinical rabies shortly after the virus is present in saliva. Bite exposure should not be treated if a healthy dog (or cat) is captured; the animal should be observed for 10 days. If the animal develops signs of rabies, treatment in the human should be commenced immediately. If the animal is a stray, it should be sacrificed immediately and the head removed and shipped to an appropriate laboratory. Treatment is delayed pending laboratory testing. The same approach is recommended for nonbite exposures.

Group 3: Rabies is not endemic in the animal species involved in the exposure and is uncommon in other wild animals in the region. This incudes most domestic cats and dogs and wild land animals in Idaho, Washington, Utah, Nevada, and Colorado, where the proportion of rabid animals is very low. For bite or nonbite exposures from Group 3 animals, either consult the local health department or do not treat.

Postexposure treatment consists of:

1. Vigorous wound cleaning – this has been shown to decrease the risk of rabies.
2. Administration or rabies vaccine, either human diploid-cell rabies vaccine or rabies vaccine adsorbed. For persons not previously vaccinated, rabies vaccine should be given 1 mL I.M. on days 0, 3, 7, 14, and 28. Abbreviated regimens have been described. For persons previously vaccinated, the rabies vaccine should be given 1 mL I.M. on days 0 and 3.
3. Administration of rabies immunoglobulin. For persons not previously vaccinated, this should be given at 20 IU/kg of body weight. If possible, one-half the dose should be injected locally near the original wound and the rest given I.M. (using a new needle). For persons previously vaccinated, rabies immunoglobulin is not recommended.

Diagnostic Tests/Procedures

Rabies Identification *on page 1345*

Additional Information

Epidemiology:

Rabies remains primarily a disease of animals, not humans. In many areas of Asia, Africa, and Latin America, canine rabies is poorly controlled, and dogs account for up to 90% of animal rabies cases. In contrast, in Europe and the United States, dogs account for a much lower percentage of cases. In the United States, different species of animals are involved in well-defined geographic areas. For example, raccoons are important in two regions, the Eastern seaboard states (New York, New Jersey, Delaware, Maryland, Virginia) and some Southeastern states (Florida, South Carolina, Georgia, Alabama). Skunks predominate in the North Central states and California, gray foxes in Texas and Arizona, and coyotes in southern Texas. A total of ten distinct geographic areas in the United States have been identified; one terrestrial animal predominates and one antigenic variant of the rabies virus predominates. Bats remain an important reservoir of rabies and cause sporadic cases.

Human rabies is distinctly unusual in the United States although it is still problematic in some areas worldwide. In large part, this is due to the control of canine rabies in this country. Between 1980 and 1993, there were 18 reported cases of rabies in the United States with 10 of these acquired outside the country. Of the rabies cases reported since 1960, the great majority involved males younger than 16 years of age or older than 50 years of age. Most cases in the United States are now reported from the following groups:

* U.S. travelers to foreign countries who sustain a dog bite in a rabies-endemic region
* persons bitten by wild animals in the U.S.
* persons with unknown exposure history

A few cases of "nonbite rabies" have been reported. These include:

* laboratory exposure to rabies virus (aerosolized virus)
* rabies contracted from corneal transplant from an infected donor (4 cases)
* inhalation of aerosolized virus in caves with high concentrations of bat secretions (rare)
* contact of virus on mucous membranes, scratches, or eyes (rare)

Diagnosis: Currently, there are no tests available to detect rabies prior to the development of symptoms. The virus is felt to be immunologically "protected" in the muscle cells or nerve cells near the inoculation site, and antibody production occurs late in infection. Rabies encephalitis may be difficult to distinguish from other forms of viral encephalitis. Laboratory tests available include:

* rabies neutralizing antibody
* rabies viral culture of saliva, cerebrospinal fluid, urine, respiratory secretions
* brain biopsy – specimens may be submitted for rabies viral culture; immunofluorescent rabies antibody staining of brain cells; and pathologic examination for Negri bodies, which are cytoplasmic inculsions characteristic of rabies encephalitis seen in 20% to 30% of cases.

(Continued)

Rabies Virus *(Continued)*

Specific References

Bernard KW and Fishbein DB, "Rabies Virus," *Principles and Practice of Infectious Diseases*, 3rd ed, Mandell GL, Douglas RG Jr, and Benett JE, eds, New York, NY: Churchill Livingstone, 1990, 1291-303.

Center for Disease Control, Human Rabies, California - 1994," *MMWR Morb Mortal Wkly Rep*, 1994, 43(25):455-8.

Center for Disease Control, Mass Treatment of Humans Exposed to Rabies - New Hampshire 1994," *MMWR Morb Mortal Wkly Rep*, 1995, 44:484-6.

Fishbein DB and Robinson LE, "Rabies," *N Engl J Med*, 1993, 329(22):1632-8.

Ramaria formosa *see* Mushrooms, Toxic (Group VII) *on page 1116*

***Ramaria gelantinosa* ("Oregon Gelatinous Coral")** *see* Mushrooms, Toxic (Group VII) *on page 1116*

Ranunculus aquatilis *see* Buttercup *on page 1063*

Rattlesnakes

Scientific Name *Crotalus adamanteus*; *Crotalus atrox*; *Crotalus horridus*; *Crotalus lepidus*; *Crotalus molossus*; *Crotalus scutulatus*; *Crotalus viridis*; *Sistrurus catenatus*; *Sistrurus miliarius*

Synonyms Banded Rock Rattlesnake; Black-Tailed Rattlesnake; Canebrake Rattlesnake; Carolina Pygmy Rattlesnake; Dusky Pygmy Rattlesnake; Eastern Diamondback Rattlesnake; Eastern Massasauga; Mojave Rattlesnake; Mottled Rock Rattlesnake; Prairie Rattlesnake; *Sistrurus* (Pygmy Rattler, Massasauga); Timber Rattlesnake; Western Diamondback Rattlesnake; Western Massasauga; Western Pygmy Rattlesnake

Mechanism of Toxic Action Venom; quality and potency vary among species; composition: 90% water with 5-15 enzymes, 3-12 nonenzymatic proteins, as well as other unidentified substances

Signs & Symptoms of Acute Overdose Local signs include tenderness, edema, erythema, ecchymoses, hemorrhage, bullae, lymphangitis, and rarely a compartment syndrome. Systemic signs and symptoms include hypotension, asthenia, sweating, chills, paresthesia, nausea, vomiting, fasciculations, and CNS depression; coagulopathy can occur including thrombocytopenia, hypofibrinogenemia, increased PT and PTT. Shock, hypotension, lactic acidosis, hemoconcentration, hypoproteinemia, proteinuria, and hematuria are also potential complications. Neurotoxic effects of Mojave rattlesnake venom may be delayed in onset

Overdosage Treatment

Decontamination: Rapid transport to medical facility; immobilize area; if negative pressure suction device is available, this may be used; do not incise the wound; constriction band may be applied, **not** a tourniquet

Wyeth Crotalid Polyvalent antivenin; treat moderate to severe envenomations with increments of 5-10 vials at a time; skin test per manufacturer's instructions; if positive skin test develops, may prophylax with H_1- and H_2-receptor blockers; give until local injury has stopped and coagulopathy is reversed; complications include allergic reactions, anaphylaxis, and delayed serum sickness

Supportive therapy: ABC assessment, physical exam; mark the extent of local edema with skin marking pen; repeat CBC, platelets, PT, PTT, fibrinogen, CPK, UA every 3-4 hours for at least first 12 hours; I.V. fluids, tetanus prophylaxis, and analgesics may be given as needed; treat infected wounds with antibiotics. Snakes' mouths contain primarily gram-negative and anaerobic organisms.

Antidote(s)

Antivenin (Crotalidae) Polyvalent *on page 1392*

Additional Information Family: *Crotalidae* (Pit Viper)

Banded Rock Rattlesnake: *Crotalus lepidus klauberi*
Black-Tailed Rattlesnake: *Crotalus molossus molossus*
Canebrake Rattlesnake: *Crotalus horridus atricaudatus*
Carolina Pygmy Rattlesnake: *Sistrurus miliarius miliarius*
Dusky Pygmy Rattlesnake: *Sistrurus miliarius barbouri*
Eastern Diamondback Rattlesnake: *Crotalus adamanteus*
Eastern Massasauga: *Sistrurus catenatus catenatus*
Mojave Rattlesnake: *Crotalus scutulatus scutulatus*
Mottled Rock Rattlesnake: *Crotalus lepidus lepidus*
Prairie Rattlesnake: *Crotalus viridis viridis*
Timber Rattlesnake: *Crotalus horridus horridus*
Western Diamondback Rattlesnake: *Crotalus atrox*
Western Massasauga: *Sistrurus catenatus tergeminus*
Western Pygmy Rattlesnake: *Sistrurus miliarius streckeri*

Specific References

Hassen LB, "Reptile and Arthropod Envenomations," *Occup Med*, 1991, 6(3):447-61.

Sullivan JB Jr and Wingert WA, "Reptile Bites," *Management of Wilderness and Environmental Emergencies*, 2nd ed, Auerbach PS and Geehr EC, eds, St Louis, MO: CV Mosby Co, 1989, 479-511.

Rattlesnake Weed *see* Corn Lily *on page 1074*

Red Berried Elder *see* Elderberry *on page 1081*

Red Flame *see* Shamrock *on page 1140*

"Red-Footed Bolete" Mushroom *see* Mushrooms, Toxic (Group VII) *on page 1116*

"Red Milkcap" Mushroom *see* Mushrooms, Toxic (Group VII) *on page 1116*

"Red-Pored Bolete" Mushroom *see* Mushrooms, Toxic (Group III) *on page 1112*

"Red-Pored Bolete" Mushroom *see* Mushrooms, Toxic (Group VII) *on page 1116*

Red Sage *see* Lantana *on page 1096*

Reduvids

Scientific Name *Reduviidae* Family; *Triatoma sanguisuga*

Synonyms Assassin Bugs; "Kissing Bugs"; Mexican Bed Bug

Signs & Symptoms of Acute Overdose Multiple, essentially painless bites; dermal lesions may be papular, vesicular, or rash; nausea, vomiting, lymphangitis, may also occur; laryngeal and oropharyngeal edema may occur in sensitive individuals

Overdosage Treatment Supportive therapy: Ice to area decreases edema and pain; antihistamine may be useful for rash, lesions

Additional Information

Characteristics: Almost 1" in length, *Triatoma sanguisuga* is dark brown with orange markings along the posterior two-thirds of its body

Range: Located on the Pacific coast; habits are nocturnal; generally found in South America

Triatoma species are the vectors (through insect waste material) of Chagas' disease by transmission of *Trypanosoma cruzi*

Specific References

Burnett JW, Calton GJ, and Morgan RJ, "*Triatoma*: The 'Kissing Bug'," *Cutis* 1987, 39(5):399.

Hoffman DR, "Allergy to Biting Insects," *Clin Rev Allergy*, 1987, 5(2):177-90.

***Reduviidae* Family** *see* Reduvids *on this page*

Redwood Sorrel *see* Shamrock *on page 1140*

Revebjelle *see* Foxglove *on page 1085*

Revienta Caballos *see* Star-of-Bethlehem (*Hippobroma longiflora*) *on page 1145*

Rhamnus cathartica *see* Buckthorn *on page 1062*

Rheum rhaponticum *see* Rhubarb *on next page*

Rhodactis howesii *see* Sea Anemones *on page 1138*

Rhododendron

Scientific Name *Rhododendron*

Mechanism of Toxic Action Contains grayanotoxin which binds to a subset of sodium channels causing structural modifications which cause slow opening of these channels which leads to cell depolarization

Signs & Symptoms of Acute Overdose Hypotension, ataxia, bradycardia, sweating, asthenia, dermatitis, nausea, vomiting, oral numbness or burning, paresthesia; transient blindness and visual changes; seizures

Toxic Dosage Three whole leaves or flowers likely nontoxic; consider decontamination if more; toxicity is unpredictable, variable among rhododendron types

Overdosage Treatment

Decontamination: Avoid ipecac, vagal stimulation increases toxicity; lavage/activated charcoal with cathartic

Supportive therapy: Atropine for bradycardia, I.V. fluids should be sufficient for hypotension

Antidote(s)

Atropine Sulfate *on page 1395*

Additional Information Whole plant toxic, foliage especially; contaminated honey may cause systemic symptoms

Rhododendron *see* Azalea *on page 1055*

Rhododendron *see* Rhododendron *on this page*

Rhododendron nudiflorum *see* Azalea *on page 1055*

Rhubarb

Scientific Name *Rheum rhaponticum*

Mechanism of Toxic Action Leaves are toxic and contain soluble and insoluble oxalates; contains soluble and insoluble sodium and potassium oxalates

Signs & Symptoms of Acute Overdose

Dermal pain, irritation, swelling; sap may cause ocular pain, lacrimation, photophobia, corneal abrasion; oxalate crystals may be deposited on cornea; may also cause dermatitis reaction; seizures; edema, vomiting, diarrhea, salivation, feces discoloration (yellow-green), dysphonia; hypocalcemia, renal injury due to calcium oxalate precipitation

Overdosage Treatment

Decontamination: Oral: Dilute; ipecac/lavage/activated charcoal not likely necessary; milk/water to rinse crystals

Supportive therapy: For treatment of soluble oxalates, which may cause systemic oxalate toxicity, keep well hydrated, monitor renal function, fluid/electrolytes; hypocalcemia may occur which can be treated with calcium gluconate, monitor urine for crystals; treat other symptoms supportively

Rivea corymbosa *see* Morning Glory *on page 1109*

Robinia pseudoacacia *see* Black Locust *on page 1057*

Rosary Bean *see* Jequirity Bean *on page 1093*

Rosary Pearls (Nontoxic Plant)

Scientific Name *Senecio lereianus; Senecio rowleyanus*

Synonyms String of Pearls

Additional Information Nontoxic species only include houseplants with round green pea-like leaves; poisonous species contain toxic pyrrolizidine alkaloid

Contact botanist for differentiation if any question on identification exists

Rosary Plant (Nontoxic Plant)

Rosebay *see* Oleander *on page 1120*

Rosy Anemone *see* Sea Anemones *on page 1138*

Rubber Plant (Nontoxic Plant)

Adverse Reactions May cause mild dermatitis

Rubber Vine

Scientific Name *Cryptostegia grandiflora*

Synonyms Indian Rubber Vine; Pink *Allamanda*; Purple *Allamanda*

Mechanism of Toxic Action All parts of the plant contain potentially cardioactive substances

Signs & Symptoms of Acute Overdose Likely gastrointestinal irritation only, but has potential to cause digitalis-like toxicity, including gastrointestinal upset, vomiting, dizziness, bradycardia, hypotension, arrhythmias

Overdosage Treatment

Decontamination: Ipecac may be beneficial if given within 30 minutes of ingestion; lavage and multidose activated charcoal enhance total body clearance of digitalis; whole bowel irrigation is also beneficial in removing plant debris from the GI tract and is recommended for ingestions of large amounts of plant material

Supportive therapy: Monitor cardiac status and serum potassium levels; bradycardia will frequently respond to atropine; phenytoin is the recommended treatment for ventricular arrhythmias because it will also improve conduction through the A-V node; lidocaine can also be used to treat ventricular arrhythmias, but will not have an effect on A-V conduction; other antiarrhythmics which have been used in arrhythmias resistant to the above therapy include magnesium, amiodarone, and bretylium; a pacemaker should be considered for bradycardia and A-V nodal blocks resistant to medical management

Antidote: Digoxin immune Fab has been shown to interact with several different plant cardiac glycosides and may be beneficial in cases resistant to conventional treatment; indications for its use include ventricular arrhythmias resistant to conventional treatment, severe bradycardia and/or second or third degree heart block resistant to atropine and phenytoin

Antidote(s)

Digoxin Immune Fab *on page 1411*

Additional Information Cases of death from these plants have been reported in India; GI irritant

Toxin: Cardiac glycoside

Russula emetica *see* Mushrooms, Toxic (Group VII) *on page 1116*

***Sagartia* Species** *see* Sea Anemones *on page 1138*

Salmonella enteritidis *see Salmonella* Food Poisoning *on this page*

Salmonella Food Poisoning

Synonyms *Salmonella enteritidis*; *Salmonella typhi*

Commonly Found in Unpasteurized milk, raw eggs, meat (poultry), pet turtles, pet chicks

Mechanism of Toxic Action Gram-negative rod which is invasive to the intestines (endotoxin); incubation period: ~8 hours postingestion

Signs & Symptoms of Acute Overdose Vomiting, abdominal cramps; green, bloody diarrhea, loose stools; fever, headache, photophobia, asthenia; may last 3-5 days

Overdosage Treatment Note: *Salmonella* species resistant to multiple antimicrobials are increasing in frequency. *In vitro* susceptibility studies should be performed, particularly in severe cases. Treatment guidelines vary with the type of syndrome, as follows:

1. Enterocolitis: The majority of cases are self-resolving and do not need antibiotics. Clinical trials have demonstrated that a variety of antibiotics fail to influence the course of mild infections and may prolong excretion of the organisms. For severe cases, or in the immunosuppressed host, a number of antibiotics are usually effective including ampicillin, chloramphenicol, co-trimoxazole, and third-generation cephalosporins.
2. Typhoid fever: Cases should be treated promptly. Chloramphenicol and ampicillin are effective and have been the most extensively studied. Recent studies show that ciprofloxacin is highly active. Third-generation cephalosporins and co-trimoxazole are useful in organisms that are resistant to standard agents.
3. Bacteremia: Ampicillin, chloramphenicol, co-trimoxazole, and third-generation cephalosporins are all effective. However, chloramphenicol should be avoided in endocarditis or mycotic aneurysms. Ciprofloxacin is effective in treating recurrent *Salmonella* bacteremia in AIDS.
4. Chronic carriage: Ampicillin or amoxicillin for 6 weeks, although relapses are common; if there is underlying gallbladder disease, cholecystectomy may be an option with repeated relapses. Ciprofloxacin may also be effective.

Diagnostic Tests/Procedures

Blood Culture, Aerobic and Anaerobic *on page 1204*
Complete Blood Count *on page 1236*
Electrolytes, Blood *on page 1254*
Fecal Leukocyte Stain *on page 1263*
Stool Culture *on page 1356*

Additional Information Outbreaks occur most commonly in summer months; *Salmonella enteritidis* is the most common in the U.S.; killed by heat (72°C); can cause carrier state, septic arthritis

Microbiology:

Salmonella species are gram-negative bacilli which are important causes of bacterial gastroenteritis, septicemia, and a nonspecific febrile illness called typhoid fever. Unfortunately, the classification system for the different *Salmonella* species is complex and confusing to most clinicians. Over 2000 separate serotypes have been identified; and, in the past and currently, each is named as if it was a species. Most experts agree that there are 7 distinct subgroups of *Salmonella* (1, 2, 3a, 3b, 4, 5, and 6), each of which contain many serotypes ("species"). The main pathogens in humans are serotypes, *S. choleraesuis*, *S. typhi*, and *S. paratyphi*, (all in subgroup 1).

Salmonella is an aerobic gram-negative bacillus in the family *Enterobacteriaceae*. It is almost always associated with disease when isolated from humans, and is not considered part of the normal human flora. As with other members of this family, *Salmonella* carries the endotoxin lipopolysaccharide on its outer membrane, which is released upon cell lysis.

Epidemiology:

It is estimated that about 3 million new cases of salmonellosis occur each year. *Salmonella* species are found worldwide. Many are easily recovered from animals such as chickens, birds, livestock, rodents, and reptiles (turtles). Some serotypes cause disease almost exclusively in man (*S. typhi*) while others are primarily seen in animals but can cause severe disease when infecting humans (*S. choleraesuis*). Transmission is via ingestion of contaminated materials, particularly raw fruits and vegetables, oysters and other shellfish, and contaminated water. Eggs, poultry, and other dairy products are important sources. Outbreaks have been described in the summer months where children consume contaminated egg salad. Other outbreaks have been associated with pet turtles, other pets, marijuana, and rarely food handlers. The incubation period is about 1-3 weeks. The period of communicability lasts until all *Salmonella* have been eradicated from the stool or urine. Reptile-associated

(Continued)

Salmonella Food Poisoning *(Continued)*

Salmonellosis (lizards, snakes, turtles, and especially iguanas), can be quite hazardous to pregnant women, children <5 years of age, or immunocompromised patients. The Centers for Disease Control has recommended that reptiles should not be kept in child care centers and may not be appropriate pets in the above patient categories. Individuals should always wash hands after handling reptiles or reptile cages and reptiles should be kept out of food preparation areas.

Clinical infection is favored when there is a high inoculum of bacteria in the ingested food, since experimental models suggest that 10^6 bacteria are needed for clinical disease. Contaminated food improperly refrigerated will allow such multiplication. Host factors are important; and disease is more likely in immunocompromised individuals, sickle cell disease, or achlorhydria (gastric acid decreases the viable bacterial inoculum). Although salmonellosis can occur at any age, children are most commonly infected.

Clinical Syndromes: The following are the major syndromes associated with salmonellosis. It should be emphasized that these syndromes are often overlapping.

- **Gastroenteritis:** The most common manifestation of *Salmonella* infection. After ingestion of contaminated food, the bacteria are absorbed in the terminal portion of the small intestine. The organisms then penetrate into the lamina propria of the ileocecal area. Following this, there is reticuloendothelial hypertrophy with usually a brisk host immune response. As the organisms multiply in the lymphoid follicles, polymorphonuclear leukocytes attempt to limit the infection. There is release of prostaglandins and other mediators, which stimulates cyclic AMP. This results in intestinal fluid secretion which is nonbloody. Clinically, the patient complains of nausea, vomiting, and diarrhea from several hours to several days after consumption of contaminated food. Other symptoms include fever, malaise, muscle aches, and abdominal pain. Symptoms usually resolve from several days to 1 week, even without antibiotics.
- **Typhoid fever:** Also known as enteric fever, this febrile illness is caused classically by *S. typhi.* Following ingestion of the bacteria, the organisms pass into the ileocecal area where intraluminal multiplication occurs. There is a mononuclear host cell response, but the organisms remain viable within the macrophages. The bacteria are carried to the organs of the reticuloendothelial system (spleen, liver, bone marrow) by the macrophages; and clinical signs of infection become apparent. Patients complain of insidious onset of fever, myalgias, headache, malaise, and constipation, corresponding to this phase of bacteremia. A pulse-temperature dissociation may be present. A characteristic rash may be seen in about 50% of patients, called "rose spots", which are 2-4 mm pink maculopapular lesions that blanch with pressure, usually on the trunk. Symptoms last for 1 or more weeks. During this time, bacteria multiply in the mesenteric lymphoid tissue; and these areas eventually exhibit necrosis and hemorrhage. There are microperforations of the abdominal wall. *Salmonella* spreads from the liver through the gallbladder and eventually back into the intestines. This phase of intestinal reinfection is characterized by prominent gastrointestinal symptoms including diarrhea. Overall, fatality with treatment is <2%. A similar, but milder syndrome, can occur with *S. paratyphi*, called paratyphoid fever.
- **Chronic carrier state:** Following infection with *S. typhi*, up to 5% of patients will excrete the bacteria for over 1 year. Such patients are termed chronic carriers and are asymptomatic. Millions of viable bacteria are present in the biliary tree and are shed into the bile and into the feces. Urinary carriage can also occur, particularly in patients who are co-infected with *Schistosoma haematobium*. The chronic carrier state is less important for other *Salmonella* species, where the carriage rate is <1%.

Diagnosis:

Laboratory confirmation is generally required, since the major syndromes are seldom distinctive enough to be diagnosed solely on clinical criteria. *Salmonella* grows readily on most media under standard aerobic conditions. Cultures from blood, joint aspirations, and cerebrospinal fluid can be plated on routine media. Specimens which are likely to contain other organisms, such as stool or sputum, require selective media; and the laboratory should be appropriately notified. Recovery of *Salmonella* from the stool is the most common means of establishing the diagnosis, and enrichment media are available to maximize the yield. Other laboratory findings may suggest salmonellosis, including a profound leukopenia often seen with typhoid fever.

Recent antimicrobial therapy may render blood and stool cultures negative. In such cases, proctoscopy with biopsy and culture of ulcerations may establish the diagnosis in the enterocolitis syndrome. Serologic tests are not particularly useful in this instance. When typhoid fever is suspected but the patient has already received antimicrobial agents, bone marrow biopsies as well as skin biopsies of any rose spots may yield *Salmonella typhi* in culture. Serologic studies are more helpful in diagnosing typhoid fever, but >50% of patients will fail to show the expected rise in agglutinins against the typhoid O antigen.

Specific References

Baird-Parker AC, "Foodbourne Salmonellosis," *Lancet*, 1990, 336(8725):1231-5.

Barkin RM, "Acute Infectious Diarrheal Disease in Children," *J Emerg Med*, 1985, 3(1):1-9.

CDC, "African Pygmy Salmonellosis - Washington 1994," *MMWR Morb Mortal Wkly Rep*, 1995, 44:462-3.

CDC, "Reptile-Associated Salmonellosis," *MMWR Morb Mortal Wkly Rep*, 1995, 44(17):347-50.

Levine WC, Buehler JW, Bean NH, et al, "Epidemiology of Nontyphoidal *Salmonella* Bacteremia During the Human Immunodeficiency Virus Epidemic," *J Infect Dis*, 1991, 164(1):81-7.

"Outbreaks of *Salmonella enteritidis* Gastroenteritis – California 1993," *MMWR Morb Mortal Wkly Rep*, 1993, 42(41):793-7.

Telzak EE, Budnick LD, Greenberg MS, et al, "A Nosocomial Outbreak of *Salmonella enteritidis* Infection Due to the Consumption of Raw Eggs," *N Engl J Med*, 1990, 323(6):394-7.

Salmonella typhi *see* *Salmonella* Food Poisoning *on page 1135*

Sambucus *see* Elderberry *on page 1081*

Sand Corn *see* Death Camas *on page 1078*

Sarcoptes scabiei *see* Mites *on page 1107*

Sarothaminum scoparius *see* Scotch Broom *on next page*

"Satan's Bolete" Mushroom *see* Mushrooms, Toxic (Group III) *on page 1112*

"Satan's Bolete" Mushroom *see* Mushrooms, Toxic (Group VII) *on page 1116*

"Scaly Chanterelle" Mushroom *see* Mushrooms, Toxic (Group VII) *on page 1116*

Scarlet Berry *see* Deadly Nightshade *on page 1078*

Schefflera (Nontoxic Plant)

Synonyms Umbrella Tree

Adverse Reactions Minimal risk of contact dermatitis

Additional Information Does not include umbrella tree of *Musanga* genus

Scilla maritima *see* Squill *on page 1143*

Scombroid Food Poisoning

Synonyms Mahi Mahi Flush

Commonly Found in Skipjack, mackerel, bluefish, mahi mahi, salmon, Japanese saury, kingfish, tuna (usually poorly refrigerated)

Mechanism of Toxic Action Histidine found in fish musculature causes clinical syndrome; onset develops within 1 hour (often with 10 minutes); resolves within 36 hours

Signs & Symptoms of Acute Overdose Erythematous flushing, pruritus, slurred speech, watery diarrhea (explosive), nausea, vomiting, facial edema, palpitations, wheezing, and headache

Overdosage Treatment Supportive therapy: Fluids for dehydration; diphenhydramine (25-50 mg) with cimetidine (300 mg) or ranitidine (50 mg) can cause resolution of symptoms

Diagnostic Tests/Procedures

Histamine Level *on page 1273*

Additional Information Heat stable; refrigeration prevents scombroid poisoning; fish may have a peppery taste; can cause elevated blood and urine histamine levels; cultures are not useful; isoniazid may exacerbate symptoms

Specific References

Blakesley ML, "Scombroid Poisoning: Prompt Resolution of Symptoms With Cimetidine," *Ann Emerg Med*, 1983, 12(2):104-6.

Hughes JM and Potter ME, "Scombroid – Fish Poisoning," *N Engl J Med*, 1991, 324(11):766-8.

Uragodu CG and Kottegoda SR, "Adverse Reaction to Isoniazid and Ingestion of Fish With a High Histamine Content," *Tubercle* 1977, 58(2):83-9.

Scorpion *see* Arizona Bark Scorpion *on page 1053*

Scorpion Fish

Mechanism of Toxic Action Fish contains spines covered with integumentary sheaths from which venom is released through grooves on the spine as it travels from glands located at the base; venom is composed of high-molecular weight, heat labile, nondialyzable proteins; potency between the scorpionfish and other species is similar; the difference in clinical presentation may lie in the amount and way in which the venom is delivered; venom is a muscle toxin affecting cardiac, involuntary, and skeletal muscles

(Continued)

Scorpion Fish *(Continued)*

Signs & Symptoms of Acute Overdose Severity depends on number of stings, species, amount of venom, and patient age and health; severe pain peaking in 60-90 minutes and lasting 6-12 hours up to 24 hours. Wound may become ischemic and cyanotic with erythema, edema, warmth, and vesicle formation; systemic signs and symptoms include anxiety, headache, tremor, dyspnea, rash, nausea, vomiting, diarrhea, and abdominal pain; also sweating, pallor, delirium, seizures, paralysis, paresthesia, lymphangitis, arthritis, fasciculations, fever, hypertension, bradycardia, tachycardia, A-V block, ventricular fibrillation, CHF, pericarditis, hypotension, syncope, and respiratory distress; death usually occurs within the first 6-8 hours from respiratory paralysis

Overdosage Treatment

Decontamination: Immerse wound in hot water to tolerance to inactivate heat labile components of the venom for 30-90 minutes as needed for pain relief, repeat if pain reoccurs; remove pieces of spine from wound; surgical removal of the spines may be necessary

Supportive therapy: Local pain may be treated with tissue infiltration with lidocaine; systemic symptoms should be treated with supportive care (fluids for hypotension)

Antidote: Antivenin for stonefish envenomations does exist (Commonwealth Serum Laboratories, Melbourne, Australia); bites from other members of the *Scorpaenidae* family usually do not require this antivenin

Additional Information

Family: Scorpaenidae; three groups separated by different genera based on the venom apparatus

Pterois (zebrafish, turkeyfish, lionfish, butterfly cod)

Scorpaena (scorpionfish, sculpin)

Synanceja (stonefish)

Range: Bottom dwellers found in shallow water, bays, and among coral reef and rocky coastlines; camouflaged by their shape and color; found in tropical and sometimes temperate oceans

Specific References

Auerbach PS and Halsted BW, "Hazardous Aquatic Life," *Management of Wilderness and Environmental Emergencies*, 2nd ed, Auerbach PS and Geehr EC, eds, St Louis, MO: CV Mosby Co, 1989, 979-83.

Bogomolski-Yahalom V, Amitai Y, and Stalnikowicz R, "Paresthesia in Envenomation by the Scorpion *Leiurus quinquestriatus*," *Clin Toxicol*, 1995, 33:79-82.

Kizer KW, McKinney HE, and Auerbach PS, "*Scorpaenidae* Envenomation: A Five Year Poison Center Experience," *JAMA*, 1985, 253(6):807-10.

Scotch Broom

Scientific Name *Cytisus*; *Genista scopafia*; *Sarothaminum scoparius*; *Spartium scoparium*

Synonyms Basam; Bisom; Bizzom; Breeam; Broom Tops; Browme; Brum; Green Broom; Irish Tops

Mechanism of Toxic Action Contains cytisine which has effects similar to nicotine

Signs & Symptoms of Acute Overdose Nausea, vomiting, asthenia, headache, pallor, drowsiness, ataxia, mydriasis, tachycardia, hypotension, paralysis, seizures; may also cause dermatitis

Toxicodynamics/Kinetics Onset of symptoms: Within 15 minutes to 4 hours

Overdosage Treatment

Decontamination: Ipecac relatively contraindicated because of risk of seizures occurring rapidly with large ingestion; lavage/activated charcoal with cathartic if large amounts ingested

Supportive care: Maintain respiration and blood pressure in symptomatic patient

Specific References

Galloway JH, Farmer K, Weeks GR, et al, "Potentially Hazardous Compound in a Herbal Slimming Remedy," *Lancet*, 1992, 340(8812):179.

Scotch Lanburnum *see* Golden Chain Tree *on page 1087*

***Scyphozoa* Class** *see* Box Jellyfish *on page 1060*

Sea Anemones

Scientific Name *Actinia* Species; *Actinodendron* Species; *Adamsia* Species; *Anemonia* Species; *Anthea* Species; *Anthoptreura* Species; *Chondylactis* Species; *Physobrachia* Species; *Rhodactis howesii*; *Sagartia* Species; *Stichactis* Species; *Triactis* Species

Synonyms Hell's Fire Anemone; Malu-Malu; Rosy Anemone; Stinging Anemone

Mechanism of Toxic Action Hemolysis through phospholipase A activity; thalassin, congestin, hypnotoxin; toxic proteins: equinatoxin, possible potassium channel blockers, sodium channel blockers, cytolysin activity

Signs & Symptoms of Acute Overdose

Dermal: Stinging (burning, ulceration, necrosis, vomiting, abdominal pain, thirst, malaise, headache, chills, fever, myalgias)

Hepatic failure may occur from the sting of the genus *Chondylactis*

Ingestion of *R. howesii*: Agitated hemolysis can also be seen with coelenterate venoms

Overdosage Treatment

Decontamination: If ingested, gastric decontamination including charcoal/lavage; irrigate if eye exposure; hot water generally recommended, though heat will denature

Supportive therapy: Pain control, wound care, antihistamines (oral and topical), topical steroids

Toxin neutralization:

Dilute ammonium hydroxide, sodium bicarbonate, olive oil, sugar, ethyl alcohol with varying success

Irrigate with sea water and then topical acetic acid 5% (vinegar) recommended; shave area

Antidote: No specific antidote; antihistamines (oral and topical), topical steroids

Pregnancy Implications Not known to be teratogenic

Additional Information

Phylum: Coelenterata

Class: Anthozoa

Rhodactis howesii (brown or green anemone)

Specific References

Garcia PJ, Schein RM, and Burnett JW, "Fulminant Hepatic Failure From a Sea Anemone Sting," *Ann Intern Med*, 1994, 120(8):665-6.

Halstead BW, "Dangerous Marine Animals," 2nd ed, Centrevil, MD: Cornell Maritime Press, 1980.

McGoldrick J and Marx JA, "Marine Envenomations, Part 2: Invertebrates," *J Emerg Med*, 1992, 10(1):71-7.

Tu AT, ed, "Handbook of Natural Toxins, V3: Marine Toxins and Venoms," New York, NY: Marcel Dekker Inc, 1988.

Seagull *see* Caladium *on page 1063*

Sea Onion *see* Squill *on page 1143*

Sea Urchins

Scientific Name *Arbacia punctulata*

Signs & Symptoms of Acute Overdose Stinging, burning, violet dye harmless, pain, redness, swelling, myalgias, reports of paralysis, hypersensitivity

Overdosage Treatment

Decontamination: Remove spines, if possible; hot water soaks (<113°F for 30-90 minutes); surgical removal may be necessary, especially if located in or near a joint

Supportive therapy: 2-hour infections, tetanus

Antidote: No specific antidote

Sea Wasp

Related Information

Box Jellyfish *on page 1060*

Scientific Name *Chironex fleckeri*

Commonly Found in Australia *Chiropsalmus quadrigatus* – Philippines

Signs & Symptoms of Acute Overdose Erythema, edema, vesiculations, pain, necrosis; systemic effects include myocardial and respiratory depression, nausea, vomiting, fatality

Overdosage Treatment

Decontamination: Sheep antivenins, fluids, vasopressors, antiarrhythmics as needed; immobilize affected area, inactivate nematocysts with alcohol or vinegar; immediately rinse with seawater, should then prevent further envenomation by applying acetic acid 5% (vinegar) to any tentacles still adhering to tissue; if acetic acid is not available, use isopropyl alcohol 40% to 70% or finally may use aluminum sulfate; shave envenomated area after initial treatment, then repeat local decontamination therapy. Ocular exposures are to be decontaminated by water irrigation only. Do not rub affected area. Wear gloves during decontamination. Meat tenderizers have been used, however they are not preferred decontamination measures and should not have prolonged contact times (>10 minutes).

Sheep antivenin (Commonwealth Serum Laboratories, Melbourne, Australia): Dose: I.V.: 20,000 units (1 vial) over 5 minutes after skin testing

Additional Information Invertebrate, most venomous sea creature

Specific References

Comis A, Hartwick RF, and Howden ME, "Stabilization of Lethal and Hemolytic Activities of Box Jellyfish (*Chironex fleckeri*) Venom," *Toxicon*, 1989, 27(4):439-47.

Kizer KW, "Marine Envenomations," *J Toxicol Clin Toxicol*, 1983-84, 21(4-5):527-55.

Sedum

Synonyms Christmas Cheer; Live Forever; Orphine

Signs & Symptoms of Acute Overdose No evidence plant is toxic internally; some species have product contact dermatitis

Overdosage Treatment

Decontamination: Wash, irrigate

Supportive therapy: Corticosteroids or antihistamines may be used

Seeds of Oak Trees *see* Acorns *on page 1050*

Seminole Bead *see* Jequirity Bean *on page 1093*

Senecio lereianus *see* Rosary Pearls (Nontoxic Plant) *on page 1134*

Senecio rowleyanus *see* Rosary Pearls (Nontoxic Plant) *on page 1134*

"Sensitive" *Boletus* Mushroom *see* Mushrooms, Toxic (Group VII) *on page 1116*

Sensitive Plant (Nontoxic Plant)

"Shaggy Bear" Mushroom *see* Mushrooms, Toxic (Group VII) *on page 1116*

"Shaggy Scalecap" Mushroom *see* Mushrooms, Toxic (Group VII) *on page 1116*

Shamrock

Scientific Name *Oxalis hedysaroides*

Synonyms Alleluia; Cuckoo's Meat; Fire Fern; Good Luck Leaf; Good Luck Plant; Irish Shamrock; Julicla; Lucky Clover; Red Flame; Redwood Sorrel; Sorrel; Sour Sob; Tree Oxalis; Violet Wood Sorrel; Wood Sour; Xanthoxalis Species

Mechanism of Toxic Action Contains soluble and insoluble oxalates; soluble oxalates may cause damage to the kidney, brain, liver, or heart

Signs & Symptoms of Acute Overdose Renal damage, tetany, hypocalcemic arrhythmia, metabolic acidosis, hypocalcemia, dermatitis

Toxicodynamics/Kinetics Onset: Within 2-12 hours

Toxic Dosage Unclear, but unlikely due to large amount necessary

Overdosage Treatment

Decontamination: Dilute; ipecac/lavage/activated charcoal not likely necessary; milk/water to rinse crystals

Supportive therapy: For treatment of soluble oxalates, which may cause systemic oxalate toxicity, keep well hydrated, monitor renal function, fluid/electrolytes; hypocalcemia may occur which can be treated with calcium gluconate, monitor urine for crystals; treat other symptoms supportively

Additional Information Family: Oxalis

Specific References

James LF, "Oxalate Toxicosis," *Clin Toxicol*, 1972, 5(2):231-43.

Sheep Laurel *see* Mountain Laurel *on page 1110*

Shellfish/Atlantic Mussel Food Poisoning

Synonyms Domoic Acid Poisoning

Commonly Found in Shellfish, mussels

Mechanism of Toxic Action Toxin involves domoic acid structurally similar to glutamate which can cause neuronal necrosis in the amygdaloid nucleus and hippocampus; incubation period: 5 hours

Signs & Symptoms of Acute Overdose Nausea, short-term memory loss, bronchorrhea, facial grimacing; can cause seizures, hypotension, headache, myoclonus, and piloerection; long-term anterograde memory loss (10%), vomiting, abdominal cramps

Overdosage Treatment

Decontamination: Avoid ipecac; activated charcoal with cathartic may be used; lavage may be used

Supportive therapy: Diazepam is useful for seizures, fluids for hypotension

Test Interactions Can result in elevated serum creatinine

Additional Information Heat stable toxin which is not destroyed by cooking; neurologic symptoms may be more pronounced in the elderly; domoic acid activates glutamate receptors thus causing seizures; mortality rate: 2%

Specific References

Cendes F, Andermann F, Carpenter S, et al, "Temporal Lobe Epilepsy Caused by Domoic Acid Intoxication: Evidence For Glutamate Receptor-Mediated Excitotoxicity in Humans," *Ann Neurol*, 1995, 37(1):123-6.

Gray C, "Mussel Mystery: The More You Know, the More You Don't Know," *Can Med Assoc J*, 1988, 138(4):350-1.

Kizer KW, "Domoic Acid Poisoning," *West J Med*, 1994, 161(1):59-60.
Perl TM, Bedard L, Kosatsky T, et al, "An Outbreak of Toxic Encephalopathy Caused by Eating Mussels Contaminated With Domoic Acid," *N Engl J Med*, 1990, 322(25):1775-80.
Teitelbaum JS, Zatorre RJ, Carpenter S, et al, "Neurologic Sequelae of Domoic Acid Intoxication Due to the Ingestion of Contaminated Mussels," *N Engl J Med*, 1990, 322(25):1781-7.

Shellfish Food Poisoning

Synonyms Diarrheic Shellfish Poisoning (DSP); DSP

Commonly Found in Shellfish, blue mussel

Mechanism of Toxic Action May contain either clinophysistoxin (okadaic acid), pectenotoxin, or yessotoxin which can cause fluid secretion in the intestines; incubation period: 4-12 hours postingestion

Signs & Symptoms of Acute Overdose Diarrhea, nausea, slurred speech, fasciculations, vomiting, abdominal cramping, and chills

Overdosage Treatment

Decontamination: Do not use ipecac or laxatives; activated charcoal is of little use

Supportive therapy: Fluid and electrolyte replacement therapy

Diagnostic Tests/Procedures

Electrolytes, Blood *on page 1254*

Additional Information Heat stable toxin

Specific References

Hamano Y, Kinoshita Y, and Yasomoto T, "Enteropathogenicity of Diarrhetic Shellfish Toxins in Intestinal Models. Studies on Diarrhetic Shellfish Toxins I," *J Food Hyg Soc JPN*, 1986, 27:375-9.

Shigella dysenteriae *see Shigella* Food Poisoning *on this page*

Shigella Food Poisoning

Synonyms *Shigella dysenteriae*; *Shigella sonnei*

Commonly Found in Potatoes, milk products, tossed salad, meat salad, stewed apples, raw oysters

Mechanism of Toxic Action Can produce an enterotoxin along with a shiga toxin (*S. dysenteriae*) which stimulates fluid secretion from the intestines; intestinally invasive gram-negative bacteria; incubation period: 1-3 days postingestion

Signs & Symptoms of Acute Overdose Watery, mucoid, bloody diarrhea, feces discoloration (yellow/green) and bloody stools; can cause coughing, high fever, dementia, nausea, and vomiting

Overdosage Treatment Many cases of *Shigella* dysentery are self-resolving. Some have suggested that antibiotics be reserved for severe cases, but this does not eliminate the reservoir for infection in the community. Antibiotics have been shown to shorten the period of excretion of the organism in the feces as well as decreasing morbidity. The antibiotic of choice is co-trimoxazole for both children and adults. However, some strains are resistant to trimethoprim, particularly in Africa and Southeast Asia, and *in vitro* susceptibility testing should be performed on all isolates. The quinolones have been effective for shigellosis in clinical trials and are useful alternatives. Antimotility agents such as opiates, paregoric, and diphenoxylate (Lomotil®) should be avoided, because of the potential for worsening the dysentery and for predisposing to toxic megacolon.

Test Interactions WBCs have a marked shift to the left (bandemia)

Diagnostic Tests/Procedures

Electrolytes, Blood *on page 1254*

Fecal Leukocyte Stain *on page 1263*

Stool Culture *on page 1356*

Additional Information Outbreaks occur most commonly in the summer; large amount of fecal leukocytes (polymorphonuclear) are noted; monitor electrolytes

Microbiology: *Shigella* species are gram-negative rods which cause a severe diarrheal syndrome, called shigellosis or bacillary dysentery. *Shigella* species belong to the family *Enterobacteriaceae*, and are, for all practical purposes, biochemically and genetically identical to *E. coli*. Four species of *Shigella* have been identified: *S. dysenteriae*, *S. flexneri*, *S. boydii*, and *S. sonnei*. There are approximately 40 serotypes. *Shigella sonnei* is most common in the industrial world and accounts for about 64% of the cases in the United States. *S. flexneri* is seen primarily in underdeveloped countries. Shigellosis can be seen following ingestion of as few as 200 organisms.

Epidemiology: Infection with *Shigella* sp is primarily a problem in the pediatric population, with most infections in the 1- to 4-year age group. Outbreaks of epidemic proportions have been described in day care centers and nurseries. The reservoir for the bacteria is in humans. Transmission is by direct or indirect fecal-oral transmission from patient or carrier. Hand transmission is important. Less commonly, transmission occurs by consumption of contaminated water, milk, and food. The organism is able to produce outbreaks in areas of poor sanitation, in part due to the low number of organisms required to produce disease. Shigellosis is the most communicable of the bacterial diarrheas.

(Continued)

Shigella Food Poisoning *(Continued)*

Clinical Syndromes:

Shigella species invade the intestinal mucosa wherein they multiply and cause local tissue damage. The organisms rarely penetrate beyond the mucosa and thus the isolation in blood cultures is unusual, even with the toxic patient. Mucosal ulcerations are common. Some strains are known to elaborate a toxin (the shiga-toxin), which contributes to mucosal destruction and probably causes the watery diarrhea seen initially.

- **Dysentery:** Initially, the patient complains of acute onset of fever, abdominal cramping, and large volumes of very watery diarrhea. This phase is enterotoxin mediated and reflects small bowel involvement. Within 24-48 hours, the fever resolves but the diarrhea turns frankly bloody, with mucous and pus in the stools as well. Fecal urgency and tenesmus are common. This phase reflects direct colonic invasion. This two-phased "descending infection" is suggestive of dysentery. Diarrhea and abdominal pain are almost universally present, but the other symptoms may be absent. Physical examination is variable and patients may be comfortable or frankly toxic. Rectal examination is often painful due to friable and inflamed rectal mucosa. The course may be complicated from dehydration from diarrhea and vomiting, particularly in the elderly and in infants. Normally, the infection is self limited and resolves within about 1 week even without antibiotics. Complications are unusual and include febrile seizures (particularly in infants), septicemia, and the hemolytic uremic syndrome (usually from the shiga-toxin from *S. dysenteriae* 1).
- **Reactive arthritis:** Following dysentery from *Shigella*, a postinfectious arthropathy resembling Reiter's syndrome has been described, particularly in patients who are HLA-B27 positive

Diagnosis: Dysentery from *Shigella* should be suspected in any patient presenting with fever and bloody diarrhea. A history of a "descending infection" as described above is further suggestive. However, the differential diagnosis of fever with bloody diarrhea is broad and includes salmonellosis, *Campylobacter* enteritis, infection with *E. coli* 0157:H7, and inflammatory bowel disease. The WBC count may show either a leukocytosis, leukopenia, or be normal.

There are two important laboratory tests indicated in suspected cases.

1. Stool exam for fecal leukocytes: Numerous white blood cells will be present during the colonic phase of the infection. Note that this is not diagnostic for *Shigella* infections; it indicates that the colonic mucosa is inflamed, from whatever cause. The finding of sheets of fecal leukocytes on smear narrows the differential diagnosis of infectious diarrheas considerably.
2. Stool culture for *Shigella*: Recovery of the organism from stool is more easily performed early in the illness when the concentration in the stool is highest. Samples should be brought to the laboratory as soon as possible to maximize viability, and specific culture for *Shigella* sp should be requested.

Specific References

Ashkenazi S, Amir J, Waisman Y, et al, "A Randomized, Double-Blind Study Comparing Cefixime and Trimethoprim-Sulfamethoxazole in the Treatment of Childhood Shigellosis," *J Pediatr*, 1993, 123(5):817-21.

Baskin DH, Lax JD, and Barenberg D, "*Shigella* Bacteremia in Patients With the Acquired Immune Deficiency Syndrome," *Am J Gastroenterol*, 1987, 82(4):338-41.

Bennish ML, "Potentially Lethal Complications of Shigellosis," *Rev Infect Dis*, 1991, 13(Suppl 4):S319-24.

Halpern Z, Dan M, Giladi M, et al, "Shigellosis in Adults: Epidemiologic, Clinical, and Laboratory Features," *Medicine (Baltimore)*, 1989, 68(4):210-7.

Pichler HET, Diridl G, Stickler K, et al, "Clinical Efficacy of Ciprofloxacin Compared With Placebo in Bacterial Diarrhea," *Am J Med*, 1987, 82(4A):329-32.

Reeve G, Martin DL, Pappas J, et al, "An Outbreak of Shigellosis Associated With the Consumption of Raw Oysters," *N Engl J Med*, 1989, 321(4):224-7.

Salam MA and Bennish ML, "Antimicrobial Therapy for Shigellosis," *Rev Infect Dis*, 1991, 13(Suppl 4):S332-41.

Tauxe RV, Puhr ND, Wells JG, et al, "Antimicrobial Resistance of *Shigella* Isolates in the USA: The Importance of International Travelers," *J Infect Dis*, 1990, 162(5):1107-11.

Shigella sonnei *see* *Shigella* Food Poisoning *on previous page*

"Showy Flamecap" Mushroom *see* Mushrooms, Toxic (Group VI) *on page 1115*

"Silly Putty" *see* Mushrooms, Toxic (Group VI) *on page 1115*

Sisal *see* Century Plant *on page 1067*

Sistrurus catenatus *see* Rattlesnakes *on page 1132*

***Sistrurus catenatus* (Pygmy Rattler, Massasauga)** *see Crotalidae on page 1075*

Sistrurus miliarius *see* Rattlesnakes *on page 1132*

***Sistrurus* (Pygmy Rattler, Massasauga)** *see* Rattlesnakes *on page 1132*

Skunk Cabbage *see* Corn Lily *on page 1074*

"Slender Death Angel" Mushroom *see* Mushrooms, Toxic (Group I) *on page 1111*

"Smooth" *Lepiota* Mushroom *see* Mushrooms, Toxic (Group VII) *on page 1116*

Snake Lily *see* Iris *on page 1092*

Snake Plant (Nontoxic Plant)

Adverse Reactions Minimal risk for mild poisoning; may cause GI upset

Snake Root *see* Water Hemlock *on page 1156*

"Snow Morel" Mushroom *see* Mushrooms, Toxic (Group II) *on page 1112*

Sodium Bisulfite *see* Sulfite Food Poisoning *on page 1148*

Sodium Glutamate *see* Monosodium Glutamate Food Poisoning *on page 1109*

Sodium Metabisulfite *see* Sulfite Food Poisoning *on page 1148*

Sodium Sulfite *see* Sulfite Food Poisoning *on page 1148*

Solanum *see* Christmas Cherry *on page 1068*

Solanum *see* Tomato (Leaves and Stems) *on page 1150*

Solanum dulcamara *see* Deadly Nightshade *on page 1078*

Solanum nigrum *see* Black Nightshade *on page 1057*

Solanum tuberosum *see* Potato (Leaves, Stems, Tubercles) *on page 1128*

Soldier's Buttons *see* Marsh Marigold *on page 1105*

Soldier's Cap *see* Monkshood *on page 1108*

Solenopsis invicta *see* Fire Ants *on page 1084*

Solenopsis richteri *see* Fire Ants *on page 1084*

Solomon Island Ivy *see* Devil's Ivy *on page 1079*

Sorrel *see* Shamrock *on page 1140*

Sour Sob *see* Shamrock *on page 1140*

Southern Tree Yew *see* Yew *on page 1159*

Spartium scoparium *see* Scotch Broom *on page 1138*

Spider Aralia (Nontoxic Plant)

Spider Plant (Nontoxic Plant)

"Splendid Webcap" Mushroom *see* Mushrooms, Toxic (Group VIII) *on page 1117*

Spoonwood Ivy *see* Mountain Laurel *on page 1110*

Spotted Hemlock *see* Poison Hemlock *on page 1126*

Spotted Octopus *see* Blue-Ringed Octopus *on page 1059*

"Spotted-Stemmed" Mushroom *see* Mushrooms, Toxic (Group VII) *on page 1116*

Spurge Laurel *see* Daphne *on page 1077*

Spurge Olive *see* Daphne *on page 1077*

Squill

Scientific Name *Scilla maritima*; *Urginea maritima*

Synonyms Sea Onion

Mechanism of Toxic Action Contains scillaren-A, scillaren-B, glucoscillaren A, scillaridin A, and scilliroside which are cardiac glycosides

Adverse Reactions

Cardiovascular: Ventricular arrhythmias, bradycardia
Central nervous system: Seizures
Endocrine & metabolic: Hyperkalemia
Gastrointestinal: Nausea, vomiting
Miscellaneous: Hypothyroidism

Overdosage Treatment

Decontamination: Lavage and multidose activated charcoal enhance total body clearance of digitalis; whole bowel irrigation is also beneficial in removing plant

(Continued)

Squill *(Continued)*

debris from the GI tract and is recommended for ingestions of large amounts of plant material

Supportive therapy: Monitor cardiac status and serum potassium levels; bradycardia will frequently respond to atropine; phenytoin is the recommended treatment for ventricular arrhythmias because it will also improve conduction through the A-V node; lidocaine can also be used to treat ventricular arrhythmias, but will not have an effect on A-V conduction; other antiarrhythmics which have been used in arrhythmias resistant to the above therapy include magnesium, amiodarone, and bretylium; a pacemaker should be considered for bradycardia and A-V nodal blocks resistant to medical management

Antidote: Digoxin immune Fab has been shown to interact with several different plant cardiac glycosides and may be beneficial in cases resistant to conventional treatment; indications for its use include ventricular arrhythmias resistant to conventional treatment, severe bradycardia and/or second or third degree heart block resistant to atropine and phenytoin

Antidote(s)

Digoxin Immune Fab *on page 1411*

Test Interactions Serum digoxin level can be detectable by enzyme immunoassay method

Additional Information Found in Eastern Mediterranean and South Africa; bulbs (which resemble onions) can weigh as much as 2 mg and often are used as a folk remedy

Specific References

Tuncok V, Kozan O, Cavdar C, et al, "*Urginea maritima* (Squill) Toxicity," *Clin Toxicol*, 1995, 33:83-6.

Wax PM, "Squill Through the Ages," *Clin Toxicol*, 1995, 33:86.

Squirting Cucumber

Scientific Name *Ecballium elaterium*

Mechanism of Toxic Action Irritant; contains alkaloid resins and glycosides; also a purgative and has anti-inflammatory effects

Signs & Symptoms of Acute Overdose Mucosal irritation, renal failure, laryngeal edema, facial edema, vomiting, diarrhea, dyspnea, tachycardia, neurotoxicity

Overdosage Treatment Supportive therapy: Corticosteroids can be used for edema; hemodialysis can be utilized for renal failure

Additional Information

Region: Endemic to the Mediterranean region; has been used medicinally in Crete and Greece for constipation, rheumatic diseases, and sinusitis, although a death has recently been reported by its use for sinusitis through aspiration. Similar toxins also found in colocynth (bitter apple).

Toxic parts: All parts of the plant are toxic, especially the ovoid green fruit

Specific References

Vlachos P, Kanitsakis NN, and Kokonas N, "Fatal Cardiac and Renal Failure Due to *Ecballium elaterium* (Squirting Cucumber)," *J Toxicol Clin Toxicol*, 1994, 32(6):737-8.

Stagger Weed *see* Bleeding Heart *on page 1058*

Staphylococcus Food Poisoning

Commonly Found in Ham, pork, poultry, potato salad, egg salad, and foods stored at room temperature

Mechanism of Toxic Action Heat stable enterotoxin; incubation period: 1-6 hours

Signs & Symptoms of Acute Overdose Abdominal pain, nausea, vomiting, low-grade fever, bloody diarrhea

Overdosage Treatment Supportive therapy: Fluid/electrolyte replacement

Diagnostic Tests/Procedures

Electrolytes, Blood *on page 1254*

Stool Culture *on page 1356*

Additional Information

Microbiology: Staphylococci derives its name from the Greek word staphyle meaning "bunch of grapes". On Gram's stain, staphylococci are gram-positive cocci, 0.7-1.2 μm, nonspore forming, occurring singly, in pairs, in short 4-5 cocci chains or clusters. Staphylococci grow rapidly both as an aerobe and anaerobe on blood agar. The colonies are sharply defined, smooth, and 1-4 mm in diameter. Staphylococci are catalase-positive and differ from micrococci by the following: anaerobic acid production from glucose, sensitivity <200 mg/mL lysostaphin, and production of acid from glycerol in the presence of 0.4 mg/mL erythromycin.

Staphylococcus aureus may have a golden pigmentation secondary to carotenoid and produce β-hemolysis on horse, sheep, or human blood agar after an incubation of 24-48 hours. *Staphylococcus epidermidis* and coagulase-negative staph (CNS) are often used interchangeably but recognize that there are over 30 species of CNS of which *S. epidermidis* is the most common. It is important to distinguish three clinically relevant species: *S. aureus*, *S. epidermidis*, and *S. saprophyticus*.

Clinical Syndromes:

- **Food poisoning:** Usually caused by ingestion of heat stable enterotoxin B. Second most common cause of acute food poisoning. May occur by person-to-person transmission. Incubation 2-6 hours after ingestion of toxin contained in custard-filled bakery goods, canned foods, processed meats, potato salads, and ice cream. Patients present with acute salivation, nausea, vomiting progressing to abdominal cramps, and watery, nonbloody diarrhea (risk of dehydration).

Diagnosis: Diagnosis is made by Gram's stain and culture with sensitivities of appropriate site. Semiquantitation roll technique by Dennis Maki in which catheter is rolled over surface of blood agar plate is useful in suggesting a true intravascular catheter sepsis when both blood culture grows MSSE and count >15 colonies on blood agar plate.

Specific References

Holmberg SD and Blake PA, "Staphylococcal Food Poisoning in the United States: New Facts and Old Misconceptions," *JAMA*, 1984, 251(4):487-9.

Starch Wort *see* Jack-in-the-Pulpit *on page 1093*

Star-of-Bethlehem (*Hippobroma longiflora*)

CAS Number 90-69-7; 134-63-4

Scientific Name *Hippobroma longiflora*; *Isotoma longiflora*; *Laurentia longiflora*

Synonyms Cipril; Feuilles Crabe; Ginbey; Horse Poison; Madame Fate; Pua Hoku; Revienta Caballos; Tibey

Mechanism of Toxic Action All parts of the plant, especially seed capsules and roots, contain the toxin diphenyl lobelidiol; this toxin produces primary stimulation and secondary depression of autonomic ganglia; also acts as a central stimulant, affecting medullary centers for respiration and vomiting; high concentrations have a curare-like effect

Signs & Symptoms of Acute Overdose Low doses cause nausea, vomiting, diarrhea, abdominal pain, metallic taste, increased salivation, sweating, hypothermia, tachypnea, dermatitis; high doses cause seizures, paralysis, coma, bradycardia, and hypertension

Toxicodynamics/Kinetics

Onset of symptoms: Following S.C. injection, within minutes

Absorption: Well absorbed orally, cutaneously, and by inhalation

Toxic Dosage In cats: 0.4-4 mg/kg: Nausea, vomiting; 60 mg/kg: Convulsions and death; 80 mg/kg: Respiratory paralysis; toxicity is very unlikely with the houseplants which are available; dried material has little activity; lobeline is used in many homeopathic medicines (antiasthmatic, spasmolytics, and emetics); toxicity is possible from these preparations due to the narrow therapeutic margin

Overdosage Treatment

Decontamination: Ipecac is generally not necessary for houseplant ingestions; ipecac is controversial for other preparations which contain lobeline, but probably not advisable secondary to the rapid onset of symptoms and the possibility of seizures; lavage and activated charcoal with cathartic are the treatment of choice for symptomatic patients

Supportive therapy: Respiratory status and seizures

Additional Information

Family: Lobeliaceae

Range: Native to the tropics, but found throughout the West Indies, Hawaii, and Guam

Toxin: Lobeline

Star-of-Bethlehem (*Ornithogalum pyrenaicum*)

Related Information

Amaryllis *on page 1052*

Indian Tobacco *on page 1091*

Poinsettia *on page 1126*

Scientific Name *Ornithogalum pyrenaicum*

Synonyms Prussian Asparagus

Mechanism of Toxic Action All parts of the plant, especially the bulb, contain the digitalis-like glycosides convallatoxin and convalloside

Signs & Symptoms of Acute Overdose GI effects (nausea and vomiting) usually precede the cardiovascular effects by several hours; bradycardia; first, second, and third degree heart block; asystole, hypotension, A-V block, ventricular arrhythmias, atrial fibrillation, decreased Q-T interval and prolonged P-R interval; fatigue,

(Continued)

Star-of-Bethlehem (*Ornithogalum pyrenaicum*) (*Continued*)

confusion, headache, dizziness, contact dermatitis, seeing yellow halos, and hyperkalemia have also been reported

Overdosage Treatment

Decontamination: Ipecac may be beneficial if given within 30 minutes of ingestion; lavage and multidose activated charcoal enhance total body clearance of digitalis; whole bowel irrigation is also beneficial in removing plant debris from the GI tract and is recommended for ingestions of large amounts of plant material

Supportive therapy: Monitor cardiac status and serum potassium levels; bradycardia will frequently respond to atropine; phenytoin is the recommended treatment for ventricular arrhythmias because it will also improve conduction through the A-V node; lidocaine can also be used to treat ventricular arrhythmias, but will not have an effect on A-V conduction; other antiarrhythmics which have been used in arrhythmias resistant to the above therapy include magnesium, amiodarone, and bretylium; a pacemaker should be considered for bradycardia and A-V nodal blocks resistant to medical management

Antidote: Digoxin immune Fab has been shown to interact with several different plant cardiac glycosides and may be beneficial in cases resistant to conventional treatment; indications for its use include ventricular arrhythmias resistant to conventional treatment, severe bradycardia and/or second or third degree heart block resistant to atropine and phenytoin

Antidote(s)

Digoxin Immune Fab *on page 1411*

Additional Information Toxin: Cardiac glycoside

Star-of-Bethlehem (*Ornithogalum umbellatum*)

Related Information

Amaryllis *on page 1052*

Indian Tobacco *on page 1091*

Poinsettia *on page 1126*

Scientific Name *Ornithogalum umbellatum*

Synonyms Dove's Dung; Fuglestjerne; Nap-at-Noon; Summer Snowflake

Mechanism of Toxic Action All parts of the plant, especially the bulb, contain digitalis-like glycosides similar to those seen in Lily-of-the-Valley

Signs & Symptoms of Acute Overdose GI effects (nausea and vomiting) usually precede the cardiovascular effects by several hours; bradycardia; first, second, and third degree heart block; asystole, hypotension, A-V block, ventricular arrhythmias, atrial fibrillation, decreased Q-T interval and prolonged P-R interval; fatigue, confusion, headache, dizziness, contact dermatitis, seeing yellow halos, and hyperkalemia have also been reported

Overdosage Treatment

Decontamination: Ipecac may be beneficial if given within 30 minutes of ingestion; lavage and multidose activated charcoal enhance total body clearance of digitalis; whole bowel irrigation is also beneficial in removing plant debris from the GI tract and is recommended for ingestions of large amounts of plant material

Supportive therapy: Monitor cardiac status and serum potassium levels; bradycardia will frequently respond to atropine; phenytoin is the recommended treatment for ventricular arrhythmias because it will also improve conduction through the A-V node; lidocaine can also be used to treat ventricular arrhythmias, but will not have an effect on A-V conduction; other antiarrhythmics which have been used in arrhythmias resistant to the above therapy include magnesium, amiodarone, and bretylium; a pacemaker should be considered for bradycardia and A-V nodal blocks resistant to medical management

Antidote: Digoxin immune Fab has been shown to interact with several different plant cardiac glycosides and may be beneficial in cases resistant to conventional treatment; indications for its use include ventricular arrhythmias resistant to conventional treatment, severe bradycardia and/or second or third degree heart block resistant to atropine and phenytoin

Antidote(s)

Digoxin Immune Fab *on page 1411*

Additional Information Toxin: Cardiac glycosides

***Stichactis* Species** *see* Sea Anemones *on page 1138*

Stinging Anemone *see* Sea Anemones *on page 1138*

Stinking Elder *see* Elderberry *on page 1081*

Stink Weed *see* Jimson Weed *on page 1094*

St Joseph's Lily *see* Amaryllis *on page 1052*

Stonefish

Mechanism of Toxic Action Fish contains spines covered with integumentary sheaths from which venom is released through grooves on the spine as it travels from glands located at the base; venom is composed of high-molecular weight, heat labile, nondialyzable proteins; potency between the scorpionfish and other species are similar, the difference in clinical presentation may lie in the amount and way in which the venom is delivered; venom is a muscle toxin affecting cardiac, involuntary, and skeletal muscles

Signs & Symptoms of Acute Overdose Severity depends on number of stings, species, amount of venom, and patient age and health; severe pain peaking in 60-90 minutes and lasting 6-12 hours up to 24 hours. Wound may become ischemic and cyanotic with erythema, edema, warmth, and vesicle formation; systemic signs and symptoms include anxiety, headache, tremor, rash, nausea, vomiting, diarrhea, and abdominal pain; also sweating, pallor, delirium, seizures, paralysis, peripheral neuropathies, lymphangitis, arthritis, fever, hypertension, bradycardia, tachycardia, A-V block, ventricular fibrillation, CHF, pericarditis, hypotension, syncope, and respiratory distress; death usually occurs within the first 6-8 hours from respiratory paralysis.

Overdosage Treatment

Decontamination: Immerse wound in hot water to tolerance to inactivate heat labile components of the venom for 30-90 minutes as needed for pain relief, repeat if pain reoccurs; remove pieces of spine from wound; surgical removal of the spines may be necessary

Supportive therapy: Local pain may be treated with tissue infiltration with lidocaine; systemic symptoms should be treated with supportive care (fluids for hypotension)

Antidote:

Antivenin for stonefish envenomations does exist (Commonwealth Serum Laboratories, Melbourne, Australia); bites from other members of the *Scorpaenidae* family usually do not require this antivenin

Antivenin is available in 2 mL vials; made of hyperimmune horse serum; 10 mg of dried antivenin neutralized by 1 mL; dilute in 50-100 mL NS and give slow I.V.; skin test before administration; adverse reactions include anaphylaxis and serum sickness; available from Sea World, San Diego (619-222-6363, ext 2201); Sea World, Aurora, OH (216-562-8101); and Steinhart Aquarium, San Francisco, CA (415-770-7171).

Additional Information

Family: Scorpaenidae; three groups separated by different genera based on the venom apparatus

Pterois (zebrafish, turkeyfish, lionfish, butterfly cod)

Scorpaena (scorpionfish, sculpin)

Synanceja (stonefish)

Range: Found in shallow waters, very motionless, near rocks, coral, or buried in sand

Specific References

Auerbach PS and Halsted BW, "Hazardous Aquatic Life," *Management of Wilderness and Environmental Emergencies*, 2nd ed, Auerbach PS and Geehr EC, eds, St Louis, MO: CV Mosby Co, 1989, 979-83.

Gopalakrishnakone P and Gwee MC, "The Structure of the Venom Gland of Stonefish *Synanceja horrida*," *Toxicon*, 1993, 31(8):979-88.

Lehmann DF and Hardy JC, "Stonefish Envenomation," *N Engl J Med*, 1993, 329(7):510-1.

Stoplight *see* Caladium *on page 1063*

Storkjelm *see* Monkshood *on page 1108*

"Straw-Colored Fiberhead" Mushroom *see* Mushrooms, Toxic (Group III) *on page 1112*

"Straw-Colored Fiberhead" Mushroom *see* Mushrooms, Toxic (Group V) *on page 1114*

Streptococcus Food Poisoning

Commonly Found in Eggs/dairy products, steamed lobster, meat, sausage

Mechanism of Toxic Action Groups A, D, or G *Streptococcus* onset: 1-4 days postingestion

Signs & Symptoms of Acute Overdose Headache, diarrhea, vomiting, fever, pyoderma, asthenia, myalgia, enlarged cervical adenopathy, sore throat

Overdosage Treatment Supportive therapy: Fluid/electrolyte therapy; penicillin may prevent secondary attacks

Diagnostic Tests/Procedures

Electrolytes, Blood *on page 1254*

Additional Information Heat sensitive

Specific References

Berkley SF, Rigau-Perez JG, Facklam R, et al, "Foodbourne Streptococcal Pharyngitis After a Party," *Public Health Rep*, 1986, 101(2):211-5.

Decker MD, Lavely GB, Hutcheson RH Jr, et al, "Foodborne Streptococcal Pharyngitis in a Hospital Pediatrics Clinic," *JAMA*, 1985, 253(5):679-81.

Stricted Cone *see* Cone Shells *on page 1073*

String of Pearls *see* Rosary Pearls (Nontoxic Plant) *on page 1134*

Striped Blister Beetles

CAS Number 56-25-7

Scientific Name *Epicauta* Species (*Meloidae*)

Mechanism of Toxic Action Cantharidin causing a dermatitis manifesting several hours post exposure; average concentration: 2.6% to 4.3%

Signs & Symptoms of Acute Overdose Contact with beetle is painless; blisters appear 2-5 hours with contact; unless broken or rubbed, they are not painful

Adverse Reactions

Dermatologic: Blisters, vesiculobullae

Ocular: Conjunctivitis

Renal: Nephritis, renal failure

Overdosage Treatment

Decontamination: Wash skin with soap and water

Supportive therapy: Steroid cream may be helpful to decrease inflammation

Additional Information Range: Eastern U.S., Nova Scotia, Saskatchewan

Specific References

Brown SG, "Cantharidin Poisoning Due to Blister Beetle," *Br Med J*, 1960, 2(5208):1290-1.

Nicholls DS, Christmas TI, and Greig DE, "Oedemerid Blister Beetle Dermatosis: A Review," *J Am Acad Dermatol*, 1990, 22(5 Pt 1):815-9.

***Stropharia coronilla* ("Crown" Toadstool)** *see* Mushrooms, Toxic (Group VI) *on page 1115*

***Stropharia semiglobata* ("Halfglobe Mushroom" or "Manure Roundhead")** *see* Mushrooms, Toxic (Group VI) *on page 1115*

"Stumper" Mushroom *see* Mushrooms, Toxic (Group VII) *on page 1116*

"Stuntz's Blue Legs" Mushroom *see* Mushrooms, Toxic (Group VI) *on page 1115*

Sulfite *see* Sulfite Food Poisoning *on this page*

Sulfite Food Poisoning

CAS Number 4429-42-9; 7446-09-5; 7631-90-5; 7757-74-6; 7757-83-7; 7790-56-9; 10196-04-0; 10257-55-3

Synonyms Ammonium Sulfite; Calcium Sulfite; Metabisulfites; Potassium Metabisulfite; Sodium Bisulfite; Sodium Metabisulfite; Sodium Sulfite; Sulfite; Sulfur Dioxide

Commonly Found in Sausages, fruits, vegetables, wine, beer, soft drinks, bronchodilator aerosols, injectable preparation of metoclopramide, epinephrine, aminophylline, photography, metal lubricants, lidocaine, dexamethasone, phenylephrine, isoproterenol, dopamine

Mechanism of Toxic Action Preservative in food as an antioxidant; can cause type I hypersensitivity reaction due to a cholinergic reflex mechanism. Onset of symptoms: Within 1 hour

Signs & Symptoms of Acute Overdose Nausea, watery diarrhea, abdominal cramps, hypotension, wheezing, flushing, sweating, tachycardia, seizures, vomiting, rash, hand eczema

Overdosage Treatment

Decontamination: Avoid ipecac; dilute with 4-8 oz of milk or water

Supportive therapy: Fluid/electrolyte replacement; epinephrine or diphenhydramine for allergic manifestations

Antidote(s)

Epinephrine *on page 1422*

Diagnostic Tests/Procedures

Electrolytes, Blood *on page 1254*

Pregnancy Implications Atrophied testes have been noted as a teratogenic effect in rats

Additional Information Primary route of exposure is by ingestion, inhalation, or intravenous; minimum dose for CNS toxicity is 6 mg/kg

Specific References

Acosta R, Granados J, Mourelle M, et al, "Sulfite Sensitivity: Relationship Between Sulfite Plasma Levels and Bronchospasm – Case Report," *Ann Allergy*, 1989, 62(5):402-5.

Dalton-Bunnow MF, "Sulfite Content of Drug Products," *Am J Hosp Pharm*, 1985, 42(10):2196-201.

Riggs BS, Harchelroad FP Jr, and Poole C, "Allergic Reaction to Sulfiting Agents," *Ann Emerg Med*, 1986, 15(1):77-9.

Sulfur Dioxide *see* Sulfite Food Poisoning *on this page*

"Sulphur Tuft" Mushroom *see* Mushrooms, Toxic (Group VII) *on page 1116*

Summer Snowflake *see* Star-of-Bethlehem (*Ornithogalum umbellatum*) *on page 1146*

Swamp Hellebore *see* Corn Lily *on page 1074*

"Sweater" Mushroom *see* Mushrooms, Toxic (Group III) *on page 1112*

Swedish Ivy (Nontoxic Plant)

Sweet Pea

Scientific Name *Lathyrus odoratus*

Signs & Symptoms of Acute Overdose Bradycardia, paralysis, respiratory depression, and seizures

Overdosage Treatment Large quantities must be ingested chronically to result in toxicity

Exclude cathyrus peas from the diet

Symptomatic and supportive treatment

Additional Information

Toxin: Beta-aminopropionitrite

Range: Found throughout the U.S.

Toxic part: All parts, particularly the seeds

Sweet Root *see* Licorice *on page 1098*

"Sylvan" Mushroom *see* Mushrooms, Toxic (Group VII) *on page 1116*

Syngonium *see* Nephthytis *on page 1118*

Syngonium podophyllum *see* Nephthytis *on page 1118*

Sysport *see Clostridium botulinum* Food Poisoning *on page 1070*

Tahitian Bridal Veil (Nontoxic Plant)

Taro *see* Caladium *on page 1063*

Taro Vine *see* Devil's Ivy *on page 1079*

Tartar Yellow S *see* Tartrazine Food Poisoning *on this page*

Tartrazine Food Poisoning

CAS Number 1934-21-0

Synonyms Acid Yellow T; Acilan Yellow GG; Cake Yellow; Food and Drug Coloring No. 5; Tartar Yellow S; Wool Yellow

Mechanism of Toxic Action Coloring agent in foods can cause hypersensitivity reactions (not IgE-related); incubation period: 30 minutes

Signs & Symptoms of Acute Overdose Angioedema, wheezing, rash, anaphylaxis; can last several hours

Overdosage Treatment Supportive therapy: Epinephrine/diphenhydramine for allergic manifestations

Antidote(s)

Epinephrine *on page 1422*

Additional Information 8% to 15% of affected individuals are intolerant of salicylates

Specific References

Murdoch RD, Pollock I, and Naeem S, "Tartrazine-Induced Histamine Release *In Vivo* in Normal Subjects," *J R Coll Physicians Lond*, 1987, 21(4):257-61.

"Tartrazine: A Yellow Hazard," *Drug Ther Bull*, 1980, 18(14):53-5.

Taxus **Species** *see* Yew *on page 1159*

Tetraodon *see* Tetrodotoxin Food Poisoning *on this page*

Tetrodotoxin Food Poisoning

Synonyms Puffer Poisoning; Tetraodon; TTX

Commonly Found in Pufferfish, blow fish, botefe, tambores, swell fish, *Taricha* newt, blue-ringed octopus, Atelopus frogs, xanthid crab, starfish, and fugu

Mechanism of Toxic Action A neurotoxin on the motor axons and skeletal muscle tissue (inhibits sodium conductance of nerve cells); incubation time: 10 minutes to 3 hours postingestion

Signs & Symptoms of Acute Overdose Tingling of the lips with mydriasis, blurred vision, hypotension following apnea, lacrimation; respiratory depression can occur within 2 hours as can paralysis, seizures, fasciculation, headache, slurred speech, dysarthria, ataxia, dyspnea, asthenia, dysphagia, vomiting, salivation, watery diarrhea, sweating, and hypothermia. Hypertension has also been observed.

(Continued)

Tetrodotoxin Food Poisoning *(Continued)*

Toxicodynamics/Kinetics
Half-life: ~3 hours
Elimination: In the urine

Toxic Dosage Fatal dose: 10 mcg/kg (200,000 mouse units of tetrodotoxin)

Overdosage Treatment
Decontamination: Lavage with 2% bicarbonate solution/activated charcoal with laxative; avoid ipecac
Supportive therapy: Fluids, norepinephrine (8-12 mcg/minute in adults, 0.1-0.2 mcg/kg/minute in children) for hypotension. Atropine is useful for bradycardia; mechanical ventilation may be required for respiratory support

Additional Information Can produce total paralysis with fixed mydriasis; when pronouncing patients dead, caution is advised; not heat labile; heat stable, water soluble toxin

Specific References

Bradley SG and Klika LJ, "A Fatal Poisoning From the Oregon Rough-Skinned Newt (*Taricha granulosa*)," *JAMA*, 1981, 246(3):247.
Laobhripatr S, Limpakarnjanarat K, Sangwonloy O, et al, "Food Poisoning Due to Consumption of the Freshwater Puffer Tetraodon Fangi in Thailand," *Toxicon*, 1990, 28(11):1372-5.
Sims JK and Ostman DC, "Pufferfish Poisoning: Emergency Diagnosis and Management of Mild Human Tetrodotoxication," *Ann Emerg Med*, 1986, 15(9):1094-8.
Sun K, Wat J, and So P, "Puffer Fish Poisoning," *Anaesth Intensive Care*, 1994, 22(3):307-8.
Torda TA, "Pufferfish (Tetrodotoxin) Poisoning: Clinical Record and Suggested Management," *Med J Aust*, 1973, 1(12):599-602.

Texas Blue Bonnet *see* Lupine *on page 1102*
Texas Wonder *see* Caladium *on page 1063*
Textile Cone *see* Cone Shells *on page 1073*
Thelotornis kirtlandi *see* Colubrids *on page 1073*
Thevitia *see* Oleander *on page 1120*
Thorn Apple *see* Jimson Weed *on page 1094*
Three-Leaved Indian Turnip *see* Jack-in-the-Pulpit *on page 1093*
Thymelaeaceae *see* Daphne *on page 1077*
Tibey *see* Star-of-Bethlehem (*Hippobroma longiflora*) *on page 1145*
Tickleweed *see* Corn Lily *on page 1074*
Timber Rattlesnake *see* Rattlesnakes *on page 1132*

Tin Plant (Nontoxic Plant)

Tobacco

Scientific Name *Nicotiana tabacum*

Synonyms Cultivated Tobacco

Mechanism of Toxic Action All parts of the plant contain the toxin nicotine which stimulates motor endplates, ganglionic sites, and smooth muscles by a direct acetylcholine-like action

Signs & Symptoms of Acute Overdose Low doses can cause nausea, vomiting, oral irritation, headache, thirst, sweating, and asthenia; higher doses can cause hallucinations, confusion; CNS stimulation followed by depression, seizures, hyperthermia, hypertension, and tachycardia followed by hypotension, bradycardia, and an irregular pulse

Toxicodynamics/Kinetics
Onset of action: 15-60 minutes
Duration: 3-12 hours
Absorption: Well absorbed by all routes
Half-life: 0.8-2.2 hours

Toxic Dosage Human fatalities have been seen at 0.8 mg/kg of nicotine, but depend largely on the extent of spontaneous vomiting

Overdosage Treatment
Decontamination: Ipecac is contraindicated due to the risk of seizures; lavage and multidose activated charcoal may enhance total body clearance of nicotine
Supportive therapy: Seizures usually respond to diazepam; hypotension generally resolves with I.V. fluids

Additional Information Toxin: Nicotine

Tolguacha *see* Jimson Weed *on page 1094*

Tomato (Leaves and Stems)

Scientific Name *Lycopersicon*; *Lycopersicon lycopersicum*; *Solanum*

Synonyms Gold Apple; Love Apple; Pear Tomato

Mechanism of Toxic Action Contains toxic alkaloids, solanine most significant structurally similar to cardioglycoside, causes hemolytic and hemorrhagic damage to GI tract similar to saponins; some plants may also contain alpha-cholinergic alkaloids

Signs & Symptoms of Acute Overdose Nausea, vomiting, diarrhea, headache, visual changes, drowsiness, fever, sweating, asthenia, hallucinations, anticholinergic effects may or may not be present to varying degrees

Toxicodynamics/Kinetics Toxicity occurs within 2-24 hours, diarrhea may last 3-6 days, anticholinergic effects may delay GI emptying and produce delayed effects

Toxic Dosage Unclear, toxicity reported in livestock

Overdosage Treatment

Decontamination: Ipecac if vomiting has not already occurred, lavage and/or charcoal may be beneficial if patient presents symptomatic

Supportive therapy: Maintain fluid and electrolyte balance as necessary, support vital signs; physostigmine will reverse anticholinergic toxicity that may be associated with exposure

Antidote(s)

Physostigmine *on page 1457*

Additional Information Green fruit and entire plant excluding ripe fruit potentially toxic

Tom Thumb *see* Christmas Cherry *on page 1068*

"Torn-Capped Fiberhead" Mushroom *see* Mushrooms, Toxic (Group III) *on page 1112*

"Torn-Capped Fiberhead" Mushroom *see* Mushrooms, Toxic (Group V) *on page 1114*

Toxicodendron guercifolium *see* Poison Oak *on page 1127*

Toxicodendron radicans *see* Poison Ivy *on page 1126*

Toxicodendron vernex *see* Poison Sumac *on page 1127*

Travelers' Diarrhea (Enterotoxin) *see Escherichia coli* Food Poisoning *on page 1082*

Tree Cobra *see* Cobras *on page 1072*

Tree Oxalis *see* Shamrock *on page 1140*

Tree Tobacco *see* Mustard Tree *on page 1117*

***Triactis* Species** *see* Sea Anemones *on page 1138*

Triatoma sanguisuga *see* Reduvids *on page 1133*

Trichinella spiralis Food Poisoning

Synonyms Trichinosis

Commonly Found in Dogs, swine, cats, rats, bear meat, pork

Mechanism of Toxic Action Ingestion of *Trichinella* cysts which will eventually produce mucosal invasive larvae; incubation period: About 1 week

Signs & Symptoms of Acute Overdose Fever, myalgia, rash, periorbital edema, cranial nerve palsies, abdominal cramps, headache, malaise

Overdosage Treatment

Decontamination: Majority of symptomatic patients need supportive care only as infection is self-limited. Benzimidazole carbonates may be given. Mebendazole 200-400 mg 3 times/day for 3 days followed by 400-500 mg 3 times/day for 10 days is active against both invasive and encystment stages. Mebendazole does not cross the blood-brain barrier. Thiabendazole 25 mg/kg twice daily for 7 days is indicated to eliminate gut-dwelling adult worms. It is not effective against larval stages in tissue. Not well tolerated secondary to increased gastrointestinal side effects. Albendazole is still under investigation. Steroids (prednisone 40-60 mg/day) may reduce inflammation and are recommended in serious infections.

Overall prognosis is related to severity and intensity of initial infection as well as effectiveness of antiparasitic agents, anti-inflammatory agents, patient's immune status, and whether any end-organ damage was rendered. Mortality related to pulmonary, cardiac, and CNS involvement.

All patients traveling outside the United States should receive pre-travel counseling. Smoking, microwaving, and freezing are not reliable means of eliminating trichinosis.

Diagnostic Tests/Procedures

Creatine Kinase, Blood *on page 1242*

Electrolytes, Blood *on page 1254*

Eosinophil Count *on page 1259*

Muscle Biopsy *on page 1301*

Additional Information Dissemination to striated muscles can occur in the second week. Can cause myocarditis or meningitis. Prevalent on both coasts in the U.S., Australia, and the Pacific islands.

Microbiology: *Trichinella spiralis*, a nematode, is the infectious agent of human trichinosis. The adult male worm measures 1.5 mm in length and the adult fe-

(Continued)

Trichinella spiralis Food Poisoning *(Continued)*

male measures 2-4 mm. The average lifespan is 4 months. Identification is made by demonstration of the characteristic encapsulated larvae in biopsy specimens of infected muscles. The cyst wall is derived from the host cell muscle. The larva may incite an inflammatory reaction characterized by surrounding lymphocytes and eosinophils and eventual larval calcification.

Epidemiology:

Trichinella is found worldwide except Australia and several Pacific islands. Trichinosis results from consumption of undercooked pork, unsanitary cooking practices and contaminated meats. Its reservoirs include pigs, horses, bears, and arctic mammals. The three subspecies reflect three sylvatic cycles – arctic, temperate, and tropical.

The incidence in the United States continues to decline probably because of increased public awareness, commercial freezing, and legislature prohibiting feeding of raw garbage to swine. From 1982-1986, approximately 57 cases per year were reported with three associated deaths. From 1987-1990, 206 cases were reported to the CDC. Most of the cases reported in the U.S. are associated with improperly cooked game animals and travel to Mexico, Asia, and other endemic areas.

Trichinosis results from ingestion of encysted larvae in the contaminated meat. The acid-pepsin environment in the stomach digest the cyst wall, releasing the infectious larvae which burrow and attach to the mucosa at the base of the villi. Over a 6- to 10-day period, the larvae molt four times to become sexually mature adult worms which attach to the duodenal and jejunal mucosa producing between 200-1500 larvae over the next 2 weeks. The newborn or first-stage larvae penetrate the gut mucosa into the lamina propria. An immunologic reaction partially mediated by IgE-mast cell system results in release of vasoactive substances that promote intestinal motility and secretion (diarrhea). The larvae then migrate into the draining lymphatics and blood vessels and have a high predilection to invade muscles of increased use and blood flow (ie, diaphragm, extraocular muscles, masseters, tongue, deltoids, and gastrocnemius). Once penetrated into the skeletal muscle, the larvae elicit a host inflammatory response which surrounds the larvae and creates granulomas and calcifications. Only larvae that encyst mature. Larvae may remain viable and infective for many years even in calcified cysts.

The severity of the symptoms is directly related to the larvae load. Patients usually remain asymptomatic with 1-10 larvae per gram muscle and systemic illness occurs with 50-100 larvae per gram.

Clinical Syndromes:

- **Asymptomatic:** 90% to 95% infections are asymptomatic
- **Self-limited:** 1-2 weeks after ingestion, patients experience enteric phase associated with nonbloody diarrhea and abdominal cramps. Approximately 2-4 weeks later, patients experience fever, intense myalgia especially extraocular and masseters, periorbital edema, conjunctivitis, headache, and/or subconjunctival and subungual petechia. Ninety percent will have peripheral eosinophilia which peaks at 3-4 weeks. Absence of eosinophilia is a poor prognostic sign. Approximately 50% will have elevated CK and LDH enzymes.
- **Arctic trichinosis:** Described in Northern Canada and Alaska in which patients have eaten contaminated walruses or seals. Associated with diarrhea lasting up to 14 weeks, mild and transitory myalgia without fever, peripheral eosinophilia, and no pathogens isolated in stools to explain etiology.
- **Myocarditis:** Incidence of approximately 5% of symptomatic patients. Typically occurs 3 weeks after larvae migration and presents with tachycardia and chest pain mimicking infarction. Patients have myocardium invasion without encystment. EKG reveals benign, reversible nonspecific EKG changes. May develop nonspecific inflammatory myocarditis predominantly eosinophilic and sometimes associated with pericarditis. Fewer than 0.1% patients die from cardiac complications (ie, congestive heart failure).
- **Pulmonary:** Up to 6% symptomatic patients may develop cough and dyspnea on exertion presumed secondary to larvae migration associated with infiltrates, hemorrhage, and allergic granulomatous reactions
- **CNS:** Prevalence of 10% to 24% in symptomatic patients. In the first 2 weeks when larvae migration is maximal, can result in CNS invasion which appears as meningoencephalitis with delirium and confusion. Larvae encystment may result in focal neurological deficits, anal/urinary sphincter dysfunction, cranial nerve palsies especially VI and VII, seizures, dizziness, anisocoria, tinnitus, diminished auditory acuity, or ataxia. Papilledema, hemianopia, aphasia, and paresis have been reported. CNS and peripheral nerve deficits generally resolve in 4-6 months but may persist up to 10 years. May also cause eosinophilic meningitis. CT scan is usually normal but may see multiple nodular or ring enhancing lesions 3-8 mm and calcification. EEG reveals nonspecific abnormalities consistent with diffuse encephalopathy.

Diagnosis: CDC case definition must fit one of two criteria:

1. Positive muscle biopsy or positive serology titer in a patient with clinical symptoms compatible with trichinosis including eosinophilia, fever, myalgias or periorbital edema
2. In an outbreak (at least one person must fit above criteria), must have either a positive serology titer or clinical symptoms compatible with trichinosis in a person who shared the implicated meat source

IgM and IgE serology tests are helpful in distinguishing active from previous infection

Specific References

Bailey TM and Schantz PM, "Trends in the Incidence and Transmission Patterns of Trichinosis in Humans in the United States: Comparisons of the Periods 1975-1981 and 1982-1986," *Rev Infect Dis*, 1990, 12(1):5-11.

Compton SJ, Celum CL, Lee C, et al, "Trichinosis With Ventilatory Failure and Persistent Myocarditis," *Clin Infect Dis*, 1993, 16(4):500-4.

Levin ML, "Treatment of Trichinosis With Mebendazole," *Am J Trop Med Hyg*, 1983, 32(5):980-3.

Mawhorter SD and Kazura JW, "Trichinosis of the Central Nervous System," *Semin Neurol*, 1993, 13(2):148-52.

McAuley JB, Michelson MK, and Schantz PM, "*Trichinella* Infection in Travelers," *J Infect Dis*, 1991, 164(5):1013-6.

Trichinosis *see* *Trichinella spiralis* Food Poisoning *on page 1151*

Tricholoma pardinum *see* Mushrooms, Toxic (Group VII) *on page 1116*

Tricholoma pessundatum *see* Mushrooms, Toxic (Group VII) *on page 1116*

Trombicula irritans *see* Mites *on page 1107*

Trumpet Lily *see* Jimson Weed *on page 1094*

TTX *see* Tetrodotoxin Food Poisoning *on page 1149*

Tuft Root *see* Dieffenbachia *on page 1079*

Tulip

Scientific Name *Tulipa*

Mechanism of Toxic Action Allergic dermatitis

Signs & Symptoms of Acute Overdose Tingling sensation of fingers may be an early indication of symptoms; symptoms are not necessarily restricted to area of direct exposure, dust may produce symptoms; rash, possibly with erythema, hyperkeratosis, fissuring, blistering, crusting, brittle nails

Toxicodynamics/Kinetics Dermal reaction may be delayed 12 hours

Overdosage Treatment

Decontamination: Wash thoroughly

Supportive therapy: Corticosteroids or antihistamines may be useful

Tulipa *see* Tulip *on this page*

Tulip Cone *see* Cone Shells *on page 1073*

"Turban Fungus" Mushroom *see* Mushrooms, Toxic (Group II) *on page 1112*

Turkey Fish

Mechanism of Toxic Action Fish contains spines covered with integumentary sheaths from which venom is released through grooves on the spine as it travels from glands located at the base; venom is composed of high-molecular weight, heat labile, nondialyzable proteins; potency between the scorpionfish and other species are similar, the difference in clinical presentation may lie in the amount and way in which the venom is delivered; venom is a muscle toxin affecting cardiac, involuntary, and skeletal muscles

Signs & Symptoms of Acute Overdose Severity depends on number of stings, species, amount of venom, and patient's age and health; severe pain peaking in 60-90 minutes and lasting 6-12 hours up to 24 hours. Wound may become ischemic and cyanotic with erythema, edema, warmth, and vesicle formation; systemic signs and symptoms include anxiety, headache, tremor, rash, nausea, vomiting, diarrhea, and abdominal pain; also sweating, pallor, delirium, seizures, paralysis, paresthesia, lymphangitis, arthritis, fever, hypertension, bradycardia, tachycardia, A-V block, ventricular fibrillation, CHF, pericarditis, hypotension, syncope, and respiratory distress; death usually occurs within the first 6-8 hours from respiratory paralysis

Overdosage Treatment

Decontamination: Immerse wound in hot water to tolerance to inactivate heat labile components of the venom for 30-40 minutes; remove pieces of spine from wound; surgical removal of the spines may be necessary

(Continued)

Turkey Fish *(Continued)*

Supportive therapy: Local pain may be treated with tissue infiltration with lidocaine; systemic symptoms should be treated with supportive care (fluids for hypotension)

Antidote: Antivenin for stonefish envenomations does exist (Commonwealth Serum Laboratories, Melbourne, Australia); bites from other members of the *Scorpaenidae* family usually do not require this antivenin

Additional Information

Family: Scorpaenidae; three groups separated by different genera based on the venom apparatus

Pterois (zebrafish, turkeyfish, lionfish, butterfly cod)

Scorpaena (scorpionfish, sculpin)

Synanceja (stonefish)

Range: Very beautiful coral reef fish found in Asia; usually single or paired in shallow water; contains vertical dark stripes with lengths up to 35"

Specific References

Auerbach PS and Halsted BW, "Hazardous Aquatic Life," *Management of Wilderness and Environmental Emergencies*, 2nd ed, Auerbach PS and Geehr EC, eds, St Louis, MO: CV Mosby Co, 1989, 979-83.

Ellenhorn MJ and Barceloux DG, "Envenomations From Bites and Stings," *Medical Toxicology Diagnosis and Treatment of Wyman Poisoning*, New York, NY: Elsevier, 1988, 1153-65.

Kizer KW, McKinney HE, and Auerbach PS, "*Scorpaenidae* Envenomation: A Five Year Poison Center Experience," *JAMA*, 1985, 253(6):807-10.

Turkeyfish (*Pterois*) *see* Lionfish *on page 1099*

Tyramine Hydrochloride Food Poisoning

CAS Number 51-67-2; 60-19-5

Synonyms Tyrosamine Hydrochloride

Commonly Found in Cheeses (especially aged cheeses), yeast extracts, spoiled (decaying) meats, pickled herring, smoked fish, alcohol-containing beverages, broad bean pods (fava beans)

Mechanism of Toxic Action Can precipitate the release of norepinephrine

Signs & Symptoms of Acute Overdose Palpitations, hypertension, hypotension, headache, sweating, mydriasis, vertigo; can cause intracerebral hemorrhage

Overdosage Treatment Supportive therapy: Phentolamine mesylate to treat hypertensive crises (I.V.: 2.5-5 mg; titrate as necessary)

Additional Information Should not consume tyramine-containing foods within 14 days of MAO ingestion; can cause hypertensive crisis when given with MAO inhibitors or amphetamines; when given in combination with chlorpromazine, hypotension can result. Tyramine hydrochloride is not noted in cottage cheese or cream cheese. Milk and cream are also safe; cooking does not inactivate tyramine.

Specific References

Hannah P, Glover V, and Sandler M, "Tyramine in Wine and Beer," *Lancet*, 1988, 1(8590):879.

Lippman SB and Nash K, "Monoamine Oxidase Inhibitor Update: Potential Adverse Food and Drug Interactions," *Drug Saf*, 1990, 5(3):195-204.

McCabe BJ and Tsuang M, "Dietary Considerations in MAO Inhibitor Regimens," *J Clin Psychiatry*, 1982, 43(5):178-81.

Tyrosamine Hydrochloride *see* Tyramine Hydrochloride Food Poisoning *on this page*

Ulgastrin Neo *see* Licorice *on page 1098*

Umbrella Leaf *see* Mayapple *on page 1105*

Umbrella Tree *see* Schefflera (Nontoxic Plant) *on page 1137*

Urginea maritima *see* Squill *on page 1143*

Variegated Philodendron *see* Devil's Ivy *on page 1079*

Venusvogn *see* Monkshood *on page 1108*

Vibrio cholerae and *Vibrio parahaemolyticus* Food Poisoning

Commonly Found in Uncooked shellfish and raw seafood

Mechanism of Toxic Action *Vibrio parahaemolyticus* and *Vibrio cholerae* are motile, gram-negative rods; *V. parahaemolyticus* produces shiga toxin; *V. cholerae* produces cholera toxin (an enterotoxin) which inhibits absorption and enhances intestinal secretion; incubation period: 12-14 hours

Signs & Symptoms of Acute Overdose Grayish, watery diarrhea [rice-water stools] (profuse); fluid losses may exceed 1 L/hour

Overdosage Treatment

Vibrio cholerae: Early and rapid replacement of fluid and electrolytes can decrease the mortality to <1%. Oral rehydration is usually successful, but in severe cases, intravenous replacement is required. When fluid and electrolyte imbalances are corrected, cholera is a short, self-limiting disease lasting a few days. According to the *MMWR*, doxycycline, tetracycline, co-trimoxazole, erythromycin, and furazolidone have all demonstrated effectiveness in decreasing the diarrhea and bacterial shedding in this disease. The usual recommendation is doxycycline 300 mg as a single dose for adults, and co-trimoxazole 5 mg/kg as trimethoprim, twice daily for 3 days.

Vibrio parahaemolyticus: Tetracycline: 500 mg 4 times/day for 5 days

Diagnostic Tests/Procedures

Electrolytes, Blood *on page 1254*

Stool Culture *on page 1356*

Additional Information Immunity with cholera vaccines is relatively short-lived; can cause hypokalemia; toxin is heat labile; in 1993-94, a total of 69 cholera cases were reported to the CDC with 65 cases (94%) being associated with foreign travel

Microbiology:

Vibrio cholerae is an oxidase-positive, fermentative, gram-negative rod that can have a comma-shaped appearance on initial isolation. *V. cholerae* can be subdivided by the production of endotoxin and agglutination in 0-1 antisera with the nomenclature of *V. cholerae* 0-1, atypical or nontoxigenic 0-1, or non-0-1. The serogroup 0-1 can further be subdivided into the El Tor and Classic cholera biotypes which can be further subdivided into a variety of serotypes. The major virulence factor of *V. cholerae* is the extracellular enterotoxin produced by the 0-1 strain, although nontoxin-producing organisms have been implicated in some outbreaks.

V. cholerae is a facultative anaerobe which grows best at a pH of 7.0 and at a wide temperature range (18°C to 37°C). *Vibrio* species can be differentiated from other gram-negative bacilli by their sensitivity to 0129 and may be speciated by a variety of biochemical tests.

Epidemiology:

Cholera is usually spread by contamination of water and food by infected feces, with fecal contamination of water being the principal vehicle of transmission. Person-to-person transmission is less common due to the large organism load necessary for infection. Asymptomatic carriers play a minor role in cholera outbreaks. Outbreaks may be seasonally dependent based on either temperature or rainfall. Transmission by food can be eliminated by thorough cooking. Adequate sanitation is the best means of cholera prevention.

There have been several pandemics of cholera reported since 1817, originating in Bengal and subsequently spreading to a variety of geographic locations, responsible for hundreds of thousands of deaths. The latest pandemic originated in Indonesia in 1961 and moved to the Western hemisphere. In 1991, a cholera outbreak in Peru and 20 other countries in the Western hemisphere accounted for over 600,000 cases with 5000 deaths caused by El Tor 0-1.

Clinical Syndromes: After a 2- to 5-day incubation period, classic cholera is characterized by an abrupt onset of vomiting and profuse watery diarrhea with flecks of mucus (rice water stool). Fluid losses can be significant (up to 20 L/day). Hypovolemic shock and metabolic acidosis can cause death within a few hours of onset, especially in children. Mortality, in untreated cases, is as high as 60%. Milder forms of the disease also occur, especially with the non-0-1 cholera.

Diagnosis: Organisms can be identified by darkfield microscopy showing large numbers of comma-shaped organisms with significant motility. However, this test is relatively insensitive and is nonspecific. Thiosulfate-citrate-bile salt-sucrose agar (TCBS) or alkaline peptone broth are used to facilitate growth and identification. Positive identification depends on serologic and biochemical testing.

Specific References

"Cholera Associated With Food Transported From El Salvador - Indiana, 1994," *MMWR Morb Mortal Wkly Rep*, 1995, 44:385-6.

"Cholera Associated With International Travel, 1992," *MMWR Morb Mortal Wkly Rep*, 1992, 41(36):664-7.

Falkow S and Mekalanos J, "The Enteric Bacilli and *Vibrios*," *Microbiology*, 4th ed, Davis BD, Dulbecco R, Eisen HN, et al, eds, Philadelphia, PA: JB Lippincott Co, 1990, 561-87.

Johnston JM, Becker SF, McFarland LM, "*Vibrio vulnificus*: Man and the Sea," *JAMA* , 1985, 253(19):2850-3.

Levine WC and Griffin PM, "*Vibrio* Infections on the Gulf Coast: The Results of a First Year of Regional Surveillance Gulf Coast *Vibrio* Working Group," *J Infect Dis*, 1993, 167(2):479-83.

Morris JG Jr and Black RE, "Cholera and Other *Vibrioses* in the United States," *N Engl J Med*, 1985, 312(6):343-50.

Rabbani GH, "Cholera," *J Clin Gastroenterol*, 1986, 15(3):507-28.

Tacket CO, Brenner F, Blake PA, "Clinical Features and an Epidemiological Study of *Vibrio vulnificus* Infections," *J Infect Dis*, 1984, 149(4):558-61.

"Update: Cholera -- Western Hemisphere, and Recommendations for Treatment of Cholera," *MMWR Morb Mortal Wkly Rep*, 1991, 40(32):562-5.

"Update: *Vibrio cholerae* 01-Western Hemisphere, 1991-1994, and *V. cholerae* 0139-Asia, 1994," *MMWR Morb Mortal Wkly Rep*, 1995, 44(11):215-9.

(Continued)

Vibrio cholerae and *Vibrio parahaemolyticus* Food Poisoning *(Continued)*

"*Vibrio vulnificus* Infections Associated With Raw Oyster Consumption – Florida, 1981-1992," *MMWR Morb Mortal Wkly Rep*, 1993, 42(21):405-7.
Zwadyk P, "Vibrionaceae," *Zinsser Microbiology*, 20th ed, Joklik WK, Willett HP, Amos DB, et al, eds, Norwalk, CT: Appleton & Lange, 1992, 566-76.

***Viola* Species** *see* Pansy *on page 1121*

Violet Bloom *see* Deadly Nightshade *on page 1078*

Violet Wood Sorrel *see* Shamrock *on page 1140*

Violin Brown Recluse Spider *see* Brown Recluse Spider *on page 1061*

Viscum album *see* Mistletoe *on page 1107*

"Vomit Wort" *see* Indian Tobacco *on page 1091*

Wake Robin *see* Jack-in-the-Pulpit *on page 1093*

Wandering Jew (Nontoxic Plant)

Warneckei (Nontoxic Plant)

Water Buttercup *see* Buttercup *on page 1063*

Water Goggles *see* Marsh Marigold *on page 1105*

Water Hemlock

Scientific Name *Cicuta bulbifera*; *Cicuta douglasii*; *Cicuta maculata*

Synonyms Cowbane; False Parsley; Snake Root; Wild Carrot; Wild Parsnip

Signs & Symptoms of Acute Overdose Nausea, vomiting, diarrhea, mydriasis, tachycardia, hypotension, acidosis, myoglobinuria, rhabdomyolysis, renal failure, seizures, and death

Overdosage Treatment

Decontamination: Activated charcoal with cathartic for recent ingestions

Supportive therapy: Provide symptomatic and supportive therapy; manage seizures with diazepam or lorazepam; recurring seizures may need barbiturate or phenytoin treatment; sodium bicarbonate can be given for acidosis

Additional Information

Family: Umbelliferae

Toxin: Cicutoxin

Toxic part: Whole plant, especially the root

Range: Found in swamps in Western U.S. and Alaska

Fatal dose: 1 square inch piece of root may be fatal upon ingestion

Specific References

Landers D, Seppi K, and Blauer W, "Seizures and Death on a White River Float Trip. Report of Water Hemlock Poisoning," *West J Med*, 1985, 142(5):637-40.
Robson P, "Water Hemlock Poisoning," *Lancet*, 1965, 2:1274-5.
Starreveld E and Hope E, "Cicutoxin POisoning (Water Hemlock)," *Neurology*, 1975, 25:730-4.

Weanling Diarrhea *see* *Escherichia coli* Food Poisoning *on page 1082*

Weather Plant *see* Jequirity Bean *on page 1093*

Weedy Nightshade *see* Deadly Nightshade *on page 1078*

Weeping Fig (Nontoxic Plant)

Western Coral Snake (*Micrurus euryxanthus*) *see* Elapids *on page 1080*

Western Diamondback Rattlesnake *see* Rattlesnakes *on page 1132*

Western Massasauga *see* Rattlesnakes *on page 1132*

Western Pygmy Rattlesnake *see* Rattlesnakes *on page 1132*

Western Yew *see* Yew *on page 1159*

White Hellebore *see* Corn Lily *on page 1074*

"White" *Lepiota* Mushroom *see* Mushrooms, Toxic (Group VII) *on page 1116*

Wicky *see* Mountain Laurel *on page 1110*

Wild Carrot *see* Water Hemlock *on this page*

Wild Cucumber

Scientific Name *Echinocystis oregana*; *Marah oreganus*

Synonyms Bigroot; Mock Cucumber

Mechanism of Toxic Action Contains cucurbitacin which is a cytotoxic substance

Signs & Symptoms of Acute Overdose Leg cramps, abdominal pain, DIC, hypotension, mydriasis, cyanosis

Toxicodynamics/Kinetics Symptoms can occur within 9 hours

Overdosage Treatment Supportive therapy: Treat hypotension with fluids, colloids, and pressor solutions

Additional Information An ovoid fruit found on a perennial vine; usually located in Western North America; similar spiny pods as Jimson weed

Specific References

Hugelmeyer CD, Putnam TS, and Burton BT, "Fatal Poisoning Due to Ingestion of Wild Cucumber Seed Tea," *AAPCC/AACT/ABMT Scientific Meeting*, Vancouver BC, 1987.

Wild Licorice *see* Jequirity Bean *on page 1093*

Wild Mustard

Scientific Name *Brassica* Species

Synonyms California Rape; Charlock

Signs & Symptoms of Acute Overdose Contact dermatitis, nausea, vomiting

Toxic Dosage No specific cases of human toxicity have been reported

Overdosage Treatment

Decontamination: Dermal: Decontaminate area, remove any foreign bodies which remain, topical steroids may be of benefit

Supportive therapy:

Dermal: Observe for any signs of infection

Oral: Supportive care and fluid replacement is seldom required

Additional Information

Family: Cruciferae

Range: Seen over much of the temperate zones of the U.S.

Toxin: Hairs of the plant can cause mechanical injury and seeds contain GI irritants

Wild Parsnip *see* Water Hemlock *on previous page*

Wild Pepper *see* Daphne Mezereum *on page 1077*

Wild Sage *see* Lantana *on page 1096*

Wild Strawberry (Nontoxic Plant)

Wild Tobacco *see* Indian Tobacco *on page 1091*

Wild Turnip *see* Jack-in-the-Pulpit *on page 1093*

Willow-Leaves Foxglove *see* Foxglove *on page 1085*

Winter Cherry *see* Christmas Cherry *on page 1068*

Winter Fern *see* Poison Hemlock *on page 1126*

Wistaria *see* Wisteria *on this page*

Wisteria

Scientific Name *Wisteria*

Synonyms Kidney Bean Tree; Wistaria

Mechanism of Toxic Action Contains glycosides which cause GI upset

Signs & Symptoms of Acute Overdose Oral burning, nausea, vomiting, abdominal pain, minimal diarrhea, fluid loss, shock

Toxicodynamics/Kinetics Unclear, but duration reported to be 24 hours

Toxic Dosage Two seeds or pods can be toxic

Overdosage Treatment

Decontamination: Consider ipecac if early after ingestion and patient is asymptomatic; activated charcoal with cathartic may be beneficial

Supportive therapy: Maintain fluid and electrolyte balance

Additional Information Toxic parts: All, pods and seeds mostly

Wisteria *see* Wisteria *on this page*

Wolfsbane *see* Monkshood *on page 1108*

Wonderberry *see* Black Nightshade *on page 1057*

Wonderbulb *see* Autumn Crocus *on page 1054*

Wood Laurel *see* Mountain Laurel *on page 1110*

"Wood-Loving" Mushroom *see* Mushrooms, Toxic (Group VII) *on page 1116*

Wood Sour *see* Shamrock *on page 1140*

"Woods" *Psalliota* Mushroom *see* Mushrooms, Toxic (Group VII) *on page 1116*

"Wooly Chanterelle" Mushroom *see* Mushrooms, Toxic (Group VII) *on page 1116*

Wool Yellow *see* Tartrazine Food Poisoning *on page 1149*

"Wooly Milkcap" Mushroom *see* Mushrooms, Toxic (Group VII) *on page 1116*

Xanthoxalis Species *see* Shamrock *on page 1140*

Yanpon *see* Holly *on page 1089*

Yaxci *see* Century Plant *on page 1067*

"Yellow-Juiced" *Lactarius* Mushroom *see* Mushrooms, Toxic (Group VII) *on page 1116*

Yellow Oleander *see* Oleander *on page 1120*

Yellow Parilla *see* Moonseed *on page 1109*

Yellow Sage *see* Lantana *on page 1096*

Yersinia enterocolitica Food Poisoning

Commonly Found in Milk, tofu

Mechanism of Toxic Action *Yersinia enterocolitica* is a gram-negative bacillus which is invasive and produces a heat stable toxin

Signs & Symptoms of Acute Overdose Mesenteric lymphadenitis, arthritis, erythema nodosum, fever, abdominal pain (may resemble appendicitis), diarrhea

Overdosage Treatment Many cases of enterocolitis and mesenteric adenitis secondary to *Yersinia* are self-resolving, and the role of antibiotics is unclear. Patients with *Yersinia* septicemia, however, definitely require antibiotic therapy since the mortality approaches 50%. The organism is susceptible *in vitro* to a number of agents, including third-generation cephalosporins, piperacillin, co-trimoxazole, and aminoglycosides. Most isolates are resistant to penicillin, ampicillin, and first-generation cephalosporins. The optimal drug regimen *in vivo* has not been defined in the literature. For serious infections it seems reasonable to treat initially with a combination (eg, third-generation cephalosporin and aminoglycoside) until the patient has stabilized.

Diagnostic Tests/Procedures

Electrolytes, Blood *on page 1254*

Additional Information Infection rate increased with prolonged (over 36 hours) deferoxamine use

Microbiology: *Yersinia enterocolitica* is a gram-negative bacillus named in honor of the French bacteriologist Alexander Yersin, who discovered *Yersinia pestis* (the cause of plague) in 1894. *Y. enterocolitica* is an unusual cause of enterocolitis, terminal ileitis mimicking acute appendicitis, and septicemia. The organism is an aerobic gram-negative rod, nonlactose fermenting, which is motile at 25°C. It is unusual in that it grows better at somewhat cooler temperatures than do other pathogenic gram-negative rods (25°C to 32°C). It also is able to grow well at 4°C, which is the basis for CEM.

Epidemiology:

Yersinia enterocolitica is endemic in many animals which serve as reservoirs: cattle, pigs, dogs, cats, and others. The usual route of human infection is via ingestion of contaminated food, milk, and water. There have been three major foodborne epidemics in the United States:

1. June 1982, outbreak in several states linked to consumption of milk pasteurized at a plant in Memphis, Tennessee; 172 positive cultures from cases in Tennessee, Arkansas, and Mississippi, where patients presented with diarrhea, fever, abdominal pain. It also included 24 cases of extraintestinal infections including throat, blood, urinary tract, central nervous system, and wounds.
2. 1976, contaminated chocolate milk in New York state
3. 1982, contaminated tofu in Washington state

Clinical Syndromes:

- **Enterocolitis:** *Yersinia enterocolitica* is a rare cause of enterocolitis. The severity of symptoms can be quite variable and can range from mild fever, diarrhea and abdominal pain, to fulminant colitis with spiking fevers and rectal hemorrhage.
- **Mesenteric adenopathy with or without terminal ileitis:** This form of *Yersinia* infection is known to mimic acute appendicitis. Patients present with right lower quadrant pain, fever, and leukocytosis. Upon laparotomy, the appendix is normal; but enlarged mesenteric lymph nodes are palpable and

when cultured will yield the organism. This has been described primarily in adolescents, although cases have been reported in adults.

- **Polyarthritis:** This has been described as the sole manifestation of *Yersinia enterocolitica* infection or as a secondary manifestation of gastrointestinal infection. Well documented cases have been described in Scandinavia, where up to 30% of cases develop erythema nodosum; and 10% to 30% develop polyarthritis (especially associated with HLA-B27 haplotype). *Yersinia* antigens have recently been found in synovial fluid cells from patients suffering from reactive arthritis following *Yersinia* infection.
- **Liver abscess:** *Yersinia* is a rare, but reported cause of liver abscess in the absence of typical enterocolitis symptoms
- **Ascending infection of an extremity:** Recently cases of infections of the hand and upper extremity due to *Yersinia enterocolitica* have been described. These infections occurred in adults preparing contaminated chitterlings (pig intestines) with local inoculation into the hand via small cuts.
- **Septicemia:** *Yersinia* is an unusual cause of community-acquired septicemia, but may occur following ingestion of heavily contaminated food. Risk factors for septicemia are cirrhosis, malignancy, diabetes mellitus, and patients with iron overload syndromes (such as hemachromatosis, frequent blood transfusions). Typically, there is fever, myalgias, confusion, and possibly hypotension. Symptoms of enterocolitis, such as diarrhea and abdominal pain, may be completely absent, adding to the diagnostic confusion. Elevated liver enzymes and muscle enzymes may occur. Blood cultures are often positive for the organism.
- **Miscellaneous:** Other manifestations of *Yersinia* infection include osteomyelitis, meningitis, pharyngitis (without enterocolitis), intra-abdominal abscess

Diagnosis: In the absence of an outbreak, the diagnosis of enterocolitis due to *Yersinia* is difficult to make on clinical grounds alone. Thus, laboratory confirmation is important in most cases. Appropriate specimens for culture include stool, blood, lymph node, pharyngeal exudates, ascites fluid, and cerebrospinal fluid. Joint aspiration fluid may be sent for *Yersinia* culture in the appropriate clinical setting (ie, reactive polyarthritis following a diarrheal illness), but the yield is extremely low. The laboratory should be notified if a stool specimen is being examined for *Yersinia*. Serologic tests for specific antibody production to *Yersinia enterocolitica* are available in some laboratories.

Specific References

Bottone E and Sheehan DJ, "*Yersinia enterocolitica*: Guidelines for Serologic Diagnosis of Human Infections," *Rev Infect Dis*, 1983, 5(5):898-906.

Centers for Disease Control, "*Yersinia enterocolitica* Bacteremia and Endotoxin Shock Associated With Red Blood Cell Transfusions - United States, 1991," *JAMA*, 1991, 256(17):2174-5.

Cohen JI and Rodday P, "*Yersinia enterocolitica* Bacteremia in a Patient With the Acquired Immunodeficiency Syndrome," *Am J Med*, 1989, 86(2):254-5.

Cover TL and Aber RC, "*Yersinia enterocolitica*," *N Engl J Med*, 1989, 321(1):16-24.

Gayraud M, Scavizzi MR, Mollaret HH, et al, "Antibiotic Treatment of *Yersinia enterocolitica* Septicemia: A Retrospective Review of 43 Cases," *Clin Infect Dis*, 1993, 17(3):405-10.

Granfors K, Jalkanen S, von Essen R, et al, "*Yersinia* Antigens in Synovial-Fluid Cells From Patients With Reactive Arthritis," *N Engl J Med*, 1989, 320(4):216-21.

Naqvi SH, Swierkosz EM, and Gerard J, "Presentation of *Yersinia enterocolitica* Enteritis in Children," *Pediatr Infect Dis J*, 1993, 12(5):386-9.

Tacket CO, Ballard J, Harris N, et al, "An Outbreak of *Yersinia enterocolitica* Infections Caused by Contaminated Tofu (Soybean Curd)," *Am J Epidemiol*, 1985, 121(5):705-10.

Yew

Scientific Name *Taxus* Species

Synonyms American Yew; Chinese Yew; English Yew; Florida Yew; Ground Hemlock; Japanese Yew; Pacific Yew; Southern Tree Yew; Western Yew

Mechanism of Toxic Action All parts of the plant are toxic except the red fleshy aril; the toxin appears to inhibit sodium and calcium current in cardiac cells causing a block of the distal portion of the conduction tissue of the heart; the hard seed coat is resistant to digestive enzymes and is nontoxic unless chewed or broken

Signs & Symptoms of Acute Overdose Nausea, vomiting, abdominal pain, mydriasis, pale complexion, cyanotic lips, contact dermatitis, A-V block, dizziness, headache, asthenia, seizures, coma, tachycardia, respiratory distress/arrest, cardiac arrhythmias (sinus bradycardia, tachycardia (ventricular), ventricular fibrillation, and heart block), hypotension, death is usually secondary to either arrhythmias, circulatory collapse, or respiratory failure

Toxicodynamics/Kinetics Onset of symptoms: Generally within 1-3 hours; in large ingestions, cardiovascular collapse can occur within 30 minutes

Toxic Dosage Literature suggests that <6 berries produce minimal symptoms, and ingestion of 150 leaves can produce death within 5 hours; LD_{50} in mice and rats is ~20 mg/kg

Overdosage Treatment

Decontamination: Ipecac is contraindicated secondary to rapid onset of symptoms; lavage is of questionable benefit, due to the large size of the seeds, un-

(Continued)

Yew *(Continued)*

less the seeds are chewed well; activated charcoal with sorbitol is recommended; whole bowel irrigation is beneficial for ingestions of large amounts of plant material

Supportive therapy: Hypotension can be resistant to dopamine and dobutamine, and may require norepinephrine; bradycardia and complete heart block has on occasion been resistant to atropine; external pacing and/or digoxin immune Fab may be of benefit; monitor electrolytes

Antidote(s)

Digoxin Immune Fab *on page 1411*

Norepinephrine Bitartrate *on page 1451*

Additional Information

Family: Taxaceae

Range: Located deep in the woods of Western North Carolina to Northcentral and Northeastern U.S.

Toxin: Taxine

Yucca Plant (Nontoxic Plant)

Zantedeschia aethiopica *see* Calla *on page 1064*

Zebrafish *see* Lionfish *on page 1099*

Zebra Plant (Nontoxic Plant)

Zigadenus nuttrallii *see* Death Camas *on page 1078*

Zigadenus paniculatus *see* Death Camas *on page 1078*

Zigadenus venenosus *see* Death Camas *on page 1078*

LABORATORY TESTS

DRUG TESTING IN THE 90s

DRUG USE AND ABUSE IN THE USA

The number of people who currently use or admit to having used an illicit drug has increased markedly over the last 20 years. In 1989, approximately 20 million people in the USA admitted to using cocaine and of those, 5 million used it on a regular basis.

A recent survey of hospital emergency rooms by the Drug Abuse Warning Network (DAWN) showed heroin-related cases rose in every age group by 44% (21,400 to 30,800) between the first half of 1992 and the first half of 1993. During the same period, cocaine-related incidents rose from 57,700 to 61,000; there were also increases in the use of marijuana (19%), methamphetamine (61%), and phencyclidine combinations (45%).[1]

Abuse of prescription drugs such as benzodiazepines (eg, diazepam, chlordiazepoxide, nitrazepam), tricyclic antidepressants (eg, amitriptyline, imipramine), or synthetic analgesics (eg, meperidine) is also a problem, with 1% of all physicians being drug dependent. In 1976, over 2.8 billion prescriptions and drug orders were written. Today, at least 250,000 drugs and commercial products are readily available for ingestion.[2]

OBJECTIVES AND GUIDELINES FOR DRUG TESTING

Analysis of body fluids is a necessary step in determining whether or not an individual has ingested illegal drugs or an excessive amount of prescription drugs. It is important to note that at this time, the amount of drug found does not give any direct information about the amount of drug ingested, the route of ingestion, the degree of impairment, or the extent of drug dependence of the individual. However, studies and research are ongoing to provide as much interpretive data as possible.

Some questions need to be considered before the implementation of any drug testing program[3] and these include:

- which drugs should be included in the test?
- how sensitive should the screening procedure be?
- how sensitive and specific should the confirmation be?
- is an adequate chain-of-custody present?
- how will the results be used?

In 1986, the National Institute on Drug Abuse (NIDA) which is now known as the Substance Abuse and Mental Health Services Administration (SAMHSA) addressed some of these issues and developed urine drug testing proficiency guidelines leading to laboratory certification.[4] The guidelines provide for accurate analysis of urine samples by proficiency testing followed by satisfactory laboratory inspections carried out by qualified personnel. Laboratories are required to adhere to Good Laboratory Practice (GLP) as well as establish defensible sample handling (chain-of-custody), reporting, and data reviewing.

The guidelines require the screening and confirmation capability to the levels shown in Table 1 for cocaine metabolite (benzoylecgonine), opiates (codeine and morphine), phencyclidine (PCP), marijuana metabolite (THC-COOH), and amphetamines (amphetamine and methamphetamine).

Table 1. Screening and Confirmation Levels for the NIDA 5

	Screening (ng/mL)	Confirmation (ng/mL)
Cocaine metabolite (benzoylecgonine)	300	150
Opiates (codeine & morphine)	300	300
Phencyclidine	25	25
Amphetamines	1000	250
Marijuana metabolite (THC-COOH)	50	15

Additional testing is allowed in some cases:

- to determine adulteration
- to determine 6-monoacetylmorphine (a metabolite specific to heroin use) at the discretion of the Medical Review Officer (MRO)
- when conducting reasonable suspicion, accident, or unsafe practice testing, a federal agency may test for any drug listed in Schedules I or II of the Controlled Substances Act. The laboratory can only test for drugs specifically requested by the federal agency.

Other agencies such as the Centers for Disease Control, the American Association of Clinical Chemistry, and the American Society of Bioanalysts have administered drug testing programs. The College of American Pathologists (CAP) continues to run and monitor regular proficiency testing services for laboratories involved in drug analysis.[5]

TECHNIQUES IN DRUG TESTING

DRUG SCREENING

The technology of drug screening has greatly improved throughout the 1980s and into this decade. Screening tests are designed for maximum sensitivity at the expense of selectivity. It is important, however, that screening tests do not give false-negative results since this terminates the testing process. False-positives at this stage are acceptable because all presumptive positive samples are re-extracted and analyzed by a confirmatory technique.

For example, a urine sample from a poppy seed bagel eater may well give a positive screening level for opiates;[6,7] a urine sample from a Vicks® inhaler user may give a positive amphetamine screen. Therefore, a confirmatory procedure is essential.

Color or Spot Tests

These tests were developed 30-40 years ago, but still find occasional application in emergency room toxicology.[8,9] A small amount of urine is added to a reagent and the resulting mixture shows a specific color if a drug is present. Spot tests are quick, easy, cheap, and can be performed directly upon the urine sample. They are also nonspecific (drugs and metabolites of similar structures will produce the same color) and require a high concentration of drug to produce a color change. These tests find most application in the testing of salicylates[10] and ethchlorvynol.[11]

Methods based on paper chromatography have recently been introduced but so far have not been favorably received.[12]

Thin-Layer Chromatography (TLC)

TLC is an old but still widely used technique for the separation and identification of drugs. Essentially, the drug is extracted from urine and concentrated onto a silica plate. The plate is then placed in a solvent tank of chosen polarity. As the solvent rises up the plate, it "elutes" the drugs and carries them to various distances depending upon the affinity of the drug for the plate and for the solvent (or mobile phase). The plate is then sprayed with suitable reagents which allow the drugs to be identified by color and specific positioning relative to drug standards.[13,14]

The technique is cheap, relatively simple, and there are many choices of stationary and mobile phases making complex separations possible.

Disadvantages include interpretation due to interference from endogenous substances. Also, the technique involves lengthy extraction and concentration steps, difficulties in saving data (spots on plates fade with time and photographic representations do not reproduce colors well), and a need for operator experience and skill in spotting and spraying plates. A commercial TLC kit for THC determination is available and has adequate sensitivity for the detection of the metabolite (11-nor-Δ^9-THC-9-carboxylic acid) in urine. However, TLC is not very specific and results require further confirmation.

Immunoassays

Immunoassay techniques are now the most widely used screening procedures in drug testing. Popular versions of these tests include radioimmunoassay (RIA), enzyme-multiplied immunoassay technique (EMIT), enzyme-linked immunosorbent assay (ELISA), and fluorescence polarization immunoassay (FPIA).

These techniques use antibodies specific to the drug being assayed and a labeled form of the same drug. The label itself may be a radioactive isotope (RIA), an active enzyme (EMIT and ELISA), or a fluorescent label (FPIA) which is incorporated synthetically. A fixed quantity of antibody and labeled drug are added to the test sample. The binding sites on the antibody attract both labeled drug and the unlabeled drug in the sample. The amount of labeled drug bound is inversely proportional to the number of unlabeled drug molecules present.

In RIA, a radioactively labeled drug competes for the antibody binding site as the unlabeled drug. The analytical measurement of radioactivity remaining in the solution determines the amount of unlabeled drug in the sample. The method is used to detect opiates, cannabinoids, benzoylecgonine, amphetamines, and phencyclidine.

In EMIT and FPIA testing, the analytical measurement is of an optically detected change such as UV absorption, fluorescence, or luminescence. These systems avoid the use of radioactive isotopes but also have reduced sensitivity when compared to RIA because the optical signal is measured in the presence of the original biological fluid.[15,16] The application of these assays to forensic blood work has recently been described.[17]

Additional antibody kits are also available expanding the uses of these systems to include methadone, benzodiazepines, methaqualone, and barbiturates. Advantages include high sensitivity, no extraction steps, and applicability to large numbers of samples.[18]

All immunoassay tests are susceptible to false-positive results due to cross-reactivity of the antibodies with legal or prescription drugs (Table 2).[19]

Table 2. Possible Cross-Reactive Substances in RIA or EMIT

Test	Cross-Reactors
Amphetamines	Cathinone; diethylpropion; dopamine; ephedrine; p-hydroxyamphetamine; isoxsuprine; labetalol; methylphenidate; l-methamphetamine; nylidrin; phenmetrazine; phentermine; phenylephrine; phenylpropanolamine; propylhexedrine; pseudoephedrine; ranitidine; sergiline
Barbiturates	Glutethimide; phenytoin
Cocaine (benzoylecgonine)	Salicylate
Opiates	Chlorpromazine; codeine; dextromethorphan; dihydrocodeine; diphenoxylate; hydromorphone; levorphanol; meperidine; oxycodone; d-propoxyphene
Phencyclidine	Amitriptyline; chlorpromazine; dextromethorphan; diphenhydramine; doxylamine; meperidine; thioridazine
THC-COOH	Ibuprofen; promethazine; riboflavin

DRUG CONFIRMATIONS

High Performance Liquid Chromatography (HPLC)

HPLC allows the separation of nonvolatile substances from each other or from other components of an extraction residue. When a mixture of substances is injected onto the column, each component is partitioned between the stationary phase (column) and the liquid (mobile) phase. Molecules with greater affinity for the column spend more time in that phase and, therefore, take longer to reach the detector. The time taken from injection to the peak maximum is known as the retention time. The detector responds in direct proportion to the concentration of material passing through it, hence peak heights and areas shown on the chromatogram are directly related to the concentration of each analyte.

HPLC shows good sensitivity and high specificity depending upon the detection system used. The most common detectors utilize absorption of UV light by the drug. A diode array detector will allow a full UV spectrum of the analyte to be obtained. This can be compared to a standard spectrum of the drug, and identification is then based both on retention time and UV spectra. Most instruments also include the facility to obtain first and second derivative spectra to provide an additional means of identification. Postcolumn reactions for increased sensitivity have also been described[20] (Figure 1).

Figure 1.

HPLC Chromatogram from Roy IM, Jefferies TM, Threadgill MD, and Dewar GH, School of Pharmacy and Pharmacology, University of Bath, United Kingdom.

Peaks:

1: Cocaine 0.6 µg/mL
2: Ethylcocaine 0.44 µg/mL
3: N-butylnorcocaine 0.4 µg/mL
4: Butylbenzoylecgonine 0.5 µg/mL
5: Methadone 0.3 µg/mL
6: t-butyldimethylsilyl ecgonine methyl ester 0.6 µg/mL
7: Hexylbenzoylecgonine 2 µg/mL

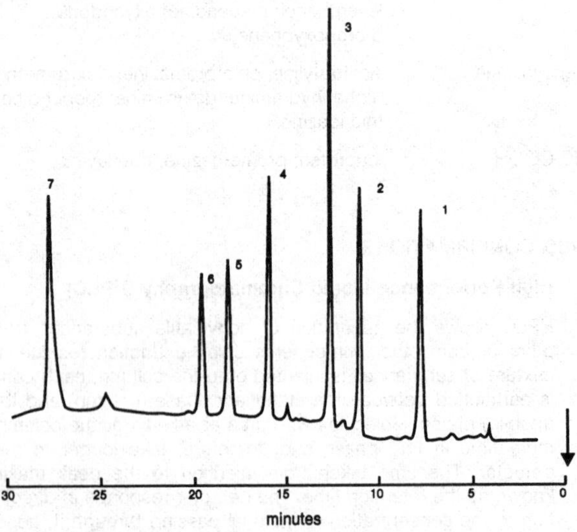

Reprinted from "Analysis of Cocaine, Benzoylecgonine, Ecgonine Methyl Ester, Ethylcocaine and Norcocaine in Human Urine Using HPLC With Post Column Ion Pair Extraction and Fluorescence Detection," *J Pharm Biomed Anal*, 1992, 10(10-12):943-8, with permission.

HPLC is expensive and can be used for confirmations[21], but is not completely forensically defensible as a single technique.

Gas Chromatography (GC)

Gas chromatography is also a method of separating substances of analytical interest. It is one of the most sensitive techniques available for detecting drugs in body fluids. The separation is carried out on an analytical column containing a stationary phase (liquid or solid, depending on temperature) which is maintained at a given temperature inside an oven. The whole GC system comprises six components: gas supply and flow controllers, injector, oven, column, detector, and recording device. In drug testing, GC capillary (rather than packed) columns are commonly used. A compound is identified by matching its retention time (the time between injection and peak maximum) with that of a drug standard under the same conditions (gas flow rate, temperature, column length, etc).

GC equipment is expensive and experienced personnel are required to run and maintain instruments and interpret chromatograms. Additionally, while GC is fairly specific, its use with nonspecific detectors such as flame ionization (FID), nitrogen-phosphorus (NPD), or electron capture (ECD) does not absolutely identify a compound.

Gas Chromatography/Mass Spectrometry (GC/MS)

GC/MS is the so-called "gold standard" of forensic and drug testing work. The use of GC with a mass spectrometric detection system is forensically defensible as an absolute identification procedure.

When a molecule is injected into the chromatographic system, it is separated from other components of the extraction residue on the basis of its degree of affinity for and interaction with the stationary phase. Upon elution from the chromatographic column, it is bombarded with electrons which cause it to break apart. The fragments produced are separated on the basis of their mass to charge ratio. Under the same conditions, a molecule will fragment in exactly the same way every time, producing the same spectrum. This spectrum or "fingerprint" can then be compared to that of a drug standard for absolute identification (Figure 2).

Figure 2.

a. GC/MS Chromatogram
Drug test mixture containing cocaine (retention time 5.8 minutes)

b. GC/MS Spectrum
Spectrum of peak at 5.8 minutes

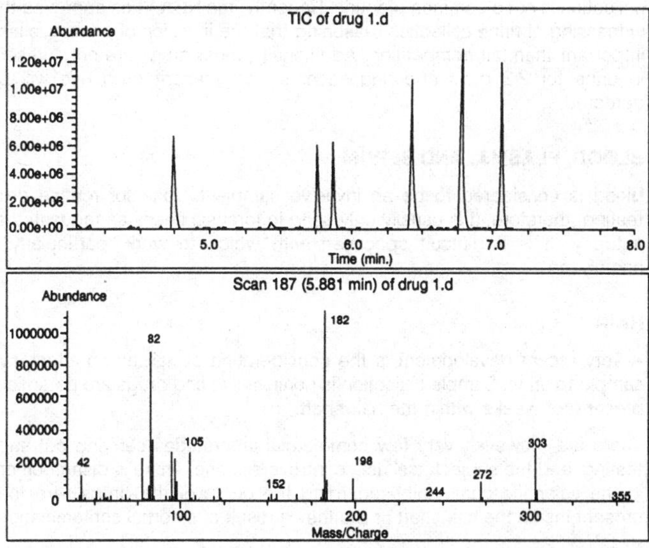

GC/MS is an expensive technique but is necessary in every laboratory which is carrying out confirmatory testing for drugs of metabolites in biological fluids.[22,23] Experienced operators and interpreters are also needed in order to produce good data.

Gas Chromatography-Fourier Transform Infra Red

GC-FTIR is also a forensically acceptable and defensible technique. It is more expensive and less common than GC/MS because it is more difficult to interpret the spectra requiring skilled and experienced operators and reviewers.

Other Hyphenated Techniques

Other hyphenated techniques include high-performance liquid chromatography/mass spectrometry (LC/MS); gas chromatography/mass spectrometry/mass spectrometry (GC/MS/MS); gas chromatography/infrared/mass spectrometry (GC/IR/MS). All these techniques have high sensitivity and specificity. All are considered forensically defensible, but are extremely expensive requiring highly skilled operators to produce quality data.

ALTERNATIVE SPECIMENS FOR DRUG TESTING

Urine is the most common specimen chosen for drug analysis and is the only matrix to which the NIDA guidelines apply. NIDA (SAMHSA) approved laboratories are **not** certified to carry out drug analysis in plasma, serum, blood, meconium, amniotic fluid, hair, or any other tissue or fluid.

Urine is chosen for many reasons:

- it is easy to collect
- it is not considered an invasive sample to request
- large volumes can often be collected
- drugs and metabolites are often present in higher concentrations than in other body fluids
- it is easier to analyze than other fluids or tissues
- drugs and metabolites are usually stable in frozen urine allowing long-term storage of positive samples

Urine, however, can be easily adulterated[24,25] since observed specimen collection is not a common practice. Recently, the NCAA has approved the witnessing of urine collection reasoning that the invasion of privacy is less important than fair competition. Additionally, most drugs are only present in urine for 2-3 days after ingestion, so only recent drug use will be detected.

BLOOD, PLASMA, AND SERUM

Blood is considered to be an invasive sample to take for routine drug testing; therefore, it is usually only used in forensic cases as requested at autopsy. It is a difficult specimen with which to work, particularly if hemolyzed.

HAIR

A very recent development is the consideration of hair as an alternative sample to urine. Sample collection is noninvasive and drugs are potentially present for weeks within the hair shaft.

There are, however, very few commercial laboratories carrying out such testing, and the subject itself is a controversial one. There is disagreement in the scientific community regarding the origin of the drugs. Are they present inside the hair shaft or are they a result of external contamination?

Experts disagree, some claiming that external contamination can be removed by washing;[26-28] others claim that washing removes drugs from inside the shaft and does not completely remove external contaminants.[29]

Additionally, dark, African American or Asian hair has been shown to absorb more drug than the same amount of light, Caucasian hair, so the potential for racial bias in hair testing is a major pitfall. However, the long-term stability of drugs in hair make it an attractive specimen for analysis. There are far less problems associated with storage and preservation of hair compared to other biological samples. Experts disagree on the ability of hair to provide diagnostic information regarding rate of growth and dose response.

Hair is currently used in pre-employment drug testing, clinical studies, and occasionally fetal hair is tested for the determination of drug use *in utero*.

Compounds reported in hair include:

Predominantly Forensic Purposes	Predominantly Clinical Purposes
Cocaine, benzoylecgonine, cocaethylene	Ephedrine, pseudoephedrine
Amphetamine, methamphetamine	Buprenorphine
Codeine, morphine,[30] monoacetylmorphine, heroin	Fentanyl
Phencyclidine	Haloperidol
THC and THC-COOH	Caffeine
Fentanyl	Nicotine
Haloperidol[31]	Antidepressants
Phenobarbital	
Antidepressants	
Meprobamate	

Overall, hair is a good matrix for the isolation of lipophilic basic drugs, but is difficult to test for acidic, polar drugs. The evaluation of analytical methods and the development of suitable reference materials for hair analysis is still being studied by the National Institute of Standards (NIST, Gaithersburg, MD).

SWEAT

The presence of alcohol, as well as a number of drugs, in sweat has been reported, but it is not yet considered a sample of choice for drug testing. This is because the collection of sweat from various parts of the body is difficult and unequal, since sweat production depends on temperature, adrenalin level, and degree of physical activity. About 50% of the body's sweat is produced by the torso, with about 25% produced by the head and legs.

However, there are many reports of drugs being detected in sweat and these include methadone, phencyclidine, amphetamine, phenobarbital, morphine, cocaine.[32]

The most recent development in the determination of drugs in sweat is the "Sweat Patch" manufactured by Sudormed (Santa Ana, CA), consisting of polyurethane adhesive, a cellulose blotter, and a cellulose release liner. The patch, which has apparently overcome problems associated with previous patches such as skin hydration, irritation, and perspiration leaks, is intended primarily for use in the parole system, whereby parolees wear the patch between parole visits. The use of illicit drugs is a violation of parole, so the patches are tested at each visit and a new one is applied.

Advantages to this type of testing include noninvasive sample collection (the patch is worn on the back, biceps, or chest), ability to carry out normal activities including swimming and showering without removing the patch, and the ability to tell if a patch has been removed and reapplied, so preventing adulteration.[33]

The predominant species found in sweat are parent compounds, not drug metabolites. Analysis of duplicate patches in controlled studies have reported that intrasubject variability is low but intersubject variability is high.[32]

SALIVA

Saliva is considered a possible alternative specimen to urine for drug testing because it is an easy and a noninvasive sample to collect. Additionally, it offers and advantage over urine testing if impairment determination is required. Generally, drug concentrations in saliva are lower than those found in urine or plasma and the major compound detected is the parent drug, not the metabolites. Initially, oral, intranasal, or smoking drugs may produce high concentrations in saliva for a few hours. However, later, the concentration of drug in saliva is thought to reflect free drug fraction in blood.

Drug excretion in saliva depends on pH and salivary flow, leading to highly variable saliva/plasma ratios for drugs of abuse.

A comprehensive review of saliva testing for drugs of abuse which includes information on alcohol, amphetamines, barbiturates, benzodiazepines, caffeine, cocaine, inhalants, LSD, marijuana, opioids, phencyclidine, and tobacco products is available.[34]

MECONIUM AND AMNIOTIC FLUID

NIDA's 1991 National Household Survey on Drug Use indicates that of the 59.2 million women of childbearing age (15-44 years), over 4.5 million (7.6%) are estimated to have used illicit drugs in the past month. About 601,000 women in this age group appear to be cocaine users.

The drug use of this population group will have an effect upon the next generation, and urine testing for neonates and pregnant women is common.

Drug-, alcohol-, and tobacco-exposed babies suffer from a variety of adverse effects at birth including low birth weight and head size, and in later life, possible learning disabilities.[35-39]

Progressive pediatricians and nurses are now requesting the analysis of neonatal meconium rather than urine. Studies show meconium to be a better indicator of drug use during pregnancy than urine.[40,41] As previously discussed, the half-life of drugs and metabolites in urine only allows fairly recent use of a drug to be detected. Meconium begins to form after about 16 weeks of gestation and is cumulative thereafter.

Meconium as a matrix presents unique extraction problems. Therefore, there are only a few commercial laboratories willing and able to carry out this type of testing.

Amniotic fluid, umbilical cord, and cord blood have also been suggested as alternative samples. Amniotic fluid is present throughout gestation and is constantly diluted due to fetal urination. Fetal swallowing of amniotic fluid may also contribute to the recirculation of drug metabolites through the baby.[42,43]

Substances Most Frequently Reported Being Used by Pregnant Women in 1992

Substances*	Percentage of Pregnant Women Who Used During Pregnancy	Estimated Number of Pregnant Users†
Cigarettes	20.4%	819,700
Alcohol	18.8%	756,900
Prescription analgesics	7.6%	305,200
Prescription sedatives	3.6%	144,100
Marijuana	2.9%	118,700
Prescription tranquilizers	1.4%	55,400
Nonprescription analgesics	1.2%	48,700
Cocaine	1.1%	45,100
Any illicit drug‡	5.5%	220,900

*Excludes substances used by <1% of all pregnant women.
†Based on an estimated 4 million women giving birth in the U.S. in 1992.
‡Use of all marijuana, cocaine, methamphetamine, heroin, methadone, inhalants, hallucinogenics, or nonmedical use of psychotherapeutics.

Adapted from "Dawn Briefings," Vol X, No 4, Dec 1994, 1-7 by the Center for Substance Abuse Research from the National Institute on Drug Abuse (NIDA) Press Briefing, September 12, 1994.

FUTURE TRENDS

POTENCY OF ILLICIT DRUGS AND PHARMACEUTICALS

1. **LSD**
   The recent resurgence of lysergic acid diethylamide (LSD) as a drug of choice poses particular problems for the physician in diagnosis and the analyst in determination. The amounts ingested in order to produce the desired effect are extremely low and, therefore, very difficult to detect in biological specimens. There are no FPIA or EMIT kits readily available to screen for LSD; in fact, RIA is the only method which may be used as a screening procedure. For confirmation, some papers have suggested using electron impact GC/MS[44] (the most common approach) but it is likely that the sensitivity of GC/MS/MS systems will be required, or chemical ionization procedures[45]. Such techniques are somewhat complicated and not currently used in the majority of routine hospital laboratories.

2. **Fentanyl**
   Fentanyl (N-phenyl-N-[1-(2-phenylethyl)-4-piperidinyl] (propanamide)) is a potent, fast-acting, synthetic narcotic analgesic. Its potency is considered to be 100-200 times that of morphine[46,47], but its effects are shorter. It was developed as an intravenous anesthetic, marketed in the USA as Sublimaze® and as Innovar® when used with droperidol. However, a number of fentanyl analogues are also available, specifically alphamethylfentanyl (twice the potency of fentanyl), sufentanil, carfentanil, alfentanil, thienylfentanyl, lofentanil, 3-methylfentanyl, and p-fluorofentanyl. These are mostly sold for surgical and veterinary purposes, but are increasingly appearing on the street as "designer drugs," "synthetic heroin," and "China White."

   Most of the screening for these drugs is currently carried out using RIA[48,49]. Confirmation is by GC/MS and the levels present are detectable using electron impact GC/MS.

3. **Benzodiazepines**
   The extremely potent new benzodiazepines such as alprazolam, flunitrazepam, and triazolam are administered at very low doses. Detection of the parent drug in biological fluids is extremely difficult and the

majority of laboratories search for metabolites. Benzodiazepine immunoassays do cross-react well with metabolites as well as parent drugs, but the confirmation procedures become more difficult. Different modes of detection are usually employed such as negative or positive ion chemical ionization GC/MS.

ANABOLIC STEROIDS

The use of anabolic steroids among teenagers and young adults is becoming increasingly popular, particularly in those involved in sports requiring great strength such as weight lifting and body building.

All anabolic steroids are derivatives of the male hormone testosterone and all are intended for "tissue building" and increasing masculinizing effects.

Over 100 anabolic steroids are widely available in oral or injectable form. They are used for many medical reasons including the treatment of some breast cancers, growth promotion, and delayed puberty. Reported psychological side effects associated with their use include aggression, psychosis, and changes in libido.

In 1974, they were added to the list of doping agents banned by the International Olympic Committee (IOC). Extensive metabolic pathways, as well as natural occurrence, makes the detection of these substances difficult. However, athletic drug testing laboratories are routinely able to detect many of the anabolic steroids in urine samples by using gas chromatography/mass spectrometry (GC/MS) methods.

Athletes have frequently turned to using exogenous administration of the naturally occurring anabolic steroid testosterone for its potent anabolic effects. The IOC has thus mandated testing for the ratio of testosterone to epitestosterone (T/E ratio). Epitestosterone is a naturally occurring epimer of testosterone thought to be of extratesticular origin and having no biological activity. A T/E ratio $\geq$6 is considered evidence of testosterone doping. To further foil ingenious athletes from taking exogenous epitestosterone to titrate their T/E ratios to $\leq$6, a maximum allowable urine concentration of 150 ng/mL of epitestosterone has been established.

CONCLUSIONS

1. It is important to be aware of the limitations of screening and confirmatory drug testing techniques. Even though GC/MS instrumentation is expensive, it is the cheapest way to absolutely identify the contents of a biological sample, ensuring the analysis is forensically defensible.

2. Drug levels do not give any information about possible drug abuse or dependence, route or amount of drug ingestion, or degree of impairment. It is recommended that readers familiarize themselves with metabolic routes and pharmacokinetics of the drugs in question.

3. Urine is still the most commonly tested biological fluid although the search continues for a noninvasive, adulterant-free sample which will provide a history of drug use.

4. The increasing potency of new "designer drugs" and pharmaceuticals, as well as the increasing number of drugs will place new demands on the laboratory. A wider range of immunoassay kits with better sensitivity and specificity will be required, as will increasingly sensitive confirmation instrumentation.

FOOTNOTES

1. Drug Detection Report, *Pace Publications*, April 20, 1994, 5.

2. Goldfrank LR, General Perspective in *Goldfrank's Toxicologic Emergencies*, 4th ed, Norwalk, CT: Appleton and Lange, 1990, 3-4.

3. Schnoll SH and Lewis DE, "Drug Screening in the Workplace: Pros and Cons," *Semin Occup Med*, 1986, 1(4):243-51.

4. NIDA and DHSS Mandatory Guidelines for Federal Workplace Drug Testing Programs, *Fed Reg*, 1988, 53/69.

5. Substance-Abuse Testing Committee, "Critical Issues in Urinalysis of Abused Substances," *Clin Chem*, 1988, 34(3):605-32.

6. Struempler RE, "Excretion of Codeine and Morphine Following Ingestion of Poppy Seeds," *J Anal Toxicol*, 1987, 11(3):97-9.

7. Zebelman AM, Troyer BL, Randall GL, et al, "Detection of Morphine and Codeine Following Consumption of Poppy Seeds," *J Anal Toxicol*, 1987, 11(3):131-2.

8. Fiegl F, *Spot Tests in Organic Analysis*, 7th ed, Amsterdam, The Netherlands: Elsevier Publishers, 1966.

9. Johnson CA and Thornton-Jones AD, eds, *Drug Identification*, London, England: The Pharmaceutical Press, 1966.

10. Trinder P, "Rapid Determination of Salicylate in Biological Fluids," *Biochem J*, 1954, 57:301-3.

11. Frings CS and Cohen PS, "Rapid Colorimetric Method for the Quantitative Determination of Ethchlorvynol (Placidyl) in Serum and Urine," *Am J Clin Pathol*, 1970, 54(6):833-6.

12. Schwartz RH, Bogema S, and Thorne MM, "Evaluation of the Keystone Diagnostic Quiktest: A Paper Chromatography Test for Drugs of Abuse in Urine," *Arch Pathol Lab Med*, 1989, 113(4):363-4.

13. Heaton AM and Blumberg AG, "Thin-Layer Chromatographic Detection of Barbiturates, Narcotics, and Amphetamines in Urine of Patients Receiving Psychotropic Drugs," *J Chromatogr*, 1969, 41(3):367-70.

14. Kaistha KK, and Jaffe JH, "TLC Techniques for Identification of Narcotics, Barbiturates and CNS Stimulants in a Drug Abuse Urine Screening Program," *J Pharm Sci*, 1972, 61(5):679-89.

15. Walters R, "An Abused Drug Assay System," *Am Clin Prod Rev*, March, 1987.

16. Popelka SR, Miller DM, Holen JT, et al, "Fluorescence Polarization Immunoassay. II. Analyzer for Rapid, Precise Measurement of Fluorescence Polarization With Use of Disposable Cuvettes," *Clin Chem*, 1981, 27(7):1198-201.

17. Gjerde H, Christophersen AS, Skuterud B, et al, "Screening for Drugs in Forensic Blood Samples Using EMIT Urine Assays," *Forensic Sci Int*, 1990, 44(2-3):179-85.

18. Cooke C Edgar, "Critical Overview on Immunological and Chromatographic Analytical Methods," *Proceedings of 1st International Symposium - Current Issues in Drug Testing*, Seguar J and de la Torre R, eds, 1990, Ch 14:73-82.

19. Baselt RC, "Urine Drug Screening by Immunoassay: Interpretation of Results," *Advances in Analytical Toxicology*, Baselt RC, ed, Foster City, CA: BioMedical Publications, 1984, 1:81-123.

20. Roy IM, Jefferies TM, Threadgill MD, et al, "Analysis of Cocaine, Benzoylecgonine, Ecgonine Methyl Ester, Ethylcocaine, and Norcocaine in Human Urine Using HPLC With Post-Column Ion-Pair Extraction and Fluorescence Detection," *J Pharm Biomed Anal*, 1992, 10(10-12):943-8.

21. Posey BL and Kimble SN, "High-Performance Liquid Chromatographic Study of Codeine, Norcodeine, and Morphine as Indicators of Codeine Ingestion" *J Anal Toxicol*, 1984, 8(2):68-74.

22. Park J, Park S, Lho D, et al, "Drug Testing at the 10th Asian Games and 24th Seoul Olympic Games," *J Anal Toxicol*, 1990, 14(2):66-72.

23. Lillsunde P and Korte T, "Comprehensive Drug Screening in Urine Using Solid-Phase Extraction and Combined TLC and GC/MS Identification," *J Anal Toxicol*, 1991, 15(2):71-81.

24. Pearson SD, Ash KO, and Urry FM, "Mechanism of False-Negative Urine Cannabinoid Immunoassay Screens by Visine Eyedrops," *Clin Chem*, 1989, 35(4):636-8.

25. Warner A, "Interference of Common Household Chemicals in Immunoassay Methods for Drugs of Abuse," *Clin Chem*, 1989, 35(4):648-51.

26. Baumgartner WA, Hill VA, and Blahd WD, "Hair Analysis for Drugs of Abuse," *J Forensic Sci*, 1989, 34:1433-53.

27. Arnold W, "Radioimmunological Hair Analysis for Narcotics and Substitutes," *J Clin Chem Clin Biochem*, 1987, 25(10):753-7.

28. Marigo M, Tagliaro F, Poiesi C, et al, "Determination of Morphine in the Hair of Heroin Addicts by High Performance Liquid Chromatography With Fluorimetric Detection," *J Anal Toxicol*, 1986, 10(4):158-61.

29. Cone EJ, Yousefnejad D, Darwin WD, et al, "Testing Human Hair for Drugs of Abuse. II. Identification of Unique Cocaine Metabolites in Hair of Drug Abusers and Evaluation of Decontamination Procedures," *J Anal Toxicol*, 1991, 15(5):250-5.

30. Cone EJ, "Testing Human Hair for Drugs of Abuse. Individual Dose and Time Profiles of Morphine and Codeine in Plasma, Saliva, Urine, and Beard Compared to Drug-Induced Effects on Pupils and Behavior," *J Anal Toxicol*, 1990, 14(1):1-7.

31. Selavka CM, "The Schizophrenic, the Transvestites and the Growth Rate of Hair," *Tox Talk*, 1994, 18(2):6-8.

32. Cone EJ, Hillsgrove MJ, Jenkins AJ, et al, "Sweat Testing for Heroin, Cocaine, and Metabolites," *J Anal Toxicol*, 1994, 18(6):298-305.

33. Burns and Baselt RC, "Monitoring Drug Use With a Sweat Patch: An Experiment With Cocaine," *J Anal Toxicol*, 1995, 19(1):41-8.

34. Cone EJ, "Saliva Testing for Drugs of Abuse," *Annals of the New York Academy of Sciences*, 1993, 694:91-127.

35. Fried PA and Watkinson B, "36 and 48-Month Neurobehavioural Follow-up of Children Prenatally Exposed to Marijuana, Cigarettes and Alcohol," *J Dev Behav Pediatr*, 1990, 11(2):49-58.

36. Spohr HI, Willms J, and Steinhausen HC, "Prenatal Alcohol Exposure and Long-Term Developmental Consequences," *Lancet*, 1993, 341:907-10.

37. Rush D, Andrews J, and Kristal A, "Maternal Cigarette Smoking During Pregnancy, Adioposity, Social Class, and Perinatal Outcome in Cardiff, Wales, 1965-1977," *Am J Perinatology*, 1990, 7(4):319-26.

38. Streissguth AP, Aase JM, Clarren SK, et al, "Fetal Alcohol Syndrome in Adolescents and Adults," *JAMA*, 1991, 265(15):1961-7.

39. Dusick AM, Covert RF, Schreiber MD, et al, "Risk of Intracranial Hemorrhage and Other Adverse Outcomes After Cocaine Exposure in a Cohort of 323 Very Low Birth Weight Infants," *J Pediatr*, 1993, 122(3):438-45.

40. Ostrea EM, Jr, Brady MJ, Parks PM, et al, "Drug Screening of Meconium in Infants of Drug Dependent Mothers: An Alternative to Urine Testing," *J Pediatr*, 1989, 115(3):474-7.

41. Browne SP, Tebbett IR, Moore CM, et al, "Analysis of Meconium for Cocaine in Neonates," *J Chromatogr*, 1992, 575(1):158-61.

42. Moore CM, Brown S, Negrusz A, et al, "Determination of Cocaine and Its Major Metabolite Benzoylecgonine, in Amniotic Fluid, Umbilical Cord Blood, Umbilical Cord Tissue, and Neonatal Urine: A Case Study," *J Anal Toxicol*, 1993, 17(1):62.

43. Jain L, Meyer W, Moore C, et al, "Detection of Fetal Cocaine Exposure by Analysis of Amniotic Fluid," *Obstet Gynecol*, 1993, 81(5 Pt 1):787-90.

44. Francom P, Andrenyak D, Lim HK, et al, "Determination of LSD in Urine by Capillary Column Gas Chromatography and Electron Impact Mass Spectrometry," *J Anal Toxicol*, 1988, 12(1):1-8.

45. Papac DI and Foltz RL, "Measurement of Lysergic Acid Diethylamide (LSD) in Human Plasma by Gas Chromatography/Negative Ion Chemical Ionization Mass Spectrometry," *J Anal Toxicol*, 1990, 14(3):189-90.

46. Hammargren WR and Henderson GL, "Analyzing Normetabolites of the Fentanyls by Gas Chromatography/Electron Capture Detection," *J Anal Toxicol*, 1988, 12(4):183-91.

47. Henderson GL, "Designer Drugs: Past History and Future Prospects," *J Forensic Sci*, 1988, 33(2):569-75.

48. Henderson GL, Harkey MR, and Jones AD, "Rapid Screening of Fentanyl (China White) Powder Samples by Solid-Phase Radioimmunoassay," *J Anal Toxicol*, 1990, 14(3):172-5.

49. Levi V, Scott JC, White PF, et al, "Improved Radioreceptor Assay of Opiate Narcotics in Human Serum: Application to Fentanyl and Morphine Metabolism," *Pharm Res*, 1987, 4(1):46-9.

— This introductory text was written by
Christine M. Moore, PhD
U.S. Drug Testing, Chicago, IL

ETHANOL AND BLOOD ALCOHOL DETERMINATION: WHAT DOES IT REALLY MEAN?

The association of alcohol (ethanol) use and traumatic events is so well established that alcohol use is considered a major risk factor in the etiology of accidents. It has been estimated that at least 52% of victims of head injury, 55% of drivers, and 77% of car passengers involved in fatal car accidents will have measurable blood alcohol levels in their bodies. As a result, emergency department physicians will now routinely obtain a blood alcohol level in a multiple traumatized patient.

However, when one attempts to extrapolate these specific blood alcohol levels to certain times or events, confusion can occur. It is in these circumstances that medical/scientific knowledge and legal interpretation can often diverge to two different conclusions.

One area of confusion is centered on the term "blood alcohol level." Simply put, a blood alcohol level may not be an alcohol level originating from blood. Essentially, alcohol can be measured from several sites in the body: blood, serum, eye (vitreous), bile, urine, kidney, saliva, bone marrow, or breath. Each of these sites has specific applications with respect to alcohol determination. For example, a urinary alcohol level is usually performed in conjunction with a blood alcohol level. When the urinary alcohol to blood alcohol ratio is >1.3, this indicates that the alcohol has been absorbed into the bloodstream and is dissipating (postabsorptive state).

A second example is that of determination of a blood alcohol level in the postmortem state. The alcohol level derived from blood can be falsely elevated when extensive decomposition or putrefaction has taken place. The eye (vitreous) can serve as a reliable site for postmortem alcohol determinations in that it is stable for prolonged intervals after death and that it may be closely related to the brain alcohol levels at time of death.

While breath alcohol testing has been utilized since 1938, the interpretation of results derived by these instruments is constantly being challenged. It has been alleged that radio frequency interference, burping, severe emphysema or diabetes mellitus, gasoline or acetone vapors, aerosolized mouth sprays, paint thinner fumes, or mouthwash can interfere with its results. While most of these scenarios will (at most) only mildly affect the instrument, certain procedures should be followed by the operator of the unit to alleviate these concerns. Calibration of the instrument along with obtaining two separate breath sample (3-5 minutes apart) from a cooperative subject taking a deep breath is essential to proper interpretation of the method. It should be remembered that the value obtained from these instruments is then converted to a blood alcohol concentration (using a blood:breath ratio of 2100:1). If any discrepancy results, sampling from other sites should occur.

Saliva alcohol testing is a relatively new and simple technique which essentially entails the use of a cotton swab to sample saliva from a subject's mouth. While it correlates closely with blood alcohol levels, it should be performed at least 10 minutes after alcohol ingestion. Collection of specimens from patients with dry mouth may be particularly difficult.

While it may be obvious from medical or autopsy records where the origin of the specimen is, it is the difference between serum or plasma and whole blood alcohol levels that causes confusion. Some clinical laboratories may measure alcohol levels from blood utilizing serum or plasma. Since alcohol distributes easily into a water medium and since there is a higher percentage of water in serum or plasma, the concentration of alcohol is about 12% to 20% higher in plasma or serum than in whole blood. Thus, one would need to divided the serum ethanol level (often described in units/dL or mmol/L) by 1.12-1.2 in order to obtain the equivalent blood alcohol concentration (often described as a percentage). It is in this way that an alcohol level derived from blood is not the same as "blood alcohol level." However, this discrepancy is rarely of any clinical importance and its relevance is questionable (see reference 10). For ethanol analysis from vitreous humor specimens, the blood alcohol concentration would be approximately 90% of the vitreous humor alcohol concentration.

The quantitative analysis of a blood alcohol concentration (BAC) can also lead to misinterpretation. In my opinion, most of the disputes regarding specific BAC center on the magic number of 0.1%. Since the first "per se" law was enacted by Nebraska in 1963, 42 states have established the "per se" BAC at 0.10%. Thus, chemical test evidence for alcohol intoxication has often centered on a specific level rather than merely it's presence (unlike cocaine or marijuana abuse).

Clearly we are entering an age of "zero tolerance" to the adverse effects of toxins. For example, the Centers of Disease Control (CDC) has been a leader in reducing lead exposure to virtually zero; the Federal Government has initiated random and pre-employment urine drug testing to eliminate substance abuse from its employees; new campaigns are initiated by the Environmental Protection Agency against not only cigarette smoking but also the effects of inhaling passive smoke.

This zero tolerance attitude is making its way to the field of driving-under-the-influence (DUI) enforcement. The National Safety Council, American Medical Association, Surgeon General, the Association for the Advancement of Automotive Medicine, and the American College of Emergency Physicians all have supported a lowering of "per se" BAC limits.

Certainly, the scientific data is plentiful in support of this attitude. It is clear that the crash risk increases as the level of the BAC of the driver increases. Deleterious effects of alcohol at a BAC at the range of 0.05% to 0.06% include impairment of curve-negotiating "driving" tasks, deterioration of information processing, and impairment in driving through narrow spaces. It has been estimated that 15% to 38% of drivers in injury-causing accidents had BAC of 0.05% or greater (see Figure 1 and Figure 2).

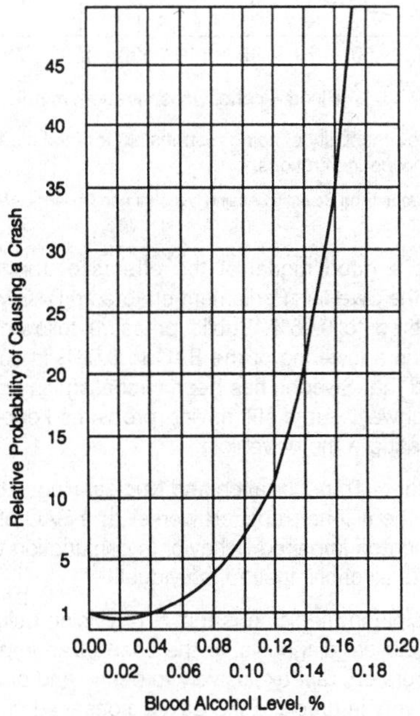

Figure 1. Relative probability of causing a crash rises with rising blood alcohol levels.

Reprinted from the Council on Scientific Affairs, "Alcohol and Driver," *JAMA*, 1992, 255:523, with permission.

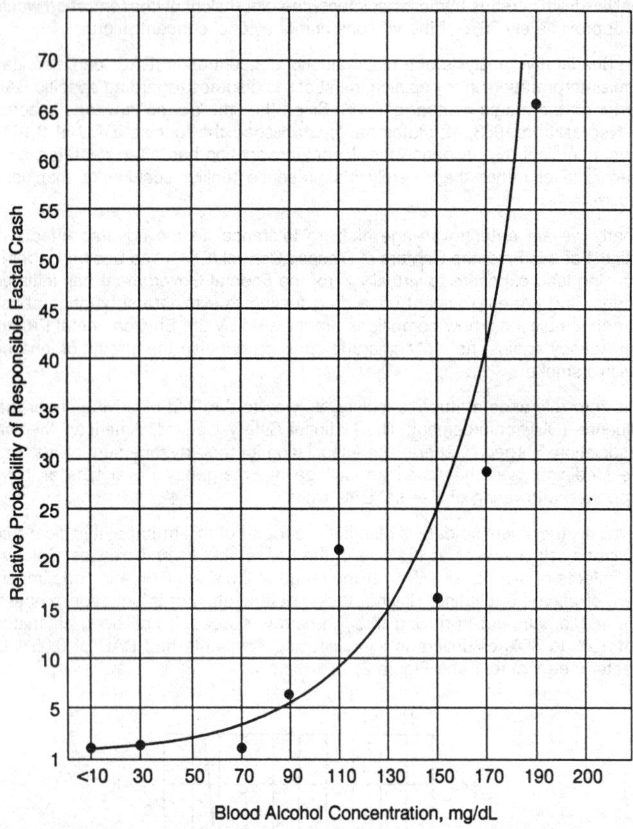

Figure 2. Relative probability of being responsible for fatal crash rises with rising blood alcohol concentrations.

Reprinted from the Council on Scientific Affairs, "Alcohol and Driver," *JAMA*, 1986, 255:523, with permission.

Sweden gives us a good model of the effects of this "zero tolerance" attitude. In 1941, the Swedish Parliament enacted a BAC limit of 0.08%; by 1957, it was lowered to 0.05%. Public pressure following Parliamentary hearings resulted in a lowering of the BAC to 0.02% in July, 1990. Essentially, it is believed that Sweden has been successful in keeping the social drinker off the highway, but is still having problems keeping the problem drinker from operating a motor vehicle.

Recent Department of Transportation and Nuclear Regulatory Commission guidelines define the alcohol-impaired worker at a BAC of 0.04%. Clearly, reliance of documented impaired behavior in conjunction with measurable BAC will define the alcohol-impaired individual.

One guiding principle in medicine is that a physician utilizes a laboratory test to confirm a clinical diagnosis. In the case of an impaired driver, we have used the laboratory test exclusively to define and diagnose. This has often led to other very imprecise BAC calculations – such as in the area of "back dating" the BAC to a specific time. When one considers the metabolism of alcohol to be somewhat variable (anywhere from 10-30 mg/dL/hour), it is apparent that this practice is fraught with hazards. Furthermore, the issue of disinfectant (isopropyl alcohol) use affecting BAC is truly extraneous with virtually no scientific basis. Additionally, food coingestion is a variable which has questionable measurable clinical impact. Multiple traumatic injury with resultant paralytic ileus may also result in a delay of ethanol absorption. Misinterpretation of BAC will be minimized if one is cognizant of the intent of obtaining the specimen, site from which the level is obtained along with the circumstances and nature of the impairment.

REFERENCES

1. American College of Emergency Physicians, "Blood Alcohol Concentration and Driving," *Ann Emerg Med*, 1988, 17(11):1252.
2. Angell M and Kassirer JP, "Alcohol and Other Drugs - Toward a More Rational and Consistent Policy," *N Engl J Med*, 1994, 331:537-8.
3. Brewer RD, Morris PD, Cole TB, et al, "The Risk of Dying in Alcohol-Related Automobile Crashes Among Habitual Drunk Drivers," *N Engl J Med*, 1994, 331:513-7.
4. Coe JI and Sherman RE, "Comparative Study of Postmortem Vitreous Humor and Blood Alcohol," *J Forensic Sciences*, 1970, 15(2):185-90.
5. Council on Scientific Affairs, "Alcohol and the Driver," *JAMA*, 1986, 255(4):522-7.
6. Chang J and Kollman SE, "The Effect of Temperature on the Formation of Ethanol by *Candida albicans* in Blood," *J Forensic Sci*, 1989, 34(1):105-9.
7. Hedlund JH, "If They Didn't Drink, Would They Crash Anyway? The Role of Alcohol in Traffic Crashes," *Alcohol, Drugs, and Driving*, 1994, 10(2):115-25.
8. Laurell H, "The Swedish Experience: Changes in BAC Legislation," *Alcohol, Drugs, and Driving*, 1991, 7:261-5.
9. Lundberg GD, "Lets Stop Driving After Drinking and Using Other Psychoactive Drugs," *JAMA*, 1986, 255(4):529-30.
10. Orsay E and Doan-Wiggins L, "Serum Alcohol Is Not the Same as Blood Alcohol Concentration," *Ann Emerg Med*, 1995, 25:430-1.
11. Tagliaro F, Lubli G, and Ghielmi S, "Chromatographic Methods for Blood Alcohol Determination," *J Chromatogr*, 1992, 580(1-2):161-90.
12. Voas RB, "Enforcement of DUI Laws," *Alcohol, Drugs, and Driving*, 1991, 7:173-96.
13. Watson WA and Garriott JC, "Alcohol and Motorcycle Riders: A Comparison of Motorcycle and Car/Truck DWIs," *Vet Hum Toxicol*, 1992, 34(3):213-5.

— This introductory text was written by
Jerrold B. Leikin, MD
Associate Medical Director, Emergency Services
Medical Director, Rush Poison Control Center
Rush-Presbyterian-St. Luke's Medical Center, Chicago, IL

ABGs *see* Blood Gases, Arterial *on page 1207*

Absolute Eosinophil Count *see* Eosinophil Count *on page 1259*

Abuse Screen *see* Drugs of Abuse Screen, Urine *on page 1252*

Acetaminophen, Serum

Synonyms Anacin-3®; Datril®; Liquiprin®; Panadol®; Panex®; Paracetamol; Phenaphen®; Tempra®; Tylenol®

Abstract Acetaminophen is an analgesic-antipyretic widely used as a replacement for aspirin. It is frequently seen in the deliberate overdose situation.

Specimen Blood

Volume 10 mL

Minimum Volume 3 mL

Container Red top tube

Reference Range Acetaminophen, serum: 20-110 μg/mL (SI: 43-240 μmol)

Critical Values Toxic: >150 μg/mL (SI: >990 μmol/L) (within 4 hours); >50 μg/mL (SI: >330 μmol/L) (within 12 hours)

Use Therapeutic monitoring; evaluate acetaminophen toxicity

Methodology UV spectrophotometry, immunoassay, gas-liquid chromatography (GLC), or high performance liquid chromatography (HPLC)

Additional Information Acetaminophen is an analgesic and antipyretic with little anti-inflammatory properties. It is used for headache, fever, relief of pain in patients who cannot tolerate aspirin or those with bleeding disorders or peptic ulcers. Acetaminophen is the analgesic/antipyretic of choice in children 13 years of age or younger due to the association of aspirin with the possible development of Reye's syndrome.

Acetaminophen is rapidly absorbed from the GI tract. Peak plasma concentrations are reached in 30-60 minutes. Steady-state concentrations are reached in 10-20 hours. However, prolonged (more than 10 days in adults; more than 5 days in children) treatment is to be avoided. Acetaminophen is metabolized to several conjugated forms, glucuronide (45% to 55%), sulfate (20% to 30%), and cysteine and mercaptopurine (20%). Acetanilide and phenacetin owe much of their analgesic effect to their metabolite, acetaminophen.

One indicator of acetaminophen toxicity may be to measure the drug half-life by analyzing a blood level taken 4 hours postingestion, then a second level 3-4 hours later. Expected half-life is 1-3 hours. Half-lives exceeding 4 hours are consistent with hepatic necrosis. The Rumack nomogram is useful for estimation of toxicity from serum level at 6 hours or later after ingestion. See nomogram. Nomogram is not to be utilized for extended release preparations.

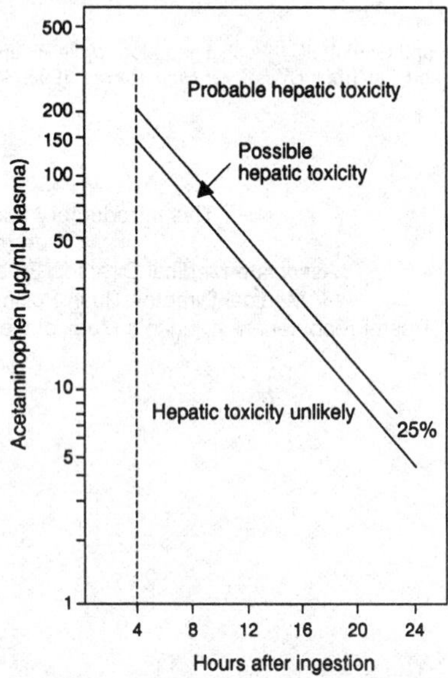

The Rumack-Matthew nomogram, relating expected severity of liver toxicity to serum acetaminophen concentrations. (From Smilkstein MJ et al, *Ann Emerg Med*, 1991, 10:1058.)

Hepatic toxicity may appear 3-5 days after ingestion of a toxic dose. Toxic levels require monitoring liver function with AST (SGOT), ALT (SGPT), and bilirubin with study also of glucose, creatinine, prothrombin time, and electrolytes. Serum levels drawn before 4 hours may not represent peak levels. The hepatotoxicity of acetaminophen is related to the formation of one or more highly reactive metabolites in the liver. Impaired hepatic metabolism may be found in the elderly. Orally administered N-acetylcysteine (Mucomyst®) has been shown to provide rather dramatic protection against acetaminophen hepatotoxicity. Early treatment is especially recommended in pregnant subjects.

Specific References

Ashbourne JF, Olson KR, and Khayam-Bashi H, "Value of Rapid Screening for Acetaminophen in All Patients With Intentional Drug Overdose," *Ann Emerg Med*, 1989, 18(10):1035-8.

Baselt RC and Cravey RH, "Acetaminophen," *Disposition of Toxic Drugs and Chemicals in Man*, 3rd ed, Chicago, IL: Year Book Medical Publishers Inc, 1989, 2-5.

Kumar S and Rex DK, "Failure of Physicians to Recognize Acetaminophen Hepatotoxicity in Chronic Alcoholics," *Arch Intern Med*, 1991, 151(6):1189-91.

Montamat SC, Cusack BJ, and Vestal RE, "Management of Drug Therapy in the Elderly," *N Engl J Med*, 1989, 321(5):303-9.

Rumack BH and Matthew H, "Acetaminophen Poisoning and Toxicity," *Pediatrics*, 1975, 55(6):871-6.

Stewart MJ and Watson ID, "Analytical Reviews in Clinical Chemistry: Methods for the Estimation of Salicylate and Paracetamol in Serum, Plasma, and Urine," *Ann Clin Biochem*, 1987, 24(Pt 6):552-65.

Veltri JC and Rollins DE, "A Comparison of the Frequency and Severity of Poisoning Cases For Ingestion of Acetaminophen, Aspirin, and Ibuprofen," *Am J Emerg Med*, 1988, 6(2):104-7.

Acetoacetate *see* Ketone Bodies, Blood *on page 1277*

Acetoacetic Acid, Urine *see* Ketones, Urine *on page 1278*

Acetone *see* Ketone Bodies, Blood *on page 1277*

Acetone *see* Volatile Screen *on page 1378*

Acetone, Semiquantitative, Urine *see* Ketones, Urine *on page 1278*

Acetylcholinesterase, RBC *see* Acetylcholinesterase, Red Blood Cell *on this page*

Acetylcholinesterase, Red Blood Cell

Related Information

Pseudocholinesterase, Serum *on page 1340*

Synonyms Acetylcholinesterase, RBC; Cholinesterase, Erythrocytic; Erythrocyte Cholinesterase; Red Cell Cholinesterase; True Cholinesterase

Specimen Blood

Minimum Volume 2 mL whole blood

Container Green top (heparin) tube or heparinized capillary tubes

Storage Instructions Stable at 4°C to 25°C for 1 week only.

Reference Range Not well established, varies with method, age, sex, and use of oral contraceptives. Normally absent in amniotic fluid. Usual range in healthy individuals: 4000-12,000 unit/L. While neonatal levels are initially low, adult levels are achieved after 2 months of age. Mild poisoning usually results in acetylcholinesterase levels 20% to 50% of normals; moderate poisoning results in a depression to 10% to 20% of normal, while severe poisoning results in a depression of $<10\%$ of normal.

Use Erythrocyte cholinesterase is measured to diagnose organophosphate and carbamate toxicity and to detect atypical forms of the enzyme. Cholinesterase is irreversibly inhibited by organophosphate insecticides and reversibly inhibited by carbamate insecticides. Serum or plasma pseudocholinesterase is a better measure of acute toxicity, while erythrocyte levels are better for chronic exposure. (Serum level returns to normal prior to normalizing of red cell level.) Acetylcholinesterase is increased in amniotic fluid in cases of neural tube defect. Persons with an atypical form of the enzyme (with low enzyme activity) exhibit prolonged apnea following the use of certain suxamethonium-type muscle relaxants in anesthesia (succinylcholine sensitivity – AA phenotype). These atypical forms may be detected by the use of fluoride or dibucaine inhibition. In amniotic fluid, it is used for the evaluation of neural tube defects in conjunction with alpha-fetoprotein.

Limitations Values decrease as erythrocytes become senescent.

Methodology Methods are based on determination of result (rate) of hydrolysis of an ester catalyzed by the enzyme acetylcholinesterase and include colorimetry, fluorometry, spectrophotometry based systems. Polyacrylamide gel electrophoresis is used for the qualitative demonstration of acetylcholinesterase in amniotic fluid. Screening methods are available.

Additional Information The cholinesterase activity in human red cells is highly but not exclusively specific for acetylcholine. It is referred to as true or specific cholinesterase. Cholinesterase activity present in the serum/plasma hydrolyses both choline and aliphatic esters, has a broader range of esterolytic activity and is referred to as "pseudo-" or "nonspecific" cholinesterase. It hydrolyses acetylcholine only slowly. The systematic name for acetylcholinesterase is acetylcholine acetyl-

(Continued)

Acetylcholinesterase, Red Blood Cell *(Continued)*

hydrolase. Systematic name for cholinesterase (serum/plasma) is acylcholine acylhydrolase. The different nature of the cholinesterases was first described in 1940. The plasma enzyme is synthesized by the liver, the red cell enzyme during erythropoiesis.

Cholinesterase activity is low at birth and higher in adult males than females. The enzyme is a large complex protein. There is evidence that it has a multiple subunit structure, four peptide chains that form two dimers. Because of the many constituent amino acids, many molecular variants are possible. The RBC level is **increased** in hemolytic states such as the thalassemias, spherocytosis, hemoglobin SS, and acquired hemolytic anemias. It is **decreased** in paroxysmal nocturnal hemoglobinuria and in relapse of megaloblastic anemia. (It returns to normal with therapy.)

Potent inhibitors of cholinesterase may present important clinical toxicological problems. Systemic insecticides (eg, organophosphates or carbamates) are examples. Both RBC acetylcholinesterase and plasma cholinesterase are usually inhibited. The effect on the plasma enzyme is more marked, however, and serum levels are usually utilized in diagnosis and assessment of recovery. Recovery is best determined by looking for a plateau in erythrocyte cholinesterase activity. Toxic potency may vary, plasma versus red cell cholinesterase, such that in some cases erythrocyte levels may be needed for diagnosis and/or monitoring. If there is suspicion that a decrease in cholinesterase activity may not relate to the inhibitor effect of an organophosphate then red cell level of acetylcholinesterase should be obtained. If both serum and RBC levels are significantly decreased, findings are those of exogenous toxic effect.

True cholinesterase (acetylcholinesterase-RBC cholinesterase) is not normally present in amniotic fluid. Presence of acetylcholinesterase activity and increased levels of alpha-fetoprotein in amniotic fluid are presumptive evidence of an open neural tube defect (eg, anencephaly, open spina bifida, or omphalocele) in the fetus.

Specific References

King ME, "Cholinesterase," *Methods in Clinical Chemistry*, Pesce AJ and Kaplan LA, eds, St Louis, MO: Mosby-Year Book Inc, 1987, 161-8.

Kobayashi K, Sakoguchi T, and Matsuoka A, "Stimulating Effects of Calcium and Magnesium on Serum Pseudocholinesterase Activity," *Clin Chem*, 1988, 34(1):173-4.

Phillip AT, "Cholinesterases: Assay Methods and Significance," *Clin Toxicol Rev*, 1995, 17:7.

Whittaker M, "Cholinesterase," *Monographs in Human Genetics*, Vol 11, Beckman L, ed, Basel: Karger, 1986.

Acetylsalicylic Acid, Blood *see* Salicylate, Blood *on page 1347*

Ac-Globulin *see* Factor V, Plasma *on page 1262*

Acid-Base Status Evaluation *see* Carbon Dioxide, Blood *on page 1220*

Acid-Fast Stain, Modified, *Cryptosporidium* *see Cryptosporidium* Diagnostic Procedures, Stool *on page 1244*

Acute Phase Reactants *see* Fibrinogen, Plasma *on page 1265*

Adapin® *see* Doxepin, Blood *on page 1251*

Advil® *see* Ibuprofen, Serum *on page 1273*

Aerobic Culture, Blood *see* Blood Culture, Aerobic and Anaerobic *on page 1204*

Aerosol Lung Scan *see* Lung Scan, Ventilation *on page 1288*

Ag, Blood *see* Silver, Serum *on page 1351*

Ag, Urine *see* Silver, Urine *on page 1351*

Albumin, Urine *see* Protein, Semiquantitative, Urine *on page 1337*

Alcohol, Semiquantitative, Urine

Synonyms Ethyl Alcohol, Urine; Urine Alcohol Level; Urine Ethanol

Test Includes Ethyl alcohol for medical purpose only, not for legal use. Assay also measures methyl alcohol, isopropyl alcohol, and paraldehyde. Results reported as ethanol unless another alcohol is requested.

Specimen Random urine

Volume 15 mL

Minimum Volume 1 mL

Container Plastic urine container

Collection Freshly voided random urine

Reference Range Negative

Methodology Dichromate diffusion

Additional Information Ethanol is absorbed rapidly from the GI tract. Peak blood levels usually occur within 30-60 minutes on an empty stomach. Food in the stomach can delay the absorption of alcohol. Ethanol is metabolized by the liver to acetaldehyde. Once peak blood ethanol levels are reached, disappearance is linear; a 70 kg man metabolizes 7-10 g alcohol/hour (20±10 mg/dL/hour). The average urine/blood ratio is 1.35 in the postabsorptive state. Symptoms of intoxication in the presence of low alcohol levels could indicate a serious acute medical problem requiring immediate attention. The half-lives and effectiveness of certain drugs (eg, barbiturates, etc) are increased in the presence of ethanol.

Alcohol, Serum

Synonyms Ethanol, Blood; Ethyl Alcohol, Blood; EtOH

Abstract Alcohol is the single most abused drug in the United States. Whole blood values are required for legal use.

Patient Preparation Do not use alcohol wipe to clean venipuncture site for forensic samples. While it should be noted that the possibility of an isopropyl-based swab significantly interfering with an ethanol-based assay is negligible, this aspect may be challenged in court, and therefore, it may be best to avoid this argument by using a nonalcohol-based swab. Hexachlorophene-based, iodine-based, or mercury-based antiseptics not containing alcohol may be used.

Specimen Blood

Volume 5 mL

Minimum Volume 2 mL serum or plasma

Container Red top tube; gray top (sodium fluoride) tube is recommended for medicolegal specimens and prolonged storage.

Collection Do not prepare venipuncture site with an alcohol swab for forensic samples. When police agencies bring an individual in for blood alcohol levels, medical and laboratory people should at all times be aware of their state statutes.

Storage Instructions Refrigerate in a tightly stoppered tube.

Special Instructions Concentrations of ethanol are 10% to 15% higher in serum and plasma versus whole blood. For forensic purposes, only whole blood values are used.

Reference Range Blood: negative. In most laboratories, values <10 mg/dL (SI: <2.0 mmol/L) are considered negative. Signs of intoxication can be observed at levels of 30-100 mg/dL (SI: 6.6-21.7 mmol/L).

Critical Values Fatal concentration is usually considered to be >400 mg/dL (SI: >86.8 mmol/L). Whole blood levels of 300 mg/dL (SI: 65.1 mmol/L) are associated with coma. In most states, levels ≥100 mg/dL are considered evidence of impairment for driving.

Possible Panic Range ≥300 mg/dL (SI: ≥65.1 mmol/L)

Use Quantitation of alcohol level for medical or legal purposes; screen unconscious patients; used to diagnose alcohol intoxication and determine appropriate therapy; screen for alcoholism and monitor ethanol treatment for methanol intoxication. Must be tested as possible cause of coma of unknown etiology since alcohol intoxication may mimic diabetic coma, cerebral trauma, and drug overdose.

Limitations Certain other alcohols (in high concentration) can interfere with enzymatic methods. The rate of dehydrogenation of isopropanol (2-propanol) is 6% and that of n-propanol (1-propanol) is 36% of that of ethanol. Methanol does not interfere. Gas chromatography is the most specific methodology because it can separate, identify, and quantitate each type of alcohol present. Freezing point osmometry and enzymatic analysis can together determine the presence of volatile intoxicants and can determine causes of metabolic intoxication.

Methodology Enzymatic analysis (alcohol dehydrogenase), freezing point osmometry, gas chromatography (GC)

Additional Information For more information, see introduction. Ethanol is absorbed rapidly from the GI tract. Peak blood levels usually occur within 30-60 minutes on an empty stomach. Food in the stomach can delay the absorption of alcohol. Ethanol is metabolized by the liver to acetaldehyde. Once peak blood ethanol levels are reached, disappearance is linear; a 70 kg man metabolizes 7-10 g of alcohol/hour (20±10 mg/dL/hour). The urine/blood ratio is considered to be about 1:35 but is quite variable. The average saliva/blood ratio is 1:20. Symptoms of intoxication in the presence of low alcohol levels could indicate a serious acute medical problem requiring immediate attention. The half-lives and effectiveness of certain drugs (eg, barbiturates, etc) are increased in the presence of ethanol. Urine alcohol can be measured by immunoassay and gas chromatography and is tested for in abused drug screening programs. Only in Europe are urine ethanol levels accepted as legal evidence. Breath alcohol analyzers are used by law enforcement personnel and the results are accepted as legal evidence of intoxication. They must not be used less than 15 minutes after the last alcohol ingestion. Elevated serum lactate and lactate dehydrogenase levels may interfere with enzymatic ethanol assays.

Specific References

Blume SB, "Women and Alcohol. A Review," *JAMA*, 1986, 256(11):1467-70.

(Continued)

Alcohol, Serum *(Continued)*

Gadsden RH and Terry CS, "Alcohols in Biological Fluids by Gas Chromatography," *Selected Methods of Emergency Toxicology*, Frings CS and Faulkner WR, eds, Washington, DC: American Association of Clinical Chemistry Press, 1986, 40-3.
Jones AW, "Observations on the Specificity of Breath-Alcohol Analyzers Used for Clinical and Medicolegal Purposes," *J Forensic Sci*, 1989, 34(4):842-7.
Keim ME, Bartfield JM, Raccio-Robak N, et al, "Use of Enzymatic Assay Device for Serum Ethanol Measurement," *Acad Emerg Med*, 1995, 2:402.
Lovejoy FH, "Ethanol Intoxication," *Clin Toxicol Rev*, 1981, 4:1-2.
Macchia T, Mancinelli R, Gentili S, et al, "Ethanol in Biological Fluids: Headspace GC Measurement," *J Anal Toxicol*, 1995, 19:241-6.
Mendenhall CL and Weesner RE, "Alcoholism," *Clin Chem*, Kaplan LA and Pesce AJ, eds, St Louis, MO: Mosby-Year Book Inc, 1984, 594-610.
Nine JS, Moraca M, Virji MA, et al, "Serum-Ethanol Determination: Comparison of Lactate and Lactate Dehydrogenase Interference in Three Enzymatic Assays," *J Anal Toxicol*, 1995, 19:192-6.
Wilkinson PK, "Pharmacokinetics of Ethanol: A Review," *Alcohol Clin Exp Res*, 1980, 4(1):6-21.

Alkaline Phosphatase, Serum

Synonyms ALP; Phosphatase, Alkaline

Abstract Serum alkaline phosphatase (ALP) activity normally originates from liver and bone. ALP is excreted in bile. Serum total ALP level provides a useful but nonspecific indication of liver or bone disease. With biliary tract obstruction, the rise in ALP parallels increase in serum bilirubin. Heating serum at 56°C causes significant inactivation of ALP of bone origin.

Patient Preparation Patient should be fasting.

Specimen Blood

Volume 1 mL

Minimum Volume 0.5 mL serum

Container Red top tube or capillary tube

Storage Instructions Refrigerate. Serum alkaline phosphatase increases slowly with storage. Increases of 5% to 10% can be expected after less than 4 hours storage at 4°C. For this reason, it is best to analyze on the day of collection.

Reference Range Normal values are higher for pediatric patients and in pregnancy. Levels are two to three or more times adult range in children and are increased in puberty compared to adult range. During episodes of very rapid growth, levels as high as 1000 units/L may be normal. The high level of ALP in childhood results from increase in bone fraction. Postpuberty, serum ALP is mostly of liver origin. Adult normal range is approximately 35-100 units/L. Values in adult males are slightly higher than in adult females. With menopause and after, values in women increase, are similar to or higher than those in men, and are higher than in younger subjects.

Use Causes of **high alkaline phosphatase** include nonfasting specimen; elevations occur especially 2-4 hours after a fatty meal, especially in people who are Lewis positive secretors of blood type O or B. (See Additional Information.) Standing of blood specimen before analysis; up to 30% increase with storage of serum. Bone growth, healing fracture, acromegaly, osteogenic sarcoma, liver or bone metastases, leukemia, myelofibrosis, and rarely myeloma. Alkaline phosphatase is used as a tumor marker.

In rickets and osteomalacia, serum calcium and phosphorus are low to normal; and alkaline phosphatase may be normal or increased.

Hypervitaminosis D may cause elevations in alkaline phosphatase.

In Paget's disease of bone, there is often isolated elevation of serum alkaline phosphatase. Some of the highest levels of serum ALP are seen in Paget's disease.

Hyperthyroidism, by its effects upon bone, may elevate alkaline phosphatase. There is evidence that thyroid hormone (T_3) acts to stimulate bone alkaline phosphatase activity through an osteoblast nuclear receptor-mediated process.

Hyperparathyroidism, in some patients.

Pseudohyperparathyroidism.

Chronic alcohol ingestion (in chronic alcoholism, alkaline phosphatase may be normal or increased, but often with high AST (SGOT) and/or high bilirubin and especially with high GGT; MCV may be high).

Biliary obstruction (tenfold increase may be seen with carcinoma of the head of pancreas, choledocholithiasis); cholestasis; GGT also high. Cholecystitis with cholangitis. (In most patients with cholecystitis and cholangitis who do not have a common duct stone, alkaline phosphatase is within normal limits or only slightly increased.) Sclerosing cholangitis (eg, with ulcerative colitis), although importantly, 3% of cases of symptomatic sclerosing cholangitis may have normal serum ALP. Endoscopic retrograde cholangiography might be considered then in patients with diseases known to be associated with primary sclerosing cholangitis and with appropriate symptomatology even though ALP level is normal. With primary or metastatic tumor in the liver, there may be a marked increase in alkaline phosphatase and GGT. Only three laboratory markers were consistently abnormal, in screening for metastatic carcinoma of breast, prior to clinical detectability of metastases: these were alkaline phosphatase, GGT, and CEA.

Cirrhosis, especially in primary biliary cirrhosis, in which fivefold or more increases are seen.

Gilbert's syndrome: Increase in intestinal alkaline phosphatase is seen.

Hepatitis: Moderate increases in alkaline phosphatase occur in viral hepatitis, but greater elevations of the transaminases (AST (SGOT), ALT (SGPT)) are usually found.

Fatty metamorphosis of liver (moderate increase occurs in acute fatty liver).

Diabetes mellitus, diabetic hepatic lipidosis.

Infiltrative liver diseases (eg, sarcoid, TB, amyloidosis, abscess).

Sepsis and certain viral diseases including infectious mononucleosis and cytomegalovirus infections.

Postoperative cholestasis – pancreatitis, carcinoma of pancreas, cystic fibrosis.

Pulmonary infarct (1-3 weeks after embolism. Healing infarcts in other organs, including kidney, may also cause increased alkaline phosphatase); other situations in which angiofibroplasia occurs, such as healing in a large decubitus ulcer.

Tumors, especially hypernephroma; neoplastic ectopic production (Regan, Nagao isoenzymes).

Fanconi syndrome.

Peptic ulcer, erosion; intestinal strangulation or obstruction, or ulcerative lesion; steatorrhea, malabsorption (from bone, secondary to vitamin D deficiency); ulcerative colitis with pericholangitis, other erosive lesions of colon.

Congestive heart failure.

Parenteral hyperalimentation of glucose, intravenous albumin administration.

Familial hyperphosphatasemia.

Idiopathic.

Drugs – estrogens (large doses), birth control agents, methyltestosterone, phenothiazines, oral hypoglycemic agents, erythromycin, or any drug producing hypersensitivity or toxic cholestasis. Many commonly and uncommonly used drugs elevate alkaline phosphatase, and tenfold increases may be seen with drug cholestasis.

Causes of **low alkaline phosphatase** are said to include hypothyroidism – but most hypothyroid patients have normal alkaline phosphatase.

Pernicious anemia – in very few patients.

Hypophosphatasia: Very low alkaline phosphatase values are found in the presence of normocalcemia or hypocalcemia. This diagnosis may be confirmed by quantitation of urinary phosphoethanolamine.

Malnutrition has been reported to relate to low values, but in practice, diseases causing malnutrition relate often to high alkaline phosphatase results (eg, disseminated neoplasia).

Some drugs (clofibrate, azathioprine, estrogens and estrogens in combination with androgens) lower serum ALP activity.

Limitations Normal ranges dependent upon methodology, age, and sex. Used alone, alkaline phosphatase may be misleading. Fluoride salts can interfere with the assay resulting in a false depression.

Methodology Some original spectrophotometric methods and their modifications (eg, King-Armstrong, described in 1934 and using the substrate phenylphosphate) have been largely supplanted by more recent end point, kinetic spectrophotometric or fluorescent procedures. Most current assays use *p*-nitrophenyl phosphate (pNPP) as substrate (eg, Bessay-Lowry-Brock). More recent techniques utilize chromogenic substrates (eg, methylumbelliferyl phosphate) and improved buffer systems with resultant increased sensitivity. A reference method using pNPP as substrate has been proposed by the American Association of Clinical Chemistry.

Additional Information Serum alkaline phosphatase is a member of a family of zinc metalloprotein enzymes that function to split off a terminal phosphate group from an organic phosphate ester. This enzyme functions in an alkaline environment (optimum pH of 10). Active center of ALP enzymes includes a serine residue. Magnesium and zinc ions are required for minimal activity. Enzyme activity is localized in the brush border of the proximal convoluted tubule of the kidney, intestinal mucosal epithelial cells, hepatic sinusoidal membranes, vascular endothelial cells, and osteoblasts of bone. There are distinctive forms of ALP in the placenta and small intestine; hepatic, renal, and osteoblast (bone) ALP are similar molecules.

(Continued)

Alkaline Phosphatase, Serum *(Continued)*

Serum ALP activity of intestinal origin occurs only in individuals of ABO blood type O or A. They are secretors of ABH RBC antigens and also carry the Lewis red cell antigen. Serum intestinal ALP level increases in these individuals about 2 hours following consumption of a fatty meal.

Liver alkaline phosphatase is increased in cholestasis and inflammatory liver disease as well as in infiltrative liver disease. The enzyme is sensitive to obstructive biliary processes, even small secondary bile duct obstruction, and thus may be increased in those patients when the bilirubin is normal due to compensatory bilirubin excretion by the rest of the liver. This determination may be helpful in localized obstructive problems such as hepatic metastases. An electrophoretically slow moving isoenzyme with high relative mass may occur in some patients with bile duct obstruction and hepatic metastases and may result in false elevation of CK-MB.

To confirm biliary abnormality, an additional useful test is GGT. GGT is elevated in hepatobiliary disease, not in uncomplicated bone disease.

Serum ALP is increased during pregnancy. Marked decline of high ALP of pregnancy is seen with placental insufficiency and imminent fetal demise.

Specific References

Batsakis JG, "Serum Alkaline Phosphatase. Refining an Old Test for the Future," *Diagn Med*, 1982, 25-33.

Epstein S, "Serum and Urinary Markers for Bone Remodeling: Assessment of Bone Turnover," *Endocr Rev*, 1988, 9(4):437-49.

Kazmierczak SC and Lott JA, "Alkaline Phosphatase," Chapter 138, *Methods in Clinical Chemistry*, Pesce AJ and Kaplan LA, eds, St Louis, MO: Mosby-Year Book Inc, 1987.

Kihn L, Dinwoodie A, and Stinson RA, "High-Molecular-Weight Alkaline Phosphatase in Serum Has Properties Similar to the Enzyme in Plasma Membranes of the Liver," *Am J Clin Pathol*, 1991, 96(4):470-8.

Reichling JJ and Kaplan MM, "Clinical Use of Serum Enzymes in Liver Disease," *Dig Dis Sci*, 1988, 33(12):1601-14.

Van Hoof VO, Hoylaerts MF, Geryl H, et al, "Age and Sex Distribution of Alkaline Phosphatase Isoenzymes by Agarose Electrophoresis," *Clin Chem*, 1990, 36(6):875-8.

Vincent-Viry M and Galteau MM, "Alkaline Phosphatases," *Drug Effects on Laboratory Test Results Analytical Interferences and Pharmacological Effects*, Siest G and Galteau MM, eds, Littleton, MA: PSG Publishing Co Inc, 1988, 67-90.

Wilson JW, "Inherited Elevation of Alkaline Phosphatase Activity in the Absence of Disease," *N Engl J Med*, 1979, 301(18):983-4.

ALP *see* Alkaline Phosphatase, Serum *on page 1184*

Aluminum, Serum

Specimen Blood, dialysis fluid, urine, cerebrospinal fluid

Volume 5 mL

Container Special metal-free Sherwood Monoject™ trace element blood collection tube #8881-307006 for serum separation; acid-washed plastic vials for other samples.

Collection Use B-D #5175 20-gauge stainless steel needle, or Terumo or Abbot butterfly needle. Draw any trace metal tube prior to any other type of blood sample to prevent contamination of needle by regular rubber stoppers.

Causes for Rejection Contamination by aluminum contact, dust, or ordinary collection tubes or stoppers. Urine must not be contaminated by stool.

Special Instructions The patient should take no aluminum containing antacids or medicines (such as Basaljel®, Gelusil®, Maalox®, Amphojel®, Sucralfate) for 24 hours prior to blood test.

Reference Range Serum (normal patient): 0-10 ng/mL (SI: 0-0.37 μmol/L) (may vary with laboratory); serum (dialysis patients): up to 40 ng/mL (SI: <1.48 μmol/L) without apparent acute effects, >100 ng/mL (SI: >3.7 μmol/L) possible CNS toxicity, >200 ng/mL (SI: >7.4 μmol/L) probable multisystem toxicity; urine: 0-32 ng/day (SI: 0-1.2 μmol/day); dialysate: <0.01 mg/L (AAMI standards)

Use Monitor patients for prior and ongoing exposure to aluminum. Patients at risk include:

- infants on parenteral fluids, particularly parenteral nutrition
- burn patients through administration of intravenous albumin, particularly with coexisting renal failure
- adult and pediatric patients with chronic renal failure, who accumulate aluminum readily from medications and dialysate
- adult parenteral nutrition patients (less so, recently)
- patients with industrial exposure

Monitor dialysate and water to prepare dialysate to prevent aluminum toxicity in dialysis patients. Research use: investigation of amyotrophic lateral sclerosis (in Guam) and Alzheimer's disease.

Limitations Serum levels rise and fall after each dose of aluminum-containing phosphate binder or sucralfate. If renal function is normal, renal clearance of aluminum is prompt with urine levels rising quickly after a course of aluminum-containing antacid is begun and elevated levels persisting for over a week. Urine levels rise after a dose of desferrioxamine given for any reason. The degree of rise in serum aluminum after desferrioxamine is regarded as reflecting total body aluminum burden.

Methodology Atomic absorption (AA), inductively coupled plasma atomic emission spectrometry

Additional Information Aluminum toxicity has been recognized in many settings where exposure is heavy or prolonged, where renal function is limited, or where a previously accumulated bone burden is released in stress or illness. Toxicity may include:

- encephalopathy (stuttering, gait disturbance, myoclonic jerks, seizures, coma, abnormal EEG)
- osteomalacia or aplastic bone disease (associated with painful spontaneous fractures, hypercalcemia, tumorous calcinosis)
- proximal myopathy
- increased risk of infection
- increased left ventricular mass and decreased myocardial function
- microcytic anemia
- with very high levels, sudden death

Aluminum is ubiquitous in our environment; it is the third most prevalent element in the earth's crust. The gastrointestinal tract is relatively impervious to aluminum, absorption normally being only about 2%. Aluminum is absorbed by a mechanism related to that for calcium. Gastric acidity and oral citrate favors absorption, and H_2-blockers reduce absorption. As is true for several trace elements, transferrin is the primary protein binder and carrier for aluminum in the plasma, where 80% is protein bound and 20% is free or complexed to small molecules such as citrate. Cells appear to take up aluminum from transferrin rather than from citrate. Purified preparations of ferritin from brain and liver have been found to contain aluminum. It is not known if ferritin has a specific binding site for aluminum. Factors regulating the migration of aluminum across the blood-brain barrier are not well understood. Serum aluminum correlates with encephalopathy; red cell aluminum correlates with microcytic anemia; and bone aluminum correlates with aluminum bone disease. Basal PTH when elevated appears to protect bone and thereby favor CNS toxicity. Other factors favoring one form of toxicity over another are not well understood. Aluminum toxicity has been reported to impair the formation and release of parathyroid hormone. The parathyroid glands concentrate aluminum above levels in surrounding tissues. Treatment of aluminum toxicity in renal failure patients often reactivates hyperparathyroidism, which to a certain extent is helpful for bone remodeling and healing.

Specific References

Alfrey AC, LeGendre GR, and Kaehny WD, "The Dialysis Encephalopathy Syndrome: Possible Aluminum Intoxication," *N Engl J Med*, 1976, 294(4):184-8.

Chappuis P, Poupon J, and Rousselet F, "A Sequential and Simple Determination of Zinc, Copper, and Aluminum in Blood Samples by Inductively Coupled Plasma Atomic Emission Spectrometry," *Clin Chim Acta*, 1992, 206(3):155-65.

Ellenberg R, King AL, Sica DA, et al, "Cerebrospinal Fluid Aluminum Levels Following Deferoxamine," *Am J Kidney Dis*, 1990, 16(2):157-9.

Gruskin AB, "Aluminum: A Pediatric Overview," *Adv Pediatr*, 1988, 35:281-330.

Klein GL, "Aluminum in Parenteral Products: Medical Perspective on Large and Small Volume Parenterals," *J Parenter Sci Technol*, 1989, 43(3):120-4.

Monteagudo FS, Cassidy MJ, and Folb PI, "Recent Developments in Aluminum Toxicology," *Med Toxicol Adverse Drug Exp*, 1989, 4(1):1-16.

Tzamaloukas AH, "Diagnosis and Management of Bone Disorders in Chronic Renal Failure and Dialyzed Patients," *Med Clin North Am*, 1990, 74(4):961-74.

Wills MR and Savory J, "Aluminum and Chronic Renal Failure: Sources, Absorption, Transport, and Toxicity," *Crit Rev Clin Lab Sci*, 1989, 27(1):59-107.

Alurate® *see* Barbiturates, Quantitative, Blood *on page 1201*

Aminophylline *see* Theophylline, Blood *on page 1359*

Aminotransferases *see* Aspartate Aminotransferase *on page 1199*

Amitriptyline, Blood

Synonyms Elavil®; Endep®; Etrafon®; Limbitrol®; Triavil®

Applies To Pamelor®

Test Includes Nortriptyline levels

Abstract Amitriptyline is a tricyclic antidepressant. Nortriptyline is a major active metabolite.

Specimen Blood

Volume 5 mL

Minimum Volume 3 mL serum or plasma

Container Red top tube, green top (heparin) tube

Sampling Time Trough levels at steady-state

Reference Range Amitriptyline and nortriptyline 100-250 ng/mL (SI: 360-900

(Continued)

Amitriptyline, Blood *(Continued)*

nmol/L); nortriptyline 50-150 ng/mL (SI: 190-570 nmol/L). Metabolism may be impaired in the elderly.

Critical Values >300 ng/mL (SI: >1080 nmol/L)

Use Therapeutic monitoring; toxicity assessment

Methodology Immunoassay, high performance liquid chromatography (HPLC), gas chromatography (GC)

Additional Information Amitriptyline is a tricyclic antidepressant that blocks the reuptake of serotonin at nerve endings and possesses high anticholinergic activity and cardiovascular toxicity. The drug is extensively metabolized to many polar compounds, the chief of which is nortriptyline; also an antidepressant. Both drugs are prescribed for depression and a range of other disorders.

Amitriptyline has a peak serum concentration 2-6 hours postoral dose, and steady-state is achieved after 3-8 days of chronic oral dosing. The half-life is 17-40 hours and the usual therapeutic range (predose sample at steady-state) includes nortriptyline and is 100-250 ng/mL. Nortriptyline is administered orally, has a half-life of 15-90 hours, and peak serum values 2-6 hours postoral dose. Steady-state is achieved after 4-20 days of chronic dosing. Therapeutic levels of nortriptyline alone are 50-150 ng/mL. Moderate intoxication occurs at plasma levels of 50-430 ng/mL and toxic symptoms at levels >300 ng/mL; fatal blood concentrations range: 500-16,000 ng/mL.

All the tricyclic antidepressants have significant **drug interactions**: hydrocortisone methylphenidate and phenothiazines increase tricyclic levels; barbiturates, chloral hydrate, phenytoin, and glutethimide lower serum tricyclic levels; tricyclics impair the antihypertensive effectiveness of clonidine and guanethidine; tricyclics and alcohol produce additive sedative effects; tricyclics and antiparkinsonism agents have potent anticholinergic side effects; and tricyclics and MAO inhibitors should not be coadministered because of the potential for antihypertensive and CNS crises.

Tricyclics should be avoided in pregnant and lactating women because these drugs have not been established as safe. Geriatric patients are especially prone to postural hypotension, urinary retention, and sedation. Red blood cell metabolite assays may be the best predictor for cardiac conduction abnormalities.

Specific References

Amitai Y, Erickson T, Kennedy EJ, et al, "Tricyclic Antidepressants in Red Cells and Plasma: Correlation With Impaired Intraventricular Conduction in Acute Overdose," *Clin Pharmacol Ther*, 1993, 54(2):219-27.

Katz IR, Curlik S, and Lesher EL, "Use of Antidepressants in the Frail Elderly. When, Why and How," *Clin Geriatr Med*, 1988, 4(1):203-22.

Katz MM, Koslow SH, Maas JW, et al, "Identifying the Specific Clinical Actions of Amitriptyline: Interrelationships of Behavior, Affect, and Plasma Levels in Depression," *Psychol Med*, 1991, 21(3):599-611.

Knudsen K, Ricksten SE, and Heath A, "Clonidine Interaction in Amitriptyline Poisoning," *J Toxicol Clin Toxicol*, 1988, 26(3-4):223-32.

Lukey BJ, Jones DR, Wright JH, et al, "Relationships Among Nortriptyline, 10-OH (E) Nortriptyline and 10-OH (Z) Nortriptyline Steady-State Plasma Levels and Nortriptyline Dosage," *Ther Drug Monit*, 1989, 11(3):221-7.

Preskorm SH, Dorey RC, and Jerkovich GS, "Therapeutic Drug Monitoring of Tricyclic Antidepressants," *Clin Chem*, 1988, 34(5):822-8.

Svensson C, Nyberg G, and Martensson E, "High Performance Liquid Chromatographic Quantitation of Amitriptyline and Nortriptyline in Dialysate From Plasma or Serum Using On-line Solid-Phase Extraction," *J Chromatogr*, 1988, 432:363-9.

Wong SH, "Measurement of Antidepressants by Liquid Chromatography: A Review of Current Methodology," *Clin Chem*, 1988, 34(5):848-55.

Ammonia, Blood

Synonyms NH_3, Blood

Applies To Ammonia, Cerebrospinal Fluid

Patient Preparation Patient should avoid smoking prior to sampling.

Specimen Blood

Volume 7 mL

Minimum Volume 4 mL plasma

Container Green top (sodium or lithium heparin) tube or lavender top (EDTA) tube. One author, however, suggests that heparin will produce false low results.

Collection Tube must be filled completely and kept tightly stoppered at all times. Specimen must be placed on ice immediately and rotated, then centrifuged at 4°C. Plasma should be very promptly separated from the cells. Test must be performed within 20 minutes of the venipuncture, or the plasma frozen immediately. Concentration rapidly increases on standing. Never freeze whole blood.

Storage Instructions Ammonia is stable for several days at -70°C.

Causes for Rejection Improper collection tube, not stoppered, delayed delivery to the laboratory

Special Instructions Avoid hemolysis, which increases plasma ammonia.

Reference Range Variations of reference ranges between laboratories exist for

Ammonia, Blood

Age	µg/dL	SI: µmol/L
Neonates	90–150	64–107
<2 wk	79–129	56–92
Children	29–70	21–50
Adults	15–45	11–32

Note: Values are somewhat higher in capillary blood.

ammonia. See table for approximate ranges. Ammonia level in cerebrospinal fluid is about 33% to 50% of that in arterial blood.

Use Ammonia is elevated in liver disease, urinary tract infection with distention and stasis, Reye's syndrome, inborn errors of metabolism including deficiency of enzymes in the urea cycle, HHH syndrome (hyperornithinemia, hyperammonemia-homocitrullinuria), some normal neonates (usually returning to normal in 48 hours), total parenteral nutrition, ureterosigmoidostomy, and sodium valproate therapy. Ammonia determination is indicated in neonates with neurological deterioration, subjects with lethargy and/or emesis not explained, and in patients with possible encephalopathy.

The diagnostic utility of ammonia measurements is limited. They are mainly of use in the diagnosis of urea cycle deficiencies (any neonate with unexplained nausea, vomiting, or neurological deterioration appearing after first feeding); and they play an important part in the detection of Reye's syndrome.

In Reye's syndrome, threefold increases in AST, ALT, and serum ammonia are required for diagnosis with/or the diagnostic liver biopsy findings. Ammonia levels increase characteristically early; serum ammonia ≥100 µg/dL (SI: ≥59 µmol/L) reflects severe hepatic changes. Prothrombin time is increased in essentially all patients, prototypically three seconds longer than the control. Bilirubin is usually normal. Glucose should be monitored; hypoglycemia may develop. Hyperosmolality and acid-base imbalance may develop, lactate may increase, CK may increase and CK-MB may be elevated. Uric acid may increase. Increased ammonia and prolonged prothrombin time provide indicators of disease progression.

Limitations The correlation between blood ammonia levels and hepatic coma is poor. Ammonia determinations are not reliable predictors of impending hepatic coma. Ammonia levels are not always high in all patients with urea cycle disorders. High protein diet may cause increased levels. Ammonia levels may also be elevated with gastrointestinal hemorrhage. If portal hypertension develops with cirrhosis, hepatic blood flow is altered, leading to elevated blood ammonia levels. Drugs that can cause a decrease in blood ammonia include oral kanamycin, lactulose, oral neomycin, and oral potassium salts.

Methodology Laboratory contamination by NH_4OH, tobacco smoke, urine, formaldehyde must be avoided. Ion-selective electrode (ISE) methods are preferred; Ektachem® dry film method is also recommended. A number of methods for ammonia are found in standard texts. Many are in use. Some are obsolete. A recommendation to soak glassware in hypochlorite, 52.5 g/L and to then rinse it thoroughly with deionized water is provided to Paramax™ users.

Additional Information Ammonia and alpha-ketoglutarate with NADH yield glutamate; glutamate and ammonia yield glutamine. Cerebrospinal fluid glutamine levels are useful in hepatic encephalopathy and with Reye's syndrome. In the HHH syndrome hyperammonemia is intermittent; it presents in infancy often, but symptoms can be delayed.

Specific References

Cascino GD, Jensen JM, Nelson LA, et al, "Periodic Hyperammonemic Encephalopathy Associated With a Ureterosigmoidostomy," *Mayo Clin Proc*, 1989, 64(6):653-6.

Diamond DA, Blight A, Samuell CT, et al, "Ammonia Levels in Paediatric Ureterosigmoidostomy Patients: A Screen for Hyperammonaemia?" *Br J Urol*, 1991, 67(5):541-4.

Fine P, Adler K, and Gerstenfeld D, "Idiopathic Hyperammonemia After High-Dose Chemotherapy," *Am J Med*, 1989, 86(5):629, (letter).

Fishman RA, *Cerebrospinal Fluid in Diseases of the Nervous System*, 2nd ed, Philadelphia, PA: WB Saunders Co, 1992, 238-9.

Gambino R, "When and How Should Ammonia Be Measured?" *Lab Report for Physicians,*™ 1988, 10:78-80.

Giacoia GP and Padilla-Lugo A, "Severe Transient Neonatal Hyperammonemia," *Am J Perinatol*, 1986, 3(3):249-54.

Green A, "When and How Should We Measure Plasma Ammonia?" *Ann Clin Biochem*, 1988, 25(Pt 3):199-204.

Hurwitz ES, "Reye's Syndrome," *Epidemiol Rev*, 1989, 11:249-53.

Ammonia, Cerebrospinal Fluid *see* Ammonia, Blood *on previous page*

Amobarbital *see* Barbiturates, Quantitative, Blood *on page 1201*

Amobarbital, Urine *see* Barbiturates, Qualitative, Urine *on page 1200*

Amoxapine, Blood

Synonyms Asendin®

Test Includes 8-OH-amoxapine

Abstract Amoxapine is a tricyclic antidepressant.

Specimen Blood

Volume 5 mL

Minimum Volume 3 mL serum or plasma

Container Red top tube or green top (heparin) tube

Sampling Time Trough level at steady-state. Time to steady-state is 35-50 hours.

Reference Range Amoxapine: 20-100 ng/mL (SI: 64-319 nmol/L); 8-OH-amoxapine: 150-400 ng/mL (SI: 478-1275 nmol/L); both: 200-500 ng/mL (SI: 637-1594 nmol/L)

Critical Values Both: >500 ng/mL (SI: >1594 nmol/L)

Use Therapeutic monitoring; toxicity assessment

Methodology High performance liquid chromatography (HPLC), gas chromatography (GC)

Additional Information Amoxapine is a tricyclic antidepressant that is chemically distinct from amitriptyline and imipramine. The drug is a demethylated derivative of loxapine, a neuroleptic used to treat schizophrenia. Half-life is 8 hours. Time to peak in blood after dose is 1-2 hours. Amoxapine is metabolized by the liver to 7-hydroxy and 8-hydroxy metabolites. The 8-hydroxy derivative is an active antidepressant with a half-life of 30 hours. The 7-hydroxy derivative has neuroleptic potency. Both acute and chronic toxicities of amoxapine are different from other tricyclics; its cardiotoxicity is very low.

Specific References

Anton RF Jr and Burch EA Jr, "Amoxapine Versus Amitriptyline Combined With Perphenazine in the Treatment of Psychotic Depression," *Am J Psychiatry*, 1990, 147(9):1203-8.

Coccaro EF and Siever LJ, "Second Generation Antidepressants: A Comparative Review," *J Clin Pharmacol*, 1985, 25(4):241-60.

Osiewicz RJ and Middleburg R, "Detection of a Novel Compound After Overdoses of Aspirin and Amoxapine," *J Anal Toxicol*, 1989, 13(2):97-9.

Amphetamines, Qualitative, Urine

Related Information

Methamphetamines, Urine *on page 1294*

Synonyms Bennies; Crystal; Dexies; Ice; Speed; Uppers

Test Includes Amphetamine, methamphetamine

Abstract Amphetamine and methamphetamine are major drugs of abuse. They have limited medical use and are DEA schedule II drugs.

Specimen Random urine

Volume 50-60 mL

Minimum Volume 5 mL

Container Plastic urine container

Collection If forensic, observe precautions.

Storage Instructions Refrigerate

Causes for Rejection If forensic, failure to meet temperature requirements and/or tests for unusual urine dilution (specific gravity or creatinine) or alteration

Special Instructions If forensic, use chain-of-custody form.

Reference Range Negative (less than cutoff)

Critical Values Cutoff: screen: 1000 ng/mL; confirmation: 500 ng/mL

Use Drug abuse evaluation; toxicity assessment

Limitations Some over-the-counter cold and antiallergy medications may cross react in certain immunoassay screens; confirmation by a different, more sensitive method (eg, GC/MS) is necessary. Clobenzorex hydrochlorate (an anoretic) can give a positive urine result for amphetamine by immunoassay and GC/MS. A labetalol metabolite (3-amino-1-phenylbutane or APB) may cause a false-positive result with amphetamine/methamphetamine by thin layer chromatography or immunoassay.

Methodology Screen: fluorescence polarization immunoassay (FPIA), radioimmunoassay (RIA), enzyme immunoassay (EIA), gas chromatography (GC), thin-layer chromatography (TLC), high performance liquid chromatography (HPLC); confirmation: gas chromatography/mass spectrometry (GC/MS)

Additional Information For the amphetamine class, the material detected is the parent drug. Amphetamines are stimulants that tend to increase alertness and physical activity. Methamphetamine is more frequently the abused drug because its more pronounced central effects are preferred. Some drivers use amphetamines to counteract the drowsiness or "down" feeling caused by sleeping pills or alcohol. In pure form, they are yellowish crystals that are manufactured into tablets or capsules. Abusers also sniff the crystals, make a solution and inject it, or smoke the form known as "ice." Can be detected in urine 3 hours after use. Half-life is 10-20 hours. Usually detectable 24-48 hours after use.

Amphetamines increase the heart and breathing rate and blood pressure, dilate pupils, and decrease appetite. The user can experience a dry mouth, sweating, headache, blurred vision, dizziness, sleeplessness, and anxiety. Extremely high doses can cause people to flush or become pale; they can cause a rapid or irregular heartbeat, tremors, loss of coordination, and even physical collapse. People who use a large dose over a long period of time may develop an amphetamine psychosis: seeing, hearing, and feeling things that do not exist, having irrational thoughts or beliefs and feeling that people are out to get them. People in this extremely suspicious state frequently exhibit bizarre and sometimes violent behavior. Tolerance to the drug is developed after repeated use. Life-threatening overdoses are rare.

Specific References

Blandford DE and Desjardins PR, "Detection and Identification of Amphetamine and Methamphetamine in Urine by GC/MS," *Clin Chem*, 1994, 40(1):145-7.

Bost RO, "3,4 Methylenedioxymethamphetamine (MDMA) and Other Amphetamine Derivatives," *J Forensic Sci*, 1988, 33(2):576-87.

Ellenhorn MJ and Barceloux DG, "Amphetamines," *Medical Toxicology*, New York, NY: Elsevier, 1988, 625-42.

Gan BK, Baugh D, Liu RH, et al, "Simultaneous Analysis of Amphetamine, Methamphetamine, and 3,4-Methylenedioxymethamphetamine (MDMA) in Urine Samples by Solid-Phase Extraction, Derivatization, and Gas Chromatography/Mass Spectrometry," *J Forensic Sci*, 1991, 36(5):1331-41.

Gibert RB, Peng PI, and Wong D, "A Labetalol Metabolite With Analytical Characteristics Resembling Amphetamines," *J Anal Toxicol*, 1995, 19:84-6.

Gillogley KM, Evans AT, Hansen RL, et al, "The Perinatal Impact of Cocaine, Amphetamine, and Opiate Use Detected by Universal Intrapartum Screening," *Am J Obstet Gynecol*, 1990, 163(5 Pt 1):1535-42.

Grinstead GF, "Ranitidine and High Concentrations of Phenylpropanolamine Cross React in the EMIT Monoclonal Amphetamine/Methamphetamine Assay," *Clin Chem*, 1989, 35(9):1998-9.

Hurst PM, "Amphetamines and Driving," *Alcohol, Drugs, and Driving*, 1987, 3:9-11.

Martz W and Schutz HW, "Synthetic Sweetener Cyclamate as a Potential Source of False-Positive Amphetamine Results in the TDx System," *Clin Chem*, 1991, 37(11):2016-7.

Poklis A and Moore KA, "Stereoselectivity of the TDxADx/FLx Amphetamine/Methamphetamine II Amphetamine/Methamphetamine Immunoassay-Response of Urine Specimens Following Nasal Inhaler Use," *J Toxicol Clin Toxicol*, 1995, 33(1):35-41.

Tarver JA, "Amphetamine-Positive Drug Screens From Use of Clobenzorex Hydrochloride," *J Anal Toxicol*, 1994, 18(3):183.

Amylase, Serum

Synonyms 1,4-α-D Glucanohydrolase, Serum

Abstract Amylase is a group of enzymes (hydrolases) from the exocrine pancreas.

Specimen Blood

Volume 1 mL

Minimum Volume 0.5 mL serum

Container Red top tube

Collection Anticoagulants other than heparin diminish amylase activity

Storage Instructions Amylase is stable for 1 week at 25°C and 2 months at 4°C.

Special Instructions Dilution of lipemic sera may cause amylase values to increase.

Reference Range 23-85 units/L. Method dependent. Newborns' serum shows little amylase activity. Much of this activity is apparently of salivary origin. Children up to 2 years of age have virtually no pancreatic isoamylase. Markedly low values may not rise to adult values until the end of the second year of life.

Possible Panic Range Over three times the upper limit of normal for a given method probably indicates a significant increase.

Use Work up abdominal pain, epigastric tenderness, nausea, and vomiting. Such findings characterize acute pancreatitis as well as acute surgical emergencies such as gastrointestinal perforation (eg, peptic ulcer with perforation) or bowel infarct. Amylase is used in the differential diagnosis of acute or chronic pancreatitis, which may or may not in an individual be related to alcoholism. Hypercalcemia related to pancreatitis is described with hyperparathyroidism and other entities. About 80% of subjects with acute pancreatitis have increased serum amylase within 24 hours.

Limitations Poor specificity. Oxalate or citrate depress results. Chloride salts and fluoride salts can interfere with the assay resulting in a false elevation. Lipemic sera (hypertriglyceridemia) may contain inhibitors which falsely depress results. About 20% of patients with acute pancreatitis have abnormal lipids. Normal serum amylase may occur in pancreatitis, especially relapsing and chronic pancreatitis. (Subjects in whom pseudocysts complicate chronic pancreatitis often do have elevations of the pancreatic enzymes.) The entire pancreas can be destroyed in pancreatitis; in such cases serum amylase will derive from other structures (eg, the salivary glands). Urinary amylase increases often persist longer than do those of serum. High levels in alcoholics, in pregnancy, and in diabetic ketoacidosis are of salivary rather than pancreatic origin. Salivary type amylase makes up about 60% of the enzyme, while it is the pancreatic fraction that is of clinical interest. The

(Continued)

Amylase, Serum *(Continued)*

expression "salivary amylase" includes other nonpancreatic sources of the enzyme. Serum amylase is cleared by renal excretion. Serum amylase may increase one to two times upper limit of normal in renal failure without diagnostic significance. In such cases, urine amylase is normal or low.

Methodology Amyloclastic, saccharogenic, chromolytic; up to 200 methods exist

Additional Information Causes of **high serum amylase** include acute pancreatitis, pancreatic pseudocyst, pancreatic ascites, pancreatic abscess, neoplasm in or adjacent to pancreas, trauma to pancreas, and common duct stones.

Nonpancreatic causes of hyperamylasemia include inflammatory salivary lesions (eg, mumps), perforated peptic ulcer involving pancreas or not, intestinal obstruction and infarction, afferent loop syndrome, biliary tract disease including stones, aortic aneurysm, peritonitis, acute appendicitis, cerebral trauma, burns and traumatic shock, the postoperative state (with and without pancreatitis), diabetic ketoacidosis, and extrapancreatic carcinomas (especially of esophagus, lung, ovary). Amylase levels more than 25-fold the upper limit of normal are often found when metastatic tumors produce ectopic amylase. Such levels are higher than those usually found in cases of pancreatitis. In renal insufficiency amylase is usually not more than three times the upper limit of normal. Moderate increases may be reported in normal pregnancy. Increases may be found with tubo-ovarian abscess, ruptured ectopic pregnancy, macroamylasemia, and with a substantial number of drugs, including morphine. Relationships between pancreatitis and hyperlipidemias types I, IV, and V are described. Amylasemia may be associated with hyperparathyroidism.

Macroamylase is a high molecular weight material, normal amylase complexed to high molecular weight protein such as immunoglobulin. It is characterized by high serum amylase and low to normal urine amylase. Macroamylase occurs in normal as well as abnormal subjects.

Other tests: In **pancreatitis**, varying percentages of patients have the following other abnormalities in varying combinations: elevation of triglyceride, alkaline phosphatase, AST (SGOT), total bilirubin, white blood cell count, left shift. Calcium levels should be followed in fulminant pancreatitis, since extremely low serum calcium levels can evolve. **Serum lipase and 2-hour urine amylase** may both be extremely valuable. Although determination of serum methemalbumin has been advocated as a test for acute hemorrhagic pancreatitis, it is cumbersome and is not done in many American laboratories.

Isoenzymes of amylase exist: pancreatic and salivary type, as noted under Limitations. They can be separated by polyacrylamide gel or agarose film electrophoresis, isoelectric focusing, ion exchange chromatography, and plant isoamylase inhibitors. A monoclonal antibody approach is described. Amylase isoenzymes are separated in few laboratories. Where available the procedure is an expensive one. It is useful in assessing the decrease of pancreatic function in cystic fibrosis, in children older than 5 years of age, who may be candidates for enzyme replacement.

Specific References

Aderka D, Tene M, Graff E, et al, "Amylase-Creatinine Clearance Ratio: A Simple Test to Predict Gentamicin Nephrotoxicity," *Arch Intern Med*, 1988, 148(5):1093-6.

Agarwal N, Pitchumoni CS, and Sivaprasad AV, "Evaluating Tests for Acute Pancreatitis," *Am J Gastroenterol*, 1990, 85(4):356-66.

Barnett JL and Wilson JA, "Alcoholic Pancreatitis and Parotitis: Utility of Lipase and Urinary Amylase Clearance Determinations," *South Med J*, 1986, 79(7):832-5.

Borgström A and Bohe M, "Severe Acute Pancreatitis and Normal Serum Amylase Activity Due to Pancreatic Isoamylase Deficiency," *Dig Dis Sci*, 1989, 34(4):644-6.

Clavien PA, Burgan S, and Moossa AR, "Serum Enzymes and Other Laboratory Tests in Acute Pancreatitis," *Br J Surg*, 1989, 76(12):1234-43.

Dougherty SH, Saltzstein EC, Peacock JB, et al, "Rapid Resolution of High Level Hyperamylasemia as a Guide to Clinical Diagnosis and Timing of Surgical Treatment in Patients With Gallstones," *Surg Gynecol Obstet*, 1988, 166(6):491-6.

Dubick MA, Conteas CN, Billy HT, et al, "Raised Serum Concentrations of Pancreatic Enzymes in Cigarette Smokers," *Gut*, 1987, 28(3):330-5.

Eckfeldt JH and Kershaw MJ, "Hyperamylasemia Following Methyl Alcohol Intoxication: Source and Significance," *Arch Intern Med*, 1986, 146(1):193-4.

Feintuch TA, "Amylase: Review of Methods," *ASCP Check Sample®*, Chicago, IL: American Society of Clinical Pathologists, 1986, 2:1-12.

Gumaste VV, Dave PB, Weissman D, et al, "Lipase/Amylase Ratio. A New Index That Distinguishes Acute Episodes of Alcoholic From Nonalcoholic Acute Pancreatitis," *Gastroenterology*, 1991, 101(5):1361-6.

Hayakawa T, Kameya A, Mizuno R, et al, "Hyperamylasemia With Papillary Serous Cystadenocarcinoma of the Ovary," *Cancer*, 1984, 54(8):1662-5.

Humphries LL, Adams LJ, Eckfeldt JH, et al, "Hyperamylasemia in Patients With Eating Disorders," *Ann Intern Med*, 1987, 106(1):50-2.

Kleinman DS and O'Brien JF, "Macroamylase," *Mayo Clin Proc*, 1986, 61(8):669-70.

Lang E, Afilalo M, Dankoff J, et al, "The Prognostic Significance of Moderate Hyperamylasemia in the Evaluation of the Emergency Department Patient," *J Emerg Med*, 1995, 13:107-12.

Lott JA and Lu CJ, "Lipase Isoforms and Amylase Isoenzymes: Assays and Application in the Diagnosis of Acute Pancreatitis," *Clin Chem*, 1991, 37(3):361-8.

Moss DW, Henderson AR, and Kachmar JF, "Enzymes," Tietz NW, ed, *Fundamentals of Clinical Chemistry*, 3rd ed, Philadelphia, PA: WB Saunders Co, 1987, 346.
Rattner DW, Gu Z-Y, Vlahakes GJ, et al, "Hyperamylasemia After Cardiac Surgery – Incidence, Significance, and Management," *Ann Surg*, 1989, 209(3):279-83.
Ruzena S, "Normal Serum Amylase in Acute Pancreatitis," *Dig Dis Sci*, 1989, 34(6):960-1, (letter).
Spechler ST, "How Much Can We Know About Acute Pancreatitis?" *Ann Intern Med*, 1985, 102(5):704-5.
Steinberg WM, Goldstein SS, Davis ND, et al, "Diagnostic Assays in Acute Pancreatitis: A Study of Sensitivity and Specificity," *Ann Intern Med*, 1985, 102(5):576-80.
Tietz NW and Shuey DF, "Determination of P-Type Amylase in Serum Using a Selective Inhibitor," *Lab Med*, 1986, 17:739-41.
Wilson C and Imrie CW, "Amylase and Gut Infarction," *Br J Surg*, 1986, 73(3):219-21.

Amytal® *see* Barbiturates, Quantitative, Blood *on page 1201*

Anacin-3® *see* Acetaminophen, Serum *on page 1180*

Anaerobic Culture, Blood *see* Blood Culture, Aerobic and Anaerobic *on page 1204*

Angel Dust *see* Phencyclidine, Qualitative, Urine *on page 1319*

Angel Dust *see* Phencyclidine, Quantitative, Serum *on page 1319*

Anion Gap, Blood

Synonyms Electrolyte Gap; Gap; Ion Gap

Applies To Urinary Anion Gap

Test Includes A calculation from electrolytes, sodium, potassium, HCO_3^-, and chloride to ascertain quantities of unmeasured cations and anions

Abstract The anion gap is useful in evaluation of patients with acid-base abnormalities. The sum of anions and cations must be equal in the blood.

Specimen Blood

Container Red top tube

Reference Range 6-16 mmol/L (SI: 6-16 mmol/L); slight differences may be established in different laboratories. Electrolytes until recently were done mostly by flame photometry. As ion-selective electrodes have come into wider use, reference ranges for anion gap will probably change.

Use Extensively used for quality control in the laboratory, the widest clinical application of the anion gap is in the diagnosis of types of metabolic acidosis. Unmeasured cations include calcium and magnesium. Unmeasured anions include protein, PO_4^{3-}, SO_4^{2-}, and organic acids. Organic acidosis includes lactic acidosis and ketoacidosis.

A marked elevation of anion gap, >30 mmol/L, bears a strong implication of metabolic acidosis. Increased anion gaps are found in states such as renal failure and toxic ingestions. Above 30 mmol/L gap increase is commonly secondary to lactic acidosis or ketoacidosis but can be caused also by rhabdomyolysis or nonketotic hyperglycemic coma.

In diabetic ketoacidosis plasma glucose is high, often much >300 mg/dL (SI: >16.7 mmol/L), pH is <7.3, and ketones are found in blood and urine. Increased serum osmolality and increased calculated osmolality (osmolar gap) are found, and serum sodium is often decreased.

In alcoholic ketoacidosis glucose may be increased, normal or low, but a high alcohol level may be found, and amylase and uric acid may be increased.

Limitations Minor differences in formula are used by different laboratories. A spurious increase may follow excessive exposure of the sample to room air as well as underfilling the Vacutainer® tube. Some gaps remain unexplained. All metabolic abnormalities are not detected by abnormal gaps (eg, isopropanol ingestion is accompanied by normal gap, but ketone bodies are positive). There are a number of causes of normal anion gap acidosis associated with hyperchloremia. Anion gap is unsuitable as a quick screen for lactic acidosis. Still useful, the anion gap should not replace assay for lactate, creatinine, ketone bodies, or osmolality. In one study, only 66% of patients with an anion gap of 20-29 mmol/L could be proven to have an organic acidosis.

Methodology Calculation: $(Na^+ + K^+) - (Cl^- + HCO_3^-)$ or $Na^+ - (Cl^- + HCO_3^-)$ = anion gap; actually determined by the difference between concentrations of anions and cations.

Additional Information Anion gap represents approximately the sum of the unmeasured anions charges of which with chloride and HCO_3^-, balance sodium. (Measured anions are chloride and bicarbonate. Measured cations are sodium.)

Anion gap high ("unmeasured anions"): With **pH high:** extracellular volume contraction; massive transfusion (with renal failure and/or volume contraction); carbenicillin, penicillin (large doses), salts of organic acids such as citrate. With **pH low:** uremia: most common cause; abnormal anion gap in uremia is usually seen only when creatinine is >4.0 mg/dL (SI: >354 µmol/L). Uremic acidosis is rare without hyperphosphatemia. Nonketotic hyperglycemic coma and rhabdomyolysis

(Continued)

Anion Gap, Blood *(Continued)*

may cause high anion gap metabolic acidosis. Lactic acidosis and diabetic or alcoholic ketoacidosis characteristically fall into this group. With **normal osmolal gap**: salicylate and paraldehyde toxicity; with **increased osmolal gap**: methanol and ethylene glycol toxicity.

High anion gap metabolic acidosis without elevated lactic acid or acetone; consider: ketoacidosis with negative or slightly positive "acetone" if patient is hypoxic and/or has alcoholic ketoacidosis, such ketoacidosis may be life-threatening; salicylate toxicity; methanol toxicity (paint thinners); ethylene glycol toxicity (antifreeze) – urinary sediment contains abundant calcium oxalate and/or hippurate crystals; paraldehyde intoxication (may have positive ketone reactions); toluene toxicity (transmission fluid, paint thinner inhalation or sniffing).

Anion gap low: Caused by retained unmeasured anions. Most common cause is hypoalbuminemia (eg, in nephrosis, cirrhosis), dilution, hypernatremia, very marked hypercalcemia, very severe hypermagnesemia, IgG myeloma and polyclonal gamma globulin increases – hyperviscosity with certain lab instruments, lithium toxicity, bromism (low anion gap may not be present). Decreased anion gap with spurious hyperchloremia and with hyponatremia is reported in hyperlipidemia. Dilution of extracellular fluid may cause a decreased gap. The finding of a low anion gap is perceived as an unreliable diagnostic parameter and may indicate potential laboratory error.

Normal anion gap may occur with **metabolic acidosis,** causes have been published. They include diarrhea, renal tubular acidosis, hyperalimentation, ureteroileostomy, ureterosigmoidostomy, external drainage of pancreaticobiliary fluids, NH_4Cl and other drugs.

The urinary anion gap is used in the diagnosis of hyperchloremic metabolic acidosis and evaluation of renal potassium wasting.

Specific References

Adams SL, "Alcoholic Ketoacidosis," *Emerg Med Clin North Am*, 1990, 8(4):749-60.

Baker RJ, "Biochemical Gaps: Osmolal and Anion," *Curr Surg*, 1987, 44(5):378-81.

Cembrowski GS, Westgard JO, and Kurtycz DF, "Use of the Anion Gap for the Quality Control of Electrolyte Analyzers," *Am J Clin Pathol*, 1983, 79(6):688-96.

Hertford JA, McKenna JP, and Chamovitz BN, "Metabolic Acidosis With an Elevated Anion Gap," *Am Fam Physician*, 1989, 39(4):159-68.

Rothenberg DM, Berns AS, Barkin R, et al, "Bromide Intoxication Secondary to Pyridostigmine Bromide Therapy," *JAMA*, 1990, 263(8):1121-2.

"Urinary Anion Gap in Hyperchloremic Metabolic Acidosis," *N Engl J Med*, 1988, 319(9):585-6.

Wrenn K, "The Delta (Delta) Gap: An Approach to Mixed Acid-Base Disorders," *Ann Emerg Med*, 1990, 19(11):1310-3.

Wrenn KD, Slovis CM, Minion GE, et al, "The Syndrome of Alcoholic Ketoacidosis," *Am J Med*, 1991, 91(2):119-28.

Antibiotic Level, Serum

Synonyms Antimicrobial Assay

Abstract Assays for antimicrobial agents in serum are performed for two primary reasons: 1. to ensure therapeutic levels, and 2. to monitor for potentially toxic levels. In most situations, it is not necessary to monitor antimicrobial levels because serum levels are relatively predictable based on dosing; *in vitro* susceptibility testing uses those predictable levels to determine clinical efficacy. Similarly, toxicity is not always related to serum levels. It may be more appropriate to monitor for toxicity by following determinants of hematologic, renal, or hepatic function. In certain situations however (eg, aminoglycoside antibiotics which have a narrow therapeutic range and a high potential for toxicity), it is essential to follow serum levels.

Specimen Serum

Container Red top tube or serum separator tube

Sampling Time Peak: 30 minutes after 30 minute I.V. infusion; 1 hour after I.M. dose. Trough: immediately prior to next dose.

Collection Keep frozen if not assayed immediately.

Causes for Rejection Incomplete clinical information (eg, specific antimicrobial, dosage and schedule, other concurrent antimicrobials)

Reference Range Therapeutic range depends on agent being tested for, and minimal inhibitory concentration of drug against organism. Selected ranges in μg/mL are presented as a guide only.

Use Evaluate adequacy of serum antibiotic level; detect toxic levels

Limitations May not be technically possible in a patient taking more than one antibiotic

Methodology Bioassay: cephalosporins, clindamycin, erythromycin, metronidazole, penicillins, polymyxin, tetracycline, trimethoprim. High performance liquid chromatography: chloramphenicol, flucytosine, mezlocillin. Fluorescence polarization immunoassay (FPIA): amikacin, gentamicin, tobramycin, kanamycin, streptomycin, vancomycin, neomycin, netilmicin.

Additional Information With the increasing availability of *in vitro* sensitivity testing expressed as the minimal inhibitory or bactericidal concentration of an antibi-

Antibiotic Level, Serum

Drug	Peak		Trough	
	μg/mL	SI: μmol/L	μg/mL	SI: μmol/L
Amikacin	15–25	26–43	<10	<17
Chloramphenicol	25	77		
Flucytosine	100	775		
Gentamicin	4–10	8–21	<2	<4
Netilmicin	4–8	8.0–17.0	1–2	0.7–1.4
Streptomycin	5–20	9–34	<5	<9
Tobramycin	4–10	8–21	<2	<4
Trimethoprim	≥5	17		
Sulfamethoxazole	≥100	395		
Vancomycin	20–40	13.6–27.2	5–10	3.4–6.8

Selected ranges in μg/mL are presented as a guide only.

otic, measurement of serum levels of these drugs has taken on practical clinical importance. This is especially true for agents with narrow therapeutic ranges and significant toxicity. It should be remembered, however, that in most patients, cure of infection depends on numerous host factors as well as on antibiotics. Therefore, antibiotic levels should not be relied on as the sole guide to therapy.

Specific References

Donowitz GR and Mandell GL, "Drug Therapy. Beta-Lactam Antibiotics," *N Engl J Med*, 1988, 318(8):490-500.

Rosenblatt JE, "Laboratory Tests Used to Guide Antimicrobial Therapy," *Mayo Clin Proc*, 1991, 66(9):942-8.

Smith AL and Opheim E, "Comparison of Methods for Clinical Quantitation of Antibiotics," *Curr Clin Top Infect Dis*, 1983, 4:333-57.

Anticoagulants, Oral *see* Warfarin, Blood *on page 1379*

Anticonvulsant Drugs, Blood

Synonyms Antiepileptic Drugs

Test Includes Carbamazepine, ethosuximide, phenobarbital, phenytoin, primidone, valproic acid

Specimen Blood

Volume 7 mL

Minimum Volume 1 mL serum

Container Red top tube

Special Instructions Individual tests can be ordered separately.

Reference Range Carbamazepine: 5-12 mg/L; ethosuximide: 50-100 mg/L; phenobarbital: 10-25 mg/L; phenytoin: 10-20 mg/L; primidone: 6-12 mg/L; valproic acid: 50-100 mg/L

Use Monitor therapeutic drug level; evaluate toxicity

Methodology High performance liquid chromatography (HPLC)

Antidepressants *see* Tricyclic Antidepressants, Blood *on page 1368*

Antiepileptic Drugs *see* Anticonvulsant Drugs, Blood *on this page*

Antifreeze *see* Ethylene Glycol, Blood *on page 1262*

Antifungal Therapy *see page 1496*

Antiglobulin Test, Direct

Synonyms Anti-human Globulin Test, Direct; Anti-human Serum Test, Direct; Broad Spectrum Direct Antiglobulin; Coombs' Test, Direct; DAT; Direct Antiglobulin Test; Direct Coombs'; Polyspecific Direct Antiglobulin

Test Includes Direct antiglobulin testing with polyspecific anti-human globulin serum. It may include use of monospecific reagents (anti-IgG, anticomplement) when indicated. Eluates from coated red cells may be prepared for antibody identification (eg, specimens from cord bloods, recently transfused patients, hemolytic anemia work-up).

Specimen Blood

Volume 5 mL

Minimum Volume 3 mL

Container One lavender top (EDTA) tube and one red top tube

(Continued)

Antiglobulin Test, Direct *(Continued)*

Causes for Rejection Gross hemolysis, sample placed in a serum separator tube, specimen tube not properly labeled

Special Instructions Indicate diagnosis, transfusion history, and pertinent medications on the requisition form.

Reference Range Negative

Use Polyspecific antiglobulin serum detects immunoproteins, IgG, or complement on red cells (ie, detection of sensitization of erythrocytes *in vivo*). Coated red cells are said to be "sensitized." Used to detect autoimmune hemolytic anemias caused by antibody and/or complement components being bound to patient's red cells (including drug-induced), transfusion reaction, and erythroblastosis fetalis (hemolytic disease of the newborn). In warm autoimmune hemolytic anemias, the antibody is usually IgG. In cold hemolytic anemias, the cell coating is usually with complement components.

Limitations False-positives may occur with cold agglutinins. Use of red top tubes or serum separator tubes may cause false-positive reactions particularly if tubes have been refrigerated. Newborn's cells may have negative direct antiglobulin test in ABO hemolytic disease. Wharton's jelly from cord samples can cause problems. Technical factors can cause false-positive and false-negative reactions; lists of technical causes of misleading results are published and include saline stored improperly, cold autoagglutinins, and contaminated glassware. Drugs which can cause a positive antiglobulin test include chlorpromazine, chlorpropamide, ethosuximide, hydralazine, isoniazid, levodopa, mefenamic acid, methyldopa, penicillins, quinidine, and quinine.

Methodology Antiglobulin serum. In the **direct antiglobulin test**, one examines for antibody attached to the patient's red cells *in vivo*. In the **indirect antiglobulin test**, the antigen-antibody reaction occurs *in vitro* and one tests patient's serum for antibody with reagent red cells (the antigen).

Additional Information Drugs, including the penicillins and cephalosporins, α-methyldopa, levodopa, quinidine, insulin, mefenamic acid, sulfonamides, tetracycline, and others may cause positive direct antiglobulin tests. Many positive direct antiglobulin tests are due to methyldopa. Methyldopa antibodies are predominantly IgG; about 1% of patients on methyldopa develop hemolytic anemia, but as many as 15% develop a positive DAT. Although drugs and alloantibodies may cause a positive direct antiglobulin test, the majority have no such association. It is unusual to find a significant antibody in the eluate from a positive direct antiglobulin test. Broad spectrum or polyspecific antisera contain both anti-IgG and anti-C3d. Anti-IgG may be used to determine if the cells are coated with IgG. If indicated, an indirect test and antibody identification are included in the work-up of a positive direct antiglobulin test. In cases of autoimmune hemolytic anemia, an eluate from the patient's red cells can indicate antibody specificity. Elution is also indicated when the DAT on the patient's red cells is positive within 14 days of transfusion and in newborns.

Specific References

Canadian Red Cross Society, *Serological and Immunological Methods of the Canadian Red Cross Blood Transfusion Service*, 8th ed, Toronto: The Canadian Red Cross Society, 1980.

Freedman J, "False-Positive Antiglobulin Tests in Healthy Subjects and in Hospital Patients," *J Clin Pathol*, 1979, 32(10):1014-8.

Garratty G, "The Clinical Significance (and Insignificance) of Red-Cell-Bound IgG and Complement," *Current Applications and Interpretations of the Direct Antiglobulin Test*, Arlington, VA: American Association of Blood Banks, 1988.

Hansten PD, "Drugs in the Production of Direct Coombs' Test Positivity," *Am J Hosp Pharm*, 1971, 28(8):629-32.

Huh YO, Liu FJ, Rogge K, et al, "Positive Direct Antiglobulin Test and High Serum Immunoglobulin G Values," *Am J Clin Pathol*, 1988, 90(2):197-200.

Judd WJ, Barnes BA, Steiner EA, et al, "The Evaluation of a Positive Direct Antiglobulin Test (Autocontrol) in Pretransfusion Testing Revisited," *Transfusion*, 1986, 26(3):220-4.

Snyder EL and Falast GA, "Significance of the Direct Antiglobulin Test," *Lab Med*, 1985, 16:89-96.

Walker RH, ed, *Technical Manual*, 10th ed, Arlington, VA: American Association of Blood Banks, 1990, 147-57.

Anti-human Globulin Test, Direct *see* Antiglobulin Test, Direct *on previous page*

Anti-human Serum Test, Direct *see* Antiglobulin Test, Direct *on previous page*

Antimicrobial Assay *see* Antibiotic Level, Serum *on page 1194*

Antimicrobial Removal Device (ARD) Blood Culture *see* Blood Culture, Aerobic and Anaerobic *on page 1204*

Aprobarbital *see* Barbiturates, Quantitative, Blood *on page 1201*

Aquachloral®, Urine *see* Chloral Hydrate, Qualitative, Urine *on page 1224*

ARD, Blood Culture *see* Blood Culture, Aerobic and Anaerobic *on page 1204*

Arsenic, Blood

Related Information

Heavy Metal Screen, Blood *on page 1271*

Abstract Arsenic is a toxic heavy metal. The largest source of human exposure is arsenic in food resulting from broad use of arsenical pesticides.

Specimen Blood

Volume 30 mL

Minimum Volume 10 mL

Container Trace metal-free container

Causes for Rejection Containers not metal-free

Reference Range <5 μg/dL (SI: <93.5 nmol/g)

Critical Values 10-50 μg/dL (SI: 133.5-667.5 nmol/g) in chronic poisoning; >60 μg/dL (SI: >801 nmol/g) in acute poisoning

Use Blood arsenic is for diagnosis of acute poisoning only

Limitations Short half-life in blood

Methodology Electrothermal atomic absorption spectrometry (AA)

Additional Information Heparinized whole blood and serum have been used for arsenic determination. Blood levels of arsenic have a short half-life and are useful only within a few days of exposure. Urine arsenic concentration is a better measure of arsenic poisoning. In addition to pesticides, rodenticides, weed killers, paint, and wood preservatives contain arsenic. See following listing.

Specific References

Bryson PD, "Arsenic," *Comprehensive Review in Toxicology*, 2nd ed, Rockville, MD: Aspen Publishers, 1989, 501-8.

Campbell JP and Alvarez JA, "Acute Arsenic Intoxication," *Am Fam Physician*, 1989, 40(6):93-7.

Goyer RA, "Toxic Effects of Metals," *Casarett and Doull's Toxicology*, 4th ed, Klassen CD, Amdur MO, and Doull J, eds, New York, NY: Macmillan Publishing, 1991, 623-80.

Arsenic, Gastric Content *see* Arsenic, Urine *on this page*

Arsenic, Hair *see* Arsenic, Hair, Nails *on this page*

Arsenic, Hair, Nails

Synonyms Arsenic, Hair; Arsenic, Nails

Abstract This is a toxic heavy metal that is incorporated into hair and nails. Its presence there in abnormal concentrations is a sign of chronic poisoning.

Specimen Clean hair or nails

Volume 0.5 g

Container Clean envelope or heavy metal-free screw top plastic container

Collection Extreme care is necessary to avoid surface contamination; pubic hair is preferable as are toenails.

Special Instructions Hair should be clean, free of oil and tonic; clip close. Nails should be thoroughly washed, dried, and clipped close to cuticle.

Reference Range Hair: up to 65 μg/100 g (SI: 8.7 nmol/g); nail: 90-180 μg/100 g (SI: 12-24 nmol/g)

Critical Values Values >100 μg/100 g (SI: >13.4 nmol/g) of hair are considered toxic

Use Diagnose chronic arsenic intoxication

Limitations Curly hair may pose problems in dating. Not useful for diagnosing acute toxicity. Urine arsenic concentration is a better indication of recent exposure.

Methodology Electrothermal atomic absorption spectrometry (AA), neutron activation analysis

Additional Information Arsenic accumulates in bones, hair, and nails and is used to detect chronic exposure, since arsenic is laid down in keratin soon after ingestion. Arsenic binds to protein sulfhydryl groups. Variations in arsenic hair levels may be due to geographic location and exposure to industrial waste and drinking water.

Specific References

Bryson PD, *Comprehensive Review in Toxicology*, 2nd ed, Rockville, MD: Aspen Publishers Inc, 1989, 501-8.

Robertson WO, "Arsenic and Other Heavy Metals," *Clinical Management of Poisoning and Drug Overdose*, Haddad LM and Winchester JF, eds, Philadelphia, PA: WB Saunders Co, 1983, 656-64.

Arsenic, Nails *see* Arsenic, Hair, Nails *on this page*

Arsenic, Urine

Related Information

Heavy Metal Screen, Urine *on page 1272*

(Continued)

Arsenic, Urine *(Continued)*

Synonyms As, Quantitative, Urine

Applies To Arsenic, Gastric Content

Abstract This toxic heavy metal appears in urine, and its excretion rate is used to determine toxicity.

Specimen 24-hour urine

Volume Entire collection

Container Acid-washed plastic container, no preservative

Collection Collect a 24-hour urine specimen, on ice, with care to avoid specimen contact with metal. Container must be securely closed and properly labeled.

Storage Instructions Refrigerate

Causes for Rejection Specimen not collected on ice, specimen in contact with metal during collection

Reference Range Ranges for urine arsenic levels can be variable among different laboratories. A general guideline is given: normal: 0-50 μg/L (SI: 0-0.65 μmol/L); chronic industrial exposure: >100 μg/L (SI: >1.3 μmol/L). The 24-hour urinary excretion rate should be <50 μg/24 hours.

Critical Values Toxic: >850 μg/L (SI: >11.3 μmol/L).

Use Evaluate recent exposure to arsenic, arsenic toxicity

Methodology Atomic absorption spectrometry (AA)

Additional Information 25 mL acidified gastric washing is acceptable for arsenic analysis; gastric content normally contains no arsenic. Random urine samples are acceptable.

Specific References

Amdur MO, Doull J, and Klaasen CD, eds, *Casarett and Doull's Toxicology*, 4th ed, New York, NY: Pergammon Press, 1991, 623-80.

Le XC, Cullen WR, and Reimer KJ, "Human Urinary Arsenic Excretion After One Time Ingestion of Seaweed, Crab, and shrimp," *Clin Chem*, 1994, 40(4):617-24.

Nixon DE, Mussmann GV, Eckdahl SJ, et al, "Total Arsenic in Urine: Palladium-Persulfate vs Nickel as a Matrix Modifier for Graphite Furnace Atomic Absorption Spectrophotometry," *Clin Chem*, 1991, 37(9):1575-9.

Arterial Blood Gases *see* Blood Gases, Arterial *on page 1207*

Arterial CO-Oximetry *see* CO-Oximetry Arterial *on page 1241*

Arthropod Identification

Synonyms Ectoparasite Identification; Insect Identification

Applies To Bed Bugs Identification; Body Lice Identification; *Cimex* Identification; Crab Lice Identification; Deer Tick Identification; Flea Identification; Head Lice Identification; *Ixodes dammini* Identification; Lice Identification; Mite Identification; Nits Identification; *Pediculus humanus* Identification; *Phthirus pubis* Identification; Pubic Lice Identification; *Sarcoptes scabiei* Skin Scrapings Identification; Skin Scrapings for *Sarcoptes scabiei* Identification; Tick Identification

Specimen Gross arthropod, skin scrapings

Container Screw cap tube or screw cap jar

Collection Arthropods (gross) are to be submitted in alcohol (70%) or formaldehyde in tube or container with secure closure. To establish the diagnosis of scabies, skin scrapings may be collected with a scalpel and a drop of mineral oil. The liquid may be examined directly or alternatively the organism may be teased away from its burrow or papule with a needle or scalpel.

Storage Instructions Room temperature, fill the container with preservative as completely as possible to avoid damage to the specimen by air bubbles in the container

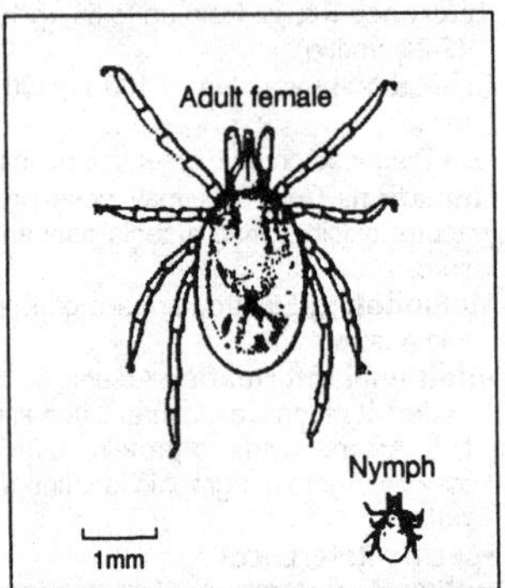

Deer tick (*Ixodes dammini*)

Reference Range No arthropod identified

Use Identify arthropods affecting humans; establish the presence of ectoparasite infestation

Methodology Macroscopic evaluation

Specific References

Hobbs GD and Harrell RE Jr, "Brown Recluse Spider Bites: A Common Cause of Necrotic Arachnidism," *Am J Emerg Med*, 1989, 7(3):309-12.

Nelson JA and Bouseman JK, "Human Tick-Borne Illnesses: United States," *Clin Microbiol Newslett*, 1992, 14(14):105-12.

Pratt HD and Smith JW, "Arthropods of Medical Importance," *Manual of Clinical Microbiology*, 5th ed, Balows A, Hausler WJ Jr, Herrmann KL, et al, eds, Washington, DC: American Society for Microbiology, 1991, 796-810.

ASA, Blood *see* Salicylate, Blood *on page 1347*
Asendin® *see* Amoxapine, Blood *on page 1190*

Aspartate Aminotransferase

Synonyms AST; Glutamic Oxaloacetic Transaminase, Serum; GOT; L-Aspartate; 2-Oxoglutarate Aminotransferase; SGOT
Applies To Aminotransferases
Specimen Blood
Volume 7 mL
Minimum Volume 1 mL serum
Container Red top tube
Storage Instructions Stable 3 days at 25°C and 1 week at 4°C; fairly stable refrigerated or frozen.
Causes for Rejection Hemolysis
Reference Range Levels in infancy are two to three times those found in adults. Ranges decrease during childhood years. Typical adult reference range: 8-45 units/L. AST reference values are higher in males.
Use A wide range of disease entities alters AST (SGOT), with origin from many organs. When an increased AST is from the liver, it is more likely to relate to disease of the hepatocyte. Other enzymes, including alkaline phosphatase and GGT, are more sensitive indicators of biliary obstruction.

Causes of low AST: uremia, vitamin B_6 deficiency (this can be corrected), metronidazole, trifluoperazine.

Causes of high AST: chronic alcohol ingestion, not limited to overt chronic alcoholism; cirrhosis. In alcoholic hepatitis, AST values usually are <300 units/L. In viral hepatitis, look for high AST/LD (LDH) ratio, >3, and very high AST peaking at 500-3000 units/L in acute viral hepatitis (ie, in clinical acute viral hepatitis the transaminases may be increased ten times or more above their upper limits of normal). AST increases are found in other types of liver disease, including earlier stages of hemochromatosis and chemical injury, (eg, necrosis related to toxins such as carbon tetrachloride). Some instances of cholecystitis cause increased AST.

AST and ALT (SGPT) are increased in Reye's syndrome. In infectious mononucleosis, LD (LDH) is commonly considerably higher than AST. Trauma (including head trauma and including surgery) and other striated muscle diseases, including dystrophy, dermatomyositis, trichinosis, polymyositis, and gangrene cause AST increases. Both AST and ALT elevations are found with Duchenne's muscular dystrophy. Look for high CK in myositis, high LD_5 (or isomorphic pattern in some instances of polymyositis) on LD isoenzymes.

In myocardial infarction AST peaks about 24 hours after infarct and returns to normal 3-7 days later. In acute MI without shock or heart failure, ALT is not apt to increase significantly. AST increases in congestive failure with centrilobular liver congestion, in which high LD_5 on LD isoenzymes is found, and in pericarditis, myocarditis, pancreatitis, and other inflammatory states including Legionnaires' disease. In renal infarction LD is usually high, out of proportion to AST. Lung infarction and other disease entities leading to necrosis including large, necrotic tumors cause increased AST; LD is commonly also increased in such instances. Shock (LD also usually increased); hypothyroidism (LD and/or CK not infrequently increased in myxedema); hemolytic anemias (LD high with increased LD_1) and certain CNS diseases may increase AST.

Very high AST levels usually are caused by liver disease and/or by shock.

Drugs: A large number of commonly used drugs have been reported to elevate AST: isoniazid, phenothiazines, erythromycin, progesterone, anabolic-androgenic steroids, halothane, methyldopa, opiates, indomethacin, salicylates in children, and other drugs. Hepatotoxicity from drugs may cause high aminotransferase activity with elevation of AST/ALT ratio.

Acetaminophen hepatotoxicity deserves special mention. In alcoholics, apparently moderate doses of the analgesic have caused severe hepatotoxicity. Doses of 2.6-16.5 g/24 hours are reported with total bilirubin 1.3-23.9 mg/dL (SI: 22-409 μmol/L), AST 1960-29,700 units/L, and ALT 12,000-12,550 units/L. The characteristic pattern included mild to severe coagulopathy and AST greater than ALT by a considerable margin.

Macroenzyme causing unexplained increase of AST is described with normal levels of CK and ALT.
Limitations Only gross hemolysis may cause falsely high values.
Methodology Spectrophotometry, kinetic assay, malate dehydrogenase; like ALT, AST can be measured at 25°C, 30°C, 32°C, and 37°C.

(Continued)

Aspartate Aminotransferase *(Continued)*

Additional Information AST has origin from heart, liver, skeletal muscle, kidney, pancreas, spleen, and lung. Very high values, >500 units/L, usually suggest hepatitis or other kinds of hepatocellular necrosis but can also be found with large necrotic tumors, other types of necrosis or extensive hypoxia, congestive failure, and shock. Unexplained AST elevations should first be investigated with ALT and GGT. Mitochondrial AST (m-AST) may be useful in the diagnosis of alcoholic liver disease.

Specific References

Faulkner WR, "Best First Tests for Reye Syndrome," *Lab Report for Physicians*, 1987, 9:76-8.

Rosenthal P and Haight M, "Aminotransferase as a Prognostic Index in Infants With Liver Disease," *Clin Chem*, 1990, 36(2):346-8.

Rotenberg Z, Weinberger I, Davidson E, et al, "Does Determination of Serum Aspartate Aminotransferase Contribute to the Diagnosis of Acute Myocardial Infarction?" *Am J Clin Pathol*, 1989, 91(1):91-4.

Schölmerich J, Gross V, Johannesson T, et al, "Detection of Biliary Origin of Acute Pancreatitis. Comparison of Laboratory Tests, Ultrasound, Computed Tomography, and ERCP," *Dig Dis Sci*, 1989, 34(6):830-3.

Vincent-Viry M and Delwaide P, "Aspartate Aminotransferase and Alanine Aminotransferase," *Drug Effects on Laboratory Test Results Analytical Interferences and Pharmacological Effects*, Siest G and Galteau MM, eds, Littleton, MA: PSG Publishing Co Inc, 1988, 91-130.

Williams AL and Hoofnagle JH, "Ratio of Serum Aspartate to Alanine Aminotransferase in Chronic Hepatitis. Relationship to Cirrhosis," *Gastroenterology*, 1988, 95(3):734-9.

Aspirin, Blood *see* Salicylate, Blood *on page 1347*

As, Quantitative, Urine *see* Arsenic, Urine *on page 1197*

AST *see* Aspartate Aminotransferase *on previous page*

Athrombin-K® *see* Warfarin, Blood *on page 1379*

Ativan® *see* Lorazepam, Blood *on page 1288*

Aurothioglucose *see* Gold Level *on page 1270*

Aventyl® *see* Nortriptyline, Blood *on page 1309*

Azidothymidine *see* Zidovudine, Blood *on page 1381*

AZT *see* Zidovudine, Blood *on page 1381*

Bactec® *see* Blood Culture, Aerobic and Anaerobic *on page 1204*

Barbiturates, Qualitative, Urine

Applies To Amobarbital, Urine; Butalbital, Urine; Mephobarbital, Urine; Pentobarbital, Urine; Secobarbital, Urine

Test Includes Identification and confirmation of barbiturates in urine

Abstract This test is usually used to detect barbiturate as a drug of abuse.

Specimen Random urine

Volume 20 mL

Minimum Volume 10 mL

Container Plastic urine container

Collection If forensic, observe precautions

Storage Instructions Refrigerate

Causes for Rejection If forensic, failure to meet temperature requirements or test for unusual urine dilution

Special Instructions Chain-of-custody documentation required for samples submitted for pre-employment, random employee testing, and forensic purposes.

Reference Range Less than cutoff

Critical Values Cutoff: screen: 300 ng/mL, confirmation: 300 ng/mL

Use Urine drugs of abuse testing, pre-employment screens, random drug testing

Limitations Short- and intermediate-acting barbiturates can be detected in urine 24-72 hours following ingestion, longer-acting drugs up to 7 days.

Methodology Enzyme immunoassay (EIA), gas chromatography/mass spectrometry (GC/MS)

Additional Information Barbiturates are nonselective CNS depressants that may be used as sedative-hypnotics or anticonvulsants. They are capable of producing all levels of CNS mood effects from sedation to hypnosis to deep coma and anesthesia. Sensory cortex functions, cerebellar functions, and motor activity are decreased. Secobarbital and pentobarbital are short-term hypnotics and lose effectiveness after about 2 weeks of continued usage. Withdrawal symptoms from any barbiturate may be severe and may include convulsions and delirium. The presence of barbiturates in urine is presumptively positive at a level >300 ng/mL using secobarbital as a standard and can indicate prescribed or abused intake of this class of drugs. The presence of these drugs should be confirmed.

Specific References

Pesce AJ, "Barbiturates," *Clinical Chemistry – Theory, Analysis, and Correlation*, 2nd ed, Kaplan LA and Pesce AJ, eds, St Louis, MO: Mosby-Year Book Inc, 1989, 1081-7.

Maurer HH, "Identification and Differentiation of Barbiturates and Their Metabolites in Urine," *J Chromatogr*, 1990, 530:307-26.

Barbiturates, Quantitative, Blood

Related Information

Butabarbital, Quantitative *on page 1213*
Mephobarbital, Blood *on page 1291*
Metharbital, Quantitative *on page 1296*
Pentobarbital, Blood *on page 1317*

Applies To Alurate®; Amobarbital; Amytal®; Aprobarbital; Blue Angels; Butalbital; Butisol Sodium®; Fiorinal®; Lotusate®; Luminal®; Nembutal®; Red Devils; Talbutal; Yellow Jackets

Test Includes Quantitation of barbiturates present in blood

Abstract Measurement of barbiturates as a class is usually used for drug-of-abuse testing or as evidence for toxicity.

Specimen Blood

Volume 7 mL

Minimum Volume 5 mL plasma or serum

Container Lavender top (EDTA) tube, green top (heparin) tube, red top tube; avoid serum separator tube for pentobarbital.

Reference Range Negative. Therapeutic: short-acting (secobarbital): 1-5 μg/mL (SI: 4.2-21.0 μmol/L); intermediate-acting (amobarbital): 5-15 μg/mL (SI: 22-66 μmol/L); long-acting (phenobarbital): 15-40 μg/mL (SI: 65-172 μmol/L); for seizure control, phenobarbital therapeutic levels: 10-30 μg/mL (SI: 43-129 μmol/L)

Critical Values Toxic: short-acting: >10 μg/mL (SI: >43 μmol/L); intermediate-acting: >20 μg/mL (SI: >86 μmol/L); long-acting: >40 μg/mL (SI: >172 μmol/L)

Use Evaluate barbiturate toxicity, drug abuse, therapeutic levels; if barbiturates are suspected in a drug overdose, determination of long-, medium-, or short-acting may influence treatment.

Limitations Only barbiturates will be identified and quantitated; individual agents cannot be identified by screening tests, particularly if there has been a mixed ingestion

Methodology Gas chromatography (GC), high performance liquid chromatography (HPLC), immunoassay

Additional Information To monitor therapeutic phenobarbital level see listing for Phenobarbital, Blood. Barbiturates are sedative hypnotics and frequent drugs of abuse, alone and in combination with alcohol and/or amphetamines. If overdosage occurs, coma and death may result. The implication of any concentration is more serious for short-acting barbiturates than for phenobarbital. The toxic or lethal blood level varies with many factors and cannot be stated with certainty. Lethal blood levels determined at autopsy may be as low as 60 μg/mL (SI: 258 μmol/L) for long-acting (barbital and phenobarbital) and 10 μg/mL (SI: 43 μmol/L) for intermediate- and short-acting barbiturates (amobarbital, butabarbital, butalbital, pentobarbital, secobarbital). In presence of alcohol or other depressant drugs, the lethal concentrations may be lower. Addicts, however, may tolerate with no ill effect levels which would be acutely toxic to a nonaddicted individual. The long-acting drugs are metabolized slowly and depend primarily on the kidney for elimination, the short- and intermediate-acting drugs are metabolized primarily by the liver and are much less dependent on the kidney for excretion. Except for barbital, all barbiturates are primarily transformed by the liver. Only barbital is dependent mainly on renal excretion for termination of its pharmacological action. Individual barbiturates can be identified and separated from each other by HPLC.

Barbiturates can be assayed in **urine** or **gastric contents**. The presence of barbiturates in urine is presumptively positive at a level ≥300 ng/mL using secobarbital as a standard and can indicate prescribed or abused intake of this class of drugs. The presence of these drugs should be confirmed. The most commonly abused barbiturates are secobarbital (red devils), pentobarbital (yellow jackets), and amobarbital (blue angels). Short- and intermediate-acting barbiturates can be detected in urine 24-72 hours following ingestion, longer-acting drugs up to 7 days.

Specific References

Chen XH, "Solid-Phase Extraction for Screening of Acidic, Neutral, and Basic Drugs in Plasma Using a Single-Column Procedure on Bond Elut Certify," *J Chromatogr*, 1990, 529:161-6.

Pesce AJ, "Barbiturates," *Clinical Chemistry – Theory, Analysis, and Correlation*, 2nd ed, Kaplan LA and Pesce AJ, eds, St Louis, MO: Mosby-Year Book Inc, 1989, 1081-7.

Pocci R, Dixit V, and Dixit VM, "Solid-Phase Extraction and GC/MS Confirmation of Barbiturates From Human Urine," *J Anal Toxicol*, 1992, 16(1):45-7.

Bed Bugs Identification *see* Arthropod Identification *on page 1198*

Benadryl® *see* Diphenhydramine, Blood *on page 1250*

Bennies *see* Amphetamines, Qualitative, Urine *on page 1190*

Benzene, Blood

Specimen Blood

Minimum Volume 7 mL

Container Lavender top (EDTA) tube

(Continued)

Benzene, Blood *(Continued)*

Storage Instructions Refrigerate

Reference Range None detected; blood benzene level of 0.2 mg/L is consistent with exposure of 25 ppm

Use Evaluate benzene toxicity

Methodology Gas-liquid chromatography (GLC)

Additional Information Benzene, a known carcinogen, is a common solvent used in the manufacture of many organic compounds. Chronic exposure to even low concentrations may cause fatal poisoning, aplastic anemia, or a form of leukemia. Acute cases of exposure may result in respiratory or ventricular failure that leads to death. Benzene poisoning, caused by inhalation of benzene fumes or exposure through the skin, is characterized by nausea, headache, dizziness, and incoordination.

Benzodiazepines Comparison *see page 1643*

Benzodiazepines, Qualitative, Urine

Related Information

Benzodiazepines Comparison *on page 1643*

Synonyms Tranquilizers (Valium®, Librium®, etc)

Abstract This group of drugs is used as antianxiety agents (tranquilizers). They are used by more Americans than any other single prescription drug.

Specimen Random urine

Volume 50 mL

Minimum Volume 10 mL

Container Clean plastic urine container

Storage Instructions Refrigerate or freeze if not analyzing immediately

Reference Range None present unless prescribed. When used as drug-of-abuse screen, negative (less than cutoff).

Critical Values Cutoff: screen: 300 ng/mL (as oxazepam); confirmation: 200 ng/mL

Use Drug abuse evaluation; toxicity assessment

Methodology Immunoassay, thin-layer chromatography (TLC), high performance liquid chromatography (HPLC), gas chromatography (GC), gas chromatography/mass spectrometry (GC/MS)

Additional Information The benzodiazepines are a class of chemically-related central nervous depressants used as sedative-hypnotics to treat sleep disorders, anxiety, alcohol withdrawal, and seizure disorders. The drug class in low doses can cause sedation, drowsiness, blurred vision, fatigue, mental depression, and loss of coordination. In higher doses or used chronically, they can cause confusion, slurred speech, hypotension, and diminished reflexes. Chronic use may produce a physical dependence and a withdrawal syndrome which can last for weeks. Urine should be screened for benzodiazepines in suspected overdose cases, or as part of an abused drug program. These drugs have a relatively low potential for abuse. They are, however, frequently found with other drugs in emergency room drug screens. Immunoassay screens detect a broad range of drugs and their metabolites in this class using either oxazepam or nordiazepam as positive controls. Using the latter, the test is more specific and more sensitive for detecting flurazepam. Positive screen results (usually >300 ng/mL of urine metabolites) should be confirmed by an alternate technique. High concentrations of fenoprofen, flurbiprofen, indomethacin, ketoprofen, and tolmetin may give a false-positive result by a TDx assay. Oxaprozine may cause false-positive urine benzodiazepine result by immunoassay.

Specific References

"Abuse of Benzodiazepines: The Problem and the Solutions," *Am J Drug Alcohol Abuse*, 1988, 14(Suppl 1):1-69.

Baker MI and Oleen MA, "The Use of Benzodiazepines Hypnotics in the Elderly," *Pharmacotherapy*, 1988, 8(4):241-7.

Beck O, Lafolie P, Hjemdahl P, et al, "Detection of Benzodiazepine Intake in Therapeutic Doses by Immunoanalysis of Urine: Two Techniques Evaluated and Modified for Improved Performance," *Clin Chem*, 1992, 38(2):271-5.

Jones CE, Wians FH Jr, Martinez LA, et al, "Benzodiazepines Identified by Capillary Gas Chromatography-Mass Spectrometry With Specific Ion Screening Used to Detect Benzophenone Derivatives," *Clin Chem*, 1989, 35(7):1394-8.

Joseph R, Dickerson S, Willis R, et al, "Interference by Nonsteroidal Anti-inflammatory Drugs in EMIT® and TDx® Assays for Drugs of Abuse," *J Anal Toxicol*, 1995, 19:13.

Matuch-Hite T, Jones P, and Moriarity J, "Interference of Oxaprozin With Benzodiazepines via Enzyme Immunoassay Technique," *J Anal Toxicol*, 1995, 19:130.

Meatherall R, "GC-MS Confirmation of Urinary Benzodiazepine Metabolites," *J Anal Toxicol*, 1994, 18(7):369-81.

Montamat SC, Cusack BJ, and Vestal RE, "Management of Drug Therapy in the Elderly," *N Engl J Med*, 1989, 321(5):303-9.

Smith DE and Landry MJ, "Benzodiazepine Dependency Discontinuation: Focus on the Chemical Dependency Detoxification Setting and Benzodiazepine-Polydrug Abuse," *J Psychiatr Res*, 1990, 24(Suppl 2):145-56.

Beta-Hydroxybutyrate *see* Ketone Bodies, Blood *on page 1277*

Beta-Hydroxybutyric Acid, Urine *see* Ketones, Urine *on page 1278*

Beta-Subunit Human Chorionic Gonadotropin, Urine or Serum *see* Pregnancy Test *on page 1330*

Bilirubin, Total

Synonyms Total Bilirubin

Specimen Blood

Volume 3 mL

Minimum Volume 0.1 mL serum

Container Red top tube; capillary tube for babies

Collection Blood drawn from a heelstick for babies.

Storage Instructions Protect sample from light.

Causes for Rejection Grossly hemolyzed specimen, specimen not protected from light

Reference Range Adults: 0.3-1.0 mg/dL (SI: 5-17 μmol/L)

Use Causes of **high bilirubin:** Liver disease: hepatitis, cholangitis, cirrhosis, other types of liver disease (including primary or secondary neoplasia); alcoholism (usually with high AST (SGOT), GGT, MCV, or some combination of these findings); biliary obstruction (intrahepatic or extrahepatic); infectious mononucleosis (look also for increased LD (LDH), lymphocytosis); Dubin-Johnson syndrome; Gilbert's disease (familial hyperbilirubinemia) is encountered as a moderate elevation with otherwise unremarkable chemistries.

Anorexia or prolonged fasting: 36 hours or more may cause moderate rise.

Pernicious anemia, hemolytic anemias, erythroblastosis fetalis, other neonatal jaundice, hematoma and following a blood transfusion, especially if several units are given in a short time.

Pulmonary embolism and/or infarct, congestive heart failure.

Drugs: A large number of drugs can cause jaundice by *in vivo* action or by chemistry methodology. Drugs causing cholestasis and/or hepatocellular damage include diphenylhydantoin, azathioprine, phenothiazines, erythromycin, penicillin, sulfonamides, oral contraceptives, anabolic-androgenic steroids, halothane, aminosalicylic acid, isoniazid, methyldopa, indomethacin, pyrazinamide, and others.

Limitations Differential diagnosis of liver diseases requires total and direct bilirubin values, as well as other tests. Visibly hemolyzed sera and lipemia can produce erroneous results. Ascorbic acid, dextran, epinephrine, methyldopa, and rifampin can interfere with bilirubin assays resulting in false elevation. Total serum bilirubin assays can be decreased by barbiturates or pindolol.

Methodology Diazo reaction for adults, differential spectrophotometry for neonates

Additional Information Total bilirubin is commonly available in chemistry multitest profiling instruments, in which it is a useful parameter. Interpretation of increased bilirubin is greatly enhanced by other chemistry results. In acute viral hepatitis with jaundice, for instance, the transaminases ALT (SGPT) and AST (SGOT) are consistently increased, while an isolated elevation of bilirubin is seen in Gilbert's disease. **Obstruction** causes increases in bilirubin and alkaline phosphatase greater than and out of proportion to the transaminases. Amylase and lipase are useful in differential diagnosis of obstructive jaundice. In **intrahepatic cholestasis,** the transaminases are not as increased, relative to bilirubin, as they are in hepatitis. Work-up of jaundice has been outlined.

Nicotinic acid increases the formation of bilirubin in the spleen, leading to a rise in unconjugated bilirubin. This can be used as a test for Gilbert's disease in which there is a decreased hepatic clearance of unconjugated bilirubin. Although the indirect bilirubin level is increased in normal controls when nicotinic acid is given, the increase is much greater in patients with Gilbert's disease. In the Crigler-Najjar syndrome type I, the unconjugated bilirubin is >20 μg/dL. In type II, the level is <20 μg/dL.

Specific References

Adachi Y, Katoh H, Fuchi I, et al, "Serum Bilirubin Fractions in Healthy Subjects and Patients With Unconjugated Hyperbilirubinemia," *Clin Biochem*, 1990, 23(3):247-51.

Donnachie EM, Seccombe DW, Urquhart NI, et al, "Indocyanine Green Interference in the Kodak Ektachem® Determination of Total Bilirubin," *Clin Chem*, 1989, 35(5):899-900, (letter).

Frank BB, "Clinical Evaluation of Jaundice – A Guideline of the Patient Care Committee of the American Gastroenterological Association," *JAMA*, 1989, 262(21):3031-4.

Helzberg JH and Spiro HM, "LFTs Test More Than the Liver," *JAMA*, 1986, 256(21):3006-7.

Lepage L and Trivin F, "Total Bilirubin," *Drug Effects on Laboratory Test Results Analytical Interferences and Pharmacological Effects*, Siest G and Galteau MM, eds, Littleton, MA: PSG Publishing Co Inc, 1988, 131-47.

Westwood A, "The Analysis of Bilirubin in Serum," *Ann Clin Biochem*, 1991, 28(Pt 2):119-30.

Biotin *see* Lactic Acid, Blood *on page 1281*

Bishydroxycoumarin, Blood

Synonyms Dicumarol

Specimen Blood

Volume 10 mL

Collection Blood must be accurately added to special tube.

Storage Instructions Transport specimen to the laboratory immediately. Do not store.

Causes for Rejection Excessive delay in transport, improper specimen collection

Reference Range 20-30 μg/mL

Critical Values Toxic: 70 μg/mL

Use Evaluate toxicity. It is helpful when surreptitious ingestion is suspected or when a possible medication error is involved. It should **not** be used for TDM.

Limitations This test does not quantitate warfarin and should not be used to monitor any other anticoagulant. Warfarin may be ordered separately.

Additional Information This test should be ordered only if the patient's prothrombin time is prolonged. It is not as useful for TDM as the prothrombin time.

Blood Cell Profile *see* Complete Blood Count *on page 1236*

Blood Count *see* Complete Blood Count *on page 1236*

Blood Culture, Aerobic and Anaerobic

Synonyms Aerobic Culture, Blood; Anaerobic Culture, Blood; Culture, Blood

Applies To Antimicrobial Removal Device (ARD) Blood Culture; ARD, Blood Culture; Bactec®; Blood Culture, Isolator™; Blood Culture, Lysis Centrifugation; Blood Culture, *Mycobacterium avium-intracellulare*; Blood Culture With Antimicrobial Removal Device (ARD); Blood Mycobacteria Culture; Isolator™ Blood Culture; Mycobacteria Culture, Blood

Test Includes Isolation of both aerobic and anaerobic microorganisms and susceptibility testing on all significant isolates

Patient Preparation The major difficulty in interpretation of blood cultures is potential contamination by skin flora. This difficulty can be markedly reduced by careful attention to the details of skin preparation and antisepsis prior to collection of the specimen. After location of the vein by palpation, the venipuncture site should be cleansed with 70% alcohol (isopropyl or ethyl) and then swabbed in a circular motion concentrically from the center outward using tincture of iodine or a povidone iodine solution. The iodine should be allowed to dry before the venipuncture is undertaken. If palpation is required during the venipuncture, the glove covering the palpating finger tip should be disinfected. In iodine sensitive patients, a double alcohol, green soap, or acetone alcohol preparation may be substituted.

Aftercare Iodine used in the skin preparation should be carefully removed from the skin after venipuncture.

Specimen Venous blood. The yield of positives is not increased by culturing arterial blood even in endocarditis. It is optimal to collect blood specimens from at least two separate venipuncture sites.

Volume 10 mL; 5 mL per bottle

Minimum Volume Pediatrics 1 mL in vented bottle. If more than 1 mL is available, divide equally between two bottles.

Container Bottles of trypticase soy broth or other standard medium, one vented (for aerobes), one unvented (for anaerobes). Recovery may be enhanced by lysis filtration or concentration.

Collection Blood cultures should be drawn prior to initiation of antimicrobial therapy. If more than one culture is ordered, the specimens should be drawn from separately prepared sites. A syringe and needle, transfer set, or pre-evacuated set of tubes containing culture media may be used to collect blood. Collection tubes should be held below the level of the venipuncture to avoid reflux. A sample volume of 10-20 mL in adults or 1-5 mL in pediatric patients is usually collected for each set. The likelihood of recovering a pathogen increases as the volume of blood sampled increases. If a syringe and needle or transfer set is used, the top of the blood culture bottles should also be aseptically prepared. See following table.

Transient bacteremia caused by brushing teeth, bowel movements, etc or by local irritations caused by scratching of the skin may cause positive blood cultures as can contamination by skin flora at the time of collection. Interpretation of results can be enhanced by collecting blood cultures from more than one site and after a time interval (15-30 minutes). Cultures should be taken as early as possible in the course of a febrile episode.

Storage Instructions Specimens collected in tubes with SPS (sodium polyanetholesulfonate) should be processed without delay. The specimen should be

Blood Culture Collection

Clinical Disease Suspected	Culture Recommendation	Rational
Sepsis, meningitis osteomyelitis, septic arthritis, bacterial pneumonia	Two sets of cultures – one from each of two prepared sites, the second drawn after a brief time interval, then begin therapy.	Assure sufficient sampling in cases of intermittent or low level bacteremia. Minimize the confusion caused by a positive culture resulting from transient bacteremia or skin contamination.
Fever of unknown origin (eg, occult abscess, empyema, typhoid fever, etc)	Two sets of cultures – one from each of two prepared sites, the second drawn after a brief time interval (30 minutes). If cultures are negative after 24–48 hours obtain two more sets, preferably prior to an anticipated temperature rise.	The yield after four sets of cultures is minimal. A maximum of three sets per patient per day for 3 consecutive days is recommended.
Endocarditis:		
Acute	Obtain three blood culture sets within 2 hours, then begin therapy.	95% to 99% of acute endocarditis patients (untreated) will yield a positive in one of the first three cultures.
Subacute	Obtain three blood culture sets on day 1, repeat if negative after 24 hours. If still negative or if the patient had prior antibiotic therapy, repeat.	Adequate sample volume despite low level bacteremia or previous therapy should result in a positive yield.
Immunocompromised host (eg, AIDS):		
Septicemia, fungemia, mycobacteremia	Obtain two sets of cultures from each of two prepared sites; consider lysis concentration technique to enhance recovery for fungi and mycobacteria.	Low levels of fungemia and mycobacteremia frequently encountered.
Previous antimicrobial therapy:		
Septicemia, bacteremia; monitor effect of antimicrobial therapy	Obtain two sets of cultures from each of two prepared sites; consider use of antimicrobial removal device (ARD) or increased volume >10 mL/set.	Recovery of organisms is enhanced by dilution, increased sample volume, and removal of inhibiting antimicrobials.

transferred to appropriate culture media to avoid any possible decrease in yield due to storage or prolonged contact with SPS.

Causes for Rejection Unlabeled bottles are not acceptable.

Special Instructions The requisition should indicate current antibiotic therapy and clinical diagnosis.

Reference Range Negative

Use Isolate and identify potentially pathogenic organisms causing bacteremia, septicemia, enteric fever, meningitis, pneumonia, and other disease states caused by microorganisms

Limitations Three sets of blood cultures in the absence of antimicrobial therapy provide optimal yield for detection of bacteremia; one set is seldom ever sufficient. Prior antibiotic therapy may cause negative blood cultures or delayed growth. Blood cultures from patients suspected of having *Brucella* or *Leptospira* must be requested as special cultures. Consultation with the laboratory for special culture procedures for the recovery of these organisms prior to collection of the specimen is recommended. Yeast often are isolated from routine blood cultures. However, if yeast or other fungi are specifically suspected, a separate fungal blood culture should be drawn along with each of the routine blood culture specimens. *Mycobacterium avium-intracellulare* (MAI) is frequently recovered from blood of immunocompromised patients, particularly those with acquired immunodeficiency syndrome (AIDS). Special procedures are required for the recovery of these organisms (ie, lysis filtration concentration or use of a special mycobacteria blood culture medium). Radiometric methods facilitate the recovery of mycobacteria from blood.

A substantial fraction of blood culture isolates are not clinically significant. Many of the false-positives involve coagulase-negative staphylococci, however, such organisms can cause serious infections.

(Continued)

Blood Culture, Aerobic and Anaerobic *(Continued)*

Blood culture contamination (ie, false-positives) cause substantial negative financial impact when laboratory costs, hospital stay, and other costs are considered.

Contraindications Use of a 2% iodine preparation is contraindicated in patients sensitive to iodine. Green soap may be substituted for the iodine or alcohol acetone alone may be used.

Methodology Early subculture of aerobic bottle; visual, radiometric, or infrared monitoring. Aerobic and anaerobic culture in broth media usually with subculture to blood agar and chocolate agar. The antimicrobial removal device procedure (ARD) includes use of an adsorbent resin in the aerobic bottle. Other vendors also provide resin-containing bottles for use in radiometric or infrared automated detection systems. In the lysis centrifugation procedure, blood is lysed and centrifuged using a Wampole Isolator™ tube or similar method. The sediment is inoculated to media appropriate for growing aerobic and anaerobic bacteria, fungi, and mycobacteria. A new method of continuously monitoring media for increased CO_2 content is available.

Additional Information Sequential blood cultures in nonendocarditis patients using a 20 mL sample resulted in an 80% positive yield after the first set, a 90% yield after the second set, and a 99% yield after the third set. Volume of blood cultured seems to be more important than the specific culture technique being employed by the laboratory. The isolation of *Staphylococcus epidermidis* (coagulase-negative *Staphylococcus*) poses a critical and difficult clinical dilemma. Although *S. epidermidis* is the most commonly isolated organism from blood cultures, only a few (6.3%) of the isolates represent "true" clinically significant bacteremia. Conversely, *S. epidermidis* is well recognized as a cause of infections involving prosthetic devices, cardiac valves, CSF shunts, dialysis catheters, and indwelling vascular catheters. Ultimately, the physician is responsible for determination of whether an organism is a contaminant or a pathogen. The decision is based on both laboratory and clinical data. Patient data including patient history, physical examination, body temperatures, clinical course, and laboratory data (ie, culture results, white blood cell count, and differential) are relevant. Clinical experience and judgment may play a significant role in resolution of this clinical dilemma. Various sources of contamination include the patient's own skin flora, transient benign bacteremias, and perhaps, disinfection materials.

The use of a lysis centrifugation system has been reported to increase the recovery rate and decrease the time of fungal recovery compared to traditional or biphasic blood culture systems. Recovery of mycobacteria, atypical mycobacteria, and *Legionella* may also be enhanced by lysis filtration. In patients who have received antimicrobial drugs, four to six blood cultures may be necessary. Any organism isolated from the blood is usually tested for susceptibility.

The use of antimicrobial removal devices (ARD) or resin bottles to attempt to increase the yield of blood cultures drawn from patients on antimicrobial therapy is controversial. Some microorganisms are occasionally not recovered with the use of ARD blood cultures. It is, therefore, advised that at least one culture in a series of three be requested without the use of the ARD bottles. ARD blood cultures are substantially more expensive than routine blood cultures. There is no consensus as to the effectiveness of the ARD cultures in enhancing recovery of organisms. A recent study reports no significant increase in recovery of organisms with the device. Selective use of the ARD with consideration of the clinical setting has been recommended.

The diagnosis of bacterial meningitis is accomplished by blood culture as well as culture and examination of the cerebrospinal fluid. Most children with bacterial meningitis are initially bacteremic.

Interpretation of Positive Blood Cultures

Virtually **any** organism, including normal flora, **can** cause bacteremia.

A negative culture result does not necessarily rule out bacteremia; false-negative results occur when pathogens fail to grow.

A positive culture result does not necessarily indicate bacteremia; false-positive results occur when contaminants grow.

Gram-negative bacilli, anaerobes, and fungi should be considered pathogens until proven otherwise.

The most difficult interpretation problem is to determine whether an organism that is usually considered normal skin flora is a true pathogen.

From Flournoy DJ and Adkins L, "Understanding the Blood Culture Report," *Am J Infect Control*, 1986, 14:41-6, with permission.

Specific References

MacLowry JD, "Clinical Microbiology of Bacteremia: An Overview," *Am J Med*, 1983, 75(1B):2-6.

Mermel LA and Maki DG, "Detection of Bacteremia in Adults: Consequences of Culturing an Inadequate Volume of Blood," *Ann Intern Med*, 1993, 119(4):270-2.
Murray PR, Traynor P, and Hopson D, "Critical Assessment of Blood Culture Techniques: Analysis of Recovery of Obligate and Facultative Anaerobes, Strict Aerobic Bacteria, and Fungi in Aerobic and Anaerobic Blood Culture Bottles," *J Clin Microbiol*, 1992, 30(6):1462-8.
Salfinger M, Stool EW, Piot D, et al, "Comparison of Three Methods for Recovery of *Mycobacterium avium* Complex From Blood Specimens," *J Clin Microbiol*, 1988, 26(6):1225-6.
Schifman RB and Pindur A, "The Effect of Skin Disinfection Materials on Reducing Blood Culture Contamination," *Am J Clin Pathol*, 1993, 99(5):536-8.
Wilson ML, Weinstein MP, Reimer LG, et al, "Controlled Comparison of the BacT/Alert™ and Bactec® 660/730 Nonradiometric Blood Culture Systems," *J Clin Microbiol*, 1992, 30(2):323-9.

Blood Culture, Isolator™ *see* Blood Culture, Aerobic and Anaerobic *on page 1204*

Blood Culture, Lysis Centrifugation *see* Blood Culture, Aerobic and Anaerobic *on page 1204*

Blood Culture, *Mycobacterium avium-intracellulare* *see* Blood Culture, Aerobic and Anaerobic *on page 1204*

Blood Culture With Antimicrobial Removal Device (ARD) *see* Blood Culture, Aerobic and Anaerobic *on page 1204*

Blood Gases, Arterial

Related Information

Oxygen Saturation, Blood *on page 1313*
pH, Blood *on page 1318*

Synonyms ABGs; Arterial Blood Gases; Gases, Arterial

Applies To Oxygen Content; pCO_2; pO_2

Test Includes Measured results include pH, pCO_2 ($PaCO_2$), pO_2 (PaO_2), hematocrit, and may also include electrolytes and ionized calcium. Calculated values include total carbon dioxide (TCO_2), bicarbonate (HCO_3^-), oxygen saturation, oxygen content, base excess, alveolar-arterial (A-a) gradient, and P_{50} offered by some laboratories. Standard bicarbonate concentration (SBc), base excess of extracellular fluid, carboxyhemoglobin, methemoglobin, normalized calcium, hemoglobin content, and anion gap and osmolality (if electrolytes measured) may also be provided as calculations.

Patient Preparation Patient should be supine, relaxed. The patient's temperature should be recorded.

Aftercare Watch for bleeding, hematoma. Ideally, extremity punctured should be kept up for 10 minutes with pressure applied to the puncture site if the patient is not on anticoagulants. If patient is receiving heparin, pressure must be applied to puncture site for a minimum of 15 minutes. Arterial puncture may be especially hazardous in the anticoagulated patient. However, there is frequently simultaneous need for arterial blood gases and for anticoagulation.

Specimen Whole blood

Volume 2 mL

Minimum Volume 0.5 mL

Container Heparinized syringe or through an indwelling arterial line

Collection Very small diameter needles are used, usually 25-gauge. Specimen is drawn into air-free heparinized syringe, then stoppered. The radial artery is commonly used, utilizing the Allen test. The Allen test is used to assess the presence of normal collateral circulation. The brachial artery is the second choice. **All specimens should be on ice and brought to the laboratory immediately.** Mode of oxygen delivery or room air must be indicated. Rapid changes may occur if collected immediately after exercise. Avoid excessive heparin. Strict anaerobiosis must be maintained. Blood drawn from a vein or capillary can provide helpful information including pH, pCO_2, and, occasionally, pO_2.

Storage Instructions Place on ice. The following *in vitro* changes occur in blood gas parameters: pH, 0.001/10 minutes at 4°C, pCO_2, 0.1 mm Hg/10 minutes at 4°C, pO_2, 3 mm Hg/10 minutes at 4°C. No difference exists between glass and newer plastic syringes.

Causes for Rejection Specimen **not** received on ice, air bubbles or clots in syringe

Special Instructions Sample obtained just after a change in FiO_2 (eg, room air or quantity of therapeutic oxygen delivered) is apt to generate confusing results.

Reference Range pH: 7.35-7.45; TCO_2: 23-29 mmol/L; pCO_2: 35-45 mm Hg; pO_2: adults: 80-95 mm Hg, newborns: 60-70 mm Hg; O_2: 95% to 99% saturation. Such normal ranges must be interpreted in light of the FiO_2 and other parameters.

Possible Panic Range pH <7.2, >7.55; pCO_2 <20 mm Hg, >60 mm Hg; pO_2 <40 mm Hg

Use Evaluate oxygen and carbon dioxide gas exchange, respiratory function including hypoxia, and acid-base status; assess asthma, chronic obstructive pulmonary disease (COPD), and other types of lung disease, embolism including fat embolism, and coronary arterial bypass surgical cases.

(Continued)

Blood Gases, Arterial *(Continued)*

ARTERIAL BLOOD GAS QUALITY ASSURANCE AND APPROPRIATENESS REVIEW:

In the following lists, clinical judgment is required. Many of the clinical entities listed do not necessarily require blood gas analysis.

Criteria:

Severe cardiorespiratory disturbances:

- shock
- cardiac arrest
- coma
- acute respiratory failure
- acute infarct, myocardium with complications
- severe congestive heart failure
- pulmonary edema
- serious disturbances of cardiac rhythm
- unexplained right heart failure
- suspected R-L shunt evaluation
- evaluate V/Q abnormality

Investigate cardiorespiratory, metabolic, central nervous system disturbances:

- shortness of breath by history, if indicated
- unexplained tachypnea, if indicated
- unexplained dyspnea, if indicated
- lung disease, if indicated
- decompensated established lung disease
- deep vein thrombus
- pulmonary embolism, including fat embolism
- pneumonia
- unexplained polycythemia, erythrocytosis
- unexplained mental status abnormalities
- cyanosis
- smoke inhalation, possibly with CO intoxication
- toxin ingestion (CN, ASA, methanol, ethylene glycol)
- rule out carboxyhemoglobinemia or methemoglobinemia
- monitor oxygen therapy as medically needed
- home oxygen management, selected instances
- exercise, oxygen therapy
- fracture
- metabolic acidosis and alkalosis, selected instances
- electrolyte disturbances (abnormal bicarbonate level, anion gap), selected cases
- change in patient's clinical status
- rest and exercise pulmonary function testing
- sleep disorder work-up

Miscellaneous medical/surgical conditions:

- change in ventilatory settings, if indicated
- contemplated prolonged anesthesia
- contemplated major abdominal surgery, if indicated
- contemplated pulmonary resection
- chest pain, pleurisy, if indicated
- abnormal chest x-ray with clinical indications
- follow-up abnormal ABG, if indicated
- follow O_2 prescription if needed
- during surgery, if indicated
- abnormal oxygen saturation, if indicated
- during dialysis, if needed
- after prescription of $NaHCO_3$ or Na citrate, if indicated
- Kussmaul respirations
- uncontrolled diabetes with suspected acidosis as medically indicated
- previous pH <7.35 or 7.30, if indicated
- renal failure (creatinine >4 mg/dL (SI: >353 μmol/L) or creatinine clearance <25 mL/min), if indicated
- profuse diarrhea, if indicated
- history of renal tubular acidosis (RTA), if indicated
- ureterosigmoidostomy, if indicated
- pancreatic, small bowel or biliary drainage, if indicated
- nausea/vomiting, if indicated
- nasogastric drainage, if indicated
- hypokalemia, if indicated

- diuretic use, if indicated

In ill adults who are stable, blood gas analysis is considered when a change in clinical management is considered or when an alteration in the patient's clinical status develops.

Limitations Arterial puncture may be extremely difficult in some individuals. O_2 saturation is calculated on assumption of 100% A hemoglobin. Reported value may be misleading when hemoglobins with different dissociation curves are present. Calculations commonly assume body temperature of 37°C.

When hemoglobin is reported with blood gases, it usually is a screening hemoglobin, which is less reliable than a conventional hemoglobin ordered as such.

Variability of results occurs; changes in pO_2 in isolated reports must be interpreted cautiously and in light of data trends, oxygen delivery, and the patient's clinical appearance. Such variation occurs without change in FiO_2 or the patient's clinical status.

Correlation of arterial gases with pulmonary function testing in asthma was reported as poor. Correlation with severity of asthma is suboptimal.

ABGs are of little value in treatment decisions for carbon monoxide poisoning.

Complications of arterial puncture potentially include hematoma, bleeding, arterial occlusion, infection, and, very rarely, gangrene.

Although normal pO_2 diminishes the likelihood of pulmonary embolism, the former does not rule out the latter. (Alveolar-arterial gradient usually is widened in pulmonary embolism.)

Methodology Specific electrodes

Additional Information The pH, pCO_2 and pO_2 are measured directly while the hemoglobin, carboxyhemoglobin, and methemoglobin are measured and calculated using spectrophotometric analysis at specific wavelengths and electronic representation of mathematical relationships. It is assumed that largely normal A hemoglobin is present (most importantly that there are no significant levels of fetal hemoglobin.) Methemoglobin levels <10% are subject to about a 1% error; but with methemoglobin levels >10%, the error is at about the 10% level. High serum bilirubin levels do not contribute to error. Methylene blue (used in treatment of some forms of methemoglobinemia) may interfere and result in nonrepresentative methemoglobin and other hemoglobin measurements. Sulfhemoglobin is a cause of spectral interference.

"Hypoxemia" can be defined as pO_2 <80 mm Hg, but other, more sophisticated definitions are available.

Raffin points out that few studies are available to indicate how many arterial samples are actually indicated. He observes that a complete list of clinical settings involving ill patients in whom blood gas studies might be indicated would include much of the tables of contents of general medicine texts.

The combination of pH values <7.25 without elevation of pCO_2 may indicate need for a lactic acid determination.

Nonsurvivors in a group of COPD patients had lower arterial oxygen tension and higher carbon dioxide tension.

Assessment of acid-base status of tissues in patients in circulatory failure may be misleading if only arterial blood gas data is available. Information on mixed venous, as well as arterial gases, in care of critically ill patients should be collected.

Specific References

Anderson S, "ABGs. Six Easy Steps to Interpreting Blood Gases," *Am J Nurs*, 1990, 90(8):42-5.

Courtney SE, Weber KR, Breakie LA, et al, "Capillary Blood Gases in the Neonate. A Reassessment and Review of the Literature," *Am J Dis Child*, 1990, 144(2):168-72.

Eichhorn JH, "Performance Characteristics for Devices Measuring pO_2 and pCO_2 in Blood Samples," *National Committee for Clinical Laboratory Standards*, 1989.

Hansen JE, "Arterial Blood Gases," *Clin Chest Med*, 1989, 10(2):227-37.

Hibbard JU, Hibbard MC, and Whalen MP, "Umbilical Cord Blood Gases and Mortality and Morbidity in the Very Low Birth Weight Infant," *Obstet Gynecol*, 1991, 78(5 Pt 1):768-73.

Meyer BA, Dickinson JE, Chambers C, et al, "The Effect of Fetal Sepsis on Umbilical Cord Blood Gases," *Am J Obstet Gynecol*, 1992, 166(2):612-7.

Pierson DJ, "Pulse Oximetry Versus Arterial Blood Gas Specimens in Long-Term Oxygen Therapy," *Lung*, 1990, 168(Suppl):782-8.

Ribbert LS, Snijders RJ, Nicolaides KH, et al, "Relation of Fetal Blood Gases and Data From Computer-Assisted Analysis of Fetal Heart Rate Patterns in Small for Gestation Fetuses," *Br J Obstet Gynaecol*, 1991, 98(8):820-3.

Blood Lactate *see* Lactic Acid, Blood *on page 1281*

Blood Mycobacteria Culture *see* Blood Culture, Aerobic and Anaerobic *on page 1204*

Blood, Occult, Urine *see* Blood, Urine *on next page*

Blood pH *see* pH, Blood *on page 1318*

Blood Urea Nitrogen *see* Urea Nitrogen, Blood *on page 1370*

Blood, Urine

Synonyms Blood, Occult, Urine; Hemoglobin, Urine; Occult Blood, Urine

Test Includes Dipstick method for occult blood is usually a part of urinalysis.

Abstract Positive dipstick usually indicates hematuria, hemoglobinuria, or myoglobinuria

Specimen Random urine

Volume 10 mL

Minimum Volume 2 mL

Container Plastic urine container

Storage Instructions If test not performed immediately, specimen should be refrigerated.

Causes for Rejection Improper labeling. Standing for more than 2 hours at room temperature may be a reason to consider a specimen unacceptable.

Reference Range Negative by dipstick; 2-3 red cells/hpf are generally accepted as normal by microscopy.

Use Detect myoglobin, hemoglobin, or red blood cells in urine (detect hematuria, microhematuria, hemoglobinuria, or erythrocyturia). See table.

Blood, Urine

Causes of Hematuria	Causes of Hemoglobinuria
Renal diseases including: glomerulonephritis Goodpasture's syndrome lupus nephritis arteritis Wegener's granulomatosis stone tumor polycystic kidney infarct infection, including pyelonephritis necrotizing papillitis trauma Blood diseases including: thrombocytopenia thrombotic thrombocytopenic purpura Henoch-Schönlein purpura infective endocarditis leukemia hemophilias sickle cell trait Bladder diseases including: cystitis carcinoma papilloma Prostatic diseases including: prostatitis BPH (benign nodular and glandular hyperplasia) prostatic adenocarcinoma Urethral diseases including: urethritis tumor Trauma Drugs including: Coumadin® heparin salicylates many others (see Appendix)	Hemolysis associated with: parasites (ie, malaria) drugs chemicals antibodies March hemoglobinuria — secondary to severe exercise Transfusion reactions incompatible blood Burns Crush injury Poisoning snake or spider bite Paroxysmal nocturnal hemoglobinuria Paroxysmal cold hemoglobinuria

Limitations Dipstick methods detect myoglobin as hemoglobin. Both intact erythrocytes and free hemoglobin give a positive reaction. Iodine solutions in urine, or applied to patient's skin, are reported to cause false-positives. Certain oxidizing agents such as hypochlorite (bleach) may produce false-positive results if present in the collection vessel. Microbial peroxidase, associated with urinary tract infection and leukocyte peroxidase, may cause a false-positive reaction. Pyridium® (phenazopyridine) and Serenium® (ethoxazene hydrochloride) metabolites may mask the dipstick reaction. Large amounts of nitrite may delay reactions. The sensitivity of the occult blood test is reduced in urines with high specific gravity and/or high ascorbic acid content. High urine protein and formalin are reported to cause false-negatives. Prolonged air exposure of the dipstick (dipstick jar left uncapped) reduces the sensitivity of the dipstick for blood. Transient hematuria can reflect menstruation, catheterization, and strenuous exercise. Urine sediment microscopy should be used to confirm a diagnosis of hematuria suggested by positive dipstick.

Methodology Dipstick is based on the pseudoperoxidase activity of hemoglobin. Microscopy is used for recognition of red blood cells and red cell casts.

Additional Information The test will detect 0.03 mg/dL free hemoglobin or 10 intact red blood cells/μL. Further tests to work-up hematuria may include CBC, platelet count, urine culture, ESR, ANA, prothrombin time, PTT, serum BUN, creatinine, and other examinations as appropriate. More than 3 g of protein in a 24-hour urine collection provides indication of glomerular disease; more than 1 g of protein is suggestive.

The number of red cells (grade of microhematuria) does not necessarily correlate with the degree or significance of urologic pathologic findings (ie, a patient with more than 5 unexplained red cells in urine may have an important urologic lesion). Additional studies (such as urine culture, cytology, excretory urography, cystoscopy) may be indicated. Patients on anticoagulants exhibiting gross or microscopic hematuria should be carefully evaluated. A recent review by Schuster and Lewis indicated the high likelihood (16 of 24 cases) of identifying significant pathologic findings in subjects with gross hematuria, which included carcinoma and calculi. The use of nonsteroidal anti-inflammatory drugs including aspirin may be associated with a significant incidence of hematuria.

A positive dipstick test for blood without red cells in the urine sediment may indicate hemoglobinuria, myoglobinuria, or the presence of porphyrins. Drugs causing hematuria are listed. Algorithms for diagnosis of hematuria are published for children and adults. Phenytoin does not cause urine to appear red, but uric acid and urate crystals in acid urine may cause a pink to red-brown color.

Daum and coworkers studied correlation between dipsticks and microscopy in abdominal trauma. If the dipstick is positive, they decided that microscopy is needed to determine whether or not an IVP is indicated, although others have recommended urine microscopy in all cases of blunt abdominal traumas. Kennedy et al report false-negatives and false-positives but conclude that the safety of dipsticks for hematuria in subjects sustaining blunt or penetrating abdominal trauma is acceptable. Messing and coworkers found that hematuria, even in the presence of significant disease such as urinary tract malignancy, often was intermittent. They have proposed home dipstick screening based upon their study of asymptomatic men older than 50 years of age; others disagree.

An important response to the paper reporting inaccurate results of urine dipstick results is that by Cadoff, who emphasizes the need for quality control and addresses the exemption of tests waivered under CLIA '88 by the Health Care Finance Administration. Cadoff perceives the need for laboratory testing to be performed by those well versed in good laboratory practice.

Specific References

Abarbanel J, Benet AE, Lask D, et al, "Sports Hematuria," *J Urol*, 1990, 143(5):887-90.

Abuelo JG, "Evaluation of Hematuria," *Urology*, 1983, 21(3):215-25.

Bee DE, James GP, and Paul KL, "Hemoglobinuria and Hematuria: Accuracy and Precision of Laboratory Diagnosis," *Clin Chem*, 1979, 25(10):1696-9.

Bloom KJ, "An Algorithm for Hematuria," *Clin Lab Med*, 1988, 8(3):577-84.

Copley JC, "Isolated Asymptomatic Hematuria in the Adult," *Am J Med Sci*, 1986, 291(2):101-11, (review).

Mohr DN, Offord KP, Owen RA, et al, "Asymptomatic Microhematuria and Urologic Disease. A Population-Based Study," *JAMA*, 1986, 256(2):224-9.

Moore GP and Robinson M, "Do Urine Dipsticks Reliably Predict Microhematuria? The Bloody Truth!" *Ann Emerg Med*, 1988, 17(3):257-60.

Smith RF, Mohr DN, Torres VE, et al, "Renal Insufficiency in Community Patients With Mild Asymptomatic Microhematuria," *Mayo Clin Proc*, 1989, 64(4):409-14.

Yoshikawa N, Matsuyama S, Iijima K, et al, "Benign Familial Hematuria," *Arch Pathol Lab Med*, 1988, 112(8):794-7.

Blue Angels *see* Barbiturates, Quantitative, Blood *on page 1201*

Body Lice Identification *see* Arthropod Identification *on page 1198*

Botulism Diagnostic Procedure

Synonyms *Clostridium botulinum* Toxin Identification Procedure; Infant Botulism, Toxin Identification

Applies To Sudden Infant Death Syndrome

Specimen Vomitus or feces, gastric washings, cerebrospinal fluid or autopsy tissue, blood, food samples

Volume 50 g vomitus or feces, gastric washings, cerebrospinal fluid or autopsy tissue, 15-20 mL serum; infant botulism: 25 g feces

Container Sterile wide-mouth, leakproof, screw cap jar; serum: red top tube

Storage Instructions Refrigerate specimen at 4°C except for unopened canned foods.

(Continued)

Botulism Diagnostic Procedure *(Continued)*

Special Instructions Laboratory must be notified prior to obtaining specimen in order to prepare for transport of the specimen to the State Health Laboratory.

Reference Range No toxin identified, no *Clostridium botulinum* isolated

Use Diagnose infant botulism, sudden death syndrome, floppy baby syndrome, classic botulism in adults

Limitations Test invalid if patient has been treated with botulism antitoxin

Contraindications Due to the difficulty in performance of the diagnostic test and because of the extensive epidemiological studies initiated upon receipt of the specimen, State Department of Health Laboratories require specific clinical symptomatology for infant botulism and therefore should be consulted early to optimize handling of the suspect case.

Methodology Toxin neutralization test in mice

Additional Information The classic presentation of infant botulism is hypotonia (floppy baby syndrome), constipation, difficulty in feeding, and a weak cry. Some cases of sudden death syndrome have been traced to ingesting honey containing *C. botulinum*. Both *C. botulinum* and *C. butyricum* have been identified as species capable of toxin production. Autointoxication may occur from toxin production during organism growth in tissue, the intestinal tract in both adults and infants, and in wounds.

Brain, CT *see* Computed Transaxial Tomography, Head Studies *on page 1240*

Broad Spectrum Direct Antiglobulin *see* Antiglobulin Test, Direct *on page 1195*

Bromide, Serum

Abstract Inorganic bromide salts were formerly used as antiepileptics. They are no longer available as nonprescription items in the United States.

Specimen Blood

Volume 5 mL

Minimum Volume 3 mL serum

Container Red top tube

Reference Range Normal: <20 mg/dL (SI: <2.5 mmol/L); therapeutic: 20-120 mg/dL (SI: 2.5-15.0 mmol/L)

Critical Values Toxic: >120 mg/dL (SI: >15.0 mmol/L)

Use Evaluate bromide toxicity. This test is seldom ordered.

Limitations Patients on iodide therapy will have falsely elevated serum bromide levels. A high level of bromide in the serum will falsely elevate the chloride level.

Methodology Reaction of bromide in a protein-free filtrate with gold chloride

Additional Information In order to convert mg/dL to mEq/L (the same units in which serum or plasma chlorides are reported), multiply the bromide values in mg/dL by 0.125. Both chloride and bromide react identically to titrimetric chloride methods (chloridometer). Many ion selective chloride electrodes give a response to bromide which is double that for chloride. A reported "chloride" value will equal the true sum of chloride and bromide. Bromism may be suspected in the presence of a history of ingestion of proprietary bromide preparations, fever, skin rash, and neurologic symptoms. Over-the-counter former bromide-containing preparations such as Bromo-Seltzer® and Nervine® have not contained bromide in the U.S. since 1971.

Specific References

Svirbely J, "Bromide," *Methods in Clinical Chemistry*, Pesce AJ and Kaplan LA, eds, St Louis, MO: Mosby-Year Book Inc, 1987, 342-5.

Bromide, Urine

Synonyms Br, Urine

Specimen Urine

Minimum Volume 75 mL

Container Plastic urine container

Reference Range <0.25 mg/dL

Use Evaluate bromide toxicity

Additional Information Bromide, a CNS depressant, is commonly used as a sedative. Bromide is accumulative and slowly excreted from the body. Such nonprescription drugs as Bromo-Seltzer®, Nytol®, and Sominex®, contain bromide, thus making it easily available to patients prone to drug abuse. Bromism may be suspected in the presence of a history of ingestion of proprietary bromide preparations, fever, skin rash, and neurologic symptoms.

Bromomethane *see* Methylbromides, Blood *on page 1298*

Br, Urine *see* Bromide, Urine *on this page*

BSP *replaced by* Alkaline Phosphatase, Serum *on page 1184*

BUN *see* Urea Nitrogen, Blood *on page 1370*

Butabarbital, Quantitative

Related Information

Barbiturates, Quantitative, Blood *on page 1201*

Synonyms Buticaps®; Butisol Sodium®

Specimen Blood

Volume 7 mL

Minimum Volume 0.5 mL serum

Container Red top tube

Collection Collect specimen immediately prior to next dose unless specified otherwise by physician. Put time of last dose on requisition, if it is available.

Reference Range Therapeutic: mildly sedated 3-25 μg/mL

Critical Values Toxic: mildly comatose 20-40 μg/mL; severely comatose >40 μg/mL

Use Monitor therapeutic drug level; evaluate toxicity

Limitations Can only be performed if patient is not taking other barbiturates

Contraindications Presence of other barbiturates

Methodology Enzyme immunoassay (EIA)

Additional Information Butabarbital, an intermediate-acting barbiturate, is used as a sedative to manage anxiety, for the short-term treatment of insomnia and as a preoperative sedative. Effects are achieved in 40-60 minutes and last 6-8 hours. The half-life is 66-140 hours. Adverse effects include drowsiness, "hangover", nausea, and vomiting.

Butalbital *see* Barbiturates, Quantitative, Blood *on page 1201*

Butalbital, Urine *see* Barbiturates, Qualitative, Urine *on page 1200*

Buticaps® *see* Butabarbital, Quantitative *on this page*

Butisol Sodium® *see* Butabarbital, Quantitative *on this page*

Butisol Sodium® *see* Barbiturates, Quantitative, Blood *on page 1201*

Ca, Blood *see* Calcium, Serum *on next page*

Cadmium, Blood

Related Information

Heavy Metal Screen, Blood *on page 1271*

Synonyms Cd, Blood

Abstract This toxic heavy metal is used in industry in alloys and metal platings

Specimen Whole blood

Volume Entire specimen

Container Metal-free tube

Collection Blood must be collected into metal-free tubes with a plastic syringe.

Causes for Rejection Specimen allowed to contact metal

Special Instructions Requisition must state date and time urine collection started and date and time collection finished.

Reference Range Whole blood: <1 μg/L

Possible Panic Range Levels >10 μg/L (SI: >88.97 μmol/L) in whole blood probably reflect excessive exposure.

Use Evaluate cadmium toxicity in industrial exposure to cadmium fumes or cadmium ingestion

Methodology Flameless atomic absorption spectrophotometry (AA); electrothermal atomization atomic absorption

Additional Information Inhalation of cadmium fumes produces an acute pneumonitis. Long-term exposure may lead to emphysema (with decreased α_1-antitrypsin). Increased cadmium is reported to be associated with hypertension and (perhaps) prostatic cancer. Cadmium ingestion may result from contact of acid foods with metal containers. There is exposure of the general populace to cadmium from food, water, and air contamination. Because of slow excretion and constant exposure cadmium values increase with age. Body cadmium elimination half-life may be as long as 30 years. Chronic cadmium exposure can cause proteinuria and a degree of renal insufficiency.

Specific References

Baselt RC, *Disposition of Toxic Drugs and Chemicals in Man;* 2nd ed, Davis, CA: Biomedical Publications, 1982, 105-8.

Tonks DB, "Cadmium," *Methods in Clinical Chemistry*, Pesce AJ and Kaplan LA, eds, St Louis, MO: Mosby-Year Book Inc, 1987, 346-61.

Cadmium, Hair

Synonyms Cd, Hair

Specimen Hair

Container Envelope or plastic Petri dish

(Continued)

Cadmium, Hair *(Continued)*

Collection Clip lock of hair at nape of neck extending to a distance of 20 mm. Place in an envelope or plastic Petri dish.

Use Evaluate chronic cadmium toxicity; hair analysis can reflect chronic cadmium poisoning for long-term exposure.

Limitations Hair analysis does not reflect cadmium concentration in the body at the time the sample is collected, but at some prior time.

Methodology Flameless atomic absorption spectrophotometry (AA)

Cadmium, Urine

Related Information

Heavy Metal Screen, Urine *on page 1272*

Synonyms Cd, Urine

Patient Preparation Patient should be instructed to use a plastic bedpan or urinal if necessary.

Specimen Random urine

Volume Entire collection

Minimum Volume 100 mL aliquot

Container Plastic urine container

Collection Freshly voided random urine

Storage Instructions Keep specimen on ice or refrigerate.

Causes for Rejection Specimen allowed to contact metal, specimen not kept chilled

Reference Range Nonexposed: 0-20 μg/L; exposed: 10-580 μg/L

Use Evaluate cadmium toxicity in industrial exposure to cadmium fumes or cadmium ingestion

Additional Information Cadmium is a nonessential, highly toxic metal which accumulates in human tissues. Chronic exposure produces a wide variety of effects and affects the kidneys, lungs, heart, bones, and gonads. Cadmium ingestion may result from contact of acidic foods with metal containers. Inhalation of fumes is the main route of occupational exposure and produces an acute pneumonitis. Long-term exposure may lead to emphysema (with decreased α_1-antitrypsin). Increased cadmium is reported to be associated with hypertension and (perhaps) prostatic cancer.

Caffeine, Blood

Abstract The principle intake is from drinking coffee and tea. Some soft drinks may also contain moderate amounts of caffeine. It is a metabolite of theophylline in infants.

Specimen Blood

Minimum Volume 1 mL serum

Container Red top tube

Collection Indicate exact time blood drawn and relationship to last theophylline or caffeine dose on requisition.

Reference Range None present. Caffeine is one of the most widely used mind-altering substances and is found in numerous beverages (cocoa, coffee, cola, tea) and prescription and nonprescription medications. The therapeutic range in the treatment of neonatal apnea is 8-14 μg/mL (SI: 41-72 μmol/L).

Possible Panic Range Toxic concentration: >30 μg/mL (SI: >155 μmol/L)

Use Monitor total xanthine concentration in newborns receiving theophylline

Limitations Not often ordered

Methodology High performance liquid chromatography (HPLC)

Additional Information Theophylline is used to treat neonatal apnea. Unlike its metabolism in adults, theophylline in neonates is extensively metabolized to caffeine. Plasma elimination half-life in adults is 3-6 hours. In neonates caffeine has a half-life of 30 hours. Caffeine overdoses are rare. The clinical presentation is similar to that of theophylline.

Specific References

Bryson PD, "Stimulants," *Comprehensive Review in Toxicology*, 2nd ed, Rockville, MD: Aspen Publishers, 1989, 374-9.

Moyer TP, Pippinger CE, Blanke RV, et al, "Therapeutic Drug Monitoring," *Clin Chem*, Tietz NW, ed, New York, NY: WB Saunders Co, 1986, 1647-9.

Calcium, Serum

Synonyms Ca, Blood; Total Calcium, Serum

Test Includes Disorders of calcium metabolism are initially evaluated with measurements of serum phosphorus, alkaline phosphatase, albumin, chloride, total protein and commonly, parathormone assays as well as serum and often 24-hour urine calcium levels.

Abstract The two most common causes of hypercalcemia (beyond slight increases from dehydration) are primary hyperparathyroidism and malignancy.

Specimen Blood
Volume 1 mL
Minimum Volume 0.5 mL serum
Container Red top tube
Sampling Time Morning, fasting sample is desirable, since some diurnal variation exists (which may reflect postural changes).
Collection Pediatrics: Blood drawn from heelstick for capillary. Since about half of serum calcium is bound to proteins, there is variation with posture. Venous stasis in sampling causes misleading results.
Storage Instructions Refrigerate in stoppered vials, not in sample cups.
Causes for Rejection Gross hemolysis
Reference Range Infant to 1 month: 7.0-11.5 mg/dL (SI: 1.75-2.87 mmol/L); 1 month to 1 year: 8.6-11.2 mg/dL (SI: 2.15-2.79 mmol/L) normal range slowly descends; up to 30 years: 8.2-10.2 mg/dL (SI: 2.05-2.54 mmol/L); decreases slightly in older years
Possible Panic Range <7.0 mg/dL (SI: <1.75 mmol/L) may lead to tetany. Calcium >12.0 mg/dL (SI: >2.99 mmol/L) may induce coma, although some patients tolerate higher levels. Possibly life-threatening levels: ≤6.0 mg/dL (SI: ≤1.50 mmol/L), ≥14.0 mg/dL (SI: ≥3.49 mmol/L). Extremely high levels may be found with primary parathyroid carcinomas, which are very uncommon.
Use Work-up for coma, pancreatitis and other gastrointestinal problems, nephrolithiasis, polydipsia, polyuria, azotemia, multiple endocrine adenomatosis.

Causes of high calcium:

- Hyperparathyroidism – look also for high ionized calcium, measured or calculated. Hyperparathyroidism may coexist with other endocrine tumors (multiple endocrine adenomatosis syndromes).
- Carcinoma, with or without bone metastases. Humoral hypercalcemia of malignancy (HHM), (tumor induced hypercalcemia) is seen especially in primary squamous cell carcinoma of lung, head and neck, but other important tumors include primaries in the kidney, liver, bladder, and ovary. It is probably caused by parathormone-like peptides. The most common solid tumors causing bone metastases are primaries in the breast and lung. Other neoplasms may also cause hypercalcemia. Differences between HPT and humoral hypercalcemia of malignancy include low dihydroxyvitamin D, reduced calcium absorption, and the presence of a nonparathyroid tumor. Hypercalcemia with alkaline phosphatase more than twice its upper limit is more suggestive of **cancer** than of hyperparathyroidism. Especially if there is only a brief duration of symptoms, anemia, hypoalbuminemia, and other findings suggestive of malignant disease, chloride/phosphorus ratio <29 mmol/L, chloride <100 mmol/L, high serum LD (LDH) and/or phosphorus, think first of malignant neoplasm. **The chloride/phosphorus ratio** is predominantly of value when it is <29 mmol/L, to provide evidence **against** a diagnosis of primary hyperparathyroidism. Laboratory results which would favor malignancy include anemia, increased LD and alkaline phosphatase, decreased serum albumin and chloride, and chloride/phosphorus ratio <29 mmol/L. **Parathyroid hormone-related protein** was recently purified and identified by molecular cloning as a 141-amino acid peptide with limited homology to PTH itself. Both peptides activate the PTH receptor to produce hypercalcemia. PTH-related protein is now recognized as the cause of hypercalcemia in most solid tumors, particularly squamous, and renal carcinomas.
- Myeloma
- Leukemia, lymphoma; especially T-cell lymphoma/leukemia and Burkitt's lymphoma.
- Dehydration is an extremely common cause of slight increases of calcium.
- Sarcoidosis (a fraction of patients have high serum calcium; usually without low serum phosphorus). More have hypercalciuria.
- Chronic hypervitaminosis D. Vitamin A intoxication, isotretinoin (a vitamin A derivative).
- Prolonged immobilization (probably uncommon), in patient with increased bone turnover (eg, Paget's disease of bone, malignancy, children).
- TB, histoplasmosis, coccidioidomycosis, berylliosis
- Milk-alkali syndrome: prolonged use of calcium-containing materials and alkali (eg, $CaCO_3$ or other absorbable alkali ulcer remedies with high milk intake – now rare).
- Idiopathic hypercalcemia of infancy (uncommon)
- Endocrine: hyperthyroidism; Addison's disease; acromegaly; pheochromocytoma (rare cause of hypercalcemia)
- Advanced chronic liver disease
- Bacteremia
- Familial hypocalciuric hypercalcemia (dominant inheritance); the best test for familial benign hypercalciuria (FBH) is a plot of fasting serum PTH against fasting urine calcium excretion
- Aluminum induced renal osteomalacia

(Continued)

Calcium, Serum *(Continued)*

- Rhabdomyolysis
- Several commonly used drugs cause *in vivo* elevation, including calcium salts, lithium, thiazide/chlorthalidone therapy, other diuretics; vitamins D and A and estrogens (rapid increase in patients with breast carcinoma). Hydralazine can interfere with the calcium assay resulting in a false elevation.

In any case of hypercalcemia, it is desirable to measure magnesium and potassium levels. A helpful mnemonic for the differential diagnosis of the more common causes of hypercalcemia is DCHIMPS (drugs, cancer, hyperparathyroidism, intoxication with vitamin D or A, milk alkali syndrome, Paget's disease of bone, sarcoidosis).

Causes of low calcium:

- Low albumin and low total protein relate to common, usually slight decreases of calcium. The routine method measures **total** calcium, about half of which is bound to plasma proteins. Since the metabolically active form of calcium is the ionized state, the patient's serum protein level should be considered when interpreting a calcium result. For example, a patient's ionized calcium may be normal when the total calcium is elevated in the presence of elevated proteins and, conversely, may also be normal when the total calcium is low and the proteins are low.
- High phosphorus: renal insufficiency, hypoparathyroidism, pseudohypoparathyroidism
- Vitamin D deficiency, rickets, osteomalacia (Alkaline phosphatase is a screening test for osteomalacia. Calcium, phosphorus, and alkaline phosphatase can all be normal in osteomalacia.)
- Milkman's syndrome
- Malabsorption or malnutrition with interference with vitamin D and/or calcium absorption
- Renal tubular acidosis
- Pancreatitis, acute
- Dilutional: I.V. fluids
- Bacteremia
- Hypomagnesemia
- Anticonvulsants and other common drugs, most by *in vivo* action, can depress calcium. Barbiturates in elderly may cause calcium decrease; other drugs including calcitonin, corticosteroids, gastrin, glucagon, glucose, insulin, magnesium salts, methicillin, and tetracycline in pregnancy. Salicylates, heparin, or sulfisoxazole can interfere with the assay, thus resulting in a false depression.

The differential diagnosis is shown in a graph presented in the listing Parathyroid Hormone, in which PTH is plotted against calcium.

Limitations Sodium citrate, EDTA, and NaF/potassium oxalate interfere. Gross hemolysis falsely elevates results.

Methodology Cresolphthalein complexone; complexone is required to minimize effect of hemolysis; atomic absorption (AA) is not used extensively, but remains the reference method.

Additional Information In the differential diagnosis of hypercalcemia serum calcium should be measured on at least three occasions. In **primary hyperparathyroidism** (HPT), parathyroid hormone, serum chloride, and urine calcium are increased. Rarely, in HPT the hypercalcemia is accompanied by a low-normal PTH. In HPT, calcium rises, then phosphorus falls, then alkaline phosphatase rises. Alkaline phosphatase is usually not more than twice its upper limit in HPT. Measured ionized calcium and calculated ionized calcium may be helpful.

Twenty-four hour urinary calcium is increased in HPT, low in **familial hypocalciuric hypercalcemia** (FHH) which is characterized by hypercalcemia and hypocalciuria. An autosomal dominant, it apparently has no complications. Ratio of renal calcium clearance to creatinine clearance <0.01 suggests this genetic disease. The calcium/creatinine clearance ratio is said to discriminate between FHH and hyperparathyroidism. Family studies are highly desirable.

Hypocalcemia, then hypercalcemia occur with rhabdomyolysis – induced acute renal failure.

Specific References

Aderka D, Schwartz D, Dan M, et al, "Bacteremic Hypocalcemia. A Comparison Between the Calcium Levels of Bacteremic and Nonbacteremic Patients With Infection," *Arch Intern Med*, 1987, 147(2):232-6.

Balland M and Trivin F, "Total Calcium," *Drug Effects on Laboratory Test Results Analytical Interferences and Pharmacological Effects*, Siest G and Galteau MM, eds, Littleton, MA: PSG Publishing Co Inc, 1988, 148-64.

Bourke E and Delaney V, "Assessment of Hypocalcemia and Hypercalcemia," *Clin Lab Med*, 1993, 13(1):157-81.

Broadus AE, Mangin M, Ikeda K, et al, "Humoral Hypercalcemia of Cancer: Identification of a Novel Parathyroid Hormone-Like Peptide," *N Engl J Med*, 1988, 319(9):556-63.

Budayr AA, Nissenson RA, Klein RF, et al, "Increased Serum Levels of a Parathyroid Hormone-like Protein in Malignancy-Associated Hypercalcemia," *Ann Intern Med*, 1989, 111(10):807-12.

Cadeau BJ and MacKay JS, "Serum Calcium: Review of Methods," *ASCP Check Sample®*, Chicago, IL: American Society of Clinical Pathologists, 1988.
Chasan SA, Pothel LR, and Huben RP, "Management and Prognostic Significance of Hypercalcemia in Renal Cell Carcinoma," *Urology*, 1989, 33(3):167-70.
Gerhardt A, Greenberg A, Reilly JJ Jr, et al, "Hypercalcemia: A Complication of Advanced Chronic Liver Disease," *Arch Intern Med*, 1987, 147(2):274-7.
Jayabose S, Iqbal K, Newman L, et al, "Hypercalcemia in Childhood Renal Tumors," *Cancer*, 1988, 61(4):788-91.
Klee GG, Kao PC, and Heath H 3d, "Hypercalcemia," *Endocrinol Metab Clin North Am*, 1988, 17(3):573-600.
Ladenson JH and Bowers GN Jr, "Free Calcium in Serum. I. Determination With the Ion-Specific Electrode, and Factors Affecting the Results," *Clin Chem*, 1973, 19(6):565-74.
Lobaugh B, Neelon FA, Oyama H, et al, "Circadian Rhythms for Calcium, Inorganic Phosphorus, and Parathyroid Hormone in Primary Hyperparathyroidism: Functional and Practical Considerations," *Surgery*, 1989, 106(6):1009-16.
Sanchez GJ, Venkataraman PS, Pryor RW, et al, "Hypercalcitoninemia and Hypocalcemia in Acutely Ill Children: Studies in Serum Calcium, Blood Ionized Calcium, and Calcium-Regulating Hormones," *J Pediatr*, 1989, 114(6):952-6.
Walter RM Jr and Greenberg BR, "Hypercalcemia in the Accelerated Phase of Chronic Myelogenous Leukemia," *Cancer*, 1980, 46(5):1174-8.
Zaloga GP, Chernow B, and Eil C, "Hypercalcemia and Disseminated Cytomegalovirus Infection in the Acquired Immunodeficiency Syndrome," *Ann Intern Med*, 1985, 102(3):331-3.

Cannabinoid Confirmation

Test Includes Confirmation of positive screen test; measurement of THC-9-carboxy metabolite by gas chromatography/mass spectrometry.

Specimen Random urine

Volume 50 mL aliquot

Minimum Volume 25 mL

Container Plastic urine container

Collection Freshly voided random urine

Storage Instructions Refrigerate or freeze specimen.

Reference Range Levels >10 ng/mL reported as confirmed positive

Use Confirm positive screen result by an alternate, specific method

Limitations Limit of detection for THC-9-carboxy metabolite is 10 ng/mL.

Methodology Gas chromatography/mass spectrometry (GC/MS)

Additional Information A marijuana cigarette is made from the dried particles of the plant, *Cannabis sativa*. The immediate effects of smoking marijuana include a faster heartbeat and pulse rate, bloodshot eyes, and a dry mouth and throat. The drug can impair or reduce short-term memory, alter sense of time and reduce the ability to do things which require concentration, swift reactions and coordination, such as driving and operating machinery.

A positive screen for cannabinoids indicates the presence of cannabinoid metabolites (11-nor-9-carboxy-delta-9-THC is the major one) in urine but is not related to source, time of exposure, amount, or impairment. Unless the screen is confirmed by GC/MS, a positive result is presumptive and an unconfirmed screen should not be used to test employees.

Specific References

Congost M, de la Torre R, and Segura J, "Optimization of the Quantitative Analysis of the Major Cannabis Metabolite (11-nor-9-COOH-delta 9-tetrahydrocannabinol) in Urine by Gas Chromatography/Mass Spectrometry," *Biomed Environ Mass Spectrom*, 1988, 16(1-12):367-72.
Wimbish GH and Johnson KG, "Full Spectral GC/MS Identification of Δ^9-Carboxytetrahydrocannabinol in Urine With the Finnegan ITS40," *J Anal Toxicol*, 1990, 14(5):292-5.

Cannabinoids, Qualitative

Synonyms Cannabis; Carboxy THC; Grass; Hashish; Hemp; Herb and Al; Marijuana; 11-Nor-9-Carboxy-Delta-9-Tetrahydrocannabinol; Pot; THC (Delta-9-Tetrahydrocannabinol); Weed

Abstract The main active ingredient of marijuana (cannabinoids) is tetrahydrocannabinol (THC). It is metabolized to THC-carboxylic acid which is detected in the urine. The name comes from the source of marijuana, the plant *Cannabis sativa*. It is a DEA schedule I drug and a widely used drug of abuse.

Specimen Random urine

Volume 20 mL

Minimum Volume 10 mL

Container Plastic urine container

Collection For employee screening or forensic purpose, use precautions during collection.

Causes for Rejection Evidence of urine dilution or alteration

Special Instructions If forensic, use chain-of-custody protocol and form.

Reference Range Negative (less than cutoff)

Critical Values Cutoff: screen (NIDA): 100 ng/mL. Some laboratories use 50 ng/mL and a few use 20 ng/mL; confirmation: 15 ng/mL.

(Continued)

Cannabinoids, Qualitative *(Continued)*

Use Drug abuse evaluation; toxicity assessment

Limitations Cannabinoids are rapidly metabolized from blood. Urine is the best specimen for screening although blood (serum or plasma) and saliva have been used. Cannabinoids can adhere to plastic.

Methodology Enzyme immunoassay (EIA), fluorescence polarization immunoassay (FPIA), thin-layer chromatography (TLC), gas chromatography/mass spectrometry (GC/MS)

Additional Information A positive screen for cannabinoids indicates the presence of cannabinoid metabolites, 11-nor-9-carboxy-delta-9-THC is the major one (carboxy THC), in urine but is not related to source, time of exposure, amount, or impairment. Unless the screen is confirmed by GC/MS, a positive result is presumptive and an unconfirmed screen should not be used to test employees. Urine may contain carboxy THC for a week or 10 days after light or moderate use and as long as a month to 6 weeks after heavy use. Elimination half-life of carboxy THC is 35-40 hours. Rapid storage of THC metabolites in body fat occurs after use. These substances are then released from storage sites slowly over time.

A marijuana cigarette is made form the dried particles of the plant, *Cannabis sativa*. The immediate effects of smoking marijuana include a faster heartbeat and pulse rate, bloodshot eyes, and a dry mouth and throat. The drug can impair or reduce short-term memory, alter sense of time, and reduce the ability to do things which require concentration, swift reactions and coordination, such as driving and operating machinery.

While positive urine FPIA screen virtually will not occur due to passive inhalation at a cutoff of 100 ng/mL, there may be positive EMIT screen in children at threshold of 10 ng/mL.

Driving experiments show that marijuana affects a wide range of skills needed for safe driving. Thinking and reflexes are slowed, making it hard for drivers to respond to sudden unexpected events. Furthermore, a driver's ability to "track" through curves, brake quickly, and maintain speed and proper distance between vehicles is affected. Research shows that these skills are impaired for at least 4-6 hours after smoking a single marijuana cigarette. If a driver drinks alcohol along with using marijuana, the risks of a vehicular collision greatly increase.

Small amounts of hypochlorite (household bleach: 8-64 μL/mL of urine) can cause a significant decrease in cannabinoid urinary level as measured by immunoassay and GC/MS

Tolmetin may give false-negative results by EMIT® assay.

Specific References

Baiker C, Serrano L, and Lindner B, "Hypochlorite Adulteration of Urine Causing Decreased Concentration of Δ^9-THC-COOH by GC/MS," *J Anal Toxicol*, 1994, 18(2):101-3.

Bhushan V, Ng S, Spiller D, et al, "Detecting Children's Passive Exposure to Cocaine and Marijuana," *Am J Public Health*, 1994, 84(4):675-6.

Chiang CN and Barnett G, "Marijuana Pharmacokinetics and Pharmacodynamics," *Cocaine, Marijuana, Designer Drugs: Chemistry, Pharmacology and Behavior*, Redda KK, Walker CA, and Barnell G, eds, Boca Raton, FL: CRC Press, 1989, 113-26.

Congost M, de la Torre R, and Segura J, "Optimization of the Quantitative Analysis of the Major Cannabis Metabolite (11-nor-9-COOH-delta 9-tetrahydrocannabinol) in Urine by Gas Chromatography/Mass Spectrometry," *Biomed Environ Mass Spectrom*, 1988, 16(1-12):367-72.

ElSohly MA and ElSohly HN, "Marijuana: Analysis and Detection of Use Through Urinalysis," *Cocaine, Marijuana, Designer Drugs: Chemistry, Pharmacology and Behavior*, Redda KK, Walker CA, and Barnett G, eds, Boca Raton, FL: CRC Press, 1989, 145-62.

Hailer M, Glienke Y, Schwab IM, et al, "Modification and Evaluation of Abuscreen On Line Assays for Drug Metabolites in Urine Performed on a COBAS FARA 11 in Comparison With EMIT® d.a.u. Cannabinoid 20," *J Anal Toxicol*, 1995, 19:99-103.

Hawks RL and Chiang CN, "Examples of Specific Drug Assays: Marijuana/Cannabinoids," *Urine Testing for Drugs of Abuse*, NIDA Research Monograph 73, Rockville, MD, 1986, 85-92.

Joseph R, Dickerson S, Willis R, et al, "Interference by Nonsteroidal Anti-inflammatory Drugs in EMIT® and TDx® Assays for Drugs of Abuse," *J Anal Toxicol*, 1995, 19:13.

Kudo K, Nagata T, Kumura K, et al, "Sensitive Determination of Delta-9-Tetrahydrocannabinol in Human Tissues by GC-MS," *J Anal Toxicol*, 1995, 19:87-90.

Schucket MA, "Cannabinols," *Drug and Alcohol Abuse*, New York, NY: Plenum, 1989, 143-57.

Wells DJ and Barnhill MT Jr, "Comparative Results With Five Cannabinoid Immunoassay Systems at the Screening Threshold of 100 Micrograms/L," *Clin Chem*, 1989, 35(11):2241-3.

Wimbish GH and Johnson KG, "Full Spectral GC/MS Identification of Δ^9-Carboxytetrahydrocannabinol in Urine With the Finnegan ITS40," *J Anal Toxicol*, 1990, 14(5):292-5.

Zuckerman B, Frank DA, Hingson R, et al, "Effects of Maternal Marijuana and Cocaine Use on Fetal Growth," *N Engl J Med*, 1989, 320(12):762-8.

Cannabis *see* Cannabinoids, Qualitative *on previous page*

Carbamates, Quantitative, Serum *see* Cholinesterase Inhibitors, Quantitative, Serum *on page 1230*

Carbamazepine-10,11-Epoxide

Related Information

Carbamazepine, Blood *on this page*

Synonyms Carbamazepine Metabolite

Test Includes Carbamazepine and carbamazepine-10,11-epoxide

Abstract Occasional cases of carbamazepine toxicity occur with normal levels of carbamazepine due to accumulation of the active metabolite, 10,11-epoxide.

Specimen Blood

Volume 7 mL

Minimum Volume 1 mL serum

Container Red top tube

Reference Range 0.8-3.2 mg/L. High level: In patients on chronic carbamazepine therapy, the addition of valpromide or progabide produces clinical toxicity with high levels of metabolite and normal levels of parent compound.

Limitations Valproic acid, a compound chemically related to valpromide, may increase the epoxide/carbamazepine ratio by eliminating excretion of the epoxide. Since most cases of fatal valproate hepatotoxicity occur in young children on multiple anticonvulsants, the combination of valproate and carbamazepine is not recommended. Phenytoin may also increase the ratio of epoxide/parent compound.

Methodology High performance liquid chromatography (HPLC), fluorescence polarization immunoassay (FPIA); enzyme multiplied immunoassay (EMIT)

Additional Information Carbamazepine-10,11-epoxide has been shown to be pharmacologically active in animals.

Specific References

Bonato PS, Lanchote VL, de Carvalho D, et al, "Measurement of Carbamazepine and its Main Biotransformation Products in Plasma by HPLC," *J Anal Toxicol*, 1992, 16(2):88-92.

Contin M, Riva R, Albani F, et al, "Determination of Total and Free Plasma Carbamazepine Concentration by Enzyme Multiplied Immunoassay: Interference With the 10,11-Epoxide Metabolite," *Ther Drug Monit*, 1985, 7(1):46-50.

Monaco F and Piredda S, "Carbamazepine 10,11-Epoxide Determined by EMIT Carbamazepine Reagent," *Epilepsia*, 1980, 21(5):475-7.

Carbamazepine, Blood

Related Information

Carbamazepine-10,11-Epoxide *on this page*

Synonyms Tegretol®

Applies To P-450 System Inhibitor

Abstract Carbamazepine is a first-line antiepileptic drug for generalized and partial seizures. It is used for control of pain in trigeminal neuralgia and in treatment of bipolar affective disorder.

Patient Preparation Levels should be drawn before next oral dose with patient at steady-state.

Specimen Blood

Volume 5 mL

Minimum Volume 1 mL serum

Container Red top tube

Sampling Time A consistent sampling time, ideally a trough level, should be used to monitor patients on chronic therapy.

Reference Range 6-12 μg/mL (SI: 25-51 μmol/L). Low level: The most common cause of a low level is noncompliance. The addition of anticonvulsants which induce the P-450 system, such as phenytoin, primidone, and phenobarbital, may decrease carbamazepine levels without causing seizures. (The P-450 system is a liver enzymatic system which degrades drugs.) The withdrawal of phenytoin from the regimen of a patient on carbamazepine may lower the level and cause seizures. Because of autoinduction of metabolism, patients in the first 2 months of therapy may have diminishing levels and be at risk for seizures. Occasionally, patients may have toxicity when levels are within the reference range. High level: Drugs which inhibit the P-450 system, including isoniazid, fluoxetine, propoxyphene, verapamil, and stiripentol can cause a precipitous rise in carbamazepine levels and clinical toxicity, usually within 48 hours. Danazol may cause a delayed toxicity. The addition of cimetidine, erythromycin, lithium, triacetyloleandomycin, and valproic acid also can cause toxicity.

Critical Values Toxic: >20 μg/mL

Possible Panic Range Central nervous system toxicity occurs progressively with levels near or above high end of reference range.

Use Monitor for compliance, efficacy, or possible toxicity

Limitations See Carbamazepine-10,11-Epoxide listing.

Contraindications Half-life of warfarin is shortened; monoamine oxidase inhibitors not recommended.

Methodology Enzyme immunoassay (EIA), gas-liquid chromatography (GLC), high performance liquid chromatography (HPLC)

Additional Information Leukopenia may be dose related and necessitates stopping the drug if the absolute neutrophil count falls <1000/mm^3. Hyponatremia may

(Continued)

Carbamazepine, Blood *(Continued)*

occur, especially in older patients. Patients in the first month of pregnancy are at increased risk of neural tube defects. Carbamazepine may interfere with the actions of theophylline, oral contraceptives, oral anticoagulants, or doxycycline.

Specific References

Bertilsson L and Tomson T, "Clinical Pharmacokinetics and Pharmacological Effects of Carbamazepine and Carbamazepine-10, 11-Epoxide. An Update," *Clin Pharmacokinet*, 1986, 11(3):177-98.

Grimsley SR, Jann MW, Carter JG, et al, "Increased Carbamazepine Concentrations After Fluoxetine Coadministration," *Clin Pharmacol Ther*, 1991, 50(1):10-5.

Levy RH, Dreifuss FE, Mattson RH, et al, *Antiepileptic Drugs*, 3rd ed, New York, NY: Raven Press, 1989.

Perry PJ, Alexander B, and Liskow BI, *Psychotropic Drug Handbook*, Cincinnati, OH: Harvey Whitney Books, 1988.

Carbamazepine, Free

Synonyms Tegretol®, Free

Test Includes Free and total carbamazepine

Specimen Blood

Volume 2 mL

Minimum Volume 1 mL

Container Red top tube

Collection Draw just prior to next dose.

Reference Range Therapeutic free: 1.6-2.4 μg/mL; therapeutic total: 6.0-12.0 μg/mL

Methodology Ultrafiltrate assayed by fluorescence polarization immunoassay (FPIA)

Specific References

Contin M, Riva R, Albani F, et al, "Determination of Total and Free Plasma Carbamazepine Concentration by Enzyme Multiplied Immunoassay: Interference With the 10,11-Epoxide Metabolite," *Ther Drug Monit*, 1985, 7(1):46-50.

Carbamazepine Metabolite *see* Carbamazepine-10,11-Epoxide *on previous page*

Carbolic Acid *see* Phenol, Quantitative, Urine *on page 1321*

Carbon Dioxide, Blood

Synonyms CO_2 Content; CO_2T; TCO_2

Applies To Acid-Base Status Evaluation

Specimen Whole blood

Container Green top (heparin) tube

Collection Specimen should be kept tightly closed, as CO_2 will diffuse out, causing erroneous values. This loss may amount to 6 mmol/hour. Anaerobic conditions are best.

Reference Range Infancy to 2 years: 18-28 mmol/L (SI: 18-28 mmol/L); 2 years and older: arterial: 23-29 mmol/L (SI: 23-29 mmol/L); venous: 22-26 mmol/L (SI: 22-26 mmol/L)

Possible Panic Range <15 mmol/L (SI: <15 mmol/L), >50 mmol/L (SI: >50 mmol/L)

Use Evaluate the total carbonate buffering system in the body, acid-base balance. High results may represent respiratory acidosis with CO_2 retention, or metabolic alkalosis (eg, prolonged vomiting). Low value may indicate respiratory alkalosis as in hyperventilation or metabolic acidosis, (eg, diabetes with ketoacidosis).

Limitations Interpretation requires clinical information and the other electrolytes. Can be elevated by loop or thiazide diuretics.

Methodology Colorimetry, enzyme assay, or pCO_2 electrode. Organic acids interfere (positively) in the total carbon dioxide as measured on the Kodak Ektachem® 700.

Additional Information "Total carbon dioxide" consists of CO_2 in solution or bound to proteins, HCO_3^-, CO_3^{2-}, and H_2CO_3. In practice, 80% to 90% is present as bicarbonate (HCO_3^-). "Hypercapnia" means excessive carbon dioxide in the blood. Impaired elimination of CO_2 reflects interaction of abnormalities in respiratory drive, the muscles of respiration, and the function of the lung. Elimination of carbon dioxide from the lung involves alveolar ventilation but not dead-space ventilation. Partitioning of these spaces is expressed as a ratio between dead space and total volume per breath: the tidal volume. The tidal volume normally is <0.30. These and other aspects of pulmonary gas exchange, ventilation and their consequences are addressed as the partial pressure of arterial carbon dioxide, $PaCO_2$, a part of arterial blood gases.

Specific References

Henneman PL, Gruber JE, and Marx JA, "Development of Acidosis in Human Beings During Closed-Chest and Open-Chest CPR," *Ann Emerg Med*, 1988, 17(7):672-5.

McLain BI, Evans J, and Dear PR, "Comparison of Capillary and Arterial Blood Gas Measurements in Neonates," *Arch Dis Child*, 1988, 63(7 Spec No):743-7.

O'Leary TD and Langton SR, "Calculated Bicarbonate or Total Carbon Dioxide?" *Clin Chem*, 1989, 35(8):1697-700.
Rifai N, Hyde J, Iosefsohn M, et al, "Organic Acids Interfere in the Measurement of Carbon Dioxide Concentration by the Kodak Ektachem® 700," *Ann Clin Biochem*, 1992, 29(Pt 1):105-8.
Tietz NW, Pruden EL, and Siggaard-Andersen O, "Electrolytes, Blood Gases, and Acid-Base Balance," *Textbook of Clinical Chemistry*, Tietz NW, ed, Philadelphia, PA: WB Saunders Co, 1986, 1172-253.
Weinberger SE, Schwartzstein RM, and Weiss JW, "Hypercapnia," *N Engl J Med*, 1989, 321(18):1223-31.

Carbon Monoxide *see* Carboxyhemoglobin, Blood *on this page*

Carboxyhemoglobin, Blood

Synonyms Carbon Monoxide; CO; COHb

Test Includes COHb is sometimes included in blood gases but may be ordered as a separate test.

Patient Preparation In suspected carbon monoxide poisoning, the specimen should be collected immediately.

Specimen Blood

Minimum Volume 1 mL whole blood

Container Green top (heparin) tube or lavender top (EDTA) tube, depending upon laboratory

Sampling Time Draw before the patient is started on oxygen if possible.

Collection Keep tube capped

Storage Instructions Refrigerate immediately after collection. Do not remove cap. Carboxyhemoglobin is stable 4 months in filled, well-capped tube.

Reference Range Nonsmokers: <3%; smokers: 1-2 packs/day: 4% to 5%, >2 packs/day: 8% to 9%. Carboxyhemoglobin in the **newborn** may run to 10% to 12%. Carbon monoxide is a metabolic product of hemoglobin catabolism. The increased turnover of hemoglobin in the newborn together with decreased efficiency of the infant's respiratory system may and does lead to higher levels of carboxyhemoglobin. Venous and arterial samples are equivalent.

Critical Values Toxic concentration is 20%; lethal is >40%

Possible Panic Range Disturbance of judgment, headache, and dizziness occur at 10% to 30%; coma at 50% to 60%; fatality occurs at ≥60%, and rapid death at level of 80%.

Use Determine the extent of carbon monoxide poisoning, toxicity; check on the effect of smoking on the patient; work up headache, irritability, nausea, vomiting, vertigo, dyspnea, collapse, coma, convulsions; work up persons exposed to fires and smoke inhalation

Limitations Carbon monoxide levels are of limited value in screening for smoking, since it is cleared rapidly. The half-life of carboxyhemoglobin in individuals with normal cardiopulmonary function is 1-2 hours on 100% oxygen. Urinary nicotine, if available, is preferable as a screening test for tobacco use. Arterial blood gases may be of limited value in treatment decisions for carbon monoxide poisoning. Pulse oximetry is of no use.

Methodology Spectrophotometric, gas-liquid chromatography (GLC), pulse oximetry

Additional Information Carboxyhemoglobin is useful in judging the extent of carbon monoxide toxicity and in considering the effect of smoking on the patient. A direct correlation has been claimed between CO level and symptoms of atherosclerotic diseases, intermittent claudication, angina, and myocardial infarction. Exposure may occur not only from smoking but also from garage exposure and from various engines. This test may be included when blood gases are ordered, when there is sufficient sample, and when such instrumentation is available.

A danger of missed diagnosis of CO intoxication is continued exposure of the patient and others to a toxic environment. The cherry red color of CO poisoning is not consistently seen. CO intoxication may contribute to the risk of myocardial infarction.

A strong correlation is present between carboxyhemoglobin levels and psychometric testing abnormalities. Psychometric testing measures actual neurologic disability and may therefore better define carboxyhemoglobin poisoning severity than blood CO level. The half-life with O_2 administration is 80 minutes. With O_2 at three atmospheres, the half-life is 24 minutes.

Also elevated in methylene chloride intoxications due to endogenous hepatic metabolism to carbon monoxide.

Specific References

Fechner GG and Gee DJ, "Study on the Effects of Heat on Blood and on the Postmortem Estimation of Carboxyhemoglobin and Methaemoglobin," *Forensic Sci Int*, 1989, 40(1):63-7.
Heckerling PS, Leikin JB, Maturen A, et al, "Screening Hospital Admissions From the Emergency Department for Occult Carbon Monoxide Poisoning," *Am J Emerg Med*, 1990, 8(4):301-4.
Krantz T, Thisted B, Strøm J, et al, "Acute Carbon Monoxide Poisoning," *Acta Anaesthesiol Scand*, 1988, 32(4):278-82.

(Continued)

Carboxyhemoglobin, Blood *(Continued)*

Thom SR and Keim LW, "Carbon Monoxide Poisoning: A Review Epidemiology, Pathophysiology, Clinical Findings, and Treatment Options Including Hyperbaric Oxygen Therapy," *J Toxicol Clin Toxicol*, 1989, 27(3):141-56.

Touger M, Gallagher EJ, and Tyrell J, "Relationship Between Venous and Arterial Carboxyhemoglobin Levels in Patients With Suspected Carbon Monoxide Poisoning," *Ann Emerg Med*, 1995, 25:481-3.

Variend S and Forrest AR, "Carbon Monoxide Concentrations in Infant Deaths," *Arch Dis Child*, 1987, 62(4):417-8.

Zijistra WG, Buursma A, and Meeuwsen-van-der-Roest WP, "Absorption Spectra of Human Fetal and Adult Oxyhemoglobin, Deoxyhemoglobin, Carboxyhemoglobin, and Methemoglobin," *Clin Chem*, 1991, 37(9):1633-8.

Carboxy THC *see* Cannabinoids, Qualitative *on page 1217*

Cardiogram, Electro *see* Electrocardiography *on page 1253*

Cardioquin® *see* Quinidine, Serum *on page 1344*

Carisoma® *see* Carisoprodol, Quantitative *on this page*

Carisoprodol, Quantitative

Synonyms Carisoma®; Flexartal®; Mioxom®; Rela®; Soma®

Specimen Blood

Volume 10 mL

Minimum Volume 3 mL serum

Container Red top tube

Collection Collect specimen immediately prior to next dose unless specified otherwise by physician.

Storage Instructions Refrigerate blood.

Reference Range Therapeutic: 10-40 μg/mL

Critical Values Toxic: ≥60 μg/mL

Use Monitor therapeutic drug level; evaluate toxicity

Limitations Does not include meprobamate metabolite

Methodology Gas chromatography (GC), gas chromatography/mass spectrometry (GC/MS)

Additional Information Carisoprodol is a propanediol derivative used as a skeletal muscle relaxant. It is rapidly absorbed from the GI tract; therapeutic effects usually appear within 30 minutes. The plasma half-life is approximately 8 hours. Carisoprodol has a low incidence of toxicity and adverse effects include drowsiness, dizziness, tachycardia, postural hypotension, hypersensitivity, and extreme weakness. Metabolized to meprobamate, hydroxymeprobamate, and their glucuronides.

Specific References

Adams HR, Kerzee T, and Morehead CD, "Carisoprodol-Related Death in a Child," *J Forensic Sci*, 1975, 20(1):200-2.

Casts, Urine *see* Urinalysis *on page 1373*

Catecholamines, Fractionation, Urine

Synonyms Free Catecholamine Fractionation, Urine

Applies To Dopamine, Urine; Epinephrine, Urine; Norepinephrine, Urine

Patient Preparation Avoid patient stress, exercise, smoking, and pain. Many drugs (reserpine and α-methyldopa, levodopa, monoamine oxidase inhibitors, and sympathomimetic amines) may interfere and should be discontinued 2 weeks prior to specimen collection. Nose drops, sinus and cough medicines, bronchodilators and appetite suppressants, α_2-agonists, calcium channel blockers, converting enzyme inhibitors, bromocriptine, phenothiazine, tricyclic antidepressants, alpha and beta blockers, labetalol may interfere. Mandelamine® interferes, but thiazides do not. Caffeine products should be avoided before and during collection. The patient should not be subjected to hypoglycemia or exertion. Increased intracranial pressure and clonidine withdrawal can also cause false-positive results.

Specimen 24-hour urine

Volume Entire collection

Container Brown urine container. Adjust to pH 4 with acetic or hydrochloric acid.

Collection 24-hour urine collection

Storage Instructions Refrigerate during and after collection.

Reference Range Adults: approximate range, urine: epinephrine: 0-20 μg/24 hours (SI: 0-118 nmol/day); norepinephrine: 15-80 μg/24 hours (SI: 89-473 nmol/day); dopamine: 65-400 μg/24 hours (SI: 384-2364 nmol/day). Ranges given here are not identical among all laboratories.

Critical Values >50 μg/24 hours (SI: >297 nmol/day) of epinephrine secretion may be the only abnormality in subjects who have the multiple endocrine adenomatosis syndrome.

Use Work up neuroblastoma; diagnose pheochromocytoma. Pheochromocytomas and occasional paragangliomas may cause persistent or paroxysmal hypertension. Work up of palpitation, severe headache, diaphoresis. Urine collections are preferred to blood sampling when there is suspicion for tumor (eg, family history of MEA II) when hypertension is not paroxysmal. Evaluate possible multiple endocrine adenomatosis type II.

Limitations False-negatives and false-positives occur. False elevation of urinary catecholamine assay can be caused by acetaminophen, chloral hydrate, erythromycin, labetalol, niacin and tetracyclines. Iodinated contrast media can cause false depression of catecholamine assay. Many interfering substances exist for fluorometric assays. Urine collections for metanephrines are among the best screening tests for pheochromocytoma. Sheps et al use urinary catecholamine fractionation as confirmation, following a metanephrine screen. Neuroblastoma is better worked up with urinary collections for HVA and VMA. MHPG (3-methoxy-4-hydroxyphenylethylene glycol) is a major metabolite of norepinephrine in the central nervous system; it is a metabolite of some neuroblastomas.

Methodology High performance liquid chromatography (HPLC) with electrochemical detection, trihydroxyindole methods after boric acid elution or resin exchange column extraction. Alumina absorption methods displayed the poorest intralaboratory precision in a CAP urine chemistry survey.

Additional Information The expression "free" in free catecholamine fractionation means unconjugated. This assay is of most value for pheochromocytoma when specimen is collected during a hypertensive episode. Since a 24-hour urine collection represents a longer sampling time than a random, or symptom-directed serum sample, and because catecholamine secretion by pheochromocytomas is intermittent, the urine test may detect some cases missed by a blood level.

Specific References

"Case Records of the Massachusetts General Hospital. Weekly Clinicopathological Exercises. Case 45-1989. A 48 Year-Old Woman With Acute Respiratory Failure and a Left Suprarenal Mass," *N Engl J Med*, 1989, 321(19):1316-29.

Cleland JG and Dargie HJ, "Arrhythmias, Catecholamines and Electrolytes," *Am J Cardiol*, 1988, 62(2):55A-9A.

Davidson DF, "Urinary Free Catecholamines-Diagnostic Application of an HPLC Technique to the Investigation of Neural Crest Tumors," *Ann Clin Biochem*, 1987, 24(Pt 5):494-9.

Graham-Pole J, Salmi T, Anton AH, et al, "Tumor and Urine Catecholamines (CATs) in Neurogenic Tumors. Correlations With Other Prognostic Factors and Survival," *Cancer*, 1983, 51(5):834-9.

Knight JA and Wu JT, "Catecholamines and Their Metabolites: Clinical and Laboratory Aspects," *Lab Med*, 1987, 18:153-8.

Landsberg L and Young JB, "Pheochromocytoma," *Harrison's Principles of Internal Medicine*, Braunwald E, Isselbacher KJ, Petersdorf RG, et al, eds, New York, NY: McGraw-Hill Inc, 1987, 1775-8.

Rosano TG, Swift TA, and Hayes LW, "Advances in Catecholamine and Metabolite Measurements for Diagnosis of Pheochromocytoma," *Clin Chem*, 1991, 37(10 Pt 2):1854-67.

Sheps SG, Jiang N-S, Klee GG, et al, "Recent Developments in the Diagnosis and Treatment of Pheochromocytoma," *Mayo Clin Proc*, 1990, 65(1):88-95.

Weaver DK and Glenn GC, "The Urine Chemistry Survey – Series 2: 5 Years Experience With and Interlaboratory Comparison Program," *Arch Pathol Lab Med*, 1989, 113(7):713-22.

Weinkove C, "Measurement of Catecholamines and Their Metabolites in Urine," *J Clin Pathol*, 1991, 44(4):269-75.

CBC *see* Complete Blood Count *on page 1236*

Cd, Blood *see* Cadmium, Blood *on page 1213*

Cd, Hair *see* Cadmium, Hair *on page 1213*

Cd, Urine *see* Cadmium, Urine *on page 1214*

Celontin® *see* Methsuximide, Blood *on page 1298*

Cephalin Flocculation *replaced by* Aspartate Aminotransferase *on page 1199*

Cerebrospinal Fluid Methotrexate *see* Methotrexate, Blood *on page 1297*

Chain-of-Custody Protocol

Synonyms Specimen Chain-of-Custody Protocol

Applies To Medical Legal Specimens

Abstract A procedure to ensure sample integrity from collection through transport, receipt, sampling, and analysis. It is associated with a chain-of-custody form.

Causes for Rejection Sample cup or bag containing sample cup not sealed

Reference Range Normal: all seals intact and Chain-of-Custody form completed.

Use Chain-of-custody is a legal term that describes a method to maintain sample integrity in the collection, handling, and storage of urine samples.

Additional Information The chain-of-custody protocol is a clerical and custodial service offered by the laboratory to document specimen transfer and provide for extended specimen storage. A written record of specimen transfer from patient,

(Continued)

Chain-of-Custody Protocol *(Continued)*

to analyst, to storage and disposal is maintained on all specimens covered by chain-of-custody. All drug screens, blood alcohols, or any other tests that have medicolegal significance should be accompanied by Chain-of-Custody form and a written release form. (Department of Transportation collections or any collection involving Medical Review officers.)

Specific References

Smith ML, Bronner WE, Shimomura ET, et al, "Quality Assurance in Drug Testing Laboratories," *Clin Lab Med*, 1990, 10(3):503-16.

Chest Films

Synonyms CXR; PA; PA and Lateral CXR

Test Includes PA and lateral exposures of the chest. Sagel and his colleagues published an article in 1974 questioning the efficacy of screening examinations of the chest and whether or not lateral views should be obtained. Both medical and economic factors were considered. The study was based on a review of PA and lateral views of the chest in 10,597 examinations and reached the following conclusions.

- Routine screening for hospital admission or for surgery was not warranted for patients younger than 20 years of age.
- Lateral projection could be eliminated in routine screening of patients 20-39 years of age.
- Lateral projection should be obtained at any age when disease of the chest is suspected.
- Lateral projection should be obtained in screening examinations of patients older than 40 years of age.

Patient Preparation Remove medals, lockets, and other jewelry from neck. Arrange hair, when long, high on head so that no locks hang over chest or shoulders.

Special Instructions The chest x-ray can be modified in various ways to answer specific questions. For example, while the standard PA view of the chest is obtained in full inspiration, a pneumothorax will be more readily appreciated when the film is exposed in expiration. Decubitus films are helpful in differentiating mobile fluid in the pleural space from fluid loculations or pleural thickening. A lordotic view of the chest may be helpful in evaluating the apices. Oblique views of the chest done with 45° angulation in the right anterior oblique projection and 60° angulation in the left anterior oblique projection with barium opacifying the esophagus at the time of exposure are helpful in evaluating the size of the various cardiac chambers. A standard radiographic examination of the chest in addition to the modifications mentioned may be scheduled by calling the Radiology Department.

Use Evaluate lungs and thoracic bones for presence of metastatic and primary neoplasm, infectious disease, degenerative and reactive processes, trauma, and surgical change. The chest film is also used to evaluate the heart and great vessels.

Specific References

Sagel SS, Evens RG, Forrest JV, et al, "Efficacy of Routine Screening and Lateral Chest Radiographs in a Hospital-Based Population," *N Engl J Med*, 1974, 291(19):1001-4.

Chloral Hydrate, Plasma

Synonyms Noctec®, Plasma; Trichloroethanol, Plasma

Specimen Blood

Volume 10 mL

Minimum Volume 1 mL plasma

Container Gray top (sodium fluoride) tube

Storage Instructions Separate plasma and refrigerate.

Reference Range Therapeutic: 2-12 μg/mL

Critical Values Toxic: >100 μg/mL

Use Monitor therapeutic drug level; evaluate toxicity

Methodology Gas-liquid chromatography (GLC)

Additional Information Chloral hydrate is used as a short-term sedative and hypnotic (2 weeks), for sedation pre- and postsurgery, and to decrease drug and alcohol withdrawal symptoms. Rapidly absorbed, the hypnotic dose produces sleep within 30 minutes to 1 hour. The plasma half-life is 8-11 hours. Adverse reactions include nausea, vomiting, diarrhea, dizziness, headache, urticaria, leukopenia, and eosinophilia.

Chloral Hydrate, Qualitative, Urine

Synonyms Aquachloral®, Urine; Trichloroacetic Acid, Urine; Trichloroethanol, Urine; Trichloroethylene, Urine

Specimen Random urine

Volume 25 mL

Minimum Volume 5 mL

Container Stoppered test tubes

Collection Random urine sample collection

Reference Range Results reported as positive or none detectable

Use Evaluate toxicity

Limitations This procedure is a rapid qualitative test to rule out the ingestion of chlorinated compounds. Therefore, it is not specific for chloral hydrate.

Methodology Difficult to detect in body fluids after normal doses; UV spectrophotometry, GC-ECD (gas chromatography-electron capture detection)

Additional Information Chloral hydrate is used as a short-term sedative and hypnotic (2 weeks), for sedation pre- and postsurgery, and to decrease drug and alcohol withdrawal symptoms. Rapidly absorbed, the hypnotic dose produces sleep within 30 minutes to 1 hour. The plasma half-life is 8-11 hours. Adverse reactions include nausea, vomiting, diarrhea, dizziness, headache, urticaria, leukopenia, and eosinophilia.

Specific References

McBay AJ, Boiling VR, and Reynolds PC, "Spectrophotometric Determination of Trichloroethanol in Chloral Hydrate Poisoning," *J Anal Toxicol*, 1980, 4(2):99-101.

Meyer E, Van Bocxlaer JF, Lambert WE, et al, "Determination of Chloral Hydrate and Metabolites in a Fatal Intoxication," *J Anal Toxicol*, 1995, 19:124-6.

Chloramphenicol, Serum

Synonyms Chloromycetin®; Mychel-S®

Abstract Chloramphenicol is an antimicrobial agent whose use has been greatly reduced in recent years because of the introduction of a wide variety of less toxic alternative agents. It is still appropriately used to treat certain rickettsial infections or penicillin-allergic patients with bacterial meningitis. Life-threatening bone marrow toxicity is not closely associated with high serum levels.

Specimen Blood

Volume 7 mL

Minimum Volume 1 mL serum

Container Red top tube or serum separator tube

Sampling Time Collect for trough level immediately before next dose; for peak level about 2 hours after oral dose, 30 minutes after I.V. dose (time to peak can be variable)

Storage Instructions Freeze processed specimen

Reference Range Therapeutic: 10-25 μg/mL (SI: 31-77 μmol/L), trough <5 μg/mL (SI: <15 μmol/L)

Critical Values Toxic: >25 μg/mL (SI: >77 μmol/L)

Use Monitor drug therapy; monitor potential toxicity

Limitations Reversible dose related bone marrow depression may occur when serum/plasma concentration >25 μg/mL (SI: >77 μmol/L). Idiosyncratic bone marrow aplasia is a rare event that usually occurs weeks to months after completing therapy, but approximately 25% occur during the course of therapy. Hematologic studies should be performed before and during therapy.

Methodology High performance liquid chromatography (HPLC), gas-liquid chromatography (GLC), immunoassay

Additional Information Chloramphenicol is an extremely effective antibacterial agent which unfortunately has both idiosyncratic and dose-related toxicities. Half-life is 1.6-3.3 hours longer in infants and patients with hepatic and renal disease. The dose related toxicity is, in adults, bone marrow suppression. "Gray syndrome," a type of circulatory collapse, occurs primarily in infants whose livers are unable to metabolize chloramphenicol effectively. Idiosyncratic aplastic anemia occurs in between 1 in 20,000 and 1 in 40,000 exposures. There are a number of chloramphenicol drug interactions since chloramphenicol can inhibit hepatic microsomal metabolism, increasing the serum concentration of phenytoin, tolbutamide, and dicumarol. Phenobarbital may be elevated in the presence of chloramphenicol.

Specific References

Baselt RC, *Analytical Procedures for Therapeutic Drug Monitoring and Emergency Toxicology*, Davis, CA: Biomedical Publications, 1980, 71-5.

de Louvois J, Mulhall A, and Hurley R, "Comparison of Methods Available for Assay of Chloramphenicol in Clinical Specimens," *J Clin Pathol*, 1980, 33(6):575-80.

Smilack JD, Wilson WR, and Cockerill FR 3d, "Tetracyclines, Chloramphenicol, Erythromycin, Clindamycin, and Metronidazole," *Mayo Clin Proc*, 1991, 66(12):1270-80.

Chlordiazepoxide, Blood

Synonyms Librax®; Librium®

Abstract This is a benzodiazepine drug used as a sedative-hypnotic (tranquilizer). It is widely prescribed.

Specimen Blood

Volume 5 mL

Minimum Volume 2 mL serum

Container Red top tube

Sampling Time Collect for trough level prior to next dose; collect for peak level 4 hours after oral dosing.

(Continued)

Chlordiazepoxide, Blood *(Continued)*

Storage Instructions Process immediately; avoid exposure to light; freeze if not analyzed immediately.

Reference Range Therapeutic: 0.1-3.0 μg/mL (SI: 0-10 μmol/L)

Critical Values Toxic (stupor): >20.0 μg/mL (SI: >77 μmol/L)

Use Monitor therapeutic drug level; determine toxic level

Methodology High performance liquid chromatography (HPLC), thin-layer chromatography (TLC), gas chromatography (GC), fluorometry

Additional Information This drug is an antianxiety agent commonly used in suicide attempts. Chlordiazepoxide is slowly absorbed and may take several hours to reach a peak plasma level. Distribution after intramuscular administration is poor. Drug half-life in blood ranges from 16-27 hours. The drug is highly (90%) protein bound. Overdosage with the benzodiazepines is frequent, but serious sequelae are rare. However, there is an additive effect when used with other CNS depressants (eg, ethanol). If a patient is comatose after a drug ingestion, chlordiazepoxide **alone** is not a sufficient explanation. Metabolism results in the production of four active metabolites, including desmethyldiazepam and oxazepam which are also metabolites of diazepam (Valium®).

Specific References

Baselt RC and Cravey RH, *Disposition of Toxic Drugs and Chemicals in Man*, 3rd ed, Chicago, IL: Year Book Medical Publishers Inc, 1989, 155.

Minder EI, "Toxicity in a Case of Acute and Massive Overdose of Chlordiazepoxide and its Correlation to Blood Concentration," *J Toxicol Clin Toxicol*, 1989, 27(1-2):117-27.

Moore CM, Sato K, and Katsumata Y, "Rapid Monitoring of Benzodiazepines in Clinical Samples by Using On-Line Column Switching HPLC," *Clin Chem*, 1991, 37(6):804-8.

Chloride, Blood

Synonyms Cl, Blood

Specimen Blood

Volume 10 mL

Minimum Volume 1 mL serum

Container Red top tube; green top (heparin) tube is acceptable but use of anticoagulants other than heparin may alter electrolyte composition.

Collection Pediatrics: Blood drawn from heelstick for capillary.

Storage Instructions Refrigerate

Reference Range Premature: 95-110 mmol/L (SI: 95-110 mmol/L); full-term: 96-106 mmol/L (SI: 96-106 mmol/L); children and adults: 97-107 mmol/L (SI: 97-107 mmol/L)

Possible Panic Range <80 mmol/L (SI: <80 mmol/L), >115 mmol/L (SI: >115 mmol/L)

Use Evaluate electrolytes, acid-base balance, water balance. Chloride generally increases and decreases with plasma or serum sodium.

Chloride is **increased** in dehydration, with ammonium chloride administration, with renal tubular acidosis (hyperchloremic metabolic acidosis), and with excessive infusion of normal saline. Differential diagnosis of acidemias and alkalemias. Chloride is higher in hyperparathyroidism than in some of the other causes of hypercalcemia, but a great deal of overlap exists.

Chloride is **decreased** with overhydration, congestive failure, syndrome of inappropriate secretion of ADH, vomiting, gastric suction, chronic respiratory acidosis, Addison's disease, salt-losing nephritis, burns, metabolic alkalosis, and in some instances of diuretic therapy.

An important use of chloride is in application of the anion gap. Consult that listing for more information.

Limitations Interference from bromide occurs in hospital patients, in some of whom bromide concentrations are detectable. Iodine can interfere with assay resulting in false elevation. Chloride is not used independently but commonly with sodium, potassium, and a measurement of carbon dioxide.

Methodology Coulometry, colorimetry, mercuric thiocyanate, ion-specific electrode (ISE)

Additional Information Like other electrolytes, chloride cannot be interpreted without clinical knowledge of the patient. A diagnostic approach to the evaluation of hyperchloremic metabolic acidosis includes use of the urinary anion gap in conjunction with measurement of plasma potassium and urinary pH.

Specific References

Batlle DC, Hizon M, Cohen E, et al, "The Use of the Urinary Anion Gap in the Diagnosis of Hyperchloremic Metabolic Acidosis," *N Engl J Med*, 1988, 318(10):594-9.

Koch SM and Taylor RW, "Chloride Ion in Intensive Care Medicine," *Crit Care Med*, 1992, 20(2):227-40.

Lowe RA, Wood AB, Burney RE, et al, "Rational Ordering of Serum Electrolytes: Development of Clinical Criteria," *Ann Emerg Med*, 1987, 16(3):260-9.

McCleane GJ, "Urea and Electrolyte Measurement in Preoperative Surgical Patients," *Anaesthesia*, 1988, 43(5):413-5.

Rehak NN and Andersen TE, "Evaluation of Gilford Chemistry Control Analyzer: Cumulative Effect of Bromide on Chloride Results," *Clin Chem*, 1989, 35(7):1538.

Rothenberg DM, Berns AS, Barkin R, et al, "Bromide Intoxication Secondary to Pyridostigmine Bromide Therapy," *JAMA*, 1990, 263(8):1121-2.

Wenk RE, Lustagarten JA, Pappas NJ, et al, "Serum Chloride Analysis, Bromide Detection, and the Diagnosis of Bromism," *Am J Clin Pathol*, 1976, 65(1):49-57.

Wrenn KD, Slovis CM, Minion GE, et al, "The Syndrome of Alcoholic Ketoacidosis," *Am J Med*, 1991, 91(2):119-28.

Chloromycetin® *see* Chloramphenicol, Serum *on page 1225*

Chlorpiprazine *see* Perphenazine, Blood *on page 1317*

Chlorpromazine *see* Methamphetamines, Urine *on page 1294*

Cholesterol

Patient Preparation To support proper interpretation of lipid analysis:

- For optimum patient condition at the time of blood drawing: no change in diet for 3 weeks, stable body weight, and fasting (no food, except water and possibly black coffee without sugar in the morning) for 12 hours.
- Posture may be a significant factor: cholesterol values may be 10% to 15% lower after 20 minutes in a recumbent position. From standing to a sitting position values are about 6% lower after 20 minutes.
- Increases of 2% to 5% in cholesterol may be seen if tourniquet is applied for 2 minutes during sampling. Emotional and physical stress may also be factors influencing cholesterol levels.
- Abstinence from alcohol for 72 hours may be desirable, but only inconclusive information is available.

Specimen Blood

Volume 1 mL

Minimum Volume 0.5 mL serum

Container Red top tube

Reference Range Sharp inconsistencies are obvious when one studies published normal ranges of serum cholesterol in the United States through the 1970s and much of the 1980s. Cholesterol levels have decreased from 1980 to 1987 in a study by the Minnesota Heart Survey.

Cord blood cholesterol: <100 mg/dL (SI: <2.59 mmol/L); >100 mg/dL (SI: >2.59 mmol/L) is indicative of type II hyperlipoproteinemia. 0-1 month: 45-100 mg/dL (SI: 1.16-2.59 mmol/L). Adults 20 years and older: Although 100-210 mg/dL (SI: 2.59-5.43 mmol/L) would be regarded as a low normal range for American adults, an increase between ages 25 and 45 of about 25 mg/dL (SI: 0.65 mmol/L) is recognized. Levels >180 mg/dL (SI: >4.65 mmol/L) are not desirable, but are commonplace in the United States. Percentile values are provided in a LRC report.

Cholesterol <115 mg/dL (SI: <2.97 mmol/L) in youthful subjects is in the 5th percentile for males, <119 mg/dL (SI: <3.08 mmol/L) for females 0-19 years. Cholesterol levels <50 mg/dL (SI: <1.29 mmol/L) are found in the Bassen-Kornzweig syndrome with triglycerides <30 mg/dL. Cholesterol levels <100 mg/dL are found in Tangier disease without low triglycerides. Each is an autosomal recessive disease. Severe liver disease, severe acute illness, and abetalipoproteinemia may lower cholesterol dramatically.

Cholesterol >240 mg/dL (SI: >6.21 mmol/L) may indicate need for dietary or other intervention. This level is excessive for young adults and even 220 mg/dL (SI: 5.69 mmol/L) is somewhat high for young adults, depending on LDL, HDL, family history, and other factors.

A national effort is underway to identify patients at risk for coronary heart disease due to elevated cholesterol levels. A key facet is standardization of cholesterol measurements traceable to the National Reference System for Cholesterol, rather than the customary instrument/method dependent "reference ranges." NBS (National Bureau of Standards) Standard Reference Material for Cholesterol in Human Serum was released to general laboratories in the first half of 1988 and has been valuable. A collaborative study between the CAP and CDC to evaluate reference materials has been of great utility in the effort to determine specific instrument bias.

Plasma cholesterol values are up to 10% lower than serum values. This difference should be considered when comparing patient values to published reference tables.

Use Evaluate risk of coronary arterial occlusion, atherosclerosis, myocardial infarction, and complications including the demise of the patient. **Increased** in primary hypercholesterolemia, secondary hyperlipoproteinemias including nephrotic syndrome, hypothyroidism, primary biliary cirrhosis, and some cases of diabetes mellitus. **Low levels** have been found in cases of malnutrition, malabsorption, hyperthyroidism, myeloma, macroglobulinemia of Waldenström, polycythemia vera, myeloid metaplasia, myelofibrosis, chronic myelocytic leukemia,

(Continued)

Cholesterol *(Continued)*

analphalipoproteinemia (Tangier disease), abetalipoproteinemia (Bassen-Kornzweig syndrome) (acanthocytosis), and in some individuals who subsequently present with carcinoma. Levy points out that the weak inverse relationship with cancer, mostly colon carcinoma, is limited to cholesterol levels <190 mg/dL (SI: <4.91 mmol/L) and is limited to men. Hypocholesterolemia may occur with sideroblastic anemia or in the thalassemias.

Cholesterol relates to coronary heart disease risk. Since premature mortality from coronary arterial disease is rampant and since cholesterol levels are available as a test which can detect a modifiable risk factor, serum cholesterol remains a critical and genuinely newsworthy topic and an important screening test. Effective intervention is available when cholesterol studies identify subjects likely to benefit, asymptomatic persons as well as those with recognized coronary disease. A report of the Lipid Research Clinics (LRC) is available with reference ranges.

Limitations Other risk factors for coronary arterial disease include hypertension, family history of premature coronary arterial disease, use of cigarettes, obesity, physical inactivity, low HDLC, diabetes mellitus, prior myocardial infarct, prior cerebrovascular or occlusive peripheral vascular disease, *vide infra*. Many heart attacks occur at levels of cholesterol considered "within normal limits." In fact, a majority of cases of heart disease are found in persons whose cholesterol levels are not worse than moderately elevated. The curves of those without and those with a coronary event heavily overlap when plotted against cholesterol levels. Random testing of TC, HDLC, and LDLC may fail to detect wide fluctuations in these levels (±20%). Variations of more than ±20% were seen in 75%, 65%, and 95% of a tested group.

Cholesterol values are altered by weight loss, pregnancy and (like HDL and apolipoproteins) acute illness, as well as by acute myocardial infarct. Inconsistencies exist between the serum cholesterol, the proportion of younger individuals who experience coronary occlusion, and the severity of atherogenesis. Nevertheless, cholesterol determinations done in good, well-standardized laboratories on samples from well subjects provide reliable information. The serum total cholesterol is insufficient as a screening tool for detection of elevated levels of low density lipoprotein cholesterol in children and adolescents.

Drugs which interfere with assays causing a false elevation include ascorbic acid, salicylates, phenothiazines, and vitamins A and D. Nitroglycerin can cause a false depression.

Methodology Enzymatic, ferric chloride-sulfuric acid, Leibermann-Burchardt reaction

Additional Information About 50% to 80% of plasma/serum cholesterol is carried as low density lipoprotein cholesterol (LDLC) (β-lipoprotein). Much of the remainder is found in HDL, with small quantities as VLDL and as chylomicrons. Cholesterol is a component of cell membranes and organelles. It is the precursor of steroid hormones.

Cholesterol is included in lipid profiles. For optimal prediction of coronary atherosclerosis, some do not regard cholesterol alone as an adequate evaluation of all adults' blood lipids. However, relationships have been shown between diet, serum cholesterol, and long-term risk of death from coronary arterial disease in middle-aged American men. Rifkind and Segal point out that male subjects in the upper quintile of cholesterol levels had more than 50% of excessive coronary events related to high cholesterol. Hyperlipoproteinemia type II (hypercholesterolemia) is recognizable at any age and can be recognized at birth from cord blood cholesterol. Cholesterol levels should not be drawn immediately after a myocardial infarct has occurred.

The National Cholesterol Education Program (NCEP) has defined a classification based on cholesterol. Unfortunately, this program did not provide age-adjusted normal ranges. Palumbo, reacting to the NCEP recommendations, wrote his opinions regarding the data and the recommendations. He went on to discuss the disconcerting lack of data on older persons. Palumbo, writing the Mayo editorial, compares proposals of the NCEP with those of the Consensus Conference of 1985 for serum cholesterol levels. Dr. Palumbo recommends that "...the most prudent advice seems to be to adhere to the recommendations of the Consensus Conference of 1985" and use the 75th and 90th percentile for serum cholesterol levels based on age as guidelines. See table. Palumbo's editorial should itself be read through. He writes that there is no quibble that hyperlipidemia, especially hypercholesterolemia, is associated with an increased risk for cardiovascular morbidity and mortality and that treatment of hypercholesterolemia will reduce such risks.

"Hyperlipoproteinemia" indicates increased cholesterol and/or triglyceride. Intervention levels from the Lipid Research Clinics Data were presented by Kuske and Feldman. See table.

Male					Female				
Age (y)	Percentile				Age (y)	Percentile			
	75th		90th			75th		90th	
0–19	170	(4.40)	185	(4.80)	0–19	175	(4.50)	190	(4.90)
20–24	185	(4.80)	205	(5.30)	20–24	190	(4.90)	215	(5.55)
25–29	200	(5.15)	225	(5.80)	25–34	195	(5.05)	220	(5.70)
30–34	215	(5.55)	240	(6.20)	35–39	205	(5.30)	230	(5.95)
35–39	225	(5.80)	250	(6.45)	40–44	215	(5.55)	235	(6.05)
40–44	230	(5.95)	250	(6.45)	45–49	225	(5.80)	250	(6.45)
45–69	235	(6.05)	260	(6.70)	50–54	240	(6.20)	265	(6.85)
70+	230	(5.95)	250	(6.45)	55+	250	(6.45)	275	(7.10)

Values in mg/dL (mmol/L).

*From the Lipid Research Clinics Data, with permission. *Arch Intern Med,* 1987, 147:357–60.

Palumbo, writing an editorial in *JAMA*, emphasizes that for individuals older than 60 years intervention should be based on the judgment of the physician and patient preference. Calculating 24 million Americans eligible for antilipid medications, he discusses costs and benefits. Sempos et al also examine prevalence and project about 60 million Americans' candidacy for medical advice and intervention.

Portable chemistry analyzers have appeared in places such as shopping malls. A relevant paper addresses a perceived need for further evaluation of the instruments as well as recommendation for training of the personnel who use them regarding maintenance and quality assurance procedures. A Health and Human Services inspector general's report was reiterated by Rep Ron Wyden (D, Oregon), that the accuracy and usefulness of public cholesterol screening may be compromised by need for quality assurance, improved on site counseling and referral to a physician when appropriate, according to American Medical News. In 1993, the FDA approved a "home" cholesterol test.

Specific References

American Academy of Pediatrics Committee on Nutrition, "Indications for Cholesterol Testing in Children," *Pediatrics*, 1989, 83(1):141-2.

Anderson KM, Castelli WP, and Levy D, "Cholesterol and Mortality: 30 Years of Follow-Up From the Framingham Study," *JAMA*, 1987, 257(16):2176-80.

Austin GE, Hollman J, Lynn MJ, et al, "Serum Lipoprotein Levels Fail to Predict Postangioplasty Recurrent Coronary Artery Stenosis," *Cleve Clin J Med*, 1989, 56(5):509-14.

Bak AA and Grobbee DE, "The Effect on Serum Cholesterol Levels of Coffee Brewed by Filtering or Boiling," *N Engl J Med*, 1989, 321(21):1432-7.

Benfante R and Reed D, "Is Elevated Serum Cholesterol Level a Risk Factor for Coronary Heart Disease in the Elderly?" *JAMA*, 1990, 263(3):393-6.

Borhani NO, "Prevention of Coronary Heart Disease in Practice: Implications of the Results of Recent Clinical Trials," *JAMA*, 1985, 254(2):257-62.

Bowers GN Jr, "Accuracy and Blood Cholesterol Measurements," *Clin Chem*, 1988, 34(1):192.

Christenson RH, Roeback JR Jr, Watson TE, et al, "Improving the Reliability of Total and High-Density Lipoprotein Cholesterol Measurements. Four Testing Strategies Compared in a High-Risk Population," *Arch Pathol Lab Med*, 1991, 115(12):1212-6.

Copeland BE, "Serum Cholesterol Methodology: 100 Years of Development," *Ann Clin Lab Sci*, 1990, 20(1):1-11.

Garber AM, "Where to Draw the Line Against Cholesterol," *Ann Intern Med*, 1989, 111(8):625-7.

Garber AM, Sox HC Jr, and Littenberg B, "Screening Asymptomatic Adults for Cardiac Risk Factors: The Serum Cholesterol Level," *Ann Intern Med*, 1989, 110(8):622-39.

Goodman DS, "New Guidelines for Lowering Blood Cholesterol," *Clin Lab Med*, 1989, 9(1)17-27.

Goodman DS, Bradford RH, Brewer HB Jr, et al, "AHA Conference Report on Cholesterol. Diagnosis, Evaluation, and Treatment: Current Status and Issues," *Circulation*, 1989, 80(3):735-8.

Isles CG, Hole DJ, Gillis CR, et al, "Plasma Cholesterol, Coronary Heart Disease, and Cancer in the Renfrew and Paisley Survey," *Br Med J [Clin Res]*, 1989, 298(6678):920-4.

Iso H, Jacobs DR Jr, Wentworth D, et al, "Serum Cholesterol Levels and Six-Year Mortality From Stroke in 350,977 Men Screened for the Multiple Risk Factor Intervention Trial," *N Engl J Med*, 1989, 320(14):904-10.

Koch DD, Hassemer DJ, Wiebe DA, et al, "Testing Cholesterol Accuracy. Performance of Several Common Laboratory Instruments," *JAMA*, 1988, 260(17):2552-7.

Laemmle P, Unger L, McCray C, et al, "Cholesterol Guidelines, Lipoprotein Cholesterol Levels, and Triglyceride Levels: Potential for Misclassification of Coronary Heart Disease Risk," *J Lab Clin Med*, 1989, 113(3):325-33.

Marshall WJ and Ballantyne FC, "Clinical Topics: Current Clinical Laboratory Practice: Investigation of Plasma Lipids – Which Tests and When?" *Br Med J (Clin Res)*, 1986, 292(6536):1652-4.

McManus BM, "Reference Ranges and Ideal Patient Values for Blood Cholesterol. Can There be Reconciliation?," *Arch Pathol Lab Med*, 1986, 110(6):469-73.

(Continued)

Cholesterol *(Continued)*

McManus BM, Toth AB, Engel JA, et al, "Progress in Lipid Reporting Practices and Reliability of Blood Cholesterol Measurement in Clinical Laboratories in Nebraska," *JAMA*, 1989, 262(1):83-8.

Naito HK, "Cholesterol: Review of Methods," *ASCP Check Sample®*, Chicago, IL: American Society of Clinical Pathologists, 1988, 4:1-20.

Naito HK, "The Need for Accurate Total Cholesterol Measurement: Recommended Analytical Goals, Current State of Reliability, and Guidelines for Better Determinations," *Clin Lab Med*, 1989, 9(1):37-60.

Shekelle RB, Shryock AM, Paul O, et al, "Diet, Serum Cholesterol, and Death From Coronary Heart Disease. The Western Electric Study," *N Engl J Med*, 1981, 304(2):65-70.

Stamler J, Wentworth D, and Neaton JD, "Is Relationship Between Serum Cholesterol and Risk of Premature Death From Coronary Heart Disease Continuous and Graded? Findings in 356,222 Primary Screens of Multiple Risk Factor Intervention Trial (MRFIT)," *JAMA*, 1986, 256(20):2823-8.

Steinmetz J, Jouanel P, and Delattre J, "Total Cholesterol," *Drug Effects on Laboratory Test Results Analytical Interferences and Pharmacological Effects*, Siest G and Galteau MM, eds, Littleton, MA: PSG Publishing Co Inc, 1988, 165-84.

Vanderlinde RE, Bowers GN Jr, Schaffer R, et al, "The National Reference System for Cholesterol," *Clin Lab Med* , 1989, 9(1):89-104.

Cholinesterase, Erythrocytic *see* Acetylcholinesterase, Red Blood Cell *on page 1181*

Cholinesterase Inhibitors, Quantitative, Serum

Synonyms Carbamates, Quantitative, Serum

Test Includes Neostigmine, pyridostigmine, physostigmine

Specimen Blood

Volume 15 mL

Minimum Volume 2 mL serum

Container Red top tube

Collection Routine venipuncture

Reference Range 559-1493 units/L

Use Evaluate exposure to organophosphate and carbamate insecticides; preoperative screening of patients who are at risk for prolonged paralysis following surgical choline administration during anesthesia

Limitations May be decreased in a number of advanced chronic diseases.

Methodology UV spectrophotometry

Additional Information Organophosphate and carbamate insecticides inhibit both serum and erythrocyte cholinesterase. Serum cholinesterase falls and returns to normal more rapidly than erythrocyte levels. Decreases in activity are best evaluated by comparison to baseline levels established before exposure. Patients with atypical variants of serum cholinesterase, which are autosomal recessively inherited, may be unable to effectively hydrolyze certain muscle relaxants such as succinylcholine, which may be administered during anesthesia, resulting in prolonged paralysis. Most patients with such variants will have low plasma cholinesterase activity and resistance to dibucaine inhibition.

Cholinesterase, Serum *see* Pseudocholinesterase, Serum *on page 1340*

Chord Compliance *see* Pulmonary Compliance (Dynamic) *on page 1342*

Chromium, Serum

Related Information

Chromium, Urine *on next page*

Synonyms Cr, Serum

Patient Preparation The patient should be fasting for basal level.

Specimen Blood

Container Special metal-free, Sherwood Monoject™ trace element blood collection tube #8881-307006

Sampling Time In the nocturnal total parenteral nutrition patient, the sample will be drawn "fasting" in the afternoon, before the nocturnal solution is started for the evening.

Collection Follow specific instructions of laboratory to which sample will be submitted. Contact with steel, dust, ordinary glassware, or plastic is to be avoided. Draw blood through indwelling plastic intracath needle. Some siliconized stainless steel needles have also been found to be acceptable as is the B-D #5175 20-gauge stainless steel needle, or the Terumo or Abbot butterfly needles. Draw trace metal sample prior to any other blood samples. Remove serum with an all-plastic pipette (no internal metal parts) and store serum in plastic vial. Leeching plastic containers in 10% nitric acid for 48 hours removes trace metal contamination if special purpose vials are not available. The containers are then rinsed three times with twice distilled water and air dried in a dust-free environment prior to use.

Storage Instructions Some reference laboratories request specimens to be frozen and sent on dry ice.

Causes for Rejection Improper collection or storage with contact by steel, dust, or ordinary Vacutainer® tubes

Reference Range 0.05-0.15 ng/mL (SI: 1-3 nmol/L). Some laboratories report much higher "normals" because the methods they use or the collection technique is not adequate to prevent substantial contamination. If a laboratory reports "<1 ng/mL" or some similar figure without a lower level for normal, the value can be relied upon to discover toxic states, perhaps, but not deficiency states. Serum levels of 10 ng/mL correspond to short-term atmospheric exposure limit of 0.1 mg/m^3 of chromium trioxide. Serum levels even higher would be expected in acute systemic toxicity. Almost a twofold diurnal variation is noted in serum chromium levels, with the level highest in the morning and falling after each meal as insulin levels rise. Serum chromium levels are about 60% of normal in diabetic patients, which overlaps the normal range.

Use Evaluate suspected chromium toxicity or exposure; follow patients receiving chromium in their parenteral nutrition; evaluate acquired glucose intolerance in refeeding programs, or in parenteral or enteral nutrition; evaluate insulin resistance in the nonseptic patient during parenteral nutrition

Limitations Extreme attention to detail is needed to achieve reliable results; for many laboratories even now a high serum level more often reflects sample contamination rather than excess chromium exposure.

Methodology Any reported levels in biological materials prior to about 1979 are suspect, as the available methods did not have the sensitivity to separate normal values from the "blank." Reported levels were tenfold or more too high. Accurate and independently verified values have been reported with:

- stable isotope dilution, isotope ratio mass spectroscopy
- graphite furnace atomic absorption spectroscopy

All pipettes must have plastic tips and no exposed internal metal parts. Work is done in the laboratory under a laminar flow class 100 work station, free from exposed stainless steel to avoid airborne contamination. This is essential to reduce contamination sufficiently to detect "normal levels" in human serum or urine. Even with these precautions, different laboratories report different normal values.

Additional Information Iron competitively inhibits the binding of chromium III to transferrin. Iron overloaded patients with hemochromatosis poorly retain a radioactive tracer dose of chromium III. It has been suggested that chromium deficiency at a cellular level may play a role in the development of diabetes in hemochromatosis.

Specific References

Brown RO, Forloines-Lynn S, Cross RE, et al, "Chromium Deficiency After Long-Term Total Parenteral Nutrition," *Dig Dis Sci*, 1986, 31(6):661-4.

Hopkins LL Jr, Ransome-Kuti O, and Majaj AS, "Improvement of Impaired Carbohydrate Metabolism by Chromium 3 in Malnourished Infants," *Am J Clin Nutr*, 1968, 21(3):203-11.

Morris BW, Blumsohn A, Mac Neil S, et al, "The Trace Element Chromium – A Role in Glucose Homeostasis," *Am J Clin Nutr*, 1992, 55(5):989-91.

Schermaier AJ, O'Connor LH, and Pearson KH, "Semiautomated Determination of Chromium in Whole Blood and Serum by Zeeman Electrothermal Atomic Absorption Spectrophotometry," *Clin Chim Acta*, 1985, 152(1-2):123-34.

Veillon C, "Chromium," *Methods Enzymol*, 1988, 158:334-43.

Chromium, Urine

Related Information

Chromium, Serum *on previous page*

Synonyms Cr, Urine

Abstract Urine chromium levels are extremely low, and until recently, not reliable. Urine chromium assay is used to look for chromium toxicity in cases of potential exposure. As testing becomes more reliable, new applications of the test will arise to determine chromium III nutritional adequacy or deficiency states. There are also potential uses in the follow-up of patients with mild glucose intolerance. See listing, Chromium, Serum for signs and symptoms of toxicity and deficiency states, and for additional references.

Specimen 24-hour urine

Container Plastic metal-free container. To prepare, leech 48 hours in 10% nitric acid and wash with distilled water that has had no contact with metal. Dry in quiet air in a metal-free environment.

Collection Care must be taken to avoid contact with metal. Use plastic urinal, prepared as above. Stool contamination must be avoided.

Causes for Rejection Improper collection, contact with metal, ordinary containers, or stool contamination

Reference Range <1.8 μg/L. Levels vary with the laboratory and have declined with improved methods of avoiding contamination. Levels two- to threefold above this may reflect supplementation or excess losses. Levels elevated tenfold and higher have been seen in exposed asymptomatic tannery workers. Spot levels of

(Continued)

Chromium, Urine *(Continued)*

chromium in urine of 30 ng/g creatinine correspond to the short-term atmospheric exposure limit of 0.1 mg/m^3 of chromium trioxide in industrial exposure situations.

Use Evaluate industrial exposure, suspected toxicity; or in conjunction with serum levels, to attempt to detect suspected chromium deficiency, especially in a recent onset of glucose intolerance

Limitations Levels are so low in normal people (on the order of one part in 10 billion in urine) that many laboratories are not able to detect the lower limit of normal, and thus report "less than" some set level as being normal. Thus, for many laboratories, the test can only be used to detect toxicity. Contamination of the specimen may result in a tenfold or more increase in urine concentration being reported, making potential contamination the major limiting factor in the test.

Methodology Atomic absorption (AA) or neutron activation

Additional Information The main excretory pathway for chromium III is renal. Estimated safe and adequate, oral intake recommended by the U.S. National Academy of Sciences range from 50-200 μg/day, but in the U.S. 90% of people eat less, the mean intake being 25-33 μg/day. Such intake recommendations likely derive from the 1980s when average estimated intake was determined to be 50-100 μg/day. With increasingly accurate assays, new recommended ranges may be set lower. Absorption of chromium III is on the order of 0.5%, by radioisotope studies. One hospital pharmacy supplies 12 μg of chromium from MTE5® trace mineral parenteral nutrition supplement per day. We are unaware of a large survey.

As improved methods have progressively reduced the lower level of detection, urine chromium levels have been found to be related to glucose metabolism. Recent studies have demonstrated the metabolic relationships between serum insulin, serum glucose, and serum chromium III in the fasting and postprandial states and the relationship of the postprandial state to urine chromium concentration. Briefly, diabetic patients lose threefold more chromium in the urine than nondiabetics, and despite increased intestinal absorption, diabetic patients on ordinary diets develop and maintain lower serum levels. Chromium loss is not specifically related to micro- or macroalbuminuria and precedes the onset of diabetic nephropathy. Urine chromium rises threefold 40 minutes after a carbohydrate meal and more so with carbohydrates that stimulate higher insulin levels. Serum levels fall after a meal, more so than can be explained by urine loss. Thus, glucose stimulates insulin to take chromium to a cellular location, which favors increased renal excretion.

Chrysotherapy *see* Gold Level *on page 1270*

***Cimex* Identification** *see* Arthropod Identification *on page 1198*

CK *see* Creatine Kinase, Blood *on page 1242*

Cl, Blood *see* Chloride, Blood *on page 1226*

Clonazepam, Serum

Synonyms Klonopin™; Rivatril®

Abstract The drug is in the class of benzodiazepines which are used as tranquilizers.

Specimen Blood

Volume 10 mL

Minimum Volume 5 mL serum

Container Red top tube

Storage Instructions Separate serum and freeze. Protect from sunlight.

Reference Range Therapeutic: 10-50 ng/mL (SI: 32-158 nmol/L)

Possible Panic Range Toxic: >100 ng/mL (SI: >317 nmol/L)

Use Monitor drug level and toxicity

Methodology Gas-liquid chromatography (GLC)

Additional Information Serum peak levels occur approximately 2 hours after oral administration. The apparent half-life after a single oral dose is 20-40 hours. Active metabolites have longer half-lives than the parent drug. Half-lives are increased in the elderly. Therapeutic effect is not well correlated with serum levels. Effect of CNS depressants may be augmented by concomitant use of this agent. This drug is used as an anticonvulsant. It is useful in reducing tardive dyskinesia.

Specific References

Baselt RC and Cravey RH, *Disposition of Toxic Drugs and Chemicals in Man*, Chicago, IL: Year Book Medical Publishers Inc, 1989, 199-201.

Doran TC, "Liquid Chromatographic Assay for Serum Clonazepam," *Ther Drug Monit*, 1988, 10(4):474-9.

Lin WN, "Determination of Clonazepam in Serum by High-Performance Liquid Chromatography," *Ther Drug Monit*, 1987, 9(3):337-42.

Clorazepate, Blood

Synonyms Tranxene®

Specimen Blood

Volume 10 mL

Minimum Volume 3 mL serum
Container Red top tube
Collection Collect specimen immediately prior to next dose unless specified otherwise by physician.
Storage Instructions Separate serum and refrigerate.
Reference Range Therapeutic: 123-2175 ng/mL
Critical Values Toxic: 1000-7000 ng/mL
Use Monitor therapeutic drug level; evaluate toxicity
Limitations Severely hemolytic, lipemic, or icteric samples may cause decreased recovery and poor reproducibility.
Methodology High performance liquid chromatography (HPLC)
Additional Information Clorazepate is a psychotherapeutic drug similar to chlordiazepoxide in actions, uses, and interactions but with less side effects. It is used in the treatment of anxiety and management of alcohol withdrawal and may also be used as an anticonvulsant in the management of simple partial seizures. Clorazepate is decarboxylated in the stomach and absorbed as desmethyldiazepam, the active metabolite. Peak serum levels are achieved in 1 hour. Adverse effects of this drug include drowsiness, dizziness, headache, and nausea. Long-term use may be associated with renal or hepatic injury and a reduced hematocrit.

***Clostridium botulinum* Toxin Identification Procedure** *see* Botulism Diagnostic Procedure *on page 1211*

CN⁻ *see* Cyanide, Blood *on page 1246*

CO *see* Carboxyhemoglobin, Blood *on page 1221*

CO_2 Content *see* Carbon Dioxide, Blood *on page 1220*

CO_2T *see* Carbon Dioxide, Blood *on page 1220*

Cobalt, Serum

Related Information
Heavy Metal Screen, Blood *on page 1271*
Synonyms Co, Blood
Specimen Blood
Minimum Volume 7 mL
Container Red top tube
Storage Instructions Refrigerate serum.
Reference Range 0.4-1.0 μg/100 mL
Use Evaluate cobalt toxicity, nutritional status
Additional Information Cobalt, a metallic element, is a component of vitamin B_{12}, and is found in most foods. The daily requirement is unknown, as is deficiency in humans. Cobalt has the capacity to cause polycythemia, and for that reason, cobaltous chloride is used to successfully treat certain types of anemia. Accidental overdose of cobaltous chloride, especially in children, may lead to cyanosis, coma, and death. Cobalt dust inhaled in industrial settings may produce asthma and pulmonary symptoms. Long-term exposure may result in accumulation and cause polycythemia, goiter, cardiomyopathy, and nerve damage.

Cobalt, Urine

Related Information
Heavy Metal Screen, Urine *on page 1272*
Synonyms Co, Urine
Patient Preparation Patient should be instructed to use a plastic bedpan or urinal if necessary.
Specimen 24-hour urine
Volume Entire collection
Minimum Volume 100 mL
Container Plastic urine container, no preservative
Collection Instruct the patient to void at 8 AM and discard the specimen. Then collect all urine including the final specimen voided at the end of the 24-hour collection period (ie, 8 AM the next morning). Avoid contact with metal during collection. Screw the lid on securely. Transport the specimen promptly to the laboratory. Container **must** be labeled with patient's full name, room number, date and time collection started, and date and time collection finished.
Special Instructions Requisition **must** state date and time collection started and date and time collection finished.
Reference Range Diet dependent, normals not established
Use Evaluate cobalt toxicity
Additional Information Cobalt, a metallic element, is a component of vitamin B_{12} and is found in most foods. The daily requirement is unknown, as is deficiency in humans. Cobalt has the capacity to cause polycythemia, and for that reason, cobaltous chloride is used to successfully treat certain types of anemia. Accidental

(Continued)

Cobalt, Urine *(Continued)*

overdose of cobaltous chloride, especially in children, may lead to cyanosis, coma, and death. Cobalt dust inhaled in industrial settings may produce asthma and pulmonary symptoms. Long-term exposure may result in accumulation and cause polycythemia, goiter, cardiomyopathy, and nerve damage.

Co, Blood *see* Cobalt, Serum *on previous page*

Cocaine (Cocaine Metabolite), Qualitative

Synonyms Coke; Crack; Snow

Test Includes Cocaine is detected in urine as its metabolite, benzoylecgonine; see chart.

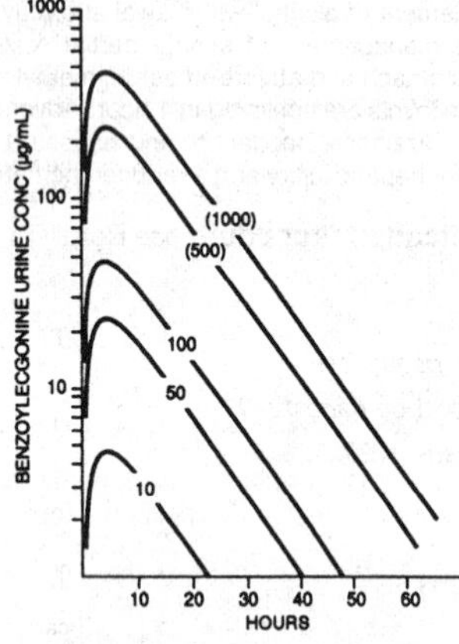

A nomogram for relating benzoylecgonine urine concentrations to the size of and time interval since the cocaine dose. The cocaine dose may be single or repeated and cumulative, if taken within a relatively short period (relative to BZ excretion) of a few hours. Extrapolate between curves for other doses. Doses of 500 mg and above are in parentheses to indicate that although kinetics are probably similar above 200 mg, there is no data available at the present time.

Reprinted with permission from Ambre J, "The Urinary Excretion of Cocaine and Metabolites," *Journ Anal Tox*, 1985, 9:245.

Abstract A prominent metabolite of cocaine is benzoylecgonine, which is the substance measured in urine to detect the presence of cocaine. Cocaine is a heavily abused drug which has legitimate medical uses in some ENT procedures.

Specimen Urine

Volume 50 mL

Minimum Volume 10 mL

Container Plastic urine container

Collection If forensic, observe precautions concerning surreptitious dilution or alteration.

Storage Instructions Refrigerate; optimal storage conditions for urine specimens with cocaine and benzoylecgonine are at 18°C and a pH of 5.0; unsilanized glass is a favorable container material

Causes for Rejection If forensic, failure to meet temperature requirements immediately after collection and/or tests for unusual dilution (specific gravity, urine creatinine) or alteration.

Special Instructions If forensic, use chain-of-custody protocol and form.

Reference Range Negative (less than cutoff)

Critical Values Cutoff: screen: 300 ng/mL; confirmation: 150 ng/mL

Use Evaluate cocaine use

Methodology Screen: immunoassay, fluorescence polarization immunoassay (FPIA), thin-layer chromatography (TLC); confirmation: gas chromatography/mass spectrometry (GC/MS)

Additional Information Cocaine is a highly abused drug which is most frequently detected in the urine as the metabolite, benzoylecgonine and usually as part of a multiclass drug panel. In pre-employment drug screening, the presence of cocaine (benzoylecgonine) should be confirmed by GC/MS.

Cocaine is a central nervous system stimulant. It usually appears as a fine crystal-like powder which is the hydrochloride or sulfate salt and as such is "snorted" (inhaled through the nose). When mixed with sodium bicarbonate and converted to free base, it appears as hard pieces called "crack" which can be smoked. This is currently a very prevalent form of the drug.

The effects of the drug begin within minutes and peak within 15-20 minutes. These effects include dilated pupils, increase in blood pressure, heart rate, breathing rate, and body temperature. The dangers of cocaine use vary, depending on how the drug is taken, the dose, and the individual. Some regular users report feelings of restlessness, irritability, anxiety, and sleeplessness. In some people even low doses of cocaine may create psychological problems. People who use high doses of cocaine over a long period of time may become paranoid or experience what is called a cocaine psychosis. This may include hallucinations of touch, sight, taste, and smell. Cocaine itself has a half-life of 1-2 hours while benzoylecgonine has a half-life of 7-9 hours. Benzoylecgonine is detectable in urine within 2-3 hours and for a period of 2-3 days after a single use.

Positive urine screen due to passive inhalation of cocaine virtually will not occur at cutoff of 300 ng/mL by FPIA, but is possible in children if test by EMIT with a cutoff of 30 ng/mL.

Ecgonine urinary levels >50 ng/mL can increase sensitivity of cocaine assays. Urine cocaine metabolites levels may be elevated after a series of sauna treatments.

Specific References

Bailey DN, "Cocaethylene (Ethylcocaine) Detection During Toxicological Screening of a University Medical Center Patient Population," *J Anal Toxicol*, 1995, 19:247-50.

Bhushan V, Ng S, Spiller D, et al, "Detecting Children's Passive Exposure to Cocaine and Marijuana," *Am J Public Health*, 1994, 84(4):675-6.

Cone EJ, "Validity Testing of Commercial Urine Cocaine Metabolite Assays: III. Evaluation of an Enzyme-Linked Immunosorbent Assay (ELISA) for Detection of Cocaine and Cocaine Metabolite," *J Forensic Sci*, 1989, 34(4):991-5.

Cone EJ, Menchen SL, Paul BD, et al, "Validity Testing of Commercial Urine Cocaine Metabolite Assays: I. Assay Detection Times, Individual Excretion Patterns, and Kinetics After Cocaine Administration to Humans," *J Forensic Sci*, 1989, 34(1):15-31.

Cone EJ and Mitchell J, "Validity Testing of Commercial Urine Cocaine Metabolite Assays: II. Sensitivity, Specificity, Accuracy, and Confirmation by Gas Chromatography/Mass Spectrometry," *J Forensic Sci*, 1989, 34(1):32-45.

Gawin FH and Ellinwood EH Jr, "Cocaine and Other Stimulants. Actions, Abuse, and Treatment," *N Engl J Med*, 1988, 318(18):1173-82.

Karch SB, "The History of Cocaine Toxicity," *Hum Pathol*, 1989, 20(11):1037-9.

Hippenstiel MJ and Gerson B, "Optimization of Storage Conditions for Cocaine and Benzoylecgonine in Urine: A Review," *J Anal Toxicol*, 1994, 18(2):104-9.

Hornbeck CL, Barton KM, and Czarny RJ, "Urine Concentrations of Ecgonine From Specimens With Low Benzoylecgonine Levels Using a New Ecgonine Assay," *J Anal Toxicol*, 1995, 19:133-8.

Lewis DE, Moore CM, Leikin JB, et al, "Meconium Analysis for Cocaine: A Validation Study and Comparison With Paired Urine Analysis," *J Anal Toxicol*, 1995, 19:148-50.

Zuckerman B, Frank DA, Hingson R, et al, "Effects of Maternal Marijuana and Cocaine Use on Fetal Growth," *N Engl J Med*, 1989, 320(12):762-8.

Codeine, Blood

Specimen Blood

Minimum Volume 20 mL

Container Gray top (sodium fluoride) tube

Storage Instructions Refrigerate

Reference Range Therapeutic: 13-33 ng/mL

Critical Values Lethal: >1000 ng/mL

Use Evaluate codeine toxicity

Methodology Radioimmunoassay (RIA), gas chromatography (GC), high performance liquid chromatography (HPLC)

Additional Information Codeine, made by the methylation of morphine, is similar to morphine in uses, actions, contraindications, and adverse reactions. Not as potent as morphine, it is used to manage mild to moderate pain. In low doses, it is an antitussive. After oral dose, the onset of action is 15-30 minutes, and peak levels are reached in 1-1.5 hours. The half-life is 2.5-4 hours. Codeine is excreted mainly in the urine as norcodeine and free and conjugated morphine. Adverse effects of codeine include miosis, increased intracranial pressure, antidiuretic hormone release, and physical and psychological dependence.

Specific References

Pearce D, Wiersema S, Kuo M, et al, "Simultaneous Determination of Morphine and Codeine in Blood by Use of Select Ion Monitoring and Deuterated Internal Standards," *Clin Toxicol*, 1979, 14(2):161-8.

Stubbs RJ, Chiou R, and Bayne WF, "Determination of Codeine in Plasma and Urine by Reversed Phase High-Performance Liquid Chromatography," *J Chromatogr*, 1986, 377:447-53.

Codeine, Urine

Related Information

Opiates, Qualitative, Urine *on page 1309*

Test Includes Part of opiate screen

Abstract Codeine occurs naturally in opium but is produced commercially by 3-O-methylation of morphine. It is used as a narcotic analgesic. It is present in numerous proprietary preparations combined with non-narcotic analgesics and antihistamines. It is a drug of abuse.

Specimen Random urine

Volume 20 mL

Minimum Volume 10 mL

Container Plastic urine container

(Continued)

Codeine, Urine *(Continued)*

Storage Instructions Refrigerate

Special Instructions If forensic, use precautions in collection and Chain-of-Custody form.

Reference Range Negative (below cutoff)

Critical Values Cutoff: screen: 300 ng/mL (for drug-of-abuse screen), confirmation: 300 ng/mL

Use Evaluate codeine toxicity; detect drug-of-abuse

Methodology Enzyme immunoassay (EIA); thin-layer chromatography (TLC)

Additional Information Codeine, made by the methylation of morphine, is similar to morphine in uses, actions, contraindications, and adverse reactions. About $\frac{1}{6}$ to $\frac{1}{10}$ as potent as morphine, it is used to manage mild to moderate pain. In low doses, it is an antitussive. After oral dose, the onset of action is 15-30 minutes, and peak levels are reached in 1-1.5 hours. The half-life is 2.5-4 hours. Codeine is excreted mainly in the urine as norcodeine and free and conjugated morphine. Adverse effects of codeine include miosis, increased intracranial pressure, antidiuretic hormone release, and physical and psychological dependence.

Urine codeine/morphine ratio is usually >1.0 during first the 24 hours postingestion, decreases <1.0 from 24-30 hours and usually only morphine is detectable after 30 hours. Poppyseed ingestion can result in urine codeine levels as high as 4.5 mg/L and urine morphine levels as high as 0.2 mg/L; urine drug screen remains positive for 2-4 days.

Specific References

Barsan W, "Narcotic Agents," *Ann Emerg Med*, 1986, 15:1019-20.

Blanke RV and Decker WJ, "Analysis of Toxic Substances," *Textbook of Clinical Chemistry*, Tietz NW, ed, Philadelphia, PA: WB Saunders Co, 1986, 1735-9.

Romberg RW and Lee L, "Comparison of the Hydrolysis Rates of Morphine-3-Glucuronide and Morphine-6-Glucuronide With Acid and Beta-Glucuronidase," *J Anal Toxicol*, 1995, 19:157-62.

COHb *see* Carboxyhemoglobin, Blood *on page 1221*

Coke *see* Cocaine (Cocaine Metabolite), Qualitative *on page 1234*

Comatose Profile *see* Toxicology Drug Screen, Blood *on page 1364*

Compazine® *see* Prochlorperazine, Blood *on page 1333*

Complete Blood Count

Synonyms Blood Cell Profile; Blood Count; CBC; Hemogram

Test Includes WBC and differential count, Hct, Hgb, RBC, WBC and RBC morphology, RBC indices, platelet estimate, platelet count, RDW, and histograms. Although RBC, WBC, and platelet histograms are not usually available on patient charts, they are helpful to the technologist in detecting problems with patients and quality control. Even though the histograms are not on the chart, they can be viewed in the laboratory along with the blood smear. New analyzers also provide automated 5-part white cell differentials: granulocytes, monocytes, lymphocytes, eosinophils, and basophils.

Abstract The standard broadly inclusive automated test for evaluation of RBC, WBC, and platelets. The majority of CBC results are generated by highly automated electronic and pneumatic multichannel analyzers based on aperture-impedance and/or laser beam cell sizing and counting (see reference by Koepke).

Specimen Whole blood

Volume 5 mL

Minimum Volume 1 mL

Container Lavender top (EDTA) tube

Collection Mix specimen 10 times by gentle inversion. If specimen is not brought to the laboratory immediately refrigeration is required. If the anticipated delay in arrival is more than 4 hours, two blood smears should be prepared immediately after the venipuncture and submitted with the blood specimen.

Causes for Rejection Improper tube, clotted specimen, hemolyzed specimen, dilution of blood with I.V. fluid

Reference Range Accompanying tables summarize differences in red cell parameter normal ranges, note especially important age and sex variances. Refer to tables.

Critical Values Critical values: Hematocrit: <18% or >54%; hemoglobin: <6.0 g/dL or >18.0 g/dL; WBC on admission: <2500/mm^3 or >30,000/mm^3; platelets: <20,000/mm^3 or >1,000,000/mm^3

Use Evaluate anemia, leukemia, reaction to inflammation and infections, peripheral blood cellular characteristics, state of hydration and dehydration, polycythemia, hemolytic disease of the newborn; manage chemotherapy decisions

Limitations Hemoglobin may be falsely high if the plasma is lipemic or if the white count is >50,000 cells/mm^3. "Spun" (manual centrifuged) microhematocrits are approximately 3% higher (due to plasma trapping) compared to automated hematocrit levels. The increase is especially pronounced in cases of polycythemia (increased Hct levels) and when the cells are hypochromic and microcytic. The spun Hct level (as compared to Coulter S) may be 12% higher at Hct levels of 70% and MCV of 48 fL with decrease in change to 3% higher at Hct levels of 70% with MCV of 100 fL. Cold agglutinins (high titer) may cause spurious macrocytosis and low RBC count. This results when RBC couplets are "seen" and processed as single cells by the detection circuitry. Keeping the blood warm and warming the diluent prior to and during counting can correct this problem.

Methodology Varies considerably between institutions. Most laboratories have high capacity multichannel instruments in place (available from multiple commercial sources). The majority measure RBC and WBC parameters on the basis of changes in electrical impedance as cells and platelets are pulled through a tiny aperture. These are highly automated devices with extensive computer processing of the electrical signals after analog/digital conversion. Accuracy (with proper standardization) and precision (usually in the 0.5% to 2% range) is significantly improved over older manual and semiautomated methods. Some instruments count light impulses that are generated as cells flow across a laser beam. Proper calibration is a prime requisite (see references by Koepke, Lewis et al, and Rowan et al).

Additional Information Presence of one or more of the following may be indications for further investigation: hemoglobin <10 g/dL, hemoglobin >18 g/dL, MCV >100 fL, MCV <80 fL, MCHC >37%, WBC >20,000/mm³, WBC <2000/mm³, presence of sickle cells, significant spherocytosis, basophilic stippling, stomatocytes,significant schistocytosis, oval macrocytes, tear drop red blood cells, eosinophilia (>10%) monocytosis (>15%), nucleated red blood cells in other than the newborn, malarial organisms or the possibility of malarial organisms, hypersegmented (five or more nuclear segments) PMNs, agranular PMNs, Pelger-Huët anomaly, Auer rods, Döhle bodies, marked toxic granulation, mononuclears in which apparent nucleoli are prominent (blast type cells), presence of metamyelocytes, myelocytes, promyelocytes, neutropenia, presence of plasma cells, peculiar atypical lymphocytes, significant increase or decrease in platelets. Some quantitative elements of the CBC are related to each other, normally, such that examination of the results of any individual analysis allow for the application of a simple but effective case individualized quality control maneuver. The RBC count, hemoglobin, and hematocrit may be analyzed by applying a "rule of three." If red cells are normochromic/normocytic, the RBC count times 3 should approximately equal the hemoglobin and the hemoglobin multiplied by 3 should approximate the hematocrit. If there is significant deviation from this relation, one should check for supporting abnormalities in RBC indices and peripheral smear. The indices themselves offer a quick quality control check of the CBC. If patient transfusion can be excluded, then RBC indices should vary little consecutively from day to day.

Anemias have been classified on the basis of their MCV and RDW (RBC heterogeneity). This classification has been especially helpful in the separation of iron deficiency from thalassemia. Heterozygous thalassemia (thalassemia minor) when associated with normal hemoglobin has a normal RDW (13.4 ±1.2%) while RDW is high with iron deficiency (16.3 ±1.8%). RDW will be increased slightly in cases of thalassemia with slight anemia. Some studies have found that the RDW does not reliably separate iron deficiency from thalassemia minor unless, possibly, a higher cutoff value of 17.0% is utilized.

In patients who do not have disorders known to result in anisocytosis (eg, liver disease, alcoholism, combined nutritional deficiency) and who have not received a recent blood transfusion, it has been claimed RDW may be helpful in separating the anemia of chronic disease (RDW in normal range) from iron deficiency (RDW in-

Red Cell Values on First Postnatal Day*

Gestational Age (wk)	24–25	26–27	28–29	30–31	32–33	34–35	36–37	Term
RBC (x 10⁶/mm³)	4.65 ±0.43	4.73 ±0.45	4.62 ±0.75	4.79 ±0.74	5.0 ±0.76	5.09 ±0.5	5.27 ±0.68	5.14 ±0.7
Hgb (g/dL)	19.4 ±1.5	19.0 ±2.5	19.3 ±1.8	19.1 ±2.2	18.5 ±2.0	19.6 ±2.1	19.2 ±1.7	19.3 ±2.2
Hct (%)	63 ±4	62 ±8	60 ±7	60 ±8	60 ±8	61 ±7	64 ±7	61 ±7.4
MCV (fL)	135 ±0.2	132 ±14.4	131 ±13.5	127 ±12.7	123 ±15.7	122 ±10.0	121 ±12.5	119 ±9.4
Retic (%)	6.0 ±0.5	9.6 ±3.2	7.5 ±2.5	5.8 ±2.0	5.0 ±1.9	3.9 ±1.6	4.2 ±1.8	3.2 ±1.4

*Mean values ± SD.

From Zaizov R and Matoth Y, "Red Cell Values on the First Postnatal Day During the Last 16 Weeks of Gestation," *Amer J Hematol,* 1976, 1:2, 275–8, with permission.

(Continued)

Mean Hematologic Values for Full-Term Infants, Children, and Adults*

Age	Hemoglobin (g/dL)	Hematocrit (%)	RBC ($10^6/mm^3$)	MCV (fL)	MCH (pg)	MCHC (g/dL)
Birth (cord blood)	17.1±1.8	52.0±5	4.64±0.5	113±6	37±2	33±1
1 d	19.4±2.1	58.0±7	5.30±0.5	110±6	37±2	33±1
2-6 d	19.8±2.4	66.0±8	5.40±0.7	122±14	37±4	30±3
14-23 d	15.7±1.5	52.0±5	4.92±0.6	106±11	32±3	30±2
24-37 d	14.1±1.9	45.0±7	4.35±0.6	104±11	32±3	31±3
40-50 d	12.8±1.9	42.0±6	4.10±0.5	103±11	31±3	30±2
2-2.5 mo	11.4±1.1	38.0±4	3.75±0.5	101±10	30±3	30±2
3-3.5 mo	11.2±0.8	37.0±3	3.88±0.4	95±9	29±3	30±2
5-7 mo	11.5±0.7	38.0±3	4.21±0.5	91±9	27±3	30±2
8-10 mo	11.7±0.6	39.0±2	4.35±0.4	90±8	27±3	30±1
11-13.5 mo	11.9±0.6	39.0±2	4.44±0.4	88±7	27±2	30±1
1.5-3 y	11.8±0.5	39.0±2	4.45±0.4	87±7	27±2	30±2
5 y	12.7±1.0	37.0±3	4.65±0.5	80±4	27±2	34±1
10 y	13.2±1.2	39.0±3	4.80±0.5	81±6	28±3	34±1
Male	15.5±1.1	46.0±3.1	5.11±0.38	—	—	—
Female	13.7±1.0	40.9±3	4.51±0.36	—	—	—
Male and female	—	—	—	90.1±4.8	30.2±1.8	33.7±1.1

*Mean ± 1 SD.

From Johnson TR, "How Growing Up Can Alter Lab Values in Pediatric Laboratory Medicine," *Diag Med* (special issue), 1982, 5:13-8, with permission.

Mean Hematologic Values for Low-Birth-Weight Infants*

Weight and Gestational Age at Birth	Age at Testing	Hemoglobin (g/dL)	Hematocrit (%)	Reticulocytes (%)
<1500 g 28-32 wk	3 d	17.5±1.5	54±5	8.0±3.5
	1 wk	15.5±1.5	48±5	3.0±1.0
	2 wk	13.5±1.1	42±4	3.0±1.0
	3 wk	11.5±1.0	35±4	—
	4 wk	10.0±0.9	30±3	6.0±2.0
	6 wk	8.5±0.5	25±2	11.0±3.5
	8 wk	8.5±0.5	25±2	8.5±3.5
	10 wk	9.0±0.5	28±3	7.0±3.0
1500-2000 g 32-36 wk	3 d	19.0±2.0	59±6	6.0±2.0
	1 wk	16.5±1.5	51±5	3.0±1.0
	2 wk	14.5±1.1	44±5	2.5±1.0
	3 wk	13.0±1.1	39±4	—
	4 wk	12.0±1.0	36±4	3.0±1.0
	6 wk	9.5±0.8	28±3	6.0±2.0
	8 wk	9.5±0.5	28±3	5.0±1.5
	10 wk	9.5±0.5	29±3	4.5±1.5
2000-2500 g 36-40 wk	3 d	19.0±2.0	59±6	4.0±1.0
	1 wk	16.5±1.5	51±5	3.0±1.0
	2 wk	15.0±1.5	45±5	2.5±1.0
	3 wk	14.0±1.1	43±4	—
	4 wk	12.5±1.0	37±4	2.0±1.0
	6 wk	10.5±0.9	31±3	3.0±1.0
	8 wk	10.5±0.9	31±3	3.0±1.0
	10 wk	11.0±1.0	33±3	3.0±1.0

*Mean ± 1 SD.

From Johnson TR, "How Growing Up Can Alter Lab Values in Pediatric Laboratory Medicine," *Diag Med* (special issue), 1982, 5:13-8, with permission.

Proposed Classification of Anemic Disorders Based on Red Cell Mean (MCV) and Heterogeneity (RDW)

MCV Low RDW Normal (microcytic homogeneous)	MCV Low RDW High (microcytic heterogeneous)	MCV Normal RDW Normal (normocytic homogeneous)	MCV Normal RDW High (normocytic heterogeneous)	MCV High RDW Normal (macrocytic homogeneous)	MCV High RDW High (macrocytic heterogeneous)
Heterozygous thalassemia*	Iron deficiency*	Normal	Mixed deficiency*	Aplastic anemia	Folate deficiency*
Chronic disease*	S/β-thalassemia	Chronic disease* chronic liver disease*†	Early iron or folate deficiency*	Preleukemia†	Vitamin B_{12} deficiency
	Hemoglobin H	Nonanemic hemoglobinopathy (eg, AS, AC)	Anemic hemoglobinopathy (eg, SS, SC)*		Immune hemolytic anemia
	Red cell fragmentation	Transfusion†	Myelofibrosis		Cold agglutinins
		Chemotherapy	Sideroblastic*		Chronic lymphocytic leukemia, high count
		Chronic lymphocytic leukemia			
		Chronic myelocytic leukemia†			
		Hemorrhage			
		Hereditary spherocytosis			

*MCV alone <90% sensitive.
†RDW alone <90% sensitive.

From Bessman JD Jr, Gilmer PR, and Gardner FH, "Improved Classification of Anemias by MCV and RDW," *Am J Clin Pathol,* 1983, 80:324, with permission. The data for sensitivity of RDW and MCV in each disease category can be obtained from the authors.

(Continued)

Complete Blood Count *(Continued)*

creased) thereby reducing the need for marrow study to determine iron stores. It has also been reported, however, on the basis of serum ferritin levels in relatively undefined patient populations that RDW is not clinically useful in distinguishing the anemia of chronic disease from iron deficiency.

Bessman claims that the RDW is increased before the MCV decreases in iron deficiency. Although this is somewhat controversial, perhaps even a simple marketing tool copied by all hematology instrument manufacturers, it serves as an inexpensive screen for the common iron deficiency anemia. See tables.

As might be anticipated, the RDW is an insensitive parameter for the diagnosis of vitamin B_{12} deficiency, as well as for the diagnosis of folate deficiency, and the RDW has no value in separating alcohol-related macrocytosis from B_{12}/folate deficiency. It has been found that in a hospitalized urban patient population, zidovudine treatment of AIDS is the most common cause of macrocytosis (44%) and B_{12}/folate deficiency are relatively decreased (3% and 4%, respectively).

Specific References

Burgess PR, Kershaw GW, Coleman RH, et al, "A Computerized Expert System for Handling the Output of the Technicon H1 Haematology Analyzer," *Clin Lab Haematol*, 1993, 15(1):21-32.

Fraser CG, Wilkinson SP, Neville RG, et al, "Biologic Variation of Common Hematologic Laboratory Quantities in the Elderly," *Am J Clin Pathol*, 1989, 92(4):465-70.

Koepke J, "Quantitative Blood Cell Counting," *Practical Laboratory Hematology*, Chapter 3, Koepke J, ed, New York, NY: Churchill Livingstone, 1991, 43-60.

Lee GR, "Microcytosis and the Anemias Associated With Impaired Hemoglobin Synthesis," *Wintrobe's Clinical Hematology*, 9th ed, Vol 1, Chapter 25, Lee GR, Bithell TC, Foerster J, et al, eds, Philadelphia, PA: Lea & Febiger, 1993, 791-807.

Lewis SM, England JM, and Rowan RM, "Current Concerns in Haematology 3: Blood Count Calibration," *J Clin Pathol*, 1991, 44(11):881-4.

Penn D, Williams PR, Dutcher TF, et al, "Comparison of Hematocrit Determinations by Microhematocrit and Electronic Particle Counter," *Am J Clin Pathol*, 1979, 72(1):71-4.

Rowan RM and England JM, "Special Aspects in Haematology," *Evaluation Methods in Laboratory Medicine*, Chapter 7, Haeckel R, ed, New York, NY: VCH Publishers, 1993, 141-51.

Second National Health and Nutrition Examination Survey, "Hematological and Nutritional Biochemistry Reference Data for Persons 6 Months-74 Years of Age: United States, 1976-80," *Vital Health Stat*, DHHS Publication No (PHS) 83-1682, 1982.

Computed Transaxial Tomography, Head Studies

Synonyms Brain, CT; Head Studies, CT

Test Includes CT scan of the brain

Patient Preparation The examination should be ordered and a requisition with information pertaining to the reason for the request and the clinical history should be completed by the referring physician. If there is the slightest possibility that intravenous contrast material will be administered, the patient's oral intake should be limited to liquids for at least 4 hours prior to the examination. Care must be taken to ensure the patient does not become dehydrated and medications should not be interrupted. A recent serum creatinine is requested on patients with preexisting renal disease, diabetes mellitus, significant atherosclerotic disease, and advancing age (60 years and older). Agitated patients and children may require sedation prior to the examination. In these cases, an order for the appropriate sedative and dose should be recently recorded within the patient's chart. Sedatives should be administered by a physician within the Radiology Department.

Equipment Any commercially available computed tomographic scanner

Technique CT scans of the head are usually obtained at 15° angulation to the orbitomeatal line, a line connecting the lateral canthus of the eye with the external auditory canal. Contiguous slices 8 or 10 mm in thickness are obtained from the vertex of the skull to the foramen magnum. The orbital roof should be included. The patient is positioned supine for the examination. The head is placed securely in a head holder. The chin is flexed comfortably towards the chest. The appropriate 15° angulation can be obtained by angulation of the gantry if necessary.

Use Evaluate known/suspected primary or secondary neoplasm, cystic lesions, hydrocephalus, head trauma, seizure disorder, multiple sclerosis, atrophy, Alzheimer's disease, normal pressure hydrocephalus, Parkinson's disease, dementia, depression, organic brain syndrome, etc

Contraindications Assuming a cooperative or quiescent patient, there are no absolute contraindications to a CT scan of the head. A decision must be taken, however, as to whether the study is to be done with or without intravenous contrast material. While each case must be assessed individually, the following broad guidelines may be helpful. Those studies indicated by virtue of a recent infarct, cerebrovascular accident or stroke, or those being done for assessment of atrophy, Alzheimer's disease, normal pressure hydrocephalus, Parkinson's disease, hydrocephalus, evaluation of an intraventricular shunt, assessment of ventricular size, subdural hematoma, or suspected dementia are examined without contrast material. Patients for whom the indication is headache, psychiatric condition (such as anorexia or bulimia), tumor follow-up, rule out tumor, rule out metastasis, multiple sclerosis, seizure disorders, depression, and organic brain syndrome are generally studied with contrast material. Patients in whom the indication is one of infection, abscess, meningitis, transient ischemic attack, arteriovenous malformation, remote subdural hematoma, or who have recently undergone a craniotomy and are being studied for postoperative evaluation are best studied with and without contrast material. Patients with a known diagnosis of plasmacytoma or multiple myeloma should not receive intravenous contrast material. Patients with compromised renal function may or may not benefit from intravenous contrast material. A recent serum creatinine and BUN will be helpful in deciding whether or not the latter group of patients receive contrast material.

Coombs' Test, Direct *see* Antiglobulin Test, Direct *on page 1195*

CO-Oximetry Arterial

Synonyms Arterial CO-Oximetry

Test Includes % carboxyhemoglobin (COHb), % methemoglobin (MetHb), % O_2Hb = oxyhemoglobin and O_2 saturation, total hemoglobin (THb), and volume % O_2 = O_2 content

Patient Preparation Patient should be supine and relaxed

Aftercare Watch for bleeding, hematoma. Ideally, extremity punctured should be kept up for 10 minutes with pressure (4 x 4) applied to the puncture site. If patient is receiving heparin, pressure must be applied to puncture site for a minimum of 15 minutes.

Specimen Arterial blood

Volume 2 mL

Minimum Volume 0.5 mL

Container Preheparinized sampler, heparinized syringe, heparinized capillary tube, or lavender top (EDTA) tube

Collection Specimen drawn into air-free heparinized syringe with stopper. All specimens should be on ice and brought to the laboratory immediately. For capillary collection the skin area to be punctured should be warmed a full 10 minutes. The puncture should be deep enough to allow a free flow of blood. Blood is then collected in heparinized capillary tubes, which should be filled as much as possible, capped and mixed well. All specimens must be labeled with patient's name and hospital number. Indicate on the requisition mode of oxygen delivery or room air if applicable. Also indicate capillary specimen type (heel or digital) if applicable.

Storage Instructions Place specimen in ice water.

Causes for Rejection Specimen not received on ice, air bubbles or clots in syringe

Special Instructions Requisition must indicate source (ie, arterial) and time sample was drawn.

Reference Range Calculated THb: 12% to 15%; % COHb: $\leq$1.5 nonsmokers, 1.5-5 smokers; % MetHb: 0.4-1.5; vol % O_2: 15-23

Use Evaluate fractional components of hemoglobin in arterial blood; evaluate the extent of carbon monoxide poisoning

Limitations Arterial punctures may be extremely difficult in some individuals

Methodology CO-Oximeter™, spectrophotometry

Additional Information Patients on methylene blue or sulfhemoglobin may have erroneous results due to spectral interferences.

CO-Oximetry Venous

Synonyms Venous CO-Oximetry

Test Includes % O_2Hb = oxyhemoglobin and O_2 saturation, % carboxyhemoglobin (COHb), % methemoglobin (MetHb), volume % O_2 = O_2 content, and total hemoglobin (THb)

Patient Preparation Patient should be supine and relaxed

Aftercare Watch for bleeding, hematoma. Ideally, extremity punctured should be kept up for 10 minutes with pressure applied to the puncture site. If patient is receiving heparin, pressure must be applied to puncture site for a minimum of 15 minutes.

Specimen Venous blood

Volume 2 mL

Minimum Volume 0.5 mL

Container Pharmaseal preheparinized sampler, heparinized syringe, or heparinized capillary tube

Collection Specimen drawn into air-free heparinized syringe with needle stoppered. All specimens should be on ice and brought to the laboratory immediately. For capillary collection the skin area to be punctured should be warmed a full 10 minutes. The puncture should be deep enough to allow a free flow of blood. Blood is then collected in heparinized capillary tubes, which should be filled as much as possible, capped and mixed well. All specimens must be labeled with patient's name and hospital number. Indicate on the requisition mode of oxygen delivery or room air if applicable. Also indicate capillary specimen type (heel or digital) if applicable.

(Continued)

CO-Oximetry Venous *(Continued)*

Storage Instructions Place specimen in ice water.

Causes for Rejection Specimen not received on ice, air bubbles or clots in syringe

Use Evaluate fractional components of hemoglobin in venous blood

Additional Information Patients on methylene blue or sulfhemoglobin may have erroneous results due to spectral interference.

Coproporphyrin Screen, Urine

Related Information

Porphyrins, Quantitative, Urine *on page 1326*

Specimen Random urine

• **Volume** 10 mL

Minimum Volume 5 mL

Container Plastic urine container wrapped in aluminum foil

Storage Instructions Transport specimen within 1 hour. Protect from light.

Causes for Rejection Excessive delay in transport, specimen not protected from light

Reference Range Negative

Use Evaluate porphyrias, including those involving deficiencies of enzymes which are needed for heme synthesis and chemical porphyrias

Limitations Certain drugs may cause interference

Additional Information Porphyrins are the byproducts of porphyrinogens. Accumulations of either cause porphyrias, which are characterized by increased excretion of porphyrins, porphyrinogens, or their precursors. The following conditions result in an increase of coproporphyrins: congenital erythropoietic porphyria, acute intermittent porphyria (mild increases), hereditary coproporphyria (markedly increased), and lead poisoning.

Coumadin® *see* Warfarin, Blood *on page 1379*

Co, Urine *see* Cobalt, Urine *on page 1233*

CPAP Titration *see* Pulse Oximetry *on page 1342*

CPK *see* Creatine Kinase, Blood *on this page*

Crab Lice Identification *see* Arthropod Identification *on page 1198*

Crack *see* Cocaine (Cocaine Metabolite), Qualitative *on page 1234*

Creatine Kinase, Blood

Synonyms CK; CPK; Creatine Phosphokinase, Total, Serum

Patient Preparation Avoid exercise before venipuncture. Increases may be anticipated in the immediate postoperative period following surgical procedures involving incision through muscle.

Specimen Blood

Volume 1 mL

Minimum Volume 0.5 mL serum

Container Red top tube

Storage Instructions Separate serum from red cells. Store in refrigerator. Avoid hemolysis.

Causes for Rejection Hemolyzed specimen

Reference Range Method dependent, but usually 0-250 units/L. Females have levels 20% to 25% less than males. Infants to 1 year of age may have levels two times adult. On average, black females have higher levels than white males.

Use Test for acute myocardial infarct and for skeletal muscular disease or damage; elevated in some patients with myxedema (hypothyroidism); elevated in patients with malignant hyperthermia syndrome. Elevated in muscular dystrophy: CK is a marker for Duchenne's muscular dystrophy, with elevations of 20-200 times normal. CK is increased in female carriers of this X-linked disease, and in muscular stress, in polymyositis, dermatomyositis, and with muscle trauma. Elevated in myocarditis. Documentation of postictal state (recent grand mal seizure). Extremely high values are seen in some instances of myositis and in the postictal state. CK may be elevated in a number of entities, including the eosinophilia-myalgia syndrome. Marked increases occur with rhabdomyolysis including that with cocaine intoxication. CK is sometimes increased with cerebrovascular accident. Malignancy (advanced) may show increased CK. Cardioversion with multiple shocks may release CK-MB and may result in a false-positive diagnosis of myocardial infarction. Low CK may reflect decreased muscle mass. It has been reported with a number of entities, including metastatic neoplasia, patients with steroid therapy, with alcoholic liver disease and with connective tissue diseases. Overnight bedrest may lower CK 10% to 20%.

Limitations Intramuscular injections increase serum CK activity. Elevated following exercise. Increases in CK and CK-MB must be interpreted cautiously during the peripartum period. **Normal at onset of acute MI** unless the subject has been exercising or doing physical work. Elevation of CK following acute MI may not be observed until 6 or more hours after onset. CK returns to normal early in approximately 48-72 hours after acute MI. Total CK can be normal early in acute MI, when CK-MB is increased. Newer tests (CK isoforms, human ventricular myosin light chains and Troponin A) may allow for earlier detection of myocardial injury/infarction than routine CK and CK-MB measurements. Low CK does not rule out myositis in patients with the connective tissue diseases. Decreased with pregnancy.

Methodology Kinetic – UV spectrophotometric

Additional Information High CK is found after trauma, surgery, and exercise; these entities are not accompanied by elevation of CK-MB. To distinguish myoglobinuria from hemoglobinuria, serum CK and LD may be helpful. CK is normal with uncomplicated hemolysis but LD and LD_1 usually are increased. When myoglobin is released, 40-fold elevation of CK may be anticipated with only moderate increase in serum LD and increased LD_5.

Specific References

Beek AM, Verheugt FW, and Meyer A, "Usefulness of Electrocardiographic Findings and Creatine Kinase Levels on Admission in Predicting the Accuracy of the Interval Between Onset of Chest Pain of Acute Myocardial Infarction and Initiation of Thrombolytic Therapy," *Am J Cardiol*, 1991, 68(13):1287-90.

Crisp DE, Ziter FA, and Bray PF, "Diagnostic Delay in Duchenne's Muscular Dystrophy," *JAMA*, 1982, 247(4):478-80.

Leung FY, Griffith AP, Jablonsky G, et al, "Comparison of the Diagnostic Utility of Timed Serial (Slope) Creatine Kinase Measurements With Conventional Serum Tests in the Early Diagnosis of Myocardial Infarction," *Ann Clin Biochem*, 1991, 28(Pt 1):78-82.

Lott JA, "Serum Enzyme Determinations in the Diagnosis of Acute Myocardial Infarction: An Update," *Hum Pathol*, 1984, 15(8):706-16.

Schneider CM, Dennehy CA, Rodearmel SJ, et al, "Effects of Physical Activity on Creatine Phosphokinase and the Isoenzyme Creatine-Kinase-MB," *Ann Emerg Med*, 1995, 25(4):520-4.

Creatine Phosphokinase, Total, Serum *see* Creatine Kinase, Blood *on previous page*

Creatinine, Serum

Patient Preparation Fasting may be desirable. Certain cephalosporins, especially cefoxitin, cause misleading (high) results.

Specimen Blood

Volume 10 mL

Minimum Volume 1 mL serum

Container Red top tube

Collection Pediatrics: Blood drawn from heelstick.

Causes for Rejection Hemolysis

Reference Range Children: 1-5 years: 0.3-0.5 mg/dL (SI: 27-44 µmol/L), 5-10 years: 0.5-0.8 mg/dL (SI: 44-71 µmol/L); adults: male: up to 1.2 mg/dL (SI: 106 µmol/L), female: up to 1.1 mg/dL (SI: 97 µmol/L). Variation between sources for serum creatinine normal ranges is perhaps greater than for many other important tests. There are slight differences between the sexes with males higher, since the range relates to the amount of muscle mass present. The glomerular filtration rate increases in pregnancy; thus, serum creatinine should be slightly less during that period. In older patients, decrease of muscle mass must be considered in interpretation of results; the elderly have reduced creatinine generation. Similarly, other patients may have creatinine levels in which muscle abnormalities must be considered, including long-term corticosteroid therapy, hyperthyroidism, muscular dystrophy and paralysis, and dermatomyositis and polymyositis.

Use The most common clinical renal function test, providing a rough approximation of glomerular filtration.

Causes of high creatinine include renal diseases and insufficiency with decreased glomerular filtration (uremia or azotemia if severe); urinary tract obstruction; reduced renal blood flow including congestive heart failure, shock and dehydration; rhabdomyolysis causes high serum creatinine, which may be elevated out of proportion to BUN, or to the reduction in renal function.

Causes of low creatinine include small stature, debilitation, decreased muscle mass, some complex cases of severe hepatic disease. In advanced liver disease, low creatinine may result from decreased hepatic production of creatinine and inadequate dietary protein as well as reduced muscle mass.

Index of fetal maturity in amniotic fluid analysis.

Limitations With reduced renal blood flow, creatinine rises less quickly than urea nitrogen. Concentration of creatinine only becomes abnormal when about half or more of the nephrons have stopped functioning in chronic progressive renal disease.

Increased serum creatinine results may occur from noncreatinine substances, including meat ingestion, glucose, pyruvate, uric acid, fructose, guanidine, ke-

(Continued)

Creatinine, Serum *(Continued)*

tonemia (acetoacetate), hydantoin, ascorbic acid, and numerous cephalosporin antibiotics, especially cefoxitin. Cefoxitin levels fall in patients with normal kidney function, such that a sample can be drawn 2 hours after a dose but preferably, 4 hours or more afterwards. With severe renal disease, creatinine is not reliable in the presence of cefoxitin therapy. There is less interference reported from the cephalosporins cephalothin, cephaloridine, cephadrile sodium, and cephaloglycin dihydrate. Cefazolin and cefamandole may cause increased colorimetric values. Cephapirin and moxalactam are described as not causing interference. Differences in the interference of such cephalosporins between assay systems are published.

Methyldopa and trimethoprim may increase serum creatinine levels. Lipemia, hemolysis, and bilirubin may interfere. High creatinine in serum has been reported with methanol intoxication.

An antifungal drug, 5-flucytosine, and glucose interfere with the imidohydrolase method. Cefoxitin and cefpirome interfere with the Jaffé method causing a false elevation.

Tagamet® interferes with creatinine excretion in the renal tubule, causing a rise in creatinine without reduction in renal function. It may also cause an allergic nephritis with reduced renal function.

Moderate variation of results exists between chemistry analyzer systems.

Serum creatinine is only a crude guide to the progress of renal disease. Moderate changes in the glomerular filtration rate (GFR) may not be detected by serum creatinine levels. Levey et al and others emphasize that the serum creatinine does **not** provide an adequate estimate of GFR. A fraction of urine creatinine is from tubular secretion. Such tubular secretion increases with declining renal function.

Methodology Alkaline picrate (Jaffé reaction), *o*-nitrobenzaldehyde (Sakaguchi reaction), imidohydrolase (Ektachem®). Many interference problems are still unresolved in the Jaffé reaction.

Additional Information Serum creatinine level is proportional to lean body muscle mass. It is unaffected by most diet or activity and is freely filtered by the glomerulus. Both BUN and creatinine are often ordered to follow renal problems. Creatinine overall is the more reliable index, but each has pitfalls. As creatinine increases in chronic renal failure, the hematocrit decreases, total carbon dioxide and bicarbonate fall, and serum phosphate and BUN increase. When serum creatinine increases postoperatively, a group of patients may be identified who are at risk for more severe renal failure. Creatinine clearances have a role in such investigations. Serum creatinine has a role in determination of dosages of some drugs (eg, the aminoglycosides and digoxin), especially in elderly subjects.

Specific References

Abuelo JG, "Benign Azotemia of Long-Term Hemodialysis: Increase in Blood Urea Nitrogen and Serum Creatinine Concentrations After the Initiation of Dialysis," *Am J Med*, 1989, 86(6 Pt 1):738-9.

Duarte CG and Preuss HG, "Assessment of Renal Function: Glomerular and Tubular," *Clin Lab Med*, 1993, 13(1):33-52.

Grotsch H and Hajdu P, "Interference by the New Antibiotic Cefpirome and Other Cephalosporins in Clinical Laboratory Test, With Special Regard to the 'Jaffé' Reaction," *J Clin Chem Clin Biochem*, 1987, 25(1):49-52.

Lemann J, Bidani AK, Bain RP, et al, "Use of the Serum Creatinine to Estimate Glomerular Filtration Rate in Health and Early Diabetic Nephropathy. Collaborative Study Group of Angiotensin Converting Enzyme Inhibition in Diabetic Nephropathy," *Am J Kidney Dis*, 1990, 16(3):236-43.

Lepage L and Galimany R, "Creatinine," *Drug Effects on Laboratory Test Results Analytical Interferences and Pharmacological Effects*, Siest G and Galteau MM, eds, Littleton, MA: PSG Publishing Co Inc, 1988, 198-210.

Narayanan S, "Creatinine: Review of Methods," *ASCP Check Sample®*, Gambino SR and Batsakis JG, eds, Chicago, IL: American Society of Clinical Pathologists, 1988, 4:1-10.

Cr, Serum *see* Chromium, Serum *on page 1230*

Cr, Urine *see* Chromium, Urine *on page 1231*

Cryptosporidium Diagnostic Procedures, Stool

Synonyms Acid-Fast Stain, Modified, *Cryptosporidium*

Test Includes Examination of stool for the presence of *Cryptosporidium* by phase contrast microscopy and/or modified acid-fast stain, or fluorescent labeled antibody

Abstract *Cryptosporidium*, a parasite, may cause severe diarrhea, predominantly in immunocompromised individuals.

Specimen Fresh stool; stool preserved with 10% formalin or sodium acetate-acetic acid formalin preservative

Container Plastic stool container

Collection Transport fresh specimen to the laboratory promptly following collection. Specimen on outside of container poses excessive risk of contamination to laboratory personnel.

Special Instructions Procedures for the detection of *Cryptosporidium* in humans have recently become available in most clinical laboratories. Consult the laboratory regarding availability of the procedure and specific specimen collection instructions before collecting the specimen.

Reference Range Negative

Use A part of the differential work-up of diarrhea, particularly in immunocompromised hosts and suspected AIDS patients; establish the diagnosis of cryptosporidiosis by demonstration of the oocysts. A recent outbreak in healthy individuals from a contaminated water supply was noted.

Limitations *Cryptosporidium* is not detected by standard methods used to examine stool specimens for other ova and parasites; special stains are required for its detection, and in many laboratories, must be specifically requested. The organisms are most readily demonstrated in concentrated diarrheal stools. Forms of *Blastocystis hominis* may cause confusion if Giemsa stain is used. Most recommended procedures cannot be performed on polyvinyl alcohol (PVA) preserved specimens.

Methodology Phase contrast microscopy after sucrose floatation concentration technique (Sheather's); modified acid-fast stain on air-dried, methanol-fixed smears (decolorization with 1% H_2SO_4). Auramine and carbol-fuchsin stain is used by some laboratories for screening. A technique utilizing formalin-ethyl acetate and floatation over hypertonic saline is reported to enhance detection of *Cryptosporidium* oocysts. Fluorescent-labeled IgG monoclonal anti-*Cryptosporidium* antibodies are commercially available.

Additional Information *Cryptosporidium* (similar to *Isospora belli*) is a coccidian parasite of the intestines and respiratory tract of many animals including mice, sheep, snakes, turkeys, chickens, cows, monkeys, and domestic cats. The first reported human case occurred in 1976. The prevalence of cryptosporidial infection in the U.S. is estimated to be 2.6%. It is a cause of severe and chronic diarrhea in patients with hypogammaglobulinemia and the acquired immune deficiency syndrome. The organism is widely recognized as a disease of the immunocompromised patient, however, it can also cause disease in immunocompetent subjects. Animal contact, travel to endemic areas, living in a rural environment, and day care attendance by toddlers have been recognized as risk factors for the development of cryptosporidiosis. Perinatal infection has been reported. Children are more prone to develop infection than are adults. In these patients, the disease is a self-limited gastroenteritis, but in immunocompromised patients, a profound enteropathy results. A seasonal variation in incidence exists with the highest frequency reported in summer and autumn. The organism can be demonstrated in biopsies of small bowel and colon, adherent to surface of the epithelial cells (Giemsa stain) and by demonstration in feces by floatation with modified acid-fast stain (cold Kinyoun stain) or smear. Most therapeutic regimens for cryptosporidiosis are not successful unless immunosuppression is reversed. Enteric precautions should be taken. Transmission of *Cryptosporidium* can occur via swimming pools; *Cryptosporidium* oocysts are chloride-resistant.

Specific References

Baron EJ, Schenone C, and Tanenbaum B, "Comparison of Three Methods for Detection of *Cryptosporidium* Oocysts in a Low-Prevalence Population," *J Clin Microbiol*, 1989, 27(1):223-4.

Casemore DP, Armstrong M, and Sands RL, "Laboratory Diagnosis of Cryptosporidiosis," *J Clin Pathol*, 1985, 38(12):1337-41.

Current WL, "The Biology of *Cryptosporidium*," *Am Soc Microbiol News*, 1988, 54:605-11, (review).

Dale BA, Gordon G, Thomson R, et al, "Perinatal Infection With *Cryptosporidium*," *Lancet*, 1987, 1(8540)1042-3.

Ferrera PC and Cirillo LA, "Cryptosporidiosis in an Immunocompetent Host," *Am J Emerg Med*, 1995, 13:378-80.

Garcia LS, Brewer TC, and Brucker DA, "Incidence of *Cryptosporidium* in All Patients Submitting Stool Specimens for Ova and Parasite Examination: Monoclonal Antibody IFA Method," *Diagn Microbiol Infect Dis*, 1988, 11(1):25-7.

Garcia LS, Shum AC, and Bruckner DA, "Evaluation of a New Monoclonal Antibody Combination Reagent for Direct Fluorescence Detection of *Giardia* Cysts and *Cryptosporidium* Oocysts in Human Fecal Specimens," *J Clin Microbiol*, 1992, 30(12):3255-7.

Koch KL, Shankey TV, Weinstein GS, et al, "Cryptosporidiosis in a Patient With Hemophilia, Common Variable Hypogammaglobulinemia and the Acquired Immunodeficiency Syndrome," *Ann Intern Med*, 1983, 99:337-40.

Kocoshis SA, "Diagnosis and Treatment of Cryptosporidiosis in Children," *Compr Ther*, 1986, 12(4):56-61.

Koneman EW, Allen SD, Janda WM, et al, *Color Atlas and Textbook of Diagnostic Microbiology*, 4th ed, Philadelphia, PA: JB Lippincott Co, 1992.

Millard PS, Gensheimer KF, Addiss DG, et al, "An Outbreak of Cryptosporidiosis From Fresh Pressed Apple Cider," *JAMA*, 1994, 272(20):1592-6.

Petersen C, "Cryptosporidiosis in Patients Infected With the Human Immunodeficiency Virus," *Clin Infect Dis*, 1992, 15(6):903-9.

Reisberg B, *Common Intestinal Parasites, in the Biologic and Clinical Basis of Infectious Diseases*, 4th ed, Shulman ST, Phair JB, Summers HM, eds, Philadelphia, PA: WB Saunders Co, 1992, 305-6.

(Continued)

Cryptosporidium Diagnostic Procedures, Stool *(Continued)*

Soave R and Armstrong D, "*Cryptosporidium* and Cryptosporidiosis," *Rev Infect Dis*, 1986, 8(6):1012-23.

Weber R, Bryan RT, and Juranek DD, "Improved Stool Concentration Procedure for Detection of *Cryptosporidium* Oocysts in Fecal Specimens," *J Clin Microbiol*, 1992, 30(11):2869-73.

Crystal *see* Amphetamines, Qualitative, Urine *on page 1190*

Crystal *see* Methamphetamines, Urine *on page 1294*

Crystals, Urine

Related Information

Urinalysis *on page 1373*

Synonyms Urine Crystals

Test Includes Test is part of a routine urinalysis; includes checking for uric acid, cystine, tyrosine, leucine, cholesterol, sulfa, oxalate, and phosphate crystals

Specimen Random urine, catheterized urine

Volume 12 mL

Minimum Volume 2 mL

Container Plastic urine container, tightly capped

Storage Instructions Refrigerate specimen if test cannot be performed immediately.

Causes for Rejection Quantity not sufficient, improperly labeled specimen, specimen not brought to the laboratory within 1 hour of collection

Use Diagnose metabolic disorders, calculus formation, regulation of medication

Methodology Microscopic examination

Additional Information Crystalluria is uncommon despite maximal concentrations in warm, fresh urine because of the normal presence of crystal inhibitors, the lack of available nidus, and the time factor. When properly observed in fresh urine, crystals are diagnostically useful for a physician evaluating microhematuria, nephrolithiasis, or toxin ingestion.

In abundance, calcium oxalate and/or hippurate crystals may suggest ethylene glycol ingestion (can be accompanied by neurological abnormalities, appearance of drunkenness, hypertension, and a high anion gap acidosis).

Calcium magnesium ammonium phosphate may be present in massive quantities in alkaline urine. They usually are associated with urine infected by urea splitting bacteria which cause "infection," or "triple phosphate" stones.

Tyrosine and leucine crystals are found in acid urine, indicating abnormal metabolism. These crystals occur together in acute yellow atrophy and in other destructive diseases of the liver.

Crystals may also provide a clue to the composition of renal stones not yet passed.

Crystodigin® *see* Digitoxin, Blood *on page 1249*

Culture, Blood *see* Blood Culture, Aerobic and Anaerobic *on page 1204*

CXR *see* Chest Films *on page 1224*

Cyanide, Blood

Synonyms CN^-; Hydrocyanic Acid; Potassium or Sodium Cyanide

Abstract This highly toxic substance is one of the oldest poisons known. It binds to cytochrome oxidase and prevents cellular respiration.

Specimen Blood

Volume 10 mL

Minimum Volume 7 mL whole blood or 5 mL serum

Container Lavender top (EDTA) tube or red top tube

Storage Instructions Fill tube to capacity and keep tightly closed; analyze as soon as possible. Refrigerate whole blood, gastric contents or tissue.

Reference Range

Whole blood levels: Smoker: ≤0.5 mg/L

Flushing and tachycardia seen at 0.5-1.0 mg/L; obtundation at 1.0-2.5 mg/L

Coma and death occur at >2.5 mg/L

Plasma cyanide:

- Normal: 4-5 μg/L
- Asymptomatic (with metabolic acidosis): 80 μg/L
- Death: >260 μg/L

Red blood cell cyanide:

- Normal: <26 μg/L

Metabolic acidosis: 1040 μg/L
Symptomatic: 5200 μg/L
Fatal: >10,400 μg/L

Critical Values In whole blood, values >2.5 μg/mL are potentially fatal although subjects with higher values have survived.

Possible Panic Range Toxic: >1.0 μg/mL (SI: >77 μmol/L); >2.0 μg/mL (SI: >115 μmol/L) is lethal

Use Establish the diagnosis of cyanide poisoning

Methodology Conway diffusion, color reaction, ion specific potentiometry

Additional Information Cyanide is present in insecticides, rodenticides, vermicides, metal polishes, and electroplating baths. Symptoms of toxicity include headache, agitation, vomiting, and confusion. A scent of bitter almonds is suggestive, but not all individuals can detect it. Treatment with nitrites is effective. Nitrites produce methemoglobin which binds cyanide ions and thus removes them from cytochrome oxidase. Half-life of cyanide in whole blood is 45-65 hours. Cyanide is metabolized by rhodanase to thiocyanate. Thiosulfate is given along with nitrites to promote the conversion of cyanide to thiocyanate which is much less toxic and is excreted. Cyanide itself blocks cellular metabolism by inhibiting cytochrome oxidase.

Whole blood cyanide determination by acidification usually provides an overestimation of levels by about 70%; it is most correlated with thiocyanate levels. Most accurate tissue cyanide levels concentration are reflected by plasma cyanide levels. Ratio of red blood cell to plasma cyanide concentration is 60:1. Signs or symptoms due to thiocyanate toxicity usually do not occur at plasma or serum levels <100 mg/L.

Specific References

Lundquist P and Sorbo B, "Rapid Determination of Toxic Cyanide Concentrations in Blood," *Clin Chem*, 1989, 35(4):617-9.

Moore SJ, Ho IK, and Hume AS, "Severe Hypoxia Produced by Concomitant Intoxication With Sublethal Doses of Carbon Monoxide and Cyanide," *Toxicol Appl Pharmacol*, 1991, 109(3):412-20.

Cyclosporine A *see* Cyclosporine, Blood *on this page*

Cyclosporine, Blood

Synonyms Sandimmune®

Applies To Cyclosporine A

Abstract This drug is widely used as an immunosuppressant, especially after organ transplants.

Specimen Whole blood, plasma, or serum

Container Lavender top (EDTA) tube (whole blood), green top (heparin) tube (plasma), red top tube (serum)

Sampling Time Trough levels should be obtained 12-18 hours after oral dose (chronic usage), 12 hours after intravenous dose, or immediately prior to next dose.

Reference Range RIA: immediately following transplant: 150-250 ng/mL (SI: 125-210 nmol/L) (plasma levels), 450-750 ng/mL (SI: 374-624 nmol/L) (whole blood levels). Maintenance levels months after transplant: 50-150 ng/mL (SI: 40-125 nmol/L) (plasma levels), 150-450 ng/mL (SI: 125-375 nmol/L) (whole blood levels). Reference ranges are method dependent and specimen dependent.

Use Monitor blood level in management of immunosuppression of organ transplant recipients

Limitations Results are method dependent – some measure multiple metabolites as well as parent drug. It is not yet clearly established whether whole blood or plasma/serum levels are clinically most appropriate. Single assays are not as informative as a series over time.

Methodology Radioimmunoassay (RIA), high performance liquid chromatography (HPLC), fluorescence polarization immunoassay (FPIA)

Additional Information Cyclosporine is an immunosuppressive agent derived from *Tolypocladium inflatum gams*, a fungus originally isolated from a Norwegian soil sample. The agent is used extensively to control rejection of organ transplants, especially of liver, heart, or kidney. The exact mechanism of action of the drug is not known, but it appears to interfere with T-helper cell function and secretion of lymphokines. It is not myelosuppressive.

Monitoring of blood levels is imperative because the pharmacokinetics of cyclosporine are not only complex, but vary over time in the same patient; thus, blood levels cannot be well predicted from dosing schedules. Furthermore, this drug has a narrow therapeutic window and significant toxicity at levels above that range.

Renal toxicity with eventual renal failure is the most severe complication. Other assays to assess renal function (ie, BUN, creatinine clearance) should be ordered along with cyclosporine level, since toxicity may begin even with "acceptable"

(Continued)

Cyclosporine, Blood *(Continued)*

blood levels. Other toxicities include hypertension, convulsions, tremors, pulmonary edema, and an increased risk of lymphoma.

Drugs which enhance the potential toxicity of cyclosporine, and which are also likely to be administered to a transplant recipient, include aminoglycoside antibiotics, cephalosporins, trimethoprim-sulfa, amphotericin B, acyclovir, ketoconazole, and furosemide. Agents which raise cyclosporine levels by decreasing biotransformation include methylprednisolone, amphotericin B, cimetidine, and erythromycin. Drugs which increase hepatic metabolism and thus lower cyclosporine levels include phenobarbital, phenytoin, rifampin, and trimetheprim-sulfa.

Because results will vary depending on whether the assay is done on whole blood or serum/plasma and on the method and cyclosporine antibody employed (monospecific or polyspecific), it is best for a given patient's specimens to be analyzed at a single laboratory to eliminate as many assay-dependent variables as possible. If switching of laboratories is unavoidable, it is advisable to have a few specimens run in parallel in the second laboratory prior to changing.

The clinical use of cyclosporine is difficult and requires experience and judgment. A drug blood level is only one of many pieces in the puzzle of transplant medicine.

Specific References

Canafax DM and Ascher NL, "Cyclosporine Immunosuppression," *Clin Pharm*, 1983, 2(6):515-24.

Frey FJ, Horber FF, and Frey BM, "Trough Levels and Concentration Time Curves of Cyclosporine in Patients Undergoing Renal Transplantation," *Clin Pharmacol Ther*, 1988, 43(1):55-62.

Gerson B, "Cyclosporine Controversies," *Clin Lab Med*, 1987, 7(3):669-86.

Giesbrecht, EE, Soldin SJ, and Wong PY, "A Rapid, Reliable High Performance Liquid Chromatographic Micromethod for the Measurement of Cyclosporine in Whole Blood," *Ther Drug Monit*, 1989, 11(3):332-36.

Hayashi Y, Shibata N, Minouchi T, et al, "Evaluation of Fluorescence Polarization Immunoassay for Determination of Cyclosporine in Plasma," *Ther Drug Monit*, 1989, 11(2):205-9.

Hooks MA, Millikan WJ, Henderson JM, et al, "Comparison of Whole-Blood Cyclosporine Levels Measured by Radioimmunoassay and Fluorescence Polarization in Patients Post Orthotropic Liver Transplant," *Ther Drug Monit*, 1989, 11(3):304-9.

Kahan BD, "Cyclosporine," *N Engl J Med*, 1989, 321(25):1725-38.

Kahan BD, "Individualization of Cyclosporine Therapy Using Pharmacokinetics and Pharmacodynamic Parameters," *Transplantation*, 1985, 40(5):457-76.

Lindholm A and Henricsson S, "Simultaneous Monitoring of Cyclosporine in Blood and Plasma With Four Analytical Methods: A Clinical Evaluation," *Transplant Proc*, 1989, 21(1 Pt 2):1472-4.

Martinez L, Foradori A, Vaccarezza A, et al, "Monitoring of Cyclosporine Blood Levels With Polyclonal and Monoclonal Assays During Episodes of Renal Graft Dysfunction," *Transplant Proc*, 1989, 21(1 Pt 2):1490-1.

McBride JH, Rodgerson DO, Allin RE, et al, "Comparison of Four Immunoassays for the Measurement of Cyclosporine and Metabolites in Plasma," *Clin Chem*, 1988, 34(6):1259.

Moyer TP, Johnson P, Faynor SM, et al, "Cyclosporine: A Review of Drug Monitoring Problems and Presentation of a Simple, Accurate Liquid Chromatographic Procedure That Solves These Problems," *Clin Biochem*, 1986, 19(2):83-9.

Ptachcinski R, Venkataramanan R, and Burckart GJ, "Clinical Pharmacokinetics of Cyclosporin," *Clin Pharmacokinet*, 1986, 11(2):107-32.

Sanghvi A, Diven W, Seltman H, et al, "Abbott's Fluorescence Polarization Immunoassay for Cyclosporine and Metabolites Compared With the Sandoz "Sandimmune®" RIA," *Clin Chem*, 1988, 34(9):1904-6.

Cytochrome b_5 Reductase *see* Methemoglobin, Blood *on page 1296*

Cytokines *see* Eosinophil Count *on page 1259*

Dalmane® *see* Flurazepam, Blood *on page 1268*

Darvocet-N® *see* Propoxyphene, Blood or Urine *on page 1334*

Darvon® *see* Propoxyphene, Blood or Urine *on page 1334*

DAT *see* Antiglobulin Test, Direct *on page 1195*

Datril® *see* Acetaminophen, Serum *on page 1180*

DAU *see* Drugs of Abuse Screen, Urine *on page 1252*

DAU-10 *see* Drugs of Abuse Screen, Urine *on page 1252*

DDC *see* Zalcitabine, Blood or Urine *on page 1380*

DDI *see* Didanosine, Blood *on next page*

Deer Tick Identification *see* Arthropod Identification *on page 1198*

Delta Aminolevulinic Acid Dehydratase *see* Lead, Blood *on page 1282*

Depakene® *see* Valproic Acid, Blood *on page 1377*

Depakote® (Enteric-Coated Divalproex Sodium) *see* Valproic Acid, Blood *on page 1377*

Depamide® *see* Valproic Acid, Blood *on page 1377*

Desaturation Oximetry *see* Pulse Oximetry *on page 1342*

Desipramine *see* Imipramine, Blood *on page 1274*

Desoxyn® *see* Methamphetamines, Serum *on page 1294*

Desoxyn® *see* Methamphetamines, Urine *on page 1294*

Desyrel® *see* Trazodone, Blood *on page 1367*

Dexies *see* Amphetamines, Qualitative, Urine *on page 1190*

1,4-α-D Glucanohydrolase, Serum *see* Amylase, Serum *on page 1191*

Diazepam, Blood

Synonyms Valium®

Abstract This is a benzodiazepine used as a sedative-hypnotic (tranquilizer).

Specimen Blood

Volume 10 mL

Minimum Volume 1 mL serum

Container Red top tube

Sampling Time For peak level, 1 hour after oral dose or 15 minutes after I.V.

Storage Instructions Do not freeze

Reference Range Diazepam: therapeutic: 0.2-1.5 μg/mL (SI: 0.7-5.3 μmol/L); N-desmethyldiazepam (nordiazepam): therapeutic: 0.1-0.5 μg/mL (SI: 0.35-1.80 μmol/L)

Critical Values Toxic: sum of diazepam plus N-desmethyldiazepam >3.0 μg/mL

Possible Panic Range Total of diazepam and nordiazepam >5.0 μg/mL (SI: >18 μmol/L) is toxic.

Use Therapeutic monitoring; toxicity assessment

Methodology Enzyme immunoassay (EIA), high performance liquid chromatography (HPLC), UV spectrophotometry, gas-liquid chromatography (GLC)

Additional Information Diazepam is a muscle relaxant and antianxiety drug. Peak blood levels are achieved within 1 hour after oral dose. Half-life in adults is 21-37 hours. The major metabolite (N-desmethyldiazepam) has a half-life in adults of 50-99 hours. It is the major metabolite also of Tranxene® and prazepam. Diazepam may exhibit synergism with barbiturates, tricyclic antidepressants, and amine oxidase inhibitors. Toxicity may be additive with other central nervous system depressants, and ethanol enhances the absorption of diazepam itself. Many cases of overdose are seen but few fatalities result from use of this drug alone. A frequent finding is a combination of this drug and ethanol.

Specific References

Greenblatt DJ, Ehrenberg BL, Gunderman J, et al, "Pharmacokinetic and Electroencephalographic Study of Intravenous Diazepam, Midazolam, and Placebo," *Clin Pharmacol Ther*, 1989, 45(4):356-65.

Dicumarol *see* Bishydroxycoumarin, Blood *on page 1204*

Didanosine, Blood

Synonyms DDI

Abstract HIV reverse transcriptase inhibitor; metabolizes to uric acid and hypoxanthine

Patient Preparation Interacts with quinolone and tetracycline antibiotics

Specimen Blood

Volume 5-10 mL

Reference Range No therapeutic range established

Use AIDS therapy; slows progression

Methodology Radioimmunoassay (RIA); high performance liquid chromatography (HPLC)

Additional Information Half-life: Oral: 0.6-1.6 hours; dose: 125-375 mg twice daily; minor side effects: rash, constipation, mild myositis

Specific References

Faulds D and Brogden RN, "Didanosine: A Review of Its Antiviral Activity, Pharmacokinetic Properties and Therapeutic Potential in Human Immunodeficiency Virus Infection," *Drugs*, 1992, 44(1):94-116.

Knupp CA, Stancato FA, Papp EA, et al, "Quantitation of Didanosine in Human Plasma and Urine by High-Performance Liquid Chromatography," *J Chromatogr*, 1990, 533:282-90.

Stretcher BN, "Current AIDS Therapies," *Ther Drug Monit & Toxic In-Service Training and Continuing Education*, 1994, 15(3):51-61.

Digacin® *see* Digoxin, Blood *on next page*

Digitalis *see* Digitoxin, Blood *on this page*

Digitoxin, Blood

Synonyms Crystodigin®; Digitalis; Lanotoxin®; Purodigin®

Abstract One of a group of plant glycosides used in the treatment of congestive heart failure, digitoxin is infrequently used compared to digoxin. It must not be confused with digoxin when serum levels are ordered.

(Continued)

Digitoxin, Blood *(Continued)*

Specimen Blood

Minimum Volume 3 mL serum

Container Red top tube

Sampling Time 6-12 hours after dose

Storage Instructions Separate serum and store in refrigerator.

Reference Range Therapeutic: 18-22 ng/mL (SI: 23-28 nmol/L)

Critical Values Levels >35 ng/mL (SI: >46 nmol/L) are associated with clinical toxicity in 80% of patients.

Use Therapeutic monitoring; toxicity assessment

Limitations **Do not order digitoxin level on a patient receiving digoxin**. Digitoxin is not commonly used. Digoxin immune Fab can increase digitoxin levels by assay.

Contraindications Patient on **digoxin**; recent radioactive tracer

Methodology Radioimmunoassay (RIA), gas-liquid chromatography (GLC), high performance liquid chromatography (HPLC)

Additional Information Optimal sampling time after dosage is 6 hours. Optimal resampling time after change in dosage is 48-96 hours. Elimination half-life is 5-7 days. Be sure the patient is not on digoxin instead of digitoxin. There is cross reactivity between the two drugs and the levels reported will not be valid, and in fact could be misleading and catastrophic. Digitalis leaf has both digoxin and digitoxin as active components. Digitoxin is the best test for evaluation of toxicity in a patient taking digitalis leaf, but neither test is truly satisfactory. There is considerable overlap in the upper therapeutic ranges with levels which may be toxic. **Digitoxin levels must be correlated with clinical and other chemical data.** Numerous factors modify the effect of cardiac glycosides, including serum potassium, calcium, magnesium, and cardiac blood flow. Hypokalemia, hypomagnesemia, and hypercalcemia all potentiate toxicity from cardiac glycosides. Agents with significant interactions with digitoxin include cholestyramine, heparin, phenobarbital, phenytoin, rifampin, and possibly quinidine.

Specific References

Bayer MJ, "Recognition and Management of Digitalis Intoxication: Implications for Emergency Medicine," *Am J Emerg Med*, 1991, 9(2 Suppl 1):29-34.

Kulick DL and Rahimtoola SH, "Current Role of Digitalis Therapy in Patients With Congestive Heart Failure," *JAMA*, 1991, 265(22):2995-7.

Digoxin, Blood

Synonyms Digacin®; Digoxosodium; Lanoxin®

Specimen Blood

Container Red top tube

Reference Range Therapeutic: 0.5-2.0 ng/mL

Critical Values Toxic effects: Serum: >2.0 ng/mL

Possible Panic Range Fatalities: 1.5-300.0 ng/mL

Use Cardiac glycoside

Limitations Digoxin immune Fab fragments can interfere with assay. Endogenous digoxin-like immunoreactive substances (DLIS) may cause artificial elevation of serum digoxin level. Chinese toad venom used in medicinals also cross-reacts with FPIA technique.

Methodology High performance liquid chromatography (HPLC), radioimmunoassay (RIA); fluorescence polarisation immunoassay with ultra filtration (FPIA-UF) accurately measures free digoxin in the presence of immune Fab fragments

Specific References

Aruna AS and Jue SG, "Digoxin Immune Fab Administration Following an Unexplained Increase in Serum Digoxin Concentration," *J Pharm Sci Technol*, 1994, 10:246-9.

Koobatian TJ and Roberts JR, "Falsely Elevated Serum Digoxin Levels Secondary to Endogenous Digoxin-Like Immunoreactive Substances," *Acad Emerg Med*, 1995, 2:322-6.

Digoxosodium *see* Digoxin, Blood *on this page*

Dilantin® *see* Phenytoin, Blood *on page 1321*

Diphenhydramine, Blood

Synonyms Benadryl®; Isomer of Phenyltoloxamine

Specimen Blood

Volume 20 mL

Minimum Volume 5 mL plasma

Container Two green top (heparin) tubes

Storage Instructions Refrigerate plasma

Reference Range Therapeutic: 0.1-1.0 μg/mL

Critical Values Toxic: >10.0 μg/mL

Use Monitor therapeutic drug level; evaluate toxicity

Methodology Colorimetric, high performance liquid chromatography (HPLC), UV spectrophotometry, gas chromatography/mass spectrometry (GC/MS)

Additional Information Diphenhydramine, an ethanolamine antihistamine, works by blocking histamine release by competing for H_1 receptor sites on effector cells. It is used for the symptomatic relief of allergic symptoms caused by histamine release, which include nasal allergies and allergic dermatosis. It is also used as a mild nighttime sedative, for the prevention of motion sickness, and as an antitussive. Maximal effects are felt in 1-3 hours, and the half-life is 2-7 hours. Adverse effects of diphenhydramine include sedation, dizziness, hypotension, nausea, vomiting, blurred vision, insomnia, and tremor.

Diphenylhydantoin *see* Phenytoin, Blood *on page 1321*

Direct Antiglobulin Test *see* Antiglobulin Test, Direct *on page 1195*

Direct Coombs' *see* Antiglobulin Test, Direct *on page 1195*

Disopyramide, Blood

Synonyms Norpace®

Abstract Disopyramide is an antiarrhythmic agent which is frequently monitored.

Specimen Blood

Volume 7 mL

Minimum Volume 4 mL serum or plasma

Container Red top tube, green top (heparin) tube, or lavender top (EDTA) tube

Sampling Time Collect specimen 2-3 hours after an oral dose of disopyramide for peak. Draw trough just before next dose. Trough level is the best guide for dosing.

Special Instructions Specify other cardiac medications on requisition.

Reference Range Therapeutic: 2-5 μg/mL (SI: 5.9-14.7 μmol/L)

Critical Values Fatalities are seen with concentrations >16 μg/mL.

Possible Panic Range Toxic: >7 μg/mL (SI: >20.6 μmol/L)

Use Therapeutic monitoring

Limitations Arrhythmias may occur at low levels

Methodology Enzyme immunoassay (EIA), high performance liquid chromatography (HPLC)

Additional Information Disopyramide shares electrophysiologic properties with quinidine and procainamide. Up to 80% of oral dose is absorbed. Half-life is 4-10 hours. Eighty percent of the drug is excreted in the urine. Dosage must be modified (dosage intervals prolonged) in patients with renal failure. Serious toxic effects are depression of myocardial contractility and disturbances in myocardial conduction. Other effects include dry mouth, constipation, urinary hesitancy, and blurred vision. Metabolite N-desisopropyl disopyramide is also pharmacologically active. Concomitant treatment with phenytoin may lead to decreased serum levels of disopyramide. There may be cumulative effects with other class I antiarrhythmic drugs (lidocaine, procainamide).

Specific References

Duff HJ, Mitchell LB, Nath CF, et al, "Concentration-Response Relationships of Disopyramide in Patients With Ventricular Tachycardia," *Clin Pharmacol Ther*, 1989, 45(5):542-7.

Ragosta M, Weihl AC, and Rosenfeld LE, "Potentially Fatal Interaction Between Erythromycin and Disopyramide," *Am J Med*, 1989, 86(4):465-6.

d-Methamphetamine *see* Methamphetamines, Urine *on page 1294*

Doe *see* Methamphetamines, Urine *on page 1294*

Dolophine® *see* Methadone, Quantitative, Serum *on page 1293*

Dolophine® *see* Methadone, Urine *on page 1293*

Dopamine, Urine *see* Catecholamines, Fractionation, Urine *on page 1222*

Doriden® *see* Glutethimide, Blood *on page 1270*

Doxepin, Blood

Synonyms Adapin®; Sinequan®

Test Includes Desmethyldoxepin

Abstract This is a tricyclic antidepressant. It is not a drug of abuse.

Specimen Blood

Container Red top tube or green top (heparin) tube

Sampling Time Trough levels at steady-state

Reference Range Doxepin and desmethyldoxepin 110-250 ng/mL (SI: 4-9 nmol/L)

Critical Values >300 ng/mL (SI: >11 nmol/L); fatal cases associated with values >10,000 ng/mL

Use Therapeutic monitoring; toxicity assessment

Methodology High performance liquid chromatography (HPLC), gas chromatography (GC)

Additional Information Doxepin, a tricyclic antidepressant, is a tertiary amine structural analog of amitriptyline with similar but less potent neurotransmitter ef-

(Continued)

Doxepin, Blood *(Continued)*

fects and considerably less cardiotoxicity. Doxepin is metabolized to the active metabolite desmethyldoxepin (nordoxepin); its half-life is 45 hours. Doxepin serum levels peak at 2-6 hours after an oral dose and the half-life is 8-25 hours (average is 15 hours). The parent drug has a low bioavailability and steady-state is reached in 2-8 days. Geriatric patients respond well to doxepin.

Specific References

Ereshefsky L, Tran-Johnson T, Davis CM, et al, "Pharmacokinetic Factors Affecting Antidepressant Drug Clearance and Clinical Effect: Evaluation of Doxepin and Imipramine – New Data and Review," *Clin Chem*, 1988, 34(5):863-80.

Milstein S, Buetikofer J, Dunnigan A, et al, "Usefulness of Disopyramide for Prevention of Upright Tilt-Induced Hypotension-Bradycardia," *Am J Cardiol*, 1990, 65(20):1339-44.

2,3-DPG *see* Oxygen Saturation, Blood *on page 1313*

Drug Analysis, Not Specifically Listed *see* Toxicology Studies, Not Specifically Listed *on page 1367*

Drug Levels, Not Specifically Listed *see* Toxicology Studies, Not Specifically Listed *on page 1367*

Drug Screen, Comprehensive Panel or Analysis *see* Toxicology Drug Screen, Blood *on page 1364*

Drug Screen, Comprehensive Panel or Analysis, Urine *see* Toxicology Drug Screen, Urine *on page 1365*

Drug Screen, Meconium *see* Meconium Drug Screen *on page 1291*

Drugs of Abuse Screen, Urine

Synonyms Abuse Screen; DAU; DAU-10; Pre-employment Drug Screen

Test Includes Screens for common classes of abused drugs – amphetamines, barbiturates, benzodiazepines, cannabinoids, cocaine, methadone, methaqualone, opiates, phencyclidine, propoxyphene. In some laboratories, urine ethanol is included.

Abstract The usual drug-of-abuse screening panel consists of the 10 drugs listed above under "test includes".

Specimen Urine

Volume 50 mL

Minimum Volume 5 mL

Container Plastic urine container

Collection If forensic, observe precautions.

Storage Instructions Refrigerate

Causes for Rejection If forensic, failure to meet temperature requirements and tests for unusual urine dilution or alteration

Special Instructions Specify the drug or drugs suspected in an emergency situation. If forensic, use chain-of-custody protocol and form.

Reference Range Negative (less than cutoff)

Use Screen for drug overdose and toxicity; screen for the presence of drugs of abuse

Limitations This test provides only **qualitative** detection of drugs. Quantitation of drug levels is not included and is not recommended because urine levels are time and clearance dependent and are not directly related to toxic symptoms seen clinically. In a nonclinical setting (eg, pre-employment drug screening, etc), the sample should be collected under chain-of-custody, and all positive screens must be confirmed by a different, more sensitive method, preferably GC/MS. The transportation industry [Department of Transportation (DOT)] tests certain employees by screening for five classes of drugs only (amphetamines, cannabinoids, cocaine, opiates, phencyclidine) and confirms all positive results with GC/MS. National Institute on Drug Abuse (NIDA) certification required to perform tests for DOT. (See Federal Register 54(230), December 1, 1989.) Chain-of-custody protocol must be followed for these specimens. Any agent identified in a screening test **should be confirmed** by a test specific for that drug (usually GC/MS).

Methodology Screen: immunoassay, gas chromatography (GC), thin-layer chromatography (TLC), high performance liquid chromatography (HPLC); confirmation: gas chromatography/mass spectrometry (GC/MS)

Specific References

Caplan YH, "Drug Testing in Urine," *J Forensic Sci*, 1989, 34:1417-21.

Chia DT and Gere JA, "Rapid Drug Screening Using Toxi-Lab® Extraction Followed by Capillary Gas Chromatography/Mass Spectroscopy," *Clin Biochem*, 1987, 20(5):303-6.

Council on Scientific Affairs, "Alcohol and the Driver," *JAMA*, 1986, 255(4):522-7.

De Cresce R, Mazura A, Lifshitz M, et al, *Drug Testing in the Workplace*, Chicago, IL: ASCP Press, 1989.

Hawks RL and Chiang CN, "Urine Testing for Drugs of Abuse," NIDA Research Monograph 73, 1986.

Lillsunde P and Korte T, "Comprehensive Drug Screening in Urine Using Solid-Phase Extraction and Combined TLC and GC/MS Identification," *J Anal Toxicol*, 1991, 15(2):71-81.

McBay AJ and Mason AP, "Forensic Science Identification of Drugs of Abuse," *J Forensic Sci*, 1989, 34:1471-6.

Nice A, Leikin JB, Maturen A, et al, "Toxidrome Recognition to Improve Efficiency of Emergency Urine Drug Screens," *Ann Emerg Med*, 1988, 17(7):676-80.

Schwartz RH, "Urine Testing in the Detection of Drugs of Abuse," *Arch Intern Med*, 1988, 148(11):2407-12.

Simpson D, Jarvie DR, and Heyworth R, "An Evaluation of Six Methods for the Detection of Drugs of Abuse in Urine," *Ann Clin Biochem*, 1989, 26(Pt 2):172-81.

Wells VE, Halperin W, Thun M, "The Estimated Predictive Value of Screening for Illicit Drugs in the Workplace," *Am J Public Health*, 1988, 78(7):817-9.

Ear Oximetry *see* Pulse Oximetry *on page 1342*

ECG *see* Electrocardiography *on this page*

Ectoparasite Identification *see* Arthropod Identification *on page 1198*

E.E.S.® *see* Erythromycin, Blood *on page 1260*

EKG *see* Electrocardiography *on this page*

Elavil® *see* Amitriptyline, Blood *on page 1187*

Electrocardiography

Synonyms Cardiogram, Electro; ECG; EKG

Test Includes The electrocardiogram (EKG) remains the basic cardiologic test and is widely applied in patients with suspected or known heart disease and as a basic reference for most other cardiologic tests. Although 1-lead EKG is used as reference for most other cardiologic diagnostic procedures, the electrocardiogram, in the present context, will be the full 12-lead EKG recording.

Patient Preparation No special patient preparation is needed, patients do not need to fast before the EKG is taken and no special time of the day is preferable.

Technique After checking the appropriateness and type of EKG to be taken, a brief description of the procedure is provided to the patient. With the patient in a supine and relaxed position, the wrists and ankles are prepared for the extremity leads. The precordium is prepared and marked for the precordial leads and the electrodes are put in place with contact gel and supported by elastic straps in the extremities and suction cups in the precordium. After making sure the calibration settings are adequate, registration of the 12 leads is accomplished. This can be done by selecting lead by lead or, with the newer EKG recorders, by simultaneous recordings of 3-6 leads. The recordings are usually made at a paper speed of 25 mm/second. Usually one copy is left in the chart or is given to the patient and one copy goes to the EKG Laboratory for interpretation and findings.

Special Instructions Inpatients will have a bedside EKG and outpatients will go to the EKG Laboratory. Patients can be scheduled to have a routine EKG (to be done within 24 hours of request) or stat EKG to be done immediately. The reason for the request should be noted in the chart or in the requisition form. Additional information of interest includes patient's age, sex, and race, as well as any cardiac medications they may be taking. Situations that require special lead placement should be noted. These include use of back leads if a posterior myocardial infarction is suspected and use of right precordial leads if a right ventricular infarction is suspected. If the patient has a rhythm disturbance a rhythm strip may be requested.

Reference Range Proper interpretation of electrocardiograms is essential for all physicians and especially for those who take care of patients with potential heart problems. The interpretation of the normal electrocardiogram and its variants needs to be emphasized at all levels of medical training and continued interpretation and education is required if a person is to maintain proficiency in EKG interpretation. Distinct abnormalities exist in the EKG in the presence of chamber dilatation or hypertrophy, in the presence of acute or remote myocardial infarction, pericarditis, ventricular aneurysms, and conduction abnormalities.

Use In patients without known heart disease, the EKG is used as a screening test for occult coronary artery disease, cardiomyopathies, or left ventricular hypertrophy. EKG is used as a baseline for future reference and comparison and preoperatively, to rule out silent coronary artery disease. The EKG may also provide useful insight in the presence of metabolic alterations, such as hypercalcemia and hypocalcemia and hyperkalemia and hypokalemia. In patients with known heart disease, the EKG serves as a useful marker for the severity and progression of the disease process. The EKG is invaluable in the evaluation of patients with chest pain and in the management of patients with suspected or known to have acute myocardial infarction or coronary insufficiency. Most patients with myocardial, valvular, and congenital heart disease will eventually demonstrate EKG abnormalities and an EKG is warranted in these cases for diagnostic as well as management purposes. Rhythm disorders can be evaluated through EKG rhythm strips. In toxicology, the EKG is particularly useful in tricyclic antidepressant poisoning (widened QRS, prolonged PR and QT intervals, sinus tachycardia) along with antiarrhythmic toxicity. Various drugs can cause QT interval prolongation along with torsade de pointes.

(Continued)

Electrocardiography *(Continued)*

Contraindications There are no contraindications for EKG recordings.

Specific References

Grauer K and Curry RW, *Clinical Electrocardiography: A Primary Care Approach*, Oradell, NJ: Medical Economics Books, 1986.

Wilson RF, Marcus ML, Christensen BV, et al, "Accuracy of Exercise Electrocardiography in Detecting Physiologically Significant Coronary Arterial Lesions," *Circulation*, 1991, 83(2):412-21.

Electrodiagnostic Study *see* Electromyography *on next page*

Electrolyte Gap *see* Anion Gap, Blood *on page 1193*

Electrolytes, Blood

Synonyms Plasma Electrolytes; Serum Electrolytes

Test Includes Sodium, potassium, chloride; often total CO_2, but in some laboratories pH and pCO_2 are measured and bicarbonate (HCO_3) and CO_2T are calculated. Anion gap is reported with electrolytes by some laboratories.

Specimen Blood

Volume 10 mL

Minimum Volume 3 mL serum or plasma

Container Red top tube or green top (heparin) tube

Collection Best to collect without tourniquet if possible. Do **not** allow patient to clench-unclench his/her hand.

Storage Instructions Do not freeze.

Use Monitor electrolyte status; screen water balance; diagnose respiratory and metabolic acid-base balance; evaluate hydrational status, diarrhea, dehydration, ketoacidosis in diabetes mellitus and other disorders; evaluate alcoholism and other toxicity states

Limitations Hemolysis and prolonged contact of serum with cells produces elevation of potassium. The usual order for "electrolytes" does not include magnesium, osmolality, phosphorus, or lactic acid.

Methodology Ion-selective electrodes (ISE) or flame photometry are used for sodium and potassium. Sodium and potassium may also be measured by inductively-coupled plasma emission spectrometry.

Additional Information May be performed on heparinized plasma but not on EDTA plasma. Knowledge of pertinent clinical criteria allows for more cost effective ordering of blood electrolytes in patients in whom the information will be clinically significant. The anion gap, calculated $Na^+ - (Cl^- + HCO_3^-)$, provides useful information for interpreting acid-base disorders and may be useful for establishing a differential diagnosis in some conditions.

Specific References

Cleland JG and Dargie HJ, "Arrhythmias, Catecholamines and Electrolytes," *Am J Cardiol*, 1988, 62(2):55A-9A.

Ford HC, Lim WC, Chisnall WN, et al, "Renal Function and Electrolyte Levels in Hyperthyroidism: Urinary Protein Excretion and the Plasma Concentrations of Urea, Creatinine, Uric Acid, Hydrogen Ion, and Electrolytes," *Clin Endocrinol (Oxf)*, 1989, 30(3):293-301.

Graber M and Corish D, "The Electrolytes in Hyponatremia," *Am J Kidney Dis*, 1991, 18(5):527-45.

Kapsner CO and Tzamaloukas AH, "Understanding Serum Electrolytes. How to Avoid Mistakes," *Postgrad Med*, 1991, 90(8):151-4, 157-8, 161.

Lowe RA, Arst HF, and Ellis BK, "Rational Ordering of Electrolytes in the Emergency Department," *Ann Emerg Med*, 1991, 20(1):16-21.

McCleane GJ, "Urea and Electrolyte Measurement in Preoperative Surgical Patients," *Anaesthesia*, 1988, 43(5):413-5.

Olshaker JS and Mason JD, "The Usefulness of Serum Electrolytes in the Evaluation of Acute Adult Gastroenteritis," *Ann Emerg Med*, 1989, 18(3):258-60.

Electrolytes, Serum or Plasma *see* Potassium, Blood *on page 1328*

Electrolytes, Urine

Related Information

Osmolality, Urine *on page 1311*

Synonyms Urine Electrolytes

Test Includes Sodium, potassium, and chloride on random or timed collections. Osmolality must be ordered as such.

Specimen Random, 12-, or 24-hour urine

Volume 10 mL

Container Clean urine container

Collection Specify whether random or timed collection.

Causes for Rejection Blood in urine

Special Instructions Urine osmolality may be ordered with urine electrolytes, usually it must be specifically ordered.

Reference Range There is a large diurnal variation in range for spot samples. Na/K ratio: 0.90-3.88; borderline Na/K ratio: 0.3-6.0.

Use Monitor kidney function, fluid and electrolyte balance, water balance, acid-base balance; evaluate electrolyte composition of urine, correlation with renin and aldosterone studies. Urine sodium levels are appropriate in patients with volume depletion, with acute oliguria, and with decreased plasma sodium. Urine potassium levels are needed in work-up of hypokalemia of unknown etiology (eg, possible Conn's syndrome (primary aldosteronism), adrenal hyperplasia, Bartter's syndrome, renal tubular acidosis, Fanconi's syndrome). Urine chloride is helpful to work up metabolic alkalosis in patients who are not on diuretics; assess dietary salt restriction. Urine electrolytes are used in work-up with aldosterone and renin assays.

Additional Information If a 24-hour timed specimen is collected, other tests which may be ordered simultaneously include Protein, Quantitative, 24-hour Urine and/or Creatinine Clearance, (all of which can be collected together). Aldosterone and other adrenocortical steroids enhance reabsorption of sodium and promote excretion of potassium. In subjects with hyponatremia, normal blood volume, and urine Na and Cl >40 mmol/L, the differential diagnosis includes hypothyroidism and the syndrome of inappropriate secretion of antidiuretic hormone. See Osmolality, Urine listing. Metabolic alkalosis, urinary chloride excretion, and relationships to Cushing's, Conn's, and Bartter's syndromes are discussed in the references following. Fetal (amniotic fluid) electrolytes are not predictive of ultimate renal function.

Specific References

Kamel KS, Ethier JH, Richardson RM, et al, "Urine Electrolytes and Osmolality: When and How to Use Them," *Am J Nephrol*, 1990, 10(2):89-102.

Kamel KS, Magner PO, Ethier JH, et al, "Urine Electrolytes in the Assessment of Extracellular Fluid Volume Contraction," *Am J Nephrol*, 1989, 9(4):344-7.

Knuiman JT, van Poppel G, Burema J, et al, "Multiple Overnight Urine Collections May Be Used for Estimating the Excretion of Electrolytes and Creatinine," *Clin Chem*, 1988, 34(1):135-8.

Sherman RA and Eisinger RP, "The Use (and Misuse) of Urinary Sodium and Chloride Measurements," *JAMA*, 1982, 247(22):3121:4.

Electromyography

Synonyms Electrodiagnostic Study; EMG

Test Includes Insertion of a needle electrode into skeletal muscle to measure electrical activity and assess physiologic function. In this procedure, percutaneous, extracellular needle electrodes are placed into a selected muscle group. Muscle action potentials (AP) are detected by these electrodes, amplified, and displayed on a cathode ray oscilloscope. In addition, fluctuations in voltage are heard as "crackles" over a loudspeaker, permitting both auditory and visual analysis of the muscle APs. Testing is performed with the muscle at rest, with a mild voluntary contraction, and with maximal muscle contraction (where recruitment pattern and interference are noted). Unlike nerve conduction studies, EMG does not involve external electrical stimulation. Muscle APs (normal or abnormal) are physiologically generated. In various diseases of the motor system, typical electrical abnormalities may be present: increased insertional activity, abnormal motor unit potentials, fibrillations, fasciculations, positive sharp waves, decreased recruitment pattern, and others. EMG assesses the integrity of upper motor neurons, lower motor neurons, the neuromuscular junction, and the muscle itself. However, EMG is seldom diagnostic of a particular disease entity. Its major use lies in differentiating between the following disease classes: primary myopathy, peripheral motor neuron disease, and disease of the neuromuscular junction. As with nerve conduction velocity studies (with which EMG is usually paired), EMG should be considered an extension of the history and physical examination.

Patient Preparation Details of procedure are reviewed with the patient. Considerable patient apprehension often accompanies "needle tests" and calm reassurance from the medical team will go far in allaying such anxieties. Aspirin products should be discontinued 5-7 days beforehand. Nonsteroidal agents should also be stopped several days in advance. Routine medications may be taken on the morning of the examination. If coagulopathy is suspected, appropriate hematologic tests should be ordered (PT/PTT, CBC, bleeding time, etc). If a primary muscle disease is suspected, creatine phosphokinase (CPK) level should be drawn prior to needle examination. Routine EMG testing may cause minor elevations in CPK up to one and one-half times baseline. However, striking elevations in CPK, as seen with polymyositis or muscular dystrophy, are not associated with EMG testing.

Aftercare No specific activity restrictions are necessary. Patient may resume previous activity level.

Equipment EMG is performed in a specially equipped procedure room, usually reserved for electrodiagnostic studies. Basic instrumentation includes:

- needle electrodes; these may be monopolar (sharpened, coated steel wires), coaxial, or bipolar (two wires within a needle). These needles record electrical activity from muscle fibers directly contacting the tip, as well as fibers within a several millimeter radius.
- amplifier with filters

(Continued)

Electromyography *(Continued)*

- cathode ray oscilloscope with the vertical axis measuring voltage, the horizontal axis measuring time. This device usually has an audio amplifier and loudspeaker, which converts APs to sound energy.
- data storage apparatus (eg, magnetic tape recorder)

Technique A brief neurologic examination is performed prior to the start of the procedure. For EMG of the extremities, patient lies recumbent on the examination table. When paraspinal muscles are tested, the patient adopts a prone position. No intravenous sedatives or pain medications are used. Local anesthesia is also not required despite the generous number of needle insertions. The skin is cleansed thoroughly with alcohol pads, as necessary. Patient is instructed to relax as much as possible. The following steps are carried out.

- Recording needle electrode is inserted percutaneously into the muscle under consideration. The initial electrical activity of the muscle, as seen on the oscilloscope screen and heard over the loudspeaker, is termed the **insertional activity**.
- Next, the needle is held stationary and the muscle action potentials during voluntary relaxation are recorded.
- Patient performs a mild, submaximal contraction of the test muscle. The summed muscle action potentials - the motor unit potential - are observed on the oscilloscope.
- Finally, a maximal muscle contraction is carried out. The compound action potentials generated during this maneuver are studied for **interference** and **recruitment pattern**.

Needle examination is, by nature, a slow and labor-intensive process. Numerous muscles must be tested individually including both symptomatic and clinically asymptomatic muscles. Within a specific muscle, several independent sites may need to be examined, particularly when the muscle has a large surface area. A number of myopathic processes are focal and sampling errors even within an individual muscle are possible (ie, disease process may effect proximal portion of a muscle, sparing distal fibers).

Special Instructions Requisition from ordering physician should include brief clinical history, tentative neurologic diagnosis, and the specific limb(s) or muscle group(s) in question. Physician should also state whether nerve conduction studies are desired, although in some centers these may be added at the neurologist's discretion.

Reference Range Results are interpreted by neurologist or physiatrist with preliminary impression written in chart immediately. A formal, typed report is completed several days later. The fundamental principles underlying test interpretation are as follows.

- Insertional activity: Immediately upon needle insertion, there is a brief burst of electrical activity lasting <300 msec. This "insertional activity" is heard over the loudspeaker and may be increased or decreased in various disease states.
- Electrical activity at rest: Muscle tissue is normally silent at rest. No action potentials are seen on the oscilloscope.
- Minimal muscle contraction: When a minimal contraction is performed, several motor unit potentials (MUPs) are activated. Several individual APs are normally visible on the oscilloscope at a rate of 4-5/second. The idealized configuration of a single MUP is depicted in the following figure (see normal column).

EMG FINDINGS

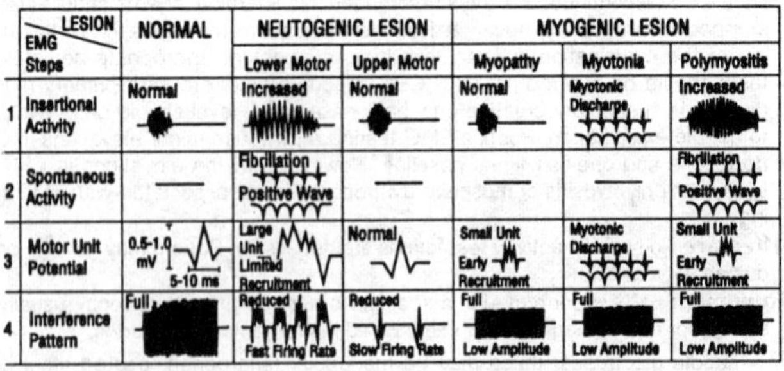

	EMG Steps / LESION	NORMAL	NEUTOGENIC LESION		MYOGENIC LESION		
			Lower Motor	Upper Motor	Myopathy	Myotonia	Polymyositis
1	Insertional Activity	Normal	Increased	Normal	Normal	Myotonic Discharge	Increased
2	Spontaneous Activity		Fibrillation Positive Wave				Fibrillation Positive Wave
3	Motor Unit Potential	0.5-1.0 mV 5-10 ms	Large Unit Limited Recruitment	Normal	Small Unit Early Recruitment	Myotonic Discharge	Small Unit Early Recruitment
4	Interference Pattern	Full	Reduced Fast Firing Rate	Reduced Slow Firing Rate	Full Low Amplitude	Full Low Amplitude	Full Low Amplitude

Idealized EMG findings, normal, neurogenic lesions, and myogenic lesions. Reproduced with permission from Kimura J, Chapter 13, "Types of Abnormality," *Electrodiagnosis in Diseases of Nerve and Muscle: Principles and Practice*, 2nd ed, Philadelphia, PA: FA Davis, 1989, 263.

- Full voluntary contraction: As the strength of the muscle contraction increases, further muscle units are "recruited". On the oscilloscope the APs appear more disorganized and individual APs can no longer be recognized. At the peak of a contraction the "complete recruitment pattern" is seen, which represents a compilation of motor unit potentials firing asynchronously. The normal interference pattern is considered "full," that is, the amplitude of APs is high (≤5 mV) and firing rate is fast (40/second).

Critical Values Abnormalities in one or more of the previously stated parameters may be seen.

Insertional activity: Increased in both neurogenic disorders (eg, lower motor nerve disease) and myogenic disorders (eg, polymyositis), and thus is considered nonspecific. Decreased insertional activity is less common, but may be associated with far advanced denervation or myopathy, especially when muscle is replaced by fat or collagen. A distinctive insertional pattern is seen with myotonia, an unusual neurologic disorder, and is termed "myotonic discharge".

Abnormal activity at rest: Instead of the electrical silence which characterizes the muscle at rest, spontaneous action potentials in single muscle fibers ("fibrillation potentials") may be observed in several disease states.

Fibrillations are seen 1-3 weeks after destruction of a lower motor neuron. Denervated muscle fibers develop heightened chemosensitivity and individual muscle fibers contract spontaneously. The phenomenon of "positive sharp waves" may also be seen. Fibrillations may also occur with severe polymyositis when extensive areas of necrosis interrupt nerve innervation. The naked eye is unable to perceive fibrillations.

Fasciculations represent random contractions of a full motor unit, often visible through the skin. (A motor unit is comprised of an anterior horn cell, axon, neuromuscular junction, and the numerous muscle fibers supplied by the axon.) Fasciculations may be benign, with no other EMG abnormalities observed. They may also be associated with amyotrophic lateral sclerosis, other anterior horn cell diseases, nerve root compression, herniated nucleus pulposus syndrome, acute polyneuropathy, and others.

Abnormalities in the motor unit potential (MUP): Individual motor unit potentials are distinguishable during a submaximal muscle contraction. Abnormalities in amplitude, shape (number of phases, serrations, configuration), and duration are possible. Increased MUP amplitude is seen in lower motor neuron disease but is normal in upper motor neuron disease. Decreased MUP amplitude is characteristic of polymyositis and other myopathies and duration of the MUP is also decreased.

Abnormalities in interference pattern: The normal "full recruitment" pattern seen during maximal muscle contraction is often compromised in disease states. In myogenic lesions, such as polymyositis and myotonia, the amplitude of the MUPs is significantly decreased but the recruitment pattern is normal (ie, the number of activated motor units is normal but the number of muscle fibers per motor unit is diminished). In LMN lesions, the number of motor units recruited is decreased. In severe cases of neuropathy, the maximum interference pattern resembles that of a single MUP, with individual potentials visible. Amplitude of MUPs may be normal. These findings are summarized in the previous figure.

Use In the neurologic literature, EMG has been performed in a wide variety of clinical situations, many of which are experimental or highly specialized in nature. Common indications for EMG in general practice include:

Evaluation of the patient with clinical features of primary muscle disease (symmetric and proximal weakness, muscle atrophy, intact sensory system, etc). Examples include:

- muscular dystrophy
- glycogen storage disease
- myotonia
- inflammatory myopathies (systemic lupus, sarcoidosis, infectious myopathies)
- polydermatomyositis
- alcoholic myopathy
- endocrine myopathies, and others

Evaluation of the patient with lower motor neuron disease, including:

- suspected peripheral nerve lesions, such as diffuse peripheral neuropathies, spinal root lesions, and trauma
- suspected disease of the anterior horn cells (characterized by asymmetric weakness, muscle atrophy, fasciculations), as in amyotrophic lateral sclerosis or poliomyelitis

In clinical toxicology, EMG may be of some use in evaluation of botulism.

Assessment of the patient with suspected upper motor neuron disease, when prior imaging studies are inconclusive. This includes occult lesions of the corti-

(Continued)

Electromyography *(Continued)*

cospinal tract (syringomyelia, tumor) and, less commonly, lesions of the cerebral tract (tumor, CVA). Evaluation of the patient with suspected neuromuscular junction disease (NMJ). This includes myasthenia gravis and the paraneoplastic Eaton-Lambert syndrome. Conventional EMG, as described here, is not the diagnostic test of choice for myasthenia gravis. However, other forms of EMG such as single fiber EMG and repetitive stimulation tests are highly specific for NMJ disease. Assessment of the patient with severe and persistent muscle cramps. Serial documentation of response to therapy for known cases of myopathy or neuropathy. Identification of significantly diseased muscle groups to help guide muscle biopsy (if clinical examination is not inconclusive). EMG is less useful in:

- the restless legs syndrome
- transient, self-resolving muscle cramps
- uncomplicated cases of polymyalgia rheumatica unless the diagnosis is in doubt or underlying myositis is suspected
- routine cases of fibrositis/fibromyalgia (EMG abnormalities have recently been documented in the medical literature but needle examination is not routinely indicated)

Contraindications The following situations represent relative contraindications:

- severe coagulopathy, including hemophilia and marked thrombocytopenia. It should be noted that EMG has been performed safely with platelet counts as low as 20,000/mm^3, but this is not recommended.
- systemic anticoagulation (eg, intravenous heparin, oral Coumadin®)
- patients with an unusual susceptibility to systemic infections (EMG has been known to cause transient bacteremia)
- patients undergoing a muscle biopsy after EMG require special consideration. It is well known that needle insertion and manipulation during EMG may cause local microscopic tissue damage on a traumatic basis. Histologically, this damage may be confused with a focal myopathy. Thus, some experts avoid detailed needle examinations of the specific muscle group which will be biopsied (although EMG testing of surrounding muscle groups is frequently performed).

Specific References

Adams RD and Victor M, *Principles of Neurology*, 4th ed, New York, NY: McGraw-Hill Book Co, 1989, 1009-27.

Aminoff MJ, *Electromyography in Clinical Practice*, 2nd ed, New York, NY: Churchill-Livingston, 1987.

Goodgold J and Eberstein A, *Electrodiagnosis of Neuromuscular Diseases*, 3rd ed, Baltimore, MD: Williams & Wilkins, 1983.

Griggs RC, Bradley WG, and Shahani B, "Approach to the Patient With Neuromuscular Disease," *Harrison's Principles of Internal Medicine*, 12th ed, Wilson JD, Braunwald E, Isselbacher KJ, et al, eds, New York, NY: McGraw-Hill Book Co, 1991, 2088-96.

Johnson EW and Wiechers D, "Electrodiagnosis," *Krusen's Handbook of Physical Medicine and Rehabilitation*, 3rd ed, Kottke FJ, Stillwell GK, and Lehmann JF, eds, Philadelphia, PA: WB Saunders Co, 1982, 56-85.

Kimura J, *Electrodiagnosis in Diseases of Nerve and Muscle: Principles and Practice*, 2nd ed, Philadelphia, PA: FA Davis Co, 1989.

Elephant Tranquilizers *see* Phencyclidine, Qualitative, Urine *on page 1319*

Elixophyllin® *see* Theophylline, Blood *on page 1359*

EMG *see* Electromyography *on page 1255*

E-Mycin® *see* Erythromycin, Blood *on page 1260*

Encainide, Blood

Synonyms Enkaid®

Test Includes 3-methoxy-O-desmethylencainide (MODE), O-desmethylencainide (ODE)

Abstract Encainide is an antiarrhythmic used to suppress premature ventricular contractions and ventricular tachycardia. It undergoes extensive metabolism to two very active metabolites, which must also be measured.

Specimen Blood

Container Red top tube

Storage Instructions Centrifuge, separate, and freeze if not analyzing immediately.

Reference Range At steady-state encainide: 50-85 μg/L (SI: 130-220 nmol/L); ODE: 180-220 μg/L (SI: 460-565 nmol/L); MODE: 140-185 μg/L (SI: 360-475 nmol/L) (normal phenotype)

Possible Panic Range Not well established; side effects at ODE levels of 300-500 μg/L (SI: 770-1285 nmol/L)

Use Therapeutic monitoring; toxicity assessment

Contraindications Cimetidine significantly increases serum concentration of parent and metabolites

Methodology High performance liquid chromatography (HPLC)

Additional Information Encainide is a class 1C antiarrhythmic drug approved for the suppression of premature ventricular contractions and life-threatening ventricular tachycardia. It undergoes extensive first-pass metabolism. The metabolites O-desmethyl (ODE) and 3-methoxy-O-desmethylencainide (MODE) have greater activity than the parent drug. In normal metabolizers, therapeutic effect correlates with combined concentration of two metabolites and the parent drug; in poor metabolizers there are small amounts of metabolites and effect correlates with parent drug concentration. Drug can worsen arrhythmias or induce new tachycardias. Minor side effects (dizziness and blurred vision) can be minimized by administering drug with food. Coadministration with other cardioactive drugs is well tolerated. Can cause adverse effects in patients with severe chronic heart failure.

Specific References

Bartek MJ, Mayol RF, Boarman MP, et al, "Analysis of Encainide and Metabolites in Plasma and Urine by High-Performance Liquid Chromatography," *Ther Drug Monit*, 1988, 10(4):446-51.

Fish FA, Gillette PC, and Benson DW Jr, "Proarrhythmia, Cardiac Arrest and Death in Young Patients Receiving Encainide and Flecainide. The Pediatric Electrophysiology Group," *J Am Coll Cardiol*, 1991, 18(2):356-65.

Roden DM and Woosley RL, "Clinical Pharmacokinetics of Encainide," *Clin Pharmacokinet*, 1988, 14(3):141-7.

Turgeon J and Roden DM, "Pharmacokinetic Profile of Encainide," *Clin Pharmacol Ther*, 1989, 45(6):692-4.

Woosley RL, Wood AJ, and Roden DM, "Drug Therapy. Encainide," *N Engl J Med*, 1988, 318(17):1107-15.

Endep® *see* Amitriptyline, Blood *on page 1187*

Enkaid® *see* Encainide, Blood *on previous page*

Enteric Pathogens Culture, Routine *see* Stool Culture *on page 1356*

Eos Count *see* Eosinophil Count *on this page*

Eosinophil Count

Synonyms Absolute Eosinophil Count; Eos Count; Total Eosinophil Count

Applies To Cytokines; Granulocyte/Macrophage Colony Stimulating Factor; Interleukin-3; Interleukin-5

Abstract Manual (using phloxine stain) or automated absolute eosinophil count is requested in certain clinical situations because of expected greater precision/accuracy than is usually obtained using the relative number of eosinophils from the manual differential count. Eosinophil count is increased in a wide variety of conditions including especially, allergy, drug reaction, parasitism, collagen vascular disease, and some malignant states. Eosinophils are decreased with hyperadrenalism.

Specimen Whole blood

Volume 5 mL

Minimum Volume 1 mL

Container Lavender top (EDTA) tube

Causes for Rejection Clotted specimen, specimen more than 4 hours old

Reference Range 50-350/mm^3

Use Aid in the diagnosis of allergy, drug reaction, parasitic infestations, collagen disease, Hodgkin's disease, and myeloproliferative diseases. Increased also in a broad range of less common conditions including the acute hypereosinophilic syndrome, angioneurotic edema, acute renal allograft rejection, eosinophilic nonallergic rhinitis, anisakiasis, eosinophilic gastroenteritis, eosinophilia myalgia syndrome, and others. Decrease in eosinophils occurs in Cushing's disease (hyperadrenalism).

Limitations Manual method is subject to an inherent error of 20% to 30%.

Methodology Manual, using Fuchs-Rosenthal or Speirs-Levy special large volume hemocytometer and eosinophil stain diluent (eg, Pilot's solution or phloxine B solution as used in the Unopette™ Brand System, Becton Dickinson, Rutherford, NJ). Automated method (eg, Technicon®, Coulter, Sysmex) should provide greater precision/accuracy and is recommended for obtaining an absolute eosinophil count.

Additional Information Toxocaral disease (visceral larva migrans) is a typical parasitic disease in which eosinophil counts (eosinophils >30% on differential) are usually elevated. Taylor et al point out, however, that up to 27% of children with toxocariasis have normal eosinophil counts. Thus, normal eosinophil counts do not rule out toxocaral disease or other parasitic infestations. The T-cell produced cytokines interleukin-3, granulocyte/macrophage colony stimulating factor, and interleukin-5 (IL-5) stimulate eosinophil production *in vitro*. Murine eosinophil differentiation factor (IL-5) has its most specific effect on eosinophil growth in culture with no significant effect on growth/development of other myeloid cell lines. IL-5 appears to be the prime mediator of eosinophilia in patients with certain parasitic diseases.

(Continued)

Eosinophil Count *(Continued)*

An important although rare cause of increased eosinophils in the peripheral blood is the acute hypereosinophilic syndrome (HES). Reported mortalities range from 81% to 95% in 1-3 years. The HES syndrome includes high peripheral WBC count, circulating early eosinophil forms without blast cells, mental confusion, delusions, near coma, and severe cardiac symptoms. Consistently associated with a poor prognosis are WBC count ≥90,000/mm³, blast forms in blood, heart failure, and severe CNS symptoms (confusion, organic psychosis and coma). This condition may not be a true leukemic myeloproliferative disease, although concepts of HES are controversial.

Infiltrative lung diseases, in which peripheral blood eosinophils may be increased, include eosinophilic pneumonia, Löffler's syndrome (often related to *Ascaris* infestation), and tropical eosinophilia (usually related to filariasis).

Eosinophilic gastroenteritis may occur with blood eosinophilia.

Eosinophilia myalgia syndrome (EMS) characterized by an eosinophil count ≥1000 cells/mm³ and severe often incapacitating myalgia is possibly associated with the use of L-tryptophan-containing products (LTCPs). Further definition of this syndrome, causal association between LTCPs and EMS, and modifying etiologic factors/cofactors has been recommended and is being pursued by CDC. An EMS-like syndrome has been considered to result from several factors including ingestion of tryptophan, inactivation of indoleamine-2,3-dioxygenase, and possible impairment of the hypothalamic-pituitary-adrenal axis. The differential diagnosis of EMS (causes other than L-tryptophan) is discussed by Dicker et al (see Specific References). Sarcoidosis, granulomatous myositis, collagen vascular diseases, neoplastic myositis, and other entities should be considered. EMS is potentially fatal (Guillain-Barré like ascending polyneuropathy) with a clinical course resembling the toxic oil syndrome that was epidemic in Spain in 1981.

Specific References

Dicker RM, James N, and Cunha BA, "The Eosinophilia-Myalgia Syndrome With Neuritis Associated With L-Tryptophan Use," *Ann Intern Med*, 1990, 112(12):957-8.

Duffy J, "Eosinophilia-Myalgia Syndrome," *Mayo Clin Proc*, 1992, 67(12):1201-2.

Mahmond, AAF, Austen, KF, and Simon, AS, *The Eosinophil in Health and Disease*, New York, NY: Grune and Stratton Inc, 1980.

Martin RW, Duffy J, Engel AG, et al, "The Clinical Spectrum of the Eosinophilia-Myalgia Syndrome Associated With L-Tryptophan Ingestion. Clinical Features in 20 Patients and Aspects of Pathophysiology," *Ann Intern Med*, 1990, 113(9):124-34.

Mayeno AN, Belongia EA, Lin F, et al, "3-(Phenylamino)alanine, a Novel Aniline-Derived Amino Acid Associated With the Eosinophilia-Myalgia Syndrome: A Link to the Toxic Oil Syndrome?" *Mayo Clin Proc*, 1992, 67(12):1134-9.

Randolph TG, "Differentiation and Enumeration of Eosinophils in the Counting Chamber With a Glycol Stain; A Valuable Technique in Appraising ACTH Dosage," *J Lab Clin Med*, 1949, 34:1696-1701.

Shurin SB, "Eosinophil and Basophil Structure and Function," *Hematology Basic Principles and Practice*, Chapter 41, Hoffman R, Benz EJ Jr, Shattil SJ, et al, eds, New York, NY: Churchill Livingstone, 1991, 538-42.

Van Slyck EJ and Adamson TC III, "Acute Hypereosinophilic Syndrome. Successful Treatment With Vincristine, Cytarabine, and Prednisone," *JAMA*, 1979, 242(2):175-6.

Smith H and Cook RM, *Immunopharmacology of Eosinophils, The Handbook of Immunopharmacology*, Page C, ed, San Diego, CA: Academic Press, 1993, 1-250.

Epilim® *see* Valproic Acid, Blood *on page 1377*

Epinephrine, Urine *see* Catecholamines, Fractionation, Urine *on page 1222*

Equagesic® *see* Meprobamate, Blood *on page 1291*

Equanil® *see* Meprobamate, Blood *on page 1291*

Ergenyl® *see* Valproic Acid, Blood *on page 1377*

Erythrocyte Cholinesterase *see* Acetylcholinesterase, Red Blood Cell *on page 1181*

Erythromycin, Blood

Synonyms E.E.S.®; E-Mycin®; Ilotycin®; Robimycin®

Specimen Blood

Volume 10 mL

Minimum Volume 2 mL serum

Container Red top tube

Collection Routine venipuncture

Storage Instructions Refrigerate serum.

Special Instructions Must indicate time and date collected.

Reference Range Single oral dose of 0.5 g after 1-4 hours: 2-20 mg/L

Contraindications Erythromycin is contraindicated in patients with hypersensitivity to this drug.

Methodology High performance liquid chromatography (HPLC)

Additional Information Erythromycin, one of the safest antibiotics in use today, is produced by a strain of *Streptomyces erythraeus*. It is used in the treatment of susceptible bacterial infections of the upper and lower respiratory tract, otitis media, pelvic inflammatory disease, and other infections in patients allergic to penicillin. The peak plasma levels are achieved in about 4 hours, and the half-life is 0.8-3 hours. Administration every 6 hours is needed to achieve adequate blood levels. Adverse effects include abdominal pain, nausea, vomiting, diarrhea, hepatic dysfunction, rash, and ototoxicity.

Eskalith® *see* Lithium, Blood *on page 1285*

1,2-Ethanediol *see* Ethylene Glycol, Blood *on next page*

Ethanol *see* Volatile Screen *on page 1378*

Ethanol, Blood *see* Alcohol, Serum *on page 1183*

Ethchlorvynol, Blood

Synonyms Placidyl®

Abstract This is a sedative hypnotic which is considered dangerous if not carefully monitored.

Specimen Blood

Volume 10 mL

Container Red top tube or green top (heparin) tube

Sampling Time The peak blood level is attained in 1.5 hours

Reference Range 2-8 μg/mL (SI: 14-55 μmol/L)

Possible Panic Range Toxic: levels >20 μg/mL (SI: >138 μmol/L) are associated with severe sedation, coma, respiratory depression, hypotension, bradycardia, and hypothermia

Use Monitor therapeutic drug level

Methodology High performance liquid chromatography (HPLC), gas chromatography (GC), spectrophotometry

Additional Information Ethchlorvynol is a nonbarbiturate sedative-hypnotic drug. The peak blood level is attained in 1.5 hours. The half-life is 10-20 hours and increases to 100 hours when high levels of drug are present. Most of the drug is metabolized in the liver. Exaggerated hypnotic effects occur if taken with ethanol. Can be detected in urine but only small amounts of the parent drug are present. Should be used cautiously in combination with oral anticoagulants. Effect is potentiated by alcohol.

Specific References

Baselt RC and Cravey RH, *Disposition of Toxic Drugs and Chemicals in Man*, 3rd ed, Year Book Medical Publishers Inc, 1989, 326.

Gomolin I, "Ethchlorvynol," *Clin Toxicol Rev*, 1980, 2:1-2.

Winek CL, Wahba WW, and Winek CL Jr, "Body Distribution of Ethchlorvynol," *J Forensic Sci*, 1989, 34(3):687-90.

Yell RP, "Ethchlorvynol Overdose," *Am J Emerg Med*, 1990, 8(3):246-50.

Ethosuximide, Blood

Synonyms Suxinutin®; Zarontin®; Zartalin®

Abstract Ethosuximide is a drug of choice for absence seizures not accompanied by other seizure types.

Specimen Blood

Volume 5 mL serum or plasma

Container Red top tube or green top (heparin) tube

Sampling Time Peak or trough levels may be used to monitor therapy because blood levels are fairly constant.

Reference Range 40-100 μg/mL (SI: 284-710 μmol/L)

Possible Panic Range >100 μg/mL (SI: >710 μmol/L); toxicity may manifest with lethargy or psychotic behavior; significant drug interactions are uncommon.

Use Monitor for compliance, efficacy, or possible toxicity

Limitations Ethosuximide has relatively few serious adverse effects with chronic administration. Dose-related adverse effects, including photophobia and lethargy, sometimes may be avoided by slowly titrating the drug to effective levels. Blood dyscrasias may occur and respond to decreasing dose or stopping the drug. If patients have other seizure types in addition to absence seizures, ethosuximide may exacerbate the other seizure types. Therefore, valproic acid is the drug of choice in that situation. Other succinimides, notably methsuximide and phensuximide, have been used adjunctively for absence seizures but are less effective and more toxic.

Methodology Enzyme immunoassay (EIA), gas-liquid chromatography (GLC), high performance liquid chromatography (HPLC)

Specific References

Baselt RC and Cravey RH, "Ethosuximide," *Disposition of Toxic Drugs and Chemicals in Man*, 3rd ed, Chicago, IL: Year Book Medical Publishers Inc, 1989, 332-4.

Kabra PM, Nelson MA, and Marton LJ, "Simultaneous Very Fast Liquid-Chromatographic Analysis of Ethosuximide, Primidone, Phenobarbital, Phenytoin, and Carbamazepine in Serum," *Clin Chem*, 1983, 29(3):673-6.

(Continued)

Ethosuximide, Blood *(Continued)*

Wad N, "Rapid Extraction Method for Ethosuximide and Other Antiepileptics in Serum for Determination by High-Performance Liquid Chromatography," *J Chromatogr*, 1985, 338(2):460-2.

Ethyl Alcohol, Blood *see* Alcohol, Serum *on page 1183*

Ethyl Alcohol, Urine *see* Alcohol, Semiquantitative, Urine *on page 1182*

Ethyl and Methyl Thiocyanate (Thanite® and Lethane®) *see* Thiocyanate, Blood or Urine *on page 1360*

Ethylene Glycol, Blood

Synonyms 1,2-Ethanediol

Applies To Antifreeze

Test Includes Propylene glycol

Abstract A commercial chemical used as a radiator antifreeze and for commercial chemical synthesis.

Specimen Blood

Container Red top tube or green top (heparin) tube

Reference Range Negative

Possible Panic Range Values between 0.3-4.0 g/L have been observed in fatal cases; levels at 0.5 g/L indicate hemodialysis.

Use Detect and quantitate ingestion of ethylene glycol

Methodology Gas-liquid chromatography (GLC), photometry, fluorometry, enzymatic assay (automated)

Additional Information Ethylene glycol is a colorless, odorless, sweet tasting compound used commercially in antifreeze. It has been utilized in suicide attempts, as a substitute for ethanol, and in accidental poisonings in both children and domestic pets. 100 mL is lethal; rapid treatment can prevent damage. Half-life is 3-5 hours. Toxicity is manifested by CNS depression (1-12 hours after ingestion), cardiopulmonary symptoms (12-24 hours after ingestion), and renal damage (24-72 hours after ingestion). Oxalate is a minor metabolite of ethylene glycol and crystals are commonly seen in urine. In addition to blood levels of ethylene glycol, hypocalcemia, anion gap metabolic acidosis, and osmolal gap elevation are observed. **Precaution:** Toxicity may be manifested without osmolal gap changes and osmolal and anion gap increases can be present with very low levels of glycol. Metabolizes to lactic and oxalic acid.

Specific References

Burkhart KK and Kulig KW, "The Other Alcohols. Methanol, Ethylene Glycol, and Isopropanol," *Emerg Med Clin North Am*, 1990, 8(4):913-28.

Cheng JT, Beysolow TD, Kaul B, et al, "Clearance of Ethylene Glycol by Kidneys and Hemodialysis," *J Toxicol Clin Toxicol*, 1987, 25(1-2):95-108.

Doedens DJ, "Review of Assay Methods," *Vet Hum Toxicol*, 1983, 25:96-101.

Jarvie DR and Simpson D, "Simple Screening Tests for the Emergency Identification of Methanol and Ethylene Glycol in Poisoned Patients," *Clin Chem*, 1990, 36(11):1957-61.

Mahly M, Lardet G, and Vallon JJ, "Automated Cobas Mira Kinetic Enzymatic Assay for Ethylene Glycol Applied to Emergency Situations," *J Anal Toxicol*, 1994, 18(5):269-71.

Ryder KW, Glick MR, and Jackson SA, "Emergency Screening of Ethylene Glycol in Serum," *Clin Chem*, 1986, 32(8):1574-7.

Ochs ML, Glick MR, Ryder KW, et al, "Improved Method for Emergency Screening for Ethylene Glycol in Serum," *Clin Chem*, 1988, 34(7):1507-8.

Porter GA, "The Treatment of Ethylene Glycol Poisoning Simplified," *N Engl J Med*, 1988, 319(2):109-10.

EtOH *see* Alcohol, Serum *on page 1183*

Etrafon® *see* Amitriptyline, Blood *on page 1187*

Exercise ABG *replaced by* Pulse Oximetry *on page 1342*

Factor V, Plasma

Synonyms Ac-Globulin; Labile Factor; Proaccelerin

Patient Preparation Avoid Coumadin® therapy for 2 weeks and heparin therapy for 2 days prior to test.

Specimen Plasma

Minimum Volume 4.5 mL

Container Blue top (sodium citrate) tube

Collection Routine venipuncture. If multiple tests are being drawn, draw coagulation studies last. If only coagulation tests are being drawn, draw 1-2 mL into another Vacutainer®, discard, and then collect coagulation tests. This collection procedure avoids contamination of the specimen with tissue thromboplastins.

Storage Instructions Deliver specimen immediately to the laboratory on ice. Centrifuge (in refrigerated centrifuge at 4°C) and separate plasma. Keep refrigerated and test immediately, preferably within 1-2 hours.

Causes for Rejection Tube not full, specimen hemolyzed, specimen clotted, specimen received more than 2 hours after collection

Special Instructions Not available in most general clinical laboratories. Communicate with laboratory for scheduling and referral as required.

Reference Range 50% to 150% of normal. Homozygous factor V deficient patients have <10% (often <5%) activity.

Use Document specific factor deficiency

Limitations Interpretation of results may be limited if patient is receiving anticoagulant therapy or if test is done more than 2 hours after collection.

Methodology Modified one-stage prothrombin time using commercially available factor V deficient preparation, known factor V deficient patient plasma or artificially prepared factor V deficient plasma. Chromogenic substrate assay.

Additional Information Factor V, a glycoprotein with molecular weight of 300,000, is synthesized in the liver. It is converted in the plasma from a single chain to a two chain molecule under the influence of thrombin activation. Activated V (Va) is a part of the prothrombin converting complex. Va is inactivated by protein Ca. The molecular characterization of Va, in particular identification of the structural determinants responsible for acceleration of prothrombin activation and those that bind to phospholipid surfaces, have been described. Factor V deficiency is inherited as an autosomal recessive, males and females are equally affected. Only homozygotes have bleeding symptoms; heterozygotes are largely asymptomatic. Symptoms include ecchymoses, epistaxis, menorrhagia, and bleeding following trauma and tooth extraction. GI hemorrhage and hemarthrosis may occur. Severity of bleeding does not correlate directly with factor V level, and symptoms are often mild, even in homozygotes. Cases of apparent combined factor V and factor VIII deficiency appear to be due to inherited deficiency of a plasma protein that inhibits activated protein C. Protein C is yet another vitamin K dependent serine protease zymogen coagulation protein, an anticoagulant that when activated (by thrombin, trypsin, or plasmin) destroys activated factors V and VIII. Homozygous V deficient individuals usually have prolonged whole blood clotting time, prothrombin time, and APTT. Platelet factor V is present in α-granules of platelets and is necessary to the binding of Xa to the platelet surface. Factor V deficient patients have varying levels of platelet factor V (may not be fully deficient). Platelet transfusion may have a role in the treatment of factor V deficient patients. It has been shown that commercial preparations of bovine thrombin may contain bovine factor V and patients exposed to topical thrombin (bovine) may develop antibodies to factor V. Antithrombin antibodies may also develop and mask the factor V inhibitor of activity that is responsible in part for clinical bleeding.

Specific References

Mammen EF, "Factor V Deficiency; Congenital Coagulation Disorders," *Semin Thromb Hemost*, New York, NY: Thieme-Stratton Inc, 1983, 9:17-8.

Factor I *see* Fibrinogen, Plasma *on page 1265*

Fe and TIBC *see* Iron and Total Iron Binding Capacity/Transferrin *on page 1275*

Fecal Leukocyte Stain

Test Includes Methylene blue, Gram's, or Wright stain of stool smear

Patient Preparation Collect specimen prior to barium procedures if possible.

Specimen Fresh random stool, rectal swab

Volume One rectal swab, 1 mL stool

Container Culturette®, sealed plastic stool container

Collection Transport specimen to laboratory as soon as possible after collection, significant deterioration of the specimen occurs with prolonged storage.

Storage Instructions Refrigerate

Causes for Rejection Insufficient specimen volume. Specimens which are delayed in transit are less than optimal.

Reference Range Few, if any, leukocytes

Use Assist in the differential diagnosis of diarrheal disease

Limitations Ten percent to 15% of stools which yield an invasive bacterial pathogen have an absence of fecal leukocytes. Many bacterial intestinal pathogens do not elicit a leukocyte response in stool. Fecal leukocytes are present in idiopathic inflammatory bowel disease.

Methodology Smear of stool (preferably mucus) with one drop methylene blue (or other stain), coverslip, and observe the presence of leukocytes.

Additional Information Conditions associated with varying degrees of fecal leukocytes, blood and/or mucus include diffuse antibiotic associated colitis, ulcerative colitis, shigellosis, *Campylobacter*, *Yersinia*, amebiasis, and some diarrheagenic *E. coli* infection. Conditions associated with an absence of fecal leukocytes include toxigenic bacterial infection, giardiasis, and viral infections. In a review the methylene blue stain for polymorpholeukocytes had a high sensitivity (85%) and specificity (88%) for bacterial diarrhea (*Shigella*, *Salmonella*, *Campylobacter*). Positive predictive value was poor (59%). Negative predicative value was 97%. In the presence of a history of abrupt onset, greater than four stools per day and no vom-

(Continued)

Fecal Leukocyte Stain *(Continued)*

iting before the onset of diarrhea, the methylene blue stain for fecal polymorphonuclear leukocytes was a very effective presumptive diagnostic test for bacterial diarrhea. A positive occult blood test may also be suggestive of acute bacterial diarrhea. Neither method is sufficiently sensitive or specific to pre-empt the use of culture. Similar findings including a sensitivity of 81% and specificity 74% were observed when both tests were positive.

Specific References

Bishop WP and Ulshen MH, "Bacterial Gastroenteritis," *Pediatr Clin North Am*, 1988, 35(1):69-87.

Harris JC, Dupont HL, and Hornick RB, "Fecal Leukocytes in Diarrheal Illness," *Ann Intern Med*, 1972, 76(5):697-703.

Siegel D, Cohen PT, Neighbor M, et al, "Predictive Value of Stool Examination in Acute Diarrhea," *Arch Pathol Lab Med*, 1987, 111(8):715-8.

Felbamate, Blood

Abstract FDA approved in August, 1993 for epilepsy treatment which does not respond to monotherapy or polypharmacy with other anticonvulsants.

Specimen Blood

Volume 5 mL

Reference Range None established; normal: 20-100 mg/L plasma concentrations during clinical trials

Use Monitor therapeutic and toxic levels

Methodology Thin-layer chromatography (TLC), high performance liquid chromatography (HPLC)

Additional Information

Distribution: V_d: 0.7-1.0 L/kg

Metabolizes to 2-hydroxy felbamate, *p*-phenylhydroxyfelbamate,and 2-phenyl-1,3-propanediol monocarbamate

Half-life: 20-23 hours

Primarily used as an anticonvulsant in epilepsy treatment; Lennox-Gastaut syndrome; wide therapeutic index, few significant side effects; significant interactions with valproic acid, carbamazepine, and phenytoin; low toxicity, reversible side effects include anorexia and insomnia

Specific References

Remmel RP, Miller SA, and Graves NM, "Simultaneous Assay of Felbamate Plus Carbamazepine, Phenytoin and Their Metabolites by Liquid Chromatography With Mobile Phase Optimization," *Ther Drug Monit*, 1990, 12(1):90-6.

Schmidt D, "Felbamate: Successful Development of a New Compound for the Treatment of Epilepsy," *Epilepsia*, 1993, 34(Suppl 7):S30-3.

Stone JA, "Felbamate: Analyte of the Month," *Ther Drug Monit and Toxi In-Service Training and Continuing Education*, 1994, 15(3):47-8.

Fentanyl, Blood or Urine

Synonyms Innovar® (fentanyl plus droperidol); Sublimaze®

Abstract Highly potent, fast-acting analgesic; approximately 100 times more potent than morphine

Specimen Blood, urine

Volume 6 mL

Minimum Volume 2 mL

Container Lavender top (EDTA) tube, do not use separator tube; plastic urine container

Storage Instructions Centrifuge and store at room temperature.

Causes for Rejection Specimen collected in separator tube, request form not accurately completed

Special Instructions Do not use separator tubes.

Reference Range Therapeutic: 2.0-200.0 μg/L

Use Monitor therapeutic and toxic plasma levels of fentanyl citrate

Methodology Gas chromatography (GC) – nitrogen phosphorus detection (GC-NPD); gas chromatography/mass spectrometry (GC/MS); radioimmunoassay (RIA); gas chromatography – electron capture detection (GC-ECD)

Additional Information Fentanyl is a potent, opioid, narcotic analgesic used as an adjunct to anesthesia. Toxic effects include respiratory depression, apnea, rigidity and bradycardia. Fentanyl is also used in combination with droperidol, a neuroleptic (major tranquilizer) for surgical and diagnostic procedures.

Specific References

Buchanan JF and Brown CR, "Designer Drugs - A Problem in Clinical Toxicology," *Med Toxicol Adverse Drug Exp* 1988, 3(1):1-17.

Fung DL and Eisele JH, "Fentanyl Pharmacokinetics in Awake Volunteers," *J Clin Pharmacol*, 1980, 20(11-12):652-8.

Hammargren WR and Henderson GL, "Analyzing Normetabolites of the Fentanyls by Gas Chromatography/Electron Capture Detection," *J Anal Toxicol*, 1988, 12(4):183-91.

Henderson GL, "Designer Drugs: Past History and Future Prospects," *J Forensic Sci*, 1988, 33(2):569-75.

McClain DA and Hug CC, "Intravenous Fentanyl Kinetics," *Clin Pharmacol Ther*, 1980, 28(1):106-14.

FEP *see* Protoporphyrin, Free Erythrocyte *on page 1339*

Fibrinogen Level *see* Fibrinogen, Plasma *on this page*

Fibrinogen, Plasma

Synonyms Factor I; Fibrinogen Level; Quantitative Fibrinogen

Applies To Acute Phase Reactants

Abstract Precursor of fibrin, major contributor to the meshwork of blood clots. Meaningful assay of fibrinogen is uniquely challenging. Fibrinogen is an acute phase reactant as well as the focal point in the coagulation process. Consumption of fibrinogen is a major and clinically threatening aspect of disseminated intravascular coagulation.

Specimen Plasma

Minimum Volume 4.5 mL

Container Blue top (sodium citrate) tube

Collection If multiple tests are being drawn, draw coagulation studies last. If only a fibrinogen is being drawn, draw 1-2 mL into another Vacutainer® or syringe (two-syringe technique), discard, and then collect the fibrinogen tube. This collection procedure avoids contamination of the specimen with tissue thromboplastin.

Storage Instructions Separate and freeze plasma as soon as possible if test is not run immediately.

Causes for Rejection Tube not full, tube clotted, specimen improperly labeled, specimen hemolyzed, specimen more than 1 hour old, stored specimen not frozen

Reference Range Quantitative: 200-400 mg/dL. The normal range in childhood (ages 1-16) is similar to that in adults (see reference by Andrew et al).

Possible Panic Range <100 mg/dL

Use Identify congenital afibrinogenemia, disseminated intravascular coagulation, and fibrinolytic activity

Limitations Increased in patients on oral contraceptives. Interpretations of results may be limited if patient is receiving anticoagulant therapy depending upon method of analysis. In cases of dysfibrinogenemia, results of fibrinogen determination will vary widely (method dependent). Individual methods may very widely (see following information) and suffer specific, occasionally significant, limitation.

Contraindications Patient receiving heparin less than 1 hour prior to specimen collection (depending upon method of analysis)

Methodology The many tests for fibrinogen proposed and in use over the past generation are a reflection of difficulties encountered in their clinical application. Generally, the most useful clinical information is obtained from "functional" based methods (ie, those that determine clottable plasma protein). These, however, are dependent upon fibrinogen activation with subsequent assessment of fibrin (which may or may not be contaminated with other protein). Functional methods are "blind" to the presence of nonclottable fibrinogen (molecular aberrant forms – dysfibrinogens). Most immunologic-based methods give misleading high results (from the vantage point of availability in the patient of useable-clottable fibrinogen). They will usually detect altered molecular forms but may include breakdown products (largely fragment X). Consideration should be given to employing two different methodologies depending on the clinical situation. Functional methods with different modes of activation and/or end point detection or one "functional" and one immunologic-based method, as available in the individual laboratory situation.

Earlier literature describes many methods based on harvesting the fibrin clot from plasma, washing, and determining the protein in the clot (by weight or chemically). These methods are generally time consuming, technically difficult, and suffer from inaccuracy due to inclusion of nonfibrinogen proteins in the clot, loss of clot fragments, and inaccuracies in measuring the clot protein. They will not measure the nonclottable fibrinogen derived protein.

Modified thrombin time method, the Clauss assay (in which a high concentration of thrombin is added to diluted plasma, resultant clotting time then proportional to the fibrinogen concentration) has the advantage that the endpoint is measured as a rate reaction. It is a rapid and simple procedure. The Clauss assay, however, depends upon the reliable maintenance of an accurate reference dilution curve and may give falsely low results in patients with circulating FBPs or paraproteins.

A method similar to the Clauss assay is growing in use due to its adaptation to several automated instruments. Thrombin and calcium are added to citrated plasma, and the change in resultant turbidity is measured. The extent of fibrin polymerization rather than the rate of fibrinogen conversion is the parameter utilized.

A variety of immunologic-based tests have been and continue to be developed. The FI™ test was a screening procedure utilizing antibody coated latex particles. When modified, it was used as a screen for FBP, a forerunner of the Thrombo-Wellcotest®. Radioimmunoassays have been developed for fibrinogen fragments, monomers, and fibrinopeptides A and B. Interest exists in RIA for released fibrinopeptide A as an indication of presence of thromboembolic process.

(Continued)

Fibrinogen, Plasma *(Continued)*

A number of less well established (and uncommonly available) approaches to the determination of fibrinogen have been proposed. As an example, the method of Frigola et al combines electrophoresis and thrombin clotting of fibrinogen. Following protein electrophoresis of plasma, thrombin is applied to "fix" fibrinogen (it is converted to fibrin on the cellulose acetate electrophoretic membrane) and nonclotted proteins are washed away with saline. The membrane is then stained and quantitated by densitometry.

Additional Information Fibrinogen is a complex polypeptide which upon enzyme action (physiologically by thrombin but pathologically by other substances such as occur in snake venom, eg, Reptilase®-R) is converted to fibrin that forms along with platelets the meshwork of the common blood clot. Fibrinogen is formed of three different pairs of polypeptide chains (α, β, γ) linked by disulfide bonds and forming a dimer. With conversion to fibrin, two pairs of peptides are released from the N-terminals of the α- and β-chains (fibrinopeptides A are released from the α-chains, fibrinopeptides B from the β-chains). The detailed and intricate molecular biochemistry has been explored, and the primary structure completely established. Fibrinogen levels are decreased with hereditary afibrinogenemia, intravascular coagulation, primary and secondary fibrinolysis, and liver disease. Increased levels may be seen with inflammation, pregnancy, and in women taking oral contraceptives. Very high levels of heparin or fibrin breakdown products may affect results of some assays. See Methodology for discussion of clinical implications of assay method. Some clinical problems may benefit from application of more than one test method (eg, in the assessment of cardiovascular risk).

Fibrinogen, while of primary importance as a coagulation protein, is also an acute-phase protein reactant. As such, it is increased in disease processes involving tissue damage/inflammation. It is not often employed clinically as a measure of acute phase response as concurrent hemorrhage (fibrinogen concentration rises initially) and DIC (rise or fall in fibrinogen depending on method) renders interpretation problematic. Fibrinogen is one of the major determinants of the ESR/ZSR (sedimentation rate) phenomenon. Changes in fibrinogen may impair the reliability of erythrocyte sedimentation measurements. There is evidence that increase in dietary fish oils results in decreased fibrinogen levels.

Congenital hypofibrinogenemia may be responsible for mild hemorrhagic symptoms, fibrinogen levels are usually <100 mg/dL, and screening tests (eg, PT, APTT) may be normal or only slightly prolonged. There are a growing number of patients with fibrinogen variants. About 150 varieties of such dysfibrinogenemia have been recorded. These individuals are usually detected when prolonged clotting times are discovered as a result of routine laboratory testing. Over 50% of the cases are asymptomatic; only in about 33% of the cases has a mild bleeding tendency been noted. Some 20 cases have been associated with thrombocytopenia, recurrent thrombosis, or spontaneous abortion. Most cases show a pattern of autosomal dominant inheritance. Most are heterozygous, but in some there is a negative family history. Most cases of dysfibrinogenemia show discrepancy between the results of fibrinogen assays based on the thrombin clotting time (functional) and immune or chemical based methods.

Specific References

Andrew M, Vegh P, Johnston M, et al, "Maturation of the Hemostatic System During Childhood," *Blood*, 1992, 80(8):1998-2005.

Bovill EG, McDonagh J, Triplett DA, et al, "Performance Characteristics of Fibrinogen Assays – Results of the College of American Pathologists Proficiency Testing Program 1988-1991," *Arch Pathol Lab Med*, 1993, 117(1):58-66.

Galanakis DK, "Dysfibrinogenemia: A Current Perspective," *Clin Lab Med*, 1984, 4(2):395-418.

Hermans J and McDonagh J, "Fibrin: Structure and Interactions," *Semin Thromb Hemost*, 1982, 8(1):11-24.

Hollensead SC and Triplett DA, "Review of Fibrinogen Methods: Clinical Considerations," *ASCP Check Sample®*, Chicago, IL: American Society of Clinical Pathologists, 1988.

Palareti G, Maccaferri M, Manotti C, et al, "Fibrinogen Assays: A Collaborative Study of Six Different Methods," *Clin Chem*, 1991, 37(5):714-9.

Finger Oximetry *see* Pulse Oximetry *on page 1342*

Fiorinal® *see* Barbiturates, Quantitative, Blood *on page 1201*

Flea Identification *see* Arthropod Identification *on page 1198*

Flecainide, Blood

Synonyms Tambocor®

Abstract An antiarrhythmic drug not significantly metabolized. When coadministered, can affect activity of other antiarrhythmic drugs.

Specimen Blood

Container Red top tube (preferred) or green top (heparin) tube; do not use serum separator tube.

Sampling Time Draw sample 3 hours after last dose.

Storage Instructions Separate serum or plasma within 2 hours of specimen draw.

Special Instructions Draw immediately prior to next dose for trough levels.

Reference Range Therapeutic: 0.2-1.0 μg/mL (SI: 0.4-2.0 μmol/L)

Possible Panic Range >1.0 μg/mL (SI: >2.0 μmol/L)

Use Therapeutic monitoring; toxicity assessment (toxic effects – hypotension, asystole – proportional to dose and concentration)

Methodology High performance liquid chromatography (HPLC), fluorescence polarization immunoassay (FPIA)

Additional Information Flecainide is a class 1C antiarrhythmic drug approved for the suppression of ventricular arrhythmias. The drug is well absorbed orally. Plasma half-life averages 20 hours (range 12-27 hours) in adults although in children it has been reported to be 8 hours. Steady-state concentrations are achieved in 3-5 days. Since 10% to 50% of the drug is eliminated in the urine as unchanged drug, impaired renal function will significantly prolong the plasma half-life. Clearance of flecainide can be accelerated by phenobarbital and rifampin. There are no significant metabolites of flecainide. Coadministration with digoxin increases serum digoxin by 20%; coadministration with propranolol increases both by 20% in serum and creates an additive pharmacological effect.

Specific References

Perry JC, McQuinn RL, Smith RT Jr, et al, "Flecainide Acetate for Resistant Arrhythmias in the Young: Efficacy and Pharmacokinetics," *J Am Coll Cardiol*, 1989, 14(1):185-93.

Roden DM and Woosely RL, "Drug Therapy. Flecainide," *N Engl J Med*, 1986, 315(1):36-41.

Flexartal® *see* Carisoprodol, Quantitative *on page 1222*

Fluoride, Serum

Synonyms Sodium Fluoride

Abstract Fluoride is added at low levels to toothpaste and is added to drinking water in many areas at a level of 1 ppm. It is present in high concentrations in insecticides and rodenticides.

Specimen Blood

Container Red top tube

Reference Range Diet dependent, approximately 1.9-7.6 μg/dL (SI: 1-4 μmol/L)

Possible Panic Range Toxic concentration: >28.5 μg/dL (SI: >15 μmol/L)

Use Evaluate fluoride toxicity; work up ant poison and roach poison intoxication

Methodology Fluoride-specific electrode

Additional Information Fluoride poisoning can occur from ingestion of ant or roach poisons; death is usually from cardiovascular collapse. Fatal dose is 5-10 g orally. Half-life is 2-9 hours.

Specific References

Frink EJ Jr, Ghantous H, Malan TP, et al, "Plasma Inorganic Fluoride With Sevoflurane Anesthesia: Correlation With Indices of Hepatic and Renal Function," *Anesth Analg*, 1992, 74(2):231-5.

Gruber HE and Baylink DJ, "The Effects of Fluoride on Bone," *Clin Orthop*, 1991, 267:264-77.

Whitford GM, "The Physiological and Toxicological Characteristics of Fluoride," *J Dent Res*, 1990, 69:539-49.

Fluoride, Urine

Synonyms F, Urine

Patient Preparation Patient should be instructed that specimen must not come in contact with glass containers.

Specimen Random urine

Minimum Volume 10 mL

Container Plastic urine container

Causes for Rejection Specimen received in a glass container

Reference Range Diet dependent

Critical Values Toxic: >10 mg/L

Use Evaluate fluoride toxicity; work up poisoning with insecticides, rodenticides, and delousing powders; monitor industrial exposure

Additional Information Continued exposure to fluoride can lead to toxicity manifested by respiratory distress, neurological abnormalities, gastrointestinal pain, muscular fibrillation and excessive calcification of bone. Death from fluoride poisoning is usually from cardiovascular collapse.

Fluoxetine, Blood

Synonyms Prozac®

Test Includes Fluoxetine and norfluoxetine

Abstract This is a new nontricyclic antidepressant with a long half-life and an active metabolite.

Specimen Blood

Container Red top tube or green top (heparin) tube; do not use serum separator tube.

(Continued)

Fluoxetine, Blood *(Continued)*

Sampling Time Trough just prior to next dose

Reference Range Fluoxetine: 100-800 ng/mL (SI: 289-2314 nmol/L); norfluoxetine: 100-600 ng/mL (SI: 289-1735 nmol/L)

Critical Values Fluoxetine and norfluoxetine: >2000 ng/mL (SI: >5784 nmol/L)

Use Therapeutic monitoring; toxicity assessment

Methodology High performance liquid chromatography (HPLC), gas chromatography (GC), gas chromatography/mass spectrometry (GC/MS)

Additional Information Fluoxetine is a new antidepressant that is a potent, selective inhibitor of serotonin reuptake. It is metabolized via demethylation to the active norfluoxetine. The parent drug has a long half-life of 24-96 hours which facilitates maintenance of steady-state concentrations (2-6 weeks to steady-state). The therapeutic efficiency as an antidepressant is comparable to the tricyclics but not for the relief of sleep disorders. The overall toxicity of the drug is considerably less than that of the tricyclics.

Specific References

Benfield P, Heel RC, and Lewis SP, "Fluoxetine: A Review of its Pharmacodynamic and Pharmacokinetic Properties and Therapeutic Efficacy in Depressive Illness," *Drugs*, 1986, 32(6):481-508.

Bergstrom RF, Lemberger L, Farid NA, et al, "Clinical Pharmacology and Pharmacokinetics of Fluoxetine: A Review," *Br J Psychiatry Suppl*, 1988, 153(3):47-50.

Borys DJ, Setzer SC, Ling LJ, et al, "The Effects of Fluoxetine in the Overdose Patient," *J Toxicol Clin Toxicol*, 1990, 28(3):331-40.

el Maanni A, Combourieu I, Bonini M, et al, "Fluoxetine, an Antidepressant, and Norfluoxetine, Its Metabolite, Determined by HPLC With a C8 Column and Ultraviolet Detection," *Clin Chem*, 1993, 39(8): 1749-50.

Pary R, Tobias CR, and Lippmann S, "Fluoxetine: Prescribing Guidelines for the Newest Antidepressant," *South Med J*, 1989, 82(8):1005-9.

Tacke U, "Fluoxetine: An Alternative to the Tricyclics in the Treatment of Major Depression?" *Am J Med Sci*, 1989, 298(2):126-9.

Fluphenazine, Blood

Synonyms Lyogen®; Pacinol®; Permitil®; Prolixin®

Abstract Fluphenazine is a phenothiazine antipsychotic active at low dosage.

Specimen Blood

Container Red top tube

Reference Range 5-20 ng/mL (SI: 10-40 nmol/L)

Critical Values >50 ng/mL (SI: >98 nmol/L)

Use Therapeutic monitoring; toxicity assessment

Methodology High performance liquid chromatography (HPLC), gas chromatography (GC), radioimmunoassay (RIA)

Additional Information Fluphenazine is a phenothiazine derivative (piperazine) used in the treatment of psychotic disorders. Its dose in milligrams equivalent to 100 mg of chlorpromazine is 0.6-1.2 mg. As a high potency antipsychotic it may have a high potential for causing extrapyramidal side effects. This would be in addition to the usual adverse effects of antipsychotic drugs (neurologic, anticholinergic, hypotension). Elderly patients should be observed for these occurrences. The half-life of fluphenazine is formulation-dependent. (The decanoate is 5-12 days; the hydrochloride 12-60 hours.) Fluphenazine is also used to alleviate pain and in childhood development disorders.

Specific References

Chouinard G, Annable L, and Campbell W, "A Randomized Clinical Trial of Haloperidol Decanoate and Fluphenazine Decanoate in the Outpatient Treatment of Schizophrenia," *J Clin Psychopharmacol*, 1989, 9(4):247-53.

Cooper JK, Hawes EM, Hubbard JW, et al, "An Ultrasensitive Method for the Measurement of Fluphenazine in Plasma by High Performance Liquid Chromatography With Coulometric Detection," *Ther Drug Monit*, 1989, 11(3):354-60.

Levinson DF, Simpson GM, Singh H, et al, "Fluphenazine Dose, Clinical Response, and Extrapyramidal Symptoms During Acute Treatment," *Arch Gen Psychiatry*, 1990, 47(8):761-8.

Marder SR, Midha KK, Van Putten T, et al, "Plasma Levels of Fluphenazine in Patients Receiving Fluphenazine Decanoate. Relationship to Clinical Response," *Br J Psychiatry*, 1991, 158:658-65.

Mendel CM, Klein RF, Chappell DA, et al, "A Trial of Amitriptyline and Fluphenazine in the Treatment of Painful Diabetic Neuropathy," *JAMA*, 1986, 255(5):637-9.

Midha KK, McKay G, Edom R, et al, "Kinetics of Oral Fluphenazine Disposition in Humans By GC-MS," *Eur J Clin Pharmacol*, 1983, 25(5):709-11.

Flurazepam, Blood

Synonyms Dalmane®

Abstract This drug is a sedative-hypnotic of the benzodiazepine class with a rather wide therapeutic window.

Specimen Blood

Volume 5 mL

Container Red top tube

Reference Range Therapeutic: 0-4 ng/mL (SI: 0-9 nmol/L); N-desalkylflurazepam (metabolite): 20-110 ng/mL (SI: 43-240 nmol/L)

Possible Panic Range Toxic: 2000 ng/mL (SI: 4300 nmol/L)

Use Monitor therapeutic drug level (rarely); toxicity assessment

Methodology Thin-layer chromatography (TLC), high performance liquid chromatography (HPLC)

Additional Information Half-life of parent drug is 2-3 hours. Half-life of active metabolite, N-desalkylflurazepam, is 50-100 hours. Most common side effect is daytime drowsiness. The major urinary metabolite is N-1-hydroxyethyl flurazepam.

Specific References

Greenblatt DJ, Harmatz JS, Engelhardt N, et al, "Pharmacokinetic Determinants of Dynamic Differences Among Three Benzodiazepine Hypnotics. Flurazepam, Temazepam, and Triazolam," *Arch Gen Psychiatry*, 1989, 46(4):326-32.

Kales A, "Benzodiazepine Hypnotics and Insomnia," *Hosp Pract (Off Ed)*, 1990, 25(Suppl 3):7-23.

Fortral® *see* Pentazocine, Urine *on page 1316*

Free Catecholamine Fractionation, Urine *see* Catecholamines, Fractionation, Urine *on page 1222*

Free Erythrocyte Protoporphyrin *see* Protoporphyrin, Free Erythrocyte *on page 1339*

F, Urine *see* Fluoride, Urine *on page 1267*

Gap *see* Anion Gap, Blood *on page 1193*

Gardenal® *see* Phenobarbital, Blood *on page 1320*

Gases, Arterial *see* Blood Gases, Arterial *on page 1207*

Gastric Aspirate, Drug Screen *see* Toxicology, Drug Screen, Gastric *on page 1364*

Gemonil® *see* Metharbital, Quantitative *on page 1296*

Globulin *see* Protein, Total, Serum *on page 1338*

Glucose, Random

Specimen Blood

Volume 10 mL

Minimum Volume 5 mL plasma or serum

Container Gray top (sodium fluoride) tube preferred; red top tube acceptable

Collection Pediatrics: Draw blood from heelstick.

Causes for Rejection Blood stored overnight on clot

Reference Range Dependent on time and content of last meal. Glucose of >200 mg/dL (SI: >11.1 mmol/L) in a nonstressed, ambulatory subject supports the diagnosis of diabetes mellitus. Values in term neonates are published.

Possible Panic Range Neonates: <40 mg/dL (SI: <2.2 mmol/L); adults: male: <50 mg/dL (SI: <2.8 mmol/L), >400 mg/dL (SI: >22.2 mmol/L); adults female: <40 mg/dL (SI: <2.2 mmol/L), >400 mg/dL (SI: >22.2 mmol/L)

Use Evaluate carbohydrate metabolism, acidosis and ketoacidosis, dehydration; work up alcoholism, or apparent alcoholism; work-up of coma, neuroglycopenia. Hypoglycemia if present should be investigated with insulin levels as well. For the diagnosis of diabetes mellitus in nonpregnant adult subjects, random glucose >200 mg/dL (SI: >11.1 mmol/L) is required. Other criteria exist. Determination of blood glucose on admission in patients who have had an out-of-hospital cardiac arrest can serve as a predictor of neurologic recovery. Higher levels are indicative of more severe brain ischemia and difficult resuscitation. In pregnant women, a value >105 mg/dL usually prompts further investigation.

Limitations Glucose will decrease in samples left on the clot and in tubes other than fluoride prior to analysis. Acetaminophen can cause a false elevation of serum glucose when the neocuprione method is utilized.

Methodology Hexokinase, glucose oxidase, oxygen rate, ortho-toluidine

Additional Information Recall that **blood glucose** values are not equivalent to **plasma glucose**. If glucose is >400 mg/dL (SI: >22.2 mmol/L), an acetone (ketone body) examination probably should be done. A fasting and a 2-hour postprandial specimen is preferable to a random specimen for evaluation of possible diabetes mellitus. The incidence of hypoglycemia in hospitalized patients appears to be significant, but may be better controlled if frequent monitoring of glucose levels is employed. Wider utilization of bedside glucose testing may allow for closer patient monitoring, but the establishment of uniform quality control procedures is necessary to ensure valid results from this type of testing. Evaluation of glycated hemoglobin and self-monitoring of blood glucose are two relatively new means of assessing glycemia which have become widely available.

Specific References

Brandt KR and Miles JM, "Relationship Between Severity of Hyperglycemia and Metabolic Acidosis in Diabetic Ketoacidosis," *Mayo Clin Proc*, 1988, 63(11):1071-4.

Carter PE, Lloyd DJ, and Duffty P, "Glucagon for Hypoglycemia in Infants Small for Gestational Age," *Arch Dis Child*, 1988, 63(10):1264-6.

(Continued)

Glucose, Random *(Continued)*

Palardy J, Havrankova J, Lepage R, et al, "Blood Glucose Measurements During Symptomatic Episodes in Patients With Suspected Postprandial Hypoglycemia," *N Engl J Med*, 1989, 321(21):1421-5.

Service FJ, "Hypoglycemia and the Postprandial Syndrome," *N Engl J Med*, 1989, 321(21):1472-4.

Service FJ, "Hypoglycemic Disorders," *N Engl J Med*, 1995, 332:1144-52.

Weiner CP, Faustich M, Burns J, et al, "The Relationship Between Capillary and Venous Glucose Concentration During Pregnancy," *Am J Obstet Gynecol*, 1986, 155(1):61-4.

Glutamic Oxaloacetic Transaminase, Serum *see* Aspartate Aminotransferase *on page 1199*

Glutethimide, Blood

Synonyms Doriden®; Loads

Abstract This drug is a sedative hypnotic which has been in use for some time. The pharmacological effect is similar to that of barbiturates.

Specimen Blood

Volume 5 mL

Container Red top tube

Reference Range Therapeutic: 5 μg/mL (variable) (SI: 23 μmol/L)

Possible Panic Range Toxic: >10 μg/mL (SI: >46 μmol/L); fatalities have occurred with serum levels between 10-100 μg/mL (average, 50 μg/mL).

Use Monitor therapeutic drug level; determine toxic level

Limitations Serum levels obtained during dialysis may not reflect tissue levels

Methodology Gas-liquid chromatography (GLC), high performance liquid chromatography (HPLC), thin-layer chromatography (TLC); a spot test has been described

Additional Information Glutethimide is a nonbarbiturate sedative-hypnotic. The drug is erratically absorbed from the gastrointestinal tract and undergoes extensive metabolism to pharmacologically active and inactive metabolites. An important active metabolite in 4-hydroxy-2-ethyl-2-phenylglutarimide. This metabolite has twice the potency of glutethimide and a longer half-life. Peak blood levels are at 2-3 hours postingestion. The half-life is biphasic, ranging from 5-22 hours. The average plasma half-life is 10 hours. Serious toxic effects are respiratory depression and circulatory collapse. Glutethimide and codeine ("packs" or "loads") in combination are frequently used by drug abusers.

Specific References

Bailey DN and Shaw RF, "Blood Concentrations and Clinical Findings in Nonfatal and Fatal Intoxications Involving Glutethimide and Codeine," *J Toxicol Clin Toxicol*, 1985-86, 23(7-8):557-70.

Gold Level

Synonyms Aurothioglucose; Chrysotherapy; Gold Sodium Thiomalate; Myochrysine®; Solganal®

Abstract Gold is used as a treatment for rheumatoid arthritis, but its value is being questioned.

Specimen Blood, urine

Volume 7 mL blood or entire collection urine

Container Red top tube for blood, acid-washed polyethylene container for urine

Reference Range Normal: 0-0.1 μg/mL (SI: 0-0.5 μmol/L); therapeutic: 1.0-3.0 μg/mL (SI: 5.1-15.2 μmol/L); urine <0.1 μg/24 hours

Limitations Blood levels do not correlate with therapeutic or toxic effects. No relationship between serum gold levels and efficacy is established. Serum gold concentrations have not been helpful in monitoring adverse reactions. A relationship is not recognized between urinary gold and response to therapy. Hair and nail gold concentrations have not been helpful.

Methodology Atomic absorption spectrometry (AA)

Additional Information Complex gold compounds are used in the treatment of severe, progressive rheumatoid arthritis which is not controlled by other medical therapy. It is also used selectively for juvenile rheumatoid arthritis and for psoriatic arthritis affecting peripheral joints. The mechanism of action is not clear, but may be due to reticuloendothelial system blockade, and/or effects on lymphocyte proliferation and antibody production. Elimination is mainly renal and the half-life is 5.5 days. Gold toxicity may be manifested by dermatitis, pruritus, stomatitis, metallic taste, eosinophilia, leukopenia, anemia, thrombocytopenia, hematuria, proteinuria, nephrosis, and bone marrow suppression, among other possible effects.

Specific References

Bendix G and Bjelle A, "Outcome of Parenteral Gold Therapy in RA Patients: A Comparison Between Two Periods Using Life-Table Analysis," *Br J Rheumatol*, 1991, 30(6):407-12.

Epstein WV, Henke CJ, Yelin EH, et al, "Effect of Parenterally Administered Gold Therapy on the Course of Adult Rheumatoid Arthritis," *Ann Intern Med*, 1991, 114(6):437-44.

Gold Sodium Thiomalate *see* Gold Level *on this page*

GOT *see* Aspartate Aminotransferase *on page 1199*

Granulocyte/Macrophage Colony Stimulating Factor *see* Eosinophil Count *on page 1259*

Grass *see* Cannabinoids, Qualitative *on page 1217*

GX *see* Lidocaine, Blood *on page 1284*

H1-Antihistamine Comparison *see page 1649*

Halcion® *see* Triazolam, Blood *on page 1368*

Haldol® *see* Haloperidol, Blood *on this page*

Haloperidol, Blood

Synonyms Haldol®

Abstract This drug is an antipsychotic agent which is extensively metabolized and should be monitored.

Specimen Blood

Container Red top tube or green top (heparin) tube

Reference Range 5-15 ng/mL (SI: 10-40 nmol/L) (psychotic disorders – less for Tourette's and mania)

Critical Values >50 ng/mL (SI: >130 nmol/L) (variable)

Use Therapeutic monitoring; toxicity assessment

Methodology High performance liquid chromatography (HPLC), gas chromatography (GC)

Additional Information Half-life is 15-40 hours. Haloperidol is an antipsychotic tranquilizer used to control acute and chronic psychotic disorders, for the control of Tourette's syndrome, and for the treatment of severe behavior problems in hyperactive children. Haloperidol is metabolized by dealkalization, oxidation, and conjugation; the hydroxy derivative is active but concentrations are very low. Haloperidol should be monitored to assess and optimize dosing regimens and maintenance therapy since the relationship between dosage and serum levels at steady-state can be highly variable. The drug should also be monitored to assess adverse reactions and changes associated with coadministered drugs. Haloperidol may increase serum tricyclic concentrations, increase the toxicity of lithium, inhibit hypertensive action, and antagonize the stimulant effect of amphetamines.

Specific References

Cannon DJ, McMillan DE, Newton JE, et al, "Serum Haloperidol and Neuroleptic Receptor Levels in Chronic Psychosis," *Ann Clin Lab Sci*, 1988, 18(5):378-83.

Derlet RW, Albertson TE, and Rice P, "The Effect of Haloperidol in Cocaine and Amphetamine Intoxication," *J Emerg Med*, 1989, 7(6):633-7.

Goff DC, Midha KK, Brotman AW, et al, "Elevation of Plasma Concentrations of Haloperidol After the Addition of Fluoxetine," *Am J Psychiatry*, 1991, 148(6):790-2.

Hemstrom CA, Evans RL, and Lobeck FG, "Haloperidol Decanoate: A Depot Antipsychotic," *Drug Intell Clin Pharm*, 1988, 22(4):290-95.

Rifkin A, Doddi S, Karajgi B, et al, "Dosage of Haloperidol for Schizophrenia," *Arch Gen Psychiatry*, 1991, 48(2):166-70.

Volavka J and Cooper TB, "Review of Haloperidol Blood Levels and Clinical Response," *J Clin Psychopharmacol*, 1987, 7(1):25-30.

Hashish *see* Cannabinoids, Qualitative *on page 1217*

hCG, Slide Test, Stat *see* Pregnancy Test *on page 1330*

hCG, Urine *see* Pregnancy Test *on page 1330*

Head Lice Identification *see* Arthropod Identification *on page 1198*

Head Studies, CT *see* Computed Transaxial Tomography, Head Studies *on page 1240*

Heavy Metal Screen, Blood

Synonyms Metals, Blood; Poisonous Metals, Blood; Toxic Metals, Blood

Test Includes Antimony, arsenic, bismuth, boron, cadmium, cobalt, copper, lead, mercury, selenium, tellurium, thallium, zinc

Abstract Used principally to detect arsenic, cadmium, mercury, and lead poisoning.

Specimen Whole blood (EDTA) plus serum

Volume 20 mL

Container Special metal-free tube and red top tube

Storage Instructions Refrigerate: do not spin down.

Special Instructions Check with laboratory performing the assay to determine what elements will be detected and for any special instructions.

Reference Range Varies with metal detected.

Use Screen for heavy metal poisoning

Methodology Atomic absorption spectrometry (AA)

Specific References

Gerson B, "Lead," *Clin Lab Med*, 1990, 10(3):441-73.

(Continued)

Heavy Metal Screen, Blood *(Continued)*

Malachowski ME, "An Update on Arsenic," *Clin Lab Med*, 1990, 10(3):459-72.

Heavy Metal Screen, Hair *see* Heavy Metal Screen, Urine *on this page*

Heavy Metal Screen, Urine

Synonyms Metal Screen; Metals, Toxic; Poisonous Metals, Urine; Toxic Metals, Urine

Applies To Heavy Metal Screen, Hair

Test Includes Arsenic, mercury, lead (could also include nickel and cadmium)

Abstract Used to detect arsenic, mercury, lead, and cadmium poisoning

Specimen 24-hour urine

Volume Entire collection

Minimum Volume 150 mL aliquot

Container Plastic, acid-washed urine container (preferably polyethylene), no preservative, 20-25 mL 6N HCl (low metal content)

Collection 24-hour collection

Storage Instructions Refrigerate

Special Instructions Include volume of urine

Reference Range Arsenic: <50 μg/L; lead: <80 μg/L; mercury: <20 μg/L; nickel: <25 μg/L; cadmium: <10 μg/L

Use Screen for heavy metal poisoning and toxic exposure; urine lead analysis is useful for organic lead exposure and to monitor chelation. Blood is preferred for inorganic lead exposure monitoring.

Limitations Hair analysis should be used for arsenic and mercury poisoning or exposure especially if one is interested in determining chronic exposure. Hair should be clean, free of oil, and clipped (0.5 g for As; 2 g for Hg) as close as possible. Recent ingestion of seafood can cause misleading increases of urine arsenic.

Methodology Atomic absorption spectrometry (AA)

Specific References

Gerson B, "Lead," *Clin Lab Med*, 1990, 10(3):441-73.
Malachowski ME, "An Update on Arsenic," *Clin Lab Med*, 1990, 10(3):459-72.

Hemoglobin, Qualitative, Urine

Test Includes Dipstick screening of urine for hemoglobin

Abstract Test for hemoglobin in urine. This also screens for blood in urine, which must be confirmed microscopically.

Specimen Random urine

Volume 20 mL

Minimum Volume 10 mL

Container Plastic urine container

Reference Range Negative

Use Determine the presence of hemoglobinuria

Limitations Menstrual or other uterine bleeding may appear as a contaminant in the urine. False-positives to dipsticks occur with oxidizing contaminants or Betadine® (povidone-iodine). False-negatives occur with large amounts of ascorbic acid. Formalin in urine can cause false-negative results. Urine dipsticks for blood that are exposed to air lose sensitivity over time. To prevent this, keep dipstick jar tightly capped.

Methodology The peroxidase-like activity of hemoglobin catalyzes the reaction of cumene hydroperoxide and 3,3',5,5'-tetramethylbenzidine.

Additional Information Hemoglobinuria, the presence of free hemoglobin in the urine, may result from hemolysis. It occurs if the serum haptoglobin binding capacity (100-200 mg/dL Hgb (SI: 1.0-2.0 g/L)) is exceeded and if the renal threshold for tubular reabsorption of hemoglobin (90-140 mg/dL Hgb (SI: 0.9-1.4 g/L)) is exceeded. Hemoglobin is catabolized in the renal tubular cells, and the iron is stored as hemosiderin. The urine in hemoglobinuria may be clear red, clear red-brown, or dark brown. Myoglobinuria also produces a dark or red-orange urine. Both hemoglobin and myoglobin produce positive dipstick tests for blood and must be identified by additional tests. In hematuria, red cells or ghosts (lysed red cells) are observed microscopically. Algorithms for medical work-up of hematuria have been published.

Hemoglobin Saturation, Percent *see* Oxygen Saturation, Blood *on page 1313*

Hemoglobin, Urine *see* Blood, Urine *on page 1210*

Hemogram *see* Complete Blood Count *on page 1236*

Hemp *see* Cannabinoids, Qualitative *on page 1217*

Herb and Al *see* Cannabinoids, Qualitative *on page 1217*

Heroin *see* Opiates, Qualitative, Urine *on page 1309*

Heroin Metabolite, Blood *see* Morphine, Blood *on page 1300*

Heroin Metabolite, Urine *see* Morphine, Urine *on page 1300*

Hg, Blood *see* Mercury, Blood *on page 1292*

Hg, Urine *see* Mercury, Urine *on page 1292*

Histamine Level

Patient Preparation Patient must be on a diet of microbially processed foods, such as cheeses or sauerkraut.

Specimen Blood, urine, or cerebrospinal fluid

Volume 10 mL

Container Special vial is required for blood

Collection Collect 10 mL blood without preservative and transfer immediately to vial containing 20 mg potassium oxalate; 24-hour urine collection, send 50 mL aliquot

Storage Instructions Store blood or urine frozen.

Special Instructions Test is ordinarily available only from a few reference laboratories.

Reference Range Blood: 3-9 μg/dL (SI: 98-293 nmol/L); urine: 17-68 μg/24 hours (SI: 553-2210 nmol/L); considerably method variable

Use Evaluate possible systemic mastocytosis

Limitations Test not very sensitive. There are false-positive results associated with urinary tract infections. Histamine level alone may not fully reflect the role of histamine in a disease process. Measurement of histamine and its metabolites may be necessary.

Methodology Gas chromatography (GC), fluorometry, radioisotope enzymatic, high performance liquid chromatography (HPLC), chemical ionization mass spectrometry

Additional Information Mast cells produce numerous biologically active materials, including histamine. Histamine is often, but not consistently, elevated in cases of systemic mastocytosis, and also in other myeloproliferative disorders such as chronic myelogenous leukemia and polycythemia vera. Some carcinoid tumors (particularly of gastric origin) produce excessive amounts of histamine. Measurement of urinary methylated and other histamine metabolites may be more sensitive and specific. In a study of 25 patients with urticaria pigmentosa, methylimidazoleacetic acid, the major histamine metabolite, was able to identify all cases of systemic mastocytosis (>4.1 mg/24 hours) while histamine was elevated in only half of cases. In another study of systemic mast cell disease urinary histamine was elevated in only 1 of 26 cases. Histamine release from basophils and mast cells in response to allergen and reagin complex is generally recognized. There is also evidence that histamine is synthesized by T cells/macrophages *de novo* through the action of histidine decarboxylase. There is evidence suggesting that basophils have an interleukin 1 receptor that can modulate the response to IgE-related signals.

Serum histamine levels are decreased with HIV infection, a finding of possible prognostic significance. Splenectomy results in a rise in histamine levels in AIDS patients with thrombocytopenic purpura. Histamine levels have been reported decreased in some 60% of patients with malignant disease.

Specific References

Jacobs R, Kaliner M, Shelhamer JH, et al, "Blood Histamine Concentrations Are Not Elevated in Humans With Septic Shock," *Crit Care Med*, 1989, 17(1):30-5.

Keyzer JJ, de Monchy JG, van Doormaal JJ, et al, "Improved Diagnosis of Mastocytosis by Measurement of Urinary Histamine Metabolites," *N Engl J Med*, 1983, 309(26):1603-5.

Hog *see* Phencyclidine, Qualitative, Urine *on page 1319*

Hog *see* Phencyclidine, Quantitative, Serum *on page 1319*

Human Chorionic Gonadotropin, Urine *see* Pregnancy Test *on page 1330*

Hydrocyanic Acid *see* Cyanide, Blood *on page 1246*

β-Hydroxybutyrate *see* Ketone Bodies, Blood *on page 1277*

Hypnotics and Tranquilizers, Toxicology, Blood *see* Toxicology, Hypnotics and Tranquilizers, Serum *on page 1365*

Ibuprofen, Serum

Synonyms Advil®; Motrin®

Specimen Blood

Volume 7 mL

Minimum Volume 1 mL serum

Container Red top tube or serum separator tube

(Continued)

Ibuprofen, Serum *(Continued)*

Storage Instructions Refrigerate serum.

Reference Range Therapeutic: 10-50 μg/mL

Critical Values Toxic: >100 μg/mL

Use Ibuprofen has analgesic, anti-inflammatory, and antipyretic actions. It relieves mild to moderate postoperative pain (eg, dental, episiotomy), dysmenorrhea, and headache. Its effectiveness is comparable to or greater than that of acetaminophen, aspirin, codeine, aspirin with codeine, or propoxyphene.

Methodology High-performance liquid chromatography (HPLC)

Additional Information About 85% of an oral dose is absorbed. Peak plasma concentrations are attained within 0.5-1.5 hours if the drug is taken on an empty stomach. Metabolites of ibuprofen are eliminated; only 1% of a dose is excreted in the urine unchanged. The urinary metabolites include 2-(2-carboxypropyl)-phenylpropionic acid (37%), 2-(*p*-2-hydroxy-2-methyl propyl)-phenylpropionic acid (25%), and conjugated ibuprofen (14%). The drug is tightly bound to plasma protein (99%). It is not excreted in breast milk. The elimination half-life is 2-2.5 hours. The pharmacokinetics are not altered in the elderly or in alcoholics with severe liver disease. Dosage adjustment is not required for these patients.

Ice *see* Amphetamines, Qualitative, Urine *on page 1190*

Ilotycin® *see* Erythromycin, Blood *on page 1260*

Imipramine, Blood

Synonyms Presamine®; Tofranil®

Applies To Desipramine; Norpramin®; Pertofrane®

Test Includes Desipramine levels

Abstract This drug is a tricyclic antidepressant. It has an active metabolite which should also be monitored.

Specimen Blood

Container Red top tube or green top (heparin) tube

Sampling Time Trough levels at steady-state

Reference Range Imipramine and desipramine: 150-250 ng/mL (SI: 530-890 nmol/L); desipramine: 150-300 ng/mL (SI: 560-1125 nmol/L). Metabolism may be impaired in geriatric patients.

Critical Values >300 ng/mL (SI: >1070 nmol/L)

Possible Panic Range 1000 ng/mL (SI: 3570 nmol/L)

Use Therapeutic monitoring; toxicity assessment

Methodology Immunoassay, high performance liquid chromatography (HPLC), gas chromatography (GC)

Additional Information Imipramine is a tertiary tricyclic antidepressant prescribed for the treatment of various depressive disorders. Imipramine is metabolized to desipramine which is pharmacologically active and marketed separately. Both drugs have anticholinergic and antihistamine effects and are cardiotoxic. Imipramine reaches a peak serum concentration in 1-2 hours (desipramine 2-6 hours), has a half-life of 9-24 hours (desipramine 12-54 hours) and reaches steady-state levels in 2-5 days (desipramine 3-11 days). Drug interactions and effects in geriatric patients are the same as listed under amitriptyline. Red blood cell assays for metabolites of imipramine may be a more effective marker for cardiac conduction disturbances.

Specific References

Amitai Y, Erickson T, Kennedy EJ, et al, "Tricyclic Antidepressants in Red Cells and Plasma: Correlation With Impaired Intraventricular Conduction in Acute Overdose," *Clin Pharmacol Ther*, 1993, 54(2):219-27.

Amsterdam JD, Brunswick DJ, Potter L, et al, "Desipramine and 2-Hydroxydesipramine Plasma Levels in Endogenous Depressed Patients. Lack of Correlation With Therapeutic Response," *Arch Gen Psychiatry*, 1985, 42(4):361-4.

Ereshefsky L, Tran-Johnson T, Davis CM, et al, "Pharmacokinetic Factors Affecting Antidepressant Drug Clearance and Clinical Effect: Evaluation of Doxepin and Imipramine – New Data and Review," *Clin Chem*, 1988, 34(5):863-80.

Gawin FH, Kleber HD, Byck R, et al, "Desipramine Facilitation of Initial Cocaine Abstinence," *Arch Gen Psychiatry*, 1989, 46(2):117-21.

Siegel DM, "Bulimia, Tricyclic Antidepressants and Mania," *Clin Pediatr (Phila)*, 1989, 28(3):123-6.

Inderal® *see* Propranolol, Blood *on page 1334*

Infant Botulism, Toxin Identification *see* Botulism Diagnostic Procedure *on page 1211*

INH *see* Isoniazid, Blood *on page 1277*

Innovar® (fentanyl plus droperidol) *see* Fentanyl, Blood or Urine *on page 1264*

Insect Identification *see* Arthropod Identification *on page 1198*

Interleukin-3 *see* Eosinophil Count *on page 1259*

Interleukin-5 *see* Eosinophil Count *on page 1259*

Ion Gap *see* Anion Gap, Blood *on page 1193*

Iron and Total Iron Binding Capacity/Transferrin

Synonyms Fe and TIBC; Iron Binding Capacity; Iron Profile; TIBC; Total Iron Binding Capacity

Test Includes Serum iron, total iron binding capacity and/or transferrin, percent of saturation

Patient Preparation Specimen should be drawn fasting in the morning (circadian rhythm affects iron; levels are lower in the evening). Sample should be drawn before patient is given therapeutic iron or blood transfusion. Iron determinations on patients who have had blood transfusions should be delayed several days.

Specimen Blood

Volume 10 mL

Minimum Volume 7 mL serum

Container Red top tube

Sampling Time Morning; marked daily variation occurs

Collection Serum iron levels are 30% higher in the morning and blood levels should be determined on fasting AM samples. Blood should be drawn before other specimens which require anticoagulated tubes. Separate serum from cells as soon as possible.

Storage Instructions Stable 1 week at 4°C

Reference Range A variety of approaches to the estimation of serum iron, TIBC, and transferrin are in use. Expect normal ranges to vary between laboratories as they are in part method dependent. Iron: 50-160 μg/dL (SI: 9.0-28.8 μmol/L) for adult males; slightly lower (5% to 10%) values for adult females. Iron binding capacity: 250-350 μg/dL (SI: 45-63 μmol/L). Percent saturation (transferrin saturation): 20% to 50%. TIBC is a chemical approximation of transferrin. Quantitative assays for transferrin are widely available. A mathematical relationship between TIBC and transferrin can be derived, depending on methodology, in which transferrin can be measured, then TIBC calculated.

Use Differential diagnosis of anemia, especially with hypochromia and/or low MCV. The **percent saturation** sometimes is more helpful than is the iron result to estimate iron stores and iron deficiency anemia. Evaluate thalassemia and possible sideroblastic anemia; work up hemochromatosis, in which iron is increased and iron saturation is high. Decrease in iron level after performance of a Schilling test supports the diagnosis of vitamin B_{12} deficiency, *vide infra*. Evaluate iron poisoning (toxicity) and overload in renal dialysis patients or patients with transfusion dependent anemias. Use of TIBC in iron toxicity may be less useful than previously believed. TIBC or transferrin is a useful index of nutritional status, but is not useful for evaluating iron poisoning.

Uncomplicated iron deficiency: Serum transferrin (and TIBC) high, serum iron low, saturation low. Usual causes of depleted iron stores include blood loss, inadequate dietary iron. RBCs in moderately severe iron deficiency are hypochromic and microcytic. The red cell distribution width increases and MCV decreases. Stainable marrow iron is absent. Serum ferritin decrease is the earliest indicator of iron deficiency if inflammation is absent.

Anemia of chronic disease: Serum transferrin (and TIBC) low to normal, serum iron low, saturation low or normal. Transferrin decreases with many inflammatory diseases. With chronic disease there is a block in movement to and utilization of iron by marrow. This leads to low serum iron and decreased erythropoiesis. Examples include acute and chronic infections, malignancy, and renal failure.

Sideroblastic anemia: Serum transferrin (and TIBC) normal to low, serum iron normal to high, saturation high.

Hemolytic anemias: Serum transferrin (and TIBC) normal to low, serum iron high, saturation high.

Hemochromatosis: Serum transferrin (and TIBC) slightly low, serum iron high, saturation very high.

Protein depletion: Serum transferrin (and TIBC) may be low, serum iron normal or low (if patient also is iron deficient). This may occur as a result of malnutrition, liver disease, renal disease (eg, nephrosis) or other entities.

Liver disease: Serum transferrin variable; with acute viral hepatitis, high along with serum iron and ferritin. With chronic liver disease (eg, cirrhosis), transferrin may be low. Patients who have cirrhosis and portacaval shunting have saturated TIBC/transferrin as well as high ferritin.

Chronic dialysis for renal failure: Monitor iron levels in patients undergoing dialysis. To follow treatment of iron overload with deferoxamine or with regimen of recombinant human erythropoietin and phlebotomy.

Limitations Except for iron poisoning, a serum iron without TIBC or transferrin is of limited value. Ferritin levels are also useful for iron deficiency. Low iron level may

(Continued)

Iron and Total Iron Binding Capacity/Transferrin

(Continued)

not indicate iron deficiency in acute infection with leukocytosis. Low iron levels may be misleading in chronic infection, inflammation, and malignancy; high ferritin levels occur in many such states. TIBC and transferrin are increased in patients on oral contraceptives, with normal saturation. Gross hemolysis may interfere with serum iron.

Contraindications Parenteral iron before sample is drawn will cause misleading high iron results. Recent blood transfusion may have only a small positive effect on iron.

Methodology Ferrozine, bathophenanthroline (iron); nephelometry (transferrin); $MgCO_3$ column, other methods (TIBC); atomic absorption (iron, TIBC), anodal stripping; inductively coupled plasma atomic emission spectroscopy

Additional Information Serum iron is **increased** in hemosiderosis, hemolytic anemias especially thalassemia, sideroachrestic anemias, hepatitis, acute hepatic necrosis, hemochromatosis, and with inappropriate iron therapy. Iron may reach high levels with iron poisoning. Some patients who receive multiple transfusions (eg, some hemolytic anemias, thalassemia, renal dialysis patients) will have increased serum iron levels. Patients receiving chloramphenicol, estrogens, and methyldopa can have elevated iron levels.

Serum iron is **decreased** with insufficient dietary iron, chronic blood loss (including the hemolytic anemias, paroxysmal nocturnal hemoglobinuria), inadequate absorption of iron and impaired release of iron stores as in inflammation, infection, and chronic diseases. Cholestyramine and colchicine can cause a decrease in serum iron. Deferoxamine may interfere with colorimetric iron and total iron binding capacity assays. The combination of low iron, high TIBC and/or transferrin, and low saturation indicates iron deficiency. Without all of these findings together, iron deficiency is unproven. Low ferritin supports the diagnosis of iron deficiency. **Detection of iron deficiency may lead to detection of adenocarcinoma of gastrointestinal tract, a point which cannot be overemphasized.** In recovery from pernicious anemia, especially just after B_{12} dose, iron levels are low. In fact, the drop in serum iron 1 to several days after the Schilling test flushing dose of vitamin B_{12} may be more useful in diagnosis than the radioactivity of the 24-hour urine collection. Serum iron is reported to drop with acute infarct of myocardium.

TIBC is increased in iron-deficiency, use of oral contraceptives, and in pregnancy.

TIBC decreased in hypoproteinemia from many causes, and in a number of inflammatory states. Also, chloramphenicol and corticotropin can decrease TIBC.

Increased saturation occurs with HLA-related (classical) hemochromatosis before ferritin is greatly increased, and also with iron overload (eg, cirrhosis and portacaval shunt), in hemolytic anemias, and with iron therapy. Saturation >70% in females, >80% in males is described as prerequisite for parenchymal loading. However, sample contamination and the vagaries of fluctuation in serum iron levels can make such criteria misleading on occasion.

The serum ferritin is a more sensitive test than the serum iron or TIBC for iron deficiency and for iron overload. When all these tests are used together, as is often necessary, they usually can distinguish between iron deficiency anemia and the anemia of chronic disease. The best and most reliable evaluation of total body iron stores is by bone marrow aspiration and biopsy. The best evaluation of iron deficiency in childhood (unless lead toxicity is suspected) is free erythrocyte porphyrins.

With recombinant erythropoietin therapy serum iron, transferrin saturation, and ferritin levels decline due to rapid utilization by stimulated erythropoiesis with resultant decrease in storage iron.

While iron is usually considered in relation to hematopoiesis and oxygen transport functions of red cells, it is also of prime import to the lymphomyeloid systems.

Specific References

Brown EB, "Iron Metabolism: A 40 Year Overview," *Am J Med*, 1989, 87(3N):35-9.

Burns ER, Goldberg SN, Lawrence C, et al, "Clinical Utility of Serum Test for Iron Deficiency in Hospitalized Patients," *Am J Clin Pathol*, 1990, 93(2):240-5.

Finch CA and Huebers H, "Perspectives in Iron Metabolism," *N Engl J Med*, 1982, 306(25):1520-8.

Oski FA, "Iron Deficiency in Infancy and Childhood," *N Engl J Med*, 1993, 329(3):190-3.

Iron Binding Capacity *see* Iron and Total Iron Binding Capacity/Transferrin *on previous page*

Iron Profile *see* Iron and Total Iron Binding Capacity/Transferrin *on previous page*

Isolator™ Blood Culture *see* Blood Culture, Aerobic and Anaerobic *on page 1204*

Isomer of Phenyltoloxamine *see* Diphenhydramine, Blood *on page 1250*

Isoniazid, Blood

Synonyms INH
Specimen Blood
Volume 10 mL
Minimum Volume 4 mL serum
Container Red top tube
Collection Put time of last dose on requisition, if it is available.
Storage Instructions Transport specimen to the laboratory immediately. Separate serum and freeze immediately.
Reference Range 1-7 μg/mL (SI: 7-51 μmol/L)
Critical Values Toxic: >20 μg/mL (SI: >146 μmol/L)
Use Monitor therapeutic drug level; evaluate toxicity
Methodology Gas chromatography (GC), high performance liquid chromatography (HPLC), UV spectrophotometry, gas chromatography/mass spectrometry (GC/MS)
Additional Information Isoniazid is a hydrazide of isonicotinic acid and used in the treatment of susceptible tuberculosis infections and prophylactically for those individuals exposed to tuberculosis. Peak blood levels are achieved in 1-2 hours after injection and the rate of metabolization is determined genetically. In "slow" inactivators, the half-life is 2-5 hours. In fast inactivators, it is 0.5-1.6 hours. Adverse effects of isoniazid include peripheral neuritis, seizures, ataxia, tinnitus, dizziness, psychosis, hepatitis, blood dyscrasias, vomiting, and optic neuritis. Severe and sometimes fatal hepatitis may occur or develop even after many months of treatment.
Specific References

Holdiness MR, *J Liq Chromatogr*, 1982, 5:707-14.

Isopropanol, Blood

Related Information
Volatile Screen *on page 1378*
Synonyms 2-Propanol; Propyl Alcohol; Rubbing Alcohol
Specimen Blood
Volume 7 mL
Minimum Volume 2 mL
Container Red top tube
Collection Do not prepare venipuncture site with any alcohol-containing swab; send immediately to the laboratory.
Storage Instructions Refrigerate specimen at 4°C.
Reference Range None detected
Critical Values Lethal dose: ~240 mL; twice as toxic as ethanol, similar symptoms of intoxication
Use Assess isopropanol toxicity
Limitations Isopropanol is rapidly cleared from the blood
Methodology Gas chromatography (GC)
Additional Information Isopropyl alcohol or rubbing alcohol, if accidentally ingested, causes hypothermia, vomiting, dizziness, deep coma, and hypotension. Large quantities can be fatal. Isopropanol is metabolized to acetone which will appear in large quantities in the urine and blood.
Specific References

Alexander CB, McBay AJ, and Hudson RP, "Isopropanol and Isopropanol Deaths – Ten Years' Experience," *J Forensic Sci*, 1982, 27(3):541-8.

***Ixodes dammini* Identification** *see* Arthropod Identification *on page 1198*

Ketone Bodies, Blood

Synonyms Ketones, Blood; Nitroprusside Reaction, Blood
Applies To Acetoacetate; Acetone; Beta-Hydroxybutyrate; β-Hydroxybutyrate
Abstract Carbohydrate deprivation and increased catabolism of fatty acids leads to increases in the ketone bodies (acetoacetate and acetone). β-hydroxybutyrate is also increased and is usually listed with the "ketone" bodies although it is not a ketone.
Specimen Blood
Volume 7 mL
Minimum Volume 1 mL serum
Container Red top tube
Collection Capillary tubes should be filled as much as possible using technique to avoid air bubbles. Free flowing heelstick. Avoid hemolysis.

(Continued)

Ketone Bodies, Blood *(Continued)*

Causes for Rejection Hemolysis

Special Instructions Placement of peripheral venous catheter on admission may be useful in selected cases, such as instances of ketoacidosis. Lactic acid, glucose, electrolytes, urea nitrogen, venous or arterial pH should also be measured in possible ketoacidosis, with alcohol level, CBC, and urinalysis if clinically indicated. Serum osmolality is often needed.

Reference Range Negative in normal nutritional states by semiquantitative screening tests.

Possible Panic Range Positivity in 1:32 dilution indicates severe ketosis.

Use Diagnose ketonemia, ketoacidosis resulting from diabetes mellitus, alcoholism, stress, starvation, intestinal disorders including emesis, glycogen storage disease (von Gierke's), infantile organic acidemias, and other metabolic disorders; determining the presence of ketone bodies is useful when isopropanol ingestion is suspected.

Limitations False-negatives or falsely weak reactions may occur. Up to 33% of cases of diabetic ketoacidosis also have lactic acidosis. Acidosis shifts ketone bodies to β-hydroxybutyrate. However, β-hydroxybutyrate is not measured by nitroprusside, which reacts with both acetoacetic acid and acetone. The reagent is 5-20 times more sensitive to acetoacetic acid than to acetone and does not react with β-hydroxybutyrate. Thus, as ketoacidosis is treated, an apparent positive Acetest® is found while there is an actual reduction of total plasma ketone body concentration. Acidosis shifts equilibrium toward β-hydroxybutyrate (unmeasured), but treatment of ketoacidosis results in increased acetoacetate (measured) and thus a more positive "acetone" reaction, before ketone bodies decrease. Ketostix® false-positives occur with large amounts of levodopa. Nonketotic coma in diabetes may be caused by hyperosmolarity.

Methodology Nitroprusside reaction (colorimetry); gas chromatography (GC) and enzymatic methods are used in some institutions, but fast laboratory response is usually needed.

Additional Information Strongly positive serum acetone without severe acidosis, with normal anion gap, bicarbonate, and plasma glucose suggests the possibility of rubbing alcohol intoxication. Look for dehydration with ketosis. Ketoacidosis in diabetes usually occurs with decreased plasma pH and bicarbonate, increased glucose and other abnormalities. As ketoacidosis and metabolic acidosis are treated, hypokalemia may become evident. A normal or low potassium on admission of a patient with ketoacidosis may indicate severe potassium depletion. Thus, potassium is especially important among the parameters to follow in treatment of ketoacidosis. Hypophosphatemia may evolve. Acetone may be elevated due to absolute or relative starvation, especially in children. A significant mortality rate exists; in children younger than 10 years of age, diabetic ketoacidosis is reported to account for 70% of diabetes related deaths. A multipoint kinetic method allows determination of acetoacetate plus β-hydroxybutyrate and lactate plus pyruvate in a single cuvette.

Specific References

Caraway WT and Watts NB, "Carbohydrates," *Fundamentals of Clinical Chemistry*, 3rd ed, Tietz NW, ed, Philadelphia, PA: WB Saunders Co, 1987, 438-40.

Kaplan LA, "Ketones," *Clinical Chemistry – Theory, Analysis, and Correlation*, 2nd ed, Kaplan LA and Pesce AJ, eds, St Louis, MO: Mosby-Year Book Inc, 1989, 856-8.

Monaghan MS, Olsen KM, Ackerman BH, et al, "Measurement of Serum Isopropanol and the Acetone Metabolite by Proton Nuclear Magnetic Resonance: Application to Pharmacokinetic Evaluation in a Simulated Overdose Model," *J Toxicol Clin Toxicol*, 1995, 33(2):141-9.

Shaffer PA, "Antiketogenesis: Its Mechanism and Significance. 1932 (Classical Article)," *Medicine (Baltimore)*, 1990, 69(5):317-23.

Ketones, Blood *see* Ketone Bodies, Blood *on previous page*

Ketones, Urine

Synonyms Nitroprusside Reaction for Ketones, Urine; Urine Ketones

Applies To Acetoacetic Acid, Urine; Acetone, Semiquantitative, Urine; Beta-Hydroxybutyric Acid, Urine

Specimen Random urine

Volume Entire specimen

Minimum Volume 3 mL

Container Plastic urine container

Storage Instructions If sample cannot be tested immediately, it should be refrigerated.

Special Instructions Transport specimen to the laboratory promptly following collection.

Reference Range Negative; in starvation diets or in other instances of abnormal carbohydrate metabolism, ketones appear in the urine in excessively large amounts before serum ketones are elevated

Use Semiquantitative test to evaluate ketonuria, detect acidosis, ketoacidosis of alcoholism and diabetes mellitus, fasting, starvation, high protein diets, and isopropanol ingestion. Remains useful as a monitor in known diabetics, in type I patients when ill and during marked hyperglycemia and in type II diabetics during acute illness. In pregnancy, the risk of ketosis is increased; all pregnant type I diabetics are advised to monitor urine for ketosis in first morning urine and when blood glucose is >150 mg/dL.

Limitations Specimens containing large amounts of ascorbic acid or levodopa metabolites, valproic acid, phenazopyridine (Pyridium®), PSP dye, phenylketones, or phthalein compounds such as are administered for liver and kidney function tests may cause false-positives. Beta-hydroxybutyric acid (the third of the three ketone bodies) is not detected. N-acetylcysteine, levodopa, mesna, phenazopyridine, phenothiazines, and salicylates cause false-positive ketone results. Isoniazid can result in a true positive urinary ketone result.

Methodology Nitroprusside reaction, Ketostix® or Acetest®; acetoacetic acid and acetone react with nitroprusside to create a color change, especially the former.

Additional Information In infants and children, ketonuria can occur with febrile illnesses, toxic states with marked vomiting or diarrhea. Genetic disorders resulting in ketonuria include propionyl CoA carboxylase deficiency, glycogen storage disease, branched chain ketonuria and methylmalonic aciduria. In adult healthy men, a fast of 18 hours or longer produces ketonemia at a level that would result in detectable ketonuria. Aging is associated with increased susceptibility to fasting-induced hyperketonemia. Ketonuria may be noted in normal pregnancy. Acetoacetic acid, beta-hydroxybutyric acid, and acetone are ketone bodies. In ketosis, usually 80% of total ketones are beta-hydroxybutyric acid. Acetoacetic acid comprises most of the remainder with acetone present in trace amounts. Urine ketones should generally be determined in patients with a positive urine test for urine glucose and followed during the management of diabetes mellitus and ketoacidosis.

Specific References

Foster DW, "Banting Lecture 1984. From Glycogen to Ketones and Back," *Diabetes*, 1984, 33(12):1188-99.

McGarry JD, "New Perspectives in the Regulation of Ketogenesis," *Diabetes*, 1979, 28(5):517-23.

Kidney Profile

Synonyms Renal Panel; Renal Profile

Test Includes Urea nitrogen (BUN), creatinine, glucose, electrolytes

Abstract A test grouping ordered on a regular basis by nephrologists caring for patients with renal diseases.

Specimen Blood

Container Red top tube

Collection Routine venipuncture.

Use Evaluate renal diseases

Additional Information Electrolytes are needed to evaluate renal problems. The rationale for this test grouping is that patients who require frequent monitoring of renal function also require monitoring of serum electrolytes. Hyponatremia may indicate hyperglycemia. Many of these patients are diabetic and others are on intravenous glucose infusions, another reason to monitor glucose. Finally, interpretation and correction of potassium fluctuations are aided by current knowledge of glucose concentration.

Specific References

Andreoli TE, "Approach to the Patient With Renal Disease," *Cecil's Textbook of Medicine*, Wyngaarden JB, Smith LH, and Bennett JC, eds, 19th ed, Vol 1, Philadelphia, PA: WB Saunders Co, 1992, 477-82.

Dennis VW, "Investigations of Renal Function," *Cecil's Textbook of Medicine*, Wyngaarden JB, Smith LH, and Bennett JC, eds, 19th ed, Vol 1, Philadelphia, PA: WB Saunders Co, 1992, 492-9.

Klahr S, "Structure and Function of the Kidneys," *Cecil's Textbook of Medicine*, Wyngaarden JB, Smith LH, and Bennett JC, eds, 19th ed, Vol 1, Philadelphia, PA: WB Saunders Co, 1992, 482-92.

Killer Weed *see* Phencyclidine, Qualitative, Urine *on page 1319*

Killer Weed *see* Phencyclidine, Quantitative, Serum *on page 1319*

Klonopin™ *see* Clonazepam, Serum *on page 1232*

K^+, Plasma *see* Potassium, Blood *on page 1328*

K^+, Serum *see* Potassium, Blood *on page 1328*

Labile Factor *see* Factor V, Plasma *on page 1262*

Lactate, Blood *see* Lactic Acid, Blood *on page 1281*

Lactate Dehydrogenase, Blood

Synonyms Lactic Acid Dehydrogenase; LD; LDH

Abstract This enzyme catalyzes the interconversion of lactate and pyruvate. It is found in all cells of the body and exists in five molecular forms (isoenzymes).

(Continued)

Lactate Dehydrogenase, Blood *(Continued)*

Specimen Blood

Volume 7 mL

Minimum Volume 2 mL serum

Container Red top tube; serum separator tube is acceptable. Green top (heparin) tube is also acceptable.

Storage Instructions Avoid hemolysis. Stable 2-3 days at room temperature.

Causes for Rejection Hemolysis

Reference Range Normal ranges for serum LD (LDH) vary among methods. They are higher in childhood. For adults, in most laboratories, the range is up to approximately 200 units/L. See following table for approximate ranges.

Lactate Dehydrogenase

Age	units/L
0–2 y	125–275
2–3 y	166–232
3–4 y	112–221
4–5 y	108–206
5–6 y	104–205
6–7 y	100–204
7–8 y	95–203
8–12 y	90–201
12–14 y	90–199
14–16 y	Up to 168
16–17 y	Up to 161
17–43 y	90–156
≥43 y	90–176

Use Causes of **high LD:** Neoplastic states (especially with high alkaline phosphatase, very high total LD, and isomorphic pattern of LD isoenzymes); hypoxic cardiorespiratory diseases; hemolytic anemia; megaloblastic anemias, including pernicious anemia (levels may be >2000 units/L and LD isoenzymes reveal LD_1:LD_2 flip); infectious mononucleosis; inflammation; hypothyroidism (some cases); myocardial infarct: LD begins to rise about 12 hours after infarct and usually returns to normal after CK (CPK) and AST (SGOT) levels return to normal, isoenzymes usually most useful 48 hours from onset of infarct to reveal LD_1:LD_2 inversion; pulmonary infarct (rarely, triad of LD, bilirubin, AST increases occurs); other lung diseases.

Diseases of liver, including cirrhosis. Total LD in cirrhosis is usually not greatly increased. In acute viral hepatitis, LD is not greatly elevated and AST is usually three or more times higher (in relation to the upper limit of normal) than LD; chronic alcoholism is usually associated with some combination of elevated MCV (mean corpuscular volume), triglyceride, alkaline phosphatase, AST (SGOT), ALT (SGPT), GGT, and bilirubin and low folate.

Renal infarct – high LD, out of proportion to AST and alkaline phosphatase; seizures, other CNS diseases; acute pancreatitis; collagen diseases; excessive destruction of cells; fracture, other trauma, including head trauma, muscle damage; muscular dystrophy; focal necrosis; shock, hypotension; intestinal obstruction.

LD isoenzymes may be useful in the diagnosis of a number of the disease states mentioned above including myocardial infarction, neoplastic states, hemolytic anemia, megaloblastic anemias including pernicious anemia, infectious mononucleosis, some cases of hypothyroidism, diseases of the liver, renal infarct, and excessive destruction of cells

Other causes of increased LD include specimen tube artifact, such as serum contact with clot or exposure to heat. Chemistry profile with very high LD and no glucose may relate to unseparated serum and cells in a tube at room temperature or higher. Since LD is found in virtually every tissue in the body, the diagnostic value of an elevated level is limited.

Limitations Hemolysis elevates LD results, oxalate inhibits LD, ascorbic acid can decrease LD values.

Methodology Lactate to pyruvate monitored at 340 nm is predominant method but pyruvate to lactate is used. Pyruvate to lactate assay results in values about twice those of the lactate to pyruvate method. The temperature is usually 37°C but 30°C is also used.

Additional Information In **infectious mononucleosis**, LD is usually more elevated than AST, and there is usually an isomorphic pattern of LD isoenzymes. In **viral hepatitis**, by contrast, AST and ALT (the transaminases) are much more increased than is LD, about three or more times higher than total LD, and LD_5 is high. The differential diagnosis of acute infarct of myocardium includes pericarditis and angina, entities in which enzymes are usually not substantially increased. LD is useful in selected settings as a tumor marker, but LD is not helpful as a screening test for cancer. (Other applications as a tumor marker are included in the subsequent listing.) Bovine or porcine heparin therapy can cause increases of AST, ALT, and LD with elevated LD hepatic fractions.

Specific References

Gulbis B, Unger P, Lenaers A, et al, "Mass Concentration of Creatine Kinase MB Isoenzyme and Lactate Dehydrogenase Isoenzyme 1 in Diagnosis of Perioperative Myocardial Infarction After Coronary Bypass Surgery," *Clin Chem*, 1990, 36(10):1784-8.

Kagawa FT, Kirsch CM, Yenokida GG, et al, "Serum Lactate Dehydrogenase Activity in Patients With AIDS and *Pneumocystis carinii* Pneumonia: An Adjunct to Diagnosis," *Chest*, 1988, 94(5):1031-3.

Reis GJ, Kaufman HW, Horowitz GL, et al, "Usefulness of Lactate Dehydrogenase and Lactate Dehydrogenase Isoenzymes for Diagnosis of Acute Myocardial Infarction," *Am J Cardiol*, 1988, 61(10):754-8.

Schiele F, "Lactate Dehydrogenase," *Drug Effects on Laboratory Test Results Analytical Interferences and Pharmacological Effects*, Siest G and Galteau MM, eds, Littleton, MA: PSG Publishing Co Inc, 1988, 269-306.

Lactic Acid, Blood

Synonyms Blood Lactate; Lactate, Blood

Applies To Biotin; Phenformin

Abstract Hypoperfusion is the most common cause of lactic acidosis, and hyperlactacidemia may be the only marker of tissue hypoperfusion.

Specimen Whole blood, arterial or venous, or plasma

Volume 7 mL

Minimum Volume 4 mL whole blood

Container Gray top (sodium fluoride) tube

Collection Avoid hand-clenching and use of a tourniquet. A tourniquet or a patient clenching and unclenching his/her hand will lead to build-up of potassium and lactic acid from the hand muscles. Commonly needed with or as stat follow-up to venous or arterial pH. Serial determinations are often valuable. Send specimen on ice.

Storage Instructions Centrifuge immediately and take off plasma (unless laboratory uses a whole blood method). Keep plasma on ice or at 2°C to 8°C, analyze promptly. A recent study of blood handling techniques and their effect on lactate concentration has been published.

Causes for Rejection Specimen not received on ice

Special Instructions Keep tube on ice until delivered to the laboratory. Tube must be in laboratory within 15 minutes of being drawn.

Reference Range Plasma values: venous: 4.5-19.8 mg/dL (SI: 0.5-2.2 mmol/L); arterial: 4.5-14.4 mg/dL (SI: 0.5-1.6 mmol/L)

Possible Panic Range ≥45.0 mg/dL

Use Suspect lactic acidosis when unexplained anion gap metabolic acidosis is encountered, especially if azotemia or ketoacidosis are not present. Evaluate metabolic acidosis, regional or diffuse tissue hypoperfusion, hypoxia, shock, congestive heart failure, dehydration, complicated postoperative state, ketoacidosis or nonketotic acidosis in diabetes mellitus, patients with infections, inflammatory states, postictal state, certain myopathies, acute leukemia and other neoplasia, enzyme defects, glycogen storage disease (type I), thiamine deficiency, and hepatic failure. A spontaneous form of lactic acidosis occurs. It is a prognostic index in particular clinical settings, especially in critically ill patients in shock. A relationship to renal disease also exists. With skin rash, seizures, alopecia, ataxia, keratoconjunctivitis, and lactic acidosis in children, consider defective biotin metabolism. Phenformin, ethanol, methanol, and salicylate and ethylene glycol poisoning may cause lactic acidosis. Acetaminophen toxicity causes lactic acidosis, sometimes with hypoglycemia. Cyanide, isoniazid, and propylene glycol are among the causes of lactic acidosis. Lactic acidosis may be due to inborn errors of metabolism.

Limitations Gross hemolysis depresses results. Intravenous injections or infusions which modify acid-base balance, may cause alterations in lactate levels. Epinephrine and exercise elevate lactate, as may I.V. sodium bicarbonate, glucose, and hyperventilation. False low values with a high LD (LDH) value. Normal L-lactate occurs with high D-lactate in D-lactic acidosis. Metabolic acidosis following bypass for obesity, related to altered gastrointestinal flora, is a feature of subjects who develop mental changes as well, in whom D-lactate is the causative anion.

Contraindications Lack of acidosis is **not** a contraindication for this test.

Methodology Enzymatic; other methods include gas chromatography (GC)

(Continued)

Lactic Acid, Blood *(Continued)*

Additional Information Phosphorus is sometimes significantly abnormal in lactic acidosis. Creatinine is higher in ketoacidosis than in lactic acidosis, by interference produced by acetoacetic acid on creatinine. Causes of lactic acidosis (usually <45 mg/dL (SI: <5.0 mmol/L)) include carbohydrate infusions, exercise, diabetic ketosis, alcohol. Causes of lactic acidosis (>45 mg/dL) include shock (in which lactic acidosis may occur early, before fall in blood pressure, decrease in urine output), hypoxia (including congestive failure, severe anemia, hypotension) and malignancies. Severe lactic acidosis can develop in minutes. Lactic acidosis can accompany dehydration. Blood lactate concentration correlates negatively with survival in patients with acute myocardial infarction, with persistent elevation, >36 mg/dL (SI: >4.0 mmol/L) for more than 12 hours, being associated with poor prognosis. At a given bicarbonate level, the average pCO_2 is lower in lactic acidosis than in diabetic ketoacidosis. Lactic acid determination is generally indicated if anion gap is >20 mmol/L and if pH is <7.25 and the pCO_2 is not elevated. (Mizock uses pH 7.35 as a diagnostic criterion). The measurement of lactate levels may be indicated in the clinical setting of metabolic acidosis. Serum salicylate, ethanol level, and osmolality may be helpful. Spontaneous lactic acidosis may be fatal. Protocols are available for measurement of lactate in cord blood.

Specific References

Gau N, "Lactic Acid," *Methods in Clinical Chemistry*, Pesce AJ and Kaplan LA, eds, St Louis, MO: Mosby-Year Book Inc, 1987, 78-82.

Kreisberg RA, "Lactate Homeostasis and Lactic Acidosis," *Ann Intern Med*, 1980, 92(2 Pt 1):227-37.

Lactic Acid Dehydrogenase *see* Lactate Dehydrogenase, Blood *on page 1279*

Lanotoxin® *see* Digitoxin, Blood *on page 1249*

Lanoxin® *see* Digoxin, Blood *on page 1250*

L-Aspartate *see* Aspartate Aminotransferase *on page 1199*

Latency Studies *see* Nerve Conduction Studies *on page 1304*

LD *see* Lactate Dehydrogenase, Blood *on page 1279*

LDH *see* Lactate Dehydrogenase, Blood *on page 1279*

Lead, Blood

Related Information

Heavy Metal Screen, Blood *on page 1271*

Synonyms Pb, Blood

Applies To Delta Aminolevulinic Acid Dehydratase

Abstract Blood lead concentrations are used to detect recent lead exposure. Does not necessarily measure lead body burden from chronic exposure in the past.

Specimen Whole blood

Volume 10 mL

Container Special lead-free tube with heparin

Storage Instructions Do not separate red cells.

Special Instructions Avoid contact with leaded glass during collection

Reference Range <10 μg/dL (whole blood) (SI: <0.97 μmol/L). See accompanying CDC chart for evaluating blood lead concentrations in children.

CDC Classification of Blood Lead in Children

Class	Blood Lead Level* (μg/dL)	Comment
I	<10	Not lead-poisoned
IIA	10–14	Rescreen frequently and consider prevention activities
IIB	15–19	Institute nutritional and educational interventions
III	20–44	Evaluate environment and consider chelation therapy
IV	45–69	Institute environmental intervention and chelation therapy
V	>69	A medical emergency

*Due to possible contamination during collection, elevated levels should be confirmed with a second specimen before action is instituted.

Possible Panic Range >80 μg/dL (SI: >3.86 μmol/L) in acute lead poisoning; toxicity at lower levels in chronic poisoning

Use Evaluate lead toxicity, poisoning

Limitations Lead poisoning is not ruled out by normal blood levels; clinical findings and heme synthetic enzymes must also be evaluated.

Methodology Electrothermal atomic absorption spectrometry (AA), photometry, anodic stripping voltammeter

Additional Information Great care is required to avoid contamination in the collection of specimens for lead analysis. Lead can be measured in tissue and urine. Another test that may be used to evaluate lead intoxication is **free erythrocyte protoporphyrin (FEP)**. FEP concentrations >35 μg/dL are consistent with undue absorption of lead. However, FEP is also elevated in iron deficiency, sickle cell anemia, and chronic infection. **Erythrocyte zinc protoporphyrin** is a more specific indicator of lead toxicity and, therefore, superior to FEP. Normal values for erythrocyte zinc protoporphyrin are <100 ng/dL. Inhibition of erythrocyte **delta aminolevulinic acid dehydratase** is a very sensitive measure of lead toxicity. However, a blood lead assay is the definitive test for recent acute exposure if sample collection is meticulous. Blood lead concentrations are evidence of **recent** exposure but do not indicate the body burden from past exposure. Lead poisoning causes renal damage. Capillary tube collections of fingerstick blood provides adequate samples for atomic absorption spectrophotometry; false-positive rates per this method (19%) are comparable to conventional venous blood sampling (13%).

Specific References

Bernard BP and Becker CE, "Environmental Lead Exposure and the Kidney," *J Toxicol Clin Toxicol*, 1988, 26(1-2):1-34.

Braithwaite RA and Brown SS, "Clinical and Subclinical Lead Poisoning: A Laboratory Perspective," *Hum Toxicol*, 1988, 7(5):503-13.

Goyer RA, "Mechanisms of Lead and Cadmium Nephrotoxicity," *Toxicol Lett* 1989, 46(1-3):153-62.

Markowitz ME and Rosen JF, "Need for the Lead Mobilization Test in Children With Lead Poisoning," *J Pediatr*, 1991, 119(2):305-10.

Mushak P, Davis JM, Crocetti AF, et al, "Prenatal and Postnatal Effects of Low-Level Lead Exposure: Integrated Summary of a Report to the U.S. Congress on Childhood Lead Poisoning," *Environ Res*, 1989, 50(1):11-36.

Rempel D, "The Lead-Exposed Worker," *JAMA*, 1989, 262(4):532-4.

Schonfeld DJ, Cullen MR, Rainey PM, et al, "Screening for Lead Poisoning in an Urban Pediatric Clinic Using Samples Obtained by Fingerstick," *Pediatrics*, 1994, 94(2 Pt 1):174-9.

Staessen JA, Lauwerys RR, Buchet J-P, et al, "Impairment of Renal Function With Increasing Blood Lead Concentrations in the General Population," *N Engl J Med*, 1992, 327(3):151-6.

Lead Excretion Ratio *see* Lead, Urine *on this page*

Lead, Quantitative, Hair or Nails

Synonyms Pb, Quantitative

Specimen Hair, nails

Volume 0.5 g

Container Bottle

Collection Nails: Clip all patient's fingernails and toenails. Place clippings in a small bottle. Do not transmit to laboratory in an envelope.

Hair: Clip several locks of hair, place in a small bottle. Do not send in same container as nails or in an envelope.

Reference Range Negative

Use Establish the diagnosis of lead poisoning

Methodology Anodic-strip voltametry

Additional Information Hematologic consequences ascribed to lead toxicity may be basophilic stippling, mild anemia, and reticulocytosis. Other characteristics of toxicity may include increased urine delta aminolevulinic acid, increased erythrocyte porphyrins, and decreased aminolevulinic acid dehydrase. Lead-lines on gums or at the metaphyses of long bones in children may also be present.

Early symptoms of lead poisoning include anorexia, apathy or irritability, fatigue and anemia. Toxic effects include GI distress, joint pain, colic, headache, stupor, convulsions, and coma. Another test that may be used to evaluate lead intoxication in free erythrocyte protoporphyrin. However, a blood lead assay is the definitive test.

Lead, Urine

Related Information

Heavy Metal Screen, Urine *on page 1272*

Synonyms Pb, Urine

Applies To Lead Excretion Ratio

Abstract This test is used to assess lead body burden (lead mobilization test), not to diagnose lead poisoning.

Patient Preparation Patient should be instructed to use a specially cleaned plastic urinal or bedpan

Specimen Random or 24-hour urine

Volume 50 mL random, entire 24-hour collection

(Continued)

Lead, Urine *(Continued)*

Container Plastic (preferably polyethylene) acid-washed urine container

Storage Instructions Record total volume. Acidify to pH 2 with concentrated HCl or add 20 mL 6N HCl to the 24-hour volume.

Causes for Rejection Specimen allowed to contact glass or metal, specimen not collected in acid-washed containers

Special Instructions Indicate if a chelating agent has been administered

Reference Range ≤80 μg/24 hours (SI: ≤0.39 μmol/day)

Possible Panic Range >125 μg/24 hours (SI: >0.60 μmol/day) is considered excessive and associated with toxicity; values of 80-125 μg/24 hours (SI: 0.39-0.60 μmol/day) are inconclusive

Use Evaluate lead toxicity and chelation therapy

Methodology Electrothermal atomic absorption (AA)

Additional Information Lead is poorly excreted and is found in lower concentrations in urine versus blood. Urine is not the specimen for screening potential toxicity. Urine lead mobilization tests (postchelation therapy) are good indicators of lead body burden. Children with blood lead levels between 25-40 μg/dL should be evaluated by a lead mobilization test to determine need for chelation therapy. Those with levels >40 μg/dL should receive chelation therapy. A lead mobilization test is carried out by giving Ca EDTA and measuring the lead excreted in the next 24-hour urine. The lead excretion ratio (LER) is calculated by dividing the amount of lead excreted (in μg/24 hours) by the amount of Ca EDTA given (in mg). A ratio >0.60 is considered positive for the LER. Unstimulated urinary excretion at rates >0.19 μg lead/mg creatinine may also be used to indicate need for chelation therapy.

Specific References

Bryson PD, *Comprehensive Review in Toxicology*, 2nd ed, Rockville, MD: Aspen Publishers Inc, 1989, 487-500.

Cory-Slechta DA, "Lead Exposure During Advanced Age: Alterations in Kinetics and Biochemical Effects," *Toxicol Appl Pharmacol*, 1990, 104(1):67-78.

D'Haese PC, Lamberts LV, Liang L, et al, "Elimination of Matrix and Spectral Interferences in the Measurement of Lead and Cadmium in Urine and Blood by Electrothermal Atomic Absorption Spectrometry With Deuterium Background Correction," *Clin Chem*, 1991, 37(9):1583-8.

Leukocyte Count *see* White Blood Count *on page 1380*

Librax® *see* Chlordiazepoxide, Blood *on page 1225*

Librium® *see* Chlordiazepoxide, Blood *on page 1225*

Lice Identification *see* Arthropod Identification *on page 1198*

Lidocaine, Blood

Synonyms Lignocaine; Xylocaine®

Applies To GX; MEGX

Abstract Lidocaine is a local anesthetic which more recently has been used as an antiarrhythmic. The most active metabolite is MEGX.

Specimen Blood

Volume 10 mL

Container Red top tube, green top (heparin) tube, or lavender top (EDTA) tube

Sampling Time Draw specimens 12 hours after initiating therapy for arrhythmia prophylaxis, then every 24 hours thereafter. Obtain specimens every 12 hours when cardiac or hepatic insufficiency exists.

Collection Avoid collection tubes with stoppers containing the plasticizer, TBEP.

Reference Range Therapeutic: 1.5-5.0 μg/mL (SI: 6.4-21.4 μmol/L), up to 6.0 μg/mL (SI: 25.6 μmol/L) if necessary.

Possible Panic Range At levels >6.0 μg/mL (SI: >25.6 μmol/L), there may be seizure activity.

Use Monitor therapeutic drug level. Lidocaine is used especially in acute arrhythmias.

Limitations Cross reactions with other drugs occur. Certain blood collection tubes have been shown to lead to falsely low results. See Collection.

Methodology Enzyme immunoassay (EIA), gas-liquid chromatography (GLC), high performance liquid chromatography (HPLC)

Additional Information This drug is used in therapy of ventricular but not supraventricular arrhythmias. Following initial parenteral administration of a bolus, lidocaine is rapidly cleared with a short half-life of approximately 10 minutes (first-pass effect). After approximately 30 minutes, there is a slower elimination phase about 90 minutes long. With continuous intravenous administration, a half-life of about 1.5-2 hours may be achieved, hence, prolonged administration by the I.V. route is often necessary to achieve the desired therapeutic result. Time to reach steady-state by I.V. is 6-12 hours. In most cases, a relatively constant plasma level may be maintained by slow intravenous infusion administered over a period of 6-10 hours. Blood levels are also elevated by impaired cardiac or hepatic function. The drug is metabolized by the liver to two active metabolites, monoethylglycinexylidide (MEGX) and glycinexylidide (GX). Both accumulate and MEGX most likely contributes to toxicity. Toxic symptoms may include confusion, respiratory depression, seizures, dizziness, drowsiness, paresthesias, hypotension, bradycardia, and double vision. Convulsions, cardiac and respiratory arrest may occur. Barbiturates and phenytoin seem to enhance drug metabolism and lower serum levels, whereas propranolol, cimetidine, and norepinephrine increase levels. Lidocaine is approximately 70% bound to plasma proteins, especially alpha$_1$ acid glycoprotein (the concentration of which is variable) and to albumin.

Specific References

Gumucio CA, Bennie JB, Fernando B, et al, "Plasma Lidocaine Levels During Augmentation Mammoplasty and Suction-Assisted Lipectomy," *Plast Reconstr Surg*, 1989, 84(4):624-7.

Montamat SC, Cusack BJ, and Vestal RE, "Management of Drug Therapy in the Elderly," *N Engl J Med*, 1989, 321(5):303-9.

Palmisano JM, Meliones JN, Crowley DC, et al, "Lidocaine Toxicity After Subcutaneous Infiltration in Children Undergoing Cardiac Catheterization," *Am J Cardiol*, 1991, 67(7):647-8.

Lignocaine *see* Lidocaine, Blood *on previous page*

Limbitrol® *see* Amitriptyline, Blood *on page 1187*

Liquiprin® *see* Acetaminophen, Serum *on page 1180*

Lithium, Blood

Synonyms Eskalith®; Lithonate®

Abstract Lithium is used in the treatment of depression and particularly for manic-depressive psychosis. It should be monitored.

Aftercare Follow urine osmolality, EKGs, thyroid profile, BUN, creatinine, and sodium. Avoid sodium depletion.

Specimen Blood

Volume 7 mL

Minimum Volume 2 mL serum

Container Red top tube

Collection Collect at a standard time from last dose, 6-12 hours is recommended.

Storage Instructions Refrigerate a minimum of 2 mL serum. Serum specimens are stable for 24 hours at room temperature. Separate serum immediately.

Causes for Rejection Specimen collected in tube containing lithium heparin, hemolysis

Reference Range Therapeutic: 0.6-1.2 mEq/L (SI: 0.6-1.2 mmol/L), for acute mania; 0.8-1.0 mEq/L (SI: 0.8-1.0 mmol/L) for protection against future episodes in most patients with bipolar disorder. A higher rate of relapse is described in subjects who are maintained at levels $<$0.4 mEq/L (SI: 0.4 mmol/L).

Possible Panic Range Toxic: $>$1.5 mEq/L (SI: $>$1.5 mmol/L). Toxicity can become serious when levels rise to levels $\geq$2.0 mEq/L (SI: $\geq$2.0 mmol/L). Levels $>$4.0 mEq/L (SI: $>$4.0 mmol/L) are associated with coma, death. A narrow therapeutic index exists for lithium.

Use Monitor therapeutic drug level; evaluate coma

Limitations Lithium toxicity can occur with normal serum lithium levels. Thiazides can cause significant rise in serum lithium.

Methodology Flame photometry, atomic absorption spectrophotometry (AA), ion-selective electrode (ISE)

Additional Information Lithium as lithium carbonate is used as a psychoactive agent in the treatment of manic depressive disorders. Lithium therapy demands daily monitoring of serum lithium levels until the proper dose schedule is determined. Serum half-life ranges from 20-60 hours. Insomnia in a low-range group is described. Tremor, gastrointestinal symptoms, urinary frequency, and weight gain were less frequent at lower levels. Intoxication never occurs suddenly. Several days to a week before full-blown symptoms develop, a patient will experience lethargy, drowsiness, tremor, muscle twitching, dysarthria, anorexia and vomiting or diarrhea. A fully developed case of intoxication shows coma to semicoma, rigidity, hyperactive reflexes and seizures at times. There is a high incidence of pulmonary complications. It is advisable to perform periodic plasma sodium determinations. Low plasma sodium levels are associated with lithium retention; high levels with lithium elimination. Varying degrees of nephrogenic diabetes insipidus have been reported to occur in 33% of lithium treated patients. Lithium significantly inhibits antidiuretic-hormone-induced water transport in kidney. Lithium interferes with solute and water absorption from the gastrointestinal system producing nausea, vomiting, diarrhea, and abdominal pain. These symptoms may occur at any time, at any serum level. They most commonly occur during early treatment stages and usually clear spontaneously or by adjustment of dosage. Chronic lithium administration has a goitrogenic effect on 4% of lithium-treated patients, with or without hypothyroidism. In general, lithium administration results in slightly decreased serum T_4 levels and transiently elevated levels of TSH in nearly 33% of these patients. Lithium affects the cardiac conduction system by incomplete substitution

(Continued)

Lithium, Blood *(Continued)*

for other cations, especially sodium and potassium. These electrolyte changes account for the usually unimportant and reversible T-wave depressions observed in 10% to 20% of patients on lithium therapy.

Specific References

Chamberlain S, Hahn PM, Casson P, et al, "Effect of Menstrual Cycle Phase and Oral Contraceptive Use on Serum Lithium Levels After a Loading Dose of Lithium in Normal Women," *Am J Psychiatry*, 1990, 147(7):907-9.

Krishel S and Jackimczyk K, "Cyclic Antidepressants, Lithium, and Neuroleptic Agents. Pharmacology and Toxicology," *Emerg Med Clin North Am*, 1991, 9(1):53-86.

Manji HK, Hsiao JK, Risby ED, et al, "The Mechanisms of Action of Lithium. I. Effects on Serotoninergic and Noradrenergic Systems in Normal Subjects," *Arch Gen Psychiatry*, 1991, 48(6):505-12.

Murray RL, "Lithium," *Clinical Chemistry – Theory Analysis, and Correlation*, 2nd ed, Kaplan LA and Pesce AJ, eds, St Louis, MO: Mosby-Year Book Inc, 1989, 1108-10.

Schweyen DH, Sporka MC, and Burnakis TG, "Evaluation of Serum Lithium Concentration Determinations," *Am J Hosp Pharm*, 1991, 48(7):1536-7.

Lithium RBC/Plasma Ratio

Test Includes Plasma lithium, RBC lithium, and RBCs/plasma ratio

Specimen Blood

Volume 10 mL

Minimum Volume 2 mL

Container Lavender top (EDTA) tube

Storage Instructions Do not refrigerate.

Causes for Rejection Gross hemolysis, clotted specimen

Reference Range RBC lithium: 0.10-0.40 mEq/L; plasma lithium; 1.00-1.50 mEq/L; RBC plasma/ratio: none defined

Methodology Atomic absorption spectrophotometry (AA)

Lithonate® *see* Lithium, Blood *on previous page*

Liver Battery *see* Liver Profile *on this page*

Liver Panel *see* Liver Profile *on this page*

Liver Profile

Synonyms Liver Battery; Liver Panel

Test Includes Liver profile most often includes total bilirubin, conjugated bilirubin, alkaline phosphatase, LD (LDH), AST (SGOT), ALT (SGPT), and GGT (GGTP). It may also include serum protein electrophoresis, prothrombin time, HB_sAg, perhaps LAP (leucine aminopeptidase) or 5' nucleotidase. Alpha$_1$-antitrypsin phenotype and quantitation on occasion explains cases otherwise difficult to classify but is rarely if ever included in liver profiles.

Abstract Characterization of liver disease requires intelligent correlation of the medical history, physical examination, and laboratory test results.

Specimen Blood

Volume 10 mL

Minimum Volume 2 mL serum

Container Red top tube

Storage Instructions Protect bilirubin specimens from light.

Causes for Rejection Hemolysis interferes with certain tests.

Special Instructions The specimen should be handled with extra precaution, especially if there is a greater than usual possibility of hepatitis. Prothrombin time tube should be spun down immediately, plasma separated from cells, placed in special plastic tube, kept refrigerated, and analyzed within 4 hours.

Use Evaluate liver disease, biliary disease, hepatoma, chronic active hepatitis, cirrhosis, including biliary cirrhosis; investigate otherwise unexplained increases in such tests as AST, ALT, alkaline phosphatase, or prolongation of the prothrombin time; work up possible alcoholism

Limitations A number of useful tests include those to work up pancreatitis, such as serum amylase and lipase and urine 2-hour amylase. Other tests helpful in evaluation of liver disease include 5' nucleotidase; immunoglobulins IgG, IgA, IgM; ANA; antimitochondrial antibody; smooth muscle antibody; LD isoenzymes; alpha-fetoprotein, and 2-hour urine urobilinogen. Ammonia is useful only in selected cases, (eg, Reye's syndrome).

Use of blood alcohol determinations for investigation of liver disease has been advocated, because the test is cheap and simple. Other tests useful in alcoholism include MCV and folate levels, triglycerides as well as GGT, AST, and bilirubin. Prothrombin time is often helpful. False-positive tests occur in asymptomatic patients. Repeat testing on initial abnormalities is important. Viral hepatitis serological tests additional to HB_sAg may be indicated. Liver disease related to alpha$_1$-antitrypsin deficiency and to Wilson's disease must be considered.

Contraindications Many physicians prefer to order tests individually, as clinically indicated. Among the problems with such profiles, tests appropriate for specific clinical indications may not be included. Few physicians recall accurately the content of a liver profile offered by a specific clinical laboratory.

Additional Information Liver profile interpretation can be considered as follows:

Cholestasis and biliary tract: alkaline phosphatase (very rarely, isoenzymes of alkaline phosphatase), GGT, leucine aminopeptidase, 5' nucleotidase, total bilirubin, conjugated bilirubin, eosinophil count, urine bile (as part of urinalysis) are used. In extrahepatic biliary obstruction the serum alkaline phosphatase is increased two to three times or more while AST remains <300 units/L. Very high alkaline phosphatase levels may be found with intrahepatic cholestasis, such that alkaline phosphatase which is high out of proportion to the severity of jaundice, may indicate an intrahepatic disease. Serum and urine amylase and lipase are often relevant. Viral, alcoholic, or drug-related cholestatic hepatitis may give rise to chemistry tests indistinguishable from those of extrahepatic obstruction.

Liver excretory function: urine urobilinogen, total bilirubin, conjugated bilirubin.

Hepatoma and other tumors: alkaline phosphatase, GGT, total LD, CEA, HB_sAg (hepatitis B surface antigen). $Alpha_1$-fetoprotein may increase moderately in nonmalignant liver diseases; rising or high levels may indicate hepatoma. Such clinical laboratory tests do not prove tumor without imaging and biopsy.

Hepatocellular disease: AST, ALT (more specific than AST), LD, LD_4, LD_5 (fractions related to liver in LD isoenzymes), liver biopsy, HB_sAg (hepatitis B surface antigen), anti-HB_s (antibody to hepatitis B surface antigen), anti-HB_c (antibody to hepatitis B core antigen), HB_eAg (hepatitis B "e" antigen), anti-HB_e (antibody to hepatitis B_e antigen), anti-HAV, IgM (antibody to hepatitis A virus, IgM).

Liver metabolic function: Serum ammonia may increase in liver necrosis and cirrhosis.

Hemochromatosis: Mild abnormalities in liver profile tests (AST, ALT, ALP) may occur in hemochromatosis.

Immunologic stimulation: Protein electrophoresis: features suggestive of cirrhosis but not always present in that disease include low albumin, low $alpha_2$, polyclonal or oligoclonal gammopathy, and beta/gamma bridging. Many but not all cases of conventional hepatic cirrhosis are accompanied by polyclonal gammopathy, sometimes with beta/gamma bridging. Oligoclonal gammopathy is found in <50% of cases of chronic active hepatitis (CAH).

Immunoglobulins: IgM: very helpful in primary biliary cirrhosis; high in acute and chronic hepatitis, cholangitis, and CAH. $Alpha_1$-globulin tends to fall with serum albumin. Both alpha and beta globulins may decrease in hepatocellular failure.

Antibodies: ANA: A portion of cases of CAH have positive ANA and/or positive LE prep. **Antimitochondrial antibody**: Extremely useful in primary biliary cirrhosis; high more often in cholangitis than in cholecystitis. **Smooth muscle antibody:** Hepatitis and conventional as well as biliary cirrhosis; especially useful for CAH (chronic active hepatitis). Antibodies usually negative in drug jaundice and nonfebrile extrahepatic obstruction. In intrahepatic or extrahepatic biliary obstructive disease, the tests listed under Cholestasis and Biliary Tract are more abnormal than those listed under Hepatocellular Disease.

In **viral hepatitis**, AST is usually three to five times or more higher (as multiples of the upper limit of normal) than LD; in cases which clinically resemble hepatitis, but in which LD equals or exceeds AST, LD isoenzymes may be useful. LD_4 and LD_5 are the hepatic fractions. An isomorphic pattern, if detected, may suggest infectious mononucleosis, CMV infection, neoplasm, or cirrhosis/alcoholism, depending on clinical setting. Appropriate positive serological tests support a diagnosis of viral hepatitis, while negative ones provide support for drug-induced hepatitis. Resolution of liver disease with removal of the offending agent enhances the latter diagnosis.

Hepatic functional reserve: Both albumin and prothrombin time are useful in evaluation of the liver, but they are nonspecific. Representing hepatic synthesis, albumin reflects also nutritional status and is lost in a variety of gastrointestinal and renal diseases.

Liver biopsy is not replaced by such testing. Liver biopsy remains a vital diagnostic modality. Its interpretation commonly requires and is supported by clinical laboratory investigation. Results of testing must be provided to the histopathologist who works up and holds responsibility for interpretation of the liver biopsy.

Specific References

Sherwin JE, "Liver Function," *Clinical Chemistry Theory Analysis and Correlation*, Chapter 23, Kaplan LA and Pesce AJ, eds, St Louis, MO: Mosby-Year Book Inc, 1989, 359-72.

l-Methamphetamine *see* Methamphetamines, Urine *on page 1294*

Loads *see* Glutethimide, Blood *on page 1270*

Lorazepam, Blood

Synonyms Ativan®
Specimen Blood
Volume 10 mL
Minimum Volume 3 mL serum
Container Red top tube
Storage Instructions Separate serum from clot and refrigerate.
Reference Range 0.05-0.24 μg/mL (SI: 156-746 nmol/L)
Critical Values 0.30-0.60 μg/mL
Use Monitor therapeutic drug level; evaluate toxicity
Methodology High performance liquid chromatography (HPLC)
Additional Information Lorazepam is a benzodiazepine derivative and similar to chlordiazepoxide in its actions, uses, limitations, and interactions. It is used for the management of anxiety and to provide preoperative sedation and amnesia; it is a potent benzodiazepine. Peak plasma levels are achieved in 2 hours after oral dose and 1-1.5 hours after I.M. injection. Half-life is 10-16 hours. Adverse effects include CNS confusion, depression, lethargy, dizziness, bradycardia, transitory hallucinations, nausea and vomiting, respiratory depression, and hyper- or hypotension.

Lotusate® *see* Barbiturates, Quantitative, Blood *on page 1201*
LSD *see* Lysergic Acid Diethylamine Level *on next page*
Lude® *see* Methaqualone Level *on page 1295*
Luminal® *see* Phenobarbital, Blood *on page 1320*
Luminal® *see* Barbiturates, Quantitative, Blood *on page 1201*

Lung Scan, Ventilation

Synonyms Aerosol Lung Scan; Radionuclide Ventilation Lung Scan; Ventilation Lung Scan; Xenon Lung Scan
Applies To Quantitative Ventilation Lung Scan; Ventilation-Perfusion Lung Scan
Test Includes The patient inhales a radioactive gas or nebulized aerosol and multiple images of the lungs are then acquired to assess lung ventilation. **Special note:** This procedure is almost always combined with a lung perfusion scan to detect a characteristic pattern of segmental perfusion deficits with normal corresponding regional ventilation that is the hallmark of pulmonary emboli.
Patient Preparation Patient should have all RIA blood work performed, or at least drawn, prior to injection of any radioactive material. The patient does not need to be fasting or NPO for this procedure. The patient should have a routine chest radiograph performed within 12 hours prior to imaging or receive one immediately after. Notify the Nuclear Medicine Department if patients require high flow oxygen or respirator assistance.
Causes for Rejection Other recent Nuclear Medicine procedure may interfere. If uncertain, call the Nuclear Medicine Department.
Special Instructions Requisition must state the current patient diagnosis in order to select the most appropriate radiopharmaceutical and/or imaging technique. The duration of the procedure is 30 minutes to 1 hour. See table for radiopharmaceuticals.

Radiopharmaceuticals for Lung Ventilation Imaging

Agent	Isotope Half-Life	Timing vs Perfusion Scan	Advantages	Disadvantages
^{99m}Tc DTPA aerosol	6 hours	Before	Multiple views of ventilation	Turbulent air flow can cause patchy distribution; no washout phase
^{133}Xe gas	5 days	Before	Single view with equilibrium and washout phases	Requires good single-breath effort; single view (usually posterior)
^{127}Xe gas	36 days	After	Single view with equilibrium and washout phases; may be performed after perfusion scan	
^{81m}Kr gas	13 seconds	During	Multiple views of ventilation; no gas trap required	Nonavailability on 24-hour basis; expense

Reference Range Homogeneous distribution of activity throughout the lungs
Use The primary indication for lung ventilation and perfusion imaging is the detection of acute pulmonary emboli. These procedures together provide an accurate noninvasive screening test both for the detection of emboli and for documentation of resolution during and after therapy. Lung ventilation imaging is also helpful in

quantifying regional pulmonary ventilation in patients with severe obstructive lung disease or who are being considered for lung resection surgery. Useful for acute toxic inhalation; retention of xenon indicative of parenchymal lung damage.

Limitations Patients must be able to cooperate in performing this test. They will be required to breathe through a mouthpiece, remain still for approximately 15 minutes, (usually in the supine position) and if xenon gas is used, hold their breath for 10 seconds or longer. The procedure is somewhat nonspecific in the presence of underlying lung conditions such as pneumonia or chronic obstructive disease. A same day chest radiograph is necessary for review and comparison with scan findings.

Additional Information Patients on high flow oxygen or respirator assistance can undergo ventilation scans with radioactive aerosols using special nebulizer adaptors.

Specific References

Butler SP, Alderson PO, Greenspan RL, et al, "The Utility of Technetium-99m DTPA Inhalational Scans in Artificially Ventilated Patients," *J Nucl Med*, 1990, 31(1):46-51.

Kahn D, Bushnell DL, Dean R, et al, "Clinical Outcome of Patients With a "Low Probability" of Pulmonary Embolism on Ventilation-Perfusion Lung Scan," *Arch Intern Med*, 1989, 149(2):377-9.

PIOPED Investigators, "Value of the Ventilation/Perfusion Scan in Acute Pulmonary Embolism. Results of the Prospective Investigation of Pulmonary Embolism Diagnosis (PIOPED)," *JAMA*, 1990, 263(20):2753-9.

Lyogen® *see* Fluphenazine, Blood *on page 1268*

Lysergic Acid Diethylamine Level

Synonyms LSD

Specimen Blood or urine

Volume 10 mL blood, 10 mL urine

Container Royal blue top tube, plastic urine container

Reference Range None detected

Use Evaluate LSD toxicity; confirm suspected overdose or abuse

Methodology Gas chromatography/mass spectrometry (GC/MS)

Additional Information Lysergic acid diethylamine, LSD, is a synthetic hallucinogen that acts on multiple sites in the CNS. Ingestion of this drug may result in sensory distortions, hallucinations, delusions, euphoria or dysphoria, dizziness, and paresthesia. Prolonged use may lead to psychological dependence and significant hazards such as panic, serious depression, paranoid behavior, and a persistent psychotic state.

Specific References

McCarron MM, Walberg CB, and Baselt RC, "Confirmation of LSD Intoxication by Analysis of Serum and Urine," *J Anal Toxicol*, 1990, 14(3):165-7.

Lim HK, Andrenyak D, Francom P, et al, "Quantification of LSD and N-Demethyl LSD in Urine by Gas Chromatography/Resonance Electron Capture Ionization Mass Spectrometry," *Anal Chem*, 1988, 60(14):1420-5.

Papac DI and Foltz RL, "Measurement of Lysergic Acid Diethylamide (LSD) in Human Plasma by Gas Chromatography/Negative Ion Chemical Ionization Mass Spectrometry," *J Anal Toxicol*, 1990, 14(3):189-90.

Magnesium, Serum

Synonyms Mg, Serum

Abstract Magnesium is one of the major inorganic cations; the others are sodium, potassium, and calcium. Intracellular magnesium concentrations are much higher than extracellular (serum) values. Most intracellular magnesium is complexed.

Specimen Blood

Volume 7 mL

Minimum Volume 2 mL serum

Container Red top tube

Collection Draw without venous stasis, separate serum from red cells as soon as possible.

Storage Instructions Refrigerate. Serum separated from cells is stable at 2°C to 6°C for several days.

Causes for Rejection Hemolysis

Reference Range 1.5-2.8 mg/dL (SI: 0.6-1.1 mmol/L or 1.2-2.3 mEq/L), not consistent among published papers, laboratories, and geographic areas. Four sets of units are in use to express concentration of magnesium: 1.0 mEq/L = 1.22 mg/dL = 0.5 mmol/L = 12.2 mg/L. Magnesium, like calcium, is partly protein bound. Slightly low values in the presence of hypoalbuminemia or hypoproteinemia should not, therefore, be of major concern.

Critical Values In patients with acute myocardial infarct, serum magnesium <2.0 mg/dL (SI: <0.82 mmol/L) may increase the risk of ventricular arrhythmia in the presence of hypokalemia.

Possible Panic Range Symptoms appear at <1.2 mg/dL (SI: <0.5 mmol/L); <1.2 mg/dL is severe depletion. Slightly low levels should be repeated on a new speci-

(Continued)

Magnesium, Serum *(Continued)*

men. Hospital diet often improves magnesium levels, especially in those who have not been on a normal diet. Toxic symptoms appear >4.9 mg/dL (SI: >2.0 mmol/L). Possible death from respiratory failure >14.6 mg/dL (SI: >6.0 mmol/L).

Use **Magnesium deficiency** produces neuromuscular disorders. It may cause weakness, tremors, tetany, and convulsions. **Hypomagnesemia** is associated with hypocalcemia, hypokalemia, long-term hyperalimentation, intravenous therapy, diabetes mellitus, especially during treatment of ketoacidosis; alcoholism and other types of malnutrition; malabsorption; hyperparathyroidism; dialysis; pregnancy; and hyperaldosteronism. Renal loss of magnesium occurs with cisplatinum therapy. Alfrey also adds amphotericin toxicity to the causes of hypomagnesemia.

Magnesium deficiency is described with cardiac arrhythmias. The concept that magnesium deficiency may cause arrhythmias is repeatedly expressed.

Increased magnesium levels relate mostly to patients in renal failure. Marked increases may be found in such patients who take magnesium salts (eg, as antacids which contain magnesium). Increased serum magnesium is also found with Addison's disease and in pregnant patients with severe pre-eclampsia or eclampsia who are receiving magnesium sulfate as an anticonvulsant. Hypermagnesemia may occur in patients using magnesium-containing cathartics. High magnesium levels are manifested by decreased reflexes, somnolence, and heart block.

Indications for measurement of serum magnesium include the presence of unexplained hypocalcemia, instances in which hypokalemia is unresponsive to potassium supplementation, and in patients who have cardiac disorders in which hypomagnesemia may be especially hazardous such as congestive failure, ventricular ectopy, digitalis use, or left ventricular hypertrophy. Serum magnesium is indicated only selectively in patients on diuretics: those on high dose thiazides, loop diuretics or hydrochlorothiazide in doses >50 mg/day.

Because an association between aminoglycoside therapy and severe hypomagnesemia is described, a recommendation is published to measure serum magnesium in subjects receiving aminoglycosides. Recommendations also exist to measure it in patients on cyclosporine.

Limitations Hemolysis will yield elevated results as levels in erythrocytes are two to three times higher than serum. Bilirubin and calcium salts may cause falsely low values.

Methodology Spectrophotometry using calmagite dye, methylthymol blue; atomic absorption spectrophotometry. These methods were found to correlate, although a slight bias to higher values was reported with the Du Pont aca®, for levels >2.4 mg/dL (SI: >1.0 mmol/L).

Additional Information Parathormone enhances tubular reabsorption of magnesium. Measure magnesium in patients with hypocalcemia, of whom 23%, without renal failure, were found in one study to have hypomagnesemia. Magnesium-containing drugs can cause toxic levels in patients with impaired renal function. A causal relation between decreased magnesium content of cardiac muscle/coronary arteries and nonocclusive sudden-death ischemic heart disease has been proposed. Serum magnesium constitutes only a small fraction of total body stores and may not predict magnesium status correctly. Magnesium acts as a metallic cofactor in over 300 enzymatic reactions. A positive correlation between normomagnesemia and successful resuscitation is reported. Serum magnesium has prognostic importance in congestive heart failure.

Specific References

Castelbaum AR, Donofrio PD, Walker FO, et al, "Laxative Abuse Causing Hypermagnesemia, Quadriparesis, and Neuromuscular Junction Defect," *Neurology*, 1989, 39(5):746-7.

Farrell EC Jr, "Magnesium," *Clinical Chemistry – Theory, Analysis, and Correlation*, 2nd ed, Kaplan LA and Pesce AJ, eds, St Louis, MO: Mosby-Year Book Inc, 1989, 875-9.

Gottlieb SS, "Importance of Magnesium in Congestive Heart Failure," *Am J Cardiol*, 1989, 63(14):39G-42G, (review).

Gren J and Woolf A, "Hypermagnesemia Associated With Catharsis in a Salicylate-Intoxicated Patient With Anorexia Nervosa," *Ann Emerg Med*, 1989, 18(2):200-3.

Lum G, "Hypomagnesemia in Acute and Chronic Care Patient Populations," *Am J Clin Pathol*, 1992, 97(6):827-30.

Quamme GA, "Laboratory Evaluation of Magnesium Status: Renal Function and Free Intracellular Magnesium Concentration," *Clin Lab Med*, 1993, 13(1):209-23.

Ryan MF, "The Role of Magnesium in Clinical Biochemistry: An Overview," *Ann Clin Biochem*, 1991, 28(Pt 1):19-26.

Sipes SL, Weiner CP, Gellhaus TM, et al, "The Plasma Renin-Angiotensin System in Preeclampsia: Effects of Magnesium Sulfate," *Obstet Gynecol*, 1989, 73(6):934-7.

Weber CA and Santiago RM, "Hypermagnesemia. A Potential Complication During Treatment of Theophylline Intoxication With Oral Activated Charcoal and Magnesium-Containing Cathartics," *Chest*, 1989, 95(1):56-9.

Majsolin® *see* Primidone, Blood *on page 1332*

Marijuana *see* Cannabinoids, Qualitative *on page 1217*

MDMA *see* Methamphetamines, Urine *on page 1294*

Mebaral® *see* Mephobarbital, Blood *on this page*

Meconium Drug Screen

Synonyms Drug Screen, Meconium

Specimen 1 g first meconium

Container Small plastic vial with cap

Collection Sample must be first specimen, second accepted but less desirable

Storage Instructions Refrigerate

Causes for Rejection Specimen later than the second meconium, specimen mixed with stool

Use Drugs of abuse screen (amphetamines, opiates, cocaine, marijuana, phencyclidine)

Methodology Fluorescent polarization immunoassay (FPIA) confirmed by gas chromatography/mass spectrometry (GC/MS) is most effective assay method.

Additional Information Can detect maternal drug usage during the final 20 weeks of gestation. May detect three times higher rate of drugs of abuse then maternal urinary screening at time of birth. Cocaethylene can also be detected.

Specific References

Dusick AM, Covert RF, Schreiber MD, et al, "Risk of Intracranial Hemorrhage and Other Adverse Outcomes After Cocaine Exposure in a Cohort of 323 Very Low Birth Weight Babies," *J Pediatr*, 1993, 122(3):438-45.

Murphey LJ, Olsen GD, and Konkol RJ, "Quantitation of Benzoylnorecgonine and Other Cocaine Metabolites in Meconium by High Performance Liquid Chromatography," *J Chromatogr*, 1993, 613(2):330-5.

Ostrea EM Jr, Brady MJ, Parks PM, et al, "Drug Screening of Meconium in Infants of Drug-Dependent Mothers: An Alternative to Urine Testing," *J Pediatr*, 1989, 115(3):474-7.

Schutzman DL, Frankenfield-Chernicoff M, Clatterbaugh HE, et al, "Incidence of Intrauterine Cocaine Exposure in a Suburban Setting," *Pediatrics*, 1991, 88(4):825-7.

Medical Legal Specimens *see* Chain-of-Custody Protocol *on page 1223*

MEGX *see* Lidocaine, Blood *on page 1284*

Mellaril® *see* Thioridazine, Quantitative *on page 1360*

Mephobarbital, Blood

Related Information

Barbiturates, Quantitative, Blood *on page 1201*

Synonyms Mebaral®

Specimen Blood

Volume 7 mL

Minimum Volume 3 mL serum

Container Red top tube

Collection Collect specimen immediately prior to next dose unless specified otherwise.

Storage Instructions Separate serum and refrigerate.

Reference Range Mephobarbital: therapeutic: 8-15 mg/L; phenobarbital metabolite: therapeutic: 10-30 mg/L; total: therapeutic: 15-40 mg/L; notification level: >50 mg/L

Use Monitor therapeutic drug level; evaluate toxicity

Limitations Mephobarbital is not measured; instead, its metabolite phenobarbital is quantitated

Additional Information Mephobarbital is an anticonvulsant used in prophylactic management of grand mal and petit mal epilepsy in those patients who must discontinue phenobarbital due to side effects. It is also useful for the management of anxiety states, delirium tremens, and acute agitation due to its sedative effect. The half-life of mephobarbital is 34 hours. Approximately 75% is metabolized to phenobarbital in the liver within 24 hours. Toxic effects include CNS and respiratory depression, hypothermia, tachycardia, and renal failure.

Mephobarbital, Urine *see* Barbiturates, Qualitative, Urine *on page 1200*

Meprobamate, Blood

Synonyms Equagesic®; Equanil®; Meprospan®; Miltown®

Abstract Meprobamate is a sedative-anxiolytic producing effects similar to the benzodiazepines and barbiturates.

Specimen Blood

Volume 5 mL

Container Red top tube

Reference Range Sedative dose: 8-24 μg/mL (SI: 37-110 μmol/L)

(Continued)

Meprobamate, Blood *(Continued)*

Possible Panic Range Toxic: >50 μg/mL (SI: >229 μmol/L); lethal: 200 μg/mL (SI: 916 μmol/L)

Use Therapeutic monitoring; toxicity assessment

Methodology Gas-liquid chromatography (GLC)

Additional Information Meprobamate is a propanediol carbamate sedative and tranquilizer, having pharmacological effects similar to barbiturates. It is well absorbed from the gastrointestinal tract and reaches its peak concentration in 2-3 hours. Its half-life is 6-15 hours. Respiratory depression, coma, and cardiovascular collapse characterize overdosage. It may also be detected in urine or gastric juice.

Specific References

Bertino JS Jr and Reed MD, "Barbiturate and Nonbarbiturate Sedative Hypnotic Intoxication in Children," *Pediatr Clin North Am*, 1986, 33(3):703-22.

Dennison J, Edwards JN, and Volans GN, "Meprobamate Overdosage," *Hum Toxicol*, 1985, 4(2):215-7.

Meprospan® *see* Meprobamate, Blood *on previous page*

Mercury Analysis, Hair *see* Mercury, Blood *on this page*

Mercury, Blood

Related Information

Heavy Metal Screen, Blood *on page 1271*

Mercury, Urine *on this page*

Synonyms Hg, Blood

Applies To Mercury Analysis, Hair

Abstract This metal is toxic in any of its three forms: elemental, inorganic, and organic. The mode of entry into the body varies among the three forms.

Specimen Whole blood

Volume 7 mL

Container Special metal-free EDTA tube

Special Instructions Whole blood is analyzed.

Reference Range 0.020-0.080 μg/mL (SI: 0.10-0.80 μmol/L)

Possible Panic Range >0.10 μg/mL

Use Evaluate for mercury toxicity, neurological findings related to organic mercurials, inhalation of mercury vapors

Limitations Methyl mercury must be measured in whole blood or erythrocytes.

Methodology Electrothermal atomic absorption (AA), gold electrode deposition, gas chromatography (GC)

Additional Information Organic methyl mercury is a new important environmental mercurial contaminant. It was discovered that inorganic mercurial industrial wastes dumped into Minimata Bay (Japan) could be organified by plankton and incorporated into fish, and thus, the human food chain. Ingestion of mercury-laden fish leads to severe neurologic deficits. Inhalation of mercury vapors can lead to pneumonitis. Inorganic mercurials deposit in kidneys, liver, heart, striated muscle, marrow, brain, and lungs. Gastrointestinal symptoms, stomatitis, colitis, anemia, and peripheral neuritis can relate to mercury poisoning. Ingestion of inorganic mercurials results in a serious medical emergency. Mercury exposure from a brand of interior latex paint was recently described. Half-life of inorganic mercury is 24 days and of methyl mercury (organic mercury) is 54 days. Hair analysis can be used for poisoning or exposure. It should be clean and clipped as close to the scalp as possible. Mercurial salts can cause renal failure.

Specific References

Bryson PD, *Comprehensive Review in Toxicology*, 2nd ed, Rockville, MD: Aspen Publishers Inc, 1989, 477-86.

Snapp KR, Boyer DB, Peterson LC, et al, "The Contribution of Dental Amalgam to Mercury in Blood," *J Dent Res*, 1989, 68(5):780-5.

Mercury, Urine

Related Information

Heavy Metal Screen, Urine *on page 1272*

Mercury, Blood *on this page*

Synonyms Hg, Urine

Abstract This metal is toxic in elemental, inorganic, and organic forms. Urine mercury is used for evaluation of inorganic and possibly elemental forms.

Specimen 24-hour urine

Volume Entire collection

Minimum Volume 50 mL aliquot

Container Plastic (preferably polyethylene) acid-washed container, no preservative

Storage Instructions Store in special metal-free container

Reference Range 10-50 μg/24 hours (SI: 0.05-0.25 μmol/day)

Possible Panic Range >100 μg/24 hours (SI: >0.50 μmol/day)

Use Inorganic mercury toxicity is best evaluated by urine mercury levels.

Limitations Organic mercury is found mostly in red cells; see Mercury, Blood listing. Urine mercury would not be useful for organic mercury poisoning.

Methodology Electrothermal atomic absorption (AA), gold electrode deposition, gas chromatography (GC)

Additional Information Industrial and agricultural exposure includes inhalation of vapor and ingestion.

Specific References

Bryson PD, *Comprehensive Review in Toxicology*, 2nd ed, Rockville, MD: Aspen Publishers Inc, 1989, 477-86.

Gothe CJ, Langworth S, Carleson R, et al, "Biological Monitoring of Exposure to Metallic Mercury," *J Toxicol Clin Toxicol*, 1985, 23(4-6):381-9.

Piikivi L and Ruokonen A, "Renal Function and Long-Term Low Mercury Vapor Exposure," *Arch Environ Health*, 1989, 44(3):146-9.

Metabolites of Primidone *see* Primidone, Blood *on page 1332*

Metals, Blood *see* Heavy Metal Screen, Blood *on page 1271*

Metal Screen *see* Heavy Metal Screen, Urine *on page 1272*

Metals, Toxic *see* Heavy Metal Screen, Urine *on page 1272*

Methadone, Quantitative, Serum

Synonyms Dolophine®; Phenadone, Serum

Specimen Blood

Volume 10 mL

Minimum Volume 3 mL serum

Container Red top tube

Storage Instructions Refrigerate serum.

Reference Range For narcotic stabilization: 0.3-1.0 μg/mL

Possible Panic Range 1.0-2.0 μg/mL; >2.0 μg/mL is lethal

Use Monitor patient compliance; evaluate toxicity

Additional Information Methadone is a synthetic diphenylheptanone derivative. It produces less sedation and euphoria than morphine and its effects are cumulative. Methadone is highly addictive, but the withdrawal symptoms are less intense. This drug is used in the management of severe pain and in narcotic detoxification maintenance programs. Onset of action is 30-60 minutes after oral dose and 10-20 minutes following parenteral administration. The half-life is 15-25 hours. Adverse effects include marked sedation after repeated administration, CNS and respiratory depression, nausea and vomiting, bradycardia, hypotension, increased intracranial pressure, miosis, antidiuretic hormone release, and physical and psychological dependence.

Methadone, Urine

Synonyms Dolophine®

Abstract This drug is a synthetic opiate agonist used during World War II as a morphine substitute. It is used for detoxification of opiate addicts. It is a drug of abuse.

Specimen Urine

Volume 50 mL

Minimum Volume 20 mL

Container Plastic urine container

Storage Instructions Refrigerate

Special Instructions If forensic, use chain-of-custody protocol and form.

Reference Range Negative (less than cutoff); when used therapeutically for pain, plasma levels are in the range of 0.05-0.10 μg/mL

Critical Values Cutoff for screening: 0.30 μg/mL; confirmation: 0.20 μg/mL

Use Evaluate toxicity; detect drugs of abuse

Methodology Thin-layer chromatography (TLC) and enzyme immunoassay (EIA) for screening; gas chromatography/mass spectrometry (GC/MS) for confirmation

Additional Information Methadone is a synthetic diphenylheptane derivative. It produces less sedation and euphoria than morphine and its effects are cumulative. Methadone is highly addictive, but the withdrawal symptoms are less intense. This drug is used in the management of severe pain and in narcotic detoxification maintenance programs. Onset of action is 30-60 minutes after oral dose and 10-20 minutes following parenteral administration. The half-life is 15-25 hours. Adverse effects include marked sedation after repeated administration, CNS and respiratory depression, nausea and vomiting, bradycardia, hypotension, increased intracranial pressure, miosis, antidiuretic hormone release, and physical and psychological dependence. Methadone is a drug of abuse and is included in most drug-of-abuse screening panels. Patients on methadone maintenance protocols will test above cutoff in urine drug screens.

Specific References

Baselt RC and Cravey RH, *Disposition of Toxic Drugs and Chemicals in Man*, 3rd ed, Chicago, IL: Year Book Medical Publishers Inc, 1989, 512-5.

(Continued)

Methadone, Urine *(Continued)*

Bryson PD, *Comprehensive Review in Toxicology*, 2nd ed, Rockville, MD: Aspen Publishers Inc, 1989, 329.
Calsyn DA, Saxon AJ, and Barndt DC, "Urine Screening Practices in Methadone Maintenance Clinics. A Survey of How the Results Are Used," *J Nerv Ment Dis*, 1991, 179(4):222-7.
Wolff K, Hay AW, and Raistrick D, "Plasma Methadone Measurements and Their Role in Methadone Detoxification Programs," *Clin Chem*, 1992, 38(3):420-5.
Wolff K, Sanderson M, Hay AW, et al, "Methadone Concentrations in Plasma and Their Relationship to Drug Dosage," *Clin Chem*, 1991, 37(2):205-9.

Methamphetamines, Serum

Synonyms Desoxyn®
Specimen Blood
Volume 20 mL
Minimum Volume 5 mL serum
Container Red top tube
Storage Instructions Refrigerate
Reference Range Therapeutic: 20-30 ng/mL
Use Evaluate toxicity; detect abuse
Methodology Gas-liquid chromatography (GLC)
Additional Information Methamphetamine is sympathomimetic amine chemically related to ephedrine and amphetamine. It is used in the management of obesity, to treat certain depressive reactions, and as adjunctive therapy for narcolepsy, epilepsy, attention deficit disorders, and postencephalitic parkinsonism. Methamphetamine is readily absorbed by the GI tract and the effects last from 6-12 hours. Adverse effects include tremor, insomnia, nervousness, anxiety, euphoria or dysphoria, hyper- or hypotension, arrhythmias, circulatory collapse, and nausea and vomiting.

Methamphetamines, Urine

Related Information
Amphetamines, Qualitative, Urine *on page 1190*
Synonyms Crystal; Desoxyn®; Doe; Methedrine®; Speed
Applies To Chlorpromazine; d-Methamphetamine; l-Methamphetamine; MDMA; Methylenedioxymethamphetamine; Phentermine; Phenylpropanolamine; Pseudoephedrine; Ranitidine
Test Includes Amphetamine
Abstract The D-isomer of this drug is used therapeutically as an anorectic agent and for treatment of hyperactive children. It is also a drug of abuse.
Specimen Random urine
Volume 50 mL
Minimum Volume 5 mL
Container Plastic urine container
Collection If forensic, observe precautions.
Storage Instructions Refrigerate
Causes for Rejection If forensic, failure to meet temperature check and reasonable urine creatinine concentration
Special Instructions If forensic, use chain-of-custody protocol and form.
Reference Range Negative (less than cutoff)
Critical Values Cutoff: screen: 1000 ng/mL; confirmation: 500 ng/mL
Use Evaluate for drug abuse; assess toxicity
Limitations Screening test may give false-positives with common cold and antiallergy medications. Qualitative results only (positive or negative). A labetalol metabolite (3-amino-1-phenylbutane or APB) may cause a false-positive result with amphetamine/methamphetamine by thin-layer chromatography or immunoassay.
Methodology Screening: enzyme immunoassay (EIA), fluorescence polarization immunoassay (FPIA), thin-layer chromatography (TLC); confirmation: gas chromatography/mass spectrometry (GC/MS), gas-liquid chromatography (GLC), high performance liquid chromatography (HPLC)
Additional Information The most abused drug in this class is d-methamphetamine. The optical isomer, L-methamphetamine, has less pronounced central effects and is used as a nasal decongestant in Vicks Inhaler® (legal, over-the-counter). Amphetamine isomers are present in Dexedrine® and Benzedrine®. These drugs are self-administered orally, I.V., or by smoking. Half-life is 10-20 hours and it can be detected in urine within 3 hours of use. The parent drugs are the substances detected by the screening tests. Over-the-counter medication for colds and allergies (Contac®, Dimetapp®, Sine-Off®, Sudafed®) contain phenylpropanolamine or pseudoephedrine which give a positive EIA screening test when the polyclonal antibody is used. This antibody also detects methylenedioxymethamphetamine (MDMA), a controlled substance classed as an hallucinogen and "designer" drug. With the monoclonal EIA test, the above medications are not detected, but phentermine (Adipex®, Fastin®), ranitidine (Zantac®), and chlor-

promazine (Thorazine®) give a positive test. Confirmation by GC/MS rules out these false-positives. In order to rule out the false-positive given by L-methamphetamine (legal nasal decongestant), a chiral column or procedure, which separates the "L" and "D" isomers, must be used in the GC/MS confirmation. Famprofazone (which metabolizes to methamphetamine and amphetamine) can give a positive immunoassay and GC/MS assay for methamphetamine for up to 56 hours.

Methamphetamine is a sympathomimetic amine chemically related to ephedrine and amphetamine. It is used in the management of obesity, to treat certain depressive reactions, and as adjunctive therapy for narcolepsy, epilepsy, attention deficit disorders, and postencephalitic parkinsonism. Methamphetamine is readily absorbed by the GI tract and the effects last from 6-12 hours. Adverse effects include tremor, insomnia, nervousness, anxiety, euphoria or dysphoria, hyper- or hypotension, arrhythmias, circulatory collapse, and nausea and vomiting.

Specific References

Baselt RC and Cravey RH, *Disposition of Toxic Drugs and Chemicals in Man*, 3rd ed, Chicago, IL: Year Book Medical Publishers Inc, 1989, 516-9.

Bryson PD, *Comprehensive Review in Toxicology*, 2nd ed, Rockville, MD: Aspen Publishers Inc, 1989, 369-79.

DePace A, Verebey K, and elSohly M, "Capillary Gas-Liquid Chromatography Separation of Phenethylamines in Amphetamine-Positive Urine Samples," *J Forensic Sci*, 1990, 35(6):1431-5.

Derlet RW and Heischober B, "Methamphetamine. Stimulant of the 1990s?" *West J Med*, 1990, 153(6):625-8.

Ellenhorn MJ and Barceloux DG, "Amphetamines," *Medical Toxicology*, New York, NY: Elsevier, 1988, 625-42.

Gan BK, Baugh D, Liu RH, et al, "Simultaneous Analysis of Amphetamine, Methamphetamine, and 3,4-Methylenedioxymethamphetamine (MDMA) in Urine Samples by Solid-Phase Extraction, Derivatization, and Gas Chromatography/Mass Spectrometry," *J Forensic Sci*, 1991, 36(5):1331-41.

Gibert RB, Peng PI, and Wong D, "A Labetalol Metabolite With Analytical Characteristics Resembling Amphetamines," *J Anal Toxicol*, 1995, 19:84-6.

Grinstead GF, "Ranitidine and High Concentrations of Phenylpropanolamine Cross React in the EMIT Monoclonal Amphetamine/Methamphetamine Assay," *Clin Chem*, 1989, 35(9):1998-9.

Poklis A and Moore KA, "Stereoselectivity of the TDxADx/FLx Amphetamine/Methamphetamine II Amphetamine/Methamphetamine Immunoassay-Response of Urine Specimens Following Nasal Inhaler Use," *J Toxicol Clin Toxicol*, 1995, 33(1):35-41.

Sukbuntherng J, Hutchaleelaha A, Chow H-H, et al, "Separation and Quantitation of the Enantiomers of Methamphetamine and Its Metabolites in Urine by HPLC: Precolumn Derivatization and Fluorescence Detection," *J Anal Toxicol*, 1995, 19:139-47.

Yoo Y, Chung H, and Choi H, "Urinary Methamphetamine Concentration Following Famprofazone Administration," *J Anal Toxicol*, 1994, 18(5):265-8.

Methanol, Blood

Related Information

Volatile Screen *on page 1378*

Synonyms Methyl Alcohol; Wood Alcohol

Specimen Blood

Volume 14 mL

Minimum Volume 5 mL serum or plasma

Container Red top tube or gray top (sodium fluoride) tube

Collection Routine venipuncture

Special Instructions Note if methanol ingested.

Reference Range Normal: <0.005%

Critical Values Toxic: >0.02%; lethal: >0.04%

Use Determine methanol toxicity

Methodology Gas-liquid chromatography (GLC)

Additional Information Methanol is oxidized by liver alcohol dehydrogenase at about one-tenth the rate of ethanol. The highly toxic formaldehyde that is formed does not accumulate, but is oxidized to formic acid, which is 6 times more toxic than methanol and which is primarily responsible for the severe metabolic acidosis and ocular toxicity of methanol. The initial narcotic effects of methanol are much milder than those of ethanol, and the characteristic toxic syndrome may not appear until 6-30 hours after ingestion. The clinical effects of methanol ingestion include convulsions, coma, drunkenness without alcohol on the breath, and blindness. Treatment may include administration of ethanol to inhibit methanol metabolism, administration of folate to induce formic acid intoxication and hemodialysis for the removal of methanol and formic acid. A blood methanol concentration of 40 mg/dL is believed to be a minimum lethal level in individuals receiving no medical treatment.

Methaqualone Level

Synonyms Lude®

Abstract This drug is a sedative-hypnotic but is currently a DEA schedule II drug. It is a drug of abuse.

Specimen Blood, urine

Volume 5 mL

(Continued)

Methaqualone Level *(Continued)*

Container Red top tube, plastic urine container

Special Instructions If forensic, use chain-of-custody protocol and form.

Reference Range Urine: negative (less than cutoff); serum: 1-5 μg/mL (SI: 4-20 nmol/L)

Critical Values Cutoff for urine: screen: 300 ng/mL; confirmation: 200 ng/mL

Possible Panic Range Serum values >8 μg/mL (SI: >32 nmol/L) associated with unconsciousness; toxic: >10 μg/mL (SI: >40 nmol/L)

Use Evaluate for toxicity; evaluate for drug abuse

Methodology Immunoassay, gas-liquid chromatography (GLC), UV spectrophotometry, fluorometry

Additional Information Methaqualone is a nonbarbiturate sedative-hypnotic. It is rapidly absorbed from the GI tract. Hyperexcitability, coma, and cardiovascular and respiratory depression characterize overdosage. It is a common drug of abuse, and "street" preparations may be adulterated with other pharmacoactive substances. Half-life is 20-60 hours. It is extensively metabolized and screening methods must detect metabolites. Enzyme-multiplied immunoassay technique (EMIT) detects four of the most common metabolites.

Specific References

Baselt RC and Cravey RH, *Disposition of Toxic Drugs and Chemicals in Man*, 3rd ed, Chicago, IL: Year Book Medical Publishers Inc, 1989, 524-7.

Beebe DK and Walley E, "Substance Abuse: The Designer Drugs," *Am Fam Physician*, 1991, 43(5):1689-98.

Buckner JC and Mandell W, "Risk Factors for Depressive Symptomatology in a Drug Using Population," *Am J Public Health*, 1990, 80(5):580-5.

Metharbital, Quantitative

Related Information

Barbiturates, Quantitative, Blood *on page 1201*

Synonyms Gemonil®; Metharbitone

Specimen Blood

Volume 10 mL

Minimum Volume 3 mL serum

Container Red top tube

Collection Collect specimen immediately prior to next dose unless specified otherwise.

Storage Instructions Separate serum and refrigerate.

Reference Range Therapeutic: 5-10 μg/mL

Possible Panic Range Lethal dose: 2 g

Use Monitor therapeutic drug level; evaluate toxicity

Methodology High performance liquid chromatography (HPLC), gas chromatography/mass spectrometry (GC/MS)

Additional Information Metharbital is a long-acting barbiturate. The sedative effect is greater than that of phenobarbital, but the anticonvulsant activity is less. The onset of effects is 2-4 hours and they last 6-12 hours. Toxic effects are rare and mild, including dizziness, drowsiness, and increased irritability. Metabolizes to barbitone (~10%).

Metharbitone *see* Metharbital, Quantitative *on this page*

MetHb *see* Methemoglobin, Blood *on this page*

Methedrine® *see* Methamphetamines, Urine *on page 1294*

Methemoglobin, Blood

Synonyms MetHb; NADH-MetHb Reductase

Applies To Cytochrome b_5 Reductase

Abstract This pigment is hemoglobin in which the iron is in the trivalent state. It cannot act as an oxygen carrier.

Specimen Blood

Volume 5 mL

Minimum Volume 1 mL whole blood

Container Green top (heparin) tube

Storage Instructions Keep tube on ice. pH dependent. Should be run within 8 hours, or false-negatives may occur. Run as promptly as possible after draw. Studies have shown up to 10% drop in 4 hours, up to 16% drop in 8 hours, in samples kept on ice. Such studies have not been extensive. May be drawn into sodium fluoride-containing tubes and immediately frozen at 0°C to -4°C prior to analysis.

Reference Range Up to 1.5% of total hemoglobin. Smokers have a slightly higher percent methemoglobin than do nonsmokers.

Possible Panic Range Headache and other symptoms occur at levels >30%. Methemoglobinemia can be fatal, particularly >70% saturation levels.

Use Evaluate cyanosis, especially in the presence of normal arterial gases; evaluate polycythemia and hemoglobinopathies; work up dyspnea and headache; work up "poppers" and "sniffers"; evaluate drug or chemical toxicity, since most instances of methemoglobinemia are so acquired; monitor patients on high dose nitrate therapy; measurement in CSF may detect small cerebral and subdural hematomas.

Limitations Sulfhemoglobin, methylene blue, and Evans blue dye may interfere. Methemoglobin exhibits pH sensitivity.

Methodology Spectrophotometry; Hb M variants are best detected by electrophoresis because spectrophotometry is unreliable due to their abnormal ferrihemoglobin spectra.

Additional Information Methemoglobin is an inactive, oxidized form of hemoglobin resulting in decreased oxygen-carrying capacity of blood. Concentrations of methemoglobin of over 10% to 15% of hemoglobin will cause cyanosis. Sulfhemoglobin will interfere with methemoglobin determined by the above method. Methemoglobinemia may be hereditary or acquired. Polycythemia is occasionally present as a compensatory mechanism. Elevations of methemoglobin lead to dyspnea and headache, and can be lethal. Most instances of methemoglobinemia are acquired, from drugs and chemicals. Nitro and amino groups are especially involved, eg, aniline and derivatives, nitrites, nitroglycerin, nitrate salts in burn patients, dapsone (perhaps the most common cause of drug-induced methemoglobinemia), acetophenetidin, phenacetin and some sulfonamides, chlorates, quinones, large doses of ferrous sulfate, and many other drugs and some intestinal bacteria. Well water containing nitrate is the most common cause of methemoglobinemia in the newborn. Methemoglobinemia has been reported after exposure to automobile exhaust fumes.

Hereditary methemoglobinemia is uncommon. It may be due to a deficiency of red cell NADH-methemoglobin reductase (diaphorase, also termed cytochrome b_5 reductase), which has an autosomal recessive mode of inheritance. It may also be the result of presence of certain hemoglobinopathies, members of the Hb M family including Hb M Saskatoon, Boston, Iwate, Hyde Park, and Milwaukee. These have autosomal dominant mode of inheritance and may be associated with clinical cyanosis. Hb Seattle and other hemoglobinopathies also show increase in the *in vitro* rate of methemoglobin formation. A recently identified new hemoglobin variant, Hb Warsaw, is also characterized by elevated blood levels of methemoglobin.

A study of postmortem methemoglobin levels showed a range of 0.8% to 57% in individuals who, clinically, should have had normal antemortem concentrations. There was no correlation with antemortem circumstances, autopsy findings, or interval of time from death to autopsy.

Specific References

Beutler E and Gelbart T, "Carboxyhemoglobin, Methemoglobin, and Sulfhemoglobin Determinations," *Hematology*, 4th ed, Chapter A16, Williams WT, Beutler E, Erslev AJ, et al, eds, New York, NY: McGraw-Hill Inc, 1990, 1732-4.

Dean BS, Lopez G, and Krenzelok EP, "Environmentally-Induced Methemoglobinemia in an Infant," *J Toxicol Clin Toxicol*, 1992, 30(1):127-33.

Fechner GG and Gee DJ, "Study on the Effects of Heat on Blood and on the Postmortem Estimation of Carboxyhemoglobin and Methaemoglobin," *Forensic Sci Int*, 1989, 40(1):63-7.

Jaffé ER and Hultquist DE, "Cytochrome b_5 Reductase Deficiency and Enzymopenic Hereditary Methemoglobinemia," Chapter 92, *The Metabolic Basis of Inherited Disease*, 6th ed, Scriver CR, Beaudet AL, Sly WS, et al, eds, New York, NY: McGraw-Hill Inc, 1989, 2267-80.

Johnson WS, Hall AH, and Rumack BH, "Cyanide Poisoning Successfully Treated Without Therapeutic Methemoglobin Levels," *Am J Emerg Med*, 1989, 7(4):437-40.

Weatherall DJ, Clegg JB, Higgs DR, et al, "The Hemoglobinopathies," Chapter 93, *The Metabolic Basis of Inherited Disease*, 6th ed, Scriver CR, Beaudet AL, Sly WS, et al, eds, New York, NY: McGraw-Hill Inc, 1989, 2304-5.

Methotrexate, Blood

Synonyms Mexate®; MTX, Blood

Applies To Cerebrospinal Fluid Methotrexate; Methotrexate, CSF

Abstract This is a widely used anticancer drug acting as an antimetabolite in DNA synthesis. It must be monitored.

Specimen Blood

Volume 7 mL

Minimum Volume 2 mL serum or plasma

Container Red top tube, green top (heparin) tube, or lavender top (EDTA) tube

Sampling Time Will vary according to dosing protocol

Storage Instructions Separate and freeze

Special Instructions Advise laboratory if patient is also on trimethoprim.

Reference Range Therapeutic range is dependent upon therapeutic approach. "High dose" regimens produce drug levels between 10^{-6} M and 10^{-7} M 24-72 hours after drug infusion.

Possible Panic Range >2.27 μg/mL (SI: >5 μmol/L) 24 hours after high dose therapy

(Continued)

Methotrexate, Blood *(Continued)*

Use Monitor therapeutic drug level of methotrexate; evaluate potential toxicity

Methodology Enzyme immunoassay (EIA), radioimmunoassay (RIA), high performance liquid chromatography (HPLC)

Additional Information Methotrexate is an antimetabolite that combines with dihydrofolate reductase and therefore interferes with the synthesis of tetrahydrofolic acid necessary for DNA synthesis. From 40% to 50% of a small dose and up to 90% of a larger dose is excreted unchanged in the urine in 48 hours, a major portion of it during the first 8 hours. Toxicity consists of bone marrow depression with megaloblastosis. Concomitant salicylate administration increases incidence of toxicity, due to diminished renal tubular excretion. The effect of methotrexate on normal cells may be reversed by administration of 5-formyltetrahydrofolate, also called citrovorum factor or leucovorin. This "rescue" makes possible administration of much higher doses of methotrexate than the body would otherwise survive. The initial half-life is 2-4 hours but the total body clearance (terminal) half-life is 8-15 hours.

Specific References

Brooks PJ, Spruill WJ, Parish RC, et al, "Pharmacokinetics of Methotrexate Administered by Intramuscular and Subcutaneous Injections in Patients With Rheumatoid Arthritis," *Arthritis Rheum*, 1990, 33(1):91-4.

Fossa SD, Heilo A, and Bormer O, "Unexpectedly High Serum Methotrexate Levels in Cystectomized Bladder Cancer Patients With an Ileal Conduit Treated With Intermediate Doses of the Drug," *J Urol*, 1990, 143(3):498-501.

Moore MJ and Erlichman C, "Therapeutic Drug Monitoring in Oncology. Problems and Potential in Antineoplastic Therapy," *Clin Pharmacokinet*, 1987, 13(4):205-27.

Olsen EA, "The Pharmacology of Methotrexate," *J Am Acad Dermatol*, 1991, 25(2 Pt 1):306-18.

Wallace CA, Bleyer WA, Sherry DD, et al, "Toxicity and Serum Levels of Methotrexate in Children With Juvenile Rheumatoid Arthritis," *Arthritis Rheum*, 1989, 32(6):677-81.

Wernick R and Smith DL, "Central Nervous System Toxicity Associated With Weekly Low-Dose Methotrexate Treatment," *Arthritis Rheum*, 1989, 32(6):770-5.

Methotrexate, CSF *see* Methotrexate, Blood *on previous page*

Methsuximide, Blood

Synonyms Celontin®

Test Includes Methsuximide and active metabolite normethsuximide

Specimen Blood

Volume 15 mL

Minimum Volume 4 mL serum

Container Red top tube

Collection Collect specimen immediately prior to next dose unless specified otherwise.

Storage Instructions Separate serum and refrigerate.

Reference Range Methsuximide: 0.1-1.4 μg/mL; normethsuximide: 10-40 μg/mL

Critical Values Toxic: normethsuximide: >60 μg/mL

Use Monitor therapeutic drug level

Additional Information Methsuximide is a succinimide derivative used to control absence (petit mal) seizures and as an adjunct in refractory, partial complex seizures. Its actions are similar to those of ethosuximide. Methsuximide is rapidly absorbed and metabolized to its active form, N-desmethylmethsuximide. It is this metabolite that probably accounts for the anticonvulsant action. Peak levels are achieved in 1-3 hours and the plasma half-life is 2-4 hours. Adverse effects include eosinophilia, leukopenia, monocytosis, pancytopenia, Stevens-Johnson syndrome, nervousness, headaches, mental confusion, and nausea and vomiting.

Methyl Alcohol *see* Methanol, Blood *on page 1295*

Methylbromides, Blood

Synonyms Bromomethane; Monobromomethane

Specimen Blood

Minimum Volume 14 mL

Container Two lavender top (EDTA) tubes

Storage Instructions Refrigerate

Reference Range Methyl bromide: not established after low level occupational exposure; baseline blood bromide (inorganic): 1-5 mg/L

Use Evaluate industrial exposure

Additional Information Methylbromide is a gaseous chemical that is frequently employed as a fumigant for large enclosed industrial and agricultural areas. Methylbromide is extremely toxic and can be absorbed through the skin, inhaled, or ingested. The toxic effects include narcosis, pulmonary edema, CNS depression, and kidney damage.

Methylenedioxymethamphetamine *see* Methamphetamines, Urine *on page 1294*

Methylphenidate, Blood

Synonyms Ritalin®

Specimen Blood

Volume 10 mL

Minimum Volume 3 mL serum

Container Red top tube

Collection Date and time must accompany the specimen.

Reference Range After oral administration of 20 mg/day, concentration in plasma after 1 hour is 20 ng/mL; therapeutic level: 5-40 ng/mL

Possible Panic Range Toxic values (urine): 0.8-40 μg/mL

Use Monitor therapeutic drug level; evaluate toxicity

Methodology High performance liquid chromatography (HPLC), UV spectrophotometry, gas chromatography (GC)

Additional Information Methylphenidate is a piperidine derivative used to treat attention deficit disorder and symptomatic management of narcolepsy. Its actions are similar to those of amphetamines. Methylphenidate is absorbed well from the GI tract and effects last from 3-6 hours. Adverse effects include nervousness, insomnia, anorexia, dizziness, palpitation, cardiac arrhythmias, fever, hypersensitivity reactions, thrombocytopenia, and hypertension. Its abuse potential is similar to that of amphetamines.

Specific References

Allen HW and Sedgwick B, "Detection of Ritalinic Acid in Urine by Thin-Layer Chromatography and Gas Chromatography," *J Anal Toxicol*, 1984, 8(2):61-2.

3-(1-Methylpyrrolidine-2-yl)pyridine *see* Nicotine Level *on page 1308*

Methyl Salicylate *see* Salicylate, Blood *on page 1347*

Methyprylon, Blood

Synonyms Noludar®

Test Includes Metabolite of methyprylon

Specimen Blood

Volume 20 mL

Minimum Volume 5 mL plasma

Container Two green top (heparin) tubes

Collection Collect specimen immediately prior to next dose unless specified otherwise.

Storage Instructions Separate plasma and refrigerate.

Reference Range Therapeutic: 8-10 μg/mL

Critical Values Toxic: ≥30 μg/mL

Use Monitor therapeutic drug level; evaluate toxicity

Methodology Colorimetric

Additional Information Methyprylon, a derivative of piperidine, is used as a nonbarbiturate hypnotic to aid simple insomnia. The dependency and withdrawal are similar to barbiturates. Sleep is induced within 45 minutes when a hypnotic dose is administered. The duration is 5-8 hours. The adverse effects of acute toxicity include somnolence, confusion, hyperpyrexia, hypothermia, respiratory depression, coma, and death.

Mexate® *see* Methotrexate, Blood *on page 1297*

Mexiletine, Blood

Synonyms Mexitil®

Abstract Mexiletine is an antiarrhythmic used to treat ventricular arrhythmia.

Specimen Blood

Container Red top tube

Sampling Time Draw 2-4 hours after last dose for peak level. Draw immediately prior to next dose for trough levels.

Reference Range Therapeutic 0.75-2.00 μg/mL (SI: 4-9 μmol/L)

Possible Panic Range >2.00 μg/mL (SI: >9 μmol/L)

Use Therapeutic monitoring; toxicity assessment

Methodology Fluorometry, high performance liquid chromatography (HPLC), gas chromatography (GC)

Additional Information Mexiletine is a class I antiarrhythmic approved for treatment of ventricular arrhythmias. It has no active metabolites. Toxic effects include dizziness, vomiting, confusion, tremor, bradycardia, and hypotension. Metabolism of mexiletine is accelerated by rifampin, phenobarbital, and phenytoin and retarded by cimetidine and ketoconazole. Half-life is 8-17 hours and is urine pH dependent. Acidic urine accelerates elimination.

(Continued)

Mexiletine, Blood *(Continued)*

Specific References

Gottlieb SS and Weinberg M, "Comparative Hemodynamic Effects of Mexiletine and Quinidine in Patients With Severe Left Ventricular Dysfunction," *Am Heart J*, 1991, 122(5):1368-74.

Grech-Belanger O, Barbeau G, Kishka P, et al, "Pharmacokinetics of Mexiletine in the Elderly," *J Clin Pharmacol*, 1989, 29(4):311-5.

Kempton J, Manoukian A, Levine B, et al, "A Mexiletine Intoxication," *J Anal Toxicol*, 1994, 18(6):346-7.

Manolis AS, Deering TF, Cameron J, et al, "Mexiletine: Pharmacology and Therapeutic Use," *Clin Cardiol*, 1990, 13(5):349-59.

Rohrig TP and Harty LE, "Postmortem Distribution of Mexiletine in a Fatal Overdose," *J Anal Toxicol*, 1994, 18(6):354-6.

Skluth H, Grauer K, and Gums J, "Ventricular Arrhythmias. An Assessment of Newer Therapeutic Agents," *Postgrad Med*, 1989, 85(6):137-8, 141-8, 153.

Mexitil® *see* Mexiletine, Blood *on previous page*

Mg, Serum *see* Magnesium, Serum *on page 1289*

Miltown® *see* Meprobamate, Blood *on page 1291*

Mioxom® *see* Carisoprodol, Quantitative *on page 1222*

Mite Identification *see* Arthropod Identification *on page 1198*

Monobromomethane *see* Methylbromides, Blood *on page 1298*

Morphine, Blood

Synonyms Heroin Metabolite, Blood

Specimen Blood

Minimum Volume 15 mL

Container Green top (heparin) tube or gray top (sodium fluoride) tube

Storage Instructions Refrigerate

Reference Range Therapeutic: 65-80 ng/mL (SI: 227-280 nmol/L)

Critical Values Toxic: >200 ng/mL (SI: >700 nmol/L)

Use Evaluate toxicity; detect drugs of abuse. Heroin is metabolized to morphine, therefore morphine detection may indicate heroin use.

Additional Information Morphine, the major phenanthrene alkaloid of powdered opium, is used for relief of moderate to severe acute and chronic pain after nonnarcotic analgesics have failed. It is also used as preanesthetic medication, to relieve the pain of myocardial infarction and to relieve the dyspnea of acute left ventricular failure and pulmonary edema. Peak analgesia is achieved 50-90 minutes after subcutaneous administration and 20 minutes after I.V. injection. The half-life is 2.5-3 hours. Ninety percent of morphine is found in the urine after 24 hours, either free, or the majority in the glucuronide conjugated form. Adverse effects include CNS depression, nausea and vomiting, hypotension, bradycardia, histamine release, increased intracranial pressure, miosis, antidiuretic hormone release, and physical and psychological dependence. High 6-acetyl morphine levels in serum associated with fatalities in heroin overdose.

Specific References

Aderjan R, Hofmann S, Schmitt G, et al, "Morphine and Morphine Glucuronidines in Serum of Heroin Consumers and in Heroin-Related Deaths Determined by HPLC With Native Fluorescene Detection," *J Anal Toxicol*, 1995, 19:163-8.

Brunk SF and Delle M, "Morphine Metabolism in Man," *Clin Pharmacol Ther*, 1974, 16(1):51-7.

Goldberger BA, Darwin WD, Grant TM, et al, "Measurement of Heroin and its Metabolites by Isotope-Dilution Electron-Impact Mass Spectrometry," *Clin Chem*, 1993, 39(4):670-5.

Morphine, Urine

Synonyms Heroin Metabolite, Urine

Test Includes Codeine, Demerol®, heroin, hydromorphone (Dilaudid®), morphine, and morphine glucuronide

Abstract This drug is widely used therapeutically as an analgesic. Morphine itself is not an extensively used drug of abuse but two derivatives, heroin and codeine, are.

Specimen Urine

Volume 50 mL

Minimum Volume 20 mL

Container Plastic urine container

Storage Instructions Refrigerate

Special Instructions If forensic, use chain-of-custody protocol and form.

Reference Range Negative (less than cutoff)

Critical Values Cutoff: screen (total opiates): 300 ng/mL; confirmatory: 300 ng/mL

Use Evaluate toxicity or detect drug of abuse. Heroin is metabolized to morphine, therefore morphine detection may suggest heroin use. To **prove** heroin use, 6-O-acetyl morphine must be identified in the urine.

Methodology Immunoassays, gas-liquid chromatography (GLC), high performance liquid chromatography-electrochemical detection (HPLC-ECD)

Additional Information Morphine, the major phenanthrene alkaloid of powdered opium, is used for relief of moderate to severe acute and chronic pain after non-narcotic analgesics have failed. It is also used as preanesthetic medication to relieve the pain of myocardial infarction and to relieve the dyspnea of acute left ventricular failure and pulmonary edema. Peak analgesia is achieved 50-90 minutes after subcutaneous administration and 20 minutes after I.V. injection. The half-life is 2.5-3 hours. Ninety percent of morphine is found in the urine after 24 hours, either free, or the majority in the glucuronide conjugated form. Adverse effects include CNS depression, nausea and vomiting, hypotension, bradycardia, histamine release, increased intracranial pressure, miosis, antidiuretic hormone release, and physical and psychological dependence. Naloxone is a specific antidote.

Urine codeine/morphine ratio usually exceeds 1.0 during the first 24 hours post-ingestion, decreases <1.0 from 24-30 hours and usually only morphine is detectable after 30 hours. Poppyseed ingestion can result in urine codeine levels as high as 4.5 mg/L and urine morphine levels as high as 0.2 mg/L; urine drug screen remains positive for 2-4 days.

Specific References

Baselt RC and Cravey RH, *Disposition of Toxic Drugs and Chemicals in Man*, 3rd ed, Chicago, IL: Year Book Medical Publishers Inc, 1989, 575-9.

McQuay HJ, Carroll D, Faura CC, et al, "Oral Morphine in Cancer Pain: Influences on Morphine and Metabolite Concentration," *Clin Pharmacol Ther*, 1990, 48(3):236-44.

Moore RA, Baldwin D, McQuay HJ, et al, "HPLC of Morphine With Electrochemical Detection: Analysis in Human Plasma," *Ann Clin Biochem*, 1984, 21(Pt 2):125-30.

Osborne R, Joel S, Trew D, et al, "Morphine and Metabolite Behavior After Different Routes of Morphine Administration: Demonstration of the Importance of the Active Metabolite Morphine-6-Glucuronide," *Clin Pharmacol Ther*, 1990, 47(1):12-9.

Portenoy RK, Khan E, Layman M, et al, "Chronic Morphine Therapy for Cancer Pain: Plasma and Cerebrospinal Fluid Morphine and Morphine-6-Glucuronide Concentrations," *Neurology*, 1991, 41(9):1457-61.

Portenoy RK, Thaler HT, Inturrisi CE, et al, "The Metabolite Morphine-6-Glucuronide Contributes to the Analgesia Produced by Morphine Infusion in Patients With Pain and Normal Renal Function," *Clin Pharmacol Ther*, 1992, 51(4):422-31.

Romberg RW and Lee L, "Comparison of the Hydrolysis Rates of Morphine-3-Glucuronide and Morphine-6-Glucuronide With Acid and Beta-Glucuronidase," *J Anal Toxicol*, 1995, 19:157-62.

Sear JW, Hand CW, Moore RA, et al, "Studies on Morphine Disposition: Influence of Renal Failure on the Kinetics of Morphine and its Metabolites," *Br J Anaesth*, 1989, 62(1):28-32.

"Toxicity and Pharmacokinetics of Morphine and Morphine-6-Glucuronide," *Br J Anaesth*, 1991, 67(3):362-3.

Zakowski MI, Ramanathan S, Sharnick S, et al, "Uptake and Distribution of Bupivacaine and Morphine After Intrathecal Administration in Parturients: Effects of Epinephrine," *Anesth Analg*, 1992, 74(5):664-9.

Motrin® *see* Ibuprofen, Serum *on page 1273*

MTX, Blood *see* Methotrexate, Blood *on page 1297*

Murphy-Pattee *replaced by* Thyroxine, Blood *on page 1361*

Muscle Biopsy

Synonyms Skeletal Muscle Biopsy

Test Includes For state-of-the-art muscle biopsy, indeed to make the surgical procedure worthwhile, enzyme histochemistry of the biopsied specimens must be included.

Abstract Diagnosis and classification of muscle disease

Patient Preparation Clinical data is required and should include the patient's age and sex; the pattern, severity, and tempo of the muscle involvement; relevant laboratory results (ie, CPK, ESR); electromyographic (EMG) findings; and the presence of significant related conditions (ie, dermatitis, neoplasm, steroid/AZT therapy, AIDS).

Sampling Time The biopsy should be performed early in the day as the specimen will immediately require special handling and should arrive when histotechnical personnel are available. The requisition should state a brief clinical history, pertinent laboratory findings, the biopsy site, and the name of the referring internist or neurologist.

Collection Selection of muscle biopsy site: The site for muscle biopsy should be one that is familiar to the pathologist (ie, quadriceps, deltoid, biceps, or gastrocnemius). Unusual muscle groups such as oculomotor or pharyngeal muscles should be avoided, as they have several unique and potentially confusing features. Biopsy should be from a muscle that is involved by the disease but has not reached "end-stage" atrophy. EMG/injection sites and sites near the myotendinous junction should be avoided as these biopsies will commonly exhibit artifactual changes.

Surgical technique: Except for children or exceptional adult cases, the procedure is done with local anesthesia. Ideally, the biopsied muscle should not be allowed to contract because this creates severe microscopic artifacts. To achieve an isometric specimen, it is best to use a surgical muscle clamp that prevents contraction. If no clamp is available, the specimen may be pinned to a tongue blade

(Continued)

Muscle Biopsy *(Continued)*

to prevent contraction. A portion of the muscle, in continuity with that held in the clamp, should extend from the clamp so it may be cut off for freezing and histochemistry. A small piece should be placed in 1% glutaraldehyde for electron microscopy. Deliver on a saline-moistened gauze pad immediately to the Pathology Department. Moistened gauze is used to prevent drying. The specimen must not become saturated as this will cause severe ice crystal artifact during snap freezing. **The tissue should not be placed in fixative or frozen.** It should ideally reach the Pathology Laboratory within 30 minutes to retain enzyme activity.

Storage Instructions At least a small portion of the fresh material will be stored deep frozen for possible later use in biochemical assays (eg, quantitation of glycogen, enzymes, or dystrophin levels).

Use Evaluate muscle disease in terms of neurogenic atrophy, muscular dystrophies, myositis (infectious and "idiopathic," or autoimmune), endocrine myopathies, and congenital myopathies and enzyme deficiencies. A muscle biopsy may shed light on a systemic condition such as systemic vasculitis in the absence of overt clinical muscle disease.

Methodology A portion of the clamped muscle is oriented, frozen in isopentane/liquid nitrogen, and transverse sections are obtained for H & E, trichrome, and various histochemical preparations, some of which are listed below.

- Adenosine triphosphate (ATPase): At differing pHs, used to differentiates type I, IIa, and IIb myofibers and reveals abnormal fiber type distributions and diseases that selectively involve certain myofiber types.
- Succinate dehydrogenase (SDH): Stains mitochondria and shows abnormal aggregates or loss. Nicotinamide adenine dinucleotide-tetrazolium reductase (NADH-TR) may be used, but it is less sensitive.
- Oil red O: Stains lipids to detect abnormal accumulations.
- Periodic acid-Schiff (PAS): Used to detect glycogen in glycogenoses (ie, McArdle's disease, Pompe's disease, etc).

Extra frozen sections should be obtained and held in case additional more specific, enzyme preparations are needed (ie, cytochrome C oxidase, phosphofructokinase, phosphorylase). The remaining muscle tissue is formalin-fixed, paraffin-embedded, and stained with H & E and trichrome. Such preparations are used to detect small foci of myositis or vasculitis which may be missed on cryostat-cut sections, which are, of necessity, much smaller.

Specific References

Brooke MH, "Disorders of Skeletal Muscle," *Neurology in Clinical Practice*, Bradley WG, Daroff RB, Fenichel GM, et al, eds, Boston, MA: Butterworth-Heinemann, 1991, 1843-86.

DeGirolami U, Smith TW, Chad D, et al, "Skeletal Muscle," *Principles and Practice of Surgical Pathology*, Silverberg SG, ed, New York, NY: Churchill Livingstone, 1990, 545-92.

Heffner RR Jr, "Muscle Biopsy in Neuromuscular Disorders," *Diagnostic Surgical Pathology*, Sternberg SS, ed, New York, NY: Raven Press, 1989, 119-39.

Heffner RR Jr, "Skeletal Muscle," *Histology for Pathologists*, Sternberg SS, ed, New York, NY: Raven Press, 1992, 81-108.

Plotz PH, "Not Myositis: A Series of Chance Encounters," *JAMA*, 1992, 268(15):2074-7.

Mychel-S® *see* Chloramphenicol, Serum *on page 1225*

Mycobacteria Culture, Blood *see* Blood Culture, Aerobic and Anaerobic *on page 1204*

Mylepsin® *see* Primidone, Blood *on page 1332*

Myochrysine® *see* Gold Level *on page 1270*

Myoglobin, Qualitative, Urine

Synonyms Myoglobin Screen, Urine

Specimen Random urine

Volume 20 mL

Container Clean, chemical-free, plastic (preferable) urine container

Reference Range Negative

Use Determine the presence of myoglobinuria; investigate myositis and other entities which damage muscle. See table.

Limitations Urine tests for myoglobin may not be reliable. Presence of hypochlorite or microbial peroxidase or other oxidizing contaminants may cause false-positive reactions. Presence of ascorbic acid (high concentrations) may decrease sensitivity. Serum testing is recommended.

Methodology Qualitative or screening methods are based on the oxidation of a chromogen (eg, ortho-toluidine) with production of a colored compound. This reaction is catalyzed by hemoglobin or myoglobin. Test sensitivity is about 0.3 mg/dL (SI: 3 mg/L). Specificity for myoglobin can be obtained by the ammonium sulfate test. If initial testing is positive for blood (or myoglobin), preparation of an 80% saturated urine solution of ammonium sulfate will precipitate hemoglobin. On filtering or centrifugation myoglobin stays in solution. Color in the supernatant indicates presence of myoglobin pigment. Electrophoresis can provide definitive differentia-

Causes of Myoglobinuria

Metabolic — impaired substrate utilization for energy metabolism	Enzyme deficiencies (LD and others), substrate deficiency, hypokalemia, hypophosphatemia, hypomagnesemia
Excessive muscle use	Severe/unaccustomed exercise, seizures, march hemoglobinuria with myoglobinuria
Hyperpyrexia	Heat stroke, exertional hyperthermia, hyperthermia associated with drug use (eg, cocaine), heat injury
Postinfections viral	Influenza A, herpes simplex, Epstein-Barr, coxsackie
bacterial	Fever and sepsis, clostridial with gangrene
Primary muscle disease	Muscular dystrophy, McArdle's disease, polymyositis, dermato-myositis, familial paroxysmal myoglobinuria
Poisoning drug	Carbon monoxide, alcohol, barbiturate, cocaine, amphetamine, phencyclidine, neuroleptic malignant syndrome
animal	Hoff's disease (fish poisoning), sea snake bite (*Enhydrina schistosa*), trichinosis
Ischemia	Arterial occlusion, myocardial infarction, thromboembolism, infarction of large muscle, anterior tibial syndrome
Traumatic	Crush injury, wounds, surgical muscle trauma, beatings, electro-cution, limb compression with prolonged immobilization due to sleep or coma

tion between hemoglobin and myoglobin. Immunoassays (immunodiffusion (ID), isoelectric focusing (IEF), radioimmunoassay (RIA), immunoprecipitation; immunonephelometric; hemagglutination inhibition (HAI)) can also be used in the determination of myoglobin.

Additional Information Myoglobin (MW approximately 17,000) is released from cardiac/skeletal muscle, filtered by renal glomeruli and excreted in the urine. Resultant urine, depending upon the amount of excreted myoglobin varies in hue and intensity of red/brown/black color and is often referred to as cola colored. Myoglobin causes a false-positive reaction for urine hemoglobin on dipsticks. Serum myoglobin is not bound to haptoglobin and has a renal threshold of 2 mg/dL (SI: 20 mg/L). Muscle injury (metabolic or traumatic, see table) releases myoglobin into the circulation from which it is rapidly cleared into the urine.

Myoglobinuria has been associated with renal failure. Renal failure itself may cause high serum myoglobin level. Myoglobinuric renal failure commonly complicates rhabdomyolysis of either traumatic and metabolic origin. The mechanism of renal injury is unknown but does not appear to be solely due to nephrotoxicity of myoglobin. The combined effects of toxic products released in rhabdomyolysis with dehydration, hypotension, and electrolyte imbalance may play a role in pathogenesis of the renal failure. Cases associated with the use of cocaine may develop as a result of cocaine-induced renal artery vasoconstriction, renal ischemia, and tubular damage. Myoglobinuria may occur with myocardial infarction. Myoglobin deposits in the kidney are demonstrable by immunofluorescent techniques. There are a few reports of rhabdomyolysis-induced renal failure occurring in cases of child abuse. Use of neuroleptic agents in individuals with or without predisposing factors (exhaustion, dehydration, others) may result in the neuroleptic malignant syndrome, a hyperpyrexic syndrome that may be fatal, and associated with myoglobinuria. The dark urine color associated with myoglobinuria develops on standing or in the bladder at acid pH.

The pathophysiology of cocaine- (and other drugs of abuse) induced rhabdomyolysis is not clearly established. In addition to presence of serum and urine myoglobin, there is striking increase in serum CK and elevations of LD (LDH), AST (SGOT), and ALT (SGPT). Cocaine blocks presynaptic reuptake of neurotransmitters at postsynaptic receptor sites. In some cases, rhabdomyolysis subsequent to

(Continued)

Myoglobin, Qualitative, Urine *(Continued)*

use of cocaine may relate to ischemia of arterial vasoconstriction, to muscle activity associated with dysphoric agitation, and/or to hyperthermia. The most common cause, however, of rhabdomyolysis related to use of abused drugs is limb compression during sleep or coma. Serum CK is usually normal with hemolysis, in which serum LD is generally increased with high LD_1. With circulating myoglobin, serum CK is usually very high, serum LD may be moderately increased, but it is LD_5 that is usually elevated on LD isoenzyme electrophoresis. An isomorphic pattern of LD isoenzymes may also be seen. When no specific cause of rhabdomyolysis is apparent, or when precipitating physical exercise was not extreme, or when CPK does not return to baseline, muscle biopsy with measurement of specific muscle enzymes may be indicated. In 77 such muscle biopsies, enzyme deficiencies were noted in 36 patients.

Specific References

Engel AG, "Disease of Muscle (Myopathies) and Neuromuscular Junction," *Cecil's Textbook of Medicine*, Wyngaarden JB and Smith LH Jr, eds, 18th ed, Philadelphia, PA: WB Saunders Co, 1988, 2282-3.

Penn AS, "Myoglobinuria," *Myology*, Engel AG and Banker BQ, eds, New York, NY: McGraw-Hill Inc, 1986, 1785-1803.

Schumann GB and Schweitzer SC, "Examination of Urine," *Clinical Diagnosis and Management by Laboratory Methods*, Chapter 17, Henry JB, ed, Philadelphia, PA: WB Saunders Co, 1991, 410-2.

Myoglobin Screen, Urine *see* Myoglobin, Qualitative, Urine *on page 1302*

Mysoline® *see* Primidone, Blood *on page 1332*

Na⁺ *see* Sodium, Blood *on page 1352*

N-Acetyl Procainamide *see* Procainamide, Blood *on page 1332*

NADH-MetHb Reductase *see* Methemoglobin, Blood *on page 1296*

NAPA *see* Procainamide, Blood *on page 1332*

Narcotics *see* Opiates, Qualitative, Urine *on page 1309*

Narcotics Drug Screen, Urine *see* Toxicology Drug Screen, Urine *on page 1365*

Na, Urine *see* Sodium, Urine *on page 1353*

Navane® *see* Thiothixene, Blood *on page 1361*

NCV *see* Nerve Conduction Studies *on this page*

Nembutal® *see* Pentobarbital, Blood *on page 1317*

Nembutal® *see* Barbiturates, Quantitative, Blood *on page 1201*

Nerve Conduction Studies

Synonyms Latency Studies; NCV; Nerve Conduction Velocity

Test Includes Electrical stimulation of a peripheral nerve and recording of the evoked action potentials. Nerve conduction studies may be performed on either sensory nerves or mixed sensorimotor nerves. Following percutaneous electrical stimulation of an axon, a physiologic action potential (AP) is generated. This signal propagates down the axon, where it is detected at a distant site by surface electrodes. If a motor nerve is tested, the AP of the corresponding muscle is recorded. If a sensory nerve is examined, the AP of the identical nerve is recorded. In either case, the evoked AP is displayed on an oscilloscope screen where amplitude (in mV) and duration (in msec) are read directly. From this, several important parameters are calculated including the **latency time** (the time interval between stimulus presentation and initiation of action potential) and maximum **nerve conduction velocity** (speed of impulse propagation). This technique provides objective information regarding nerve function not obtainable from conventional electromyography alone. NCV testing is considered the procedure of choice in evaluating the patient with peripheral nerve dysfunction and should be considered an extension of the history and physical examination.

Patient Preparation Risks and benefits of the procedure are discussed with the patient and informed consent is obtained. As a general rule, patient should be seen and evaluated by physician prior to this procedure. The accuracy of this test depends in part on the accuracy of the clinician's impression. Patient may take usual medications on the morning of examination including pain medications as needed.

Aftercare No specific activity restrictions are required postprocedure. Patient may resume prior level of activity.

Equipment NCV testing is performed with commercial EMG equipment adaptable to a nerve stimulator. Surface electrodes are round silver plates (0.5-1 cm diameter) placed directly on the skin for nerve stimulation. When two electrodes are contacted by the nerve stimulator, one will act as the cathode and the other as the anode, and current will flow between these negative and positive poles respectively, depolarizing the underlying nerve. The nerve stimulator itself is available in a variety of designs. Commonly it is a bipolar device with two metal prongs, 2-3 cm apart, attached to an insulated handle. The electrical impulse produced is a square wave of short duration (0.5-1 msec) and variable intensity (0-600 V). All stimulators are capable of generating either a threshold stimulus (evoked action in potential in a few axons) or a supramaximal stimulus (all axons in a nerve stimulated). Stimuli may be delivered in pairs or as a constant train. The stimulation and cathode ray oscilloscope are coordinated so that the "sweep" on the oscilloscope precedes the stimulus by a variable delay. In this way, a marker indicating the precise moment of stimulus delivery is always visible. The evoked action potentials, whether muscle or nerve, are preferably recorded on surface electrodes. (Occasionally, needle electrodes may be needed, especially when evaluating small, atrophic muscle fibers.) The compound action potentials detected by the recording electrodes are amplified 1000 times for muscle action potentials and approximately 100,000 times for sensory action potentials. Due to this magnitude of amplification, surrounding "noise" must be reduced, primarily through the use of high frequency, low-pass filters and amplifiers with a high signal-to-noise ratio (100,000:1) and high impedance (megaohm range). The amplified action potential is displayed on a cathode ray oscilloscope (frequency range 10 Hz to 10 kHz). Action potentials may be photographed using a synchronized shutter mechanism and/or stored onto magnetic tape. The oscilloscope is also capable of displaying multiple, serial action potentials on the screen for simultaneous comparison (each succeeding AP is placed on a higher baseline). The oscilloscope screen is calibrated for electric potential on the vertical axis (eg, 1 cm = 1 volt) and time on the horizontal axis (in msec). Some devices calculate the values for latency automatically and provide an automatic digital readout.

Technique Technique differs somewhat amongst laboratories. The following outlines common principles only. A brief neurologic examination is conducted by the examiner prior to the procedure. Patient is asked to rest comfortably with muscles relaxed. For evaluation of a motor nerve, the axon must be stimulated at two (or more) sites (ie, a distal and proximal site). For example, when testing the median nerve the electrical stimulus is delivered to the wrist (distal site) and the antecubital fossa (proximal site); each site is tested separately. The cathodic lead of the bipolar stimulator depolarizes the nerve and the resultant action potential propagates down the axon in one direction (the anode hyperpolarizes the nerve and blocks conduction in the opposite direction). Recording electrodes located over the innervated muscle (eg, thenar muscle with median nerve testing) sense the compound muscle action potential which eventually results. This entire sequence (or "sweep") is displayed on the oscilloscope, starting from the original stimulus presentation (indicated by a "stimulus artifact" marker), followed by a delay prior to the start of the muscle action potential. Paired stimuli or a train of stimuli are presented. These steps are repeated at separate sites along the same axon. The **latency** (in msec) is defined as the time delay between the stimulus artifact and the first (negative) deflection of the muscle action potential. Values for latency are determined for both the proximal and distal stimulation sites with the recording electrode sites kept constant. Latency in motor nerve testing reflects the sum of pure nerve conduction time and the delay at the neuromuscular junction (NMJ). Since conduction velocity for the nerve alone is desired, the delay at the NMJ must be factored out. This is the basis for testing at both proximal and distal stimulating sites. Maximum NCV is calculated by the following:

- NCV (motor nerve) = distance (in mm) between proximal and distal sites / proximal latency (msec) – distal latency (msec)

NCV is an estimation of action potential propagation between the two sites of electrical stimulation. It does not measure nerve function past the distal site (eg, the hand) or closer than the proximal site (eg, spinal root). The nerve conduction time from stimulus presentation at the distal electrode to the start of the muscle action potential, the **distal** or **terminal latency**, is often recorded separately from maximum NCV. Distal latency reflects both nerve conduction and NMJ transmission. Sensory nerves may be tested in an analogous fashion. NCVs may be obtained in two ways: (1) orthodromic testing – stimulating electrodes are placed distally (eg, over digital nerves) and sensing electrodes placed proximally (eg, forearm), or (2) antidromic testing – stimulating electrodes placed proximally and sensing electrodes distally; this mimics physiologic impulse propagation. **Latency** is the time delay between electrical stimulation and appearance of the nerve action potential at the sensing electrode. Testing of sensory nerves does not involve muscle action potentials or NMJ delays. Calculation of sensory nerve latencies is more simple than motor latencies, since stimulation is required at only one site along the axon:

- NCV (sensory) = distance (mm) between stimulation point and recording electrode / sensory latency (msec)

Other important variables are the **amplitude** of the action potentials (in mV), **dispersion** of the action potentials, and the presence of **conduction blocks**. NCV

(Continued)

Nerve Conduction Studies *(Continued)*

may be determined for any peripheral nerve accessible to surface electrical stimulation. Only a limited number of nerves can be tested, in practicality, and the examination must be tailored to the clinical impression. In most centers, nonaffected limbs are also screened for generalized neuropathy (or to serve as internal controls). Commonly evaluated nerves include:

- upper extremity – median, ulnar, radial nerves (both sensory and motor)
- lower extremity – peroneal, tibial, superficial peroneal, sural nerves

Less accessible nerves in the upper extremity include the brachial plexus and shoulder girdle nerves. In the lower extremity the lumbosacral plexus, saphenous nerve, and lateral femoral cutaneous nerve are relatively difficult to test and are not usually used for asymptomatic screening.

Special Instructions Requisition from ordering physician should include brief clinical history, pertinent neurologic findings, specific disease conditions sought, and specific limbs to be tested. Ordering physician should also state if electromyography (or other electrophysiologic testing) is desired.

Reference Range Preliminary written impression is given by neurologist or physiatrist usually on the same day. Normal values for distal latency, conduction velocity, and amplitude of evoked action potential have been established. These values are dependent on age and gender. Since equipment and technique vary from one laboratory to another, each laboratory develops its own set of normal values. Published normal values for median nerve motor conduction are:

- distal latency, 3.7 msec
- conduction velocity, elbow to wrist, 58 msec
- amplitude (wrist stimulation), 13.2 mV

Of course, normal values vary for each peripheral nerve.

Critical Values In addition to objectively confirming the existence of a peripheral neuropathy, NCV testing can usually distinguish between the two major pathologic forms of neuropathy – axonal and demyelinating neuropathy. It is difficult to distinguish these disorders on the basis of history and physical examination alone. In addition, management strategies for these disorders are quite divergent. NCV testing allows initial categorization of a neuropathic process as a mononeuropathy, mononeuritis multiplex, or polyneuropathy. Within these broad categories, the pathologic process may be further divided into axonal or demyelinating lesions. In general, demyelinating diseases are characterized by decreased conduction velocities, markedly prolonged distal latencies, and normal (or slightly decreased) AP amplitude. In addition, two may be variably present: (1) AP dispersion (temporal variability of APs), and (2) conduction block (markedly decreased or absent AP amplitude with proximal nerve stimulation but not with distal site stimulation). NCV testing is often effective in diagnosing demyelinating disorders. Polyneuropathies due to demyelinating diseases include Guillain-Barré syndrome, diphtheric polyneuritis, demyelinating neuropathy associated with carcinoma, and several rare genetic neuropathies, Dejerine-Sottas disease, metachromatic leukodystrophy, and others. Axonal neuropathies are characterized by normal conduction velocity but decreased AP amplitude. Usually only a fraction of the axons in a nerve undergo degeneration. The fastest conducting axons in a nerve may be relatively spaced (unless disease is severe). Since nerve conduction velocities reflect only the fast fibers, and not the slow or medium velocity fibers, conduction velocities are typically normal despite extensive axonal degeneration. Polyneuropathies due to axonal degeneration are common and include neuropathies due to systemic disease (uremia, porphyria, vitamin B_{12} deficiency, systemic amyloidosis, severe hypothyroidism, chronic liver disease), medications (cis-platinum, vincristine, metronidazole), toxins (alcohol, arsenic, lead, and others), and hereditary neuropathies (ataxia-telangiectasia syndrome, Friedreich's ataxia). Many neuropathies are due to mixed axonal-demyelinating processes. Examples include diabetic neuropathy, neuropathy associated with multiple myeloma or lymphoma, and several drugs. Characteristic features of the neuropathies are shown in the following table. NCV testing is also useful in the diagnosis of mononeuropathy multiplex, a condition in which neuropathy develops in multiple, but noncontiguous nerves, either simultaneously or over a prolonged period of time. Individual nerve trunks appear to be afflicted in a random fashion. NCV testing can determine if mononeuritis multiplex is being caused by an axonal or demyelinating neuropathy. Axonal processes potentially leading to mononeuritis multiplex are polyarteritis nodosum and vasculitic syndromes associated with connective tissue diseases (systemic lupus erythematosus, rheumatoid arthritis, and others). Demyelinating mononeuritis multiplex is most often due to chronic inflammatory demyelinating polyradiculoneuropathy (CIDP). Again, the distinction between axonal and demyelinating processes is crucial in clinical decision making. Focal involvement of a single nerve or mononeuropathy is frequently encountered in general practice. This implies local nerve compression usually from trauma or entrapment. NCV testing reveals localized slowing of nerve conduction at the point of compression due to localized demyelination (which precedes distal axon degeneration). Carpal

Nerve Conduction Studies

	Axonal Neuropathy	Severe Axonal Neuropathy	Demyelinating Neuropathy
Conduction velocity	N	N or ↓	↓↓
Distal latency	N or ↑	↑	↑↑
Action potential amplitude	↓	↓↓	N
Dispersion of APs	—	—	Possible
Conduction blocks	—	—	Possible
Examples	Uremic, alcoholic		Guillain–Barré syndrome

tunnel syndrome is a common entrapment syndrome involving the median nerve. Testing can localize the lesion, exclude polyneuropathy, and assess severity. The presence of axonal degeneration distal to the compression site may warrant surgical intervention.

Use NCV testing is useful in the following situations:

- confirm the presence of a sensory deficit in an objective manner, especially when the physical examination is inconclusive (or malignancy is suspected)
- evaluate the patient with diffuse polyneuropathy to determine severity and extent of disease and to distinguish demyelinating from axonal processes
- assess the patient with muscle weakness in order to distinguish a neuropathic process from primary muscle disease
- evaluate the patient with acute ascending paralysis to confirm the diagnosis of Guillain-Barré syndrome rapidly prior to plasmapheresis
- confirm the diagnosis of mononeuritis multiplex
- assess nerve entrapment syndromes (mononeuropathies) such as carpal tunnel syndrome; to determine the lesion site, differentiate entrapment from diffuse neuropathy, assess severity, and evaluate response to surgical interventions

Conventional NCV testing may often be **normal** in the following:

- primary muscle disease
- radiculopathies
- disease involving very proximal segments of a peripheral nerve (if suspected clinically, "H reflex" testing is indicated)
- most axonal-type neuropathies, unless the so-called "fast-fibers" are severely damaged
- anterior horn cell disease, such as any atrophic lateral sclerosis, NCVs are typically normal, or only marginally abnormal
- peripheral nerve lesions of any type, if examined early in the disease course. For example, in the first 1-2 weeks of acute Guillain-Barré syndrome, NCVs are usually normal. Even with complete transection of a peripheral nerve (eg, trauma), NCVs distal to the lesion remain normal for several days.

Despite these potentially "normal" test results, NCV testing may still provide valuable information. For example, in the patient with possible amyotrophic lateral sclerosis, it is important to document a normal NCV study in addition to the more typical EMG abnormalities.

Contraindications Relative contraindications include:

- the agitated, uncooperative patient
- presence of a cardiac pacemaker (or implantable cardiac defibrillation device). The pacemaker may be effected by the electrical current delivered to the skin.
- presence of an indwelling cardiac catheter, such as Swan-Ganz or central venous line.

Specific References

Adams RD and Victor M, *Principles of Neurology*, 4th ed, New York, NY: McGraw-Hill Book Co, 1989, 1009-27.

Aminoff MF, *Electrodiagnosis in Clinical Neurology*, 2nd ed, New York, NY: Churchill-Livingstone, 1986.

Asbury AK, "Disease of the Peripheral Nervous System," *Harrison's Principles of Internal Medicine*, 12th ed, JD Wilson, ed, New York, NY: McGraw-Hill Book Co, 1991, 2096-107.

Johnson EW and Wiechers D, "Electrodiagnosis," *Krusen's Handbook of Physical Medicine and Rehabilitation*, 3rd ed, FJ Kottke, GK Stillwell, and JF Lehmann, eds, Philadelphia, PA: WB Saunders Co, 1982, 56-85.

Kimura J, *Electrodiagnosis in Diseases of Nerve and Muscle: Principles and Practice*, 2nd ed, Philadelphia, PA: FA Davis Co, 1989.

Nerve Conduction Velocity *see* Nerve Conduction Studies *on page 1304*

NH_3, Blood *see* Ammonia, Blood *on page 1188*

Nickel, Urine

Synonyms Ni, Urine

Patient Preparation Instruct patient to use plastic urinal or bedpan if necessary.

Specimen 24-hour urine

Volume Entire collection

Minimum Volume 100 mL

Container Plastic container, kept on ice

Collection Instruct the patient to void at 8 AM and discard the specimen. Then collect all urine including the final specimen voided at the end of the 24-hour collection period (ie, 8 AM the next morning). Avoid contact with metal during specimen collection. Screw the lid on securely. Transport the specimen promptly to the laboratory. Container **must** be labeled with patient's full name, room number, date and time collection started, and date and time collection finished.

Storage Instructions Keep on ice or refrigerate. Laboratory will measure urine volume and remove 120 mL aliquot.

Causes for Rejection Specimen in contact with metal

Special Instructions Requisition **must** state date and time collection started and date and time collection finished.

Reference Range ≤25 μg/L

Use Evaluate nickel toxicity

Additional Information Elemental nickel causes little human toxicity, but nickel carbonyl is extremely toxic. Acute inhalation can cause severe pulmonary edema, often delayed, and liver necrosis. Chronic industrial exposure is associated with increased incidence of nasal and lung carcinoma.

Nicotine Level

Synonyms 3-(1-Methylpyrrolidine-2-yl)pyridine

Specimen Blood

Reference Range Plasma nicotine levels peak rapidly after each cigarette (from 0.03-0.05 mg/L); moderate accumulation over a longer time period. In pipe smokers, average plasma levels average 0.004 mg/L; nicotine gum chewers (2 mg size) average 0.012 mg/L. Plasma concentrations of cotinine in children living with smokers are four times higher than those in children from nonsmoking environments.

Critical Values Lethal dose: 40-60 mg; blood concentrations >5 mg/L may be fatal. Dermal exposure has caused nonfatal poisoning. Postmortem blood concentrations: 11-600 mg/L; postmortem urine concentrations: 17-58 mg/L.

Methodology Spectrophotometry, thin-layer chromatography (TLC), high performance liquid chromatography (HPLC), fluorescence polarization immunoassay (FPIA), gas chromatography (GC); confirmation: gas chromatography/mass spectrometry (GC/MS)

Additional Information Highly toxic alkaloid causing stimulation of the autonomic ganglia and the central nervous system. Small doses produce nausea, tachycardia, dizziness, sweating, and hypertension. Present in tobacco at amounts of ~0.5% to 0.8% by weight, the average cigarette in the U.S. contains 1.5% nicotine.

Nicotine is extensively transformed to inactive metabolites (eg, cotinine). Cotinine is further oxidized to hydroxycotinine. Other metabolites include nornicotine and nicotine-1'-N-oxide. Plasma half-life of nicotine in cigarette smokers: 0.5-2 hours (average 40 minutes); cotinine: 6-16 hours (average 11 hours). Twenty-four hours after nicotine dosing, 5% is excreted unchanged in urine, 10% as cotinine, and 4% as other metabolites. Excretion is decreased if the urine is alkaline.

Specific References

Barlow RD, Thompson PA, and Stone RB, "Simultaneous Determination of Nicotine, Cotinine and Five Additional Metabolites in the Urine of Smokers Using Pre-Column Derivatisation and High Performance Liquid Chromatography," *J Chromatogr*, 1987, 419:375-80.

Baselt RC and Cravey RH, *Disposition of Toxic Drugs and Chemicals in Man*, 3rd ed, Chicago, IL: Year Book Medical Publishers Inc, 591.

Kogan MJ, Verebey K, Jaffee JH, et al, "Simultaneous Determination of NIcotine and Cotinine in Human Plasma by Nitrogen Detection Gas-Liquid Chromatography," *J Forensic Sci*, 1981, 26:6-11.

Pattishall EN, Strope GL, Etzel RA, et al, "Serum Cotinine as a Measure of Tobacco Smoke Exposure in Children," *Am J Dis Child*, 1985, 139(11):1101-4.

Nipride® *see* Thiocyanate, Blood or Urine *on page 1360*

Nitroprusside *see* Thiocyanate, Blood or Urine *on page 1360*

Nitroprusside Reaction, Blood *see* Ketone Bodies, Blood *on page 1277*

Nitroprusside Reaction for Ketones, Urine *see* Ketones, Urine *on page 1278*

Nits Identification *see* Arthropod Identification *on page 1198*

Ni, Urine *see* Nickel, Urine *on previous page*

Noctec®, Plasma *see* Chloral Hydrate, Plasma *on page 1224*

Noludar® *see* Methyprylon, Blood *on page 1299*

Nonsteroidal Anti-Inflammatory Comparison *see page 1655*

11-Nor-9-Carboxy-Delta-9-Tetrahydrocannabinol *see* Cannabinoids, Qualitative *on page 1217*

Norepinephrine, Urine *see* Catecholamines, Fractionation, Urine *on page 1222*

Norpace® *see* Disopyramide, Blood *on page 1251*

Norpramin® *see* Imipramine, Blood *on page 1274*

Norpropoxyphene *see* Propoxyphene, Blood or Urine *on page 1334*

Nortriptyline, Blood

Synonyms Aventyl®; Pamelor®

Abstract This is a tricyclic antidepressant.

Specimen Blood

Volume 7 mL

Minimum Volume 3 mL serum

Container Red top tube

Collection Collect specimen immediately prior to next dose unless specified otherwise.

Storage Instructions Separate serum and refrigerate.

Reference Range Therapeutic: 50-150 ng/mL

Critical Values Toxic: >1000 ng/mL

Use Monitor therapeutic drug level; evaluate toxicity

Limitations Results not valid if patient receiving imipramine or desipramine

Methodology High performance liquid chromatography (HPLC)

Additional Information Nortriptyline, a tricyclic antidepressant, is a derivative and metabolite of amitriptyline and is used to treat endogenous depression. The half-life of nortriptyline is 20-80 hours. Nortriptyline may be associated with cholestasis and cholestatic jaundice. Hematological consequences include agranulocytosis, purpura, and thrombocytopenia. Other side effects include a host of GI, endocrinologic, allergic, anticholinergic, cardiovascular, and neurologic disorders. Red cell levels of metabolites may be a more sensitive indicator of myocardial toxicity.

Specific References

Baselt RC and Cravey RH, *Disposition of Toxic Drugs and Chemicals in Man*, 3rd ed, Chicago, IL: Year Book Medical Publishers Inc, 1989, 613-5.

Brasfield KH, "Practical Psychopharmacologic Considerations in Depression," *Nurs Clin North Am*, 1991, 26(3):651-63.

Shapiro PA, "Nortriptyline Treatment of Depressed Cardiac Transplant Recipients," *Am J Psychiatry*, 1991, 148(3):371-3.

O_2 Capacity *see* Oxygen Saturation, Blood *on page 1313*

O_2 Content *see* Oxygen Saturation, Blood *on page 1313*

Occult Blood, Urine *see* Blood, Urine *on page 1210*

Oil of Wintergreen *see* Salicylate, Blood *on page 1347*

Opiates, Qualitative, Urine

Related Information

Codeine, Urine *on page 1235*

Applies To Heroin; Narcotics; Poppy Seeds

Test Includes Morphine, codeine, hydrocodone (Hycodan®), hydromorphone (Dilaudid®)

Abstract The qualitative detection of urine opiates is used almost exclusively to show presence of drugs of abuse in this class. Morphine and codeine are used therapeutically for pain.

Specimen Random urine

Volume 50-60 mL

Container Plastic urine container

Collection If forensic, observe precautions.

Storage Instructions Refrigerate

Special Instructions If forensic, use chain-of-custody protocol and form.

Reference Range Negative (less than cutoff)

Critical Values Cutoff: screen: 300 ng/mL; confirmation: 300 ng/mL of specific opiates

(Continued)

Opiates, Qualitative, Urine *(Continued)*

Use Evaluate drug abuse; assess toxicity

Limitations In most immunoassays a number of narcotic drugs can cross react to give a positive screen. Every effort should be made to confirm, by an analytically different and more sensitive method, all presumptive, positive opiate screens. Hydromorphone, hydrocodone, oxymorphone, and oxycodone usually will test negative after 48 hours by gas chromatography-mass spectrometric methods. EMIT immunoassays may not detect oxymorphone. Hydromorphone, hydrocodone, and oxycodone may become negative by immunoassay after one day. See Test Commonly Includes.

Methodology Screening: immunoassay, thin-layer chromatography (TLC), high performance liquid chromatography (HPLC), gas chromatography (GC); confirmation: gas chromatography/mass spectrometry (GC/MS)

Additional Information A qualitative urine screen for opiates is performed in suspected overdose cases or as part of a drugs-of-abuse program. The test is most sensitive for morphine and codeine, but other drugs will cross react in an immunoassay and give positive results (eg, hydrocodone, hydromorphone). All presumptive positive assays should be confirmed, preferably by GC/MS. Morphine is a prescribed drug for pain relief, a metabolite of heroin, a metabolite of codeine, and a constituent of poppy seeds. Its presence in urine, even after confirmation, must be interpreted very carefully. Ingestion of poppy seeds (bagels, Danish) can cause positive opiate screens at a 300 ng/mL cutoff. The intake of heroin by the user can only be proved by the detection of 6-O-acetyl morphine by the urine confirmatory test.

Opiates in general are a group of drugs (commonly referred to as narcotics) which are used medically to relieve pain, but which also have a high potential for abuse. Some opiates come from a resin taken from the seed pod of the Asian poppy. This group of drugs includes opium, morphine, and codeine. Other opiates are synthesized or manufactured (eg, heroin). Opium appears as dark brown chunks or as a powder, and is usually smoked or eaten. Heroin can be a white or brownish powder which is usually dissolved in water and injected.

Opiates tend to relax the user. When the opiates are injected, the user feels an immediate "rush." Other initial and unpleasant effects include restlessness, nausea, and vomiting. The user may go "on the nod," going back and forth from feeling alert to drowsy. With very large doses, the user cannot be awakened, pupils become smaller, and the skin becomes cold, moist, and bluish in color. Furthermore, breathing slows down and death may occur. Clearance may be slower in geriatric patients.

Tolmetin can give false-negative results by EMIT® assay.

Specific References

Barsan W, "Narcotic Agents," *Ann Emerg Med*, 1986, 15:1019-20.

Gillogley KM, Evans AT, Hansen RL, et al, "The Perinatal Impact of Cocaine, Amphetamine, and Opiate Use Detected by Universal Intrapartum Screening," *Am J Obstet Gynecol*, 1990, 163(5 Pt 1):1535-42.

Joseph R, Dickerson S, Willis R, et al, "Interference by Nonsteroidal Anti-inflammatory Drugs in EMIT® and TDx® Assays for Drugs of Abuse," *J Anal Toxicol*, 19:13.

Kulberg A, "Substance Abuse: Clinical Identification and Management," *Pediatr Clin North Am*, 1986, 33(2):325-61.

Montamat SC, Cusack BJ, and Vestal RE, "Management of Drug Therapy in the Elderly," *N Engl J Med*, 1989, 321(5):303-9.

Pettitt BC Jr, Dyszel SM, and Hood LV, "Opiates in Poppy Seed: Effect on Urinalysis Results After Consumption of Poppy Seed Cake-Filling," *Clin Chem*, 1987, 33(7):1251-2.

Smith ML, Hughes RO, Levine B, et al, "Forensic Drug Testing for Opiates. VI. Urine Testing for Hydromorphone, Hydrocodone, Oxymorphone, and Oxycodone With Commercial Opiate Immunoassays and Gas Chromatography-Mass Spectrometry," *J Anal Toxicol*, 1995, 19:18-19.

Trevilla PH, Jimenez O, and Tena T, "Presence of Rifampicin in Urine Causes Cross-Reactivity With Opiates Using the KIMS Method," *J Anal Toxicol*, 1995, 19:200.

Osmolal Gap *see* Osmolality, Serum *on this page*

Osmolal Gap, Urine *see* Osmolality, Urine *on next page*

Osmolality, Serum

Synonyms Serum Osmolality

Applies To Osmolal Gap

Abstract The osmolality of a solution is defined as the number of molecules or ions (particles) in a solution of water. Osmolality is independent of particle size or charge. Nonpolar solutions yield one molecule (eg, glucose) while polar solutions yield multiples of the number of ions solubilized (eg, sodium chloride yields two ions while magnesium chloride yields three ions).

Specimen Blood

Volume 7 mL

Minimum Volume 4 mL serum

Container Red top tube

Collection Pediatrics: Blood drawn from heelstick

Storage Instructions Refrigerate or freeze serum if not run within 4 hours.

Reference Range 275-295 mOsm/kg (SI: 275-295 mmol/kg) H_2O. Some consider normal to be 280-290 mOsm/kg (SI: 280-290 mmol/kg) H_2O and others within 270-310 mOsm/kg (SI: 270-310 mmol/kg) H_2O.

Possible Panic Range <265 mOsm/kg (SI: <265 mmol/kg), >320 mOsm/kg (SI: >320 mmol/kg). Result of 385 mOsm/kg (SI: 385 mmol/kg) relates to stupor in hyperglycemia. Values 400-420 mOsm/kg (SI: 400-420 mmol/kg) can relate to grand mal seizures. Values >420 mOsm/kg (SI: >420 mmol/kg) may be lethal.

Use Evaluate electrolyte and water balance, hyperosmolar status and hydration status, dehydration, acid-base balance, seizures; evaluate antidiuretic hormone function, liver disease, hyperosmolar coma. Osmolality measures the concentration of particles in solution. Freezing point depression serum osmolality with calculated osmolal gap, is useful in screening for and approximating the serum concentrations of certain low molecular weight toxins, such as ethanol, ethylene glycol, isopropanol, and methanol, especially as a rapid approximation for emergent situations. See Limitations.

High serum osmolality may result from hypernatremia, dehydration, hyperglycemia, mannitol therapy, azotemia, ingestion of ethanol, methanol, ethylene glycol. Thus, osmolality has a role in toxicology and in coma evaluation. Very low birth weight infants may have elevated serum osmolality for the first week of life.

Low serum osmolality may be secondary to overhydration, hyponatremia, syndrome of inappropriate antidiuretic hormone secretion (SIADH) with carcinoma of lung and other entities. Chlorpropamide use can also result in a low serum osmolality.

Causes of hyperosmolality, hypo-osmolality, and of factors affecting ADH are published. Serum osmolality measurements do not measure the fraction of serum that is water. Osmolality measurement by freezing point depression is also indifferent to permeability of solutes to cell membranes.

Limitations When vapor pressure osmometry is used, volatile solutes (eg, alcohols and glycols) may remain in the vapor phase and not be detected.

Methodology Freezing point depression (more often used) or vapor pressure. (Do not use for toxicologic determination.)

Additional Information Measured osmolality is usually more than calculated osmolality. If measured osmolality is >15 mOsm/kg (SI: >15 mmol/kg) greater than calculated, consider methanol, ethylene glycol, or ethanol ingestion or other toxicity; shock; or trauma. Elevated serum osmolality with normal sodium suggests possible hyperglycemia, uremia, or alcoholism. Both serum and urine values and calculated osmolality (see previous listing) are sometimes needed. Although lactic acidosis theoretically should not contribute to the osmolal gap, increases in the osmolal gap in lactic acidosis have been reported. Drugs including thiazide diuretics, steroids, cimetidine, and others have been implicated in the development of hyperosmolar hyperglycemic nonketotic coma. Slight elevation of serum osmolality over expected values have been reported in the elderly. After overnight dehydration, urine/serum ratio is usually ≥3.

Specific References

Baker RJ, "Biochemical Gaps: Osmolal and Anion," *Curr Surg*, 1987, 44(5):378-81.

Fraser CL and Arieff AI, "Fatal Central Diabetes Mellitus and Insipidus Resulting From Untreated Hyponatremia: A New Syndrome," *Ann Intern Med*, 1990, 112(2):113-9.

Leech S and Penney MD, "Correlation of Specific Gravity and Osmolality of Urine in Neonates and Adults," *Arch Dis Child*, 1987, 62(7):671-3.

Maffly RH, "Renal Function and Disorders of Water, Sodium, and Potassium Balance," *Scientific American Medicine*, Section 10, Chapter 1, Rubenstein E and Federman DD, eds, New York, NY: Scientific American Inc, 1990, 2-34.

Nose H, Mack GW, Shi XR, et al, "Role of Osmolality and Plasma Volume During Rehydration in Humans," *J Appl Physiol*, 1988, 65(1):325-31.

Penney MD and Walters G, "Are Osmolality Measurements Clinically Useful?" *Ann Clin Biochem*, 1987, 24(Pt 6):566-71.

Snyder H, Williams D, Zink B, et al, "Accuracy of Blood Ethanol Determination Using Serum Osmolality," *J Emerg Med*, 1992, 10(2):129-33.

Worthley LI, Guerin M, and Pain RW, "For Calculating Osmolality, the Simplest Formula Is the Best," *Anaesth Intensive Care*, 1987, 15(2):199-202.

Osmolality, Urine

Related Information

Electrolytes, Urine *on page 1254*

Synonyms Urine Osmolality

Applies To Osmolal Gap, Urine; U/P Ratio

Abstract Osmolality is a definitive measure of urine concentration.

Specimen Random urine or timed specimen

Volume Entire collection

Minimum Volume 5 mL

Container Clean urine container

Storage Instructions Refrigerate during collection and storage.

(Continued)

Osmolality, Urine *(Continued)*

Reference Range Random urine: neonates: 75-300 mOsm/kg (SI: 75-300 mmol/kg); children and adults: 250-900 mOsm/kg (SI: 250-900 mmol/kg). Normal range of serum sodium (mmol/L) to osmolality (mOsm/kg) ratio is 0.43-0.50. Patients with normal renal function after 14-hour restriction of fluids should be able to concentrate to >800 mOsm/kg (SI: >800 mmol/kg); <400 mOsm/kg (SI: <400 mmol/kg) is interpreted by Weisberg as severe renal impairment. Prolonged dehydration may be dangerous for some patients.

Possible Panic Range <100 mOsm/kg (SI: <100 mmol/kg) in overhydration, >800 mOsm/kg (SI: >800 mmol/kg) in dehydration

Use Evaluate concentrating ability of the kidneys (eg, in acute and chronic renal failure); evaluate electrolyte and water balance; used in work-up for renal disease, syndrome of inappropriate antidiuretic hormone secretion (SIADH), and diabetes insipidus; may be used with urinalysis when patient has had radiopaque substances, has glycosuria or proteinuria; evaluate dehydration, amyloidosis; estimate urinary ammonium concentrations using the urine osmolal gap and detect increased osmolality due to the presence of unusual molecules. Osmolality is desirable in examination of neonatal urine when protein or glucose are present.

Limitations Serum osmolality is often needed to interpret urine osmolality.

Methodology Freezing point depression

Additional Information Osmolality is a better measurement of urine concentration than specific gravity. Osmolality is a measure of renal tubular concentration, depending on the state of hydration. Simultaneous determination of urine and serum osmolalities facilitates interpretation of results. High urinary/plasma ratio is seen in concentrated urine. Normal ranges for the U/P ratio are given by Weisberg as approximately 0.2-4.7, and >3.0 with overnight dehydration. With poor concentrating ability the ratio is low but still ≥1.0. In SIADH urine sodium and urine osmolality are high for plasma osmolality. Neonatal urine osmolality is discussed in a 1987 paper. Specifically derived regression equations are advocated to predict urine osmolality from specific gravity measurements. Low birthweight infants have been reported to have increased serum osmolality with normal urine osmolality.

The urine osmolal gap is described as the sum of urinary concentrations of sodium, potassium, bicarbonate, chloride, glucose, and urea compared to measured urine osmolality. The gap is normally 80-100 mOsm/kg (SI: 80-100 mmol/kg) H_2O. Determination of the urine osmolal gap is used to characterize metabolic acidosis. High urine osmolal gap can be used semiquantitatively.

Specific References

Fraser CL and Arieff AI, "Fatal Central Diabetes Mellitus and Insipidus Resulting From Untreated Hyponatremia: A New Syndrome," *Ann Intern Med*, 1990, 112(2):113-9.

Halperin ML and Skorecki KL, "Interpretation of the Urine Electrolytes and Osmolality in the Regulation of Body Fluid Tonicity," *Am J Nephrol*, 1986, 6(4):241-5.

Osmolarity *replaced by* Osmolality, Serum *on page 1310*

Oxazepam, Serum

Synonyms Serax®

Abstract Oxazepam is a benzodiazepine used as an antianxiety agent. It is an active metabolite of several other benzodiazepines that are used therapeutically.

Specimen Blood

Volume 15 mL

Minimum Volume 5 mL serum

Container Red top tube

Sampling Time Collect specimen immediately prior to next dose unless specified otherwise.

Storage Instructions Separate serum and refrigerate.

Reference Range 0.2-1.4 μg/mL (SI: 0.7-4.9 μmol/L)

Possible Panic Range <2.0 μg/mL

Use Monitor therapeutic drug level; evaluate toxicity

Methodology High performance liquid chromatography (HPLC)

Additional Information Oxazepam, a benzodiazepine derivative, is related to chlordiazepoxide and shares many of its qualities. It does, however, have a shorter duration of action and causes fewer adverse effects. It is rapidly eliminated by urinary excretion as a glucuronide conjugate. Oxazepam is used to manage tension and anxiety and to aid in the control of acute withdrawal symptoms in chronic alcoholism. Peak plasma levels are achieved in 2-4 hours and the half-life is 4-12 hours. Adverse effects are mild and infrequent. They include drowsiness, vertigo, ataxia, headache, tremor, slurred speech, nausea, hypotension, and leukopenia. Simultaneous alcohol ingestion potentiates some of the effects of benzodiazepines.

Specific References

Baselt RC and Cravey RH, *Disposition of Toxic Drugs and Chemicals in Man*, Chicago, IL: Year Book Medical Publishers Inc, 1989, 622-3.

Craig CR and Stitzel RE, *Modern Pharmacology*, 3rd ed, Boston, MA: Little, Brown and Co, 1990, 440-6.

2-Oxoglutarate Aminotransferase *see* Aspartate Aminotransferase *on page 1199*

Oxycodone, Blood or Urine

Synonyms Percocet®; Percodan®; Tylox®

Specimen Blood, urine

Volume 10 mL blood, 20 mL urine

Minimum Volume 2 mL serum, 10 mL urine

Container Red top tube, plastic urine container

Storage Instructions Refrigerate serum and urine.

Critical Values Blood level of 5 mg/L associated with fatality

Possible Panic Range Lethal dose: 500 mg

Use Detect Percodan® abuse or toxicity

Methodology High performance liquid chromatography (HPLC) for serum, enzyme immunoassay (EIA) and thin-layer chromatography (TLC) for urine

Additional Information Oxycodone, a semisynthetic derivative of the opium alkaloid thebaine, is used for the management of moderate to severe pain. This drug is 10 times more potent than codeine and equally as potent as morphine. Analgesic action of oxycodone is achieved in 10-15 minutes and lasts for 4-5 hours. The adverse effects include CNS and respiratory depression, nausea and vomiting, hypotension, bradycardia, increased intracranial pressure, miosis, drowsiness, and physical and psychological dependence.

Oxygen Content *see* Blood Gases, Arterial *on page 1207*

Oxygen-Hemoglobin Dissociation Curve (ODC) *see* Oxygen Saturation, Blood *on this page*

Oxygen Saturation, Blood

Related Information

Blood Gases, Arterial *on page 1207*

Synonyms Hemoglobin Saturation, Percent; SaO_2; SO_2

Applies To 2,3-DPG; O_2 Capacity; O_2 Content; Oxygen-Hemoglobin Dissociation Curve (ODC); Transcutaneous Pulse Oximetry

Test Includes A part of blood gas determination in many laboratories.

Abstract The partial pressure of oxygen physically dissolved in plasma determines the amount of oxygen bound to hemoglobin = the oxygen saturation.

Specimen Whole blood, arterial

Container Heparinized syringe, capillary tubes, or green top (heparin) tube

Collection Draw specimen into heparinized syringe, avoid air bubbles, and stopper tightly, knotting scalp vein infusion set tubing, fitting shank of syringe with a special closure or other means of insuring an airtight fit. Place heparinized specimen on ice. Take to the laboratory immediately.

Causes for Rejection Specimen received with clots or air bubbles in the syringe, specimen not on ice, specimen not tightly stoppered

Special Instructions If capillaries are used to collect the specimen, warm skin 10-15 minutes prior to puncture, obtain free flow of blood with a sufficiently deep puncture ("arterialized capillary blood"), fill heparinized capillaries completely full (enough capillaries to provide at least 0.5 mL whole blood), cap and mix.

Reference Range Children and adults: 95% to 99%. Arterial pO_2 of 80 mm Hg, SO_2 of 95% are normal for the aged. Arterial pO_2 of 100 mm Hg, SO_2 of 97% are normal for the young.

Possible Panic Range Arterial pO_2 of 20 mm Hg, SO_2 of 35% are critically low, life-endangering levels; the same values from mixed venous blood indicate tissue hypoxia. Arterial pO_2 of 40 mm Hg, SO_2 of 75% are panic values that correlate with cyanosis, but these values are normal for mixed venous blood.

Use Evaluate the extent of oxygenation of hemoglobin and adequacy of tissue oxygenation, together with pO_2. Allows evaluation of oxygenation and oxyhemoglobin dissociation of blood with use of the oxygen dissociation curve (ODC). The dissociation curve expresses relationships between pO_2 and oxyhemoglobin saturation. Diagnose hypoxia; monitor respiratory function during mechanical ventilation. Central venous oxygen saturation may also be used in detection of blood loss in cases of acute injury.

Limitations Accuracy and precision may be affected by the presence of other pigments in the blood, including especially other heme derivatives (eg, carboxyhemoglobin), low hemoglobin concentrations, plasma turbidity (ie, as with lipemia), and presence of cell fragments. Interpretation is more meaningful if the nature of patient's inspired gas is recorded (ie, room air or mixture of gases with a controlled oxygen content).

(Continued)

Oxygen Saturation, Blood *(Continued)*

Contraindications Contraindications of arterial puncture

Methodology Spectrophotometric analysis of hemolysate with current automated analyzers directly measuring SO_2. Alternatively, a calculated SO_2 may be derived from the Hill equation using measured pH and pO_2. In the latter method, blood is analyzed at two wavelengths, one with a large difference in absorbance between oxygenated and deoxygenated hemoglobin, the other at the isobestic point (molar absorbance identical for the oxygenated and deoxygenated forms). Transcutaneous pulse oximetry measures the absorption of different wavelengths of light passed through living tissue.

Additional Information The terms "O_2 content," "O_2 capacity," and "O_2 saturation" refer to various definitions of the amount of oxygen carried in the blood. **Oxygen content** is the total amount of oxygen present (bound to hemoglobin and dissolved in plasma) in the blood. Normally hemoglobin exists in blood in the oxygen-bound state (oxyhemoglobin) and in some unoxygenated forms (reduced hemoglobin, methemoglobin, carboxyhemoglobin, and sulfhemoglobin). Inactive forms account for about 4% of the total hemoglobin. **Oxygen capacity** is the amount of O_2 that would bind to hemoglobin if all the hemoglobin were oxygenated. **Oxygen saturation** is the ratio (in %) of oxyhemoglobin to the total amount of hemoglobin present.

The large pool of hemoglobin allows blood to transport 65 times the amount of oxygen dissolved in plasma. This relationship is dependent upon (primarily) pH (and thereby CO_2 parameters that contribute to the control of pH), temperature, the concentration of 2,3-diphosphoglycerate (2,3-DPG), and the molecular species of hemoglobin. When graphed, the relationship results in a sigmoid (S-shaped) oxygen-hemoglobin dissociation curve (ODC). The oxygen saturation (in %) is represented on the Y axis, the partial pressure of oxygen (in mm Hg) on the X axis with the curve shifted to the right or left (isobars) by changes in pH or other parameters. This is a physicochemically fixed relation such that if any two of the three determinants, pH, pO_2, or O_2 saturation are known, the other may be predicted. With the ODC in hand one can verify the accuracy of laboratory performance by assuring that the three reported values are consistent with each other as defined by the ODC (assuming normal molecular species of hemoglobin, concentration of 2,3-DPG, and constant temperature).

Red cell 2,3-DPG concentration plays an important role in regulation of hemoglobin's affinity for oxygen. 2,3-DPG binds to the β chains of deoxyhemoglobin and results in displacement of O_2 by the following equation: Hgb O_2 + 2,3-DPG = Hgb - 2,3-DPG + O_2. An increase in 2,3-DPG will cause a shift of the reaction to the right. Greater affinity of fetal hemoglobin for oxygen has been ascribed to the poor binding of 2,3-DPG by the γ chains of fetal hemoglobin. Increased erythrocyte 2,3-DPG concentrations decrease intracellular pH resulting in a further reduction in oxygen affinity. 2,3-DPG is increased with hypoxia. Red cells of newborns contain approximately 80% hemoglobin F. Hemoglobin F has a slightly lower oxygen affinity compared to hemoglobin A (normal adult hemoglobin) and binds 2,3-DPG less strongly than hemoglobin A. Following birth, O_2 affinity decreases as red cell 2,3-DPG concentrations rise (20% during the first week of life). At 1-4 weeks, healthy prematures have P-50 values approaching those of normal adults.

Decreased oxygen saturation relates to impaired cardiorespiratory function at the macro-organ level of heart and/or lungs (due to a variety of diseases) or at the intracellular chemical respiratory level (a number of pathologic mechanisms resulting in methemoglobinemia). The four mechanisms of abnormal gas exchange are hypoventilation, ventilation-perfusion disturbance, diffusion defect, and venous admixture. The hypoxemia accompanying right-to-left shunting in cardiac diseases (venous admixture) is preferentially evaluated with oxygen saturation. O_2 saturation provides a more direct indication of the size of the shunt than the pO_2 value. Decreased central venous oxygen saturation was found to correlate better with estimated blood loss volumes in 26 trauma patients than vital signs including heart rate, blood pressure, central venous pressure, pulse pressure, and urine output. In this series of trauma patients, all had normal vital signs upon admission and a significant percentage of these patients had serious injuries and ongoing blood loss that required immediate attention.

In some clinical situations, measurement of pO_2 alone may give misleading information as to sufficiency of the blood's oxygen-carrying ability. Partial pressure of oxygen may be normal or even increased while O_2 saturation may be decreased as the result of an abnormal heme compound (eg, carboxyhemoglobin as in cases of carbon monoxide poisoning). Oxygen saturation gap (calculated oxygen saturation - measured oxygen saturation) $>5\%$ can occur in carbon monoxide poisoning. Oxygen saturation is preferably measured directly (spectrophotometrically) and not derived from the pH and pO_2 values by use of the ODC relationships. Derived SO_2 values would give false normal results in the above example.

Arterial oxygen desaturation occurs after sedation for peritoneoscopy with resultant hypoxemia, hypercarbia, and acidosis.

There is growing use of **transcutaneous pulse oximetry** to determine oxygen saturation, particularly in premature and in critically ill newborns and children. This noninvasive technique avoids the rigors of arterial puncture, necessity of subsequent proper sample handling, and can provide continual monitoring. This technique has generally been found reliable and useful in monitoring adequacy of oxygenation, effectiveness of resuscitative efforts, detection of development of prolonged periods of decreased SO_2 in neonates, and monitoring preterm infant's response to physical therapy. Pulse oximetry has also been applied to detection of hyperoxemia in newborns but has low specificity. Limitations of pulse oximetry have included overestimation of SO_2 at values $\leq$65%, and variation from *in vitro* determined SO_2 in samples with >50% fetal hemoglobin as compared with samples having <25% fetal hemoglobin. Furthermore, it is not useful in carbon monoxide or methemoglobin intoxication because false elevations of saturation may occur. A study of pulse oximeter determined oxygen saturation in pregnant patients and their newborns has found that SO_2 in neonates is commonly $\leq$90% within 10 minutes after birth and may not always be indicative of pathologic hypoxia. Specialized devices (eg, balloon-tipped, thermodilution, fiberoptic, pulmonary arterial catheter) have been developed for the intraoperative monitoring of mixed venous oxygen saturation.

Specific References

Chripko D, Bevan JC, Archer DP, et al, "Decreases in Arterial Oxygen Saturation in Paediatric Outpatients During Transfer to the Postanaesthetic Recovery Room," *Can J Anaesth*, 1989, 36(2):128-32.

Grebstad JA, Svendsen L, and Gulsvik A, "Precision of Arterial Blood Gases and Cutaneous Oxygen Saturation in Healthy Nonsmokers," *Scand J Clin Lab Invest*, 1989, 49(3):265-8.

Kwant B, Oeseburg B, and Zijistra WG, "Reliability of the Determination of Whole-Blood Oxygen Affinity by Means of Blood-Gas Analyzers and Multi-Wavelength Oximeters," *Clin Chem*, 1989, 35(5):773-7.

Porter KB, "Evaluation of Arterial Oxygen Saturation of the Newborn in the Labor and Delivery Suite," *J Perinatol*, 1987, 7(4):337-9.

Woolf CR, "Respiratory Disorders," *Applied Biochemistry of Clinical Disorders*, 2nd ed, Gornall AG, ed, Philadelphia, PA: JB Lippincott Co, 1986, 129-38.

Oxygen Titration Test *see* Pulse Oximetry *on page 1342*

P-450 System Inhibitor *see* Carbamazepine, Blood *on page 1219*

PA *see* Chest Films *on page 1224*

PA and Lateral CXR *see* Chest Films *on page 1224*

Pacinol® *see* Fluphenazine, Blood *on page 1268*

Pamelor® *see* Nortriptyline, Blood *on page 1309*

Pamelor® *see* Amitriptyline, Blood *on page 1187*

Panadol® *see* Acetaminophen, Serum *on page 1180*

Panex® *see* Acetaminophen, Serum *on page 1180*

Panwarfin® *see* Warfarin, Blood *on page 1379*

Paracetamol *see* Acetaminophen, Serum *on page 1180*

Paradione® *see* Paramethadione, Blood *on this page*

Paral® *see* Paraldehyde, Serum *on this page*

Paraldehyde, Serum

Synonyms Paral®

Specimen Blood

Volume 15 mL

Minimum Volume 5 mL serum

Container Red top tube

Storage Instructions Refrigerate serum.

Reference Range Therapeutic: 1-10 mg/100 mL

Critical Values Toxic: >27 mg/100 mL

Use Monitor therapeutic drug level; evaluate toxicity

Additional Information Paraldehyde, a cyclic ether, is a potent CNS depressant. It is used to control convulsions arising from tetanus, status epilepticus, eclampsia, and drug poisoning. It is also used to treat acute agitation due to alcohol withdrawal. Paraldehyde is absorbed well and achieves hypnotic effects within 10-15 minutes. The half-life is 7.5 hours. Adverse effects include gastric irritation, erythematous rash, hepatitis, corrosion of the rectum, metabolic acidosis, coughing, and pulmonary edema.

Paramethadione, Blood

Synonyms Paradione®

Specimen Blood

Volume 7 mL

(Continued)

Paramethadione, Blood *(Continued)*

Container Red top tube
Reference Range Therapeutic: 5-50 μg/mL
Possible Panic Range Lethal dose: 5 g
Use Monitor therapeutic drug level; evaluate toxicity
Methodology Gas chromatography (GC)
Additional Information Paramethadione is an oxazolidinedione (dione-type) anticonvulsant agent. It has many qualities similar to trimethadione (ie, actions, uses, contraindications, and adverse effects). It is used in the management of absence (petit mal) seizures that do not respond to other drugs. Paramethadione is rapidly absorbed after oral ingestion and metabolized by the liver. Adverse effects include sedation and drowsiness, headache, dizziness, changes in blood pressure, lymphadenopathy, abnormal liver function tests, albuminuria, GI distress, and alopecia.

Paraquat, Blood

Specimen Blood
Volume 14 mL
Minimum Volume 10 mL whole blood
Container Two gray top (sodium fluoride) tubes
Reference Range <0.25 μg/mL
Use Evaluate exposure to paraquat
Additional Information Paraquat is a herbicide, heavy exposure to which may cause heavy respiratory failure. Low dose exposure results in pulmonary fibrosis and edema.
Specific References

Hart TB, Nevitt A, and Whitehead A, "A New Statistical Approach to the Prognostic Significance of Plasma Paraquat Concentrations," *Lancet*, 1984, 2(8413):1222-3.
Jarvie DR, Fell AF, and Stewart MJ, "A Rapid Method for the Emergency Analysis of Paraquat in Plasma Using a Second Derivative Spectroscopy," *Clin Chim Acta*, 1981, 117(2):153-65.
Smith NB, Mathialagan S, and Brooks KE, "Simple Sensitive Solid-Phase Extraction of Paraquat From Plasma Using Cyanopropyl Columns," *J Anal Toxicol*, 1993, 17(3):143-5.

Pb, Blood *see* Lead, Blood *on page 1282*
PBI *replaced by* Thyroxine, Blood *on page 1361*
Pb, Quantitative *see* Lead, Quantitative, Hair or Nails *on page 1283*
Pb, Urine *see* Lead, Urine *on page 1283*
PCE *see* Pseudocholinesterase, Serum *on page 1340*
pCO_2 *see* Blood Gases, Arterial *on page 1207*
PCP *see* Phencyclidine, Qualitative, Urine *on page 1319*
PCP *see* Phencyclidine, Quantitative, Serum *on page 1319*
Peace Pills *see* Phencyclidine, Qualitative, Urine *on page 1319*
***Pediculus humanus* Identification** *see* Arthropod Identification *on page 1198*
PEMA *see* Primidone, Blood *on page 1332*
Pentazine® *see* Trifluoperazine, Blood *on page 1369*

Pentazocine, Urine

Synonyms Fortral®; Talwin®
Specimen Random urine
Volume 50 mL
Minimum Volume 20 mL
Container Plastic urine container
Reference Range Not established for urine
Possible Panic Range Blood: 1 μg/mL; lethal dose: 0.3 g
Use Evaluate toxicity
Methodology Gas-liquid chromatography (GLC)
Additional Information Pentazocine, a synthetic benzomorphan analgesic, is used for the relief of moderate to severe pain. It is also a sedative used prior to surgery and as a supplement to surgical anesthesia. The onset of action is achieved 2-3 minutes after an I.V. dose and 15-30 minutes following all other routes of administration. Within 24 hours, 60% of the dose is lost in the urine. Adverse reactions include CNS and respiratory depression, nausea and vomiting, bradycardia, histamine release, seizures in predisposed patients, increased intracranial pressure, miosis, drowsiness, antidiuretic hormone release, and physical and psychological dependence.

Pentobarbital, Blood

Related Information

Barbiturates, Quantitative, Blood *on page 1201*

Synonyms Nembutal®; Pentobarbitone

Specimen Blood

Volume 15 mL

Minimum Volume 5 mL serum

Container Red top tube

Collection Collect specimen immediately prior to next dose unless specified otherwise. Routine venipuncture.

Storage Instructions Separate serum and refrigerate.

Reference Range Therapeutic: 1-10 μg/mL

Critical Values Toxic: 11 μg/mL; lethal: 20 μg/mL

Use Monitor therapeutic drug level; evaluate toxicity

Methodology High performance liquid chromatography (HPLC), gas chromatography (GC)

Additional Information Pentobarbital, a short-acting barbiturate, is used for the short-term treatment of insomnia and as a preoperative sedative. Onset of action is 15-30 minutes after oral ingestion and peak plasma levels are achieved in 30-60 minutes. I.V. administration delivers onset of action within 1 minute. The adverse effects of pentobarbital include hypotension, hypothermia, oliguria, cardiac arrhythmias, respiratory depression, CNS excitement or depression, nausea and vomiting, and impaired judgment.

Pentobarbital, Urine *see* Barbiturates, Qualitative, Urine *on page 1200*

Pentobarbitone *see* Pentobarbital, Blood *on this page*

Percocet® *see* Oxycodone, Blood or Urine *on page 1313*

Percodan® *see* Oxycodone, Blood or Urine *on page 1313*

Permitil® *see* Fluphenazine, Blood *on page 1268*

Perphenazine, Blood

Synonyms Chlorpiprazine; Trilafon®

Test Includes Chlorpromazine, mesoridazine, perphenazine, prochlorperazine, promazine, promethazine, thioridazine

Specimen Blood

Volume 10 mL

Minimum Volume 3 mL serum

Container Red top tube

Storage Instructions Refrigerate serum.

Reference Range 0.004-0.064 mg/L

Possible Panic Range 3.000 μg/mL

Use Monitor therapeutic drug level; evaluate toxicity

Methodology High performance liquid chromatography (HPLC), gas chromatography (GC)

Additional Information Perphenazine, a piperazine phenothiazine, is used to manage the manifestations of psychotic disorders. It is also used to control hiccups, nausea and vomiting, and violent retching during surgery. Adverse effects include convulsions, xerostomia, nasal congestion, tachycardia, bradycardia, hypotension, and photosensitivity.

Pertofrane® *see* Imipramine, Blood *on page 1274*

Pesticide Screen, Chlorinated

Test Includes Aldrin, chlordane, DDT, dieldrin, heptachlor, lindane, methoxychlor

Specimen Urine, blood, or gastric contents

Volume 100 mL urine, 20 mL whole blood, 50 mL gastric contents

Container Two royal blue top (heparin) tubes

Special Instructions Requisition must state date and time of specimen collection. Specify suspected pesticide. Specify if quantitation of a positive screen result is desired.

Reference Range None detected

Use Screen aids in identification or confirmation of exposure to common polychlorinated hydrocarbon compounds used as pesticidal sprays or dusts.

Pesticide Screen, Organophosphate

Test Includes Diazinon; Dicapthon; Malathion; Parathion; Trichlorfon; Dichloron

Specimen Urine, blood, or gastric contents

Volume 100 mL urine, 20 mL whole blood, 50 mL gastric contents

(Continued)

Pesticide Screen, Organophosphate *(Continued)*

Container Two royal blue top (heparin) tubes

Special Instructions Requisition must state date and time of specimen collection. Specify suspected pesticide. Specify if quantitation of a positive screen result is desired.

Reference Range None detected

Use Screen aids in identification or confirmation of exposure to common organophosphate compounds used as pesticidal sprays or dusts

pH, Blood

Related Information

Blood Gases, Arterial *on page 1207*

Synonyms Blood pH

Abstract Blood pH is an expression of acidity or acidemia.

Specimen Blood

Volume 2 mL

Minimum Volume 1 mL whole blood

Container Green top (heparin) tube or heparinized syringe

Collection For venous sample, it is best to collect without tourniquet if possible. **Do not allow patient to clench/unclench his/her hand**. This builds up lactic acid. Draw specimen into air-free heparinized syringe with needle quickly stoppered, making sure that no air bubbles remain. Capillary tubes should be filled as much as possible, metal flea inserted, capped, and mixed well with magnet. All specimens should be on ice and brought to the laboratory immediately. For capillary collection, the skin area to be punctured should be warmed 10-15 minutes. The puncture should be deep enough to allow a free flow of blood. Place arterial or venous blood on ice and transport to the laboratory immediately.

Storage Instructions Keep on ice in a syringe. pH changes 0.01/10 minutes at 37°C and 0.001/10 minutes at 4°C.

Causes for Rejection Specimen with clots, air bubbles, not iced, needle not tightly stoppered

Reference Range Pediatrics: newborns, with arterialized capillary blood (heel, fingertip, big toe) or arterial blood; 7.32-7.49; 2 months to 2 years, arterialized capillary or arterial blood: 7.34-7.46; children and adults: arterial: 7.35-7.45, venous: 7.32-7.43. Blood pH can be measured from either arterial or venous blood samples, usually with only very small differences in normal range.

Possible Panic Range <7.20, >7.60. Occasionally, patients with acidosis as severe as pH 6.80 survive. Many of these present with diabetic ketoacidosis, for which effective therapy is available.

Use Diagnose acidosis (eg, ketoacidosis), alkalosis (eg, emesis with loss of gastric juice); evaluate acid-base balance, significance of serum or plasma potassium levels; work up hypokalemia; use of oxyhemoglobin dissociation curves. May be useful for assessment of birth asphyxia in the depressed newborn. **Increased** with uncompensated metabolic and respiratory alkalosis, **decreased** with uncompensated metabolic and respiratory acidosis.

Limitations pH values are sensitive to sampling technique. Concurrent metabolic acidosis and respiratory alkalosis may result in normal pH, pCO_2, HCO_3, and anion gap, but abnormality might be detected by potassium level and blood volume measurement. Organic acidemias of infancy are beyond the scope of this manual.

Methodology Glass pH electrode

Additional Information pH should be judged in relation to other parameters such as pCO_2, HCO^-_3, sodium, potassium, chloride, glucose, ketone bodies, phosphorus, and lactic acid, BUN, creatinine, and osmolality of serum and urine. A small amount of information about some acid base disorders is provided in the Anion Gap listing and the references which are included.

Methanol, ethylene glycol, paraldehyde, and salicylate toxicity, diabetic ketoacidosis, alcoholic ketoacidosis, lactic acidosis, renal failure, and starvation are causes of **high anion gap metabolic acidosis**.

Additional to electrolytes and other tests listed above, relevant laboratory findings in acidemia may also include ketones, ethanol concentration, uric acid, albumin, CBC, urinalysis with examination for oxalate crystals, and salicylate concentration. Hypoproteinemia causes a metabolic alkalosis.

Umbilical artery pH may be useful in the assessment of birth asphyxia of the depressed neonate. Others contend that infants must be severely depressed with Apgar scores ≤ 3 at 1 and 5 minutes to be reflected in a decreased serum pH. Blood may be obtained from a clamped umbilical segment up to 1 hour after delivery.

In hypotensive patients, tissue hypoxia may be assessed by measurements of arterial pH, mixed venous pH, and bicarbonate concentrations. Such measurements do not appear to reliably assess tissue hypoxia in patients with fulminant hepatic failure. For such patients, oxygen flux (the difference between arterial and venous oxygen) remains the best way to detect the presence of covert tissue hypoxia.

Specific References

Adrogué HJ, Wilson H, Boyd AE 3d, et al, "Plasma Acid-Base Patterns in Diabetic Ketoacidosis," *N Engl J Med*, 1982, 307(26):1603-10.

Preuss HG, "Fundamentals of Clinical Acid-Base Evaluation," *Clin Lab Med*, 1993, 13(1):103-16.

Shapiro BA, "pH and Blood Gas Measurements: Discerning Innovation From Sophistication," *Crit Care Med*, 1989, 17(9):966.

Shapiro BA, Cane RD, Chomka CM, et al, "Preliminary Evaluation of an Intra-arterial Blood Gas System in Dogs and Humans," *Crit Care Med*, 1989, 17(5):455-60.

Wang F, Butler T, Rabbani GH, et al, "The Acidosis of Cholera. Contributions of Hyperproteinemia, Lactic Acidemia, and Hyperphosphatemia to an Increased Serum Anion Gap," *N Engl J Med*, 1986, 315(25):1591-5.

Phenadone, Serum *see* Methadone, Quantitative, Serum *on page 1293*

Phenaphen® *see* Acetaminophen, Serum *on page 1180*

Phencyclidine, Qualitative, Urine

Synonyms Angel Dust; Elephant Tranquilizers; Hog; Killer Weed; PCP; Peace Pills; Rocket Fuel

Abstract This is a widely used drug of abuse which was formerly sold as a veterinary tranquilizer. All legal manufacture and sale has been stopped. It is classified by DEA as a Schedule II controlled substance.

Specimen Random urine

Volume 100 mL

Minimum Volume 5 mL

Container Plastic urine container

Collection If forensic, observe precautions.

Special Instructions If forensic, use chain-of-custody protocol and form.

Reference Range Negative (less than cutoff)

Critical Values Cutoff: screen: 25 ng/mL; confirmation: 25 ng/mL (SI: 100 nmol/L)

Use Evaluate presence of phencyclidine, drug abuse, PCP toxicity; determine phencyclidine involvement in unexplained psychoses

Methodology Immunoassay, thin-layer chromatography (TLC), gas chromatography (GC), gas chromatography/mass spectrometry (GC/MS). Immunoassays are very specific and detect PCP at 25 ng/mL

Additional Information Phencyclidine is most often called "angel dust." It was first developed as an anesthetic in the 1950s. It was taken off the market for human use because it sometimes caused hallucinations. PCP is available in a number of forms. It can be a pure white crystal-like powder, a tablet or capsule, and it can be swallowed, smoked (alone or with marijuana), sniffed, or injected. Although PCP is illegal, it is easily manufactured.

Effects depend on how much of the drug is taken, the way it is used, and the individual. Small amounts act as a stimulant, speeding up body functions. For many users, PCP changes how they see their own bodies and things around them. Speech, muscle coordination, and vision are affected; sense of touch and pain are dulled; and body movements are slowed. Time seems to "space out." Effects include increased heart rate and blood pressure, flushing, sweating, dizziness, and numbness. When large doses are taken, effects include drowsiness, convulsions, and coma. Taking large amounts of PCP can also cause death from repeated convulsions, heart and lung failure, or ruptured blood vessels in the brain. PCP can be detected for 7 days after administration; 2-4 weeks in chronic users. Half-life is 7-46 hours.

Dextromethorphan can give a false-positive on an immunoassay screen; ketamine is not expected to give a positive immunoassay.

Specific References

Ellenhorn MJ and Barceloux DG, "Phencyclidine," *Medical Toxicology*, New York, NY: Elsevier, 1988, 763-78.

Milhorn HT Jr, "Diagnosis and Management of Phencyclidine Intoxication," *Am Fam Physician*, 1991, 43(4):1293-302.

Wessinger WD and Owens SM, "Phencyclidine Dependence: The Relationship of Dose and Serum Concentrations to Operant Behavioral Effects," *J Pharmacol Exp Ther*, 1991, 258(1):207-15.

Phencyclidine, Quantitative, Serum

Synonyms Angel Dust; Hog; Killer Weed; PCP; Rocket Fuel; Sernyl®

Specimen Blood

Volume 10 mL

Minimum Volume 3 mL serum

Container Gray top (sodium fluoride) tube

Use Detect drug abuse; evaluate toxicity

Additional Information Phencyclidine, most often called "angel dust," is available

(Continued)

Phencyclidine, Quantitative, Serum *(Continued)*

in a number of forms. It can be a pure white crystal-like powder, a tablet or capsule, and it can be swallowed, smoked (alone or with marijuana), sniffed, or injected. Although PCP is illegal, it is easily manufactured and is a legitimate veterinary tranquilizer.

Effects depend on how much of the drug is taken, the way it is used, and the individual. Small amounts act as a stimulant, speeding up body functions. For many users, PCP changes how they see their own bodies and things around them. Speech, muscle coordination and vision are affected; sense of touch and pain are dulled; and body movements are slowed. Time seems to "space out." Effects include increased heart rate and blood pressure, flushing, sweating, dizziness, and numbness. When large doses are taken effects include drowsiness, convulsions, and coma. Taking large amounts of PCP can also cause death from repeated convulsions, heart and lung failure or ruptured blood vessels in the brain. PCP can be detected for 7 days after administration; 2-4 weeks in chronic users.

Dextromethorphan can give a false-positive on an immunoassay screen; ketamine is not expected to give a positive immunoassay.

Phenemal *see* Phenobarbital, Blood *on this page*

Phenemalum *see* Phenobarbital, Blood *on this page*

Phenformin *see* Lactic Acid, Blood *on page 1281*

Phenobarb *see* Phenobarbital, Blood *on this page*

Phenobarbital, Blood

Related Information

Barbiturates, Quantitative, Blood *on page 1201*

Synonyms Gardenal®; Luminal®; Phenemal; Phenemalum; Phenobarb; Phenobarbitone; Stental Extentabs®

Abstract Phenobarbital is indicated for generalized tonic-clonic and partial seizures.

Specimen Blood

Volume 7 mL

Minimum Volume 1 mL serum or plasma

Container Red top tube, green top (heparin) tube, or lavender top (EDTA) tube

Sampling Time Consistent sampling time is desirable but less important than for other anticonvulsants due to its long half-life.

Reference Range Infants and children: 15-30 μg/mL (SI: 65-129 μmol/L); adults: 20-40 μg/mL (SI: 86-172 μmol/L). Low level: Most common cause is noncompliance. Other causes include drug interactions, including antipsychotic medication, chloramphenicol, acetazolamide, and phenytoin. Some patients are fast metabolizers, such as infants and children. High level: addition of valproic acid to regimen inhibits phenobarbital metabolism (parahydroxylation) and should be accompanied by a cut in phenobarbital dosage. Newborns, unlike older infants, have very long half-lives which may be associated with high levels.

Critical Values Toxic: >40 μg/mL (SI: >172 μmol/L) but if given intravenously, life-threatening side effects can occur with much lower levels, and patients should be monitored. Toxic effects are mostly neurologic. Adults present with lethargy and coma; children may present with irritability or hyperactivity.

Use Monitor patients for compliance, efficacy, and possible toxicity. Mephobarbital and primidone are metabolized to phenobarbital and, therefore, patients taking these drugs will have detectable levels of phenobarbital on therapeutic monitoring.

Methodology Enzyme immunoassay (EIA), gas-liquid chromatography (GLC), high performance liquid chromatography (HPLC)

Additional Information Phenobarbital has a half-life of 84-108 hours. Phenobarbital can affect the metabolism of phenytoin, ethosuximide, and increase the clearance and elimination of chloramphenicol, theophylline, oral anticoagulants (warfarin), cyclosporine, and oral contraceptives; where appropriate, the use of these drugs in patients on phenobarbital should be monitored clinically and through the laboratory.

Specific References

Bertino JS Jr and Reed MD, "Barbiturate and Nonbarbiturate Sedative-Hypnotic Intoxication in Children," *Pediatr Clin North Am*, 1986, 33(3):703-22.

Kutt H, "Phenobarbital: Interactions With Other Drugs," *Antiepileptic Drugs*, 3rd ed, Levy RH, Dreifuss FE, Mattson RH, et al, eds, New York, NY: Raven Press, 1989, 313-27.

Phenobarbital, Free, Blood

Test Includes Total and free phenobarbital

Specimen Blood

Volume 2 mL

Minimum Volume Two plain Microtainer™ tubes
Container Red top tube
Collection Draw just prior to the next dose.
Reference Range Therapeutic free: 7.5-20.0 μg/mL; therapeutic total: 15-40 μg/mL
Critical Values Toxic total: >60 μg/mL
Use Monitor therapeutic drug level; evaluate toxicity
Methodology Ultrafiltrate assayed by fluorescence polarization immunoassay (FPIA) or enzyme immunoassay (EIA)
Additional Information Phenobarbital, a long-acting barbiturate, is used in the treatment of grand mal and partial seizures and febrile seizures in children. It is used as a preoperative sedative and a hypnotic. Phenobarbital lowers bilirubin by inducing the production of glucuronyl transferase and is therefore used to prevent and treat neonatal hyperbilirubinemia and for the lowering of bilirubin in chronic cholestasis. Phenobarbital is slowly absorbed and peak serum concentrations are achieved in 8-12 hours. The half-life is 53-116 hours. Adverse effects include respiratory depression, hypotension, circulatory collapse, hyperkinetic activity, megaloblastic anemia, hepatitis, and exfoliative dermatitis.

Phenobarbitone *see* Phenobarbital, Blood *on previous page*

Phenol, Quantitative, Urine

Synonyms Carbolic Acid
Patient Preparation Patient should be instructed to use a plastic urinal or bedpan if necessary.
Specimen Urine
Minimum Volume 50 mL
Container Plastic urine container
Collection Freshly voided random urine
Storage Instructions Refrigerate
Critical Values Toxic: >75 mg/L, corrected to specific gravity 1.024
Use Evaluate toxicity
Additional Information Phenol, is a caustic, highly poisonous derivative of coal tar. It is a powerful disinfectant used in topical antiseptics and as an antimicrobial agent in solutions of low concentrations. Phenol is commonly used in industry, especially plastic manufacturing. Ingestion of amounts as small as 1 g can be fatal, as is skin absorption when large portions of the body are contaminated. Chronic poisoning can cause liver and kidney damage. The symptoms of acute poisoning include nausea and vomiting, dark-colored urine, necrosis of the mouth and GI tract, paralysis, convulsions, coma, respiratory depression, and cardiac arrest.

Phenothiazines *see* Thioridazine, Quantitative *on page 1360*
Phentermine *see* Methamphetamines, Urine *on page 1294*
Phenylethylmalonamide *see* Primidone, Blood *on page 1332*
Phenylpropanolamine *see* Methamphetamines, Urine *on page 1294*

Phenytoin, Blood

Synonyms Dilantin®; Diphenylhydantoin
Abstract Phenytoin is effective for generalized tonic-clonic and partial seizures.
Specimen Blood, saliva
Volume 7 mL
Minimum Volume 1 mL serum or plasma; 1 mL saliva
Container Red top tube or lavender top (EDTA) tube
Sampling Time In monitoring patients maintained on chronic therapy, a trough level or consistent sampling time should be used.
Reference Range 10-20 μg/mL (SI: 40-79 μmol/L). Patients treated for status epilepticus should have levels at or slightly above the upper limit of range. Low level: The most common cause of a low level is noncompliance. Absorption problems are most important in young infants (younger than 3 months) or occasionally in patients given phenobarbital, charcoal, or antacids at the same time as the phenytoin. Pediatric and some adult patients (fast metabolizers), who have breakthrough seizures at the end of the day, require more than once daily dosing. Some formulations other than Kapseals® may require more than once daily dosing, and changing formulations can cause changes in levels. Pregnancy or intercurrent illness such as mononucleosis can cause subtherapeutic levels with seizures. The addition of carbamazepine to a patient taking phenytoin can lower or raise phenytoin level but usually does not cause seizures. Disulfiram administration can increase phenytoin metabolism, lower levels, and may cause seizures. Patients can have lower than expected values if intravenous formulations are given with fluids containing glucose, which precipitates in solution with phenytoin. High levels: In patients chronically controlled on phenytoin who become clinically toxic without a

(Continued)

Phenytoin, Blood *(Continued)*

change in dose, toxicity can be brought on by a change in formulation, drug interaction, or intercurrent infection. Drugs which can precipitate phenytoin toxicity include chloramphenicol, tricyclic antidepressants, fluconazole, and levodopa. Small dose changes or changes in formulation (including change from one brand to another or to a generic) can cause large changes in antiepileptic drug (AED) levels and toxicity, because phenytoin manifests zero-order kinetics.

Possible Panic Range Toxicity may manifest progressively above 20 μg/mL (SI: >79 μmol/L) with ataxia, dizziness, nystagmus, and diplopia. Patients can have life-threatening complications with intravenous administration with normal levels; such patients should be placed on a cardiac monitor during intravenous administration of drug. Lethal dose: 5 g.

Use Monitor for compliance, efficacy, and possible toxicity

Methodology Routine: Enzyme-multiplied immunoassay technique (EMIT), enzyme-linked immunosorbent assay (ELISA), and fluorescence polarization immunoassay (FPIA). For physician's office testing, apoenzyme reactive immunoassay (ARIS; Ames Seralyzer®) is rapid, accurate, and may become increasingly important.

Additional Information Ninety percent of phenytoin is bound to serum proteins. Only the unbound fraction is biologically active. Primary site of action is thought to be the motor cortex, where the promotion of a sodium "efflux" from neurons probably stabilizes the threshold of the neuron against hyperexcitability. Most of a dose of phenytoin is excreted into the bile as inactive metabolites which are then reabsorbed from the intestines and excreted into the urine. Despite normal levels, phenytoin may interfere with the actions of other drugs, including cyclosporine, oral anticoagulants, oral contraceptives, and theophylline; appropriate laboratory monitoring of some of these agents is advised. The half-life of phenytoin in adults is 20-40 hours; in children, it is around 10 hours. Teratogenic effects of phenytoin have been proposed but not confirmed; the risks in women of childbearing age should be balanced against the risks of increased seizures.

Specific References

Engel J, *Seizures and Epilepsy*, Contemporary Neurology Series, Philadelphia, PA: FA Davis Co, 1989.

Lu Steffes M, Pittluck GW, Jolley ME, et al, "Fluorescence Polarization Immunoassay IV. Determination of Phenytoin and Phenobarbital in Human Serum and Plasma," *Clin Chem*, 1982, 28(11):2278-82.

Phosphatase, Alkaline *see* Alkaline Phosphatase, Serum *on page 1184*

Phosphorus, Serum

Synonyms PO_4, Blood

Abstract With exclusion of factitious types of hyperphosphatemia, causes of increased phosphate include diminished glomerular filtration, increased absorption in the renal tubules, and/or increased exogenous or endogenous phosphate loads. Hypophosphatemia and its complications are outlined.

Patient Preparation Ideally, patient should be fasting. Phosphate levels are lower following meals.

Specimen Blood

Volume 7 mL

Minimum Volume 1 mL serum

Container Red top tube

Collection Pediatrics: Blood drawn from heelstick for capillary

Storage Instructions Serum should be promptly separated from the clot to avoid false elevations.

Causes for Rejection Observable hemolysis

Reference Range Both low and high ends of the normal range are higher in children than in adults. Children: approximately 4.0-6.0 mg/dL (SI: 1.29-1.94 mmol/L). Adults: 2.5-4.5 mg/dL (SI: 0.81-1.45 mmol/L). Some variation exists among authorities.

Possible Panic Range <1.0 mg/dL is critical

Use Causes of **high phosphorus:** Youth; exercise; dehydration and hypovolemia; high phosphorus content enema; acromegaly; hypoparathyroidism; pseudohypoparathyroidism; bone metastases; hypervitaminosis D; sarcoidosis; milk-alkali syndrome; liver disease, such as portal cirrhosis; catastrophic events such as cardiac resuscitation, pulmonary embolism, renal failure; diabetes mellitus with ketosis; serum artifact – sample not refrigerated; overheated, hemolyzed sample, or serum allowed to remain too long on the clot.

Although phosphate accumulation occurs as renal disease progresses, hyperphosphatemia is not a feature of early renal failure; it does not usually develop before renal function has diminished to about 25% of normal. Osteitis fibrosa in uremic subjects, from excessive bone turnover, relates to hyperphosphatasia. The role of hyperphosphatemia in promotion of such secondary hyperparathyroidism is well established. A relationship to osteomalacia in hemodialysis patients exists.

Causes of **low phosphorus:** (Hypophosphatemia may occur with or without phosphate depletion. Serum levels vary as much as 2.0 mg/dL (SI: 0.65 mmol/L) during the day.)

Very severely malnourished subjects may have low phosphate levels, but even in starvation, phosphorus levels usually are normal. Antacids, diuretics, and long-term steroids are among the common agents bearing a relationship to severe hypophosphatemia. Recent carbohydrate ingestion decreases phosphorus, as does intravenous glucose administration; cases of hypophosphatemia relate to I.V. carbohydrate, dialysis, hyperalimentation, prolonged intravenous administration of phosphate-free fluids, metabolic states involving glucose, potassium, and pH. Depletion of phosphate occurs in diabetic ketoacidosis. Like potassium, phosphorus returns to the cell with therapy of diabetic ketoacidosis, and serum levels may diminish significantly during treatment. Osmotic diuresis induced by glycosuria in poorly controlled diabetes may lead to urinary phosphate losses with negative phosphorus balance. PO_4 levels may prove useful in initiation of insulin therapy, in diabetic ketoacidosis and other situations of insulin lack; with hyperglucagonemia, corticosteroid and epinephrine use, and in respiratory alkalosis. Association of hypophosphatemia with impaired glucose metabolism is thought to reflect decreased tissue sensitivity to insulin. Alcoholism and other hepatic disorders are found very frequently among patients with low PO_4. Alcoholic ketosis and alcohol withdrawal are among causes of hypophosphatemia. There is a slight decrease in serum phosphorus in the last trimester of pregnancy.

Primary hyperparathyroidism and other causes of calcium elevation, including ectopic hyperparathyroidism (pseudohyperparathyroidism).

Patients with sepsis, including Legionnaires' disease and other respiratory infections. Twenty-two percent of instances of respiratory infections had serum phosphorous $\leq$2.4 mg/dL.

Vitamin D deficiency; osteomalacia, inherited and sporadic forms of hypophosphatemic rickets. In work-up for osteomalacia, look for decreased calcium and phosphorus and increased alkaline phosphatase. Biopsy, however, can be abnormal even when these biochemical parameters are within normal limits.

Renal tubular disorders (Fanconi syndrome, renal tubular acidosis); use of antacids that bind phosphorus (look for hypercalciuria, low urinary phosphorus, high alkaline phosphatase); dialysis, vomiting; saline or lactate I.V.; steatorrhea, malabsorption, severe diarrhea, nasogastric suction; hypokalemia; negative nitrogen balance; decreased dietary PO_4 intake; recovery from severe burn injury; salicylate poisoning; acute gout; tumor-related: described as including hemangiopericytomas (uncommon pathologic entities) and neurofibromatosis; transfusion of blood; arteriography.

The signs and symptoms of phosphate depletion may include neuromuscular, neuropsychiatric, gastrointestinal, skeletal, and cardiopulmonary systems. Manifestations usually are accompanied by serum levels <1.0 mg/dL (SI: <0.32 mmol/L).

Severe hypophosphatemia is most common in elderly patients and is often found in postoperative subjects.

Complications of hypophosphatemia: Effect on RBC 2,3-diphosphoglycerate and oxygen dissociation. Depression of myocardial function (contractibility), decreased cardiac output; respiratory failure and respiratory muscle weakness; increased incidence of sepsis, impairment of bactericidal activities. CNS consequences: polyradiculopathy, paresthesias, tremor, ataxia, weakness, slurred speech, stupor, coma, seizure; joint stiffness; myopathy; renal stones, hypercalciuria secondary to renal phosphate leak; insulin resistance, glucose intolerance. Rhabdomyolysis may complicate marked hypophosphatemia. A mortality rate of 20% is described in patients whose phosphorus concentration was 1.1-1.5 mg/dL (SI: 0.36-0.48 mmol/L).

Limitations Ninety-seven percent of hyperparathyroid subjects with normal renal function have <3.3 mg/dL serum phosphate, 80% <3.0 mg/dL and 40% <2.5 mg/dL. Collection of multiple data points throughout the day may help to establish the diagnosis of primary hyperparathyroidism in patients with borderline serum biochemistries. Thus, some hyperparathyroid patients have serum phosphorus levels within normal limits. Hemolysis, glassware contaminated with detergents, hyperbilirubinemia, or dysproteinemia may cause increased results. Spurious hyperphosphatemia may be due to increased serum triglycerides. Phosphorus measurement on the Du Pont aca® was reported to be low with I.V. mannitol administration. Falsely elevated serum phosphate concentrations have been reported in patients with multiple myeloma using a molybdate colorimetric assay on the Hitachi® 717. Drug effects have been summarized.

Contraindications Sampling not long after a phosphorus-containing enema can provide startlingly high PO_4 levels.

(Continued)

Phosphorus, Serum *(Continued)*

Methodology Phosphomolybdate – colorimetric; modified molybdate – enzymatic, colorimetric

Additional Information Increasing dietary intake of potassium has been reported to increase serum phosphate concentrations apparently by decreasing renal excretion of phosphate. During the last trimester of pregnancy, there is a sixfold increase in calcium and phosphorus accumulation as the fetus triples its weight. Plasma phosphorus concentrations may provide a useful means to assess response to phosphate supplements in the premature infant.

Specific References

Bourke E and Yanagawa M, "Assessment of Hyperphosphatemia and Hypophosphatemia," *Clin Lab Med*, 1993, 13(1):183-207.

Chan GM, Mileur L, and Hansen JW, "Calcium and Phosphorus Requirements in Bone Mineralization of Preterm Infants," *J Pediatr*, 1988, 113(1 Pt 2):225-9.

Gravelyn TR, Brophy N, Siegert C, et al, "Hypophosphatemia-Associated Respiratory Muscle Weakness in a General Inpatient Population," *Am J Med*, 1988, 84(5):870-6.

Hanukoglu A, Chalew SA, Sun CJ, et al, "Surgically Curable Hypophosphatemic Rickets. Diagnosis and Management," *Clin Pediatr (Phila)*, 1989, 28(7):321-5.

Laaban J-P, Waked M, Laromiguiere M, et al, "Hypophosphatemia Complicating Management of Acute Severe Asthma," *Ann Intern Med*, 1990, 112(1):68-9.

O'Connor LR, Klein KL, and Bethume JE, "Hyperphosphatemia in Lactic Acidosis," *N Engl J Med*, 1977, 297(13):707-9.

Peach H, Compston JE, Vedi S, et al, "Value of Plasma Calcium, Phosphate, and Alkaline Phosphatase Measurements in the Diagnosis of Histological Osteomalacia," *J Clin Pathol*, 1982, 35(6):625-30.

Tieder M, Modai D, Samuel R, et al, "Hereditary Hypophosphatemic Rickets With Hypercalciuria," *N Engl J Med*, 1985, 312(10):611-7.

Watchko J, Bifano EM, and Bergstrom WH, "Effect of Hyperventilation on Total Calcium, Ionized Calcium, and Serum Phosphorus in Neonates," *Crit Care Med*, 1984, 12(12):1055-6.

Weintraub Z, Iancu TC, Sheinfeld M, et al, "Urinary and Blood Levels of Adenosine 3',5'-Monophosphate, Phosphorus, and Calcium in Infants," *Biol Neonate*, 1989, 55(4-5):233-7.

***Phthirus pubis* Identification** *see* Arthropod Identification *on page 1198*

pH, Urine

Test Includes pH is part of a routine urinalysis.

Specimen Random urine

Volume 5 mL

Minimum Volume 2 mL

Container Plastic urine container

Storage Instructions If the specimen cannot be processed promptly, it should be refrigerated.

Causes for Rejection Improper labeling, specimen not refrigerated

Reference Range 4.5-7.8; normal kidneys can produce urine with pH from 4.5-8.2, but with ordinary diet, urine pH is about 6.0. Urine becomes more alkaline after meals and is most acidic fasting in the morning.

Use Urine pH is a crude measure of the acid-base balance of the body. It may be helpful in determining subtle presence of distal renal tubular disease or pyelonephritis. Urine pH is useful for identifying crystals in urine and determining predisposition to form a given type of stone. See table. When an accurate pH assessment of acid-base status and renal response is desired, the urine should be collected under circumstances more controlled than is usual. Attention is given to the time of day, the fasting status of the patient, and transfer of sample so as to prevent degaussing of sample or growth of bacteria; rapid analysis by pH meter rather than dipstick is indicated. Usually simultaneous serum pH is then also ordered.

Conditions Associated With Acid Urine	Conditions Associated With Alkaline Urine	
Metabolic acidosis	Respiratory alkalosis	Postprandial alkaline tide (1 hour after meal)
Diabetes mellitus	Metabolic alkalosis	Fanconi's syndrome and Milkman's syndrome (increased urinary loss of bicarbonate)
Diarrhea	Urea-splitting bacteria (*Proteus* sp)	Alkali therapy (citrate, bicarbonate)
Starvation	Vegetable diet	
Respiratory acidosis	Gastric suction and vomiting	
Emphysema	Diuretic therapy	
Sleep		
Renal failure with lack of NH_3 buffer		

Limitations On standing urine becomes alkaline due to the action of urea splitting bacteria (*Proteus* sp).

Methodology Dipstick double indicator principle (methyl red and bromthymol blue) which gives a broad range of colors covering the urinary pH range 5-9 ±0.5 pH units. A pH meter is the back-up and most accurate method.

Additional Information Dietary factors affect urine pH. Alkaline urine is observed in persons who eat large quantities of citrus fruit and vegetables. Acid urine is observed with high meat intake. Pyridium® metabolites may mask the pH reaction. Urine pH >6.5 indicates presence of bicarbonate while pH <5.5 indicates absence of bicarbonate. Consistently acid urine, pH <5.5, is associated with xanthine, cystine, and uric acid stones. Calcium oxalate and apatite stones are not associated with any particular disturbance of urine pH. Alkaline urine (pH >7) is associated with calcium carbonate, calcium phosphate, and especially magnesium ammonium phosphate stones. In conjunction with serum pH and bicarbonate levels, urine pH may be applied to the study of renal tubular acidification.

Specific References

Cogan MG and Rector FC Jr, "Acid-Base Disorders," *Kidney*, Chapter 18, Brenner BM and Rector FC Jr, eds, Philadelphia, PA: WB Saunders Co, 1991, 737-804.

Schumann GB and Schweitzer SC, "Examination of Urine," *Clinical Diagnosis and Management by Laboratory Methods*, Chapter 17, Henry JB, ed, Philadelphia, PA: WB Saunders Co, 1991, 398-400.

Ziyadeh FN and Goldfarb S, "XII Nephrolithiasis," *Sci Am*, 1993, 1-10.

Placidyl® *see* Ethchlorvynol, Blood *on page 1261*

Plasma Cholinesterase *see* Pseudocholinesterase, Serum *on page 1340*

Plasma Electrolytes *see* Electrolytes, Blood *on page 1254*

Platinum, Blood

Synonyms Pt, Blood

Specimen Blood

Volume 10 mL

Minimum Volume 1 mL serum or plasma

Container Red top tube or green top (sodium heparin) tube

Storage Instructions Refrigerate specimen. Do not separate.

Use Evaluate platinum toxicity, usually from the use of cis-platinum for cancer chemotherapy and occasionally from industrial exposure

Methodology Flameless atomic absorption spectrophotometry (AA)

Additional Information Since normal biological fluids are free from detectable platinum, quantitation enables direct correlation between exposure and distribution in the body. Symptoms of platinum toxicity include impaired renal function, sensorineural hearing loss, anemia, and peripheral neuropathies.

Platinum, Urine

Synonyms Pt, Urine

Specimen Random urine

Volume 100 mL

Minimum Volume 5 mL

Container Plastic urine container

Storage Instructions Refrigerate.

Use Monitor platinum excretion during chemotherapy or industrial exposure

Methodology Flameless atomic absorption spectrophotometry (AA), high performance liquid chromatography (HPLC), voltametry

Additional Information Since normal biological fluids are free from detectable platinum, quantitation enables direct correlation between exposure and distribution in the body. Symptoms of platinum toxicity include impaired renal function, sensorineural hearing loss, anemia, and peripheral neuropathies.

Specific References

Drummer OH, Proudfoot A, Howes L, et al, "High Performance Liquid Chromatographic Determination of Platinum (II) in Plasma Ultrafiltrate and Urine: Comparison With a Flameless Atomic Absorption Spectrometric Method," *Clin Chim Acta*, 1984, 136(1):65-74.

Schmid GM and Atherton DR, "Voltammetric Determination of Platinum From Aqueous Solutions and Urine," *Anal Chem*, 1986, 58(9):1956-9.

pO_2 *see* Blood Gases, Arterial *on page 1207*

PO_4, Blood *see* Phosphorus, Serum *on page 1322*

Poisonous Metals, Blood *see* Heavy Metal Screen, Blood *on page 1271*

Poisonous Metals, Urine *see* Heavy Metal Screen, Urine *on page 1272*

Polyspecific Direct Antiglobulin *see* Antiglobulin Test, Direct *on page 1195*

Poppy Seeds *see* Opiates, Qualitative, Urine *on page 1309*

Porphobilinogen *see* Porphyrins, Quantitative, Urine *on this page*

Porphyrins, Erythrocytes *see* Porphyrins, Quantitative, Urine *on this page*

Porphyrins, Feces *see* Porphyrins, Quantitative, Urine *on this page*

Porphyrins, Plasma *see* Porphyrins, Quantitative, Urine *on this page*

Porphyrins, Quantitative, Urine

Related Information

Coproporphyrin Screen, Urine *on page 1242*
Protoporphyrin, Free Erythrocyte *on page 1339*

Applies To Porphobilinogen; Porphyrins, Erythrocytes; Porphyrins, Feces; Porphyrins, Plasma; Uroporphyrins

Test Includes Uroporphyrins (octacarboxylporphyrins), heptacarboxylporphyrins, hexacarboxylporphyrins, pentacarboxylporphyrins, coproporphyrins (tetracarboxylporphyrins)

Abstract Porphyrins are byproducts of porphyrinogens. Accumulations of either cause porphyrias, which are characterized by increased excretion of porphyrins, porphyrinogens, or their precursors. Such precursors include delta aminolevulinic acid and porphobilinogen. The disease entities relate to specific enzyme defects.

Patient Preparation Avoid alcohol and excessive fluid intake during collection. Phenothiazines may cause misleading porphobilinogen results.

Specimen 24-hour urine

Volume Entire collection

Container Clean, dark container. Must be kept covered.

Collection Check with laboratory; 5 g sodium bicarbonate is usually added to container before collection. Instruct the patient to void at 8 AM and discard the specimen. Then collect all urine including the final specimen voided at the end of the 24-hour collection period (ie, 8 AM the next morning). Specimen should be kept cool during collection. Container must be labeled with patient's name, date and time collection started, and date and time collection finished. Transport specimen immediately to the laboratory upon completion of collection. Adjust to pH 6-7 with sodium bicarbonate.

Storage Instructions Refrigerate during collection. Protect collection from light.

Special Instructions Do **not** expose to light.

Reference Range See literature from individual laboratory.

Use Evaluate porphyrias, including those involving deficiencies of enzymes which are needed for heme synthesis and chemical porphyrias.

In **congenital erythropoietic porphyria**, elevations of urinary uroporphyrin and coproporphyrin occur, with the former exceeding the latter.

In **acute intermittent porphyria**, porphobilinogen and delta aminolevulinic acid are elevated in acute attacks, and mild increases of urinary uroporphyrin and coproporphyrin may be found. Porphobilinogen is increased in many but not all patients with acute intermittent porphyria in latent periods. Quantitative porphobilinogen is a better test than delta aminolevulinic acid overall for acute intermittent porphyria, but both are used (as well as the Watson-Schwartz test).

Coproporphyrin and porphobilinogen excretion in urine are markedly increased during acute attacks of **hereditary coproporphyria**, increase of urinary uroporphyrin may be found, and increased fecal coproporphyrin III is described.

In **variegate porphyria** in acute attacks, results are similar to those of acute intermittent porphyria. Porphobilinogen and ALA are prone to become normal between attacks. Urine coproporphyrin exceeds uroporphyrin excretion during acute attacks.

Chemical porphyrias occur. Porphyrinogenic chemicals include certain halogenated hydrocarbons which cause the excretion of increased uroporphyrin.

In **lead poisoning** elevation of delta aminolevulinic acid greater than that of porphobilinogen occurs and porphobilinogen may be normal. Urinary coproporphyrin characteristically is increased. Free erythrocyte protoporphyrin is increased. Toxins such as lead interfere with heme synthesis and cause porphyrinuria.

Increased urine excretion of uroporphyrinogen, uroporphyrin, and coproporphyrin occurs in **porphyria cutanea tarda**. It is found in middle-aged men who like ethanol, young women on oral contraceptives, and in subjects on dialysis. These patients do not excrete increased porphobilinogen, but may have slight elevations of delta aminolevulinic acid.

Limitations Increased porphobilinogen may occur in patients on oral contraceptives. This test and delta aminolevulinic acid will not detect protoporphyria. Coproporphyrinuria alone lacks specificity and sensitivity for lead screening. Erythrocyte uroporphyrinogen-I-synthase is decreased in latent acute intermittent porphyria, and is needed in patients with possible latent acute intermittent porphyria. Quantitative porphobilinogen is of value in active and in many cases of latent acute intermittent porphyria, but will miss some of the latter when compared to red cell uroporphyrinogen-I-synthase.

Increased urine porphyrin excretion may be secondary to other diseases (eg, hepatobiliary diseases), especially coproporphyrin excretion. These are secondary porphyrinurias. They lack increased urinary porphobilinogen or Δ-ALA, with the important exception of lead poisoning.

Methodology Chromatography, fluorometry, high performance liquid chromatography (HPLC)

Additional Information The table provides an abbreviated overview of the porphyrias. Porphyrin fractionation of plasma can be done. Increases of urine porphyrins are found with congenital erythropoietic porphyria, acute intermittent porphyria, hereditary coproporphyria, variegate porphyria, and porphyria cutanea tarda.

Porphyrias: Overview of Some Clinical Aspects and Chemical Findings

Disorder	Inheritance	Age of Clinical Onset	Primary Organ Involvement	Useful Tests	Primary Symptoms
Congenital erythropoietic porphyria Günther's disease	Autosomal recessive Rare	Birth — 5 y	Erythroid cells	Urinary porphyrins Fecal porphyrins Red cell porphyrins sometimes useful	Severe photosensitivity Red urine Stains diapers Hemolytic anemia
Acute intermittent porphyria Precipitating causes include barbiturates, hydantoins, sulfonamides	Autosomal dominant Most common acute hepatic porphyria in U.S.	Adults	Hepatic, probably erythroid cells	Urine porphobilinogen Urine porphyrins Urinary delta aminolevulinic acid Erythrocyte uroporphyrinogen-1-synthase Fecal porphyrins	Mild to severe neurologic/visceral symptoms Acute attacks
Hereditary coproporphyria	Autosomal dominant	Adults	Hepatic, possibly erythroid cells	Urine porphobilinogen Urine porphyrins including coproporphyrin Fecal porphyrins Erythrocyte uroporphyrinogen-1-synthase Plasma porphyrins	Similar to variegate porphyria Acute attacks
Variegate porphyria	Autosomal dominant	Adults	Hepatic, possibly erythroid cells	Urine porphobilinogen Urine porphyrins Fecal porphyrins Plasma porphyrins Erythrocyte uroporphyrinogen-1-synthase	Mild to severe photosensitivity and neurologic/visceral symptoms Acute attacks
Porphyria cutanea tarda	Unknown Most common porphyria in U.S.	Adults	Hepatic, possibly erythroid cells	Urine porphyrins Plasma porphyrins	Similar to variegate porphyria Photosensitization Liver damage
Protoporphyria	Autosomal dominant	Usually childhood	Erythroid cells, probably liver	Erythrocytic, plasma and fecal porphyrins	Photosensitization Liver damage
Acquired (intoxication) porphyria	Acquired	Children and adults	Hepatic, erythroid cells	Erythrocyte porphyrins Urinary delta aminolevulinic acid Urine porphobilinogen Urine porphyrins Fecal porphyrins	Mild photosensitivity

From Bauer JD, *Clinical Laboratory Methods*, 9th ed, St Louis, MO: Mosby-Year Book Inc, 1982, 707, with permission.

(Continued)

Porphyrins, Quantitative, Urine *(Continued)*

Fecal porphyrin examination for hereditary coproporphyria, variegate porphyria, and protoporphyria can be used for adult patients. Stool examination for coproporphyrin and protoporphyrin is recommended for diagnosis of variegate porphyria.

Neurologic dysfunction occurs in the **hepatic porphyrias**, the types of porphyria in which acute attacks develop: acute intermittent porphyria, variegate porphyria, hereditary coproporphyria, and ALA dehydrase deficiency. Abdominal pain, caused by autonomic neuropathy, occurs with acute attacks (eg, acute intermittent porphyria). It is the most common symptom of acute intermittent porphyria.

Cutaneous aspects of the porphyrias are caused by photosensitization (eg, porphyria cutanea tarda, protoporphyria).

Hepatic complications are found with **porphyria cutanea tarda** and **protoporphyria**. Fluorescence is demonstrable in liver biopsies from patients with the former, as well as siderosis. Crystalline deposits may be found in protoporphyria. The amount of porphobilinogen excreted in acute intermittent porphyria is usually greater than the excretion of delta aminolevulinic acid (Δ-ALA). When there is more Δ-ALA, another diagnosis should be considered, including lead poisoning, another type of porphyria, or hereditary tyrosinemia. See also Protoporphyrin, Free Erythrocyte, which pertains to lead poisoning, and erythropoietic protoporphyria. The differential diagnosis of lead poisoning is relevant.

Specific References

Billett HH, "Porphyrias: Inborn Errors in Heme Production," *Hosp Pract (Off Ed)*, 1988, 23(9A):40-2, 44-5, 50.

Deacon AC, "Performance of Screening Tests for Porphyria," *Ann Clin Biochem*, 1988, 25(Pt 4):392-7.

Elder GH, "Recent Advances in the Identification of Enzyme Deficiencies in the Porphyrias," *Br J Dermatol*, 1983, 108(6):729-34.

Elder GH, Urquhart AJ, De Salamanca RE, et al, "Immunoreactive Uroporphyrinogen Decarboxylase in the Liver in Porphyria Cutanea Tarda," *Lancet*, 1985, 2(8449):229-33.

Ellefson RD, "Porphyrinogens, Porphyrins, and the Porphyrias," *Mayo Clin Proc*, 1982, 57(7):454-8.

Galbraith RA, Sassa S, and Kappas A, "A Comparison of the Utility of Dowex Resin and Polybenzimidazole Aurorez Resin in the Determination of Urinary Porphobilinogen Concentrations," *Clin Chim Acta*, 1987, 164(2):235-9.

Kimbrough RD, "Porphyrins and Hepatotoxicity," *Ann N Y Acad Sci*, 1987, 514:289-96.

Leahy DT and Brien TG, "A Simple Method for the Separation and Quantification of Urinary Porphyrins," *J Clin Pathol*, 1982, 35(11):1232-5.

Ostrowski J, "Urinary Excretion of Porphyrins and Their Precursors in Chronic Liver Disease," *Mater Med Pol*, 1985, 17(4):240-5.

Pimstone NR, Gandhi SN, and Mukerji SK, "Therapeutic Efficacy of Oral Charcoal in Congenital Erythropoietic Porphyria," *N Engl J Med*, 1987, 316(7):390-3.

Rose IS, Young GP, St John DJ, et al, "Effect of Ingestion of Hemoproteins on Fecal Excretion of Hemes and Porphyrins," *Clin Chem*, 1989, 35(12):2290-6.

Scully RE, Mark EJ, and McNeely BU, "Case 39-1984: (Coproporphyria With Neuropathy), Presentation of Case," *Case Records of the Massachusetts General Hospital*, 1984, 839-47.

Stevens JF, "A Regional Quality Control Scheme for Urine Porphyrins," *Ann Clin Biochem*, 1989, 26(Pt 2):189-90.

Strik JJ, "Porphyrins in Urine as an Indication of Exposure to Chlorinated Hydrocarbons," *Ann N Y Acad Sci*, 1987, 514:219-21.

Toback AC, Sassa S, Poh-Fitzpatrick MB, et al, "Hepatoerythropoietic Porphyria: Clinical, Biochemical, and Enzymatic Studies in a Three-Generation Family Lineage," *N Engl J Med*, 1987, 316(11):645-50.

Westerlund J, Pudek M, and Schreiber WE, "A Rapid and Accurate Spectrofluorometric Method for Quantification and Screening of Urinary Porphyrins," *Clin Chem*, 1988, 34(2):345-51.

Pot *see* Cannabinoids, Qualitative *on page 1217*

Potassium, Arterial *see* Potassium, Blood *on this page*

Potassium, Blood

Synonyms K^+, Plasma; K^+, Serum

Applies To Electrolytes, Serum or Plasma; Potassium, Arterial

Abstract The major intracellular cation, potassium is very commonly measured as one of the serum or plasma electrolytes and as a urinary electrolyte as well.

Specimen Blood

Volume 10 mL

Minimum Volume 1 mL serum or plasma

Container Red top tube or green top (heparin) tube

Collection Avoid very small needles if possible. Avoid stasis, use of tourniquet, and hand-clenching if possible. Avoid potassium-containing tubes such as potassium oxalate. Potassium can be reported from arterial as well as from venous blood. If arterial puncture is done for pO_2, plasma can be tested for sodium, potassium, and chloride so long as lithium and not potassium heparinate anticoagulant is used.

Storage Instructions Remove plasma or serum from red cells within 4 hours before specimen is refrigerated.

Causes for Rejection Hemolyzed specimen, serum specimen not removed from clot in patient with high platelet count. Such specimens may be analyzed but the likelihood of a falsely high potassium level must be recognized and stated in report. Preferably, sample should be rejected.

Reference Range Plasma: 3.5-5.0 mmol/L (SI: 3.5-5.0 mmol/L). Add **approximately** 0.1 to normal ranges if serum is sampled rather than plasma. Pediatric ranges are sometimes reported as slightly higher than adult levels. Differences may well relate to the amount of hemolysis in specimens used to establish normal ranges. In daily practice some degree of hemolysis may occur in neonatal and pediatric specimens. Although grossly hemolyzed specimens are usually rejected, the acceptability of samples with slight hemolysis is debatable. Even slight hemolysis can increase potassium results; red cells have an intracellular concentration of 100-120 mmol/L or more potassium.

Possible Panic Range Newborns: <2.5 mmol/L (SI: <2.5 mmol/L), >7.0 mmol/L (SI: >7.0 mmol/L); adults: <2.5 mmol/L (SI: <2.5 mmol/L), >6.5 mmol/L (SI: >6.5 mmol/L). With unanticipated high or low potassium, EKG may be indicated. If potassium is high and serum was used, examine peripheral blood smear for thrombocytosis and/or leukocytosis; obtain platelet and white count if indicated.

Use Evaluate electrolyte balance; potassium level should be followed especially in elderly patients, those on intravenous hyperalimentation, in patients on diuretic therapy and in cases of renal disease, particularly renal failure, patients on hemodialysis, and those with interstitial nephritis or nephropathy. Evaluate hypertension. Hyperkalemia may occur in and be caused by renal failure. Potassium should be monitored during treatment of acidosis, including ketoacidosis in diabetes mellitus. As one of the major electrolytes, potassium levels are a portion of regular assessment of acid-base balance and management of intravenous therapy.

Evaluate muscular weakness and irritability, mental confusion, weakness; manage leukemia, diseases of gastrointestinal tract including laxative abuse, large villous tumors, hepatic encephalopathy, emesis, fistulas and tube drainage; evaluate and prevent cardiac arrhythmias; evaluate alcoholism with delirium tremens; detect, diagnose, and manage mineralocorticoid excess (primary aldosteronism, Cushing's syndrome, tumor with ectopic ACTH production, some cases of congenital adrenal hyperplasia), heat stroke, licorice ingestion mineralocorticoid effect.

Limitations Inadequate sodium intake may mask the hypokalemia of aldosteronism; sodium loading in that setting may make hypokalemia recognizable. Heparinized plasma is probably the specimen of choice for potassium, because clotting causes cytolysis and may elevate serum values, usually but not always only slightly.

Since platelets release potassium during coagulation, samples from patients who have thrombocytosis (eg, some cases of polycythemia vera and other myeloproliferative diseases) will yield spuriously elevated potassium concentrations. Such "pseudohyperkalemia" may also occur in cases of leukemia with high WBC count (notably chronic myelogenous leukemia) as potassium is released from WBCs and platelets during clot formation. For such patients it is best to assay potassium on a heparinized sample. Pseudohyperkalemia in rheumatoid arthritis may be due to increased platelets. Graber et al conclude that serum potassium increases with the platelet count in normal subjects and in those with thrombocytosis, and that the increment is an artifact.

Methodology Flame emission photometry or ion-selective electrode (ISE)

Additional Information **Hypokalemia (low potassium)** has been found in >90% of hypertensive patients with primary aldosteronism (Conn's syndrome). This uncommon entity is a curable cause of hypertension. Low potassium occurs with endogenous or exogenous increase in other corticosteroids, including that in Cushing's syndrome as well as with dietary or parenteral deprivation of potassium (eg, parenteral therapy without adequate potassium replacement). Hypokalemia occurs with vomiting, diarrhea, fistulas, laxatives, diuretics, burns, excessive perspiration, Bartter's syndrome, some cases of alcoholism and folic acid deficiency, in alkalosis and in renal tubular acidosis, as well as in other entities. Drugs resulting in hypokalemia include beta agonists, theophylline, insulin, chloroquine, and barium.

Low potassium is much more significant with a low pH than with a high pH. When pH increases by 0.1, potassium decreases approximately 0.6 mmol/L. With low pH, as in ketoacidosis, as therapeutic adjustment towards normal is made, plasma/serum potassium levels will decrease. Phosphorus levels tend to follow potassium levels downwards during therapy of diabetic ketoacidosis; both are largely intracellular. With insulin therapy (and increased utilization of carbohydrate), potassium moves into cells and serum/plasma level falls. Hyperalimentation may have a similar effect. Hypokalemia has been reported in slightly >50% of a series of 32 patients with acute myelogenous leukemia, but thrombocytosis can increase serum potassium levels, *vide supra*.

Thiazide/chlorthalidone therapy may cause hyperuricemia and hypercalcemia as well as hypokalemia.

(Continued)

Potassium, Blood *(Continued)*

The watery diarrhea-hypokalemia-achlorhydria (WDHA) syndrome most often is related to vasoactive intestinal polypeptide (VIP).

Consider magnesium status in patients who have hypokalemia.

Hyperkalemia (high potassium) reflects generally inadequate renal excretion, mobilization of potassium from the tissues, or excessive intake or administration. Hyperkalemia occurs with hemolysis, trauma, with administration of potassium salts of some drugs, Addison's disease, acidosis, insulin lack, with increased osmolality (eg, glucose, mannitol), and in other entities as well as with renal diseases. Increased potassium can occur with potassium-sparing diuretics, nonsteroidal anti-inflammatory drugs, especially in the presence of renal disease. Systemic heparin therapy can suppress aldosterone release and increase potassium, especially in the presence of other factors. Digitalis poisoning can also result in hyperkalemia.

Specific References

Alpern RJ and Toto RD, "Hypokalemic Nephropathy - A Clue to Cystogenesis?" *N Engl J Med*, 1990, 322(6):398-9.

Bradberry SM and Vale JA, "Disturbances of Potassium Homeostasis in Poisoning," *J Toxicol Clin Toxicol*, 1995, 33(4):295-310.

Brem AS, "Disorders of Potassium Homeostasis," *Pediatr Clin North Am*, 1990, 37(2):419-27.

Corr LA, Grounds RM, Beacham JL, et al, "Effects of Circulating Endogenous Catecholamines on Plasma Glucose, Potassium, and Magnesium," *Clin Sci*, 1990, 78(2):185-91.

Jensen MD, Braun JS, Vetter RJ, et al, "Measurement of Body Potassium With a Whole-Body Counter: Relationship Between Lean Body Mass and Resting Energy Expenditure," *Mayo Clin Proc*, 1988, 63(9):864-8.

Kassirer JP and Harrington JT, "Fending Off the Potassium Pushers," *N Engl J Med*, 1985, 312(12):785-7.

Latta K, Hisano S, and Chan JC, "Perturbations in Potassium Balance," *Clin Lab Med*, 1993, 13(1):149-56.

Maffly RH, "Renal Function and Disorders of Water, Sodium, and Potassium Balance," *Scientific American Medicine*, Section 10, Chapter 1, Rubenstein E and Federman DD, eds, New York, NY: Scientific American Inc, 1990, 2-34.

Pierson RN Jr and Wang J, "Body Composition Denominators for Measurements of Metabolism: What Measurements Can Be Believed?" *Mayo Clin Proc*, 1988, 63(9):947-9.

Quamme GA, "Laboratory Evaluation of Magnesium Status: Renal Function and Free Intracellular Magnesium Concentration," *Clin Lab Med*, 1993, 13(1):209-23.

Solomon R, Weinberg MS, and Dubey A, "The Diurnal Rhythm of Plasma Potassium: Relationship to Diuretic Therapy," *J Cardiovasc Pharmacol*, 1991, 17(5):854-9.

Tietz NW, Pruden EL, and Siggaard-Anderson O, "Electrolytes," *Fundamentals of Clinical Chemistry*, 3rd ed, Tietz NW, ed, Philadelphia, PA: WB Saunders Co, 1987, 616-20.

Torres VE, Young WF Jr, Offord KP, et al, "Association of Hypokalemia, Aldosteronism, and Renal Cysts," *N Engl J Med*, 1990, 322(6):345-51.

Young WF Jr, Hogan MJ, Klee GG, et al, "Primary Aldosteronism: Diagnosis and Treatment," *Mayo Clin Proc*, 1990, 65(1):96-110.

Potassium or Sodium Cyanide *see* Cyanide, Blood *on page 1246*

Potassium Thiocyanate (KCN) *see* Thiocyanate, Blood or Urine *on page 1360*

Pre-employment Drug Screen *see* Drugs of Abuse Screen, Urine *on page 1252*

Pregnancy Test

Synonyms Beta-Subunit Human Chorionic Gonadotropin, Urine or Serum; hCG, Slide Test, Stat; hCG, Urine; Human Chorionic Gonadotropin, Urine; β-Subunit of hCG

Specimen Urine or blood; first voided morning specimen is preferred if urine is tested (to obtain most concentrated specimen).

Volume 5 mL

Minimum Volume 2 mL

Container Plastic urine container or red top tube

Storage Instructions Urine stable 4 hours at 25°C and 3 days at 4°C. Serum should be frozen at -20°C if not run within 48 hours.

Causes for Rejection Urine specimen grossly contaminated with blood or bacteria, inadequate labeling, low specific gravity, proteinuria, gross lipemia or turbidity

Special Instructions Centrifuge turbid urine specimens prior to testing.

Reference Range Normal males and nonpregnant females: negative; normal pregnant females: positive. Sensitivity and specificity of β-subunit two point RIA or EIA tests may allow early diagnosis of pregnancy, within 6 days after conception.

Use Diagnose pregnancy; screen for women at risk of being pregnant prior to performance of x-ray, sterilization, menstrual regulation, and curettage procedures and/or prior to the initiation of gestation/embryo/fetal potentially injurious medication; detect and/or evaluate incomplete/complete abortions; detect ectopic gestation; screen for gestational trophoblastic neoplasia or ectopic hCG producing tumor. (A sensitive and quantitative test for the presence of hCG is preferable for these applications.)

Limitations Results may be negative in early pregnancy or whenever specific gravity is low. Large amounts of protein or phenothiazines may result in false-positive results with use of some earlier slide/tube tests, depending upon commercial supplier and technical characteristics of the test. In early pregnancy, incomplete abortion, recent complete abortion, ectopic pregnancy (in which hCG level is low), slide test end points may be difficult to interpret. Tube tests are generally more easily read than slide tests. Methods using covalent bonded latex particles and tests producing macroagglutination are more reliably interpreted.

Methodology Slide or tube agglutination-inhibition tests (urine), false-negative and false-positive results may occur. β-Subunit hCG by radioimmunoassay (serum or urine); immunoradiometric (IRMA) (eg, Tandem® hCG which incorporates two monoclonal antibodies, each with immunospecificity for different sites on the hCG molecule, one coated on a plastic bead on which the solid phase develops). Enzyme immunoassay, including sensitive (to 20-40 mIU/mL level of hCG, SI: 20-40 IU/L) two-point urine or serum qualitative/quantitative membrane based tests of which Tandem® ICON® is most well known.

Additional Information Pregnancy testing is usually performed on urine. It is based on the the detection of human chorionic gonadotropin (hCG). Levels of hCG in the urine approach those seen in serum. In normal pregnancy, hCG levels rise at implantation and peak at 8-12 weeks. Although newer urine pregnancy tests are quite sensitive, false-negatives can occur early in gestation. In such cases, if ectopic pregnancy is suspected, serum hCG assays may be of value.

Early in the first trimester of pregnancy (1-2 weeks) serum hCG levels are from 50-500 mIU/mL (SI: 50-500 IU/L). Current generation sensitive tests can detect pregnancy shortly (2-3 days) after implantation of the ovum. By 3-4 weeks of gestation, hCG is at the 500-10,000 mIU/mL level (SI: 500-10,000 IU/L). Serum hCG level peaks during the second to third month of gestation (30,000-100,000 mIU/mL) (SI: 30,000-100,000 IU/L). Use of serum for pregnancy testing may provide greater sensitivity, of special value in cases of early pregnancy, and is of greater value in serial testing for follow-up of an abnormal gestation (eg, ectopic pregnancy or a gestational trophoblastic neoplasm). If serum (or urine) hCG levels do not appear to correlate with the anticipated clinical situation, periodic repeat hCG determinations may be helpful. If there is demise of the developing embryo/fetus (eg, ectopic pregnancy), hCG levels will fall. Because of slow clearance from the serum, hCG may be detected in serum/urine for as long as 4 weeks following abortion.

Currently, the tests most commonly used to screen for pregnancy are two-point EIA "concentration" methods. A variety of different forms are commercially available. An antibody (frequently monoclonal) is immobilized on a membrane or other solid phase and the sample hCG is "concentrated" in a small central area of the surface (a membrane, bead, paddle, tube, or dipstick). Color development occurs within minutes of addition of enzyme tagged monoclonal anti-β-hCG. These tests are sensitive, specific, and fast. They have largely supplanted slide/tube screening procedures.

A study of specificity (six commercially available ELISA urine pregnancy tests) utilizing specimens from men and postmenopausal females found variable performance by the different methods, not explained by review of the medical records. Test systems with provision for a negative reference area gave fewer false-positive results (had greater specificity). Correlation was found between mucous content of the postmenopausal female group's urine samples and the incidence of false-positive hCG results.

One year of routine use of Tandem® ICON® system for urine pregnancy testing (University of Texas) did not result in a report of known false-positive results. Stability of color development after addition of color reagents and presence or absence of a built in positive control could influence choice of a test system for routine use.

Serum progesterone levels used with beta-hCG levels may assist in differentiating normal intrauterine from abnormal intrauterine or ectopic pregnancy (cutoff point 15 ng/mL) (SI: 48 nmol/L). Beta-hCG and progesterone levels are lower in abnormal pregnancies. Less overlap occurs, however, between progesterone (as compared to beta-hCG) values in normal versus ectopic and abnormal pregnancies. When a positive pregnancy test is obtained, differential considerations should include the possibility of simultaneous intrauterine and extrauterine gestations (albeit unlikely) and the possibility of passively acquired hCG as in an individual recently transfused with fresh frozen plasma prepared from pregnant donors.

A number of commercially successful home pregnancy tests have been introduced. They have been found to vary widely in performance (optimal accuracy, sensitivity, specificity, human factor useability). A study of the use of such home pregnancy test kits has resulted in the suggestion that pharmacists have an opportunity in taking a more active role in promoting the appropriate use of such self-testing products.

Specific References

Aziz K, "Sensitivity and Specificity of Pregnancy Tests," *Am Clin Lab*, 1989, 8:12, 5-6.

(Continued)

Pregnancy Test *(Continued)*

Bandi ZL, Schoen I, and DeLara M, "Enzyme-Linked Immunosorbent Urine Pregnancy Tests: Clinical Specificity Studies," *Am J Clin Pathol*, 1987, 87(2):236-42.

Boutiette LA and Anderson GV Jr, "Heterotopic Pregnancy," *J Emerg Med*, 1989, 7(1):33-5.

Christensen H, Thyssen HH, Schebye O, et al, "Three Highly Sensitive "Bedside" Serum and Urine Tests for Pregnancy Compared," *Clin Chem*, 1990, 36(9):1686-8.

Coons SJ, "A Look at the Purchase and Use of Home Pregnancy Test Kits," *Am Pharm*, 1989, NS29(4):46-8.

Fields SA and Toffler WL, "Pregnancy Testing – Home and Office," *West J Med*, 1991, 154(3):327-8.

Hohnadel DC and Kaplan LA, "Hormones and Their Metabolites; β-hCG (β-Human Chorionic Gonadotropin)," *Clinical Chemistry – Theory, Analysis, and Correlation*, 2nd ed, Kaplan LA and Pesce AJ, eds, St Louis, MO: Mosby-Year Book Inc, 1989, 938-44.

Kruskall MS, Owings DV, Donovan LM et al, "Passive Transfusion of Human Chorionic Gonadotropin from Plasma Donated During Pregnancy," *Vox Sang*, 1989, 56(2):71-4.

Latman NS and Bruot BC, "Evaluation of Home Pregnancy Test Kits," *Biomed Instrum Technol*, 1989, 23(2):144-9.

Lee T, "Human Chorionic Gonadotropin Assays and Their Uses," *Obstet Gynecol Clin North Am*, 1988, 15:457-75.

Norman RJ, "Analytical and Clinical Sensitivity and Specificity in Pregnancy Testing," *Am J Obstet Gynecol*, 1989, 161(3):835-6.

Norman RJ, Gilmore TA, and McLoughlin JW, "Simple Quantitative Measurement of Serum Choriogonadotropin Compared With Immunoradiometric, Immunoenzymometric, and Chemiluminescent Assays," *Clin Chem*, 1992, 38(1):144-7.

Riss PA, Radivojevic K, and Bieglmayer C, "Serum Progesterone and Human Chorionic Gonadotropin in Very Early Pregnancy: Implications for Clinical Management," *Eur J Obstet Gynecol Reprod Biol*, 1989, 32(2):71-7.

Taylor CA Jr, Overstreet JW, Samuels SJ, et al, "Prospective Assessment of Early Fetal Loss Using An Immunoenzymometric Screening Assay for Detection of Urinary Human Chorionic Gonadotropin," *Fertil Steril*, 1992, 57(6):1220-4.

Presamine® *see* Imipramine, Blood *on page 1274*

Primidone, Blood

Synonyms Majsolin®; Mylepsin®; Mysoline®; Prysolin®

Applies To Metabolites of Primidone; PEMA; Phenylethylmalonamide

Test Includes Phenobarbital, PEMA

Abstract Primidone is indicated for generalized tonic-clonic and partial seizures.

Specimen Blood

Volume 5 mL

Minimum Volume 2 mL serum or plasma

Container Red top tube, green top (heparin) tube, or lavender top (EDTA) tube

Sampling Time Trough or consistent sampling time. Levels of phenobarbital and PEMA can be measured simultaneously.

Reference Range Children younger than 5 years of age: 7-10 μg/mL (SI: 32-46 μmol/L); adults: 5-12 μg/mL. Phenobarbital concentration can also be used to guide dosing.

Critical Values At levels >12 μg/mL (SI: >55 μmol/L) primidone produces CNS depression, vertigo, visual disturbances, areflexia, somnolence, and lethargy. Clinical toxicity correlates with primidone rather than metabolite concentrations. In overdosage, a biphasic peak may be seen with highest toxicity a few hours after ingestion and again 48 hours afterwards. Crystalluria is a feature of overdosage.

Possible Panic Range >12 μg/mL (SI: >55 μmol/L)

Use Monitor efficacy, compliance, and possible toxicity

Methodology Enzyme immunoassay (EIA), gas-liquid chromatography (GLC), high performance liquid chromatography (HPLC)

Additional Information Plasma half-life of primidone usually ranges from 6-8 hours with rapid elimination (24-40 hours). Since phenobarbital requires a longer interval (48 hours) to achieve therapeutic blood levels, checking both levels can be used to determine chronic compliance. The phenobarbital/primidone ratio normally is 2.5, can be higher (4.3 mean) in patients on other anticonvulsants (phenytoin, carbamazepine) and lower than normal among patients discontinued from those medicines or who are chronically noncompliant. Primidone decreases the effects of oral anticoagulants.

Specific References

Kutt H, "Phenobarbital: Interactions With Other Drugs," *Antiepileptic Drugs*, 3rd ed, Levy RH, Dreifuss FE, Mattson RH, et al, eds, New York, NY: Raven Press, 1989, 313-27.

Schafer H, "Primidone: Chemistry and Methods of Determination," *Antiepileptic Drugs*, 3rd ed, Levy RH, Dreifuss FE, Mattson RH, et al, eds, New York, NY: Raven Press, 1989, 379-90.

Proaccelerin *see* Factor V, Plasma *on page 1262*

Procainamide, Blood

Synonyms Pronestyl®

Applies To N-Acetyl Procainamide; NAPA

Test Includes Procainamide and its metabolite, N-acetyl procainamide (NAPA)

Abstract This drug is an antiarrhythmic with an active metabolite, N-acetyl procainamide. Both should be measured when TDM is used.

Specimen Blood

Volume 10 mL

Container Red top tube

Sampling Time Oral treatment: peak: 75 minutes after dose; trough: immediately before next dose. I.V. treatment: immediately after loading dose; 2, 6, 12, and 24 hours after starting I.V. maintenance.

Special Instructions One sample is an inadequate basis for evaluating dosing. Three steady-state levels should be obtained during one dosing interval. For therapeutic drug monitoring, consistently use the same time interval between sampling and dose administration when comparing results from serial samples.

Reference Range Therapeutic: procainamide: 4.0-10.0 μg/mL (SI: 17-42 μmol/L); sum of procainamide and N-acetyl procainamide: <30.0 μg/mL (SI: <127 μmol/L). Optimal ranges must be ascertained for individual patients with EKG monitoring.

Possible Panic Range Toxic: procainamide: >20.0 μg/mL (SI: >85 μmol/L); sum of procainamide and N-acetyl procainamide: >30.0 μg/mL (SI: >127 μmol/L).

Use Monitor therapeutic drug level

Limitations Severely hemolyzed, lipemic, or icteric specimens interfere with methods other than HPLC and GC. **Evaluation of toxicity must be made with consideration of patient's clinical status**.

Methodology Enzyme immunoassay (EIA), fluorescence polarization immunoassay (FPIA), enzyme-multiplied immunoassay (EMIT); high performance liquid chromatography (HPLC), gas chromatography (GC)

Additional Information The cardiac actions of this drug are similar to those of quinidine. It is used in a variety of arrhythmias. Procainamide usually is rapidly absorbed from the gastrointestinal tract. Peak blood levels are reached within 1 hour. Optimal plasma sampling time after oral dosage is 1-2 hours. Optimal sampling time after I.V. administration of dose is 30 minutes. The drug is converted by the liver to its active metabolite, N-acetyl procainamide (NAPA). The half-life of procainamide is 2-6 hours and for NAPA is 8 hours. Rate of metabolism is genetically determined (slow and fast acetylator types) contributing to significant interindividual variability. Impairment of renal function has pronounced effect on drug disposition, especially for NAPA. Patients with severe renal dysfunction generally have prolonged and highly variable half-life characteristics. Elimination half-life may be prolonged in geriatric subjects.

Specific References

Funck-Brentano C, Light RT, Lineberry MD, et al, "Pharmacokinetic and Pharmacodynamic Interaction of N-Acetyl Procainamide and Procainamide in Humans," *J Cardiovasc Pharmacol*, 1989, 14(3):364-73.

Gottlieb SS, Kukin ML, Medina N, et al, "Comparative Hemodynamic Effects of Procainamide, Tocainide, and Encainide in Severe Chronic Heart Failure," *Circulation*, 1990, 81(3):860-4.

Interian A Jr, Zaman L, Velez-Robinson E, et al, "Paired Comparisons of Efficacy of Intravenous and Oral Procainamide in Patients With Inducible Sustained Ventricular Tachyarrhythmias," *J Am Coll Cardiol*, 1991, 17(7):1581-6.

Yamaji A, Kataoka K, Oishi M, et al, "Simultaneous Determination of Procainamide and N-Acetylprocainamide in Serum by Gas Chromatography With Nitrogen-Selective Detection," *J Chromatogr*, 1987, 415(1):143-7.

Prochlorperazine, Blood

Synonyms Compazine®

Specimen Blood

Volume 10 mL

Minimum Volume 3 mL serum

Container Red top tube

Storage Instructions Refrigerate serum.

Reference Range None detected

Critical Values Toxic: >1 μg/mL

Use Monitor therapeutic drug level; evaluate toxicity

Methodology High performance liquid chromatography (HPLC)

Additional Information Prochlorperazine, a piperazine phenothiazine derivative, is used for the management of acute and chronic psychosis and to control severe nausea and vomiting. The onset of action for oral ingestion is 30-40 minutes, with a duration of 3-4 hours. The most notable adverse effect is extrapyramidal reactions, which are relatively high, especially in children. Other adverse effects include sedation, anxiety, pseudoparkinsonian signs and symptoms, seizures, urinary retention and constipation, hypotension, tachycardia, agranulocytosis, leukopenia, amenorrhea, galactorrhea, gynecomastia, and photosensitivity.

Prolixin® *see* Fluphenazine, Blood *on page 1268*

Pronestyl® *see* Procainamide, Blood *on previous page*

2-Propanol *see* Isopropanol, Blood *on page 1277*

Propoxyphene, Blood or Urine

Synonyms Darvocet-N®; Darvon®

Applies To Norpropoxyphene

Test Includes Quantitation of propoxyphene and metabolite norpropoxyphene

Abstract Propoxyphene is a narcotic analgesic and is also a drug of abuse.

Specimen Blood (TDM), urine (DAU)

Volume 7 mL

Container Red top tube, plastic urine container

Special Instructions If forensic, use chain-of-custody protocol and form.

Reference Range Therapeutic: serum: 0.1-0.4 μg/mL (SI: 0.3-1.2 μmol/L) (therapeutic ranges published vary between laboratories and may not correlate with clinical effect); urine (for DAU): negative (less than cutoff)

Critical Values Cutoff for urine: screen: 0.3 μg/mL; confirmation: 0.2 μg/mL

Possible Panic Range Toxic: serum: >0.5 μg/mL (SI: >1.5 μmol/L); minimal fatal: 1.0 μg/mL (SI: 2.9 μmol/L)

Use Therapeutic monitoring; toxicity assessment; drug-of-abuse testing

Methodology Immunoassay, gas chromatography (GC), high performance liquid chromatography (HPLC)

Additional Information Propoxyphene is an analgesic structurally similar to methadone. Its metabolite, norpropoxyphene is also pharmacologically active. Toxic effects include nausea, vomiting, and progressive central nervous system depression. Toxicity is additive with ethanol. Toxicity can be neutralized by narcotic antagonists. Peak serum level occurs 2 hours postoral dose, half-life is 8-24 hours. Propoxyphene can also be measured in urine as part of a drug of abuse screen.

Specific References

Gilman AG, Goodman LS, Rall TW, et al, *The Pharmacological Basis of Therapeutics*, 7th ed, New York, NY: Macmillan Publishing, 1985, 519-20.

Hartmann B, Miyada DS, Pirkle H, et al, "Serum Propoxyphene Concentrations in a Cohort of Opiate Addicts on Long-Term Propoxyphene Maintenance Therapy. Evidence for Drug Tolerance in Humans," *J Anal Toxicol*, 1988, 12(1):25-9.

Kurlan R, Majumdar L, Deeley C, et al, "A Controlled Trial of Propoxyphene and Naltrexone in Patients With Tourette's Syndrome," *Ann Neurol*, 1991, 30(1):19-23.

Oles KS, Mirza W, and Penry JK, "Catastrophic Neurologic Signs Due to Drug Interaction: Tegretol® and Darvon®," *Surg Neurol*, 1989, 32(2):144-51.

Propranolol, Blood

Synonyms Inderal®

Abstract A relatively short-acting beta blocker. Propranolol is used as an antiarrhythmic and antihypertensive.

Specimen Blood

Volume 5 mL

Container Red top tube

Sampling Time Trough: immediately prior to next dose

Special Instructions The stoppers of some blood collection tubes contain TBEP plasticizers that affect drug distribution in sample. Check with local laboratory.

Reference Range Therapeutic: 50-100 ng/mL (SI: 190-390 nmol/L) at end of dose interval

Possible Panic Range >1000 ng/mL (SI: >3860 nmol/L)

Use Monitor therapeutic drug level in patients with cardiac arrhythmias, angina pectoris, and hypertension; evaluate for potential toxicity

Methodology Fluorometry, fluorescence polarization immunoassay (FPIA), enzyme immunoassay (EIA), gas-liquid chromatography (GLC), high performance liquid chromatography (HPLC)

Additional Information Propranolol is well absorbed after oral administration. Its plasma half-life is 2-4 hours. For therapeutic drug monitoring, consistently use the same time interval between sampling and dose administration when comparing results from serial samples. A number of metabolites have been identified with at least one, 4-hydroxyl propranolol, having pharmacologic activity. Adverse effects of this drug include precipitation of heart failure, bronchospasm, bradycardia, and hypoglycemia. Hyperthyroidism exerts an age-dependent inducing effect on the metabolism of propranolol.

Specific References

Hall ST, Harding SM, Hassani H, et al, "The Pharmacokinetic and Pharmacodynamic Interaction Between Lacidipine and Propranolol in Health Volunteers," *J Cardiovasc Pharmacol*, 1991, 18(Suppl 11):S13-7.

Harrison PM, Tonkin AM, Dixon ST, et al, "Determination of Alpha-Naphthoxylactic Acid, A Major Metabolite of Propranolol, in Plasma by High-Performance Liquid Chromatography," *J Chromatogr*, 1986, 374(1):223-5.

Nace GS and Wood AJ, "Pharmacokinetics of Long-Acting Propranolol. Implications for Therapeutic Use," *Clin Pharmacokinet*, 1987, 13(1):51-64.

Walle T, Walle UK, Cowart TD, et al, "Pathway-Selective Sex Differences in the Metabolic Clearance of Propranolol in Human Subjects," *Clin Pharmacol Ther*, 1989, 46(3):257-63.

Propyl Alcohol *see* Isopropanol, Blood *on page 1277*

Protein, Quantitative, Urine

Test Includes Concomitant creatinine clearance is often indicated. Total urine creatinine should be included to help assure that a complete 24-hour collection was tested.

Abstract Quantitation of urinary protein loss.

Specimen 24-hour urine

Volume Entire collection

Minimum Volume 10 mL urine aliquot

Container Plain urine container

Collection Instruct patient to void at 8 AM and discard the specimen. Then collect all urine including the final specimen voided at the end of the 24-hour collection period (ie, 8 AM the next morning). Label the container with the patient's name and date and time collection started and finished.

Storage Instructions Refrigerate aliquot.

Reference Range 30-150 mg/24 hours (SI: 0.03-0.15 g/day) (method dependent) Proteinuria has been defined as 24-hour urine protein excretion >150 mg/24 hours (SI: >0.15 g/day). In infants and children, different ranges apply and have been published; proteinuria >100 mg/day (SI: >0.10 g/day) in children younger than 10 years of age is regarded as abnormal.

Use Evaluate proteinuria (eg, following urinalysis in which proteinuria is detected); evaluate renal diseases, including proteinuria complicating diabetes mellitus, the nephrotic syndromes (eg, lipoid nephrosis, membranous, proliferative glomerulopathies), metal poisoning (eg, gold, lead, and cadmium), renal vein thrombosis, systemic lupus erythematosus (SLE), constrictive pericarditis, and amyloidosis; work up other renal diseases including malignant hypertension, glomerulonephritis, Goodpasture's syndrome, Henoch-Schönlein purpura, thrombotic thrombocytopenic purpura, collagen diseases, cryoglobulinemia, toxemia of pregnancy, drug nephrotoxicity, hypersensitivity reactions, allergic reactions, and renal tubular lesions; management of myeloma and macroglobulinemia of Waldenström (Bence Jones proteinuria); evaluate hypoproteinemia; tubular proteinurias include Wilson's disease and Fanconi syndrome. Even in the table shown, some renal lesions are not easily categorized (eg, the glomerular lesions of chrysotherapy) and of toxemia of pregnancy.

Limitations Although evaluation for proteinuria may be the best single test to work up chronic renal disease, proteinuria may wax and wane. In toxemia of pregnancy (pre-eclampsia/eclampsia), magnesium sulfate is used therapeutically. This may result in high urine magnesium levels, which cause spurious Du Pont aca® urine protein levels by a method which otherwise seems excellent. Toxemia is a state in which urine protein excretion is commonly measured. The standard for most methodologies is albumin. Different methods are more or less sensitive to globulin than to albumin. Thus, for nonselective proteinurias, in which a variety of proteins are present, different methodologies yield different results. Twenty-four hour urine collections are subject to collection errors. The laboratory method, depending on an aliquot and varying dilutions, is subject to calculation errors. When protein is determined by precipitation methods, x-ray contrast media, tolbutamide, penicillin or cephalosporin analogs, aminosalicylic acid, bicarbonate salts, carbonic anhydrase inhibitors, and sulfonamides may cause false-positives. Pyridium® interferes with the reaction by causing color interference. Functional and postural proteinuria occur.

Methodology A number of methods are in use including trichloroacetic acid, sulfosalicylic acid precipitation, biuret method with phosphotungstic acid, and Coomassie blue dye binding.

Additional Information Normal urine protein consists of albumin (up to 35 mg/24 hours), other plasma proteins (ie, globulins, haptoglobin, beta$_2$-microglobulin, and light chains), and Tamm-Horsfall glycoprotein secreted by renal tubular cells (may contribute up to 50 mg/24 hours). Urinary protein normally tends to increase with age, exercise, and standing posture.

Tests requiring a 24-hour urine collection with no preservative, such as creatinine, may also be performed on the same specimen. Although quantitative protein can be run on a random specimen or timed collections less than 24 hours, 24-hour collections are preferable for evaluation of the nephrotic states and inflammatory renal disorders. Creatinine, creatinine clearance, BUN, serum protein electrophoresis, ANA, anti-DNA antibodies, HIV, hepatitis C antibody, hepatitis B antigen, and complement levels (including total complement, C3, C4) are among useful tests to work up patients with proteinuria. Urine electrophoresis, immunofixation and immunoelectrophoresis are useful in patients older than 35 years of age to investigate possible diagnosis of amyloidosis, myeloma, and Waldenström's macroglobulinemia.

Some patients exhibit orthostatic proteinuria (ie, recumbent urine protein 100-180 mg in a 12-hour overnight urine collection and up to 1 g in the subsequent 12

(Continued)

Protein, Quantitative, Urine *(Continued)*

Outline of Causes of Proteinuria

Normal proteinuria	Albumin ≤35 mg/24 h	
	Tamm–Horsfall ≤50 mg/24 h	
Prerenal proteinuria	Congestive heart failure	
	Orthostatic proteinuria	
	Transient, associated with febrile illness, surgery, anemia, hyperthyroidism, stroke, exercise, seizures	
	Bence Jones proteinuria associated with myeloma, Waldenström's macroglobulinemia, amyloidosis	
	Lysozyme associated with myelocytic leukemia	
Renal proteinuria	Renovascular hypertension	
	Malignant hypertension of any cause	
	Glomerular	Membranous nephropathy and proliferative glomerulonephritis
		Chronic pyelonephritis
		Polycystic disease
		Diabetic nephropathy
		Amyloidosis
		Lupus erythematosus (SLE)
		Goodpasture's syndrome
		Renal vein thrombosis
		Minimal change nephropathy
		Proteinuria >3.5 g/24 h usually reflects a glomerular lesion
		High molecular weight proteinuria
	Tubular	Fanconi syndrome
		Wilson's disease
		Renal tubular acidosis
		Heavy metal poisoning: lead, mercury, cadmium
		Galactosemia
		Low molecular weight (<60,000) proteinuria
		Beta$_2$-microglobulinemia (molecular weight 11,800)
		<1 g/24 h
	Interstitial	Bacterial pyelonephritis
		Uric acid, urate, or calcium deposition
		Idiosyncratic drug reaction: methicillin, phenindione, sulfonamides, phenytoin, others
		Interstitial diseases generally reflected as tubular defects or mixed tubular interstitial
Postrenal	Tumors of the bladder or renal pelvis <1 g/24 h, IgM excretion significant marker, amount of proteinuria related to size and spread of tumor Cystitis, severe	

hours while ambulatory). The presence of urinary protein >200 mg in the overnight specimen or equally increased amounts of urine protein in both specimens indicates a need for further work-up.

Nephrotic syndromes are the causes of the most severe urinary protein losses. Nephrotic syndrome is defined now usually by degree of proteinuria (ie, proteinuria >50 mg/kg/day). After time, additional signs and symptoms occur including hypoproteinemia, hypoalbuminemia, elevation of alpha$_2$-globulin with decreased gamma globulin on electrophoresis, hyperlipidemia, and edema. Urinary albumin is a more sensitive marker of progression and regression of renal disease than urine total protein, especially when urine total protein is <300 mg/g creatinine. In most laboratories, urine albumin is available from protein electrophoresis following concentration procedures. However, this method is not sensitive to low concentrations of albumin.

Specific References

Burke EC and Stickler GB, "Proteinuria in Children. Review and Evaluation," *Clin Pediatr (Phila)*, 1982, 21(12):741-3.

Ginsberg JM, Chang BS, Matarese RA, and Garella S, "Use of Single Voided Urine Samples to Estimate Quantitative Proteinuria," *N Engl J Med*, 1983, 309(25):1543-6.

Glassock RJ, "The Nephrotic Syndrome," *Hosp Pract*, 1979, 14(11):105-9.

Levey AS, Madaio MP, and Perrone RD, "Laboratory Assessment of Renal Disease: Clearance, Urinalysis, and Renal Biopsy," *Kidney*, Brenner BM and Rector FC Jr, eds, Philadelphia, PA: WB Saunders Co, 1991, 919-68.

Ward PC, "Renal Dysfunction, 2, Proteinuria," *Postgrad Med*, 1981, 69(6):91-9.

Protein Screen, Urine *see* Protein, Semiquantitative, Urine *on this page*

Protein, Semiquantitative, Urine

Synonyms Albumin, Urine; Protein Screen, Urine; Protein, Urine, Sulfosalicylic Acid; Urine Screen for Albumin; Urine Screen for Protein

Test Includes Screening for urine protein by dipstick and, in many laboratories, sulfosalicylic acid method for confirmation. This is part of a routine urinalysis.

Abstract Screening test for urinary protein loss. Dipstick methods are relatively insensitive to globulins such as light chains. They may be unreliable in unusually colored urines, when the specimen is highly alkaline or when a great deal of sediment is present. The precipitation methods include sulfosalicylic acid and trichloroacetic acid. These are more sensitive to globulins.

Specimen Random urine

Volume 10 mL

Minimum Volume 2 mL for sulfosalicylic acid test; 2 drops (if no more can be obtained) for dipstick

Container Plastic urine container

Collection Early morning specimen is recommended. This will provide maximally concentrated urine when Bence Jones urine protein (light chain) detection is important. For other renal disease, daytime urine is satisfactory or even preferred. Transport specimen to the laboratory within 2 hours of collection. Container should state date and time of collection.

Storage Instructions If not run promptly, specimen should be refrigerated.

Causes for Rejection Improper labeling, specimen not refrigerated

Reference Range <20 mg/dL (SI: <0.2 g/L). The sensitivity of the dipstick is in the range of 150-300 mg/L. It is sensitive mostly for albumin.

Use Detect protein in the urine; screen for nephrotic syndromes, including complications of diabetes mellitus, glomerulonephritis, amyloidosis, and other renal diseases. Proteinuria is probably the single most important indicator of renal disease.

Limitations The dipstick method is sensitive to negatively charged proteins but much less so to positively charged proteins and so commonly will not detect Bence Jones (light chain) or myeloma protein, to which sulfosalicylic acid procedures are usually sensitive. False-positive results may be obtained with highly alkaline (pH ≥7) urines on dipsticks, and false-negatives on such urines may be found with sulfosalicylic acid. Positive protein dipstick results, especially in very alkaline urines, should be confirmed by sulfosalicylic acid testing. Contaminating quaternary ammonium groups or chlorohexidine present in disinfectants may also give false-positive dipstick results. The test area on dipsticks is more sensitive to albumin than to globulin, hemoglobin, Bence Jones protein, or mucoprotein. A negative result, therefore, does not rule out the presence of these other proteins. Pyridium® metabolites may mask the reaction. X-ray contrast media, tolbutamide, nafcillin, massive doses of penicillin, sulfisoxazole (Gantrisin®), para-aminosalicylic acid, and high levels of cephalosporins may cause false-positive reactions with the sulfosalicylic acid method. The detection limit of Albustix® (Ames Division, Miles Laboratories) is reported as 300 mg/L or 500 mg/day protein. Since normal albuminuria is <20 mg/L, the screening dipstick lacks sensitivity for early detection of protein loss in diabetic nephropathy.

Methodology Dipstick, and in some laboratories sulfosalicylic acid, are run on all urinalyses. The dipstick test is based on the color development of indicators. The sulfosalicylic acid test is based on the acid precipitation of protein. Immunofixation or immunoelectrophoresis is indicated when Bence Jones protein is suspected.

Additional Information If the dipstick for protein is negative and the sulfosalicylic acid test is positive, Bence Jones proteinuria may be present. If clinically indicated, in this situation a urine for electrophoresis and immunoelectrophoresis for light chains or immunofixation should be considered. Normal newborns may have increased levels of proteinuria during first 3 days of life. Subclinical increased uri-

(Continued)

Protein, Semiquantitative, Urine *(Continued)*

nary albumin excretion is thought to be predictive of emergence subsequently of diabetic nephropathy. A report suggests that in many situations, additional to diabetes, urine albumin by a specific method is much more sensitive to progressing renal disease than is urinary total protein (eg, hypertension, systemic lupus erythematosus). Urine albumin is easier to standardize and should be more sensitive to specific glomerular disease. Following exercise, proteinuria relates more to intensity of exercise than to its duration. Discrepancies between protein methods can be recognized in some settings by skilled microscopy of the urinary sediment.

Specific References

Burke EC and Stickler GB, "Proteinuria in Children. Review and Evaluation," *Clin Pediatr (Phila)*, 1982, 21(12):741-3.

Schwab SJ, Christensen RL, Dougherty K, et al, "Quantitation of Proteinuria by the Use of Protein-to-Creatinine Ratios in Single Urine Samples," *Arch Intern Med*, 1987, 147(5):943-4.

Viberti G and Keen H, "The Patterns of Proteinuria in Diabetes Mellitus. Relevance to Pathogenesis and Prevention of Diabetic Nephropathy," *Diabetes*, 1984, 33(7):686-92, (review).

Protein, Total, Serum

Synonyms Total Protein, Serum

Applies To Globulin

Test Includes Total protein, albumin, A/G ratio

Specimen Blood

Volume 10 mL

Minimum Volume 3 mL serum

Container Red top tube

Collection Pediatrics: Blood drawn from heelstick for capillary.

Storage Instructions Separate serum from cells and refrigerate.

Reference Range Adults: 6.0-8.0 g/dL (SI: 60-80 g/L) in later childhood and adults. Lower ranges occur in early childhood. Ambulatory values are slightly higher than are those found in recumbency. If normal ranges are set for inpatients, then many outpatients appear to be a little above the upper limit.

Use Evaluate nutritional status; investigate edema.

In the entities which follow, the diseases listed are sometimes increased or decreased as indicated, but are not always so.

Causes of **high total protein:** dehydration; some cases of chronic liver disease, including chronic active hepatitis and cirrhosis; neoplasms, especially myeloma; macroglobulinemia of Waldenström; tropical diseases (eg, kala-azar, leprosy, and others); granulomatous diseases, such as sarcoidosis; diseases in which total protein is sometimes high include collagen disease (eg, lupus erythematosus (SLE), and other instances of chronic infection/inflammation).

Causes of **low total protein:** pregnancy; intravenous fluids; cirrhosis or other liver disease, including chronic alcoholism; prolonged immobilization; heart failure; nephrotic syndromes; glomerulonephritis; neoplasia; protein losing enteropathies; Crohn's disease and chronic ulcerative colitis; starvation, malabsorption, or malnutrition; hyperthyroidism; burns; severe skin disease; and other chronic diseases. Very low total protein (<4.0 g/dL (SI: <40 g/L)) and low albumin cause edema (eg, nephrotic syndromes).

Limitations Venous stasis during venipuncture can lead to increased values. Hyperviscosity was reported to cause error in total protein through a discrete laboratory sampler-dilutor. Hemolysis can falsely elevate total protein. Clinical interpretation is greatly enhanced by examination of the fractions composing total protein, when such separation is clinically indicated (ie, serum protein electrophoresis, quantitative immunodiffusion or other methods for IgG, IgA, IgM, immunofixation, immunoelectrophoresis). Serum protein can also be elevated by phenazopyridine.

Methodology Biuret for total protein, refractometry, BCG for albumin

Additional Information Total protein and albumin normally decrease by 5% to 10% upon recumbency, as in hospitalization. "Globulin" may be provided as a calculation, total protein – albumin = globulin. Such a result is a screening test much less definitive than other methods. Total protein and albumin are commonly measured on chemistry profiling instruments.

Specific References

Chan KM and Ladenson JH, "Sample Viscosity Can Be a Source of Analytical Error When Discrete Sampler-Dilutors Are Used," *Clin Chem*, 1981, 27(11):1896-8.

Dawnay AB, Hirst AD, Perry DE, et al, "A Critical Assessment of Current Analytical Methods for the Routine Assay of Serum Total Protein and Recommendations for Their Improvement," *Ann Clin Biochem*, 1991, 28(Pt 6):556-67.

Camara PD, Wright C, Dextraze P, et al, "Comparison of a Commercial Method for Total Protein With a Candidate Reference Method," *Ann Clin Lab Sci*, 1991, 21(5):335-9.

Herbeth B, Diemert MC, and Galli A, "Total Proteins," *Drug Effects on Laboratory Test Results Analytical Interferences and Pharmacological Effects*, Siest G and Galteau MM, eds, Littleton, MA: PSG Publishing Co Inc, 1988, 375-90.

Koller A and Kaplan LA, "Total Serum Protein," *Methods in Clinical Chemistry*, Pesce AJ and Kaplan LA, eds, St Louis, MO: Mosby-Year Book Inc, 1987, 1134-8.

Protein, Urine, Sulfosalicylic Acid *see* Protein, Semiquantitative, Urine *on page 1337*

Protoporphyrin, Free Erythrocyte

Related Information

Porphyrins, Quantitative, Urine *on page 1326*

Synonyms FEP; Free Erythrocyte Protoporphyrin; Protoporphyrins, Fractionation, Erythrocytes; RBC Protoporphyrin

Abstract Free erythrocyte protoporphyrin expresses the amount of nonheme protoporphyrin in red cells.

Specimen Whole blood (test done on washed erythrocytes)

Volume 7 mL

Minimum Volume 1 mL whole blood

Container Lavender top (EDTA) tube or green top (heparin) tube

Collection Pediatrics: Blood drawn from heelstick for capillary.

Storage Instructions Stable 3 weeks at 4°C. Do not freeze.

Special Instructions Current hematocrit must be measured or specified.

Reference Range Depends on method; ascertain ranges for individual testing laboratory. The FEP is considered unreliable in infants younger than 6 months of age. Pediatric upper limit is 50 μg/dL (SI: 0.89 μmol/L) RBC. Adults: male: <30 μg/dL (SI: <0.53 μmol/L), female: <40 μg/dL (SI: <0.71 μmol/L) by hematofluorometer; 11-45 (SI: 0.20-0.80 μmol/L) for adult men and 19-52 (SI: 0.34-0.92 μmol/L) for adult women by Piomelli FEP expressed as μg/dL blood.

Possible Panic Range >190 μg/dL (SI: >3.38 μmol/L)

Use Differential diagnosis of disorders of heme production versus diseases of globin synthesis. FEP is increased in lead poisoning, protoporphyria, in iron deficiency, anemia of chronic disease and with some sideroblastic anemias. FEP levels are also reported increased in entities characterized by marked increase in erythropoiesis, such as severe hemolytic anemias. Thus, FEP is useful in work-up of the microcytic anemias. FEP is increased with lead poisoning but not in acute intermittent porphyria. FEP is reported normal with presumed alpha thalassemia trait, hemoglobin H, beta thalassemia trait, and hemoglobin E.

Limitations Fluorescent substances in plasma may interfere with hematofluorometer results. Elevated FEPs should be verified by retesting washed RBCs or by microextraction. Skin contamination may lead to false elevations. Both this test and blood lead are needed for full evaluation.

Methodology Hematofluorometer, extraction method, and high performance liquid chromatography (HPLC). The hematofluorometer measures porphyrins unbound in erythrocytes. With iron deficiency and diminished heme synthesis, free porphyrin accumulates in the red blood cell.

Additional Information "Free" protoporphyrin is not complexed, nonheme protoporphyrin. **Lead poisoning** is characterized by elevated plasma and urine delta aminolevulinic acid and increased urinary coproporphyrin. Urinary porphobilinogen and uroporphyrin are normal to slightly increased. Free erythrocyte protoporphyrin is a sensitive test for lead toxicity or chronic exposure, **although, a careful study based on receiver operator curves showed that erythrocyte protoporphyrin levels should not be used as a screening test for lead poisoning in children**. The diagnosis of lead exposure or poisoning includes consideration of environmental exposure, as well as symptoms and abnormal erythrocyte protoporphyrin. FEP is given as 92-288 μg/dL (SI: 1.63-5.12 μmol/L) RBC in level II increased lead absorption, with higher FEP results in level III. Increased lead absorption is reported in the presence of iron deficiency. Increased erythrocyte protoporphyrin exists as free protoporphyrin in protoporphyria, not as a zinc chelate, in contrast to lead poisoning and iron deficiency. These two compounds, zinc protoporphyrin and metal free protoporphyrin, can be distinguished from each other by spectrophotofluorometry.

Specific References

Bird TD, Wallace DM, and Labbe RF, "The Porphyria, Plumbism, Pottery Puzzle," *JAMA*, 1982, 247(6):813-4.

Houk VN, "Protoporphyrins," *Lab Report for Physicians*, 1986, 8:60-1, (letter).

Schreiber WE, "Iron, Porphyrin, and Bilirubin Metabolism," *Clinical Chemistry – Theory, Analysis, and Correlation*, 2nd ed, Kaplan LA and Pesce AJ, eds, St Louis, MO: Mosby-Year Book Inc, 1989, 496-511.

Zanella A, Gridelli L, Berzuini A, et al, "Sensitivity and Predictive Value of Serum Ferritin and Free Erythrocyte Protoporphyrin for Iron Deficiency," *J Lab Clin Med*, 1989, 113(1):73-8.

Protoporphyrins, Fractionation, Erythrocytes *see* Protoporphyrin, Free Erythrocyte *on this page*

Protoporphyrin, Zinc, Blood

Synonyms Zinc Protoporphyrin; ZPP

Abstract Zinc protoporphyrin measurement may be a useful adjunct in the diagnosis of nonanemic iron deficiency but is not useful in screening programs for lead intoxication.

(Continued)

Protoporphyrin, Zinc, Blood *(Continued)*

Specimen Whole blood

Volume 3 mL

Minimum Volume 1 mL whole blood

Container Lavender top (EDTA) tube, green top (heparin) tube

Collection Routine venipuncture

Storage Instructions Do not centrifuge. Refrigerate and protect from light. Stable 1 week at 4°C.

Causes for Rejection Specimen not protected from light, specimen improperly collected, hemolysis, icterus

Reference Range 17-77 μg/dL (SI: 0.27-1.23 μmol/L). Results may be obtained as ZPP/heme ratio; reference range: 30-80 μmol/mol heme.

Critical Values >100 μg/dL (SI: >1.6 μmol/L)

Use Evaluate iron deficiency, especially nonanemic iron deficiency. ZPP is superior to hemoglobin in identifying female blood donors with nonanemic iron deficiency.

Limitations Zinc protoporphyrin may also be increased in lead poisoning, anemia of chronic disease, and erythropoietic protoporphyria. ZPP should **not** be used to screen or diagnose lead poisoning.

Methodology Hematofluorometry (front-face); if washed erythrocytes are used, the assay becomes more specific and sensitive

Additional Information Zinc protoporphyrin levels increase as blood lead levels increase. Various authorities caution using ZPP as a screening test for lead poisoning. The Center for Disease Control has lowered the cutoff level for lead intoxication in children younger than 6 years of age to **10 μg/dL (SI: 0.48 μmol/L)**, and this level is so low that **ZPP is not useful** in this context because it is insensitive to such a lead level. Therefore, it is mandatory to measure lead levels in any screening program, rather than ZPP. ZPP appears only in new RBCs and remains for the life of the RBC; therefore, ZPP does not increase until several weeks after the onset of lead exposure and remains high long after exposure to lead. It is a reasonable indicator of total body burden of lead and remains a useful adjunct to the diagnosis of iron deficiency, particularly in nonanemic or questionably anemic patients. It reflects iron depletion in the bone marrow.

Specific References

Cone DC, "Lead Screening and Follow-Up in an Urban Pediatric Clinic," *N Y State J Med*, 1992, 92(8):338-42.

Labbe RF, "Clinical Utility of Zinc Protoporphyrin," *Clin Chem*, 1992, 38(11):2167-8.

Zwennis WC, Franssen AC, and Wijnans MJ, "Use of Zinc Protoporphyrin in Screening Individuals for Exposure to Lead," *Clin Chem*, 1990, 36(8 Pt 1):1456-9.

Protriptyline, Blood

Synonyms Vivactil®

Specimen Blood

Volume 20 mL

Minimum Volume 4 mL serum

Container Red top serum separator tube preferred, plain red top tube acceptable

Storage Instructions Freeze serum.

Reference Range Therapeutic: 70-260 ng/mL

Critical Values Toxic: >500 ng/mL

Use Monitor therapeutic drug level; evaluate toxicity

Methodology Gas-liquid chromatography (GLC)

Additional Information Protriptyline, a tricyclic antidepressant, is used to treat endogenous depression. The drug is very similar to imipramine in actions, limitations, and interactions. The half-life is 54-98 hours and peak serum levels are reached in 24-30 hours. Adverse reactions include CNS stimulation, tachycardia, and strong anticholinergic activity. Orthostatic hypotension frequently occurs.

Prozac® *see* Fluoxetine, Blood *on page 1267*

Prysolin® *see* Primidone, Blood *on page 1332*

Pseudocholinesterase, Serum

Related Information

Acetylcholinesterase, Red Blood Cell *on page 1181*

Synonyms Cholinesterase, Serum; PCE; Plasma Cholinesterase

Abstract Two types of cholinesterase are found in blood: "true" cholinesterase (acetylcholinesterase) in red cells and "pseudocholinesterase" (acylcholine acylhydrolase) in serum (plasma).

Specimen Blood

Volume 7 mL

Minimum Volume 1 mL serum

Container Red top tube

Storage Instructions Cholinesterase is stable in separated serum for 80 days at room temperature and 3 years at -20°C. However, specimens submitted to evaluate possible pesticide toxicity should be collected on ice, separated in a refrigerated centrifuge, and frozen until analyzed.

Reference Range Low in infancy, then increasing in early childhood. Ranges vary between methods and laboratories.

Possible Panic Range Less than lower limit of normal

Use Screen preoperative patients for succinylcholine (suxamethonium) anesthetic sensitivity, genetic or secondary to insecticide exposure, in appropriate circumstances. Prevent or evaluate prolonged anesthetic effect, prolonged apnea, after surgery. Very small amounts (0.04-0.06 mg/kg) of succinylcholine are needed to obtain 90% of neuromuscular blockade in patients with low levels of plasma cholinesterase activity.

Monitor organophosphorous or carbamate insecticide poisoning, in which level is decreased; establish patient's baseline value before exposure. Indications include such pesticide exposure, especially with miosis, blurred vision, muscle weakness, twitching, and fasciculation, bradycardia, nausea, diarrhea, vomiting, salivation, sweating, pulmonary edema, arrhythmias, and convulsions. The value of assessing risk status in persons exposed to organophosphate insecticides on the basis of plasma cholinesterase levels alone has been called into question. Are normal levels indicative of no exposure or of a genetic variant with or without exposure? There are interpretive problems with low or high values.

Family studies may be done when an individual with a genetically abnormal type is documented by serum pseudocholinesterase deficiency and, ideally, confirmed by phenotyping.

Limitations Serum pseudocholinesterase may be decreased in patients on estrogens and oral contraceptives. Fluoride interferes. Pseudocholinesterase is low also in some instances of liver disease, including decompensated cirrhosis, hepatitis, metastatic carcinoma, CHF, and in malnutrition, but not sufficiently consistently enough to be a useful clinical test for such disorders. Genetic atypical enzyme does not explain every instance of prolonged postsurgical apnea. Red cell cholinesterase is more useful for chronic insecticide exposure. Carbamate-poisoned persons can appear to have near normal or normal levels of pseudocholinesterase. Plasma cholinesterase is lower and red blood cell cholinesterase higher in pregnant women than in nonpregnant women. Thus, a low red blood cell cholinesterase in pregnant women is more consistent with a possible overexposure to anticholinesterases than a low plasma cholinesterase.

Contraindications Not useful to screen for toxicity from chlorinated insecticides.

Methodology Colorimetry, kinetic enzyme utilizing different substrates, fluorometry

Additional Information Low serum cholinesterase activity may relate to exposure to insecticides or to one of a number of variant genotypes. Dibucaine and fluoride numbers are useful to phenotype such homozygous and heterozygous individuals, who are genetically sensitive to succinylcholine.

One patient in 1500 is susceptible to succinyldicholine anesthetic mishap.

Plasmapheresis has been noted to decrease the level of plasma cholinesterase. Patients with abnormally low cholinesterase activity after transfusion of blood or plasma will experience temporary augmentation of enzyme level. In estimating the duration of this enhanced activity, measures of plasma cholinesterase half-life have been utilized. The true half-life value has, however, been uncertain. A half-life value determined by measuring the rate of disappearance after intravenous injection of human cholinesterase has provided an average value of 11 days.

A low level of activity of pseudocholinesterase has been demonstrated in cerebrospinal fluid, at about 1/20 to 1/100 the activity present in the corresponding plasma. With clinical conditions characterized by bleeding into the CSF, pseudocholinesterase activity increases 25% to 50% that of plasma.

Patients with a variety of carcinomas have been reported to accumulate an embryonic type of cholinesterase activity in their sera. Such novel cholinesterase activity was found only in the sera of patients undergoing antitumor therapy (eg, chemotherapy or radiation therapy and/or hormone therapy).

Increase in acetylcholinesterase activity, notably, in an acetylcholinesterase to butyrylcholine esterase ratio (histochemical study, not as measured in serum) has provided discriminatory diagnostic value in some cases of Hirschsprung's disease.

Specific References

de Peyster A, Willis WO, and Liebhaber M, "Cholinesterase Activity in Pregnant Women and Newborns," *Clin Toxicol*, 1994, 32(6):683-96.

Hoffman RS, Henry GC, Howland MA, et al, "Association Between Life-Threatening Cocaine Toxicity and Plasma Cholinesterase Activity," *Ann Emerg Med*, 1992, 21(3):247-53.

Newman MA and Que Hee SS, "Interconversion and Comparison of Three Methods for Cholinesterase in Serum," *Clin Chem*, 1984, 30(2):308-10.

Pseudoephedrine *see* Methamphetamines, Urine *on page 1294*

Pt, Blood *see* Platinum, Blood *on page 1325*

Pt, Urine *see* Platinum, Urine *on page 1325*

Pubic Lice Identification *see* Arthropod Identification *on page 1198*

Pulmonary Compliance (Dynamic)

Applies To Chord Compliance

Test Includes Pulmonary compliance reported in units of $liter_{BTPS}/cm\ H_2O$, maximum static elastic recoil pressure reported in units of cm H_2O, dynamic compliance at 60 breaths/minute reported as a percentage of the static compliance measurement ($Cdyn_{60}$).

Patient Preparation Patient should not take anything by mouth for 2-3 hours prior to testing. Nasal passage should be treated with a topical Xylocaine®/epinephrine solution to widen nasal passage and minimize discomfort. Patient should take small sips of ice water (if not contraindicated) before and during passage of a nasogastric balloon.

Aftercare Usually none, occasionally patient will experience vagal stimulation during passage of the nasogastric balloon. Placement in a feet up supine position may aid in the treatment of hypotension, dizziness and nausea.

Technique With the patient in a seated position, an uninflated, 10 cm x 1 cm, thin walled, latex balloon-catheter set-up attached to a pressure transducer is inserted transnasally after topical anesthesia and positioned in the lower third of the esophagus. Sips of water will aid in the passage of the balloon. The patient is instructed to perform a Valsalva maneuver with the end of the balloon catheter open to a loose fitting glass syringe. The balloon is then inflated with approximately 0.2-0.5 mL air. Several volume histories are obtained (inhalation to TLC) prior to making any measurement. Measurement of maximal static recoil pressure may be made while holding breath at TLC for several seconds. Peak pressure should be ignored and stable pressure recorded. After several static recoil measurements are made, relaxed shutter interrupted exhalations from TLC to FRC (or RV if the entire pressure volume curve is desired) are made while plotting transpulmonary pressure (pleural pressure minus mouth pressure) against exhaled volume. Compliance measurements (so-called "chord compliance") are made along the exhalation pressure volume curve from points corresponding to FRC and FRC plus 0.5 $liter_{BTPS}$. Patients are then asked to increase their breathing rate 10 breaths/minute to a maximum rate of 100 breaths/minute. Measurement of transpulmonary pressure and volume are plotted on an X-Y plotter. Dynamic compliance is measured by dividing volume change by pressure change at points of zero flow. Dynamic compliance is typically reported as a percentage of the static compliance or $Cdyn_{60}$ = dynamic compliance measured during 60 breaths/minute panting/static compliance x 100.

Specimen Transpulmonary pressures (mouth pressure minus esophageal (**pleural**) pressures) are plotted against volumes obtained from an interrupted, passive, expiratory volume history from TLC to RV. Compliance measurements are made along the recorded pressure lines at points corresponding to FRC and FRC + 1 $liter_{BTPS}$.

Collection Measurement is made by recording mouth pressure and pressures recorded from an esophageal balloon inserted transnasally into the lower one-third of the thorax of an upright seated patient. Volume should be measured from a device that meets standards recommended by the American Thoracic Society (ATS).

Causes for Rejection Wide variations in baseline level of FRC. Active expiratory efforts made against the shutter during interrupted passive exhalation.

Special Instructions Balloon should be coated with a topical anesthetic treated lubricant to aid in minimizing the gag reflex. Balloon should contain a small amount (usually 0.5 mL) of air. If excessive amounts of air are used esophageal pressures will be overstated resulting in an erroneously low pulmonary compliance.

Reference Range Normal value for pulmonary compliance can be derived from the following equation:

$$C_{st} \text{ in } liter_{BTPS} = (0.00343 \times \text{height in cm}) - 0.425$$

Use Assess small airways dysfunction

Limitations Technically difficult secondary to correct placement of the balloon and the need for the patient to relax against an obstruction while maintaining an open glottis. Patients often find transnasal passage of the esophageal balloon unpleasant.

Contraindications Patients that are unable to follow instructions and relax, patients in whom placement of an esophageal balloon is contraindicated

Specific References

Vollmer WM, McCamant LE, Johnson LR, et al, "Long-Term Reproducibility of Tests of Small Airways Function. Comparisons With Spirometry," *Chest*, 1990, 98(2):303-7.

Pulse Oximetry

Synonyms CPAP Titration; Desaturation Oximetry; Oxygen Titration Test

Applies To Ear Oximetry; Finger Oximetry

Test Includes Report generally includes baseline heart rate and functional O_2 saturation, heart rate and lowest functional O_2 saturation during whatever event may be taking place: exercise, sleep or therapeutic intervention such as nasal CPAP or oxygen therapy.

Patient Preparation Fingernail polish should be removed with acetone. Permanent or disposable sensors should be applied according to the manufacturer's instructions. When finger probes are used, the patient should be instructed not to grip treadmill rail or handlebars tightly to avoid reduction of circulation to the digits. Preparation depends on the type of test being performed. Exercise patients should wear loose comfortable clothing. Patients should refrain from smoking 24 hours prior to test to avoid functional versus fractional O_2 saturation discrepancy that occurs with elevated carboxyhemoglobin levels. If possible, an arterial blood gas should be drawn and pH, pCO_2, pO_2, Hemoglobin, oxyhemoglobin ($O_2Hb\%$), carboxyhemoglobin (COHb%) and methemoglobin (metHb%) should be measured. Draw the heparinized arterial blood sample while the pulse oximetry sensor is in place and is stable. Correlation of oxyhemoglobin ($O_2Hb\%$) (measured by blood oximetry) and $SpO_2\%$ (measured by pulse oximetry) should be made. The discrepancy between the $O_2Hb\% - SpO_2\%$ should be used to determine the endpoint of the maneuver inducing arterial desaturation. For example, if the pulse oximeter displays a SpO_2 reading of 93% and a simultaneously obtained arterial blood sample shows an $O_2Hb\%$ of 91%, 2% should be subtracted from subsequent SpO_2 measurements during exercise for a more valid estimate of arterial oxygen saturation. This adjustment should also be made to determine the therapeutic endpoint when titrating supplemental oxygen therapy at rest, during sleep, or exercise.

Aftercare After exercise, allow patient to walk slowly on level treadmill or pedal bicycle ergometer at zero load slowly to allow gradual cool down period. Monitor EKG, blood pressure, and patient status frequently during the first 5 minutes after a maximum exercise test.

Technique Methodology may differ widely depending on the type of challenge or intervention planned. Basic methodology should include correlation with blood oximetry as outlined in Patient Preparation. External EKG should correlate within 5 beats/minute of the pulse oximeter's pulse display. Record baseline functional saturation, external EKG rate and pulse oximeter heart rate along with patient status, workload, and supplemental oxygen given at each stage of the test.

Specimen Spectrophotometric measurement is made by passing light at two specific wavelengths through a pulsing capillary bed (finger, toe, bridge of nose, and ear are the most common sites for sensor placement). Light collection on the other side of the site is proportional to the amount of oxyhemoglobin present in the arterial capillary bed relative to the amount of hemoglobin available for binding with oxygen (exclusive of the dyshemoglobins: carboxyhemoglobin and methemoglobin).

Causes for Rejection Unstable readings secondary to any cause: external light, poor peripheral circulation, or skin pigmentation are common causes.

Special Instructions Poor collateral circulation may be compensated for by warming the hands with warm towels. Fluctuation $\pm 1\%$ is acceptable. Range of fluctuation should be noted.

Reference Range Normal adult oxyhemoglobin saturation is >95%. Drops in oxyhemoglobin are usually the result of cardiac, pulmonary, or combined cardiopulmonary disease. Significant declines (>5%) during exercise or sleep are abnormal.

Possible Panic Range Values <90% indicate the need for oxygen therapy. Values <85% are require immediate attention. If available, add the measured carboxyhemoglobin and methemoglobin to the values listed to adjust for nonfunctioning dyshemoglobins.

Use Determine an estimate of the level of arterial oxygenation at rest and in the presence of positive and negative intervention. These include exercise, sleep, and during procedures such as surgery, bronchoscopy, ventilator assist/support therapy, etc.

Limitations Test does not measure or take into consideration total hemoglobin or the dyshemoglobins, carboxyhemoglobin, and methemoglobin. May overestimate total oxygen delivery (oxygen content) if not correlated with blood oximetry. Not accurate in the presence of poor peripheral circulation. Accuracy at most units is $\pm 2\%$, standard deviation is usually 1%.

Contraindications Not to be used in the presence of flammable anesthetics. Contraindications for exercise may be found in the section on cardiopulmonary exercise testing.

Additional Information Guidelines for reimbursement of home oxygen therapy state that a resting arterial pO_2 <55 torr or a resting oxygen saturation ($SpO_2\%$) <88% with evidence of improvement with oxygen therapy qualify a patient for continuous oxygen therapy reimbursement. Guidelines for reimbursement for nocturnal and exercise oxygen therapy state that O_2 saturations during exercise or sleep that fall to <88% that improve with oxygen therapy will be reimbursed. Because of the limitations of pulse oximetry, decisions regarding discontinuing oxygen therapy should **not** be made on the basis of pulse oximetry alone. Assessment of the PaO_2 by arterial blood gas and/or $O_2Hb\%$ by arterial blood oximetry should be

(Continued)

Pulse Oximetry *(Continued)*

done before such decisions are made. Carlin et al has shown that patients with PaO_2 ≤55 torr may be denied oxygen therapy if the decision was based on pulse oximetry measurements alone (a significant number of these patients had SpO_2% measurements >88%).

Specific References

Buckley RG, Aks SE, Eshom JL, et al, "The Pulse Oximetry Gap in Carbon Monoxide Intoxication," *Ann Emerg Med*, 1994, 24(2):252-5.

Carlin BW, Clausen JL, and Ries AL, "The Use of Cutaneous Oximetry in the Prescription of Long-Term Oxygen Therapy," *Chest*, 1988, 94(2):239-41.

Escourrou PJ, Delaperche MF, and Visseaux A, "Reliability of Pulse Oximetry During Exercise in Pulmonary Patients," *Chest*, 1990, 97(3):635-8.

Joyce WP, Walsh K, Gough DB, et al, "Pulse Oximetry: A New Non-Invasive Assessment of Peripheral Arterial Occlusive Disease," *Br J Surg*, 1990, 77(10):1115-7.

Jubran A and Tobin MJ, "Reliability of Pulse Oximetry in Titrating Supplemental Oxygen Therapy in Ventilator-Dependent Patients," *Chest*, 1990, 97(6):1420-5.

Kumar A, Chawla R, Ahuja S, et al, "Nitrobenzene Poisoning and Spurious Pulse Oximetry," *Anaesthesia*, 1990, 45(11):949-51.

Pierson DJ, "Pulse Oximetry Versus Arterial Blood Gas Specimens in Long-Term Oxygen Therapy," *Lung*, 1990, 168(Suppl):782-8.

Purodigin® *see* Digitoxin, Blood *on page 1249*

Quantitative Fibrinogen *see* Fibrinogen, Plasma *on page 1265*

Quantitative Ventilation Lung Scan *see* Lung Scan, Ventilation *on page 1288*

Quinidex® *see* Quinidine, Serum *on this page*

Quinidine, Serum

Synonyms Cardioquin®; Quinidex®; Quinora®

Abstract Quinidine is an antiarrhythmic that is frequently monitored.

Specimen Blood

Volume 7 mL

Minimum Volume 1 mL serum

Container Red top tube. The stoppers on some tubes contain plasticizers which affect measured drug levels.

Sampling Time Collect just before next dose.

Special Instructions Serum concentration **must be correlated** with patient's clinical status.

Reference Range Therapeutic: 2-5 μg/mL (SI: 6.2-15.4 μmol/L). Patient dependent therapeutic response occurs at levels of 3-6 μg/mL (SI: 9.2-18.5 μmol/L). Optimal therapeutic level is method dependent.

Possible Panic Range Toxic: >8 μg/mL (SI: >24.7 μmol/L).

Use Therapeutic monitoring for quinidine to provide documentation for adequate dosage; toxicity assessment

Limitations An assay method should be used which also detects active metabolites, in particular dihydroquinidine. Cross reactions occur with EMIT and fluorescence polarization methods.

Methodology Enzyme-multiplied immunoassay technique (EMIT), fluorometry, high performance liquid chromatography (HPLC), gas chromatography (GC)

Additional Information Optimal resampling time after change in dosage is 1-2 days. Biologic half-life is about 6-8 hours. **Doses >250 mg/day of quinidine result in increased serum digoxin concentrations about 2.5 times the digoxin concentration before quinidine was added.** The new steady-state of digoxin concentration occurs in 7-14 days, with signs of toxicity beginning to appear in 3-7 days after initiation of quinidine therapy. Therefore, **serum digoxin concentrations should be measured before initiation of quinidine therapy and again in 4-6 days.** Measure trough because of variability of peak interval. **Renal failure** prolongs apparent half-life, perhaps through accumulation of fluorescent metabolites. Severe heart failure also prolongs half-life, as does liver disease. Concomitant administration of **phenytoin** increases hepatic metabolism, and therefore decreases half-life and serum quinidine concentrations. Clearance may be diminished in the elderly.

Specific References

Giardina EG and Wechsler ME, "Low Dose Quinidine-Mexiletine Combination Therapy Versus Quinidine Monotherapy for Treatment of Ventricular Arrhythmias," *J Am Coll Cardiol*, 1990, 15(5):1138-45.

Kavanagh KM, Wyse DG, Mitchell LB, et al, "Contribution of Quinidine Metabolites to Electrophysiologic Responses in Human Subjects," *Clin Pharmacol Ther*, 1989, 46(3):352-8.

Kessler KM, Wozniak PM, McAuliffe D, et al, "The Clinical Implication of Changing Unbound Quinidine Levels," *Am Heart J*, 1989, 118(1):63-9.

Quinora® *see* Quinidine, Serum *on this page*

Rabid Animals *see* Rabies Identification *on next page*

Rabies Identification

Synonyms Rabid Animals

Test Includes Examination of animal brain for Negri bodies or inoculation of mice with suspension of brain tissue

Specimen Head of large animal or entire small animal suspected of rabies. Use gloves and mask when handling an animal carcass suspected of rabies.

Container Sealed container

Storage Instructions Ideally, animal brain should be examined in the fresh state. Transport using wet ice or place in absorbent material, then in two plastic bags, or, place half the brain in 50% glycerol, half in 10% formalin, depending on instructions from state laboratory. Local state laboratory must be consulted. Rabies virus may also be demonstrated by immunofluorescence in skin biopsies of patients suspected of having rabies (*vide infra*).

Causes for Rejection Unlabeled or improperly packaged specimen

Use Diagnose rabies; evaluate animal bites

Limitations Negri bodies are found in about 90% of rabid animals.

Contraindications Formalin fixation precludes fluorescent antibody application

Methodology Fluorescent antibody examination (but Negri bodies can be seen in H & E)

Additional Information Antemortem rabies virus has been isolated from human saliva, brain tissues, CSF, urine sediment, and tracheal secretions. Rabies virus may also be demonstrated by immunofluorescent rabies antibody staining of skin biopsy tissue. The most reliable and reproducible of the immunofluorescent studies that can aid in patient diagnosis is biopsy of the neck skin. A 6-8 mm full thickness wedge or punch biopsy specimen from the neck containing as many hair follicles as possible should be sampled, snap frozen, and shipped frozen at -70°C to a reference laboratory. Consult with reference laboratory for shipping instructions. False-negative results do occur especially after the development of neutralizing antibodies. Six rabies associated deaths reported in U.S. in 1994. Reported cases of animal rabies in U.S. in 1993 was 9495 cases.

Rabies immune globulin (RIG) may be obtained through Connaught Laboratories (800-822-2463) or through Miles Pharmaceutical Division (203-937-2242 or 800-288-8371); RIG has been tested negative for HCV-RNA

Specific References

Bussereau F, Vincent J, Coudrier D, et al, "Monoclonal Antibodies to Mokola Virus for Identification of Rabies and Rabies-Related Viruses," *J Clin Microbiol*, 1988, 26(12):2489-94.

Center for Disease Control, "Compendium of Animal Rabies Control, 1990," *MMWR Morb Mortal Wkly Rep*, 1990, 39(RR-4):1-8.

Center for Disease Control, "Human Rabies – Alabama, Tennessee, and Texas, 1994," *MMWR Morb Mortal Wkly Rep*, 1995, 44:269-72.

Center for Disease Control, "Human Rabies – Oregon," *MMWR Morb Mortal Wkly Rep*, 1989, 38(19):335-7.

Center for Disease Control, "Rabies Prevention – United States, 1991 – Recommendations of the Immunization Practices Advisory Committee (ACIP)," *MMWR Morb Mortal Wkly Rep*, 1991, 40(RR-3):1-19.

Dietzschold B, Tollis M, Rupprecht CE, et al, "Antigenic Variation in Rabies and Rabies-Related Viruses: Cross-Protection Independent of Glycoprotein-Mediated Virus-Neutralizing Antibody," *J Infect Dis*, 1987, 156(5):815-22.

Fishbein DB and Baer GM, "Animal Rabies: Implications for Diagnosis and Human Treatment," *Ann Intern Med*, 1988, 109(12):935-7.

Fushimi R, Yamamsiti H, Inoue M, et al, "Digoxin Immunoassay That Avoids Cross-Reactivity From Chinese Medicines," *Clin Chem*, 1995, 44:621.

Grabenstein JD, "Rabies: Americas Only Overused Immunization," *Hosp Pharm*, 1995, 30(4):323-8.

Mrak, RE and Young L, "Rabies Encephalitis in a Patient With No History of Exposure," *Hum Pathol*, 1992, 24(1):109-10.

Smith JS, Fishbein DB, Rupprecht CE, et al, "Unexplained Rabies in Three Immigrants in the United States. A Virologic Investigation," *N Engl J Med*, 1991, 324(4):205-11.

Whitley RJ and Middlebrooks M, "Rabies," *Infections of the Central Nervous System*, Scheld WM, Whitley RJ, and Durack DT, eds, New York, NY: Raven Press, 1991, 134.

Radionuclide Ventilation Lung Scan *see* Lung Scan, Ventilation *on page 1288*

Ranitidine *see* Methamphetamines, Urine *on page 1294*

RBC Protoporphyrin *see* Protoporphyrin, Free Erythrocyte *on page 1339*

Rectal Swab Culture *see* Stool Culture *on page 1356*

Red Cell Cholinesterase *see* Acetylcholinesterase, Red Blood Cell *on page 1181*

Red Devils *see* Barbiturates, Quantitative, Blood *on page 1201*

Rela® *see* Carisoprodol, Quantitative *on page 1222*

Renal Panel *see* Kidney Profile *on page 1279*

Renal Profile *see* Kidney Profile *on page 1279*

Retic Count *see* Reticulocyte Count *on this page*

Reticulocyte Count

Synonyms Retic Count

Specimen Whole blood

Volume 7 mL for venipuncture specimens; one heparinized capillary tube ¾ full for capillary specimen

Minimum Volume 1 mL

Container Lavender top (EDTA) tube or green top (heparin) tube for venipuncture specimen; heparinized capillary tube for capillary specimen

Storage Instructions Store EDTA anticoagulated blood at room temperature for up to 48 hours.

Causes for Rejection Clotted or hemolyzed specimen

Reference Range Adults: 0.5% to 1.5%; newborns: ≤7%, expressed as a percentage of 1000 RBCs. Normal values at birth: 2.5% to 6.5%, falling to normal adult level by the end of the second week. The elderly (older than 70 years of age) have a slightly higher percent of reticulocytes than young individuals but still fall within the normal range.

Use Evaluate erythropoietic activity. Increased in acute and chronic hemorrhage, hemolytic anemias. Evaluate erythropoietic response to therapy of various anemias. **The test is underutilized, especially when one considers it is at a pivotal decision-making conjuncture.** The reticulocyte production index will decide if one is working with a hyperproliferative or nonproliferative anemia, and thus, which tests should be subsequently ordered.

Limitations In recently transfused patients reticulocytes may decrease on a dilutional basis due to transfusion.

Contraindications Patients receiving a large number of blood transfusions

Methodology Vital stains, new methylene blue is commonly used; brilliant cresyl blue may be used. Recently, flow cytometric methods have been developed that have the advantage of reproducibility. The disadvantage is that not every laboratory has a flow cytometer. The assay may be adapted to standard hematology instruments in the future.

Additional Information Demonstration of an increase in the number of circulating reticulocytes provides reliable and inexpensive evidence of increased red cell production. Care should be exercised during interpretation of results that an apparent increase in reticulocytes is not the result of decrease in the number of nonreticulated RBCs (ie, anemia with fewer mature red cells). A variety of corrections have been proposed and are in use. Absolute reticulocyte count = reticulocytes (%) x RBC count. This gives the number of reticulocytes per mm^3 of blood. Reticulocyte index (RI) = reticulocytes (%) x patient Hct/normal Hct or patient RBC/normal RBC or patient Hgb/normal Hgb. This corrects the reticulocyte count for anemia. Reticulocyte production index (RPI) = RI x (1/maturation time), or RPI = patient's absolute reticulocyte count/normal absolute reticulocyte count x (1/maturation time). Maturation time is usually taken as 2. RPI corrects for the premature release of reticulocytes from the marrow as might occur in cases of brisk hemolysis or significant bleeding. RPI gives a reticulocyte percent value that reliably estimates RBC production. Failure of marrow production would be reflected by anemia with absence of the expected increase in RPI. Reticulocyte count should be performed prior to transfusion. Image recognition and flow cytometry methods of reticulocyte determination appear to provide greater precision and comparable accuracy compared to the manual method for reticulocyte counting.

Specific References

Brecher G, "New Methylene Blue as a Reticulocyte Stain," *Am J Pathol*, 1949, 19:895.

Brown BA, *Hematology: Principles and Procedures*, 6th ed, Philadelphia, PA: Lea & Febiger, 1993, 111-6, 279-80, 386-90.

Davis BH and Bigelow NC, "Flow Cytometric Reticulocyte Analysis and the Reticulocyte Maturity Index," *Ann N Y Acad Sci*, 1993, 677:281-92.

Houwen B, "Reticulocyte Maturation," *Blood Cells*, 1992, 18(2):167-86.

Lee GR, "The Hemolytic Disorders: General Considerations," *Wintrobe's Clinical Hematology*, 9th ed, Chapter 32, Lee GR, Bithell TC, Foerster J, et al, eds, Philadelphia, PA: Lea and Febiger, 1993, 944-64.

Retrovir® *see* Zidovudine, Blood *on page 1381*

Ritalin® *see* Methylphenidate, Blood *on page 1299*

Rivatril® *see* Clonazepam, Serum *on page 1232*

Robimycin® *see* Erythromycin, Blood *on page 1260*

Rocket Fuel *see* Phencyclidine, Qualitative, Urine *on page 1319*

Rocket Fuel *see* Phencyclidine, Quantitative, Serum *on page 1319*

Routine Culture, Rectal Swab *see* Stool Culture *on page 1356*

Rubbing Alcohol *see* Isopropanol, Blood *on page 1277*

Salicylate, Blood

Synonyms Acetylsalicylic Acid, Blood; ASA, Blood; Aspirin, Blood; Salicylic Acid, Blood

Applies To Methyl Salicylate; Oil of Wintergreen

Abstract This is the active product produced from aspirin (acetylsalicylic acid) in the body. It is an analgesic, antipyretic, and anti-inflammatory drug.

Specimen Blood

Volume 7 mL

Minimum Volume 2 mL serum or plasma

Container Red top tube or lavender top (EDTA) tube

Reference Range Therapeutic: <10 mg/dL (SI: <0.72 mmol/L) for analgesic; 15-20 mg/dL (SI: 1.09-1.45 mmol/L) for anti-inflammatory

Possible Panic Range Mild toxicity: 30 mg/dL (SI: 2.17 mmol/L) (tinnitus, dizziness); severe toxicity: >80 mg/dL (SI: >3.62 mmol/L) (CNS effects)

Use Monitor therapeutic drug level; evaluate aspirin toxicity

Limitations Bilirubin (at concentrations of 5-20 mg/dL) has been shown to depress salicylate results by 1-5 mg/dL. Sodium azide will increase results significantly; anticoagulants interfere.

Methodology Photometry, fluorometry, high performance liquid chromatography (HPLC), gas-liquid chromatography (GLC)

Additional Information Optimal sampling time after dosage is 2-6 hours. Serum half-life is 2-3 hours on low dose therapy, 15-30 hours on high dose treatment. Optimal resampling time after change in dosage is 6 hours. In patients on chronic therapy, small dose changes may produce disproportionate changes in serum level. Use of antacids, which increase renal excretion, can lower serum levels. Steady-state concentrations for an individual patient are not adequately predicted from nomograms or standard dose schedules. In salicylate poisoning the following symptoms may occur: initial alkalosis followed by acidosis in the blood, ketosis, and possible elevated plasma glucose. Glucose should be measured when levels >25 mg/dL (SI: >1.81 mmol/L) are detected. Salicylate can be done on urine or gastric juice. The Done nomogram is used to estimate blood level and prognosis following a single dose ingestion. See nomogram. The level measured 6 hours or

SERUM SALICYLATE LEVEL AND SEVERITY OF INTOXICATION SINGLE DOSE ACUTE INGESTION NOMOGRAM

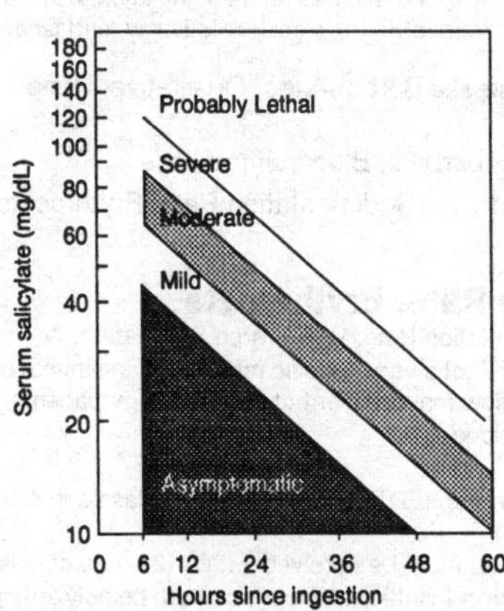

Done nomogram for salicylate poisoning. Note that this nomogram is not accurate for chronic ingestions. (From Done AK, "Salicylate Intoxication: Significance of Measurements of Salicylate in Blood in Cases of Acute Ingestions," *Pediatrics*, 1960, 26:800; copyright American Academy of Pediatrics, 1960.)

more following ingestion is plotted. Specimens drawn earlier may not reflect the peak. The nomogram is not useful when accumulation over several ingestions exists. Urine pH and volume hourly is advocated with plasma pH, potassium and other electrolytes, prothrombin time, AST, ALT, serum bilirubin and arterial blood gases for care of serious pediatric salicylate poisoning. Salicylate hepatitis, usually at blood levels of 20-25 mg/dL (1.45-1.81 mmol/L), occurs. Salicylates are believed to play a role in the hepatonecrosis of Reye's syndrome in children. They are no longer recommended for use in children.

Specific References

Bailey RB and Jones SR, "Chronic Salicylate Intoxication. A Common Cause of Morbidity in the Elderly," *J Am Geriatr Soc*, 1989, 37(6):556-61.

(Continued)

Salicylate, Blood *(Continued)*

Chapman BJ and Proudfoot AT, "Adult Salicylate Poisoning: Deaths and Outcome in Patients With High Plasma Salicylate Concentrations," *Q J Med*, 1989, 72(268):699-707.

Done AK, "Aspirin Overdosage: Incidence, Diagnosis, and Management," *Pediatrics*, 1978, 62(5 Pt 2 Suppl):890-7.

Mayer AL, Sitar DS, and Tenenbein M, "Multiple-Dose Charcoal and Whole-Bowel Irrigation Do Not Increase Clearance of Absorbed Salicylate," *Arch Intern Med*, 1992, 152(2):393-6.

Pierce RP, Gazewood J, and Blake RL Jr, "Salicylate Poisoning From Enteric-Coated Aspirin. Delayed Absorption May Complicate Management," *Postgrad Med*, 1991, 89(5):61-2, 64.

Sallis RE, "Management of Salicylate Toxicity," *Am Fam Physician*, 1989, 39(3):265-70.

Sullivan J and Lander D, "Planning an Effective Therapeutic Strategy in Salicylate Poisoning," *Emerg Med*, 1986, 7:89-96.

Salicylic Acid, Blood *see* Salicylate, Blood *on previous page*

Sandimmune® *see* Cyclosporine, Blood *on page 1247*

SaO_2 *see* Oxygen Saturation, Blood *on page 1313*

***Sarcoptes scabiei* Skin Scrapings Identification** *see* Arthropod Identification *on page 1198*

Secobarbital, Blood

Related Information

Barbiturates, Quantitative, Blood *on page 1201*

Synonyms Seconal™

Specimen Blood

Volume 15 mL

Minimum Volume 5 mL serum

Container Red top tube

Collection Collect specimen immediately prior to next dose unless specified otherwise.

Storage Instructions Separate serum and refrigerate.

Reference Range Therapeutic: 3-5 μg/mL

Critical Values Toxic: 5-15 μg/mL; lethal: ≥20 μg/mL

Use Monitor therapeutic drug level; evaluate toxicity

Additional Information Secobarbital is a short-acting barbiturate used in short-term treatment of insomnia and as a preanesthetic agent. It is also effective in the management of acute agitated states. The half-life is 30 hours and effectiveness is reached as quickly as 1-3 minutes after I.V. injection. Adverse effects include fall in blood pressure, respiratory depression, lethargy, and laryngospasm.

Secobarbital, Urine *see* Barbiturates, Qualitative, Urine *on page 1200*

Seconal™ *see* Secobarbital, Blood *on this page*

Sedimentation Rate *see* Sedimentation Rate, Erythrocyte *on this page*

Sedimentation Rate, Erythrocyte

Synonyms Sedimentation Rate; Westergren Sed Rate

Abstract This test is not a very specific measure of inflammation and infection. It is used mainly to follow management of rheumatology patients.

Specimen Whole blood

Volume 4.5 mL

Container Lavender top (EDTA) tube or citrated plasma in 4:1 dilution (9:1 dilution is **not** acceptable)

Collection Specimen must be received within 12 hours of collection.

Causes for Rejection Insufficient blood, clotted, hemolyzed specimen

Reference Range Male: younger than age 50: 0-15 mm/hour, older than age 50: 0-20 mm/hour; female: younger than age 50: 0-25 mm/hour, older than age 50: 0-30 mm/hour by Westergren method

Use Evaluate the nonspecific activity of infections, inflammatory states, autoimmune disorders, and plasma cell dyscrasias

Limitations Anemia and paraproteinemia invalidate results; some procedural methods may be associated with hazardous exposure of medical technologists to fresh whole blood. Drugs which can elevate erythrocyte sedimentation rate (ESR) include dextran, methyldopa, methysergide, penicillamine, theophylline, and vitamin A. Quinine and salicylates can decrease the ESR.

Methodology Red cell sedimentation rate expressed in mm/hour, utilizing Westergren type sedimentation tubes. A validation procedure and method for the in laboratory production of a sedimentation rate reference material has been developed for and can be used for quality assurance programs.

Additional Information Elevations in fibrinogen, alpha- and beta-globulins (acute phase reactants), and immunoglobulins increase the sedimentation rate of red cells through plasma. The test is important in the diagnosis of temporal arteritis, as well as its management. Use of the ESR, ZSR, and/or CRP may aid in the differential diagnosis of the anemia of chronic disease from iron deficiency anemia.

Specific References

Gambino R, DiRe JJ, Monteleone M, et al, "The Westergren Sedimentation Rate, Using K_3 EDTA," *Am J Clin Pathol*, 1965, 43:173-80.

Johnson MA, "Iron: Nutrition Monitoring and Nutrition Status Assessment," *J Nutr*, 1990, 120(Suppl 11):1486-91.

Singer JI, Buchino JJ, and Chabali R, "Selected Laboratory in Pediatric Emergency Care," *Emerg Med Clin North Am*, 1986, 4(2):377-96.

Stuart J and Nash GB, "Technological Advances in Blood Rheology," *Crit Rev Clin Lab Sci*, 1990, 28(1):61-93.

Thomas RD, Westengard JC, Hay KL, et al, "Calibration and Validation for Erythrocyte Sedimentation Tests. Role of the International Committee on Standardization in Hematology Reference Procedure," *Arch Pathol Lab Med*, 1993, 117(7):719-23.

Wong RL and Korn JH, "Temporal Arteritis Without an Elevated Erythrocyte Sedimentation Rate. Case Report and Review of the Literature," *Am J Med*, 1986, 80(5):959-64.

Selenium, Serum

Related Information

Heavy Metal Screen, Blood *on page 1271*

Synonyms Se, Serum

Abstract The essential nature of selenium in human nutrition is beyond dispute. The element is part of the enzyme that converts T_4 to the active thyroid hormone T_3. It is also part of selenium-dependant glutathione peroxidase, an important antioxidant in blood and tissue. Multiple cases of selenium deficiency have been reported, mostly among patients given parenteral nutrition with no added selenium. Deficiency also occurs endemically in places where soil selenium is low, and low levels are thus present throughout the food chain. Endemic cretinism, Balkan nephropathy, Keschan disease (endemic dilated cardiomyopathy), and Kashin-Bek disease (endemic deforming osteoarthritis) are probably all caused by endemic selenium deficiency conditioning the host to poorly tolerate an additional environmental stress (cretinism: iodine deficiency; the others: unknown local toxins). Simple deficiency is marked by whitening of the nailbeds, erythrocyte macrocytosis, cardiomyopathy, painful weak muscles, skin and hair depigmentation, and elevations of transaminase and creatinine kinase. The cardiomyopathy may be mild and asymptomatic or fulminant and fatal. Selenium toxicity can occur endemically, again due to high soil levels, or through accidental or industrial exposure. Symptoms include garlic breath, odor, thick brittle fingernails, dry brittle hair, red swollen skin of the hands and feet, and nervous system abnormalities of numbness, convulsions, or paralysis.

Specimen Blood

Container Sherwood Monoject™ trace element blood collection tube #8881-307006 or #8881-307022 with EDTA for whole blood

Collection Draw blood through B-D #5175 stainless steel needle into special trace metal vacuum tube. Centrifuge and pour serum into special plastic metal-free vial for transport.

Reference Range Serum: 95-165 ng/mL. Approximately 40% higher for whole blood. Serum reflects recent intake; red cells reflect more remote intake. Whole blood therefore reflects an average of recent and remote intake of selenium. (Selenium-dependent glutathione peroxidase activity reflects selenium available for enzyme synthesis – see below.) Levels are depressed in HIV infection, critical illness, kwashiorkor, inflammatory bowel disease, renal failure, hemodialysis status, low protein diet, phenylketonuria, maple syrup urine disease, (possibly all in part related to poor protein intake), low birth weight, and premature infants with inadequate selenium intake. Levels are increased mostly with the use of glucocorticoids. Levels >500 ng/mL are associated with toxicity.

Use Monitor selenium nutritional status in long-term parenteral nutrition. Studies have indicated no factor or factors that can accurately predict serum selenium levels to preclude need for measurement. May be used diagnostically in cardiomyopathy of unknown cause, especially where nutritional factors are suspected.

Limitations Some controversy exists regarding the "best" marker for selenium status. Since selenium as selenomethionine is incorporated nonspecifically into protein, serum and whole blood selenium concentration increases with increasing selenium intake to different degrees depending on inorganic or organic sources of selenium. Glutathione peroxidase activity is more sensitive to deficiency but the test is not well standardized and therefore not reproducible from laboratory to laboratory. Hair selenium may be contaminated by selenium-containing shampoo. Serum selenium level correlates best with intake and therefore with both deficiency and toxicity states, but a wide range of serum levels is compatible with apparent good health.

Methodology Atomic absorption, fluorometric methods

Additional Information Selenium is excreted in feces from the bile, in sweat and skin losses, and the remaining 50% to 70% in the urine. Significant breath losses

(Continued)

Selenium, Serum *(Continued)*

occur only in toxic states. Dosages in renal failure need not be modified. The deficiency syndrome may be rapidly induced under surgery or other stress after a long asymptomatic phase.

Specific References

Fleming CR, Lie JT, McCall JT, et al, "Selenium Deficiency and Fatal Cardiomyopathy in A Patient on Home Parenteral Nutrition," *Gastroenterology*, 1982, 83(3):689-93.

Koller LD and Exon JH, "The Two Faces of Selenium-Deficiency and Toxicity – Are Similar in Animals and Man," *Can J Vet Res*, 1986, 50(3):297-306.

Mathias PM and Jackson AA, "Selenium Deficiency in Kwashiorkor," *Lancet*, 1982, 1(8284):1312-3.

Pentel P, Fletcher D, and Jentzen J, "Fatal Acute Selenium Toxicity," *J Forensic Sci*, 1985, 30(2):556-62.

Vinton NE, Dahlstrom KA, Strobel CT, et al, "Macrocytosis and Pseudoalbinism: Manifestations of Selenium Deficiency," *J Pediatr*, 1987, 111(5):711-7.

Selenium, Urine

Synonyms Se, Urine

Abstract Urine selenium is used in conjunction with serum selenium to assess selenium nutrition or potential toxic exposure. Like any other 24-hour urine collection of an essential element, this reflects recent intake, assuming the patient is in selenium balance. In the case of selenium, skin and stool losses are significant and amount to 30% to 50% of total losses; nevertheless, urine losses often represent overflow losses and can help indicate whether recent intake has been adequate or possibly toxic. When selenium intake is low to normal, less than approximately 140 μg/day, 24-hour urine may not reflect the 24-hour intake of the previous day. This is especially true when the body stores are low and selenium is retained to fill body stores. At higher levels of intake, the 24-hour urine is well correlated with intake and can be used as evidence of excess intake, adequate intake, or prior toxic exposure. Twenty-four hour urine selenium reflects recent intake. When selenium supplementation normalizes serum selenium and whole blood selenium, and then selenium supplementation is stopped, urine selenium falls back toward baseline much faster than blood or serum levels. Urine selenium has recently been found to be correlated with 24-hour urine urea in critically ill patients. This probably reflects catabolism of protein and release of body stores of selenium, though details of the selenium intake of the patients (proportional to protein intake in tube-fed patients) were not provided.

Specimen 24-hour urine

Container Acid-washed plastic urine container

Collection Avoid contamination by hair since some patients use selenium-containing shampoos.

Reference Range Levels <15 μg/L or >150 μg/L probably represent unusually low or high intake without necessarily representing illness. Values vary widely and in apparently healthy U.S. citizens they have been reported to vary from 7 μg/L (24-hour sample) to 231 μg/L. Intake is partly determined by local soil content of selenium and use of local vegetables as food. Healthy persons in New Guinea have been reported with levels as low as 0.9 μg/L but similar patients have rapidly developed symptomatic selenium deficiency when placed on total parenteral nutrition lacking selenium. Urine levels of 7 μg/L have been reported from China in areas where selenium deficiency is symptomatic. Levels >880 μg/L have been seen in chronic selenosis and >600 μg/L during the first 24 hours after acute selenium intoxication. Levels >500 μg/L probably represent toxicity. See the comprehensive review by Robberecht and Deelstra. Some authors or laboratories report as μg/day.

Use Monitor nutritional therapy, especially parenteral nutrition; monitor potential toxic exposure

Limitations Selenomethionine is incorporated into body protein nonspecifically as methionine, so it is not as quickly excreted in the urine as inorganic selenium (selenite). Thus, the form of selenium ingested will affect short-term balance estimates. Spot urine selenium is of little value, as urine selenium goes up after each meal related to selenium intake and probably other factors, and dilution in spot urine samples varies.

Methodology Fluorometry, atomic absorption (AA)

Additional Information In addition to serum and urine levels of selenium, red cell glutathione peroxidase can be monitored as an example of the activity of a selenoenzyme. Levels will be depressed in deficiency but will not monitor toxicity.

Specific References

Levander OA, "A Global View of Human Selenium Nutrition," *Annu Rev Nutr*, 1987, 7:227-50.

Mathias PM and Jackson AA, "Selenium Deficiency in Kwashiorkor," *Lancet*, 1982, 1(8284):1312-3.

Pentel P, Fletcher D, and Jentzen J, "Fatal Acute Selenium Toxicity," *J Forensic Sci*, 1985, 30(2):556-62.

Thomson CD, "Clinical Consequences and Assessment of Low Selenium Status," *N Z Med J*, 1991, 104(919):376-7.

Serax® *see* Oxazepam, Serum *on page 1312*

Sernyl® *see* Phencyclidine, Quantitative, Serum *on page 1319*

Sertraline, Blood

Synonyms Zoloft™

Abstract Antidepressant with fewer adverse side effects than Prozac®; metabolizes to desmethylsertraline which has 10% of the activity of sertraline

Specimen Blood

Volume 5 mL

Minimum Volume 1 mL serum or plasma

Container Red top tube

Reference Range Postmortem blood: sertraline: 0.4-0.84 mg/L; desmethylsertraline: 1.3-1.5 mg/L; therapeutic clinical trials: sertraline: 0.03-0.19 mg/L

Use Antidepressant used when undesirable side effects noted with Prozac®; therapeutic monitoring and toxicity assessment

Methodology High performance liquid chromatography (HPLC), gas chromatography (GC), gas chromatography/mass spectrometry (GC/MS)

Specific References

Heym J and Koe BK, "Pharmacology of Sertraline. A Review," *J Clin Psychiatry*, 1988, 49(Suppl):40-5.

Rogowsky D, Marr M, Long G, et al, "Determination of Sertraline and Desmethylsertraline in Human Serum Using Copolymeric Bonded-Phase Extraction, HPLC and GC/MS," *J Chromatogr B Biomed Appl*, 1994, 655(1):138-41.

Serum Electrolytes *see* Electrolytes, Blood *on page 1254*

Serum Osmolality *see* Osmolality, Serum *on page 1310*

Se, Serum *see* Selenium, Serum *on page 1349*

Se, Urine *see* Selenium, Urine *on previous page*

SGOT *see* Aspartate Aminotransferase *on page 1199*

Silver, Serum

Synonyms Ag, Blood

Specimen Blood

Volume 5 mL

Container Red top tube

Reference Range Nondetectable

Use Evaluate silver toxicity

Additional Information Argyria is the result of inhalation or ingestion of silver or silver salts. Insoluble silver salts are deposited in the elastic fibers of the dermis and other organs, particularly the lungs. Patchy blue-black pigmentation of the skin, cornea, conjunctiva of the eye, vomiting, abdominal pain, dizziness, and convulsions are characteristic of this condition.

Silver, Urine

Synonyms Ag, Urine

Patient Preparation Patient should be instructed to use a plastic urinal or bedpan is necessary.

Specimen 24-hour urine

Volume Entire collection

Minimum Volume 100 mL aliquot

Container Plastic urine container, no preservative

Collection Instruct the patient to void at 8 AM and discard the specimen. Then collect all urine including the final specimen voided at the end of the 24-hour collection period (ie, 8 AM the next morning). Avoid contact with metal during collection. Screw the lid on securely. Transport the specimen promptly to the laboratory. Container **must** be labeled with patient's full name, room number, date and time collection started, and date and time collection finished.

Storage Instructions Keep on ice or refrigerate. Laboratory will measure urine volume and remove 120 mL aliquot.

Causes for Rejection Specimen allowed to contact metal

Special Instructions Requisition **must** state date and time collection started and date and time collection finished.

Reference Range Negative

Use Evaluate silver toxicity

Additional Information Argyria is the result of inhalation or ingestion of silver or silver salts. Insoluble silver salts are deposited in the elastic fibers of the dermis and other organs, particularly the lungs. Patchy blue-black pigmentation of the skin, cornea, conjunctiva of the eye, vomiting, abdominal pain, dizziness, and convulsions are characteristic of this condition.

Sinequan® *see* Doxepin, Blood *on page 1251*

Skeletal Muscle Biopsy *see* Muscle Biopsy *on page 1301*

Skin Scrapings for *Sarcoptes scabiei* Identification *see* Arthropod Identification *on page 1198*

Slo-Phyllin® *see* Theophylline, Blood *on page 1359*

Snow *see* Cocaine (Cocaine Metabolite), Qualitative *on page 1234*

SO_2 *see* Oxygen Saturation, Blood *on page 1313*

Sodium, Arterial Blood *see* Sodium, Blood *on this page*

Sodium, Blood

Related Information

Urea Nitrogen, Blood *on page 1370*

Synonyms Na^+

Applies To Sodium, Arterial Blood; Sodium, Corrected

Abstract Sodium with its accompanying anions is the most important extracellular osmotically active solute.

Specimen Blood

Volume 10 mL

Minimum Volume 2 mL serum or plasma

Container Red top tube or green top (lithium heparin) tube

Collection Pediatrics: Blood drawn from heelstick for capillary sample. Sodium, with potassium and chloride, can be reported from arterial or venous blood. If an arterial puncture is done for pO_2, lithium heparin anticoagulant must be used.

Reference Range Adults: 135-145 mmol/L

Possible Panic Range $<$120 mmol/L, $>$160 mmol/L

Use Evaluate electrolytes, acid-base balance, water balance, water intoxication, and diagnose dehydration.

Hypernatremia occurs in dehydration. For instance, nasogastric protein feeding with insufficient fluids may cause hypernatremia. Hypernatremia without obvious cause may relate to Cushing's syndrome, central or nephrogenic diabetes insipidus with insufficient fluids, primary aldosteronism, and other diseases. Severe hypernatremia may be associated with volume contraction, lactic acidosis, azotemia, weight loss, and increased hematocrit as evidence of dehydration. The corrected serum sodium is often high in nonketotic hyperosmolar coma. (A corrected sodium is calculated by increasing sodium by 1.3-1.6 mmol/L for each 100 mg/dL increment in serum or plasma glucose). 100 mg = 5.56 mmol/L. The corrected serum sodium level should be calculated in nonketotic hyperosmolar coma. Apparent mild hyponatremia with very high glucose may actually mean hypernatremia.

Hyponatremia occurs with nephrotic syndrome, cachexia, hypoproteinemia, intravenous glucose infusion, congestive heart failure, and other clinical entities. Serum sodium is a predictor of cardiovascular mortality in patients with severe congestive heart failure. **Hyponatremia** without congestive heart failure or dehydration may occur with hypothyroidism, the syndrome of inappropriate secretion of antidiuretic hormone (SIADH), renal failure, or renal sodium loss.

The differential diagnosis of hyponatremia includes Addison's disease, hypopituitarism, liver disease including cirrhosis, hypertriglyceridemia, and psychogenic polydipsia. Diuretics and other drugs may cause hyponatremia. Sodium decreasing to levels $<$115 mmol/L can lead to significant neurological dysfunction with cerebral edema and increased intracranial pressure.

The differential diagnosis of hyponatremia includes determination of urine sodium and osmolality and serum urea nitrogen (BUN). BUN is often decreased in SIADH.

Limitations Care should be taken that one is not dealing with "pseudohyponatremia." See the following comments.

Methodology Flame emission photometry, ion-selective electrode (ISE)

Additional Information The ratio of serum sodium to osmolality is normally 0.43-0.50; a decreased ratio is found in uremia and other states in which there are increased substances with osmotic activity.

See Urea Nitrogen, Blood regarding hyponatremia with sodium $<$128 mmol/L, hypo-osmolality, low BUN, and the syndrome of inappropriate secretion of antidiuretic hormone.

A number of situations result in "pseudohyponatremia." In these circumstances, treatment may be undesirable. With pseudohyponatremia serum sodium is decreased but the serum is not hypotonic (serum osmolality is normal or even increased). This may occur as the result of other molecules replacing water in relation to sodium. The water content is effectively lowered – sodium is "diluted." In severe hypertriglyceridemia or paraprotein-related marked increase in protein, the concentration of sodium in relation to water is normal but the analytic result is determined as mmol/L of serum. Osmolality in this situation is determined as amount of particles per kg of water and will be normal. It has been shown that analyses by sodium electrode of the direct potentiometric type (requires no dilution) are not artifactually low in patients with hyperlipidemia. If large amounts of solute, such as glucose or mannitol, are present, movement of intracellular water into the extracellular space may produce dilutional hyponatremia. In this case, sodium concentration in relation to water is actually low. "Osmolal gap" however exists between measured and calculated serum osmolality. Other substances capable of increasing serum osmolality (eg, ethanol) may also cause increase in the osmolal gap. Yet another cause of pseudohyponatremia is increased serum viscosity due to increased globulin proteins, occurring particularly in Waldenström's macroglobulinemia. The sodium analyzer may aspirate too little sample when viscosity is so high, leading to a factitious low sodium concentration. See discussion of "pseudohyponatremia" by Epstein and Oster.

Hyponatremia may manifest lethal neurological complications (water intoxication with brain edema).

Specific References

Aw TC and Kiechle FL, "Pseudohyponatremia," *Am J Emerg Med*, 1985, 3(3):236-9.

Daugirdas JT, Kronfol NO, Tzamaloukas AH, et al, "Hyperosmolar Coma: Cellular Dehydration and the Serum Sodium Concentration," *Ann Intern Med*, 1989, 110(11):855-7, (review).

DeVita MV and Michelis MF, "Perturbations in Sodium Balance: Hyponatremia and Hypernatremia," *Clin Lab Med*, 1993, 13(1):135-48.

Epstein M and Oster JR, "Disorders of Hyponatremia and Hypernatremia," *The Laboratory in Clinical Medicine. Interpretation and Application*, 2nd ed, Halsted JA and Halsted CH, eds, Philadelphia, PA: WB Saunders Co, 1981, 289-95.

Fogh-Andersen N, Wimberley PD, Thode J, et al, "Determination of Sodium and Potassium With Ion-Selective Electrodes," *Clin Chem*, 1984, 30(3):433-6.

Hitz J and Trivin F, "Sodium," *Drug Effects on Laboratory Test Results Analytical Interferences and Pharmacological Effects*, Siest G and Galteau MM, eds, Littleton, MA: PSG Publishing Co Inc, 1988, 391-404.

Kaplan LA and Pesce AJ, eds, *Clinical Chemistry: Theory, Analysis, and Correlation*, St Louis, MO: Mosby-Year Book Inc, 1984.

Lee WH and Packer M, "Prognostic Importance of Serum Sodium Concentration and Its Modification by Converting Enzyme Inhibition in Patients With Severe Chronic Heart Failure," *Circulation*, 1986, 73(2):257-67.

Leehey DJ, Daugirdas JT, Manahan FJ, et al, "Prolonged Hypernatremia Associated With Azotemia and Hyponatruria," *Am J Med*, 1989, 86(4):494-6.

Maffly RH, "Renal Function and Disorders of Water, Sodium, and Potassium Balance," *Scientific American Medicine*, Section 10, Chapter 1, Rubenstein E and Federman DD, eds, New York, NY: Scientific American Inc, 1990, 2-34.

McCleane GJ, "Urea and Electrolyte Measurement in Preoperative Surgical Patients," *Anaesthesia*, 1988, 43(5):413-5.

Votey SR, Peters AL, and Hoffman JR, "Disorders of Water Metabolism: Hyponatremia and Hypernatremia," *Emerg Med Clin North Am*, 1989, 7(4):749-69.

Sodium, Corrected *see* Sodium, Blood *on previous page*

Sodium Fluoride *see* Fluoride, Serum *on page 1267*

Sodium, Urine

Synonyms Na, Urine; Urine Na

Specimen Timed or random urine

Volume 0.5 mL

Container Plain urine container

Causes for Rejection Improper labeling

Reference Range 24-hour urine: 27-287 mmol/d, varies markedly with dietary intake of sodium. There is diurnal variation (output is lower at night). A European study provides average sodium excretion: male: 162 mmol/day, range: 143-208 mmol/day; female: 134 mmol/day, range: 119-165 mmol/day; within person CV: male: 30%, female: 34%.

Use Work up volume depletion, acute renal failure, acute oliguria, and differential diagnosis of hyponatremia. Division of hyponatremia into hypervolemia or not, edema or not, and urinary sodium less than or greater than 10 mmol/L provides a classification of hyponatremia. History of diuretics, other drug intake, setting of osmotic diuresis or not, serum/plasma electrolytes, and other factors are needed.

Limitations It is often advantageous to request urine potassium and creatinine along with sodium measurement. High urine sodium does not necessarily indicate that total body sodium is increased (eg, salt-losing nephritis). This area is complex; the reader is referred to the footnotes and references.

Methodology Flame emission photometry or ion-selective electrode (ISE)

Additional Information In cases of hyponatremia, random urine sodium <10 mmol/L may indicate extrarenal depletion: dehydration (gastrointestinal or sweat loss), congestive heart failure, liver disease or nephrotic syndromes.

Random urine sodium >10 mmol/L may indicate diuretics, emesis, intrinsic renal diseases, Addison's disease, hypothyroidism, or syndrome of inappropriate antidi-

(Continued)

Evaluation and Treatment of the **Hypernatremic** Patient

CONDITION		ETIOLOGY	URINARY ELECTROLYTES	TREATMENT
Hypovolemic	Renal losses	Osmotic diuresis	Urinary sodium >30 mmol/L	Isotonic saline (0.9 NaCl) until hemodynamically stable, then hypotonic fluids
	Extrarenal losses	Sweating Diarrhea in children	Urinary sodium <30 mmol/L	
Euvolemic	Renal losses	Central diabetes insipidus Nephrogenic diabetes insipidus Partial diabetes insipidus Hypodipsia	Variable urinary sodium	Administer vasopressin and water replacement. If urine volume decreased, diagnosis is central diabetes insipidus or partial diabetes insipidus. If no response, diagnosis is nephrogenic diabetes insipidus. Give trial of hydrochlorothiazide.
	Extrarenal losses	Respiratory or skin losses		
Hypervolemic	Increased total body sodium	Primary or secondary aldosteronism Cushing's syndrome Hypertonic I.V. infusion I.V. sodium bicarbonate administration Sodium chloride tablets	Urinary sodium >30 mmol/L	Diuretics and water replacement

From Devita MV and Michelis MF, "Perturbations in Sodium Balance: Hyponatremia and Hypernatremia", *Clinics in Laboratory Medicine*, Vol 13, Preuss HG, ed, Philadelphia, PA: WB Saunders Co, 1993, 135-48, with permission.

Evaluation and Treatment of **Hyponatremic** Patient

CONDITION	CLINICAL PRESENTATION	URINARY ELECTROLYTES	ETIOLOGY	TREATMENT
Hypovolemic	Orthostatic hypotension Tachycardia Azotemia	Urinary sodium >30 mmol/L	Diuretics, RTA, mineralocorticoid deficiency, salt-wasting nephritis	0.9 NaCl I.V.
		Urinary sodium <30 mmol/L	Extrarenal losses: vomiting, diarrhea, burns, sequestration	0.9 NaCl I.V.
Euvolemic	No evidence of volume depletion or overload. Subclinical increase in TBW may be present.	Urinary sodium >20 mmol/L	Hypothyroidism	Thyroid replacement
			Glucocorticoid deficiency	I.V. glucocorticoids
			SIADH, drugs, acute water intoxication	Fluid restriction
Hypervolemic	Volume excess Edema	Urinary sodium >30 mmol/L	Acute and chronic renal failure	Fluid restriction; treat renal failure
		Urinary sodium <10 mmol/L	Cirrhosis Cardiac failure Nephrotic syndrome	Fluid restriction; sodium restriction; treat underlying disorders

From Devita MV and Michelis MF, "Perturbations in Sodium Balance: Hyponatremia and Hypernatremia," *Clinics in Laboratory Medicine*, Vol 13, Preuss HG, ed, Philadelphia, PA: WB Saunders Co, 1993, 135-48, with permission.

(Continued)

Sodium, Urine *(Continued)*

uretic hormone (SIADH). In hypothyroidism and in SIADH, sodium and chloride may be >40 mmol/L. (Depending on intake, such results also can be found in normal individuals.) In SIADH, random urinary sodium usually is >20 mmol/L. Inappropriate secretion of antidiuretic hormone (SIADH) was found in 7% of 250 patients with small cell lung cancer. Such patients have hyponatremia, often severe, with hypo-osmolar serum, high urinary sodium excretion with urine osmolality greater than that of serum. Acute and subacute diseases of the CNS, TB, and other chronic pulmonary diseases may also cause SIADH. SIADH may also be caused by acute intermittent porphyria, LE, occasional malignant neoplasms other than small cell carcinoma of the lung, and a number of drugs.

The classification as presented here is overly abbreviated for clinical application. Pitfalls exist (eg, increase of sodium necessary to balance excretion of penicillin).

Urine sodium >40 mmol/L in oliguria suggests acute tubular necrosis. (However, spot urine sodiums without other data have been criticized for their applicability to this diagnosis.)

Low sodium excretion may be found with early obstructive uropathy and with the oliguria of acute glomerulonephritis and in some patients with x-ray contrast acute renal failure.

Silver et al recommend measurement of urinary sodium excretion in patients with nephrolithiasis and hypercalciuria.

It is important to know the urinary sodium level in patients with unexplained hyperchloremic metabolic acidosis when the diagnosis of distal renal tubular acidosis is being considered.

Specific References

Batlle DC, von Riotte A, and Schlueter W, "Urinary Sodium in the Evaluation of Hyperchloremic Metabolic Acidosis," *N Engl J Med*, 1987, 316(3):140-4.

Brown MA, Gallery ED, Ross MR, et al, "Sodium Excretion in Normal and Hypertensive Pregnancy: A Prospective Study," *Am J Obstet Gynecol*, 1988, 159(2):297-307.

DeVita MV and Michelis MF, "Perturbations in Sodium Balance: Hyponatremia and Hypernatremia," *Clin Lab Med*, 1993, 13(1):135-48.

Hainsworth JD, Workman R, and Greco FA, "Management of the Syndrome of Inappropriate Antidiuretic Hormone Secretion in Small Cell Lung Cancer," *Cancer*, 1983, 51(1):161-5.

Harrington JT and Cohen JJ, "Measurement of Urinary Electrolytes – Indications and Limitations," *N Engl J Med*, 1975, 293(24):1241-3.

Intersalt Cooperative Research Group, "Intersalt: An International Study of Electrolyte Excretion and Blood Pressure. Results for 24-Hour Urinary Sodium and Potassium Excretion," *BMJ*, 1988, 297(6644):319-28.

Kamel KS, Ethier JH, Richardson RM, et al, "Urine Electrolytes and Osmolality: When and How to Use Them," *Am J Nephrol*, 1990, 10(2):89-102.

Knuiman JT, Hautvast JG, van der Heijden L, et al, "A Multi-Centre Study on Within-Person Variability in the Urinary Excretion of Sodium, Potassium, Calcium, Magnesium, and Creatinine in 8 European Centres," *Hum Nutr Clin Nutr*, 1986, 40(5):343-8.

Preuss HG, Podlasek SJ, and Henry JB, "Evaluation of Renal Function and Water, Electrolyte, and Acid-Base Balance," *Clinical Diagnosis and Management by Laboratory Methods*, 18th ed, Henry JB, ed, Philadelphia, PA: WB Saunders Co, 1991, 118-39.

Schrier RW, "Acute Renal Failure," *JAMA*, 1982, 247(18):2518-22, 2524.

Sherman RA and Eisinger RP, "The Use (and Misuse) of Urinary Sodium and Chloride Measurements," *JAMA*, 1982, 247(22):3121-4.

Silver J, Rubinger D, Friedlaender MM, et al, "Sodium-Dependent Idiopathic Hypercalciuria in Renal-Stone Formers," *Lancet*, 1983, 2(8348):484-6.

Streeten DHP and Moses AM, "Disorders of the Neurohypophysis," *Harrison's Principles of Internal Medicine*, Braunwald E, Isselbacher KJ, Petersdorf RG, et al, eds, New York, NY: McGraw-Hill Inc, 1991, 1682-91.

Solganal® *see* Gold Level *on page 1270*

Soma® *see* Carisoprodol, Quantitative *on page 1222*

Specimen Chain-of-Custody Protocol *see* Chain-of-Custody Protocol *on page 1223*

Speed *see* Amphetamines, Qualitative, Urine *on page 1190*

Speed *see* Methamphetamines, Urine *on page 1294*

Stelazine® *see* Trifluoperazine, Blood *on page 1369*

Stental Extentabs® *see* Phenobarbital, Blood *on page 1320*

Steroid Drug Screen, Urine *see* Toxicology, Steroid Drug Screen, Urine *on page 1367*

Stool Culture

Synonyms Enteric Pathogens Culture, Routine; Stool for Culture

Applies To Rectal Swab Culture; Routine Culture, Rectal Swab

Test Includes Screening culture for *Salmonella*, *Shigella*, *Helicobacter*, and, if requested, *Staphylococcus*.

Specimen Fresh random stool, rectal swab

Volume 5 mL

Container Plastic stool container, Culturette®

Collection If stool is collected in a clean bedpan, it must not be contaminated with urine, residual soap, or disinfectants. Swabs of lesions of the rectal wall during proctoscopy or sigmoidoscopy are preferred.

Rectal swab: Insert the swab past the anal sphincter, move the swab circumferentially around the rectum. Allow 15-30 seconds for organisms to adsorb onto the swab. Withdraw swab, place in Culturette® tube, and crush media compartment.

Storage Instructions Refrigerate if the specimen cannot be processed promptly.

Causes for Rejection Because of risk to laboratory personnel, specimens sent on diaper or tissue paper, specimen contaminating outside of transport container may not be acceptable to the laboratory. Specimen containing interfering substances (eg, castor oil, bismuth, Metamucil®, barium), specimens delayed in transit and those contaminated with urine may not have optimal yield.

Special Instructions The laboratory should be informed of the specific pathogen suspected if not *Salmonella*, *Shigella*, or *Campylobacter*.

Reference Range Negative for *Salmonella*, *Shigella*, and *Campylobacter*. In endemic areas the isolation of a pathogen may not indicate the cause or only cause of diarrhea.

Use Screen for common bacterial pathogenic organisms in the stool; diagnose typhoid fever, enteric fever, bacillary dysentery, *Salmonella* infection.

Indications for stool culture include:

- bloody diarrhea
- fever
- tenesmus
- severe or persistent symptoms
- recent travel to a third world country
- known exposure to a bacterial agent
- presence of fecal leukocytes

Limitations *Yersinia* species and *Vibrio* species may not be isolated unless specifically requested.

Contraindications A rectal swab culture is not as effective as a stool culture for detection of the carrier state.

Methodology Aerobic culture on selective media

Additional Information Stool cultures on patients hospitalized ≥3 days **are not productive and should not be ordered** unless special circumstances exist.

In enteric fever caused by *Salmonella typhi*, *S. choleraesuis*, or *S. enteritidis*, blood culture may be positive before stool cultures, and blood cultures are indicated early. Diarrhea is common in patients with the acquired immunodeficiency syndrome (AIDS). Diarrhea in AIDS is frequently caused by the classic bacterial pathogens; however, parasitic infestation is also common with *Giardia* and *Cryptosporidium*. Rectal swabs are useful for the diagnosis of *Neisseria gonorrhoeae* and *Chlamydia* infections.

In acute or subacute diarrhea, three common syndromes are recognized: gastroenteritis, enteritis, and colitis (dysenteric syndrome). With colitis, patients have fecal urgency and tenesmus. Stool are frequently small in volume and contain blood, mucus, and leukocytes. External hemorrhoids are common and painful. Diarrhea of small bowel origin is indicated by the passage of few large volume stools. This is due to accumulation of fluid in the large bowel before passage. Leukocytes indicate colonic inflammation rather than a specific pathogen. Bacterial diarrhea may be present in the absence of fecal leukocytes and fecal leukocytes may be present in the absence of bacterial or parasitic agents (ie, idiopathic inflammatory bowel disease). See table. Although most bacterial diarrhea is tran-

Diarrhea Syndromes Classified by Predominant Features

Syndrome (anatomic site)	Features	Characteristic Etiologies
Gastroenteritis (stomach)	Vomiting	Rotavirus Norwalk virus Staphylococcal food poisoning *Bacillus cereus* food poisoning
Enteritis (small bowel)	Watery diarrhea Large–volume stools, few in number	Enterotoxigenic *E. coli* *Vibrio cholerae* Any enteric microbe
Dysentery, colitis (colon)	Small–volume stools containing blood and/or mucus and many leukocytes	*Shigella* *Campylobacter* *Salmonella* Invasive *E. coli* *Plesiomonas shigelloides* *Aeromonas hydrophila* *Vibrio parahaemolyticus* *Clostridium difficile* *Entamoeba histolytica* Inflammatory bowel disease

(Continued)

Stool Culture *(Continued)*

sient (1-30 days) cases of persistent symptoms (10 months) have been reported. The etiologic agent in the reported case was *Shigella flexneri* diagnosed by culture of rectal swab. In infants younger than 1 year of age, a history of blood in the stool, more than 10 stools in 24 hours, and temperature greater than 39°C have a high probability of having bacterial diarrhea.

Specific References

Bishop WP and Ulshen MH, "Bacterial Gastroenteritis," *Pediatr Clin North Am*, 1988, 35(1):69-87.
Farmer RG, "Infectious Causes of Diarrhea in the Differential Diagnosis of Inflammatory Bowel Disease," *Med Clin North Am*, 1990, 74(1):29-38.
Gracey M, "Bacterial Diarrhea," *J Clin Gastroenterol*, 1986, 15(1):21-37.
Guerrant RL, Wanke CA, Barrett LJ, et al, "A Cost Effective and Effective Approach to the Diagnosis and Management of Acute Infectious Diarrhea," *Bull N Y Acad Med*, 1987, 63(6):484-99.
Pickering LK, "Therapy for Acute Infectious Diarrhea in Children," *J Pediatr*, 1991, 118(4 Pt 2):S118-28.
Radetsky M, "Laboratory Evaluation of Acute Diarrhea," *Pediatr Infect Dis*, 1986, 5(2):230-8.

Stool for Culture *see* Stool Culture *on previous page*

Strychnine, Quantitative

Specimen Blood
Volume 15 mL
Minimum Volume 5 mL serum
Container Red top tube
Critical Values Toxic: >2 μg/mL
Use Evaluate toxicity
Additional Information Strychnine is used in commercial rodent poison. Its ingestion results in tonic convulsions that last approximately 1 minute and death soon after due to respiratory paralysis. Treatment includes artificial respiration and O_2 administration to prevent respiratory failure and short-acting barbiturates or benzoidazepine administration.

Sublimaze® *see* Fentanyl, Blood or Urine *on page 1264*
β-Subunit of hCG *see* Pregnancy Test *on page 1330*
Sudden Infant Death Syndrome *see* Botulism Diagnostic Procedure *on page 1211*

Sulfhemoglobin

Specimen Blood
Volume 10 mL
Minimum Volume 1 mL whole blood
Container Amber top tube
Storage Instructions Maintain specimen at room temperature.
Reference Range None detectable
Use Evaluate cyanosis
Methodology Spectrophotometry
Additional Information The term sulfhemoglobin refers to a poorly characterized hemoglobin derivative which can be produced *in vitro* from the action of hydrogen sulfide on hemoglobin. Sulfhemoglobinemia may occur in association with the administration of various drugs, including sulfonamides, phenacetin, metoclopropramide, and acetanilide but has been reported also in the absence of exposure to drugs or toxins. The symptoms are few but the cyanosis is intense even though the concentration is seldom >10%. Once formed, sulfhemoglobin is stable and cannot be reduced back to hemoglobin. It disappears as the red cells become senescent and are destroyed.

Surmontil® *see* Trimipramine, Semiquantitative, Urine *on page 1370*
Sustaire® *see* Theophylline, Blood *on next page*
Suxinutin® *see* Ethosuximide, Blood *on page 1261*
T_4 *see* Thyroxine, Blood *on page 1361*
T_4 by EIA *see* Thyroxine, Blood *on page 1361*
T_4 CPB *replaced by* Thyroxine, Blood *on page 1361*
T_4 (RIA) *see* Thyroxine, Blood *on page 1361*
TAD *see* Tricyclic Antidepressants, Blood *on page 1368*
Talbutal *see* Barbiturates, Quantitative, Blood *on page 1201*
Talwin® *see* Pentazocine, Urine *on page 1316*
Tambocor® *see* Flecainide, Blood *on page 1266*
TCA *see* Tricyclic Antidepressants, Blood *on page 1368*

TCO_2 *see* Carbon Dioxide, Blood *on page 1220*

Tegretol® *see* Carbamazepine, Blood *on page 1219*

Tegretol®, Free *see* Carbamazepine, Free *on page 1220*

Tempra® *see* Acetaminophen, Serum *on page 1180*

Tetracyclic Antidepressants *see* Tricyclic Antidepressants, Blood *on page 1368*

Tetraiodothyronine *see* Thyroxine, Blood *on page 1361*

Thallium, Urine or Blood

Related Information

Heavy Metal Screen, Blood *on page 1271*

Abstract Thallium salts are components of insecticides and rodenticides.

Patient Preparation The patient should be instructed to use a plastic bedpan or urinal if necessary

Specimen 24-hour urine, blood

Volume Entire collection

Container Plastic urine container, red top tube

Causes for Rejection Specimen allowed to contact metal

Reference Range Urine: <10 μg/24 hours; serum: <10 ng/mL (SI: <49 nmol/L)

Use Diagnose thallium toxicity in patients exposed to insecticides and rat poisons

Methodology Atomic absorption spectrometry (AA)

Additional Information Thallium salts have been used in the past as a depilatory. Alopecia may occur several weeks after poisoning. Thallium is an ingredient in rodenticides and insecticides. Poisoning causes GI symptoms, rash, polyneuritis, encephalitis, delirium, convulsions, shock, and coma. Lethal dose is 1 g. Half-life is 2 days.

Specific References

Baselt RC and Cravey RH, *Disposition of Toxic Drugs and Chemicals in Man*, 3rd ed, Chicago, IL: Year Book Medical Publishers Inc, 1989, 786-8.

THC (Delta-9-Tetrahydrocannabinol) *see* Cannabinoids, Qualitative *on page 1217*

Theo-Dur® *see* Theophylline, Blood *on this page*

Theolair™ *see* Theophylline, Blood *on this page*

Theophylline, Blood

Synonyms Aminophylline; Elixophyllin®; Slo-Phyllin®; Sustaire®; Theo-Dur®; Theolair™; Theospan®

Abstract Theophylline is an antiasthmatic which is frequently monitored.

Specimen Blood

Volume 7 mL

Minimum Volume 3 mL serum

Container Red top tube

Sampling Time Measure **trough** (just before the next dose) and **peak**. Ideally, to measure peak serum theophylline **no** missed doses for previous 48 hours; blood drawn at 2 hours after most recent dose for rapid dissolution preparations; 4-6 hours after sustained release preparations.

Storage Instructions Refrigerate (do not freeze) a minimum of 0.5 mL serum.

Causes for Rejection Stored specimen not refrigerated

Reference Range Therapeutic: 10-20 μg/mL (SI: 56-111 μmol/L)

Possible Panic Range >20 μg/mL (SI: >111 μmol/L); neonates: >10 μg/mL (SI: >56 μmol/L); high probability of seizures when levels are >40 μg/mL.

Use Monitor therapeutic drug level; detect noncompliance and subtherapeutic levels; attempt to predict theophylline toxicity if possible

Methodology Enzyme immunoassay (EIA), high performance liquid chromatography (HPLC), gas chromatography (GC)

Additional Information Theophylline is prescribed for bronchial asthma, for chronic obstructive pulmonary disease, and for newborn apnea. The drug is extensively metabolized with peak serum levels reached 4 hours after oral dose. Troleandomycin and erythromycin may slow theophylline elimination. Heart failure, liver disease, prolonged fever, certain infections, and obesity may have similar effects. Prolonged half-life occurs in premature infants. **Dosage should be reduced in these situations.**

By contrast, half-life is shortened in smokers, variable with phenobarbital administration; higher doses tolerated also in acidemia. Smokers on the average are reported to need 1.5 to 2 times as much of the drugs as nonsmokers to achieve the same effects. Optimal resampling time after change in dosage is 48 hours for adults, 1-2 days for children. The half-life of theophylline is from 3-10 hours for adults and 1.4-7.9 hours for children, but varies between individuals.

(Continued)

Theophylline, Blood *(Continued)*

Studying serum concentrations and toxic effects, Bertino et al found toxicity with peak theophylline concentrations as low as 19.4 mg/L (SI: 108 μmol/L). Recognizing theophylline toxicity over a wide range of theophylline levels, these authors questioned the association between the severity of toxic effects and serum concentrations.

Blood levels should be interpreted in light of the patient's clinical status and use of other medications.

Toxic effects include nausea, vomiting, diarrhea, headache, atrial and ventricular arrhythmias, tremors, and convulsions.

Specific References

Anderson W, Youl B, and Mackay IR, "Acute Theophylline Intoxication," *Ann Emerg Med*, 1991, 20(10):1143-5.

Bryson PD, "Theophylline," *Comprehensive Review in Toxicology*, 2nd ed, Rockville, MD: Aspen Publications, 1989, 105-16.

Butts JD, Secrest B, and Berger R, "Nonlinear Theophylline Pharmacokinetics. A Preventable Cause of Iatrogenic Theophylline Toxic Reactions," *Arch Intern Med*, 1991, 151(10):2073-7.

Emerman CL, Devlin C, and Connors AF, "Risk of Toxicity in Patients With Elevated Theophylline Levels," *Ann Emerg Med*, 1990, 19(6):643-8.

Greenberger PA, Cranberg JA, Ganz MA, et al, "A Prospective Evaluation of Elevated Serum Theophylline Concentrations to Determine if High Concentrations are Predictable," *Am J Med*, 1991, 91(1):67-73.

Meatheral R and Ford D, "Isoeratic Liquid Chromatographic Determination of Theophylline, Acetaminophen, Caffeine, Chloramphenicol, Anticonvulsants and Barbiturates in Serum," *Ther Drug Monit*, 1988, 10(1):101-15.

Paloucek FP and Rodvold KA, "Evaluation of Theophylline Overdoses and Toxicities," *Ann Emerg Med*, 1988, 17(2):135-44.

Poe RH and Utell MJ, "Theophylline in Asthma and COPD: Changing Perspectives and Controversies," *Geriatrics*, 1991, 46(4):55-6, 61-5.

Rowe DJ, Watson ID, and Williams J, "The Clinical Use and Measurement of Theophylline," *Ann Clin Biochem*, 1988, 25(Pt 1):4-26.

Ruff F, Santais MC, Callens E, et al, "Effect of Temafloxacin on the Pharmacokinetics of Theophylline," *Am J Med*, 1991, 91(6A):76S-80S.

Sessler CN, "Theophylline Toxicity: Clinical Features of 116 Consecutive Cases," *Am J Med*, 1990, 88(6):567-76.

Tsiu SJ, Self TH, and Burns R, "Theophylline Toxicity: Update," *Ann Allergy*, 1990, 64(2 Pt 2):241-57.

Theospan® *see* Theophylline, Blood *on previous page*

Thiocyanate, Blood or Urine

Synonyms Ethyl and Methyl Thiocyanate (Thanite® and Lethane®); Potassium Thiocyanate (KCN)

Applies To Nipride®; Nitroprusside

Abstract Thiocyanate is a metabolite of the antihypertensive drug, nitroprusside. It is also a product of cyanide metabolism.

Specimen Blood, urine

Volume 7 mL

Container Red top tube, lavender top (EDTA) tube, plastic urine container

Reference Range Serum, therapeutic: 1-4 μg/mL (SI: 0.02-0.07 mmol/L), smokers: 3-12 μg/mL (SI: 0.05-0.21 mmol/L); urine: 1-4 mg/24 hours, smokers: 7-17 mg/24 hours

Possible Panic Range Serum: >35 μg/mL (SI: >0.60 mmol/L); 200 μg/mL (SI: 3.44 mmol/L) is lethal

Use Evaluate thiocyanate toxicity, nitroprusside poisoning, smoking. Toxic manifestations are psychotic behavior, agitation, and convulsions.

Limitations Because of rapid metabolism of the drug, results are usually meaningless in the clinical setting by the time they are reported.

Methodology Photometry/chromatography

Additional Information Thiocyanate is a major metabolite of cyanide produced in the liver by the enzyme rhodanase. Thiocyanate is present in healthy subjects. It is a component of cigarette smoke, and it can arise from the drug nitroprusside.

Specific References

Balistreri WF, A-Kader HH, Setchell KD, et al, "New Methods for Assessing Liver Function in Infants and Children," *Ann Clin Lab Sci*, 1992, 22(3):162-74.

Hall AH and Rumack BH, "Clinical Toxicology of Cyanide," *Ann Emerg Med*, 1986, 15(9):1067-74.

Thioridazine, Quantitative

Synonyms Mellaril®

Applies To Phenothiazines

Specimen Blood

Volume 15 mL

Minimum Volume 5 mL

Container Three yellow top (ACD) tubes

Collection Collect specimen immediately prior to next dose unless specified otherwise.

Storage Instructions Separate and refrigerate.

Reference Range <1 μg/mL

Critical Values 2 μg/mL

Possible Panic Range Lethal dose: 1 g

Use Monitor therapeutic drug level; evaluate toxicity

Additional Information Thioridazine, a piperidine phenothiazine, is used to manage the manifestations of psychotic disorders, depressive neurosis, alcohol withdrawal, dementia in the elderly, and attention deficit disorders in children. Thioridazine shares many characteristics with chlorpromazine, but EKG changes and retinal pigmentation is more common than with chlorpromazine. Extrapyramidal effects are rare, and sedation and anticholinergic effects are more pronounced. The half-life is 26-36 hours. Adverse effects include anxiety, extrapyramidal reactions, pseudoparkinsonian signs and symptoms, seizures, hypotension, tachycardia and arrhythmias, agranulocytosis, leukopenia, amenorrhea, galactorrhea, and gynecomastia.

Specific References

Poklis A, Wells CE, and Juenge EC, "Thioridazine and Its Metabolites in Post Mortem Blood, Including Two Stereoisomeric Ring Sulfoxides," *J Anal Toxicol*, 1982, 6(5):250-2.

Thiothixene, Blood

Synonyms Navane®

Specimen Blood

Volume 10 mL

Minimum Volume 3 mL serum

Container Red top tube

Storage Instructions Refrigerate serum.

Reference Range Therapeutic: 10-40 ng/mL

Possible Panic Range >200 ng/mL

Methodology High performance liquid chromatography (HPLC)

Additional Information Thiothixene, a thioxanthene derivative, is used to manage psychotic disorders. It is similar pharmacologically and chemically to chlorprothixene and the piperazine phenothiazines. Therapeutic effects are achieved 1-6 hours after an I.M. injection and the half-life is 34 hours. Adverse effects include anticholinergic effects, tachycardia, hypotension, and EKG changes, drowsiness, insomnia, seizures, nonreversible tardive dyskinesia, gynecomastia, amenorrhea, and transient leukopenia.

Specific References

Baselt RC, *Disposition of Toxic Drugs and Chemicals in Man*, 2nd ed, Davis, CA: Biomedical Publications, 1982, 734-6.

Thymol Turbidity *replaced by* Aspartate Aminotransferase *on page 1199*

Thyroxine, Blood

Synonyms T_4; T_4 by EIA; T_4 (RIA); Tetraiodothyronine; Thyroxine by RIA

Abstract Thyroxine (T_4) is the major secretory product of the thyroid gland. It is carried through the blood bound (in equilibrium) to thyroxine binding globulin (TBG), prealbumin, and albumin. T_4 secretion is stimulated by thyroid stimulating hormone (TSH).

Patient Preparation Avoid radioisotope administration prior to collection of specimen.

Specimen Blood

Volume 7 mL

Minimum Volume 1 mL serum

Container Red top tube

Storage Instructions Separate serum within 48 hours and refrigerate. Separated serum stable 1 week at 25°C.

Reference Range Pediatrics: Cord T_4 and values in the first few weeks are much higher, falling over the first months and years; 10 years and older: approximately 5.8-11.0 μg/dL (SI: 75-142 nmol/L), varying somewhat between laboratories. Borderline low is ≤4.5-5.7 μg/dL (SI: ≤58-73 nmol/L); low is ≤4.4 μg/dL (SI: ≤57 nmol/L); results <2.5 μg/dL (SI: <32 nmol/L) are strong evidence for hypothyroidism.

Approximate adult normal range is given by Ingbar as 4.0-12.0 μg/dL (SI: 51-154 nmol/L) and by Larsen as 5.0-11.0 μg/dL (SI: 64-142 nmol/L); borderline high is 11.1-13.0 μg/dL (SI: 143-167 nmol/L); high is ≥13.1 μg/dL (SI: ≥169 nmol/L). High is sometimes given as ≥8-10 μg/dL (SI: ≥103-129 nmol/L). Normal range is increased in women on birth control pills, owing to increased TBG. Free thyroxine index will still be within the normal range. Normal range in pregnancy: approximately 5.5-16.0 μg/dL (SI: 71-206 nmol/L).

Possible Panic Range At values <2.0 μg/dL (SI: <26 nmol/L), myxedema coma is possible. At values >20.0 μg/dL (SI: >257 nmol/L), thyroid storm is possible.

(Continued)

Thyroxine, Blood *(Continued)*

Use Best general thyroid function screening test. **Decreased** in hypothyroidism, in genetically decreased TBG, and in the third stage of (painful) subacute thyroiditis; **increased** with hyperthyroidism, with subacute thyroiditis in its first stage, with thyrotoxicosis due to Graves' disease, with increased TBG (pregnancy, genetically increased TBG, acute intermittent porphyria, primary biliary cirrhosis), thyrotoxicosis factitia, and occasionally in euthyroid patients with familial dysalbuminemic hyperthyroxinemia. Used to diagnose T_4 thyrotoxicosis.

Primary hypothyroidism (hypometabolism) is caused by Hashimoto's thyroiditis, idiopathic myxedema, prior radioactive iodine therapy for hyperthyroidism, prior thyroid surgery, endemic goiter and other entities. Congenital causes include enzyme blocks and agenesis. Causes of **secondary hypothyroidism** include primary pituitary disease (eg, postpartum pituitary necrosis (Sheehan's syndrome) and pituitary tumors). The expression "myxedema" indicates advanced clinical hypothyroidism, with dermal mucopolysaccharide deposits. Comprehensive lists of causes of hypothyroidism are published. A diagnosis of primary hypothyroidism should be confirmed by a TSH assay.

Graves' disease is classical thyrotoxicosis (hypermetabolism) caused by an immune or autoimmune disorder. Other causes of **hyperthyroidism** include toxic multinodular or uninodular goiter, phases of thyroiditis and a number of uncommon to rare entities, which cause increased T_4. Tabulations of causes of hyperthyroidism are widely available.

T_4 and other tests are used to investigate goiter, an expression for thyroid enlargement, which may be found with hypothyroidism, euthyroidism, or hyperthyroidism.

Limitations T_4 may be increased with excess intake of iodine or or with surreptitious use of thyroxine. T_4 levels may be abnormal in the presence of systemic nonthyroidal disease. Alterations in binding capacity or quantity of TBG may increase or decrease total thyroxine without causing symptoms. A common cause of elevated T_4 in nonthyroidal disease is said to be liver disease.

Serum thyroxine and free thyroxine (FT_4) are increased in familial dysalbuminemic hyperthyroxinemia, a euthyroid syndrome in which an abnormal binding site has affinity for thyroxine. The T_3 is usually normal in this entity, as is T_3 uptake. Thus, T_3 uptake is commonly ordered with T_4.

T_4 is less sensitive than TSH in the diagnosis of hypothyroidism.

Euthyroid hyperthyroxinemia has been reviewed. It is an expression used as a collective term for nonthyroidal diseases and states which increase thyroxine levels with normal thyroid tissue and metabolism. In addition to thyroid hormone binding globulin changes and drug related phenomena, peripheral resistance to thyroid hormones and increases related to medical and acute psychiatric illness are described. Hyperemesis gravidarum and hyponatremia may cause euthyroid hyperthyroxinemia. Extensive tabulations of thyroid tests and some causes of changes in them have been published.

Anti-T_4 antibodies may exist, interfering with T_4 and free T_4 determinations.

Heparin can cause false readings by interfering with assays.

Methodology Radioimmunoassay (RIA), enzyme-linked immunosorbent assay (ELISA), fluorescence polarization immunoassay (FPIA), chemiluminescence assay (CIA)

Additional Information The combination of the serum T_4 and T_3 uptake as an assessment of TBG, helps to determine whether an abnormal T_4 value is due to alterations in serum thyroxine binding globulin or to changes of thyroid hormone levels. Deviations of both tests in the same direction usually indicate that an abnormal T_4 is due to abnormalities in thyroid hormone. Deviations of the two tests in opposite directions provide evidence that an abnormal T_4 may relate to alterations in TBG.

Thyroid Tests With Disease and Varying TBG

Diagnosis	T_4	FT_4 (or FT_4I)	TSH
Normal	Normal	Normal	Normal
Hyperthyroid	Increased	Increased	Decreased
Hypothyroid	Decreased	Decreased	Increased
Increased TBG	Increased	Normal	Normal
Decreased TBG	Decreased	Normal	Normal

Causes of increased TBG binding include neonatal state, molar and conventional pregnancy, estrogens, oral contraceptives, heroin, methadone, 5-fluorouracil, clofibrate, infectious hepatitis, chronic active hepatitis, and primary biliary cirrhosis, acute intermittent porphyria, lymphoma, and hereditary TBG increase.

Causes of decreased TBG binding include abnormal protein states. These include nephrotic syndrome, androgens, anabolic steroids, prednisone, acromegaly, liver or other systemic illness, severe stress, and hereditary TBG deficiency. Salicylates and diphenylhydantoin may lower T_4 significantly. Amiodarone may cause increased thyroxine levels and can cause hypothyroidism or hyperthyroidism.

Lithium carbonate may cause goiter with or without hypothyroidism.

Carbamazepine (Tegretol®) is reported to cause decreased values in thyroid function tests.

This brief review must point out that clinical interpretation of patients' signs and symptoms has primary significance. Definitive treatment based on insufficient laboratory tests is condemned.

The sensitive TSH assay has been advocated as a single screening test for thyroid disease. Such proposals are controversial; others find it difficult to accept one test as adequate for screening and warn that a single test cannot adequately, in all settings, reflect thyroid status. An inverse relationship exists between thyroxine and TSH. While the former represents thyroid hormone concentration, the latter is a test of thyroid regulation.

Specific References

de los Santos ET and Mazzaferri EL, "Thyroid Function Tests. Guidelines for Interpretation in Common Clinical Disorders," *Postgrad Med*, 1989, 85(5):333-40, 345-52, (review).

Franklyn JA, Davis JR, Ramsden DB, et al, "Phenytoin and Thyroid Hormone Action," *J Endocrinol*, 1985, 104(2):201-4.

Gharib H and Klee GG, "Familial Euthyroid Hyperthyroxinemia Secondary to Pituitary and Peripheral Resistance to Thyroid Hormones," *Mayo Clin Proc*, 1985, 60(1):9-15.

Griffin JE, "Hypothyroidism in the Elderly," *Am J Med Sci*, 1990, 299(5):334-45.

Gruhn JG, Barsano CP, and Kumar Y, "The Development of Tests of Thyroid Function," *Arch Pathol Lab Med*, 1987, 111(1):84-100.

Klee GG, Young WF, and Hay ID, "Biochemical Tests of Thyroid and Pituitary Function," *ASCP National Meeting*, Chicago, IL: American Society of Clinical Pathologists, 1990.

Larsen PR, Alexander NM, Chopra IJ, et al, "Revised Nomenclature for Tests of Thyroid Hormones and Thyroid-Related Proteins in Serum," *Arch Pathol Lab Med*, 1987, 111(12):1141-5.

Miller MJ, Pan C, and Barzel US, "The Prevalence of Subclinical Hypothyroidism in Adults With Low-Normal Blood Thyroxine Levels," *N Y State J Med*, 1990, 90(11):541-4.

Rallison ML, Dobyns BM, Meikle AW, et al, "Natural History of Thyroid Abnormalities: Prevalence, Incidence, and Regression of Thyroid Diseases in Adolescents and Young Adults," *Am J Med*, 1991, 91(4):363-70.

Schectman JM and Pawlson LG, "Screening for Thyroid Disease," *Ann Intern Med*, 1990, 113(11):896.

Schectman JM and Pawlson LG, "The Cost-Effectiveness of Three Thyroid Function Testing Strategies for Suspicion of Hypothyroidism in a Primary Care Setting," *J Gen Intern Med*, 1990, 5(1):9-15.

Staub JJ, Althaus BU, Engler H, et al, "Spectrum of Subclinical and Overt Hypothyroidism: Effect on Thyrotropin, Prolactin, and Thyroid Reserve, and Metabolic Impact on Peripheral Target Tissues," *Am J Med*, 1992, 92(6):631-42.

Surks MI, "Guidelines for Thyroid Testing," *Lab Med*, 1993, 24(5):270-4.

Wolf PG and Meek JC, "Practical Approach to the Treatment of Hypothyroidism," *Am Fam Physician*, 1992, 45(2):722-31.

Thyroxine by RIA *see* Thyroxine, Blood *on page 1361*

TIBC *see* Iron and Total Iron Binding Capacity/Transferrin *on page 1275*

Tick Identification *see* Arthropod Identification *on page 1198*

Tocainide, Blood

Synonyms Tonocard®

Abstract Tocainide is an antiarrhythmic closely related to lidocaine.

Specimen Blood

Container Red top tube or green top (heparin) tube; avoid serum separator tube

Sampling Time Peak: 1-1.5 hours after administration; trough: just before next dose

Reference Range Therapeutic: 4-10 μg/mL (SI: 18-43 μmol/L)

Possible Panic Range >12 μg/mL (SI: >52 μmol/L)

Use Therapeutic monitoring; toxicity assessment

Methodology High performance liquid chromatography (HPLC), gas chromatography (GC)

Additional Information Tocainide is an analog of lidocaine used in the treatment of ventricular antiarrhythmias (class 1B). Adverse effects of tocainide are mainly neurological (faintness, tremor) and following overdose coma, seizures, edema and respiratory arrest can occur. Tocainide has a plasma half-life of 12-18 hours and metabolites are inactive.

Specific References

Gottlieb SS, Kukin ML, Medina N, et al, "Comparative Hemodynamic Effects of Procainamide, Tocainide, and Encainide in Severe Chronic Heart Failure," *Circulation*, 1990, 81(3):860-4.

(Continued)

Tocainide, Blood *(Continued)*

Manolis AS, Smith E, Payne D, et al, "Randomized Double-Blind Study of Intravenous Tocainide Versus Lidocaine for Suppression of Ventricular Arrhythmias After Cardiac Surgery," *Clin Cardiol*, 1990, 13(3):177-81.
Roden DM and Woosley RL, "Drug Therapy. Tocainide," *N Engl J Med*, 1986, 315(1):41-5.
Sperry K, Wohlenberg N, and Standefer JC, "Fatal Intoxication by Tocainide," *J Forensic Sci*, 1987, 32(5):1440-6.

Tofranil® *see* Imipramine, Blood *on page 1274*

Tonocard® *see* Tocainide, Blood *on previous page*

Total Bilirubin *see* Bilirubin, Total *on page 1203*

Total Calcium, Serum *see* Calcium, Serum *on page 1214*

Total Eosinophil Count *see* Eosinophil Count *on page 1259*

Total Iron Binding Capacity *see* Iron and Total Iron Binding Capacity/ Transferrin *on page 1275*

Total Protein, Serum *see* Protein, Total, Serum *on page 1338*

Total Urinary Catecholamines *replaced by* Catecholamines, Fractionation, Urine *on page 1222*

Total WBC *see* White Blood Count *on page 1380*

Toxic Metals, Blood *see* Heavy Metal Screen, Blood *on page 1271*

Toxic Metals, Urine *see* Heavy Metal Screen, Urine *on page 1272*

Toxicology Drug Screen, Blood

Related Information

Toxicology Drug Screen, Urine *on next page*

Synonyms Drug Screen, Comprehensive Panel or Analysis

Applies To Comatose Profile

Test Includes Amobarbital, butabarbital, butalbital, chlordiazepoxide, diazepam, ethchlorvynol, glutethimide, meprobamate, methaqualone, pentobarbital, phenobarbital, secobarbital, ethanol, methanol, acetone, isopropanol, acetaminophen, phenytoin, salicylates, tricyclics, other drugs could also be analyzed.

Abstract This toxicology screen is carried out by performing individual quantitative tests for each drug. Many times urine qualitative screening is faster and more useful in toxicologic emergencies but both may be needed. Recent introduction of systems such as the Remedi® make an automated approach to this screen possible.

Specimen Blood

Volume 10 mL

Minimum Volume 5 mL serum or plasma

Container Red top tube or lavender top (EDTA) tube; do **not** collect blood in heparinized tubes.

Causes for Rejection Specimen collected in heparinized tube

Use Monitor toxic/overdose situations; most desirable to analyze in conjunction with urine toxicology testing; used to quantitate drug identified qualitatively in urine

Limitations Evidence for presence of a drug/drug metabolite (screening, qualitative) in the case of most groups of therapeutic agents and drugs of abuse will be found in urine rather than serum. See Toxicology Drug Screen, Urine. **All agents identified in a screening test should be confirmed with a specific test.**

Methodology Immunoassay, thin-layer chromatography (TLC), gas chromatography (GC), high performance liquid chromatography (HPLC), colorimetry, spectrophotometry

Additional Information If only documentation of exposure to toxic drugs or drugs of abuse is desired, a urine drug screen is the most economical approach. See listing for Toxicology Drug Screen, Urine. When Toxicology Drug Screen, Blood is ordered, the individual drugs are quantitated in serum. When Toxicology Drug Screen, Urine is ordered, qualitative identification is carried out.

Specific References

Bryson PD, *Comprehensive Review in Toxicology*, 2nd ed, Rockville, MD: Aspen Publishers Inc, 1989, 43-52.
Hepler B, Sutheimer C, and Sunshine I, "Role of the Toxicology Laboratory in Suspected Ingestions," *Pediatr Clin North Am*, 1986, 33(2):245-60.
Puopolo PR, Volpicelli SA, Johnson DM, et al, "Emergency Toxicology Testing (Detection, Confirmation, and Quantification) of Basic Drugs in Serum by Liquid Chromatography With Photodiode Array Detection," *Clin Chem*, 1991, 37(12):2124-30.
Schwartz JG, Zollars R, Okorodudu AO, et al, "Accuracy of Common Drug Screen Tests," *Am J Emerg Med*, 1991, 9(2):166-70.

Toxicology, Drug Screen, Gastric

Synonyms Gastric Aspirate, Drug Screen

Test Includes Amobarbital, amphetamine, butabarbital, codeine, heroin (as morphine), meperidine, methadone, methamphetamine, pentobarbital, phencyclidine (PCP), phenobarbital, phenothiazines, propoxyphene, quinine, secobarbital

Specimen Gastric aspirate
Volume 50 mL
Minimum Volume 30 mL
Container Plastic urine container
Special Instructions Specify the drug or drugs suspected.
Reference Range None detected
Use Detect drug abuse; evaluate toxicity
Methodology Thin-layer chromatography (TLC)

Toxicology Drug Screen, Urine

Related Information
Toxicology Drug Screen, Blood *on previous page*
Synonyms Drug Screen, Comprehensive Panel or Analysis, Urine
Applies To Narcotics Drug Screen, Urine
Test Includes A variety of qualitative screens are in use. Sensitivity and specificity vary and are method dependent. Screens should detect drugs (qualitatively) in the following classes: amphetamines, analgesics, anticonvulsants, antidepressants, antihistamines, cardiacs, narcotics, sedative/hypnotics, tranquilizers, volatiles, and drugs of abuse.
Abstract This is a qualitative screen which in the case of thin-layer chromatography or automated high performance liquid chromatography can detect any of several hundred drugs.
Specimen Random urine. The use of meconium samples from newborns has been shown to be useful.
Volume 50-100 mL
Minimum Volume 50 mL
Container Plastic urine container
Storage Instructions Keep refrigerated
Special Instructions Specify the drug or drugs suspected.
Reference Range None detected or negative (less than cutoff for drugs of abuse)
Use Screen for drug abuse, drug toxicity alone or in conjunction with serum/plasma testing
Limitations Test provides **only** qualitative detection of drugs, unless laboratory automatically confirms and quantitates drugs detected as a part of the "screening" procedure. Quantitation of urine drug levels is usually not included and is not recommended because urine levels are time and clearance dependent and are not directly related to toxic symptoms seen clinically. Some drugs and/or metabolites are not detected or optimally detected in urine, again relating to method. Serum may be preferable because of clinical and at times technical/kinetic factors (eg, barbiturates, phenytoin). Sensitivity is of the order of 0.5-1.0 μg/mL for TLC of urine. Some substances should be quantitated in blood or serum (eg, iron overdose, methanol, acetaminophen, salicylate, carbon monoxide, ethanol, digoxin, lithium, theophylline, and methemoglobin).
Methodology A variety of methods or combination of methods are in fairly common use and include thin-layer chromatography (TLC), colorimetry/spectrophotometry, enzyme immunoassay technique (EIA), enzyme-multiplied immunoassay technique (EMIT), gas chromatography (GC), gas chromatography/mass spectrometry (GC/MS), high performance liquid chromatography (HPLC).
Additional Information Some toxins (eg, metals, volatiles, gaseous compounds) may require specific methodology (eg, atomic absorption spectrophotometry, gas chromatography). Also see Toxicology Drug Screen, Blood test listing.
Specific References

Bryson PD, *Comprehensive Review in Toxicology*, 2nd ed, Rockville, MD: Aspen Publishers Inc, 1989, 43-52.

Caplan YH, "Drug Testing in Urine," *J Forensic Sci*, 1989, 34:1417-21.

Logan BK, Stafford DT, Tebbett IR, et al, "Rapid Screening for 100 Basic Drugs and Metabolites in Urine Using Cation Exchange Solid-Phase Extraction and High-Performance Liquid Chromatography With Diode Array Detection," *J Anal Toxicol*, 1990, 14(3):154-9.

Osterloh JD, "Utility and Reliability of Emergency Toxicologic Testing," *Emerg Med Clin North Am*, 1990, 8(3):693-723.

Osterloh JD and Lee BL, "Urine Drug Screening in Mothers and Newborns," *Am J Dis Child*, 1989, 143(7):791-3.

Toxicology, Hypnotics and Tranquilizers, Serum

Synonyms Hypnotics and Tranquilizers, Toxicology, Blood
Test Includes Amobarbital, butabarbital, chlordiazepoxide, diazepam, ethchlorvynol, glutethimide, meprobamate, methaqualone, methyprylon, pentobarbital, phenobarbital, secobarbital
Specimen Blood
Volume 10 mL
Minimum Volume 5 serum
Container Red top tube; do **not** collect blood in heparinized tube

(Continued)

Toxicology, Hypnotics and Tranquilizers, Serum *(Continued)*

Causes for Rejection Specimen collected in heparinized tube

Special Instructions Specify the drug or drugs suspected.

Reference Range Therapeutic:

- amobarbital: 7-15 μg/mL
- butabarbital: mildly sedated 3-25 μg/mL
- chlordiazepoxide: 0.1-3.0 μg/mL
- diazepam: 105-1540 ng/mL
- ethchlorvynol: 0.5-6.5 μg/mL
- glutethimide: 4-12 μg/mL
- meprobamate: 10-20 μg/mL
- methaqualone 0.9-8.0 μg/mL
- pentobarbital: 4-6 μg/mL
- phenobarbital: 15-40 μg/mL
- secobarbital: 3-5 μg/mL

Critical Values Toxic: amobarbital 30 μg/mL, lethal: 60 μg/mL; butabarbital: mildly comatose 20-40 μg/mL, severely comatose >40 μg/mL; chlordiazepoxide: >3 μg/mL; diazepam: 3000 ng/mL; ethchlorvynol: >20 μg/mL; glutethimide: >10 μg/mL; meprobamate: >50 μg/mL, lethal: 200 μg/dL; methaqualone: >5 μg/mL; methyprylon: >10 μg/mL; pentobarbital: 15-20 μg/mL, lethal: 30 μg/mL; phenobarbital: >40 μg/mL; secobarbital: 10-15 μg/mL, lethal: 20 μg/mL. Great variability in small children in serum levels during the day. Toxic effects mostly neurological, beginning about 35 μg/mL. Coma without reflexes noted at 100 μg/mL.

Use Detect drug abuse; evaluate toxicity; most desirable to analyze in conjunction with urine toxicology testing to quantitate drug identified qualitatively in urine

Limitations Evidence for presence of a drug/drug metabolite (screening, qualitative) in the case of most groups of therapeutic agents and drugs of abuse will be found in urine rather than serum.

Additional Information If only documentation of exposure to toxic drugs or drugs of abuse is desired, a urine drug screen is the most economical approach.

Toxicology, Opiates Drug Screen, Urine With Confirmation

Test Includes Codeine, Darvon®, Demerol®, Dolophine®, heroin, meperidine, methadone, morphine, oxycodone, pentazocine, Percodan®, propoxyphene, Talwin®

Specimen Random urine

Volume 50 mL

Minimum Volume 10 mL aliquot

Container Plastic urine container

Collection Freshly voided random urine

Storage Instructions Refrigerate

Special Instructions Specify the drug or drugs suspected.

Critical Values Toxic propoxyphene: 0.4-14.0 μg/mL

Use Detect drug abuse; evaluate toxicity

Limitations This test provides **only** qualitative detection of drugs. Quantitation of urine drug levels is not included and is not recommended because urine levels are time and clearance dependent and are not directly related to toxic symptoms seen clinically.

Methodology Thin-layer chromatography (TLC) and enzyme immunoassay (EIA), gas chromatography (GC) for confirmation

Additional Information Opiates in general are a group of drugs (commonly referred to as narcotics) which are used medically to relieve pain, but which also have a high potential for abuse.

A qualitative urine screen for opiates is performed in suspected overdose cases or as part of a drug of abuse program. The test is most sensitive for morphine and codeine but other drugs will cross react in an immunoassay and give positive results (eg, hydrocodone, hydromorphone). All presumptive positive assays are confirmed by GC/MS. Morphine is a prescribed drug for pain relief, a metabolite of heroin, a metabolite of codeine and a constituent of poppy seeds. Its presence in urine, even after confirmation must be interpreted very carefully.

Opiates tend to relax the user. When the opiates are injected, the user feels an immediate "rush". Other initial and unpleasant effects include restlessness, nausea, and vomiting. The user may go "on the nod," going back and forth from feeling alert to drowsy. With very large doses, the user cannot be awakened, pupils become smaller, and the skin becomes cold, moist, and bluish in color. Furthermore, breathing slows down and death may occur. Clearance may be slower in geriatric patients.

Toxicology, Steroid Drug Screen, Urine

Synonyms Steroid Drug Screen, Urine

Test Includes Anabolic steroids screen and testosterone/epitestosterone ratio; confirmation of positive results is available.

Patient Preparation Sample collection should be observed and specimen chain of custody should be documented.

Specimen Random urine

Volume 100 mL

Minimum Volume 50 mL

Container Glass bottle

Collection Freshly voided random urine

Special Instructions Specify the drug or drugs suspected.

Use Detect anabolic steroid use in athletes

Methodology Chromatography

Toxicology, Stimulant Panel, Urine

Synonyms Urine Stimulant Drug Screen

Test Includes Qualitative identification of D-amphetamine, methamphetamine, phentermine, phenmetrazine, phenylpropanolamine, cocaine, phencyclidine

Specimen Random urine

Volume 30 mL

Minimum Volume 20 mL

Container Plastic urine container

Collection Freshly voided random urine

Special Instructions Specify the drug or drugs suspected.

Reference Range None detected

Use Detect drug abuse; evaluate toxicity

Limitations This test provides **only** qualitative detection of drugs. Quantitation of urine drug levels is not included and is not recommended because urine levels are time and clearance dependent and are not directly related to toxic symptoms seen clinically.

Methodology Enzyme immunoassay (EIA), gas chromatography (GC)

Toxicology Studies, Not Specifically Listed

Synonyms Drug Analysis, Not Specifically Listed; Drug Levels, Not Specifically Listed

Specimen Blood, urine, gastric washings

Volume 30 mL blood, 100 mL urine, 100 mL gastric washings

Minimum Volume As much of specified volume as possible

Container Gray top (sodium fluoride) tube, plastic urine container, 100 mL plastic gastric washing bottle

Special Instructions Specify the drug or drugs suspected.

Reference Range None detected

Use Confirm toxicity due to a specific drug; detect drug abuse

Limitations Analysis will be limited to those drugs specifically requested. Toxicologic screening for drugs is extremely expensive and seldom results in modification of the patients therapy. The potential effect of the data obtained on the patients course and therapy should be carefully considered before the studies are requested.

Contraindications Suspect drug identity doubtful or unknown

Toxicology, Volatiles *see* Volatile Screen *on page 1378*

Tranquilizers (Valium®, Librium®, etc) *see* Benzodiazepines, Qualitative, Urine *on page 1202*

Transcutaneous Pulse Oximetry *see* Oxygen Saturation, Blood *on page 1313*

Tranxene® *see* Clorazepate, Blood *on page 1232*

Trazodone, Blood

Synonyms Desyrel®

Abstract This drug is an antidepressant chemically unrelated to the tricyclic or tetracyclic antidepressants.

Specimen Blood

Container Red top tube or green top (heparin) tube

Sampling Time Trough: just before next dose

Reference Range Therapeutic: 0.5-2.5 μg/mL (SI: 1-6 μmol/L)

Critical Values >2.5 μg/mL (SI: >6 μmol/L)

Possible Panic Range 4 μg/mL (SI: 10 μmol/L)

(Continued)

Trazodone, Blood *(Continued)*

Use Therapeutic monitoring; toxicity assessment

Methodology High performance liquid chromatography (HPLC), gas chromatography (GC)

Additional Information Trazodone is a structurally unique antidepressant that is pharmacologically different from other drugs of this class. The toxicities observed in tricyclic overdose (neuro- and cardiotoxicity and respiratory depression) are not seen with trazodone. Chronic toxicity is very low with trazodone although it does have unique side effects including akathisia, allergic reactions, chest pain, delayed urine flow, early and delayed menses, hypersalivation and hypomania, among others. The half-life of trazodone is 4-7 hours, peak plasma concentrations with average daily dosing is reached in 2-4 hours.

Specific References

Aranow AB, Hudson JI, Pope HG Jr, et al, "Elevated Antidepressant Plasma Levels After Addition of Fluoxetine," *Am J Psychiatry*, 1989, 146(7):911-3.

Carson CC 3d and Mino RD, "Priapism Associated With Trazodone Therapy," *J Urol*, 1988, 139(2):369-70.

Fabre LF, "United States Experience and Perspectives With Trazodone," *Clin Neuropharmacol*, 1989, 12(Suppl 1):S11-7.

Spar JE, "Plasma Trazodone Concentrations in Elderly, Depressed Inpatients: Cardiac Effects and Short-Term Efficacy," *J Clin Psychopharmacol*, 1987, 7(6):406-9.

Triavil® *see* Amitriptyline, Blood *on page 1187*

Triazolam, Blood

Synonyms Halcion®

Specimen Blood

Volume 20 mL

Minimum Volume 5 mL serum

Container Red top tube

Storage Instructions Refrigerate

Critical Values Fatalities associated with postmortem levels >47 nmol/L.

Use Monitor therapeutic drug level; evaluate toxicity

Additional Information Triazolam, a benzodiazepine derivative, is used for the short-term treatment of insomnia. Its hypnotic effects are similar to those of flurazepam, but the residual daytime effects are fewer. The onset of action is rapid, 15-30 minutes, and the half-life is 1.7-3 hours. Adverse effects include drowsiness, ataxia, anterograde amnesia, dizziness, agitation, nausea and vomiting, and jaundice. If discontinued abruptly, withdrawal and rebound insomnia can result.

Trichloroacetic Acid, Urine *see* Chloral Hydrate, Qualitative, Urine *on page 1224*

Trichloroethanol, Plasma *see* Chloral Hydrate, Plasma *on page 1224*

Trichloroethanol, Urine *see* Chloral Hydrate, Qualitative, Urine *on page 1224*

Trichloroethylene, Urine *see* Chloral Hydrate, Qualitative, Urine *on page 1224*

Tricyclic Antidepressants, Blood

Synonyms Antidepressants; TAD; TCA; Tetracyclic Antidepressants

Abstract Drugs in this class are widely used as antidepressants. They are frequently involved in suicidal ingestion and responsible for a large percentage of drug-related deaths.

Specimen Blood

Volume 7 mL

Container Red top tube, green top (heparin) tube; avoid serum separator tubes and the plasticizer, TBEP.

Sampling Time Steady-state specimen after 1 week of dose schedule; draw specimen 12 hours after the last dose.

Storage Instructions Remove serum within 2 hours of drawing; refrigerate or freeze if not analyzed immediately.

Special Instructions Order individual drug level or tricyclic overdose screen

Reference Range Therapeutic:

- amitriptyline: 100-250 ng/mL (SI: 360-900 nmol/L)
- amoxapine: 50-400 ng/mL
- desipramine: 150-300 ng/mL (SI: 563-1126 nmol/L)
- doxepin: 100-200 ng/mL (SI: 360-720 nmol/L)
- imipramine: 75-250 ng/mL (SI: 279-890 nmol/L)
- maprotiline: 150-400 ng/mL (SI: 541-1442 nmol/L)
- nortriptyline: 50-150 ng/mL (SI: 190-570 nmol/L)

- protriptyline: 50-150 ng/mL (SI: 190-570 nmol/L)
- trazodone: 300-1600 ng/mL

Possible Panic Range >500 ng/mL; toxicity observed at ≥300 ng/mL

Use Therapeutic monitoring; toxicity assessment

Limitations Immunoassays for tricyclic antidepressants (toxic overdose) do not distinguish between parent compounds and active metabolites. Immunoassays are available for amitriptyline, nortriptyline, desipramine, and imipramine. Drug-drug interactions occur; hydrocortisone, neuroleptics, methylphenidate, cimetidine, and oral contraceptives produce higher levels by inhibiting metabolism of tricyclics by the liver. Barbiturates, chloral hydrate, and glutethimide lower plasma tricyclic levels by stimulating liver microsomal activity. Cigarette smoking also lowers steady-state plasma levels, apparently by a similar hepatic enzyme induction mechanism. Red blood cell metabolite assays may be a more sensitive biomarker for cardiac conduction disturbances.

Contraindications Patient taking more than one tricyclic antidepressant, patient taking phenothiazines or monoamine oxidase inhibitors

Methodology Immunoassay, gas chromatography (GC), gas chromatography/mass spectrometry (GC/MS), high performance liquid chromatography (HPLC)

Additional Information Tricyclic antidepressants (TADs) are metabolized to secondary active compounds. These agents are useful in treating clinical depression, and enuresis (imipramine). However, they show a narrow therapeutic window, and great individual variations in blood levels associated with dosage. Blacks usually have 50% greater blood level than whites for same dose schedule. Symptoms of overdose may mimic those of condition for which agent was prescribed. The most important of the more serious or toxic effects of TADs is cardiotoxicity. Arrhythmias and conduction defects with precipitation of congestive heart failure and possibly myocardial infarction are common at combined levels >1000 ng/mL. Widening of the QRS interval to >100 msec is highly suggestive of a TAD overdose.

Tricyclic antidepressant drugs represent a frequent and serious problem in both unintentional and intentional overdosage. Reports of poor correlations between plasma levels and toxic clinical manifestations indicate that QRS duration >100 msec may provide the most reliable indicator of toxicity. It has been reported that levels of parent to metabolite (P/M) ratios >2 are associated with acute overdosage. In contrast, P/M ratios <2 are more consistent with high steady-state plasma levels following "therapeutic" dosages although EKG or other clinical evidence of toxicity may be present. Variations in blood levels between doses are comparatively small. Peak levels occur 4-8 hours after oral ingestion. A level dose of medication should be prescribed for at least 2 weeks to obtain steady plasma levels. Monitoring of tricyclic antidepressant plasma levels is useful in a number of situations. Older patients may develop higher steady-state plasma levels than younger individuals. In geriatric patients conventional doses may lead to toxic levels. Toxic plasma levels of tricyclic drugs may be dangerous in cardiac disease patients. Recommended lower and higher plasma levels for the different tricyclic drugs are evolving and are discussed in the literature. A recent study of tricyclic levels in children and adolescents has emphasized the lack of correlation between oral dose and plasma concentration and has found that the incidence of side effects and therapeutic effect in treatment of enuresis relates to concentration of circulating drug.

Specific References

Beaumont G, "The Toxicity of Antidepressants," *Br J Psychiatry*, 1989, 154:454-8.

Bergstrom RF, Peyton AL, and Lemberger L, "Quantification and Mechanism of the Fluoxetine and Tricyclic Antidepressant Interaction," *Clin Pharmacol Ther*, 1992, 51(3):239-48.

Brasfield KH, "Practical Psychopharmacologic Considerations in Depression," *Nurs Clin North Am*, 1991, 26(3):651-63.

Frommer DA, Kulig KW, Marx JA, et al, "Tricyclic Antidepressant Overdose. A Review," *JAMA*, 1987, 257(4):521-6.

Hantsen PH, *Drug Interactions*, 5th ed, Philadelphia, PA: Lea & Febiger, 1985, 366-7.

Krishel S and Jackimczyk K, "Cyclic Antidepressants, Lithium, and Neuroleptic Agents. Pharmacology and Toxicology," *Emerg Med Clin North Am*, 1991, 9(1):53-86.

Lavoie FW, Gansert GG, and Weiss RE, "Value of Initial ECG Findings and Plasma Drug Levels in Cyclic Antidepressant Overdose," *Ann Emerg Med*, 1990, 19(6):696-700.

Sorisky A and Watson DC, "Positive Diphenhydramine Interference in the EMIT-ST Assay for Tricyclic Antidepressants in Serum," *Clin Chem*, 1986, 32(4):715.

Trifluoperazine, Blood

Synonyms Pentazine®; Stelazine®

Specimen Blood

Volume 10 mL

Minimum Volume 3 mL serum

Container Red top tube

Reference Range Therapeutic level: 0.002-0.060 mg/L

Use Monitor therapeutic drug level; evaluate toxicity

Methodology High performance liquid chromatography (HPLC)

Additional Information Trifluoperazine, a piperazine phenothiazine, is used to

(Continued)

Trifluoperazine, Blood *(Continued)*

manage the manifestations of psychotic disorders. It is rapidly absorbed after oral ingestion and peak levels are achieved in 2-4 hours after oral intake and 15-20 minutes after I.M. injection. Adverse effects include blurred vision, drowsiness, dizziness, extrapyramidal effects, agranulocytosis, tachycardia, hypotension, gynecomastia, and galactorrhea.

Trilafon® *see* Perphenazine, Blood *on page 1317*

Trimipramine, Semiquantitative, Urine

Synonyms Surmontil®

Specimen Urine

Volume 5 mL

Container Plastic urine container

Collection Freshly voided random urine

Use Monitor therapeutic drug level; evaluate toxicity

Methodology Visual color reaction

Additional Information Trimipramine, a tricyclic antidepressant, is used for the treatment of various forms of depression, often in conjunction with psychotherapy. It is most effective in the treatment of endogenous depression and is useful in treating depression accompanied by sleep disturbances due to its strong sedative effect. Imipramine is well absorbed from the GI tract and the principle active metabolite is desipramine. Half-life is 6-20 hours. Adverse effects include blurred vision, hyperthermia, weakness, fatigue, seizures, arrhythmias, hypotension, blood dyscrasias, and psychiatric consequences.

True Cholinesterase *see* Acetylcholinesterase, Red Blood Cell *on page 1181*

Tylenol® *see* Acetaminophen, Serum *on page 1180*

Tylox® *see* Oxycodone, Blood or Urine *on page 1313*

UA *see* Urinalysis *on page 1373*

Uppers *see* Amphetamines, Qualitative, Urine *on page 1190*

U/P Ratio *see* Osmolality, Urine *on page 1311*

Urate *see* Uric Acid, Serum *on next page*

Urea Nitrogen, Blood

Related Information

Sodium, Blood *on page 1352*

Synonyms Blood Urea Nitrogen; BUN

Abstract Urea nitrogen reflects the ratio between urea **production** and **clearance**. Increased BUN may be due to increased production or decreased excretion. Although we commonly use the expression "BUN," most laboratories use serum, occasionally plasma but never whole blood.

Specimen Blood

Volume 10 mL

Minimum Volume 3 mL serum or plasma

Container Red top tube. Avoid fluoride and sodium citrate tubes if urease reaction is used and ammonium heparin tubes when conductometric method is used. EDTA is suitable as well as lithium heparin for young children.

Collection Pediatrics: Blood drawn from heelstick for capillary (lithium heparin tube)

Storage Instructions Stable 1 day at room temperature, 3 days at 4°C to 8°C, and 3 months at -20°C.

Reference Range Birth to 1 year: 4-16 mg/dL (SI: 1.4-5.7 mmol/L); 1-40 years: 5-20 mg/dL (SI: 1.8-7.1 mmol/L); gradual slight increase subsequently occurs over 40 years of age.

Possible Panic Range BUN >100 mg/dL (SI: >35.7 mmol/L) has been used in the definition of uremia.

Use High BUN occurs in chronic glomerulonephritis, pyelonephritis, and other causes of chronic renal disease; with acute renal failure, decreased renal perfusion (prerenal azotemia) as in shock. With urinary tract obstruction BUN increases (postrenal azotemia), for example as caused by neoplastic infiltration of the ureters, hyperplasia, or carcinoma of the prostate. BUN is useful to follow hemodialysis and other therapy. "Uremia" was defined by Luke as an expression of a constellation of signs and symptoms in patients with severe azotemia secondary to acute or chronic renal failure. Causes of increased BUN include severe congestive heart failure, increased protein catabolism, tetracyclines with diuretic use, hyperalimentation, ketoacidosis, and dehydration as in diabetes mellitus, but even moderate dehydration can cause BUN to increase. Corticosteroids tend to increase BUN by causing increased protein catabolism. Bleeding from the gastrointestinal tract is an important cause of high urea nitrogen, commonly accompanied by elevation of BUN/creatinine ratio. Nephrotoxic drugs must be considered. Chloral hydrate or chloramphenicol can cause false elevation.

Borderline high values may occur after recent ingestion of high protein meal and muscle wasting may cause an elevation as well.

With creatinine, BUN is used to monitor patients on dialysis.

Low BUN occurs in late normal pregnancy, decreased protein intake, with intravenous fluids, with some antibiotics, and in severe liver damage.

As described by DeCaux et al in 1980, in the syndrome of inappropriate secretion of antidiuretic hormone (SIADH), findings include hyponatremia with serum or plasma sodium ≤128 mmol/L, serum hypo-osmolality, <260 mOsm/kg, with urine osmolality >300 mOsm/kg (SI: >300 mmol/kg) with low BUN. Such findings occur in situations in which patients are overhydrated. Clinical findings included absence of edema or evidence of heart, liver, thyroid, renal or adrenal disease. Hypouricemia, with uric acid levels in 16 of 17 patients <4 mg/dL (SI: <238 μmol/L), is reported with the syndrome of inappropriate secretion of antidiuretic hormone. SIADH can be seen with higher serum sodiums and higher osmolalities. Urine osmolality is greater than serum osmolality in SIADH. Chloramphenicol or streptomycin can cause false depression.

Osmolality (mOsm/kg H_2O) may be calculated as follows: Osmolality = [Na^+ (mmol/L) x 2] + urea N (mg/dL)/2.8 + glucose (mg/dL)/18.

Limitations Uremia is best evaluated with creatinine as well as urea nitrogen. In both prerenal and postrenal azotemia, for instance, BUN is apt to be increased somewhat more than is creatinine. However, in a series of dehydrated children with gastroenteritis who had metabolic acidosis and increased anion gap, 88% had BUN concentration ≤18 mg/dL (SI: ≤6.4 mmol/L). The authors found bicarbonate and anion gap more sensitive indices in this setting. In chronic progressive renal disease, about 75% of renal parenchyma must be damaged or destroyed before azotemia develops. BUN lacks sensitivity and specificity, but still remains a useful test.

Methodology Diacetyl monoxime; urease, Berthelot reaction; rate conductivity

Additional Information Although creatinine is generally considered a more specific test to evaluate renal function, they are commonly used together. Luke points out that clinical renal failure is variable between individual patients. Drug effects have been summarized.

Specific References

Abuelo JG, "Benign Azotemia of Long-Term Hemodialysis: Increase in Blood Urea Nitrogen and Serum Creatinine Concentrations After the Initiation of Dialysis," *Am J Med*, 1989, 86(6 Pt 1):738-9.

Bidani A and Churchill PC, "Acute Renal Failure," *Dis Mon*, 1989, 35(2):57-132.

Comtois R, Bertrand S, Beauregard H, et al, "Low Serum Urea Level in Dehydrated Patients With Central Diabetes Insipidus," *Can Med Assoc J*, 1988, 139(10):965-9.

Uric Acid, Serum

Synonyms Urate

Abstract Uric acid, the end product of purine metabolism, is increased in a variety of clinicopathologic entities in addition to gout.

Patient Preparation Ideally, patient should be fasting. Diurnal variations occur. Uric acid concentration is usually higher in the morning and lower in the evening.

Specimen Blood

Volume 3 mL

Minimum Volume 1 mL serum

Container Red top tube

Collection Separate serum. Do not collect in lavender top (EDTA) tube or gray top (sodium fluoride) tube for urease method.

Storage Instructions Urate is stable in serum for 3 days at 25°C, 3-7 days at 4°C, and 6-12 months at -20°C.

Reference Range An increase occurs during childhood. Adults: male: 3.4-7.0 mg/dL (SI: 202-416 μmol/L), female: 2.4-6.0 mg/dL (SI: 143-357 μmol/L). Values >7.0 mg/dL (SI: >416 μmol/L) are sometimes arbitrarily regarded as hyperuricemia, but there is no sharp line between normals on the one hand, and the serum uric acid of those with clinical gout. Normal ranges cannot be adjusted for purine ingestion, but high purine diet increases uric acid. Uric acid may be increased with body size, exercise, and stress.

Possible Panic Range "Severe hyperuricemia" has been classified as uric acid >12.0 mg/dL (SI: >714 μmol/L)

Use An increased uric acid level does not necessarily translate to a diagnosis of gout; about 10% to 15% of instances of hyperuricemia are caused by gout. The overlap between uric acid levels in those with and without gout is shown in a study in which the lowest level in a gouty subject was 6.0 mg/dL (SI: 357 μmol/L), while the highest uric acid in a nongouty person was 9.5 mg/dL (SI: 565 μmol/L).

(Continued)

Uric Acid, Serum *(Continued)*

Elevations of uric acid occur in renal diseases with renal failure and prerenal azotemia (eg, dehydration) as well as gout. Other drugs causing increased uric acid concentration include diuretics, pyrazinamide, ethambutol, nicotinic acid, and aspirin in low doses.

Excessive cell destruction: neoplasia, even before as well as following chemotherapy and radiation therapy, especially lymphoma and leukemia; hemolytic anemia, resolving pneumonia and other inflammation; polycythemia, myeloma, pernicious anemia, infectious mononucleosis, congestive heart failure, large myocardial infarct.

Endocrine: hypothyroidism, hypoparathyroidism, hyperparathyroidism, pseudohypoparathyroidism; diabetes insipidus of nephrogenic type, Addison's disease.

Lead poisoning (saturnine gout) from paint, batteries, and moonshine. A causal relationship between plumbism and gout was recognized before 1876. Gout as a common complication of subclinical lead poisoning is described among the Roman aristocracy.

Acidosis: lactic acidosis, diabetic ketoacidosis, recent alcohol ingestion, alcoholic ketosis. Shock and hypoxia relate to hyperuricemia. Attention has been directed at the cause of hyperuricemia in the intensive care unit; severely increased uric acid levels in acutely ill patients is explained by degradation of ATP with degradation of accumulated nucleotides to purine metabolites, uric acid among them. Such ATP degradation may occur with strenuous exercise and the adult respiratory distress syndrome. With metabolism of ethanol to acetyl CoA, the degradation of ATP explains the hyperuricemia of alcohol use. Hyperuricemia becomes then a marker for cell injury crisis.

Toxemia of pregnancy, diet, weight loss, fasting, or starvation. Decreased urate clearance: cyclosporine-induced hyperuricemia.

Triglyceride increase bears an association with hyperuricemia, as do diabetes mellitus and obesity. Hyperuricemia bears an association with obesity, hypertension and statistical association with myocardial infarct.

Hereditary gout: Lesch-Nyhan (X-linked) with deficiency of hypoxanthine-guanine phosphoribosyltransferase. Gout with partial absence HPRT. Increased 5-phosphoribosyl-1-pyrophosphate synthetase. Glycogen storage disease type I.

Only a minority of individuals with hyperuricemia develop gout.

Three types of kidney disease are caused by precipitation: acute uric acid nephropathy, nephrolithiasis, and chronic urate nephropathy.

Hyperuricemia in early essential hypertension correlates with renal vascular resistance and inversely with renal blood flow. Increased serum uric acid may indicate renal involvement.

Low uric acid: Drugs: Drugs apparently bearing a relationship to low serum uric acid levels included aspirin (high doses), x-ray contrast agents, glyceryl guaiacolate or allopurinol. Corticosteroids and probenecid cause low uric. Massive doses of vitamin C are uricosuric.

Poor dietary intake of purines and protein; tea, coffee.

Renal tubular defects, Fanconi syndrome, late in Wilson's disease, outdated tetracycline, cystinosis, galactosemia, heavy metal poisoning, malignant neoplasms, hypereosinophilic syndrome.

Xanthinuria (deficiency of xanthine oxidase).

Hypouricemia is reported with acute intermittent porphyria, severe liver disease (especially obstructive biliary disease), and as an isolated defect in the tubular transport of uric acid.

With increased renal clearance of urate, hypercalciuria, and decreased bone density, diabetes, and in SIADH.

With hyponatremia, serum hypo-osmolarity: Beck has described low uric acid with the syndrome of inappropriate secretion of antidiuretic hormone (SIADH): 16 of 17 patients with this syndrome were hypouricemic, with serum urate $\leq$4.0 mg/dL (SI: $\leq$238 μmol/L). All 13 patients with other causes of hyponatremia had serum urate $\geq$5.0 mg/dL (SI: $\geq$297 μmol/L). Volume expansion, as with SIADH, causes decreased uric acid. The combination of low uric and low sodium may also be found in instances of liver disease and was anticipated with ticrynafen.

Azlocillin is reported to cause decrease of serum uric acid levels. Drug effects on uric acid metabolism are published in tabular form.

Idiopathic hypouricemia commonly is transient. Familial hypouricemia has been described.

Limitations Positive interferences may be caused by ascorbic acid, caffeine, epinephrine, levodopa, methyldopa, and theophylline.

Methodology Phosphotungstate, uricase, high performance liquid chromatography (HPLC)

Specific References

Conger JD, "Acute Uric Acid Nephropathy," *Med Clin North Am*, 1990, 74(4):859-71.

Devgun MS and Dhillon HS, "Importance of Diurnal Variations on Clinical Value and Interpretation of Serum Urate Measurements," *J Clin Pathol*, 1992, 45(2):110-3.

Dykman D and Simon EE, "Hyperuricemia and Uric Acid Nephropathy," *Arch Intern Med*, 1987, 147(7):1341-5.

Fievet P, Pleskov L, Desailly I, et al, "Plasma Renin Activity, Blood Uric Acid and Plasma Volume in Pregnancy-Induced Hypertension," *Nephron*, 1985, 40(4):429-32.

Fox IH, Palella TD, and Kelley WN, "Hyperuricemia: A Marker for Cell Energy Crisis," *N Engl J Med*, 1987, 317(2):111-2, (editorial).

German DC and Holmes EW, "Gout and Hyperuricemia: Diagnosis and Management," *Hosp Pract (Off Ed)*, 1986, 21(11):119-26, 131-2.

Gores PF, Fryd DS, Sutherland DE, et al, "Hyperuricemia After Renal Transplantation," *Am J Surg*, 1988, 156(5):397-400.

Langford HG, Blaufox MD, Borhani NO, et al, "Is Thiazide-Produced Uric Acid Elevation Harmful?" *Arch Intern Med*, 1987, 147(4):645-9.

Lin HY, Rocher LL, McQuillan MA, et al, "Cyclosporine-Induced Hyperuricemia and Gout," *N Engl J Med*, 1989, 321(5):287-92.

Mejías E, Navas J, Lluberes R, et al, "Hyperuricemia, Gout, and Autosomal Dominant Polycystic Kidney Disease," *Am J Med Sci*, 1989, 297(3):145-8.

Menon RK, Mikhailidis DP, Bell JL, et al, "Warfarin Administration Increases Uric Acid Concentrations in Plasma," *Clin Chem*, 1986, 32(8):1557-9.

Nunez BD, Frohlich ED, Garavaglia GE, et al, "Serum Uric Acid in Renovascular Hypertension: Reduction Following Surgical Correction," *Am J Med Sci*, 1987, 294(6):419-22.

O'Connor JP and Emmerson BT, "The Treatment of Hyperuricaemia and Gout," *Aust Fam Physician*, 1985, 14(3):193-8.

Rock RC, Walker WG, and Jennings CD, "Nitrogen Metabolites and Renal Function," *Textbook of Clinical Chemistry*, Tietz NW, ed, Philadelphia, PA: WB Saunders Co, 1986, 1254-1316.

Shichiri M, Iwamoto H, and Shiigai T, "Diabetic Renal Hypouricemia," *Arch Intern Med*, 1987, 147(2):225-8.

Tammes AR, "Uric Acid," *Quality Assurance Service*, CAP Computer Center, 1986.

Zhiri A and Jouanel P, "Urates," *Drug Effects on Laboratory Test Results Analytical Interferences and Pharmacological Effects*, Siest G and Galteau MM, eds, Littleton, MA: PSG Publishing Co Inc, 1988, 423-38.

Urinalysis

Related Information

Crystals, Urine *on page 1246*

Synonyms UA

Applies To Casts, Urine

Test Includes Opacity, color, appearance, specific gravity, pH, protein, glucose, occult blood, ketones, bilirubin, and in some laboratories, urobilinogen and microscopic examination of urine sediment. Some laboratories include screening for leukocyte esterase and nitrite and do not perform a microscopic examination unless one of the chemical screening (macroscopic) tests is abnormal or unless a specific request for microscopic examination is made.

Abstract The examination of urine is one of the oldest practices in medicine. A carefully performed urinalysis still provides a wealth of information about the patient, both in terms of differential diagnosis, and by exclusion of many conditions when the urinalysis is "normal."

Patient Preparation Instructions should be given in method of collection. Both males and females need instruction in cleansing the urethral meatus. "Midstream collections" are performed by initiating urination into the toilet, then bringing the collection device into the urine stream to catch the midportion of the void.

Specimen Urine

Volume 5 mL

Minimum Volume 2 mL

Container Plastic urine container

Collection A voided specimen is usually suitable. If the specimen is likely to be contaminated by vaginal discharge or hemorrhage, a clean catch specimen is desirable. If the specimen is collected by catheter, it should be so labeled. The timing of urine collection will vary with the purpose of the test. To check for casts or renal concentration ability, a first voided morning specimen may be preferred. For screening purposes, this is also the best time, as a later and more dilute specimen may make small increases in protein, RBC, or WBC excretion harder to detect. The upright position increases protein excretion by hemodynamic factors. Midmorning urine is likely to give the highest albumin excretion, but early morning urine is best when attempting to detect Bence Jones protein.

Storage Instructions Transport specimen to the laboratory as soon as possible after collection. If the specimen cannot be processed immediately by the laboratory it should be refrigerated. Refrigeration preserves formed elements in the urine, but may precipitate crystals not originally present.

Causes for Rejection Specimen delayed in transport, fecal contamination, decomposition, or bacterial overgrowth

(Continued)

Urinalysis *(Continued)*

Reference Range See table. **Crystals** are interpreted by the physician. Warm, freshly voided urine sediment from normal subjects almost never contains crystals, despite maximal concentration. Xanthine, cystine, and uric acid crystal (and stone) formation is favored by a consistently acid urine (pH <5.5-6). Calcium oxalate and apatite stones are associated with no particular disturbance of urine pH. Calcium carbonate, calcium phosphate, and especially magnesium ammonium phosphate stones are associated with pH >7. Urine pH >7.5 may briefly follow meals (alkaline tide) but more commonly indicate systemic alkali intake ($NaHCO_3$, etc) or urine infected by bacteria which split urea to ammonia.

Urinalysis

Test	Reference Range
Specific gravity	1.003–1.029
pH	4.5–7.8
Protein	Negative
Glucose	Negative
Ketones	Negative
Bilirubin	Negative
Occult blood	Negative
Leukocyte osterase	Negative
Nitrite	Negative
Urobilinogen	0.1–1.0 EU/dL
WBCs	0–5/hpf
RBCs	male: 0–3/hpf female: 0–5/hpf
Casts	0–4/lpf hyaline
Bacteria	Negative

hpf = high power field
lpf = low power field
EU = Ehrlich units

Possible Panic Range The presence of massive amounts of oxalate crystals in fresh urine should be reported promptly to the physician, as this finding may represent ethylene glycol intoxication.

Use Screen for abnormalities of urine; diagnose and manage renal diseases, urinary tract infection, urinary tract neoplasms, systemic diseases, and inflammatory or neoplastic diseases adjacent to the urinary tract

Limitations Insufficient volume, less than 2 mL, may limit the extent of procedures performed. Metabolites of Pyridium® may interfere with the dipstick reactions by producing color interference. High vitamin C intake may cause an underestimate of glucosuria, or a false-negative nitrate test. Survival of WBCs is decreased by low osmolality, alkalinity, and lack of refrigeration. Formed elements in the urine including casts disintegrate rapidly, therefore the specimen should be analyzed as soon as possible after collection. Specific gravity is affected by glucosuria, mannitol infusion, or prior administration of iodinated contrast material for radiologic studies (IVP dye). Some brands of test strips give a "trace positive" protein indication if not stored in dry atmosphere (cap of test strip bottle not on tight). Ambient humidity exposure of the test strips over time also causes some reduction of sensitivity for occult blood and nitrate and increased sensitivity for glucose (false-positive). This can be detected by using tap water as a negative control. False-positive tests for protein can also be due to contamination of the urine by an ammonium-containing cleansing solution.

Methodology The chemical portion of the urinalysis is done by test strip, with confirming chemical method for protein (sulfosalicylic acid precipitation).

Additional Information

MICROSCOPY:

Crystalluria is frequently observed in urine specimens stored at room temperature or refrigerated. Such crystals are diagnostically useful when observed in warm, fresh urine by a physician evaluating microhematuria, nephrolithiasis, or toxin ingestion.

In abundance, **calcium oxalate** and/or **hippurate crystals** may suggest ethylene glycol ingestion (especially if known to be accompanied by neurological abnormalities, appearance of drunkenness, hypertension, and a high anion gap acidosis.) Urine is usually supersaturated in calcium oxalate, often in calcium phosphate, and acid urine is often saturated in uric acid. Yet crystalluria is uncommon (in warm, fresh urine) because of the normal presence of crystal inhibitors, the lack of available nidus, and the time factor. When properly observed in fresh urine, crystals may provide a clue to the composition of renal stones even not yet passed, the nidus for such stones, or, as such, have been associated with microhematuria.

Uric acid crystals are reddish brown, rectangular, rhomboidal, or flower-like structures of narrow rectangular petals. **Ammonium urates,** in alkaline urine, are irregular blobs and crescents, sometimes resembling fragmented red cell shapes.

Calcium oxalate crystals are fairly uniform small double pyramids, base to base, which under the microscope look like little crosses on a square.

Calcium phosphate crystallizes in urine as flowers of narrow rectangular needles.

Cystine crystals, uniquely in urine, form large irregular hexagonal plates, which may dissolve if alkalinized. They occur only in the urine of subjects with cystinuria.

Calcium magnesium ammonium phosphate, or "triple phosphate," forms unique "coffin lid" angularly domed rectangles which may be present in massive quantities in alkaline urine. They usually are associated with urine infected by urea splitting bacteria which cause "infection," or "triple phosphate" stones.

Leukocyturia may indicate inflammatory disease in the genitourinary tract, including bacterial infection, glomerulonephritis, chemical injury, autoimmune diseases, or inflammatory disease adjacent to the urinary tract such as appendicitis or diverticulitis.

White cell casts indicate the renal origin of leukocytes, and are most frequently found in acute pyelonephritis. White cell casts are also found in glomerulonephritis such as lupus nephritis, and in acute and chronic interstitial nephritis. When nuclei degenerate, such leukocyte casts resemble renal tubular casts.

Red cell casts indicate renal origin of hematuria and suggest glomerulonephritis, including lupus nephritis. Red cell casts may also be found in subacute bacterial endocarditis, renal infarct, vasculitis, Goodpasture's syndrome, sickle cell disease, and in malignant hypertension. Degenerated red cell casts may be called **"hemoglobin casts"**. Orange to red casts may be found with myoglobinuria as well.

Dysmorphic red cells are observed in glomerulonephritis. "Dysmorphic" red cells refer to heterogeneous sizes, hypochromia, distorted irregular outlines and frequently small blobs extruding from the cell membrane. Phase contrast microscopy best demonstrates RBC and WBC morphology. Nonglomerular urinary red blood cells resemble peripheral circulating red blood cells. Schramek et al have used the presence or absence of dysmorphic red cells to direct the degree of work-up for hematuria and for follow-up.

Crenated RBCs provide no implication regarding RBC source.

Dark brown or smoky urine suggests a renal source of hematuria.

A **pink or red urine** suggests an extrarenal source.

Hyaline casts occur in physiologic states (eg, after exercise) and many types of renal diseases. They are best seen in phase contrast microscopy or with reduced illumination.

Renal tubular (epithelial) casts are most suggestive of tubular injury, as in acute tubular necrosis. They are also found in other disorders, including eclampsia, heavy metal poisoning, ethylene glycol intoxication, and acute allograft rejection.

Granular casts: Very finely granulated casts may be found after exercise and in a variety of glomerular and tubulointerstitial diseases.; coarse granular casts are abnormal and are present in a wide variety of renal diseases.

"Dirty brown" granular casts are typical of acute tubular necrosis.

Waxy casts are found especially in chronic renal diseases, and are associated with chronic renal failure; they occur in diabetic nephropathy, malignant hypertension, and glomerulonephritis, among other conditions. They are named for their waxy or glossy appearance. They often appear brittle and cracked.

Fatty casts are generally found in the nephrotic syndromes, diabetic nephropathy, other forms of chronic renal diseases, and glomerulonephritis. The fat droplets originate in renal tubular cells when they exceed their capacity to reabsorb protein of glomerular origin. Their inclusions have the features and significance of oval fat bodies.

Broad casts originate from dilated, chronically damaged tubules or the collecting ducts. They can be granular or waxy. **Broad waxy casts** are called "renal failure casts."

Spermatozoa may be seen in male urine related to recent or retrograde ejaculation. In female urine, the presence of spermatozoa may provide evidence of vaginal contamination following recent intercourse.

(Continued)

Urinalysis *(Continued)*

Automation of the urinalysis is routine in many laboratories. Some authors wish to abandon microscopic evaluation of the urine, which is not easily automated, on urine samples testing "normal" by dipstick screening. A urine sample that is normal to inspection and dipstick will be normal to microscopic exam 95% of the time.

One instrument for automating the entire urinalysis, the Yellow IRIS®, includes a module that automates the microscopic sediment exam. This has been found to be more consistent than the manual method for routine urinalysis and has increased the number of abnormal urines detected.

Specific References

Carlson D and Statland BE, "Automated Urinalysis," *Clin Lab Med*, 1988, 8(3):449-61.

Cohen HT and Spiegel DM, "Air-Exposed Urine Dipsticks Give False-Positive Results for Glucose and False-Negative Results for Blood," *Am J Clin Pathol*, 1991, 96(3):398-400.

Freeman JA and Beeler MF, *Laboratory Medicine/Urinalysis and Medical Microscopy*, 2nd ed, Philadelphia, PA: Lea & Febiger, 1983.

Haber MH, "Quality Assurance in Urinalysis," *Clin Lab Med*, 1988, 8(3):431-47.

Haber MH, *Urinary Sediment: A Textbook Atlas*, American Society of Clinical Pathologists, 1981.

Kiel DP and Moskowitz MA, "The Urinalysis: A Critical Appraisal," *Med Clin North Am*, 1987, 71(4):607-24.

Mariani AJ, Luangphinith S, Loo S, et al, "Dipstick Chemical Urinalysis: An Accurate Cost-Effective Screening Test," *J Urol*, 1984, 132(1):64-6.

Rizzoni G, Braggion F, and Zacchello G, "Evaluation of Glomerular and Nonglomerular Hematuria by Phase-Contrast Microscopy," *J Pediatr*, 1983, 103(3):370-4.

Roe CE, Carlson DA, Daigneault RW, et al, "Evaluation of the Yellow IRIS®. An Automated Method for Urinalysis," *Am J Clin Pathol*, 1986, 86(5):661-5.

Schramek P, Schuster FX, Georgopoulos M, et al, "Value of Urinary Erythrocyte Morphology in Assessment of Symptomless Microhaematuria," *Lancet*, 1989, 2(8675):1316-9.

Schumann GB, "Cytodiagnostic Urinalysis for the Nephrology Practice," *Semin Nephrol*, 1986, 6(4):308-45.

Schumann GB, *Urine Sediment Examination*, Baltimore, MD: Williams and Wilkins, 1980.

Scott JH 3d, Amin M, and Harty JI, "Abnormal Urinalysis in Appendicitis," *J Urol*, 1983, 129(5):1015.

Segasothy M, Lau TM, Birch DF, et al, "Immunocytologic Dissection of the Urine Sediment Using Monoclonal Antibodies," *Am J Clin Pathol*, 1988, 90(6):691-6.

Sheets C and Lyman JL, "Urinalysis," *Emerg Med Clin North Am*, 1986, 4(2):263-80.

Shenoy UA, "Current Assessment of Microhematuria and Leukocyturia," *Clin Lab Med*, 1985, 5(2):317-29.

Wargotz ES, Hyde JE, Karcher DS, et al, "Urine Sediment Analysis by the Yellow IRIS® Automated Urinalysis Workstation," *Am J Clin Pathol*, 1987, 88(6):746-8.

Yager HM and Harrington JT, "Urinalysis and Urinary Electrolytes," *The Principles and Practice of Nephrology*, Chapter 28, Jacobson HR, Striker GE, and Klahr S, eds, Philadelphia, PA: BC Decker Inc, 1991, 167-77.

Urinary Anion Gap *see* Anion Gap, Blood *on page 1193*

Urine Alcohol Level *see* Alcohol, Semiquantitative, Urine *on page 1182*

Urine Crystals *see* Crystals, Urine *on page 1246*

Urine Electrolytes *see* Electrolytes, Urine *on page 1254*

Urine Ethanol *see* Alcohol, Semiquantitative, Urine *on page 1182*

Urine Ketones *see* Ketones, Urine *on page 1278*

Urine Na *see* Sodium, Urine *on page 1353*

Urine Osmolality *see* Osmolality, Urine *on page 1311*

Urine Screen for Albumin *see* Protein, Semiquantitative, Urine *on page 1337*

Urine Screen for Protein *see* Protein, Semiquantitative, Urine *on page 1337*

Urine Stimulant Drug Screen *see* Toxicology, Stimulant Panel, Urine *on page 1367*

Urobilinogen, 2-Hour Urine

Synonyms Urobilinogen, Quantitative, Urine

Abstract This urine screening test detects some but not all instances of hemolytic anemia and liver diseases such as hepatitis and cirrhosis. It is not widely used.

Patient Preparation Alkalinization of the urine by sodium bicarbonate administration increases excretion of urobilinogen. A marked diurnal peak in excretion occurs; therefore an afternoon collection ideally should be scheduled.

Specimen 2-hour urine

Volume Entire collection

Container Dark urine container or foil wrapped container

Collection Have patient void at 2 PM and discard urine. Give patient 500 mL of water to be ingested at once. Collect all urine from 2 PM – 4 PM. Transport promptly to the laboratory. Urobilinogen is sensitive to room temperature and light.

Storage Instructions Refrigerate specimen and protect from light.

Causes for Rejection Completed 2-hour specimen not received, specimen exposed to light or not refrigerated

Reference Range Male: 0.3-2.1 mg/2 hours (SI: 0.5-3.6 μmol/2 hours); female: 0.1-1.1 mg/2 hours (SI: 0.2-1.9 μmol/2 hours). Results are sometimes expressed in Ehrlich units, 1 mg urobilinogen = 1 EU.

Use Screen for biliary and liver disease, obstructive jaundice; increased in hemolytic anemia, hepatitis, liver damage with or without jaundice (eg, cirrhosis, congestive heart failure)

Limitations Antibiotics supressing intestinal flora may cause very low levels. Levels may be normal with incomplete obstructive jaundice. Patients with acute porphyria may have an increased value because porphobilinogen also gives a positive result with Ehrlich's aldehyde reagent, as does para-aminosalicylic acid. The absence of or low urobilinogen cannot be determined by dipsticks, a serious drawback, since detection of decreased urine urobilinogen would enhance diagnosis of common duct obstruction. Drugs containing azo dyes may mask the reaction. Mefenamic acid, phenazopyridine, and phenothiazines can cause false elevation by interfering with assays. Like urine bile detection, screen for urobilinogen in urine has fairly good specificity. However, the two tests lack great sensitivity when compared with a variety of serum tests related to liver disease.

Methodology Urobilistix®, Watson's method, Ehrlich's aldehyde reagent; para-diethylaminobenzaldehyde reacts with urobilinogen with a color enhancer

Additional Information Urobilinogen is formed in the intestine by the action of bacteria on excreted conjugated (direct) bilirubin. A portion of the urobilinogen is absorbed from the gastrointestinal tract into the bloodstream. It returns to the liver where some is re-excreted in bile (enterohepatic circulation), and the rest (via the general circulation) is excreted into the urine. Urine urobilinogen can be increased as an early indicator of moderate hepatic parenchymal damage. Early toxic injury or hepatitis may also cause increased urine urobilinogen. However, if no bilirubin enters the bile no urobilinogen will be produced; thus, with complete common bile duct obstruction, both urine and fecal urobilinogen will be decreased. Collection time is important because of diurnal variation in urobilinogen excretion. Alkaline pH of urine increases clearance of urobilinogen and increases reliability of results.

Urobilinogen, 24-Hour Urine *replaced by* Urobilinogen, 2-Hour Urine *on previous page*

Urobilinogen, Quantitative, Urine *see* Urobilinogen, 2-Hour Urine *on previous page*

Uroporphyrins *see* Porphyrins, Quantitative, Urine *on page 1326*

Valium® *see* Diazepam, Blood *on page 1249*

Valproic Acid, Blood

Synonyms Depakene®; Depakote® (Enteric-Coated Divalproex Sodium); Depamide®; Epilim®; Ergenyl®

Abstract Valproic acid is a first-line anticonvulsant for absence seizures. It is useful for many other seizure types, including primary generalized tonic-clonic, myoclonic, atonic, and mixed seizures. It is the drug of choice for mixed absence and generalized seizures and for the epileptic syndromes of juvenile myoclonic epilepsy and generalized tonic-clonic seizures on awakening.

Specimen Blood

Volume 5 mL

Minimum Volume 3 mL serum or plasma

Container Red top tube or green top (heparin) tube

Sampling Time Trough values drawn just before next dose or consistent sampling time in chronic monitoring

Reference Range 50-100 μg/mL (SI: 350-690 μmol/L). Low levels: The most important cause is noncompliance. Phenytoin, phenobarbital, primidone, and carbamazepine decrease the half-life of valproic acid. High levels: Carbamazepine and phenytoin can increase the level of valproic acid.

Critical Values Toxic concentration >200 μg/mL (SI: >1390 μmol/L). Seizure control may improve at levels >100 μg/mL (SI: >690 μmol/L), but toxicity may occur at levels of 100-150 μg/mL (SI: 690-1040 μmol/L).

Use Monitor for compliance, efficacy, and possible toxicity

Limitations Since valproic acid is highly bound, drugs that compete for protein binding sites can increase the amount of free valproic acid (biologically active fraction). These include dicumarol, high dose salicylates, and phenylbutazone. If toxicity is suspected, a free valproic acid level should be obtained.

Methodology Enzyme immunoassay (EIA), gas-liquid chromatography (GLC), high performance liquid chromatography (HPLC)

Additional Information Hepatic failure has occurred during the first 6 months of therapy. Hepatotoxicity may be preceded by nonspecific symptoms such as mal-

(Continued)

Valproic Acid, Blood *(Continued)*

aise, weakness, lethargy, anorexia, and vomiting. Hepatotoxicity may be fatal, but is idiosyncratic and not preventable by routinely monitoring liver enzymes. Hepatotoxicity occurs in very young children, most often those on multiple anticonvulsants. Valproate-induced cytopenias may be dose-related and warrant monitoring of complete blood counts during therapy. Encephalopathy with hyperammonemia without liver function test abnormalities may occur. Pregnant women in first month are at risk for neural tube defects.

Specific References

Engel J, *Seizures and Epilepsy*, Contemporary Neurology Series, Philadelphia, PA: FA Davis Co, 1989.

Levy RH, Dreifuss FE, Mattson RH, et al, *Antiepileptic Drugs*, 3rd ed, New York, NY: Raven Press, 1989.

Vancocin® *see* Vancomycin Level *on this page*

Vancomycin Level

Synonyms Vancocin®

Abstract Vancomycin is an antimicrobial agent with potent activity against most gram-positive bacteria. Its use has occasionally been associated with nephrotoxicity and/or ototoxicity, though the frequency of these toxicities has decreased as vancomycin preparations have become more purified.

Specimen Blood, body fluid

Volume 10 mL blood or 2 mL body fluid

Container Red top tube, sterile fluid container

Sampling Time Peak: 30 minutes following dose; trough: immediately prior to next dose

Storage Instructions Separate serum using aseptic technique and place in freezer

Causes for Rejection Specimen more than 4 hours old

Reference Range Therapeutic concentration: peak: 20-40 μg/mL (SI: 14.0-27.0 μmol/L) (depends in part on minimum inhibitory concentration of organism being treated); trough: 5-10 μg/mL (SI: 3.4-6.8 μmol/L)

Possible Panic Range Toxic: >80 μg/mL (SI: >54.0 μmol/L)

Use Monitor therapeutic levels and potential toxicities, particularly in patients with impaired renal function and in patients also being treated with aminoglycoside antibiotics

Methodology High performance liquid chromatography (HPLC), gas-liquid chromatography (GLC), immunoassay

Additional Information Vancomycin is currently being used in its intravenous form to treat a variety of gram-positive bacterial infections, particularly those due to methicillin-resistant staphylococci. Additionally, vancomycin is often used in its oral form to treat pseudomembranous colitis due to *Clostridium difficile*. When administered orally, serum vancomycin levels are undetectable due to poor absorption from the gastrointestinal tract. When administered intravenously, vancomycin may be ototoxic and nephrotoxic, though nephrotoxicity is rare with newer preparations. Ototoxicity is seen primarily in patients with extremely high serum concentrations (80-100 μg/mL) and rarely occurs when serum concentrations are maintained at ≤30 μg/mL. Both oto- and nephrotoxicity is enhanced by concurrent administration of aminoglycosides.

Specific References

Fogarty KA and McClain WJ, "Vancomycin: Current Perspectives and Guidelines for Use in the NICU," *Neonatal Netw*, 1989, 7(5):31-5.

Ingerman MJ and Santoro J, "Vancomycin. A New Old Agent," *Infect Dis Clin North Am*, 1989, 3(3):641-51.

Levine JF, "Vancomycin: A Review," *Med Clin North Am*, 1987, 71(6):1135-45.

Miceli JN, "Chloramphenicol and Vancomycin," *Clin Lab Med*, 1987, 7(3):531-40.

Wilhelm MP, "Vancomycin," *Mayo Clin Proc*, 1991, 66(11):1165-70.

Venous CO-Oximetry *see* CO-Oximetry Venous *on page 1241*

Ventilation Lung Scan *see* Lung Scan, Ventilation *on page 1288*

Ventilation-Perfusion Lung Scan *see* Lung Scan, Ventilation *on page 1288*

Vivactil® *see* Protriptyline, Blood *on page 1340*

Volatile Screen

Synonyms Toxicology, Volatiles

Applies To Acetone; Ethanol

Test Includes Determination of volatiles by GLC including acetone, ethanol, isopropanol, and methanol. Note: Ethylene glycol in not considered to be a volatile alcohol.

Abstract This screening profile measures ethanol and other possible volatiles.

Specimen Blood, urine, gastric fluid

Volume 7 mL blood, 25 mL urine, 25 mL gastric washing

Minimum Volume 3 mL serum or plasma

Container Red top tube, gray top (sodium fluoride) tube; tightly stoppered container for urine and gastric fluid

Collection All containers should be tightly stoppered and transported on ice. The gray (oxalate/fluoride) tube top is recommended for medicolegal collections and if storage is prolonged. Sodium fluoride (50 mg) can be added as a preservative to urine and gastric samples. Other anticoagulants (eg, heparin EDTA) are acceptable.

Causes for Rejection Specimen leakage

Reference Range None detected

Possible Panic Range Blood: acetone, methanol, isopropanol >500 μg/mL (SI: acetone: >8610 μmol/L, methanol: >15.6 mmol/L, isopropanol: >8.32 mmol/L), ethanol: >2000 μg/mL (SI: >43.4 mmol/L); urine: acetone, methanol, isopropanol >500 μg/mL (SI: acetone: >8610 μmol/L, methanol: >15.6 mmol/L, isopropanol: 8.32 mmol/L), ethanol: >1600 μg/mL (SI: >34.7 mmol/L)

Use Evaluate methanol and isopropanol toxicity, and alcohol drug abuse

Methodology Gas-liquid chromatography (GLC)

Additional Information Both methanol and isopropanol are more intoxicating than ethanol. Methanol is converted to formaldehyde and formic acid which causes retinal damage leading to blindness and metabolic acidosis. Isopropanol is converted to acetone.

Specific References

Burkhart KK and Kulig KW, "The Other Alcohols. Methanol, Ethylene Glycol, and Isopropanol," *Emerg Med Clin North Am*, 1990, 8(4):913-28.

Jarvie DR and Simpson D, "Simple Screening Tests for the Emergency Identification of Methanol and Ethylene Glycol in Poisoned Patients," *Clin Chem*, 1990, 36(11):1957-61.

Lacouture PG, Heldreth DD, Shannon M, et al, "The Generation of Acetonemia/Acetonuria Following Ingestion of a Subtoxic Dose of Isopropyl Alcohol," *Am J Emerg Med*, 1989, 7(1):38-40.

Litovitz T, "The Alcohols: Ethanol, Methanol, Isopropanol, Ethylene Glycol," *Pediatr Clin North Am*, 1986, 33(2):311-23.

Warfarin, Blood

Synonyms Athrombin-K®; Coumadin®; Panwarfin®

Applies To Anticoagulants, Oral

Abstract Warfarin is an oral anticoagulant. Serum warfarin concentrations are seldom used to manage therapy; rather, typically, prothrombin time is used.

Specimen Blood

Volume 7 mL

Container Red top tube, lavender top (EDTA) tube

Reference Range Therapeutic: 2-5 μg/mL (SI: 6.5-16.2 μmol/L); free warfarin level: 5-23 ng/mL

Possible Panic Range Toxic: >10 μg/mL (SI: >32.4 μmol/L)

Use Therapeutic monitoring; toxicity assessment

Limitations This test **does not** measure bishydroxycoumarin and should not be used to monitor this drug.

Methodology High performance liquid chromatography (HPLC), gas-liquid chromatography (GLC), UV spectrophotometry

Additional Information Warfarin is used for chronic oral anticoagulation in a variety of clinical settings. Management of warfarin therapy is usually done by following the **prothrombin time and international normalized ratio (INR)**, rather than by measuring serum drug concentrations. Warfarin is subject to a bewildering number and variety of drug interactions, producing increased or decreased clinical effect of itself or other drugs. Many of these effects are due to changes in protein binding or hepatic metabolism. Reductions in dosage may be indicated for aging subjects treated for venous thromboembolic or coronary arterial disease, but not in those with peripheral vascular disease, deep vein thrombosis, or valvular heart disease.

Specific References

Bick RL, "Antithrombolytic Therapy," *Disorders of Thrombosis and Hemostasis: Clinical Laboratory Practice*, Chapter 14, Chicago, IL: ASCP Press, 1992, 291-312.

Mortensen ML, "Management of Acute Childhood Poisonings Caused By Selected Insecticides and Herbicides," *Pediatr Clin North Am*, 1986, 33(2):421-45.

Redwood M, Taylor C, Bain BJ, et al, "The Association of Age With Dosage Requirement for Warfarin," *Age-Ageing*, 1991, 20(3):217-20.

Schreiber TL, Miller DH, Silvasi D, et al, "Superiority of Warfarin Over Aspirin Long-Term After Thrombolytic Therapy for Acute Myocardial Infarction," *Am Heart J*, 1990, 119(6):1238-44.

WBC *see* White Blood Count *on next page*

Weed *see* Cannabinoids, Qualitative *on page 1217*

Westergren Sed Rate *see* Sedimentation Rate, Erythrocyte *on page 1348*

White Blood Count

Synonyms Leukocyte Count; Total WBC; WBC; White Count

Abstract This procedure determines the white blood cell concentration in a body fluid, usually blood. The count is most commonly generated by an automated analyzer using aperture-impedance and/or laser beam technology. Different types of white blood cells (eg, granulocytes, monocytes, lymphocytes, etc) are included in the total count. The results have widespread application to the diagnosis and monitoring of a variety of clinical conditions including infectious, neoplastic, and immunologic disease states.

Specimen Whole blood or other body fluid

Volume 5 mL

Minimum Volume 1 mL

Container Lavender top (EDTA) tube

Causes for Rejection Clotted specimen, hemolyzed specimen

Reference Range Peripheral blood: 4500-11,000/mm^3 (SI: 4.5-11.0 x 10^9/L)

Possible Panic Range On admission <2500/mm^3 (SI: 2.5 x 10^9/L) or >30,000/mm^3 (SI: >30.0 x 10^9/L)

Use White cell enumeration; evaluate myelopoiesis, bacterial and viral infections, toxic metabolic processes; diagnose/evaluate leukemic states

Limitations If nucleated RBCs are found in differential count, the white blood count should be corrected. Electronic counters are subject to spurious high WBC counts in cases where clumped platelet aggregates are "seen" as white cells.

Methodology Manual – hemocytometer counting chambers. Most WBC count determinations are obtained from one channel of a highly automated multichannel electronic and pneumatic analyzer using aperture-impedance and/or aperture conductance and/or laser light scattering technologies. WBC differential determination is provided by recent generations of analyzers. Excellent performance (precision, linearity, and lack of carryover) has been found on field evaluation of a commonly utilized multichannel device.

Additional Information In newborn infants, WBC counts from different vascular sources (ie, capillary vs venous vs arterial blood) should not necessarily be considered equivalent. WBC counts from actively crying babies may show leukocytosis with left shift, possibly erroneously suggesting bacterial infections. Any stressful situation in newborns, children, or adults which leads to increase in endogenous epinephrine production may cause a rapid (15-30 minutes) increase in WBC count. In the evaluation of infection in newborns and young children, it is recommended that several counts be obtained from a consistent vascular source in resting individuals. A study of within subject and between subject variation has reaffirmed that hematologic parameters have significant individuality. Screening using conventional reference limits may be misleading. Subject specific reference values are likely to have greater clinical utility. There is modest progressive leukocytosis (due to neutrophils) throughout pregnancy into the third trimester with subsequent decline in white count after about 34 weeks gestation. Included in the broad differential consideration for the cause of neutropenia is collagen-vascular disease, notably lupus erythematosus and other autoimmune neutropenias (see Specific References). Many drugs result in leukopenia including bezafibrate, an antihyperlipidemic fibric acid.

Specific References

Christensen RD and Rothstein G, "Pitfalls in the Interpretation of Leukocyte Counts of Newborn Infants," *Am J Clin Pathol*, 1979, 72(4):608-11.

Second National Health and Nutrition Examination Survey, "Hematological and Nutritional Biochemistry Reference Data for Persons 6 Months to 74 Years of Age: United States, 1976-80," *Vital Health Stat*, DHHS Publication No (PHS) 83-1682, 1982.

Shastri KA and Logue GL, "Autoimmune Neutropenia," *Blood*, 1993, 81(8):1984-95.

White Count *see* White Blood Count *on this page*

Wood Alcohol *see* Methanol, Blood *on page 1295*

Xenon Lung Scan *see* Lung Scan, Ventilation *on page 1288*

Xylocaine® *see* Lidocaine, Blood *on page 1284*

Yellow Jackets *see* Barbiturates, Quantitative, Blood *on page 1201*

Zalcitabine, Blood or Urine

Synonyms DDC

Specimen Blood, urine

Volume 5 mL

Reference Range <10 ng/mL

Use AIDS therapy; therapeutic monitoring

Limitations Only used in combination with zidovudine; not approved for use in children; if used concurrently with drugs causing renal clearance problems, do so with caution

Methodology Radioimmunoassy (RIA), gas chromatography/mass spectrometry (GC/MS), high performance liquid chromatography (HPLC)

Additional Information Potential toxicities include congestive heart failure, cardiomyopathy. No liver metabolites have been identified in humans; half-life: 8.5 hours.

Specific References

Rubio FR, Crews T, Garland WA, et al, "Quantification of Dideoxycytidine in Human Plasma by Gas Chromatography/Mass Spectrometry," *Biomed Environ Mass Spectrom*, 1988, 17(5):399-404.

Shelton MJ, O'Donnell AM, and Morse GD, "Zalcitabine," *Ann Pharmacother*, 1993, 27(4):480-9.

Zarontin® *see* Ethosuximide, Blood *on page 1261*

Zartalin® *see* Ethosuximide, Blood *on page 1261*

Zidovudine, Blood

Synonyms Azidothymidine; AZT; Retrovir®

Abstract Azidothymidine (AZT) is the first FDA approved drug for the treatment of human immunodeficiency virus (HIV) infection, the cause of AIDS. The drug is a competitive inhibitor of HIV reverse transcriptase; it is incorporated into the viral DNA in place of thymidine and interrupts viral replication because the DNA can no longer elongate.

Specimen Blood

Minimum Volume Volume needed is method dependent (0.1-1 mL serum or plasma)

Container Red top tube preferred, green top (heparin) tube acceptable

Sampling Time Trough level, just before next dose

Causes for Rejection Incorrect specimen sampling time

Reference Range Not established

Use Not established for routine clinical use. Monitoring should probably be limited to studies on pharmacokinetics and efficacy of antiretroviral therapy.

Methodology High performance liquid chromatography (HPLC), radioimmunoassay (RIA), fluorescence polarization immunoassay (FPIA)

Additional Information Zidovudine is usually administered at a total daily dose of 500 mg (100 mg orally, every 4 hours while the patient is awake); optimal dosing, however, has not been established. Peak serum concentrations are attained within 30-40 minutes after ingestion. The drug has a half-life of approximately 1 hour; the main metabolite is a glucuronide derivative with no antiviral activity that is excreted by the kidneys. The major toxicity associated with zidovudine use is hematologic suppression which may manifest as anemia, leukopenia, and/or granulocytopenia. Monitoring hematologic parameters is the most reasonable approach toward evaluating toxicity; serum levels currently contribute little to evaluating toxic effects of zidovudine. Coadministration of probenecid results in increased serum levels due to competition for glucuronidation pathways. Hepatic and renal failure increases serum levels.

Specific References

Amin NM, "Zidovudine for Treating AIDS. What Physicians Need to Know," *Postgrad Med*, 1989, 86(1):195-6, 201-8.

Collins JM and Unadket JD, "Clinical Pharmacokinetics of Zidovudine. An Overview of Current Data," *Clin Pharmacokinet*, 1989, 17(1):1-9.

Granich GG, Eveland MR, and Krogstad DJ, "Fluorescence Polarization Immunoassay for Zidovudine<" *Antimicrob Agents Chemother*, 1989, 33(8):1275-9.

Langtry HD and Campoli-Richards DM, "Zidovudine. A Review of its Pharmacodynamic and Pharmacokinetic Properties, and Therapeutic Efficacy," *Drugs*, 1989, 37(4):408-50.

Stretcher BN, "Current AIDS Therapies," *Therapeutic Drug Monitoring and Toxicology In-Service Training and Continuing Education*, 1994, 15(3):51-61.

Wilde MI and Langtry HD, "Zidovudine: An Update of its Pharmacodynamic and Pharmacokinetic Properties and Therapeutic Efficacy," *Drugs*, 1993, 46(3):515-78.

Zinc Protoporphyrin *see* Protoporphyrin, Zinc, Blood *on page 1339*

Zoloft™ *see* Sertraline, Blood *on page 1351*

ZPP *see* Protoporphyrin, Zinc, Blood *on page 1339*

ANTIDOTES

EFFECTIVE USE OF ANTIDOTES

The use of agents to reverse the effects of a poisoning probably began with the initial recognition that xenobiotics caused toxicity. It is popular to label an agent used therapeutically in the treatment of a poisoning victim as an antidote but there exists no consensual definition. A common definition for an antidote is "an agent that increases the median lethal dose (LD_{50}) of a toxin" or more simply "an agent which reverses or neutralizes a poison." A definition using pharmacodynamic and pharmacokinetic terms for an antidote is an agent that reduces toxicity by inhibiting the translocation of the toxin at an effector site or reducing toxin concentration and/or action at the effector site. The clinical toxicology literature has classified agents used therapeutically in treating poison by the terms supportive, adjunct, or antidote therapy. These terms are not mutually exclusive and agents in any classification meet the above definitions of antidote. This virtually guarantees that no single table, article, or book describing antidotes is likely to be complete in its list of "antidote", as it requires the inclusion of any agent capable of decreasing absorption, altering distribution or metabolism, enhancing elimination, acting as a partial or complete receptor antagonist, acting via pharmacologically competitive physiologic systems, and chelating or immunologically binding a toxin. This section contains a number of agents classified as antidotes. This does not preclude the need to refer to additional agents not classified as antidotes, found in the medicinal toxins section which have a role as an antidote/adjunct or supportive therapy. The classification was empiric and generally dependent on the individual agent's relative importance as a cause or cure for toxicity.

Review of the annual summary of the American Association of Poison Control Center (AAPCC) Toxic Exposure Surveillance System (TESS) reveals some interesting data regarding antidotal therapy of poisoning. Compilation of reports of this data for 1983-1991 yields the following top 10 toxin classes resulting in fatalities (in descending order):

1. analgesics
2. antidepressants
3. sedative/hypnotics
4. street drugs
5. cardiovascular agents
6. alcohols
7. fumes
8. asthma therapies (theophylline)
9. chemicals
10. hydrocarbons

Similar review yields the following top ten antidotes (in descending order) provided as therapy for poisonings:

1. oral and intravenous N-acetylcysteine (intravenous would be 10th most used alone)
2. naloxone
3. atropine
4. deferoxamine
5. antivenins
6. ethanol
7. hydroxocobalamin (investigational)
8. Digibind®
9. pralidoxime

The two lists do not match on the basis of rankings of toxin and intended antidote. Several of the toxin classes have no clearly recognized single antidote (sedative/hypnotics, street drugs, cardiovascular, theophylline as example). Others, like antidepressants, have a clearly accepted "antidote" (sodium bicarbonate) which is more commonly found as supportive care and thus not listed in the antidote rankings. Equally important to note from the AAPCC TESS data is the relative infrequency with which antidotes are used. The following table (adapted) summarizes the total number of poison calls recorded for the listed years and the number of times antidotal therapy was provided.

Incidence of Antidote Use Recorded by AAPCC TESS

Year	Total Calls to TESS	# of Cases in Which an Antidote Was Provided
1990	1,713,462	16,536 (0.9%)
1991	1,837,939	19,272 (1.0%)
1992	1,864,188	19,839 (1.1%)
1993	1,751,476	21,949 (1.3%)

The optimal use of an antidote should be guided by the principles of pharmaceutical care and the prevention of drug-related problems. The consideration of the eight commonly accepted drug-related problems provides a structure to the consideration and use of an antidote. A regional poison control center and/or a clinical toxicology service should be consulted with consideration of antidotal therapy to assist in this process. It is important to note that recommendations vary greatly between individuals and/or poison centers reflecting local idiosyncracies, circumstances, or practice philosophies. Also, there are few prospective controlled trials evaluating an antidote's performance *in vivo*, thus treatment recommendations are often very empiric. Always remember to stabilize the patient first. The eight drug-related problems to avoid are:

1. untreated indications
2. improper drug selection
3. failure to receive medication
4. subtherapeutic dosing
5. supratherapeutic dosing
6. adverse reactions
7. drug use without indication
8. interactions

UNTREATED INDICATIONS

While it may seem obvious that an antidote should be reserved until an indication is recognized, the issue is more complex than having a presumptive diagnosis based on initial evaluation. There should be a high degree of correlation of history, physical exam, and laboratory findings. The possibility of competing or misleading coingestants has to be addressed. When treating an unknown ingestant and relying on a presumptive diagnosis based on a specific toxidrome, all potential toxins capable of that toxidrome need consideration and potential treatment. The choice of antidote in such a setting may be dependent on adverse effect profile, frequency, or toxin exposures, availability, staff familiarity, and even cost. Factors such as laboratory turnaround time may require empiric initiation of an antidote whose duration is dependent on the pending laboratory test. An example would be initiation of N-acetylcysteine in a patient with a significant historical ingestion for whom a serum acetaminophen concentration will be unavailable until more than 8 hours after ingestion.

IMPROPER DRUG SELECTION

As for untreated indications above, carefully consider the presentation. Are all etiologies accounted for, are potential concomitant ingestants present which may impair antidotal effects or increase the frequency of adverse effects or outcomes? An example would be concomitant benzodiazepine ingestion in a severe cyclic antidepressant overdose being reversed by flumazenil and thus unmasking seizures from the antidepressant. Another example would be the difficulty in approaching a patient presenting with the "hypotensive/bradycardia" toxidrome. This can be caused by beta-blockers, calcium channel blockers, cholinesterase inhibitors, cyanide, cyclic antidepressants, digitalis, and clonidine. Most are not detectable readily by laboratory methods and have unique antidotes that may be contraindicated for the alternative toxins (calcium indicated for calcium channel blockers but contraindicated for digitalis). The failure to consider the basic pharmacology of a toxin can lead to improper antidote selection. Dopamine is less likely than norepinephrine to ameliorate hypotension in the acute ingestion of cyclic antidepressants of a chronically maintained rather than in a previously unexposed patient. Another example would be choosing physostigmine for cyclic antidepressant poisoning, neglecting to consider that the toxic effects of a cyclic antidepressant are ameliorated by mechanism in addition to anticholinergic.

FAILURE TO RECEIVE MEDICATION

Many institutions fail to maintain sufficient antidotes or amount of any specific antidote to treat the severe poisoning. In a recent survey, only 7 of 124 responding hospitals maintained sufficient amounts of 10 common antidotes to treat a 2-dose supply for an adult. Another avenue is to consult the regional poison control center which should maintain or have access to an antidote depot. The American Academy of Clinical Toxicology has proposed criteria for Regional Toxicology Treatment Centers. One of the criteria was a list of required antidotes to be maintained by the Center. That list is included in the Appendix located in the back of this handbook. Complications of the toxin or its treatment may result in the failure to receive an antidote. An example is patients with persistent vomiting due to toxins or gastric decontamination procedures failing to receive oral antidotes (eg, N-acetylcysteine).

SUB- OR SUPRATHERAPEUTIC DOSING

As a general rule, an antidote should be dosed on the basis of the amount of toxin or the patient's size dependent on the antidote's mechanism of action. If the antidote acts by binding to the toxin (eg, activated charcoal), then the amount of toxin is most important. If the antidote reverses pharmacologic activity, sodium bicarbonate for cyclic antidepressant or other sodium channel blockers, then patient size is most important. There are examples of using the patient's size and laboratory findings, digoxin serum concentrations, to determine the amount of toxin an antidote should be dosed to reverse (Digibind®). It is most important to note that antidotes are intended to override the effects of a poison, this may require dosing in excess of conventional uses. Specifically, relying on dosing guidelines found in product labeling or practice guidelines such as Advanced Cardiac Life Support (ACLS) will lead to subtherapeutic dosing of the severely poisoned patient. Atropine and deferoxamine are good examples of this occurrence. Supratherapeutic dosing is possibly less common although the amount of activated charcoal necessary to achieve elimination enhancement is not known and patients are likely given too much on occasion.

ADVERSE REACTIONS

The use of antidotes which have alternative common indications often requires unusual dosing, as described above, (which can be in excess of product labeling) and exposes the patient to a greater incidence or number of adverse reactions. The clinical toxicology of most antidotes is not well determined secondary to the inability to separate toxin from treatment effects. Consider the presence of salts (salicylate salts of the oral cholinergic agents, eg, physostigmine), excipients/diluents (phenol in glucagon diluent), and dosage form (intravenous agents and fluid overload with infusions) as causes or potential sources of adverse effects of antidotes, especially once high dose and/or prolonged administration occurs.

DRUG USE WITHOUT INDICATION

The initiation of antidotal therapy on the basis of an uncorroborated history, inconsistent physical findings, or isolated laboratory tests (especially urine "tox screens") should generally be considered drug use without indication. The selection and initiation of an antidote should be based on consistent patient specific signs, symptoms, and/or laboratory findings that contribute or provide a presumptive diagnosis.

INTERACTIONS

Many antidotes have effects on lab tests used to monitor poisonings. For these agents, once antidotal therapy is initiated, routine interpretation of laboratory findings is not appropriate. Examples would be serum iron concentrations after deferoxamine administration or serum digoxin concentrations after Digibind® use. The reader is cautioned to refer to the test interactions section of each antidote monograph.

SUMMARY

Always stabilize the patient first and consider consulting clinical toxicology personnel. Double check the dosing of the antidote which should ultimately be based on mechanism of action, clinical symptomatology, lab values, and adverse effects. Consider availability and potential duration of effect with available supplies. Anticipate the need to acquire additional stock, it does no good to stabilize a patient for 30 minutes (total supply of antidote) when the toxin can have persistent life-threatening effects for more than 24 hours.

REFERENCES

The American Academy of Clinical Toxicology, "Facility Assessment Guidelines for Regional Toxicology Treatment Center," *J Toxicol Clin Toxicol*, 1993, 31:211-7.

Bolgiano EB and Barish RA, "Use of New and Established Antidotes," *Emerg Med Clin North Am*, 1994, 12(2):317-34.

Chyka PA and Conner HG, "Availability of Antidotes in Rural and Urban Hospitals in Tennessee," *Am J Hosp Pharm*, 1994, 51:1346-8.

Litovitz TL, Clark LR, and Soloway RA, "1993 Annual Report of the American Association of Poison Control Center Toxic Exposure Surveillance System," *Am J Emerg Med*, 1994, 12:546-84.

Schauben J and Frenia ML, "Update on Antidotal Therapy," *J Pharm Pract*, 1993, 6:63-73.

Scharman EJ, and Rosencrane JG, "Isoniazid Toxicity: A Survey of Pyridoxine Availability," *Am J Emerg Med*, 1994, 12(3):386-8.

Scherrman JM, "Antibody Treatment of Toxic Poisoning - Recent Advances," *J Toxicol Clin Toxicol*, 1994, 32:363-75.

Scherrman JM, Terrien N, Urtizberra M, et al, "Immunotoxicotherapy: Present Status and Future Trends," *J Toxicol Clin Toxicol*, 1989, 27:1-35.

Smilkstein MJ, "A Rational Approach to the Unknown Ingestion," *Emerg Med*, 1993, 73-88.

— This introductory text was written by Frank P. Paloucek, PharmD
University of Illinois at Chicago

Acetylcysteine (a se teel sis' tay een)

CAS Number 616-91-1; 19542-74-6 (Acetylcysteine Sodium)

Brand Names Acetyst®; Airbron®; Alveolex®; Bromuc®; Brunac®; Exomuc®; Mucolator®; Mucomyst®; Mucosol®; Mucret®; Siran®; Solmucol®; Tamuc®; Tixair®

Synonyms Mercapturic Acid; NAC; *N*-Acetylcysteine; *N*-Acetyl-L-cysteine

Use Antidote for acute acetaminophen toxicity; for hepatic failure/encephalopathy following delayed presentation (>24 hours) of an acute acetaminophen overdose; possibly beneficial as a free radical scavenger for any significant acute hepatotoxic exposures including carbon tetrachloride and other drugs; see following listing

Acute acetaminophen ingestions:

- >7.5 g ingested in an adult or >200 mg/kg in a child if no serum acetaminophen level is available
- Serum acetaminophen 4-hour level >150 mcg/mL
- Evidence of hepatotoxicity or measurable acetaminophen levels >24 hours post-acute ingestion
- Unknown quantity ingested and >24 hours have elapsed since time of ingestion or unable to obtain serum acetaminophen levels with 12 hours of ingestion

Antidote Useful For

Acetaminophen *on page 79*
Carbon Tetrachloride *on page 882*
Cobalt *on page 895*
Oxycodone and Acetaminophen *on page 584*
Propoxyphene and Acetaminophen *on page 656*

Mechanism of Action Exerts mucolytic action through its free sulfhydryl group which opens up the disulfide bonds in the mucoproteins thus lowering the viscosity. The exact mechanism of action in acetaminophen toxicity is unknown. It may act by maintaining or restoring glutathione levels or by acting as an alternative substrate for conjugation with the toxic metabolite.

Adverse Reactions

Cardiovascular: Hypotension (in acetylcysteine overdose)

Central nervous system: Drowsiness, clamminess, fever/pyrexia, chills, headache

Dermatologic: Generalized urticaria

Gastrointestinal: Stomatitis, nausea, vomiting

Hepatic: Mild increases in liver function tests have occurred after oral therapy

Local: Irritation

Otic: Tinnitus

Respiratory: Bronchospasm, wheezing, rotten egg breath, cough, rhinorrhea, hemoptysis

Miscellaneous: Anaphylactoid reactions with I.V. use (0.3% to 3.0%); chills

Toxicodynamics/Kinetics

Onset of action: Upon inhalation, within 1 minute; direct instillation, immediate peak within 5-10 minutes

Duration: Can persist for longer than 1 hour

Absorption: Mostly acts directly on mucus in lungs; remainder is absorbed by pulmonary epithelium; after oral administration, absorbed from GI tract

Distribution: Unknown

Protein binding: 50%

Metabolism: Hepatic; undergoes rapid deacetylation *in vivo* to yield cysteine or oxidation to yield diacetylcysteine

Half-life: V_d: 0.5 L/kg

- Reduced acetylcysteine: 2 hours
- Total acetylcysteine: 5.5 hours

Elimination: Unknown; renal clearance may account for 30% elimination

Usual Dosage

Acetaminophen poisoning (initiate treatment within 24 hours): Children and Adults: Oral: 140 mg/kg followed by 17 doses of 70 mg/kg every 4 hours or until acetaminophen assay reveals nontoxic levels; repeat dose if emesis occurs within 1 hour of administration. For treatment of acetaminophen overdosage, administer orally as a 5% solution [dilute the 20% solution 1:3 with a cola, orange juice or other soft drink and use within 1 hour of preparation]; unpleasant odor becomes less noticeable as treatment progresses.

I.V.: Two protocols for acute overdose:

- Intermittent bolus: Same as oral regimen; 140 mg/kg followed by 70 mg/kg every 4 hours for 17 doses; infuse dose over 1 hour
- Continuous infusion: Total 300 mg/kg given as follows: 150 mg/kg over 15 minutes, then 50 mg/kg over 4 hours, then 100 mg/kg over 16 hours

For late presentation or hepatic failure, give acetylcysteine via appropriate route by any dosing protocol until biochemical evidence of significant hepatic failure resolves

DRUGS OR DISEASE STATES IN WHICH N-ACETYLCYSTEINE IS INVESTIGATIONAL FOR CYTOPROTECTIVE EFFECTS

AIDS
Acetaminophen (definite antidote)*
Acrolein
Acrylonitrile
Arsenic
Benzo(a)pyrene (BaP)
Bromobenzene
Carbon monoxide (delayed neuropsychiatric toxicity prevention)*
Carbon tetrachloride (hepatoprotective)*
Chloramphenicol (bone marrow toxicity)
Chloroform
Chromium (nephroprotective)*
Cobalt
Corneal alkali exposure
Cyclophosphamide/ifosfamide (protective against hemorrhagic cystitis)*
Dichlorodiethyl sulfide (mustard gas)
1,2 Dichloropropane
Doxorubicin (cardiomyopathy)*
Ethylene dichloride
Gold (aplastic anemia)*
Keratoconjunctivitis sicca
Methyl bromide
Methyl iodide
Methyl mercury*
Mustard gas*
Paraquat (lung toxicity)
Pennyroyal oil (pulegone)
Radiation therapy (topical administration-reduction of skin reaction)*
Sodium hydroxide (caustic ingestion)
Sulfasalazine*
Thallium (preventing corneal ulceration)
Zinc chloride (chelation)*
Zinc sulfate (chelation)

*Denotes human experience.

REFERENCES

Banner W, Koch M, Hopf S, et al, "N-Acetylcysteine in the Chelation of Zinc Sulfate," *Vet Hum Toxicol*, 1985, 28:293.

Crystal RG and Bast A, "Oxidants and Antioxidants: Pathophysiologic Determinants and Therapeutic Agents," *Am J Med*, 1991, (Suppl-3C)1S-145S.

Flanagan RJ, "The Role of Acetylcysteine in Clinical Toxicology," *Med Toxicol*, 1987, 2(2):93-104.

Flanagan RJ and Meredith TJ, "Use of N-Acetylcysteine in Clinical Toxicology," *Am J Med*, 1991, 91(3C):131S-139S.

Hjortso E, Qvist J, Bud M, et al, "ARDS After Accidental Inhalation of Zinc Chloride Smoke," *Intensive Care Med*, 1988, 14:17-24.

Howard RJ, Blake DR, Pall H, et al, "Allopurinol/N-Acetylcysteine for Carbon Monoxide Poisoning," *Lancet*, 1987, 2(8559):628-9.

Liu A, Richardson M, and Robertson WO, "Effects of N-Acetylcysteine on Caustic Burns," *Vet Hum Toxicol*, 1985, 28:316.

Llobet JM, Domingo JL, and Corbella J, "Comparative Effects of Repeated Parenteral Administration of Several Chelators on the Distribution and Excretion of Cobalt," *Res Commun Chem Pathol Pharmacol*, 1988, 60:225-33.

Meggs WJ, Morasco R, Shih RD, et al, "Effects of Prussian Blue and N-Acetylcysteine on Thallium Toxicity in Mice," *Vet Hum Toxicol*, 1994, 36:364.

Messner K and Leibowitz HM, "Acetylcysteine Treatment of Keratitis Sicca," *Arch Ophthalmol*, 1971, 86:357-9.

Roederer M, Ela SW, Staal FJ, et al, "N-Acetylcysteine: A New Approach to Anti-HIV Therapy," *AIDS Res Hum Retroviruses*, 1992, 8(2):209-17.

Slansky HH, Berman MB, et al, "Cysteine and Acetylcysteine in the Prevention of Corneal Ulcerations," *Ann Ophthalmol*, 1970, 2:488-91.

Yarbro JW, "N-Acetylcysteine (NAC): A Significant Chemoprotective Adjunct," *Semin Oncol*, 1983, 10(Suppl):1-89.

(Continued)

Acetylcysteine *(Continued)*

Inhalation: Acetylcysteine 10% and 20% solution (Mucomyst®) (dilute with water or 0.9% sodium chloride):

Infants: 2 mL of 5% solution nebulized given 3-4 times/day

Children: 3-5 mL of 5% to 10% solution nebulized given 3-4 times/day

Adolescents: 5-10 mL of 5% to 10% solution nebulized given 3-4 times/day

Note: Patients should receive an aerosolized bronchodilator 10-15 minutes prior to acetylcysteine

Meconium ileus equivalent: Children and Adults: 100-200 mL of 5% to 10% solution by irrigation or orally **or** 5-30 mL of 10% solution administered 3-6 times/24 hours orally or rectally

Contraindications Known hypersensitivity to acetylcysteine

Dosage Forms Solution, as sodium: 10% [100 mg/mL] (4 mL, 10 mL, 30 mL); 20% [200 mg/mL] (4 mL, 10 mL, 30 mL, 100 mL)

Reference Range Determine acetaminophen level as soon as possible, but no sooner than 4 hours after ingestion (to ensure peak levels have been obtained); toxic concentration with possible hepatotoxicity >150 μg/mL (probably hepatotoxicity >200 μg/mL) at 4 hours or 50 μg/mL at 12 hours; serum N-acetylcysteine levels are ~500 mg/L 15 minutes after a loading dose of 150 mg/kg

Drug Interactions Adsorbed by activated charcoal; clinical significance is minimal, though, once a pure acetaminophen ingestion requiring N-acetylcysteine is established; further charcoal dosing is unnecessary once the appropriate initial charcoal dose is achieved (5-10 g:g acetaminophen)

Pregnancy Risk Factor B

Pregnancy Implications Does not appear to cross the placenta

Nursing Implications Assess patient for nausea, vomiting, and skin rash following oral administration for treatment of acetaminophen poisoning; intermittent aerosol treatments are commonly given when patient arises, before meals, and just before retiring at bedtime

Additional Information Oral therapy is preferred; I.V. route is investigational in U.S. if nonparenteral dosage form is to be used; for I.V. administration, filter with 0.22-micron filter needle; unpleasant odor becomes less noticeable as treatment progresses

Specific References

Harrison PM, Wendon JA, Gimson AE, et al, "Improvement by Acetylcysteine of Hemodynamics and Oxygen Transport in Fulminant Hepatic Failure," *N Engl J Med*, 1991, 324(26):1852-7.

Henderson A and Hayes P, "Acetylcysteine as a Cytoprotective Antioxidant in Patients With Severe Sepsis: Potential New Use for an Old Drug," *Ann Pharmacother*, 1994, 28:1086-8.

Keays R, Harrison PM, Wendon JA, et al, "Intravenous Acetylcysteine in Paracetamol Induced Fulminant Hepatic Failure: A Prospective Controlled Trial," *BMJ*, 1991, 303(6809):1026-9.

Mohammed S, Jamal AZ, and Robison LR, "Serum Sickness-Like Illness Associated With N-Acetylcysteine Therapy," *Ann Pharmacother*, 1994, 28(2):285.

Prescott LF, Donovan JW, Jarvie DR, et al, "The Disposition and Kinetics of Intravenous N-acetylcysteine in Patients With Paracetamol Overdosage," *Eur J Clin Pharmacol*, 1989, 37(5):501-6.

Smilkstein MJ, Knapp GL, Kulig KW, et al, "Efficacy of N-Acetylcysteine in the Treatment of Acetaminophen Overdose: Analysis of the National Multicenter Study (1976 to 1985)," *N Engl J Med*, 1988, 319(24):1557-62.

Acetyst® *see* Acetylcysteine *on page 1388*

Actidose-Aqua® [OTC] *see* Charcoal *on page 1403*

Actidose® With Sorbitol [OTC] *see* Charcoal *on page 1403*

Adrenalin® Chloride *see* Epinephrine *on page 1422*

Adrenergic Agonists, Cardiovascular Comparison *see page 1638*

Adrenergic Agonists Drug Infusions Comparison *see page 1638*

Airbron® *see* Acetylcysteine *on page 1388*

AllerMax® Oral [OTC] *see* Diphenhydramine Hydrochloride *on page 1415*

Alphamin® Injection *see* Hydroxocobalamin *on page 1433*

Aludrin® *see* Isoproterenol *on page 1436*

Alveolex® *see* Acetylcysteine *on page 1388*

Amylis Nitris *see* Amyl Nitrite *on this page*

Amyl Nitrite (am' il)

CAS Number 110-46-3; 463-04-7

Brand Names Amyl Nitrite Aspirols®; Amyl Nitrite Vaporole®; Nitrit®

Synonyms Amylis Nitris; Isoamyl Nitrite; Isopentyl Nitrite; Pentyl Nitrite; Poppers

Use Coronary vasodilator in angina pectoris; an adjunct in treatment of cyanide poisoning; also used to produce changes in the intensity of heart murmurs

Antidote Useful For
Acetonitrile *on page 850*
Acrylonitrile *on page 853*
Cyanide *on page 899*
Hydrogen Sulfide *on page 942*

Mechanism of Action Vasodilator (vascular smooth muscle relaxant)

Adverse Reactions
Cardiovascular: Postural hypotension, cutaneous flushing of head, neck, and clavicular area, palpitations, tachycardia
Central nervous system: Headache, incoherent speech
Dermatologic: Contact dermatitis
Gastrointestinal: Nausea, colitis, vomiting
Genitourinary: Penile erection is enhanced, ejaculation (retarded)
Hematologic: Heinz body hemolysis/hemolytic anemia
Ocular: Increased intraocular pressure, blurred vision, yellow vision
Respiratory: Tracheobronchitis

Signs & Symptoms of Acute Overdose Tachycardia, methemoglobinemia, coma, stupor, cyanosis, dyspnea, ataxia, bradycardia

Toxicodynamics/Kinetics
Onset of action: Within 30 seconds
Duration: 5 minutes
Absorption:
Readily through the respiratory tract
Rapidly with oral ingestion
Metabolism: Hepatic; metabolized by liver to form inorganic nitrates (less potent)
Half-life:
Parent: <1 hour
Methemoglobin: 1 hour
Elimination: Renal: ~33%

Usual Dosage 1-6 inhalations from 1 capsule are usually sufficient to produce the desired effect

Contraindications Severe anemia; hypersensitivity to nitrates

Dosage Forms Inhalant, crushable glass perles: 0.18 mL, 0.3 mL

Stability Store in cool place, protect from light; insoluble in water; inflammable

Drug Interactions Alcohol

Pregnancy Risk Factor X

Monitoring Parameters Monitor blood pressure during therapy or have patient lie down during inhalation; methemoglobin levels; arterial blood gas
Methemoglobin levels:
15%: Chocolate-colored blood
20%: Symptomatic
40%: Tachycardia
50%: Stupor
70%: Lethal

Nursing Implications Administer by nasal inhalation; patient should be sitting; crush ampul in woven covering between fingers and then hold under patient's nostrils

Additional Information Weak methemoglobin agent when inhaled

Specific References

Dudley MJ and Solomon T, "A Case of Methaemoglobinaemia," *Arch Emerg Med*, 1993, 10(2):117-9.
Laaban JP, Bodenan P, and Rochemaure J, "Amyl Nitrate Poppers and Methemoglobinemia," *Ann Intern Med*, 1985, 103(5):804-5.
Osterloh J and Olson K, "Toxicities of Alkyl Nitrites," *Ann Intern Med*, 1986, 104(5):727.
Schwartz RH, "When to Suspect Inhalant Abuse," *Patient Care*, 1989, 23:39-64.

Amyl Nitrite Aspirols® *see* Amyl Nitrite *on previous page*

Amyl Nitrite Vaporole® *see* Amyl Nitrite *on previous page*

Ana-Kit® *see* Insect Sting Kit *on page 1434*

Antidigoxin Fab Fragments *see* Digoxin Immune Fab *on page 1411*

Antilirium® Injection *see* Physostigmine *on page 1457*

Antitoxin Botulinin Types A, B, and E

Brand Names Lioserio®

Use Prophylaxis or active treatment of individuals who have eaten food known or strongly suspected of being infected with *Clostridium botulinum*

Antidote Useful For
Clostridium botulinum Food Poisoning *on page 1070*

Adverse Reactions
Cardiovascular: Tachycardia, cardiovascular collapse, flushing, cyanosis
(Continued)

Antitoxin Botulinin Types A, B, and E *(Continued)*

Dermatologic: Urticaria

Respiratory: Wheezing, bronchospasm, apnea

Miscellaneous: Signs or symptoms of anaphylaxis (typically occur within 20-60 minutes); serum sickness may occur within 14 days of administration and is more likely to follow a repeat injection of equine serum

Administration Administer 1-2 vials slowly I.V. in a 1:10 dilution with 0.9% normal saline (may also give a dose of 1 vial I.M.), and then subsequent doses every 2-4 hours I.V. based on clinical findings

Contraindications History of anaphylaxis to equine-derived serums is a relative contraindication

Warnings Always precede treatment with a skin test for sensitivity, as described in the dosage section; when administering this agent, have ready access to drugs of resuscitation, including epinephrine and ventilatory support equipment. Botulism equine antitoxin does not limit the microbial spread of *C. botulinum.* Likewise, antibiotics do not decrease adverse effects to the toxin. Botulinum toxoid is required to confer long-lasting immunity. The preparation contains 0.25% phenol and 0.005% thimerosal in antivenin, and 1:100,000 phenylmercuric nitrate in bacteriostatic water for diluent. Not effective for botulinum type C toxicity.

Dosage Forms Package contains one vial containing drug, equivalent to 7500 IU of type A, 5500 IU of type B, and 8500 IU of type E antitoxin

Stability Excessive agitation or shaking of the reconstituted vial may cause foaming, which may lead to denaturation of the antivenin

Pregnancy Risk Factor C

Pregnancy Implications Use only if the potential benefits outweigh the risks; it is not known if botulinum antitoxin antibodies cross the placenta

Monitoring Parameters Resolution of symptoms of botulism, or emergence of symptoms of sensitivity to the antitoxin

Additional Information Trivalent botulinum antitoxin will not neutralize toxin that is already bound to the synaptic cleft, and will therefore not reverse established paralysis. Antitoxin is only available from the Immunobiologics Unit, Clinical Medicine Branch, Division of Host Factors, Center for Infectious Diseases, Centers for Disease Control, Atlanta, GA. To order this product, call (404) 639-3334 or (404) 639-3670 Monday through Friday, 8 AM to 4:30 PM EST, or (404) 639-2206 or (404) 639-3670 weekends and after working hours (emergency requests only). Additional information may be obtained through the CDC Drug Information Services at (404) 639-3356.

Specific References

Grabenstein JD, "Immunoantidotes: II. One Hundred Years of Antitoxins," *Hosp Pharm*, 1992, 27:637-46.

Antivenin (Crotalidae) Polyvalent

(an tee ven' in (kroe tal' ih day) pol ee vay' lent)

Synonyms Crotaline Antivenin, Polyvalent; North and South American Antisnake-bite Serum; Snake (Pit Vipers) Antivenin

Use Neutralization of venoms of North and South America crotalids: rattlesnake, copperhead, cottonmouth, tropical moccasins, fer-de-lance, bushmaster

Antidote Useful For

Bushmaster *on page 1063*

Copperhead Snake *on page 1074*

Crotalidae on page 1075

Rattlesnakes *on page 1132*

Mechanism of Action Enhances venom elimination but has no effect on local tissue injury

Adverse Reactions

Cardiovascular: Shock, edema of the face

Central nervous system: Apprehension, peripheral neuritis

Dermatologic: Urticaria

Neuromuscular & skeletal: Muscle weakness

Respiratory: Dyspnea

Miscellaneous: Anaphylaxis, serum sickness (83% of patients receiving more than 8 vials) usually 7-14 days after initial administration; treat with steroids

Usual Dosage Initial intradermal sensitivity test. The entire initial dose of antivenin should be administered as soon as possible to be most effective (within 4 hours after the bite). False-negative rate with skin testing is 20%. Dosage is based on severity of clinical picture; see table.

Children and Adults: I.V.:

Minimal envenomation: 20-40 mL

Moderate envenomation: 50-90 mL

Severe envenomation: 100-150 mL

Additional doses of antivenin is based on clinical response to the initial dose. If swelling continues to progress, symptoms increase in severity, hypoten-

Antivenin Therapy for Pit Viper Bites

Clinical Severity		No. of Vials
Minimal	Symptoms confined to bite area; absent or insignificant systemic symptoms	0
Mild	Edema progressing slowly; bite site reveals small amount of ecchymosis; only systemic sign is metallic taste	5
Moderate	Tissue damage beyond immediate bite area; moderate laboratory changes; perioral fasciculation, paresthesias	10
Severe	Tissue damage to entire extremity; major systemic symptoms; significant laboratory abnormalities	>15

Adapted from Howland MA and Smilkstein MI, "Primer on Immunology With Applications to Toxicology," *Crit Care Toxicol,* 1991, 1(3):135.

sion occurs, or decrease in hematocrit appears, an additional 10-50 mL should be administered.

For I.V. infusion: 1:1-1:10 dilution of reconstituted antivenin in normal saline or D_5W should be prepared. Infuse the initial 5-10 mL of diluted antivenin over 3-5 minutes monitoring closely for signs of sensitivity reactions.

Administration Antivenin may be given I.M. for minimal envenomation. I.V. administration of antivenin is preferred for moderate to severe envenomation or in the presence of shock; for I.V. infusion, prepare a 1:1 to 1:10 dilution of reconstituted antivenin in normal saline or D_5W; infuse the initial 5-10 mL dilution over 3-5 minutes while carefully observing the patient for signs and symptoms of sensitivity reactions. If no reaction occurs, continue infusion at a safe I.V. fluid delivery rate.

Contraindications Not effective against the venoms of coral snakes

Dosage Forms Injection: Lyophilized serum, diluent (10 mL); one vacuum vial to yield 10 mL of serum

Stability Store in refrigerator, avoid temperatures >37°C; reconstituted solutions should be used within 48 hours

Pregnancy Risk Factor C

Pregnancy Implications Not a contraindication for antivenin therapy

Monitoring Parameters Vital signs, hematocrit

Nursing Implications Do **not** inject into a finger or toe; epinephrine should be available. Desensitization may need to be performed on patients with positive skin test reaction or history of sensitivity to equine serum; 1% of patients with negative skin test may still react when antivenin is administered; skin test should not be done unless antivenin is to be used.

Additional Information Intradermal skin test: 0.02-0.03 mL of a 1:10 dilution of antivenin in normal saline; if patient has a history of equine serum sensitivity, administer a 1:100 or greater dilution skin test. May contain 0.25% phenol and 0.005% thimerosal as a preservative.

Specific References

Bush SP and Jansen PW, "Severe Rattlesnake Envenomation With Anaphylaxis and Rhabdomyolysis," *Ann Emerg Med,* 1995, 25:845-8.

Gold BS and Wingert WA, "Snake Venom Poisoning in the United States: A Review of Therapeutic Practice," *S Med J,* 1994, 87:579-87.

Jurkovich GJ, Luterman A, McCullan K, et al, "Complications of Crotalidae Antivenin Therapy," *J Trauma,* 1988, 28(7):1032-7.

Nelson BK, "Snake Envenomation: Incidence, Clinical Presentation, and Management," *Med Toxicol Adverse Drug Exp,* 1989, 4(1):17-31.

Rydel JJ, Aks S, Lewis RB, et al, "Management Considerations in Copperhead Envenomation," *J Emerg Nurs,* 1993, 19(3):193-6.

Smith TA 2d and Figge HL, "Treatment of Snakebite Poisoning," *Am J Hosp Pharm,* 1991, 48(10):2190-6.

Antivenin *(Latrodectus)*

Use Symptoms of envenomation by the black widow spider (*Latrodectus mactans*) including severe hypertension or pain refractory to analgesia, calcium, or sedation; and/or abdominal muscle spasm in pregnancy, threatening spontaneous abortion or early onset labor

Antidote Useful For

Black Widow Spider *on page 1058*

Mechanism of Action Refined, concentrated, and lyophilized preparation of serum globulins from horses immunized with black widow spider (*Latrodectus mactans*) venom

(Continued)

Antivenin *(Latrodectus)* *(Continued)*

Adverse Reactions

Cardiovascular: Tachycardia, cardiovascular collapse, flushing, cyanosis

Dermatologic: Urticaria

Respiratory: Wheezing, bronchospasm, apnea

Miscellaneous: Other signs or symptoms of anaphylaxis (typically occur within 20-60 minutes); serum sickness may occur within 14 days of administration, and is more likely to follow a repeat injection of equine serum

Administration After one test dose, give 1-2 vials I.V. diluted in normal saline (50-100 mL) infused over a 1-hour period; pretreatment with an antihistamine may prevent allergic reactions

Contraindications History of anaphylaxis to equine-derived serums is a relative contraindication

Warnings When administering this agent, have ready access to drugs of resuscitation, including epinephrine, and ventilatory support equipment; antivenin; the preparation contains 1:10,000 thimerosal

Dosage Forms Package containing one vial of 6000 antivenin units/vial, one 2.5 mL vial of sterile water for injection, and one 1 mL vial of 1:10 normal horse serum for sensitivity testing

Stability Excessive agitation or shaking of the reconstituted vial may cause foaming, which may lead to denaturation of the antivenin

Pregnancy Risk Factor C

Pregnancy Implications Use only if the potential benefits outweigh risks; it is not known if *L. mactans* antivenin antibodies cross the placenta

Monitoring Parameters Resolution of symptoms of *L. mactans* intoxication or emergence of symptoms of sensitivity to the antivenin

Nursing Implications Patient should be closely monitored for symptoms of hypersensitivity or anaphylaxis during skin or eye testing, desensitization, drug administration, and for 24 hours following administration

Specific References

Binder LS, "Acute Arthropod Envenomation: Incidence, Clinical Features, and Management," *Med Toxicol Adverse Drug Exp*, 1989, 4(3):163-73.

Clark RF, Wetherm-Kestner S, Vance MV, et al, "Clinical Presentation and Treatment of Black Widow Spider Envenomation: A Review of 163 Cases," *Ann Emerg Med*, 1992, 21(7):782-7.

Rauber A, "Black Widow Spider Bites," *J Toxicol Clin Toxicol*, 1984, 21:473-85.

Suntorntham S, Roberts JR, and Nilsen GJ, "Dramatic Clinical Response to the Delayed Administration of Black Widow Spider Antivenin," *Ann Emerg Med*, 1994, 24(6):1198-9.

Antivenin *(Micrurus fulvius)*

Use Envenomation by the eastern coral snake (*Micrurus fulvius fulvius*) or the Texas coral snake (*M. fulvius tenere*); antivenin therapy should be instituted as soon as the biting snake is identified as *M. fulvius fulvius* or *M. fulvius tenere*, because systemic symptoms may be impossible to reverse at a later time

Antidote Useful For

Elapids *on page 1080*

Mechanism of Action Refined, concentrated, and lyophilized preparation of serum globulins from horses immunized with eastern coral snake (*M. fulvius fulvius*) venom

Administration Similar scheme as per antivenin for Crotalidae; usually less amount of vials need to be administered; average dose: 4-6 vials; rarely more than 10 vials are necessary; can treat allergic reactions with antihistamines and corticosteroids

Contraindications History of anaphylaxis to equine-derived serums is a relative contraindication

Warnings When administering this agent, have ready access to drugs of resuscitation, including epinephrine and ventilatory support equipment. The absence of a skin hypersensitivity reaction does not exclude anaphylaxis or hypersensitivity following antivenin administration. False-negative rate for skin testing is 20%. Conversely, hypersensitivity is not an absolute contraindication in a significantly envenomated patient. The preparation contains 0.25% phenol and 0.005% thimerosal in antivenin and 1:100,000 phenylmercuric nitrate in bacteriostatic water for diluent.

Dosage Forms Package containing one vial antivenin and one vial bacteriostatic water for diluent

Stability Excessive agitation or shaking of the reconstituted vial may cause foaming, which may lead to denaturation of the antivenin

Pregnancy Risk Factor C

Pregnancy Implications Use only if the potential benefits outweigh risks; it is not known if *M. fulvius* antivenin antibodies cross out the placenta

Monitoring Parameters Resolution of symptoms of *M. fulvius* intoxication or emergence of symptoms of sensitivity to the antivenin; also monitor respiratory function and oxygenation, as well as the urine for hemoglobinuria

Nursing Implications Patient should be closely monitored for symptoms of hypersensitivity or anaphylaxis during skin or eye testing, desensitization, drug administration, and for 24 hours following administration

Additional Information Antivenin preparation will neutralize the venom of the eastern coral snake (*M. fulvius fulvius*) and the Texas coral snake (*M. fulvius tenere*), but not the venom of the Arizona or Sonoral coral snake (*M. euryxanthus*); each vial of antivenom neutralizes 2 mg of venom

Specific References

Gold BS and Wingert WA, "Snake Venom Poisoning in the United States: A Review of Therapeutic Practice," *S Med J*, 1994, 87:579-89.

Kitchens CS and Van Mierop LH, "Envenomation by the Eastern Coral Snake (*Micrurus fulvius fulvius*). A Study of 39 Victims," *JAMA*, 1987, 258(12):1615-8.

Kunkel DB, Curry SC, Vance MV, et al, "Reptile Envenomations," *J Toxicol Clin Toxicol*, 1984, 21:503-26.

AquaMEPHYTON® *see* Phytonadione *on page 1458*

ASL 279 *replaced by* Dopamine Hydrochloride *on page 1418*

AsthmaHaler® Mist [OTC] *see* Epinephrine *on page 1422*

AsthmaNefrin® [OTC] *see* Epinephrine *on page 1422*

Atropair® *see* Atropine Sulfate *on this page*

Atropine-Care® *see* Atropine Sulfate *on this page*

Atropine Sulfate (a' troe peen)

Related Information

Cycloplegic Mydriatics Comparison *on page 1648*

CAS Number 51-55-8; 55-48-1; 5908-99-6

Brand Names Atropair®; Atropine-Care®; Atropisol®; Atropt®; Eumydrin®; Eyesule®; Isopto® Atropine; I-Tropine®; Ocu-Tropine®; Steropine®

Use Preoperative medication to inhibit salivation and secretions; treatment of sinus bradycardia; management of peptic ulcer; treat exercise-induced bronchospasm; antidote for organophosphate pesticide poisoning, anticholinesterase, cholinergic medication poisoning, and muscarinic symptoms of mushroom poisoning (*Clitocybe*, *Inocybe*); used to produce mydriasis and cycloplegia for examination of the retina and optic disk and accurate measurement of refractive errors; uveitis; also useful in antihistamine and methyldopa cardiac toxicities

Antidote Useful For

Aldicarb *on page 855*
Azalea *on page 1055*
Baclofen *on page 143*
Bethanechol Chloride *on page 154*
Bisoprolol Fumarate *on page 157*
Bromophos *on page 873*
Carbaryl *on page 877*
Chlorfenvinphos *on page 886*
Chloroform *on page 890*
Chlorpyrifos *on page 891*
Diazinon *on page 904*
Dicrotophos *on page 909*
Dioxathion *on page 916*
Disulfoton *on page 919*
Edrophonium Chloride *on page 309*
Fensulfothion *on page 928*
Fenthion *on page 929*
Malathion *on page 950*
Malathion (Topical Lotion) *on page 489*
Methidathion *on page 959*
Methiocarb *on page 961*
Methomyl *on page 962*
Mushrooms, Toxic (Group III) *on page 1112*
Nerve Gases *on page 974*
Nicotine *on page 556*
Parathion *on page 988*
Profenofos *on page 998*
Propoxur *on page 1000*
Rhododendron *on page 1133*
Tacrine Hydrochloride *on page 719*
Terbufos *on page 1020*
Tetraethyl Pyrophosphate *on page 1024*

(Continued)

Atropine Sulfate *(Continued)*

Mechanism of Action Blocks the action of acetylcholine at parasympathetic sites in smooth muscle, secretory glands, and the central muscarinic receptors; increases cardiac output, dries secretions, antagonizes histamine and serotonin

Adverse Reactions

Cardiovascular: Tachycardia, palpitations, impotence, hypertension, hypotension (orthostatic)

Central nervous system: Fatigue, delirium, seizures, ataxia; lilliputian hallucinations, dizziness, disorientation, hypothermia or hyperthermia, headache, ataxia, restlessness

Dermatologic: Dry skin, eczema

Gastrointestinal: Impaired GI motility, thirst, dry mouth

Neuromuscular & skeletal: Tremors

Ocular: Blurred vision, photophobia, intraocular pressure (increased), blindness, mydriasis with cycloplegia

Otic: Ototoxicity

Renal: Urinary retention

Respiratory: Tachypnea

Signs & Symptoms of Acute Overdose Dilated, unreactive pupils; blurred vision; flushing; dryness of mucous membranes; ileus; difficulty in swallowing, foul breath, diminished or absent bowel sounds, urinary retention, tachycardia, hyperthermia, hypertension, respiratory rate (increased), hallucinations (lilliputian), seizures/seizures, ataxia, coma, flushing, tinnitus, ototoxicity (deafness)

Toxicodynamics/Kinetics

Onset of action: I.V.: Effects on heart rate peak within 2-4 minutes

Duration:

Oral: 4-6 hours

Parenteral: Brief

Absorption: Well absorbed from all dosage forms

Distribution: V_d: 2.3 L/kg; widely distributed; crosses the blood-brain barrier

Protein binding: Moderate 18%

Metabolism: Liver to tropic acid, atropine

Half-life: 2-3 hours (10 hours in elderly)

Time to peak serum concentration: I.M.: 30-45 minutes

Elimination: Into urine of both metabolites and unchanged drug (30% to 50%); clearance: 660 mL/minute

Usual Dosage

Children:

Preanesthetic: I.M., I.V., S.C.:

<5 kg: 0.02 mg/kg/dose 30-60 minutes preop then every 4-6 hours as needed

>5 kg: 0.01-0.02 mg/kg/dose to a maximum 0.4 mg 30-60 minutes preop; minimum dose: 0.1 mg

Bradycardia: I.V., intratracheal: 0.02 mg/kg every 5 minutes

Minimum dose: 0.1 mg (if administered via endotracheal tube, dilute to 1-2 mL with normal saline prior to endotracheal administration)

Maximum single dose: 0.5 mg (adolescents: 1 mg)

Total maximum dose: 1 mg (adolescents: 2 mg)

When using to treat bradycardia in neonates, reserve use for those patients unresponsive to improved oxygenation

Organophosphate or carbamate poisoning: I.V.: 0.02-0.05 mg/kg every 10-20 minutes until atropine effect (dry flushed skin, tachycardia, mydriasis, fever) is observed then every 1-4 hours for at least 24 hours

Bronchospasm: Inhalation: 0.03-0.05 mg/kg/dose 3-4 times/day; maximum: 1 mg

Ophthalmic, 0.5% solution: Instill 1-2 drops twice daily for 1-3 days before the procedure

Adults (doses <0.5 mg have been associated with paradoxical bradycardia):

Asystole: I.V.: 1 mg; may repeat every 3-5 minutes as needed; may give intratracheal in 1 mg/10 mL dilution only, intratracheal dose should be 2-2.5 times the I.V. dose

Preanesthetic: I.M., I.V., S.C.: 0.4-0.6 mg 30-60 minutes preop and repeat every 4-6 hours as needed

Bradycardia: I.V.: 0.5-1 mg every 5 minutes, not to exceed a total of 3 mg or 0.04 mg/kg; may give intratracheal in 1 mg/10 mL dilution only, intratracheal dose should be 2-2.5 times the I.V. dose

Neuromuscular blockade reversal: I.V.: 25-30 mcg/kg 30 seconds before neostigmine or 10 mcg/kg 30 seconds before edrophonium

Organophosphate or carbamate poisoning: I.V.: 1-2 mg/dose every 10-20 minutes until atropine effect (dry flushed skin, tachycardia, mydriasis, fever) is observed, then every 1-4 hours for at least 24 hours; up to 50 mg in first 24 hours and 2 g over several days may be given in cases of severe intoxication; over 30 g has been given to manage this toxicity

Bronchospasm: Inhalation: 0.025-0.05 mg/kg/dose every 4-6 hours as needed (maximum: 5 mg/dose)

Ophthalmic solution: 1%: Instill 1-2 drops 1 hour before the procedure

Uveitis: 1-2 drops 4 times/day

Ophthalmic ointment: Apply a small amount in the conjunctival sac up to three times daily; compress the lacrimal sac by digital pressure for 1-3 minutes after instillation

Administration Administer undiluted by rapid I.V. injection; slow injection may result in paradoxical bradycardia

Contraindications Hypersensitivity to atropine sulfate or any component; narrow-angle glaucoma; tachycardia; thyrotoxicosis; obstructive disease of the GI tract; obstructive uropathy

Warnings Use with caution in children with spastic paralysis; use with caution in elderly patients. Low doses cause a paradoxical decrease in heart rates. Some commercial products contain sodium metabisulfite, which can cause allergic-type reactions; use with caution in patients with autonomic neuropathy, prostatic hypertrophy, hyperthyroidism, congestive heart failure, cardiac arrhythmias, chronic lung disease, biliary tract disease; with massive dosing in treatment of severe pesticide poisoning, hemolysis from free water dilution can occur.

Dosage Forms

Injection: 0.05 mg/mL (5 mL); 0.1 mg/mL (5 mL, 10 mL); 0.3 mg/mL (1 mL, 30 mL); 0.4 mg/mL (1 mL, 20 mL, 30 mL); 0.5 mg/mL (1 mL, 5 mL, 30 mL); 0.8 mg/mL (0.5 mL, 1 mL); 1 mg/mL (1 mL, 10 mL)

Ointment, ophthalmic: 0.5% (3.5 g); 1% (3.5 g)

Solution, ophthalmic: 0.5% (1 mL, 5 mL); 1% (1 mL, 2 mL, 5 mL, 15 mL); 2% (1 mL, 2 mL); 3% (5 mL)

Tablet: 0.4 mg

Tablet, soluble: 0.4 mg, 0.6 mg

Stability Store injection below 40°C, avoid freezing

Reference Range Peak serum atropine level after a 1 mg I.V. dose: ~0.003 mg/L (within 30 minutes of administration); blood level (postmortem) of 0.2 mg/L and urine level of 1.5 mg/L associated with fatality

Drug Interactions Phenothiazines, amantadine, antiparkinsonian drugs, glutethimide, meperidine, tricyclic antidepressants, antiarrhythmic agents, some antihistamines; all have anticholinergic activity; not compatible with alkali solutions

Pregnancy Risk Factor C

Pregnancy Implications Crosses the placenta; trace amounts appear in breast milk

Monitoring Parameters Heart rate (EKG), respiratory status

Nursing Implications Give by rapid I.V. injection since slow infusion may cause a paradoxical bradycardia; may give intratracheal in 1 mg/10 mL dilution only

Additional Information Response to atropine may not be observed until after I.V. calcium administration. In New York City, emergency medical ambulances stock up to 52 mg of atropine (an increase from 4 mg prior to the Tokyo nerve gas attack in March, 1995)

Specific References

Afzaal S, Shakoor A, Rabbani MU, et al, "High Dose Atropine in Organophosphorus Poisoning," *Postgrad Med J*, 1990, 66(771):70-1.

Amitai Y, Singer R, Almog S, et al, "Atropine Poisoning in Children During the Persian Gulf Crisis," *JAMA*, 1992, 268(5):642-4.

Berman JM and Bertoldi IM, "Preparation of Atropine Sulfate Ampuls for High-Dose Therapy," *Am J Hosp Pharm*, 1985, 42(5):1046.

Howarth DM, Dawson AH, Smith AJ, et al, "Calcium Channel Blocking Drug Overdose: An Australian Series," *Hum Exp Toxicol*, 1994, 13(3):161-6.

Meerstadt PW, "Atropine Poisoning in Early Infancy Due to Eumydrin Drops," *Br Med J [Clin Res]*, 1982, 285(6336):196-7.

Michelson EA, Schneider SM, and Martin TG, "Adult Inadvertent Massive Oral Atropine Overdose," *Vet Hum Toxicol*, 1991, 33:360.

Shockley LW, "The Use of Inhaled Nebulized Atropine for the Treatment of Malathion Poisoning," *J Toxicol Clin Toxicol*, 1989, 27(3):183-92.

Atropisol® *see* Atropine Sulfate *on page 1395*

Atropt® *see* Atropine Sulfate *on page 1395*

BA-33112 *see* Deferoxamine Mesylate *on page 1407*

Baking Soda *see* Sodium Bicarbonate *on page 1467*

BAL *see* Dimercaprol *on page 1414*

BAL in Oil® *see* Dimercaprol *on page 1414*

Banophen® Oral [OTC] *see* Diphenhydramine Hydrochloride *on page 1415*

Baritop® *see* Sodium Bicarbonate *on page 1467*

Beesix® *see* Pyridoxine Hydrochloride *on page 1465*

Belix® Oral [OTC] *see* Diphenhydramine Hydrochloride *on page 1415*

Bena-D® Injection *see* Diphenhydramine Hydrochloride *on page 1415*

Benadryl® *see* Diphenhydramine Hydrochloride *on page 1415*

Benahist® Injection *see* Diphenhydramine Hydrochloride *on page 1415*

Benoject® Injection *see* Diphenhydramine Hydrochloride *on page 1415*

Benylin® Cough Syrup [OTC] *see* Diphenhydramine Hydrochloride *on page 1415*

Bilkaby, K® *see* Phytonadione *on page 1458*

Bonusunit® *see* Pyridoxine Hydrochloride *on page 1465*

British Anti-Lewisite *see* Dimercaprol *on page 1414*

Bromocriptine Mesylate (broe moe krip' teen mess' a late)

CAS Number 25614-03-3; 22260-51-1

Brand Names Lactismine®; Parlodel®; Pravidel®; Serocryptin®

Use Approved for the treatment of idiopathic or postencephalitic parkinsonism; has also been used to decrease drug craving following discontinuation of cocaine abuse, to decrease symptoms of neuroleptic malignant syndrome, and to block postpartum lactation or hyperprolactinemia

Mechanism of Action Semisynthetic ergot alkaloid derivative with direct dopaminergic agonist activity at striatal receptors

Adverse Reactions

Cardiovascular: Hypertension then hypotension, syncope

Central nervous system: Headache, dizziness, insomnia, auditory and visual hallucinations, seizures, extrapyramidal symptoms, chorea (extrapyramidal), dyskinesias

Dermatologic: Alopecia

Endocrine & metabolic: Hyponatremia, impotence

Gastrointestinal: Nausea, vomiting, abdominal cramps, anorexia

Hematologic: Leukopenia, coagulopathy, thrombocytopenia

Ocular: Myopia

Respiratory: Pleuropulmonary fibrosis

Miscellaneous: Clitoral hypertrophy

Toxicodynamics/Kinetics

Absorption: Oral: Complete and rapid

Distribution: V_d: 13 L/kg; rapid tissue distribution

Protein binding: 90% to 96%

Metabolism: Hepatic

Half-life:

Initial: 6-8 hours

Terminal: 50 hours

Time to peak serum concentration: Oral: Within 1-2 hours

Elimination: In bile with only 2% to 6% unchanged in urine; clearance: 4.4 L/hour/kg

Usual Dosage Oral: 1.25-2.5 mg/day increasing in 2.5 mg/day increments every 14 days

Neuroleptic malignant syndrome: Initial: 5 mg 3 times/day, then increase to 10 mg 3 times/day

Contraindications Known hypersensitivity to bromocriptine, severe ischemic heart disease or peripheral vascular disease; women of childbearing age should use mechanical contraceptive means

Warnings Use with caution in patients with impaired renal or hepatic function

Dosage Forms

Capsule: 5 mg

Tablet: 2.5 mg

Reference Range Peak plasma level of 24.6 ng/mL achieved after a dose of 100 mg

Test Interactions Bromocriptine may increase blood urea nitrogen, serum AST, serum ALT, serum CPK, alkaline phosphatase, and serum uric acid

Drug Interactions Ergot alkaloids increase cardiovascular and peripheral vascular side effects

Pregnancy Risk Factor C

Pregnancy Implications Use only if the potential benefits outweigh the risks

Nursing Implications Patient should be monitored for signs of postural hypotension, sedation, and hallucinations

Additional Information Adverse reactions, especially GI distress, are common during the first few days of treatment or after dosage increases

Specific References

Dackis CA and Gold MS, "Bromocriptine as Treatment of Cocaine Abuse," *Lancet*, 1985, 1(8438):1151-2.

LeJoyeux M, et al, "Serotonin Syndrome: Incidence, Symptoms, and Treatment," *CNS Drugs*, 1994, 2:132-43.

Melmed S and Braunstein GD, "Bromocriptine and Pleuropulmonary Disease," *Arch Intern Med*, 1989, 149(2):258-9.

Mueller PS, Vester JW, and Fermaglich J, "Neuroleptic Malignant Syndrome. Successful Treatment With Bromocriptine," *JAMA*, 1983, 249(3):386-8.

Parkes D, "Drug Therapy: Bromocriptine," *N Engl J Med*, 1979, 301(16):873-8.

Bromuc® *see* Acetylcysteine *on page 1388*

Bronitin® Mist [OTC] *see* Epinephrine *on page 1422*

Bronkaid® Mist [OTC] *see* Epinephrine *on page 1422*

Brown Acetate *see* Calcium Acetate *on this page*

Brunac® *see* Acetylcysteine *on page 1388*

Butyrylcholinesterase

Use Treatment of postsurgical apnea; also experimental use for reduction and clearance of cocaine in an overdose situation

Antidote Useful For

Cocaine Hydrochloride *on page 236*

Mechanism of Action Cleavage of the ester linkage of cocaine

Toxicodynamics/Kinetics

Distribution: V_d: 0.085 L/kg

Half-life: 7.8 hours

Dosage Forms Injection: 5 mg/mL, 10 mg/mL

Additional Information May reduce cocaine-induced seizure frequency or adverse effects of cocaine on cardiovascular system; experimental

Specific References

Hoffman RS, Marasco R, and Goldfrank LR, "Human Plasma Cholinesterase Protects Against Cocaine Toxicity in Mice," *Vet Hum Toxicol*, 1993, 35:349.

Bydramine® Cough Syrup [OTC] *see* Diphenhydramine Hydrochloride *on page 1415*

Calcium Acetate (kal' see um as' e tate)

CAS Number 62-54-4

Brand Names Phos-Ex®; PhosLo®

Synonyms Brown Acetate; Lime Acetate

Use Control of hyperphosphatemia in end stage renal failure and does not promote aluminum absorption; used in dialysis solutions and as a food preservative; also in drying, tanning of skins, corrosive inhibitor, and in manufacture of acetone and acetic acid

Mechanism of Action Moderates nerve and muscle performance via action potential excitation threshold regulation

Adverse Reactions

Central nervous system: Headache, fatigue

Endocrine & metabolic: Hypophosphatemia, hypercalcemia

Gastrointestinal: Anorexia, vomiting, abdominal pain, thirst, constipation

Signs & Symptoms of Acute Overdose Hypercalcemia, lethargy, nausea, vomiting, thrombocytopenia, coma, bradycardia, hypotension, decreased reflexes, renal insufficiency, coagulopathy

Toxicodynamics/Kinetics

Absorption: I.M. and I.V. calcium salts are absorbed directly into the bloodstream, absorption from the GI tract requires vitamin D

Protein binding: 40% to 45%

Elimination: Mainly in feces as unabsorbed calcium with 20% eliminated by the kidneys

Usual Dosage Adults: Oral: 2 tablets with each meal; dosage may be increased to bring serum phosphate value to <6 mg/dL; most patients require 3-4 tablets with each meal

Contraindications Hypercalcemia

Warnings No other calcium supplements should be given concurrently; progressive hypercalcemia due to overdose may be severe as to require emergency measures; chronic hypercalcemia may lead to vascular calcification and other soft tissue calcification. The serum calcium level should be monitored twice weekly during the early dose adjustment period. The serum calcium times phosphate product should not be allowed to exceed 66.

(Continued)

Calcium Acetate *(Continued)*

Dosage Forms Elemental calcium listed in brackets
Capsule: 500 mg [125 mg]
Tablet: 250 mg [62.5 mg], 667 mg [169 mg], 1000 mg [250 mg]

Reference Range Normal serum levels: 9-10.4 mg/dL (2.2-2.6 mmol/L); toxicity noted at levels >12 mg/dL

Test Interactions Elevates prothrombin in overdose

Drug Interactions May decrease the bioavailability of tetracyclines; administer cautiously to a digitalized patient, may precipitate arrhythmias; calcium may antagonize the effects of verapamil; renders tetracycline antibiotics inactive

Pregnancy Risk Factor C

Pregnancy Implications Crosses the placenta; appears in breast milk

Monitoring Parameters Serum calcium levels, renal function, EKG

Additional Information Calcium acetate binds phosphorus in the GI tract better than other calcium salts due to its lower solubility and subsequent reduction in calcium or phosphorus absorption. 3.95 g of calcium acetate is equivalent to 1 g of calcium.

Specific References

Kaiser W, Biesenbach G, Kramar R, et al, "Calcium Free Hemodialysis: An Effective Therapy in Hypercalcemic Crisis – Report of Four Cases," *Intensive Care Med*, 1989, 15(7):471-4.
Texier D, Chevallier P, Perrotin D, et al, "Hypercalcemia Associated With Resorbable Haemostatic Compresses," *Lancet*, 1982, 1(8273):688-9.

Calcium Chel 330 (Ca-DTPA) *see* Diethylene Triamine Penta-acetic Acid *on page 1411*

Calcium Chloride (kal' see um klor' ide)

CAS Number 10035-04-8; 10043-52-4; 7774-34-7

Use Cardiac resuscitation when epinephrine fails to improve myocardial contractions, cardiac disturbances of hyperkalemia, hypocalcemia or calcium channel blocking agent toxicity; also used for fluoride, hydrogen fluoride, ethylene glycol, magnesium sulfate, oxalate, and black widow spider bites

Antidote Useful For
Black Widow Spider *on page 1058*
Ethylene Glycol *on page 925*
Fluoride *on page 355*
Hydrogen Fluoride *on page 941*
Nifedipine *on page 558*
Nimodipine *on page 560*
Verapamil Hydrochloride *on page 787*

Mechanism of Action Moderates nerve and muscle performance via action potential excitation threshold regulation

Adverse Reactions
Cardiovascular: Vasodilation, hypotension, bradycardia, cardiac arrhythmias, ventricular fibrillation, syncope
Central nervous system: Lethargy, coma
Dermatologic: Erythema
Endocrine & metabolic: Elevated serum amylase, hypomagnesemia, hypercalcemia
Local: Tissue necrosis (more irritant than calcium gluconate)
Neuromuscular & skeletal: Muscle weakness
Renal: Hypercalciuria

Signs & Symptoms of Acute Overdose Lethargy, nausea, vomiting, coma

Toxicodynamics/Kinetics
Absorption: I.V. calcium salts are absorbed directly into the bloodstream
Elimination: Mainly in feces as unabsorbed calcium with 20% eliminated by the kidneys

Usual Dosage I.V. (calcium chloride is 3 times as potent as calcium gluconate):
Cardiac arrest in the presence of hyperkalemia or hypocalcemia, magnesium toxicity, or calcium antagonist toxicity:
Infants and Children: 10-20 mg/kg; may repeat in 10 minutes if necessary
Adults: 2.5-5 mL/dose every 10 minutes

Hypocalcemia:
Infants and Children: 10-20 mg/kg/dose, repeat every 4-6 hours if needed
Adults: 500 mg to 1 g at 1- to 3-day intervals

Tetany:
Neonates: 2.4 mEq/kg/day
Infants and Children: 10 mg/kg over 5-10 minutes; may repeat after 6 hours or follow with an infusion with a maximum dose of 200 mg/kg/day
Adults: 1 g over 10-30 minutes; may repeat after 6 hours

Hypocalcemia secondary to citrated blood transfusion give 0.45 mEq **elemental** calcium for each 100 mL citrated blood infused

Administration Generally, I.V. infusion rates should not exceed 0.7-1.5 mEq/minute (0.5-1 mL/minute); stop the infusion if the patient complains of pain or discomfort; do not inject calcium chloride I.M. or administer S.C. since severe necrosis and sloughing may occur. Do not use scalp vein or small hand or foot veins for I.V. administration. Warm to body temperature; administer slowly, do not exceed 1 mL/minute (inject into ventricular cavity – not myocardium).

Contraindications Ventricular fibrillation during cardiac resuscitation, and in patients with risk of digitalis toxicity, renal or cardiac disease

Warnings Avoid too rapid I.V. administration; avoid extravasation; use with caution in digitalized patients, respiratory failure or acidosis; acidifying effect; give only 2-3 days then change to another calcium salt

Dosage Forms Injection: 10% [100 mg/mL] (10 mL)

Stability Admixture incompatibilities: Carbonates, phosphates, sulfates, tartrates

Reference Range Serum 9-10.4 mg/dL; due to a poor correlation between the serum ionized calcium (free) and total serum calcium, particularly in states of low albumin or acid/base imbalances, direct measurement of ionized calcium is recommended. In low albumin states, the corrected **total** serum calcium may be estimated by this equation (assuming a normal albumin of 4 g/dL); corrected total calcium = total serum calcium + 0.8 (4- measured serum albumin).

Test Interactions ↑ calcium (S); ↓ magnesium

Drug Interactions Administer cautiously to a digitalized patient, may precipitate arrhythmias; calcium may antagonize the effects of verapamil; renders tetracycline antibiotics inactive

Pregnancy Risk Factor C

Pregnancy Implications Crosses the placenta; appears in breast milk

Monitoring Parameters EKG

Nursing Implications Monitor EKG if calcium is infused faster than 2.5 mEq/minute (occasionally necessary in treating hyperkalemia)

Extravasation: Give hyaluronidase (1:10 dilution of a 150 unit vial in saline equivalent to 15 units/mL) S.C. in multiple (usually about 5) injections of 0.2 mL each to help increase absorption

Additional Information 14 mEq/g/10 mL; 270 mg elemental calcium/g (27% elemental calcium)

Specific References

Bilezikian JP, "Management of Acute Hypercalcemia," *N Engl J Med*, 1992, 326(18):1196-215.

Binder LS, "Acute Arthropod Envenomation: Incidence, Clinical Features, and Management," *Med Toxicol Adverse Drug Exp*, 1989, 4(3):163-73.

Chin RL, Garmel GM, and Harter PM, "Development of Ventricular Fibrillation After Intravenous Calcium Chloride Administration in a Patient With Supraventricular Tachycardia," *Ann Emerg Med*, 1995, 25:416-9.

McIvor ME, "Acute Fluoride Toxicity. Pathophysiology and Management," *Drug Saf*, 1990, 5(2):79-84.

Pearigen PD and Benowitz NL, "Poisoning Due to Calcium Antagonists. Experience With Verapamil, Diltiazem, and Nifedipine," *Drug Saf*, 1991, 6(6):408-30.

Worthley LI and Phillips PJ, "Intravenous Calcium Salts," *Lancet*, 1980, 2(8186):149.

Calcium Disodium Versenate® *see* Edetate Calcium Disodium *on page 1419*

Calcium Edetate-Heyl® *see* Edetate Calcium Disodium *on page 1419*

Calcium EDTA *see* Edetate Calcium Disodium *on page 1419*

Calcium Gluconate (gloo' koe nate)

CAS Number 299-28-5; 18016-24-5

Brand Names Kalcinate®

Use Treatment and prevention of hypocalcemia, treatment of tetany, cardiac disturbances of hyperkalemia, cardiac resuscitation when epinephrine fails to improve myocardial contractions, hypocalcemia, or calcium channel blocker toxicity

Antidote Useful For

Bepridil Hydrochloride *on page 152*
Black Widow Spider *on page 1058*
Diltiazem *on page 287*
Fluoride *on page 355*
Hydrogen Fluoride *on page 941*
Nifedipine *on page 558*
Nimodipine *on page 560*
Phosphine *on page 993*
Verapamil Hydrochloride *on page 787*

Mechanism of Action Moderates nerve and muscle performance via action potential excitation threshold regulation

Adverse Reactions

Cardiovascular: Vasodilation, hypotension, bradycardia, cardiac arrhythmias, ventricular fibrillation, syncope

(Continued)

Calcium Gluconate *(Continued)*

Central nervous system: Lethargy, coma, mental confusion
Dermatologic: Erythema
Endocrine & metabolic: Elevated serum amylase, hypomagnesemia, hypercalcemia
Local: Tissue necrosis
Neuromuscular & skeletal: Muscle weakness
Renal: Hypercalciuria

Signs & Symptoms of Acute Overdose Lethargy, nausea, vomiting, coma

Toxicodynamics/Kinetics

Absorption: I.M. and I.V. calcium salts are absorbed directly into the bloodstream; absorption from the GI tract requires vitamin D

Elimination: Mainly in feces as unabsorbed calcium with 20% eliminated by the kidneys

Usual Dosage Dosage is in terms of elemental calcium

Recommended daily allowance (RDA):
- Children:
  - <6 months: 360 mg/day
  - 6-12 months: 540 mg/day
  - 1-10 years: 800 mg/day
  - 10-18 years: 1200 mg/day
- Adults: 800 mg/day

Calcium gluconate electrolyte requirement in newborn period:
- Premature: 200-1000 mg/kg/24 hours
- Term:
  - 0-24 hours: 0-500 mg/kg/24 hours
  - 24-48 hours: 200-500 mg/kg/24 hours
  - 48-72 hours: 200-600 mg/kg/24 hours
  - >3 days: 200-800 mg/kg/24 hours

Hypocalcemia:
- Oral:
  - Children: 200-500 mg/kg/day divided every 6 hours
  - Adults: 500 mg to 2 g 2-4 times/day
- I.V.:
  - Neonates: 200-400 mg/kg/day as a continuous infusion or in 4 divided doses
  - Infants and Children: 200-1000 mg/kg/day as a continuous infusion or in 4 divided doses
  - Adults: 2-15 g/24 hours as a continuous infusion or in divided doses

Calcium antagonist toxicity, magnesium intoxication; cardiac arrest in the presence of hyperkalemia or hypocalcemia: I.V.:
- Infants and Children: 100 mg/kg/dose
- Adults: 1-3 g

Tetany: I.V.:
- Neonates: 100-200 mg/kg/dose, may follow with 500 mg/kg/day in 3-4 divided doses or as an infusion
- Infants and Children: 100-200 mg/kg/dose over 5-10 minutes; may repeat after 6 hours or follow with an infusion of 500 mg/kg/day
- Adults: 1-3 g may be administered until therapeutic response occurs

Cardiac resuscitation: I.V.:
- Infants and Children: 100 mg/kg/dose (1 mL/kg/dose) every 10 minutes
- Adults: 500-800 mg/dose (5-8 mL) every 10 minutes

Hypocalcemia secondary to citrated blood infusion; give 0.45 mEq **elemental** calcium for each 100 mL citrated blood infused

Exchange transfusion:
- Neonates: 100 mg/100 mL of citrated blood exchanged
- Adults: 300 mg/100 mL of citrated blood exchanged

Maintenance electrolyte requirements for total parenteral nutrition: I.V.: Daily requirements: Adults: 10-20 mEq/1000 kcals/24 hours

Administration I.M. injections should be administered in the gluteal region in adults, usually in volumes <5 mL; avoid I.M. injections in children and adults with muscle mass wasting; do not use scalp veins or small hand or foot veins for I.V. administration; generally, I.V. infusion rates should not exceed 0.7-1.5 mEq/minute (1.5-3.3 mL/minute); stop the infusion if the patient complains of pain or discomfort. Warm to body temperature; administer slowly, usually no faster than 1.5-3.3 mL/minute, do not inject into the myocardium when using calcium during advanced cardiac life support.

Contraindications Ventricular fibrillation during cardiac resuscitation and in patients with risk of digitalis toxicity, renal or cardiac disease

Warnings Avoid too rapid I.V. administration; use with caution in digitalized patients, respiratory failure or acidosis; avoid extravasation; may produce cardiac arrest. The serum calcium level should be monitored twice weekly during the early dose adjustment period. The serum calcium times phosphate product should not be allowed to exceed 66.

Dosage Forms
Injection: 10% [100 mg/mL] (10 mL, 50 mL, 100 mL, 200 mL)
Tablet: 500 mg, 650 mg, 975 mg, 1 g

Stability Admixture incompatibilities: Carbonates, phosphates, sulfates, tartrates; store at room temperature; do not use if precipitate occurs

Reference Range Serum: 9-10.4 mg/dL; due to a poor correlation between the serum ionized calcium (free) and total serum calcium, particularly in states of low albumin or acid/base imbalances, direct measurement of ionized calcium is recommended. If ionized calcium is unavailable, in low albumin states, the corrected **total** serum calcium may be estimated by this equation (assuming a normal albumin of 4 g/dL); corrected total calcium = total serum calcium + 0.8 (4- measured serum albumin).

Test Interactions ↑ calcium (S); ↓ magnesium

Drug Interactions Administer cautiously to a digitalized patient, may precipitate arrhythmias; calcium may antagonize the effects of verapamil; renders tetracycline antibiotics inactive

Pregnancy Risk Factor C

Pregnancy Implications Crosses the placenta; appears in breast milk

Monitoring Parameters Serum calcium

Nursing Implications Do not administer I.M. or S.C.
Extravasation: Give hyaluronidase (1:10 dilution of a 150 unit vial in saline equivalent to 15 units/mL) S.C. in multiple (usually about 5) injections of 0.2 mL each to help increase absorption

Additional Information 4.65 mEq/g; 93 mg elemental calcium/g (9.3% elemental calcium)

Specific References

Bilezikian JP, "Management of Acute Hypercalcemia," *N Engl J Med*, 1992, 326(18):1196-215.
Binder LS, "Acute Arthropod Envenomation: Incidence, Clinical Features, and Management," *Med Toxicol Adverse Drug Exp*, 1989, 4(3):163-73.
McIvor ME, "Acute Fluoride Toxicity. Pathophysiology and Management," *Drug Saf*, 1990, 5(2):79-84.
Pearigen PD and Benowitz NL, "Poisoning Due to Calcium Antagonists: Experience With Verapamil, Diltiazem, and Nifedipine," *Drug Saf*, 1991, 6(6):408-30.
Worthley LI and Phillips PJ, "Intravenous Calcium Salts," *Lancet*, 1980, 2(8186):149.

Calcium Leucovorin *see* Leucovorin Calcium *on page 1437*

Carbex® *see* Sodium Bicarbonate *on page 1467*

Centruroides Scorpion Venom Antisera

Use Severe *Centruroides* scorpion envenomation (grade IV)

Antidote Useful For
Arizona Bark Scorpion *on page 1053*

Mechanism of Action Made by lyophilizing micron-filtered hypersensitized goat serum

Adverse Reactions Delayed allergic reactions (58%) include rash, urticaria, serum sickness

Usual Dosage One vial I.V.; give second vial I.V. in 1 hour if symptoms not improved; do not administer I.M.

Additional Information May be obtained from the Arizona Poison Control Center (602-253-3334 or 602-253-0813) or Good Samaritan Poison Control Center in Phoenix, Arizona (602-626-6016). Full resolution of neurologic respiratory and cardiovascular symptoms can occur rapidly; not subjected to FDA testing or approval at present time.

Specific References

Binder LS, "Acute Arthropod Envenomation: Incidence, Clinical Features, and Management," *Med Toxicol Adverse Drug Exp*, 1989, 4(3):163-73.
Bond GR, "Antivenin Administration for *Centruroides* Scorpion Sting: Risks and Benefits," *Ann Emerg Med*, 1992, 21(7):788-91.

Charcoaid® [OTC] *see* Charcoal *on this page*

Charcoal (char' kole)

CAS Number 16291-96-6

Brand Names Actidose-Aqua® [OTC]; Actidose® With Sorbitol [OTC]; Charcoaid® [OTC]; Charcocaps® [OTC]; Insta-Char® [OTC]; Liqui-Char® [OTC]; SuperChar® [OTC]

Use Emergency treatment in poisoning by drugs and chemicals; repetitive doses for gastrointestinal dialysis for drug overdose and in uremia to adsorb various waste products; also used for hyperbilirubinemia

Antidote Useful For

Anticoagulant Rodenticide *on page 859*

Manganese *on page 952*

Strychnine *on page 1016*

Mechanism of Action Adsorbs toxic substances or irritants, thus inhibiting GI absorption and for selected drugs increasing clearance by interfering with enterohepatic recycling or dialysis across intestinal vascular membranes; adsorbs intestinal gas; the addition of sorbitol results in hyperosmotic laxative action causing catharsis

Adverse Reactions

Gastrointestinal: Emesis, diarrhea with sorbitol, constipation, intestinal obstruction can occur

Miscellaneous: Stools will turn black; aspiration usually does not cause major problems in adults, but can cause tracheal obstruction in infants

Toxicodynamics/Kinetics

Absorption: Not absorbed from GI tract

Metabolism: Not metabolized

Elimination: As charcoal in feces

Usual Dosage Oral: Ideally achieving a 10 g charcoal:1 g toxin dose is desired outcome

Acute poisoning: Single dose: Charcoal with sorbitol (**Note:** Check product label for sorbitol content):

Children and Adults: At least 5-10 times the weight of the ingested poison on a g:g ratio; minimum dose is probably 15-30 g; in young children sorbitol dose should not exceed 1.5 g/kg/day

Adults: 30-100 g

Charcoal in water: Same as above, but sorbitol should be added in appropriate daily doses

Single dose:

Infants and Children 1-12 years: 15-30 g

Adults: 30-100 g

Multiple dose (use only one dose of cathartic daily):

Infants <1 year: 15-30 g every 4-6 hours

Children 1-12 years: 20-60 g every 2-6 hours until clinical observations and serum drug concentration have returned to a subtherapeutic range or the development of absent bowel sounds or ileus

Adults: 20-60 g every 2-6 hours

Contraindications Not effective for cyanide, mineral acids, caustic alkalis, organic solvents, iron, ethanol, methanol poisoning, lithium; do not use charcoal with sorbitol in patients with fructose intolerance; charcoal with sorbitol is not recommended in children <1 year of age

Warnings If charcoal in sorbitol is administered, doses should be limited to prevent excessive fluid and electrolyte losses

Dosage Forms

Capsule (Charcocaps®): 260 mg

Liquid, activated:

Actidose-Aqua®: 12.5 g (60 mL); 25 g (120 mL)

Liqui-Char®: 12.5 g (60 mL); 15 g (75 mL); 25 g (120 mL); 30 g (120 mL); 50 g (240 mL)

SuperChar®: 30 g (240 mL)

Liquid, activated, with propylene glycol: 12.5 g (60 mL); 25 g (120 mL)

Liquid, activated, with sorbitol:

Actidose® With Sorbitol: 25 g (120 mL); 50 g (240 mL)

Charcoaid®: 30 g (150 mL)

SuperChar®: 30 g (240 mL)

Powder for suspension, activated:

15 g, 30 g, 40 g, 120 g, 240 g

SuperChar®: 30 g

Stability Adsorbs gases from air, store in closed container

Pregnancy Risk Factor C

Nursing Implications Instruct patient to drink slowly, rapid administration appears to increase frequency of vomiting; for persistent vomiting, activated charcoal can be administered as a continuous enteral infusion at doses of 10-25 g/hour; fluid volume and sorbitol dosing must be reviewed carefully; too concentrated of slurries may clog airway; stools will turn black; vigorous shaking of product is suggested

Additional Information 75-90 mL is approximately equal to 30 g of activated charcoal; charcoal in water with extemporaneous addition of cathartic is preferred; variation exists in adsorptive surface area between commercial products, importance is not known at this time

Specific References

Cooney DO, "Evaluation of the U.S. Pharmacopeia Adsorption tests for Activated Charcoal and Proposals for Changes," *Vet Hum Toxicol*, 1995, 37(4):371-7.

Cooney DO, "*In vitro* Adsorption of Phenobarbital, Chlorpheniramine Maleate, and Theophylline by Four Commercially Available Activated Charcoal Suspensions," *Clin Toxicol*, 1995, 33(3):213-7.

MacFarland AF and Chyka PA, "Selection of Activated Charcoal Products for the Treatment of Poisonings," *Ann Pharmacother*, 1993, 27(3):358-61.

Mauro LS, Nawarskas JJ, and Mauro VF, "Misadventures With Activated Charcoal and Recommendations for Safe Use," *Ann Pharmacother*, 1994, 28(7-8):915-24.

Neuvonen PJ, "Clinical Pharmacokinetics of Oral Activated Charcoal in Acute Intoxications," *Clin Pharmacokinet*, 1982, 7(6):465-89.

Palatnick W and Tenebein M, "Activated Charcoal in the Treatment of Drug Overdose: An Update," *Drug Saf*, 1992, 7(1):3-7.

Charcocaps® [OTC] *see* Charcoal *on page 1403*

Chealamide® *see* Edetate Disodium *on page 1421*

Chelante® *see* Edetate Calcium Disodium *on page 1419*

Chelintox® *see* Edetate Calcium Disodium *on page 1419*

Chemet® *see* Succimer *on page 1473*

Cholestyramine Resin (koe less' tir a meen)

CAS Number 11041-12-6

Brand Names Lismol®; Quantalan®; Questran®; Questran® Light; Resincolestiramina®

Use Adjunct in the management of primary hypercholesterolemia; pruritus associated with elevated levels of bile acids; diarrhea associated with excess fecal bile acids; binding toxicologic agents, such as digitoxin, possibly phenobarbital, warfarin, lindane, lorazepam, methotrexate, chlordecone; pseudomembraneous colitis (*Clostridium difficile*), oxaluria

Antidote Useful For

Dicumarol *on page 277*
Digitoxin *on page 283*
Digoxin *on page 284*
Hexachlorobenzene *on page 936*
Lindane *on page 470*
Organochlorines *on page 983*
Warfarin Sodium *on page 800*

Mechanism of Action Forms a nonabsorbable complex with bile acids in the intestine, releasing chloride ions in the process; inhibits enterohepatic reuptake of intestinal bile salts and thereby increases the fecal loss of bile salt-bound low density lipoprotein cholesterol; an anion-exchange resin (chloride form)

Adverse Reactions

Dermatologic: Rash, irritation of perianal area, skin, or tongue

Endocrine & metabolic: Hyperchloremic acidosis, hypoprothrombinemia, hypernatremia from free water loss due to diarrhea

Gastrointestinal: Constipation, nausea, vomiting, abdominal distention and pain, malabsorption of fat-soluble vitamins, fecal impaction

Genitourinary: Increased urinary calcium excretion

Hepatic: increases in alkaline, phosphatase, and liver function tests

Signs & Symptoms of Acute Overdose GI obstruction/concretion

Toxicodynamics/Kinetics

Onset of action: Reduction of plasma cholesterol concentrations generally occurs within 24-48 hours after initiation of cholestyramine therapy, but may continue to fall for up to 1 year; in some patients after the initial decrease, serum cholesterol concentrations return to or exceed baseline levels with continued therapy; relief of pruritus associated with biliary stasis usually occurs within 2-3 weeks after initiation of therapy; relief of diarrhea associated with bile acids occurs within 24 hours

Duration:

Reduction of plasma cholesterol concentration: After withdrawal of cholestyramine, cholesterol concentrations return to baseline in about 2-4 weeks

Relief of pruritus associated with biliary stasis: Pruritus returns within 1-2 weeks when medication is withdrawn

Absorption: Not absorbed from the GI tract

Distribution: None

Metabolism: None

Elimination: In the feces as an insoluble complex with bile acids

Usual Dosage Oral (dosages are expressed in terms of anhydrous resin):

Children: 240 mg/kg/day in 3 divided doses; need to titrate dose depending on indication

(Continued)

Cholestyramine Resin *(Continued)*

Adults: 4 g 1-6 times/day to a maximum of 16-32 g/day

Contraindications Avoid using in complete biliary obstruction

Dosage Forms

Powder: 4 g of resin/9 g of powder (9 g, 378 g)

Powder, for oral suspension, with aspartame: 4 g of resin/5 g of powder (5 g, 210 g)

Stability Suspension may be used for up to 48 hours after refrigeration

Test Interactions Increases prothrombin time (S); decreases cholesterol (S), iron (B)

Drug Interactions Decreased absorption (oral) of digitalis glycosides, warfarin, thyroid hormones, thiazide diuretics, loperamide, phenylbutazone, propranolol, phenobarbital, fat soluble vitamins, amiodarone, methotrexate, NSAIDs, and other drugs by binding to the drug in the intestine

Pregnancy Risk Factor C

Nursing Implications Do not administer the powder in its dry form; just prior to administration, mix with fluid or with applesauce; administer warfarin at least 1-2 hours prior to, or 6 hours after cholestyramine because cholestyramine may bind warfarin and decrease its total absorption. (**Note:** Cholestyramine itself may cause hypoprothrombinemia in patients with impaired enterohepatic circulation.)

Additional Information Questran® Light contains aspartame

Specific References

Cohn WJ, Boylan JJ, Blanke RV, et al, "Treatment of Chlordecone (Kepone) Toxicity With Cholestyramine," *N Engl J Med*, 1978, 298(5):243-8.

Pieroni RE and Fisher JG, "Use of Cholestyramine Resin in Digitoxin Toxicity," *JAMA*, 1981, 245(19):1939-40.

Citramag® *see* Magnesium Citrate *on page 1439*

Citrate of Magnesia *see* Magnesium Citrate *on page 1439*

Citro-Mag® *see* Magnesium Citrate *on page 1439*

Citrovorin Rescue *see* Leucovorin Calcium *on page 1437*

Citrovorum Factor *see* Leucovorin Calcium *on page 1437*

Codroxomin® Injection *see* Hydroxocobalamin *on page 1433*

Co-Lav® *see* Polyethylene Glycol *on page 1460*

Colon Electrolyte Lavage Preparation *see* Polyethylene Glycol *on page 1460*

Colovage® *see* Polyethylene Glycol *on page 1460*

CoLyte® *see* Polyethylene Glycol *on page 1460*

Crotaline Antivenin, Polyvalent *see* Antivenin (Crotalidae) Polyvalent *on page 1392*

Cuprid® *replaced by* Trientine Dihydrochloride *on page 1474*

Cuprimine® *see* Penicillamine *on page 1454*

Cupripen® *see* Penicillamine *on page 1454*

Cyanide Antidote Kit (sye' a nide)

Related Information

Amyl Nitrite *on page 1390*

Sodium Nitrite *on page 1469*

Sodium Thiosulfate *on page 1470*

Use Treatment of cyanide poisoning

Antidote Useful For

Acrylonitrile *on page 853*

Apricot *on page 1052*

Cyanide *on page 899*

Hydrangea *on page 1090*

Nitroprusside Sodium *on page 568*

Peach *on page 1123*

Usual Dosage For cyanide poisoning, a 0.3 mL ampul of amyl nitrite is crushed every minute and vapor is inhaled for 15-30 seconds until an I.V. sodium nitrite infusion is available. Following administration of 300 mg I.V. sodium nitrite, inject 12.5 g sodium thiosulfate I.V. (over ~10 minutes), if needed; injection of both may be repeated at $\frac{1}{2}$ the original dose.

Contraindications Hypersensitivity to any component

Dosage Forms Kit: Sodium nitrite 300 mg/10 mL (#2); sodium thiosulfate 12.5 g/50 mL (#2); amyl nitrite 0.3 mL (#12); also disposable syringes, stomach tube, tourniquet and instructions

Reference Range Blood cyanide levels with symptoms:

Flushing and tachycardia: 0.5-1.0 μg/mL

Obtundation: 1.0-2.5 μg/mL

Coma and respiratory depression: >2.5 μg/mL

Death: >3.0 μg/mL

Specific References

Way JL, "Cyanide Intoxication and Its Mechanism of Antagonism," *Annu Rev Pharmacol Toxicol*, 1984, 24:451-81.

Cycloplegic Mydriatics Comparison *see page 1648*

Cystosol® *see* Sorbitol *on page 1472*

Cytospray® *see* Polyethylene Glycol *on page 1460*

D-3-Mercaptovaline *see* Penicillamine *on page 1454*

D_5W *see* Dextrose *on page 1409*

$D_{10}W$ *see* Dextrose *on page 1409*

$D_{20}W$ *see* Dextrose *on page 1409*

$D_{50}W$ *see* Dextrose *on page 1409*

$D_{70}W$ *see* Dextrose *on page 1409*

DDC *see* Diethyldithiocarbamate Trihydrate *on page 1410*

DDTC *see* Diethyldithiocarbamate Trihydrate *on page 1410*

Deferiprone

CAS Number 30652-11-0

Synonyms 1,2-Dimethyl-3-Hydroxypyrid-4-One; L_1

Use Investigational: Prevention of chronic iron overload in patients with transfusion-dependent beta-thalassemia

Mechanism of Action Orally active iron chelator

Adverse Reactions

Hematologic: Bone marrow depression, thrombocytopenia, leukopenia

Neuromuscular & skeletal: Arthritis, arthralgia

Toxicodynamics/Kinetics

Absorption: Delayed by food

Half-life: 3-4 hours

Usual Dosage Oral: 75-100 mg/kg/day in 3 divided doses

Dosage Forms Capsule: 300 mg

Reference Range Oral dose of 25 mg/kg produces a peak plasma level of 14-17 μg/mL

Test Interactions Decreases serum ferritin level; increases urinary excretion of iron

Additional Information Criteria proposed for effective chronic chelation in thalassemia major is hepatic iron concentration <80 μmol/g and serum ferritin level <2500 μg/L; 3 molecules of deferiprone binds one molecule of iron

Specific References

Klein J, Damani LA, Chung D, et al, "A High Performance Liquid Chromatographic Method for the Measurement of the Iron Chelator 1,2-Dimethyl-3-Hydroxypyridin-4-One in Human Plasma," *Ther Drug Monit*, 1991, 13(1):51-4.

Kontoghiorghes GJ and Hoffbrand AV, "Clinical Trials With Oral Iron Chelator," *Lancet*, 1989, 2(8678-8679):1516-7.

Matsui D, Hermann C, Klein J, et al, "Critical Comparison of Novel and Existing Methods of Compliance Assessment During a Clinical Trial of an Oral Iron Chelator," *J Clin Pharmacol*, 1994, 34(9):944-9.

Matsui D, Klein J, Hermann C, et al, "Relationship Between the Pharmacokinetics and Iron Excretion Pharmacodynamics of the New Oral Iron Chelator 1,2-Dimethyl-3-Hydroxypyridin-4-One in Patients With Thalassemia," *Clin Pharmacol Ther*, 1991, 50(3):294-8.

Nathan DG, "An Orally Active Iron Chelator," *N Engl J Med*, 1995, 322:953-4.

Olivieri NF, Brittenham GM, Matsui D, et al, "Iron Chelation Therapy With Oral Deferiprone in Patients With Thalassemia Major," *N Engl J Med*, 1995, 332:918-22.

Deferoxamine Mesylate (de fer ox' a meen)

CAS Number 70-51-9; 138-14-7; 1950-39-6

Brand Names Desferal® Mesylate; Desferin®

Synonyms BA-33112; DFM Mesylate; DFO

Use Acute iron intoxication (>350 μg/dL); chronic iron overload secondary to multiple transfusions; diagnostic test for iron overload

Investigational: Treatment of aluminum accumulation in renal failure; iron overload secondary to congenital anemias; hemochromatosis; removal of corneal rust rings following surgical removal of foreign bodies; has also been used for porphyria cutanea tarda and rheumatoid arthritis, aluminum toxicity

Antidote Useful For
Iron *on page 439*

Mechanism of Action Complexes with trivalent ions (ferric ions) to form ferrioxamine, which is removed by the kidneys

Adverse Reactions
Cardiovascular: Flushing, hypotension, tachycardia, shock, swelling
Central nervous system: Fever, seizures
Dermatologic: Erythema, urticaria, pruritus, rash, cutaneous wheal formation
Gastrointestinal: Abdominal discomfort, diarrhea
Local: Pain and induration at injection site, macular edema
Neuromuscular & skeletal: Leg cramps
Ocular: Blurred vision, cataract, visual field defects, night blindness
Otic: Hearing loss, tinnitus
Renal: Renal insufficiency, dysuria
Miscellaneous: Anaphylaxis, possible increased risk of fungal and *Y. enterocolitica* infections; phycomycosis; thrombocytopenia, toxicity and fibrosis and edema at high doses (over 24 hours) – restrictive lung pathology has been noted

Signs & Symptoms of Acute Overdose Seizures

Toxicodynamics/Kinetics
Absorption: Oral: <15%
Distribution: V_d: 2.6 L/kg in healthy individuals; 1.9 L/kg in patients with chronic iron overload; distributed widely into body
Metabolism: In the liver to ferrioxamine
Half-life:
- Deferoxamine: 6.1 hours
- Ferrioxamine: 5.8 hours
- Hemochromatosis patients: 5.6 hours

Elimination: Renal excretion of the metabolite and unchanged drug (tubular reabsorption can occur)
- Clearance:
  - Healthy patients: 0.296 L/hour/kg
  - Hemochromatosis patients: 0.234 L/hour/kg
  - Thalassemic children: 1.8-2.4 L/hour/kg

Usual Dosage Oral use is probably not effective; 100 mg DFO binds 10 mg iron
Children:
- Acute iron intoxication (I.M. is preferred route for patients not in shock). Treat until urine is no longer pink salmon (vin rosé) colored:
  - I.M.: 90 mg/kg/dose every 8 hours; maximum: 6 g/day
  - I.V.: 15 mg/kg/hour (up to 35 mg/kg/hour with caution in severe poisoning); maximum: 6 g/day
- Chronic iron overload:
  - I.V.: 15 mg/kg/hour
  - S.C.: 20-40 mg/kg/day over 8-12 hours
- Aluminum-induced bone disease: 20-40 mg/kg every hemodialysis treatment, frequency dependent on clinical status of the patient

Adults:
- Acute iron intoxication (I.M. is preferred route for patients not in shock). Treat until urine is no longer pink salmon (vin rosé) colored:
  - I.M.: 1 g stat, then 0.5 g every 4 hours for two doses, then 0.5 g every 4-12 hours up to 6 g/day
  - I.V.: 15 mg/kg/hour, up to 6-8 g/day; maximum given 16 g/day without side effects
- Chronic iron overload:
  - I.M.: 0.5-1 g every day
  - S.C.: 1-2 g every day over 8-24 hours

Contraindications Patients with anuria

Warnings Use with caution in patients with severe renal disease, pyelonephritis; may increase susceptibility to *Yersinia enterocolitica*, phycomycosis, *Cunninghamella bertholletiae*, *Pneumocystis carinii*, and *Staphylococcus aureus*

Dosage Forms Powder for injection: 500 mg

Stability Protect from light; reconstituted solutions (sterile water) may be stored at room temperature for 7 days

Test Interactions May interfere with colorimetric iron assays along with total iron binding capacities.

Drug Interactions Can cause loss of consciousness when administered with prochlorperazine

Pregnancy Risk Factor C

Pregnancy Implications Do not withhold chelation treatment for iron overdose solely due to pregnancy; has caused fetal skeletal abnormalities in animal models but is probably safe to use in the gravid patient

Monitoring Parameters Serum iron, total iron binding capacity; ophthalmologic exam and audiometry with chronic therapy

Nursing Implications Iron chelate colors urine salmon pink; I.M. is preferred route; maximum I.V. rate is 35 mg/kg/hour; incompatible with heparin

Additional Information One proposed endpoint of therapy after standard (15 mg/kg/hour) dose of deferoxamine is to obtain a urine iron to creatinine ratio; a value >12.5 indicates need for continued therapy of deferoxamine; hypotension (with rapid I.V. administration: >15 mg/kg/hour); one molecule of deferoxamine binds to one molecule of iron

Specific References

Allain P, Mauras Y, Chaleil D, et al, "Pharmacokinetics and Renal Elimination of Desferrioxamine and Ferrioxamine in Healthy Subjects and Patients With Haemochromatosis," *Br J Clin Pharmacol*, 1987, 24(2):207-12.

Bentur Y, McGuigan M, and Koren G, "Deferoxamine (Desferrioxamine): New Toxicities for an Old Drug," *Drug Saf*, 1991, 6(1):37-46.

Cheney K, Gumbiner C, Benson B, et al, "Survival After a Severe Iron Poisoning Treated With Intermittent Infusions of Deferoxamine," *Clin Toxicol*, 1995, 33:61-6.

Jackson TW, Ling LJ, and Washington V, "The Effect of Oral Deferoxamine on Iron Absorption in Humans," *J Toxicol Clin Toxicol*, 1995, 33(4):325-9.

Shannon M, "Desferrioxamine in Acute Iron Poisoning," *Lancet*, 1992, 339(8809):1601.

Voest EE, Vreugdenhil G, and Marx JJ, "Iron-Chelating Agents in Non-Iron Overload Conditions," *Ann Intern Med*, 1994, 120(6):490-9.

Winship KA, "Toxicity of Aluminum: A Historical Review, Part 2," *Adverse Drug React Toxicol Rev*, 1993, 12(3):177-211.

Yatscoff RW, Wayne EA, and Tenenbein M, "An Objective Criterion for the Cessation of Deferoxamine Therapy in the Acutely Iron Poisoned Patient," *J Toxicol Clin Toxicol*, 1991, 29(1):1-10.

Demo 6® *see* Pyridoxine Hydrochloride *on page 1465*

Depen® *see* Penicillamine *on page 1454*

Desferal® Mesylate *see* Deferoxamine Mesylate *on page 1407*

Desferin® *see* Deferoxamine Mesylate *on page 1407*

Desmoidpillen® *see* Methylene Blue *on page 1444*

Dextran 1 (dex' tran)

CAS Number 9004-54-0

Brand Names Promit®; Promiten®

Synonyms Dextranum 1

Use Prophylaxis of serious anaphylactic reactions to I.V. infusion of dextran in a dose-dependent manner; can prevent clot formation due to ergotism

Mechanism of Action Produces plasma volume expansion by virtue of its highly colloidal starch structure, similar to albumin

Adverse Reactions

Cardiovascular: Mild hypotension, bradycardia, tightness of chest
Central nervous system: Fever
Dermatologic: Urticaria
Gastrointestinal: Nausea, vomiting
Hematologic: Coagulopathy
Neuromuscular & skeletal: Arthralgia
Respiratory: Wheezing, nasal congestion
Miscellaneous: Anaphylaxis

Signs & Symptoms of Acute Overdose Bradycardia, hypotension

Usual Dosage I.V. (time between dextran 1 and dextran solution should not exceed 15 minutes):

Children: 0.3 mL/kg 1-2 minutes before I.V. infusion of dextran
Adults: 20 mL 1-2 minutes before I.V. infusion of dextran

Contraindications Marked cardiac decompensation, oliguria or anuria, known hypersensitivity to dextrans

Dosage Forms Injection: 150 mg/mL (20 mL)

Pregnancy Risk Factor C

Nursing Implications Do not dilute or admix with dextrans

Specific References

Renck H, Ljungstrom KG, Hedin H, et al, "Prevention of Dextran-Induced Anaphylactic Reactions by Hapten Inhibition," *Acta Chir Scand*, 1983, 149(4):355-60.

Dextranum 1 *see* Dextran 1 *on this page*

Dextrose (dex' trose)

CAS Number 50-99-7; 5996-10-1

Synonyms D_5W; $D_{10}W$; $D_{20}W$; $D_{50}W$; $D_{70}W$; Glucose

Use Patients with altered mental status due to hypoglycemia

Antidote Useful For

Acetohexamide *on page 86*
Akee Fruit Food Poisoning *on page 1050*
Chlorpropamide *on page 207*
Glipizide *on page 382*
Glyburide *on page 384*
Insulin Preparations *on page 426*
Metformin *on page 507*
Tolazamide *on page 756*
Tolbutamide *on page 757*
Troglitazone *on page 777*

Mechanism of Action A carbohydrate substrate for aerobic metabolism

Adverse Reactions

Endocrine & metabolic: Hypokalemia, hyperglycemia, hypomagnesemia, hypophosphatemia

Miscellaneous: Vein irritation, thrombophlebitis; hyperosmolar solution which can cause a Volkmann's contraction of an extremity if extravasation occurs; has been associated with worsening of ischemic strokes

Toxicodynamics/Kinetics Metabolism: To carbon dioxide and water

Usual Dosage Dextrose 50% solution (parenteral administration)

Children: Dilute to 10% to 25% and given 2-4 mL/kg body weight

Adults: 50-100 mL

Warnings Do not administer within same tubing as whole blood in that hemolysis can occur; administer thiamine (50-100 mg I.V.) to prevent Wenicke's encephalopathy

Monitoring Parameters Serum glucose

Additional Information Has been used as a sclerosing agent (for varicose vein treatment or to produce adhesive pleuritis)

Specific References

Browning RG, Olson DW, Stueven HA, et al, "50% Dextrose: Antidote or Toxin?" *Ann Emerg Med*, 1990, 19(6):683-7.

DFM Mesylate *see* Deferoxamine Mesylate *on page 1407*

DFO *see* Deferoxamine Mesylate *on page 1407*

Diethyldithiocarbamate Trihydrate

CAS Number 148-18-5

Synonyms DDC; DDTC; Dithiocarb Sodium; DTC

Use Investigational: Chelating agent for nickel; a metabolite of disulfiram, it has also been used to treat thallium poisoning, but is not effective; shown to be active against HIV *in vitro*

Antidote Useful For

Nickel *on page 976*
Nickel Carbonyl *on page 977*

Mechanism of Action Binds to nickel, the nickel-diethyldithiocarbamate complex is lipophilic thus enhancing its elimination

Adverse Reactions Gastrointestinal: Nausea

Toxicodynamics/Kinetics

Metabolism: To carbon disulfide and diethylamine
Half-life: 15.5 hours
Elimination: Urine and feces

Usual Dosage

Mild or doubtful nickel exposure (urine nickel <100 mcg/L): Oral: 2 g in divided doses (every 4 hours)

Severe nickel exposure (levels 100-500 mcg/L): Oral: Initial: 2 g with 1 g sodium bicarbonate, then 1 g at 4 hours, 600 mg at 8 hours, 400 mg at 16 hours, and 400 mg every 8 hours thereafter

Alternatively, 50 mg/kg/day on day one, then 400 mg every 8 hours until symptoms are resolved or urine nickel levels are <100 mcg/L

Urinary nickel levels >500 mcg/L: Give 25-100 mg/kg/day

Dosage Forms Capsule: 200 mg

Additional Information May facilitate nickel GI absorption; may actually cause an increase in CNS levels of thallium; can cause disulfiram reaction with ethanol. Dr FW Sunderman has IND for this agent (215-922-6554). Not useful to treat ocular copper nitrate toxicity; probably not useful to treat nickel dermatitis. Sodium bicarbonate dosage is used to prevent nausea; experimental use (in rodents) to remove cadmium bound to metallothione

Specific References

Hersh EM, Brewton G, Abrams D, et al, "Dithiocarb Sodium (Diethyldithiocarbamate) Therapy in Patients With Symptomatic HIV Infection and AIDS: A Randomized, Double-Blind, Placebo-Controlled, Multicenter Study," *JAMA*, 1991, 265(12):1538-44.

Kojima S, Ono H, Kiyozumi M, et al, "Effect of N-Benzyl-D-Glucamine Dithiocarbamate on Renal Toxicity Produced by Subacute Exposure to Cadmium in Rats," *Toxicol Appl Pharmacol*, 1989, 98(1):39-48.
Nogue S, et al, "Acute Thallium Poisoning: An Evaluation of Different Forms of Treatment," *J Toxicol Clin Toxicol*, 1982-83, 19:1015-21.
Sunderman Jr FW, "The Treatment of Acute Nickel Carbonyl Poisoning With Sodium Diethyldithiocarbamate," *Ann Clin Res*, 1971, 3:182-5.
Sunderman Sr FW, "Chelation Therapy in Nickel Poisoning," *Ann Clin Lab Sci*, 1981, 11:1-8.

Diethylene Triamine Penta-acetic Acid

CAS Number 67-43-6

Synonyms Calcium Chel 330 (Ca-DTPA); DPTA: Pentetic Acid; DTPA; IND 4041 (Ca-DTPA); IND-14603 (Zn-DTPA)

Use Chelating absorbed multivalent radioisotopes of the actinide series (plutonium, neptunium, americium) as well as cesium and actinide; may be useful for uranium, curium, californium, cerium, yttrium, lanthanum, scandium, promethium, niobium, manganese, thorium, lutetium, zirconium, and zinc; on IND status

Antidote Useful For

Plutonium *on page 995*

Mechanism of Action Chelation for multivalent radioisotopes

Adverse Reactions

Central nervous system: Chills, fever
Dermal: Pruritus
Gastrointestinal: Transient nausea, vomiting, diarrhea
Neuromuscular & skeletal: Muscle cramps in first day of therapy
Renal: Nephrotoxicity
Miscellaneous: Ca-DTPA may cause zinc depletion leading to transient anosmia

Toxicodynamics/Kinetics

Half-life, plasma: 20-60 minutes
Elimination: Renal, fecal is <3%

Usual Dosage 1 g of the calcium salt diluted in 250 mL of 5% dextrose in water infused over 60-90 minutes; may be repeated daily for 5 days; zinc salt can be used for pregnant patients; may be aerosolized through nebulization

Contraindications Ca-DTPA: Do not use in pregnant females, children, patients with nephrotic syndrome or patients with bone marrow depression (Zn-DTPA may be used in above circumstances); neither Zn-DTPA nor Ca-DTPA should be used for uranium (due to nephrotoxic effects) or neptunium (due to increased bone deposition)

Dosage Forms

Ca-DTPA: 1 g ampul (0.5 M in 4 mL [25%] sterile water)
Zn-DTPA: 1.1 g ampul (0.5 M in 4.4 mL [25%] sterile water)

Stability Store in cool environment and away from sunlight

Pregnancy Risk Factor C (Zn-DTPA); D (Ca-DTPA)

Monitoring Parameters Urine analysis, radioassay, renal function and blood counts during therapy, pulse and blood pressure

Additional Information Calcium salt appears to more effective than zinc salt during first hours postexposure; combination with dimercaprol has been demonstrated to be effective in rodents to enhance the elimination of cadmium; may be obtained from Radiation Emergency Assistance Center/Training Site (REAC/TS) in Oak Ridge, TN (615-576-3131 or 615-576-1004 or 615-481-1000)

Zinc replacement (with 220 mg of zinc sulfate tablets) may be required if long-term Ca-DTPA treatment is performed; IND forms need to be followed. Questions regarding use of these agents may be directed to Robert C Ricks, PhD (615-576-3131), Shirley A Fry, MPH (615-576-3480), WW Burr, MD, PhD (615-576-5262), Dale E Minner, MD (615-576-2124), or AS Garrett, MD (615-576-7431) at the Medical Sciences Division of Oak Ridge Associated Universities, PO Box 117, Oak Ridge, TN 37831-0117.

Specific References

Ca-DTPA/Zn-DTPA: Informational Material Package Insert; Oak Ridge Institute for Science and Education (ORISE), July, 1994.
Cherian M and Rogers K, "Chelation of Cadmium From Metallothionein *In Vivo* and Its Excretion in Rats Repeatedly Injected With Cadmium Chloride," *Pharmacol Exp Ther*, 1982, 222:699-704.

Digibind® *see* Digoxin Immune Fab *on this page*

Digoxin Immune Fab (di jox' in i myun' fab)

Brand Names Digibind®

Synonyms Antidigoxin Fab Fragments

Use Treatment of potentially life-threatening digoxin or digitoxin intoxication in carefully selected patients with ventricular arrhythmias, progressive bradycardia with or without heart block or hyperkalemia; useful to treat delirium due to digitalis; effective for oleander, lanatoside C ingestions also

Antidote Useful For

Digitoxin *on page 283*
Digoxin *on page 284*
Foxglove *on page 1085*
Lily-of-the-Valley *on page 1099*
Oleander *on page 1120*
Rubber Vine *on page 1134*
Squill *on page 1143*
Star-of-Bethlehem (*Ornithogalum pyrenaicum*) *on page 1145*
Star-of-Bethlehem (*Ornithogalum umbellatum*) *on page 1146*
Yew *on page 1159*

Mechanism of Action Binds with molecules of digoxin or digitoxin and then is excreted by the kidneys and removed from the body; promotes egress of free intracellular digoxin into extracellular fluid whereupon it is rapidly bound; prevents reassociation to membrane receptors

Adverse Reactions

Cardiovascular: Worsening of low cardiac output or congestive heart failure, rapid ventricular response in patients with atrial fibrillation as digoxin is withdrawn
Dermatologic: Urticarial rash
Endocrine & metabolic: Hypokalemia, hypoglycemia in neonates
Respiratory: Transient apnea
Miscellaneous: Recrudescent toxicity can develop within 3 days, facial swelling and redness, allergic reactions

Toxicodynamics/Kinetics

Onset of action: I.V.: Improvement in signs and symptoms occur within 2-30 minutes
Distribution: V_d: 0.5-54 L/kg; appears to distribute rapidly throughout extracellular space into both plasma and interstitial fluid
Affinity constant: 10^{9} to 10^{10} M-1 (digoxin) 10^{8} M-1 (digitoxin)
Half-life: 16-20 hours; prolonged in patients with renal impairment
Time to peak serum concentration: Occurs at completion of I.V. infusion
Elimination: Renal with levels declining to undetectable amounts within 5-7 days; renal clearance: 13.6 mL/minute; can be removed by plasmapheresis but not hemodialysis or CAVH

Usual Dosage See package insert. To determine the dose of digoxin immune Fab, first determine the total body load of digoxin (TBL) as follows (using either an approximation of the amount ingested or a postdistribution serum digoxin concentration):

TBL of digoxin (in mg) = C (in ng/mL) x 5.6 x body weight (in kg)/1000 or TBL = mg of digoxin ingested (as tablets or elixir) x 0.8; C = postdistribution digoxin concentration

Dose of digoxin immune Fab (in mg) I.V. = TBL x 66.7 or dose of digoxin immune Fab (in number of 38 mg vials) = [C of digoxin (in ng/mL) x body weight (in kg)]/100

If neither ingestion amount or serum level is known: Adult dosage is 20 vials (760 mg) I.V. infusion; see tables.

Contraindications Hypersensitivity to sheep products

Warnings Monitor serum potassium levels, allergic reactions possible; epinephrine should be immediately available, Fab fragments may be eliminated more slowly in patients with renal failure, heart failure may be exacerbated as digoxin level is reduced, monitor potassium levels

Dosage Forms Powder for injection, lyophilized: 40 mg

Stability Use reconstituted product promptly; if not used immediately, may be kept in refrigerator for up to 4 hours only

Reference Range Digoxin toxic concentration: >2.0 ng/mL

Test Interactions Increases digoxin level by 50-fold; decreases potassium; may decrease glucose in patients with low glycogen stores

Drug Interactions Cardiac glycosides; does not cross react with spironolactone, cortisone, or cholesterol; decreases potassium, increases digoxin levels

Pregnancy Risk Factor C (no animal reproduction studies conducted)

Monitoring Parameters Serum potassium, serum digoxin concentration priot to first dose of digoxin immune Fab

Nursing Implications Continuous I.V. infusion over 15-30 minutes is preferred; digoxin immune Fab is reconstituted by adding 4 mL sterile water, resulting in 10 mg/mL for I.V. infusion, the reconstituted solution may be further diluted with normal saline to a convenient volume (eg, 1 mg/mL)

Additional Information Serum digoxin levels drawn prior to therapy may be difficult to evaluate if 6-8 hours have not elapsed after the last dose of digoxin (time to equilibration between serum and tissue); digoxin immune Fab fragments may

Approximate Digibind® Dose for Reversal of a Single Ingestion Digoxin Overdose

# of Digoxin Tablets or Capsules Ingested*	Digibind® Dose	
	mg	# of Vials
25	340	8.5
50	680	17
75	1000	25
100	1360	34
150	2000	50
200	2680	67

*0.25 mg tablets with 80% bioavailability or 0.2 mg Lanoxicaps® capsules.

Adult Dose Estimate of Digibind® (in # of Vials) From Serum Digoxin Concentration

Patient Weight (kg)	Serum Digoxin Concentration (ng/mL)						
	1	2	4	8	12	16	20
40	0.5 v*	1 v	2 v	3 v	5 v	7 v	8 v
60	0.5 v	1 v	3 v	5 v	7 v	10 v	12 v
70	1 v	2 v	3 v	6 v	9 v	11 v	14 v
80	1 v	2 v	3 v	7 v	10 v	13 v	16 v
100	1 v	2 v	4 v	8 v	12 v	16 v	20 v

* v = vials.

Infants and Children Dose Estimates of Digibind® (in mg) From Serum Digoxin Concentration

Patient Weight (kg)	Serum Digoxin Concentration (ng/mL)						
	1	2	4	8	12	16	20
1	0.4 mg*	1 mg*	1.5 mg*	3 mg	5 mg	6 mg	8 mg
3	1 mg*	2 mg*	5 mg	9 mg	14 mg	18 mg	23 mg
5	2 mg*	4 mg	8 mg	15 mg	23 mg	30 mg	38 mg
10	4 mg	8 mg	15 mg	30 mg	46 mg	61 mg	76 mg
20	8 mg	15 mg	30 mg	61 mg	91 mg	122 mg	152 mg

*Dilution of reconstituted vial to 1 mg/mL may be desirable.

interfere with digoxin measurements depending upon the assay used; has reversed thrombocytopenia induced by digoxin. For individuals at increased risk of sensitivity, an intradermal or scratch technique skin test using a 1:100 dilution of reconstituted digoxin immune Fab diluted in normal saline has been used; skin test volume is 0.1 mL of 1:100 dilution; evaluate after 20 minutes. Each vial of Digibind® contains 38 mg of protein content and will bind 0.5 mg of digoxin; also contains 75 mg of sorbitol and 28 mg of sodium chloride. Digoxin therapy can be instituted 1-3 days after Fab use in patients with normal renal function. Questions of its use can be directed to Drug Information, Burroughs Wellcome: (800) 443-6763.

Specific References

Antman EM, Wenger TL, Butler VP Jr, et al, "Treatment of 150 Cases of Life-Threatening Digitalis Intoxication With Digoxin-Specific Fab Antibody Fragments," *Circulation*, 1990, 81(6):1744-52.

Aruna AS and Jue SG, "Digoxin Immune Fab Administration Following an Unexplained Increase in Serum Digoxin Concentration," *J Pharm Sci Technol*, 1994, 10:246-9.

Kaufman J, Leikin J, Kendziershi D, et al, "Use of Digoxin Fab Immune Fragments in a Seven-Day-Old Infant," *Pediatr Emerg Care*, 1990, 6(2):118-21.

Leikin J, Vogel S, Graft J, et al, "Use of Fab Fragments of Digoxin-Specific Antibodies in the Therapy of Massive Digoxin Poisoning," *Ann Emerg Med*, 1985, 14(2):175-8.

Martiny SS, Phelps SJ, and Massey KL, "Treatment of Severe Digitalis Intoxication With Digoxin-Specific Antibody Fragments, A Clinical Review," *Crit Care Med*, 1988, 16(6):629-35.

Shumaik GM, Wu AW, and Ping AC, "Oleander Poisoning: Treatment With Digoxin-Specific Fab Antibody Fragments," *Ann Emerg Med*, 1988, 17(7):732-5.

Ujhelyi MR and Robert S, "Pharmacokinetic Aspects of Digoxin-Specific Fab Therapy in the Management of Digitalis Toxicity," *Clin Pharmacokinet*, 1995, 28:483-93.

(Continued)

Digoxin Immune Fab *(Continued)*

Varriale P and Mossavi A, "Rapid Reversal of Digitalis Delirium Using Digoxin Immune Fab Therapy," *Clin Cardiol*, 1995, 18:351-2.

Dimercaprol (dye mer kap' role)

CAS Number 59-52-9

Brand Names BAL in Oil®; Sulfactin Homburg®

Synonyms BAL; British Anti-Lewisite; 2,3-Dimercaptupropan-1-ol; Dithioglycerol

Use Antidote to gold, arsenic, mercury, methyl bromide, methyl iodide, or trivalent antimony poisoning; adjunct to edetate calcium disodium in lead poisoning; possibly effective for bismuth, polonium, chromium, copper, nickel, tungsten, or zinc

Antidote Useful For

Antimony *on page 862*
Arsenic *on page 862*
Cobalt *on page 895*
Copper *on page 896*
Gold Compounds *on page 386*
Lead *on page 945*
Mercury *on page 954*
Methyl Bromide *on page 964*

Mechanism of Action Sulfhydryl group combines with ions of various heavy metals to form relatively stable, nontoxic, soluble chelates which are excreted in bile and urine

Adverse Reactions

Cardiovascular: Hypertension, tachycardia, chest pain
Central nervous system: Nervousness, fever, headache, seizures
Gastrointestinal: Vomiting, nausea
Hematologic: Transient neutropenia, hemolysis in G-6-PD deficiency
Local: Pain at injection site
Ocular: Blepharospasm
Renal: Nephrotoxicity
Respiratory: Rhinorrhea
Miscellaneous: Salivation, burning sensation of the lips, mouth, throat, eyes, diaphoresis

Toxicodynamics/Kinetics

Duration of action: ~4 hours; frequent doses at 3- to 4-hour intervals over prolonged periods are necessary to maintain therapeutic effect
Absorption: Slow through the skin
Distribution: To all tissues including the brain; highest concentrations in liver and kidneys
Metabolism: Rapid to inactive products
Half-life: Short
Time to peak serum concentration: Obtained in 30-60 minutes
Elimination: In the urine within 4 hours

Usual Dosage Children and Adults:

I.M.:
- Mild arsenic and gold poisoning: 2.5 mg/kg/dose every 6 hours for 2 days, then every 12 hours on the third day, and once daily thereafter for 10 days
- Severe arsenic and gold poisoning: 3 mg/kg/dose every 4 hours for 2 days then every 6 hours on the third day, then every 12 hours thereafter for 10 days
- Mercury poisoning: Initial: 5 mg/kg followed by 2.5 mg/kg/dose 1-2 times/day for 10 days
- Lead poisoning (use with edetate calcium disodium):
  - Mild: 3-5 mg/kg/dose every 4 hours for 2 days, then 2.5-3 mg/kg/dose every 6 hours for 2 days, then 2.5-3 mg/kg/dose every 12 hours for 1 week
  - Severe: 4 mg/kg/dose every 4 hours for 5-7 days
  - Acute encephalopathy: Initial: 4 mg/kg/dose, then every 4 hours

Topical dermal/ocular dose for Lewisite exposure: <20% solution

Contraindications Hepatic insufficiency; do not use on iron, cadmium, or selenium poisoning; contraindicated in patients allergic to peanuts

Warnings Potentially a nephrotoxic drug, use with caution in patients with oliguria; keep urine alkaline to protect kidneys; use with caution in patients with hypertension or with glucose 6-phosphate dehydrogenase deficiency; give all injections deep I.M. at different sites. Also may contain benzl benzoate and peanut oil. (Do not use in patients allergic to peanuts.)

Dosage Forms Injection: 100 mg/mL (3 mL)

Test Interactions Iodine I 131 thyroidal uptake values may be decreased

Drug Interactions Toxic complexes with iron, cadmium, selenium, or uranium

Pregnancy Risk Factor C

Nursing Implications Administer deep I.M. only; urine should be kept alkaline

Additional Information Preadministration with ephedrine or antihistamines may reduce side effects; nephrotoxic effects can be minimized by maintaining an alkaline urine flow; effectiveness questionable for arsenic-induced liver damage or short-chain organic mercury compounds; ineffective for thallium, tellurium, or vanadium

Specific References

Cantilena LR Jr and Klaassen CD, "The Effect of Chelating Agents on the Excretion of Endogenous Metals," *Toxicol Appl Pharmacol*, 1982, 63(3):344-50.

Committee on Drugs, American Academy of Pediatrics, "Treatment Guidelines for Lead Exposure in Children," *Pediatrics*, 1995, 96:155-60.

Kosnett MJ, "Unanswered Questions in Metal Chelation," *J Toxicol Clin Toxicol*, 1992, 30(4):529-47.

2,3-Dimercaptosuccinic Acid *see* Succimer *on page 1473*

2,3-Dimercaptupropan-1-ol *see* Dimercaprol *on previous page*

1,2-Dimethyl-3-Hydroxypyrid-4-One *see* Deferiprone *on page 1407*

β,β-Dimethylcysteine *see* Penicillamine *on page 1454*

Diphenhydramine Hydrochloride (dye fen hye' dra meen)

Related Information

H1-Antihistamine Comparison *on page 1649*

Therapeutic Drugs Associated With Hallucinations *on page 1558-1559*

CAS Number 147-24-0

Brand Names AllerMax® Oral [OTC]; Banophen® Oral [OTC]; Belix® Oral [OTC]; Bena-D® Injection; Benadryl®; Benahist® Injection; Benoject® Injection; Benylin® Cough Syrup [OTC]; Bydramine® Cough Syrup [OTC]; Diphen® Cough [OTC]; Dormin® Oral [OTC]; Genahist® Oral; Gen-D-phen® Cough Syrup [OTC]; Hydramine® Oral [OTC]; Hydramyn® Syrup [OTC]; Maximum Strength Nytol® [OTC]; Nidryl® Oral [OTC]; Nordryl® Injection; Nordryl® Oral; Nytol® Oral [OTC]; Phendry® Oral [OTC]; Silphen® Cough [OTC]; Sleep-eze 3® Oral [OTC]; Sleepinal® [OTC]; Sominex® Oral [OTC]; Tusstat® Syrup; Twilite® Oral [OTC]; Uni-Bent® Cough Syrup; Wehdryl® Injection

Use Reversal of toxin-induced extrapyramidal reactions or serum sickness secondary to antivenin

Antidote Useful For

Monosodium Glutamate Food Poisoning *on page 1109*

Paclitaxel *on page 589*

Mechanism of Action Competes with histamine for H_1-receptor sites on effector cells in the gastrointestinal tract, blood vessels, and respiratory tract

Adverse Reactions

Cardiovascular: Hypotension, palpitations

Central nervous system: Sedation, disorientation, dizziness, paradoxical excitement, extrapyramidal symptoms, fatigue, insomnia, visual hallucinations, acute dystonia

Gastrointestinal: Nausea, vomiting

Neuromuscular & skeletal: Tremors

Ocular: Blurred vision

Renal: Urinary retention, impotence

Respiratory: Bronchospasm

Miscellaneous: Dry mucous membranes, dental erosion

Signs & Symptoms of Acute Overdose CNS stimulation or depression; overdose may result in death in infants and children

Toxicodynamics/Kinetics

Onset of action:

- I.M.: 20-30 minutes
- Rectal: 30-45 minutes

Duration: 4-7 hours

Absorption: Oral: ~65%

Distribution: V_d: 4.5 L/kg; distributed widely throughout the body including the CNS

Protein binding: 98% to 99%

Metabolism: Extensive in the liver and to smaller degrees in the lung and kidney

Half-life: 8 hours (15 hours in cirrhotic patients)

Time to peak serum concentration: Within 2-4 hours

Elimination: Renal; clearance: 0.37 L/kg/hour

Usual Dosage

Children: Oral, I.M., I.V.: 5 mg/kg/day or 150 mg/m^2/day in divided doses every 6-8 hours, not to exceed 300 mg/day

Adults:

- Oral: 25-50 mg every 4-6 hours
- I.M., I.V.: 10-50 mg in a single dose every 2-4 hours, not to exceed 400 mg/day

Contraindications Hypersensitivity to diphenhydramine or any component; should not be used in acute attacks of asthma

(Continued)

Diphenhydramine Hydrochloride *(Continued)*

Dosage Forms

Capsule: 25 mg, 50 mg
Cream: 1%, 2%
Elixir: 12.5 mg/5 mL (5 mL, 10 mL, 20 mL, 120 mL, 480 mL, 3780 mL)
Injection: 10 mg/mL (10 mL, 30 mL); 50 mg/mL (1 mL, 10 mL)
Lotion: 1% (75 mL)
Solution, topical spray: 1% (60 mL)
Syrup: 12.5 mg/5 mL (5 mL, 120 mL, 240 mL, 480 mL, 3780 mL)
Tablet: 25 mg, 50 mg

Stability Protect from light

Reference Range Therapeutic: Not established; Toxic: >0.1 μg/mL; plasma diphenhydramine levels >50 μg/L (0.17 μmol/L) associated with sedation; blood diphenhyrdramine level of 12.8 mg/L associated with fatality

Test Interactions May suppress the wheal and flare reactions to skin test antigens

Drug Interactions CNS depressants, monoamine oxidase inhibitors, syrup should not be given to patients taking drugs that can cause disulfiram reactions (ie, metronidazole, chlorpropamide) due to alcohol content; adsorbed by charcoal

Pregnancy Risk Factor C

Pregnancy Implications Crosses placenta

Nursing Implications I.V. must be given slowly

Additional Information Has antinauseant and topical anesthetic properties

Specific References

Corre KA, Niemann JT, Bessen HA, et al, "Extended Therapy for Acute Dystonic Reactions," *Ann Emerg Med*, 1984, 13(3):194:7.
Doenecke AL and Heuermann RC, "Treatment of Haloperidol Abuse With Diphenhydramine," *Am J Psychiatry*, 1980, 137(4):487-8.
Lindsay CA, Williams GD, and Levin DL, "Fatal Adult Respiratory Distress Syndrome After Diphenhydramine Toxicity in a Child: A Case Report," *Crit Care Med*, 1995, 23:777-81.
Weston MV, "Lovelorn and Snakebit," *Hosp Pract (Off Ed)*, 1986, 21(3A):140-3.

Diphen® Cough [OTC] *see* Diphenhydramine Hydrochloride *on previous page*

Disotate® *see* Edetate Disodium *on page 1421*

Distamine® *see* Penicillamine *on page 1454*

Dithiocarb Sodium *see* Diethyldithiocarbamate Trihydrate *on page 1410*

Dithioglycerol *see* Dimercaprol *on page 1414*

DMSA *see* Succimer *on page 1473*

Dobutamine Hydrochloride (doe byoo' ta meen)

Related Information

Adrenergic Agonists, Cardiovascular Comparison *on page 1638*
Adrenergic Agonists Drug Infusions Comparison *on page 1638*

CAS Number 49745-95-1

Brand Names Dobutrex®

Use Short-term management of patients with cardiac decompensation; useful for hypotension induced by tricyclic antidepressants, beta-adrenergic blockers, doxazosin, calcium channel blockers, or sedative-hypnotic toxicity

Antidote Useful For

Doxazosin *on page 300*

Mechanism of Action Stimulates $beta_1$-adrenergic receptors, causing increased contractility and heart rate, with little effect on $beta_2$- or alpha-receptors

Adverse Reactions Symptoms can occur for up to 2 hours

Cardiovascular: Ectopic beats, chest pain, angina, tachycardia, atrial fibrillation, hypertension, palpitations, elevation in blood pressure; in higher doses tachycardia (ventricular) or cardiac arrhythmias may be seen; patients with atrial fibrillation or flutter are at risk of developing a rapid ventricular response
Central nervous system: Tingling sensation, headache
Endocrine and Metabolic: Hypokalemia
Gastrointestinal: Nausea, vomiting, emesis
Hematologic: Coagulopathy, platelet inhibition
Neuromuscular & skeletal: Mild leg cramps, neuropathy (peripheral), paresthesia
Renal: Urinary incontinence
Respiratory: Dyspnea, tachypnea

Signs & Symptoms of Acute Overdose Fatigue, nervousness

Toxicodynamics/Kinetics

Onset of action: I.V.: Within 1-10 minutes

Duration: A few minutes
Distribution: Wide throughout the body
Metabolism: In tissues and the liver to inactive metabolites
Time to peak serum concentration: Within 10-20 minutes
Half-life: 2 minutes
Elimination: Urine

Usual Dosage I.V. infusion:
Neonates and Children: 2.5-15 mcg/kg/minute, titrate to desired response
Adults: 2.5-15 mcg/kg/minute; maximum: 40 mcg/kg/minute, titrate to desired response

Infusion Rates of Various Dilutions of Dobutamine

Desired Delivery Rate (mcg/kg/min)	Infusion Rate (mL/kg/min)	
	500 mcg/mL*	1000 mcg/mL†
2.5	0.005	0.0025
5.0	0.01	0.005
7.5	0.015	0.0075
10.0	0.02	0.01
12.5	0.025	0.0125
15.0	0.03	0.015

* 500 mg per liter or 250 mg per 500 mL of diluent.
†1000 mg per liter or 250 mg per 250 mL of diluent.

Maximum I.V. dose: 40 mcg/kg/minute
Maximum survivable dose on record: 130 mcg/kg/minute for 30 minutes

Contraindications Hypersensitivity to sulfites (commercial preparation contains sodium bisulfite) and/or dobutamine; patients with idiopathic hypertrophic subaortic stenosis

Warnings Hypovolemia should be corrected prior to use; infiltration causes local inflammatory changes, extravasation may cause dermal necrosis; use with extreme caution following myocardial infarction; potent drug, must be diluted prior to use; patient's hemodynamic status should be monitored

Dosage Forms Injection: 250 mg (20 mL)

Stability Remix solution every 24 hours; incompatible with sodium bicarbonate solutions; store reconstituted solution under refrigeration for 48 hours or 6 hours at room temperature; pink discoloration of solution indicates slight oxidation but **no** significant loss of potency

Drug Interactions General anesthetics (ie, halothane or cyclopropane) and usual doses of dobutamine have resulted in ventricular arrhythmias in animals. In animals, the cardiac effects of dobutamine are antagonized by beta-adrenergic blockers, resulting in predominance of alpha-adrenergic effects and increased peripheral resistance.

Pregnancy Risk Factor C

Monitoring Parameters Blood pressure, EKG, heart rate, CVP, RAP, MAP, urine output; if pulmonary artery catheter is in place, monitor CI, PCWP, and SVR

Nursing Implications Alkaline solutions (sodium bicarbonate); do not give through same I.V. line as heparin, hydrocortisone sodium succinate, cefazolin, or penicillin; administer into large vein; use infusion device to control rate of flow

Extravasation: Use phentolamine as antidote; mix 5 mg with 9 mL of normal saline; inject a small amount of this dilution into extravasated area; blanching should reverse immediately. Monitor site; if blanching should recur, additional injections of phentolamine may be needed.

Additional Information
Standard diluent: 250 mg/500 mL D_5W
Minimum volume: 500 mg/250 mL D_5W

Specific References

Leier CV, Webel J, and Bush CA, "The Cardiovascular Effects of the Continuous Infusion of Dobutamine in Patients With Severe Cardiac Failure," *Circulation*, 1977, 56:468-78.

Paulman PM, Cantral K, Meade JG, et al, "Dobutamine Overdose," *JAMA*, 1990, 264(18):2386-7.

Wirtz CE, "Sustained Atrial Fibrillation After Dobutamine Stress Echocardiography in an Older Patient With Left Atrial Enlargement," *West J Med*, 1995, 162:268-9.

Dobutrex® *see* Dobutamine Hydrochloride *on previous page*

Dopamine Hydrochloride (doe' pa meen)

Related Information

Adrenergic Agonists, Cardiovascular Comparison *on page 1638*

Adrenergic Agonists Drug Infusions Comparison *on page 1638*

CAS Number 51-61-6; 62-31-7

Brand Names Dopastat®; Giludop®; Inovan®; Intropin®; Revivan®

Synonyms 3-Hydroxytyramine

Replaces ASL 279

Use Adjunct in the treatment of shock which persists after adequate fluid volume replacement; dose-related inotropic and vasopressor effects; stimulates dopaminergic, beta- and alpha-receptors; increased renal blood flow at low to moderate doses; useful for antidysrhythmia, antihistamine, arsenic, beta-adrenergic blocking agents, calcium channel blockers, phenytoin, sedative-hypnotic, clonidine, cholinergic agents, opioids, or magnesium-induced hypotension

Antidote Useful For

Autumn Crocus *on page 1054*

Copper *on page 896*

Dantrolene Sodium *on page 258*

Ethchlorvynol *on page 330*

Mushrooms, Toxic (Group III) *on page 1112*

Torsemide *on page 761*

Mechanism of Action Stimulates both adrenergic and dopaminergic receptors, lower doses are mainly dopaminergic stimulating and produces renal and mesenteric vasodilation, higher doses also are both dopaminergic and beta$_1$-adrenergic and produces cardiac stimulation and renal vasodilation, large doses stimulate alpha-adrenergic receptors. A metabolic precursor to norepinephrine.

Adverse Reactions

Cardiovascular: Ectopic heartbeats, tachycardia, vasoconstriction, hypotension, cardiac conduction abnormalities, widened QRS complex, bradycardia, hypertension, ventricular arrhythmias, gangrene of the extremities (with high doses for prolonged periods or even with low doses in patients with occlusive vascular disease), palpitations, facial flushing

Central nervous system: Anxiety, headache, dizziness, vertigo, piloerection

Gastrointestinal: Nausea, vomiting

Ocular: Mydriasis

Renal: Decreased urine output, azotemia

Respiratory: Dyspnea

Signs & Symptoms of Acute Overdose Fixed, dilated pupils, tachycardia, severe hypertension

Toxicodynamics/Kinetics

Children: With medication changes, may not achieve steady-state for ~1 hour rather than 20 minutes

Adults:

Onset of action: 5 minutes

Duration: <10 minutes

Metabolism: In the plasma, kidneys, and liver 75% to inactive metabolites by monoamine oxidase and 25% to norepinephrine (active)

Half-life: 2 minutes

Elimination: Metabolites are excreted in the urine; neonatal clearance varies and appears to be age related; clearance is more prolonged with combined hepatic and renal dysfunction

Dopamine has exhibited nonlinear kinetics in children

Usual Dosage I.V. infusion:

Neonates: 1-20 mcg/kg/minute continuous infusion, titrate to desired response

Children: 1-20 mcg/kg/minute, maximum: 50 mcg/kg/minute continuous infusion, titrate to desired response

Adults: 1-5 mcg/kg/minute up to 50 mcg/kg/minute, titrate to desired response; infusion may be increased by 1-4 mcg/kg/minute at 10- to 30-minute intervals until optimal response is obtained

If dosages >20-30 mcg/kg/minute are needed, a more direct-acting pressor may be more beneficial (ie, epinephrine, norepinephrine)

The hemodynamic effects of dopamine are dose-dependent:

Low-dose: 1-5 mcg/kg/minute, increased renal blood flow and urine output

Intermediate-dose: 5-15 mcg/kg/minute, increased renal blood flow, heart rate, cardiac contractility, and cardiac output

High-dose: >15 mcg/kg/minute, alpha-adrenergic effects begin to predominate, vasoconstriction, increased blood pressure

Administration Administer into large vein to prevent the possibility of extravasation; use infusion device to control rate of flow; due to short half-life withdrawal of drug is often only necessary treatment

Extravasation: Use phentolamine as antidote; mix 5 mg with 9 mL of normal saline; inject a small amount of this dilution into extravasated area; blanching should reverse immediately. Monitor site; if blanching should recur, additional injections of phentolamine may be needed.

Contraindications Hypersensitivity to sulfites (commercial preparation contains sodium bisulfite); pheochromocytoma, or ventricular fibrillation

Warnings Potent drug; must be diluted prior to use. Patient's hemodynamic status should be monitored; patients with peripheral vascular disease may develop gangrene. Not effective for hypotension induced by ethanol-disulfiram interaction; avoid tricyclic antidepressants; alpha$_1$-adrenergic antagonist, phenothiazine, or hydrocarbon toxicity.

Dosage Forms

Infusion, in D_5W: 0.8 mg/mL (250 mL, 500 mL); 1.6 mg/mL (250 mL, 500 mL); 3.2 mg/mL (250 mL, 500 mL)

Injection: 40 mg/mL (5 mL, 10 mL, 20 mL); 80 mg/mL (5 mL, 20 mL); 160 mg/mL (5 mL)

Stability Protect from light; solutions that are darker than slightly yellow should not be used; incompatible with alkaline solutions or iron salts; compatible when coadministered with dobutamine, epinephrine, isoproterenol, and lidocaine

Drug Interactions Dopamine's effects are prolonged and intensified by MAO inhibitors, alpha- and beta-adrenergic blockers, general anesthetics, phenytoin. Paradoxical hypotension can develop when tolazoline is also given; concomitant use with ergometrine can cause gangrene.

Pregnancy Risk Factor C

Pregnancy Implications Not known if it crosses the placenta

Monitoring Parameters Potassium, glucose, blood pressure, EKG, heart rate, CVP, RAP, MAP, urine output; if pulmonary artery catheter is in place, monitor CI, PCWP, SVR, and PVR

Nursing Implications Monitor continuously for free flow

Extravasation: Use phentolamine as antidote; mix 5 mg with 9 mL of normal saline; inject a small amount of this dilution into extravasated area; blanching should reverse immediately. Monitor site; if blanching should recur, additional injections of phentolamine may be needed.

Additional Information Phentolamine can be used for the treatment of hypertension or tissue necrosis due to extravasation of dopamine; compatible with heparin, lidocaine, potassium chloride, and calcium chloride

Specific References

Bania TC, Sauter D, and Hoffman RS, "Management of Hemodynamic Compromise in the Poisoned Patient. Contemporary Management in Critical Care," *Crit Care Toxicol*, 1991, 1(3):179-202.

Chan TYK, "Low-Dose Dopamine in Severe Right Heart Failure and Chronic Obstructive Pulmonary Disease," *Ann Pharmacother*, 1995, 29:493-6.

Papazian MC, Perrin G, et al, "Norepinephrine or Dopamine for the Treatment of Hyperdynamic Septic Shock?" *Chest*, 1993, 103:1826-31.

Strauss R, "Accidental Dopamine in the Eye," *West J Med*, 1985, 142(3):397-8.

Dopastat® *see* Dopamine Hydrochloride *on previous page*

Dormin® Oral [OTC] *see* Diphenhydramine Hydrochloride *on page 1415*

D-Penamine® *see* Penicillamine *on page 1454*

D-Penicillamine *see* Penicillamine *on page 1454*

DPTA: Pentetic Acid *see* Diethylene Triamine Penta-acetic Acid *on page 1411*

Drugs and Chemicals Proven to be Teratogenic in Humans *see page 1572*

DTC *see* Diethyldithiocarbamate Trihydrate *on page 1410*

DTPA *see* Diethylene Triamine Penta-acetic Acid *on page 1411*

Edathamil Disodium *see* Edetate Disodium *on page 1421*

Edetate Calcium Disodium (ed' e tate)

CAS Number 23411-34-9; 62-33-9

Brand Names Calcium Disodium Versenate®; Calcium Edetate-Heyl®; Chelante®; Chelintox®; Ledclair®

Synonyms Calcium EDTA; Sodium Calcium Edetate

Use Treatment of acute and chronic lead, manganese, scandium, lanthanum, plutonium, or zinc poisoning; an aid in the diagnosis of lead poisoning

Investigational: Cholelitholytic agent (through biliary duct infusion) for pigment bile duct stones

Antidote Useful For

Cobalt *on page 895*

Copper *on page 896*

Hexachlorobenzene *on page 936*

Lead *on page 945*

Manganese *on page 952*

Mechanism of Action Calcium is displaced by divalent and trivalent heavy metals, forming a nonionizing soluble complex that is excreted in urine

Adverse Reactions

Cardiovascular: Hypotension, arrhythmias, EKG changes

Central nervous system: Numbness, tingling, fever, headache, chills

Dermatologic: Skin lesions, exfoliative dermatitis, dermatitis

Endocrine & metabolic: Hypercalcemia

Gastrointestinal: GI upset, diarrhea

Hematologic: Transient marrow suppression

Local: Pain at injection site following I.M. injection, thrombophlebitis following I.V. infusion (when concentration >5 mg/mL)

Ocular: Lacrimation

Renal: Renal tubular necrosis (3%), proteinuria, microscopic hematuria

Respiratory: Sneezing, nasal congestion

Miscellaneous: Chills

Toxicodynamics/Kinetics

Distribution: Into extracellular fluid

Metabolism: Not metabolized

Elimination: Rapid in urine; urinary excretion of chelated lead begins in 1 hour and peak excretion of chelated lead occurs within 24-48 hours

Usual Dosage

Children: I.M. (preferred route of administration as rapid I.V. infusion may be lethal), I.V., S.C.:

Asymptomatic lead poisoning: (Blood lead concentration >55 μg/dL or blood lead concentrations of 25-55 μg/dL with blood erythrocyte protoporphyrin concentrations ≥35 μg/dL and positive mobilization test) or **symptomatic lead poisoning without encephalopathy** with lead level <100 μg/dL: 1 g/m^2/day I.M./I.V. in divided doses every 8-12 hours for 3-5 days (usually 5 days) with dimercaprol; maximum: 1 g/24 hours or 50 mg/kg/day

Symptomatic lead poisoning with encephalopathy with lead level >100 μg/dL (treatment with calcium EDTA and dimercaprol is preferred): 250 mg/m^2 I.M. or intermittent I.V. infusion 4 hours after dimercaprol, then at 4-hour intervals thereafter for 5 days (1.5 g/m^2/day); dose (1.5 g/m^2/day) can also be given as a single I.V. continuous infusion over 12-24 hours/day for 5 days; maximum: 1 g/24 hours or 75 mg/kg/day

Note: Course of therapy may be repeated in 2-3 weeks until blood lead level is normal

Adults: Treatment: I.M., I.V.: 2-4 g/day or 1.5 g/m^2/day in divided doses every 12-24 hours for 5 days; may repeat course one time after at least 2 days (usually after 2 weeks) not more than 2 courses of therapy are recommended

Dosing adjustment/comments in renal impairment: Calcium disodium EDTA is almost exclusively eliminated in urine and should not be administered during periods of anuria

Administration For intermittent I.V. infusion, administer the dose I.V. over at least 1 hour in asymptomatic patients, 2 hours in symptomatic patients; for I.V. continuous infusion, dilute to 2-4 mg/mL in D_5W or normal saline and infuse over at least 8 hours, usually over 12-24 hours; for I.M. injection, 1 mL of 1% procaine hydrochloride may be added to each mL of EDTA calcium to minimize pain at injection site

Contraindications Severe renal disease, anuria

Warnings Potentially nephrotoxic; monitor BUN, creatinine, urinalysis, I & O during therapy; acidosis (renal tubular) and fatal nephrosis may occur, especially with high doses; EKG changes may occur during therapy; do not exceed recommended daily dose; avoid rapid I.V. infusion in the management of lead encephalopathy, may increase intracranial pressure to lethal levels. If anuria, increasing proteinuria, or hematuria occurs during therapy, discontinue calcium EDTA. Can also chelate zinc and iron.

Dosage Forms Injection: 200 mg/mL (5 mL)

Stability Dilute with 0.9% sodium chloride or D_5W; physically **incompatible** with $D_{10}W$, lactated Ringer's, Ringer's

Test Interactions If calcium EDTA is given as a continuous I.V. infusion, stop the infusion for at least 1 hour before blood is drawn for lead concentration to avoid a falsely elevated value

Drug Interactions Do not use simultaneously with zinc insulin preparations, do not mix in the same syringe with dimercaprol

Pregnancy Risk Factor C

Monitoring Parameters BUN, creatinine, urinalysis, I & O, and EKG during therapy

Specific References

Moel DI and Kumar K, "Reversible Nephrotic Reactions to a Combined 2,3-Dimercapto-1-propanol and Calcium Disodium Ethylenediaminetetraacetic Acid Regimen in Asymptomatic Children With Elevated Blood Lead Levels," *Pediatrics*, 1982, 70(2):259-62.

Osterloh J and Becker CE, "Pharmacokinetics of $CaNa_2$ EDTA and Chelation of Lead in Renal Failure," *Clin Pharmacol Ther*, 1986, 40(6):686-93.

Edetate Disodium (ed' e tate)

CAS Number 139-33-3; 6381-92-6; 150-38-9 (Trisodium Edetate)

Brand Names Chealamide®; Disotate®; Endrate®; Limclair®; Murine®; Tracémate®

Synonyms Edathamil Disodium; EDTA; Sodium Edetate

Use Emergency treatment of hypercalcemia; also used as contact lens cleaner; also used as a 0.05 molar topical solution for alkali ocular exposure due to calcium hydroxide (lime) from motor or cement exposures; also chelates lead, copper, manganese, zinc, lanthanum, plutonium, scandium, or yttrium; useful in treating extravasation due to mithramycin

Mechanism of Action Chelates with divalent or trivalent metals to form a soluble complex that is then eliminated in urine

Adverse Reactions

Cardiovascular: Arrhythmias, transient hypotension

Central nervous system: Seizures, numbness, fever, headache, chills

Dermatologic: Skin eruptions, exfoliative dermatitis, dermatitis, dermatologic lesions

Endocrine & metabolic: Hypocalcemic tetany, hypomagnesemia, hypokalemia

Gastrointestinal: Nausea, vomiting, abdominal cramps, diarrhea

Hematologic: Anemia

Local: Pain at the site of injection, thrombophlebitis

Neuromuscular & skeletal: Back pain, muscle cramps, paresthesia

Renal: Nephrotoxicity, acute tubular necrosis

Respiratory: Death from respiratory arrest

Miscellaneous: Chills

Toxicodynamics/Kinetics

Metabolism: Not metabolized

Half-life: 20-60 minutes

Elimination: Following chelation, 95% excreted in urine as chelates within 24-48 hours

Usual Dosage Hypercalcemia: I.V.:

Children: 40-70 mg/kg/day slow infusion over 3-4 hours or more to a maximum of 3 g/24 hours; administer for 5 days and allow 5 days between courses of therapy

Adults: 50 mg/kg/day over 3 or more hours to a maximum of 3 g/24 hours; a suggested regimen of 5 days followed by 2 days without drug and repeated courses up to 15 total doses

Mithramycin extravasation: 150 mg of sodium edetate either through offending I.V. catheter of through multiple S.C. injections; apply ice to affected area

Administration Must be diluted before use in 500 mL D_5W or normal saline to <30 mg/mL

Contraindications Severe renal failure or anuria

Warnings Monitor cardiac function (EKG monitoring), blood pressure during infusion; renal function should be assessed before and during therapy; monitor calcium, magnesium, potassium levels; use of this drug is recommended only when the severity of the clinical condition justifies the aggressive measures associated with this type of therapy. Use with caution in patients with intracranial lesions, seizure disorders, coronary or peripheral vascular disease, or patients with tuberculosis.

Dosage Forms Injection: 150 mg/mL (20 mL)

Drug Interactions May decrease blood glucose concentrations and reduce insulin requirements in diabetic patients treated with insulin

Pregnancy Risk Factor C

Monitoring Parameters Serum calcium

Nursing Implications Avoid extravasation; patient should remain supine for a short period after infusion

Additional Information Sodium content of 1 g: 5.4 mEq

Specific References

Committee on Drugs, American Academy of Pediatrics, "Treatment Guidelines for Lead Exposure in Children," *Pediatrics*, 1995, 96:155-60.

MacCara ME, "Extravasation – A Hazard of Intravenous Therapy," *Drug Intell Clin Pharm*, 1983, 17:713.

(Continued)

Edetate Disodium *(Continued)*

Pfister RR, "Chemical Injuries of the Eye," *Ophthalmology*, 1983, 90(10):1246-53.

EDTA *see* Edetate Disodium *on previous page*

Electrolyte Lavage Solution *see* Polyethylene Glycol *on page 1460*

Endrate® *see* Edetate Disodium *on previous page*

Epinephrine (ep i nef' rin)

Related Information

Adrenergic Agonists, Cardiovascular Comparison *on page 1638*
Adrenergic Agonists Drug Infusions Comparison *on page 1638*
Insect Sting Kit *on page 1434*

CAS Number 51-43-4

Brand Names Adrenalin® Chloride; AsthmaHaler® Mist [OTC]; AsthmaNefrin® [OTC]; Bronitin® Mist [OTC]; Bronkaid® Mist [OTC]; EpiPen®; EpiPen® Jr; Medihaler-Epi® [OTC]; microNefrin® [OTC]; Primatene® Mist [OTC]; S-2® [OTC]; Sus-Phrine®; Vaponefrin® [OTC]

Use Bronchospasms, anaphylactic reactions, bradycardia, cardiac arrest, management of open-angle (chronic simple) glaucoma, hypotension, allergic reactions to antivenin, specifically improved mortality secondary to chloroquine overdose

Antidote Useful For

Autumn Crocus *on page 1054*
Chloroquine Phosphate *on page 202*
Fire Ants *on page 1084*
Penicillin G, Parenteral, Aqueous *on page 600*
Sulfite Food Poisoning *on page 1148*
Tartrazine Food Poisoning *on page 1149*
Zileuton *on page 811*

Mechanism of Action Stimulates alpha-adrenergic, $beta_1$- and $beta_2$-adrenergic receptors; small doses can causes vasodilation via $beta_2$ vascular receptors; decreases production of aqueous humor and increases aqueous outflow; dilates the pupil by contracting the dilator muscle

Adverse Reactions

Cardiovascular: Pallor, tachycardia, hypertension, myocardial oxygen consumption (increased), cardiac arrhythmias, sudden death, chest pain
Central nervous system: Anxiety, headache
Endocrine & metabolic: Lactic acidosis
Gastrointestinal: Nausea
Local: Tissue ischemia and necrosis with extravasation; allergic reactions
Neuromuscular & skeletal: Weakness
Ocular: Precipitation of or exacerbation of narrow-angle glaucoma
Renal: Decreased renal and splanchnic blood flow, hyperglycemia, acute urinary retention in patients with bladder outflow obstruction

Signs & Symptoms of Acute Overdose Hypertension which may result in subarachnoid hemorrhage and hemiplegia; cardiac arrhythmias, unusually large pupils, pulmonary edema, renal failure, metabolic acidosis, hyperglycemia

Toxicodynamics/Kinetics

Onset of action:
- Inhalation: Within 1 minute
- S.C.: Within 3-5 minutes

Following conjunctival instillation intraocular pressures fall within 1 hour with a maximal response occurring within 4-8 hours; ocular effects persist for 12-24 hours
Absorption: Absorbed well; rapid and prolonged following administration of aqueous suspension
Distribution: Does not cross blood-brain barrier; distributes throughout the body
Metabolism: Following administration, drug is taken up into the adrenergic neuron and metabolized by monoamine oxidase and catechol-o-methyltransferase, circulating drug is metabolized in the liver; inactive metabolites (metanephrine and the sulfate and hydroxy derivatives of mandelic acid)
Elimination: Small amount of unchanged drug excreted in urine

Usual Dosage

Children:
- Bronchodilator: S.C.: 10 mcg/kg (0.01 mL/kg of 1:1000) (single doses not to exceed 0.5 mg); injection suspension (1:200): 0.005 mL/kg/dose (0.025 mg/kg/dose) to a maximum of 0.15 mL (0.75 mg for single dose) every 6 hours
- Cardiac arrest:
  - Neonates: I.V. or intratracheal: 0.01-0.03 mg/kg (0.1-0.3 mL/kg) of 1:10,000 solution every 3-5 minutes as needed
  - Children: 0.01 mg/kg (0.1 mL/kg) of 1:10,000 solution (to maximum 5 mL) every 3-5 minutes as needed

Refractory hypotension (refractory to dopamine/dobutamine): Children: Infusion rate 0.1-4 mcg/kg/minute

Start infusion 0.1 mcg/kg/minute, titrate to desired effect

Hypersensitivity reaction: S.C.: 0.01 mg/kg every 15 minutes for 2 doses then every 4 hours as needed (single doses not to exceed 0.5 mg)

Nebulization:

Children <2 years: 0.25 mL of 1:1000 diluted in 3 mL normal saline with treatments ordered individually

Children >2 years and Adolescents: 0.5 mL of 1:1000 concentration diluted in 3 mL normal saline

Children >2 years and Adults (racemic epinephrine):

<10 kg: 2 mL of 1:8 dilution over 15 minutes every 1-4 hours

10-15 kg: 2 mL of 1:6 dilution over 15 minutes every 1-4 hours

15-20 kg: 2 mL of 1:4 dilution over 15 minutes every 1-4 hours

>20 kg: 2 mL of 1:3 dilution over 15 minutes every 1-4 hours

Adults:

Bronchodilator:

I.M., S.C. (1:1000): 0.1-0.5 mg every 10-15 minutes to 4 hours

I.V.: 0.1-0.25 mg (single dose maximum 1 mg)

Suspension (1:200) S.C.: 0.1-0.3 mL (0.5-1.5 mg)

Nebulizer: Instill 8-15 drops into nebulizer reservoirs; administer 1-3 inhalations 4-6 times/day

Cardiac arrest:

I.V.: Intermediate dose: 2-5 mg every 3-5 minutes; escalating dose: 1 mg – 3 mg – 5 mg, 3 minutes apart; high dose: 0.1 mg/kg I.V. push every 3-5 minutes; each dose given by peripheral injection should be followed by a 20 mL flush of I.V. fluid

I.V., intracardiac: 0.1-1 mg (1-10 mL of 1:10,000 dilution) every 3-5 minutes as needed

Intratracheal: 1 mg; higher doses (0.1 mg/kg every 3-5 minutes) should be considered, but only after 1 mg doses have failed

Hypotension: I.V. infusion: 1 mg in 250 mL NS/D_5W at 1-4 mcg/minute

Hypersensitivity reaction: I.M., S.C.: 0.2-0.5 mg every 20 minutes to 4 hours (single dose maximum: 1 mg)

Intranasal: Children ≥6 years and Adults: Apply locally as drops or spray or with sterile swab

Contraindications Hypersensitivity to epinephrine or any component (particularly sulfites); cardiac arrhythmias; angle-closure glaucoma

Warnings Rapid I.V. infusion may cause death from cerebrovascular hemorrhage or cardiac arrhythmias; often preserved with sulfites

Dosage Forms

Aerosol, oral:

Bitartrate (AsthmaHaler® Mist, Bronitin® Mist, Medihaler-Epi®, Primatene® Mist Suspension): 0.3 mg/spray [epinephrine base 0.16 mg/spray] (10 mL, 15 mL, 22.5 mL)

Bronkaid® Mist: 0.5% (10 mL, 15 mL, 22.5 mL)

Primatene® Mist: 0.2 mg/spray (15 mL, 22.5 mL)

Emergency kit, auto-injector:

EpiPen®: Delivers 0.3 mg I.M. of epinephrine 1:1000 (2 mL)

EpiPen® Jr.: Delivers 0.15 mg I.M. of epinephrine 1:2000 (2 mL)

Solution:

Inhalation:

Adrenalin®: 1% [10 mg/mL – 1:100] (7.5 mL)

AsthmaNefrin®, microNefrin®, Nephron®, Racepinephrine®, S-2®: Racepinephrine 2.25% [epinephrine base 1.125%] (7.5 mL, 15 mL, 30 mL)

Vaponefrin®: Racepinephrine 2% [epinephrine base 1%] (15 mL, 30 mL)

Injection: 0.01 mg/mL [1:100,000] (5 mL); 0.1 mg/mL [1:10,000] (3 mL, 10 mL); 1 mg/mL [1:1000] (1 mL, 2 mL, 30 mL)

Adrenalin®: 1 mg/mL [1:1000] (1 mL, 30 mL)

Nasal (Adrenalin®): 0.1% [1 mg/mL – 1:1000] (30 mL)

Topical (Adrenalin®): 0.1% [1 mg/mL, 1:1000] (30 mL, 10 mL)

Suspension for injection (Sus-Phrine®): 5 mg/mL [1:200] (0.3 mL, 5 mL)

Stability Protect from light, oxidation turns drug pink, then a brown color; solutions should not be used if they are discolored or contain a precipitate; stability of injection of parenteral admixture at room temperature and refrigeration: 24 hours; unstable in alkaline solution; do not use D_5W as a diluent; D_5W is incompatible with epinephrine

Reference Range Therapeutic: 31-95 pg/mL (SI: 170-520 pmol/L); norepinephrine level of 438 pg/mL associated with myocardial ischemia in children

Test Interactions Increases bilirubin (S), catecholamines (U), glucose, uric acid (S)

(Continued)

Epinephrine *(Continued)*

Drug Interactions Increased cardiac irritability if administered concurrently with halogenated inhalational anesthetics; in presence of beta-blockers, an exaggerated increase in blood pressure can occur; avoid if possible concomitant infusion with sodium bicarbonate

Pregnancy Risk Factor C

Pregnancy Implications Crosses the placenta; appears in breast milk

Monitoring Parameters Heart rate, blood pressure

Nursing Implications Protect from light; oxidation turns dark pink, then brown – solutions should not be used if they are discolored or contain a precipitate. Epinephrine is unstable in alkaline solution.

Extravasation: Use phentolamine as antidote; mix 5 mg with 9 mL of normal saline; inject a small amount of this dilution into extravasated area; blanching should reverse immediately. Monitor site; if blanching should recur, additional injections of phentolamine may be needed.

Specific References

Davis C and Wax P, "Subcutaneous Epinephrine O.D. in a Child Resulting in Dysrhythmias and Myocardial Ischemia," *Vet Hum Toxicol*, 1994, 36:367.

Klein JS, Rich MR, and Yunginger JW, "Myocardial Ischemia Without Coronary Artery Disease After Epinephrine Overdose for Insect Sting Reaction," *J Allergy Clin Immunol*, 1995, 95(2):371.

Kuracheck SC and Rockoff MA, "Inadvertent Intravenous Administration of Racemic Epinephrine," *JAMA*, 1984, 253(10):1441-2.

Murphy FT, Manown TJ, Knuttson SW, et al, "Epinephrine-Induced Lactic Acidosis in the Setting of Status Asthmaticus," *South Med J*, 1995, 88:577-9.

Nicholson KE and Rogers JE, "Cocaine and Adrenaline Paste: A Fatal Combination?," *Br Med J*, 1995, 311:250-1.

Riou B, Barriot P, Rimailho A, et al, "Treatment of Severe Chloroquine Poisoning," *N Engl J Med*, 1988, 318(1):1-6.

EpiPen® *see* Epinephrine *on page 1422*

EpiPen® Jr *see* Epinephrine *on page 1422*

Ethanol

Related Information

Ethanol and Blood Alcohol Determination *on page 1176-1179*

Commonly Includes Whiskey; Vodka

Use Antidotal therapy for methanol and ethylene glycol intoxication

Antidote Useful For

Ethylene Glycol *on page 925*

Methanol *on page 957*

Mechanism of Action Competitive antagonism with methanol and ethylene glycol as substrate alcohol dehydrogenase; the interaction thereby results in decreased formation of toxic metabolites and metabolic acidosis

Adverse Reactions

Cardiovascular: Postural hypotension, palpitations, hypotension (orthostatic)

Central nervous system: Inebriation, sedation, coma

Endocrine and metabolic: Hypoglycemia

Gastrointestinal: Nausea, vomiting, gastritis

Respiratory: Respiratory sedation

Miscellaneous: Osmolal gap

Toxicodynamics/Kinetics Specific gravity: 0.79 g/mL

Usual Dosage

Oral: Loading dose: 1 g/kg (may be diluted in juice), then for maintenance: 0.1 g/kg/hour (in nondrinkers) or 0.2 g/kg/hour (in a chronic drinker); on dialysis, double the maintenance dose

I.V.: Administer 750 mg/kg as a loading dose, followed by 100-150 mg/hour; increase to 175-200 mg/kg in chronic alcoholics, or during hemodialysis; see table.

	5% I.V.	**10% I.V.**	**50% P.O.**
Loading	15 mL/kg	7.5 mL/kg	1.5 mL/kg
Maintenance	2–4 mL/kg	1–2 mL/kg	0.2–0.4 mL/kg/h
Maintenance during hemolysis	4–7 mL/kg	2–3.5 mL/kg	0.4–0.7 mL/kg/h

Contraindications Concurrent administration of CNS depressants or of drugs causing disulfiram-like reaction including disulfiram, chlorpropamide, metronidazole, etc

Warnings In the event of too rapid a loading or maintenance dose, slow the infusion; monitor blood glucose throughout the treatment interval

Dosage Forms 5% ethanol in 5% dextrose in water, 1000 mL for parenteral use; 10% ethanol in 5% dextrose in water, 1000 mL for parenteral use; vodka or whiskey for oral consumption (40% to 50% ethanol for oral use)

Pregnancy Risk Factor C

Pregnancy Implications Use only if the potential benefits outweigh the risks; ethanol crosses the placenta readily and enters fetal circulation

Monitoring Parameters Respiration rate, blood pressure

Nursing Implications Patients receiving ethanol by infusion or mouth, may become obtunded and inebriated; they may pose health hazards to themselves and others and should be cared for in a carefully monitored environment

Additional Information Desired blood concentration of ethanol for methanol or ethylene glycol intoxication is 100 mg/dL, or a 1:4 ratio of ethanol to ethylene glycol or methanol; ethanol exhibits zero order kinetics, with healthy, nondrinking volunteers clearing approximately 15 mg/dL/hour; ethanol clearance may also be enhanced by hemodialysis; contribution of a serum concentration level of 100 mg/dL to elevation of osmolar gap: 22

Specific References

Fuchs CS, Stampfer MJ, Colditz GA, et al, "Alcohol Consumption and Mortality Among Women," *N Engl J Med*, 1995, 332:1245-50.

Jacobsen D and McMartin KE, "Methanol and Ethylene Glycol Poisonings: Mechanism of Toxicity, Clinical Course, Diagnosis and Treatment," *Med Toxicol*, 1986, 1(5):309-34.

Jones AW, "Measuring Ethanol in Saliva With the QED® Enzymatic Test Device: Comparison of Results With Blood- and Breath-Alcohol Concentrations," *J Anal Toxicol*, 1995, 19:169-74.

Peterson CD, "Oral Ethanol Doses in Patients With Methanol Poisoning," *Am J Hosp Pharm*, 1981, 38(7):1024-7.

Rembert AM, Sklar DP, Cutler PV, et al, "Two Point Discrimination in Ethanol Intoxicated Patients," *Acad Emerg Med*, 1995, 2:464.

Tamaszewski C, Cline DM, Whitley TW, et al, "Effect of Acute Ethanol Ingestion on Orthostatic Vital Signs," *Ann Emerg Med*, 1995, 25:636-41.

Ethanol and Blood Alcohol Determination *see page 1176*

Eumydrin® *see* Atropine Sulfate *on page 1395*

Evac-Q-Mag® [OTC] *see* Magnesium Citrate *on page 1439*

Exomuc® *see* Acetylcysteine *on page 1388*

Eyesule® *see* Atropine Sulfate *on page 1395*

Filgrastim (fil gra' stim)

Brand Names Neupogen® Injection

Synonyms G-CSF; Granulocyte Colony Stimulating Factor

Use These guidelines were created in August 1992 and reflect the consensus of the expert panel of clinicians from University Hospital Consortium (UHC) member institutions with expertise in the use of colony-stimulating factors. The agents considered appropriate for each indication is included in parenthesis (G-CSF: Filgrastim; GM-CSF: Sargramostim)

Decrease incidence of and to prevent infection as manifested by febrile neutropenia following myelosuppressive chemotherapy in nonmyeloid malignancies (G-CSF)

Myeloid reconstitution after autologous bone marrow transplantation (G/GM-CSF)

Bone marrow transplantation engraftment failure or delay (GM-CSF)

Chronic neutropenia, including cyclic, idiopathic, and congenital neutropenia (G-CSF)

Peripheral stem cell harvesting prior to bone marrow transplantation (G/GM-CSF)

Allogeneic bone marrow transplantation

AIDS drug-induced neutropenia (ie, zidovudine and ganciclovir) with ANC <500 x 10^6 cells/L (G/GM-CSF)

Aplastic anemia with ANC <500 x 10^6 cells/L and history of at least one documented serious infection requiring antibiotic therapy (G/GM-CSF)

Myelodysplastic syndrome in a clinical trial protocol; or when there is no access to a clinical trial, with blasts <25%, ANC <500 x 10^6 cells/L, and a history of at least one documented serious infection requiring antibiotic therapy (G/GM-CSF)

Unproven uses:

Treatment of established febrile neutropenia (eg, with infection)

Peripheral stem cell transplantation

Inappropriate uses:

Neutropenia associated with the AIDS disease process

Non-neutropenic infectious disease

Burns

(Continued)

Filgrastim *(Continued)*

Extensive surgery
Chemotherapy dose intensification outside clinical trial protocol

Antidote Useful For

Clozapine *on page 235*
Colchicine *on page 240*
Zidovudine *on page 807*

Mechanism of Action Stimulates the production, maturation, and activation of neutrophils, G-CSF activates neutrophils to increase both their migration and cytotoxicity. Natural proteins which stimulate hematopoietic stem cells to proliferate, prolong cell survival, stimulate cell differentiation, and stimulate functional activity of mature cells. CSFs are produced by a wide variety of cell types. Specific mechanisms of action are not yet fully understood, but possibly work by a second-messenger pathway with resultant protein production. Specific activity: 1 x 10^8 units/mg; neutrophil production rate increases 9.4-fold.

Adverse Reactions

Cardiovascular: Chest pain, transient supraventricular arrhythmia, pericarditis, fluid retention
Central nervous system: Fever, headache
Dermatologic: Alopecia, skin rash
Gastrointestinal: Nausea, vomiting, diarrhea, anorexia, stomatitis, constipation
Neuromuscular & skeletal: Skeletal pain, weakness
Respiratory: Dyspnea, cough, sore throat, mucositis
Miscellaneous: Neutropenic fever, pain at injection site, leukocytosis, anaphylactic reaction, lymphoma, thrombophlebitis, thrombocytopenia

Toxicodynamics/Kinetics

Onset of action: Rapid elevation in neutrophil counts within the first 24 hours, reaching a plateau in 3-5 days; immature neutrophils (bands) may be elevated within 1 hour
Duration: ANC decreases by 50% within 2 days after discontinuing G-CSF; white counts return to the normal range in 4-7 days
Absorption: S.C.: 100%; peak plasma levels can be maintained for up to 12 hours
Distribution: V_d: 0.15 L/kg; no evidence of drug accumulation over a 11- to 20-day period
Metabolism: Systemic
Bioavailability: Oral: Not bioavailable
Half-life: 1.3-7.2 hours (longer with doses exceeding 10 mcg/kg)
Time to peak serum concentration: S.C.: Within 2-6 hours

Usual Dosage Children and Adults:

Initial dosing recommendations: 5 mcg/kg/day administered S.C. or I.V. as a single daily infusion over 20-30 minutes

Doses may be increased in increments of 5 mcg/kg for each chemotherapy cycle, according to the duration and severity of the absolute neutrophil count (ANC) nadir. In phase III trials, efficacy was observed at doses of 4-6 mcg/kg/day. Discontinue therapy if the ANC count is >10,000/mm³ after the ANC nadir has occurred.

Length of therapy:

Bone marrow transplant patients: G-CSF should be administered daily for up to 30 days, until the ANC has reached 1000/mm³ for 3 consecutive days following the expected chemotherapy-induced neutrophil nadir.

Chemotherapy-treated patients: G-CSF may be administered daily for up to 2 weeks until the ANC has reached 10,000/mm³ following the expected chemotherapy-induced neutrophil nadir. Duration of therapy needed to attenuate chemotherapy-induced neutropenia may be dependent on the myelosuppressive potential of the chemotherapy regimen employed. Duration of therapy in clinical studies has ranged from 2 weeks to 3 years. Safety and efficacy of chronic administration have not been established.

Premature discontinuation of G-CSF therapy prior to the time of recovery from the expected neutrophil is generally not recommended. A transient increase in neutrophil counts is typically seen 1-2 days after initiation of therapy.

Colchicine overdose: Daily doses of 300 mg S.C. for 5 days has been used in adults

Administration The UHC Colony-Stimulating Factors Expert Panel has made the following clinical and administrative recommendations:

Clinical:

Very few data are available to support the therapeutic interchangeability of G-CSF and GM-CSF. On the basis of the panel's clinical experience and in the absence of conclusive data, interchangeability is acceptable in limited situations, as indicated in the UHC CSF guidelines.

For most indications, an ANC of <500 x 10^6 cells/L can be recommended as a starting point for the initiation of therapy. Stopping CSF therapy is based on a biologic endpoint, and the panel felt that CSF therapy could be discontinued in most patients at an ANC ≥5000 x 10^6 cells/L, depending on the expected nadir of chemotherapy. Several panel members suggested an ANC endpoint to CSF therapy at 2000 x 10^6 cells/L.

Food and Drug Administration labeling recommends daily dosing of G-CSF at 5 mcg/kg, but panel members felt that doses as low as 2 mcg/kg might be effective for some indications. Daily doses of >10 mcg/kg were considered not appropriate for any chemotherapy regimens. Overall, CSF dosing on the basis of patient weight has not been well studied.

In general, patients should not receive CSFs with their first cycle of cancer chemotherapy. Patients who have previously demonstrated febrile neutropenia following chemotherapy or have had a previous positive response to CSF therapy following chemotherapy would be appropriate for CSF therapy.

Certain chemotherapeutic regimens may warrant CSF use for every patient. These clinical situations should be determined at each UHC member institution. Some examples cited by the panel include patients in the following categories: adult acute lymphocytic leukemia, induction therapy; previously radiated Hodgkin's disease; previous pelvic radiation; adjuvant breast cancer chemotherapy (to avoid any treatment delays caused by neutropenia); and AIDS lymphoma treatment with myelosuppressive chemotherapy.

Administrative:

CSF guidelines developed by an institution for inpatient use should apply to the outpatient setting

Several examples of strategies for CSF cost-containment were offered by the panel, including requiring blood count results prior to dispensing CSF doses; strictly enforced inpatient and outpatient use guidelines; institutional reimbursement precertification for CSF patients; accessing pharmaceutical company reimbursement assistance/indigent programs; forming biotechnology review committees; and dosing based on vial size, rather than on a mcg/kg basis, using the smallest vial size that is clinically acceptable.

Contraindications Hypersensitivity to *E. coli* derived proteins or G-CSF

Warnings Complete blood count and platelet count should be obtained prior to chemotherapy. Do not use G-CSF in the period 24 hours before to 24 hours after administration of cytotoxic chemotherapy because of the potential sensitivity of rapidly dividing myeloid cells to cytotoxic chemotherapy. Precaution should be exercised in the usage of G-CSF in any malignancy with myeloid characteristics. G-CSF can potentially act as a growth factor for any tumor type, particularly myeloid malignancies. Tumors of nonhematopoietic origin may have surface receptors for G-CSF.

Dosage Forms Injection, preservative free: 300 mcg/mL (1 mL, 1.6 mL)

Stability Store at 2°C to 8°C (36°F to 46°F); do not expose to freezing or dry ice. Prior to administration, filgrastim may be allowed to be at room temperature for a maximum of 24 hours. It may be diluted in dextrose 5% in water to a concentration ≥15 mcg/mL for I.V. infusion administration. Minimum concentration is 15 mcg/mL; concentrations <15 mcg/mL require addition of albumin (1 mL of 5%) to the bag to prevent absorption. This diluted solution is stable for 7 days under refrigeration or at room temperature. **Filgrastim is incompatible with 0.9% sodium chloride (normal saline)**.

Standard diluent: ≥375 mcg/25 mL D_5W

Reference Range Peak plasma level as high as 600 ng/mL achieved after I.V. doses of 3-60 mcg/kg

Test Interactions Increases uric acid, lactate dehydrogenase, alkaline phosphatase; may cause a decrease in cholesterol

Drug Interactions Acts with synergy with interleukin-3 to increase megacaryocyte and platelet production

Pregnancy Risk Factor C

Monitoring Parameters Complete blood cell count and platelet count should be obtained twice weekly. Leukocytosis (white blood cell counts ≥100,000/mm^3) has been observed in ~2% of patients receiving G-CSF at doses >5 mcg/kg/day. Monitor platelets and hematocrit regularly. Monitor patients with pre-existing cardiac conditions closely as cardiac events (myocardial infarctions, arrhythmias) have been reported in premarketing clinical studies.

Patient Information Possible bone pain

Nursing Implications Do not mix with sodium chloride solutions

Additional Information Reimbursement hotline: 1-800-28-AMGEN; monitor CBC at least twice weekly when used in conjunction with chemotherapy; analgesic agents can be used to control skeletal pain

Specific References

Couderc LJ, Philippe B, Franck N, et al, "Necrotizing Vasculitis and Exacerbation of Psoriasis After Granulocyte Colony-Stimulating Factor for Small Cell Lung Carcinoma," *Respir Med*, 1995, 89:237-8.

Duhrsen U, Ranges H-H, Mayer U, et al, "Leukemia Nodules at the Site of G-CSF Injection in Acute Myelomonoacytic Leukemia," *Eur J Haematol*, 1995, 54:51-2.

(Continued)

Filgrastim *(Continued)*

Gerson SL, Gullion G, Yeh HS, et al, "Granulocyte Colony-Stimulating Factor for Clozapine-Induced Agranulocytosis," *Lancet*, 1992, 340(8827):1097.

Lieschke GJ and Burgess AW, "Granulocyte Colony-Stimulating Factor and Granulocyte-Macrophage Colony-Stimulating Factor," *N Engl J Med*, 1992, 327(1):28-35.

Mulligan SP, Wegman A, and Cooke B, "Leucocytoclastic Vasculitis Occurring With the Second Dose of Granulocyte-Colony Stimulating Factor for Severe Chronic Neutropenia," *Aust N Z J Med*, 1995, 25:75.

Nagy LC, De Roos F, Hoffman RS, et al, "Colchicine-Induced Neutropenia Treated With Granulocyte Colony Stimulating Factor," *Vet Hum Toxicol*, 1994, 36:366.

Reale MA, Yen Y, Strair RK, et al, "Pseudoleukemia After Granulocyte Colony Stimulating Factor Therapy," *South Med J*, 1995, 88:462-4.

Weisbart RH, Gasson JC, and Golde DW, "Colony-Stimulating Factors and Host Defense," *Ann Intern Med*, 1989, 110(4):297-303.

Yim JM, Matuszewski KA, Vermeulen LC, et al, "Surveillance of Colony-Stimulating Factor Use in U.S. Academic Health Centers," *Ann Pharmacother*, 1995, 29:475-81.

Flumazenil (floo' may ze nil)

CAS Number 78755-81-4

Brand Names Romazicon™ Injection

Replaces Mazicon™

Use Benzodiazepine antagonist – reverses sedative effects of benzodiazepines used in general anesthesia; for management of benzodiazepine or zolpidem overdose; flumazenil does **not** antagonize the CNS effects of other GABA agonists (such as ethanol, barbiturates, or general anesthetics), **does not** reverse narcotics

Antidote Useful For

Alprazolam *on page 99*
Chlordiazepoxide *on page 198*
Clobazam *on page 224*
Clonazepam *on page 229*
Clorazepate Dipotassium *on page 232*
Diazepam *on page 271*
Estazolam *on page 324*
Ethyl Alcohol *on page 336*
Flunitrazepam *on page 354*
Lorazepam *on page 482*
Midazolam Hydrochloride *on page 532*
Nitrazepam *on page 562*
Oxazepam *on page 582*
Prazepam *on page 637*
Quazepam *on page 665*
Temazepam *on page 724*
Triazolam *on page 767*
Zolpidem Tartrate *on page 814*

Mechanism of Action Antagonizes the effect of benzodiazepines on the GABA/benzodiazepine receptor complex, including synergistic effects with the other GABA agonists. Flumazenil is benzodiazepine specific and does not antagonize other nonbenzodiazepine GABA agonists (including ethanol, barbiturates, general anesthetics); flumazenil does not reverse the effects of opiates.

Adverse Reactions

Cardiovascular: Cardiac arrhythmias, bradycardia, tachycardia, chest pain, hypertension, ventricular extrasystoles, altered blood pressure (increases and decreases)

Central nervous system: Convulsions (more common in patients physically dependent on benzodiazepines or with tricyclic antidepressant overdoses), fatigue, dizziness/vertigo, amnesia, delirium, dysphoria, fear, headache, agitation, emotional liability, hot flashes, anxiety, nervousness, malaise, shivering, sensation of coldness, abnormal crying, euphoria, depression, somnolence, asthenia

Gastrointestinal: Nausea, vomiting, dry mouth

Local: Pain at injection site

Neuromuscular & skeletal: Tremors

Ocular: Blurred vision, vision disorders

Respiratory: Dyspnea, hyperventilation

Miscellaneous: Abnormal hearing, thick tongue, withdrawal syndrome, hiccups, increased sweating

Toxicodynamics/Kinetics

Onset of benzodiazepine reversal: Within 1-3 minutes

Peak effect: 6-10 minutes

Duration: Usually <1 hour; duration is related to dose given and benzodiazepine plasma concentrations; reversal effects of flumazenil may wear off before effects of benzodiazepine

Distribution: Adults:
Initial V_d: 0.5 L/kg
V_{dss}: 0.77-1.6 L/kg
Protein binding: ~50%
Half-life: Adults:
Alpha: 7-15 minutes
Terminal: 41-79 minutes
Elimination: Clearance dependent upon hepatic blood flow, hepatically eliminated; <1% excreted unchanged in urine

Usual Dosage I.V.:

Children:

Reversal of conscious sedation or general anesthesia: Minimal information available; an initial dose of 0.01 mg/kg (maximum dose: 0.2 mg), then 0.005 mg/kg (maximum dose: 0.2 mg) given every minute to a maximum total dose of 1 mg has been used to reverse midazolam after circumcision in 40 children 3-12 years of age (mean: 7 years); mean total dose required: 0.024 mg/kg; further studies are needed

Management of benzodiazepine overdose: Minimal information available; a few cases have reported an initial dose of 0.01 or 0.02 mg/kg (maximum dose: 0.125 mg) with repeat doses of 0.01 mg/kg or follow up continuous infusions of 0.05 mg/hour (0.004 mg/kg/hour) or 0.05 mg/kg/hour (n=1) for 2-6 hours; further studies are needed

Adults:

Reversal of conscious sedation or general anesthesia: 0.2 mg over 15 seconds; may repeat 0.2 mg every 60 seconds up to a total of 1 mg, usual dose: 0.6-1 mg. In event of resedation, may repeat doses at 20-minute intervals with maximum 1 mg/dose given as 0.2 mg/minute, maximum of 3 mg in 1 hour.

Management of benzodiazepine overdose: 0.2 mg over 30 seconds; may give 0.3 mg dose after 30 seconds if desired level of consciousness is not obtained; additional doses of 0.5 mg can be given over 30 seconds at 1-minute intervals up to a cumulative dose of 3 mg, usual cumulative dose: 1-3 mg; rarely, patients with partial response at 3 mg may require additional titration up to total dose of 5 mg; if patient has not responded 5 minutes after cumulative dose of 5 mg, the major cause of sedation is likely not due to benzodiazepines. In the event of resedation, may repeat doses at 20-minute intervals with maximum of 1 mg/dose (given at 0.5 mg/minute); maximum: 3 mg in 1 hour.

Contraindications Known hypersensitivity to flumazenil or benzodiazepines; patients given benzodiazepines for control of potentially life-threatening conditions (eg, control of intracranial pressure or status epilepticus); patients who are showing signs of serious tricyclic antidepressant overdosage

Warnings Monitor patients for return of sedation or respiratory depression. Flumazenil should be used with caution in the intensive care unit because of increased risk of unrecognized benzodiazepine dependence in such settings. Flumazenil may produce severe withdrawal reactions in patients physically dependent on benzodiazepines.

Dosage Forms Injection: 0.1 mg/mL (5 mL, 10 mL)

Stability For I.V. use only; compatible with D_5W, lactated Ringer's or normal saline; once drawn up in the syringe or mixed with solution use within 24 hours; discard any unused solution after 24 hours

Reference Range Plasma flumazenil levels between 10-20 µg/L for 1-2 hours reverse benzodiazepine-induced CNS depression

Drug Interactions Increased toxicity: Use with caution in overdosage involving mixed drug overdose; toxic effects may emerge (especially with tricyclic antidepressants) with the reversal of the benzodiazepine effect by flumazenil

Pregnancy Risk Factor C

Monitoring Parameters Respiratory rate, level of sedation

Nursing Implications Flumazenil does not effectively reverse hypoventilation, even in alert patients

Additional Information Flumazenil does **not** antagonize the CNS effects of other GABA agonists (such as ethanol, barbiturates, or general anesthetics), nor does it reverse narcotics or tricyclic antidepressants unless benzodiazepines are also present; reverses benzodiazepine-induced depression of ventilatory responses to hypercapnia and hypoxia. Does not decrease antiepileptic effect of diazepam when given concomitantly and may have intrinsic anti-epileptic properties.

Specific References

Chern CH, Chern TL, Hu SC, et al, "Complete and Partial Response to Flumazenil in Patients With Suspected Benzodiazepine Overdose," *Am J Emerg Med*, 1995, 13:372-5.

Geller E, Crome P, Schaller MD, et al, "Risks and Benefits of Therapy With Flumazenil (Anexate®) in Mixed Drug Intoxications," *Eur Neurol*, 1991, 31(4):241-50.

Ghouri AF, Ramirez Ruiz MA, and White PF, "Effect of Flumazenil on Recovery After Midazolam and Propofol Sedation," *Anesthesiology*, 1994, 81(2):330-9.

(Continued)

Flumazenil *(Continued)*

Haverkos GP, DiSalvo RP, and Imhoff TE, "Fatal Seizures After Flumazenil Administration in a Patient With Mixed Overdose," *Ann Pharmacother*, 1994, 28:1347-9.
Hojer J, Baehrendtz S, Magnusson A, et al, "A Placebo-Controlled Trial of Flumazenil Given by Continuous Infusion in Severe Benzodiazepine Overdosage," *Acta Anaesthesiol Scand*, 1991, 35(7):584-90.
McDuffee AT and Tobias JD, "Seizure After Flumazenil Administration in a Pediatric Patient," *Pediatr Emerg Care*, 1995, 11(3):186.
Reisner-Keller LA and Pham Z, "Oral Flumazenil in the Treatment of Epilepsy," *Ann Pharmacother*, 1995, 29:530-1.
Spivey WH, "Flumazenil and Seizures: Analysis of 43 Cases," *Clin Ther*, 1992, 14(2):292-305.

Folacin *see* Folic Acid *on this page*

Folate *see* Folic Acid *on this page*

Folic Acid (foe' lik)

CAS Number 59-30-3; 6484-89-5

Brand Names Folvite®

Synonyms Folacin; Folate; Pteroylglutamic Acid

Use Treatment of megaloblastic and macrocytic anemias due to folate deficiency; used in methanol toxicity, methotrexate toxicity, chronic alcoholism

Antidote Useful For

Methanol *on page 957*
Methotrexate *on page 515*
Trimetrexate Glucuronate *on page 773*

Mechanism of Action Necessary for normal erythropoiesis

Adverse Reactions

Central nervous system: Irritability, difficulty sleeping, confusion
Gastrointestinal: GI upset
Miscellaneous: Hypersensitivity reactions

Toxicodynamics/Kinetics

Peak effect: Oral: Within 30-60 minutes
Absorption: In the proximal part of the small intestine

Usual Dosage Oral, I.M., I.V., S.C.:

Minimal daily requirement: 50 mcg; pregnant/critically ill: 100-200 mcg
Infants: 0.1 mg/day

Children: Initial: 1 mg/day
- Deficiency: 0.5-1 mg/day
- Maintenance dose:
  - <4 years: Up to 0.3 mg/day
  - >4 years: 0.4 mg/day

Adults: Initial: 1 mg/day
- Deficiency: 1-3 mg/day
- Maintenance dose: 0.5 mg/day
- Pregnant and lactating women: 0.8 mg/day

Administration Oral, but may also be administered by deep I.M., S.C., or I.V. injection; a diluted solution for oral or for parenteral administration may be prepared by diluting 1 mL of folic acid injection (5 mg/mL), with 49 mL sterile water for injection; resulting solution is 0.1 mg folic acid/1 mL

Contraindications Pernicious, aplastic, or normocytic anemias

Warnings Doses >0.1 mg/day may obscure pernicious anemia; patients with pernicious anemia may show hematologic improvement with doses as low as 0.25 mg/day with continuing irreversible nerve damage progression; resistance to treatment may occur with depressed hematopoiesis, alcoholism, deficiencies of other vitamins; injection contains benzyl alcohol (1.5%) as preservative

Dosage Forms

Injection, as sodium folate: 5 mg/mL (10 mL); 10 mg/mL (10 mL)
- Folvite®: 5 mg/mL (10 mL)

Tablet: 0.1 mg, 0.4 mg, 0.8 mg, 1 mg
- Folvite®: 1 mg

Stability Incompatible with oxidizing and reducing agents and heavy metal ions

Reference Range Therapeutic: 0.005-0.015 μg/mL

Test Interactions Falsely low serum concentrations may occur with the *Lactobacillus casei* assay method in patients on anti-infectives (ie, tetracycline)

Drug Interactions In folate-deficient patients, folic acid therapy may increase phenytoin metabolism resulting in decreased phenytoin serum concentrations. Concurrent administration of chloramphenicol and folic acid in these patients may result in antagonism of the hematopoietic response to folic acid. Oral contraceptives may impair folate metabolism and produce folate depletion; may interfere with the antimicrobial actions of pyrimethamine against toxoplasmosis.

Pregnancy Risk Factor A (C if dose exceeds RDA recommendation)

Monitoring Parameters Hemoglobin

Nursing Implications Oral, but may also be administered by deep I.M., S.C., or I.V. injection; a diluted solution for oral or for parenteral administration may be prepared by diluting 1 mL of folic acid injection (5 mg/mL), with 49 mL sterile water for injection; resulting solution is 0.1 mg folic acid per 1 mL

Additional Information Water-soluble vitamin with a wide margin of safety

Specific References

Davis RE, "Clinical Chemistry of Folic Acid," *Adv Clin Chem*, 1986, 25:233-94.

Lambie DG and Johnson RH, "Drugs and Folate Metabolism," *Drugs*, 1985, 30(2):145-55.

Folinic Acid *see* Leucovorin Calcium *on page 1437*

Folvite® *see* Folic Acid *on previous page*

Fomepizole *see* 4-Methylpyrazole *on page 1446*

5-Formyl Tetrahydrofolate *see* Leucovorin Calcium *on page 1437*

G-CSF *see* Filgrastim *on page 1425*

Genahist® Oral *see* Diphenhydramine Hydrochloride *on page 1415*

Gen-D-phen® Cough Syrup [OTC] *see* Diphenhydramine Hydrochloride *on page 1415*

Giludop® *see* Dopamine Hydrochloride *on page 1418*

Glucagon (gloo' ka gon)

CAS Number 16941-32-5

Use Hypoglycemia; diagnostic aid in the radiologic examination of GI tract when a hypotonic state is needed; useful in esophageal food impaction, cardiogenic shock; used with some success as a cardiac stimulant in management of severe cases of beta-adrenergic or calcium channel blocking agent, calcium channel blocker, or oral hypoglycemia overdosage; may be useful in treating hypotension due to imipramine toxicity; noninsulin-dependent diabetes mellitus

Antidote Useful For

Acetohexamide *on page 86*
Bisoprolol Fumarate *on page 157*
Celiprolol Hydrochloride *on page 191*
Diltiazem *on page 287*
Glipizide *on page 382*
Glyburide *on page 384*
Insulin Preparations *on page 426*
Metformin *on page 507*
Nebivolol *on page 551*
Nifedipine *on page 558*
Pindolol *on page 627*
Propranolol Hydrochloride *on page 657*
Sotalol Hydrochloride *on page 703*
Tolazamide *on page 756*
Tolbutamide *on page 757*
Verapamil Hydrochloride *on page 787*

Mechanism of Action Stimulates adenylate cyclase to produce increased cyclic AMP, which promotes hepatic glycogenolysis and gluconeogenesis, causing a raise in blood glucose levels

Adverse Reactions

Cardiovascular: Hypotension
Central nervous system: Dizziness/vertigo
Dermatologic: Urticaria, erythema multiforme, Stevens-Johnson syndrome
Endocrine & metabolic: Hyperglycemia, hypoglycemia, hypokalemia
Gastrointestinal: Nausea, vomiting
Neuromuscular & skeletal: Weakness
Respiratory: Respiratory distress
Miscellaneous: Thrombophlebitis

Signs & Symptoms of Acute Overdose Hypokalemia, nausea, vomiting, hyperglycemia, allergic reactions, hypertension, hypotension, weakness, dizziness, hyperglycemia

Toxicodynamics/Kinetics

Onset of action: Effects on blood glucose levels occur within 5-20 minutes following parenteral administration
Duration: 60-90 minutes
Absorption: Destroyed in the GI tract
Distribution: Not fully understood
Metabolism: In the liver with some inactivation occurring in the kidneys and plasma

(Continued)

Glucagon *(Continued)*

Half-life: 3-10 minutes
Elimination: Renal

Usual Dosage

Hypoglycemia or insulin shock therapy: I.M., I.V., S.C.:
Neonates: 0.3 mg/kg/dose; maximum: 1 mg/dose
Children: 0.025-0.1 mg/kg/dose, not to exceed 1 mg/dose, repeated in 20 minutes as needed
Adults: 0.5-1 mg, may repeat in 20 minutes as needed

Cardiotoxic agent toxicity: I.V.: 0.05 mg/kg (up to 10 mg) over 1 minute, then continuous infusion of 2-5 mg/hour in 5% dextrose

Diagnostic aid: Adults: I.M., I.V.: 0.25-2 mg 10 minutes prior to procedure

Administration Reconstitute powder for injection by adding 1 or 10 mL of sterile diluent to a vial containing 1 or 10 units of the drug, respectively, to provide solutions containing 1 mg of glucagon/mL; if dose to be administered is <2 mg of the drug → use only the diluent provided by the manufacturer; if >2 mg → use sterile water for injection; use immediately after reconstitution

Contraindications Hypersensitivity to glucagon or any component

Warnings Use with caution in patients with a history of insulinoma and/or pheochromocytoma

Dosage Forms Powder for injection, lyophilized: 1 mg [1 unit]; 10 mg [10 units]

Stability After reconstitution, use immediately; may be kept at 5°C for up to 48 hours if necessary

Reference Range Normal range: 50-60 pg/mL

Drug Interactions Oral anticoagulant – hypoprothrombinemic effects may be increased possibly with bleeding

Pregnancy Risk Factor B

Monitoring Parameters Blood pressure, blood glucose, potassium, and glucose

Additional Information 1 unit = 1 mg; the diluent contains 2 mg of phenol/mL as a preservative; normal basal levels 50-60 pg/mL; I.V. infusion contains phenol; 1 mg glucagon (I.M.) used to remove orogastric tube due to esophageal (distal) spasm; glucagon may be quite effective for treatment of beta-blocker induced anaphylaxis

Specific References

Lang DM, "Anaphylactoid and Anaphylactic Reactions: Hazards of Beta-Blockers," 1995, *Drug Saf*, 1995, 12(5):299-304.

Lvoff R and Wilcken D, "Glucagon in Heart Failure and in Cardiogenic Shock – Experience in 50 Patients," *Circulation*, 1972, 45(3):534-42.

Pollack CV Jr, "Utility of Glucagon in the Emergency Department," *J Emerg Med*, 1993, 11(2):195-205.

Thoma ME and Glauser JM, "Use of Glucagon for Removal of an Orogastric Lavage Tube," *Am J Emerg Med*, 1995, 13:219-22.

Glucose *see* Dextrose *on page 1409*

Go-Evac® *see* Polyethylene Glycol *on page 1460*

GoLYTELY® *see* Polyethylene Glycol *on page 1460*

Granulocyte Colony Stimulating Factor *see* Filgrastim *on page 1425*

H1-Antihistamine Comparison *see page 1649*

Hyaluronidase (hye al yoor on' i dase)

CAS Number 9001-54-1

Use Enhance diffusion of locally irritating or toxic drugs in the management of I.V. due to aminophylline, calcium solutions, dextrose (≥10% solution), nafcillin, parenteral nutrition solutions, potassium solutions, radiocontrast media, and *Vinca* alkaloid agents

Antidote Useful For

Potassium Chloride *on page 634*
Vinblastine Sulfate *on page 790*
Vincristine Sulfate *on page 792*

Mechanism of Action Modifies the permeability of connective tissue through hydrolysis of hyaluronic acid, one of the chief ingredients of tissue cement which offers resistance to diffusion of liquids through tissues

Adverse Reactions

Cardiovascular: Tachycardia, hypotension
Central nervous system: Dizziness, chills
Dermatologic: Urticaria, erythema
Gastrointestinal: Nausea, vomiting

Signs & Symptoms of Acute Overdose Local edema, urticaria, erythema, chills, nausea, vomiting, hypotension; treat with epinephrine

Toxicodynamics/Kinetics Treatment of extravasation:
Onset of action: S.C., I.D.: Immediate
Duration: 24-48 hours

Usual Dosage
Infants and Children:
Management of I.V. extravasation: Reconstitute the 150 unit vial of lyophilized powder with 1 mL normal saline; take 0.1 mL of this solution and dilute with 0.9 mL normal saline to yield 15 units/mL; using a 25- or 26-gauge needle, five 0.2 mL injections are made subcutaneously or intradermally into the extravasation site at the leading edge, changing the needle after each injection
Hypodermoclysis: S.C.: 15 units are added to each 100 mL of I.V. fluid to be administered

Adults: Absorption and dispersion of drugs: 150 units are added to the vehicle containing the drug

Contraindications Hypersensitivity to hyaluronidase or any component; do not inject in or around infected, inflamed, or cancerous areas

Warnings Drug infiltrates in which hyaluronidase is contraindicated: dopamine, alpha agonists

Stability Reconstituted hyaluronidase solution remains stable for only 24 hours when stored in the refrigerator; do not use discolored solutions

Drug Interactions Salicylates, cortisone, ACTH, estrogens, antihistamines

Pregnancy Risk Factor C

Nursing Implications Administer hyaluronidase within the first few minutes to 1 hour after the extravasation is recognized; do not administer I.V.

Additional Information The USP hyaluronidase unit is equivalent to the turbidity-reducing (TR) unit and the International Unit; each unit is defined as being the activity contained in 100 mcg of the International Standard Preparation

Specific References
Dorr RT, "Vinca Alkaloid Ulceration: Experimental Mouse Model and Effects of Local Antidotes," *Proc Am Soc Clin Oncol*, 1982, 1:428.
Zenk KE, "Management of Intravenous Extravasations," *Infusion*, 1981, 5:77-9.
Zenk KE, "Treating I.V. Extravasations With Hyaluronidase," *ASHP Signal*, 1986, 10:25,29.

Hybalamin® Injection *see* Hydroxocobalamin *on this page*

Hydramine® Oral [OTC] *see* Diphenhydramine Hydrochloride *on page 1415*

Hydramyn® Syrup [OTC] *see* Diphenhydramine Hydrochloride *on page 1415*

Hydrobexan® Injection *see* Hydroxocobalamin *on this page*

Hydro-Cobex® Injection *see* Hydroxocobalamin *on this page*

Hydro-Crysti-12® Injection *see* Hydroxocobalamin *on this page*

Hydroxocobalamin (hye drox oh koe bal' a min)

CAS Number 13422-52-1

Brand Names Alphamin® Injection; Codroxomin® Injection; Hybalamin® Injection; Hydrobexan® Injection; Hydro-Cobex® Injection; Hydro-Crysti-12® Injection; LA-12® Injection

Synonyms Vitamin B_{12}

Use Treatment of pernicious anemia, vitamin B_{12} deficiency, increased B_{12} requirements due to pregnancy, thyrotoxicosis, hemorrhage, malignancy, liver or kidney disease

Antidote Useful For
Acrylonitrile *on page 853*
Cyanide *on page 899*
Nitroprusside Sodium *on page 568*

Mechanism of Action Coenzyme for various metabolic functions, including fat and carbohydrate metabolism and protein synthesis, used in cell replication and hematopoiesis

Adverse Reactions
Dermatologic: Itching, urticaria
Endocrine and Metabolic: Hypokalemia
Gastrointestinal: Diarrhea, feces discoloration (red)
Local: Pain at injection site
Respiratory: Pulmonary edema
Miscellaneous: Anaphylactoid reactions, polycythemia, red color of urine

Usual Dosage Vitamin B_{12} deficiency: I.M.:
Children: 1-5 mg given in single doses of 100 mcg over 2 or more weeks, followed by 30-50 mcg/month

Adults: 30 mcg/day for 5-10 days, followed by 100-200 mcg/month

Cyanide overdose: 50 g of hydroxocobalamin required to bind 1 g cyanide infused at doses of 4 g associated with sodium thiosulfate

(Continued)

Hydroxocobalamin *(Continued)*

Contraindications Hypersensitivity to cyanocobalamin or any component, cobalt; patients with hereditary optic nerve atrophy

Warnings Some products contain benzoyl alcohol; avoid use in premature infants; an intradermal test dose should be performed for hypersensitivity; use only if oral supplementation not possible or when treating pernicious anemia; appropriate doses for cyanide poisoning requires excessive fluid administration

Dosage Forms Injection: 1000 mcg/mL (10 mL, 30 mL)

Reference Range Normal vitamin B_{12} plasma levels: 200-800 pg/mL

Test Interactions In therapeutic concentrations, hydroxocobalamin falsely elevates bilirubin and magnesium and falsely lowers AST and creatinine

Pregnancy Risk Factor C

Nursing Implications Administer I.M. only; may require coadministration of folic acid

Additional Information An investigational combination of hydroxocobalamin (4 g) and sodium thiosulfate (8 g) is under study in the U.S. and is possibly available from the manufacturer (EVREKA)

Specific References

Cottrell JE, Casthely P, Brodie JD, et al, "Prevention of Nitroprusside-Induced Cyanide Toxicity With Hydroxocobalamin," *N Engl J Med*, 1978, 298(15):809-11.

Curry SC, Connor DA, and Raschke RA, "Effect of the Cyanide Antidote Hydroxocobalamin on Commonly Ordered Serum Chemistries," *Ann Emerg Med*, 1994, 24:65-7.

Holland MA and Kozlowski LM, "Clinical Features and Management of Cyanide Poisoning," *Clin Pharm*, 1986, 5(9):737-41.

Kayser SR and Kurisu S, "Hydroxocobalamin in Nitroprusside Induced Cyanide Toxicity," *Drug Intell Clin Pharm*, 1986, 20:365-6.

3-Hydroxytyramine *see* Dopamine Hydrochloride *on page 1418*

Hyperbaric Oxygen *see* Oxygen (Hyperbaric) *on page 1453*

Hyposulfene® *see* Sodium Thiosulfate *on page 1470*

Hypotears® *see* Polyethylene Glycol *on page 1460*

Imuprel® *see* Isoproterenol *on page 1436*

IND 4041 (Ca-DTPA) *see* Diethylene Triamine Penta-acetic Acid *on page 1411*

IND-14603 (Zn-DTPA) *see* Diethylene Triamine Penta-acetic Acid *on page 1411*

Ingelan® *see* Isoproterenol *on page 1436*

Inovan® *see* Dopamine Hydrochloride *on page 1418*

Insect Sting Kit

Related Information

Epinephrine *on page 1422*

Brand Names Ana-Kit®

Use Anaphylaxis; emergency treatment of insect bites or stings (ie, yellow jacket, honeybee, hornet, wasp, deerfly, kissing bug) by the sensitive patient when self-treatment may occur within minutes of insect sting or exposure to an allergenic substance

Usual Dosage Children and Adults:

Epinephrine:
- <2 years: 0.05-0.1 mL
- 2-6 years: 0.15 mL
- 6-12 years: 0.2 mL
- >12 years : 0.3 mL

Chlorpheniramine:
- <6 years: 1 tablet
- 6-12 years: 2 tablets
- >12 years: 4 tablets

Contraindications Hypertensive or hyperthyroid patients

Warnings Use caution in elderly patients, patients with diabetes mellitus or cardiovascular diseases and/or history of sensitivity to sympathomimetic amines; epinephrine should be used with caution in patients also taking beta-adrenergic blockers as unopposed alpha-adrenergic effects may occur (primarily hypertension)

Dosage Forms Kit: Epinephrine hydrochloride 1:1000 (1 mL syringe), chlorpheniramine maleate chewable tablet 2 mg (4), sterile alcohol pads (2), tourniquet

Stability Protect from light, store at room temperature, prevent from freezing

Patient Information Physician should instruct patient on proper use of kit

Additional Information Not intended for I.V. use (I.M. or S.C. only); not intended as a substitute for professional medical treatment; hypotension due to a systemic allergic reaction does not respond well to epinephrine; not effective for skin reactions due to fire ant bites

Specific References

Fortenberry JE, Laine J, Shalit M, et al, "Use of Epinephrine for Anaphylaxis by Emergency Medical Technicians in a Wilderness," *Ann Emerg Med*, 1995, 25:785-7.

Klein JS, Rich MR, and Yunginger JW, "Myocardial Ischemia Without Coronary Artery Disease After Epinephrine Overdose for Insect Sting Reaction," *J Allergy Clin Immunol*, 1995, 95:371.

Valentine MD and Lichtenstein LM, "Anaphylaxis and Stinging Insect Hypersensitivity," *JAMA*, 1987, 258(20):2881-5.

Insta-Char® [OTC] *see* Charcoal *on page 1403*

Intrastigmina® *see* Neostigmine *on page 1450*

Intropin® *see* Dopamine Hydrochloride *on page 1418*

Invite B$_6$® *see* Pyridoxine Hydrochloride *on page 1465*

Ipecac Syrup (ip' e kak)

CAS Number 8012-96-2

Use Treatment of acute oral drug overdosage and in certain poisonings

Antidote Useful For

Anticoagulant Rodenticide *on page 859*

Mechanism of Action Irritates the gastric mucosa and stimulates the medullary chemoreceptor trigger zone to induce vomiting

Adverse Reactions

Cardiovascular: Cardiotoxicity, tachycardia, heart block, congestive heart failure, pericarditis, hypotension

Central nervous system: Lethargy, hypotonia

Gastrointestinal: Protracted vomiting, diarrhea, pneumomediastinum, gastric rupture, Mallory-Weiss tear, hemorrhagic colitis

Hepatic: Hepatomegaly, elevated liver enzyme

Neuromuscular & skeletal: Myopathy, myalgia

Signs & Symptoms of Acute Overdose Diarrhea, persistent vomiting, hypotension, cardiomyopathy, atrial fibrillation

Toxicodynamics/Kinetics

Onset of action: Within 15-30 minutes

Duration: 20-25 minutes; can last longer, 60 minutes in some cases

Absorption: Significant amounts, mainly when it does not produce emesis

Distribution: Unknown

Metabolism: Unknown

Elimination: Emetine (alkaloid component) may be detected in urine 60 days after excess dose or chronic use

Usual Dosage Oral:

Children:

- 6-12 months: 5-10 mL followed by 10-20 mL/kg of water; repeat dose one time if vomiting does not occur within 20 minutes
- 1-12 years: 15 mL followed by 10-20 mL/kg of water; repeat dose one time if vomiting does not occur within 20 minutes

Adults: 15-30 mL followed by 200-300 mL of water; repeat dose one time if vomiting does not occur within 20 minutes

Contraindications Do not use in unconscious patients, patients with absent gag reflex; ingestion of strong bases or acids, volatile oils; seizures

Dosage Forms Syrup: 70 mg/mL (15 mL, 30 mL, 473 mL, 4000 mL)

Reference Range Blood emetine levels within hours of a 30 mL oral dose of ipecac range from 0-75 μg/L

Drug Interactions Activated charcoal, milk, carbonated beverages

Pregnancy Risk Factor C

Nursing Implications Do **not** administer to unconscious patients; if vomiting does not occur after second dose, gastric lavage may be considered to remove ingested substance

Specific References

Colletti RB and Wasserman RC, "Recurrent Infantile Vomiting Due to Intentional Ipecac Poisoning," *J Pediatr Gastroenterol Nutr*, 1989, 8(3):394-6.

Day L, Kelly C, Reed G, et al, "Fatal Cardiomyopathy: Suspected Child Abuse by Chronic Ipecac Administration," *Vet Hum Toxicol*, 1989, 31(3):225-7.

Klein-Schwartz W, Gorman RL, Oderda GM, et al, "Ipecac Use in the Elderly: The Unanswered Question," *Ann Emerg Med*, 1984, 13(12):1152-4.

Kunkel DB, "The Toxic Toll of Keeping Thin," *Emerg Med*, 1985, 17:176-80.

Manno BR and Manno JE, "Toxicology of Ipecac: A Review," *Clin Toxicol*, 1977, 10:221-42.

Moran DM, Crouch DC, Finkle BS, et al, "Absorption of Ipecac Alkaloids in Emergency Room Patients," *Vet Hum Toxicol*, 1983, 25:286.

Isoamyl Nitrite *see* Amyl Nitrite *on page 1390*

Isopentyl Nitrite *see* Amyl Nitrite *on page 1390*

Isoprenaline Hydrochloride *see* Isoproterenol *on this page*

Isoproterenol (eye soe proe ter' e nole)

Related Information

Adrenergic Agonists, Cardiovascular Comparison *on page 1638*

Adrenergic Agonists Drug Infusions Comparison *on page 1638*

CAS Number 7683-59-2; 51-30-9; 299-95-6; 6700-39-6

Brand Names Aludrin®; Imuprel®; Ingelan®; Isuprel®; Medihaler-Iso® Inhalation Aerosol; Saventrine®; Vapo-iso®

Synonyms Isoprenaline Hydrochloride; Isoproterenol Hydrochloride; Isoproterenol Sulfate

Use Asthma or COPD (reversible airway obstruction); A-V nodal block; hemodynamically compromised bradyarrhythmias or atropine-resistant bradyarrhythmias, temporary use in third degree A-V block until pacemaker insertion; low cardiac output; vasoconstrictive shock states; torsade de pointes; useful for beta-adrenergic blocker toxicity; calcium channel blocker overdose

Mechanism of Action Relaxes bronchial smooth muscle by action on $beta_2$-receptors; causes increased heart rate and contractility by action on $beta_1$-receptors

Adverse Reactions

Cardiovascular: Hypertension, tachycardia, arrhythmias, chest pain, ventricular arrhythmia, cardiomyopathy, cardiomegaly, flushing of face

Central nervous system: Insomnia, restlessness, weakness, dizziness, lightheadedness, parotid gland swelling (prolonged use)

Gastrointestinal: Dry mouth or throat, vomiting, nausea

Neuromuscular & skeletal: Trembling

Respiratory: Paradoxical bronchospasm

Miscellaneous: Discoloration of saliva (pinkish-red), eosinopenia, thrombocytopenia, increased sweating

Toxicodynamics/Kinetics

Distribution: V_d: 0.5 L/kg

Protein binding: 65%

Metabolism: Metabolized by conjugation in many tissues including the liver and lungs by catecholamine-O-methyltransferase (COMT) to 3-O-methylisoproterenol (weak beta-blocker activity)

Half-life: Biphasic: First phase: 2.5-5 minutes; second phase: 3-7 hours

Time to peak serum concentration: Oral: Within 1-2 hours

Elimination: Principally in urine as sulfate conjugates

Usual Dosage

Children:

- Bronchodilation: Inhalation: Metered dose inhaler: 1-2 metered doses up to 5 times/day
- Bronchodilation (using 1:200 inhalation solution) 0.01 mL/kg/dose every 4 hours as needed (maximum: 0.05 mL/dose) diluted with normal saline to 2 mL
- Sublingual: 5-10 mg every 3-4 hours, not to exceed 30 mg/day
- Cardiac arrhythmias: I.V.: Start 0.1 mcg/kg/minute (usual effective dose 0.2-2 mcg/kg/minute)

Adults:

- Bronchodilation: Inhalation: Metered dose inhaler: 1-2 metered doses 4-6 times/day
- Bronchodilation: 1-2 inhalations of a 0.25% solution, no more than 2 inhalations at any one time (1-5 minutes between inhalations); no more than 6 inhalations in any hour during a 24-hour period; maintenance therapy: 1-2 inhalations 4-6 times/day. Alternatively: 0.5% solution via hand bulb nebulizer is 5-15 deep inhalations repeated once in 5-10 minutes if necessary; treatments may be repeated up to 5 times/day.
- Sublingual: 10-20 mg every 3-4 hours; not to exceed 60 mg/day
- Cardiac arrhythmias: I.V.: 5 mcg/minute initially, titrate to patient response (2-20 mcg/minute)
- Shock: I.V.: 0.5-5 mcg/minute; adjust according to response

Administration I.V. infusion administration requires the use of an infusion pump. To prepare infusion:

$$\frac{\text{6 x weight (kg) x desired dose (mcg/kg/min)}}{\text{I.V. infusion rate (mL/h)}} = \text{mg of drug to be added to 100 mL of I.V. fluid}$$

Contraindications Angina, pre-existing cardiac arrhythmias (ventricular); tachycardia or A-V block caused by cardiac glycoside intoxication; allergy to sulfites or isoproterenol or other sympathomimetic amines; avoid in hydrocarbon exposure

Warnings Elderly patients, diabetics, renal or cardiovascular disease, hyperthyroidism; excessive or prolonged use may result in decreased effectiveness

Dosage Forms

Inhalation: Aerosol: 0.2% [2 mg/mL = 1:500] (15 mL, 22.5 mL); 0.25% [2.5 mg/mL = 1:400] (15 mL)

Injection: 0.02% [0.2 mg/mL = 1:5000] (1 mL, 5 mL, 10 mL)

Solution for nebulization: 0.031% (4 mL); 0.062% (4 mL); 0.25% (0.5 mL, 30 mL); 0.5% (0.5 mL, 10 mL, 60 mL); 1% (10 mL)

Tablet, sublingual: 10 mg, 15 mg

Stability Do not use discolored solutions; limit exposure to heat, light or air; stability of parenteral admixture at room temperature (25°C) and at refrigeration temperature (4°C): 24 hours; **incompatible** when mixed with aminophylline, furosemide; **incompatible** with alkaline solutions

Reference Range Peak plasma isoproterenol level of 0.0004 mg/L achieved after an I.V. injection of 0.063 mcg/kg postmortem level of 0.1 mg/L noted following a death in an asthmatic patient relatable to isoproterenol use

Drug Interactions Increased toxicity with sympathomimetics (increased blood pressure and headache), general anesthetics (arrhythmias); increases clearance of theophylline

Pregnancy Risk Factor C

Monitoring Parameters EKG, heart rate, respiratory rate, arterial blood gas, arterial blood pressure, CVP

Nursing Implications Give around-the-clock to promote less variation in peak and trough serum levels

Additional Information

Isoproterenol hydrochloride: Aerolone®, Dey-Dose® isoproterenol, Dispos-a-Med® isoproterenol, Isopro®, Isuprel®, Norisodrine®, Vapo-Iso®

Isoproterenol sulfate: Medihaler-Iso®

Specific References

Almquist A, Goldenberg IF, Milstein S, et al, "Provocation of Bradycardia and Hypotension by Isoproterenol and Upright Posture in Patients With Unexplained Syncope," *N Engl J Med*, 1989, 320(6):346-51.

Hemstreet MP, Miles MV, and Rutland RO, "Effect of Intravenous Isoproterenol on Theophylline Kinetics," *J Allergy Clin Immunol*, 1982, 69(4):360-4.

Lang CC, Stein M, Brown RM, et al, "Attenuation of Isoproterenol-Mediated Vasodilitation in Blacks," *N Engl J Med*, 1995, 333:155-60.

Isoproterenol Hydrochloride *see* Isoproterenol *on previous page*

Isoproterenol Sulfate *see* Isoproterenol *on previous page*

Isopto® Atropine *see* Atropine Sulfate *on page 1395*

Isopto® Eserine Ophthalmic *see* Physostigmine *on page 1457*

Isotol® *see* Mannitol *on page 1442*

Isuprel® *see* Isoproterenol *on previous page*

I-Tropine® *see* Atropine Sulfate *on page 1395*

Kaergona® *see* Phytonadione *on page 1458*

Kalcinate® *see* Calcium Gluconate *on page 1401*

Kayexalate® *see* Sodium Polystyrene Sulfonate *on page 1469*

Kaywan® *see* Phytonadione *on page 1458*

Kelatin® *see* Penicillamine *on page 1454*

Konakion® *see* Phytonadione *on page 1458*

L_1 *see* Deferiprone *on page 1407*

LA-12® Injection *see* Hydroxocobalamin *on page 1433*

Lactismine® *see* Bromocriptine Mesylate *on page 1398*

Ledclair® *see* Edetate Calcium Disodium *on page 1419*

Leucovorin Calcium (loo koe vor' in)

CAS Number 1492-18-8; 58-05-9; 41926-89-3

Brand Names Wellcovorin®

Synonyms Calcium Leucovorin; Citrovorin Rescue; Citrovorum Factor; Folinic Acid; 5-Formyl Tetrahydrofolate

Use Antidote for folic acid antagonists (trimethoprim, pyrimethoprim, pyrimethamine), prevention of hematopoietic effects of folic acid antagonists, treatment of anemia (megaloblastic)s when folate is deficient as in infancy, sprue, pregnancy, and nutritional deficiency when oral folate therapy is not possible and I.V. folic acid cannot be used; in combination with fluorouracil in the treatment of malignancy; trimetrexate possibly effective for vinblastine

Antidote Useful For

Methanol *on page 957*

Methotrexate *on page 515*

Pyrimethamine *on page 664*

Trimetrexate Glucuronate *on page 773*

Mechanism of Action Reduced form of folic acid, but does not require a reduction reaction by an enzyme for activation, allows for purine and thymidine synthesis, a necessity for normal erythropoiesis

Adverse Reactions Dermatologic: Rash, pruritus, erythema

Signs & Symptoms of Acute Overdose EKG changes

Toxicodynamics/Kinetics

Onset of action:

Oral: Within 30 minutes

I.V.: Within 5 minutes

Duration: All routes: 3-6 hours

Absorption: Oral, I.M.: Rapid

Distribution: Crosses blood-brain barrier in moderate amounts; largely concentrated in liver

Metabolism: Rapidly converted to (5MTHF) 5-methyl-tetrahydrofolate (active) following administration in the intestinal mucosa and by the liver

Bioavailability: 97% for 25 mg dose; 75% for 50 mg dose; 37% for 100 mg dose

Half-life:

Leucovorin: 15 minutes

5MTHF: 33-35 minutes

Elimination: Primarily in urine (80% to 90%) with small losses appearing in feces (5% to 8%)

Usual Dosage Children and Adults:

Adjunctive therapy with antimicrobial agents (pyrimethamine): Oral: 2-15 mg/day for 3 days or until blood counts are normal or 5 mg every 3 days; doses of 6 mg/day are needed for patients with platelet counts $<100{,}000/mm^3$

Rescue dose: I.V.: 10 mg/m^2 to start, then 10 mg/m^2 every 6 hours orally for 72 hours; if serum creatinine 24 hours after methotrexate is elevated 50% or more **or** the serum MTX concentration is $>5 \times 10^{-6}$M (see graph), increase dose to 100 mg/m^2/dose every 3 hours until serum methotrexate level is $<1 \times 10^{-8}$M

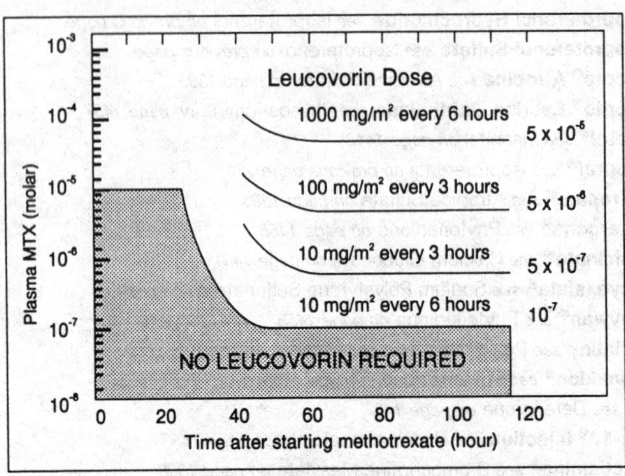

Investigational: Post I.T. methotrexate: Oral, I.V.: 12 mg/m^2 as a single dose; post high-dose methotrexate: 100-1000 mg/m^2/dose until the serum methotrexate level is $<1 \times 10^{-7}$ molar; with 5FU: Oral: 500 mg/m^2/day divided into 4 doses for 5 days

Methanol poisoning: 1 mg/kg; may repeat in 4 hours; further therapy should be with folic acid (secondary to cost and availability)

Plasma MTX concentration as a therapeutic guide to high-dose MTX therapy with leucovorin factor rescue. Leucovorin is continued until the plasma MTX level is $<1 \times 10^{-7}$ molar. Each dose of leucovorin is increased if the plasma MTX concentration is excessively high, according to the guidelines. With 4- to 6-hour high-dose MTX infusions, plasma drug values $>5 \times 10^{-5}$ and 10^{-6} molar at 24 and 48 hours after starting the infusion, respectively, are often predictive of delayed MTX clearance. See graph.

The drug should be given parenterally instead of orally in patients with GI toxicity, nausea, vomiting, and when individual doses are >25 mg.

Dosage Forms
Injection: 3 mg/mL (1 mL)
Powder for injection: 25 mg, 50 mg, 100 mg, 350 mg
Powder for oral solution: 1 mg/mL (60 mL)
Tablet: 5 mg, 10 mg, 15 mg, 25 mg

Stability Protect from light; store intact vials at room temperature
Stability of parenteral admixture at room temperature (25°C): 24 hours
Stability of parenteral admixture at refrigeration temperature (4°C): 7 days
Reconstituted I.V. solutions are stable 24 hours at room temperature

Drug Interactions I.V. administration of fluorouracil and leucovorin are not compatible

Pregnancy Risk Factor C

Nursing Implications I.V. infusion should not exceed 160 mg of leucovorin per minute

Specific References

Bleyer WA, "New Vistas for Leucovorin in Cancer Chemotherapy," *Cancer*, 1984, 63:4843-8.
Hansen RM, "Systemic Therapy in Metastatic Colorectal Cancer," *Arch Intern Med*, 1990, 150(11):2265-9.
Jacobsen D and McMartin K, "Methanol and Ethylene Glycol Poisonings. Mechanism of Toxicity, Clinical Course, Diagnosis and Treatment," *Med Toxicol*, 1986, 1(5):309-34.
Trissel LA, Martinez JF, and Xu QA, "Incompatibility of Fluorouracil With Leucovorin Calcium or Levoleucovorin Calcium," *Am J Health Syst Pharm*, 1995, 52:710-5.

Levarterenol Bitartrate *see* Norepinephrine Bitartrate *on page 1451*
Levophed® *see* Norepinephrine Bitartrate *on page 1451*
Limclair® *see* Edetate Disodium *on page 1421*
Lime Acetate *see* Calcium Acetate *on page 1399*
Lioserio® *see* Antitoxin Botulinin Types A, B, and E *on page 1391*
Liqui-Char® [OTC] *see* Charcoal *on page 1403*
Lismol® *see* Cholestyramine Resin *on page 1405*
Macrogol *see* Polyethylene Glycol *on page 1460*

Magnesium Citrate (mag nee' ze um sit' rate

CAS Number 3344-18-1

Brand Names Citramag®; Citro-Mag®; Evac-Q-Mag® [OTC]; Magnesium-Diasporal

Synonyms Citrate of Magnesia

Use Evacuates bowel prior to certain surgical and diagnostic procedures

Mechanism of Action A saline cathartic which promotes bowel evacuation by causing osmotic retention of fluid which distends the colon with increased peristaltic activity

Adverse Reactions
Cardiovascular: Hypotension
Gastrointestinal: Abdominal cramps, diarrhea, gas formation
Endocrine & metabolic: Hypermagnesemia
Respiratory: Respiratory depression

Signs & Symptoms of Acute Overdose Serious, potentially life-threatening electrolyte disturbances may occur with long-term use or overdosage, nausea, vomiting, diarrhea; **Serum level >12 mEq/L** may be fatal, **serum level ~10 mEq/L** may cause complete heart block

Toxicodynamics/Kinetics
Onset of action: 30 minutes to 3 hours
Absorption: Oral: 15% to 30%
Distribution: V_d: 0.2-0.4 L/kg
Protein binding: 34%
Elimination: Renal

Usual Dosage Cathartic: Oral:
Children:
<6 years: 0.5 mL/kg up to a maximum of 200 mL repeated every 4-6 hours until stools are clear
6-12 years: ⅓ to ½ bottle
Adults ≥12 years: ½ to 1 full bottle as needed

Contraindications Renal failure, appendicitis, abdominal pain, intestinal impaction, obstruction or perforation, diabetes mellitus

Warnings Use with caution in patients with impaired renal function

Dosage Forms Solution, oral: 300 mL

Reference Range Normal urinary levels: 1-6 mmol/L
Serum magnesium:
Children: 1.5-1.9 mg/dL ~1.2-1.6 mEq/L

(Continued)

Magnesium Citrate *(Continued)*

Adults: 2.2-2.8 mg/dL ~1.8-2.3 mEq/L

Test Interactions ↑ magnesium; ↓ protein, calcium (S), ↓ potassium (S)

Drug Interactions

Danthron, mineral oil, milk, antacids, salicylate, lipid soluble vitamins, decreased tetracycline, decreased digoxin absorption

Decreased absorption of chloroquine, digoxin, penicillamine, tetracyclines, quinolones

Pregnancy Risk Factor B

Patient Information Take with a glass of water, fruit juice, or citrus flavored carbonated beverage to improve taste; chill before using

Nursing Implications To increase palatability, manufacturer suggests chilling the solution prior to administration

Additional Information Magnesium content of 5 mL: 3.85-4.71 mEq; no inhibition of cathartic effect when administered with clidinium

Elderly, due to disease or drug therapy, may be predisposed to diarrhea. Diarrhea may result in electrolyte imbalance. Decreased renal function (Cl_{cr} <30 mL/minute) may result in toxicity; monitor for toxicity and Cl_{cr} <30 mL/minute

Specific References

Vuignier BI, Oderda GM, Gorman RL, et al, "Effects of Magnesium Citrate and Clidinium Bromide on the Excretion of Activated Charcoal in Normal Subjects," *DICP*, 1989, 23(1):26-9.

Magnesium-Diasporal *see* Magnesium Citrate *on previous page*

Magnesium Sulfate (mag nee' ze um sul' fate)

CAS Number 7487-88-9; 10034-99-8

Use Anticonvulsant in pre-eclampsia or eclampsia; antiarrhythmic (especially in torsade de pointes, ventricular tachyarrhythmias); tocolytic agent (controversial about its bronchodilatory properties); in its oral form, it is used as a saline laxative; as a paste, it can be applied topically to promote wound healing; useful for digitalis toxicity, chronic alcoholism, injection for hydrofluoric acid burns

Antidote Useful For

Hydrogen Fluoride *on page 941*

Phosphine *on page 993*

Mechanism of Action Essential in the synthesis of adenosine triphosphate (ATP) and other enzymes involved in muscle contractility and neuronal transmissions; promotes bowel evacuation by causing osmotic retention of fluid which distends the colon with increased peristaltic activity when taken orally; parenterally, decreases acetylcholine in motor nerve terminals and acts on myocardium by slowing rate of S-A node impulse formation and prolonging conduction time

Adverse Reactions Adverse effects with parenteral $MgSO_4$ therapy are related to the magnesium serum level

Serum magnesium levels >3 mg/dL:
- Central nervous system: Depressed CNS
- Gastrointestinal: Diarrhea

Serum magnesium >5 mg/dL:
- Cardiovascular: Flushing
- Central nervous system: Somnolence
- Gastrointestinal: Diarrhea
- Neuromuscular & skeletal: Depressed deep tendon reflexes, myalgia, blocked peripheral neuromuscular transmission leading to anticonvulsant effects

Serum magnesium >12 mg/dL:
- Cardiovascular: Complete heart block
- Endocrine & metabolic: Hypercalcemia, hypernatremia
- Gastrointestinal: Diarrhea
- Respiratory: Respiratory paralysis

Signs & Symptoms of Acute Overdose Nausea, vomiting, flushing, diuresis, lethargy, hypotension, hyporeflexia, muscle weakness, coma, respiratory depression, EKG changes, atrial fibrillation, heart block

Toxicodynamics/Kinetics

Oral: Onset of cathartic action: Within 1-2 hours

I.M.:
- Onset of action: 60 minutes
- Duration: 3-4 hours

I.V.:
- Onset of action: Immediate
- Duration: 30 minutes

Absorption: ~33% in small intestine

Elimination: Primarily in feces; absorbed magnesium is rapidly eliminated by the kidneys

Usual Dosage The recommended dietary allowance (RDA) of magnesium is 4.5 mg/kg which is a total daily allowance of 350-400 mg for adult men and 280-300 mg for adult women. During pregnancy the RDA is 300 mg and during lactation the RDA is 355 mg. Average daily intakes of dietary magnesium have declined in recent years due to processing of food. The latest estimate of the average American dietary intake was 349 mg/day. Dose represented as $MgSO_4$ unless stated otherwise.

Note: Serum magnesium is poor reflection of repletional status as the majority of magnesium is intracellular; serum levels may be transiently normal for a few hours after a dose is given, therefore, aim for consistently high normal serum levels in patients with normal renal function for most efficient repletion

Hypomagnesemia:

Neonates: I.V.: 25-50 mg/kg/dose (0.2-0.4 mEq/kg/dose) every 8-12 hours for 2-3 doses

Children:

I.M., I.V.: 25-50 mg/kg/dose (0.2-0.4 mEq/kg/dose) every 4-6 hours for 3-4 doses, maximum single dose: 2000 mg (16 mEq), may repeat if hypomagnesemia persists (higher dosage up to 100 mg/kg/dose $MgSO_4$ I.V. has been used); maintenance: I.V.: 60-125 mg/kg/day (0.25-0.5 mEq/kg/day)

For management of seizures and hypertension: I.M., I.V.: 20-100 mg/kg/dose every 4-6 hours as needed; in severe cases doses as high as 200 mg/kg/dose have been used

Oral: 100-200 mg/kg/dose 4 times/day

Adults:

I.M., I.V.: 1 g every 6 hours for 4 doses; for severe hypomagnesemia: 8-12 g $MgSO_4$/day in divided doses has been used

Oral: 3 g every 6 hours for 4 doses as needed

Eclampsia, pre-eclampsia: Adults:

I.M.: 1-4 g every 4 hours

I.V.: Initial: 4 g, then switch to I.M. or 1-4 g/hour by continuous infusion

Maximum dose should not exceed 30-40 g/day; maximum rate of infusion: 1-2 g/hour

Maintenance electrolyte requirements:

Daily requirements: 0.2-0.5 mEq/kg/24 hours or 3-10 mEq/1000 kcal/24 hours

Maximum: 8-16 mEq/24 hours

Cathartic: Oral:

Children: 0.25 g/kg every 4-6 hours

Adults: 10-15 g in a glass of water

Dosing comments in renal impairment: Cl_{cr} <25 mL/minute: Do not administer

Contraindications Heart block, serious renal impairment

Warnings Use with caution in patients with impaired renal function (accumulation of magnesium which may lead to magnesium intoxication); use with caution in digitalized patients (may alter cardiac conduction leading to heart block); monitor serum magnesium level, respiratory rate, deep tendon reflex, renal function when $MgSO_4$ is administered parenterally; avoid in botulism

Dosage Forms

Injection: 100 mg/mL (20 mL); 125 mg/mL (8 mL); 250 mg/mL (150 mL); 500 mg/mL (2 mL, 5 mL, 10 mL, 30 mL, 50 mL)

Stability Refrigeration of intact ampuls may result in precipitation or crystallization; stability of parenteral admixture at room temperature (25°C): 60 days

Reference Range Serum magnesium:

Children: 1.5-1.9 mg/dL ~1.2-1.6 mEq/L

Adults: 2.2-2.8 mg/dL ~1.8-2.3 mEq/L

Test Interactions Analytical interference by calcium salts can result in a false depression of magnesium levels

Drug Interactions

Decreased effect: Nifedipine (decreased blood pressure and neuromuscular blockade)

Increased toxicity of aminoglycoside (increased neuromuscular blockade), CNS depressants (increased CNS depression), neuromuscular antagonists, betamethasone (pulmonary edema), colistin (neuromuscular blockade), ritodrine (increased cardiotoxicity)

Pregnancy Risk Factor B

Pregnancy Implications No harmful effects regarding breast-feeding; hypermagnesemia can lead to neonatal intrauterine growth retardation, CNS respiratory depression

Monitoring Parameters Monitor for arrhythmias, hypotension, respiratory and CNS depression during rapid I.V. administration; monitor serum magnesium level to avoid overdosages

(Continued)

Magnesium Sulfate *(Continued)*

Nursing Implications Monitor blood pressure when administering $MgSO_4$ I.V.; serum magnesium levels should be monitored to avoid overdose

Additional Information Found in nuts and green vegetables; 1 g of magnesium sulfate has ~99 mg of magnesium (4.1 mmol or 8.1 mEq); lithium-induced tachycardia (ventricular) may respond to I.V. magnesium sulfate

Specific References

Bohman VR and Cotton DB, "Supralethal Magnesemia With Patient Survival," *Obstet Gynecol*, 1990, 76(5 Pt 2):984-6.
Ferroggiaro A, Walther JM, and Cairns CB, "High Doses of Magnesium Impair Cardiac Oxidative Metabolism," *Acad Emerg Med*, 1995, 2:423-9.
Lucas MJ, Leveno KJ, and Cunningham IG, "A Comparison of Magnesium Sulfate With Phenytoin for the Prevention of Eclampsia," *N Engl J Med*, 1995, 333:201-5.
Worthley LT, "Lithium Toxicity and Refractory Cardiac Arrhythmia Treated With Intravenous Magnesium," *Anaesth Intensive Care*, 1974, 4:357-60.

Mannitol (man' i tole)

CAS Number 69-65-8

Brand Names Isotol®; Osmitrol® Injection; Resectisol® Irrigation Solution

Use Reduction of increased intracranial pressure associated with cerebral edema; promotion of diuresis in the prevention and/or treatment of oliguria or anuria due to acute renal failure; reduction of increased intraocular pressure; promoting urinary excretion of toxic substances (lithium); used for ciguatera poisoning

Antidote Useful For

Ciguatera Food Poisoning *on page 1069*
Cisplatin *on page 218*
Hyoscyamine Sulfate *on page 415*
Strychnine *on page 1016*

Mechanism of Action Increases the osmotic pressure of glomerular filtrate, which inhibits tubular reabsorption of water and electrolytes and increases urinary output

Adverse Reactions

Cardiovascular: Circulatory overload, diuresis, congestive heart failure
Central nervous system: Convulsions/seizures, headache
Dermatologic: Urticaria
Endocrine & metabolic: Fluid and electrolyte imbalance, water intoxication, hypernatremia, dehydration and hypovolemia secondary to rapid diuresis, hyponatremia
Gastrointestinal: Dry mouth, diarrhea (oral ingestion), colonic perforation (oral ingestion)
Local: Tissue necrosis
Ocular: Blurred vision
Renal and genitourinary: Focal osmotic nephrosis of proximal convoluted tubules
Respiratory: Pulmonary edema
Miscellaneous: Allergic reactions, osmolal gap

Signs & Symptoms of Acute Overdose Polyuria, hypotension, renal failure, cardiovascular collapse, chest pain, headache, tinnitus, ototoxicity (deafness), chills; can cause diarrhea when taken orally; pulmonary edema has occurred after a dose of 400 g over 2.5 hours

Toxicodynamics/Kinetics

Onset of action: Following injection, diuresis occurs within 1-3 hours and reductions in intracerebral pressures occur within 15 minutes
Duration:
Reduction in CSF pressure: Persists 3-8 hours after infusion discontinued
Reduction in intraocular pressure: Persists 4-8 hours
Absorption: Variable
Distribution: Remains confined to extracellular space (except in extreme concentrations) and does not penetrate the blood-brain barrier
Metabolism: Minimal amounts in the liver to glycogen
Half-life: 1.1-1.6 hours
Time to peak serum concentration: Reduction in intraocular fluid pressure: 30-60 minutes after injection
Elimination: Primarily excreted unchanged in urine by glomerular filtration

Usual Dosage I.V.:

Children:
Test dose (to assess adequate renal function): 200 mg/kg over 3-5 minutes to produce a urine flow of at least 1 mL/kg/hour for 1-3 hours
Initial: 0.5-1 g/kg
Maintenance: 0.25-0.5 g/kg/hour given every 4-6 hours

Adults:
Test dose: 12.5 g (200 mg/kg) over 3-5 minutes to produce a urine flow of at least 30-50 mL of urine per hour over the next 2-3 hours

Initial: 0.5-1 g/kg

Maintenance: 0.25-0.5 g/kg every 4-6 hours; usual adult dose: 20-200 g/24 hours

Intracranial pressure: Cerebral edema: 1.5-2 g/kg/dose I.V. as a 15% to 20% solution over ≥30 minutes; maintain serum osmolality 310-320 mOsm/kg

Preoperative for neurosurgery: 1.5-2 g/kg administered 1-1.5 hours prior to surgery

Transurethral irrigation: Use urogenital solution as required for irrigation

Contraindications Severe renal disease, dehydration, or active intracranial bleeding, severe pulmonary edema or congestion

Dosage Forms

Injection: 5% [50 mg/mL] (1000 mL); 10% [100 mg/mL] (500 mL, 1000 mL); 15% [150 mg/mL] (150 mL, 500 mL); 20% [200 mg/mL] (150 mL, 250 mL, 500 mL); 25% [250 mg/mL] (50 mL, 500 mL)

Solution, urogenital: 0.54% [5.4 mg/mL] (2000 mL)

Stability Should be stored at room temperature (15°C to 30°C) and protected from freezing; crystallization may occur at low temperatures; do not use solutions that contain crystals, heating in a hot water bath and vigorous shaking may be utilized for resolubilization; cool solutions to body temperature before using

Test Interactions Increases or decreases inorganic phosphorus (B); lowers serum sodium; causes false-positive of ethylene glycol

Drug Interactions Lithium

Pregnancy Risk Factor C

Monitoring Parameters Renal function, daily fluid I & O, serum electrolytes, serum and urine osmolality; hyponatremia can occur, also hyperglycemia (may be cause of osmolar gap)

Nursing Implications In-line 5-micron filter set should always be used for mannitol infusion with concentrations of 20% or greater; avoid extravasation; crenation and agglutination of red blood cells may occur if administered with whole blood; appears to be compatible with furosemide

Additional Information Mannitol 20% has an approximate osmolarity of 1100 mOsm/L and mannitol 25% has an approximate osmolarity of 1375 mOsm/L; for treatment of elevated intracranial pressure, maintain serum osmolality 310-320 mOsm/kg

Specific References

Gadallah MF, Lynn M, and Work J, "Case Report: Mannitol Nephrotoxicity Syndrome: Role of Hemodialysis and Postulate of Mechanisms," *Am H Med Sci*, 1995, 309:219-22.

Goodwin WE and Latta H, "Focal Osmotic Nephrosis Due to Therapeutic Use of Mannitol: A Case of Perirenal Hematoma After Renal Biopsy," *J Urol*, 1970, 103(1):11-4.

Huff JS, "Acute Mannitol Intoxication in a Patient With Normal Renal Function," *Am J Emerg Med*, 1990, 8(4):338-9.

Moses FM, "Colonic Perforation Due to Oral Mannitol," *JAMA*, 1988, 260(5):640.

Palmquist KL, Quattrocchi FP, and Looney LL, "Compatibility of Furosemide With 20% Mannitol," *Am J Health-Syst Pharm*, 1995, 52:648-50.

Maximum Strength Nytol® [OTC] *see* Diphenhydramine Hydrochloride *on page 1415*

Mazicon™ *replaced by* Flumazenil *on page 1428*

Medihaler-Epi® [OTC] *see* Epinephrine *on page 1422*

Medihaler-Iso® Inhalation Aerosol *see* Isoproterenol *on page 1436*

Mephyton® *see* Phytonadione *on page 1458*

Mercapturic Acid *see* Acetylcysteine *on page 1388*

Mercaptyl® *see* Penicillamine *on page 1454*

Mesna (mes' na)

CAS Number 19767-45-4

Brand Names Mesnex™ Injection

Synonyms Mesnum

Use Detoxifying agent used as a protectant against cystitis (hemorrhagic) induced by ifosfamide and cyclophosphamide

Mechanism of Action Binds with and detoxifies acrolein and other urotoxic metabolites of ifosfamide and cyclophosphamide

Adverse Reactions

Cardiovascular: Hypotension

Central nervous system: Malaise, headache

Dermatologic: Skin rash

Endocrine and Metabolic: Hypokalemia

Gastrointestinal: Diarrhea, nausea, vomiting, bad taste in mouth

Neuromuscular & skeletal: Limb pain

Ocular: Conjunctivitis

(Continued)

Mesna *(Continued)*

Miscellaneous: Chills

Toxicodynamics/Kinetics

Distribution: V_d: 0.652 L/kg

Metabolism: Rapidly oxidized intravascularly to mesna disulfide

Half-life: 24 minutes; mesna disulfide: 72 minutes

Elimination: Unchanged drug and metabolite are excreted primarily in the urine; time it takes for maximum urinary mesna excretion: 1 hour after I.V. and 2-3 hours after an oral mesna dose

Usual Dosage Children and Adults (refer to individual protocols):

Ifosfamide: I.V.: 20% W/W of ifosfamide dose at time of administration and 4 and 8 hours after each dose of ifosfamide

Cyclophosphamide: I.V.: 20% W/W of cyclophosphamide dose prior to administration and 3, 6, 9, 12 hours after cyclophosphamide dose (total daily dose = 120% to 180% of cyclophosphamide dose)

Oral dose: 40% W/W of the antineoplastic agent dose in 3 doses at 4-hour intervals

Contraindications Hypersensitivity to mesna or other thiol compounds

Warnings Will not prevent or alleviate other toxicities associated with ifosfamide or cyclophosphamide and will not prevent cystitis (hemorrhagic) in all patients

Dosage Forms Injection: 100 mg/mL (2 mL, 4 mL, 10 mL)

Stability Diluted solutions are chemically and physically stable for 24 hours at room temperature; however, it is recommended that solutions be refrigerated and used within 6 hours; incompatible with cisplatin

Test Interactions False-positive urinary ketones with Multistix® or Labstix®

Pregnancy Risk Factor B

Monitoring Parameters Urinalysis

Nursing Implications Used in conjunction with ifosfamide; examine morning urine specimen for hematuria prior to ifosfamide or cyclophosphamide treatment; if hematuria develops, reduce the ifosfamide/cyclophosphamide dose or discontinue the drug

Additional Information Injection may be given orally

Specific References

Pohl J, "Toxicology, Pharmacology, and Interactions of Sodium 2-Mercaptoethane Sulfonate (Mesna)," *Curr Chemotherapy*, 1981, 2:1387-9.

Mesnex™ Injection *see* Mesna *on previous page*

Mesnum *see* Mesna *on previous page*

Mestinon® Injection *see* Pyridostigmine Bromide *on page 1463*

Mestinon® Oral *see* Pyridostigmine Bromide *on page 1463*

Methylene Blue (meth' i leen)

CAS Number 61-73-4; 7220-79-3

Brand Names Desmoidpillen®; Urolene Blue® Oral; Vitableu®

Use Antidote for G-6-PD deficiency and drug-induced methemoglobinemia, indicator dye, chronic urolithiasis; bacteriostatic genitourinary antiseptic. Has been used topically (0.1% solutions) in conjunction with polychromatic light to photoinactivate viruses such as herpes simplex; this is an unlabeled indication; has been used alone or in combination with vitamin C for the management of chronic urolithiasis; has reversed ifosfamide (Ifex®) associated encephalopathy.

Investigational: May be of use in increasing vascular tone and myocardial function (without benefiting cell function) in patients with septic shock

Antidote Useful For

Aniline *on page 858*
Bismuth Subgallate *on page 157*
Chlorate Salts *on page 884*
Cresols *on page 898*
Dapsone *on page 260*
1,3-Dinitrobenzene *on page 914*
Diuron *on page 920*
Glutethimide *on page 383*
Hydrazine *on page 939*
Isosorbide Dinitrate *on page 445*
Lidocaine and Epinephrine *on page 467*
Methyl Mercaptan *on page 968*
Metoclopramide *on page 523*
Mushrooms, Toxic (Group II) *on page 1112*
Naphthalene *on page 973*

Nitrates *on page 978*
Nitric Oxide *on page 563*
Nitrites *on page 978*
Nitrofurantoin *on page 564*
Nitrogen Oxide *on page 980*
Nitroglycerin *on page 566*
Nitrous Oxide *on page 981*
Phenol *on page 616*
Propylene Glycol Dinitrate *on page 1003*
2,4,6-Trinitrotoluene *on page 1035*

Mechanism of Action Weak germicide; in low concentrations, hastens the conversion of methemoglobin to hemoglobin; has opposite effect at high concentrations by converting ferrous iron of reduced hemoglobin to ferric iron to form methemoglobin; in cyanide toxicity, it combines with cyanide to form cyanmethemoglobin preventing the interference of cyanide with the cytochrome system; indicated for symptomatic methemoglobinemia (usually when methemoglobin levels are >20%)

Adverse Reactions

Cardiovascular: Hypertension, cyanosis, large I.V. doses have been associated with precordial pain

Central nervous system: Dizziness/vertigo, mental confusion, headache, fever/hyperreflexia/pyrexia

Dermatologic: Stains skin

Gastrointestinal: Nausea, vomiting, abdominal pain

Genitourinary: Bladder irritation, dysuria

Hematologic: Formation of methemoglobin, hemolytic anemia in patients with G-6-PD deficiency

Miscellaneous: Discoloration of urine to blue or green, sweating

Signs & Symptoms of Acute Overdose Jaundice; urine discoloration (blue), urine discoloration (blue-green), urine discoloration (green), urine discoloration (green-yellow), urine discoloration (yellow-brown), feces discoloration (black), feces discoloration (blue)

Toxicodynamics/Kinetics

Maximum effect: 30 minutes

Absorption: Oral: 53% to 97%; absorbed poorly from GI tract

Metabolism: Reduced to leukomethylene blue by the tissues

Elimination: Bile, feces, and urine

Usual Dosage

Children: NADPH-methemoglobin reductase deficiency: Oral: 1-1.5 mg/kg/day (maximum: 300 mg/day) given with 5-8 mg/kg/day of ascorbic acid

Children and Adults: Methemoglobinemia: I.V.: 1-2 mg/kg or 25-50 mg/m^2 over several minutes; may be repeated in 1 hour if necessary

Adults:

Genitourinary antiseptic: Oral: 55-130 mg 3 times/day with a full glass of water (maximum: 390 mg/day)

Septic shock (investigational): 2 mg/kg over 15 minutes

Contraindications Severe renal insufficiency; intraspinal injection; hypersensitivity to methylene blue or any component

Warnings Can cause cyanide release in patients with sodium nitrite overdosage; use will not reverse cyanosis due to sulfhemoglobinemia (as with dapsone)

Dosage Forms

Injection: 10 mg/mL (1 mL, 10 mL)

Tablet: 55 mg, 65 mg

Test Interactions Can reduce arterial lactate concentration in septic shock

Pregnancy Risk Factor C (D if injected intra-amniotically)

Monitoring Parameters Hemoglobin, methemoglobin concentrations should drop within 1 hour

Nursing Implications Inject over several minutes to avoid high concentration; S.C. injection may cause necrotic abscess; may be diluted with normal saline

Additional Information Skin stains may be removed using a hypochlorite solution; does not interfere with spectrophotometric measurement of methemoglobin

Specific References

Burnakis TG, "Inadvertent Substitution of Methylene Blue for Indigo Carmine to Detect Premature Rupture of Membranes," *Hosp Pharm*, 1995, 30(4):336-8.

Dawson AH and Whyte IM, "Management of Dapsone Poisoning Complicated by Methaemoglobinaemia," *Med Toxicol Adverse Drug Exp*, 1989, 4(5):387-92.

DiSanto AR and Wagner JG, "Pharmacokinetics of Highly Ionized Drugs II: Methylene Blue – Absorption, Metabolism, and Excretion in Man and Dog After Oral Administration," *J Pharm Sci*, 1972, 61(7):1086-90.

Harvey JW and Keitt AS, "Studies of the Efficacy and Potential Hazards of Methylene Blue Therapy in Aniline-Induced Methaemoglobinaemia," *Br J Haematol*, 1983, 54(1):29-41.

(Continued)

Methylene Blue *(Continued)*

Jahns BE, Rynn KO, and Paloucek FP, "Interference of Methylene Blue (MthB) in the Determination of Whole Blood Methemoglobin (MtHgb) Concentrations," *Vet Hum Toxicol*, 1994, 36:342.

Preiser J, Lejeune P, Roma A, et al, "Methylene Blue Administration in Septic Shock," *Crit Care Med*, 1995, 23:259-64.

Zulian GB, Tullen E, and Maton B, "Methylene Blue for Ifosfamide-Associated Encephalopathy," *N Engl J Med*, 1995, 332:1239-40.

Methylphytyl Napthoquinone *see* Phytonadione *on page 1458*

4-Methylpyrazole

CAS Number 7554-65-6

Synonyms Fomepizole; 4-MP

Use Ethylene glycol and methanol toxicity; may be useful in propylene glycol; unclear whether it is useful in disulfiram-ethanol reactions

Antidote Useful For

Ethylene Glycol *on page 925*

Methanol *on page 957*

Mechanism of Action Complexes and inactivates alcohol dehydrogenase thus preventing formation of the toxic metabolites of the alcohols

Adverse Reactions

Dermatologic: Rash

Gastrointestinal: Dose-related nausea and dizziness

Hematologic: Eosinophilia

Hepatic: Transient increases in liver transaminases (possibly due to underlying ingestion)

Toxicodynamics/Kinetics

Maximum effect: 1.5-2 hours

Absorption: Oral: Readily absorbed

Distribution: V_d: 0.6-0.7 L/kg; unknown distribution, probably very similar to ethanol

Protein binding: Negligible

Elimination: Nonlinear elimination; at suggested therapeutic doses of 10-20 mg/kg the apparent elimination rate is 4-5 μmol/L/hour; 4-MP is dialyzable

Usual Dosage Oral: 15 mg/kg followed by 5 mg/kg in 12 hours and then 10 mg/kg every 12 hours until levels of toxin are not present

Reference Range Concentrations >10 μmol/L should result in enzyme inhibition

Drug Interactions Inhibitory effects on alcohol dehydrogenase are increased in presence of ethanol; ethanol also decreases metabolism of 4-MP; 4-MPO induces cytochrome P-450 mixed function oxidases *in vitro*

Additional Information Investigational (Phase 1) orphan drug undergoing clinical trials; dialyzable in animal studies; may be useful in ethanol-disulfiram reactions

Specific References

Jacobsen D, Ostensen J, Bredegen L, et al, "4-Methylpyrazole (4-MP) Is Effectively Removed by Hemodialysis in the Pig Model," *Vet Hum Toxicol*, 1992, 34:362.

Jacobsen D, Sebastian CS, Barron SK, et al, "Effects of 4-Methylpyrazole, Methanol/Ethylene Glycol Antidote in Healthy Humans," *J Emerg Med*, 1990, 8(4):455-61.

McMartin KE and Heath A, "Treatment of Ethylene Glycol Poisoning With Intravenous 4-Methylpyrazole," *N Engl J Med*, 1989, 320(2):125.

microNefrin® [OTC] *see* Epinephrine *on page 1422*

MK-0681 *replaced by* Trientine Dihydrochloride *on page 1474*

Monosodium Carbonate *see* Sodium Bicarbonate *on page 1467*

4-MP *see* 4-Methylpyrazole *on this page*

Mucolator® *see* Acetylcysteine *on page 1388*

Mucomyst® *see* Acetylcysteine *on page 1388*

Mucosol® *see* Acetylcysteine *on page 1388*

Mucret® *see* Acetylcysteine *on page 1388*

Murine® *see* Edetate Disodium *on page 1421*

NAC *see* Acetylcysteine *on page 1388*

N-Acetyl-3-Mercaptovalline *see* N-Acetyl-D-Penicillamine *on this page*

***N*-Acetylcysteine** *see* Acetylcysteine *on page 1388*

N-Acetyl-D-Penicillamine

Related Information

Penicillamine *on page 1454*

CAS Number 15537-71-0

Synonyms N-Acetyl-3-Mercaptovalline; NAP

Additional Information Requires IND number from the FDA for special purchase; through Food and Drug Division of Aldrich Chemical Co, Milwaukee, WI (414)-273-3850 DL-isomer D/C in 1988 or Sigma Chemical, St Louis, 1-800-325-3010; D-isomer (has not been used for human use)

***N*-Acetyl-L-cysteine** *see* Acetylcysteine *on page 1388*

$NaHCO_3$ *see* Sodium Bicarbonate *on page 1467*

Nalmefene Hydrochloride (nal' me feen)

CAS Number 55096-26-9; 58895-64-0

Brand Names Revex®

Synonyms Nalmetrene

Use Investigational in U.S.: Reversal of adverse opiate effects; may be useful for pruritus

Mechanism of Action Derivative of naltrexone with opioid antagonist effects; does not produce opiate agonist effects

Adverse Reactions

Cardiovascular: Hypotension, tachycardia, hypertension
Central nervous system: Dizziness, fatigue, fever, headache
Gastrointestinal: Nausea, vomiting
Neuromuscular & skeletal: Paresthesia

Toxicodynamics/Kinetics

Onset of action: 2 minutes
Distribution: V_d: 8.5 L/kg
Protein binding: 45%
Metabolism: In the liver
Half-life:
  Oral: 11 hours
  I.V.: 8-9 hours
Elimination: Urine (clearance: 1.37 L/hour/kg)

Usual Dosage

Opiate overdose: Adults: I.V. bolus: 0.5-1 mg every 2 minutes as clinically needed up to a total dose of 2 mg; may be given I.M. or S.C.
Pruritus: Oral: 10-20 mg
Reversal of postoperative opioid depression: I.V.: 0.1-0.5 mcg/kg; may repeat up to a total dose of 1 mcg/kg

Warnings In patients with renal or hepatic failure, administer doses over a 1-minute time period; renal or hepatic failure reduces clearance by 28%

Dosage Forms I.V. ampuls at concentrations of 1 mL of 100 mcg/mL and 2 mL of 1 mg/mL

Reference Range Therapeutic plasma level: 0.5 ng/mL

Pregnancy Risk Factor B

Specific References

Barsan WG, Seger D, Danzl DF, et al, "Duration of Antagonistic Effects of Nalmefene and Naloxone in Opiate-Induced Sedation for Emergency Department Procedures," *Am J Emerg Med*, 1989, 7(2):155-61.

Dixon R, Howes J, Gentile J, et al, "Nalmefene: Intravenous Safety and Kinetics of a New Opioid Antagonist," *Clin Pharmacol Ther*, 1986, 39(1):49-53.

Fudala PJ, Heishman SJ, Henningfield JE, et al, "Human Pharmacology and Abuse Potential of Nalmefene," *Clin Pharmacol Ther*, 1991, 49(3):300-6.

Gal TJ and Difazio CA, "Prolonged Antagonism of Opiod Action With Intravenous Nalmefene in Man," *Anesthesiology*, 1986, 64:175-80.

Kaplan J and Marx J, "Effectiveness and Safety of I.V. Nalmefene for E.D. Patients With Suspected Narcotic Overdoses," *Ann Emerg Med*, 1991, 20:31.

Monroe EW, "Efficacy an Safety of Nalmefene in Patients With Severe Pruritus Caused by Chronic Urticaria and Atopic Dermatitis," *J Am Acad Dermatol*, 1989, 21(1):135-6.

Nalmetrene *see* Nalmefene Hydrochloride *on this page*

Naloxone Hydrochloride (nal ox' one)

CAS Number 465-65-6; 357-08-4; 51481-60-8

Brand Names Narcan®; Narcanti®

Use Reverses CNS and respiratory depression in suspected narcotic overdose; neonatal opiate depression; coma of unknown etiology

Investigational: Shock, alcohol ingestion; pruritus due to cholestasis; also useful in clonidine, camylofin, valproic acid, and captopril overdose; may be useful in reversing cardiac depression due to dextropropoxyphine

Antidote Useful For

Alfentanil Hydrochloride *on page 94*
Belladonna and Opium *on page 145*

Buprenorphine Hydrochloride *on page 169*
Butorphanol Tartrate *on page 174*
Captopril *on page 181*
Captopril and Hydrochlorothiazide *on page 183*
Clonidine *on page 231*
Codeine *on page 238*
Dextromethorphan Hydrobromide *on page 270*
Diphenoxylate and Atropine *on page 291*
Fentanyl Citrate *on page 347*
Gamma Hydroxybutyric Acid *on page 376*
Guanfacine Hydrochloride *on page 394*
Heroin Hydrochloride *on page 401*
Hydrocodone and Homatropine *on page 407*
Hydromorphone Hydrochloride *on page 409*
Ketobemidone Hydrochloride *on page 452*
Levomethadyl Acetate Hydrochloride *on page 463*
Levorphanol Tartrate *on page 464*
Lisinopril *on page 475*
Loperamide Hydrochloride *on page 480*
Meperidine Hydrochloride *on page 499*
Methadone Hydrochloride *on page 508*
Morphine Sulfate *on page 539*
Nalbuphine Hydrochloride *on page 546*
Nitrous Oxide *on page 981*
Opium Alkaloids (Hydrochlorides) *on page 579*
Opium Tincture *on page 580*
Oxycodone and Acetaminophen *on page 584*
Oxycodone Hydrochloride *on page 585*
Oxymorphone Hydrochloride *on page 587*
Paregoric *on page 595*
Pentazocine *on page 603*
Propoxyphene *on page 655*
Propoxyphene and Acetaminophen *on page 656*
Sufentanil Citrate *on page 711*
Tilidine Hydrochloride *on page 752*
Tramadol Hydrochloride *on page 762*
Valproic Acid and Derivatives *on page 782*
Zipeprol Hydrochloride *on page 813*

Mechanism of Action Competes and displaces narcotics at narcotic receptor sites

Adverse Reactions

Cardiovascular: Hypertension, hypotension, tachycardia, ventricular arrhythmias
Central nervous system: Insomnia, irritability, anxiety
Dermatologic: Rash
Gastrointestinal: Nausea, vomiting
Genitourinary: Urinary urgency
Hematologic: Coagulopathy
Ocular: Blurred vision
Respiratory: Pulmonary edema has been described
Miscellaneous: Narcotic withdrawal, sweating

Signs & Symptoms of Acute Overdose Irritability, agitation, anxiety, anorexia, nausea, diaphoresis at 2-4 mg/kg, hypotension, laryngospasm, bradycardia, focal seizures

Toxicodynamics/Kinetics

Onset of effect:
Endotracheal, I.M., S.C.: Within 2-5 minutes
I.V.: Within 2 minutes

Duration: 20-60 minutes; since shorter than that of most opioids, repeated doses are usually needed

Distribution: V_d: 2.7 L/kg; crosses the placenta

Metabolism: Primarily by glucuronidation in the liver to naloxone 3-glucuronide

Half-life:
Neonates: 1.2-3.5 hours
Adults: 1-1.5 hours

Elimination: In urine as metabolites

Usual Dosage I.M., I.V. (preferred), intratracheal, S.C.:

Neonates: Narcotic-induced asphyxia: 0.01-0.1 mg/kg every 2-3 minutes as needed; may need to repeat every 1-2 hours

Infants and Children: Postanesthesia narcotic reversal: 0.01 mg/kg; may repeat every 2-3 minutes as needed based on response

Opiate intoxication: Birth (including premature infants) to 5 years or <20 kg: 0.1 mg/kg; repeat every 2-3 minutes if needed; may need to repeat doses every 20-60 minutes

>5 years or ≥20 kg: 2 mg/dose; if no response, repeat every 2-3 minutes; may need to repeat doses every 20-60 minutes

Children and Adults: Continuous infusion: I.V.: If continuous infusion is required, calculate dosage/hour based on effective intermittent dose used and duration of adequate response seen, titrate dose 0.04-0.16 mg/kg/hour for 2-5 days in children, up to 0.8 mg/kg/hour in adults; alternatively, continuous infusion utilizes ⅔ of the initial naloxone bolus on an hourly basis; add 10 times this dose to each liter of D_5W and infuse at a rate of 100 mL/hour; ½ of the initial bolus dose should be readministered 15 minutes after initiation of the continuous infusion to prevent a drop in naloxone levels; increase infusion rate as needed to assure adequate ventilation

Adults: Narcotic overdose: I.V.: 0.4-2 mg every 2-3 minutes as needed; may need to repeat doses every 20-60 minutes, if no response is observed after 10 mg, question the diagnosis. **Note:** Use 0.1-0.2 mg increments in patients who are opioid dependent and in postoperative patients to avoid large cardiovascular changes

Contraindications Hypersensitivity to naloxone or any component

Warnings Use with caution in patients with cardiovascular disease; excessive dosages should be avoided after use of opiates in surgery, because naloxone may cause an increase in blood pressure and reversal of anesthesia; may precipitate withdrawal symptoms in patients addicted to opiates, including pain, hypertension, sweating, agitation, irritability, shrill cry, failure to feed

Dosage Forms

Injection: 0.4 mg/mL (1 mL, 2 mL, 10 mL); 1 mg/mL (2 mL, 10 mL)

Injection, neonatal: 0.02 mg/mL (2 mL)

Stability Protect from light; stable in 0.9% sodium chloride and D_5W at 4 mcg/mL for 24 hours; do not mix with alkaline solutions

Reference Range Plasma naloxone levels at 2 and 5 minutes after a 0.4 mg I.V. dose: 0.01 mg/L and 0.004 mg/L respectively

Test Interactions Will not give a false-positive enzymatic urine screen for opiates

Drug Interactions Decreased effect of narcotic analgesics; use with cocaine; may have caused ventricular arrhythmias and atrial fibrillation in one case report

Pregnancy Risk Factor B

Monitoring Parameters Respiratory rate, heart rate, blood pressure

Nursing Implications The use of neonatal naloxone is no longer recommended because unacceptable fluid volumes will result, especially to small neonates; the 0.4 mg/mL preparation is available and can be accurately dosed with appropriately sized syringes (1 mL)

Additional Information In Talwin® Nx to prevent abuse of tablets via parenteral administration; not compatible with alkaline solutions, bisulfite, or metabisulfite

Specific References

Gergasa NY, Alling DW, Talbot TL, et al, "Effects of Naloxone Infusions in Patients With the Pruritis of Cholestasis," *Ann Intern Med*, 1995, 123:161-7.

Chamberlain JM and Klein BL, "A Comprehensive Review of Naloxone for the Emergency Physician," *Am J Emerg Med*, 1994, 12(6):650-60.

Evans LE, Swainson CP, Roscoe P, et al, "Treatment of Drug Overdosage With Naloxone, a Specific Narcotic Antagonist," *Lancet*, 1973, 1(801):452-5.

Goldfrank L, Weisman RS, Errick JK, et al, "A Dosing Nomogram for Continuous Infusion Intravenous Naloxone," *Ann Emerg Med*, 1986, 15(5):566-70.

Hantson P, Evenepoel E, Ziade D, et al, "Adverse Cardiac Manifestations Following Dextropropoxyphene Overdose: Can Naloxone Be Helpful?" *Ann Emerg Med*, 1995, 25:263-6.

Merigian KS, "Cocaine-Induced Ventricular Arrhythmias and Rapid Atrial Fibrillation Temporally Related to Naloxone Administration," *Am J Emerg Med*, 1993, 11:96-7.

Olsen KS, "Naloxone Administration and Laryngospasm Followed by Pulmonary Edema," *Intensive Care Med*, 1990, 16(5):340-1.

Salvucci Jr AA, Eckstein M, and Iscovich AL, "Submental Injection of Naloxone," *Ann Emerg Med*, 1995, 25:719-20.

Storrow AB, Wians FH Jr, Mikkelsen SL, et al, "Does Naloxone Cause a Positive Urine Opiate Screen?" *Ann Emerg Med*, 1994, 24(6):1151-3.

Tandberg D and Abercrombie D, "Treatment of Heroin Overdose With Endotracheal Naloxone," *Ann Emerg Med*, 1982, 11(8):443-5.

NAP *see* N-Acetyl-D-Penicillamine *on page 1446*

Narcan® *see* Naloxone Hydrochloride *on page 1447*

Narcanti® *see* Naloxone Hydrochloride *on page 1447*

Natril *see* Sodium Nitrite *on page 1469*

Natrium Nitrosum *see* Sodium Nitrite *on page 1469*

Neostigmine (nee oh stig' meen)

CAS Number 59-99-4; 114-80-7; 51-60-5

Brand Names Intrastigmina®; Prostigmin® Injection; Prostigmin® Oral

Use Second-line agent for envenomation by Asian snakes or intoxication with tetradotoxin exposures if edrophonium supplies are depleted; reversal of the effects of nondepolarizing neuromuscular blocking agents after surgery

Mechanism of Action Inhibits destruction of acetylcholine by acetylcholinesterase which facilitates transmission of impulses across myoneural junction

Adverse Reactions

Cardiovascular: Bradycardia, hypotension, bradyarrhythmias, asystole (maximum effect: 90 minutes)

Central nervous system: Restlessness, agitation, seizures/seizures, slurred speech, headache, coma, ataxia

Gastrointestinal: Hyperperistalsis, nausea, vomiting, salivation, diarrhea, defecation

Neuromuscular & skeletal: Tremors, fasciculations, weakness

Ocular: Miosis, lacrimation, nystagmus

Respiratory: Bronchoconstriction, bronchial secretion (increased)

Miscellaneous: Sweating

Signs & Symptoms of Acute Overdose Muscle weakness, blurred vision, excessive sweating, tearing and salivation, nausea, vomiting, tachypnea, bradycardia

Toxicodynamics/Kinetics

Onset of action: I.V.: 1-20 minutes

Duration: 1-2 hours

Absorption: Poor from GI tract

Distribution: V_d: ~1 L/kg

Protein binding: 15% to 25%

Metabolism: In the liver

Half-life:

- Oral: 52 minutes
- I.M.: 51-90 minutes
- I.V.: 53 minutes

Elimination: 50% excreted renally as unchanged drug

Usual Dosage

Myasthenia gravis: Diagnosis: I.M.:

- Children: 0.04 mg/kg as a single dose
- Adults: 0.02 mg/kg as a single dose

Myasthenia gravis: Treatment:

- Children:
  - Oral: 2 mg/kg/day divided every 3-4 hours
  - I.M., I.V., S.C.: 0.01-.04 mg/kg every 2-4 hours
- Adults:
  - Oral: 15 mg/dose every 3-4 hours
  - I.M., I.V., S.C.: 0.5-2.5 mg every 1-3 hours

Reversal of nondepolarizing neuromuscular blockade after surgery in conjunction with atropine or glycopyrrolate: I.V.:

- Infants: 0.025-0.1 mg/kg/dose
- Children: 0.025-0.08 mg/kg/dose
- Adults: 0.5-2.5 mg; total dose not to exceed 5 mg

Bladder atony: Adults: I.M., S.C.:

- Prevention: 0.25 mg every 4-6 hours for 2-3 days
- Treatment: 0.5-1 mg every 3 hours for 5 doses after bladder has emptied

Contraindications Hypersensitivity to neostigmine, bromides or any component; GI or GU obstruction

Warnings Adequate facilities should be available for cardiopulmonary resuscitation when testing and adjusting dose for myasthenia gravis

Dosage Forms

Injection, as methylsulfate: 0.25 mg/mL (1 mL); 0.5 mg/mL (1 mL, 10 mL); 1 mg/mL (10 mL)

Tablet, as bromide: 15 mg

Test Interactions Increases aminotransferase [ALT (SGPT)/AST (SGOT)] (S), amylase (S)

Drug Interactions Neuromuscular blocking agents, when taken with digitalis glycosides, prolonged A-V node conduction time may result

Pregnancy Risk Factor C

Pregnancy Implications Does not cross placental barrier except with large doses; not distributed into breast milk

Monitoring Parameters Respiratory status/muscle weakness

Nursing Implications In the diagnosis of myasthenia gravis, all anticholinesterase medications should be discontinued for at least 8 hours before administering neostigmine

Additional Information

Neostigmine bromide: Prostigmin® tablet
Neostigmine methylsulfate: Prostigmin® injection

Specific References

Fisher DM, Cronnelly R, Miller RD, et al, "The Neuromuscular Pharmacology of Neostigmine in Infants and Children," *Anesthesiology*, 1983, 59(3):220-5.
Payne JP, Hughes R, and Al Azawi S, "Neuromuscular Blockade by Neostigmine in Anaesthetized Man," *Br J Anaesth*, 1980, 52(1):69-76.

Nestrex® *see* Pyridoxine Hydrochloride *on page 1465*
Neupogen® Injection *see* Filgrastim *on page 1425*
Neut® *see* Sodium Bicarbonate *on page 1467*
Nidryl® Oral [OTC] *see* Diphenhydramine Hydrochloride *on page 1415*
Nitris *see* Sodium Nitrite *on page 1469*
Nitrit® *see* Amyl Nitrite *on page 1390*
Nitrous Acid *see* Sodium Nitrite *on page 1469*
Noradrenaline Acid Tartrate *see* Norepinephrine Bitartrate *on this page*
Nordryl® Injection *see* Diphenhydramine Hydrochloride *on page 1415*
Nordryl® Oral *see* Diphenhydramine Hydrochloride *on page 1415*

Norepinephrine Bitartrate (nor ep i nef' rin)

Related Information

Adrenergic Agonists, Cardiovascular Comparison *on page 1638*
Adrenergic Agonists Drug Infusions Comparison *on page 1638*

CAS Number 51-41-2; 51-40-1; 6981-49-5

Brand Names Levophed®

Synonyms Levarterenol Bitartrate; Noradrenaline Acid Tartrate

Use Treatment of shock which persists after adequate fluid volume replacement; useful for hypotension induced by tricyclic antidepressants, disulfiram-ethanol interaction, phenothiazine antidysrhythmic agents

Antidote Useful For

Copper *on page 896*
Dantrolene Sodium *on page 258*
Disulfiram *on page 296*
Ethchlorvynol *on page 330*
Mushrooms, Toxic (Group III) *on page 1112*
Mushrooms, Toxic (Group IV) *on page 1114*
Prazosin Hydrochloride *on page 638*
Quinine Sulfate *on page 671*
Torsemide *on page 761*
Yew *on page 1159*

Mechanism of Action Stimulates $beta_1$-adrenergic receptors and alpha-adrenergic receptors causing increased contractility and heart rate as well as vasoconstriction, thereby increasing systemic blood pressure and coronary blood flow

Adverse Reactions

Cardiovascular: Cardiac arrhythmias, palpitations, bradycardia, tachycardia, hypertension, chest pain
Central nervous system: Anxiety, fear, headache
Dermatologic: Pallor
Endocrine & metabolic: Uterine contractions
Gastrointestinal: Vomiting
Local: Organ ischemia (due to vasoconstriction of renal and mesenteric arteries); ischemic necrosis and sloughing of superficial tissue after extravasation
Ocular: Photophobia, nystagmus
Respiratory: Respiratory distress
Miscellaneous: Diaphoresis

Signs & Symptoms of Acute Overdose Hypotension, sweating, cerebral hemorrhage, seizures/seizures

Toxicodynamics/Kinetics

Onset of action: I.M.: Very rapid acting
Duration: 1-2 minutes
Absorption: S.C.: Poor
Distribution: Localizes primarily in sympathetic tissue; does not cross the blood-brain barrier

(Continued)

Norepinephrine Bitartrate *(Continued)*

Metabolism: By catechol-o-methyltransferase (COMT) and monoamine oxidase (MAO)

Elimination: In urine (84% to 96% as inactive metabolites) and in the liver

Usual Dosage I.V. infusion (dose stated in terms of norepinephrine base):

Children: Initial: 0.05-0.1 mcg/kg/minute, titrate to desired effect

Rate (mL/hour) = dose (mcg/kg/minute) x weight (kg) x 60 minutes/hour divided by concentration (mcg/mL)

Adults: 8-12 mcg/minute as an infusion; initiate at 4 mcg/minute and titrate to desired response

Note: Dose stated in terms of norepinephrine base

Rate of infusion: 4 mg in 500 mL D_5W

2 mcg/minute = 15 mL/hour
4 mcg/minute = 30 mL/hour
6 mcg/minute = 45 mL/hour
8 mcg/minute = 60 mL/hour
10 mcg/minute = 75 mL/hour
12 mcg/minute = 90 mL/hour
14 mcg/minute = 105 mL/hour
16 mcg/minute = 120 mL/hour
18 mcg/minute = 135 mL/hour
20 mcg/minute = 150 mL/hour

Administration Administer into large vein to avoid the potential for extravasation; standard concentration: 4 mg/500 mL but 8 mg/500 mL has been used

Contraindications Hypersensitivity to norepinephrine or sulfites

Warnings Blood/volume depletion should be corrected, if possible, before norepinephrine therapy; extravasation may cause severe tissue necrosis, give into a large vein. The drug should not be given to patients with peripheral or mesenteric vascular thrombosis because ischemia may be increased and the area of infarct extended; use with caution during cyclopropane and halothane anesthesia; use with caution in patients with occlusive vascular disease; some products may contain sulfites.

Dosage Forms Injection: 1 mg/mL (4 mL)

Stability Readily oxidized, protect from light, do not use if brown coloration; dilute with D_5W or D_5NS, but not recommended to dilute in normal saline; not stable with alkaline solutions

Stability of parenteral admixture at room temperature (25°C): 24 hours

Reference Range 24-hour urinary catecholamine level: <100 µg; normal plasma basal norepinephrine level: 100-447 pg/mL

Drug Interactions Atropine sulfate may block the reflex bradycardia caused by norepinephrine and enhances the pressor response; tricyclic antidepressants, MAO inhibitors, antihistamines (diphenhydramine, tripelennamine), guanethidine, ergot alkaloids, and methyldopa may potentiate the effect of norepinephrine

Pregnancy Risk Factor D

Pregnancy Implications Crosses the placenta

Monitoring Parameters Blood pressure, heart rate, urine output, peripheral perfusion

Nursing Implications Patient hemodynamic status should be monitored

Extravasation: Use phentolamine as antidote; mix 5 mg with 9 mL of normal saline; inject a small amount of this dilution into extravasated area; blanching should reverse immediately. Monitor site; if blanching should recur, additional injections of phentolamine may be needed.

Additional Information Do not use normal saline as a diluent, normal saline is incompatible with norepinephrine; rate of infusion: 2-12 mcg/minute

Standard diluent: 4 mg/500 mL D_5W; 4 mg/250 mL D_5W

Minimum volume: 8 mg/500 mL D_5W

Specific References

Aron DC, Bravo EL, and Kapcala LP, "Erroneous Plasma Norepinephrine Levels With Radioimmunoassay," *Ann Intern Med*, 1983, 98(6):1023.

Cryer PE, "Physiology and Pathophysiology of the Human Sympathoadrenal Neuroendocrine System," *N Engl J Med*, 1980, 303(8):436-44.

Papazian MC, Perrin G, et al, "Norepinephrine or Dopamine for the Treatment of Hyperdynamic Septic Shock?" *Chest*, 1993, 103:1826-31.

North and South American Antisnake-bite Serum *see* Antivenin (Crotalidae) Polyvalent *on page 1392*

NuLYTELY® *see* Polyethylene Glycol *on page 1460*

Nytol® Oral [OTC] *see* Diphenhydramine Hydrochloride *on page 1415*

O.A.R.® *see* Sodium Nitrite *on page 1469*

OCL® *see* Polyethylene Glycol *on page 1460*

Ocu-Tropine® *see* Atropine Sulfate *on page 1395*

Osmitrol® Injection *see* Mannitol *on page 1442*

Oxygen (Hyperbaric)

Synonyms Hyperbaric Oxygen

Use Carbon monoxide, carbon tetrachloride, cyanide, hydrocarbon, hydrogen sulfide, methylene chloride, mushroom (*Amanita* toxin), brown recluse spider bite, chloroform; also decompression sickness, air emboli, and anaerobic infections; may also be useful in methemoglobinemia; treatment of helium-induced embolism

Antidote Useful For

Acrylonitrile *on page 853*
Brown Recluse Spider *on page 1061*
Carbon Monoxide *on page 880*
Carbon Tetrachloride *on page 882*
Cyanide *on page 899*
Hydrogen Sulfide *on page 942*
Mushrooms, Toxic (Group I) *on page 1111*

Mechanism of Action Displaces carbon monoxide from binding sites and increases elimination rate; also alleviates cerebral edema and CO-induced peroxidation

Adverse Reactions Miscellaneous: Temporary visual deficits, otic discomfort, ruptured tympanic membranes; also barotrauma to CNS or lung and seizures are reported with prolonged durations (greater than those used for CO poisoning)

Usual Dosage 2.5-3 atmospheres

Contraindications Absolute contraindications are pneumothorax and bowel obstruction; avoid in paraquat or bleomycin-induced pulmonary toxicity. Relative contraindications include claustrophobia, respiratory infections, seizure disorder, asthma, COPD, pneumothorax or history of spontaneous pneumothorax, thoracic or otic surgery, optic neuritis, and pulmonary lesions; also may exacerbate acetaminophen or bromobenzene-induced hepatic necrosis. Use of hyperbaric oxygen in nitrogen oxide exposure is contraindicated.

Reference Range Concentrations of CO >30% in nonpregnant patients or >20% in pregnant patients are indications for treatment

Pregnancy Implications Well tolerated in the treatment of carbon monoxide and indicated for the treatment of pregnant patients when symptomatic or with carboxyhemoglobin levels >20%

Additional Information Hyperbaric oxygen has a clear benefit in the treatment of direct and indirect (methylene chloride) CO poisoning; recent study demonstrated decreased incidence of delayed neurologic sequelae due to CO poisoning; its role in other toxins is not well defined, its relative unavailability and delays in initiating therapy preclude direct extension of promising experimental results; may be of some use in quinine or organophosphate poisoning

Specific References

Guidotti TL, "The Higher Oxides of Nitrogen: Inhalation Toxicology," *Environ Res*, 1978, 15:443-72.

McMurray B, Seger D, Bonfiglio F, et al, "Criteria Used to Recommend HBO in Carbon Monoxide Poisoning: A Survey of Poison Centers, Burn Centers, and HBO Centers," *Vet Hum Toxicol*, 1994, 36(24):344.

Olson KR and Seger D, "Hyperbaric Oxygen for Carbon Monoxide Poisoning: Does it Really Work?" *Ann Emerg Med*, 1995, 25:535-7.

Rudge FW, "Treatment of Methylene Chloride Induced Carbon Monoxide Poisoning With Hyperbaric Oxygenation," *Mil Med*, 1990, 155(11):570-2.

Sloan EP, Murphy DG, Hart R, et al, "Complications and Protocol Considerations in Carbon Monoxide-Poisoned Patients Who Require Hyperbaric Oxygen Therapy: Report From a Ten Year Experience," *Ann Emerg Med*, 1989, 18(6):629-34.

Thom SR, Taber RL, Mendiguren I, et al, "Delayed Neuropsychologic Sequelae After Carbon Monoxide Poisoning: Prevention by Treatment With Hyperbaric Oxygen," *Ann Emerg Med*, 1995, 25:474-80.

Tibbles PM and Perrotta PL, "Treatment of Carbon Monoxide Poisoning: A Critical Review of Human Outcome Studies Comparing Normobaric Oxygen With Hyperbaric Oxygen," *Ann Emerg Med*, 1994, 24(2):269-76.

Tomaszewski CA and Thom SR, "Use of Hyperbaric Oxygen in Toxicology," *Emerg Med Clin North Am*, 1994, 12(2):437-59.

Van Hoesen KB, Camporesi EM, Moon RE, et al, "Should Hyperbaric Oxygen Be Used to Treat the Pregnant Patient for Acute Carbon Monoxide Poisoning?" *JAMA*, 1989, 261(7):1039-43.

2-PAM *see* Pralidoxime Chloride *on page 1461*

Parlodel® *see* Bromocriptine Mesylate *on page 1398*

PEG *see* Polyethylene Glycol *on page 1460*

Penicillamine (pen i sil' a meen)

Related Information

Drugs and Chemicals Proven to be Teratogenic in Humans *on page 1572-1575*

N-Acetyl-D-Penicillamine *on page 1446*

CAS Number 59-53-0; 52-67-5; 2219-30-9

Brand Names Cuprimine®; Cupripen®; Depen®; Distamine®; D-Penamine®; Kelatin®; Mercaptyl®; Sufortan®; Trolovol®

Synonyms D-3-Mercaptovaline; β,β-Dimethylcysteine; D-Penicillamine

Use Treatment of Wilson's disease, cystinuria, adjunct in the treatment of rheumatoid arthritis; lead, mercury, cadmium iron poisoning; primary biliary cirrhosis

Antidote Useful For

Arsenic *on page 862*

Bismuth Subgallate *on page 157*

Copper *on page 896*

Gold Compounds *on page 386*

Lead *on page 945*

Mechanism of Action Chelates with lead, copper, mercury, iron, and other heavy metals to form stable, soluble complexes that are excreted in urine; depresses circulating IgM rheumatoid factor, depresses T-cell but not B-cell activity; combines with cystine to form a compound which is more soluble, thus cystine calculi are prevented

Adverse Reactions

Cardiovascular: Swelling of face, feet, or lower legs; periarteritis nodosa

Central nervous system: Fever, peripheral sensory and motor neuropathies, myasthenic syndrome, seizures, chills, weakness, tiredness

Dermatologic: Rash, pruritus, pemphigus, increased friability of the skin, hirsutism, epidural necrolysis, hives, itching, psoriasiform eruptions

Endocrine & metabolic: Iron deficiency, gynecomastia, weight gain

Gastrointestinal: Oral lesions, diarrhea, colitis, nausea, vomiting, hypogeusia, anorexia

Hematologic: Leukopenia, thrombocytopenia (12% to 27% in patients with rheumatoid arthritis), eosinophilia, aplastic anemia, hemolytic anemia, lymphopenia, sideroblastic anemia

Hepatic: Hepatic dysfunction

Neuromuscular & skeletal: Arthralgia, dermatomyositis, joint pain, myasthenia gravis

Ocular: Optic neuritis, ptosis, diplopia, retinopathy, photophobia

Otic: Tinnitus

Renal & genitourinary: Nephrotic syndrome, renal vasculitis, hematuria, bloody or cloudy urine, glomerulonephritis

Respiratory: Obliterative bronchiolitis, pulmonary fibrosis, interstitial pneumonitis, coughing or wheezing, rhinitis, sore throat

Miscellaneous: Lymphadenopathy, allergic reactions, dysphoria, SLE-like syndrome, polymyositis, white spots on lips or mouth

Signs & Symptoms of Acute Overdose Seizures, agitation, hemoptysis, hypertrichosis, acrodynia, dysphagia, nausea, vomiting

Toxicodynamics/Kinetics

Absorption: Oral: 40% to 70%

Protein binding: 80%

Metabolism: Small amounts of hepatic metabolism to disulfides

Half-life: 1.7-3.2 hours

Time to peak serum concentration: Within 1 hour

Elimination: Primarily (30% to 60%) in urine as unchanged drug

Usual Dosage Oral:

Rheumatoid arthritis:

Children: Initial: 3 mg/kg/day (≤250 mg/day) for 3 months, then 6 mg/kg/day (≤500 mg/day) in divided doses twice daily for 3 months to a maximum of 10 mg/kg/day in 3-4 divided doses

Adults: 125-250 mg/day, may increase dose at 1- to 3-month intervals up to 1-1.5 g/day

Wilson's disease (doses titrated to maintain urinary copper excretion >1 mg/day):

Infants <6 months: 250 mg/dose once daily

Children <12 years: 250 mg/dose 2-3 times/day

Adults: 250 mg 4 times/day

Cystinuria:

Children: 30 mg/kg/day in 4 divided doses

Adults: 1-4 g/day in divided doses every 6 hours

Lead poisoning (continue until blood lead level is <60 mcg/dL):

Children: 25-40 mg/kg/day in 3 divided doses

Adults: 250-500 mg/dose every 8-12 hours

Primary biliary cirrhosis: 250 mg/day to start, increase by 250 mg every 2 weeks up to a maintenance dose of 1 g/day, usually given 250 mg 4 times/day

Arsenic poisoning: Children: 100 mg/kg/day in divided doses every 6 hours for 5 days; maximum: 1 g/day

Mercury poisoning:
Children: 20-30 mg/kg in 4 divided doses
Adults: 250 mg 4 times/day

Dosing adjustment/comments in renal impairment: Cl_{cr} <50 mL/minute: Avoid use

N-acetyl D,L-penicillamine: Chronic elemental mercury exposure:
Children: 30 mg/kg/day on an empty stomach in 4 divided doses for up to 6 days
Adults: 250 mg 4 times/day for up to 6 days; may repeat course as needed

Can be obtained through Aldrich Chemical Co, 940 West St Paul Ave, Milwaukee, WI (414-273-3850 or 800-336-9719; Product No A-19008)

Contraindications Hypersensitivity to penicillamine; rheumatoid arthritis patients with renal insufficiency; patients with previous penicillamine-related aplastic anemia or agranulocytosis

Warnings Cross-sensitivity with penicillin is possible; therefore, should be used cautiously in patients with a history of penicillin allergy. Patients on penicillamine for Wilson's disease or cystinuria should receive pyridoxine supplementation 25 mg/day; once instituted for Wilson's disease or cystinuria, continue treatment on a daily basis; interruptions of even a few days have been followed by hypersensitivity with reinstitution of therapy. Penicillamine has been associated with fatalities due to agranulocytosis, aplastic anemia, thrombocytopenia, Goodpasture's syndrome, and myasthenia gravis; patients should be warned to report promptly any symptoms suggesting toxicity; approximately 33% of patients will experience an allergic reaction.

Dosage Forms
Capsule: 125 mg, 250 mg
Tablet: 250 mg

Stability Store in tight, well-closed containers

Test Interactions Positive ANA

Drug Interactions

Decreased absorption with iron and zinc salts, probenecid, antacids (magnesium, calcium, aluminum) and food; food, aluminum-based antacids, and ferrous sulfate reduce absorption by >50%

Decreased effect/levels of digoxin

Increased effect of gold, antimalarials, immunosuppressants, phenylbutazone (hematologic, renal toxicity), insulin (hypoglycemia)

Pregnancy Risk Factor D

Pregnancy Implications Correlated with cutis laxa in neonates

Monitoring Parameters Urinalysis, CBC with differential, hemoglobin, platelet count, liver function tests

Nursing Implications For patients who cannot swallow, contents of capsules may be administered in 15-30 mL of chilled puréed fruit or fruit juice; patients should be warned to report promptly any symptoms suggesting toxicity

Additional Information Danazol can be used to treat breast enlargement. N-acetyl form of penicillamine is less toxic but still investigational. L-isomer is the more toxic isomer. An IND process must be followed; essentially its use has been supplanted by 2,3-dimercaptosuccinic acid. Pyridoxine can be used to treat sideroblastic anemia.

Specific References

Adelman HM, Winters PR, Mahan CS, et al, "D-Penicillamine-Induced Myasthenia Gravis; Diagnosis Obscured by Coexisting Chronic Obstructive Pulmonary Disease," *Am J Med Sci*, 1995, 309:191-3.

Albert C, Aynard B, Terbe V, et al, "D-Penicillamine Induced Rapidly Progressive Glomerulonephritis With Membranous Nephropathy in a Patient With Rheumatoid Arthritis," *Clin Exp Rheumatol*, 1994, 12(Suppl 11):108.

Andonopoulos AP, Terzis E, Tsibri E, et al, "D-Penicillamine Induced Myasthenia Gravis in Rheumatoid Arthritis: An Unpredictable Common Occurrence?" *Clin Rheumatol*, 1994, 13:586-8.

Aronow R and Fleschmann LE, "Mercury Poisoning in Children," *Clin Pediatr*, 1976, 15(10):936-45.

Hryhorczuk DO, Meyers L, and Chen G, "Treatment of Mercury Intoxication in a Dentist With N-Acetyl-D,L-Penicillamine," *J Toxicol Clin Toxicol*, 1982, 19(4):401-8.

Kandola L, Swannell AJ, and Hunter A, "Acquired Sideroblastic Anaemia Associated With Penicillamine Therapy for Rheumatoid Arthritis," *Ann Rheum Dis*, 1995, 54:529-30.

Lyle WH, "Penicillamine in Metal Poisoning," *J Rheumatol Suppl*, 1981, 7:96-9.

Multz CV, "Cholestatic Hepatitis Caused by Penicillamine," *JAMA*, 1981, 246(6):674-5.

Negishi M, Matsuda A, Kaga S, et al, "A Case of Agranulocytosis Which Occurred Several Hours After the Readministration of D-Penicillamine Accompanied by Shivering-Chillness," *Arerugi*, 1995, 44(2):96-9.

(Continued)

Penicillamine *(Continued)*

Rosa FW, "Teratogen Update. Penicillamine," *Teratology*, 1986, 33(1):127-31.
Smith DB and Gallagher BB, "The Effect of Penicillamine on Seizure Threshold. The Role of Pyridoxine," *Arch Neurol*, 1970, 23(1):59-62.

Pentyl Nitrite *see* Amyl Nitrite *on page 1390*

Phendry® Oral [OTC] *see* Diphenhydramine Hydrochloride *on page 1415*

Phentolamine Mesylate (fen tole' a meen)

CAS Number 65-28-1

Brand Names Regitin®; Regitine®; Rogitine®

Use Prevention or control of hypertensive episodes that may occur in a patient with pheochromocytoma as a result of stress or manipulation during preoperative preparation and surgical excision; also used to treat hypertension caused by food/drug interactions with MAO inhibitors. Prevention or treatment of dermal necrosis and sloughing following intravenous administration or extravasation of dopamine or norepinephrine. Diagnosis of pheochromocytoma by the Regitine® blocking test; can be used for cocaine-induced vasospasm; also used for rebound hypertension due to clonidine withdrawal.

Antidote Useful For

Cocaine Hydrochloride *on page 236*

Mechanism of Action Competitively blocks alpha-adrenergic receptors to produce brief antagonism of circulating epinephrine and norepinephrine to reduce hypertension caused by these catecholamines; no inotropic activity

Adverse Reactions

Cardiovascular: Reflex tachycardia, anginal pain, myocardial infarction, hypotension (orthostatic)

Central nervous system: Fainting, flushing of face, severe headache

Gastrointestinal: Nausea, abdominal pain, diarrhea, vomiting

Neuromuscular & skeletal: Weakness

Respiratory: Nasal stuffiness

Miscellaneous: Exacerbation of peptic ulcer; hypocalcemia; can precipitate disulfiram-like reaction with ethanol; priapism with injection into corpus cavernosum

Toxicodynamics/Kinetics

Onset of action:

- I.M.: Within 15-20 minutes
- I.V.: Immediate

Metabolism: In the liver

Bioavailability: Oral: 20%

Half-life: 19 minutes

Elimination: In urine (10% as unchanged drug)

Usual Dosage

Treatment of alpha-adrenergic drug extravasation: S.C.:

- Children: 0.1-0.2 mg/kg diluted in 10 mL 0.9% sodium chloride infiltrated into area of extravasation within 12 hours
- Adults: Infiltrate area with small amount of solution made by diluting 5-10 mg in 10 mL 0.9% sodium chloride within 12 hours of extravasation
- If dose is effective, normal skin color should return to the blanched area within 1 hour

Diagnosis of pheochromocytoma: I.M., I.V.:

- Children: 0.05-0.1 mg/kg/dose, maximum single dose: 5 mg
- Adults: 5 mg

Surgery for pheochromocytoma: Hypertension: I.M., I.V.:

- Children: 0.05-0.1 mg/kg/dose given 1-2 hours before procedure; repeat as needed every 2-4 hours until hypertension is controlled; maximum single dose: 5 mg
- Adults: 5 mg given 1-2 hours before procedure and repeated as needed every 2-4 hours

Hypertensive crisis: Adults: 5-20 mg

Administration Treatment of extravasation: Infiltrate area of extravasation with multiple small injections; use 27- or 30-gauge needles and change needle between each skin entry

Contraindications Hypersensitivity to phentolamine or any component; renal impairment; coronary or cerebral arteriosclerosis; do not use in the setting of monoamine oxidase inhibitor overdose; but can be used for hypertension due to MAO inhibitor interactions with tyramine

Warnings Myocardial infarction, cerebrovascular spasm and cerebrovascular occlusion have occurred following administration; use with caution in patients with a history of cardiac arrhythmias

Dosage Forms Injection: 5 mg/mL (1 mL)

Stability Reconstituted solution is stable for 48 hours at room temperature and 1 week when refrigerated

Test Interactions ↑ LFTs rarely

Drug Interactions Increased toxicity with ethanol (disulfiram reaction); can enhance arginine-induced gastrin secretion; tachycardia may occur when combined with tolazoline

Pregnancy Risk Factor C

Monitoring Parameters Blood pressure, heart rate

Nursing Implications Infiltrate the area of dopamine extravasation with multiple small injections using only 27- or 30-gauge needles and changing the needle between each skin entry; take care not to cause so much swelling of the extremity or digit that a compartment syndrome occurs; monitor patient for orthostasis; assist with ambulation

Additional Information Injection contains mannitol 25 mg/vial

Specific References

Cooper BE, "High-Dose Phentolamine for Extravasation of Pressors," *Clin Pharm*, 1989, 8(10):689.

Gould L, Reddy CV, Chua W, et al, "Electrophysiological Properties of Phentolamine in Man," *Br Heart J*, 1977, 39(9):939-44.

Hollander JE, Carter WA, and Hoffman RS, "Use of Phentolamine for Cocaine-Induced Myocardial Ischemia," *N Engl J Med*, 1992, 327(5):361.

Roberts JR and Krisanda TJ, "Accidental Intra-Arterial Injection of Epinephrine Treated With Phentolamine," *Ann Emerg Med*, 1989, 18(4):424-5.

Seino S, Seino Y, Taminato T, et al, "Effect of Adrenergic Blocking Agents on Plasma Gastrin and Secretion Levels in Man," *Am J Gastroenterol*, 1980, 73(2):137-40.

Wespes E, Rondeux C, and Schulman CC, "Effect of Phentolamine on Venous Return in Human Erection," *Br J Urol*, 1989, 63(1):95-7.

Phos-Ex® *see* Calcium Acetate *on page 1399*

PhosLo® *see* Calcium Acetate *on page 1399*

Phylloquinone *see* Phytonadione *on next page*

Physostigmine (fye zoe stig' meen)

CAS Number 57-47-6; 64-47-1; 57-64-7

Brand Names Antilirium® Injection; Isopto® Eserine Ophthalmic

Use Second-line agent for envenomation of Asian snakes or intoxication with tetradotoxin exposures if edrophonium supplies are depleted; reverse toxic CNS effects caused by anticholinergic drugs; controversial role for baclofen and tricyclic antidepressant poisonings (virtually no role in the latter exposure)

Antidote Useful For

Baclofen *on page 143*
Belladonna and Opium *on page 145*
Black Nightshade *on page 1057*
Box Thorn *on page 1061*
Cyclobenzaprine Hydrochloride *on page 248*
Deadly Nightshade *on page 1078*
Hyoscyamine Sulfate *on page 415*
Ipratropium Bromide *on page 438*
Mecamylamine Hydrochloride *on page 492*
Mushrooms, Toxic (Group III) *on page 1112*
Mushrooms, Toxic (Group V) *on page 1114*
Potato (Leaves, Stems, Tubercles) *on page 1128*
Promethazine Hydrochloride *on page 650*
Scopolamine *on page 691*
Thioridazine Hydrochloride *on page 745*
Tomato (Leaves and Stems) *on page 1150*

Mechanism of Action Inhibits destruction of acetylcholine by acetylcholinesterase which facilitates transmission of impulses across myoneural junction

Adverse Reactions

Cardiovascular: Palpitations, bradycardia, atrial fibrillation, asystole
Central nervous system: Restlessness, hallucinations, seizures/seizures
Gastrointestinal: Nausea, vomiting, diarrhea, salivation, hyperperistalsis, defecation
Genitourinary: Urinary incontinence
Local: Topical stinging, burning, lacrimation
Neuromuscular & skeletal: Muscle twitching, weakness
Ocular: Miosis, blurred vision
Respiratory: Dyspnea, bronchospasm, respiratory paralysis, pulmonary edema
Miscellaneous: Sweating

Signs & Symptoms of Acute Overdose Muscle weakness, blurred vision, excessive sweating, tearing and salivation, nausea, laryngospasm, hypertension, fasciculations, vomiting, seizures/seizures, hypertension, hallucinations

(Continued)

Physostigmine *(Continued)*

Toxicodynamics/Kinetics

Onset of action:

Ophthalmic: Within 10-30 minutes

I.V.: within 5 minutes

Duration:

Ophthalmic: 12-48 hours

I.V.: 0.5-2 hours

Absorption: Readily following I.M. and S.C. administration; readily from mucous membranes, muscle and subcutaneous tissue

Distribution: Wide throughout body; readily passes blood-brain barrier

Half-life: 1-2 hours

Elimination: Not fully understood; only small amounts found in urine; clearance: 12.43 mL/minute

Usual Dosage

Children: Anticholinergic drug overdose: Reserve for life-threatening situations only: I.V.: 0.01-0.03 mg/kg/dose, (maximum: 0.5 mg/minute); may repeat after 5-10 minutes to a maximum total dose of 2 mg or until response occurs or adverse cholinergic effects occur

Adults:

Anticholinergic drug overdose:

I.M., I.V.: 0.5-2 mg to start, repeat every 20 minutes until response occurs or adverse effect occurs

Repeat 1-4 mg every 30-60 minutes as life-threatening signs (arrhythmias, seizures, deep coma) recur; maximum I.V. rate: 1 mg/minute

Ophthalmic:

Ointment: Instill a small quantity to lower fornix up to 3 times/day

Solution: Instill 1-2 drops into eye(s) up to 4 times/day

Contraindications Hypersensitivity to physostigmine or any component; GI or GU obstruction, asthma, diabetes, gangrene, cardiovascular disease; patients receiving choline esters or depolarizing neuromuscular blocking agents

Warnings Not intended as a first-line agent for anticholinergic toxicity, especially tricyclic antidepressant

Dosage Forms

Injection, as salicylate: 1 mg/mL (2 mL)

Ointment, ophthalmic: 0.25% (3.5 g, 3.7 g)

Solution, ophthalmic: 0.25% (15 mL); 0.5% (2 mL, 15 mL)

Stability Do not use solution if cloudy or dark brown

Reference Range After oral dose of 2 mg of physostigmine salicylate, plasma level after 15 minutes was 1.03 ng/mL

Test Interactions Increases aminotransferase [ALT (SGPT)/AST (SGOT)] (S), amylase (S); increased serum cortisol, prolactin and epinephrine levels

Drug Interactions Potentiates effects of nondepolarizing neuromuscular blockers

Pregnancy Risk Factor C

Additional Information Drug crosses the blood-brain barrier readily and reverses both central and peripheral anticholinergic effects; I.V. rate not to exceed 1 mg/minute in adults; 0.5 mg/minute in children or 0.01 mg/kg/minute; whichever is slower; have atropine on hand to control bradycardia or seizures; toxic effect is more severe than with physostigmine; physostigmine therapy of drug intoxications should be used with extreme caution in patients with asthma, gangrene, severe cardiovascular disease or mechanical obstruction of the GI tract or urogenital tract. In these patients physostigmine should be used only when life-threatening.

Specific References

Brier RH, "Physostigmine Dose for Tricyclic Drug Overdose," *Ann Intern Med*, 1978, 89(4):579.

Caine ED, "Anticholinergic Toxicity," *N Engl J Med*, 1979, 300(22):1278.

Dysken MW and Janowsky DS, "Dose-Related Physostigmine-Induced Ventricular Arrhythmia: Case Report," *J Clin Psychiatry*, 1985, 46(10):446-7.

Pentel P and Peterson CD, "Asystole Complicating Physostigmine Treatment of Tricyclic Antidepressant Overdose," *Ann Emerg Med*, 1980, 9(11):588-90.

Phytomenadione *see* Phytonadione *on this page*

Phytonadione (fye toe na dye' one)

CAS Number 84-80-0

Brand Names AquaMEPHYTON®; Bilkaby, K®; Kaergona®; Kaywan®; Konakion®; Mephyton®; Synkavite®; Thrombin®

Synonyms Methylphytyl Napthoquinone; Phylloquinone; Phytomenadione; Vitamin K_1

Use Prevention and treatment of hypoprothrombinemia caused by drug-induced treatment of anticoagulant-induced vitamin K deficiency, hemorrhagic disease of the newborn; phytonadione is more effective and is preferred to other vitamin K preparations in the presence of impending hemorrhage; oral absorption depends on the presence of bile salts

Antidote Useful For

Anticoagulant Rodenticide *on page 859*

Dicumarol *on page 277*

Warfarin Sodium *on page 800*

Mechanism of Action Promotes liver synthesis of clotting factors (II, VII, IX, X)

Adverse Reactions

Gastrointestinal: GI upset

Local: Pain, swelling, tenderness at injection site

Signs & Symptoms of Acute Overdose Hemiplegia

Toxicodynamics/Kinetics

Onset of increased coagulation factors:

Oral: Within 6-12 hours

Parenteral: Within 1-2 hours; patient may become normal after 12-14 hours

Absorption: Oral: Absorbed from the intestines in the presence of bile

Distribution: V_d: 0.024-0.81 L/kg in neonates

Metabolism: In the liver rapidly to vitamin K_1-2,3-epoxide

Half-life:

Phytonadione: 2 hours

Metabolite: 1 hour

Elimination: Bile and urine

Usual Dosage I.V. route should be restricted for emergency use only

Newborns: Hemorrhagic disease:

Prophylaxis: I.M., S.C.: 0.5-1 mg within 1 hour of birth

Treatment: I.M., S.C.: 1-2 mg/dose/day

Oral anticoagulant overdose:

Infants: I.M., S.C.: 1-2 mg/dose every 4-8 hours

Children and Adults: Oral, I.M., I.V., S.C.: 2.5-10 mg/dose; rarely up to 25-50 mg has been used; may repeat in 6-8 hours if given by I.M., I.V., S.C. route; may repeat 12-48 hours after oral route

Vitamin K deficiency: Due to drugs, malabsorption or decreased synthesis of vitamin K

Infants and Children:

Oral: 2.5-5 mg/24 hours

I.M., I.V.: 1-2 mg/dose as a single dose

Adults:

Oral: 5-25 mg/24 hours

I.M., I.V.: 10 mg

Minimum daily requirement: Not well established

Infants: 1-5 mcg/kg/day

Adults: 0.03 mcg/kg/day

Maximum tolerated dose: 1 g

Administration Dilute in 5-10 mL I.V. fluid (D_5W or normal saline) (maximum concentration: 10 mg/mL); infuse over 15-30 minutes; maximum rate of infusion: 1 mg/minute

Contraindications Hypersensitivity to phytonadione or any component

Warnings Severe reactions resembling anaphylaxis or hypersensitivity have occurred rarely during or immediately after I.V. administration (even with proper dilution and rate of administration); restrict I.V. administration for emergency use only; ineffective in hereditary hypoprothrombinemia, hypoprothrombinemia caused by severe liver disease; severe hemolytic anemia has been reported rarely in neonates following large doses (10-20 mg) of phytonadione

Dosage Forms

Injection:

Aqueous colloidal: 2 mg/mL (0.5 mL); 10 mg/mL (1 mL, 2.5 mL, 5 mL)

Aqueous (I.M. only): 2 mg/mL (0.5 mL); 10 mg/mL (1 mL)

Tablet: 5 mg

Stability Protect injection from light at all times; may be autoclaved

Reference Range Normal range: 0.09-2.12 μg/L

Drug Interactions Decreased effect of warfarin sodium, dicumarol, anisindione

Pregnancy Risk Factor C (X if used in 3rd trimester or near term)

Monitoring Parameters PT

Nursing Implications I.V. administration: Dilute in normal saline, D_5W or D_5NS and infuse slowly; rate of infusion should not exceed 1 mg/minute. **This route should be used only if administration by another route is not feasible.** The parenteral preparation has been administered orally to neonates. I.V. administration should not exceed 1 mg/minute; for I.V. infusion, dilute in PF (preservative free) D_5W or normal saline.

(Continued)

Phytonadione *(Continued)*

Additional Information Injection contains benzyl alcohol 0.9% as preservative; diet should contain less vitamin K rich foods (ie, broccoli, asparagus, cabbage, liver); cardiovascular collapse at infusion rates >1 mg/minute due to decrease in peripheral resistance, hypotension, dyspnea

Specific References

Barash P, Kitahata LM, and Mandel S, "Acute Cardiovascular Collapse After Intravenous Phytonadione," *Anesth Analg*, 1976, 55(2):304-6.

Hopkins CS, "Adverse Reaction to a Cremophor-Containing Preparation of Intravenous Vitamin K," *Intensive Therapy Clin Monit*, 1988, 9:254-5.

Martinez-Abad M, Delgado F, Palop V, et al, "Vitamin K_1 and Anaphylactic Shock," *DICP*, 1991, 25(7-8):871-2.

Pima® *see* Potassium Iodide *on this page*

Polyethylene Glycol (pol ee eth' i leen gly' kol)

CAS Number 25322-68-3

Brand Names Co-Lav®; Colovage®; CoLyte®; Cytospray®; Go-Evac®; GoLYTELY®; Hypotears®; NuLYTELY®; OCL®; Rhinaris®; Salinol®; Secaris®

Synonyms Colon Electrolyte Lavage Preparation; Electrolyte Lavage Solution; Macrogol; PEG

Use Whole bowel irrigation in acute overdoses of iron, lithium, ampicillin, heavy metals, "body packers", sustained release medications; also used in bowel cleansing procedures

Antidote Useful For

Iron *on page 439*
Lithium *on page 476*

Mechanism of Action Nonabsorbable agent which increases bowel osmotic pressure

Adverse Reactions

Cardiovascular: Ventricular ectopy
Central nervous system: Coma
Endocrine & metabolic: Metabolic acidosis, hypercalcemia
Gastrointestinal: Nausea, diarrhea, abdominal fullness, vomiting, taste disturbance

Toxicodynamics/Kinetics

Onset of effect: Oral: Within 1-2 hours
Absorption: Not absorbed
Half-life: 7.7 hours

Usual Dosage Children and Adults: Oral: 15-60 mL/kg/hour until clear rectal effluent appears

Contraindications Gastrointestinal obstruction, gastric retention, bowel perforation, toxic colitis, megacolon

Warnings May decrease the adsorptive capacity of charcoal for cocaine and/or theophylline

Dosage Forms Powder, for oral solution: PEG 3350 236 g, sodium sulfate 22.74 g, sodium bicarbonate 6.74 g, sodium chloride 5.86 g and potassium chloride 2.97 g (2000 mL, 4000 mL, 4800 mL, 6000 mL)

Drug Interactions Reduces activity of bacitracin or penicillin

Pregnancy Risk Factor C

Additional Information Use with caution in patients with coma and lethargy; a total dose of 3 L in adults may be sufficient for whole bowel irrigation; metoclopramide pretreatment does not improve efficiency of whole bowel irrigation

Specific References

Harris CR and Kingston R, "Gastrointestinal Decontamination, Which Method Is Best?" *Postgrad Med*, 1992, 92(2):116-22, 125, 128.

Olsen KM, Gurley BJ, and Davis GA, "Comparison of Fluid Volumes With Whole Bowel Irrigation in a Simulated Overdose of Ibuprofen," *Ann Pharmacother*, 1995, 29:246-50.

Porter RS and Baker EB, "Drug Clearance by Diarrhea Induction," *Am J Emerg Med*, 1985, 3(3):182-6.

Scharman EJ, Lembersky R, and Krenzelok EP, "Efficiency of Whole Bowel Irrigation With and Without Metoclopramide Pretreatment," *Am J Emerg Med*, 1994, 12:302-5.

Poppers *see* Amyl Nitrite *on page 1390*

Potassium Iodide (poe tass' y um eye' oh dide)

CAS Number 7681-11-0

Brand Names Pima®; Potassium Iodide Enseals®; SSKI®; Thyro-Block®

Use Block thyroidal uptake of radioactive isotopes of iodine in a radiation emergency

Mechanism of Action Inhibits uptake of I-131 by thyroid

Adverse Reactions

Cardiovascular: Angioedema
Central nervous system: Fever, headache

Dermatologic: Urticaria, acne
Endocrine & metabolic: Goiter with hypothyroidism
Gastrointestinal: Metallic taste, GI upset
Hematologic: Cutaneous and mucosal hemorrhage, eosinophilia
Neuromuscular & skeletal: Arthralgia
Miscellaneous: Lymph node enlargement, soreness of teeth and gums, rhinitis

Signs & Symptoms of Acute Overdose Angioedema, laryngeal edema

Toxicodynamics/Kinetics
Onset of action: 24-48 hours
Peak effect: 10-15 days after continuous therapy
Absorption: Adequate from GI tract
Elimination: If patient is euthyroid, renal clearance rate is 2 times that of the thyroid

Usual Dosage Oral: RDA:
Children: 50 mcg
Adults: 130 mcg

Contraindications Known hypersensitivity to iodine; hyperkalemia

Warnings Essentially ineffective if administered more than 6 hours after radiation exposure

Dosage Forms
Solution, oral:
SSKI®: 1 g/mL (30 mL, 240 mL)
Lugol's Solution, strong iodine: Potassium iodide 100 mg and iodine 50 mg per mL (120 mL, 473 mL, 4000 mL)
Syrup: 325 mg/5 mL (473 mL, 4000 mL)
Tablet: 130 mg

Stability Store in tight, light-resistant containers at temperature <40°C; freezing should be avoided

Test Interactions Thyroid function tests

Drug Interactions Lithium

Pregnancy Risk Factor D

Pregnancy Implications Crosses placenta

Nursing Implications Must be diluted before administration of 240 mL of water, fruit juice, milk, or broth

Additional Information 10 drops of SSKI® = potassium iodide 500 mg; tablets are radiopaque

Specific References
"Potassium Iodide as a Thyroid Blocking Agent in a Radiation Emergency: Final Recommendations on Use," Washington DC, Bureau of Radiological Health and Bureau of Drugs, Food and Drug Administration, 1982.

Potassium Iodide Enseals® *see* Potassium Iodide *on previous page*

Pralidoxime Chloride (pra li dox' eem)

CAS Number 51-15-0

Brand Names Protopam® Chloride

Synonyms 2-PAM; 2-Pyridine Aldoxime Methochloride

Use
Reverse muscle paralysis with toxic exposure to organophosphate anticholinesterase pesticides and chemicals; control of overdose of drugs used to treat myasthenia gravis; may be effective for tacrine toxicity; nerve gas agents
Not generally indicated for carbamate ingestions, although recent reports have shown a benefit in receiving nicotinic symptoms refractory to atropine; questionable efficacy for selected organophosphates (ciodrin, dimefox, dimethoate, methyl diazonin, phorate, schaadan, weesyn)

Antidote Useful For
Bromophos *on page 873*
Chlorfenvinphos *on page 886*
Chlorpyrifos *on page 891*
Diazinon *on page 904*
Dicrotophos *on page 909*
Dioxathion *on page 916*
Disulfoton *on page 919*
Edrophonium Chloride *on page 309*
Fensulfothion *on page 928*
Fenthion *on page 929*
Malathion *on page 950*
Malathion (Topical Lotion) *on page 489*
Methidathion *on page 959*
Nerve Gases *on page 974*
Parathion *on page 988*

Profenofos *on page 998*
Tacrine Hydrochloride *on page 719*
Terbufos *on page 1020*
Tetraethyl Pyrophosphate *on page 1024*

Mechanism of Action Reactivates cholinesterase that had been inactivated by phosphorylation due to exposure to organophosphate pesticides by displacing the enzyme from its receptor sites; most effective if given within 24 hours of exposure; has greater impact on reversing nicotinic effects versus muscarinic

Adverse Reactions
Cardiovascular: Tachycardia, hypertension (diastolic)
Central nervous system: Dizziness/vertigo, headache, drowsiness
Dermatologic: Rash
Gastrointestinal: Nausea
Neuromuscular & skeletal: Muscle rigidity, weakness
Ocular: Blurred vision, diplopia, mydriasis
Respiratory: Hyperventilation, laryngospasm

Signs & Symptoms of Acute Overdose Blurred vision, nausea, tachycardia, dizziness/vertigo

Toxicodynamics/Kinetics
Absorption: Variable and incomplete
Distribution: Throughout extracellular fluids; crosses blood-brain barrier very slowly, if at all
Protein binding: Not bound to plasma proteins
Metabolism: In the liver
Half-life: 90-110 hours
Time to peak serum concentration: Within 5-15 minutes
Elimination: Quickly excreted in urine, mostly as metabolites

Usual Dosage
Poisoning: I.M., I.V. (use in conjunction with atropine):
Children: 25-50 mg/kg/dose, infuse over 5-30 minutes; repeat in 1-2 hours if muscle weakness has not been relieved, then at 10- to 12-hour intervals if cholinergic signs recur
Adults: 1-2 g; repeat in 1-2 hours if muscle weakness has not been relieved, then at 10- to 12-hour intervals if cholinergic signs recur

Mild organophosphate poisoning: Oral: Initial: 1-3 g, repeat as needed in 5 hours

Dosing adjustment in renal impairment: Dose should be reduced

Contraindications Hypersensitivity to pralidoxime or any component; poisonings due to phosphorus, inorganic phosphates, or organic phosphates without anticholinesterase activity

Dosage Forms
Injection: 20 mL vial containing 1 g each pralidoxime chloride with one 20 mL ampul diluent, disposable syringe, needle, and alcohol swab
Injection: 300 mg/mL (2 mL)
Tablets: 500 mg

Reference Range Pralidoxime concentration of 4 μg/mL therapeutic *in vitro*

Drug Interactions Barbiturates (potentiated); avoid morphine, theophylline, succinylcholine, reserpine and phenothiazines in patients with organophosphate poisoning

Pregnancy Risk Factor C

Monitoring Parameters Blood or plasma cholinesterase

Specific References
de Kort WL, Kiestra SH, and Sangster B, "The Use of Atropine and Oximes in Organophosphate Poisoning: A Modified Approach," *J Toxicol Clin Toxicol*, 1988, 26(3-4):199-208.
Ekins BR and Geller RJ, "Methomyl-Induced Carbamate Poisoning Treated With Pralidoxime Chloride," *West J Med*, 1994, 161(1):68-70.
Farrar HC, Wells TG, and Kearns GL, "Use of Continuous Infusion of Pralidoxime for Treatment of Organophosphate Poisoning in Children," *J Pediatr*, 1990, 116(4):658-61.
Jovanovic D, "Pharmacokinetics of Pralidoxime Chloride. A Comparative Study in Healthy Volunteers and in Organophosphorus Poisoning," *Arch Toxicol*, 1989, 63(5):416-8.
Kurtz PH, "Pralidoxime in the Treatment of Carbamate Intoxication," *Am J Emerg Med*, 1990, 8(1):68-70.
Medicis JJ, Stork CM, Hoffman RS, et al, "Improved 2-PAM Dosing Regimen in Human Volunteers: A Pharmacokinetic Study," *Vet Hum Toxicol*, 1994, 36:377.
Murphy M and Desai H, "Pralidoxime-Induced Laryngospasm," *Vet Hum Toxicol*, 1994, 36:375.

Pravidel® *see* Bromocriptine Mesylate *on page 1398*

Primatene® Mist [OTC] *see* Epinephrine *on page 1422*

Promit® *see* Dextran 1 *on page 1409*

Promiten® *see* Dextran 1 *on page 1409*

Prostigmin® Injection *see* Neostigmine *on page 1450*

Prostigmin® Oral *see* Neostigmine *on page 1450*

Prosulf® *see* Protamine Sulfate *on this page*

Protamine Sulfate (proe' ta meen)

CAS Number 9012-00-4; 9009-65-8

Brand Names Prosulf®

Use Treatment of heparin, dalteparin, enoxaparin overdosage; neutralize heparin during surgery or dialysis procedures

Antidote Useful For

Dalteparin *on page 256*
Enoxaparin Sodium *on page 315*
Heparin *on page 398*

Mechanism of Action Weak anticoagulant; combines with strongly acidic heparin to form a stable complex (salt) neutralizing the anticoagulant activity of both drugs

Adverse Reactions

Cardiovascular: Hypotension, cyanosis, bradycardia, flushing
Central nervous system: Lassitude, numbness
Gastrointestinal: Nausea, vomiting
Hematologic: Thrombocytopenia, bleeding, coagulopathy, leukopenia
Respiratory: Pulmonary hypertension, wheezing, dyspnea
Miscellaneous: Hypersensitivity reactions (anaphylaxis and anaphylactic shock)

Signs & Symptoms of Acute Overdose Hypertension; may cause hemorrhage

Toxicodynamics/Kinetics

Onset of action: 30 seconds to 1 minute
Duration: 2 hours (dependent on body temperature)
Distribution: Not applicable
Metabolism: Unknown
Elimination: Unknown

Usual Dosage Children and Adults: I.V.: 1 mg of protamine neutralizes, 80-90 USP units of heparin (lung) and 115 USP units of heparin (intestinal); heparin neutralization occurs within 5 minutes following I.V. injection; administer 1 mg for each 100 units of heparin given in preceding 3-4 hours up to a maximum dose of 50 mg; rate should not exceed 50 mg/10 minutes

Contraindications Hypersensitivity to protamine or any component

Warnings May not be totally effective in some patients following cardiac surgery despite adequate doses; may cause hypersensitivity reaction in patients with a history of allergy to fish (have epinephrine 1:1000 available) and in patients sensitized to protamine (via protamine zinc insulin); too rapid administration can cause severe hypotensive and anaphylactoid-like reactions

Dosage Forms Injection: 10 mg/mL (5 mL, 10 mL, 25 mL)

Stability Refrigerate, avoid freezing; remains stable for at least 2 weeks at room temperature

Reference Range Protamine plasma levels of 0.02-0.5 mg/mL are associated with prolonged activated partial thromboplastin time and prothrombin time

Drug Interactions May prolong the effects of insulin

Pregnancy Risk Factor C

Monitoring Parameters Coagulation test

Nursing Implications For I.V. use only; incompatible with cephalosporins and penicillins; administer slow IVP (50 mg over 10 minutes); give over 1-3 minutes, rapid infusion causes hypotension

Specific References

Horrow JC, "Protamine: A Review of Its Toxicity," *Anesth Analg*, 1985, 64(3):348-61.
Lindblad B, "Protamine Sulfate: A Review of Its Effects – Hypersensitivity and Toxicity," *Eur J Vasc Surg*, 1989, 3(3):195-201.

Protopam® Chloride *see* Pralidoxime Chloride *on page 1461*

Pteroylglutamic Acid *see* Folic Acid *on page 1430*

Pydox® *see* Pyridoxine Hydrochloride *on page 1465*

2-Pyridine Aldoxime Methochloride *see* Pralidoxime Chloride *on page 1461*

Pyridostigmine Bromide (peer id oh stig' meen)

CAS Number 101-26-8

Brand Names Mestinon® Injection; Mestinon® Oral; Regonol® Injection

Use Second-line agent for envenomation by Asian snakes or intoxication with tetradotoxin exposures if edrophonium supplies are depleted; reversal of the effects of nondepolarizing neuromuscular blocking agents after surgery; pretreatment for chemical warfare agents (ie, Soman), thus making the use of atropine and pralidoxime more effective

Antidote Useful For
Nerve Gases *on page 974*

Mechanism of Action Inhibits destruction of acetylcholine by acetylcholinesterase which facilitates transmission of impulses across myoneural junction

Adverse Reactions
Cardiovascular: Salivation, bradycardia
Central nervous system: Headache
Dermatologic: Rash, diaphoresis
Gastrointestinal: Nausea, vomiting, diarrhea, flatus, salivation
Neuromuscular & skeletal: Muscle cramps, weakness
Ocular: Miosis
Respiratory: Increased bronchial secretions, bronchospasm
Miscellaneous: Sweating

Signs & Symptoms of Acute Overdose Muscle weakness, blurred vision, excessive sweating, tearing and salivation, nausea, vomiting

Toxicodynamics/Kinetics
Onset of action:
Oral, I.M.: Within 15-30 minutes
I.V.: Within 2-5 minutes
Duration:
Oral:
Syrup, tablets: 3-6 hours
Extended release tablets: 6-12 hours
I.M., I.V.: 2-4 hours
Absorption: Oral: Very poor (10% to 20%) from the GI tract
Distribution: Does not cross blood-brain barrier
Half-life: ~90 minutes
Metabolism: In the liver
Elimination: Renal

Usual Dosage Normally, sustained release dosage form is used at bedtime for patients who complain of morning weakness
Myasthenia gravis:
Oral:
Children: 7 mg/kg/day in 5-6 divided doses
Adults: Initial: 60 mg 3 times/day with maintenance dose ranging from 60 mg to 1.5 g/day; sustained release formulation should be dosed at least every 6 hours (usually 12-24 hours)
I.M., I.V.:
Children: 0.05-0.15 mg/kg/dose (maximum single dose: 10 mg)
Adults: 2 mg every 2-3 hours or 1/30th of oral dose
Reversal of nondepolarizing neuromuscular blocker: I.M., I.V.:
Children: 0.1-0.25 mg/kg/dose preceded by atropine
Adults: 10-20 mg preceded by atropine
Pretreatment under threat of nerve agent attack: Oral: 30 mg every 8 hours

Contraindications Hypersensitivity to pyridostigmine, bromides, or any component; GI or GU obstruction

Dosage Forms
Injection: 5 mg/mL (2 mL, 5 mL)
Syrup (raspberry flavor): 60 mg/5 mL (480 mL)
Tablet: 60 mg
Tablet, sustained release: 180 mg

Stability Protect from light

Test Interactions Increases aminotransferase [ALT (SGPT)/AST (SGOT)] (S), amylase (S)

Drug Interactions Depolarizing neuromuscular blockers (eg, succinylcholine or decamethonium)

Pregnancy Risk Factor C

Pregnancy Implications Crosses placenta

Nursing Implications Do not crush sustained release drug product

Additional Information Not a cure; patient may develop resistance to the drug; normally, sustained release dosage form is used at bedtime for patients who complain of morning weakness; atropine counteracts cholinergic effects

Specific References

Dunn MA and Sidell FR, "Progress in Medical Defense Against Nerve Agents," *JAMA*, 1989, 262(5):649-52.

Keeler JR, Hurst CG, and Dunn MA, "Pyridostigmine Used as a Nerve Agent Pretreatment Under Wartime Conditions," *JAMA*, 1991, 266(5):693-5.

Sidell FR and Borak J, "Chemical Warfare Agents: II. Nerve Agents," *Ann Emerg Med*, 1992, 21(7):865-71.

Pyridoxine Hydrochloride (peer i dox' een)

CAS Number 65-23-6; 58-56-0

Brand Names Beesix®; Bonusunit®; Demo 6®; Invite B_6®; Nestrex®; Pydox®; Rodex®; Xanturenusi®

Synonyms Vitamin B_6

Use Prevents and treats vitamin B_6 deficiency, pyridoxine-dependent seizures in infants, adjunct to treatment of acute toxicity from acrylamide, isoniazid, cycloserine, penicillamine, altretamine, or hydrazine overdose; optic neuritis due to isoniazid or chloramphenicol; hydrazine-containing mushrooms (*Gyromitra*); useful for primary oxaluria; questionable and unproven use in carbon disulfide toxicity

Antidote Useful For

Acrylamide *on page 852*
Altretamine *on page 103*
Chloramphenicol *on page 196*
Ethylene Glycol *on page 925*
Hydrazine *on page 939*
Isoniazid *on page 443*
Mushrooms, Toxic (Group II) *on page 1112*

Mechanism of Action Precursor to pyridoxal, which functions in the metabolism of proteins, carbohydrates, and fats; pyridoxal also aids in the release of liver and muscle stored glycogen, inhibits lactation

Adverse Reactions

Central nervous system: Sensory neuropathy (after chronic administration of large doses), seizures (following I.V. administration of very large doses), headache, hypotonia
Gastrointestinal: Nausea
Hematologic: Decreased serum folic acid concentration
Hepatic: Increased AST
Local: Burning or stinging at injection site
Neuromuscular & skeletal: Paresthesia
Respiratory: Respiratory distress
Miscellaneous: Allergic reactions have been reported; may suppress lactation at doses >600 mg/day

Signs & Symptoms of Acute Overdose Seizures, lethargy, ataxia, sensory neuropathy

Toxicodynamics/Kinetics

Absorption: Enteral, parenteral: Well absorbed in the jejunum
Distribution: V_d: 0.07-0.17 L/kg
Protein binding: 0%
Metabolism: In 4-pyridoxic acid, and other metabolites
Half-life: 2-3 weeks
Elimination: Urinary excretion

Usual Dosage

Pyridoxine-dependent Infants:
Oral: 2-100 mg/day
I.M., I.V.: 10-100 mg

Dietary deficiency: Oral:
Children: 5-10 mg/24 hours for 3 weeks
Adults: 10-20 mg/day for 3 weeks

Drug-induced neuritis (eg, isoniazid, hydrazine, penicillamine, cycloserine): Oral treatment:
Children: 10-50 mg/24 hours; prophylaxis: 1-2 mg/kg/24 hours
Adults: 100-200 mg/24 hours; prophylaxis: 10-100 mg/24 hours

For the treatment of seizures and/or coma from acute isoniazid toxicity, a dose of pyridoxine hydrochloride equal to the amount of INH ingested can be given I.M./I.V. in divided doses together with other anticonvulsants. Can give as much as 1 g/kg in adults or 250 mg/kg in children.

For the treatment of acute hydrazine toxicity, a pyridoxine dose of 25 mg/kg in divided doses I.M./I.V. has been used

Neuropathy may occur at doses >2 g/day

Contraindications Hypersensitivity to pyridoxine or any component

Warnings Dependence and withdrawal may occur with doses >200 mg/day

Dosage Forms

Injection: 100 mg/mL (10 mL, 30 mL)
Tablet: 25 mg, 50 mg, 100 mg
Tablet, extended release: 100 mg

Stability Protect from light

Reference Range A broad normal range is ~25-80 ng/mL (SI: 122-389 nmol/L); HPLC method for pyridoxal phosphate has normal range of 3.5-18 ng/mL (SI: 17-88 nmol/L)

(Continued)

Pyridoxine Hydrochloride *(Continued)*

Test Interactions Urobilinogen

Drug Interactions

Decreased serum levels of levodopa, phenobarbital, and phenytoin

Drugs which deplete pyridoxine: Levodopa, cycloserine, penicillamine, hydrazine, isoniazid, dimethylhydrazine, phenylhydrazine, nialamide, acrylamide, hydralazine, procarbazine, iproniazid, monomethylhydrazine-containing mushrooms

Pregnancy Risk Factor A (C if dose exceeds RDA recommendation)

Nursing Implications Burning may occur at the injection site after I.M. or S.C. administration; seizures have occurred following I.V. administration of very large doses

Specific References

Albin RL, Albers JW, Greensberg HS, et al, "Acute Sensory Neuropathy – Neuronopathy From Pyridoxine Overdose," *Neurology*, 1987, 37(11):1729-32.

de Zegher FD, Przyrembel H, Chalmers RA, et al, "Successful Treatment on Infantile Type I Primary Hyperoxaluria Complicated by Pyridoxine Toxicity," *Lancet*, 1985, 2(8451):392-3.

Glenn GM, Krober MS, Kelly P, et al, "Pyridoxine as Therapy in Theophylline-Induced Seizures," *Vet Hum Toxicol*, 1995, 37:342-5.

Harati Y and Niakan E, "Hydrazine Toxicity, Pyridoxine Therapy, and Peripheral Neuropathy," *Ann Intern Med*, 1986, 104(5):728-9.

Orlowski JP, Paganini EP, Pippenger CE, et al, "Treatment of a Potentially Lethal Dose Isoniazid Ingestion," *Ann Emerg Med*, 1988, 17(1):73-6.

Pauling L, "Sensory Neuropathy From Pyridoxine Abuse," *N Engl J Med*, 1984, 310(3):197-8.

Scharman EJ and Rosencrane JG, "Isoniazid Toxicity: A Survey of Pyridoxine Availability," *Am J Emerg Med*, 1994, 12(3):386-8.

Quantalan® *see* Cholestyramine Resin *on page 1405*

Questran® *see* Cholestyramine Resin *on page 1405*

Questran® Light *see* Cholestyramine Resin *on page 1405*

Regitin® *see* Phentolamine Mesylate *on page 1456*

Regitine® *see* Phentolamine Mesylate *on page 1456*

Regonol® Injection *see* Pyridostigmine Bromide *on page 1463*

Resectisol® Irrigation Solution *see* Mannitol *on page 1442*

Resincolestiramina® *see* Cholestyramine Resin *on page 1405*

Resinsodio® *see* Sodium Polystyrene Sulfonate *on page 1469*

Resonium® *see* Sodium Polystyrene Sulfonate *on page 1469*

Resonium A® *see* Sodium Polystyrene Sulfonate *on page 1469*

Resulax® *see* Sorbitol *on page 1472*

Revex® *see* Nalmefene Hydrochloride *on page 1447*

Revivan® *see* Dopamine Hydrochloride *on page 1418*

Rhinaris® *see* Polyethylene Glycol *on page 1460*

Rodex® *see* Pyridoxine Hydrochloride *on previous page*

Rogitine® *see* Phentolamine Mesylate *on page 1456*

Romazicon™ Injection *see* Flumazenil *on page 1428*

S-2® [OTC] *see* Epinephrine *on page 1422*

Sal de Vichy *see* Sodium Bicarbonate *on next page*

Salinol® *see* Polyethylene Glycol *on page 1460*

Saventrine® *see* Isoproterenol *on page 1436*

Secaris® *see* Polyethylene Glycol *on page 1460*

Serocryptin® *see* Bromocriptine Mesylate *on page 1398*

S-Hydril® *see* Sodium Thiosulfate *on page 1470*

Silphen® Cough [OTC] *see* Diphenhydramine Hydrochloride *on page 1415*

Siran® *see* Acetylcysteine *on page 1388*

Sleep-eze 3® Oral [OTC] *see* Diphenhydramine Hydrochloride *on page 1415*

Sleepinal® [OTC] *see* Diphenhydramine Hydrochloride *on page 1415*

Snake (Pit Vipers) Antivenin *see* Antivenin (Crotalidae) Polyvalent *on page 1392*

Sodium Acid Carbonate *see* Sodium Bicarbonate *on next page*

Sodium Bicarbonate (sow' dee um bye kar' bo nate)

CAS Number 144-55-8

Brand Names Baritop®; Carbex®; Neut®

Synonyms Baking Soda; Monosodium Carbonate; $NaHCO_3$; Sal de Vichy; Sodium Acid Carbonate; Sodium Hydrogen Carbonate

Use Management of metabolic acidosis; antacid; alkalinize urine; severe diarrhea; can reverse QRS prolongation in antidepressant overdose and propoxyphene; cardiac conduction defects due to quinidine-like action of cardiotoxic drugs; increases protein binding of tricyclic antidepressants; nebulized sodium bicarbonate is useful to treat chlorine gas exposure; also used to prevent rhabdomyolysis-induced renal failure; useful in extravasation injury due to carmustine; metformin-induced lactic acidosis

Antidote Useful For

Amitriptyline and Perphenazine *on page 115*
Amitriptyline Hydrochloride *on page 116*
Amoxapine *on page 119*
Desipramine Hydrochloride *on page 263*
Diethylene Glycol *on page 911*
Doxepin Hydrochloride *on page 301*
Ethylene Glycol *on page 925*
Formaldehyde *on page 931*
Glycol Ethers *on page 934*
Imipramine *on page 422*
Maprotiline Hydrochloride *on page 490*
Metformin *on page 507*
Methanol *on page 957*
Nortriptyline Hydrochloride *on page 571*
Potassium Chloride *on page 634*
Propylene Glycol *on page 1002*
Quinidine *on page 668*
Strychnine *on page 1016*
Trimipramine Maleate *on page 775*

Mechanism of Action Dissociates to provide bicarbonate ion which neutralizes hydrogen ion concentration and raises blood and urinary pH

Adverse Reactions

Cardiovascular: Edema, cerebral hemorrhage (especially with rapid injection of the hyperosmotic $NaHCO_3$ solution in infants)

Endocrine & metabolic: Metabolic alkalosis, hypernatremia, hypokalemia, hypocalcemia, intracranial acidosis, increased affinity of hemoglobin for oxygen-reduced pH in myocardia

Gastrointestinal: Gastric distention, flatulence may occur with oral administration, gastric rupture

Local: Tissue necrosis, ulceration after I.V. extravasation

Signs & Symptoms of Acute Overdose Hypocalcemia, hypokalemia, hypernatremia, seizures/seizures, confusion, nausea, weakness, hypokalemic/hypochloremic metabolic alkalosis, muscle cramps, tetany, cyanosis, pulmonary edema

Toxicodynamics/Kinetics

Oral:
- Onset of action: Rapid
- Duration: 8-10 minutes

I.V.:
- Onset of action: 15 minutes
- Duration: 1-2 hours

Absorption: Oral: Well absorbed

Distribution: Bicarbonate occurs naturally and is confined to systemic circulation

Elimination: Reabsorbed by kidney and <1% is excreted by urine Rapid oral onset of action and duration of action of 8-10 minutes; after I.V. administration, onset of action 15 minutes and duration of action of 1-2 hours

Usual Dosage

Cardiac arrest: **Routine use of $NaHCO_3$ is not recommended and should be given only after adequate alveolar ventilation has been established and effective cardiac compressions are provided**

- Children and Infants: I.V.: 0.5-1 mEq/kg/dose repeated every 10 minutes or as indicated by arterial blood gases
- Adults: I.V.: Initial: 1 mEq/kg/dose one time; maintenance: 0.5 mEq/kg/dose every 10 minutes or as indicated by arterial blood gases

Metabolic acidosis: I.V.:
- Neonates: 1-3 mEq/kg/dose slowly (usually over 20-60 minutes)
- Older Children and Adults: 2-5 mEq/kg/dose over 4-8 hours infusion or calculate dose based on base deficit (re-evaluate acid-base status) mEq $NaHCO_3$

(Continued)

Sodium Bicarbonate *(Continued)*

= 0.3 x body weight (kg) x base deficit (mEq/L); give up to 1 mEq/kg/dose over several minutes or dilute larger doses in maintenance fluids for slow infusion; re-evaluate acid-base status frequently

Maximum daily dose: 200 mEq in adults <60 years and 100 mEq in adults >60 years

Maintenance electrolyte requirements of sodium: Daily requirements: 3-4 mEq/kg/24 hours or 25-40 mEq/1000 kcal/24 hours

Chronic renal failure: Oral: Initiate when plasma HCO_3 <15 mEq/L

Children: 1-3 mEq/kg/day

Adults: Start with 20-36 mEq/day in divided doses, titrate to bicarbonate level of 18-20 mEq/L

Renal tubular acidosis: Oral:

Distal: Children: 2-3 mEq/kg/day; Adults: 1 mEq/kg/day

Proximal: Children: Initial: 5-10 mEq/kg/day; maintenance: Increase as required to maintain serum bicarbonate in the normal range

Urine alkalinization: Oral:

Children: 1-10 mEq (84-840 mg)/kg/day in divided doses every 4-6 hours; dose should be titrated to desired urinary pH

Adults: Initial: 48 mEq (4 g), then 12-24 mEq (1-2 g) every 4 hours; dose should be titrated to desired urinary pH; doses up to 17 g/day (200 mEq) in patients <60 years and 8 g (100 mEq) in patients >60 years

Antacid: Adults: Oral: 325 mg to 2 g 1-4 times/day

Carmustine extravasation: 5 mL of a 8.4% solution of sodium bicarbonate either through offending I.V. cannulas or through multiple S.C. injections after cannula removal; apply ice to affected area

Contraindications Alkalosis, hypocalcemia; unknown abdominal pain, inadequate ventilation during cardiopulmonary resuscitation

Warnings Use of I.V. $NaHCO_3$ should be reserved for documented metabolic acidosis and for hyperkalemia-induced cardiac arrest; routine use in cardiac arrest is not recommended. Avoid extravasation, tissue necrosis can occur due to the hypertonicity of $NaHCO_3$; may cause sodium retention especially if renal function is impaired; not to be used in treatment of peptic ulcer; use with caution in patients with CHF, edema, cirrhosis, or renal failure.

Dosage Forms

Injection: 4% [40 mg/mL = 2.4 mEq/5 mL] (5 mL); 4.2% [42 mg/mL = 5 mEq/10 mL] (10 mL); 7.5% [75 mg/mL = 8.92 mEq/10 mL] (10 mL, 50 mL); 8.4% [84 mg/mL = 10 mEq/10 mL] (10 mL, 50 mL)

Powder: 120 g, 480 g

Tablet: 300 mg [3.6 mEq]; 325 mg [3.8 mEq]; 520 mg [6.3 mEq]; 600 mg [7.3 mEq]; 650 mg [7.6 mEq]

Stability Store injection at room temperature; protect from heat and from freezing; use only clear solutions; do not mix $NaHCO_3$ with calcium salts, catecholamines, atropine

Reference Range Therapeutic (sodium): 135-145 mEq/L (SI: 135-145 mmol/L)

Drug Interactions Amphetamines, quinidine levels may increase due to urinary alkalinization reduced excretion

Pregnancy Risk Factor C

Monitoring Parameters Serum electrolytes including calcium, urinary pH, arterial blood gases (if indicated)

Nursing Implications Advise patient of milk-alkali syndrome if use is long-term; observe for extravasation when giving I.V.; incompatible with acids, acidic salts, alkaloid salts, calcium salts, catecholamines, atropine

Additional Information May cause sodium retention especially if renal function is impaired; not to be used in treatment of peptic ulcer

Baking soda contains 35-55 mEq per teaspoon of sodium; serum sodium concentrations in children with baking soda ingestions range from 155-210 mEq/L with serum bicarbonates ranging form 29-54 mEq/L; hypocalcemia may also be present; metabolic alkalosis is usually present

Sodium content of injection 50 mL, 8.4% = 1150 mg = 50 mEq; each 6 mg of $NaHCO_3$ contains 12 mEq sodium; 1 mEq $NaHCO_3$ = 84 mg mEq $NaHCO_3$ = 0.3 x body weight (kg) x base deficit (mEq/L)

Each 84 mg of sodium bicarbonate provides 1 mEq of sodium and bicarbonate ions; each gram of sodium bicarbonate provides 12 mEq of sodium and bicarbonate ions

Specific References

Del Beccaro MA and Robertson WO, "Baking Soda Poisoning," *Vet Hum Toxicol*, 1988, 30(2):164-5.

Levin T, "What This Patient Didn't Need: A Dose of Salts," *Hosp Pract (Off Ed)*, 1983, 18(7):95-8.

Linford SM and James HD, "Sodium Bicarbonate Abuse: A Case Report," *Br J Psychiatry*, 1986, 149:502-3.
MacCara ME, "Extravasation – A Hazard of Intravenous Therapy," *Drug Intell Clin Pharm*, 1983, 17:713.
Narins RG and Cohen JJ, "Bicarbonate Therapy for Organic Acidosis: The Case for Its Continued Use," *Ann Intern Med*, 1987, 106:615-8.
Nichols MH, Wason S, Del Rey JG, et al, "Baking Soda: A Potentially Fatal Home Remedy," *Pediatr Emerg Care*, 1995, 11:109-11.
Stark CM, Redd JT, Fine K, et al, "Propoxyphene-Induced Wide QRS Complex Dysrhythmia Responsive to Sodium Bicarbonate – A Case Report," *Clin Toxicol*, 1995, 33:179-83.

Sodium Calcium Edetate *see* Edetate Calcium Disodium *on page 1419*

Sodium Edetate *see* Edetate Disodium *on page 1421*

Sodium Hydrogen Carbonate *see* Sodium Bicarbonate *on page 1467*

Sodium Hyposulfate *see* Sodium Thiosulfate *on next page*

Sodium Nitrite (sow' dee um nye' trate)

CAS Number 7632-00-0

UN Number 1500

Brand Names O.A.R.®

Synonyms Natril; Natrium Nitrosum; Nitris; Nitrous Acid; Sodium Salt

Use Cyanide toxicity in conjunction with amyl nitrite pearls and sodium thiosulfate; may be of use in hydrogen sulfide poisoning

Antidote Useful For

Acetonitrile *on page 850*
Acrylonitrile *on page 853*
Cyanide *on page 899*
Hydrogen Sulfide *on page 942*

Mechanism of Action Vasodilation and methemoglobin producer

Adverse Reactions

Cardiovascular: Tachycardia, hypotension from vasodilatation, syncope, cyanosis
Central nervous system: Headache, flushing
Gastrointestinal: Nausea, vomiting
Miscellaneous: Forms methemoglobin

Signs & Symptoms of Acute Overdose Seizures, cardiovascular collapse, coma, hemolysis/hemolytic anemia

Toxicodynamics/Kinetics

Metabolism: To ammonia
Elimination: Renal (33%)

Usual Dosage

Cyanide toxicity:
- Children (without anemia): 4.5-10 mg/kg (0.15-0.33 mL/kg of a 3% solution up to 10 mL)
- Adults: 300 mg (10 mL of a 3% solution)

Acceptable daily intake: 0.4 mg/kg
Estimated adult lethal dose: 2.6 g

Dosage Forms Injection: 300 mg/10 mL

Reference Range Sodium nitrite levels associated with fatalities range from 0.5-350 mg/L

Monitoring Parameters Methemoglobin levels

Additional Information Used in photography, meat preservative (up to 200 ppm), metal corrosion inhibitor, fertilizers, manufacture of diazo dyes; arterial blood appears "chocolate brown"

Specific References

Gautami S, Rao RN, Rayhuran TC, et al, "Accidental Acute Fatal Sodium Nitrite Poisoning," *Clin Toxicol*, 1995, 33:131-3.
Hall AH and Rumack BH, "Clinical Toxicology of Cyanide," *Ann Emerg Med*, 1986, 15(9):1067-74.
Harris JC, Rumack BH, Peterson RG, et al, "Methemoglobinemia Resulting From Absorption of Nitrates," *JAMA*, 1979, 242(26):2869-71.
Kirby NG, "Sodium Nitrite Poisoning Treated by Exchange Transfusion," *Lancet*, 1955, 1(6864):594-5.
Peters JW, "Hydrogen Sulfide Poisoning in a Hospital Setting," *JAMA*, 1981, 246(14):1588-9.
Walley T and Flanagan M, "Nitrite-Induced Methaemoglobinaemia," *Postgrad Med J*, 1987, 63(742):643-4.

Sodium Oxide Sulfide *see* Sodium Thiosulfate *on next page*

Sodium Polystyrene Sulfonate (pol ee stye' reen)

CAS Number 9003-59-2; 25704-18-1

Brand Names Kayexalate®; Resinsodio®; Resonium®; Resonium A®; SPS®

Use Treatment of hyperkalemia; gastric decontamination for lithium

Antidote Useful For
Lithium *on page 476*
Potassium Chloride *on page 634*

Mechanism of Action Removes potassium by exchanging sodium ions for potassium ions in the intestine before the resin is passed from the body

Adverse Reactions
Cardiovascular: Congestive heart failure
Endocrine & metabolic: Hypokalemia, hypocalcemia, hypomagnesemia, hypernatremia
Gastrointestinal: Anorexia, nausea, vomiting, constipation, intestinal necrosis
Respiratory: Aspiration can cause pneumonitis

Toxicodynamics/Kinetics
Onset of action: Within 2-24 hours
Absorption: Remains in GI tract
Elimination: Completely excreted in feces (primarily as potassium polystyrene sulfonate)

Usual Dosage
Children:
Oral: 1 g/kg/dose every 6 hours
Rectal: 1 g/kg/dose every 2-6 hours (In small children and infants, employ lower doses by using the practical exchange ratio of 1 mEq K^+/g of resin as the basis for calculation)
Adults:
Oral: 15 g (60 mL) 1-4 times/day
Rectal: 30-50 g every 6 hours

Contraindications Hypernatremia

Warnings Avoid using the commercially available liquid product in neonates due to the preservative content, also may not be as effective in low birth weight infants. Enema may be prepared with powder and diluted with sorbitol 10% solution or oral solution with 25% sorbitol solution. Enema will reduce the serum potassium faster than oral administration, but the oral route will result in a greater reduction over several hours.

Dosage Forms Oral or rectal:
Powder for suspension: 454 g
Suspension: 1.25 g/5 mL with sorbitol 33% and alcohol 0.3% (60 mL, 120 mL, 200 mL, 500 mL)

Reference Range Serum potassium: Adults: 3.5-5.2 mEq/L

Test Interactions Increases sodium; decreases potassium (S), calcium (S), magnesium (S)

Drug Interactions Cation-donating antacids and saline cathartics should be avoided

Pregnancy Risk Factor C

Monitoring Parameters Serum electrolytes, EKG

Nursing Implications Administer oral (or NG) as ~25% sorbitol solution, never mix in orange juice; enema route is less effective than oral administration; retain enema in colon for at least 30-60 minutes and for several hours, if possible

Additional Information 1 g of resin binds approximately 1 mEq of potassium; chilling the oral mixture will increase palatability; sodium content of 1 g: 31 mg (1.3 mEq); may be useful in preventing lithium absorption

Specific References
Belanger DR, Tierney MG, and Dickinson G, "Effect of Sodium Polystyrene Sulfonate on Lithium Bioavailability," *Ann Emerg Med*, 1992, 21(11):1312-5.
Haupt HM and Hutchins GM, "Sodium Polystyrene Sulfonate Pneumonitis," *Arch Intern Med*, 1982, 142(2):379-81.
Malone TA, "Glucose and Insulin Versus Cation-Exchange Resin for the Treatment of Hyperkalemia in Very Low Birth Weight Infants," *J Pediatr*, 1991, 118(1):121-3.
Tomaszewski C, Musso C, Pearson JR, et al, "Lithium Absorption Prevented by Sodium Polystyrene Sulfonate in Volunteers," *Ann Emerg Med*, 1992, 21(11):1308-11.

Sodium Salt *see* Sodium Nitrite *on previous page*

Sodium Thiosulfate (sow' dee um thye oh sul' fate & re sor' si nole)

CAS Number 7772-98-7; 10102-17-7

Brand Names Hyposulfene®; S-Hydril®

Synonyms Sodium Hyposulfate; Sodium Oxide Sulfide

Use Alone or with sodium nitrite or amyl nitrite (or hydroxocobalamin) in cyanide poisoning; to reduce the risk of nephrotoxicity associated with cisplatin therapy; topically in the treatment of tinea versicolor; an inorganic reducing agent used as a fixative bleaching of bone; used in manufacture of leather; for selenium dioxide burns; can reduce cisplatin nephrotoxicity; oral lavage use (1% to 5%) for use in gastric decontamination for iodine exposure, can be used for mechlorethamine extravasation along with actinomycin D and mitomycin C; may be useful in chlorate salt toxicity and bromate toxicity; may be used alone in smoke inhalations and to reduce the toxicity of sodium nitroprusside

Antidote Useful For

Acetonitrile *on page 850*
Acrylonitrile *on page 853*
Chlorate Salts *on page 884*
Cisplatin *on page 218*
Cyanide *on page 899*
Iodine *on page 437*

Mechanism of Action

Cyanide toxicity: Increases the rate of detoxification of cyanide by the enzyme rhodanese by providing an extra sulfur

Cisplatin toxicity: Complexes with cisplatin to form a compound that is nontoxic to either normal or cancerous cells

Adverse Reactions

Cardiovascular: Hypotension, coma

Central nervous system: CNS depression secondary to thiocyanate intoxication, psychosis, confusion

Dermatologic: Contact dermatitis

Gastrointestinal: Nausea, vomiting, abdominal cramps, diarrhea

Local: Local irritation

Neuromuscular & skeletal: Weakness

Otic: Tinnitus

Toxicodynamics/Kinetics

Absorption: Well with parenteral administration

Distribution: V_d: 0.15 L/kg

Half-life: 0.65 hour

Elimination: 28.5% unchanged in urine

Usual Dosage

Cyanide and nitroprusside antidote: I.V.:

Children <25 kg: 50 mg/kg after receiving 4.5-10 mg/kg sodium nitrite; a half dose of each may be repeated if necessary

Children >25 kg and Adults: 12.5 g after 300 mg of sodium nitrite; a half dose of each may be repeated if necessary

Cyanide poisoning: I.V.: Dose should be based on determination as with nitrite, at rate of 2.5-5 mL/minute to maximum of 50 mL. See table.

Variation of Sodium Nitrite and Sodium Thiosulfate Dose With Hemoglobin Concentration*

Hemoglobin (g/dL)	Initial Dose Sodium Nitrite (mg/kg)	Initial Dose Sodium Nitrite 33% (mL/kg)	Initial Dose Sodium Thiosulfate 25% (mL/kg)
7	5.8	0.19	0.95
8	6.6	0.22	1.10
9	7.5	0.25	1.25
10	8.3	0.27	1.35
11	9.1	0.30	1.50
12	10.0	0.33	1.65
13	10.8	0.36	1.80
14	11.6	0.39	1.95

*Adapted from Berlin DM Jr, "The Treatment of Cyanide Poisoning in Children," *Pediatrics*, 1970, 46:793.

Cisplatin rescue should be given before or during cisplatin administration: I.V. infusion (in sterile water): 12 g/m^2 over 6 hours or a 9 g/m^2 I.V. push followed by 1.2 g/m^2 continuous infusion for 6 hours

Arsenic poisoning: I.V. 1 mL first day, 2 mL second day, 3 mL third day, 4 mL fourth day, 5 mL on alternate days thereafter

For use with nitroprusside, give 1 g of sodium thiosulfate for every 100 mg of nitroprusside administered to prevent cyanide toxicity

Extravasation injury due to actinomycin, mechlorethamine, and mitomycin mix: 4 mL of 10% sodium thiosulfate with 6 mL of sterile water, administer through either the offending I.V. catheter or through multiple S.C. injections after catheter removal; use ice to extravasated area

Children and Adults: Topical: 20% to 25% solution: Apply a thin layer to affected areas twice daily

(Continued)

Sodium Thiosulfate *(Continued)*

Contraindications Hypersensitivity to any component, hydrogen sulfide poisoning

Dosage Forms Injection: 100 mg/mL (10 mL); 250 mg/mL (50 mL)

Stability Explosive when titrated with chlorates, nitrates, or permanganates

Reference Range Serum levels of 11.13 ± 1.1 mg/L are normal in adults; levels may be decreased to 5-8 mg/L in postoperative coronary artery bypass graft patients; levels may be elevated up to 22 mg/L in patients kept NPO for 1-3 weeks

Pregnancy Risk Factor C

Monitoring Parameters Monitor for signs of thiocyanate toxicity; administer slow I.V.; chest x-ray for inhalation injuries

Nursing Implications Given I.V. as slow I.V. push only over 10 minutes

Additional Information White, odorless crystals or powder with a salty taste; normal body burden: 1.5 mg/kg

Specific References

Hall AH and Rumack BH, "Hydroxocobalamin/Sodium Thiosulfate as a Cyanide Antidote," *J Emerg Med*, 1987, 5(2):115-21.

Howell SB, Pfeifle CL, Wung WE, et al, "Intraperitoneal Cisplatin With Systemic Thiosulfate Protection," *Ann Intern Med*, 1982, 97(6):845-51.

Ignoffo RJ and Friedman MA, "Therapy of Local Toxicities Caused by Extravasation of Cancer Chemotherapeutic Drugs," *Cancer Treat Rev*, 1980, 7(1):17-27.

MacCara ME, "Extravasation – A Hazard of Intravenous Therapy," *Drug Intell Clin Pharm*, 1983, 17:713.

Pfeifle CE, Howell SB, Felthouse RD, et al, "High-Dose Cisplatin With Sodium Thiosulfate Protection," *J Clin Oncol*, 1985, 3(2):237-44.

Willhite CC, "Inhalation Toxicology of Acute Exposure to Aliphatic Nitriles," *Clin Toxicol*, 1981, 18(8):991-1003.

Solmucol® *see* Acetylcysteine *on page 1388*

Sominex® Oral [OTC] *see* Diphenhydramine Hydrochloride *on page 1415*

Sorbilande® *see* Sorbitol *on this page*

Sorbitol (sor' bi tole)

CAS Number 50-70-4

Brand Names Cystosol®; Resulax®; Sorbilande®; Sorbitur®; Sorbostyl®; Syn M.D.®

Use Genitourinary irrigant in transurethral prostatic resection or other transurethral resection or other transurethral surgical procedures; diuretic; humectant; sweetening agent; hyperosmotic laxative; facilitate the passage of sodium polystyrene sulfonate through the intestinal tract

Mechanism of Action Polyalcoholic sugar with osmotic cathartic actions

Adverse Reactions

Cardiovascular: Edema

Endocrine & metabolic: Fluid and electrolyte losses, hypernatremia, lactic acidosis

Gastrointestinal: Diarrhea, nausea, vomiting, abdominal discomfort, dry mouth

Signs & Symptoms of Acute Overdose Nausea, diarrhea, fluid and electrolyte loss, hyperglycemia, hypernatremia

Toxicodynamics/Kinetics

Onset of action: ~15-60 minutes

Absorption: Oral, rectal: Poor

Metabolism: Mainly in the liver to fructose

Usual Dosage Hyperosmotic laxative (as single dose, at infrequent intervals):

Children 2-11 years:

- Oral: 2 mL/kg (as 70% solution)
- Rectal enema: 30-60 mL as 25% to 30% solution

Children >12 years and Adults:

- Oral: 30-150 mL (as 70% solution)
- Rectal enema: 120 mL as 25% to 30% solution
- Adjunct to sodium polystyrene sulfonate: 15 mL as 70% solution orally until diarrhea occurs (10-20 mL/2 hours) or 20-100 mL as an oral vehicle for the sodium polystyrene sulfonate resin

When administered with charcoal:

- Oral:
  - Children: 4.3 mL/kg of 35% sorbitol with 1 g/kg of activated charcoal
  - Adults: 4.3 mL/kg of 70% sorbitol with 1 g/kg of activated charcoal every 4 hours until first stool containing charcoal is passed
- Topical: 3% to 3.3% as transurethral surgical procedure irrigation

Contraindications Anuria

Dosage Forms

Solution: 70%

Solution, genitourinary irrigation: 3% (1500 mL, 3000 mL); 3.3% (2000 mL)

Nursing Implications Do not use unless solution is clear

Additional Information I.V. sorbitol can cause a metabolic acidosis

Specific References

Brown AM and Masson E, "Hidden Sorbitol in Proprietary Medicines = A Cause for Concern?" *Pharm J*, 1990, 245:211.

Gazda-Smith E and Synhavsky A, "Hypernatremia Following Treatment of Theophylline Toxicity With Activated Charcoal and Sorbitol," *Arch Intern Med*, 1990, 150(3):689, 692.

Sorbitur® *see* Sorbitol *on previous page*

Sorbostyl® *see* Sorbitol *on previous page*

SPS® *see* Sodium Polystyrene Sulfonate *on page 1469*

SSKI® *see* Potassium Iodide *on page 1460*

Steropine® *see* Atropine Sulfate *on page 1395*

Succimer (sux' sim mer)

CAS Number 304-55-2

Brand Names Chemet®

Synonyms 2,3-Dimercaptosuccinic Acid; DMSA

Use Treatment of lead poisoning in children with blood levels >45 μg/dL. It is not indicated for prophylaxis of lead poisoning in a lead-containing environment. Following oral administration, succimer is generally well tolerated and produces a linear dose-dependent reduction in serum lead concentrations; also has been used for arsenic and mercury poisoning.

Antidote Useful For

Arsenic *on page 862*
Cadmium *on page 876*
Cobalt *on page 895*
Lead *on page 945*
Mercury *on page 954*

Mechanism of Action Succimer is an analog of dimercaprol. It forms water soluble chelates with heavy metals which are subsequently excreted renally. Initial data have shown encouraging results in the treatment of mercury and arsenic poisoning. Succimer binds heavy metals; however, the chemical form of these chelates is not known.

Adverse Reactions The most common events attributable to succimer have been observed in about 10% of patients treated

Dermatologic: Rash
Gastrointestinal: Nausea, vomiting, diarrhea, appetite loss, metallic taste
Genitourinary: Sulfurous odor to urine, dysuria, hemorrhoidal symptoms
Hepatic: Elevated AST, ALT, alkaline phosphatase, serum cholesterol
Miscellaneous: Flu-like symptoms, sulfurous odor to breath, thrombocytosis, eosinophilia, transient neutropenia

Signs & Symptoms of Acute Overdose Respiratory depression

Toxicodynamics/Kinetics

Absorption: Rapid but incomplete
Metabolism: Rapid and extensive to mixed succimer cysteine disulfides
Half-life, elimination: 2 days
Time to peak serum concentration: ~1-2 hours
Elimination: ~25% in urine with peak urinary excretion occurring between 2-4 hours after dosing; of the total amount of succimer eliminated in urine, 90% is eliminated as mixed succimer-cysteine disulfide conjugates; 10% is excreted unchanged; fecal excretion of succimer probably represents unabsorbed drug

Usual Dosage Children and Adults: Oral: 10 mg/kg/dose every 8 hours for an additional 5 days followed by 10 mg/kg/dose every 12 hours for 14 days

Dosing adjustment in renal/hepatic impairment: Administer with caution and monitor closely

Concomitant iron therapy has been reported in a small number of children without the formation of a toxic complex with iron (as seen with dimercaprol); courses of therapy may be repeated if indicated by weekly monitoring of blood lead levels; lead levels should be stabilized <15 mg/dL; 2 weeks between courses is recommended unless more timely treatment is indicated by lead levels

Contraindications Known hypersensitivity to succimer

Warnings Caution in patients with renal or hepatic impairment; adequate hydration should be maintained during therapy

Dosage Forms Capsule: 100 mg

Test Interactions False-positive ketones (U) using nitroprusside methods, falsely elevated serum CPK; falsely decreased uric acid measurement

Drug Interactions Not recommended for concomitant administration with edetate calcium disodium or penicillamine

(Continued)

Succimer *(Continued)*

Pregnancy Risk Factor C

Pregnancy Implications No evidence for mutagenicity

Monitoring Parameters Blood lead levels, serum amino transferases

Nursing Implications Adequately hydrate patients; rapid rebound of serum lead levels can occur; monitor closely

Additional Information This agent appears to offer advantages over existing lead chelating agents by not facilitating gastric absorption of lead, not significantly chelating other divalent minerals (iron, copper, and zinc) and safety in G-6-PD deficiency

Specific References

Committee on Drugs, American Academy of Pediatrics, "Treatment Guidelines for Lead Exposure in Children," *Pediatrics*, 1995, 96:155-60.

Dart RC, et al, "Pharmacokinetics of Meso-2,3-Dimercaptosuccinic Acid in Patients With Lead Poisoning and Healthy Adults," *J Pediatr*, 1994, 125:309-16.

Fournier L, Thomas G, Garnier R, et al, "2,3-Dimercaptosuccinic Acid Treatment of Heavy Metal Poisoning in Humans," *Med Toxicol Adverse Drug Exp*, 1988, 3(6):499-504.

Glotzer DE, "The Current Role of 2,3 Dimercaptosuccinic Acid (DMSA) in Management of Childhood Lead Poisoning," *Drug Saf*, 1993, 9(2):85-92.

Graziano JH, Lolacono NJ, Moulton T, et al, "Controlled Study of Meso-2,3-Dimercaptosuccinic Acid for the Management of Childhood Lead Intoxication," *J Pediatr*, 1992, 120(1):133-9.

Mann KV and Travers JD, "Succimer, An Oral Lead Chelator," *Clin Pharm*, 1991, 10(12):914-22.

Marcus S, Okose P, Jennis T, et al, "Untoward Effects of Oral Dimercaptosuccinic Acid in the Treatment for Lead Poisoning," *Vet Hum Toxicol*, 1991, 33:376.

Sufortan® *see* Penicillamine *on page 1454*

Sulfactin Homburg® *see* Dimercaprol *on page 1414*

SuperChar® [OTC] *see* Charcoal *on page 1403*

Sus-Phrine® *see* Epinephrine *on page 1422*

Synkavite® *see* Phytonadione *on page 1458*

Syn M.D.® *see* Sorbitol *on page 1472*

Syprine® *see* Trientine Dihydrochloride *on this page*

Tamuc® *see* Acetylcysteine *on page 1388*

Therapeutic Drugs Associated With Hallucinations *see page 1558*

Thrombin® *see* Phytonadione *on page 1458*

Thyro-Block® *see* Potassium Iodide *on page 1460*

Tixair® *see* Acetylcysteine *on page 1388*

Tracémate® *see* Edetate Disodium *on page 1421*

Trientine Dihydrochloride (trye' en teen)

CAS Number 112-24-3; 38260-01-4

Brand Names Syprine®

Replaces Cuprid®; MK-0681

Use Treatment of Wilson's disease in patients intolerant to penicillamine; possible use in copper poisoning

Antidote Useful For

Copper *on page 896*

Mechanism of Action Trientine hydrochloride is an oral chelating agent structurally dissimilar from penicillamine and other available chelating agents; an effective oral chelator of copper used to induce adequate cupriuresis

Adverse Reactions

Central nervous system: Malaise

Dermatologic: Tenderness, thickening and fissuring of skin

Endocrine & metabolic: Iron deficiency

Gastrointestinal: Heartburn, diarrhea, epigastric pain

Neuromuscular & skeletal: Muscle and pain cramps

Miscellaneous: Systemic lupus erythematosus (SLE)

Signs & Symptoms of Acute Overdose Systemic lupus erythematosus (SLE)

Usual Dosage Oral (administer on an empty stomach):

Children <12 years: 500-750 mg/day in divided doses 2-4 times/day; maximum: 1.5 g/day

Adults: 750-1250 mg/day in divided doses 2-4 times/day; maximum daily dose: 2 g

Contraindications Rheumatoid arthritis, biliary cirrhosis, cystinuria, known hypersensitivity to trientine

Dosage Forms Capsule: 250 mg

Drug Interactions Decreased effect with iron and possibly other mineral supplements

Pregnancy Risk Factor C

Monitoring Parameters Iron levels

Additional Information Water soluble

Specific References

Stavinoha MW and Soloway RD, "Current Therapy of Chronic Liver Disease," *Drugs*, 1990, 39(6):814-40.

Tankanow RM, "Pathophysiology and Treatment of Wilson's Disease," *Clin Pharm*, 1991, 10(11):839-49.

Walshe JM, "Treatment of Wilson's Disease With Trientine (Triethylene Tetramine) Dihydrochloride," *Lancet*, 1982, 1(8273):643-7.

Trolovol® *see* Penicillamine *on page 1454*

Tusstat® Syrup *see* Diphenhydramine Hydrochloride *on page 1415*

Twilite® Oral [OTC] *see* Diphenhydramine Hydrochloride *on page 1415*

Uni-Bent® Cough Syrup *see* Diphenhydramine Hydrochloride *on page 1415*

Urolene Blue® Oral *see* Methylene Blue *on page 1444*

Vapo-iso® *see* Isoproterenol *on page 1436*

Vaponefrin® [OTC] *see* Epinephrine *on page 1422*

Vitableu® *see* Methylene Blue *on page 1444*

Vitamin B_6 *see* Pyridoxine Hydrochloride *on page 1465*

Vitamin B_{12} *see* Hydroxocobalamin *on page 1433*

Vitamin K_1 *see* Phytonadione *on page 1458*

Wehdryl® Injection *see* Diphenhydramine Hydrochloride *on page 1415*

Wellcovorin® *see* Leucovorin Calcium *on page 1437*

Xanturenusi® *see* Pyridoxine Hydrochloride *on page 1465*

APPENDIX

Comparison Charts

ADIPOSE TISSUE RANGES OF TOXINS

General Population (Background)

Beta-hexachlorocyclohexane	ND* to 570 ng/g
Boron	ND
Bromoform	ND
Chlorobenzene	1-9 ng/g
Chloroform	ND to 580 ng/g
Cobalt	0.035-0.078 mg/kg
Di-(2-ethylhexyl)phthalate	ND to 850 ng/g
Diethyl phthalate	ND to 0.65 μg/g
Dibromochloromethane	ND
1,4-Dichlorobenzene	12-500 ng/g
Dieldrin	ND to 4100 ng/g
Di-N-octylphthalate	ND to 850 ng/g
Endrin	ND
Ethylbenzene	ND to 280 ng/g
Heptachlor epoxide	ND to 310 ng/g
1,2,3,4,6,7,8-Heptachlorodibenzofurans	21 ppt
Hexachlorobenzene	12-1300 ng/g
Hexachlorobutadiene	0.8-8 μg/kg
1,2,3,4,7,8-Hexachlorodibenzofurans	9.3 ppt
1,2,3,6,7,8-Hexachlorodibenzofurans	5.4 ppt
2,3,4,6,7,8-Hexachlorodibenzofurans	1.8 ppt
Manganese	0.07 μg/g
Mirex	ND to 41 ng/g
Naphthalene	ND to 63 ng/g
Octachlorodibenzofurans	60 ppt
Oxychlordane	90-120 ng/g
2,3,4,7,8-Pentachlorodibenzofurans	40 ppt
Phenanthrene	ND to 24 ng/g
Polybrominated biphenyls (in Michigan)	15-12,820 μg/kg
Polychlorinated biphenyl (PCB)	14-1700 ng/g
Polycyclic aromatic hydrocarbons (PAH)	ND
Styrene	8-350 ng/g
2,3,7,8-Tetrachlorodibenzofurans	9.1 ppt
Tin	8.7-15 μg/g
Toluene	ND to 250 ng/g
Tributyl phosphate	ND to 120 ng/g
1,1,1-Trichloroethane	ND to 830 ng/g
1,1,2-Trichloroethane	ND
Vanadium	0.7 ng/g

*Not detected.

Reference: U.S. Department of Health and Human Services, Toxicology Profile Series, ATSDR.

ALLERGIC SKIN REACTIONS TO DRUGS

Skin eruptions are the most common clinically observed form of drug "allergy." Cutaneous manifestations of hypersensitivity may include pruritus, urticaria, and angioedema; maculopapular, morbilliform, or erythematous rashes; erythema multiforme; eczema; erythema nodosum; photosensitivity reactions; and fixed drug eruptions. The most severe drug-related reactions are exfoliative dermatitis and vesiculobullous eruptions such as the Stevens-Johnson syndrome and toxic epidermal necrolysis (Lyell's syndrome). This table lists the incidence of drugs associated with cutaneous manifestations reported in 22,227 consecutive medical inpatients in the Boston Collaborative Drug Surveillance Program.

Drug	Reaction per 1000 Recipients
Sulfamethoxazole and trimethoprim	59
Ampicillin	52
Semisynthetic penicillins	36
Blood, whole human	35
Corticotropin	28
Erythromycin	23
Sulfisoxazole	17
Penicillin G	16
Gentamicin sulfate	16
Practolol	16
Cephalosporins	13
Quinidine	13
Plasma protein fraction	12
Dipyrone	11
Mercurial diuretics	9.5
Nitrofurantoin	9.1
Packed RBCs	8.1
Heparin	7.7
Chloramphenicol	6.8
Trimethobenzamide	6.6
Phenazopyridine	6.5
Methenamine	6.4
Nitrazepam	6.3
Barbiturates	4.7
Glutethimide	4.5
Indomethacin	4.4
Chlordiazepoxide	4.2
Metoclopramide	4.0
Diazepam	3.8
Propoxyphene	3.4
Isoniazid	3.0
Guaifenesin and theophylline	2.9
Nystatin	2.9
Chlorothiazide	2.8
Furosemide	2.6
Isophane insulin suspension	1.3
Phenytoin	1.1
Phytonadione	0.9
Flurazepam	0.5
Chloral hydrate	0.2

Reference: Patterson R and Anderson J, "Allergic Reactions to Drugs and Biologic Agents," *JAMA*, 1982, 248:2637-45.

AMERICAN ACADEMY OF CLINICAL TOXICOLOGY FACILITY ASSESSMENT GUIDELINES FOR REGIONAL TOXICOLOGY TREATMENT CENTERS

These guidelines were developed by the Acute and Intensive Care Section and endorsed by the Board of Directors of the American Academy of Clinical Toxicology (AACT).

Statements of Purpose

The primary rationale for regional toxicology treatment centers is to enhance the medical care provided to victims of severe or unusual poisonings or overdoses. These guidelines enhance care by promoting a systematized, multidisciplinary approach. The systematized approach encourages a health center to properly prepare for these victims by recruiting a qualified director and staff, stockpiling antidotes, and negotiating agreements with critical ancillary services such as the Psychiatry Department and the Toxicology Laboratory. Adherence to these guidelines requires a major philosophical and financial commitment by a health center. The other major rationale for regional toxicology treatment centers is to recruit a "critical mass" of patients. This critical mass is essential for high quality clinical training and research program and will facilitate the development of Medical Toxicology as a specialty. The financial commitment required and the need for a critical mass mandate that these treatment centers be established on a regional basis.

The rationale for publishing these guidelines is twofold. First, these guidelines will serve as a template for those who wish to design and promote a treatment center for their region. Secondly, by meeting these guidelines, a health center will demonstrate its commitment to the local Emergency Medicine Service system, referring physicians and poison control center. Acceptance by these groups is crucial to the successful establishment of a regional toxicology treatment center.

The establishment of regional treatment centers for other specialty care areas such as trauma, burns and spinal cord injuries has enhanced patient care and medical training and facilitated research in those areas. Regional toxicology treatment centers are intended to complement the services and not to compete with a regional poison control (information) center in enhancing the care of poisoned patients. These guidelines will be reviewed periodically by AACT and amended when appropriate.

A regional toxicology treatment center (RTTC) provides comprehensive treatment for severe or unusual cases of poisonings. All activities of the facility shall be under physician control. Treatment centers (which may be comprised of more than one facility) should meet the following general guidelines.

1. The facility must demonstrate a commitment to providing high quality medical care to poisoned patients. This commitment must be both philosophical and financial. This commitment includes but is not limited to:
   - proper organization and sufficient staffing of the Medical Toxicology service
   - ensuring timely availability of inpatient bed space appropriate for the patient's severity of illness
   - providing essential equipment and rapid laboratory analyses
   - stocking adequate types and amounts of antidotes
2. The facility must develop or adopt acute care protocols, provide acute psychiatric consultation, perform postdischarge follow-up, perform quality assurance activities, report data, perform research and provide educational programs. The details of these programs must be delineated in written policies and procedures.

3. The facility must work closely with the regional poison control (information) center, which provides poison information to health care professionals and the public. The treatment center will attempt to identify special regional needs that would require additional resources.
4. The facility shall submit to periodic review or audit if required by governmental or national professional organizations.
5. The facility must negotiate interhospital transfer agreements with referring hospitals.
6. The facility must recommend prehospital triage guidelines for poisoned victims in the regional EMS system.
7. The facility must identify and publicize the availability or restriction of services to the pediatric, obstetric, or adult population.
8. The facility must determine and declare its medical catchment areas (geographic referral base). It could consist of multiple EMS regions and may cross state lines.

The following sections will be discussed:

A. Organization
B. Medical Staff
C. Facilities
D. Capabilities
E. Quality Assurance
F. Research
G. Education
H. Data Collection

A. Organization

1. The medical director is responsible for clinical operations, quality assurance, and development of clinical protocols.
2. The medical toxicology service will provide inpatient admission and/or consultation services for poisoned victims.
3. Hospital administration will develop a regional plan to delineate the relationship of the RTTC to regional hospitals.
4. The relationship to other medical departments and essential services must be established and documented in the policy and procedure manual. The departments and services should at least include the Regional Poison Information Center, Regional Hazardous Materials Team, Nephrology, Neurology, Pulmonary, Psychiatry, Pediatrics, Intensive Care Medicine, Toxicology Laboratory, Pharmacy, Regional EMS system and local mycologists, botanists, and herpetologists.
5. A policy and procedure manual will be developed and maintained by the medical toxicology service.

B. Medical Staff

1. Medical Toxicology Staff

    a. Medical Director

    The Medical Director must demonstrate expertise and special interest in the field of medical toxicology. The Medical Director must be a physician and board certified in Medical Toxicology.

    b. Attending Physicians

    Attending physicians on the medical toxicology service should be board certified in Medical Toxicology or in Emergency Medicine, Family Medicine, Internal Medicine, Pediatrics, or Occupational Medicine with demonstrated expertise and special interest in medical toxicology as evidenced by publications, research, and meeting attendance.

2. Other Medical Staff

The following requirements may be fulfilled by senior resident physicians with special competence in the care of patients with poisoning/drug emergencies as judged by the Medical Director of the Medical Toxicology service. These residents must be capable of initiating measures directed toward stabilizing the patient and beginning the patient management process. Attending staff specialists are to be "on call" and promptly available for emergency consultation.

In-Hospital 24 Hours/Day

Anesthesiology/Nurse Anesthetist
Emergency Medicine

"On Call" and Promptly Available From Inside or Outside Hospital

Anesthesiology
Cardiology
General Surgery
GI (Endoscopy)
Hematology
Infectious Disease
Internal Medicine (adult facilities)
Medical Toxicology
Nephrology
Neurology
Obstetrics
Pathology (Analytic Toxicology)
Pediatrics (pediatric facilities)
Pediatric surgeon (pediatric facilities)
Psychiatry
Pulmonary Diseases
Radiology
Surgery

C. Facilities

1. Emergency Department

   a. Personnel

      (1) Designated Medical Director

      (2) Staffed in-house, 24 hours/day, with physicians certified by or board prepared for the American Board of Emergency Medicine or Osteopathic Emergency Medicine or American Board of Pediatrics (for pediatric facilities).

      (3) RNs 24 hours/day competent in care of poisoned patients as evidenced by CEN certification or annual continuing education in medical toxicology.

   b. Equipment — see JCAH criteria for level 1 unit

      (1) Hazardous materials decontamination unit

   c. Emergency department protocols regarding the management of the poisoned patients.

2. Intensive Care Unit (ICU) Adults and/or Children

   a. Designated Medical Director

   b. Physician competent in resuscitation and initial management of poisoned patient available in-house 24 hours/day.

   c. Nurse - patient minimum ratio of 1:3 on each shift and competence in the care of poisoned patients as evidenced by CCRN certification or annual continuing education in medical toxicology.

   d. Equipment — see JCAH criteria for level 1 unit.

D. Capabilities (available 24 hours/day)

1. Hemodialysis/Hemoperfusion
2. Radiology
   a. CAT scan
   b. Fluoroscopy
3. Clinical Laboratory
   a. Standard analyses of blood, urine, and other body fluids
   b. Blood typing and crossmatching
   c. Coagulation studies
   d. Comprehensive Blood Bank or access to community central Blood Bank and adequate hospital storage facilities
   e. Microbiology
   f. Toxicology Laboratory Services (in-house or by formal agreement — see Appendix A for required toxicology laboratory analyses)
4. Pharmacy
   a. Pharmacist available in-house 24 hours/day.
   b. Stock of all common antidotes in amounts adequate to meet regional needs. (See Appendix B.)
5. Respiratory Care (by qualified respiratory therapists)
6. Hyperbaric Oxygenation (in-house or by formal agreement)
7. Social Services Department
8. Electrophysiology Laboratory (in-house or by formal agreement)
   a. EEG
   b. EMG
9. Psychiatry

   There must be capabilities for on-site psychiatric care of suspected suicidal patients. Inpatient psychiatric care must be available within the RTTC or via transfer.
10. Endoscopy
11. Surgery

E. Programs for Quality Assurance

1. Audit all poison deaths
2. Morbidity and morality review conference
3. Case conference, multidisciplinary
4. Medical nursing audit, utilization review, lab review
5. Medical records review

F. Research

The RTTC shall conduct research and publications relating to medical toxicology.

G. Education

1. There shall be continuing education in medical toxicology for the medical and nursing staff of the RTTC.

2. Training in medical toxicology shall be made available to medical and/or PharmD students, physicians in training, and medical and nursing staff from other health care facilities in the region.

H. Data Collection

The RTTC shall maintain a registry of all patients and report all cases to the nearest poison information center participating in the American Association of Poison Control Center National Data Collection System.

These guidelines are subject to periodic review and revision by the American Academy of Clinical Toxicology.

APPENDIX A

Required Laboratory Tests for Regional Toxicology Treatment Centers

QUALITATIVE TESTS

Available within 4 hours:

Acetaminophen, aspirin, anticonvulsants, antidepressants, antihistamines, antipsychotics, barbiturates, benzodiazepines, opiates, phencyclidine, stimulants

QUANTITATIVE TESTS

Available within 2 hours:

Acetone
ABG and measured O_2 saturation
Alcohols (ethanol, ethylene glycol, isopropanol, methanol)
Analgesics — acetaminophen, salicylate
Carboxyhemoglobin
Complete blood count and differential
Creatine kinase
Electrolytes, glucose, urea, creatinine
Lactic acid
Methemoglobin
Mg, Ca, phosphate
Phenobarbital
PT, PTT, fibrin split products (or D-D dimers), fibrinogen level, platelets
Serum osmolality by freezing point determination
SGOT (AST), SGPT (ALT), LDH, total/direct bilirubin
Theophylline

Available within 4 hours:

Barbiturates
Carbamazepine
Cholinesterase, serum
Digoxin
Iron
Lidocaine
Lithium
Phenytoin
Valproic acid

Available within 48 hours:

Cyanide and thiocyanate
Blood — lead, mercury
Urine — arsenic, lead, mercury

APPENDIX B

Required Antidotes for Regional Toxicology Treatment Centers

Acetylcysteine 20% (Mucomyst®)
Activated charcoal
Antivenin, crotalidae polyvalent
Antivenin, lactrodectus mactans
Atropine sulfate
Benztropine mesylate
Bromocriptine mesylate
Calcium chloride 10%
Calcium disodium edetate
Calcium gluconate 10%
Calcium gluconate gel
Cathartic
  Magnesium citrate
  Magnesium sulfate or sodium sulfate
  Sorbitol
Cyanide antidote kit
  Amyl nitrite
  Sodium nitrite 3%
  Sodium thiosulfate
Dantrolene sodium
Deferoxamine mesylate (Desferal®)
Dextrose 50% in water
Diazepam (Valium®)
Diazoxide
Digoxin immune fab (Digibind®)
Dimercaprol (BAL®)
Dimercaptosuccinic acid (DMSA) (Succimer®, Chemet®)
Diphenhydramine hydrochloride
Droperidol or haloperidol
Esmolol
Ethyl alcohol 95%
Folic acid
Glucagon
Ipecac syrup
Lorazepam
Leucovorin (folinic acid)
Mannitol 20%
Methocarbamol
Methylene blue 1%
Naloxone hydrochloride (Narcan®)
Nitroprusside, sodium
Penicillamine
Phentolamine
Physostigmine salicylate
Polyethylene glycol (GoLYTELY®, PEG)
Pralidoxime chloride (2-PAM, Protopam®)
Propranolol
Protamine sulfate
Pyridoxine hydrochloride
Sodium bicarbonate
Starch
Thiamine hydrochloride
Vitamin K_1 (AquaMEPHYTON®)

Reprinted with permission from "Guidelines for Regional Toxicology Treatment Centers," *Clinical Toxicology*, New York, NY: Marcel Dekker, Inc, 1993, 31:209-17.

ABOUT THE AMERICAN ACADEMY OF CLINICAL TOXICOLOGY

Mission Statement

The American Academy of Clinical Toxicology (AACT) is a not-for-profit multidisciplinary organization uniting scientists and clinicians in the advancement of research, education, prevention, and treatment of diseases caused by chemicals, drugs, and other toxins.

Historical Perspective

The AACT was founded in 1968 by physicians and scientists with the specific goal of advancing the diagnosis and treatment of poisonings. The founders provided and maintained mechanisms for certification of professionals in the specialty of clinical toxicology.

In 1974, the AACT established the American Board of Medical Toxicology to certify physicians in the specialty of clinical toxicology. In 1985, a second certifying board, the American Board of Applied Toxicology (ABAT) was established for nonphysician peer recognition.

Today, the AACT is an international organization whose membership is comprised of clinical and research toxicologists, physicians, veterinarians, nurses, pharmacists, analytical chemists, industrial hygienists, poison information center specialists, and allied professionals.

The AACT, affiliated with many professional organizations, holds annual meetings in conjunction with both the American and Canadian Associations of Poison Control Centers, and the American College of Medical Toxicology. It is a charter member of the World Federation of Associations of Clinical Toxicology Centers and Poison Control Centers sponsored by the World Health Organization. In addition, the Academy is a member of the International Union of Toxicology (IUTOX) and supports the efforts of other toxicology organizations worldwide. Currently, there are over 450 members of AACT worldwide. Membership inquiries are welcomed and may be directed to: Gregory Gaar, MD; Secretary-Treasurer; American Academy of Clinical Toxicology Inc; c/o Medical Toxicology Consultants; 4 Columbia Drive, Suite 810; Tampa, FL 33606; Tel: (813) 251-6911; Fax: (813) 254-2504.

1994/95 Officers and Trustees

Future Meetings of the North American Congress of Clinical Toxicology

Portland, Oregon	October, 1996
St Louis, Missouri	September, 1997
Montreal, Canada	August, 1998

AMINOGLYCOSIDE DOSING AND MONITORING

All aminoglycoside therapy should be individualized for specific patients in specific clinical situation. The following are guidelines for initiating therapy.

1. Loading dose based on estimated ideal body weight (IBW). **All patients require a loading dose independent of renal function.**

Agent	Dose
Gentamicin	2 mg/kg
Tobramycin	2 mg/kg
Amikacin	7.5 mg/kg

Significantly higher loading doses may be required in severely ill intensive care unit patients.

2. Initial maintenance doses as a percent of loading dose according to desired dosing interval and creatinine clearance (Cl_{cr}):

$$\text{Male } Cl_{cr} \text{ (mL/min)} = \frac{(140 - \text{age}) \times \text{IBW}}{72 \times \text{serum creatinine}}$$

$$\text{Female} = 0.85 \times Cl_{cr} \text{ males}$$

Cl_{cr} (mL/min)	Dosing Interval (h) 8	12	24
90	84%	—	—
80	80%	—	—
70	76%	88%	—
60	—	84%	—
50	—	79%	—
40	—	72%	92%
30	—	—	86%
25	—	—	81%
20	—	—	75%

Patients older than 65 years of age should not receive initial aminoglycoside maintenance dosing more often than every 12 hours.

3. Serum concentration monitoring

   a. Serum concentration monitoring is necessary for **safe** and **effective** therapy, particularly in patients with serious infections and those with risk factors for toxicity.

   b. Peak serum concentrations should be drawn 30 minutes after the completion of a 30-minute infusion. Trough serum concentrations should be drawn within 30 minutes prior to the administered dose.

   c. Serum concentrations should be drawn after 5 half-lives, usually around the third dose or thereafter.

4. Desired measured serum concentrations

	Peak (μg/mL)	Trough (μg/mL)
Gentamicin	6-10	0.5-2
Tobramycin	6-10	0.5-2
Amikacin	20-30	<5
Netilmicin	4-10	<2

5. For patients receiving hemodialysis:
   - administer the **same** loading dose
   - administer ⅔ of the loading dose after each dialysis
   - **serum concentrations must be monitored**
   - watch for ototoxicity from accumulation of drug
6. For individual clinical situations the prescribing physician should feel free to consult Infectious Disease, the Pharmacology Service, or the Pharmacy.

AMINOGLYCOSIDE PENETRATION INTO VARIOUS TISSUES

Site	Extent of Distribution
Eye	Poor
CNS	Poor (<25%)
Pleural	Excellent
Bronchial secretions	Poor
Sputum	Fair (10%-50%)
Pulmonary tissue	Excellent
Ascitic fluid	Variable (43%-132%)
Peritoneal fluid	Poor
Bile	Variable (25%-90%)
Bile with obstruction	Poor
Synovial fluid	Excellent
Bone	Poor
Prostate	Poor
Urine	Excellent
Renal tissue	Excellent

From Neu HC, "Pharmacology of Aminoglycosides," *The Aminoglycosides*, Whelton E, Neu HC, eds, New York, NY: Marcel Dekker, Inc, 1981.

ANIMAL AND HUMAN BITES GUIDELINES

Wound Management

Irrigation: Critically important; irrigate all penetration wounds using 20 mL syringe, 19 gauge needle and >250 mL 1% povidone iodine solution. This method will reduce wound infection by a factor of 20. When there is high risk of rabies, use viricidal 1% benzalkonium chloride in addition to the 1% povidone iodine. Irrigate wound with normal saline after antiseptic irrigation.

Debridement: Remove all crushed or devitalized tissue remaining after irrigation; minimize removal on face and over thin skin areas or anywhere you would create a worse situation than the bite itself already has; do not extend puncture wounds surgically — rather, manage them with irrigation and antibiotics.

Suturing: Close most dog bites if <8 hours (<12 hours on face); do not routinely close puncture wounds, or deep or severe bites on the hands or feet, as these are at highest risk for infection. Cat and human bites should not be sutured unless cosmetically important. Wound edge freshening, where feasible, reduces infection; minimize sutures in the wound and use monofilament on the surface.

Immobilization: Critical in all hand wounds; important for infected extremities.

Hospitalization/I.V. Antibiotics: Admit for I.V. antibiotics all significant human bites to the hand, especially closed fist injuries, and bites involving penetration of the bone or joint (a high index of suspicion is needed). Consider I.V. antibiotics for significant established wound infections with cellulitis or lymphangitis, any infected bite on the hand, any infected cat bite, and any infection in an immunocompromised or asplenic patient. Outpatient treatment with I.V. antibiotics may be possible in selected cases by consulting with infectious disease.

Laboratory Assessment

Gram's Stain: Not useful prior to onset of clinically apparent infection; examination of purulent material may show a predominant organism in established infection, aiding antibiotic selection; not warranted unless results will change your treatment.

Culture: Not useful or cost effective prior to onset of clinically apparent infection.

X-Ray: Whenever you suspect bony involvement, especially in craniofacial dog bites in very small children or severe bite/crush in an extremity; cat bites with their long needle like teeth may cause osteomyelitis or a septic joint, especially in the hand or wrist.

Immunizations

Tetanus: All bite wounds are contaminated. If not immunized in last 5 years, or if not current in a child, give DPT, DT, Td, or TT as indicated. For absent or incomplete primary immunization, give 250 units tetanus immune globulin (TIG) in addition.

Rabies: In the U.S. 30,000 persons are treated each year in an attempt to prevent 1-5 cases. Domestic animals should be quarantined for 10 days to prove need for prophylaxis. High risk animal bites (85% of cases = bat >>skunk >racoon) usually receive treatment consisting of:

- human rabies immune globulin (HRIG): 20 units/kg I.M. (unless previously immunized with HDCV)
- human diploid cell vaccine (HDCV): 1 mL I.M. on days 0, 3, 7, 14 and 28 (unless previously immunized with HDCV — then give only first 2 doses)

Consult with Infectious Disease before ordering rabies prophylaxis.

Bite Wounds and Prophylactic Antibiotics

Parenteral vs Oral: If warranted, consider an initial I.V. dose to rapidly establish effective serum levels, especially if high risk, delayed treatment, or if patient reliability is poor.

Dog Bite:

1. Rarely get infected (~5%)
2. Infecting organisms: Staph coag negative, staph coag positive, alpha strep, diphtheroids, beta strep, *Pseudomonas aeruginosa*, gamma strep, *Pasteurella multocida*
3. Prophylactic antibiotics are seldom indicated. Consider for high risk wounds such as distal extremity puncture wounds, severe crush injury, bites occurring in cosmetically sensitive areas (eg, face), or in immunocompromised or asplenic patients.

Cat Bite:

1. Often get infected (~25% to 50%)
2. Infecting organisms: *Pasteurella multocida* (first 24 hours), coag positive staph, anaerobic cocci (after first 24 hours)
3. Prophylactic antibiotics are indicated in all cases.

Human Bite:

1. Intermediate infection rate (~15% to 20%)
2. Infecting organisms: Coag positive staph α, β, γ strep, *Haemophilus*, *Eikenella corrodens*, anaerobic streptococci, *Fusobacterium*, *Veillonella*, bacteroides.
3. Prophylactic antibiotics are indicated in almost all cases except superficial injuries.

See attached table for prophylactic antibiotic summary.

Bite Wound Antibiotic Regimens

	Dog Bite	Cat Bite	Human Bite
Prophylactic Antibiotics			
Prophylaxis	No routine prophylaxis, consider if involves face or hand, or immunosuppressed or asplenic patients	Routine prophylaxis	Routine prophylaxis
Prophylactic antibiotic	Amoxicillin	Amoxicillin	Amoxicillin
Penicillin allergy	Doxycycline if >10 y or co-trimoxazole	Doxycycline if >10 y or co-trimoxazole	Doxycycline if >10 y or erythromycin and cephalexin*
Outpatient Oral Antibiotic Treatment (mild to moderate infection)			
Established infection	Amoxicillin and clavulanic acid	Amoxicillin and clavulanic acid	Amoxicillin and clavulanic acid
Penicillin allergy (mild infection only)	Doxycycline if >10 y	Doxycycline if >10 y	Cephalexin* or clindamycin
Outpatient Parenteral Antibiotic Treatment (moderate infections — single drug regimens)			
	Ceftriaxone	Ceftriaxone	Cefotetan
Inpatient Parenteral Antibiotic Treatment			
Established infection	Ampicillin + cefazolin	Ampicillin + cefazolin	Ampicillin + clindamycin
Penicillin allergy	Cefazolin*	Ceftriaxone*	Cefotetan* or imipenem

*Contraindicated if history of immediate hypersensitivity reaction (anaphylaxis) to penicillin.

Duration of Prophylactic and Treatment Regimens

Prophylaxis: 5 days
Treatment: 10-14 days

Antibiotic Dosages

Antibiotic	Adult Dosage	Pediatric Dosage
Oral regimens		
Amoxicillin	500 mg P.O. tid	50 mg/kg/d with tid dosing
Amoxicillin/clavulanate	500/125 P.O. tid (750 mg P.O. qid if >180 lb)	50 mg/kg/d based on amoxicillin content with tid dosing
Cephalexin	500 mg P.O. qid (750 mg P.O. qid if >180 lb)	50 mg/kg/d with qid dosing
Clindamycin	450 mg P.O. tid	25-30 mg/kg/d with tid-qid dosing
Co-trimoxazole	2 tabs P.O. bid	8 mg/kg/d based on trimethoprim content with bid dosing
Dicloxacillin	500 mg P.O. qid	50 mg/kg/d with qid dosing
Doxycycline	100 mg P.O. bid	5 mg/kg/d with bid dosing
Erythromycin	500 mg P.O. qid	50 mg/kg/d with qid dosing
Penicillin VK	500 mg P.O. qid	75-100 mg/kg/d with qid dosing
Parenteral Regimens		
Ampicillin	2 g I.V. q4-6h	250-300 mg/kg/d I.V. given q6h
Ampicillin/sulbactam	2 g I.V. q6h based on ampicillin component	250-300 mg/kg/d I.V. based on ampicillin component given q6h
Cefazolin	2 g I.V.q8h	100 mg/kg/d I.V. given q8h
Cefotetan	2 g I.V. q12h	60-80 mg/kg/d I.V. given q12h
Ceftriaxone	2 g I.V. or I.M. q24h	75 mg/kg/d I.M./I.V. given q24h
Clindamycin	900 mg I.V. q8h	25-30 mg/kg/d I.V. given q8h
Imipenem	500 mg I.V. q6h	

ANTACID DRUG INTERACTIONS

Drug	Antacid			
	Aluminum Salts	Calcium Salts	Magnesium Salts	Magnesium Aluminum Combinations
Allopurinol	↓			
Benzodiazepines	↑		↓	↓
Calcitriol			x*	x*
Captopril				↓
Cimetidine				↓
Corticosteroids	↓		↓	↓
Dicumarol			↑	
Diflunisal	↓			
Digoxin	↓		↓	
Iron	↓	↓	↓	↓
Isoniazid	↓			
Ketoconazole				↓
Levodopa				↑
Nitrofurantoin			↓	
Penicillamine	↓		↓	↓
Phenothiazines	↓		↓	↓
Phenytoin		↓		↓
Quinidine		↑	↑	↑
Quinolones				↓
Ranitidine	↓			↓
Salicylates		↓		↓
Sodium polystyrene sulfonate	x†		x†	x†
Tetracyclines	↓	↓	↓	↓
Valproic acid				↑

Pharmacologic effect increased (↑) or decreased (↓) by antacids.

*Concomitant use in patients on chronic renal dialysis may lead to hypermagnesemia.

†Concomitant use may cause metabolic alkalosis in patients with renal failure.

ANTIFUNGAL THERAPY

Drugs of Choice for Specific Fungal Infections

Fungal Infection	Primary Choice	Alternative Therapy
Aspergillosis		
Allergic bronchopulmonary	None	
Aspergilloma (fungus ball)	Surgery/? itraconazole P.O.	
Pulmonary infection	Amphotericin B I.V. (± rifampin P.O.)	Itraconazole P.O.
Disseminated/extrapulmonary	Amphotericin B I.V. (± rifampin P.O.)	Itraconazole P.O.
Blastomycosis	Itraconazole P.O.	Ketoconazole P.O. or amphotericin B I.V.
Cutaneous		
Pulmonary		
Extrapulmonary		
Candidiasis		
Systemic/invasive disease	Amphotericin B I.V.	Fluconazole I.V., P.O.
Chronic mucocutaneous	Ketoconazole P.O.	Amphotericin B I.V.
Endocarditis	Surgery/amphotericin B I.V. + flucytosine P.O.	None
Oral thrush	Nystatin or clotrimazole nonabsorbable lozenges P.O.	Fluconazole P.O.
Urinary (cystitis)	None or fluconazole P.O.	Amphotericin B bladder irrigation
Cutaneous/vaginal	Topical azoles	Oral absorbable azoles
Coccidioidomycosis		
Non-CNS	Amphotericin B I.V.	Fluconazole I.V., P.O., or itraconazole P.O.
Meningitis	Amphotericin B I.V., intrathecal	Fluconazole I.V. + amphotericin B intrathecal
Cryptococcosis		
Immunocompetent		
Nonmeningeal	Amphotericin B I.V. → fluconazole P.O.	Amphotericin B I.V. + flucytosine P.O.
CNS	Amphotericin B I.V. + flucytosine P.O. → fluconazole P.O.	None
Immunocompromised		
Initial	Amphotericin B I.V.	Fluconazole I.V.
Maintenance (in AIDS)	Fluconazole P.O.	Fluconazole P.O.
Histoplasmosis		
Immunocompetent		
Non-CNS	Itraconazole P.O.	Amphotericin B I.V.
Immunocompromised or CNS		
Initial	Amphotericin B I.V.	Ketoconazole or itraconazole P.O.
Maintenance (in AIDS)	Amphotericin B I.V. intermittently	? Itraconazole P.O.
Mucormycosis	Amphotericin B I.V.	None
Paracoccidioidomycosis (South American blastomycosis)	Itraconazole or ketoconazole P.O.	Amphotericin B I.V. or sulfonamides P.O.
Sporotrichosis		
Cutaneous	Saturated solution of potassium iodide P.O.	Itraconazole P.O.
Systemic	Itraconazole P.O.	Amphotericin B I.V.

Adapted from Goyal BK and Forienza SW, "Approaches to Antifungal Therapy in the 1990s," *Hospital Medicine®*, May 1995, 19.

Adverse Effects of Antifungal Agents

Agent	Side Effect/Toxicity	Monitoring (at least weekly)
Amphotericin B	GI symptoms, headache, chills; anemia, azotemia (up to 80% of cases), renal tubular acidosis, hypokalemia, hypomagnesemia, thrombophlebitis	Complete blood count (CBC), blood urea nitrogen (BUN), serum creatinine, electrolytes, serum magnesium
Fluconazole	GI symptoms, headache; rash (rarely, exfoliative dermatitis, Stevens-Johnson syndrome), asymptomatic elevation of liver enzymes, hepatitis (rare), seizures	Liver enzymes
Flucytosine	GI symptoms, headache, confusion; pancytopenia, neutropenia (more common with abnormal renal function), asymptomatic elevation of liver enzymes, hepatitis (rare)	CBC, BUN, serum creatinine, liver enzymes
Itraconazole	GI symptoms, pruritus, edema, headache, dizziness; rash, hyponatremia, hypokalemia, asymptomatic elevation of liver enzymes, hepatitis (rare)	Serum electrolytes, liver enzymes
Ketoconazole	GI symptoms, headache, fever, chills, pruritus; rash, asymptomatic elevation of liver enzymes, hepatitis, endocrine disturbances	Liver enzymes, serum cortisol levels
Miconazole	GI symptoms, fever, psychosis; pancytopenia, hyperlipidemia, phlebitis, occasional thrombocytosis	CBC, serum cholesterol levels

Adapted from Goyal BK and Forienza SW, "Approaches to Antifungal Therapy in the 1990s," *Hospital Medicine®*, May 1995, 21.

ANTIMICROBIAL AGENTS (PHARMACOKINETICS), ADULTS

Drug	Half-life (h)		V_d (L/kg)	Protein Binding (%)	Time to Peak (h)	Bioavailability (%)
	Normal Renal Function	Impaired Renal Function				
Acyclovir	3	20	0.7-0.8	15-30	P.O.: 1.7	20
Amantadine hydrochloride	10-28	7-10 d	4-5	60-67	1-4	55-90
Amikacin sulfate	1.6-96	17-150	0.22-0.29	<5	I.M.: 0.75-2	
Amoxicillin trihydrate	0.7-1.4	7-21	0.26	15-25	2	85
Amphotericin B	15-48		4	90		
Ampicillin	1-1.8	7-20	0.17-0.31	8-20	I.M.: 1 P.O.: 2	50
Ampicillin/sulbactam	1	5-9		20-40		
Atovaquone	2.9 d			>99.9	1-8	~30
Azithromycin dihydrate	35-40		31.1	7-51	3-4	37
Aztreonam	1.3-2.6	6-8	0.1-0.2	50-60	I.M.: 0.6-1.3	
Capreomycin sulfate	4-6	55			I.M.: 1-2	
Carbenicillin	1.5	10-20	0.12-0.2	30-60	1-3	30-50
Cefaclor	0.5-1	3	0.34-0.35	25	0.5-1	95
Cefadroxil sodium	1-2	20-24	0.31	20	1.2-1.5	95
Cefamandole nafate	0.5-1	3-18	0.16-0.25	75		
Cefazolin sodium	1.5-2.4	40-70	0.13-0.22	80		
Cefixime	3-4	11.5	0.11	65-70	2-6	45
Cefonicid sodium	3.5-4.5	17-56	0.09-0.15	96		
Cefoperazone sodium	1.6-2.5	2.9	0.14-0.2	90		
Cefotaxime sodium	1-1.5	15	0.15-0.55	37		
Cefotetan disodium	3-5	13-25	0.15	85		
Cefoxitin sodium	0.75-1	13-25	0.13-0.39	41-75		
Cefpodoxime proxetil	2-3	9.8	0.46	21-29	1	40-60
Cefprozil	1-2	5.2		36	1-2	95
Ceftazidime	1-2	13-25	0.28	17		
Ceftizoxime sodium	1.6	25	0.26-0.42	28-50		
Ceftriaxone sodium	5-9	12-24	0.12-0.14	85-95		
Cefuroxime	1-2	17	0.13-1.8	33	P.O.: 3	52
Cephalexin monohydrate	0.5-1.2	20-40	0.26	10-15	1	95
Cephalothin sodium	0.5-1	20-40	0.18-0.33	15		
Cephapirin sodium	0.5-1	2.4-2.7	45-60	0.5		
Cephradine	1-2	6-15	0.25-0.33	10	1-2	95
Chloramphenicol	1.6-3.3	3-7	0.8-1.2	50	P.O.: 0.5-3	80
Chloroquine phosphate	3-5 d	5-50 d	800*	50-65	1-2	89
Cinoxacin	1.5	>10	0.24-0.26	60-80	2-3	30-40
Ciprofloxacin hydrochloride	3-5	6-9	2.1	40	P.O.: 0.5-2	70-80
Clarithromycin	3-7	22		65-75	2-4	55
Clindamycin	2-3	3-5	0.6-1.2	60-95	P.O.: 1-3	90
Clofazimine	70 d				1-6	45-62
Cloxacillin sodium	0.5-1.5	1	0.15-0.2	85-94	0.5-2	
Co-trimoxazole SMZ	9	20-50	0.21	68	P.O.: 2-4	90-100
TMP	6-17	20-40	1.2-2	68	P.O.: 1-4	90-100
Cycloserine	10		0.11-0.26		3-4	

(continued)

Drug	Half-life (h)		V_d (L/kg)	Protein Binding (%)	Time to Peak (h)	Bioavailability (%)
	Normal Renal Function	Impaired Renal Function				
Demeclocycline	10-17	40-60	1.79	91	3-6	41-50
Dicloxacillin sodium	0.6-0.8	1-2	0.13-0.19	91-98	0.5-2	80
Didanosine	0.8-2.7		0.7-1	<5	0.5-1	31
Doxycycline	12-15	24	0.75	88-90	P.O.: 1.5-4	90-100
Eflornithine	3.2-3.6		0.3-0.43			50
Enoxacin	3-6	9.4		40	1-2	90
Erythromycin	1.5-2	5-6	0.72	75-90	P.O.: 1-4	Variable
Ethambutol	2.5-3.6	7-15	1.6-2.3	10-30	2-4	75-80
Ethionamide	3		2-8	10	1.8	100
Fluconazole	25-30	<100	0.7-1	11	P.O.: 1-2	<90
Flucytosine	2.5-6	12-250	0.6	2-4	1-2	78-90
Foscarnet	3.3-6.8		0.3-0.7	14-17		
Ganciclovir	1.7-5.8	5-28	0.15-0.31	1-2		
Gentamicin sulfate	1.5-3	36-70	0.23-0.6	<30	0.5-1	
Griseofulvin	9-22				4	25-70
Imipenem/cilastatin imipenem	1	4	0.26	20		
cilastatin	1	17		40	1	
Interferon alfa-2b	2-3				3.8	
Isoniazid fast acetylizers	0.5-1.5		0.6	10-15	1.2	
slow acetylizers	2-5	22-28				
Itraconazole	21		796	99	3-4	
Ivermectin	22-28		46.8	93	3.6	
Kanamycin	2-4	40-96	0.23-0.29	<5	3.6	
Ketoconazole	1.5-3		0.36	99	1-4	37-97
Lomefloxacin	7-8	21-45	1.8-2.5	10	1.5	95-98
Loracarbef	1	≤32		25	1.2	
Mebendazole	1-11.5	35		90-95	2-4	
Mefloquine hydrochloride	21-22		20	98	7-24	85
Methenamine	3-6		0.56		2-8	
Methicillin sodium	0.4-0.5	4	0.43	35-60		
Metronidazole	6-8	21	0.25-0.85	20	P.O.: 1-2	80
Mezlocillin sodium	0.8-1.2	2.6-5.4	0.17-0.2	20-46		
Miconazole	0.8-2.1	20-24	2.1	90		
Minocycline	15	11-23	0.14-0.7	70-75	2-4	
Moxalactam disodium	2-3	18-23	0.18-0.4	35-50		
Nafcillin sodium	0.5-1.5	1.2	0.31-0.38	80-90		
Nalidixic acid	6-7	21	0.25-0.35	90	1-2	90
Neomycin sulfate	2-4	40-96	0.23-0.29	<5	3.6	
Netilmicin sulfate	2-3	24-52	0.6-1.3	<5		
Nitrofurantoin	0.3-0.6	1	0.8	60-90		60
Norfloxacin	4.8	6-9	3.2	10-15	1-2	30-70
Ofloxacin	5-7.5	30	2.4-3.5	20-25	P.O.: 1.2-2	95-100
Oxacillin sodium	0.5-0.7	1-3	0.2	90-93		
Oxamniquine	1-2.5				1-1.5	50
Oxytetracycline	8.5-9.6	47-66	0.9-1.6	35	2-4	

(continued)

Drug	Half-life (h)		V_d (L/kg)	Protein Binding (%)	Time to Peak (h)	Bioavailability (%)
	Normal Renal Function	Impaired Renal Function				
Penicillin G benzathine, parenteral	0.5	6-20	0.2	40-60	12-24	
Penicillin G, parenteral	0.3-0.9	6-20	0.2	40-60		
Penicillin G procaine, aqueous	0.3-0.9	6-20	0.2	40-60	1-4	
Pentamidine isethionate	6.4-9.4†	48	3	69		
Piperacillin sodium	0.5-1.2	3.3-5.1	0.18-0.3	20-40	0.5-0.9	
Polymyxin B	4.6-6				I.M.: <2	
Praziquantel	0.8-1.5			80	1-3	80
Primaquine	3.7-9.6		3.5		<6	
Pyrazinamide	9-10	26	0.57-0.74	10-20	1-2	~100
Pyrimethamine	111		3	87	2	
Quinacrine hydrochloride	5-14 d			80-90	8-12	
Quinidine	6-8		2-3.5	80-90	I.M.: 1	70-80
Quinine sulfate	6-14	6-14	1.2-1.7	70-95	1-1.5	
Ribavirin	24	1-40 d		0	1-1.5	45
Rifabutin	16-69		9.32	85	2-4	20
Rifampin	3-4	1.8-11	1.6	80-90	P.O.: 1.5-4	90
Spectinomycin hydrochloride	1.7	16-29	0.25	5-20	1-2	
Streptomycin sulfate	2-4.7	100	0.26	35	I.M.: 1	
Sulfadiazine	10	34	0.29	45	3-6	
Sulfadoxine	169			90	2.5-6	
Sulfamethoxazole	9-12	20-50	0.15	70	3-4	
Sulfisoxazole	4-7	6-12	0.14-0.28	85-88	2-3	
Tetracycline	6-11	57-108	1.3-1.6	65	2-3 d	
Thiabendazole	1.2				1-2	
Ticarcillin disodium	1.1-1.2	16	0.18-0.21	45-60		
Tobramycin	2.5	27-60	0.22-0.33	<5	I.M.: 0.5-1	
Trimetrexate	15-17		0.62	86-94	1.8	42
Vancomycin hydrochloride	6-8	200-250	0.47-1.25	10		
Vidarabine	1.5		0.7	20-30		
Zalcitabine	1-3	8.5	0.54	<4	1-2	80
Zidovudine	0.8-1.2	1.4	1.4-1.7	30-38	0.5-1.5	66-70

*In plasma.

†Multiphasic elimination.

APOTHECARY-METRIC CONVERSIONS

Exact Equivalents

1 gram (g) = 15.43 grains		0.1 mg = 1/600 gr	
1 milliliter (mL) = 16.23 minims		0.12 mg = 1/500 gr	
1 minim (♏) = 0.06 milliliter		0.15 mg = 1/400 gr	
1 grain (gr) = 64.8 milligrams		0.2 mg = 1/300 gr	
1 ounce (℥) = 31.1 grams		0.3 mg = 1/200 gr	
1 fluid ounce (fl℥) = 29.57 milliliters		0.4 mg = 1/150 gr	
1 pint (pt) = 473.2 milliliters		0.5 mg = 1/120 gr	
1 ounce (oz) = 28.35 grams		0.6 mg = 1/100 gr	
1 pound (lb) = 453.6 grams		0.8 mg = 1/80 gr	
1 kilogram (kg) = 2.2 pounds		1 mg = 1/65 gr	
1 quart (qt) = 946.4 milliliters			

Approximate Equivalents*

Liquids	Solids
1 teaspoonful = 5 mL	¼ grain = 15 mg
1 tablespoonful = 15 mL	½ grain = 30 mg
1 fluid ounce = 30 mL	1 grain = 60 mg
15 minims = 1 mL	1½ grains = 100 mg
	5 grains = 300 mg
	10 grains = 600 mg
	1 ounce = 30 g

*Use exact equivalents for compounding and calculations requiring a high degree of accuracy.

Metric Abbreviations

L = liter	kg = kilogram
mL = milliliter	g = gram
m = meter	mg = milligram
cm = centimeter	μg/mcg = microgram
	ng = nanogram

AVERAGE WEIGHTS AND SURFACE AREAS

Average Weight and Surface Area of Preterm Infants, Term Infants, and Children

Age	Average Weight (kg)*	Approximate Surface Area (m^2)
Weeks Gestation		
26	0.9-1	0.1
30	1.3-1.5	0.12
32	1.6-2	0.15
38	2.9-3	0.2
40 (term infant at birth)	3.1-4	0.25
Months		
3	5	0.29
6	7	0.38
9	8	0.42
Year		
1	10	0.49
2	12	0.55
3	15	0.64
4	17	0.74
5	18	0.76
6	20	0.82
7	23	0.90
8	25	0.95
9	28	1.06
10	33	1.18
11	35	1.23
12	40	1.34
Adult	70	1.73

*Weights from age three months and over are rounded off to the nearest kilogram.

BIOCONCENTRATION FACTORS (BCF)

Extent of bioaccumulation in aquatic organisms, BCF is the ratio of aquatic tissue concentration of a chemical to chemical's concentration in an aquatic environment. (BCF values over 500 are believed to be significant and over 1000 to be highly significant.)

Agent	Approximate BCF
Acetone	<1
Acrolein	0.6-344
Acrylonitrile	30
Alkene hydrocarbon	10
Anthracene	900
Antimony	0.2-390
Aromatic hydrocarbon	20-200
Arsenic	0-350
Benzene	4-24
Benzidine	44-370
2,3-Benzofuran	40-468
Benzo(a)pyrene	4900
Beryllium	19-100
Boron	52-198
Bromoform	2-10
Bromomethane	3
2-Butanone	<1
Cadmium	3-18,000
Carbon disulfide	7-26
Carbon tetrachloride	1-3
Chlordane	200-55,900
Chlordecone	333-60,200
Chlorodibenzofurans	590-7760
Chloroform	6-14
Chromium (VI)	1-192
Cobalt	40-4000
Cresols	14-19
Cumylphenyl diphenylphosphate	1156-2807
Cyanide	2.3
DDT	12,000-39,000
Diazinon	4-337
1,2-Dibromo-3-chloropropane	11
1,4-Dichlorobenzene	370-2455
1,2-Dichloroethane	2
1,2-Dichloroethene	5-23
Diethyl phthalate	117
Di(2-ethylhexyl)phthalate	54-2700
1,3-Dinitrobenzene	74
Dinitrocresol	40
Di-N-octylphthalate	2600-28,500
Disulfoton	100-110
Docosane	10-10,100
Endrin	140-49,000
Endosulfan	23-2755
Ethylbenzene	38
Heptachlor epoxide	851-2330
Hexachlorobutadiene	392
α-Hexachlorocyclohexane	1100
β-Hexachlorocyclohexane	1460
δ-Hexachlorocyclohexane	1770
γ-Hexachlorocyclohexane	63-1613

(continued)

Agent	Approximate BCF
2-Hexanone	7
Lead	42-2570
Long-chain alkane hydrocarbon	100-1500
Manganese	35-40,000
Methoxychlor	113-120,000
Methylene chloride	2.3
Methyl mercaptan	1-2
Methylmercury	6200
Methyl parathion	1-3
Methyl tert-butyl ether	1.5-3
Mirex	3200-40,000
Naphthalene	1.6-3
Nickel	36-259
Nitrobenzene	10-15
4-nitrophenol	30-57
N-nitrosodiphenylamine	217
Nonylphenyl diphenylphosphate	133-691
Pentachlorophenol	13-10,000
Plutonium	10-1000
Polybrominated biphenyls	2-1,445,440
Polychlorinated biphenyls	26,000-660,000
Pyridine	<5
RDX	1.2-6.4
Selenium	150-3975
Silver	4-26
Styrene	13.5-25
tert-Butylphenyl diphenylphosphate	785-1096
1,1,2,2-tetrachloroethane	8-49
Tetrachloroethylene	39-49
Tetryl	15
Thallium	12-1430
Thorium	465
Tin	
inorganic	100-3000
organic	12-11,400
Toluene	4.2-10.7
Toxaphene	4200-60,000
1,1,1-trichloroethane	9
Trichloroethylene	17
2,4,6-Trichlorophenol	30-100
2,4,6-Trinitrotoluene	9.5-338
Triphenyl phosphate	216-573
Uranium	38
Vinyl chloride	5.1
White phosphorus	10-100
Xylene	45-257
Zinc	4-24,000

Data from this table obtained from U.S. Department of Public Health: Toxicological Profile Series (ATSDR) and Smith RP, ed, *A Primer of Environmental Toxicology*, Philadelphia, PA: Lea and Febiger Press, 1992, 243.

BODY SURFACE AREA OF ADULTS AND CHILDREN

Calculating Body Surface Area in Children

In a child of average size, find weight and corresponding surface area on the boxed scale to the left; or, use the nomogram to the right. Lay a straightedge on the correct height and weight points for the child, then read the intersecting point on the surface area scale.

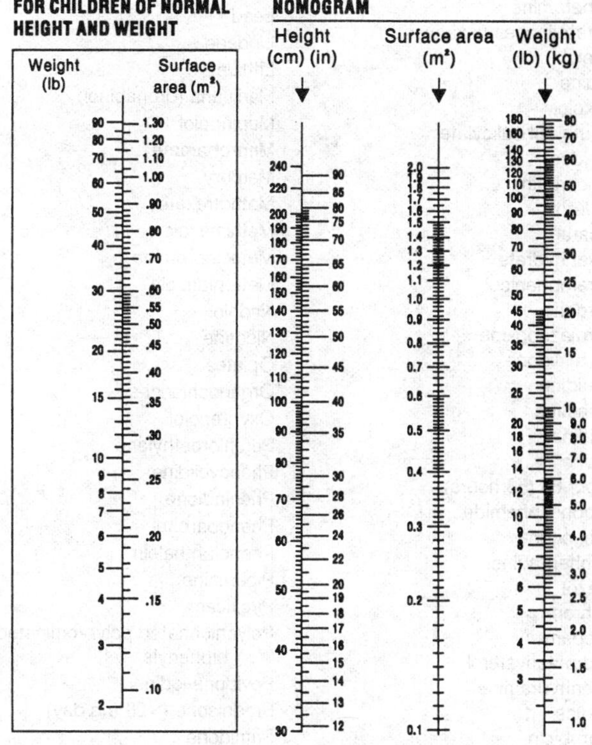

BODY SURFACE AREA FORMULA
(Adult and Pediatric)

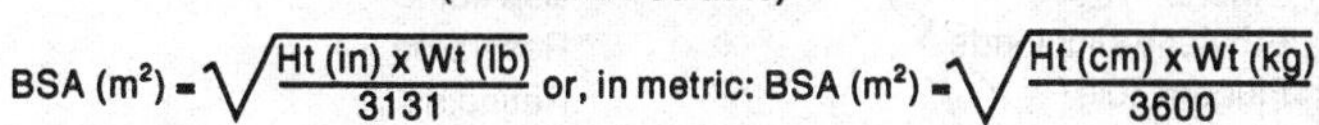

$$BSA\ (m^2) = \sqrt{\frac{Ht\ (in) \times Wt\ (lb)}{3131}}$$ or, in metric: $$BSA\ (m^2) = \sqrt{\frac{Ht\ (cm) \times Wt\ (kg)}{3600}}$$

References:

1. Mosteller RD, "Simplified Calculation of Body Surface Area", *N Engl J Med*, 1987, 317:1098.
2. Lam TK, Leung DT, (Letter to the Editor), *N Engl J Med*, 1988, 318:1130.

BREAST FEEDING

Toxins/Drugs to Be Avoided During Breast Feeding

Acebutolol
Aloe
Alprazolam
Amantadine
5-Aminosalicylic acid
Amiodarone
Amphetamine
Anthroquinones (laxatives)
Atenolol
Atropine
Betaxolol
Bismuth subsalicylate
Bromides
Bromocriptine
Calciferol
Cascara
Chloral hydrate
Chloramphenicol
Chlordane
Chlordiazepoxide
Chlorthalidone
Cimetidine
Clemastine
Clonidine
Cocaine
Copper-64 (50 hours)
Cyclophosphamide
Cyclosporine
Cyproheptadine
Danazol
Danthron
Diazepam
Dihydrotachysterol
Diphenhydramine
Diuretics
Doxorubicin
Dyphylline
Ergotamine
Ethanol
Ethylene dichloride
Fluconazole
Fluorescein
Fluoxetine
Gallium-67 (14 days*)
Gold salts
Guanfacine
Heptachlor
Heroin
Hexachlorobenzene
Hexachlorophene
Hydroxyurea
Indium-111 isotope (20 hours*)
Iodides (especially potassium iodide)
Iodine-123 (36 hours*)
Iodine-125 (12 days*)
Iodine-131 (14 days*)
Isoniazid
Ivermectin
Ketorolac
Lead
Lindane
Lithium
Marijuana (dronabinol)
Mepindolol
Meprobamate
Mercury
Methotrexate
Methimazole
Metoclopramide
Metronidazole
Nadolol
Nicotine
Opiates
Organochlorines
Oxyprenolol
Perchloroethylene
Phencyclidine
Phenindione
Phenobarbital
Phenolphthalein
Piperazine
Piroxicam
Polychlorinated/polybrominated biphenyls
Povidone-iodine
Prednisone (>20 mg/day)
Primidone
Radioactive diagnostic and therapeutic agents
Ranitidine
Reserpine
Retinoids
Salicylate (>1 g)
Sodium isotope (4 days*)
Sotalol
Sulfasalazine
Technetium-99m (1-3 days*)
Tetracycline
Theophylline (sustained release)
Thiouracil
Tilidine
Timolol
Tinidazole
Tocainide

*Duration of radioactivity excretion in breast milk.

CHEMICAL WARFARE (CW) AGENTS

BLISTER AGENTS

Blister agents primarily affect eyes, lungs, and skin. Effects may be immediate or delayed depending on the agent.

Distilled Mustard (HD) — HD is H more purified and has less odor and a slightly greater blistering power than the more impure mustard chemical. It is also more stable in storage.

Chemical name: Bis(2-chloroethyl) sulfide
Formula: $(ClCH_2CH_2)_2S$
CAS: 505-60-2
Combustible: Yes
Appearance: Colorless to yellow, oily liquid
Molecular weight: 159.08
Vapor density (compared with air): 5.4
Liquid density: 1.2685 at 25°C
Boiling point: 217°C calculated; decomposition temperature: 149°C to 177°C
Treatment: See Mustard Gas
Potential for rescuer contamination from exposed patients: High prior to decontamination
Rate of hydrolysis: Half-life: 8.5 minutes in distilled water at 25°C and 60 minutes in salt water at 25°C
Hydrolysis products: Hydrogen chloride and thiodiglycol
Stability in storage: In steel or aluminum containers
Action on metals or other materials: Very little when pure
Odor: Garlic, horseradish, or mustard
Median lethal dosage (MLD_{50}):
Inhalation: 1500 mg/min/m^3
Skin absorption (masked personnel): 10,000 mg/min/m^3
Ocular injury: 200 mg/min/m^3
Dermal absorption (masked personnel): 2000 mg/min/m^3. Wet skin absorbs more mustard than dry skin. For this reason HD exerts a casualty effect at lower concentrations in hot humid weather, since the body is moist with perspiration. The dosage given above for skin absorption applies to temperatures of approximately 21°C to 27°C, as the body would not be perspiring excessively at these temperatures. >27°C, perspiration causes increased skin absorption. The incapacitating dosage drops rapidly as perspiration increases; at 32°C, 1000 mg/min/m^3 could be incapacitating.
Rate of detoxification: Very low. Even very small, repeated exposures are cumulative in their effects or more than cumulative due to sensitization. This has been shown in the postwar case histories of workers in mustard-filling plants. Exposure to vapors from spilled HD causes minor irritative symptoms. Repeated severe exposure to such vapors can produce pulmonary damage.
Clinical effects: Eyes are very susceptible to low concentrations; higher concentrations are required to produce incapacitating effects on skin
Rate of action: Delayed; usually 4-6 hours until first symptoms appear. (Latent periods have been observed, however, up to 24 hours and, in rare cases, up to 12 days.)
Protection required: Protective mask and permeable protective clothing for vapor and small droplets; impermeable clothing for protection against large droplets, splashes, and smears
Persistency: Depends upon munition used and the weather. Heavily splashed liquid persists 1-2 days in concentrations that can cause casualties under average weather conditions, and a week to months under very cold conditions. May persist on trees and plants for weeks.

Comment: Odor threshold: 0.6 mg/m^3. Insoluble in water. Combat zone in World War I air concentrations estimated to be 3-5 ppm.

Ethyldichloroarsine (ED) — It was introduced by the Germans in March 1918 in an effort to produce a volatile agent with a short duration of effectiveness that would be quicker acting than DP or HD and that would be more lasting in its effects than PD.

Chemical name: Ethyldichloroarsine
Formula: $C_2H_5AsCl_2$
Molecular weight: 174.88
Vapor density (compared with air): 6.0
Liquid density: 1.66 at 20°C
Boiling point: 156°C
Decomposition temperature: Stable to boiling point
Rate of hydrolysis: Rapid
Hydrolysis products: Hydrogen chloride and ethylarsenious oxide
Stability in storage: Stable in steel
Action on metals or other materials: None on steel; attacks brass at 50°C; destructive to rubber and plastics
Odor: Fruity, but biting and irritating
Median lethal dosage (MLD_{50}): Inhalation: 3000-5000 mg/min/m^3, depending on the period of exposure. Since ED is detoxified by the body at an appreciable rate, the product of concentration and time is not a constant. As "time" increases, "concentration" does not decrease proportionately. For example, exposure to 40 mg/m^3 for 75 minutes might have an effect similar to that produced by exposure to 30 mg/m^3 for 166 minutes.
Skin absorption: 100,000 mg/min/m^3
Median temporarily incapacitating dosage (ICt_{50}) by inhalation: 5-10 mg/min/m^3
Clinical effects: Dermal and ocular eye toxicity. Vapor is irritating but not harmful to eyes and skin except on prolonged exposure. Liquid ED has approximately one-twentieth the blistering action of liquid lewisite. Irritating effect on nose and throat, is intolerable after 1 minute at moderate concentrations; blistering effect is less delayed than with HD, whose skin effects may be delayed 12 hours or longer.
Protection required: Protective mask and permeable protective clothing for vapor and small droplets; impermeable protective clothing for protection against large droplets, splashes, and smears
Persistency: Short

Lewisite (L)

Chemical name: Dichloro(2-chlorovinyl)arsine
Formula: ClCH:CHAsCl$_2$
CAS: 541-25-3
Molecular weight: 207.35
Vapor density (compared with air): 7.1
Liquid density: 1.89 at 20°C
Boiling point: 190°C
Decomposition temperature: >100°C
Treatment: See Arsine
- Dermal: Topical dimercaprol application may be helpful; irrigate with water
- Ocular: Application of dimercaprol (<20% concentration) to the eye within 1 hour of exposure may be helpful

Potential for rescuer contamination from exposed patients: High prior to decontamination
Rate of hydrolysis: Rapid for vapor and dissolved lewisite; low solubility in water limits hydrolysis
Hydrolysis products: Hydrogen chloride and chlorovinylarsenious oxide. The latter is a nonvolatile blister-forming solid not readily

washed away by water. Alkaline hydrolysis destroys these blister-forming properties.

Stability in storage: Stable in steel or glass container

Action on metals or other materials: None if L is dry

Odor: Very little when pure; fruity or geranium odor; usually a liquid

Median lethal dosage (MLD_{50}):

Inhalation: 1200-1500 mg/min/m^3

Dermal: 100,000 mg/min/m^3

Median incapacitating dosage:

Ocular: <300 mg/min/m^3

Dermal: >1500 mg/min/m^3

Lowest lethal dermal dose: 38 mg/kg (as little as 2 mL on skin can be lethal)

Dermal absorption (masked personnel): 100,000 mg/min/m^3. When the humidity is high, it hydrolyzes rapidly and it is difficult to maintain a concentration sufficient to blister bare skin. This difficulty is still further increased by the high vapor pressure and short duration of effectiveness of lewisite.

Median incapacitating dosage (ICt_{50}):

Ocular injury: <300 mg/min/m^3

Dermal absorption (masked personnel): >1500 mg/min/m^3

Lewisite irritates the eyes and skin and gives warning of its presence.

Clinical effects: Mainly dermal and ocular toxicity. An exposure of 1500 mg/min/m^3 produces severe corneal damage to the eyes. It has the same blistering action on the skin as HD, even though the lethal dosage for lewisite is much higher.

Rate of action: Rapid; immediate erythema followed by blister formation in 2-3 hours

Protection required: Protective mask and permeable protective clothing for vapor and small droplets; impermeable clothing for protection against large droplets, splashes, and smears

Persistency: Somewhat shorter than for HD. Very short duration under humid conditions

Mustard-Lewisite Mixture (HL) — A variable of HD and lewisite which provides a low-freezing mixture for use in cold weather operations or as high-altitude spray. Properties are listed for the eutectic mixture (the mixture having the lowest possible freezing point), which is 63% lewisite and 37% HD by weight. Other mixtures, such as 50-50, may be prepared to meet predetermined weather conditions and have advantages over the eutectic mixture because of the increased HD content.

Appearance: Dark, oily liquid

Molecular weight: 186.4 (calculated on basis of eutectic mixture 63% L and 37% HD)

Vapor density (compared with air): 6.5

Liquid density: Between the densities of the components; approximately 1.66 at 20°C

Boiling point: Indefinite, but <190°C

Decomposition temperature: >100°C

Rate of hydrolysis: Lewisite is rapidly hydrolyzed in the liquid or vapor state; HD hydrolyzes slowly at ordinary temperatures

Hydrolysis products: Hydrogen chloride, thiodiglycol, and chlorovinylarsenious oxide. Alkaline hydrolysis destroys the blistering properties.

Stability in storage: Stable in lacquered steel containers

Action on metals or other materials: Little or none if dry

Median lethal dosage (MLD_{50}):

Ocular injury: About 200 mg/min/m^3

Dermal absorption: 1500-2000 mg/min/m^3

Odor: Garlic

Clinical effects: Dermal and ocular toxicity are very high. Produces immediate burning and irritation of skin and erythema within 30 minutes; blistering delayed about 13 hours.
Protection required: Protective mask and permeable protective clothing for vapor and small droplets; impermeable protective clothing for protection against large droplets, splashes, and smears
Persistency: Depends on munitions used and the weather. Somewhat shorter than that of HD, whose heavily splashed liquid persists 1-2 days under average weather conditions and a week or more under very cold conditions.

Mustard-T Mixture (HT) — A mixture of 60% HD and 40% T, sulfur and chlorine compound similar in structure to HD. It is a clear yellowish liquid with an odor similar to that of HD. HT has a strong blistering effect, has a longer duration of effectiveness, is more stable, and has a lower freezing point than HD. Its low volatility makes effective vapor concentrations in the field difficult to obtain. Properties are essentially the same as those of HD.
Treatment: See Mustard Gas
Clinical effects: Causes blisters, irritates the eyes, and is toxic when inhaled
Protection required: Protective mask and permeable protective clothing for vapor and small droplets; impermeable clothing for protection against large droplets, splashes, and smears
Personnel decontamination: Bleach; remove clothing
Persistency: Depends on munitions used and the weather. Somewhat longer than duration of effectiveness of HD, whose heavily splashed liquid persists 1-2 days under average weather conditions, and a week or more under very cold conditions.

Nitrogen Mustard (HN-1)
Chemical name: 2,2-Dichlorotriethylamine
Formula: $(ClCH_2CH_2)_2NC_2H_5$
CAS: 538-07-8
Flammable: Very slightly
Molecular weight: 170.08
Vapor density (compared with air): 5.9
Liquid density: 1.09 at 25°C
Decomposition temperature: Decomposes before boiling point is reached
Treatment: See Mustard Gas
Potential for rescuer contamination from exposed patients: High prior to decontamination
Rate of hydrolysis: Slow due to low solubility in water
Hydrolysis products: Hydroxyl derivatives and condensation products. (Intermediate products, all of which are toxic, are produced during hydrolysis.)
Stability in storage: Polymerizes slowly and stable enough for munition use
Action on metals or other materials: Slight corrosion of steel at 65°C
Odor: Faint fishy or musty odor; may not have an odor
Median lethal dosage (MLD_{50}):
Inhalation: 1500 mg/min/m^3
Skin absorption (masked personnel): 20,000 mg/min/m^3
Median incapacitating dosage (ICt_{50}): Ocular injury: 200 mg/min/m^3
Dermal absorption (masked personnel): 9000 mg/min/m^3
Rate of detoxification: Not detoxified; cumulative
Clinical effects: Eye are susceptible to low concentration; higher concentrations are required to produce incapacitating effects by skin absorption. Toxicity may be delayed 12 hours or longer.
Protection required: Protective mask and permeable protective clothing for vapor and small droplets; impermeable clothing for protection against large droplets, splashes, and smears.

Persistency: Depends on munitions used and the weather. Somewhat shorter than duration of effectiveness for HD, whose heavily splashed liquid persists 1-2 days under average weather conditions, and a week or more under very cold conditions.

Nitrogen Mustard (HN-2) — Highly unstable and is no longer seriously considered for use as a military chemical agent. It is more toxic than HN-1.

Chemical name: 2,2′-Dichloro-N-methyldiethylamine
Formula: $(ClCH_2CH_2)_2NCH_3$
CAS: 51-75-2
Appearance: Dark liquid
Molecular weight: 156.07
Vapor density (compared with air): 5.9
Liquid density: 1.15 at 20°C
Boiling point: 75°C at 15 mm Hg; at atmospheric pressure, HN-2 decomposes below boiling point
Decomposition temperature: Decomposes before boiling point is reached. Instability of HN-2 is associated with its tendency to polymerize or condense; the reactions involved could generate enough heat to cause an explosion.
Treatment: See Mustard Gas
Potential for rescuer contamination from exposed patients: Rescuer decontamination will probably need to be performed if rescuers are exposed prior to initial decontamination
Rate of hydrolysis: Hydrolysis is slow except where alkali is present; dimerizes rapidly in water
Hydrolysis products: Complex condensates or polymers
Stability in storage: Not stable
Action on metals or other materials: None
Odor: In dilute form like soft soap; in high concentrations fruity
Median lethal dosage (MLD_{50}) (by inhalation): 3000 mg/min/m^3
Median incapacitating dosage (ICt_{50}):
Ocular injury: 100 mg/min/m^3
Dermal absorption (masked personnel): Somewhere between the values given for HN-1 and HN-3
Rate of detoxification: Not detoxified
Clinical effects: Dermal and ocular toxicity mainly. HN-2 has the greatest blistering power of the nitrogen mustards in vapor form, but is intermediate as a liquid blistering agent. Toxic eye effects are produced more rapidly than HD. Skin effects may be delayed 12 hours or longer.
Protection required: Protective mask and permeable protective clothing for vapor and small droplets; impermeable clothing for protection against large droplets, splashes, and smears.
Persistency: Depends on munitions used and the weather. Somewhat shorter than duration of effectiveness for HD, whose heavily splashed liquid persists 1-2 days under average weather conditions, and a week or more under very cold conditions.

Nitrogen Mustard (HN-3) — The most stable in storage of the three nitrogen mustards

Chemical name: 2,2′2″-trichlorotriethylamine
Formula: $N(CH_2CH_2Cl)_3$
CAS: 555-77-1
Molecular weight: 204.54
Vapor density (compared with air): 7.1
Liquid density: 1.24 at 25°C
Boiling point: 256°C calculated, decomposes; at atmospheric pressure, HN-3 decomposes below boiling point
Decomposition temperature: Decomposes before boiling point is reached; relatively high
Personnel decontamination: See Distilled Mustard

Treatment: See Mustard Gas
Rate of hydrolysis: Very slow due to low solubility in water
Hydrolysis products: $N(CH_2CH_2OH)_3$ and hydrogen chloride in dilute solutions. Dimer formation in higher concentrations.
Stability in storage: Stable enough for use as a munition even under tropical conditions. However, the agent darkens and deposits a crystalline solid in storage.
Action on metals or other materials: None if HN-3 is dry
Odor: None when pure
Median lethal dosage (MLD_{50}):
Inhalation: 1500 mg/min/m^3
Dermal absorption (masked personnel): 10,000 mg/min/m^3
Median incapacitating dosage (ICt_{50}):
Ocular injury: 200 mg/min/m^3
Dermal absorption (masked personnel): 2500 mg/min/m^3
This information is based on estimates and indicates that HN-3 closely approaches HD in vapor toxicity and that it is the most toxic of the nitrogen mustards.
Rate of detoxification: Not detoxified; cumulative
Rate of action: Most symptoms are delayed 4-6 hours (as after exposure to HD) but, in some cases, lacrimation, eye irritation, and photophobia develop immediately
Protection required: Protective mask and permeable protective clothing for vapor and small droplets; impermeable clothing for protection against large droplets, splashes, and smears
Persistency: Considerably longer than for HD (see HD)

Phenyldichloroarsine (PD) — Although phenyldichloroarsine is classed as a blister agent, it also acts as a vomiting or lacrimator compound.

Chemical name: Phenyldichloroarsine
Formula: $C_6H_5AsCl_2$
CAS: 696-28-6
UN/DOT: 1556
Molecular weight: 222.91
Vapor density (compared with air): 7.7
Liquid density: 1.65 at 20°C
Boiling point: 252°C to 255°C
Decomposition temperature: Stable to boiling point
Rate of hydrolysis: Rapid
Hydrolysis products: Hydrogen chloride and phenylarsenious oxide
Stability in storage: Very stable
Action on metals or other materials: None
Odor: None
Median concentration detectable (by nasal and throat irritation): 0.9 mg/m^3
Median lethal dosage (MLD_{50}) (by inhalation): 2600 mg/min/m^3
Median incapacitating dosage (ICt_{50}): 16 mg/min/m^3 as a vomiting agent; 1800 mg/min/m^3 as a blistering agent
Rate of detoxification: No specific information, but like related arsenicals, PD is probably rapidly detoxified in sublethal dosages
Clinical effects: Dermal and ocular toxicity: About 30% as toxic to the eyes as HD; that is 633 mg/min/m^3 would produce casualties by eye injury. On bare skin PD is about 90% as blistering as HD, but is decomposed immediately by wet clothing. Immediate effect on eyes; effects on skin delayed 30 minutes to 1 hour.
Protection required: Protective mask and permeable protective clothing for vapor and small droplets; impermeable protective clothing for protection against large droplets, splashes, and smears
Persistency: Depends on munitions used and the weather. Somewhat shorter than that of HD under dry conditions; short duration when wet. (Heavily splashed liquid HD persists 1-2 days under average weather conditions, and a week or more under very cold conditions.)

Phosgene Oxime (CX) — It may appear as a colorless, low-melting point (crystalline) solid or as a liquid. It has a high vapor pressure.

Chemical name: Dichloroformoxine; phosgene oximedichloroforoximine
Formula: CCl_2NOH
Vapor density as compared to air: 3.9
Boiling point: 53°C to 54°C at 28 mm Hg
Melting point: 35°C to 40°C, and is readily soluble in water
Decomposition temperature: Slowly decomposes at normal temperatures (depending on temperature and humidity)
Treatment: See Phosgene
Potential for rescuer contamination from exposed patients: High possibility prior to decontamination
Odor: It has a disagreeable odor
Median lethal dosage: 3200 mg/min/m^3
Clinical effects: CS is a powerful irritant which produces immediate pain varying from a mild irritancy sensation to severe local pain. Severe irritation of the mucous membranes. When CX comes in contact with the skin, the area becomes blanched in 30 seconds and is surrounded by erythema. A wheal forms in about 30 minutes and the blanched area turns brown in about 24 hours, scab formation in a week. The scab generally falls off in about 3 weeks. Itching may be present throughout healing which, in some cases, may be delayed beyond 2 months.
Protection required: A proper fitting protective mask protects the respiratory system; the remainder of the body can be protected by a complete set of protective clothing
Decontaminants: Because of the rapid reaction of CX with the skin, decontamination will not be entirely effective after pain occurs. Remove contaminated clothing. Nevertheless, decontamination should be accomplished as rapidly as possible by flushing the area with large amounts of water to remove any agent that has not reacted with the skin. Sodium bicarbonate dressings may be helpful.
Persistency: Not persistent; hydrolyzed rapidly in alkaline solutions

BLOOD AGENTS

Arsine (SA)

Chemical name: Arsenic trihydride; arsine; hydrogen arsenide
Formula: AsH_3
CAS: 7784-42-1
UN/DOT: 2188
Appearance: Colorless gas
Flammable: Yes
Molecular weight: 77.93
Vapor density (compared with air): 2.69
Liquid density: 1.34 at 20°C
Boiling point: 62.5°C
Decomposition temperature: 280°C
Treatment: See Arsine
Potential for rescuer exposure solely from treating exposed patient: None
Rate of hydrolysis: Rapid, but an equilibrium condition is reached quickly. (Under certain conditions, SA forms a solid product with water which decomposes at 30°C.)
Hydrolysis products: Arsenic acids and hydride
Stability in storage: Not stable in uncoated metal containers. Metals catalyze decomposition of arsine.
Action on metals or other materials: Reacts slowly with copper, brass, and nickel. May also be decomposed by contact with other metals.
Odor: Mild garlic-like odor
Median lethal dosage (MLD_{50}): 5000 mg/min/m^3. It is estimated that 2 mg of SA per kilogram of body weight would be lethal to a human.
Median incapacitating dosage (ICt_{50}): 2500 mg/min/m^3
Rate of detoxification: Not rapid enough to be of importance
Toxic effects: Rapid red blood cell hemolysis with potential subsequent renal failure and other target organ failure; one of the most potent hemolytic toxins
Rate of action: Effects are delayed from 2 hours to as much as 11 days

Cyanogen Bromide

Chemical name: Bromine cyanide
CAS: 506-68-3
UN/DOT: 1889
Appearance: Colorless needles
Molecular weight: 105.93
Density as compared to air: 2.02
Melting point: 52°C
Boiling point: 61.6°C
Odor: Bitter almonds
Potential for rescuer contamination from exposed patients: High before initial decontamination; low after decontamination
Lethal concentration (10 minutes): 92 ppm
Clinical effects: Similar to cyanide; also is a pulmonary irritant
Persistency: Does not concentrate in soil or food chain

Cyanogen Chloride (CK)

Chemical name: Cyanogen chloride
Formula: CNCl
CAS: 506-77-4
UN/DOT: 1589
Appearance: Colorless liquid or gas
Flammable: Yes
Molecular weight: 61.48
Vapor density (compared with air): 1.98

Liquid density: 1.18 at 20°C
Melting point: -6.5°C
Boiling point: 13.1°C
Decomposition temperature: >100°C
Treatment: See Cyanide
Potential for rescuer contamination from exposed patients: High before initial decontamination; low after decontamination
Rate of hydrolysis: Very low
Hydrolysis products: HCl and CNOH
Stability in storage: Stable at 65°C for 30 days. Tends to undergo condensation or polymerization in storage to form the solid compound 2,4,6-trichloro-*s*-triazine, $C_3N_3Cl_3$ (cyclic). Impurities promote polymerization which may occur with explosive violence.
Action on metals or other materials: None if CK is dry
Odor: Its irritating and lacrimatory properties are so great that the odor can go unnoticed
Median concentration detectable (lacrimatory effect): 12 mg/m^3
Median lethal dosage (MLD_{50}): 11,000 $mg/min/m^3$
Median incapacitating dosage (ICt_{50}): 7000 $mg/min/m^3$
Rate of detoxification: 0.02-0.1 mg/kg/min
Clinical effects: It is assumed that the effect of CK arises from its conversion to cyanide in the body. In general, CK may be considered a rapid-acting chemical agent with clinical toxic effects like cyanide.
Protection required: Protective mask. CK will break or penetrate a protective mask canister or filter element more readily than most other agents. A very high concentration may overpower the filter; high dosages will break down its protective ability.
Persistency: Short; vapor may persist in jungle and forest for some time under suitable weather conditions. Does not concentrate in food chain. Contaminated water can be treated with ozone, hydrogen peroxide, calcium, or sodium hypochlorite bleach.

Hydrogen Cyanide

Chemical name: Hydrogen cyanide or hydrocyanic acid
Formula: HCN
CAS: 74-90-8
UN/DOT: 1613, 1614
Appearance: Bluish white liquid
Flammable: Yes
Explosive: Yes
Molecular weight: 27.02
Vapor density (compared with air): 0.932
Liquid density: 0.687
Melting point: -13.2°C
Boiling point: 25.7°C
Decomposition temperature: >65.5°C (Forms explosive polymer on standing. Stabilized material can be stored up to 65°C.)
Treatment: See Cyanide
Potential for rescuer contamination from exposed patients: High before initial decontamination; low after decontamination
Rate of hydrolysis: Low under field conditions
Stability in storage: Unstable except when very pure. May form explosive polymer on long standing. Can be stabilized by addition of small amounts of phosphoric acid or sulfur dioxide. Reacts violently with acetaldehyde.
Action on metals or other materials: Little or none
Odor: Similar to bitter almonds
Clinical effects: Binds to cytochrome oxidase enzyme system and interferes with cellular respiration. Produces seizures, metabolic acidosis, hypotension, cardiovascular collapse, respiratory failure.
Median lethal dosage (MLD_{50}): Median lethal dosage varies widely with concentration because of the rather high rate at which AC is

detoxified by the body. For example, at 200 mg/m^3 concentration, the lethal dosage is approximately 2000 mg/min/m^3, whereas at 150 mg/m^3 the lethal dosage is approximately 4500 mg/min/m^3.

Median incapacitating dosage (ICt_{50}): Varies with the concentration

Dermal effects: Dermatitis

Rate of action: Very rapid; death occurs within 15 minutes after a lethal dosage has been received

Protection required: Protective mask and protective clothing

Persistency: Short; the agent is highly volatile, and in the gaseous state it dissipates quickly in the air. Does not accumulate in soil or food chain. Contaminated water can be treated with hydrogen peroxide, calcium, or sodium hypochlorite bleach.

CHOKING AGENTS

Diphosgene (DP)

Chemical name: Perchloromethyl formate

CAS: 503-38-8

UN: 1076

Molecular weight: 198

State at 20°C: Colorless liquid

Odor: New-mown hay

Vapor density as compared to air: 6.8

Liquid density at 20°C: 1.65 g/mL

Freezing point: -57°C

Treatment: See Phosgene

Median lethal dosage: 3200 mg/min/m^3

Median incapacitating dosage: 1600 mg/min/m^3

Rate of detoxification: Cumulative

Stability: Tends to convert to phosgene (unstable)

Clinical effect: Slight lacrimation; lung irritant within 12-24 hours

Field decontamination: Potential exists for rescuer contamination in treating exposed patients prior to initial decontamination

Persistency: Not persistent; decomposes easily

Phosgene (CG)

Chemical name: Carbonyl chloride

CAS: 75-44-5

UN: 1076

Molecular weight: 99

State at 20°C: Colorless gas

Odor: New-mown hay

Vapor density as compared to air: 3.4

Liquid density at 20°C: 1.37 g/mL

Freezing point: -128°C

Treatment: See Phosgene

Median lethal dosage: 3200 mg/min/m^3

Median incapacitating dosage: 1600 mg/min/m^3

Rate of detoxification: Cumulative

Clinical effect: Lung irritant within 3 hours

Field decontamination: None needed; potential for rescuer contamination is low

Persistency: Not persistent; decomposes easily to form hydrochloric acid and carbon monoxide in the presence of water

LACRIMATORS

These agents cause increased lacrimation and irritation of the skin. Since tear compounds produce only transient casualties, they are widely used for riot control, and for situations where long-term incapacitation is unacceptable. When released indoors, they can cause serious illness or death.

Bromobenzylcyanide (CA)

Chemical name: Bromobenzylcyanide; bromobenzylnitrile
Formula: $C_6H_5Ch(Br)CN$
CAS: 5748-79-8
UN/DOT: 1694
Appearance: Yellowish/white crystals or brown oily liquid
Molecular weight: 196.0
Vapor density (compared with air): 6.7
Liquid density: 1.47 at 20°C
Boiling point: 242°C, but with decomposition
Decomposition temperature: Decomposes slowly at 60°C; more rapidly as the temperature increases. Decomposes completely at 242°C. Hydrobromic acid and dicyanostilbene are formed.
Treatment: Remove to fresh air
Rate of hydrolysis: Very slow
Hydrolysis products: Complex condensation products
Stability in storage: Fairly stable in glass, leadlined, or enamelled containers
Action on metals or other materials: Vigorous corrosive action on all common metals except lead. Reaction with iron may be explosive.
Odor: Like soured fruit, but not unpleasant
Median lethal dosage (MLD_{50}): Estimated 8000-11,000 mg/min/m^3. Volatility is too low to permit attaining a lethal dosage in the field. Lethal dosage may be obtained in enclosed places.
Median incapacitating dosage (ICt_{50}): About 30 mg/min/m^3
Rate of detoxification: Rapidly detoxified at the low concentrations ordinarily encountered
Clinical effects: Dermal and ocular irritation
Rate of action: Instantaneous
Protection required: Protective mask
Persistency: Depends on munitions used and the weather. Heavily splashed liquid persists 1-2 days under average weather conditions.

Chloroacetophenone (CN)

Chemical name: Alpha-chloroacetophenone
Formula: $C_6H_5COCH_2Cl$
CAS: 532-27-4
UN/DOT: 1697
Appearance: Colorless to white vapor; clear to yellow-brown solid
Molecular weight: 154.59
Vapor density (compared with air): 5.3
Liquid density: 1.187 at 58°C
Boiling point: 248°C
Decomposition temperature: Stable to boiling point
Treatment: Remove patient to fresh air; give 100% humidified oxygen
Potential for rescuer contamination from exposed patients: High prior to decontamination
Rate of hydrolysis: Not readily hydrolyzed
Hydrolysis products: Hydrogen chloride and a hydroxyacetophenone
Stability in storage: Stable
Action on metals or other materials: Tarnishes steel slightly
Odor: Fragrant; similar to that of apple blossoms
Median lethal dosage (MLD_{50}):
7000 mg/min/m^3, dispersed from solvent
14,000 mg/min/m^3 dispersed from thermal grenade

Median incapacitating dosage (ICt_{50}): 80 mg/min/m^3
Rate of detoxification: Rapid; effects disappear in minutes. High concentrations may cause skin irritation which usually disappears within a few hours.
Clinical effects: Dermal and ocular toxicity. Irritating; not toxic in concentrations likely to be encountered in the field. Rapidly acting. Allergic contact dermatitis may occur.
Protection required: Protective mask
Persistency: Short, because the compounds are disseminated as an aerosol

CNB — It was adopted in 1920 and remained in use until it was replaced by CNS. The advantage claimed for CNB was that its lower chloroacetophenone content made it more satisfactory than CNS for training purposes. Actually, the same result can be obtained with CNC merely by using a lower concentration.

Chemical name: None; solution of chloroacetophenone in benzene and carbon tetrachloride
Formula:
CN: $C_6H_5COCH_2Cl$ (10 parts by weight)
Carbon tetrachloride: CCl_4 (45 parts by weight)
Benzene: C_6H_5 (45 parts by weight)
Molecular weight: 119.7 (on basis of components)
Vapor density (compared with air): Approximately 4
Liquid density: 1.14 at 20°C
Boiling point: Varies from 75°C to 247°C as the two solvents are vaporized
Decomposition temperature: $>$247°C
Rate of hydrolysis: None
Hydrolysis products: None
Stability in storage: Adequate
Action on metals or other materials: Very slight
Odor: Like benzene
Median lethal dosage (MLD_{50}): No specific data, but about the same as for CN (11,000 mg/min/m^3)
Median incapacitating dosage (ICt_{50}): 80 mg/min/m^3
Rate of detoxification: Rapid, if poisonous amounts of solvents have been inhaled
Clinical effects: Dermal and ocular toxicity; not toxic; instantaneous acting
Protection required: Protective mask
Persistency: Short

CNC

Chemical name: None; solution of chloroacetophenone in chloroform
Formula: Chloroform: $CHCl_3$ (70 parts by weight); CN: $C_6H_5COCH_2Cl$ (30 parts by weight)
Molecular weight: 128.17 (on basis of components)
Vapor density (compared with air): 4.4
Liquid density: 1.40 at 20°C
Boiling point: Variable. Increases as chloroform boils off and approaches the boiling point of pure CN (60°C to 247°C).
Volatility: This is an indeterminate value under field conditions because the vapor pressure of chloroform is high and the vapor pressure of CN is low. Therefore, there is no true volatility as in the case of a pure compound.
Decomposition temperature: Stable to the boiling point
Rate of hydrolysis: Not readily hydrolyzed
Hydrolysis products: Hydrogen chloride and a hydroxyacetophenone
Stability in storage: Adequate
Action on metals or other materials: Slight
Odor: Similar to that of chloroform

Median lethal dosage (MLD_{50}): The active ingredient is CN; therefore, with allowance for the diluting action of the chloroform vapor, the median lethal dosage would be similar to that of CN, about 11,000 mg/min/m^3
Median incapacitating dosage (ICt_{50}): About 80 mg/min/m^3
Rate of detoxification: Rapid for sublethal exposure
Clinical effects: Dermal and ocular toxicity. Irritating; instantaneous acting.
Protection required: Protective mask
Persistency: Short, because the compound is disseminated as an aerosol

CNS

Chemical name: None; mixture of chloroacetophenone, chloropicrin, and chloroform
Formula:
CN: $C_6H_5COCH_2Cl$ (23%)
Chloropicrin (PS): $C(NO_2)Cl_3$ (38.4%)
Chloroform: $CHCl_3$ (38.4%)
Molecular weight: 141.78 (on basis of components)
Vapor density (compared with air): About 5.0
Liquid density: 1.47 at 20°C
Boiling point: No fixed temperature; varies from 60°C to 247°C
Decomposition temperature: Stable to boiling point
Rate of hydrolysis: Not readily hydrolyzed
Hydrolysis products: Hydrogen chloride and a hydroxyacetophenone
Stability in storage: Stable
Action on metals or other materials: Very little
Odor: Like flypaper
Median lethal dosage (MLD_{50}): 11,400 mg/min/m^3
Median incapacitating dosage (ICt_{50}): 60 mg/min/m^3
Dermal and ocular toxicity: Irritating; not toxic
Rate of action: Instantaneous
Clinical effects: In addition to having effects described under CN, CNS also has the effects of chloropicrin (PS), which acts as a vomiting compound, a choking agent, and a tear compound. CNS may cause lung effects similar to those of CG and also may cause nausea, vomiting, colic, and diarrhea which may persist for weeks. The lacrimatory effects of PS are much less marked than those of CN and are relatively unimportant for CNS, as shown by the fact that these effects are no greater than with CNC, which contains no PS. Effects of CNS my be prolonged for weeks.
Protection required: Protective mask
Persistency: Short

O-chlorobenzylidene Malononitrile (CS) — For riot control CS exists as a family of three forms: CS, CS1, and CS2. CS identifies the white crystalline form. It has a minimum purity of 96%; it is insoluble in water and ethanol, but is soluble in methylene chloride. CS is thermally dispersed as a solid aerosol. CS1 is a mixture consisting of 95% crystalline CS blended with 5% silica aerogel to reduce agglomeration, and micropulverized to 3- to 10-micron size to achieve the desired respiratory effects when dispersed as a solid aerosol. CS2 is CS containing a hydrophoric compound, Cab-O-sil, which improves the physical characteristics of CS by reducing agglomeration and hydrolysis.

Chemical name: O-chlorobenzylidene malononitrile
Formula: $ClC_6H_4CHO(CN)_2$
CAS: 2698-41-1
Appearance: White crystals; gas is white
Molecular weight: 188.5
Density: 1.04 g/mL crystalline density; 0.24-0.26 g/mL bulk density
Boiling point: 310°C to 315°C (with decomposition)

Decomposition temperature: Unknown
Treatment: Intact skin decontamination with 5% to 10% sodium bicarbonate solution. Copious irrigation with cold water (at least 2 L) should be used for skin exposure. Saline can be used for nonintact skin. Irrigate eyes copiously with water.
Potential for rescuer contamination from exposed patients: High prior to decontamination
Rate of hydrolysis: Rapid for dissolved CS. CS is only slightly soluble in water (about 0.008 weight percent at 25°C); thus solid CS in water is hydrolyzed relatively slowly.
Hydrolysis products: O-chlorobenzaldehyde and malononitrile
Stability in storage: Stable
Action on metals: Very slight action on steel
Odor: Pepper-like
Median lethal dosage (MLD_{50}): 61,000 mg/min/m^3 (M7A3 grenade)
Median incapacitating dosage (ICt_{50}): 10-20 mg/min/m^3
Rate of detoxification: Quite rapid. Incapacitating dosages lose their effects in 5-10 minutes.
Clinical effects: Highly irritating
Rate of action: Very rapid
Protection required: Protection is provided by the protective mask and ordinary field clothing secured at the neck, wrist, and ankles. Personnel handling CS should wear rubber gloves for additional protection.
Persistency: Varies, depending upon amount of contamination. Water half-life is 15 minutes at 25°C.

NERVE AGENTS

GF

Chemical name: Cyclohexyl methylphosphonofluoridate
CAS: 329-99-7
Appearance: Liquid
Volatility: Low
Molecular weight: 180
Odor: Sweet, musty, peaches
Vapor density as compared to air: 6.2
Liquid density at 20°C: 1.13
Freezing point: -30°C
Boiling point: 239°C
Vapor pressure at 20°C: 0.044
Flash point: 94°C
Treatment: See Nerve Agents
Decontamination: Irrigate dermally with diluted bleach or alkali

Sarin (GB) — A colorless liquid; vapor is colorless
Chemical name: Isopropyl methyl phosphonofluoridate
Formula: Molecular — $CH_3P(O)(F)OCH(CH_3)_2$
CAS: 107-44-8
Molecular weight: 140.10
Vapor density (compared with air): 4.86
Liquid density: 1.0887 at 25°C
Boiling point: 158°C
Decomposition temperature: Complete decomposition after 2.5 hours at 150°C
Treatment: See Nerve Gas
Potential for rescuer contamination from exposed patients: See Tabun
Rate of hydrolysis: Variable with pH. Half-life: 7.5 hours at pH 1.8; 30 hours in unbuffered solution. Rapidly hydrolyzed in alkaline solutions.
Hydrolysis products: Hydrofluoric acid under acid conditions; **isopropyl alcohol and polymers under alkaline conditions**

Stability in storage: Fairly stable in steel containers at 65°C. Stability improves with increasing purity.
Action on metals or other materials: Slightly corrosive on steel
Odor: Almost none in pure state; can have a faint sweetish odor
Median lethal dosage (LCt_{50}) (respiratory):
70-100 mg/min/m^3 for resting men
35 mg/min/m^3 for men engaged in mild activity
Median incapacitating dosage (ICt_{50}):
75 mg/min/m^3 for resting men
35 mg/min/m^3 for men engaged in mild activity
Rate of detoxification: Low detoxification rate; cumulative
Clinical effects: Very high toxicity and rapidly acting toxin; much greater through eye than through skin. Vapor causes miosis and decreased vision. Irreversible inhibition of acetylcholinesterase.
Dermal effect: LD_{50} is 1.7 g/person. Liquid does not injure skin but penetrates it rapidly. Immediate decontamination of the smallest drop is essential. Vapor penetrates skin also. Skin MLD_{50} of vapor is approximately 12,000 mg/min/m^3 for naked man, and 15,000 mg/min/m^3 for man in ordinary combat clothing. Median incapacitating dosage from vapor skin is approximately 8000 mg/min/m^3 with ordinary clothing.
Long-term neurotoxic effects: Possible central nervous system and peripheral nerve damage
Persistency: Evaporates at approximately the same rate as water; depends upon munitions used and the weather (30 minutes at 15°C; 8 hours at -10°C)
Comment: 12 tons can kill 9 million individuals (entire population of Sweden). Very soluble in water.

Soman (GD) — A colorless liquid which gives off a colorless vapor
Chemical name: Pinacolyl methyl phosphonofluoridate
Formula: $CH_3P(O)(F)OCH(CH_3)$
CAS: 96-64-0; 68190-07-8
Molecular weight: 182.178
Vapor density (compared with air): 6.33
Liquid density: 1.0222 at 25°C
Boiling point: 198°C
Decomposition temperature: Unstabilized: Decomposes in 4 hours at 130°C. Stabilized: Decomposes in 200 hours at 130°C.
Treatment: See Nerve Gas
Personnel decontamination: See Tabun
Potential for rescuer contamination from exposed patients: See Tabun
Rate of hydrolysis: Varies with pH; complete in 5 minutes in 5% NaOH solutions. Half-life at pH 6.65 and 25°C: 45 hours
Hydrolysis products: Hydrofluoric acid
Stability in storage: Less stable than GA or GB
Odor: Fruity; with impurities, odor of camphor
Median lethal dosage (MLD_{50}) (respiratory): 70-100 mg/min/m^3; skin; 18 mg/kg — lowest lethal concentration known
Median incapacitating dosage (ICt_{50}): GB, GA range
Rate of detoxification: Low detoxification rate; essentially cumulative
Clinical effects: Very high toxicity and rapidly acting toxin; vapor causes miosis with decreased vision. Toxicity much greater through eye than through skin. Irreversibly binds to acetylcholinesterase.
Dermal effect: Extremely toxic by skin absorption. Liquid does not injure skin, but penetrates it rapidly. Immediate decontamination of the smallest drop is essential. Skin LCt_{50} of vapor is not known.
Long-term neurotoxic effects: Peripheral nerve damage, neurobehavioral changes
Rate of action: Very rapid; death usually occurs within 15 minutes after fatal dosage is absorbed

Protection required: Protective mask and protective clothing. Ordinary clothing degasses vapor for about 30 minutes after contact with vapor. This should be considered before unmasking. Immediately remove all liquid from clothing.

Persistency: Depends upon munitions used and the weather. Heavily splashed liquid persists 1-2 days under average weather conditions (5 hours at 15°C; 2 days at -10°C).

Comment: Pretreatment with pyridostigmine (30 mg orally every 8 hours) in an impending soman attack may be of value in decreasing lethality

Tabun (GA) — A colorless to brownish liquid giving a colorless vapor

Chemical name: Ethyl N,N-dimethyl-phosphoroamidocyanidate

Formula: $C_2H_5OP(O)(CN)N(CH_3)_2$

CAS: 77-81-6

Appearance: Colorless to brownish liquid

Flammable: Yes

Molecular weight: 162.3

Vapor density (compared with air): 5.63

Liquid density: 1.073 at 25°C

Vapor pressure: 0.070 mm Hg at 25°C

Decomposition temperature: Complete decomposition in 3¼ hours at 150°C

Treatment: See Nerve Gas

Potential for rescuer contamination from exposed patients: High before initial decontamination; low thereafter

Rate of hydrolysis: Reacts slowly with water but rapidly with strong acids or alkalies; self-buffering at pH 4-5. Autocatalytic below pH 4, due to presence of HCN. Half-life: 7 hours at pH 4-5. Hydrolysis catalyzed by phosphate.

Hydrolysis products: HCN

Stability in storage: Stable in steel containers at ordinary temperatures. No activity on metals or other materials.

Odor: Faintly fruity; none when pure

Median concentration detectable (by eye effects): 3.2 mg/m^3

Median lethal dosage (MLD_{50}) (respiratory): Approximately 200-400 $mg/min/m^3$ for resting individuals

Median incapacitating dosage (ICt_{50}) (respiratory): Approximately 300 $mg/min/m^3$ for resting individuals

Clinical effects: Very high toxicity; rapid acting, much greater toxic effects through eye than through skin. Vapor causes miosis resulting in decreased vision. Irreversibly inhibits acetylcholinesterase enzyme.

Dermal effects: LD_{50} (liquid), 1-1.5 g/person. Liquid decontamination of smallest drop is essential. Vapor penetrates skin readily. Skin LCt_{50} of vapor is not known — probably between 20,000 and 40,000 $mg/min/m^3$.

Protection required: Protective mask and protective clothing. Ordinary clothing may degas vapors for about 30 minutes after contact with vapor. Immediately remove all liquid from clothing.

Decontaminants:

Dermal: Copious wash (at least 3 times) with diluted bleach solution (1:10 with water), ethanol, or tincture of green soap

Ocular: Irrigate with water

Persistency: Depends upon munitions used and the weather. Heavily splashed liquid persists 1-4 days under average weather conditions (1 day at 15°C; 4 days at -10°C).

Comment: Generates cyanogen chloride when in contact with bleaching powder

V-Agents — The standard V-agent is VX. VX is an odorless amber colored liquid similar in appearance to motor oil.

Formula: $C_{11}H_{26}NO_2PS$
CAS: 50782-69-9
Appearance: Tasteless
Molecular weight: 267.38
Vapor density (compared with air): 9.2
Liquid density: 1.0083 g/mL at 25°C
Freezing point: Below -51°C; -39°C calculated
Boiling point: 298°C (calculated) decomposes
Vapor pressure: 0.0007 mm Hg at 25°C
Decomposition temperature: Half-life: 36 hours at 150°C, 1.6 hours at 200°C; 4 minutes at 250°C; 36 seconds at 295°C
Treatment: See Nerve Gas
Potential for rescuer contamination from exposed patients: See Tabun
Rate of hydrolysis: Half-life at 25°C pH 2-3: 100 days; pH 13: 16 minutes; pH 14: 1.3 minutes
Hydrolysis products: Diethyl methylphosphonate, 2-disopropylaminoethyl mercaptan, ethyl hydrogen methyl-phosphonate, bis(ethylmethylphosphonic) anhydride, bis *S*-(2-diisopropylaminoethyl) methylphosphonodithioate. (Toxic hydrolysis products form at pH 7-10.)
Stability in storage: Relatively stable at room temperature. Unstabilized VX of 95% purity decomposed at a rate of 5% a month at 71°C.
Action on metals or other materials: Negligible on brass, steel, and aluminum
Median lethal dosage (MLD_{50}): 30 mg/min/m^3
    Oral: Lowest toxic dose: 4 mcg/kg (GI effects)
    I.V.: Lowest toxic dose: 1500 ng/kg
    I.M.: Lowest toxic dose: 3200 ng/kg
    Dermal: Lowest toxic dose: 86 mcg/kg
Median incapacitating dosage (ICt_{50}): 50 mg/min/m^3
Rate of detoxification: Low; essentially cumulative
Dermal and ocular toxicity: Extremely toxic by skin and eye absorption. Liquid does not injure the skin or eye, but penetrates rapidly. Immediate decontamination of the smallest drop is essential.
Rate of action: Very rapid; death usually occurs within 15 minutes after fatal dosage is absorbed
Protection required: Protective masks and protective clothing
Persistency: Depends upon munitions used and the weather. Heavily splashed liquid persists for long periods of time under average weather conditions (3 days at +15°C; 8-9 days at -10°C).
Comment: 100 times as toxic as sarin; 120 kg can kill 9 million individuals (the entire population of Sweden). Metal surface contamination may still be present for up to 8 days (liquid VX) to up to 15 days (gas VX on painted metal surface).

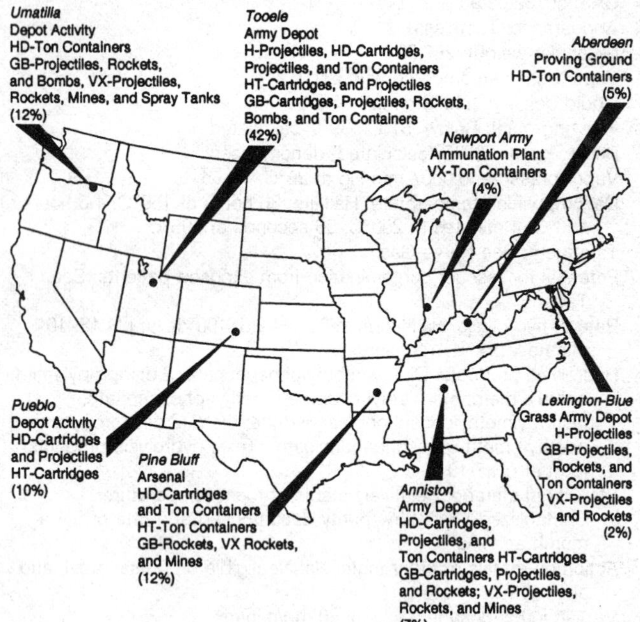

Storage sites of chemical munitions in the United States. Reprinted with permission from Stewart CE and Sullivan JB, "Military Munitions and Antipersonnel Agents," *Hazardous Materials Toxicology - Clinical Principles of Environmental Health*, Sullivan JB and Krieger GR, eds, Williams & Wilkins, Baltimore, MD: 1992, 100:986-1003.

VOMITING AGENTS

Vomiting compounds cause great discomfort to victims; when released indoors, they can cause serious illness or death.

Adamsite (DM)

Chemical name: Diphenylaminochloroarsine (also phenarsazine chloride)
Formula: $C_6H_4(AsCl)(NH)C_6H_4$
CAS: 578-94-9
UN/DOT: 1698
Appearance: Yellow or white to invisible gas; yellow to green granules
Molecular weight: 277.57
Vapor density (compared with air): Forms no appreciable vapor
Solid density: 1.65 at 20°C
Boiling point: 410°C calculated
Vapor pressure: Negligible
Action on metal: Corrodes iron/bronze
Decomposition temperature: Above melting point
Treatment: Wash skin with diluted bleach
Rate of hydrolysis: Quite rapid when in aerosol form. When solid DM is covered with water, a protective oxide coating is formed hindering further hydrolysis.
Hydrolysis products: Diphenylarsenious oxide and hydrogen chloride. The oxide is very poisonous if taken internally.
Stability in storage: Stable when pure
Action on metals or other materials: Slight when dry
Odor: No pronounced odor; may have the odor of burning fireworks
Median lethal dosage (MLD_{50}): 15,000 mg/min/m^3
Median lethal dosage: About 11,000 mg/min/m^3
Median incapacitating dosage (ICt_{50}): 22 mg/min/m^3 for 1-minute exposure, 8 mg/min/m^3 for 60-minute exposure
Rate of detoxification: Quite rapid in small amounts. Incapacitating amounts lose their effects after about 30 minutes.
Clinical effects: Dermal and ocular toxicity. Headache, nausea and vomiting, lacrimation, salivation, sneezing, and coughing. Irritating; relatively nontoxic. Rapidly acting in about 1 minute is required for temporary incapacitation at a concentration of 22 mg/min/m^3.
Protection required: Protective mask
Persistency: Short, because compounds are disseminated as an aerosol

Diphenylchloroarsine (DA)

Chemical name: Diphenylchloroarsine
Formula: $(C_6H_5)_2AsCl$
CAS: 712-48-1
UN/DOT: 1699
Appearance: Colorless crystals or dark brown liquid
Molecular weight: 264.5
Vapor density (compared with air): Forms no appreciable vapor
Liquid density: 1.387 at 50°C
Boiling point: 333°C with decomposition
Decomposition temperature: 300°C
Treatment: See Arsine
Rate of hydrolysis: Slow in mass but rapid when finely divided
Hydrolysis products: Diphenylarsenious oxide and hydrogen chloride. The oxide is very poisonous if taken internally.
Stability in storage: Stable when pure
Action on metals or other materials: None when dry
Odor: None
Median lethal dosage (MLD_{50}): 15,000 mg/min/m^3 (estimated)
Median incapacitating dosage (ICt_{50}): 12 mg/min/m^3 if received over 10-minute periods; probably higher for shorter time

Clinical effects: Dermal and ocular toxicity, vomiting. Very rapid acting, within 2-3 minutes after 1-minute exposure.

Protection required: Protective mask

Decontamination: Diluted bleach or caustic soda dermally

Persistency: Short, because compound is disseminated as an aerosol

Diphenylcyanoarsine (DC)

Chemical name: Diphenylcyanoarsine

Formula: $(C_6H_5)_2AsCN$

Molecular weight: 255.0

Vapor density (compared with air): Does not form appreciable vapor

Liquid density: 1.3338 at 35°C

Boiling point: 350°C with decomposition

Decomposition temperature: About 25% decomposed at 300°C. Largely decomposed as a result of dispersing blast.

Treatment: Wash skin with diluted bleach or alkali solution

Rate of hydrolysis: Very slow

Hydrolysis products: Hydrogen cyanide and diphenylarsenious oxide

Stability in storage: Stable at all ordinary temperatures

Action on metals or other materials: None

Odor: Similar to a mixture of garlic and bitter almonds

Median lethal dosage (MLD_{50}): 10,000 mg/min/m^3. It would be nearly impossible to build up a vapor concentration of DC which would be lethal within a practicable time.

Median incapacitating dosage (ICt_{50}): 30 mg/min/m^3 for 30-second exposure; 20 mg/min/m^3 for 5-minute exposure

Rate of detoxification: Rapid; incapacitating amounts lose their effect after about 1 hour

Clinical effects: Dermal and ocular toxicity. Irritating; very rapid acting. Higher concentrations are intolerable in about 30 seconds.

Protection required: Protective mask

Persistency: Short, because the compound is disseminated as an aerosol

Methyldichloroarsine (MD)

CAS: 593-89-5

UN/DOT: 1556

Appearance: Colorless liquid

Molecular weight: 161

Odor: None

Vapor density as compared to air: 5.5

Liquid density at 20°C: 1.836

Freezing point: -59°C

Boiling point: 13°C (little decomposition to boiling point)

Treatment: See Arsine

Median lethal dosage: 3000-5000 mg/min/m^3

Median incapacitating dosage (inhalation): 25 mg/min/m^3

Clinical effects: Immediate eye, lung irritant; can cause blisters on a delayed basis

Decontamination: Bleach or caustic soda

Rate of detoxification: Rapid

Comment: Combustible upon heating; explosive when reacts with chlorine

---

Adapted with permission from Stewart CE and Sullivan JB, "Military Munitions and Antipersonnel Agents," *Hazardous Materials Toxicology — Clinical Principles of Environmental Health*, Sullivan JB and Krieger GR, eds, Baltimore, MD: Williams & Wilkins, 1992, 986-1003.

Additional References

Borak J and Sidell FR, "Agents of Chemical Warfare: Sulfur Mustard," *Ann Emerg Med*, 1992, 21:303-8.

Cancio LC, "Chemical Casualty Decontamination by Medical Platoons in the 82nd Airborne Division," *Military Medicine*, 1993, 158:1-5.

Gunderson CH, Lehmann CR, Sidell FR, et al, "Nerve Agents: A Review," *Neurology*, 1992, 42:946-50.

Lee BH, Knopp R, and Richardson ML, "Treatment of Exposure to Chemical Personnel Protection Agents," *Annals of Emerg Med*, 1984, 13(6):487-8.

Press N, "Haber's Choice, Hobson's Choice and Biological Warfare: Perspectives in Biology and Medicine," 1985, 29:92-108.

Sidell FR and Borak J, "Chemical Warfare Agents: II. Nerve Agents," *Ann Emerg Med*, 1992, 21:865-71.

Smith WJ and Dunn MA, "Medical Defense Against Blistering Chemical Warfare Agents," *Arch Dermatol*, 1991, 127:1207-13.

Yokoyama K, Ogura Y, Kishimoto M, et al, "Blood Purification for Severe Sarin Poisoning After the Tokyo Subway Attack," *JAMA*, 274(5):379.

CHEMICALS/DRUGS IN WHICH THERAPEUTIC ANTIBODIES HAVE BEEN OR ARE BEING STUDIED AS ANTIDOTES

Arsenic
Aspirin
Cardiac glycosides (FDA approved as Digibind®)*
Colchicine*
Cyclic antidepressants
Morphine
Paraquat
Penicillin*
Pentobarbital
Phencyclidine
Ricin

*Denotes human experience.

References

Baud FJ, Sabouraud A, Vicaut E, et al, "Treatment of Severe Colchicine Overdose Fragments," *N Engl J Med*, 1995, 332:642-5.

Howland MA and Smilkstein MJ, "Primer on Immunology With Applications to Toxicology," *Contemp Management in Crit Care*, 1991, 1(3):109-46.

Keyler DE, Shelver WL, Landon J, et al, "Toxicity of High Doses of Polyclonal Drug-Specific Antibody Fab Fragments," *Vet Hum Toxicol*, 1994, 36:346.

Owens SM and Mayersohn M, "Phencyclidine Specific Fab Fragments Alter Phencyclidine Disposition in Dogs," *Drug Metab Dispos Biol Fate Chem*, 1986, 14(1):52-8.

Pentel PR, Landon J, and Sidki A, "Effects of Drug-Specific Polyclonal Fab on Desipramine Cardiotoxicity and Lethality in Rats," *Vet Hum Toxicol*, 1994, 36:362.

Scherrmann JM, "Antibody Treatment of Toxin Poisoning — Recent Advances," *J Toxicol Clin Toxicol*, 1994, 32:363-75.

CLINICAL POLICY FOR THE INITIAL APPROACH TO PATIENTS PRESENTING WITH ACUTE TOXIC INGESTION OR DERMAL OR INHALATION EXPOSURE

Adapted with permission from American College of Emergency Physicians: Clinical Policy for the Initial Approach to Patients Presenting With Acute Toxic Ingestion or Dermal or Inhalation Exposure, *Ann Emerg Med*, April 1995, 25(4):570-85.

A clinical policy on the initial approach to patients with acute toxic ingestion or dermal or inhalation exposure was selected because of the frequency with which these patients present to the emergency department and the potential for serious adverse outcomes. Initial identification, evaluation, and management of these patients are recognized as an integral part of emergency medicine clinical practice.

The complex clinical nature of these patients and the diverse toxic substances to which patients may be exposed required the development of a clinical policy that focuses on the basic clinical approach for most patients. This policy does not attempt to delineate the specific presentation of or treatments for specific toxic substances. The Clinical Policies Committee of the American College of Emergency Physicians recommends that clinicians use appropriate sources for this detailed information, when needed. This policy does not apply to all toxic substance exposures; excluded are envenomation, radiation exposure, food poisoning, parenteral exposure, and eye exposure.

Frequently, the most challenging aspect of patient care is the recognition and identification of a toxic substance exposure that has caused the patient's symptoms. Emergency physicians must maintain a high level of clinical suspicion and consider toxicologic causes for many clinical presentations. This policy does not apply to patients who have not been recognized as having a toxic exposure.

Because different institutions have different resources and capabilities in the management of these patients, the recommendation to admit a patient (or to obtain a specific consultation) may require transfer of the patient to an institution better able to deal with the patient's specific needs.

The subcommittee preparing the initial draft of this policy was composed of emergency physicians and toxicologists. This policy is based on the existing literature; where literature was not available, consensus of emergency physicians and toxicologists was used. This policy went through the ACEP clinical policy development process, including expert review and field testing. The reasons for developing clinical policies and the approaches used in their development have been enumerated.[1] After this policy was drafted, it was reviewed by experts in toxicology and emergency medicine, and their responses were used for further refinement and enhancement of the policy. Field testing was conducted in EDs differing in locales, sizes, and resources to deal with patients with acute toxic ingestion or dermal or inhalation exposure. The field testing experience resulted in further refinements to the policy.

Clinical policies are scheduled for revision every 3 years; however, interim reviews are conducted when technology or the practice environment changes significantly. The value of this policy is in establishing a benchmark based on literature and a consensus of toxicologists and emergency physicians on a general approach to the care of patients with toxic substance exposures. The Clinical Policies Committee hopes the policy will help delineate areas for future research, which will further improve patient care.

Inclusion Criteria: Patients with a presumptive diagnosis of toxic exposure.

Exclusion Criteria: This policy is **not** intended for envenomation, radiation exposure, food poisoning, parenteral exposure, or eye exposure.

[1] Schriger DL, Cantrill SV, and Green CS, "The Origins, Benefits, Harms, and Implications of Emergency Medicine Clinical Policies," *Ann Emerg Med*, 1993, 22:597-602.

Stabilization: This policy assumes that patients with life-threatening emergencies have been treated or stabilized and is not meant to apply to the unstable patient. If a patient presents in an unstable condition, initial resuscitation and stabilization must take precedence over any action in this policy.

Rationale: Patients with toxicologic problems represent an important part of the practice of emergency medicine. This policy provides rational guidelines for the initial evaluation, stabilization, and treatment of patients once a presumptive diagnosis is considered. This policy does not address patients who present without suspicion of a toxicologic exposure; nor does it address all of the conditions that might result from exposure to a toxic substance, including occult or atypical presentations. Emergency physicians should be aware of the diverse presentations of toxic exposures and carefully consider toxic substances as a cause of many patients' complaints.

Identification of the toxic substances will guide therapy. When the patient is unable to or will not provide a reliable history of exposure, emergency physicians must use their best efforts to perform good detective work. A search to determine what substances were available to the patient will create a potential toxic substance list. This history-taking may include family, friends, prehospital care providers, other witnesses, or a collection of physical evidence. The signs of toxicity of these agents then are searched for in the presentation and physical examination of the overdose patient. These steps will aid in the identification of the agent and thus guide treatment decisions.

Initial stabilization and treatment focus on removal of the toxicologic agent to prevent further exposure and toxicity. Health care workers should protect their own safety and that of others by preventing exposure to toxic substances during the care of these patients. Initial treatment of dermal or inhalation exposure begins by separating the patient from the toxic substance to prevent further exposures and toxicity. Care must be exercised during the decontamination process to prevent exposures to toxic substances by health care providers. The health care worker may be protected by surface barriers, filters, masks, contained-breathing devices, ocular protection, equipment decontamination, and appropriate disposal of contaminated equipment and supplies.

Gastrointestinal decontamination represents an area of tremendous controversy. Although some issues involving gastrointestinal decontamination are unresolved, the majority of the current literature supports the following conclusions:

- Activated charcoal adsorbs almost all commonly ingested drugs and chemicals and usually should be administered to most overdose patients as quickly as possible. Commonly ingested substances **not** adsorbed include iron, lithium, ethanol, and potassium.
- Syrup of ipecac generally is believed to be of little value in the ED.
- Gastric lavage is of unproven benefit for routine use. In general, this procedure is best reserved for patients who may have recently ingested a life-threatening overdose. In these cases, administering a dose of activated charcoal before lavage is of theoretic benefit.
- The use of cathartics is also of unproven benefit, but a single dose is commonly administered with activated charcoal to speed gastrointestinal transit and prevent charcoal inspissation. Multiple doses of any cathartics should not be used because dehydration and electrolyte imbalances may occur.
- Whole-bowel irrigation has been shown to be effective under certain conditions, especially when activated charcoal lacks efficacy.

No definitive recommendation can be made on the use of ipecac, gastric lavage, cathartics, and whole-bowel irrigation for all patients. If any of these modalities are used, the choice should be based on consideration of the offending toxic substance, time of exposure, and condition of the patient. The use of forced diuresis, hemodialysis, and charcoal hemoperfusion to eliminate toxic substances must be based on the suspected toxic substance and physiologic status of the patient.

This policy does not advocate the routine use of toxicologic drug screens in the evaluation and treatment of most patients. The lack of proven clinical usefulness of qualitative screening tests — coupled with the scientific limitations and variability of the tests available at different institutions, their expense, and the time required for results — prevents recommendation of their use in most patients. Effective treatment may be provided without a toxicologic screen after obtaining a history and physical examination focused on identifying the toxic substance, or a clinical toxic syndrome, and establishing the physiologic status of the patient. Specific treatments must be based on the patient's physiologic condition and suspected or known toxic substances. Supportive care is successfully combined with removal or elimination of the toxic substance for most cases. For some toxic substances such as acetaminophen, methanol/ethylene glycol, lithium, and salicylates, specific quantitative tests may be useful in determining appropriate treatment and disposition. The value of quantitative and qualitative toxicologic tests in patients who have ingested unknown substances must be determined by the physician for individual patients.

Some patients may be effectively treated with specific or nonspecific antidotes. The use of specific antidotes for individual toxic substances is beyond the scope of this policy. Generally, the use of antidotes should be individualized to the toxic substance and physiologic condition of the patient.

The large number of potentially toxic agents and their diverse effects may require the emergency physician to access specific expertise, information, or both. Toxicologists, poison information centers, toxicology references, and computerized data bases may aid the emergency physician in the treatment of some patients. Emergency physicians should be familiar with resources through their poison information center.

Many patients with a toxicologic problem have other injuries or illnesses. Altered mental status resulting from toxic substances may make identification of head injury or other pathologic conditions difficult. Emergency physicians should be aware of the nee to consider other etiologies for their patients' signs and symptoms.

In addition, these patients may be suicidal, have significant psychiatric illness, or be victims of abuse or neglect. After initial treatment of the toxicologic exposure, patients should be assessed for these underlying problems.

Many exposures and pediatric ingestions are accidental. The ED encounter provides an opportunity for education and other preventive measures that may minimize the risk of future incidents.

Implementing the Policy

The rules and guidelines for patient management emphasize finding with the potential for high risk to the patient. It is important that no single finding be considered independently. Some actions are separated by a slash (/), which means that either may be appropriate in a given clinical situation; the action is at the discretion of the clinician. The order in which items appear in the rules and guidelines is arbitrary and not meant to imply the order in which they should be performed. In using this clinical policy it may be helpful to think of **rules** as broad categories that should be recorded as pertinent positives or negatives and of **guidelines** as detailed or expanded lists that are meant to prompt the physician to consider many possibilities. Documentation should be sufficient to reflect the clinical decision-making process. It is unrealistic for a physician to perform or document every item in the guidelines.

Rules and Guidelines for Patient Management

Rule*	**Guideline†**
Solicit and record a history that includes:	**Consider these aspects of the history:**
History of exposure	Route of exposure, what, how much, when, why (suicidal intent), other substances, chronicity
	Corroborative history and other physical evidence (eg, pill containers) from prehospital care providers
	Time course of symptoms
	Neurologic: Seizure, alteration of consciousness, confusion, ataxia, slurred speech, tremor, headache, syncope
	Cardiopulmonary: Syncope, palpitations, cough, chest pain, shortness of breath, burning, or irritation in upper airway
	Gastrointestinal: Abdominal pain, nausea, vomiting, diarrhea, pain, or difficulty in swallowing
Past medical history	Medications including nonprescription substances, alcohol/drug abuse, psychiatric history, allergies, occupational or hobby exposures, travel, prior ingestions, social history with potential for domestic violence/neglect, last normal menstrual period, or pregnancy
Conduct and record a physical exam that includes:	**Consider these aspects of the physical exam:**
Vital signs: Blood pressure, pulse, respirations, temperature	Pulse: Rate, regularity
	Respirations: Rate, regularity, depth
	Temperature: Rectal temperature preferable
General appearance	Agitation, color, signs of trauma, diaphoresis, odor
Weight (if age <6 y)	
Neurologic mental status	Level of consciousness, orientation, affect, agitation, combativeness, hallucinations, cognition, speech
	Sensorimotor function: Strength, tremor, fasciculation, myoclonus, pain in response to light touch
	General: Cranial nerves, reflexes, coordination (cerebellar)
	HEENT: Vision, sclerae, conjunctivae, nystagmus, dysconjugate gaze, fundi, pupils (size and reactivity), hearing, nasal mucosa, breath odor, oral mucosa (burns, moisture), gag reflex
Cardiovascular	Rhythm, abnormal heart sounds, pulses
Pulmonary	Adequacy of respirations, breath sounds, rales, rhonchi, wheezes
	Gastrointestinal: Abdomen: Bowel sounds, tenderness, distention
	Genitourinary: Bladder (distention), rectal (gross or occult blood, drugs), vaginal (drugs)
	Skin: Moisture, color, temperature, signs of I.V. drug use, evidence of bleeding, lesions

*An action reflecting principles of good practice in most situations. There may be circumstances when a rule need not or cannot be followed; in these situations, it is advisable that deviation from the rule be justified in writing. Inability to comply with rules should be incorporated in institutional policies.

†An action that may be considered, depending on the patient, the circumstances, or other factors. Thus, guidelines are not always followed, and there is no implication that failure to follow a guideline is improper.

Implement ACTIONS Based on the FINDINGS for the following VARIABLES

Variable	Finding	Action	
		Rule	Guideline
History	Dermal exposure	Skin decontamination* Protection of health care worker	Complete disrobing of patient (proper disposal) Assess for systemic exposure/toxicity Copious eye irrigation with water Decontamination of skin folds/creases
	Gastrointestinal exposure		
	Caustics	Avoid emesis and gastric lavage	Dilute Endoscopy
	Hydrocarbons		Evaluate neurologic and pulmonary status
	Most other toxic substances	Charcoal	Protection of health care worker GI decontamination Specific drug or toxic substance levels Radiopaque substances: KUB Drug bezoars, body packers: contrast study
	Intentional ingestion	Evaluation for potential suicidal risk	Patient restraint Patient supervision Psychiatric consultation
	Accidental ingestion	Evaluation for abuse or neglect	Protective service referral
	Unknown potentially toxic substances	Charcoal	GI decontamination Acetaminophen level Salicylate level Toxicologic blood screen Toxicologic urine screen
	Inhalation exposure		Protection of patient and health care worker Supplemental oxygen Humidification ABG/oximetry/ co-oximetry/ methemoglobin level/ carboxyhemoglobin level Chest x-ray
Physical Examination	Pulse <60	I.V. access Cardiac monitor	Supplemental oxygen/ABG/ oximetry EKG
	>120 (≥6 y) >140 (peds <6 y)	I.V. access Cardiac monitor	Supplemental oxygen/oximetry ABG/co-oximetry/ methemoglobin level/carboxy-hemoglobin level EKG
	irregular	Cardiac monitor	I.V. access EKG
	Respirations		
	<10 (adult) <xx (peds) see Attachment A	I.V. access Supplemental oxygen Cardiac monitor	Intubate Ventilate Rapid glucose determination ABG/co-oximetry/ methemoglobin level/carboxy-hemoglobin level Pulse oximetry Opioid antagonist
	>24 (adult) >xx (peds) see Attachment A	I.V. access	Supplemental oxygen Cardiac monitor ABG/oximetry Salicylate level Chest x-ray

(continued)

Variable	Finding	Action: Rule	Action: Guideline
	Temperature		
	>40°C	I.V. access Active cooling	Supplemental oxygen Cardiac monitor Assess for neuroleptic malignant syndrome EKG
	<35°C		I.V. access Supplemental oxygen Cardiac monitor Rapid glucose determination EKG Treat hypothermia
	General appearance		
	Cyanosis	I.V. access Supplemental oxygen Cardiac monitor ABG/oximetry	Intubate Methemoglobin level Measured oxygen saturation/ co-oximetry Chest x-ray EKG
	Neurologic		
	Decreased level of consciousness with no gag reflex	I.V. access Cardiac monitor Airway management	Rapid glucose determination
	Unresponsive to painful stimuli	I.V. access Supplemental oxygen Cardiac monitor Glucose administration/rapid glucose determination ABG/oximetry	ABG/co-oximetry/ carboxyhemoglobin level Toxicologic screen Urinalysis Abdominal x-ray for radiopaque toxic substances Opioid antagonist Thiamine
	Altered level of consciousness	Frequent assessment	Rapid glucose determination Carboxyhemoglobin level Opioid antagonist Thiamine
	Female with reproductive potential		Assess for pregnancy
HEENT	Miotic pupils		I.V. access Opioid antagonist
	Oral burns of mucous membranes		Endoscopy Avoid emesis and gastric lavage
Pulmonary	Rales/rhonchi		Supplemental oxygen Cardiac monitor ABG/oximetry Chest x-ray
	Wheezes		Supplemental oxygen Cardiac monitor ABG/oximetry Peak expiratory flow Chest x-ray Beta agonist
Abdomen	Rectal/vaginal drug packets	Remove	Abdominal series x-ray Cathartics
	Distended abdomen		Rectal examination Abdominal series x-ray Orogastric tube
	Distended bladder		Bladder decompression
Skin	Pressure sores (erythema/vesicles) bullae		Assess for rhabdomyolysis/ compartment syndrome Carboxyhemoglobin level

(continued)

Variable	Finding	Action: Rule	Action: Guideline
Diagnostic Testing			
ABG	Hypercapnia	Ventilate	Intubate Opioid antagonist
	Hypoxemia	Supplemental oxygen	Intubate Chest x-ray EKG
Urinalysis	Dipstick positive for blood with few or no RBCs on microscopic analysis		Evaluate/treat for rhabdomyolysis/ hemolysis

*May be performed prehospital.

Implement ACTIONS for the Following VARIABLES

Assessment

The causes and clinical severity of toxic exposures in patients presenting to the ED are far too varied to be considered in detail in this clinical policy; however, the majority of toxic exposures are readily managed in the ED with the following:

- general supportive care
- treatment of respiratory, cardiovascular, and neurologic complications
- attempt to identify toxic substance
- appropriate decontamination techniques
- specific therapy of treatable toxic exposures
- consultation/reporting with medical toxicologists or poison information centers when appropriate
- psychiatric evaluation/referral when appropriate

Variable	Action: Rule	Action: Guideline
Disposition		
Admission	Transfer care to accepting physician	
Transfer	Follow ACEP and other applicable transfer principles*	
Discharge	Provide referral for follow-up care	
	Provide instructions regarding treatment and circumstances that require return to ED	Social services/protective services consult

*American College of Emergency Physicians: Appropriate Interhospital Patient Transfer, *Ann Emerg Med*, 1993, 22:766-7.

Attachment A

Normal Resting Respiratory Rates*

Age	Rate (breaths per minute)
Newborn	30-60
Infant	
1-6 months	30-50
6-12 months	24-46
1-4 years	20-30
4-6 years	20-25
6-12 years	16-20
>12 years	12-16

*American Academy of Pediatrics and the American College of Emergency Physicians: Respiratory Distress, *APLS: The Pediatric Emergency Medicine Course*, ed 2, Elk Grove Village, IL, and Dallas, TX: AAP and ACEP, 1993, 5.

Bibliography

The following citations are not intended to be a comprehensive review of the literature or a complete listing of all the works used in the development of this clinical policy. The purpose of this listing is to provide a sample of the kinds of documents that the Clinical Policies Committee reviewed during the development of this policy and to provide the reader with a general reading list.

Albertson TE, Derlet RW, Foulke GE, et al, "Superiority of Activated Charcoal Alone Compared With Ipecac and Activated Charcoal in the Treatment of Acute Toxic Ingestions," *Ann Emerg Med*, 1989, 18:56-9.

Amitai Y, Mitchell AA, McGuigan MA, et al, "Ipecac-Induced Emesis and Reduction of Plasma Concentrations of Drugs Following Accidental Overdose in Children," *Pediatrics*, 1987, 80:364-7.

Arnold M, "Ipecac: When Prevention Fails," *AJDC*, 1988, 142:595.

Askenasi R, Ambramowicz M, and Jeanmart J, "Esophageal Perforation: An Unusual Complication of Gastric Lavage," *Ann Emerg Med*, 1984, 13:146.

Auerbach PS, Osterloh J, Braun O, et al, "Efficacy of Gastric Emptying: Gastric Lavage Versus Emesis Induced With Ipecac," *Ann Emerg Med*, 1986, 15:692-8.

Banner W and Veltri JC, "The Case for Ipecac Syrup," *ADJC*, 1988, 142:596.

Bennett HS, Spiro AJ, Pollack NA, et al, "Ipecac-Induced Myopathy Simulating Dermatomyositis," *Neurology*, 1982, 32:91-4.

Berlinger WG, Spector R, Goldberg MJ, et al, "Enhancement of Theophylline Clearance by Oral Activated Charcoal," *Clin Pharmacol Ther*, 1983, 33:351-4.

Bessen HA and Rothstein RJ, "Sorbitol • A Safe and Effective Cathartic," *Ann Emerg Med*, 1987, 16:729.

Blake DR and Bramble MG, "Is There Excessive Use of Gastric Lavage in the Treatment of Self-Poisoning?" *Lancet*, 1978, 1362-4.

Boba A, "Rapid Whole-Gut Evacuation," *Illinois Medical Journal*, 1979, 155:156-7.

Brotman MC, Forbath N, Garfinkel PE, et al, "Myopathy Due to Ipecac Syrup Poisoning in a Patient With Anorexia Nervosa," *CMA Journal*, 1981, 125:453-4.

Burton BT and Mayer MJ, "Gastric Emptying: Initial Management of the Poisoned Patient?" *Ann Emerg Med*, 1988, 17:762-3.

Burton BT, Bayer MJ, Barron L, et al, "Comparison of Activated Charcoal and Gastric Lavage in the Prevention of Aspirin Absorption," *J Emerg Med*, 1984, 1:411-6.

Caldwell JW, Nava AJ, and DeHaas DD, "Hypernatremia Associated With Cathartics in Overdose Management," *West J Med*, 1987, 147:593-6.

Calvanese JC, "Midesophageal Kinking and Lodgement of a 34-F Gastric Lavage Tube," *Ann Emerg Med*, 1985, 14:1123-5.

Chafee-Bahamon C, Lacouture PG, and Lovejoy FH, "Risk Assessment of Ipecac in the Home," *Pediatrics*, 1985, 75:1105-9.

Comstock EG, Boisaubin EV, Comstock BS, et al, "Assessment of the Efficacy of Activated Charcoal Following Gastric Lavage in Acute Drug Emergencies," *J Toxicol Clin Toxicol*, 1982, 19:149-65.

Cupit GC and Temple AR, "Gastrointestinal Decontamination in the Management of the Poisoned Patient," *Emerg Med Clin North Am*, 1984, 2:15-28.

Curd-Sneed CD, Parks KS, Bordelon JG, et al, "*In vitro* Adsorption of Sodium Pentobarbital by Superchar, USP and Darco G-60 Activated Charcoals," *Clin Tox*, 1987, 25:1-11.

Curtis RA, Barone J, and Giacona N, "Efficacy of Ipecac and Activated Charcoal/Cathartic. Prevention of Salicylate Absorption in a Simulated Overdose," *Arch Intern Med*, 1984, 144:48-52.

Czajka PA and Konrad JD, "Saline Cathartics and the Adsorptive Capacity of Activated Charcoal for Aspirin," *Ann Emerg Med*, 1986, 15:548-51.

Czajka PA and Russell SL, "Nonemetic Effects of Ipecac Syrup," *Pediatrics*, 1985, 75:1101-4.

Danel V and Henry JA, "Activated Charcoal, Emesis, and Gastric Lavage in Aspirin Overdose," *Br J Med*, 1988, 296:1507.

Decker WJ, "Gastrointestinal Decontamination," *J Toxicol Clin Toxicol*, 1983, 20:iii-vi.

Freedman GE, Pasternak S, and Krenzelok EP, "A Clinical Trial Using Syrup of ipecac and Activated Charcoal Concurrently," *Ann Emerg Med*, 1987, 16:164-6.

Gaudreault P, McCormick MA, Lacouture PG, et al, "Poisoning Exposures and Use of Ipecac in Children Less Than 1 Year Old," *Ann Emerg Med*, 1986, 15:808-10.

Greenbaum DM, "Clinical Aspects of Drug Intoxication: The St Vincent's Hospital Symposium - Part I," *J Crit Care*, 1983, 12:109-14.

Greensher J, Mofenson HC, and Caraccio TR, "Ascendency of the Black Bottle (Activated Charcoal)," *Pediatrics*, 1987, 80:949-51.

Jones J, Heiselman D, Dougherty J, et al, "Cathartic-Induced Magnesium Toxicity During Overdose Management," *Ann Emerg Med*, 1986, 15:1214-8.
Jorden RC, "Initial Evaluation of the Patient With Altered Mental Status," *Topics in Emergency Medicine*, 1991, 13:1-9.
Katona BG, Siegel EG, and Cluxton RJ, "The New Black Magic: Activated Charcoal and New Therapeutic Uses," *J Emerg Med*, 1987, 5:9-18.
Klein-Schwartz, Gorman RL, Oderda GM, et al, "Ipecac Use in the Elderly: The Unanswered Question," *Ann Emerg Med*, 1984, 13:1152-4.
Krenzelok EP and Dean BS, "Syrup of Ipecac in Children Less Than One Year of Age," *Clin Toxicol*, 1985, 23:171-6.
Krenzelok EP, "The Contemporary Management of Poisoning Emergencies," *Pharmacy Times*, 1990, 56:132-9.
Krenzelok EP, Freedman GE, and Pasternak S, "Preserving the Emetic Effect of Syrup of Ipecac With Concurrent Activated Charcoal Administration: A Preliminary Study," *Clin Toxicol*, 1986, 24:159-66.
Krenzelok EP and Lush RM, "Container Residue After the Administration of Aqueous Activated Charcoal Products," *Am J Emerg Med*, 1991, 9:144-6.
Kulig K, Bar-Or D, Cantrill SV, et al, "Management of Acutely Poisoned Patients Without Gastric Emptying," *Ann Emerg Med*, 1985, 14:562-7.
Kulig K, "Interpreting Gastric Emptying Studies," *J Emerg Med*, 1984, 1:447-8.
Kulig K, "Gastric Lavage in Acute Drug Overdose," *JAMA*, 1989, 262:1392.
Lanphear WF, "Gastric Lavage," *J Emerg Med*, 1986, 4:43-7.
Litovitz T, "In Defense of Retaining Ipecac Syrup as an Over-the-Counter Drug," *Pediatrics*, 1988, 82:514-5.
Margulis MS, Mordashev BK, Andreiman LA, et al, "Prospects for the Use of Assisted Circulation in Cases of Poisoning," *Resuscitation*, 1982, 10:121-7.
Matthew H, Mackintosh TG, Tompsett SL, et al, "Gastric Aspiration and Lavage in Acute Poisoning," *BMJ*, 1966, 1:1333-7.
Mattila MJ, Takki S, and Jussila J, "Effect of Sodium Sulphate and Castor Oil on Drug Absorption From the Human Intestine," *Ann Clin Res*, 1974, 6:19-24.
McDougal C and Maclean MA, "Modifications in the Technique of Gastric Lavage," *Ann Emerg Med*, 1981, 10:514-7.
McNamara RM and Aaron CK, "Sorbitol Catharsis Does Not Enhance Efficacy of Charcoal in a Simulated Acetaminophen Overdose," *Ann emerg Med*, 1988, 17:243-6.
McNamara RM, Aaron CK, Gemborys M, et al, "Efficacy of Charcoal Cathartic Versus Ipecac in Reducing Serum Acetaminophen in a Simulated Overdose," *Ann Emerg Med*, 1989, 18:934-8.
Meester W, Emesis and Lavage. Presentation AACT/AAPCC Meeting, 1979.
Merigian KS, Woodard M, Hedges JR, et al, "Prospective Evaluation of Gastric Emptying in the Self-Poisoned Patient," *Am J Emerg Med*, 1990, 8:479-83.
Millar AJW, Rode H, Buchler J, et al, "Whole-Gut Lavage in Children Using an Iso-osmolar Solution Containing Polyethylene Glycol (GoLYTELY®)," *J Pediatr Surg*, 1988, 23:822-4.
Minocha A, Krenzelok EP, and Spyker DA, "Dosage Recommendations for Activated Charcoal-Sorbitol Treatment," *Clin Toxicol*, 1985, 23:579-87.
Miser JS and Robertson WO, "Ipecac Poisoning," *West J Med*, 1978, 128:440-3.
Mofenson HC and Caraccio TR, "Benefits/Risks of Syrup of Ipecac," *Pediatrics*, 1986, 77:551-2.
Mofenson HC, Caraccio TR, Greensher J, et al, "Gastrointestinal Dialysis With Activated Charcoal and Cathartic in the Treatment of Adolescent Intoxications," *Clin Pediatr*, 1985, 24:678-84.
Moran DM, Crouch DJ, and Finkle BS, "Absorption of Ipecac Alkaloids in Emergency Patients," *Ann Emerg Med*, 1984, 13:1100-2.
Muhlendahl KE, Krienke EG, and Bunjes R, "Fatal Overtreatment of Accidental Childhood Intoxication," *J Pediatr*, 1978, 93:1003-4.
Nejamn G, Hoekstra J, and Kelley M, "Gastric Emptying in the Poisoned Patient," *Am J Emerg Med*, 1990, 8:265-9.
Neuvonen PJ, Vartiainen M, and Tokola O, "Comparison of Activated Charcoal and Ipecac Syrup in Prevention of Drug Absorption," *Eur J Clin Pharmacol*, 1983, 24:557-62.
Neuvonen PJ and Olkkola KT, "Activated Charcoal and Syrup of Ipecac in Prevention of Cimetidine and Pindolol Absorption in Man After Administration of Metoclopramide as an Antiemetic Agent," *Clin Toxicol*, 1984, 22:103-14.
Olkkola KT and Neuvonen PJ, "Do Gastric Contents Modify Antidotal Efficacy of Oral Activated Charcoal?" *Br J Clin Pharmacol*, 1984, 18:633-9.
Olson KR, "Is Gut Emptying All Washed Up?" *Am J Emerg Med*, 1990, 8:560-1.
Park GD, Spector R, Goldberg MJ, et al, "Expanded Role of Charcoal Therapy in the Poisoned and Overdosed Patient," *Arch Intern Med*, 1986, 146:969-73.

Payment P, Richardson L, Siemiatycki J, et al, "A Randomized Trial to Evaluate the Risk of Gastrointestinal Disease Due to Consumption of Drinking Water Meeting current Microbiological Standards," *Am J Public Health*, 1991, 81:703-8.
Pond SM, "A Review of the Pharmacokinetics and Efficacy of Emesis, Gastric Lavage, and Single and Repeated Doses of Charcoal in Overdose Patients," *Dev Toxicol Environ Sci*, 1986, 12:315-28.
Porter RS and Baker EB, "Drug Clearance by Diarrhea Induction," *Am J Emerg Med*, 1985, 3:182-6.
Rappolt RT, Gay GR, Decker WJ, et al, "NAGD (Naloxone, Activated Charcoal, Glucagon, Doxapram) Regimen for the Coma of Drug-Related Overdose," *Ann Emerg Med*, 1980, 9:357-63.
Riegel Jm and Becker CE, "Use of Cathartics in Toxic Ingestions," *Ann Emerg Med*, 1981, 10:254-8.
Rodgers GC and Matyunas NJ, "Gastrointestinal Decontamination for Acute Poisoning," *Pediatr Clin North Am*, 1986, 33:261-85.
Rosenberg PJ, Livingstone DJ, and McLellan BA, "Effect of Whole-Bowel Irrigation on the Antidotal Efficacy of Oral Activated Charcoal," *Ann Emerg Med*, 1988, 17:681-3.
Rudolph JP, "Automated Gastric Lavage and a Comparison of 0.9% Normal Saline Solution and Tap Water Irrigant," *Ann Emerg Med*, 1985, 14:1156-9.
Rumack BH, "Emesis: Safe and Effective?" *Ann Emerg Med* 1981, 10:551.
Rumack BH, "Ipecac Use in the Home," *Pediatrics*, 1985, 75:1148.
Sarvesvaran R, "Dilute the Poison • A Case of Fatal Water Intoxications," *Med Sci Law*, 1984, 92-94.
Sketris IS, Mowry JB, Czajka PA, et al, "Saline Catharsis: Effect on Aspirin Bioavailability in Combination With Activated Charcoal," *J Clin Pharmacol*, 1982, 22:59-64.
Sorensen PM, Lindkaer-Jensen St, "The Effect of Magnesium Sulfate on the Absorption of Acetylsalicylic Acid and Lithium Carbonate From the Human Intestine," *Arch Toxicol*, 1975, 34:121-7.
Stewart JJ, "Effects of Emetic and Cathartic Agents on the Gastrointestinal Tract and the Treatment of Toxic Ingestion," *J Toxicol Clin Toxicol*, 1983, 20:199-253.
Tanberg D, Liechty EJ, and Fishbein D, "Mallory-Weiss Syndrome: An Unusual Complication of Ipecac-Induced Emesis," *Ann Emerg Med*, 1981, 10:521-3.
Tandberg D, Diven BG, and McLeod JW, "Ipecac-Induced Emesis Versus Gastric Lavage: A Controlled Study in Normal Adults," *Am J Emerg Med*, 1986, 4:205-9.
Tenenbein M, Cohen S, and Sitar DS, "Efficacy of Ipecac-Indued Emesis, Orogastric Lavage, and Activated Charcoal for Acute Drug Overdose," *Ann Emerg Med*, 1987, 16:838-41.
Tenenbein M, "Whole Bowel Irrigation for Toxic Ingestions," *Clin Toxicol*, 1985, 23:177-84.
Tenenbein M, "Inefficacy of Gastric Emptying Procedures," *J Emerg Med*, 1985, 3:133-6.
Tenenbein M, Cohen S, and Sitar DS, "Whole Bowel Irrigation as a Decontamination Procedure After Acute Drug Overdose," *Arch Intern Med*, 1987, 147:905-7.
Tenenbein M, "Whole Bowel Irrigation in Iron Poisoning," *J Pediatr*, 1987, 111:142-5.
Tenenbein M, "Whole Bowel Irrigation as a Gastrointestinal Decontamination Procedure After Acute Poisoning," *Med Toxicol*, 1988, 3:77-84.
Thompson AM, Robins JB, and Prescott LF, "Changes in Cardiorespiratory Function During Gastric Lavage for Drug Overdose," *Hum Toxicol*, 1987, 6:215-8.
Todd JW, "Do Measures to Enhance Drug Removal Save Lives?" *Lancet*, 1984, 331.
True RJ, Berman JM, and Mahutte CK, "Treatment of Theophylline Toxicity With Oral Activated Charcoal," *Crit Care Med*, 1984, 12:113-4.
Uden DL, Davison GJ, and Kohen DP, "The Effect of Carbonated Beverages on Ipecac-Induced Emesis," *Ann Emerg Med*, 1981, 10:79-81.
Vale JA, Meredith TJ, and Proudfoot AT, "Syrup of Ipecacuanha: Is It Really Useful?" *BMJ*, 1986, 293:1321-2.
Vale A, Meredith T, and Buckley B, "Eliminating Poisons," *BMJ*, 1984, 289:366-9.
Wason S, "Gastrointestinal Decontamination of the Poisoned Patient • A Critical Review," *Drugs of Today*, 1987, 23:455-65.
Watson WA, Leighton J, Guy J, et al, "Recovery of Cyclic Antidepressants With Gastric Lavage," *J Emerg Med*, 1989, 7:373-7.
Watson WA, Bradford DC, and Veltri JC, "The Volume of a Swallow: Correlation of Deglutition With Patient and Container Parameters," *Am J Emerg Med*, 1983, 3:278-81.
Wheeler-Usher DH, Wanke LA, and Bayer MJ, "Gastric Emptying: Risk Versus Benefit in the Treatment of Acute Poisoning," *Med Toxicol*, 1986, 1:142-53.
Wolowodiuk OJ, McMicken DB, and O'Brien P, "Pneumomediastinum and Retropneumoperitoneum: An Unusual Complication of Syrup of Ipecac-Induced Emesis," *Ann Emerg Med*, 1984, 13:1148-51.

Quality Assurance Form: Acute Toxic Ingestion or Dermal or Inhalation Exposure

Instructions: Use this form to review medical records of patients presenting with the problem of acute toxic ingestion or dermal or inhalation exposure.

Documentation Review

Does the medical record contain a description of the following:

	Yes	No
1. History of exposure	—	—
2. Past medical history	—	—

Is there documentation that the physical exam included the following:

	Yes	No
3. Vital signs: blood pressure, pule, respirations, temperature	—	—
4. General appearance	—	—
5. Weight (if age <6 y)	—	—
6. Neurologic mental status	—	—
7. Cardiovascular	—	—
8. Pulmonary	—	—

Comments ______________________________

____

____

____

____

____

____

Quality Assurance Form: Acute Toxic Ingestion or Dermal or Inhalation Exposure

Instructions: Draw horizontal lines across QA Form for each positive finding. Draw vertical lines down QA Form for each action taken. Count the dots that are intersected by both horizontal and vertical lines (A:____). Then count all the dots bisected by a horizontal line (B:____). Divide A by B to determine the QA ratio for this medical record.

$$\text{Ratio} = \frac{\text{Rules Followed (A)}}{\text{Rules Called for by Findings (B)}}$$

Findings: If positive, draw a horizontal line across the form

Actions: If done, draw a vertical line done the form

Findings	Skin decontamination (may be performed prehospital)	Protection of health care worker	Avoid emesis and gastric lavage	Charcoal	Evaluation for potential suicidal risk	Evaluation for abuse or neglect	IV access	Cardiac monitor	Supplemental oxygen	Active cooling	ABG/oximetry	Airway management
History												
Dermal exposure?	●	●										
Gastrointestinal exposure—caustics?			●									
Most other toxic substances?				●								
Intentional ingestion?					●							
Accidental ingestion?						●						
Unknown potentially toxic substances?				●								
Physical Examination												
Pulse <60?							●	●				
Pulse >120 (≥ 6 yr), >140(peds <6 yr)?							●	●				
Irregular pulse?								●				
Respirations												
<10 (adults), <xx(peds)? See Attachment A							●	●	●			
>24 (adults), >xx(peds)? See Attachment A							●					
Temperature >40° C?							●			●		
Cyanosis?							●	●	●		●	
Decreased level of consciousness with no gag reflex?							●	●				●

Findings: If positive, draw a horizontal line across the form

Actions: If done, draw a vertical line down the form

Findings	IV access	Supplemental oxygen	Cardiac monitor	Glucose administration/rapid glucose determination	ABG/oximetry	Frequent assessment	Remove	Ventilate	Transfer care to accepting physician	Follow ACEP & other applicable transfer principles	Provide referral for follow-up care	Provide instructions re Rx & reasons to return to ED
Physical Examination												
Unresponsive to painful stimuli?	●	●	●	●	●							
Altered level of consciousness?						●						
Rectal/vaginal drug packets?							●					
Diagnostic Testing												
ABG-hypercapnia?								●				
ABG-hypoxemia?		●										
Disposition												
Admission?									●			
Transfer?										●		
Discharge?											●	●

Totals

Total dots with intersecting horizontal and vertical lines:
A:________

Total dots with horizontal lines:
B:________

QA Ratio = ________

Quick Reference Form: Acute Toxic Ingestion or Dermal or Inhalation Exposure

Solicit and record a history that includes history of exposure and past medical history. Conduct and record a physical exam that includes vital signs (blood pressure, pulse, respirations, temperature), general appearance, weight (if age <6 years), neurologic mental status, cardiovascular, and pulmonary.

Circle line number if yes. **Bolded actions are rules.** Actions not bolded are guidelines.

1. Dermal exposure ..... **skin decontamination (may be performed prehospital)**, **protection of health care worker**, complete disrobing of patient (proper disposal), assess for systemic exposure/toxicity, perform copious eye irrigation with water, decontamination of skin folds/creases
2. Gastrointestinal exposure — caustics ..... **avoid emesis and gastric lavage**, dilute, endoscopy
3. Gastrointestinal exposure — hydrocarbons ..... evaluate neurologic and pulmonary status
4. Most other toxic substances ..... **charcoal**, protection of health care worker, GI decontamination, specific drug or toxic substance levels, radiopaque substances: KUB, drug bezoars, body packers: contrast study
5. Intentional ingestion ..... **evaluation for potential suicidal risk**, patient restraint, patient supervision, psychiatric consultation
6. Accidental ingestion ..... **evaluation for abuse or neglect**, protective service referral
7. Unknown potentially toxic substances ..... **charcoal**, GI decontamination, acetaminophen level, salicylate level, toxicologic blood screen, toxicologic urine screen
8. Inhalation exposure ..... protection of patient and health care worker, supplemental oxygen, humidification, ABG/oximetry/co-oximetry/methemoglobin level/carboxyhemoglobin level, CXR

Physical Examination

9. Pulse <60 ..... **I.V. access**, **cardiac monitor**, supplemental oxygen/ABG/oximetry, EKG
10. Pulse >120 (≥6 years), >140 (peds <6 years) ..... **I.V. access**, **cardiac monitor**, supplemental oxygen/oximetry, ABG/co-oximetry/methemoglobin level/carboxyhemoglobin level, EKG
11. Pulse — irregular ..... **cardiac monitor**, I.V. access, EKG
12. Respirations <10 (adult), <xx (peds) see Attachment A ..... **I.V. access**, **supplemental oxygen**, **cardiac monitor**, intubate, ventilate, rapid glucose determination, ABG/co-oximetry/methemoglobin level/carboxyhemoglobin level, pulse oximetry, opioid antagonist
13. Respirations >24 (adult), >xx (peds) see Attachment A ..... **I.V. access**, supplemental oxygen, cardiac monitor, ABG/oximetry, salicylate level, CXR
14. Temperature >40°C ..... **I.V. access**, **active cooling**, supplemental oxygen, cardiac monitor, assess for neuroleptic malignant syndrome, EKG
15. Temperature <35°C ..... I.V. access, supplemental oxygen, cardiac monitor, rapid glucose determination, EKG, treat hypothermia
16. General appearance — cyanosis ..... **I.V. access**, **supplemental oxygen**, **cardiac monitor**, **ABG/oximetry**, intubate, methemoglobin level, measured oxygen saturation/co-oximetry, CXR, EKG
17. Neurologic — decreased level of consciousness with no gag reflex ..... **I.V. access**, **cardiac monitor**, **airway management**, rapid glucose determination
18. Neurologic — unresponsive to painful stimuli ..... **I.V. access**, **supplemental oxygen**, **cardiac monitor**, **glucose administration/rapid glucose determination**, **ABG/oximetry**, ABG/co-oximetry/carboxyhemoglobin level, toxicologic screen, urinalysis, abdominal x-ray for radiopaque toxic substances, opioid antagonist, thiamine
19. Neurologic — altered level of consciousness ..... **frequent assessment**, rapid glucose determination, carboxyhemoglobin level, opioid antagonist, thiamine
20. Female with reproductive potential ..... assess for pregnancy
21. HEENT — miotic pupils ..... I.V. access, opioid antagonist
22. HEENT — oral burns of mucous membranes ..... endoscopy, avoid emesis and gastric lavage

23. Pulmonary — rales/rhonchi ..... supplemental oxygen, cardiac monitor, ABG/oximetry, CXR
24. Pulmonary — wheezes ..... supplemental oxygen, cardiac monitor, ABG/oximetry, peak expiratory flow, CXR, beta agonist
25. Abdomen — rectal/vaginal drug packets ..... **remove**, abdominal series x-ray, cathartics
26. Abdomen — distended abdomen ..... rectal examination, abdominal series x-ray, orogastric tube
27. Abdomen — distended bladder ..... bladder decompression
28. Skin — pressure sores (erythema/vesicles) bullae ..... assess for rhabdomyolysis/compartment syndrome, carboxyhemoglobin level

Diagnostic Testing

29. ABG — hypercapnia ..... **ventilate**, intubate, opioid antagonist
30. ABG — hypoxemia ..... **supplemental oxygen**, intubate, CXR, EKG
31. Urinalysis — dipstick positive for blood with few or no RBCs on microscopic analysis ..... evaluate/treat for rhabdomyolysis/hemolysis

Disposition

32. Admission ..... **transfer care to accepting physician**
33. Transfer ..... **follow ACEP and other applicable transfer principles**
34. Discharge ..... **provide referral for follow-up care, provide instructions regarding treatment and circumstances that require return to ED**, social services/protective services consult

Abbreviations

ABG = arterial blood gas
CXR = chest x-ray
ED = Emergency Department
EKG = electrocardiogram
GI = gastrointestinal
KUB = kidney, ureter, and bladder

COMPATIBILITY OF MEDICATIONS MIXED IN A SYRINGE

	Atropine	Chlorpromazine	Codeine	Diphenhydramine	Droperidol	Fentanyl	Glycopyrrolate	Hydroxyzine	Meperidine	Metoclopramide	Midazolam	Morphine	Pentazocine	Pentobarbital†	Prochlorperazine	Promazine	Promethazine	Trimethobenzamide
Atropine		C	•	C	C	C	C	C	C	C	C	C	C	C	C	C	C	•
Chlorpromazine	C		•	C	C	C	C	C	C	C	C	C	C	X	C	C	C	•
Codeine	•	•		•	•	•	C	C	•	•	•	•	•	X	•	•	•	•
Diphenhydramine	C	C	•		C	C	C	C	C	C	C	C	C	X	C	C	C	•
Droperidol	C	C	•	C		C	C	C	C	C	C	C	C	X	C	C	C	•
Fentanyl	C	C	•	C	C		C	C	C	C	C	C	C	X	C	C	C	•
Glycopyrrolate	C	C	C	C	C	C		C	C	•	C	C	X	X	C	C	C	C
Hydroxyzine	C	C	C	C	C	C	C		C	C	C	C	C	X	C	C	C	•
Meperidine	C	C	•	C	C	C	C	C		C	C	X	C	X	C	C	C	•
Metoclopramide	C	C	•	C	C	C	•	C	C		C	C	C	•	C	C	C	•
Midazolam	C	C	•	C	C	C	C	C	C	C		C	•	X	X	C	C	C
Morphine	C	C	•	C	C	C	C	C	C	C	C		C	X	C*	C	C	•
Pentazocine	C	C	•	C	C	C	C	C	C	C	•	C		X	C	C	C	C
Pentobarbital†	C	X	X	X	X	X	X	X	X	•	X	X	X		X	X	X	•
Prochlorperazine	C	C	•	C	C	C	C	C	C	C	X	C*	C	X		C	C	•
Promazine	C	C	•	C	C	C	C	C	C	C	C	C	C	X	C		C	•
Promethazine	C	C	•	C	C	C	C	C	C	C	C	C	C	X	C	C		•
Trimethobenzamide	•	•	•	•	•	•	C	•	•	•	C	•	C	•	•	•	•	

C = Physically compatible if used within 15 minutes after mixing in a syringe

X = Incompatible

• = No documented information

C* = Potential incompatibility produced by certain manufacturers

† = Compatibility profile is characteristic of most barbiturate salts, such as phenobarbital and secobarbital

The following combinations have been found to be compatible:

atropine / meperidine / promethazine
atropine / meperidine / hydroxyzine
meperidine / promethazine / chlorpromazine

The following drugs should not be mixed with any other drugs in the same syringe:

diazepam, chlordiazepoxide

DISCOLORATION OF FECES DUE TO TOXINS

Black
Acetazolamide
Aconitine
Alcohols
Alkalies
Aminophylline
Aminopyrine
Aminosalicylic acid
Amphetamine
Amphotericin
Amyl alcohol
Antacids
Anticoagulants
Arsenic
Aspirin
Barium
Benzene
Betamethasone
Bismuth
Bismuth sodium
Blackberries
Boric acid
Bromides
Carmine
Charcoal
Chloramphenicol
Chlorophenothane
Chlorpropamide
Chocolate
Cinchophen
Clindamycin
Copper
Corticosteroids
Cortisone
Cyclophosphamide
Cytarabine
Dicumarol
Digitalis
Dipyrone
Dithiazanine iodine
Ethacrynic acid
Fenoprofen
Ferrous salts
Floxuridine
Fluorouracil
Fluroxene
Formaldehyde
Halothane
Heparin
Hetacilline
Histamine
Huckleberries
Hydralazine
Hydrocortisone
Hypochlorites
Ibufenac
Ibuprofen
Indomethacin
Iodine drugs
Iron salts
Isopropanol
Lead
Levarterenol
Levodopa
Lincomycin
Lipomul
Manganese
Mefenamic acid
Melphalan
Methylprednisolone
Methotrexate
Methylene blue
Nitrates

Black *(cont)*
Novobiocin
Oxalate
Oxyphenbutazone
Paraldehyde
Paramethadione
Paramethasone
Phenacetin
Phenolphthalein
Phenylbutazone
Phenylephrine
Phosphorous
Potassium salts
Prednisolone
Procarbazine
Pyrazolones
Pyrvinium
Reserpine
Salicylates
Silver
Sulfonamides
Sulthiame
Tetracycline
Thallium
Theophylline
Thioglycollamate
Thiotepa
Triamcinolone
Warfarin

Blue
Boric acid (ingested)
Chloramphenicol
Diathiazine
Manganese dioxide
Methylene blue

Blue-Green
Boric acid
Dithiazanine

Clay/Putty
Barium
Carbon tetrachloride
Cocoa
Kerosene

Dark Brown
Chloride
Cocoa
Danthron
Dexamethasone
Manganese dioxide
Mercurous chloride

Gray
Cocoa
Colchicine
Dithiazanine

Green
Beets
Dithiazanine iodine
Indocyanine green
Indomethacin
Iron
Medroxyprogesterone
Mercurous chloride
Spinach

Greenish Gray
Oral antibiotics
Oxyphenbutazone
Phenylbutazone

Light Brown
Anticoagulants
Milk

Orange-Red
Phenazopyridine
Pyrivinium
Rifampin

Pink
Anticoagulants
Aspirin
Heparin
Manganese dioxide
Oxyphenbutazone
Phenylbutazone
Salicylates

Red
Anticoagulants
Aspirin
Barium
Blackberries
Carmine
Cocoa
Heparin
Hydroxocobalamin
Lead
Oxyphenbutazone
Phenolphthalein
Phenylbutazone
Pyrvinium pamoate
Salicylates
Sulfobromopthalein
Tetracycline syrup
Tomatoes

Red-Brown
Clofazimine palmitate
Hematoxylin
Oxyphenbutazone
Phenylbutazone
Rifampin

Tan
Mercury

Tarry
Ergot preparations
Ibuprofen
Salicylates
Warfarin

White/Speckling
Aluminum hydroxide
Antibiotics (oral)
Barium
Indocyanine green

Yellow
Acetanilid
Mercurous chloride
Milk
Rhubarb
Santonin
Senna

Yellow-Green
1,8-Dihydroxyanthraquinone
Gold
Mercurous chloride
Rhubarb
Santonin
Senna

Adapted from Drugdex® — Drug Consults, Micromedex, vol 81, Denver, CO: Rocky Mountain Drug Consultation Center, August, 1994, and Knoben JE and Anderson PO, *Handbook of Clinical Drug Data*, 7th ed, Hamilton, IL: Drug Intelligence Publication, 1993, 22.

DISCOLORATION OF URINE DUE TO TOXINS

Amber
Trinitrotoluene

Black
Cascara
Cresols
Fava bean
Ferrous salts
Iron dextran
Levodopa
Methocarbamol
Methyldopa
Naphthalene
Pamaquine
Phenacetin
Phenols
Pyrogallol
Rhubarb
Quinine
Sulfonamides
Thymol

Blue
Anthraquinone
Arbuth
Azuresin
Carbolic acid
Dithiazanine iodide
Evans blue
Indigo blue
Indigo carmine
Methocarbamol
Methylene blue
Mitoxantrone
Nitrofurans
Resorcinol
Tetrahydronaphthalene
Thymol
Tolonium
Triamterene

Blue-Green
Amitriptyline
Anthraquinone
Arbutin
Azuresin
Blutene
Boric acid
Carbolic acid
DeWitt's pills
Dithiazanine iodide
Doan's® pills
Indigo blue
Indigo carmine
Magnesium salicylate
Methylene blue
Resorcinol
Tetrahydronaphthalene
Thymol
Tolonium

Brown
Aminopyrine
Aniline
Anthraquinone dyes
Cascara
Chloroquine
Cinchophen
Cresols
Danthron
Dipyrone
Eosin dyes
Furazolidone
Furoxone®
Hydroquinone
Levodopa
Methocarbamol
Methyldopa

Brown *(cont)*
Metronidazole
Naphthalene
Nitrofurans
Nitrofurantoin
Pamaquin
Phenacetin
Phenols
Phenylhydrazine
Primaquine
Pyrogallol
Quinine
Rifampin
Rhubarb
Riboflavin
Senna
Sodium diatrizoate
Sulfonamides
Tannins
Thymol

Brown-Black
Quinine

Brown-Green
Hydroquinone

Dark
p-Aminosalicylic acid
Analine
Cadmium
Cascara
Chlorobenzenes
Chloronaphthalene
Dacium
Ferrous salts
Furazolidone
Furoxone®
Hydroquinone
Iron sorbitex
Levodopa
Metronidazole
Naphthol
Nitridazol
Nitrites
Nitrobenzene
Para-aminosalicylic acid
Phenacetin
Phenol
Phenyl salicylate
Primaquine
Pyrogallol
Quinine
Resorcinol
Rhubarb
Riboflavin
Senna
Thymol
Trinitrophenol
Trinitrotoluene

Fluorescent
Acriflavine (green)
Merbromin (pink)
Triamterene (blue)

Green
Acriflavine
Anthraquinone
Antipyrine
Arbutin
Azuresin
Bromeform
Carbolic acid
Creosote
DeWitt's pills
Guaiacol
Hydroquinone

Green *(cont)*
Indigo blue
Indigo carmine
Indomethacin
Methocarbamol
Methylene blue
Mitoxantrone
Nitrofurans
Phenols
Phenyl salicylate
Pyrogallo
Resorcinol
Santonin
Suprofen
Tetrahydronaphthalene
Thymol

Green-Yellow
Bromoform
DeWitt's pills
Methylene blue

Milky
Phosphates

Orange
Anisindione
Canthaxanthines
Chlorzoxazone
Chrysophanic acid
Dihydroergotamine mesylate
Diphenadione
Ethoxazene
Heparin sodium
Monnose
Paprika
Phenazopyridine
Phenindione
Rifampin
Rhubarb
Riboflavin
Salicylazosulfapyridine
Sulfasalazine
Warfarin

Orange-Brown
Furazolidone
Ethoxazene

Orange-Red
Anisindione
Chlorzoxazone
Doxidan with PSP
Ethoxazene
Phenazopyridine
Phenindione
Rifampin

Orange-Yellow
Fluorescein sodium
Riboflavin
Rifampin
Sulfasalazine

Pale
Chlorosis

Pink
Aminopyrine
Anisindione
Anthraquinone dyes
Chrysophanic acid
Cinchophen
Danthron
Deferoxamine
1,8-Dihydroxyanthraquinone
Dipyrone
Emodin
Eosin dyes

Pink *(cont)*
Ethoxazine
Merbromin
Phenindione
Phenolphthalein
Phenothiazines
Phensuximide
Phenytoin
Porphyrins
Salicylates
Santonin
Selenium
Thiazolsulfone
Urates

Red
Acetanilid
Aminopyrine
Aniline
Anthraquinone
Antipyrine
Beets
Blackberries
Cardiografin
Cascara
Chrysarobin
Chrysophanic acid
Cinchophen
Danthson
Daunorubicin
Deferoxamine mesylate
Dihydroergotamine mesylate
1,8-Dihydroxyanthraquinone
Dimethyl sulfoxide
Dipyrone
DMSO
Doxorubicin
Emodin
Eosin dyes
Ethoxazene
Fava bean
Fuscin
Heparin
Ibuprofen
Idarubicin
Logwood
Methyldopa
Naphthalene
Oxyphenbutazone
Phenacetin
Phenazopyridine
Phenolphthalein
Phenothiazines
Phensuximide
Phenylbutazone
Phenytoin
Porphyphenazone
Rhodamine
Riboflavin
Rifampin
Santonin
Senna
Selenium

Red *(cont)*
Sulfonal
Thiazolsulfone
Trinitrotoluene
Trional
Urates
Uroerythrin

Red-Brown
Aloin
Aminopyrine
Anisindione
Antipyrine
Beets
Benzene
Carbon tetrachloride
Cascara
Chrysarobin
Chrysophanic acid
Clofazimine palmitate
Danthron
1,8-Dihydroxyanthraquinone
Dinitrophenol
Dipyrone
Emodin
Fava bean
Lead
Mercury
Methyldopa
Oxyphenbutazone
Pamaquine
Phenacetin
Phenolphthalein
Phenothiazines
Phensuximide
Phenylbutazone
Phenytoin
Picric acid
Propaphenazone
Quinine
Rhubarb
Santonin
Urates

Red-Purple
Chlorzoxazone
Ibuprofen
Phenacetin
Senna

Red-Yellow
Urates

Rust
Acetanilid
Acriflavine
Aloin
Bromoform
Carrots
Cascara
Chloroquine
Furazolidone

Rust *(cont)*
Furoxone®
Metronidazole
Nitrofurantoin
Pamaquine
Phenacetin
Picric acid
Pyrogallol
Quinacrine
Rhubarb
Riboflavin
Santonin
Senna
Sulfonal
Sulfonamides
Trinitrophenol
Trional
Urates

Yellow
Acetanilid
Acriflavine
5-Aminoacridine
Bromoform
Carrots
Nitrofurantoin
Phenacetin
Picric acid
Pyrogallol
Quinacrine
Riboflavin
Santonin
Sulfasalazine
Sulfonal
Trinitrophenol
Trional

Yellow, Bright
Flavine

Yellow-Brown
Aloin
Cascara
Chloroquine
DeWitt's pills
Flurazolidone
Methylene blue
Metronidazole
Nitrofurantoin
Pamaquine
Primaquine
Quinacrine
Rhubarb
Senna
Sulfonamides

Yellow-Pink
Aloin
Cascara
Rhubarb
Senna
Urates

Changes color in contact with hypochlorite: methyldopa (black or red), levodopa (dark), aminosalicylic acid (red).

Adapted from Drugdex® — Drug Consults, Micromedex, vol 81, Rocky Mountain Drug Consultation Center, Denver, CO: August, 1994, and Knoben JE and Anderson PO, *Handbook of Clinical Drug Data*, 7th ed, Hamilton, IL: Drug Intelligence Publication, 1993, 23-4.

DRUGS THAT MAY CAUSE PHOTOSENSITIVITY REACTIONS

Drug	Comments
Amantadine	Single case report, confirmed with patch test
Amiodarone	Incidence may be as high as 76%; usually occurs within first four months of use of the drug
Benzocaine	Two cases; not confirmed in another study
Benzodiazepines	Two well-documented cases (alprazolam, chlordiazepoxide)
Carbamazepine	Photoallergic reaction; incidence is about 0.1%; **even reported with UVA light from a photocopier**
Chloroquine	An incidence of 0.3% in one large study
Clomipramine	Photoallergy confirmed in one case
Coal tar	Causes stinging and burning ("coal smart") within minutes of sun exposure, sometimes followed by hives; avoid sunlight for 24-72 hours after application
Corticosteroids	Two reports
Dacarbazine	Well-documented; a burning sensation may occur in 36%
Dapsone	Two reports
Diltiazem	Two reports
Diphenhydramine	One case reported with oral and one with topical use
Griseofulvin	Rare reaction, but well-documented
Methotrexate	May enhance sunburn if given up to 3 days after sun exposure
Minoxidil	One case report
Nifedipine	Four cases reported
Nonsteroidal anti-inflammatory drugs	Low potential for phototoxic reactions; reported with ibuprofen, aspirin, indomethacin, piroxicam, and naproxen
Phenothiazines	Reported with many drugs in this class, frequency may be highest with chlorpromazine; as high as 3%
Psoralens	Symptoms within 6-12 hours, peak aat 48 hours
Pyrazinamide	Red-brown discoloration on sun-exposed skin
Quinine or quinidine	Photoallergic reaction; cross-sensitivity between these two agents. Note: Quinine found in nonprescription drugs for leg cramps.
Quinolones	Reported with ciprofloxacin, lomefloxacin, ofloxacin, nalidixic acid; incidence may be as high as 10%
Retinoids	Increased tendency to sunburn noted in 25% to 50% of those taking etretinate and 5% taking isotretinoin
Sulfonamides	Reported with oral, topical, and ophthalmic use; low potential with silver sulfadiazine
Sulfonylureas	Three cases reported with three different agents in this class
Sunscreens	Such reactions have been well-documented after exposure to aminobenzoic acid derivatives (eg, Presun®, Tropical Blend®), avobenzone (eg, Shade UVA Guard®), benzophenones (eg, Bain de Soleil®), cinnamates (eg, Bullfrog®, Coppertone®), homosalates (eg, Coppertone®, Tropical Blend®), and methyl anthranilate (eg, Hawaiian Tropic®, Neutrogena®)
Tetracyclines	Phototoxic; incidence with minocycline may be lowest
Thiazide diuretics	Very uncommon, suggesting photoallergic reactions
Triamterene	Single case
Trimethoprim	Single case

Adapted with permission from Allen JE, "Drug-Induced Photosensitivity," *Clin Pharm*, 1993, 12:580-7.

Used with permission *New Developments in Medicine & Drug Therapy*, Glenview, IL: Physicians & Scientists Publishing Co, Inc, 1994.

EMERGENCY ADULT DRUG DOSAGES

Drug and Strength	Recommended I.V. Doses	Comments and Preparation for Infusion
Adenosine 3 mg/mL	Adult: 6 mg bolus I.V. followed by 12 mg	May repeat the 12 mg dose.
Aminophylline 500 mg/20 mL	Load 5.6 mg/kg then infusion at 0.4-0.8 mg/kg/h IBW or less based upon patient status	Give ½ loading dose if previous theophylline on board and no signs of toxicity. Give load slowly in 50-100 mL over 30-60 minutes. Max rate 25 mg/min. Can antagonize adenosine.
Amrinone	75 mg/kg over 3 minutes	2-10 mcg/kg/min. Effective against calcium channel blocker induced hypotension. Do not mix in dextrose.
Atropine 1 mg/10 mL 1 mg/1 mL	0.5 mg increments I.V. push up to 2 mg max. May give ET.	Initial slowing of rate with small doses (<0.4 mg)
Bretylium 500 mg/10 mL	For resistant ventricular fibrillation or ventricular tachycardia 5 mg/kg I.V. push. If ineffective in 10 minutes and after 1 or more DC shocks, give 10 mg/kg. May repeat to maximum of 30 mg/kg total. If effective begin drip at 1-2 mg/min.	Rapid I.V. infusion may cause nausea and vomiting. May cause transient HTN, PVCs, or other arrhythmia. Hypotension is most frequent side effect. May accumulate in renal failure. Not recommended in digitalis toxicity. Initial response may take up to 60 minutes in ventricular tachycardia. Infusion: mix 1 g/500 mL = 2 mg/mL.
Calcium salts Ca chloride 5 mL = 7 mEq (1.3 mEq/mL) Ca gluconate 10 mL = 5 mEq (0.5 mEq/mL)	0.5-1 g I.V.	May repeat every 10 minutes. Give cautiously in digitalis toxicity. Inactivated by blood products. Precipitates with sodium bicarbonate. Current ACLS guidelines do not recommend routine administration.
Dexamethasone 20 mg/5 mL	Variable. Cerebral edema: 10 mg I.V. initially.	I.V. push over 30 seconds.
Dextrose 25 g/50 mL	50 mL I.V. push for hypoglycemia	
Diazepam 10 mg/2 mL	Initially 5-10 mg. May repeat prn.	Max 5 mg/min I.V. push; propylene glycol solvent. Cardiorespiratory toxicity with rapid administration.
Digoxin 0.5 mg/2 mL	0.125-0.5 mg I.V.	Give slowly 0.25 mg/min; propylene glycol solvent. I.V. push may increase systemic vascular resistance.
Diltiazem 25 mg/5 mL 50 mg/lU/mL	0.25 mg/kg I.V. over 2 minutes	May give a second dose of 0.35 mg/kg I.V. after 15 minutes; may give continuous infusion rate of 5-15 mg/hour for no longer than 24 hours
Diphenhydramine 50 mg/mL	Max 100 mg I.V. over 60 seconds.	I.V. administration with epinephrine for anaphylaxis; or for drug induced extrapyramidal reactions.

(continued)

Drug and Strength	Recommended I.V. Doses	Comments and Preparation for Infusion
Dobutamine 250 mg/vial	Infusion only. Initial infusion 2.5-10 mcg/kg/min.	Increases cardiac output and heart rate. Titrate to patient's response. Recommend close hemodynamic monitoring. Mix 500 mg in 500 mL = 1000 mcg/mL.
Dopamine 400 mg/5 mL 800 mg/5 mL	Infusion only. 1-5 mcg/kg/min: ↑ renal blood flow only. 5-10 mcg/kg/min: ↑ CO, < >HR, ↑ RBF. >10 mcg/kg/min: ↑ CO, ↑ HR, ↓ RBF. >20 mcg/kg/min: ↑ CO, ↑ HR, ↑ SVR, ↓ RBF. Above are approximate ranges only.	Infusion: 400 mg in 250 mL = 1600 mcg/mL (double strength); titrate to BP. Increasing dose increases potential for tachyarrhythmia. Not effective for ethanol-disulfiram induced hypotension.
Epinephrine 1:10,000 10 mL 1:1000 30 mL	0.5-1 mg push every 5 min; may give intracardiac or in ET tube. Initial infusion 1-4 mcg/min.	Stimulates heart, increases BP, and coarsens ventricular fibrillation. Infusion: 2 mg in 500 mL = 4 mcg/mL; titrate to BP. Avoid in solvent exposures.
Esmolol 250 mg/mL	Loading dose 500 mcg/kg/min for 1 minute	50-300 mcg/kg/min
Furosemide 40 mg/4 mL 100 mg/10 mL	Variable	Initiate at 20-40 mg I.V. push over 1-2 minutes. Larger doses, maximum rate = 500 mg over 30 minutes diluted. Rapid administration may lead to ototoxicity.
Heparin 1000 units/mL	80 units/kg IBW I.V. push for PE or DVT. Start constant infusion — 18 units/kg IBW/h.	Caution in elderly patients or patients with bleeding potential. If patient weight is less than IBW, then base dose on actual weight.
Hydrocortisone 1 g	Variable dosing. Shock: 50 mg/kg I.V. initially.	If dose >500 mg, give over several minutes.
Isoproterenol 1 mg/5 mL 0.2 mg/mL	Infusion initial 1-4 mcg/min. I.V. push initial 0.02-0.04 mg. May repeat with up to 0.2 mg every 5 minutes. May use 0.1 mg I.V. push to counter 1 mg I.V. propranolol.	Used in complete heart block prior to pacer. May cause tachyarrhythmias. May have varied effect on BP. Infusion: mix 2 mg in 500 mL = 4 mcg/mL; titrate to BP. I.V. push: dilute 1 mg of 1:5000 with 9 mL of NS = 0.02 mg/mL.
Lidocaine 100 mg/5 mL 2 g/50 mL	Initial 0.5-1 mg/kg I.V. push — may give ET. May repeat 0.5-1.0 mg/kg every 10 min to maximum load. Begin infusion at 1-4 mg/min.	Infusion: mix 2 g in 500 mL = 4 mg/mL. Maximum load: 200-300 mg over 1 h. Severe adverse effects include respiratory depression, seizures, psychosis, and arrhythmias. May exacerbate cocaine-induced seizures.
Metaraminol 100 mg/10 mL	0.1-5.0 mg I.V. push. Initial infusion = 0.1-0.4 mg/min.	Mix 100 mg/500 mL = 0.2 mg/mL; titrate to BP. For direct I.V. push, dilute 1 mg (0.1 mL) in 9.9 mL NS (0.1 mg/mL). Direct/indirect acting alpha adrenergic agonist.

(continued)

Drug and Strength	Recommended I.V. Doses	Comments and Preparation for Infusion
Methylprednisolone 1 g	Variable	100-1000 mg given over 5-minute period.
Midazolam	0.4-0.6 mcg/kg/min	1-12 mcg/kg/min infusion
Naloxone 0.4 mg/mL	0.4 mg to 2 mg I.V. push, may repeat every 2 to 3 minutes, as needed.	Short-acting, may need to repeat frequently. If no response after 10 mg total, re-evaluate diagnosis of narcotic overdose.
Nitroglycerin	0.5-10 mcg/kg/min infusion	In glass container with special "Nitro" tubing.
Nitroprusside	0.5-10 mcg/kg/min infusion	Protect from light.
Norepinephrine 4 mg/4 mL	Infusion only: initial 1-4 mcg/min.	Infusion: mix 8 mg in 500 mL = 16 mcg/mL; titrate to BP. Infiltration causes tissue necrosis (reverse with 5-10 mg Regitine® I.V. around infiltrated site).
Phenytoin 100 mg/2 mL	Load: 15 mg/kg IBW to maximum 1 g. Maximum rate 50 mg/min I.V. push.	Reduce if phenytoin on board already. Useful in digoxin or tricyclic antidepressant toxic arrhythmias. Propylene glycol solvent can cause cardiotoxicity with rapid infusion. Must infuse with NS or ½ NS. Not soluble in D_5W.
Potassium chloride 40 mEq/20 mL	Recommend infusion only. Usual maximum by infusion 10-40 mEq/h for short periods.	Rates >10 mEq/h require EKG monitoring. Too rapid I.V. infusion may cause heart block or asystole. I.V. push not recommended.
Procainamide 100 mg/mL 1000 mg/2 mL	Maximum 50 mg/min up to total of 1 g. Initial infusion 2-6 mg/min.	Reduce loading dose if procainamide on board already. Infusion: mix 2 g in 500 mL = 4 mg/mL. Do not use in tricyclic induced ventricular arrhythmia.
Propranolol 1 mg/mL	Maximum 1 mg/min up to total dose 5 mg.	Beta blocker. Decreases AV conduction. Adverse reactions: heart block, hypotension, heart failure, and bronchospasm (may be reversed with isoproterenol). Caution in patients with verapamil on board.
Sodium bicarbonate 50 mEq/50 mL	Initially 1 mEq/kg then 0.5 mEq/kg every 10 minutes. For tricyclic induced ventricular arrhythmia, dose is 1-3 mEq/kg.	Indicated only in hypoxemic arrest. Excessive amounts lead to alkalosis, hyperosmolality. Doses should be determined by repeat ABGs.
Terbutaline	2 mcg/kg I.V. over 5 minutes. Infusion is 0.1-2 mcg/kg/min.	
Verapamil 5 mg/2 mL	2.5-10 mg slow I.V. push initial. May repeat dose every 15-30 minutes.	Give over 3 minutes in older patients. Caution in patients with beta blocker or digitalis on board. Contraindicated in patients with second or third degree AV block, sick sinus syndrome, or shock. Hypotension may be controlled with metaraminol.

EMERGENCY PEDIATRIC DRUG DOSAGES

Drug	Dose
Adenosine	40-50 mcg/kg. Increase by 40 mcg/kg increments to conversion.
Albumin 5% injection	5-10 mL/kg, may repeat in 15 min
Atropine injection 0.1 mg/mL	0.02 mg/kg q 5 min (min = 0.1 mg) Max total dose: 0.04 mg/kg or 2 mg, whichever is smaller
Bretylium injection 50 mg/mL	1st dose: 5 mg/kg 2nd dose: 10 mg/kg q 15-30 min Max total dose: 30 mg/kg
Calcium chloride injection 100 mg/mL	0.2-0.5 mL/kg q 10 min **Note:** Role in resuscitation questionable, should only be used when hyperkalemia, hypermagnesemia, hypocalcemia, or calcium channel blocker toxicity is present
Dextrose 50% injection 0.5 g/mL	0.5 g/kg or (2 mL/kg of dextrose 25%) **Warning:** Dilute to a 25% solution before administration
Diazepam 10 mg/2 mL	0.2-0.5 mg/kg
Dobutamine injection 12.5 mg/mL	I.V. infusion: 2.5-20 mcg/kg/min
Dopamine injection 40 mg/mL	I.V. infusion: 2.5-20 mcg/kg/min
Epinephrine injection 1:10,000	0.01-0.02 mg/kg q 5 min Max dose: 0.5-1 mg I.V. infusion: 0.1-1.5 mcg/kg/min
Furosemide injection	0.5-1 mg/kg as needed
Isoproterenol injection 0.2 mg/mL	I.V. infusion: 0.05-1 mcg/kg/min (rarely >0.5 mcg/kg/min)
Lidocaine injection 10 mg/mL	0.5-1 mg/kg loading dose (total dose not greater than 3 mg/kg) I.V. infusion: 20-50 mcg/kg/min
Naloxone injection 0.4 mg/mL or 1 mg/mL	Birth to 5 y or 20 kg: 0.1 mg/kg/dose >5 y or 20 kg: 2 mg/dose May repeat doses q 2-3 minutes
Propranolol 1 mg/mL	0.1 mg/kg slowly May repeat in 2 minutes
Sodium bicarbonate injection 1 mEq/mL or 0.5 mEq/mL	1 mEq/kg x 1 may repeat with 0.5 mEq/kg **Warning:** Use only the 0.5 mEq/mL solution for neonates or dilute 1 mEq/mL solution 1:1 with sterile water for injection. **Note:** $NaHCO_3$ should be used based on documented metabolic acidosis. Routine use in cardiac arrest is not recommended.
Terbutaline	2 mcg/kg over 5 minutes Infusion is 0.1-2 mcg/kg/min
Verapamil	0.1-0.2 mg/kg up to 5 mg

EMERGENCY MANAGEMENT OF CAUSTIC AGENTS

Emergency Management Outline:
(1) Household Cleaning Product Ingestion

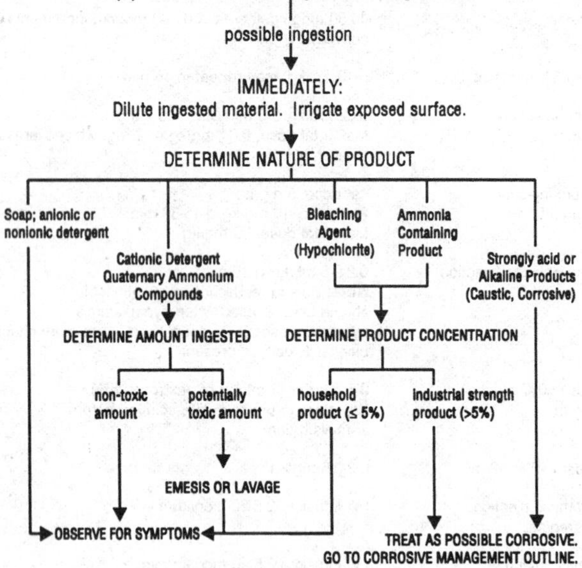

possible ingestion

IMMEDIATELY:
Dilute ingested material. Irrigate exposed surface.

DETERMINE NATURE OF PRODUCT

Soap; anionic or nonionic detergent

Cationic Detergent Quaternary Ammonium Compounds

Bleaching Agent (Hypochlorite)

Ammonia Containing Product

Strongly acid or Alkaline Products (Caustic, Corrosive)

DETERMINE AMOUNT INGESTED

DETERMINE PRODUCT CONCENTRATION

non-toxic amount

potentially toxic amount

household product (≤ 5%)

industrial strength product (>5%)

EMESIS OR LAVAGE

OBSERVE FOR SYMPTOMS

TREAT AS POSSIBLE CORROSIVE.
GO TO CORROSIVE MANAGEMENT OUTLINE.

(2) Corrosive (Caustic, Acid) Ingestion

possible ingestion

IMMEDIATELY: Dilute ingested material. Irrigate exposed surfaces.
REVIEW HISTORY: Clarify ingredients of product. Determine concentration. Determine if exposure was real.

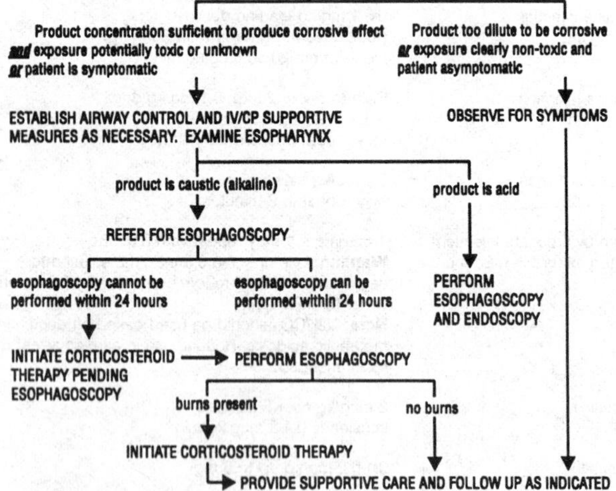

Reprinted with permission from Temple AR and Spoerke DG, "Cleaning Products and Their Accidental Exposure," The Soap and Detergent Association, New York, NY, 1989, Sixth Edition, 26-7.

EXTRAVASATION TREATMENT

Medication Extravasated	Cold/Warm Pack	Antidote
CHEMOTHERAPEUTIC AGENTS		
Anthracyclines		
Daunorubicin Doxorubicin	Cold	DMSO (Rimso®-50) Topical application of 1-2 mL of DMSO 50% Dexamethasone (4 mg) or hydrocortisone (50-200 mg) either subcutaneously or intradermally into extravasation site can also be utilized
Vinca Alkaloids		
Etoposide Vinblastine Vincristine Vindesine Vinorelbine	Warm	Hyaluronidase (Wydase®) 1. Add 1 mL NS to 150-unit vial to make 150 units/mL concentration 2. Mix 0.1 mL of above with 0.9 mL NS in 1 mL syringe to make final concentration = 15 units/mL 3. Inject 5 injections of 0.2 mL each with a 25 G needle into area of extravasation Dexamethasone (4 mg) or hydrocortisone (50-200 mg) either subcutaneously or intradermally into extravasation site can also be utilized
Alkylating and Other Vesicant Chemotherapeutic Agents		
Actinomycin D Mechlorethamine (nitrogen mustard) Mitomycin-C	Cold	Sodium thiosulfate 1/6 molar solution: mix 4 mL of 10% sodium thiosulfate with 6 mL of sterile water injected with fine hypodermic needle into area of extravasation; use ice
VASOPRESSORS		
Dobutamine Dopamine Epinephrine Norepinephrine Phenylephrine	None	Phentolamine (Regitine®) Mix 5-10 mg with 9-10 mL of NS Inject a small amount of this dilution into extravasated area. Blanching should reverse immediately. Monitor site. If blanching should recur, additional injections of phentolamine dilution may be needed.
I.V. FLUIDS AND OTHER MEDICATIONS		
Aminophylline Calcium Dextrose 10% Nafcillin Parenteral nutrition prep Potassium Radiocontrast media	Cold	Hyaluronidase (Wydase®) 1. Add 1 mL NS to 150-unit vial to make 150 units/mL concentration 2. Mix 0.1 mL of above with 0.9 mL NS in 1 mL syringe to make final concentration = 15 units/mL 3. Inject 5 injections of 0.2 mL each with a 25 G needle into area of extravasation

FACTORS AFFECTING PLASMA LEVELS OBTAINED FOR COMMON DRUGS

Agent	Increased Levels	Decreased Levels
Aminoglycosides (amikacin, gentamicin, tobramycin)	Renal dysfunction, reduced volume of distribution (VD)	Pregnancy and early postpartum, ascites, burns
Carbamazepine	Enzyme inhibitors (eg, erythromycin, INH, propoxyphene)	Pregnancy, enzyme inducers (eg, phenytoin)
Digoxin	Renal dysfunction, severe CHF, hypothyroidism, drug intoxins	Malabsorption, hyperthyroidism
Lidocaine	CHF, liver disease, severe renal failure	
Lithium	NSAIDs, thiazide diuretics	Theophylline, pregnancy (2nd and 3rd trimester)
Nortriptyline		Pregnancy, other states with increased VD
Phenytoin	Liver disease, disulfiram, INH	Renal failure (measure free levels), alcohol
Procainamide	Renal dysfunction, severe CHF, slow acetylator (NAPA/PA = 0.8 with normal renal function)	Fast acetylators (NAPA/PA = 1.2 with normal renal function)
Quinidine	Severe CHF, liver disease	Enzyme inducers (eg, phenytoin, Pb, rifampin)
Theophylline	CHF, liver disease, cor pulmonale, prolonged fever associated with viral illness, enzyme inhibitors (eg, cimetidine, cipro, verapamil, erythromycin)	Smoking, age <16, enzyme inducers (eg, rifampin, phenobarbital, carbamazepine, phenytoin)
Valproic acid	Liver cirrhosis, hypoalbuminemia	Induction of liver enzymes (Pb, phenytoin)

FOOD-DRUG INTERACTIONS, KEY SUMMARY

Drug	Food	Interaction
Aspirin Captopril Isoniazid Mercaptopurine Methotrexate Methyldopa Penicillin G and V Phenobarbital Propantheline Rifampin Tetracycline	Any food	Decreased absorption
Carbamazepine Hydralazine Lithium Metoprolol Propranolol	Any food	Increased absorption
Cefuroxime	Any food	Increased absorption
Chlorpropamide Disulfiram Griseofulvin Metronidazole Procarbazine Quinacrine Tolazoline	Alcohol	Antabuse reaction consisting of flushing, headache, nausea, and in some patients, vomiting, and chest and/or abdominal pain
Cyclosporine	Many foods Fatty foods	Decreased absorption Increased absorption
Cyclosporine Felodipine	Grapefruit juice	Increased absorption
Erythromycin stearate	Any food	Increased or decreased absorption
Furosemide	Any food	Decreased rate of absorption, potentially decreasing effect
Levodopa	High-protein diet	Decreased absorption
Lithium	Sodium	Enhanced elimination requiring higher doses
MAO inhibitors: Isocarboxazid Phenelzine Procarbazine Tranylcypromine	High-protein foods that have undergone aging, fermentation, pickling, or smoking; aged cheeses, red wines, pods of broad beans and fava beans; bananas, raisins, avocados; caffeine-containing beverages, beer, ale, and chocolate	Elevated blood pressure
Phenobarbital Phenytoin	High doses of vitamin B_6 (pyridoxine) and folic acid	Decreased absorption
Phenobarbital Phenytoin Theophylline Warfarin	Charcoal-broiled foods	Increased metabolism requiring higher doses

(continued)

Drug	Food	Interaction
Phenytoin	Most foods Pudding	Absorption increased by 25% Absorption decreased by 50%
Quinolones (eg, ciprofloxacin) Tetracycline	Iron, calcium, aluminum, zinc, magnesium (eg, dairy products)	Decreased absorption
Warfarin	Diets rich in vitamin K such as cauliflower, spinach, broccoli, turnip greens, liver, beans, rice, pork, fish, and some cheeses	Antagonism of effect

Reprinted with permission from Saltiel E, "Food-Drug Interactions," *New Developments in Medicine & Drug Therapy*, Glenview, IL: Physicians & Scientists Publishing Co, Inc, 1994, 3(4):61.

HALLUCINOGENIC DRUGS

Principal Pharmacological Properties of Hallucinogenic Drugs

Drug; Chemical Structure	Duration of Acute Effect (h)	pKa	Route of Metabolism/ Excretion	Half-Life	Protein Binding (%)	Vd (L/kg)	Urine Screen Positive for	Duration of Psychotropic Effects	Doses of Abuse	Fatal Dose
Phencyclidine (PCP); arylcyclohexylamine	4-6	8.5	Hepatic/urine	1 h	65	6.2-0.3	2 wk	Up to 1 mo	1-9 mg	1 mg/kg
Cocaine; tropane alkaloid	0.5	5.6	Plasma hydrolysis*	48-75 min	9-90	1.2-1.9	144 h	≤5-7 d	20-200 mg (intranasally)	1-1.2 g
Cannabis; monoterpenoid	0.5-3	10.6	Hepatic hydroxylation	25-57 h	97-99	10	Up to 6 d	≤6 h	5-15 mg THC	
LSD; indole alkylamine	0.7-8	7.8	Hepatic hydroxylation	2.5 h		0.27	120 h	May last for days	100-300 μg	0.2 mg/kg
Psilocybin; tryptamine	0.5-6						Not detected	12 h	20-100 mushrooms	5-15 mg of psilocybin
Mescaline; phenylalkylamine	4.6	Not known	Hepatic/urine†	6 h	None	Not known		12 h	5 mg/kg	20 mg/kg
Morphine; alkaloid/derivative of opium	4-5	8.05	Glucuronidation/ urine	1.9-3.1 h	35	3.2	48 h	≤6 h	2-20 mg	Variable — dependent on tolerance, nontolerant fatal dose is 120 mg orally or 30 mg parenterally
Heroin; diacetylmorphine	3.4	7.6	Hepatic‡	3-20 min	40	25	~40 h	≤6 h	2.2 mg	Variable — dependent on tolerance
Amphetamine; b-(phenylisopropyl)-amine	Variable	9.93	Hepatic§	12 h¶	16-20	3-6	2-4 d	Delusions may remain for months	100-1000 mg/d	Variable — dependent on tolerance

Reprinted with permission from Leikin JB et al, "Clinical Feature and Management of Intoxication Due to Hallucinogenic Drugs," *Med Toxicol Adverse Drug Exp*, 1989, 4(5):328.

*By serum cholinesterase.

†60% excreted unchanged.

‡Converted to morphine.

§Converted to phenylacetone.

¶Urine pH-dependent.

Therapeutic Drugs Associated With Hallucinations

Drug	Type of Hallucination
Acyclovir	V, T
Amantadine	A, V
Aminocaproic Acid	A
Amitriptyline	V
Amoxapine	V
Amphetamines	T, V
Asparaginase	V
Baclofen	A, V
Benztropine	V
Biperiden	V
Bromocriptine	A, V
Bupropion	V
Carbamazepine	V
Chlordiazepoxide	V
Chloroquine	V
Chlorpheniramine	A, V
Chlorpromazine	A, V
Cimetidine	A, V
Clonazepam	A, V, T
Clonidine	A, V
Corticosteroids	A, V
Cyclobenzaprine	V
Cyclosporine	V
Dantrolene	A, V
Dapsone	V
Dextromethorphan	A, V
Diethylpropion	A
Digoxin	A, V
Dimenhydrinate	A, V
Diphenhydramine	V
Disopyramide	A, V
Disulfiram	A, V
Doxepin	V
Enoxacin	V
Ephedrine	A, V, T
Erythropoietin	V
Ethambutol	V
Ethchlorvynol	V
Ethosuximide	V
Gentamicin	NS
Griseofulvin	A
Hexamethylamine	V
Hydroxytryptophan	V
Hyoscine (scopolamine)	NS
Imipramine	V
Indomethacin	V, O
Isoniazid	A, V
Isosorbide	V
Isoxsuprine	A
Ketamine	V
Levodopa	A, V
Levothyroxine	V
Lisuride	V
Lithium	V
Lorazepam	V
Maprotiline	V
Mazindol	A
Methyldopa	V
Methylphenidate	V
Methylprednisolone	V
Minocycline	V
Nalidixic Acid	V
Orciprenaline (metaproterenol)	V, G
Oxamniquine	V
Pemoline	A, V, T

(continued)

Drug	Type of Hallucination
Phenelzine	A, V
Phenobarbital	V
Phenylephrine	A, V
Phenytoin	V
Pindolol	A
Piroxicam	A, V
Primidone	V
Procainamide	V
Promethazine	V
Propoxyphene	A
Propranolol	A, V
Quinacrine	V
Quinidine	NS
Ranitidine	A, V
Salicylates	V
Streptokinase	V
Sulfasalazine	V
Tetracycline	V
Theophylline	V
Timolol	NS
Tocainide	V
Triazolam	A, V, T
Trihexyphenidyl	A, V
Vidarabine	NS
Vincristine	V
Zipeprol	A, V

Abbreviations: A = auditory; V = visual; T = tactile; G = gustatory; O = olfactory; NS = not specified.

Reprinted with permission from Leikin JB et al, "Clinical Feature and Management of Intoxication Due to Hallucinogenic Drugs," *Med Toxicol Adverse Drug Exp*, 1989, 4(5):342 and Differential Diagnostic Lists (ie, Dosing and Therapeutic Tools Database, Sullivan CA, Gelman CR, ed) and Micromedex Inc, Englewood, CO.

HEMATOLOGIC ADVERSE EFFECTS OF DRUGS

Drug	Red Cell Aplasia	Thrombo-cytopenia	Neutro-penia	Pancyto-penia	Hemolysis
Acetazolamide		+	+	+	
Allopurinol			+		
Amiodarone	+				
Amphotericin B				+	
Amrinone		++			
Asparaginase		+++	+++	+++	++
Barbiturates		+		+	
Benzocaine					++
Captopril			++		+
Carbamazepine		++	+		
Cephalosporins			+		++
Chloramphenicol		+	++	+++	
Chlordiazepoxide			+	+	
Chloroquine		+			
Chlorothiazides		++			
Chlorpropamide	+	++	+	++	+
Chlortetracycline				+	
Chlorthalidone			+		
Cimetidine		+	++	+	
Codeine		+			
Colchicine				+	
Cyclophosphamide		+++	+++	+++	+
Dapsone					+++
Desipramine		++			
Digitalis		+			
Digitoxin		++			
Erythromycin		+			
Estrogen		+		+	
Ethacrynic acid			+		
Fluorouracil		+++	+++	+++	+
Furosemide		+	+		
Gold salts	+	+++	+++	+++	
Heparin		++		+	
Ibuprofen			+		+
Imipramine			++		
Indomethacin		+	++	+	
Isoniazid		+		+	
Isosorbide dinitrate					+
Levodopa					++
Meperidine		+			
Meprobamate		+	+	+	
Methimazole			++		
Methyldopa		++			+++
Methotrexate		+++	+++	+++	++
Methylene blue					+

(continued)

Drug	Red Cell Aplasia	Thrombo-cytopenia	Neutro-penia	Pancyto-penia	Hemolysis
Metronidazole			+		
Nalidixic acid					+
Naproxen				+	
Nitrofurantoin			++		+
Nitroglycerine		+			
Penicillamine		++	+		
Penicillins		+	++	+	+++
Phenazopyridine					+++
Phenothiazines		+	++	+++	+
Phenylbutazone		+	++	+++	+
Phenytoin		++	++	++	+
Potassium iodide		+			
Prednisone		+			
Primaquine					+++
Procainamide			+		
Procarbazine		+	++	++	+
Propylthiouracil		+	++	+	+
Quinidine		+++	+		
Quinine		+++	+		
Reserpine		+			
Rifampicin		++	+		+++
Spironolactone			+		
Streptomycin		+		+	
Sulfamethoxazole with trimethoprim			+		
Sulfonamides	+	++	++	++	++
Sulindac	+	+	+	+	
Tetracyclines		+			+
Thioridazine			++		
Tolbutamide		++	+	++	
Triamterene					+
Valproate	+				
Vancomycin			+		

+ = rare or single reports.
++ = occasional reports.
+++ = substantial number of reports.

Adapted from D'Arcy PF and Griffin JP, eds, *Iatrogenic Diseases*, New York, NY: Oxford University Press, 1986, 128-30.

IMPAIRED RENAL FUNCTION DOSING, ADULTS

Drug	Cl_{cr} (mL/min)	Suggested Dosage Regimen	Supplement for Dialysis	
			Hemo-dialysis	Peritoneal Dialysis
Acyclovir (I.V.)	>50	5–10 mg/kg q8h	Yes	—
	25–50	5–10 mg/kg q12h		
	10–25	5–10 mg/kg q24h		
Amantadine (P.O.)	>80	100 mg bid	No	No
	60–80	200 mg/100 mg alternating daily		
	40–60	100 mg/d		
	30–40	200 mg 2 times/wk		
	20–30	100 mg 3 times/wk		
	10–20	200 mg/100 mg alternating weekly		
Amikacin (I.M., I.V.)	Individualize regimen with serum concentrations.		Yes	Yes
Aminosalicylic acid (P.O.)	>50	150 mg/kg/day in 2-3 divided doses	—	—
	10–50	50%–70%		
	<10	50% of dose		
Amoxicillin (P.O.)	>50	250–500 mg q8h	Yes	No
	10–50	250–500 mg q8–12h		
	<10	250–500 mg q12h		
Amoxicillin clavulanate (P.O.)	>30	250–500 mg q6h	Yes	No
	15–30	250–500 mg q8–12h		
	5–15	250–500 mg q24h		
Amphotericin B (I.V.)	Usual dose: 0.3–0.7 mg/kg q24h; a 1 mg test dose may be administered over 30 minutes with vital sign monitoring over the next hour to assure no anaphylactoid reaction; then remaining full dose may be administered.			
Ampicillin (I.V.)	>50	1–2 g q4–6h	Yes	No
	10–50	1–2 g q6–12h		
	<10	1–2 g q8–12h		
Ampicillin/sulbactam (I.V.)	≥30	1.5–3 g q6–8h	Yes	—
	15–29	1.5–3 g q12h		
	5–14	1.5–3 g q24h		
Atovaquone* (P.O.)	—	750 mg tid	—	—
Azithromycin* (P.O.)	—	500 mg day 1 then 250 mg daily	—	—
Aztreonam (I.V.)	>50	500 mg–2 g q6–8h	Yes	Yes
	10–50	50%–75% of usual dosage		
	10	25% of usual dosage		
Bismuth (P.O.)	See specific indication. Avoid use in renal failure.			
Capreomycin sulfate (I.M.)	>100	13–15 mg/kg q24h	—	—
	80–100	10–13 mg/kg q24h		
	60–80	7–10 mg/kg q24h		
	40–60	11–14 mg/kg q48h		
	20–40	10–14 mg/kg q72h		
	<20	4–7 mg/kg q72h		

*No renal dose adjustment necessary.

(continued)

Drug	Cl_{cr} (mL/min)	Suggested Dosage Regimen	Supplement for Dialysis	
			Hemo-dialysis	Peritoneal Dialysis
Carbenicillin (P.O.)	>50	382–764 mg q8–12h	Yes	—
	10–50	382–764 mg q12–24h		
	10	382–764 mg q24–48h		
Cefaclor (P.O.)	>50	250–500 mg q8h	Yes	Yes
	10–50	125–500 mg q8h		
Cefadroxil monohydrate (P.O.)	>50	500 mg–1 g q12h	Yes	No
	10–50	500 mg q24h		
	<10	500 mg q36h		
Cefamandole nafate (I.V.)	>50	1–2 g q4h	Yes	—
	25–50	1–2 g q8h		
	10–25	1 g q8h		
	<10	1 g q12h		
Cefazolin (I.V.)	>30	1–2 g q8h	Yes	No
	10–30	1 g q12h		
	<10	1 g q24h		
Cefixime (P.O.)	>60	400 mg q24h	—	—
	21–60	300 mg q24h		
	≤20	200 mg q24h		
Cefmetazole sodium (I.V.)	>50	1–2 g q12h	—	—
	30–49	1–2 g q16h		
	10–29	1–2 g q24h		
	<10	1–2 g q48h		
Cefonicid sodium (I.M., I.V.)	>20	1 g q24h	No	No
	10–20	500 mg–1 g q48h		
	<10	250 mg–1 g q72h		
Cefoperazone sodium* (I.M., I.V.)	—	1–2 g q8–12h	No	No
Cefotaxime sodium (I.M., I.V.)	>50	1–2 g q6–8h	Yes	No
	10–50	1–2 g q8–12h		
	<10	1–2 g q24h		
Cefotetan disodium (I.M., I.V.)	>30	1–2 g q12h	Yes	No
	10–30	1–2 g q24h		
	<10	1–2 g q48h		
Cefoxitin sodium (I.M., I.V.)	>50	1–2 g q6–8h	Yes	No
	30–50	1–2 g q8–12h		
	10–30	1–2 g q12–24h		
	<10	500 mg–1 g q24–48h		
Cefpodoxime proxetil (P.O.)	>30	100–200 mg q12h	Yes	—
	<30	100–200 mg q24h		
Cefprozil (P.O.)	≥30	250–500 mg q12–24h	Yes	—
	<30	125–250 mg q12–24h		

*No renal dose adjustment necessary.

(continued)

Drug	Cl_{cr} (mL/min)	Suggested Dosage Regimen	Supplement for Dialysis	
			Hemodialysis	Peritoneal Dialysis
Ceftazidime (I.V.)	>50	1 g q8–12h	Yes	Yes
	30–50	1 g q12h		
	15–30	1 g q24h		
	<15	500 mg–1 g q24h		
Ceftizoxime (I.V.)	>30	1–2 g q8–12h	Yes	—
	10–30	1 g q12h		
	<10	1 g q24h		
Ceftriaxone sodium (I.M., I.V.)*	—	1–2 g q24h	—	—
Cefuroxime (I.V.)	>20	750 mg–1.5 g q8h	Yes	No
	10–20	750 mg q12h		
	<10	750 mg q24h		
Cephalexin (P.O.)	>40	250–500 mg q6h	Yes	Yes
	10–40	250–500 mg q8–12h		
	<10	250 mg q12–24h		
Cephalothin sodium (I.M., I.V.)	>50	500 mg–2 g q4–6h	Yes	No
	10–50	500 mg–1 g q6–8h		
	<10	500 mg–1 g q12h		
Cephapirin sodium (I.M., I.V.)	>50	1 g q6h	Yes	No
	10–50	1 g q6–8h		
	<10	1 g q12h		
Cephradine (P.O.)	>50	500 mg q6h	Yes	Yes
	10–50	250 mg q6h		
	<10	250 mg q12h		
Chloramphenicol (I.V.)*	—	0.5–1 g q6h	No	No
Chloroquine (P.O.)	See monograph for dosing information.		No	—
Cinoxacin (P.O.)	>50	250 mg q6–12h	—	—
	20–50	250 mg bid		
	<20	250 mg/d		
Ciprofloxacin (P.O.)	>30	250 mg q12h, 500 mg q12h, or 750 mg q12h	No	No
	<30	500 mg q24h or 750 mg q24h		
Ciprofloxacin (I.V.)	≥30	200–400 mg q12h	No	No
	5–29	200–400 mg q18–24h		
Clarithromycin (P.O.)	>30	250–500 mg bid	—	—
	<30	500 mg loading dose, then 250 mg once daily or bid		

*No renal dose adjustment necessary.

(continued)

Drug	Cl_{cr} (mL/min)	Suggested Dosage Regimen	Supplement for Dialysis	
			Hemo-dialysis	Peritoneal Dialysis
Clindamycin (I.V.)*	—	900 mg q8h	No	No
Clindamycin (P.O.)*	—	150–450 mg q6h	No	No
Cloxacillin sodium (P.O.)*	—	250–500 mg q6h	—	—
Colistimethate (I.M., I.V.)	S_{cr} (mg/dL)		—	—
	0.7–1.2	100–125 mg bid–qid		
	1.3–1.5	75–115 mg bid		
	1.6–2.5	66–150 mg bid or once daily		
	2.6–4	100–150 mg q36h		
Co-trimoxazole† (P.O., I.V.)	>30	5 mg/kg q6–8h	Yes	No
	15–30	2.5–5 mg/kg q12h		
	<15	2.5–5 mg/kg q24h		
Cycloserine (P.O.)	>50	250 mg q12h	—	—
	10–50	250 mg q24h		
	<10	250 mg q36–48h		
Dapsone (P.O.)*	—	100 mg q24h	No	No
Demeclocycline (P.O.)	—	300 mg bid (do not use in renal impairment)		
Dicloxacillin (P.O.)*	—	500 mg q6h	No	—
Didanosine (P.O.)	>60	See individual dosing per body weight range.	—	—
	<60	Consider dosage reduction.		
Doxycycline (P.O., I.V.)	>10	100 mg q12h	No	—
	<10	100 mg q24h		
Eflornithine (P.O.)	>60	100 mg/kg q6h	—	—
	<60	Consider dosage reduction.		
Enoxacin (P.O.)	>30	400 mg bid	—	—
	<30	200 mg bid		
Erythromycin (I.V.)	>10	0.5–1 g q6h	No	No
	<10	250–500 mg q6h		
Erythromycin (P.O.)*	—	250–500 mg q6h	No	No
Ethambutol (P.O.)	>50	15–25 mg/kg q24h	Yes	Yes
	10–50	15 mg/kg q24–36h		
	<10	15 mg/kg q48h		
	—	Maximum dose: 2.5 g/d		
Ethionamide (P.O.)	>50	250–500 mg q12h	—	—
	<50	125–250 mg q12h		
Fluconazole (P.O., I.V.)	>50	100–400 mg loading dose x 1 then ½ loading dose q24h	Yes	—
	20–50	Loading dose then 50% of recommended dose		
	<20	Loading dose then 25% of recommended dose		

*No renal dose adjustment necessary.
†All doses based on trimethoprim.

(continued)

Drug	Cl_{cr} (mL/min)	Suggested Dosage Regimen	Supplement for Dialysis	
			Hemo-dialysis	Peritoneal Dialysis
Flucytosine (P.O.)	>40	12.5–37.5 mg/kg q6h	Yes	—
	20–40	12.5–37.5 mg/kg q12h		
	<20	12.5–37.5 mg/kg q24h		
Foscarnet (I.V.)# (induction)	**(mL/min/kg)**		—	—
	≥1.6	60 mg/kg q8h		
	1.5	57 mg/kg q8h		
	1.4	53 mg/kg q8h		
	1.3	49 mg/kg q8h		
	1.2	46 mg/kg q8h		
	1.1	42 mg/kg q8h		
	1.0	39 mg/kg q8h		
	0.9	35 mg/kg q8h		
	0.8	32 mg/kg q8h		
	0.7	28 mg/kg q8h		
	0.6	25 mg/kg q8h		
	0.5	21 mg/kg q8h		
	0.4	18 mg/kg q8h		
Ganciclovir (I.V.)	>80	5 mg/kg q12h	—	—
	50–80	2.5 mg/kg q12h		
	25–50	2.5 mg/kg q24h		
	<25	1.25 mg/kg q24h		
Gentamicin (I.M., I.V.)	Individualize regimen with serum concentrations.		Yes	Yes
Imipenem/cilastatin (I.V.)	>70	500 mg q6h	Yes	—
	30–70	500 mg q8h		
	20–30	500 mg q12h		
	0–20	250–500 mg q12h		
Isoniazid (P.O., I.V.)*	—	300 mg q24h	Yes	Yes
Itraconazole (P.O.)	—	200 mg once daily	—	—
Kanamycin	Avoid I.V. administration.		—	—
Ketoconazole (P.O.)*	—	200 mg q24h	No	No
Lomefloxacin (P.O.)	>40	400 mg q24h	—	—
	≤40	400 mg 1st dose, then 200 mg once a day		
Loracarbef (P.O.)	>50	200–400 mg q12h	—	—
	10–49	200–400 mg q24h		
	<10	200–400 mg q3–5d		
Mefloquine* (P.O.)	—	See individual dosing for prophylaxis vs treatment.	—	—
Methicillin sodium (I.M., I.V.)	>50	1–2 g q4–6h	No	No
	10–50	1–2 g q6–8h		
	<10	1–2 g q8–12h		
Metronidazole (P.O., I.V.)	>10	250–500 mg q6–8h	Yes	—
	<10	250–500 mg q8–12h		

*No renal dose adjustment necessary.
#See monograph for maintenance dosing.

(continued)

Drug	Cl_{cr} (mL/min)	Suggested Dosage Regimen	Supplement for Dialysis	
			Hemo-dialysis	Peritoneal Dialysis
Mezlocillin sodium (I.M., I.V.)	>30	3–4 g q4–6h	No	No
	10–30	1.5–3 g q6–8h		
	<10	3 g q8h		
Miconazole (I.V.)*	—	400–1200 mg q8h	No	No
Nafcillin sodium (I.M., I.V.)*	—	1–2 g q4–6h	No	No
Neomycin sulfate (P.O.)	Avoid I.V. administration.		—	—
Netilmicin sulfate (I.M., I.V.)	Individualize regimen with serum concentrations.		Yes	Yes
Nitrofurantoin (P.O.)	>50	50–100 mg q6h	—	—
	<50	Avoid use		
Norfloxacin (P.O.)	>30	400 mg q12h	No	—
	<30	400 mg q24h		
Ofloxacin (P.O., I.V.)	>50	200–400 mg q12h	—	—
	10–50	200–400 mg q24h		
	<10	100–200 mg q24h		
Oxacillin (I.V.)*	—	1–2 g q4–6h	No	—
Oxytetracycline (P.O.)	>10	250–500 mg q6h	—	—
	<10	Avoid use		
Penicillin G (I.V.)	>50	2–4 million units q2–4h	Yes	—
	10–50	1–2 million units q4–6h		
	<10	1–2 million units q8–12h or 0.5–1 million units q4–6h		
Penicillin V potassium (P.O.)	>10	250–500 mg q6h	Yes	—
	<10	250 mg q6h		
Pentamidine (I.V.)	>50	4 mg/kg q24h	—	—
	10–50	4 mg/kg q24–36h		
	<10	4 mg/kg q48h		
Piperacillin (I.V.)	>40	3–4 g q4–6h	Yes	—
	20–40	3–4 g q8h		
	<20	3–4 g q12h		
Piperacillin/tazobactam (I.V.)	>40	3.375 g q6h	Yes	Yes
	20–40	2.25 g q6h		
	<20	2.25 g q8h		
Polymyxin B	Avoid I.V. administration.		—	—
Pyrazinamide (P.O.)	—	15–30 mg/kg q24h	—	—
	—	Maximum dose: 2 g/d		
Pyrimethamine (P.O.)*	—	100 mg q24h	—	—
Quinacrine (P.O.)	—	See individual dosing per disease.	—	—
Quinidine*	—	See monograph.	Yes	Yes

*No renal dose adjustment necessary.

(continued)

Drug	Cl_{cr} (mL/min)	Suggested Dosage Regimen	Supplement for Dialysis	
			Hemo-dialysis	Peritoneal Dialysis
Quinine sulfate (P.O.)	>50	650 mg q6–8h	Yes	No
	10–50	650 mg q8–12h		
	<10	650 mg q24h		
Rifampin (P.O., I.V.)*	—	600 mg/d	No	—
Rimantadine (P.O.)	>10	100 mg q12h	—	—
	<10	100 mg q24h		
Spectinomycin hydrochloride (I.M.)*	—	2–4 g q24h	Yes	Yes
Streptomycin sulfate (I.M.)	—	See individual dosing per disease.	Yes	—
Sulfadiazine (P.O.)*	—	1–2 g q6h	—	—
Sulfamethoxazole (P.O.)	>50	1 g q12h	Yes	No
	10–50	1 g q12–24h		
	<10	1 g q24h		
Sulfisoxazole (P.O.)	>50	1–2 g q6h	Yes	No
	10–50	1 g q8–12h		
	<10	1 g q12–24h		
Tetracycline hydrochloride (P.O.)	>50	250–500 mg q6–12h	No	No
	10–50	250–500 mg q12–24h		
	<10	250–500 mg q24h		
Thiabendazole (P.O.)	—	See individual dosing per disease.	—	—
Ticarcillin/clavulanate (I.V.)	>60	3.1 g q4–6h	Yes	Yes
	30–60	3.1 g q8h		
	10–30	3.1 g q12h		
Ticarcillin disodium (I.M., I.V.)	>60	3 g q4h	Yes	No
	30–60	2 g q4h		
	10–30	2 g q8h		
	<10	2 g q12h		
Tobramycin	Individualize regimen with serum concentrations.		Yes	Yes
Trimethoprim (P.O.)	>50	100–200 mg q6h	Yes	—
	10–50	100 mg q12–24h		
	<10	50–100 mg q24h		
Vancomycin (I.V.)	Individualize dosing with serum concentrations; 1 g q12h is usual starting dose in patients with normal renal function.			
Vancomycin (P.O.)*	—	125–250 mg q6h	—	—
Vidarabine (I.V.)	>10	15 mg/kg/d	Yes	—
	<10	75% of usual dosage		
Zalcitabine (P.O.)	>40	0.75 mg q8h	—	—
	10–40	0.75 mg q12h		
	<10	0.75 mg q24h		
Zidovudine	—	100 mg 5 times/d	—	—

*No renal dose adjustment necessary.

INDOOR AIR POLLUTION

Diagnostic Quick Reference to Effects of Indoor Pollutants

Signs and Symptoms	Environmental Tobacco Smoke*	Other Combustion Products	Biological Pollutants	Volatile Organics	Heavy Metals†	Sick Building Syndrome‡
Respiratory						
Rhinitis, nasal congestion	●	●	●	●		●
Epistaxis				●§		
Pharyngitis, cough	●	●	●	●		●
Wheezing, worsening asthma	●	●	●	●		●
Dyspnea	●¶	●	●			●
Severe lung disease						●#
Other						
Conjunctival irritation	●	●	●	●		●
Headache or dizziness	●	●	●	●	●	●
Lethargy, fatigue, malaise		●‖	●**	●	●	●
Nausea, vomiting, anorexia		●‖	●	●	●	
Cognitive impairment, personality change		●‖		●	●	●
Rash			●	●	●	
Fever, chills			●††		●	
Tachycardia		●‖			●	
Retinal hemorrhage		●‖				
Myalgia		●‖		●**	●	●
Hearing loss				●		

Adapted from Ratner D and Carrey Z, "Medical Effects of Indoor Air Pollution," *Hosp Med*, May 1995, 41.

*In infants and children, signs and symptoms include frequent upper respiratory infections, otitis media; persistent middle-ear effusion; asthma onset, increased severity; and recurrent pneumonia, bronchitis.

†In infants and children, signs and symptoms include irritability, abdominal pain, ataxia, seizures, and loss of consciousness.

‡The signs and symptoms listed here are similar to those caused by the contaminants found in household and building materials that are discussed in the text.

§Associated especially with formaldehyde.

¶In asthma.

#Hypersensitivity pneumonitis, Legionnaires' disease.

‖Particularly associated with high CO levels.

**Hypersensitivity pneumonitis, humidifier fever.

††With marked hypersensitivity reactions and Legionnaires' disease.

INVESTIGATIONAL NEW DRUG APPLICATION

A new drug for investigational use in human subjects may not be in interstate commerce unless some responsible individual or firm sponsors clinical studies with the drug and submits an Investigational New Drug (IND) Application (Form FDA-1571)

The application should include the facts that satisfy the sponsor that the agent may be justifiably administered to man as proposed. Thus the claim for exemption should contain information on appropriate prior animal studies for safety evaluation, any available clinical data, adequate drug identification, and manufacturing information necessary to support safety and give significance to a clinical trial, and a detailed outline of the proposed clinical study to include dosage ranges, routes of administration, approximate number of patients involved, and approximate duration of treatment.

The sponsor should provide a statement of the scientific training and experience he will require investigators to demonstrate. Further, the names and a summary of the training experience of each investigator should be a part of the filed application. Where the sponsor himself is the sole investigator, submission of his curriculum vitae may be adequate.

Additionally, the sponsor is required to obtain statements from clinical investigators (Form FDA-1572 for clinical pharmacology and other clinical studies) and retain them in his files. Copies of the completed statements may be included as part of the material filed for an exemption. Specimens of these forms are included.

If a sponsor does not himself perform manufacturing and control operations for new drug substances or final dosage forms, this information (required by parts 1 through 5 of Form FDA-1571) can be furnished on his behalf by suppliers performing those operations. Similarly, a supplier may provide preclinical or clinical study data. The sponsor may forward such supporting information or arrange to have it sent directly to FDA.

The application is to be filed in triplicate with the Food and Drug Administration. The information filed may be in narrative form but should be presented as outlined in the application form. In addition to the name of the drug, please be sure to indicate the dosage form. Mail to:

Food and Drug Administration
Center for Drug Evaluation and Research
Central Documents Room
Park Building, Room 2-14
12420 Parklawn Drive
Rockville, Maryland 20852

Mail in triplicate including cover letter.

FDA Receipt of the IND

Upon receipt of the IND by the FDA, an IND number will be assigned, and the application will be forwarded to the appropriate reviewing division. The reviewing division will send a letter to the Sponsor-Investigator providing notification of the IND number assigned, date of receipt of the original application, address where future submissions to the IND should be sent, and the name and telephone number of the FDA person to whom questions about the application should be directed. Studies may not be initiated until 30 days after the FDA receives the IND.

A study placed on clinical hold may not be conducted under the IND. If the study if placed on clinical hold within the 30-day period, the sponsor will be contacted by telephone. A follow-up letter will discuss the reasons for the clinical hold.

Adapted from the FDA Instructions for Filing an Investigational New Drug Application (IND), Revision 0994 and 0694/HFD-8.

MAGNESIUM REPLACEMENT GUIDELINES

Normal magnesium serum concentrations = 1.8-2.9 mg/dL

If serum magnesium is <1.8 mEq/L, repletion should be considered.

Magnesium Formulations

$MgSO_4$ injection 1 g = 8 mEq

Magnesium gluconate 500 mg tablet (2.5 mEq/tablet)
Magnesium hydroxide (MOM) (13.7 mEq/5 mL)
Magnesium chloride 535 mg tablet (5.2 mEq/tablet)
Magnesium oxide 420 mg (20.8 mEq/capsule)
Magnesium citrate liquid (3.85-4.71 mEq/5 mL)
Mylanta®-II (13.7 mEq/5 mL)
Maalox® Plus (6.9 mEq/5 mL)

Oral Magnesium Supplementation

Oral magnesium is generally not adequate for repletion in patients with serum magnesium concentrations <1.5.

Magnesium chloride 535 mg/tab = 5.2 mEq/tab given 2 tab tid for 5-7 days.

May need **more** if renal function is good or absorptive capacity is poor. May need **less** if renal function deteriorates. Reassess to determine maintenance dose, if necessary at 0.35-0.45 mEq/kg/day.

Intravenous Repletion (available as 50% solution, 2 mL vials = 1 g or 8 mEq)

Asymptomatic or serum concentration >1 mEq/L

<50 kg	16-32 mEq/day infused over 24 hours for 5-7 days
>50 kg	24-40 mEq/day infused over 24 hours for 5-7 days

Symptomatic or serum concentration <1 mEq/L

<50 kg	24-40 mEq/day infused over 24 hours for 5-7 days
>50 kg	32-48 mEq/day infused over 24 hours for 5-7 days

Maximal rate of infusion: 2 g/hour to avoid hypotension. Doses of 4 g/hour have been given in emergencies (eclampsia, seizures).

Optimally, should add magnesium to I.V. fluids or to IVH, but bolus doses are also effective.

Follow-up Monitoring

Serum magnesium will equilibrate over 2-4 days with intracellular concentrations. Therefore, caution should be exercised in interpreting serum levels immediately after boluses.

MATERNAL-FETAL TOXICOLOGY

Drugs and Chemicals Proven to Be Teratogenic in Humans

Drug/Chemical	Fetal Adverse Effects	Relative Risk for Teratogenicity	Clinical Intervention
Alcohol	**Fetal alcohol syndrome:** Mental retardation, microcephaly, poor coordination, hypotonia, hyperactivity, short upturned nose, micrognathia or retrognathia (infancy) or prognathia (adolescence), short palpebral fissures, hypoplastic philtrum, thinned upper lips, microphthalmia, antenatal/postnatal growth retardation, occasional pathologies of eyes, mouth, heart, kidneys, gonads, skin, muscle, and skeleton	In alcoholic women consuming >2 g/kg/d ethanol over first trimester: 2- to 3-fold higher risk for congenital malformations (about 10%)	To calculate accurate dose of alcohol: **Prospective:** To discontinue exposure; if woman is alcoholic, refer to addiction center **During pregnancy:** To alleviate fears in mild or occasional drinkers who may terminate pregnancy based on unrealistic perception of risk, level 2 ultrasound to rule out visible malformation
Alkylating agents (busulfan, chlorambucil, cyclophosphamide, mechlorethamine)	Growth retardation, cleft palate, microphthalmia hypoplastic ovaries, cloudy corneas, agenesis of kidney, malformations of digits, cardiac defects, multiple other anomalies	Based on case reports, between 10% and 50% of cases were malformed for different drugs. It is possible that adverse outcome was overrepresented.	Level 2 ultrasound to rule out visible malformations. Supplement folic acid to women receiving antifolates (eg, methotrexate).
Antimetabolite agents (aminopterin azauridine, cytarabine, 5-FU, 6-MP, methotrexate)	Hydrocephalus, meningoencephalocele, anencephaly, malformed skull, cerebral hypoplasia, growth retardation, eye and ear malformations, malformed nose and cleft palate, malformed extremities and fingers **Aminopterin syndrome:** Cranial dysostosis, hydrocephalus, hypertelorism, anomalies of external ear, micrognathia, posterior cleft palate	Based on case reports 7%-75% of cases were malformed. It is possible that adverse outcome was overrepresented.	Level 2 ultrasound to rule out visible malformations.
Carbamazepine	Increased risk for neural tube defects (NTDs)	NTDs estimated at 1% with carbamazepine	Periconceptional folate; maternal and/or amniotic α-fetoprotein; ultrasound to rule out NTD.

(continued)

Drug/Chemical	Fetal Adverse Effects	Relative Risk for Teratogenicity	Clinical Intervention
Carbon monoxide	Cerebral atrophy, mental retardation, microcephaly, convulsions, spastic disorders, intrauterine or postnatal death	Based on case reports, when mother is severely poisoned, high risk for neurological sequelae; no increased risk in mild accidental exposures	Measure maternal carboxyhemoglobin levels. Treat with 100% oxygen for 5 hours after maternal carboxyhemoglobin returns to normal because fetal equilibration takes longer. If hyperbaric chamber available, should be used, as elimination half-life of CO is more rapid. Fetal monitoring by an obstetrician; sonographic follow-up.
Coumadin®	**Fetal warfarin syndrome:** Nasal hypoplasia, chondrodysplasia punctata, branchydactyly, skull defects, abnormal ears, malformed eyes, CNS malformations, microcephaly, hydrocephalus, skeletal deformities, mental retardation, optic atrophy, spasticity, Dandy Walker malformations	16% of exposed fetuses have malformation; another 3% hemorrhages; 8% stillbirths	**Prospective:** Switch to heparin for the first trimester. Deliver by a cesarean section. Women should be followed up in a high-risk perinatal unit.
Diethylstilbestrol (DES)	**Female offspring:** Clear cell vaginal or cervical adenocarcinoma in young female adults exposed in utero (before 18th week); irregular menses (oligomenorrhea), reduced pregnancy rates, increased rate of preterm deliveries, increased perinatal mortality and spontaneous abortion **Male offspring:** Cysts of epididymis, cryptorchidism, hypogonadism, diminished spermatogenesis	Exposure before 18 weeks of gestation: ≤1.4/1000 of exposed female with carcinoma. Congenital morphological changes in vaginal epithelium in 39% of exposures.	**Diagnosis:** Direct observation of mucosa and Shiller's test. **Treatment:** Mechanical excision or destruction in relatively confined area. Surgery and radiotherapy for diffused tumor.
Lead	Lower scores in developmental tests	Higher risk when maternal lead is >10 μg/dL	**Maternal lead levels >10 μg/dL:** Investigate for possible source of contamination. **Levels >25 μg/dL:** Consider chelation

(continued)

Drug/Chemical	Fetal Adverse Effects	Relative Risk for Teratogenicity	Clinical Intervention
Lithium carbonate	Possibly higher risk for Ebstein's anomaly; no detectable higher risk for other malformations		Women who need lithium should continue therapy, with sonographic follow-up. Patients may need higher doses because of increased clearance rate.
Methyl mercury, mercuric sulfide	Microcephaly, eye malformations, cerebral palsy, mental retardation, malocclusion of teeth	Women of affected babies consumed 9-27 ppm mercury; greater risk when ingested at 6-8 gestational months. Relative risk was not elucidated, but 13/220 babies born in Minamata, Japan, at time of contamination had severe disease.	Good correlation between mercury concentrations in maternal hair follicles and neurological outcome of the fetus. Hair mercury content >50 ppm was used successfully as a cut point for termination. In acute poisoning, the fetus is 4-10 times more sensitive than the adult to methylmercury toxicity.
PCBs	**Stillbirth** **Signs at birth:** White eye discharge, 30% (32/108); teeth present, 8.7% (11/127); irritated/swollen gums, 11% (11/99); hyperpigmentation ("cola" staining), 42.5% (54/127); deformed/small nails, 24.6% (30/122); acne, 12.8% (16/125) **Subsequent history:** Bronchitis or pneumonia, 27.2% (30/124); chipped or broken teeth, 35.5% (38/107); hair loss, 12.2% (14/115); acne scars, 9.6% (11/115); generalized itching, 27.8% (32/1150) **Developmental:** Do not meet milestones; lower scores than unexposed controls; evidence of CNS damage	4%-20% (6/159-8/39)	These figures, which are from cases poisoned by high consumption of PCB-contaminated rice oil, cannot be extrapolated to cases in which maternal poisoning has not been verified. Women working near PCBs (eg, hydroelectric facilities) should use effective protection.
Penicillamine	Skin hyperelastosis	Few case reports; risk unknown	

(continued)

Drug/Chemical	Fetal Adverse Effects	Relative Risk for Teratogenicity	Clinical Intervention
Phenytoin	**Fetal hydantoin syndrome:** Low nasal bridge, inner epicanthal folds, ptosis, strabismus, hypertelorism, low set or abnormal ears, wide mouth, large fontanels, anomalies and hypoplasia of distal phalanges and nails, skeletal abnormalities, microcephaly and mental retardation, growth deficiency, neuroblastoma, cardiac defects, cleft palate/lip	5%-10% of typical syndrome; about 30% of partial picture. Relative risk of 7 for offspring IQ $\leq$84.	Neurologist should consider changing to other medications. Keep phenytoin concentrations at lower effective levels. Level 2 ultrasound to rule out visible malformations, vitamin K to neonate. Epilepsy itself increases teratogenic risk.
Systemic retinoids (isotretinoin, etretinate)	Spontaneous abortions; deformities of cranium, ears, face, heart, limbs, liver; hydrocephalus, microcephalus, heart defects. Cognitive defects even without dysmorphology	For isotretinoin: 38% risk. 80% of malformation are CNS.	Treated women should have an effective method of contraception. Pregnancy termination. If diagnosed too late, sonographic follow-up to rule out confirmed malformations.
Tetracycline	Yellow, gray-brown, or brown staining of deciduous teeth, destruction of enamel	From 4 months of gestation and on, occurs in 50% of fetuses exposed to tetracycline; 12.5% to oxytetracycline	If exposure before 14-16 weeks of gestation, no known risk
Thalidomide	Limb phocomelia, amelia, hypoplasia, congenital heart defects, renal malformations, cryptorchidism, abducens paralysis, deafness, microtia, anotia	About 20% risk when exposure to drug occurs in days 34-50 of gestation.	Thalidomide is an effective drug for some forms of leprosy. Treated women should have an effective mode of contraception.
Trimethadione	**Fetal trimethadione syndrome:** Intrauterine growth retardation, cardiac anomalies, microcephaly, cleft palate and lip, abnormal ears, dysmorphic face, mental retardation, tracheoesophageal fistula, postnatal death	Based on case reports: 83% risk; 32% infantile or neonatal death	No need for this antiepileptic to date
Valproic acid	Lumbosacral spina bifida with meningomyelocele; CNS defects, microcephaly, cardiac defects	1.2% risk of neural tube defects	Level 2 ultrasound and maternal α-fetoproteins or amniocentesis to rule out neural tube defects. Epilepsy itself increases teratogenic risk.

Reprinted with permission from "Drugs and Chemicals Proven to Be Teratogenic in Humans," *Maternal-Fetal Toxicology: A Clinician's Guide*, 2nd ed, Koren G, ed, New York, NY: Marcel Dekker, Inc, 1994, 37-43.

MEDICAL EXAMINER DATA
(Drug Abuse Warning Network)

Number of Drug Abuse Deaths by Metropolitan Area: 1990-1993

Metropolitan Area	1990	1991	1992	1993	Percent Change in Numbers, 1992-1993
Atlanta, GA	110	113	120	145	20.8
Baltimore, MD	97	269	295	406	37.6
Buffalo, NY	23	20	32	10	-68.6
Chicago, IL	321	350	390	587	45.4
Cleveland, OH	60	56	84	95	13.1
Dallas, TX	100	143	194	360	85.6
Denver, CO	35	45	48	51	6.3
Detroit, MI	239	247	313	292	-6.7
Indianapolis, IN	13	23	11	29	163.6
Kansas City, KS/MO	40	60	27	35	29.6
Los Angeles, CA	985	924	1094	1083	-1.0
Miami, FL	86	151	141	178	26.2
Minneapolis, MN/WI	26	55	39	47	20.5
New Orleans, LA	63	63	61	62	1.6
New York, NY	1540	1439	1397	1465	4.9
Newark, NJ	117	194	178	187	5.1
Norfolk, VA	15	20	46	37	-19.6
Oklahoma City, OK	120	120	105	139	32.4
Philadelphia, NJ/PA	445	590	667	759	13.8
Phoenix, AZ	114	143	198	242	22.2
St Louis, IL/MO	163	195	210	236	12.4
San Antonio, TX	59	63	95	69	-27.4
San Diego, CA	245	211	270	251	-7.0
San Francisco, CA	273	268	398	340	-14.6
Seattle, WA	127	118	143	152	6.3
Washington, DC/MD/VA	223	232	212	248	17.0
Total DAWN system	5628	6099	6768	7485	10.6

Note: Excludes deaths in which AIDS was reported and deaths in which "drug unknown" was the only substance mentioned.

Adapted with permission from Office of Applied Studies, SAMHSA, "Drug Abuse Warning Network," *Annual Medical Examiner Data 1993*, 1995, 57.

Drugs Mentioned Most Frequently by Medical Examiners in 1993

(Drugs With Fewer Than 10 Mentions Are Excluded.)

Rank	Drug Name	Number of Mentions	Percent of Total Episodes
1	Cocaine	3910	45.78
2	Heroin/morphine*	3805	44.55
3	Alcohol (in combination)	3444	40.32
4	Codeine	990	11.59
5	Diazepam	605	7.08
6	Marijuana/hashish	457	5.35
7	Methadone	457	5.35
8	Amitriptyline	404	4.73
9	Methamphetamine/speed	382	4.47
10	Diphenhydramine	369	4.32
11	Nortriptyline	351	4.11
12	D-Propoxyphene	338	3.96
13	Acetaminophen	301	3.52
14	Amphetamine	259	3.03
15	PCP/PCP combinations	206	2.41
16	Doxepin	197	2.31
17	Lidocaine	192	2.25
18	Quinine	179	2.10
19	Phenobarbital	169	1.98
20	Unspec benzodiazepine	152	1.78
21	Desipramine	127	1.49
22	Fluoxetine	118	1.38
23	Hydantoin	115	1.35
24	Aspirin	113	1.32
25	Alprazolam	113	1.32
26	Hydrocodone	105	1.23
27	Imipramine	99	1.16
28	Butalbital	95	1.11
29	Chlordiazepoxide	88	1.03
30	Temazepam	76	0.89
31	Thioridazine	70	0.82
32	Meprobamate	66	0.77
33	Chlorpheniramine	65	0.76
34	Secobarbital	63	0.74
35	Doxylamine succinate	62	0.73
36	Carisoprodol	61	0.71
37	Carbamazepine	60	0.70
38	Dextromethorphan	59	0.69
39	Meperidine HCl	55	0.64
40	Oxycodone	48	0.56

(continued)

Rank	Drug Name	Number of Mentions	Percent of Total Episodes
41	Mesoridazine	47	0.55
42	Trazodone	47	0.55
43	Chlorpromazine	45	0.53
44	Flurazepam	45	0.53
45	Oxazepam	43	0.50
46	Promethazine	41	0.48
47	Pseudoephedrine	39	0.46
48	Fentanyl	36	0.42
49	Ephedrine	36	0.42
50	Pentobarbital	30	0.35
51	Lorazepam	30	0.35
52	Hydroxyzine	25	0.29
53	Lithium carbonate	25	0.29
54	Theophylline	25	0.29
55	Benztropine	25	0.29
56	Phenylpropanolamine	24	0.28
57	Clomipramine	24	0.28
58	Ibuprofen	24	0.28
59	Hydromorphone	21	0.25
60	Cyclobenzaprine	21	0.25
61	Caffeine	20	0.23
62	Propranolol HCl	20	0.23
63	Clonazepam	17	0.20
64	Brompheniramine maleate	15	0.18
65	Amoxapine	15	0.18
66	Phentermine	14	0.16
67	Glutethimide	14	0.16
68	Haloperidol	14	0.16
69	Quinidine sulfate	14	0.16
70	Amobarbital	12	0.14
71	Hydrocarbon	12	0.14
72	Glues	11	0.13
73	Loxapine	11	0.13
74	Triazolam	11	0.13
75	Valproic acid	10	0.12
76	Metoclopramide	10	0.12

Note: Percentages are based on a total raw medical examiner drug abuse case count of 8541.

*Includes opiates not specified as to type.

Adapted with permission from Office of Applied Studies, SAMHSA, "Drug Abuse Warning Network," *Annual Medical Examiner Data 1993*, 1995, 16.

MILLIEQUIVALENTS FOR SELECTED IONS

Approximate Milliequivalents — Weights of Selected Ions

Salt	mEq/g Salt	Mg Salt/mEq
Calcium carbonate ($CaCO_3$)	20	50
Calcium chloride ($CaCl_2 \cdot 2H_2O$)	14	73
Calcium gluconate (Ca gluconate$_2 \cdot 1H_2O$)	4	224
Calcium lactate (Ca lactate$_2 \cdot 5H_2O$)	6	154
Magnesium sulfate ($MgSO_4$)	16	60
Magnesium sulfate ($MgSO_4 \cdot 7H_2O$)	8	123
Potassium acetate (K acetate)	10	98
Potassium chloride (KCl)	13	75
Potassium citrate (K_3 citrate $\cdot 1H_2O$)	9	108
Potassium iodide (KI)	6	166
Sodium bicarbonate ($NaHCO_3$)	12	84
Sodium chloride (NaCl)	17	58
Sodium citrate (Na_3 citrate $\cdot 2H_2O$)	10	98
Sodium iodide (NaI)	7	150
Sodium lactate (Na lactate)	9	112
Zinc sulfate ($ZnSO_4 \cdot 7H_2O$)	7	144

Valences and Approximate Weights of Selected Ions

Substance	Electrolyte	Valence	Ionic Wt
Calcium	Ca^{++}	2	40
Chloride	Cl^-	1	35.5
Magnesium	Mg^{++}	2	24
Phosphate	PO_4^{---}	3	95*
	HPO_4^{--}	2	96
	$H_2PO_4^-$	1	97
Potassium	K^+	1	39
Sodium	Na^+	1	23
Sulfate	SO_4^{--}	2	96*

*The atomic weight of phosphorus is 31, and of sulfur is 32.

MILLIMOLE AND MILLIEQUIVALENT CALCULATIONS

Definitions

mole	= gram molecular weight of a substance (aka molar weight)
millimole (mM)	= milligram molecular weight of a substance (a millimole is 1/1000 of a mole)
equivalent weight	= gram weight of a substance which will combine with or replace 1 gram (1 mole) of hydrogen; an equivalent weight can be determined by dividing the molar weight of a substance by its ionic valence
milliequivalent (mEq)	= milligram weight of a substance which will combine with or replace 1 milligram (1 millimole) of hydrogen (a milliequivalent is 1/1000 of an equivalent)

Calculations

$$\text{moles} = \frac{\text{weight of a substance (grams)}}{\text{molecular weight of that substance (grams)}}$$

$$\text{millimoles} = \frac{\text{weight of a substance (milligrams)}}{\text{molecular weight of that substance (milligrams)}}$$

equivalents = moles x valence of ion

milliequivalents = millimoles x valence of ion

$$\text{moles} = \frac{\text{equivalents}}{\text{valence of ion}}$$

$$\text{millimoles} = \frac{\text{milliequivalents}}{\text{valence of ion}}$$

millimoles = moles x 1000

milliequivalents = equivalents x 1000

Note: Use of equivalents and milliequivalents is valid only for those substances which have fixed ionic valences (eg, sodium, potassium, calcium, chlorine, magnesium bromine, etc). For substances with variable ionic valences (eg, phosphorous), a reliable equivalent value cannot be determined. In these instances, one should calculate millimoles (which are fixed and reliable) rather than milliequivalents.

NONSTEROIDAL ANTI-INFLAMMATORY DRUGS

Some Possible NSAID-Drug Interactions in the Elderly

Agent/Drug Class	Mechanism	Management
Antihypertensive Agents		
β-Blockers ACE inhibitors Diuretics	NSAID-induced vasoconstriction, salt and water retention; antagonizes drug effect on vascular tone. (Note: Some studies suggest that sulindac causes less interference with renal function and blood pressure control.)	Use calcium channel antagonist or α-agonist, or increase dose of antihypertensive drug
	Hyperkalemia may result from combinations of NSAIDs with potassium-sparing diuretics or ACE inhibitors	Monitor potassium level
Antiseizure Agents		
Phenytoin	Inhibition of hepatic metabolism by NSAID or displacement from albumin-binding sites, resulting in higher plasma levels	Reduce dose of antiseizure drug, or monitor drug levels
Sodium valproate	Inhibition of hepatic metabolism found with high doses of aspirin	Avoid aspirin and monitor valproate drug levels with use of other NSAIDs
Oral Hypoglycemics		
Sulfonylureas	Inhibition of metabolism or displacement from albumin binding sites; increased hypoglycemic effect	Monitor blood glucose level closely
Oral Anticoagulants		
Warfarin	Inhibition of metabolism or displacement from albumin binding sites; increased anticoagulant effect	Concomitant use not recommended because of effect on platelet and protein clotting pathways
Others		
Digoxin	Inhibition of renal clearance in patients susceptible to decreases in renal blood flow when taking NSAIDs; increased levels of digoxin	Monitor digoxin and serum creatinine levels
Methotrexate	Reduction in methotrexate clearance, with increased plasma concentration of methotrexate	Not an important interaction at rheumatologic doses

Adapted from Conaway DC, "Using NSAIDs Safely in the Elderly," *Hospital Medicine®*, May 1995, 23.

NORMAL LABORATORY VALUES FOR ADULTS*

CHEMISTRY

Lab Test		Normal Values
Chemistry, Routine		
Albumin		3.5-5.0 g/dL
Bilirubin, conjugated		0-0.2 mg/dL
Bilirubin, total		0.2-1.2 mg/dL
Blood urea nitrogen		8-23 mg/dL
Calcium		8.4-10.3 mg/dL
Creatinine		0.5-1.2 mg/dL
Glucose		65-110 mg/dL
Phosphorus		2.8-4.5 mg/dL
Protein, total		6.0-8.0 g/dL
Uric acid	male	3.5-7.2 mg/dL
	female	2.6-6.5 mg/dL
Electrolytes		
Chlorides		100-110 mEq/L
CO_2		23-31 mEq/L
Potassium		3.5-5.0 mEq/L
Sodium		136-146 mEq/L
Anion gap		5-14 mEq/L
Enzymes		
Alk phos	male	34-110 units/L
	female	24-100 units/L
ALT		5-35 units/L
AST		5-35 units/L
CPK	male	0-206 units/L
	female	0-175 units/L
LDH		50-200 units/L
Sperm Analysis		
Volume		2-6 mL
Sperm concentration		20-250 (10^6/mL)
Sperm motility		>50%
Sperm vitality		≥50%
Normal forms		≥60%

Lab Test		Normal Values
Thyroid Function		
FTI (free thyroxine index)		4.5-12.0
T_3 resin uptake		25%-35%
T_3 (tri-iodothyronine) by RIA		70-200 ng/dL
T_4 (thyroxine) by RIA		4.0-11.0 μg/dL
Others		
Ammonia, plasma		20-60 μg/dL
Amylase, serum		44-128 units/L
Calcium, ionized		4.6-5.2 mg/dL
Cholesterol		140-230 mg/dL
Iron, serum		50-170 μg/dL
Lactate, serum		1.4-3.9 mEq/L
Lipase		10-208 units/L
Magnesium		1.5-2.5 mg/dL
Oncotic pressure		22-28 mm Hg
Osmolality		280-300 mOsm/kg
Serum ferritin	male	25-400 ng/mL
	female	10-150 ng/mL
TIBC		270-390 μg/dL
Triglycerides		50-150 mg/dL

BLOOD GASES

	Arterial	Venous
Base excess	-3.0 to +3.0 mEq/L	-5.0 to +5.0 mEq/L
HCO_3	18-25 mEq/L	18-25 mEq/L
O_2 saturation	90-98%	60-85%
pCO_2	34-45 mm Hg	35-52 mm Hg
pH	7.35-7.45	7.32-7.42
pO_2	80-95 mm Hg	30-48 mm Hg
TCO_2	23-29 mEq/L	24-30 mEq/L

Weight/Volume Equivalents

1 mg/dL = 10 μg/mL	1 ppm = 1 mg/L
1 mg/dL = 1 mg%	1 μg/mL = 1 mg/L

*The normal ranges for laboratory values vary with different age groups, and may change as new methodologies for the lab tests are used. These values are current for adults (age 17 years or older).

NORMAL LABORATORY VALUES FOR CHILDREN

CHEMISTRY

		Normal Values
Albumin		
	0-1 y	2-4 g/dL
	1 y to adult	3.5-5.5 g/dL
Ammonia		
	Newborns	90-150 μg/dL
	Children	40-120 μg/dL
	Adults	18-54 μg/dL
Amylase		
	Newborns	0-60 units/L
	Adults	30-110 units/L
Bilirubin, conjugated, direct		
	Newborns	<1.5 mg/dL
	1 mo to adult	0-0.5 mg/dL
Bilirubin, total		
	0-3 d	2-10 mg/dL
	1 mo to adult	0-1.5 mg/dL
Bilirubin, unconjugated, indirect		0.6-10.5 mg/dL
Calcium		
	Newborns	7-12 mg/dL
	0-2 y	8.8-11.2 mg/dL
	2 y to adult	9-11 mg/dL
Calcium, ionized, whole blood		4.4-5.4 mg/dL
Carbon dioxide, total		23-33 mEq/L
Chloride		95-105 mEq/L
Cholesterol		
	Newborns	45-170 mg/dL
	0-1 y	65-175 mg/dL
	1-20 y	120-230 mg/dL
Creatinine		
	0-1 y	≤0.6 mg/dL
	1 y to adult	0.5-1.5 mg/dL
Glucose		
	Newborns	30-90 mg/dL
	0-2 y	60-105 mg/dL
	2 y to adult	70-110 mg/dL
Iron		
	Newborns	110-270 μg/dL
	Infants	30-70 μg/dL
	Children	55-120 μg/dL
	Adults	70-180 μg/dL
Iron binding		
	Newborns	59-175 μg/dL
	Infants	100-400 μg/dL
	Adults	250-400 μg/dL
Lactic acid, lactate		2-20 mg/dL
Lead, whole blood		<30 μg/dL
Lipase		
	Children	20-140 units/L
	Adults	0-190 units/L
Magnesium		1.5-2.5 mEq/L
Osmolality, serum		275-296 mOsm/kg
Osmolality, urine		50-1400 mOsm/kg

(continued)

		Normal Values
Phosphorus		
	Newborns	4.2-9 mg/dL
	6 wk to 19 mo	3.8-6.7 mg/dL
	18 mo to 3 y	2.9-5.9 mg/dL
	3-15 y	3.6-5.6 mg/dL
	>15 y	2.5-5 mg/dL
Potassium, plasma		
	Newborns	4.5-7.2 mEq/L
	2 d to 3 mo	4-6.2 mEq/L
	3 mo to 1 y	3.7-5.6 mEq/L
	1-16 y	3.5-5 mEq/L
Protein, total		
	0-2 y	4.2-7.4 g/dL
	>2 y	6-8 g/dL
Sodium		136-145 mEq/L
Triglycerides		
	Infants	0-171 mg/dL
	Children	20-130 mg/dL
	Adults	30-200 mg/dL
Urea nitrogen, blood		
	0-2 y	4-15 mg/dL
	2 y to adult	5-20 mg/dL
Uric acid		
	Male	3-7 mg/dL
	Female	2-6 mg/dL

ENZYMES

Alanine aminotransferase (ALT) (SGPT)		
	0-2 mo	8-78 units/L
	>2 mo	8-36 units/L
Alkaline phosphatase (ALKP)		
	Newborns	60-130 units/L
	0-16 y	85-400 units/L
	>16 y	30-115 units/L
Aspartate aminotransferase (AST) (SGOT)		
	Infants	18-74 units/L
	Children	15-46 units/L
	Adults	5-35 units/L
Creatine kinase (CK)		
	Infants	20-200 units/L
	Children	10-90 units/L
	Adult male	0-206 units/L
	Adult female	0-175 units/L
Lactate dehydrogenase (LDH)		
	Newborns	290-501 units/L
	1 mo to 2 y	110-144 units/L
	>16 y	60-170 units/L

BLOOD GASES

	Arterial	Capillary	Venous
pH	7.35-7.45	7.35-7.45	7.32-7.42
pCO_2 (mm Hg)	35-45	35-45	38-52
pO_2 (mm Hg)	70-100	60-80	24-48
HCO_3 (mEq/L)	19-25	19-25	19-25
TCO_2 (mEq/L)	19-29	19-29	23-33
O_2 saturation (%)	90-95	90-95	40-70
Base excess (mEq/L)	-5 to +5	-5 to +5	-5 to +5

THYROID FUNCTION TESTS

T_4 (thyroxine)		
	1-7 d	10.1-20.9 μg/dL
	8-14 d	9.8-16.6 μg/dL
	1 mo to 1 y	5.5-16 μg/dL
	>1 y	4-12 μg/dL
FTI		
	1-3 d	9.3-26.6
	1-4 wk	7.6-20.8
	1-4 mo	7.4-17.9
	4-12 mo	5.1-14.5
	1-6 y	5.7-13.3
	>6 y	4.8-14
T_3 by RIA		
	Newborns	100-470 ng/dL
	1-5 y	100-260 ng/dL
	5-10 y	90-240 ng/dL
	10 y to adult	70-210 ng/dL
T_3 uptake		35%-45%
TSH		
	Cord	3-22 μIU/mL
	1-3 d	<40 μIU/mL
	3-7 d	<25 μIU/mL
	>7 d	0-10 μIU/mL

HEMATOLOGY VALUES

	Hgb (g/dL)	Hct (%)	MCV (fl)	MCH (pg)	MCHC (%)	RBC (mill/mm^3)	RDW	PLTS ($\times 10^3/mm^3$)
0-3 d	15-20	45-61	95-115	31-37	29-37	4-5.9	<18	250-450
1-2 wk	12.5-18.5	39-57	86-110	28-36	28-38	3.6-5.5	<17	250-450
1-6 mo	10-13	29-42	74-96	25-35	30-36	3.1-4.3	<16.5	300-700
7 mo to 2 y	10.5-13	33-38	70-84	23-30	31-37	3.7-4.9	<16	250-600
2-5 y	11.5-13	34-39	75-87	24-30	31-37	3.9-5	<15	250-550
5-8 y	11.5-14.5	35-42	77-95	25-33	31-37	4-4.9	<15	250-550
13-18 y	12-15.2	36-47	78-96	25-35	31-37	4.5-5.1	<14.5	150-450
Adult male	13.5-16.5	41-50	80-100	26-34	31-37	4.5-5.5	<14.5	150-450
Adult female	12-15	36-44	80-100	26-34	31-37	4-4.9	<14.5	150-450

WBC and Diff

	WBC (x $10^3/mm^3$)	Segmented Neutrophils	Band Neutrophils	Eosinophils	Basophils	Lymphocytes	Atypical Lymphs	Monocytes	Number of NRBCs
0-3 d	9-35	32-62	10-18	0-2	0-1	19-29	0-8	5-7	0-2
1-2 wk	5-20	14-34	6-14	0-2	0-1	36-45	0-8	6-10	0
1-6 mo	6-17.5	13-33	4-12	0-3	0-1	41-71	0-8	4-7	0
7 mo to 2 y	6-17	15-35	5-11	0-3	0-1	45-76	0-8	3-6	0
2-5 y	5.5-15.5	23-45	5-11	0-3	0-1	35-65	0-8	3-6	0
5-8 y	5-14.5	32-54	5-11	0-3	0-1	28-48	0-8	3-6	0
13-18 y	4.5-13	34-64	5-11	0-3	0-1	25-45	0-8	3-6	0
Adults	4.5-11	35-66	5-11	0-3	0-1	24-44	0-8	3-6	0

Sedimentation rate, Westergren
- Children 0-20 mm/hour
- Adult male 0-15 mm/hour
- Adult female 0-20 mm/hour

Sedimentation rate, Wintrobe
- Children 0-13 mm/hour
- Adult male 0-10 mm/hour
- Adult female 0-15 mm/hour

Reticulocyte count
- Newborns 2%-6%
- 1-6 mo 0%-2.8%
- Adults 0.5%-1.5%

PESTICIDES BY COMMON NAME WITH TOXICITY INFORMATION

Common Name	Class and Type	LD_{50} Oral (mg/kg)	Relative Toxicity
2,4-D	Chlorophenoxy herbicide	699	Low[1]
2,4-DB	Chlorophenoxy herbicide	2000	Low
Acephate	Organophosphate insecticide	980	Low
Acifluorfen-sodium	Miscellaneous herbicide	1540	High[2]
Alachlor	Anilide herbicide	930	Mod[3]
Aldicarb	Carbamate insecticide	1	High
Ametryn	Triazine herbicide	1950	Low
Anilazine	Triazine fungicide	5000	High[4]
Atrazine	Triazine herbicide	1780	Low
Azinphos-methyl	Organophosphate insecticide	4	High
Bacillus thuringiensis	Biological insecticide	≥2670	Low
Benefin	Fluorodinitrotoluidine herbicide	10,000	Low
Benomyl	Benzimidazole fungicide	10,000	Low
Bensulide	Organophosphate herbicide	271	Mod
Bentazone	Miscellaneous herbicide	2063	Low
Bromacil	Uracil herbicide	5200	Low[5]
Bromoxynil	Benzonitrile herbicide	260	Mod
Butylate	Carbamate herbicide	3500	Low
Captan	Phthalimide fungicide	9000	High[6]
Carbaryl	Carbamate insecticide	246	Mod[7]
Carbofuran	Carbamate insecticide	11	High
Chloramben	Chlorobenzoic acid herbicide	5620	Low
Chlorimuron ethyl	Urea derivative herbicide	4000	Low
Chloropicrin	Organochlorine fumigant	250	High[8]
Chlorothalonil	Benzonitrile fungicide	10,000	High[9]
Chlorpyrifos	Organophosphate insecticide	96	Mod
Clomazone	Miscellaneous herbicide	1369	Low
Copper hydroxide	Copper fungicide	1000	High[10]
Copper sulfate	Copper fungicide	472	Mod
Cu ammonium carbonate	Copper fungicide	≥501	Low
Cyanazine	Triazine herbicide	288	Mod
Cycloate	Carbamate herbicide	2000	Low
Cypermethrin	Pyrethroid insecticide	250	Mod[11]
Cyromazine	Triazine insect growth regulator	3387	Low
DCNA	Miscellaneous fungicide	5000	Low
DCPA	Phthalate herbicide	5000	Low
Diazinon	Organophosphate insecticide	300	Mod
Dicamba	Chlorobenzoic acid herbicide	1700	Low
Dichlobenil	Benzonitrile herbicide	3160	Low
Dichloropropene	Organochlorine nematicide	127	Mod
Dicofol	Organochlorine acaricide	570	Low[12]
Diethatyl ethyl	Amide herbicide	2300	Low
Dimethoate	Organophosphate insecticide	235	Mod
Dinocap	Nitrophenol fungicide	980	Low
Diquat	Dipyridyl herbicide	215	Mod
Disulfoton	Organophosphate insecticide	4	High
Diuron	Substituted urea herbicide	3400	Low
Dodine	Miscellaneous fungicide	1000	Low[13]
Endosulfan	Organochlorine insecticide	160	High[14]
Endothall	Phthalate herbicide	51	High
EPTC	Carbamate herbicide	1630	Low
Esfenvalerate	Pyrethroid insecticide	458	Mod
Ethalfluralin	Fluorodinitrotoluidine herbicide	10,000	Low[15]
Ethoprop	Organophosphate insecticide	62	High[14]
Fenamiphos	Organophosphate nematicide	3	High
Fenarimol	Miscellaneous fungicide	2500	Low[16]
Fenvalerate	Pyrethroid insecticide	458	Mod
Fluazifop-p-butyl	Miscellaneous herbicide	2712	Low[17]
Flucythrinate	Pyrethroid insecticide	67	High
Fomesafen	Miscellaneous herbicide	1858	Mod[18]
Fonofos	Organophosphate insecticide	8	High
Formetanate	Carbamate insecticide	20	High
Fosamine ammonium	Phosphonate herbicide	5000	Mod[19]
Glyphosate	Phosphonate herbicide	5000	Low

(continued)

Common Name	Class and Type	LD_{50} Oral (mg/kg)	Relative Toxicity
Hexazinone	Triazine herbicide	1690	High/Mod[10]
Imazaquin	Imidazolinone herbicide	5000	Low
Imazethapyr	Imidazolinone herbicide	5000	Low
Iprodione	Amide fungicide	4400	Low
Isoxaben	Amide herbicide	10,000	Low
Lindane	Organochlorine insecticide	88	Mod
Linuron	Urea derivative herbicide	4000	Low
Malathion	Organophosphate insecticide	2800	Low
Mancozeb	Dithiocarbamate fungicide	11200	Low
Maneb	Dithiocarbamate fungicide	7990	Low
MCPA	Chlorophenoxy herbicide	1160	High[20]
MCPB	Chlorophenoxy herbicide	680	Low
Metalaxyl	Miscellaneous fungicide	669	Low
Metaldehyde	Aldehyde molluscicide	630	Low
Metam-sodium	Dithiocarbamate fungicide	1891	Mod[21]
Methamidophos	Organophosphate insecticide	20	High
Methomyl	Carbamate insecticide	17	High
Methoxychlor	Organochlorine insecticide	6000	Low
Methyl bromide	Miscellaneous fumigant	214	High[22]
Methyl demeton	Organophosphate insecticide	48	High
Methyl isothiocyanate	Miscellaneous fumigant	305	High[23]
Methyl parathion	Organophosphate insecticide	20	High
Metiram	Dithiocarbamate fungicide	10,000	Low
Metolachlor	Amide herbicide	2780	Low
Metribuzin	Triazine herbicide	1100	Low
Mevinphos	Organophosphate insecticide	3	High
Myclobutanil	Miscellaneous fungicide	1600	Low[24]
Naled	Organophosphate insecticide	376	High[25]
Napropamide	Amide herbicide	500	Low
Naptalam	Miscellaneous herbicide	8200	Mod[26]
Norflurazon	Miscellaneous herbicide	8000	Low
Oryzalin	Dinitroaniline herbicide	10,000	Low
Oxamyl	Carbamate insecticide	6	High
Oxyfluorfen	Miscellaneous herbicide	5000	Mod[18]
Paraquat	Dipyridyl herbicide	40	High
Parathion (ethyl)	Organophosphate insecticide	2	High
PCNB	Miscellaneous fungicide	1700	Low[27]
Pebulate	Carbamate herbicide	921	Low
Pendimethalin	Dinitroaniline herbicide	3956	Low
Permethrin	Pyrethroid insecticide	430	Mod
Phenmedipham	Carbamate herbicide	8000	Low[28]
Phorate	Organophosphate insecticide	2	High
Phosmet	Organophosphate insecticide	147	Mod
Phosphamidon	Organophosphate insecticide	17	High
Piperonyl butoxide	Miscellaneous synergist	7500	Low
Primisulfuron-methyl	Substituted urea herbicide	5050	Low
Prometryn	Triazine herbicide	5235	Low
Pronamide	Amide herbicide	8350	Low
Propachlor	Anilide herbicide	500	Mod[29]
Propargite	Miscellaneous acaricide	4029	High[30]
Pyrazon	Miscellaneous herbicide	3030	Low
Quizalofop-ethyl	Miscellaneous herbicide	1670	Low
Rotenone	Miscellaneous insecticide	132	Mod
Sethoxydim	Miscellaneous herbicide	3200	Low
Simazine	Triazine herbicide	5000	Low
Streptomycin	Antibiotic bactericide	9000	Low
Sulfometuron methyl	Urea derivative herbicide	5000	Low
Sulfur	Miscellaneous fungicide	5000	Low
Tebuthiuron	Substituted urea herbicide	644	Low
Tefluthrin	Pyrethroid insecticide	79	Mod
Tenn-Cop®	Copper fungicide	≥10,000	Low[31]
Terbacil	Uracil herbicide	5000	Low
Terbufos	Organophosphate insecticide	5	High
Thiabendazole	Miscellaneous fungicide	3100	Low
Thifensulfuron methyl	Substituted urea herbicide	5000	Low
Thiodicarb	Carbamate insecticide	166	Mod

(continued)

Common Name	Class and Type	LD_{50} Oral (mg/kg)	Relative Toxicity
Thiophanate methyl	Miscellaneous fungicide	7500	Low
Thiram	Dithiocarbamate fungicide	1000	Low
Triadimefon	Triazole fungicide	1000	Mod[32]
Trichlorfon	Organophosphate insecticide	250	Mod
Triclopyr	Organochlorine herbicide	630	High[33]
Tridiphane	Miscellaneous herbicide	1740	Mod[34]
Trifluralin	Fluorodinitrotoluidine herbicide	10,000	High[35]
Triforine	Miscellaneous fungicide	16,000	High[36]
Triphenyltin hydroxide	Organotin fungicide	156	High[37]
Vinclozolin	Miscellaneous fungicide	10,000	Low

Morgan K and Ackerman J, "Pesticides by Common Name With Toxicity Information," *Pesticide Poisoning Action Guide for Agricultural Pesticides in the Midwest*, U.S. Environmental Protection Agency Region 5, 1994, 3.2-3.9.

[1]Methylamine salts of 2,4-D carry the DANGER designation.

[2]Acifluorfen-sodium **formulation** will cause severe and perhaps permanent eye injury — can be absorbed through intact skin.

[3]Alachlor is an eye irritant.

[4]Anilazine can cause severe eye damage.

[5]Liquid **formulations** of bromacil will carry the warning label.

[6]Captan is a severe eye irritant.

[7]Some **formulations** of carbaryl are classed DANGER or WARNING.

[8]Chloropicrin is rated high for inhalation hazard, and is also a severe eye irritant.

[9]Chlorothalonil in **most formulations** is an eye irritant in varying degree.

[10]Copper hydroxide and hexazinone are severe eye irritants.

[11]Certain **formulations** of cypermethrin carry a DANGER designation.

[12]Some **formulations** of dicofol are classed WARNING.

[13]Dodine will "burn" eyes.

[14]Most **formulations** of endosulfan and ethoprop have high relative toxicity.

[15]**EC formulations** of ethalfluralin are classed WARNING.

[16]Fenarimol **EC formulations** carry the WARNING designation.

[17]Some **formulations** of fluazifop-p-butyl carry WARNING designations relating to eye irritation.

[18]Fomesafen and oxyfluorfen can cause substantial, temporary eye damage.

[19]Fosamine ammonium is an eye irritant.

[20]MCPA can cause irreversible eye damage.

[21]Metam-sodium will decompose with moisture. The decomposition product is an inhalation hazard as well as an eye and skin irritant.

[22]Methyl bromide is poison by inhalation.

[23]Methyl isothiocyanate is an inhalation and eye hazard.

[24]**EC formulations** of myclobutanil carry the DANGER designation.

[25]Naled can cause permanent eye damage.

[26]Naptalam is a severe eye irritant.

[27]PCNB **formulations** show extreme relative toxicity variations; from DANGER to CAUTION.

[28]Certain **formulations** of phenmedipham carry WARNING designations relating to eye irritation.

[29]Propachlor is corrosive to skin and an eye irritant.

[30]Propargite is high risk as an inhalation hazard.

[31]Tenn-Cop's **formulation** acts as an eye irritant.

[32]Triadimefon is an inhalation hazard and an eye irritant.

[33]**Many formulations** of triclopyr carry the DANGER designation.

[34]Tridiphane can cause severe eye irritation and moderate, reversible corneal injury.

[35]Trifluralin is an eye irritant — relative hazard depends on **formulation**.

[36]**EC formulations** of triforine carry the DANGER designation.

[37]Triphenyltin can be fatal if inhaled and can cause irreversible eye damage.

PHOSPHATE REPLETION GUIDELINES

For moderate hypophosphatemia (serum PO_4 <2 mg/dL but ≥1 mg/dL):

1. Discontinue any phosphate binding antacids.
2. Give 0.08-0.16 mmol/kg I.V. in 250 mL NS or D_5W over 4-6 hours via pump.
3. Recheck serum phosphate level.
4. If still <2 mg/dL, repeat.

For severe hypophosphatemia (serum PO_4 <1 mg/dL):

1. Discontinue any phosphate binding antacids.
2. Give 0.25 mmol/kg I.V. in 250 mL NS or D_5W over 4-6 hours via pump.
3. Recheck serum phosphate level.
4. If still <1 mg/dL, repeat.
5. If ≥1 mg/dL but ≤2 mg/dL, use guidelines for moderate hypophosphatemia above.

Dosages as high as 0.5 mmol/kg over 6 hours have been used for patients with serum PO_4 levels <0.5 mg/dL. If necessary, dosages may be infused over 2 hours.

Medicinal Chemistry Notes

Inorganic phosphate solutions exist as a mixture of two valence states: HPO_4^{-2} and $H_2PO_4^-$. At pH 7.4, the molar ratio of HPO_4^{-2}:$H_2PO_4^-$ is 80:20, yielding an average valence of 1.8. Therefore:

1 mmol of phosphate = 1.8 mEq of phosphate = 31 mg elemental P.
For clinical purposes, we round off to a ratio of 1 mmol:2 mEq.

In K phosphate solutions, the mEq of K^+ does not equal the mEq of phosphorus. K phosphate I.V. solution provides:

4.4 mEq K^+/mL
6 mEq phosphorus/mL
3 mmol K & phosphorus/mL

Therefore, orders for K phosphate written as mEq are ambiguous and subject to misinterpretation.

Important: Orders for K phosphate written as mEq must be clarified with the prescribing physician.

The compatibility of calcium and phosphates in solution is conditional, dependent on the concentration of both ions. As a rule of thumb, the **sum of the mEq Ca plus the mEq phosphate should not exceed 40.**

References

Kingston M and Al-Siba'l MB, "Treatment of Severe Hypophosphatemia," *Crit Care Med* 1985, 13(1):16-8.

Lent RD, Brown DM and Kjellstrand CM, "Treatment of Severe Hypophosphatemia," *Ann Intern Med*, 1978, 89:941-4.

POTASSIUM CONTENT OF FOODS*

Beverages (8 fluid ounces)	mg	mEq
Apple juice, canned	250	6.4
Apricot juice	372	9.5
Coffee, instant, 2 g	238	6.1
Grape juice, canned, sweetened	285	7.3
Grapefruit juice, canned	360	9.2
Milk, whole (high in sodium)	352	9
Milk, nonfat (high in sodium)	408	10.4
Orange juice, fresh or canned	496	12.7
Pineapple juice, canned	379	9.7
Prune juice, canned	563	14.4
Tea	66	1.7
Tomato juice, canned (high in sodium)	544	13.9
Foods		
Apricots, raw, 2-3 medium	281	7.2
Banana, fresh, 1 medium	550	14.1
Bouillon, 1 meat extract cube (high in sodium)	108	2.8
Bouillon, 1 vegetable extract cube (high in sodium)	138	3.3
Cantaloupe, ½, 5" diameter	251	6.4
Cauliflower, raw, 1¼ cup (10 oz)	500	12.8
Dates, dried, 10 medium	648	16.6
Figs, dried, 5 medium	640	16.4
Fruit cocktail, canned sweet, 1 cup	330	8.4
Molasses, 1 tablespoonful	269	6.9
Peaches, dried, ½ cup (4 oz) uncooked	1100	28.2
Pears, raw, 1, 2½ x 2"	180	4.6
Prunes, dried, 5 large, raw	349	8.9
Raisins, dried, 2 tablespoonfuls	152	3.9
Strawberries, raw, 8 oz	246	6.3
Watermelon, ½ slice, ¾ x 10"	380	9.7
Wheat germ, 100 g	737	18.9
Salt Substitutes		
Adolph's, 1 packet	430	11
Co-Salt, 1 g	450	11.5
Diasal, 1 g	442	11.3
Lite-Salt, 1 g (high in sodium)	260	6.6
Neocurtasal, 1 g	470	12.1
Nu-Salt, 1 g	404	10.4
Salfree, 1 g	548	14.1

*Pearson RE and Fish KH Jr, "Potassium Content of Selected Medicines, Foods and Salt Substitutes," *Hosp Pharm*, 1971, 6(9):6-9.

POUNDS-KILOGRAMS CONVERSION

1 pound = 0.45359 kilograms
1 kilogram = 2.2 pounds

TEMPERATURE CONVERSION

Celsius to Fahrenheit = (°C x 9/5) + 32 = °F
Fahrenheit to Celsius = (°F - 32) x 5/9 = °C

°C	= °F	°C	= °F	°C	= °F
100.0	212.0	39.0	102.2	36.8	98.2
50.0	122.0	38.8	101.8	36.6	97.9
41.0	105.8	38.6	101.5	36.4	97.5
40.8	105.4	38.4	101.1	36.2	97.2
40.6	105.1	38.2	100.8	36.0	96.8
40.4	104.7	38.0	100.4	35.8	96.4
40.2	104.4	37.8	100.1	35.6	96.1
40.0	104.0	37.6	99.7	35.4	95.7
39.8	103.6	37.4	99.3	35.2	95.4
39.6	103.3	37.2	99.0	35.0	95.0
39.4	102.9	37.0	98.6	0	32.0
39.2	102.6				

RADIATION: BASICS OF EXPOSURE

Adapted from *ATSDR Case Studies in Environmental Medicine: Ionizing Radiation*, U.S. Department of Health & Human Services, Public Health Service Agency for Toxic Substances and Disease Registry, October 1993, 1-48.

Units of Radiation Measurement

Characteristic	Unit	Description
Energy	electron volt (eV) (also ergs, joule)	Kinetic energy of an electron as it moves through a potential difference of 1 volt.
Rate of radioactive decay	curie (Ci)	Radioactivity emitted per unit of time (1 Ci = 3.7 x 10^{10} disintegrations per second).
Air exposure	roentgen (R)	Amount of X and gamma radiation that causes ionization in air. One roentgen of exposure will produce about 2 billion ion pairs per cubic centimeter of air.
Absorbed dose	rad	Dose resulting from one roentgen of ionizing radiation deposited in any medium, typically water or tissue. One rad results in the absorption of 100 ergs of ionizing radiation per gram of medium.
Biologic effectiveness	rem	Dose of any form of ionizing radiation that produces the same biological effect as 1 roentgen; 1 rem = 1 rad x radiation weighting factor (RWF), where the value of RWF depends on the type of radiation as follows: X radiation = 1 gamma radiation = 1 beta = 1 alpha = 20 neutrons = 5-20, depending on their energy

Common Diagnostic X-ray Doses*

Examination	Mean KVP	Mean MAS (mrem)	Testes/ Ovaries (mrem)	Embryo/ Fetus
Chest (PA)	80	12	<0.5	<0.5
Skull (lateral)	72	50	<0.5	<0.5
Abdomen (KUB, AP)	78	601	13.7/146	150
Retrograde pyelogram (AP)	77	91	17.2/161	170
Thoracic spine (AP)	75	82	<0.5/0.7	0.9
Cervical spine (AP)	69	48	<0.5	<0.5
Lumbosacral spine (AP)	77	112	13.2/145	150
Pelvis (AP)	100	30	83/79	133
Barium enema (AP)	120	20	68/132	140

*KVP = kilovolt peak; MAS = milliampere second; PA = posteroanterior view; AP = anteroposterior view; mrem = millirem; KUB = kidney, ureter, bladder.

Common Radionuclides Used in Nuclear Medicine

Examination	Agent	mCi*	Whole Body (mrem)*	Target Organ (mrem)
Lung	Technetium-99†	3	10	Lung - 1000
Lung	Xenon-133 gas	15	3	Lung - 150
Heart	Thallium-201 chloride	1.5	360	Kidney - 2200
Heart	Technetium-99‡	15	200	Blood - 300
Liver	Technetium-99§	3	60	Liver - 1000
Bone	Technetium-99¶	20	200	Bone - 450
Kidney	Technetium-99#	10	233	Kidney - 5000

*mCi = millicurie, mrem = millirem.

†Radionuclide delivered in microspheres of human serum albumin.

‡Radionuclide incorporated in red blood cells.

§Radionuclide delivered as sulfur colloid.

¶Radionuclide incorporated in methylene diphosphonate.

#Radionuclide incorporated in diethylenetriaminepentaacetic acid (DTPA).

Background Radiation From Consumer Products

Product	Local Dose (mrem/year)	Portion of Body Considered
Coal combustion (fly ash)	0.03-0.3	Lungs
Oil combustion (soot)	1.6	Lungs
Gas ranges (natural gas)	5	Lungs
Tobacco products*	16,000	Lungs
Dentures and crowns†	700	Superficial layers of tissue in contact with teeth
Ophthalmic glass‡	4000	Cornea
Smoke detectors	0.008	Whole body

*Dose for cigarette smokers only; does not include doses experienced by those subjected to passive smoke.

†Due to the uranium present in glazed dental porcelain.

‡Applies to eyeglasses tinted with uranium or thorium.

Summary of Recommendations for Ionizing Radiation

Dose Limits for Workers*	ICRP, 1991†	NCRP, 1993‡
Based on stochastic effects§ (eg, cancer and genetic damage)	5 rem (50 mSv) annual effective dose limit and 10 rem (100 mSv) as 5-year cumulative effective dose limit	5 rem (50 mSv) annual effective dose limit and 1 rem (10 mSv) times age in years cumulative effective dose limit
Based on nonstochastic effects§ (eg, lens cataracts and fertility impairment)	15 rem (150 mSv) equivalent dose limit to lens of eye and 50 rem (500 mSv) annual equivalent dose limit to skin, hands, and feet	15 rem (150 mSv) annual equivalent dose limit to lens of eye and 50 rem (500 mSv) annual equivalent dose limit to skin, hands, and feet

Dose Limits for the Public*	ICRP, 1991	NCRP, 1993
Based on stochastic effects	0.1 rem (1 mSv) annual effective dose limit, and, if needed, higher values provided that the annual average over 5 years does not exceed 0.1 rem	0.1 rem (1 mSv) annual effective dose limit for continuous exposure and 0.5 rem (5 mSv) annual dose limit for infrequent exposure
Based on nonstochastic effects	1.5 rem (15 mSv) annual equivalent to lens of eye and 5 rem (50 mSv) annual equivalent dose limit to skin, hands, and feet	5 rem (50 mSv) annual equivalent dose limit to lens of eye, skin, and extremities
Embryo-fetus	2 rem (2 mSv) equivalent dose to the woman's abdomen once pregnancy has been declared	0.05 rem (0.5 mSv) equivalent dose limit in a month once pregnancy is known

*The dose limits for both workers and the public exclude medical and natural background exposures. Note that the dose limits for the public are lower, in general, than those for workers. Workers, by virtue of the ability to work, tend to be a healthier population than the public, which includes susceptible populations, the elderly, and children.

†International Commission on Radiological Protection. 1990 Recommendations of the International Commission on Radiological Protection, ICRP Publication 60, Annals of the ICRP 21, Elmsford, NY: Pergamon Press, 1991.

‡National Council on Radiation Protection and Measurements (NCRP). Limitation of exposure to ionizing radiation. Bethesda, MD: NCRP, 1993. NCRP Report No. 116.

§Stochastic effects are those effects for which the probability of occurrence, rather than the magnitude of the effect, is proportional to dose. Not all irradiated persons show such effects; however, the probability that they will can be described by a dose-response curve that extends to zero with no threshold. Nonstochastic effects are proportional in severity to the magnitude of the absorbed dose; they probably have a threshold below which no effect will be observed because simultaneous injury to many cells is required.

Types of Ionizing Radiation

Type	Charge	Atomic Mass (amu)	Source*	Shielding†
Alpha	+2	4	Radium-226 Polonium-210 Uranium-238	Sheet of paper; intact skin
Beta	±1	0.0005	Carbon-14 Strontium-90 Tritium Iodine-131	Lead; aluminium foil; a few centimeters of plastic
Neutron	0	1	Particle accelerator Nuclear reactor	High energy=paraffin Low energy=water
Proton	+1	1	Cosmic radiation Particle accelerator	Air
Gamma	0	0	Cobalt-60 Uranium-238 Iodine-131	A few centimeters of lead; many inches of steel
X	0	0	Diagnostic and therapeutic medicine	A few centimeters of lead; many inches of steel

*Familiar examples of originating source.

†In any given situation, the type and thickness of shielding is dependent on the energy and intensity of the radiation.

Treatment Summary for Internal Contamination, by Selected Radioactive Elements

The benefit from therapy recommendations in the Immediate Actions to Consider (column 2) and Drugs to Consider (column 3) will be influenced by the route of exposure: ingestion, inhalation, skin absorption, injection, or contaminated wounds. The chemical form and solubility of the radionuclide will also change markedly the efficacy of the recommended treatment. The table below lists therapeutic procedures or drug therapy that may be helpful for the listed elements in favorable circumstances.

Element	Immediate Actions to Consider	Drugs to Consider	Information and Comment
Americium (Am)	DTPA*	DTPA	Chelation should be started as soon as treatment decision can be made. CaEDTA† may be used if CaDTPA‡ is not immediately available.
Arsenic (As)	Lavage	Dimercaprol	Short-lived isotopes. Use of dimercaprol is not indicated except in massive exposures.
Barium (Ba)	Lavage, purgatives	See column 4	Use of sodium or magnesium sulfate with and after stomach lavage will precipitate insoluble barium sulfate.
Calcium (Ca)	Lavage, purgatives, calcium	Calcium, furosemide	Massive exposure may warrant use of the sodium salt of EDTA§, but with caution over a 3- to 4-hour period to avoid tetany. Furosemide enhances urinary excretion.
Californium (Cf)	DTPA, lavage, purgatives	DTPA	Same as for Americium
Carbon (C)	(None listed)	No treatment available	Low-energy beta rays of carbon-14 are not detected by survey instruments; collect samples and smears for special low-energy beta counting in laboratory.
Cerium (Ce)	DTPA, lavage, purgatives	DTPA	Same as for Americium.
Cesium (Cs)	Prussian blue, lavage, purgatives	Prussian blue	Ion exchange resins should be as effective as Prussian blue, but have not been used in humans.
Chromium (Cr)	Lavage, purgatives	No treatment available for anionic forms; DTPA or DFOA¶ for cationic forms	Antacids are contraindicated. Adsorbents, such as charcoal, may reduce intestinal tract absorption.
Cobalt (Co)	Lavage, purgatives	See column 4	Penicillamine may be considered for therapeutic trial in large exposures.
Curium (Cm)	DTPA, lavage, purgatives	DTPA	Same as for Americium
Europium (Eu)	Lavage, purgatives	DTPA	None.

(continued)

Element	Immediate Actions to Consider	Drugs to Consider	Information and Comment
Fission products	Lavage, purgatives	#	Gamma-ray spectroscopy of air or swipe samples may identify prominent radionuclides (mixed). Check also for possible alpha emitters.
Fluorine (F)	Aluminum hydroxide gel	See column 4	Very short half-life. Oral aluminum hydroxide gel will reduce absorption in the gastrointestinal (GI) tract.
Gallium (Ga)	See column 4	See column 4	Short half-life. Penicillamine can be considered for therapeutic trial.
Gold (Au)	None	Dimercaprol and penicillamine are possible therapeutic agents	No known therapy for colloidal gold.
Iodine (I)	Potassium iodide, lavage	Potassium iodide	Success of stable iodine depends on early administration.
Iron (Fe)	Lavage	DFOA	Materials that reduce GI absorption include egg yolk or adsorbents. Oral penicillamine also chelates iron.
Lanthanum (La)	Lavage, purgatives	DTPA	CaEDTA may be used if CaDTPA is not immediately available.
Lead (Pb)	Lavage	EDTA	Dimercaprol and penicillamine are less satisfactory alternative drugs.
Mercury (Hg)	Lavage	Penicillamine	Dimercaprol may be considered for alternative therapy. Gastric lavage with egg white solution or 5% sodium formaldehyde sulfoxide; if unavailable, use a 2% to 5% solution of sodium bicarbonate.
Phosphorus (P)	Lavage, aluminum hydroxide	Phosphates	Severe overdosage may be treated with parathyroid extract (intramuscular) in addition to oral phosphates.
Plutonium (Pu)	DTPA	DTPA	DFOA may be used initially if DTPA is not available. CaEDTA may also be used, but is less effective.
Polonium (Po)	Lavage, purgatives	Dimercaprol	Consider toxicity of dimercaprol before using in cases of low-level exposure. Penicillamine is an alternative treatment.
Potassium (K)	Purgatives, diuretics, aluminum hydroxide	Diuretics	Use aluminum hydroxide antacids first to reduce GI tract absorption. Use oral liquid potassium supplements for dilution.

(continued)

Element	Immediate Actions to Consider	Drugs to Consider	Information and Comment
Promethium (Pm)	DTPA	DTPA	Chelation treatment should be started as soon as possible.
Radium (Ra)	Magnesium sulfate, lavage, purgatives	See column 4	Use 10% magnesium sulfate solution for gastric lavage and as saline cathartic. Oral sulfates reduce intestinal absorption. No effective therapy after absorption.
Rubidium (Rb)	Prussian blue	Prussian blue	Chemical properties are similar to potassium, but efficacy of similar treatments is unknown.
Ruthenium (Ru)	Lavage, purgatives	See column 4	Chlorthalidone causes enhanced urinary excretion. DTPA has variable effectiveness.
Scandium (Sc)	Lavage, purgatives	DTPA	EDTA may be used in place of DTPA.
Sodium (Na)	Lavage	Diuretic	Isotopic dilution (1 L of 0.9% sodium chloride) by intravenous route, followed by furosemide or other diuretic agent.
Strontium (Sr)	Aluminum phosphate, lavage	Strontium or calcium intravenously	Corticosteroid may be considered, but adverse reactions should be balanced against probable limited effectiveness.
Technetium (Tc)	(None listed)	(None listed)	Potassium perchlorate has been used effectively to reduce thyroid dose.
Thorium (Th)	(None listed)	DTPA or DFOA for soluble compounds	Treatment not effective for thorotrast (ThO_2).
Tritium (^3H)	Forced water	Forced water	Low-energy beta rays of ^3H are not detectable by survey instruments; requires samples for special low-energy beta counting in laboratory.
Uranium (U)	DTPA	(None listed)	DTPA must be given within 4 hours to be effective. Sodium bicarbonate protects the kidneys from damage.
Yttrium (Y)	(None listed)	DTPA	CaEDTA may be used if CaDTPA is not immediately available.
Zinc (Zn)	Lavage	DTPA	Zinc sulfate or CaEDTA may be used as a diluting agent if CaDTPA is not immediately available. Penicillamine is another alternative.

*DTPA = diethylenetriaminepentaacetic acid.

†CaEDTA = calcium salt of ethylenediaminetetraacetic acid.

‡CaDTPA = calcium diethylenetriaminepentaacetic acid.

§EDTA = ethylenediaminetetraacetic acid.

¶DFOA = deferoxamine or desferrioxamine.

#Depends on major isotope(s) in mixture, which varies with age of the isotope mixture.

Treatment Scheme For Patients Receiving An Acute High-Dose Radiation Exposure

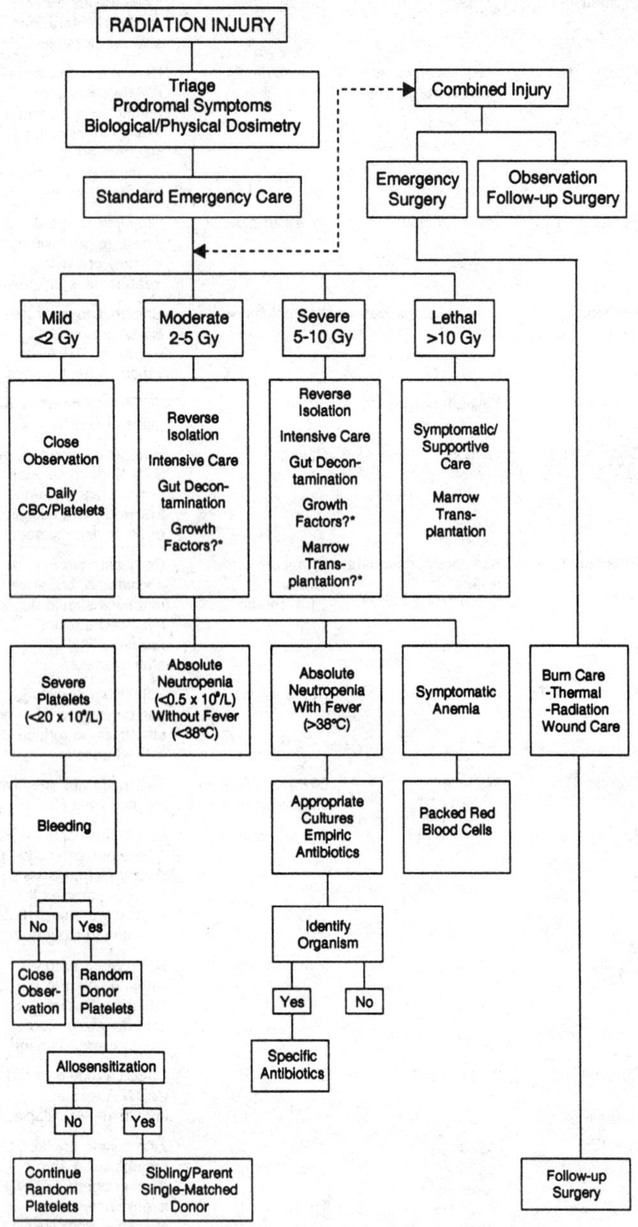

* Whole-body exposures >4 Gy may require bone marrow transplantation or administration of colony-stimulating factors or other hematopoietic growth factors that stimulate proliferation of hematopoietic stem cells. However, few data exist to support firm recommendations about the use of these treatments for radiation victims.

REPRODUCTIVE AND DEVELOPMENTAL HAZARDS

Agents Associated With Adverse Female Reproductive Capacity or Developmental Effects in Human and Animal Studies*

Agent	Human Outcomes	Strength of Association in Humans†	Animal Outcomes	Strength of Association in Animals†
Anesthetic gases‡	Reduced fertility, spontaneous abortion	1,3	Birth defects	1,3
Arsenic	Spontaneous abortion, low birth weight	1	Birth defects, fetal loss	2
Benzo(a)pyrene	None	NA§	Birth defects	1
Cadmium	None	NA	Fetal loss, birth defects	2
Carbon disulfide	Menstrual disorders, spontaneous abortion	1	Birth defects	1
Carbon monoxide	Low birth weight, fetal death (high doses)	1	Birth defects, neonatal mortality	2
Chlordecone	None	NA	Fetal loss	2,3
Chloroform	None	NA	Fetal loss	1
Chloroprene	None	NA	Birth defects	2,3
Ethylene glycol ethers	Spontaneous abortion	1	Birth defects	2
Ethylene oxide	Spontaneous abortion	1	Fetal loss	1
Formamides	None	NA	Fetal loss, birth defects	2
Inorganic mercury‡	Menstrual disorders, spontaneous abortion	1	Fetal loss, birth defects	1
Lead‡	Spontaneous abortion, prematurity, neurologic dysfunction in child	2	Birth defects, fetal loss	2
Organic mercury	CNS malformation, cerebral palsy	2	Birth defects, fetal loss	2
Physical stress	Prematurity	2	None	NA
Polybrominated biphenyls (PBBs)	None	NA	Fetal loss	2
Polychlorinated biphenyls (PCBs)	Neonatal PCB syndrome (low birth weight, hyperpigmentation, eye abnormalities)	2	Low birth weight, fetal loss	2
Radiation, ionizing	Menstrual disorders, CNS defects, skeletal and eye anomalies, mental retardation, childhood cancer	2	Fetal loss, birth defects	2
Selenium	Spontaneous abortion	3	Low birth weight, birth defects	2
Tellurium	None	NA	Birth defects	2
2,4-Dichlorophenoxy-acetic acid (2,4-D)	Skeletal defects	4	Birth defects	1
2,4,5-Trichlorophenoxy-acetic acid (2,4,5-T)	Skeletal defects	4	Birth defects	1
Video display terminals	Spontaneous abortion	4	Birth defects	1
Vinyl chloride‡	CNS defects	1	Birth defects	1,4
Xylene	Menstrual disorders, fetal loss	1	Fetal loss, birth defects	1

U.S. Department of Health & Human Services, "Reproductive and Developmental Hazards," *Case Studies in Environmental Medicine*, Agency for Toxic Substances and Disease Registry, September 1993.

*Major studies of the reproductive health effects of exposure to dioxin are currently in progress.

†1 = limited positive data. 3 = limited negative data.
2 = strong positive data. 4 = strong negative data.

‡Symbol used to designate agents that may have male-mediated effects.

§Not applicable because no adverse outcomes were observed.

Exposures Associated With Male Reproductive Dysfunction

Agent	Human Outcomes	Strength of Association in Humans*	Animal Outcomes	Strength of Association in Animals*
Boron	Decreased sperm count	1	Testicular damage	2
Benzene	None	NA†	Decreased sperm motility, testicular damage	1
Benzo(a)pyrene	None	NA	Testicular damage	1
Cadmium	Reduced fertility	1	Testicular damage	2
Carbon disulfide	Decreased sperm count, decreased sperm motility	2,3	Testicular damage	1
Carbon monoxide	None	NA	Testicular damage	1
Carbon tetrachloride	None	NA	Testicular damage	1
Carbaryl	Abnormal sperm morphology	1	Testicular damage	1
Chlordecone	Decreased sperm count, decreased sperm motility	2	Testicular damage	2
Chloroprene	Decreased sperm motility, abnormal morphology, decreased libido	2	Testicular damage	1
Dibromochloropropane (DBCP)	Decreased sperm count, azoospermia, hormonal changes	2	Testicular damage	2
Dimethyl dichlorovinyl phosphate (DDVP)	None	NA	Decreased sperm count	2
Epichlorohydrin	None	NA	Testicular damage	2,3
Estrogens	Decreased sperm count	2	Decreased sperm count	2
Ethylene oxide	None	NA	Testicular damage	1
Ethylene dibromide (EDB)	Abnormal sperm motility	1	Testicular damage	2,3
Ethylene glycol ethers	Decreased sperm count	1	Testicular damage	2
Heat	Decreased sperm count	2	Decreased sperm count	2
Lead	Decreased sperm count	2	Testicular damage, decreased sperm count, decreased sperm motility, abnormal morphology	2
Manganese	Decreased libido, impotence	1	Testicular damage	1,3
Polybrominated biphenyls (PBBs)	None	NA	Testicular damage	1
Polychlorinated biphenyls (PCBs)	None	NA	Testicular damage	1
Radiation, ionizing	Decreased sperm count	2	Testicular damage	2

U.S. Department of Health & Human Services, "Reproductive and Developmental Hazards," *Case Studies in Environmental Medicine*, Agency for Toxic Substances and Disease Registry, September 1993.

*1 = limited positive data. 3 = limited negative data.
2 = strong positive data. 4 = strong negative data.

†Not applicable because no adverse outcomes were observed.

SALIVARY FLUIDS, DRUG CONCENTRATIONS

	Saliva/Plasma* Ratio	Range
Amphetamine	2.76	
Antipurine	1	
Benzoylecgonine	0-0.5	0-51 ng/mL
	0.1-0.2	0-56 ng/mL
	0.1-0.3	0-46 ng/mL
Buprenorphine	0.05-0.41	0.1-1000 ng/mL
Caffeine	0.6-1	
Carbamazepine	0.1-0.3	1.4-3.5 mg/L†
Chlorpromazine	0.4	
Clorazepate	5.78	5-20 ng/mL
Cocaine		
crack, 42 mg	1.5-17	0-3404 ng/mL
intranasal, 42 mg	0.7 to 13,239	0-540,800 ng/mL
I.V., 25 mg	0.5-3.5 (avg 1.3)	0-531 ng/mL
Codeine	3.3-3.6	1-308 ng/mL
Cotinine		
smokers	0.8-1.4	10 to >100 ng/mL
nonsmokers		<5 ng/mL
Dehydroepiandrosterone	0.001	5 nmol/L
Delta-9-tetrahydrocannabinol	0.5 to 6	50-1000 ng/mL
Diazepam	0.013	0-20 ng/mL
Diphenylhydantoin	0.1-0.3	1-2 mg/L†
Doxorubicin	2.3	
Ethanol	1.03 to 1.08	0-210 mg/dL
Etoposide	1.0	
5-Fluorouracil	0.8	
Haloperidol	2.2	
Hexobarbital	0.34	
Hydromorphone	0.3-2.3	
Lithium	3-13	
Lysergic acid diethylamide	1.4	0.3-3.1 ng/mL
Melphalan	1.2	
Meperidine	2.6	
Methaqualone	0.1	
Morphine	0.4-0.7	0-60 ng/mL
Pentobarbital	0.36	
Phencyclidine	2.4	
Phenobarbital	0.3	5-15 mg/L†
Secobarbital	0.24-0.38	
Theophylline	0.5-1	5.6-11.3 μg/mL†
Thiocyanate		
smokers	10.6	0-220 μg/mL
nonsmokers	13.4	0-150 μg/mL

*S/P values assumed saliva pH 6.8, serum pH 7.4.

†Proposed therapeutic range.

Reference: Malamud D and Tabak L, eds, "Saliva as A Diagnostic Fluid," *Ann of NY Acad of Science*, New York, NY: 1993, vol 694.

SEIZURES, NEONATAL GUIDELINES

Approach to the Treatment of Neonatal Seizures

Drug	Loading Dose	Maintenance Dose	Half-life	Therapeutic Range
Diazepam	0.25 mg/kg I.V. (in 2 min)	Dose may be repeated several times as clinically needed	25 h preterm 31 h term	35-81 μmol/L
Lorazepam (for refractory seizures)	0.04-0.1 mg/kg I.V. over 2-5 minutes	May repeat in 15 minutes	10-40 h	50-240 ng/mL
Paraldehyde (rarely used)	0.150-0.200 mL/kg I.V.	0.020 mL/kg/h I.V.	10 h	10-40 μg/mL
Phenobarbital	20 mg/kg I.V. (in 10 min)	3-4 mg/kg divided (bid), I.V./I.M./P.O.	Age dependant: 100 h by 14 d 20 h by 28 d	16-40 μg/mL
Phenytoin	20 mg/kg I.V. (1 mg/kg/min)	4-8 mg/kg divided (bid), I.V.	Age dependant: 104 h early neonatal period to 2-7 h late neonatal period	15-20 μg/mL
Primidone	15-25 mg/kg P.O.	12-20 mg/kg/d	12 h	6-15 μg/mL

Causes of Neonatal Seizures

1. Trauma
   a. subdural hematoma
   b. intracortical hemorrhage
   c. cortical vein thrombosis
2. Asphyxia — subependymal hemorrhage
3. Congenital abnormalities (cerebral dysgenesis)
   a. lissencephaly
   b. schizencephaly
4. Hypertension
5. Metabolic
   a. hypocalcemia
      - hypomagnesemia
      - high phosphate load
      - IDM (infants of diabetic mothers)
      - hypoparathyroidism
      - maternal hyperparathyroidism
      - idiopathic
      - DiGeorge's syndrome
   b. hypoglycemia
      - galactosemia
      - IUGR (intrauterine growth retardation)
      - IDM (infants of diabetic mothers)
      - glycogen storage disease
      - idiopathic
      - methylmalonic acidemia
      - propionic acidemia
      - maple syrup urine disease
      - asphyxia
   c. electrolyte imbalance
      - hypernatremia
      - hypomagnesemia
      - hyponatremia

6. Infections
   a. bacterial meningitis
   b. cerebral abscess
   c. herpes encephalitis
   d. Coxsackie meningoencephalitis
   e. cytomegalovirus
   f. toxoplasmosis
   g. syphilis
7. Drug withdrawal
   a. methadone
   b. heroin
   c. barbiturate (short-acting, such as secobarbital and butalbital)
   d. propoxyphene
   e. benzodiazepines (chlordiazepoxide, diazepam)
   f. cocaine
   g. ethanol
   h. codeine
8. Pyridoxine dependency
9. Amino acid disturbances
   a. maple syrup urine disease
   b. urea cycle abnormalities
   c. nonketotic hyperglycinemia
   d. ketotic hyperglycinemia
   e. Leigh disease
   f. isovaleric acidemia
10. Toxins
    a. local anesthetics
    b. isoniazid
    c. lead
    d. indomethacin (from breast feeding)
11. Familial seizures
    a. neurocutaneous syndromes
       - tuberous sclerosis
       - incontinentia pigmenti
    b. genetic syndromes
       - Zellweger's
       - Smith Lemli Opitz
       - neonatal adrenoleukodystrophy
    c. benign familial epilepsy
12. Hyperbilirubinemia
13. Cerebral hemorrhage
    a. intraventricular
    b. subarachnoid
    c. subdural

Adapted from Painter MJ, Bergman I, and Crumrie P, "Neonatal Seizures," *Pediatr Clin North Am*, 1986, 33:91-107.

SODIUM CONTENT OF SELECTED MEDICINALS

Name and Dosage Unit*	Sodium mg	Sodium mEq
Antibiotics		
Amikacin sulfate, 1 g	29.9	1.3
Aminosalicylate sodium, 1 g	109	4.7
Ampicillin, suspension, 250 mg/5 mL, 5 mL	10	0.4
Ampicillin sodium, 1 g	66.7	3
Azlocillin sodium, 1 g	50	2.2
Carbenicillin disodium, 382 mg (tablet)	22	1
Cefazolin sodium, 1 g	47	2
Cefotaxime sodium, 1 g	30.5	2.2
Cefoxitin sodium, 1 g	53	2.3
Ceftriaxone sodium, 1 g	83	3.6
Cefuroxime, 1 g	54.2	2.4
Chloramphenicol sodium succinate, 1 g	51.8	2.3
Dicloxacillin, 250 mg (capsule)	13	0.6
Dicloxacillin, suspension, 65 mg/5 mL	27	1.2
Erythromycin ethyl succinate, suspension, 200 mg/5 mL	29	1.3
Erythromycin Base Filmtab®, 250 mg	70	3
Methicillin sodium, 1 g	66.7	2.9
Metronidazole, 500 mg I.V.	322	14
Mezlocillin sodium, 1 g	42.6	1.9
Moxalactam sodium, 1 g	88	3.8
Nafcillin sodium, 1 g	66.7	2.9
Nitrofurantoin, suspension, 25 mg/5 mL	7	0.3
Penicillin G potassium, 1,000,000 units I.V.	7.6	0.3
Penicillin G sodium, 1,000,000 units I.V.	46	2
Penicillin V potassium, suspension, 250 mg/5 mL	38	1.7
Piperacillin sodium, 1 g	42.6	1.8
Ticarcillin disodium, 1 g	119.6	5.2
Antacids, Liquid (content per 5 mL)		
Amphojel®	<2.3	<0.1
ALternaGEL®	2	0.1
Basaljel®	2.4	0.1
Extra Strength Maalox®-Plus	0.65	~0.05
Gaviscon®	13	0.57
Maalox®	1.3	0.06
Tums E-X™	<4.8	<0.2
Sodium Content of Miscellaneous Medicinals		
Acetazolamide sodium, 500 mg	47.2	2.05
Chlorothiazide sodium, 500 mg	57.5	2
Cisplatin, 10 mg	35.4	1.54
Edetate calcium disodium, 1 g	122	5.3
Fleet® Enema, 4.5 oz	5000†	218
Fleet® Phospho®-Soda, 20 mL	2217	96.4
Hydrocortisone sodium succinate, 1 g	47.5	2.07
Hypaque® M 75%, injection, 20 mL	200	8.7
Hypaque® M 90%, injection, 20 mL	220	9.6
Metamucil® Instant Mix (orange)	6	0.27
Methotrexate sodium, 100 mg vial	20	0.86
Methotrexate sodium, 100 mg vial (low sodium)	15	0.65
Naproxen sodium, 250 mg (tablet)	23	1
Neutra-Phos®, capsule and 75 mL reconstituted solution	164	7.13
Oragrafin® (capsule)	19	0.8
Pentobarbital sodium, 50 mg/mL, 1 mL vial	5	0.2
Phenobarbital sodium, 65 mg, 1 mL vial	6	0.3
Phenytoin sodium, 1 g	88	3.8
Promethazine expectorant, 5 mL	53	2.3
Shohl's solution modified, 1 mL	23	1
Sodium ascorbate, 500 mg acid equivalent	65.3	2.84
Sodium bicarbonate, 50 mL 8.4%	1150	50
Sodium nitroprusside, 50 mg	7.8	0.34
Sodium polystyrene sulfonate, 1 g	94.3‡	4.1
Thiopental sodium, 1 g	86.8	3.8
Valproate sodium, 250 mg/5 mL, 5 mL	23	1

*Product formulations and hence sodium content are subject to change by the manufacturer. Please contact the Pharmacy Department for current information.
†Average systemic absorption 250-300 mg.
‡Total sodium content. Only about 33% is liberated in clinical use.

SORBITOL CONTENT OF ACTIVATED CHARCOAL PRODUCTS

Product		Sorbitol Content
Acta-Char®	50 g	62 g
Actidose®	25 g	48 g
	50 g	96 g
Charcoaid®	30 g	105 g
Charcolex®	40 g	18.8 g
Liqui-Char®	25 g	27 g
	50 g	54 g
UDL	25 g	27 g

STATUS EPILEPTICUS TREATMENT ALGORITHM

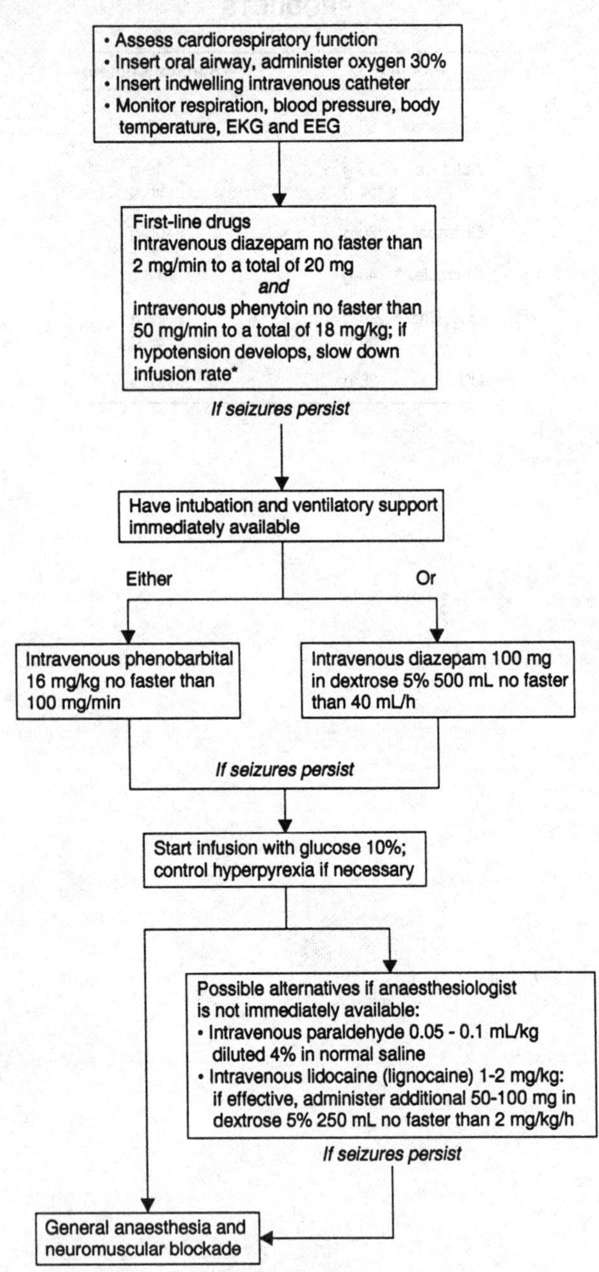

* May not be effective for xanthine or sympathomimetic overdose

Reprinted with permission from "Induced Seizures in Drug Safety," *Drug Safety*, 1990, 5(2):140.

STREET DRUG SLANG

Slang	Meaning
1 on 1	Glutethimide and codeine
1-Way	LSD
10-dollar ready rock	Cocaine
10's	Amphetamine
100x	Amphetamine-like hallucinogen
1980 supergrass	Ketamine
2 on 2	Glutethimide and codeine
20th anniversary	LSD
21	LSD
3 on 3	Glutethimide and codeine
3's & 8's	Glutethimide and codeine
357 magnum	Caffeine
4's and doors	Glutethimide and codeine
45-minute psychosis	DMT
5-dollar ready rock	Cocaine
51	Cocaine and marijuana
68	Oil of peppermint
69-69	Cocaine; heroin
712	Methaqualone
714	Methaqualone
750	Ethchlorvynol
8-ball	Cocaine
930 Porche turbo	Heroin
A boot	Under the influence of drugs
AB	Abscess at injection site
A-bomb	Marijuana and heroin
Acapulco gold	Marijuana
Ace	Marijuana
Aceite	Heroin
Acid	LSD
Adam	Methamphetamine
Afgano	Marijuana
African black	Marijuana
African tea	Cathinone
Afterburner	Amphetamines
Aimes	Amyl nitrate
Airplane	Marijuana
A.J.	Heroin
AK-47	Heroin
Alice B. Toklas brownies	Recipe using LSD and marijuana
All-American drug	Cocaine
Alley juice	Methanol
Amarillas	Pentobarbital
Ames	Amyl nitrate
Amidone	Methadone
Ammo	Amobarbital
Amp	Marijuana soaked in formaldehyde
Amps	Glass ampuls of amphetamine
A.M.T.	DMT
Anfeta	Amphetamine
Angel dust	PCP
Angel hair	PCP
Angel mist	PCP
Animal	LSD
Antifreeze	Heroin
Antilog	Peyote
Apache	Heroin
Apples	Marijuana
Arabian tea	Cathinone
A's	Amphetamine
Ashes	Marijuana
Asthmador	*Datura stramonium*
Atom bomb	Marijuana
Azucar	LSD
B	PCP

Slang	Meaning
B-bombs	Benzedrine® inhalers
Baby	Marijuana
Bacha	Marijuana
Bachica	Marijuana
Bad seed	Heroin
Bam D	Preludin® and Dilaudid®
Bamate	Meprobamate
Bambita	Methamphetamine
Bammies	Marijuana
Bammo	Meprobamate
Bams	Pure amphetamine
Banana with cheese	Marijuana and cocaine free-base cigarette
Bananas	Talwin NX® and Pyribenzamine®
Ban-apple gas	N-butyl nitrite
Bang	Isobutyl nitrite; marijuana
Bank bandit pills	Barbiturate
Bar	Marijuana
Barbs	Barbiturate
Barrels	LSD
Baseball	Freebase cocaine
Bash	Marijuana
Bathtub crank	Homemade speed
Battery acid	LSD
Bazooka	Cocaine; marijuana
Bazooka paste	Marijuana and procaine
Beam-me-up	Freebase cocaine
Bean	Benzedrine® inhalers; Doriden® and Valium® with codeine cough syrup
Beans	Amphetamines; mescaline
Beauties	Amphetamines
Beef	Heroin and cocaine
Bees	Marijuana
Belushi	Cocaine and heroin
Benz	Benzedrine®
Berkley blood	LSD
Berkley boo	Marijuana
Bernice	Cocaine
Bernies	Cocaine
Bhang	Marijuana
Big chief	Peyote
Big D	LSD
Big flake	Cocaine
Big Harry	Heroin
Big O	Opium
Big T	Talwin® and Pyribenzamine®
Bindle	Heroin
Birds	Marijuana
Bitter	Paregoric
Black and green capsules	Amitriptyline and salicylamide
Black and red capsules	Caffeine
Black beauties	Amphetamines
Black bombers	Amphetamines
Black capsules	Amphetamines
Black dex	Dextroamphetamine
Black doves	LSD
Black dust	PCP
Black glass	Heroin
Black gum	Heroin
Black gunion	Marijuana
Black hash	Marijuana and opium
Black heroin	Heroin and molasses
Black horses	Heroin
Black Jack	Paregoric
Black mollies	Amphetamines
Black mote	Marijuana

Slang	Meaning
Black pearl	Diazepam
Black pills	Opium
Black Russian	Marijuana
Black star	LSD
Black stuff	Opium
Black sunshine	LSD
Black tabs	LSD
Black widow	Biphetamine®
Blake	Cocaine
Blank	Low grade heroin
Blinky	Cocaine
Block	Marijuana
Block busters	Barbiturate
Blotter acid	LSD
Blotter cube	LSD
Blow	Heroin
Blue acid	LSD
Blue angels	Amobarbital
Blue bands	Carbital®
Blue barrels	LSD
Blue Berkely	LSD
Blue bombers	Diazepam
Blue boys	Diazepam
Blue bullets	Amobarbital
Blue caps	Mescaline
Blue cheer	LSD
Blue clouds	Amobarbital
Blue cross	Pyrilamine maleate
Blue devils	Amobarbital
Blue diamonds	Heroin
Blue dolls	Amobarbital
Blue dots	LSD
Blue dragon	LSD
Blue egg	Caffeine
Blue heaven	Isopropyl alcohol; LSD
Blue Magoo's	Diazepam
Blue microdots	LSD
Blue mist	LSD
Blue moon	LSD
Blue morphine	Numorphan®
Blue octopus	LSD
Blue speckled meth	Obetrol®
Bluebird	Heroin and cocaine
Blues	Amobarbital
Blunts	Marijuana in cigar casings
Boost	Potentiate
Bud	Marijuana
Bunk weed	Poor quality marijuana
C & H	Cocaine and heroin
C & M	Cocaine and morphine
Caballo	Heroin
Cabo	Marijuana
Caca	Heroin
Cactus	Peyote
Cactus head	Mescaline
Cadillac	PCP
Cadillac of drugs	Cocaine
Cafe	Marijuana
Cakes and syrup	Glutethimide and codeine
California glass	Methamphetamine
California sunshine	LSD
California white cross	Methamphetamine
Can	PCP; marijuana
Canadian black	Marijuana
Canary	Phenobarbital
Cancelled stick	Marijuana
Candy	Tuinal® and Seconal™
Cane	Cocaine
Canned sativa	Marijuana
Canned stuff	Opium
Capricorn tabs	Caffeine
Carga	Heroin
Carmabis	Marijuana
Carrie	Cocaine
Carry Nation	Cocaine
Cartwheels	Amphetamine
Cat	Methcathinone

Slang	Meaning
CB	Glutethimide
CC-duct	Cocaine
CD	Glutethimide
Cecil	Cocaine
Centurion	Benzodiazepine
Cha cha	Cocaine
Chafa	Marijuana
Champagne of drugs	Cocaine
Charas	Marijuana
Charge	Marijuana
Charlie	Cocaine
Chasing the dragon	Heroin
Checkboard	LSD
Checkmate	Heroin
Cheeba-cheeba	Marijuana soaked in formaldehyde
Cheva	Heroin
Chiba-chiba	Marijuana
Chicago green	Marijuana and opium
Chicarra	Marijuana and tobacco
Chicken powder	Amphetamines
Chicle	Cocaine; heroin
Chiclosa	Heroin
Chief	LSD; mescaline
China white	Fentanyl; heroin
Chinese blowing	Heroin
Chinese red	Heroin
Chinesing	Heroin
Chiva	Heroin
Chocolate	Heroin
Chocolate chips	LSD
Chocolate rock	Heroin and cocaine
Chokers	Heroin and tobacco
Cholly	Cocaine
Chris	Methamphetamine
Christmas tree	Amphetamines
Churro	Marijuana
Churus	Marijuana
Cibas	Glutethimide
Cibas and codeine	Glutethimide and codeine
Citexal	Methaqualone
CJ	PCP
Clarity	MDMA
Clear and blues	Caffeine, ephedrine, and phenylpropanolamine
Clear and green	Methapyrilene
Clear and pink	Diphenhydramine
Clear and yellow	Caffeine and phenylpropanolamine
Clear lights	LSD
Clickers	Marijuana, PCP, and formaldehyde
Clicks	Marijuana, PCP, and formaldehyde
Clickums	Marijuana and PCP
Climax	Isobutyl nitrite
Coast	Methylphenidate hydrochloride
Coast to coast	Amphetamines
Cobra	Heroin
Coca	Cocaine
Coca Cola®	Cocaine
Cocktail	Marijuana
Cocoa	Heroin
Cocoa leaf	Procaine and caffeine
Cocoa snow	Benzocaine, procaine, and caffeine
Coconuts	Cocaine
Cod cock	Cocaine mixed with other medications
Coffee	LSD
Coffin	Tobacco
Coffin nails	Tobacco
Cohete	Heroin
Cohobe	DMT in powdered seeds
Coke	Cocaine

Slang	Meaning
Cokomo	Cocaine
Cola	Glue
Colombian	Marijuana
Colonial spirit	Methanol
Colorado cocktails	Marijuana
Columbian	Marijuana
Columbian spirit	Methanol
Columbus	Marijuana
Comeback	Cocaine
Coney only	Heroin and cocaine
Contact lens	LSD
Copping	Area to procure drugs
Coral	Chloral hydrate
Corga	Heroin
Corgy	Heroin
Corrine	Cocaine
Costo	Marijuana
Courage pills	Barbiturates
Crack	Cocaine
Crackers	LSD
Crack meth	Methamphetamine
Crank	Methamphetamine
Crap	Heroin
Crazy dust	PCP
Crazy Eddie	Cocaine in formaldehyde
Crazy K	PCP
Crink	Methamphetamine
Cris	Methamphetamine
Criss-cross	Amphetamine
Cristina	Methamphetamine
Croak	Methamphetamine and cocaine
Croke	Methamphetamine and cocaine
Cross	Methamphetamine
Crossroads	Amphetamine
Cross-tops	Amphetamine
Crypt	Isobutyl nitrite
Crystal	D-methamphetamine
Crystal caine	Caffeine and phenylpropanolamine
Crystal joint	PCP
Crystal meth	Methamphetamine
Crystal THC	PCP
Cuartel	Marijuana
Cube	LSD
Cube juice	Morphine
Cucaracha	Marijuana
Cujo	Heroin and cocaine
Culley	Marijuana
Cupcakes	LSD
Cura	Heroin
Cyclone	PCP
D	LSD
Dagga	Marijuana
Dama blanca	Cocaine
Datura	Belladonna and jimson weed
Dava	Heroin
Dawamesk	Marijuana and spices in green cake
Deadly	Heroin
Dead on arrival	PCP
Deck	Narcotics
Deeda	LSD
Deep fry	Marijuana
Descontin	LSD
Det	Diethyltryptamine
Deuce	Heroin
Dex	Dexedrine®
Diablitos	Marijuana and crack
Diane	Demerol®
Dice	Methamphetamine
Dicoroma	Isobutyl nitrite
Diet pills	Amphetamines
Dillies	Dilaudid®
Dinky dows	Marijuana
Dip jimming	Marijuana dipped in PCP and formaldehyde
Dipper	PCP
Dips	Marijuana dipped in PCP
Dirt	Heroin
Disco biscuits	Methaqualone
Disco hits	LSD
Dish rag	Heroin
Ditch weed	Marijuana
Djamba	Marijuana
Djoma	Marijuana
DMA	Dimethoxyamphetamine
DMDA	Synthetic amphetamine
DMT	Dimethyltryptamine
DMZ	Benactyzine
DOA	PCP
DOM	Dimethoxyamphetamine
Doctor	MDMA
Doe	Methamphetamine
Dogie	Heroin
Dominos	Amphetamines
Doobie	Marijuana
Doojee	Heroin
Dopar	Levodopa
Dope	Marijuana
Doper	Levodopa
Doriden® load	Glutethimide, codeine, and aspirin
Dors and fours	Doriden® and Empirin® #4
Dose	Cocaine
Doses	LSD
Dot	LSD
Double cross	Amphetamines
Double dome	LSD
Double trouble	Amobarbital and secobarbital
Down head	Heroin
Downers	Depressants or sedatives
Downie	Depressants or sedatives
Downs	Depressants or sedatives
Do-wop	Heroin
Doxy	Desoxyn® (amphetamine)
DPT	Dipropyltryptamine
Dream	Cocaine
Dream dust	PCP
Dreamer	Morphine
Drivers	Amphetamine
Dry high	Marijuana
Dry whiskey	Peyote
D's & B's	Dilaudid® and Pyribenzamine®
D's & T's	Doriden® and codeine
Dubie	Marijuana
Duby	Marijuana
Duct	Cocaine
Dugie	Heroin
Dujie	Heroin
Dummy dust	PCP
Dust	Cocaine; heroin and cocaine; morphine; PCP
Dust of angels	PCP
Dusted parsley	PCP
Dynamite	Marijuana and cocaine; marijuana and heroin
Dynamites	Amphetamines
Dyno	Heroin
E	MDMA
Ecstasy	MDMA
Ectasy	MDMA
Eden	MDA

Slang	Meaning
Eight ball	Cocaine
Eight balls	1/8 ounce
Electric Kool-Aid®	LSD
Elephant	Marijuana
Elephant tranquilizer	PCP
Embalming fluid	PCP
Emsel	Morphine
Endurets®	Preludin®
E's & V's	Elavil® and Valium®
Essence	MDMA
Estasy	MDMA
Estofa	Heroin
Estuffa	Heroin
Eve	MDA
Exotic	Sinsemilla
Exotic mushroom	Psilocybin
Extasy	MDMA
Eye of horus	LSD
F-40's	Secobarbital
F-66's	Tuinal®
Face Drano®	Cocaine
Factitious air	Nitrous oxide
Fag	Tobacco
Fentanyl	Synthetic heroin
Ferry dust	Heroin
Fine stuff	Marijuana
Fingers	Marijuana
Fir	Marijuana
Fire	Heroin
First line	Morphine
Fizzies	Methadone
Flake	Cocaine
Flamethrower	Heroin, cocaine, and tobacco
Flats	LSD
Flea powder	Heroin
Flesh of the gods	Peyote
Florida	Lidocaine
Flower	Marijuana
Fly	Cocaine
Flying saucers	Morning glory seeds; PCP
Foil	Cocaine and baking soda
Foolish powder	Heroin
Footballs	Amphetamine; Elavil® and ethanol; Talwin NX® and Pyribenzamine®
Forty-five minute psychosis	DMT
Four doors	Doriden®, codeine and ASA/acetaminophen
Fours	Acetaminophen and codeine (Tylenol® #4); aspirin and codeine (Empirin® #4)
Four-way	LSD
Freedy	Ephedrine
French blue	Amphetamine and barbiturate
French fries	Cocaine
Frisco speedball	Heroin, cocaine, and PCP
Frisky powder	Cocaine
FU	Marijuana
F.U.K.	STP
Fuel	Amphetamine; marijuana
Full moon	Peyote
Fun-foon-fong	Opium
Gage	Marijuana
Gauge	Marijuana
Gammon	LSD
Ganja	Marijuana
Gangster	Marijuana
G.B.'s	Barbiturate; Doriden®; heroin

Slang	Meaning
Gee	Opium
Gekoote coke	Cocaine
Genga	Marijuana
Geronimo	Barbiturate and ethanol
Ghana	Marijuana
Ghost	LSD
Ghostbuster	Cocaine and PCP
Gift-of-the-sun-god	Cocaine
Giggle smoke	Marijuana
GI gin	Terpin hydrate with codeine elixir
Gin	Cocaine
Girl	Cocaine
Girl and boy	Heroin and cocaine
Glass	Methamphetamine
Globe	Heroin
Glory seeds	Morning glory seeds
Go	Methamphetamine
Goblet of jam	Marijuana
God's flesh	Psilosybin
God's medicine	Morphine
Gofast	Methamphetamine
Gold	Marijuana
Gold dolphin	LSD
Gold dust	Cocaine
Golden leaf	Marijuana
Gold hornet	LSD
Goma	Heroin
Gomero	Heroin
Good and Plenty	Heroin
Goofballs	Amphetamines; barbiturates; barbiturates and ethanol
Goof butt	Marijuana
Goofers	Barbiturates
Goof juice	Novahistine® DH
Goon	PCP
Gorilla biscuits	PCP
Gorilla pills	Tuinal®
Grape parfait	LSD
Grapes	Morphine; wine
Grasa	Marijuana
Grash	Marijuana
Grass	Marijuana
Grass spaghetti sauce	Marijuana
Grateful Dead	LSD
Gravel	Cocaine
Grease	Amphetamine
Green	Dexamyl®; ketamine; marijuana; PCP on parsley or mint leaves
Green and black	Librium®; cocaine
Green apples	Librium®
Green domes	LSD
Green double domes	LSD
Green dragon	LSD; barbiturate
Green frog	Chloral hydrate; phenylpropanolamine, ephedrine, and caffeine
Green gold	Cocaine
Green hearts	Dextroamphetamine and amobarbital
Greenies	Dextroamphetamine and amobarbital
Green octopus	LSD
Green single domes	LSD
Green-speckled pups	Phendimetrazine
Green weenie	Ethylchlorvynol
Greta	Marijuana
Griefo	Marijuana
Grifa	Marijuana
Griffo	Marijuana
Guarumo	Marijuana
Guato	Marijuana
Gum	Heroin; opium
Gumball	Heroin

Slang	Meaning	Slang	Meaning
Gummy	Heroin	In-betweens	Barbiturate and amphetamine
Gunga	Marijuana	Incentive	Cocaine
Gungeon	Marijuana	Indian bay	Marijuana
Gungi	Marijuana	Indian hat	Marijuana
H	Heroin	Indian hay	Marijuana
Hairy	Heroin	Indica	Marijuana
Half moon	Peyote	Instant zen	LSD
Hanhich	Marijuana	Isobutyl nitrite	Inhalant drug
Happy cigarette	Marijuana	IT 290	Alpha-methyl tryptamine
Happy dust	Cocaine	J	Marijuana
Happy sticks	Marijuana with PCP	Jac aroma	Isobutyl nitrite
Happy trails	Cocaine	Jack	Heroin
Hard candy	Heroin; cocaine	Jack up	Amobarbital
Hard stuff	Heroi; morphine	Jam	Cocaine
Hardware	Isobutyl nitrite	Jamaican	Marijuana
Harry	Heroin	Jammy whammy	Marijuana
Harry Jones	Heroin	Jane	Marijuana
Hawaiian sinsemian	Marijuana	Jay	Marijuana
Hawaiian sunshine	LSD	Jay joint	Marijuana
Hawk	LSD; vocally advertise	JB 318	Methyl piperidyl benzilate
Hay	Marijuana	JB 336	Methyl piperidyl benzilate
Haze	LSD	Jee gee	Heroin
H-caps	Heroin	Jeff	Methcathinone
H.C.P.	PCP	Jellies	Chloral hydrate
Heart on	Isobutyl nitrite	Jelly babies	Temazepam
Hearts	Amphetamine and dextroamphetamine	Jelly beans	Amphetamines
Heaven dust	Cocaine	Jerry Lewis's kids	Fentanyl analog
Heavenly blue	LSD; morning glory seeds	Jet	Ketamine
Heavenly sunshine	LSD	Jive	Marijuana
Helen	Heroin	Jive doojee	Heroin
Hemp	Marijuana	Jive stick	Marijuana
Henry	Heroin	Jock aroma	Amyl or butyl nitrite
Her	Cocaine	John Hinckley	PCP
Herb	Marijuana	Joint	Marijuana
Hessle	Heroin	Jojee	Heroin
Hi ball	Isobutyl nitrite	Jolly babies	Amphetamines
Hierba	Marijuana	Jolly beans	Amphetamines
Hierbabuena	Marijuana	Jolly greens	Ethchlorvynol (Placidyl®)
Hikori	Peyote	Joy juice	Chloral hydrate
Hikuli	Peyote	Joy plant	Opium
Hilo high	Marijuana	Joy powder	Cocaine; heroin
Him	Heroin	Joy smoke	Marijuana
Hiropong	Methamphetamine	Joy sticks	Marijuana and PCP
Hiroppon	Methamphetamine	Juana	Marijuana
Hits	Glutethimide and codeine	Juanita	Marijuana
Hocus	Morphine	Juan Valdez	Marijuana
Hog	Benactyline; choral hydrate; PCP	Jugs	Amphetamine
Home brew	Ethanol	Jugs and beans	Codeine; Darvon®; Doriden®; flurazepam
Hong Kong rock heroin	Strychnine, morphine, heroin, and caffeine	Juice	Ethanol; Novahistine® DH; PCP
Hootch	Ethanol	Jungle love tablets	Red pepper
Hooter	Marijuana	Junk	Heroin; narcotics
Hop	Opium	K2	LSD
Horse	Heroin	Kaksonjae	Methamphetamine
Horse heads	Amphetamines	K-amine	Ketamine
Horse hearts	Amphetamine; Benzedrine®; Dexedrine®	Kansas grass	Marijuana
Horse trank	PCP	Karachi	Heroin with phenobarbital
Horseweed	PCP	Kat	Methcathinone; cathinone
Hot pot fudge	LSD or marijuana	Kay	Ketamine
Hot shot	Heroin, strychnine, and potassium cyanide	Kay jay	PCP
Hot sticks	Marijuana	Keef	Marijuana
Huarache	Marijuana; barbiturate	Kentucky blue	Marijuana
Huatari	Peyote	Kerochi	Heroin
Hubba	Cocaine	Khat	Amphetamine-like stimulant; marijuana; cathinone
Human powder	Heroin	Khib	Marijuana
Hyatari	Peyote	Kibbles and Bits	Talwin® and Ritalin®
Hyke	Hycodan®	Kif	Marijuana
Ice	Methamphetamine	Killer bee	Heroin
Ice cream	Methamphetamine	Killer weed	PCP
Idiot pills	Barbiturates		
I Love New York	Heroin		

Slang	Meaning
Kilter	Marijuana
King-Kong pills	Barbiturates; glutethimide
King Tut	LSD
KJ	PCP
Knock-out drops	Chloral hydrate
Kona gold	Marijuana
Kool-Aid®	LSD
K-pot	Marijuana
Kreteks	Clove cigarette
Kristal	PCP
Kristal joint	PCP
Kryptonite	Cocaine
KW	Marijuana and PCP
La cura	Heroin
Lady	Cocaine
Lady snow	Cocaine
L.A. glass	Methamphetamine
Lambjam	Marijuana
Lamb's breath	Marijuana
La rochas	Flunitrazepam
L.A. turnabouts	Amphetamines
Laughing dust	PCP
Laughing gas	Nitrous oxide
Laughing tobacco	Marijuana
Lay back	Barbiturates
LBJ-336	Methyl piperidyl benzilate
Le power	Heroin
Leaf	Cocaine
Leapers	Amphetamines
Leather jackets	Phentermine
Lebanese	Marijuana
Lemmons	Methaqualone
Lemonade	Heroin
Leno	Marijuana
Lhesca	Marijuana
Liberty	Heroin
Lick'em	MDMA powder in Jello®
Lickum	MDMA powder in Jello®
Licorice	Codeine; paregoric
Licorice drops	Morning glory seeds
Lid	Marijuana
Lid poppers	Amphetamines
Life in death	Heroin
Lightning	Amphetamines
Lilly	Seconal™
Lime acid	LSD
Lipton tea	Narcotics
Liquid lady	Cocaine and ethanol
Little bomb	Amphetamine, heroin, and barbiturate
LL	Marijuana
Loads	Doriden® and ASA/acetaminophen with codeine
Locker room	Isobutyl nitrite
Locoweed	Marijuana
Log	Marijuana
Lords	Dilaudid®
Los ninos	Psilocybin
Love	PCP
Love drug	Methaqualone; PCP
Love lace	PCP
Love trip	MDA; mescaline
Love weed	Marijuana
Lovely	PCP
Lucy in the sky with diamonds	LSD
Ludes	Methaqualone
Luding out	Methaqualone
Luds	Methaqualone
Lumber	Marijuana
Lunch hour trip	DMT
M	Morphine
M & C	Morphine and cocaine
M & M's	MDMA
Mac	Marijuana and cocaine
Mace	Nutmeg
Machaca	Marijuana
Machine	Devices used to inject drugs
Macizo	Marijuana
Mackers	Marijuana and cocaine
Mad Dog 20-20	Wine
Madness	MDA/MDMA
Magic	PCP
Magic dust	PCP
Magic five	DMT
Magic mist	PCP
Magic mushroom	Psilocybin/psilocyn
Magic pumpkin	Mescaline
Magic pumpkin seeds	STP
Magnum 357	Caffeine
Magoo's blue	Mescaline
Mainline	Heroin
Mama poppers	Isobutyl nitrite
Mandies	Methaqualone
Manhattan silver	Marijuana
Manhattan spirit	Methanol
Maniac	Heroin and cocaine
Man-o-man	Cocaine; heroin
Manteca	Marijuana
Marathons	Amphetamines
Marax	Methaqualone and diphenhydramine
Marro	Marijuana
Marsh mallow reds	Barbiturates
Mary	Marijuana
Mary Jane	Marijuana
Mary Warner	Marijuana
Mary Weaver	Marijuana
Masa	Cocaine
Mash allah	Opium
Masterblaster	Cocaine and PCP; marijuana and PCP
Mata	Marijuana
Matchbook acid	LSD
Material	Heroin
Material negro	Opium
Mauve	Ketamine
Maze	Fentanyl derivative
McCoy	Narcotics
MDA	LSD, heroin, and cocaine; methylenedioxyamphetamine
MDM	N-methyl-3,4-methylenedioxyamphetamine
MDMA	3,4-methylenedioxymethamphetamine
Mellow drug of America	MDA
Mellow T	PCP
Mellow yellow	Dried banana skins with LSD
Melter	Morphine
Memish	Nembutal®
Mercancia	Heroin
Mercedes Benz	Heroin
Mervalon	Methaqualone
Mescal	Peyote
Mescal beans	Peyote
Mescal buttons	Peyote
Mescalito	Peyote
Mese	Mescaline
Messerole	Marijuana
Met	Methamphetamine
Meth	Methadone; methamphetamine
Metro	Heroin
Mexican brown	Heroin; marijuana
Mexican green	Marijuana
Mexican horse	Heroin
Mexican landmines	Methaqualone
Mexican locoweed	Marijuana

Slang	Meaning
Mexican mud	Heroin
Mexican mushroom	Psilocybin
Mexican tar	Heroin
Mexican valium	Flunitrazepam
Mexican yellow	Pentobarbital
Mezy	Marijuana
Mezz	Marijuana
MG	Marijuana
Mickey Finn	Chloral hydrate
Mickey Mouse	LSD
Microdot	LSD
Midnight hour	LSD
Milky trails	Lidocaine and ephedrine
Milwaukee road	Marijuana
Mind detergent	LSD
Minibennies	Amphetamine
Mini-whites	Amphetamine
Minstrel	Durophet
Mint leaves	Marijuana with formaldehyde
Mintweed	PCP
Miraa	Cathinone
Miss Emma	Morphine
Missile	Cocaine and PCP
Mist	PCP
Mister blue	Synthetic morphine
Mister jive	Heroin
Mister natural	LSD
Mister sinse	Marijuana
Mixto	Coca paste and tobacco
MJ	Marijuana
MMDA	Synthetic amphetamine
Mohasky	Marijuana
Mojaun	Marijuana
Mojo	Marijuana; morphine
Molly	Biphetamine®
Monkey	Morphine
Monkey dust	PCP
Monkey tranquilizer	PCP
Monster	Methedrine
Moocha	Marijuana
Moon 1	Marijuana; mescaline; peyote
Moon rock	Cocaine and heroin
Moonshine	Ethanol
Mooters	Marijuana
Mor-a-grifa	Marijuana
Morf	Morphine
Moroccan	Marijuana
Morph	Morphine
Morphie	Morphine
Morpho	Morphine
Morphy	Morphine
Mostaza	Marijuana
Mota	Marijuana
Mother	Marijuana
Mother Goose	LSD
Mountain Dew	Ethanol
Movie star drug	Cocaine
MPPP	Meperidine analog
Mr Clean	LSD
Mr Natural	LSD
Mrs White	Heroin
MS	Morphine
MU	Marijuana
Mud	Heroin; marijuana
Muggies	Marijuana
Muta	Marijuana
Mutah	Marijuana
Nail	Cigarettes
NASA	Heroin
Nats	Barbiturate
Narc	Narcotic agent
Narco	Narcotic agent
Narcoland	Environment of the drug user

Slang	Meaning
Narghile	Turkish water pipe
Natch trips	Highs produced by natural substances
Neat	Uncut drugs
Nebbies	Phenobarbital
Needle freak	User who enjoys the sensation of using a needle
Needle happy	Frequent user
Nembies	Pentobarbital; phenobarbital
Nemish	Phenobarbital
Nemmies	Phenobarbital
Nepal charas	Marijuana
Nepalese	Marijuana
New boy	Heroin
New heroin	Meperidine derivative
New magic	PCP
New York loads	Glutethimide and codeine
Nieve	Cocaine
Nigerian white	Heroin
Night shift	Heroin
Night train	PCP
Nimbies	Nembutal®; barbiturate
Nimby	Nembutal®
Nitroglycerin tabs	Heroin
NO	Nitric oxide
No. 1	Heroin and cocaine
No. 714	Methaqualone
Noise	Heroin
Noise candy	Cocaine
Nols	Nembutal®
Noodlars	Noludar®
Nose	Cocaine
Nose candy	Cocaine
Nova	Novahistine® DH
Nuggets	Amphetamines
Number	Marijuana
Nut	Heroin and cocaine
NY 89	Heroin
O2	Isobutyl nitrite
One on one	Doriden®, codeine, and aspirin
Oneway	LSD
Orange and blue	Methapyrilene
Orange barrels	LSD
Orange bulb acid	LSD
Orange caps	Methapyrilene
Orange hearts	Amphetamines
Orange mushrooms	LSD
Orange sunshine	LSD
Orange tabs	Caffeine, ephedrine, and phenylpropanolamine
Orange Tang® mesc	LSD
Orange wedges	LSD
Oranges	Dexedrine®
Organic mescaline	Morning glory seeds
Owskey's acid	LSD
Ozone	PCP
P	Peyote
Pack	Heroin
Packs	Glutethimide and codeine
Paid	Heroin and cocaine
Pajao rojo	Barbiturates
Pall Mall	Cigarette soaked in paregoric
Panama red	Marijuana
Panama reed	Marijuana
Panatella	Marijuana
Pancakes and syrup	Glutethimide and codeine cough syrup
Paper	Heroin; LSD; methamphetamine
Paper acid	LSD
Paradise	Cocaine
Paris 400	Methaqualone

Slang	Meaning
Pasta de coca	Coca paste
Paste lavada paste	Coca paste
Pat	Marijuana
Pata	Marijuana
Pattillo	Tobacco and coca paste cigarette
PCC	PCP analog
PCE	PCP analog
PCPY	PCP analog
P-Dope	Heroin
Pea shooter	Caffeine
Peace pills	PCP
Peace tab	LSD; PCP
Peace weed	PCP
Peaches	Amphetamines
Peanut butter	Heroin
Peanut butter crank	Methamphetamine
Peanuts	Barbiturates
Pearls	Amyl Nitrate
Pearly gates	Morning glory; LSD
Pedazo	Heroin
Pee	Heroin
Pellets	LSD
Pen yen	Opium
Pennies	Phenobarbital
Pen-Yan	Opium
Pep pills	Amphetamines
Pepaop	Meperidine analog
Percs	Percodan®
Perico	Cocaine
Perp	Crack look-alike
Persian	Heroin
Persian brown	Heroin
Peter	Chloral hydrate
Peyotl	Peyote
Pez	LSD on Pez® candies
P-Funk	Heroin
P.G.	Paregoric
Phantos	Phenobarbital and amphetamine
Phenos	Phenobarbital
Philly blunt	Marijuana
Phoenix	LSD
Pickles	Placidyl®
Pig killer	PCP
Pillows	Methaqualone
Pimp	Cocaine
Pineapple	Heroin and Ritalin®
Pink bam	Preludin®
Pink caps	Diphenhydramine; ephedrine; methapyrilene
Pink football	Caffeine, ephedrine, and phenylpropanolamine
Pink hearts	Amphetamines
Pink ladies	Barbiturates
Pink lemons	Dexedrine®
Pink passion	LSD
Pink spoon	Percodan®
Pink tablet	Caffeine
Pink wedge	DOM; LSD
Pinks	Seconal™
Piperidine	PCP
Pistola	Tobacco and cocaine
Pito	Marijuana
Pits	PCP
Placids	Placidyl®
Plants	Mescaline
P.O.	Paregoric
Polvo	Heroin; marijuana
Polvoron	Marijuana
Pop	Codeine
Poppers	Amyl nitrite; isobutyl nitrite; nitrous oxide
Porker	PCP
Porsche	Heroin
Pot	Marijuana
Potato alcohol	Ethanol
Powder	Amphetamines; heroin
Powder 95	Heroin
Powder 2000	Heroin
Powder stew	Codeine and Ritalin®
Premo	Marijuana and cocaine
President	Heroin
Primo	Heroin
Procrystal	Benzocaine
Product	Heroin
Product IV	LSD and PCP
Prope-dope	Methamphetamine
Pseudocaine	Ephedrine combination
Puke weed	Indian tobacco
Pumpkin seeds	Propoxyphene napsylate
Puna buds	Marijuana
Pure	Heroin; narcotics
Purple	Ketamine
Purple barrels	LSD
Purple dragon	LSD
Purple flats	LSD
Purple haze	LSD
Purple Jesus	Amphetamine on a microdot; LSD; PCP; PCP and LSD
Purple Owsleys	LSD
Purple ozoline	LSD
Purple ozolone	LSD
Purple splash	LSD
Purple star	PCP
Purple wedges	LSD
Q	Methaqualone
Quaas	Methaqualone
Quacks	Methaqualone
Quads	Methaqualone
Quartz	Methamphetamine
Quat	Cathinone
Quay	Methaqualone
Quick silver	Isobutyl nitrite
R-2	Flunitrazepam
R & R	Ripple® wine and Seconal™
Raggedy Andy	LSD
Raggedy Ann	LSD
Raw fusion	Heroin
Readyrock	Cocaine
Reaganomics	Cocaine; heroin
Red and black	Caffeine
Red and blues	Barbiturates; Tuinal®
Red and greys	Propoxyphene
Red birds	Seconal™
Red chicken	Heroin
Red crow beads	Amitriptyline
Red devils	Seconal™
Red lillies	Seconal™
Red pop	Novahistine® DH
Redneck cocaine	Methamphetamine
Reds	Barbiturates; chloral hydrate; Seconal™
Reefer	Marijuana
Reina	Flunitrazepam
Repro crystals	Procaine and caffeine
Rerock	Heroin
Rev Ike	PCP
Rhapsody	MDMA
Rhythm	Amphetamine
Rib	Flunitrazepam
Ribbets	Librax®
Rich man's	Cocaine
Rippers	Amphetamines
Ripple	Ripple® wine
Ripple and reds	Ripple® wine and Seconal™
Rising high	Heroin
Ritz and T	Ritalin® and Talwin®
R.J.'s	Biphetamine®
Roach	Marijuana
Roach-2	Flunitrazepam
Roaches	Flunitrazepam

Slang	Meaning
Roar	Methaqualone
Robe	Robitussin® A-C
Robin eggs	Methamphetamine
Roche	Flunitrazepam
Roches	Benzodiazepines
Rock	Cocaine
Rock crystal	Procaine and benzocaine
Rocket fuel	PCP
Rockets	Marijuana
Roofer	Marijuana
Roofies	Flunitrazepam
Rooms	Psilocybin
Root	Marijuana
Rope	Marijuana
Rophies	Flunitrazepam
Ropies	Flunitrazepam
Rose Maria	Marijuana
Roses	Amphetamines
Rot	Flunitrazepam
Roxanne	Cocaine
Royal blue	LSD
Rubber band	Cocaine
Ruby reds	Placidyl®
Ruffies	Flunitrazepam
Rufus	Heroin
Rush	Heroin; isobutyl nitrate
Rush 5	Haldol® 5 mg
STP	Amphetamines; DOM
Sacraments	LSD
Salmon River skunk	Marijuana
Salt	Heroin
Salt and peppers	Heroin in milk sugar
Sandoz	LSD
Satan's scent	Butyl nitrite
Sativa	Marijuana
Saturn	LSD
Sauce	Ethanol
Savage	Heroin
Scag	Heroin
Scarface	Heroin
Scat	Heroin
Schmack	Cocaine
Schmeck	Heroin
Schoolboy	Codeine
Schoolboy scotch	Codeine
Schrooms	Psilocybin
Scott	Heroin
Scramble	Heroin
Scratch	PCP
Scuffle	PCP
Seals	Amphetamines
Seccy	Secobarbital
Second-to-none	Heroin
Seeds	Marijuana; morning glory seeds
Seeds and stems	Marijuana; morning glory seeds
Seeds and twigs	Marijuana
Semi	Peyote
Senylan	PCP
Serenity	DOM
Serenity, tranquility, and peace	Dimethoxyamphetamine (DOM)
Sernyl	PCP
Sets	Glutethimide and codeine; Talwin® and Pyribenzamine®
Seven-fourteen	Methaqualone
Seven-fifty special	Placidyl®
Seventy-two hour bummer	STP
Shabu	Methamphetamine
Shabu-shabu	Methamphetamine
She	Cocaine
Sheets	PCP
Sherm	PCP
Silent partner	Heroin
Silly	Psilocybin

Slang	Meaning
Silly putty	Psilocybin
Simple Simon	Psilocybin
Sinsemilla	Marijuana
Sixteenths	1/16 ounce
Skag	Heroin
Skee opium	Heroin
Skot	Heroin
Skunk weed	Marijuana
Slab	Cocaine
Slamming	Intravenous injection of street drug
Sled	One ounce of heroin
Sleepers	Barbiturates
Sleigh ride	Under the influence of drugs
Smack	Cocaine; heroin
Smash	Marijuana
Smears	LSD
Smeck	Heroin
Snorts	PCP
Snow	Amphetamine; heroin
Snow cones	Cocaine
Snow pellets	Amphetamine
Snow seal	PCP
Snow seals	Amphetamine
Snow toke	Codeine and PCP
Snowbirds	Cocaine
Snowdust	Cocaine
Snowflake	Cocaine
Soapers	Methaqualone
Society high	Cocaine
Soft stuff	Marijuana
Softballs	Barbiturates
Sole	Marijuana
Solid	Heroin; marijuana
Solid gold	Heroin
Soma	PCP
Sopes	Methaqualone
Sound	Benactyzine
Soup	Talwin® and Benadryl®
Soup and beans	Glutethimide and codeine cough syrup
Sourcerer's apprentice	LSD
Spaghetti sauce	Robitussin® A-C
Sparkle plenties	Amphetamines
Spearmint	PCP
Special LA coke	Ketamine
Speckled birds	Amphetamine
Speed	Methamphetamine; methedrine
Speed for lovers	MDA
Speedball	Cocaine and heroin; cocaine and marijuana
Speedboat	PCP and heroin
Spiderman	Heroin
Splash	Amphetamines
Spliff	Marijuana
Splim	Marijuana
Splint	Marijuana
Splits	Tranquilizers
Spliven	Amphetamines
Square	Cigarette
Squirrels	LSD
Stack	Marijuana
Stamp	LSD
Stanley's stuff	LSD
Star	LSD
Star dust	Cocaine; cocaine and PCP; heroin and cocaine; PCP
Star-spangled	Cocaine
Stick	Marijuana
Stinkweed	Marijuana
Stofa	Heroin
Stoppers	Barbiturates
Straw	Marijuana
Strawberry fields	LSD
Strawberry flats	LSD

Slang	Meaning
Strawberry shortcakes	Methamphetamine and pentobarbital
Strawberry tablets	Mescaline
Street acid	LSD
Stuff	Heroin
Stumblers	Barbiturates
Suey	Opium
Sugar lump	LSD
Sugar weeds	Marijuana and sugar
Sugar	LSD
Suma caine	Phenylpropanolamine
Summer skies	Morning glory seeds
Sunny	Heroin
Sunshine	Heroin; LSD; PCP
Super acid	Ketamine
Super C	Ketamine
Super joint	Marijuana and PCP
Super K	Ketamine
Super Kools	Marijuana and PCP
Super P	Heroin
Super pot	Marijuana soaked in alcohol
Super tobacco	Tobacco and PCP
Super weed	PCP
Supergrass	Marijuana; PCP
Supra	Heroin
Surfer	PCP
Surprise	Cocaine; heroin
Survival	Cocaine; heroin
Swag	Methadone
Sweet Lucy	Marijuana; wine
Sweet lunch	Marijuana
Sweet tart	DOM
Sweeties	Phenmetrazine
Sweets	Amphetamines
Syndicate acid	2,5-Dimethoxy-4-methylamphetamine
Synth coke	Pseudoephedrine
Synthetic dope	Heroin
Synthetic marijuana	PCP
T	Marijuana; PCP
T2P	Cocaine sprayed with chlopyrifos; marijuana sprayed with chlopyrifos
TAC	PCP; THC
Talco	Cocaine
Tanks	PCP
Tar	Heroin
Tar baby	Heroin
Tar balls	Heroin
Tatto	LSD
Tchai	Cathinone
T's & B's	Talwin® and Pyribenzamine®
T-Birds	Secobarbital and amobarbital
T's & Blue's	Talwin® and Pyribenzamine®
TCH	THC
Tea	Marijuana; PCP
Teacher	LSD
Tecata	Heroin
Teddies and Betties	Talwin® and Pyribenzamine®
Teenage short	Coricidin® and beer
Teeth	Cocaine
Tens	Amphetamine 10 mg tablet
Terps	Terpin hydrate with codeine elixir
Terron	LSD
Tessies and Betties	Talwin® and Pyribenzamine®
Texas reefer	Marijuana
Texas tea	Marijuana
Thai weed	Marijuana
THC	Tetrahydrocannabinol
The bomb no. 1	Heroin
The kind	Marijuana
The pits	PCP
The white lady	Heroin
The wizard	LSD
The yuppie drug	MDMA
Thing	Cocaine; heroin
Three on three	Codeine with aspirin or acetaminophen; glutethimide
Threes and eights	Glutethimide and codeine
Thriller	Cocaine; heroin
Thrusters	Amphetamines
Thumb	Marijuana
Thunder	Heroin
Thunderbird	Wine
Tias	Barbiturates
Tic	PCP
Tic tac	PCP
Tick	THC
Tickle	Titanium
Tiger	Tiger rose wine
Time bomb	Heroin
Tin	Marijuana; opium
TMA	Trimethoxyphenylaminopropane
TMM	Trimethoxyphenylaminopropane
TNT	Heroin
Toilet water	Isobutyl nitrite
Tolley	Toluene
Toms and Bettys	Talwin® and Pyribenzamine®
Tooies	Amobarbital and secobarbital
Toot	Benzocaine and caffeine; cocaine
Tooties	Barbiturates
Tootonium	Cocaine
Tootsie Roll	Heroin
Top rank	Heroin
Tope	Marijuana
Topi	Peyote
Tops	Marijuana; peyote
Tops and bottoms	Talwin® and Pyribenzamine®
Torpedo	Drink with chloral hydrate
Tortilla discs	Marijuana
Toys	Opium
TR 8's	Amphetamines
Tranks	PCP
Tranq	PCP
Tranquility	DOM
Trees	Amytal®; Tuinal®
Triad trip	Strychnine, LSD, and methedrine
Tricycles and bicycles	Talwin® and Pyribenzamine®
Trips	LSD
Truck drivers	Amphetamines
True-1984	Heroin and cocaine
Trunks	PCP
T's	Talwin®
TS	Talwin® and Pyribenzamine®
T's and purples	Talwin® and Pyribenzamine®
T's and R's	Talwin® and Ritalin®
T shirts and blue jeans	Talwin® and Pyribenzamine®
TT's	Talwin® and Pyribenzamine®
Tui's	Tuinal®
Tuie's	Tuinal®
Turn abouts	Amphetamines
Turps	Terpin hydrate
Twenty-five	LSD
Twist Twistum	Marijuana

Slang	Meaning
Two on two	Codeine and glutethimide
Ultra caine	Ephedrine
Uncle milities	Meprobamate
Unicorn acid	LSD
Unkie	Morphine
Up-head	LSD
Uppers	Amphetamines
Up-Quaalude®	Cocaine
Uptown	Cocaine
USDA	Heroin
V	Valium®
Valleys	Valium®
Venom	Heroin
Venus	MDMA
Victory	Heroin
Viper's weed	Marijuana
Vitamin A	LSD
Vitamin Q	Methaqualone
Vomit wort	Indian tobacco
WAC	Marijuana laced with insecticides
Wack	Marijuana
Wacky weed	Marijuana
Wafer	LSD
Waimea wipeout	Marijuana
Wake-ups	Amphetamines
Water	Methamphetamine; methedrine; PCP solution
Watergate	Heroin
Weasel dust	MDMA
Wedding bells	LSD; morning glory seeds
Wedges	LSD
Weed	Marijuana
Weisels taub	MDMA
Wen-Shee	Opium
West coast	Amphetamines; methylphenidate hydrochloride
Wheat	Marijuana
When-Shee	Opium
Whippet	Nitrous oxide
White	Cocaine
White acid	LSD
White blotter	LSD
White cross	Methamphetamine; phenylpropanolamine and ephedrine
White dexies	Amphetamines
White double	LSD
White girl	Cocaine
White gold	Cocaine
White horizon	PCP
White horses	Cocaine
White junk	Heroin
White lady	Cocaine; heroin; morphine

Slang	Meaning
White light	Mescaline
White lightening	LSD
White merchandise	Morphine
White paste	Coca paste
White powder	Cocaine
White single domes	LSD
White stuff	Heroin; morphine
White tornado	Cocaine
White water	LSD
White wedge	DOM
Whites	Amphetamines; phenobarbital
Whiz bang	Cocaine and heroin; morphine and cocaine
Wickistick	PCP
Wiki stick	PCP
Wild Geronimo	Barbiturate and ethanol
Window glass	LSD
Window pane	LSD; MDMA
Wobble	PCP
Wokouri	Peyote
Wokowi	Peyote
World series	Cocaine
X	MDMA
X's	Amphetamine
XTC	MDMA
Yaamaa	Methamphetamine
Yaegermeister	Opium
Yellow bam	Methamphetamine
Yellow bullets	Pentobarbital
Yellow dimples	LSD
Yellow dolls	Pentobarbital
Yellow eggs	Temazepam
Yellow jackets	Pentobarbital; phentermine
Yellow kimples	LSD
Yellow Mollies	Phentermine
Yellow pyramid	LSD
Yellow speed	Ionamin®
Yellow submarine	Marijuana
Yellow T	PCP
Yellow tablet	Caffeine and phenylpropanolamine; ephedrine
Yellow wedge	DOM
Yellows	LSD; pentobarbital; phentermine
Yen shee suey	Opium
Yerba	Marijuana
Yesco	Marijuana
Ying gee	Marijuana
Yo-Yo	Yohimbine hydrochloride
Yocaine	Cocaine
Yuppie drug	MDMA

SULFITE — HYPERSENSITIVITY

Response

Sulfite derivatives are common antioxidant preservatives used in foods and medications. Hypersensitivity reactions to sulfites have been noted with increasing frequency, however, the reaction is still rare. Reactions occur within 2-15 minutes after ingestion or inhalation and include nasal pruritus, rhinorrhea, conjunctivitis, generalized urticaria, dyspnea, wheezing, angioedema, flushing, weakness, and anaphylaxis. Patients frequently have underlying allergic or asthmatic disease and report exacerbations when exposed to air pollution or smog. One study has suggested 5% to 10% of all asthmatics may be at risk for sulfite sensitivity. A more recent study indicates the prevalence rate for nonsteroid-dependent asthmatics is 0.8% and for steroid-dependent asthmatics 8.4%.

The mechanism of hypersensitivity has not been fully elucidated. Available data suggest the reaction is probably IgE mediated; however, IgE antibodies to sulfites have yet to be identified. Accurate diagnosis of sulfite sensitivity is obtained from oral provocative challenge. Skin tests are of no value. There is some evidence that the reaction may be dose related, since more severe reactions have occurred following ingestion of restaurant meals containing 25-100 mg sodium metabisulfite than smaller oral challenge doses. These authors suggested that bisulfites convert to sulfur dioxide in solution, which activates the tracheobronchial irritant receptors and stimulates a cholinergic reflex leading to bronchoconstriction, bradycardia, hypotension, peripheral vasodilation, and diaphoresis.

Sulfite derivatives include sodium bisulfite ($NaHSO_3$), potassium bisulfite ($KHSO_3$), sodium metabisulfite ($Na_2S_2O_5$), sodium sulfite (Na_2SO_3), potassium metabisulfite ($K_2S_2O_5$), and sulfur dioxide (SO_2). The most common food sources are fresh fruits and vegetables (particularly potatoes and green salads), shellfish, soft drinks, beer, wine, dried foods, and fruit drinks. Sympathomimetic medications are very susceptible to oxidation and frequently contain bisulfites in concentrations of 0.3% to 0.75%.

Table 1 is a list of common asthma inhalant medications and the type of preservative used.

Other drugs that contain sulfite preservatives are listed in Table 2.

Sulfite Preservatives

Table 1

Inhalation	
Epinephrine	Adrenalin® chloride 1:100 (Parke-Davis) Dey-Dose® epinephrine (Dey) microNEFRIN® (Bird)
Isoetharine HCl	Arm-a-Med® (Armour) Beta-2® (Nephron) Bronkosol® unit dose (Breon) Bronkosol® 1% (Breon) Dey-Lube® isoetharine (Dey) Dispos-a-Med® isoetharine (Parke-Davis) Isoetharine HCl (Roxane) Isoetharine HCl (Travenol)
Isoproterenol	Dispos-a-Med® isoproterenol (Parke-Davis) Isuprel® (Breon)
Metaproterenol 5% solution	Alupent® (BI)* Metaprel® (Dorsey)
Injectable	
Epinephrine	Adrenalin® chloride (Parke-Davis) Ana-Kit® (Hollister-Stier) EpiPen® (Center)
Oral	
Metaproterenol syrup	Alupent® (BI) Metaprel® (Dorsey)

*Boehringer Ingelheim has reformulated the Alupent® inhalant solution 5% and replaced the preservative sodium metabisulfite with benzalkonium chloride. This new product is available as of July 1986; however, the older product will still be on the market until all supplies are used up.

Table 2

Amikacin	Amikin® injection
Atropine	Lyopine Vari-Dose®
Bupivacaine	Marcaine® with epinephrine (except dental syringes) Sensorcaine® with epinephrine
Chloroprocaine	Nesacaine® injection

Chlorpromazine	Thorazine® injection
Codeine	Codeine phosphate (Wyeth)
Co-trimoxazole	Bactrim™ injection Septra® injection
Dexamethasone acetate	Decadron®-LA (MSD) Dexone LA® (Kay Phar) Solurex LA® (Hyrex)
Dexamethasone phosphate	AK-Dex® ophthalmic 0.1% solution
Dexamethasone sodium phosphate	Decadron® (MSD) Dexamethasone sodium phosphate (Elkins-Sinns) Solurex® (Hyrex)
Dexamethasone/ neomycin	NeoDecadron® solution NeoDecadron® topical cream
Dipivefrin	Propine® solution
Dopamine	Intropin® injection
Epinephrine	Epitrate® 1% solution
Etidocaine	Duranest® with epinephrine injection
Gallamine triethiodide	Flaxedil®
Gentamicin	Apogen® Bristagen® Garamycin® Gentamicin (various)
Hydrocortisone acetate	Hydrocortone® acetate (MSD)
Hydrocortisone acetate/neomycin	Cor-Oticin® suspension
Hydrocortisone sodium phosphate	Hydrocortone® (MSD)
Imipramine	Tofranil® injection
I.V. solutions	Aminosyn® Dialyte® with dextrose Freamine® Hepatamine® Isolyte E with D_5W in plastic container Nephramine® 5.4% Normosol® and dextrose 5% in plastic container ProcalAmine® RenAmin® electrolytes Travasol® Veinamine® 8%
Iothalamate sodium	Angio-Conray®
Kanamycin	Klebcil® injection
Lidocaine	Xylocaine® with epinephrine (Astra)
Meperidine	Demerol® injection
Mepivacaine HCl with levonordefrin	Carbocaine® with Neo-Cobefrin®
Metaraminol bitartrate	Aramine® injection
Methotrimeprazine	Levoprome® injection
Methyldopa	Aldomet® injection
Metoclopramide	Reglan® injection
Methoxamine	Vasoxyl® injection
Nalbuphine	Nubain® injection
Netilmicin	Netromycin® injection
Norepinephrine	Levophed® injection
Orphenadrine citrate	Orphenadrine citrate injection (various)
Otic preparations (combination product)	AK-Spore HC® Otic Cortisporin® Otic MY Cort Otic 1-20® Ortega Otic M® Otocort® Otoreid-HC®
Parenteral liver combinations	Reticulogen® Reticulogen Fortified®
Pentazocine	Talwin®
Perphenazine	Trilafon® injection

Phenylephrine/ scopolamine	Murocoll-2® ophthalmic drops
Phenylephrine/pyrilamine maleate/antipyrine	Prefrin™ A ophthalmic
Physostigmine	Eserine sulfate ointment Isopto® eserine 0.25%, 5% solution
Pilocarpine/epinephrine	E-Pilo-1® P_1E_1® E-Pilo-2® P_2E_1® E-Pilo-3® P_3E_1® E-Pilo-4® P_4E_1® E-Pilo-6® P_6E_1®
Pilocarpine/ physostigmine	Miocel® solution
Prednisolone acetate	Pred Forte® ophthalmic Pred Mild® ophthalmic Prednisolone acetate ophthalmic 1% suspension (Rugby) Predulose® ophthalmic 0.25% suspension
Prednisolone sodium phosphate	AK-Pred® ophthalmic 0.125%, 1% solution Hydeltrasol® (MSD) Key-Pred-SP® (Hyrex) Prednisolone sodium phosphate 0.125%, 1% solution (Rugby) Predulose® ophthalmic 0.25% suspension Solupredalone® (O'Neal)
Prilocaine	Citanest® Forte
Procainamide	Procainamide injection (ASCAT) Pronestyl®
Procaine	Novocain® 1%, 2% injection
Prochlorperazine	Compazine® injection
Promethazine	Anergan® injection Bay Meth® injection Ganphene® injection K-Phene® injection Mallergan® injection Pentazine® injection Phenazine® injection Phencen-50® injection Phenergan® injection Phenoject® injection Prometh® injection Promethazine HCl (various) Prorex® injection Prothazine® injection Provigan® injection V-Gan® injection Zipan® injection
Promethazine/ meperidine	Mepergan®
Propiomazine	Largon®
Propoxycaine/procaine	Ravocaine® and Novocain® with Neo-Cobefrin®
Reserpine	Serpasil® injection
Ritodrine	Yutopar® injection
Sodium sulfacetamide	AK-Sulf® Forte Ophthacet®
Streptomycin	Streptomycin sulfate injection (Pfipharmecs)
Sulfisoxazole	Gantrisin® injection
Tetracaine	Pontocaine® 1% injection
Thiethylperazine maleate	Torecan® injection
Tobramycin	Nebcin® injection
Trifluoperazine	Stelazine® concentrate
Tubocurarine chloride	Abbott, Lilly, Squibb

Table 3. Foods

Canned or dry soup mixes
Cider vinegar
Cornstarch
Dehydrated fruits and vegetables (75 mg)
Flour tortillas
Frozen or dried potatoes
Fruit drinks/soft drinks (25-30 mg)
Horseradish
Instant tea
Jams/jellies
Jelling agents
Molasses
Olives
Pickle/onion relish
Pie crust
Sausages (60 mg)
Seafoods (especially shellfish)
Shredded coconut
Soy protein products
Spinach pasta
Wine/beer (5-10 mg)

TABLETS THAT CANNOT BE CRUSHED OR ALTERED

There are a variety of reasons for crushing tablets or capsule contents prior to administering to the patient. Patients may have nasogastric tubes which do not permit the administration of tablets or capsules; an oral solution for a particular medication may not be available from the manufacturer or readily prepared by pharmacy; patients may have difficulty swallowing capsules or tablets; or mixing of powdered medication with food or drink may make the drug more palatable.

Generally, medications which should not be crushed fall into one of the following categories.

- **Extended-Release Products**. The formulation of some tablets is specialized as to allow the medication within it to be slowly released into the body. This is sometimes accomplished by centering the drug within the core of the tablet, with a subsequent shedding of multiple layers around the core. Wax melts in the GI tract. Slow-K® is an example of this. Capsules may contain beads which have multiple layers which are slowly dissolved with time.
- **Medications Which Are Irritating to the Stomach**. Tablets which are irritating to the stomach may be enteric-coated which delays release of the drug until the time when it reaches the small intestine. Enteric-coated aspirin is an example of this.
- **Foul Tasting Medication**. Some drugs are quite unpleasant to taste so the manufacturer coats the tablet in a sugar coating to increase its palatability. By crushing the tablet, this sugar coating is lost and the patient tastes the unpleasant tasting medication.
- **Sublingual Medication**. Medication intended for use under the tongue should not be crushed. While it appears to be obvious, it is not always easy to determine if a medication is to be used sublingually. Sublingual medications should indicate on the package that they are intended for sublingual use.
- **Effervescent Tablets**. These are tablets which, when dropped into a liquid, quickly dissolve to yield a solution. Many effervescent tablets, when crushed, lose their ability to quickly dissolve.

Recommendations

1. It is not advisable to crush certain medications.
2. Consult individual monographs prior to crushing capsule or tablet.
3. If crushing a tablet or capsule is contraindicated, consult with your pharmacist to determine whether an oral solution exists or can be compounded.

Oral Dosage Forms That Should Not Be Crushed

Drug Product	Dosage Forms	Reasons/Comments
Accutane®	Capsule	Mucous membrane irritant
Acutrim®	Tablet	Slow release
Adalat® CC	Tablet	Slow release
Aerolate® SR, JR, III	Capsule	Slow release*†
Afrinol® Repetabs®	Tablet	Slow release
Anaplex SR	Capsule	Slow release
Ansaid®	Tablet	Taste‖
Allerest® 12-Hour	Caplet	Slow release
Artane® Sequels®	Capsule	Slow release*†
Arthritis Bayer Time Release	Capsule	Slow release
Asacol®	Tablet	Slow release
ASA Enseals®	Tablet	Enteric-coated
Asbron G® Inlay	Tablet	Multiple compressed tablet†
Aspirin Delayed-Release	Tablet	Enteric-coated
Atrohist Plus	Tablet	Slow release*
Atrohist Sprinkle	Capsule	Slow release

(continued)

Drug Product	Dosage Forms	Reasons/Comments
Azulfidine® EN-tabs®	Tablet	Enteric-coated
Baros	Tablet	Effervescent tablet¶
Betachron E-R	Capsule	Slow release
Betapen®-VK	Tablet	Taste‖
Biphetamine	Capsule	Slow release
Bisacodyl	Tablet	Enteric-coated‡
Bisco-Lax®	Tablet	Enteric-coated‡
Bontril SR	Capsule	Slow release
Breonesin®	Capsule	Liquid filled§
Brexin® LA	Capsule	Slow release
Bromfed®	Capsule	Slow release†
Bromfed-PD®	Capsule	Slow release†
Calan® SR	Tablet	Slow release♦
Cama Arthritis Pain Reliever	Tablet	Multiple compressed tablet
Carbiset-TR®	Tablet	Slow release
Cardizem®	Tablet	Slow release
Cardizem® CD	Capsule	Slow release*
Cardizem® SR	Capsule	Slow release*
Carter's Little Pills®	Tablet	Enteric-coated
Cefal Filmtab®	Tablet	Enteric-coated
Charcoal Plus	Tablet	Enteric-coated
Chloral Hydrate	Capsule	Note: Product is in liquid form within a special capsule†
Chlorphedrine SR	Capsule	Slow release
Chlorpheniramine Maleate Time Release	Capsule	Slow release
Chlor-Trimeton® 12-Hour Allergy	Tablet	Slow release†
Choledyl® SA	Tablet	Slow release†
Chromagen®	Capsule	Taste‖
Cipro™	Tablet	Taste‖
Cleocin®	Capsule	Taste†‖
Codimal-LA®	Capsule	Slow release
Codimal-LA® Half	Capsule	Slow release
Colace®	Capsule	Taste‖
Comhist® LA	Capsule	Slow release*
Compazine® Spansule®	Capsule	Slow release†
Congess SR, JR	Capsule	Slow release
Contac®	Capsule	Slow release*
Cotazym-S®	Capsule	Enteric-coated*
Creon®	Capsule	Enteric-coated*
Creon® 10 Minimicrospheres	Capsule	Enteric-coated*
Creon® 25	Capsule	Enteric-coated*
Dallergy®	Capsule	Slow release†
Dallergy-D®	Capsule	Slow release
Dallergy-JR®	Capsule	Slow release
Deconamine® SR	Capsule	Slow release†
Deconsal® II	Tablet	Slow release
Deconsal® Sprinkle	Capsule	Slow release*
Demazin® Repetabs®	Tablet	Slow release†
Depakene®	Capsule	Slow-release-mucous membrane irritant†
Depakote®	Capsule	Enteric-coated
Desoxyn® Gradumets®	Tablet	Slow release
Desyrel®	Tablet	Taste‖
Dexatrim® Max Strength	Tablet	Slow release
Dexedrine® Spansule®	Capsule	Slow release
Diamox® Sequels®	Capsule	Slow release
Dilacor™ XR	Capsule	Slow release
Dilatrate SR	Capsule	Slow release
Dimetane® Extentab®	Tablet	Slow release†
Disobrom®	Tablet	Slow release
Disophrol® Chronotab®	Tablet	Slow release
Dital	Capsule	Slow release
Docusate	Capsule	Liquid filled§
Docusate with Casanthranol	Capsule	Liquid filled§
Donnatal® Extentab®	Tablet	Slow release†
Donnazyme	Tablet	Enteric-coated
Doxidan® liquigels	Capsule	Liquid filled§
Drisdol®	Capsule	Liquid filled§
Drixoral®	Tablet	Slow release†

(continued)

Drug Product	Dosage Forms	Reasons/Comments
Drixoral® Sinus	Tablet	Slow release
Dulcolax®	Tablet	Enteric-coated‡
Dura-Vent®	Tablet	Slow release
Dura-Vent®/A	Capsule	Slow release
Dura-Vent®/DA	Tablet	Slow release
Dura-Tap/PD®	Capsule	Slow release
Duratuss	Tablet	Slow release♦
Easprin®	Tablet	Enteric-coated
Ecotrin®	Tablet	Enteric-coated
E.E.S.® 400	Tablet	Enteric-coated†
Efidac/24®	Tablet	Slow release
Elixophyllin® SR	Capsule	Slow release*†
E-Mycin®	Tablet	Enteric-coated
Endafed®	Capsule	Slow release
Entex® LA	Tablet	Slow release†
Entex® PSE	Tablet	Slow release†
Entozyme	Tablet	Enteric-coated
Equanil®	Tablet	Taste‖
Ergostat®	Tablet	Sublingual form•
Eryc®	Capsule	Enteric-coated*
Ery-Tab®	Tablet	Enteric-coated
Erythrocin® Stearate	Tablet	Enteric-coated
Erythromycin Base	Tablet	Enteric-coated
Eskalith® CR	Tablet	Slow release
Fedahist® TimeCaps®	Capsule	Slow release†
Feldene®	Capsule	Mucous membrane irritant
Fenesin™	Tablet	Slow release
Feocyte	Tablet	Slow release
Feosol®	Tablet	Enteric-coated†
Feosol® Spansule®	Capsule	Slow release*†
Ferrous Gluconate	Tablet	Film-coated
Feratab®	Tablet	Enteric-coated†
Fergon®	Tablet	May cause excessive GI upset
Fero-Grad 500® mg	Tablet	Slow release
Fero-Gradumet®	Tablet	Slow release
Ferralet® SR	Tablet	Slow release
Feverall™ Sprinkle Caps	Capsule	Taste* Note: Capsule contents intended to be placed in a teaspoonful of water or soft food.
Fumatinic	Capsule	Slow release
Gastrocrom®	Capsule	Note: Contents should be dissolved in water for administration.
Geocillin®	Tablet	Taste
Gris-PEG®	Tablet	Note: Crushing may result in precipitation as larger particles.
Guaifed	Capsule	Slow release
Guaifed-PD	Capsule	Slow release
Guaimax-D	Tablet	Slow release
Halfprin	Tablet	Enteric coated
Humabid® DM	Tablet	Slow release
Humabid® DM Sprinkle	Capsule	Slow release*
Humabid® LA	Tablet	Slow release
Humabid® Sprinkle	Capsule	Slow release*
Hydergine® LC	Capsule	Note: Product is in liquid form within a special capsule†
Hydergine® Sublingual	Tablet	Sublingual route†
Hytakerol®	Capsule	Liquid filled§†
Iberet®	Tablet	Slow release†
Iberet-500®	Tablet	Slow release†
Ilotycin®	Tablet	Enteric-coated
Imdur™	Tablet	Slow release♦
Inderal® LA	Capsule	Slow release
Inderide® LA	Capsule	Slow release
Indocin® SR	Capsule	Slow release*†
Ionamin®	Capsule	Slow release

(continued)

Drug Product	Dosage Forms	Reasons/Comments
Isoclor® Timesule®	Capsule	Slow release†
Isoptin® SR	Tablet	Slow release
Isordil® Sublingual	Tablet	Sublingual form•
Isordil® Tembid®	Tablet	Slow release
Isosorbide Dinitrate Sublingual	Tablet	Sublingual form•
Isosorbide Dinitrate SR	Tablet	Slow release
Isuprel® Glossets®	Tablet	Sublingual form•
K+® 8	Tablet	Slow release†
K+® 10	Tablet	Slow release†
Kaon-Cl® 6.7 mEq	Tablet	Slow release†
Kaon-Cl® 10	Tablet	Slow release†
K + Care®	Tablet	Effervescent tablet†¶
K-Dur®	Tablet	Slow release♦
Klor-Con®	Tablet	Slow release†
Klor-Con®/EF	Tablet	Effervescent tablet†¶
Klorvess®	Tablet	Effervescent tablet†¶
Klotrix®	Tablet	Slow release†
K-Lyte®	Tablet	Effervescent tablet¶
K-Lyte/Cl®	Tablet	Effervescent tablet¶
K-Tab®	Tablet	Slow release†
Levsinex® TimeCaps®	Capsule	Slow release
Macrobid®	Capsule	Slow release
Meprospan®	Capsule	Slow release*
Mestinon® Timespan®	Tablet	Slow release†
MI-Cebrin	Tablet	Enteric-coated
MI-Cebrin T	Tablet	Enteric-coated
Micro-K®	Capsule	Slow release*†
Motrin®	Tablet	Taste†‖
Motrin® IB	Tablet	Taste†‖
Motrin® IB-sinus	Tablet	Taste†‖
MS Contin®	Tablet	Slow release†
MSC Triaminic®	Tablet	Enteric-coated
Naldecon®	Tablet	Slow release†
Nasabid™	Capsule	Slow release
Nasatab LA	Tablet	Slow release
Nico 400	Capsule	Slow release
Nicobid®	Capsule	Slow release
Nitro-Bid®	Capsule	Slow release*
Nitrocine® TimeCaps®	Capsule	Slow release
Nitroglyn®	Capsule	Slow release*
Nitrong®	Tablet	Slow release
Nitrostat®	Tablet	Sublingual route•
Nolamine®	Tablet	Slow release
Nolex® LA	Tablet	Slow release
Norflex®	Tablet	Slow release
Norpace® CR	Capsule	Slow release form within a special capsule
Novafed®	Capsule	Slow release
Novafed® A	Capsule	Slow release
Optilets-500® Filmtab®	Tablet	Enteric-coated
Optilets-M-500® Filmtab®	Tablet	Enteric-coated
Oragrafin®	Capsule	Note: Product is in liquid form within a special capsule
Ordrine® SR	Capsule	Slow release
Oramorph SR™	Tablet	Slow release†
Ornade® Spansule®	Capsule	Slow release
Oruvail®	Capsule	Slow release
Pabalate	Tablet	Enteric-coated
Pabalate SF	Tablet	Enteric-coated
Pancrease®	Capsule	Enteric-coated*
Pancrease® MT	Capsule	Enteric-coated*
Panmycin®	Capsule	Taste
Papaverine Sustained Action	Capsule	Slow release
Pathilon® Sequels®	Capsule	Slow release*
Pavabid® Plateau	Capsule	Slow release*
PBZ-SR®	Tablet	Slow release†
Pentasa®	Capsule	Slow release
Perdiem®	Granules	Wax coated
Peritrate® SA	Tablet	Slow release♦
Permitil® Chronotab®	Tablet	Slow release†

(continued)

Drug Product	Dosage Forms	Reasons/Comments
Phazyme®	Tablet	Slow release
Phazyme® 95	Tablet	Slow release
Phenergan®	Tablet	Taste†‖
Phyllocontin®	Tablet	Slow release
Plendil®	Tablet	Slow release
Pneumonist®	Tablet	Slow release†
Polaramine® Repetabs®	Tablet	Slow release†
Prelu-2®	Capsule	Slow release
Prilosec™	Capsule	Slow release
Pro-Banthine®	Tablet	Taste
Procainamide HCl SR	Tablet	Slow release
Procan® SR	Tablet	Slow release
Procardia®	Capsule	Delays absorption§#
Procardia XL®	Tablet	Slow release Note: AUC is unaffected.
Pronestyl-SR®	Tablet	Slow release
Proventil® Repetabs®	Tablet	Slow release†
Prozac®	Capsule	Slow release*
Quadra-Hist®	Tablet	Slow release
Quibron®-T SR	Tablet	Slow release†
Quinaglute® Dura-Tabs®	Tablet	Slow release
Quinalan® Lanatabs®	Tablet	Slow release
Quinalan® SR	Tablet	Slow release
Quinidex® Extentabs®	Tablet	Slow release
Respaire® SR	Capsule	Slow release
Respid®	Tablet	Slow release
Ritalin-SR®	Tablet	Slow release
Robimycin® Robitab®	Tablet	Enteric-coated
Rondec-TR®	Tablet	Slow release†
Roxanol SR™	Tablet	Slow release†
Ru-Tuss®	Tablet	Slow release
Ru-Tuss® DE	Tablet	Slow release
Seldane-D®	Tablet	Slow release
Sinemet® CR	Tablet	Slow release♦
Singlet®	Tablet	Slow release
Slo-bid™ Gyrocaps®	Capsule	Slow release*
Slo-Niacin®	Tablet	Slow release
Slo-Phyllin GG®	Capsule	Slow release†
Slo-Phyllin® Gyrocaps®	Capsule	Slow release*†
Slow FE®	Tablet	Slow release†
Slow-K®	Tablet	Slow release†
Slow-Mag®	Tablet	Slow release
Sorbitrate® SA	Tablet	Slow release
Sorbitrate® Sublingual	Tablet	Sublingual route
Sparine®	Tablet	Taste‖
S-P-T	Capsule	Note: Liquid gelatin thyroid suspension.
Stamoist E	Tablet	Slow release
Stamoist LA	Tablet	Slow release
Sudafed® 12-Hour	Caplet	Slow release†
Surfak® Liquigels	Capsule	Liquid filled§
Tavist-D®	Tablet	Multiple compressed tablet
Teldrin®	Capsule	Slow release*
Temaril® Spansule®	Capsule	Slow release†
Tepanil® Tentab®	Tablet	Slow release
Tessalon® Perles	Capsule	Slow release
Theo-24®	Tablet	Slow release†
Theobid®	Capsule	Slow release*†
Theobid® Jr	Capsule	Slow release*†
Theoclear® L.A	Capsule	Slow release†
Theochron®	Tablet	Slow release
Theo-Dur®	Tablet	Slow release†♦
Theo-Dur® Sprinkle	Capsule	Slow release*†
Theo-Sav	Tablet	Slow release♦
Theolair™ SR	Tablet	Slow release†
Theovent®	Capsule	Slow release†
Theox®	Tablet	Slow release
Therapy Bayer	Caplet	Enteric-coated
Thorazine® Spansule®	Capsule	Slow release

(continued)

Drug Product	Dosage Forms	Reasons/Comments
Toprol XL®	Tablet	Slow release♦
Touro A&H®	Capsule	Slow release*
Touro EX®	Tablet	Slow release♦
Touro LA®	Tablet	Slow release♦
T-Phyl®	Tablet	Slow release
Trental®	Tablet	Slow release
Triaminic®	Tablet	Enteric-coated†
Triaminic-12® Tablet	Slow release†	
Trilafon® Repetabs®	Tablet	Slow release†
Trinalin® Repetabs®	Tablet	Slow release
Tuss-LA®	Tablet	Slow release
Tuss-Ornade® Spansule®	Capsule	Slow release
ULR-LA®	Tablet	Slow release
Unicap®	Capsule	Liquid filled§
Uniphyl®	Tablet	Slow release
Valrelease®	Capsule	Slow release
Vanex® Forte	Caplet	Slow release
Vantin®	Tablet	Taste†‖
Verelan®	Capsule	Slow release*
Volmax®	Tablet	Slow release†
Wyamycin® S	Tablet	Slow release
Wygesic®	Tablet	Taste
Zephrex LA®	Tablet	Slow release
ZORprin®	Tablet	Slow release
Zymase®	Capsule	Enteric-coated

Adapted from Mitchell JF and Pawlicki KS, "Oral Solid Dosage Forms That Should Not Be Crushed: 1994 Revision," *Hosp Pharm*, 1994, 29(7):666-75.

*Capsule may be opened and the contents taken without crushing or chewing; soft food such as applesauce or pudding may facilitate administration; contents may generally be administered via nasogastric tube using an appropriate fluid provided entire contents are washed down the tube.

†Liquid dosage forms of the product are available; however, dose, frequency of administration, and manufacturers may differ from that of the solid dosage form.

‡Antacids and/or milk may prematurely dissolve the coating of the tablet.

§Capsule may be opened and the liquid contents removed for administration.

‖The taste of this product in a liquid form would likely be unacceptable to the patient; administration via nasogastric tube should be acceptable.

¶Effervescent tablets must be dissolved in the amount of diluent recommended by the manufacturer.

#If the liquid capsule is crushed or the contents expressed, the active ingredient will be, in part, absorbed sublingually.

•Tablets are made to disintegrate under the tongue.

♦Tablet is scored.

TOXIC DOSES OF SELECTED DRUGS REQUIRING REFERRAL TO A PHYSICIAN OR EMERGENCY DEPARTMENT UPON INGESTION BY PEDIATRIC PATIENTS(Home Decontamination and/or Observation Not Sufficient)

Agent	Dose (mg/kg)
Acetaminophen*	200
Albuterol	1
Aspirin	200
Caffeine	15
Camphor	10
Dextromethorphan*	10
Digoxin	0.05
Fluoride (elemental)	8
Ibuprofen	200
Iron (elemental)	60
Phenobarbital	8
Phenylpropanolamine	8
Propoxyphene	10
Warfarin	0.5

*Not a long-acting preparation.

TOXICITIES OF CHEMOTHERAPEUTIC AGENTS

Drug	Radiation-Recall Reactions	Ocular Toxicity	Pulmonary Toxicity	Cardiotoxicity	Hepatotoxicity	Cumulative Myelosuppression	Peripheral Neuropathy	CNS Depression
Allopurinol		x						
Altretamine							x	
Ara-C					x			x
Azathioprine					x			
BCNU (carmustine)			x		x	x		
Bleomycin	x		x					
Busulfan		x	x		x			
Carboplatin						x	x	
CCNU (lomustine)			x		x			
Chlorambucil		x	x		x			
Cisplatin		x			x		x	
Corticosteroids		x						
Cyclophosphamide		x	x	x*	x			
Cytarabine		x	x					
Dactinomycin	x		x		x			
Daunomycin				x†				
2'-Deoxycoformycin		x						
Doxorubicin	x	x	x	x†	x			
Etoposide	x		x		x			
Fludarabine			x					

(continued)

Drug	Radiation-Recall Reactions	Ocular Toxicity	Pulmonary Toxicity	Cardiotoxicity	Hepatotoxicity	Cumulative Myelosuppression	Peripheral Neuropathy	CNS Depression
5-Fluorouracil		x		x‡	x			x
G-CSF			x					
Hydroxyurea	x							
Idarubicin				x†				
Ifosfamide			x					x
Interferon		x	x					
Irinotecan						x		
L-asparaginase			x		x			x
Mechlorethamine						x		
Melphalan			x			x		
6-Mercaptopurine					x			
Methotrexate	x	x	x					
Methyl-CCNU (semustine)			x			x		
Mithramycin		x						
Mitomycin-C		x	x			x		
Mitotane		x						
Mitoxantrone				x†				
Nitrogen mustard		x						

(continued)

Drug	Radiation-Recall Reactions	Ocular Toxicity	Pulmonary Toxicity	Cardiotoxicity	Hepatotoxicity	Cumulative Myelosuppression	Peripheral Neuropathy	CNS Depression
Nitrosoureas		x						
Procarbazine			x			x		x
Streptozocin					x			
Tamoxifen		x	x					
Taxol®	x		x				x	
Teniposide			x					
Trimetrexate	x							
Vinblastine	x	x	x		x		x	
Vincristine		x	x				x	
Vinorelbine						x	x	

Reprinted with permission from Patterson W and Perry MC, "Chemotherapeutic Toxicities: A Comprehensive Overview," *Contemporary Oncology*, 1993, 3(7):58-61.

G-CSF = granulocyte-colony stimulating factor.
*At high dose.
†Dose-related.
‡Idiosyncratic.

TOXINS/DRUGS THAT CAUSE DISULFIRAM-LIKE REACTIONS WITH ETHANOL

- Aminopyrine
- Bisethylxanthogen
- 4-Bromopyrazole
- Butanol oxime
- Calcium carbamide
- Calcium cyanamide
- Carbamate fungicides
- Carbamate herbicides
- Carbon disulfide
- Carmofur (1-hexyl carbamoyl-5-fluorouracil)
- Cephalosporins
  - Cefamandole sodium
  - Cefoperazone
  - Cefotetan disodium (up to 60%)
  - Moxalactam disodium
- Chloral hydrate
- Chloramphenicol
- Chlorpropamide
- Citrated calcium cyanamid
- Cyanamide
- Cyclothiazide
- Demethylformamide (up to 20%)
- Diethylthiocarbamate
- Dimercaprol
- Dimethyl formamide
- Disulfiram
- Ethacrynic acid
- Ethylene dibromide
- Furaltadone
- Furazolidone
- Griseofulvin
- Hydrogen sulfide
- Irgopyrine
- Isoniazid
- Isosorbide dinitrate
- Mineral spirits
- Mushrooms
  - *Coprinus atramentarius*
  - *Clitocybe clavipes*
  - *Boletus luridus*
  - *Verpa bohemica*
- Metronidazole (up to 24%)
- N-butyraldoxine
- Niforoxime
- Nitrofurantoin
- Nitroglycerin
- Paraldehyde
- Pargyline
- Phenacetin
- Phenformin
- Phentolamine
- Phenylbutazone
- Procarbazine
- Procarbazine hydrochloride
- Pyrogallol
- Quinacrine hydrochloride
- Sulfonamides
- Sulfonylureas
  - Acetohexamide
  - Chlorpropamide (up to 33%)
  - Glyburide
  - Tolazamide
  - Tolbutamide
- Tetrachloroethylene
- Tetraethyl lead
- Tetraethylthiuram monosulfide
- Tetramethyl monosulfide
- Thiram
- Tolazoline
- Tranylcypromine
- Trichloroethylene

TOXINS WHICH SHOULD BE LAVAGED WITH SOLUTIONS OTHER THAN WATER

Toxin	Lavage solution
Aluminum phosphide or zinc phosphide	Avoid water due to release of phosphine Lavage with 1:5000 potassium permanganate
Barium carbonate	Magnesium sulfate or sodium sulfate
Bromates Tetrodotoxin	Sodium bicarbonate
Cesium Rubidium Thallium	Berlin/Prussian blue Potassium ferric hexayanoferrate
Chromium	Ascorbic acid 1% solution (10 g in 1 L)
Creosote	Olive oil
DDT	Mannitol
Fluoride	Calcium gluconate (10%)
Iodine	Starch/sodium thiosulfate (1%-5%)
Mercury	Sodium formaldehyde sulfoxylate (20 g in a 5% solution) A 2% to 5% solution of sodium bicarbonate can be used as an alternative therapy
Nicotine Phosphorus Physostigmine Quinine Strychnine	1:10,000 potassium permanganate (100 mg in 1 L water)
Paraquat	1-2 g/kg Fullers earth (15%) or bentonite (7%)
Radium Sodium monofluroacetate	Magnesium sulfate (10%)
Strontium	Avoid contact with water due to thermal reaction

ACE INHIBITORS COMPARISON

	Benazepril (Lotensin®)	Captopril (Capoten®)	Enalapril (Vasotec®)	Enalaprilat (Vasotec®)	Fosinopril (Monopril®)	Lisinopril (Prinivil®, Zestril®)	Quinapril (Accupril®)	Ramipril (Altace™)	Spirapril (Renormax®)
Route	P.O.	P.O.	P.O.	I.V.	P.O.	P.O.	P.O.	P.O.	P.O.
Dosing (mg)	10 20	12.5 25 50	5 10	1.25 mg/mL	10	10 20	5 10 20 40	2.5 5	3 6 12 24
Usual starting dose (mg)	10	25	5*,‡	1.25 mg/mL	10	10	10*	2.5*	1.5 (CHF) 12 (HTN)
Dosing interval	qd	bid† or tid	qd	q6h over 5 min	qd	qd	qd–bid	qd	qd–bid
Indications HTN	x	x	x	x	x	x	x	x	x
CHF		x	x				x		x
Protein binding (%)	>95	25–30	50–60	<50	~95	—	97	~73% ramipril 56% ramiprilat	86% to 91%
Active metabolites	x		x§		x		x	x§	x§
Half-life normal renal function (h)	22¶	<2	1.3	11–35	12#	12	1–3	1–2	1–2
Half-life impaired renal function (h)	Prolonged	3.5–32	No data	Prolonged•	Prolonged	Prolonged•	Prolonged	Prolonged	Prolonged
Maximum dose (mg)		450	40	20	80	40	80	20	24
GI absorption (%)	37	75	60	—	36	25	60	50–60	53–60
Absorption reduced by presence of food	No	Yes	No	—	Yes	No	Yes	Yes	Delays

(continued)

	Benazepril (Lotensin®)	Captopril (Capoten®)	Enalapril (Vasotec®)	Enalaprilat (Vasotec®)	Fosinopril (Monopril®)	Lisinopril (Prinivil®, Zestril®)	Quinapril (Accupril®)	Ramipril (Altace™)	Spirapril (Renormax®)
Elimination total	No data	>95%	95% in urine and feces	No data	50% in urine 50% in feces	No data	61% in urine 37% in feces	60% in urine 40% in feces	95%
unchanged	Trace	40%–50% in urine	54% in urine (40% enalapril)	>90% in urine	Negligible in oral dose	100%♦ in urine	5% in urine	<2%♦	Trace
Incidence of side effects cough (%)	1.9–3.4	0.5–2	1.3–2.2		2.2	2.9		12	1.5% to 4%
angioedema (%)	0.5	0.1	0.2		≤1	0.1		0.3	
rash (%)	x	4–7	1.3–1.4		≤1	1.5	0.7	x	1
headache (%)	5	0.5–2	1.8–5.2		3.2	5.3	6.9	5.4	≤10%
dizziness (%)	3.3	0.5–2	4.3–7.9		1.6	6.3	4.7	2.2	≤10%
chest pain (%)		1	2.1		≤1	1.3		<1	
hypotension (%)	0.3	2–5	6.7		≤1	1.2–5	1	0.5	
diarrhea (%)		0.5–2	1.4–2.1		1.5	3.2	1.5	<1	

*Patient not on diuretics.
†Dosing interval for heart failure 25 mg tid.
‡Dosing interval for heart failure 2.5 mg qd or bid.
§Prodrug. Enalaprilat is dialyzable.
¶Half-life accumulates after multiple dosing.
#Fosinoprilat, after I.V. administration.
•GFR ≤30 mL/min.
♦Time frame undefined.
x — reported, no incidence given.

ADRENERGIC AGONISTS, CARDIOVASCULAR COMPARISON

Drug	Hemodynamic Effects			
	CO	TPR	Mean BP	Renal Perfusion
Amrinone (Inocor®)	↑	↓	<->	↑
Dobutamine (Dobutrex®)	↑	↓	↑	<->
Dopamine (Intropin®)	↑	+/-*	<->/↑*	↑*
Epinephrine (Adrenalin®)	↑	↓	↑	↓
Isoproterenol (Isuprel®)	↑	↓	↓	+/-†
Mephentermine (Wyamine®)	↑	<->/↑	↑	+/-
Metaraminol (Aramine®)	↓	↑	↑	↓
Methoxamine	<->/↓	↑	↑	↓
Norepinephrine (Levophed®)	<->/↓	↑	↑	↓
Phenylephrine (Neo-Synephrine®)	↓	↑	↑	↓

↑ = increase ↓ = decrease, <-> = no change, * = dose dependent

† In patients with cardiogenic or septic shock, renal perfusion commonly increases, however, in the normal patient, renal perfusion may be reduced with isoproterenol.

ADRENERGIC AGONISTS DRUG INFUSIONS COMPARISON

Inotropic Agent	Dilution	Final Concentration	Usual Rate of Administration
Amrinone (Inocor®)	Reg: 250 mg/250 mL	1 mg/mL	5-20 mcg/kg/min
Dobutamine (Dobutrex®)	Reg: 250 mg/500 mL Max: 500 mg/500 mL	0.5 mg/mL 1 mg/mL	2.5-40 mcg/kg/min Titrate to therapeutic end point
Dopamine (Intropin®)	Reg: 400 mg/250 mL Max: 800 mg/250 mL	1.6 mg/mL 3.2 mg/mL	2.5-30 mcg/kg/min Titrate to therapeutic end point
Epinephrine (Adrenalin®)	Reg: 1 mg/250 mL	4 mcg/mL	Titrate Initially: 1-4 mcg/min
Isoproterenol (Isuprel®)	Reg: 2 mg/500 mL Max: 1 mg/100 mL	4 mcg/mL 10 mcg/mL	Titrate Initially: 2-10 mcg/min
Mephentermine (Wyamine®)	Reg: 600 mg/500 mL	1.2 mg/mL	1-5 mg/min
Metaraminol (Aramine®)	Reg: 100 mg/500 mL Max: 100 mg/250 mL	200 mcg/mL 400 mcg/mL	Titrate
Norepinephrine (Levophed®)	Reg: 4 mg/500 mL Max: 8 mg/500 mL	8 mcg/mL 16 mcg/mL	Titrate Initially: 2-12 mcg/min
Phenylephrine (Neo-Synephrine®)	Reg: 20 mg/250 mL	80 mcg/mL	Titrate Initially: 50-100 mcg/min

ANTIDEPRESSANT AGENTS COMPARISON

Drug	Class	Anticholinergic Side Effects	Sedation	Orthostatic Hypotension	Usual Adult Daily Dose (mg)	Cardiac Toxicity	Volume of Distribution (L/kg)	Protein Binding (%)	Bio-availability (%)
Amitriptyline	TCA	++++	++++	++	30–100	++++	8.3	96	30–60
Amoxapine	Dibenzoxazepine	+++	++	+	200–300	+	60–70	90	95–100
Bupropion	Chloropropiophenones	—	—	—	150–300	+	27–63	75–88	—
Desipramine	TCA	+	+	+	75–200	++++	33–42	92	33–51
Doxepin	TCA	++	+++	++++	75–150	++++	20	80–85	13–45
Fluoxetine	SSRI	+	+/-	+	20–80	+	27	95	100
Imipramine	TCA	++	++	+++	75–100	++++	15	86	22–77
Nefazodone	Phenylpiperazine	+	++	++	300–600	+	0.22–0.87	99	20
Sertraline	SSRI	—	—	—	50–200	+	20	98	36
Trazodone	Triazolopyridines	+	++++	++	150	+	0.8	85–95	72–91

SSRI = specific serotonin reuptake inhibitors.
TCA = tricyclic antidepressant.

ANTIEMETICS FOR CHEMOTHERAPY-INDUCED NAUSEA AND VOMITING

Basic Principles of Antiemetic Therapy

1. Rule out other causes of nausea and vomiting before prescribing antiemetics.
2. Evaluate the relative emetic potential of antineoplastic drugs and choose antiemetics accordingly.
3. Treat delayed nausea and vomiting with scheduled antiemetics for a period of several days.
4. Combination antiemetic regimens provide greater protection against chemotherapy induced emesis than do single agents.
5. Head off trouble before it starts by initiating an aggressive antiemetic regimen before giving highly emetogenic chemotherapy.

Relative Emetic Potential of Antineoplastic Drugs

Class I
Low
(<10%)

Androgens
Busulfan
Chlorambucil
Corticosteroids
Cyclophosphamide (oral)
Estrogens
Progestins
Thioguanine (oral)
Thiotepa
Vincristine

Class II
Moderately Low
(10%-30%)

Bleomycin
Cytarabine (<20 mg)
Doxorubicin (<20 mg)
Etoposide
Hydroxyurea
Melphalan
Mercaptopurine
Methotrexate (<100 mg)
Teniposide
Thiotepa
Vinblastine
Vinorelbine

Class III
Moderate
(30%-60%)

Asparaginase
Azacytidine
Cyclophosphamide (<1 g)
Daunorubicin
Doxorubicin (20-75 mg)
Fluorouracil (>1 g)
Hexamethylmelamine
Irinotecan
Methotrexate (100-250 mg)
Mitomycin-C
Teniposide
Vinblastine

Class IV
Moderately High
(60%-90%)

Actinomycin D
Carmustine (<200 mg)
Cisplatin (<75 mg)
Cyclophosphamide (1 g)
Cytarabine (250 mg - 1 g)
Dacarbazine (<500 mg)
Doxorubicin (≥75 mg)
Lomustine (<60 mg)
Methotrexate (>200 mg/m^2 or 250 mg total)
Mithramycin
Mitomycin
Procarbazine
Semustine

Class V
High
(>90%)

Carmustine (≥200 mg)
Cisplatin (≥75 mg)
Cyclophosphamide (<1 g)
Cytarabine (>500 mg/m^2 or 1 g total)
Dacarbazine (≥500 mg)
Lomustine (≥60 mg)
Pentostatin
Mechlorethamine
Streptozotocin

Doses and Administration of Several Frequently Used Antiemetic Agents

Antiemetic Agent	Route	Dose Range	Frequency of Administration	Toxicology Treatment Considerations
Serotonin antagonist				
Ondansetron	I.V. P.O.*	0.15 mg/kg†	30 min prior to chemotherapy and repeated q4h x 2 doses	Acetaminophen
Substituted benzamide				
Metoclopramide	I.V. P.O.*	1-3 mg/kg 1-3 mg/kg	q2h q2-4h	May be effective for theophylline-induced vomiting
Butyrophenones				
Haloperidol	I.V. P.O.	1-3 mg 1-2 mg	q2-6h q3-6h	
Droperidol	I.V.	0.5-2 mg	q4h	Droperidol may be effective for theophylline-induced vomiting
Corticosteroids				
Dexamethasone	I.V./P.O.	4-20 mg	Once only, or q4-6h	
Methylprednisolone	I.V.	250-500 mg	Once only, or q4-6h	
Phenothiazines				
Prochlorperazine	P.O. P.R. I.M./I.V.	5-10 mg 25 mg 10-20 mg	q2-4h q4-6h q3-6h	Do not use for seizuregenic overdoses (ie, theophylline)
Chlorpromazine	P.O. I.M./I.V.	25-50 mg 25 mg	q3-6h q3-6h	May be effective for ipecac toxicity
Benzodiazepine				
Lorazepam	I.V.	1-2 mg/m^2	q4h	
Cannabinoid				
THC	P.O.	5-10 mg/m^2	q3-4h	
Ranitidine	I.V. P.O.	50-100 mg 150 mg	q6-12h q12h	May be effective for theophylline-induced vomiting

*Using investigational.

†Fix dose (eg, 10 mg) possible since efficacy is similar within a wide dose range.

ANTIPSYCHOTIC AGENTS COMPARISON

Antipsychotic Agent	Equivalent Dosages (approx) (mg)	Usual Adult Daily Maintenance Dose (mg)	Sedation (Incidence)	Extrapyramidal Side Effects	Anticholinergic (Antimuscarinic) Side Effects	Cardiovascular Side Effects	Chemical Class
Chlorpromazine	100	200–1000	High	Moderate	Moderate	Moderate/high	Phenothiazine
Clozapine	50	50–400	High	Low	High	High	Dibenzazepine
Fluphenazine	2	5–40	Low	High	Low	Low	Phenothiazine
Haloperidol	2	5–40	Low	High	Low	Low	Butyrophenone
Loxapine	10	25–100	Moderate	High	Low	Low	Dibenzoxazepine
Mesoridazine	50	30–400	High	Low	High	Moderate	Phenothiazine
Molindone	15	25–100	Low	High	Low	Low	Dihydroindolone
Perphenazine	10	16–48	Low	High	Low	Low	Phenothiazine
Promazine	200	40–1200	Moderate	Moderate	High	Moderate	Phenothiazine
Sertindole		16–20	Low	Low	Low	Low	Imidazolidinone
Sulpiride (investigational)	400	200–400	Low	Moderate	Low/moderate	Low	Benzamide
Thioridazine	100	200–800	High	Low	High	Moderate/high	Phenothiazine
Thiothixene	5	5–40	Low	Moderate	Low	Low/moderate	Thioxanthene
Trifluoperazine	5	10–40	Low	High	Low	Low	Phenothiazine

BENZODIAZEPINES COMPARISON

	Peak Blood Levels (oral) (h)	Protein Binding %	Volume of Distribution (L/kg)	Major Active Metabolite	t½ (parent) (h)	t½* (metabolite) (h)	Usual Oral Dosage Range	Maximum Daily Dose (mg)	Bioavailability (%)
Sedative/Hypnotic									
Flurazepam (Dalmane®)	3–6	97	3.4	Yes	40–114	47–100	15–30 mg	30	100
Temazepam (Restoril®)	2–3	96	1.4	Yes	10–15	—	15–30 mg	30	>80
Triazolam (Halcion®)	0.7	89–94	0.8–1.8	No	2.3	—	0.25–1 mg	—	44–53
Anxiolytic									
Alprazolam (Xanax®)	0.7–1.6	80	0.9–1.6	No	12–15	10–15	0.75–4 mg/d	10	92
Chlordiazepoxide (Librium®)	1–4	90–98	3.3	Yes	5–25	24–96	15–700 mg/d	300	100
Diazepam (Valium®)	1–2	96	1.1	Yes	20–50	50–100	6–40 mg/d	40	100
Lorazepam (Ativan®)	0.5–3	88–92	1–1.3	No	10–16	—	2–6 mg/d	10	83–100
Oxazepam (Serax®)	2–3	86–96	0.6–2	No	5–15	—	30–120 mg/d	120	>90
Miscellaneous									
Clobazam (Frisium®)	1.3	85–90	1	Yes	10–50	77	10–30	60	—
Clonazepam (Klonopin®)	1–4	50–86	1.5–4.4	No	19–50	—	1.5–20 mg/d	20	98
Clorazepate (Tranxene®)	1	80–95	0.16–1.27	Yes	>24	48–96	15–60	90	Variable
Flunitrazepam	1–2	80–90	3.4–5.5	No	19–22	—	0.5–2	—	80–90
Midazolam (Versed®)	0.4–0.7	>95	0.8–2.5	No	1–4	—	—	—	35–44
Nitrazepam (Mogadon®)	1.4	85–86	2.4–4.8	No	24–29	—	5–10	20	78

Abstracted from Micromedex, Inc, vol 81, 1994. * = significant metabolite.

BETA-BLOCKERS COMPARISON

Agent	Adrenergic Receptor Blocking Activity	Lipid Solubility	Half-life (h)	Primary (Secondary) Route of Elimination	Starting Oral Daily Dose	Protein Binding (%)	Volume of Distribution (L/kg)	Membrane Stabilization	Partial Agonist	Oral Absorption (%)
Acebutolol (Sectral®)	$beta_1$	Low	3–4	Hepatic (renal)	400 mg	25	1.2	Yes	Yes	70
Atenolol (Tenormin®)	$beta_1$	Low	6–9*	Renal (hepatic)	50 mg	<5	0.6–1.1	No	No	50
Betaxolol (Kerlone®)	$beta_1$	Low	14–22	Hepatic (renal)	10 mg	50–60	4.9–13	Yes	No	90
Carteolol (Cartrol®)	$beta_1$ $beta_2$	Low	6	Renal (biliary)	15 mg	23–30		Yes	Yes	85
Carvedilol (Kredex®)	$alpha_1$ $beta_1$ $beta_2$†	High	6–8	Hepatic (renal)	25 mg		1–2	Yes	No	22–24
Celiprolol (Selecor®)	$alpha_2$ $beta_2$	Low	4–10	Renal (hepatic)	200 mg	25		No	Yes	30–74
Esmolol (Brevibloc®)	$beta_1$	Low	0.15	Red blood cell	NA	55	3.5	No	No	—
Labetalol (Trandate®, Normodyne®)	$alpha_1$ $beta_1$ $beta_2$	Moderate	5.5–8	Renal (hepatic)	200 mg	50	9.4	No	Yes	90
Metoprolol (Lopressor®)	$beta_1$	Moderate	3–4	Hepatic/renal	100 mg	8–12	4.2	No	No	90

(continued)

Agent	Adrenergic Receptor Blocking Activity	Lipid Solubility	Half-life (h)	Primary (Secondary) Route of Elimination	Starting Oral Daily Dose	Protein Binding (%)	Volume of Distribution (L/kg)	Membrane Stabilization	Partial Agonist	Oral Absorption (%)
Nadolol (Corgard®)	$beta_1$ $beta_2$	Low	20–24	Renal	320 mg	30	1.8–2	No	No	30
Penbutolol (Levatol®)	$beta_1$ $beta_2$	High	4.5	Hepatic (renal)	20 mg	80–97	~0.5	No	Yes	Almost 100
Pindolol (Visken®)	$beta_1$ $beta_2$	Moderate	3–4‡	Hepatic/renal	20 mg	57	1.2–2	Yes	Yes	50–95
Propranolol (Inderal®, various)	$beta_1$ $beta_2$	High	3–5	Hepatic	80 mg	93	3.9	Yes	No	90
Propranolol long-acting (Inderal-LA®)	$beta_1$ $beta_2$	High	9–18	Hepatic	80 mg	93	3.9	Yes	No	90
Sotalol (Betapace®)	$beta_1$ $beta_2$	Low	7–15	Renal (hepatic)	80 mg	0	0.2–0.7	No	No	70
Timolol (Blocadren®)	$beta_1$ $beta_2$	Low to moderate	4	Hepatic (renal)	20 mg	10	1.3–3.6	No	No	90

*Half-life increased to 16–27 h in creatinine clearances of 15–35 mL/min and >27 h in Cl_{cr} <15 mL/min.
†Calcium channel blocking effect at high concentrations (>1 μmol/L).
‡Half-life variable: 7–15 h.
NA = not applicable.
Note: All $beta_1$ selective agents will inhibit $beta_2$ receptors at higher doses.

CALCIUM CHANNEL BLOCKING AGENTS COMPARISON

	Diltiazem	Felodipine	Nicardipine	Nifedipine	Nilvadipine	Nimodipine	Nitrendipine	Verapamil
Bioavailability (%)	40	15	35	60–75	14–19	13	16–23	20–35
Protein binding (%)	77–85	99	95	95	98	95	98	83–92
Half-life	3.5–6 h (5–7 h in sustained released preparations)	10–16 h	2–4 h	2–5 h	9.8–18.2 h	1–2 h	8.6	Oral: One dose: 2.8–7.4 h Rep dose: 4.5–12 h I.V. (biphasic) Short phase: 4 min Long phase: 2–5 h
Onset of action	Oral: 60 min	2-5 h	20 min	Oral: 10–20 min	—	20 min	Within 2 h	Oral: 30 min I.V.: 1–5 min
Peak	Oral: 2–3 h	2–4 h	0.5–2 h	Oral: 0.5–6 h	—	<1 h	4 h	Oral: 1–2.2 h Oral, ext release: 5–7 h I.V.: 2 h
Duration of action	Ext release: 12 h Tablet: 6–8 h	24 h	8 h	12–24 h	—	4–6 h	7–8 h	Oral, ext release: 24 h Tablet: 8–10 h I.V.: 2 h
Elimination	Biliary/renal 96%–98% (2%–4% unchanged)	Renal 70% Biliary 30%	Renal 60% Biliary/fecal 35%	Renal 80% Biliary/fecal 20%	—	Renal 60% Biliary/fecal 32%	Renal 80% metabolites Feces 8% metabolites	Renal 70% Biliary/fecal 9%–16%
Volume of distribution (L/kg)	3.1	10	0.7	0.8–1.4	24–40	0.9	6	4.7
Activity of metabolites	Desacetyldiltiazem (25%–30%)	None	Inactive	Inactive	—	Inactive	Inactive	Norverapamil (12%)
Solubility in water	Yes		Slightly	No	—	No	—	Yes
Therapeutic blood level	50–200 ng/mL	5–10 nmol/L	24–50 ng/mL	25–100 ng/mL	—	—	—	80–300 ng/mL
Therapeutic dose	30–60 mg tid or qid for standard 180–400 mg daily for sustained release	2–10 mg daily	20–40 mg tid for standard 30–60 mg bid for sustained release	10–40 mg tid or qid for standard 90–180 mg once daily for sustained release	4–16 mg for hypertension	60 mg q4h for 21 d	10–40 mg (hypertension)	80–160 mg qid for standard 120–240 mg once daily for sustained release

(continued)

	Diltiazem	Felodipine	Nicardipine	Nifedipine	Nilvadipine	Nimodipine	Nitrendipine	Verapamil
Actions contractility	↓	0/↑	↓	↑	↑	↑	↑	↓↓
heart rate	↓	↑	↑	↑	↑	↑	↑	↓
cardiac output	↑	↑	↑↑	↑	↑	↑	↑	↓↑
peripheral vascular resistance	↓	↓↓	↓↓↓	↓↓↓	↓↓↓	↓↓	↓↓↓	↓↓
Side effects constipation	+	0	–	+	+	–	–	+
dizziness	+	+	+	++	+	+	++	+
flushing	+	++	++	++	+	–	+	–
headache	+	+	+	++	+	+	++	+
nausea	+	+	+	++	+	+	++	+
Hypotension	+	+	+	+	+	+	+	++
Breast milk excretion amount	++	ND	+	+	ND	ND	ND	+

ND = no data.
++ = most frequent
+ = less frequent
- = rare

CYCLOPLEGIC MYDRIATICS COMPARISON

Agent	Peak Mydriasis	Peak Cycloplegia	Time to Recovery
Atropine	30-40 min	1-3 h	>14 d
Cyclopentolate	25-75 min	25-75 min	24 h
Homatropine	30-90 min	30-90 min	6 h-4 d
Scopolamine	20-30 min	30 min to 1 h	5-7 d
Tropicamide	20-40 min	20-35 min	1-6 h

H_1-ANTIHISTAMINE COMPARISON

Name (Class)	Plasma Half-life (h)	Time to Peak (h)	Usual Duration (h)	Notes
Astemizole (Miscellaneous)	168-264	1	24	Torsades reported
Azatadine (Piperidine)	8	4		
Brompheniramine (Alkylamine)	12-34	2-5	4-12	Available in sustained-release capsule
Chlorpheniramine (Alkylamine)	12-24	2-6	4-12	Available in sustained-release capsule
Diphenhydramine (Ethanolamine)	2-8	2-4	4-7	
Loratadine (Miscellaneous)	12-15	8-12	24	Torsades reported
Promethazine (Phenothiazine)		3-4	4-6	
Terfenadine (Miscellaneous)	16-22	1-2	12-24	Torsades reported
Tripelennamine (Ethylenediamine)			4-8	Available in sustained-release capsule

HYPOGLYCEMIC AGENTS COMPARISON, ORAL

Sulfonylureas	Equivalent Dose	Maximum Recommended Daily Dose (mg)	Usual Regimen	Duration of Action (h)	Onset of Action (h)	Plasma Half-Life (h)	Peak Effect (h)	Peak Plasma Level (h)	Protein Binding (%)	Volume of Distribution (L/kg)	Renal Fractional Excretion %	Active Metabolite (by hepatic metabolism)
Acetohexamide	625 mg	1500	qd-bid	12–24	1	0.8–2.4	8–10	2–5	85–88		72	+
Chlorpropamide	250 mg	500	qd	24–72	1	30–42	3–6	3–4	60–90	0.09–0.27	80–90	+
Glipizide	5 mg	40	qd-bid	12–24	1–1.5	3–4	1–3	1.5–2	92–99	0.2	70	—
Glyburide	5 mg	20	qd-bid	24	1	5–10	2–4	2–4	97–99	0.3	50	—
Tolazamide	250 mg	1000	qd-bid	10–24	4–6	7	3–4	2–5	94	0.1–0.3	85	+
Tolbutamide	1 g	2000	bid–tid	6–12	⅓	6	1–3	2–5	96	0.1	100	—
Biguanide/Agent												
Metformin	2 g	3500	bid–tid	8–12	1	1.5–5	2	1–3	<5	1	90–100	—

LAXATIVES, CLASSIFICATION AND PROPERTIES COMPARISON

Laxative	Onset of Action	Site of Action	Mechanism of Action	Adverse Effects	Toxicologic Perspective for Gastric Decontamination
Bulk–Producing					
Methylcellulose Psyllium (Metamucil®) Malt soup extract (Maltsupex®)	12–24 h (up to 72 h)	Small and large intestine	Holds water in stool; mechanical distention; malt soup extract reduces fecal pH; peristalsis is stimulated reflexly	No systemic effects	Not useful for gastric decontamination
Irritant/Stimulant					
Senna (Senokot®)	6–12 h	Colon	Direct action on intestinal mucosa; stimulate myenteric plexus; alter water and electrolyte secretion (especially potassium)	Chronic use can cause hepatitis	Not useful for gastric decontamination
Bisacodyl (Dulcolax®) tablets, suppositories	0.25–1 h (rectal) 6–12 h (oral)			Chronic use can cause atonic colon; do not use suppositories in patients with hemorrhoids	
Castor oil (ricinoleic acid)	2–6 h	Small intestine		May induce labor	May reduce the absorption of dinitrocresol by 50% (nonpurgative dose). Not useful for routine gastric decontamination. May increase absorption of organochlorine agents.
Cascara aromatic fluid extract	6–8 h	Colon			
Lubricant					
Mineral oil (Agoral®)	6–8 h	Colon	Lubricates intestine; retards colonic absorption of fecal water	Lipoid pneumonia may occur with aspiration	May increase absorption of organochlorine agents. Not recommended for children <6 years due to aspiration risk. Not useful for gastric decontamination (except in phosphorus exposure)

(continued)

Laxative	Onset of Action	Site of Action	Mechanism of Action	Adverse Effects	Toxicologic Perspective for Gastric Decontamination
Miscellaneous and Combination Laxatives					
Glycerin suppository	0.25–0.5 h	Colon	Hyperosmotic action	Local irritation	Not useful for gastric decontamination
Lactulose (Cephulac®)	24–48 h	Colon	Delivers osmotically active molecules to colon		
Docusate/casanthranol (Peri–Colace®)	8–12 h	Small and large intestine	Casanthranol — mild stimulant; docusate — stool softener		
Osmotic					
Sorbitol	1–1.5 h	Small and large intestine	Increase intraluminal water volume — can stimulate peristalsis	Vomiting, hypernatremic dehydration at high doses	Dose 0.5–1.5 g/kg (0.5 g/kg in children <1 year; up to 50 g of a 35% solution) Not to be used more than once daily in combination with multiple dosing of activated charcoal. Increases elimination by about 30% when used with charcoal for decontamination
Combination macrogols with polyethylene glycol/ sodium sulphate (GoLYTELY®)	1 h	Small and large intestine	Increases osmotic pressure	Vomiting may occur (related to rate of administration); do not give in presence of GI obstruction, bowel perforation, or toxic megacolon	Drug of choice for whole bowel irrigation. Dose (PEG–3350) is 250–500 mL/h in pediatrics, 1–2 L/h in adults orally for at least 3 hours or until rectal effluent is clear

(continued)

Laxative	Onset of Action	Site of Action	Mechanism of Action	Adverse Effects	Toxicologic Perspective for Gastric Decontamination
Saline					
Magnesium citrate (Citroma®) Magnesium hydroxide (Milk of Magnesia) Magnesium sulfate (Epsom salts)	0.5–3 h	Small and large intestine	Attract/retain water in intestinal lumen increasing intraluminal pressure; cholecystokinin release (magnesium cathartics)	Do not use in renal failure Hypermagnesemia with multiple doses (99 mg or 8.1 mEq of magnesium/g)	300 mL magnesium citrate should be given for oral hydroflouric acid ingestion. Dose for decontamination: 4 mL/kg – 300 mL/dose 250 mL/kg – 30 g Do not use if botulism is suspected. Calcium gluconate (1 mL/kg of a 10% solution) can be given for magnesium intoxication Dose for gastric decontamination: 250 mg/kg (pediatric); 20–30 g (adult)
Sodium phosphate/ biphosphate enema (Fleet® Enema)	2–15 min	Colon		Can cause hypocalcemia	Do not use in children. Contraindicated in ethylene glycol ingestions
Sodium sulfate	0.5–3 h	Small and large intestine		Do not use in patient with congestive heart failure; hypernatremia may develop	Useful for barium ingestions to convert to nonabsorbable barium sulfate. Dose 250 mg/kg (pediatric); 15–20 g (adult)
Surfactants/Stool Softener					
Docusate (Colace®)	24–72 h	Small and large intestine	Detergent activity; facilitates admixture of fat and water to soften stool	Excreted in breast milk and bile	Due to slow onset, not used in gastric decontamination

NARCOTIC ANALGESIC PHARMACOKINETIC PROFILE

I.V. administration is most reliable and rapid; I.M. or S.C. use may cause delayed absorption and peak effect, especially with impaired tissue perfusion. Many agents undergo a significant first-pass effect. All are metabolized by the liver and excreted primarily in urine. Meperidine is metabolized to normeperidine, a metabolite with significant pharmacologic activity. The half-life of normeperidine is 15-30 hours and accumulates with chronic dosing, especially in patients with renal dysfunction. The accumulation of this metabolite may lead to CNS excitation (eg, tremors, twitches, seizures).

Pharmacokinetics of Narcotic Agonist Analgesics

Drug	Onset (min)	Peak (h)	Duration* (h)	t½ (h)	Equianalgesic Doses† I.M. (mg)	Equianalgesic Doses† Oral (mg)	Volume of Distribution (L/kg)	Protein Binding (%)
Alfentanil	Immediate	ND	ND	1.2‡	ND	NA	0.6-1	92
Codeine	30-60	1-1.5	4-6	3	200	120-130	3.5	7
Fentanyl	7-8	ND	1-2	1.5-6	0.1	NA	4	80-86
Heroin	5-10	0.5-1.2	3-4	0.05-1.5	3-5	60	25	40
Hydrocodone	ND	0.5-2	4-8	3.3-4.5	ND	15-20	—	—
Hydromorphone	15-30	0.5-1	4-5	2-3	1.5	7.5	1.2	—
Ketobemidone	15‡	1-3	4-5	2-2.4	3-10	ND	2-7.8	—
Levorphanol	10-30	0.5-1	6-8	12-16	2	4	—	—
Meperidine	10-45	0.5-1	2-4	3-4■	75-100	300	3.1-5	55-75
Methadone	30-60	0.5-1	4-6§	15-30	7.5-10	15	3.6	80-89
Morphine	15-60¶	0.5-1	3-7	1.5-2	10	30-40	3-4	35
Oxycodone, P.O.	15-30	1	3-6	2-5	NA	15-30	—	—
Oxymorphone	5-10	0.5-1	3-6	ND	1	10#	—	—
Pentazocine	15-30	1-3	4-5	2-3	60	180	4.4-7.8	61
Propoxyphene, P.O.	30-60	2-2.5	4-6	15⁺	ND	180/240♦	12-26	78
Sufentanil	1.3-3‡	ND	0.5-1	2.5	0.02	NA	2.9	93
Tilidine	15-30	0.5	4-6	5	100	ND	3.71	—
Tramdol, P.O.	60	2	9	6	100	ND	2.5-3	20

ND = no data available. NA = not applicable.
*After I.V. administration, peak effects may be more pronounced but duration is shorter. Duration of action may be longer with the oral route.
†Based on acute, short-term use. Chronic administration may alter pharmacokinetics and decrease the oral:parenteral dose ratio. The morphine oral:parenteral ratio decreases to ≈1.5-2.5:1 upon chronic dosing.
‡Data based on I.V. administration.
§Duration and half-life increase with repeated use due to cumulative effects.
¶Data based on intrathecal or epidural administration.
#Rectal.
•HCl salt.
♦Napsylate salt.
■Normeperidine (active metabolite) has a half-life of 14-21 hours.
⁺Norpropoxyphene (active metabolite) has a half-life of 30-36 hours.

NONSTEROIDAL ANTI-INFLAMMATORY COMPARISON

Name	Plasma Half-life (h)	Time to Peak (h)	Usual Duration (h)	Maximum Recommended Daily Dose (mg)
Diclofenac	1-2	2-3		200
Etodolac	7	1		1200
Fenoprofen	2-3	2	4-6	3200
Flurbiprofen	3-4	1.5-2		300
Ibuprofen	2	1-2	4-6	3200
Indomethacin	4.5	3-4	4-6	200
Ketoprofen	1-4	0.5-2		300
Ketorolac	5-6	1	6-8	P.O.: 40 I.M.: 120
Meclofenamate	2-3	0.5-1.5	2-4	400
Mefenamic acid	3.5	2-4	2-6	1000
Nabumetone	24	3-6		2000
Naproxen (base and sodium salt)	9-20	1-2	2-7	1500
Piroxicam	30-86	P.O.: 3-5	24	40
Sulindac	7	2-4		400
Tolmetin	5	0.5-1		2000

SYMPTOMS INDEX

ACETONE BREATH

ALOPECIA

(Continued)

ANAPHYLACTIC SHOCK *(Continued)*

BLINDNESS

BULLOUS SKIN DISEASE/PEMPHIGOID

CLITORAL HYPERTROPHY

CORTICAL BLINDNESS

COUGH

(Continued)

COUGH *(Continued)*

CRANIAL NERVE PALSIES

DELIRIUM

(Continued)

DELIRIUM *(Continued)*

DENTAL EROSION

DIABETES INSIPIDUS

DIPLOPIA

(Continued)

DIPLOPIA *(Continued)*

ECZEMA

ENURESIS

ESOPHAGEAL ULCERATION

EXTRAPYRAMIDAL REACTION

(Continued)

EXTRAPYRAMIDAL REACTION *(Continued)*

FACIAL EDEMA

FANCONI SYNDROME

FINGERNAIL LOSS

GALACTORRHEA

GINGIVAL HYPERPLASIA

GYNECOMASTIA

HEMOLYSIS

HICCUPS

HIRSUTISM

HYPERCALCEMIA

(Continued)

HYPERCALCEMIA *(Continued)*

HYPERCALCIURIA

HYPERGLYCEMIA

(Continued)

HYPOGLYCEMIA

(Continued)

HYPOGLYCEMIA *(Continued)*

HYPOKALEMIA

(Continued)

HYPOMAGNESEMIA *(Continued)*

HYPONATREMIA

HYPOPHOSPHATEMIA

IMPOTENCE

(Continued)

IMPOTENCE *(Continued)*

INSOMNIA

(Continued)

INSOMNIA *(Continued)*

LARYNGOSPASM

LEUKEMOID REACTIONS

LICHENOID ERUPTIONS

MANIA

METHEMOGLOBINEMIA

(Continued)

METHEMOGLOBINEMIA *(Continued)*

MIOSIS

MYASTHENIA GRAVIS (EXACERBATION OR PRECIPITATION OF)

MYDRIASIS

(Continued)

MYDRIASIS *(Continued)*

MYOCLONUS

(Continued)

MYOCLONUS *(Continued)*

NASAL CONGESTION

NEUROLEPTIC MALIGNANT SYNDROME

NYSTAGMUS

(Continued)

NYSTAGMUS *(Continued)*

PANCREATITIS

(Continued)

PANCREATITIS *(Continued)*

PARKINSONISM

PERIARTERITIS NODOSA

PHOTOPHOBIA

(Continued)

PHOTOPHOBIA *(Continued)*

PHOTOSENSITIVITY

PITYRIASIS (ROSEA)

PORPHYRIA

(Continued)

PORPHYRIA *(Continued)*

PREGNANCY RISK FACTOR A

PREGNANCY RISK FACTOR B

(Continued)

PREGNANCY RISK FACTOR B *(Continued)*

PREGNANCY RISK FACTOR C

(Continued)

PREGNANCY RISK FACTOR C *(Continued)*

(Continued)

PREGNANCY RISK FACTOR C *(Continued)*

PREGNANCY RISK FACTOR D

PREGNANCY RISK FACTOR (FURTHER EXPLANATION IN MONOGRAPH)

(Continued)

PREGNANCY RISK FACTOR (FURTHER EXPLANATION IN MONOGRAPH) *(Continued)*

PREGNANCY RISK FACTOR X

PRIAPISM

PSEUDOTUMOR CEREBRI

PSORIASIS

PSYCHOSIS

(Continued)

PSYCHOSIS *(Continued)*

PTOSIS

(Continued)

PTOSIS *(Continued)*

PULMONARY EDEMA

(Continued)

PULMONARY EDEMA *(Continued)*

PULMONARY FIBROSIS

PURPURA

PYLORIC STENOSIS

Q-T PROLONGATION

RADIOPAQUE

(Continued)

RADIOPAQUE *(Continued)*

RAYNAUD'S (EXACERBATION OF)

REDMAN SYNDROME

RENAL TUBULAR NECROSIS

ROTTEN EGG BREATH

SCLERODERMA

SEBORRHEIC DERMATITIS

SEIZURES

(Continued)

SEIZURES *(Continued)*

(Continued)

SEIZURES *(Continued)*

(Continued)

SEIZURES *(Continued)*

SERUM SICKNESS

SEXUAL DYSFUNCTION

(Continued)

SEXUAL DYSFUNCTION *(Continued)*

SKIN DISCOLORATION (YELLOW)

SNEEZING

STEVENS-JOHNSON SYNDROME

SYNDROME OF INAPPROPRIATE ANTIDIURETIC HORMONE (SIADH)

(Continued)

SYNDROME OF INAPPROPRIATE ANTIDIURETIC HORMONE (SIADH) *(Continued)*

SYSTEMIC LUPUS ERYTHEMATOSUS (SLE)

TARDIVE DYSKINESIA

THIRST

(Continued)

THIRST *(Continued)*

THROMBOCYTOPENIA

(Continued)

THROMBOCYTOPENIA *(Continued)*

THROMBOCYTOSIS

TINNITUS

(Continued)

TINNITUS *(Continued)*

TONGUE DISCOLORATION

TORTICOLLIS

TOURETTE'S DISEASE (EXACERBATION)

TOXIC EPIDERMAL NECROLYSIS

(Continued)

TREMOR *(Continued)*

CAS NUMERICAL INDEX

UN NUMERICAL INDEX

ALPHABETICAL INDEX

Letters in brackets signify the chapter where the agent is located.

NOTES

NOTES